CECIL

TEXTBOOK

of

MEDICINE

Editor for Neurologic and Behavioral Diseases

FRED PLUM, M.D.
Anne Parrish Titzell Professor and Chairman,
Department of Neurology, Cornell University Medical College;
Neurologist-in-Chief, The New York Hospital–Cornell Medical Center,
New York, New York

The Consulting Editors:

Renal Diseases
THOMAS E. ANDREOLI, M.D.

Professor and Chairman,
Department of Internal Medicine,
University of Arkansas College of Medicine;
Chief of Medicine, University of Arkansas Hospital,
Little Rock, Arkansas

Infectious Diseases
GERALD L. MANDELL, M.D.

Head, Division of Infectious Diseases, and
Professor of Medicine, University of Virginia,
Owen R. Cheatham Professor of the Sciences,
Charlottesville, Virginia

Respiratory Diseases
JOHN F. MURRAY, M.D.

Professor of Medicine,
University of California, San Francisco,
School of Medicine

Hematologic and Hematopoietic Diseases
DAVID G. NATHAN, M.D.

Robert G. Stranahan Professor of Pediatrics,
Harvard Medical School;
Physician-in-Chief, Children's Hospital,
Boston, Massachusetts

Diseases of the Digestive System
ROBERT K. OCKNER, M.D.

Professor of Medicine and Director, Liver Center,
University of California, San Francisco,
School of Medicine,
San Francisco, California

Cardiovascular Diseases
THOMAS W. SMITH, M.D.

Professor of Medicine, Harvard Medical School;
Chief, Cardiovascular Division,
Brigham and Women's Hospital,
Boston, Massachusetts

VOLUME 2

CECIL

TEXTBOOK of MEDICINE

19th edition

Edited by

JAMES B. WYNGAARDEN, M.D.
Professor of Medicine and
Associate Vice-Chancellor for Health Affairs,
Duke University School of Medicine,
Durham, North Carolina

LLOYD H. SMITH, Jr., M.D.
Professor of Medicine and
Associate Dean,
University of California, San Francisco,
School of Medicine,
San Francisco, California

J. CLAUDE BENNETT, M.D.
Professor and Chairman,
Department of Medicine,
University of Alabama at Birmingham,
School of Medicine,
Birmingham, Alabama

W. B. SAUNDERS COMPANY
HARCOURT BRACE JOVANOVICH, INC.
Philadelphia London Toronto Montreal Sydney Tokyo

W. B. SAUNDERS COMPANY
Harcourt Brace Jovanovich, Inc.

The Curtis Center
Independence Square West
Philadelphia, PA 19106

Library of Congress Cataloging-in-Publication Data

Cecil textbook of medicine / edited by James B. Wyngaarden,
Lloyd H. Smith, Jr., J. Claude Bennett.—19th ed.

p. cm

Rev. ed. of: Textbook of medicine / [edited by] Cecil. 18th ed.
1988.

Includes bibliographical references and index.

ISBN 0–7216–2928–8 (single v.).—ISBN 0–7216–2929–6 (v. 1).—
ISBN 0–7216–2930–X (v. 2).—ISBN 0–7216–2931–8 (set)

1. Internal medicine   I. Cecil, Russell L. (Russell La Fayette),
   1881–1965.   II. Wyngaarden, James B.   III. Smith,
   Lloyd H.   IV. Bennett, J. Claude.   V. Title: Textbook
   of Medicine.

[DNLM: 1. Medicine. WB 100 C3888]

RC46.C423 1992

616—dc20

DNLM/DLC   91–31268

Editor: John Dyson
Designer: Lorraine B. Kilmer
Production Manager: Frank Polizzano
Manuscript Editors: Donna Walker and Bonnie Boehme
Illustration Coordinator: Matt Andrews
Indexer: Donna Walker

ISBN	0–7216–2928–8	Single Volume
ISBN	0–7216–2929–6	Volume 1
ISBN	0–7216–2930–X	Volume 2
ISBN	0–7216–2931–8	Set

CECIL TEXTBOOK OF MEDICINE

CONTENTS

(Detailed table of contents begins on page vii.)

PART XX INFECTIOUS DISEASES

Section One   Introduction

Section Two   Bacterial Diseases

Streptococcal Diseases

Endocarditis

Staphylococcal Infections

Bacterial Meningitis, *Morton N. Swartz*

Osteomyelitis

Whooping Cough

Diphtheria

Clostridial Diseases, *John G. Bartlett*

Anaerobic Bacteria

Enteric Infections

Other Bacterial Infections

Diseases Due to Mycobacteria

Sexually Transmitted Diseases, *P. Frederick Sparling*

Spirochetal Diseases Other Than Syphilis

Diseases Caused by Chlamydiae, *Walter E. Stamm*

Rickettsial Diseases, *Richard B. Hornick*

Zoonoses

Section Three   Viral Diseases

Viral Infections of the Respiratory Tract

COLOR PLATES

COLOR PLATES

CECIL
TEXTBOOK
of
MEDICINE

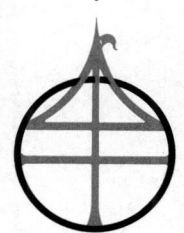

PART XV
NUTRITIONAL DISEASES

199 Nutrient Requirements
Robert M. Russell

Recommended Dietary Allowances

Recommended Dietary Allowances (RDA's) have been established for most essential nutrients by the Food and Nutrition Board of the National Academy of Sciences. A nutrient is defined as essential if its absence from the diet results in a deficiency disease. For certain nutrients, notably some trace elements, essentiality has not been established. The United States RDA's are but one set of many recommendations put out by various countries and organizations (e.g., World Health Organization, Food and Agriculture Organization). In the United States the RDA's are used as a standard upon which several food assistance programs are based. For example, the school lunch program must meet 33 per cent of the RDA's for 12-year-old children in its meal planning. It is necessary in meeting such standards, however, that planners choose foods that will be eaten and enjoyed. The RDA's (Table 199–1) do not represent nutrient requirements for individuals; they are designed as guidelines for the daily intake of nutrients sufficient to ensure that almost all members of the population are not at risk of developing nutrient deficits. Thus, the RDA's exceed the nutrient requirements for most healthy individuals. Recommendations for energy intakes are an exception in that they represent values derived by multiplying resting energy expenditure (REE) by an activity factor for particular age and sex groups.

RDA's have been determined by balance studies, measurement of the amount of a nutrient needed to result in tissue saturation, examination of the food supplies of healthy populations, examination of minimal nutrient intakes required to prevent or correct either a naturally occurring or an experimentally produced deficit, epidemiologic observations, and animal studies. Precise RDA's have not been established for some nutrients (e.g., biotin, manganese) because of limited experimental data. However, ranges of safe intakes of these nutrients have been determined by the National Academy of Sciences and are provided in Table 199–2. Continued consumption of trace minerals above the upper limit of the recommended ranges can lead to toxic effects, as is the case with most individual nutrients.

The RDA's should be met by a variety of foods for two major reasons. First, certain dietary components (e.g., carotene, fiber, and possibly others as yet undefined) that are not considered "required" may nevertheless have a beneficial effect on body functioning. For example, if an individual is limited to a diet containing only preformed vitamin A, he or she could be deprived of the alleged beneficial effects of carotene (a vitamin A precursor). Second, a monotonous diet over a prolonged period may not supply a beneficial ratio of individual nutrients (e.g., a diet of very high carbohydrate content may increase the body's need for thiamine). Although other nutrient interactions have been defined (vitamin B_{12} is necessary for the demethylation of 5-methyl tetrahydrofolate; zinc is needed for the oxidation of retinol to photochemically active retinaldehyde), many such interactions are not fully known at present.

Body growth, body size, pregnancy, and lactation alter the RDA's. Pregnancy increases nutrient needs for the expansion of blood volume and for the growth and development of the fetus, placenta, uterus, and breasts. Similarly, lactation increases nutrient needs in proportion to the quantity of milk produced. Pregnancy and lactation RDA adjustments are provided in Table

199–1. Other factors that result in an alteration of dietary needs include environmental temperature, fever, menstruation (an increased requirement for iron), disease, and medication. Disease and/or drugs may change nutrient requirements by altering nutrient absorption or bioavailability, storage capacity, or excretion or by changing a nutrient's metabolism. For example, kidney disease may result in a decreased ability to change 25-hydroxy-vitamin D to its active 1,25-dihydroxylated form (Ch. 233); drugs that stimulate microsomal cytochrome P-450-mediated enzyme activities (e.g., alcohol) cause an increased hepatic metabolism of vitamin A. The physician should remember that the RDA's were not designed for sick or traumatized patients or for individuals with metabolic disorders such as hyperthyroidism. Despite all of these caveats, the RDA's do serve as useful guidelines for the practitioner to judge the adequacy of an individual's diet. Table 199–3 provides a guide to the possible effects of medication on nutrient requirements and the mechanisms by which these interactions occur.

Nutrient requirements and dietary recommendations for adults are defined in broad age classes in Table 199–1, namely 19 to 24 years, 25 to 50 years, and 51 years and older. In the absence of adequate information, the present recommendations for the elderly are the same as for the young adult population. However, old people eat fewer calories than young people, and accompanying this diminished calorie intake is a concomitant reduction in intake of almost all other nutrients. For nutrients whose requirements are fixed (rather than relative to calories), such across-the-board reductions may result in intakes that are insufficient to meet metabolic demands; for example, the amount of dietary protein needed for nitrogen equilibrium is not reduced with age. Age-related changes affect the absorption, metabolism, and excretion of many nutrients, so that age-specific standards for the elderly are needed. In addition, chronic disability, illness, and the increased use of medications in the elderly introduce other variables. Suffice it to say that the elderly person's diet should be of high quality in terms of nutrient density (i.e., quantity of nutrients/calorie).

Since parenteral administration of some nutrients bypasses any problems due to limited absorption, nutrient requirements are generally less when delivered by the parenteral route than by the enteral route. However, the underlying cause (e.g., disease, trauma) that necessitates parenteral delivery in a patient often dictates overall higher nutrient requirements (see Ch. 207).

WATER

Owing to a high ratio of surface area to volume, infants are more prone to dehydration than adults. The average adult needs a minimum of 700 to 1000 ml of water per day in order to survive, but 2000 ml per day (1 ml per Kcal intake) provides a safe and adequate basal maintenance amount. Approximately 100 ml per day of water is lost in feces, 500 to 1000 ml in evaporation and exhalation (insensible loss), and the remainder in urine. Diets providing a high renal solute load (e.g., diets high in protein, sodium, potassium, chloride) will result in higher urinary water losses. In a sick patient additional water must be supplied if body temperature is elevated (each 1°C elevation over normal results in an additional obligatory water loss of 200 ml per day), if diarrhea is present, or if polyuria is present (e.g., from uncontrolled diabetes mellitus or kidney disease). In such cases, measured losses may be added to the maintenance requirements. Elevated environmental temperature and exercise increase insensible losses (for each 2°C rise in temperature above 32°C, 500 ml of extra water should be provided). Acute alterations in water balance can be estimated by rapid changes in body weight.

TABLE 199-1. FOOD AND NUTRITION BOARD, NATIONAL ACADEMY OF SCIENCES—NATIONAL RESEARCH COUNCIL RECOMMENDED DIETARY ALLOWANCES,[a] Revised 1989

Designed for the maintenance of good nutrition of practically all healthy people in the United States

Category	Age (years) or Condition	Weight[b] (kg)	Weight[b] (lb)	Height[b] (cm)	Height[b] (in)	Protein (g)	Vitamin A (µg RE)[c]	Vitamin D (µg)[d]	Vitamin E (mg α-TE)[e]	Vitamin K (µg)	Vitamin C (mg)	Thiamine (mg)	Riboflavin (mg)	Niacin (mg NE)[f]	Vitamin B6 (mg)	Folate (µg)	Vitamin B12 (µg)	Calcium (mg)	Phosphorus (mg)	Magnesium (mg)	Iron (mg)	Zinc (mg)	Iodine (µg)	Selenium (µg)
Infants	0.0–0.5	6	13	60	24	13	375	7.5	3	5	30	0.3	0.4	5	0.3	25	0.3	400	300	40	6	5	40	10
	0.5–1.0	9	20	71	28	14	375	10	4	10	35	0.4	0.5	6	0.6	35	0.5	600	500	60	10	5	50	15
Children	1–3	13	29	90	35	16	400	10	6	15	40	0.7	0.8	9	1.0	50	0.7	800	800	80	10	10	70	20
	4–7	20	44	112	44	24	500	10	7	20	45	0.9	1.1	12	1.1	75	1.0	800	800	120	10	10	90	20
	7–10	28	62	132	52	28	700	10	7	30	45	1.0	1.2	13	1.4	100	1.4	800	800	170	10	10	120	30
Males	11–14	45	99	157	62	45	1,000	10	10	45	50	1.3	1.5	17	1.7	150	2.0	1,200	1,200	270	12	15	150	40
	15–18	66	145	176	69	59	1,000	10	10	65	60	1.5	1.8	20	2.0	200	2.0	1,200	1,200	400	12	15	150	50
	19–24	72	160	177	70	58	1,000	10	10	70	60	1.5	1.7	19	2.0	200	2.0	1,200	1,200	350	10	15	150	70
	25–50	79	174	176	70	63	1,000	5	10	80	60	1.5	1.7	19	2.0	200	2.0	800	800	350	10	15	150	70
	51+	77	170	173	68	63	1,000	5	10	80	60	1.2	1.4	15	2.0	200	2.0	800	800	350	10	15	150	70
Females	11–14	46	101	157	62	46	800	10	8	45	50	1.1	1.3	15	1.4	150	2.0	1,200	1,200	280	15	12	150	45
	15–18	55	120	163	64	44	800	10	8	55	60	1.1	1.3	15	1.5	180	2.0	1,200	1,200	300	15	12	150	50
	19–24	58	128	164	65	46	800	10	8	60	60	1.1	1.3	15	1.6	180	2.0	1,200	1,200	280	15	12	150	55
	25–50	63	138	163	64	50	800	5	8	65	60	1.1	1.3	15	1.6	180	2.0	800	800	280	15	12	150	55
	51+	65	143	160	63	50	800	5	8	65	60	1.0	1.2	13	1.6	180	2.0	800	800	280	10	12	150	55
Pregnant						60	800	10	10	65	70	1.5	1.6	17	2.2	400	2.2	1,200	1,200	320	30	15	175	65
Lactating	1st 6 months					65	1,300	10	12	65	95	1.6	1.8	20	2.1	280	2.6	1,200	1,200	355	15	19	200	75
	2nd 6 months					62	1,200	10	11	65	90	1.6	1.7	20	2.1	260	2.6	1,200	1,200	340	15	16	200	75

[a]The allowances, expressed as average daily intakes over time, are intended to provide for individual variations among most normal persons as they live in the United States under usual environmental stresses. Diets should be based on a variety of common foods in order to provide other nutrients for which human requirements have been less well defined.

[b]Weights and heights of Reference Adults are actual medians for the designated age, as reported by NHANES II. The use of these figures does not imply that the height-to-weight ratios are ideal.

[c]Retinol equivalents. 1 retinol equivalent = 1 µg retinol or 6 µg β-carotene.

[d]As cholecalciferol: 10 µg cholecalciferol = 400 IU of vitamin D.

[e]α-Tocopherol equivalents. 1 mg D-α-tocopherol = 1 α-TE.

[f]1 NE (niacin equivalent) is equal to 1 mg of niacin or 60 mg of dietary tryptophan.

TABLE 199–2. ESTIMATED SAFE AND ADEQUATE DAILY DIETARY INTAKES OF SELECTED VITAMINS AND MINERALS[a]

Category	Age (years)	Biotin (μg)	Pantothenic Acid (mg)	Copper (mg)	Manganese (mg)	Fluoride (mg)	Chromium (μg)	Molybdenum (μg)
		Vitamins		**Trace Elements**[b]				
Infants	0–0.5	10	2	0.4–0.6	0.3–0.6	0.1–0.5	10–40	15–30
	0.5–1	15	3	0.6–0.7	0.6–1.0	0.2–1.0	20–60	20–40
Children and	1–3	20	3	0.7–1.0	1.0–1.5	0.5–1.5	20–80	25–50
adolescents	4–6	25	3–4	1.0–1.5	1.5–2.0	1.0–2.5	30–120	30–75
	7–10	30	4–5	1.0–2.0	2.0–3.0	1.5–2.5	50–200	50–150
	11 +	30–100	4–7	1.5–2.5	2.0–5.0	1.5–2.5	50–200	75–250
Adults		30–100	4–7	1.5–3.0	2.0–5.0	1.5–4.0	50–200	75–250

[a]Because there is less information on which to base allowances, these figures are not given in Table 199–1 and are provided here in the form of ranges of recommended intakes.

[b]Since the toxic levels for many trace elements may be only several times usual intakes, the upper levels for the trace elements given in this table should not be habitually exceeded.

ENERGY

Energy needs vary with body size, growth phase, age, sex, and activity. Factors that increase energy requirements are cold exposure, pregnancy, lactation, infection, fever, hyperthyroidism, and trauma. Recommended energy allowances for all ages are presented in Table 199–4. A normal variation of ± 20 per cent is accepted for younger adults, the ranges being wider for children. In pregnancy, energy allowances should be increased 300 Kcal per day for the second and third trimesters of pregnancy. Lactation increases energy requirements by 500 Kcal per day. The energy allowances for children from birth through age 10 are World Health Organization figures. The allowances for adults are based on median weights and heights from the second U.S. Health and Nutrition Examination Survey (NHANES II) for moderate work (e.g., walking, shopping, playing golf). In addition to the age groups 19 to 24 and 25 to 50 years, energy recommendations for older people are provided for those over age 50. The aging process normally results in a progressive decrease in energy needs, primarily as a result of a decrease in energy expenditure.

Protein and carbohydrate supply approximately 4 Kcal per gram, alcohol 7 Kcal per gram, and fat 9 Kcal per gram. Resting energy expenditure (REE) is the amount of oxygen consumed under resting conditions extrapolated to 24 hours. A simple rule of thumb to estimate REE is 25 Kcal per kilogram body weight. However, this formula is not useful in overweight people. Since adipose tissue is relatively inert from a metabolic point of view, the relationship between REE and body weight becomes nonlinear in overweightness. A more accurate estimate of REE for healthy individuals is the Harris-Benedict equation:

Men: REE = 66 + (13.7 weight in kg) + (5 × height in cm) − 6.8 (age in years)

Women: REE = 665 + (9.6 × weight in kg) + (1.7 × height in cm) − 4.7 (age in years)

Depending on factors such as activity level and illness, energy needs may be increased many times over the basal level. Ingestion and metabolism of food increase the caloric requirement by about 7 per cent of the REE, provided that a mixed diet is being consumed. Activity increases energy requirements over a wide range (1.1 to 10.3 Kcal per kilogram per hour) depending on the intensity and type of work being done. The number of daily calories that should be provided in addition to the REE are 400 to 800 Kcal for sedentary activity, 800 to 1200 Kcal for light activity (e.g., sewing, desk work), and 1200 to 1800 Kcal for moderate work (e.g., walking). The number of kilocalories to be added for heavy work (e.g., running, swimming) ranges from 1800 to 4500 Kcal per day. Although fasting and malnutrition reduce energy expenditure, the stress of illness increases caloric requirements. For each 1°C of fever, a 13 per cent increase in calories is required. In catabolic patients, an additional 50 to 100 per cent of the REE may be necessary to prevent further tissue breakdown.

PROTEIN

A constant supply of protein (i.e., amino acids) is needed to maintain body function and structure. On a protein-free diet, the average net loss of body protein by males is about 0.34 gram per kilogram of body weight. However, when allowance is made for incomplete utilization of dietary protein and for variability in needs, the allowance recommended for adults rises to 0.75 gram of protein per kilogram. Protein needs are dependent, in part, on energy intake. Increased energy intake results in protein conservation and decreased energy intake results in the diversion of protein to meet energy needs. Pregnancy and lactation increase the body's protein requirement.

There is a continuum of food protein quality depending on the digestibility of the protein and its amino acid composition. Nine essential amino acids must be provided in the diet, since the human body lacks the ability to synthesize them. These are lysine, leucine, isoleucine, valine, methionine, phenylalanine, tryptophan, threonine, and possibly histidine, especially for infants.

High-quality proteins are those that have a high degree of bioavailability (i.e., they are easily digested and absorbed) and have a high biologic value (a measure of the efficiency of utilization of absorbed protein, which in turn is dependent on adequate amounts and proportions of essential amino acids). The highest quality proteins are found in eggs and milk. Seeds and nuts, rice, corn, and grain proteins are of lesser quality. It is recommended that 10 to 15 per cent of caloric intake be derived from protein. Amino acids supplied in excess of the body's requirement are not

TABLE 199–3. EXAMPLES OF DRUG-NUTRIENT INTERACTIONS

Drug	Increased Requirement	Potential Mechanism	Deficiency Symptoms
Antacids (aluminum and magnesium hydroxides)	Phosphate	Formation of insoluble salts	Malaise, paresthesias, anorexia
Anticonvulsants (phenobarbital, phenytoin)	Vitamin D	Induction of hepatic microsomal enzymes resulting in inactive vitamin D metabolites	Rickets, osteomalacia
Oral contraceptives (norethindrone/mestranol)	Folic acid	Inhibition of polyglutamic folate absorption	Megaloblastic anemia
Antituberculous drugs (isoniazid, cycloserine)	Vitamin B_6	Excretion of pyridoxal hydrazone complex	Peripheral neuropathy
Anticoagulants (coumarin, warfarin)	Vitamin K	Inhibition of vitamin K recycling	Hypoprothrombinemia
Diuretics (benzothiadiazides)	Potassium	Enhancement of renal excretion	Hypokalemia

TABLE 199–4. MEDIAN REFERENCE HEIGHTS AND WEIGHTS AND RECOMMENDED ENERGY INTAKE

Category	Age (years) or Condition	Weight (kg)	Weight (lb)	Height (cm)	Height (in)	REE[a] (Kcal/day)	Average Energy Allowance (Kcal)[b] Multiples per Kg per Day[c] of REE		
Infants	0.0–0.5	6	13	60	24	320		108	650
	0.5–1.0	9	20	71	28	500		98	850
Children	1–3	13	29	90	35	740		102	1,300
	4–6	20	44	112	44	950		90	1,800
	7–10	28	62	132	52	1,130		70	2,000
Males	11–14	45	99	157	62	1,440	1.70	55	2,500
	15–18	66	145	176	69	1,760	1.67	45	3,000
	19–24	72	160	177	70	1,780	1.67	40	2,900
	25–50	79	174	176	70	1,800	1.60	37	2,900
	51+	77	170	173	68	1,530	1.50	30	2,300
Females	11–14	46	101	157	62	1,310	1.67	47	2,200
	15–18	55	120	163	64	1,370	1.60	40	2,200
	19–24	58	128	164	65	1,350	1.60	38	2,200
	25–50	63	138	163	64	1,380	1.55	36	2,200
	51+	65	143	160	63	1,280	1.50	30	1,900
Pregnant	1st trimester								+0
	2nd trimester								+300
	3rd trimester								+300
Lactating	1st 6 months								+500
	2nd 6 months								+500

[a]Calculation based on Food and Agricultural Organization equations, then rounded.
[b]In the range of light to moderate activity, the coefficient of variation is ±20%.
[c]Figure is rounded.
Source: Food and Nutrition Board, National Academy of Sciences–National Research Council, Recommended Dietary Allowances, revised 1989.

stored but are degraded to metabolic products (urea, uric acid, etc.), and the carbon skeleton is converted to carbohydrate and fat or oxidized for energy. It is important that a mixed diet be consumed so that adequate amounts of each essential amino acid are received. Some amino acids are complementary; for example, tyrosine may in part meet the body's requirement for phenylalanine, and cystine may in part meet the body's requirement for methionine. The ability of the body to utilize protein is impaired if one essential amino acid is missing, underscoring the need for mixed sources of dietary proteins.

In parenterally fed patients, zero nitrogen balance may be achieved with as little as 0.5 gram per kilogram per day of mixed amino acids (including all essential amino acids). However, patients with abnormal losses or increased demands (burns, trauma, wound repair) may require 1.2 to 1.6 grams per kilogram of desirable body weight per day.

In the clinical setting, the state of nitrogen balance can be crudely estimated by measuring the 24-hour urinary urea nitrogen excretion:

$$\text{Nitrogen balance} = \frac{\text{protein intake (g)}}{6.25} - [\text{urinary urea nitrogen (g)} + 4]$$

CARBOHYDRATE

Carbohydrate supplies 65 per cent of the world's food energy (50 per cent in developed countries, 75 per cent in developing countries), and of this 10 to 50 per cent is from simple sugars. Although a diet low in carbohydrate may result in ketosis, there is no fixed requirement for carbohydrate in the diet. Carbohydrate may be divided into available (i.e., digestible and utilizable as sugars) and unavailable (i.e., dietary fiber). The primary sources of both available and unavailable carbohydrates are of vegetable origin. Dietary fiber reaches the large intestine intact but then may undergo fermentation by bacteria, with the subsequent absorption of breakdown products and some "rescue" of calories. Dietary fiber is made up of crude fiber (cellulose, lignin), mucilages, pectins, hemicellulose, and water-soluble gums. Each type of fiber has different characteristics with regard to water holding, cation exchange, and adsorptive properties (e.g., for bile acids and drugs). For example, mucilages have a high capacity for water holding, and pectins avidly adsorb bile acids. Increases in stool weight and faster intestinal transit result from increases in dietary fiber. Primarily because of epidemiologic disease patterns (e.g., for colon cancer and diverticulitis), an increase of dietary fiber has been suggested. At least 20 to 25 grams of dietary fiber per day are needed for a therapeutic effect in the

irritable bowel syndrome. Gums and pectins have been shown to have a beneficial effect on diabetes by delaying the absorption of glucose. As with most dietary components, too much fiber may be harmful: Large amounts of dietary fiber may contribute to trace metal deficiency in certain parts of the world by adsorbing divalent cations (e.g., zinc) and making them unavailable for gastrointestinal absorption. Carbohydrate intolerance syndromes (e.g., lactose intolerance) are described in Ch. 102.

FAT

Fat, a concentrated source of calories, serves as a carrier for fat-soluble vitamins and as a source of essential fatty acids. All body cells with the exception of the central nervous system and erythrocytes can directly utilize fatty acids as a source of energy. Polyunsaturated essential fatty acids (linoleic, linolenic) and their derivatives serve as precursors for eicosanoids, which include the leukotrienes, prostaglandins, and thromboxanes. They are also needed for membrane structure and integrity. Polyunsaturated fatty acids have been shown to promote carcinogenesis in experimental animals, however, and may reduce circulating HDL cholesterol and promote gallstone formation. Thus, an upper limit of 10 per cent of calories taken in as polyunsaturated fats is advised. Monounsaturated fatty acids are effective for optimizing plasma lipoproteins. There is recent interest in the role of N-3 polyunsaturated fatty acids, derived from linolenic acid or from fish oils, in the prevention of ischemic heart disease. However, more investigation is needed on the interaction between N-6 and N-3 fatty acids in human tissue before sound dietary recommendations can be made. Linoleic acid is a prominent component of dietary fats, but deficiency has been recognized only among patients on prolonged parenteral feedings containing no fat. Two per cent of calories in the form of linoleic acid and 0.5 per cent as linolenic acid are sufficient for preventing essential fatty acid deficiency.

VITAMINS AND MINERALS

Requirements for vitamins and minerals are discussed in Ch. 204 and 205.

NUTRITIONAL RECOMMENDATIONS

The Surgeon General's Report on Nutrition and Health published in 1988 outlines prudent dietary recommendations for the United States population in order to avoid diseases and disabilities that appear to have a relation to diet. Other sets of similar recommendations have been proposed by organizations such as the American Heart Association and the National Cancer Institute. Such dietary goals include a reduction in the percentage of calories ingested as fat by the United States public from 37 per cent to 30 per cent (<10 per cent saturated, <10 per cent polyunsaturated). At least 12 per cent of total calories should be ingested as protein. Further recommendations are that total calories ingested as carbohydrate be increased to approximately 60 per cent, with an increase in complex carbohydrates (e.g., starches, fiber) and naturally occurring sugars to approximately 50 per cent. Refined and processed sugar ingestion should be decreased to about 10 per cent of the total caloric intake. With a view toward reducing coronary artery disease, the American Heart Association recommends, in addition, a restriction of dietary cholesterol to less than 300 mg per day and of sodium to less than 3 grams per day. The judicious diet is outlined in detail in Ch. 12.

Diet and Health. Washington, D.C., National Academy of Sciences, 1989. *A comprehensive analysis of the scientific literature on the role of diet in the etiology and prevention of chronic disease in the United States.*

Energy and Protein Requirements, Report of a Joint FAO/WHO/UNU Expert Consultation. Geneva, WHO, 1985.

National Research Council: Recommended Dietary Allowances, 10th ed. Washington, D.C., National Academy of Sciences, 1989.

Roe DA: Drug Induced Nutritional Deficiencies, 2nd ed. Westport, CT, AVI Publishing Company, Inc., 1985.

The Surgeon General's Report on Nutrition and Health. US Dept of Health and Human Services (DHHS) Publication No 88-50211. Washington, D.C., 1988. *This report's major conclusion is that overconsumption of fat at the expense of foods high in complex carbohydrates is detrimental to health.*

200 Nutritional Assessment

Robert M. Russell

The recognition and treatment of malnutrition that accompanies illness play important roles in optimizing patient care. New modes of delivering nutrients to sick patients by both the parenteral and enteral routes may result in reductions in morbidity and mortality and shorten the length of hospitalization for both medical and surgical patients (Ch. 206 and 207).

Methods of nutritional assessment that have been used for some time to judge the severity of malnutrition among populations in lesser developed countries (e.g., anthropometric measures) are now being applied to hospitalized patients. An unexpectedly high prevalence (up to 40 per cent) of protein-energy malnutrition has been identified among Western patients. Reasons for the lack of recognition of malnutrition in hospitalized patients include preoccupation with the treatment of the disease process, neglect of the overall nutritional status of the patient (e.g., failure to obtain regular weights or to observe a patient's dietary intake), lack of sensitivity of casual observation in the recognition of protein-energy malnutrition, absence of a single indicator for diagnosis of malnutrition, and latent onset of clinical signs of malnutrition and relative lack of specificity of these signs. A single nutrient deficiency rarely occurs in a patient; rather, a complex and confusing array of deficiencies is most often present.

The diagnosis of malnutrition should be made on the basis of several consolidated pieces of information, including dietary history, anthropometric and laboratory measurements, and clinical examination. By using all of this information in a coordinated fashion, a more accurate diagnosis of the malnourished can be achieved, and an effective plan of treatment can be instituted.

DIET

It is not expected that the physician will interpret dietary records of a patient in detail. However, a physician should be able to perform a dietary evaluation by assessing the intakes of major food groups (milk-yogurt-cheese, meat-poultry-fish-eggs, fruits-vegetables, breads-cereals-grains, alcohol, fats such as oil, butter, bacon, and gravy) and the quality of selection within these groups. This is best done by asking the patient to recall all foods eaten within the last 24 hours (including snacks) and the

approximate portion sizes. A mixed diet is a desirable goal, when advising patients on healthful diets (Ch. 12). Moreover, the clinician should be aware of the key questions to ask patients, which provide clues about whether or not the patient's dietary intake requires adjustment (Table 200–1). A detailed medical and social history can alert the physician to an existing dietary problem or the likelihood of a dietary problem occurring in the future. For example, poverty, physical or mental disability, complaints of dysphagia, anorexia, nausea, abdominal pain while eating, ill-fitting dentures, and alcoholism may all be factors that prevent adequate dietary intake. Increased nutritional requirements can result from diarrhea, fever, open wounds or burns, malabsorption, diabetes, and hyperthyroidism. The physician should be able to counsel patients regarding general dietary guidelines (Ch. 12) and recognize cases for referral to a dietitian for more detailed counseling.

The elderly are a group with an increased risk of malnutrition. The reasons for this include poverty, the inability to move around easily, the cumulative effects of chronic disease necessitating multiple medications, social isolation, and the lack of knowledge for adequate preparation of meals (particularly among elderly men). Problems often arise when interviewing the elderly person for dietary habits (e.g., by 24-hour dietary recall, food frequency questionnaires) if the individual is senile or has impaired short-term memory. Even a 3- to 7-day dietary record, wherein the patient records everything eaten during that period, has proven difficult for the elderly patient to keep. A family member may therefore be of great assistance when obtaining dietary information. Finally, appropriate standards for judging the elderly person's diet are not currently available. The Recommended Dietary Allowances (see Table 199–1) were developed as population standards (not individual requirements) and are set to meet the needs of most healthy individuals. The standards for adults are based almost exclusively on young adults. As a result, they may not be appropriate for meeting the needs of the elderly patient who has an array of chronic diseases or aging disorders, or both.

ANTHROPOMETRIC MEASUREMENTS

Sophisticated and specialized methods to assess body composition are available, e.g., underwater weighing for body density, CT scanning, neutron activation analysis, and ^{40}K counting. However, none of these methods is available for widespread clinical use. Anthropometric reference values derived from measurements on normal populations provide inexpensive, quick, and convenient estimates of a patient's nutritional status in terms of protein and fat reserves. The most useful anthropometric meas-

TABLE 200–1. KEY QUESTIONS TO ASK AS PART OF THE NUTRITIONAL ASSESSMENT OF THE ADULT

1. Is there recent weight gain or weight loss? How much?
2. Are there alterations in appetite, sense of smell, or taste?
3. Are there problems with chewing or swallowing? Does the patient have poor dentition or poorly fitting dentures?
4. Are there symptoms of gastrointestinal disorders: diarrhea, constipation, nausea, vomiting, early satiety?
5. Does the patient live alone? If not, who prepares meals? Does he/she know how to cook?
6. What type of cooking facilities and refrigeration are in the patient's home?
7. Does the patient purchase a variety of foods? If not, is it due to financial difficulties?
8. How many meals are eaten per day? How many snacks? Are one or more meals eaten outside of the home? If so, where?
9. Is the patient physically or mentally handicapped? Does this prevent the individual from shopping, cooking, or feeding herself or himself?
10. Does the patient take any dietary supplements (e.g., vitamins)?
11. How much alcohol does the patient consume?
12. Does the patient use prescription or nonprescription drugs?
13. Are there any religious or ethnic beliefs or food intolerances that prevent adequate food intake?
14. Does the patient follow a dietary restriction? Is it prescribed or self-imposed?
15. Is the patient depressed?

TABLE 200–2. REFERENCE WEIGHTS FOR VARIOUS HEIGHTS DERIVED FROM ACTUARIAL (MORTALITY EXPERIENCE) DATA OF THE 1979 BUILD AND BLOOD PRESSURE STUDY FOR USE IN AGES 20 TO 55*

Height		Weight			
		Male		Female	
in	cm	lb	kg	lb	kg
58	147.3	—	—	114	51.7
59	149.9	—	—	116.5	52.8
60	152.4	—	—	119	53.9
61	154.9	—	—	122	55.3
62	157.5	133	60.3	125	56.7
63	160.0	135	61.2	128	58.0
64	162.6	137.5	62.4	131	59.4
65	165.1	140	63.5	134	60.8
66	167.6	143	64.9	137	62.1
67	170.2	146	66.2	140	63.5
68	172.7	149	67.6	143	64.9
69	175.3	152	68.9	146	66.2
70	177.8	155	70.3	149	67.6
71	180.3	158.5	71.9	152	69.0
72	182.9	162	73.9	—	—
73	185.4	166	75.3	—	—
74	188.0	169.5	76.9	—	—
75	190.5	174	78.9	—	—

*Weights represent the midpoint of the middle frame for each height. These values correct the 1983 Metropolitan Tables to nude weights and heights.

ures include height, weight, triceps skinfold (actually fatfold) thickness, and midarm muscle area. Accurate measurements require only three simple pieces of equipment: a beam or lever balance scale with a vertical measuring rod and a headpiece, a constant tension skinfold caliper, and a flexible measuring tape, preferably with an insertion.

WEIGHT FOR HEIGHT. Single reference weights for each inch of height have been derived from United States life insurance actuarial data on longevity and have been termed "ideal" or "optimal" by some investigators. However, these single weights should not be interpreted as "ideal," since they represent the midpoint of an acceptable range for a person of medium frame and were derived from the mortality experience of only those men and women between the ages of 20 to 59 years who could afford life insurance. These weights are neither age- nor race-specific and do not represent all cultural groups. Further, these reference weights cannot be applied to patients with peripheral edema or ascites. Despite the recognized flaws in using such

TABLE 200–3. MEDIAN WEIGHT FOR VARIOUS HEIGHTS FOR AGE 55 to 74 FROM COMBINED NHANES I AND II DATA SETS

Height		Weight			
		Male		Female	
in	cm	lb	kg	lb	kg
58	147	—	—	125.4	57
59	150	—	—	136.4	62
60	152	—	—	143.0	65
61	155	—	—	140.8	64
62	157	149.6	68	140.8	64
63	160	154.0	70	143.0	65
64	163	156.2	71	145.2	66
65	165	158.4	72	147.4	67
66	168	162.8	74	145.2	66
67	170	171.6	78	158.4	72
68	173	171.6	78	154.0	70
69	175	169.4	77	158.4	72
70	178	176.0	80	160.6	73
71	180	184.8	84	—	—
72	183	178.2	81	—	—
73	185	193.6	88	—	—
74	188	209.0	95	—	—

Adapted from Frisancho AB: Am J Clin Nutr 40:808, 1984. © Am J Clin Nutr, American Society for Clinical Nutrition.

single reference weights as standards, clinicians have found the 1983 Metropolitan Life Insurance Reference Weights for Height useful for judging a patient's nutritional status reflecting caloric sufficiency. These reference weights (corrected to the nude state) are provided in Table 200–2 and may be used for judging underweightness or overweightness for the population age group 20 to 55. For people over the age of 55 it is recommended to use age-specific weight-for-height median values (medium frame size) derived from the combined data sets of the National Health and Nutrition Examination Surveys of 1971 to 1974 and 1976 to 1980 (NHANES) (Table 200–3). Body mass index (weight ÷ height squared) is another means of assessing relative body weight which has the advantage of minimizing height as a factor in estimating overweightness and underweightness. Body mass index thus partially compensates for the shrinkage in height which takes place during the adult life span (Ch. 203). A nomogram for determining and interpreting body mass index is provided in Figure 200–1. In children, weight and height are often used as separate measures to indicate malnutrition and are expressed as percentiles of a cross-section of American children. Weight and height tables for children can be found in most pediatric textbooks.

The amount of weight lost and the rate at which it was lost by

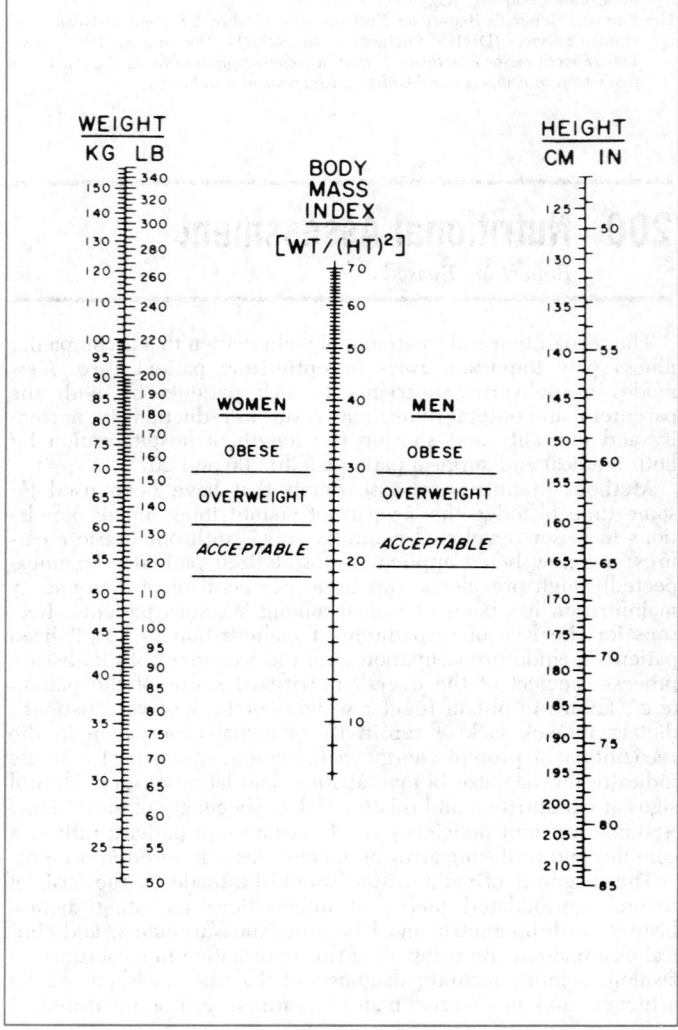

FIGURE 200–1. A nomogram for determining body mass index (BMI). To use this nomogram, place a ruler or other straight edge between the column for height and the column for weight connecting an individual's numbers for those two variables. Read the BMI in kg/m² where the straight line crosses the middle lines when the height and weight are connected. Overweight: BMI of 25–30 kg/m²; obesity: BMI above 30 kg/m². Heights and weights are without shoes or clothes. (From Bray GA: Obesity: definition, diagnoses and disadvantages. Med J Aust 142:S2–S8. Copyright 1985, The Medical Journal of Australia; reprinted with permission.)

TABLE 200–4. SUGGESTED CRITERIA TO JUDGE MALNUTRITION AND OBESITY IN THE UNITED STATES POPULATION

	Standard Male/Female	At Risk for Malnutrition (% of standard)	At Risk for Obesity (% of standard)
Weight/Height			
Age 20–55	Table 200–2	<80	>130
Age >55	Table 200–3	<80	>120
Triceps skinfold (mm)			
Age 25–54	12/23	<50	>170
Age 55–75	12/25	<50	>150
Midarm muscle area (cm²)			
Age 25–54	55/31	<70	NA
Age 55–75	52/35	<65	NA

The percentages below and above the given standards for assessing malnutrition and obesity correspond to less than the 15th percentile and greater than the 85th percentile, respectively, on the combined data sets of NHANES I and II normative values.

a patient are also important for judging an individual's nutritional status. A weight loss of 1 kg represents approximately a 7000-calorie deficit. A history of unintentional weight loss of 10 per cent or greater (6 per cent in an overweight patient) over a 6-month period can be indicative of malnutrition.

TRICEPS SKINFOLD THICKNESS. This measurement provides an estimate of the body's fat reserves. The measurement should be taken at a marked point on the right arm, halfway between the acromial process of the scapula and the olecranon process of the elbow. The patient's arm should be relaxed when the fatfold is grasped posteriorly between the thumb and forefinger of the examiner. The fold should be raised, allowing underlying muscle to fall back to the bone, and the calipers applied. The measurement is useless if arm edema or paralysis is present. Age- and sex-specific standards for triceps skinfold (TSF) thickness for all ages through 75 years are summarized in Table 200–4. A wide range on either side of the standard is considered an acceptable TSF measure, since large variances are found for fatfold thicknesses in the normal population. A patient whose TSF thickness is less than 50 per cent of the NHANES standard is considered to have depleted body fat stores, whereas the patient whose TSF thickness is more than 150 to 170 per cent of standard is considered obese.

MIDARM MUSCLE AREA. This derived value is used to estimate lean body or skeletal muscle mass. To calculate this value, the midarm circumference must first be measured at the same site as for the triceps fatfold, with the patient's right arm in a relaxed posture. The formula to calculate bone-free, upper-arm midarm muscle area (MAMA) is:

$$\frac{\{\text{midarm circumference (cm)} - [0.314 \times \text{TSF (mm)}]\}^2}{4\pi} - 10 \text{ (males)}$$
$$- 6.5 \text{ (females)}$$

Median values are summarized in Table 200–4. Thirty to 35 per cent below this standard (depending upon age) is indicative of a depletion of lean body mass. Neither TSF nor midarm muscle area standards have been derived for the very elderly (i.e., older than 75 years). A summary of criteria to judge malnutrition and obesity by anthropometric measurements is presented in Table 200–4.

CLINICAL ASSESSMENT

By noting certain physical changes in the patient (e.g., temporal muscle wasting, hair depigmentation, edema), the clinician may have the clinical impression of protein-calorie malnutrition, which objective anthropometric and laboratory measurements can confirm. However, early clinical symptoms and signs of malnutrition are rather vague and often include weakness, lethargy, irritability, and lightheadedness. Many of the symptoms and signs are nonspecific for a single nutrient deficit and may be caused by insufficiency of one of several nutrients. For example, flaking dermatitis may accompany deficiencies of protein, riboflavin, or linoleic acid. On the other hand, when certain clinical signs

TABLE 200–5. CLINICAL SIGNS AND SYMPTOMS OF NUTRITIONAL INADEQUACY IN ADULT PATIENTS

	Clinical Sign or Symptom	Nutrient
General	Wasted, skinny	Calorie
	Loss of appetite	Protein-energy
Skin	Psoriasiform rash, eczematous scaling	Zinc
	Pallor	Folate, iron, vitamin B_{12}, copper
	Follicular hyperkeratosis	Vitamin A
	Perifollicular petechiae	Vitamin C
	Flaking dermatitis	Protein-energy, niacin, riboflavin, zinc
	Bruising	Vitamin C, vitamin K
	Pigmentation changes	Niacin, protein-energy
	Scrotal dermatosis	Riboflavin
	Thickening and dryness of skin	Linoleic acid
Head	Temporal muscle wasting	Protein-energy
Hair	Sparse and thin, dyspigmentation	Protein
	Easy to pull out	
Eyes	History of night blindness (also impaired visual recovery after glare)	Vitamin A, zinc
	Photophobia, blurring, conjunctival inflammation	Riboflavin, vitamin A
	Corneal vascularization	Riboflavin
	Xerosis, Bitot spots, keratomalacia	Vitamin A
Mouth	Glossitis	Riboflavin, niacin, folic acid, vitamin B_{12}, pyridoxine
	Bleeding gums	Vitamin C, riboflavin
	Cheilosis	Riboflavin
	Angular stomatitis	Riboflavin, iron
	Hypogeusia	Zinc
	Tongue fissuring	Niacin
	Tongue atrophy	Riboflavin, niacin, iron
	Scarlet and raw tongue	Niacin
	Nasolabial seborrhea	Pyridoxine
Neck	Goiter	Iodine
	Parotid enlargement	Protein
Thorax	Thoracic rosary	Vitamin D
Abdomen	Diarrhea	Niacin, folate, vitamin B_{12}
	Distention	Protein-energy
	Hepatomegaly	Protein-energy
Extremities	Edema	Protein, thiamine
	Softening of bone	Vitamin D, calcium, phosphorus
	Bone tenderness	Vitamin D
	Bone ache, joint pain	Vitamin C
	Muscle wasting and weakness	Protein, calorie, vitamin D, selenium, sodium chloride
	Muscle tenderness, muscle pain	Thiamine
	Hyporeflexia	Thiamine
	Ataxia	Vitamin B_{12}
Nails	Spooning	Iron
	Transverse lines	Protein
Neurologic	Tetany	Calcium, magnesium
	Paresthesias	Thiamine, vitamin B_{12}
	Loss of reflexes, wrist drop, foot drop	Thiamine
	Loss of vibratory and position sense	Vitamin B_{12}
	Dementia, disorientation	Niacin
Blood	Anemia	Vitamins E, B_{12}, folate, iron, pyridoxine
	Hemolysis	Phosphorus

appear, the nutrient deficit may be very severe (e.g., scleromalacia, a leading and rapidly progressive cause of blindness due to vitamin A deficiency). Table 200–5 contains a listing of the most prevalent clinical presentations and the associated nutrient deficits that may cause them.

Functional and end-organ testing has been advocated for diagnosis of specific nutrient deficits (e.g., dark adaptation for vitamin A, taste and smell for zinc, bone density for vitamin D). However, functional tests are not available to assess the status of most nutrients, and, as with clinical signs, the functional tests are often nonspecific. For example, impairment of dark adaptation may be caused by zinc deficiency as well as vitamin A deficiency. Taste and smell may be affected by age, smoking, and drugs as well as by zinc nutriture. Bone density is diminished in both osteoporosis and vitamin D deficiency (osteomalacia).

As with dietary assessment, the elderly present a particular problem when evaluated for the presence or absence of clinical signs or symptoms of malnutrition. Some of the changes associated with malnutrition may also be a function of normal aging (e.g., hypogeusia, dry skin, sparse hair, atrophy of the tongue, bleeding gums from ill-fitting dentures). Nevertheless, as with younger patients, clinical signs should be assessed for dietary, laboratory, and anthropometric correlates vis-à-vis possible nutritional implications.

LABORATORY ASSESSMENT

Laboratory measurements are another tool that can aid the physician in making a diagnosis of malnutrition, although, once again, certain laboratory abnormalities that could reflect malnutrition can also have a non-nutritional cause (e.g., calcium, albumin, hematocrit). Modern analytical instruments (e.g., high-performance liquid chromatography), techniques (e.g., radio or enzyme immunoassays), and computerization have greatly increased the capability of nutritional biochemical testing. Currently available biochemical tests for assessing nutritional status include the direct measurement of a nutrient or nutrient metabolite in blood, other body fluids (e.g., urine, saliva), or tissues (e.g., white blood cells, hair, liver) and the measurement of a biochemical function that is nutrient specific. For example, laboratory tests for pyridoxine status may include the direct measurement of pyridoxal 5'-phosphate in plasma or the enzymatic activity of erythrocyte transaminase, for which pyridoxal 5'-phosphate is a cofactor. The latter test involves the calculation of an activity coefficient whereby red blood cell transaminase activity is determined before and after the addition of pyridoxal 5'-phosphate. An activity coefficient of greater than 2.2 is indicative of pyridoxine deficiency.

The establishment of normal nutrient values in body fluids or tissues for each sex varies from laboratory to laboratory, and the normal range usually represents a mean ± 2 SD of a normal population. Optimally, a low biochemical nutrient value in body fluids or tissue should be coupled with a specific functional abnormality before making the diagnosis of a nutrient deficiency. However, in practice this is rarely done. One guide for interpretation of laboratory values that reflects the status of various nutrients in the blood or serum of adults is presented in Table 200–6. For some nutrients (e.g., vitamin A) children have a different normal range than adults. The reader is referred to a pediatric text for children's normal values. Normal biochemical ranges have not been established for the very old (i.e., over 75 years). The physician must rely upon values derived from younger populations to judge the nutritional biochemical parameters for this group.

Many nutrient biochemical diagnostic tests are not readily available in a hospital clinical chemistry laboratory. Nevertheless, there are several laboratory tests that are routinely performed (e.g., hemoglobin level, serum protein level) that may aid the physician in assessing the nutritional status of his or her patients. In the absence of liver disease, a low serum albumin may be used as an indicator of protein nutriture. In sick patients who are obese, silent kwashiorkor (protein malnutrition) may develop (Ch. 201), as reflected by low serum protein values, although the patient may continue to look overnourished and anthropometric

TABLE 200–6. GUIDE FOR INTERPRETATION OF SERUM AND/OR BLOOD INDICES FOR SELECTED NUTRIENTS

Nutrient	Normal*	Deficient	Marginal
Albumin	3.5–5.5 grams/dl	2.8–3.2	3.2–3.5
Transferrin	200–400 mg/dl	< 200	
Transthyretin	10–40 mg/dl	< 10	
Ferritin	12–300 ng/ml	< 12	
Retinol	30–90 µg/dl	< 15	15–30
Carotene	40–240 µg/dl	< 40	
Vitamin E	0.5–1.8 mg/dl	< 0.5	0.5–0.7
Vitamin D (25-OH-D$_3$)	15–40 ng/ml		
Thiamine (erythrocyte)	0.9–1.25†	> 1.25	1.25–1.20
Riboflavin	0.9–1.39†	> 1.40	1.30–1.40
Pyridoxine	0.9–2.2†	> 2.2	
Niacin (urine 2-pyridone/N'-methyl nicotinamide—metabolite ratio)	1.0–4.0	< 1.0	
Serum folate	6–20 ng/ml	≤ 3.0	3–6
Red cell folate	150–450 ng/ml	< 150	
Vitamin B$_{12}$	>200 pg/ml	< 150	150–200
Vitamin C	0.3–2.0 mg/dl	< 0.2	0.2–0.3
Calcium	8.5–10.5 mg/dl	< 8.5	
Phosphorus	2.5–4.5 mg/dl	< 2.5	
Iron	50–170 µg/dl		
Zinc	70–130 µg/dl	≤ 65	65–70
Copper	70–160 µg/dl	< 70	
Magnesium	1.4–2.5 mg/dl	≤ 1.4	

*These normal values will vary with the method used and in different laboratories.
†An enzymatic assay. Values represent an activity coefficient.

measures may be normal or exceed the normal range. Other proteins that are synthesized in the liver and that have a more rapid turnover than albumin (e.g., transferrin, transthyretin) may also be used to diagnose protein malnutrition at an earlier stage, provided that the patient does not have liver damage. The transferrin in serum, if not directly measured, may be estimated from the total iron binding capacity (TIBC) according to the formula: $(0.8 \times TIBC) - 43$. Protein values that are more than 20 per cent below the lower limit of the normal range are generally regarded as severely substandard.

Muscle protein can be estimated from urinary creatinine excretion; this complements the anthropometric indicator MAMA. The amount of creatinine appearing in the urine over 24 hours is proportional to muscle mass. A crude standard for creatinine excretion can be derived by multiplying an individual's reference weight-for-height by 23 or 18 (for males or females, respectively). Twenty per cent below these derived values may represent muscle protein depletion. However, several factors are known to affect creatinine excretion (e.g., kidney disease, diet, fever, strenuous exercise, menstrual cycle), and the interpretation, therefore, must be carried out cautiously.

In protein-energy malnutrition, the number of circulating lymphocytes diminishes, and the patient demonstrates impaired delayed hypersensitivity to common skin antigens (e.g., mumps, Candida, tuberculin). Thus, these tests also may be used in assessing the patient's nutritional status, although anergy may result from many non-nutritional factors as well (e.g., disease, drugs). A lymphocyte count of fewer than 1200 per cubic millimeter is regarded as severely substandard. The effect of advanced age on these parameters is uncertain.

The value of nutritional assessment parameters in predicting patient outcome is unproven. A prognostic nutritional index has been derived from various nutritional assessment indices (e.g., albumin, transferrin, triceps skinfold, delayed hypersensitivity) and applied to surgical patients to predict postoperative complications and mortality. In one study a higher prognostic nutritional index score correlated with greater postoperative problems, but further evaluation is necessary. Moreover, it is not known whether this index has any value in predicting outcomes in medical patients.

Andres A: Mortality and obesity: The rationale for age specific height-weight tables. In Andres R, Bierman EL, Hazzard WR (eds.): Principles of Geriatric Medicine. New York, McGraw-Hill, 1985, pp 311–318. *This article discusses the problems with available weight-height standards and describes a U-shaped relationship between body mass index and mortality.*

Frisancho AR: New standards of weight and body composition by frame size and height for assessment of nutritional status of adults and the elderly. Am J Clin Nutr 40:808, 1984. *This article presents American standards for weight and height from ages 1 to 75, derived from the combined data sets of NHANES I (1971–1974) and II (1976–1980).*

201 Protein-Energy Malnutrition

Robert B. Baron

Protein-energy malnutrition (PEM) occurs when inadequate protein and/or calories are ingested to meet an individual's nutritional requirements. PEM may be primary, as a result of inadequate food intake, or secondary, as a result of illness. In developing nations, PEM is most often primary and affects predominantly infants and children. It is the most important nutritional disorder and one of the developing world's most important health problems. In industrialized nations, PEM is most often secondary to other diseases and affects both children and adults. In North America and Europe, 28 to 80 per cent of hospitalized patients have been reported to have secondary PEM. This chapter emphasizes clinical features of secondary PEM as seen in industrialized nations.

Pathogenesis

Secondary PEM is caused by decreased intake of calories and protein, increased nutrient losses, or increased nutrient requirements (Table 201–1). It can develop slowly owing to chronic illness or chronic semistarvation or quite rapidly owing to acute illness.

In uncomplicated starvation and semistarvation, metabolism adapts to reduce the breakdown of lean body mass. Fat and fat-derived fuels gradually replace glucose as the major energy source. During the initial phase of a complete fast, glucose requirements for the brain, bone marrow, renal medulla, and peripheral nerves are provided by glycogen. Glycogen stores, however, last for only 12 to 24 hours. As glucose levels decline, insulin levels also decline and glucagon levels increase. Amino acids, particularly alanine, are released by muscle. Hepatic gluconeogenesis from amino acids provides glucose for the central nervous system and other glycolytic tissues. The changes in insulin and glucagon also favor lipolysis. Mobilized fatty acids provide the fuel for the remaining tissues. By the second week of a complete fast, fatty acids are less completely oxidized and more of them form ketone bodies. Ketones become the primary energy source for the brain and reduce the need for glucose. The muscles catabolize less protein and release less alanine, thus conserving their protein content.

Adaptation also decreases the body's total energy requirement, by as much as 40 per cent in severe chronic undernutrition. Absolute requirements decrease as body weight diminishes owing to a decrease in body mass. More importantly, however, energy

TABLE 201–1. CAUSES OF PROTEIN-ENERGY MALNUTRITION IN HOSPITALIZED PATIENTS

Decreased Oral Intake

Anorexia	Poverty
Nausea	Old age
Dysphagia	Social isolation
Pain	Substance abuse
Gastrointestinal obstruction	Depression
Poor dentition	

Increased Nutrient Losses

Malabsorption	Nephrosis
Diarrhea	Fistula drainage
Bleeding	Protein-losing enteropathy
Glycosuria	

Increased Nutrient Requirements

Fever	Trauma
Infection	Burns
Neoplasms	Medications
Surgery	

requirements also decrease per unit of body mass. Both ingested food and circulating endogenous substrates are utilized more efficiently. More endogenous amino acids, for example, are utilized for protein synthesis than for oxidation. In addition, virtually all of the body's biochemical and physiologic processes are curtailed. Less energy is expended for the sodium potassium pump, protein turnover, temperature regulation, the inflammatory response, and the function of most body organs during chronic undernutrition.

During a severe acute illness, hormonal and inflammatory responses prevent this adaptation to starvation and result in changes in protein and energy metabolism that can rapidly lead to PEM. Circulating levels of the catecholamines, glucocorticoids, glucagon, and growth hormone are all increased. Although necessary to mediate the body's response to physical stress, these hormonal and inflammatory changes result in marked increases in energy expenditure, nitrogen loss, gluconeogenesis, and the failure of ketoadaptation. In this manner, changes in body composition, including depletion of protein and fat stores, may occur rapidly. A number of other compounds may also play important roles in the metabolic response to injury. Of particular interest are the metabolic effects of the cytokines, such as tumor necrosis factor and interleukin 1, and the eicosanoids, such as prostaglandins, thromboxane, prostacyclin, and leukotrienes.

The resting metabolic expenditure (RME) may increase significantly during the response to illness. In burns involving greater than 40 per cent of the body surface area, for example, the RME may double. In other critical illnesses such as trauma or sepsis, the RME typically increases by 20 to 50 per cent. Nitrogen losses also typically increase by 20 to 100 per cent. During the response to illness, amino acids are released by skeletal muscle at a markedly accelerated rate. Released amino acids can then be metabolized for energy or shifted to the liver or other visceral organs, where their need for protein synthesis is more immediate. During prolonged illness and continued energy and protein deficiency, however, depletion of visceral protein also occurs and functional impairment of body organs can result.

Physiologic Consequences

Virtually every organ and organ system of the body can undergo marked morphologic and functional changes during protein-energy malnutrition

BODY WEIGHT. The most obvious manifestation of chronic PEM is loss of body weight. Most patients can tolerate a loss of 5 to 10 per cent of body weight without significant consequences, but losses greater than 40 per cent below ideal weight are almost always fatal. Both adipose tissue and the lean body mass are depleted, but losses of adipose tissue are greater. Extracellular water remains nearly constant, resulting in its relative increase. In severe PEM, the body's organs also decrease in size. In experimental animals, for example, a 7-day fast results in a 40 per cent decrease in liver mass, 28 per cent decrease in the gastrointestinal tract, 20 per cent decrease in the kidneys, and 17 per cent decrease in cardiac mass. During acute PEM caused by critical illness, changes in body weight and adipose stores may be less marked despite changes in organ morphology and function. Many patients may actually gain weight owing to retention of sodium and therefore of body water.

HEART. Severe PEM results in both quantitative and qualitative changes in the heart. In the "Minnesota experiment," for example, in which 32 male volunteers were semistarved for 6 months, a 24 per cent decrease in body weight was associated with an 18 per cent decrease in cardiac stroke volume and a 38 per cent decrease in cardiac index. Animal studies have demonstrated similar findings, as well as decreases in left ventricular contractility and compliance, decreased myocardial glycogen, myofibrillar atrophy, and interstitial edema. These changes are reversed with nutritional repletion.

LUNG. The lung parenchyma is minimally affected during PEM, but marked changes in pulmonary function can occur as a result of the loss of mass and strength of the muscles of respiration. In the "Minnesota experiment," vital capacity, tidal volume, and minute volume were decreased by 8 per cent, 19 per cent, and 30 per cent, respectively, after 24 weeks of semistarvation.

The ventilatory response to hypoxia is also decreased during semistarvation, but the clinical significance of this is unclear.

GASTROINTESTINAL TRACT. During severe PEM, gastric motility is slowed and gastric acid secretion is decreased. The most significant effects of PEM on the luminal gastrointestinal tract are seen in the small intestine. Total small bowel mass is decreased, primarily owing to mucosal atrophy and loss of villi. Lymphocytic infiltration of surface epithelial cells can occur, and epithelial cell renewal is decreased. Both disaccharidase enzyme activity and the rate of absorption of amino acids are decreased. Although pancreatic endocrine activity is spared, exocrine insufficiency can occur in severe PEM. Similar changes in the gastrointestinal tract are observed in individuals fed exclusively with parenteral nutrition, suggesting that stimulation of the gut by intraluminal nutrients is necessary for normal gut structure and function.

LIVER. In typical secondary PEM, liver mass decreases but the liver histology remains normal. Fat, protein, and glycogen are depleted, but the number of hepatocytes is preserved. In contrast, children with severe, primary protein deficiency resulting in kwashiorkor have enlarged livers with fatty infiltration and excess glycogen. In both instances, serum levels of albumin and other serum transport proteins are commonly decreased owing to diminished hepatic synthesis.

KIDNEY. Renal mass is also decreased during PEM, but renal histology remains normal. Renal function is well preserved except for an impaired concentrating ability due to a lowering of the medullary osmotic gradient.

ENDOCRINE. The endocrine response to PEM is complex and greatly affected by the extent of concurrent illnesses, as discussed above. In addition, serum thyroxine is typically at the lower limits of normal or slightly decreased. Peripheral conversion of thyroxine (T_4) to triiodothyronine (T_3) is commonly decreased, favoring the conversion to reverse triiodothyronine (Ch. 216). Serum TSH and the TSH response to TRH, however, are unaltered. Gonadal hormones are also affected. In men, testosterone levels are decreased and LH and FSH levels are appropriately increased. In women, however, gonadotropin release is depressed despite low levels of circulating estrogens.

IMMUNOLOGIC FUNCTION. The effects of severe PEM on the immune system are among its most important consequences. Virtually all components of the immune system are adversely affected in rough proportion to the degree of nutritional impairment. Peripheral blood lymphocyte counts are commonly decreased, with values often less than 1200 per cubic millimeter. Both the percentage of T cells and T-cell function are depressed. Skin tests for delayed hypersensitivity reactions are often nonreactive, and lymphocyte response to phytohemagglutinin and poke weed mitogens is decreased.

Humoral immunity is also affected, but in a more variable fashion. Specific antibody responses are depressed in some instances and preserved in others. For example, antibody production following administration of poliovirus, tetanus, diphtheria, measles, and pneumococcal polysaccharide antigens is normal, whereas impaired responses have been observed after the administration of yellow fever and influenza A vaccines. In some instances, the affinities and binding capacity of antibodies are reduced.

Slight neutropenia may occur during PEM, but the usual concurrent bacterial infections cause leukocytosis. Neutrophils are normal morphologically, but some measures of neutrophil function, including chemotaxis and bacterial killing, are abnormal. Phagocytosis is usually normal.

Levels of individual complement components, other than C4, and total serum hemolytic complement activity are commonly decreased. Other nonspecific host defense mechanisms, including interferon production, opsonization, and plasma lysozyme production, may also be adversely affected by protein-calorie undernutrition. Acute phase reactants such as C-reactive proteins, α_2-macroglobulin, α_1-antitrypsin, and haptoglobin tend to be elevated. Changes in the body's anatomic barriers to infection, including atrophy of the skin and gastrointestinal mucosa, may contribute to an increased risk of infection.

It is not possible to define the exact mechanisms of enhanced susceptibility to infections observed with PEM. Each of the abnormalities of the immune response probably contributes in part. Micronutrient deficiencies may occur concurrently with PEM and can also cause significant abnormalities in the immune response.

WOUND HEALING. Almost all aspects of wound healing are adversely affected in patients with severe PEM. Neovascularization, fibroblast proliferation, collagen synthesis, and wound remodeling are delayed. Local factors, such as edema associated with hypoalbuminemia and micronutrient deficiencies, may contribute to poor wound healing in undernourished patients. In mild PEM, however, wound healing is relatively well-preserved despite negative nitrogen balance. Even during complete starvation, endogenous substrates can be effectively utilized for collagen synthesis during the early phases of wound healing.

Clinical Manifestations

The clinical manifestations of PEM are extremely diverse, ranging from mild growth retardation and weight loss to several distinct clinical syndromes. This diversity is due to differences in the relative degree of protein and energy deficiency, the cause of the deficiency, the severity and duration of the deficiency, the age of the patient, and the association with other illnesses or nutritional deficiencies. In children in the developing world with severe PEM, for example, the classic syndromes of kwashiorkor (predominant protein deficiency) and marasmus (predominant energy deficiency) may develop. Marasmic kwashiorkor, an intermediate syndrome, may be seen when protein deficiency develops in combination with chronic energy deficiency. Although these syndromes are not typically encountered in secondary PEM in industrialized nations, they serve to illustrate the range of manifestations of PEM.

KWASHIORKOR. The child with severe kwashiorkor commonly has a decreased blood pressure, bradycardia, and hypothermia. Body weight is usually low but may be normal owing to edema and anasarca. The child is usually apathetic, lethargic, and anorectic, with decreased spontaneous movement. The skin demonstrates a "flaky paint" dermatitis with dry, hyperpigmented, hyperkeratotic lesions over the face, extremities, and perineum. The hair is typically sparse, dry, and brittle and may be reddish or yellowish. The abdomen is distended owing to hepatomegaly and ascites. The extremities are commonly wasted and edematous. Clinical signs of concurrent micronutrient deficiency may also be present (Ch. 205).

The serum albumin is typically less than 2.8 grams per deciliter and the lymphocyte count less than 1200 cells per cubic millimeter. A mild anemia is common; it is usually normochromic and normocytic unless other deficiencies coexist. The serum transferrin is usually decreased but may be normal or slightly elevated if iron deficiency is also present. Other serum transport proteins, including prealbumin and retinol-binding protein, are decreased. Serum glucose and lipids are decreased. Serum levels of liver enzymes are most often normal and may be low. Blood urea nitrogen and urinary urea nitrogen are low. Fluid and electrolyte disorders are common, particularly hypokalemia, hypophosphatemia, and a hyperchloremic metabolic acidosis.

MARASMUS. Children with marasmus have less characteristic manifestations. Although the pulse, blood pressure, and body temperature may be low, patients tend to be less apathetic and lethargic and to have a good appetite. Growth is retarded and the weight is low. There is obvious muscle wasting and loss of body fat and the patient looks emaciated, but there is no edema. The skin is dry and loose with decreased turgor. The dermatitis of kwashiorkor is usually absent. The hair is thin, dry, and dull. The abdomen is thin without signs of hepatomegaly or edema. Typically, there are fewer laboratory abnormalities than in children with kwashiorkor. Serum albumin and other transport proteins are often normal. A mild anemia is common. Any of the other laboratory abnormalities of kwashiorkor may be present but are usually absent.

SECONDARY PROTEIN-ENERGY MALNUTRITION. Secondary PEM, as seen in industrialized nations, is usually due to a deficiency of both protein and energy. Clinical manifestations vary considerably, in large part reflecting the associated illness that has caused the malnutrition and the nutritional status of the patient prior to the illness. In mild forms of secondary PEM, growth retardation in children and weight loss in adults may be the only manifestation. In more severe cases, depletion of fat stores results in loss of subcutaneous fat in the face and extremities. Reduction of lean body mass is reflected in loss of skeletal muscle, most noticeably in the interosseous and temporal muscles. The skin is often dry with decreased turgor, and the hair may be brittle and thin. Serum proteins are often decreased, and if particularly low, may result in dependent edema or anasarca. Patients with low serum proteins have a poor prognosis.

Obese patients who develop secondary PEM may have persistent fat stores and adequate subcutaneous fat and may demonstrate few of the manifestations of PEM. Although skeletal muscle is usually decreased, evaluation is difficult if large amounts of body fat are present. Serum proteins may be decreased or normal.

Diagnosis

The absence of distinct clinical manifestations can make the diagnosis of PEM quite difficult. A high index of suspicion based on the patient's risk factors for malnutrition, the overall clinical setting, and close observation of the patient are often necessary.

BODY WEIGHT. The most sensitive diagnostic measure is a documented history of weight loss. Weight loss should be quantified as a per cent of original body weight. Significant changes in weight may be obscured by edema. Some patients, particularly those with a severe acute illness such as sepsis, burns, or multiple trauma, can develop severe protein depletion rapidly without significant weight loss. Unfortunately, no standard amount of weight loss occurring over an established period of time clearly indicates clinically significant PEM. Nevertheless, most authors consider a 10 per cent loss of body weight occurring during the present illness to be clinically significant.

LABORATORY TESTS. Each of the clinical abnormalities seen in patients with severe PEM can be used as a diagnostic test to detect undernutrition. Most valuable are the serum albumin, other serum transport proteins such as transferrin, prealbumin, and retinol-binding protein, anergy to skin test antigens, total lymphocyte count, blood urea nitrogen, urinary excretion of creatinine, and anthropomorphic measures of body composition, such as skinfold thickness and mid-arm muscle circumference. Each of these tests when abnormal, like a history of weight loss, has been shown to predict poor clinical outcomes in patients in a wide variety of clinical settings. Combining these tests into indices such as the prognostic nutritional index further improves their predictive accuracy. Unfortunately, it remains unclear whether the poor outcomes predicted by excessive weight loss or by abnormalities in these tests reflect the consequences of PEM or the severity of the underlying illness.

A number of other nutrition assessment methods have been developed to more specifically define abnormalities in body composition. These include isotopic measurement of body composition, densitometry, computed tomography, nuclear magnetic resonance imaging, ultrasonography, whole-body impedance, and measures of muscle function. Although many of these are useful research techniques, their application in clinical practice is limited.

CLINICAL ASSESSMENT. A thorough, nutritionally focused history and physical examination can predict outcomes as well as any of the above tests and indices. The history should emphasize recent reduction in dietary intake, changes in body weight, gastrointestinal symptoms, the underlying illness, and the patient's functional status. The physical examination should emphasize loss of subcutaneous fat, muscle wasting, volume status, and signs of micronutrient deficiencies (Ch. 205). The initial clinical assessment is often equivocal; that is, the presence of clinically significant undernutrition is uncertain. In such cases, serial evaluations of the clinical examination, body weight, and laboratory parameters and close observation of the patient's nutrient intake as a function of estimated requirements is necessary to make the diagnosis of PEM.

Treatment

The goals of treatment of PEM are to provide adequate energy, protein, and micronutrients to restore body composition to normal and to treat the underlying process that caused the deficiency to develop.

STRATEGY. Treatment should proceed in two stages. In severe PEM, the first priority should be correction of fluid and electrolyte abnormalities and treatment of acute medical problems, most commonly infections. Although any combination of electrolyte and acid-base abnormalities can occur, most common are hypokalemia, hypocalcemia, hypophosphatemia, hypomagnesemia, and a hyperchloremic metabolic acidosis.

In the second phase one must provide adequate nutritional substrate to begin repletion. Nutrients should be provided quite slowly to prevent complications of overfeeding. In most adult patients no more than 0.8 gram of protein per kilogram and 30 Kcal per kilogram of actual body weight should be provided per day. As the patient becomes stabilized, protein and energy intake can be increased to 35 to 40 Kcal per kilogram and 1.0 to 1.5 grams of protein per kilogram per day. Adequate micronutrients must also be simultaneously provided. Patients with severe, life-threatening PEM should be fed even more cautiously.

ROUTE OF THERAPY. Nutrients can be provided either enterally or parenterally. Patients whose gastrointestinal tract is functioning and who can protect their airway should be fed enterally, either by mouth, feeding tube, or tube enterostomy (Ch. 206). Patients with contraindications to enteral feeding can be given required nutrients parenterally via either peripheral or central veins (Ch. 207). An algorithm for selecting the most appropriate method of nutritional support is shown in Figure 201–1.

COMPLICATIONS OF THERAPY. Particular care must be taken to avoid complications of refeeding. Many deaths attributable to PEM occur not during starvation but during repletion.

Electrolyte abnormalities, for example, are common during refeeding. The provision of energy and protein to a severely undernourished patient may convert a catabolic state to an anabolic one. As new tissues are synthesized and old tissues replenished, potassium and other electrolytes are transported intracellularly and may precipitate an acute drop in serum levels and result in life-threatening cardiac arrhythmias.

Congestive heart failure and pulmonary edema can be precip-

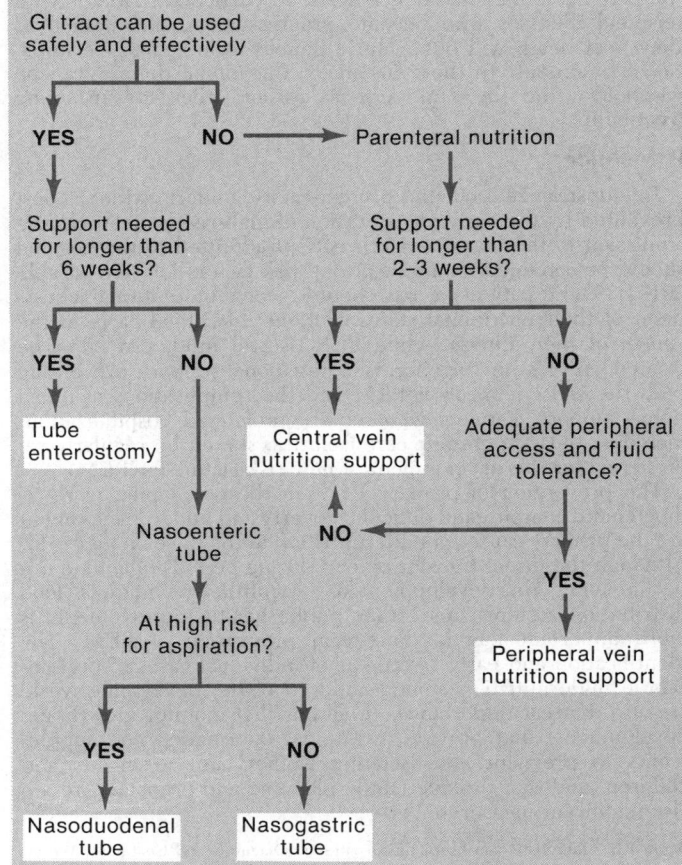

FIGURE 201–1. Decision tree concerning method of nutritional support.

itated by refeeding. As noted above, undernutrition is associated with decreased cardiac mass, decreased cardiac index and stroke volume, a slowing of the metabolic rate, and hypovolemia. The acute provision of carbohydrate, fluid, and sodium may correct the metabolic and volume abnormalities more rapidly than the depressed myocardium can handle and result in fluid overload. Should this complication occur, standard measures for the treatment of congestive heart failure should be used together with a slowing of the rate of nutritional repletion.

Benign refeeding edema must be differentiated from refeeding congestive heart failure. Many severely undernourished patients develop edema in dependent areas during refeeding without an associated increase in left ventricular filling pressures. The cause of refeeding edema is unclear. Changes in renal sodium retention, in part due to increased serum insulin, and poor venous tone have both been implicated. Treatment should include reassurance, elevation of dependent areas, and modest sodium restriction. Diuretics are rarely effective and may result in exacerbation of fluid and electrolyte abnormalities.

Diarrhea may result from enteral refeeding. Severely malnourished patients have atrophy of the gastric mucosa, decreased disaccharidase activity, and a mild deficiency of the exocrine pancreas. The provision of intraluminal nutrients can thus result in malabsorption and diarrhea. Gradual refeeding and restriction of lactose and lipid during the early refeeding phase decrease the risk of diarrhea.

REHABILITATION. Treatment of patients with PEM requires more than the provision of nutrients. Physical therapy and other measures to improve the patient's functional status are effective adjuncts to nutritional treatment. Physical therapy may result in greater repletion of muscle mass and smaller adipose tissue stores than nutritional repletion without muscle contraction.

The most important non-nutritional factor in the treatment of these patients is the resolution of the disease or social process that caused the PEM. In most instances, if the underlying process cannot be effectively treated, little benefit is derived from treating the patient's nutritional deficiencies. In particular, patients with terminal illnesses who become progressively malnourished as they near death will obtain little benefit from aggressive nutritional treatment. In these instances, nutritional therapy can be withheld using the same criteria as for other life-sustaining treatments.

Prevention

In industrialized societies protein-calorie undernutrition is best prevented by the early identification of high-risk patients during admission to the hospital. Each patient admitted to the hospital should be screened for predisposing risk factors for PEM (Table 201–1). Those patients at risk should receive more formal assessment of their nutritional status. Patients identified early in the course of their illness, while PEM is still mild, can often be treated with less invasive forms of nutritional support, preventing both the consequences of PEM and the complications of nutritional support. Patients who require prolonged hospitalization, including those in chronic care facilities, should be regularly re-evaluated for the development of new risk factors for PEM.

The prevention of primary PEM in the developing world is much more complex and difficult. Poverty and underdevelopment are the primary causes of undernutrition in the developing world. Although the direct transfer of food during periods of famine can be lifesaving, the development of agricultural techniques, food distribution systems, and other public health improvements is more important for the long-term prevention of PEM. The identification and early treatment of individual cases of protein-calorie undernutrition among children of the developing world are also of great importance. Programs that monitor growth and development, that provide nutritional information and supplements to pregnant and lactating women and to infants and children, and that provide family planning and prenatal care are also important measures.

Baron RB: Malnutrition in hospitalized patients: Diagnosis and treatment. West J Med 144:63, 1986. *A brief review of current controversies in the diagnosis and treatment of secondary protein-energy malnutrition.*

Goldstein SA, Elwyn DH: The effects of injury and sepsis on fuel utilization. Annu Rev Nutr 9:445, 1989. *A detailed review of the metabolic and hormonal alterations occurring during critical illness and their impact on nutritional status.*

Heymsfield SB, Williams PJ: Nutritional assessment by clinical and biochemical methods. *In* Shils ME, Young VR (eds.): Modern Nutrition in Health and Disease, 7th ed. Philadelphia, Lea & Febiger, 1988. *A comprehensive review of traditional and newer techniques for diagnosing protein-energy malnutrition.*

Silberman H: Parenteral and Enteral Nutrition, 2nd ed. Norwalk, CT, Appleton & Lange, 1988. *An excellent brief textbook covering theoretical and practical aspects of nutrition support of patients with protein-energy malnutrition.*

Torún B, Viteri FE: Protein-energy malnutrition. *In* Shils ME, Young VR (eds.): Modern Nutrition in Health and Disease. 7th ed. Philadelphia, Lea & Febiger, 1988. *A balanced review of the classic syndromes of primary protein-energy malnutrition.*

202 The Eating Disorders

Douglas A. Drossman

The eating disorders—anorexia nervosa, bulimia, and rumination—attract much public attention and scientific inquiry. Diagnosis and treatment require an understanding that these disorders result from a combination of biologic, psychological, and social influences.

ANOREXIA NERVOSA

DEFINITION. Anorexia nervosa is a chronic disorder characterized behaviorally by self-induced weight loss, psychologically by body-image and other perceptual disturbances, and biologically by physiologic alterations (e.g., amenorrhea) that result from nutritional depletion.

HISTORICAL NOTE. The disorder was first reported 300 years ago by Morton in describing an 18-year-old patient as a "skeleton only clad with skin" with "total suppression of her monthly courses." In 1874, Gull first used the term *anorexia nervosa* in reporting a "nervous, morbid disease" associated with loss of appetite and severe wasting. It is now recognized that these patients are not truly anorectic; they are *preoccupied* with food and struggle against hunger to achieve the desired goal of thinness.

EPIDEMIOLOGY. Anorexia nervosa afflicts predominantly young, affluent white females (95 per cent). The incidence may be increasing. In one community study the number of new cases per year over a 10-year period rose from 0.55 per 100,000 to 3.26 per 100,000. The disorder is associated with higher social class, occurring in up to 1 in 250 adolescent students in private school and with a prevalence of 1 per cent.

ETIOLOGY AND PATHOGENESIS. *Sociocultural Factors.* The cultural ideal for women's bodies has shifted in the last century from that of plumpness (formerly representing wealth, abundance, maternalism, and fertility) to a slimmer female image (representing independence, assertiveness, and success). Thinner women predominate on prime-time television and among beauty pageant contestants and high-fashion models. Social pressures from peers, particularly during adolescence, seem to influence young women and girls to engage in anorectic behaviors. These factors are probably not sufficient for the disorder to develop but may create the proper environment for its expression in the predisposed individual. Recent studies also report an association of childhood sexual abuse history among patients with anorexia nervosa. The possible relationship of abuse in the pathogenesis of the disorder needs further study.

Psychological Factors. It is believed that anorectics have an incompletely developed personal identity and struggle to maintain a sense of control over their environment. Psychiatric interviews suggest that the patient develops within a family that values outward appearance, proper behavior, and achievement more than self-actualization. In response to parental expectations, the pre-anorectic child learns to be hard working, eager to please, and attentive to family needs. In turn, the parents support and indulge in the behaviors of their model child ("best little girl in the world"). Therefore, these actions are mutually reinforced, leading to interdependence among the family members (enmeshment). However, the high standards within the family are rarely achieved by the child, who obsessively struggles for parental approval.

It follows that "negative" childhood behaviors (e.g., assertiveness, rebellion) are not permitted. These behaviors are believed necessary for the development of individual identity. As a result, the pre-anorectic child comes to rely on externally imposed ideal values to maintain self-esteem, but at the expense of self-actualization and a sense of autonomy.

It is not surprising that a distressing period for the pre-anorectic child occurs during or soon after puberty, when physical, social, and psychological events (menarche, growth spurt, school, and adolescent peer pressure) encourage separation from the family and individuation. Over 80 per cent of anorectic patients develop the disorder within 7 years of menarche. The compounded life events at this time are experienced with feelings of helplessness and ineffectiveness. The decision to diet, while not fully understood, may be a desperate attempt for control of one's body, at least, in a distressing new environment.

Biologic Factors. There is an increased risk of anorexia nervosa among siblings (6 per cent), with a four- to five-fold difference in concordance rates for monozygotic twins, suggesting a predisposing role for genetic factors. Also, there are more perinatal complications reported among anorexia nervosa patients. The higher birth weight and the increased prevalence of obesity preceding the onset of illness suggest that premorbid obesity is an influencing factor. Abnormalities in satiety, temperature regulation, and endocrine function suggest that a hypothalamic abnormality exists, although no specific lesion has been identified. It is more likely that the hypothalamus serves a modulating role. In the predisposed individual, the biologic and psychosocial events around the time of adolescence may produce neurotransmitter, endocrine, or immune changes via the hypothalamus, leading to the physiologic and behavioral changes characteristic of the disorder. The biologic findings of anorexia nervosa can be viewed as homeostatic adaptations to self-imposed energy depletion.

CLINICAL MANIFESTATIONS. There are no characteristic pathologic or physiologic findings, and no consistent psychiatric diagnosis is found. The consistency of the medical and behavioral features, however, argues for classifying the disorder as a clinical entity.

Psychological and Behavioral Features. Pursuit of Thinness. Patients are not truly anorectic, but struggle against hunger to achieve an unrealistic degree of weight loss. Interestingly, they are preoccupied with food and exhibit bizarre food preferences or elaborately prepare food for others. For most anorectics, weight loss is accomplished through dietary restriction and exercise (restrictor subgroup), although up to 50 per cent will also self-induce vomiting or take purgatives (bulimic subgroup).

Perceptual Disturbances. Anorectics overestimate their body width, insisting they are too fat despite profound weight loss. Their assessment of the body habitus of others is not affected. Anorectics may also exhibit abnormalities in the perception of enteroceptive stimuli. They distort hunger awareness, deny fatigue, and fail to recognize emotional states such as anger and depression.

Sense of Ineffectiveness. Patients feel as though they are controlled by their environment and seem unable to function separately from family or other relationships. They gauge their responses to the expectations of others.

Cognitive Deficits. Patients may exhibit deficits in conceptual thought and abstract reasoning. They may be unable to view situations in anything but extremes, and they interpret events in a rigid and highly personalized form.

Medical Features. Most of the physical, metabolic, and endocrine abnormalities of anorexia nervosa are also seen in starvation secondary to the other conditions. The severity of the findings correlates with the nutritional state.

Physical Signs. Patients may have severe loss of subcutaneous fat and exhibit bony prominences. Core temperature, blood pressure, and pulse are decreased. Examination of the skin may reveal acrocyanosis, downy hair (lanugo), and a yellow discoloration (hypercarotenemia). Elevated serum carotene and vitamin A levels are due either to an excess intake of dietary carotenoids or to an acquired defect in the utilization or metabolism of these compounds. Secondary sexual features are absent in the patient who develops anorexia nervosa before puberty.

Endocrine Abnormalities. *Gonadal.* The endocrine hallmark is gonadal dysfunction, and for women this presents as amenorrhea. Male anorectics lose libido and are infertile. Patients have decreased follicle-stimulating (FSH) and luteinizing hormone (LH) and do not exhibit secretory bursts of LH throughout the day in response to endogenous luteinizing hormone-releasing factor (LHRF), indicating an abnormality in hypothalamic regulation. This "immature" secretory pattern, characteristic of prepubertal girls, may result from the loss of a critical amount of body fat content or from the psychophysiologic effects of stress in the absence of significant weight loss. Normal menses usually recur with weight gain, when body fat content reaches 22 per cent.

Thyroid. Patients may exhibit clinical features suggestive of hypothyroidism, such as decreased vital signs, dry skin, constipation, cold intolerance, and a delayed ankle jerk, although lethargy is not usually observed. T_3 levels tend to be low, with a corresponding increase in reverse T_3, the relatively inactive isomer of T_3 (Ch. 216). Under the stress of malnutrition, the liver preferentially deiodinates T_4 to rT_3. The clinical findings of mild hypothyroidism may arise from a decreased availability of the more active T_3 isomer, which preferentially binds to the thyroid receptor. However, free thyroxine, total T_4 levels, and the TSH response to TRH are normal. Clinically significant hypothyroidism does not occur, and treatment with exogenous thyroid is not indicated.

Adrenal. Anorectic patients usually have normal or slightly elevated plasma cortisol levels with decreased urinary excretion of 17-hydroxycorticosteroids. This is due to a decrease in the metabolic clearance of cortisol from plasma with an increase in cortisol-binding capacity. The 24-hour cortisol production rate and basal ACTH secretion are normal. The response to ACTH stimulation may be increased, and the response to metyrapone stimulation is normal. Decreased libido and delayed virilization in males may be due to a shift of androgen metabolism from the 5α-reductase enzyme system (yielding testosterone and its congeners) to the 5β-reductase system, producing the weaker androgen etiocholanolone (Ch. 222).

Growth Hormone. Human growth hormone (hGH) levels are normal or slightly elevated. Concurrently there is a decrease in somatomedin levels. This growth-promoting peptide is produced by the liver and other tissues under the influence of hGH. Somatomedin mediates the anabolic effects of hGH but not its lipolytic effects. Thus, anorectic patients and other malnourished individuals maintain their adipose tissue breakdown (increased hGH) without growth effects.

Cardiovascular Abnormalities. Patients exhibit depressed cardiovascular function with a decreased cardiac O_2 consumption, left ventricular wall thickness, cardiac chamber size, and blood pressure. These are adaptive responses to malnutrition and decreased catecholamine levels. Electrocardiographic changes include bradycardia, decreased QRS amplitude, prolonged QT interval, nonspecific ST segment changes, and U waves. Patients may also develop arrhythmias (tachycardia, sinus arrest, and ectopic atrial, junctional, or ventricular rhythms) due either to the primary disorder or to metabolic disturbances secondary to purgation. Sudden death has been reported among severely emaciated patients.

Hematologic Findings. Leukopenia and decreased white cell function, anemia, thrombocytopenia, and hypocomplementemia may occur. Anorectic patients do not seem to have a greater susceptibility to infection, however.

Gastrointestinal Findings. Constipation, delayed gastric emptying, pancreatic fibrosis, and jejunal dilatation may occur. Malabsorptive diarrhea and acute gastric dilatation may develop with rapid refeeding.

DIAGNOSIS. It is difficult to know when the diagnosis should be made, since social and cultural factors promote and maintain anorectic behaviors. Five per cent of college women without weight loss display attitudes and behaviors consistent with the diagnosis. Within some population groups (e.g., high-fashion models, ballerinas) low body weight is *de rigeur* and the associated anorectic behaviors are accepted. The diagnosis of anorexia nervosa should be considered when the person voluntarily restricts food intake in the face of hunger to achieve an unrealistic degree of weight loss and becomes psychosocially dysfunctional. The diagnosis is confirmed by identifying the described behavioral features and by excluding any treatable medical disorders.

The use of clinical criteria such as those proposed by the American Psychiatric Association (Table 202–1) is recommended. The differential diagnosis in this young population includes primary endocrine disorders (panhypopituitarism, Addison's disease, hyperthyroidism, diabetes mellitus), gastrointestinal disease (Crohn's disease, celiac sprue), chronic infection (tuberculosis), neoplastic disorders (lymphoma), and, rarely, CNS disorders (hypothalamic tumor, vascular malformation).

All patients should receive a nutritional assessment to determine the severity of the malnutrition and to establish a baseline for follow-up. Height and weight are usually sufficient. Patients with marked weight loss should have other nutritional measures obtained (serum transferrin, albumin, measurement of triceps skin fold thickness, skin test reactivity to *Candida* antigen) in order to gauge the approach to nutritional treatment.

TREATMENT. There are two goals in the treatment of patients with anorexia nervosa: nutritional restitution with alleviation of medical complications, and modification of the psychological and environmental factors that promote anorectic behavior. No single treatment is superior, and a multidisciplinary approach involving medical, psychiatric/psychological, and nutritional (dietitians, pharmacists) personnel is needed.

General Medical Care. The medical physician performs the initial clinical assessment, is responsible for the medical and nutritional care of the patient, and provides psychological support. The general approach should include (1) fostering a sense of autonomy in the patient by encouraging her to take personal responsibility in the treatment plan, (2) remaining objective, consistent, and honest in order to maintain the patient's trust, (3) involving the family as part of the treatment program, (4) serving as liaison and patient advocate with the various consultants and counselors.

Nutritional Care. All anorectic patients require some dietary management, although nutritional supplementation is not needed unless the patient is at risk of medical complications. With mild degrees of weight loss (e.g., weight 80 per cent of ideal or better), nutritional and psychological counseling is sufficient. The physician's role includes personal support, education about adolescent body development and its relationship to diet, and scheduling of periodic visits to observe for clinical deterioration. With moderate malnutrition (weight 65 to 80 per cent of ideal) nutritional supplements may be necessary, but hospitalization usually is not required. Oral replacement with a palatable, nutritionally complete formulation (e.g., Ensure Plus) may help, with the goal being intake of 250 to 500 calories above daily energy requirement. In some cases metoclopramide or bethanechol may be used to improve gastric emptying and the patient's tolerance of larger meals. With severe malnutrition (weight less than 65 per cent of ideal) hospitalization is usually required. Oral replacement

TABLE 202–1. DIAGNOSTIC CRITERIA FOR ANOREXIA NERVOSA*

A. Refusal to maintain body weight over a minimal normal weight for age and height (e.g., weight loss leading to maintenance of body weight 15% below that expected) or failure to make expected weight gain during period of growth, leading to body weight 15% below that expected.
B. Intense fear of gaining weight or becoming fat, even though underweight.
C. Disturbance in the way in which one's body weight, size, or shape is experienced (e.g., claiming to "feel fat" even when emaciated or belief that one area of the body is "too fat" even when obviously underweight).
D. In females, absence of at least three consecutive menstrual cycles when otherwise expected to occur (primary or secondary amenorrhea; a woman is considered to have amenorrhea if her periods occur only following hormone [e.g., estrogen] administration).

*American Psychiatric Association Diagnostic and Statistical Manual of Mental Disorders (DSM-IIIR), 3rd ed. Washington, D.C., Copyright APA 1987. Used with permission.

may be attempted, but if the patient is unable or unwilling to comply, tube feeding into the duodenum may be necessary. The patient can receive 400 to 600 calories above daily caloric need, with the goal being no more than 1 to 2 kg weight gain per week.

If the patient is severely malnourished and tolerates a feeding tube poorly or refuses to eat, parenteral nutrition may be considered. The peripheral venous route is preferred, since central hyperalimentation is more expensive and is associated with a greater frequency of complications. If a central venous route is chosen, it should be supervised by an experienced hyperalimentation team. Caloric delivery should begin with one half of the daily requirement, progressing to full requirement by day three or four. Electrolytes, serum chemistries, and hepatic and renal function must be monitored.

The goal of enteral or parenteral supplementation is to *slowly* get the patient to a body weight out of the range of medical risk. Rapid refeeding produces excess water stores and edema, secondary metabolic disturbances, and possibly cardiac failure. Continued nutritional intervention beyond achieving a "dry weight" of 80 per cent of ideal is not recommended. These procedures are psychologically invasive and minimize the patient's involvement in treatment, thereby increasing anxiety and resistance. Furthermore, supplements interfere with appetite and with attempts to re-establish normal eating patterns.

Pharmacotherapy. No pharmacologic agent is of proven value. Chlorpromazine, amitriptyline, lithium carbonate, and cyproheptadine have been reported effective in small, short-term inpatient treatment trials. Their use should be ancillary to the long-term nutritional and behavioral approaches.

Psychotherapy. Psychotherapy is used to help the patient modify the aberrant eating behavior and to improve psychosocial function. Behavior modification is an effective means of achieving short-term weight gain. Family therapy offers the best potential for long-term benefit, since treatment is directed toward modifying the family interactions that maintain the anorectic behavior. Insight therapy may occasionally help the motivated patient.

PROGNOSIS. The short-term prognosis is generally favorable; over 75 per cent of patients will attain a body weight above 75 per cent of ideal. Menses will resume in at least half; however, less than one third of patients will resume normal eating patterns. The long-term prognosis is variable, and relapses requiring hospitalization occur in about half of the patients. The mortality rate among hospitalized patients averages 6 per cent, with the main causes of death being inanition and severe electrolyte disturbances; suicide occurs in 1 per cent. A poorer prognosis is associated with a late age of onset, self-induced vomiting or laxative abuse, long duration of illness, male sex, and the presence of associated psychiatric disturbance. A better prognosis is associated with the patient's ability to achieve a degree of social integration (e.g., with parent, spouse, and friends). It appears that anorexia nervosa is a lifelong behavioral disorder with periodic exacerbations requiring medical, psychological, and nutritional intervention.

BULIMIA

DEFINITION. Bulimia, derived from the Greek meaning "ox-eating," is a behavioral disorder characterized by episodes of overeating (binging), usually followed by acts to "undo" the threatened weight gain with self-induced vomiting, cathartic or diuretic abuse (purging), fasting, or excessive physical activity. Bulimia nervosa is sometimes used to distinguish the behavior of patients who binge and purge from that of other bulimics who binge but do not purge. Compared with anorectics, bulimics have normal body weight and tend to have less distortion of body image. Bulimics are more aware that their behavior, although secretive, is aberrant, and they may therefore be more accepting of treatment.

EPIDEMIOLOGY. Although bulimia was only first reported as a diagnostic entity in 1979, its prevalence is very high and it has probably existed a long time. Binge eating, at least once, occurs in half of the population, and weekly binge eating is reported by up to 15 per cent. Self-induced vomiting or laxative/diuretic abuse associated with binge eating occurs in up to 20 per cent of college students, and 4 per cent report this type of behavior at least weekly. Bulimia is almost exclusively diagnosed in young (<30 years) women (>95 per cent). Most bulimics carry on their activity secretly; less than one third have discussed their behavior with their physician, and in one survey only 2.5 per cent were under medical care.

ETIOLOGY AND PATHOGENESIS. Patients commonly report obesity during childhood or adolescence, and the onset of bulimia is associated with a conscious decision to diet. At some point the patients lose control of their compulsion to eat large amounts of "forbidden foods" and binge. Self-induced vomiting is discovered as a convenient method of re-establishing weight control. Thus, a binge-purge cycle becomes established.

As with anorexia nervosa, societal influences seem to play a prominent role in the desire to be thin. Also, there are historical and social precedents for self-induced vomiting. The ancient Romans ate lavishly and then induced vomiting at feasts. Socialites who must attend many dinner parties sometimes induce vomiting. Bulimics report coming from families that emphasize hearty eating and where food is used to celebrate happy times and to console during sad times. For these patients eating takes on greater meaning than simply to achieve nutritional benefit, and this may help to explain the emotional and behavioral investment present in food and eating.

A possible role for cholecystokinin (a satiety-inducing nerve-gut peptide) has been implicated in bulimia. When compared with healthy subjects, bulimic patients have a blunted meal-induced secretion of cholecystokinin.

CLINICAL MANIFESTATIONS. *Psychological and Behavioral Features.* The characteristic behavioral feature is the binge-purge cycle: an eating compulsion with a failure to achieve or to respond to normal satiety. These episodes occur secretly and are often associated with feelings of frustration, loneliness, or the sight of tempting foods. Binges are usually planned, and the preparation is associated with anxiety and excitement. During the binge, high-calorie "junk" foods are pleasurably consumed. The binge is usually terminated when feelings of guilt or physical discomfort such as nausea, abdominal pain, or headache occurs. At this point the patient self-induces vomiting and/or takes cathartics or laxatives. Bulimics generally look healthy, and their behaviors are unnoticed by friends and family. They are more outgoing than their anorectic counterparts. Some patients may exhibit impulsive or antisocial behaviors such as drug abuse, kleptomania, and sexual promiscuity. The patient who seeks help does so because of feelings of guilt, anxiety, or depression, or she is no longer able to continue the habit and still function in daily activities.

Medical Features. The medical findings of bulimia are consequences of the vomiting and laxative abuse. The physical examination may reveal parotid or salivary gland swelling due to vomiting, bruising of the knuckles from their rubbing against the upper incisors during the induction of vomiting, pharyngitis and dental erosions from reflux of gastric acid, or conjunctival hemorrhages from retching.

Frequent vomiting may also be complicated by esophagitis, Mallory-Weiss tears, or aspiration pneumonitis. Hypokalemic hypochloremic metabolic alkalosis due to loss of H^+, Cl^-, and K^+ is the most common metabolic complication, and this may lead to cardiac arrhythmias or renal injury. Secondary metabolic disturbances may produce weakness, tetany, and seizures. Emetics such as ipecac may produce cardiac conduction defects and arrhythmias. Stimulant laxatives can produce a "cathartic colon" with degeneration of Auerbach's plexus.

The majority of patients are clinically depressed by the time of clinical presentation, and 5 per cent have attempted suicide. It is believed that bulimia may be a manifestation of an underlying depressive disorder, since a large proportion of patients have first-degree relatives with major affective disorders.

DIAGNOSIS. The diagnosis of bulimia is based on recognition of the binge eating pattern and the exclusion of other medical diseases that might explain the behavior. The differential diagnosis, which is limited in this young population group, would include schizophrenia, use of oral contraceptives, seizures, and rare neurologic disorders. The latter may include *Klüver-Bucy syndrome*, a disorder of bilateral temporal lobe damage associated with indiscriminate sexual behavior, hyperphagia, and pica, and *Kleine-Levin syndrome*, a sleep disorder associated with hypersomnia and overeating.

TREATMENT. The goal of treatment is to help the patient overcome the urge to overeat. Bulimic patients recognize their behaviors as maladaptive. Compared with anorectics, they are more aware of associated psychological difficulties and are more willing to work with physicians and counselors in a treatment plan.

The current psychotherapeutic technique is cognitive-behavioral treatment in which the patient identifies the abnormal behaviors and then uses behavioral techniques to extinguish them, thereby accomplishing greater self-control. The treatment is safe and probably effective.

Antidepressants have been reported to be successful in decreasing the binge activity and in increasing the patient's sense of well-being.

RUMINATION SYNDROME

Rumination syndrome, or merycism, is an eating disorder in which the person repetitively regurgitates small amounts of food from the stomach, rechews the food, and then reswallows it. The disorder has been recognized as a medical curiosity for over 300 years, and ruminators have been known for their tendencies to offer public performances.

Infants frequently ruminate, and the disorder is described among institutionalized adults and children with emotional and intellectual deficits. No characteristic psychological profile or psychiatric diagnosis has been reported. There may be two subpopulations with the disorder, those in whom the behavior develops in childhood as a learned maladaptive habit worsening at times of stress, and those in whom rumination is associated with bulimia. A familial association is reported, although the role for genetic factors in the pathogenesis is not established.

The prevalance of rumination in adults is unknown, since generally physicians are unfamiliar with the clinical features. Patients who seek treatment report symptoms of weight loss, regurgitation, or vomiting and may express concern about there being an underlying medical disorder. Parents may bring the adolescent child to the doctor because of halitosis or dental problems.

Rumination in humans is not the same physiologic event as in ruminant animals, since reverse peristalsis does not occur. Radiographic and manometric studies indicate that an episode is initiated by a belch or swallow, at which time the lower esophageal sphincter pressure is lowered, creating a common channel between the stomach and esophagus. At the same time diaphragmatic and rectus muscle contractions raise the intra-abdominal pressure, thereby leading to regurgitation. When the upper esophageal sphincter is relaxed, food is ejected into the mouth, where it is expectorated or reswallowed.

The diagnosis depends on identifying the characteristic clinical features in the absence of other organic or psychiatric disease. Medical conditions such as esophageal stricture, reflux esophagitis, intestinal obstruction, or esophageal motor disorders (achalasia, diffuse esophageal spasm) should be excluded by radiography, video-fluoroscopy, and manometry. Since the disorder appears to be a learned maladaptive habit, behavioral modification and biofeedback techniques are recommended as approaches to treatment. However, cure may be difficult because the act is pleasurable and patients may not be motivated to change.

Balaa MA, Drossman DA: Anorexia nervosa and bulimia: The eating disorders. DM 31:1, 1985. *This monograph comprehensively reviews the epidemiology, pathophysiology, medical and psychosocial characteristics, diagnosis, and treatment of the two major eating disorders.*

Diagnostic and Statistical Manual of Mental Disorders. 4th ed (DSM-IIIR). Washington, DC, American Psychiatric Association, 1987. *This manual provides the standards of nomenclature and diagnostic criteria for anorexia nervosa and bulimia.*

Harris RT: Bulimarexia and related serious eating disorders with medical complications. Ann Intern Med 99:800, 1983. *Provides a good review of the medical complications in bulimia.*

Hsu LKG: The treatment of anorexia nervosa. Am J Psychiatry 143:573, 1986. *A review of treatment, including discussion of the approach to the patient, pharmacotherapy, psychotherapy, and behavior modification.*

Mitchell JE, Seim HC, Colon E, et al.: Medical complications and medical management of bulimia. Ann Intern Med 107:71, 1987. *This is an excellent general review documented with 86 useful references concerning this common disorder.*

Levine DF, Wingate DL, Pfeffer JM, et al.: Habitual rumination: A benign disorder. Br Med J 287:255, 1983. *Presents some of the clinical features of nine patients with rumination syndrome.*

203 Obesity

F. Xavier Pi-Sunyer

Obesity is a frustrating problem for patient and physician alike. Its underlying cause is rarely clear, and its treatment is fraught with difficulty and failure. Management of obesity therefore requires much understanding and persistence.

About 34 million adult Americans (26 per cent of those aged 20 to 75 years) are overweight, 12.4 million severely so. The per cent of adult women who are overweight (27.1 per cent) is somewhat greater than that of men (24.2 per cent).

DEFINITION

Visual inspection of a patient can give a subjective but fairly accurate estimate of the degree of obesity. More objective measures are height-weight tables, weight-related indices, and other anthropometric measurements.

The three most commonly used indices are (1) tables of average weights by height and age; (2) tables of desirable weights for height associated with lowest mortalities in insured populations; and (3) indices derived from height and weight, of which the body mass index is the most useful.

TABLES OF AVERAGE WEIGHTS. National Health and Nutrition Examination Surveys (NHANES) are periodically conducted on a representative United States population and then compiled in percentile tables as weights for height for sex. These cross-sectional data can be used for defining obesity, with a commonly made arbitrary decision that above the 85th percentile is "overweight." This comparison to a reference population makes no statement as to health risk involved at any weight level. The biggest problem is that of finding an appropriate reference population, particularly for minorities.

IDEAL WEIGHT TABLES. The Metropolitan Life Insurance Company Tables of Heights and Weights indicate the weight at which longevity is greatest, based on those insured. The 1983 tables were derived from the pooled data of 25 insurance companies in the United States and Canada, including about 4.2 million policies issued between 1950 and 1971. People with major diseases were screened out. The tables show weights based on lowest mortality for men and women at ages 25 to 59 by height and body frame.

The Metropolitan tables have been criticized as being inaccurate because (1) insured subjects do not represent a random sample of the population; (2) insured subjects are screened for illness and so are healthier than average; (3) no actual body frame measurements were taken when data were gathered so that the division into three frame categories (small, medium, and large) was a post hoc manipulation of the data; (4) about 20 per cent of the subjects used in the tables reported their heights and weights but were not actually measured (the bias being that women tend to under-report their weight and men to over-report their height); (5) the tables do not distinguish between obesity and overweight.

BODY MASS INDEX (BMI). In an effort to clear the confusion about how to classify overweight, the BMI has been computed:

$$BMI = kg/(ht \text{ in meters})^2$$
$$\text{or } BMI = lb/(ht \text{ in inches})^2 \times 703.1$$

This simple measurement correlates quite highly with other estimates of fatness, although some very muscular individuals may be classified as obese when they are not. It is also a somewhat more accurate index of fatness for males than for females.

The mean BMI (weighted for the height distribution of the United States population) taken from the mid-point of the medium frame of the 1983 Metropolitan tables is 22.4 kg/m^2 for men and 22.5 kg/m^2 for women. Patients can be divided for degree of obesity as shown in Figure 203–1. Health risks increase as BMI increases above 25.

Aging is a fattening process, so that a young and old person of comparable body weight are not comparably obese (Fig. 203–2). This has led to controversy concerning whether it is the total weight of an individual that should stay constant from 25 years

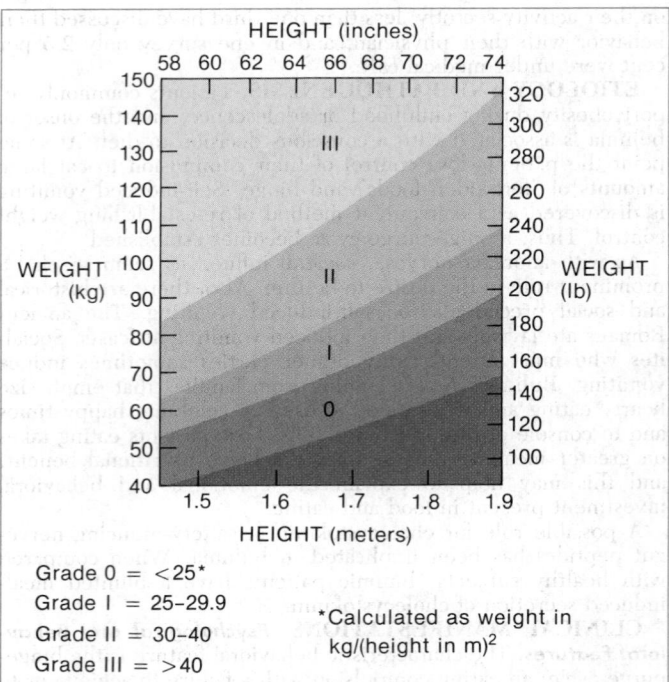

Grade 0 = <25*
Grade I = 25–29.9
Grade II = 30–40
Grade III = >40

*Calculated as weight in kg/(height in m)²

FIGURE 203–1. Grades of obesity as defined by body mass index. (Reproduced with permission from Garrow JS: Treat Obesity Seriously. Edinburgh, Churchill Livingstone, 1981, p 3.)

to 70 years or the fat-free mass, that is, the working cellular mass of the body plus the skeleton. The average weight data from the United States population show a gradually increasing weight with age, more pronounced and sustained for women than for men (Fig. 203–3). Whereas many studies suggest that an increase from one's weight at 25 years old may increase mortality, a number have suggested that for the lowest mortality, the pattern of body

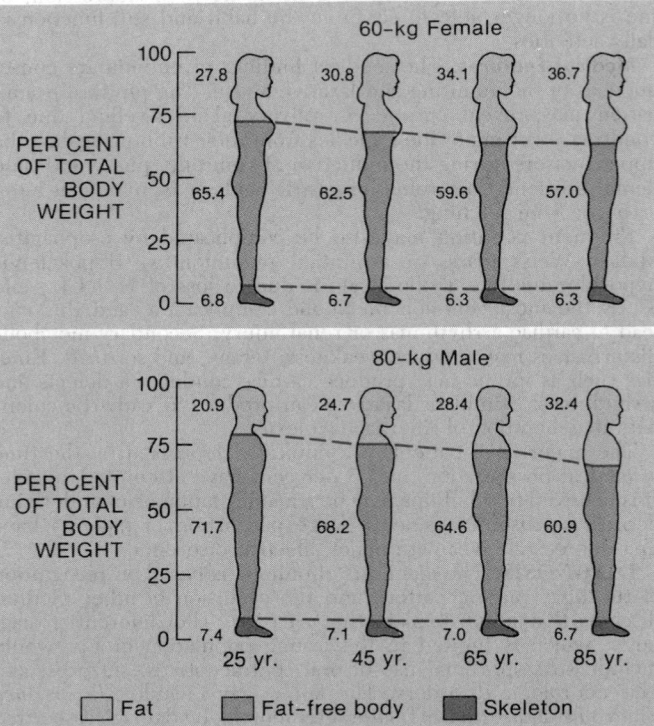

FIGURE 203–2. Body composition change with aging of representative normal adults. (Adapted from Moore FD, Olesen KH, McMurrey JE, et al.: The Body Cell Mass and Its Supporting Environment. Philadelphia, W. B. Saunders Company, 1963.)

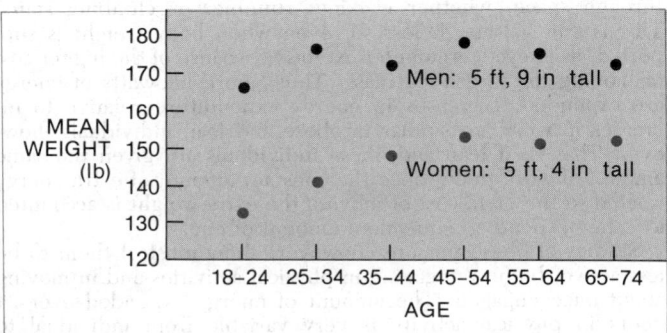

FIGURE 203–3. Weight change with aging for men and women. (Adapted from National Center for Health Statistics: Weight by height and age for adults 18–74 years, United States, 1971–1974. DHEW Publication No. [PHS] 79-1656, Series 11, No. 208, 1979.)

weight should be leanness in the twenties followed by a very moderate weight gain as one gets older. The minimal mortality points in relation to BMI for each age-sex grouping have been calculated. The regression lines, computed separately for men and women, are presented in Figure 203–4. Clearly, age strongly affects the BMI associated with the lowest mortality in this study. Also, the regression lines for men and women are nearly the same. The "best" BMI gradually increases with age in both sexes, with no consistent difference between men and women. As a result, a single set of weight goal tables (Table 203–1) can be constructed which are applicable for both men and women. The goals, which are somewhat more liberal for certain age groups than are the Metropolitan tables, are given by decade of age, with generally higher allowable weights as persons get older. Until the issue is further clarified, these goals seem to be reasonable for a physician to utilize in counseling patients in preventive medicine. Two caveats must be added. First, these tables have been derived from and are applicable primarily to white men and women in the United States. Second, the tables have been derived from populations without known risk factors. Patients with significant risk factors such as coronary artery disease, hypertension, and diabetes mellitus are better counseled

TABLE 203–1. AGE-SPECIFIC WEIGHT-FOR-HEIGHT TABLES* (GERONTOLOGY RESEARCH CENTER)

Height	Weight Range for Men and Women by Age (Years)†				
	25	35	45	55	65
ft–in			lb		
4–10	84–111	92–119	99–127	107–135	115–142
4–11	87–115	95–123	103–131	111–139	119–147
5–0	90–119	98–127	106–135	114–143	123–152
5–1	93–123	101–131	110–140	118–148	127–157
5–2	96–127	105–136	113–144	122–153	131–163
5–3	99–131	108–140	117–149	126–158	135–168
5–4	102–135	112–145	121–154	130–163	140–173
5–5	106–140	115–149	125–159	134–168	144–179
5–6	109–144	119–154	129–164	138–174	148–184
5–7	112–148	122–159	133–169	143–179	153–190
5–8	116–153	126–163	137–174	147–184	158–196
5–9	119–157	130–168	141–179	151–190	162–201
5–10	122–162	134–173	145–184	156–195	167–207
5–11	126–167	137–178	149–190	160–201	172–213
6–0	129–171	141–183	153–195	165–207	177–219
6–1	133–176	145–188	157–200	169–213	182–225
6–2	137–181	149–194	162–206	174–219	187–232
6–3	141–186	153–199	166–212	179–225	192–238
6–4	144–191	157–205	171–218	184–231	197–244

*Values in this table are for height without shoes and weight without clothes. To convert inches to centimeters, multiply by 2.54; to convert pounds to kilograms, multiply by 0.455.

†Data from Andres R: Gerontology Research Center, National Institute of Aging, Baltimore, MD.

on stricter tables, such as the Metropolitan Life Tables of 1983 (Ch. 200).

OTHER METHODS. Over half of the fat in the body is deposited under the skin. Its thickness can be measured at various sites using standard skin calipers. It is not difficult to become adept in the use of the calipers, and a running record of a patient's estimated body fat can be easily kept. The most useful and accurate tables are based on the measurement of four skinfold thicknesses—biceps, triceps, subscapular, and suprailiac. For such tables, see the British Journal of Nutrition 2:77, 1974.

Other methods of defining obesity are more difficult and expensive and therefore are used mostly for research purposes: (1) Total body water can be measured by dilution with tritiated or deuterated water. Water is then assumed to be a fixed proportion of fat-free mass (FFM = water mass/0.73), and FFM is subtracted from total body weight to obtain total body fat. (2) Body density can be measured by underwater weighing (with accurate correction for lung and abdominal air) and the amount of fat-free mass and body fat can be calculated. (3) The amount of body potassium can be estimated by measuring the amount of its naturally radioactive isotope ^{40}K in a whole-body counter. From this figure the lean body mass can be calculated as LBM = total K^+ (mmol)/68.1. Total body fat can be calculated as total weight minus LBM.

ETIOLOGY

Very little is known about the etiology of obesity. There are probably many different causes, and some may even co-exist in one individual. Obviously excess lipid deposition occurs because energy intake exceeds energy expenditure. An obese individual may have increased intake, decreased expenditure, or both.

GENETICS. Recent twin and adoption studies indicate that human fatness is under strong genetic control. From 64 to 88 per cent of the variance in skinfold thickness, body mass index, and relative weight has been attributed to genetic factors. The studies that have shown this degree of variance describe the genetic influences found in persons living under particular environmental conditions, namely those of western society. Since the environment in which heritable characteristics are expressed affects the expression, these variance ranges may not apply to all societies. Not only is there a strong genetic component to fatness, but there is also a similarly strong genetic component to regional

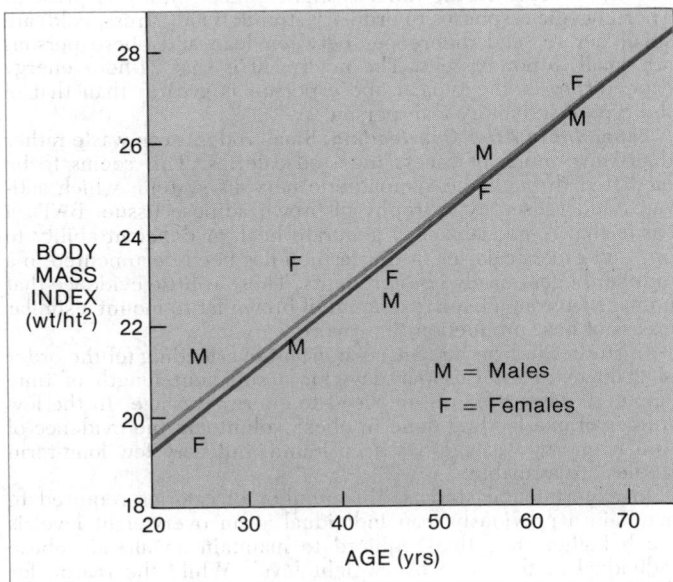

FIGURE 203–4. The effect of age on the body mass index (BMI) associated with lowest mortality. Minimal mortality points were computed for each age-sex group. The regression lines were computed separately for men (dark red line) and for women (light red line). Note that there is a strong effect of age on the BMI associated with lowest mortality and that the regression lines for men and women are nearly identical. (From The Build Study, 1979. Adapted by Andres R: In Andres R, Bierman EL, Hazzard WR, Blass JP (eds.): Principles of Geriatric Medicine. Copyright © 1990 by McGraw-Hill, Inc. Used by permission of McGraw-Hill Book Company.)

fat distribution. Thus, a person's genotype is an important determinant of how adaptation to excess energy intake occurs. Environment is also clearly important, and the interrelation of genetics to particular environments needs to be further investigated.

A number of rare genetic diseases are associated with obesity, but through unknown mechanisms: the Prader-Willi syndrome, the Laurence-Moon-Biedl syndrome, the Alstrom syndrome, the Cohen syndrome, the Carpenter syndrome, and Blount's disease. The reader is referred to textbooks on genetic disorders for further descriptions of these entities.

ENERGY INTAKE. Hyperphagia is the striking cause of obesity in a number of animal models (both genetic and brain-lesioned). The cause of human obesity is usually much less straightforward, however. Obesity has been regarded as an eating disorder for centuries, but the presumed eating abnormality has been difficult to document. Measuring food intake in a free-living environment is subject to large errors. It is also difficult to agree on what constitutes abnormal intake, since the range of caloric intake varies greatly even in lean individuals. Most studies have suggested that obese persons do overeat (at least in their weight-gaining phases). There are numerous examples of individuals who categorically deny overeating but who lose weight when brought into a metabolic ward and placed on a calculated weight-maintaining diet for their height and age.

Possibly obese persons are unduly attracted by the hedonic aspects of food, or they have impaired feedback signals registering satiety, or they have insensitive central reception centers for the feedback signals. It has also been suggested that feeding behavior is learned and that satiety is a conditioned response. Maladaptive conditioning is said to occur in obese persons. None of these theories has been scientifically validated.

ENERGY EXPENDITURE. *Resting Metabolic Expenditure.* Obese individuals may gain weight because they are "thrifty"; i.e., less ingested nutrient is spent as heat and thus more is available for storage. This argument has been put forward by those who contend that obese individuals do not eat more than lean ones and may actually eat less. Impaired thermogenesis exists in certain animal models of obesity. While it has been more difficult to document in humans, recent studies in both adults and infants have reported that a low rate of energy expenditure may predispose to obesity.

Thermogenesis can be divided into three components—resting metabolic rate (RMR), thermic effect of food (TEF), and thermic effect of exercise or activity (TEE).

RMR is the energy expended in the postabsorptive state to drive basic life-supporting processes under thermoneutral conditions. RMR, expressed as total amount of energy spent per unit time, is higher in obese persons than in lean ones. RMR can be well correlated with total weight but can be better correlated with lean body mass (LBM). This explains why men have higher RMR's than women and why RMR's decrease with age.

Obese individuals have a higher LBM than those who are lean, since they require an extra amount of sustaining cell mass to maintain the extra fat. When RMR is expressed as kilocalories per kilogram of LBM, obese persons have values equivalent to the lean. It is only when RMR is expressed as kilocalories per kilogram of body weight that they have values below those who are lean. This is because per unit of weight they have a relatively lower amount of metabolizing cell mass and a larger amount of stored fat, which is relatively inert in energy utilization. In terms of basal or resting energetics, therefore, the obese once they are obese do not have impaired RMR's and are not more "efficient" than lean persons. Some recent studies have reported, however, that in certain individuals a low RMR may predispose them to gain weight.

The RMR varies as much as ±15 per cent from individual to individual, even when they are matched for age, sex, and surface area. If a difference in metabolic rate between individuals can be as great as one third, it is clear that at a given caloric intake one individual may gain weight and another may lose it. Energy balance depends on matching intake to expenditure. It is not surprising that different individuals maintain weight on widely differing caloric intakes.

Expenditure in Activity. The obese expend more energy during physical activity, since an obese person is moving a greater load through space, whether walking, running, or climbing stairs. This is true, although less so, even when body weight is supported, as in cycle ergometer exercise, because of the higher cost of moving the larger leg mass. Thus, more kilowatts of energy are expended. Increases in energy expenditure relative to increases in work are similar in obese and lean individuals, however. That is, if lean and obese individuals are given the same amount of work to do, once the constant amount of extra energy related to the extra cost of moving the extra weight is accounted for, they expend an equivalent amount of energy.

Studies of obese persons, however, show most of them to be less active, both in engaging in physical activities and in moving about once engaged. The amount of energy expended over 24 hours in physical activity is very variable from individual to individual, however, and it is difficult to generalize.

Expenditure After Food. Food is an important thermogenic stimulant, since it generates heat as it is metabolized. Because of this, a fed person has a higher metabolic rate than a fasting one. This elevation of postcibal metabolic rate above basal has been called the thermic effect of food (TEF). With a mixed diet, about 10 per cent of the metabolizable energy ingested is lost as heat.

Obese persons may have TEF responses equivalent to lean persons, or they may have a somewhat depressed response. The impaired response appears to be related to insulin resistance. Obese persons with insulin resistance have a slower glucose disposal. The impaired utilization of glucose by the cells of the body slows down heat production. Thus, glucose loads in an insulin-resistant obese person can generate lesser amounts of heat per calorie ingested. This impaired thermogenic effect can be normalized by giving insulin, so that an equivalent thermic response to that of insulin-sensitive persons occurs. Thus, it seems likely that a thermogenic defect relating to carbohydrate disposal is found in obese patients who are insulin resistant and not found in those who are equivalently obese but insulin sensitive. Thus, there is evidence for an overall somewhat diminished thermic effect of food in obese as compared to lean individuals. However, even insulin-resistant obese persons with a decreased TEF have an overall energy expenditure greater than do lean persons for the 3- to 4-hour period after the meal, since the slight decrease in TEF is less than the inherent elevation in their RMR.

In summary, although hypometabolism may predispose to obesity in some cases, RMR is higher once obesity is present. Thermogenic responses to ordinary stimuli (food, stress, cold) are small per se, and differences between lean and obese persons are small to nonexistent. The net result is that 24-hour energy expenditure in the typical obese person is greater than that of the typical sedentary lean person.

Expenditure After Overfeeding. Small rodents can waste rather than store much of excess ingested calories. This seems to be mediated through the sympathetic nervous system, which activates and causes hypertrophy of brown adipose tissue (BAT), a tissue that is specialized to generate heat. A deficient ability to burn off excess calories in this fashion has been documented in a number of genetically obese rodents. There is little evidence that humans have an adequate amount of brown fat to mount a similar excess of heat production, however.

In studies in lean humans, significant overfeeding (of the order of 2000 extra calories per day) for a sufficient length of time (about 10 days or more) may lead to energy wastage. In the few studies of overfeeding done in obese volunteers, no evidence of similar energy wastage has been found, but very few long-term studies are available.

In experimental studies, the number of calories required to maintain a previously lean individual at an overweight level is much higher than that required to maintain an already obese individual at the same overweight level. While the reason for this is unclear, it does suggest an increased "efficiency" of at least some obese subjects.

Do obese people lack a protective mechanism, i.e., heat dissipation, that lean people possess if they overeat? There is not much convincing experimental evidence to date, although it is a tempting hypothesis that needs to be further investigated.

PATHOPHYSIOLOGY

FAT CELLS. Fat cells (adipocytes) form a reservoir of energy that expands or contracts according to the energy balance of the organism. Fat cells develop from precursor preadipocytes to accommodate excess nutrient calories. Adipocytes gradually increase in volume to about 1 μg of mass, at which point little further enlargement seems to be possible. With continuing positive energy balance, new adipocytes form from precursor cells and the total cell number increases. Adipocytes can increase their number in an unlimited fashion, so that fat mass can reach huge dimensions through hyperplasia.

Once fat cells are formed, it is difficult to dedifferentiate them. This has been termed the "ratchet effect," because a ratchet turns in only one direction. Even though weight may be lost, fat cell numbers remain fixed. As a result, fat cell size reverts toward normal and with sustained weight loss may actually go below normal (Fig. 203–5).

What the stimulus is for the differentiation of preadipocytes into adipocytes is unknown. Adipose tissue lipoprotein lipase (LPL) may be involved. LPL acts on circulating chylomicrons and very low density lipoproteins (VLDL), activating the breakdown of triglyceride to glycerophosphate and free fatty acids (FFA). The FFA can then enter adipocytes, be re-esterified to triglycerides, and be stored. Adipose tissue LPL activity is high in obesity. Whether it is primary and causative for obesity or is secondary to the obesity is unclear. While LPL activity seems to rise with weight loss and is thought to be important in the accelerated weight regain of many patients, it seems to drop after the maintenance of weight loss for a time, suggesting that its elevation in the obese patient may be secondary rather than primary.

REGIONAL DISTRIBUTION OF ADIPOSE TISSUE. Fat mass is distributed differently in men and women. The android, or male, pattern is characterized by fat distributed predominantly in the upper body above the waist, whereas the gynecoid, or female, pattern shows fat predominantly in the lower body, that is, lower abdomen, buttocks, hips, and thighs. Upper body fat has a significantly worse prognosis for morbidity and mortality than does lower body fat. The regional distribution can be measured in a variety of ways. The easiest, most common, and very useful way is by measuring body circumference at the waist and at the hips and calculating a waist:hip ratio. A ratio of greater than 0.85 in women and greater than 1.0 in males can be considered abnormal.

Fat cells from the upper body seem to be functionally different from fat cells in the lower body. They are more sensitive to catecholamines and insulin. It is likely that the greater lipolytic and lipogenic potential of the upper body cells is related to an underlying difference in sex-hormone response of the two tissues. Thus, testosterone and estrogen influences may be important and may act differently on upper and lower body fat cells.

Abdominal or android fatness carries a greater risk for hypertension, cardiovascular disease, hyperinsulinemia, diabetes mellitus, gallbladder disease, and stroke. It also carries a greater risk of overall mortality. Since more men than women have the android distribution, they are more at risk for these conditions. Also, women who deposit their excess fat in a more android manner have a greater risk than women whose fat distribution is more gynecoid. Upper body fat deposition tends to occur primarily by hypertrophy of the existing cells, whereas lower body fat deposition is by differentiation of new fat cells, i.e., hyperplasia. Reducing a normal number of enlarged fat cells to normal size is easier than reducing large numbers of the cells in the lower body hyperplastic depot to normal or below normal sized cells. This may explain the weight loss difficulties of many women with lower body obesity.

Thus, three components of body fat are associated with health risk: per cent body fat, subcutaneous truncal or abdominal fat, and visceral fat in the abdominal cavity. While partly correlated with each other, they do show independence of expression.

SET POINT. The concept of a "set point" of body weight suggests that each person has a control system that "sets" how much weight, or alternatively how much fat, he or she should have. How the control system is regulated, that is, where the feedback signals from "weight" or "fat" originate and how they might be transmitted (humoral, neural, both?) to the hypothalamic feeding and satiety areas are totally unknown.

This set-point theory suggests that people are at a given weight because they are "set" there. That is, one's set point is the weight one normally maintains. Although this is circular thinking, set-point theory has been used to suggest that weight loss programs are misguided and that the effort to lose weight is inevitably fraught with failure because set point will bring individuals up to their pre-weightloss weight.

Animals with ventromedial hypothalamus (VMH) lesions seem

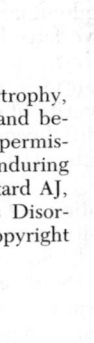

FIGURE 203–5. Fat cell hypertrophy, proliferation, and shrinkage to and below initial size. (Adapted with permission from Van Itallie TB: The enduring storage capacity of fat. *In* Stunkard AJ, Stellar E (eds.): Eating and Its Disorders. New York, Raven Press, copyright 1984.)

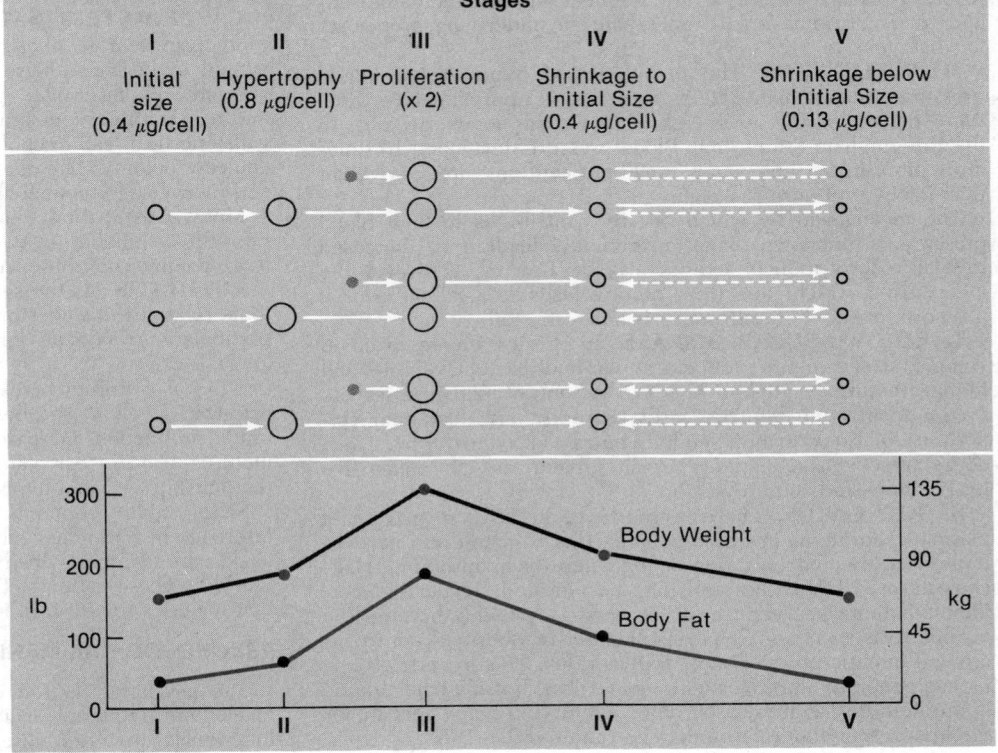

to "set" themselves at a higher prevailing weight, from which they then once more regulate their weight normally. That is, once they have attained their plateau higher weight, they gain more weight if overfed but return to previous weight if they are allowed to eat ad lib; if they are food-deprived, they lose weight and when fed ad lib also return to their previous plateau weight. In a similar manner, animals with lesions in the lateral hypothalamus are hypophagic and lose weight to a new lower weight "set point," which they then return back to from either overweight if they have been overfed or underweight if they have been further underfed. Genetically obese animals, such as the Zucker rat, also seem to defend elevated weights.

If and how these models relate to human obesity is unclear. The set-point theory has been used to suggest that exercise and some drugs lower set point and most palatable foods raise it. Once these statements have been made, however, no closer understanding of the regulation of body weight and of food intake has been attained. Certainly, if there is a "set point," it is a very movable one that seems to change easily under the influence of a number of environmental conditions.

CLINICAL MANIFESTATIONS

INSULIN RESISTANCE. Obesity induces an insulin-resistant state in man, one that is associated with both basal and stimulated hyperinsulinemia. This results from a change in β-cell insulin release rather than in the threshold to glucose stimulation. The enlarged fat cell is less sensitive to the antilipolytic and lipogenic actions of insulin. While a decreased number of insulin receptors contributes to the insulin resistance, the resistance is generally much greater than would be predicted from the magnitude of this decrease. A "postreceptor" defect is therefore presumed to occur as well. This defect in glucose utilization occurs also in other insulin-sensitive tissues, particularly muscle. The liver is also less responsive to insulin. As the insulin resistance becomes more profound, glucose uptake in peripheral tissues is impaired and glucose output by the liver is increased.

DIABETES MELLITUS. In a certain number of obese individuals, diabetes mellitus occurs, as the non-insulin-dependent (NIDDM) type (Ch. 218). The prevalence of diabetes is approximately three times higher in overweight than in nonoverweight persons. In the United States about 85 per cent of patients with NIDDM are obese. Clinically manifest diabetes develops only with the appropriate genetic legacy, but obesity, by enhancing insulin resistance, increases the demand on the pancreatic islets and tends to unmask and exacerbate an underlying propensity for diabetes.

HYPERTENSION. The prevalence of hypertension (blood pressure greater than 160/95 mm Hg) is approximately three times higher for the overweight than for the nonoverweight. In the Framingham Study, high blood pressure developed 10 times more often in persons who were 20 per cent or more overweight than in those of normal weight.

The mechanism by which obesity contributes to high blood pressure is unknown. Hyperinsulinemia leading to increased tubular reabsorption of sodium may be a factor. Whatever the mechanism, weight loss from dieting leads to a fall in arterial pressure, even when salt intake is not restricted.

CARDIOVASCULAR DISEASE. In obesity, increased blood volume, stroke volume, left ventricular end-diastolic volume, and filling pressure result in a high cardiac output. This can lead to predominantly left ventricular hypertrophy and dilatation. Hypertension also contributes to left ventricular hypertrophy. Thus, obese hypertensive patients are at greater risk for congestive heart failure and sudden death.

BLOOD LIPIDS. There seems to be an adverse pattern of plasma lipoproteins in obese people. This is manifested particularly by a low concentration of high density lipoprotein (HDL) cholesterol. LDL cholesterol may be elevated. Hypertriglyceridemia is more prevalent in obese persons, possibly because the insulin resistance and hyperinsulinemia of obesity lead to increased hepatic production of triglycerides. This hypertriglyceridemia generally improves with weight loss, but if a true genetic lipoprotein disorder coexists, more intensive therapy specific for the lipoprotein abnormality may be required (Ch. 172).

RESPIRATORY PROBLEMS. Severe obesity can lead to chronic hypoxia with cyanosis and hypercapnia. Associated with this are an increased demand for ventilation, an increased breathing workload, respiratory muscle inefficiency, and decreased functional reserve capacity and expiratory reserve volume. Peripheral lung units can close, resulting in a ventilation-perfusion mismatch.

The end-stage associated with severe obesity is the pickwickian syndrome, in which hypoventilation is so marked that hypoxia leads to long periods of somnolence. In these patients, pulmonary hypertension occurs and cardiac failure may supervene.

SLEEP APNEA. Sleep apnea is very common in severely obese patients (Ch. 70). The relationship between obesity and sleep apnea is unclear, since the most obese individuals are not necessarily the most severely affected. Apnea can be obstructive or central, and both are more prevalent in obese persons. In obese persons the upper airways may be obstructed by the large local accumulation of fat tissue, often in combination with micrognathia and enlarged tonsils and adenoids. The obstruction leads to hypoventilation and hypoxia, which somehow trigger apneic episodes that then make the hypoxia and hypercapnia worse. These patients benefit from weight loss and sometimes from surgical removal of some of the obstructive tissues. Central apnea is characterized by a cessation of ventilatory drive from brain centers, so that diaphragmatic excursions stop for periods of 10 to 30 seconds. The reason obese persons are prone to this condition is unknown. Pharmacotherapy is sometimes helpful. Daytime somnolence is common in obese patients with apnea, partly from hypoxia and partly from the continual disturbance of sleep at night, since they tend to awake after each apneic episode.

VENOUS CIRCULATORY DISEASE. Severely obese individuals often have varicose veins and venous stasis. Congestive heart failure may add to dependent edema, with the further complications of trophic changes of the skin and an increased propensity for thrombophlebitis and thromboembolism. Pulmonary embolism is much more common in the obese than in those of normal weight (Ch. 65).

CANCER. Endometrial cancer is two to three times more common in obese than in lean women. Risk of breast cancer increases with increasing BMI in postmenopausal women. It has been speculated that this increased risk is due to the stimulatory effect of increased levels of estrogens in the postmenopausal period. Obese women also have a higher incidence of cancer of the gallbladder and of the biliary system. Obese men have a higher mortality from cancer of the colon, rectum, and prostate for reasons that are unknown.

GASTROINTESTINAL DISEASE. Cholesterol gallstones are more prevalent in obesity. The pathogenetic sequence is presumed to be that of greater cholesterol production in the increased body fat depots, greater biliary excretion of cholesterol, and a resulting supersaturation of the cholesterol in bile. The gallstones can lead to cholecystitis (see Ch. 126) and the need for cholecystectomy. The obese carry a greater risk for complications and mortality from such abdominal surgery.

Many obese patients have fatty livers with modest abnormalities of liver function tests, but hepatic diseases in general are not more common in obese than in lean persons.

ARTHRITIS. As the severity of obesity increases, joint symptoms related to osteoarthritis become common. Excess stress is particularly placed on joints of the lower extremities and the lower back.

There is a strong correlation between body weight and serum uric acid level. With obesity, urate clearance is decreased and urate production increased. Since hypertension and diabetes mellitus also are correlated with elevated uric acid levels, the relationship between hyperuricemia and obesity is multifactorial.

SKIN. Skin problems are common in obesity, particularly intertrigo in redundant folds of skin. Fungal and yeast infections of skin are common. Acanthosis nigricans occurs in a minority of morbidly obese patients. These patients can manifest a syndrome that includes severe insulin resistance.

PSYCHOLOGICAL MANIFESTATIONS

The psychological toll of severe obesity is large. Poor self-image and impaired social relationships are common. Obese individuals are often discriminated against in educational and

TABLE 203–2. PATTERN OF EXCESS MORTALITY VARIATION WITH EXCESS WEIGHT (MEN AGES 15–34 YRS AT ENTRY)

Weight Relative to Average Weight (per cent)	Mortality Ratio
105–115	110
115–125	127
125–135	134
135–145	141
145–155	211
155–165	227

Adapted from Society of Actuaries and Association of Life Insurance Medical Directors of America: *Build Study 1979*. Chicago, Society of Actuaries, March 1980, p 82.

professional settings, engendering anxiety, anger, and self-doubt. There is no evidence, however, of any particular neurotic or psychotic character in obese individuals. The depression and anxiety seem to be situational rather than endogenous and often improve if the obesity can be ameliorated.

MORTALITY

Obesity is associated with increased mortality. The effect of obesity on cardiovascular mortality generally occurs through linkage with other risk factors such as hypertension, diabetes, and hyperlipidemia. However, obesity can also make independent contribution to mortality. In the Framingham Study, for every 10 per cent rise in relative weight, systolic blood pressure rose 6.5 mm Hg, plasma cholesterol 12 mg per deciliter, and fasting blood glucose 2 mg per deciliter. The causes of increased mortality for those 20 per cent or more overweight include coronary heart disease, cerebral "hemorrhage" (stroke), diabetes, digestive diseases, and cancer (Table 203–2).

OBESITY AND THE ENDOCRINE SYSTEM

Although obesity has often been described as an "endocrine" disease, less than 1 per cent of obese patients have any significant endocrine dysfunction. Hypothalamic, pituitary, thyroid, adrenal, ovarian, and possibly pancreatic endocrine syndromes have been related to obesity.

HYPOTHALAMIC DISEASE. In this type of obesity, the appetite systems or tracts located in the hypothalamus are affected. Bilateral damage in the ventromedial hypothalamus produces obesity in the rat; conversely, bilateral damage in the extreme lateral portion of the hypothalamus causes aphagia. Rather than a single balance of a "feeding center" and a "satiety center," however, it is now clear that diffuse excitatory and inhibitory neuronal systems controlling feeding course through the limbic system and the whole brain. Following trauma, inflammation, or a tumor in the hypothalamus, a few patients develop hyperphagic obesity, most of them after surgery for tumors in the hypothalamic area. Craniopharyngioma has been most commonly associated with rapidly progressive obesity. The diagnosis is usually based on history and physical findings, which may or may not include focal neurologic defects, depending on the nature and extent of the injury.

PITUITARY AND ADRENAL DYSFUNCTION. Cushing's disease is the most common form of pituitary dysfunction leading to obesity (Ch. 217). ACTH is excessively produced either by a pituitary tumor or by hyperactive pituitary cells, which leads to excess production of cortisol by the adrenal cortex. Cushing's syndrome can also have a variety of other causes, including exogenous glucocorticoids, primary disorders of the adrenal, and paraneoplastic syndromes of excess ACTH production. The hypercortisolism causes adipocytes located primarily at the center of the body to expand, while those at the extremities do so much less. With this central obesity comes hypertension and diabetes.

THYROID DISEASE. Obesity is often ascribed to "hypometabolism" caused by underactivity of the thyroid gland, but this is in fact seldom true. Severe hypothyroidism can lead to some increased fat, but most of the excess weight is actually edema, which is lost with the institution of thyroid hormone replacement.

POLYCYSTIC OVARIAN SYNDROME (Ch. 224). Mild hirsutism, irregular menses or amenorrhea, and obesity have been linked in the "polycystic ovarian syndrome." In this syndrome the ovaries have atretic follicles, the patient is anovulatory, and

menstrual disturbance (long-term amenorrhea to oligomenorrhea) is the rule. The ovaries overproduce androgens, some of which are converted to estrogens peripherally, primarily in adipose tissue. Hirsutism is common, but virilization is not. The relation of obesity to the polycystic ovarian syndrome is not clear, but the two conditions often coexist.

ENDOCRINE CONSEQUENCES OF OBESITY. One of the pathophysiologic consequences of obesity may be certain endocrine abnormalities. The sex-hormone abnormalities associated with obesity are different in males and females. While mildly obese men have no detectable abnormalities, severely obese men have mild hypogonadotropic hypogonadism, with less than two thirds the normal mean plasma levels of total testosterone, free testosterone, and follicle-stimulating hormone. Gonadotropic hormones are suppressed by elevated plasma estrogens derived from increased aromatization of adrenal precursors in the excessive body fat. Obesity may be associated with increased metabolic clearance rates of testosterone, caused partly by decreased sex hormone-binding globulin (SHBG). Spermatogenesis, libido, and potency, however, are normal.

Estrogens are not elevated in obese premenopausal women, probably because the amount of estrone conversion by the adipose tissue is small in comparison with regular ovarian estradiol production. Estrogens are elevated, however, in postmenopausal obese women, most likely owing to increased peripheral conversion of the prehormone androstenedione to estrone. This may be a partial explanation as to why there is less osteoporosis in obese women.

There are differences in the androgen-estrogen environment in persons with upper (UBO) and lower (LBO) body obesity. This is more clearly defined in women. Women with UBO have higher androgen production rates and higher concentrations of testosterone and estradiol levels than those with LBO. They also have decreased levels of SHBG, so that free testosterone concentrations are higher. Women with LBO have increased estrone from peripheral aromatization of circulating androgens.

In obesity, insulin resistance develops and hyperinsulinemia results. Whether impaired glucose tolerance or frank diabetes ensues depends on the degree of insulin resistance and the underlying genetic make-up of the individual. Triiodothyronine (T_3) may be elevated to high normal in conditions of high caloric intake with adequate carbohydrate, while thyroxine levels and TSH levels are normal. Slightly low blood cortisol levels may be present in obesity, probably because of enhanced turnover rates of cortisol. The circadian rhythm of cortisol secretion is usually normal in obesity. Urinary free cortisol levels are normal if related to the lean body mass or urinary creatinine. Also, these obese patients usually suppress normally with dexamethasone (Ch. 217).

Pseudotumor cerebri (benign intracranial hypertension) (Ch. 486) occurs most commonly in young women who are frequently obese. No intracranial pathology has been found, although headache and blurred vision occur. Why obesity is common in so many of these patients is unclear. It is possible that altered function of the ventromedial or paraventricular region of the brain occurs owing to the increased intracranial pressure. Hypothalamic control of prolactin and growth hormone is often defective in obesity, with poor response to insulin hypoglycemia. These abnormalities generally revert to normal with significant weight loss, but not always. Whether these pituitary abnormalities reflect altered hypothalamic control due to obesity or abet the obesity in some way is unclear.

TREATMENT

Obesity is very difficult to treat, because the primary emphasis must be on active patient self-control rather than on passive drug therapy. The responsibility of the physician is to be as supportive and helpful as possible. The three approaches to weight control are diet, exercise, and drugs.

DIET. A truly motivated individual will generally stay on a diet for a long time, initially for weight loss and then for weight maintenance. Crash diets for a few days or weeks generally accomplish little of permanent value. Because of the long-term requirement for a diet, it must be tailored to a person's tastes and habits.

The diet must be nutritionally adequate. It is not possible to calculate a diet under 1100 calories that contains adequate amounts of vitamins and minerals. If the diet is lower in calories than this, vitamin and mineral supplements are necessary. The goal of weight loss is loss of as much fat as possible while losing as little lean body mass as possible. A mixed, balanced diet is a sensible approach to long-term weight reduction. A diet of at least 0.8 to 1.2 grams of protein per kilogram of desirable body weight will minimize nitrogen losses. The protein should be of high quality, so that essential amino acids can be utilized to maintain lean body mass.

It is a common strategy in many popular weight-reduction programs to use very unbalanced diets that focus on particular food groups at the expense of others. The high-fat–low-carbohydrate diets that are low in calories are ketogenic, whereas the low-fat–high-carbohydrate diets are not. These diets have in common a marked imbalance of macronutrients, with a concomitant imbalance of micronutrients. They cannot be recommended. If such diets are used, careful calculations for nutritional adequacy must be made, and appropriate supplements must be taken daily by the patient. These supplements require a number of tablets and capsules each day, so that compliance becomes a greater problem that must be strictly monitored.

VERY LOW CALORIE DIETS. Very low calorie diets (VLCD) severely limit daily intake to 300 to 700 calories. Some diets are strictly limited to protein and have been called protein-supplemented modified fasts (PSMF). Others allow both protein and carbohydrate. The concept of protein-supplemented fasting arose because this regimen improves nitrogen balance over fasting programs. There is little evidence, however, that at equicaloric levels protein alone is better than protein with carbohydrate. The extra weight lost early in the diet when protein alone is given is that of water. With this water diuresis there is electrolyte loss as well. The calories can be given either in liquid formula form or as natural foods. High-quality protein must be given. It is also imperative that adequate supplements of vitamins and minerals be taken. Although these very severe diets have been given for extensive periods of time, it is dangerous to allow them for longer than 12 weeks. The heavier the patient, the safer the diet seems to be. The lighter the patient, the more LBM is lost per unit of weight loss, so that more caution, more liberal calories, and a shorter time period of diet should be followed. These diets, especially those relying on liquid formulas, have been popular because of their relative ease and because, since they are so hypocaloric, the weight loss is more rapid. However, they can have serious side effects.

Side effects of these severe diets include orthostatic hypotension (secondary to both sodium loss and impaired norepinephrine secretion), fatigue, cold intolerance, dry skin, hair loss, and menstrual irregularities. Cholelithiasis, cholecystitis, and rarely pancreatitis occur. Unfortunately, most individuals rapidly regain weight after being on these crash programs, perhaps in large measure because the very low caloric content and the liquid form of the diet do not educate the patient to make the adjustments in lifestyle and eating behavior necessary to maintain the weight loss.

BEHAVIOR MODIFICATION. Psychoanalysis and psychotherapy have not been very helpful in weight control. An extended change in eating behavior requires a great change in life style, however, so behavior modification programs have proliferated. Behavior therapy is a fundamental departure from the traditional "dietary" training of the past, in which a list of foods, the allowable quantities, and specific menus were supplied. In behavior modification the patient is first made aware of what and how much he or she eats as a background for changing that behavior. Many persons eat quite unconsciously, with little thought of how much they eat and with little or no knowledge of its caloric content. Initially, in the education process, careful food intake diaries are kept. Patients record not only what was eaten, but where, with whom, how, their feelings, and their degree of hunger. These diaries are analyzed, and nutrient densities of foods are discussed. New modes of eating are suggested, including not eating between meals, eating always at table, eating only three times per day, watching the portions of food eaten, not doing other activities while eating, and eating slowly with con-

centration. Behavior modification also strives at stimulus control and environmental management. The aim is to break learned associations between environmental cues and food intake. Particular situations that trigger eating are avoided or controlled. Behavior modification therapy is usually done in groups, with continued dialogue between the trained group leader (psychologist, nutritionist, physician), the other group members, and the patient.

EXERCISE. Obesity is a consequence of greater energy intake than energy expenditure. To lose weight, the imbalance must be tipped the other way, with expenditure becoming greater than intake. This is done not only by hypocaloric dieting, but also by increasing activity. Obese persons tend to be inactive; it is therefore important to increase caloric utilization. The patient should be taught the approximate number of calories being expended over basal level in individual activities. Most patients are surprised at how much exercise it takes to expend just a few calories (Table 203–3).

Moderate exercise only transiently increases the metabolic rate. The calories expended are the calories of work done. In the obese, moderate exercise does not actually lower food intake, but intake does not increase to keep pace with the extra expenditure, as it does in lean persons. This is helpful in inducing weight loss.

DRUG THERAPY. Drugs in weight control have been used as short-term adjunctive therapy to diet and exercise. Over the long term the use of drugs has been disappointing, owing to small effects on weight loss or adverse side effects. In general, drugs affect appetite modestly. The anorectic drugs act centrally through brain catecholamine, dopaminergic, or serotoninergic pathways. For example, amphetamine and its derivatives seem to produce anorexia through stimulating the central hypothalamic neurochemical pathways in which norepinephrine and/or dopamine is the principal neurotransmitter.

Amphetamine not only decreases appetite; it also elevates mood and increases arousal, probably mediated through making norepinephrine and dopamine more abundant at synapses. In

TABLE 203–3. APPROXIMATE ENERGY EXPENDITURE IN SELECTED ACTIVITIES FOR PEOPLE OF DIFFERENT WEIGHTS (CALORIES PER 30 MINUTES)*

Activity	Weight (pounds)					
	110	130	150	170	190	210
Aerobic dancing						
"walking pace"	99	114	132	150	168	186
"jogging pace"	159	186	213	243	270	300
"running pace"	204	240	276	315	351	387
Basketball	207	243	282	318	357	396
Canoeing—leisure	66	78	90	102	114	126
Canoeing—racing	156	183	210	237	267	294
Carpentry	78	93	105	120	135	147
Cycling—5.5 mph	96	114	132	147	165	183
Cycling—9.4 mph	150	177	204	231	258	285
Dancing—ballroom	78	90	105	117	132	144
Dancing—disco	156	183	210	237	267	294
Gardening	150	177	204	231	258	285
Golf	129	150	174	195	219	243
Judo	294	345	399	450	504	558
Lying or sitting down	33	39	45	51	57	63
Mopping floor	96	105	120	138	153	171
Running						
11.5 minutes per mile	204	240	276	315	351	387
9 minutes per mile	291	342	393	447	498	552
7 minutes per mile	366	417	468	522	573	624
5.5 minutes per mile	435	513	591	669	747	828
Skiing, cross-country	216	252	291	330	369	408
Standing quietly	39	45	51	57	66	72
Swimming						
backstroke	255	300	345	390	435	486
crawl	192	228	261	297	330	366
Table tennis	102	120	138	156	174	195
Tennis	165	192	222	252	282	312
Walking						
3 mph	102	114	126	138	153	165
4 mph	120	141	162	186	207	228

*Adapted from The High Energy Factor, by Bernard Gutin. Copyright © 1983 by Bernard Gutin and Gail Kessler. Reprinted by permission of Random House, Inc.

contrast, fenfluramine is thought to increase brain serotonin. Mazindol probably works through a dopaminergic mechanism. It therefore appears that increasing the activity of norepinephrine, dopamine, and/or serotonin at certain central nervous system sites can lead to anorexia and weight loss.

All of the drugs mentioned have a greater effect on appetite control than do placebos. Problems arise, however, from abuse potential and side effects. Amphetamine has clearly addictive properties. Amphetamine and phenmetrazine have disturbing side effects, such as sleep disturbances, agitation, and psychosis. Irritability and insomnia have been reported with diethylpropion, mazindol, and phentermine. Fenfluramine often causes depression, sedation, and diarrhea. Contraindications include severe hypertension, coronary artery disease, glaucoma, and history of drug abuse.

These drugs are generally prescribed for short periods of time, in an effort to help patients over difficult weight "plateaus" or crisis periods. Some experts, however, suggest that certain of the drugs lower "set point" of weight and should be given chronically. This is not, however, generally accepted practice.

GOALS. Very often the patient, and sometimes the physician, has unrealistic goals of what can be accomplished. One pound of fat is equivalent to 4000 kilocalories. With a deficit of 400 kilocalories per day, losing one pound takes 10 days. The more accurate the knowledge of daily energy expenditure and energy intake is, the closer a physician can predict the rate of weight loss. This may prevent unrealistic goals and disappointment by both patient and therapist.

SURGERY. Certain patients have severe obesity (greater than 100 per cent of desirable weight), have tried weight control programs without success, and often have complications like sleep apnea, heart failure, phlebitis, and arthritis. Their life expectancy is much lower than normal. These patients may be candidates for surgery for obesity, since nonoperative management rarely leads to permanent weight reduction.

Surgery for obesity should be considered experimental, as there is no one accepted procedure and all carry significant risks and complications. Short bowel procedures (jejunoileal bypass) generally leave about 50 cm of small bowel between the ligament of Treitz and the ileocecal valve, with the bypassed portion of bowel draining directly into the ileal remnant (end-to-end or end-to-side) or into the colon. Jejunoileal bypass generally produces weight loss but is fraught with complications, including diarrhea, electrolyte losses, vitamin deficiencies, hepatic toxicity, calcium oxalate kidney stones, intestinal pseudo-obstruction, and polyarthritis. As a result, it cannot be recommended.

Because of the severe side effects of intestinal surgery, gastric surgical procedures have become popular. In these operations, no part of the stomach is resected, so that the operation is theoretically reversible. A small fundic pouch or reservoir is created so that the individual is severely limited in the amount of food that he or she can eat. The pouch is generally created by stapling across the stomach, leaving a very small reservoir. The distal stoma created for the pouch has variably been designed to empty into the rest of the stomach or into a loop of jejunum, with the rest of the stomach and duodenum becoming a blind loop. Alternatively, in vertical banded gastroplasty, as opposed to horizontal banding, only a small tubular reservoir remains for food entering from the esophagus. Side effects include gastric distress and vomiting. If vomiting is severe enough, electrolyte disturbances can occur. Also, some patients do not lose much weight, because many eat "around" the small reservoir with frequent servings of liquid or semisolid foods. A mean weight loss of two thirds of excess weight has been reported, but failure is not uncommon. Dilatation of the gastric pouch, stomal dilation, stomal obstruction, and staple line dehiscence can occur as complications.

Surgery is still unsatisfactory and experimental, but it may be advisable in some cases. Because life-long follow-up and vitamin and mineral supplementation are necessary, a responsible and cooperative patient and an experienced surgeon are a requisite duo.

WEIGHT REGAIN

The most difficult problem in the treatment of obesity is the maintenance of a reduced body weight. The ability to maintain weight loss may depend on the severity of obesity and the amount of hypercellularity of the adipocytes in a given individual.

A person who is modestly overweight with enlarged adipocytes but little proliferation of extra adipocytes can more easily maintain weight loss. The adipocyte hyperplasia of greater obesity is likely to create a much greater problem in maintenance of weight loss. The degree of filling of adipocytes is very likely a regulated factor in energy balance. Obese persons with adipocyte hyperplasia begin to decrease the mass of each adipocyte as they lose weight. If the adipocyte mass drops below a normal lower level of about 0.5 µg per cell, individuals seem to have greater difficulty in maintaining weight reduction. Adipocyte mass seems to be a regulated factor with a feedback effect on energy intake, so that the reduced obese seem to experience strong food intake cues that they have trouble resisting.

Lipogenic enzyme activities increase when a hypocaloric diet is liberalized as a patient goes from a weight-loss to a weight-maintenance period. This is consequent to an increase in caloric intake rather than being primarily caused by the reduction in weight. It is not clear whether an increased food efficiency is present, but reduced obese individuals have been reported to require about 25 per cent fewer calories per square meter of surface area to maintain their body weight than do either normal persons or obese individuals who have not dieted and lost weight. Thus, reduced obese persons have energy requirements typical of a semifasted state despite their taking sufficient calories to maintain weight at a level that is still above normal.

PREVENTION

The propensity toward obesity is partially inherited, but a large component is also environmental. Obesity leads to an increased morbidity and mortality from a number of diseases, especially for those who are under 45 years old. Being overweight in early adult life is more dangerous than it is at older ages.

It is incumbent on physicians to make their patients aware of these risks and try to keep patients at a body mass index of grade 0 to grade 1 (see Fig. 203–1). This is particularly true for those patients who already have, or have a family history of, the diseases that are precipitated and abetted by obesity.

Hubert HB, Feinleib M, McNamara PM, et al.: Obesity as an independent risk factor for cardiovascular disease: A 26-year follow-up of participants in the Framingham Heart Study. Circulation 67:968, 1983. A re-examination of the relationship of the degree of obesity and the incidence of cardiovascular disease over 26 years in more than 5200 men and women indicates that obesity is a significant independent predictor, particularly among women.
Kissebah AH, Vydelingum N, Murray R, et al.: Relation of body fat distribution to metabolic complications of obesity. J Clin Endocrinol Metab 54:254, 1982. A study in women of the sites of fat predominance as an important prognostic marker for glucose intolerance, hyperinsulinemia, and hypertriglyceridemia.
Krotkiewski M, Bjorntorp P, Sjostrom L, et al.: Impact of obesity on metabolism in men and women. Importance of regional adipose tissue distribution. J Clin Invest 72:1150, 1983. A study of the regional differences between the sexes with regard to adipose tissue distribution and of the differential risk of upper and lower body obesity as it relates to lipid and carbohydrate metabolism.
Lew EA, Garfinkel L: Variations in mortality by weight among 750,000 men and women. J Chron Dis 32:563, 1979. A description of the mortality experience of men and women in a long-term prospective study by the American Cancer Society, documenting that individuals 30 to 40 per cent heavier than average had a mortality rate 50 per cent higher than those of average weight. Mortality comparisons as a function of weight for all common diseases are included.
National Institutes of Health Consensus Development Panel on the Health Implications of Obesity: Health implications of obesity. Ann Intern Med 103:147, 1985. A statement on the risks of obesity.
Ravussin E, Lillioja MB, Knowler WC, et al.: Reduced rate of energy expenditure as a risk factor for body-weight gain. N Engl J Med 318(8):467–471, 1988. A report of hypometabolism as a predisposing cause of obesity.
Segal KR, Pi-Sunyer FX: Exercise, resting metabolic rate, and thermogenesis. Diabetes/Metab Rev 2:19, 1986. A review of the differences in thermogenic response to food and to exercise in lean and obese persons.
Sims EA: Mechanisms of hypertension in the overweight. Hypertension 4:43, 1982. A review of the pathophysiology of hypertension in the obese.
Sims EAH, Danforth E: Expenditure and storage of energy in man. J Clin Invest 79:1019, 1987. An excellent, up-to-date review of energy balance in man with a useful bibliography of 71 references.
Stunkard AJ, Sorensen TIA, Harris C, et al.: An adoption study of human obesity. N Engl J Med 314:193, 1986. A study of the contributions of genetic factors and the family environment to human fatness, concluding that genetic influences have an important role in determining human fatness in adults.
Van Itallie TB, Yang MU: Diet and weight loss. N Engl J Med 297:1158, 1977. A review and a careful metabolic study of the effects of macronutrient composition of low-calorie reducing diets on body composition.

Wadden TA, Van Itallie TB, Blackburn GL: Responsible and irresponsible use of very low calorie diets in the treatment of obesity. JAMA 263:83–85, 1990. *A useful and responsible commentary on treatment with very low calorie diets.*

204 Disorders of Vitamin Metabolism: Deficiencies, Metabolic Abnormalities, and Excesses

Richard S. Rivlin

In approaching disorders of vitamin metabolism, several considerations should be kept in mind about the properties of vitamins, their roles in medicine, and the evolving patterns of their deficiency syndromes as commonly encountered.

Although generations of students are familiar with the syndrome of pellagra (niacin deficiency) as involving four D's (dermatitis, diarrhea, dementia, and death), in clinical practice in the United States such a classic syndrome is encountered only rarely. Rather, the typical picture one sees in severely ill patients with protein-calorie malnutrition is that of multiple vitamin deficiencies without manifestations of any single classic deficiency syndrome. Overt vitamin deficiencies caused by diet are seldom isolated for several reasons. First, a diet poor in one vitamin is usually poor in several others. In addition, one vitamin is often required for the metabolism of another. An example is riboflavin, which is involved in the metabolism of folic acid, pyridoxine, vitamin K, and niacin. Thus a vitamin deficiency may develop secondary to the inadequate dietary intake of a related nutrient.

The clinical development of vitamin deficiencies is typically gradual; the physical examination is usually not useful in detecting deficiencies of specific vitamins early in their development. For example, by the time that perifollicular hemorrhages characteristic of scurvy have developed, vitamin C deficiency is already far advanced. Even the abnormalities detected by physical examination late in the course of the deficiency state are often not pathognomonic. Cheilosis and glossitis, typically attributed to deficiency of riboflavin, can be observed with deficiencies of a number of other B vitamins. Finding an abnormality of this kind on physical examination helps to establish the diagnosis of malnutrition but usually does not identify a specific nutrient as missing from the diet.

Increasing attention is now being paid to drugs and alcohol as significant causes of specific vitamin deficiencies. Drug-induced vitamin deficiencies often are poorly recognized and become evident most frequently in chronically ill patients requiring long-term treatment who have a marginally adequate diet. The elderly are particularly vulnerable to the deleterious effects of ethanol. This commonly used and abused substance is now established as the major cause of deficiencies of folate and thiamine among individuals 65 years of age and older, and probably in many younger age groups as well.

In general, most vitamins must be acquired from dietary sources because they cannot be synthesized in the body. There are several exceptions to this rule in that certain vitamins are synthesized in the body but in very small amounts. An example is niacin, which is formed in vivo from an essential amino acid, tryptophan. A tryptophan-poor diet, such as that consumed when corn is the major food staple, cannot provide sufficient precursor to meet the metabolic needs for niacin, and pellagra may develop. Other examples of vitamins synthesized by the body, or more correctly by the intestinal microflora, are vitamin K and biotin. Deficiency of these vitamins often results from long-term antibiotic therapy, which eliminates the bacterial sources. Under the usual circumstances, however, bacterial synthesis of vitamin K and biotin is not sufficient, and some must be obtained from food sources. Vitamin D is synthesized in the skin in considerable amounts after exposure to light (Ch. 233), and constitutes a source of the vitamin which is at least as important as its dietary intake.

The B vitamins as a group function as essential coenzymes required in intermediary metabolism. The dietary form of each vitamin is first converted into its active derivatives before serving as a coenzyme. Examples include dietary thiamine and its coenzyme derivative, thiamine pyrophosphate, pyridoxine and pyridoxal phosphate, and riboflavin and flavin mononucleotide (riboflavin-5'phosphate) and flavin adenine dinucleotide. Vitamin deficiencies may arise not only because of dietary deficiencies but also because conversion of the dietary form of the vitamin to its coenzyme derivatives is diminished by drugs, disease, or other factors. Vitamin deficiencies may also be caused by abnormalities of intestinal absorption, plasma transport, tissue storage, binding to proteins, or excretion. Ensuring adequate vitamin status involves exogenous factors, such as dietary adequacy and food processing, preparation, and storage, as well as endogenous factors, such as hormones, that control vitamin utilization by the body.

The rate at which stores of vitamins are depleted following restriction of their dietary intake varies widely among vitamins. The body stores of vitamin B_{12} may not be depleted for years, whereas folic acid, thiamine, and niacin may be depleted within weeks or months of reduced dietary intake. In general, the body's capacity for storage of water-soluble vitamins is limited, and when the storage capacity is exceeded, the excess is usually excreted rapidly rather than stored; their tissue concentrations often cannot be increased beyond a certain point even by massive doses. By contrast, body stores of fat-soluble vitamins may become very great with prolonged administration of doses greatly exceeding their recommended dietary allowances (RDA).

At present, many individuals are consuming vitamins in doses far in excess of the RDA. More than one third of individuals 65 years of age and older in the United States are estimated to be taking some kind of nutritional supplement. Left to their own judgment, many persons will not select supplements appropriately. Supplement use is greater among females than males, whites than blacks, and well educated than poorly educated; vitamin C is the most commonly consumed individual supplement. Serious toxicity may develop with prolonged use of vitamins A and D at 5 to 10 times the RDA, particularly in children. Individuals vary considerably in the rate at which they develop toxicity with prolonged use of megadoses of vitamins. Certain conditions predispose to early symptoms. For example, individuals who become dehydrated may be at increased risk for developing hypercalcemia from large doses of vitamin D, and the onset of acute liver disease may precipitate vitamin A toxicity in a stable patient who previously had taken megadoses of this vitamin.

Vitamins increasingly may play specific roles in prevention of disease. Examples include vitamin A and β-carotene in possible prevention of certain malignancies and B vitamins and vitamin C in the possible prevention of neural tube defects when consumed during pregnancy. These subjects are under active investigation at the present time and remain controversial. It is still too early to make firm recommendations on either subject.

For certain disorders vitamins may be used quite appropriately as drugs. For example, ascorbic acid is widely employed to acidify the urine in cases of refractory urinary tract infections. Certain derivatives of vitamin A, in particular the 13-*cis* isomer of retinoic acid, have potent antikeratinizing effects that have been applied to the treatment of cystic acne. Nicotinic acid is widely utilized in the management of severe hyperlipoproteinemia. Certain pyridoxine-dependency syndromes require pharmacologic doses of vitamin B_6. In these and other vitamin-responsive inborn errors of metabolism, therapy must be specific and targeted. Thus, the therapeutic applications of vitamins extend far beyond their roles in correcting dietary deficiency. Both the therapeutic role of vitamins and their potential for toxicity should be kept in mind by the practicing physician.

While the emphasis in clinical medicine is appropriately on the correction of vitamin deficiencies, under certain conditions decreased vitamin intake may confer certain advantages. In malaria, vitamin supplementation programs have been observed to worsen parasitemia, and deficiencies of vitamin E and riboflavin appear to have antimalarial actions. Dietary deficiency of riboflavin, as well as of structural analogues, drugs, and diseases that interfere with the metabolism of this vitamin, all exert antimalarial effects.

Elsas LJ, McCormick DB: Genetic defects in vitamin utilization. Part 1: General aspects and fat-soluble vitamins. Vitam Horm 43:103, 1986. *Review of inherited disorders with special vitamin requirements.*

Machlin LJ (ed.): Handbook of Vitamins, 2nd ed. New York, Marcel Dekker, 1990. *Recently updated volume covering new research and therapeutic applications of vitamins.*

Rivlin RS: Vitamin deficiency. In Samiy A, Douglas RG Jr, Barondess J (eds.): Therapeutic Medicine for Practicing Physicians. Philadelphia, Lea and Febiger, 1990, in press. *Discussion of vitamin deficiency syndromes and their therapies.*

VITAMIN B₁ (THIAMINE)

Structure and Biochemical Function

The thiamine molecule is shown in Figure 204–1. The principal biochemical role of thiamine is that of precursor of thiamine pyrophosphate, a coenzyme required for oxidative decarboxylation of α-ketoacids to aldehydes. These reactions are widely distributed in intermediary metabolism and are an important source of energy generation. In addition, thiamine pyrophosphate serves as the coenzyme for transketolase, which catalyzes the conversions of the two 5-carbon sugars, xylulose-5-PO_4 and ribose-5-PO_4, to the 7-carbon sugar, sedoheptulose-7-PO_4 and the 3-carbon sugar, glyceraldehyde-3-PO_4. This reaction is used as a functional index of thiamine nutritional status, as discussed later in this chapter.

It has been suggested that thiamine may have an additional role in conduction of impulses in peripheral nerves apart from its function as a coenzyme in intermediary metabolism. The initiation of nerve impulses is associated with hydrolysis of thiamine diphosphate and thiamine triphosphate.

Normal Physiology

Dietary thiamine is absorbed from the intestinal tract both by passive diffusion (at high concentrations) and by active transport (at low concentrations.) The absorptive process is associated with phosphorylation of the thiamine molecule within the mucosal cell. In folate deficiency the absorption of thiamine is diminished. About 30 per cent of thiamine is bound to serum proteins normally. Muscle serves as the major storage organ for thiamine; most of the body stores are in the form of thiamine pyrophosphate, with lesser amounts stored as thiamine triphosphate, thiamine monophosphate, and thiamine itself. The degradation and excretion pathways of thiamine are not known with certainty, and more than 25 metabolites of the vitamin have been recovered from urine.

Requirements and Dietary Sources

The RDA for thiamine in adult males is 1.2 to 1.5 mg per day and in adult women, 1.0 to 1.1 mg per day, depending upon age, with a 50 per cent increase during pregnancy and lactation. The allowance is generally related to caloric intake, expressed as 0.5 mg per 1000 kcal, although it is recommended that thiamine intake not go below 1.0 mg per day even with a caloric intake reduced below 2000 kcal. The best dietary sources of thiamine are beef, pork, whole grains, enriched cereal grains, peas, beans, and nuts. The milling and polishing of rice, unless it is subsequently fortified, greatly reduces the thiamine content. Thiamine is rapidly destroyed at alkaline pH and is also heat sensitive when not under strongly acid conditions. Some food items, particularly raw fish, coffee, tea, betel nuts, and many plants, have been shown to contain thiaminases, enzymes that destroy the dietary supply of thiamine. A number of antithiamine factors have been identified from both plant and animal sources, and their consumption in large amounts has resulted in frank deficiency.

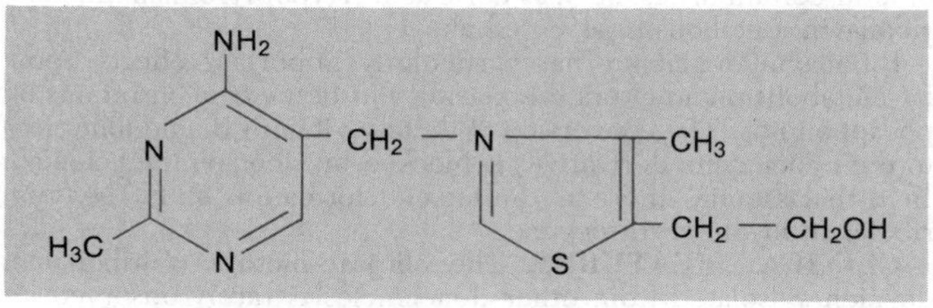

FIGURE 204–1. Structural formula of thiamine.

Deficiency

PATHOGENESIS. In addition to being caused by a poor diet, thiamine deficiency in the United States most commonly occurs as a result of alcoholism. Thiamine absorption is exquisitely sensitive to ingested ethanol, which significantly interferes with thiamine absorption even in healthy individuals. Repeated drinking throughout the day prevents most of the dietary thiamine from being absorbed, particularly in alcoholic patients in whom some degree of malabsorption is quite common. Approximately 25 per cent of alcoholic patients admitted to general hospitals in the United States have some evidence of thiamine deficiency by either clinical or biochemical criteria. Alcoholism is clearly the most important cause of thiamine deficiency in older age groups and probably in younger age groups as well. There is some evidence that alcohol also adversely affects the intermediary metabolism of thiamine, and chronic liver disease secondary to alcoholism may diminish the conversion of thiamine to thiamine pyrophosphate. Refeeding an alcoholic patient without additional thiamine may precipitate thiamine deficiency.

In developing countries that rely on polished rice as a staple in the diet, beriberi prevalence remains very high. It is likely that other factors, such as heavy coffee consumption, possibly may diminish the intestinal absorption of thiamine. Thiamine deficiency is also observed with diabetes, cancer, and other chronic illnesses and with long-term parenteral nutrition or use of intravenous fluids not containing thiamine.

CLINICAL FEATURES. Early thiamine deficiency is characterized by anorexia, irritability, and weight loss. Later, patients experience weakness, peripheral neuropathy, headache, and tachycardia. Advanced thiamine deficiency presents with involvement of two major organ systems predominantly: the cardiovascular system (the syndrome known as "wet beriberi," i.e., beriberi heart disease) and the nervous system, both central and peripheral (known as "dry beriberi").

The following criteria are generally accepted for the diagnosis of beriberi heart disease: absence of other known etiologic factors, history of at least 3 months of documented dietary thiamine deficiency, associated peripheral neuritis, enlarged heart with normal sinus rhythm (usually tachycardia), peripheral edema, nonspecific ST- and T-wave changes, and rapid therapeutic response to thiamine administration. Beriberi heart disease is well recognized as a cause of high-output failure, which is a consequence of the profound peripheral vasodilation. Resting tachycardia, weakness, and weight loss often resemble the clinical features of apathetic hyperthyroidism, with which it is frequently confused.

The central nervous system manifestations of thiamine deficiency consist primarily of the Wernicke-Korsakoff syndrome (Ch. 456). The Wernicke's component is an acute disorder consisting of variable degrees of vomiting, horizontal nystagmus, ophthalmoplegia caused by weakness of the rectus muscles, fever, ataxic gait, and progressive mental impairment. Patients have died when the disease has been unrecognized and allowed to progress. The Korsakoff syndrome typically has loss of memory and confabulation as prominent features.

The peripheral nervous system abnormalities of thiamine deficiency typically consist of a symmetric lesion that involves motor, sensory, and reflex responses. The legs are usually involved earlier and more completely than the arms. Pain and paresthesias may be particularly disabling to afflicted patients. An abnormal transketolase with high Km for thiamine pyrophosphate has been described, which may predispose certain alcohol abusers to severe neurologic impairment when thiamine deficiency develops.

DIAGNOSIS. Thiamine status can be evaluated using bioassays, microbiologic techniques, chemical analyses, and functional enzyme assays. The most sensitive method for analyzing thiamine in small quantities in body fluids, tissues, and foods is high performance liquid chromatography (HPLC). In actual practice, the two most widely used assays are urinary thiamine excretion and the transketolase activity coefficient. Urinary thiamine can be determined accurately, but the results may be misleading if there has been recent thiamine intake in a previously deficient patient or if the patient has recently taken diuretics, which promote thiamine excretion. The results obtained under those circumstances would not yield the expected low value.

Transketolase, as noted above, requires thiamine pyrophosphate as its coenzyme. In thiamine deficiency, the erythrocyte apoenzyme is not fully saturated with its cofactor, and addition of the cofactor in vitro to an erythrocyte hemolysate results in an increase in measured enzyme activity. The degree of increase in the activity coefficient (i.e., enzyme activity after incubation with the coenzyme in vitro compared to that before, expressed as per cent increase) is an indication of the degree of unsaturation of the apoenzyme with thiamine pyrophosphate. The degree of unsaturation, in turn, is indicative of the magnitude of depletion of body stores of thiamine. An activity coefficient of 15 to 20 per cent or greater is generally regarded as reflecting significant thiamine deficiency. If these assays are unavailable, a therapeutic trial of thiamine, which provides rapid improvement (in 12 hours or less) in cardiovascular function and in ophthalmoplegia, may be regarded as supportive evidence for the diagnosis of thiamine deficiency. In a patient with beriberi, cardiac output may diminish and vascular resistance increase within 30 minutes of intravenous administration of a single 100-mg dose of thiamine.

TREATMENT. If thiamine deficiency is suspected, rapid treatment with large doses of the vitamin is essential. Generally, 50 to 100 mg are administered intramuscularly or intravenously every day for the first few days, after which lower doses in the range of 5 to 10 mg may be given orally. Other therapeutic applications for which pharmacologic doses of thiamine are required include several rare inborn errors of metabolism: thiamine-responsive branched-chain ketoaciduria (maple syrup urine disease), as well as subacute necrotizing encephalomyelopathy (Leigh's syndrome), a condition in which thiamine triphosphate is deficient in the brain.

Toxicity

Thiamine can be given safely by mouth in very large amounts without fear of toxicity. When given by the intravenous route, large doses of thiamine on very rare occasions have been associated with poorly understood reactions resembling anaphylactic shock. Fortunately, these reactions occur so rarely that intravenous therapy with thiamine should not be withheld from a seriously ill patient in whom thiamine deficiency is suspected.

Gubler CJ: Thiamin. In Machlin LJ (ed.): Handbook of Vitamins, 2nd ed. New York, Marcel Dekker, 1990, p 233. Comprehensive review of biochemical and nutritional aspects of thiamine.

Haas RH: Thiamin and the brain. Ann Rev Nutr 8:483, 1988. Review of effects of thiamine deficiency on brain function.

Iber FL, Blass JP, Brin M, et al.: Thiamin in the elderly—Relation to alcoholism and to neurological degenerative disease. Am J Clin Nutr 36(Suppl):1067, 1982. Discussion of prevalence of thiamine deficiency and effects of alcohol and drugs upon thiamine bioavailability.

Mukherjee AB, Svoronos S, Ghazanfari A, et al.: Transketolase abnormality in cultured fibroblasts from familial chronic alcoholic men and their male offspring. J Clin Invest 79:1039, 1987. Confirmatory description of an inborn error of transketolase predisposing to severe consequences of thiamine deficiency.

VITAMIN B₂ (RIBOFLAVIN)

Structure and Biochemical Functions

Riboflavin (Fig. 204–2) must be converted to its coenzyme derivatives, flavin mononucleotide (riboflavin-5'-PO_4, FMN) and flavin adenine dinucleotide (FAD), in order to be metabolically active. These coenzymes are formed sequentially from dietary riboflavin after reacting with ATP and function as cofactors for a wide variety of enzymes in intermediary metabolism, particularly those involving oxidation-reduction reactions. FAD-dependent enzymes include α-glycerophosphate dehydrogenase, xanthine oxidase, and NADPH-cytochrome c reductase. A small fraction of tissue flavins is found in covalent linkage with proteins and includes the enzymes monoamine oxidase (MAO) and succinic dehydrogenase.

Normal Physiology

Riboflavin and FMN are absorbed from the upper gastrointestinal tract by a specific and saturable transport process. FAD, the predominant form in foods such as meat, must first be degraded to riboflavin and FMN prior to being absorbed. Cova-

lently bound flavins are largely unavailable as nutritional sources of riboflavin. A number of metals and drugs form complexes or chelates with dietary riboflavin and may influence the bioavailability of this vitamin. Such agents include copper, zinc, iron, saccharin, tryptophan, ascorbic acid, and dietary fiber. Dietary fiber in the form of psyllium but not wheat bran decreases the apparent intestinal absorption of a single 30-mg dose of riboflavin; effects of fiber on usual amounts of dietary riboflavin are not known.

After absorption, riboflavin is bound loosely to serum albumin and more tightly to immunoglobulins, particularly IgA and IgG. The amount of riboflavin bound to serum proteins varies widely in normal individuals. In pregnancy there are specific riboflavin-binding proteins that appear to be essential to normal fetal development. The renal tubule transports riboflavin in both directions, and in urine the predominant form detected is riboflavin rather than the coenzyme derivatives. There are additional metabolites of riboflavin in human urine including 7-hydroxymethylriboflavin, 8-α-sulfonylriboflavin, and trace amounts of other substances.

Thyroid and adrenal hormones regulate the conversion of riboflavin to FMN, FAD, and covalently bound flavins, and riboflavin metabolism is impaired in adult hypothyroid patients. Analogues of riboflavin interfere with certain actions of aldosterone.

Requirements and Dietary Sources

The RDA for riboflavin in adult males is 1.4 to 1.7 mg per day and in adult females, 1.2 to 1.3 mg per day, depending upon age. Allowances are increased during pregnancy and lactation and probably should be increased with heavy exercise. When riboflavin is consumed in amounts greater than the RDA, increased urinary excretion occurs promptly. In the United States, milk and dairy products supply close to half the daily intake of riboflavin, with meat, fish, poultry, eggs, and legumes providing other important sources; the remainder comes largely from green leafy vegetables, fruits, and grain products. In developing countries, the principal sources are cereals, roots, and tubers. Riboflavin is light-, acid-, and alkali-sensitive and rapidly loses biologic activity when exposed to sunlight or when treated with sodium bicarbonate, a common but unfortunate practice used to retain the color of green vegetables.

Deficiency

PATHOGENESIS. Riboflavin deficiency arises not only because of an inadequate diet but also when hormones, drugs, or disease impair the absorption, utilization, metabolic transformations, binding, or excretion of this vitamin. In experimental animals, the psychotropic drugs chlorpromazine, imipramine, and amitriptyline and the antitumor agent doxorubicin, as well as several antimalarial agents, all diminish the conversion of riboflavin to its active coenzyme derivatives, FMN and FAD. Chlorpromazine treatment greatly accelerates the development of riboflavin deficiency. The underlying mechanism of this effect appears to be inhibition of flavokinase, the enzyme that converts riboflavin to FMN, the first of two steps in the biosynthesis of FAD.

Phototherapy of newborn infants with hyperbilirubinemia leads to some decomposition of riboflavin because of its light sensitivity. Ethanol diminishes both the intestinal absorption of riboflavin and its bioavailability from food sources. Deficiency of riboflavin likely results also after severe trauma, burns, surgery, chronic debilitating diseases, dialysis, and severe and prolonged diarrhea. Increased riboflavin excretion occurs under conditions of negative nitrogen balance, including diabetes, after withdrawal of insulin, or after certain drugs, such as boric acid. Hypothyroidism impairs riboflavin metabolism, as noted above.

Riboflavin deficiency has particularly important effects upon fat metabolism and alters the plasma and tissue concentrations of phospholipids. The conversion of dietary vitamin B₆ and folic acid to their coenzyme derivatives is blocked by riboflavin deficiency. In β-thalassemia, there is diminished formation of FMN from riboflavin in the erythrocyte.

CLINICAL FEATURES. The clinical picture of riboflavin deficiency isolated from other deficiencies is rarely observed as noted above. Early symptoms of riboflavin deficiency include

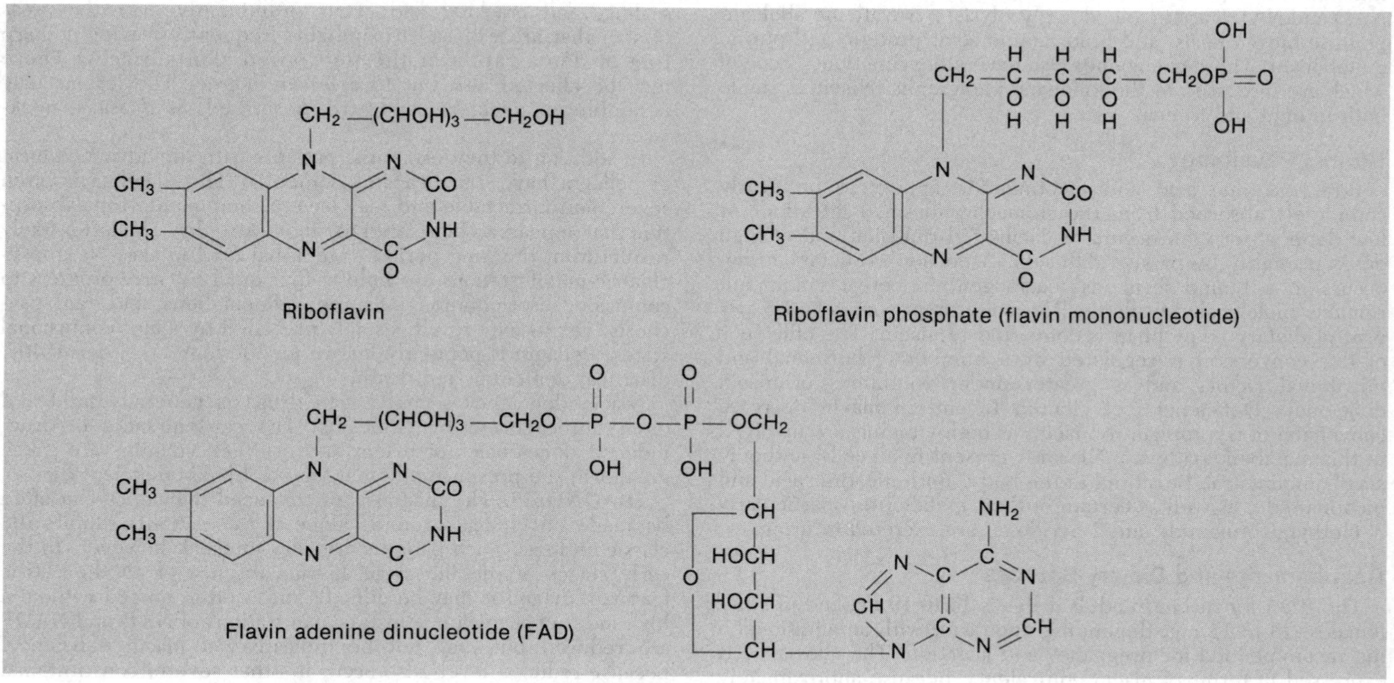

CH2—(CHOH)3—CH2OH

Riboflavin

Riboflavin phosphate (flavin mononucleotide)

Flavin adenine dinucleotide (FAD)

FIGURE 204–2. Structural formulae of riboflavin (vitamin B_2) and its coenzyme derivatives.

soreness of the mouth, burning and itching of the eyes, and personality deterioration. Advanced riboflavin deficiency produces a constellation of findings that include cheilosis, angular stomatitis, seborrheic dermatitis, glossitis, corneal vascularization, reticulocytopenia and anemia, and retarded intellectual development. Cheilosis and angular stomatitis, once thought to be specific for riboflavin deficiency, are now known to occur frequently in other nutritional deficiencies, particularly B_6 deficiency. Riboflavin deficiency is a major cause of congenital malformations in experimental animals, but it is unclear at present whether malformations result from human maternal riboflavin deficiency. The rate of metabolism of a number of drugs is altered in riboflavin deficiency, at least in part because the microsomal hydroxylase system requires flavin coenzymes. There is evidence that riboflavin deficiency antagonizes *Plasmodium* infection in both animals and humans.

DIAGNOSIS. In riboflavin deficiency, there is a reduction in urinary excretion of riboflavin as well as a reduction in the concentrations of various flavins in plasma and in erythrocytes. Assays of urinary excretion of riboflavin in longstanding deficiency may be misleading if there has been some recent intake of this vitamin. A useful functional test of riboflavin status is the activity coefficient of erythrocyte glutathione reductase, an FAD-requiring enzyme. When FAD is added in vitro to an erythrocyte hemolysate, the increase in activity measured is much greater in erythrocytes from riboflavin-deficient than from riboflavin-replete individuals. As with transketolase and thiamine pyrophosphate (referred to above), this assay reflects the lesser degree of saturation of the apoenzyme with its cofactor in deficient compared with normal individuals. Results are expressed as the activity coefficient, i.e., the ratio of enzyme activity after incubation with FAD in vitro to that before incubation. Activity coefficients greater than 1.2 to 1.3 are generally considered to be indicative of a riboflavin-deficient state.

TREATMENT. Riboflavin deficiency can be treated satisfactorily with food sources high in riboflavin, such as milk, liver, meat, eggs, and green, leafy vegetables, or with the vitamin itself. Deficient patients treated with 10 to 15 mg per day of riboflavin undergo healing of skin lesions within days to weeks of initiation of therapy. The intravenous administration of riboflavin, which may be needed in debilitated patients or in those with serious disorders of the gastrointestinal tract, is greatly restricted by its limited solubility in aqueous solution.

Riboflavin in large doses has been utilized to treat several rare inborn errors of metabolism, including congenital methemoglobinemia, pyruvate kinase deficiency, glutaryl-CoA dehydrogenase deficiency, and defects of β-oxidation.

Toxicity

Riboflavin, FMN, and FAD are completely free of any known clinical toxicity. There is a theoretical possibility that the photosensitizing properties of riboflavin may constitute some risk.

Cooperman JM, Lopez R: Riboflavin. *In* Machlin LJ (ed.): Handbook of Vitamins, 2nd ed. New York, Marcel Dekker, 1990, p 283. *Update on riboflavin metabolism, sources, and deficiency.*

McCormick DB: Riboflavin. *In* Brown ML (ed.): Present Knowledge in Nutrition, 6th ed. Washington, D.C., International Life Sciences Institute, The Nutrition Foundation, 1990, p 146. *Discussion of the physiology, sources, functions, and metabolic roles of riboflavin.*

Pinto JT, Huang YP, Rivlin RS: Mechanisms underlying the differential effects of ethanol upon the bioavailability of riboflavin and flavin adenine dinucleotide. J Clin Invest 79:1343, 1987. *Study showing how alcohol causes riboflavin deficiency.*

Rivlin RS: Medical aspects of vitamin B_2. *In* Muller F (ed.): Chemistry and Biochemistry of Flavins. Boca Raton, CRC Press 1990, in press. *Review of diseases that disturb riboflavin metabolism clinically and their treatment.*

NIACIN (UNOFFICIALLY CALLED VITAMIN B₃)

Structure and Biochemical Function

The term "niacin" is used generally to refer to nicotinic acid and nicotinamide and other biologically active pyridine derivatives, as shown in Figure 204–3. The term "niacin" is sometimes used loosely to refer to nicotinic acid only. Niacin is a precursor of two coenzymes, nicotinamide adenine dinucleotide (NAD) and nicotinamide adenine dinucleotide phosphate (NADP), which

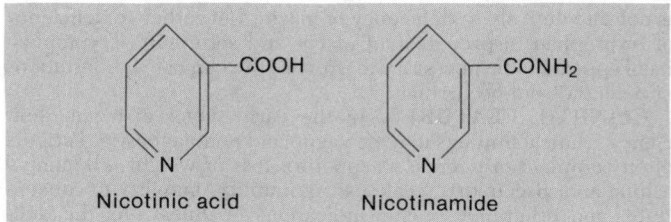

FIGURE 204–3. Structural formulae of nicotinic acid and nicotinamide.

function in a wide number of oxidation and reduction reactions. NAD and NADP are involved in glycolysis, pyruvate metabolism, pentose biosynthesis, and lipid, amino acid, protein, and purine metabolism. These coenzymes also have other functions, some of which are discussed in the following paragraphs. Niacin is stable both to light and to heat.

Normal Physiology

Both nicotinic acid and nicotinamide appear to be nearly completely absorbed from the stomach and small intestine. At low doses absorption occurs by facilitated diffusion and at high doses primarily by passive diffusion. A portion of dietary niacin occurs in a bound form (as niacinogen) in cereal grains but remains biologically available. Normally, approximately 1.5 per cent of dietary tryptophan is converted to niacin. The efficiency of this conversion is regulated by a number of hormonal and nutritional factors and is greater under conditions of niacin deficiency. Deficiencies of vitamin B_6 and riboflavin decrease conversion of tryptophan to niacin, as both vitamins are involved in this metabolic pathway. Niacin is present in all cells, and only small amounts can be stored in the body. Both nicotinic acid and nicotinamide, as well as certain of their metabolites, particularly N-methylnicotinamide and 2-pyridone, are excreted in urine.

Requirements and Dietary Sources

The RDA for niacin in adult males is 15 to 19 mg and in adult females, 13 to 15 mg, depending upon age, with an additional 5 mg recommended for pregnancy and lactation. The allowance is expressed in terms of niacin equivalents, because approximately 60 mg of dietary tryptophan are needed to form 1 mg of niacin. Proteins of animal origin such as meat, milk, and eggs have a relatively high tryptophan content and therefore are good sources of endogenously generated niacin. Vegetable proteins also supply tryptophan, but the concentration is lower than in animal proteins. Diets dependent heavily upon corn are a particular problem because the tryptophan content is low. Niacin from wheat sources has limited bioavailability. Pyridoxine deficiency and riboflavin deficiency increase the dietary requirement for niacin, because they are required for the biosynthesis of niacin from tryptophan, as noted above.

Deficiency

PATHOGENESIS. Niacin deficiency or pellagra may develop because of a number of factors. First, dietary deficiency develops when corn is the major staple of the diet. Pellagra caused by consumption of corn was once very common in the southeastern United States but fortunately has largely disappeared at the present time. Secondly, niacin deficiency may arise as a result of alcoholism, a condition in which diet is often poor and erratic. It is likely that in prolonged alcoholism, particularly in the presence of other nutrient deficiencies, the absorption and metabolism of niacin may be impaired. In addition, certain drugs interfere with niacin metabolism to a clinically significant degree, the best known of which is isonicotinic acid hydrazide (INH). The neurologic symptoms occurring with INH treatment can be ameliorated by administration of pyridoxine. Certain anticancer drugs, particularly 6-mercaptopurine, may produce niacin deficiency. In the rare inborn error of Hartnup's disease, pellagra may develop because of a defect in the intestinal and renal tubular transport of tryptophan and of several other amino acids (Ch. 176). Malnourished patients with the malignant carcinoid syndrome have been known occasionally to exhibit manifestations of pellagra because of diversion of dietary tryptophan to serotonin (Ch. 230). Some authorities believe that the symptom complex of pellagra is not due entirely to deficiency of niacin, but rather to deficiency of tryptophan, a precursor of niacin and serotonin. Tryptophan itself appears to be necessary to prevent the clinical manifestations of pellagra from occurring.

CLINICAL FEATURES. In the early stages of niacin deficiency, clinical findings may be vague and nondiagnostic. Patients often complain of decreased appetite, loss of weight, abdominal aching and discomfort, weakness, irritability, inability to concentrate, and other nonspecific indications of illness. As the deficiency progresses, there may be epithelial changes that include glossitis, stomatitis, soreness and pain in the mouth (particularly the tongue), and eventually development of the characteristic skin lesions. These lesions, when well established, are dark, scaling, and cracking and occur prominently over the areas of skin that are exposed to sunlight, frequently leaving a sharp line of demarcation at the unexposed skin surfaces. These may be affected also but to a lesser degree. The lesions may resemble a necklace and are described as Casal's necklace.

In addition to the dermatitis, patients with the advanced form of pellagra have diarrhea and dementia. The diarrhea is often severe and intractable and may have a component of malabsorption that appears to be related to villous atrophy. The latter likely results from the long period of minimal food intake. Neuropsychiatric manifestations are mild at first but later may progress to confusion, disorientation, seizures, hallucinations, and frank psychosis. Death may result, usually preceded by major confusional states. Pellagra is popularly known for the four D's—dermatitis, diarrhea, dementia, and death.

Niacin deficiency secondary to drugs is generally mild and often unrecognized by clinicians. The consequences of drug-induced deficiencies of niacin and of other vitamins are much greater in the presence of a marginal or frankly deficient diet.

DIAGNOSIS. The diagnosis of advanced deficiency can often be made on clinical grounds alone if the patient exhibits the classic findings. Such patients are very unusual, however. In the early stages of the illness or in the absence of all the classic features, diagnosis may be difficult and is often missed without a high index of suspicion. Blood concentrations of NAD and NADP are reduced but may not be indicative of niacin deficiency, because reduced levels also occur in other severe, constitutional illnesses that are unrelated to niacin intake. Attention has therefore turned to assay of urinary metabolites of niacin as indices of niacin nutriture. The most widely used is N-methylnicotinamide. Low urinary levels are interpreted as indicative of niacin deficiency. The excretion of another metabolite, 2-pyridone, is less widely used and requires a cumbersome assay. Some investigators have considered the ratio of these two metabolites in urine to be the most accurate index of niacin nutriture. Urinary metabolites can now be measured accurately by HPLC.

TREATMENT. The treatment of advanced pellagra can be accomplished satisfactorily by administering large oral doses (approximately 50 to 150 mg) of nicotinamide (the form present in most commercial vitamin formulations). The exact dose given is somewhat empiric. The therapeutic response is often dramatic, and patients may show marked improvement within several days after the start of therapy. Maintenance levels are then given together with dietary repletion. Nicotinamide is usually well tolerated under these conditions. Nicotinic acid is also effective against pellagra.

Other therapeutic applications of niacin include its use as nicotinic acid in the control of an elevated serum cholesterol level in daily doses of 3 grams or more (Ch. 172). Nicotinic acid may be useful in treating patients with types II, IV, and V hyperlipoproteinemia. The mechanism of the therapeutic effect on lipid metabolism is not known with precision, and this property is not shared by nicotinamide. With nicotinic acid treatment, HDL levels tend to rise because of a slight decrease in synthetic rate with a large decrease in degradative rate. Therapy is generally initiated with low doses of nicotinic acid and gradually increased with frequent monitoring of appropriate laboratory tests.

Doses in the range of those used to treat pellagra are also needed to treat niacin deficiency in Hartnup disease and in the carcinoid syndrome. Massive doses of niacin have not proven useful in the treatment of schizophrenia and other psychiatric disorders, despite the claims of food faddists and "orthomolecular" therapists.

Toxicity

At the doses of nicotinamide used to treat niacin deficiency (described previously) there is little if any toxicity. When nicotinic acid in doses of 3 grams or more is used in the treatment of a lipid disorder, the most common side effect observed is flushing of the face due to vascular dilation. Administering one tablet of aspirin prior to the dose of nicotinic acid often ameliorates the flushing. Other common side effects of nicotinic acid may include dryness, itching, and increased pigmentation of the skin and abdominal pain. Rarely, hepatotoxicity, hyperuricemia, and worsening of peptic ulcer and glucose tolerance have been observed. Abnormalities in liver function tests are common toxicities, but both biochemical and histologic findings generally regress with discontinuation of nicotinic acid. There is some evidence that so-called sustained-release capsules of nicotinic acid may be more toxic than crystalline nicotinic acid.

Henderson LaVM: Niacin. *In* Darby WJ, Broquist HP, Olson RE (eds.): Annual Review of Nutrition. Vol. 3. Palo Alto, Annual Reviews Inc, 1983, p 289. *This review covers transport, metabolism, and physiologic and pharmacologic effects of niacin.*
Krieger I, Statter M: Tryptophan deficiency and picolinic acid: Effect on zinc metabolism and clinical manifestations of pellagra. Am J Clin Nutr 46:511, 1987. *Report providing evidence that pellagra is due to tryptophan deficiency.*
Van Eys J: Nicotinic acid. *In* Machlin LJ (ed.): Handbook of Vitamins, 2nd ed. New York, Marcel Dekker, 1990, p 312. *Recent review stressing metabolism, pharmacology, and toxicity of niacin.*

VITAMIN B₆ (PYRIDOXINE)

Structure and Biochemical Function

The term "vitamin B_6" or "pyridoxine" is often used to refer to three closely interrelated compounds—pyridoxine, pyridoxamine, and pyridoxal—together with their phosphate derivatives. Of all these compounds, pyridoxal-5'-phosphate (Fig. 204–4) is the most important, because it constitutes the major coenzyme involved in the intermediary metabolism of amino acids, including aminotransferases, decarboxylases, racemases, and synthetases. Pyridoxal phosphate is involved in metabolism of several vitamins and in biosynthesis of heme and sphingosine. It is estimated that more than 100 reactions involve pyridoxal-5'-phosphate as a cofactor. In certain circumstances pyridoxamine phosphate can also fulfill a coenzyme function. Pyridoxine is the major dietary source found in plants, whereas pyridoxal and pyridoxamine constitute the major forms in foods from animal sources. Pyridoxine is stable in acid solutions in the absence of light but is highly light-sensitive in acid or neutral solutions. Pyridoxal and pyridoxamine are destroyed at high temperatures, particularly by autoclaving and in the presence of protein or amino acids.

Normal Physiology

Dietary pyridoxine and related compounds are absorbed from the upper gastrointestinal tract, probably by simple diffusion. The vitamin is widely distributed in the body; muscle constitutes an important storage organ, in which it is bound to phosphorylase a, thus serving to stabilize the enzyme molecule. The various forms of pyridoxine are readily interconverted to one another by the liver and erythrocytes. Under ordinary circumstances only very small amounts of dietary pyridoxine are converted to pyridoxal phosphate. In urine, pyridoxine, pyridoxal, and pyridoxamine can all be detected but at low concentrations; the major metabolite of pyridoxine, 4-pyridoxic acid, is found in urine in high concentrations, particularly in alcoholic patients.

Thyroid hormones reduce the concentrations of vitamin B_6 in various tissues, and increased sensitivity to insulin is demonstrable during B_6 deficiency.

Requirements and Dietary Sources

The RDA for vitamin B_6 is 2.0 mg per day for adult males and 1.6 per day for adult females, regardless of age, with a 0.5 mg

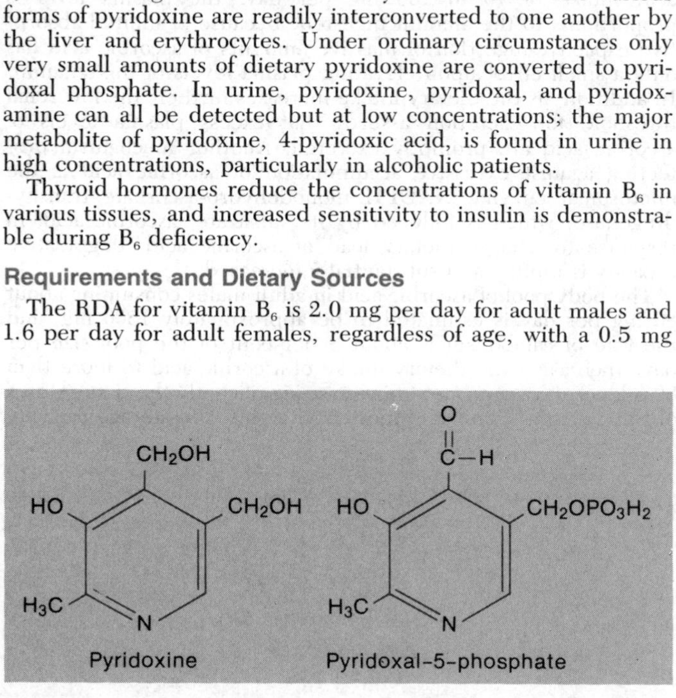

FIGURE 204–4. Structural formulae of pyridoxine and its phosphate derivative.

per day increase during pregnancy and lactation. The requirement for vitamin B_6 is greater with a higher protein intake.

Vitamin B_6 is widely distributed in the food supply and can be derived from both plants and animals. Sources of vitamin B_6 are similar to those of other B vitamins and include liver, meat, wheat, nuts, beans and other vegetables, fruits, and cereals. Considerable losses occur during prolonged cooking, particularly pressure cooking. The bioavailability of vitamin B_6 from dietary sources varies widely, averaging about 70 per cent; bananas and walnuts have nearly 80 per cent B_6 bioavailability, spinach only 22 per cent, and orange juice 9 per cent. Bioavailability is low when there is high glycosylated B_6 in the food item.

Deficiency

PATHOGENESIS. Dietary deficiency of pyridoxine may occur occasionally despite its widespread sources in the food supply. Deficiency of pyridoxine is recognized increasingly as a consequence of prolonged therapy with certain medications. Foremost among these drugs is isoniazid, which complexes with pyridoxal phosphate to a clinically significant degree. Individuals with the genetic trait of inactivating isoniazid at a slow rate are particularly susceptible to B_6 deficiency from this drug. Isoniazid induces peripheral neuritis and diarrhea in adult patients; in children it produces anemia and seizures that can be prevented by coincident administration of pyridoxine. Cycloserine, another drug widely used for tuberculosis, is also a vitamin B_6 antagonist. With the widespread use of penicillamine for the treatment of rheumatoid arthritis, its B_6 antagonistic properties are of increasing clinical importance. Pyridoxine deficiency occurs frequently in alcoholism in association with deficiencies of other vitamins, particularly folic acid. The principal effect of ethanol is to accelerate catabolism of pyridoxal phosphate. The increased urinary excretion of certain tryptophan metabolites, particularly xanthurenic acid, in women treated with oral contraceptives has been interpreted as indicating vitamin B_6 deficiency, because B_6 is needed for conversion of tryptophan to niacin. L-Dopa, used for Parkinson's disease, may also cause B_6 deficiency over a prolonged period of time.

CLINICAL FEATURES. Deficiency of vitamin B_6 is not thought to produce a characteristic syndrome. As with deficiencies of other B vitamins, dermatitis, glossitis, cheilosis, and stomatitis may be manifestations of pyridoxine deficiency. Markedly B_6-deficient patients may have irritability, weakness, depression, dizziness, peripheral neuropathy, and seizures. As noted previously, deficiency in infants and children is typically characterized by diarrhea, anemia, and seizures. The rapidity with which drug-induced deficiency of B_6 occurs depends upon the adequacy of the patient's diet as well as the dosage and duration of drug therapy. Chronic vitamin B_6 deficiency also leads to secondary hyperoxaluria, increasing the risk of kidney stone formation (Ch. 88).

In addition to the deficiency syndromes of vitamin B_6 caused by diet or drugs or both, there is a group of disorders in which the affected patients do not display manifestations of deficiency yet require pharmacologic doses of this vitamin for adequate treatment. These disorders are known as dependency syndromes and include such diverse entities as pyridoxine-dependent convulsions, pyridoxine-responsive anemia, homocystinuria caused by cystathionine synthetase deficiency, cystathioninuria, xanthurenic aciduria, and some cases of primary hyperoxaluria.

Of these dependency syndromes, pyridoxine-responsive anemia requires special mention because it is often confused with iron-deficiency anemia; both disorders are characterized by hypochromic, microcytic red cells. In the pyridoxine-responsive anemia, however, serum iron is generally elevated with an increase in saturation of transferrin and an increase in iron absorption from the intestinal tract. There is evidence of iron overload, with hemosiderin deposits in bone marrow, liver, and other organs. Many patients have hepatosplenomegaly, and a hemolytic component may contribute to the anemia. It is important to differentiate this syndrome from iron-deficient anemia, because inadvertent administration of iron worsens pyridoxine-responsive anemia. The blood count rises satisfactorily in response to pharmacologic doses of vitamin B_6. In patients with cystathionine synthetase deficiency, the greatly elevated serum concentrations of homocysteine and methionine can be normalized with doses of pyridoxine of several hundred milligrams per day.

DIAGNOSIS. The diagnosis of pyridoxine deficiency can be made by direct assay of vitamin B_6 in blood (normal levels generally are greater than 50 ng per milliliter) or by determining the urinary excretion of the main metabolite of pyridoxine, 4-pyridoxic acid. The excretion of less than 1.0 mg per day of this compound is generally considered suggestive of deficiency. Less frequently, the excretion of pyridoxine in urine is also determined. Functional enzyme assays, similar to those in use for diagnosing thiamine and riboflavin deficiencies, have also been developed for vitamin B_6 using aspartate aminotransferase or alanine aminotransferase in erythrocyte hemolysates. Enzyme activity is determined with and without the addition of pyridoxal phosphate in vitro. When activity coefficients (as defined previously) are greater than 1.5 for aspartate aminotransferase and 1.2 for alanine aminotransferase, they are considered indicative of pyridoxine deficiency. These procedures have generally supplanted the tryptophan load test, in which the increased excretion of xanthurenic acid is taken as an index of B_6 nutriture. Probably the most widely accepted index of vitamin B_6 nutriture at present is the direct measurement of pyridoxal phosphate concentrations in blood.

TREATMENT. Dietary deficiency of pyridoxine can be treated satisfactorily with oral doses in the general range of 2 to 10 mg per day; doses of 10 to 20 mg per day may be needed in pregnancy. Pyridoxine deficiency occurring in association with specific drugs that inhibit pyridoxine metabolism, such as isoniazid, cycloserine, and penicillamine, requires higher doses, perhaps up to 100 mg per day, to ameliorate peripheral neuropathy. Rather than administer B_6 when symptoms develop, it may be much more beneficial to attempt to prevent these side effects by administering vitamin B_6 at the time when therapy with a B_6-antagonizing drug is initiated and particularly when a prolonged course of treatment is anticipated. Since iatrogenic vitamin B_6 deficiency is entirely preventable, B_6 is now routinely prescribed for patients receiving INH. Treatment with high doses of vitamin B_6 is contraindicated in patients receiving L-dopa, however, as it may interfere with the efficacy of the drug.

Treatment of a pyridoxine-dependency syndrome requires much higher doses of B_6, and amounts in the range of 300 to 500 mg per day generally have been prescribed. In patients with gyrate atrophy, a rare genetic eye disease in which progressive visual loss develops as a result of chorioretinal degeneration, there is a deficiency of the mitochondrial enzyme ornithine aminotransferase. The elevated serum ornithine in these patients can be corrected by treatment with pyridoxal phosphate, the cofactor of this enzyme. In common with homocystinuria and several other genetic disorders, gyrate atrophy occurs in a vitamin B_6-responsive and vitamin B_6-unresponsive form.

The possible effectiveness of pyridoxine in the management of the carpal tunnel syndrome and premenstrual tension is controversial. In some women on contraceptive steroids, vitamin B_6 has appeared to ameliorate depression. Pyridoxine is regarded as ineffective in treating schizophrenia, autism, and childhood hyperactivity, as well as peripheral neuropathies in which there is no known B_6 deficiency, such as in diabetes.

Toxicity

A sensory neuropathy has been described in a small number of patients receiving 2 grams or more of pyridoxine per day, and some subjects have had symptoms on 500 mg or possibly less per day. This potentially important finding requires confirmation and extension. At the present time, there are probably no indications for treatment of any disorder, even a pyridoxine-dependency syndrome, with doses of this magnitude. Thus, pyridoxine appears to be safe when prescribed in the appropriate milligram amounts needed to correct deficiency and to treat vitamin B_6-dependency states.

McCormick DB: Two interconnected B vitamins: riboflavin and pyridoxine. Physiol Rev 69:1170, 1989. *Review of the interrelations between vitamins B_2 and B_6.*

Ramesh V, McClatchey AI, Ramesh N, et al.: Molecular basis of ornithine aminotransferase deficiency in B_6-responsive and -nonresponsive forms of gyrate atrophy. Proc Natl Acad Sci USA 85:3777, 1988. *Report that pyridoxine-responsive and nonresponsive forms of gyrate atrophy result from mutations in the ornithine aminotransferase structural gene.*

Reynolds RD, Leklem JE: Vitamin B_6: Its Role in Health and Disease. New York, Alan R. Liss, 1986. *Volume covering the proceedings of a conference on this vitamin in nutrition and metabolism.*

Schaumburg H, Kaplan J, Winderbank A, et al.: Sensory neuropathy from pyridoxine abuse. A new megavitamin syndrome. N Engl J Med 309:445, 1983. *Description of B_6 toxicity.*

VITAMIN B_{12} (COBALAMIN) AND FOLIC ACID

The structure, function, pathophysiology, and therapeutic use of vitamin B_{12} and folic acid are discussed in Ch. 132 in association with the megaloblastic anemias.

VITAMIN C (ASCORBIC ACID)

Structure and Biochemical Function

Ascorbic acid resembles glucose in having several polyhydroxyl groups adjacent to one another (Fig. 204–5). Ascorbic acid can be oxidized to dehydro-L-ascorbic acid, which is also biologically active, and can be generated from the latter by reacting with reduced glutathione. Ascorbic acid is a precursor of oxalate, an important component of kidney stones.

Ascorbic acid participates in oxidation-reduction reactions and in hydrogen ion transfer. This vitamin is a powerful reducing agent or antioxidant, particularly in lipid and vitamin metabolism, and is especially important in preventing oxidation of tetrahydrofolate. In addition, ascorbic acid enhances the intestinal absorption of nonheme iron. This vitamin is involved in collagen metabolism, and defects in collagen biosynthesis are believed to be the basis for many of the symptoms of scurvy. In the absence of vitamin C, dopamine-B-hydroxylase activity is reduced, impairing the biosynthesis of neurotransmitters. Ascorbic acid is also involved in carnitine biosynthesis, tyrosine metabolism, wound healing, and immune function and is a component of drug-metabolizing enzyme systems.

Prolonged storage or excessive cooking diminishes the biologic activity of ascorbic acid. This highly water-soluble vitamin is also destroyed by oxidation, particularly by exposure to air in the presence of copper ion and an alkaline medium.

Normal Physiology

Ascorbic acid is absorbed by a limited-capacity mechanism in the distal small intestine. As dietary intake of ascorbic acid increases, a progressively smaller proportion is absorbed—that is, about 95 per cent at 100 mg, 75 per cent at 1 gram, and 20 per cent at 5 grams. Within the usual range of dietary ascorbic acid intake of 10 to 130 mg per day, the plasma level is proportional to the amount ingested. Because of limited absorptive capacity, ingestion of massive amounts of ascorbic acid has only a small effect upon elevating plasma levels of this vitamin. In addition, as the dietary intake increases further, the low renal threshold for excretion assures that excess plasma levels of ascorbic acid are promptly excreted. Another mechanism protecting against excessive accumulation of ascorbic acid is the microsomal enzyme NADPH monodehydro-ascorbate transhydrogenase, which is induced by its substrate, ascorbic acid; in response to a large dietary load of ascorbic acid, degradative capacity is rapidly and substantially increased.

The body pool of ascorbic acid in adult males consuming about 80 mg per day is estimated to be approximately 1500 mg, and the rate of catabolism is about 3 per cent of the pool size per day. Increasing the dietary intake of ascorbic acid to more than 80 mg per day seems not to increase significantly the tissue stores of this vitamin. Similar to most B vitamins, the storage capacity

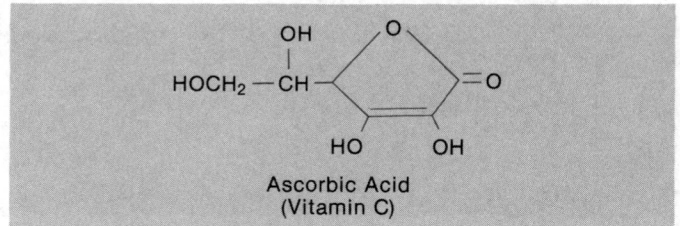

FIGURE 204–5. Structural formula of ascorbic acid.

for vitamin C is limited. Urinary excretion is in the form of ascorbic acid and dehydro-L-ascorbic acid, as well as several metabolites, including a sulfated derivative, ascorbate-2-sulfate, and oxalic acid, as noted above.

Requirements and Dietary Sources

The RDA for ascorbic acid is 60 mg per day for healthy adult males and females regardless of age. This allowance is generally regarded as quite generous inasmuch as amounts as low as 10 mg per day prevent scurvy. Amounts greatly in excess of the RDA have potential for toxicity. The recommended dietary allowance is increased to 70 mg per day during pregnancy and to 90 to 95 mg per day during lactation. Human milk contains about 30 to 55 mg per liter. It is especially important for women to maintain an adequate intake of ascorbic acid during lactation, because the vitamin concentration in milk is closely dependent upon dietary intake.

Serum ascorbic acid levels are lowered in smokers, possibly as a result of accelerated metabolism or diminished intake, and in users of oral contraceptive drugs, but the implications of these findings are unclear. The decreases are quantitatively small and can be corrected with a modest increase in consumption of ascorbic acid from dietary sources (about 40 mg for smokers, the amount contained in a glass of fresh orange juice). Patients who are exposed to cold or heat stress or who are febrile, undergoing surgery, or subjected to trauma may have increased requirements for vitamin C. Patients receiving parenteral nutrition exclusively have higher requirements because of urinary losses.

The best dietary sources of ascorbic acid appear to be citrus fruits and green vegetables, especially broccoli, green peppers, tomatoes, cabbage, oranges, grapefruits, and lemons. Care must be taken during food preparation in order to avoid losses of the vitamin. Much smaller amounts are contained in milk, meats, and cereals. As noted above, ascorbic acid is heat-sensitive and is destroyed by alkali. Some decreased vitamin content is also observed with prolonged storage.

Deficiency

PATHOGENESIS. Urban poor, particularly the elderly, are at increased risk for dietary deficiency of ascorbic acid, in large measure because economic deprivation prevents them from obtaining the richest sources, namely citrus fruits, leafy vegetables, and tomatoes.

An increasingly important cause of ascorbic acid deficiency in the United States today is food faddism and bizarre nutritional practices. The strict macrobiotic diet may lead to scurvy, particularly with pressure cooking of food items that have little ascorbic acid to begin with. Elderly individuals following a "tea and toast" diet are vulnerable to a number of deficiencies, particularly of ascorbic acid, as these sources are grossly inadequate. Children may develop scurvy when fed unsupplemented cow's milk exclusively for the first year of life. Vitamin C deficiency progressing to scurvy is common in chronic alcoholic patients, probably because the diet is notably deficient in vitamin C–containing food items. Vitamin C deficiency, however, is not generally as prevalent as deficiencies of B vitamins in chronic alcoholism. Scurvy was not prominent during the famine in Ireland in the nineteenth century, as people subsisted on raw potatoes, a good source of vitamin C.

CLINICAL FEATURES. In the early stages of deficiency, symptoms and signs may be nonspecific and include general malaise, lethargy, and weakness. As the disease progresses, probably 1 to 3 months after onset, patients may complain of dyspnea and pain in bones and joints, due predominantly to hemorrhages below the periosteum. Perifollicular hemorrhages, particularly about hair follicles, are indicative of advanced deficiency. Petechiae often are prominent and may appear over the arms after application of a sphygmomanometer. This finding is known as the Rumpel-Leed test. With progressive vitamin C depletion, ecchymoses and purpura may develop initially at areas of trauma, irritation, or pressure. Joints, muscles, and subcutaneous tissues may become sites of hemorrhage. Swollen, bleeding gums are characteristic of advanced deficiency. Pallor and anemia may be the result of prolonged bleeding or associated folic acid deficiency, with which scurvy commonly occurs. In children, disturbances of growth occur, and teeth, bones, blood vessels,

and other collagen-rich structures develop abnormally. Preformed teeth may become loose and fall out because of alveolar bone resorption.

Wounds heal poorly, and previously healed wounds may open up again. In very advanced deficiency, edema, oliguria, and neuropathy are prominent. Should intracerebral bleeding occur, serious neurologic sequelae and even death may result.

DIAGNOSIS. The diagnosis of advanced scurvy can be made on clinical grounds alone because the skin changes often are quite characteristic. These classic presentations occur rarely, however. Capillary fragility is commonly abnormal. Radiographs are useful in demonstrating subperiosteal elevation, disturbances of calcification of the cartilage matrix, fractures and dislocations, ground glass appearance of the cortex, alveolar bone resorption, and other findings.

Plasma ascorbic acid levels are greatly reduced in scurvy, usually to 0.1 mg per deciliter or lower. Some depression of plasma ascorbic acid levels occurs, however, in a variety of other conditions, including cigarette smoking, tuberculosis, rheumatic fever, and many chronic disorders and in some women using oral contraceptive drugs. These conditions must be considered when a low ascorbic acid level is detected.

The assay of ascorbic acid in serum or plasma can be accomplished with titrimetric, spectrophotometric, or fluorometric methods. Some laboratories prefer to make the diagnosis of scurvy by assay of platelet or white blood cell ascorbic acid content.

TREATMENT. As little as 10 mg per day of ascorbic acid can completely prevent the clinical manifestations of scurvy. Even far-advanced cases of scurvy respond rapidly to ascorbic acid in the range of 100 to 200 mg per day. Marked improvement is to be expected within several days. Patients should also be instructed in the importance of a proper diet to prevent further recurrences.

Patients with rare inborn errors of metabolism, including tyrosinemia, osteogenesis imperfecta, and Chédiak-Higashi syndrome, have had some apparent benefit from the use of ascorbic acid in the range of 50 to 200 mg per day. Certain forms of the Ehlers-Danlos syndrome are disorders in which pharmacologic doses (4 grams) have been reported to be effective.

Special mention must be made of two conditions in which the use of megadoses of ascorbic acid has attracted wide attention in the popular press: the common cold and advanced cancer. Many studies have been performed on the possible benefits of 2 grams and higher per day of ascorbic acid on the prevention of colds and on the alleviation of symptoms once colds develop. On balance, the predominance of evidence favors the view that while some individuals may receive slight benefit in terms of symptoms, probably as a result of a mild antihistamine action of ascorbic acid, no consistent, reproducible improvements occur in the frequency, duration, or severity of illness in the great majority of cases.

With respect to treatment of cancer, there is some theoretical basis for the view that maintenance of immune function may depend upon the adequacy of vitamin C nutriture, as may wound healing, collagen formation, and cytotoxicity of a number of chemotherapeutic drugs. Nevertheless, treatment of patients with advanced colon cancer with megadoses of vitamin C after chemotherapy and radiation has been ineffective when evaluated in an objective manner. The use of vitamin C under no circumstances should replace established methods of treating cancer with chemotherapy, surgery, or radiation.

Vitamin C at a dose level of approximately 0.5 to 3 grams per day has long been used empirically to acidify the urine in cases of refractory urinary tract infections. Ascorbic acid is only a weak acidifying agent, and its efficacy under these circumstances is difficult to evaluate.

Ascorbic acid in amounts ordinarily contained in food may be useful in facilitating the intestinal absorption of nonheme iron. To be effective, the ascorbic acid and the iron sources must be consumed together. As little as 100 ml of orange juice, which contains 40 to 50 mg of ascorbic acid, has been reported to increase the absorption of iron from vegetable sources more than threefold. Iron from meat is not absorbed more efficiently by ascorbic acid.

A potentially useful application of ascorbic acid lies in its ability to inhibit the conversion of nitrites and secondary amines to the carcinogenic nitrosoamines in vitro, and, under certain circumstances, in vivo. Whether ascorbic acid can achieve this effect in vivo under ordinary circumstances of food consumption is important to determine. It is of interest that consumption of foods high in vitamin C is associated with reduced risk of gastric and esophageal cancer. The antioxidant effect of ascorbic acid may be synergistic with that of vitamin E and β-carotene, and trials of cancer prevention with a combination of antioxidants are now in progress in patients at high risk.

Another potential therapeutic role for vitamin C may lie in diabetes. Doses of 500 to 2000 mg per day of ascorbic acid have been reported to reduce erythrocyte concentrations of sorbitol possibly implicated in the pathogenesis of complications of diabetes. There is recent evidence that ascorbic acid alone or in combination with zinc, iron, calcium, or EDTA may reduce the body burden of lead.

Toxicity

At the dose range of approximately 1 to 2 grams per day and higher there is potential for some adverse side effects. There is great variability among individuals in regard to their susceptibility to the adverse effects of large doses of ascorbic acid. In the intestinal tract, large doses (2 grams and higher) of ascorbic acid may produce pain, discomfort, and an osmotic diarrhea. Doses of ascorbic acid above 1 gram may give a false-negative guaiac test for blood, thereby obscuring recognition of occult bleeding. Urine tests for glucose also may be misleading when very large doses of ascorbic acid are ingested, producing a false-negative glucose oxidase reaction (Tes-Tape) and false-positive copper-reduction reaction (Clinitest) and making urine strips more difficult to read. At daily doses of 3 grams and higher, automated measurements of alanine aminotransferase, lactate dehydrogenase, and uric acid may be affected.

As oxalate is a degradative product of ascorbic acid, large amounts of this vitamin are expected to increase biosynthesis and renal excretion of oxalate, posing the potential risk of formation of oxalate stones in susceptible individuals. The increase in oxalate excretion is small in magnitude, however, and in most cases still falls within the normal range. There is recent evidence that patients with recurrent formation of kidney stones exhibit increased production and urinary excretion of oxalate following a 2-gram load of ascorbic acid. Uricosuria and uric acid stones are also believed to occur with increased frequency after large doses of ascorbic acid. Nevertheless, the real risk of kidney stone formation in users of large doses of ascorbic acid is not known with precision at the present time. Precipitation of calcium oxalate stones is favored by an alkaline urine. With chronic consumption of large doses of ascorbic acid, there is a likelihood of exacerbating systemic acidosis in those disorders with failure of urinary acidification, such as chronic renal disease and renal tubular acidosis. Certain patients with diminished glucose-6-phosphate dehydrogenase activity may be at increased risk for hemolytic episodes with large doses of ascorbic acid therapy. There is some concern that indiscriminate use of ascorbic acid, which increases intestinal absorption of iron, may put patients with hemochromatosis at risk for hyperabsorption of iron. Vitamin C may also increase the risk of iron overload in patients with β-thalassemia and other disorders that require frequent long-term blood transfusions.

Block G, Menkes M: Ascorbic acid in cancer prevention. In Moon TE, Micozzi MC (eds.): Nutrition and Cancer Prevention. Investigating the Role of Micronutrients. New York, Marcel Dekker, 1989, p 341. Current status of epidemiology of vitamin C intake and cancer prevalence.
Burns JJ, Rivers JM, Machlin LJ (eds.): Third conference on vitamin C. NY Acad Sci Vol. 498, 1987. Proceedings of a recent symposium on advances in understanding of vitamin C metabolism.
Hathcock JN, Rader J: Micronutrient safety. In Bendich A, Chandra R (eds.): Micronutrients and Immune Function. New York, Academy of Sciences, 1990, Vol. 587, p 257. Recent review of toxicities of vitamins and minerals.
Levine M: New concepts in the biology and biochemistry of ascorbic acid. N Engl J Med 314:892, 1986. Important update of biochemistry, physiology, and nutritional applications of vitamin C.

VITAMIN A
Structure and Biochemical Function

Vitamin A refers to retinol, although the term is often used loosely to indicate all related compounds (Fig. 204–6). The term "retinoids" has been used to designate all the natural and synthetic isomers and derivatives of vitamin A. Retinol is oxidized to vitamin A aldehyde (retinal), which is critical to vision. Retinoic acid (vitamin A acid) is the major oxidative metabolite of retinol. Retinoic acid can fulfill the growth-promoting and epithelium-differentiating roles of retinol but cannot fully maintain its function in reproduction, nor can retinoic acid fulfill the functions of retinal in vision. Carotenoids are larger precursor molecules that undergo cleavage to yield retinal. The most important of the more than 30 carotenoids with pro-vitamin A activity is β-carotene.

Of the various metabolic roles of vitamin A, the best understood is the visual process. Retinal is the prosthetic group of all the visual pigments that capture light. The human retina contains four kinds of visual pigments: rhodopsin in rods and three iodopsins in cones. In the dark-adapted retina, rhodopsin is activated by photons of light. This event initiates the visual cycle, during which retinal changes its conformation from a cis to a trans isomer and other conformational changes occur in the protein. During dark adaptation, these processes are reversed and rhodopsin is regenerated. In view of the absolute requirement for retinal, it is not surprising that loss of highly sensitive night vision is an early symptom of vitamin A deficiency. Vitamin A probably serves additional roles in the normal functioning of the retina.

The mechanism of action of vitamin A in growth and differentiation is not known. One hypothesis is that vitamin A is similar to steroid hormones in influencing events in the genome following attachment to specific cellular binding proteins. The striking effects of vitamin A upon differentiation, particularly of epithelial tissues, underlie the current concept that this vitamin and its derivatives may have a role in the prevention of certain cancers, particularly of epithelial origin.

Retinol is fat soluble, sensitive to acid and heat, and rapidly oxidized upon exposure to light and oxygen. β-Carotene is relatively less heat-sensitive than retinol. β-Carotene is capable of quenching singlet oxygen and is a powerful antioxidant, protecting cell membranes from damage caused by free radicals.

Normal Physiology

Foods containing vitamin A (largely in the form of retinyl esters) or carotenoids are digested by gastric and intestinal enzymes, and then both forms are absorbed by the intestinal mucosa. About 80 to 90 per cent of dietary vitamin A is absorbed. The rate of absorption of dietary β-carotene is much slower, and only 40 to 60 per cent is absorbed, the percentage decreasing at higher doses. Absorption of β-carotene is more dependent than vitamin A upon interactions with bile salts.

Within the intestinal mucosa, β-carotene is cleaved to two molecules of retinal, which are then reduced to retinol (Fig. 204–6). The retinol generated from β-carotene, as well as that absorbed directly, is esterified subsequently. The retinyl esters formed are incorporated into chylomicrons and transported via lymph to the general circulation, where the triglycerides in the chylomicrons are degraded by lipoprotein lipase. The smaller chylomicron remnants remaining are then cleared by the liver, the major storage organ for vitamin A, which contains approximately 90 per cent of the total body reserves. Retinyl esters, mostly in the form of retinyl palmitate, are stored in the liver, and their hydrolysis generates retinol, which binds to a specific hepatic apo-retinol binding protein (RBP). The holo-RBP is secreted into the plasma, where it forms a 1:1 molar complex with a tetrameric protein, formerly called prealbumin, which also binds thyroxine and triiodothyronine. In recognition of both roles, this protein is now named transthyretin.

Cell surfaces recognize the RBP-retinol complex rather than retinol, and once inside the cell, all trans-retinol binds to a specific protein, cellular retinol binding protein (CRBP). CRBP may deliver retinol to intranuclear binding sites that mediate genomic expression and/or transport retinol across cellular membranes. CRBP concentrations are increased in certain animal and human tumors. A cellular retinoic acid binding protein (CRABP) has also been detected in a number of neonatal tissues and epithelial tumors that are sensitive to retinoic acid therapeutically.

Retinoic acid does not accumulate in liver, and it fulfills some but not all of the physiologic functions of retinol. In vitamin A deficiency, hepatic concentrations of vitamin A are nearly completely depleted before total plasma RBP levels begin to fall. With vitamin A repletion, the liver apo-RBP becomes more saturated, and levels of holo-RBP begin to rise in blood.

The degradative metabolism of retinol and its derivatives proceeds by a series of chain-shortening steps to yield a group of compounds of little if any intrinsic biologic activity.

Requirements and Dietary Sources

The RDA for vitamin A is currently 1000 µg of retinol equivalents (RE) for adult males and 800 µg for adult females. One RE is defined as 1 µg of retinol or 6 µg of β-carotene. The allowances are calculated in this fashion because the overall utilization of β-carotene is only about one sixth that of retinol, as a result of the relative inefficiency with which β-carotene is absorbed and converted to vitamin A.

Vitamin A allowances were formerly expressed in terms of international units (IU), and this nomenclature still appears on most commercial vitamin bottles. One RE is equal to 3.33 IU retinol and 10 IU β-carotene. The RDA for vitamin A expressed in terms of IU is 5000 for adult males and 4000 for adult females. These figures are based upon the estimate that the American diet contains approximately equal amounts of β-carotene (2500 IU = 250 RE, for males) and retinol (2500 IU = 750 RE, for males).

β-Carotene is derived from plant sources, including vegetables such as carrots and sweet potatoes, leafy green vegetables, and some fruits, such as cantaloupe and papaya. Preformed vitamin A is derived almost exclusively from animal sources. Liver obviously is a rich source, followed by kidney, milk and milk products, and fish. Fish liver oils have unusually high concentrations of vitamin A.

Deficiency

PATHOGENESIS. Vitamin A deficiency is a very common problem worldwide, particularly in developing countries, as a consequence of famine or shortages of vitamin A–rich foods. The ocular manifestations of vitamin A deficiency are such a serious problem that half a million preschool children become blind every year as a result. In such situations, a diet high in rice, wheat, maize, and tubers contains little if any β-carotene. Breast and cow's milk do not provide enough vitamin A to meet the needs of the growing child.

In the United States, vitamin A deficiency may be encountered among the urban poor, the elderly, alcohol abusers, patients with malabsorption, and other individuals on a marginal diet. In alcoholism, vitamin A deficiency may develop for several reasons. Zinc deficiency, which frequently coexists in alcoholism, impairs the release of holo-RBP from liver, thereby interfering with vitamin A mobilization from storage sites. Thus, alcohol-associated zinc deficiency may intensify sequelae of dietary vitamin A

deficiency. In addition, in alcoholism the degradative enzyme, alcohol dehydrogenase, which also converts retinol to retinal in the retina, may be so saturated with ethanol that retinal production is sharply diminished. Furthermore, as malabsorption develops in chronic alcoholism, dietary carotenes and vitamin A may be lost in increasing amounts in the stool.

Vitamin A deficiency may occur after long-term use of mineral oil, because this fat-soluble vitamin is dissolved in the oil. Other laxatives may result in vitamin A deficiency because of rapid intestinal transit and diminished intestinal absorption. Vitamin A deficiency may result also after prolonged use of certain drugs, such as cholestyramine, colestipol, neomycin, and colchicine.

CLINICAL FEATURES. Night blindness, as noted previously, may be an early manifestation of vitamin A deficiency. It has been suggested that the frequent episodes of falling and of traffic accidents involving chronic alcoholic persons at night may be due to some degree to underlying night blindness. In addition, dryness or xerosis of the conjunctivae and later of the cornea may develop (xerophthalmia), leading to softening and perforation of the cornea and development of Bitot's spots (small, white patches) on the sclerae. Because of the role of vitamin A in maintaining differentiated epithelium, dietary deficiency leads to abnormalities of epithelial tissue and keratinization, particularly in the eye, lung, sweat glands, and gastrointestinal tract. Loss of taste may also occur. Vitamin A deficiency leads to increased frequency, severity, and mortality rate of infectious diseases.

It has been suggested that decreased intake of β-carotene or vitamin A–rich foods or both may be associated with an increased prevalence of epithelial cancers, particularly lung cancers, among smokers. In some studies, intake of β-carotene but not vitamin A has had a strong negative correlation with cancer risk. Also, vitamin A–deficient animals have an increased risk of chemical carcinogenesis; administration of retinoids can prevent chemically induced cancers in animals.

DIAGNOSIS. The demonstration of abnormal dark adaptation is important evidence for the diagnosis of vitamin A deficiency. Techniques are being developed that can be carried out under field conditions without expensive equipment. Retinol can be detected directly in serum by immunoassay. Normal levels are in the range of 30 to 65 µg per deciliter. Serum levels may be increased by hypothyroidism, nephrotic syndrome, oral contraceptives, and disorders of lipid metabolism. By the time serum levels of retinol begin to decrease from dietary deficiency, liver reserves are already nearly completely depleted. A new technique, conjunctival impression cytology, may be useful in detecting early histologic abnormalities in the cornea.

TREATMENT. The extensive eye problems of vitamin A deficiency that are encountered in developing countries are best

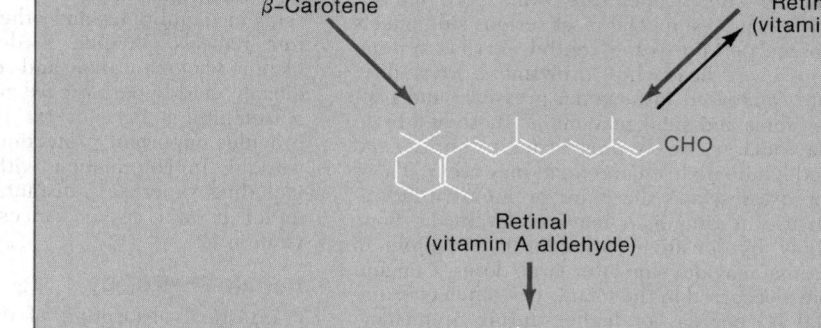

FIGURE 204–6. Structural formulae and interconversions of retinol, retinal, retinoic acid, and β-carotene.

approached through a systematic plan of prevention. Such programs are increasing in scope and magnitude. Injections of vitamin A in large doses (50,000 to 100,000 IU) every 4 to 6 months are highly effective and are tolerated remarkably well. In children from population groups that have a high prevalence of vitamin A deficiency, capsules containing 200,000 IU given every 6 months have reduced mortality markedly, particularly from infectious diseases. In the United States, only when dietary deficiency is far advanced should it be treated with similar doses and for several days only; then maintenance doses should be administered. Water-soluble forms of vitamin A should provide great assistance in patient management.

Derivatives of vitamin A (referred to as retinoids), particularly 13-*cis*-retinoic acid (isotretinoin), have been used to treat cystic acne with considerable success. Investigations are continuing in other dermatologic disorders, including psoriasis, actinic keratosis, leukoplakia, and pityriasis rosea. The mechanism of action of this derivative may lie in inhibition of keratinization, suppression of sebaceous gland secretion, or possibly a direct anti-inflammatory effect.

The use of β-carotene or retinoids or both, especially the less toxic forms, for the possible prevention of epithelial cancers is under intense study. Smokers should be expected to benefit particularly by increasing their intake of carotenoids, but no amounts of these agents are large enough to protect completely against the harmful effects of smoking. Consumption of foods rich in carotenes and vitamin A is not a substitute for failure to stop smoking. The exact doses necessary to achieve preventive effects are not known at present.

A new therapeutic application for vitamin A is in children with severe measles infection. Measles depresses the serum levels of vitamin A, and vitamin A deficiency greatly increases risk of pneumonia, diarrhea, and death in infected patients. Treatment with large doses of water-miscible retinyl palmitate reduces severity of complications and death rate in severely ill children with malaria.

Toxicity

β-Carotene is entirely without toxicity when consumed in food or as a nutritional supplement. Because only limited amounts of β-carotene can be converted to vitamin A by the body, consumption of β-carotene in amounts several-fold above the RDA does not lead to vitamin A toxicity. Consumption of β-carotene in large amounts from foods such as carrots may stain the skin a yellow-orange color, but this phenomenon is entirely benign and may even be beneficial in providing protection against solar exposure. The sclerae remain white in carotenemia; thus, the condition can easily be differentiated from jaundice.

Vitamin A (retinol), on the other hand, can be quite toxic when taken continuously for a few days to several weeks in large amounts (particularly at 100,000 IU and higher) or for periods of several months or more at lower doses of 25,000 to 50,000 IU per day. The skin may become dry, pruritic, coarse, and scaly with fissures; hair loss may occur. Both vitamin A excess and deficiency have adverse effects upon the skin. Sore mouth, anorexia, and vomiting may ensue. The most serious side effects of vitamin A overdosage pertain to the central nervous system: patients may develop severe headaches, drowsiness, irritability, failure to concentrate, increased intracranial pressure, and papilledema. These symptoms and signs may mimic those of a brain tumor. The liver may enlarge, rarely progressing to fibrosis and cirrhosis. Generalized lymph node enlargement may occur. There may be painful hyperostoses, and there are preliminary indications that long-term use of vitamin A may accelerate the bone loss of aging, possibly by sensitizing vitamin D receptors to calcitriol. Hypercalcemia may develop after large doses. Congenital malformations have occurred in the infants of women consuming 25,000 to 50,000 IU per day or higher during pregnancy. Symptoms of acute vitamin A toxicity are shown in Table 204–1.

In cases of vitamin A toxicity, serum vitamin A levels are increased, particularly in the form of retinyl esters. In an asymptomatic patient consuming megadoses of vitamin A, the onset of liver disease, such as viral or alcoholic hepatitis, may precipitate overt clinical toxicity, presumably by releasing stored retinol into

TABLE 204–1. SIGNS AND SYMPTOMS OF ACUTE VITAMIN A TOXICITY

Children	Adults
Anorexia	Abdominal pain
Bulging fontanelles	Anorexia
Drowsiness	Blurred vision
Increased intracranial pressure	Drowsiness
Irritability	Headache
Vomiting	Hypercalcemia
	Irritability
	Muscle weakness
	Nausea, vomiting
	Peripheral neuritis
	Skin desquamation

From Hathcock JN, Hattan DG, Jenkins MY, et al.: Evaluation of vitamin A toxicity. Am J Clin Nutr 52:183, 1990. © Am J Clin Nutr, American Society for Clinical Nutrition.

the general circulation. With discontinuation of large doses of vitamin A, the symptoms gradually recede. Low-protein diets enhance hepatic toxicity of vitamin A, and treatment with tetracycline may increase the risk for increased intracranial pressure. Treatment with zinc may facilitate mobilization of vitamin A from the liver, a useful adjunct when there is hepatotoxicity.

The development of synthetic retinoids with lower toxicities and greater uptake in target organs is expected to facilitate the safe application of these agents to the possible chemoprevention of cancer. At present it is essential to realize that derivatives of vitamin A such as 13-*cis*-retinoic acid may cause birth defects and other manifestations of vitamin A toxicity.

Goodman DS: Vitamin A and retinoids in health and disease. N Engl J Med 310:1023, 1984. *This comprehensive review highlights advances relating vitamin A and retinoids to clinical medicine and public health, particularly ophthalmology, nutrition, dermatology, and cancer.*

Hathcock JN, Hattan DG, Jenkins MY, et al: Evaluation of vitamin A toxicity. Am J Clin Nutr 52:183, 1990. *Review of vitamin A toxicity, particularly with respect to causing birth defects.*

Hussey GD, Klein M: A randomized controlled trial of vitamin A in children with severe measles. N Engl J Med 323:160, 1990. *Large doses of vitamin A reduce death rate and severity of complications.*

Olson JA: Vitamin A. *In* Brown ML (ed.): Present Knowledge in Nutrition, 6th ed. Washington, D.C., International Life Sciences Institute, The Nutrition Foundation, 1990, p 96. *Review of physiology, binding proteins, metabolism, and function of vitamin A.*

Ziegler RG: A review of epidemiological evidence that carotenoids reduce the risk of cancer. J Nutr 119:116, 1989. *Documents evidence that low intake of fruits and vegetables is associated with increased risk for certain cancers.*

VITAMIN D

Vitamin D is discussed in Chapter 233 in association with calcium metabolism and metabolic bone diseases.

VITAMIN E

Structure and Biochemical Function

Vitamin E activity is derived from a series of dietary tocopherols and tocotrienols, the most potent of which is D-α-tocopherol (Fig. 204–7). At least eight compounds with vitamin E activity have been isolated from plants. The most widely accepted function of this vitamin is as an antioxidant, protecting polyunsaturated fatty acids in membranes and other cellular structures from attack by free radicals. Vitamin E deficiency in animals increases the likelihood of membrane and cellular damage from ozone, nitrogen dioxide, and hyperbaric oxygen. Dietary selenium is a precursor of selenite, a cofactor for glutathione peroxidase, which also provides important protection against lipid peroxidation in vivo, working in conjunction with vitamin E and other enzymes, including superoxide dismutase and catalase. Dietary selenium under certain circumstances may spare the requirement for vitamin E.

Normal Physiology

Intestinal absorption of dietary vitamin E requires normal mechanisms of digestion and absorption of fat, particularly bile acids. About 20 to 50 per cent of tocopherols are absorbed normally, with lower percentages at higher doses. Medium-chain triglycerides enhance absorption of tocopherols, and polyunsaturated fatty acids inhibit absorption. Tocopherols are absorbed as micelles primarily from the mid-small intestine. Vitamin E in blood is bound to all the lipoproteins, and levels correlate with those of lipoproteins to which they are bound both normally and in various disease states. In contrast to vitamin A, there does not appear to be a specific carrier protein in blood for vitamin E, nor a specific organ in which it is stored. Some vitamin E is also transported in erythrocytes. The most important storage sites of the vitamin are fat, liver, and muscle. Recent reports raise the possibility of specific binding proteins for E in tissues. Vitamin E undergoes little metabolic transformation after absorption. The major excretory route is through the feces.

Since dietary deficiency occurs only under very unusual circumstances, cases of vitamin E deficiency have usually been identified primarily in patients with prolonged and severe fat malabsorption. Vitamin E deficiency has also been detected in patients receiving parenteral nutrition without adequate E replacement.

Requirements and Dietary Sources

The dietary allowance for vitamin E is expressed in terms of milligrams of α-tocopherol equivalents (α-TE) and is 10 mg per day (15 IU) for adult males and 8 mg per day (12 IU) for adult females, with increases of 2 mg per day for pregnancy and 3 to 4 mg per day for lactation. The increased requirement for vitamin E with diets high in polyunsaturated fatty acids is thought not to be clinically relevant, since the items highest in vitamin E content—soybean, corn, cottonseed, wheat germ, and safflower oils and their derivatives—are also high in polyunsaturated fatty acids. As a group, the tocopherols and tocotrienols are widely distributed in the food supply. They are relatively unstable and lose significant activity during storage and cooking.

Deficiency

PATHOGENESIS. Clinical deficiency of vitamin E is generally encountered in the setting of severe malabsorption. The most serious deficiency is associated with a genetic disorder, abetalipoproteinemia, in which there is failure both of intestinal absorption and of serum transport of vitamin E. Vitamin E deficiency occurs in children with biliary atresia, cystic fibrosis, and chronic cholestasis, as well as in adults who survive these diseases or who have celiac disease, Crohn's disease, or other serious forms of malabsorption (Ch. 102).

An apparent inborn error of vitamin E metabolism, named familial isolated vitamin E deficiency, has recently been identified. Affected patients have a common pattern of neurologic abnormalities, are vitamin E deficient despite consuming an adequate diet, have no evidence of vitamin E malabsorption, and can achieve normal serum levels as well as neurologic improvement after treatment with large doses of the vitamin (800 to 1000 mg per day). The defect appears to reside in inability to incorporate dietary vitamin E into VLDL, resulting in very rapid clearance from plasma.

CLINICAL FEATURES. Deficiency of vitamin E has generally not been recognized as a clearly definable syndrome. The red cell half-life may be shortened, although anemia is uncommon in the absence of other causes. Most importantly, clinical and neuropathologic evidence of posterior column and spinocerebellar tract abnormalities have been described, with areflexia, ophthalmoplegia, and disturbances of gait, proprioception, and vibration. In premature infants, vitamin E deficiency is associated with hemolytic anemia, thrombocytosis, edema, intraventricular hem-

orrhage, and increasing risk of retrolental fibroplasia and bronchopulmonary dysplasia, both of which are related to oxygen toxicity.

DIAGNOSIS. Diagnosis of vitamin E deficiency is usually made by measurement of plasma vitamin E levels; normal levels are generally 0.50 to 0.70 mg per deciliter and higher. In several of the hemolytic anemias, such as sickle cell anemia and G-6-PD deficiency, serum vitamin E levels tend to be low. Serum vitamin E concentration should be expressed in relation to serum lipid levels when vitamin E nutritional status is being evaluated, inasmuch as serum vitamin E levels correlate with those of serum cholesterol and total lipids and may be elevated in diabetes and primary lipid disorders.

TREATMENT. The therapeutic role of vitamin E remains controversial at the present time. Although vitamin E has been advocated by food faddists as an "anti-aging" vitamin, there is no evidence that it prolongs life in man. This vitamin has been claimed to enhance sexual performance, an attribute that also has not been substantiated. Some patients with intermittent claudication appear to have improved after therapy with vitamin E. Hemolytic anemia in the premature newborn is generally benefited by vitamin E therapy, and the severity but not the incidence of retrolental fibroplasia may be reduced. Administration of vitamin E has reduced the incidence of intraventricular hemorrhage in premature infants. Large doses of vitamin E have diminished the neurologic complications in abetalipoproteinemia, cholestatic liver disease, and cystic fibrosis.

There are a number of other effects of vitamin E demonstrable in vitro in experimental animals and in some instances in humans, but their clinical relevance remains unresolved. These effects include reducing platelet aggregation, inhibiting conversion of nitrites to nitrosamines, inhibiting prostaglandin synthesis, improving immune function, protecting against environmental toxicants and pollutants, and diminishing progression of cataracts, among others. There is much interest in the potential therapeutic role of vitamin E as an antioxidant. Vitamins E and C are synergistic in their antioxidant activities in vitro. A number of studies have found that elevated serum levels of vitamin E are associated with lower risk of cancer, as noted above. Such relationships possibly may relate to the antioxidant properties of vitamin E. Current investigations are seeking to determine whether vitamin E delays the emergence of cancer, heart disease, and other major health problems.

Toxicity

Vitamin E is far less toxic than vitamins A and D, and a daily intake in the range of 200 to 800 mg per day (20 to 80 times the RDA) is generally considered safe. Nausea, flatulence, and diarrhea have been reported at doses in excess of 1000 mg. In animals the intestinal absorption of vitamin A and K is reduced at high doses of E, which may be clinically significant in patients on marginal diets. Vitamin E appears to increase the vitamin K requirement, and megadoses of vitamin E administered together with the anticoagulant drug warfarin may result in overt bleeding.

Bieri JG, Corash L, Hubbard VS: Medical uses of vitamin E. N Engl J Med 308:1063, 1983. *This article reviews the rationale for treatment with vitamin E in various clinical disorders, limitations of treatment, and toxicities encountered.*

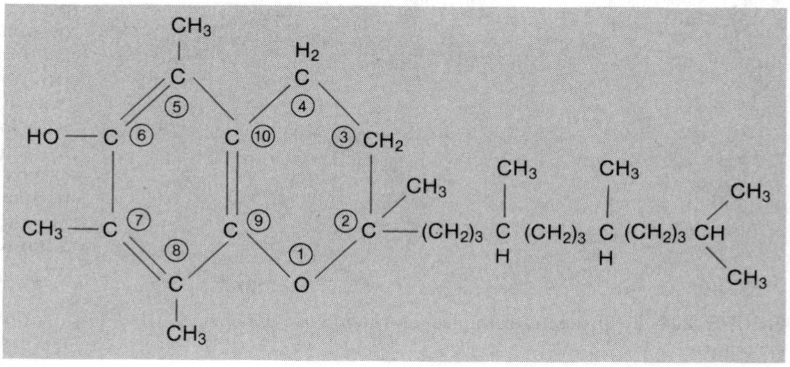

FIGURE 204–7. Structural formula of D-alpha tocopherol (vitamin E).

Machlin LJ: Vitamin E. *In* Machlin LJ (ed.): Handbook of Vitamins, 2nd ed. New York, Marcel Dekker, 1990, p 99. *Up-to-date review of physiology and medical uses of vitamin E.*

Murphy SP, Subar AF, Block G: Vitamin E intakes and sources in the United States. Am J Clin Nutr 52:361, 1990. *Survey identifying sources of dietary intake of E.*

Traber MG, Somol RJ, Burton GW, et al.: Impaired ability of patients with familial isolated vitamin E deficiency to incorporate α-tocopherol into lipoproteins secreted by the liver. J Clin Invest 85:397, 1990. *Research into mechanism of vitamin E deficiency in a familial disorder.*

VITAMIN K

Structure and Biochemical Functions

Vitamin K occurs naturally in two forms, differing from one another only in their side chains. Vitamin K_1 (now called phylloquinone) is made by plant sources; vitamin K_2 (menaquinone) is synthesized by normal intestinal flora. It is also contained in some animal tissues. Vitamin K_3 (menadione) is an artificial provitamin that can be converted to menaquinone by the liver (Fig. 204–8). Compounds with vitamin K activity are sensitive to ultraviolet light and alkali.

It has been proposed that the mechanism of action of vitamin K consists of a post-translational γ-carboxylation of glutamic acid moieties in inactive precursor proteins, which confers calcium-binding properties to the proteins. The most widely known of these proteins are involved in blood coagulation. Four clotting factors are dependent upon vitamin K for this important action: prothrombin (Factor II), proconvertin (Factor VII), Christmas factor (Factor IX), and Stuart-Prower factor (Factor X). Lack of vitamin K may result in death from uncontrolled hemorrhage.

The anticoagulant drugs warfarin and dicoumarol inhibit the vitamin K–dependent γ-carboxylation by interfering with activation of vitamin K to its metabolically active hydroquinone form. As a result of this inhibition, the activation of the four clotting factors is greatly reduced.

Proteins that are involved in the mineralization of bone (osteocalcin) and possibly also in calcium resorption from the renal tubule also require vitamin K for their synthesis. Other vitamin K–dependent proteins have been identified (protein C, protein S). The vitamin K antagonists warfarin and dicoumarol also cause a marked decrease in formation of osteocalcin, presumably by interfering with γ-carboxylation.

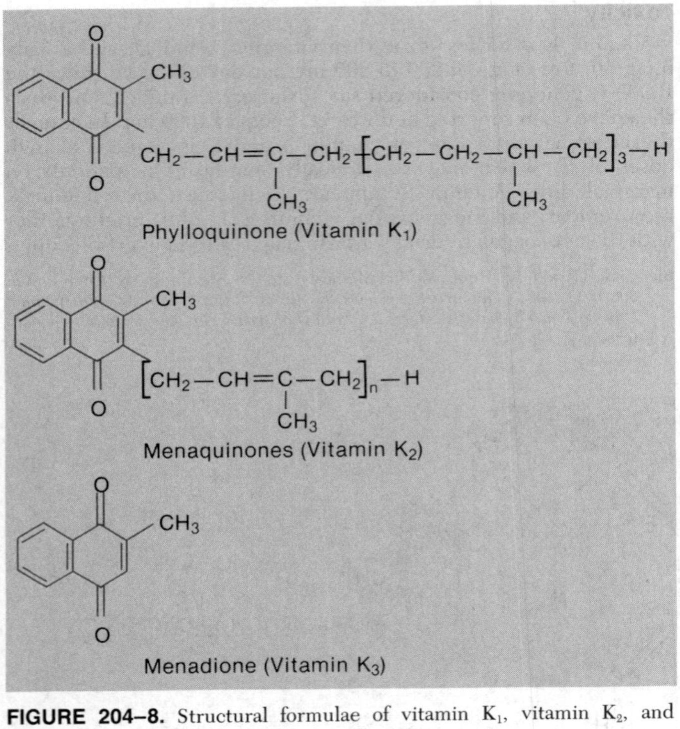

FIGURE 204–8. Structural formulae of vitamin K_1, vitamin K_2, and vitamin K_3.

Normal Physiology

The intestinal absorption of various forms of vitamin K resembles that of vitamin E in requiring bile salts and other normal mechanisms of fat absorption and in being incorporated into micelles. Vitamin K_1 is absorbed principally in the proximal segment via a saturable energy-dependent process, whereas vitamin K_2 is absorbed by the small intestine and by the colon via a non–carrier-mediated, non–energy-dependent process. Liver and other parenchymal organs store vitamin K, but apparently only to a limited degree. The efficiency of absorption varies greatly and is markedly diminished by mineral oil, other fat solvents, and laxatives. In patients who have fat malabsorption that is severe and prolonged, as in sprue, regional ileitis, and other disorders, or in patients with obstruction to bile flow, vitamin K deficiency commonly develops. Deficiency also may occur after prolonged antibiotic therapy, destroying the intestinal synthesis of vitamin K.

After absorption, vitamin K is transported via the lymphatic system in association with chylomicrons. Liver is probably the most important storage site for vitamin K; high concentrations are also found in the adrenal glands, lungs, bone marrow, kidneys, and lymph nodes. The main excretory products of vitamin K in urine are glucuronide derivatives that have undergone chain shortening and beta oxidation.

Requirements and Dietary Sources

The best sources of vitamin K are green leafy vegetables, particularly turnip greens, broccoli, brussels sprouts, spinach, and lettuce. There are moderate amounts in liver, bacon, cheese, butter, coffee, and green tea. Significant amounts are synthesized by intestinal bacteria. There may be discrepancies in the analysis of foods by several different methods. In 1989 for the first time a recommended dietary allowance was made for vitamin K by the National Academy of Sciences. It is recommended that normal adult males consume 70 to 80 μg per day and normal adult females 60 to 65 μg per day. No increase is recommended for either pregnancy or lactation. Dietary deficiency based upon consuming less than this amount is uncommon at the present time in the United States, because the usual diet contains ample amounts of vitamin K.

Deficiency

PATHOGENESIS. Vitamin K deficiency occurs frequently in newborn infants for several reasons. First, fetal stores tend to be low because very little of this vitamin is transported across the placenta. In addition, the fetal gut is sterile, and therefore the newborn lacks the supply of vitamin K that can be provided by normal intestinal flora. As the intestinal tract becomes colonized postnatally, the synthesis of vitamin K becomes appreciable. Deficiency generally does not develop unless there is an abnormality of intestinal function or antibiotic therapy.

CLINICAL FEATURES. Vitamin K deficiency may be manifested clinically as increased tendency to hemorrhage. Such bleeding episodes may be particularly severe in newborn infants.

DIAGNOSIS. The only practical and reliable method for diagnosis of vitamin K deficiency is direct assay of one or more of the four vitamin K–dependent clotting factors. Hypothyroidism inhibits both the synthesis and degradation of these four clotting factors.

TREATMENT. Vitamin K deficiency responds rapidly to the administration of vitamin K, provided that liver function is normal. A number of preparations of vitamin K are available, some of which are water soluble, e.g., menadiol sodium diphosphate. These forms are more toxic than the lipid-soluble phylloquinone form. In patients with advanced liver disease, the serum prothrombin is decreased and responds poorly if at all to administration of vitamin K. Patients with low serum prothrombin caused by vitamin K deficiency can be distinguished from those with low prothrombin caused by liver disease because in vitamin K deficiency the prothrombin precursor in blood is not γ-carboxylated; usually γ-carboxylated prothrombin is found in patients with liver disease. When vitamin K is given orally to patients with malabsorption, bile salts may also need to be administered to achieve optimal results.

Toxicity

Consumption of large quantities of foods rich in vitamin K is not believed to produce clinical toxicity. Certain water-soluble derivatives administered parenterally have caused hemolytic anemia and jaundice.

Olson RE: Vitamin K. *In* Goodhart RS, Shils ME (eds.): Modern Nutrition in Health and Disease, 6th ed. Philadelphia, Lea & Febiger, 1980, pp 170–180. *Thorough discussion of nutritional aspects of vitamin K, with emphasis upon biochemical mechanisms.*

Suttie JW: Current concepts of the mechanism of action of vitamin K and its antagonist. *In* Lindenbaum J (ed.): Nutrition in Hematology. Contemporary Issues in Clinical Nutrition. Vol. 5. New York, Churchill Livingstone, 1983, pp 245–270. *Discussion of the basic biochemistry of vitamin K and its relation to clotting factors.*

Suttie JW: Vitamin K. *In* Machlin LJ (ed.): Handbook of Vitamins, 2nd ed. New York, Marcel Dekker, 1990, p 145. *Comprehensive review of nutritional aspects of vitamin K.*

205 Disturbances of Trace Mineral Metabolism

Clifford Tasman-Jones

The bulk of living material is formed by 11 elements, all of which are from the lower atomic numbers of the periodic table (H, C, N, O, Na, Mg, P, S, Cl, K, and Ca). In addition to these, there are essential minerals that are present in trace amounts. These include F, Si, V, Cr, Mn, Fe, Co, Ni, Cu, Zn, Se, Mo, Sn, and I.

While deficiencies of trace minerals and vitamins are uncommon in humans eating a variety of foods, trace mineral deficiencies can occur in premature infants and in those with disordered eating habits owing to physical or psychological causes and with the use of enteral and parenteral feeding. Deficiencies developing during parenteral nutrition have stimulated interest in trace mineral function in human metabolism.

Trace minerals essential for life act as essential cofactors of enzymes and as organizers of the molecular structures of the cell (e.g., mitochondria) and its membrane. There is an optimal tissue concentration for trace minerals; excess can be toxic and insufficiency leads to metabolic failure.

Trace mineral bioavailability is affected by the physiologic status of the person (intrinsic factors), as well as by dietary availability (extrinsic factors). The absorptive mechanisms in the intestine vary with the trace mineral. Once in the plasma they are bound either to specific proteins or to albumin for transportation. The excretory path varies, but most are excreted into the gastrointestinal tract, many by way of bile; some are excreted into the urine and some by sweat glands. Not all trace minerals have been shown to be clinically important. Some, such as iron and iodine, are so important in specific disorders that they are covered separately in this volume.

ZINC

METABOLISM. Although zinc represents only 0.003 per cent (1.4 to 2.3 grams) of the human body, it is an intrinsic part of at least 110 metalloenzymes and other cellular components and is essential for the synthesis of protein, DNA, and RNA. Zinc is an important stabilizing component of macromolecules and biomembranes. It is required for growth at all stages of life, particularly during fetal growth in pregnancy.

Zinc is widely available from food of both animal and vegetable origin. Zinc from flesh food is generally more available than that from cereals.

Zinc is absorbed from the small intestine, although the exact mechanism for this remains uncertain. Its absorption is influenced by dietary factors and is inhibited by phytate, high dietary fiber, oxalate, iron, copper, and tin but enhanced by animal protein. A low molecular weight zinc-binding ligand, possibly secreted from the pancreas, is a postulated mechanism for absorption.

The highest concentrations of zinc are in the prostate, the skin and its appendages, the brain choroid, liver, pancreas, bone, and blood. In blood approximately 80 per cent of zinc is in erythrocytes, 16 per cent in plasma, 3 per cent in leukocytes, and the remaining 1 per cent in platelets. Plasma zinc is normally 12 to 20 μmol per liter. Zinc is excreted mainly in the feces, but small amounts (between 4.0 and 12.0 μmol per 24 hours) are secreted in the urine.

DEFICIENCY SYNDROMES (Table 205–1). In man zinc deficiency has been described in a chronic and an acute form. In Iran and Egypt hypogonadal dwarfism in males is associated with deficiency of zinc and dietary protein. Additionally, many of these children usually eat clay, which may bind zinc, making it unavailable for absorption.

Acrodermatitis enterohepatica, a rare autosomal recessive inherited disorder of zinc metabolism, represents a chronic form of pure zinc deficiency. This entity is characterized by diarrhea; an unpleasant skin rash of the extremities, face, and perineum; alopecia; mental irritability; muscle wasting; and depression. Although the nature of the disease remains in doubt, it may be caused by an absence of the ligand essential for zinc absorption. This ligand is present in human milk but not in cow's milk.

Acute zinc deficiency has been described in patients receiving parenteral nutrition. This syndrome is characterized by diarrhea; disturbance of the central nervous system with mental irritability and depression; skin lesions of the face, perineum, limbs, and skin folds; alopecia; loss of taste; and defects in the immunologic mechanisms. Treatment with zinc supplementation, usually in the form of zinc sulfate, results in a dramatic response.

The true importance of zinc in premature and young infants has still to be fully evaluated. A scaly erythema of the cheeks and diaper areas can be caused by zinc deficiency and incorrectly diagnosed as an eczematous rash. Many of the artificial milk formulas have added zinc, and it is suggested that zinc in human milk may sometimes be inadequate.

Zinc deficiency may occur in a number of conditions, including AIDS, diabetes, uremia, inflammatory bowel disease, malabsorption, cirrhosis, and alcoholism. The potential causes of zinc deficiency are indicated in Table 205–2.

In Crohn's disease, when there is severe catabolism, zincuria may be severe, depleting body stores that are needed during metabolism.

Individuals with sickle cell anemia may have delayed puberty, decreased hair, poor growth, and roughened skin related to zinc deficiency.

EXCESS. Zinc taken in excess may cause gastrointestinal upset with nausea and vomiting.

COPPER

The best-described function of copper is its effect on erythropoiesis. Ceruloplasmin ferroxidase transports iron essential for hemoglobin formation. Copper-containing monoamine oxidase enzymes explain its role in pigmentation and in central nervous system function. Copper-containing lysyl oxidase is necessary for elastin and collagen cross-linking in connective tissues. Cytochrome c oxidase and superoxide dismutase play key roles in the defenses against free radicals.

TABLE 205–1. CLINICAL FEATURES OF ZINC DEFICIENCY

Symptoms	Signs	Laboratory	Treatment
Growth retardation in adolescent males	Failure to thrive	Low plasma zinc	Oral 1 mg zinc/kg body weight as sulfate or acetate
Reduced taste (hypoguesia)	Hypogonadism in males	Hypercholesterolemia	
Reduced smell (hyposmia)	Skin rash of face, perineum, and extremities		
Irritability and depression, diarrhea	Alopecia		

TABLE 205–2. CAUSES OF ZINC DEFICIENCY

Inadequate dietary intake
    Anorexia
        Total parenteral nutrition
        Eating disorders (e.g., anorexia nervosa)
Increased requirement
    Growth
    Wound healing
    Infection
Decreased absorption
    Inflammatory bowel disease
    Surgical resection
    Intestinal fistulae
    Competing minerals (e.g., iron)
    Reduced availability (e.g., dietary fiber)
Increased loss
    Zincuria
    Fecal loss
    Skin loss

Usually copper is excreted in the bile as a metallocomplex. There is an additional copper loss in the urine (0.16 to 0.95 μmol per day) and saliva (0.006 to 0.008 μmol per day).

The highest concentrations of copper occur in the liver, brain, heart, spleen, kidneys, and blood. The mean daily requirement of copper is estimated to be between 5 and 15 μmol when given intravenously and between 30 and 40 μmol when given orally.

The copper content of plant foods is influenced by the copper content of the soil. Similarly, foods derived from animals vary according to their diet. The richest source of copper is liver, but nuts, peas and beans, soy beans, wheat germ, and bran provide good sources. Milk, both human and cow's milk, is a poor source of copper.

DEFICIENCY SYNDROMES. Hypocupremia occurs in a number of inherited disorders such as Wilson's disease (a disease of copper excess), Menkes' kinky hair syndrome (a syndrome of neurologic disorder with hypocupremia), and familial hypoceruloplasminemia. It may also be found with decreased copper intake, as in parenteral nutrition, or with the poor absorption or increased loss associated with protein-losing enteropathy, the nephrotic syndrome, cystic fibrosis, and other malabsorptive diseases such as celiac disease and sprue. Premature and underweight infants may manifest a deficiency of copper, the importance of which is still undefined.

SELENIUM

METABOLISM. Selenocysteine in the enzyme glutathionine peroxidase is important in protecting lipids of cell membranes, proteins, and nucleic acids against oxidant damage.

In the United States, the blood level of selenium is 1.90 to 3.17 μmol per liter. A low blood selenium concentration reflecting a low soil content has been noted in Finland, China, New Zealand, Sweden, and Denmark.

The daily requirement for selenium is estimated to be 0.72 μmol for women and 1.02 μmol for men. It probably depends on the supply of other trace minerals, including zinc, copper, magnesium, and iron and also the supply of other antioxidant substances, such as vitamin E and vitamin C. In the United States the intake is 0.76 to 2.79 μmol per day.

DEFICIENCY (Table 205–3). *Keshan disease* is a syndrome of endemic cardiomyopathy in the People's Republic of China that is alleviated by giving oral sodium selenite. In the areas of China where Keshan disease is prevalent, the dietary intake is estimated to be less than 0.38 μmol.

Selenium deficiency has been associated with intravenous feeding when the patient has developed muscle pain and tenderness associated with a very low blood selenium level. These symptoms are alleviated by giving selenomethionine.

Decreased levels of selenium in patients who have had acute myocardial infarction have been reported, and in Finland a reduced serum selenium concentration has been shown to correlate with cardiovascular death and acute coronary artery disease. The significance and importance of this remain to be confirmed.

A moderate drop in the selenium levels has been reported in patients with diseases of the gastrointestinal tract, particularly celiac disease and ulcerative colitis. Because of the importance of selenium in immune function, such a decrease may have clinical significance.

In newborn infants the level of selenium is about one-half that of the average adult. Because of a reduced selenium level in patients with malignant disease, there is interest in the possibility of a relationship between this trace mineral and cancer.

EXCESS. Selenium is a cell toxin and, as such, should be given with considerable care. Selinosis occurs with daily intake in excess of 6.35 μmol.

FLUORINE

METABOLISM. Fluorine is universally present in body fluids, tissues, and the skeleton. The environmental water and soil content of fluoride is the principal determinant of the fluoride status of the body.

Fluorine is readily absorbed in the intestine after release into its ionic form. It is retained in the body, mainly deposited in bones, and is excreted principally in the urine.

The principal health-related importance of fluorine is its ability to maintain the structure of the teeth. Fluoride, taken regularly throughout life, enhances the resistance of teeth to acidic dental plaque–related caries. Its role in the maintenance of normal bone calcification is not clear but may be important.

As water is a major source of fluoride, beverages provide a major source of fluoride intake. All foods, however, contain traces of fluoride, with plant foods containing more than animal foods.

CLINICAL FEATURES. The principal clinical importance of fluoride deficiency is in dental caries and possibly in the development of osteoporosis. Where the food and water sources of fluoride are deficient, fluoride can be given either by water fluoridation or by use of fluoride tablets, with further supplementation through toothpastes, dentifrices, and mouth rinses.

EXCESS. There is a risk of overexposure, and this manifests itself by fluorosis with defects of the tooth enamel.

TRACE MINERALS OF MINOR CLINICAL IMPORTANCE

Manganese

METABOLISM. Manganese, a trace element essential for life, is present in an amount of approximately 12 to 20 mg in the average adult. Maximally absorbed in the duodenum by an unknown transport mechanism, manganese is bound to transmanganin, a specific β-globulin transport protein. Manganese is concentrated in tissues rich in mitochondria and is widely distributed in the body, with maximal concentrations in the brain, kidneys, pancreas, bone, and liver. The blood and serum levels vary widely. Manganese is excreted principally in bile.

Manganese is an activator of many enzymes, but pyruvate carboxylase is the only manganese metalloenzyme. Manganese appears to be intimately involved in the synthesis of DNA, RNA, and protein.

DEFICIENCY. A syndrome has been described with impaired growth, skeletal abnormalities, abnormal reproductive function, ataxia, convulsions, and anomalies of fat metabolism. This deficiency is very rare.

EXCESS. Manganese poisoning, which usually occurs after industrial exposure, induces a syndrome that closely resembles Parkinson's disease.

Chromium

METABOLISM. Chromium is an essential micronutrient required for the maintenance of normal blood glucose levels. The

TABLE 205–3. CLINICAL FEATURES OF SELENIUM DEFICIENCY

Symptoms	Signs	Diagnosis	Treatment
Heart failure Skeletal muscle weakness	Cardiac dilatation	Selenium levels 0.55 μ mol/L	Oral selomethionine 100–200 g/day

recommended daily intake is 50 to 200 μg, and the normal serum level is 0.5 to 9.0 μg per liter. Chromium is present in yeast, meat, and grain. The chromium glucose tolerance factor is postulated to facilitate insulin receptor activity.

DEFICIENCY. Chromium deficiency is characterized by impaired glucose tolerance, encephalopathy, and neuropathy. Because of impaired insulin activity, patients may develop hyperglycemia with hyperosmolar nonketotic coma. Chromium deficiency may give a confusional state similar to hepatic encephalopathy with ataxia and peripheral neuropathy. A suggested association between chromium deficiency and coronary artery disease awaits confirmation.

EXCESS. If too much chromium is given, symptoms of nausea, vomiting, gastrointestinal ulceration, liver damage, kidney damage, and central nervous system abnormalities with convulsions may occur.

Vanadium

Analysis of vanadium is difficult. The total body vanadium content is about 100 μg. Blood levels are very low, 0.005 to 8.4 μmol per liter.

Vanadium depresses plasma cholesterol levels, Na^+, K^+-ATPase, myosin, Ca^{2+} ATPase, adenylate kinase, and phosphofructokinase and stimulates adenyl cyclase. Vanadium deficiency has been postulated to play a role in nutritional edema, and vanadium excess has been postulated to be a factor in manic-depressive illness. Neither of these suggestions has been confirmed.

Silicon

Silicon is found in high concentrations in tendons, aorta, and eye tissues. It is necessary for mammalian bone growth and calcification. In experimental animals, silicon appears to inhibit atheroma development. Chronic inhalation of silicon as silica (SiO_2) produces lung disease, as described in Ch. 527.

Cousins RJ: Absorption, transport and hepatic metabolism of copper and zinc. Special reference to metallothionein and ceruloplasmin. Physiol Rev 65:238, 1985. *A comprehensive review of copper and zinc metabolism, with particular reference to the key role of the liver.*

Featherstone JDB: The mechanism of dental decay. Nutr Today 22:10–16, 1987. *The role of fluoride in stabilizing enamel.*

Fitzgerald FT, Tierney IM: Trace metals in human disease. Adv Intern Med 30:337, 1984. *An overall introduction to trace metals in human disease.*

Nève J, Vertongen F, Molle L: Selenium deficiency. Clin Endocrinol Metab 14:629, 1985. *A useful review emphasizing the current knowledge and areas of poor understanding.*

O'Dell BL: Bioavailability of trace elements, Nutr Rev 42:301, 1984. *A useful review of problems of determining and understanding trace mineral availability.*

Prasad AS: Clinical manifestations of zinc deficiency. Am Rev Nutr 5:341, 1985. *A full review of the etiological and clinical features of zinc deficiency.*

Robinson MF: Selenium in human nutrition in New Zealand. Nutr Rev 47:99–107, 1989. *Blood selenium concentrations reflect low selenium soil content. Intravenous feeding may also be associated with a low selenium blood level and muscle pain responsive to selenomethionine.*

Wallach S: Clinical and biochemical aspects of chromium deficiency. J Am Coll Nutr 4:107, 1985. *A comprehensive readable review of chromium metabolism indicating its importance in clinical medicine.*

Williams DG: Copper deficiency in humans. Semin Hematol 20:118, 1983. *Major features of normal copper metabolism and copper deficiency are summarized in a very readable form.*

206 Principles of Nutritional Support: Enteral Nutritional Therapy

David H. Alpers

Enteral nutritional therapy implies modification of the usual diet and is used for two major general indications. The first is supplementation of protein and calories in a wide variety of situations with the intention of providing part or all of the daily requirements. This use is not disease-specific. The second and more traditional indication involves the use of diets for specific

TABLE 206–1. STRATEGY FOR CALORIE AND PROTEIN SUPPLEMENTATION

Route of Delivery	Incomplete Provision	Complete Provision
Enteral	Oral supplementation Table foods, e.g., milk, peanut butter, egg Commercial supplements Individual macronutrients (e.g., protein, fat, carbohydrate) Nutritionally complete supplement	Forced enteral feeding Nutritionally complete commercial diets Blenderized formulas
Parenteral	Peripheral (e.g., 3 per cent amino acids, 5 to 10 per cent dextrose, 10 per cent lipid emulsion)	Central (e.g., 4.25 per cent amino acid, 25 per cent dextrose, vitamins, minerals, fatty acids)

diseases or pathophysiologic situations. The diets used involve restricting a particular element of the diet (e.g., fat, lactose), adding a nutrient that may be required in larger amounts than are available from a well-balanced diet (e.g., calcium, potassium), or altering the consistency of the diet (e.g., high-fiber, full-liquid). These two major indications are discussed in this chapter. Also included is a discussion about formulating a plan for calorie and protein supplementation, which places this and the following chapter on parenteral nutrition in proper perspective.

PROTEIN AND CALORIE SUPPLEMENTATION

Initial Decisions: Completeness of Nutrient Provision and Route of Administration

The range of methods for providing protein and calorie supplements has expanded greatly beyond table foods in recent years, and likewise the range of available products for this use is very great. For many patients all that may be needed is a careful history of dietary intake, estimation of protein and caloric requirements, and adjustment of the diet to provide the needed nutrients. Whether table foods or commercial supplements are used, there are two major considerations for the physician to provide the most appropriate therapy for each patient: (1) Is the supplement intended as a partial fulfillment of daily needs (incomplete provision) or a total replacement of calories and protein (complete provision)? (2) Are the nutrients to be delivered by the enteral or the parenteral route? Table 206–1 summarizes these major choices. Forced enteral feeding refers to the delivery of nutrients to the small intestine via a small (7 to 8 French) polyurethane or silicone catheter placed through the nose or percutaneously via the endoscope (percutaneous endoscopic gastrostomy) or by a surgical procedure. Parenteral supplementation by peripheral or central vein will be discussed in Ch. 207. The options listed in Table 206–1 are not mutually exclusive. For example, sometimes forced enteral feeding can be used together with peripheral vein feeding; nutritionally complete commercial supplements can be used orally in some patients to supply total macronutrient requirements; central vein feeding can be supplemented by oral intake.

Formulating a Protein-Calorie Support Plan

Figure 206–1 illustrates a flow diagram used for selecting patients in negative protein and calorie balance for intensive nutritional support. The correct choice for nutritional support (enteral versus parenteral, oral versus forced enteral) depends largely upon the four key questions outlined in the figure. The physician should estimate protein and caloric requirements for the individual patient. Methods for making these estimates are available in a number of handbooks. While the estimates are fairly crude, they are clinically useful, because they provide some quantitative guidelines for deciding the magnitude of supplementation needed. The most commonly used formulas for determining basal requirements are those of Harris and Benedict:

$$BMR_{women} = 655 + (9.6 \times W) + (1.8 \times H) - (4.7 \times A)$$
$$BMR_{men} = 66 + (13.7 \times W) + (5 \times H) - (6.8 \times A)$$

where BMR is basal metabolic requirement in kcal; W is ideal weight in kg; H is height in cm; A is age in years. For ambulatory patients the basal requirements can be estimated at two thirds of their total caloric need. This equation underestimates BMR in malnourished patients by up to 10 per cent and overestimates it in obesity. Most ill hospitalized patients do not require calories in excess of their estimated basal requirement, based on their usual weight. Hospitalized patients receiving protein of high biologic value (egg, milk, meat) need only 0.6 gram per kilogram body weight per day for mild illness if body protein is not depleted by prior chronic or acute illness. For ambulatory patients this figure becomes 0.8 to 0.9 gram per kilogram per day to allow for the protein content of a mixed animal and vegetable diet. For severely ill patients, even if depleted of protein, the requirement rarely exceeds 1.2 grams per kilogram per day. Larger amounts of protein cannot be assimilated by sick patients, largely because of increased catabolism and the high caloric requirement needed to retain amino acids as protein. In general, calorie and protein requirements for ill or hospitalized patients have been overestimated in the past.

If the diet is meeting requirements (question 1), no further therapy is needed. If the diet is inadequate, an assessment of the patient's present nutritional status is then obtained. Caloric reserves are monitored most easily by body weight and protein reserves by serum albumin levels. Other available methods are discussed in Ch. 200. If the degree of depletion (question 2) as assessed by body weight is mild (about 5 per cent decreased) and the gastrointestinal tract is intact, oral supplements may be used. If the degree of depletion is moderate (5 to 10 per cent decreased) to severe (over 10 per cent decreased) and the anticipated duration of support is long (question 3), intensive therapy may be needed. As is apparent in the algorithm in Figure 206–1, the definition of *long* is crucial for decision making. If the patient can be expected to lose up to 10 per cent of body weight during the illness, the needed duration of treatment is considered to be long. Alternatively, an arbitrary number of days with inadequate intake can be considered "long": 7 to 10 days for normally nourished patients, 3 to 5 days for poorly nourished patients. Whether forced enteral feeding or total parenteral nutrition (TPN) via a central vein is chosen depends on the availability or adequacy of the gastrointestinal tract (question 4). The gastrointestinal tract is usually evaluated by history (the presence or absence of diarrhea or malabsorption), physical examination (normal motility or ileus), and barium radiographs. Some patients are selected for TPN because of the need for complete bowel rest. Data to support the use of this therapy have been obtained in the acute management of Crohn's disease and ulcerative colitis and in the postoperative adaptive period of the short-bowel syndrome, and severe pancreatitis (see Ch. 106). Some patients with these disorders can be treated with forced enteral feeding. Often, however, bowel rest will control symptoms more rapidly. Other considerations (social, economic) may play a role in the final choice of therapy for a given patient. The patient may be unwilling to maintain a nasal or gastric feeding tube, or hospitalization may not be possible because of cost restrictions. Finally, some patients may need to be fed via gastrostomy or jejunostomy.

The percutaneous gastrostomy has allowed relatively simple establishment of this feeding route and has expanded the indications for gastrostomy. Gastrostomy feeding is now used, especially in the United States, when the anticipated time for enteral supplementation is long, and the patient cannot swallow. The tube is placed endoscopically or radiographically if the esophagus is patent (e.g., stroke) or surgically if it is not. Complications include pneumoperitoneum, abdominal and gastric wall hematomas, and subcutaneous emphysema. A more detailed discussion of the indications for TPN can be found in the following chapter (Ch. 207).

The following categories of patients are commonly considered for enteral nutrition therapy: (1) chronically ill patients with anorexia, (2) patients with chronic inflammatory illnesses who

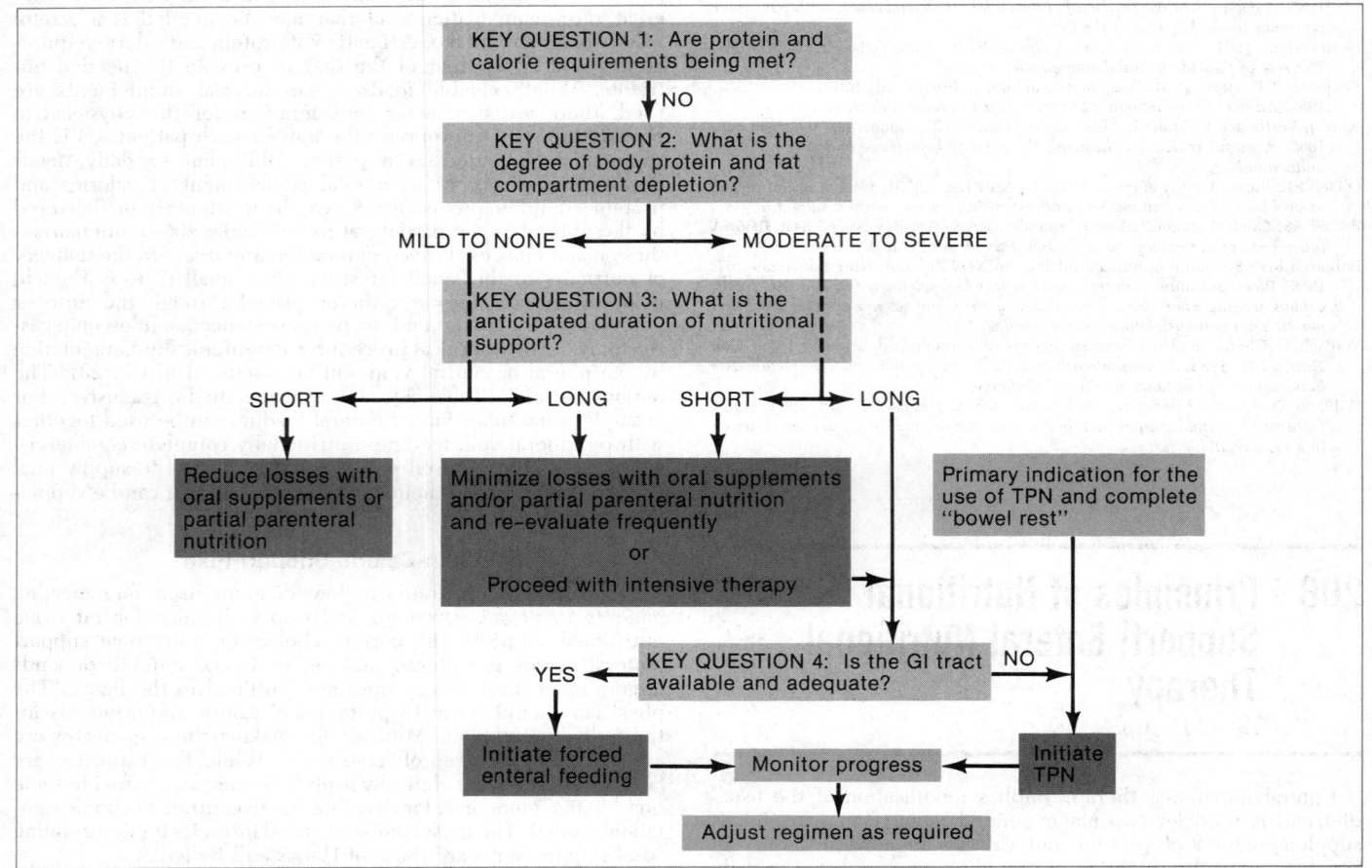

FIGURE 206–1. Flow diagram useful for selecting patients in negative protein and calorie balance for intensive nutritional support. TPN = total parenteral nutrition; GI = gastrointestinal.

have increased requirements but who can tolerate only a usual caloric intake for their size, (3) poor or marginally nourished patients preparing for tests or intestinal surgery, and (4) patients with specific dietary needs that benefit from the special characteristics of some commercial supplements (e.g., low-residue, lactose-free). Forced enteral feeding typically is used for those patients who have moderate to severe anorexia, those who cannot maintain a calorie and protein intake commensurate with their needs (e.g., burn patients), or those whose illnesses prevent them from satisfactory oral feeding (e.g., patients with cervical spine fractures or swallowing disorders).

Delivery of Enteral Supplements

TABLE FOODS

If requirements are not great and appetite is good, table foods can be recommended as protein and calorie supplements. Each ounce of meat, fish, poultry, or cheese contains about 7 grams of protein, an egg 6 to 7 grams, and one cup of milk 8 grams. One-half cup of dried beans, peas, or nuts contains 5 grams or more of protein, but these sources contain protein of a lower biologic value (sustains growth less well) and are not usually recommended for a major role in "catch up" therapy in nutritionally depleted patients. Milk products are very useful, provided that lactose intolerance is not a problem. Meat and fish are helpful if fat is well tolerated. Otherwise, poultry without skin or tuna canned in water should be selected. Peanut butter contains 8 grams of fat and 4.2 grams of protein per tablespoon and is a good source of concentrated calories and protein. Table foods remain an excellent choice for oral supplementation, because they are tasty, esthetically and socially appealing, reasonable in cost, easily obtained, and available in a wide variety of choices. If well tolerated and adequate for the requirements, they should not be supplemented by commercial supplements unless the supplements exhibit specific properties that make them preferable.

COMMERCIAL SUPPLEMENTS

Commercial supplements, like table foods, display a diversity of characteristics that help the physician determine the choice for each patient. They are available as sources of single macronutrients (protein, carbohydrate, or lipid) or as nutritionally complete supplements, containing all necessary macronutrients and micronutrients. These products are of high caloric density and precisely defined nutrient composition but have the disadvantages of limited esthetic and taste appeal, taste fatigue with constant use, frequent occurrence of diarrhea, and higher cost than table foods. The nutritionally incomplete supplements can be used when the deficiency is specific (protein or calorie) or the deficiency is anticipated only for a short time, as in preparation for surgery. Protein is not wisely provided without another source of calories, since about 25 to 40 nonprotein kilocalories are needed per gram of protein to maintain positive nitrogen balance. Otherwise, a portion of the amino acids in the protein is converted to carbohydrate to provide the energy needed for amino acid assimilation.

The nutritionally complete supplements are largely distinguished by four major characteristics: (1) the presence or absence of lactose, (2) the use of intact protein or hydrolyzed protein (or amino acids), (3) the presence of small or large amounts of fat as caloric sources, and (4) isotonic or hypertonic osmolality. Supplements that are isotonic or nearly so contain less available carbohydrate and more lipid, which is osmotically less active. This characteristic is of greatest importance when forced enteral feeding is used, but any of the hypertonic solutions may be diluted or infused at a slower rate. The other three characteristics are more important for patients with abnormal intestinal absorption. Hydrolyzed protein may be useful for patients with pancreatic insufficiency, lactose-free supplements for patients with lactose intolerance, and low-fat supplements for those with limited intestinal fat absorption. The nutritionally complete supplements just described are designed to be the sole source of daily nutrients and thus contain all needed micronutrients in adequate quantities, if deficiencies are not present and if requirements are usual. Nonprescription milk-based products also provide good sources of protein and calories in a wide variety of flavors. If the patient is lactose tolerant, they may be used very successfully.

COMPLICATIONS OF ENTERAL FEEDING USING

COMMERCIAL SUPPLEMENTS. The use of enteral feeding with highly concentrated supplements can be limited by side effects. The most common is diarrhea, which can be due to intolerance to one of the macronutrients (fat, lactose) or intolerance to the osmotic load. Altering the rate of delivery or the concentration of the supplement is often helpful, but may compromise the delivery of adequate calories. Complications of forced enteral feeding alone include esophagitis and tracheobronchial aspiration. Volume or sodium overload can occur, especially in the edema-prone patient.

THERAPEUTIC DIETS FOR SPECIFIC DISORDERS OR PATHOPHYSIOLOGIC STATES

The diets most commonly used to control symptoms are those that restrict one or another element in the diet. Diets restricted for each of the major macronutrients (fat, carbohydrate, and protein) have their individual uses (Table 206–2). As expected, these diets are helpful in altering pathophysiologic states and are not specific for any disease. Any condition causing steatorrhea can be improved symptomatically by limiting fat (triacylglyceride) intake. Care must be taken with any restrictive diet to supplement any nutrients that have been secondarily limited with fat restriction. However, levels of intake that improve symptoms in most cases (40 to 50 grams per day) still supply sufficient fat sources so that deficiency of fat-soluble vitamins does not occur. A fat-restricted diet can be made isocaloric only by increasing carbohydrate intake, because most food sources of fat also contain protein. For this diet to be successful the patient must not have any generalized carbohydrate intolerance. Similarly, the low-lactose or low-available-carbohydrate diet is low in calcium.

Most restrictive diets do not eliminate the nutrient whose content is altered. A low-lactose diet is much easier to achieve than a truly lactose-free one and is usually sufficient to relieve symptoms. Control of symptoms is the usual goal of dietary management, and restriction of the appropriate nutrient to the point at which symptoms are altered is an acceptable goal. Thus, a low-protein diet for hepatic encephalopathy should still deliver the estimated daily protein allowance (0.5 to 0.8 gram per kilogram of body weight) to avoid protein deficiency. This concept is especially important in the management of chronic renal failure, a situation in which the protein requirement may be actually increased. When the glomerular filtration rate (GFR) falls below 25 ml per minute, the protein allowance should not be more than 1.3 grams per kilogram per day (referring to ideal body weight) and falls to 0.6 gram per kilogram per day for a GFR of 4 to 10 ml per minute. Over 50 per cent of the protein intake should be of high biologic value (with high essential amino acid content). Requirements actually increase with dialysis because of the loss of amino acids in the dialysate. The allowance rises with hemodialysis to 1 gram per kilogram per day, and to 1.2 to 1.5 grams per kilogram per day with chronic peritoneal dialysis.

TABLE 206–2. THERAPEUTIC DIETS CHARACTERIZED BY RESTRICTION OF DIETARY COMPONENTS

Diet	Typical Indication
Low fat (60–75 grams/day)	Steatorrhea, mild (see Ch. 102)
Low fat (40–60 grams/day)	Steatorrhea, severe (see Ch. 102)
Low oxalate	Enteric hyperoxaluria (see Ch. 102)
Low lactose	Lactose intolerance (see Ch. 102)
Gluten free	Celiac sprue (see Ch. 102)
Low fiber	Acute diarrhea, bowel preparation (see Ch. 101)
Low protein	Hepatic encephalopathy (see Ch. 123)
	Chronic renal failure (see Ch. 77)
Elimination	Food allergies
Controlled carbohydrate	Diabetes mellitus (see Ch. 218)
Calorie restricted	Obesity (see Ch. 203)
Low sodium	Edematous states (see Ch.75)
Low fat, cholesterol, or carbohydrate according to type	Hyperlipidemia (see Ch. 172)
Low copper	Wilson's disease (see Ch. 121)
Low phosphate	Chronic renal failure (see Ch. 77)

Some of the diets used for therapy control or modify the content of macronutrients rather than restrict them. The diet for diabetes mellitus is a good example of this principle (see Ch. 218). Successful management of the obese diabetic combines a weight reduction diet with regulation of the carbohydrate content. The prudent diet recommended by the American Diabetes Association still contains 40 to 55 per cent of calories as carbohydrates, with relatively less (5 to 15 per cent) as simple sugars (requiring no pancreatic digestion) and more (30 to 45 per cent) as starch. There is also less cholesterol and saturated fats to reduce blood lipids. These latest recommendations contain relaxed restrictions on carbohydrate intake. High-starch diets are well tolerated by diabetics as long as total caloric intake is controlled. Many patients require diets that may utilize elements from diets designed specifically for weight reduction, diabetes mellitus, hyperlipidemias, and chronic renal failure.

Diets That Supplement Dietary Components

Although less commonly required, diets that add a component to the normal diet are often employed (Table 206–3). A high fiber intake has not been clearly shown to have a beneficial effect on the symptoms of all patients with irritable bowel syndrome and on the recurrence of attacks of acute diverticulitis, although supplementation with fiber is now commonly used for these disorders. The reasons for the uncertainty are that (1) these disorders are identified mostly by clinical criteria, (2) the irritable bowel syndrome is probably a heterogeneous group of motility disorders, (3) the definition of fiber and estimation of its intake are imperfectly developed, and (4) many types of fiber supplements are used, containing different components of dietary fiber. Dietary fiber is useful in the prevention and treatment of constipation not associated with laxative abuse. A diet low in fiber (see Table 206–2) is useful in acute diarrheal illness and as a preparation for barium enema, colonoscopy, and intestinal surgery. The diet is then additionally modified in the form of a clear liquid diet for further reduction in ileal residue.

There are limited data on the food content of the major components of dietary fiber, i.e., cellulose, hemicelluloses, pectin, mucilage and gums, and lignins. Thus, it is not always clear when an individual patient is ingesting a low-fiber diet, although total daily average fiber intake in the United States is probably about 12 to 15 grams lower than what is considered ideal. Most often fiber is supplemented by ingestion of commercial preparations containing psyllium seed or by the use of bran. Psyllium is rich in hemicelluloses, while bran contains more cellulose. Present practice recommends the addition of 6 to 10 grams of fiber per day (2 teaspoons of psyllium seed or three-quarters cup of bran) for the irritable bowel syndrome (characterized by alternating diarrhea and constipation) and for recurrent diverticulitis. Benefits of high fiber intake (type and amount variable) have also been reported for diabetes mellitus, maintenance of lower calorie intake, lowering of serum cholesterol, and prevention of colon cancer. At present the data do not clearly support a specific role for a fiber-supplemented diet in any of these disorders.

The best treatment for postmenopausal osteoporosis is still debatable, but it is no longer agreed that increased calcium intake needs to be an important component of the treatment plan (Ch. 238). Published reports show only a modestly positive relationship between dietary calcium and cortical bone mass, but no correlation with trabecular bone where rapid turnover occurs, and which comprises up to 50 per cent of bone in the spine. Calcium supplementation appears to be inferior to estrogen therapy in slowing bone loss in postmenopausal women. The probable long-term effects of calcium, however, are not clear, because most studies have been for 2 years or less.

When diuretics and low-sodium diets are used, potassium is frequently replaced as an inorganic salt, but dietary supplementation can often be used and would be more palatable. For instance, the salt substitutes often used with low-sodium diets contain about 12 mEq of potassium per gram, and potassium is present in fairly high concentration in most fruits and vegetables and their juices (Table 206–4). Eight ounces of frozen orange or tomato juice contains 12 mEq potassium and one medium orange or banana 6 to 8 mEq. Milk is also a good source of potassium, but because of its high sodium content would be an inappropriate supplement for a patient taking diuretics. Only some patients taking diuretics daily in appropriate doses develop hypokalemia. Urinary potassium loss can be measured; if not excessive, it can be matched by table foods. Therefore, for many patients, advice on dietary potassium supplements will be sufficient.

Protein supplements are needed for conditions characterized by excessive protein loss, such as protein-losing enteropathy, dialysis, and burns. These supplements can be supplied as table food or as commercial supplements. For each 10 grams of protein added, another 250 kcal from nonprotein sources must also be ingested to ensure that the amino acids will be converted into body protein.

Diets That Alter the Consistency of Food

One of the most common dietary manipulations used in hospitalized patients is the *liquid diet*. The *clear* liquid diet provides the daily requirement for water mostly in the form of juices, bouillons, and gelatins, and requires minimal digestion and intestinal motility, but it does not provide adequate amounts of protein, calories, vitamins, or minerals. It is also a low-fiber diet. If the patient who requires such a diet is already protein and calorie malnourished, the diet needs to be supplemented with carbohydrate, protein, or both, and with micronutrients. Even so, it is difficult to provide much more than 1000 kcal per day. For long-term use the *full* liquid diet is more often prescribed, including milk and other dairy products, cereals, and eggs. If table foods from all food groups are used or the diet is enriched with commercial supplements, the diet can be nutritionally complete. Care should be given to determining the actual food ingested, however, because a full liquid diet is often used for a patient who has some difficulty in swallowing table food. Thus, the ingested food may not equal what is ordered. This precaution, of course, should be exercised when any diet is used for therapy, but it is particularly important when impairment of food ingestion or anorexia is the reason for the prescribed diet.

The *bland diet* restricts spicy foods and is often combined with a mechanical soft diet for the treatment of peptic ulcer disease. Despite this widespread use, there are no data that clearly support the value of such a diet for any clinical condition, and present practice does not favor its use (see Ch. 98). Restriction of seasonings makes the food less palatable and discourages the successful use of whichever diet is being presented.

Alpers DH, Clouse RE, Stenson WF: Manual of Nutritional Therapeutics, 2nd ed. Boston, Little, Brown and Company, 1988. *A detailed practical account of the use of diets and enteral therapy. Includes nutritional characteristics of most commercial supplements and diets.*

American Dietetic Association: Handbook of Clinical Dietetics. New Haven, Yale University Press, 1982. *A comprehensive and carefully outlined source of obtaining the details of most diets.*

TABLE 206–4. SODIUM AND POTASSIUM CONTENT OF COMMON FOODS*

Food	Portion	Sodium Content (mg)	Potassium Content (mg)
Milk	cup	120	350
Meat, fish, poultry	ounce	25	100–180
Most fruits and their juices	cup	4–10	300–490
Most vegetables	½ cup	5–9	300–500

*Content refers to uncooked or unprocessed foods.

TABLE 206–3. THERAPEUTIC DIETS CHARACTERIZED BY SUPPLEMENTATION OF DIETARY COMPONENTS

Diet	Typical Indication
High fiber	Irritable bowel, prevention of recurrent diverticulitis
High calcium (milk products, CaCO₃, or combination)	Postmenopausal osteoporosis
High protein (high biologic value)	Chronic hemodialysis or peritoneal dialysis
High protein	Malabsorption
Supplemental potassium	Diuretic use
High calorie	Weight loss due to illness

Diet and Health: Implications for reducing chronic disease risk. Committee on Diet and Health, Food and Nutrition Board; Commission on Life Sciences, National Research Council. Washington, D.C., National Academy Press, 1989. *An up-to-date extensive survey of dietary patterns and guidelines pertaining to chronic disease, including suggestions for future research. Its conclusions are general and may not apply in all clinical situations.*

Garrow JS: Treat Obesity Seriously. London, Churchill Livingstone, 1981. *A sensible and multifaceted approach to the therapy of obesity, especially for use of diet.*

Gorlin R. The biological actions and potential clinical significance of dietary ω-3 fatty acids. Arch Intern Med 148:2043, 1988. *A judicious review of the potential uses of fish oil.*

Kabadi UM: Nutritional therapy in diabetics. Postgrad Med 79:145, 1986. *A balanced review of carbohydrate restriction.*

Physiological Effects and Health Consequences of Dietary Fiber. Washington, D.C., Life Sciences Research Office, Federation of American Societies for Experimental Biology, 1987. *Summarizes the evidence for the role of fiber in human disease.*

Report of the National Cholesterol Education Program Expert Panel on Detection, Evaluation, and Treatment of High Blood Cholesterol in Adults. Arch Intern Med 148:36, 1988. *The most definitive statement available on the rationale for and use of altered fat diets for atherosclerosis.*

The Surgeon General's Report on Nutrition and Health. U.S. Dept of Health and Human Services. DHHS (PHS) Publication No. 88–80210, 1988. *Focus is on the relationship of diet to chronic diseases, more from the point of view of nutritional policy makers than individual physicians.*

Taylor TV: Miscellaneous problems in the stomach and duodenum: Percutaneous endoscopic gastrostomy. Curr Opinion Gastroenterol 5:874, 1989. *A brief summary of recent experience with this technique.*

207 Parenteral Nutrition

Ray E. Clouse

Parenteral nutrition includes delivery of micronutrients and macronutrients, and all recognized human nutrients can be provided. Those nutrients that rapidly become depleted in disease, such as water and major minerals, are administered routinely by vein to the hospitalized patient. Concentrated solutions are needed to provide protein and calories, and central venous access is often required. The complications associated with these solutions and with the access catheters become important limiting factors in the routine use of more comprehensive parenteral nutrition for the average patient. Although parenteral nutrition could be utilized in much the same way as enteral supplements or forced enteral feeding when an appropriate nutritional support plan is designed (see Ch. 206), parenteral nutrition is usually reserved for those requiring the total daily administration of protein and calories by the intravenous route.

PARENTERAL ENERGY AND PROTEIN DELIVERY

Protein and calorie requirements are closely linked. Positive nitrogen balance, reflecting net positive endogenous protein synthesis, is most successfully accomplished when positive energy balance has been achieved. If parenteral nonprotein calories are provided for the average hospitalized patient in a ratio of calories to amino acid nitrogen (in grams) of greater than or equal to 150:1, delivered amino acids are likely to be utilized for protein synthesis. The required ratio decreases in more intense catabolic states (e.g., major burns) and increases in less stressed situations.

ENERGY (CALORIE) SOURCES. Both carbohydrate and lipid are used as parenteral calorie sources (Table 207–1). The monohydrate form of dextrose used in most commercial intravenous solutions provides 3.4 kcal per gram, in contrast to 4 kcal per gram for the carbohydrate alone. Dextrose can be used as the sole nonprotein calorie source. Aproximately 50 per cent of patients require insulin supplementation in the parenteral infusion if dextrose is used to meet all daily calorie requirements. Lipid emulsions contain a source of calories in the form of emulsified droplets of soybean or safflower oil, which provide 9 kcal per gram, supplemented slightly by the caloric contribution of the emulsifiers (Table 207–1). Lipid emulsions may be used to supply the essential fatty acid linoleic acid as well as up to 70 per cent of the daily caloric requirement. A contraindication to the use of the emulsions is pre-existing hyperlipidemia. Complications related to the lipids are uncommon but may limit their use (see below).

The preferred parenteral energy source or combination of sources varies with different patient situations. Positive energy balance and nitrogen balance can be achieved if dextrose is used alone to provide daily calories, as long as adequate amino acids are also supplied. This fact is of importance to the patient intolerant to the lipid emulsions. Lipid emulsions reduce the likelihood of hyperglycemia, the volume of fluid needed, and the metabolic response to the infusion. They also are utilized for their essential fatty acid content. Thus, a combination of lipids and dextrose is usually employed as the energy source. Lipids also have theoretical and practical advantages in patients with respiratory compromise because they have a lower respiratory quotient (0.7) than carbohydrates (1.0): Less carbon dioxide is produced from delivery of a lipid-dextrose combination than from an equicaloric dextrose solution.

Lipid emulsions are somewhat more expensive than dextrose and usually necessitate additional intravenous equipment. The use of a combination of lipid and dextrose with other nutrients in a single infusion bag has eliminated some of the cumbersome equipment required for lipid infusion, but not all patients are in stable enough condition to make this technique practical.

PROTEIN DELIVERY. Protein requirements are met in parenteral nutrition by infusion of amino acids. Amino acid profiles in standard commercial products are based largely on normal plasma amino acid concentrations, with modifications to stimulate anabolism. The amino acid content (in grams) is roughly comparable to the dietary protein in the RDA, except for differences due to absorption efficiency and slight differences related to dissimilarities of amino acid profiles in average dietary proteins and in the solutions.

Amino acid ratios in specialized commercial products have been modified for use in renal failure, liver failure, and increased metabolic stress. Relatively reduced concentrations of essential amino acids are found in the plasma profiles of patients with renal failure, possibly as a result of the catabolic state of uremia. Blood urea nitrogen levels are reduced yet positive nitrogen balance is attained if a large percentage of the protein requirement is provided as essential amino acids in these patients. The parenteral formulation employed depends on the conditions of the renal failure. In chronic stable renal failure without dialysis, a modified commercial solution with higher proportions of essential amino acids may prevent worsening of uremia yet accomplish positive nitrogen balance. Once dialysis is employed, a more balanced, standard amino acid solution should be used. Consistent benefit of commercial solutions with increased proportions of essential amino acids has not been demonstrated in acute renal failure, but outcome of these patients depends upon many variables. The use of essential amino acids alone in relatively low quantities in conjunction with concentrated dextrose is being studied. In principle, the dextrose should partially inhibit amino acid use for gluconeogenesis, thereby slowing urea formation and forcing reutilization of nonessential amino acids for protein synthesis. Both essential and nonessential amino acids are ultimately necessary, however, for sustained anabolism.

Parenteral solutions favoring the branched-chain amino acids (isoleucine, leucine, valine) are used in some cases of liver failure and in metabolic stress. Routine use of these formulas remains controversial because of their expense in relation to their documented benefits. In liver failure, blood levels of aromatic amino acids (phenylalanine, tyrosine, tryptophan) are elevated, whereas levels of branched-chain amino acids are decreased; the cause for this alteration is unclear. Aromatic amino acids enter the brain and participate in encephalopathy. In order to meet protein

TABLE 207–1. PROTEIN AND CALORIE SOURCES UTILIZED IN PARENTERAL NUTRITION

Macronutrient Category		Parenteral Form of Macronutrient	Nonprotein Caloric Value
Protein		Crystalline amino acids	
Calories	Carbohydrate	Dextrose monohydrate	3.4 kcal/g
	Fat	Lipid emulsion	10% emulsion—1.1 kcal/ml 20% emulsion—2.0 kcal/ml

requirements without further promoting encephalopathy, parenteral formulations with increased ratios of branched-chain amino acids to aromatic amino acids can be used (branched-chain amino acids increased to 35 to 45 per cent of total from the usual of 20 to 25 per cent in standard solutions). Besides not promoting encephalopathy, the branched-chain amino acids do not require any hepatic processing as metabolic substrates. Best use of modified amino acid solutions in liver disease may be in mildly encephalopathic patients with acute exacerbations of chronic liver failure. The branched-chain amino acids are oxidized extrahepatically in skeletal muscle, heart, and kidney and serve as a fuel source for muscle in the injured state. These amino acids also appear to have a regulatory role in preventing protein degradation and stimulating protein synthesis both in liver and muscle. Because of these observations, parenteral formulas with branched-chain amino acids composing 45 to 50 per cent of total amino acids have been suggested for use in cases of sepsis or extreme metabolic stress, situations of marked catabolism resistant to reversal.

PRACTICAL APPLICATIONS. A combination of dextrose, amino acids, and water provides the base solution to which vitamins and minerals can be added. Parenteral nutrition solutions that provide all energy and protein requirements are administered through a central vein in most cases because they are so hyperosmotic. For example, a formulation made from 500 ml of 50 per cent dextrose (2500 mOsm per liter) and 500 ml of 8.5 per cent amino acids (850 mOsm per liter) would provide 850 kcal (from nonprotein sources) and 42.5 grams of amino acids with a resultant osmolarity of 1675 mOsm per liter. All additives, particularly major minerals (e.g., sodium, potassium), further raise the final osmolarity. Lipid emulsions are infused in parallel with the base solution or are added directly to the solution bag. If lipids, dextrose, and amino acids are combined ("3-in-1" solutions), compatibility restrictions limit the range of formulations. Macronutrient delivery can be shortened for patients in stable condition to a 10- to 12-hour period, e.g., at night. Both methods of calorie and protein delivery are effective in achieving positive energy and nitrogen balance. Gradual conversion over 2 to 3 days is required from a 24-hour schedule to the cyclic schedule. Once conversion is effected, the base solution (and lipid emulsion, if used as a daily energy source) is discontinued each morning by reducing the rate in two or three 30-minute steps. The rate is similarly increased at the reinitiation of infusion in the evening. These precautions are effective in preventing hypoglycemia for most patients. Patients on cyclic regimens are then free from infusion in the daytime.

Macronutrients may also be provided through peripheral veins. Lesser concentrations of dextrose and amino acids are required to keep the final osmolarity less than 600 to 800 mOsm per liter and thereby reduce the likelihood of thrombophlebitis. Continuous coadministration of isotonic lipid emulsion reduces the osmolarity yet allows for the total energy and protein requirement to be infused. For this reason, lipid emulsions are regularly used as daily energy sources in peripheral vein parenteral nutrition. Parenteral prescriptions that provide fewer calories than the daily energy requirement can serve as supplements to an inadequate enteral regimen or can be used alone to reduce negative nitrogen balance. Even with excessive amino acid infusion (greater than 2 grams per kilogram per day), however, sustained positive nitrogen balance is not accomplished without adequate energy supply. Thus this parenteral nutrition practice is not a substitute for more intensive support, if nutritional restoration is the goal.

TOTAL PARENTERAL NUTRITION

Besides amino acids and calorie sources, all other recognized nutrients can be provided by a parenteral route. Total parenteral nutrition (TPN) is required for short or long periods by patients with either temporarily or permanently unusable or inadequate small intestines. In most instances, a central venous access is employed. Detailed techniques of TPN are beyond the scope of this textbook and are described in many monographs and handbooks. The most successful TPN programs involve direction by a knowledgeable physician and the cooperation of informed and interested colleagues in the pharmacy, nursing, and dietetics departments.

INDICATIONS. A small number of patients require lifelong TPN because of extensive resection (e.g., from mesenteric vascular accidents, Crohn's disease, trauma) or advanced small bowel disease (e.g., scleroderma, radiation enteritis). The majority of patients with short-bowel syndrome from resection, however, can eventually be managed with oral feeding after an initial adaptation period. More commonly TPN is indicated as a temporary nutritional therapy for two patient groups: (1) those selected for intensive nutritional support in whom the intestinal tract is not usable for forced enteral feeding (see Ch. 206) and (2) those in whom a nothing-by-mouth regimen ("bowel rest") would be beneficial to a primary gastrointestinal disease. The majority of patients placed on a TPN regimen are those with the first indication. Figure 206–1 gives a flow diagram incorporating the various questions used in deciding which patients are indeed candidates for intensive nutritional support. In general, this group (a) has moderate to severe protein compartment depletion at the initial evaluation and is expected to suffer significant additional losses with the current illness, or (b) will be undergoing a surgical intervention or specialized treatment (e.g., radiation) that will predictably interfere with enteral nutritional support.

Gastrointestinal Diseases. Parenteral nutrition has two potential roles in patients with gastrointestinal diseases: (1) to provide nutritional restoration and (2) to assist disease regression by allowing the bowel to remain in an unstimulated state (bowel rest). The ability of TPN to reverse malnutrition associated with gastrointestinal disease is not disputed, and TPN is indicated for any patient selected for intensive nutritional support by the conventional algorithm. Thus, patients with nutritional deterioration from severe inflammatory bowel disease may well benefit from TPN for nutritional restoration. The value of bowel rest, in contrast, remains controversial, particularly for inflammatory bowel disease. A summary of reported responses to TPN and bowel rest for a variety of gastrointestinal diseases is listed in Table 207–2. In most of these disorders, enteral dietary treatment is also effective, other treatments (such as corticosteroids for inflammatory bowel disease) have influenced the reported results, and overall efficacy of the bowel rest regimen remains unproven. Because of these observations, the primary indication for TPN in gastrointestinal disease is for nutritional support when enteral treatment is not feasible. Bowel rest regimens are generally reserved for patients who fail other conventional treatments. In the case of inflammatory bowel disease, colonic disorders are less likely than small intestinal disorders to respond to bowel rest.

TPN with or without bowel rest is also often indicated in gastrointestinal disorders associated with severe symptoms, especially if the patient would also be selected for intensive nutritional support. Such conditions include severe diarrhea,

TABLE 207–2. SUMMARY OF THE EFFECTS OF TOTAL PARENTERAL NUTRITION (TPN) WITH BOWEL REST IN VARIOUS DISEASES

Disease	Nutritional Maintenance or Repletion Achieved	Short-Term (In-Hospital) Disease Regression	Long-Term Disease Regression
Ulcerative colitis*	Majority	30–50%	20–30%
Crohn's disease*	Yes	60–80%	50–60%
Subgroup with fistulas†	Yes	30–40%	10–30%
Subgroup with colitis†	Yes	60%	NA‡
Enterocutaneous fistulas (not Crohn's disease)	Yes	30–70% closure§	NA
Severe pancreatitis	Yes¶	NA	NA

*Many patients in reported series are treated with corticosteroids as well as TPN and bowel rest.

†Small patient series; subgroups not always designated.

‡Adequate data not available.

§Many patients eventually managed with surgical therapy; wide range of reported success rates.

¶Parenteral nutrition is successful and does not contribute to morbidity of pancreatitis despite theoretical concern regarding pancreatic stimulatory effects.

intractable vomiting, and small intestinal disorders that interfere significantly with enteral feeding (e.g., radiation enteritis, obstruction from inflammatory adhesions, following small bowel resection).

Perioperative Management. A strong correlation exists between nutritional status and postoperative morbidity and mortality. Advantages from routine use of preoperative TPN, however, have not been established. One large and well-designed study has demonstrated the value of 10 days of preoperative TPN in malnourished patients undergoing surgery for gastrointestinal tract malignancies. Guidelines for choosing patients for preoperative TPN remain incomplete, but 7 to 10 days of preoperative treatment for malnourished subjects needing a major abdominal or thoracic operation are now recommended. Data are also absent to support the use of TPN in managing postoperative complications. However, TPN prevents nutritional deterioration in subjects with complications that interfere with eating (e.g., prolonged ileus, mechanical obstruction) or that increase metabolic demands (e.g., wound dehiscence, intra-abdominal abscess). In some of these instances, forced enteral feeding may be successful and more cost effective.

Other Diseases. When TPN is utilized in management of patients with disease not involving the gastrointestinal tract, bowel rest is not enforced. Use of TPN with modified amino acid formulas in patients with hepatic and renal disease has been mentioned. Despite intuitive impressions that TPN should reduce mortality and could improve organ function in these disorders, results from clinical studies have not been conclusive. In patients with cancer, nutritional status can be maintained or improved with an adequate TPN program, but this has not proved to be of overall benefit in enhancing tumor responsiveness to antineoplastic agents. The best candidates for intensive nutritional support are those who have tumors potentially responsive to anticancer therapy, but who could not receive optimal management because of the combined detrimental effects of the planned therapy and malnutrition. Patients undergoing allogeneic bone marrow transplantation for leukemia often typify this situation. Some patients can be managed with forced enteral nutrition rather than TPN. Patients who are severely catabolic or who will likely need major surgery may also be candidates for intensive nutritional support. Such candidates would be selected by following the algorithm outlined in Ch. 206.

Home TPN. Home administration should be considered for patients with irreversible gastrointestinal disease or for patients whose conditions are relatively stable and who need TPN for a month or more. The cyclic method of macronutrient delivery and long central catheters burrowed through a subcutaneous tunnel on the anterior chest are employed. Approximately one third of patients requiring home TPN have malignant disease or intestinal complications related to therapy for malignant disease (resection or radiation). One third have inflammatory bowel disease, and the remainder have a variety of intestinal disorders, including severe gastrointestinal motility disturbances (such as scleroderma bowel) and short-bowel syndrome following trauma or ischemic insult.

NUTRIENTS PROVIDED DURING TPN (Table 207–3). Protein requirements (as described in Ch. 199) are met with crystalline amino acids in commercially available solutions. Nonprotein calories are provided by concentrated dextrose and by lipid emulsions. Two liters of a base solution composed of equal amounts of 8.5 per cent amino acids and 50 per cent dextrose in conjunction with 500 ml of a 10 per cent lipid emulsion is a feasible daily protein-calorie prescription. This provides approximately 80 grams of protein as amino acids, 1680 carbohydrate calories, and 550 fat calories. The resultant nonprotein calorie–nitrogen ratio is 170:1, with 25 per cent of the daily calories provided by fat. An alternate regimen would provide all the nonprotein calories as dextrose. The daily protein and calorie prescription should be tailored to a patient's requirements or exceed them by 20 to 40 grams of protein and 500 to 1000 kcal, if restoration of depleted compartments is a goal. Water requirement varies, depending on the capability of the patient to excrete an osmotic load, 30 ml per kilogram (or approximately 1 ml per kilocalorie delivered) being typical. Increased water delivery is necessary for fever (360 ml per day per degree Celsius elevation) and anabolism (300 to 400 ml per day).

Major mineral requirements vary considerably from patient to

TABLE 207–3. TYPICAL DAILY NUTRIENT PROVISIONS DURING TOTAL PARENTERAL NUTRITION (TPN) FOR STABLE ADULT PATIENTS WITHOUT CARDIAC, HEPATIC, OR RENAL FAILURE

Calories	Dextrose	60–80% of requirement (see Ch. 199)
	Lipid emulsion*	20–40% of requirement
Protein	Crystalline amino acids	100% of requirement (see Ch. 199)
Minerals	Sodium	90–120 mEq
	Potassium	90–150 mEq
	Chloride	90–150 mEq
	Calcium	12–16 mEq
	Phosphorus	20–40 mmol
	Magnesium	12–16 mEq
	Iron†	
	Zinc‡	2.5–4 mg
	Copper	300–500 μg
	Chromium	10–20 μg
	Manganese	0.15–4 mg
	Selenium§	40–80 μg
	Iodine§	70–140 μg
	Molybdenum§	100–200 μg
Vitamins	A	3300 IU
	D	200 IU
	E	10 IU
	B_1 (thiamine)	3.0 mg
	B_2 (riboflavin)	3.6 mg
	Pantothenic acid	15.0 mg
	Niacin	40.0 mg
	B_6 (pyridoxine)	4.0 mg
	Biotin	60.0 μg
	Folic acid	400.0 μg
	B_{12} (cobalamin)**	5.0 μg
	C (ascorbic acid)	100.0 mg††
	K	5 mg/wk‡‡
Essential Fatty Acid§§	Linoleic acid	4% of total calories

*See text for a discussion of the use of lipid emulsion as a daily calorie source. May be co-administered with the base sodium.

†The daily requirement (not taking phlebotomy losses into consideration) is about 1.5 mg and can be met by giving 1 ml (50 mg Fe) of iron-dextran solution intramuscularly per month. Replacement is usually dictated by indices of iron stores.

‡Requirements are increased if intestinal fluid losses are great (see Ch. 205).

§Additive usually reserved for patients on long courses of TPN.

**May be given by monthly intramuscular injection.

††Daily provision often increased to 500 mg or more during periods of catabolic stress.

‡‡Not provided by multivitamin preparation; given by separate injection.

§§Provided by lipid emulsions on a biweekly or triweekly basis. Linolenic acid is also present in some emulsions and may be required during long-term TPN (see text).

patient and during any one patient's course of TPN. In particular, potassium requirements may be initially large because of extracellular to intracellular fluxes with glucose (and possibly insulin) infusion and because of reversal of the catabolic state. The ranges of major mineral requirements listed in Table 207–3 are typical for the average adult patient, but careful monitoring of serum levels is always necessary to determine the correct provision, especially in the first few weeks of TPN.

Deficiencies of trace elements are rarely observed in patients receiving oral feedings because these nutrients are widely distributed among foods and the requirements are low. Deficiencies of zinc, chromium, copper, molybdenum, and selenium may occur during long courses of TPN, however. Such deficiencies are now prevented by supplementing TPN fluid with trace elements from the outset. Zinc, copper, chromium, and manganese are commonly provided; selenium and iodine (and occasionally molybdenum) are usually given only to patients receiving long courses of TPN, as during home TPN. Manganese deficiency has not yet been reported in TPN patients. See Ch. 205 for further discussion of the trace elements.

Recommendations for vitamin supplementation are given in

Table 207–3; few detrimental effects have appeared when these guidelines have been followed. More commonly, vitamin deficiency results from the inadvertent omission of folate or cobalamin, which may not be included in the multivitamin preparation used, or from omission of vitamin K, which is not included in any parenteral multivitamin formulation. Less vitamin D than the recommendation is necessary for patients undergoing long-term therapy.

Linoleic, linolenic, and arachidonic acids cannot be synthesized by humans. However, essential fatty acid (EFA) deficiency can usually be prevented by supplying adequate quantities of linoleic acid alone. EFA deficiency is rarely observed as an isolated deficiency except during TPN. A large amount (8 to 10 per cent) of the fat in adipose tissue contains the EFA's. However, the high insulin levels observed during TPN with concentrated dextrose are believed to impair access to this store through inhibition of lipolysis. Manifestations of EFA deficiency include dry, cracked skin, coarsening of the hair, hair loss, and impaired wound healing. It is estimated that 4 to 5 per cent of the daily energy requirement should be provided by linoleic acid to prevent deficiency, and lipid emulsions (500 ml of 10 per cent emulsion triweekly) satisfy this requirement. A report of linolenic acid deficiency in a child receiving a lipid emulsion low in this fatty acid during long-term TPN suggests that linoleic acid alone may not always be adequate to prevent EFA deficiency in humans. Use of a lipid emulsion with both linoleic and linolenic acid is currrently recommended to avoid EFA deficiency during long courses of TPN.

COMPLICATIONS OF PARENTERAL NUTRITION

Both administration-related and metabolic complications may occur with parenteral nutrition (Table 207–4). Several complications can be detected by a chest radiograph (in expiration if pneumothorax is suspected) after central-vein catheter insertion, a practice that should always be followed. Some degree of clinically inapparent catheter-related thrombosis may occur in as many as 50 per cent of patients. At present, only symptomatic patients (certainly less than 5 per cent of those with subclavian vein catheters) are observed and treated for noninfected thrombosis along the catheter path. Thrombophlebitis from hyperos-

TABLE 207–4. COMPLICATIONS OF PARENTERAL NUTRITION

Administration-related Complications
Central vein catheter
  Infection
  Inappropriate tip placement
  Pneumothorax
  Venous thrombosis
  Hemothorax
  Air embolus
  Arterial laceration
  Brachial plexus injury
  Catheter fragmentation and embolization
Peripheral vein catheter
  Thrombophlebitis
  Infection

Metabolic Complications
More frequent
  Hyperglycemia and hyperosmolarity
  Hypoglycemia
  Electrolyte disturbances
  BUN elevation
  Liver dysfunction
  Fatty liver
  Hypercapnia
  Cholelithiasis (long-term treatment)
  Hyperlipidemia from lipid emulsion
Rare
  Vitamin and trace mineral deficiency (Fig. 207–1)
  Essential fatty acid deficiency
  Metabolic bone disease
  Other adverse reaction to lipid emulsion
  Hyperammonemia

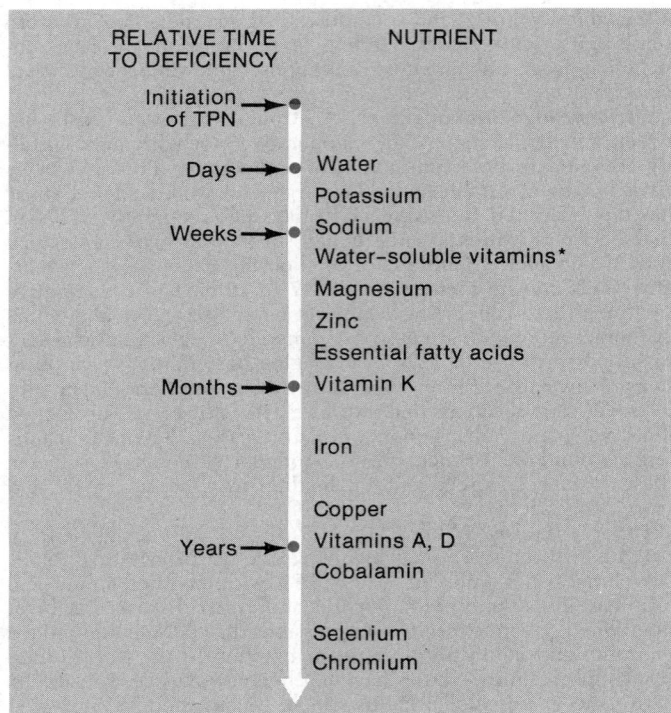

FIGURE 207–1. Relative time to the development of nutrient deficiencies during inadequately supplemented total parenteral nutrition (TPN). The time is proportional to body stores and inversely related to the fractional catabolic rate of the nutrient in an individual patient. Thus, the relative times given are only estimates. (*Excluding cobalamin.)

molar solutions is the most frequent administration-related complication when a peripheral vein is used.

Catheter-related sepsis can be held to no more than 5 per cent of patients treated with TPN of varying course length in a typical hospital-based program if maximal efforts are being made to prevent infection. Contamination from the catheter hub is often responsible for catheter-related infection. Culturing of material from removed catheter tips indicates whether the source of fever was actually an infected catheter.

Metabolic complications include the appearance of nutritional deficiencies resulting from inadequately prescribed TPN. Figure 207–1 shows the relative time to appearance of deficiencies under these circumstances. Each deficiency, of course, becomes more quickly apparent if body stores of that nutrient were originally depleted. Deficiencies are rare if nutrients are attentively prescribed.

Hyperglycemia is common in patients given concentrated dextrose by central vein. Regular insulin should be added to the base solution to keep serum glucose below 200 mg per deciliter. *Hypoglycemia* is not likely to occur if (1) exogenous insulin is added to the base solution rather than given subcutaneously, (2) the base solution is not interrupted abruptly, and (3) parenteral nutrition is terminated slowly over 24 hours or more with a stepwise reduction in the rate of glucose delivery. Incorrect provisions of major minerals can also be detected by regular laboratory monitoring, especially during the first 2 weeks of parenteral nutrition therapy.

Hepatic dysfunction not infrequently occurs. Increases in serum levels of liver enzyme activities are frequently noted following initiation of TPN. Transaminase increases usually do not persist. Delayed or persistent increases (> 20 days) may indicate toxic hepatitis related to the amino acid infusion or, more likely, a process not related to parenteral nutrition. Elevations of alkaline phosphatase values (up to two times normal) are noted in half of patients receiving TPN for more than 20 days. In some patients this represents fat accumulation from excessive carbohydrate feeding. Painful hepatomegaly may occur in these circumstances; fatty liver may be detected by computed tomography. Prevention or correction of increases of liver enzymes has been observed in some patients treated with metronidazole. Reduction in overgrowth of intestinal organisms and their toxic by-products in the portal stream has been speculated as the mechanism of this effect.

Periarticular, long-bone, and back pain, a syndrome that usually appears months into a course of TPN, is of unclear cause, but is likely related to altered vitamin D metabolism. Other factors contributing to bone disease include hypercalciuria observed during the TPN infusion (probably related to glucose loading and/or increased organic sulfate burden) and possibly improper trace mineral administration. Patients respond to discontinuation of TPN and removal of vitamin D from the TPN fluid.

Early or immediate *reactions to lipid emulsions* (dyspnea, cyanosis, cutaneous allergic phenomena, nausea, headache, back pain, autonomic discharge) occur with an incidence of less than 1 per cent. Hyperlipidemia resulting from the infusion should clear within 4 hours after the infusion. Poor lipid clearance is common with renal or hepatic failure. Delayed adverse reactions include hepatomegaly, jaundice, splenomegaly, thrombocytopenia, and leukopenia. Alterations in pulmonary function studies may occur in patients receiving lipid emulsions. A reduction in pulmonary diffusing capacity may be the most significant change, a change that has been seriously detrimental to premature infants with hyaline membrane disease, but less clinically significant to adults with respiratory disease.

As many as one third of patients treated with TPN for a period of 2 years have detectable *gallstones*. The prevalence is even higher (50 per cent) in the subset with ileal disease (Crohn's disease or prior resection or both). Gallbladder stasis and an increase in bile saturation with fasting are possible explanations for these higher than expected prevalences.

Alpers DH, Clouse RE, Stenson WF: Manual of Nutritional Therapeutics, 2nd ed. Boston, Little, Brown and Company, 1988. *This manual outlines parenteral nutrient requirements and describes techniques of parenteral nutrition in a chapter devoted to the subject. It is also a reference source for nutrient composition of proprietary products.*

A.S.P.E.N. Board of Directors: Guidelines for use of local parenteral nutrition in the hospitalized adult patient. J Parent Enteral Nutr 10:441, 1986. *A more comprehensive list of current recommendations for the use of parenteral nutrition in various disease settings.*

Berger R, Adams L: Nutritional support in the critical care setting. Chest 96:139, 1989. *A review of the principles and practical applications of parenteral nutrition in the intensive care unit.*

Detsky AS, Baker JP, O'Rourke K, Goel V: Perioperative parenteral nutrition: A meta-analysis. Ann Intern Med 107:195, 1987. *A comprehensive review of the trials examining TPN in the perioperative setting.*

Seidman EG: Nutritional management of inflammatory bowel disease. Gastroenterol Clin North Am 17:129, 1989. *Comparison of parenteral and enteral nutrition management strategies in patients with inflammatory bowel disease.*

PART XVI
ENDOCRINE AND REPRODUCTIVE DISEASES

208 Principles of Endocrinology

Gordon N. Gill

Communication is essential for all life processes. Accurate sensing of the environment and appropriate coordinated responses depend on the nervous and endocrine systems, which are tightly interwoven. Nervous system functions are mediated by hormones, and the endocrine system is centrally controlled by the nervous system. Communication between cells is necessary for development from a single fertilized egg to a mature adult, for an orderly reproductive cycle, and for homeostatic adjustments to a constantly changing environment. Hormones, distinct chemical messengers, transmit information from one cell to another to coordinate homeostatic adaptations, growth, development, and reproduction. Hormones, a word derived from Greek meaning "excite" or "set in motion," bind with high affinity and specificity to receptors, which are allosteric proteins. Receptor proteins have two essential functional characteristics: a recognition site, which binds hormone with high specificity and affinity, and an activity site, which transduces the information received into a biochemical message. Allosteric receptor proteins adopt various conformational states; binding of the hormone ligand results in the active conformation. The initial event in hormone action is thus a bimolecular reaction dependent on the concentration of hormone, the concentration of receptor, and the affinity of receptor for hormone.

$$[\text{Hormone}] + [\text{Receptor}] \underset{k_{-1}}{\overset{k_1}{\rightleftharpoons}} [\text{Hormone-Receptor}]$$

Inactive   Active

Factors that control the concentration of both hormone and receptor determine biologic responses of cells, of organs, and of the whole organism.

Traditional endocrinology dealt with the glands that produce hormones and the concentrations of hormone to which cells expressing receptors are exposed. Biosynthesis, secretion, transport of hormone to target cells, and metabolic inactivation determine the effective hormone concentration. Diseases of endocrine glands that impair hormone production result in deficiency states, while diseases that cause excessive production result in hormone excess states. Expression of receptor is equally important in forming the active hormone-receptor complex. Genetic and acquired diseases that impair receptors result in deficiency states even though hormone concentrations are compensatorily increased. Increased receptor expression results in an excess state, an event that occurs with growth factor receptors in malignant transformation.

Hormones are produced not only by the glands of internal secretion but by a variety of cells throughout the body. Neurohormones, produced in the hypothalamus, are also produced in cells throughout the nervous system to modulate neuronal function. Gastrointestinal hormones are produced within the nervous system. Hormones that regulate production and maturation of cells of the hematopoietic and immune systems are made in cells of these lineages and in endothelial and mesenchymal cells. Growth-promoting and -inhibiting hormones (growth factors and

growth inhibitors) are produced by macrophages and mesenchymal cells. Many of these signaling molecules do not travel long distances through the blood to reach target cells as do classic hormones (endocrine), but act on target cells in the vicinity of the producer cell (paracrine) or even on the producer cell itself (autocrine). During development, cell surface hormones may act on the cell surface receptor of a neighbor cell as a cell-cell communication system. Regardless of signaling distance, the same principles of hormone-receptor interactions operate.

HOW HORMONES WORK

Two classes of hormones operate via two types of receptors (Fig. 208–1). Peptide hormones are synthesized as parts of larger protein molecules and are processed as secretory proteins. They act via receptors located in the cell membrane with the recognition/binding site exposed on the cell surface and the activity domain facing the inside of the cell. Activated cell surface receptors use a variety of strategies to transduce signal information, often activating second messengers, which amplify and distribute the molecular information. Many peptide hormones ultimately signal via regulation of protein phosphorylation. In this most common process through which proteins are covalently modified, a phosphate group is donated to the protein by adenosine triphosphate. This allows peptide hormones to change rapidly the conformation and thus the function of existing cell enzymes. It also allows somewhat slower changes in gene tran-

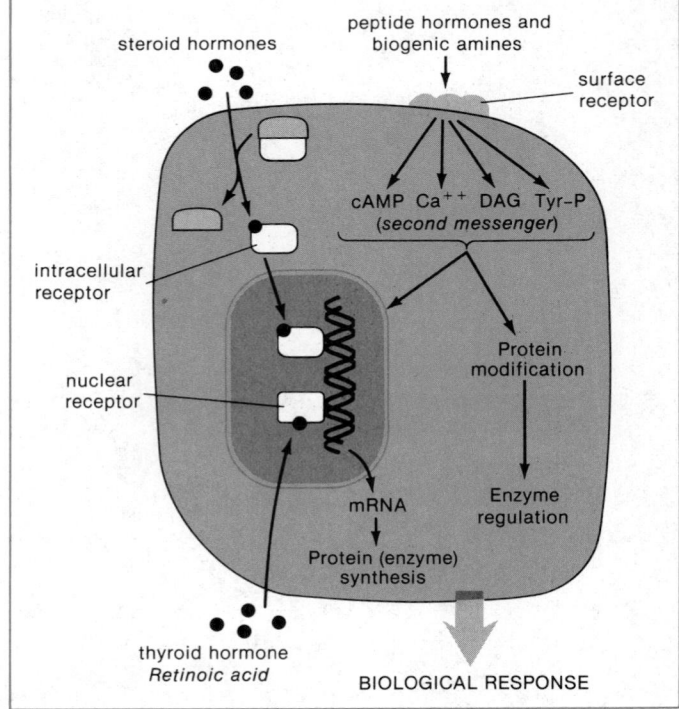

FIGURE 208–1. Mechanisms by which peptide and steroid hormones signal.

scription to regulate the concentration of enzyme proteins. Biogenic amines function like peptide hormones.

Steroid hormones are synthesized from precursor cholesterol. Thyroid hormone, retinoic acid (vitamin A), and vitamin D are synthesized via separate pathways but act through the same family of receptors and mechanisms as do steroid hormones. This group of hormones acts via structurally related receptors that bind to DNA recognition sites to regulate transcription of target genes. They change the concentration of cell proteins, primarily enzymes, and thus the metabolic activity underlying the physiologic response.

Peptide Hormones Act Via Cell Surface Receptors

HORMONE BINDING AND SIGNAL TRANSDUCTION. Peptide hormone receptors have one of three general structures (Fig. 208–2): (1) a seven membrane–spanning structure, in which the recognition site is formed by exterior sequences between membrane-spanning helices and the activity site is formed by interhelical regions inside the cell, (2) a single membrane-spanning helical structure separating the recognition domain from the cytoplasmic domain, which contains an intrinsic enzyme activity, and (3) a single membrane-spanning helix that separates the recognition domain from an intracellular domain that couples to second messenger systems as do the seven member–spanning receptors. The protein coupled may be an intracellular tyrosine kinase or other enzyme.

Hormone ligands and receptors bind with high affinities (equilibrium dissociation constants (K_D) of nM to pM), thus providing the specificity necessary for cells to decode the information provided by the low concentration of hormone present among the many other circulating and extracellular proteins. Measurements of hormone binding to cell surface receptors yield complex functions. These are likely due to interaction of hormone-receptor complexes with cell proteins but may arise from receptor aggregation, receptor modification, or cooperativity in binding.

The conformational change resulting from peptide hormone binding activates receptors to signal from the cell surface. Removal of receptors from the cell surface results in down-regulation and attenuation of the response. Binding affinities and dose-response curves for the initial event in cell signaling are the same. For example, binding of ACTH and production of cAMP occur with similar affinities and saturation; binding of insulin and activation of protein tyrosine kinase also occur with the same affinity and saturation. Biologic responses consequent to these initial events occur via a series of amplifications, each with its own affinity. The result is a dose-response curve for biologic

activities which is more sensitive than that for binding and activation of the initial response. Full biologic responses may thus occur at a low concentration of hormone that results in occupancy of only 10 per cent or less of receptors. This provides high sensitivity to small changes in hormone concentration. It also provides significant reserve. Hormone-induced down-regulation may remove 90 per cent of receptors from the cell surface. This renders the cell refractory to the initial hormone concentration, but if the need is great enough, hormone concentrations can increase 10-fold and fully activate the residual 10 per cent of receptors to give full biologic responses. Such a response system provides high initial sensitivity, buffering via down-regulation against excessive hormone responses, but a reserve that can operate when the signal is strong enough.

Receptors are mobile in the plane of the membrane. Ligand binding not only transduces signals but also induces down-regulation by removing receptors from the cell surface. Ligand binding may induce sequestration of receptors and their retention inside the cell via interactions with cell proteins, as occurs with rhodopsin and adrenergic receptors. Ligand binding may induce endocytosis via clathrin-coated pits with ultimate degradation via lysosomal enzymes, as occurs with insulin and epidermal growth factor receptors. The concentration of cell surface receptors is regulated by interaction with hormone ligand and by other signals that regulate its synthesis and affinity. The concentration of receptors determines the cells' responsiveness. Antagonists occupy receptors but in general do not induce desensitization. When antagonists are removed, receptor concentrations are high and cells are very responsive to hormone exposure. Effects on receptor concentration are seen clinically as up-regulation (e.g., as excessive adrenergic responses when β blockers are rapidly withdrawn) and as down-regulation (e.g., insulin resistance in type II diabetes). Regulation of receptor synthesis is an important mechanism by which one hormone regulates responsiveness to another to coordinate biologic effects.

A class of cell surface receptors serves a nutrient delivery rather than an informational function. These molecules include the low density lipoprotein (LDL) receptor, the transferrin receptor, and the asialoglycoprotein receptor. LDL and transferrin receptors, which are clustered in coated pits, internalize, deliver LDL (cholesterol) and iron to the cell interior, and then recycle to the cell surface. Such receptors do not down-regulate, but undergo recycling to provide the cell with essential nutrients.

INTRACELLULAR SECOND MESSENGERS. cAMP and cGMP. The concept of second messengers was established by

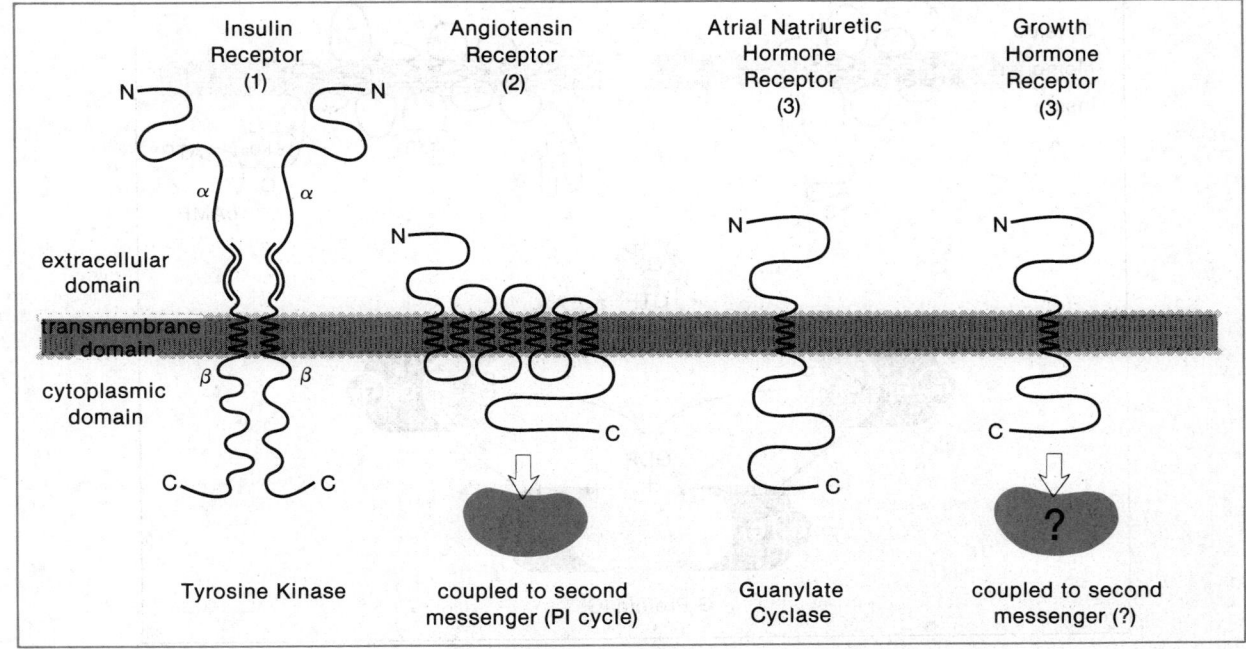

FIGURE 208–2. Structures of peptide hormone receptors.

Earl Sutherland, who discovered cAMP, an intracellular allosteric effector that mediates the action of many peptide hormones. Hormone receptors are coupled to catalytic adenylate cyclase via guanosine nucleotide binding (G) proteins, the β-adrenergic receptor being a paradigm for this signaling pathway (Fig. 208–3). This receptor belongs to the seven membrane–spanning class. On ligand binding, the receptor interacts with a G protein trimer consisting of α, β, and γ subunits. G proteins are ancient signaling molecules involved in regulating many cell processes, including initiation and elongation of protein synthesis, protein transport between membrane compartments, and signal transduction. In all cases binding of GDP results in an inactive conformation, whereas binding of GTP results in an active conformation. The activity of G proteins is thus regulated by the ratio of GTP to GDP, which is, in turn, linked to the energy state of the cell. Because G proteins bind GDP with higher affinity than GTP, guanine nucleotide exchange is triggered by proteins that facilitate exchange of GTP for GDP. Activity is reversed by hydrolysis of GTP to GDP. Binding of hormones to receptors that operate through the cAMP second messenger system results in a conformational change causing receptors to bind to G proteins. Ligand-activated receptors facilitate exchange of GTP for GDP so that the activated $G_\alpha s$ (stimulating α GTP-binding subunit) dissociates from the β and γ subunits. The [ligand-hormone receptor]-[$G_\alpha s$-GTP] complex activates adenylate cyclase to catalyze formation of cAMP from ATP. Each hormone ligand induces formation of multiple cAMP molecules via this mechanism. Inhibitory G proteins operate in a similar manner to decrease cAMP formation. In both cases ligand-activated receptors act to exchange GTP for GDP, analogous to proteins that catalyze this process to regulate protein synthesis.

Adenylate cyclase is a large complex molecule with a 12 membrane–spanning structure resembling the family of glucose transporters, sodium and calcium channels, and the mutated gene in cystic fibrosis. The two large cytoplasmic domains have internal sequence similarities and are related to sequences in guanylate cyclase. Four adenylate cyclases have been identified, and their channel-like structure suggests that they may function as transporters in addition to catalyzing formation of cAMP.

Activation of adenylate cyclase is buffered and terminated by several mechanisms: (1) Hormone dissociates from receptor. Binding of G_α-GTP to the receptor decreases affinity for hormone about one order of magnitude to facilitate this dissociation. (2)

Receptors desensitize and are removed from the cell surface by a process involving phosphorylation and interaction with cell proteins termed "arrestins." (3) Most importantly, G_α proteins possess intrinsic GTPase activity so that GTP is hydrolyzed to GDP and, on GDP binding, G_α is inactivated and reassociates with the β/γ subunits. If hormone exposure is short, receptors are dephosphorylated and reappear on the cell surface; if exposure is prolonged, receptors are degraded and resensitization requires new receptor synthesis.

There are many consequences when this mechanism of signal transduction is perturbed. Continuous exposure to hormone results in desensitization or tachyphylaxis. Deficiency of G protein, which occurs in certain forms of pseudohypoparathyroidism, results in insensitivity to hormone. Cholera toxin, which activates ADP ribosylation of $G_\alpha s$, inhibits GTPase activity, interfering with reversibility so that profound and prolonged elevations in cAMP occur. Mutations in G_α proteins that are predicted to impair GTPase activity have been described in tumors. The *ras* family of G proteins is frequently mutated and oncogenic in human tumors. Mutations impair interaction of these proteins with GTPase-activating proteins, so that, by analogy to cholera toxin, the mutant *ras* proteins remain in the GTP-bound active conformation. *ras* proteins are presumed to couple a signaling pathway different from adenylate cyclase because *ras* cannot substitute for mammalian G_α.

cAMP, an intracellular allosteric effector, binds to the regulatory subunit of cAMP-dependent protein kinase. A-kinase is a tetrameric protein consisting of two regulatory and two catalytic subunits. Binding of cAMP dissociates the inhibitory regulatory subunits as a dimer from the two catalytic subunits. The latter then catalyze the transfer of the γ phosphate of ATP to serine and threonine residues in proteins. This covalent modification by phosphorylation causes an allosteric conformational change in the substrate protein that results in a change in its activity. The hormonal signal is transduced into an alteration in enzyme activity and thus in cell function.

cAMP actions are reversed by hydrolysis of cAMP by phosphodiesterase to 5' AMP, and protein phosphorylation is reversed by the action of phosphatases. Phosphodiesterases are regulated and are a frequent target of inhibitor drugs, such as methyl xanthines, which prolong cAMP action by blocking its degradation. Phosphatases are regulated by phosphatase inhibitor proteins, which are fine tuned by phosphorylation of these molecules.

A conceptually similar but structurally distinct system provides

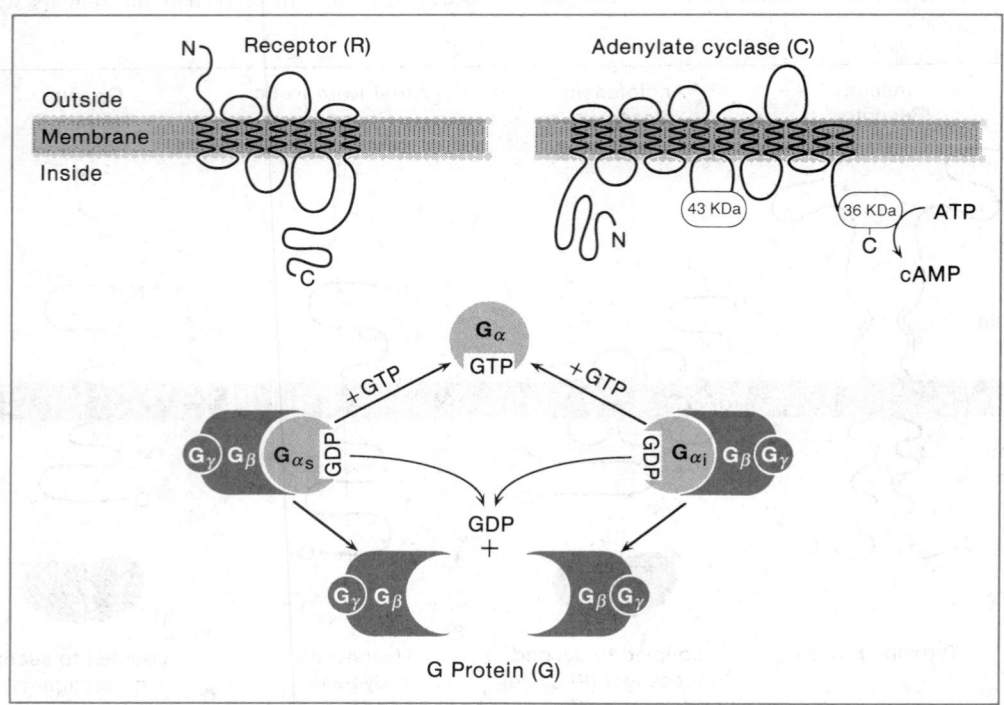

FIGURE 208–3. Hormone-regulated adenylate cyclase.

signal transduction via the second messenger cGMP. Two forms of guanylate cyclase catalyze formation of cGMP from GTP. The best characterized mammalian enzyme is the receptor for atrial natriuretic hormone (ANH) (Ch. 211). The binding site for ANH is located on the extracellular portion of its receptor separated by a single membrane–spanning domain from the cytoplasmic guanylate cyclase (see Fig. 208–2). In contrast to adenylate cyclase, receptor and catalytic activities reside in the same molecule. Activity is regulated primarily by ligand binding but also depends on phosphorylation of the enzyme, with dephosphorylation causing desensitization. A cytoplasmic form of guanylate cyclase contains a heme moiety and is activated by nitrous oxide and free radicals.

cGMP acts by binding to the regulatory domain of cGMP-dependent protein kinase. G-kinase, a dimeric enzyme that is evolutionarily related to A-kinase, is allosterically activated on cGMP binding. Like A-kinase, it catalyzes protein phosphorylation to alter enzyme function and physiologic responses. Reactions are terminated by cGMP phosphodiesterase and protein phosphatases. cGMP phosphodiesterase is activated by binding of calcium-calmodulin, a mechanism providing biochemical communication between two signaling systems.

Calcium and Diacylglycerol. Hormone receptors that activate the phosphatidylinositol (PI) cycle transmit information to the interior of the cell via two second messengers: calcium (Ca^{2+}) and diacylglycerol (DAG) (Fig. 208–4). The cycle of PI metabolism consists of synthesis of this phospholipid, its breakdown, and its resynthesis. PI is composed of a three-carbon glycerol backbone with long-chain fatty acids esterified at carbons 1 and 2 and an inositol ring esterified via a phosphoester bond at carbon 3. Distinct kinase enzymes catalyze phosphorylation of the inositol ring at positions 3, 4, and 5. Quantitatively the principal phosphorylations occur sequentially at position 4 and then 5 (PI 4-kinase and PI 4(P)-5-kinase). Although both kinases are regulated, the principal function of activated hormone receptors is to stimulate phosphoinositidase (phospholipase C), which releases the phosphorylated inositol to generate inositol triphosphate (IP_3, inositol 1,4,5 P_3) and DAG (the glycerol backbone with fatty acids attached at carbons 1 and 2). IP_3 increases the concentration of cytoplasmic [Ca^{2+}]. It mobilizes stored intracellular Ca^{2+} by binding to specific receptors on intracellular membranes and by facilitating opening of calcium channels. The concentration of basal cytoplasmic Ca^{2+} is at least 1000-fold less than that in storage sites and outside the cell. The release from intracellular stores or entry of Ca^{2+} into the cell rapidly increases cytoplasmic [Ca^{2+}].

Ca^{2+} plays a regulatory role in muscle contraction, in neuromuscular transmission, and in hormone signaling. Ca^{2+} binds to calmodulin and alters its conformation, causing the Ca^{2+}-calmodulin complex to bind to a variety of enzymes to regulate their activities. Ca^{2+}-calmodulin regulates protein kinases, including myosin light chain kinase involved in smooth muscle contraction, phosphorylase kinase involved in breakdown of glycogen, and calmodulin-dependent protein kinase important in synaptic transmission. Ca^{2+}-calmodulin regulates cyclic nucleotide phosphodiesterase and adenylate and guanylate cyclases to influence cAMP and cGMP concentrations, and it is involved in microtubule assembly and disassembly. Ca^{2+}-calmodulin is thus able to bind to a variety of other proteins and to alter their activity in response to information provided by the cytoplasmic Ca^{2+} concentration. This provides for diffusion and integration of information received at the cell surface.

DAG acts as a second messenger by binding to protein kinase C to activate this important regulatory enzyme. Protein kinase C also requires Ca^{2+} for activation, so both second messengers of this pathway cooperate to increase the activity of this enzyme. Tumor promoters, such as active phorbol esters, are DAG analogues and act via protein kinase C.

The components of this second messenger system are diverse and complex. There are multiple isoenzyme forms of protein kinase C and of phosphoinositidase. Additional kinases phosphorylate alternate positions on the inositol ring; PI 3-kinase appears to be activated by certain tyrosine kinases to yield unique PI metabolites with functions distinct from Ca^{2+} mobilization. Sphingosine, a component of glycosphingolipid metabolism, inhibits protein kinase C, which provides dual regulation of this protein. Specific phosphatases remove the phosphate groups from the inositol ring to terminate its activity; lithium blocks the activity of one of these phosphatases to enhance accumulation of the biologically active inositol phosphates. Like other information pathways, this one is diffused to generate coordinated cellular responses and is buffered and ultimately turned off when the signal strength decreases.

Protein Tyrosine Kinases. A group of peptide hormone receptors contains intrinsic protein tyrosine kinase activity. Ligand binding to the extracellular domain results in an allosteric change that is

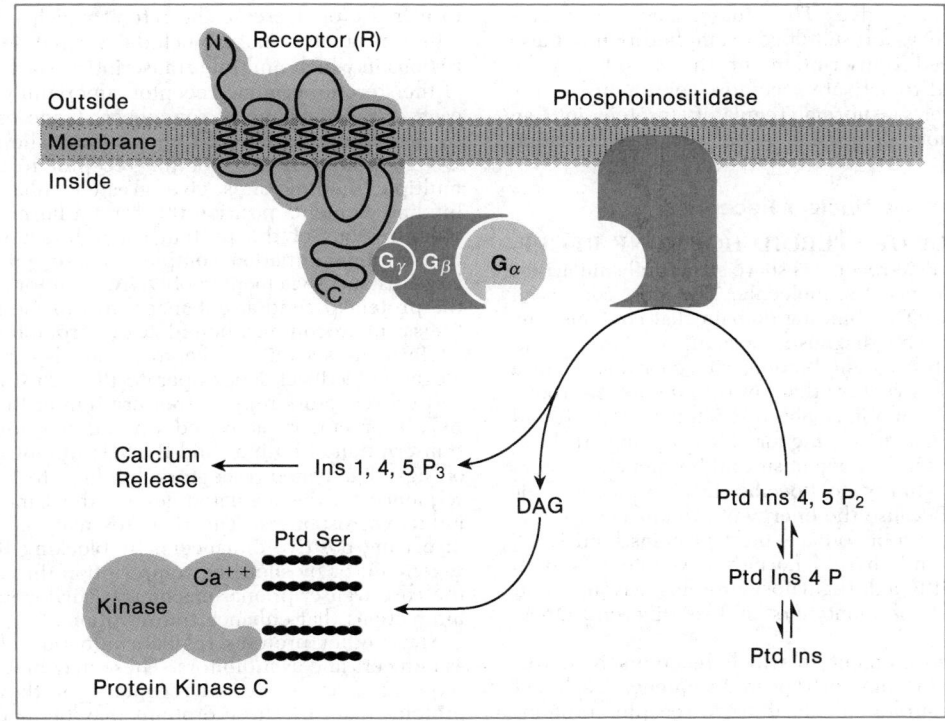

FIGURE 208–4. The phosphatidylinositol signaling pathway.

transmitted across the single membrane-spanning segment to activate the cytoplasmic kinase domain (see Fig. 208–2). In a second structural motif a transmembrane receptor is coupled to a distinct cytoplasmic tyrosine kinase subunit. The lymphocyte receptor CD4 and cellular p56[lck] belong to this second class.

Within the cell the great majority of protein-bound phosphate is attached to serine and threonine residues; only a small fraction (3 to 10 parts per 10,000) is attached to tyrosine. Numerous kinases, however, covalently modify tyrosine residues in proteins as a central regulatory function in cell proliferation, developmental processes, and differentiated function. Historically, this was revealed by the discovery that tyrosine kinase activity is intrinsic to the transforming protein of the Rous sarcoma virus. Several transforming retroviruses presumably "captured" cellular tyrosine kinases in the past and have disarmed their regulatory features or have constitutively expressed them under strong retroviral promoters. When introduced into cells, these retroviruses result in unregulated excessive tyrosine kinase activity and transformation of cells from normal to unrestrained malignant proliferation (Ch. 376).

The extracellular ligand-binding domains of receptors of this class contain cysteine-rich regions that create the binding sites either as monomers (epidermal growth factor [EGF] receptor) or as dimers (insulin receptor), or contain immunoglobulin-like structures (platelet-derived growth factor [PDGF] and fibroblast growth factor [FGF] receptors). The cytoplasmic protein tyrosine kinase domains are highly homologous, containing ATP and substrate-binding sites, but different receptors recognize distinct substrates to give specific biologic responses. For example, insulin stimulates glucose uptake while EGF stimulates cell proliferation. The tyrosine kinases contain variable domains on both sides of the tyrosine kinase core as well as inserts within the kinase domain which provide regulatory sites that modulate ligand-activated tyrosine kinase activity.

Increased tyrosine kinase activity is reversed by three principal mechanisms: (1) by ligand-induced endocytosis and down-regulation of surface receptors, (2) by tyrosine phosphatases, which specifically remove phosphate from tyrosine residues, and (3) by reversal of the kinase reaction to transfer the phosphate from tyrosine residues in protein to ADP.

Regulation and reversibility of ligand-activated tyrosine kinases are very important. Mutations involving these proteins occur frequently in cells transformed from normal to cancerous patterns of growth. Mutations may bypass regulatory features so that the kinases are constitutively active. The kinases may be overexpressed, most frequently as a result of gene amplification but also as a result of enhanced transcription; or the ligand may be constitutively expressed to activate receptors continuously. Any of these changes converts a normal regulatory protein into an oncoprotein, one capable of causing neoplastic transformation (Ch. 157).

Steroid Hormones Act Via Nuclear Receptors

THE SUPERFAMILY OF STEROID HORMONE RECEPTORS. All steroid hormone receptors share structural similarities indicative of a common ancestral molecule. The most conserved structural feature is the DNA-binding domain that contains zinc "fingers" (Fig. 208–5). The diagnostic spacing of cysteine and histidine residues creates a tight binding site coordinated to a Zn^{2+} atom and a peptide structure that binds to the major groove of DNA. This structural motif is not restricted to the steroid receptor gene family nor is it specific for DNA binding. It does, however, create the protein surface in steroid hormone receptors that binds with high affinity to specific DNA sequences or recognition elements. Because the energy of protein-DNA interaction depends on the area of contact, most proteins bind DNA as complexes. Steroid and thyroid hormone receptors bind to DNA as homodimers, although regulatory proteins may also bind as heterodimers formed of monomers of two different DNA-binding proteins.

The DNA recognition element to which receptors bind frequently consists of a palindrome or repeated sequence, each half binding one monomer surface of the dimeric receptor protein. Small variations in the DNA-binding domain and in the DNA

recognition element provide specificity for hormone action. Cortisol receptors bind to glucocorticoid DNA response elements (GRE's) but not to estrogen DNA response elements (ERE's). Specificity is quantitative, not absolute. For example, progesterone receptors bind to GRE's, and retinoic acid receptors bind to thyroid hormone receptor DNA response elements (TRE's). Specificity is sufficient for generating hormone-specific responses but may permit overlapping functions, as in ligand-activated progesterone receptor induction of glucocorticoid-regulated genes. Targeting via DNA-binding domains can be clearly demonstrated by swapping the DNA-binding domain of one receptor for another. Replacing the DNA-binding domain of the estrogen receptor with that of the cortisol receptor targets the hybrid receptor to GRE's, resulting in estrogen-inducing genes normally regulated by cortisol.

Hormone binding activates the biologic function of the receptor. Cortisol receptors exist in inactive complexes with other proteins; cortisol binding induces an allosteric change that facilitates dissociation, allowing the ligand-bound receptor to bind to GRE DNA. Thyroid hormone and retinoic acid receptors exist bound to DNA rather than complexed to protein; hormone binding results in an allosteric change that activates the receptor, so it interacts with other components of the transcription machinery.

The steroid hormone receptor family is a large one, extending to include receptors for $1,25(OH)_2$ vitamin D, thyroid hormone, and retinoic acid. There are also subfamilies of receptors—at least four for retinoic acid, two for thyroid hormone, and a group of "orphans" whose ligands remain to be identified. This structural motif is an important one, which in evolution has diverged to specify responses to many hormonal signals and to control expression of numerous genes. Identifying the orphan receptors will expand understanding of ligand molecules that can signal metabolic and developmental information.

REGULATION OF GENE TRANSCRIPTION. Hormone-activated receptor proteins bound to their DNA response element targets act as *cis*-active enhancers. They act from various positions relative to the start of transcription and in various combinations with other regulatory proteins to control the rate of initiation of gene transcription. Gene promoters lie upstream of the site where eukaryotic RNA polymerase II initiates transcription of messenger RNA. The best-characterized promoter contains a TATA box that binds a protein, transcription factor II D (TFIID), which directs accurate transcription by RNA polymerase II approximately 30 base pairs downstream. A variety of regulatory proteins interact with the basic transcription initiation complex to increase or decrease the rate at which mRNA is synthesized. Other promoter motifs include a basal initiator and GC-rich regions in which multiple transcription start sites exist. Members of the steroid hormone receptor superfamily regulate genes with each of these promoter sequences. Gene expression is induced by increasing the rate of transcription. The gene must contain a DNA binding element for the receptor to generate a response; multiple binding sites give greater enhancement. The DNA binding elements position the steroid hormone receptors so that other regions of the protein can interact with proteins in the transcription initiation complex. These enhancers can act over large distances via looping of DNA. Adaptor proteins may connect the proteins bound at enhancer sites to the proteins of the basal transcription complex bound at the promoter.

Hormone-activated receptors can also repress transcription. Negative feedback loops operate through this process. Activated cortisol receptors repress transcription of the gene encoding the ACTH precursor; activated thyroid hormone receptors inhibit transcription of both α- and β-TSH subunit genes. The principle of ligand-activated receptors binding to specific DNA target sequences in the regulated gene is the same as that required for inductive responses. The receptor may inhibit transcription by displacing positive enhancers, by blocking RNA polymerase engagement, or by silencing transcription through interactions with the core transcriptional machinery, analogous to protein-protein interactions that enhance transcription.

Many other proteins regulate initiation of transcription, both as inducers and as inhibitors. These may bind to DNA via specific sequences, as do steroid receptors, or they may interact with proteins that do. These proteins may be modified in response to hormonal signals initiated at the cell surface. Such alterations account for the changes in gene transcription due to hormones acting via surface receptors. Genes regulated by cAMP contain DNA sequences that specify binding of a specific nuclear transcription regulator, the cAMP response element binding protein (CREB). This protein, which is a member of a family of related transcriptional regulators, is a required final mediator of gene induction by peptide hormones that act at the cell surface to activate adenylate cyclase and cAMP-dependent protein kinase. This chain of effects alters transcription of mRNA's and cell protein concentrations to dictate changes in cell function and organ physiology.

BIOSYNTHESIS OF HORMONES AND RECEPTORS
Synthesis and Delivery of Peptide Hormones

Peptide hormones are small secretory proteins; their biosynthesis and secretion occur via the same processes as other nonhormonal secretory proteins. In general, peptide hormones are synthesized as part of larger precursor proteins that contain additional information. Within the endoplasmic reticulum space, the precursor protein is cleaved, covalently modified, and folded into the form that will ultimately be secreted.

The precursor structure may have a variety of functions. Precursors for antidiuretic hormone and oxytocin contain specific neurophysins that serve as carriers of the peptides from the site of synthesis in the hypothalamus to storage granules in axon terminals in the posterior pituitary (Ch. 214). The ACTH precursor, pro-opiomelanocortin, contains information for several peptides that may be coordinately involved in stress responses (Ch. 209). The precursor for gonadotropin-releasing hormone contains a potent prolactin-inhibitory peptide, a structure that allows reciprocal regulation of lactation and reproductive function. Structures in the precursor protein may serve to fold the peptide correctly. The connecting peptide in the insulin precursor between the β and the α subunits facilitates folding for formation of mature insulin with correctly formed disulfide bonds between and within the two chains (Ch. 218). The connecting peptide is then excised and removed from mature α-β insulin.

Within the endoplasmic reticulum and Golgi apparatus, glycosylation of TSH, LH, FSH, and hCG occurs. Secretory granules containing highly concentrated hormone accumulate in the unstimulated cell. During secretion the membrane of the secretory granule fuses with the plasma membrane and stored hormone is discharged into the circulation, a process termed exocytosis. Rapid release of hormone in response to stimuli reflects discharge of secretory granules, whereas prolonged secretion reflects release of newly synthesized hormone.

Peptide hormones may also be derived from precursors with receptor-like structures or from circulating forms. EGF and transforming growth factor α (TGF-α) are made as a part of the surface domain of a transmembrane protein with a receptor-like structure. These are released by proteolysis, although they may act on adjacent cells without processing to provide cell-to-cell

communication. Renin, an enzyme released from juxtaglomerular cells, acts on angiotensinogen secreted from liver. Active angiotensin is synthesized by progressive extracellular proteolysis of a precursor: renin to yield angiotensin I and angiotensin-converting enzyme to yield angiotensin II.

Secreted peptide hormones have a short half-life of about 3 to 7 minutes in the circulation. Glycoprotein hormones have longer half-lives of 1 to 4 hours. The short circulating half-life and peptide degradation by gastric acid and intestinal enzymes have precluded oral use of this class of hormones. Several attempts to prolong half-lives have met with partial success: Complexing with Zn^{2+} and protamine creates a slowly absorbed and longer-acting form of injectable insulin; removing the amino group from the N' terminal amino acid and substituting a D-arginine creates a longer-acting ADH which can be absorbed from nasal mucous membranes. At present direct use of peptide hormones is limited to injectable forms. Prolonged action results in receptor desensitization, so recapitulation of normal cyclic secretion typical of endogenous production presents a second difficulty. Use of GnRH must be both by parental routes and pulsatile in nature to induce ovulation and successful pregnancy.

Synthesis and Transport of Steroid Hormones

Steroid hormones are derived from cholesterol provided by de novo cellular synthesis from acetate or by uptake of circulating cholesterol made in the liver and delivered to cells via low density lipoprotein particles. Because synthesized steroid hormones are not stored, secretory rates directly reflect production rates. In adrenal and gonadal tissues the rate-limiting step for increased steroid hormone biosynthesis is transfer of substrate cholesterol to the side chain cleavage enzyme located in the inner mitochondrial membrane. Cleavage of the side chain of cholesterol is catalyzed by a cytochrome P-450 enzyme that resembles other steroid hydroxylases. These enzymes progressively modify the cholesterol nucleus by the sequential addition of hydroxyl groups to specific sites. The rate-limiting step is stimulated in target cells by ACTH, LH, and FSH to result in rapid increases in steroid hormone biosynthesis. The trophic stimulatory hormones also maintain the structure of the target glands and induce each of the enzymes involved in hormone biosynthesis. With hypophysectomy or feedback inhibition of pituitary hormone production, the entire steroid biosynthetic pathway decreases and the adrenal, ovary, and testis atrophy. Addition of trophic hormones induces enzymes and regrowth of target glands. Induction of biosynthetic enzymes appears directly mediated via second messenger pathways, primarily cAMP, but growth requires coordinated provision of growth factors because cAMP, in general, inhibits growth.

The pattern of biosynthetic enzymes expressed during cell differentiation determines which steroid hormone is produced

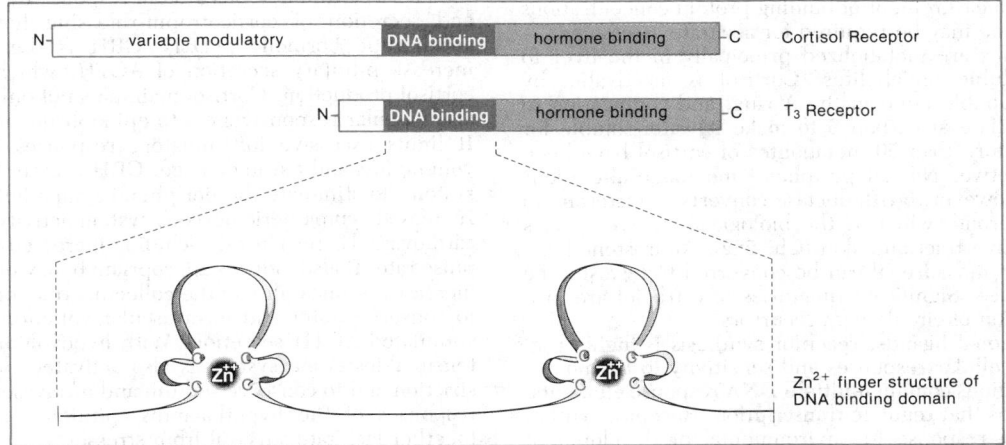

FIGURE 208–5. Structural features of steroid hormone receptors. The cortisol and T₃ receptors have variable modulatory domains but highly conserved DNA-binding domains. The DNA-binding domains contain two Zn²⁺ fingers.

and is the basis of the differentiated function of adrenal and gonads. The fascicularis zones of the adrenal cortex express cytochrome P-450 enzymes that catalyze hydroxylations at carbons 21, 17, and 11. They also express 3β-hydroxysteroid dehydrogenase, $\Delta^{4,5}$ isomerase which forms cortisol. The zona glomerulosa of the adrenal cortex makes aldosterone through a similar series of reactions, but the pathway lacks 17α-hydroxylase and contains an activity that acts at carbon 18. The testis lacks 21- and 11β-hydroxylases, so reactants flow to testosterone. Ovarian synthesis of estradiol requires cooperation between adjacent theca interna and granulosa cells. Granulosa cells express aromatase, the enzyme that catalyzes placement of three double bonds in the A ring of estrogens but cannot provide precursor androstenedione, which is synthesized in the theca interna cell located adjacent to the granulosa cell. Granulosa cells efficiently convert precursor androstenedione provided by the theca interna to estrone and estradiol.

The active form of vitamin D, $1,25(OH)_2D$, is also made from cholesterol, but the biosynthetic enzymes are located in three separate organs: skin, liver, and kidney (Ch. 233). Vitamin D_3 is formed from 7-dehydrocholesterol by ultraviolet irradiation of skin. D_3 is then hydroxylated at carbon-25 in the liver to yield $25(OH)D$. This is converted by 1α-hydroxylase to $1,25(OH)_2D$ in proximal tubule cells of the kidney. In this unique endocrine system, the major site for regulation is the final 1α-hydroxylation in renal proximal tubule cells, a step controlled by parathyroid hormone and phosphate.

In contrast to peptide hormones, steroid hormones have longer circulating half-lives and may be active when administered orally. Following secretion into the circulation, steroid hormones are bound to transport glycoproteins made in the liver. The transport proteins, which have a binding but not an activity site, provide a reservoir of hormone, protected from metabolism and renal clearance, which can be released to cells. Three transport proteins have been characterized: corticosteroid-binding globulin (CBG) which binds cortisol and progesterone, sex steroid hormone–binding globulin (SHBG) which binds testosterone with greater affinity than estradiol, and vitamin D–binding protein which binds precursor $25(OH)D$ with greater affinity than $1,25(OH)_2D$. Thyroid-binding globulin (TBG) binds L-thyroxine to provide its uniquely long half-life of 7 days. Estrogen induces and androgens inhibit synthesis of these transport proteins. Albumin provides a large carrier system that weakly binds hormones.

Free steroid hormone, which is in equilibrium with that bound to transport protein, enters cells to bind intracellular receptors and generate biologic responses. The free fraction is also the active one in feedback regulation, so it is the concentration of free hormone that is altered in homeostatic responses. The free fraction is very small compared to the bound fraction, but total hormone concentrations from both fractions are measured in most clinical assays. Conditions, such as pregnancy, that alter binding protein concentrations alter total measured hormone but not the biologically relevant free hormone concentrations. In special clinical situations measurement of binding protein concentrations and of free hormone may be required for accurate assessment.

Steroid hormones are metabolized principally in the liver to inactive water-soluble metabolites. Cortisol is inactivated by reduction of the double bond in the A ring, and conjugation to glucuronide or sulfate at carbon 3 to make it water-soluble for renal excretion. More than 50 metabolites of cortisol have been identified, all inactive. Not all peripheral metabolic alterations are inactivating, however. 5α-Reductase converts testosterone to 5α-dihydrotestosterone, which is the biologically active species in male reproductive tract and skin (Ch. 222). Androstenedione produced in ovary and adrenal can be converted to testosterone in peripheral tissues. Significant quantities of estradiol are produced by conversion of circulating precursors.

Like their hormonal ligands, receptor synthesis is highly regulated to control cellular responses and sensitivity to hormones. Gene promoter regions contain multiple DNA response elements, which bind proteins that regulate transcription. Receptor synthesis is increased in response to environmental or development need or is repressed in negative feedback loops and during stages of development. Receptor concentration is as important as hormone concentration in determining cell responses. Regulation of

receptor synthesis is therefore central to providing coordinated and appropriate endocrine responses.

INTEGRATION OF ENDOCRINE RESPONSES
Feedback Loops

A number of hormones cooperate to coordinate development, reproduction, and homeostasis. When a hormone has elicited an appropriate response, the signal must be terminated. In addition to the buffering that occurs in target cells, feedback control is the principal mechanism through which this occurs (Fig. 208–6). Feedback loops are especially important for communication between organs that are spatially separated. The hormonal products of peripheral endocrine glands, such as thyroid, adrenal cortex, ovary, and testis, exert negative feedback control over the synthesis and secretion of the stimulatory pituitary hormone. Feedback, which occurs at the level of the pituitary cell and in the hypothalamus, operates via control of several essential steps. The neurohormone TRH stimulates thyrotropes of the anterior pituitary to synthesize and secrete TSH, which in turn increases synthesis and secretion of thyroid hormone. Increased production of thyroid hormone induces appropriate metabolic responses in target organs; it also inhibits production of TSH to return the system to baseline. The prohormone L-thyroxine (T_4) is converted in the pituitary thyrotrope to active T_3, and T_3 binds to nuclear T_3 receptors to inhibit transcription of both α- and β-TSH subunit genes. T_3-bound receptors also decrease synthesis of TRH receptors, rendering cells less responsive to stimulatory TRH. In addition, T_3 inhibits hypothalamic production of TRH. Conversely, when thyroid hormone concentrations are low, feedback inhibition is relieved and TRH stimulates increased production of TSH, which increases production of T_4 and thus re-establishes homeostasis. Feedback principles provide an exquisitely sensitive system for making appropriate changes and then returning to the homeostatic set-point.

Feedback operates not only via steroid and thyroid hormones but also through peptides and ions. Pituitary FSH production is feedback regulated by the ovarian steroid hormone estrogen and by the ovarian peptide hormone inhibin. Parathyroid hormone regulates serum Ca^{2+} concentrations; with hypocalcemia PTH increases and re-establishes normocalcemia. The increase in serum $[Ca^{2+}]$ feedback inhibits PTH synthesis and secretion to re-establish serum PTH concentrations appropriate to normocalcemia (Ch. 235).

Recruitment of Coordinate Responses

Physiologic responses result from many different cell types and organs acting in concert. The necessary coordination is provided both by a hormone acting at multiple sites and by each hormone eliciting multiple responses, which sum to give the overall effect. Integrated responses require that one hormone regulate the synthesis or action of another; the nervous system is integrated into the overall response. Paradigms of such coordinated responses include stress, fasting, and reproduction.

A major stress, such as trauma with pain and hypovolemia, initiates a central nervous system response that includes synthesis and secretion of corticotropin-releasing hormone (CRH) and antidiuretic hormone (ADH). CRH is the major stimulus to increase pituitary secretion of ACTH, which increases adrenal cortisol production. Cortisol maintains not only blood glucose but also vascular responsiveness to epinephrine and norepinephrine. It limits excessive inflammatory responses to prevent further volume loss and tissue damage. CRH acts, in the central nervous system, to stimulate the peripheral sympathetic nervous system. Increased sympathetic nervous system activity mediates adaptive cardiovascular responses, including increased blood pressure and pulse rate. It also induces appropriate behavioral responses. ADH increases permeability of the collecting duct of the distal nephron to conserve water and intravascular volume. It facilitates CRH-stimulated ACTH secretion. With hypovolemia the renin-angiotensin-aldosterone system is also activated to enhance vasoconstriction and to conserve sodium and intravascular volume. These responses of the hypothalamus, pituitary, and adrenal cortex together facilitate survival from stresses.

With fasting, blood glucose concentrations are maintained for 12 to 24 hours by glucagon- and epinephrine-mediated release of glucose from glycogen stores. With more prolonged fasting cortisol-stimulated gluconeogenesis is the major mechanism that sustains blood glucose. Insulin secretion is suppressed. Metabolic demands are decreased by inhibition of 5′ deiodinase to decrease conversion of T_4 to active T_3 in peripheral tissues. Growth-promoting hormones, such as insulin-like growth factor I, are also suppressed under conditions of substrate lack. With starvation gonadotropin secretion decreases and reproductive capacity is diminished.

Female reproductive cycles result from coordinated signaling by hypothalamic, pituitary, and ovarian hormones. Pulsatile secretion of GnRH stimulates pituitary production of LH and FSH. During the follicular phase of the menstrual cycle these peptide hormones regulate ovarian secretion of estrogen and direct maturation of follicles, one of which increases 1000-fold in diameter and becomes dominant for ovulation (Ch. 224). FSH induces LH receptors in ovarian granulosa cells, and both LH and FSH induce aromatase as part of the mechanism that enhances estrogen production. LH and FSH increase during the follicular phase and, with follicle development, estrogen secretion rises. Positive feedback effects of estrogen result in the mid-cycle surge of LH and FSH, which induces ovulation. The remaining granulosa and theca cells reorganize to form the corpus luteum, which produces progesterone as well as estrogen. Concentrations of these hormones negatively inhibit FSH and LH production and induce additional uterine changes necessary for implantation. Ovarian inhibin also feedback inhibits FSH production. If fertilization and implantation occur, the corpus luteum is regulated by hCG until placental steroidogenesis is established. If fertilization does not occur, negative feedback of estrogen and progesterone inhibits LH and FSH, and the luteal phase of the menstrual cycle ends after about 10 days when the corpus luteum, now deprived of trophic stimulation, decreases estrogen and progesterone production. Menstruation occurs and, in the absence of negative feedback, FSH and LH again rise to initiate a subsequent reproductive cycle.

Cycles and Rhythms

Nervous system rhythms are evident within feedback loops and coordinate hormonal responses. Several pituitary hormones are secreted with a frequency of 15 to 60 minutes owing to pulsatile secretion of hypothalamic hormones. Longer rhythms are superimposed on these pulses. Pulsatile secretion of peptide hormones maximizes target cell responses by preventing excessive receptor down-regulation. ACTH and consequently cortisol exhibit a diurnal rhythm with early morning secretion exceeding evening secretion at least twofold. Growth hormone is entrained to deep sleep, with maximal daily production occurring coincident with EEG-defined slow wave sleep. Cycles also occur at different stages of development. At puberty nocturnal increases in gonadotropins occur, a rhythm much less pronounced in adult life. Measured hormone levels must be interpreted relative to these rhythms and cycles, as well as to stages of the menstrual cycle, when assaying reproductive hormones.

ASSESSMENT OF ENDOCRINE FUNCTION

Quantitation of Circulating Hormones and Metabolic Products

Endocrine function is assessed by accurately measuring the concentration of hormones present in blood. Even though circulating concentrations are low (nM to μM for steroid hormones and thyroxine and pM to nM for peptide hormones), precise assays based on competitive protein binding are widely available. Most clinical assays use antibodies that bind the hormone of interest with high affinity and high specificity. Both polyclonal and monoclonal antibodies are used; monoclonal antibodies have the advantage of purity and virtually unlimited supply. As originally developed, radioimmunoassays (RIA) mix radiolabeled hormone with specific antibody in the presence of increasing con-

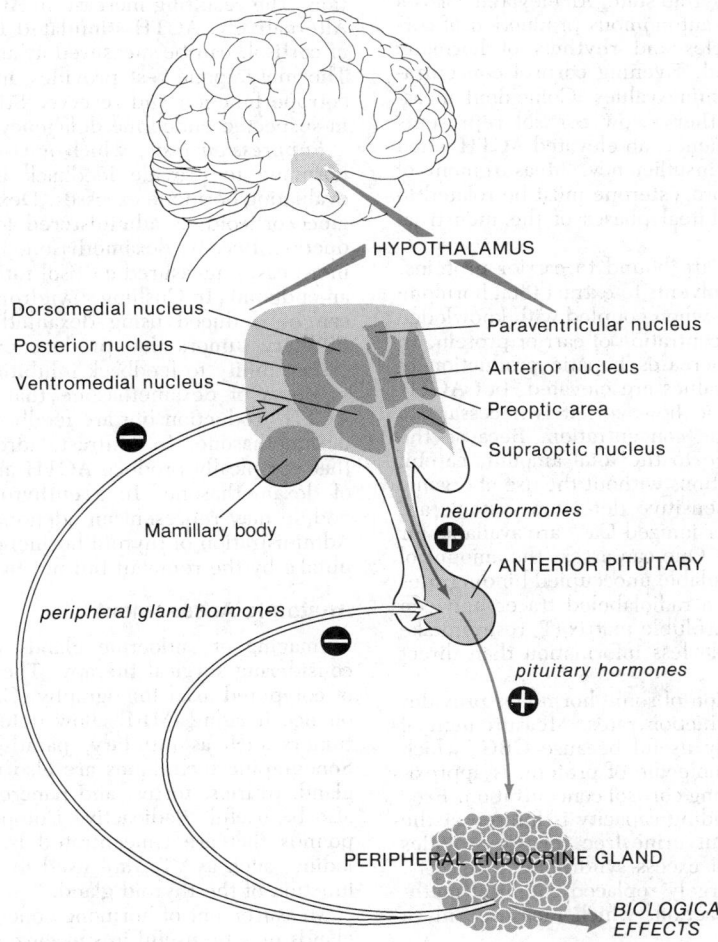

FIGURE 208–6. Forward regulation and negative feedback.

centrations of standard unlabeled hormone. Unlabeled hormone competes with radiolabeled hormone for binding to antibody to generate a standard curve of decreasing radioactive hormone bound to antibody. Samples for assay are mixed with radiolabeled hormone and antibody, and the extent of displacement of radiolabeled hormone from subsequently isolated antibody can be directly compared to displacement by known amounts of hormone. For a sensitive, precise assay a specific high-affinity antibody, a radiolabeling procedure that does not damage the hormone, and unlabeled pure hormone are required. To avoid radioactivity, enzyme-linked immunoabsorbent assays (ELISA) have been increasingly adapted. These assays use enzyme activity to generate a color change that can be quantitated with a spectrophotometer. Two antibodies directed against different epitopes in the same hormone molecule may be used. The first antibody binds hormone and is immobilized; the second antibody with an attached enzyme is then added and the amount of antibody-bound enzyme activity provides a measure of the amount of hormone attached to the first antibody. Other assays use fluorescent dyes attached to either the hormone standard or to a second antibody. Improved sensitivity and accuracy of hormone measurements reduce the need to perform more complex stimulation and suppression tests.

Even with sensitive and precise assays of hormone concentration, clinical assessment is essential. Measured values must be interpreted in relation to clinical signs and symptoms. It is also extremely helpful to measure both arms of a feedback loop. Most hormone concentrations exhibit a gaussian distribution of normal values, so an individual measurement at either end of the normal range may be normal or abnormal for that individual. Coincident measurement of TSH and T_4, LH and testosterone, ACTH and cortisol, PTH and Ca^{2+} gives greater information than either alone. A T_4 at the lower end of the normal range with an elevated TSH indicates thyroid gland failure, whereas the same T_4 with a normal TSH likely indicates a euthyroid state. An elevated cortisol with suppressed ACTH indicates autonomous production of cortisol by an adrenal tumor. Cycles and rhythms of hormone secretion must also be considered. Evening cortisol concentrations are half or less of peak morning values. Coincident measurement of ACTH clarifies whether a low cortisol represents diurnal rhythm or adrenal insufficiency; an elevated ACTH when cortisol is low suggests adrenal insufficiency. Measurement of gonadotropins and estradiol and progesterone must be related to normal values for follicular and luteal phases of the menstrual cycle.

Steroid and thyroid hormones are bound to carrier proteins. Most measurements use organic solvents to extract total hormone for assay. This is usually sufficient when coupled with knowledge of effects of hormones on the concentration of carrier protein. In pregnancy, in which estrogen increases hepatic production of carrier proteins, cortisol and T_4 values are elevated, but ACTH and TSH are normal. On occasion, however, it is necessary to measure the free, active hormone concentration. Because the free fraction is very small relative to the total amount, careful separation of bound from free fractions without the use of organic solvents is necessary, and very sensitive detection systems are required. Assays for free T_4 and for ionized Ca^{2+} are available for specialized clinical circumstances. One can assess the amount of binding globulin by RIA or the available unoccupied binding sites by measuring the distribution of a radiolabeled tracer between soluble binding globulin and an insoluble matrix (T_3 resin uptake tests). These indirect tests provide less information than direct measurements of free hormone.

Measurement of urinary excretion of some hormones provides an integrated value for daily production rates. Measurement of urinary free cortisol is particularly useful because CBG, which binds one cortisol molecule per molecule of protein, is approximately saturated at the peak morning cortisol concentration. Free unbound cortisol that exceeds binding capacity is filtered at the glomerulus, so an elevated 24-hour urine free cortisol provides an accurate assessment in cortisol excess syndromes (Ch. 217). Precise RIA's or ELISA's have largely replaced chemical methods, such as the Porter-Silber reaction, which measure only a fraction of cortisol metabolites.

Measurement of metabolic effects is an essential component of endocrine evaluation. Insulin function is assessed by measuring plasma and urine glucose concentrations, PTH by measuring serum $[Ca^{2+}]$, aldosterone by measuring serum $[K^+]$, and ADH by measuring serum and urine osmolalities.

Stimulation and Suppression Tests

Measurement of both arms of a feedback loop provides sufficient laboratory information in most endocrine deficiency or excess states. Additional diagnostic information can be gained, however, by perturbing the feedback system through administration of hormones.

For *stimulation tests* a hormone is administered and the ability of the target gland to respond is assessed by measuring its product. This provides an estimate of the ability of the target gland to synthesize hormone, of its trophic maintenance, and of its exposure to feedback inhibition. Baseline measurements are made before hormone administration and at the established normal time of peak target gland response. Ranges of normal responses have been established for comparison. Examples include TRH stimulation tests, in which serum levels of pituitary-produced TSH are measured. In hypopituitarism, serum TSH fails to rise in response to a standard intravenous injection of TRH. In primary hypothyroidism, in which feedback inhibition by thyroid hormone is small, TSH rises excessively, whereas in hyperthyroidism excessive feedback inhibition results in minimal or no increases in TSH. For ACTH stimulation tests $ACTH_{1-24}$ is administered as an intravenous injection to assess the ability of the adrenal cortex to produce cortisol. A low baseline cortisol that fails to rise indicates adrenal insufficiency. Interpretation requires integration of clinical information because failure to respond to ACTH may also occur when the adrenal cortex has been suppressed as a result of treatment with synthetic glucocorticoids. A variation of stimulation tests involves interruption of the feedback loop by metabolic inhibitors of hormone biosynthesis. Metyrapone, an inhibitor of 11β-hydroxylase, decreases serum cortisol, relieving feedback suppression of ACTH production. The resulting increase in ACTH can be measured directly. Alternatively, ACTH-stimulated 11-desoxycortisol, the precursor of cortisol, can be measured as an indicator of increased ACTH. The metyrapone test provides an assessment of pituitary corticotrope function and reserve. Stimulation tests are most useful in suspected endocrine deficiency states.

Suppression tests, which measure the ability of administered hormone to provide feedback inhibition, are most useful in evaluating hormone excesses. Dexamethasone, a potent synthetic glucocorticoid, is administered to feedback inhibit ACTH production. Because dexamethasone is not detected in cortisol assays, more easily measured cortisol rather than ACTH can be used as an endpoint. In Cushing's syndrome, the source of cortisol excess can be deduced using dexamethasone suppression (Ch. 217). Pituitary tumors that produce excess ACTH frequently retain susceptibility to feedback inhibition. These tumors are resistant to doses of dexamethasone that suppress normal corticotrope ACTH production but are feedback inhibited by higher doses of dexamethasone. In contrast, adrenal gland tumors and tumors that ectopically produce ACTH are resistant to even high doses of dexamethasone. In a euthyroid patient a hyperfunctioning nodule may represent an adenoma or a thyroid gland remnant. Administration of thyroid hormone suppresses radioactive iodine uptake by the remnant but not by the adenoma.

Anatomic Assessment

Imaging of endocrine glands is important, especially when considering surgical therapy. The high sensitivity and precision of computed axial tomography (CAT) and nuclear magnetic resonance imaging (MRI) allow detection of even small endocrine tumors such as pituitary, parathyroid, and adrenal adenomas. Sonographic techniques are also useful for imaging the thyroid gland, ovaries, testes, and pancreas. Radionuclide imaging may also be useful. Radioactive isotopes of iodine (^{123}I, ^{131}I) or compounds that are concentrated by the thyroid gland similar to iodine, such as ^{99}Tc, are used to determine anatomy and imply function of the thyroid gland.

Measurement of hormone concentrations in venous effluent of glands may be useful in specialized circumstances to localize the source of abnormal production. Measurement of ACTH in petrosal sinus blood may be useful in localizing pituitary tumors, PTH in neck and chest veins in localizing unusually located parathyroid adenomas, and insulin in mesenteric venous drainage in localizing pancreatic insulinomas.

Cytologic and immunocytochemical techniques are important. Fine-needle aspiration of thyroid nodules with cytologic examinations analogous to those used in Papanicolaou smears has become the procedure of choice to distinguish benign and malignant thyroid nodules. Staining of surgical tissues with antihormone antibodies provides proof of hormone production and serves as a guide to future therapy.

Receptors are not routinely measured but can be quantitated using immunologic techniques. Recombinant DNA technologies can be used to define inherited defects in receptors. When oncogenes are identified in specific endocrine neoplasms, these can be measured and mutations identified using DNA hybridization techniques. Autoimmune endocrine diseases can be documented by quantitating antibodies directed against specific organs (thyroid-stimulating immunoglobulin, anti–islet cell antibodies, antiadrenal antibodies).

ABERRATIONS IN DISEASE

Deficiency States

The most prevalent endocrine disorders result from hormone deficiencies. A variety of disease states impair or destroy endocrine glands: defects in organ development, genetic defects in biosynthetic enzymes, immune-mediated destruction, neoplasia, infections, hemorrhage, nutritional deficits, and vascular insufficiency. Endocrine gland failure may be acute with rapid development of symptoms or chronic with slower development of symptoms but more pronounced physical changes. Defects in a gland such as the thyroid may result in a multisystem disorder due to failure to produce a single hormone, whereas defects in the hypothalamus or pituitary may result in a multisystem disorder, including thyroid deficiency, due to failure to produce many hormones. Multiple endocrine gland deficiencies may also result from autoimmune-mediated mechanisms in the polyglandular autoimmune deficiency syndromes (Ch. 228). Because hormones participate in coordinated responses, secondary changes in other endocrine responses often result from deficiency of a single hormone.

Deficiency states also result from defects in hormone receptors and in signaling mechanisms. Defects may be inherited or acquired. Genetic abnormalities in androgen receptors result in unresponsiveness to androgens and an XY male with a female phenotype (Ch. 221); defects in vitamin D receptors result in vitamin D–resistant rickets (Ch. 233); defects in thyroid hormone receptors result in the resistance to thyroid hormone of Refetoff's syndrome (Ch. 216); defects in growth hormone receptors result in ateliotic dwarfism of Laron's syndrome (Ch. 213). Acquired receptor defects most often result from immunologic mechanisms whereby antibodies bind to receptors, blocking ligand access. Postreceptor defects may occur. A defect in $G_{\alpha}s$ results in pseudohypoparathyroidism with unresponsiveness to PTH. Such patients fail to respond normally to other hormones whose receptors couple to adenylate cyclase (TSH, glucagon, LH). Type II diabetes mellitus, which is inherited, is characterized by insulin resistance (Ch. 218). The molecular defect has not yet been characterized, but understanding this pathophysiology underlies therapeutic approaches directed at reducing resistance to and augmenting secretion of insulin. Because receptor and postreceptor defects are characterized by hormone resistance, feedback does not occur and producer glands enlarge and circulating hormone concentrations are high despite clinical evidence for deficiency.

Excess States

Excessive production of hormone and clinical evidence of such excess imply failure of normal feedback mechanisms. This occurs most commonly with neoplasia and with autoimmunity, in which antireceptor antibodies act as hormone agonists. Tumors of endocrine glands characteristically produce excessive amounts of the hormone made by the cell of origin but are no longer subject to normal feedback controls. Some tumors, such as pituitary adenomas that produce ACTH, retain feedback but require higher

concentrations of cortisol to suppress ACTH. Prolactinomas retain dopamine suppression, and both their function and growth can be inhibited by dopamine agonists. Tumors arising in peripheral endocrine glands that are under pituitary trophic hormone regulation are autonomous because they are not normally subject to negative feedback. More undifferentiated tumors may also be insensitive to feedback regulation.

Hormones may be produced in excess by tumors arising from cells that do not normally produce the hormone (Ch. 161). Ectopic production of peptide hormones is common in a variety of neoplasms, and symptoms due to the hormone excess may contribute significantly to morbidity. Because steroid hormones are made via a multienzyme pathway, excesses of these hormones occur only with tumors arising in the producer gland or when there is excessive production of the trophic peptide hormone. Cortisol excess may result from adrenocortical tumors or from excessive stimulation by ACTH produced by pituitary or ectopic neoplasms.

The most prevalent disease due to agonistic antibodies is Graves' disease, in which antibodies are produced that activate the TSH receptor (Ch. 216). Because many hormones are available as therapeutic agents, some patients take excessive amounts and present with an endocrine excess syndrome.

Genetic Determinants of Disease

Many endocrine diseases result from genetic mutations, although only a minority of these have been characterized. Genetic defects in biosynthetic enzymes may result in deficiency states: Hypothyroidism may result from thyroid peroxidase or deiodinase enzyme defects; adrenal insufficiency may result from 21-hydroxylase deficiency or a defect in other steroid biosynthetic enzymes; a form of male hypogonadism may result from 5α-reductase deficiency. Receptor defects are thought to be uncommon, but methods to define these have only recently become available. Type II diabetes, the most common endocrine abnormality, is inherited but its molecular basis is not yet known. Autoimmune endocrine disease also has a genetic basis involving an inherited defect in immune surveillance. Multiple endocrine neoplasia syndromes are likely due to defects in tumor suppressor genes analogous to that which occurs in retinoblastoma (Ch. 228).

As normal structures become defined, mutations can be identified. Once these are defined, precise diagnostic methods using nucleic acid probes can be used to make precise diagnoses in disease states and to provide predictive information before overt disease develops. Because genetic defects are present in all DNA, peripheral blood cells or skin fibroblasts provide a ready source of material for assay. Development of such assays will improve precision in diagnosis of endocrine disorders.

Alberts B, Bray D, Lewis J, et al. (eds.): Molecular Biology of the Cell. New York, Garland Publishing Inc., 1989. *Chapter 12 gives an excellent overview of hormonal signaling mechanisms.*

Beato M: Gene regulation by steroid hormones. Cell 56:335, 1989. *Concise review of mechanisms of steroid hormone action.*

Berridge MJ, Irvine RF: Inositol phosphates and cell signalling. Nature 341:197, 1989. *Review of this second messenger signaling system.*

Bourne HR, Sanders DA, McCormick F: The GTPase superfamily: A conserved switch for diverse cell functions. Nature 348:125, 1990. *Thoughtful review of how the large number of G proteins work.*

Felig F, Baxter JD, Broadus AE, et al. (eds.): Endocrinology and Metabolism, 2nd ed. New York, McGraw-Hill, 1987. *Textbook of endocrinology containing six introductory chapters on principles of endocrinology and pathophysiology of diseases affecting the endocrine system.*

Gilman AG: G proteins and regulation of adenylyl cyclase. JAMA 262:1819, 1989. *Albert Lasker Award lecture concisely reviewing G protein function.*

Levitzki A: From epinephrine to cyclic AMP. Science 241:800, 1988. *Summary of signaling by β-adrenergic receptors; a good model for receptors that signal via cAMP.*

Weinberg RA (ed.): Oncogenes and the Molecular Origins of Cancer. Cold Spring Harbor, New York, Cold Spring Harbor Laboratory Press, 1989. *Monograph that provides a precise summary of concepts of regulation of growth and how normal control mechanisms are disordered in malignancy.*

West JB (ed.): Best and Taylor's Physiological Basis of Medical Practice, 12th ed. New York, Williams & Wilkins, 1990. *Sections 7 and 8, Metabolism and Endocrine Systems, detail physiologic principles of each of the major endocrine glands and metabolic systems.*

209 The Endorphin Family of Opioid Peptides: Biochemistry, Anatomy, and Physiology

Stanley J. Watson

Many structures throughout the central and peripheral nervous system contain cells that secrete peptides. Major among these is a family of endogenous neuropeptides capable of mimicking many actions of opiate alkaloids, such as morphine and heroin. These peptides have a common pentapeptide sequence at their amino terminus [Tyr-Gly-Gly-Phe-Met (or-Leu)], which is important for their opiate activity. All such *endogenous opioid peptides* carry the generic name of endorphins (*endogenous morphines*). There are actually three main families of endorphins, each with its own separate protein precursor, mRNA, and gene (Fig. 209–1). (1) *Pro-Opio-Melano-Cortin* (or POMC), (2) *Pro-Enkephalin*, and (3) *Pro-Dynorphin/Neo-Endorphin*. POMC produces one opiate peptide, β-endorphin, and several nonopioid products, e.g., ACTH and α-, β-, and γ-melanocyte-stimulating hormones (MSH). In contrast, pro-enkephalin has seven repeated opioid sequences, and pro-dynorphin has three.

The discovery of three families of endorphins with their many active peptides grew out of a rich set of pharmacologic tools and behavioral paradigms. Briefly, the structural pharmacology of the opiate alkaloids allowed the description of active and inactive stereoisomers of both opiate agonists and antagonists. The introduction of radiolabeled versions of the active alkaloids made it possible, in the early 1970's, to describe the existence of opiate receptors in brain. A search for their natural ligands followed, and more than 20 active peptide fragments were extracted and sequenced during the next decade—chief among these are β-endorphin, met- and leu-enkephalin, and dynorphin. Gene and mRNA information radically improved our knowledge of the sequences of the endorphins within their precursors and provided better understanding of their relationships with their nonopiate fragments. The availability of peptide and precursor sequences then allowed the production of antibodies and nucleic acid probes for studying the anatomy, peptide biochemistry, nucleic acid biochemistry, receptors, and physiology of all three endorphin families.

All three members of the endorphin family are widely distributed, including being found in brain, heart, lung, adrenal, ovary, pituitary, testes, and gut. Each endorphin originates in a separate set of cells and rarely coexists in the same neuron or endocrine cell with other endorphins. Specifically, POMC is found in the corticotrophs of the anterior lobe of the pituitary, in the arcuate nucleus in the base of the hypothalamus, and in the nucleus tractus solitarius in the brain stem. POMC fibers project heavily through limbic, autonomic, and pain systems. The dynorphin system, more widespread both within the brain and in the periphery, is found in testes, ovary, gut wall, adrenal cortex, and LH and FSH cells of anterior pituitary. In brain the dynorphin system is linked through a very complex fiber network to sympathetic tone, pain systems, motor systems, endocrine control, limbic system, and cortical functions. The enkephalin system, even more widespread than dynorphin and POMC, is found with the catecholamine cells of the adrenal medulla; it is also in heart, lung, gut wall, sympathetic ganglia, and pituitary and shows many brain fiber systems. In brain it is extremely widespread, so that currently only very few circuits linking enkephalin cells and fibers have been described. The most obvious systems impacted by enkephalin are motor, pain, endocrine, autonomic, limbic (reward), cortex, and hippocampus.

As the structure of the endorphin peptides and precursors became clear, major questions arose concerning the biosynthetic processing of the peptides in different neural and endocrine tissue. The most obvious example of tissue-specific processing of the endorphins is found with POMC in the pituitary of the rat. In the anterior lobe the corticotrophs produce, among other peptides, the stress hormone ACTH (1-39). In contrast, in the intermediate lobe (found in most species, but in humans present only in pregnant women and fetuses) that same molecule is further processed to make α-melanocyte-stimulating hormone [or N-acetyl ACTH 1-13 amide and ACTH (18-39)]. Similar tissue-specific processing patterns are found for other POMC peptides, such as β-endorphin, as well as for pro-dynorphin– and pro-enkephalin–produced peptides. For example, pro-enkephalin in adrenal is cleaved into larger fragments, whereas in brain it is actively processed to much smaller peptides.

Several principles have emerged about the processing of neuropeptides. A given precursor can give rise to one set of products in one tissue and a different set of products in another tissue.

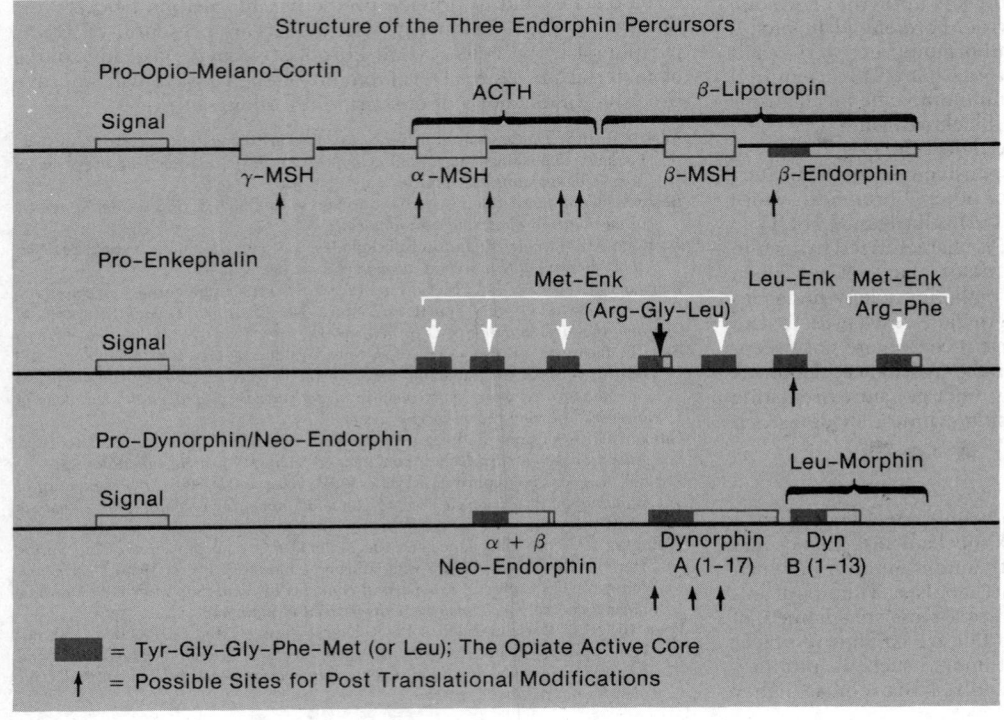

FIGURE 209–1. Simplified schematic of the precursors for all three endorphin families. Note the many peptides produced from each precursor, their similar size, and in the case of pro-enkephalin and pro-dynorphin, the multiple copies of opioid peptides produced by each.

General processing differences are due to the cleavage site chosen, indicated by the presence of a dibasic peptide bond (e.g., lysine-arginine). In a second type of processing variant other chemical moieties are added to a given site in a peptide sequence, e.g., amidation, acetylation, sulfation, or phosphorylation. Both types of processing choices can alter the nature and potency of these molecules. For example, the addition of an acetyl group to the amino terminal tyrosine of β-endorphin decreases its opiate activity by more than 1000-fold. Thus, two of the largest problems in peptidergic systems, especially in brain, are in understanding the precursor-processing pathways and the final structure of the peptides produced by each precursor, in a tissue of interest. Figure 209–1 provides a simplified version of this information for each precursor.

Peptidergic cells have a range of control over the materials that they secrete. To add further complexity, several peptides arise from each of the three endorphin precursors, and nonopioid peptides can be co-produced and co-secreted along with the endorphins (e.g., ACTH and β-endorphin from anterior lobe).

Three main opiate receptor subclasses, each with a different distribution pattern in brain, gut, pituitary, adrenal, and reproductive tissues, have been described (μ, κ, δ).

The μ receptor is very sensitive to morphine; the δ receptor seems to prefer enkephalin-like peptides; the κ receptor was characterized by the action of dynorphin-like peptides. In addition, an ε receptor has been suggested for β-endorphin, although it has been demonstrated only in peripheral tissue. The selectivity of the receptors is not absolute. For example, dynorphin, while κ preferring, is also a potent μ agonist, and enkephalins, while δ preferring, can also interact with the μ site. More accurate characterization of these receptors and their biochemistry, structure, and ligand preferences will depend on the cloning of their respective genes and on study of post-translational modifications of gene products in specific tissues. In addition, there is not a one-to-one anatomic link between κ receptors and dynorphin-producing cells and fibers; nor is there one for the δ receptor and pro-enkephalin systems. Rather, one tends to see two or even three opiate receptor subtypes associated with the terminal systems of the peptidergic neurons. It is conceivable that the processing choices of a cell, by altering the peptide products, can alter the receptor preference of the materials secreted. In effect, it is possible that the cell modulates its products as a function of physiologic or pharmacologic demand, to act on different receptor subtypes at the synapse. Thus, such a system would be extremely flexible in the way it modulates its synaptic transmission.

With a multiplicity of peptides and receptors across a variety of tissues, it is clear that endorphins do not have a single physiologic role. Furthermore, multiple active transmitters and modulators may exist in the same cell. A particularly clear example of "co-transmission" can be found with the pro-dynorphin peptides in the hypothalamus. Pro-dynorphin peptides (and mRNA) are found in the same cells that produce vasopressin. Consistent with this finding, arginine vasopressin (AVP) and dynorphin are co-released from the posterior pituitary with the same stimuli. It is hypothesized that dynorphin provides local feedback inhibition on further AVP secretion. Other examples of co-transmission among the endorphins include enkephalin and catecholamines in the adrenal medulla, enkephalin and catecholamines in the sympathetic nervous system, and dynorphin and LH/FSH in the anterior pituitary.

Table 209–1 summarizes the main physiologic observations associated with the endorphins. The endorphins have been classically associated with modulation of stress and pain. The neuronal and endocrine systems involved in these responses are, in the case of stress, the hypothalamic-pituitary-adrenal system and the limbic system. In fact, each major component of the stress-response system contains endorphins. For example, the hippocampus, a main site of corticosteroid feedback, contains enkephalin and dynorphin neurons; the hypothalamus contains all three opioid families; the anterior pituitary contains POMC and enkephalin; and the adrenal medulla produces enkephalin and the adrenal cortex, dynorphin. A similar pattern is seen in pain-modulatory systems in the spinal cord, periaqueductal central gray, thalamus, and the limbic system. It seems clear that stress and pain responses are, in several ways, dependent on endorphin physiology.

TABLE 209–1. PROPOSED FUNCTIONS AND KNOWN ANATOMIC LOCALIZATIONS OF THE ENDOGENOUS OPIOID SYSTEMS

Function	Anatomic Localization
Appetite modulation and eating behavior	Limbic system, including hypothalamus and amygdala
Cardiovascular regulation	NTS, parabrachial nucleus
Drinking and water balance	Subfornical organ, magnocellular hypothalamic-pituitary system
Endocrine responses	Hypothalamic-pituitary-peripheral axis
Stimulatory effects on Growth hormone Melanocyte-stimulating hormone Prolactin	Hypothalamus and anterior lobe
Inhibitory effects on Follicle-stimulating hormone Luteinizing hormone Thyroid-stimulating hormone	Hypothalamus and anterior lobe
Inhibition of release of vasopressin and oxytocin	Hypothalamus and posterior lobe
Gastrointestinal motility	NTS, area postrema, and GI nervous plexi
Pain inhibition	Thalamus, periaqueductal gray, substantia gelatinosa, NTS, spinal cord
Respiration	Parabrachial nucleus, NTS
Response to stress	Hypothalamic-pituitary-adrenal axis
Sensory-motor integration	Nigrostriatal system, globus pallidus, inferior and superior colliculi
Thermoregulation	Hypothalamus

NTS = Nucleus tractus solitarius.

The physiology of the endorphins presents certain patterns in Table 209–1: (1) These peptides are implicated in a wide variety of physiologic events. (2) Many of these events correlate fairly well with the anatomy of the opioid peptides. For example, all three endorphins are found in the nucleus tractus solitarius and are implicated in cardiovascular regulation; gut motility is controlled from the brain and gut opiatergic loci; respiration is regulated partially by the parabrachial nucleus, an area with both opiate peptides and receptors; and motor integration actively involves the nigrostriatal system, rich in opioid anatomy. (3) The functions associated with the endorphins are basic, homeostatic, limbic, "core" functions; they do not seem to be primarily cognitive but may be more affective or drive related. (4) There are a few "unexpected" physiologic links, such as appetite modulation, drinking, and thermoregulation.

The current state of endorphin biology does not allow precise links between particular peptides, neural circuits or receptors, and specific behaviors. Only a few such inferences can be made. For example, dynorphin in posterior pituitary may play a role in thirst regulation, or anterior pituitary POMC may be involved in stress responses.

Finally, perhaps the most exciting set of advances has come from the study of the regulation of the transcription of pro-enkephalin and POMC genes. Several enhancer and repressor DNA sequences have been identified in the 5' untranslated flanking regions of both genes. Among these are sequences that respond to A and C kinase second messenger systems, and to glucocorticoids. The specific proteins that bind to those sites have been described and in some cases sequenced.

It is clear that the next decade will be one of consolidation and organization of the great wealth of biologic data on these important systems. One of the main foci will be a clearer view of the physiology-peptide-receptor interface; the other will be an increased understanding of the genetic regulation of these systems. With the increasing clarity will come an improved appreciation of the regulation of a whole series of critical basic brain functions.

Akil H, Bronstein D, Mansour A: Overview of the endogenous opioid systems. In Rodgers RJ, Cooper SJ (eds.): Endorphins, Opiates and Behavioral Processes.

Chichester, John Wiley and Sons Limited, 1988, pp 1–23. *A general overview of the biochemistry, anatomy, and physiology of endorphins.*

Herbert E, Seasholtz A, Comb M, et al.: Study of the regulation of expression of neuropeptide genes by gene transfer methods. *In* Psychopharmacology: The Third Generation of Progress. New York, Raven Press, 1987, pp 373–384. *A summary of the gene structure and promoter elements of several peptide genes.*

Holoday JW: Endogenous opioids and their receptors. *In* Current Concepts. Kalamazoo, Mich. Upjohn Company, 1984, pp 4–64. *A summary of some of the physiologic functions attributable to the endogenous opioid systems. It is particularly recommended for the novice who wishes to have a general summary of opioid systems and their possible function.*

Khachaturian H, Lewis ME, Schafer MK, et al.: Anatomy of the CNS opioid systems. Trends Neurosc 8(3):111, 1985. *A summary of the cells and circuits that contain endorphin peptides in brain.*

Mansour A, Khachaturian H, Lewis ME, et al.: Anatomy of CNS opioid receptors. Trends Neurosc 11(7):308, 1988. *A summary of the distribution of the three types of opioid receptors in rat brain.*

Mansour A, Schafer MKH, Newman SW, et al.: Central distribution of opioid receptors: A cross-species comparison of the multiple opioid systems of the basal ganglia. *In* Almeida OFX, Shippenberg TS (eds.): Opioid Peptides and Receptors. Berlin, Springer-Verlag, in press.

Martin WR: Pharmacology of opioids. Pharmacol Rev 32:283, 1984. *An authoritative and comprehensive review of opiate pharmacology. The author presents an in-depth analysis of how different classes of opiates may influence analgesia, respiration, cardiovascular function, pupil dilation, temperature, EEG, and dependence.*

Millan MJ, Herz A: The endocrinology of the opioids. Int Rev Neurobiol 26:1, 1985. *A comprehensive review of the role of the opioid peptides and receptors in neuroendocrine responses. The authors have worked many years in this area and provide a thoughtful review of this field.*

210 Prostaglandins and Related Compounds

Garret A. FitzGerald

Arachidonic acid, derived from dietary sources, is transported in plasma in both esterified and nonesterified forms, primarily bound to lipoproteins and albumin, respectively. The relative importance of these two sources for cellular delivery is poorly understood. Esterified arachidonic acid in low density lipoproteins is taken up by cells by a process dependent on the low density lipoprotein receptor. The fatty acid is compartmentalized in the phospholipid domain of cell membranes. This localization appears relevant to the availability of arachidonate for release (in response to specific stimuli as well as to nonspecific physical and chemical perturbation of membranes) for subsequent oxygenation by either cyclo-oxygenase or lipoxygenase to give rise to biologically active compounds. A third pathway of metabolism via cytochrome P-450 also exists (Fig. 210–1).

All cells can release arachidonic acid, but the predominant enzymatic products that are formed are highly cell specific. Because they are derived from a polyunsaturated eicosanoic (C_{20}) fatty acid, these compounds—thromboxane A_2, the prostaglandins (PG's), epoxygenases, leukotrienes, and lipoxins—are collectively known as eicosanoids. Because of their diverse biologic properties and rapid metabolism to inactive products, the eicosanoids have

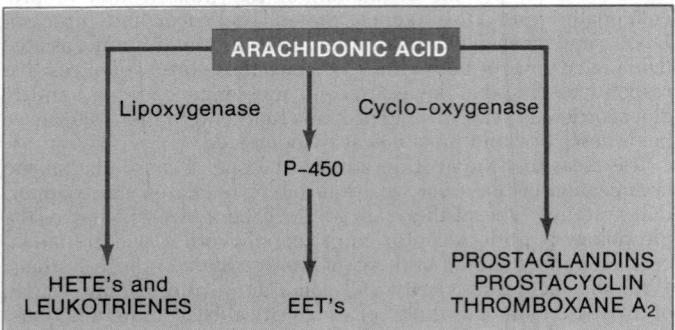

FIGURE 210–1. Major pathways of metabolism of arachidonic acid.

been implicated as local mediators of receptor-dependent events in a range of physiologic processes and in diverse human diseases, including bronchial asthma, inflammation, and unstable coronary disease. Arachidonic acid itself and its metabolites may also function as intracellular second messengers, particularly in the modulation of ion channels.

THE CYCLO-OXYGENASE PATHWAY (Fig. 210–2)

The biotransformation of arachidonic acid into thromboxane (Tx)A_2, prostacyclin (PGI$_2$), PGE$_2$, PGF$_{2\alpha}$, and PGD$_2$ is catalyzed by a common enzyme, the fatty acid cyclo-oxygenase. The product of the cyclo-oxygenase reaction is an unstable endoperoxide, PGG. A second oxygen molecule is then introduced at C_{15}; this results in the 15-hydroperoxy endoperoxide PGH, and liberates a free radical. The cyclo-oxygenase and peroxidase activities reside in a single membrane-associated protein, PGG/H synthase, for which the human gene has been cloned and localized to chromosome 9.

PGH is metabolized by cell-specific enzymes to form either the "classic" prostaglandins of the D, E, and F series, PGI$_2$, or TxA$_2$. Arachidonic acid contains four double bonds ($\Delta^{5,8,11,14}$). It is apparent from the sequence of biosynthesis (Fig. 210–2) that two double bonds remain in its (bisenoic) cyclo-oxygenase products. This is denoted by the subscript 2, as in TxA$_2$ and PGE$_2$. Analogous metabolism of other fatty acid substrates gives rise to monoenoic or trienoic prostaglandins and thromboxanes (Fig. 210–3). For example, metabolites of eicosatrienoic acid ($C_{20:3}$n-6) contain only one (Δ^{13}) double bond. Eicosapentaenoic acid (EPA) ($C_{20:5}$n-3), which is prevalent in certain fish and aquatic mammals, is transformed by cyclo-oxygenase to metabolites with three ($\Delta^{5,13,17}$) double bonds, such as PGI$_3$ and TxA$_3$. Structurally, prostaglandins of the D, E, and F series possess a cyclopentane ring and differ only in their substituent groups. The F series prostaglandins are referred to as PGF$_{1\alpha}$, PGF$_{2\alpha}$, and PGF$_{3\alpha}$. In man, many of the metabolites formed from PGD$_2$ contain an F ring and one of these, 9α,11β-PGF, contracts bronchial and vascular smooth muscle and inhibits platelet aggregation.

THROMBOXANE A$_2$. TxA$_2$, the predominant cyclo-oxygenase product formed by platelets, stimulates aggregation of these cells and constricts vascular and bronchial smooth muscle. These biologic properties are shared by the PG endoperoxides. Use of analogues of PGH$_2$ and/or TxA$_2$ has identified specific binding sites for these eicosanoids on many tissues, including platelets, vascular smooth muscle cells, and glomerular mesangial cells. A cDNA encoding a placental TxA$_2$ receptor has been cloned. The relative rank order potency of different ligands suggests that distinct receptors mediate platelet aggregation and smooth muscle cell contraction. Indeed, it appears that different forms of the receptor (or distinct receptors) transduce the platelet shape change and aggregation responses to these eicosanoids. The relative affinity of these receptors for PGH$_2$ and TxA$_2$ is unknown. Platelet aggregation is induced via receptors linked to a G protein (that is insensitive to pertussis toxin) to activate phospholipase (PL) C. TxA$_2$ is very evanescent at physiologic pH; its half-life has been estimated at 30 seconds.

In addition to initiating aggregation of platelets, TxA$_2$ that is generated by platelets aggregated in response to epinephrine, adenosine diphosphate (ADP), and platelet-activating factor (PAF) is responsible for a "secondary wave" of aggregation. Aspirin inhibits platelet aggregation by preventing the formation of TxA$_2$, although the capacity of platelets to form TxA$_2$ must be inhibited by greater than 95 per cent for even modest inhibition of platelet function.

PROSTACYCLIN. Prostacyclin (PGI$_2$), the predominant cyclo-oxygenase product of arachidonic acid formed by vascular endothelium and also by subendothelium, both inhibits the aggregation of platelets by all recognized agonists and disaggregates previously aggregated platelets. PGI$_2$ inhibits the adherence of platelets and neutrophils to foreign surfaces and damaged endothelium and dilates both bronchial and vascular smooth muscle. PGI$_2$ acts at specific binding sites to activate adenylate cyclase via the stimulatory G protein, G$_s$. Another important property of PGI$_2$ is the modulation of cholesterol efflux from arterial walls. Nanomolar quantities of PGI$_2$ stimulate the activity of both the lysosomal and cytoplasmic cholesterol ester hydrolases when added experimentally to vascular smooth muscle cells but have

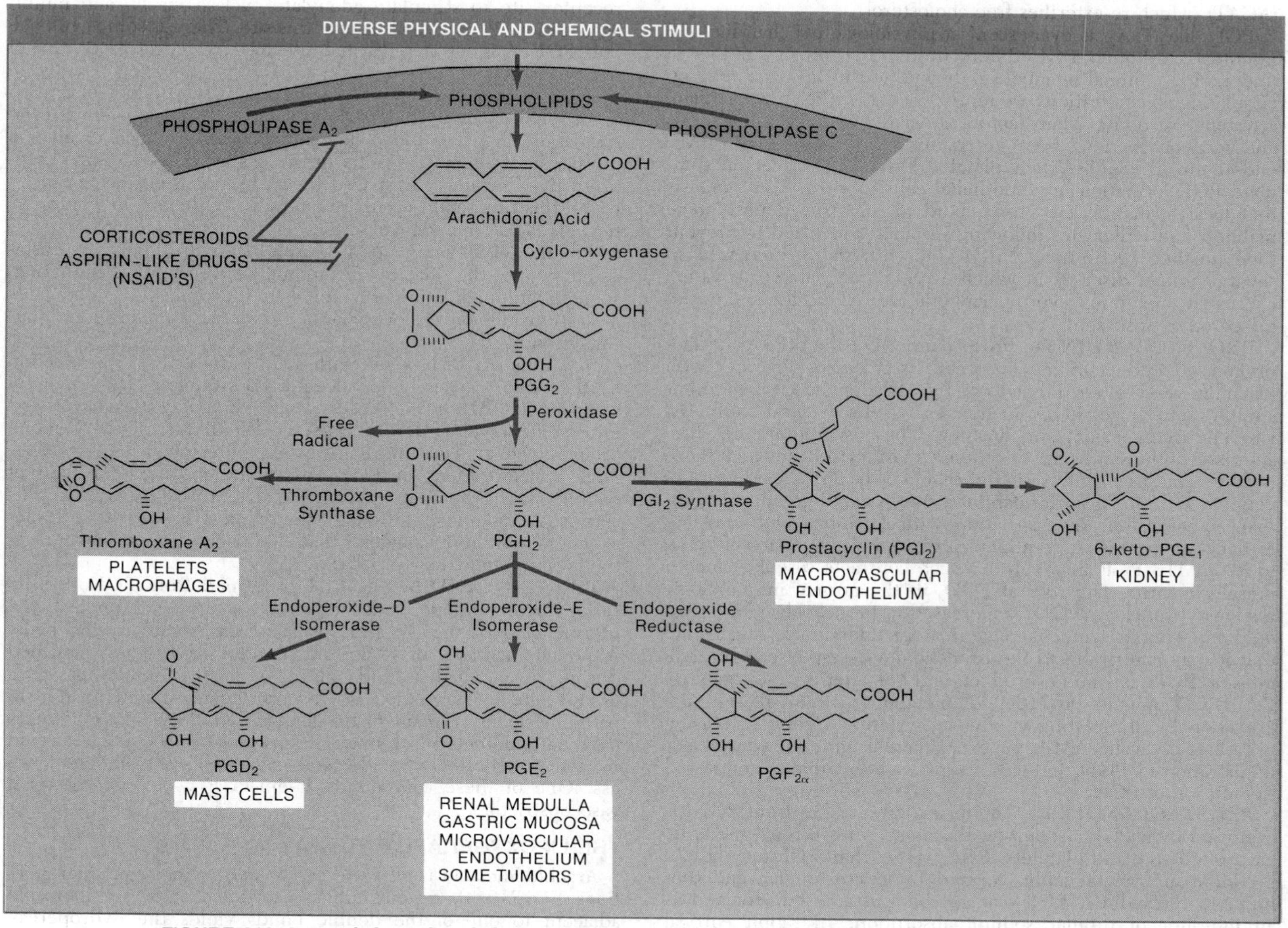

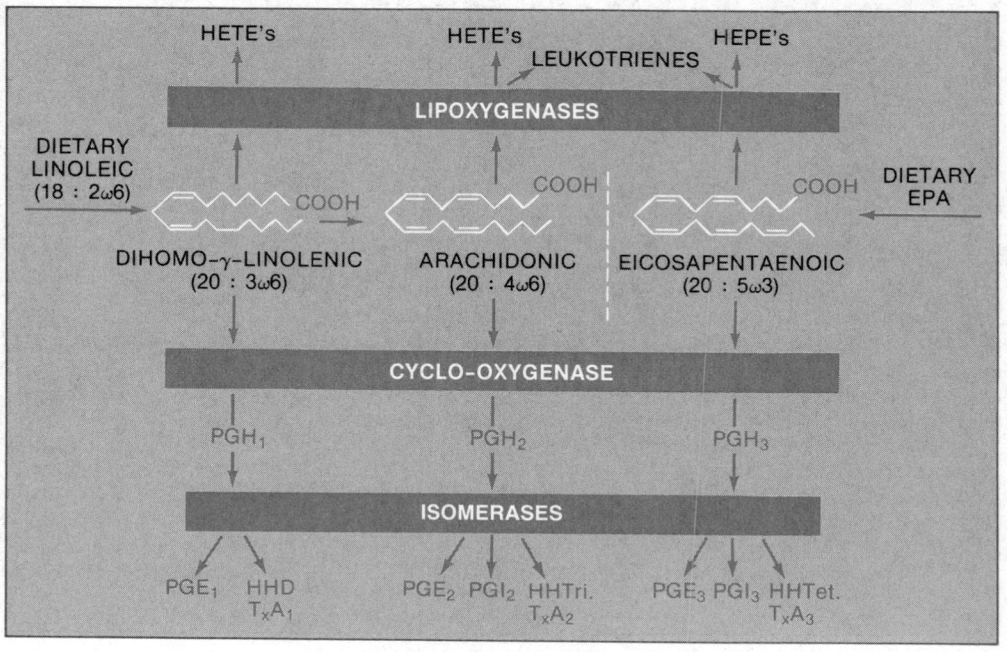

FIGURE 210–2. Metabolism of arachidonic acid by fatty acid cyclo-oxygenase. The major tissues of origin of the eicosanoids are shown.

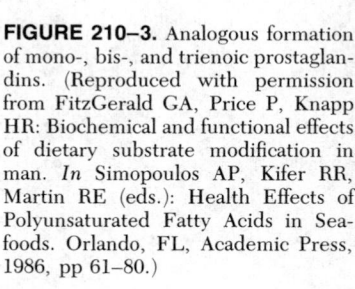

FIGURE 210–3. Analogous formation of mono-, bis-, and trienoic prostaglandins. (Reproduced with permission from FitzGerald GA, Price P, Knapp HR: Biochemical and functional effects of dietary substrate modification in man. *In* Simopoulos AP, Kifer RR, Martin RE (eds.): Health Effects of Polyunsaturated Fatty Acids in Seafoods. Orlando, FL, Academic Press, 1986, pp 61–80.)

no effect on the microsomal acyl-CoA cholesterol acyl transferase (ACAT), which re-esterifies free cholesterol.

PGI_2, like TxA_2, is evanescent at physiologic pH (half-life of 3 minutes). Although PGI_2 differs from other prostaglandins in undergoing minimal metabolism during transit through the lung, circulating concentrations are rarely, if ever, sufficient to mediate a systemic response. Many factors associated with thrombogenesis and vasoconstriction, such as trauma, thrombin, ADP, PAF, endothelin, PGH_2/TxA_2, and platelet-derived growth factor, stimulate PGI_2 formation by endothelial cells in vitro. This suggests that local formation may serve both to limit the deposition of platelets and leukocytes following vascular injury and to prevent their further recruitment. PGI_2 biosynthesis is increased in several human diseases in which evidence of platelet activation is present, including severe peripheral arterial disease and unstable coronary disease.

PROSTAGLANDIN D_2. Prostaglandin D_2, the principal cyclo-oxygenase product of the mast cell, is released, together with histamine and other mediators, by IgE-dependent and other stimuli. Infusion of PGD_2 in humans results in nasal stuffiness, systemic hypotension, and flushing. These symptoms are characteristic of the syndrome of systemic mastocytosis in which there is diffuse mast cell infiltration of tissues (Ch. 252). A minority of patients with this disorder exhibit a rise in blood pressure, rather than hypotension, in association with flushing. One possible explanation for this observation is preferential conversion of PGD_2 to its $9\alpha,11\beta$-PGF metabolite, which contracts vascular smooth muscle in vitro. The role of PGD_2 in the normal immunologic response is unclear. PGD_2 is increased in bronchoalveolar lavage fluid following antigen challenge in atopic individuals, suggesting that it may contribute to the bronchomotor response in allergic asthma. PGD_2 is a minor product of the platelet cyclo-oxygenase. Both PGD_2 and its $9\alpha,11\beta$-PGF metabolite inhibit platelet aggregation by stimulating adenylate cyclase, thereby increasing intraplatelet cyclic AMP. In experimental animals, central administration of PGD_2 induces sleep, an event that is countered by infusion of PGE_2.

PROSTAGLANDIN E_2. The formation of PGE_2 from PGH_2 is catalyzed by a PGE_2 isomerase that is present in renal medulla, gastric mucosa, and platelets. PGE_2 rather than PGI_2 may be the predominant prostaglandin formed by microvascular endothelium. In the kidney, PGE_2 can act both as a vasodilator and as an inhibitor of tubular sodium absorption. In rabbit cortical collecting tubular cells, PGE_2 acts via distinct receptors to stimulate and inhibit adenylate cyclase via G_s and G_i, respectively. In human platelets, PGE_1 and PGI_2 apparently act at an identical receptor site to stimulate adenylate cyclase via G_s and inhibit aggregation. PGE_2 can also act at this site. There is some evidence that PGE_2 can act at a distinct site to exert negative control of the cyclase via G_i.

PGE_2 is the predominant cyclo-oxygenase product of arachidonic acid formed in gastric mucosa. It participates in the regulation of gastric blood flow and limits the effects of diverse physical and chemical insults to the gastric mucosa. This "cytoprotective" property is shared by PGI_2, but the mechanism by which this protection occurs is unknown. Other biologic properties of PGE_2 include relaxation of bronchial smooth muscle, contraction of uterine smooth muscle (19-hydroxylated E prostaglandins are the major arachidonic acid products in human semen), and modulation of lymphocyte function. PGE_2 modulates neurotransmission via presynaptic receptors on adrenergic neurons in vitro.

In a minority of patients with solid tumors, PGE_2 production by the tumor causes hypercalcemia via stimulation of osteoclast activity (Ch. 161). In such cases, suppression of PGE_2 biosynthesis lowers the level of serum calcium. When metastases to bone occur, however, local mechanisms for hypercalcemia supervene. High concentrations of PGE_2 are found in the joint fluid of patients with rheumatoid arthritis. The role of PGE_2 in this setting is unknown, although the clinical response to cyclo-oxygenase inhibitors suggests that eicosanoids are of relevance to the local inflammatory process.

PROSTAGLANDIN $F_{2\alpha}$. $PGF_{2\alpha}$, formed from PGH_2 by the action of an endoperoxide reductase, contracts bronchial and uterine smooth muscle and vasoconstricts some uterine beds. Although increases in $PGF_{2\alpha}$ metabolites have been described during dysmenorrhea and allergen-evoked bronchospasm, a unique site for formation of this prostaglandin and its role in pathophysiology remain to be determined. Novel PGF isomers have been detected in human plasma and urine that are formed by a free radical–catalyzed, cyclo-oxygenase-independent process. One of these compounds, 8-epi-$PGF_{2\alpha}$, is a potent renal vasoconstrictor.

THE LIPOXYGENASE PATHWAY (Fig. 210–4)

Arachidonic acid is also widely subject to lipoxygenation reactions (Fig. 210–4). In neutrophils, insertion of an oxygen molecule adjacent to one of the double bonds yields the hydroperoxy

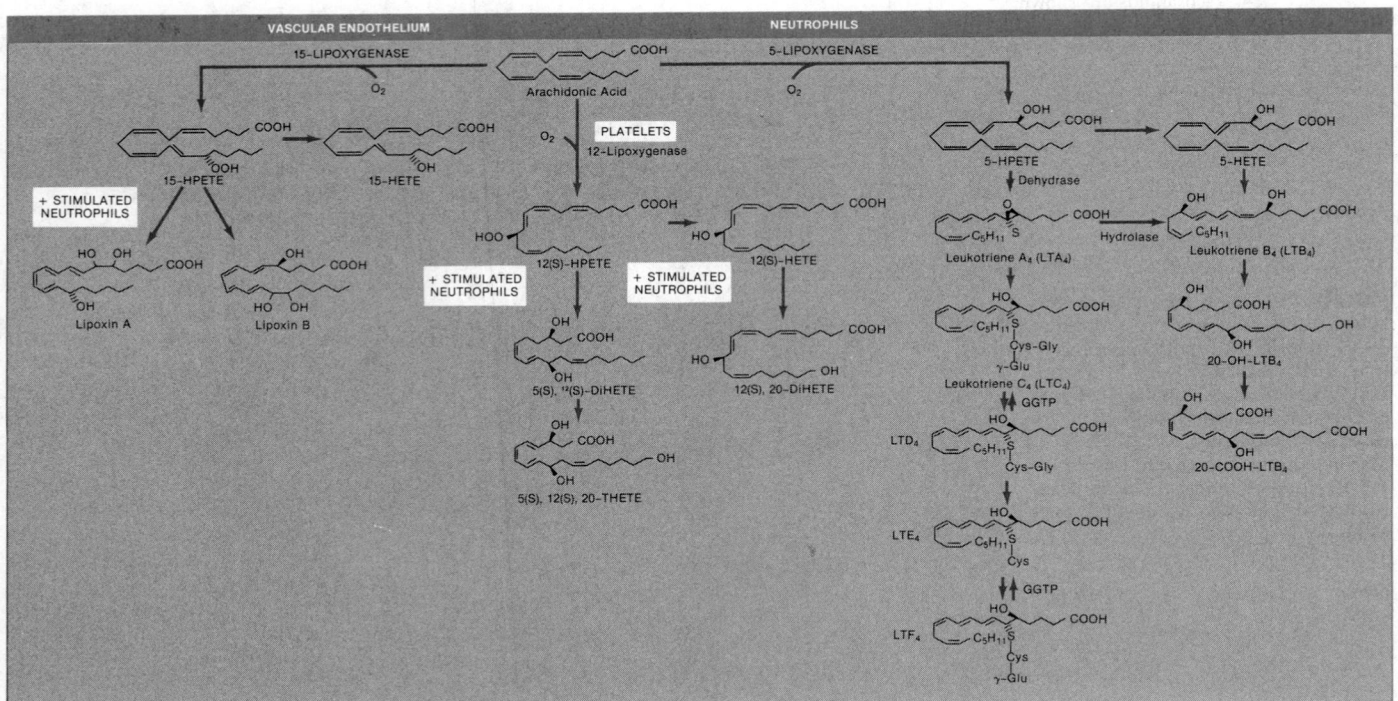

FIGURE 210–4. Metabolism of arachidonic acid by lipoxygenase enzymes.

derivative, 5-hydroperoxyeicosatetraenoic acid (5-HPETE). This can undergo further metabolism to either a 5-hydroxyeicosatetraenoic acid (5-HETE) or to an unstable 5,6-epoxide intermediate, leukotriene (LT)A$_4$. This compound can be hydrolyzed to 5,12-dihydroxyeicosatetraenoic acids, one of which is LTB$_4$. The subscript 4 refers to the number of double bonds. Thus, analogous to the nomenclature for cyclo-oxygenase products, substitution of eicosapentaenoic acid for arachidonic acid as a substrate would result in formation of LTB$_5$. The site of the initial lipoxygenation reaction tends to vary with cell type. Thus, 12-HETE is formed predominantly in platelets, 5-HETE by polymorphonuclear leukocytes, and 5-HETE, 11-HETE, and 15-HETE by endothelial cells as measured in culture.

The 5-lipoxygenase of human neutrophils, a cytosolic enzyme, is translocated to the membrane for metabolism of arachidonic acid. It requires an 18K protein, termed the five lipoxygenase activating protein (FLAP), to achieve full activation. The development of both 5-lipoxygenase inhibitors and of a translocation inhibitor is likely to elucidate the role of the products of this pathway in human physiology and disease. Analogous activating proteins do not appear necessary for expression of 12- and 15-lipoxygenase activity. The primary structures of two distinct 12-lipoxygenases have been reported. One, in porcine leukocytes, is immunologically identical to that in porcine brain and human tracheal cells. It is closely related to the 15-lipoxygenase. The human platelet 12-lipoxygenase is a distinct gene product. The role of 12-HETE in platelets is unknown. Platelet 12-lipoxygenase is translocated from the cytosol to the membrane in a calcium-dependent manner, and 12-HETE inhibits the mobilization of a glycoprotein IIb/IIIa complex in tumor cell lines. This complex is analogous to that which serves as a receptor for adhesive macromolecules, such as fibrinogen, in activated platelets. 12-Lipoxygenase products regulate potassium channel flux in Aplysia. Formation of 15-HETE is reportedly increased in atherosclerotic blood vessels, and recent in situ hybridization studies suggest that expression of the enzyme is increased and colocalized with oxidized low density lipoproteins in human atherosclerotic plaques.

LTA$_4$ is conjugated enzymatically with glutathione to yield LTC$_4$. This compound is metabolized to LTD$_4$ and LTE$_4$ by successive elimination of a γ-glutamyl residue and glycine. The cysteinyl-containing leukotrienes are powerful bronchoconstrictors and vasoconstrictors. In addition, they have been shown to be identical with "slow-reacting substance of anaphylaxis"—a product first identified following immunologic challenge or addition of cobra venom to guinea pig ileum. These compounds also dilate microvessels, increase vascular permeability, and stimulate mucus secretion. LTC$_4$ causes pulmonary bronchoconstriction, an effect that is partially blocked by cyclo-oxygenase inhibitors. This implies that LTC$_4$ may mediate this effect via the release of a bronchoconstrictor prostaglandin, such as thromboxane A$_2$. LTC$_4$ may cooperate with luteinizing hormone–releasing hormone (LHRH) in the control of LH release by cells of the anterior pituitary, judged by in vitro studies.

LTB$_4$ stimulates adhesion, migration, aggregation, enzyme release, and generation of superoxide by polymorphonuclear leukocytes. These biologic properties strongly suggest a role for lipoxygenase products in both inflammation and antigen-evoked bronchoconstriction. DiHETE's can be formed via transcellular metabolism, at least in vitro. Examples include 12,20-DiHETE formed by a mixed suspension of platelets and polymorphonuclear leukocytes. Leukocytes can utilize erythrocyte LTA$_4$ to generate LTB$_4$ and endothelial cells can utilize platelet-derived PGH$_2$ to generate PGI$_2$.

Stimulated human leukocytes can convert 15-HPETE to products termed lipoxins (LX) containing a characteristic tetraenoic structure (Fig. 210–4). The two major products are identified as LXA and LXB. LXA is a potent stimulus to superoxide generation by neutrophils and contracts pulmonary tissue. Both LXA and LXB inhibit natural killer cell cytotoxicity in vitro, by a mechanism distinct from that of PGE$_2$, which decreases the binding between target and effector cells. Another series of compounds with potent biologic properties in vitro are the hepoxilins, formed by an intramolecular rearrangement of 12-HETE. Glutathione conjugates of hepoxilin A$_3$ cause hyperpolarization of rat brain neurons at nanomolar concentrations. Definitive evidence for the formation of either LX's or hepoxilins in vivo has yet to be provided.

THE EPOXYGENASE PATHWAY (Fig. 210–5)

In addition to metabolism by cyclo-oxygenase and lipoxygenase enzymes, arachidonic acid is subject to ω and ω-1 oxidation by cytochrome P-450 enzymes in microsomal preparations. This results in the formation of 19-OH and 19-oxo-eicosatetraenoic acid (by ω-1-oxidation) and 20-OH-eicosatetraenoic and eicosatetraene-1,20-dioic acids (by ω oxidation). In addition, a series of epoxides 14(15)-epoxy-, 11(12)-epoxy-, 8(9)-epoxy-, and 5(6)-epoxy-eicosatrienoic acids (EET's) can be formed by this enzyme from arachidonic acid. These compounds can then be further transformed to vicinyl diols by epoxide hydrolases. One such compound, 11,12-dihydroxyeicosatrienoic acid, inhibits the Na$^+$-K$^+$-ATPase enzyme in vascular smooth muscle. 5(6)-EET inhibits sodium absorption and potassium secretion by the rabbit cortical collecting duct, and synthetic 5(6)-EET stimulates the release of LH and somatostatin by pituitary cells in culture. Interestingly, 8,9-EET and 14,15-EET stereospecifically inhibit human platelet cyclo-oxygenase. By contrast, all EET's studied inhibit platelet aggregation in vitro by a nonspecific mechanism, independent of an effect on thromboxane formation. EET's weakly inhibit monocyte and platelet adherence to endothelial cells. Finally, 5(6)-EET is metabolized to epoxides of PGG$_1$, PGH$_1$, and PGE$_1$ and to the 5S, 6S and 5R, 6R isomers of 5-hydroxy-PGI$_1$. The biosynthesis of EET's has recently been confirmed in vivo. Urinary excretion of their vicinyl diols (DHET's) is increased in normal pregnancy, and further increments, particularly of 14(15)-DHET, are observed in patients with pregnancy-induced hypertension.

PHARMACOLOGIC AND DIETARY REGULATION OF BIOSYNTHESIS

With the exception of P-450–derived metabolites, none of the oxygenated products of arachidonic acid are stored in significant quantities for subsequent release by cells. Release is equivalent to biosynthesis. Arachidonate release may occur by several mechanisms. Phosphatidylinositol (PI) may be hydrolyzed by a PI-specific PLC, yielding diacylglycerol (DAG) and inositol phosphate. DAG is then further hydrolyzed, yielding free arachidonic acid and other fatty acids. Alternatively, phosphatidylcholine (PC) may be hydrolyzed by phospholipase A$_2$(PLA$_2$), yielding arachidonic acid from the sn-2 position. PLA$_2$ may also liberate arachidonic acid from phosphatidylethanolamine. Selectivity of phospholipid compartmentalization and phospholipase action permits some HETE's and EET's to modulate second messenger formation. Thus, 15-HETE incubated with endothelial cells is selectively incorporated into PI, and agonist-evoked activation of PLC results in release of a 1-stearoyl-2(15-HETE)-DAG. Similarly, PLD-catalyzed formation of a modified phosphatidic acid has been demonstrated.

CORTICOSTEROIDS. The effects of steroids on eicosanoid biosynthesis are complex. It is thought that they induce formation of a phospholipase-inhibitory protein, variously named lipocortin, macrocortin, lipomodulin, and renomodulin (see Fig. 210–2). It is hypothesized that initially steroids bind to specific cytosolic receptors and that the complex is then transferred to the nucleus where steroids regulate the expression of genes and subsequently the synthesis of a PLA$_2$-inhibitory protein (Ch. 208). The lipocortin family is derived from a monomeric 40K protein, phosphorylation of which by protein kinases results in its activation as an inhibitor. Interestingly, there is a striking sequence homology between this protein and the 40K protein that is phosphorylated following the binding of epidermal growth factor to its receptor. The amino acid sequence of one member of the family, lipocortin III, is identical to that of inositol 1,2-cyclic phosphate 2 phosphohydrolase. It is possible that other lipocortins are also enzymes that regulate the intracellular levels of inositol phosphate messages during cellular activation. Prevention of protein synthesis blocks the inhibitory effect of steroids on the release of radiolabeled arachidonate by neutrophils with the chemoattractant peptide, f-Met-Leu-Phe. A cDNA has been isolated and cloned that encodes for a 40K protein that inhibits arachidonic acid release from prelabeled cells. Such a role for lipocortin has been disputed, however, especially as lipocortins bind nonspecifically to phospholipids. The effects of steroids on eicosanoid biosynthesis in vivo are complex and appear to exhibit cellular specificity. Although steroids do not affect the activity of constitutively expressed PGG/H synthase, they block its induction in several systems by agents such as interleukin-1, bacterial lipopolysaccharide, and DMSO. There is also some evidence that steroids regulate stimulated increases in phospholipase mRNA. Further studies are necessary to elucidate the contribution of these mechanisms to the therapeutic efficacy of corticosteroids in man.

CYCLO-OXYGENASE INHIBITORS. Nonsteroidal anti-inflammatory drugs (NSAID's) prevent the formation of prostaglandins by inhibiting the enzyme cyclo-oxygenase. This group of drugs includes aspirin, salicylates, indomethacin, ibuprofen, piroxicam, fenoprofen, paracetamol, phenylbutazone, oxyphenbutazone, bolmetin, sulfinpyrazone, and sulindac. Paracetamol (acetaminophen) is a considerably less potent inhibitor than the other compounds, except perhaps in the brain. Aspirin is also unlike the other compounds in that it acetylates a serine residue at position 529, close to the active site of the platelet PGG/H synthase, and inhibits the enzyme irreversibly. This accounts for the unique effects of aspirin on the platelet. While other cells have the capacity for de novo protein synthesis, the anucleate platelet does not; thus inhibition of TxA_2 formation by aspirin persists for the lifetime of the platelet. By contrast, the effects of aspirin on eicosanoid formation by other cells (e.g., prostacyclin biosynthesis by vascular endothelium) are not so prolonged. The irreversible actions of aspirin on platelet cyclo-oxygenase also account for the cumulative inhibition of platelet TxA_2 formation by the repeated administration of low dosages of aspirin (20 to 40 mg per day; a regular aspirin tablet contains 325 mg). This results in partial inhibition of platelet cyclo-oxygenase after single-dose administration. Even though low doses of aspirin tend to depress PGI_2 formation, its effect is more pronounced on platelet TxA_2 biosynthesis during long-term therapy. This relative "biochemical selectivity" for TxA_2 may result from partial recovery of PGI_2 formation or pharmacokinetic properties of the drug. A differential sensitivity of the enzyme in platelets and endothelial cells is a superficially unlikely explanation, given the identity of the deduced primary structures of the PGG/H synthases in the two tissues. Aspirin is subject to extensive first-pass metabolism by the liver, and its deacylated product, salicylic acid, is a weak inhibitor of platelet cyclo-oxygenase. Reduction in the rate of drug delivery in a controlled release preparation permits more efficient hepatic extraction of aspirin. This still permits cumulative inhibition of platelet cyclo-oxygenase in the presystemic circulation, while protecting the cyclo-oxygenase in the systemic vasculature from aspirin exposure.

Tissue-selective inhibition of cyclo-oxygenase may also be possible with sulindac and sulfinpyrazone. These compounds are prodrugs that are converted by the intestinal flora to their sulfide derivatives, which are potent cyclo-oxygenase inhibitors. Renal tissue possesses the capacity to retroconvert these sulfides to their inactive sulfones, and evidence suggests that renal prostaglandin synthesis may be spared by doses of these drugs that completely inhibit TxA_2 formation by platelets.

THROMBOXANE SYNTHASE INHIBITORS AND RECEPTOR ANTAGONISTS. Many imidazole and pyridine analogues selectively inhibit thromboxane synthase. These compounds depress TxA_2 formation without coincidental inhibition of PGI_2 synthesis, as seen with NSAID's. Indeed, following Tx synthase inhibition, accumulated platelet PGH_2 can be utilized by vascular PGI_2 synthase. Tx synthase inhibitors increase the biosynthesis of platelet-inhibitory, vasodilator prostaglandins, such as PGI_2 and PGE_2, at the platelet-vascular interface in man. Although limited clinical trials have failed to demonstrate benefit from these compounds, this may reflect incomplete suppression of TxA_2 biosynthesis throughout the dosing interval with these reversible inhibitors and/or substitution for the action of TxA_2 by accumulated PGH_2. In this regard, antagonists of the shared TxA_2-PGH_2 receptor are currently under study in man. Synergy of these compounds with Tx synthase inhibitors has been demonstrated in animal models of thrombosis, and several drugs that combine both properties are under study in man.

DIETARY SUBSTRATE MODIFICATION. Mortality from coronary heart disease seems to be lower in populations who consume large quantities of n-3 fatty acids, such as EPA, from aquatic mammals or fish. One hypothesis has been that a shift toward the formation of TxA_3 (which is less biologically active than TxA_2) and PGI_3 (which is a platelet-inhibitory, vasodilator compound like PGI_2) may favorably influence platelet–vessel wall interactions (see Fig. 210–3). Although fish oil supplementation of the western diet has only modest effects on platelet function, it has caused apparent regression of atherosclerosis in several animal models. The biologic properties of many eicosanoids suggest their relevance to the evolving atherosclerotic lesion. It is possible that the altered biologic activity of their trienoic analogues, together with other properties of marine oils, such as

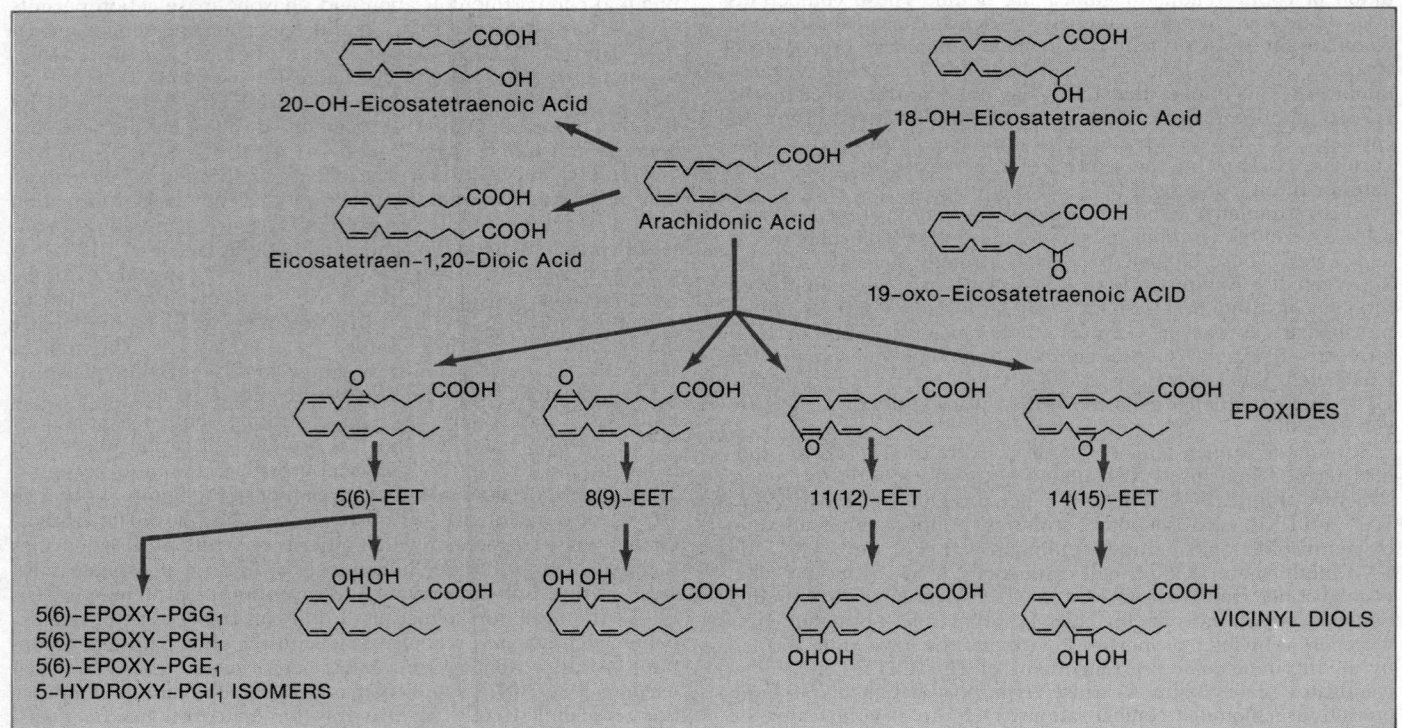

FIGURE 210–5. Metabolism of arachidonic acid by cytochrome P-450.

their ability to influence plasma lipids and cell membrane fluidity, may facilitate plaque regression.

Supplementation of the diet with n-3 fatty acids lowers blood pressure in patients with mild essential hypertension. This effect is not obviously related to altered eicosanoid formation. Similarly, it has been hypothesized that marine oils might modulate inflammatory or immune diseases by altering the profile of lipoxygenase product formation.

LIPOXYGENASE INHIBITORS AND ANTAGONISTS. Several selective 5-lipoxygenase inhibitors are bioavailable and well tolerated in man, and preliminary evidence of efficacy has been obtained using surrogate endpoints in both ulcerative colitis and allergic rhinitis. Prototype sulfidopeptide leukotriene antagonists diminish the early- and late-phase bronchoconstrictor response to allergen challenge in asthmatic patients. No selective inhibitors of epoxygenase product formation are currently available for use in humans.

FUNCTIONS OF ARACHIDONIC ACID METABOLITES IN VIVO

The evidence implicating arachidonate metabolites in mechanisms of some human diseases includes measurements of their biosynthesis and the effects of drugs that prevent their formation or antagonize their actions. Because of the evanescence of the primary compounds, estimates of in vivo synthesis have largely been based upon measurement of long-lived but biologically inactive metabolites. Quantitative assays for the major urinary metabolites of primary prostaglandins, PGI_2 and TxA_2, have been useful in identifying potential targets for drugs designed to modulate their actions. Similar methodology is now available to explore lipoxygenase and epoxygenase product formation in vivo. The capacity of tissues to generate arachidonic acid metabolites greatly exceeds the actual production rates in vivo. Thus, artifacts related to sample collection (for example, platelet activation ex vivo during blood sampling, catheter-induced vascular trauma, or formation of free radical–catalyzed derivatives during sample storage) can seriously confound attempts to measure these compounds in the bloodstream. Measurement of metabolite excretion in urine has been favored as a noninvasive, albeit indirect, approach. The most specific and sensitive method for measurement of eicosanoid metabolites is gas chromatography–mass spectrometry, which has been used to validate radioimmunoassays and enzyme immunoassays for selected compounds.

THE CARDIOVASCULAR SYSTEM. TxA_2 is one of many platelet agonists generated in vivo. While aspirin inhibits Tx-dependent aggregation, other agonists, such as thrombin and high doses of collagen, can induce aggregation in vitro despite the presence of aspirin. In view of these properties, it is superficially surprising that aspirin has been shown to influence clinical outcome in a variety of trials in cardiovascular disease, presumably because of its effects on TxA_2 formation. This may reflect the importance of TxA_2 as an amplifying signal for other platelet agonists.

Aspirin reduces significantly the incidence of stroke in patients suffering transient ischemic attacks and those with nonvalvular atrial fibrillation, the incidence of thrombotic occlusion following coronary artery bypass graft implantation, and the incidence of myocardial infarction and death in patients with unstable coronary disease. The risk of a combined endpoint of myocardial infarction, stroke, and vascular death is reduced by about 25 per cent in aspirin-treated patients. The most convincing evidence that aspirin reduces mortality in patients who have suffered an acute myocardial infarction is provided by the ISIS-2 study of more than 17,000 patients. The reduction in mortality achieved by aspirin and the thrombolytic agent streptokinase were comparable and additive.

Clear-cut evidence of the benefit of aspirin has been obtained in smaller trials of patients with unstable angina. This may reflect the early initiation of aspirin therapy and the more prominent role of thrombosis in determining outcome in these patients. Angioscopic and angiographic evidence of thrombosis is present in unstable angina, and phasic increases of TxA_2 formation coincide with episodes of cardiac ischemia. By contrast, the alteration of TxA_2 formation after myocardial infarction is transient, and there is no evidence of platelet activation in patients with chronic stable angina. Thus, if entry to the trial is delayed after a

myocardial infarction, patients represent a more "dilute" population potentially susceptible to benefit from antiplatelet therapy. Although aspirin has been used in combination with dipyridamole in many of these studies, there is little evidence that this latter drug contributes to the antithrombotic efficacy of aspirin in humans. The lowest dose of aspirin that has been shown to be effective in unstable angina has been 75 mg per day.

The use of PGI_2 and its analogues as a platelet-inhibitory drug has been restricted by the need to administer it as an infusion and its steep dose-response relationship. Doses that inhibit platelet function are close to those that cause side effects, such as gastric cramping and hypotension. Nonetheless, its potential efficacy as a platelet inhibitor is illustrated by its effects on platelet adhesion and aggregation in extracorporeal circuits, such as pump oxygenators and hemodialysis units, a setting in which aspirin is markedly less effective. Attempts to assess the efficacy of PGI_2 in atherosclerotic disease involving major vessels in the lower limb have been confounded by a high placebo response rate, but preliminary results look more convincing in thromboangiitis obliterans (Buerger's disease).

Infusion of PGE_1 may reduce the incidence of reocclusion following coronary thrombolysis. Several prototype, orally available PGI and PGE analogues are under investigation.

THE RESPIRATORY SYSTEM. While preliminary evidence indicates that sulfidopeptide antagonists blunt both the early- and late-phase bronchoconstrictor responses to inhaled allergen, the utility of these compounds in the treatment of asthma remains to be defined. Although TxA_2 as well as LT biosynthesis is increased coincident with the bronchoconstrictor response to inhaled allergen, experiments with aspirin and thromboxane antagonists suggest that its functional importance is marginal. A minority of asthmatics, perhaps 10 per cent, exhibit bronchoconstrictive, hypersensitivity reactions to aspirin. This appears to reflect a role for prostaglandins, TxA_2, or leukotrienes, as these attacks are provoked by a range of structurally distinct inhibitors of cyclo-oxygenase but rarely by salicylate, which resembles aspirin but is a weak inhibitor of that enzyme. No evidence currently supports an allergic basis for this condition. Drug-induced reactions in such patients may be quite severe and often feature profuse rhinorrhea and flushing in addition to bronchospasm. Whether such attacks are mediated by differential inhibition of bronchoconstrictor versus bronchodilator prostaglandins, by a shunting of the arachidonate substrate toward lipoxygenation and the formation of bronchoconstrictor leukotrienes, or by reduced formation of a prostaglandin that normally inhibits release of other mediators of bronchoconstriction is unknown.

Aspirin may also trigger a hypersensitivity response in which alterations in blood pressure, flushing, tachycardia, and diarrhea predominate over bronchospasm. Some of these patients have systemic mastocytosis (Ch. 252).

THE GASTROINTESTINAL SYSTEM. Both PGI_2 and PGE_2 are cytoprotective of gastric mucosa in vitro and are thought to contribute to the regulation of mucosal blood flow. The dose-related gastrointestinal side effects of NSAID's are thought to reflect increased susceptibility to local injury (e.g., H^+ backdiffusion) due to inhibition of these prostaglandins. Oral dimethyl PGE analogues have been approved for use as an adjunct to NSAID therapy. The watery diarrhea associated with multiple endocrine neoplasia often responds to treatment with prostaglandin inhibitors. Excessive formation of LTB_4 has been demonstrated in colonic mucosa and rectal dialysates obtained from patients with inflammatory bowel disease.

RENIN RELEASE AND RENAL FUNCTION. While sympathoadrenal activity is the principal regulator of renin release, it appears to be via a cyclo-oxygenase metabolite of arachidonic acid. PGI_2 is the most potent of the prostaglandins as a renin secretagogue. Inhibition of cyclo-oxygenase by NSAID's has implications for the diagnostic application of renin measurements. The associated reduction in aldosterone production may be deleterious for patients with hyperkalemia.

Metabolites of arachidonic acid contribute little to the regulation of renal blood flow under physiologic circumstances. Under conditions of increased vasoconstrictor tone, however, preservation of renal blood flow becomes increasingly dependent upon the generation of vasodilator prostaglandins. This is particularly so in patients with chronic glomerulonephritis, Bartter's syndrome, the nephropathy of systemic lupus erythematosus, congestive heart failure, or combined hepatic and renal dysfunction. It has been proposed that the decline in renal function in such patients following administration of NSAID's is less likely to occur with sulindac as a result of retroconversion of the sulfide to the sulfone.

The kidney possesses the capacity to generate TxA_2 in addition to vasodilator prostaglandins. Renal biosynthesis of TxA_2 is increased in some patients with severe nephropathy in association with systemic lupus erythematosus, and infusion of a PGH_2-TxA_2 receptor antagonist improves indices of renal function in such patients. Increased TxA_2 biosynthesis by the kidney has been demonstrated in animal models in response to ureteric obstruction, renal vein thrombosis, and development of hypertension following partial renal ablation and coincident with the development of cyclosporine-induced nephrotoxicity. Increased TxA_2 formation during renal allograft rejection has been reported in humans; however, it is unknown whether this is an epiphenomenon or of primary importance in the rejection process. 16,16-Dimethyl PGE_2 delays renal allograft rejection in man, although the mechanism is unknown.

PGE_2 is the major product formed from arachidonic acid in the renal medulla, where it appears to inhibit sodium reabsorption in the distal tubule. The consequent sodium retention caused by administration of a cyclo-oxygenase inhibitor persists only for a day or two, after which sodium balance is reversed despite continued treatment. Prostaglandins may also influence free water clearance. Indomethacin diminishes the excessive water elimination in nephrogenic and lithium-induced diabetes insipidus.

Although P-450–catalyzed metabolism of arachidonate occurs in renal tissue and several of the compounds influence tubular ion flux, glomerular filtration rate, and vascular tone, their precise role in renal physiology and pathology remains to be established.

THE REPRODUCTIVE SYSTEM. Both PGE_2 and $PGF_{2\alpha}$ are potent stimulants of myometrial contraction. Both they and their methylated analogues have been utilized as abortifacients and in the induction of labor, usually as an adjunct to low amniotomy. Cyclo-oxygenase inhibitors are currently being evaluated in the treatment of premature labor. A potential hazard of this approach has been premature closure of the ductus arteriosus, although the incidence of the complication is unknown. Closure of a persistent ductus arteriosus can be achieved with indomethacin in the neonatal period. This implies that a cyclo-oxygenase metabolite contributes to ductal patency. Infusion of PGE_1 has been used to maintain an open ductus in infants with pulmonary atresia until corrective surgery is performed.

Biosynthesis of the prostaglandins increases during pregnancy, particularly during labor. In the case of PGI_2, biosynthesis is increased markedly from as early as the first trimester. Interestingly, this increment is less pronounced in patients with pregnancy-induced hypertension (PIH). Indeed, diminished PGI_2 biosynthesis is apparent prior to the rise in blood pressure. Studies of TxA_2 biosynthesis indicate that platelet activation is present in normal pregnancy and is further increased in patients with severe PIH. TxA_2 is a potent vasoconstrictor in the placental bed and may contribute to the depressed placental blood flow that is a hallmark of PIH. Encouraging results from several small studies have prompted the initiation of multicenter trials to determine if aspirin will reduce the incidence of PIH in women at risk of developing the disease. It has been difficult to document a teratogenic risk from maternal consumption of aspirin in the first trimester.

FEVER AND INFLAMMATION. Cyclo-oxygenase inhibitors share antipyretic, analgesic, and anti-inflammatory actions. Paracetamol differs from the other compounds in being an efficient antipyretic despite weak anti-inflammatory properties in the periphery. The prostaglandins that mediate fever are unknown. Vasodilator prostaglandins seem to act in concert with other mediators to augment the inflammatory response. Among these may be the leukotrienes, which enhance capillary permeability and function as chemoattractants and leukocyte activators. These properties suggest that combined cyclo-oxygenase and lipoxygenase inhibitors may be more effective anti-inflammatory agents than aspirin-like drugs.

Fitzpatrick F, Murphy R: Cytochrome P450 metabolism of arachidonic acid: Formation and biological actions of "epoxygenase" derived eicosanoids. Pharmacol Rev 40:229, 1989. *A comprehensive review of this pathway of arachidonic acid metabolism.*

Hennekens MD, Buring JE, Sandercock P, et al.: Aspirin and other antiplatelet agents in the secondary and primary prevention of cardiovascular disease. Circulation 80:749, 1989. *A comprehensive review of clinical trials of aspirin, including ISIS-2.*

Hirata M, Hayashi Y, Ushikube F, et al.: Cloning and expression of cDNA for a human thromboxane A_2 receptor. Nature 349:617, 1991. *The first cloning of a receptor for an eicosanoid.*

Kerins D, Murray R, FitzGerald GA: Prostacyclin and PGE_1: Molecular mechanisms and therapeutic utility. Prog Hemostasis 10:307, 1991. *A comprehensive review of basic and clinical knowledge about these prostaglandins.*

Leaf A, Weber PC: Cardiovascular effects of n-3 fatty acids. N Engl J Med 318:549, 1988. *A review of the biochemistry and potential benefits of fish oils in cardiovascular disease.*

Samuelsson B: Leukotrienes: Mediators of immediate hypersensitivity and inflammation. Science 220:568, 1983. *A review that concentrates on the biosynthesis and metabolism of these compounds and their role in inflammation.*

Vane JR: The road to prostacyclin. Adv Prostaglandin Thromboxane Leukotriene Res 15:11, 1985. *An account of the discovery and pharmacology of this prostaglandin.*

211 Natriuretic Hormones

Dennis A. Ausiello

In the last decade, considerable interest has focused on endogenous factors that play a role in the regulation of water and electrolyte balance. The isolation and cloning of the cardiac-derived atrial natriuretic peptide (ANP) has led to a rapid definition of its biosynthesis, storage, release response, and action. Although there are still some uncertainties, a picture of its role in physiology and pathophysiology and a possible therapeutic agent have been developed. A second compound (or compounds), called natriuretic hormone (NH), whose presumed structure and function are distinct from those of ANP, has not yet been completely characterized. Therefore, its physiology, pathophysiology, and therapeutic potential are still unclear.

NATRIURETIC HORMONE (NH)

Experimental observations led to the concept of the existence of an endogenous regulator of mammalian Na^+-K^+-ATPase (the Na^+ pump) more than 25 years ago. At that time intravascular expansion with saline in dogs produced a brisk natriuresis with no change in renal perfusion pressure, glomerular filtration rate, or mineralocorticoid activity. The natriuretic effects of extracellular fluid volume expansion in one animal also occurred in a second animal cross-circulated with the blood of the first. The presumption was that the natriuresis was due to a circulating substance that exerted its effects directly on the renal tubular Na^+ reabsorptive process without affecting renal hemodynamics. Further experiments confirmed that active extracts from plasma, urine, and tissue sources that were natriuretic in vivo had a direct effect on transepithelial sodium transport. These substances have digitalis-like characteristics, although there is no reason to assume a structural identity between the postulated endogenous Na^+-K^+-ATPase inhibitor and the cardiac glycosides. Digitalis is a potent inhibitor of Na^+-K^+-ATPase and causes both natriuresis and an increase in vascular resistance, although these are not its major pharmacologic effects. Using the digoxin radioimmunoassay, digitalis-like immunoactivity has been found in the urine and plasma of sodium-loaded normal human subjects and in uremic and hypertensive subjects. Whether NH and digitalis-like compounds are the same endogenous Na^+-K^+-ATPase inhibitors remains to be defined.

BIOLOGIC ACTIVITIES. The biologic effects that have been claimed for the putative NH include (a) natriuresis in vivo, (b) inhibition of sodium transport in vitro, (c) Na^+-K^+-ATPase inhibition, (d) positive cardiac inotropism, and (e) increased vascular reactivity.

BIOCHEMICAL CHARACTERIZATION. Controversy still exists about the chemical nature of the substance. Some maintain that it is a peptide, whereas others have found its properties inconsistent with this class of compounds and propose a steroidal nature.

SITE OF ORIGIN. The site of origin of the NH also remains uncertain, but the brain has been favored, since the natriuretic effects of extracellular fluid volume expansion appear to depend on an intact central nervous system. In addition, Na^+-K^+-ATPase inhibitory activity has been extracted and partially purified from cerebral and hypothalamic tissue. A ouabain-like compound has been isolated from human cerebrospinal fluid. The hypothalamus represents an enriched source of an endogenous inhibitor of Na^+-K^+-ATPase, if not the site of its production.

NH AND THE PATHOPHYSIOLOGY OF ESSENTIAL HYPERTENSION. NH may play a role in normal volume regulation and in the pathophysiology of hypertension and secondary edema states. NH may have an extrarenal action leading to enhanced vascular reactivity. The hypothesis proposed is that in hereditary forms of hypertension, there is a persistent tendency toward renal retention of sodium. This may be due to increased Na^+-K^+ cotransport or Na^+-H^+ exchange in the proximal tubule, occurring as a manifestation of a generalized genetic defect in Na^+-Na^+ (Na^+-Li^+) countertransport. This defect exists in the erythrocytes of some patients with essential hypertension and in their first-degree normotensive relatives. The renal sodium retention leads to a transient increase in extracellular fluid volume, which serves as a stimulus for the release of a Na^+-K^+-ATPase inhibitor. The sodium pump inhibitor acts on the renal tubule to promote sodium excretion, thus restoring extracellular fluid volume to normal levels. It has similar inhibitory effects on the Na^+-K^+-ATPase in vascular smooth muscle cells, resulting in a tonic increase in vascular tone, increased total peripheral resistance, and hypertension. It is assumed that Na^+-K^+-ATPase inhibition in vascular smooth muscle results in an increase in cytosolic free calcium concentration, which must occur to produce the arterial vasoconstriction. How this occurs is unclear. One of the hypotheses is that altered Na^+-Ca^{2+} exchange resulting from partial sodium-pump inhibition may account for an increase in intracellular free Ca^{2+} concentration. At this time, this hypothesis remains attractive but unproven.

ATRIAL NATRIURETIC PEPTIDE (ANP)

ANP, a peptide hormone, is secreted primarily by the cardiac atria and produces natriuresis, diuresis, smooth muscle relaxation, and inhibition of renin and aldosterone secretion. Its major sites of action include the cardiovascular, renal, and endocrine systems. Although the exact mechanisms triggering the release of ANP are not clear, stretch of the atria appears to be the principal stimulus.

It has been known for several decades that membrane-bound secretory granules exist in the cardiac atria. In 1981 in a pioneering report, DeBold and his colleagues observed that bolus injection of crude extracts of rat atria, but not ventricles, produced a rapid, massive, and short-lasting diuresis and natriuresis and a modest kaliuresis. This suggested the existence of a natriuretic hormone in the atrial granules. Subsequently, this unique hormonal system has been thoroughly studied. The amino acid sequence of the active circulating peptide and its prehormone forms have been defined together with their gene structure, target tissue receptors, and signal transduction pathways.

STRUCTURE, BIOSYNTHESIS, AND SECRETION. The atrium first produces a pre-pro ANP (151 amino acids), the final 126 amino acids of which are pro ANP. The pro ANP, the principal storage form of the hormone in the atrial granules, is the immediate precursor of the biologically active 28 amino acid ANP, the predominant circulatory peptide. Circulatory ANP has a cysteine-cysteine disulfide crosslink that is essential for its activity.

The human gene for pre-pro ANP is located on the short arm of chromosome 1. Transcription of the pre-pro ANP gene proceeds at a high rate in the cardiac atria, estimated to be 1 to 3 per cent of all mRNA in the atrial cardiocytes. ANP gene expression is transcriptionally regulated by dexamethasone and thyroid hormone. ANP is also expressed at very low levels in other tissues, such as brain, anterior pituitary, adrenal medulla, lung, kidney, thyroid, and submandibular gland. The major site of ANP synthesis is the myocytes of the right cardiac atrium, with lesser production in the left atrium. Pro ANP is cleaved by a specific atrial protease, probably at the time of exocytotic fusion of atrial granules with the plasma membrane and possibly even soon after secretion from the myocyte, resulting in ANP as the predominant form entering the coronary sinus blood.

STIMULI FOR RELEASE. Atrial stretch, measured as atrial transmural pressure, is the principal stimulus for ANP secretion into the circulation. Atrial pressure is also correlated with release of ANP. During infusion of isotonic saline in humans, plasma ANP increases in parallel with the increase of right atrial pressure. This results from rapid conversion of pro ANP to ANP and/or release of ANP. With cardiovascular or pulmonary disease, a significant correlation exists between circulating ANP levels and the right and left atrial pressures.

Mineralocorticoids, as well as glucocorticoids administered in high doses, increase mRNA encoding for pre-pro ANP and circulating ANP levels, indicating an increase in ANP production and release. In addition, adrenalectomized rats do not respond to increased atrial pressure with increased atrial and circulating ANP levels in the absence of glucocorticoid or mineralocorticoid replacement. Thus these hormones may play a permissive role in the volume response mediating ANP release as well as inducing ANP secretion directly.

BIOLOGIC AND PLASMA HALF-LIFE. A sensitive radioimmunoassay, generally specific for the mid to C-terminal peptides of ANP, will detect levels of 1 to 10 pg of the peptide in plasma. In subjects on varied sodium diets, the plasma ANP levels range from 10 to 40 pg per milliliter.

After release from the atrium or after intravenous administration, ANP is rapidly cleared with a plasma half-life between 2 and 4 minutes in humans. Biologic activity of ANP critically depends on the intact ring structure and carboxy-terminal residues. The rank order of tissue degradative potency appears to be kidney > liver > lung > plasma > heart.

ANP RECEPTORS. ANP receptors are localized on the cell surface of target tissues, including most notably adrenal, kidney, and the vasculature. They are also found, to a lesser extent, in the central nervous system, hepatocytes, colonic smooth muscle, and lung. In kidney, ANP binding sites are most prevalent in large vessels, glomeruli, and the renal medulla. In the adrenal, ANP binding is limited primarily to the zona glomerulosa.

Molecular cloning has defined three ANP receptors: (a) the ANP-C (or ANP-R2) clearance receptor, which is not coupled to cGMP production, the signal transduction pathway involved in ANP action. Clearance receptors do not mediate any known physiologic effect. The receptors for ANP in the kidney and vascular smooth muscle are predominantly clearance receptors. Their abundance accounts for the short half-life of circulatory ANP. It seems probable that the atrial peptide system has a novel receptor-mediated sequestration and clearance mechanism that is responsible, at least in part, for maintaining plasma levels of the hormone. (b) Two structurally similar plasma membrane receptors, ANP-R1 and ANP-R3, are the biologically active receptor forms. ANP binding to the extracellular domain of R1 or R3 activates the cytoplasmic domain of the receptor, which is a guanylate cyclase responsible for the generation of the second messenger, cGMP.

CELLULAR ACTION. The most apparent action of ANP is to increase intracellular cGMP concentration. ANP is a unique peptide hormone in its use of cGMP as a second messenger, which mediates most of the physiologic actions of the hormone. ANP also influences intracellular calcium homeostasis, which may be responsible for some of its biologic effects.

The physiologic responses to ANP include (a) relaxation of vascular and other smooth muscles, (b) increase in glomerular filtration rate and inhibition of tubular water and sodium transport in the kidney, and (c) inhibition of hormone secretion (Fig. 211–1).

KIDNEY ACTION. The kidney is the primary target organ for ANP. ANP causes natriuresis and diuresis by a concerted action at several nephron segments. The primary sites of action of ANP are the glomerulus, the renal vasculature, and the inner medullary collecting duct, although other nephron segments may be involved in the response to ANP. ANP can increase glomerular filtration rate by raising the glomerular hydraulic pressure gradient from capillary lumen to Bowman's space through differential effects on afferent and efferent arteriole tone. By relaxing glomerular mesangial cells, ANP also increases the glomerular ultrafiltration coefficient, Kf. The combined effects result in an increased filtration pressure and thus an increased filtration fraction, with a higher load of salt and water being delivered to the tubules for excretion.

The increased quantity of sodium filtered is not completely reabsorbed. There is an increased delivery of sodium to the distal tubule and collecting duct, where ANP reduces sodium reabsorption and vasopressin-induced water reabsorption, leading to a profound natriuresis. In addition, redistribution of blood flow from the cortex to inner medulla, which dilutes the papillary interstitium, results in an increase in sodium and water excretion.

CARDIOVASCULAR ACTION. ANP directly relaxes arterial vascular smooth muscle through the action of its second messenger, cGMP. This ANP-induced vasorelaxation occurs independent of the presence of endothelium. ANP most effectively relaxes large-caliber arteries, such as the aorta, renal, and iliac arteries. The more peripheral vascular segments of the arterial tree are less sensitive to the hormone. ANP causes vasorelaxation of the aorta constricted with norepinephrine or angiotensin II, compatible with its role as one of the most potent vasodilators known and as a functional antagonist of a variety of vasoconstrictors.

ANP at pharmacologic concentrations reduces mean arterial pressure in man by reducing peripheral vascular resistance and decreasing intravascular volume. This is followed by a decrease in cardiac output attributed to (1) a shift of volume from the intravascular to extravascular space, probably due to alteration in capillary permeability or an increase in resistance to venous return at the site of postcapillary circulation; hemoconcentration, secondary to a decreased plasma volume, may occur in humans in response to ANP; and (2) preload reduction due to relaxation of venous smooth muscle, leading to an augmentation of venous capacitance and a reduction of venous return.

ENDOCRINE ACTION. ANP modulates renin-angiotensin-aldosterone secretion. Administration of ANP causes a prompt decline in circulatory renin and aldosterone levels. ANP blocks both basal and agonist-stimulated (angiotensin II, ACTH, K⁺)

secretion of aldosterone in isolated adrenal zona glomerulosa cells. This appears to be a direct action of ANP on these cells. In addition, ANP decreases the biosynthesis and release of vasopressin. The decrease in vasopressin may potentiate a decrease in vascular tone and augment the diuresis and natriuresis induced by ANP.

SIGNIFICANCE OF ANP IN BODY FLUID HOMEOSTASIS

It is not yet possible to describe definitively the physiologic relevance of ANP. Some evidence suggests that ANP exerts a trivial influence on the normal regulation of body fluid homeostasis: (1) Infusion of ANP into conscious animals and normal human subjects results in plasma concentrations slightly above the physiologic range but produces only a slowly developing and relatively modest natriuresis. (2) Ingestion of food containing salt does not increase plasma ANP, yet a natriuresis routinely occurs postprandially. (3) In a number of common physiologic and experimental conditions, circulating ANP levels do not correlate with renal sodium excretion.

Other evidence suggests that ANP plays a significant role in regulation of body fluid homeostasis: (1) ANP is potent, has a short duration of action, and the hormone responds to physiologically relevant stimuli in a feedback-controlled system. (2) The peptide circulates at nanomolar concentrations, which is consistent with its Kd for receptor binding and second messenger activation in target cells. (3) Long-term, low-dose ANP infusion directly into the renal artery of conscious dogs supports a physiologic action of ANP to promote urinary sodium excretion. (4) The role played by ANP in volume regulation is highly complex and the kidney responds with increased sodium excretion only when a constellation of natriuretic forces is appropriately assayed. Therefore, a rise in ANP levels may be a necessary, but not sufficient, condition to induce natriuresis.

ROLE OF ANP IN PATHOPHYSIOLOGY
Diseases of Disordered Volume Regulation (Edematous States)

CONGESTIVE HEART FAILURE (CHF). CHF is associated with increased atrial pressure and elevated ANP levels. Despite

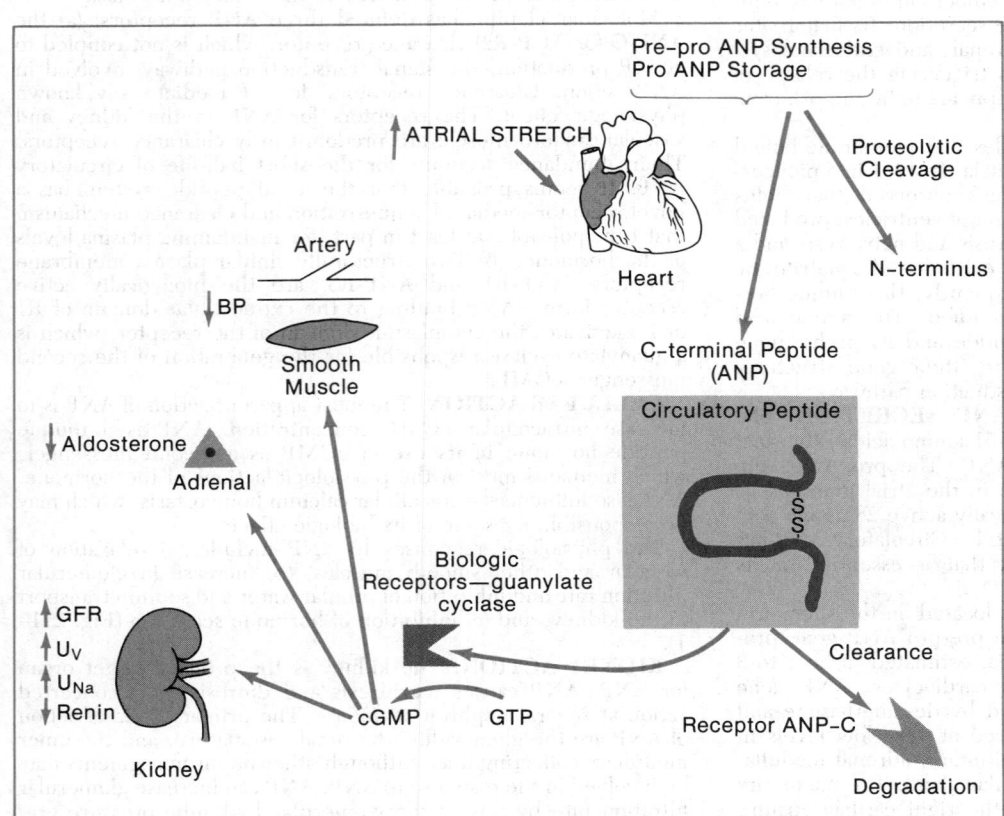

FIGURE 211–1. Major target organs and actions of atrial natriuretic peptide (ANP).

high circulating ANP, however, these patients retain salt and water. CHF is associated with a decreased response of the kidney to ANP, which could result from receptor down-regulation due to high plasma ANP concentrations. These high levels of circulating ANP appear to play a role in the maintenance of sodium excretion by modulating the renal, hemodynamic, and endocrine effects of CHF. The degree of ANP elevation increases with the severity of the clinical disease, as measured by the New York Heart Association functional classification. Class I patients have normal or only moderately elevated levels; class III and IV patients have dramatic elevations. The direct correlation between the severity of the heart failure and plasma ANP has allowed the use of ANP levels to serve as a marker for CHF in adults and children, including those with congenital heart disease. ANP levels correlate directly with right atrial pressure, pulmonary capillary wedge pressure, and pulmonary artery pressure and inversely with cardiac output and cardiac index.

CIRRHOSIS. Progressive cirrhosis of the liver is accompanied by renal sodium and water retention with the development of ascites and edema. This state is usually accompanied by elevated plasma ANP levels, consistent with the "overflow" theory of ascites formation. As in CHF, raised ANP plasma concentrations in the presence of total body volume expansion implies a "refractory" or "reset" response to ANP. This hyporesponsiveness to ANP in cirrhosis is supported by the observation that ANP levels can be stimulated to increase further by water immersion, peritoneovenous shunting, and acute volume expansion with a resultant natriuresis in some patients. It is probable that a complex balance between ANP and antinatriuretic factors is responsible for renal sodium retention in early and late cirrhosis. In the former, hepatic venous outflow obstruction results in renal salt retention and intravascular volume expansion (overflow hypothesis). This in turn leads to an elevation in ANP levels counterbalanced by antinatriuretic factors such that the net effect is ascites formation. In late cirrhosis, with loss of intravascular volume into the peritoneal compartment (underfill hypothesis), there is a reduced stimulus for ANP secretion such that ANP plasma levels no longer offset antinatriuretic processes.

NEPHROTIC SYNDROME. Why edema forms in the nephrotic syndrome is not completely understood. Traditionally it has been suggested that renal sodium and water retention is a consequence of the lower plasma oncotic pressure from hypoalbuminemia and the resultant reduction in plasma volume. Consistent with this hypothesis, nephrotic syndrome is found to be associated with normal or diminished circulatory levels of ANP that can be stimulated to rise after intravascular volume expansion. Head-out water immersion conducted on patients with nephrotic syndrome demonstrated that ANP levels increased, but renal salt and water excretion was blunted. There thus appears to be an impaired renal response to ANP in the nephrotic syndrome.

ESSENTIAL HYPERTENSION. Patients with essential hypertension have a wide range of plasma ANP concentrations, suggesting that the contribution of ANP may vary in the heterogeneous population of patients with this disease. This finding precludes the use of ANP levels to differentiate among the various causes of hypertension.

RENAL DISEASE. Progressive renal disease is frequently associated with plasma volume expansion and elevated ANP levels. In patients undergoing regular dialysis, ANP levels can be used as an indicator of volume status. Decreased levels correlate with the amount of weight loss and fluid removal in dialysis patients.

THERAPEUTIC POTENTIAL

ANP may have a role as a therapeutic agent, especially in critical care situations. Intervention, in general, is limited by a lack of an effective oral agent. ANP must be administered intravenously. Its potency as a pharmacologic agent in altering cardiovascular and renal function makes it potentially attractive in treating patients with diseases associated with edema (CHF, cirrhosis, nephrotic syndrome), hypertension, and ischemic renal injury: (a) In patients with CHF, the natriuretic and diuretic effects of pharmacologic concentrations of ANP are often limited, but the effect on augmenting cardiac output is quite favorable; (b) in cirrhosis, the renal hyporesponsiveness together with a

relative increased sensitivity to hypotension make the therapeutic use of ANP problematic; (c) in patients with nephrotic syndrome, ANP infusion may result in a natriuresis; (d) variable short-term benefits have been reported in patients with hypertension. The use of low-dose ANP with other agents may prove effective if a satisfactory oral agent is developed; and (e) a potentially important therapeutic action of ANP may be the prevention and reversal of acute renal failure (Ch. 76). In various animal models of acute renal failure, ANP given prophylactically or immediately following the hemodynamic insult restores GFR. The therapeutic potential of ANP in human acute renal failure still needs to be assessed.

ANP infusion in all human studies has not exceeded a duration of a few hours. Therefore all reported responses to ANP in humans are acute. Prolonged administration of ANP with a nonparenteral analogue will be necessary to evaluate its therapeutic potential in chronic human diseases.

Blain EH: Atrial natriuretic factor plays a significant role in body fluid homeostasis. Hypertension 15:2, 1990. *Debate on the role ANP plays in body fluid homeostasis.*
Brenner BM, Ballermann BY, Gunning ME, et al.: Diverse biological actions of atrial natriuretic peptide. Physiol Rev 70:665, 1990. *Comprehensive review of the current understanding of the structure of ANP, its synthesis, secretion, cellular and target organ action, and its role in various pathophysiologic states.*
Cogan MG: Atrial natriuretic peptide. Kidney Int 37:1148, 1990. *Comprehensive review of the renal properties of ANP.*
Floras JS: Sympathoinhibitory effects of atrial natriuretic factor in normal humans. Circulation 81:1860, 1990. *Integrative cardiovascular responses to ANP in normal humans.*
Goetz KL: Evidence that atriopeptin is not a physiological regulator of sodium excretion. Hypertension 15:9, 1990. *Debate on the role ANP plays in body fluid homeostasis.*
Haupert GT: Sodium pump regulation by endogenous inhibition. Curr Top Membrane Transport 34:345, 1989. *Review of current knowledge of the hypothalamic ouabain-like factor.*

ACKNOWLEDGMENT: I would like to thank Eliezer Holtzman for his invaluable help in preparing this chapter.

212 Neuroendocrine Regulation and Its Disorders

Lawrence A. Frohman

NEUROENDOCRINE REGULATION

The central nervous system exerts profound regulatory control over hormonal secretion and metabolic processes. The integration of this control is focused in the region of the ventral hypothalamus and consists of three major systems:

1. A neuronal pathway descending through the base of the brain, the autonomic nervous system pathways of the spinal cord, and terminating in the liver, gastrointestinal tract, pancreas, adrenal medullae, and adipose tissue. This pathway, which consists of bidirectional fibers, participates in neurometabolic regulation, and its greatest effects are on blood glucose and fatty acid regulation and on metabolic homeostasis, i.e., appetite control (satiety), temperature control (thermoregulation), and body fat stores (nutrient regulation).

2. A neurosecretory pathway from the anterior hypothalamus that traverses the floor of the ventral hypothalamus and pituitary stalk and terminates in specialized neuronal elements called pituicytes, located in the posterior pituitary. This system is involved in osmoregulation, through the production of vasopressin, and in parturition and nursing, through the secretion of oxytocin. A detailed discussion of this system is provided in Ch. 214.

3. A neuroendocrine system involving clusters of peptide- and monoamine-secreting cells in the anterior and mid-portion of the ventral hypothalamus whose products are transported along nerve fibers to terminals in the outer layer of the median eminence, from which they are released into the capillary vessels of the

hypothalamic-hypophyseal portal system and transported to the pituitary to regulate the secretion of the hormones of the anterior pituitary.

Neuroendocrine Anatomy

The *neurometabolic function* of the hypothalamus can be divided into those components associated with the sympathetic or the parasympathetic branches of the autonomic nervous system. Although medial sympathetic and lateral parasympathetic zones of the hypothalamus can be distinguished, the cellular elements (neuronal perikarya) involved in a particular function cannot be precisely localized to one specific nuclear region. Neurons involved in the inhibitory control of food intake (satiety) are located medially, and those responsible for appetite stimulation are located laterally. This distinction probably explains why destructive lesions of the hypothalamus, which frequently occur in the midline, are more likely to result in obesity than in starvation. A second reason is that fibers from the hypothalamic controlling centers cross the midline, and thus bilateral hypothalamic destruction is necessary for interruption of normal regulatory control.

Neurons of the *neurohypophyseal system* constitute a more anatomically distinct entity with cell bodies located in the paraventricular and supraoptic hypothalamic nuclei. Within these areas are also neurons producing other neuropeptides. The posterior pituitary hormones, oxytocin and vasopressin, along with their specific carrier proteins (neurophysins), are synthesized in the cell bodies as part of a single precursor molecule and transported along axonal fibers through the ventral hypothalamus and pituitary stalk, during which time the hormones are cleaved from the precursor. In the pituicytes of the posterior pituitary they are packaged into storage granules to be released in response to stimulation (e.g., osmotic, barometric) of receptors on the cell bodies in the hypothalamus. The posterior pituitary is therefore functionally an integral part of the brain.

The cell bodies of the neuroendocrine system are diffusely distributed throughout the mediobasal hypothalamus in an area known as the hypophysiotropic region. Although the hypothalamic hormone-secreting neurons receive input from other brain regions in response to changes in the external environment, they continue to function even in the absence of extrahypothalamic input, indicating that their most important homeostatic stimuli are blood borne. Cells secreting thyrotropin releasing hormone (TRH) and somatotropin release inhibiting factor (SRIF) that regulate pituitary function are located in the anterior hypothalamus, while those secreting growth hormone releasing hormone (GRH) are concentrated in the region of the arcuate nuclei. Cells secreting gonadotropin releasing hormone (GnRH) are more widely distributed, with cell bodies in both the anterior hypothalamus and the arcuate nuclei. Cell bodies of corticotropin releasing hormone (CRH) neurons terminating in the median eminence are located predominantly in the paraventricular nucleus. A prolactin inhibiting factor (PIF) exhibits a distribution identical to that of GnRH.

The releasing and inhibiting hormones are stored in nerve terminals in the median eminence. Since the portal blood flow to the pituitary is not compartmentalized, i.e., various cell types in the pituitary are distributed throughout the gland, releasing and inhibiting factors secreted into the portal system have access to all cell types of the anterior pituitary. Specificity of action is achieved by the presence of specific receptors on individual pituitary cell types.

The cells of both the neuroendocrine and neurohypophyseal systems have been called transducer cells, containing both neuronal and endocrine characteristics. They respond to classic neurotransmitter-mediated signals, yet they release peptide hormones into a regional or systemic circulation.

PORTAL VASCULAR SYSTEM. The vascular supply of the anterior pituitary has no direct connections with the arterial system. All of the arterial blood flows through the hypothalamic arteries and forms a capillary plexus within the outer layer of the median eminence in juxtaposition to nerve terminals of the hypophysiotropic neurons. In contrast to most other brain regions, the blood-brain barrier in the area of the median eminence is incomplete, permitting protein and peptide hormones as well as other charged particles access to the intercapillary spaces and the nerve terminals contained therein. These terminals (and/or their perikarya) respond to changes in concentrations of circulating hormones and metabolic signals as well as to neuronal stimuli by secreting releasing and inhibiting factors into the portal system. The portal capillaries coalesce into a series of veins that descend through the pituitary stalk and form a second capillary plexus that bathes the cells of the anterior pituitary. Venous drainage from the anterior pituitary passes through the posterior pituitary and from there into systemic veins.

Releasing and Inhibiting Hormones

The hypothalamic hormones that control the secretion of anterior pituitary hormones and their effects on pituitary hormone secretion are shown in Figure 212–1. Several different patterns of control exist: (1) multiple hypothalamic hormones stimulating release of a single pituitary hormone (CRH and vasopressin [VP]: ACTH), (2) a single hypothalamic hormone stimulating release of several pituitary hormones (GnRH:luteinizing hormone [LH] and follicle-stimulating hormone [FSH], TRH:thyroid-stimulating hormone [TSH] and prolactin), and (3) dual stimulatory/inhibitory influences of hypothalamic hormones on pituitary hormones (GRH and SRIF:growth hormone [GH]).

With one exception, the predominant influence of the hypothalamic hormones on the pituitary is stimulatory. Interference with the integrity of the hypothalamic-pituitary connection results in decreased secretion of all pituitary hormones except for prolactin, the secretion of which is increased when hypothalamic influence is removed.

All of the recognized hypothalamic hormones whose structures have been determined are, with one exception, peptides with sequence length ranging from 3 to 44 amino acids. As the length of the structures increases, both multiple forms of the peptide (see section on somatostatin and GRH) and marked species variation in sequence occur. Whereas the sequences of TRH, GnRH, and SRIF are identical in all mammalian species studied to date, those of GRH and CRH exhibit marked species specificity. The existence of a separate PRF is still controversial, although a candidate for this title is vasoactive intestinal polypeptide (VIP). The one nonpeptide hypophysiotropic hormone is dopamine. In addition to its major role as a neurotransmitter, dopamine is the most important physiologic inhibitor of prolactin. A 56-amino acid prolactin-inhibiting peptide has been identified as a carboxy-terminal extension on the GnRH precursor molecule. The physiologic roles of this GnRH-associated peptide (GAP), as well as other less fully characterized prolactin-releasing factors, remain to be confirmed.

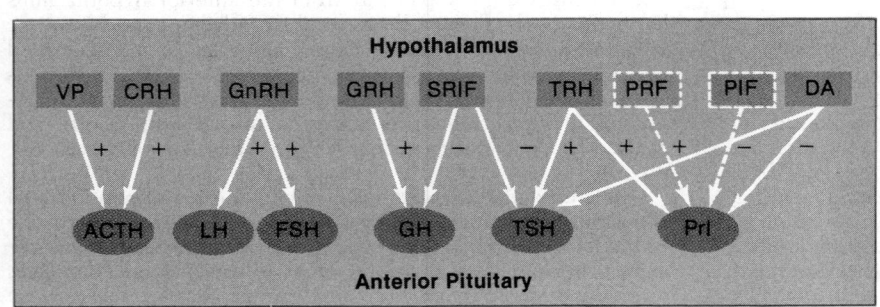

FIGURE 212–1. Interrelationships between hypothalamic and pituitary hormones. Solid lines denote hormones, the structures of which have been determined. Interrupted line indicates factors, the identity of which is still unknown.

ROLE OF BIOGENIC AMINES AND NEUROPEPTIDES IN THE REGULATION OF HYPOTHALAMIC HORMONE SECRETION.

The major neurotransmitter systems utilized for intercellular communication within the central nervous system consist of monoamines and peptides. Neurotransmitters can influence the hypothalamic hormone-secreting neurons at several sites (Fig. 212–2). These include axodendritic connections (site 1) and axoaxonic connections involving presynaptic receptors on the hormone-containing nerve terminals (site 3). Multiple neurotransmitters may also participate in the regulation of hormone secretion through intermediary neurons (site 2), and neurotransmitters may be released directly into the portal system to modify the effect of hypothalamic hormones on the pituitary (site 4). Major advances in the understanding of hypothalamic-pituitary function have occurred as a consequence of the availability of neuropharmacologic compounds that selectively alter neurotransmitter function.

Catecholamines (Dopamine, Norepinephrine, Epinephrine). The common precursor for the catecholamines is tyrosine, which is actively transported from the blood into catecholaminergic neurons in the CNS. Tyrosine is converted to dihydroxyphenylalanine (L-dopa) by tyrosine hydroxylase, which, because of its low concentration, represents the rate-limiting step in catecholamine biosynthesis. It is therefore the enzyme most susceptible to pharmacologic blockage by tyrosine analogues such as α-methylparatyrosine. L-dopa is rapidly decarboxylated to dopamine (5-hydroxytryptamine). This enzyme can be inhibited by L-dopa analogues such as α-methyldopa and α-methyldopahydrazine (carbidopa). In dopaminergic neurons, dopamine is stored in secretory granules and released as a neurotransmitter, while in noradrenergic and adrenergic neurons it is further hydroxylated by dopamine β-hydroxylase to form norepinephrine. Copper-chelating agents such as disulfiram are potent inhibitors of this step and impair the conversion of dopamine to norepinephrine. In noradrenergic neurons, this transmitter is packaged similarly to that of dopamine, whereas in selective neurons it is converted to epinephrine

by phenylethanolamine-N-methyltransferase. See Ch. 229 also for a discussion of catecholamine metabolism.

In nerve endings, newly synthesized catecholamines are stored in secretory granules that protect them from enzymatic degradation. There are at least two distinct pools of neurotransmitters that are differentially susceptible to releasing stimuli. A long-lasting depletion of catecholamines can be produced by reserpine, which causes a slow but constant release of the monoamines and inhibits reuptake. Catecholamine release occurs in response to nerve stimulation by fusion of the secretion vesicle membrane with the cell membrane and extrusion of the amine directly into the intercellular space. Once released, catecholamines bind to postsynaptic receptors that appear to be similar in the hypophysiotropic neurons to those demonstrated in other neural sites. In addition, they bind to presynaptic receptors on the nerve terminals to effect a feedback regulation. Alterations in presynaptic and postsynaptic receptor activity are accomplished by the use of receptor agonists and antagonists. Catecholamine action terminates primarily by reuptake of the neurotransmitter into the presynaptic neuron, but also by removal into the circulation and metabolic degradation. Drugs such as cocaine, tricyclic antidepressants, or nomifensine inhibit reuptake, resulting in enhancement of catecholamine effects. Metabolic degradation occurs by two enzymes: monoamine oxidase (MAO) and catechol-O-methyltransferase. Catecholamine action is therefore enhanced by MAO inhibitors such as pargyline and tranylcypromine.

Indolamines (Serotonin, Melatonin). Tryptophan, the precursor of serotonin, is actively transported from blood to brain. Since tryptophan hydroxylase activity is not saturated at physiologic concentrations, fluctuations in plasma tryptophan levels determine the rate of brain serotonin synthesis. After hydroxylation, 5-hydroxytryptophan is converted to serotonin by aromatic L-amino acid decarboxylase. Serotonin functions as a neurotransmitter and, in the pineal, also serves as a precursor of melatonin. Serotonin synthesis can be inhibited by p-chlorophenylalanine, which inhibits tryptophan hydroxylase, and by L-dopa, which competes with 5-hydroxytryptophan for decarboxylation. The storage, release, and uptake of serotonin are similar to those of norepinephrine, with many of the same agents (i.e., amphetamine) releasing both compounds. Tricyclic antidepressants inhibit serotonin uptake, although in contrast to norepinephrine, imipramine and amitriptyline are more potent than their desmethyl derivatives (desmethylimipramine and nortriptyline). Alteration of serotonin receptor activity can be produced by agonists such as quipazine and LSD and by antagonists (methysergide and cyproheptadine). Termination of serotonin effects occurs by presynaptic reuptake and metabolic degradation involving MAO. Drugs interfering with MAO activity also enhance serotonin effects.

Acetylcholine. Acetylcholine is synthesized from acetyl-CoA and choline. The source of choline is probably phosphatidylcholine which, after crossing the blood-brain barrier, is partially degraded to choline. Choline is then converted to acetylcholine by choline acetyltransferase. There are two types of acetylcholine receptors, muscarinic and nicotinic, which have different anatomic distribution and physiologic function. Arecoline and atropine, a muscarinic agonist and antagonist, respectively, cross the blood-brain barrier and modify acetylcholine receptor activity. Inhibitors of acetylcholinesterase, such as pyridostigmine, enhance cholinergic tone.

Gamma-Aminobutyric Acid (GABA). In the mammalian hypothalamus GABA is an inhibitory neurotransmitter. It is formed by the decarboxylation of L-glutamate and is metabolized by transamination. Numerous agents inhibit GABA synthesis and metabolism, but only one, valproate, an inhibitor of GABA degradation, has been shown to be useful clinically in altering neuroendocrine function.

Histamine. Histamine is synthesized within the CNS from histidine by a specific decarboxylase and the nonspecific aromatic L-amino acid decarboxylase. Alteration of histamine effects is brought about primarily by histamine receptor antagonists. There are two classes of histamine receptors: H_1 and H_2. Drugs such as diphenhydramine and cyproheptadine inhibit H_1 receptors, while cimetidine and ranitidine inhibit H_2 receptors.

Neuropeptides. A large number of neuropeptides have been

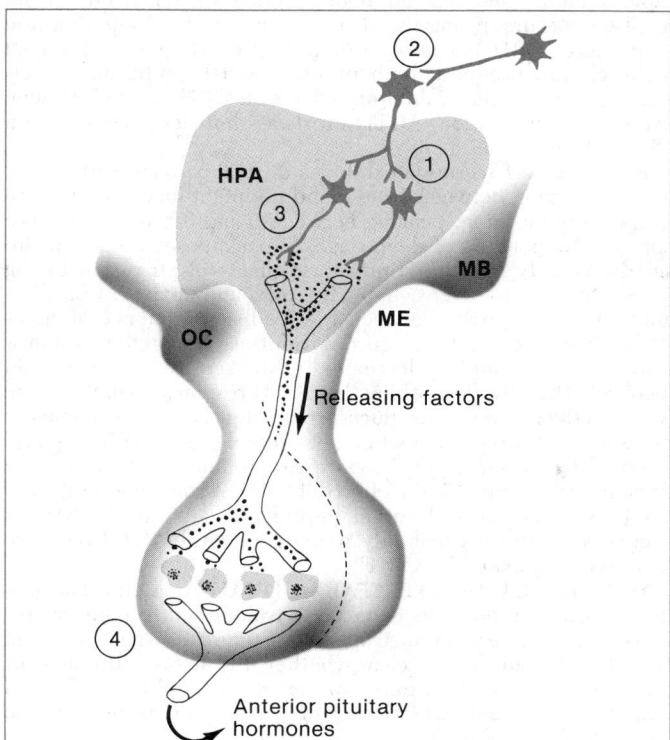

FIGURE 212–2. Sites of potential neurotransmitter effects on hypothalamic releasing and inhibiting hormone secretion and function. HPA = Hypophysiotropic area; OC = optic chiasm; ME = median eminence; MB = mamillary body. Refer to text for description of effects at each site. (From Frohman LA: Clinical neuropharmacology of hypothalamic releasing factors. N Engl J Med 286:1391, 1972. Reprinted by permission of the New England Journal of Medicine.)

identified in the hypothalamus, and their role in the regulation of neuroendocrine function is, at present, only incompletely understood. A list of neuropeptides with potential effects on releasing and inhibiting hormones is provided in Table 212–1. Many of these peptides are widely distributed in extrahypothalamic CNS and function as neurotransmitters or neuromodulators in other pathways. Of particular significance is a group of peptides common to both the CNS and the gastrointestinal tract. Although the function of many of these peptides within the CNS remains to be determined, they appear to have a role in integrative systems relating to homeostatic mechanisms. Their presence throughout evolution and as far back as unicellular organisms underscores their essential role in intercellular communication. With the exception of analogues of enkephalin capable of crossing the blood-brain barrier and of TRH, neuroendocrine effects of peptides other than hypophysiotropic hormones have not been convincingly documented in man. Limited information is available concerning biosynthesis, storage, secretion, and local metabolism of hypothalamic neuropeptides. The hypothalamus also contains numerous lymphokines and monokines, and these immunoregulatory signals are capable of affecting neuroendocrine function. Interleukin (IL)-1, IL-6, and thymic peptides release both hypothalamic and pituitary hormones.

MECHANISM OF ACTION OF HYPOTHALAMIC HORMONES.

Hypophysiotropic hormones affect pituitary hormone secretion by several mechanisms. Specific, high-affinity receptors are present on the anterior pituitary target cells, and evidence now points to the participation of several intracellular mediator or second messenger systems, including adenylate cyclase–cyclic AMP, calcium-calmodulin, and phosphatidylinositol–protein kinase C. In addition, at least some releasing hormones stimulate pituitary hormone gene expression and exhibit mitogenic effects, since stimulation can lead to cellular hyperplasia and even tumor formation.

The mechanism of action of the inhibitory hormones somatostatin and dopamine is less well understood. Somatostatin inhibits cyclic AMP formation and enhances phosphodiesterase activity, both of which actions impair hormone release mediated by cyclic AMP. Somatostatin also inhibits transmembrane Ca^{2+} transport and may have other effects on exocytosis. The inhibitory effects of dopamine appear to be independent of cyclic AMP levels, and, like somatostatin, occur at a late stage in the secretory process. Dopamine also exhibits inhibitory effects on gene expression in lactotrophs.

The effects of all the hypophysiotropic hormones studied to date are modified by target gland hormones, i.e., thyroxine, cortisol, estrogens, androgens, inhibin, and insulin-like growth factors. These hormones alter the number of releasing or inhibiting hormone receptors, but also exhibit effects at postreceptor sites.

Regulation of Hypophysiotropic and Pituitary Hormone Secretion

The control of hypophysiotropic hormone secretion is best appreciated when considered in conjunction with that of the five major pituitary hormone systems they regulate: ACTH, LH and FSH, TSH, GH, and prolactin. Each consists of feedback (closed loop) systems involving primarily blood-borne signals on which are superimposed other neurotransmitter-mediated signals mostly originating within the CNS (open loop) and representing environment (temperature, light-dark), stress (pain, fear, psychic), and intrinsic rhythmicity (ranging from ultradian or short-term to diurnal, monthly, and seasonal). Thus, both internal and external environmental factors are important determinants of the activity of these systems. A summary of neurotransmitter effects on pituitary hormone secretion is provided in Table 212–2.

HYPOTHALAMIC-PITUITARY-ADRENOCORTICAL AXIS. Nearly all of the monoamine neurotransmitters affect CRH release. Acetylcholine stimulates CRH release predominantly through nicotinic receptors and appears to be the primary neurotransmitter mediating stress-induced CRH release. Serotonin also stimulates CRH release, but the effect is likely mediated through a cholinergic interneuron, since it can be blocked by atropine. Norepinephrine inhibits the cholinergic effects on CRH release through an α-adrenergic receptor, and GABA exerts a similar effect. Melatonin inhibits CRH and may be responsible for the circadian pattern of CRH release that is entrained to the light-dark cycle. Enkephalins exert inhibitory effects on the pituitary-adrenal axis. This effect is believed to occur within the hypothalamus at the level of CRH release, although an additional action on the pituitary has not been excluded. Interleukin-1 (IL-1), a neuroimmunomodulator, also stimulates CRH release.

CRH stimulates ACTH release, which in turn stimulates the secretion of glucocorticoids and mineralocorticoids from the adrenal cortex. Glucocorticoids inhibit ACTH secretion by both rapid (minutes) and delayed (hours) feedback mechanisms. Rapid feedback occurs primarily at the pituitary by inhibiting the response to CRH but also by inhibiting CRH release. Delayed feedback also occurs at both pituitary and hypothalamic levels and appears to reflect inhibitory effects on CRH and ACTH gene expression. In addition, ACTH exerts a "short-loop feedback" on CRH release.

Plasma ACTH secretion exhibits a diurnal pattern, with lowest levels occurring between 10 P.M. and midnight followed by a rise in the early morning, peaking between 6 and 8 A.M. The pattern appears independent of sleep stage. Superimposed on this intrinsic rhythmicity are the stimulatory effects of stress, including severe trauma, pyrogens, hypoglycemia, and anxiety. Considerable interaction exists between the feedback influence of circulating corticosteroids and neurotransmitters. Phenytoin administration, for example, decreases CNS sensitivity to steroid feedback, thereby diminishing the ACTH response to metyrapone (which reduces circulating glucocorticoid levels) but also enhances pulsatile ACTH secretion while not affecting the ACTH response to stress and vasopressin. Vasopressin stimulates ACTH release directly and potentiates the effects of CRH. A role for endogenous vasopressin and possibly other peptides as additional CRH's is suggested by the fact that only 80 per cent of the ACTH response to stress is mediated by CRH.

HYPOTHALAMIC-PITUITARY-GONADAL AXIS. The major neurotransmitter effects on GnRH identified to date involve dopamine and serotonin. Dopamine stimulates the release of GnRH, although it is not clear whether this involves the tonic or cyclic release of GnRH. Serotonin exerts an inhibitory effect on both cyclic and tonic GnRH secretion. Norepinephrine may also stimulate GnRH release.

The regulation of the hypothalamic-pituitary-gonadal axis varies with age and sex. LH and FSH are present in circulation from birth, and through the early stages of puberty FSH levels gradually increase to a greater degree than do LH levels. During this period, FSH responses to GnRH are greater than are LH responses, a pattern opposite to that seen after puberty, and the hypothalamus is exceedingly sensitive to the suppressive effects

---

TABLE 212–1. NEUROPEPTIDES WITH POTENTIAL EFFECTS ON HYPOTHALAMIC RELEASING HORMONES

Gastroenteropancreatic peptides
Cholecystokinin
Galanin
Gastrin
Gastrin-releasing peptide
Glucagon
Insulin
Motilin
Neuropeptide PHI/PHM
Neurotensin
Pancreatic polypeptide
Secretin
Substance P
Vasoactive intestinal peptide

Hypothalamic hormones
Corticotropin-releasing hormone
Growth hormone–releasing hormone
Somatostatin
Thyrotropin-releasing hormone
Vasopressin

Endorphin-enkephalin peptides
α-Melanocyte stimulating hormone
β-Endorphin
Dynorphin
Methionine/leucine enkephalin

Immunomodulators
Interleukin-1
Interleukin-6
Thymosin fraction 5

Others
Angiotensin
Bradykinin
Calcitonin
Calcitonin gene–related product
Neuropeptide PYY

of gonadal steroids. In the later prepubertal period (7 to 9 years) sleep-related pulsatile LH secretion begins, and synchronization occurs between LH and FSH pulses. These pulses stimulate the secretion of testosterone in boys and estradiol in girls that initiates the clinical characteristics of puberty. At the same time, evidence for lessening sensitivity of hypothalamic GnRH secretion in response to steroid feedback can be demonstrated. In females, development of positive feedback on LH and FSH by gonadal steroids generates the cyclic preovulatory gonadotropin surge resulting in the establishment of cyclic ovulation by the mid-teens. In adult males the LH secretory pattern is characterized by eight to ten pulses occurring at regular intervals through the day, and the teenage relationship to the sleep-wake pattern disappears. Similar pulsatile secretion of LH and FSH occurs in mature women, the frequency and magnitude of the pulses varying with the phase of the menstrual cycle. When ovarian follicles disappear at menopause, secretion of the major ovarian hormones decreases, and the loss of negative feedback of these hormones enhances secretion of FSH and, to a lesser extent, LH. A similar increase in LH and FSH is observed in men in the seventh and eighth decades in response to decreasing testicular function.

In men, surgical stress results in a transitory rise in the level of LH followed by a prolonged fall, accompanied by a fall in testosterone levels. No changes have been observed in women, although hypothalamic anovulation is frequently seen during periods of stress. Pheromones or other environmental factors have been implicated as the cause for the synchronization of menstrual cycles seen in women living in close association.

Steroid hormones regulate LH and FSH secretion by two major mechanisms. Gonadal steroids regulate tonic secretion by a negative feedback mechanism. Testosterone appears to be more potent than estrogen in this negative feedback effect, while progesterone has an intermediate effect. Inhibin, a peptide produced by ovarian granulosa cells and testicular Sertoli cells, has a selective action in inhibiting FSH release, possibly by impairing the effects of GnRH. Cyclic release of LH and FSH is stimulated by a positive feedback effect of ovarian steroids during the final phases of follicular growth prior to ovulation. The preovulatory surge of LH is preceded by an increase in circulating estrogen levels in the presence of low or decreasing progesterone levels. The positive effects occur at both the hypothalamic and pituitary levels, although the latter appear to be more important. GnRH is released in a tonic pulsatile manner by the hypothalamus approximately every 90 minutes, and this pattern of secretion is critical for its effects on the pituitary. In an individual deficient in GnRH secretion, pulsatile administration of GnRH allows restoration of normal cyclic ovulation. In contrast, constant infusion of GnRH leads to down-regulation of pituitary GnRH receptors and a suppression of gonadotropin secretion. This phenomenon has resulted in major advances in therapy aimed at enhancing or preventing fertility.

HYPOTHALAMIC-PITUITARY-THYROID AXIS. TSH secretion by the pituitary is regulated by TRH, dopamine, and somatostatin. For a discussion of the control of somatostatin secretion, the reader is referred to the section on the regulation of GH secretion. TRH secretion is stimulated by norepinephrine and dopamine and is inhibited by serotonin. TRH stimulates TSH secretion, which in turn enhances the release of thyroxine and triiodothyronine by the thyroid. The feedback effects of these hormones, primarily triiodothyronine, occur principally in the pituitary, where they inhibit the TSH response to TRH. A reduction in circulating thyroid hormone levels leads to a prompt rise in TSH levels. TRH is not required for this acute response, although it is necessary for the full expression of TSH hypersecretion over a long time. In addition, TRH is required for maintaining basal TSH secretion. In addition to its effects on the pituitary, triiodothyronine exerts an inhibitory effect on TRH gene expression in the hypothalamus.

Acute changes in environmental conditions requiring increased metabolic activity, such as cold exposure, lead to a TRH-mediated increase in TSH secretion. This effect is readily demonstrable in infants but not in adults, in whom other mechanisms of thermogenesis (mediated by the autonomic nervous system and resulting in shivering and free fatty acid mobilization) are more important. Agents inhibiting adrenergic neurotransmission block the TSH response to cold.

Dopaminergic agents exert an inhibitory effect on TSH release by the pituitary which is most pronounced in patients with elevated TSH levels but is also seen in normal individuals. A role of endogenous dopamine in suppressing TSH secretion has also been demonstrated.

Somatostatin inhibition of TSH secretion exerts a relatively minor physiologic role under normal circumstances, but increases in hypothalamic somatostatin release as a result of elevated GH levels can suppress TSH secretion to subnormal levels. Somatostatin, however, is a less potent inhibitor of TSH than of GH.

HYPOTHALAMIC-PITUITARY-SOMATOTROPH AXIS. GH secretion is regulated by releasing and inhibiting hormones: GRH and SRIF (somatostatin). GH is secreted in a pulsatile pattern with basal levels at or beneath the level of detection, superimposed on which are pulses of GH related to an inherent neural rhythmicity resulting in pulsatile release of both GRH and SRIF. The majority of pulsatile GH secretion occurs about 1 hour after the onset of sleep and is associated with sleep stages 3 and 4. With age, GH secretion changes dramatically, both qualitatively and quantitatively. Extremely high levels seen in the first few days of life decrease by 2 weeks of age. During the pubertal period levels comparable to or greater than those of adults are seen, and the GH surges occur more frequently. After the fourth decade, there is a gradual and progressive decrease in spontaneous GH secretion and responses to GH releasing stimuli also decrease. Neurotransmitter regulation of GH secretion has been extensively defined. Dopamine, norepinephrine (through the α receptor), epinephrine, serotonin, GABA, and acetylcholine have all been shown to stimulate GH secretion. Melatonin has both stimulatory and inhibitory effects, TRH and CRH exhibit inhibitory effects (both peptides stimulate SRIF release), and endorphins-enkephalins have stimulatory effects, all mediated within the CNS.

GH secretion is profoundly affected by nutrients. Elevations of amino acid levels, decreases in free fatty acids, and hypoglycemia all stimulate GH secretion, while hyperglycemia inhibits GH release. GH secretion is increased by exercise, anxiety, and emotional or physical stress. Many hormones affect GH secretion. Estrogen administration increases GH responsiveness, while corticosteroid and thyroid hormone deficiency and excess decrease responsiveness. In pubertal and prepubertal males, androgen

TABLE 212–2. EFFECTS OF AMINERGIC AND PEPTIDERGIC NEUROTRANSMITTERS ON ANTERIOR PITUITARY HORMONE SECRETION

	Norepinephrine	Dopamine	Serotonin	Acetylcholine	Histamine	GABA	Other
ACTH	α ↑	−	↑	↑	−	−	Enkephalins ↓
LH and FSH	(↑)	↓	−	−	−	−	−
TSH	↑	↓	↑	−	−	−	Neurotensin ↓
GH	α ↑ β ↓	↑	↑	↑	−	(↑)	Neurotensin ↓ Substance P ↓ Enkephalins ↑
Prolactin	−	↓	↑	−	↑	↑	Neurotensin ↓ Enkephalins ↑ VIP ↑

NOTE: ↑ = stimulates; ↓ = inhibits; − = no effect or insufficient data; ( ) = conflicting data exist. All effects reflect CNS rather than pituitary sites of action (with the exception of dopamine). The data are derived (whenever possible) from studies in humans.

administration also enhances GH responses. GH secretion is sexually dimorphic: Women have higher basal levels and smaller pulses than do men. These differences may, in part, contribute to sex-related differences in growth patterns and selected enzyme activity.

In addition to these "open-loop" stimuli is a closed-loop feedback system. GH stimulates the production of somatomedin C (insulin-like growth factor [IGF-I]) by numerous tissues, and both GH and IGF-I exhibit feedback effects. IGF-I stimulates the release of somatostatin, inhibits that of GH, and also inhibits basal and GRH-stimulated GH synthesis and release by the pituitary. GH itself stimulates SRIF secretion and inhibits GRH gene expression and secretion.

HYPOTHALAMIC-LACTOTROPH-BREAST AXIS. Prolactin secretion is predominantly controlled by inhibitory CNS influences, with dopamine being the major prolactin-inhibiting factor. Two peptides, TRH and vasoactive intestinal polypeptide (VIP), appear to have physiologic prolactin-releasing factor (PRF) activity, although their relative importance is not yet clear. Neurotransmitter influences on prolactin secretion are extensive. Serotonin stimulates prolactin release by effects on PRF. Melatonin and histamine have stimulatory effects within the CNS, as do opioid peptides and GABA. The effect of the latter two agents appears due to their inhibitory effects on the tuberoinfundibular dopaminergic system.

Prolactin secretion is increased by tactile stimulation of the breast via receptors in the nipple and areola that reach the spinal cord by the intercostal nerves. During pregnancy, prolactin levels increase as a result of estrogen stimulation. Following parturition, the rapid decline in estrogen and progesterone levels allows the unopposed action of prolactin to stimulate lactation from the estrogen-primed breast. The suckling stimulation of prolactin secretion is in part controlled by VIP. Prolactin levels return to normal after several months even during continual lactation. Prolactin is a stress-responsive hormone, and increased secretion is observed after surgical stress, exercise, and insulin hypoglycemia. Prolactin secretion is increased in states of thyroid hormone deficiency and decreased in the presence of thyroid hormone excess.

Bateman A, Singh A, Kral T, et al.: The immune-hypothalamic-pituitary-adrenal axis. Endocr Rev 10:92, 1989. *A critical review of the developing field of neuroendoimmunology. The interaction of cytokines with the neuroendocrine system, while not yet completely understood, is likely to become of major importance.*

Frohman LA, Krieger DT: Neuroendocrine physiology and disease. In Felig P, Baxter JD, Broadus AE, et al. (eds.): Endocrinology and Metabolism, 2nd ed. New York, McGraw-Hill Book Company, 1987, pp 185–247. *A systematic in-depth presentation of the anatomy and physiology of human neuroendocrinology, along with the clinical manifestations, diagnosis, and therapy of anatomic and functional disorders. Designed for the medical student, clinical trainee, and practicing physician.*

Krieger DT, Brownstein M, Martin JB (eds.): Brain Peptides. Vol 2. New York, John Wiley & Sons, 1987. *A comprehensive collection of monographs on the role of brain peptides as transmitters, hypophysiotropic hormones, and messengers throughout the nervous system. This is a definitive reference volume. Of interest to the medical student, neurobiologist, and clinical trainee.*

Marshall JC, Kelch RP: Gonadotropin-releasing hormone: Role of pulsatile secretion in the regulation of reproduction. N Engl J Med 315:1215, 1986. *An excellent discussion of the importance of pulsatility in the biologic effects of gonadotropin-releasing hormone on the pituitary.*

Morley JE: Neuropeptide regulation of appetite and weight. Endocr Rev 8:256, 1987. *The regulation of food intake is a complex issue that involves several distinct brain regions and neurochemical mediators. This review provides an up-to-date assessment of the importance of various brain peptides in this activity.*

Muller EE: Neural control of somatotropic function. Physiol Rev 67:962, 1987. *An excellent review of the current knowledge of neuroendocrine regulation of growth hormone secretion.*

Nieman LK, Loriaux DL: Corticotropin-releasing hormone: Clinical applications. Annu Rev Med 40:331, 1989. Taylor AL, Fishman LM: Corticotropin-releasing hormone. N Engl J Med 319:213, 1988. *Two excellent reviews of the physiology, pathology, and clinical utility of the releasing hormone.*

DISEASES OF THE CENTRAL NERVOUS SYSTEM WITH ALTERED NEUROENDOCRINE AND NEUROMETABOLIC FUNCTION

The frequent association of altered hormone secretion with disorders of the CNS has been recognized for many decades. Although attention was initially focused on the hypothalamus

because of its crucial role in neuroendocrine regulation, diseases localized to extrahypothalamic brain regions as well as nonlocalized CNS disorders can also produce disturbances in neuroendocrine function. The clinical and laboratory manifestations of these disorders are frequently indistinguishable from those of hypothalamic origin, since their mediation is usually via the hypothalamus. Similarly, the distinction between hypothalamic and pituitary causes of certain pituitary hormone secretory disorders may be difficult for other reasons.

Because of the reticular organization of the anatomic structure of the hypothalamus, only certain functions can be localized to a precise site. In addition, neurons within a specific hypothalamic locus may be involved in several separate regulatory functions. Consequently the extent of endocrine or metabolic disturbance is more dependent on the location than the size of the hypothalamic lesion. Furthermore, slowly growing lesions tend to be silent until they have reached considerable size, whereas rapidly enlarging lesions, depending on location, can cause dramatic clinical and laboratory manifestations even when quite small.

Acute hypothalamic damage is associated with impairment of consciousness, sustained hyperthermia, and severe disturbances of cardiovascular, gastrointestinal, or respiratory function. In contrast, persistent disease in the hypothalamus results in alterations in cognition and complex homeostatic functions. Although disorders of neuroendocrine regulation can be produced by acute lesions that destroy the median eminence or the pituitary stalk, they generally tend to be seen with chronic disorders and often result in an inability of the endocrine system to adapt to environmental changes rather than in an alteration of basal hormone secretion. Because hypothalamic neuronal projections, in contrast to those involving sensory and motor function, are generally not lateralized, unilateral damage seldom results in significant or prolonged symptoms. Thus disturbances of hypothalamic function are most commonly seen with diffuse infiltrative or inflammatory diseases, with tumors of the midline that expand bilaterally, or with disorders affecting the median eminence, the final common effector pathway to the pituitary.

Etiology of Hypothalamic Disease

Anatomically defined disorders of the hypothalamus vary in frequency with age groups and are summarized in Table 212–3. In addition, disturbances of neuroendocrine or neurometabolic function are frequently unassociated with anatomic evidence of hypothalamic disease using available neuroradiologic techniques. Many have been attributed to disorders of neurochemical function, although precise mechanisms are currently not known.

TUMORS. Hypothalamic tumors are frequently located in the region of the third ventricle. Those tumors located in the inferior portion of the third ventricle or the anterior mediobasal hypothalamus commonly produce disturbances in neuroendocrine and neurometabolic regulation. The most frequent hypothalamic tumors are craniopharyngiomas (see next section) and their variants (ependymomas and epidermoid cysts), followed by astrocytomas and dysgerminomas. Two other tumor types, hypothalamic pinealomas and hamartomas, are considered separately because of their association with specific neuroendocrine disorders. Since they are frequently of developmental origin, the majority of hypothalamic tumors occur in patients under 25 years of age. Endocrine disturbances generally result from destruction of those neuronal elements required for normal pituitary function. The most frequently occurring manifestations are diabetes insipidus, hypogonadism, and growth retardation. Disturbances in thyroid and adrenal function are less common. The diagnosis of a hypothalamic tumor is made by magnetic resonance imaging and visual field measurement. The combination of an atypical visual field defect (i.e., loss of inferior visual fields), normal sellar anatomy, and intact responses to releasing hormones in a patient with hypopituitarism points to primary hypothalamic disease. It is difficult to remove hypothalamic tumors completely without destroying normal tissue critical for maintaining homeostasis. Many of these tumors, because of their developmental origin, tend to be slow growing and may even undergo spontaneous growth arrest or regression. Cystic tumors can be aspirated or marsupialized into the cerebroventricular system. Radiotherapy is also effective in many of these tumors. The loss of endocrine function is, however, rarely reversible, and replacement hormone therapy is required.

Neonates
  Intraventricular hemorrhage
  Meningitis: bacterial
  Tumors: glioma, hemangioma
  Trauma
  Hydrocephalus, hydranencephaly, kernicterus

1 Month–2 Years
  Tumors: glioma, especially optic glioma, histiocytosis X, hemangiomas
  Hydrocephalus, meningitis
  "Familial" disorders: Laurence-Moon, Bardet-Biedl, Prader-Labhart-Willi

2–10 Years
  Tumors: craniopharyngioma, glioma, dysgerminoma, hamartoma, histiocytosis X, leukemia, ganglioneuroma, ependymoma, medulloblastoma
  Meningitis: bacterial, tuberculous
  Encephalitis: viral and demyelinating, various viral encephalitides and exanthematous demyelinating encephalitides, disseminated encephalomyelitis
  "Familial" disorders: diabetes insipidus, etc.
  Damage from nasopharyngeal radiation therapy

10–25 Years
  Tumors: craniopharyngioma, pituitary tumors, glioma, hamartoma, dysgerminoma, histiocytosis X, leukemia, dermoid, lipoma, neuroblastoma
  Trauma
  Subarachnoid hemorrhage, vascular aneurysm, arteriovenous malformation
  Inflammatory diseases: meningitis, encephalitis, sarcoidosis, tuberculosis
  Associated with midline brain defects: agenesis of corpus callosum
  Chronic hydrocephalus or increased intracranial pressure

25–50 Years
  Nutritional: Wernicke's disease
  Tumors: glioma, lymphoma, meningioma, craniopharyngioma, pituitary tumors, angioma, plasmacytoma, colloid cysts, ependymoma, sarcoma, histiocytosis X
  Inflammatory: sarcoidosis, tuberculosis, viral encephalitis
  Subarachnoid hemorrhage, vascular aneurysms, arteriovenous malformation
  Damage from pituitary radiation therapy

50 Years and Older
  Nutritional: Wernicke's disease
  Tumors: sarcoma, glioblastoma, lymphoma, meningioma, colloid cysts, ependymoma, pituitary tumors
  Vascular: infarct, subarachnoid hemorrhage, pituitary apoplexy
  Infectious: encephalitis, sarcoidosis, meningitis

Adapted from Plum F, Van Uitert R: Non-endocrine diseases of the hypothalamus. *In* Reichlin S, Baldessarini RJ, Martin JB (eds.): The Hypothalamus. New York, Raven Press, 1978, p 415.

Hamartomas. One type of hypothalamic tumor, the hamartoma, has been associated with increased, rather than decreased, hypothalamic function. Hamartomas consist of masses of redundant, partially disoriented glial and neuronal cells or an abnormally lodged collection of normal nerve tissue. Hamartomas associated with precocious puberty consist of encapsulated nodules in the posterior hypothalamus containing membrane-bound secretion granules similar to those in hypothalamic neurosecretory cells. Vessels in the hamartoma have fenestrations characteristic of those in the median eminence, suggesting a secretory process similar to that in the median eminence. These vessels are presumed to connect to the pituitary portal system. The secretion granules contain GnRH, which is found in high concentrations in CSF from patients with this disorder. Hamartomatous cells are believed to secrete GnRH in a pulsatile manner, but are not under normal prepubertal inhibitory influences. The resultant hormonal effects produce pubertal changes that in girls lead to menarche and cyclic ovulatory menses as early as the second year of life.

Hamartomas are present in one third of all children with this form of precocious puberty. Specific therapy aimed at the hamartoma appears unnecessary, since its course is benign with no other neuroendocrine disturbances and no loss of nonendocrine hypothalamic structure or function. Therapy of the precocious

puberty, however, is of great importance both for psychological reasons and for prevention of premature epiphyseal fusion and stunted growth. Optimal therapy is currently achieved with the use of a GnRH agonist to down-regulate pituitary GnRH receptors, resulting in diminished gonadotropin secretion and suppression of bone growth.

Hypothalamic hamartomas have also been associated with gigantism, acromegaly, and GH-secreting pituitary tumors. They have been shown to contain GRH, which is secreted into the portal system, resulting in GH hypersecretion and somatotroph hyperplasia and tumor formation.

Gangliocytomas. A closely related tumor, the gangliocytoma, consists of randomly oriented large ganglion cells similar to those in the hypothalamic magnocellular (large cell) nuclei. Intrapituitary gangliocytomas are also seen in association with acromegaly and GH-secreting tumors of the pituitary and contain GRH. In contrast to hypothalamic hamartomas, the axons of the intrapituitary tumors directly contact the somatotropic cells. A CRH-containing pituitary gangliocytoma has also been described in association with ACTH hypersecretion and Cushing's disease.

Pineal Tumors. Pineal tumors constitute less than 1 per cent of all intracranial neoplasms and consist of three separate tumor types: pinealomas (pineal parenchymal tumor [20 per cent]), glial tumors (25 per cent), and germinomas (also called ectopic pinealomas or teratomas [55 per cent]). The neuroendocrine effects (precocious puberty) of the first two types are most likely a consequence of destruction of the normal pineal by tumor, leading to loss of pineal secretory products (possibly melatonin, arginine vasotocin, or another factor) that normally inhibit the initiation of sexual maturation. Only a small percentage of pineal tumors cause sexual precocity and usually not until they extend beyond the pineal region. Some pineal tumors are associated with delayed puberty, which may be mediated by production of an antigonadotropic factor. Precocious puberty associated with germinomas, which are similar both histologically and functionally to ovarian and testicular germ cell tumors, is caused by the production of chorionic gonadotropin. Levels as high as those seen during the first month of pregnancy are often present. Many of the "ectopic" pinealomas occur in the midline of the ventral hypothalamus and result in loss of other endocrine functions. Surgical treatment of pinealomas is generally unsatisfactory although the tumors consisting of germinal elements are exquisitely radiosensitive. Many tumors, however, contain nongerminal elements (teratomas) that are relatively radioresistant. See also Ch. 215.

INFILTRATIVE AND INFLAMMATORY DISEASES. **Histiocytosis X** (see also Ch. 149). This granulomatous disease of the histiocytic type, with eosinophilic elements, involves the ventromedial hypothalamus and is associated with diabetes insipidus, anterior hypopituitarism due to destruction of releasing hormone-secreting neurons, or both. The three clinical subgroups of the disease are Hand-Schüller-Christian disease, the most common type, characterized by polyuria, exophthalmos, and skull defects; Letterer-Siwe disease, a more rapidly progressive form; and eosinophilic granuloma, in which similar pathologic findings are present in bones. The disease may begin with diabetes insipidus, which is present in nearly 50 per cent of patients with Hand-Schüller-Christian disease. Less commonly, growth failure, hypogonadism, and panhypopituitarism are seen. The diagnosis is established by bone or intracranial biopsy. The CNS forms of the disease may respond to high-dose glucocorticoid therapy or chemotherapy, but the impairment in neuroendocrine function appears irreversible.

Sarcoidosis (see Ch. 67). Involvement of the CNS by sarcoidosis is uncommon. When it is present, however, the hypothalamus and pituitary are frequently involved with infiltrating granulomatous nodules. Patients may develop diabetes insipidus, galactorrhea due to hyperprolactinemia, partial or total anterior pituitary insufficiency, and neurometabolic and neurovegetative symptoms such as somnolence or hyperphagia. In general, the usual treatment with glucocorticoids does not improve the endocrine dysfunction. Granulomatous hypothalamic disease, producing the same endocrine disturbances, can also occur in the absence of peripheral manifestations of sarcoidosis.

TRAUMA. Basal skull fractures are frequently accompanied by shearing of the pituitary stalk, leading to panhypopituitarism and diabetes insipidus. In patients who become comatose following skull fractures, impairment in the pituitary-thyroid and pituitary-gonadal axes has been reported in the absence of stalk damage. Gonadal and thyroid hormones generally return to normal upon recovery.

RADIATION-INDUCED HYPOTHALAMIC DYSFUNCTION. Radiation therapy for intracranial neoplasms, including pituitary tumors, and for nasopharyngeal and maxillary sinus carcinomas frequently leads to hypopituitarism. The interval between therapy and appearance of hormone deficiencies ranges from 1 to 10 years or possibly longer. Children appear more susceptible than adults, and the critical dose is believed to be about 4000 rads. In children, growth failure associated with reduced GH secretion, hypogonadotropic hypogonadism, and hypothyroidism is seen. The site of the defect appears to be variable, with some patients exhibiting hypothalamic and others pituitary damage. In some, but not all, patients, pituitary hormone responses to the injection of hypothalamic releasing hormones may distinguish the anatomic site of the defect.

FUNCTIONAL DISEASES OF THE CENTRAL NERVOUS SYSTEM WITH NEUROENDOCRINE DISTURBANCES

Disturbances in neuroendocrine function manifested by both decreased and increased pituitary hormone secretion can occur in the absence of structurally detectable disease in the pituitary or CNS. With the aid of releasing hormones to test specifically the pituitary component and other stimuli to test the hypothalamic-pituitary unit, some degree of discrimination can be made as to the source of the disordered hormone secretion. The following are recognized functional disturbances that have been attributed to hypothalamic (or possibly other CNS) disease. The specific biochemical defect responsible remains to be determined.

HYPOTHALAMIC HYPOGONADISM. This disorder is defined as an impairment in pituitary-gonadal function caused by deficient or disordered secretion of GnRH. The manifestations vary according to the age at presentation (see also Ch. 222 and 224).

Prepubertal. The presence of hypothalamic hypogonadism prior to puberty results in failure of normal sexual maturation. Other pituitary hormone deficiencies, also attributed to hypothalamic dysfunction, may coexist. A major subgroup of this disorder, most frequently seen in boys, includes anosmia or hyposmia (*Kallmann's syndrome* or olfactory-genital dysplasia). This syndrome may be associated with other neurologic defects such as color blindness and nerve deafness. The disorder is frequently familial, although sporadic cases have also been reported. Midline developmental defects occasionally occur, and hypoplasia in the region of the anterior commissure, olfactory bulb, and hypothalamus has been found. In some patients there is an additional defect characterized by decreased testicular response to LH. The gonadotropin responses to a single injection of GnRH are markedly impaired or absent, indicating a lack of prior GnRH function. Repeated administration of GnRH, given to prime the gonadotrophs, eventually produces a normal or supranormal gonadotropin response and serves to differentiate this disorder from that of primary gonadotroph failure. Standard therapy consists of the use of gonadal steroids for the development and maintenance of secondary sexual characteristics. GnRH can produce similar effects and promote fertility if administered by an intermittent infusion pump to simulate endogenous gonadotropin secretion.

Postpubertal. Postpubertal hypothalamic hypogonadism is more frequently seen in women but also affects men. In women, it is manifested clinically by secondary amenorrhea or oligomenorrhea and occasionally by infertility associated with anovulatory cycles. The terms *functional* or *psychogenic amenorrhea* and *infertility* have also been used for this disorder. Patients may exhibit normal basal levels of gonadotropins and estradiol, resulting in maintenance of secondary sexual characteristics, although pulsatile secretion of LH is absent, and the cyclic ovulatory surge of gonadotropins does not occur. The gonadotropin responses to a single injection of GnRH reveal enhancement of the FSH rather than the LH response. These women respond normally to clomiphene, an estrogen receptor antagonist, suggesting that the defect is related to a functional derangement in

the positive estrogen feedback mechanism. The disorder is usually self-limited. In men, the presenting symptoms are decreased libido and impotency. Therapy consists of testosterone alone unless there is also a desire for fertility.

Hyperprolactinemia exerts an inhibitory effect on the positive feedback effect of estradiol on GnRH secretion that has been attributed to enhanced tuberoinfundibular dopamine secretion. The negative estrogen feedback mechanism appears intact, since elevated FSH and LH levels are maintained in postmenopausal women with hyperprolactinemia. In men, hyperprolactinemia produces hypogonadism, manifested most frequently by diminished libido and potency and occasionally by gynecomastia.

In severe cases, basal estradiol levels and serum gonadotropin responses to GnRH are reduced, implying a defect in tonic as well as cyclic GnRH secretion. Similar physiologic disturbances are seen in some patients with hyperprolactinemia irrespective of cause. Marked increases and decreases in body weight are often accompanied by amenorrhea, as occurs with severe obesity and in professional ballet dancers, female athletes, and anorexia nervosa (see details later in this section). Evidence for decreased GnRH secretion has also been found in male athletes.

Treatment of this disorder depends on the extent of hypogonadism and the patient's desire for fertility. Restoration of ovulatory menses may be accomplished by cycles of clomiphene administration, cyclic estrogen-progestin (oral contraceptive) therapy, gonadotropin administration, or GnRH infusions, depending on the desired goal. In hypoestrogenemic women, decreased vaginal secretions, leading to dyspareunia and decreased libido, and the long-term consequences of osteopenia and metabolic bone disease warrant replacement therapy. In men, testosterone replacement therapy is indicated if endogenous hormone levels are subnormal.

Polycystic Ovary Syndrome (see also Ch. 224). The polycystic ovary (Stein-Leventhal) syndrome is characterized by amenorrhea, obesity, hirsutism, and consistently elevated LH levels. It is occasionally associated with a history of childhood CNS injury or "encephalitis." The altered hormonal secretory pattern of polycystic ovaries appears to be secondary to the increased LH secretion. This syndrome is occasionally seen in patients with hyperprolactinemia, but the causal relationship remains to be established.

HYPOTHALAMIC HYPOTHYROIDISM. This is an uncommon disorder manifested by hypothyroidism, a low or normal plasma TSH level, and an exaggerated and delayed response of TSH to TRH. In patients with this disorder, peak TSH responses occur at 90 to 120 minutes, in contrast to the 15- to 30-minute peak response time seen in normal subjects. Some patients have elevated basal TSH levels with decreased biologic activity, but in most, basal levels are normal. Hypothalamic hypothyroidism can occur as an isolated defect or, more commonly, is seen in association with deficiencies of gonadotropin, GH, or ACTH secretion. Treatment of this disorder is with thyroxine.

HYPOTHALAMIC-ADRENAL DYSFUNCTION. Decreased ACTH secretion on the basis of hypothalamic or other CNS disorders is relatively rare. It is seen most commonly in association with other pituitary hormone deficiencies during childhood and, by inference, has been attributed to a CNS cause. Disturbances of ACTH diurnal rhythm and suppressibility of ACTH are common in patients with a variety of intracranial diseases and reflect disturbances in neuroendocrine control mechanisms. They do not have major clinical significance, but subtle effects on behavior cannot be excluded. In particular, patients with affective disorders (unipolar depression) or experiencing bereavement exhibit a lack of normal glucocorticoid suppressibility similar to that seen in Cushing's disease.

IDIOPATHIC HYPERPROLACTINEMIA. Idiopathic hyperprolactinemia (IH) is a disorder in which prolactin levels are elevated in the absence of demonstrable pituitary or CNS disease and of any other recognized cause of increased prolactin secretion (see Ch. 226). The clinical manifestations of IH consist of galactorrhea and amenorrhea. In some patients, oligomenorrhea is present, and in a few, sporadic ovulation persists. Prolactin levels are elevated, but rarely exceed 150 ng per milliliter. The disease is confined to women of child-bearing age. The diagnosis remains inferential and based on exclusion of a pituitary microadenoma.

Many patients in whom IH was previously diagnosed have subsequently been found by magnetic resonance imaging to harbor microadenomas. Extensive testing using neuropharmacologic probes has failed to distinguish patients with IH from those with microadenomas, suggesting that the same pathophysiologic mechanism underlies both disorders. IH has been attributed to a CNS neurotransmitter defect related to dopamine metabolism, based on the observations that drugs impairing dopaminergic neurotransmission (i.e., neuroleptic dopamine receptor antagonists) increase prolactin secretion. The major action of these drugs in elevating prolactin levels, however, appears to be at the pituitary rather than within the CNS. IH is a benign condition, since less than 5 per cent of patients observed over a period of years subsequently show evidence of a pituitary tumor.

Therapy depends on the level of symptoms and the degree of inconvenience they produce. Bromocriptine (2.5 mg two or three times a day) is a dopamine receptor agonist that suppresses prolactin levels, eliminates galactorrhea, and restores cyclic menses and fertility. Nearly 80 per cent of patients experience menses within 2 months of initiating therapy, and 65 per cent become fertile. The effect of the drug is of short duration, however, and hyperprolactinemia recurs following its discontinuation. In some patients, hyperprolactinemia may remit spontaneously or following a pregnancy subsequent to bromocriptine administration. There is no evidence that long-term bromocriptine therapy per se restores prolactin secretory dynamics to normal. Even in the absence of a desire for fertility, the increased risk of osteopenia in hyperprolactinemic, hypoestrogenemic women provides the rationale for therapy.

HYPOTHALAMIC DISORDERS OF GROWTH HORMONE SECRETION. *Idiopathic Growth Hormone Deficiency.* Idiopathic GH deficiency (IGHD) occurs as either an isolated hormone deficiency or in association with other anterior pituitary hormone deficiencies and as both a familial and sporadic disorder. It is a disease of childhood, the diagnosis frequently being made because of impaired linear growth when the child is between 2 and 3 years of age. Impairment in GH secretion may be complete, with basal levels barely detectable, or partial, with subnormal responses to stimuli. The absence of radiologic abnormalities of the pituitary and the frequent coexistence of TRH- and GnRH-responsive deficiencies of TSH and gonadotropins suggest that the defect is located in the hypothalamus. Limited histologic studies of the pituitary or hypothalamus are available because of the generally benign nature of the disease. It is assumed to be due to a deficiency of GRH secretion, most likely on the basis of a neurotransmitter or biosynthetic abnormality, rather than to a structural defect in the hypothalamus. Approximately 75 per cent of patients with IGHD exhibit an intact GH response to GRH, indicating that the disorder has a heterogeneous etiology. Several other subgroups of GH deficiency are now also recognized, including one in which partial deletion of the GH gene results in complete absence of the hormone and another in which there is spontaneous recovery of GH secretion. In addition, other defects may be present in the pituitary, rendering it unresponsive to GRH. Therapy of IGHD should be initiated as soon as the diagnosis is established and consists of administration of biosynthetic human GH. Preliminary results using GRH as therapy indicate that this releasing hormone may effectively substitute for GH in about half of the patients with IGHD. Hypothyroidism, if present, must also be treated. If gonadotropin deficiency is present, therapy with gonadal steroids is postponed as long as possible to avoid accelerating bone growth and producing epiphyseal closure before acceptable linear bone growth is achieved by GH.

Psychosocial Dwarfism. A pattern indistinguishable from IGHD is seen occasionally in children reared in environments with deficient maternal care and affection. Children with this disorder, also termed the emotional deprivation syndrome, exhibit impaired GH responses to stimuli when studied. Within a short time in an improved environment, however, GH secretion returns to normal, and linear growth is restored. It is presumed that the impaired GH secretion is secondary to a behaviorly associated alteration in neurotransmitter metabolism impairing normal GRH-SRIF interrelationships.

Cerebral Gigantism. This childhood disease is characterized by rapid growth, accelerated bone age, and mental retardation. Ventricular enlargement is present, although no focal CNS lesions have been detected. GH secretion has been normal in the few patients described with this disorder. A variant of the syndrome

is associated with lipodystrophy, hyperpigmentation, hypertrichosis, hepatosplenomegaly, increased adrenal steroid production, and hyperlipemia.

CENTRAL NERVOUS SYSTEM DISORDERS OF WATER REGULATION. Organic lesions of the CNS and drug therapy can lead to "cerebral hyponatremia" or "cerebral hypernatremia," which are entities distinct from diabetes insipidus (see Ch. 214).

Hyponatremia. The syndrome of inappropriate secretion of antidiuretic hormone (ADH) results from the autonomous secretion of vasopressin, resulting in hyponatremia, renal sodium loss, and inability to excrete dilute urine in the presence of normal renal, pituitary, adrenal, and thyroid function; resistance to correction by hypertonic saline; and reversibility following restriction of water (see Ch. 75). The increased renal sodium excretion occurs secondary to expanded extracellular volume. When measured, plasma vasopressin levels have been increased.

This syndrome has been reported in patients with carcinoma metastatic to the brain, primary brain tumors, cerebral infarction, basal skull fracture, subarachnoid hemorrhage, meningoencephalitis, and acute intermittent porphyria, but it may also occur in the absence of any underlying structural disease. Certain hypoglycemic and antineoplastic drugs can produce the same syndrome. The former, including chlorpropamide and tolbutamide, augment ADH action on the renal tubule and also stimulate ADH release. Vincristine and cyclophosphamide have direct neurotoxic effects on neurohypophyseal tissue. Other agents such as carbamazepine (Tegretol), amitriptyline (Elavil), thioridazine (Mellaril), and clofibrate (Atromid-S) also produce the syndrome, presumably by affecting endogenous vasopressin release.

Hypernatremia. Patients with intracranial lesions with or without disturbances of consciousness may exhibit hypernatremia in the presence of normal renal function, adequate fluid intake, absence of thirst, and failure of forced fluid intake to correct the hyperosmolality. This syndrome has been attributed to impaired regulation of thirst as well as vasopressin secretion and has been described in association with histiocytosis, craniopharyngioma, optic nerve glioma, pineal tumor, encephalitis, and ruptured intracranial aneurysm. The treatment of this disorder, above and beyond that of the specific causative lesion, is similar to that for diabetes insipidus.

DISORDERS OF NEUROMETABOLIC REGULATION. *Acute Disorders.* Acute disturbances of metabolic regulation occur most commonly in states of stress that activate the sympathetic nervous system. Thus, patients with hyperthermia, trauma, sepsis, and burns, and undergoing general anesthesia, may exhibit hyperglycemia and hyperglucagonemia along with impaired insulin secretion. In most instances these changes represent merely an extension of normal physiologic processes, do not result in significant clinical problems, and resolve spontaneously when the stress disappears. However, when stress is prolonged, as in severe burns, the responses can produce a severe catabolic state that can be life threatening.

Stress diabetes, seen frequently in the same clinical disorders, may have several causes. Some patients may manifest true diabetes mellitus for the first time under circumstances in which there is enhanced secretion of cortisol, glucagon, catecholamines, and GH, but in other patients the marked hyperglycemia may be unrelated to true diabetes. A syndrome indistinguishable from nonketotic hyperglycemia with or without coma is associated with severe head injury, cerebral thrombosis, encephalitis, and heat stroke. The severity of the hyperglycemia and its duration predict the probability of survival following head injury. Treatment consists of hydration and small doses of insulin.

Hypoglycemia is seen only rarely with hypothalamic disease. It has been reported in association with subdural hemorrhage.

Chronic Disorders. Destruction of the ventromedial hypothalamus leads to a syndrome of obesity, while damage to the ventrolateral hypothalamus results in anorexia and inanition. Because bilateral destruction is necessary, inanition is infrequently observed, since the concomitant loss of other important homeostatic mechanisms is usually incompatible with prolonged survival. An anatomically identifiable hypothalamic lesion is present in only a small percentage of patients with extensive obesity or inanition. However, the remarkable similarity of clinical and biochemical features in patients with and without definable lesions suggests that many "functional" disorders of caloric homeostasis ("essential" obesity and anorexia nervosa) are caused by biochemical disturbances in hypothalamic function that are currently undefined.

Hypothalamic Obesity. Ventromedial hypothalamic destruction resulting from encephalitis, infiltrative diseases (leukemia or histiocytosis X), trauma, vascular accidents, and tumors has been associated with obesity. Oxygen consumption, insulin secretion, body composition, and adipose metabolism are similar in patients with hypothalamic obesity and those with essential obesity. Adipose tissue mass increases primarily as the result of hypertrophy rather than hyperplasia. Marked insulin resistance is present, and diabetes may develop in some patients. GH secretion is impaired, and hypogonadism is common.

A number of familial disorders (Laurence-Moon, Bardet-Biedl, Alstrom-Hallgren, Prader-Willi) are associated with extreme obesity and evidence of other hypothalamic disturbances, including hypogonadism, temperature intolerance, and loss of diurnal rhythms; and of extrahypothalamic disturbances, such as deafness, pigmentary retinopathy, hypotonia, and mental retardation.

Therapy of hypothalamic obesity is not very successful. Once true destruction has occurred, the functional alterations are almost always irreversible. In children with hypothalamic leukemic infiltrates, successful chemotherapy can lead to cessation of hyperphagia and reduction of weight to normal. In general, therapeutic measures are aimed at treatment of the morbidly obese patient.

Anorexia Nervosa. This disorder is seen almost exclusively in young women and consists of weight loss, amenorrhea, and behavioral disturbances. Bulimia may also be present (see Ch. 202).

Almost every neuroendocrine system is affected by the disorder. Gonadotropin secretion "regresses" to a prepubertal stage characterized by absence of pulsatile secretion of LH and altered FSH-LH responses to GnRH. GH levels are normal or, at times, elevated, particularly in the presence of severe malnutrition, in which a paradoxic response to glucose may be observed. TSH responses to TRH are reduced, but thyroid function tends to be normal. Plasma cortisol levels are elevated, but diurnal variation is generally preserved. Patients tend to be poikilothermic, exhibiting difficulty in maintaining body temperature in response to changes in the environment. Impaired vasopressin secretion can be demonstrated but is rarely of clinical importance.

Most of the endocrine metabolic disturbances can be attributed to the severe malnutrition, and successful therapy resulting in weight gain is usually accompanied by restoration of normal neuroendocrine responses. One exception is gonadotropin secretion, which frequently remains abnormal and results in persistence of amenorrhea in up to one third of patients. Another is osmoregulation, which is accompanied by dysregulated vasopressin secretion for prolonged periods.

Prognosis for the reversal of cachexia and weight loss is reasonably good. Mortality is currently less than 5 per cent, and the majority of patients return to within 10 per cent of original body weight. Only 40 per cent of patients maintain their weight over a long term; the remainder exhibit moderate to severe weight loss with time.

CENTRAL NERVOUS SYSTEM BEHAVIORAL DISORDERS AFFECTING NEUROENDOCRINE FUNCTION. Disturbances of endocrine function have been observed in patients with a variety of psychiatric illnesses. The association is presumably through disordered neurotransmitter metabolism, although it is still unclear whether the same defect underlies both the behavioral and neuroendocrine dysfunction or whether altered behavior itself secondarily affects neuroendocrine function.

Of all the conditions studied, depressive affective behavior and the manic-depressive state have been most clearly shown to exhibit endocrine changes. Cortisol secretion in depressed patients is enhanced, and they are relatively resistant to dexamethasone suppression. This abnormality reverts to normal with successful treatment. In manic-depressive patients, cortisol secretion tends to be decreased during manic states and elevated during depressive periods.

Brown WA (ed.): Endocrinology of neuropsychiatric disorders. Endocrinol Metab Clin North Am 17:1–239, 1988. *An excellent collection of review articles on the variety of behavioral and other CNS disorders that have effects on neuroendocrine function.*

Goldman MB, Luchins DJ, Robertson GL: Mechanisms of altered water metabolism in psychotic patients with polydipsia and hyponatremia. N Engl J Med 318:397, 1988. *A carefully conducted study of the mechanisms underlying altered water metabolism in association with behavioral disease.*

Kopelman PG: Neuroendocrine function in obesity. Clin Endocrinol (Oxf) 28:675, 1988. *Obesity is associated with a number of neuroendocrine disturbances, some of which appear to be secondary and others primary. This article reviews the most important aspects.*

Lamberts SWJ: The role of somatostatin in the regulation of anterior pituitary hormone secretion and the use of its analogs in the treatment of human pituitary tumors. Endocrinol Rev 9:417, 1988. *This hypothalamic hormone and its superactive analogue have now become important in the suppression of many endocrine and exocrine functions. Its physiology and clinical use are reviewed in relation to pituitary tumors.*

Manasco PK, Pescovitz OH, Hill SC, et al.: Six-year results of luteinizing hormone releasing hormone (LHRH) agonist treatment in children with LHRH-dependent precocious puberty. J Pediatr 115:105, 1989. *The most comprehensive results available demonstrating the efficacy of an analogue in blocking the pituitary responses to endogenous GnRH and markedly affecting outcome of a significant neuroendocrine disorder.*

Sano T, Asa SL, Kovacs K: Growth hormone-releasing hormone–producing tumors: Clinical, biochemical, and morphological manifestations. Endocrinol Rev 9:357, 1988. *A comprehensive review of tumors that secrete a hypothalamic hormone and cause growth hormone hypersecretion and acromegaly. Although uncommon, the disorder requires treatment that is different from that of the typical patient with acromegaly.*

Whitcomb RW, Crowley WF Jr: Clinical review 4: Diagnosis and treatment of isolated gonadotropin-releasing hormone deficiency in men. J Clin Endocrinol Metab 70:3, 1990. *The understanding of the physiology of GnRH secretion has permitted the use of the hormone in treating endogenous GnRH deficiency. The authors review their extensive experience with this agent.*

213 The Anterior Pituitary

Lawrence A. Frohman

ANATOMY

The pituitary is located in a saddle-shaped cavity, the *sella turcica,* which is an integral portion of the sphenoid bone. Its anterior boundary is the midline *tuberculum sellae* and the anterior clinoid processes that project posteriorly from the sphenoid wings. The posterior limit is the *dorsum sellae,* which projects laterally to form the posterior clinoid processes. The lateral boundaries of the sella are nonosseous and consist of the medial wall of the cavernous sinus, in which is contained the internal carotid artery. The *diaphragma sellae,* a thickened reflection of the *dura mater,* forms the roof of the sella and is attached to the clinoid processes. Only the external layer of the dura extends into the sella as a periosteal lining, and thus the pituitary is normally extradural and not in direct communication with cerebrospinal fluid. The pituitary stalk and its blood vessels pass through a foramen in this membrane that may be incomplete or fenestrated.

The shape of the sella varies from ovoid to spheroid, resulting in considerable variation in normal pituitary dimensions. The average dimensions of the pituitary are 10 mm (anterior-posterior) by 13 mm (transverse) by 6 mm (height). Pituitary weight varies from 0.5 to 0.7 gram, being slightly greater in women. The anterior lobe constitutes about 75 per cent of the total pituitary weight and during pregnancy can increase up to twofold in size.

The arterial blood supply of the pituitary originates from the internal carotid artery via branches from the circle of Willis and hypophyseal arteries. Whereas the posterior lobe is supplied directly by the inferior hypophyseal artery, the blood supply of the anterior lobe is derived entirely from the portal vascular system (see Ch. 212). Venous drainage from the anterior lobe enters the posterior pituitary capillary bed and then the cavernous sinus. The nerve supply of the anterior pituitary consists of postganglionic sympathetic fibers that accompany and terminate on arteriolar vessels and nerve fibers connecting the posterior and anterior lobes. Their function is currently unknown.

EMBRYOLOGY

The glandular portion of the pituitary (*adenohypophysis*) is derived from Rathke's pouch, an ectodermal evagination of the oropharynx that fuses with a diencephalic outpouching of the region of the third ventricle in the developing embryo that eventually differentiates into the *neurohypophysis,* or posterior lobe. That portion of Rathke's pouch not in contact with the diencephalon differentiates to form the *pars anterior,* or anterior lobe. Two lateral outgrowths from the anterior lobes fuse in the midline and extend forward along the hypophyseal stalk to form the *pars tuberalis,* which in humans is limited to a small group of cells along the anterior region of the stalk. The portion of Rathke's pouch contiguous with the neurohypophysis develops less extensively and forms the *pars intermedia,* or intermediate lobe. This structure is not well defined in humans and tends to become intermingled with the anterior lobe. This combined structure has been called the *pars distalis.*

Differentiation of the pars anterior results in cells that secrete growth hormone (GH), prolactin, corticotropin (ACTH), thyroid-stimulating hormone (TSH), luteinizing hormone (LH), and follicle-stimulating hormone (FSH) as well as non–hormone-secreting cells. Cells of the pars intermedia secrete ACTH, lipotropin, and endorphins. Pituitary tumors developing in various regions of the pars distalis tend to reflect the predominant cell types in each region.

The lumen of Rathke's pouch is obliterated during development, although remnants may persist at the boundary of the neurohypophysis as either a cleft or small colloid-filled cysts. The connection with the oropharynx disappears early in development, because of growth of the sphenoid bone, although a few cells in the lower portion of the pouch may persist along the tract, occasionally within the sphenoid bone, and are known as the pharyngeal pituitary. These cells contain secretory granules for GH and prolactin, can be a source of "ectopic" pituitary tumor development, and conceivably could exhibit significant endocrine function subsequent to destruction or removal of the pars distalis.

Pituitary hormones are detected immunochemically as early as the seventh week of fetal life, and some CNS control of anterior pituitary hormone secretion occurs early in gestation. In contrast, true functional maturation, including aspects of feedback regulation, do not develop until postnatal life.

CELL TYPES

The anterior pituitary contains many cell types, the predominant function of which is the synthesis, storage, and release of a specific hormone(s). The frequency of heterogeneous cell type clustering suggests the presence of paracrine effects on hormone secretion.

SOMATOTROPHS. Originally identified as acidophilic cells, these cells secrete GH and are located predominantly in the lateral portions of the anterior lobe where they constitute up to 50 per cent of all cells. Tumors derived from this cell type lead to acromegaly.

LACTOTROPHS. Lactotrophs are also acidophilic and secrete prolactin. They are slightly less numerous than somatotrophs, tend to be located more peripherally than somatotrophs, and have smaller secretion granules. During pregnancy and fetal life, lactotrophs are increased in number, reflecting the effects of increased estrogen levels. Virtually all of the increase in pituitary size during pregnancy can be accounted for by lactotroph proliferation. Both lactotrophs and somatotrophs appear to be derived from a common stem cell, the somatomammotroph, tumors of which may secrete both GH and prolactin.

THYROTROPHS. The basophilic staining cells that secrete TSH occur most frequently at the anterior edge of the pituitary near the midline, although they are also present in deeper portions of the gland. Their secretory granules are smaller than GH and prolactin granules. Thyrotrophs normally constitute only about 6 per cent of anterior lobe cells. In primary hypothyroidism they undergo marked hypertrophy.

GONADOTROPHS. These cells are located deep in the lateral portion of the gland in association with lactotrophs and secrete both LH and FSH. Although constituting only 3 to 4 per cent of anterior pituitary cells normally, they increase in number following castration and decrease during pregnancy as a result of placental gonadotropin production.

CORTICOTROPHS. Cells of this type, which can be chromophobic or basophilic, are found in two separate locations. One group of cells resides most commonly in the medial mucoid region of the anterior lobe. A second group migrates during development to the junctional region of the anterior and posterior lobes and also to the pars tuberalis. Anterior lobe corticotrophs exhibit sparse granulation, whereas those in the pars tuberalis–posterior lobe region contain large, electron-dense granules. The same precursor molecule is present in both cell types, although processing enzyme activity varies, resulting in different ratios of hormones derived from the precursor (ACTH, melanocyte-stimulating hormone [MSH], lipotropins, and endorphins) in the two different regions. Anterior lobe corticotrophs increase in number with glucocorticoid deficiency, whereas those in the intermediate-posterior lobe region decrease, suggesting that only the former are physiologically important ACTH-secreting cells.

OTHER CELL TYPES. As many as 15 to 20 per cent of anterior pituitary cells cannot be stained by antibodies to any of the recognized anterior pituitary hormones. Some of these may represent resting degranulated cells or undifferentiated primitive secretory cells. However, others may be responsible for the secretion of as yet uncharacterized pituitary hormones such as tissue-specific growth factors. One such cell type is stellate, with cellular processes extending into the perivascular spaces in a manner suggestive of primitive follicle formation. These *folliculostellate* cells generally do not contain secretory granules but have recently been shown to produce an endothelial cell growth factor.

ANTERIOR PITUITARY HORMONES

The anterior pituitary secretes six well-recognized hormones, all of which are readily measurable in serum. They can be divided into three general categories: corticotropin and related peptides, glycoprotein hormones, and somatomammotropin hormones. The chemical characteristics of these hormones are given in Table 213–1.

CORTICOTROPIN-RELATED PEPTIDES. ACTH and its related family of peptides are synthesized as a single precursor molecule, pro-opiomelanocortin, with a molecular weight of approximately 29,000. Following glycosylation, the molecule is differentially cleaved into an NH_2-terminal fragment of uncertain biologic activity; a midportion, which contains ACTH; and a COOH-terminal portion, β-lipotropin (LPH). Subsequent processing, which varies in the different groups of corticotrophs, may also cleave ACTH into α-MSH and corticotropin-like intermediate lobe peptides. β-LPH is also differentially processed further to β-endorphin and other endorphin-related peptides (see Ch. 212). Although the structures of β-MSH and met-enkephalin are contained within the β-LPH sequence, the former is not synthesized in postnatal human pituitaries, and the biosynthesis of the latter occurs through a separate precursor.

ACTH. The primary effects of ACTH are stimulation of secretion of glucocorticoid, mineralocorticoid, and androgenic steroids by the adrenal cortex. ACTH binds to specific receptors on adrenocortical cell membranes and stimulates steroidogenesis through a cyclic AMP–mediated mechanism by enhancing cholesterol conversion to pregnenolone. ACTH also stimulates adrenal protein synthesis, leading to cellular growth and hyperplasia.

Extra-adrenal effects of ACTH include stimulation of lipolysis in adipose tissue, insulin-releasing effects on the pancreatic B cell, stimulation of GH secretion, and enhancement of glucose and amino acid transport into muscles. Except in patients with ACTH-secreting tumors, it is unlikely that plasma ACTH levels sufficient to produce these effects are ever achieved. Although ACTH has less potent pigmenting effects than α-MSH or β-MSH, it has long been considered the major pigmenting hormone in man. Recent studies, however, have indicated control of pigmentation to be a complex process, and the importance of ACTH has come under question.

Plasma levels of ACTH exhibit great variability, in part because of its episodic secretion. Levels in normal adults range from undetectable to 80 pg per milliliter (the lower limit of detection in most assays is approximately 10 pg per milliliter). In addition to its episodic secretion, a diurnal rhythm can be detected with lowest levels in the evening and peak levels in the early morning. Changes in plasma ACTH levels can be shown to precede those of plasma cortisol with a short lag period. With stress, plasma

ACTH levels can reach several hundred picograms per milliliter. In patients with ectopic ACTH production, immunoreactive ACTH levels may be exceedingly high and consist in part of larger molecular sized forms ("big" ACTH) believed to represent partially processed but biologically inactive precursor molecules. ACTH is rapidly eliminated from plasma; its half-life is 3 to 9 minutes, leading to an estimated secretion rate of 25 μg per day, which represents approximately 5 per cent of pituitary hormone content.

β-LPH, Endorphins, and Related Peptides. β-LPH and β-endorphin are secreted in an equimolar ratio to ACTH in response to all types of stimulation. The presence of both molecules in the same precursor as ACTH provides an explanation for this observation. The plasma levels of β-LPH and β-endorphin, however, do not necessarily parallel those of ACTH because of their slower metabolic clearance rates. β-LPH is cleared primarily by the kidneys, and its levels rise disproportionately to those of ACTH in renal failure. Since ACTH secretion is normal in this disorder, β-LPH must exert relatively little feedback effect on its own secretion or that of ACTH. β-LPH and β-endorphin have not been shown to have any effects peripherally at the levels normally seen in plasma.

GLYCOPROTEIN HORMONES. The pituitary glycoprotein hormones consist of an α and β subunit, each containing a peptide core with branched carbohydrate side chains that are required for biologic activity and for stability in plasma. The α subunits of the glycoprotein hormones are identical, whereas the β subunits vary, thereby providing the biologic specificity of each hormone. There is considerable homology between β subunits of the different hormones as well as cross-species homology of both α and β subunits, which explains why bovine or ovine glycoprotein hormones are active in humans. The isolated subunits have no intrinsic biologic activity. Hormone heterogeneity, related to the degree of glycosylation, has been suggested as the explanation for the reported variations in glycoprotein bioactivity at different times in the menstrual cycle. The genes encoding the individual subunits are located on different chromosomes, and the rate-limiting step in glycoprotein hormone secretion is regulated by β subunit production. Elevations in plasma α subunit levels can be seen after both TRH and GnRH stimulation and occasionally in pituitary tumors.

TSH. TSH effects on the thyroid cells are largely analogous to those of ACTH on the adrenal cortex. High-affinity receptors are present on cell membranes, and TSH binding leads to activation of adenylate cyclase, enhanced iodine transport and binding to protein, increased thyroglobulin and thyroid hormone synthesis, and increased thyroglobulin proteolysis with release of thyroid hormones. RNA and protein synthesis are also stimulated, leading to an increase in thyroid size and vascularity.

TSH is measured by a specific assay utilizing an antibody directed to antigenic determinants on the β subunit that exhibit little or no cross-reactivity with other glycoprotein hormones. Normal levels of plasma TSH are from 0.5 to 5 μU per milliliter, with most assays exhibiting a sensitivity of 0.1 μU per milliliter. In primary hypothyroidism, TSH levels may increase to greater than 100 μU per milliliter and responses to thyrotropin-releasing hormone (TRH) are enhanced. A few patients have been described with hypothyroidism and only slightly elevated TSH levels in whom administration of TRH results in an exaggerated TSH increase and a concomitant increase in thyroxine. Evidence for a biologically less potent TSH due to altered glycosylation has been found in such individuals. TSH is cleared from circulation with a half-life of 75 to 80 minutes, and the secretion rate of the hormone is 100 to 200 mU per day. In hypothyroidism, secretion rates may be increased 10 to 15 times that in normals.

LH and FSH. Gonadal function is regulated by two pituitary hormones: (1) FSH, which stimulates ovarian follicular growth, testicular growth, and spermatogenesis, and (2) LH, which promotes ovulation and follicular luteinization, stimulates testicular interstitial cell function, and enhances production of steroids in both ovary and testis. In the ovary, FSH promotes growth and maturation of the primordial follicle, and LH stimulates progesterone production by the corpus luteum by enhancing the conversion of cholesterol to pregnenolone. In the testis, FSH acts on the Sertoli cell, where, in conjunction with testosterone, the production of an androgen-binding protein is stimulated. The target cell of LH is the Leydig cell, leading to enhanced testosterone production. The androgen binding protein serves to transport testosterone in high concentrations into tubular cells to stimulate spermatogenesis. (See also discussion in Ch. 222.) Inhibin, a glycoprotein produced by ovarian granulosa cells and testicular Sertoli cells in response to both FSH and testosterone, exerts a preferential inhibitory feedback effect on FSH secretion.

The gonadotropin assays exhibit a slight degree of cross-reactivity between the hormone and the subunits, although this is not a practical problem at present. Of importance, however, is the cross-reactivity due to the great similarity between LH and chorionic gonadotropin β subunits. While chorionic gonadotropin assays are quite specific, most LH assays do not discriminate between the two hormones.

Plasma levels of FSH and LH in women vary with the menstrual cycle. FSH levels rise slightly and then decline progressively during the early follicular phase of the cycle, during which time LH levels are generally stable or rise slightly. An abrupt rise in LH at midcycle, initiated by increasing estrogen secretion by the developing follicle and accompanied by an FSH

TABLE 213–1. ANTERIOR PITUITARY HORMONES IN HUMANS

Class	Members	Molecular Weight	Amino Acids	Carbohydrate	Other Features
Corticotropin-lipotropin	ACTH	4,500	39		All members of class derived from a single precursor
	α-MSH	1,800	13		N-terminal 13 amino acids of ACTH. In humans, found only in fetal life and in tumors
	β-Lipotropin	11,200	91		
	β-Endorphin	4,000	31		C-terminal (amino acids 61–91) portion of β-LPH
Glycoprotein	LH	29,000	α subunit: 89 β subunit: 115	1% sialic acid	All have two subunits, with the α subunit being identical or nearly identical and the β subunit conferring biologic specificity
	FSH	29,000	α subunit: 89 β subunit: 115	5% sialic acid	
	TSH	29,000	α subunit: 89 β subunit: 112	1% sialic acid	
	Chorionic gonadotropin*	46,000	α subunit: 92 β subunit: 139	12% sialic acid	
Somatomammotropin	Growth hormone	21,800	191		All single-chain proteins with two or three disulfide bridges
	Prolactin	22,500	198	†	
	Placental lactogen*	21,800	191		

Adapted from Frohman LA: Diseases of the anterior pituitary. *In* Felig P, Baxter JD, Broadus AE, et al. (eds.): Endocrinology and Metabolism, 2nd ed. Copyright © 1987 by McGraw-Hill, Inc. Used by permission of McGraw-Hill Book Company.

*Of placental origin and included for comparison purposes.

†Carbohydrate-containing forms of prolactin have been identified.

rise, triggers ovulation. Both hormone levels decline during the luteal phase. Levels of FSH and LH in males are similar to those in females during the follicular phase. FSH and LH levels increase in response to age-related decreases in gonadal function in both sexes. In women this occurs at menopause, and in men a gradual increase is seen during the sixth to eighth decades. The half-life of LH in circulation is approximately 30 minutes, whereas that of FSH is twice as long, the difference being attributed to the varying sialic acid content of the hormones. This permits clear detection of a pulsatile pattern of LH secretion but less so for FSH.

SOMATOMAMMOTROPIC HORMONES. This hormonal class consists of GH, prolactin, and a structurally similar placental hormone, chorionic somatomammotropin, or placental lactogen. Extensive interspecies homology exists for both GH and prolactin, suggesting relatively limited changes in gene duplication during evolution. Despite the similarity, subprimate growth hormones are biologically inactive in humans. GH and placental lactogen exhibit 83 per cent homology, in contrast to only 16 per cent homology between GH and prolactin. Despite these differences, each hormone has both intrinsic lactogenic and growth-promoting activity. Large-molecular-weight–sized hormones ("big" GH and prolactin) have been identified in both pituitary and plasma. The big hormones appear to be dimers connected by interchain disulfide linkages. They are secreted by the pituitary, bind to the hormone target cell receptors, and exhibit reduced biologic activity as compared to the monomer. Some of the large molecular weight GH is actually GH bound to its binding protein, which represents the extracellular domain of the GH receptor. There are four or five additional GH variants, including proteolytically modified forms, electrophoretic variants, and a smaller molecule ("20K variant") lacking amino acids 32 to 46, which is encoded by a separate mRNA species derived from the authentic GH gene and formed by differential splicing of pre-mRNA to mRNA. This variant, while representing 10 per cent of pituitary GH, constitutes less than 5 per cent of secreted GH, and levels in circulation do not change in response to GH secretagogues. It appears to have the same biologic effects as 22K GH. The GH-placental lactogen family consists of five genes, one of which encodes a GH variant that is secreted by the placenta. It is biologically active and most likely accounts for the suppression of pituitary GH secretion during pregnancy.

Growth Hormone. GH is important for linear growth and regulation of metabolic processes. GH administration results in positive nitrogen balance, decreased urea production, decreased body fat stores, and enhanced carbohydrate utilization. Biphasic effects on circulating glucose, amino acid, and free fatty acid levels occur in response to GH with an initial decrease and subsequent return to normal or an increase. The acute effects of GH in isolated tissues resemble those of insulin and include increased amino acid uptake and incorporation into protein, stimulation of RNA synthesis, and enhanced glucose utilization. GH also antagonizes the lipolytic effect of catecholamines in adipose tissue. These acute effects disappear within 3 to 4 hours, by which time a series of delayed effects appears. These include enhanced triglyceride lipolysis, increased sensitivity to catecholamine-mediated lipolysis, and inhibition of glucose uptake and utilization secondary to impaired pyruvate decarboxylation. These effects form the basis of the diabetogenic action of the hormone. GH also exhibits multiphasic effects on insulin secretion. There is an acute direct stimulatory effect on the β cell, a subsequent inhibitory effect, and a late and persistent stimulation of insulin release that occurs secondary to the impairment of carbohydrate utilization. The last effect has the greatest pathophysiologic significance in the development of diabetes secondary to GH hypersecretion.

Many GH effects cannot be produced by acute exposure of tissues to the hormone and are mediated by a group of GH-dependent growth factors that are synthesized in numerous tissues. GH binds to a specific cell-membrane receptor to stimulate their production. The most important of these factors is somatomedin C or insulin-like growth factor I (IGF-I), a peptide of about 7500 daltons that has many similarities to insulin, including structural resemblance to proinsulin and binding to insulin receptors. Somatomedin C receptors are present in many tissues, including cartilage, where sulfate incorporation into proteoglycan and amino acid uptake and incorporation are stimulated.

The importance of IGF-I in the growth-promoting effects of GH is illustrated by the Laron dwarf, in whom a mutation of the GH receptor impairs GH stimulation of IGF-I production, resulting in severe growth retardation. IGF-I may be synthesized in the same cell in which it acts (autocrine) or in neighboring cells (paracrine). Thus, while circulating IGF-I levels are a measure of GH secretion, they most likely reflect local IGF-I production rather than serving as a source for tissue uptake even though systemically administered IGF-I can enhance growth. It is currently believed that cell differentiation and growth require both GH and IGF-I, with GH serving to commit a precursor cell to a specific pathway of differentiation and IGF-I enhancing growth and replication. Other growth factors, such as IGF-II platelet-derived growth factor and epidermal growth factor, do not appear to be GH dependent although GH does stimulate production of the EGF receptor. GH also stimulates cardiac and renal hypertrophy and production of specific hormones such as renin and aldosterone and conversion of thyroxine to triiodothyronine.

Immunoreactive measurements of GH are valid indicators of GH bioactivity. Mean GH levels during adolescence and adult life are generally less than 3 ng per milliliter, although the spontaneous secretory pulses of GH can produce elevations as great as 30 to 50 ng per milliliter in young adult subjects. Levels in women during the childbearing age are generally greater than in men, particularly in response to exercise or other stimuli. GH is cleared from plasma primarily by the liver and to a lesser extent by the kidney. The half-time of GH disappearance from circulation is 20 minutes, and the overall secretion in normal adults ranges from 300 to 500 μg per square meter per day.

Prolactin. The major effect of prolactin is to stimulate the synthesis of milk constituents, including lactalbumin, casein, lipids, and carbohydrates (see Ch. 226). Prolactin receptors are present on alveolar surfaces of mammary cells and, in addition, have been identified in liver and kidney. Prolactin is not required for normal breast development in humans, and pathologic elevations of the hormone are not generally associated with an increase in breast size. During pregnancy, prolactin, in conjunction with estrogen, progesterone, and placental lactogen, results in further breast development and milk formation. Following parturition, the abrupt decrease in estrogen and progesterone derived from the placenta permits initiation of lactation. This effect underlies the previous use of estrogens to inhibit lactation in the postpartum period and explains the frequent onset of galactorrhea in hyperprolactinemic women after discontinuance of oral contraceptives. Continued prolactin secretion is required to maintain lactation once initiated, and the return of prolactin to normal levels in the postpartum period is delayed in women who nurse for prolonged periods. The actual milk let-down reflex is mediated by the release of oxytocin rather than by prolactin. Oxytocin stimulates contraction of myoepithelial cells surrounding the terminal acinar lobules that expel their milk into the lobular ducts. Although prolactin has numerous effects on behavior and on fluid and electrolyte metabolism in lower species, no such effects have been convincingly demonstrated in humans.

Normal prolactin levels do not exceed 15 ng per milliliter in men or 20 ng per milliliter in women. There are no significant changes during the menstrual cycle, but levels decrease at menopause. During pregnancy, prolactin levels rise continuously from early gestation to values of 150 to 200 ng per milliliter at term. Prolactin is cleared from circulation with a half-time of approximately 50 minutes. The liver and, to a lesser extent, the kidney are the major sites of prolactin removal.

TESTS OF ANTERIOR PITUITARY HORMONE FUNCTION

ACTH. Since ACTH levels in normal subjects may be undetectable at times, random measurements of the hormone are of limited value. In a patient with signs and symptoms of adrenocortical insufficiency and low plasma cortisol levels, a low or even normal ACTH level is suggestive of hypothalamic-pituitary disease. The most useful test at present for evaluating ACTH function is that of insulin hypoglycemia. A dose of insulin, generally 0.1 U per kilogram, to decrease the fasting blood glucose to 40 mg per deciliter is given intravenously, and plasma cortisol levels are measured over a 2-hour period. A rise greater than 10 μg per deciliter or a peak level greater than 20 μg per deciliter is indicative of a normal hypothalamic-pituitary-adrenal axis. The dose of insulin should be decreased by 50 per cent when hypopituitarism is strongly suspected and increased by 50 per cent in patients with anticipated insulin resistance (i.e., obesity). No treatment is necessary for catecholamine-mediated symptoms of hypoglycemia, but those of central glucopenia (impaired mentation or altered states of consciousness) require immediate therapy. This test must not be performed in patients with suspected primary adrenal insufficiency.

Corticotropin-releasing hormone (CRH) is a safe and specific means of assessing ACTH secretory function. Ovine CRH is more potent than human CRH, presumably because of its longer plasma half-life. When given at a dose of 1 μg per kilogram, CRH elicits both an ACTH and cortisol response. A rise in ACTH without a corresponding increase in cortisol suggests a chronically unstimulated adrenal gland and therefore a hypothalamic dysfunction. In contrast, absence of an ACTH response indicates primary pituitary disease. CRH has not yet been approved for use in the United States. When available, it should eliminate the need for the use of insulin hypoglycemia in most cases. Impairment of normal cortisol feedback using metyrapone, an 11β-hydroxylase inhibitor, at a dose of 750 mg orally every 4 hours for six doses, with measurement of plasma 11-desoxycortisol or urinary 17-hydroxycorticoids, is an alternative way to test the entire hypothalamic-pituitary-adrenal axis. This test is less useful than insulin hypoglycemia in predicting normal responsiveness of the axis to stress. ACTH stimulation has also been used as an indirect method of assessing endogenous ACTH secretory activity.

The best test of suspected excessive ACTH and cortisol secretion is by dexamethasone suppression. The rapid dexamethasone suppression test involves administration of 1 mg dexamethasone orally at 11 P.M. and measurement of plasma cortisol at 8 o'clock the following morning. A level of less than 5 μg per deciliter indicates normal suppressibility. In patients in whom normal suppression is not demonstrated, a standard low-dose dexamethasone suppression test (0.5 mg orally every 6 hours for 48 hours) is performed. Plasma cortisol will be suppressed to less than 5 μg per deciliter, and urinary free cortisol levels will be suppressed to less than 20 μg per 24 hours in normal subjects but not in patients with ACTH hypersecretion or primary adrenocortical hypersecretion. In patients in whom suppression fails, a high-dose dexamethasone suppression test (2 mg orally every 6 hours for 48 hours) is then used to distinguish between pituitary and adrenal causes.

TSH. Impaired TSH secretion should be suspected in hypothyroid patients when plasma TSH levels are not elevated. Differentiation of pituitary from hypothalamic causes of TSH deficiency can usually, but not always, be accomplished by administering TRH, 500 μg (intravenously), and measuring plasma TSH levels. In normal persons, plasma TSH increases to at least 8 μU per milliliter after TRH administration, and peak levels usually occur at 15 to 30 minutes. In hypothalamic hypothyroidism, the response may be exaggerated and is frequently prolonged, with peak values at 90 to 180 minutes. Since thyroxine impairs the TSH response to TRH, it is not possible to assess TSH function in patients receiving thyroid hormone replacement therapy until at least a month after discontinuation of medication.

LH AND FSH. LH and FSH deficiency should be suspected in patients with clinical evidence of hypogonadism and subnormal testosterone or estradiol levels in whom gonadotropin levels are not elevated. Administration of gonadotropin-releasing hormone (GnRH) may be useful in distinguishing between hypothalamic and pituitary causes of hypogonadism. In normal subjects, a single GnRH injection increases LH levels three- to fivefold. Multiple injections may be necessary to distinguish between hypothalamic and pituitary causes, since impaired responses may be seen after a single injection in both disorders. Clomiphene, an estrogen antagonist, stimulates gonadotropin levels in some patients with hypothalamic hypogonadism.

GROWTH HORMONE. The most frequently employed stimulus for GH secretion is insulin hypoglycemia. The details of testing and the cautions required are as described under ACTH testing. Peak GH levels usually occur at 60 or 90 minutes, and a

peak level of 9 ng per milliliter or greater is considered normal. Up to 30 per cent of normal subjects may not respond to insulin hypoglycemia. L-Arginine (0.5 gram per kilogram intravenously during a 30-minute period), L-dopa (0.5 gram orally), and clonidine (25 μg orally) are other effective stimuli used to test GH secretory reserve and may be used in series with insulin. The responses are comparable in magnitude to those after insulin. Other stimuli (glucagon plus propranolol, endotoxin, vasopressin, ACTH) have no advantage over those described. Although still investigational, GRH is often useful in distinguishing between hypothalamic and pituitary causes for GH deficiency. Lack of an adequate GH response, however, may also be due to excessive somatostatin secretion.

Suppressibility of GH secretion in patients with elevated GH levels is evaluated with a standard glucose tolerance test. A decrease in GH levels to less than 2 ng per milliliter is seen in normal subjects. TRH is also used in distinguishing between types of suspected GH hypersecretion. TRH has no effect on GH levels in normal subjects, whereas a rapid increase in GH levels occurs in most patients with acromegaly.

PROLACTIN. Impaired prolactin secretion is rarely a clinical problem. It should be suspected in patients with levels of less than 2 ng per milliliter, and the diagnosis is confirmed by the absence of a response to TRH. Elevated prolactin levels in nearly all patients, with the exception of occasional patients with prolactin-secreting tumors and patients with chronic renal failure, can be suppressed by dopamine infusions, L-dopa, or other dopaminergic agents. These tests are not useful in the differential diagnosis of hyperprolactinemia.

Brook CGD, Hindmarsh PC, Stanhope R: Growth and growth hormone secretion. J Endocrinol 119:179, 1988. *A clearly written review of the role of GH secretion in promoting growth.*

Chin WW: Hormonal regulation of thyrotropin and gonadotropin gene expression. Clin Res 36:484, 1988. *An up-to-date review of the hormonal control of TSH and LH using techniques of molecular biology.*

Frohman LA: Diseases of the anterior pituitary. *In* Felig P, Baxter JD, Broadus E, et al. (eds.): Endocrinology and Metabolism, 2nd ed. New York, McGraw-Hill Book Company, 1987, pp 247–338. *A detailed systematic description of the chemistry, physiology, and pathophysiology of the pituitary. Of particular use to the clinical trainee and practicing physician.*

Frohman LA, Jansson J-O: Growth hormone-releasing hormone. Endocrinol Rev 7:223, 1986. *A review of basic and clinical aspects of GRH, its use as a diagnostic and therapeutic agent, and disorders of GRH secretion.*

Gold PW, Kling MA, Whitfield HJ, et al.: The clinical implications of corticotropin-releasing hormone. Adv Exp Med Biol 245:507, 1988. *An excellent review of the recent advances in knowledge of the hypothalamic-pituitary axis resulting from the use of CRH in humans.*

Grave GD, Cassorla FG (eds.): Disorders of Human Growth: Advances in Research and Treatment. Springfield, IL, Charles C Thomas, 1988, pp 1–386. *A review of the therapeutic potentials for treatment of growth hormone deficiency along with an up-to-date review of studies on the physiologic regulation of growth hormone secretion.*

Gross KM, Matsumoto AM, Bremner WJ: Differential control of luteinizing hormone and follicle-stimulating hormone secretion by luteinizing hormone-releasing hormone pulse frequency in man. J Clin Endocrinol Metab 64:675, 1987. Sauder SE, Frager MS, Case GD, et al.: Effects of changing gonadotrophin-releasing hormone pulse frequency on gonadotrophin secretion in men. Clin Endocrinol (Oxf) 28:647, 1988. *Two excellent physiologic studies demonstrating the importance of pulsatile GnRH secretion on pituitary gonadotropin secretion in humans.*

Kovacs K, Horvath E, Ezrin C: Anatomy and histology of the normal and abnormal pituitary gland. *In* Degroot LJ, Besser LJ, Cahill GF Jr, et al. (eds.): Endocrinology, 2nd ed. Philadelphia, W. B. Saunders Company, 1989, pp 264–283. *A well-organized and referenced presentation of pituitary structure with emphasis on changes in human disease.*

Sheldon W Jr, DeBold CR, Evans WS, et al.: Rapid sequential intravenous administration of four hypothalamic releasing hormones as a combined anterior pituitary function test in normal subjects. J Clin Endocrinol Metab 60:623, 1985. *Description of a rapid, simple, and safe method of testing pituitary hormone secretory reserve.*

Spratt DI, O'Dea LSL, Schoenfeld D, et al.: Neuroendocrine-gonadal axis in men: Frequent sampling of LH, FSH, and testosterone. Am J Physiol 254:E658, 1988. *A carefully conducted study of the pulsatile nature of gonadotropin and testosterone secretion in men.*

HYPOPITUITARISM

DISEASE STATES ASSOCIATED WITH HYPOPITUITARISM (Table 213–2). The subject's age, rapidity of onset of the disorder, and the extent of impaired hormone secretion as well as the specific pathologic process all influence the clinical manifestations. When acute and complete, the disease can be life threatening, but in a mild form it can remain undetected for many years. Hypopituitarism can occur as a result of a *primary*

A. Primary
  Pituitary tumors
    Primary intrasellar (chromophobe adenoma, craniopharyngioma)
    Parasellar (meningioma, optic nerve glioma)
  Ischemic necrosis of the pituitary
    Postpartum (Sheehan's syndrome)
    Diabetes mellitus
    Other systemic diseases (temporal arteritis, sickle cell disease
      and trait, arteriosclerosis, eclampsia)
  Aneurysm of intracranial internal carotid artery
  Pituitary apoplexy (almost always related to a primary pituitary
    tumor)
  Cavernous sinus thrombosis
  Infectious disease (tuberculosis, syphilis, malaria, meningitis,
    fungal disease)
  Infiltrative disease (hemochromatosis)
  Immunologic (granulomatous or lymphocytic hypophysitis)
  Iatrogenic
    Irradiation to nasopharynx
    Irradiation to sella
    Surgical destruction
  Primary empty sella syndrome
  Metabolic disorders (chronic renal failure)
  Idiopathic (frequently monohormonal and occasionally familial)

B. Secondary
  Destruction of pituitary stalk
    Trauma
    Compression by tumor or aneurysm
    Iatrogenic (surgical)
  Hypothalamic or other central nervous system disease
    Inflammatory (sarcoidosis)
    Infiltrative (lipid storage diseases)
    Trauma
    Toxic (vincristine)
    Hormone induced (glucocorticoids, gonadal steroids)
    Tumors (primary, metastatic, lymphomas, leukemia)
    Idiopathic (frequently congenital or familial, often restricted to
      one or two hormones, and may be reversible)
    Nutritional (starvation, obesity)
    Anorexia nervosa
    Psychosocial dwarfism

Adapted from Frohman LA: Diseases of the anterior pituitary. *In* Felig P, Baxter JD, Broadus AE, et al. (eds.): Endocrinology and Metabolism, 2nd ed. Copyright © 1987 by McGraw-Hill, Inc. Used by permission of McGraw-Hill Book Company.

pituitary disorder or *secondary* to CNS disease. In the latter, pituitary hormone deficiency occurs because of a lack of appropriate releasing hormones.

The classic example of *primary hypopituitarism* is ischemic postpartum pituitary necrosis, first associated with the clinical features of hypopituitarism by Simmonds and characterized by Sheehan. The mechanism of acute ischemic necrosis is believed to relate to vasospasm of hypophyseal vessels, possibly influenced by estrogen-induced sensitivity to the vasoconstrictive stimulus of hypoxia. This disorder occurs most frequently in the immediate postpartum period associated with severe hemorrhage and hypotension. Some degree of hypopituitarism occurs in up to one third of women experiencing severe hemorrhage during delivery. The disorder is recognized by absence of lactation in the postpartum period and failure of normal cyclic menstruation to resume. Because of the slowly progressive nature of this disease the presence of postpartum lactation does not preclude development of the disorder at a later time. Since complete hypopituitarism requires at least 90 per cent destruction of the pituitary, the diagnosis may never be made in many patients with pituitary necrosis and minimal evidence of hypopituitarism. The disease is currently much less common than previously, because of the marked improvement in obstetric care during the past half century. Ischemic pituitary necrosis can be seen with other disorders, although much less commonly.

The most common cause of hypopituitarism is a pituitary tumor (discussed in the following section). Other parasellar mass lesions, including CNS tumors and internal carotid aneurysms, can also invade the sella and destroy the pituitary. Intrapituitary hemorrhage (*pituitary apoplexy*) associated with pituitary tumors may produce varying degrees of hypopituitarism. If bleeding occurs gradually, the pituitary is compressed and symptoms of hypopituitarism predominate. If the hemorrhage is sudden, presenting symptoms include headache, visual field defects or blindness, ophthalmoplegia, and subarachnoid irritation. Hemorrhage within a pre-existing pituitary tumor may cause its sudden expansion. Immediate glucocorticoid therapy is essential in such patients. Most recover without the need for surgical intervention, but it may be necessary in some to restore visual function.

Radiation therapy for treatment of malignant tumors of the head and neck frequently causes primary or secondary hypopituitarism. Growth disturbances are the most common manifestations in children, whereas hypogonadism is more common in adults. Hypopituitarism may occur at any time from 6 months to more than 5 years after a dose of 3000 rads or greater, and children appear to be more susceptible than adults. Lymphocytic hypopituitarism, a recently recognized disorder, tends to occur in the postpartum period and may present as an expanding pituitary mass lesion associated with hypopituitarism (and occasionally hyperprolactinemia). Destruction of pituitary tissue with lymphocyte infiltration has been found histologically, but the cause is unknown. Hypopituitarism may occur without detectable underlying disease and may be limited to one or two hormones. Both autosomal and X-linked recessive forms have been reported. Partial hypopituitarism also occurs in patients with chronic renal failure and is reversible after renal transplantation.

Secondary hypopituitarism can be caused by diverse CNS disorders, all of which disrupt the delivery of releasing factors to the pituitary. The distinction between CNS and pituitary causes can frequently, but not always, be made on the basis of responses to the hypothalamic releasing hormones. Diseases of the pituitary stalk are most frequently due to trauma. Basilar skull fractures often shear the stalk, rupturing both neural and vascular connections. Parasellar tumors and aneurysms can compress the stalk sufficiently to impair blood flow to portal vessels. Disorders of the CNS, primarily the hypothalamus, that impair releasing hormone secretion are described in Ch. 212.

CLINICAL FEATURES. In the most dramatic form of hypopituitarism, panhypopituitarism occurring after surgical hypophysectomy, severe pituitary apoplexy, or withdrawal of hormone replacement therapy, clinical features are noted within a few hours (diabetes insipidus) to a few days (adrenal insufficiency). In partial hypopituitarism the signs and symptoms develop slowly and may be vague and nonspecific.

Hormone-specific Features. ACTH. Manifestations of ACTH deficiency are similar to those of adrenocortical deficiency. Weakness, postural hypotension, malaise, dehydration, and cold intolerance are common, although a true addisonian crisis is infrequent because some aldosterone secretion is maintained through the renin-angiotensin mechanism, which is independent of ACTH. Nausea, vomiting, and severe hypothermia can occur, and hypoglycemia associated with prolonged fasting or alcohol ingestion may be seen as a result of impaired gluconeogenesis. In contrast to Addison's disease, in which hyperpigmentation occurs, patients with ACTH deficiency frequently exhibit depigmentation and decreased tanning after exposure to sunlight. If ACTH secretion is partially impaired, symptoms may be experienced only during periods of stress. Adrenal androgen deficiency contributes to decreased libido and to loss of axillary and pubic hair in women although in men it is of little consequence if testicular function is preserved.

TSH. The features of primary and secondary TSH deficiency are quite similar with the exception of severity. Patients experience cold intolerance, dry skin, pallor, mental slowing, bradycardia, hoarseness, and constipation. True myxedema and hypercholesterolemia are seen only infrequently. Menstrual flow may be increased or more likely decreased because of associated gonadotropin deficiency. During childhood, TSH deficiency results in growth retardation that is unresponsive to GH treatment.

LH and FSH. In women, gonadotropin deficiency results in amenorrhea and signs of estrogen deficiency, including breast atrophy, skin dryness, decreased vaginal secretions, and, occasionally, decreased libido. In males, the testes decrease in size and become softened. Decreased androgen production results in a loss of libido and potency, decreased rate of growth of secondary sexual hair, and reduced muscular strength. If the deficiency occurs prior to puberty there is total or partial impairment of secondary sexual development. If GH secretion is unaltered, failure of sex steroid–induced epiphyseal closure of the long bones produces excessive growth of limbs, leading to a eunuchoid appearance.

Growth Hormone. GH deficiency in the adult is unassociated with clinically recognized symptoms. Carbohydrate tolerance is impaired in GH-deficient subjects, but this disorder is distinct from diabetes mellitus and is not associated with microangiopathy. In children, GH deficiency results in growth retardation. Fasting hypoglycemia is often seen, particularly when ACTH deficiency is also present.

Prolactin. Prolactin deficiency results only in the absence of postpartum lactation.

Vasopressin. Deficiency of vasopressin results in diabetes insipidus, described in detail in Ch. 214. The impairment of water reabsorption by the kidneys results in polyuria and polydipsia, and, if fluid intake is not maintained, severe dehydration. Extreme thirst may be present that is preferentially relieved by ice water. Polyuria may not occur when ACTH deficiency coexists because of the requirement of cortisol for free water excretion. The appearance of polyuria during ACTH or glucocorticoid administration is highly suggestive of combined vasopressin and ACTH deficiency.

Oxytocin. Oxytocin deficiency is unassociated with any clinically apparent disease in humans. In particular, in women with panhypopituitarism who become pregnant, initiation of labor is normal, as is parturition.

General Clinical Features. The skin of hypopituitary patients often exhibits decreased turgor and a waxy character. Perioral and periorbital wrinkling is common, giving the appearance of premature aging. Nutrition, in general, is quite well preserved. Moderate anemia is common; it is usually normochromic and normocytic, but it may be hypochromic or macrocytic and is attributed to a combination of thyroid, testosterone, and erythropoietin deficiencies. Mental slowing and apathy are common, as are other psychiatric symptoms, including delusions and occasionally paranoid psychosis. Carbohydrate metabolism is generally intact in nondiabetics, but in insulin-requiring diabetics, hypopituitarism necessitates reduction of insulin dosage, frequently to less than half of the original level; there is also an increased tendency for hypoglycemic reactions. These changes may persist even with full glucocorticoid replacement therapy.

The sequence of pituitary hormone loss varies among patients with hypopituitarism. In general, deficiencies of GH and gonadotropins are the earliest to occur and thus the most frequently observed. ACTH and TSH deficiencies are less common and are seen at a later stage in the natural history of the disease. The pattern, however, is not predictable in individual patients, thus precluding the usefulness of evaluating pituitary function by measurement of only one or two hormones.

DIFFERENTIAL DIAGNOSIS. The major categories of disease with which hypopituitarism can be confused include (1) disorders of multiple target glands or of the CNS and (2) diseases that share the generalized features of hypopituitarism that are unassociated with endocrine dysfunction.

While measurement of pituitary hormones is indispensable in the differential diagnosis, certain clinical features have discriminatory value. Primary adrenal insufficiency is associated with hyperkalemia, hyperpigmentation, and salt craving, all of which are absent in hypopituitarism. Some patients with primary gonadal failure exhibit a discrepancy between the loss of gonadal steroid production and the loss of spermatogenesis or ovulation. Both components of gonadal function are diminished to the same extent in hypopituitarism. Primary ovarian failure results in characteristic symptoms (hot flashes) that are usually not seen when ovarian failure is secondary to gonadotropin deficiency.

Patients with chronic malnutrition or liver disease exhibit weakness, lethargy, cold intolerance, and decreased libido, frequently raising the possibility of hypopituitarism. The presence of cachexia is important in suggesting a nonpituitary disease. Although anorexia nervosa may often be confused with hypopituitarism, the severe weight loss, psychiatric symptoms, and preservation of axillary and pubic hair are all useful discriminating factors (see Ch. 202).

DIAGNOSIS. The diagnosis of hypopituitarism should be carefully and appropriately established because therapeutic decisions imply lifelong hormonal replacement therapy. In addition, neuroanatomic studies directed at determining the etiology of the hypopituitarism are an integral part of the workup and are discussed in the section on pituitary tumors.

Functional studies of each of the anterior pituitary hormones have been described in the previous section, where the specific testing details are provided. Certain general concepts used in testing are described here.

In evaluation of ACTH secretion, it is important to consider the practical implications. Testing is performed to identify patients with suspected partial adrenal insufficiency in whom an inadequate response to stress may occur. The best stimulus for this purpose is insulin hypoglycemia, in which the response to cortisol correlates well with that to surgical stress. The same test can also be used to evaluate GH responsiveness. Insulin hypoglycemia can be dangerous and should not be used in patients suspected of primary adrenal insufficiency. Recent administration of glucocorticoid therapy can complicate the workup of a patient with suspected hypopituitarism. The suppressive effects of glucocorticoids on the hypothalamic-pituitary-adrenal axis can result in a subnormal response or absence of response to any of the stimuli used. Glucocorticoids should be discontinued for at least 1 month, if possible, prior to definitive testing.

A similar problem occurs in evaluating TSH function in patients who have been receiving long-term thyroid hormone therapy, which can impair the TSH response to TRH for at least 1 month.

In patients with gonadotropin deficiency, a single GnRH challenge is frequently of little help in distinguishing between hypothalamic and pituitary causes and is useful primarily when neuroanatomic evidence of pituitary disease is present and the status of the gonadotrophs is being questioned.

Documentation of GH deficiency is important primarily in children of short stature when therapy with exogenous GH is being considered. The high frequency (> 75 per cent) of GH responses to GRH in children with no anatomic evidence of hypothalamic-pituitary disease argues for a hypothalamic etiology in most GH-deficient children. Decisions concerning GH therapy require careful assessment because of the effort and expense involved. Failure of response to at least two stimuli, usually insulin hypoglycemia and arginine, is generally required before institution of GH therapy. However, the use of exogenous GH in treating partial GH deficiency states is considered by some to be of value. In addition, hypothyroidism, if present, must be corrected prior to GH testing. In adults, GH deficiency serves as a marker for acquired hypopituitarism, particularly for pituitary tumors. In children and adults with obesity, GH responses to all stimuli tested are impaired, even in the presence of seemingly normal growth.

THERAPY. Hormonal replacement therapy must be determined individually and treatment goals specifically defined. The therapeutic use of pituitary hormones is restricted to GH for correcting growth retardation and gonadotropins for inducing fertility. GnRH may be used for introduction of puberty and treatment of infertility and GRH can be substituted for GH when the cause of hormone deficiency is hypothalamic rather than pituitary. For the most part, target organ hormones are used because of their cost advantage, ease of administration, and prolonged action.

ACTH. ACTH deficiency is treated with glucocorticoids. Cortisone (25 mg orally), hydrocortisone (20 mg orally), or prednisone (5 mg orally) given in two divided doses provides adequate therapy for most patients under normal conditions. Supplemental mineralocorticoid therapy is unnecessary because of the partial preservation of aldosterone secretion. The use of prednisone is preferred because of its lower cost. Occasional patients may require full glucocorticoid replacement therapy (a dose 50 per cent greater than those listed), but in most patients this dose is excessive. The clinical assessment of the adequacy of therapy relates to the patient's sense of well-being and the absence of excessive weight gain. During stress, the dose should be increased two- to threefold and then gradually tapered. If oral medication cannot be retained, injectable steroids (hydrocortisone hemisuccinate [Solu-Cortef] for initial emergency use, 100 mg intramuscularly or intravenously), or cortisone acetate for long-term use (50 to 100 mg intramuscularly every 12 hours) is indicated. Treatment of the acutely ill hypopituitary patient requires the same dosage of hydrocortisone (100 to 300 mg per day) as used in primary adrenal insufficiency. Preoperatively, patients should receive hydrocortisone hemisuccinate 50 mg intramuscularly every 6 hours beginning the night prior to surgery and continuing through the immediate postoperative period, followed by gradual tapering to maintenance dosage. Treatment of patients with partial ACTH deficiency without symptoms in the nonstressed state is more controversial. With adequate education, many patients do not need maintenance replacement therapy except in times of stress. Such patients in particular should wear appropriate medical identification bracelets.

TSH. TSH deficiency is treated with L-thyroxine 0.125 mg per day, although a lower dose may suffice in occasional patients. Clinical assessment of the patient and serum thyroxine levels during initiation of therapy are used to establish the appropriate dose. Adrenal insufficiency must be corrected first, although patients with partial adrenal insufficiency may require glucocorticoid replacement only after thyroid hormone replacement is started. The use of triiodothyronine, particularly as long-term therapy, is not recommended, because its shorter biologic half-life results in more rapid appearance of thyroid deficiency in the event therapy is omitted.

LH and FSH. Treatment of gonadotropin deficiency requires consideration of both gonadal steroid replacement and treatment of infertility. The subjects are considered in greater detail in Ch. 222 and 224.

Women. Estrogen replacement therapy is indicated in premenopausal women to maintain secondary sex characteristics and to reduce the risk of osteoporosis and possibly coronary artery disease. This can be accomplished with ethinyl estradiol 5 to 20 μg per day or conjugated estrogens (Premarin) 0.6 to 1.25 mg per day. The lowest possible dose that produces the desired clinical effects should be used. To induce cyclic bleeding, estrogen should be given for 25 days each month, accompanied on the last 5 days by a progestinic agent such as medroxyprogesterone 5 to 10 mg per day. Alternatively, an oral contraceptive preparation containing no more than the equivalent of 25 μg estradiol per day can be used. The advantage of replacement therapy after the menopause is still controversial, and the potential risks and benefits should be discussed with the patient to help make an appropriate decision. Estrogen therapy usually corrects the dyspareunia attributable to local estrogen deficiency in women with hypopituitarism, but decreased libido due to the absence of adrenal androgens often persists. This can be corrected by injection of a small dose of long-acting androgen such as testosterone enanthate 50 mg every 1 to 2 months or by oral administration of fluoxymesterone 5 to 10 mg once or twice weekly.

Restoration of fertility is possible in a large percentage of women with clomiphene or GnRH therapy (the latter given in a pulsatile manner by an intermittent infusion pump) if the cause of the disorder is hypothalamic or with combined FSH-LH preparations if pituitary disease is present. An FSH-rich preparation from postmenopausal urine is used to initiate follicular growth and maturation; it is monitored by measurement of plasma estradiol levels. Human chorionic gonadotropin is then injected to induce ovulation. This therapy is expensive, entails the risk of superovulation and multiple pregnancy, and should be undertaken only under the direction of an experienced physician.

Men. Testosterone replacement therapy in adult males is accomplished by intramuscular injection of a long-acting testosterone preparation (testosterone enanthate or cypionate, 200 mg every 3 weeks). The endpoints are restoration of full androgenization, including beard growth, and improvement in muscular strength, libido, and potency. Androgen therapy should be withheld as long as possible in the adolescent with growth retardation to avoid premature epiphyseal closure, which limits the potential for future linear growth. Testosterone therapy may be required for many months before full restoration of libido and performance. If gonadotropin deficiency has developed before puberty, full androgenization may never occur. In patients with longstanding hypogonadism, psychosocial behavioral changes affecting the patient's entire lifestyle may be disrupted by initiation of testosterone therapy, leading to major adjustment problems with both sexual and nonsexual relationships.

Infertility in men with hypopituitarism can be corrected with a combination of FSH and human chorionic gonadotropin (hCG), although therapy is required for several months, and the success rate is less than 50 per cent. GnRH, given intermittently as in women, is an alternate method of therapy in individuals with hypothalamic hypogonadism.

Growth Hormone. GH therapy is indicated for the correction of impaired linear growth, and its use is thus confined almost exclusively to childhood and adolescent years. Early establishment of the diagnosis is critical, since the probability of successful long-term therapy is inversely related to the extent of growth retardation. Treatment requires the use of human GH, which was originally extracted and purified from human pituitaries obtained at autopsy. The association of pituitary GH therapy with Creutzfeldt-Jakob disease led to a discontinuation in its use in 1985 and substitution of GH produced by recombinant DNA technology. GH is administered intramuscularly or subcutaneously at a dose of 0.1 mg per kilogram three times weekly; its use is continued until the final height is achieved, coincident with long-bone epiphyseal closure. A goal of 5 feet 4 inches is generally pursued but not always achieved. Careful attention must be given to concomitant thyroid hormone deficiency. Glucocorticoids should be used sparingly because of their interference with growth-promoting effects of GH. Small doses of oral androgens may be used simultaneously to increase growth velocity, although this has not gained widespread acceptance. Estrogens are to be avoided because of their greater effect on epiphyseal closure. Gonadal steroid therapy is usually initiated during the years of puberty to avoid psychosocial problems. However, if significant catch-up growth is required, its use should be delayed. GH therapy increases height age more rapidly than bone age, may initially be associated with a decrease in body fat, and also corrects the fasting hypoglycemia of GH-deficient children. GRH, or one of its analogues, may be useful in treatment of at least 50 per cent of children with isolated GH deficiency and in the future may be administered by noninjectable routes. Recent studies have suggested that metabolic disturbances and muscle work performance impairment of adults with GH deficiency can be improved with GH therapy. However, the use of GH in adults must still be considered experimental.

Guay AT, Agnello V, Tronic BC, et al.: Lymphocytic hypophysitis in a man. J Clin Endocrinol Metab 64:631, 1987. Scanarini M, D'Avella D, Rotilio A, et al.: Giant-cell granulomatous hypophysitis: A distinct clinicopathological entity. J Neurosurg 71:681, 1989. *Two unusual forms of hypopituitarism that can mimic a pituitary tumor.*

Komatsu M, Kondo T, Yamauchi K, et al.: Antipituitary antibodies in patients with the primary empty sella syndrome. J Clin Endocrinol Metab 67:633, 1988. Bjerre P, Lindholm J, Videbaek H: The spontaneous course of pituitary adenomas and occurrence of an empty sella in untreated acromegaly. J Clin Endocrinol Metab 63:287, 1986. *The spectrum of the empty sella syndrome is reflected in these two reports of primary and secondary forms of the disease.*

Lam KSL, Tse VKC, Wang C, et al.: Early effects of cranial irradiation on hypothalamic-pituitary function. J Clin Endocrinol Metab 64:418, 1987. Littley MD, Shalet SM, Beardwell CG, et al.: Hypopituitarism following external radiotherapy for pituitary tumours in adults. Q J Med 70:145, 1989. *Hypopituitarism following cranial irradiation for both pituitary and nonpituitary disease is being recognized more frequently in adults as well as children.*

Libber SM, Plotnick LP, Johanson AJ, et al.: Long-term follow-up of hypopituitary patients treated with human growth hormone. Medicine (Baltimore) 69:46, 1990. Binnerts A, Wilson JHP, Lamberts SWJ: The effects of human growth hormone administration in elderly adults with recent weight loss. J Clin Endocrinol Metab 67:1312, 1988. *An excellent review of the long-term effects of GH treatment of hypopituitary children, in which the results are encouraging, if not completely satisfying, contrasted with a report of acute effects in adults, the long-term significance of which is unknown.*

Phillips JA III, Vnencak-Jones CL: Genetics of growth hormone and its disorders. Adv Hum Genet 18:305, 1989. *A current review of genetic aspects of GH deficiency from clinical and molecular levels.*

Sheehan HL, Summers VK: The syndrome of hypopituitarism. Q J Med 42:319, 1949. *The classic monograph describing the clinical-pathologic correlations of hypopituitarism. Its lucid and detailed presentation makes it worthwhile reading even after more than four decades.*

Whitcomb RW, Crowley WF Jr: Diagnosis and treatment of isolated gonadotropin-releasing hormone deficiency in men. J Clin Endocrinol Metab 70:3, 1990. Blunt SM, Butt WR: Pulsatile GnRH therapy for the induction of ovulation in hypogonadotropic hypogonadism. Acta Endocrinol (Copenh) 119:58, 1988. *Pulsatile GnRH therapy is useful in the treatment of both men and women with gonadotropin deficiency, as reviewed in these articles.*

PITUITARY TUMORS

CLASSIFICATION. Pituitary tumors are subdivided by their histologic characteristics and also by their functional activity.

Specific considerations of hormone-secreting pituitary tumors are found in the next section. The two major histologic types of primary pituitary tumors are the adenoma and the craniopharyngioma. In addition, parasellar tumors such as optic nerve glioma, meningioma, chordoma, sphenoid wing sarcoma, as well as metastatic tumors, can also be present within the sella turcica.

Pituitary Adenomas. This cell type constitutes greater than 90 per cent of all pituitary tumors. The classic subdivision into chromophobic and chromophilic tumors has given way to more specific identification on the basis of immunohistochemical stains for individual hormones. Using these techniques, only 10 to 20 per cent of pituitary adenomas appear to be nonfunctioning. Pituitary tumors account for 6 to 18 per cent of all brain tumors, and small adenomas, many of which are functioning, have been detected in up to 30 per cent of unselected autopsy series. The growth pattern of pituitary adenomas appears unrelated to hormone secretion. Rapidly enlarging tumors are often recognized because of their mass effects, whereas slowly growing tumors tend to allow for greater expression of the hormone hypersecretory effects. The peak incidence of nonfunctioning pituitary adenomas is between 40 and 50 years, and the frequency is uninfluenced by sex. Many "nonfunctioning" tumors actually produce portions of hormones (e.g., the glycoprotein α subunit common to TSH, LH, and FSH) or may synthesize but be incapable of releasing the hormone. Although pituitary adenomas are almost always histologically benign, they may exhibit aggressive growth behavior with invasion of surrounding structures, making their total removal impossible. Adenomas are generally solid with a well-defined capsule, although they may on occasion be cystic and hemorrhagic. Calcification, if present, results from organization of a previous hemorrhage.

Craniopharyngiomas. These tumors are of congenital origin, may be partly or entirely cystic, and are always benign. The cyst fluid may be cholesterol rich. Calcification, generally concentric, is present in 50 per cent. The tumors grow at variable rates and may remain dormant for many years. Although half of the tumors are seen during childhood, they may appear at any time during life. The site of origin of most tumors is in the midline at the upper portion of the pituitary stalk, and approximately 15 per cent involve the upper portion of the anterior lobe and are therefore intrasellar. Variations of craniopharyngiomas include ependymomas and epidermoid cysts.

CLINICAL FEATURES. The manifestations of pituitary tumors are neuroanatomic, endocrinologic, and radiologic. Presenting symptoms of pituitary tumors have changed in frequency over the years with refinements in diagnostic procedures. Whereas nearly 90 per cent of patients diagnosed 30 years ago exhibited visual disturbances, only 25 per cent do so at present. In contrast, the most common presentation today relates to impaired gonadal function, frequently associated with prolactin-secreting pituitary tumors. A small percentage of patients (less than 5 per cent) are discovered accidentally on review of head-imaging procedures obtained for other purposes.

Neuroanatomic manifestations occur secondary to tumor growth causing pressure on the overlying dura and the diaphragma sellae. This results in headaches that are variable in nature, imprecisely located, generally of dull quality, unassociated with nausea or visual symptoms, unrelated to position, and inconsistently relieved by analgesics. Disappearance of headache is frequently a sign of rupture of the dura. With continued suprasellar expansion the tumor exerts pressure on the optic chiasm, leading to the classic findings of bitemporal hemianopsia. At early stages the field defects may be asymmetric and involve only the superior temporal fields. Eventually, blindness and optic atrophy occur. Anterior growth of the tumor may cause symptoms limited only to one eye. Papilledema occurs in one fourth of craniopharyngiomas but rarely in pituitary adenomas. Further growth results in hypothalamic compression leading to temperature instability, hyperphagia, altered sleep patterns, and emotional disturbances. Pressure on the third ventricle results in internal hydrocephalus. Rarely, temporal or frontal lobe compression may cause behavioral changes and seizures, and midbrain compression may produce long-tract signs. Lateral extension is more common and leads to compression of the third, fourth, and sixth cranial nerves in the cavernous sinus, resulting in ophthalmoplegia and diplopia. Expansion inferiorly into the sphenoid sinus may result in cerebrospinal fluid rhinorrhea. Hemorrhage into the tumor, *pituitary apoplexy,* may result in rapid expansion of the tumor and lead to the sudden appearance of headache of varying intensity that subsides after a few days. If the tumor is intrasellar, hypopituitarism often results; if extrasellar, there may be rapid deterioration of vision. "Spontaneous" cures of hormone-secreting pituitary tumors may also occur as the result of hemorrhagic tumor necrosis.

Neuroradiologic presentations consist of a deformed or enlarged sella seen on standard skull roentgenography or a mass lesion seen on computed tomography (CT) or magnetic resonance imaging (MRI).

Endocrine symptoms include diminished function secondary to destruction of normal pituitary tissue by tumor or interference with portal blood supply and hyperfunction due to tumor or hyperplasia. The two may be combined. In addition, diminished function may occur secondary to the effects of hormone hypersecretion (i.e., hypogonadism secondary to hyperprolactinemia). The frequency of presentation and the manifestations are described in the previous section.

DIAGNOSTIC PROCEDURES. Diagnosis of a pituitary tumor necessitates differentiation from other parasellar disorders, determination of the tumor size and extent of extrasellar extension, and assessment of hormone deficiencies and/or hypersecretion. Endocrine evaluation should be performed prior to definitive therapy, if possible, because the extent of hypopituitarism and presence of hormone hypersecretion may influence the type and extent of therapy. Patients with pituitary tumors undergoing stressful procedures must be considered to have panhypopituitarism unless proven otherwise and pretreated with glucocorticoids.

Neuroradiologic procedures have improved remarkably during the past decade, and MRI today constitutes the definitive study. This technique provides exquisite anatomic resolution and, using a combination of coronal and sagittal images, defines the tumor in relation to the sellar contents as well as the extrasellar structures (Fig. 213–1). Precise information concerning displacement of the pituitary stalk (if present) and relationship of the tumor to the optic chiasm and cavernous sinus usually provides sufficient data for deciding on a surgical approach, if indicated, or the need for other procedures. As an alternative, CT performed with contrast media also provides high-quality imaging of the pituitary (Fig. 213–2). Despite its lower cost, CT provides resolution inferior to that of MRI and subjects the patient to radiation exposure. If repeat imaging studies are necessary, the radiation dose may become considerable.

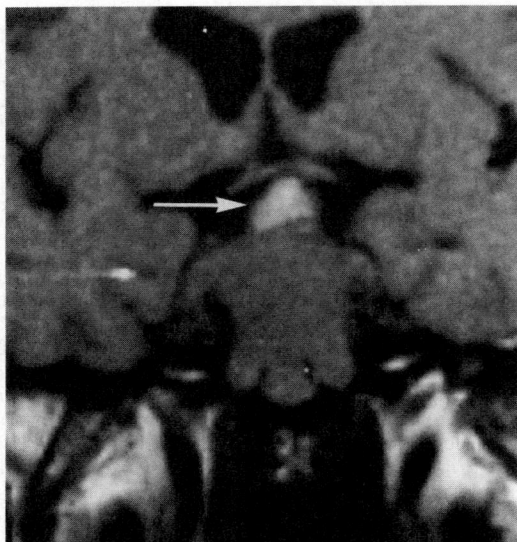

FIGURE 213–1. Magnetic resonance image (MRI) of a pituitary adenoma (coronal view). The large tumor mass extends inferiorly and superiorly. The intense (white) signal (*arrow*) in the dorsal portion of the tumor represents recent hemorrhage. The superiorly displaced optic chiasm is seen just above the tumor.

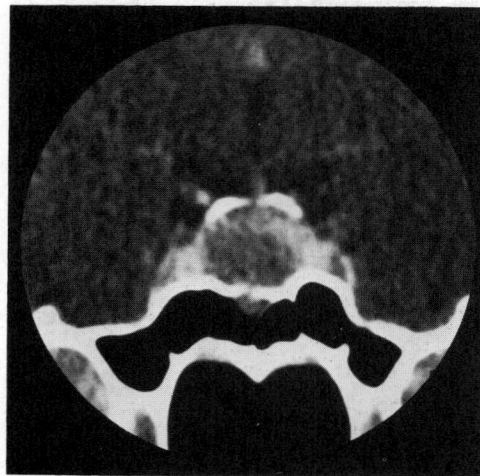

FIGURE 213–2. Computed tomographic (CT) scan of pituitary (coronal view) demonstrating a pituitary tumor with suprasellar extension and erosion of the sellar floor with inferior extension of the tumor into the sphenoid sinus.

The most important neuro-ophthalmologic study is evaluation of visual fields. Test objects of varying sizes and colors can provide an excellent assessment of both central and peripheral fields. The technique is reproducible and sensitive and useful in observing patients for serial changes. Bitemporal field defects are, however, not specific for pituitary tumors; they may occur with parasellar tumors, vascular abnormalities, arachnoiditis, or rarely with chiasmal prolapse into the sella associated with the empty sella syndrome. Atypical field defects may also occur, even those suggesting superior rather than inferior pressure.

DIFFERENTIAL DIAGNOSIS. Disorders that must be differentiated from pituitary tumors include the empty sella syndrome, parasellar diseases, and pituitary enlargement associated with other endocrine disorders.

The *empty sella* is partly or nearly completely filled with CSF and results from extension of the subarachnoid space into the intrasellar region. The pituitary gland is flattened along the posterior portion of the floor and the dorsum. Primary empty sella syndrome is unassociated with prior surgical or irradiation therapy and has been found in up to one quarter of autopsy series, usually unassociated with endocrine disease. The etiology is unknown, but the syndrome has been postulated to be due to incomplete formation of the diaphragma sella, permitting CSF pressure to be transmitted to the sella and gradually leading to herniation of the arachnoid and remodeling of the sella. Nearly all patients are asymptomatic, although some may have nonspecific headaches. The syndrome is seen commonly in obese women and in association with systemic hypertension, benign intracranial hypertension (pseudotumor cerebri), and CSF rhinorrhea. The sella is usually symmetrically enlarged or ballooned and may be deformed. Endocrine function is generally normal, although diminished TSH and gonadotropin secretion, hyperprolactinemia, and rarely panhypopituitarism or diabetes insipidus may be present. The diagnosis is established by CT or MRI. The empty sella may coexist with a pituitary tumor, which is usually hyperfunctional. The secondary empty sella syndrome is seen in patients following pituitary surgery or irradiation or intratumoral bleeding.

The signs and symptoms of parasellar disorders may mimic those of pituitary tumors. Parasellar disorders include inflammatory and granulomatous diseases (sarcoidosis, eosinophilic granuloma), degenerative disorders (aneurysms), and neoplasms (meningiomas, hamartomas, chordomas, and metastatic tumors). Suprasellar tumors usually present with the neurologic manifestations of increased intracranial pressure, hypothalamic symptoms, visual impairment, and internal hydrocephalus. Endocrine manifestations tend to follow rather than precede neurologic symptoms. CT and MRI are extremely valuable in differentiating these disorders from primary pituitary tumors.

Longstanding primary hypothyroidism or hypogonadism can result in sellar enlargement, increased TSH or gonadotropin secretion, hyperplasia of tropic hormone–producing cells, and in some patients, hormone-secreting tumors. Institution of appropriate replacement hormone therapy can reverse the hypersecretory and hyperplastic (although not neoplastic) changes.

THERAPY. Treatment of nonfunctioning pituitary tumors is indicated to prevent or limit the loss of pituitary function and the consequences of extrasellar extension. The two therapeutic methods are surgery and radiation therapy.

Pituitary surgery is the conventional therapy for pituitary tumors. The transsphenoidal approach is currently used for all tumors except those with extensive suprasellar extension, particularly when separated from the intrasellar portion by a narrow neck. Tumors encircling optic nerves or encasing cerebral vessels can be removed only by a transfrontal approach. Currently the operative mortality is less than 1 per cent. The transsphenoidal approach includes the use of modern fluoroscopic aids and microsurgical techniques. It provides better visualization of the sellar contents and permits selective adenomectomy to be performed. If preoperative evaluation reveals preservation of anterior pituitary function, a conservative approach is indicated to preserve remaining pituitary hormone secretion, since a small rim of adenohypophyseal tissue is often sufficient to maintain adequate pituitary function. Glucocorticoid coverage is essential for the perioperative period even for patients with intact pituitary-adrenal function and is accomplished with parenteral administration of hydrocortisone, 50 mg intramuscularly every 6 hours. Postoperatively the patient must be carefully observed for the development of diabetes insipidus, particularly since an obtunded patient may not perceive thirst. Transient polyuria and increased plasma osmolality commonly occur in the immediate postoperative period as a result of mild trauma to the pituitary stalk. Persistence of these findings beyond the first 48 hours usually indicates significant destruction of the stalk or posterior pituitary and permanent impairment of function. However, fluctuations in posterior pituitary function may occur for a period of several weeks, and recovery has been observed as late as many months postoperatively. Initially the patient should be treated with aqueous vasopressin (5 U subcutaneously) or desmopressin (DDAVP) (1 or 2 μg subcutaneously) rather than with a long-acting preparation so the natural history of the process can be observed.

Radiation therapy can be used as an alternative to surgical excision of the pituitary tumor or as adjunct therapy. Although less popular as primary therapy, because of its delayed effects, radiation therapy using conventional high-energy sources (supravoltage) or heavy-particle (proton beam) sources is an effective method of treatment. Radiation therapy is to be avoided in patients with significant suprasellar extension or in the presence of marked visual field defects.

The recurrence rate of pituitary tumors following surgical treatment alone ranges from 25 to nearly 100 per cent in different series. Since postoperative radiographic and endocrine studies indicate that intraoperative assessment of the extent of pituitary tumor removal is often inaccurate, postoperative irradiation is indicated in all patients with nonfunctioning pituitary adenomas unless specifically contraindicated. The dose currently employed is 4500 to 5000 rads, which can be given with minimal side effects. Some late loss of pituitary function occurs in 15 to 25 per cent of patients. Thus, if preservation of fertility is desired, radiation therapy should be delayed.

Cardoso ER, Peterson EW: Pituitary apoplexy: A review. Neurosurgery 14:363, 1984. *A thorough discussion of the varied manner in which this disorder presents and a rationale for management.*
Davis PC, Hoffman JC Jr, Spencer T, et al.: MR imaging of pituitary adenoma: CT, clinical, and surgical correlation. AJR 148:797, 1987. Peck WW, Dillon WP, Norman D, et al.: High-resolution MR imaging of pituitary microadenomas at 1.5 T: Experience with Cushing disease. AJR 152:145, 1989. L'Huillier F, Combes C, Martin N, et al.: MRI in the diagnosis of so-called pituitary apoplexy: Seven cases. J Neuroradiol 16:221, 1989. *The availability of MRI has markedly improved the diagnostic accuracy in suspected pituitary tumors and increased the likelihood of appropriate therapy.*
Grigsby PW, Simpson JR, Fineberg B: Late regrowth of pituitary adenomas after irradiation and/or surgery: Hazard function analysis. Cancer 63:1308, 1989.
Harris PE, Afshar F, Coates P, et al.: The effects of transsphenoidal surgery on endocrine function and visual fields in patients with functionless pituitary tumours. Q J Med 71:417, 1989. *Nonfunctioning tumors of the pituitary*

continue to remain a vexing therapeutic problem as reflected by these two reports that examine outcome and long-term sequelae.

Heshmati HM, Turpin G, Kujas M, et al.: The immunocytochemical heterogeneity of silent pituitary adenomas. Acta Endocrinol (Copenh) 118:533, 1988. Kovacs K, Lloyd R, Horvath E, et al.: Silent somatotroph adenomas of the human pituitary: A morphologic study of three cases including immunocytochemistry, electron microscopy, in vitro examination, and in situ hybridization. Am J Pathol 134:345, 1989. *Studies of "nonfunctioning" tumors of the pituitary gland reveal that many exhibit evidence of hormone storage and in vitro secretion. These reports illustrate the variety of such observations.*

Klibanski A, Zervas NT: Diagnosis and management of hormone-secreting pituitary adenomas. N Engl J Med 324:822, 1991. *This is a valuable, succinct general review of pituitary tumors; with 114 up-to-date references.*

PITUITARY HYPERFUNCTION: HORMONE-SECRETING PITUITARY TUMORS

Pituitary hormone hypersecretion generally involves overproduction of only a single hormone except in the case of certain hormone-secreting tumors. Hormone overproduction occurs in response to altered feedback signals (i.e., hyperprolactinemia due to increased estrogen secretion in pregnancy; ACTH, TSH, and gonadotropin hypersecretion in response to diminished target organ feedback in primary hypofunction of the adrenal, thyroid, and gonads; and GH hypersecretion associated with caloric deprivation). Whereas these changes begin as functional alterations, prolonged stimulation can result in hyperplastic as well as hypersecretory changes. Pathologic hyperfunction occurs in association with pituitary hyperplasia or tumor unrelated to regulatory feedback mechanisms. These disorders involve primarily somatotrophic, lactotrophic, and corticotrophic cells, although all cell types may be affected.

Growth Hormone–Secreting Tumors: Acromegaly

GH hypersecretion is most commonly associated with a pituitary somatotroph tumor or rarely somatotroph hyperplasia. These tumors previously were considered eosinophilic (due to GH storage granules) or chromophobic (when little hormone was stored). Tumors with abundant hormone storage tend to be better differentiated and more slowly growing, resulting in more pronounced clinical features of GH hypersecretion, whereas the less differentiated nonhormone–storing tumors tend to grow more rapidly, leading to more pronounced effects of an expanding tumor mass.

CLINICAL FEATURES. The clinical manifestations of GH hypersecretion depend on the age of onset. During childhood and prior to epiphyseal fusion, GH hypersecretion produces proportional skeletal growth leading to gigantism. Hypogonadism is frequently present, leading to delayed epiphyseal closure and thus a more prolonged growth period. The tallest reported patient with gigantism reached a height of nearly 9 feet. It is more common for patients to exhibit features of both gigantism and acromegaly, reflecting persistence of GH hypersecretion into adult life.

Signs and symptoms of GH hypersecretion beginning during adult life develop slowly. Soft tissue swelling and hypertrophy involving the extremities and face are the earliest findings (Fig. 213–3). These changes are usually best documented by comparing photographs taken over a one- to two-decade span. Spadelike changes develop in the fingers, and increased soft tissue volume necessitates ring enlargement and increases in glove and shoe sizes. The skin becomes thickened and leathery, and skin folds increase in prominence. A generalized increase in hair growth and pigmentation often occurs. Fibroma molluscum (pedunculated epithelial tags) and acanthosis nigricans are common. The skin becomes oily, and sebaceous cyst formation is common. Increased sweating occurs in most patients and is a sensitive biologic indicator of disease activity.

Bony changes occur more slowly and include cortical thickening, tufting of terminal phalanges, and osteophyte proliferation. Degenerated articular cartilages and ligamentous hypertrophy produce a hypertrophic arthropathy that eventually leads to deforming and crippling arthritis. Prognathism results from mandibular enlargement and causes a significant overbite of the lower incisors and increased spacing of the teeth. Bony overgrowth of the frontal, malar, and nasal bones occurs; increase in size of the paranasal sinuses together with vocal cord hypertrophy leads to

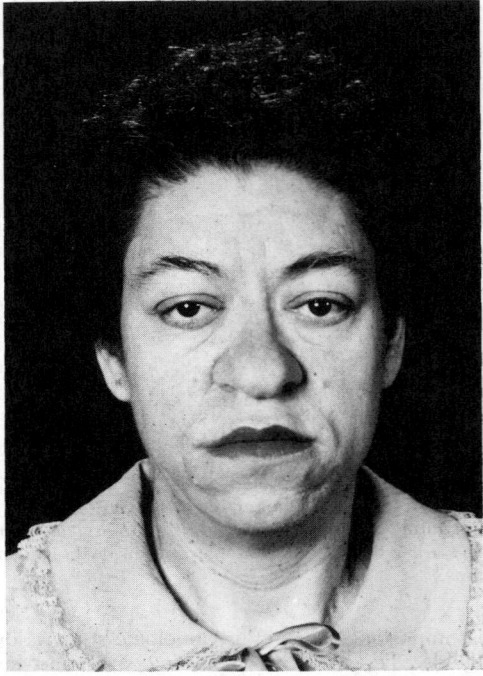

FIGURE 213–3. Clinical features of a 43-year-old patient with acromegaly of 15 years' duration. Coarsened features result from soft tissue overgrowth about the eyes, nose, and mouth. Lacrimal overgrowth, thickening of skin folds, and fibroma molluscum are also present. (From Frohman LA: *In* Felig P, Baxter JD, Broadus AE, et al. (eds.): Endocrinology and Metabolism, 2nd ed., p 301. Copyright © 1987 by McGraw-Hill, Inc. Used by permission of McGraw-Hill Book Company.)

deepening of the voice. Eustachian tube mucosal hypertrophy often produces obstruction and serous otitis media and that of the nasopharynx may lead to sleep apnea.

Peripheral neuropathy commonly occurs because of nerve entrapment by surrounding tissue overgrowth, most commonly affecting the median nerve and producing the carpal tunnel syndrome. Axonal demyelinization of peripheral nerves associated with perineural and subepineural proliferation results in palpable nerve fibers. Paresthesias, sensory losses, and proximal muscle weakness occur frequently.

Prolonged hypersecretion of GH leads to generalized visceromegaly involving salivary glands, liver, spleen, and kidneys. Salivary gland enlargement is detectable clinically whereas that of the other organs is not, and significant hepatosplenomegaly usually implies the presence of a coexisting disease. Both secretory and reabsorptive functions of the kidney are increased in acromegaly.

Thyroid enlargement with nodule formation is common, but true hyperfunction is infrequent. Parathyroid hyperplasia and adenoma may occur, often reflecting the multiple endocrine neoplasia syndrome (Type I), leading to hypercalciuria and nephrolithiasis. Elevations of prolactin levels occur in one third of patients, resulting in galactorrhea, amenorrhea, and decreased libido.

The effects of GH on the cardiovascular system are controversial. Hypertension is common but generally mild and responsive to drug therapy. Cardiomegaly is routinely found, but there is no characteristic form of acromegalic heart disease. Cardiac failure, when it occurs, appears related to hypertension and not to the effects of GH hypersecretion. Yet the incidence of cardiovascular disease is increased in acromegalics, as is mortality. Weight gain is uncommon, but carbohydrate intolerance and diabetes are seen in 25 per cent of acromegalics, primarily in those with a family history of diabetes. Insulin resistance is common and occasionally associated with ketosis. Diabetic microangiopathy, however, is extremely uncommon, even in longstanding disease.

LABORATORY STUDIES. The diagnosis of acromegaly is established by the finding of elevated plasma GH levels that do not respond normally to physiologic suppression and stimulation;

in adults, a GH value greater than 2 ng per milliliter in males or 5 ng per milliliter in females after oral glucose administration is confirmatory. Randomly obtained samples with markedly elevated levels are also diagnostic. However, in normal children and young adults, GH levels as high as 50 ng per milliliter are sporadically exhibited, thereby necessitating dynamic studies of GH secretion in many patients. TRH stimulates GH secretion in 70 to 80 per cent of acromegalics but not in normal subjects, and this procedure is also useful in following patients after therapy. GH secretion in acromegalics differs in other ways from that in normal persons, including absence of a sleep-associated increase in GH and a tendency for wide spontaneous fluctuations in GH levels, indicating intermittent secretory activity. Plasma GH levels increase after GRH in most acromegalics, but the test is not of diagnostic help.

Plasma IGF-I (somatomedin C) levels are also increased in acromegaly and provide good correlation with the clinical manifestations of GH hypersecretion. Determination of IGF-I levels for assessing disease activity after therapy is useful, particularly when GH levels are borderline.

DIFFERENTIAL DIAGNOSIS. The clinical features of acromegaly are not confused with those of other diseases. The question commonly raised is whether features suggestive of the disease are associated with active disease, inactive disease, or no disease. Dynamic studies of GH secretion are required to differentiate these possibilities. Gigantism during childhood occasionally occurs in the absence of GH hypersecretion (cerebral gigantism) through a yet to be determined mechanism. GH levels are elevated in patients with renal failure, cirrhosis, protein-calorie malnutrition, and anorexia nervosa and in the Laron dwarf (growth retardation caused by a genetic defect in the GH receptor), but in these conditions the clinical features of acromegaly are absent.

PATHOGENESIS. Acromegaly occurs nearly always as a primary tumor of somatotrophs within the pituitary, although rarely it may be secondary to excessive somatotroph stimulation by an ectopic GRH-secreting tumor, hypersecretion of GRH from the CNS, or an ectopic GH-secreting tumor. Selective removal of the GH-secreting adenoma is followed in most patients not only by restoration of normal GH values but by normal responses to dynamic testing.

GH-secreting tumors are monoclonal (as judged by X chromosome inactivation analyses). In addition, a genetic point mutation has been found in the guanine nucleotide regulatory protein ($G_s \alpha$) in 40 per cent of GH-secreting pituitary adenomas, the result of which is autonomous GH hypersecretion and cell growth. These studies therefore support the concept of a primary pituitary disease. In some patients, however, GH-secreting tumors have been associated with GRH-secreting carcinoid tumors of the bronchus and foregut, pancreatic islet tumors, and small cell carcinoma of the lung. Removal of the extrapituitary tumor has resulted in a return of GH levels to normal and regression of the pituitary tumor. Pituitary histology in patients with secondary acromegaly ranges from local or generalized somatotroph hyperplasia to actual tumor formation. In addition, neuronal tumors present in the hypothalamus (hamartomas) or in the pituitary, contiguous with the somatotroph adenoma (gangliocytoma or choristoma), may also be the source of GRH production in a few patients with acromegaly. Since excessive stimulation by GRH is capable of inducing adenomas as well as hyperplasia, it is possible that some patients now considered to have primary pituitary disease actually have a hypothalamic disorder characterized by excessive GRH production from nontumorous tissue.

Comparison of the limited numbers of reported patients with secondary acromegaly does not provide any evidence of differences in either clinical manifestations or responses to dynamic studies of GH secretion, with the possible exception of decreased frequency of GH responses to GRH. In patients with ectopic GRH production or even with CNS overproduction, immunoreactive plasma GRH levels are readily detectable, in contrast to patients presumed to have primary pituitary disease in whom levels are near or beneath the limits of detectability.

THERAPY. Therapy for patients with acromegaly involves three potential methods: surgery, irradiation, and medical (pharmacologic). Considerations of the space-occupying mass and of hypopituitarism are similar to those described for nonfunctioning pituitary tumors. Prior to initiation of therapy to the pituitary itself, consideration should be given to the possibility of an extrapituitary tumor, removal of which may reverse the GH hypersecretion.

Surgical treatment of GH-secreting pituitary tumors is currently the treatment of choice. Transsphenoidal or, if necessary, transfrontal adenomectomy is indicated once the presence of the disease has been established, even though the radiologic findings are minimal. The results in published series vary. The described "success" or "cure" rate varies considerably, depending on the criteria used for defining normal GH levels as well as on the initial size of the tumor. Using a criterion of 5 ng per milliliter, success rates of up to 90 per cent have been reported with small tumors. Using a more stringent and widely accepted criterion of 2.5 ng per milliliter, however, the success rate is probably not more than 50 to 60 per cent. Normalization of GH levels is inversely related to the size of the tumor; less favorable results occur with tumors greater than 2 cm in diameter or plasma GH levels greater than 100 ng per milliliter. The clinical features of GH, however, are frequently improved even without complete restoration of GH values to normal. In patients whose GH levels return to the normal range, tumor recurrence is infrequent (approximately 5 per cent), but with incomplete removal the recurrence rate is greater than 50 per cent if no further therapy is administered.

Radiation therapy, using methods similar to those for nonfunctioning tumors, is effective as a primary means of treatment of acromegaly. The reduction in GH hypersecretion is, however, slow, the response is inversely related to the initial GH level, and achievement of normal levels may require 5 or even 10 years, although about half of patients exhibit normal GH levels after 2 to 4 years. Postoperative irradiation is indicated when GH levels remain elevated and, used in conjunction with surgery, offers the best prognosis.

Pharmacologic therapy in acromegaly is of limited value. Bromocriptine, a dopamine receptor agonist, lowers GH levels to normal in only 25 per cent and decreases tumor size in only 5 per cent of patients. Dosages of up to 60 mg per day may be required, and side effects are frequent. Octreotide, a somatostatin analogue, is effective in reducing GH levels to normal in nearly half of acromegalics and in decreasing tumor size in nearly the same percentage. The drug must be injected three to four times daily or given by constant subcutaneous infusion and is associated with a number of side effects (acholic stools, mild carbohydrate intolerance), the most worrisome of which is the development of cholelithiasis in more than 40 per cent of patients. Neither of the drugs is tumoricidal, and each is effective only during continued administration. They should, therefore, be considered only as adjunct therapy or in patients who are not surgical candidates.

Frohman LA: Therapeutic options in acromegaly. J Clin Endocrinol Metab, 1991, in press. *A current review of the relative advantages and limitations of the various forms of therapy of this disorder.*

Frohman LA, Downs TR: Ectopic GRH syndrome. *In* Robbins RJ, Melmed S (eds.): Acromegaly. New York, Plenum Press, 1987, pp 115–125. Sano T, Asa SL, Kovacs K: Growth hormone-releasing hormone-producing tumors: Clinical, biochemical, and morphological manifestations. Endocr Rev 9:357, 1988. *The spectrum of acromegaly secondary to excess secretion of growth hormone–releasing hormone is reviewed from the clinical, laboratory, histologic, and therapeutic aspects in these two reviews.*

Lamberts SWJ: The role of somatostatin in the regulation of anterior pituitary hormone secretion and of its analogs in the treatment of human pituitary tumors. Endocrinol Rev 9:417, 1988. Page MD, Millward ME, Taylor A, et al.: Long-term treatment of acromegaly with a long-acting analogue of somatostatin, octreotide. QJ Med 74:189, 1990. Ho KY, Weissberger AJ, Marbach P, et al.: Therapeutic efficacy of the somatostatin analog SMS 201–995 (octreotide) in acromegaly. Ann Intern Med 112:173, 1990. *Three excellent series summarizing the use of octreotide in treatment of acromegaly.*

Macleod AF, Clarke DG, Pambakian H, et al.: Treatment of acromegaly by external irradiation. Clin Endocrinol (Oxf) 30:303, 1989. Littley MD, Shalet SM, Swindell R, et al.: Low-dose pituitary irradiation for acromegaly. Clin Endocrinol (Oxf) 32:261, 1990. *The role of irradiation in therapy of acromegaly is clearly described in these two reviews.*

Melmed S: Acromegaly. N Engl J Med 322:966, 1990. *An excellent review of current knowledge of acromegaly from the standpoint of pathogenesis and therapy.*

Ross DA, Wilson CB: Results of transsphenoidal microsurgery for growth hormone-secreting pituitary adenoma in a series of 214 patients. J Neurosurg 68:854, 1988. Oyen WJG, Pieters GFFM, Meijer E, et al.: Which factors predict the results of pituitary surgery in acromegaly? Acta Endocrinol (Copenh) 117:491, 1988. *Large surgical series indicating the effectiveness (and limitations) of the surgical treatment of acromegaly and a careful assessment of the predictors of surgical outcome.*

Prolactin-Secreting Tumors: Amenorrhea-Galactorrhea Syndrome

Hyperprolactinemia is the most common form of pituitary hyperfunction. It is present in as many as 25 per cent of infertile women. The incidence in men is much lower. In patients with pituitary tumors the incidence of elevated prolactin levels ranges from 60 to 80 per cent and is greater than that of any other pituitary hormone. The distinction between patients with *idiopathic hyperprolactinemia* and those with *prolactin-secreting tumors* is currently made on the basis of CT or MRI examination of the pituitary. Thus, changes in the relative frequency of the two diagnoses reflect primarily recent improvements in radiologic technology.

CLINICAL FEATURES. In women, hyperprolactinemia causes galactorrhea, oligomenorrhea or amenorrhea, and infertility (see Ch. 226 for a discussion of galactorrhea). Galactorrhea requires near-normal levels of ovarian steroids and is therefore not seen in all patients. It frequently occurs in association with oral contraceptive use, usually following its discontinuation. The reported incidence of galactorrhea in patients with prolactin-secreting tumors varies from 50 to 90 per cent. Oligomenorrhea or amenorrhea occurs in a similar percentage of patients and in nearly all with radiographic evidence of a pituitary tumor. The development of amenorrhea and the development of galactorrhea are not necessarily related to one another and are of no diagnostic importance. The cause of amenorrhea is related to effects of altered CNS neurotransmitters, principally dopamine, as a result of hyperprolactinemia, which interferes with the positive feedback effect of estradiol on GnRH secretion and the self-priming effect of GnRH. The effects of anovulation include hypoestrogenemia, which results in decreased vaginal secretion, and dyspareunia, which may be responsible for diminished libido. Mild hirsutism may also occur in association with increased dehydroepiandrosterone sulfate production by the adrenals. Longstanding hyperprolactinemia has, in some women, been associated with decreased bone density, only part of which may be attributed to the hypoestrogenemia. Whether such women are at increased risk for the development of clinically significant osteoporosis is controversial.

In men, hyperprolactinemia results in impotence and diminished libido and, rarely, gynecomastia and galactorrhea. A defect in endogenous GnRH secretion is present, along with diminished testosterone secretion. The decreased libido is, however, not explained entirely on this basis, since it often persists despite testosterone replacement therapy. In some men oligospermia is also present.

LABORATORY STUDIES. Plasma prolactin levels in patients with prolactin-secreting tumors vary from slightly above normal (15 to 20 ng per milliliter) to values greater than 10,000 ng per milliliter. Levels less than 200 ng per milliliter are of little use in distinguishing between the various causes of the disorder, whereas levels greater than 200 ng per milliliter are invariably associated with prolactin-secreting tumors. Since prolactin is a stress-responsive hormone and levels fluctuate in normal subjects, repeated sampling in patients with moderate degrees of hyperprolactinemia is essential.

A large number of dynamic studies of prolactin secretion reveal differences between normal persons and those with pathologic hyperprolactinemia, but none is reliable in distinguishing between idiopathic hyperprolactinemia and prolactin-secreting tumors. Prolactin responses to submaximally suppressive infusions of dopamine are impaired in such patients, as compared to those with known extrapituitary disorders causing hyperprolactinemia, although the latter can usually be distinguished on clinical grounds. Patients with prolactin-secreting tumors and idiopathic hyperprolactinemia have impaired responses to dopamine receptor–blocking agents, to stimulation with TRH, and to a combination of L-dopa plus the dopa decarboxylase inhibitor, carbidopa.

In some patients with pituitary tumors and mild hyperprolactinemia (i.e., less than 100 ng per milliliter) the tumor may not secrete prolactin, but rather appears to increase prolactin secretion by interruption of hypothalamic-pituitary portal blood flow.

DIFFERENTIAL DIAGNOSIS. Consideration should be given to an extrapituitary cause for hyperprolactinemia in all patients, since subtle changes on CT or MRI studies may not indicate the presence of a pituitary tumor. This is particularly true in patients with prolactin levels less than 200 ng per milliliter. The differential diagnosis of hyperprolactinemia is given in Table 213–3. If none of the disorders listed is present and there is no history of drug ingestion, the patient with a normal radiographic examination is considered to have idiopathic hyperprolactinemia.

The many similarities between patients with idiopathic hyperprolactinemia and those with small prolactin-secreting pituitary tumors (microadenomas) have led to the belief that these entities represent different stages of the same disorder. Follow-up evaluation of idiopathic hyperprolactinemia suggests that only a small percentage of cases (less than 5 per cent) progress to demonstrable pituitary tumor formation and that among cases of microadenoma the vast majority remain stable for years with respect to both prolactin levels and tumor size.

Some patients with galactorrhea have normal or borderline elevation of prolactin levels, normal dynamic studies of prolactin secretion and ovulatory menses, and normal fertility. These patients represent the most common type of nonpuerperal galactorrhea, termed *normoprolactinemic galactorrhea*, which is attributed to enhanced sensitivity of the breast to prolactin. The disorder often presents as persistence of postpartum galactorrhea or following discontinuation of oral contraceptives.

PATHOGENESIS. As with GH-secreting tumors, a controversy currently exists about whether prolactin-secreting tumors represent a primary pituitary disease or are secondary to altered hypothalamic influence. Using X-chromosome inactivation studies, prolactin-secreting adenomas also appear to be monoclonal, favoring a pituitary etiology. Prolactinomas may also occur in association with other tumors, in particular pancreatic islet tumors and parathyroid tumors/hyperplasia as part of the multiple endocrine neoplasia syndrome (Type I) (Ch. 220).

A hypothalamic etiology (or component) is supported by a large number of pharmacologic studies suggesting impaired CNS dopaminergic tone. However, evidence for prolactin resistance to dopamine has also been demonstrated, although this appears to be unrelated to altered dopamine receptors. Oral contraceptives do not exert a pathogenic role, although the possibility of a role for a yet unidentified prolactin-releasing factor still exists.

THERAPY. The treatment of prolactin-secreting tumors has undergone considerable change in the past decade. Although surgery has been the therapy of choice in the past, many prolactinomas can now be treated as effectively by medical

TABLE 213–3. DIFFERENTIAL DIAGNOSIS OF NONPHYSIOLOGIC HYPERPROLACTINEMIA

A. **Pharmacologic Agents**
    Monoamine synthesis inhibitors (α-methyldopa)
    Monoamine depletors (reserpine)
    Dopamine receptor antagonists (phenothiazines, butyrophenones, thioxanthines)
    Estrogens (oral contraceptives)
    Narcotics (morphine, heroin)

B. **Central Nervous System Disorders**
    Inflammatory/infiltrative (sarcoidosis, histiocytosis)
    Traumatic (stalk section)
    Neoplastic (hypothalamic or parasellar tumors)

C. **Pituitary Disorders**
    Prolactin-secreting tumors
        Macroadenomas
        Microadenomas
    Empty sella syndrome

D. **Idiopathic Hyperprolactinemia**

E. **Other**
    Hypothyroidism
    Renal failure
    Cirrhosis
    Granulomatous or lymphocytic hypophysitis
    Chest wall/breast disease or surgery
    Thoracic spinal lesions

(pharmacologic) means. Prolactinomas are divided into three subgroups when therapy is considered:

1. *Macroadenomas with only slightly elevated prolactin levels* (i.e., <100 to 150 ng per milliliter). This tumor (also called a *pseudoprolactinoma*) is composed primarily of nonprolactin-secreting cells and should be managed similarly to the nonfunctioning tumor, i.e., surgical removal of tumor mass with preservation of pituitary function.

2. *Microadenomas*. Primary surgical therapy of microadenomas has resulted in up to 90 per cent "cure" rates as judged by restoration of cyclic menses and fertility. However, growth of microadenomas is infrequently observed (5 to 10 per cent become macroadenomas), and this, plus their presence in one third of unselected autopsies, raises the question of whether their removal is indeed necessary in most patients. Furthermore, long-term follow-up of presumably cured patients indicates recurrence of hyperprolactinemia in up to 25 per cent. The most frequent reason for treatment of microadenomas is infertility. The most rapid and effective means of reducing prolactin levels to normal in such patients is by use of the dopamine agonist bromocriptine, which suppresses prolactin secretion in all forms of hyperprolactinemia by an action directly on the lactotroph. Prolactin levels are decreased by more than 90 per cent, and galactorrhea is improved or eliminated in most patients, even if prolactin levels remain slightly elevated. Similarly, cyclic menses and fertility may return without complete normalization of prolactin levels. The dosage required for most patients is 5 to 7.5 mg per day in divided doses although some may require up to 15 mg per day. Side effects consist primarily of nausea and vomiting due to stimulation of the emesis center, occasionally hypotension due to a CNS-mediated mechanism, and mood changes. The side effects may be minimized by initiating therapy with a small dose and gradually increasing it, although 5 to 10 per cent of patients are unable to tolerate the drug. Even when given throughout pregnancy bromocriptine appears to be safe. It is, in fact, the recommended therapy for women who develop signs and symptoms of a prolactin-secreting tumor during pregnancy. Even when fertility is not of concern, reduction of prolactin levels is warranted to restore normal estrogen levels and possibly to correct osteopenia and prevent subsequent symptomatic osteoporosis. The same rationale is used for treating idiopathic hyperprolactinemia.

3. *Macroadenomas with markedly elevated prolactin levels*. This tumor is composed almost exclusively of lactotrophs. In addition to the above considerations, the tumor size can be markedly decreased by bromocriptine, most dramatically when the tumor is very large. In about two thirds of patients, bromocriptine reduces tumor size by 50 to 75 per cent. The effects are usually quite rapid, occurring within days, but in some patients, tumor shrinkage may require several months. The reduction in size continues for as long as therapy is continued, even for more than a decade. Discontinuation of the drug after 1 year or less of therapy may be associated with rapid regrowth of the tumor, and symptoms may recur within days. However, after several years, drug dosage can be markedly reduced and in occasional patients, discontinued without evidence of tumor regrowth. Bromocriptine is useful in reducing the size of very large tumors prior to surgery, in postoperative treatment of patients in whom only partial tumor removal was accomplished, and in patients who are not candidates for surgery.

Bromocriptine is also effective in males with prolactinomas. Restoration of serum testosterone levels and of libido and potency follows institution of therapy and normalization of prolactin levels.

Another dopamine agonist, pergolide, recently approved for treatment of Parkinson's disease, is also useful as a prolactin-suppressive agent.

Kleinberg DL, Boyd AE, Wardlaw S, et al.: Pergolide for the treatment of pituitary tumors secreting prolactin or growth hormone. N Engl J Med 309:704, 1983. *This agent, a dopamine agonist like bromocriptine, is useful in treatment of both prolactin- and growth hormone–secreting tumors.*

Mehta AE, Reyes FI, Faiman C: Primary radiotherapy of prolactinomas. Am J Med 83:49, 1987. *This modality of therapy is effective. Its onset is slow, however, and the long-term risks of hypopituitarism must be considered.*

Molitch ME: Management of prolactinomas. Annu Rev Med 40:225, 1989. Dalkin AC, Marshall JC: Medical therapy of hyperprolactinemia. Endocrinol Metabol Clin North Am 18:259, 1989. *Two excellent reviews that discuss the role of pharmacotherapy in the treatment of prolactinomas.*

Schlechte J, Dolan K, Sherman B, et al.: The natural history of untreated hyperprolactinemia: A prospective analysis. J Clin Endocrinol Metab 68:412, 1989. *This article shows that untreated hyperprolactinemia is generally a stable and minimally progressive disorder.*

Schlechte J, El-Khoury G, Kathol M, et al.: Forearm and vertebral bone mineral in treated and untreated hyperprolactinemic amenorrhea. J Clin Endocrinol Metab 64:1021, 1987. Klibanski A, Biller BMK, Rosenthal DI, et al.: Effects of prolactin and estrogen deficiency in amenorrheic bone loss. J Clin Endocrinol Metab 67:124, 1988. *Patients with prolactinomas have decreased bone mineral density, although controversy exists as to whether the effects are specific to prolactin and the nature of the long-term risk associated with the finding.*

ACTH-Secreting Tumors: Cushing's Disease

Basophilic adenomas of the pituitary associated with bilateral adrenocortical hyperplasia and the features of hypercortisolism constitute a disorder first described by Cushing. The tumors, which tend to be located in the midline or near the anterior-posterior pituitary junction, are usually benign, but in contrast to other pituitary tumors, often exhibit more aggressive growth behavior, may have true malignant potential, and on rare occasions metastasize within and without the CNS. Corticotroph tumors may first become clinically apparent following bilateral adrenalectomy in patients with Cushing's disease (Nelson's syndrome). They may also be chromophobic and are found in 5 to 7 per cent of pituitaries at autopsy in patients without evidence of ACTH hypersecretion during life. Defects in the hormone secretory process may be responsible for these nonfunctioning tumors.

CLINICAL FEATURES. The clinical features of corticotroph tumors consist of those related to hypercortisolism and those caused by hypersecretion of ACTH and related peptides. The signs and symptoms of hypercortisolism are indistinguishable from those associated with adrenocortical adenomas or exogenous hormone administration and include centripetal obesity, hypertension, diabetes, amenorrhea, hirsutism, acne, osteoporosis and compression fractures, muscle atrophy, violaceous striae, capillary fragility, impaired wound healing, decreased resistance to infection, and behavioral changes. These are discussed in greater detail in Ch. 217. Increased secretion of ACTH and β-LPH produces pigmentation similar to that seen in Addison's disease. In addition to generalized pigmentation, the pressure points (knuckles, elbows, knees, belt or brassiere strap regions), areolae, genitalia, mucous membranes, and recently healed scars are particularly affected. Because ACTH production is only partially autonomous in this disease, hyperpigmentation is mild or moderate in the early stages but may be more pronounced after adrenalectomy or in very large tumors.

LABORATORY STUDIES. Randomly obtained plasma cortisol levels are elevated in only about half of the patients with Cushing's disease. The 24-hour urinary free cortisol is the most reliable screening measurement for distinguishing patients with increased adrenocortical function. Normal values are less than 100 μg per 24 hours. Of the dynamic tests, dexamethasone suppressibility is the most reliable and widely used. In normal subjects, low-dosage dexamethasone (0.5 mg every 6 hours for 2 days) decreases urinary free cortisol to less than 20 μg per 24 hours and plasma cortisol to less than 5 μg per deciliter. Patients with corticotroph tumors exhibit impaired suppression with the low dosage but at least 50 per cent suppression with the high dosage (2.0 mg every 6 hours for 2 days). In some patients, however, larger doses may be required to demonstrate suppression. An overnight dexamethasone suppression test (1 mg orally at 11 P.M. with a plasma cortisol measurement at 8 A.M. the next morning) provides comparable screening sensitivity except in obese subjects, in whom false-positive results are more frequent. Dexamethasone at any dose does not suppress cortisol secretion in patients with adrenal adenomas or ectopic ACTH. These conditions can be distinguished by measurement of plasma ACTH levels, which are absent in the former and very high in the latter. Patients with Cushing's disease exhibit ACTH hyperresponsiveness to CRH; those with adrenal adenomas or ectopic ACTH production do not respond to CRH. CT and MRI of the pituitary demonstrate the adenoma in only 60 to 70 per cent of patients with Cushing's disease. If the tumor location is unclear, petrosal sinus catheterization and sampling for ACTH levels, preferably in combination with CRH administration, often provide definitive information.

DIFFERENTIAL DIAGNOSIS. ACTH-secreting tumors are responsible for approximately 80 per cent of cases of endogenous hypercortisolemia. Adrenal tumors are present in about 15 per cent, and the remainder are caused by ectopic ACTH-secreting or, rarely, by CRH-secreting tumors. The differential diagnosis of these disorders is discussed in greater detail in Ch. 217. Ectopic ACTH production can occur in a variety of tumors, most commonly small cell lung carcinomas, carcinoids, and pancreatic islet tumors (see Ch. 161). The disease can mimic that of corticotroph tumors, although in patients with malignant diseases, weight gain is often absent and severe hypokalemia is a prominent feature. Some of these tumors have been shown to secrete CRH alone or in combination with ACTH, explaining the occasional similarity in responses to dynamic hormone testing to those in patients with corticotroph tumors. Ectopic ACTH secretion should be suspected when the clinical and biochemical features of hypercortisolism occur on a periodic or intermittent basis.

Mild elevations of plasma cortisol, loss of diurnal variation, and absence of dexamethasone suppressibility are seen in patients under stress, during periods of bereavement, and in patients with depressive illness. Biochemically it is frequently impossible to distinguish these patients from those with ACTH-secreting tumors, although the clinical features of hypercortisolism are generally absent.

PATHOGENESIS. Arguments have been made for both a hypothalamic and a pituitary cause of ACTH-secreting tumors. Hypothalamic tumors have been identified in association with Cushing's disease, suggesting tumorous overproduction of CRH. Patients with ACTH-secreting tumors generally respond to CRH, as does tumor tissue tested in vitro. Basophilic hyperplasia, rather than tumor, is occasionally found in patients with Cushing's disease. In addition, cyproheptadine, a serotonin-receptor blocker, suppresses ACTH secretion in some patients with the disorder, providing strong support for a primary CNS role. The major argument for a primary pituitary disorder is based on the successful treatment by transsphenoidal adenomectomy, which includes re-establishment not only of normal quantitative cortisol secretion but of diurnal periodicity and glucocorticoid suppressibility. It is possible that two subgroups of the disease exist that are not readily distinguishable by clinical or laboratory methods currently available. Several lines of evidence suggest the presence of two subgroups, including the ultradian pattern of ACTH and cortisol secretion and the biochemical responses of the tumor in vivo and in vitro. In support of this, X-chromosome inactivation studies reveal about half of ACTH-secreting tumors to be monoclonal and the remainder polyclonal. The latter group could represent responses to increased CRH stimulation. Both groups, however, have a common characteristic: diminished sensitivity to feedback inhibition by cortisol.

THERAPY. Definitive treatment of ACTH-secreting pituitary tumors is indicated as soon as the diagnosis has been established. Once ectopic ACTH or CRF production has been excluded, surgical removal of the pituitary ACTH-secreting tumor is indicated. Tumors may be extremely small and difficult to identify. If the tumor cannot be located or if the patient remains hypercortisolemic following surgery, anterior hypophysectomy or bilateral total adrenalectomy is necessary, the decision being influenced by the patient's age, desire for subsequent pregnancy, and overall general health. Following pituitary adenomectomy, adrenocortical hypofunction requiring glucocorticoid replacement therapy may persist for as long as 2 years. A success rate of up to 85 per cent has been reported in patients with small ACTH-secreting tumors, although in those with large tumors this figure is reduced to about 30 per cent.

Radiation is also effective as primary therapy in ACTH-secreting tumors, although its use is generally limited to patients who are not surgical candidates. Cure rates have been reported of 80 per cent in children and 60 per cent in adults with either conventional radiotherapy or proton beam therapy. Some long-term loss of other pituitary function has been noted after radiotherapy.

Pharmacologic therapy of Cushing's disease is directed at suppression of cortisol biosynthesis by the adrenals, using aminoglutethimide, metyrapone, or mitotane (o,p'-DDD) or ketoconazole; at neurotransmitter metabolism within the CNS; or at the pituitary directly. Detailed discussion of drugs acting on the adrenal is provided in Ch. 217. They have been used, together with radiotherapy, as an alternative to surgical treatment in selected patients. The serotonin-receptor blocker cyproheptadine and the GABA agonist sodium valproate have been successful in a small number of patients with Cushing's disease in restoring both ACTH and cortisol secretion to normal. Responses have also been seen in patients with Nelson's disease. A few patients also exhibit decreases in ACTH secretion during bromocriptine therapy. There is no evidence for regression of tumor size by these agents.

Howlett TA, Plowman PN, Wass JAH, et al.: Megavoltage pituitary irradiation in the management of Cushing's disease and Nelson's syndrome: Long-term follow-up. Clin Endocrinol (Oxf) 31:309, 1989. *The use of radiotherapy alone has proven disappointing in terms of its results, although this form of therapy is of value in patients with inadequate responses to pituitary surgery.*

Loli P, Berselli ME, Tagliaferri M: Use of ketoconazole in the treatment of Cushing's syndrome. J Clin Endocrinol Metab 63:1365, 1986. Schteingart DE: Cushing's syndrome. Endocrinol Metabol Clin North Am 18:311, 1989. *The use of pharmacotherapy is discussed in these articles and is most effective when directed at the inhibition of adrenocortical hormone biosynthesis.*

McCance DR, McIlrath E, McNeill A, et al.: Bilateral inferior petrosal sinus sampling as a routine procedure in ACTH-dependent Cushing's syndrome. Clin Endocrinol (Oxf) 30:157, 1989. *Widespread experience with this procedure has made it useful in confirming the pituitary origin of the disease when radiographic imaging studies are nondiagnostic; it is also frequently of help in lateralizing the tumor.*

Nieman LK, Cutler GB Jr, Oldfield EH, et al.: The ovine corticotropin-releasing hormone (CRH) stimulation test is superior to the human CRH stimulation test for the diagnosis of Cushing's disease. J Clin Endocrinol Metab 69:165, 1989. *This procedure is of greatest help in differentiating a pituitary tumor from ectopic production of ACTH.*

Tindall GT, Herring CJ, Clark RV, et al.: Cushing's disease: Results of transsphenoidal microsurgery with emphasis on surgical failures. J Neurosurg 72:363, 1990. Guilhaume B, Bertagna X, Thomsen M, et al.: Transsphenoidal pituitary surgery for the treatment of Cushing's disease: Results in 64 patients and long term follow-up studies. J Clin Endocrinol Metab 66:1056, 1988. *Two surgical series representative of the overall success that has been achieved in treatment of Cushing's disease by selective pituitary adenomectomy.*

Other Hormone-Secreting Tumors

TSH and gonadotropin secretion by pituitary tumors is extremely rare. TSH-secreting tumors are detected during the workup of hyperthyroid patients with elevated rather than suppressed TSH levels. The clinical manifestations consist of hyperthyroidism and a pituitary tumor mass. Occasionally mixed pituitary cell types are present with coexisting GH or prolactin hypersecretion. TSH secretion is not completely autonomous, since suppression of thyroxine production by methimazole frequently results in an increase of TSH secretion. Treatment must be directed to removal of the tumor mass, although medical therapy to suppress the elevated thyroxine levels is required preoperatively. Octreotide also suppresses TSH secretion in these patients, but no reduction in tumor size has been observed.

FSH- and FSH/LH-secreting pituitary tumors are very rare and often associated with longstanding hypogonadism. Many tumors otherwise considered to be nonfunctioning, however, may secrete the isolated glycoprotein α subunit, which lacks any biologic activity and serves primarily as a tumor marker. Some of these tumors may respond to either bromocriptine or octreotide.

Gesundheit N, Petrick PA, Nissim M, et al.: Thyrotropin-secreting pituitary adenomas: Clinical and biochemical heterogeneity: Case reports and follow-up of nine patients. Ann Intern Med 111:827, 1989. *This article illustrates the range of settings in which TSH-secreting tumors are seen and the long-term history of the tumors.*

Heseltine D, White MC, Kendall-Taylor P, et al.: Testicular enlargement and elevated serum inhibin concentrations occur in patients with pituitary macroadenomas secreting follicle stimulating hormone. Clin Endocrinol (Oxf) 31:411, 1989. Klibanski A, Deutsch PJ, Jameson JL, et al.: Luteinizing hormone–secreting pituitary tumor: Biosynthetic characterization and clinical studies. J Clin Endocrinol Metab 64:536, 1987. *Clinical and biochemical characterizations of gonadotropin-secreting tumors emphasize the effect on reproductive hormone physiology.*

Ishibashi M, Yamaji T, Takaku F, et al.: Secretion of glycoprotein hormone alpha-subunit by pituitary tumors. J Clin Endocrinol Metab 64:1187, 1987. Demura R, Jibiki K, Kubo O, et al.: The significance of α-subunit as a tumor marker for gonadotropin-producing pituitary adenomas. J Clin Endocrinol Metab 63:564, 1986. *Glycoprotein α-subunit may be secreted independently of glycoprotein hormones by tumors. Although the monomeric subunit is bioinactive, it defines the tumor cell type as of thyrotroph/gonadotroph origin.*

214 The Posterior Pituitary

Thomas E. Andreoli

ANTIDIURETIC HORMONE

The neurohypophysis of humans elaborates two hormones: *arginine vasopressin* (AVP), which exhibits vasopressor and antidiuretic activity, and *oxytocin*, which is galactobolic and uterotonic. Both hormones are octapeptides of approximately 1100 daltons, with a 20-member ring structure created by disulfide bonds. The antidiuretic and vasopressor activities of AVP are each approximately 100 times as great as those of oxytocin, a difference that is related to the different tertiary conformations of the two peptides.

The posterior pituitary gland contains terminal axons whose cell bodies lie in hypothalamic cell clusters known as the *supraoptic* and *paraventricular nuclei*. Synthesis of posterior pituitary hormones occurs in these hypothalamic nuclei rather than in the posterior pituitary gland: (1) AVP can be demonstrated immunochemically in cells of both the supraoptic and the paraventricular nuclei; and (2) neurosecretory granules accumulate only on the hypothalamic side of a sectioned hypophyseal stalk.

The cardinal steps in the biosynthesis of antidiuretic hormone (ADH) are illustrated in Figure 214–1. Neurohypophyseal hormones, including vasopressin, are synthesized as prohormones in conjunction with specific carrier proteins called neurophysins. Vasopressin, specifically, is synthesized as a prohormone in conjunction with neurophysin II, and the complex is sometimes termed the van Dyke protein. Both vasopressin and neurophysin II come from a common precursor gene, located on human chromosome 20 (Fig. 214–2). The hormone precursor contains three peptide regions: a signal peptide and ADH at the N-terminal, a neurophysin II region, and a C-terminal glycoprotein region of unknown significance. Each region of the precursor protein is, in turn, coded for by one of three different exons on the vasopressin precursor gene. Thus, the main steps in the biosynthesis of ADH are transcription of the vasopressin precursor mRNA; translation of the mRNA to a pre-prohormone; and removal of the signal peptide sequence while the peptide is still attached to the ribosome, yielding the prohormone. The prohormone peptide is transported in neurosecretory granules to the posterior pituitary gland. During transport, the prohormone peptide is cleaved to neurophysin II and ADH. In the posterior pituitary gland, the neurosecretory granules rest in terminal projections of axonal plasma membranes, juxtaposed to systemic circulation capillaries. Other pituicyte nerve fibers terminate in the median eminence and along the third ventricle, thus allowing access of vasopressin to cerebrospinal fluid.

There are two pools of AVP-containing neurosecretory granules in pituicytes: one adjacent to the cell membrane and therefore available for immediate release, and a second storage pool removed from immediate contact with the plasma membrane.

Release of hormone occurs by an exocytotic process involving fusion of neurosecretory granules with pituicyte plasma membranes. In other words, AVP release is quantal. A stimulus to the hypothalamic pituicyte cell body is transmitted to the site of granule storage, where it causes cell membrane depolarization, an associated increase in calcium permeability, and rapid calcium entry into the pituicytes. This influx of calcium activates the exocytosis of AVP-containing neurosecretory granules.

RELEVANT PHYSIOLOGY. Detailed accounts of the renal and pituitary processes resulting in the formation of dilute or concentrated urine are presented in Ch. 73 and 75. ADH exerts major physiologic effects on discrete regions of the nephron and also affects vascular smooth muscle tone. There are two distinct receptors for these ADH effects. Those in smooth muscle, also found on hepatocytes, are denoted V_1 receptors. Those within epithelia, for example, collecting ducts, are designated V_2 receptors. The V_2 receptors have a greater affinity for ADH than do V_1 receptors.

In all epithelia that respond to ADH, the hormone binds to V_2 receptors on the basolateral plasma membrane of the cell and, in so doing, activates the enzyme adenylate cyclase. Adenylate cyclase increases the production of 3',5'-cyclic adenosine monophosphate (cAMP) from its substrate adenosine triphosphate (ATP). Cyclic AMP then acts as a second messenger to activate a cell-specific protein kinase, protein kinase A, which induces the final cellular response to the hormone (see Ch. 208). ADH-stimulated adenylate cyclase is present in the collecting duct and in the medullary, but not cortical, thick ascending limb of Henle (mTALH) of mammalian kidneys.

The *cardinal* physiologic effect of ADH is to promote the formation of hypertonic urine, which depends particularly on two sets of events operating in parallel within the renal medulla. First, in the thick ascending limb of Henle, approximately 15 to 20 per cent of the filtered load of sodium chloride is absorbed. Since the mTALH is water impermeable, this process contributes simultaneously to the maintenance of a hypertonic medullary interstitium and to the formation of dilute urine. Under normal circumstances, the osmolality of the renal medullary interstitium rises from isotonic, at the corticomedullary junction, to very hypertonic, approximately 1200 mOsm per kilogram of H_2O, at the papillary tip. Since the enrichment of medullary interstitial osmolality and dilution of tubular fluid both depend on sodium chloride absorption by the water-impermeable mTALH, the latter region of the nephron is commonly termed the medullary diluting segment. Approximately 10 per cent of fluid filtered at the glomerulus, or about 18 liters daily, reaches the early distal tubule with an osmolality of approximately 50 mOsm per kilogram of H_2O.

When ADH is absent, the water permeability of collecting ducts is at a minimum. Thus there is reduced osmotic equilibration of fluid passing through collecting ducts with the medullary interstitium, and most of the fluid escapes unchanged as hypotonic urine. Since only 10 per cent of filtered water normally

FIGURE 214–1. Flow diagram for the pathway of posterior pituitary hormone biosynthesis. (From Reeves WB, Andreoli TE: The posterior pituitary and water metabolism. *In* Foster DW, Wilson JD [eds.]: Williams Textbook of Endocrinology, 8th ed. Philadelphia, W.B. Saunders Company, 1991.)

Form	Molecular Weight	Synthetic Step
Preprohormone	≈21,000	Protein synthesis; magnocellular neuron ribosomes
Prohormone	≈23,000	Glycosylation and membrane packaging; magnocellular neuron; Golgi apparatus
Neurosecretory Granule (NSG)	(23,000)ₙ	Transport down supraopticohyophyseal tract as osmotically inactive granules
Neurophysin + Hormone	≈10,000 ≈1,100	Storage in posterior pituitary; cleavage within NSG

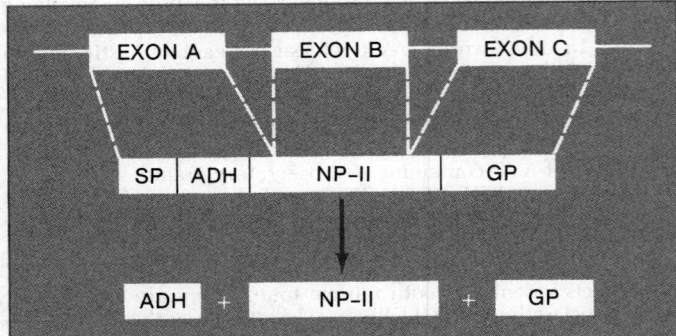

FIGURE 214–2. A schematic representation of the organization of the ADH gene and its relation to the pre-prohormone and final peptide products. SP = Signal peptide; NP-II = neurophysin II; GP = glycoprotein.

reaches the collecting duct system, the maximal degree of polyuria in a patient with complete pituitary diabetes insipidus (or complete nephrogenic diabetes insipidus) is therefore approximately 18 liters daily. During normal antidiuresis, ADH, by way of cAMP, increases the water permeability of luminal (urinary) cell membranes of cortical and outer medullary collecting ducts. Thus in the presence of ADH, there is osmotic equilibration of hypotonic luminal fluid in collecting ducts with the hypertonic medullary interstitium and, consequently, water absorption, a reduction in urine volume, concentration of urine, and conservation of body water.

The ADH-dependent increase in the water permeability of collecting ducts is due to a hormone-dependent increase in the number of water-specific channels available for water transport through luminal membranes. These channels are rather narrow, approximately 2 Å in radius, and therefore exclude urea and NaCl. As a consequence, the luminal fluid concentrations of these two solutes increase when water is abstracted from cortical and outer medullary collecting ducts during antidiuresis. In turn, the increase in luminal urea concentration creates a favorable gradient for passive urea diffusion out of inner medullary (papillary) collecting ducts into the interstitium, thereby maintaining interstitial hypertonicity. ADH also causes a slight increase in papillary duct urea permeability, thus favoring passive movement of urea down its concentration gradient for recirculation through the medullary interstitium.

A *second ADH-mediated* event in the antidiuretic response is to increase the rate of NaCl transport in medullary, but not cortical, mTALH. This process involves a furosemide-sensitive electroneutral cotransport of $Na^+:K^+:2Cl^-$ from luminal fluid into cells; virtually all of the potassium entering cells through this process is recycled back into luminal fluid via potassium-specific channels in luminal membranes. Consequently, ADH increases urinary concentrating power in two ways: by enhancing the water permeability of collecting ducts and by increasing the net rate of salt absorption by the mTALH, thus enriching medullary interstitial osmolality.

This latter effect of ADH on medullary diluting segments is opposed by at least three other factors. (1) As interstitial NaCl concentrations increase, the backleak of NaCl into the tubular lumen of the mTALH also increases and thereby tends to reduce net NaCl absorption by the mTALH. (2) Increases in interstitial osmolality down-regulate the ADH stimulation of NaCl cotransport. (3) Prostaglandins of the E series, which are produced in the renal medullary interstitium in response to increasing interstitial osmolality, inhibit competitively the ADH-mediated increases in the rate of intracellular cAMP formation.

These three processes have a negative feedback on ADH enhancement of active NaCl absorption in the mTALH, so that the diluting power of the mTALH remains constant during either antidiuresis or water diuresis.

Finally, prostaglandins of the E series also antagonize the ADH-dependent enhancement of collecting-duct water permeability. This effect may be produced either by prostaglandins synthesized endogenously by collecting-duct cells or by prostaglandins synthesized within the medullary interstitium. Thus prostaglandins blunt urinary concentrating power by offsetting ADH effects in at least two loci, the mTALH and the collecting duct.

At levels of hormone that exceed those necessary for antidiuresis, ADH also has pressor activity (this was the first known effect of posterior pituitary extract and provided the basis for the name vasopressin) that is the result of a direct constricting effect on vascular smooth muscle via the V_1 receptors described above. At all but high pharmacologic doses, this pressor effect is easily overcome by compensatory vasodilatory reflexes, so that hypertension is not routinely seen during AVP replacement therapy. Lesser doses may, however, cause significant vasoconstriction of coronary arteries. Another effect of vasopressin, seen at levels that supersede those necessary for antidiuresis, is stimulation of intestinal motility. Finally, AVP released into the CSF and thalamic centers may play a role in such diverse processes as memory and regulation of corticotropin release.

OSMOTIC REGULATION OF ADH RELEASE. Verney's elegant studies demonstrated a strong antidiuretic response to perfusion of carotid vessels with hypertonic solutions of various solutes, including sodium salts and glucose; hypertonic urea solutions elicited no such response. Therefore he concluded that specific cells that acted as osmoreceptors were present within the distribution of the carotid circulation and that the plasma membranes of these cells were impermeable to sodium salts and glucose but permeable to urea. In the presence of extracellular hyperosmolality induced by impermeable species, these osmosensing cells reached osmotic equilibrium by losing water to the hypertonic plasma. In other words, Verney deduced that osmoreceptor shrinkage, produced by raising plasma osmolality with solutes restricted to the extracellular compartment, was the stimulus for ADH release.

When the anterior wall of the third ventricle is exposed to hypertonic saline, neurons in both the anterior hypothalamus and the preoptic area have increased rates of depolarization. Concomitantly, about half of the pituicytes in hypothalamic nuclei show a characteristic depolarization pattern, and plasma antidiuretic activity increases. Therefore it is probable that the neurons in the anterior hypothalamus and preoptic areas, which depolarize in response to hypertonic saline, represent Verney's osmoreceptors.

In normal man, plasma AVP levels are undetectable below a plasma osmolality of 280 mOsm per kilogram of H_2O. Since the usual plasma osmolality in man is approximately 287 mOsm per kilogram of H_2O, secretion of AVP is tonic; the average circulating hormone levels are between 2.0 and 2.5 pg per milliliter. Vasopressin levels increase in a linear fashion with increasing plasma osmolality, such that a rise in plasma osmolality of only 1 per cent (2.9 mOsm per kilogram of H_2O) evokes a 1 pg per milliliter rise in AVP. Parallel examinations of plasma AVP and urine osmolality indicate that each unit increase in AVP allows an increase of 250 mOsm per kilogram of H_2O in urinary concentration. Since the maximal concentrating ability of the human kidney is approximately 1200 mOsm per kilogram of H_2O, maximal water conservation is therefore achieved at a plasma AVP level of 5.0 pg per milliliter.

Combining these relations yields a measure of the efficiency of the water homeostatic mechanism: for each 1 mOsm per kilogram of H_2O change in plasma osmolality there is a change in urinary concentration of 95 mOsm per kilogram of H_2O, which represents a gain of almost 100-fold. The ingestion of water sufficient to decrease plasma osmolality by only 1 mOsm per kilogram of H_2O reduces urinary concentration by 95 mOsm per kilogram of H_2O, thus allowing the water to be excreted and osmotic balance to be restored. The opposite effect, water loss, results in stimulation of ADH release, increase in urinary concentration, and conservation of body water by the same magnification phenomenon.

NONOSMOTIC REGULATION OF ADH RELEASE. Isotonic or hypotonic volume depletion results in an antidiuretic state. Evidence now exists for stretch receptors, or baroreceptors, that sense changes in vascular wall tension in both the venous (low pressure) and arterial (high pressure) circulations. Immersion and negative pressure breathing, i.e., maneuvers that augment intrathoracic blood volume, as well as balloon distension of the left atrium, all produce water diuresis that can be overcome by

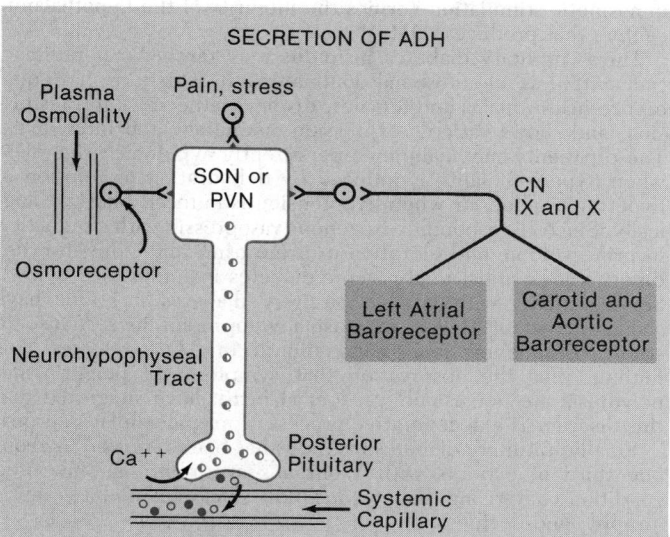

FIGURE 214–3. Secretory stimuli for calcium-dependent ADH release: van Dyke protein (◑), vasopressin (●), neurophysin II (○). SON = Supraoptic neuron, PVN = paraventricular neuron.

administering ADH. Conversely, positive pressure breathing and upright posture, which reduce intrathoracic blood volume, or left atrial collapse, produce antidiuresis. These observations indicate that the left atrium and the pulmonary vasculature are the major loci for low pressure baroreceptors that modulate ADH release.

Hypotension, or selective clamping of major systemic arterial vessels, also produces profound antidiuresis. These data indicate the presence of a baroreceptor system in the arterial circulation, localized to the carotid bifurcations and aortic arch, that also modulates ADH release. This type of nonosmotic ADH release is modulated by stimulatory or inhibitory signals arriving from the baroreceptors via parasympathetic pathways in the vagus and glossopharyngeal nerves. The low pressure baroreceptors are more sensitive regulators of ADH release than those in high pressure regions of the circulation. These relations are summarized in Figure 214–3.

Circulating levels of ADH rise with vascular volume depletion. However, volume-mediated, nonosmotic ADH release has a "threshold" requiring more than 7 per cent blood volume depletion, with greater degrees of blood volume contraction eliciting exponential rises in circulating ADH levels. Thus nonosmotic ADH release differs strikingly from osmotically mediated ADH release, which occurs with only a 1 to 2 per cent increase in plasma osmolality and rises linearly with further increases in plasma osmolality. With less than a 7 per cent decrease in blood volume, ADH release is governed wholly by plasma osmolality. At greater reductions in blood volume, ADH release is increasingly dominated by nonosmotic, volume-dependent stimuli. This observation explains the finding of progressive fluid dilution in patients with hypovolemia or states of decreased cardiac output.

Finally, the vasoconstrictor peptide endothelin-1 is also released from the posterior pituitary following water depletion. Since administered endothelin-1 increases plasma ADH levels, endothelin-1 may also play a role in ADH release.

Input from higher cortical functions also appears to influence ADH release. Pain, emotion, stress, and some psychotic states are associated with ADH stimulation or inhibition. Most common is the transient antidiuresis that occurs postoperatively.

PATHOLOGIC ALTERATION OF ADH RELEASE. A wide variety of agents and conditions are known to affect ADH activity (Table 214–1). Nicotine, as a stimulant of ADH release, and acute alcohol ingestion, as an inhibitor of ADH release, have figured prominently in devising means to assess neurohypophyseal integrity. Stimulatory drugs such as clofibrate and chlorpropamide have been utilized to treat states of partial ADH insufficiency. Other drugs, such as lithium and demeclocycline, are prominent for their effect on the renal collecting duct, making it unresponsive to ADH and thereby producing nephrogenic diabetes insipidus.

TABLE 214–1. CONDITIONS THAT ALTER ANTIDIURETIC HORMONE ACTIVITY

Enhance	Suppress
Drugs and Conditions That Modify Release of ADH	
Surgical stress	Phenytoin
Vincristine	Alcohol
Cyclophosphamide	Narcotic antagonists
Clofibrate	α-Adrenergic agents
Carbamazepine	
Barbiturates	
Morphine and narcotic analogues	
Nicotine	
β-Adrenergic agents	
Hypoxia	
Hypercapnia	
Drugs That Modify the ADH Effect on Collecting Ducts	
Chlorpropamide	Lithium
Biguanides	Methoxyflurane
Indomethacin	Demeclocycline

The syndrome of inappropriate antidiuretic hormone secretion (SIADH) is characterized by persistent hyponatremia, an inappropriately elevated urine osmolality, and no discernible stimulus for ADH release. A common cause for this condition is neoplastic, most notably oat cell carcinoma of lung; SIADH is due to ectopic production of ADH by the tumor, with persistent release of hormone independent of regulatory influences. Inflammatory disorders of the lung, such as pneumonia or cavitary tuberculosis, provide other sites for ectopic ADH production. The syndrome also occurs in patients with head trauma or with other diseases of the central nervous system and often terminates with recovery of neurologic function. The SIADH syndrome is discussed in detail in Ch. 75.

THIRST REGULATION. Body water content is governed not only by ADH modulation of renal water excretion but also by regulation of water intake through thirst. Both systems operate in parallel under the influence of osmotic and volume mediators. Thirst also requires an intact cerebral cortex, which transforms the urge to drink into appropriate behavior to secure water.

Hyperosmolality, and presumably shrinkage of thirst receptors, is the primary stimulus for thirst and requires only a 2 per cent rise in plasma osmolality. The thirst "threshold" in conscious humans is about 294 mOsm per kilogram, the same osmolality at which maximal urinary concentration under ADH is achieved. Hypovolemia also stimulates thirst via an angiotensin II–mediated mechanism. Indeed, hyperreninemic states such as malignant hypertension are often accompanied by pathologic thirst. Phenothiazines enhance thirst and contribute to the hyponatremia seen in some patients treated with these drugs for affective disorders. Finally, prostaglandin E also stimulates thirst. The polydipsia that accompanies hypokalemia probably depends on increased production of prostaglandin E.

WATER REPLETION REACTION. The positive limb of the water repletion reaction has two cardinal features—redundancy and variable gain. Thus two sets of stimuli—osmotic and nonosmotic—stimulate both thirst and antidiuresis. The osmotic stimuli represent, especially for antidiuresis, the system that is activated by 2 per cent changes in effective plasma osmolality and has a linear gain. In contrast, nonosmotic stimuli enhance thirst and antidiuresis only in response to rather large (that is, more than 7 per cent) reductions in effective circulatory volume. Moreover, particularly with respect to antidiuresis, greater degrees of volume contraction provide exponential rather than linear increases in concentrating power.

SUPPRESSION OF WATER REPLETION. At least two separate factors suppress both ADH release and thirst. First, water ingestion, via the *oropharyngeal reflex*, promptly suppresses ADH release, even prior to absorption of the ingested water. Passage of water through the pharynx also suppresses thirst, even when an esophageal fistula prevents net water absorption. These anticipatory responses for both thirst and ADH secretion are accompanied by reduced electrical activity in the hypothalamus and probably involve a neural mechanism.

Second, atrial natriuretic peptide, or atriopeptin, may have a central role in the negative feedback limb of the water repletion reaction. The factors responsible for the biosynthesis and release of atriopeptin are described in detail in Ch. 211. Stated briefly, atriopeptin is released from atrial granules in response to increases in effective circulating volume. Moreover, immunoreactive atriopeptin is produced in the anterolateral periventricular areas of the hypothalamus. In the present context, two actions of either circulating or centrally released atriopeptin have particular relevance: blunting of ADH release in response to osmotic or nonosmotic stimuli and suppression of angiotensin-mediated thirst. These effects suggest a central role for atriopeptin in negative feedback regulation of the water repletion reaction.

Reeves WB, Andreoli TE: The posterior pituitary and water metabolism. In Foster DW, Wilson JD: Williams Textbook of Endocrinology, 8th ed. Philadelphia, W. B. Saunders Company, 1990. A complete analysis of the physiology of the water repletion reaction.

Schmale H, Fehr S, Richter D: Vasopressin biosynthesis—from gene to peptide hormone. Kidney Int 32:S8, 1987. A summary of vasopressin biosynthesis.

Thrasher TN, Keil LC, Ramsay DJ: Drinking, oropharyngeal signals, and inhibition of vasopressin secretion in dogs. Am J Physiol 253:R509, 1987. The role of the oropharyngeal reflex in modulating thirst and ADH release.

DIABETES INSIPIDUS
Pituitary Diabetes Insipidus

DEFINITION. Pituitary diabetes insipidus is a polyuric syndrome that results from a lack of sufficient ADH to effect appropriate concentration of the urine or water conservation. The disease is identified by the persistence of an inappropriately dilute urine in the presence of strong osmotic or nonosmotic stimuli to ADH secretion, and in the absence of renal concentrating defects, and a rise in urine osmolality upon the administration of vasopressin. Pituitary diabetes insipidus may result either from destruction of the centers of ADH synthesis or from failure of the mechanisms effecting ADH release.

ETIOLOGY. Trauma to the neurohypophysis, either accidental or as a result of hypophysectomy, is the major identifiable cause of diabetes insipidus. A second major cause for pituitary diabetes insipidus is an intracranial tumor, which may be primary, as in craniopharyngioma, or metastatic, among which breast carcinoma is the most likely cause. Less frequent causes of pituitary diabetes insipidus are granulomatous lesions of the central nervous system, including tuberculosis and sarcoidosis, the histiocytoses, encephalomeningitis, or vascular lesions. There is a rare familial form of pituitary diabetes insipidus which affects either sex, occurs at any age, and is associated with extensive gliosis of neurohypophyseal nuclei. Finally, 30 to 40 per cent of all patients with pituitary diabetes insipidus have no identifiable cause for the disorder.

PATHOGENESIS. Pituitary diabetes insipidus depends on one of at least four different pathogenic mechanisms. Most commonly the disorder occurs when there is atrophy or destruction of the hypothalamic centers responsible for hormone production. In experimental circumstances, preservation of as few as 15 per cent of magnocellular neurons prevents polyuria, whereas evident diabetes insipidus occurs when only 6 to 8 per cent of neurons remain. Neither removal of the posterior pituitary gland alone nor low section of the neurohypophyseal tract with preservation of hypothalamic nuclei is sufficient to produce a permanent polyuric state. Rather, direct trauma to the pituitary gland or low section of the neurohypophyseal tract results in transient diabetes insipidus; for example, the polyuric state following low stalk section lasts for only 1 to 2 weeks postsurgery. Since the anterior and posterior lobes of the pituitary gland have totally separate blood supplies, infarction of the anterior pituitary gland does not disrupt posterior pituitary function.

A second group of cases has been identified, often classed under the heading essential hypernatremia, in which osmotic stimuli fail to elicit ADH release, while nonosmotic stimuli result in antidiuresis. Although euvolemic, these patients are polyuric and excrete hypotonic urine, and water deprivation alone fails to elicit an antidiuretic response. However, when volume contraction occurs in these patients, significant antidiuresis ensues. Thus, in this disorder there is selective failure of osmoreceptors to stimulate ADH release. The intact response of ADH release to nonosmotic stimulation verifies the integrity of the hypothalamic centers that produce ADH.

Third, pituitary diabetes insipidus may rarely be hereditary, transmitted as an autosomal dominant trait. This form has equal occurrence in males and females, displays father-to-son transmission, and shows variable expression among affected individuals. These patients may maintain a persistently hypotonic urine even when hyperosmolality is induced by dehydration or infusion of hypertonic saline, or when hypotension is induced pharmacologically. Since all respond to exogenous vasopressin with a reduction in urine volume and elevation of urine osmolality, this disorder differs from familial nephrogenic diabetes insipidus (see below). Some patients with familial pituitary diabetes insipidus have shown detectable levels of plasma vasopressin in response to strong osmotic or nonosmotic stimuli to ADH release. This finding, plus the observation that symptoms of polyuria and polydipsia are not usually present at birth, have suggested that this disorder is a degenerative process of magnocellular neurons.

Finally, pituitary diabetes insipidus has been reported in about one third of patients with Wolfram's syndrome, an inherited condition comprising diabetes insipidus, diabetes mellitus, optic atrophy, and deafness.

Nephrogenic Diabetes Insipidus

DEFINITION. The term nephrogenic diabetes insipidus should be applied to disorders in which renal tubular unresponsiveness to ADH, without disturbances either in solute delivery to the loop of Henle or in countercurrent multiplication or exchange processes, is responsible for polyuria and hyposthenuria. Thus nephrogenic diabetes insipidus may be due to inability of ADH to raise cellular cAMP concentrations, to inability of cAMP to increase the water permeability of luminal membranes of collecting ducts, or to a combination of these two disorders.

FAMILIAL NEPHROGENIC DIABETES INSIPIDUS. This familial disorder occurs primarily in males and exhibits a hereditary pattern of X-linked transmission with variable penetrance in females. In normal individuals or patients with pituitary diabetes insipidus, exogenous ADH can increase the rate of urinary cAMP excretion. In the majority of patients with familial nephrogenic diabetes insipidus, comparable doses of ADH do not increase rates of urinary cAMP excretion. However, in two groups of children with nephrogenic diabetes insipidus, both basal and ADH-stimulated rates of urinary cAMP excretion exceeded those of normal children. These disparate results led to the postulate that familial nephrogenic diabetes insipidus is a heterogeneous disorder produced by either a defect in hormone receptor adenylate cyclase stimulation or a defect beyond the generation of cAMP.

The lack of response to ADH in familial nephrogenic diabetes insipidus is restricted to those responses mediated by the V_2 receptor, since V_1 receptor–mediated effects such as vasoconstriction are normal. The V_2 receptor defect appears to be generalized. For example, extrarenal effects mediated by V_2 receptors include an increase in von Willebrand factor and Factor VIII, a fall in diastolic blood pressure, and stimulation of renin release. In most patients with familial nephrogenic DI, these extrarenal V_2-mediated responses are absent, indicating a generalized defect in the V_2 receptor signal transduction pathway.

ACQUIRED NEPHROGENIC DIABETES INSIPIDUS. Vasopressin-resistant hyposthenuria associated with otherwise normal or nearly normal renal function may occur as a complication of drug therapy or in association with systemic diseases. This acquired nephrogenic diabetes insipidus is to be distinguished from the rare familial disorder described earlier.

Vasopressin-unresponsive hyposthenuria occurs in patients receiving demeclocycline; both the concentrating defect and vasopressin-unresponsiveness are reversible and disappear shortly after discontinuance of antibiotic therapy. The glomerular filtration rate in these patients is generally normal, as is the ability for maximal urinary dilution (positive free water formation), indicating that solute abstraction from the loop of Henle is probably unimpaired.

In human renal medulla, demeclocycline noncompetitively inhibits basal adenylate cyclase activity, ADH-stimulated adenylate cyclase activity, and cAMP-dependent protein kinase activity, but does not affect nucleotide phosphodiesterase activity. These data suggest that demeclocycline may inhibit both cAMP accumulation and cAMP effects on renal tubular membranes.

Nephrogenic diabetes insipidus may also be produced by volatile fluorocarbon anesthetics. Methoxyflurane anesthesia is complicated by a full spectrum of renal injury, ranging from vasopressin-resistant polyuria and hyposthenuria to acute tubular necrosis. Both fluoride and oxalic acid, which are metabolic products of methoxyflurane, contribute to the nephrotoxicity of the anesthetic. However, the polyuric state is related to the markedly increased serum concentration and urinary excretion of inorganic fluoride. Sodium fluoride causes vasopressin-resistant polyuria in dogs, and in rats inorganic fluoride seems to reduce collecting duct water permeability without affecting salt transport in the ascending limb.

Serum lithium concentrations of 0.5 to 1.5 mEq per liter, which are generally regarded as being in the therapeutic range for affective disorders, produce vasopressin-resistant diabetes insipidus. Nephrogenic diabetes insipidus has been observed in 12 to 30 per cent of patients receiving lithium therapy; the defect is usually reversible, and urinary concentrating ability returns toward normal when lithium is discontinued. This defect may be due to a lithium-dependent inhibition of ADH-stimulated cAMP accumulation in collecting ducts. Finally nephrogenic diabetes insipidus characterized by persistent, vasopressin-resistant hyposthenuria and polyuria occurs rarely in certain systemic diseases, including most notably sarcoidosis and Sjögren's syndrome.

ACQUIRED POLYURIC STATES. Other disorders may present with polyuria and relative vasopressin resistance, although not necessarily with profound hyposthenuria. Rather, these polyuric disturbances are generally characterized by inability to concentrate urine maximally in response to vasopressin, either stimulated endogenously or administered exogenously; random urine samples are ordinarily not profoundly hypotonic but are usually only slightly hypotonic or modestly hypertonic.

In general, such polyuric disorders occur most commonly in association with hypokalemic nephropathy (Ch. 75) or hypercalcemic nephropathy (Ch. 235), or as a consequence of diseases that disrupt medullary architecture and consequently impair the generation and maintenance of a hypertonic medullary interstitium. The latter disorders include those diseases that affect particularly the renal interstitium, such as sickle cell disease, pyelonephritis, analgesic nephropathy, and multiple myeloma. These diseases are considered in Ch. 80.

Finally, states characterized by osmotic, or solute, diuresis, for example, in diabetic ketoacidosis and hyperglycemic nonketotic states, may result in polyuria with isotonic urine formation and unresponsiveness to vasopressin. In these disorders, the fraction of isotonic glomerular filtrate delivered to the loop of Henle is greatly increased because of failure to absorb solute, for example, glucose, in the proximal nephron. Thus the amount of solute and water reaching the loop of Henle becomes large with regard to the diluting or concentrating ability of the loop of Henle and collecting ducts, respectively, and vasopressin-resistant polyuria and isosthenuria ensue. Consequently the polyuric state in osmotic diuresis differs from that in nephrogenic diabetes insipidus in two respects; urinary solute excretion is dramatically increased in osmotic diuresis but not in nephrogenic diabetes insipidus; and the urine osmolality is nearly isotonic in solute diuresis but rather hypotonic in nephrogenic diabetes insipidus.

Pituitary or Nephrogenic Diabetes Insipidus

CLINICAL MANIFESTATIONS. The foremost clinical feature of either pituitary or nephrogenic diabetes insipidus is *polyuria*, with urine volumes ranging from 3 to 15 liters per day. Along with polyuria there is near-continuous thirst, often with a preference for ice cold water. The disease is almost always accompanied by *nocturia*, in contrast to persons with primary polydipsia (compulsive water drinking), in whom nocturia is usually absent. The onset of polyuria in pituitary diabetes insipidus is most often abrupt, with peak urine flow reached in 1 or 2 days. Therefore, polyuria developing over weeks or months suggests a disease other than pituitary diabetes insipidus. The polyuria of familial nephrogenic diabetes insipidus is present from birth.

The polyuria in complete diabetes insipidus, either pituitary or nephrogenic, has an upper limit of approximately 18 liters daily, or about 10 per cent of filtered water, since 90 per cent of the glomerular filtrate is normally absorbed by the nephron prior to reaching the collecting system. In partial diabetes insipidus, the daily urine volume may be considerably smaller. In contrast, persons afflicted with compulsive water drinking, often referred to as primary or psychogenic polydipsia, not infrequently ingest more than 20 liters of fluid daily. Therefore, the daily urine volume in these patients may also exceed 20 liters.

Modest degrees of volume depletion may curtail polyuria, even in complete diabetes insipidus, for two reasons. First, volume contraction increases the fraction of glomerular filtrate absorbed by the proximal nephron, so that a smaller volume of hypotonic fluid reaches the collecting duct system. Second, even in the absence of ADH, or when collecting ducts are unresponsive to ADH, collecting ducts have a slight permeability to water; consequently, a small fraction of the water reaching the collecting duct system can be absorbed even without ADH. Since the volume of glomerular filtrate reaching the collecting duct system is reduced during volume contraction, the further absorption of relatively small volumes of water by collecting ducts during the volume-contracted state can result in dramatic reductions in polyuria.

Aside from the discomfort and inconvenience of polyuria and polydipsia, patients with pituitary or nephrogenic diabetes insipidus suffer no ill effects unless they are *deprived of access to water*. When this happens, *circulatory collapse* or *hypertonic encephalopathy* may occur. Because of the high rates of urine flow in some patients with diabetes insipidus, these complications may develop in a period of hours. For example, a patient with pituitary diabetes insipidus might excrete 5 per cent of his glomerular filtrate daily, or about 9 liters of urine. In a 70-kg man having 42 kg of body water, this loss, if not continually replenished, would result in a 20 per cent reduction in body water in only 24 hours.

Hypertonic Encephalopathy. Acute increases in intracellular fluid osmolality to levels exceeding 350 mOsm per kilogram of H_2O produced by solutes such as NaCl or glucose (in diabetes), which cross cell membranes poorly, result in central nervous system dysfunction ranging from lethargy to frank coma. Since comparable elevations of plasma osmolality produced by urea, which permeates cell membranes freely, do not produce the disorder, it is evident that hyperosmolality per se is not the basis for the disturbance. Rather, acute hypertonic encephalopathy occurs because cell membranes, being freely permeable to water, are in virtually constant osmotic equilibrium with extracellular fluid. When hypernatremia develops acutely, cellular water loss produces brain shrinkage, and the increase in brain solute content is accounted for entirely by a rise in intracellular Na^+, K^+, and Cl^- concentrations.

In children who develop acute hypernatremia and attain a serum sodium concentration above 160 mEq per liter in 24 hours, the mortality exceeds 40 per cent; about two thirds of the survivors have permanent neurologic sequelae. At autopsy, cerebral vessels are markedly congested and engorged, hemorrhages are evident both in subcortical brain parenchyma and subarachnoid spaces, and venous thrombosis occurs.

When hypernatremia develops gradually, the incidence of hypertonic encephalopathy is greatly reduced, both in man and in experimental animals. This occurs because brain cells adapt to gradually developing hypernatremia by accumulating solutes intracellularly. The sum of brain Na^+, K^+, and Cl^- accounts for approximately 40 to 50 per cent of intracellular solutes; the remaining solutes include amino acids, myoinositol, betaine, and urea. Thus in chronic hypernatremia, the accumulation of idiogenic osmoles in the brain minimizes the extent of water loss and consequently brain shrinkage. This in turn reduces the frequency with which encephalopathy develops.

Posthypophysectomy Course. The acute diabetes insipidus following hypophysectomy has a characteristic triphasic response. For a few hours to days following the insult, there exists a polyuric, hyposthenuric phase that depends on inhibition of ADH release. Next, there follows a period with reduced urine volume and a rise in urine osmolality. During this phase, there is persistent release of ADH from atrophying neurons, an inability to excrete a water load, and the risk of progressive hypotonicity with continued parenteral administration of large volumes of hypotonic fluids. The final phase, if the diabetes insipidus becomes permanent, is marked by recurrence of polyuria and hyposthenuria.

LABORATORY MANIFESTATIONS. Persistent hyposthenuria, with urine specific gravity of 1.005 or less and urine osmolality less than 200 mOsm per kilogram of H_2O, is the hallmark of the diabetes insipidus syndromes. In euvolemic patients, the glomerular filtration rate (GFR) is normal. Since patients with diabetes insipidus ingest water in response to plasma hypertonicity, random plasma osmolality determinations in these patients will be, on the average, above the usual norm of 287 mOsm per kilogram of H_2O. The serum sodium concentrations are also elevated and account quantitatively for the increases in plasma osmolality. In contrast, persons with primary polydipsia have a primary aberration of the thirst mechanism and ingest water independent of physiologic stimuli. These patients often have mild dilutional hyponatremia.

In patients whose diabetes insipidus, either pituitary or nephrogenic in origin, begins in childhood, considerable dilation of the urinary bladder, ureters, and renal pelvis may occur. This dilation has led to a reduction in GFR in some patients.

DIAGNOSIS. Based on the underlying pathophysiology, the polyuric syndromes may be grouped into the following general categories: (1) pituitary diabetes insipidus, in which there is absence or diminished production and secretion of ADH; (2) solute diuresis, in which excessively high rates of solute delivery to the loop of Henle overwhelm quantitatively the ability of distal nephron segments to dissociate solute and water absorption; (3) nephrogenic diabetes insipidus, either familial or acquired, in which collecting duct cells are partially or completely unresponsive to ADH; (4) renal concentrating disorders, in which there is impaired generation of a hypertonic medullary interstitium by renal countercurrent multiplication and exchange processes; and (5) primary polydipsia, in which the ingestion of unusually large volumes of water results in polyuria, the appropriate physiologic response.

Disorders such as diabetes mellitus, which produces solute diuresis, are characterized by isotonic urine and by glycosuria. The history and laboratory data are adequate to identify disorders such as sickle cell disease or interstitial nephritis, both of which impair the ability to generate a hypertonic medullary interstitium. Routine laboratory screening readily identifies the presence of hypercalcemia or hypokalemia. Finally, congenital nephrogenic diabetes insipidus is identified by a history of having been present since birth, generally in males, and by *persistent* unresponsiveness to exogenous ADH. Acquired nephrogenic diabetes insipidus is recognized by ADH unresponsiveness combined with a history of exposure to agents, such as lithium, demeclocycline, or meth-oxyflurane anesthesia, which antagonize the action of ADH on collecting ducts.

The more difficult diagnostic problem is the differentiation of patients with partial or complete deficiency of ADH from those with primary polydipsia. Certain factors may point toward the most likely diagnosis. For example, a 24-hour urine volume greater than 18 liters, a random plasma osmolality determination below 285 mOsm per kilogram of H_2O, and a history of episodic polyuria all suggest compulsive water drinking as the underlying disorder. A history of head trauma or neoplasm, a history of sudden onset of unrelenting polyuria, and a random plasma osmolality determination greater than 290 mOsm per kilogram of H_2O all suggest pituitary diabetes insipidus.

The basis of all tests for pituitary diabetes insipidus rests on the ability of the kidney to excrete hypertonic urine after an osmotic stimulus. The simplest maneuver is to produce hypertonicity of body fluids by water deprivation. The absolute level of urine concentration achieved with water deprivation is nondiagnostic, since maximal concentrating ability depends on the degree of medullary hypertonicity as well as the presence of adequate amounts of ADH. For example, the maximal urine osmolality produced by water deprivation in a group of randomly selected hospitalized patients was found to be 764 mOsm per kilogram of H_2O as compared with 1067 mOsm per kilogram of H_2O in healthy volunteers. Presumably the lower value for maximal urine concentrating ability in hospitalized patients reflects a reduction in medullary interstitial hypertonicity with respect to that present in normal volunteers.

Even in patients with a reduced medullary interstitial tonicity, the maximal urine osmolality achieved with water deprivation depends on maximal degrees of endogenous ADH release in response to dehydration. Therefore, in those with intact mechanisms for ADH production and release, the administration of exogenous ADH will not produce an increase in the maximal urine osmolality achieved via water deprivation. This rationale forms the framework for a test scheme, illustrated in Figure 214–4, for distinguishing complete or partial pituitary diabetes insipidus from other polyuric syndromes.

In patients with mild polyuria, water deprivation may begin the night preceding the test; patients with severe polyuria should have water restricted during the day, to allow for close observation. The test begins with paired measurements of urine and plasma osmolality. All water intake is then withheld and hourly measurements of urine osmolality and body weight are made. When two sequential urine osmolalities vary by less than 30 mOsm per kilogram of H_2O, or when 3 to 5 per cent body weight is lost, 5 units of aqueous vasopressin is injected subcutaneously. A final urine osmolality is measured 60 minutes later.

The time required to achieve a maximal urine concentration varies from 4 to 18 hours. In normal persons, water deprivation results in urine osmolality two to four times greater than that of plasma. More important, the subsequent administration of ex-

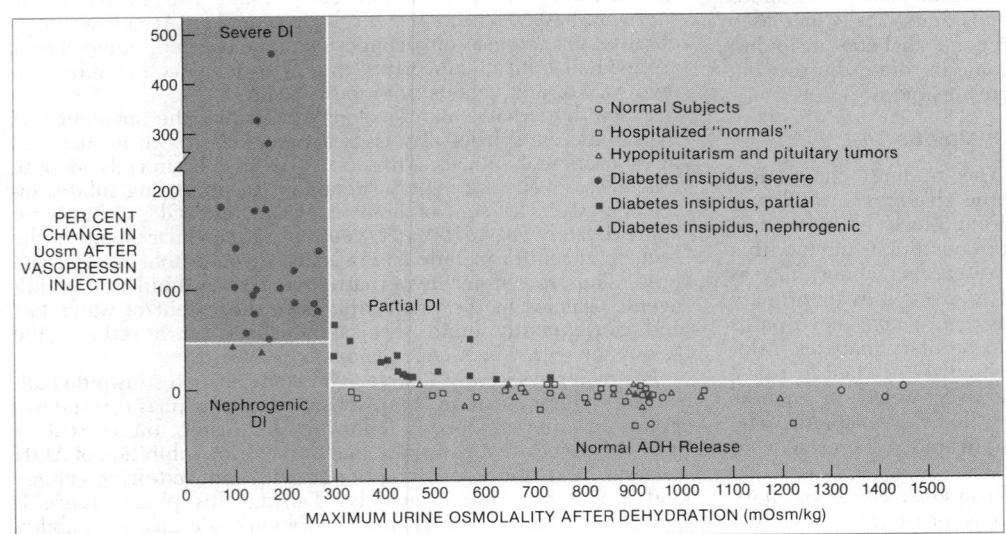

FIGURE 214–4. Maximal urine osmolality after dehydration versus the percentage change in urine osmolality induced by subsequent vasopressin injection. DI = Diabetes insipidus; ADH = antidiuretic hormone. (From Miller M, et al.: Ann Intern Med 73:721, 1970. Reprinted with permission of the publisher.)

ogenous ADH results in a less than 5 per cent further increase in urine osmolality. In patients with primary polydipsia, who have reduced medullary interstitial tonicity as a result of prolonged water diuresis, the urine may concentrate only slightly after water deprivation. However, they too will have stimulated endogenous ADH release maximally and will exhibit a less than 5 per cent rise in urine osmolality with supplemental ADH.

In patients with complete pituitary diabetes insipidus urine osmolality does not rise above that of plasma in response to water deprivation but shows a greater than 50 per cent increase in response to injection of ADH. In patients with partial pituitary diabetes insipidus the urine may concentrate to some degree in response to water deprivation, but urine osmolality also increases by at least 10 per cent after ADH injection. An interesting observation is that patients with partial pituitary diabetes insipidus often show a peak urine osmolality that decreases with further water restriction. This suggests a limited reserve of neurohypophyseal hormone that is depleted after an initial secretory burst. Finally, in patients with nephrogenic diabetes insipidus deprived of water, the urine osmolality fails to rise above that of plasma even when they are given exogenous ADH. When a diagnosis of pituitary diabetes insipidus is made, a careful evaluation for neoplasm involving the hypothalamus or neurohypophyseal tract is mandatory.

Levels of circulating vasopressin measured by radioimmunoassay have heretofore been available only for research purposes. A commercial assay is now marketed for clinical use, but its utility is, as of now, undefined. Hypertonic saline infusions have also been utilized to test for release of ADH. This procedure is hazardous in patients with limited cardiac reserve, in whom volume expansion may precipitate cardiac decompensation. Moreover, the results of the test are uninterpretable if the patient develops salt diuresis, thus fixing urine osmolality near isotonicity.

Nicotine, a nonosmotic stimulus to ADH secretion, has been used to elicit antidiuresis in those patients who have "essential hypernatremia," i.e., ADH release in response to volume contraction but not to hypertonicity. A better diagnostic approach in these patients is to assess the antidiuretic response to mild volume contraction.

TREATMENT. Patients with diabetes insipidus, either pituitary or nephrogenic, may require emergency treatment of hypertonic encephalopathy or maintenance therapy for polyuria.

Hypertonic Encephalopathy. The goal in treating this medical emergency is to replenish body water, thereby restoring osmotic balance and replenishing cell volume, at a rate that avoids significant complications. Since the brain adjusts to hypertonicity, at least in part, by increasing intracellular osmolar content, rapid repletion of body water with extracellular fluid dilution, causes translocation of water into cells to achieve osmotic equilibrium. The result of this water movement is cell swelling and cerebral edema. Seizures occur in up to 40 per cent of patients treated for severe hypernatremia by rapid infusions of hypotonic solutions. If water repletion is undertaken at a slower rate, brain cells lose the accumulated intracellular solutes and osmotic equilibration can occur without cell swelling. Consequently, a good rule of thumb is to administer fluids at a rate that reduces the serum sodium concentration to normal over a 36- to 48-hour period, or to reduce the serum sodium concentration by about 1 mEq per liter every 2 hours.

The choice of fluid to be administered in the diabetes insipidus syndromes depends in large part on three factors: the extent to which circulatory collapse may be present; the rate at which hypernatremia has developed; and the magnitude of hypernatremia. Hypotonic NaCl solutions are best used as initial therapy in patients with modest volume contraction and only modest elevations of serum sodium concentrations, that is, less than 160 mEq per liter. However, in more advanced cases of hypernatremia, particularly if the hypernatremia has developed gradually, that is, over a period greater than 24 hours, and is accompanied by signs of circulatory collapse, more prudent initial therapy is to administer normal saline solutions. The reasons for this choice are twofold: in advanced hypernatremia, a normal saline solution is dilute relative to the patient's body fluid osmolality and thus dilutes the latter while minimizing the risk of iatrogenic cerebral swelling; at the same time, the normal saline solution provides an effective means of volume expansion. Finally, 5 per cent glucose solutions may be used to replenish body water in acute hypernatremia without significant circulatory collapse. However, the glucose infusion rate must be less than the rate of glucose metabolism to avoid glycosuria. Otherwise, the resulting osmotic diuresis will thwart attempts to replenish body free water. The treatment of drug-induced nephrogenic diabetes insipidus consists of removal of the offending agent.

Polyuria. Patients with partial hormonal deficiency and volumes of urine output between 2 and 6 liters daily may require no treatment as long as they are assured access to water. Specific therapy for pituitary diabetes insipidus is some form of ADH replacement. A variety of hormone preparations are available which differ in the ratio of antidiuretic to vasopressor activity and the duration of biologic effect. These relations are depicted in Table 214–2.

Early preparations of dried posterior pituitary extract, termed pituitary snuff, were given by nasal insufflation, had an effective biologic life of only a few hours, and inevitably produced chronic rhinitis, which often led to inadequate absorption of hormone. Aqueous vasopressin injection, having an activity span of only a few hours, is not practical for long-term use. It is useful, however, for diagnostic testing or for acute management of polyuria following central nervous system trauma or surgery.

Nasal sprays of aqueous lysine vasopressin may provide intermittent relief of polyuria. Rhinitis, although not so severe as with dried extract, is also a frequent concomitant to this form of therapy.

The most widely used preparation has been Pitressin Tannate in Oil, which is given intramuscularly. As little as 0.5 ml per day may provide adequate hormone for 24 to 48 hours. Great care must be exercised in preparing the injection by careful warming and mixing of the ampule so as to suspend the pellet of hormone in the oil. Failure to do so may result in injection of the oil vehicle alone and apparent "vasopressin resistance." Pain at injection sites and sterile abscesses are frequent complaints with this preparation. Persistent abdominal pain from the effect of ADH on intestinal motility is a not uncommon problem.

A synthetic analogue of vasopressin, dDAVP (1-deamino,8-D-arginine vasopressin), provides antidiuretic activity for 8 to 20 hours with negligible pressor effect, can be taken as a nasal spray, and is the current drug of choice. The drug is best started at night to find the lowest dose that will prevent nocturia. This dose, usually 5 to 10 μg, can be given twice daily or doubled as a single morning dose. A nasal catheter is provided, which is measured for convenient dosing in the 5 to 24 μg range. Headache

TABLE 214–2. COMPARISON OF NEUROHYPOPHYSEAL HORMONES AND SYNTHETIC ANALOGUES

Preparation	Activity					Duration of Activity	Route of Administration
	Antidiuretic	:	Vasopressor	:	Oxytocic		
8-Arginine vasopressin							
Pitressin, aqueous	100	:	100	:	5	2–6 hours	Intravenous
Pitressin tannate in oil						24–48 hours	Intramuscular
8-Lysine vasopressin							
Lypressin	60	:	70	:	1	2–6 hours	Nasal insufflation
1-Deamino, 8-D-arginine vasopressin							
(dDAVP), desmopressin	290	:	0.14			6–20 hours	Nasal insufflation
Oxytocin	1	:	1	:	100		

may be a troublesome side effect with large doses but usually disappears with a reduction of dosage.

For patients having some residual ADH production, the oral hypoglycemic agent chlorpropamide may provide adequate amelioration of symptoms. This drug stimulates ADH secretion and augments the activity of residual ADH on the collecting duct. Doses of 250 to 500 mg daily are sufficient to reduce polyuria in most patients with partial pituitary diabetes insipidus, but the side effect of hypoglycemia limits the drug's usefulness.

Thiazide diuretics may reduce the volume of urine in patients with all forms of diabetes insipidus, that is, either pituitary or nephrogenic, by causing a state of mild salt depletion. This results in a secondary increase in isotonic proximal tubular fluid absorption and a decrease in the volume of fluid delivered to the collecting duct. The effect is produced by 50 to 100 mg of hydrochlorothiazide daily, is sustained even in the absence of diuretics by salt restriction, and can be abolished by salt loading even with continued diuretic administration.

Vasopressin infusions have also been used to treat bleeding esophageal varices by reducing splanchnic blood flow. Desmopressin, a synthetic analogue of arginine vasopressin, stimulates the production of clotting Factor VIII. These other actions are discussed elsewhere in this textbook.

Nephrogenic Diabetes Insipidus. The therapeutic considerations outlined above, particularly with respect to the treatment of hypertonic encephalopathy and to the value of a chronic mild salt-depleted state in minimizing polyuria, apply equally well to the care of patients with pituitary or nephrogenic diabetes insipidus. In patients with nephrogenic diabetes insipidus acquired as a consequence of drug therapy (for example, lithium or demeclocycline), the offending agent should be discontinued.

Finally, it is important to stress the need to minimize the extent of polyuria in children with congenital nephrogenic diabetes insipidus, since there is a close correlation between repeated bouts of dehydration during childhood and mental dullness in adulthood. Alternatively, in patients in whom episodes of dehydration have been minimal, both mental and physical growth retardation can be avoided.

Barlow ED, DeWardener HE: Compulsive water drinking. Q J Med 28:235, 1959. *A thorough examination of the clinical course and pathophysiology of urinary concentration in a group of patients with primary polydipsia.*
Bichet DG, Razi M, Arthus M-F, et al.: Epinephrine and dDAVP administration in patients with congenital nephrogenic diabetes insipidus. Evidence for a pre-cyclic AMP V_2 receptor defective mechanism. Kidney Int 36:859, 1989. *Analysis of the V_2 receptor defect in familial nephrogenic diabetes insipidus.*
Cunnah D, Ross G, Besser GM: Management of cranial diabetes insipidus with oral desmopressin (dDAVP). Clin Endocrinol 24:253, 1986. *The use of dDAVP in pituitary diabetes insipidus.*
Knoers N, van der Heyden H, van Oost BA, et al.: Three-point linkage analysis using multiple DNA polymorphic markers in families with X-linked nephrogenic diabetes insipidus. Genomics 4:434, 1989. *Linkage analysis in familial nephrogenic diabetes insipidus.*
Miller M, Dalakos T, Moses AM, et al.: Recognition of partial defects in antidiuretic hormone secretion. Ann Intern Med 72:721, 1970. *A concise guide to testing procedures for states of ADH insufficiency and a rational scheme for interpreting the test results.*
Reeves WB, Andreoli TE: The posterior pituitary and water metabolism. In Foster DW, Wilson JD (eds.): Williams Textbook of Endocrinology, 8th ed. Philadelphia, W. B. Saunders Company, 1991. *A full review of the polyuric syndromes, their differential diagnosis and treatment; extensively referenced.*

THE SYNDROME OF INAPPROPRIATE ADH PRODUCTION (SIADH)

For convenience SIADH has been discussed in Ch. 75 as a major disorder producing hyponatremia.

OXYTOCIN

Oxytocin is produced in the same hypothalamic nuclei and by the same synthetic mechanism as vasopressin. AVP and oxytocin are produced in both the paraventricular and the supraoptic nuclei of the hypothalamus. However, a given neuron in these nuclei produces only one hormone. Neurophysin I is the specific carrier protein synthesized with oxytocin and has been used as a marker for oxytocin release.

PHYSIOLOGY. The primary stimuli for oxytocin secretion are nipple stimulation (suckling) and deformation of the reproductive tract (especially the vagina) in females and muscular contraction of the reproductive organs in the male. The neural arcs serving these stimuli are not well defined, but some evidence suggests that the final synaptic transmitter is dopamine. Estrogens appear to influence secretion directly, based on observations of increased neurophysin I in blood during estrogen peaks of the menstrual cycle, or permissively, based on findings of a graded response to vaginal distension over the period of a menstrual cycle and an enhanced response with exogenous estradiol. Progesterones inhibit response to mechanical stimuli. Hypertonicity of body fluids also appears to cause oxytocin secretion. For example, in congenitally vasopressin-deficient Brattleboro rats, hypertonicity causes degranulation of the neurohypophysis, indicating sustained secretion of oxytocin, a relatively weak antidiuretic principle. Finally, relaxin, an ovarian peptide that suppresses uterine contraction and relaxes pelvic connective tissue during parturition, suppresses oxytocin release.

BIOLOGIC ACTIVITY. In females, oxytocin initiates its primary effect by binding to specific myometrial receptors, the affinity of which increases strikingly in the presence of estrogen. Exogenously administered oxytocin elicits contractions of the fundus indistinguishable from those of labor. However, the initiation of labor is apparently oxytocin independent, with increasing secretions seen only with dilation of the birth canal. Oxytocin may play a key role in final expulsion of the fetus and placenta. The total absence of oxytocin does not prevent parturition, although prolonged labor is seen in such women. The cellular events leading to uterine contraction are unknown but parallel an oxytocin-induced increase in ion permeability with depolarization of the myometrial cell membrane.

The milk-ejection reflex is also mediated via oxytocin. Contraction of mammary myoepithelium is stimulated, leading to a rise in intramammary pressure and expulsion of milk from alveolar channels to large sinuses, where it is accessible to the suckling infant. A true galactogenic effect of oxytocin leading to increased milk production has not been convincingly demonstrated. Absence of oxytocin abolishes the milk-ejection reflex.

In the male, oxytocin increases ejection of sperm into the semen in response to stimulation of the reproductive organs. Oxytocin retains some antidiuretic activity, about 1 per cent that of AVP, but exerts no significant antidiuretic effect at physiologic levels of secretion. Vascular smooth muscle is relaxed by oxytocin, causing a decrease in blood pressure, cutaneous flushing, and increased limb blood flow. Reflex tachycardia and sympathetic responses quickly restore hemodynamics to normal except when such reflexes are rendered inactive as in deep anesthesia.

THERAPEUTIC USE. The primary use of oxytocin (Pitocin) is to induce or to improve the quality of labor. The uterus is relatively resistant to oxytocin in early pregnancy, but infusions given with hypertonic saline injections may speed abortions of later pregnancy.

With long-term infusion of oxytocin, patients may experience sufficient antidiuretic effects to be at risk of water intoxication. Antidiuresis may be detected at oxytocin infusion rates of 15 mU per minute, and maximal urinary concentration is usually attained at rates of 45 mU per minute. Infusions for delivery and control of postpartum uterine hemorrhage may reach 20 to 40 mU per minute, and infusions for therapeutic abortions range from 20 to 100 mU per minute.

Feeney JG: Water intoxication and oxytocin. Br Med J 285:243, 1982. *An account of water intoxication following oxytocin administration.*
Roberts JS: Oxytocin, Vol I. Montreal, Eden Press, 1977. *This review covers the extensive work in oxytocin physiology and chemistry; very readable and fully referenced.*

215 The Pineal Gland

Alfred J. Lewy

The mammalian pineal is located in the "center" of the brain (above the quadrigeminal plate, just behind the posterior commissure) but is actually outside of the "blood-brain barrier." Postganglionic neurons from the superior cervical ganglia release norepinephrine, which in turn stimulates β_1-adrenergic receptors on the pinealocytes (Fig. 215–1). This results in the synthesis and release into the CSF and venous circulation of melatonin, the principal putative hormone of the pineal gland. The (paired) suprachiasmatic nuclei are the source of an approximately 24-hour rhythm in melatonin production that persists in conditions of constant darkness or blindness. Photic input, conveyed to the suprachiasmatic nuclei (SCN) via the retinohypothalamic tracts, synchronizes (entrains) the SCN and its output circadian rhythms to the 24-hour light-dark cycle. Between the SCN and the cell bodies of the preganglionic sympathetic neurons in the spinal cord, there are synapses in the paraventricular nuclei.

Melatonin production by the human pineal is decreased by β-blockers and α_2 agonists and is increased by certain tricyclic antidepressants that block reuptake of norepinephrine. Melatonin production is also increased by extreme physical exercise, norepinephrine, and psoralen. In general, diet and activity have no effect. Increased melatonin in manic states and decreased melatonin in depression probably occur but most likely represent epiphenomena following changes in adrenergic activity.

FUNCTION OF MELATONIN

The function of melatonin in humans remains elusive. In some fish and reptiles melatonin coalesces melanin-containing melanosomes and in this way causes blanching, but this effect has been lost in most animals. Melatonin may possibly have this effect on the mammalian retinal pigmented epithelium. The association of pineal tumors with disorders of puberty is most

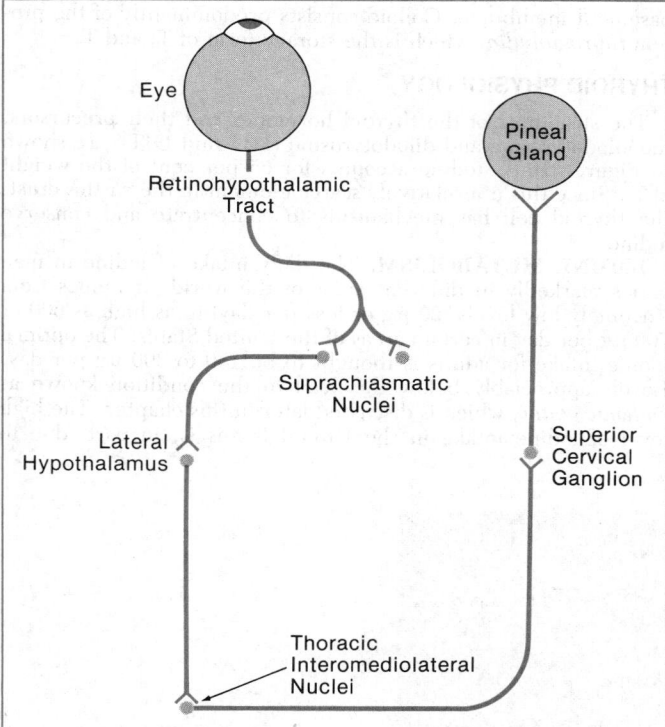

FIGURE 215–1. Schematic diagram for the neuroanatomic regulation of the timing of mammalian melatonin production. Norepinephrine, released by postganglionic sympathetic neurons, stimulates β_1-adrenergic receptors on the pinealocytes, resulting in a sequence of biochemical events which culminates in the synthesis and activation of N-acetyltransferase (the rate-limiting enzymatic step in the synthesis of melatonin and its precursor, N-acetylserotonin) and the release of melatonin into the CSF and venous circulation. The (paired) suprachiasmatic nuclei (SCN) are the source of an approximately 24-hour rhythm in melatonin production that persists in conditions of constant darkness or blindness. Photic input, conveyed to the SCN via the retinohypothalamic tracts, synchronizes (entrains) the SCN and its output circadian rhythms to the 24-hour light-dark cycle. Between the SCN and the cell bodies of the preganglionic sympathetic neurons in the spinal cord, there are synapses located in the paraventricular nuclei of the lateral hypothalamus. (Adapted by permission of the publisher from "Biochemistry and regulation of mammalian melatonin production" by AJ Lewy, in *The Pineal Gland*, edited by RM Relkin, pp 77–128. Copyright 1983 by Elsevier Science Publishing Co., Inc.)

likely explained by compression of the hypothalamus, since no melatonin-secreting tumor has yet been found. Furthermore, it now appears that the main effect of melatonin on the reproductive system lies in its ability to communicate the time of the year to animals that are seasonal breeders. In such animals it can have either anti- or progonadal activity depending on whether the species is a spring or fall breeder, respectively. Reproductive and endocrine effects of exogenous melatonin administration, not to mention endogenous melatonin secretion, have not been well documented in humans.

CHRONOBIOLOGY OF MELATONIN

Melatonin is produced only during nighttime darkness in both diurnal and nocturnal animals with an approximately 12-hour "on" phase and a 12-hour "off" phase. These phases persist even in constant darkness, although several days in constant darkness cause the melatonin rhythm to free run, beating in and out of phase with the sleep-wake cycle. Many blind people with a complete absence of light perception have free-running endogenous circadian rhythms. When these individuals are out of phase with their sleep-wake cycles (which have remained more or less synchronized to clock time), they are symptomatic (nighttime insomnia and daytime sleepiness). A pattern of insomnia that recurs every few weeks is almost pathognomonic for free-running circadian rhythms in totally blind individuals.

Darkness does not induce melatonin production. In sighted people, exposure to sufficiently bright light during the night immediately suppresses melatonin production. Two models have been proposed to explain how the nightly melatonin profile is shaped. In the *two-pacemaker model*, it is hypothesized that separate endogenous pacemakers control the onset and offset of melatonin production, cued primarily to dusk and dawn, respectively. In the *"clock-gate" model*, the suppressant effect of light (probably unique to melatonin) participates in the shortening of the duration of nighttime melatonin production during long photoperiods. Both models attempt to explain the shorter duration of melatonin secretion during the briefer summer nights compared to the longer winter nights.

The changing duration of nighttime melatonin secretion during the calendar year seems to be responsible for the reproductive effects of the light-dark cycle in seasonal breeders. Seasonal rhythms have not been well documented in humans, but it is clear that humans have most, if not all, of the circadian rhythms found in other higher animals. Whereas seasonal rhythms respond to the duration of the photoperiod or scotoperiod, circadian rhythms respond to the 24-hour light-dark cycle. In animals, the light-dark cycle's phase-shifting effects on circadian rhythms can be described by a phase response curve (PRC). This appears to be the case in humans as well. The PRC can be explained in the following way. Delay responses (shifts to a later time) result when exposure to light occurs during the first part of the night; advance responses (shifts to an earlier time) result when the exposure occurs during the latter part of the night. These phase shifts are greatest in magnitude in the middle of the night and are least during the middle of the day.

Although the suppressant effect of light is probably unique to melatonin, phase-shifting by light affects the endogenous circadian pacemaker (SCN) and all of its driven rhythms. In fact, the timing of the SCN's circadian rhythms is best measured by the circulating levels of melatonin. In some species injections of exogenous melatonin are capable of causing phase shifts and/or entrainment. In some instances, a PRC for melatonin has been described that is more or less the opposite of the PRC for light; that is, the melatonin PRC resembles a dark-pulse PRC. In humans, orally administered melatonin appears to have circadian phase-shifting effects, which can be described by a PRC that resembles a dark-pulse PRC. Thus, melatonin—which is produced only during the night—may be the chemical messenger of darkness. Therefore, human melatonin production may normally have a role, however small, in the entrainment of the SCN's circadian rhythms. Not being seasonal breeders, perhaps humans have retained the suppressant effect of light in order to use endogenous melatonin to more effectively augment entrainment and phase-shifting effects of the light-dark cycle. The melatonin PRC may also provide the rationale for precise scheduling of exogenous melatonin administration for therapeutic purposes, such as to treat chronobiologic sleep and mood disorders and to facilitate adaptation to shift work and air travel.

PINEAL TUMORS

Four main types of tumors arise that are usually malignant in the pineal: (1) pineoblastomas or pineocytomas, the term used depending on the degree of differentiation of this tumor of the pineal parenchyma, (2) germinomas, (3) embryonal carcinomas, and (4) glial tumors. Invasion of the pineal by cysts has also been reported. Destruction of pineal tissue can reduce or even ablate melatonin production, but increased circulating levels of melatonin have not been conclusively associated with pineocytomas. Melatonin production decreases with age, but this does not seem to be related to pineal calcification. By occluding the cerebral aqueduct, pineal tumors can produce symptoms associated with increased intracranial pressure, sometimes necessitating a shunt. Through pressure on the quadrigeminal plate, pineal tumors can produce Parinaud's syndrome, which includes paresis of upward conjugate gaze. Some germinomas and embryonal carcinomas secrete human chorionic gonadotropin, which has been implicated in cases of delayed onset of puberty. Treatment modalities include surgical extirpation, radiation, and chemotherapy, depending on tumor type and location and the absence or degree of metastases.

Lewy AJ, Sack RL, Singer CM, et al.: Winter depression and the phase shift hypothesis for bright light's therapeutic effects: History, theory and experimental evidence. J Biol Rhythms 3:121, 1988.
Lewy AJ, Wehr TA, Goodwin FK, et al.: Light suppresses melatonin secretion in humans. Science 210:1267, 1980.
Neuwelt EA (ed.): Diagnosis and Treatment of Pineal Region Tumors. Baltimore, Williams & Wilkins, 1984.
Reiter RJ: The pineal gland. In DeGroot LJ, Besser GM, Cahill GF Jr (eds.): Endocrinology, 2nd ed. Philadelphia, W. B. Saunders Company, 1989, pp 240–253.
Relkin R (ed.): The Pineal Gland. New York, Elsevier Biomedical, 1983.

216 The Thyroid

P. Reed Larsen

The thyroid gland secretes thyroxine, 3,5,3',5'-tetraiodothyronine (abbreviated T_4) and small amounts of 3,5,3'-triiodothyronine (abbreviated T_3). The principal role of these substances is to regulate tissue metabolism. In infants, adequate supplies of thyroid hormone are necessary for the development of the normal central nervous system in the first 1 to 2 years of life. The absence of thyroid hormone during this period results in irreversible mental retardation, a syndrome known as *cretinism*. The hormone is also required for normal growth and bone maturation in children. Despite these important functions, the body can withstand marked reductions in thyroid hormone for long periods, although at the cost of abnormal function of many organ systems.

EMBRYOLOGY AND ANATOMY

The thyroid develops from a combination of pharyngeal midline and bilateral primitive tissues from the fourth branchial pouch. These primitive thyroid cells migrate from the pharyngeal floor, leaving behind a residual thyroglossal duct that normally becomes obliterated. The major portion of the thyroid cell mass is derived from the median mid-pharyngeal tissue. The lateral thyroid anlagen migrate medially to fuse with median-derived thyroid tissue, but primarily contribute the *parafollicular* or *C cells*. The C cells secrete calcitonin, not thyroid hormone, and do not play a role in thyroid physiology (see Ch. 236). The evolution of thyroid function occurs over the first 10 to 12 weeks of fetal life, with definite appearance of T_4 in the gland by 10 to 11 weeks. The placenta is impermeable to T_3 and T_4; the fetus depends on its own thyroid for its supply of these hormones. The adult size (15 to 20 grams) of the thyroid is reached at about age 15. The thyroid gland has the configuration of a butterfly, with the two lobes measuring about 5 × 2 cm. The lobes are composed of spherical structures called *follicles*, consisting of *colloid* surrounded by a single layer of epithelial cells enclosed by a basement membrane. Colloid consists predominantly of the protein *thyroglobulin*, which is the storage form of T_4 and T_3.

THYROID PHYSIOLOGY

The structures of the thyroid hormones and their precursors, monoiodotyrosine and diiodotyrosine (MIT and DIT), are shown in Figure 216–1. Iodine accounts for 65 per cent of the weight of T_4. Since this is a relatively scarce element in the earth's crust, the thyroid cell has mechanisms to concentrate and conserve iodine.

IODINE METABOLISM. The daily intake of iodine in man varies markedly in different areas of the world. It ranges from extremely low levels (20 μg or less per day) to as high as 600 or 700 μg per day in certain areas of the United States. The optimal iodine intake for adults is thought to be 150 to 300 μg per day. Levels appreciably below this lead to the condition known as *endemic goiter*, which is discussed later in this chapter. The high level of iodine intake in the United States is, in part, due to

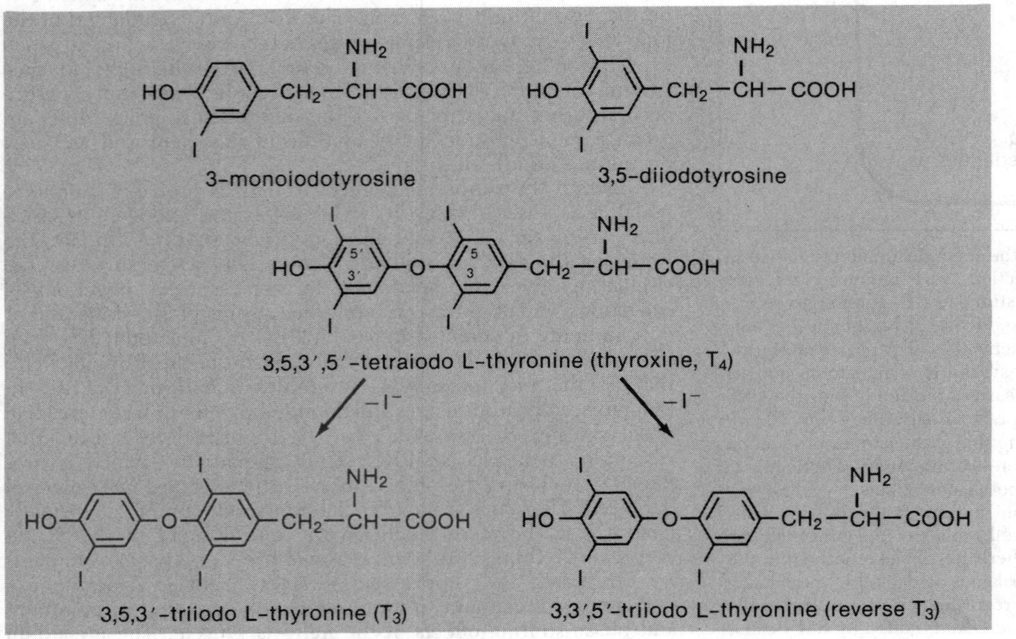

FIGURE 216–1. Structure of the thyroid hormones and their precursors.

iodination of salt. Iodine in all forms is reduced to iodide (I^-) in the gastrointestinal tract and absorbed within 30 minutes of ingestion. I^- leaves the blood via two mechanisms. It is concentrated by the thyroid or excreted in the urine. There is a wide variation in the fraction of I^- concentrated by the thyroid per 24 hours, depending on iodine uptake. In the United States, iodine uptake by the thyroid varies from about 5 to 30 per cent.

INTRATHYROIDAL IODIDE METABOLISM. In Figure 216-2 are shown the steps involved in the synthesis of the thyroid hormones. Because the concentrations of I^- in the plasma are so low, the thyroid cell concentrates I^-, the cell-plasma ratio being about 20 to 40:1. The trapped I^- is rapidly oxidized and incorporated into protein. As a consequence, there is little I^- per se in the thyroid gland. The process of I^- oxidation and its incorporation into tyrosine is known as *organification*. The substrate for iodine is the 660,000 molecular weight glycoprotein thyroglobulin. Only about 25 per cent of the tyrosine residues of this specialized protein are available for iodination. Both MIT and DIT are formed. In a typical molecule of fully iodinated human thyroglobulin, there are approximately 6 to 7 residues of MIT, 4 to 5 of DIT, 3 to 4 of T_4, and 0.2 to 0.3 of T_3. The T_4 and T_3 arise from the coupling of either 2 DIT residues or 1 MIT and 1 DIT residue, a reaction that requires thyroid peroxidase. This process is known as *coupling*. Both organification and coupling are inhibited by *thiourea compounds*, which are used in the treatment of patients with hyperthyroidism (see below). The thyroglobulin is iodinated at the apical border of the cell and is then exocytosed into the colloid. Under normal circumstances, T_4 and T_3 secretion occurs from this pool. The thyroid secretory process starts with phagocytosis of thyroglobulin by the apical cell membrane, leading to the formation of a *colloid droplet*. This is combined with a lysosome, and as the colloid droplet traverses the thyroid cell, proteolysis occurs with eventual release of T_4 and T_3 at the basal cell border. Deiodination of T_4 to T_3 also occurs during this process, resulting in a ratio of T_4 to T_3 in thyroid secretion that is somewhat less than the 15:1 value found in the thyroglobulin itself. To conserve iodine for reuse in the thyroid cell, a *deiodinase* is present that removes the iodine from MIT and DIT, allowing it to recycle.

CIRCULATING T_4 AND T_3. Thyroid hormones in plasma exist in two forms, free and protein bound. Although only about 0.02 per cent of total plasma T_4 and 0.3 per cent of plasma T_3 are free, it is the free hormone concentration that is maintained constant by the feedback regulatory system and that appears to parallel the rate of cellular uptake of these hormones. It is, therefore, the free hormone concentration that determines the thyroid status irrespective of the total plasma concentration. In the euthyroid person the total hormone is determined by the quantity and affinity of certain thyroid hormone–binding proteins, which are *thyroxine-binding globulin* (TBG), transthyretin (formerly termed thyroxine-binding prealbumin), and albumin. TBG is by far the most important of these, transporting about 75 per cent of serum T_4 and T_3. It is a glycoprotein, with a molecular weight of 55,000, which is synthesized in the liver. TBG has a high affinity for both T_4 and T_3, although the affinity for T_4 is about 10- to 15-fold higher than that for T_3. There is normally sufficient TBG in serum to bind approximately 20 μg of T_4 per deciliter at a molar ratio of 1:1. The serum TBG concentrations change under many circumstances, which are listed in Table 216-1. It is important to recognize these conditions, since the resultant changes in total T_4 and T_3 may duplicate abnormalities that are found in patients with thyroid dysfunction. For example, during pregnancy, serum total T_4 and T_3 are increased but serum free T_4 and T_3 concentrations remain constant. The relationships are described in the following equation:

$$[\text{TH}] \text{ is proportional to } \frac{[\text{TH-TBG}]}{[\text{TBG}]}$$

where TH = free T_4 or T_3, [TH-TBG] = TBG-bound T_4 or T_3, and TBG = unoccupied TBG. When [TBG] increases, the bound hormone also increases until a new steady state is achieved at which [TH] is again normal. This occurs through both decreased metabolism and increased secretion of T_4 and T_3. To interpret a total serum T_4 or T_3 measurement accurately it is necessary to know the fraction of the hormone that is free; alternatively the free hormone can be measured directly or estimated (see Direct Tests of Thyroid Function later in this chapter). Certain compounds compete with T_4 and T_3 for binding to TBG. Two such drugs are salicylates and phenytoin. About a 20 to 30 per cent reduction in serum T_4 and T_3 is observed when 300 mg of phenytoin or salicylates in excess of 2 grams per day are given.

KINETICS OF T_4 AND T_3. Deiodination of the iodothyronines is the most significant metabolic transformation of the thyroid hormones. In the case of T_4, deiodination of the distal ring, occurring predominantly in liver and kidney, gives rise to T_3, which has approximately three to four times the metabolic potency of the parent hormone (Fig. 216-1). About 30 to 40 per cent of the 80 μg of T_4 produced per day is metabolized via this pathway (Table 216-2), giving rise to about 80 per cent of the T_3 produced daily. Loss of an iodine in the proximal ring of T_4 leads to formation of *reverse T_3* (3,3′,5′-triiodothyronine), a compound that appears to have no metabolic effect. About 40 per cent of T_4

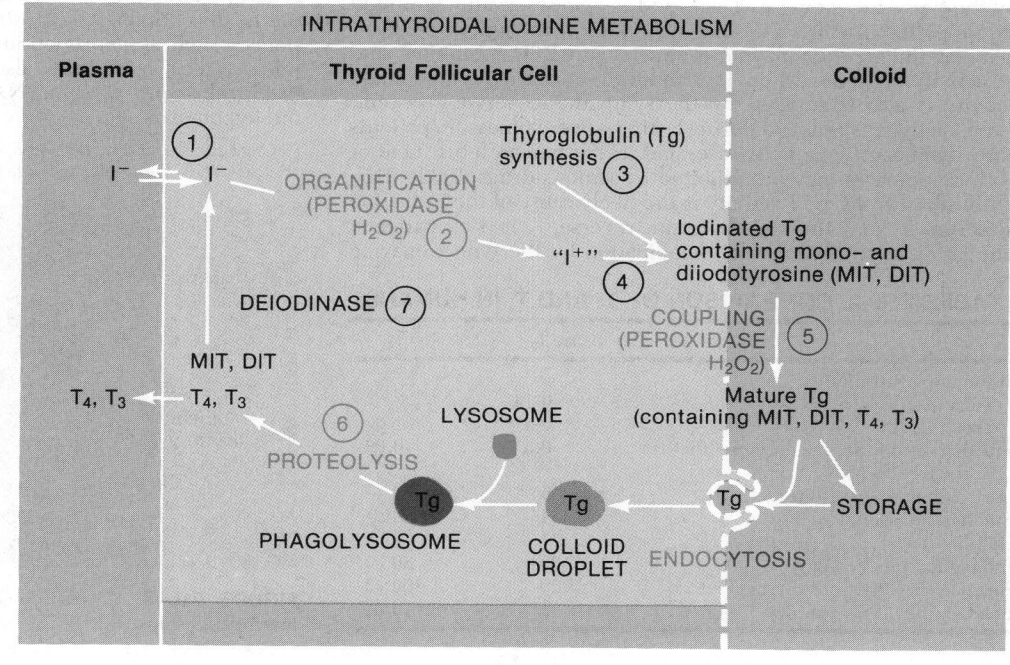

FIGURE 216-2. Principal steps in the synthesis and secretion of thyroid hormones. MIT = Monoiodotyrosine; DIT = diiodotyrosine. The steps denoted by the numbers are those in which defects have been identified in patients with inherited abnormalities in thyroid hormone biosynthesis (see Sporadic and Endemic Goiter, later in this chapter).

TABLE 216–1. CIRCUMSTANCES ASSOCIATED WITH CHANGES IN THE CIRCULATING CONCENTRATION OF THYROXINE-BINDING GLOBULIN (TBG)

Increased TBG
1. Pregnancy
2. Treatment with supraphysiologic amounts of estrogens, including oral contraceptives
3. In some patients with cirrhosis or acute hepatitis
4. As a congenital abnormality
5. In acute intermittent porphyria
6. After administration of heroin, methadone
7. After administration of clofibrate

Decreased TBG
1. Protein malnutrition, hepatic failure, chronic illness
2. Nephrotic syndrome
3. After administration of L-asparaginase
4. As a congenital abnormality (usually X-linked)
5. During treatment with androgenic steroids or pharmacologic doses of glucocorticoids

is metabolized via this pathway, the remainder being excreted via the biliary tract into the feces following conjugation with glucuronide. T_3 and reverse T_3 are, in turn, deiodinated in both proximal and distal rings, giving rise to the predicted monoiodothyronines and diiodothyronines, none of which has physiologic effects. T_4 to T_3 conversion and reverse T_3 deiodination appear to be catalyzed by the same enzyme. If this reaction is inhibited, as it is under diverse circumstances, a reduction in serum T_3 and an increase in the serum reverse T_3 concentrations occur.

The differences between T_3 and T_4 in terms of distribution volume, the intracellular fraction, and half-life can be attributed principally to the differences in the affinities of these two hormones for the plasma-binding proteins (Table 216–2). The higher intracellular T_3 content explains in part its higher potency relative to T_4. Given the 3 to 4:1 ratio of metabolic potency of T_3 and T_4 and the fact that approximately one third of T_4 is converted to T_3, it appears that T_4 has little intrinsic metabolic activity in man.

REGULATION OF T_4 TO T_3 CONVERSION. Two classes of enzymes convert T_4 to T_3 (iodothyronine 5'-deiodinases). One of these (type I), most active in liver and kidney, provides the bulk of the T_3 to the plasma pool. Plasma T_3 is the source of most of the intracellular T_3 for the liver, kidney, heart, and skeletal muscle. A second enzyme (type II), present in the central nervous system, pituitary, brown adipose tissue (BAT), and placenta, selectively provides T_3 to the cells of these tissues. For example, about 80 per cent of intracellular T_3 in cerebral cortex and 50 to 60 per cent of T_3 in the anterior pituitary or BAT are provided by the type II deiodinase. The type I enzyme is readily inhibited by propylthiouracil (PTU) and decreases with hypothyroidism, whereas the type II enzyme is resistant to PTU inhibition, and its activity increases when T_4 is reduced. In BAT the deiodinase activity is also stimulated by the sympathetic nervous system. Type I activity is reduced during fasting, severe illness, in patients with significant hepatic disease, and in the human fetus. One or both deiodinases may be inhibited by various drugs (Table 216–3). Inhibition of type I activity is the likely cause of the reduction in serum T_3 and the rise in serum reverse T_3 in sick patients. The latter occurs because 5'-deiodination by the type I enzyme

TABLE 216–2. COMPARISON OF T_3 AND T_4 IN HUMANS

	T_3	T_4
Serum concentration		
Total (µg/dl)	0.14	8
Free (ng/dl)	0.4	1.6
Fraction of total serum hormone that is in the free form (%)	0.3	0.02
Distribution volume (liters)	35	10
Fraction intracellular (%)	64	10–20
Half-life (days)	1	7
Production rate (µg/day)	33	80
Fraction directly from thyroid (%)	20	100
Relative metabolic potency	1	0.3

TABLE 216–3. DRUGS THAT CAN INFLUENCE THYROID FUNCTION OR ALTER TEST RESULTS

Type of Effect	Common Examples
Suppress TSH secretion	Dopamine, L-dopa, glucocorticoid excess
Inhibit thyroid hormone synthesis or release	Iodide, lithium carbonate, phenylbutazone, sulfonylureas
Decrease hormone-protein binding	Salicylates, phenytoin, fenclofenac, furosemide
Inhibit T_4 to T_3 conversion	
Type I 5'-deiodinase	Propylthiouracil, not methimazole (Tapazole)
	Propranolol (not other β-adrenergic antagonists)
	Glucocorticoid excess
Types I and II 5'-deiodinase	Amiodarone (Cordarone), Iopanoic acid (Telepaque), ipodate (Oragrafin)

is a rate-limiting step in reverse T_3 degradation. The increase in type II activity during hypothyroxinemia acts as a homeostatic mechanism to maintain normal intracellular T_3 concentrations in certain tissues when T_4 production is reduced. The capacity for PTU and glucocorticoid to inhibit type I activity is important in short-term treatment of severe hyperthyroidism.

MECHANISM OF ACTION OF THYROID HORMONE. Thyroid hormone regulation of protein synthesis occurs through effects on gene transcription and messenger RNA stabilization. A DNA- and T_3-binding nucleoprotein, the T_3 receptor, has about tenfold higher affinity for T_3 than for T_4, explaining in part why T_3 is the active hormone. There are two genes coding for similar thyroid hormone receptor proteins, which are both members of the erb A-related hormone receptor superfamily. Effects of thyroid hormone in many tissues can be related to the degree of saturation of these receptors by T_3. Other direct effects of thyroid hormone at the cell membrane or mitochondria may also occur. The regulation of the type II deiodinase by T_4 does not require protein synthesis, but the mechanism for this action is not understood.

REGULATION OF THYROID FUNCTION. The feedback loop for regulation of thyroid function is presented in Figure 216–3. *Thyrotropin-releasing hormone* (TRH) is secreted by hypothalamic cells and stimulates synthesis and release of thyrotropin (TSH, thyroid-stimulating hormone). This hormone in turn stimulates all of the steps involved in thyroid hormone synthesis and release through activation of adenylate cyclase. T_4 and smaller amounts of T_3 are released from the gland with monodeiodination of T_4 to T_3 in liver and kidney. Both serum T_3 and T_4 (via its intrapituitary conversion to T_3) suppress the synthesis and release of TSH competing with TRH to complete the feedback loop. *Somatostatin* (SRIF) and possibly other substances such as neuropeptides and dopamine also inhibit TSH release (see Ch. 212). T_3 also has a direct suppressive effect on the level of pro TRH mRNA in the paraventricular nucleus of the hypothalamus.

DeGroot LJ, Larsen PR, Refetoff S, et al.: The Thyroid and Its Diseases, 5th ed. New York, John Wiley & Sons, 1984. *A basic text.*

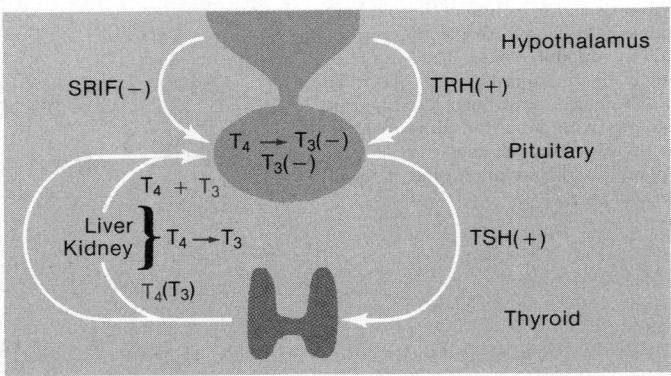

FIGURE 216–3. Current concepts of hypothalamic-pituitary-thyroid interrelationships.

Ingbar SH, Braverman LE: *In* Werner's The Thyroid, 5th ed. Philadelphia, J. B. Lippincott Company, 1986. *A basic text.*

Kaplan MM, Larsen PR (eds.): Symposium on thyroid disease. Med Clin North Am 69:847, 1985. *This issue contains chapters directed at the most important clinical aspects of thyroid disease authored by experts in their respective fields.*

Larsen PR: Feedback regulation of thyrotropin secretion by hormones. N Engl J Med 306:23, 1982. *A detailed, but clinically oriented, discussion of the feedback regulation of TSH secretion by thyroid hormones.*

Sakurai A, Takeda K, Ain K, et al.: Generalized resistance to thyroid hormone associated with a mutation in the ligand-binding domain of the human thyroid hormone receptor β. Proc Natl Acad Sci USA 86:8977, 1989. *Evidence that thyroid hormone resistance is caused by point mutations in the human gene coding for the β form of the thyroid hormone receptor.*

TESTING FOR SUSPECTED THYROID DYSFUNCTION

The thyroid gland is unique among the endocrine organs in that symptoms may arise from two general types of problems. Hyperfunction of the thyroid (*hyperthyroidism* or *thyrotoxicosis*) or decreased secretion of thyroid hormone (*hypothyroidism* or *myxedema*) may cause the patient to seek medical help. Alternatively, physical enlargement of the thyroid (*goiter*) may cause respiratory embarrassment or dysphagia or, more commonly, cosmetic abnormalities. Goiter may exist in the absence of any functional abnormality. Although the most severe forms are dramatic and unmistakable, milder degrees of thyroid dysfunction lead to many symptoms that are nonspecific, requiring biochemical tests for diagnostic confirmation.

PHYSICAL EXAMINATION OF THE THYROID

The high prevalence of thyroid disease, particularly in the female (5 to 10 per cent), makes a careful examination of the thyroid gland an important part of the general physical examination. Thyroid enlargement may be the first clue to thyroid functional abnormalities in a patient with otherwise nonspecific symptoms. A cup of water is a necessity, and the patient should first be asked to swallow with the neck moderately extended while the anterior area of the neck is inspected. Significant thyroid enlargement and thyroid nodules can often be discerned by this maneuver. The position of the trachea should then be determined, followed by palpation of the thyroid. The isthmus of the thyroid is first identified and is usually found just inferior to the cricoid cartilage. The left and right thumbs are then employed in turn to palpate the left and right lobe of the gland as the patient swallows. The normal thyroid gland is palpable in a large proportion of younger persons, although in the elderly patient it is not surprising to find the cricoid cartilage at or below the sternal notch. The pyramidal lobe, a small cylinder of tissue extending vertically from the isthmus to the thyroid cartilage to the left or right of the midline, can often be palpated as well.

DIRECT TESTS OF THYROID FUNCTION

MEASUREMENT OF TOTAL SERUM THYROID HORMONE CONCENTRATIONS. Serum T_4 and T_3 are both readily quantitated by specific radioimmunoassays that require 200 μl or less of serum. Typical normal ranges for the total T_4 and T_3 concentrations are presented in Table 216–4, as well as the values in patients with alterations in TBG and in those with thyroid dysfunction.

SERUM FREE T_4 AND T_3 AND THE FREE T_4 INDEX. Since the concentration of free, rather than total, thyroid hormones parallels the thyroid status, the ideal thyroid function test

TABLE 216–4. SERUM THYROID HORMONE CONCENTRATIONS IN NORMAL PERSONS AND PATIENTS WITH THYROID DISEASE

	Serum T_4 (μg/dl)		Serum T_3 (ng/dl)	
	Mean	*Range*	*Mean*	*Range*
Euthyroid				
Normal TBG	8	5–11	140	80–220
Increased TBG	12	8–20	190	120–320
Reduced TBG	2	<1–5	60	20–100
Infants				
Cord serum	11	8–15	48	20–80
Age 6 weeks	10	7–14	163	120–220
Hyperthyroidism	21	8–35	480	200–1600
Hypothyroidism	2	<1–5	50	<20–150

would be the direct determination of free thyroid hormones. The absolute serum free T_4 and T_3 can be measured either by immunoassay of a dialysate of human serum or by estimating the dialyzable (free) fraction of T_3 and T_4, multiplying this by the total hormone concentration (see Table 216–2). In patients who have abnormal total T_4 and T_3 concentrations caused by changes in serum TBG concentration but who are euthyroid, the free hormone concentrations are normal. Unfortunately, such determinations are time consuming.

An indirect estimate of the free fraction of T_4 and T_3 can be obtained by estimating the thyroid hormone–binding ratio (THBR). These tests, formerly termed T_3 or T_4 uptake tests, are performed by analyzing the distribution of tagged T_3 or T_4 in a sample of dilute serum. A common method has been to add charcoal or resin to this sample and quantitate the fraction of the tagged iodothyronine bound to this matrix. The result should be expressed as the ratio of matrix-bound counts to serum protein-bound counts, with a typical normal range of 33 to 50 per cent. To improve reproducibility, this result should be normalized to that obtained in samples of normal sera assayed simultaneously, such that the normal range is 0.85 to 1.15. The ratio of tracer thyroid hormone bound to the inert matrix to that bound to serum protein is directly proportional to the free fraction of thyroid hormone. While the relative distribution of T_3 on the serum-binding proteins is slightly different from that of T_4 (T_3 is only weakly bound to transthyretin), its distribution is sufficiently similar so that in many laboratories it is used instead of T_4. The similarity between the free fraction of thyroid hormones and the THBR can be formalized by calculating the free T_4 (or T_3) index. This is the product of a normalized THBR value and the total serum T_4 or T_3 concentration. The normal range for these indices in units is approximately the same as that for the total thyroid hormone concentrations. In my laboratory, the normal free T_4 index is 4.7 to 10.5. The free T_4 index is an excellent approximation of the free T_4.

An alternative estimate of the free T_4 may be obtained by using one of several commercial kits. While there are some technical advantages to these tests, they do not measure the free T_4 directly, but provide only an estimate of its concentration, as does the free T_4 index. One notable clinical situation in which both methods often provide falsely high estimates of the free T_4 is in patients with familial dysalbuminemic hyperthyroxinemia. In patients with this syndrome a portion of the serum albumin binds T_4, but not T_3, with abnormally high affinity. The total T_4 value is elevated, but the free fraction of T_4 by dialysis is reduced; therefore the free T_4 concentration is normal. Since T_3 does not bind to the abnormal albumin with increased avidity, estimation of THBR employing T_3 is normal, and therefore a free T_4 index calculated using this value is elevated. Other artifacts in the analogue method kits result in the same falsely high estimate of free T_4. The use of T_4 in estimation of THBR would solve the problem in this syndrome and in other situations such as severe illness in which the changes in the binding of T_3 and T_4 are not identical. The terms T_3 *uptake* and T_3 *resin* are sometimes confused with the direct immunoassay of serum T_3 concentrations, and these terms should be discarded in favor of the THBR.

COMPARISON OF THE UTILITY OF T_4 AND T_3 DETERMINATIONS. The free T_4 index is the best screening test for thyroid dysfunction. It is superior to the free T_3 index by virtue of the fact that the principal thyroid secretory product is T_4. About 80 per cent of circulating T_3 derives from T_4 to T_3 conversion. Therefore, in patients who are sick or who have received any of the drugs listed in Table 216–3, which inhibit T_4 to T_3 conversion, the serum T_3 is invariably reduced relative to the serum T_4, but this does not imply thyroid disease. In hypothyroidism, serum T_3 may be normal despite significant impairment of thyroid function. On the other hand, in hyperthyroidism there is a small fraction of patients in whom serum T_4 is not elevated but the concentration of serum T_3 is. This condition is called T_3 *thyrotoxicosis* (see below).

SERUM REVERSE T_3 AND OTHER IODOTHYRONINES. The normal concentration of reverse T_3 is 15 to 30 ng per deciliter. It derives exclusively from peripheral metabolism of T_4, and its concentration in the blood reflects a combination of that process and the rate of its degradation. Its measurement is not generally useful clinically, although it is an excellent barometer of the rate of T_4 to T_3 conversion. Immunoassays have been developed for both monoiodinated and diiodinated thyronines, but these measurements do not have clinical applicability.

SERUM THYROID HORMONE–BINDING PROTEIN CONCENTRATIONS. The normal concentration of circulating TBG and transthyretin can be measured by immunoassay or by determination of the binding capacity. The normal concentration of TBG is 1.5 mg per deciliter. This quantity of protein binds approximately 20 μg of T_4 (1 mole T_4 per 1 mole TBG). The binding capacity of transthyretin is approximately 250 μg T_4 per deciliter. These measurements are rarely necessary for clinical purposes. Estrogen treatment increases the glycosylation of human TBG. This reduces its metabolic clearance rate and accounts for the two- to threefold increase in the circulating TBG during pregnancy or exogenous hyperestrogenism.

RADIOACTIVE IODINE UPTAKE (RAI UPTAKE). The normal 24-hour thyroidal uptake of radioiodine ranges from 5 to 30 per cent. All the radioiodine in the thyroid at this time is in the organified form. Because of the broad normal range for this test, it is not a reliable method for determining thyroid status. Its major diagnostic use is in separating patients who have hyperthyroidism caused by subacute thyroiditis in whom the uptake is reduced or absent from those with Graves' disease (see next section). It is contraindicated in pregnancy.

TESTS OF THYROID REGULATION

SERUM THYROTROPIN. The normal range for serum TSH is 0.5 to 5.0 μU per milliliter. In patients with thyroid hypofunction, TSH increases, and when thyroid function is autonomous, TSH is reduced, as expected from the normal feedback relationships (Fig. 216–3). Newer TSH assays can discriminate between normal TSH concentrations and those that are reduced. Previously it was necessary to employ the TRH infusion test to make this differentiation. With this immunometric assay (TSH-IMA), so called because a combination of monoclonal antibodies is usually employed, serum TSH values less than 0.1 μU per milliliter correlate well with absence of a TSH increase in response to TRH (see below). The TSH-IMA should prove to be useful in monitoring the status of hypothyroid patients receiving replacement therapy and those patients in whom TSH suppression is desired, such as those with thyroid carcinoma or TSH-dependent nodular goiter. It may also be used as a screening test in patients suspected of thyroid disease as an alternative to the free T_4 index (Fig. 216–4). Virtually all patients with clinical symptoms attributable to primary hypothyroidism have serum TSH concentrations greater than 20 μU per milliliter, and many subjects with minimal symptoms or goiter alone have results between 10 and 20 μU per milliliter. An elevation of the serum TSH concentration almost always indicates that thyroid function is impaired. It is also the critical test for separating patients with primary thyroid disease from those with hypothyroidism resulting from hypothalamic or pituitary dysfunction.

THYROTROPIN-RELEASING HORMONE INFUSION TEST. TRH can be infused intravenously and TSH measured in serum to determine whether TSH is present in the pituitary. Pituitary TSH is reduced in patients with hyperthyroidism and in those with autonomous thyroid hormone production and often in patients with hypothalamic pituitary disease. This test has been superseded by the TSH-IMA described above. Typical normal and pathologic responses are shown in Figure 216–5. In practice, a basal serum sample is obtained, followed by intravenous infusion of 400 μg of TRH over 1 minute. A second serum sample is obtained 30 minutes after the infusion, and both are assayed for TSH. In normal persons the minimal TSH increment is 2 μU per milliliter except in males over the age of 40, in the seriously ill, or in patients with depression or exogenous or endogenous glucocorticoid excess in whom the normal response can be lower. The response is amplified (30-minute value greater than 25 μU per milliliter) in patients with primary hypothyroidism. A significant increment in TSH eliminates the diagnosis of hyperthyroidism except in the extremely rare patient with the TSH-induced form of this disease.

METABOLIC INDICES OF THYROID STATUS

BASAL METABOLIC RATE (BMR). Since thyroid hormone is an important factor in the regulation of the rate of oxygen consumption, this test should theoretically be useful in evaluating thyroid status. However, it has given way to serum measurements, since these are more specific and usually more accurate. The normal range for the BMR is usually from −15 to +5 per cent.

DEEP TENDON REFLEX CONTRACTION AND RELAXATION TIMES. Thyroid status is reflected in the rate (not amplitude) of contraction and relaxation of skeletal muscle. These rates are more rapid in hyperthyroidism and slowed in hypothyroidism. Some clinicians have employed a kinemometer tracing to quantitate these events and have observed as high as 70 per cent diagnostic accuracy with this test. Like the BMR, it is less specific than serum hormone measurements, since hypothermia, peripheral neuropathy, gross edema, and many other conditions may slow the rate of relaxation. However, a clinically apparent delay in the relaxation phase of the deep tendon reflexes is almost invariably present in patients with significant hypothyroidism, although the more rapid relaxation in hyperthyroidism is difficult to appreciate visually.

ANATOMIC EVALUATION OF THE THYROID GLAND

THE THYROID SCAN. The capacity of the thyroid gland to trap ions such as I^- or molecules with a similar charge and configuration has provided a useful method for correlating structure and function. Of the iodine isotopes either ^{123}I or ^{131}I can be used. ^{123}I, although more expensive, is preferred for scanning, particularly in younger persons, since the radiation dose to the thyroid is 7.5 mrads per microcurie administered, as opposed to 800 mrads per microcurie for ^{131}I. Another isotope that gives a low radiation dose is $^{99m}TcO_4^-$ (pertechnetate), which is trapped, but not organified, by the thyroid. For this reason, a scan is obtained 30 minutes after intravenous injection of this isotope. The thyroid scan is usually used to determine the functional state

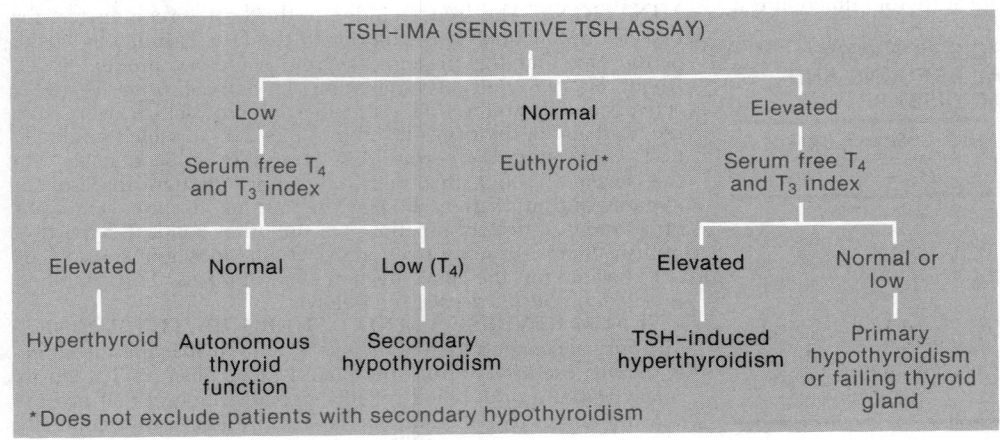

FIGURE 216–4. Proposed schema for evaluation of patients based on the TSH-IMA. The TSH-IMA is capable of differentiating the lower limit of normal from the TSH concentration in the sera of patients with autonomous thyroid hyperfunction as well as quantifying elevated levels. The current experience suggests that this approach would not be useful in patients with nonthyroidal illness in whom TSH may be suppressed by factors other than thyroid hyperfunction.

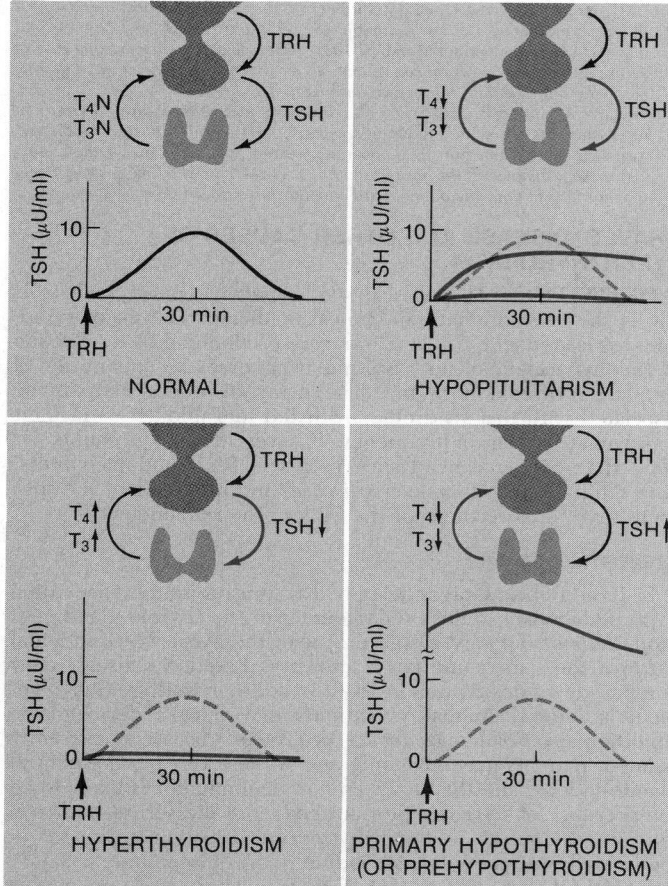

FIGURE 216–5. Typical responses to the infusion of TRH in patients with hyperthyroidism and primary and secondary hypothyroidism. In patients with hypopituitarism or hypothalamic disease virtually any TRH response pattern can be seen. The most pertinent diagnostic information is that serum TSH is not increased in a patient with a reduced serum free T_4 index.

of a palpable thyroid nodule (see later in chapter) or in evaluating masses in the neck or upper part of the chest to see if thyroid tissue is present.

THYROID ULTRASOUND. Whether a given thyroid mass is solid or cystic can be determined by ultrasonography. Ultrasound is now sufficiently sensitive to allow identification of 1- to 3-mm nodules that are too small to be palpated. Such nodules are present in as many as 40 per cent of the population and have unknown clinical significance. Ultrasound may serve as a useful objective method for following the response of a thyroid nodule to TSH suppressive therapy.

NEEDLE BIOPSY OR ASPIRATION. Either a fine (23 to 25 gauge) or cutting needle (Vim-Silverman) can be used to obtain a sample of thyroid cells for histologic examination. These techniques have received increased attention in recent years as a method for evaluation of thyroid nodules. Accurate interpretation of a fine-needle aspirate requires an experienced cytologist.

OTHER TESTS SPECIFICALLY RELATED TO THYROID FUNCTION OR DISEASE

ANTITHYROID ANTIBODIES. In autoimmune thyroid disease (Hashimoto's thyroiditis or Graves' disease), antibodies that bind to various antigens of thyroid tissue are present in the serum. The most important of these is the *thyroid microsomal antibody (TMAb).* Thyroid peroxidase is the principal antigen in thyroid microsomes. TMAb is found in approximately 95 per cent of patients with Hashimoto's thyroiditis and in only about 10 per cent of adults with no apparent thyroid disease. The test is generally performed by a tanned red cell hemagglutination technique, and the results are reported as the highest titer causing agglutination. Titers in excess of 1:100 are significant. About 55 per cent of patients with Graves' disease also have circulating

TMAb's. *Thyroglobulin antibodies* (TgAb's) are also present in the serum of about 60 per cent of patients with Hashimoto's disease.

Antibodies directed against the thyroid TSH receptor (TRAb's), present in the sera of patients with Graves' disease, can be measured by many techniques that quantitate their interaction with the TSH receptor on thyroid cells. These immunoglobulins are usually stimulatory at the receptor level but may block TSH-TSH receptor interaction without causing stimulation (see Graves' Disease and Other Causes of Hyperthyroidism).

SERUM THYROGLOBULIN. The normal serum thyroglobulin (Tg) concentration is 2 to 20 ng per milliliter. Serum Tg may be increased in any patient with an enlarged thyroid or following acute trauma to the thyroid, whether a consequence of inflammation, surgery, or radiation. Thyroglobulin determinations are most useful in the follow-up of patients with metastatic thyroid carcinoma following thyroidectomy. An increase in serum Tg indicates the presence of tumor tissue, although a normal value does not eliminate this possibility. Serum thyroglobulin concentrations are generally reduced in patients who have *thyrotoxicosis factitia,* and this measurement may be useful in separating this group of patients from those with hyperthyroidism due to thyroid inflammation.

THE EFFECTS OF NONTHYROIDAL ILLNESS AND COMMON DRUGS ON THYROID FUNCTION TESTS

ILLNESS. The physiologic response to illness changes a number of aspects of thyroid function. With moderate to severe illness, T_4 deiodination to T_3 is impaired, leading to a decrease in the serum T_3 concentration. Since the type I deiodinase that converts T_4 to T_3 is also involved in reverse T_3 degradation, the metabolic clearance of reverse T_3 decreases and reverse T_3 concentrations rise, sometimes markedly so. In many patients, the binding of thyroid hormones to the normal serum hormone-binding proteins is reduced, which decreases serum T_4 concentrations and, depending on the degree of illness, increases the free fraction of both T_3 and T_4. It is not certain whether the increase in the free hormone fractions is due to the presence of a binding inhibitor in the serum or an intrinsic change in the binding affinity of the circulating thyroid hormone–binding proteins. Whatever the cause of this decreased thyroid hormone binding, it is not recognized by the simpler techniques used to assess this binding, such as the resin or charcoal T_3 uptake, nor by the current T_4-analogue–based estimates of free T_4. The clinical relevance of this difficulty is that the free thyroxine index may be artifactually low in sick patients. If the free thyroxine is measured by equilibrium dialysis or ultrafiltration, the free thyroxine concentrations are normal. With chronic illness, the serum TBG and albumin concentrations may be lowered and the free fraction of thyroid hormones and the THBR rise. This is especially true in patients with severe hepatic disease or nephrotic syndrome.

Serum TSH concentrations are generally normal in patients with critical illness, although a normal value is not physiologically appropriate for a patient with a substantive reduction in the serum free T_3. This observation has been used as evidence that there is hypothalamic or pituitary suppression of TSH release during illness which contributes to the abnormalities of thyroid function. Paradoxically, in rare patients the TSH may be elevated, although this is more common during recovery from severe illness. Since dopamine or glucocorticoid can directly suppress TSH, individuals receiving these agents may have an additional reason to develop transient pituitary hypothyroidism. Dopamine can suppress the appropriately elevated serum TSH of a patient with primary hypothyroidism, theoretically even into the normal range. Thus, the evaluation of patients receiving dopamine infusions is complex.

The goal of thyroid function testing in ill patients should be to rule out pre-existing hypothyroidism or hyperthyroidism. The sooner after admission estimates of serum thyroid hormone levels and TSH are obtained, the more effective the results are in achieving this goal. Thus, the clinician should have a low threshold for ordering thyroid function tests during the initial evaluation of the sick patient. In the presence of a markedly reduced free thyroxine index in an extremely ill patient, the concentration of serum TSH is very important. If this is not above 5 μU per milliliter, it is quite likely that the apparent thyroid dysfunction is due to the illness and/or its treatment. If TSH is elevated, parenteral replacement therapy with thyroxine should be provided, except for patients with symptomatic coronary artery disease (see below). Since it is usually impossible to evaluate critically ill patients endocrinologically or radiographically for hypothalamic-pituitary disease, it may be necessary to treat some empirically with replacement thyroxine and to provide glucocorticoid as well if the plasma cortisol concentration is not appropriate for the patient's physiologic stress (>15 μg per deciliter). Such patients are then evaluated for underlying thyroid/pituitary disease after recovering from their acute illness.

Occasionally a patient may have severe illness and an elevated level of serum T_4. Such patients should be suspected of having underlying autonomous thyroid function and often must be treated for hyperthyroidism if the serum TSH is less than 0.1 μU per milliliter. This phenomenon may also occur in patients with *acute psychiatric illness* and *hyperemesis gravidarum*. Serum T_3 determinations are usually not useful in patients with systemic illness owing to the impairment of T_4 to T_3 conversion. As with the patient suspected of thyroid hypofunction, definitive evaluation for underlying hyperthyroidism is performed when the patient's clinical condition permits.

DRUGS. Many therapeutic agents interfere (or appear to interfere) with thyroid function. The most commonly used and troublesome agents are listed in Table 216–3. The suppression of TSH secretion by dopamine or pharmacologic administration of glucocorticoids can transiently suppress TSH concentrations and may contribute to the reduced serum T_4 often seen in the seriously ill patient. Lithium carbonate may cause goiter or hypothyroidism, especially in individuals with mild underlying Hashimoto's thyroiditis. Phenylbutazone and sulfonylurea drugs inhibit normal thyroid gland function if given in sufficient dosage. In addition to the agents listed in Table 216–1, salicylates (>2 grams per day), phenytoin, fenclofenac, and furosemide all inhibit thyroid hormone-protein binding. Because these agents are weak binding inhibitors, they do not usually cause an abnormality in the THBR, and therefore the free T_4 index is mildly reduced. Agents that inhibit the type I 5'-deiodinase generally cause a reduction in serum T_3. If this is severe and prolonged enough, a compensatory increase in TSH secretion occurs, and the serum T_4 concentration rises. In patients receiving more than 200 mg propranolol, mild elevations in the serum free T_4 index are not uncommon.

Amiodarone has complex effects on thyroid function. Since this drug is about 30 per cent iodine by weight, it may produce all of the effects of iodide, that is, either hypothyroidism or hyperthyroidism. Even after discontinuation of this agent, tissue stores of iodine are significantly increased for 6 to 9 months. In addition, amiodarone seems to inhibit both pathways for T_4 to T_3 conversion and causes compensatory hyperthyroxinemia. There is some question whether it might also be a peripheral antagonist of thyroid hormone action, a further stimulus to a compensatory increase in TSH secretion. Iopanoic acid and ipodate, radiographic agents used for visualization of the gallbladder, are also effective inhibitors of T_4 to T_3 conversion. Their effect is transient and disappears within 3 to 4 weeks. All agents that inhibit peripheral T_4 to T_3 conversion raise the ratio of serum T_4 to T_3. In a patient receiving these agents, a TSH-IMA or a TRH test may be required to determine if hyperthyroidism is present.

Ain KB, Refetoff S: Relationship of oligosaccharide modification to the cause of serum thyroxine–binding globulin excess. J Clin Endocrinol Metab 66:1037, 1988. *Evidence that changes in serum TBG during pregnancy or estrogen therapy are a consequence of altered glycosylation and the resultant reduced hepatic clearance of this protein.*

Kaplan MM: Clinical and laboratory assessment of thyroid abnormalities. Med Clin North Am 69:863, 1985. *A detailed examination of the clinical application of thyroid function tests and a review of the effects of drugs that can influence these.*

Spencer CA, Lai-Rosenfeld AO, Guttler RB, et al.: Thyrotropin secretion in thyrotoxic and thyroxine-treated patients: Assessment by a sensitive immunoenzymometric assay. J Clin Endocrinol Metab 63:349, 1986. *The performance of a TSH-IMA in monitoring patients undergoing thyroid hormone replacement or with thyrotoxicosis.*

Surks MI, Hupart KH, Pan C, et al.: Normal free thyroxine in critical nonthyroidal illnesses measured by ultrafiltration of undiluted serum and equilibrium dialysis. J Clin Endocrinol Metab 67:1031, 1988. *Evidence showing that during severe illness free thyroxine concentrations are normal or even elevated despite markedly lowered total thyroxine concentrations.*

Wiersinga WM, Endert E, Trip MD, et al.: Immunoradiometric assay of thyrotropin in plasma: Its value in predicting response to thyroliberin stimulation and assessing thyroid function in amiodarone-treated patients. Clin Chem 32:433, 1986. *An example of the utility of the TSH-IMA in that most challenging diagnostic situation, the patient with amiodarone-induced thyroid dysfunction.*

GRAVES' DISEASE AND OTHER CAUSES OF HYPERTHYROIDISM

DEFINITION. The clinical syndrome of hyperthyroidism is one of the most dramatic in clinical medicine. The major symptoms associated with this syndrome are predominantly a reflection of the hypermetabolism resulting from excessive quantities of circulating thyroid hormone. The many disorders that can be associated with this syndrome are listed in Table 216–5 in their approximate order of frequency. Graves' disease accounts for more than 85 per cent of such patients. Toxic nodular goiters, both multinodular (*Plummer's disease*) and uninodular, and subacute thyroiditis account for the bulk of the remainder.

Graves' Disease

In 1835, Robert Graves described a clinical syndrome including hypermetabolism, diffuse enlargement of the thyroid gland, and *exophthalmos* (forward displacement of the eyes). In continental Europe, the same condition is known as Basedow's disease after von Basedow's description in 1840. In addition to thyroid involvement and ophthalmopathy, patients may have a dermatologic condition, *pretibial myxedema*. As Graves' disease is currently defined, patients may have only one of these three major clinical manifestations, and the only common denominator is likely to be the presence of TSH receptor antibodies in the serum. *Jodbasedow* disease refers to hyperthyroidism (Basedow's disease) in iodine-deficient patients after iodine (jod) replacement.

ETIOLOGY AND PATHOGENESIS. The precise etiology of Graves' disease is still not known, but it seems likely that it is an autoimmune disorder. Hyperthyroidism is its principal manifestation, yet TSH is suppressed and no intrinsic regulatory abnormalities in the thyroid have been identified. Thus the thyroid stimulation seems likely to be a consequence of a circulating, non-TSH, thyroid stimulator. This "stimulator" is now thought to be a γ globulin or a family of γ globulins.

It is postulated, with increasing evidence, that in Graves' disease, for reasons as yet unclear, B lymphocytes secrete antibodies directed against the TSH receptor. These antibodies, termed TRAb, are generally polyclonal and may be stimulatory or inhibitory at the receptor, depending on the nature of their interaction with the receptor site. The reason for the appearance of TRAb and their perpetuation in Graves' disease has not been elucidated. Assays for the presence of TRAb depend either on the capacity of the serum to activate adenylate cyclase in thyroid cell membranes or thyroid cell lines or to compete with labeled TSH for binding to the TSH receptor on thyroid cells or on guinea pig adipocyte membranes. TRAb are found in 85 to 90 per cent of patients with clinical evidence of Graves' disease.

The etiology of Graves' exophthalmopathy is not known. Patients with exophthalmos and particularly those with dermopathy almost invariably have high titers of circulating TRAb, suggesting

TABLE 216–5. DISEASES OR CLINICAL SYNDROMES ASSOCIATED WITH THYROTOXICOSIS

Graves' disease
Toxic multinodular goiter
Toxic adenoma
Iodide-induced hyperthyroidism
Subacute thyroiditis
Factitious (exogenous) thyrotoxicosis
Neonatal thyrotoxicosis (mother with Graves' disease)
TSH-secreting pituitary tumor
Nontumorigenic pituitary-induced hyperthyroidism
Choriocarcinoma (uterine or testicular origin) or hydatidiform mole
Struma ovarii
Hyperfunctioning thyroid carcinoma (usually metastatic)

that these two clinical manifestations represent the most severe form of this disease. Antibodies to soluble human eye muscle antigens were found in 17 of 23 patients with Graves' ophthalmopathy, but not in Graves' patients without this manifestation and rarely in those with Hashimoto's thyroiditis. This suggests a similar autoimmune etiology for ophthalmopathy and for hyperthyroidism. It has also been proposed that Tg-anti-Tg circulating immune complexes may bind to eye muscles and play a pathogenic role. Further studies will be required to resolve this question.

Emotional Factors in the Etiology of Hyperthyroidism. The emotional lability of the patient with hyperthyroidism has led many clinicians to question the role of psychologic trauma in the pathogenesis of this disease. Numerous anecdotes have been cited to suggest that emotional trauma may somehow trigger the onset of overt hyperthyroidism. If this is so, it would still appear to require participation of the immune system, since circulating TRAb are such a constant feature of the clinical picture. In my mind, it seems more likely that an episode of physical or emotional trauma brings the patient to medical attention, at which time pre-existing hyperthyroidism is recognized.

INCIDENCE. Graves' disease is common, affecting as many as 1.9 per cent of the female population and about a tenth that number of males, according to a population survey in northern England. It reaches its peak incidence in the third and fourth decades. The reason for the female predominance in this as in all thyroid diseases is not known. There is a strong familial component to Graves' disease with a family history of autoimmune thyroid disease (Graves' disease, Hashimoto's thyroiditis, or "goiter") in a significant fraction of patients. The importance of genetic inheritance in the predisposition to this syndrome has been confirmed by finding a higher relative risk of this condition in patients with the histocompatibility antigens HLA-B8 (Caucasians), HLA-B35 (Japanese), and HLA-Bw46 (Chinese).

PATHOLOGY. The thyroid of the patient with Graves' disease is diffusely enlarged and hypercellular. In patients undergoing thyroidectomy without prior treatment with antithyroid drugs or iodine, a diffusely hyperplastic epithelium is noted with little or no colloid present and often with lymphocytic infiltration, varying from minimal to extensive. In some specimens it is impossible to distinguish the microscopic picture from Hashimoto's thyroiditis (a condition sometimes called hashitoxicosis). If the patient receives iodide preoperatively, the gland contains large amounts of colloid, cells are of normal height, and the vascularity is markedly reduced. Other tissues show no specific changes except in severely hyperthyroid patients. In those situations there may be edema and focal necrosis in the liver with cellular infiltration.

In hyperthyroid patients with mild eye manifestations of Graves' disease such as lid retraction and stare, no significant orbital pathology is found, and these changes probably are due to the hyperthyroidism per se. In more severe cases, edema of the extraocular muscles occurs in association with infiltration with lymphocytes, plasma cells, and neutrophils. In addition, hydrophilic mucopolysaccharide collects in the orbital tissues. The conjunctivae may show perivascular lymphocytic infiltration and edema (*chemosis*). The end stage of these processes is fibrosis, which most often involves the inferior eye muscles, causing restriction of upward globe movement.

CLINICAL PICTURE. The common clinical symptoms of thyrotoxicosis are listed in Table 216–6. These occur in any

TABLE 216–6. COMMON SYMPTOMS AND SIGNS OF HYPERTHYROIDISM (THYROTOXICOSIS)

Symptoms	Signs
Nervousness and/or tremor	Tachycardia or atrial fibrillation
Weight loss (usually with increased appetite)	Widened pulse pressure with increased systolic and decreased diastolic pressures
Palpitations	Hyperdynamic precordium and accentuated S1
Heat intolerance and excessive perspiration	Warm, smooth skin
Emotional lability	Tremor
Muscle weakness	Proximal muscle weakness
Hyperdefecation	Thyroid enlargement or abnormality

patient with excessive thyroid hormone secretion whether due to Graves' disease or some other cause. They are a consequence of the stimulatory effect of thyroid hormone on the metabolic rate and on many other tissues, especially the heart and central nervous system. The typical patient with Graves' disease is in her mid-20's with symptoms that can often be dated to 6 to 12 months previously. The patient is nervous, anxious, and fidgeting, and speaks rapidly. She complains of her agitated fatigue, palpitations, and, in warmer climates, heat intolerance. There may be weight loss despite increased appetite, or the patient may merely report success in her efforts at weight control. An increased frequency of bowel movements and, rarely, diarrhea may be noted. Emotional lability is often apparent during the interview, and a history of deteriorating domestic or occupational relationships may be obtained. A history of neck swelling (often not noted first by the patient) may be present. Amenorrhea or oligomenorrhea is not uncommon. Rarer manifestations of hyperthyroidism include pruritus and urticaria. About 5 per cent of males may experience gynecomastia, and even less commonly *hypokalemic periodic paralysis* may occur. For unknown reasons, this condition is much more common in males of Oriental extraction.

Apathetic or Masked Hyperthyroidism. The symptoms given in Table 216–6 are those generally found in the younger patient. The clinician should be aware that in some patients, particularly the elderly, the clinical symptoms and signs of hypermetabolism may not be so dramatic. Rather than appearing agitated, the elderly patient with hyperthyroidism may be depressed. Weight loss and symptoms of congestive heart failure can be the predominant manifestations of the hypermetabolic syndrome. Often this is complicated by atrial fibrillation or other supraventricular tachyarrhythmia, leading to suspicion that the heart, rather than the thyroid, is the source of the problem. Because of the subtlety of this clinical form of hyperthyroidism it is recommended that any patient with the recent onset of atrial fibrillation have tests of thyroid function. In this way a reversible cause of congestive heart failure and/or recurrent arrhythmias may be recognized and appropriate treatment instituted.

Graves' Ophthalmopathy. Eye symptoms are present in more than 50 per cent of patients with Graves' disease but, except for modest lid lag and stare, are rare in patients with other causes of hyperthyroidism. This is a useful point in establishing the diagnosis. Common complaints are protruding eyes; easy tearing, especially on exposure to wind or cold; photophobia; a gritty foreign body sensation in the eyes; and, less commonly, diplopia (Fig. 216–6). The patient with significant *proptosis* (exophthalmos) may complain of irritation, particularly on arising, since the eyelids do not completely cover the sclera when the patient is sleeping *(lagophthalmos)*. Rarely, severe chemosis, inflammation, and periorbital edema occur (malignant exophthalmos). Eye complaints are usually bilateral, but may be unilateral, and Graves' disease is one of the most common causes of unilateral exophthalmos.

Pretibial Myxedema. In a few patients with Graves' disease (1 to 2 per cent) a brawny, nonpitting swelling of the pretibial area, ankles, and/or feet is present. This can appear in plaques. It has an orange-skin appearance and is usually not tender. This dermopathy, found exclusively in Graves' disease, is termed *pretibial myxedema*. The name derives from the histologic similarity of the mucopolysaccharide infiltration of the subcutaneous tissues to that found in advanced hypothyroidism (myxedema).

Euthyroid Graves' Disease. In a small fraction of patients with Graves' disease, eye manifestations (unilateral or bilateral) with or without pretibial myxedema appear, but hyperthyroidism is not present. This can arise because of destruction of the thyroid as a result of coexistent Hashimoto's disease, or hyperthyroidism may be delayed in its appearance for months or years after the first eye symptoms. In many such patients, appropriate testing often reveals subtle evidence of thyroid dysfunction.

PHYSICAL SIGNS. In younger patients, tachycardia is almost universal. The systolic blood pressure is elevated primarily because of the increased inotropic effect of thyroid hormone on the heart. The diastolic pressure is reduced owing to a decrease in peripheral vascular resistance associated with increased skin capillary blood flow. Body temperature is usually normal. The

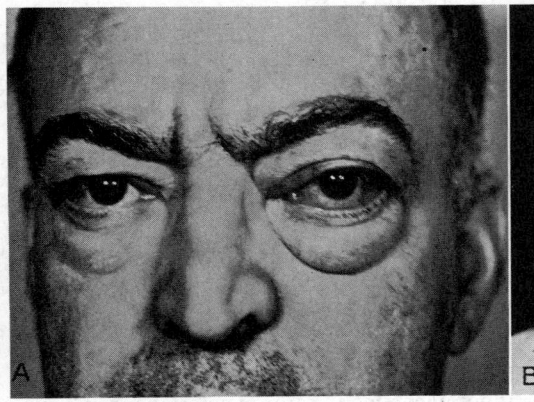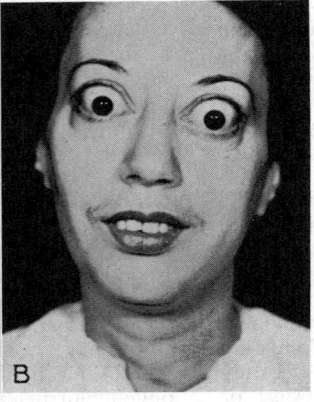

FIGURE 216–6. Two patients showing the typical ophthalmopathy characteristic of Graves' disease. Patient A demonstrates marked periorbital swelling, exophthalmos, chemosis, and conjunctival injection. The proptosis, limitation of extraocular movements, and other manifestations of ophthalmopathy are much more severe in Patient A than in Patient B. Patient B has marked widening of the palpebral fissures owing to lid retraction and also has significant proptosis. Patient A is euthyroid; Patient B is mildly hyperthyroid. (From Williams RH (ed.): Textbook of Endocrinology, 6th ed. Philadelphia, W. B. Saunders Company, 1981, p 189.)

skin is smooth, warm, and moist, and the patient may radiate heat. A fine tremor of the outstretched hands and occasionally *onycholysis* of the fourth and fifth fingers or clubbing (*thyroid acropachy*) are observed. The thyroid is almost always diffusely enlarged from 1.5 to 5 to 6 times normal. One third of elderly patients do not have a detectable goiter. The gland may be soft or firm, depending on the degree of hyperthyroidism and the level of iodine intake. Auscultation of the neck may reveal a multitude of sounds. In the younger patients a *venous hum* may be heard over the external jugular vein, particularly with the patient in the sitting position. Third or fourth heart sounds are heard easily in the neck, and a carotid bruit is not uncommon. In addition, a bruit over the thyroid gland is present in some patients, a manifestation of the high blood flow to this organ. A diffuse lymphadenopathy may be present in hyperthyroidism, and splenomegaly is found in 10 per cent of patients. The liver is not enlarged except in elderly patients with congestive failure. The neurologic examination shows tremor and proximal muscle weakness. Eye signs include lid lag, a failure of the upper lid to cover the upper margin of the iris as the globe traverses from upward to downward gaze, a widened palpebral fissure so that the sclera is visible above and/or below the iris, conjunctival injection and chemosis, periorbital swelling, and proptosis. The last-named finding is determined by measuring the distance from the lateral portion of the bony orbit to the cornea, using the *exophthalmometer*. In the white population this distance is 17 mm or less, with an upper limit of normal of 20 mm (22 mm for the black population). The difference between the two eye measurements should not be more than 3 mm. In addition to these moderate abnormalities, there may be impairment of globe movement. The most common restriction is in upward and/or outward gaze. This is due not to weakness of the superior eye muscles but to swelling and fibrosis of the inferior rectus and inferior oblique muscles beneath the globe. In addition, abduction and convergence may also be affected. Eye signs may be absent or mild, are usually bilateral when present, but may be asymmetric.

Laboratory Diagnosis of Hyperthyroidism

The various steps to be followed in establishing the laboratory diagnosis of hyperthyroidism are outlined in Figure 216–7. The initial screening test is to determine the free T_4 index. In virtually all patients an elevation in the free T_4 index is present. In the hospitalized patient the diagnosis may be somewhat more complicated if the patient is severely ill or has received any of the agents listed in Table 216–3, which cause inhibition of T_4 to T_3 conversion. In these patients an impairment of T_4 clearance or inhibition of T_4 to T_3 conversion may lead to an elevation in the serum free T_4 index without hyperthyroidism. Other causes of an elevated free T_4 index not necessarily indicating hyperthyroidism are familial dysalbuminemia (see Direct Tests of Thyroid Function), hyperemesis gravidarum, and acute psychosis. In the last two conditions the increase in the free T_4 index is usually transient. An alternate approach is to use the strategy depicted in Figure 216–4. Except in seriously ill patients this approach should be equally effective.

In such patients and in patients in whom the clinical suspicion of hyperthyroidism is present but the free T_4 index is normal or equivocal, a serum T_3 measurement is required. The ratio of T_3 to T_4 is increased in the thyroid gland in patients with Graves' disease. As a consequence, the T_3 production rate and the fraction of T_3 coming directly from the thyroid are increased. Thus the serum T_3 is elevated to a greater extent than is the serum T_4 (see Table 216–4). Patients in whom serum T_3 is elevated but the serum free T_4 index is not have *T_3 thyrotoxicosis*, which occurs in 3 to 5 per cent of patients in the United States but is more common in areas where dietary iodine is lower. The diagnosis of hyperthyroidism cannot be eliminated until the free T_3 index (as well as the free T_4 index) has been found to be normal. Even in hyperthyroidism, a substantial fraction of T_3 derives from periph-

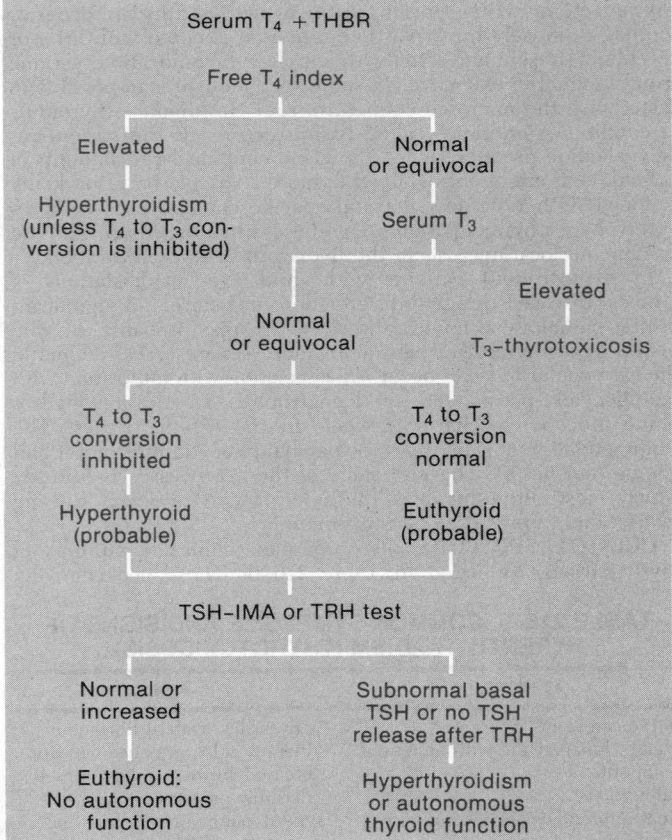

FIGURE 216–7. Laboratory diagnosis of hyperthyroidism. THBR refers to the thyroid hormone–binding ratio (formerly termed T_3 or T_4 uptake). TSH-IMA refers to the serum TSH measured by an immunometric assay that can discriminate between normal and suppressed as well as elevated TSH concentrations.

eral T_4 to T_3 conversion. Impairment of this process from any cause (illness or drugs) can lead to a reduction in serum T_3. However, in hyperthyroidism, even with severe illness, the serum T_3 is rarely depressed to less than 100 ng per deciliter. To eliminate the possibility of a TSH-producing pituitary tumor and to confirm the hyperthyroid state, the serum TSH should be measured. A normal TSH-IMA eliminates all forms of hyperthyroidism except the patient with increased TSH secretion (see Fig. 216–4). Since patients with fixed or autonomous, but not supranormal, thyroid hormone production also have a reduced serum TSH, an abnormal test does not always indicate the presence of hypermetabolism and the need for treatment.

In patients with a classic history and laboratory abnormalities, an RAI uptake and thyroid scan are not necessary to establish the diagnosis. However, if the hyperthyroidism is of brief (less than 3 months') duration, if the thyroid is not enlarged or if it is tender, subacute thyroiditis must be considered, and an uptake and scan should be performed after pregnancy has been excluded. These tests are also required when nodular goiter or factitious thyrotoxicosis is suspected (see Table 216–5).

Unilateral Ophthalmopathy. Since Graves' ophthalmopathy may be unilateral and not associated with frank hyperthyroidism, local pathology such as orbital tumor, pseudotumor of the orbit, cavernous sinus-carotid aneurysm, and sphenoid ridge meningioma must be considered. In addition to the free T_4 index, serum T_3, and TRH test, such patients require orbital radiography, ultrasonography, and computed tomography. In almost all patients with Graves' ophthalmopathy, bilateral involvement of the extraocular muscles is found even though clinically the process appears unilateral. Positive serum tests for TRAb or TMAb provide further support for this diagnosis.

OTHER CHEMICAL ABNORMALITIES ASSOCIATED WITH HYPERTHYROIDISM. In 5 to 20 per cent of patients with hyperthyroidism any of the following may be found: modest hypercalcemia, increased alkaline phosphatase (bone or hepatic isozyme), increased direct bilirubin, and a mild anemia of "chronic disease." Modest neutropenia may occur (1000 to 2000 per cubic millimeter).

Differential Diagnosis of Hyperthyroidism

Few clinical syndromes mimic hyperthyroidism. Pheochromocytoma and neurocirculatory asthenia may cause some clinical confusion, but appropriate laboratory testing eliminates these from consideration. Differentiation of patients with Graves' disease from those with other forms of hyperthyroidism is rarely difficult based solely on the history and physical examination (see Table 216–5). The use of the RAI uptake and scan to identify patients with subacute thyroiditis or nodular disease has been discussed. Iodine-induced hyperthyroidism is due to either multinodular goiter or Graves' disease (jodbasedow). Factitious thyrotoxicosis, the ingestion of excess thyroid hormone, should be considered particularly in paramedical personnel in whom symptoms and laboratory manifestations are associated with a nonpalpable thyroid gland. TSH-induced hyperthyroidism is diagnosed by finding an elevated or normal TSH in the presence of an increased free T_4 or T_3 index. It can be associated with either pituitary resistance to thyroid hormone or a thyrotroph tumor. Chorionic gonadotropin–induced hyperthyroidism is confirmed by the elevation in serum hCG in association with molar pregnancy or choriocarcinoma.

Treatment

TREATMENT OF HYPERTHYROIDISM OF GRAVES' DISEASE. The treatment of patients with Graves' disease must be considered in the context of its natural history. In 10 to 50 per cent of patients, depending on the series, thyroid function returns to normal (remission) in association with (but probably not because of) drug treatment directed at the thyroid, not at the apparent primary defect in the immune system. If the patient destined for remission could be identified, a rational treatment approach for this disease could be developed. At present this is not possible, although a reduction in circulating TRAb titers generally accompanies remission, and it may be possible to employ such assays in the future to guide therapy. Early studies suggested that if patients were given antithyroid drugs for 12 to 18 months, approximately 50 per cent would remain euthyroid

after discontinuation of the drugs. More recently that fraction may have decreased to 10 to 20 per cent. The reason for the apparent change in the natural history of hyperthyroidism in the United States is not clear. One possible explanation is the recent increase in iodine intake. Since antithyroid drugs markedly deplete thyroidal iodine, the capacity to re-establish excessive secretion of thyroid hormone could be influenced by the iodine supply. In patients with Graves' disease who undergo a remission, hypothyroidism may occur some 20 to 30 years later. This is presumably autoimmune in origin, further emphasizing the similarities between Graves' disease and Hashimoto's thyroiditis. Lastly, in patients whose condition is in remission, relapse may occur months to years later.

As the underlying cause for Graves' disease is not known, no specific therapy for this condition is available. There are two phases of the treatment of the hyperthyroidism of Graves' disease. The first is acute therapy with the goal of re-establishing euthyroidism. The second phase is definitive therapy, the induction of a permanent alteration in thyroid function.

Short-Term Treatment of Hyperthyroidism. Antithyroid Drugs. In a typical patient with hyperthyroidism caused by Graves' disease, the first step in management is to suppress the elevated thyroid hormone secretion rate. The drugs of choice for this purpose are derivatives of thiourea. In the United States, propylthiouracil (PTU) and methimazole (Tapazole) are used. Both inhibit the organification of iodine by the thyroid gland as their major mechanism of action. Neither drug affects I^- trapping, nor does either inhibit the release of preformed thyroid hormone. PTU, but not methimazole, is an inhibitor of T_4 to T_3 conversion, giving it a modest therapeutic advantage over the latter agent. This drug has special importance in the short-term treatment of hyperthyroidism. Carbimazole, rapidly converted to methimazole in the body, is used in Europe and is equal in potency to methimazole.

PTU and methimazole are rapidly absorbed and are probably concentrated by the hyperactive thyroid. Although the plasma half-life is relatively short, suggesting the need for frequent dosage, in practice it is often possible to maintain satisfactory suppression of thyroid hormone synthesis by administration of these drugs twice or even only once per day. Methimazole is approximately 15 times as potent as PTU. Initial treatment consists of 300 to 450 mg of PTU per day (or the equivalent of methimazole) divided into three doses. Rarely as much as 1600 mg per day of PTU is required, but problems with compliance are common at such dosages. Since there is a 5- to 10-day half-time for the disappearance of the metabolic effects induced by excess thyroid hormone, it is not unusual for the serum level of T_4 to fall before the patient begins to obtain relief from the symptoms of hyperthyroidism. It is my practice to see the patient 3 to 4 weeks after the initial visit, obtaining a free T_4 index and serum T_3 at that point to ascertain the progress of therapy. If clinical improvement has not occurred, the serum T_4 has not decreased, and compliance has been maintained, the dose of antithyroid drug should be increased. After the first months of treatment, the dose of antithyroid drug can be reduced to a level of 100 to 300 mg per day of PTU, and the patient seen at 2- to 3-month intervals. In patients to be treated for 6 to 18 months, therapy can be monitored by both clinical and laboratory parameters. The serum T_3-T_4 ratio is increased because of intrathyroidal iodine deficiency and the increased thyroidal T_3-T_4 ratio in Graves' disease. Therefore both serum T_3 and the free T_4 index should be monitored. Serum TSH may increase if the serum T_4 falls below normal even if serum T_3 is normal. This is undesirable, since it can lead to further thyroid enlargement and possibly an exacerbation of eye symptoms.

Thiourea derivatives have several side effects. A maculopapular rash occurs in 2 to 8 per cent of patients but does not usually require discontinuation of the drug. Both agents can rarely cause hepatocellular damage, and PTU can cause vasculitis. The most serious side effect of both agents is agranulocytosis. This occurs in 2 to 5 of 1000 patients and can be fatal if not recognized. Since this reaction may be abrupt in onset and is so rare, it is not, in the opinion of many experts, necessary to monitor the white blood count (WBC) at frequent intervals. Instead, a baseline WBC and differential are obtained, and the patient is cautioned on each visit about the symptoms and significance of agranulocytosis. The patient is instructed to report immediately if infection occurs and to stop the medication. The WBC and differential are repeated and the drug discontinued permanently if indicated. The reaction may appear at any time during therapy and does not appear to be dose related (except at extremely high doses). It is seen most commonly in the first few months of therapy. If such a reaction occurs, the drug should be withdrawn and appropriate supportive care provided. Recovery occurs in almost all patients, and an alternative treatment method should then be used. Special precautions about the use of antithyroid drugs in pregnancy are discussed below. Iodide (saturated solution of potassium iodide, 1 gram KI per milliliter) 3 drops twice a day or Lugol's solution (125 mg I⁻ per milliliter) 10 drops three times a day is the most effective antithyroid drug for short-term use, since it inhibits both thyroid hormone release and thyroid hormone synthesis (through the Wolff-Chaikoff effect). Iodide alone can be given to patients with allergies to thiourea drugs to suppress thyroid function for periods of 10 to 28 days. Since the initially depressed hormone release increases gradually during treatment, iodide administration should not be prolonged beyond 2 to 3 weeks. Iodide is often used to decrease the vascularity of the thyroid gland in the preparation of patients who are to have surgery. Since it interferes with the subsequent administration of ^{131}I, it should not be used in the weeks prior to this treatment.

The benefits of bed rest, adequate diet, and the extrication of the patient from the usual occupational or domestic pressures cannot be overemphasized. Remarkable clinical improvement is often noted within 1 to 2 days simply as a result of hospitalization. The short-term treatment of severe hyperthyroidism is discussed below under Thyroid Storm.

β-Adrenergic Blocking Agents and Other Drugs. The similarity of the symptoms of hyperthyroidism to those of catecholamine excess is striking. The molecular basis for this similarity is not clearly established. Although animal studies have shown thyroid hormone–induced increases in β-adrenergic receptors in cardiac tissue, the receptor number is normal in lymphocytes from patients with thyrotoxicosis. Plasma catecholamine concentrations are normal in hyperthyroidism. Nevertheless, blockade of β-adrenergic receptors by propranolol or other β-receptor antagonists may result in symptomatic improvement prior to a decrease in serum thyroid hormones. A dose of 20 to 40 mg of propranolol every 4 to 6 hours may be used, but patients with congestive heart failure or bronchial asthma should not receive this therapy. In most patients with mild to moderate hyperthyroidism this adjunctive therapy is not necessary and may complicate the therapeutic regimen. In patients with more profound tachycardia or with thyroid storm (see below), it may have an important beneficial effect. Propranolol, although decreasing pulse rate and cardiac output in patients with hyperthyroidism, does not alter the elevated basal metabolic rate. Therefore the tissues continue to consume oxygen at a high rate in the presence of a decrease in cardiac output.

Lithium inhibits release of preformed thyroid hormone from the thyroid gland, probably by inhibiting hydrolysis of thyroglobulin, and may also inhibit peripheral T_4 degradation. In patients with allergies to thiourea drugs and iodide, lithium carbonate 0.9 to 1.5 grams per day (serum lithium concentrations of 0.5 to 1.0 mEq per liter) may be of value in the treatment of acute hyperthyroidism. Serum lithium levels must be closely monitored, as some of the toxic effects of lithium are similar to those of thyrotoxicosis.

Iopanoic acid (Telepaque) and ipodate (Oragrafin) contain iodide and also are potent inhibitors of type I and type II 5'-deiodinase activities. These agents therefore appear to be ideal for short-term treatment of hyperthyroidism. However, both remain in the body for long periods, which may prohibit subsequent ^{131}I therapy. They can be used in emergency situations, especially if surgery is contemplated as definitive therapy, and might also be as effective as PTU for blocking T_4 to T_3 conversion, such as might be required in the rare patient with severe exogenous thyrotoxicosis.

The Second Phase of Hyperthyroidism Treatment. If the symptoms of hyperthyroidism are not severe or after short-term treatment of symptoms with thiourea drugs, a decision must be made as to long-term therapy. There are three choices: further antithyroid drugs with hopes of a spontaneous remission, surgery, or radioiodine. None of these is ideal, and the choice for each patient must be made individually.

Long-Term Antithyroid Drug Therapy. If long-term antithyroid drug therapy is undertaken in anticipation of a remission, it should be continued for 6 to 18 months. If the quantities of drug required to maintain euthyroidism remain relatively large (e.g., 200 mg of PTU or greater) and serum T_3 and T_4 rise when the dosage is reduced, then a remission has not occurred. If the thyroid becomes smaller and the required amount of antithyroid drug lower, then a remission is probable. Some authorities recommend a TSH assay at this juncture, but I prefer to determine serum T_3 and T_4, to discontinue the treatment, and to repeat these tests in 4 weeks. The serum T_3 is especially important, since it may become elevated prior to the T_4 when a relapse occurs. If thyroid hormones remain normal, the patient should be seen at bimonthly intervals for 1 year, at which time the visits can be reduced in frequency.

Surgery. Surgical removal of a portion of the thyroid gland to regulate hyperthyroidism is a time-honored and effective treatment in the hands of expert surgeons. Hyperthyroidism rarely recurs, although roughly 50 to 60 per cent of patients eventually become hypothyroid. In most patients, hyperthyroidism is controlled by antithyroid drugs for 1 to 2 months prior to surgery. About 7 to 10 days before surgery, saturated solution of potassium iodide or Lugol's solution should be given to reduce the vascularity of the thyroid (see above).

Alternatively, propranolol alone may be used to prepare the patient, or it may be combined with I⁻. One to 2 weeks of pretreatment with 40 mg of propranolol every 6 hours has been given. This approach should not be employed for patients who can undertake standard preoperative therapy with thiourea drugs. Aside from hypothyroidism, other potential complications of surgery include neck hemorrhage, recurrent laryngeal nerve damage, and hypoparathyroidism. In highly experienced clinics, such complications are quite rare (<1 per cent).

Radioiodine. Treatment of hyperthyroidism with ^{131}I has been used since the late 1940's. The principal complication of this treatment is hypothyroidism, which occurs in about 10 per cent of patients in the first year and increases about 5 per cent per year thereafter over 20 years. Depending on the dose given, about 20 per cent of patients require a second treatment. No increased risk of thyroid carcinoma or leukemia occurs after such treatment. For many years, there was a reluctance to employ ^{131}I in the treatment of women in the childbearing age group, but the ovarian dose from a typical 10-mCi treatment is approximately 2 to 4 rads, which is in the same range as that from hysterosalpingography or a barium enema. Although any unnecessary radiation is to be avoided, the calculated increase in the gamete mutation rate from exposure in this range is only a small fraction of the spontaneous mutation rate. Thus ^{131}I therapy does not appear to offer a significant risk of fetal malformation, although it is recommended that pregnancy not be undertaken for 6 months after this therapy to avoid transient radiation-induced changes in the gametes.

I generally pretreat patients who are to have ^{131}I therapy with thiourea derivatives to provide symptomatic relief and avoid the remote chance of an exacerbation of hyperthyroidism from radiation thyroiditis. These are discontinued 4 days prior to determining the 24-hour ^{131}I uptake. My practice is to administer orally an amount of ^{131}I which when multiplied by the RAI uptake will result in thyroidal accumulation of 6 mCi ^{131}I. This results in an average dose of 80 to 90 µCi per gram, or 6000 to 7000 rads, which is associated with resolution of hyperthyroidism in about 80 per cent of patients within 6 months. Therapy with thiourea drugs may be restarted after 1 week, although it is not usually required. Patients are seen monthly thereafter with appropriate diagnostic and therapeutic measures to maintain the euthyroid state. At least 6 months is allowed to elapse before considering a second treatment. Since radioiodine crosses the placenta and would be concentrated by the thyroid of the fetus at 12 weeks and older, it is imperative that the possibility of pregnancy be eliminated before radioiodine is administered.

The therapist administering radioiodine is committed to the planning of adequate follow-up. This consists of thoroughly informing the patient about the risks of delayed hypothyroidism (occurring in 80 to 100 per cent), providing written documentation of the treatment and its complications, and maintaining proper communication with referring physicians as to the need for indefinite follow-up. Patients are alerted to the symptoms of hypothyroidism and instructed that after the acute phase of treatment they should be seen at least every 4 to 6 months for appropriate thyroid function testing until hypothyroidism appears and treatment is initiated.

Choice of Therapy. None of the three long-term therapies for hyperthyroidism is ideal. Some thyroidologists do not use radioiodine in patients under the age of 35 or 40 because of the fear of long-term complications, whereas others employ radioiodine routinely in the treatment of hyperthyroidism in children. On balance, from the point of view of lack of immediate complications and effectiveness, radioiodine treatment is the most effective approach currently available. My approach is to inform the patient of all treatment options and to recommend antithyroid drugs only to patients who have goiters less than three times normal or in patients who are hesitant regarding radioiodine therapy. In women in whom pregnancy is planned, a requirement for high doses of antithyroid drugs indicates the need for definitive treatment prior to undertaking pregnancy. Surgery is recommended only for patients with extreme thyroid enlargement or those who have coexisting nonfunctioning thyroid nodules. The physician advising patients regarding this decision must consider not only these theoretical arguments and the patient's preferences but also the availability of an experienced surgeon.

Graves' Disease and Pregnancy. The peak incidence of Graves' disease occurs in women during the reproductive period. Therefore, it is not uncommon to find hyperthyroidism in a pregnant patient or for pregnancy to occur during therapy with antithyroid drugs. There is a tendency for Graves' disease to exacerbate during the first trimester of pregnancy and to ameliorate during the third trimester. One to 2 months after delivery, an exacerbation is not uncommon. Since PTU and methimazole cross the placenta, whereas thyroid hormones do not do so in appreciable amounts, minimal quantities of these agents must be used during pregnancy. PTU crosses the placenta less well than does methimazole. While pregnant patients tolerate moderate degrees of hyperthyroidism quite well, uncontrolled thyrotoxicosis is associated with an increased risk of spontaneous abortion and may be associated with thyroid storm at the time of delivery.

With these facts in mind, pregnant patients with hyperthyroidism should be seen at monthly intervals, with careful clinical examination supplemented by measurements of serum T_3, T_4, and THBR. It should be recalled that the normal range for both serum T_4 and T_3 is higher during pregnancy (see Table 216–4). PTU should be given at the lowest dosage that maintains the patient at an acceptable euthyroid state. I do not employ supplemental thyroid hormones in the treatment of most pregnant hyperthyroid patients. An attempt to reduce the antithyroid drug dose should be made as the third trimester approaches. If the patient's hyperthyroid symptoms cannot be controlled on less than 300 to 400 mg of PTU per day, then subtotal thyroidectomy should be considered during the second trimester. Iodides can be given for 7 to 10 days in preparation for surgery but should not be given over a long period during pregnancy, since the fetus may develop hypothyroidism because of transplacental iodide transfer and the Wolff-Chaikoff effect.

The newborn infant of the mother with Graves' disease should be examined carefully for either hypothyroidism as a consequence of excessive antithyroid drug or hyperthyroidism resulting from transplacental passage of TRAb. In either situation goiter may be present, which may lead to respiratory embarrassment. Even the most meticulously managed patients may have infants with modest reductions in serum T_4 that quickly normalize in the first week of life. Neonatal hyperthyroidism is transient but occasionally must be treated with antithyroid drugs and digitalis for tachycardia.

The quantities of PTU in the milk of mothers receiving 200 to 300 mg PTU per day are not great enough to cause impairment of an infant's thyroid function. It seems likely that nursing mothers could take PTU at low doses, although the infant could still be at risk for nonthyroidal complications of this drug. Methimazole (and presumably carbimazole) is present in milk in significant amounts and should not be given to nursing mothers.

Thyroid Storm. Some patients with hyperthyroidism develop

severe manifestations that are exaggerations of many of the symptoms listed in Table 216–6. Often these occur because of superimposed stress or infection. The patient may be febrile, have abdominal pain, and become delirious, obtunded, or psychotic. This condition, called *thyroid storm*, has a mortality of 20 to 40 per cent. It should be suspected in any patient with severe hyperpyrexia, or extreme tachycardia, particularly if goiter is present. Patients with suspected thyroid storm should be hospitalized and treated with a protocol such as is outlined in Table 216–7. I^- is the most effective agent for inhibiting release of preformed thyroid hormone. If it is thought that the patient has a surgical abdomen, intravenous propranolol may be used intraoperatively to control tachycardia, assuming that there are no contraindications. The line between severe hyperthyroidism and thyroid storm is nebulous. In patients with severe symptoms but without fever, I^- should be added to PTU therapy to achieve a more rapid decrease in thyroid hormones. The I^- can be discontinued after 1 week.

Treatment of Ophthalmopathy. In most patients with ophthalmopathy no specific therapy is needed. Return of the patient to the euthyroid state often results in amelioration of many of the minor symptoms, including stare and lid lag. It is important to avoid hypothyroidism, as anecdotal data suggest that this may be associated with an exacerbation of eye symptoms. The patient may note periorbital edema, especially on arising in the morning. An extra pillow or elevation of the head of the bed will relieve this. Alternatively, a diuretic can be administered at bedtime. In patients with more severe symptoms, artificial tears or 1 per cent methylcellulose are prescribed.

A small fraction of patients with Graves' disease have more severe problems than can be relieved by these minor therapeutic measures. In patients with severe proptosis, desiccation of the sclera or cornea may occur at night because of lagophthalmos. Taping the lids closed at night may alleviate this symptom, although lateral tarsorrhaphy is a more permanent solution. Diplopia may be treated by prisms or, if permanent, by muscle repositioning or relief of fibrous adhesions. This procedure should not be performed until the eye disease has stabilized, often a matter of 2 to 3 years. In the patient with severe inflammation and chemosis (*malignant exophthalmos*), prednisone is required. Although 15 to 20 mg per day may be sufficient, in many patients

TABLE 216–7. MANAGEMENT OF PATIENTS WITH THYROID STORM

Diagnostic
1. Serum T_3 and T_4 concentrations, resin or charcoal T_3 uptake
2. Appropriate evaluation for underlying precipitating causes such as infection, acute surgical abdomen, central nervous system lesions, or psychological trauma
3. Baseline WBC and differential, electrolytes, Ca, P
4. Plasma cortisol

Therapeutic
1. Intravenous fluids—dextrose with or without electrolytes as indicated, multivitamins
2. Propylthiouracil, 400 mg every 6 hours (by nasogastric tube, if necessary), to inhibit thyroid hormone synthesis and block T_4 to T_3 conversion
3. Sodium iodide, 250 mg every 6 hours (orally or intravenously)
4. Hydrocortisone, 50 to 100 mg every 6 hours intravenously
5. External cooling and acetaminophen (300 to 600 mg) every 4 to 6 hours for severe hyperpyrexia (do not use salicylates, which increase free thyroid hormones and oxygen consumption)
6. Propranolol—in patients without asthma, chronic bronchitis, or nonarrhythmia-related, congestive heart failure, 10 to 40 mg may be given every 4 to 6 hours orally; a slow intravenous infusion of 1 mg per minute for 2 to 10 minutes with careful monitoring of blood pressure and ECG may be used if oral therapy is not feasible; propranolol may precipitate pulmonary edema in a few patients with hyperthyroidism; reserpine or guanethidine do not appear to have any advantages over propranolol in this situation
7. Oxygen may be helpful
8. Digitalis glycosides should be employed for therapy of congestive failure and for blockade of a rapid ventricular response to an atrial tachyrhythmia
9. Appropriate treatment of precipitating event if any

as much as 100 mg per day is necessary with the attendant complications of treatment. Such patients should have frequent measurements of visual acuity and visual fields. Deterioration of either test is an emergency requiring steroid treatment and ophthalmologic consultation. An alternative treatment is orbital irradiation, 2000 rads being given to the retro-orbital region to suppress local lymphocytic infiltration. This is usually used in conjunction with glucocorticoid administration. In the case of optic compression or persistent corneal ulceration, surgical decompression may be required. Fortunately, in most patients the severity of the eye manifestations abates after 12 to 18 months, although in many the proptosis never reverts to normal.

Pretibial Myxedema. The lesions of pretibial myxedema are not generally incapacitating but may be cosmetically disfiguring. They may be treated with topical application of glucocorticoids, with enhancement of absorption by occlusive dressings if necessary.

PROGNOSIS. In most patients, Graves' disease is a benign disorder in which the physician can play an important role in providing considerable relief to the patient. Because of the complications of treatment and the possibility of hypothyroidism even in patients with a spontaneous remission, patients with Graves' disease require lifelong observation.

TREATMENT OF OTHER CAUSES OF HYPERTHYROIDISM. The short-term treatment of hyperthyroidism associated with toxic multinodular goiter or toxic adenoma does not differ from that of patients with Graves' disease. These entities are discussed in detail later in the chapter. The hyperthyroidism associated with subacute thyroiditis (particularly the lymphocytic variety) is discussed in the section Thyroiditis.

TSH-secreting pituitary tumor must be treated by surgery. Patients with this condition are identified and separated from the group with nontumorigenic TSH-induced hyperthyroidism by finding an elevation of the serum α-TSH subunit as well as of TSH. Nontumorigenic hypersecretion of TSH is thought to be due to a reduction in feedback sensitivity to T_3 and T_4 at the pituitary level. Such patients are treated with antithyroid drugs. In patients with choriocarcinoma or hydatidiform mole, removal of the tumor relieves these symptoms. Extremely rare is the ovarian teratoma containing thyroid tissue, *struma ovarii*. This should be treated surgically. In general, thyroid carcinoma does not function well enough to lead to hyperthyroidism. Hyperthyroidism can occur if extensive metastases that retain a significant degree of function are present, as may be seen occasionally in follicular carcinoma. This condition is readily diagnosed and is treated with [131]I.

Burrow GN: The management of thyrotoxicosis in pregnancy. N Engl J Med 313:562, 1985. *A review of factors to be considered when managing the pregnant patient with active Graves' disease.*

Cohen JH, Ingbar SH, Braverman LE: Thyrotoxicosis due to ingestion of excess thyroid hormone. Endocr Rev 10:113, 1989. *A review of the approach to the patient suspected of ingesting excess thyroid hormone.*

Davis PJ, Davis FB: Hyperthyroidism in patients over the age of 60 years. Medicine 53:161, 1974. *An excellent summary of the clinical syndrome of hyperthyroidism in the elderly patient.*

Gesundheit N, Petrick PA, Nissim M, et al.: Thyrotropin-secreting pituitary adenomas: Clinical and biochemical heterogeneity. Ann Intern Med 111:827, 1989. *Thorough description of a rare but important cause of hyperthyroidism—thyrotropin-secreting pituitary tumors.*

Henneman G, Krenning EP, Sankaranarayanan K: Place of radioactive iodine in treatment of thyrotoxicosis. Lancet 1:1369, 1986. *The author makes a persuasive argument for the use of radioiodine as the first-line treatment for patients with Graves' disease. A brief but thorough review of the pros and cons of this approach to therapy.*

McKenzie JM, Zakarija M: Clinical review 3: The clinical use of thyrotropin receptor antibody measurements. J Clin Endocrinol Metab 69:1093, 1989. *A review of when and when not to request thyrotropin receptor antibody measurements in patients suspected of Graves' disease.*

Silva JE: Effects of iodine and iodine containing compounds on thyroid function. Med Clin North Am 69:881, 1985. *The author reviews all aspects of iodine excess and deficiency. The discussion of iodide-induced hyperthyroidism is particularly relevant for this section.*

Smallridge RC, Parker RA, Wiggs EA, et al.: Thyroid hormone resistance in a large kindred: Physiologic, biochemical, pharmacologic, and neuropsychologic studies. Am J Med 86:289, 1989. *A review of the clinical manifestations of thyroid hormone resistance in a large family.*

Smith BR, McLachlan SM, Furmaniak J: Autoantibodies to the thyrotropin receptor. Endocr Rev 9:106, 1988. *Studies of the etiology of Graves' disease are reviewed.*

HYPOTHYROIDISM AND MYXEDEMA

DEFINITION. *Hypothyroidism* is the clinical syndrome that results from a deficiency of thyroid hormone. In severe hypothyroidism a hydrophilic mucopolysaccharide substance accumulates in subcutaneous tissues, causing a nonpitting edema referred to as *myxedema.* Some authorities use the terms *hypothyroidism* and *myxedema* interchangeably, whereas others reserve the latter term for the severe form of this syndrome.

ETIOLOGY. A list of causes to be considered in patients with hypothyroidism is given in Table 216–8. *Primary hypothyroidism,* that caused by thyroid gland malfunction, accounts for over 95 per cent of such cases, of which Hashimoto's thyroiditis, idiopathic myxedema (probably a variant of Hashimoto's thyroiditis), and thyroid destruction resulting from ^{131}I therapy or surgery for hyperthyroidism account for the greatest proportion. Hashimoto's and subacute thyroiditis are discussed in the next section. Hypothyroidism after therapeutic irradiation to the thyroid area for lymphoma or Hodgkin's disease is found in 10 to 30 per cent of these patients, usually within 1 to 2 years of treatment.

Hypothyroidism can also occur with normal or nearly normal thyroid tissue when there is a superimposed stress on thyroid hormone synthesis. Hypothyroidism may be caused either by severe iodine deficiency (<25 μg iodine per day) or by naturally occurring goitrogens such as have been found in Colombia or are generated by eating the cassava plant in Africa (see Sporadic Goiter and Endemic Goiter). In patients with Graves' disease, especially after RAI treatment, or in those with mild Hashimoto's thyroiditis, iodine excess may cause hypothyroidism through the Wolff-Chaikoff effect (I⁻-induced inhibition of organification). These glands are unable to reduce I⁻ uptake in the presence of an elevated plasma I⁻ as normally occurs. The drugs listed in Table 216–8 inhibit organification of thyroidal I⁻. In most cases the hypothyroidism associated with these drugs is mild.

Screening of newborns for hypothyroidism is now widely practiced, and the incidence of this condition is about 1 in 4000 births. About 65 per cent of infants with congenital hypothyroidism in North America have thyroid agenesis or hypoplasia, 25 per cent have ectopic thyroid glands, and about 10 per cent have

TABLE 216–8. CAUSES OF HYPOTHYROIDISM

I. Primary hypothyroidism
  A. Acquired
    1. Destructive lesions
      a. Hashimoto's thyroiditis
      b. Idiopathic myxedema (probably the end-stage of Hashimoto's thyroiditis)
      c. [131]I therapy for hyperthyroidism
      d. Subtotal thyroidectomy, especially for Graves' disease
      e. Therapeutic external x-ray treatment to the neck for other diseases
      f. After subacute thyroiditis (may be transient)
      g. Cystinosis
    2. Impaired function of a normal or nearly normal gland
      a. Endemic goiter—iodine deficiency or naturally occurring goitrogens
      b. Iodine excess (>6 mg per day) in patients with underlying thyroid disease
      c. Drug-induced: lithium carbonate, para-aminosalicylic acid, thiourea drugs, sulfonamides, phenylbutazone, and others
  B. Congenital
    1. Defects in enzymes required for thyroid hormone synthesis (congenital goiter)
    2. Thyroid agenesis
    3. Thyroid dysgenesis or ectopy
    4. Maternal iodide or antithyroid drugs
II. Secondary hypothyroidism
  A. Hypothalamic dysfunction
    1. Neoplasms
    2. Eosinophilic granuloma
    3. Therapeutic irradiation
  B. Pituitary dysfunction
    1. Neoplasms
    2. Pituitary surgery or irradiation
    3. Idiopathic hypopituitarism
    4. Sheehan's syndrome (postpartum pituitary necrosis)
    5. Dopamine infusion and/or severe illness(?)
III. Tissue resistance to thyroid hormone

defects in one of the steps required for thyroid hormone synthesis (see Sporadic Goiter and Endemic Goiter).

Secondary hypothyroidism occurs as a result of hypothalamic or pituitary dysfunction. Dopamine infusion and/or severe illness may suppress TSH release sufficiently to cause a modest, transient hypothyroidism. A rare cause of hypothyroidism is tissue resistance to thyroid hormones, which is usually due to an abnormality in the nuclear receptor for these hormones.

INCIDENCE. Hypothyroidism is common in adults. In one epidemiologic survey, 1.4 per cent of adult females and about 0.1 per cent of adult males were affected. Autoimmune destruction of the thyroid gland is the most common cause of thyroid gland failure in adults. This generally affects women over the age of 40 but can occur at any age. Hypothyroidism is also a common congenital disease, occurring in about 1 of 4000 neonates in North America and Western Europe and more frequently in areas of iodine deficiency.

PATHOLOGY. The pathology of the thyroid gland in hypothyroidism depends on the etiology of the syndrome. In "idiopathic myxedema," the thyroid tissue is generally replaced by fat with few intact follicles and lymphocytic infiltration (see also Thyroiditis). When the thyroid cells remain partly functional, the elevated serum TSH leads to hyperplasia and hypertrophy. In secondary hypothyroidism, the number of follicular cells is low and considerable colloid is present. The gland is small in contrast to the goiter found when thyroid cell dysfunction is present and TSH secretion is increased.

The nonthyroidal pathology of the hypothyroid state is the same regardless of its etiology. The longer the duration and the more severe the deficiency, the greater are the changes. The accumulation of mucopolysaccharide in connective tissues has already been mentioned. This material may also appear in muscle. Effusions, which often have a high protein content, occur in various serous cavities.

CLINICAL MANIFESTATIONS. The common clinical manifestations of this syndrome in the adult are summarized in Table 216–9. These symptoms and signs can be attributed to either deceleration of cellular metabolic processes or the accumulation of the hygroscopic mucopolysaccharide in the vocal cords or oropharynx, as well as the more obvious changes in the subcutaneous tissues. The symptoms are nonspecific, particularly in the early phases, and may either pass unnoticed by the patient or be attributed to advancing age. Characteristically, the patient becomes aware of their multiplicity and severity only after thyroid hormone replacement leads to a return of normal function. This is particularly true of younger patients. In the elderly, hearing impairment, somnolence, and decreased memory and ability to calculate may occur. These may lead to an apparent psychological withdrawal and paranoia at times requiring hospitalization. The term *myxedema madness* has been used to describe this syndrome, which can be mistaken for cerebrovascular insufficiency or senile dementia. Alternatively, the patient may confabulate or respond with humorous non sequiturs to draw the interviewer's attention from his or her limited recall of recent events. This behavior has been termed *myxedema wit*. A variety of menstrual disorders may be present, although menorrhagia is said to be the most common pattern. Pregnancy may occur in patients with hypothyroidism, and the increased hormone requirements of that condition may cause a previously borderline functioning thyroid to decompensate. Despite the developmental abnormalities associated with congenital hypothyroidism, the symptoms of hypothyroidism in infants are few. Severe thyroid hormone deficiency is associated with growth retardation in the older infant

TABLE 216–9. COMMON SYMPTOMS OF HYPOTHYROIDISM

Weakness, fatigue, lethargy
Dry, coarse skin
Swelling of the hands, face, and extremities
Cold intolerance, decreased sweating
Coarsening or huskiness of the voice
Modest weight gain (~10 lbs) with anorexia
Decreased memory, hearing impairment
Arthralgia, paresthesias
Constipation
Muscle cramps

and child. In the adolescent, thyroid enlargement, *adolescent goiter*, may be the only manifestation and is usually seen in the pubertal female. In some patients in whom the hypothyroidism is of rapid onset, cramps in large muscle groups may be a prominent symptom. Such symptoms usually occur after a rapid change from a hyperthyroid to a hypothyroid state, such as after surgery for Graves' disease, a second RAI treatment for hyperthyroidism, or even vigorous antithyroid drug therapy.

Many of the common signs of hypothyroidism are the opposite of those seen in the hyperthyroid patient. Bradycardia is common and is sometimes associated with hypothermia. Systolic pressure is generally reduced and diastolic pressure increased, the latter resulting from increased peripheral vascular resistance. Myxedema is manifested by a puffy, nonpitting swelling of the subcutaneous tissue, which may particularly collect in the periorbital area. Body and scalp hair are reduced; the skin may be coarse, the texture of sandpaper, and is usually cool and sallow. The yellow complexion is due to the accumulation of carotene in the serum in patients with significant hypothyroidism. The thyroid may be enlarged, of normal size, or not palpable, depending on the cause. The heart sounds are distant, and the heart shadow is often enlarged. The latter can be a manifestation of pericardial effusion, which is common but rarely leads to tamponade. In addition to the cortical dysfunction previously mentioned, cerebellar ataxia may be present. Other neurologic signs, including delayed relaxation of the deep tendon reflexes, peripheral neuropathy, and carpal tunnel syndrome, can completely resolve with treatment.

Certain physiologic abnormalities are characteristic of hypothyroidism. Cardiac output is reduced, although not out of proportion to the decrease in O_2 consumption. Glomerular filtration is also subnormal, leading to an impairment of the capacity to excrete free water. In addition, inappropriate antidiuretic hormone (ADH) secretion may lead to hyponatremia. Gastrointestinal motility is reduced, and occasionally the patient may develop an apparent obstruction, *myxedema megacolon*. There are important abnormalities in the respiratory center. The sensitivity to both hypercarbia and hypoxia is reduced, and such patients may readily develop CO_2 narcosis or cardiac arrhythmias associated with hypoxia. This is one of the chief causes of death in the severe form of myxedema, *myxedema coma*. Pituitary function is impaired in severe hypothyroidism even of the primary variety. Hypoglycemic stress does not elicit normal growth hormone or cortisol responses in such patients, so that testing pituitary function must be delayed until the hypothyroid state has been corrected. Serum prolactin is increased in moderate to severe primary hypothyroidism, and this may lead to galactorrhea in a small percentage of patients.

LABORATORY DIAGNOSIS. The diagnosis of hypothyroidism can be easily confirmed by using the scheme outlined in Figures 216–4 and 216–8. When the diagnosis is not made, it is usually because the nonspecificity of signs and symptoms does not immediately suggest this cause. This disease is one of the "great imitators," and a high index of suspicion should be maintained, as the condition is so readily diagnosed and treated. In all patients with hypothyroidism, the free T_4 index is reduced. Serum T_3 concentrations are often in the normal range in hypothyroid patients, and this test is not useful in the diagnosis of this condition. It is unlikely that significant symptoms are present in patients with an equivocal reduction in this hormone. Once a reduced free T_4 index has been found, it is imperative to determine whether the cause of the disease is primary, i.e., owing to thyroid disease, or secondary, involving the hypothalamic-pituitary axis. An increase in serum TSH establishes the diagnosis of primary hypothyroidism. If the serum TSH concentration is normal or borderline, then the diagnosis of pituitary or hypothalamic hypothyroidism is made, and further steps are taken to evaluate the possibility of a deficiency of other pituitary hormones. It is extremely important that this be done prior to the onset of therapy, since thyroid replacement exacerbates mild ACTH insufficiency associated with hypothalamic or pituitary disease. *If unrecognized, such patients may have an addisonian crisis provoked by thyroid hormone replacement.* There are two circumstances in which primary hypothyroidism is not associated with TSH elevation. This may be the case when hypothyroidism follows shortly after a period of hyperthyroidism, since the latter causes suppression of pituitary TSH synthesis lasting 4 to 5 weeks. Dopamine infusion may also cause suppression of an elevated TSH concentration into the normal range.

In the patient whose symptoms are nonspecific or borderline and in whom an equivocally reduced free T_4 index is obtained, the serum TSH may be significantly elevated. Elevated serum TSH is the most sensitive index of impairment of thyroid gland function. Whether or not such patients are actually metabolically hypothyroid cannot be determined by using present tests. This condition has been called *subclinical hypothyroidism*.

There are a few clinical situations in which the free T_4 index is reduced but serum TSH is not elevated in the absence of hypothalamic or pituitary disease. This may occur in severely ill patients without thyroid disease, but who presumably have transient hypothalamic-pituitary hypothyroidism. In such patients, a serum cortisol determination is indicated to eliminate the possibility of ACTH deficiency. If clinically indicated, therapy can then be initiated with both thyroxine and glucocorticoid. Patients receiving 2 to 3 grams per day of salicylate or 300 mg per day of phenytoin may have a reduction in the free T_4 index without hypothyroidism (see Table 216–3), and also patients ingesting replacement quantities (25 μg or more) of triiodothyronine (Cytomel) have reduced serum T_4 due to suppression of TSH, even if the thyroid gland is normal. A 24-hour RAI uptake test may not separate hypothyroidism from the euthyroid state and is not useful in diagnosis.

Other Biochemical Abnormalities and Associated Diseases in Patients with Hypothyroidism. Serum cholesterol and triglycerides, creatine phosphokinase (MM isozyme), aldolase, lactic dehydrogenase, and SGOT may all be elevated in the patient with moderate to severe hypothyroidism. Hyponatremia with or without the inappropriate ADH syndrome is seen. There is often a modest anemia of chronic disease that may be macrocytic. Serum vitamin B_{12} should be measured in these patients because of the 3 to 6 per cent coexistence of pernicious anemia with Hashimoto's thyroiditis. Other conditions found with increased frequency in patients with autoimmune thyroid disease include idiopathic adrenocortical deficiency, diabetes mellitus, hypoparathyroidism, myasthenia gravis, vitiligo (Ch. 228), and mitral valve prolapse.

DIFFERENTIAL DIAGNOSIS. There are few conditions that can masquerade as hypothyroidism in its classic form. However, patients with nephrotic syndrome or hypoalbuminemia and associated peripheral edema may be suspected of this diagnosis. Although the serum T_4 in these conditions is reduced because of hypoproteinemia, the THBR is generally quite elevated with a consequent normal free T_4 index. Patients with chronic renal disease may have symptoms entirely similar to those of hypothyroidism (including hypothermia), and laboratory tests are required to evaluate the possible coexistence of these two diseases. In patients with spontaneous primary hypothyroidism, the tests for autoantibodies to either thyroglobulin or microsomal components

of the thyroid cell are generally positive. This is true even if the typical thyroid enlargement of Hashimoto's thyroiditis is not present. The other causes of hypothyroidism have already been discussed (see Table 216–8), and reversible causes should be eliminated.

THERAPY. Hypothyroidism is a readily treatable disease. The preparations available for thyroid replacement are listed in Table 216–10. Levothyroxine is most frequently used as replacement therapy, since it provides stable and easily measureable serum concentrations for use in monitoring therapy and allows physiologic regulation of extrathyroidal T_3 production. Ideally, both serum T_3 and T_4 concentrations should be normalized for satisfactory replacement. Since in the euthyroid individual, 20 per cent of T_3 is derived directly from the thyroid gland (see Table 216–2), one would predict that normalization of serum T_3 in hypothyroid individuals would be associated with a serum free T_4 index that is about 60 per cent above the euthyroid value. Because intrapituitary T_3 is derived independently from both serum T_4 *and* serum T_3, this could well result in a subnormal TSH-IMA. At present the data are too incomplete to allow an informed decision whether serum T_3 or serum TSH concentrations should be normalized, assuming that both goals cannot be achieved simultaneously. It is recognized that excessive thyroid hormone replacement may be deleterious to cardiac function and to bone mineralization. At present, I use a combination of clinical evaluation and the TSH-IMA test as the guidelines for adequate replacement, although serum T_3 is measured periodically. The dose of levothyroxine required to achieve symptomatic and biochemical replacement in most patients is about 1.5 μg T_4 per kilogram (about 0.7 μg T_4 per pound). This is a significantly lower requirement than previously used because of improvements in tablet formulation. In most female patients a dose of 87 to 100 μg is quite adequate. The difference between this amount and the T_4 production rate of 1.1 μg per kilogram per day is due to the incomplete absorption of orally administered levothyroxine. In patients who become hypothyroid after ^{131}I treatment for Graves' disease, the requirement may be lower because of residual, nonsuppressible T_4 or T_3 secretion.

In patients who are in good health otherwise or whose hypothyroidism is very modest, therapy can be initiated with half-replacement doses immediately on establishment of the diagnosis. This can be increased to full replacement after 1 month. In patients with more severe hypothyroidism, elderly patients, or those with a history of cardiovascular disease, I prefer to begin therapy with smaller amounts (25 μg of thyroxine per day) and to increase these by 25-μg increments at 4-week intervals (with due attention to symptoms) until a replacement dose is achieved. In patients with primary hypothyroidism there may rarely be associated primary autoimmune hypoadrenalism (*Schmidt's syndrome*). Such patients require adequate replacement of glucocorticoid prior to institution of thyroid hormone replacement. A similar procedure must be employed in patients in whom hypothalamic-pituitary disease is a cause of hypothyroidism.

Long-term monitoring of thyroid hormone replacement should

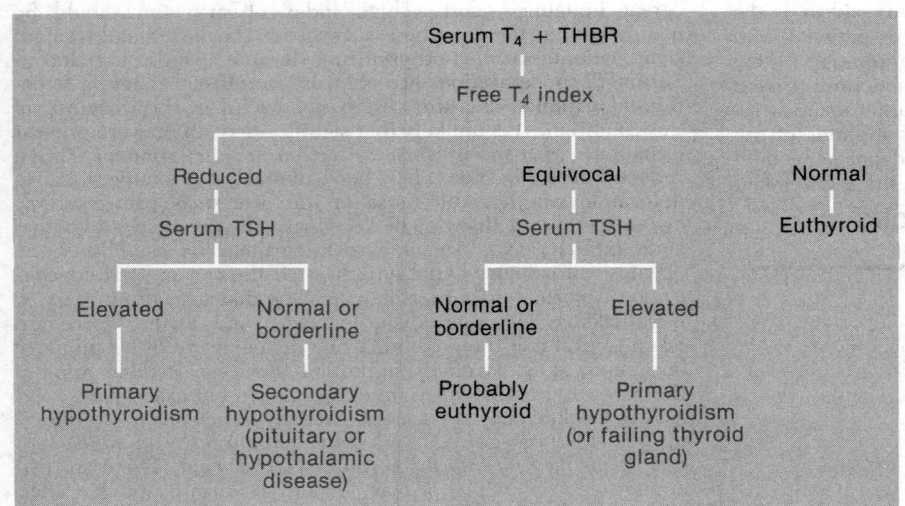

FIGURE 216–8. Laboratory diagnosis of hypothyroidism. THBR refers to the thyroid hormone–binding ratio (formerly termed T_3 or T_4 uptake).

TABLE 216–10. HORMONE CONTENT OF THYROID REPLACEMENT PREPARATIONS
(AMOUNTS APPROXIMATELY EQUIVALENT TO 1 GRAIN [65 mg] OF DESICCATED THYROID)

| | Levothyroxine | Liotrix | | Desiccated Thyroid (1-Grain Tablets) | | Levotriiodothyronine |
		Euthroid-1	Thyrolar-1	Armour	Proloid	
T_4 (μg)	100	60	50	63	55	0
T_3 (μg)	0	15	12.5	12	16	25

include annual measurements of the serum free T_4 index, TSH, and serum T_3. The replacement dose of T_4 may be 20 to 40 per cent lower in elderly patients. Thyroxine requirements increase about 25 to 50 per cent in most pregnant women with primary hypothyroidism, decreasing again immediately after delivery. Serum hormone and TSH concentrations should be monitored at monthly intervals during the first trimester and the dosage of thyroxine adjusted as needed to maintain the serum TSH in the normal range.

Special Problems in Hypothyroid Patients. The patient who presents simultaneously with angina and hypothyroidism poses a serious therapeutic problem. In some patients with coronary artery disease, reintroduction of thyroid hormones results in increased myocardial oxygen demands without an adequate increase in myocardial blood flow. A trial of propranolol with small increments of thyroxine may reduce myocardial oxygen consumption without decreasing the pulse rate to unacceptably low levels. If an exacerbation of angina occurs during thyroxine therapy, T_4 to T_3 conversion may be acutely reduced in peripheral tissues with propylthiouracil (see Graves' Disease and Other Causes of Hyperthyroidism). In patients with localized coronary artery disease in whom bypass graft surgery is indicated, the frequent adverse effects of thyroxine replacement have raised the possibility that surgery should be performed prior to thyroid hormone replacement. The overall morbidity may be lower in patients operated on in the hypothyroid state than in patients in whom replacement is attempted prior to surgery.

Although theoretical considerations suggest that hypothyroidism would impair the physiologic response to surgical stress, patients with mild to moderate hypothyroidism do not appear to have more perioperative complications with major surgery than do euthyroid patients, at least as assessed in retrospective studies. While elective surgery should not be performed in the untreated hypothyroid patient, a moderate degree of hypothyroidism does not preclude carefully managed emergency procedures.

Patients with subclinical hypothyroidism (low-normal free T_4 index and TSH >10 μU per milliliter) may benefit from therapy even though their symptoms are not obvious. This biochemical pattern together with a small goiter and positive antithyroid microsomal antibodies indicates the presence of Hashimoto's thyroiditis (see below), and it is my practice to treat such patients to prevent further thyroid enlargement.

Treatment of Myxedema Coma. In severe myxedema the patient may lapse into coma. This serious complication (mortality, 20 to 50 per cent) occurs most commonly in patients with severe hypothyroidism who are subjected to an additional physiologic stress. This may occur spontaneously, following cold exposure, or during infection, but in all too many instances it is iatrogenic. The administration of sedatives to hypothyroid patients may precipitate coma, as drugs are not metabolized as rapidly in these patients. The reduced sensitivity of the respiratory center to changes in blood gases may lead to inappropriately small ventilatory responses. In other situations, surgery may be performed in a patient who is not recognized to be severely hypothyroid, and postoperative opiates or sedatives lead to clinical deterioration. In Table 216–11 are shown the important steps in management of patients with myxedema coma. In these emergent situations it is important to institute treatment immediately. If the serum free T_4 index is reduced, treatment is begun even if the cause of the hypothyroidism (primary versus secondary) has not been identified. Accordingly, testing for adrenal function is carried out immediately, followed by institution of glucocorticoid replacement. Because of the irregularities of either intramuscular or gastrointestinal absorption in hypothyroidism, medications should be given intravenously. Glucocorticoid replacement

should not be given in pharmacologic quantities, since this impairs T_4 to T_3 conversion.

PROGNOSIS. The prognosis of hypothyroidism is excellent, provided that thyroid hormone replacement is maintained at an appropriate level.

Withdrawal of Thyroid Hormone After Prolonged Replacement. The question sometimes arises whether thyroid hormone therapy is indicated in a patient already receiving it. If, based on the history, the physician is skeptical of the need for replacement, the dosage of thyroxine may be reduced to about 50 per cent of the estimated maintenance dose. Measurements of serum free thyroxine index and TSH are then performed at monthly intervals. If these remain normal for 2 months, the thyroxine may be discontinued and monitoring continued for an additional 2 months. If the free T_4 index and TSH are normal at that time, one can exclude the diagnosis of significant hypothyroidism.

Becker C: Hypothyroidism and atherosclerotic heart disease: Pathogenesis, medical management, and the role of coronary artery bypass surgery. Endocr Rev 6:432, 1985. *A review of clinical experience in treating patients with a combination of hypothyroidism and coronary artery disease.*
Gow SM, Caldwell G, Toft AD, et al.: Relationship between pituitary and other target organ responsiveness in hypothyroid patients receiving thyroxine replacement. J Clin Endocrinol Metab 64:364, 1987. *A correlation of serum TSH-IMA and thyroid hormones with various other markers of thyroid status in hypothyroid patients receiving levothyroxine.*
Mandel SJ, Larsen PR, Seely EW, et al.: Increased need for thyroxine during pregnancy in women with primary hypothyroidism. N Engl J Med 323:91, 1990.
Rees-Jones RW, Rolla AR, Larsen PR: Hormonal content of thyroid replacement preparations. JAMA 243:459, 1980. *Analyses of desiccated thyroid tablets show that some generic preparations have reduced quantities of T_4 and T_3 relative to those contained in brand-name products.*
Vulsma T, Gons MH, de Vijlder JJM: Maternal-fetal transfer of thyroxine in congenital hypothyroidism due to a total organification defect or thyroid agenesis. N Engl J Med 321:13, 1989. *Convincing evidence of transplacental passage of maternal thyroxine to the congenitally hypothyroid fetus.*

THYROIDITIS

Thyroiditis is classified into three types: acute, subacute, and chronic. Despite the common factor of inflammation in all of these entities, there are marked differences in their clinical presentations and etiology.

Acute Thyroiditis

Acute thyroiditis results from a bacterial infection of the thyroid gland with typical symptoms of such involvement, including a

TABLE 216–11. MANAGEMENT OF PATIENTS WITH MYXEDEMA COMA

Diagnostic
1. Serum T_4, T_3 uptake (or equivalent), TSH
2. CBC, glucose, electrolytes, blood gases, BUN, creatinine, CPK
3. Plasma cortisol before and 30 and 60 minutes after cosyntropin (Cortrosyn), 0.25 mg, intravenous bolus
4. Careful evaluation for concomitant disease; continuous ECG and temperature monitoring

Therapeutic
1. Levothyroxine, 2 μg per kilogram intravenously over 5 to 10 minutes initially, and 100 μg intravenously every 24 hours thereafter
2. Cover to conserve body heat; do not rewarm externally
3. Tracheal intubation and mechanical ventilation as required
4. Intravenous fluids as determined by initial blood glucose and electrolytes and by the state of hydration; watch for water retention
5. Hydrocortisone, 100 mg by intravenous bolus, then 25 mg every 6 hours as a continuous intravenous drip
6. Vigorous treatment of associated and precipitating conditions such as infection

fever, local tenderness, and swelling. This condition is quite rare. The infection may involve the whole gland or only a portion of it. Laboratory studies generally show normal thyroid function, but there is an elevated leukocyte count with a polymorphonuclear predominance. The thyroid scan may show an area of decreased uptake corresponding to the involved portion, but the 24-hour RAI uptake is usually normal. Treatment of this condition requires proper identification of the causative agent and appropriate antimicrobial drugs. This may require a needle aspiration. If localized abscess formation occurs, the abscess should be drained. The process usually responds rapidly to these measures.

Subacute (Nonsuppurative) Thyroiditis

This condition is also referred to as *giant cell thyroiditis*, *granulomatous thyroiditis*, or *de Quervain's thyroiditis*. In the classic form of this disease the patient presents with an exquisitely tender thyroid, which is pathologically characterized by follicular cell destruction and by a lymphocytic and polymorphonuclear leukocyte infiltration, together with multinucleate giant cells. In recent years, a different type of subacute thyroiditis has appeared, which is often painless and associated with hyperthyroidism. It shares some pathologic features with Hashimoto's thyroiditis (see below). This condition, which will be denoted *subacute lymphocytic thyroiditis*, is discussed separately below because of its unique features. The disease described by de Quervain will be referred to as *subacute granulomatous thyroiditis*.

INCIDENCE. The incidence of subacute granulomatous thyroiditis is not known, but it is not rare. It is most common in the third to fifth decades, and females are affected about three to four times more commonly than males. It occurs with increased frequency in HLA-B35–positive individuals.

ETIOLOGY. The granulomatous form of subacute thyroiditis often follows a viral infection by several weeks. At the time of the acute illness, elevated titers of antibody to influenza virus, coxsackievirus, or adenovirus can be found. Over the next few months these fall in many patients, suggesting that an acute infection has recently occurred. In only two cases has a virus been cultured from thyroid tissue, which in both cases was mumps. Some authorities interpret the thyroiditis as being a consequence of a process set in motion by the viral illness but not representing a direct infection of the gland. The precise etiology is unknown.

PATHOLOGY. The classic pathologic picture includes the cellular infiltrate described above, along with severe destruction of the normal follicular architecture. Fibrosis appears in the latter phases. Despite the extensive destruction, complete restoration of the normal thyroid structure generally occurs.

CLINICAL MANIFESTATIONS. Subacute granulomatous thyroiditis is characterized by an often exquisitely painful two- to threefold enlargement of the thyroid gland together with systemic symptoms, including fever, chills, and malaise. Patients often complain of neck or ear pain or dysphagia and may have had evaluation for pharyngeal infection. Symptoms of hyperthyroidism may also be present. The patient may report a prior viral illness. If symptoms of hyperthyroidism are present, they are generally of very short duration (less than 2 months) and are due to the release of thyroid hormones resulting from thyroid destruction. Physical examination may show fever, tachycardia, and exquisite tenderness of the slightly enlarged thyroid gland. This generally involves the whole gland but may be asymmetric.

DIAGNOSIS. The leukocyte count is mildly elevated, but there is characteristically a marked elevation of the erythrocyte sedimentation rate (ESR). This has been one of the hallmarks of this disease. The free T_4 index may be normal or increased. As would be expected from the pathology, the RAI uptake is low and the thyroid is poorly visualized on scan. The RAI uptake is the principal test for separating patients with this disease from those with hyperthyroidism resulting from Graves' disease. There may be an asymmetric involvement of the thyroid with decreased function in that area. Antimicrosomal and antithyroglobulin antibodies are absent or low in titer, although the serum thyroglobulin may be increased, reflecting the destructive process.

TREATMENT. Since this is a self-limited disease, treatment is symptomatic. Mild analgesics such as aspirin (2 to 4 grams per day) should be given for neck discomfort. In a significant fraction of patients, this is not sufficient, and prednisone, 20 to 40 mg per day, is required. The immediate relief associated with this therapy is almost diagnostic. The glucocorticoid should be continued for 2 to 3 weeks and then tapered over the next 3 weeks. There may be an exacerbation of the original symptoms during discontinuation of glucocorticoid requiring reinstitution of this therapy. Eventually this will not occur. The hyperthyroidism is usually mild but may require propranolol. Antithyroid drugs are of no use, as the serum T_4 and T_3 decrease when the glandular supply is exhausted.

There may be transient hypothyroidism following subacute granulomatous thyroiditis, and this may be severe enough to require treatment in some patients. Therefore it is important for these patients to be followed closely during the recovery period to ascertain whether or not this complication has occurred. Replacement thyroxine can be discontinued after 3 to 6 months with appropriate biochemical monitoring to establish that thyroid function has returned to normal. In 5 to 10 per cent of patients, permanent hypothyroidism supervenes. Occasionally a patient will be seen initially in the hypothyroid phase of this illness. An elevation in serum TSH and low thyroid hormones in the absence of antimicrosomal or antithyroglobulin antibodies should alert the physician to this possibility.

Subacute Lymphocytic Thyroiditis

This disease has been referred to by a variety of descriptive terms, including *painless thyroiditis*, *lymphocytic thyroiditis*, *lymphocytic thyroiditis with spontaneously resolving hyperthyroidism*, *hyperthyroiditis*, and *atypical subacute thyroiditis*. This confused nomenclature reflects the principal clinical and pathologic features of the disease: hyperthyroidism that is self-limited and lymphocytic infiltration of the thyroid.

ETIOLOGY. The etiology of the disease is unknown. There is little suggestion of a prior viral illness in these patients. The pathologic features are much closer to those of Hashimoto's disease than to those of granulomatous thyroiditis, suggesting an autoimmune etiology.

INCIDENCE. The precise incidence is not known, but one suspects that it has been increasing over the last 5 to 10 years. This condition may account for 5 to 20 per cent of patients with hyperthyroidism. About two thirds of reported cases are in women, with patients ranging from 13 to over 80 years of age.

PATHOLOGY. Lymphocytic infiltration is the common feature in all specimens studied. Destruction of follicular architecture and fibrosis similar to that of subacute granulomatous thyroiditis is seen, but foreign body giant cells are rare. Germinal centers characteristic of Hashimoto's disease are rarely seen.

CLINICAL MANIFESTATIONS. The principal symptoms of this form of subacute thyroiditis are those of hyperthyroidism, as described in the section Graves' Disease and Other Causes of Hyperthyroidism. Nonthyroidal stigmata of Graves' disease, exophthalmos and pretibial myxedema, are not present, although a stare and widened palpebral fissure may occur as a consequence of the hyperthyroidism per se. The duration of the hyperthyroid phase is short (usually less than 3 months), and it is generally modest in severity. Physical signs include those typical of hyperthyroidism and a normal or slightly enlarged thyroid gland which is not tender. The gland may be firm.

The natural history of thyroid function in a patient who had a typical episode of this disease is presented in Figure 216–9. The acute phase of hyperthyroidism resolved rapidly and spontaneously and was followed by a period of transient hypothyroidism requiring treatment. This was discontinued after 3 months, and after an initial period of thyroidal resistance to TSH, normal function returned. A phase of significant hypothyroidism such as this follows the hyperthyroidism in about one third of patients. For obscure reasons, this form of thyroiditis occurs with increased frequency in the first few months post partum.

LABORATORY DIAGNOSIS. Serum T_4 and T_3 concentrations are generally elevated, the TSH subnormal, the leukocyte count normal, and the ESR normal or only slightly elevated (<50 mm at 1 hour, Westergren). This is in marked contrast to the results in the granulomatous form of the disease. The 24-hour RAI uptake is reduced and will not increase even after TSH injection. Serum thyroglobulin is increased in the acute phase of the disease, and the titers of TMAb and TgAb may be low or elevated, depending on the clinical pattern. In postpartum thyroiditis, these antibody titers are elevated, and the condition appears to be associated with underlying Hashimoto's thyroiditis. In such patients, repeated episodes of hyperthyroidism followed by transient hypothyroidism should be anticipated with each pregnancy.

This disease must be separated from other causes of hyperthyroidism, notably Graves' disease. The best test for this is the 24-hour RAI uptake. A low uptake may occasionally also be observed in a patient with Graves' disease who has received excess iodide. This may be obvious from the history or can be eliminated by measuring the urinary iodide, which must be considerably elevated (>2 mg per 24 hours) to suppress the uptake in hyperthyroidism associated with thyroid hyperfunction. A needle biopsy will also be diagnostic. In *factitious hyperthyroidism*, the serum thyroglobulin is reduced in the presence of a low serum TSH concentration. This finding distinguishes this condition from subacute lymphocytic thyroiditis.

TREATMENT. As with subacute granulomatous thyroiditis, treatment is symptomatic. β-Adrenergic blockade may be required for the hyperthyroid phase, but propylthiouracil is of no value except to inhibit T_4 to T_3 conversion. Glucocorticoid is not required because there is no tenderness, but more rapid resolution of the hyperthyroidism has been reported in patients given a 4-week course of prednisone starting at 40 mg per day. A hypothyroid phase should be treated for 3 to 6 months, followed by withdrawal of the therapy.

PROGNOSIS. The hyperthyroid phase usually remits within a few months, and the entire history of this disease lasts less than a year. However, the potential for subsequent hypothyroidism indicates the need for annual examination of thyroid function in these patients.

CHRONIC THYROIDITIS

There are two types of chronic thyroiditis: Hashimoto's and Riedel's thyroiditis *(Riedel's struma).*

Hashimoto's Thyroiditis

This is an apparently autoimmune disease of the thyroid gland. It appears to be closely related to Graves' disease. Synonyms for this condition are *chronic lymphocytic thyroiditis* and *lymphadenoid goiter.*

ETIOLOGY. The sera of patients with this condition contain antibodies to one or more thyroid antigens, including thyroid peroxidase (antithyroid microsomal antibodies), thyroglobulin, or

a colloid antigen that can be separated from thyroglobulin. At present it is not certain whether these antibodies are the cause or the result of this disease. The pathologic features of the condition can be reproduced in laboratory animals by immunization with thyroid tissue. However, the experimental disease is not sustained once immunizations have been discontinued, nor can the injury be induced by serum from immunized animals. Since the disease can be transferred by sensitized lymphocytes, it has been proposed that the destruction is produced by cell-mediated processes. On exposure to thyroid tissue antigens in vitro, lymphocytes of patients with Hashimoto's thyroiditis (and Graves' disease) produce substances causing inhibition of leukocyte migration. This response is not found in patients with other forms of thyroid disease or by exposure to extracts of other tissues. Similar observations have been made in patients with idiopathic myxedema, suggesting that the atrophic thyroid found in this condition is affected by a similar process. Other evidence supporting the autoimmune hypothesis is the increased prevalence of many of the so-called autoimmune diseases in patients with Hashimoto's thyroiditis. These include Sjögren's syndrome, lupus erythematosus, idiopathic thrombocytopenic purpura, and pernicious anemia. As many as 6 per cent of patients with Hashimoto's disease have been reported to have pernicious anemia. Although rare, involvement of other endocrine glands by this immunopathologic process may occur. Idiopathic Addison's disease and Hashimoto's disease may appear in the same patients. This combination is called Schmidt's syndrome (see Ch. 228). The parathyroids, the β cells of the pancreatic islets, the pituitary, and the gonads may also be involved. There are a few reports of transplacental passage of maternal thyroid antibodies leading to transient impairment of thyroid function in neonates, but such cases are the exception rather than the rule. An increased risk of the atrophic form of Hashimoto's thyroiditis is present in patients who are HLA-DR3 or HLA-B8 positive.

INCIDENCE. Women are affected four to five times more frequently than men. The incidence increases with increasing age. TMAb have been found in about 10 per cent and 3 per cent of asymptomatic adult females and males, respectively. Thyroid peroxidase is now recognized to be the antigen in thyroid microsomes. Ten to 20 per cent of these persons can be expected to have biochemical evidence of thyroid disease. This disease is probably the most common cause of goiter in adolescents, although the incidence is not as high as in older women.

PATHOLOGIC FINDINGS. The thyroid gland is normal or

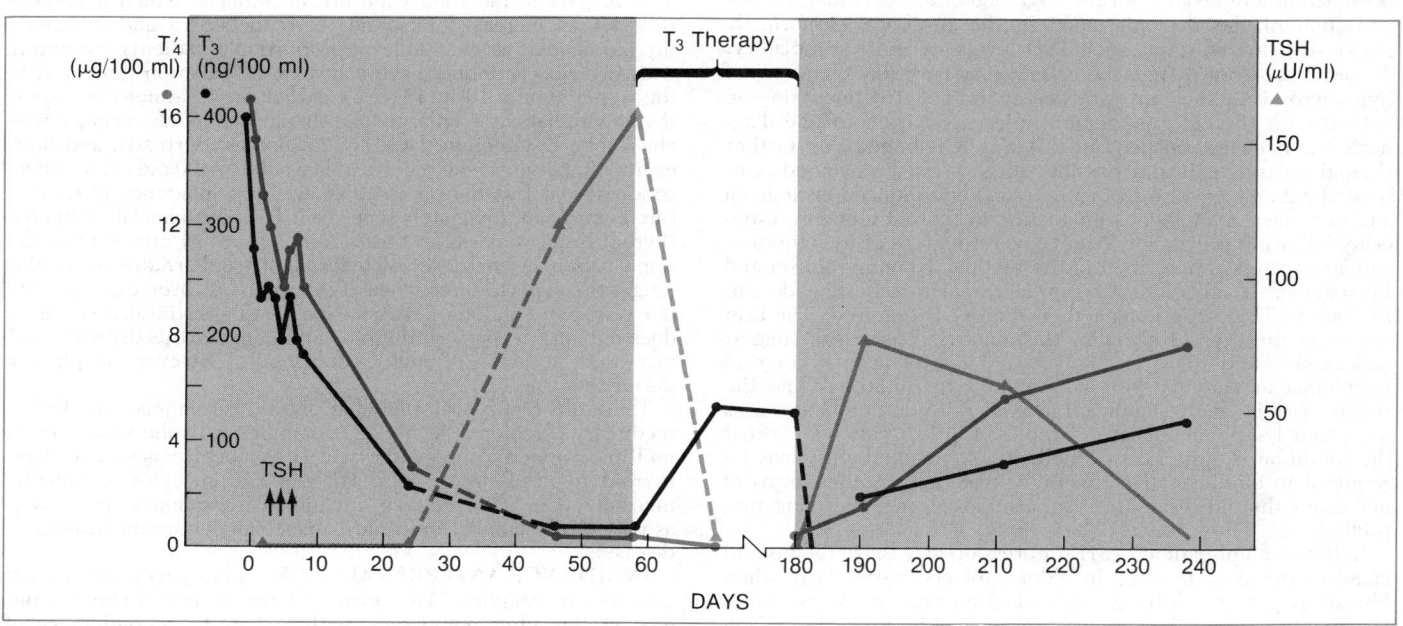

FIGURE 216–9. Changes in serum T_3, T_4, and TSH in a patient with subacute lymphocytic thyroiditis. The rapid decrease in serum T_3 and T_4 in the first 5 days is due to exhaustion of thyroidal stores as a consequence of the destructive process. Transient T_3 replacement was employed because of prolonged hypothyroidism. Normal thyroid function had returned by 8 months after the initial episode. (From Larsen PR: Serum triiodothyronine, thyroxine, and thyrotropin during hyperthyroid, hypothyroid, and recovery phases of subacute nonsuppurative thyroiditis. Metabolism 23:467, 1974. © 1974, The Williams & Wilkins Company, Baltimore.)

may be enlarged two- to fivefold, depending on the degree of fibrosis. Microscopic examination reveals that varying degrees of infiltration with lymphocytes and plasma cells, fibrosis, and, in many cases, germinal centers are present. An oxyphilic change may be present in the cytoplasm of the residual thyroid follicular cells. It may occasionally be difficult to differentiate Hashimoto's disease from primary lymphoma of the thyroid gland.

CLINICAL MANIFESTATIONS. Two clinical forms of thyroid involvement are described. In the so-called atrophic form the gland is normal or reduced in size, and hypothyroidism is the prominent symptom (see Table 216–9). This may well be the same syndrome as idiopathic myxedema. In other patients, variable degrees of thyroid enlargement and hypothyroidism occur, but goiter is the most common chief complaint. The gland is generally symmetrically enlarged, and often the pyramidal lobe is quite prominent, suggesting generalized hypertrophy. The thyroid is firm and may feel lobular or diffusely enlarged. Occasionally Hashimoto's disease presents as a single nodule in the thyroid gland, which represents the residual functioning thyroid tissue in a gland, the remainder of which has been destroyed by this disease. The patient may have a family history of Graves' or Hashimoto's disease, pernicious anemia, or other autoimmune phenomena. As mentioned in the discussion of *lymphocytic thyroiditis,* as many as 5 to 10 per cent of women may have postpartum episodes of transient hyperthyroidism followed by transient hypothyroidism associated with elevated TMAb.

LABORATORY DIAGNOSIS. The serum free T_4 index is reduced and serum TSH increased in many patients with this syndrome. Approximately 95 per cent of patients have positive TMAb tests, and about 50 to 60 per cent have positive TgAb. The RAI uptake may be reduced, normal, or even increased, depending on the residual thyroid cell function and the serum TSH. The thyroid scan generally reveals a heterogeneous uptake of the isotope. Occasionally a single island of functioning tissue remains. This can be differentiated from a functioning adenoma of the thyroid by appropriate tests of thyroid function. If the diagnosis remains in doubt, a needle biopsy can be performed and will reveal the characteristic changes of lymphocytic infiltration in the majority of cases.

TREATMENT. In the early phases of Hashimoto's thyroiditis, goiter may be present and the serum TSH mildly increased, but the free T_4 index is in the lower normal range. Nevertheless, the presence of an elevated serum TSH suggests substantial decompensation of the thyroid, since in the presence of normally responsive thyroid tissue such TSH levels are quite stimulatory. Accordingly, even though the patient may have few symptoms of hypothyroidism, it is my practice to initiate treatment in the patient with thyroid enlargement once a secure serologic diagnosis has been established. In this way it is hoped that further thyroid enlargement and possibly surgery can be avoided. Untreated patients are also susceptible to iodide-induced myxedema and may have spontaneous fluctuation in thyroid function, especially following pregnancy. More severe degrees of hypothyroidism are treated as described in the section, Hypothyroidism and Myxedema. If obstructive symptoms appear and they do not respond to TSH suppression, then surgery is required. The firm nature of the thyroid gland in Hashimoto's disease can suggest malignancy, and there is an increased risk of primary thyroid lymphoma in patients with Hashimoto's thyroiditis. While the relative risk is highly significant in this group, in one large series malignant lymphoma occurred in only 4 of 829 patients, so that the condition is quite rare. Nonetheless, a needle biopsy may be required to eliminate the possibility that this or other forms of malignant thyroid disease are superimposed on underlying thyroiditis.

In the younger patient, TSH suppression may cause the thyroid gland to decrease in size. In older subjects, particularly when fibrosis is present, little if any reduction occurs. Occasionally, Hashimoto's thyroiditis may present with hyperthyroidism ("hashitoxicosis"), which should be treated as is Graves' disease. Appropriate observation of the patient for the involvement of other tissues by autoimmune disease should be carried out as indicated.

PROGNOSIS. The prognosis of this condition is excellent as long as thyroid hormone therapy is provided when indicated. In patients with serologic evidence of Hashimoto's thyroiditis but normal thyroid function, an annual evaluation for hypothyroidism is indicated.

Riedel's Thyroiditis

This is a rare disorder of unknown cause in which a sclerosing fibrous infiltration of the thyroid gland occurs, causing the gland to become extremely firm. As the disease progresses, local muscles in the neck and the trachea are infiltrated and hypothyroidism appears. This condition may be difficult to differentiate from carcinoma of the thyroid. It is clinically associated with both retroperitoneal fibrosis and sclerosing cholangitis. Obstruction of the trachea may occur as the fibrosis proceeds, and a surgical approach is the only satisfactory method of treatment to relieve tracheal obstruction. Glucocorticoid therapy can be beneficial to some patients.

Amino N, Mori H, Iwatani Y, et al.: High prevalence of transient post-partum thyrotoxicosis and hypothyroidism. N Engl J Med 306:14, 849, 1982. *A prospective survey showing a 5.5 per cent incidence of transient thyrotoxicosis or hypothyroidism post partum.*

DeGroot LJ, Quintans J: The causes of autoimmune thyroid disease. Endocr Rev 10:537, 1989. *A review of current concepts regarding the etiology of autoimmune thyroid diseases.*

Holm L-E, Blomgren H, Lowhagen T: Cancer risks in patients with chronic lymphocytic thyroiditis. N Engl J Med 312:601, 1985. *An extensive epidemiologic study showing that while the relative risk of lymphoma is increased in individuals with chronic lymphocytic thyroiditis, the incidence of this complication is extremely low.*

Tunbridge WMG, Evered DC, Hall R, et al.: The spectrum of thyroid disease in a community: The Whickham survey. Clin Endocrinol 7:481, 1977. *The epidemiology of thyroid disease in an English community; this study provides a firm basis for estimates of the prevalence of Hashimoto's and Graves' disease as well as nodular goiter.*

BENIGN AND MALIGNANT TUMORS OF THE THYROID: THE SOLITARY THYROID NODULE

In this section are discussed those benign and malignant tumors that usually present as a solitary thyroid nodule. Multinodular goiter is discussed in the next section, Sporadic and Endemic Goiter. Virtually all tumors of the thyroid arise from glandular cells and are therefore adenomas or carcinomas. A scheme for evaluation of the patient with a solitary thyroid nodule is presented at the end of this chapter.

ETIOLOGY. The fundamental cause of thyroid tumors is unknown. However, two factors, exposure to ionizing radiation and the presence of TSH, have been found to be important for inducing thyroid tumors in animals. Similar data are available with respect to radiation exposure in humans, which is responsible for an increased incidence of both benign and malignant thyroid neoplasms. A significant proportion of patients presenting with thyroid carcinoma have a history of radiation delivered to the upper thorax 10 to 15 years earlier for treatment of "status thymolymphaticus," enlarged tonsils and adenoids, acne, eustachian tube dysfunction, facial hemangiomas, pertussis, and tinea capitis. In patients who receive at least 300 to 400 rads of thyroidal irradiation at less than 5 years of age, the incidence of thyroid carcinoma is approximately 6 per cent 10 to 20 years later. Benign thyroid tumors are about three to four times as prevalent in the same patients. For doses of external thyroid irradiation in this range, the expected incidence of carcinoma is three cases per rad per year per 1 million persons exposed. TSH stimulation per se does not appear to cause thyroid carcinoma, as this disease is not increased in areas of iodine deficiency; however, it plays a permissive role.

There are two types of familial thyroid carcinoma. The first is medullary carcinoma occurring in families with the syndrome of multiple endocrine neoplasia type II (pheochromocytoma, parathyroid hyperplasia) or type III (pheochromocytoma, mucosal neuroma) (Ch. 228). Papillary or follicular carcinoma may occur as part of the familial multiple hamartoma syndrome (Cowden's disease).

INCIDENCE AND PREVALENCE. Solitary palpable thyroid nodules are common. The estimated prevalence is about 4 per cent of the adult population, with a 2 to 1 preponderance of females. There is some difficulty in obtaining precise figures in this area, since a significant number of nodules that seem to be solitary by palpation are found to be dominant nodules in multinodular goiters at surgery or autopsy. This estimate represents a relatively small fraction of the true prevalence of thyroid nodules, which is about 40 to 50 per cent as revealed by autopsy studies or high-resolution ultrasonography. Such nodules are rarely true neoplasms. The estimated incidence of thyroid nodules is 0.1 per cent per year, but since many nodules are found at autopsy that were not suspected clinically the true incidence may be higher. The incidence of thyroid carcinoma is estimated to be 36 new cases per year per 1 million persons. These two estimates suggest that about 3 or 4 per cent of patients who develop solitary thyroid nodules have thyroid carcinoma. Many surgical series report thyroid carcinoma in 10 to 30 per cent of resected solitary nodules, which indicates that the screening procedures employed to identify high-risk patients are effective. Various autopsy series have reported an incidence of thyroid carcinoma ranging from 0.1 to 6 per cent. The higher figures are from studies in which an extremely careful search was made for microscopic carcinomas, virtually all being less than 5 mm in diameter. The clinical significance of such lesions is negligible, and this "background" of asymptomatic microscopic lesions should be kept in mind when evaluating this literature.

Benign Neoplasms

PATHOLOGY. The *follicular adenoma* is by far the most common benign thyroid tumor. It varies from microscopic to 8 to 10 cm in size and is composed of a normal-appearing thyroid epithelium arranged in a follicular structure. An intact capsule surrounds these tumors, and there is often evidence of compression of surrounding normal thyroid tissue. The follicles may range from extremely small with little colloid (*fetal adenoma* or *microfollicular adenoma*) to large distended structures (*macrofollicular adenoma*). The *embryonal* adenoma is an even more primitive-appearing structure possessing very little colloid. On occasion, the tumors may be composed of oxyphils (*oxyphil adenoma* or *Hürthle cell adenoma*). None of these differences in microscopic picture appears to bear on the functional characteristics of these nodules, nor do such nodules appear to become malignant. The hypercellular adenomas may be extremely difficult to differentiate from follicular carcinomas, especially when only a needle biopsy sample is available. Follicular adenomas have specific receptors for TSH, and these cells respond to TSH normally. However, many of these tumors do not possess the capacity for concentrating iodide or other similar substances. Since such nodules do not concentrate isotopes, they are referred to as *nonfunctioning* or *cold*.

CLINICAL MANIFESTATIONS. Thyroid adenomas fall into two categories: those that produce significant quantities of thyroid hormones and those that do not. The latter are the more common (90 to 95 per cent). Patients with these tumors present with an asymptomatic mass in the neck. The patient may be discovered to have this tumor on routine physical examination and often is completely unaware of its existence. The tumor usually becomes palpable by the time it reaches 1 cm in diameter, but it may reach 5 to 10 cm without being noticed by the patient. Thyroid function studies in patients with nonfunctioning follicular adenomas are normal, and the thyroid scan generally reveals an area of decreased or absent uptake of $^{123}I^-$ or $^{99m}TcO_4^-$ (a "cold" nodule). The precise diagnosis can be made only by obtaining a tissue specimen by aspiration biopsy, cutting needle biopsy (Vim-Silverman needle or its equivalent), or excision of the nodule. As these nodules may outgrow their blood supply, cystic degeneration may occur. Ultrasonography of such a lesion reveals a cystic cavity within the nodule.

Functioning follicular adenomas may present with or without symptoms of hyperthyroidism, largely depending on their size. Lesions over 3 cm in diameter tend to cause thyrotoxicity and constitute about 50 per cent of these adenomas in patients 60 years and older. T_3 thyrotoxicosis was found in 46 per cent of such patients in one large series. More commonly the patient is asymptomatic, and a thyroid scan shows that the only area concentrating radioactivity is the nodule itself. Such patients generally have normal or high-normal serum thyroid hormone levels, the serum TSH-IMA is subnormal, and TRH infusion will not cause TSH release. Such nodules are functioning autonomously at a rate sufficient to suppress TSH synthesis in the pituitary (hence the lack of function in the remainder of the thyroid) but not at a sufficiently high level to cause metabolic hyperthyroidism. Functional lesions that have suppressed TSH

synthesis but not caused hyperthyroidism are denoted *warm* nodules, whereas those associated with hyperthyroidism are called *hot* nodules. Assessment of the thyroid functional state is necessary for proper evaluation of these lesions, since the thyroid scan is identical. This is especially important, since Hashimoto's disease may present as a solitary focus of functioning thyroid tissue, as may congenital absence of one lobe of the thyroid. The presence of potentially functioning thyroid tissue can be demonstrated by injection of 10 units of bovine TSH, followed in 24 hours by a thyroid scan. Unlike multinodular goiters, follicular adenomas of the thyroid rarely grow large enough to cause significant physical encroachment on the trachea or esophagus.

TREATMENT. The finding of an autonomously functioning nodule virtually eliminates the diagnosis of thyroid carcinoma. Treatment at that point depends on the thyroid status. If the patient is euthyroid (a warm thyroid nodule), nothing more than an annual follow-up with appropriate thyroid function tests (including a serum T_3) is necessary. In the hyperthyroid patient, surgery or ^{131}I is available for definitive treatment, although antithyroid drugs may be necessary to control symptomatic hyperthyroidism prior to definitive therapy. The choice of treatment depends on the age of the patient and the size of the nodule. In patients under the age of 20, surgical resection should be performed, as the radiation delivered to extranodular tissue after radioiodine therapy may reach a level that is considered carcinogenic. In older patients with cosmetically disfiguring lesions or those that are compressing vital structures in the neck, surgery is also preferred. For the rest, ^{131}I is indicated. I attempt to deliver 10 mCi of ^{131}I into the nodule. Following either surgery or radioactive iodine treatment, a period of 4 to 6 weeks is required for re-establishment of pituitary TSH secretion, following which function of the previously suppressed normal thyroid tissue should occur. The patient may need to receive thyroxine supplementation during this interim period but may not require indefinite replacement. The approach to the *nonfunctioning thyroid nodule* is described below under Clinical Manifestations and Diagnosis of Thyroid Carcinoma—The Solitary Nodule.

Malignant Thyroid Tumors

Four types of malignancy are found in the thyroid gland. *Papillary carcinoma* comprises the largest fraction, about two thirds of all cases of thyroid malignancy. *Follicular carcinoma* accounts for another 20 per cent, including the *Hürthle cell* variant with *medullary*, and *poorly differentiated* carcinomas about 5 per cent each. Another 5 per cent is accounted for by *non-Hodgkin's lymphoma*, which has become more common in recent years. Medullary carcinoma is a tumor of calcitonin-producing C cells and has no relationship to the thyroid follicular epithelium.

PATHOLOGY AND NATURAL HISTORY. *Papillary carcinoma* is the most benign and the most common form of thyroid carcinoma. It is two to three times more common in women than in men and occurs with equal frequency in the third to seventh decades. Since the less well-differentiated forms of carcinoma increase with age, papillary carcinoma is the most common malignant thyroid tumor in younger patients. The size of these tumors varies from microscopic to several centimeters in diameter. Of the clinically apparent variety, the *occult* tumors (defined as those less than 1.5 cm in diameter) are differentiated from the *intrathyroidal* tumors, which are larger but do not extend through the thyroid surface. The tumor is classified as *extrathyroidal* if it extends through the thyroid capsule and involves surrounding tissues. Microscopically, papillary carcinoma consists of well-differentiated thyroid epithelium covering papillary fibrovascular stalks. The nuclei are frequently clear, as opposed to the denser appearance of normal nuclei. A virtually pathognomonic feature in about 40 per cent of papillary thyroid carcinomas is the so-called *psammoma body*. These calcific globules are 5 to 100 μ in diameter and are often present in the tips of the papillary projections. Their etiology is unknown, but their presence in the thyroid tumor raises the high likelihood of its carcinomatous nature. Cervical lymphatic involvement even with occult thyroid tumors is common, occurring in as many as 50 per cent. Blood-borne metastases are uncommon. The presence or absence of lymph node metastases does not seem to alter the prognosis. In a large series studied at the Mayo Clinic, the 20-year survival of patients with occult or intrathyroid papillary carcinoma was not significantly different from that of a control group. However, the 20-year survival for patients with extrathyroidal carcinoma was about 40 per cent, and this dropped to 20 per cent over the next 10 years. Many thyroid cancers have areas of follicular as well as papillary structure, and blood-borne metastases may occur that have a follicular pattern even though the primary tumor is papillary. Thus, many predominantly papillary tumors have follicular elements, but the biologic behavior of these lesions seems to be a function of the predominant microscopic appearance.

Follicular carcinomas also are more common in women than in men but tend to increase in incidence with increasing age. The tumors vary from well-differentiated, virtually normal-appearing thyroid tissue to nearly solid sheets of follicular epithelium with little evidence of follicle formation. The former are differentiated from follicular adenomas only by demonstration of capsular and vascular invasion. Such a diagnosis generally cannot be made without the entire nodule for examination, and even at frozen section the carcinomatous nature of the lesion may not be recognized. Cyst formation may occur as it does in benign follicular tumors, and calcification may occur centrally. Follicular carcinomas tend to metastasize via blood vessel invasion and not, in general, via lymphatics. Metastases may not be evident at the time of initial evaluation but may appear years later despite apparent complete excision of the tumor. It is not unusual for the follicular carcinoma to concentrate radioiodine, although it does so considerably less well than does normal thyroid tissue. Thus, it is only in the absence of normal thyroid tissue and in the presence of increased TSH that this potential is appreciated. However, it is useful in treatment in some of these tumors (see below). Patients who have had removal of well-encapsulated, noninvasive follicular carcinomas appear to have a normal lifespan. On the other hand, patients with tumors that show extensive local involvement and angioinvasion at the time of initial surgery have an approximately 30 per cent 10-year survival, which is decreased to less than 20 per cent at 20 years.

The most aggressive form of thyroid epithelial carcinoma, anaplastic or undifferentiated, may appear in *giant* or *spindle cell* forms. The small cell variety of this lesion has proven to be a lymphoma in most cases. Undifferentiated thyroid carcinoma is the most highly malignant tumor of the thyroid gland. It is found almost exclusively in patients over the age of 60. The average prognosis from diagnosis to death in the giant cell tumors is less than 6 months, whereas patients with small cell carcinoma may have 5-year survival of 20 to 25 per cent. Both tend to extend locally and often cause tracheal obstruction. Distant metastases may occur with either type.

Medullary carcinoma of the thyroid is a malignant tumor of the C cell and produces thyrocalcitonin. Its occurrence in association with multiple endocrine neoplasia syndromes has been mentioned. It may also occur spontaneously. These tumors are characterized by sheets of tumor cells separated by a hyaline-amyloid–containing stroma. The amyloid is formed by the tumor cells and deposited in the stroma. The tumors may also produce ACTH, prostaglandin, or carcinoembryonic antigen. In familial syndromes, the penetrance of this tumor is complete, so that screening of family members is indicated by use of calcium and/or pentagastrin infusions to stimulate calcitonin release from pathologic cells (see Ch. 236).

Lymphoma is usually the nodular histiocytic form and generally arises in a gland affected by Hashimoto's thyroiditis. It should be considered diagnostically in patients with Hashimoto's disease who present with a rapidly enlarging mass in the thyroid gland, and a core or aspiration biopsy should be performed with appropriate cytochemical stains. Depending on the clinical stage, these lesions may respond quite well to radiotherapy, with or without chemotherapy. Complete cure by surgical resection of small lesions has also been reported.

CLINICAL MANIFESTATIONS AND DIAGNOSIS OF THYROID CARCINOMA—THE SOLITARY NODULE. The approach to the patient with a solitary thyroid nodule is a matter of considerable disagreement among clinicians. For some, thyroid carcinoma is sufficiently serious to require a surgical approach to all potentially carcinomatous lesions; others believe that considerable selection should be used prior to surgery. The benign nature of the common forms of thyroid carcinoma and the relatively large number of benign nodules make a conservative approach rational. There are several clinical characteristics that dictate an open surgical approach to a nonfunctioning thyroid nodule. This includes a history of prior irradiation. Nodules in such patients carry a 20 to 25 per cent risk of carcinoma. A history of rapid growth, evidence of recurrent nerve paresis, obvious involvement of lymph nodes, or fixation of the nodule to surrounding tissues should also lead to serious consideration of immediate surgery. Statistically, the risk of a solitary cold nodule being malignant is higher in a male than in a female, since benign disease of the thyroid is much more common in females. Thyroid nodules in children are more likely to be carcinoma than those in adults.

In the absence of specific signs pointing to a diagnosis of thyroid carcinoma, there are two avenues of approach (Fig. 216–10A and B). If there is no obvious thyroid dysfunction (either hyperthyroidism or hypothyroidism) and an experienced cytopathologist is available, a needle aspiration can be performed (Fig. 216–10A). If the lesion is a simple cyst, this will be curative; otherwise the cytologic report guides therapy. If carcinoma is found, surgical exploration is indicated. If a cellular follicular aspirate is obtained that is consistent with a benign or a malignant lesion, a ^{123}I (or ^{131}I) scan is performed. If the lesion is hypofunctional, surgical exploration is advised. If it is warm or hot,

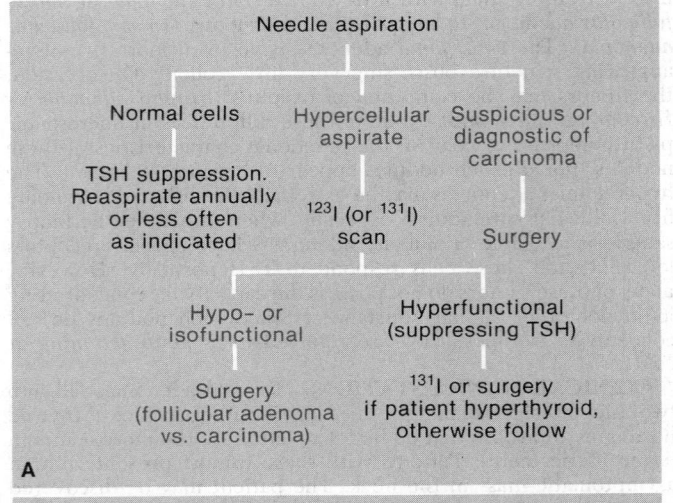

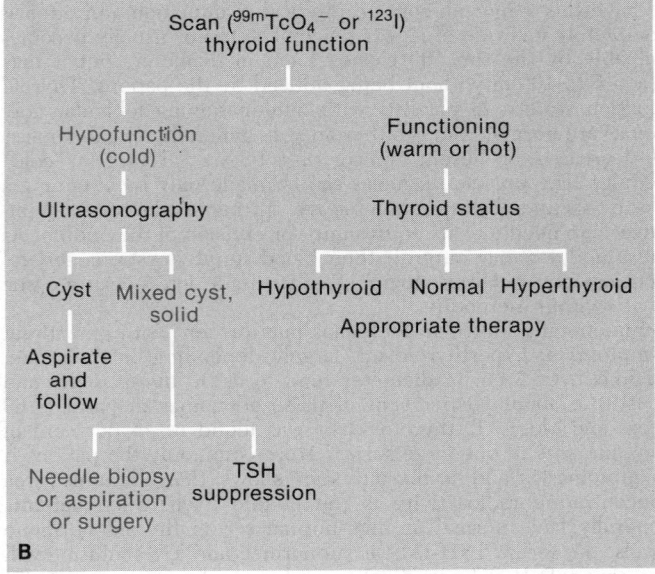

FIGURE 216–10. *A* shows a schema for the diagnostic evaluation of a patient with a solitary thyroid nodule based on aspiration biopsy cytology. *B* presents an alternative solution to the same problem starting with a thyroid scintiscan.

management is as discussed earlier under autonomous nodules. If the cytologic report indicates that the lesion is benign, thyroxine is given to suppress TSH, and this is monitored by TSH-IMA measurement. The need for surgery is then determined by the subsequent course of the individual patient. Aspiration biopsy cytology yields false-positive results (i.e., papillary carcinoma) very rarely, and false-negative results, that is, a benign diagnosis in a patient with a malignant lesion, should occur in only 2 to 3 per cent of patients. This figure, however, may be higher during the early experience with this technique in a given center. A number of patients are referred for surgery because of a cytologic picture that is suspicious but not clearly diagnostic. Nonetheless, in most clinics, aspiration cytology has reduced the apparent need for surgical exploration by 50 to 60 per cent. In other words, approximately 40 per cent of patients with solitary nodules require surgical exploration because of frankly or suspiciously malignant lesions.

If a trained cytopathologist is not available, then thyroid scanning is performed followed by ultrasonography if the nodule is not hyperfunctioning (Fig. 216–10B). Rarely a malignant nodule will be warm by $^{99m}TcO_4^-$ but cold by iodide scan. This should be suspected and tested for when warm lesions do not suppress function in the remainder of the gland. Ultrasonography of hypofunctioning nodules is performed. A cystic lesion can be treated by aspiration and the procedure repeated twice more if the fluid reaccumulates before surgery is indicated. In the nonfunctioning solid nodule, needle aspiration cytology, cutting needle biopsy, or surgical exploration is advised. I recommend surgical excision for patients under 20 and for those high-risk patients with familial carcinoma and radiation exposure. The availability of experienced thyroid surgeons plays an important role in this approach, since serious morbidity attends inadvertent resection of the parathyroid glands or recurrent laryngeal nerve paresis. In the other patients, the approach is dictated by the response to TSH suppression. Most nodules do not change in size, and therapy is individualized, whereas patients with nodules that increase during TSH suppression are referred for surgery, and those patients with nodules that decrease in size are followed with continued suppression. None of these responses clearly differentiates a benign from a malignant lesion.

At the time of initial surgery a frozen section should be obtained from all solitary thyroid nodules and an attempt made to provide definitive treatment. A reasonable approach to intrathyroidal papillary carcinoma is to perform a lobectomy with isthmectomy and explore for and remove any involved lymph nodes. An examination of the other lobe should be made for tumor, but, except in the irradiated patient, bilateral lobectomy is not required. With extrathyroidal extension of papillary carcinoma or bilateral lymph node metastases, a total thyroidectomy is performed with great care to preserve the recurrent laryngeal nerves and parathyroid glands. A follicular carcinoma is approached as are the papillary lesions, except that the presence of distant lymph node metastases or extensive capsular and vascular invasion in the initial frozen section should lead to consideration of bilateral thyroidectomy. This is done to remove residual normal tissue to facilitate radioiodine therapy (see below). Radical neck dissection does not offer any advantage over the less mutilating procedures described above. Medullary carcinoma of the sporadic variety may be treated as papillary carcinoma, but the familial form requires bilateral lobectomy. It is, of course, important to determine that pheochromocytoma and hyperparathyroidism are not present before undertaking surgery. Anaplastic carcinoma is rarely restricted enough to lend itself to surgical therapy, except for palliation to prevent tracheal compression. Lymphoma should be treated by radiotherapy and chemotherapy in consultation with a hematologist.

RADIATION THERAPY. I⁻ may be concentrated to a sufficient degree to be useful by as many as 50 to 60 per cent of well-differentiated thyroid tumors. This can be demonstrated only after the establishment of hypothyroidism with an increase in serum TSH. In general, prophylactic therapy with radioiodine in patients with papillary carcinoma does not appear to be beneficial, although metastases may respond to this method. In follicular carcinoma with evidence of vascular invasion or in patients with follicular metastases, particularly to the lungs, significant amelioration of symptoms and dramatic changes in the radiographic picture may be associated with this therapy. It does not appear

to be as useful for patients with bone metastases. To be weighed against these beneficial effects is the increased incidence of leukemia, which is 2 to 3 per cent in patients treated with large doses of ^{131}I (300 mCi and more).

The usual approach to evaluation of the feasibility of this therapeutic method is to remove residual functioning thyroid tissue surgically or by ^{131}I administration. After this, the patient is switched to triiodothyronine (50 µg per day) for a period of approximately 2 weeks, following which administration of the hormone is discontinued. Within 2 to 3 weeks, most patients show the maximal uptake in metastatic tissue. At that time, a tracer dose of ^{131}I should be given with appropriate dosimetry of the tumor mass, bone marrow, and lungs. Following this, the maximal tolerable ^{131}I dose should be given and the patient started on TSH-suppressive therapy with thyroxine 1 day later. Local recurrences of papillary carcinoma can often be treated surgically by removal of involved lymph nodes. In such patients this is preferable to ^{131}I, which should be reserved for a nonresectable lesion.

Despite the poor function of thyroid tumors in terms of radioiodine trapping, carcinomatous thyroid cells have TSH receptors and respond to TSH in vitro. Accordingly, efforts should be made to suppress TSH below normal, as monitored by TSH-IMA or by demonstrating that TRH does not increase TSH into the measurable range of a conventional assay. In patients who have had total thyroidectomy and radioiodine ablation, serum thyroglobulin concentrations should be monitored, since normal or increased levels of this protein then indicate the presence of residual thyroid tumor.

Hay ID, Grant CS, Taylor WF, et al.: Ipsilateral lobectomy versus bilateral lobar resection in papillary thyroid carcinoma: A retrospective analysis of surgical outcome using a novel prognostic scoring system. Surgery 102:1088, 1987. *An evaluation of the difficult issue of the appropriate surgery for patients with papillary thyroid carcinoma.*
Kaplan MM, Garnick MB, Gelber R, et al.: Risk factors for thyroid abnormalities after neck irradiation for childhood cancer. Am J Med 74:272, 1983. *This study shows that both benign and malignant thyroid nodules, as well as hypothyroidism, may appear 5 to 35 years after therapeutic irradiation to the neck.*
McConahey WM, Hay ID, Woolner LB, et al.: Papillary thyroid cancer treated at the Mayo Clinic 1946 through 1970: Initial manifestations, pathologic findings, therapy, and outcome. Mayo Clin Proc 61:978, 1986. *An update of a large retrospective evaluation of the results of various treatment modalities in patients with well-differentiated thyroid carcinoma.*
Pottern LM, Kaplan MM, Larsen PR, et al.: Thyroid nodularity after childhood irradiation for lymphoid hyperplasia: A comparison of questionnaire and clinical findings. J Clin Epidemiol 43:449, 1990. *An evaluation of the effect of radiation for tonsillar disease on thyroid nodularity in a large group of patients treated at Boston Children's Hospital. There is about a two- to threefold increase in the prevalence of thyroid nodules in the irradiated population compared with a large group of similarly examined controls.*

SPORADIC AND ENDEMIC GOITER

DEFINITION. *Sporadic goiter* refers to thyroid enlargement, which is found in a relatively small fraction of a given population. The cause for the thyroid enlargement may be different from patient to patient. The term *endemic goiter* refers to a condition seen in a much larger fraction of the population, which is presumably a consequence of one or several environmental influences, most commonly iodine deficiency. Although the causes of sporadic and endemic goiter are, by definition, different, the pathophysiology and pathology underlying these conditions are probably quite similar, and they are therefore grouped together.

ETIOLOGY. The common factor that is thought to lead to thyroid enlargement is *hypersecretion of TSH*. TSH increases in response to decreased production of thyroid hormones, especially T_4, as a consequence of an intrinsic abnormality in the process of thyroid hormone synthesis in the case of sporadic goiter, or the lack of adequate quantities of iodine in the diet or the presence of a goitrogen in the environment in endemic goiter. TSH increases as T_4 falls. As a consequence of the increased TSH secretion, iodine turnover by the thyroid is accelerated, the T_3 to T_4 ratio in thyroid secretion is increased, and serum T_3 may remain entirely normal. Such patients appear to be clinically euthyroid at the expense of an elevated serum TSH concentration and an enlarged thyroid gland.

PATHOLOGY. In the early phases, the thyroid gland may be diffusely enlarged with cellular hyperplasia as a result of TSH stimulation. Later, large follicles form with low epithelium. As the process continues, there is further stimulation of some thyroidal areas and atrophy of others with concomitant fibrosis. These multiple nodules have markedly varying activity. The accumulation of thyroglobulin, particularly in the iodine-deficient patients, may occur because poorly iodinated thyroglobulin is relatively resistant to digestion by endogenous proteases. To some extent, the same phenomenon may be occurring in the multinodular goiters which are sporadic and in which a specific cause has not been identified.

Sporadic Goiter

Sporadic goiter affects about 5 per cent of the population in the United States. Females outnumber males by a 3:1 ratio. In some patients an enzymatic defect in one of the steps in thyroid hormone synthesis can be identified (see Fig. 216–2). However, in most patients no specific cause can be isolated, but it is possible that milder forms of similar enzymatic deficiencies may be present.

CONGENITAL GOITER. This condition is sometimes referred to as *sporadic cretinism,* a syndrome of infantile myxedema characterized by growth failure, mental retardation, diffuse myxedema, and many of the signs and symptoms of hypothyroidism outlined in the section Hypothyroidism and Myxedema. Goitrous hypothyroidism can be due to a defect in any of the steps leading to the formation of thyroid hormone synthesis already discussed in the introduction. Defects have been identified in (1) iodide transport; (2) organification of iodide due to reduction in or absence of peroxidase, to an abnormal enzyme, or to diminished peroxide generation; (3) synthesis of an abnormal thyroglobulin molecule; (4) a structural abnormality in peroxidase, impairing its function as an iodine acceptor; (5) abnormal interrelationships of iodotyrosine; (6) impaired thyroglobulin proteolysis; and (7) a defect in iodotyrosine deiodination. The numbers given refer to the specific steps shown in Fig. 216–2. In some disorders of thyroglobulin synthesis the formation of an iodinated albumin-like protein has been described. All of these defects are rare. In North America and Europe they constitute less than 10 per cent of the approximately 1 in 4000 infants with congenital hypothyroidism.

A detailed description of each of these various defects is beyond the scope of this general text. The most common defect is the inability to organify iodine (defects in steps 2, 3, or 4). Such patients accumulate large amounts of I^- in the thyroid. This can be demonstrated by performance of a *perchlorate (ClO_4^-) discharge test.* In some patients this condition has been found in association with eighth nerve deafness and has the eponym *Pendred's syndrome.*

Regardless of the specific defect, these patients present with goiter and hypothyroidism, the serum T_4 index is reduced, and serum TSH is elevated. Further evaluation for the type of biochemical defect requires careful laboratory investigation. The treatment of such patients is with exogenous thyroid hormone. Thyroxine treatment causes regression of the enlarged thyroid, and mental retardation may be ameliorated or prevented if treatment is started before 3 months of age. Genetic counseling is desirable so that these patients are aware of the risk of hypothyroidism in subsequent offspring.

MULTINODULAR GOITER IN THE ADULT. The hypothesis that adults with multinodular goiter have mild defects in thyroid hormone synthesis similar to the more complete forms found in infants remains to be proved. If this is the case, then the goiter could be explained by modest increases in TSH, which is secreted by the pituitary in response to the reduced serum T_4. A significant physiologic increase in TSH may be as little as 2 to 3 μU per milliliter, often below the sensitivity of the TSH immunoassay that is clinically available. The compensatory increase in the size of the thyroid gland under these circumstances results in adequate rates of thyroid hormone formation, so that the vast majority of patients with this abnormality are euthyroid.

CLINICAL MANIFESTATIONS. Patients with multinodular goiter may come to the physician because of respiratory obstruction or dysphagia. More often the patient is asymptomatic and

the enlarged multinodular thyroid is discovered on a routine physical examination. Such patients should be questioned carefully for symptoms of respiratory obstruction. The goiter often extends retrosternally; this may be demonstrated by having the patient extend the arms directly over the head. If a significant substernal goiter is present, jugular venous distention and suffusion of the face occur (*Pemberton's sign*). Aside from physical obstruction, the most significant clinical aspect of the multinodular goiter is the tendency for hyperthyroidism to develop late in life (*Plummer's disease*). It is postulated that after decades of stimulation by TSH one or more of the nodular hyperplastic areas become autonomous. Since this condition generally appears in the elderly patient, the resulting hyperthyroidism may be of the apathetic variety (see the section Graves' Disease and Other Causes of Hyperthyroidism). In one series, administration of 50 to 100 mg of KI per day to eight patients with multinodular goiter resulted in hyperthyroidism in four patients, which required definitive treatment. The etiology of this form of iodide-induced thyrotoxicosis (probably not jodbasedow) is not clear, but caution is needed before the administration of iodide or iodine-containing drugs, such as amiodarone, to patients with multinodular goiter.

LABORATORY DIAGNOSIS. The physician must investigate both the anatomic and the functional nature of the thyroid pathology. Anatomic information is gained by chest or esophageal radiography, from a scintiscan, and when indicated by computed tomography of the neck and upper thorax. ^{131}I is recommended for thyroid scanning of these patients because the γ rays emitted by $^{99m}TcO_4^-$ and $^{123}I^-$ may not be strong enough to penetrate the sternum. The scintiscan image shows patchy focal uptake of radioactivity in an enlarged thyroid gland. The significance of the nonfunctioning areas in such scintiscans is discussed below. Measurements of serum free T_4 index, T_3, TSH, and TMAb and TgAb should be obtained, especially since Hashimoto's thyroiditis may present as a multinodular goiter. A TSH-IMA or a TRH test is especially important if Plummer's disease is suspected.

TREATMENT. The proper treatment depends on the clinical manifestations in the individual patient. Hyperthyroidism associated with multinodular goiter is best treated with radioactive iodine. However, because of the heterogeneity of the tissue uptake of radioiodine, a larger dose of radioiodine is necessary (180 μCi per gram or 10 mCi in a typical gland). The not uncommon coexistence of cardiac or pulmonary disease in this age group, together with the large size of the thyroid gland and the possibility of radiation thyroiditis, has led me to pretreat most elderly hyperthyroid patients with antithyroid drugs prior to radiotherapy. The antithyroid drugs are discontinued approximately 4 to 5 days prior to treatment. If a high plasma I^- (low RAI uptake) does not permit the use of radioiodine, then surgical treatment must be undertaken after appropriate preparation with antithyroid drugs.

Hypothyroid patients require treatment with thyroxine as described in the section Hypothyroidism and Myxedema. Young euthyroid patients with diffuse thyroid enlargement may be started on thyroxine replacement therapy to suppress TSH, particularly if this is slightly elevated. One may block further thyroid enlargement by this treatment as well as cause regression of goiter in some. In patients over the age of 40, it is unlikely that significant amelioration in physical symptoms will occur with TSH suppression, but this hormone may be administered on a trial basis. Great care must be exercised, particularly in the elderly, since one or more of the hyperplastic thyroid nodules may be functioning autonomously. In all patients with multinodular goiter it is suggested that a TSH-IMA or TRH test be performed prior to initiation of therapy with thyroid hormone to avoid iatrogenic hyperthyroidism. When autonomous function is present, well-meaning attempts to suppress TSH can cause iatrogenic hyperthyroidism. If physical symptoms of obstruction are present or there is evidence of recurrent laryngeal nerve dysfunction, surgical treatment is generally in order.

The Multinodular Goiter and Thyroid Carcinoma. Nodular disease of the thyroid is common and thyroid carcinoma is relatively rare. Poorly functioning areas may be present in the thyroid scintiscans of multinodular goiters, but this is not an indication for surgery for malignant disease. As heterogeneity of function is the rule, other criteria must be employed for recognition of malignancy in the multinodular goiter. Factors that raise this possibility include previous exposure to therapeutic thyroidal irradiation in childhood, a family history of thyroid carcinoma or enlargement of cervical lymph nodes, recurrent laryngeal nerve palsy, or the continuing enlargement of a single "cold" nodule in an otherwise stable gland. In situations in which doubt exists, needle biopsy may provide the requisite microscopic diagnosis to reassure the patient and the physician that conservative therapy is the appropriate course of action.

PROGNOSIS. Patients with euthyroid multinodular goiter should have thyroid function and physical findings evaluated at annual intervals. Most do not require surgery.

Endemic Goiter

Iodine deficiency is the most common cause of thyroid disease in the world population, although iodination of salt has eliminated this problem in North America. Areas in which iodine intake remains low include mountainous regions such as the Andes and Himalayas. In addition, there are areas of endemic goiter in central Africa, New Guinea, and Indonesia. Iodine prophylaxis, either in foodstuffs or in the form of iodized oil injection, has been successful in many of these countries, but iodine deficiency remains a considerable public health problem. In a few geographic locations, ingestion of a goitrogen has been implicated in the high incidence of goiter. Examples include a thiocyanate derivative from the cassava, which is eaten in large quantities in central Africa, and a goitrogenic hydrocarbon found in the water supply in parts of Colombia and in Chile.

CLINICAL MANIFESTATIONS IN ADULTS. The minimal quantity of iodine required for normal thyroid function is approximately 100 μg per day. As the level of iodine in the diet decreases below this level, there is a progressive fall in serum T_4 and a progressive rise in serum TSH. Serum T_3 concentrations remain normal or slightly elevated, a persistently elevated TSH being required for this compensation. Serum TSH concentrations may exceed 100 μU per milliliter. In the presence of lifelong stimulation of this degree, enormous hypertrophy and hyperplasia of the thyroid gland can occur. Such glands may weigh 1 to 5 kg, producing considerable physical impairment.

EFFECTS OF IODINE DEFICIENCY IN INFANTS. In areas of endemic goiter, cretinism is not uncommon. Despite the capacity of the placenta to transport I^-, in areas where iodine intake is severely reduced (25 μg per day or less) the 24-hour maternal RAI uptake is virtually 100 per cent. Infants in these areas may be born with congenital hypothyroidism as a consequence of iodine deficiency.

In areas such as the Andes or New Guinea where iodine intake may be less than 20 μg per day, a different form of *endemic cretinism* may be seen. As opposed to dwarfism and mental retardation, some children in these areas have spastic diplegia, squint, and deafness. The etiology of this syndrome is still not clarified. It may be a manifestation of the effect of iodine deficiency per se on the embryologic development of the central nervous system. Fetal or maternal hypothyroidism as a consequence of severe iodine deficiency may also contribute to this problem.

TREATMENT. The treatment of iodine deficiency is to supply this element either as a food additive or by direct injections of iodinated oil. This has often been difficult because of the inaccessibility and restricted governmental resources of those countries in which iodine deficiency is a problem. The *jodbasedow phenomenon* (iodine-induced hyperthyroidism) occurs in some patients receiving iodine supplementation. These presumably are patients with underlying Graves' (Basedow's) disease who are given adequate supplies of the substrate for thyroid hormone synthesis.

Dumont JE, Vassart G, Refetoff S: Thyroid disorders. *In* Scriver CR, Beudet A, Sly WS, et al.: The Metabolic Basis of Inherited Disease, 6th ed. New York, McGraw-Hill Book Company, 1989, pp 1843–1879. *The emphasis is on the emzymology of pathogenesis.*

Lever EG, Medeiros-Neto GA, DeGroot LJ: Inherited disorders of thyroid metabolism. Endocr Rev 4:213, 1983. *A comprehensive review of this topic.*

Studer H, Peter HJ, Gerber H: Natural heterogeneity of thyroid cells: The basis for understanding thyroid function and nodular goiter growth. Endocr Rev 10:125, 1989. *A careful study of the probable cause of hyperthyroidism in nodular goiter.*

Thilly CH, Delange F, Lagasse R, et al.: Fetal hypothyroidism and maternal thyroid status in severe endemic goiter. J Clin Endocrinol Metab 47:354, 1978. *The*

effects of iodine deficiency on mother and newborn are described, comparing treated and untreated patients.

Wolff J: Congenital goiter with defective iodide transport. Endocr Rev 4:240, 1983. *The clinical, pathophysiologic, and biochemical findings in patients with this form of sporadic goiter.*

217 Disorders of the Adrenal Cortex

J. Blake Tyrrell and John D. Baxter

217.1 STRUCTURE AND DEVELOPMENT OF THE ADRENAL CORTEX

John D. Baxter

The major function of the adrenal cortex is to produce glucocorticoid and mineralocorticoid hormones, of which cortisol and aldosterone, respectively, are the most important in humans. The glucocorticoids, named for their carbohydrate-regulating properties, are essential for survival, at least in times of stress, and regulate intermediary metabolism, hemodynamic functions, and developmental processes. The mineralocorticoids regulate sodium, potassium, and hydrogen ion balance and secondarily affect the blood pressure. Either an excess or a deficiency of these steroids can have deleterious effects. Glucocorticoid excess is termed Cushing's syndrome. Adrenocortical insufficiency due to destruction of the adrenal gland is called Addison's disease. Aldosterone excess and deficiency are referred to as aldosteronism and hypoaldosteronism, respectively. Whereas diseases of the adrenal cortex are relatively uncommon, their clinical stigmata are part of the differential diagnosis of common problems. In addition, iatrogenic glucocorticoid excess is a common clinical problem due to the widespread usage of glucocorticoids in therapy. Secondary hyperaldosteronism is also a common problem sometimes requiring antimineralocorticoid therapy.

The human adrenal cortex produces at least 50 other steroids. This gland is a major source of androgenic steroids in the female (see Ch. 224) but is a trivial source of these steroids in the male compared to the testes (see Ch. 222). The adrenal production of dehydroepiandrosterone (DHEA) and its sulfate derivative is about half that of cortisol. Although these steroids typically are designated "adrenal androgens," they may have other, as-yet-undefined actions. The adrenal produces only minute quantities of estrogens and progestins. Some other adrenal steroids (e.g., deoxycorticosterone or testosterone) can cause clinical abnormalities when they are produced in excess in certain pathologic states.

STRUCTURE. There are two adrenal glands, located extraperitoneally at the upper poles of each kidney lateral to the eleventh thoracic to first lumbar vertebrae. The right gland tends to be higher and more lateral than the left. The average gland weighs 4 grams and is 2 to 3 cm wide and 4 to 6 cm long. A series of small arteries arising from the abdominal aorta, from renal and phrenic arteries, and occasionally from ovarian or spermatic arteries, feed the gland. Because of this, arterial infarction is unusual. The venous drainage of the gland on the left is ordinarily into the renal vein and on the right into the inferior vena cava. The gland is innervated by autonomic fibers.

The adrenal cortex comprises about 90 per cent of the gland and surrounds the centrally located medulla that produces catecholamines. The cortex has three zones. The ill-defined zona glomerulosa, about 15 per cent of the cortex, is present under the capsule and contains foci of cells, with a small cytoplasmic volume and lipid content, that produce aldosterone. The remainder of the cortex, the zonae reticularis and fasciculata, can be considered a single unit involved predominantly in cortisol and androgen production. Cells of the zona fasciculata, about 75 per cent of the cortex, appear vacuolated or clear on stained sections because of their high cholesterol content. The cells of the inner zona reticularis are more compact with less lipid.

The morphology of the gland is influenced by corticotropin (ACTH), angiotensin II, and potassium. Elevations of ACTH levels increase adrenal blood flow within minutes and adrenal weight within hours; the clear fasciculata cells lose their lipid, attain the compact morphology and ultrastructural features of reticularis cells, and produce cortisol. Prolonged stimulation results in hyperplasia and hypertrophy. Increases in angiotensin II and potassium result in hypertrophy and hyperplasia of the glomerulosa cells and increased aldosterone production. Deficiency of angiotensin II leads to atrophy of the zona glomerulosa, and deficiency of ACTH to atrophy of the zonae fasciculata and reticularis; this is reversible upon restimulation. Occasionally, accessory adrenal glands may be present in a variety of locations in the abdomen or pelvis and can assume significant function in states of ACTH excess.

DEVELOPMENT. The adrenal cortex is derived from mesenchymal tissue. Cortical cells emerge to form a primitive fetal cortex around the sixth week of development. This evolves into a fetal zone involved predominantly in synthesis of androgen and estrogen precursors, and a definitive zone destined to become the adult gland. The fetal zone, the major bulk of the adrenal cortex at birth, begins to recede by the last intrauterine month and disappears around the end of the first year. The permanent cortex is formed from cells of the outer portion of the fetal gland and is not developed completely until around 3 years of age.

217.2 SYNTHESIS, CIRCULATION, AND METABOLISM OF ADRENAL STEROIDS

John D. Baxter

SYNTHESIS

The structures and steps in biosynthesis of a number of steroid hormones are shown in Figure 217–1. The letter designation for the carbon rings and the number designation of the carbon atoms are shown for pregnenolone, a key biosynthetic intermediate. α- and β- designate positions of the side groups above (β) or below (α) the plane of the molecule. The various steroids differ in (1)

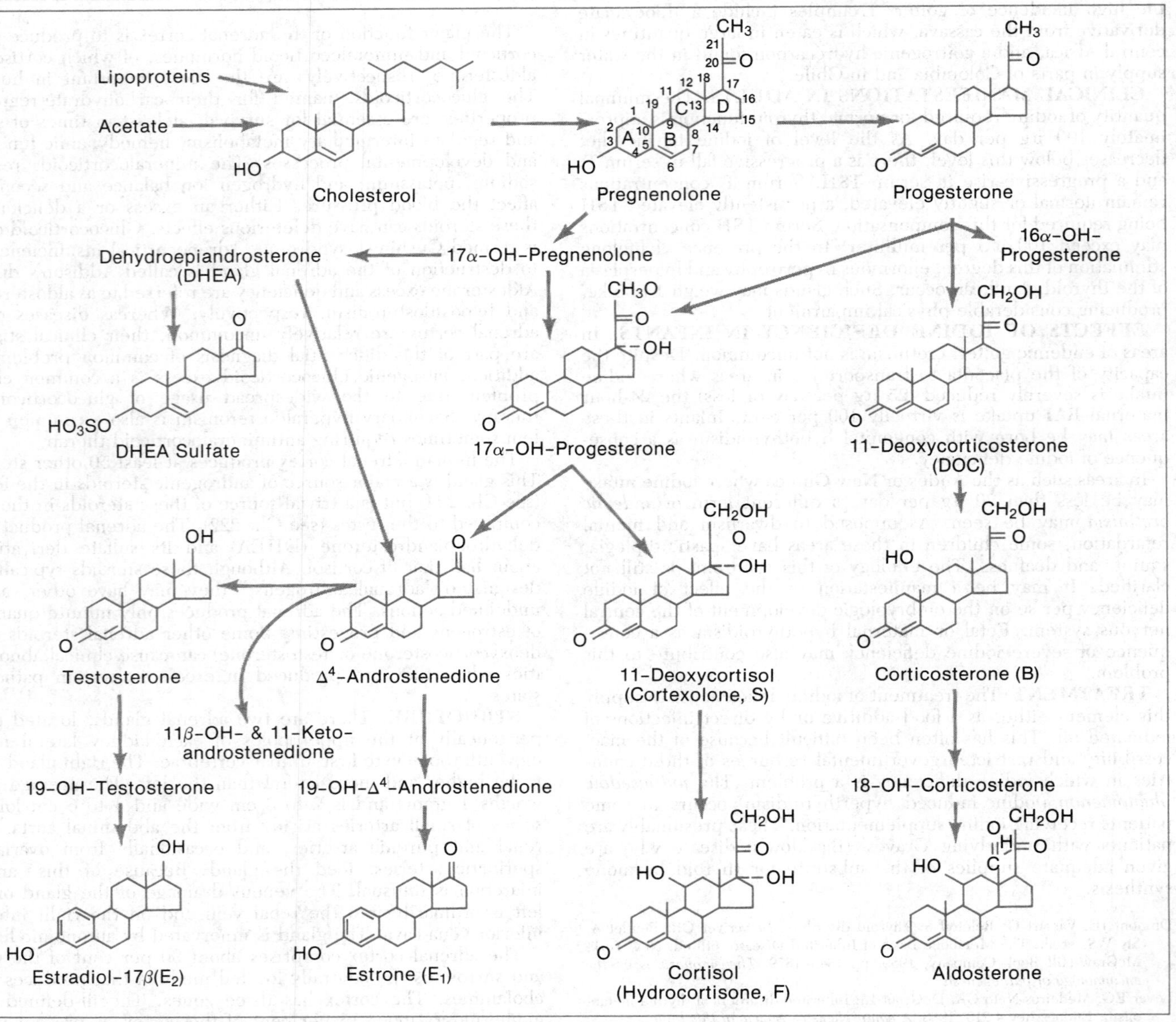

FIGURE 217–1. Steps in adrenal steroid biosynthesis. The numbers for the carbon atoms and the letters designating the rings of the steroid molecule are shown for pregnenolone. Arrows indicate the conversion pathways; the use of two arrows between intermediates indicates that more than one step is involved in the interconversion. (Adapted from Baxter JD, Tyrrell JB: *In* Felig P, Baxter JD, Broadus AE, et al. (eds.): Endocrinology and Metabolism, 2nd ed. New York, McGraw-Hill Book Company, 1987, p 516.)

TABLE 217–1. SECRETION RATES AND PLASMA CONCENTRATIONS OF ADRENAL STEROIDS*

Steroid	24-hr Secretion (mg)	Mean Plasma Concentration (ng/ml)
Aldosterone	0.15	0.16
Androstenedione	2.4	1.5
Corticosterone	2.5	3
Cortisol	16	100
11-Deoxycorticosterone (DOC)	0.6	0.16
11-Deoxycortisol	0.4	1.7
DHEA	0.7(F), 3.0(M)	5.4
DHEA-S	7	1200
Progesterone	nil	0.2(M,F), 12(F)†
17α-Hydroxyprogesterone	nil	0.2(M), 0.6(F), 2.0(F)†
Testosterone	0.2	5.6(M), 0.5(F)

Modified from Baxter JD, Tyrrell JB: The adrenal cortex. *In* Felig P, Baxter JD, Broadus AH, et al. (eds.): Endocrinology and Metabolism, 2nd ed. New York, McGraw-Hill Book Company, 1987, p 521, where references to primary source material can be found.

*Mean values are reported for adults. Individual female (F) and male (M) values are reported only when these differ by more than twofold.

†Refers to the luteal phase of the menstrual cycle.

the saturation of the A ring (Δ indicates a double bond); (2) hydroxyl and ketone groups at positions 3, 11, 17, and 21; (3) the presence of a three-carbon side chain at position 17; and (4) an aldehyde group at position 18. Since the chemical nomenclature is cumbersome, trivial names for the steroids are used most frequently.

All steroids are derived from cholesterol that is obtained mostly by receptor-mediated internalization of plasma low density lipoproteins and to a lesser extent from synthesis by the gland. This uptake mechanism is increased when the adrenal is stimulated.

Subsequent steps occur in the mitochondrion or endoplasmic reticulum. The first step is the conversion of cholesterol to pregnenolone. This rate-limiting step is regulated by the major factors (ACTH, angiotensin II, and potassium) that stimulate steroid biosynthesis. This conversion involves several steps, catalyzed by the enzyme 20,22-desmolase (cholesterol side chain cleavage enzyme). Pregnenolone is then modified either (1) by converting its 5,6 to a 4,5 double bond with the use of 3β-hydroxysteroid dehydrogenase and Δ⁵-oxysteroid isomerase, resulting in progesterone; or (2) by addition of a 17α-hydroxyl group with the use of 17α-hydroxylase, resulting in 17α-hydroxypregnenolone. The former pathway occurs in the glomerulosa, which lacks 17α-hydroxylase activity; although controversial, the latter pathway probably predominates in the fasciculata-reticularis, with subsequent conversion of 17α-hydroxypregnenolone to 17α-hydroxyprogesterone.

CORTISOL. Cortisol is synthesized by two successive hydroxylations of 17α-hydroxyprogesterone. The first is at the 21 position, catalyzed by 21-hydroxylase, and results in 11-deoxycortisol (also called compound S). The second, at the 11 position of 11-deoxycortisol, is catalyzed by 11β-hydroxylase and yields cortisol (also called hydrocortisone or compound F). These hydroxylations also require a flavoprotein dehydrogenase and a cytochrome P-450.

ALDOSTERONE. Aldosterone is produced by 21-hydroxylation of progesterone to form deoxycorticosterone (DOC); 11β-hydroxylation of DOC to form corticosterone; 18-hydroxylation of the latter to form 18-hydroxycorticosterone (18-OHB); and oxidation of the 18 CH₂OH group to an aldehyde to form aldosterone with the use of 18-hydroxycorticosteroid hydroxylase. This step is unique to the glomerulosa.

ANDROGENS. The adrenal androgens have 19 carbon atoms (C-19 steroids) and serve as precursors for more potent androgens produced in peripheral tissues. These are DHEA and its sulfate (DHEA-S), androstenedione, and testosterone. DHEA is derived from 17α-hydroxypregnenolone by removal of its C-17 side chain, that leaves a keto group, with the use of C-17,20-lyase, and 17β-hydroxysteroid dehydrogenase. The sulfation of DHEA at the 3 position to DHEA-S is catalyzed by a sulfokinase. Androstenedione can be derived from either 17α-hydroxyprogesterone or DHEA, as illustrated. The adrenal synthesizes minute quantities of the C-18 steroids estradiol and estrone (Fig. 217–1). However,

DHEA and DHEA-S synthesized by the fetal adrenal account for substantial amounts of maternal production of estriol, estradiol, estrone, testosterone, and androstenedione.

PRODUCTION RATES. The production rates and the blood levels under basal conditions of the major adrenal steroids are shown in Table 217–1. More cortisol is produced than any other steroid; much less aldosterone is produced. The production of DHEA plus DHEA-S is about half that of cortisol; although the plasma levels of DHEA are only a fraction of those of cortisol, plasma levels of DHEA-S are severalfold higher than those of cortisol because of the slow metabolism of DHEA-S. Corticosterone has substantial glucocorticoid activity but is produced at much lower levels than cortisol. Similarly, DOC has substantial mineralocorticoid activity, and more DOC than aldosterone is produced, but free levels of this steroid in plasma are much lower than those of aldosterone even though total levels are similar. The adrenal production of progesterone and 17α-hydroxyprogesterone is minimal. The production of testosterone is at levels similar to those of aldosterone.

INHIBITORS. Several compounds can inhibit adrenal steroid biosynthesis at various steps. They can be useful for diagnosis and therapy of adrenal disorders (discussed below). Of these, metyrapone (SU-4885), aminoglutethimide, and mitotane (o,p'-DDD) have been used most commonly. Metyrapone predominantly inhibits 11β-hydroxylation and to a lesser extent 21-hydroxylation. Aminoglutethimide blocks the early steps in conversion of cholesterol to pregnenolone (cholesterol to 20α-hydroxycholesterol). Mitotane blocks adrenal mitochondrial functioning and results in generalized inhibition of steroid biosynthesis and adrenal atrophy. Ketoconazole, an antifungal agent, also inhibits steroid biosynthesis by inhibiting the actions of cytochrome P-450 enzymes. Spironolactone can block aldosterone biosynthesis by inhibiting the 11β- and 18-hydroxylation steps; these actions may add to the antimineralocorticoid actions of this compound.

PLASMA BINDING OF ADRENAL STEROIDS

GLUCOCORTICOIDS. Approximately 90 to 93 per cent of the circulating cortisol is bound by plasma proteins. About 80 per cent of this binding is due to specific and high-affinity association of cortisol with corticosteroid-binding globulin (CBG, also termed transcortin). A lesser quantity is bound by albumin and a negligible amount by other plasma proteins. CBG is synthesized in the liver and at its usual concentrations in plasma has a capacity for binding cortisol of around 25 μg per deciliter; thus, when cortisol levels begin to exceed this saturation capacity, the proportion of free cortisol is increased. Although several other steroids (e.g., corticosterone, progesterone) can bind to CBG, under most circumstances such occupancy is minimal.

CBG concentrations in plasma vary on a genetic basis and are also regulated by hormones and other factors. CBG levels are increased in pregnancy (by almost twofold during the third trimester), in hyperthyroidism, in diabetes, and by estrogens and oral contraceptives. Such effects can be maximal in 3 to 5 days and reversed by 2 to 3 weeks after cessation of the stimulus. CBG levels can be low congenitally and in liver disease (decreased protein production), multiple myeloma, obesity, hypothyroidism, and the nephrotic syndrome (through urinary loss).

The physiologic role of the plasma steroid-binding proteins is unknown. CBG is not required to transport cortisol, as it is soluble at physiologically effective concentrations. CBG is also not required for cortisol action. For instance, tissue culture cells respond to cortisol in the absence of detectable CBG. Further, the free rather than the plasma-bound steroid is physiologically active, and physiologic mechanisms that regulate cortisol levels respond to the free rather than the total steroid concentration. Thus, when the CBG levels are primarily elevated or depressed, there are elevations or depressions, respectively, of the total cortisol in plasma, but the free cortisol concentration remains the same. This point is critical for evaluation of states of glucocorticoid excess or deficiency.

That CBG may have some importance is suggested by its ubiquity in mammals, even though plasma levels vary enormously, and by the fact that congenital absence of CBG in humans has never been found. A possible role for CBG is to provide a more even distribution of cortisol within larger organs. The free steroid is immediately available for tissue uptake. Thus, when blood enters a large organ such as the liver, the proximal portions of the tissue (outer hepatocytes in the lobule) could sequester most of the free hormone, making it unavailable for more distal uptake (closer to the central vein). In the presence of CBG-bound cortisol, however, the uptake of free hormone by cells would lead to the release of bound hormone to reestablish the equilibrium. Since the blood is moving, such dissociation would occur more distally, where the newly derived free cortisol would then be available for uptake. Such binding may also slow the degradation of steroids as they pass through the liver by reducing the rate at which they are taken up. In addition, CBG or CBG-like proteins can be located intracellularly, and in the kidney they may sequester cortisol and prevent it from occupying the mineralocorticoid receptors. This would preserve the latter for occupancy by aldosterone as the major salt-regulating hormone. Finally, the protein binding of steroids in the blood may buffer rapid changes in plasma free cortisol levels that would otherwise occur as a result of episodic release of cortisol from the adrenal gland.

MINERALOCORTICOIDS. Under physiologic conditions, about 60 per cent of the total plasma aldosterone is protein bound, largely to albumin. The binding is weaker than that of cortisol with CBG, and the free plasma aldosterone seems to be physiologically active.

DOC has potent mineralocorticoid activity, and its plasma levels are similar to those of aldosterone. However, DOC is not normally a physiologically important mineralocorticoid, since over 95 per cent of it is bound to plasma proteins and thus its free levels are much lower than those of aldosterone.

METABOLISM OF ADRENAL STEROIDS

The hydrophobic steroids, although filtered by the renal glomerulus and excreted into the urine, are mostly reabsorbed. For example, only about 1 per cent of the cortisol produced daily is excreted unchanged in the urine. Nevertheless, the kidneys account for over 90 per cent of the excretion of metabolized steroids (DOC and corticosterone are exceptions); the remainder is lost in the gut. To promote their renal elimination, the steroids are inactivated and made more water soluble through enzymatic modifications. These involve hydroxylation of the keto groups, reduction of the double bond in the A ring, and conjugation at the 3 or 21 positions with glucuronide or sulfate. These conversions occur mostly in liver, although during pregnancy the placenta assumes metabolic importance. The conversions alter the steroids so that the renal clearance of a major cortisol metabolite, tetrahydrocortisone glucuronide, is around 70 per cent that of the creatinine clearance. More than 50 metabolites of cortisol and aldosterone have been detected in humans. The pathways shown in Figure 217–2 appear generally to be dominant.

GLUCOCORTICOIDS. Cortisol is cleared from the plasma with a half-life of 80 to 120 minutes. About 70 per cent of infused cortisol, and presumably of that secreted, is eliminated within 24 hours. The 11β-hydroxyl group of cortisol can be oxidized by the enzyme 11β-hydroxysteroid dehydrogenase to the ketone, forming cortisone, which is devoid of glucocorticoid activity. Cortisone can also be converted to cortisol by 11-oxo-steroid reductase. Thus, administered cortisone is largely converted to active cortisol in the liver. Conversely, however, in parts of the kidney cortisol is predominantly converted to cortisone. This prevents cortisol from binding to the mineralocorticoid receptor, which in turn allows aldosterone to serve as the major mineralocorticoid. In other tissues, such as brain, where cortisol is not efficiently converted to cortisone, cortisol does occupy and act through mineralocorticoid receptors.

Cortisol and cortisone have similar subsequent metabolic fates, and overall roughly equivalent quantities of metabolites of these steroids are produced. Quantitatively the most important subsequent modification involves reduction of the 3-keto moiety to form dihydrocortisol and dihydrocortisone, followed by a reduction of the 4,5 double bond to form tetrahydrocortisol and tetrahydrocortisone. When the 3-hydroxyl group is formed, over 95 per cent of the products are conjugated at this position to form the glucuronide and to a lesser extent the sulfate derivatives. Conjugates of these two steroids make up around 30 per cent of

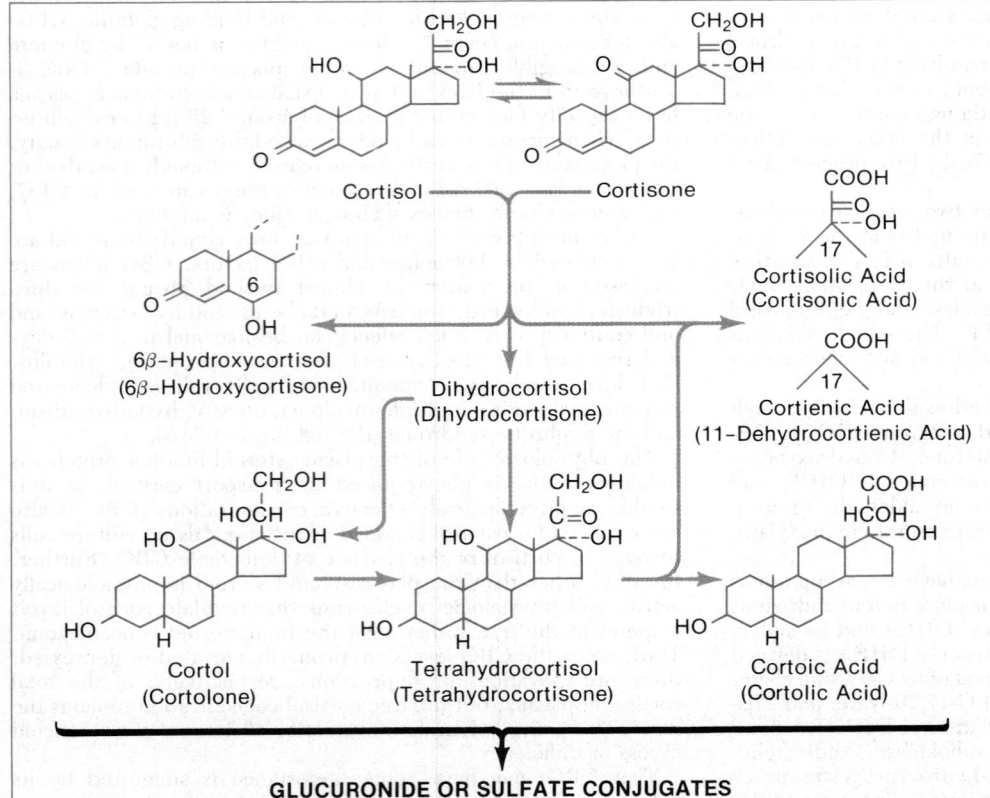

FIGURE 217–2. Metabolism of cortisol. See text. The interconversion of cortisol to cortisone is shown. The other steroid metabolites can be derivatives of either cortisol or cortisone. Structures shown and names are for the cortisol derivatives. The names of the cortisone derivatives are shown in parentheses. In some cases, only part of the steroid molecule is shown; in these cases numbers refer to the steroid carbons for orientation. For tetrahydrocortisol, tetrahydrocortisone, and their derivatives, the 3-hydroxyl and 5-hydrogen are shown in the α and β configurations, respectively, but both α and β orientations occur at both positions. For a more extensive discussion and references, see Baxter JD, Tyrrell JB: In Felig P, Baxter JD, Broadus AE, et al. (eds.): Endocrinology and Metabolism, 2nd ed. New York, McGraw-Hill Book Company, 1987, p 544.

Cortisol — Cortisone

Cortisolic Acid (Cortisonic Acid)

6β–Hydroxycortisol (6β–Hydroxycortisone)

Dihydrocortisol (Dihydrocortisone)

Cortienic Acid (11-Dehydrocortienic Acid)

Cortol (Cortolone)

Tetrahydrocortisol (Tetrahydrocortisone)

Cortoic Acid (Cortolic Acid)

GLUCURONIDE OR SULFATE CONJUGATES

the urinary cortisol metabolites. The second major site for modification involves the reduction of the 20-ketone to a hydroxyl, with subsequent reduction of the A ring, resulting in cortol (11-OH) or cortolone (11-keto). These account for approximately 25 per cent of the cortisol metabolites. Alternatively, there can be conversion of the 21-hydroxyl to a COOH to form cortisolic or cortisonic acid from cortisol and cortisone, respectively. Cortoic (11-hydroxyl) or cortolonic (11-keto) acid results from this modification of tetrahydrocortisone and tetrahydrocortisol, respectively, and these metabolites account for about 10 per cent of the cortisol metabolites. Other minor pathways involve the C-17 modifications discussed above without A-ring reduction, removal of the C-17 side chain with formation of 17-keto or 17-COOH moieties, formation of the C-21 COOH (without C-20-keto) and 6β-hydroxylation. The latter modification constitutes a major pathway in infants in whom the esterification mechanism has not been developed and for the synthetic glucocorticoids used in therapy.

MINERALOCORTICOIDS. Aldosterone is cleared with a half-life of around 15 minutes. Its conversion to metabolites is so effective that very little aldosterone survives passage through the liver. This is in part due to the weak plasma binding of aldosterone which allows it to be taken up by the liver (discussed above). Less than 0.5 per cent of the aldosterone appears in the urine in the free state. The metabolism of aldosterone is similar to that of cortisol. About 35 per cent of the steroid appears as tetrahydroaldosterone glucuronide (3 position). However, two major differences are that there is much less 11β-hydroxy to 11-keto conversion, and 15 to 20 per cent of the aldosterone appears as a C-18 glucuronide that is acid labile; measurements of the urinary "aldosterone" usually reflect this metabolite.

ANDROGENS. The metabolism of androgens is discussed in Ch. 222.

VARIATIONS IN RATES OF METABOLISM. The rate of steroid metabolism can be altered in certain clinical states and by various drugs. Agents that affect plasma steroid-binding proteins secondarily affect metabolism because of inhibitory influences of plasma binding on clearance. In chronic liver disease, hypothyroidism, infancy, very old age, anorexia nervosa, and protein-calorie malnutrition, the rate of steroid metabolism is decreased. The converse occurs in hyperthyroidism. These states are in general not associated with abnormal free steroid levels (anorexia nervosa is an exception) because the regulatory systems tend to compensate by altering steroid production. The conversion of cortisone to cortisol is not substantially impaired in liver disease. The conversion of prednisone to prednisolone may be impaired, however, and prednisolone rather than prednisone is recommended for glucocorticoid therapy in patients with severe liver disease. Also, there is no major effect of renal disease (even though it does affect the clearance of some metabolites) or of most chronic diseases, obesity, and stress.

Drugs that affect steroid metabolism usually increase 6β-hydroxylation. This is a minor pathway in adults, and these drugs do not have a major effect on endogenous cortisol. They have a greater effect on the clearance of synthetic glucocorticoids such as dexamethasone and prednisone, and this is therefore an important consideration with steroid therapy or with the use of glucocorticoids to assess the hypothalamic-pituitary-adrenal axis. These drugs include mitotane, phenytoin, rifampicin, aminoglutethimide, and barbiturates. Glycyrrhetinic acid, present in licorice, and carbenoxolone, used for treatment of peptic ulcer disease, block 11β-hydroxysteroid dehydrogenase and thereby the conversion of cortisol to cortisone. This leads to increased actions of cortisol through mineralocorticoid receptors and a hypermineralocorticoid state.

217.3 REGULATION OF ADRENAL STEROID PRODUCTION

John D. Baxter

Adrenal cortisol and androgen production is regulated by the hypothalamic-pituitary-adrenal axis, whereas aldosterone production is regulated predominantly by the renin-angiotensin system and by potassium (Fig. 217–3). These systems allow for basal and circadian steroid production, regulation of plasma steroid levels in normal circumstances, and increased or decreased steroid production in response to a number of specific stimuli.

REGULATION OF GLUCOCORTICOID PRODUCTION

The hypothalamus, pituitary, and adrenal comprise a neuroendocrine axis concerned with regulation of cortisol production (see

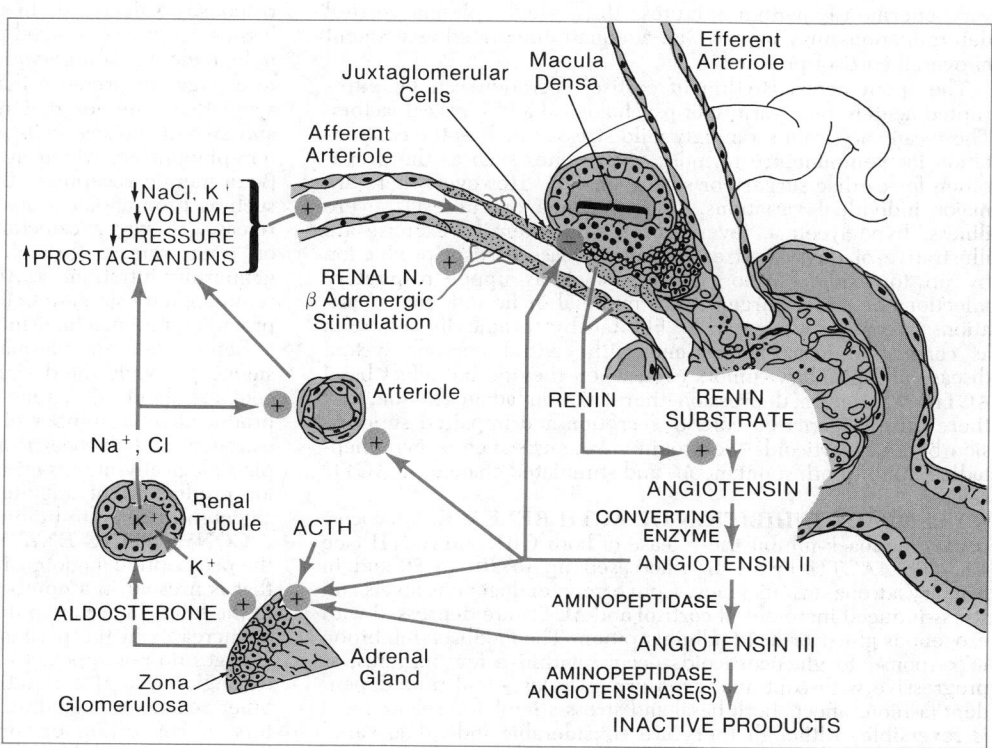

FIGURE 217–3. Renin-angiotensin system. The plus and minus signs indicate stimulation and inhibition, respectively. (Reprinted from Baxter JD, Perloff D, Hsueh W, et al.: *In* Felig P, Baxter JD, Broadus AE, et al. (eds.): Endocrinology and Metabolism, 2nd ed. New York, McGraw-Hill Book Company, 1987, p 701.)

Ch. 212). Corticotropin-releasing factor (CRF) and arginine vasopressin (AVP) are elaborated by the hypothalamus and travel through its portal system to the anterior pituitary where they stimulate the release of ACTH, which in turn increases adrenal cortisol production.

Three major types of mechanisms are involved in regulating cortisol release: (1) circadian rhythms of secretion are established by the brain, (2) a number of types of excitatory factors can increase cortisol production, and (3) production of CRF and ACTH is regulated negatively by glucocorticoids.

ACTH AND RELATED PEPTIDES. ACTH circulates free in the plasma with a half-life of around 10 minutes. It is derived from the proteolysis of pro-opiomelanocortin, a larger precursor pituitary protein of about 290 amino acids that also contains the sequences of several other proteins, including β-endorphin, α-, β-, and γ-melanocyte-stimulating hormones (MSH), β-lipotropin (β-LPH), and an amino-terminal fragment (see Ch. 208). Although MSH itself has the greatest pigment-stimulating activity, this activity in humans is due predominantly to MSH sequences contained within ACTH (α-MSH), β-LPH (β-MSH), and the amino-terminal fragment (γ-MSH), as very little MSH is present in the circulation. ACTH stimulates cortisol release within 2 to 3 minutes. This is due to increased cortisol synthesis primarily through stimulation of cholesterol to pregnenolone conversion, rather than through effects on secretion of stored hormone. More prolonged stimulation results in increased protein, RNA, and DNA synthesis with both hypertrophy and hyperplasia. ACTH binds to surface receptors and activates adenylate cyclase. This results in increased cyclic AMP generation with consequent stimulation of protein phosphorylation and of the production of phospholipids that may be involved in the stimulation of steroidogenesis. The actions of ACTH are also Ca^{2+} dependent. These effects increase cholesterol side chain cleavage and cholesterol esterase and lipoprotein uptake and block cholesterol ester synthesis with a resulting stimulation of the conversion of cholesterol to pregnenolone.

SPONTANEOUS RHYTHMS. The circadian rhythm of ACTH and cortisol results in decreasing release through the afternoon and evening. Secretion begins to increase around 3 to 4 A.M., peaks by around 8 A.M., and then begins to decline. This release occurs in pulses with intervals between them of 40 minutes to hours; the changes in overall cortisol production are due to the number of pulses that occur. These result in cortisol levels that vary enormously within minutes; thus, single plasma cortisol determinations may not give an adequate integrated assessment of overall cortisol production.

The spontaneous rhythm of cortisol secretion can be interrupted acutely by a variety of psychological and physical factors. These can vary from seemingly mild stresses such as the confrontation for venipuncture to more severe ones such as the preparation for cardiac surgery or severe anxiety. However, there are major individual variations. Major trauma or surgery, severe illness, hypoglycemia, fever, burns, and intensive exercise are illustrative of physical stresses that increase cortisol production by up to sixfold. Minor illnesses such as upper respiratory infections or minor surgery have minimal or no influence. Variations in cortisol levels can be blunted by chronic diseases such as congestive heart failure and with central nervous system disease and pituitary tumors even when they do not affect basal ACTH release. In depression there is a circadian rhythm, but there can be increased cortisol secretion and impaired suppression by glucocorticoids. Serotonin antagonists such as cyproheptadine inhibit both spontaneous and stimulated changes in ACTH release.

FEEDBACK INHIBITION OF ACTH RELEASE. Glucocorticoids feedback-inhibit the release of both CRF and ACTH (see Ch. 208). ACTH levels are increased up to 10- to 20-fold in primary adrenal insufficiency. Conversely, endogenous levels and stress-induced increases of cortisol and ACTH are depressed with exogenous glucocorticoid administration. The feedback inhibition in response to glucocorticoids occurs within a few minutes, is progressive with continual exposure in a dose- and time-dependent fashion, affects both basal and stress-stimulated release, and is reversible. Although there are considerable individual variations, administration of a large dose of glucocorticoids for a few days does not, in general, result in suppression of pituitary function for more than a few hours; more prolonged exposure is accompanied by substantial suppression. Thus after several years of glucocorticoid therapy and then withdrawal of steroid administration or following surgical removal of a tumor causing Cushing's syndrome, a year or more may be required for the hypothalamic-pituitary-adrenal axis to return to normal functioning. Although significant suppression occurs at both the hypothalamic and pituitary levels, the quantitative contribution of each of them has not been clarified.

REGULATION OF MINERALOCORTICOID PRODUCTION

Aldosterone production is controlled predominantly by the renin-angiotensin system and potassium, although other factors such as sodium, ACTH, dopamine, and serotonin also affect aldosterone secretion (Fig. 217–3). The renin-angiotensin system is important for adaptive blood pressure changes and is involved in the pathogenesis of some forms of hypertension.

RENIN. Renin, a glycoprotein of 340 amino acids, is produced in the juxtaglomerular cells of the afferent renal arteriole as a precursor protein (prorenin) that is cleaved to yield active renin. These cells release renin into the circulation where it has a half-life of around 15 minutes. Prorenin is also made in a number of other tissues, and in some of these, including the adrenal, it may be converted to active renin. The role of extrarenal renin-angiotensin systems is currently a subject of intense study. However, extrarenal prorenin does not contribute to the plasma renin, and conditions that result in impaired renal release of renin lead to aldosterone deficiency. The release of renin is stimulated by lowering the blood pressure, assumption of the erect posture, salt depletion, β-adrenergic or central nervous system stimulation, and certain prostaglandins. It is inhibited by increases in blood pressure (except with malignant hypertension), salt loading, angiotensin II, vasopressin, potassium, calcium, β-adrenergic antagonists, α-methyldopa, clonidine, and inhibitors of prostaglandin synthesis such as indomethacin.

Four factors mediate most of the changes in renin release: (1) Changes in renal tubular sodium chloride concentration are detected by the macula densa, a specialized segment of the distal tubule that makes contact with the juxtaglomerular cells of the afferent arteriole just before it enters the glomerulus. This information is transmitted to the juxtaglomerular cells so that factors that reduce volume or lower the plasma sodium and chloride levels (e.g., dehydration, fluid or blood loss) increase renin release. (2) Renal baroreceptors stimulate renin release in response to decreases in renal perfusion pressure as with fluid loss or decreases in blood pressure. These receptors can function independently of innervation and salt delivery and respond more to changes in pressure than to the absolute pressure. (3) Renal sympathetic nerves that terminate in the juxtaglomerular cells and smooth muscle cells of the renal afferent arterioles secrete norepinephrine, which in turn stimulates renin release through β-adrenergic receptors. Blockage of this mechanism by agents such as propranolol probably explains how they decrease renin release. However, catecholamines can have other indirect effects on renin release through influences on renal blood flow and glomerular filtration. (4) Angiotensin II, the major product of the renin-angiotensin system (discussed below), blocks renin release, providing one mechanism for feedback inhibition of the system.

Renin acts in the plasma and cleaves renin substrate (angiotensinogen) to yield the decapeptide angiotensin I. Angiotensinogen contains about 450 amino acids, is secreted by the liver, and is produced by a number of tissues; its level can be increased by estrogens and glucocorticoids. Angiotensin I is not known to have physiologically important actions; instead it serves as a substrate for production of angiotensin II. Normally the production of angiotensin I is rate limiting for angiotensin II generation.

CONVERTING ENZYME. The conversion of angiotensin I to the octapeptide angiotensin II is catalyzed by converting enzyme that is present in a number of tissues and in high concentrations in the lung. In certain pulmonary diseases there can be decreases or increases in the plasma levels of the enzyme, although these changes do not appear to have a physiologically important effect on angiotensin II generation. Converting enzyme also catalyzes other reactions, including the inactivation of bradykinin. Inhibitors of converting enzyme, such as captopril, enalapril, and lisinopril, are widely used to treat hypertension and heart failure.

ANGIOTENSIN II. Angiotensin II is a potent vasoconstrictor with direct effects on arterioles. It inhibits renin release as described above. It is a potent stimulator of aldosterone release, and stimulates both early and late steps in aldosterone biosynthesis, resulting in increased conversion of cholesterol to pregnenolene and of corticosterone to 18-hydroxycorticosterone. Angiotensin II binds to cell surface receptors and stimulates Ca^{2+} influx and phospholipid turnover but does not activate adenylate cyclase. Angiotensin II also has a tropic influence on the adrenal zona glomerulosa, and it may also stimulate the proliferation of smooth muscle and other cells of the body. The hormone also has other complex effects on the kidney that affect salt balance, possibly through influences on kallikreins and prostaglandins. Plasma concentrations of angiotensin II can vary up to 25-fold; the hormone has a half-life of only 1 to 2 minutes. There are several breakdown products of angiotensin II. One of these, angiotensin III, a polypeptide of seven amino acids, has angiotensin II activity, but its biologic importance is probably less than that of angiotensin II.

POTASSIUM. Increased potassium stimulates and decreased potassium inhibits aldosterone production. These effects are elicited by changes in potassium of as little as 0.1 mEq per liter in the physiologic range and are independent of sodium or angiotensin II. Prolonged hyperkalemia, like excess angiotensin II, has a tropic influence on the adrenal.

OTHER FACTORS. Other factors of lesser importance also affect aldosterone release. ACTH has a transient effect, and, rarely, aldosterone production can be blunted with chronic ACTH deficiency. Atrial natriuretic peptide blocks and other pituitary factors may stimulate aldosterone release. Sodium deficiency decreases and sodium loading increases aldosterone release, but these influences are probably mediated through effects on renin. Dopamine agonists can inhibit and dopamine antagonists can increase plasma aldosterone. Aldosterone release is episodic and shows a tendency to a circadian rhythm that is similar to but much less prominent than that of cortisol.

REGULATION OF ADRENAL ANDROGEN PRODUCTION

Adrenal androgen production is regulated by ACTH in a manner similar to that of cortisol. Plasma levels of these hormones also show the same circadian periodicity as cortisol, although this is masked in the case of DHEA-S because of its prolonged plasma half-life. Adrenal androgen release is also altered during prepuberty (adrenarche) by poorly understood mechanisms. Further, it should be remembered that androgens released by the testes and ovaries contribute to plasma androgen levels.

217.4 ACTIONS OF ADRENAL STEROIDS

John D. Baxter

GLUCOCORTICOIDS

Glucocorticoids have diverse actions that affect most mammalian tissues and are also essential for survival, at least in times of stress.

INTERMEDIARY METABOLISM. Glucocorticoids have multiple influences on glucose metabolism with diverse secondary effects (Fig. 217-4). In most tissues these steroids inhibit glucose uptake. Liver, heart, brain, and erythrocytes are exceptions. In many of these tissues the steroids also block protein and nucleic acid synthesis and stimulate turnover of these macromolecules. In adipose tissue the steroids inhibit lipolysis and block lipogenesis. In liver the steroids stimulate glycogen deposition, gluconeogenesis, the ability of other hormones to stimulate gluconeogenesis, and lipoprotein synthesis. Gluconeogenesis is further facilitated because of increased availability of glycerol and amino acid substrate due to the effects in peripheral tissues. The steroids also tend to stimulate the appetite, and in adrenal insufficiency there is anorexia. Finally, glucocorticoids tend to blunt the actions of insulin and decrease the affinity for insulin binding to its receptors.

The net effect of these influences is a glucocorticoid-induced tendency to hyperglycemia, ketosis, and hyperlipidemia. How-

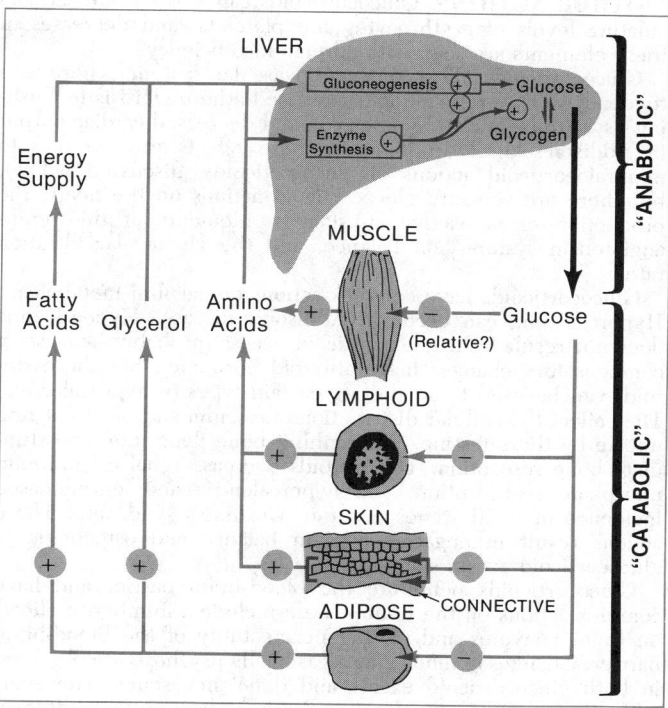

FIGURE 217-4. Glucocorticoid influences on intermediary metabolism. Plus and minus signs refer to stimulation and inhibition, respectively. (Modified from Baxter JD, Forsham PH: Tissue effects of glucocorticoids. Am J Med 53:579, 1972.)

ever, in normal subjects the elevated levels of glucose increase insulin release that in turn blunts the effects of the steroid. However, in diabetes or latent diabetes, significant hyperglycemia and insulin resistance can ensue. Lipogenesis induced by secondary increases in plasma insulin levels along with the increased food intake due to appetite stimulation may explain the truncal and sometimes generalized obesity seen in Cushing's syndrome. Conversely, in adrenal insufficiency there is a tendency to hypoglycemia; usually this is not marked in the adult, but it can be significant if there is concomitant fasting. Many of the actions of glucocorticoids on intermediary metabolism can be perceived as a protection against fasting; there is peripheral catabolism with sparing of essential tissues (heart, brain, blood cells) to make available substrate for maintenance of the blood sugar levels.

These actions of glucocorticoids on intermediary metabolism also explain many other effects of glucocorticoid excess. Thus inhibition of metabolic functions in peripheral tissues may explain glucocorticoid-induced myopathy, inhibition of immunologic and inflammatory responses, poor wound healing, thinning of the skin, striae, and osteoporosis.

INFLAMMATORY AND IMMUNOLOGIC RESPONSES. In excess, glucocorticoids suppress inflammatory and immunologic responses, but it is not clear whether they normally modulate immunologic systems. In excess, glucocorticoids inhibit antigen processing; T cell function; synthesis of cellular mediators of the inflammatory response such as interleukins, plasminogen activator, lymphokines, other active peptides, and prostaglandins and other eicosanoids; cellular migration and action at sites of inflammation; and inflammatory reactions themselves. In general they do not affect most antibody responses, although there are a few exceptions. Some populations of lymphocytes are killed by glucocorticoids; this explains the efficacy of these steroids in treating certain leukemias such as acute lymphoblastic leukemia of childhood. The steroids also affect mononuclear cell trafficking, tend to decrease blood monocyte, lymphocyte, and eosinophil levels, and increase polymorphonuclear leukocytes; there are reciprocal changes during adrenal insufficiency. Interestingly, glucocorticoids do not produce any permanent impairment of the immunologic system.

OTHER ACTIONS. Glucocorticoids can also elevate the circulating levels of erythrocytes and platelets, and decreases in these elements are seen with adrenal insufficiency.

Glucocorticoids affect the cardiovascular system. There is a tendency to hypertension and increased atherosclerosis in Cushing's syndrome and to hypotension and decreased cardiac output in Addison's disease. Some of these effects can be due to mineralocorticoid actions of glucocorticoids (discussed below), but there are separate glucocorticoid actions on the heart, the production of vasoactive substances, elements of the renin-angiotensin system, ion balance, and the glomerular filtration rate.

Glucocorticoids have complex actions on calcium metabolism. Hypercalcemia can occur in Addison's disease. Hypocalcemia does not result from glucocorticoid excess (probably because of compensatory changes in parathyroid hormone), but these steroids can be used to ameliorate certain types of hypercalcemia. They affect the cellular distribution of calcium and block calcium uptake by the intestine. They inhibit bone deposition and stimulate bone resorption. The steroids decrease renal calcium and phosphate reabsorption, and hypercalciuria and an increased incidence of renal stones occur in Cushing's syndrome. These actions result in negative calcium balance and osteopenia in glucocorticoid excess states.

Glucocorticoids penetrate the blood-brain barrier and have complex actions on the brain. These include a number of effects on brain enzymes and on the permeability of the blood-brain barrier. Changes in mood and occasionally psychosis are observed in both glucocorticoid excess and deficiency states. However, with glucocorticoid therapy, euphoria is common. Addisonian subjects commonly have increased sensitivity to a variety of sensory stimuli such as smell or taste. The mechanisms of these influences are poorly understood. Glucocorticoids increase intraocular pressure, probably by blocking fluid uptake by the trabecular meshwork. Glucocorticoid therapy can precipitate glaucoma in susceptible individuals and can enhance cataract formation.

In the gastrointestinal tract glucocorticoids inhibit DNA synthesis and tend to enhance stimuli to gastric acid secretion. They probably also enhance the tendency to form duodenal ulcers and, in high doses, the tendency to develop gastritis.

In excess, glucocorticoids inhibit linear growth, as a result of their inhibitory influences on a number of tissues. However, glucocorticoid action is required for a number of developmental processes. One particularly important process is the synthesis of surfactant in the lung. Lack of glucocorticoid induction of this factor in premature birth contributes to the respiratory distress syndrome of the newborn.

Complex interrelationships exist between glucocorticoids and other hormones. Glucocorticoids inhibit vasopressin release; conversely, ACTH deficiency can lead to hyponatremia with water intoxication. Glucocorticoids secondarily increase insulin and parathyroid hormone (PTH) levels and in some cases blunt the production of growth hormone, prolactin, insulin, glucagon, thyroid-stimulating hormone (TSH), and testosterone. Multiple synergisms and antagonisms between glucocorticoids and other hormones also exist at the cellular level. For example, they are synergistic with epinephrine and glucagon in stimulating hepatic gluconeogenesis. These effects are sometimes termed permissive glucocorticoid actions.

STRESS. Why glucocorticoids are essential for survival in times of stress is poorly understood. Two factors are probably operative. First, stress increases the production of a number of biologically active substances such as catecholamines, prostaglandins and other arachidonic acid metabolites, proteases, and kinins. Glucocorticoids, by contrast, tend to blunt the production and actions of these substances, which, if left unchecked during stress, would lead to shock and vascular decompensation. Second, the stimulation of cardiovascular functions by glucocorticoids may be critical in times of stress when other compensatory systems may be less effective.

MOLECULAR MECHANISMS OF ACTION. Glucocorticoids penetrate cells and bind to intracellular receptors. The receptors that mediate most actions of the glucocorticoids are termed "glucocorticoid" receptors. These bind active glucocorticoids with high affinity and have a much lower affinity for other classes of steroids. Glucocorticoids can also bind to the "mineralocorticoid" receptors that mediate the actions of aldosterone. As mentioned earlier, metabolic conversion of cortisol to cortisone prevents cortisol actions through mineralocorticoid receptors in the kidney, but cortisol does act through these in the brain, hypothalamus, heart, and other sites. The complexes of the glucocorticoids with either of these classes of receptors then bind to specific sites on the DNA where they either enhance or inhibit the ability of RNA polymerase to stimulate transcription of glucocorticoid-responsive genes (see Ch. 208). These actions result in changes in the levels of specific mRNA's transcribed by these genes with consequent fluctuations in the levels of their protein products that in turn mediate the glucocorticoid responses. Also, some glucocorticoid effects occur by mechanisms that do not involve stimulation of transcription.

MINERALOCORTICOIDS

Mineralocorticoid hormones act on kidney, gut, salivary glands, and sweat glands to affect the balance of electrolytes. Direct actions on other tissues including brain, mammary gland, placenta, and pituitary can occur, but the physiologic importance of these is unknown. Thus the spectrum of mineralocorticoid action is more restricted than that of glucocorticoid action.

In the kidney, the most important target organ, mineralocorticoids promote the reabsorption of sodium ion and secretion of potassium ion in the cortical collecting tubules, and possibly in the connecting segment of the nephron, and stimulate the secretion of hydrogen ion in the medullary collecting tubules. Thus, with mineralocorticoid excess, there is sodium retention, hypokalemia, and alkalosis. In primary mineralocorticoid excess, hypertension develops with time. With mineralocorticoid deficiency there is sodium ion loss and a tendency to hyperkalemia and acidosis. The overall effects of mineralocorticoids on both sodium and potassium ions also depend on the level of salt intake. Increased sodium intake results in more tubular sodium for reabsorption; this enhances potassium secretion. Conversely, sodium restriction diminishes aldosterone-induced kaliuresis. In most circumstances with persistent mineralocorticoid excess, the sodium retention that occurs reaches a limit such that the body "escapes" from further sodium retention. This is due to secondary increases in the secretion of other factors or hormones such as atrial natriuretic factor (ANF) and changes in renal hemodynamics with compensating influences of sodium excretion. Exceptions are the secondary hyperaldosteronism of heart failure and of cirrhosis with ascites in which sodium retention is progressive. As noted, hyperkalemia directly stimulates aldosterone secretion, which in turn enhances renal potassium excretion. This servomechanism forms an important component of the body's defense against hyperkalemia.

Mineralocorticoid actions are mediated through molecular mechanisms similar to those described above for cortisol and in Ch. 208. The mineralocorticoid receptors bind aldosterone and DOC with high affinity; they also bind cortisol with around 10 per cent of the affinity for aldosterone. Since plasma free cortisol concentrations are around 100-fold higher than those of aldosterone, there is a need to modulate occupancy of mineralocorticoid receptors by cortisol, as mediated through renal conversion of cortisol to cortisone, as discussed above. The synthetic steroid 9α-fluorocortisol binds tightly to mineralocorticoid receptors and is used for mineralocorticoid replacement therapy, since it is more stable than aldosterone after oral administration. Mineralocorticoid antagonists such as spironolactone bind to these receptors and block aldosterone action.

Aldosterone stimulates the synthesis of several renal proteins that result in increases in (1) sodium permeability in the apical membrane exposed to the tubular lumen; (2) various mitochondrial enzymes that increase cellular ATP and thereby enhance the actions of the Na^+-K^+-ATPase; (3) the Na^+-K^+-ATPase; and (4) probably other as yet unidentified factors of the basolateral membrane. These combined actions result in Na^+ reabsorption. Potassium ion secretion increases secondarily to the Na^+-K^+ exchange because of the pumping action of the Na^+-K^+-ATPase; however, other mechanisms must also operate because there can be independent actions of aldosterone on Na^+ and K^+.

Aldosterone-stimulated renal tubular transport of hydrogen ion, about which little is known, can probably occur independently of the effects on Na$^+$ and K$^+$. However, potassium ion deficiency decreases Na$^+$-K$^+$ exchange, which in turn increases the Na$^+$-H$^+$ exchange and hydrogen ion excretion. As in the case of potassium, hydrogen ion loss can be blunted with sodium restriction. The mineralocorticoid-induced alkalosis is also promoted by hydrogen ion movement into cells in exchange for losses in potassium.

The major known extrarenal targets for aldosterone are the sweat and salivary glands, ileum, and colon where the steroid promotes potassium loss and sodium retention. These actions are ordinarily minor in terms of overall salt balance.

217.5 LABORATORY EVALUATION OF ADRENOCORTICAL FUNCTION

J. Blake Tyrrell

The function of the adrenal cortex is best assessed by plasma assays of the major steroids and measurement of their trophic hormones, e.g., ACTH and related peptides or renin and angiotensin. Certain urinary assays remain useful, however, despite the disadvantage of 24-hour collections. The following considerations must be remembered when using these assays: (1) Current assays for plasma steroids measure total hormone concentration, not bioactive free hormone. (2) Plasma levels of cortisol and ACTH vary greatly because of episodic secretion and many other factors (see below); thus single determinations should not in general be relied upon for a definitive diagnosis. (3) In assessing adrenal function, stimulation and suppression testing provide the most definitive information.

GLUCOCORTICOID FUNCTION

ACTH AND RELATED PEPTIDES. Immunoassays for ACTH are extremely useful but are technically difficult. ACTH is unstable in plasma and adheres to glass; specimens should be collected in anticoagulated plastic or silicon-coated tubes on ice, centrifuged in the cold without delay, and frozen until assayed. The normal range of plasma ACTH in the morning (8 to 9 A.M.) is 20 to 100 pg per milliliter in most assays. Values at other times of the day are lower, but marked episodic variation may occur.

Plasma ACTH levels are used primarily to differentiate pituitary, adrenal, and other causes of adrenal dysfunction. Thus, in patients with cortisol deficiency elevated ACTH levels (generally greater than 250 pg per milliliter) confirm the diagnosis of primary adrenal insufficiency (Addison's disease). Conversely, with secondary adrenal insufficiency due to hypothalamic or pituitary disease or steroid therapy, ACTH levels are low normal or subnormal (usually <20 pg per milliliter). In states of cortisol excess (Cushing's syndrome), a suppressed or undetectable ACTH level (<20 pg per milliliter) is diagnostic of an adrenal tumor hypersecreting cortisol or of exogenous glucocorticoid administration. With ACTH-producing pituitary tumors (Cushing's disease), plasma ACTH levels are normal to modestly elevated (40 to 200 pg per milliliter), whereas in the ectopic ACTH syndrome they are usually elevated markedly (100 to >1000 pg per milliliter). ACTH levels in the two latter conditions may overlap, but very high (>300 pg per milliliter) values strongly suggest an ectopic tumor. Plasma ACTH levels are also elevated in congenital adrenal hyperplasia proportional to the extent of cortisol deficiency and are markedly elevated in pituitary tumors that arise following bilateral adrenalectomy (Nelson's syndrome).

Immunoassays for other peptides derived from pro-opiomelanocortin are also available. The antisera usually measure both β-LPH and β-endorphin. Reported normal morning values of immunoreactive β-LPH/β-endorphin are 20 to 200 pg per milliliter. Levels of these peptides vary similarly to those of ACTH, but because of its longer plasma half-life, β-LPH levels show less episodic variability than ACTH, and β-LPH is considerably more stable than ACTH in plasma.

PLASMA CORTISOL AND RELATED STEROIDS. Plasma cortisol is most frequently measured by radioimmunoassay; current antisera show little cross-reactivity with other natural or synthetic steroids. Competitive protein binding and high-performance liquid chromatography assays are also in use. Normal

TABLE 217–2. CONDITIONS CAUSING ELEVATED CORTISOL LEVELS

Increased CBG	Increased Secretion
Estrogen therapy	Spontaneous Cushing's syndrome
Pregnancy	Exercise
Hyperthyroidism	Physical stress
Diabetes mellitus	Anxiety
Hematologic disorders	Depression
Congenital	Starvation
	Anorexia nervosa
	Alcoholism
	Chronic renal failure

values of plasma cortisol vary with the circadian rhythm of ACTH. Mean levels at 8 A.M. are 10 to 12 μg per deciliter with a range of 3 to 20 μg per deciliter. Values at 4 to 6 P.M. are approximately 50 per cent of the morning levels, although there is great variability. Values obtained between 10 P.M. and 2 A.M. are less than 3 μg per deciliter and may be unmeasurable. Episodic variability and the numerous conditions increasing cortisol secretion or CBG concentrations (Table 217–2) limit the utility of single cortisol determinations.

Measurement of plasma 11-deoxycortisol (compound S) by radioimmunoassay is used in metyrapone testing of pituitary-adrenal reserve (see below) and in the assessment of patients with congenital adrenal hyperplasia or adrenal tumors.

URINARY CORTICOSTEROIDS. Measurements of urinary steroids have been traditionally used to evaluate adrenal function and provide an integrated assessment of steroid production and excretion. With the exception of urinary free cortisol, these methods are less advantageous and have been largely supplanted by plasma measurements of cortisol or other steroids.

Urine free cortisol, although less than 1 per cent of total adrenal cortisol secretion, is a useful measurement in the diagnosis of hypercortisolism. The steroid is measured by radioimmunoassay or competitive protein binding. Normal values range from 20 to 100 μg per 24 hours. Elevated levels are almost always present in Cushing's syndrome but not in simple obesity; this ability to separate these conditions is a major advantage. Urinary cortisol excretion is increased by any condition that increases adrenal cortisol secretion (Table 217–2) and is decreased in renal failure.

Urinary 17-hydroxycorticosteroids (17-OHCS) and 17-ketogenic steroids (17-KGS) measure steroid metabolites, predominantly those of cortisol and 11-deoxycortisol. These methods are currently not recommended in most situations, because the methods are not specific, the levels are altered in many disease states, and the assays are subject to interference by many commonly used drugs and medications.

SUPPRESSION TESTS. Suppression tests evaluate the ability of dexamethasone, a potent synthetic glucocorticoid not measured in current cortisol assays, to inhibit ACTH and cortisol secretion. In Cushing's syndrome glucocorticoids do not normally inhibit ACTH release. There are two types of dexamethasone suppression tests: (1) Low-dose tests are used to document the abnormal responsiveness of the hypothalamic-pituitary-adrenal axis that is characteristic of Cushing's syndrome. (2) High-dose tests are used to distinguish the various causes of Cushing's syndrome. The techniques for performing these tests and the expected responses are summarized in Table 217–3.

Low-Dose Dexamethasone Tests. The overnight 1-mg dexamethasone suppression test is an excellent screening procedure for Cushing's syndrome. The test can be used on an ambulatory basis, and in this setting abnormal responses occur in about 95 per cent of patients with Cushing's syndrome. False-positive responses occur in 25 per cent of hospitalized and chronically ill patients, in 15 per cent of obese patients, and in a number of other conditions, including acute illness, anxiety, depression, alcoholism, anorexia nervosa, estrogen therapy, and uremia. Drugs that accelerate dexamethasone metabolism, especially phenytoin and phenobarbital, also cause false-positive results. The 2-day low-dose test provides the same information as the 1-mg

TABLE 217–3. DEXAMETHASONE SUPPRESSION TESTS

Low-Dose Tests

Overnight test
Dexamethasone 1 mg p.o. at 11 P.M.; plasma cortisol at 8 to 9 A.M. Normal response—plasma cortisol <5 µg/dl

2-day test
Dexamethasone 0.5 mg p.o. q6h for 8 doses; plasma cortisol 1 hr after last dose and 24-hr urine free cortisol and/or 17-OHCS during second day of dexamethasone

Normal response—plasma cortisol <5 µg/dl; urine free cortisol <25 µg/24 hr; urine 17-OHCS <4 mg/24 hr or <1 mg/gram urine creatinine

High-Dose Tests

Overnight test
Dexamethasone 8 mg p.o. at 11 P.M.; plasma cortisol before and at 8 to 9 A.M. after dexamethasone

Response—Cushing's disease; suppression of cortisol to <50% of baseline; ectopic ACTH/adrenal tumors: no cortisol suppression

2-day test
Dexamethasone 2.0 mg p.o. q6h for 8 doses; plasma cortisol before dexamethasone and 1 hr after last dose; 24-hr urine free cortisol and/or 17-OHCS before dexamethasone and during second day
Response—Cushing's disease; suppression of plasma or urine steroids to <50% of baseline; ectopic ACTH/adrenal tumors: no steroid suppression

---

overnight test. It is most useful when the results of other tests are equivocal or inconclusive.

High-Dose Dexamethasone Tests. Glucocorticoids in pharmacologic doses suppress ACTH and cortisol secretion in most patients with ACTH-producing pituitary tumors, but not in patients with adrenal and ectopic tumors. Two tests are available (Table 217–3). The overnight high-dose test is simpler and more accurate than the 2-day high-dose test. Approximately 90 per cent of patients with pituitary ACTH-producing tumors have suppression of cortisol levels to less than 50 per cent of baseline levels, whereas about 95 per cent of those with adrenal tumors or the ectopic ACTH syndrome do not achieve this degree of suppression. With the 2-day high-dose test about 25 per cent of patients with Cushing's disease fail to achieve greater than 50 per cent suppression of urine 17-OHCS, urine free cortisol, or plasma cortisol.

STIMULATION TESTS. These procedures assess the reserve capacity of the hypothalamic-pituitary-adrenal axis and its ability to respond appropriately to stressful situations. These tests act at different sites of the axis and thus can be used to assess its different functions.

CRF Testing. Corticotropin-releasing factor (CRF) testing is utilized in the diagnosis of adrenal insufficiency and Cushing's syndrome. CRF is generally administered intravenously in a dose of 1 µg per kilogram of body weight. ACTH and cortisol secretion peak at 30 to 60 minutes and may be sustained for several hours. Flushing and occasionally hypotension have been observed; thus the test should be performed with the patient supine. Subnormal ACTH and cortisol responses occur in secondary adrenocortical insufficiency due either to hypothalamic-pituitary disorders or to glucocorticoid therapy, and a subnormal cortisol response with high ACTH levels occurs in primary adrenocortical insufficiency. Most but not all patients with pituitary ACTH-producing tumors have supranormal ACTH and cortisol responses, whereas there is no response in patients with cortisol-producing adrenal tumors and in most patients with ectopic ACTH-producing tumors.

ACTH Testing. The administration of ACTH, which allows direct assessment of adrenal glucocorticoid reserve, is useful in the diagnosis of both primary and secondary adrenal insufficiency. The rapid ACTH stimulation test is performed with synthetic human α1-24 ACTH (Cosyntropin [Cortrosyn]), which has full

biologic potency and a lesser incidence of allergic reactions than previously used ACTH preparations. Cortrosyn, 250 µg, is administered intravenously or intramuscularly; plasma cortisol levels are obtained prior to and at 30 or 60 minutes after ACTH administration. Normally the peak plasma cortisol level is greater than 15 to 20 µg per deciliter, depending on the laboratory, and increases by at least 5 µg per deciliter. Subnormal responses to ACTH stimulation establish the diagnosis of adrenal insufficiency. A normal response excludes primary adrenal failure and complete secondary insufficiency, but it does not exclude partial secondary adrenal insufficiency. A normal response to ACTH in the latter case occurs when there is sufficient basal ACTH secretion to prevent adrenal atrophy but not enough pituitary reserve to respond to stress. When this infrequent situation is suspected, the issue can be resolved with the use of metyrapone or insulin hypoglycemia testing.

The rapid ACTH stimulation test gives no information regarding the cause of adrenal dysfunction. This distinction can be made by measuring either the basal plasma ACTH level, which is elevated in primary adrenal insufficiency and is low in secondary adrenal insufficiency, or the aldosterone response to ACTH stimulation (normally an increment in the plasma aldosterone of at least 4 ng per deciliter above baseline). The latter test is based on the fact that the zona glomerulosa responds acutely to ACTH and that this response is preserved in secondary adrenal insufficiency, but is deficient in the primary form in which the entire adrenal cortex is destroyed.

Metyrapone Testing. Metyrapone inhibits the synthesis of cortisol predominantly by blocking 11β-hydroxylation. As a result, ACTH secretion increases and drives the production of steroids proximal to the site of the block. Thus, measurement of plasma 11-deoxycortisol following metyrapone administration can be used to assess the functional reserve of both the adrenal and pituitary. The test is most useful when secondary adrenal insufficiency is suspected in the setting of a normal ACTH stimulation test. The overnight test is most commonly used because of its rapidity and simplicity; because of the short duration of inhibition of cortisol synthesis there is little risk of precipitating acute adrenal insufficiency. Metyrapone is given at midnight with food, and plasma for 11-deoxycortisol and cortisol determinations is obtained at 8 A.M. The dose of metyrapone* is 2 grams for patients less than 70 kg; 2.5 grams for those 70 to 90 kg; and 3 grams for patients weighing more than 90 kg. A plasma cortisol value less than 10 µg per deciliter indicates adequate 11β-hydroxylase inhibition, and in normal persons plasma 11-deoxycortisol increases to greater than 7 µg per deciliter. A normal response to metyrapone indicates adequate function of both the pituitary and adrenals. A subnormal response establishes the diagnosis of adrenal insufficiency and correlates well with deficient responses to stress and hypoglycemia. The test per se does not differentiate primary and secondary causes. However, in the presence of a normal response to the rapid ACTH stimulation test a subnormal response to metyrapone indicates secondary adrenal insufficiency.

Insulin Hypoglycemia Testing (see Ch. 219). Hypoglycemia elicits a stress response that stimulates CRF and ACTH secretion and, as a consequence, cortisol release. A normal cortisol response to hypoglycemia indicates a normal hypothalamic-pituitary-adrenal axis and rules out adrenal insufficiency or decreased pituitary ACTH reserve. This test is most often utilized in the evaluation of suspected hypothalamic or pituitary disorders, since growth hormone reserve can be assessed simultaneously with that of ACTH.

MINERALOCORTICOID FUNCTION

PLASMA RENIN. Assessment of plasma renin is essential in the diagnosis of states of excess and deficient mineralocorticoid secretion; it is also helpful in the evaluation of other types of hypertension (see Ch. 44). Currently used assays do not measure the plasma renin concentration directly, but instead measure the plasma renin activity (PRA) by quantifying the amount of angiotensin I (AI) generated over time in the patient's plasma. The normal values of PRA depend on the salt intake and postural status. In subjects with moderate salt intake (around 110 mEq Na^+ per day) and in the supine and standing positions, for 1

---

*This dose is not listed in the manufacturer's directive.

hour, the plasma renin activity ranges, respectively, from 1 to 3 and 3 to 6 ng of AI generated per milliliter per hour. In individuals in whom salt has been restricted (20 mEq Na^+ per day) for 4 days and who have been in the upright posture for 2 hours the values range from 5 to 10 ng AI per milliliter per hour. In clinical practice, diuretic therapy is the most commonly observed factor that increases the PRA. In patients with primary hyperaldosteronism the PRA is characteristically suppressed. With most aldosterone-producing adenomas and in a small subset of patients with hyperplasia (primary adrenal hyperplasia), the PRA is unresponsive or only weakly responsive to provocative stimuli, whereas in those with primary aldosteronism with bilateral hyperplasia (idiopathic hyperaldosteronism), and in a small subset of patients with adenoma (renin-responsive adenoma), the PRA, although suppressed, usually responds to such stimuli.

In patients with borderline low PRA in whom primary aldosterone excess is suspected, stimulation tests with measurement of PRA may be necessary. Patients can be subjected to salt restriction (10 to 20 mEq of sodium per day for 5 days), given 40 to 60 mg of furosemide intravenously, or given 50 mg of captopril orally; blood samples are then taken after 1 to 4 hours in the upright posture. If the plasma renin does not increase under these conditions and the plasma and/or urinary aldosterone levels are elevated, primary aldosteronism is probable. Caution should be exercised in performing these tests, since severe and life-threatening volume depletion or hypokalemia could ensue; these risks must be weighed before the test is performed.

ALDOSTERONE AND 18-HYDROXYCORTICOSTERONE MEASUREMENTS. These measurements are utilized in the diagnosis of primary aldosteronism and in the differentiation of its subtypes of adenoma and hyperplasia. Plasma measurements ordinarily involve extraction and chromatography of the steroid followed by radioimmunoassay. The urine measurements ordinarily quantify by radioimmunoassay the 18-glucuronide metabolite of aldosterone (about 15 per cent of the total aldosterone production). Less commonly, urinary tetrahydroaldosterone is measured.

Measurements should be made after adequate sodium repletion (a sodium intake of at least 120 mEq per 24 hours for 4 days) and withdrawal of diuretics for at least 2 to 3 weeks, and in the case of plasma measurements after at least 6 hours of recumbency. Normal values for aldosterone excretion are 4 to 17 µg per 24 hours; elevated values are typically seen with both adrenal adenoma and hyperplasia causing primary aldosteronism. Basal plasma values in the supine patient are usually 4 to 12 ng per deciliter. Plasma aldosterone levels are almost always elevated above 20 ng per deciliter in patients with an aldosterone-producing adenoma. By contrast, with primary aldosteronism due to bilateral adrenal hyperplasia, plasma aldosterone levels are usually less than 20 ng per deciliter and are commonly in the normal range. Plasma and urinary aldosterone values must be interpreted with caution in the presence of hypokalemia that results in decreased aldosterone production; normal aldosterone levels may be found in patients with primary aldosteronism and hypokalemia.

Plasma 18-hydroxycorticosterone (18-OHB) measurements (normal range 10 to 30 ng per deciliter) are also especially useful in the differential diagnosis of primary aldosteronism. When sampled at 8 A.M. after overnight recumbency and during a high-salt diet as described above, plasma 18-OHB levels almost always exceed 100 ng per deciliter in patients with an aldosterone-producing adenoma. Levels are less than this with primary aldosteronism due to bilateral hyperplasia.

The use of both aldosterone and 18-OHB measurements has greatly simplified the diagnosis and differential diagnosis of primary aldosteronism. However, in circumstances in which plasma renin values are suppressed and aldosterone values are normal or borderline, suppression tests can be performed. These include (1) high-sodium diet (300 mEq per day for 5 days), (2) fludrocortisone acetate (9α-fluorocortisol) 0.3 mg per day for 3 days, or (3) 2 liters of saline intravenously over 4 hours. These maneuvers reduce plasma aldosterone levels to less than 5 ng per deciliter in normal subjects, but the levels ordinarily exceed 10 ng per deciliter in patients with primary aldosteronism.

Two additional methods for differentiating primary aldosteronism due to an adenoma from that due to hyperplasia take advantage of the fact that plasma aldosterone and 18-OHB levels in hyperplasia, but not adenoma, are under control of the renin-

angiotensin system. The first involves postural studies. The plasma aldosterone is initially measured in the supine position at 8 A.M. after 4 days of a sodium intake of at least 120 mEq per 24 hours and then subsequently after 2 to 4 hours in the upright posture. In patients with an adenoma there is generally either no increase or an actual decrease in plasma aldosterone in the upright position, whereas with hyperplasia, there is almost always an increase in plasma aldosterone concentrations after 2 to 4 hours in the upright position. The second test involves a saline infusion. Patients receiving 120 mEq of sodium per day receive an intravenous infusion of 1250 ml of isotonic saline between 8 A.M. and 10 A.M. after overnight recumbency. The ratio of 18-OHB to cortisol is measured in plasma samples taken before and immediately after the infusion. This ratio generally increases in patients with an aldosterone-producing adenoma but decreases in patients with hyperplasia.

ADRENAL ANDROGENS

Plasma levels of the predominant adrenal androgens, DHEA, DHEA-S, and androstenedione, can be measured. These assays plus that of testosterone are most frequently used for the evaluation of hirsutism. Stimulation and suppression tests have not been as useful as in other pituitary and adrenal disorders. Plasma free testosterone measurements usually provide a better index of total androgenicity than total levels of the hormone, since androgen excess decreases sex hormone–binding globulin levels and can result in a normal total level in the presence of an elevated free testosterone concentration. Measurement of androstanediol and its glucuronide, metabolic products of dihydrotestosterone, provides an index of peripheral androgen production and may provide the best index of androgen excess.

Urinary 17-ketosteroid excretion assesses adrenal androgen production and reflects metabolites of DHEA and DHEA-S. However, this test has limited utility, since the more potent androgens such as testosterone and dihydrotestosterone contribute less than 1 per cent of the total urinary 17-ketosteroids. Furthermore, 17-ketosteroids are increased in obesity without androgen excess, and there is interference by multiple drugs and medications.

217.6 ADRENOCORTICAL HYPOFUNCTION
J. Blake Tyrrell

Adrenal insufficiency is defined by deficient production of glucocorticoids or mineralocorticoids or both. Primary adrenocortical insufficiency (Addison's disease) is due to destruction of the adrenal cortex, whereas in secondary adrenocortical insufficiency impaired cortisol production is due to deficient ACTH production. Hyporeninemia causes selective aldosterone deficiency. Selective adrenal defects due to congenital enzyme deficiencies also occur (see Ch. 221).

PRIMARY ADRENOCORTICAL INSUFFICIENCY

ETIOLOGY. Primary adrenocortical insufficiency has multiple causes. In the United States over 80 per cent of the cases are due to autoimmune destruction of the adrenal. Tuberculosis is the second most frequent cause and remains a common cause of the disease in underdeveloped countries. Acquired immunodeficiency syndrome (AIDS) has become a more frequent cause of the disorder. Other rare causes include hemorrhage due to sepsis, anticoagulation, coagulopathies, trauma, surgery, and pregnancy; bilateral infarction, e.g., due to thrombosis or arteritis; fungal infection; invasive disorders such as lymphoma, metastatic tumors, amyloidosis, sarcoidosis, and hemochromatosis; surgery; cytotoxic agents such as mitotane; and congenital hypoplasia and hyporesponsiveness to ACTH. Primary adrenocortical insufficiency due to any cause is a rare disease with an estimated incidence in Western countries of around 50 per million population.

The idiopathic autoimmune form of adrenal insufficiency is two- to threefold more common in females and is usually diagnosed in the third to fifth decades of life. Early in the disease there is lymphocytic infiltration of the glands, and there is a high association (40 to 53 per cent of patients) with disorders of other endocrine glands or with pernicious anemia or vitiligo. Antibodies to the adrenal cortex are commonly present, and there is evidence for abnormal cell-mediated immunity.

The association of Addison's disease with the other disorders has been referred to as *Schmidt's syndrome*, autoimmune endocrine failure, and the polyglandular failure syndromes (Ch. 228). Approximate associations are ovarian failure, 25 per cent of female patients (testicular failure in males is unusual); hyperthyroidism, 7 per cent (mostly female); hypothyroidism or Hashimoto's thyroiditis with goiter, 9 per cent; subclinical thyroiditis, up to 80 per cent; diabetes mellitus (type I), 12 per cent; vitiligo, 9 per cent, presumably due to immunologic destruction of melanocytes; hypoparathyroidism, 6 per cent; and pernicious anemia, 4 per cent. The development of autoimmune adrenocortical insufficiency shows some hereditary predisposition, and an autosomal recessive pattern of inheritance has been suggested. About 40 per cent of patients have first- or second-degree relatives with one of the associated disorders. Further, there is an increased incidence of histocompatibility antigen (HLA) types B8, Dw3 and of the haplotype HLA-A1,B8.

Patients with AIDS commonly have subtle abnormalities of adrenal function which are not clinically significant. However, a small percentage of these patients develop frank adrenocortical insufficiency.

CLINICAL MANIFESTATIONS. The development of clinical manifestations of adrenocortical insufficiency requires loss of more than 90 per cent of the adrenal cortices. The rate of destruction varies, depending on the cause, but with the idiopathic variety this usually requires several months. With gradual destruction, increases in ACTH secondary to the lower cortisol levels tend to stimulate the gland maximally. Thus in the period prior to complete destruction there may be normal plasma cortisol levels but absence of responsiveness to stress. In about 25 per cent of patients symptoms first appear in a crisis or impending crisis. However, in the majority of cases destruction becomes more complete, and the patient experiences symptoms that lead to medical evaluation before a crisis occurs. The destruction of the gland results in loss of both glucocorticoid and mineralocorticoid functions and secondary increases in ACTH and in renin.

The clinical presentation depends on the rate and degree of adrenal destruction, the presence of stressful influences, and the pathology of associated or causative conditions. For these reasons it is convenient to discuss separately the chronic and acute presentations.

Chronic primary adrenocortical insufficiency develops gradually over months to years. The major clinical features (Table 217–4) are generalized weakness and fatigue, weight loss, anorexia, hyperpigmentation, hypotension, gastrointestinal upset (including vague discomfort, nausea, vomiting, and less commonly diarrhea), salt craving, and postural dizziness. Weight loss is due both to dehydration secondary to salt loss and to anorexia. The blood glucose concentration is ordinarily in the low-normal range, although hypoglycemia can occur with fasting, vomiting, or illness and in children. Female patients can also have amenorrhea and loss of axillary hair, the latter due to decrease of adrenal androgens. Although dehydration can be significant, this may be compensated for by increased salt intake. Hyponatremia is present in most patients, although it may be masked somewhat

TABLE 217–4. CLINICAL FEATURES OF CHRONIC PRIMARY ADRENOCORTICAL INSUFFICIENCY

Feature	%	Feature	%
Weakness and fatigue	100	Hypotension	88
Weight loss	100	Gastrointestinal symptoms	56
Anorexia	100	Salt craving	19
Hyperpigmentation	92	Postural symptoms	12

Data from Nerup J: Acta Endocrinol 76:127, 1974 and Thorn GW: The Diagnosis and Treatment of Adrenal Insufficiency. Springfield, IL, Charles C Thomas, 1951, and reprinted in Baxter JD, Tyrrell JB: The adrenal cortex. *In* Felig P, Baxter JD, Broadus AH, et al. (eds.): Endocrinology and Metabolism, 2nd ed. New York, McGraw-Hill Book Company, 1987, p 587.

if there is dehydration. Mild hyperkalemia is also usually present; the presence of severe hyperkalemia should suggest concomitant renal or other disease. A normocytic, normochromic anemia is common but can also be masked by dehydration and hemoconcentration. There tends to be neutropenia, lymphocytosis, and eosinophilia. Dehydration when present leads to increases in blood urea nitrogen and creatinine, and there may be mild acidosis. The heart tends to be small and vertical on radiographic examination; the abdominal radiograph is usually normal but can show adrenal calcification in about 50 per cent of those cases due to tuberculosis. Calcification of the ear lobes sometimes occurs in longstanding cases.

Hyperpigmentation, an important diagnostic feature, may precede other manifestations. It is generalized; but is accentuated in sun-exposed areas; pressure points such as the elbows, knees, knuckles, and toes; and on palmar creases, nail beds, buccal mucosa, tongue, nipples, areolae, and perivaginal or perianal mucosa; and in recent surgical scars. In blacks, pigmentation of the tongue is of diagnostic helpfulness. Hyperpigmentation is commonly misinterpreted as an excessive suntan and the "healthy" appearance of the patient may lead to a dismissal of other symptoms.

Acute adrenocortical insufficiency is seen most commonly in a patient with either undiagnosed or diagnosed adrenocortical insufficiency who is exposed to one of the stresses discussed earlier and who therefore has an increased requirement for glucocorticoids. It can also be seen with acute adrenal destruction secondary to hemorrhage, most commonly associated with septicemia or anticoagulant therapy (adrenal apoplexy). In these cases, anorexia is often profound with nausea and vomiting that exaggerates volume depletion and dehydration. Abdominal pain is frequent and may mimic a surgical condition of the abdomen; however, these symptoms are usually vague. The blood pressure falls, and hypovolemic shock develops that is incompletely responsive to fluid replacement. Fever is common and may or may not be due to the precipitating event. Hyperpigmentation will be present or absent, depending on the duration of the disease; when present it is an important diagnostic sign. The presence of hyperkalemia, lymphocytosis, and eosinophilia should also suggest the diagnosis. Severe hypoglycemia is uncommon and is more likely to occur in children or in adults with secondary adrenal insufficiency (see below). The diagnosis of acute adrenocortical insufficiency should be considered in any patient with unexplained shock, and the consideration of this should not be diverted by the presence of an accompanying disorder such as infection or diabetic ketoacidosis.

SECONDARY ADRENOCORTICAL INSUFFICIENCY. Secondary adrenocortical insufficiency results from inadequate ACTH production. The causes are discussed in Ch. 213. Pituitary and hypothalamic tumors are the most common spontaneous causes. In these cases there is progressive loss of ACTH such that cortisol production and responses to stress are decreased, but mineralocorticoid production is usually normal. Chronic suppression of ACTH production with exogenous glucocorticoids followed by their withdrawal also causes the syndrome and is by far the most frequent cause.

The development of clinical manifestations is usually gradual, but like primary adrenocortical insufficiency can be acute. The presenting features are similar to those of primary adrenocortical insufficiency with four exceptions: (1) Since hypersecretion of ACTH and related peptides is absent, there is no hyperpigmentation; in fact, patients with hypopituitarism commonly exhibit pallor of the skin. (2) The electrolyte abnormalities of hyponatremia, hyperkalemia, and mild acidosis are absent because of preservation of aldosterone secretion. Hyponatremia, if present, is due to decreased glomerular filtration rate, hypothyroidism, or increased vasopressin release and not to dehydration. (3) Other features of hypopituitarism (see Ch. 213) may be present. (4) Hypoglycemia is more common because of the combined ACTH and growth hormone deficiency.

DIAGNOSIS. The clinical suspicion of adrenocortical insufficiency should be confirmed by laboratory testing. Since the rapid ACTH stimulation test (discussed below) requires only 30 minutes, it is unusual that testing cannot be performed before initiating therapy, even in sick patients. However, in seriously ill patients, in whom the diagnosis is suspected, therapy should not be delayed by prolonged diagnostic measures; if means for a rapid diagnosis are unavailable, therapy should be initiated and diagnostic testing performed at a later date. Although an elevated plasma cortisol level (e.g., greater than 20 µg per deciliter) makes the diagnosis unlikely, cortisol levels below 20 µg per deciliter can be present with impaired adrenal responsiveness to stress. Thus, in circumstances when the plasma cortisol is less than 22 µg per deciliter, the adrenal reserve should be tested.

Figure 217–5 shows a diagnostic strategy. If adrenocortical insufficiency is suspected, the rapid ACTH stimulation test should be performed. This test requires only 30 minutes and can be done even in most acute situations. A normal response excludes the diagnosis of primary adrenocortical insufficiency; an abnormal response establishes the presence of adrenocortical insufficiency. Rare patients with secondary adrenocortical insufficiency respond normally. The basal plasma ACTH level, determined prior to ACTH administration, is measured to distinguish between primary and secondary adrenocortical insufficiency. In primary adrenocortical insufficiency, the levels exceed 250 pg per milliliter and usually are greater than 400 pg per milliliter. By contrast, plasma ACTH levels in secondary adrenocortical insufficiency are inappropriately low, ranging from 0 to 20 pg per milliliter. The plasma aldosterone response to ACTH can also be used to differentiate primary from secondary adrenocortical insufficiency, but there is less extensive experience with this procedure.

Further diagnostic procedures are needed only in exceptional cases, for example, in suspected secondary adrenocortical insufficiency with a normal response to ACTH or in cases in which plasma ACTH measurements are unavailable. In these cases the metyrapone or insulin hypoglycemia tests can be helpful. The latter test is usually performed in suspected hypopituitarism, since simultaneous assessment of both growth hormone and ACTH can be carried out (see Ch. 213). The metyrapone test is performed in patients in whom hypoglycemia is contraindicated or in those who have had prior glucocorticoid therapy, since it provides essentially the same information and is of less potential risk to the patient. An abnormal response to metyrapone or insulin hypoglycemia establishes the diagnosis of secondary adre-

nocortical insufficiency when the primary form has been excluded by the ACTH stimulation test. The presence of low-normal or low ACTH levels further confirms this diagnosis.

In spontaneous adrenocortical insufficiency of any type, the clinical evaluation should include an assessment of associated disorders or precipitating factors. In primary adrenocortical insufficiency the laboratory evaluation should include blood glucose and serum calcium and phosphorus; thyroid function tests, including TSH and thyroid antibody determinations; and testing for tuberculosis and HIV infection. If there is oligomenorrhea or amenorrhea, FSH and LH levels should be determined. First- and second-degree relatives should be screened for endocrine deficiency syndromes because of the increased risk in these individuals. In secondary adrenocortical insufficiency, patients should be examined for other pituitary dysfunction, pituitary or hypothalamic tumors, and prior glucocorticoid therapy (see Ch. 213). In acute adrenocortical insufficiency, the precipitating cause should be determined, since this is often infectious.

TREATMENT. *Acute Adrenocortical Insufficiency.* In an acute crisis, therapy should be instituted as soon as the diagnosis is suspected (Table 217–5). A soluble glucocorticoid, such as cortisol hemisuccinate or phosphate, should be given intravenously. Volume depletion, electrolyte abnormalities, and hypoglycemia should be corrected and general supportive measures instituted. Precipitating factors should be assessed and corrected. If recovery is satisfactory, the glucocorticoid dose can be reduced on the second day and then tapered to oral maintenance doses by the fourth to fifth day. Mineralocorticoid replacement is unnecessary when high doses of cortisol are given, but should be given when the cortisol dose has been tapered to near-maintenance levels (40 to 60 mg per 24 hours).

Chronic Adrenocortical Insufficiency. The treatment of the primary form of this condition requires both glucocorticoid and mineralocorticoid replacement, whereas the secondary form usually requires only glucocorticoid replacement (Table 217–5). Patients must be made aware that a lifetime of replacement is necessary and of the need to increase glucocorticoid replacement in times of stress. Each patient should carry an identification bracelet or card. Cortisol at levels similar to physiologic production is given in a way that approximates the circadian rhythm. Thus, for ordinary maintenance, 15 to 20 mg of cortisol are given in the early morning and 5 to 10 mg in the late afternoon. An equivalent amount of prednisolone or prednisone (about 5 mg per day) or cortisone acetate (37.5 mg per day) is also acceptable; however, the potency of dexamethasone has probably been underestimated, and this steroid is not recommended. For mineralocorticoid replacement, 9α-fluorocortisol (fludrocortisone) 0.05 to 0.2 mg orally per day, is recommended. Follow-up is mainly by clinical assessment of a feeling of well-being, examination of signs of glucocorticoid or mineralocorticoid excess or deficiency, and measurements of serum electrolytes. The serum potassium and in some cases the plasma renin levels (evaluated in conjunction with a 24-hour urinary sodium determination) can be particularly helpful for evaluating the adequacy of mineralocorticoid replacement. Measurements of cortisol and ACTH are

TABLE 217–5. THERAPY OF ADRENAL INSUFFICIENCY

Acute Crisis

1. Cortisol (hydrocortisone) 100 mg IV, every 6 hr for 24 hr. If stable, reduce to 50 mg every 6 hr and then taper to oral maintenance in 4 to 5 days. Maintain or increase dose to 200 to 400 mg per 24 hr if complications persist or occur.
2. Correct volume depletion, dehydration, hypotension, and hypoglycemia with intravenous saline and glucose.
3. Correct precipitating factors, especially infection.

Maintenance

1. Cortisol 15 to 20 mg p.o. q. A.M.; 5 to 10 mg at 4 to 6 P.M.
2. 9α-Fluorocortisol 0.05 to 0.1 mg q. A.M. (primary).
3. Follow weight, blood pressure, and electrolytes.
4. Educate patient to increase cortisol dosage during stress.

Modified from Tables 12–17 and 12–18 in Baxter JD, Tyrrell JB: The adrenal cortex. *In* Felig P, Baxter JD, Broadus AH, et al. (eds.): Endocrinology and Metabolism, 2nd ed. New York, McGraw-Hill Book Company, 1987.

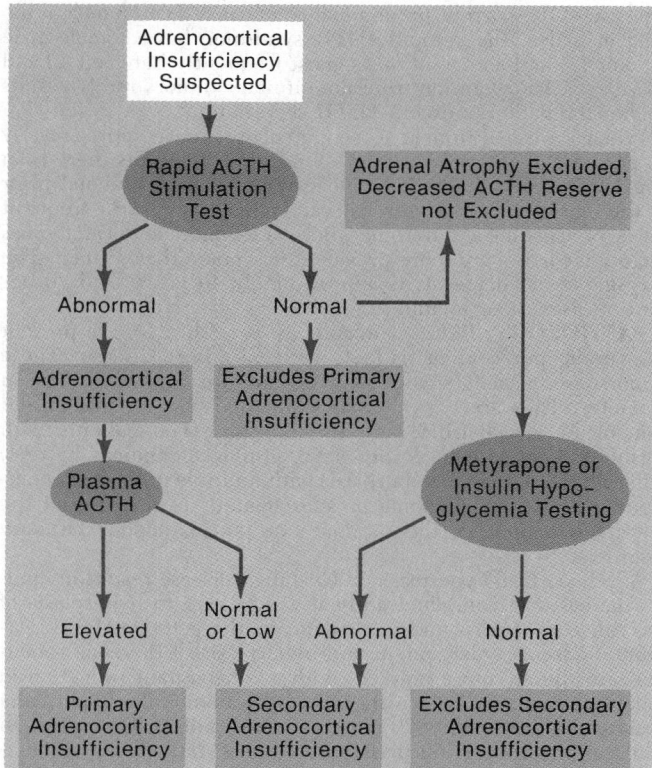

FIGURE 217–5. Evaluation of suspected primary or secondary adrenocortical insufficiency. Boxes enclose clinical decisions and ovals enclose diagnostic tests. (Reprinted from Baxter JD, Tyrrell JB: The adrenal cortex. *In* Felig P, Baxter JD, Broadus AE, et al. (eds.): Endocrinology and Metabolism, 2nd ed. New York, McGraw-Hill Book Company, 1987, p 593.)

usually less helpful. The doses may need to be adjusted somewhat. Many of the subjective complaints of Addison's disease can be reversed within a few days; a somewhat longer time is required before strength returns to normal and hyperpigmentation subsides.

In times of stress, it is sometimes difficult to predict the need for increased glucocorticoid administration. It is best to err on the side of overreplacement rather than underreplacement. For minor illnesses such as significant upper respiratory infections, the cortisol dose should be doubled or tripled and then tapered over a few days. It is not usually necessary to change the 9α-fluorocortisol dose. Patients with vomiting and diarrhea should seek medical attention and receive parenteral cortisol. Patients who may not have early access to medical attention should keep injectable cortisol available and be instructed in its use.

In the event of major trauma or severe illness, treatment should be similar to that for adrenal crisis discussed above. In the case of elective major surgery the protocol described in Table 217–6 has been shown to be effective.

PROGNOSIS. Survival of patients in whom adrenocortical insufficiency is adequately diagnosed and treated now approximates that of the normal population. This is in sharp contrast to the period before steroids were available or when only mineralocorticoid replacement was available, at which time the survival rate was usually 2 years or less.

HYPOALDOSTERONISM

PATHOGENESIS. Hypoaldosteronism can occur in association with hypocortisolism or as an isolated defect. The major cause of isolated hypoaldosteronism is defective renal renin secretion (hyporeninemic hypoaldosteronism) (see Ch. 75). Other rarer causes include isolated adrenal biosynthetic defects (18-hydroxylase syndrome) and focal destruction of the adrenal glomerulosa (hyperreninemic hypoaldosteronism), transient deficiency following removal of an aldosterone-producing tumor, unresponsiveness to aldosterone (pseudohypoaldosteronism) with normal or increased aldosterone production, marked potassium depletion, and heparin administration.

HYPORENINEMIC HYPOALDOSTERONISM. This is seen generally in older patients with renal disease. It is most commonly due to diabetic nephropathy but can also occur with other renal diseases such as interstitial nephritis or multiple myeloma. It has also been observed following removal of an aldosterone-producing tumor or rarely without any apparent cause in association with hypertension. The hyporeninemia leads to decreased aldosterone production and impaired ability of the zona glomerulosa to respond to stimuli. However, the gland usually retains some capacity to secrete aldosterone through stimulation by potassium. Hypoaldosteronism results secondarily in hyperkalemia, which is disproportionate to the extent of renal disease. Chronic renal disease per se ordinarily does not lead to hyperkalemia unless the glomerular filtration rate is severely impaired (e.g., less than 10 ml per minute). In fact, hyporeninemic hypoaldosteronism is the most common cause of hyperkalemia in patients with renal disease and creatinine clearance rates greater than 10 ml per minute. Although these patients can develop hyponatremia, in adults this is less common, probably because of the fact that the primary disease tends to favor sodium retention. These patients

TABLE 217–6. STEROID COVERAGE FOR SURGERY

1. Correct electrolytes, blood pressure, and hydration if necessary.
2. Hydrocortisone phosphate or hemisuccinate, 100 mg IM, on call to operating room.
3. Hydrocortisone phosphate or hemisuccinate, 50 mg IM or IV, in recovery room and every 6 hr for the first 24 hr.
4. If progress is satisfactory, reduce dosage to 25 mg every 6 hr for 24 hr; then taper to maintenance dosage over 3 to 5 days. Resume previous 9α-fluorocortisol dose when patient is taking oral medications.
5. Maintain or increase cortisol dosage to 200 to 400 mg per 24 hr if fever, hypotension, or other complications occur.

Modified from Baxter JD, Tyrrell JB: The adrenal cortex. *In* Felig P, Baxter JD, Broadus AH, et al. (eds.): Endocrinology and Metabolism, 2nd ed. New York, McGraw-Hill Book Company, 1987, p 596.

also tend to develop a metabolic acidosis due to the lack of H^+-secreting actions of aldosterone; this can be accentuated by a decreased glomerular filtration rate. This form of acidosis has been classified as type IV renal tubular acidosis (see Ch. 82).

TREATMENT. The treatment of hypoaldosteronism involves therapy for the primary condition plus mineralocorticoid replacement as described above for primary adrenocortical insufficiency. However, in some patients with hypertension, treatment with 9α-fluorocortisol is not indicated and diuretics are used instead. Conversely, some patients require higher doses of mineralocorticoids, probably because the renal disease renders them more refractory to the steroid. Therapy is monitored by measuring serum potassium levels.

217.7 CUSHING'S SYNDROME
J. Blake Tyrrell

Cushing's syndrome is the result of chronic glucocorticoid excess. It occurs most commonly in patients receiving supraphysiologic doses of glucocorticoids. Spontaneously occurring Cushing's syndrome, a rare disorder, occurs as a result of either primary tumors of the adrenal gland that hypersecrete cortisol or from excess ACTH secretion that may be of pituitary or nonpituitary (ectopic ACTH syndrome) sources. In addition, Cushing's syndrome can be due to excessive CRF secretion from hypothalamic or ectopic tumors.

Cushing's disease (spontaneous hypercortisolism due to excessive pituitary ACTH secretion) accounts for two thirds of reported cases. This disorder is most common in women 20 to 40 years old, with a female-male ratio of 8:1.

Secretion of ACTH from ectopic tumors accounts for about 15 per cent of cases of Cushing's syndrome. The true incidence of this disorder is probably higher, since many patients lack the typical clinical features of cortisol excess because of the dominance of the manifestations of cancer and the rapidity of progression. Because of the current predominance of oat cell carcinoma of the lung in males, the ectopic ACTH syndrome has a female-male ratio of 1:3 and an age of onset most frequently between 40 and 60 years. CRF secretion from nonpituitary tumors rarely results in the stimulation of excess ACTH secretion.

Primary adrenal tumors secreting cortisol cause approximately 15 per cent of cases of Cushing's syndrome. In adults there is an equal frequency of adenoma and carcinoma. In childhood prior to the age of 10 years, adrenal carcinoma is the most frequent cause of Cushing's syndrome. Both adenomas and carcinomas secreting cortisol are more prevalent in women than in men. The average age at diagnosis is approximately 40 years, and 70 per cent of cases occur in adults.

PATHOLOGY. Pituitary adenomas (see Ch. 213) are present in over 90 per cent of patients with Cushing's disease. These tumors are usually small; 50 per cent are 5 mm or less in diameter. They are typically basophilic and unencapsulated and contain ACTH, β-LPH, and β-endorphin. The patients with Cushing's disease who do not have pituitary adenomas have (1) diffuse hyperplasia; (2) hyperplasia with multiple nests of adenomatous cells; (3) an adenoma or adenomatous hyperplasia of the intermediate lobe of the pituitary; or (4) no obvious pituitary disorder.

Adrenocortical hyperplasia in Cushing's disease results in modest increases in combined adrenal weight due to hyperplasia of the zonae reticularis and fasciculata. In the ectopic ACTH syndrome, adrenal enlargement and hyperplasia of the zona reticularis are usually more marked, with a concomitant reduction in the number of zona fasciculata cells. Bilateral nodular hyperplasia occurs in approximately 20 per cent of cases of ACTH excess. In addition to diffuse hyperplasia of the zonae reticularis and fasciculata, there are multiple nodules that vary from microscopic to several centimeters in diameter and that contain clear cells similar to those of the zona fasciculata.

Cortisol-secreting adenomas are usually encapsulated, range from 2 to 6 cm in diameter, typically secrete cortisol alone, and are usually composed of zona fasciculata–like cells. Adrenal carcinomas that secrete cortisol are usually large at the time of diagnosis, may be palpable as abdominal masses, and usually secrete a number of steroids. Histologically these tumors may appear benign or exhibit considerable pleomorphism, and the histologic appearance does not predict benign or malignant behavior. Therefore the diagnosis of adrenal carcinoma is dependent on the demonstration of either local tumor invasiveness or metastatic spread. Extension of these tumors occurs locally, and common sites of metastases are the liver and lung.

ETIOLOGY AND PATHOGENESIS. The etiology of Cushing's disease is unknown. It is possible that primary pituitary tumors arise spontaneously. In the uncommon cases in which diffuse or adenomatous hyperplasia is present, excessive secretion of CRF or some other factor may stimulate the pituitary. Rarely hypothalamic or ectopic CRF-producing tumors have been reported. The ectopic ACTH syndrome occurs in a relatively small number of tumor types. Oat cell carcinoma of the lung accounts for approximately 50 per cent of cases. The greatly increased production of cortisol and 11-deoxycorticosterone (DOC) stimulated by very high ACTH levels commonly results in manifestations of both mineralocorticoid and glucocorticoid excess.

Other ACTH-secreting tumors include thymomas and thymic carcinoids, islet cell tumors of the pancreas, carcinoid tumors, medullary carcinomas of the thyroid, and pheochromocytomas. Many other tumors may secrete ACTH, but this occurs very rarely.

Cortisol-producing adrenal tumors arise spontaneously and are not under normal control by the hypothalamic-pituitary axis; their secretion of cortisol and the other steroids is autonomous, episodic, and random.

Nodular adrenocortical hyperplasia is usually due to ACTH excess, but rare cases have been described with persistently suppressed ACTH levels.

CLINICAL FEATURES. The classic features, most typically seen in Cushing's disease (Fig. 217–6, Table 217–7) usually develop insidiously over several years. The most common mani-

TABLE 217–7. INCIDENCE OF CLINICAL FEATURES OF CUSHING'S SYNDROME

Feature	%
Obesity	94
Facial plethora	84
Hirsutism	82
Menstrual disorders	76
Hypertension	72
Muscular weakness	58
Back pain	58
Striae	52
Acne	40
Psychological symptoms	40
Bruising	36
Congestive heart failure	22
Edema	18
Renal calculi	16
Headache	14
Polyuria/polydipsia	10
Hyperpigmentation	6

Data from Plotz CM, et al.: Am J Med 13:597, 1952, and Ross EJ, et al: Q J Med 35:149, 1966, and reprinted from Baxter JD, Tyrrell JB: The adrenal cortex. In Felig P, Baxter JD, Broadus AE, et al. (eds.): Endocrinology and Metabolism, 2nd ed. New York, McGraw-Hill Book Company, 1987, p 606.

festation is central obesity with rounding of the face and fat accumulation around the trunk, supraclavicular areas, and dorsocervical spine. Serial photographs are helpful in recognizing these gradual changes. Classically this pattern of obesity spares the extremities; however, generalized obesity including the extremities occurs in about 50 per cent of patients. Atrophy of the skin and underlying connective tissue is frequent. This leads to facial plethora, easy bruisability, and red to purple depressed striae. The last occur most commonly over the lower abdomen, but can also be more generalized on the trunk and upper legs. Patients also have poor healing of minor or major injuries and abrasions and an increased incidence of superficial fungal infections. Hirsutism is present in approximately 80 per cent of female patients as a result of excessive adrenal androgen secretion. Hypertension is present in the majority of patients; it is rarely accompanied by hypokalemia in Cushing's disease, although this is common in the ectopic ACTH syndrome or adrenal carcinoma. Hypertension contributes greatly to the mortality of untreated Cushing's syndrome.

Additional common manifestations include hypogonadism in both male and female patients, psychological disturbances (usually depression), which occur in the majority, and proximal muscle weakness. Osteopenia is present in virtually all patients and may progress to frank osteoporosis (see Ch. 238). Back pain is common, and compression fractures of the spine occur in approximately 20 per cent. Renal stones, secondary to hypercalciuria, and thirst and polyuria, which may be due to hyperglycemia, can also occur. Routine laboratory abnormalities include high normal or modestly elevated values for the hematocrit, slightly elevated white cell counts, and a depressed percentage of lymphocytes and eosinophils. Electrolyte abnormalities occur only rarely in Cushing's disease, but hypokalemia occurs commonly with the ectopic ACTH syndrome or adrenal carcinoma.

DIAGNOSIS. A suggested plan for the evaluation of suspected Cushing's syndrome is shown in Figure 217–7. If the syndrome is suspected, the 24-hour urine free cortisol should be measured and the overnight 1-mg dexamethasone suppression test performed.

If results of both of these tests are normal, the diagnosis of Cushing's syndrome is excluded, with two exceptions: (1) Rare patients whose disease activity is episodic can have normal tests during periods of inactivity. In these cases, repeated evaluation during periods of disease activity establishes the diagnosis. (2) Rare patients with Cushing's disease have delayed clearance of dexamethasone and therefore have normal responses to low-dose dexamethasone. However, these patients have elevated urine free cortisol levels.

If the 24-hour urine free cortisol level is elevated and the 1-mg overnight dexamethasone suppression test is abnormal, then

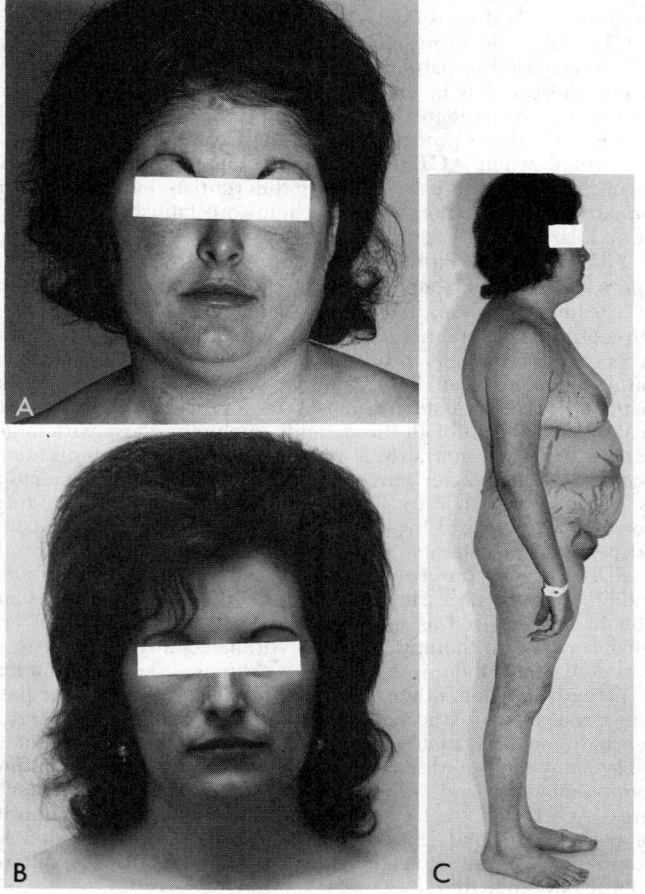

FIGURE 217–6. The appearance of a patient with Cushing's syndrome (A) before and (B) 1 year after removal of an adrenal adenoma. (C) Profile, before treatment.

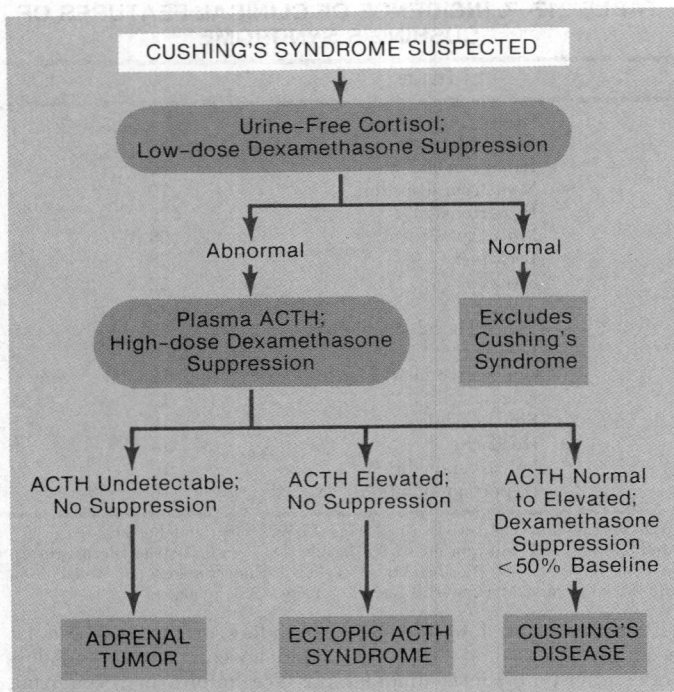

FIGURE 217–7. Evaluation of Cushing's syndrome. Boxes enclose clinical decisions and ovals enclose diagnostic tests. See the text for details and the potential for false-positive and false-negative results. (Reprinted from Baxter JD, Tyrrell JB: The adrenal cortex. *In* Felig P, Baxter JD, Broadus AE, et al. (eds.): Endocrinology and Metabolism, 2nd ed, New York, McGraw-Hill Book Company, 1987, p 609.)

spontaneous Cushing's syndrome is present provided that several abnormalities that lead to false-positive responses can be excluded. Results of the dexamethasone suppression test can be abnormal in obesity, estrogen therapy, drug therapy that increases dexamethasone metabolism (listed in Ch. 27), and chronic renal failure, although the 24-hour urine free cortisol is almost always in the normal range. In the case of obesity or estrogen therapy, the 2-day low-dose dexamethasone test should be performed; the results are almost always normal in the absence of Cushing's syndrome. Response to both the 24-hour urine free cortisol and the 1-mg dexamethasone suppression tests can be abnormal in alcoholism, acute and chronic illness, depression and other states of substantial emotional stress, and anorexia nervosa. In these cases, in the absence of spontaneous Cushing's syndrome the abnormalities subside following cessation of the condition.

ETIOLOGIC DIAGNOSIS. Once the diagnosis of Cushing's syndrome has been established, it is essential to determine its specific cause. The two most useful procedures are (1) the measurement of basal plasma ACTH levels and (2) the high-dose dexamethasone suppression test. In Cushing's disease, ACTH levels are normal to modestly elevated (50 to 200 pg per milliliter), and in 90 per cent of these patients, plasma or urinary steroid levels are suppressed to less than 50 per cent of baseline values in response to the high-dose dexamethasone test. In the ectopic ACTH syndrome, plasma ACTH values are often markedly elevated and are more than 200 pg per milliliter in two thirds of patients. In about 95 per cent of these patients, hypothalamic-pituitary control of ACTH and cortisol secretion is absent, and there is no response to high-dose dexamethasone suppression. Exceptions occur mostly in patients with relatively benign tumors, especially carcinoids, in whom ACTH levels may be only modestly elevated and in whom the high dose of dexamethasone may suppress ACTH release. With glucocorticoid-secreting adrenal tumors, plasma ACTH levels are suppressed to either low normal or undetectable levels, and dexamethasone suppression testing produces no reduction in cortisol levels.

Two major problems are encountered in determining the cause: (1) In approximately 10 per cent of patients with Cushing's disease

the cortisol levels are not suppressed adequately in response to dexamethasone, and (2) approximately 5 per cent of patients with ectopic tumors have suppression in response to high-dose dexamethasone and thus may appear to have Cushing's disease. In some cases, lack of suppression with pituitary adenomas occurs with larger tumors that are apparent when computed tomographic (CT) or magnetic resonance imaging (MRI) is performed. Also, this problem is more frequent when there is nodular adrenal hyperplasia. With these cases it is necessary to use additional procedures to establish the diagnosis. These include the use of head and body imaging studies to search for an ectopic tumor, selective venous sampling of the petrosal sinuses that drain the anterior pituitary and of other suspected regions with plasma ACTH determinations to identify the site of increased ACTH release, and utilization of higher doses of dexamethasone to suppress the activity of the pituitary tumor.

Tumor Localization. In Cushing's disease MRI is the current procedure of choice and allows excellent resolution of the hypothalamus and pituitary with better definition of parasellar structures (cavernous sinuses, pituitary stalk, and optic chiasm) than does CT (Fig. 217–8). However, the ability of MRI to detect the 50 per cent of tumors that are less than 5 mm in diameter is still limited even with gadolinium enhancement. In the absence of a radiologically evident lesion consistent with an adenoma it is recommended that selective venous sampling for ACTH be performed prior to surgical intervention. This technique is very useful in establishing a pituitary cause of Cushing's syndrome in those patients with normal neuroradiologic studies and in those with dexamethasone-nonsuppressible Cushing's disease. This procedure also excludes a pituitary etiology of ACTH excess when an occult ectopic ACTH-secreting tumor is present. The technique requires an experienced radiologist, since sampling from the inferior petrosal sinuses is required to assess pituitary ACTH secretion adequately. A gradient of 2:1 of central to peripheral ACTH levels establishes the presence of Cushing's disease. The most accurate results are obtained if the petrosal sinuses are sampled simultaneously and if CRF stimulation is utilized to maximize ACTH secretion.

CT, MRI, and ultrasonographic imaging of the adrenal (Fig. 217–9) are used in patients with suspected adrenal tumors or in whom the cause is in doubt. Adrenal tumors are usually larger than 2 cm in diameter when diagnosed and thus are readily visible with those procedures. Adrenal scanning should also be performed when ACTH levels or dexamethasone studies are inconclusive. In this case they help differentiate hyperplasia from primary adrenal tumors and may help to establish the diagnosis of nodular adrenal hyperplasia.

TREATMENT. Pituitary microsurgery with a transsphenoidal approach is the current method of choice for the initial therapy of Cushing's disease. It is critical that it be performed by a surgeon with substantial experience with the technique because it is not a common procedure. Under ideal circumstances, pituitary tumors can be located at surgery in 90 per cent of patients, and successful responses to surgery occur in approximately 80 per cent of all the patients, including those with larger tumors. Surgical mortality is rare, and significant complications occur in less than 2 per cent of patients. Heavy-particle irradiation is also effective therapy for Cushing's disease, with long-term correction of cortisol hypersecretion occurring in approximately 80 per cent of patients. Unfortunately this therapy is currently available in only one center in the United States. Conventional radiotherapy is successful in only 15 to 25 per cent of adults and should not be used as initial therapy because it precludes any further radiation therapy. Bilateral adrenalectomy, previously an accepted initial therapy for Cushing's disease, should be limited to patients in whom other therapies are unsuccessful. In the past, this procedure was accompanied by a high degree of surgical morbidity and mortality and the subsequent development of Nelson's syndrome (discussed below). Reserpine, bromocriptine, cyproheptadine, and valproate sodium have been used to suppress ACTH and treat Cushing's syndrome, but only a minority of patients respond. In general their use is recommended for adjunctive therapy in patients who have had unsuccessful responses to other therapy.

Drugs that inhibit adrenal cortisol secretion can also be used as adjunctive therapy or in patients in whom more definitive treatments have been unsuccessful. Ketoconazole, the current drug of choice, is effective in most patients, has a gradual onset of action, and has relatively few side effects. The effective dosage is 400 to 500 mg given twice daily, and cortisol levels gradually decline over 1 to 2 weeks. The major adverse effect is hepatic toxicity, which is only rarely severe. Alternatively, metyrapone* (ordinarily 2 grams per day) and aminoglutethimide (1 gram per day) are given simultaneously in four divided doses. These drugs are expensive, have frequent side effects (predominantly gastrointestinal), and result in secondary increases in ACTH levels that sometimes are sufficient to overcome the enzyme inhibition. They are not usually used for long-term therapy of Cushing's disease. Mitotane, 3 to 6 grams per day in divided doses, can be used if tolerated. Although remission rates with the drug in Cushing's disease are approximately 80 per cent, relapse occurs following discontinuation of therapy. In addition, the response to mitotane is slow, requiring weeks to months to control cortisol excess, and side effects that include nausea, vomiting, diarrhea, somnolence, and skin rash occur in the majority of patients. Since the use of these drugs may produce hypoadrenalism, careful monitoring of steroid levels and glucocorticoid replacement are required.

In the ectopic ACTH syndrome the tumor hypersecreting ACTH should be removed. This may be possible in the minority of patients with the more benign tumors such as thymoma, bronchial carcinoid, or pheochromocytoma. Unfortunately in the majority of patients the tumors are malignant and metastasize prior to the diagnosis of cortisol excess. In such patients, drug therapy as discussed above is used to control cortisol excess. Ketoconazole, metyrapone, and aminoglutethimide are preferred to mitotane because of their more rapid onset of action; multiple drugs may be required if the hypercortisolism is severe. Hypokalemia should be corrected, and spironolactone therapy may be useful in blocking the mineralocorticoid effects of cortisol and 11-deoxycorticosterone. Bilateral adrenalectomy may be considered in a rare patient in whom drug therapy is inadequate and the cortisol excess rather than the tumor is life threatening.

The treatment of adrenal tumors is primarily surgical. Patients

---

*This use is not listed in the manufacturer's directive.

with unilateral adrenal adenoma should undergo resection of the affected adrenal. Although surgical cure of adrenocortical carcinoma is unusual, surgical removal of the primary tumor is indicated to reduce cortisol secretion even when metastases are present. Mitotane, 6 to 12 grams per day in divided doses, if tolerated, is recommended for patients with residual or nonresectable carcinoma, and approximately 75 per cent of patients achieve reduced steroid secretion. Only about one third of patients undergo reduction in tumor bulk, however, and it is not clear whether the drug prolongs survival. Ketoconazole, metyrapone, and aminoglutethimide can be used in patients who do not respond to or tolerate mitotane. The prognosis is poor with adrenal carcinoma; most patients survive less than 5 years following the onset of symptoms.

The normal hypothalamic-pituitary-adrenal axis is suppressed in Cushing's syndrome of all causes, and months to sometimes 2 years are required for it to recover following removal of an adrenal, pituitary, or ectopic tumor. Thus, following the resection of a cortisol- or ACTH-producing tumor, glucocorticoid replacement therapy, as described above for secondary adrenocortical insufficiency, is required until normal pituitary and adrenal function recovers.

NELSON'S SYNDROME. Defined as the clinical progression of an ACTH-secreting pituitary adenoma following bilateral adrenalectomy for Cushing's disease, this syndrome appears to occur in at least one third of such patients. Fortunately the incidence of this disorder has dropped dramatically because of the decreased use of bilateral adrenalectomy for treatment of Cushing's disease.

The syndrome probably results when cortisol feedback inhibition is removed by bilateral adrenalectomy, thus allowing progression of the adenoma. Nelson's syndrome is characterized by increasing hyperpigmentation, usually within 1 to 2 years following adrenalectomy. In addition, these patients frequently exhibit local manifestations, including hypopituitarism, visual loss, headache, cavernous sinus invasion with extraocular muscle palsies, and rarely malignant changes with metastatic spread. Plasma ACTH levels are dramatically elevated and usually range from 1000 to 10,000 pg per milliliter. The majority of these tumors

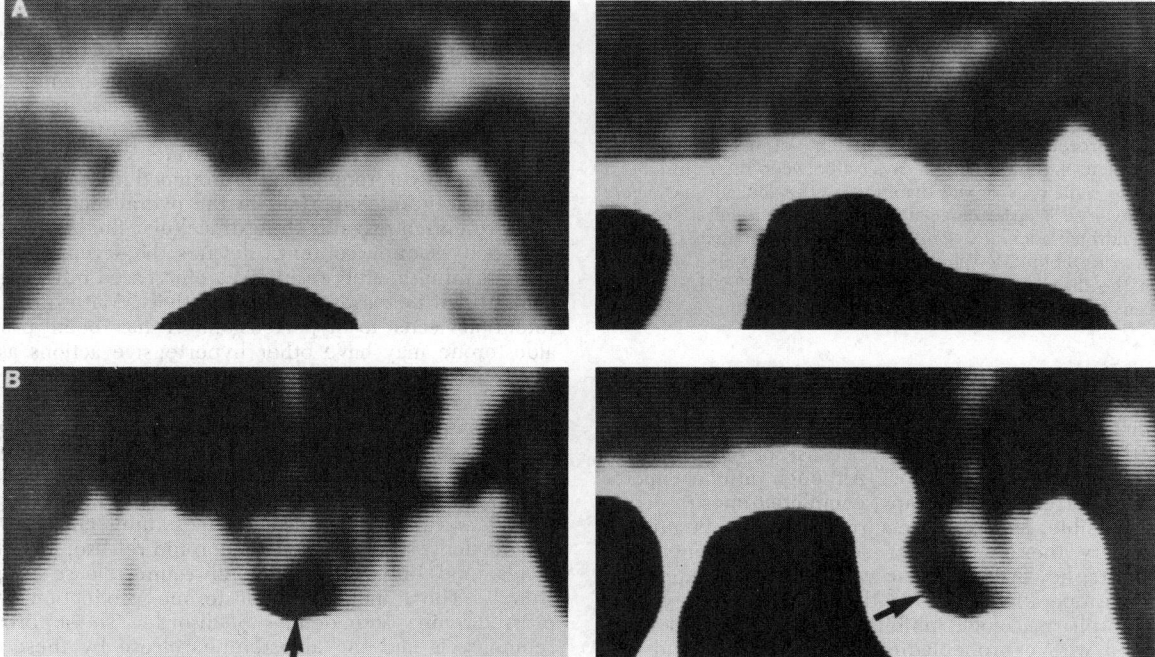

FIGURE 217–8. CT scans of normal and abnormal pituitary glands. The sections shown are computer re-formations derived from 1.5-mm axial sections through the sella turcica. Coronal re-formations are shown on the left and sagittal ones on the right. A, Normal pituitary gland. The upper border is flat; the pituitary stalk (seen on the coronal section) is midline; and the gland is relatively homogeneous in density. The lateral margins of the sella turcica (see coronal section) are formed by the contrast-enhancing cavernous sinuses. B, In a patient with Cushing's disease, a 3- to 4-mm pituitary adenoma is visualized as a low-density lesion in the anterior inferior portion of the anterior lobe (*arrows*). (Reprinted from Findling JW, Tyrrell JB: In Greenspan FS, Forsham PH (eds.): Basic and Clinical Endocrinology, 2nd ed. Los Altos, Calif., Lange Medical Publications, 1986, p 65.)

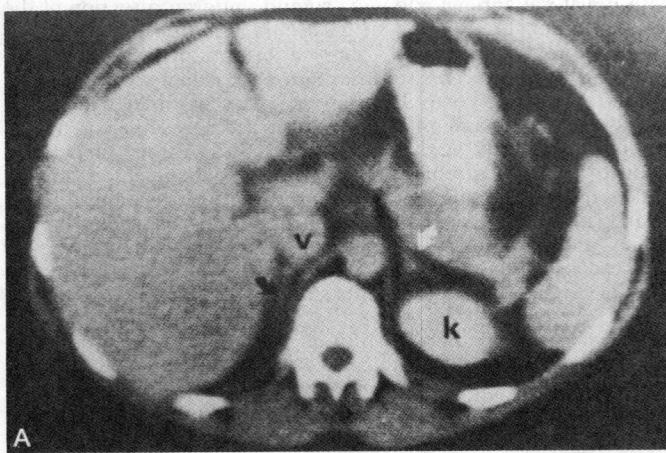

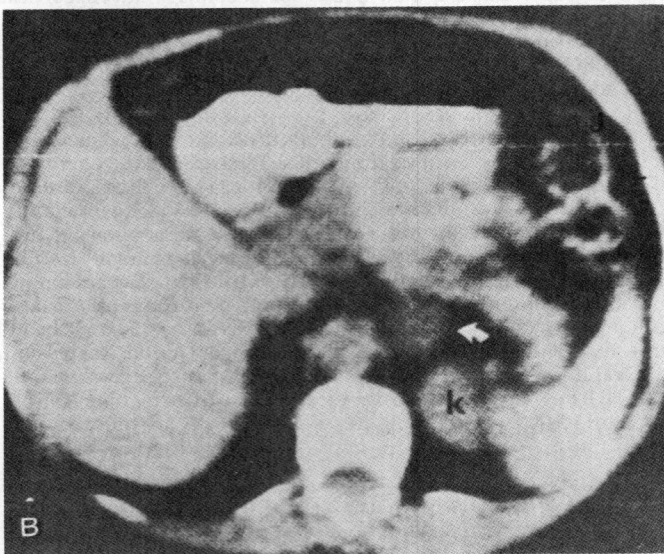

FIGURE 217–9. CT scans in Cushing's syndrome. *A,* Patient with ACTH-dependent Cushing's syndrome. The adrenal glands are not detectably abnormal by this procedure. The curvilinear right adrenal (*black arrow*) is shown posterior to the inferior vena cava (v) between the right lobe of the liver and the right crus of the diaphragm. The left adrenal (*white arrow*) has an inverted Y appearance anteromedial to the left kidney (k). *B,* A 3-cm left adrenal adenoma (*white arrow*) anteromedial to the left kidney (k). (From Korobkin M, White EA, Kressel HY, et al.: Computed tomographs in the diagnosis of adrenal disease. AJR 132:231, 1979. © 1979, American Journal of Roentgenology, The Williams & Wilkins Company.)

are greater than 1 cm in diameter and are readily localized by MRI or CT of the sella turcica.

The treatment of Nelson's syndrome is considerably less successful than that of Cushing's disease because of the large size and aggressive nature of these tumors. Although pituitary microsurgery is the preferred initial therapy, complete tumor resection is usually not possible. Heavy-particle irradiation may be utilized either as primary therapy or after surgery in patients with intrasellar tumors; however, in those with extrasellar extension, conventional postoperative radiation therapy should be undertaken. Although pharmacologic inhibition of ACTH secretion has been attempted with cyproheptadine, bromocriptine, and valproic acid, it appears that only a minority of patients respond. Nevertheless, trials of these medications are indicated if surgical treatment and radiotherapy are unsuccessful.

INCIDENTAL ADRENAL MASSES

The routine use of CT, MRI, and ultrasonography for the evaluation of intra-abdominal conditions has led not infrequently to the incidental detection of unilateral adrenal masses or less

commonly of bilateral adrenal enlargement. The great majority of such patients with unilateral lesions have benign nonfunctional adrenocortical adenomas or cysts; a few patients have functioning adenomas or rarely carcinomas of the adrenal cortex or medulla. When such lesions are identified, the patient should undergo screening tests for pheochromocytoma, Cushing's syndrome, aldosterone excess, and adrenal carcinoma. If a functioning tumor is present, it should be resected regardless of its size. Nonfunctioning lesions less than 6 cm in diameter should be re-imaged in 6 and 18 months; if growth occurs, resection is recommended. Nonfunctioning lesions greater than 6 cm should be resected because adrenal carcinoma is more common with larger lesions. The incidental discovery of bilateral adrenal enlargement is very unusual and presents a difficult diagnostic challenge. These patients may have a variety of infectious, metastatic, invasive, or hemorrhagic lesions that may ultimately lead to adrenal insufficiency (Ch. 217.6). Rare lesions are bilateral adrenal carcinomas, bilateral pheochromocytomas, and congenital adrenal hyperplasia. In such cases, if screening tests for adrenal hyper- and hypofunction are negative, needle biopsy of the adrenal should be considered to establish a histologic diagnosis and direct appropriate therapy.

217.8 MINERALOCORTICOID EXCESS STATES
John D. Baxter

PRIMARY ALDOSTERONISM

Increased and inappropriate production of aldosterone from the adrenal is known as primary aldosteronism and leads to sodium retention with hypertension, suppression of plasma renin, and hypokalemia and its manifestations. It is due mainly to an adrenocortical adenoma, bilateral adrenocortical hyperplasia, or rarely to an adrenal carcinoma. The disease occurs in all age groups, with a peak incidence during the third and fourth decades. About 70 per cent of the adenomas occur in women. Although primary aldosteronism almost always results in hypertension (normotensive primary hyperaldosteronism is extremely rare), the syndrome is present in less than 2 per cent of patients with hypertension. Nevertheless, this largely reversible form of hypertension should be considered in all hypertensive patients.

ALDOSTERONE-PRODUCING ADENOMAS. With an aldosterone-producing adenoma (Conn's syndrome), aldosterone excess leads to sodium retention and potassium and hydrogen loss. Other steroids that are normally synthesized in the zona glomerulosa (i.e., deoxycorticosterone, corticosterone, and 18-hydroxycorticosterone) are also produced in excess, although they are probably not important in the overall pathophysiology. Sodium retention expands the extracellular fluid volume, increases total body sodium content, elevates the serum sodium concentration and ultimately results in an increased intracellular sodium content that increases vascular reactivity. With time, the sodium retention leads to hypertension. It has been proposed that aldosterone may have other hypertensive actions as well. The hypokalemia results in muscular weakness, a tendency to cardiac irritability and arrhythmia, carbohydrate intolerance, resistance to vasopressin (nephrogenic diabetes insipidus), and abnormalities in baroreceptor function. The latter results in a more volume-dependent hypertension. The expansion of the extracellular fluid and plasma volume is registered by the stretch receptors at the juxtaglomerular apparatus and by sodium chloride flux at the macula densa with suppression of renin release, low plasma renin levels, and unresponsiveness of renin release to provocative stimuli. Thus, increased aldosterone production with a suppressed renin system defines the disorder. The suppressed plasma renin levels and the aldosterone release by these tumors are generally unresponsive to the usual stimuli such as posture or diuresis, although they are responsive in a small subset of patients (renin-responsive adenoma).

The sustained hypertension leads to compensatory effects that act to decrease the plasma volume, which can be normal or increased. However, an increased sodium and extracellular fluid volume persists, and the hypertension continues to be aldosterone dependent. The hypertension can also lead to many complications, such as renal damage, stroke, and myocardial infarction.

BILATERAL ADRENAL HYPERPLASIA. Bilateral adrenal hyperplasia can be diffuse or nodular, and selectively involves the glomerulosa cells. It accounts for perhaps 30 per cent of the patients in whom primary aldosteronism is diagnosed; however, its precise incidence is not known, since there is a gradient between what is termed low-renin essential hypertension without frank aldosterone excess and this syndrome. Adrenal hyperplasia does not in general precede development of an adenoma.

The pathophysiology of the most common form of hyperplasia (idiopathic hyperaldosteronism) shows several differences from that of adenoma: (1) Although the plasma renin is suppressed, it does respond to postural and other stimuli. (2) The adrenal is hypersensitive to angiotensin II, exhibiting a marked increase in aldosterone production rather than insensitivity. (3) The aldosterone hypersecretion is less than with the adenoma, a feature that is useful in the differential diagnosis. By contrast, the blood pressure in the two groups tends to be similar. (4) The hypertension in most patients does not respond to adrenalectomy, implying that common factors produce both hypertension and enhanced adrenal sensitivity to angiotensin II. The mechanisms for the development of hyperplasia are unknown. There is active inquiry whether there is abnormal production (or loss) of factor(s) that enhance adrenal and vascular sensitivity to angiotensin II.

There are also subgroups of hyperplasia. A few per cent of patients have what has been termed primary adrenal hyperplasia. In these patients the plasma aldosterone and 18-OHB levels tend to be higher; the aldosterone and renin responses to provocative stimuli resemble those with aldosterone-producing adenomas; the hypertension commonly responds to adrenalectomy; and the hyperplasia is typically nodular, being either unilateral or bilateral. In rare patients the hypertension and aldosterone excess respond to glucocorticoid therapy.

CLINICAL PRESENTATION. Patients present with elevated blood pressure detected on routine screening or, less commonly, because of hypokalemia. The blood pressure elevations range from mild to severe, with mean presenting pressures in the range of 200 mm Hg systolic and 120 mm Hg diastolic. Malignant hypertension is rare. A history of hypertension in pregnancy is common with female patients who develop the disorder. When present, symptoms of hypokalemia include tiredness, loss of stamina, weakness, nocturia, and lassitude. Symptoms of more severe depletion include alkalosis; rarely tetany with a positive Trousseau or Chvostek sign; increased thirst and polyuria with low urine specific gravity and unresponsiveness to vasopressin; paresthesias; cardiac arrhythmias such as ventricular tachycardia; and postural hypotension with dizziness. Headache is a frequent incidental complaint. There are no characteristic physical findings. In spite of fluid overload, edema is only rarely present. The heart is usually only mildly enlarged, if at all, and electrocardiographic changes are usually those of moderate left ventricular hypertrophy and potassium depletion. There tend to be fewer funduscopic changes than in other forms of hypertension of comparable severity. These patients are particularly sensitive to the potassium-wasting effects of diuretics.

DIAGNOSIS. The hallmarks of the disorder are hypertension with hypokalemia, suppression of the renin-angiotensin system, and increased aldosterone production. The serum sodium is rarely less than 139 mEq per liter in the absence of diuretic therapy. A suggested evaluation plan is shown in Figure 217–10. The initial step is to determine whether hypokalemia is present, since this is the primary clue to mineralocorticoid excess. All patients with hypertension should be screened, especially those with spontaneous hypokalemia, after diuretics have been withheld for at least 3 weeks.

The evaluation of hypokalemia requires control of the sodium balance, since sodium depletion from decreased intake or diuretics can decrease urinary potassium excretion and thus mask hypokalemia. Random serum potassium levels may be normal in up to 20 per cent of patients with primary aldosteronism, but salt loading unmasks hypokalemia in virtually all patients with adenoma and in most patients with hyperplasia. In the latter group the serum potassium levels are almost always below 4 mEq per liter. If according to the dietary history the patient's usual sodium intake is 120 mEq or greater per 24 hours, measurement of normal potassium levels on three occasions obviates the need

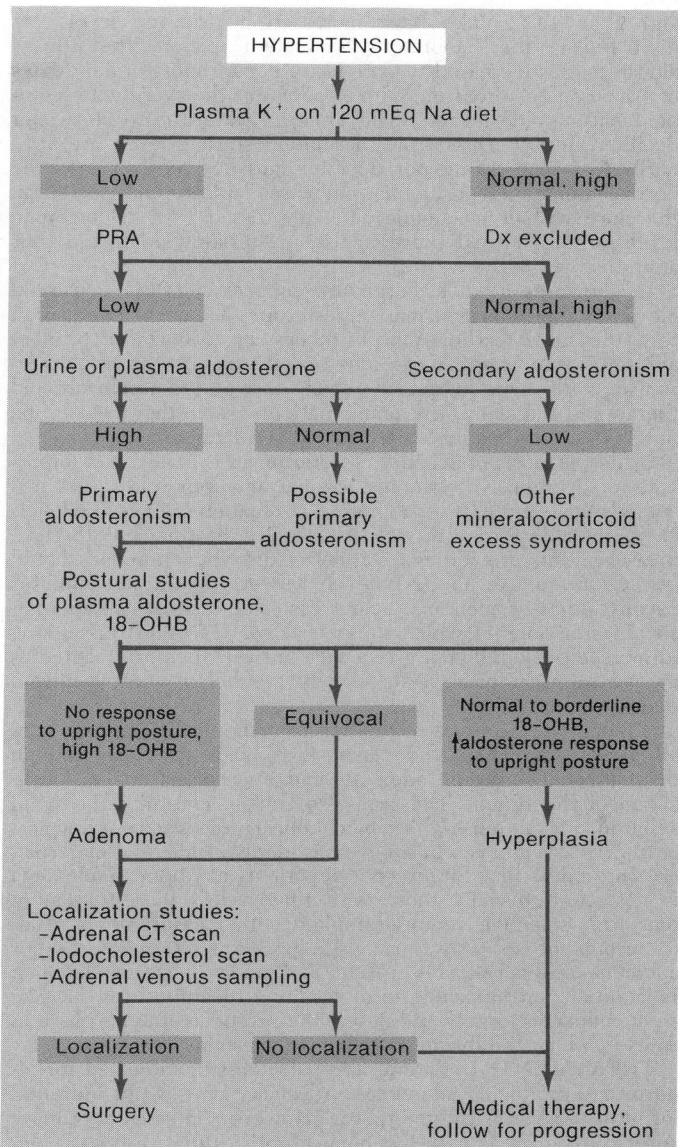

FIGURE 217–10. Flow diagram for diagnosis of primary aldosteronism and differentiation of adrenal adenoma from hyperplasia. (Adapted from Baxter JD, Perloff D, Hsueh W, et al.: *In* Felig P, Baxter JD, Broadus AE, et al. (eds.): Endocrinology and Metabolism, 2nd ed. New York, McGraw-Hill Book Company, 1987, p 756.)

for further evaluation. If dietary intake is inadequate or unclear, the patient is instructed to consume a normal diet supplemented with 1 gram of NaCl with each meal for 4 days, and the serum potassium is then measured.

If the plasma potassium value is low, other causes of hypokalemia should be ruled out: diuretic therapy, gastrointestinal loss due to vomiting or diarrhea, other mineralocorticoid excess syndromes (discussed below), starvation, insulin and glucose therapy, metabolic acidosis, renal disease, and renovascular and accelerated hypertension.

Random unstimulated plasma renin activity (PRA) or plasma renin concentration (PRC) should be determined as the next step in diagnosis. In primary aldosteronism this is suppressed even after short-term diuretic therapy, salt restriction, assumption of erect posture, or exercise, although other causes of low renin must be excluded. If PRA is normal or high, primary aldosteronism is unlikely.

If the plasma renin value is low or marginally low, 24-hour urinary aldosterone and plasma aldosterone levels should be measured. It is critical to monitor the salt intake and posture, as discussed earlier, because patients with essential hypertension and a low-salt intake have increased aldosterone levels. As discussed in the Laboratory Evaluation section, the urinary aldosterone is increased to over 17 μg per 24 hours in most cases of primary aldosteronism. With an adenoma the overnight recumbent plasma aldosterone levels almost always exceed 20 ng per deciliter. In hyperplasia the plasma aldosterone levels are ordinarily less than 20 ng per deciliter and frequently are in the normal range. Hypokalemia decreases aldosterone secretion; therefore with hypokalemia and suppressed PRA, aldosterone levels in the normal range are inappropriately high and thus abnormal.

In the presence of marginally suppressed PRC and mild elevation of plasma or urinary aldosterone, one of the stimulation tests (discussed earlier) may be necessary to diagnose primary aldosteronism. Marginal cases are usually due to primary aldosteronism with hyperplasia, in which case antimineralocorticoid therapy is indicated. In many patients such therapy can be initiated and the patient re-evaluated at a later time.

If the diagnosis of primary aldosteronism is made, it is important to distinguish between adenoma and hyperplasia. As discussed above and in the Laboratory Evaluation section, the levels of plasma aldosterone provide an initial indication, but 18-OHB measurements provide an even better discrimination and should be performed. An 18-OHB level of over 100 ng per milliliter usually indicates adenoma; below this value it suggests hyperplasia. In situations in which these tests, or CT or MRI scanning (discussed below), do not give a clear answer, the postural studies or the saline infusion tests usually are helpful in reaching a decision.

CT or MRI scanning of the adrenals should be performed in all patients in whom the diagnosis is made; this can help in distinguishing between adenoma and hyperplasia and in localization of the tumor. The scan also usually identifies the small subgroup of adenomas whose biochemical indices are more typical of hyperplasia and can in some cases identify unilateral hyperplasia. In the less than 20 per cent of patients in whom an adenoma is not found, usually those with tumors less than 1.4 cm in diameter, selective venous sampling with measurements of aldosterone-cortisol ratios is usually helpful, can determine whether adenoma or hyperplasia is present, and can lateralize an adenoma. In addition, an iodocholesterol scanning technique can localize an adenoma accurately and detect the presence of hyperplasia in cases in which the diagnosis remains uncertain.

TREATMENT. Unilateral adrenalectomy is indicated for aldosterone-producing adenomas. Adrenalectomy is not indicated for most patients with hyperplasia. However, in cases of primary adrenal hyperplasia with biochemical indices that resemble adenoma, removal of a unilaterally hyperplastic gland or of one gland (preferably the left because of surgical considerations) in patients with bilateral hyperplasia is frequently effective. However, these patients also respond to antimineralocorticoid therapy. Prior to surgery the blood pressure and serum potassium should be normalized by treatment with the mineralocorticoid antagonist spironolactone (200 to 400 mg per day) or the potassium-sparing diuretic amiloride (20 to 40 mg per day). These dosages of spironolactone can be reduced to around 100 to 150 mg per day once normalization of blood pressure and hypokalemia has occurred. Medical therapy can be continued in the rare patient in whom surgery is contraindicated or in patients in whom the etiologic diagnosis is uncertain. This form of treatment also tends to reactivate the suppressed renin-angiotensin system so that the incidence of postoperative hypoaldosteronism is reduced. Also the response of the blood pressure to this therapy provides an excellent indication of the anticipated response to surgery.

Following surgery the blood pressure returns to normal in around 50 per cent of patients, with reduction of hypertension in another 25 per cent. However, hypertension, but not hyperaldosteronism, returns in about 40 per cent by 10 years postoperatively.

Medical therapy is recommended for most patients with bilateral hyperplasia. Spironolactone in doses described above or amiloride corrects the hypokalemia but not the hypertension in most cases. Additional antihypertensive medications are usually necessary. Although treatment with a glucocorticoid is effective in the rare subgroup of patients with glucocorticoid-hyperplasia,

it is debatable whether patients should be screened for this responsiveness.

OTHER FORMS OF HYPERTENSION ASSOCIATED WITH MINERALOCORTICOID EXCESS

There are several other mineralocorticoid-excess conditions. DOC excess can occur in the 11β- and 17α-hydroxylase syndromes (see Ch. 221), in patients with Cushing's syndrome, especially with ectopic ACTH-producing carcinoma, and with adrenal adenomas and carcinoma. In these cases the PRC is suppressed as it is in primary aldosteronism; however, plasma aldosterone levels are usually suppressed as well. Rarely mineralocorticoid-excess hypertension results from excessive ingestion of licorice or carbenoxolone (discussed in Ch. 217.2), 9α-fluorocortisol used for treating postural hypotension, or mineralocorticoid-containing nasal sprays. It can be present in rare cases of insensitivity to glucocorticoids when elevated cortisol levels have mineralocorticoid actions. There are rare syndromes (predominantly observed in children) in which there are hypertension, hypokalemia, and suppressed PRC with no detectable elevations of known mineralocorticoids; in some instances these syndromes are due to 11β-hydroxysteroid dehydrogenase deficiency, which impairs renal cortisol to cortisone conversion with a consequent cortisol-induced mineralocorticoid excess state. In all of these conditions there are hypertension, hypokalemia, and suppression of PRC without an associated increase of aldosterone.

SECONDARY HYPERALDOSTERONISM

Secondary hyperaldosteronism results from stimulation of the adrenal glomerulosa by extra-adrenal factors, usually the renin-angiotensin system. It can be physiologic or contribute to the pathology of disease states. A physiologic increase occurs during excessive potassium intake as part of the body's defense against hyperkalemia. Secondary hyperaldosteronism can occur during the luteal phase of the menstrual cycle and occasionally during oral contraceptive use. Aldosterone secretion increases progressively during normal pregnancy; levels reach 10 times those of nonpregnant women by the third trimester. This is presumably due to an increase in renin and angiotensin, possibly due to a decrease in blood pressure. Interestingly, renin levels are more elevated during the first trimester, whereas plasma aldosterone levels are highest during the third trimester. This may be due to a progressive increase in sensitivity of the adrenal glomerulosa to angiotensin II. Aldosterone secretion increases when there is excessive sodium loss and when there is dietary restriction of sodium. Aldosterone increases in some patients with congestive heart failure and with significant hypoalbuminemia such as with nephrotic syndrome. In heart failure the aldosterone levels result from counterbalancing influences of decreased renal perfusion secondary to reduced cardiac output that increases renin and aldosterone release, and of sodium retention that suppresses renin and aldosterone levels. Renin and aldosterone levels are commonly elevated in cirrhosis when ascites is present; this is accentuated by decreased clearance of aldosterone. The increased aldosterone further promotes sodium retention and potassium loss. Elevated aldosterone levels are found in Bartter's syndrome (see Ch. 82). Finally, secondary hyperaldosteronism and hypertension can occur with renal artery stenosis, unilateral renal ischemia, accelerated hypertension, and renin-secreting tumors. Since secondary aldosteronism occurs in response to other primary processes and is an adaptive response, treatment is usually not indicated. However, in certain situations such as heart failure or cirrhosis, in which the excessive sodium retention and potassium loss are deleterious, antimineralocorticoid therapy, such as spironolactone, can be helpful.

Baxter JD, Tyrrell JB: The adrenal cortex. *In* Felig P, Baxter JD, Broadus AE, et al. (eds.): Endocrinology and Metabolism, 2nd ed. New York, McGraw-Hill Book Company, 1987, pp 511–650. *An extensive review of the physiology and pathology of the adrenal cortex.*

Baxter JD, Perloff D, Hsueh W, et al.: The endocrinology of hypertension. *In* Felig P, Baxter JD, Broadus AE, et al. (eds.): Endocrinology and Metabolism, 2nd ed. New York, McGraw-Hill Book Company, 1987, pp 693–788. *A description of the renin-angiotensin system and an analysis of the pathophysiology and approaches to diagnosis and treatment not only of primary aldosteronism but also of other types of endocrine hypertension.*

Crapo L: Cushing's syndrome: A review of diagnostic tests. Metabolism 28:955, 1979. *This paper, although published over a decade ago, still provides an excellent overview of the approaches to the diagnosis of Cushing's syndrome.*

Dluhy RG: The growing spectrum of HIV-related endocrine abnormalities. J Clin Endocrinol Metab 70:563, 1990. *An overview of adrenal and other abnormalities in AIDS.*

Findling JW: The Cushing syndromes: An enlarging clinical spectrum. N Engl J Med 321:1677, 1989. *An overview of causes of and diagnostic approaches to Cushing's syndrome.*

Funder JW, Pearce PT, Smith R, et al.: Mineralocorticoid action: Target tissue specificity is enzyme, not receptor, mediated. Science 242: 583, 1988. *An examination of the role of cortisol-to-cortisone conversion in the actions of cortisol and aldosterone.*

Hall PF: Tropic stimulation of steroidogenesis: In search of the elusive trigger. Recent Prog Horm Res 41:1, 1985. *A review of the mechanisms regulating steroid biosynthesis.*

Irony I, Kater CE, Biglieri EF, et al.: Correctable subsets of primary aldosteronism: Primary adrenal hyperplasia and renin responsive adenoma. Am J Hypertens 3:576, 1990. *An analysis of the types of primary aldosteronism and how to manage them.*

Kaye TB, Crapo L: The Cushing syndrome. An update in diagnostic tests. Ann Intern Med 112:434, 1990. *This updates and complements the 1979 paper by Dr. Crapo listed above.*

Keller-Wood ME, Dallman M: Corticosteroid inhibition of ACTH secretion. Endocr Rev 5:1, 1984. *A review of the kinetics and mechanisms whereby glucocorticoids block both CRF and ACTH release.*

Marver D, Kokko JP: Renal target sites and the mechanism of action of aldosterone. Miner Electrolyte Metab 9:1, 1983. *A review of the actions of aldosterone.*

May RE, Carey RM: Rapid adrenocorticotrophic test in practice. Am J Med 79:679, 1985. *An assessment of the usefulness of this test.*

Melby JC: Primary aldosteronism. Kidney Int 26:769, 1984. *An overview of mineralocorticoid-excess syndromes.*

Munck A, Guyre P, Holbrook NJ: Physiological functions of glucocorticoids in stress and their relation to pharmacological actions. Endocr Rev 5:25, 1984. *A proposal that explains how glucocorticoids are useful in the body's response to stress.*

Parker LN, Odell WD: Control of adrenal androgen secretion. Endocr Rev 1:392, 1980. *An excellent examination of the factors that regulate adrenal androgen production.*

Re NJ: Cellular biology of the renin-angiotensin systems. Arch Intern Med 144:2037, 1984. *An excellent overview of the renin-angiotensin system.*

218 Diabetes Mellitus

Jerrold M. Olefsky

DEFINITION. Diabetes mellitus is a heterogeneous primary disorder of carbohydrate metabolism with multiple etiologic factors that generally involve absolute or relative insulin deficiency or insulin resistance or both. All causes of diabetes ultimately lead to hyperglycemia, which is the hallmark of this disease syndrome.

CLASSIFICATION AND DIAGNOSIS

The currently accepted classification and the criteria for the diagnosis of diabetes mellitus are summarized in Table 218–1. Diabetes can be separated into two general disease syndromes: (1) *Type 1,* or *insulin-dependent diabetes mellitus* (IDDM), is present in patients with little or no endogenous insulin secretory capacity. These patients develop extreme hyperglycemia, ketosis, and the associated symptomatology unless treated with insulin, and they are therefore entirely dependent on exogenous insulin

TABLE 218–1. CLASSIFICATION OF DIABETES

1. Insulin-dependent, or type I diabetes (IDDM). Formerly called juvenile-onset or ketosis-prone diabetes.
2. Non–insulin-dependent, or type II diabetes (NIDDM). Formerly called adult-onset, maturity-onset, or nonketotic diabetes.
   A. Obese (~80%)
   B. Nonobese (~20%)
3. Secondary diabetes
   A. Pancreatic disease (e.g., pancreatectomy, pancreatic insufficiency, hemochromatosis)
   B. Hormonal (excess counterinsulin hormones, e.g., Cushing's syndrome, acromegaly, pheochromocytoma)
   C. Drug-induced (e.g., thiazide diuretics, steroids, phenytoin)
   D. Associated with specific genetic syndromes (e.g., lipodystrophy, myotonic dystrophy, ataxia-telangiectasia)
4. Impaired glucose tolerance (IGT). Formerly called chemical, latent, borderline, or subclinical diabetes.
5. Gestational diabetes: glucose intolerance with onset during pregnancy.

therapy for immediate survival. This form of the disease usually, but not always, develops prior to early adulthood. Older terms for this syndrome are juvenile onset, ketosis prone, or brittle diabetes. (2) *Type II,* or *non–insulin-dependent diabetes mellitus* (NIDDM), occurs in patients who retain significant endogenous insulin secretory capacity. Although treatment with insulin may be necessary for control of hyperglycemia, these patients do not develop ketosis in the absence of insulin therapy and are not dependent on exogenous insulin for immediate survival. Previous terms for this form of the disease are maturity or adult onset, nonketotic, and stable diabetes. The diagnosis of diabetes in patients with the insulin-dependent form of the disease is usually unequivocal, and the distinction between type I and type II diabetes can usually be made on clinical grounds. However, there are occasional patients with minimal, but clearly detectable, endogenous insulin secretion in whom the disease is difficult to categorize initially. Usually these are lean adult, sometimes elderly, patients who at the time of initial diagnosis retain sufficient insulin secretory function so that the disease meets the classification of type II diabetes; with time, insulin secretion diminishes to the point that the disease merges into the category of type I diabetes.

The diagnosis of NIDDM is based on a distinction between normal and abnormal levels of glycemia and therefore is less precise. Prior to the report of the National Diabetes Data Group, oral glucose tolerance tests were commonly used to establish this diagnosis. This approach is fraught with difficulties because oral glucose tolerance is affected by numerous other variables that can cause mild abnormalities of glucose metabolism independent of diabetes. Concomitant illness, stress, physical inactivity, hypocaloric or low carbohydrate intake, various drugs, and aging are among those factors that can adversely influence glucose tolerance. Therefore, when employed, glucose tolerance testing must be rigorously controlled by administering a standard oral glucose load (75 grams), ensuring an appropriate antecedent diet (eucaloric with at least 200 grams of carbohydrate per day), adequate physical activity, and the absence of drugs affecting carbohydrate metabolism. Even with these precautions, only a minority (15 to 25 per cent) of individuals who have normal fasting plasma glucose levels with abnormal glucose tolerance tests go on to develop overt diabetes. In recognition of the above facts, relatively stringent criteria for establishing the diagnosis of NIDDM have been recommended: (1) fasting venous plasma glucose concentration greater than 140 mg per deciliter on at least two separate occasions, or (2) in the absence of fasting hyperglycemia, a diagnosis of NIDDM can be made following ingestion of the standard 75-gram oral glucose tolerance test if the 2-hour venous plasma glucose and one other sample (the 30-, 60-, or 90-minute sample) exceed 200 mg per deciliter.

Impaired glucose tolerance exists if the fasting plasma glucose level is less than 140 mg per deciliter and if the 30-, 60-, or 90-minute plasma glucose concentration exceeds 200 mg per deciliter along with a 2-hour plasma glucose level between 140 and 200 mg per deciliter. Microvascular complications of diabetes rarely occur in individuals with impaired glucose tolerance, and the great majority of these cases do not deteriorate to overt diabetes in long-term follow-up. Most instances of impaired glucose tolerance, therefore, are probably unrelated to the disease syndrome of NIDDM. Almost all patients who meet the criteria for NIDDM during oral glucose tolerance testing show fasting hyperglycemia (greater than 140 mg per deciliter) when evaluations are repeated. Furthermore, in those few patients who meet the criteria for NIDDM in the absence of fasting hyperglycemia, many do not develop fasting hyperglycemia during prolonged follow-up, and clinical symptoms of diabetes are unusual. Thus, the clinical significance of impaired glucose tolerance is unclear. As previously mentioned, only a minority (2 to 35 per cent, depending on the population examined) of these patients go on to develop overt NIDDM when followed for up to 20 years. The real challenge is to develop markers to detect which patients with impaired glucose tolerance have a benign nonprogressive abnormality of glucose intolerance and which have a prediabetic state. Patients with impaired glucose tolerance who secrete low amounts of insulin, compared to normal individuals, have a much higher risk of developing overt diabetes (perhaps up to 40 per cent), whereas those who secrete high amounts of insulin seldom (about 5 per cent) progress to frank diabetes. In brief, glucose tolerance testing is unnecessary for patient management in the absence of clinical signs and symptoms of diabetes, although this is still a highly useful procedure for epidemiologic or research purposes. An exception to this would be in a pregnant subject suspected of having gestational diabetes, since criteria for this diagnosis are less stringent and vigorous management of minimal degrees of hyperglycemia is important.

Glucose tolerance declines with age. Insulin secretion is not decreased in aging, whereas insulin resistance due to a postreceptor defect in insulin action is a common finding in aged populations. Age-related variables such as inadequate diet, increasing adiposity with decreased lean body mass, and physical inactivity can contribute to this insulin-resistant state, but the aging process itself also plays a significant role. The glucose intolerance of aging tends to be mild and is most easily detected following an oral glucose challenge. When mild abnormalities of oral glucose tolerance tests were used to diagnose diabetes, age-adjusted criteria for these tests had to be employed. However, with the current more stringent criteria noted above, this problem is largely obviated, since the glucose intolerance of aging does not cause significant fasting hyperglycemia (more than 140 mg per deciliter) and only rarely would cause glucose intolerance severe enough to meet the new criteria in the absence of hyperglycemia.

EPIDEMIOLOGY AND CLINICAL PRESENTATION

Overall, in the United States the prevalence of diabetes is probably between 2 and 4 per cent, with IDDM comprising 7 to 10 per cent of all cases. The prevalence of IDDM (0.2 to 0.3 per cent) is probably more accurate than the estimates for NIDDM, because of the relative ease of ascertainment and the fact that many patients with NIDDM are asymptomatic and the disease is undiagnosed.

The prevalence of diabetes has been difficult to quantitate accurately because the criteria for the diagnosis of NIDDM have varied from survey to survey over the years; the less stringent the criteria the greater the prevalence and vice versa. Furthermore, the prevalence of diabetes differs widely among different populations, depending on ethnic group constituents, age, economic conditions, and probably other environmental factors. For example, the prevalence of diabetes is extremely high among Pima Indians (about 35 per cent) and certain Micronesian cultures (about 35 per cent). Indians, particularly after emigrating from their country, have a higher rate of diabetes than other ethnic groups. Thus, Indians living in South Africa, Trinidad, Singapore, Malaysia, and Fiji exhibit a higher prevalence of diabetes than the local population and than those living on the Indian subcontinent. A low prevalence of diabetes has been noted in Eskimos, Athabascan Indians (Alaska), and Chinese (although prevalence increases in Chinese populations living in Western countries). The proportion of IDDM to NIDDM also differs widely among different populations; IDDM is extremely rare in Pima Indians, Micronesians, and Eskimos, but is more common in Caucasian populations.

A few facts concerning the prevalence of major diabetes-related complications serve to underscore the enormous impact of this disease. Approximately 25 per cent of all new cases of end-stage renal failure occur in patients with diabetes. About 20,000 amputations (primarily of toes, feet, and legs) are carried out in patients with diabetes, representing approximately half of the nontraumatic amputations performed in the United States. Furthermore, diabetes is the leading cause of new cases of blindness, with approximately 5000 new cases occurring each year.

INSULIN-DEPENDENT DIABETES MELLITUS (IDDM, TYPE I). These patients have little or no endogenous insulin and usually present with relatively abrupt clinical symptoms of *polyuria, polydipsia,* and *polyphagia. Weight loss,* fatigue, and infection can often accompany the initial presentation. Because of the extreme hypoinsulinemia and hyperglucagonemia, these patients readily develop *ketosis,* and the initial onset of this disease may be clinically evident as full-blown ketoacidosis. At the time of the first clinical presentation, symptoms can usually be traced back for several days to a few weeks; however, in most cases β cell destruction began months and usually years prior to the onset of clinical symptoms. In some cases, detection of this preclinical state may be possible by assessing the presence of circulating antibodies to islet cells or insulin. Unfortunately, proven methods to delay or prevent the full-blown disease are not available. The peak age of onset of IDDM is 11 to 13 years, coinciding with early adolescence and puberty. A secondary peak is noted at age 6 to 8 years, and by the third decade of life the incidence falls to a steady but still substantial level. It is unusual for IDDM to begin past age 40. Once IDDM is diagnosed, insulin therapy is required to achieve initial metabolic control. In many patients a "honeymoon" period follows initial treatment in which the disease remits and little or no insulin is required. This remission is due to a partial return of endogenous insulin secretion, which may last for several weeks or months and occasionally 1 to 2 years; ultimately, however, the disease recurs, and insulin therapy is required permanently.

NON–INSULIN-DEPENDENT DIABETES MELLITUS (NIDDM, TYPE II). Patients with NIDDM typically present with polyuria and polydipsia of several weeks' to months' duration. Polyphagia can occur but is less common, whereas weight loss, weakness, and fatigue are frequent. Dizziness, headaches, and blurry vision are common accompanying complaints. In many patients no symptoms are apparent and the disease is diagnosed by routine blood or urine testing. In others, diabetes is advanced, and the presenting complaints are related to neuropathic, retinopathic, or vascular complications. NIDDM patients are usually but not always older than 40 at presentation. Obesity is a frequent feature of NIDDM, at least in Western cultures; in the United States 80 to 90 per cent of NIDDM patients are obese. Obesity by itself leads to insulin resistance and predisposes or exacerbates the NIDDM state. The mechanisms of obesity-induced insulin resistance are unclear, but the linkage between obesity and NIDDM is indisputable. Certain patterns of distribution of excess adipose tissue may be metabolically more deleterious. Abdominal, or upper body, obesity is more closely associated with NIDDM than is lower body obesity (adipose tissue deposits mainly around the hips and thighs). Endogenous insulin secretion is relatively preserved and may even be excessive; thus, ketosis is rare, explaining why NIDDM is categorized as nonketotic or ketosis resistant.

SECONDARY DIABETIC STATES. In addition to the major categories of diabetes (IDDM and NIDDM), many secondary forms of diabetes exist when some other readily identifiable primary disease entity or pathophysiologic state causes or is strongly associated with the diabetic state (Table 218–1). These cases comprise only a small proportion of the total cases of diabetes. Any disease process that limits insulin secretion or impairs insulin action can cause secondary diabetes. Disorders that lead to pancreatic destruction such as chronic pancreatitis, cystic fibrosis, or hemochromatosis can reduce insulin secretion enough to cause diabetes. Conditions in which excess amounts of counterinsulin hormones are secreted, such as Cushing's disease, acromegaly, pheochromocytoma, and glucagonoma, can also produce diabetes. A number of drugs such as thiazide diuretics, glucocorticoids, and adrenergic agents can lead to, or at least exacerbate, diabetes. Many unusual genetic diseases are associated with a higher than normal incidence of diabetes through unknown mechanisms; these include muscular dystrophy, myotonic dystrophy, Friedreich's ataxia, Turner's syndrome, and others.

Finally, several rare syndromes have been identified, the biochemical mechanisms of which are well described and which primarily involve abnormalities of insulin-glucose physiology. Certain patients with extreme insulin resistance, acanthosis nigricans, and diabetes have circulating anti-insulin receptor antibodies. These antibodies are part of a more generalized autoimmune process, since proteinuria, leukopenia, and antinuclear and anti-DNA antibodies also exist. Other patients with the triad of acanthosis nigricans, insulin resistance, and diabetes do not have antireceptor antibodies, but instead have a profound decrease in cellular insulin receptors. Typically these are young females with hirsutism and polycystic ovaries. In some of these patients, family members also have decreased insulin receptors and insulin resistance, suggesting that this disorder is due to a genetically mediated decrease in insulin receptors. In a few subjects, molecular cloning has revealed mutations in insulin receptor gene alleles, demonstrating the genetic nature of these unusual cases. In some patients, abnormal insulin products are synthesized and secreted. For example, familial hyperproinsulinemia involves a defect in the proinsulin molecule that prevents normal cleavage of proinsulin to insulin in the pancreatic β cell. This leads to the secretion of large amounts of proinsulin (which is biologically less active than insulin) instead of insulin. This disorder can lead to impaired glucose tolerance, but has not yet been associated with overt fasting hyperglycemia. Rarely patients carry mutations in the insulin structural gene itself that lead to the secretion of insulin species with single amino acid substitutions resulting in markedly reduced biologic activity. These patients have a clinical picture of typical NIDDM. These mutant insulins are immunologically reactive and are secreted in large quantities in response to the hyperglycemic state. The clinical hallmark of this condition is the presence of hyperglycemia and marked hyperinsulinemia in a patient with normal sensitivity to exogenous insulin.

GENETICS

Diabetes has long been termed a geneticist's nightmare. The disease clearly aggregates in families and has a strong familial component. However, the precise genetic contribution to diabetes has been difficult to ascertain for at least four reasons: (1) No specific genetic marker has been identified. Glucose tolerance is the currently used method of diagnosis, but because of differences in the way tests are performed and the criteria used, it is difficult to compare one study to another. (2) There is a great deal of etiologic heterogeneity between IDDM and NIDDM and within these categories. This indicates genetic heterogeneity even though the phenotype (hyperglycemia) is comparable. It is also possible that, depending on environmental factors, there can be variable phenotypic expression of a common genotype. (3) It is likely that "diabetogenic genes" interact with external factors as well as with other genetic components, making the specific genetic influences underlying the final phenotypic expression of the diabetes hard to detect. (4) Actual transmission rates of diabetes from generation to generation are low.

Genetic factors are clearly important in the etiology of diabetes. This is demonstrated by classic twin studies. When twins below the age of 40 years are studied, if one twin has diabetes (mostly IDDM based on age) then the other twin develops diabetes only 30 to 50 per cent of the time. If the two pairs are concordant, the second twin usually develops diabetes within a couple of years of the first. For a purely genetic disease, concordance should be 100 per cent. This suggests that while genetic factors are important in IDDM, they are only predisposing and must interact with environmental influences if diabetes is to develop. This does not exclude the possibility that in some patients IDDM occurs entirely because of genetic or environmental factors. In twins over 40 years the concordance rate for diabetes (almost all NIDDM based on age) approaches 100 per cent. This suggests that genetic factors are more important in this form of diabetes and may be causal or closely associated with causal mechanisms.

Despite the contribution of genetic factors, direct transmission of diabetes from parent to offspring is surprisingly low. If one parent has IDDM, the risk to the offspring of developing IDDM is on the order of 2 to 5 per cent. If one child has IDDM, the average risk for another sibling is 5 to 10 per cent. However, the risk is much greater if the second sibling is HLA (human leukocyte antigen)-identical to the first, intermediate if HLA-haploidentical, and very low if HLA-nonidentical. The risk for developing diabetes in a monozygotic twin of an IDDM patient is 30 to 50 per cent. Not only does this indicate the importance of nongenetic "triggering" factors in the etiology of IDDM but it also defines the maximal predictive value that could be achieved by tests based on genetic characteristics. The risk for IDDM is less in HLA-identical siblings than in monozygotic twins: This indicates that genes outside of, or not linked to, the HLA region contribute to the etiology of IDDM, pointing to the multigenic nature of this disease. The type of diabetes tends to run true in families, and the incidence of NIDDM in the offspring of an IDDM parent is probably not greater than normal. If one parent has NIDDM, the risk is 10 to 15 per cent for offspring developing the disease. When both parents have NIDDM, the transmission risk increases, but adequate data are not available to quantitate the

increase in risk. If one sibling has NIDDM, the risk for another sibling is 10 to 15 per cent. These low rates of transmission make it difficult to trace models of inheritance in family studies, but the facts are clinically important in counseling and reassuring diabetic patients who wish to have children.

Strong associations have been identified between IDDM and specific HLA's encoded by the major histocompatibility complex region located on the short arm of the sixth chromosome (see Ch. 250) At each of these loci numerous alleles (genes) exist, some of which confer increased risk for the development of IDDM. These high-risk alleles include: HLA-DR3, HLA-DR4, HLA-B8, and HLA-B15. The HLA-A, B, and C antigens are present on virtually all nucleated cell types, whereas the HLA-DR antigens show tissue restriction and are predominantly expressed on B lymphocytes and macrophages. It is possible that DR antigens are also expressed on islet cells, but this is unproven at the current time.

An HLA haplotype refers to a particular set of alleles at the four closely linked HLA loci A, B, C, and D, on one of the sixth chromosomes (each person inherits two haplotypes, one from each parent). In this system, some of the alleles are in linkage disequilibrium. This means that certain HLA antigens encoded by alleles at the diffeent HLA loci occur together more frequently within the same haplotype than would be predicted by random statistical chance, taking gene (allele) frequency into account. The antigens encoded by the HLA alleles associated with higher risk for IDDM do not directly cause or predispose to the disease. Rather, these alleles are believed to be in linkage disequilibrium with genes in the HLA region (possibly certain immune response genes) that are directly related to the etiology of IDDM. In other words, through linkage disequilibrium one "looks" at the "diabetogenic gene" via the more easily measured HLA antigens.

The D locus appears to be more important than the B locus because it is more closely linked to the etiologically important genes. The increased risk for IDDM development imparted by inheritance of HLA-B8 and B15 is most likely a result of linkage disequilibrium between these HLA B locus alleles and the HLA alleles DR3 and DR4, respectively. Likewise, the risk imparted by HLA-DR4 is probably due to linkage disequilibrium with HLA-DQ B. HLA-DR and DQ molecules are heterodimers composed of α and β subunits. Both subunits are transmembrane molecules and are associated with each other in a noncovalent manner. Specific alleles at the DQ B locus may define at least one proximate diabetes risk gene encoding an immune system antigen that directly participates in IDDM etiology. A specific DQ B allele, missing the aspartic acid codon at position 57 of the B chain, can be detected by direct DNA analysis, and this allele is in linkage disequilibrium to the DR4 allele and directly predisposes to IDDM. The DR3 association with IDDM is linked to some other gene not associated with the DQ locus, and this gives evidence for the multigenic etiology of this disease. Interestingly, homozygosity at any of these alleles (i.e., DR3/DR3) does not lead to greater risk than when the allele occurs on only one haplotype. However, if both sixth chromosomes bear two different diabetes-associated alleles at a particular locus (i.e., DR3/DR4), the increase in risk is more than additive. The diabetes-associated HLA antigens are quite frequent in the nondiabetic population (although clearly less frequent than in IDDM). For example, 30 to 35 per cent of normal persons are positive for DR3 or DR4. Thus, far more people who are positive for these antigens are normal than have IDDM (e.g., if the average risk for IDDM in a population is 0.2 per cent, and if a particular HLA haplotype confers a 10-fold increase in risk, then the risk would still be only 2 per cent for those with this haplotype). This is an important point to realize in thinking about HLA typing for screening or predictive value in a practical or clinical sense.

Despite all this information, the model of inheritance for IDDM is obscure, although it is clearly not autosomal dominant. The low penetrance of the diabetes-associated genes combined with the relative degrees of HLA associations suggests that the genetic predisposition must interact with specific environmental factors for IDDM to occur. Additionally, the disease could be multigenic, with at least two genes necessary for IDDM to develop. With this model, environmental factors would still be necessary.

In NIDDM no HLA associations have been identified, demonstrating the differences in etiology between the two major forms of diabetes. Although the location of the genetic component for NIDDM is not known, possible changes have been noted on the eleventh chromosome, which contains the insulin gene. A 1.5 to 3.4 kilobase insertion of extra DNA, about 500 base pairs upstream from the 5' flanking end of the insulin gene, has been described by some workers as a polymorphism more frequent in patients with NIDDM than in normal persons or patients with IDDM. However, the association is slight and has not been found by all workers. Restriction fragment length polymorphisms have also been observed in the insulin receptor as well as glucose transporter genes, some of which have a statistically significant association with the NIDDM phenotype. However, the potential importance of any of these associations is unknown at present. Identification of the NIDDM gene(s) is of major interest, with enormous diagnostic and therapeutic potential. Since this is most likely a heterogeneous multigenic disease, the search will be a most difficult task.

PATHOGENESIS

Before discussion of the pathogenetic aspects of diabetes it is important to review briefly some of the essential features of insulin and glucose physiology. Insulin is produced in the pancreatic B cell as the primary biosynthetic product preproinsulin containing 109 amino acid residues (MW $\sim$ 11,500). This peptide is rapidly converted to proinsulin (86 amino acid residues, MW $\sim$ 9000) by cleavage of the amino terminal 23 amino acid "pre" sequence. Within the B cell secretory granules, proinsulin is converted by proteolytic cleavage to insulin (51 amino acids, MW $\sim$ 6000) and C peptide (31 amino acids, MW $\sim$ 3000). Thus, the final B cell secretory product is 95 per cent insulin and C peptide in equimolar amounts and 5 per cent unconverted proinsulin. In familial hyperproinsulinemia, mutations in the proinsulin sequence prevent proteolytic conversion within the secretory granule, leading to release of large amounts of proinsulin having only 7 to 10 per cent of insulin's biologic activity. The regulation of insulin release is extremely complex, being influenced by glucose, amino acids, gut insulinogenic hormones, glucagon, neural influences, and other factors. However, glucose is the most important stimulus for insulin secretion.

After a brief circulating time ($t_{1/2}$ 4 to 8 minutes) insulin interacts with target tissues to exert its biologic effects. At the target cell, insulin action is initiated by binding of the hormone to specific cell surface insulin receptors. The complete amino acid structure of the insulin receptor has been elucidated. Following formation of the insulin receptor complex one or more signals are propagated (second messengers) that interact with a variety of cellular effector systems such as enzymes and glucose transport proteins to produce insulin's ultimate biologic effects. Insulin exerts its major effects on carbohydrate homeostasis by stimulating peripheral glucose disposal and inhibiting hepatic glucose production. A variety of abnormalities in insulin biosynthesis, secretion, and action can lead to diabetes.

A number of other hormones, termed anti-insulin or counterregulatory hormones (glucagon, growth hormone, cortisol, and catecholamines), affect carbohydrate homeostasis. Among these, glucagon is probably most important in terms of the pathophysiology of diabetes. Glucagon is 29 amino acids (MW $\sim$ 3000) in length and is synthesized in the pancreatic α cells as proglucagon (MW $\sim$ 9000 to 11,000). Its release is stimulated by hypoglycemia, amino acids, neural influences, and stress. Its major effect on glucose metabolism is exerted at the liver where it binds to surface receptors, stimulates cyclic AMP generation, and promotes glycogenolysis, gluconeogenesis, and ketogenesis. Its lipolytic effects are minimal in man, and glucagon has little if any effect on peripheral glucose uptake. Thus, glucagon affects glucose metabolism by influencing hepatic glucose production, and glucagon levels are absolutely or relatively increased in both IDDM and NIDDM.

NIDDM. Abnormalities of insulin and, to a lesser extent, glucagon secretion and action are central to the pathogenesis of NIDDM. Syndromes involving abnormalities of insulin biosynthesis have already been discussed. These include familial hy-

perproinsulinemia and mutations in the structural gene for insulin leading to secretion of a biologically defective insulin molecule. These rare syndromes lead to mild degrees of glucose intolerance or a clinical picture indistinguishable from NIDDM. Beyond these unusual syndromes, however, insulin biosynthesis is qualitatively normal in NIDDM.

Secretion of insulin is not normal in NIDDM. In some patients with impaired glucose tolerance, substantially reduced amounts of insulin are secreted in response to a glucose load. These subjects are not insulin resistant and the defect in insulin secretion appears adequately to account for their abnormal glucose metabolism. These patients have a relatively high propensity to develop overt NIDDM (up to 50 per cent) and should be followed for progression. Other patients with impaired glucose tolerance secrete normal or increased amounts of insulin, although in some cases the dynamics of secretion may be altered a delay in release of insulin following a glucose stimulus. These patients are insulin resistant primarily because of decreased insulin receptors. This is true in both the obese and nonobese categories of this classification. In relatively few (about 5 per cent) of the hyperinsulinemic insulin-resistant patients with impaired glucose tolerance is there progression to fasting hyperglycemia.

The great majority of patients with NIDDM are both insulin deficient and insulin resistant. The decrease in insulin action exists whether they are obese or nonobese (although approximately 80 per cent are obese). Patients with NIDDM may have normal or elevated fasting insulin levels, but they almost always secrete decreased amounts of insulin following oral glucose or meals. Other functional abnormalities that have been identified include a marked decrease in early release of insulin (first phase) after intravenous administration of glucose, and much greater blunting of the insulin response to glucose compared to other insulin stimuli (amino acids, sulfonylureas, glucagon, or β agonists). These latter findings have given rise to the idea that β cell dysfunction in NIDDM may be characterized by a defect in glucose recognition by islet cells. Insulin deficiency tends to be more severe in patients with longstanding disease. Interestingly, amyloid-like proteinaceous deposits are found in the islet interstitium of many such patients. A peptide termed "islet amyloid polypeptide (IAPP)," or amylin, has been isolated from this islet amyloid material. IAPP is cosecreted with insulin from β cells, but its physiologic function is unknown. Possibly, deposition of IAPP to form these amyloid deposits has a deleterious impact on β cell function in longstanding NIDDM.

In addition to these abnormalities of insulin secretion, patients with NIDDM are also insulin resistant. Insulin action is a complex sequence of events beginning with binding to surface receptors; insulin resistance can be due to any abnormality at any step along the insulin action pathway. For convenience, the cellular causes of insulin resistance can be broadly divided into binding and postbinding defects (Fig. 218–1). A binding defect involves a decrease in insulin binding due to a decrease in either receptor number or affinity or to both. A postbinding defect refers to any biologically significant abnormality in the activity of effector proteins (such as insulin sensitive enzymes or transport proteins) or an impairment in the coupling or transducing mechanisms between insulin receptor complexes and effector units. In subjects with impaired glucose tolerance who are insulin resistant, binding defects exist (decreased receptor number), but postbinding function is normal. In NIDDM, insulin resistance exists in the great majority of patients. Although a receptor defect (decreased number) is present in most insulin-resistant NIDDM patients, this does not appear to be the major abnormality. Postbinding defects also exist, and these appear to play the predominant role in causing the insulin-resistant state. As far as glucose homeostasis is concerned, several postbinding defects have been described in NIDDM; e.g., these patients exhibit decreased β subunit tyrosine kinase activity, decreased rates of cellular glucose transport, and diminished glycogen synthase activity.

Insulin deficiency and insulin resistance both contribute to the hyperglycemia of NIDDM. In addition, another abnormality also contributes to the hyperglycemia. Hepatic glucose production rates are increased in NIDDM, and the magnitude of this increase is proportional to the level of fasting hyperglycemia. This hepatic abnormality is, at least partially, due to resistance to insulin's normal restraining effect on liver glucose production. Additionally, glucagon levels are often elevated, either absolutely or

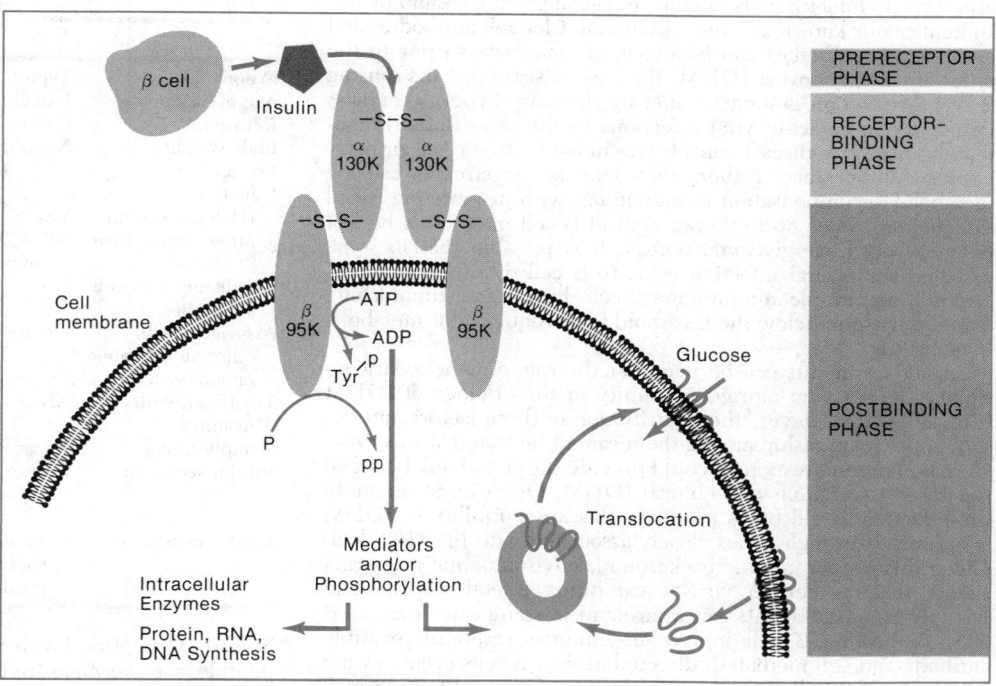

FIGURE 218–1. Model of insulin action and categories of insulin resistance. Insulin binds to the extracellular α-subunits of its receptor, stimulating tyrosine autophosphorylation of the transmembrane β subunits. This is followed by mediation of insulin's pleiotropic biologic effects, including recruitment of intracellular glucose transport proteins to the cell surface to facilitate glucose uptake. Abnormalities can occur at the prereceptor phase, involving biosynthesis and secretion of abnormal β cell products; at the receptor binding phase, involving decreased insulin binding to receptors due to decreased receptor number or affinity; or at the postbinding phase, involving any defect in the insulin action cascade distal to the initial binding event.

relatively, in NIDDM, and it is possible that excess glucagon stimulation also contributes to the increase in glucose production.

Thus, insulin deficiency, insulin resistance, and accelerated hepatic glucose production all exist in NIDDM, and all contribute to the hyperglycemia (Fig. 218–2). It is tempting to suggest a unifying pathogenetic hypothesis in which one metabolic lesion is primary and the others are secondary. Unfortunately it is not possible to choose any particular sequence at this time. All three abnormalities can be generated in animal models by inducing hyperglycemia and hypoinsulinemia, and all three are at least partially reversible with weight loss, oral sulfonylureas, or insulin therapy.

IDDM. *Autoimmunity* plays a major role in the etiology of IDDM. Circulating antibodies to thyroid, gastric mucosa, and the adrenal are far more common in patients with IDDM than in normal persons. More importantly, up to 90 per cent of patients with new-onset IDDM have demonstrable serum titers of islet cell antibodies. These antibodies are heterogeneous, some binding to cytoplasmic antigens common to all islet cells and others directed against the β cell surface. The latter lyse β cells

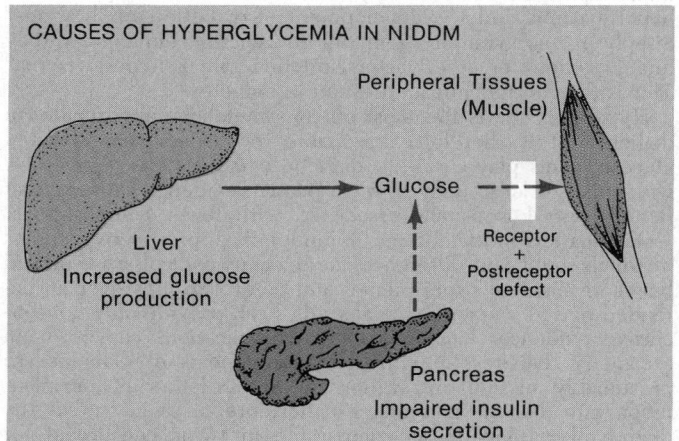

FIGURE 218–2. Summary of the metabolic abnormalities in NIDDM which contribute to the hyperglycemia. Increased hepatic glucose production, impaired insulin secretion, and insulin resistance due to receptor and postreceptor defects all combine to generate the hyperglycemic state.

in culture in the presence of complement, consistent with a pathophysiologic role in vivo. These islet cell antibodies are also observed in BB rats, an animal model that spontaneously develops an IDDM-like syndrome. Anti-insulin antibodies are also present with high frequency in IDDM sera. In humans, islet cell and anti-insulin antibodies can be detected at least several years prior to IDDM onset. Titers of these antibodies fall after the onset of clinical disease; by 5 years only 20 per cent of patients have demonstrable titers, and by 10 to 20 years the prevalence falls to 5 to 10 per cent. Patients who continue to demonstrate antibodies after several years may be examples of heterogeneity within IDDM. In these patients IDDM may represent a primary autoimmune disease, since they are largely female, show a great prevalence of other organ-specific antibodies, and have a strong family history of autoimmune disease. Patients with onset of IDDM at an older age tend to fall into this group. Genetically, they may also be different, since they have a greater prevalence of HLA-B8 and DR3. In cases of IDDM in which islet cell antibodies are cleared within 1 year of the disease's onset, patients are more often male, do not typically show signs of other autoimmune phenomena, experience onset of disease at a younger age, and have a higher association with HLA-B15 and HLA-DR4. Circulating antibodies may not be the only component of the immune response associated with IDDM; a cell-mediated immune response may also be involved. Increased K cells (killer lymphocytes) have been reported in IDDM along with alterations in T lymphocyte subpopulations. Both antibody-induced and cell-mediated immune phenomena may be involved in the pathogenesis of IDDM.

A strong genetic component is involved in the etiology of IDDM, but extragenetic factors must also contribute, at least in most patients. Several lines of evidence suggest a role for viruses in IDDM: (1) Autopsies of IDDM patients dying within a few months of the disease's onset have revealed an "insulitis" consisting of round cell infiltration of islet tissue. (2) A modest seasonal variation to the incidence of IDDM has been noted in some studies. (3) A clinical history of preceding viral-type illness, particularly coxsackie B and mumps, is often reported at the onset of IDDM. (4) Increased viral titers, including coxsackievirus B4, have been reported in IDDM patients at or near the time of the disease's onset. (5) Certain diabetogenic viruses (encephalomyocarditis M, coxsackievirus B, and rheovirus) can cause diabetes when inoculated into rodents. Further, the susceptibility of different rodent strains to develop virus-induced diabetes appears to be under genetic control. (6) Diabetogenic viruses can also directly infect β cells in culture, causing cell lysis and death. In light of our knowledge that circulating islet cell antibodies and anti-insulin antibodies can be detected many years prior to the onset of clinically overt IDDM, the basic disease process causing β cell destruction is longstanding by the time hyperglycemia is detected. Thus, acute viral infections in the time frame immediately prior to disease onset are unlikely to be of primary etiologic importance; rather, they may act as stresses causing metabolic decompensation in individuals with pre-existing β cell destruction. Since 80 to 90 per cent of β cell mass must be lost before overt hyperglycemia occurs, it is possible that in some cases an acute viral infection leads to β cell dysfunction superimposed on chronic autoimmune β cell destruction, diminishing insulin secretion below the threshold level required for metabolic homeostasis.

Strong arguments can be made for the role of genetic susceptibility viruses, and altered immunity in the etiology of IDDM (Fig. 218–3). However, the contribution of these factors and the sequential relationship among them cannot be stated at this time. Clearly, immune responses could provide the causal link between the HLA associations and clinical IDDM. One way to integrate these factors would be to postulate that susceptibility to IDDM is inherited through genes closely associated with the HLA loci. Given this proper genetic background, environmental triggering agents such as certain viruses exhibiting β cell tropism and possibly chemical agents can injure and in some cases destroy β cells. Following β cell injury, an immune response (possibly antibody and cell mediated) directed against β cells occurs owing to release of β cell antigens into the circulation, alteration of β cell antigens, cross-reactivity with viral antigens, or primary modulation of the immune response. In any event, the immune response would then exacerbate or complete the initial viral or chemical β cell injury. Of course this is only one of several sequences that can be proposed. IDDM is probably heterogeneous, and no single sequence of pathogenetic events necessarily explains all cases. For example, IDDM patients who are HLA-B8/DR3 display other organ-specific autoantibodies and probably have a primary autoimmune disease and do not need an environmental factor to trigger the disease. Regardless of the exact nature of the intertwining of genetic, viral, and immune influences, it is clear that β cell destruction is gradual, even though the clinical onset of metabolic decompensation is usually abrupt when destruction of β cell mass reaches a critical point or an intercurrent illness occurs. This raises the possibility of intervention therapies following the onset of β cell injury but prior to clinical manifestations of IDDM, since by the time IDDM appears β cell destruction may be too far advanced for effective preventive therapy. Such an approach would require a method to detect preclinical IDDM. Using a combination of autoantibody measurements and tests of insulin secretion, prediction of IDDM development is now possible in certain first-degree relatives of IDDM patients. This has allowed investigators to initiate clinical trials aimed at IDDM prevention in these selected individuals.

C peptide is secreted in equimolar amounts compared to insulin. Since C peptide has a much longer half-life than insulin, it provides an excellent measure of insulin secretory capacity, especially in those patients with circulating anti-insulin antibodies that interfere with usual insulin radioimmunoassays. In patients with IDDM who have been treated with insulin for longer than

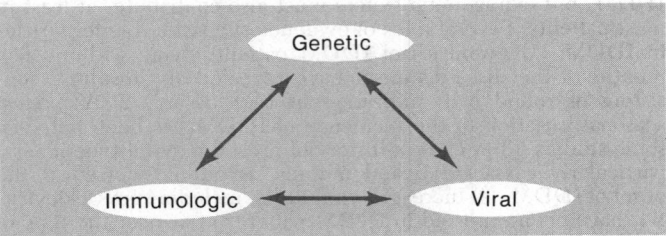

FIGURE 218–3. An interplay of genetic, immunologic, and viral etiologies contributes to the pathogenesis of NIDDM. The importance of each factor probably differs in subpopulations of IDDM, demonstrating the heterogeneity of this disease.

TABLE 218–2. SOME FEATURES DISTINGUISHING INSULIN-DEPENDENT FROM NON–INSULIN-DEPENDENT DIABETES

	IDDM	NIDDM
Synonym	Type I	Type II
Age of onset	Usually <30	Usually >40
Ketosis	Common	Rare
Body weight	Nonobese	Obese (80%)
Prevalence	0.2%–0.3%	2%–4%
Genetics		
HLA association	Yes	No
Monozygotic twin studies	40%–50% concordance rate	Concordance rate near 100%
Circulating islet cell antibodies	Yes	No
Associated with other autoimmune phenomena	Occasional	No
Treatment with insulin	Always necessary	Usually not required
Complications	Frequent	Frequent
Insulin secretion	Severe deficiency	Variable: moderate deficiency to hyperinsulinemia
Insulin resistance	Occasional: with poor control or excessive insulin antibodies	Usual: due to receptor and postreceptor defects

5 years, C peptide levels are usually undetectable. However, C peptide may be measured in many of these patients during the first years of their disease. This shows that complete loss of β cell secretion in IDDM is not abrupt, but progresses for several years after the diabetes becomes clinically apparent. For the most part, ease of diabetic management and stability of metabolic control in IDDM are correlated with the degree of residual insulin secretion. Those patients with the highest levels of circulating C peptide are easier to treat, and in those with undetectable levels the disease is more unstable. Some of the major clinical and pathophysiologic distinctions between IDDM and NIDDM are listed in Table 218–2.

TREATMENT

In this section, details concerning the various methods of diabetic management are discussed. However, since the severity and clinical picture of diabetes are quite variable, therapeutic methods are also varied. In particular, major differences exist in the approach to NIDDM versus IDDM, and whenever possible therapeutic distinctions for these two forms of diabetes will be made.

RELATIONSHIP BETWEEN HYPERGLYCEMIA AND COMPLICATIONS. It is important to start with more general principles and to identify overall therapeutic goals. A consideration of therapeutic goals involves one of the most important questions in the field, that is, what is the relationship between hyperglycemia and the development of diabetic complications? Simply put, are complications due to hyperglycemia or are they due to genetic or other factors independent of hyperglycemia? This is the central clinical question in diabetes.

Hyperglycemia is the most obvious metabolic abnormality in diabetes. It is therefore reasonable to suspect that elevated glucose levels play a role in diabetic complications. Consistent with this is a large body of retrospective evidence showing that better control is usually associated with fewer complications. Unfortunately, in the absence of randomized, prospective studies in which significant differences in glycemic control are achieved between matched experimental and control groups over an extended period, current clinical studies can provide only nonconclusive evidence. Classic diabetic complications can occur in secondary diabetes (in which genetic aspects of diabetes are presumably missing) and in normal kidneys following transplantation into diabetic patients. Furthermore, in twin studies the degree of retinopathy is comparable in twins concordant for IDDM, whereas in discordant pairs the nondiabetic twin does not have retinopathy. Certain abnormalities seen in diabetes, such as retinal capillary leakage (as demonstrated by fluorescein angiography), slowed motor nerve conductive velocity, and mi-

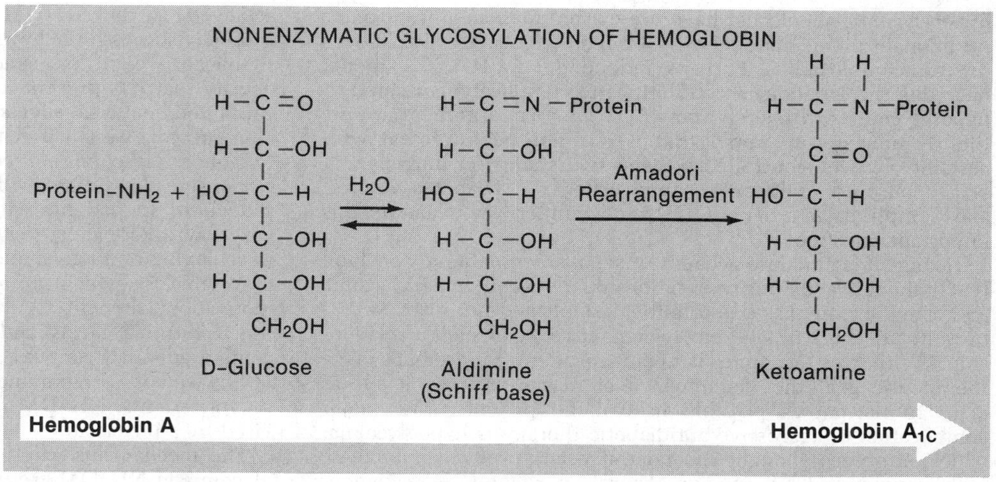

NONENZYMATIC GLYCOSYLATION OF HEMOGLOBIN

FIGURE 218–4. Chemical reactions underlying the nonenzymatic glycosylation of hemoglobin A to hemoglobin A_{1c}.

croalbuminuria, can be reversed by intensive insulin therapy, but the relationship between these physiologic abnormalities and clinically significant complications has not been demonstrated. In animal experiments a number of studies have shown good correlation between the level of hyperglycemia and microvascular complications similar (but perhaps not identical) to those seen in human diabetes. In animals, these complications can also be prevented or reversed with insulin therapy.

Several biochemical mechanisms have been proposed that may link hyperglycemia to complications. Proteins can be nonenzymatically glycosylated in vivo, and the degree of this glycosylation is directly related to the degree of hyperglycemia. Chromatography of red blood cell hemolysates shows four minor components (HbA_{1a1}, HbA_{1a2}, HbA_{1b1}, HbA_{1c}) of HbA, referred to as the HbA_1 fraction or "fast" hemoglobins (because of their more rapid elution from columns). HbA_1 is due to post-translational, nonenzymatic modification of HbA and comprises about 6 per cent of total hemoglobin in normal persons. HbA_{1c} comprises approximately two thirds of these minor components and is increased in the presence of hyperglycemia. To form HBA_{1c}, glucose combines with the N terminal valine of β chains to form a Schiff base aldimine (Fig. 218–4). This compound is relatively unstable, and the reaction is readily reversible. The aldimine undergoes an Amadori rearrangement to form the more stable ketoamine. HbA can also be glycosylated through the same chemical reaction at the N terminus of the α chain and ε amino groups of lysines. HbA_{1c} can be measured by various chromatographic techniques, and total glycosylated hemoglobin can be measured chemically. Glycosylation occurs continuously within the red cell and is a direct reflection of the average glucose concentration to which the cell is exposed throughout its 120-day lifespan. Measurement of glycosylated hemoglobin content therefore provides a useful means to assess the chronic degree of hyperglycemia that existed in a given patient over the preceding several weeks and is not affected by acute changes in plasma glucose level. Additionally, the nonspecific and nonenzymatic nature of hemoglobin glycosylation raises the possibility that glycosylation of other body proteins can occur, leading to structural or functional changes that may be related to chronic diabetic complications. Increased amounts of glycosylated low-density lipoprotein (LDL) molecules, for example, circulate in hyperglycemic diabetic patients and do not bind normally to LDL receptors. Since abnormal glycosylation may affect all tissues, this mechanism could be related to a variety of diabetic complications.

Additional biochemical lesions related to hyperglycemia have been proposed for nervous tissue. *Sorbitol* is a polyhydroxyl alcohol (polyol) produced from glucose by aldose reductase in nerve tissue; once formed, sorbitol can be converted to fructose (Fig. 218–5). It is theorized that this polyol pathway is particularly active in diabetes because of the hyperglycemia. This could lead to increased intracellular osmolarity (due to accumulation of sorbitol and fructose) with water influx, swelling of Schwann cells, anoxia, and demyelination. Consistent with this, an increase

in sorbitol content has been found in nerve tissue of diabetic rats, and it is reversible with insulin therapy. However, Schwann cell swelling and increased water content have not yet been demonstrated, and further testing of the polyol pathway hypothesis is necessary. Another hyperglycemia-related metabolic lesion in nervous tissue has been proposed involving *myoinositol*. Concentrations of this compound are decreased in peripheral nerves of diabetic rats, and this is associated with a decrease in nerve conduction velocity. These abnormalities can be prevented by insulin or oral myoinositol supplements. It is possible that uptake of myoinositol by nerves is inhibited by hyperglycemia, leading to depletion and pathologic sequelae. A link may exist between polyol and myoinositol metabolism in that increased activity of the polyol pathway contributes to the reduction in nerve myoinositol content.

The above discussion cites clinical and biochemical evidence supporting the relationship between hyperglycemia and complications. On the other hand, there is evidence against this relationship. For example, patients have been reported with diabetic complications at the time of onset of IDDM, when

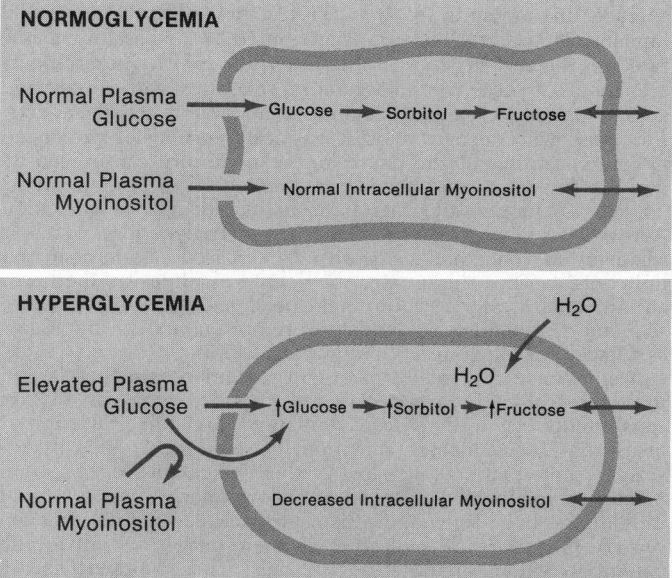

FIGURE 218–5. Metabolic theories for the pathogenesis of diabetic neuropathy secondary to hyperglycemia. This demonstrates the suggested effects of hyperglycemia to increase intracellular sorbitol and fructose concentrations, leading to an osmotic increase in intracellular water content. In addition, it has been suggested that hyperglycemia depletes intracellular myoinositol content by competitively inhibiting the uptake of myoinositol from the extracellular space.

hyperglycemia should not have pre-existed for a significant time. Additionally, some patients with very poor glycemic control never develop complications. Perhaps, independent of IDDM, patients have differing genetic susceptibilities to complications related to hyperglycemia. Ultimately, however, the main argument against the relationship is simply that it has not been proven with certainty by well-controlled, prospective studies in humans. An NIH-sponsored multicenter study called the Diabetes Control and Complications Trial (DCCT) is now under way to answer this important question.

Taking all factors into account, it seems reasonable to conclude that although a definitive relationship between hyperglycemia and complications has been neither established nor disproved at present, the bulk of evidence weighs in favor of such a relationship. With this in mind it seems prudent to establish as a therapeutic goal the maintenance of plasma glucose levels as close to normal as possible in diabetic patients. The major complication of aggressive antidiabetic therapy is hypoglycemia, which, if severe enough, can unequivocally produce immediate and irreversible CNS damage. Therefore, diabetic management should be pushed until glucose levels are normal or near normal, unless recurrent, overt episodes of hypoglycemia develop. If this occurs, then compromises are necessary in the degree of glycemic control achieved. Other therapeutic goals include (1) normal growth and development in children, (2) normal pregnancy and childbirth in females, (3) reduction of diabetes-related atherosclerosis risk factors, especially in adult diabetic patients, and (4) minimal interference with normal lifestyle in all diabetics.

DIETARY TREATMENT. Dietary treatment is an integral part of the overall therapeutic plan in all diabetic patients. In many NIDDM patients dietary therapy can be the predominant method of treatment. Dietary therapy is concerned with the total number of calories ingested, the distribution of calories throughout the day, the individual food sources that make up these calories, and maintenance of proper nutrition. Dietary therapy is much different in NIDDM and IDDM, because patients in the former are usually obese, whereas in the latter they are not, and NIDDM patients retain endogenous insulin secretion while IDDM patients do not.

Total Caloric Intake. Since most NIDDM patients are overweight, caloric restriction is advisable and can be of great benefit. The essential tenet of weight reduction is straightforward: If caloric expenditure exceeds intake, weight will be lost. There are many ways to calculate daily caloric expenditure, but on the average this amounts to 30 to 35 kcal per kilogram in normal humans; 25 kcal per kilogram is attributed to the basal metabolic rate and the rest to physical activity. Daily caloric requirements are about 30 kcal per kilogram in sedentary individuals and approximately 35 kcal per kilogram in moderately active subjects. For those who engage in brisk physical exertion for prolonged intervals throughout the day caloric expenditure can exceed 35 kcal per kilogram. Another factor affecting caloric requirements (at least on a per kilogram basis) is the degree of adiposity. Adipose tissue is predominantly storage triglyceride, which is relatively inert metabolically with a decreased caloric need per unit weight. Thus the greater the degree of adiposity, the lower an individual's caloric requirement per kilogram. In very obese, sedentary individuals, daily caloric requirements can be as low as 25 kcal per kilogram of body weight.

A number of approaches to weight reduction exist that vary in the degree of caloric restriction and rate of weight loss, dietary constituents, as well as behavioral and psychological support measures. These include nutritionally sound and modestly restricted diets that achieve slow gradual weight loss over several months, nutritionally balanced very low calorie diets for rapid weight loss, behavior modification, pharmacologic aids, and even surgical procedures (i.e., gastric plication) in the morbidly obese patient in whom medical therapy fails. These approaches are discussed in detail in Ch. 203.

For all these methods, inducing the initial period of weight loss is not the major problem in weight reduction, but, rather, the major problem is weight regain or recidivism. Motivated patients can usually successfully lose weight over the initial dietary period, but it is the unusual patient who successfully keeps the pounds off. The major challenge in weight reduction

therapy is to develop a proper supportive environment and patient motivation to maintain weight loss after it has been achieved. In the NIDDM patient, significant caloric restriction is usually successful in lowering plasma glucose levels even before significant weight loss is achieved. Depending on the degree of obesity that was present initially and the amount of weight loss, continued beneficial effects on glycemic control can be maintained after the goal weight is achieved and a eucaloric diet is initiated. In general, the more recent the onset of NIDDM, the more responsive the patient will be to the beneficial effects of weight reduction. In patients with pronounced fasting hyperglycemia, very low calorie diets (300 to 600 kcal per day) are often useful in achieving rapid glycemic control as well as an initial rapid rate of weight loss (which can often be of important psychological and motivational benefit). Very low calorie diets usually consist of liquid formula meals and should not be utilized unless they contain adequate amounts (a minimum 30 to 40 grams per day) of high-quality protein and are supplemented with vitamins and micronutrients. NIDDM patients on such diets should be supervised by a physician.

The mechanisms whereby weight reduction improves hyperglycemia in NIDDM are not completely clear. Weight loss leads to a reduction in the accelerated rates of hepatic glucose production, ameliorates the degree of insulin resistance by increasing insulin receptors and reducing the magnitude of the postreceptor defect in insulin action, and possibly improves β cell secretion. However, the precise cellular mechanisms leading to these effects are not known. Patients with IDDM are seldom obese, and an important nutritional goal is maintenance of adequate nutrition, particularly to assure normal growth and development in children and pregnant women.

Distribution of Calories. In addition to total caloric consumption, attention should also be paid to the distribution of calories throughout the day in any dietary prescription. Two principles should be kept in mind: (1) calories should be spread as evenly as possible throughout the major daily meals to avoid a large concentration of calories at any one meal and not to overwhelm the diabetic patient's impaired capacity to metabolize food; and (2) in those patients receiving exogenous insulin, caloric intake should be temporally adjusted to coincide with the time course of action of the administered insulin. The latter point highlights a major difference in dietary consideration between patients with IDDM and those with NIDDM. In NIDDM, endogenous insulin secretion is still present and the β cell can respond at the appropriate times (albeit to a limited degree) to food ingestion, regardless of when it occurs throughout the day. This is even true, although to a lesser extent, in NIDDM subjects who are treated with insulin. Thus, in these patients it is sufficient to balance calories throughout the day, but the patient has a good deal of leeway to determine the timing of specific meals as long as calories are ingested at times of peak exogenous insulin action. For practical purposes, the only insulin present in patients with IDDM is that which is administered exogenously. Therefore, patients must pay close attention to the timing of meals and must be certain that there is reasonable concordance between meal ingestion and the time course of action of the insulin they have taken. To a certain extent the patient can elect a temporal pattern suitable to his lifestyle and preference and the insulin therapy regimen can then be tailored appropriately. In this way greater flexibility is allowed that improves overall patient compliance and quality of life.

Nutrient Content of Diet. A great deal of attention is currently being paid to the individual components comprising the diabetic diet. When patients consume eucaloric diets, it is important that they be properly balanced and nutritionally sound. A generally accepted protein requirement is 0.8 gram per kilogram per day for adults, but larger amounts are usually consumed in Western diets. Thus, protein usually comprises about 15 per cent of total caloric consumption. With this as a base, the proportions of fat and carbohydrate (CHO) are inversely related. Previous attempts to restrict total CHO intake are no longer deemed advisable, and most authorities now advocate liberalization of CHO intake to 50 to 55 per cent of total calories. This means that total fat intake should not exceed 30 to 35 per cent, and because diabetic patients are predisposed to macrovascular disease, saturated fat (primarily animal fat) intake should be reduced so that the polyunsaturated-saturated fat ratio is equivalent to 1:0. Ideally, cholesterol intake should not exceed 450 mg per day, and even lower levels of intake are advisable. The recommendation of a low saturated fat, low cholesterol diet is particularly important in NIDDM patients because of the high prevalence of concomitant hyperlipidemias. The makeup of the CHO portion of the diet also requires attention. In the past it was believed that diabetics should rigorously avoid sucrose because it is rapidly absorbed and raises the blood glucose level inordinately. Although this may be true when sucrose is consumed as the sole nutritive component, as in soft drinks or certain candies, it is less of a problem when modest amounts of sucrose are eaten in a mixed meal setting. Because of this, up to 5 per cent of total CHO can be consumed as added sucrose, as long as it is taken in the context of a mixed meal and spaced out through the day. This allows the diabetic a wider variety of food choices, making the diet more palatable; a side benefit of this approach is that it improves patient adherence to the dietary prescription and to the other elements of the overall therapeutic plan. The remainder of the CHO should consist predominantly of starches. All complex CHO cannot be lumped together as a single food group because the glycemic response to different starches differs widely, being lowest for lentils and pasta and highest for wheat and potatoes. More work needs to be done to determine the glycemic potency of a large number of foods, singly and together, in diabetic patients before the precise composition of the CHO in the diet can be recommended with certainty. At this stage it is advisable for the diabetic to consume 50 to 55 per cent of calories as CHO with a modest restriction in sucrose intake and emphasis on ingestion of those complex CHOs with low glycemic potency.

Fructose is a nutritive sweetener that may also have a place in the diabetic diet. This simple CHO is somewhat sweeter than sucrose and has similar properties when prepared in foods. Thus, fructose can be substituted for sucrose in most foods with little change in taste or texture. The advantage is that fructose is absorbed from the gastrointestinal tract more slowly than sucrose and is predominantly taken up and metabolized by the liver through non–insulin-dependent mechanisms. Within the liver, fructose is phosphorylated and eventually converted to glycogen or triglyceride through the triose phosphate intermediates. Thus, little fructose escapes hepatic uptake to enter the peripheral circulation, and only a small amount of fructose is converted to glucose for release from the liver. Ingestion of fructose leads to a minimal postprandial rise in plasma glucose or insulin levels in normal persons and in diabetics when taken alone or as part of a mixed meal. For these reasons, fructose offers some advantage in the diabetic diet, and amounts up to 75 grams per day can be safely consumed. The major exception occurs in patients with severely uncontrolled NIDDM or in poorly insulinized IDDM patients. In these conditions glycogen production is inhibited and fructose enters the gluconeogenic pathway and is ultimately released as glucose, causing hyperglycemia.

Dietary fiber can also influence CHO absorption. Glycemic excursions are reduced and insulin secretion diminished when normal persons and subjects with NIDDM consume fiber-enriched diets. This effect is mediated through delayed gastric emptying and overall slowing of the rate of CHO digestion and absorption. Since large amounts of fiber (10 to 15 grams per meal) are needed to observe these effects, major changes in dietary patterns would be necessary to achieve beneficial results. Nevertheless, when fiber is consumed as natural foods, there do not seem to be any untoward effects of increased fiber ingestion, and some studies indicate that increased fiber intake can lower serum triglyceride levels. The only potential caveat to this statement involves growing children and pregnant women, since subtle undesirable changes in micronutrient absorption due to high fiber ingestion have not been ruled out.

A minority of diabetic patients adhere to the recommended dietary regimens. To a large extent this is due to inadequate understanding on the part of the patient as well as the physician regarding dietary goals and methods. An additional factor is that dietary therapy must be individualized, taking into account each patient's lifestyle, economic status, food preferences, and social needs. This can be a time-consuming process, and few physicians have the time or training to participate with patients in this type of detailed dietary management. For this reason it is critical to incorporate a dietitian or nutritionist trained in the principles of dietary therapy of diabetes as part of the health care team. One cannot simply give pamphlets, instructional aids, and meal plans and expect even motivated patients to adhere to the necessary regimens. Detailed instruction by a nutrition counselor is necessary to tailor the diet to each patient's special needs. Dietary therapy is a means of long-term treatment, and therefore the longer view is important. Occasional deviations from recommended meal plans for special occasions are acceptable, provided that the patient has a clear understanding of how this should be managed. Often this allows for better patient compliance with the overall diet plan. Periodic meetings with a nutrition counselor are necessary to implement and maintain individualized dietary regimens.

ORAL HYPOGLYCEMIC AGENTS. Oral hypoglycemic agents are often therapeutically effective in NIDDM patients. In patients who do not respond satisfactorily to diet and do not have severe hyperglycemia (i.e., plasma glucose levels consistently greater than 250 mg per deciliter), oral agents are an appropriate therapeutic choice. In patients with severe hyperglycemia, insulin therapy is preferable, at least initially, to gain more rapid control of clinical symptoms and to prevent hyperosmolarity. While sulfonylureas are effective in patients with NIDDM, they are ineffective in IDDM. Some have suggested that combinations of oral agents with insulin can reduce insulin requirements of IDDM; however, this has not been proven, and would be of minor clinical importance anyway.

The mechanism of action of sulfonylureas is complex. In the short term, they augment β cell insulin secretion. However, after several months of therapy, insulin levels return to pretreatment values while glucose levels remain improved. These findings led to the demonstration that sulfonylureas exert extrapancreatic effects on glucose metabolism: (1) They reduce the accelerated rates of hepatic glucose production in NIDDM; (2) they partially reverse the postbinding defect in insulin action; and (3) they increase the number of cellular insulin receptors. These all represent significant components of the insulin resistance of NIDDM, so sulfonylureas can improve glycemia by improving insulin's effectiveness at target cells. The relative importance of each of these actions in ameliorating hyperglycemia is unclear, but it is likely that the pancreatic and extrapancreatic effects of these agents combine to produce the hypoglycemic action of these drugs.

There are several different kinds of sulfonylureas, differing primarily in potency, pharmacokinetics, and modes of metabolism as outlined in Table 218–3. *Tolbutamide* is metabolized to inert products by the liver and has a relatively short half-life, necessi-

TABLE 218–3. CHARACTERISTICS OF SULFONYLUREAS

Generic Name	Brand Name	Dosage Range (mg)	Duration of Action (hr)	Comments
Tolbutamide	Orinase	500–3000	6–12	Metabolized by liver to inert products, given 2–3 ×/day
Chlorpropamide	Diabinese	100–500	60	Metabolized by liver (~70%) to less active metabolite, and excreted intact (~30%) by kidneys; can potentiate ADH action, given 1×/day
Acetohexamide	Dymelor	250–1500	12–24	Metabolized by liver to active metabolite, given 1–2×/day
Tolazamide	Tolinase	100–1000	10–18	Metabolized by liver to active product, given 1–2×/day
Glyburide	Micronase	2.5–30	10–30	Metabolized by liver to inert products, given 1×/day
Glipizide	Glucotrol	5–40	18–30	Metabolized by liver to inert products, given 1×/day

tating administration two to three times a day. Although it is the least potent of the available sulfonylureas on a weight basis, it has not been clearly demonstrated that any sulfonylurea produces greater hypoglycemic potency at maximal doses in diabetic patients. Therefore, for practical purposes, the differences in relative potency of the different drugs simply mean that more or less of a given agent should be used. *Tolazamide* and especially *acetohexamide* are metabolized by the liver to biologically active products that are then excreted by the kidneys. These drugs have intermediate half-lives and are usually given twice (but sometimes once) a day. *Chlorpropamide* also undergoes considerable hepatic degradation into less active metabolites excreted in the urine. This compound can cause significant water retention and hyponatremia by potentiating ADH action on the kidney. Chlorpropamide has the longest circulating half-life and duration of action (about 60 hours) and is given only once a day. Hypoglycemia is the major complication of sulfonylureas, and this can be particularly severe with chlorpropamide because of its long duration of action. Elderly NIDDM subjects are more susceptible to hypoglycemia, especially those prone to skip meals. The route of metabolism of the different compounds may influence the choice of agent. One should be cautious about the use of chlorpropamide, acetohexamide, and, to a lesser extent, tolazamide in patients with compromised renal function because of the route of excretion. Second-generation sulfonylureas, such as *glibenclamide* (or glyburide) and *glipizide*, have rapidly assumed a major share of the market, largely displacing the first-generation agents. These compounds are metabolized by the liver and have a relatively long duration of action. They can often be given once a day, although twice a day dosing is usually required in patients with initial fasting glucose levels greater than 220 mg per deciliter. A general guideline would be to progress up to 10 mg per day in the A.M. for either drug and if satisfactory control is not achieved then add a P.M. dose. It is claimed, but not rigorously demonstrated, that the second-generation sulfonylureas are more effective than the first-generation drugs.

The other major category of oral hypoglycemic agents consists of the biguanides, such as *phenformin*. The exact mechanism of action of these drugs is not clear, although they may interfere with hepatic gluconeogenesis. However, these drugs were strongly implicated in the development of lactic acidosis and have been prohibited from clinical use in the United States by the Food and Drug Administration.

In NIDDM, the usual practice is to begin with a low dose of a given sulfonylurea, advancing the dose until the therapeutic response is satisfactory or a maximal dose is reached. Occasionally patients who do not respond to one drug can be switched to another with beneficial effect. Most patients who do not achieve a therapeutic response with a given sulfonylurea will not respond satisfactorily by switching to another. Enough patients do respond to this approach, however, so that it is an appropriate tactic before it is concluded that oral hypoglycemic drugs are not effective in a specific patient. Certain drug interactions occur with sulfonylureas, that is, phenylbutazone and anticoagulants compete for hepatic removal mechanisms with sulfonylureas. A disulfiram (Antabuse)-like reaction can occasionally occur following alcohol consumption by patients taking sulfonylureas. This is most frequently reported with chlorpropamide and has not yet been noted with the second-generation agents. Potential interactions of this sort should always be kept in mind in the appropriate clinical context.

Approximately 10 to 20 per cent of NIDDM patients do not respond to oral agents, and treatment is termed primary failure. Secondary failure occurs when a patient responds initially to an oral agent, but then ceases to respond in the next year or two. This occurs in 5 to 20 per cent of patients, but these proportions obviously depend on the particular NIDDM population studied. For example, patients with new-onset diabetes respond better than those with longstanding disease. In some cases, secondary failure is due to dietary noncompliance in a patient who previously successfully adhered to a dietary regimen. However, this is often not the case, and the mechanisms of secondary failure in many patients with NIDDM remain unknown.

Debate exists as to which patients with NIDDM are appropriate candidates for oral sulfonylurea therapy. In view of the evidence implicating hyperglycemia with diabetic complications, the therapeutic goal with oral agents should be the maintenance of glucose levels as near to normal as possible. In patients with mild to moderate fasting hyperglycemia (140 to 230 mg per deciliter), dietary therapy should be tried first; if the above therapeutic goals are not achieved with this approach, then a sulfonylurea can be added. The problem arises in patients with more severe fasting hyperglycemia (more than 230 mg per deciliter) who have pronounced clinical symptoms despite dietary treatment. In these patients, some would advise an initial period of sulfonylurea therapy, and if satisfactory control is not achieved, then insulin treatment should be substituted. Others would suggest an initial period of insulin therapy following which the patient is switched to sulfonylureas; if satisfactory control is achieved, the drug is continued. Alternatively, insulin can be used indefinitely in these patients. Clearly this is a gray area, and the particular approach should be individualized to each patient, taking into account the total clinical context of the patient's disease, acceptance of the various therapeutic methods, level of diabetes education, and motivation. In a patient in whom severe fasting hyperglycemia is maintained, with marked clinical symptoms and incipient hyperosmolarity, oral agents are probably not appropriate, at least initially. In these patients insulin therapy should be the primary mode of treatment and can be continued indefinitely, or a therapeutic trial of sulfonylureas can be substituted once the hyperglycemia has been brought under control by the initial period of insulin treatment. In general, response to sulfonylurea therapy is best if the onset of diabetes is recent and the patient is over 40 years of age and not thin.

INSULIN TREATMENT. Insulin is the primary mode of therapy in all patients with IDDM and in many with NIDDM (see above). The goals of therapy include (1) normal growth and development in children, (2) normal pregnancy, delivery, and conceptus in women, (3) minimal interference with psychosocial adjustment, (4) acceptable glycemic control, with minimal hypoglycemia, and (5) prevention of complications. Little disagreement exists concerning goals 1 to 3; however, different views exist of how best to achieve goals 4 and 5. There are many different methods of insulin therapy, and the method chosen is highly dependent on one's views of goals 4 and 5. If a physician holds closely to the important relationship between control and complications, then "acceptable control" will be much more rigorously defined and a method of insulin treatment that is designed to produce the desired response will be chosen. On the other hand, those who question the link between hyperglycemia and complications are advocates of looser control and utilize a less intensive method of insulin delivery. In general, it is quite easy to eliminate overt symptoms of hyperglycemia with any method of insulin therapy, but it is extremely difficult, and probably impossible, to achieve euglycemia on a 24-hour basis. How close one comes to this ideal depends on the method of insulin delivery chosen, which in turn depends on one's philosophy of diabetic management.

At this time, the prevailing opinion among diabetologists is that hyperglycemia contributes substantially to complications. With this view, treatment of hyperglycemia (with any therapeutic modality) should be undertaken with specific glycemic target ranges in mind in order to bring the plasma glucose as close to normal as possible without unacceptable hypoglycemia. Target glucose levels recommended by the American Diabetes Association for NIDDM management are: fasting blood glucose less than 140 mg per deciliter and 2-hour postprandial blood glucose less than 200 mg per deciliter.

Insulin Preparations. To begin a discussion of the methods of insulin treatment, let us first consider the many different kinds of insulin available. Commercial insulin comes in concentrations of 100 units per milliliter (U-100) and 500 units per milliliter (U-500). The various insulin preparations differ in their time course of action (rapid, intermediate, and long acting), degree of purity, and source (beef, pork, beef-pork, or human synthetic insulin); these properties are outlined in Table 218–4. By adjustment of pH during preparation, the size of the zinc-insulin crystal can be modified; the larger the crystals, the slower the release after subcutaneous injection, and this accounts for the differences in time of action between semilente (rapid-acting) and ultralente (long-acting) insulin. Lente (intermediate-acting) insulin is simply a 30:70 mixture of semilente and ultralente, respectively. The

TABLE 218–4. PROPERTIES OF VARIOUS INSULIN PREPARATIONS

Class	Type	Peak Effect (hr)	Duration of Action (hr)
Rapid	Regular crystalline insulin (CZI)	2–4	6–8
	Semilente	2–6	10–12
Intermediate	Neutral protamine (NPH)	6–12	18–24
	Lente	6–12	18–24
Long Acting	Protamine zinc (PZI)	14–24	36
	Ultralente	18–24	36

other method to delay the onset of action of injected insulin is to mix it with a protein (protamine) and adjust the pH. This results in NPH (intermediate-acting) and PZI (long-acting) preparations. It should be cautioned that the values for peak onset and duration of action listed in Table 218–4 are simply estimates. There is a great deal of variability in these values from patient to patient as a result of circulating anti-insulin antibodies that alter the pharmacokinetics of insulin, variation in subcutaneous absorption, individual responses, and other factors. Additionally, absorption of insulin may be quite variable within a single patient from day to day, since absorption of subcutaneous insulin is markedly increased by vigorous exercise of the injected extremity, or by heating or massage of the injection site. Differences in purity also exist. Conventional insulin preparations contain less than 10,000 parts per million (ppm) of impurities; improved single peak insulin, less than 50 ppm; and "purified" insulin, 1 to 10 ppm. The impurities mentioned are predominantly proinsulin, with smaller amounts of insulin dimers, proinsulin-like products, glucagon, pancreatic polypeptide, somatostatin, and vasoactive polypeptide. For practical purposes, commercially available insulin preparations are labeled as purified (1 to 10 ppm); if they are not specifically labeled, they contain 20 to 50 ppm. The older, less pure forms are no longer widely distributed. Essentially all preparations can be obtained as purified pork, beef, or beef-pork mixtures. Finally, highly purified human insulin is now available as a product of recombinant DNA biosynthesis or chemical conversion of pork to human insulin.

Methods of Treatment. The insulin regimen can be more or less intensive, depending on the number of injections per day, types of insulin used, and frequency and method of assessing control. Many NIDDM patients, and occasional IDDM patients, can achieve excellent glycemic control with a single daily (morning) injection of an intermediate-acting insulin. Because of post-breakfast hyperglycemia, it is often necessary to mix a short-acting preparation with this single dose. In most patients who realize excellent control with this regimen, endogenous insulin secretion is retained. A somewhat more intensive method to regulate glycemia involves a split-dosage regimen. This includes morning (before breakfast) and evening (before dinner) injection of mixtures of intermediate- and rapid-acting insulin. About two thirds of the total daily dose is usually given in the morning and about one third in the evening; the proportion of intermediate-to rapid-acting insulin at each injection is usually two thirds to one third. In patients receiving single-dose therapy who require more than 50 to 60 units per day a split-dose regimen should usually be tried. In a 70-kg man, normal 24-hour insulin output has been estimated at 25 units per day. Therefore, in normal-sized diabetic subjects starting insulin therapy, it is reasonable to begin with a total daily dose of about 20 units per day with upward adjustments every several days based on the level of blood glucose. In mildly obese IDDM patients, starting doses can be 5 to 10 units per day higher. Because of insulin resistance, obese NIDDM patients requiring insulin often need 60 to 90 units per day. With the availability of highly purified insulins (both human and animal) that are less antigenic, it is probably advisable to start all new patients with one of these insulin preparations. With the above methods of insulin delivery, assessment of glycemic control can be carried out in several ways. Measurements of urinary glucose and ketones can be obtained before breakfast and once or twice throughout the day. Patients should be instructed to void 30 minutes before obtaining urine for glucose determination (double voiding), particularly for the morning sample, so that the urinary glucose is more representative of the corresponding blood glucose. Regardless of how carefully urinary glucose is determined, it provides only a rough approximation of blood glucose levels. Factors such as renal threshold, renal blood flow, and urine volume greatly affect the meaning of urine glucose measurements (i.e., a 4+ reaction in a concentrated urine sample is of little significance compared to a 4+ reaction in a dilute sample). For these reasons, urinary glucose is a poor way to monitor diabetic control and if at all possible should not be relied upon as the sole guide on which to base the insulin regimen. Twenty-four-hour urinary glucose excretion can be periodically assessed to provide a better estimate of daylong control (less than 5 grams per day is excellent control). Glycosylated hemoglobin can be measured and provides an excellent assessment of the overall state of glycemic control during the preceding few weeks. The best current method to assess glycemic control is home-, or self-, monitoring of glucose (see below). This requires the patient to assess his own blood glucose level daily and to make appropriate adjustments in insulin dosage. This approach places a large part of the management responsibility in the hands of the patient and emphasizes the need for a continuous outpatient education program.

When patients with new-onset IDDM are started on insulin therapy, after an initial period of stabilization, insulin requirements frequently decrease dramatically over the ensuing few weeks. This is the so-called honeymoon phenomenon, and it is sometimes possible to maintain nearly normal levels of glycemia without administering any insulin. This honeymoon phase may last for a few weeks and sometimes as long as 1 to 2 years. It is invariably followed by worsening of metabolic control with permanent recrudescence of the insulin-dependent state. Some experts have recommended that during this honeymoon period insulin administration should never be completely stopped, even if dosages have to be reduced to homeopathic levels. The reason for this is the fear that if there is a prolonged period in which insulin is not administered, once insulin therapy is reinstituted an anamnestic response with rising titers of anti-insulin antibodies might occur. However, with use of the highly purified insulin preparations now available, or with biosynthetic human insulin, this may be less of a problem.

If more intensive insulin management is required to achieve closer to normal glycemic control, then multiple daily injections of insulin or continuous subcutaneous insulin infusion (CSII) are used. At the current time these approaches are generally limited to patients with IDDM. However, if ideal control of glycemia is the therapeutic goal, there is no reason these methods could not be used in patients with NIDDM whose disease cannot be satisfactorily controlled by other means. Multiple injections involve administration of regular insulin before each meal, with the dose adjusted to the anticipated meal size. This is usually combined with either a long-acting or an intermediate-acting preparation in the evening.

The most intensive method of insulin delivery is CSII. This consists of constant insulin delivery into a subcutaneous site in the abdominal wall via an open loop delivery device consisting of a small insulin pump that must be worn by the patient essentially 24 hours a day. The key to this method of therapy is the constant delivery of basal insulin. The basal insulin infusion is supplemented by a preprandial bolus of insulin given 15 minutes prior to meal ingestion. This gives the patient a fair degree of flexibility in the timing and content of meals, since the preprandial bolus is given at the patient's discretion in an amount picked to match meal size. In general, the basal insulin infusion accounts for about 50 per cent of the total daily insulin dose and usually averages 0.5 to 1 unit per hour. Typically, preprandial boluses are 5 to 10 units, depending on meal size, time of day, and proximity to time of exercise. To be successful, intensive insulin therapy regimens must be combined with home- (or self-) monitoring of glucose. This requires the patient to obtain capillary blood by finger prick for glucose measurement, using a reflectance meter. There are numerous devices and algorithms for constant insulin delivery and various approaches to the frequency and method of glucose self-measurements. A detailed discussion of these issues is beyond the scope of this chapter. With properly motivated and educated patients and physicians, excellent control can be achieved in nearly all subjects. Patients generally accept this mode of therapy quite well and report an increased feeling of well-being. However, CSII should not be used indiscriminately, since pump dysfunction does occur, and hypoglycemia is a real problem, especially nocturnally. Additionally, a great deal is asked of patients when they participate in these programs in terms of dedication, education, and changes in lifestyle.

Many other insulin treatment schedules have been proposed, all of which represent variations on the above common themes. Some of these are listed in Table 218–5. No single method is inherently superior to any other, and it is probably best for a physician to become accustomed to one or two methods and use them more or less exclusively so that he will be familiar with problems associated with insulin therapy and its individualization. All of these approaches are meant as guidelines rather than rigid algorithms.

Regardless of the insulin regimen employed, an established daily dose in a given patient must not be considered to be fixed. Even long-established insulin dosages may need to be increased because of changes in growth status, subtle intercurrent illness or stress, or development of anti-insulin antibodies. Dosages may need to be decreased because of consistent increases in physical activity, dietary changes, or changes in concomitant drug therapy (e.g., stopping steroids). Additionally, absorption may vary from one anatomic site to another, and the rate of absorption of insulin can be augmented by exercise involving a particular injection site. This simply means that the physician and the patient must constantly review the treatment program and be prepared to make changes when indicated.

Complications of Insulin Therapy. The most significant complication of insulin treatment is *hypoglycemia*. This is because even the best mode of insulin delivery is still an imperfect method to mimic the homeostatic mechanisms in normal subjects. Normal persons respond to food ingestion, exercise, and stress in such a way as to keep the blood glucose level within narrowly defined limits. One can hope to approach this, but not match it, with the methods used for delivery of exogenous insulin. For example, when normal individuals exercise, peripheral glucose uptake increases, and this is matched by a corresponding increase in hepatic glucose production. A decrease in insulin secretion allows the increase in hepatic glucose production to occur. Obviously this degree of fine tuning is difficult to achieve with exogenous insulin administration. Consequently hypoglycemia is a common complication of insulin therapy as the result of overzealous insulin administration or inappropriate timing. Most often this occurs in a situation in which tight control is attempted. Occasional mild episodes of hypoglycemia are probably acceptable if they appear in a patient in whom excellent control is generally achieved and who is fully aware of their occurrence and of methods to abort

them. However, frequent and severe hypoglycemic reactions are unacceptable. These are serious and occasionally can be fatal. Furthermore, the long-term effects on the central nervous system of frequent hypoglycemic episodes have not been determined. If satisfactory control cannot be achieved without recurrence of such reactions, then compromises in the overall therapeutic plan must be made. It would seem imprudent to expose patients to known complications of hypoglycemia in the hope that superior control will prevent chronic diabetic complications in the future. Some IDDM patients are particularly susceptible to hypoglycemia, seemingly because of impaired secretion of counter-regulatory hormones, particularly glucagon.

An interesting aspect of hypoglycemic episodes is the so-called *Somogyi phenomenon.* This involves rebound hyperglycemia due to excessive secretion of counter-regulatory hormones following a previous episode of hypoglycemia. The classic situation involves nocturnal hypoglycemia followed by marked hyperglycemia prior to breakfast. This can induce a self-defeating cycle in which the insulin dose is progressively raised in response to the fasting hyperglycemia when a reduction in insulin dose, to prevent the nocturnal hypoglycemia, would be more appropriate.

A minority of patients beginning insulin therapy experience a variety of local allergic reactions at the injection site. Manifestations include local itching; erythematous, indurated lesions; and occasional small, discrete subcutaneous nodules. These local reactions are usually self-limited and eventually disappear with continued insulin treatment. Antihistamines may be used for symptomatic relief if necessary. The frequency of these problems has decreased significantly with the use of the newer more highly purified insulins. Rare patients may develop systemic reactions, including generalized urticaria and even anaphylactic reactions. This usually occurs when insulin therapy has been stopped for a time and then reinstituted. If these symptoms cannot be controlled by antihistamines, and if insulin treatment is mandatory for the patient's well-being, then formal desensitization regimens are necessary. Other local reactions at the injection site include lipoatrophy and hypertrophy. Lipoatrophy at the injection site is a benign condition usually due to impurities in the insulin preparation. It can usually be corrected by changing to a highly purified pork insulin and injecting this into the lipoatrophic areas, which then fill in with subcutaneous fat in a normal fashion. Most likely the new highly purified human insulin preparations will also be suitable for this purpose. Insulin hypertrophy is attributed to the local lipogenic effects of the injected insulin. In advanced cases the underlying tissue can be fibrous and less vascular, making the overlying skin anesthetic. This explains why many patients prefer these areas as sites of injection. This problem can usually be corrected by carefully rotating injection sites.

FUTURE MODES OF THERAPY

Even with the most meticulous mode of insulin therapy in the most motivated patients, euglycemic control is difficult to achieve for prolonged periods. Thus the search for better, more effective, and, in some cases, curative forms of therapy continues. Transplantation of the pancreas or islet cells continues to receive extensive study. Numerous logistic, immunologic, and technical problems need to be overcome before such therapies become available for routine clinical purposes, but there are signs that some positive results might be seen in the next several years. This is the one mode of therapy that might actually be considered curative.

Efforts continue to be expended in developing newer and better external or implantable insulin-delivery devices. Unquestionably the mechanical and engineering aspects of insulin-delivery devices will continue to improve dramatically over the next several years, and pumps that are smaller, safer, and more flexible will be produced. It also seems likely that reliable implantable devices are in the offing. However, unless such devices can be used to administer insulin via the portal route, the advantage of implantable pumps appears to be mostly aesthetic. An additional hope for internal devices is that a closed-loop system can be designed. This would require development of a reliable, fail-safe glucose sensor integrated into the appropriate algorithms for insulin delivery. If such artificial pancreases become readily available, they would obviously have wide applicability. Finally, since hyperglucagonemia has been implicated

TABLE 218–5. DIFFERENT INSULIN REGIMENS

Split dose intermediate (NPH or lente) + regular insulin
A.M. dose: ⅔ TDD
~70% intermediate
~30% regular
P.M. dose: ⅓ TDD
50%–70% intermediate
30%–50% regular

Intermediate + preprandial regular insulin
Breakfast: Regular, 25%–40% TDD
Lunch: Regular, 25%–30% TDD
Dinner: Regular, 25%–30% TDD
Night: NPH or lente, 15%–25% TDD

Ultralente + preprandial regular insulin
Breakfast: Regular, 15%–25% TDD
Lunch: Regular, 15%–25% TDD
Dinner: Regular, 15%–25% TDD
Ultralente, 40%–60% TDD

Triple A.M. mixture: regular, lente + ultralente insulin

Double A.M. mixture: regular + NPH (or lente) insulin

TDD = total daily dose

in the pathogenesis of the hyperglycemia in diabetes, agents that specifically suppress glucagon secretion have been sought. Attempts to develop a glucagon-specific somatostatin derivative continue; such a compound might be a useful adjunctive therapy in the management of diabetes.

ACUTE COMPLICATIONS

The acute metabolic complications of diabetes are diabetic ketoacidosis, hyperosmolar nonketotic coma, lactic acidosis, and hypoglycemia.

Diabetic Ketoacidosis (DKA)

DKA is due to insulin deficiency. Before consideration of the pathogenesis of the metabolic derangement, it is important to review the normal physiologic effects of insulin on carbohydrate, protein, and fat metabolism, since DKA simply represents a reversal of these normal insulin-stimulated processes.

PHYSIOLOGY OF FED AND FASTED STATE. When food is ingested, insulin functions as the major anabolic hormone facilitating the disposition of carbohydrate, protein, and fat and their synthesis into macromolecules for storage (Fig. 218–6A). Glucose is absorbed into the portal vein, and approximately 60 per cent of the ingested glucose-derived carbons end up in liver glycogen in the postprandial period. A significant portion of this is probably not a result of direct hepatic glucose uptake, but is due to peripheral metabolism of glucose to three-carbon fragments (lactate, pyruvate) that are then recycled to the liver where they enter the gluconeogenic pathway and are synthesized into glycogen. Glycogen then serves as the storage form of carbohydrate for later release. When glucose is metabolized via the glycolytic (anaerobic) pathway, 2 moles of ATP are generated per mole of glucose. Aerobic, or oxidative, metabolism (Krebs' cycle) is far more efficient as an energy-producing process and generates 12 moles of ATP per mole of glucose. Insulin exerts multiple anabolic effects on this process. It stimulates glucose uptake and glycogen synthesis by muscle and inhibits glycogenolysis. In liver, insulin does not directly stimulate glucose uptake, but it does actively promote glycogenesis and inhibit glycogenolysis. Although most of the ingested glucose, or glucose-derived carbon, ends up in the liver in the postprandial period, over a 24-hour day the central nervous system (CNS) (primarily brain) is the predominant tissue of glucose consumption, accounting for about 70 per cent of total glucose utilization. Glucose is the primary source of energy for brain, and glucose uptake and metabolism in this tissue are independent of insulin. A major purpose of glucose homeostasis is to store glucose as liver glycogen postprandially when glucose and insulin levels are high, so that it can be released in the interprandial period for CNS consumption. Protein digestion and absorption lead to a postprandial rise in circulating amino acid levels. Insulin plays a dominant role in converting amino acids to protein by stimulating amino acid uptake in muscle and liver and by augmenting protein synthesis and inhibiting proteolysis. Fat is absorbed as chylomicrons that enter the circulation via the lymphatic system. Insulin affects fat assimilation in a number of ways. Lipoprotein lipase, an enzyme synthesized primarily by fat and muscle tissue, is secreted into the extracellular space and incorporated into the surface of nearby endothelial cells. In this location, lipoprotein lipase hydrolyzes fatty acids from triglyceride-rich lipoproteins (chylomicrons and very low density lipoproteins). These fatty acids are then taken up, predominantly by adipose tissue, where they are esterified into triglyceride for storage in the fat droplets of adipocytes. Insulin stimulates the synthesis and secretion of lipoprotein lipase and also strongly inhibits lipolysis of triglycerides stored in adipose tissue. Additionally, by promoting glucose uptake, insulin increases the supply of glycerol within adipocytes for esterification of fatty acids. Insulin is also lipogenic and stimulates the synthesis of fatty acids from glucose or other substrates that form pyruvate.

Many of these insulin effects are antagonized by the counter-regulatory hormones, glucagon, epinephrine, cortisol, and growth hormone. When mild (fasting) or severe (DKA) insulin deficiency exists, the processes outlined in Figure 218–6A are reversed, and characteristic metabolic derangements occur. This is illustrated in Figure 218–6B. A 24-hour fast causes mild insulin deficiency, and this results in a marked decrease in peripheral glucose uptake. This is accompanied by a decrease in synthesis of

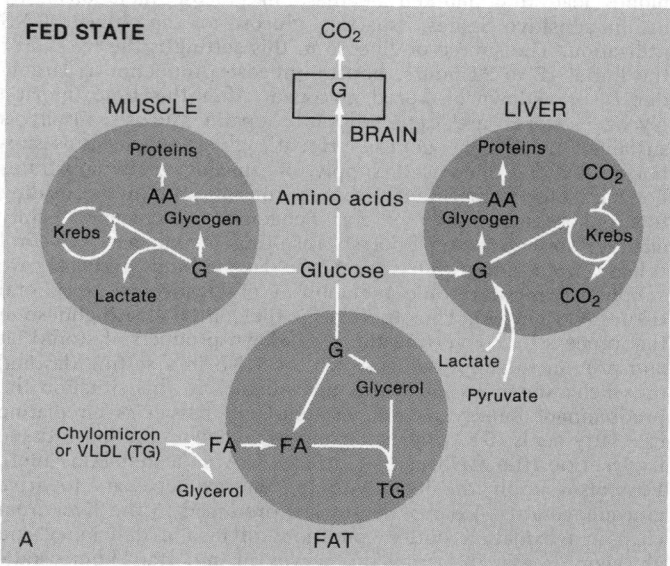

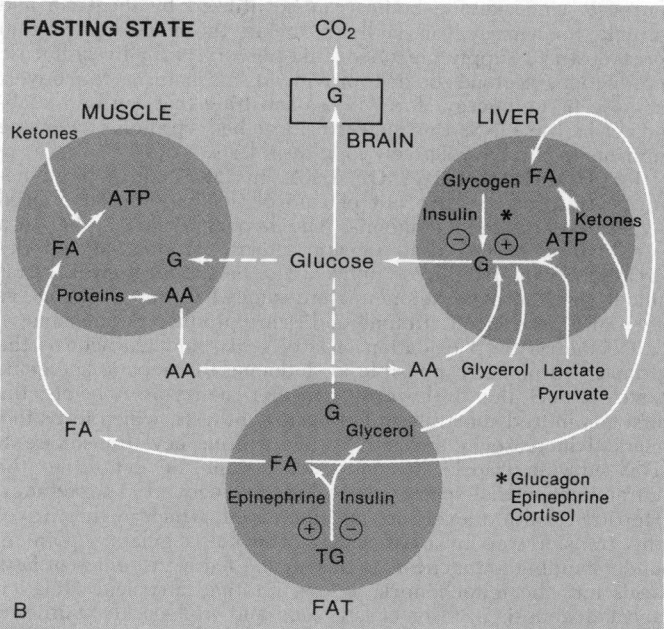

FIGURE 218–6. *A,* Fuel homeostasis during the immediate postprandial fed state. The key features of this diagram are the storage of glucose (G), amino acids (AA), and fatty acids (FA) as the macromolecules glycogen, protein, and triglyceride (TG) in tissue depots; each of these processes is facilitated by the anabolic effects of insulin. *B,* Reversal of the anabolic effects of insulin during the insulinopenic fasting state. The major purpose of these homeostatic responses is to maintain a supply of glucose for obligate glucose uptake by the CNS while other tissues cease their consumption of glucose in favor of fatty acids from adipose tissue depots.

glycogen, protein, and triglyceride, along with increased breakdown of these storage macromolecules by accelerated glycogenolysis, proteolysis, and lipolysis. These catabolic processes increase as a result of the lack of insulin effect, but breakdown of macromolecules is also augmented by increased concentrations of counter-regulatory hormones. Thus, glucagon stimulates glycogen breakdown and is also strongly ketogenic, but has no in vivo effect on glucose uptake, lipolysis, or proteolysis. Epinephrine promotes glycogenolysis and lipolysis and also inhibits peripheral glucose uptake. Cortisol probably has effects that are additive or possibly synergistic with the other counter-regulatory hormones and may independently stimulate proteolysis. Growth hormone probably plays a minor role in these events mediated through inhibition of glucose uptake. Taken together, fasting-induced insulin deficiency plus increased counter-regulatory hormones lead to a marked decrease in glucose metabolism by insulin-sensitive tissues, "sparing" glucose for the obligate CNS utilization. The source of glucose in this setting is the liver. For the initial 12 to 24 hours, hepatic glucose production is largely due to breakdown of stored glycogen. After this time, hepatic glycogen stores are depleted and hepatic glucose output is sustained by gluconeogenesis. Hepatic gluconeogenesis is supported by the increased supply of gluconeogenic substrates flowing from the periphery, that is, muscle proteolysis, leading to an increased supply of gluconeogenic amino acids (mainly alanine) and increased lipolysis resulting in enhanced glycerol release from adipose tissue. Some lactate and pyruvate are supplied from anaerobic metabolism of glucose in peripheral tissues (Cori cycle). Thus the liver is the central clearinghouse in this process by converting the breakdown products of stored fat and protein to supply glucose for the CNS in a setting (fasting) in which exogenous glucose is unavailable. In this situation the predominant energy source for non-CNS tissues is circulating free fatty acids (FFA) derived from breakdown of adipose tissue triglyceride (the CNS cannot utilize FFA as a metabolic fuel). FFA also supply the liver with the energy necessary to drive gluconeogenesis. Ketone bodies are produced in the liver from fatty acid oxidation under conditions of insulin deficiency and glucagon excess. In fasting this serves an important homeostatic purpose, since ketone bodies can be utilized by the CNS and muscle for energy, markedly reducing the need for protein breakdown to supply gluconeogenic precursors for liver glucose production. Ketone bodies provide a mechanism to convert adipose tissue energy stores into a substrate that can be metabolized in the CNS; this spares critical body proteins, allowing humans to survive relatively long-term fasts.

PATHOPHYSIOLOGY OF DKA. In DKA, all of these homeostatic processes are out of control, leading to pronounced hyperglycemia and ketonemia. The hyperglycemia is due to a combination of increased hepatic glucose production and decreased peripheral glucose uptake. The biochemical mechanisms underlying the hyperketonemia are somewhat more complex, as seen in Figure 218–7. Ketone bodies are produced in hepatocyte by β oxidation of fatty acids, and glucagon is the primary hormone responsible for inducing the hepatic ketogenic state. It does this by lowering malonyl coenzyme A levels, the first committed substrate in fatty acid synthesis, which leads to a marked increase in the activity of carnitine acyl transferase I. This enzyme translocates fatty acids from the cytosol to the intramitochondrial space, where they are converted to ketones. Hepatic carnitine levels are also increased, which further drives this transfer step by mass action. The key regulatory point in understanding ketogenesis is that in the fed state, entry of fatty acids into the mitochondria is low, limiting fatty acid oxidation and ketogenesis in favor of fatty acid and triglyceride synthesis; thus the liver is rate limiting in ketone body formation. When the level of insulin is low and glucagon high (as in starvation or DKA), fatty acids freely enter mitochondria to be converted to ketones, and therefore the supply of fatty acids to the liver is rate limiting for ketogenesis. Fatty acids are freely permeable across the hepatocyte plasma membrane, and thus the plasma concentration of FFA drives ketogenesis. In starvation, fatty acid levels are only moderately increased, leading to enhanced, but controlled, ketogenesis; in DKA, FFA levels are much higher, leading to uncontrolled ketogenesis. Another factor enhancing ketonemia in DKA is related to ketone body utilization. Insulin normally stimulates ketoacid uptake by peripheral tissues, and this is inhibited in DKA; additionally, very high levels of ketones may saturate the uptake mechanisms, further limiting utilization.

All of the pathophysiologic sequelae of DKA follow from hyperglycemia and hyperketonemia (Fig. 218–8). Thus, acidosis and ketonuria are directly due to the buildup of the ketoacids β-hydroxybutyrate and acetoacetate. The hyperglycemia and hyperketonemia produce an osmotic diuresis that causes intravascular volume depletion and dehydration and urinary electrolyte loss. The hyperosmolarity further exaggerates intracellular dehydration.

CLINICAL PICTURE. Diabetic ketoacidosis can be a life-threatening situation, and the clinical presentation is often dramatic. An antecedent history of polyuria and polydipsia for one

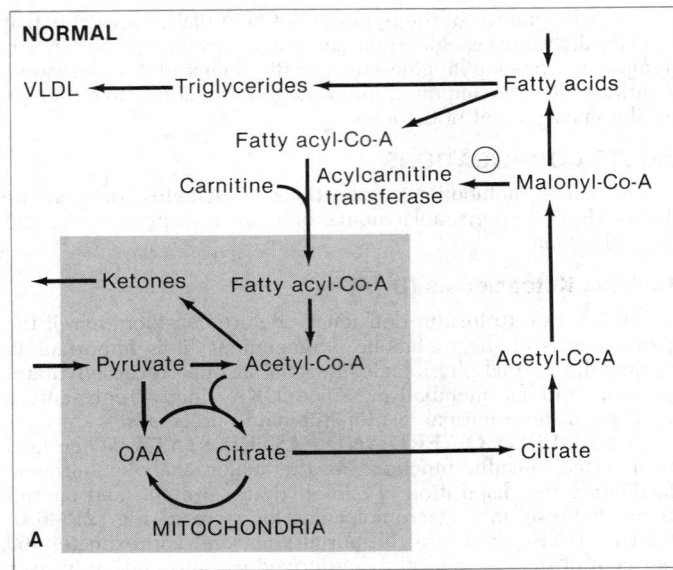

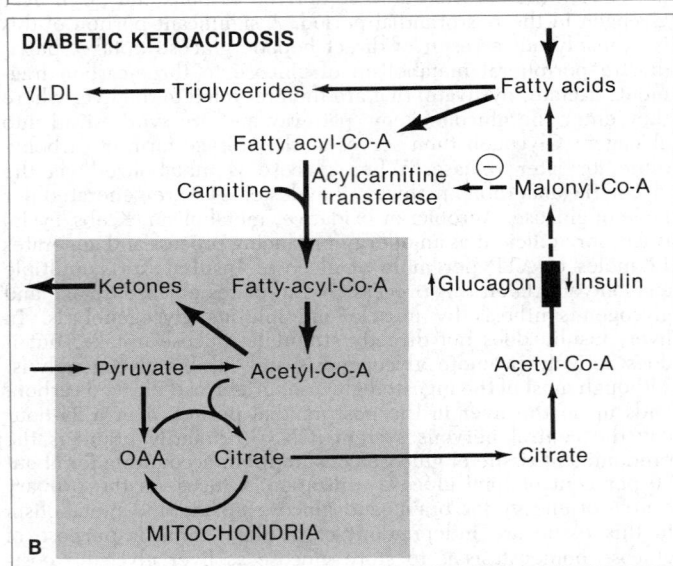

FIGURE 218–7. Hepatic fatty acid and ketoacid metabolism in the normal state *(upper panel)* and insulinopenic diabetic ketoacidotic state *(lower panel)*. Malonyl-Co-A is a key regulatory intermediate in this scheme, competitively inhibiting the ability of acyl carnitine transferase to translocate fatty acyl-Co-A molecules from the cytosol to the intramitochondrial space in the normal state. In diabetic ketoacidosis, glucagon excess and insulin deficiency inhibit the generation of malonyl-Co-A, releasing the inhibition of acyl carnitine transferase. See text for further details. VLDL = Very low density lipoproteins; OAA = oxaloacetic acid.

to several days is typical, and nausea, vomiting, and anorexia are frequent accompanying symptoms. Occasionally, abdominal pain is a predominant feature, sometimes mimicking an acute abdominal condition. Often this is due to gastric stasis and distention. In the obtunded patient with gastric distention, nasogastric suction should be considered to avoid vomiting with aspiration. Physical findings include tachypnea, dehydration, and disorientation, or even coma. If systemic acidosis is severe, Kussmaul respirations are present. Precipitating causes of DKA include failure of the patient to take insulin, infection, intercurrent illness, trauma, or emotional stress. When a known diabetic presents with signs and symptoms of DKA, the diagnosis is usually straightforward. However, DKA can also be the initial presenting episode of diabetes. DKA is a disease of IDDM, only rarely occurring in NIDDM, and only when precipitating causes are extreme.

Although the diagnosis of DKA can be strongly suspected on a clinical basis, confirmation is based on laboratory analyses. The diagnosis is made by demonstrating hyperglycemia and hyper-

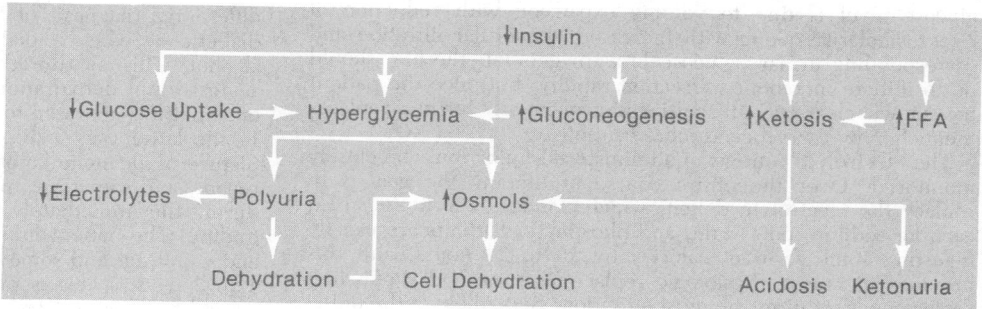

FIGURE 218–8. Pathophysiology of diabetic ketoacidosis. Severe insulin deficiency leads to hyperglycemia and ketonemia, and from this all of the other pathophysiologic sequelae result. FFA = free fatty acids.

ketonemia in the presence of acidosis. However, the severity of these abnormalities can vary over a wide range. Occasionally the presenting episode may be severe ketonemia and acidosis and only mild hyperglycemia (200 to 400 mg per deciliter). Other patients may have severe hyperglycemia and only mild ketonemia and acidosis. Occasionally, alcoholic patients have ketonemia and hyperglycemia, and this condition, termed alcoholic ketoacidosis, must be differentiated from DKA (see next section). Direct quantitative measurements of acetoacetate and β-hydroxybutyrate are not usually readily available, and most physicians rely on reagent strips (Ketostix) or tablets (Acetest) for measurements. With this method, a nitroprusside reaction is the indicator; nitroprusside reacts mainly with acetoacetate, to a lesser extent with acetone, and not at all with β-hydroxybutyrate. Since β-hydroxybutyrate levels are much higher than acetoacetate levels in DKA, this method can sometimes be confusing. For example, when concomitant lactic acidosis exists, acetoacetate production may be inhibited in the presence of very high levels of β-hydroxybutyrate. In this setting the nitroprusside reaction may not be strongly positive. During the course of insulin therapy for DKA, β-hydroxybutyrate levels may fall out of proportion to acetoacetate levels, giving the impression that therapy is less effective than it actually is. Serum sodium levels are usually mildly decreased. This is due to the hyperglycemia- and hyperketonemia-induced hyperosmolarity, which attracts extracellular water from the intracellular space, leading to dilution of serum sodium. It should be kept in mind that the osmolar contribution of the hyperketonemia can often approach the contribution of the hyperglycemia. Serum bicarbonate levels are depressed, and the magnitude of decrease is in proportion to the degree of acidosis. BUN levels are usually modestly elevated as a result of dehydration and a component of prerenal azotemia. Serum potassium levels can be high, low, or normal, depending on the degree of dehydration and acidosis. In all cases, severe total body and intracellular potassium depletion exists. Because of cellular buffering mechanisms, which exchange intracellular potassium for extracellular hydrogen ion, extracellular potassium levels are often maintained in acidotic states. Nevertheless, greater than 95 per cent of total body potassium is intracellular, so in the presence of acidosis, extracellular potassium levels do not reflect total body potassium stores unless the potassium concentration is plotted on a nomogram related to serum pH (Fig. 218–9).

TREATMENT OF DKA. The treatment of DKA should be started as soon as it is diagnosed. The goals of therapy are to increase the rate of glucose utilization by insulin-dependent tissues, to reverse ketonemia and acidosis, and to correct the depletion of water and electrolytes. To accomplish this, treatment can be divided into four general areas: (1) insulin administration, (2) replacement of fluid and electrolytes, (3) treatment of any precipitating problems, and (4) avoidance of complications.

A variety of *insulin* regimens are possible, ranging from constant intravenous infusion to intermittent administration of intravenous, subcutaneous, or intramuscular boluses. The aim of all forms of insulin administration is to achieve a rapid and maximal insulin effect. In vivo insulin action is near maximal at an insulin concentration of about 200 μU per milliliter, and achieving higher levels has little further benefit. Since insulin is rapidly cleared from the circulation ($t_{1/2}$ = 7 minutes), boluses must be given frequently (every 30 to 60 minutes) to maintain maximally effec-

tive insulin levels. With constant intravenous administration, serum insulin levels are maintained at a steady state throughout the infusion. In normal subjects, an infusion rate of 10 units per hour results in an insulin level of approximately 200 μU per milliliter by 30 minutes, and if this mode of treatment is chosen a priming dose (10 to 20 units) should be given initially. Advocates of constant intravenous infusion maintain that the rate of metabolic improvement is smoother and more predictable and hypoglycemia is less common. Additionally, problems of variable or inadequate absorption from subcutaneous or intramuscular sites are avoided. One difficulty with this method occurs in the occasional patient with severe insulin resistance due to sepsis or high titers of insulin antibodies. If clear-cut metabolic improvement is not seen within the first few hours of constant insulin infusion, a bolus of insulin (20 to 30 units) should be given and the rate of insulin infusion increased.

Fluid replacement should also be started immediately. Patients with DKA are dehydrated and hypovolemic and usually have fluid deficits of 5 to 8 liters or more. Thus, rapid expansion of intravascular volume is essential, and this is achieved by an initial infusion of 1 to 2 liters of normal saline, or equivalent, over the first 1 to 2 hours. Of course, caution should be used in those patients with underlying cardiovascular or oliguric renal disease. Following initial rapid fluid administration, the rate of replacement can be slowed to restore estimated losses by 16 to 24 hours, depending on the patient's degree of dehydration and underlying cardiovascular-renal status. Much of the initial decline in plasma

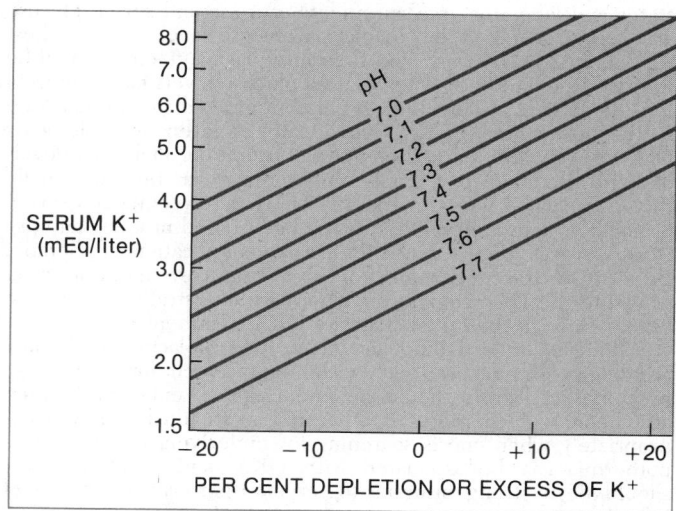

FIGURE 218–9. Nomogram depicting the relationship between total body potassium depletion, serum potassium, and serum pH. Per cent potassium depletion or excess is calculated by drawing a horizontal line from the ordinate intercept of the serum potassium concentration to the intersection of the diagonal line corresponding to the coexisting serum pH. From this intersection a vertical line is dropped to the abscissa and per cent potassium depletion or excess is read from the abscissal intercept. For example, at a serum potassium concentration of 4.0, at a concomitant serum pH of 7.2, an approximate 10 per cent depletion of total body potassium stores exists.

glucose level is due to volume expansion with reduction of hyperosmolarity, along with increased glomerular filtration and corresponding urinary glucose loss. In general, the aim should be to initiate metabolic correction rapidly, but once the patient has shown clear-cut substantial improvement, further replacement therapy can proceed more cautiously.

The electrolyte content of administered fluids must be closely monitored. Over the entire course of therapy the goal is to replace the electrolyte deficit, which averages 200 to 400 mEq each for sodium, potassium, and phosphate. Patients are usually ingesting some form of calories by 16 to 24 hours, and this provides the most physiologic replacement method. Potassium replacement requires the most attention. Regardless of the initial serum potassium level, total body reserves are depleted and serum levels fall dramatically as acidosis and hyperglycemia are corrected. As glucose is taken up by cells under the influence of insulin, potassium is also transported intracellularly, and as acidosis is reversed the cellular buffering process exchanging intracellular potassium for extracellular hydrogen ion diminishes. To prevent hypokalemia, potassium should be included in the intravenous fluids once it is established that renal perfusion and urine flow are adequate following initial intravascular fluid expansion. To accomplish this, 40 mEq of potassium can be added to each liter of intravenous fluids as the phosphate salt. Phosphate depletion is also uniform in DKA, and some replacement is advisable, particularly if serum phosphate levels are low. This can be accomplished by administering 10 to 20 mmol per hour and can be accomplished along with potassium replacement by giving potassium phosphate. Since excessive phosphate repletion can cause hypocalcemia, ongoing phosphate administration should be guided by the serum phosphorus and calcium levels. Bicarbonate replacement should be initiated in patients with severe acidosis (pH < 7.0). This can be administered at the rate of 44 mEq per liter with appropriate monitoring of pH until it rises above 7.0. Three to four ampules of bicarbonate (44 mEq per ampule) usually suffice to achieve this goal. Excessive bicarbonate replacement is contraindicated because it exacerbates the tendency toward hypokalemia and may also result in rebound CNS acidosis. The latter occurs because carbon dioxide is more rapidly diffusible across the blood-brain barrier than is bicarbonate ion, causing CNS pH to fall at a time when peripheral pH is rising. This can lead to stupor and worsening of CNS status at a time when metabolic improvement is occurring.

Therapy should be monitored by frequent assessment of clinical status and laboratory measurements of urine and serum glucose and ketone levels. A fall in plasma glucose level is the earliest sign of effective therapy, and therefore plasma glucose should be frequently monitored. Once plasma glucose levels fall to approximately 250 mg per deciliter, 5 per cent glucose should be added to the intravenous fluids. Occasionally children or adolescents with DKA exhibit marked mental deterioration, including development of coma 4 to 6 hours after therapy has begun. Usually this is associated with a marked fall in hyperglycemia and serum osmolality, and cerebral edema has been noted in a few autopsy cases. Overall this is probably a rare complication of therapy. Because of the importance of plasma glucose monitoring in assessing the effectiveness of therapy, administration of glucose has no place in the initial stages of DKA treatment.

While insulin and fluid and electrolyte replacement therapy are being administered, a concomitant search for underlying precipitating factors should be undertaken. Leukocytosis often accompanies uncomplicated DKA and so should be viewed appropriately when one is searching for underlying infection. Hypothermia can be associated with DKA, and therefore fever should be a strong impetus to screen rigorously for a site of infection.

The major complications of DKA are mostly the result of treatment and include *hypokalemia, late hypoglycemia, rebound CNS acidosis*, and *CNS deterioration* (possibly due to cerebral edema). However, with proper attention to therapeutic details the former two can always be avoided, and the latter are fortunately rare. Recurrence of DKA can occur in the hospital if the vigorous phase of therapy is relaxed too soon. Maintenance of a flow chart with all therapies and laboratory tests recorded is an important means of coordination so that unexpected results do not go undetected and inappropriate therapies are not given.

Alcoholic Ketoacidosis

Alcoholic ketoacidosis can sometimes present a problem in the differential diagnosis of DKA when the patient is not a known diabetic or when a diabetic patient ingests large amounts of alcohol. This syndrome is characterized by hyperketonemia, acidosis, and dehydration. Serum glucose levels can be normal or sometimes elevated to the lower range of values seen in DKA. In the latter case a diagnostic problem can occur. The clinical picture of alcoholic ketoacidosis occurs in alcoholics following a recent, and sometimes prolonged alcoholic debauch; abstinence during the immediately preceding 12 to 24 hours is a common finding. The patient is usually anorexic, sometimes with nausea and vomiting, and some degree of starvation over the preceding 1 to 3 days is always present. The starvation, perhaps accompanied by stress-related hyperglucagonemia, creates a ketogenic state in the liver. This is accompanied by elevated FFA levels similar to those seen in starvation, which are perhaps augmented by adrenergic activation related to alcohol withdrawal, creating the metabolic environment for ketoacidosis. It is unusual for these patients to have hyperglycemia, but it can occur. When it does, the pathogenesis is unclear. In some patients, abnormalities of glucose tolerance exist after therapy, and thus the hyperglycemia may be stress related in previously glucose-intolerant patients. Alternatively, adrenergic mechanisms related to alcohol withdrawal could suppress residual endogenous insulin secretion, facilitating mild hyperglycemia. Regardless of the underlying mechanisms, the metabolic abnormalities are rapidly reversed by intravenous administration of fluids and glucose. Only occasionally is insulin needed in the early stages of treatment.

Nonketotic Hyperosmolar Syndrome

The term *nonketotic hyperosmolar coma* has frequently been applied to this syndrome, but by no means do all patients display coma or even mental obtundity. Rather, this syndrome comprises a spectrum ranging from mild degrees of hyperosmolarity with minimal CNS symptoms to severe hyperosmolarity with minimal CNS symptoms to severe hyperosmolarity with accompanying coma. The biochemical hallmarks are extreme hyperglycemia (mean 1000 mg per deciliter, range 600 to 2400 mg per deciliter) in the absence of overt ketoacidosis. Dehydration, hypovolemia, and disorientation are accompanying features. This syndrome usually develops over a much longer interval than DKA, with symptoms of polyuria antedating clinical presentation by several days and sometimes weeks. This syndrome usually occurs in elderly patients with NIDDM (often not previously diagnosed) who for some reason are unable to keep up with the osmotic diuresis by adequate water ingestion and this results in severe dehydration. The severe hyperglycemia is at least partly caused by decreased renal glucose excretion due either to intrinsic underlying renal disease or to decreased glomerular filtration and prerenal azotemia secondary to the marked hypovolemia and dehydration. Frequently this condition is associated with steroid, diuretic, or phenytoin therapy as a precipitating cause. Other precipitating factors include infections, cerebrovascular events, or therapeutic maneuvers such as hypertonic peritoneal dialysis or parenteral nutrition.

Serum sodium and potassium levels are usually normal while serum bicarbonate levels are often somewhat depressed. This is usually not associated with significant ketonemia and probably reflects an underlying component of lactic acidosis due to hypovolemia. The BUN is uniformly elevated because of hypovolemia and prerenal azotemia. In these cases, however, acidosis is mild, and serum osmolality can be approximated by the formula:

$$\text{serum osmolality (mOsm/L)} = 2 \times [\text{Na}^+ + \text{K}^+ \text{ (mEq/L)}] + \frac{\text{plasma glucose (mg/dl)}}{18} + \frac{\text{BUN (mg/dl)}}{2.8}$$

Since urea is freely diffusible across cell membranes, it does not alter the effective serum osmolality, which is the clinically important factor to consider in this hyperosmolar condition. Most experts do not consider BUN levels in this calculation and prefer to estimate effective serum osmolarity as:

$$\text{Osm}_E = 2 \times [\text{Na}^+ + \text{K}^+ \text{ (mEq/L)}] + \frac{\text{plasma glucose (mg/dl)}}{18}$$

Values above 300 mOsm per liter are abnormal and above 320 mOsm per liter are indicative of clinically significant hyperosmolarity.

The reason ketosis is not a feature of this condition has not been satisfactorily explained. FFA levels are not as high in this syndrome as they are in DKA, and most investigators attribute the relatively lower FFA levels and decreased rates of ketogenesis to higher residual insulin levels in patients with the hyperosmolar syndrome. This answer is not entirely satisfactory, however, since measured peripheral insulin levels overlap with those reported in DKA. On the other hand, peripheral insulin levels do not always reflect portal insulin concentrations, and significant differences in portal insulin levels may exist in DKA versus hyperosmolar syndrome, with the higher levels in hyperosmolar syndrome restraining hepatic ketogenesis.

In some series, the mortality has ranged up to 50 per cent. However, the relatively high mortality reflects selection criteria because mortality tends to be higher with greater severity of the hyperosmolality. The first priority of treatment should be intravascular volume expansion to restore circulatory integrity. This is accomplished by infusion of 1 to 2 liters of normal saline, or equivalent, over 1 to 2 hours, provided that absolute cardiovascular contraindications do not exist. Even normal saline is hypotonic relative to serum in these patients, and therefore this therapy initiates the correction of the hyperosmolality. As in DKA, insulin can be administered by constant intravenous infusions or bolus therapy. Since absorption of insulin administered subcutaneously or intramuscularly is variable because of dehydration and hypovolemia, and since late hypoglycemia is a more common complication of the hyperosmolar syndrome, constant intravenous administration of insulin can be very effective in this condition, leading to a predictable and fairly constant, smooth decline in plasma glucose levels. Once plasma glucose begins to decrease, and provided that acceptable volume expansion and urine flow have been established, potassium phosphate salts should be added to the intravenous fluids. Subsequent to the initial volume expansion, intravenous fluids can consist of 0.5 normal saline with added potassium phosphate. Once plasma glucose levels decline to approximately 250 mg per deciliter, 5 per cent glucose should be added to the intravenous fluids. The above comments are meant more as guidelines than hard and fast rules, since, as in DKA, therapy must be individualized as far as replacement of fluids and electrolytes is concerned. This is best done by maintaining an organized flow chart with frequent measurements of plasma glucose, electrolytes, blood pressure, and urine volume. Despite even the best therapy, morbidity and mortality are high in this condition. Thrombosis and embolic events as well as infections, particularly pneumonia with accompanying adult respiratory distress syndrome, contribute significantly to adverse outcomes. In summary, rigorous but carefully monitored hydration and re-establishment of circulatory integrity are critical for successful therapy. These goals should be pursued while hyperosmolarity is corrected by administration of relatively hypotonic fluids with adequate free water along with insulin to reduce the hyperglycemia. Concomitantly a careful workup should be instituted to uncover precipitating factors with appropriate therapy when necessary.

CHRONIC OR LATE COMPLICATIONS OF DIABETES

Retinopathy (See Color Plate 14E)

Eye disease is common in diabetes, and permanent loss of vision is one of the most striking and feared complications. Approximately 25 per cent of all newly reported cases of blindness are attributed to diabetes. When diabetics of all ages and types are considered together, the incidence of blindness from diabetic retinopathy is 0.2 per cent per year in all diabetics and 0.6 per cent per year in diabetics with retinopathy. This is 11 and 29 times greater, respectively, than the incidence of blindness from all other causes combined in the general population.

The major form of diabetic eye disease is diabetic retinopathy. Two general categories exist: nonproliferative or background retinopathy and proliferative retinopathy. Nonproliferative retinopathy can include venous abnormalities, microaneurysms, retinal hemorrhages, retinal edema, and exudates. This may progress to proliferative retinopathy, characterized by neovascularization, glial proliferation, and vitreoretinal traction. In general, diabetic

retinopathy is progressive and tends to worsen with the duration of disease. However, most diabetics do not develop proliferative retinopathy. The incidence of this complication is substantially lower in NIDDM then in IDDM, even when corrected for duration of disease. However, since there are many more patients with NIDDM than IDDM, the absolute numbers of NIDDM and IDDM patients with proliferative retinopathy are roughly comparable.

NONPROLIFERATIVE RETINOPATHY. Probably the earliest retinal change is increased capillary permeability seen on fluorescein angiography. This abnormality can be readily reversed by effective glycemic control, but the relationship of this form of capillary permeability to retinopathy is unknown. Nonperfusion of retinal capillaries occurs early in diabetic retinopathy (so-called capillary dropout), and this leads to areas of retinal ischemia and infarction. Microaneurysms are small (15 to 50 μm diameter) excrescences along capillaries and are particularly prominent along the edges of areas of capillary nonperfusion. Fusiform aneurysms, or general dilatation of capillary loops, can also occur. Retinal veins are often tortuous and dilated; dilatation can be segmental, giving rise to a beaded or "sausage string" appearance. Exudates can be of two types: (1) Hard, waxy exudates are white to yellowish, shiny, with defined borders but without surrounding pigmentation. These exudates are due to lipid- and protein-containing fluid that has leaked from surrounding capillaries. (2) Cotton-wool, or soft, exudates are really areas of nonperfusion representing retinal microinfarcts and are often surrounded by microaneurysms. Clinically, an increase in cotton-wool areas indicates progressive capillary dropout and is a poor prognostic sign. Subretinal hemorrhages tend to be small and dot shaped and may resorb within a few weeks. Larger, flame-shaped hemorrhages occur in the superficial retinal layers and resorb more slowly. Preretinal hemorrhages are more serious and can impair vision if they are large or if they impinge on the macula. Following resorption, scarring and vitreous retraction or retinal detachment can occur. Edema of the retina is due to abnormal capillary permeability and ischemia. When persistent macular edema exists, vision is seriously impaired, and usual forms of therapy (photocoagulation) may not be effective. The primary pathogenetic events underlying these changes of nonproliferative background retinopathy are unclear, but loss of supporting capillary pericytes, endothelial proliferation, and hyperviscosity with red cell aggregation, together or alone, have all been proposed.

PROLIFERATIVE RETINOPATHY. The hallmark of proliferative retinopathy is new vessel formation or neovascularization. These capillary fronds or loops can grow on the surface of the retina or extend into the vitreous. Often this is accompanied by proliferation of glial elements in the region of the optic disc or along the new vessel arcades. Traction between the vitreous and the neovascular and glial elements can ultimately develop, leading to retinal detachment or large-scale hemorrhage into the vitreous. These events lead to serious loss of vision or blindness. It has been suggested that the stimulus for neovascularization is retinal ischemia with local release of growth-promoting factors.

Photocoagulation is the therapy of choice for proliferative diabetic retinopathy. With this therapy, a light beam is focused on the retina to produce a burn or coagulum in a precisely defined area. By this means, one can selectively destroy microaneurysms, leaky vessels, neovascular elements, and areas of microinfarction or edema. Destruction of vessels prone to hemorrhage or causing traction directly prevents further deterioration. Destroying areas of retina that are poorly perfused and hypoxic may curtail the ischemic stimulus for neovascularization, preventing further proliferative changes. Regardless of the mechanism, the cooperative trial of the Diabetic Retinopathy Study Research Group clearly showed that photocoagulation decreases the incidence of retinal detachment, hemorrhage, and loss of vision. Thus, photocoagulation involves selective treatment of new vessels as well as panretinal treatment to destroy 20 to 30 per cent of the remaining retinal tissue. Photocoagulation therapy may also be useful for proliferative retinopathy as indicated by results from the Early Treatment Diabetic Retinopathy Study. All patients with significant diabetic retinopathy should be followed by an ophthalmologist and photocoagulation considered when new vessel formation or preretinal hemorrhage occurs.

Photocoagulation early in the course of diabetic retinopathy can also be advisable. In the past, hypophysectomy was used as treatment for proliferative retinopathy. However, the therapeutic responses to this maneuver are quite variable, and significant complications exist. With the advent of photocoagulation, use of hypophysectomy has been largely abandoned. In patients with severe vitreal involvement, total vitrectomy may offer some possibility of improvement and preservation of vision.

Other Complications of Diabetes Affecting Vision

In addition to retinopathy, the eyes are affected in other ways by diabetes mellitus. Diabetics may experience temporary blurring of vision and *changes in refraction*, most likely due to osmotic changes in lens shape as a result of fluctuations in hyperglycemia. These changes can be disconcerting, but patients should be advised not to seek new refractions until a stable period of metabolic control is produced. It may take 6 to 8 weeks before the hyperglycemia-induced changes in visual acuity subside. *Glaucoma* is also more frequent in diabetics. Rubeosis iridis is due to capillary neovascularization of the iris, which can produce closed-angle glaucoma. Usually occurring when diabetic retinopathy is advanced, this form of glaucoma is generally refractory to treatment. Open-angle glaucoma is also more frequent in diabetics, and this may relate to fibrosis or scarring of the canals of Schlemm, which drain the anterior chamber. Although *cataracts* are common in diabetics, it has not been rigorously demonstrated that the incidence of cataracts is increased in this condition. For the most part, cataracts in diabetics are indistinguishable from senile cataracts in nondiabetic patients, and the indications for surgery are the same as in nondiabetics. It is possible that the presence of diabetes accelerates the development of senile cataracts so that they occur at an earlier age than in nondiabetics. It has been postulated that hyperglycemia leads to increased sorbitol production in the lens, resulting in osmotic changes that accelerate cataract formation. While evidence in favor of this theory exists, it still remains to be proved. Opacities in the lens termed snowflake cataracts are occasionally noted in young patients whose diabetes is in poor control. This form of cataract is more specific for diabetes but can occur in other conditions and, unlike the senile cataract, can regress when glycemic control is achieved.

Nephropathy

Kidney disease is common in diabetes (see also Ch. 83 for an extensive discussion of the kidney in diabetes), and renal failure is one of the major causes of death.

PATHOLOGY. The dominant form of diabetic nephropathy is microvascular disease affecting the renal glomerulus. A number of distinct morphologic and functional abnormalities characterize diabetic glomerulopathy. Early in diabetes the kidney increases in size, and the associated glomerular hypertrophy leads to an increased glomerular filtration rate with hyperfiltration and microalbuminuria in up to 50 per cent of patients with new-onset IDDM. The hyperfiltration and increased kidney size revert to normal following effective insulin therapy and are unassociated with other glomerular lesions. Later in the disease, diffuse thickening of the glomerular basement membrane is noted along with increased mesangial volume. Patients with substantial histologic changes can exhibit normal renal function; however, impaired renal function probably does not occur in the absence of morphologic changes. Later in the disease, when decreased renal function is evident, the mesangium further expands and occupies a greater proportion of the glomerular volume while the thickness of the glomerular basement membrane is not necessarily increased. Glomerular occlusion accompanies this picture. Often characteristic nodular hyaline-like deposits, termed nodular glomerulocapillary sclerosis or Kimmelstiel-Wilson lesions, are evident in the center of peripheral glomerular capillary lobules.

CLINICAL AND FUNCTIONAL ASPECTS. The manifestations of diabetic nephropathy are quite heterogeneous. Asymptomatic, mild proteinuria can remain constant for many years. In other patients proteinuria may increase and be followed by progressive reduction in glomerular filtration and renal function. Persistent proteinuria (3 to 5 grams per day or greater) is a poor prognostic sign, usually heralding renal failure within 5 years. However, exceptions exist. The proteinuria may progress to include all of the classic features of the nephrotic syndrome. Once azotemia develops, progression to renal failure and uremia is inevitable within a few months to 2 to 3 years.

The diagnosis of diabetic nephropathy is usually made on clinical grounds, and renal biopsy is rarely indicated. Invasive diagnostic procedures should be aimed at detection of reversible features such as infection or obstruction. Contrast studies should not be conducted without clear indications, since rapid deterioration of renal function with acute renal failure sometimes follows intravenous pyelography or angiography in azotemic diabetic patients. When the study is performed, patients should be well hydrated before testing.

If renal failure develops in a diabetic, dialysis or transplantation must be considered. As recently as 10 to 15 years ago, uremic diabetics were thought to be extremely poor risks for dialysis, with very low survival rates and high rates of complications, particularly infections and deterioration of vision. However, in recent years, results have been much better with a first-year survival of over 80 per cent and 3-year survival of over 60 per cent. Additionally, far fewer cases of progressive visual impairment and blindness occur. Thus, in the absence of other negative factors, the presence of diabetes should not be considered a contraindication to dialysis, and decisions to initiate this form of therapy should generally proceed as in nondiabetic uremic patients. Chronic ambulatory peritoneal dialysis (CAPD) has been tried in some patients, but overall experience is still limited. Indications for CAPD vary widely among treatment centers, as does enthusiasm for this mode of therapy. Recent experience with renal transplantation has also been encouraging. Regardless of donor source (cadaver or related donor), survival rates after renal transplantation in diabetics approach those in nondiabetics. Interestingly, diabetic-type glomerular changes have been noted in biopsy specimens from the transplanted kidney in many of these patients.

Neuropathy (See also Ch. 498)

Diabetic neuropathy is perhaps the most common disabling chronic complication of diabetes. Although death seldom results from neuropathic changes alone, a great deal of morbidity and reduced quality of life can be attributed to diabetic neuropathy. The incidence and severity of neuropathy generally progress with duration of diabetes, and severe neuropathy can often exist in the absence of other chronic diabetic complications. A number of different classification schemes have been proposed, but none is entirely satisfactory, primarily because the causes of diabetic neuropathy are not known, and therefore classification must be descriptive in nature rather than based on pathogenetic mechanisms. Table 218–6 provides a simplified method of classification that may prove useful. Polyneuropathy is a diffuse symmetric disorder of peripheral nerve function. Asymmetric neuropathy implies a cluster of signs and symptoms that can be anatomically related to dysfunction of a single nerve trunk (mononeuropathy) or to more than one nerve trunk (mononeuropathy multiplex) either simultaneously or successively. It has been proposed that the symmetric or diffuse neuropathies are due to "metabolic" abnormalities of the neurons or the Schwann cells, whereas the asymmetric or focal neuropathies are due to vascular occlusion and ischemia. Diabetic neuropathy is very common in both IDDM and NIDDM, and mild to severe disease can exist in up to 50 per cent of patients. The incidence of symmetric neuropathy is comparable in IDDM and NIDDM when corrected for duration of disease, but focal neuropathies are more common in older NIDDM patients, suggesting a vascular contribution to the etiology.

TABLE 218–6. CLASSIFICATION OF DIABETIC NEUROPATHY

1. Symmetric distal polyneuropathy
2. Asymmetric neuropathy
   A. Cranial mononeuropathy and mononeuropathy multiplex
   B. Peripheral mononeuropathy and mononeuropathy multiplex
   C. Neuromuscular syndromes
3. Autonomic neuropathy

NEUROPATHIC LESIONS AND THE DIABETIC FOOT.

Loss of sensation can lead to the development of a Charcot joint as a result of repeated undetected trauma. More commonly, neuropathic ulcers develop, particularly on the plantar aspect of the foot. This can be due to weakness of the intrinsic muscles of the foot secondary to neuropathy, leading to abnormal pressure distribution. Weight bearing is then accentuated on the metatarsal heads, causing degeneration of the underlying fat pads and eventually leading to the typical open, draining neuropathic ulcer. Ulcers can also result from penetrating wounds caused by stepping on tacks or other sharp objects the patient does not feel. The best therapy is preventive. All diabetics should be trained to examine their feet daily for callous formation, blisters, or trauma. Shoes should be properly fitted; orthotic or other devices to aid in proper weight distribution are sometimes helpful. Patients should be advised never to walk barefoot. In all cases the feet should be kept clean and dry, and professional trimming of toenails and callosities is often advisable. Neuropathic foot ulcers can lead to gangrene and the requirement for amputation. Meticulous foot care substantially decreases the incidence of these ulcers and is a major form of preventive therapy that all diabetics should receive. Once open ulcers develop, healing can still occur if peripheral circulation is adequate. A high index of suspicion should be maintained for underlying osteomyelitis. Treatment is supportive with bed rest, elevation of the foot, warm (but not hot) foot soaks, debridement, and in some cases antibiotics. Protective plaster casts are sometimes advised. If these therapies fail and gangrene develops, amputation is the only recourse.

SYMMETRIC DISTAL POLYNEUROPATHY.

This form of diabetic neuropathy can be divided into two types: (1) relatively asymptomatic and (2) painful. The first form is diffuse, distal, usually in the lower extremities with a stocking type of distribution. It is characterized by numbness, tingling, or pins-and-needles sensation, often worse at night. Although the course may wax and wane, it is generally progressive and irreversible. Symptoms of the painful form can range from burning or dull aching sensations to cramping or excruciating, lancinating pain. The pain is often worse at night and partially relieved by movement. Hyperesthesia can be so marked that even light touch is so painful that the patient cannot tolerate bed covers. Physical examination is similar in both types and is often rather unremarkable. The single most common finding is absence of deep tendon reflexes in the lower extremities (i.e., loss of knee and ankle jerks).

ASYMMETRIC NEUROPATHY.

Diabetic mononeuropathies of the cranial nerves usually involve the third, sixth, or fourth cranial nerve in order of frequency. This gives rise to extraocular muscle paralysis with diplopia. The most common syndrome is isolated third nerve palsy accompanied in 80 per cent of cases by sparing of the pupillary reflex. Mononeuropathies of peripheral nerves most frequently occur at sites of external pressure or entrapment (i.e., carpal tunnel). Manifestations include footdrop, wristdrop, or other symptoms related to the particular nerve involved.

Another diabetic neuropathic syndrome involves *radiculopathy*. This syndrome is characterized by dysesthesias and painful hyperesthesia localized to the anatomic distribution of one or more spinal nerves. Symptoms can resemble herpes zoster, although skin lesions are seldom noted.

Diabetic neuropathic cachexia is a syndrome of elderly male diabetics characterized by marked weight loss, painful peripheral polyneuropathy, and depression. The weight loss is so marked that patients appear cachectic, leading to a diagnosis of suspected underlying malignant disease. Other complications of diabetes are typically absent, and patients spontaneously recover in about 1 year.

For a thorough discussion of diabetic symmetric distal polyneuropathy, asymmetric neuropathy, and autonomic neuropathy, see Ch. 498.

Cardiovascular Disease

Cardiovascular disease is the major cause of death in diabetic patients and is far more prevalent than in the nondiabetic population because of accelerated atherogenesis. Not only is cardiovascular disease more frequent, but onset is at an earlier age, and manifestations are more severe. The etiology of the accelerated atherosclerosis in diabetes is incompletely understood, but the causes are probably multifactorial. Most forms of hyperlipoproteinemia are more common in diabetic subjects, and high-density lipoprotein levels tend to be decreased in patients with uncontrolled diabetes. Furthermore, in patients with chronic hyperglycemia, circulating lipoproteins become glycosylated, adversely altering their turnover and sites of tissue deposition. This phenomenon might contribute to the increased risk of atherosclerosis in the absence of grossly elevated circulating lipid levels. Abnormalities of endothelial cell function have also been proposed that would enhance the susceptibility of arterial walls to injury. Increased platelet aggregation and hyperviscosity have also been proposed. Medical management of these risk factors is similar to that in nondiabetic subjects. Thus, specific diet and drug therapy for the various hyperlipoproteinemias should be used when indicated (Ch. 172). On occasion, lipid-lowering drugs such as nicotinic acid may accentuate glucose intolerance. Because of the high risk for atherogenesis, diabetics should be strongly encouraged to abstain from cigarette smoking. Arterial hypertension is a frequent concomitant of diabetes and should be treated promptly. Interestingly, epidemiologic studies have suggested that the existence of hypertension causes little in the way of additive risk for atherosclerosis in diabetics. The diabetic has a substantially greater risk for the development of all forms of cardiovascular disease even when hypertension and hyperlipoproteinemia are taken into account.

The pattern of coronary artery disease (CAD) has been reported to be different in diabetics and nondiabetics, exhibiting in diabetics a greater tendency toward diffuse distal lesions in addition to the usual proximal lesions. However, systematic studies have not uniformly confirmed this notion, suggesting that if this is a feature of CAD in diabetes, then only a minority of patients show diffuse distal occlusive disease. This is important, since one would expect coronary artery bypass surgery to be less successful in patients with distal disease and poor runoff. Overall the indications for myocardial revascularization are probably no different in diabetics and nondiabetics, although a greater incidence of postoperative complications is seen in diabetics. The presence of diabetes substantially eliminates the sex differences in CAD, since the incidence of CAD is roughly comparable in premenopausal diabetic women and age-matched diabetic men. Complications of myocardial infarction are more frequent in diabetics, and postinfarction survival is less. Although angina pectoris is common in diabetic patients, atypical anginal syndromes are seen more frequently than in nondiabetics. Various atypical pain patterns have been described. Painless myocardial infarction has been described in diabetics, probably due to disturbance of afferent nerve fibers. The diagnosis should be suspected in diabetic patients with the sudden onset of left ventricular failure. A syndrome of diabetic cardiomyopathy has been described and is characterized by congestive heart failure in the absence of proximal CAD. It is thought that this syndrome is due to small-vessel occlusive disease. Whether a distinct cardiomyopathy exists in diabetes in the absence of any CAD is still being debated.

Peripheral vascular disease is far more frequent in the diabetic than in the nondiabetic population, and this is particularly so for distal vascular insufficiency of the lower limbs. When combined with the neuropathic complications of diabetes, this unfortunately presents an ideal setting for the development of ischemia and gangrene, necessitating amputation. Because of the marked distal small-vessel disease, vascular bypass surgery is often satisfactory. Most forms of cerebrovascular disease and stroke are also seen more frequently in diabetes.

Dermatologic Lesions

Dermatologic abnormalities are common in diabetes. For example, these patients are more prone to various skin infections such as carbuncles and furuncles. These can often be extensive and difficult to treat. Vaginal candidiasis is frequent in hyperglycemic glycosuric women. Antifungal agents are effective in treating this disorder, but recurrences are common until glycosuria is effectively controlled. Necrobiosis lipoidica diabeticorum consists of round or oval, sharply defined, plaque-like lesions on the anterior surface of the lower legs. The borders of these lesions are frequently elevated, and the center may be depressed. The centers tend to be yellowish, while the borders are hyperpigmented. Although this lesion is uncommon in diabetics, when it does occur, the plaques can ulcerate upon minimal trauma. Diabetic dermopathy (shin spots) is the most frequent dermatologic lesion seen in diabetic patients, occurring in 60 per cent of males and 30 per cent of females. These lesions are common over the tibial area, but also can be observed on forearms and thighs. They begin as small reddish papules that gradually heal, leaving thin hyperpigmented atrophic areas behind. Typical xanthomatoses can occur secondary to hyperlipoproteinemia. In insulin-dependent diabetic subjects, tight waxy skin over the dorsum of the hands in conjunction with joint contractions has been observed. This may be an important clinical observation, since these patients appear to have accelerated development of other microangiopathic complications.

SUMMARY

Diabetes mellitus is a chronic disease and therefore the approach to the patient and methods of management must encompass a long-term view. Patients with diabetes will be interacting with health care providers for the remainder of their lives. The patient must become well educated concerning the disease and eventually learn to individualize all the various components of therapy to his or her own personal circumstances. Ultimately many of the day-to-day therapy and management decisions rest in the hands of the patient. Since much of the treatment of diabetes involves intensive self-care, in a very real sense the patient may be his or her own most important physician. This requires education, motivation, and psychological adjustment.

Brand PW: The diabetic foot. In Ellenberg M, Rifkin H (eds.): Diabetes Mellitus. Theory and Practice, 3rd ed. New Hyde Park, NY, Medical Examination Publishing Co., 1983, pp 829–849. An in-depth review of the clinical manifestations and management of diabetic foot problems.

Bunn HF: Evaluation of glycosylated hemoglobin in diabetic patients. Diabetes 30:613, 1981. A review of the biochemistry, clinical significance, and use of glycosylated hemoglobin in diabetes.

Early Treatment Diabetic Retinopathy Study Research Group: Photocoagulation for diabetic macular edema. Arch Ophthalmol 103:1796, 1985. A report of the multicenter study designed to determine at what point photocoagulation is appropriate therapy for diabetic retinopathy.

Feingold KR: Hypoglycemia: A pitfall of insulin therapy. West J Med 139:688, 1983. An excellent clinical discussion of this important complication of the therapy of diabetes, with 56 references.

Felig PU, McCurdy DK: The hypertonic state. N Engl J Med 297:1444, 1977. A discussion of the pathophysiology and clinical treatment of the hyperosmolar syndrome.

Geffner ME, Lippe BM: The role of immunotherapy in Type I diabetes mellitus. West J Med 146:337, 1987. A recent review covering the pros and cons of the various forms of immunotherapy which have been used or considered for the early treatment of IDDM.

Given BD, Mako ME, Tager H, et al.: Circulating insulin with reduced biological activity in a patient with diabetes. N Engl J Med 302:129, 1980. The first description of a patient producing a biologically defective insulin molecule.

Goetz FC: Recent progress in the management of end-stage diabetic nephropathy. Clin Endocrinol Metab 11:579, 1982. A good discussion of the relative success rates of dialysis and transplantation in end-stage diabetic neuropathy.

Greene DA, Lattimer S, Ulbrecht J, Carroll P: Glucose-induced alterations in nerve metabolism: Current perspective on the pathogenesis of diabetic neuropathy and future directions for research and therapy. Diabetes Care 9:290, 1985. A comprehensive review article discussing current concepts about the pathogenesis of diabetic neuropathy with a view toward therapy.

Kreisberg RA: Diabetic ketoacidosis. In Rifkin H, Porte D Jr (eds.): Ellenberg and Rifkin's Diabetes Mellitus, 4th ed. New York, Elsevier Science Publishing Co., Inc., 1990, pp 591–603. A thorough and current review of the pathogenesis and treatment of this disorder.

Kroc Collaborative Study Group: Blood glucose control and the evolution of diabetic retinopathy and albuminuria. N Engl J Med 311:365, 1984. A report of a well-designed multicenter clinical trial to examine the effect of intensive diabetic control on diabetic complications.

Lernmark A, Baekkeskov S: Islet cell antibodies—Theoretical and practical implications. Diabetologia 21:431, 1981. A discussion of the potential role of autoantibodies directed against β cells in the pathogenesis of diabetes.

L'Esperance FA Jr, James SA Jr: The eye and diabetes mellitus. In Ellenberg M, Rifkin H (eds.): Diabetes Mellitus. Theory and Practice, 3rd ed. New Hyde Park, NY, Medical Examination Publishing Co., 1983, pp 727–757. A general review of the ocular complications of diabetes mellitus with particular emphasis on retinopathy.

McGarry JD, Foster DW: Regulation of hepatic fatty acid oxidation and ketone body production. Ann Rev Biochem 49:395, 1980. Detailed review of the intermediary metabolism of ketogenesis and the pathogenesis of diabetic ketoacidosis.

National Diabetes Data Group: Classification and diagnosis of diabetes mellitus and other categories of glucose intolerance. Diabetes 63:843, 1977. A description of the unified classification system and methods and criteria for diagnosis of diabetes mellitus.

Olefsky JM, Molina JM: Insulin resistance. In Rifkin H, Porte D Jr (eds.): Ellenberg and Rifkin's Diabetes Mellitus, 4th ed. New York, Elsevier Science Publishing Co., Inc., 1990, pp 121–153. A review of the pathogenesis and mechanisms of insulin resistance in NIDDM and their contribution to the overall diabetic state.

Peacock I, Tattersall R: Methods of self monitoring of diabetic control. Clin Endocrinol Metab 11:485, 1982. A review of the rationale and technique of self-monitoring of glucose in diabetes mellitus.

Rotter JI, Rimoin DL: The genetics of diabetes. Hosp Pract 22:79, 1987. A useful general discussion of the genetics of the various types of diabetes mellitus, with a tabular summary of a large number of genetic syndromes associated with it.

Rotter JI, Anderson CE, Rimoin DL: Genetics of diabetes mellitus. In Ellenberg M, Rifkin H (eds.): Diabetes Mellitus. Theory and Practice, 3rd ed. New Hyde Park, NY, Medical Examination Publishing Co., 1983, pp 481–503. A review of the inheritance patterns and the genetic contributions to the etiology of type I and type II diabetes mellitus.

Schade DS, Santiago JV, Skyler JS, et al.: Intensive Insulin Therapy. Princeton, Excerpta Medica, 1983. A monograph outlining the physiologic principles and methods of administering intensive therapy by multiple injections as well as CSII.

Segall M: HLA and genetics of IDDM. Holism vs. reductionism? Diabetes 37:1005, 1988. A review of the interrelationships between the genetic predisposition to IDDM, immunologic abnormalities, and their relationship to the HLA system.

Unger RH, Orci L: Glucagon and the A cell. Physiology and pathophysiology. N Engl J Med 304:1518, 1575, 1981. A review of the physiology of glucagon secretion and action as well as its role in the pathophysiology of diabetes.

Zata R, Brenner BM: Pathogenesis of diabetic microangiopathy. Am J Med 80:443, 1986. A discussion of the role of hemodynamic abnormalities in the pathogenesis of diabetic microangiopathy.

Ziegler AG, Herskowitz RD, Jackson RA, et al.: Predicting Type I diabetes. Diabetes Care 13:762, 1990. A state-of-the-art summary of the current methods that might be useful in predicting the eventual development of type I diabetes. This is particularly important in view of the emergency concepts concerning new therapies that might be useful early in the course of this disease, before clinical manifestations appear.

219 Hypoglycemic Disorders

F. John Service

Hypoglycemia is a pathophysiologic state and not a disease. Just as pain, fever, or vomiting requires identification of the underlying condition, hypoglycemia warrants diagnosis of the primary disorder causing the low plasma glucose concentration.

Hypoglycemia could be considered to be present at glucose concentrations below the lower limit of normal fasting plasma glucose, e.g., below 70 mg per deciliter. However, because hypoglycemic disorders are usually symptomatic clinical syndromes, hypoglycemia is usually defined as a glucose concentration below the level at which symptoms are expected to occur, e.g., below 45 mg per deciliter.

PHYSIOLOGY

Plasma glucose is maintained within narrow bounds, in spite of intermittent food ingestion and periods of fasting, as the net balance between the rates of glucose production and utilization. Following food ingestion, the increase in plasma glucose, in concert with an incretion effect from enteric factors, results in an increase in plasma insulin, which accelerates glucose utilization and suppresses hepatic glucose production. As the plasma glucose concentration falls early in the postabsorptive state, plasma insulin decreases, which restores glucose utilization and production to the preprandial rates. There is then a transition from a state of glucose storage to one of carefully husbanded glucose production at rates designed to satisfy the obligatory needs of the body (see Fig. 218–6). A more extensive discussion of glucose homeostasis is given in Ch. 218.

Glycogenolysis

In the postabsorptive period 4 to 6 hours after food ingestion, plasma glucose concentrations are generally 80 to 90 mg per deciliter, and glucose is produced and utilized at a rate of approximately 2 mg per kilogram per minute. About half of the glucose produced is metabolized by the central nervous system. At this time most glucose (70 to 80 per cent) is produced from hepatic glycogenolysis, with a small contribution (20 to 25 per cent) from gluconeogenesis. Hepatic glycogen stores become exhausted after 24 to 36 hours of fasting.

Glycogenolysis is stimulated by epinephrine and glucagon and inhibited by insulin. Several enzymes are involved in the cleavage of glucose moieties from glycogen and the final appearance of free glucose in the circulation. Abnormalities of these enzymes may result in hypoglycemia. For example, deficient activity of glucose-6-phosphatase (von Gierke's disease) may cause severe hypoglycemia, whereas deficient activities of glycogen phosphorylase and debrancher enzyme cause milder degrees of hypoglycemia (Ch. 169). Deficiency of glycogen synthetase results in severe hypoglycemia in newborns.

Gluconeogenesis

Gluconeogenesis is the generation of new glucose from non-carbohydrate substrates. Defects in this process result in hypoglycemia after prolonged fasting when glycogen stores have been depleted. Lactate and pyruvate, glycerol, and amino acids account for approximately 58 per cent, 13 per cent, and 29 per cent, respectively, of the glucose produced via gluconeogenesis. Defects in gluconeogenesis may arise from (1) diminished substrate availability, e.g., hypoglycemia in renal failure; (2) altered redox state, which inhibits several important gluconeogenic enzymes, e.g., alcohol hypoglycemia; and (3) inhibition of fatty acid oxidation, which diminishes the energy source for gluconeogenesis, e.g., poisoning from the unripe ackee fruit.

Alanine and glutamine are the most important amino acids that act as glucose precursors. The carbon source of alanine is muscle-derived pyruvate, and the nitrogen source for the transamination of pyruvate to alanine is thought to be branched-chain amino acids. Impaired metabolism of leucine, a branched-chain amino acid, observed in maple syrup urine disease, is associated with reduced alanine production and sometimes with hypoglycemia (Ch. 181). After 3 days of fasting, glucose production is derived primarily from hepatic gluconeogenesis. During starvation, renal gluconeogenesis may account for approximately 50 per cent of glucose production.

Hormonal Control of Glucose Homeostasis

The effects of insulin, glucagon, catecholamines, cortisol, and growth hormone on glucose homeostasis and recovery from hypoglycemia are shown in Table 219–1. Insulin is the primary hypoglycemic hormone; the others act by a variety of mechanisms to elevate glucose concentrations. Although glucagon, catecholamines, cortisol, and growth hormone increase in response to insulin-induced hypoglycemia, glucagon makes the major contribution to the acute recovery from hypoglycemia. Catecholamines can modestly elevate glucose concentration in the presence of glucagon deficiency or severe hypoglycemia.

CLINICAL EVALUATION

Defects of many of the mechanisms that maintain plasma glucose in the normal range are associated with readily recognizable clinical syndromes. In some instances the symptoms and signs of the primary disorder predominate over those of hypoglycemia, or at least point to the existence of the primary disorder causing hypoglycemia. In some patients with multisystem disease, poor nutrition, or multiple drug use, the causes of hypoglycemia may be uncertain and the patient too ill to undergo extensive evaluation.

When a patient is observed with symptoms of hypoglycemia, 10 to 20 ml of blood should be drawn in addition to that for glucose determination. Additional analyses (which should include measurement of sulfonylurea if plasma glucose proves to be low) can be determined by the clues generated from the history and physical examination. Such an opportunity may provide sufficient data to establish the cause of the hypoglycemic disorder or to narrow the diagnostic possibilities. Glucose or glucagon should be administered, following blood withdrawal, to any patient suspected of being hypoglycemic. Prompt treatment shortens the duration of hypoglycemia, and, if the patient is not hypoglycemic, no harm is done.

In patients with asymptomatic hypoglycemia one must be alert to artifactual hypoglycemia. Whole blood glucose values may be spuriously low in polycythemia vera because of the unequal distribution of glucose between erythyrocyte and plasma and excessive glycolysis by erythrocytes and in leukemia from excessive glycolysis by leukocytes. Prompt measurement of glucose in plasma in these conditions should provide accurate results.

An uncommon and challenging problem is the low plasma glucose concentration in an asymptomatic patient in whom laboratory error and spurious result have been ruled out. Such patients may have adapted to longstanding hypoglycemia or have mild symptoms that have been completely unrecognized.

A flow diagram of a clinical approach to the evaluation of a suspected hypoglycemic disorder is presented in Figure 219–1. Note that the evaluation is directed to patients who appear healthy. For those who do not appear healthy, the results of the history and physical examination determine the direction of the investigation.

Hypoglycemic disorders cause a constellation of symptoms that usually recur as discrete episodes at irregular intervals. A useful but not infallible historical aid is the timing of symptoms in relation to food intake: Those occurring within 5 hours of food intake are the food-stimulated hypoglycemias and those occurring 5 or more hours after food intake are the food-deprived hypoglycemias (Fig. 219–2).

Considerable effort should be expended to obtain from the patient and family members a detailed description of symptoms, and careful attention should be paid to their occurrence in relation to food intake. The food-stimulated hypoglycemias usually cause symptoms mediated by the autonomic nervous system—sweating, shakiness, anxiety, palpitations, and weakness—and rarely those of impairment of central nervous system function. The food-deprived hypoglycemias, on the other hand, usually result in impairment of central nervous system function—reduced intellectual capacity, confusion, irritability, abnormal behavior, convulsions, and coma. Hypothermia may be observed. Often the autonomic symptoms that precede the central nervous system symptoms go unrecognized. Symptoms of hypoglycemia usually occur at plasma glucose concentrations of about 45 mg per deciliter or less. They are not related to the rate of fall in glucose concentration. The symptoms of hypoglycemia are nonspecific. For this reason it is necessary to demonstrate a low plasma glucose concentration concomitant with symptoms and subsequent relief of symptoms by correction of the hypoglycemia, i.e., *Whipple's triad*. This triad should be demonstrated before hypoglycemia can be considered to be the basis for a patient's symptoms, regardless of the cause of the hypoglycemia. Since persons without a hypoglycemic disorder may feel better after eating, it is imperative to confirm that symptoms are due to hypoglycemia. Every medication used by the patient, including nonprescription drugs, must be examined.

TABLE 219–1. HORMONAL CONTROL OF GLUCOSE HOMEOSTASIS

Hormone	Hepatic Glucose Production	Extrahepatic Glucose Utilization	Basal Glucose Production	Relative Importance to Recovery from Insulin-induced Hypoglycemia
Insulin	↓	↑	↓	+ + +
Glucagon	↑	—	↑	+
Catecholamine*	↑	↓	↑	—
Cortisol	↑	↓	↑	—
Growth hormone†	↑	↓	—	—

↑ = increase; ↓ = decrease; — = no effect.
*Epinephrine is approximately 10 times more potent than norepinephrine. Its action is primarily through a β-adrenergic mechanism. In the presence of glucagon deficiency, catecholamines make a modest contribution to the recovery from hypoglycemia.
†Has an acute and transient hypoglycemic effect.

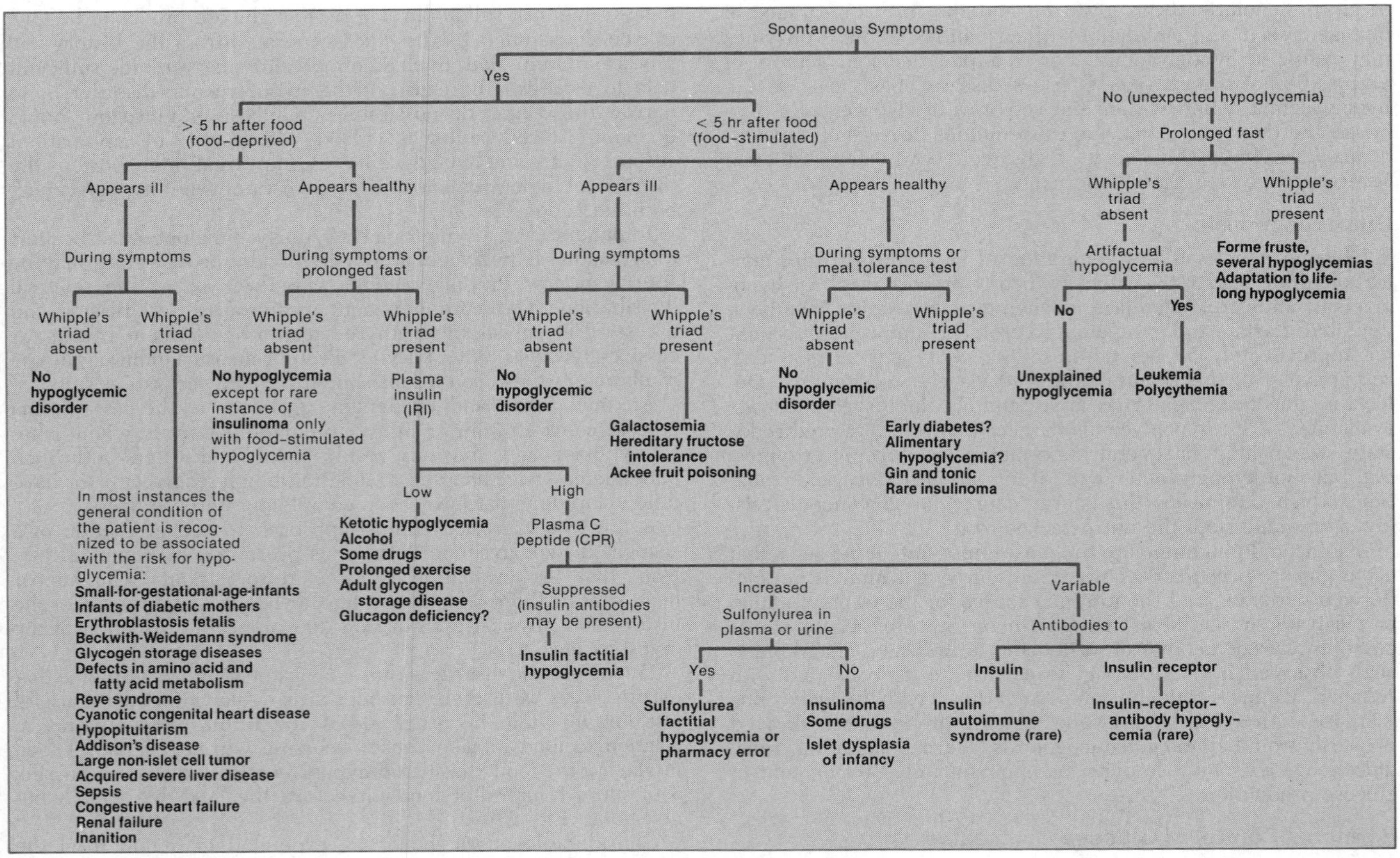

Spontaneous Symptoms

FIGURE 219–1. Evaluation of hypoglycemic disorders.

Because of the erratic occurrence of symptoms of hypoglycemia, glucose determination from a venipuncture specimen may not be feasible. Prompt provision by the patient of a capillary blood sample from a lancet puncture of a fingertip during the occurrence of spontaneous symptoms may be useful. Such a sample may be placed on filter paper or into a capillary tube for subsequent measurement of glucose in a laboratory. Reflectance meter measurement of glucose may be inaccurate in the hypoglycemic range.

FOOD-STIMULATED (POSTPRANDIAL) HYPOGLYCEMIAS

Many patients with postprandial symptoms suggestive of hypoglycemia have normal concomitant blood glucose concentra-

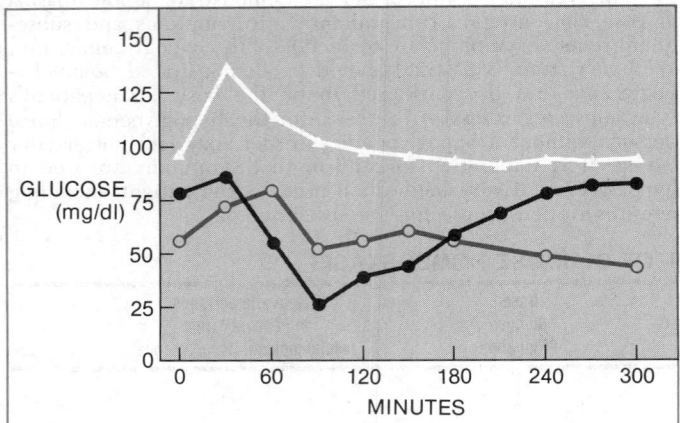

FIGURE 219–2. Differential plasma glucose responses to a mixed meal between patients with food-stimulated hypoglycemia (*closed circles*) and food-deprived hypoglycemia (*open circles*) in contrast to healthy subjects (*triangles*). (Modified from Service FJ: Hypoglycemias. *In* Smith LH Jr (ed): Cecil Textbook of Medicine Update. Philadelphia, WB Saunders Company, 1990.)

tions. For such cases the term "functional hypoglycemia" was coined. Eventually reliance on Whipple's triad was replaced by use of the oral glucose tolerance test (OGTT). If the symptoms experienced during ordinary daily activities were reproduced and a glucose nadir of 50 mg per deciliter or less was documented during the OGTT, the presence of a food-stimulated hypoglycemic disorder was considered to have been confirmed. Use of the OGTT is often misleading, however, since (1) in at least 10 per cent of healthy persons the plasma glucose nadir is less than 50 mg per deciliter; (2) there is no correlation between the nadir of plasma glucose concentrations and the occurrence of symptoms of hypoglycemia in patients with symptoms suggestive of food-stimulated hypoglycemia; (3) the results of OGTT are variable upon repeated testing; (4) subjects with symptoms during an OGTT may have similar symptoms during a placebo OGTT; and (5) glycemia less than 50 mg per deciliter after oral glucose cannot usually be reproduced after a mixed meal despite the presence of symptoms during both. Measurement of plasma cortisol responses, calculation of rates of glucose descent, and hypoglycemic indices have not improved the accuracy of the OGTT.

Unfortunately, reliance on the OGTT for the diagnosis of food-stimulated hypoglycemia has led to extensive literature, not on disorders of hypoglycemia but on the test itself. Although there undoubtedly are patients with true postprandial hypoglycemia, most persons with symptoms following meals have psychoneurosis. Low carbohydrate–high protein diets, sulfonylureas, biguanides, and anticholinergic agents have not been shown to be effective treatment for such patients.

Hypoglycemia following the ingestion of substances that are toxic to susceptible persons may be considered in the category of postprandial hypoglycemias. The ingestion of large amounts (equivalent of three highballs) of ethanol and carbohydrate (gin and tonic) may cause hypoglycemia within 3 to 4 hours in some healthy persons. The unripe ackee fruit may result in hypoglycemia in children or adults with chronic malnutrition by inhibiting the transport of long-chain fatty acids into mitochondria, thereby suppressing their oxidation and depressing gluconeogenesis. Postprandial hypoglycemia occurs in children with galactosemia (Ch.

TABLE 219–2. SYMPTOMS OF HYPOGLYCEMIA

Autonomic nervous system dysfunction
Sweating
Shakiness
Anxiety
Palpitations
Weakness

Central nervous system dysfunction
Diplopia
Blurred vision
Confusion
Abnormal behavior
Amnesia
Unconsciousness
Seizures

168) and hereditary fructose intolerance (Ch. 170) should the relevant offending hexose be eaten.

FOOD-DEPRIVED (FASTING) HYPOGLYCEMIAS

Drug-Induced Hypoglycemias

Drugs constitute the most common cause of hypoglycemia, when treatment of diabetic persons with insulin and sulfonylureas is included. Errors in filling prescriptions by substitution of a sulfonylurea for the intended medication and drug administration errors by hospital staff or the patient are increasingly common causes of hypoglycemia. Factors increasing the risk of drug-induced hypoglycemia are extremes of age, antecedent food deprivation, and impaired renal and hepatic function. Other drugs implicated as the cause of hypoglycemia are salicylates (in children), propranolol (in patients with other conditions having the potential to cause hypoglycemia), ethanol, disopyramide (Norpace), sulfamethoxazole and trimethoprim (Bactrim, Septra) (in the presence of renal failure), pentamidine (Lomidine), and quinine (when used for cerebral malaria). Since a wide variety of drugs has been implicated as the cause of hypoglycemia, the reader is referred to review articles on this subject.

Ethanol-induced hypoglycemia arises from inhibition of gluconeogenesis as a result of the increase in the NADH-NAD ratio in instances of depleted hepatic glycogen. The increased NADH-NAD ratio suppresses the conversions of lactate to pyruvate, glycerophosphate to dihydroxyacetone phosphate, and glutamate to ketoglutarate and several tricarboxylic cycle reactions. Infusion of ethanol into healthy subjects for 4 hours results in hypoglycemia, reduced rates of hepatic glucose production, suppressed plasma insulin concentrations, increased plasma lactate, β-hydroxybutyrate, glycerol, and free fatty acid concentrations, and increased lactate-pyruvate and β-hydroxybutyrate-acetoacetate ratios. Hypoglycemia usually develops within 6 to 36 hours of the ingestion of even moderate amounts of ethanol by persons chronically malnourished or by healthy persons who have missed one or two meals. Healthy children are especially susceptible to ethanol hypoglycemia. Blood ethanol levels may not be elevated when the patient is hypoglycemic.

INSULINOMA

Insulinoma is a rare disorder; its incidence is approximately 1 patient per 250,000 person-years. Insulinoma may occur slightly more commonly in women. It is uncommon in persons less than 20 years of age and rare in those less than 5 years of age. The median age at diagnosis is about 50 years, except in patients with the multiple endocrine neoplasia syndrome type 1 (MEN 1), in which it is in the mid 20's.

Of patients with insulinoma, approximately 87 per cent have single benign tumors, approximately 7 per cent have multiple benign tumors, and approximately 6 per cent have malignant tumors. Eight per cent of insulinoma patients have MEN 1 (Ch. 228). Sixty per cent of patients with MEN 1 have multiple tumors. Fifty per cent of patients with multiple insulinomas have MEN 1.

Some tumors secrete hormones in addition to insulin: gastrin, 5-hydroxyindoles, ACTH, glucagon, and somatostatin. In rare instances, insulinomas have occurred in non–insulin-dependent diabetic persons but have never been documented in an insulin-dependent patient.

Clinical Picture

Symptoms may be present for many years prior to the diagnosis. In one series 85 per cent of patients had various combinations of diplopia, blurred vision, sweating, palpitations, and weakness; 80 per cent had confusion or abnormal behavior; 53 per cent had unconsciousness or amnesia; and 12 per cent had grand mal seizures (Table 219–2). Twenty per cent of cases may be misdiagnosed, the belief being that the patient has a neurologic or psychiatric disorder.

Hypoglycemia usually occurs 5 or more hours after any meal. In rare instances, symptoms may occur solely in the postprandial period (2 to 4 hours after eating) and never during fasting. Symptoms may be aggravated by exercise, alcohol use, a high protein–low carbohydrate diet, treatment with sulfonylureas, and fasts. Less than 20 per cent of patients with insulinoma gain weight.

Diagnosis

The diagnosis of insulinoma is based on the demonstration of Whipple's triad and nonsuppressed plasma insulin and C-peptide levels, either with spontaneous hypoglycemia or with that induced by a prolonged fast. A simplified diagnostic scheme is shown in Figure 219–3. Insulin antibodies are usually undetectable but may be present in low titers. In lieu of demonstrating Whipple's triad during the spontaneous occurrence of symptoms, useful diagnostic tests are the prolonged supervised fast, the intravenous tolbutamide test, and the C-peptide suppression test.

SUPERVISED FAST. The prolonged supervised fast is the classic test for the diagnosis of insulinoma. During the fast the patient should be active during the day. Noncaloric beverages may be consumed. The frequency of blood sampling should be guided by the patient's history of tolerance to food withdrawal

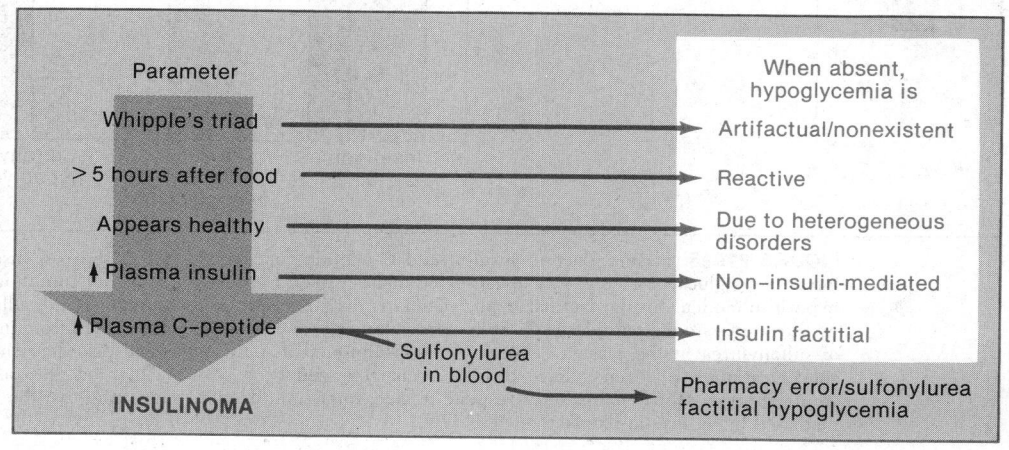

FIGURE 219–3. Important parameters for the diagnosis of insulinoma.

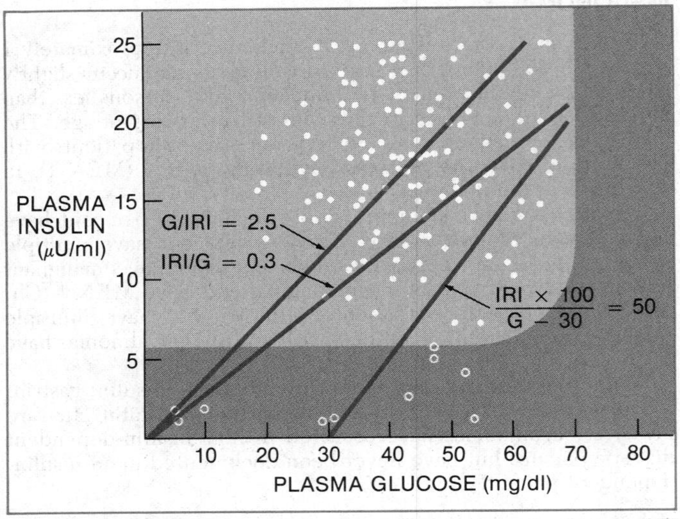

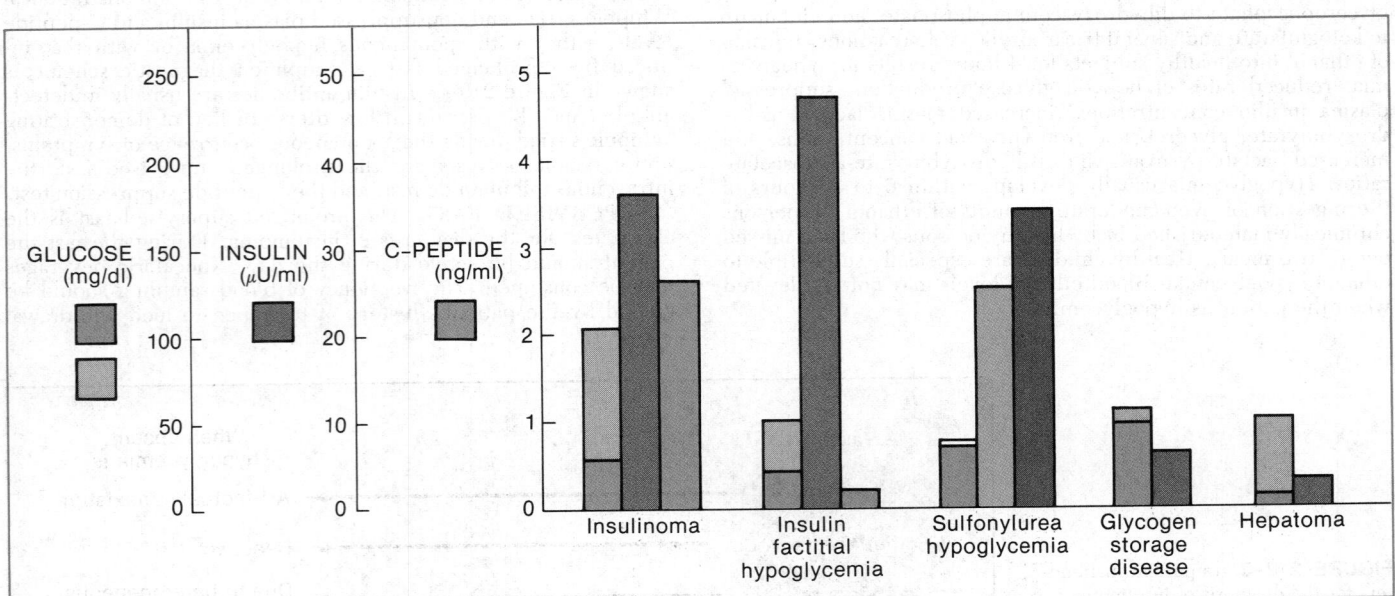

FIGURE 219-4. Simultaneously measured plasma glucose and insulin concentrations in patients with histologically confirmed insulinoma (*closed circles*) and in patients with non–insulin-mediated hypoglycemia (*open circles*). Various ratios: Glucose/insulin = 2.5, insulin/glucose = 0.3, and insulin × 100/glucose − 30 = 50, designed to establish relative hyperinsulinemia, are much less useful than using a value of plasma insulin of 6 μU per milliliter as a discriminator. (Reprinted with permission from Service FJ: Clinical presentation and laboratory evaluation of hypoglycemic disorders in adults. *In* Service FJ (ed.): Hypoglycemic Disorders. Boston, GK Hall, 1983, pp 73–95.)

and be increased as the plasma glucose approaches the hypoglycemic range. Whenever blood is withdrawn for glucose determination, plasma insulin and C-peptide should be measured. Plasma should also be submitted for detection of sulfonylurea, especially if accidental or surreptitious ingestion of this drug is suspected. The patient's mental status should be checked regularly. During prolonged fasting healthy women experience lower plasma glucose concentrations than do healthy men: Values as low as 42 mg per deciliter in men and 34 mg per deciliter in women may be unaccompanied by symptoms. Therefore, it is essential to continue the fast to the point at which symptoms develop, or to 72 hours. Upon demonstration of Whipple's triad, either during the prolonged fast or spontaneously, glucagon, 1 mg, should be injected intravenously. Whereas a prompt increase in glucose concentration indicates an insulin-mediated hypoglycemic disorder such as insulinoma, a blunted glucose response indicates glycogen storage disease or a disorder that impairs glycogenesis or glycogenolysis.

Plasma insulin concentrations frequently are "normal" when the plasma glucose is in the hypoglycemic range (Fig. 219–4). Since patients with insulinoma have been observed to have plasma insulin levels as low as 6 μU per milliliter during hypoglycemia, relative hyperinsulinemia (nonsuppressed insulin levels) may be considered as values of 6 μU per milliliter or more. Glucose-insulin ratios are less helpful in confirming relative hyperinsulinemia (Fig. 219–4). The patterns of plasma glucose, insulin, and C-peptide during hypoglycemia and the plasma glucose response to intravenous glucagon, 1 mg, are shown in Figure 219–5 for insulinoma and other causes of food-deprived hypoglycemia.

In a large series, Whipple's triad was demonstrated within 12 hours of the last meal in 29 per cent of patients, within 24 hours in 71 per cent, within 36 hours in 79 per cent, within 48 hours in 92 per cent, within 60 hours in 97 per cent, and within 72 hours in 98 per cent. In rare instances, patients with insulinoma may not develop hypoglycemia during prolonged fasting of even up to 96 hours. At the time of hypoglycemic symptoms, plasma glucose concentrations were 46 mg per deciliter or less in 100 per cent of patients, 39 mg per deciliter or less in 75 per cent, 35 mg per deciliter or less in 50 per cent, and 28 mg per deciliter or less in 25 per cent.

THE INTRAVENOUS TOLBUTAMIDE TEST. This test (tolbutamide, 1 gram intravenously over 3 minutes) should be performed only in persons for whom the fasting plasma glucose is known to exceed 50 mg per deciliter immediately prior to the test and who have not been food deprived for several days preceding the test. The best criterion for the interpretation of the tolbutamide test is the mean of the values at 120, 150, and 180 minutes (Fig. 219–6). The criterion of 55 mg per deciliter for lean persons and 62 mg per deciliter for obese persons provides 95 per cent and 100 per cent sensitivity, respectively,

FIGURE 219-5. Plasma glucose, insulin, and C-peptide concentrations and the response of plasma glucose to intravenous glucagon (1 mg) in five causes of food-deprived hypoglycemia. Three conditions are characterized by hyperinsulinemia: Insulin factitial hypoglycemia is distinguished from insulinoma and sulfonylurea hypoglycemia by the suppressed C-peptide level. Sulfonylurea hypoglycemia can be distinguished from insulin only by detection of sulfonylurea in the plasma. The two non–insulin-mediated hypoglycemic disorders show low plasma insulin concentrations. Glycogen storage disease is characterized by a severely blunted glucose response to glucagon administration. Hepatoma patients respond to glucagon administration, suggesting that the hypoglycemia is in part mediated by an insulin-like factor—IGF II?

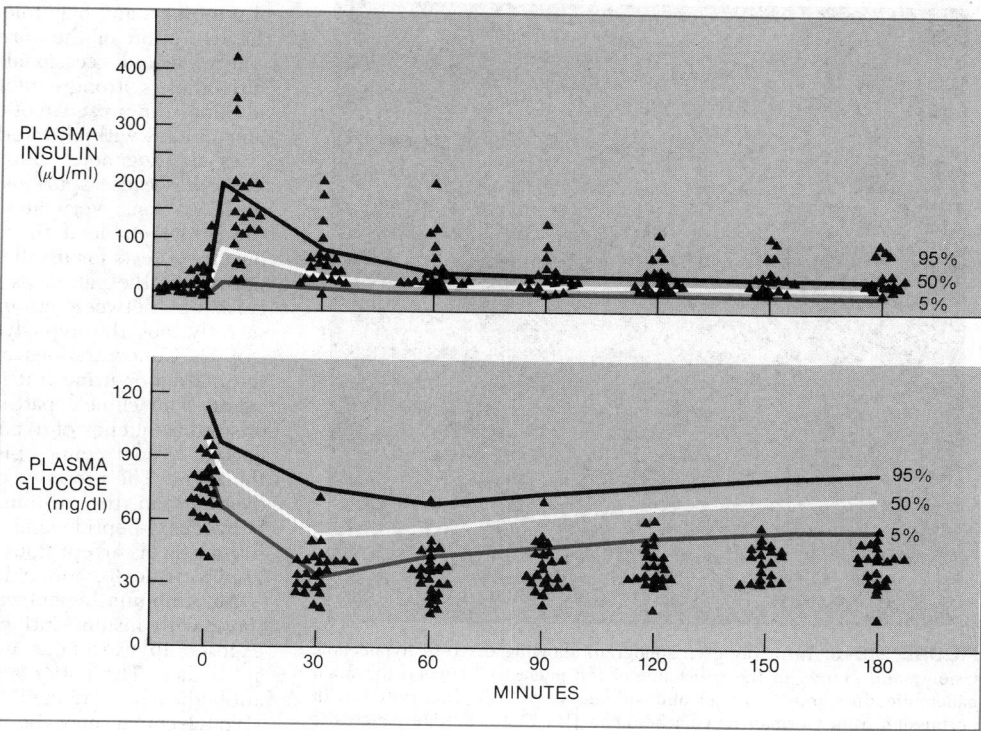

FIGURE 219–6. Plasma glucose and insulin responses to the intravenous tolbutamide test in 261 lean, healthy persons shown as the 5th, 50th, and 95th percentiles and 27 lean patients with insulinoma shown as triangles. (Modified from McMahon MM, et al.: Diagnostic interpretation of the intravenous tolbutamide test for insulinoma. Mayo Clin Proc 64:1481, 1989.)

at 95 per cent specificity. Plasma insulin responses are less sensitive diagnostic discriminators. If the plasma glucose responses to intravenous tolbutamide are normal, the insulin values should be ignored.

THE C-PEPTIDE SUPPRESSION TEST. This test (insulin 0.125 unit per kilogram over 60 minutes or an equivalent total dose given at a slower rate over 3 hours) is based on the observation that hypoglycemia induced by exogenous insulin fails to suppress C-peptide concentration normally in those with insulinomas (Fig. 219–7). The criteria for normal C-peptide suppression are influenced by age and body mass index. The euglycemic C-peptide suppression test involves maintenance of euglycemia during insulin infusion. This approach relies on inhibition of insulin release by insulin itself and has the advantage of avoiding hypoglycemia. It is difficult to know how useful this approach to C-peptide suppression is because it has been used in only a few patients. Furthermore, if the patient is hypoglycemic prior to the test, the test is virtually in process: Measurement of plasma glucose, insulin, and C-peptide will provide a diagnosis. If the patient is not hypoglycemic, the standard test (insulin infusion without maintaining euglycemia) can be conducted.

THE INTRAVENOUS GLUCAGON TEST. This test (glucagon, 1 mg intravenously) has an accuracy of 50 to 80 per cent using criteria of peak insulin of 130 μU per milliliter or more or an increase above basal level of 100 μU per milliliter or more when conducted after an overnight fast. Unfortunately, many medications influence the response to glucagon.

OTHER TESTS. The utility of other tests such as glycosylated hemoglobin, human pancreatic polypeptide, and infusions of alcohol, calcium, epinephrine and propranolol, diazoxide, and somatostatin-tolbutamide in the diagnosis of insulinoma is unproven or inadequate. Human chorionic gonadotropin or one of its subunits may be a marker for functioning malignant insulinomas. Eighty per cent of patients with insulinoma may have elevated proinsulin concentrations (>20 per cent of total immunoreactive insulin). Recently improved assays for proinsulin may enhance its diagnostic accuracy.

Localization

Only after the diagnosis of insulinoma has been confirmed biochemically should a localization procedure be done. Pancreatic

angiography has been reported to have a high rate of success if stereoscopy, magnification, and subtraction are used. Insulinomas appear as homogeneous, intensely vascular, sharply circumscribed masses within the substance of the pancreas.

Computed tomography has had limited success in localization. Real-time high-resolution ultrasonography performed by a skilled operator is the preferred localization procedure. Success at finding the tumor is 68 per cent for preoperative ultrasonography and 86 per cent for intraoperative ultrasonography (Fig. 219–8). Percutaneous transhepatic portal venous sampling for insulin has the disadvantage of being highly invasive. It is usually unnecessary if a skilled ultrasonographer is available. Failure to localize an insulinoma preoperatively should not deter pancreatic exploration in a patient for whom the diagnosis has been firmly established, because the combination of a skilled surgeon and an ultrasonographer experienced with insulinomas is highly successful in finding the tumor.

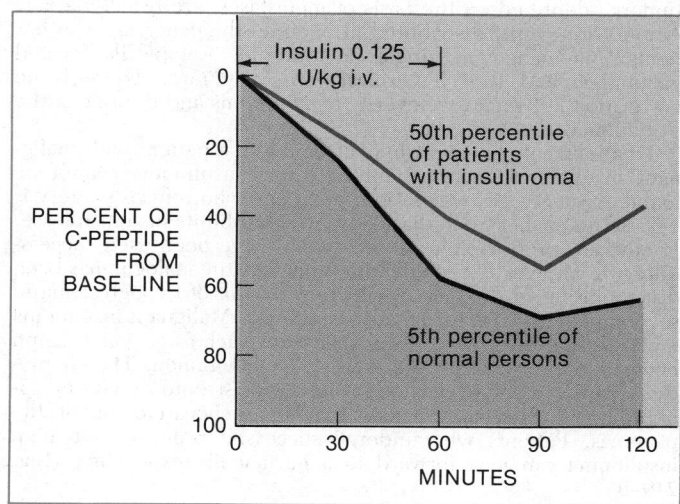

FIGURE 219–7. C-peptide suppression test shows less suppression of C-peptide in a typical patient with insulinoma in contrast to normal persons.

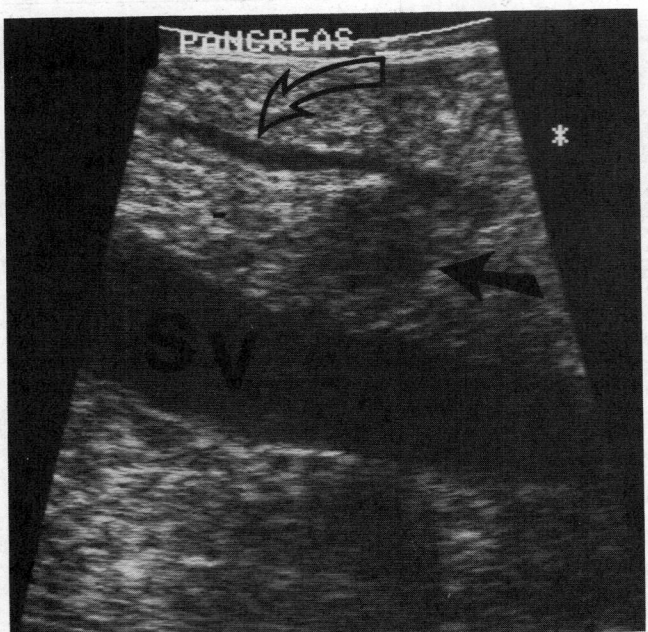

FIGURE 219–8. Intraoperative sonogram showing discrete hypoechoic lesion (*solid arrow*) in the substance of the pancreas between the main pancreatic duct (*open arrow*) and splenic vein (SV). (Reprinted with permission from Gorman B, Charbonneau JW, et al.: Benign pancreatic insulinoma: Preoperative and intraoperative sonographic localization. AJR 147:929, 1986. © 1986, American Roentgen Ray Society.)

Treatment

Surgical removal is the preferred treatment for insulinoma. In a large series, 58 per cent of subjects underwent successful enucleation of the tumor; 33 per cent, partial pancreatectomy; and the remainder, a variety of other procedures. In the series, 88 per cent were cured, 2 per cent had diabetes, and the remainder required medical treatment to control persistent hypoglycemia from malignant insulinoma, islet hyperplasia, or a tumor missed during surgery. Operative mortality has not been observed for many decades. The postoperative complication rate is about 10 per cent. The risk of recurrence is 8 per cent at 20 years following initial successful resection.

Intraoperative glucose monitoring should not be relied upon for surgical management, since there is a high (23 per cent) incidence of failure of plasma glucose to increase after successful insulinoma removal.

The median diameter of benign tumors is 1.5 cm. Malignant tumors (identified on the basis of metastases) are usually larger. Tumors are evenly distributed throughout the pancreas, whether benign or malignant, single or multiple. Ectopically located insulinoma and islet hyperplasia are very rare. There is no correlation between the severity of symptoms and the size of the insulinoma.

Treatment of persistent hypoglycemia in a patient with malignant insulinoma, in a patient in whom insulinoma cannot be found at pancreatic exploration, or in one who refuses surgery is best accomplished with diazoxide, which inhibits insulin release. Phenytoin, propranolol, and verapamil have been used successfully in some cases. A long-acting somatostatin analogue has been disappointing in the lack of effective control of hypoglycemia in several patients with malignant insulinoma. Malignant insulinoma metastasizes primarily to local structures such as regional lymph nodes and liver; distant metastases are uncommon. The chemotherapeutic regimen of choice consists of streptozotocin and 5-fluorouracil. Survival exceeds that in adenocarcinoma of the pancreas. Patients who undergo successful removal of benign insulinoma can look forward to a normal life expectancy (Fig. 219–9).

FACTITIAL AND AUTOIMMUNE HYPOGLYCEMIA

Nondiabetic persons who secretly take insulin or sulfonylureas are predominantly women in the third and fourth decades of life who are employed in health-related occupations. Patients with factitial hypoglycemia have an erratic pattern in the occurrence of symptoms and may tolerate prolonged periods of fasting. With the exception of the rare instance of the insulin autoimmune syndrome and occasional insulinomas, the presence of insulin antibodies is strong evidence of repeated injection of insulin. In addition, the presence of low plasma concentrations of C-peptide concomitant with elevated insulin levels and hypoglycemia indicates an exogenous source of insulin (see Fig. 219–5). Insulin antibodies cause spurious radioimmunoassayable plasma insulin concentrations: very high if the double-antibody assay is used and undetectable if the charcoal-coated dextran assay is used. Results of tests for insulinoma (including the C-peptide suppression test if the patient is taking a sulfonylurea) may be indistinguishable between an insulinoma patient and a patient who secretly took the hypoglycemic agent prior to the test (see Fig. 219–5). Concentrations of sulfonylurea should be measured in the plasma or urine if it is suspected of being the hypoglycemic agent. The clinical pattern in diabetic subjects consists of increased frequency of hypoglycemia during treatment and persistence of hypoglycemic episodes after complete cessation of use of the agent. The presence of insulin antibodies is of no help in the diagnosis in the insulin-treated patient. An inverse relation between C-peptide and insulin levels during hypoglycemia is diagnostic of surreptitious insulin administration. Insulin has been used for suicide, homicide, and child abuse.

Autoimmune hypoglycemia comprises two classes of patients, those with insulin antibodies who have apparently never been exposed to exogenous insulin and those with insulin receptor antibodies. The patients with spontaneous generation of insulin antibodies have ranged in age from a few days old to elderly. Hypoglycemia may be severe, may occur during fasting or postprandially, and is often self-limited. During episodes of hypoglycemia, plasma free insulin levels have been found to be elevated and plasma C-peptide concentrations have varied from elevated to suppressed. Distinguishing between insulin antibody autoimmune hypoglycemia and factitial hypoglycemia may be very difficult. The observation of intermittent production of an abnormal insulin that is immunogenic has not been supported by other studies. Species specificity, association constants, and binding capacities for human, porcine, and bovine insulins of the antibodies from patients with autoimmune hypoglycemia are not different from those of antibodies from insulin-treated diabetics. However, there are sufficient differences in the frequency and duration of insulin administration between patients with factitial hypoglycemia and insulin-treated diabetics to require full characterization of the insulin, proinsulin, and C-peptide antibodies in proved factitial hypoglycemia for comparison with those of the autoimmune hypoglycemic syndrome. Distinction between autoimmune and factitial hypoglycemia by antibody characteristics may become even more difficult now that human insulin has come into common use. Neither the biochemical characteristics of this syndrome nor the mechanism of the hypoglycemia has been fully elucidated.

Hypoglycemia has been observed in persons with insulin receptor antibodies. During hypoglycemia, plasma insulin levels have been found to be elevated and C-peptide levels have been suppressed. Most of the patients with hypoglycemia had preexisting insulin-resistant diabetes and evidence for autoimmune disease prior to the development of hypoglycemia. Antagonist and agonist action of insulin receptor antibodies may be due to different populations of insulin receptor antibodies which recognize different antigenic sites. This syndrome may respond to glucocorticoid therapy or methylpalmoxinate, an inhibitor of free fatty acid oxidation, but is not improved by immunosuppressive agents or plasmapheresis.

NON–BETA CELL TUMOR HYPOGLYCEMIA

A wide variety of tumors of mesenchymal or epithelial origin and some malignant hematologic diseases have been associated with hypoglycemia.

Mesenchymal tumors account for 45 to 64 per cent of the reported cases. Approximately one third of the tumors are located in the chest and two thirds are in the abdomen, usually in the retroperitoneum. They usually are large and therefore readily detectable. Hepatomas account for 22 per cent of cases.

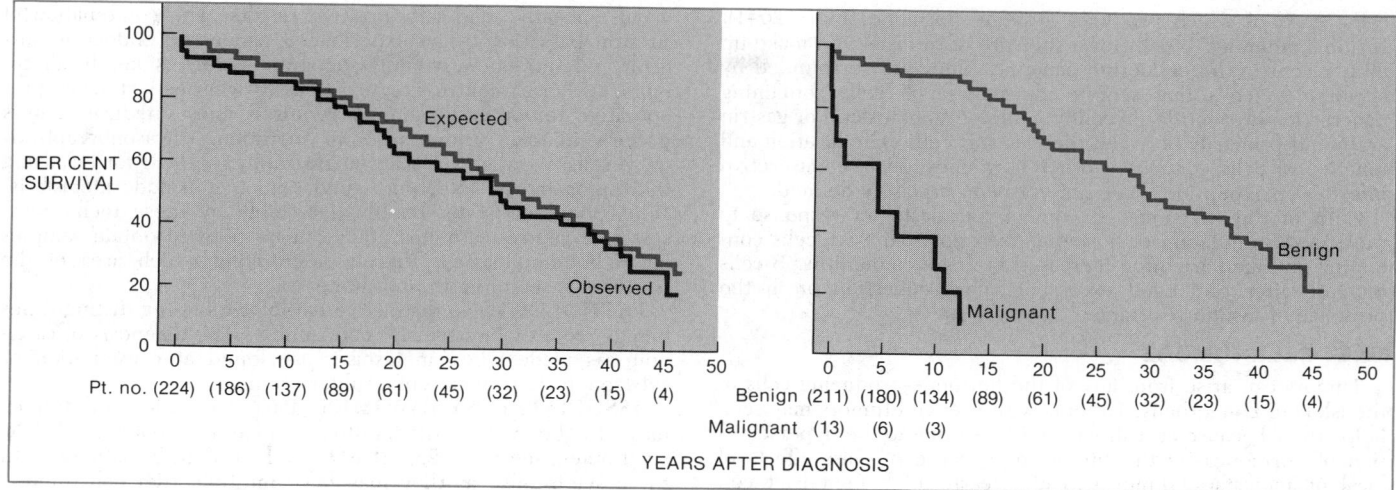

FIGURE 219–9. Survival (%) after histologic confirmation of insulinoma observed in 224 patients over 45 years in contrast to expected survival, and in benign versus malignant insulinoma. (Reprinted with permission from Service FJ, et al.: Functioning insulinoma—Incidence, recurrence and long-term survival of patients: A 60-year study. Mayo Clin Proc 66:711–719, 1991.)

No single pathogenetic mechanism satisfactorily explains all cases of tumor-related hypoglycemia. In some, more than one mechanism may be involved. Metastatic destruction of the adrenals or pituitary and extensive metastatic involvement of the liver can impair glucoregulatory mechanisms. Some tumors evince a high rate of glucose utilization. In others, substances such as tryptophan metabolites may impair gluconeogenesis. There has not been convincing documentation of insulin secretion by a non–islet cell tumor, although hyperinsulinism resolved following tumor removal in one patient. Although elevated levels of insulin-like growth factor II (IGF II) and IGF II mRNA have been observed in some patients with non–islet cell tumor hypoglycemia, there is controversy regarding the role of the polypeptide in the genesis of hypoglycemia. Total or partial surgical removal of the tumor usually results in amelioration of the hypoglycemia.

HYPOGLYCEMIA IN HEPATIC, RENAL, AND ENDOCRINE DISORDERS AND MISCELLANEOUS CONDITIONS

Symptomatic hypoglycemia is uncommon in liver disease because glucose homeostasis can be maintained with as little as 20 per cent of healthy parenchymal cells, but biochemical hypoglycemia has been reported in a wide variety of acquired hepatic diseases. The hypoglycemia of congestive heart failure, sepsis, and Reye's syndrome is considered to be due to hepatic mechanisms. During hypoglycemia, plasma insulin and C-peptide concentrations are suppressed.

Hypoglycemia is uncommon in adrenocortical insufficiency. Hypoglycemia in hypopituitarism is common in children under 6 years of age but less so beyond that age. Asymptomatic hypoglycemia has been observed in isolated growth hormone deficiency after prolonged fasting. Spontaneous hypoglycemia has been reported to be a frequent finding in isolated ACTH deficiency. Adults surgically deprived of epinephrine are not subject to hypoglycemia.

Hypoglycemia in nondiabetic persons with renal failure may be due to inadequate gluconeogenic substrate availability. Glucagon deficiency is a theoretic mechanism for hypoglycemia, but the existence of this disorder has not been confirmed.

Hypoglycemia is a concomitant of starvation. It has been observed in persons with protein-calorie malnutrition as a result of anorexia nervosa or extreme food faddism. Inanition may be one of several factors in the genesis of hypoglycemia in patients with multisystem disease and prolonged intravenous fluid therapy. Prolonged, severe exercise may provoke hypoglycemia in untrained persons but is less likely to do so in athletes.

Garber AJ, Bier DM, Cryer PE, et al.: Hypoglycemia in compensated chronic renal insufficiency. Substrate limitation of gluconeogenesis. Diabetes 23:982, 1974. *Data are presented indicating that hypoglycemia in chronic renal failure may be due to inadequate availability of alanine.*

Hogan MJ, Service FJ, Sharbrough F, et al.: Oral glucose tolerance test compared with a mixed meal in the diagnosis of reactive hypoglycemia. A caveat on stimulation. Mayo Clin Proc 58:491, 1983. *The authors demonstrated the inadequacy of the oral glucose tolerance test for the diagnosis of postprandial symptoms. Patients considered to have food-stimulated hypoglycemia after oral glucose tolerance testing had no hypoglycemia after a mixed meal despite the presence of postprandial symptoms. In addition, EEG monitoring during postprandial symptoms showed no changes.*

Lowe WL, Roberts CT Jr, LeRoith D, et al.: Insulin-like growth factor-II in nonislet cell tumors associated with hypoglycemia: Increased levels of messenger ribonucleic acid. J Clin Endocrinol Metab 69:1153, 1989. *Nonislet cell tumors associated with hypoglycemia were found to produce large amounts of IGF-II mRNA.*

Marks V: Hypoglycemia. Oxford, Blackwell Scientific Publications, Ltd., 1981. *An authoritative reference work on hypoglycemic disorders.*

Palardy J, Havrankova J, Lepage R, et al.: Blood glucose measurements during symptomatic episodes in patients with suspected postprandial hypoglycemia. N Engl J Med 321:1421, 1989. *The importance of measuring glucose during the occurrence of spontaneous symptoms of hypoglycemia is clearly demonstrated by the data in this paper. When self-collected capillary blood specimens on filter paper were analyzed for glucose, only 5 per cent had values less than 2.8 mM per liter (50 mg per deciliter).*

Scarlett JA, Mako ME, Rubenstein AH, et al.: Factitious hypoglycemia. Diagnosis and measurement of serum C-peptide immunoreactivity and insulin-binding antibodies. N Engl J Med 297:1029, 1977. *Seven cases of surreptitious injection of insulin are described. The authors emphasize the importance of the triad of low plasma glucose and high plasma insulin levels and suppression of plasma C-peptide for diagnosis of this condition. In addition, there is a useful discussion of characteristics of antibodies to insulin, proinsulin, and C-peptide of human, porcine, and bovine origin for the distinction between factitial and autoimmune hypoglycemia.*

Seltzer HS: Severe drug-induced hypoglycemia: A review. Comp Ther 5:21, 1979. *An excellent reference source regarding the drugs implicated and the conditions conducive to drug-induced hypoglycemia.*

Service FJ, McMahon MM, O'Brien PC, et al.: Incidence, recurrence and survival of insulinoma. A sixty-year study. In preparation. *This paper provides new information on the natural history of insulinoma generated from experience over a 60-year period with 224 patients with insulinoma.*

Taylor SI, Greenberger J, Marcus-Samuels B, et al.: Hypoglycemia associated with antibodies to the insulin receptor. N Engl J Med 307:1422, 1982. *The authors report a nondiabetic patient with fasting hypoglycemia ascribed to the action of autoantibodies to the insulin receptor. Although the few other patients with this syndrome had a history of prior diabetes, evidence for coexistent autoimmune disease is a clue to the presence of antireceptor antibodies.*

220 Pancreatic Islet Cell Tumors

Carl Grunfeld

THE ISLETS OF LANGERHANS

Dispersed throughout the exocrine pancreas are nests of endocrine cells, the islets of Langerhans. The islet itself is a miniature organ with a distinctive organization of individualized cells, each of which produces a single hormone (Fig. 220–1). Insulin-containing B cells form the core of the islet and make up 60 per cent of the endocrine pancreas. They are surrounded by a rim of A cells that secrete glucagon or F cells containing pancreatic polypeptide. D cells containing somatostatin or gastrin are found primarily between the A and B cells. The location and function of cells containing other hormones, such as vasoactive intestinal polypeptide, have not yet been precisely defined.

Cells of the islets may become hyperplastic in response to prolonged stimulation of hormone secretion. Thus, A cells containing glucagon are often increased in diabetes mellitus. B cells increase after prolonged excessive caloric ingestion or in the presence of insulin resistance.

ISLET CELL TUMORS

Tumors can arise from any of the hormone-producing cells of the islets of Langerhans. Patients with islet cell tumors may seek help either because of distinct syndromes due to the hypersecretion of hormones by the tumors or because of mass effects of local or metastatic tumor spread. Nearly all benign islet cell tumors and more than 80 per cent of carcinomas secrete clinically significant amounts of hormone; some secrete multiple hormones. Clinical presentation usually reflects the dominance of one hormone (Table 220–1).

The tumor is named after the hormone responsible for the syndrome or, in asymptomatic patients, the hormone found in highest concentration in the circulation or in the tumor. For example, a tumor producing insulin is known as an insulinoma, and one producing glucagon is a glucagonoma. Tumors may also secrete human chorionic gonadotropin or chromogranin A and B.

DIAGNOSIS. Diagnosis of islet cell tumors is usually made by detecting elevated basal or fasting levels of the suspected hormone in the presence of the characteristic syndrome. Provocative tests have also been developed that use pharmacologic agents to discriminate between secretion from a tumor and from normal pancreas. In addition, tumors usually secrete a larger proportion of prohormone or other species of high molecular weight than do normal islet cells.

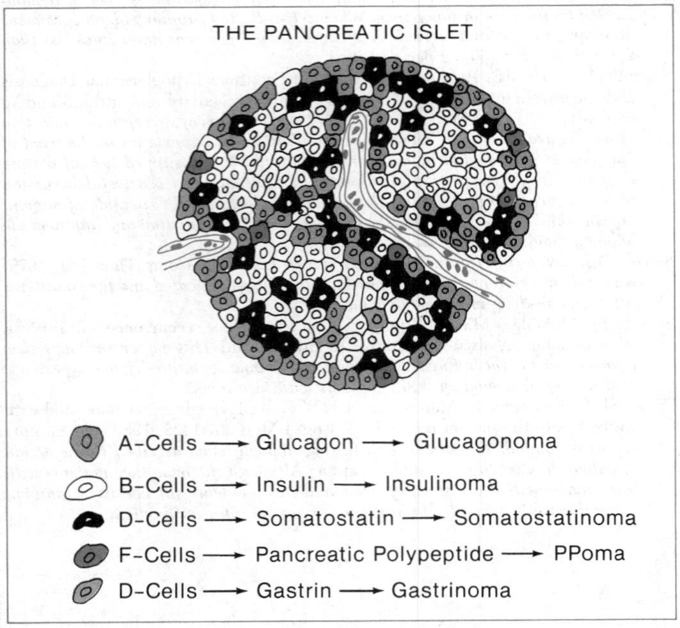

THE PANCREATIC ISLET

A-Cells ⟶ Glucagon ⟶ Glucagonoma
B-Cells ⟶ Insulin ⟶ Insulinoma
D-Cells ⟶ Somatostatin ⟶ Somatostatinoma
F-Cells ⟶ Pancreatic Polypeptide ⟶ PPoma
D-Cells ⟶ Gastrin ⟶ Gastrinoma

FIGURE 220–1. Morphology of the islets of Langerhans. This schematic representation of a typical islet demonstrates the distinctive distribution of hormone-secreting cells within the islet. Insulin-containing B cells, forming the core of the islet, are surrounded by glucagon-containing A cells. D cells are interspersed. In the posterior portion of the head of the pancreas, the proportion of cells containing pancreatic polypeptide is increased and the number of glucagon-secreting cells is strikingly decreased. (Modified from Unger RH, Orci L: Glucagon and the A cell: Physiology and pathophysiology. N Engl J Med 304:1518, 1981. Reprinted by permission of the New England Journal of Medicine.)

Imaging techniques should not be relied upon to make the diagnosis of an islet cell tumor, as there are a significant number of false-negative and false-positive results. The combination of surgical palpation by an experienced pancreatic endocrine surgeon and intraoperative ultrasonography detects nearly all tumors. Although controversy exists as to whether extensive preoperative tumor localization is required, most medical centers perform imaging studies prior to operation. Ultrasonography is more sensitive than CT scan, angiography, or MRI for localizing the tumor and in detecting hepatic and lymph node metastasis. When a tumor is not readily detectable by these techniques, selective venous catheterization can be used to obtain samples for radioimmunoassay, thereby identifying which area of the pancreas is secreting the hormone.

PATHOLOGY. No distinctive pathologic finding distinguishes benign from malignant islet cell tumors. The diagnosis of carcinoma is made when metastases are found at presentation or subsequent to resection of a solitary tumor.

ASSOCIATED SYNDROMES. Pancreatic islet cell tumors may also be part of the multiple endocrine neoplasia (MEN) syndromes (see Ch. 228). It is critical to identify patients with these syndromes, as they may have multiple islet cell tumors. Identification of the tumor or area of the pancreas responsible for excess secretion is essential to allow limited pancreatic resection. Unfortunately in patients with an MEN syndrome, tumors may recur, necessitating total pancreatectomy. The presence of hypercalcemia in patients with islet cell tumors is suggestive of the MEN 1 syndrome, as 85 per cent of patients with MEN type 1 have hyperparathyroidism at some time.

THERAPY. The primary therapy of solitary islet cell tumors is surgical resection. Therapy for islet cell carcinoma with metastasis is directed toward ameliorating the symptoms of the presenting syndrome and may include pharmacologic inhibitors of hormone secretion and action, chemotherapeutic agents, radiotherapy, or surgical debulking. Octreotide, a long-acting analogue of somatostatin approved for treatment of VIP (vasoactive intestinal polypeptide)-omas and carcinoids, is effective at reversing the symptoms of most islet cell tumors. Symptomatic relief may occur without complete suppression of circulating hormone levels. Although octreotide has become the mainstay for treating the hormone-produced syndromes, symptoms eventually recur with growth of tumor. Specific agents are discussed under each tumor.

Similar syndromes resulting from hypersecretion of pancreatic hormones occasionally occur secondary to diffuse hyperplasia of islet cells. The treatment of hyperplastic syndromes is partial or near-total pancreatectomy.

Insulinoma

The most common islet cell tumor is the insulinoma, which may produce life-threatening hypoglycemia. Insulinoma is reviewed in Ch. 219.

Gastrinoma

The second most common islet cell tumor is the gastrinoma associated with Zollinger-Ellison syndrome, producing recurrent peptic ulcers due to hypersecretion of gastric acid. This syndrome is discussed in Ch. 98.

VIPoma or the Diarrheogenic Syndrome

CLINICAL PRESENTATION. VIPoma or the diarrheogenic syndrome, associated with islet cell tumors, severe watery diarrhea, and hypokalemia, is also called pancreatic cholera, Verner-Morrison syndrome, WDHA (water diarrhea, hypokalemia, achlorhydria) syndrome, or WDHH (water diarrhea, hypokalemia, hypochlorhydria) syndrome. Patients have profound but intermittent secretory diarrhea; peak diarrhea output exceeds 3 liters per day in 80 per cent. A more general discussion of secretory diarrhea is contained in Ch. 101. Unlike the diarrheal discharge of long-term laxative abuse, the discharge in VIPoma is rich in electrolytes; fecal potassium loss can reach 300 mEq per day. Serum potassium is usually less than 3 mEq per liter and is accompanied by acidosis due to severe loss of bicarbonate.

The severe hypokalemia may lead to profound weakness, to flaccid paralysis, and to renal failure due to hypokalemic nephropathy. More than half of the patients have frank diabetes or glucose intolerance, which is probably secondary to hypokalemia, a known inhibitor of insulin secretion (see Ch. 75 for a discussion of hypokalemia). Hypercalcemia is found in half of the patients during attacks and is not usually indicative of hyperparathyroidism (and the MEN 1 syndrome), as parathyroid hormone levels are suppressed and the hypercalcemia remits with resection of the primary islet cell tumor. Despite hypercalcemia, tetany due to hypomagnesemia has been described. Flushing of the skin has been reported.

DIFFERENTIAL DIAGNOSIS. Secretory diarrhea may result from three other endocrine tumors (gastrinoma, carcinoid, and somatostatinoma), but peak volume of diarrhea rarely exceeds 3 liters per day in these syndromes. Further, the diarrhea in Zollinger-Ellison syndrome is caused by hypersecretion of gastric acid and can be reversed by gastric suction or with cimetidine. The diarrheogenic syndrome is almost always accompanied by achlorhydria or hypochlorhydria; decreased gastric acid secretion persists when the diarrhea is in remission and the serum potassium is normal.

PATHOLOGY. Eighty per cent of the patients with the diarrheogenic syndrome have islet cell tumors. Nearly half are malignant. Patients without islet cell tumors often have diffuse islet cell hyperplasia. The diarrheogenic syndrome has also been reported with bronchial tumor, pheochromocytoma, and ganglioneuroblastoma.

The diarrhea probably results from excess secretion of VIP. Infusion of VIP into laboratory animals and humans results in secretory diarrhea, hypokalemia, inhibition of gastric acid secretion, and hypercalcemia. Increased plasma VIP levels have been found in patients in whom islet cell tumor, islet cell hyperplasia, bronchogenic carcinoma, ganglioneuroblastoma, or pheochromocytoma was found to be the cause of the syndrome. VIP is difficult to detect in the circulation of normal humans; therefore the absence of VIP does not rule out the diagnosis. VIPomas also synthesize and secrete peptide histidine methionine (PHM), a peptide produced by the same mRNA as VIP that also enhances intestinal fluid secretion. Islet cell tumors producing only pancreatic polypeptide (another presumed hormone of unknown normal function) or prostaglandin E_2 have also been reported to be associated with this syndrome.

THERAPY. Treatment of the diarrheogenic syndrome is primarily by surgery. Because of the profound systemic effects of this tumor, resection is considered even in the presence of metastases. When no tumor is found, subtotal pancreatectomy is usually attempted. If hyperplasia is then identified on histopathologic examination and symptoms persist, total pancreatectomy should be considered. Octreotide is useful in preparing patients for surgery or as a palliative for metastatic disease. The tumors may also be transiently responsive to steroids, indomethacin, metoclopramide, lithium carbonate, or trifluoperazine. Radiotherapy, streptozotocin and interferon-α have been reported to reduce the size of metastases and volume of diarrhea.

Glucagonoma

CLINICAL PRESENTATION. The glucagonoma syndrome is characterized by a waxing and waning skin rash (necrolytic migratory erythema), diabetes, hypoaminoacidemia, weight loss, and anemia. The classic cutaneous lesion begins as an erythematous base, becomes indurated, and develops superficial central blistering. The blisters then erode and crust over. Healing may be accompanied by hyperpigmentation. This process takes 7 to 14 days, with lesions developing in one area while others are resolving. The rash is most prominent on the perineum, along intertriginous folds, and around the mouth and nose. Glossitis, stomatitis, and cheilitis are common. Onycholysis and brittle nails may be present.

Although cutaneous lesions were the hallmark of the first reported cases, the rash is actually present in only two thirds of patients with glucagonoma. The remainder usually present because of widespread metastatic disease.

Frank diabetes occurs in 60 per cent of patients with glucagonoma, and an additional 30 per cent have glucose intolerance. Even in patients with severe hyperglycemia, diabetic ketoacidosis is rarely observed in the glucagonoma syndrome, despite the known ability of glucagon to stimulate hepatic ketogenesis. There appear to be adequate levels of insulin to suppress lipolysis, limiting the free fatty acid substrates for hepatic ketone production.

Weight loss and anemia are found at the time of diagnosis in half of the patients with glucagonoma. Gastrointestinal symptoms include diarrhea, abdominal pain, and nausea and vomiting. Thromboembolic disease has also been described.

Glucagonoma is infrequently found in the MEN 1 syndrome. However, rare MEN 1 kindreds have been reported in which some members have glucagonoma and others have hyperglucagonemia without clinically detectable tumors. In addition, a familial glucagonoma syndrome has been reported in the absence of other endocrine tumors.

DIAGNOSIS. The diagnosis of glucagonoma is made by detecting elevated levels of glucagon and excluding other conditions associated with hyperglucagonemia, including diabetic ketoacidosis and hyperosmolar syndromes, chronic renal failure, cardiovascular collapse, and cirrhosis of the liver. Normal circulating levels of glucagon are 50 to 150 pg per milliliter. Most patients with glucagonoma have levels in excess of 500 pg per milliliter (occasionally as high as 10,000 pg per milliliter), while glucagon levels in the previously mentioned syndromes average 200 to 500 pg per milliliter. At the time of presentation 60 per cent of glucagonomas have metastasized, most commonly to the liver and local lymph nodes.

THERAPY. Surgery is the treatment of choice for glucagonoma confined to the pancreas. Surgery may also be indicated with

TABLE 220–1. SYNDROMES ASSOCIATED WITH ISLET CELL TUMORS

Tumor	Major Findings	Minor Findings	Other Hormones in Tumor or Plasma	Per Cent Malignancy	Hyperplasia	MEN Syndrome
Insulinoma	Adrenergic: palpitations, tremor, hunger, sweating; Neuroglycopenic: confusion, seizures, transient focal deficit, coma	Ischemic cardiovascular disease, permanent neurologic deficits	Gastrin, glucagon, pancreatic polypeptide, somatostatin, GRF*	10	Occasional	10%
Gastrinoma	Peptic ulcers, enhanced acid secretion	Diarrhea, malabsorption, weight loss, dumping	ACTH, insulin, glucagon, VIP, 5-HIAA, MSH, somatostatin, calcitonin, pancreatic polypeptide	40–60	10%	25%
VIPoma	Watery diarrhea, hypokalemia, hypochlorhydria	Hypercalcemia, hyperglycemia, weakness, hypomagnesemia	PHM, pancreatic polypeptide, prostaglandins (?), GRF, gastrin	40	20%	Rare
Glucagonoma	Rash, diabetes, weight loss, anemia	Diarrhea, abdominal pain, thromboembolic disease	Pancreatic polypeptide, VIP, 5-HIAA, gastrin, insulin	60	Occasional	Occasional
Somatostatinoma	Diabetes, cholelithiasis, steatorrhea, malabsorption, weight loss	Indigestion, abdominal pain, anemia, diarrhea, ductal obstruction, hypoglycemia	ACTH, gastrin, calcitonin, PGE₂, glucagon, GRF, pancreatic polypeptide, VIP, 5-HIAA, substance P	66	None reported	One case (MEN 3)
PPoma	None	Watery diarrhea, hypokalemia, achlorhydria; abdominal pain, weight loss	Glucagon, insulin, somatostatin, VIP	40	Occasional	25%

*GRF = growth hormone–releasing factor; 5-HIAA = 5-hydroxyindoleacetic acid; MSH = melanocyte-stimulating hormone; PGE₂ = prostaglandin E₂; PHM = peptide histidine methionine.

metastatic disease, as debulking of the tumor mass may ameliorate the glucagonoma syndrome. Octreotide usually decreases glucagon secretion from glucagonomas and improves symptoms. It can be used to prepare patients for surgery or to ameliorate symptoms from metastatic disease. Streptozotocin, with or without 5-fluorouracil and dacarbazine (DTIC), may induce significant remission. Phenoxybenzamine may also inhibit glucagon secretion from tumors. The skin rash often resolves within a few days of successful surgery or octreotide therapy.

Somatostatinoma

CLINICAL PRESENTATION. Somatostatinomas are not common; most are found incidentally during laparotomy or during the workup of obstructive jaundice or abdominal pain, with identification made retrospectively on the basis of elevated concentrations of somatostatin in the tumor or in the patient's plasma. The tumors contain granules characteristic of D cells. The primary tumor is located in the duodenum or jejunum in 40 per cent of cases.

A syndrome associated with hypersomatostatinemia includes diabetes mellitus, cholelithiasis, steatorrhea with malabsorption, dyspepsia, and significant weight loss. Patients may also have hypochlorhydria, watery diarrhea, anemia, and flushing. The diabetes is usually mild.

The pathophysiology of the syndrome is consistent with the known effects of somatostatin. Infusion of somatostatin in humans inhibits the release of multiple hormones, including insulin, glucagon, secretin, gastrin, and motilin. Hyperglycemia results from suppression of insulin secretion, but ketosis is infrequent, presumably because of the concomitant inhibition of glucagon secretion. Suppression of secretin, motilin, and gastrin, which decreases hydrochloric acid secretion, gastric emptying, and duodenal motility, may cause indigestion and abdominal pain. Inhibition of gallbladder contraction may predispose to cholelithiasis. Malabsorption is produced by inhibition of pancreatic exocrine function.

It is difficult to make the prospective diagnosis of somatostatinoma, as all of these symptoms are nonspecific and are found more commonly in other disorders. The incidence of cholelithiasis is increased in patients with diabetes. Malabsorption may occur in diabetics with chronic pancreatitis. This diagnostic difficulty is further compounded, as many patients with documented somatostatinoma have none of the components of the proposed syndrome. Some patients had severe hypoglycemia and were suspected to have insulinomas. Their tumors also contained insulin, and secretion of small amounts of insulin from the tumors with concomitant suppression of compensatory release of glucagon from the normal pancreas may have resulted in hypoglycemia.

Somatostatinomas may secrete additional hormones that modify the clinical syndrome. Striking elevations of serum calcitonin can cause watery diarrhea due to the effects of calcitonin on water and electrolyte transport in the gut. Somatostatinomas can produce ACTH, causing Cushing's syndrome, or prostaglandin E$_2$, causing flushing. Hyperplasia of cells containing pancreatic polypeptide (resulting in excess secretion of this hormone) has been reported in the presence of somatostatinoma.

DIAGNOSIS. The diagnosis of somatostatinoma is made by detecting elevated basal or stimulated levels of circulating somatostatin. Tolbutamide or calcium-pentagastrin infusion results in marked elevation of somatostatin in patients with somatostatinoma and normal basal somatostatin levels but not in controls.

THERAPY. Two thirds of patients with somatostatinoma have metastases at presentation; this may reflect the difficulty in the clinical diagnosis of this syndrome. Surgical resection should be performed if possible. Streptozotocin therapy reduces tumor size and plasma somatostatin levels.

Other Hormones Produced by Islet Cell Tumors

PANCREATIC POLYPEPTIDE. Many endocrine tumors of the pancreas and gut produce pancreatic polypeptide (PP) as a secondary hormone, allowing it to serve as a marker for islet cell tumors. Increasing numbers of islet cell tumors that produce PP as their major hormone are being identified; these may account for some of the tumors previously identified as "nonfunctional."

The role of PP in normal islet physiology is not apparent, and no clinical syndrome has been definitively associated with PPomas. A few cases of islet cell tumors associated with watery diarrhea, hypokalemia, and achlorhydria have been accompanied by elevated serum levels of PP with normal VIP levels.

ACTH. Pancreatic islet cell tumors producing ACTH account for nearly 10 per cent of cases of Cushing's syndrome due to ectopic ACTH production. Such tumors are usually found to secrete multiple hormones, including insulin, gastrin, serotonin, or somatostatin. However, it is more common to find Cushing's *disease* due to a pituitary adenoma associated with other islet cell tumors in patients with MEN type 1.

GROWTH HORMONE–RELEASING FACTOR. Acromegaly has been reported in patients with islet cell tumors secreting growth hormone–releasing factor. Although these patients often have hyperplasia of the growth hormone–secreting cells of the pituitary, it is very difficult to distinguish them from patients with classic acromegaly due to a pituitary adenoma (see Ch. 213). In either case the sella may be normal or enlarged, and growth hormone levels may show paradoxic responses to provocative testing.

Bloom SR, Polak JM: Glucagonoma syndrome. Am J Med 82(5B):25, 1987. *A comprehensive and useful general review, with 44 references.*
Berelowitz M: Somatostatin-producing tumors. Adv Exp Med Biol 188:475, 1985. *Only 6 of 21 patients with pancreatic somatostatinoma and none of 13 patients with a small intestine primary tumor showed clinical symptoms of the proposed somatostatinoma syndrome.*
Jensen RT (ed.): Gastrointestinal endocrinology. Gastroenterol Clin North Am 18(4): December, 1989. *This volume has eight articles covering the clinical presentation, localization, and treatment of islet cell tumors as well as four articles on the properties of the hormones.*
Krejs GJ: VIPoma syndrome. Am J Med 82(5B):37, 1987. *An excellent general review of this interesting entity, with 120 references. A good place to start.*

221 Disorders of Sexual Differentiation

Julianne Imperato-McGinley

NORMAL SEXUAL DIFFERENTIATION

The fetus is bipotential for sexual differentiation. The bipotentiality includes the gonad, the internal sex structures, and the external genitalia.

Development of the Bipotential Gonad

In fetuses of both sexes an undifferentiated gonad develops during the fifth week of fetal life. A thickened area of coelomic or germinal epithelium on the medial aspect of the mesonephros proliferates and with the underlying mesenchyme produces a prominence designated the gonadal ridge. Then cords of cells known as primary sex cords proliferate from the epithelium into the mesenchyme. The primordial germ cells are visible early in the third week among the endodermal cells of the wall of the yolk sac. During folding of the embryo, they multiply and migrate by a combination of ameboid movement and passive transfer along the dorsal mesentery to the gonadal ridges and later into the underlying mesenchyme. By the end of the sixth week the bipotential gonad is formed (Fig. 221–1). The primordial germ cells develop into spermatogonia in the male and ova in the female, the sex cords become either seminiferous tubules or primary ovarian follicles, and the mesenchymal cells form either the Leydig cells or the theca and stromal cells in the female.

Gonadal Differentiation—Development of the Testes and Ovaries

Testicular differentiation begins with the evolution of the *testicular or seminiferous cords* from primary sex cords of the indifferent gonad at approximately the seventh week of gestation (Fig. 221–1). The Sertoli cells differentiate within each cord, enlarge, aggregate, and engulf the germ cells. The distal ends of the cords interconnect to form the rete testes, which is in contact with the wolffian (mesonephric) ducts. By the sixth month the

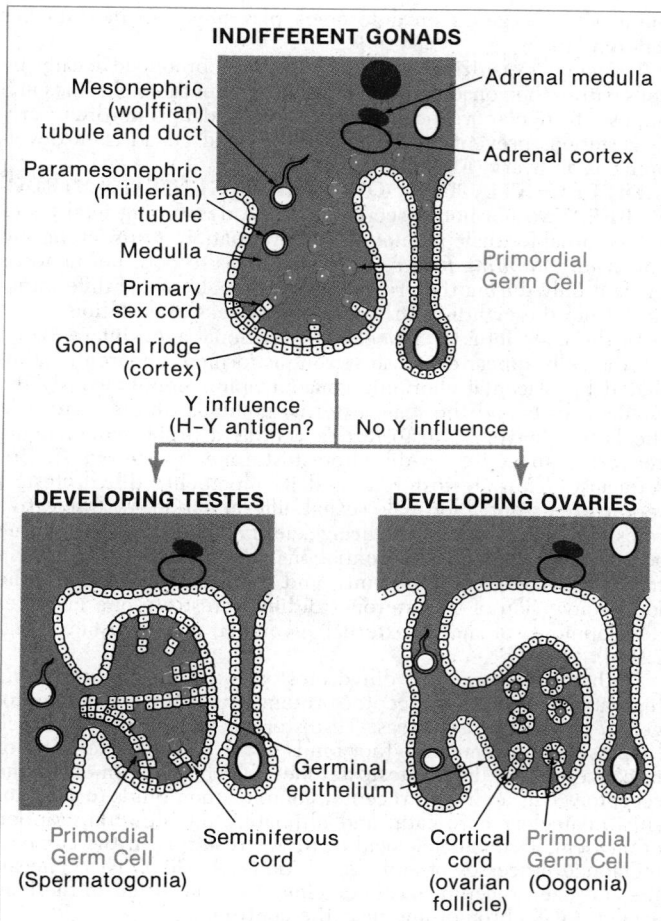

FIGURE 221–1. Development of the bipotential gonad from coelomic epithelium (primary sex cords) underlying mesenchymal tissue and primordial germ cells and its differentiation to either a testis or an ovary.

ends of the rete testes develop a lumen continuous with the mesonephric tubules, which develop into the ductuli efferentia. The fetal Leydig cells, apparent by 8 weeks of fetal life, fill the interstitial spaces at 3 months of gestation.

Ovarian differentiation from the indifferent gonad begins at approximately 50 days of gestation (Fig. 221–1). The primary sex cords form irregular groups of cells called medullary cords containing primitive granulosa cells that engulf primordial oogonia. As the oogonia differentiate, the primitive granulosa cells organize around them and form a single layer constituting the primordial follicle. At 18 to 20 weeks of gestation, there are approximately 7 million oogonia and oocytes, whereas by birth the number decreases to approximately 2 million.

Phenotypic Differentiation

DUCTAL DEVELOPMENT

Every fetus has both *wolffian (mesonephric) ducts,* which develop into epididymis, vas deferens, and seminal vesicles in the male, and *müllerian (paramesonephric) ducts,* which develop into fallopian tubes, uterus, and upper third of the vagina in the female (Fig. 221–2). In the male as the initial event the müllerian ducts regress by about 7½ weeks of gestation, following which the mesonephric wolffian ducts differentiate to form the epididymis, vas deferens, seminal vesicles, and ejaculatory ducts. In the female the wolffian ducts regress at approximately 10½ weeks, and the müllerian ducts differentiate to form the fallopian tubes, uterus, and upper portion of the vagina.

DEVELOPMENT OF THE EXTERNAL GENITALIA

The external genitalia of both sexes (like the gonad) develop from common primordia, the urogenital tubercle, urogenital folds, and urogenital swellings (Fig. 221–2). In the male, external genital masculinization begins shortly after wolffian ductal differ-

entiation and is completed by 14 weeks of gestation. The urogenital tubercle elongates to become the glans penis, the urogenital folds fuse to become the shaft of the penis, and the urogenital swellings become the scrotum. The prostate arises from endodermal buds in the urethral lining at 10 weeks and grows into the mesenchyme, which forms the muscular and connective tissue components. Descent of the testes and growth of the penis occur between 20 weeks of gestation and term. In the female the urogenital tubule becomes the clitoris, the urogenital swellings the labia majora, and the urogenital folds the labia minora. Female differentiation occurs after the embryo has reached 10½ weeks.

Determinants of Phenotypic Differentiation

Since the fetus is bipotential, what are the determinants of the male or female phenotype?

FEMALE PHENOTYPIC DIFFERENTIATION

Ovarian tissue containing primary follicles is found in human abortuses with a 45 XO complement. Thus, ovarian differentiation

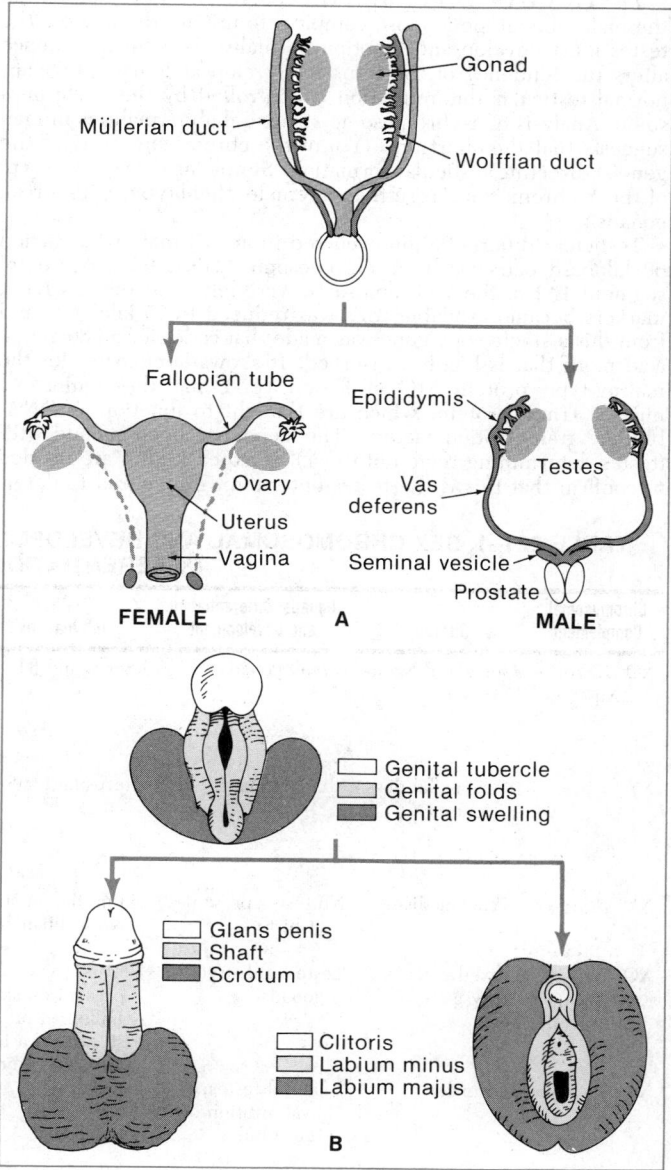

FIGURE 221–2. Summary of male and female sexual differentiation. *A,* Internal sexual differentiation from wolffian and müllerian ducts. *B,* Development of male and female external genitalia from common primordia.

does not appear to require a 46 XX chromosomal complement. Adults, however, with a 45 XO complement have only streak gonads made of whorls of connective tissue. A complete 46 XX complement, therefore, although not necessary for ovarian differentiation, is essential for maintenance of normal ovarian follicular development. Deletion of either the long or short arm of the X chromosome results in streak gonads. Deletion of the short arm of the X chromosome (XXp-) is associated with streak gonads and the skeletal and somatic anomalies of subjects with 45 XO Turner's syndrome. In contrast, long arm deletions (XXq-) are usually associated with streak gonads and none of the stigmata of Turner's syndrome (Table 221–1). See Ch. 224 for a complete discussion of XO and XX gonadal dysgenesis.

In the absence of gonads, either ovaries or testes, the wolffian anlagen regress and the müllerian ducts differentiate to form fallopian tubes, uterus, and upper portion of the vagina, and the external genital primordia differentiate as female (Fig. 221–2). Thus, femaleness is the innate tendency of every fetus and does not require gonadal influence.

MALE PHENOTYPIC DIFFERENTIATION

TESTICULAR DIFFERENTIATION. The development of the male phenotype is more complex; to initiate the process the testes must develop and function normally. Testicular influence alters the tendency of the fetus to develop as female. In man, normal testicular differentiation is controlled by the Y chromosome. Analysis of Y chromosome structural abnormalities in man suggests that the short arm (Yp) of the chromosome carries the gene(s) directing testicular formation. Simple absence of the (Yp) of the Y chromosome results in a female phenotype, with streak gonads.

Testicular differentiation occurred in an XX male who carried 60 kilobase pairs of the Y chromosome. Thus, 60 kilobases of segment 1A1 of the Y chromosome were left to search. As DNA markers became available, this was reduced to 35 kilobases and from this a single copy gene was made that codes for an 80 amino acid motif that is highly conserved. It shows homologies for the mating-type protein MC of fission yeast and the nonhistone nuclear HmG protein, which are thought to function as DNA-binding transcription factors. The gene has been named SRY (testes determining region of the Y). Further studies are needed to confirm that this is the testes-determining gene and to determine whether genes on autosomes play any role in testicular differentiation.

Testicular organizing factor or substance produced locally by cells within the gonad and under the control of the Y chromosome imposes testicular organogenesis on the gonadal primordium early in gestation, preventing the undifferentiated gonad from developing as an ovary (Fig. 221–3).

DIFFERENTIATION OF MALE GENITAL STRUCTURES. Two hormones secreted by the developing fetal testes are essential for male phenotypic differentiation, *testosterone* and *müllerian inhibiting factor*. Responsiveness to both hormones is present only during the critical period of male sexual differentiation, from the eighth to the fourteenth weeks of gestation.

In the male fetus at 8 weeks of gestational age, differentiated Leydig cells appear and testosterone is formed, apparently stimulated by placental chorionic gonadotropin. Simultaneously the wolffian ducts and the male external genitalia differentiate. For the latter, however, testosterone acts as a prohormone, being converted to active 5α-dihydrotestosterone by steroid Δ^4 5α-reductase. Thus, testosterone and its metabolite dihydrotestosterone are essential for male sexual differentiation, with selective roles for each hormone during embryogenesis. Testosterone acting locally mediates differentiation of the wolffian ductal system to the vas deferens, epididymis, and seminal vesicles, while the local conversion of testosterone to dihydrotestosterone mediates development of male external genitalia and prostate (Fig. 221–4).

Both testosterone and dihydrotestosterone bind to the same high-affinity androgen receptor protein within the cells of androgen-dependent target areas. Testosterone enters the target cell by passive diffusion and either binds to the androgen receptor or is converted to dihydrotestosterone, which then binds to the receptor. This androgen receptor complex then binds to acceptor sites in nuclear chromatin and ultimately initiates transcription of messenger ribonucleic acid (mRNA), resulting in the complex metabolic processes of androgen action (Ch. 208). The gene for the androgen receptor has been cloned and localized to the long arm of the X chromosome near the centromere.

The inhibition of the müllerian anlage is under the control of müllerian inhibiting factor, a high-molecular-weight glycoprotein, a product of the Sertoli cells of the seminiferous tubules. The human gene for müllerian inhibiting factors has been cloned and localized to the tip of the short arm of chromosome 19. Its secretion begins shortly after the initiation of seminiferous tubular differentiation. The müllerian ducts are receptive to this hormone

TABLE 221–1. SEX CHROMOSOMAL AND DEVELOPMENTAL ABNORMALITIES LEADING TO ABNORMAL SEXUAL DIFFERENTIATION AND DEVELOPMENT

Chromosomal Complement	Disorder	Gonadal Differentiation and Development	Internal Sex Structures	External Genitalia	Pubertal Development	Comments
XO, XXp-, XXq-	Gonadal dysgenesis	Streak gonads	Uterus and fallopian tubes	Female	None	XO to XXp- associated with short stature. Can be XX with abnormal X chromosome at the molecular level.
XY	XY gonadal dysgenesis	Streak gonads	Uterus and fallopian tubes	Female	None	A spectrum. See Table 221–3. Abnormality at the molecular level affecting testes determining gene.
XY	XY agonadism	No testes present at birth	No müllerian structures. No wolffian structures.	Female		Part of a spectrum. Mildest form normal male without testes.
XO/XY	Mixed gonadal dysgenesis	Testes and streak gonads	Uterus, vas deferens, if present on side of testes. Fallopian tube on side of streak, occasionally next to vas deferens.	Most commonly ambiguous (range— female to normal male)	Male	Most common cause of ambiguity in the newborn after congenital adrenal hyperplasia.
XX	XX males	Bilateral testes; hyalinization of the tubules	Normal	Usually normal. Can have ambiguous genitalia.	Male	X chromosome contains testes determining region of the Y chromosome.
XX, XX/XY, XY	True hermaphroditism	Ovary and testes; ovotestis	Uterus almost invariably present. Vas deferens on side of testes. Fallopian tube on side of ovary.	Most commonly ambiguous		May be familial. XX male in same family.

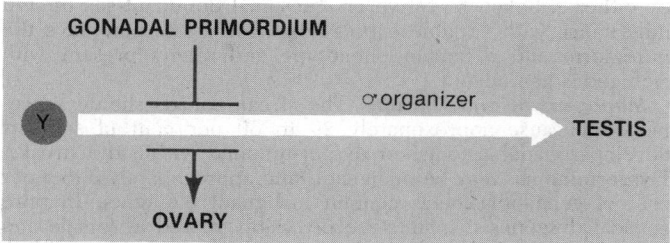

FIGURE 221–3. Testicular organizing substance under Y chromosome control imposing testicular organogenesis on the indifferent gonad.

before 8 weeks of gestation. Postnatally, the levels are high in normal boys prior to 2 years of age. They fall progressively in older boys and decrease sharply at puberty.

In summary, male phenotypic development requires normal testicular differentiation and function, so that at a critically isensitive period in utero (8 to 14 weeks) müllerian inhibiting factor, secreted by the Sertoli cells, and testosterone, secreted by the Leydig cells, are produced in sufficient amounts. Müllerian inhibiting factor, acting locally, suppresses the müllerian anlage, and testosterone, also acting locally, causes differentiation of the wolffian anlage to epididymis, vas deferens, and seminal vesicles. Testosterone is converted by the enzyme 5α-reductase to dihydrotestosterone in the anlage of the external genitalia, resulting in male external genital differentiation (Fig. 221–4). Depending upon specific target tissue, either testosterone or dihydrotestosterone complexes with the androgen receptor, to initiate androgen action at the nuclear level.

Genetic Control of Male Sexual Differentiation

Male sexual differentiation is under complex genetic control. Testicular differentiation requires gene(s) normally found on the Y chromosome. The enzymes involved in testosterone biosynthesis, as well as the enzyme 5α-reductase converting testosterone to dihydrotestosterone, are regulated by genes located on the autosomes. A gene located on the X chromosome codes for the androgen receptor at the androgen-dependent target areas. Inherited forms of müllerian inhibiting factor deficiency are transmitted as a recessive trait, either autosomal or X linked.

Thus, male phenotypic development is regulated by multiple genes located on the autosomes as well as on both X and Y chromosomes.

Byskov AG: Differentiation of mammalian embryonic gonad. Physiol Rev 66:71, 1986. *All aspects of gonadal differentiation are covered, from formation of the gonadal primordium to theories of gonadal differentiation. Excellent bibliography.*

ABNORMALITIES OF SEXUAL DIFFERENTIATION

Male Pseudohermaphroditism

The known etiologic factors in male pseudohermaphroditism or incomplete masculinization can be divided into three categories: (1) disorders of testicular differentiation; (2) disorders of testicular function; and (3) disorders of function at the androgen-dependent target areas. Table 221–2 lists the specific clinical entities within each category.

DISORDERS OF TESTICULAR DIFFERENTIATION AND DEVELOPMENT

XY GONADAL DYSGENESIS. *Clinical Presentation.* Subjects with pure gonadal dysgenesis have a 46 XY chromosomal complement but are phenotypic females with primary amenorrhea, tall stature, eunuchoidal proportions, and scant axillary and pubic hair. The uterus and fallopian tubes are present, and streak gonads are found. The incomplete forms of this condition have variable amounts of functional testicular tissue, and consequently at birth the subjects frequently have clitoromegaly, ambiguous genitalia, or, rarely, a penile urethra. The degree of virilization at puberty is also variable. In pure gonadal dysgenesis, postpubertal gonadotropins are increased to the castrate range with castrate levels of testosterone. However, when functioning testicular tissue is present, testosterone can vary from castrate levels to low-normal male levels. Additionally, if müllerian inhibiting factor is produced there may be partial or complete absence of müllerian structures (Table 221–1; Fig. 221–5).

Pathophysiology. In pure gonadal dysgenesis the testes do not

FIGURE 221–4. Schematic representation of the factors involved in male and female sexual differentiation.

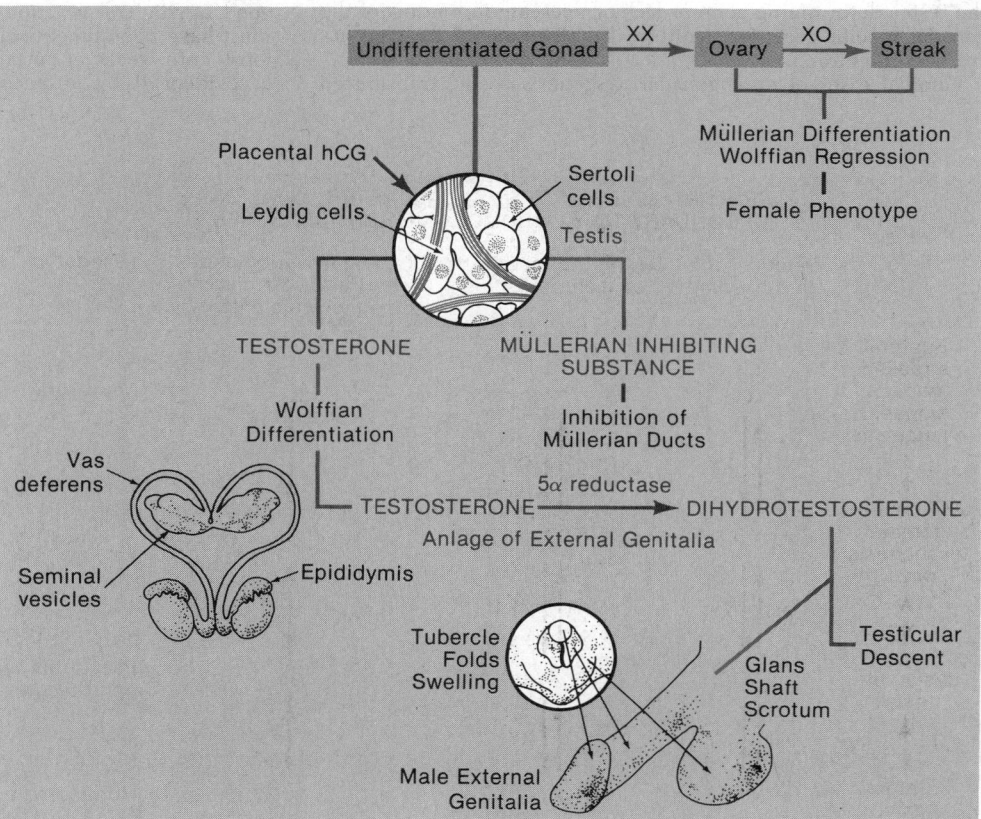

TABLE 221–2. CLASSIFICATION OF THE CAUSES OF MALE PSEUDOHERMAPHRODITISM

I. Disorders of testicular differentiation and development
  A. Testicular dysgenesis, affecting both Leydig cell and seminiferous tubule development
    1. Y chromosomal abnormalities
    2. XY gonadal dysgenesis
    3. XO/XY gonadal dysgenesis
    4. Testicular regression syndrome
  B. Leydig cell agenesis or dysgenesis—selective absence or decrease in Leydig cell differentiation and function—seminiferous tubule embryogenesis occurring normally
    1. Abnormality of the hCG-LH receptor: absence of precursor Leydig cell

II. Disorders of testicular function
  A. Abnormalities of müllerian inhibiting factor synthesis or action—persistent müllerian duct syndrome
  B. Enzyme deficiencies affecting testosterone biosynthesis
    1. Cholesterol 20,22-desmolase
    2. 17α-Hydroxylase
    3. 17,20-Desmolase
    4. 3β-Hydroxysteroid dehydrogenase:Δ^{5-4} isomerase
    5. 17β-Hydroxysteroid dehydrogenase

III. Disorders of function at the androgen-dependent target areas
  A. Disorders of androgen action (complete and partial androgen insensitivity)
    1. Cytosol androgen-receptor binding abnormalities
    2. Post cytosol androgen-receptor binding abnormalities
  B. Disorders of testosterone metabolism
    1. 5α-Reductase deficiency

differentiate at all, and in the absence of a functional testis phenotypic development is female, with wolffian duct regression and müllerian differentiation. In the incomplete forms there are varying degrees of testicular development and of fetal masculinization. The etiology of this condition could be due to a number of theoretical causes involving testicular organizing substance. Deletion of gene (SRY) on the Y chromosome near the centromere results in streak gonads. Thus, this gene is purported to code for the testicular organizing substance. There could also be abnormalities in its structure, due to deletions or point mutations of the testes determining gene or lack or decrease in binding of the gonadal specific receptor. Neither the receptor nor its gene has yet been identified.

Familial cases of pure gonadal dysgenesis occur, transmitted by either X-linked recessive or autosomal dominant-sex limited inheritance with variable expressivity. Some sibs may have the pure form and a female phenotype and others present with ambiguous genitalia.

Management and Therapy. The streak gonads should be removed because approximately 20 to 30 per cent of subjects develop gonadoblastomas or dysgerminomas within the streaks. Dysgerminomas may be malignant, and approximately 5 to 8 per cent of gonadoblastomas contain malignant elements. In pure gonadal dysgenesis, infants are invariably reared as female and come to the attention of the physician at puberty because of lack of secondary sexual development. Estrogen and progesterone replacement therapy should be instituted at the time of puberty and after prophylactic removal of the streak gonads. In incomplete forms of testicular dysgenesis, the child should be reared in the sex that will be more functional, and appropriate surgical correction of the genitalia carried out. Intra-abdominal testicular tissue should always be removed because of the increased risk of malignancy. This necessitates the use of testosterone replacement therapy at puberty, if the child is being reared as a male.

MIXED GONADAL DYSGENESIS. Clinical Presentation. Subjects with mixed gonadal dysgenesis usually have a streak gonad on one side, a testis on the contralateral side, and XO/XY mosaicism on chromosomal analysis. The phenotypic spectrum ranges from phenotypic females, with or without the clinical characteristics of Turner's syndrome, to subjects with ambiguous genitalia, to normal phenotypic males. The genitalia are sufficiently ambiguous that approximately two thirds are raised as girls, with the stigmata of Turner's syndrome occurring in one third. Affected subjects have a uterus, and most have bilateral fallopian tubes. The vas deferens, if present, is on the side of the testis, and frequently a fallopian tube also exists adjacent to the vas deferens. Virilization generally occurs at puberty. The testes appear histologically normal before puberty. However, after puberty the seminiferous tubules demonstrate thickened walls with few if any germ cells. Consequently, affected subjects are infertile. If pubertal gynecomastia occurs, a gonadal tumor should be suspected.

Pathogenesis. XO/XY mosaicism in subjects with this condition can be best explained as resulting from mitotic nondisjunction or anaphase lag, resulting in loss of the Y chromosome. Perhaps the lack of testicular differentiation of the streak gonad is related to the preponderance of the XO cell line in that gonad. Despite good Leydig cell function with virilization at puberty, the testis must have been functionally dysgenetic (between the eighth and fourteenth weeks of gestation—the critically responsive period), as evidenced by absence of or incomplete virilization of the

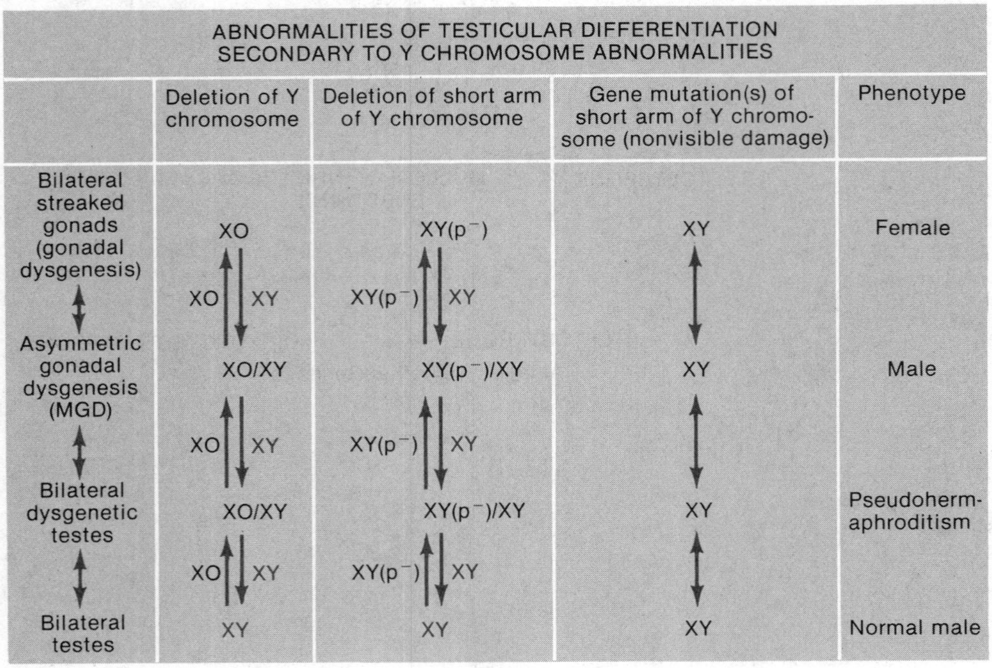

ABNORMALITIES OF TESTICULAR DIFFERENTIATION SECONDARY TO Y CHROMOSOME ABNORMALITIES				
	Deletion of Y chromosome	Deletion of short arm of Y chromosome	Gene mutation(s) of short arm of Y chromosome (nonvisible damage)	Phenotype
Bilateral streaked gonads (gonadal dysgenesis)	XO	XY(p⁻)	XY	Female
↕	XO ↕ XY	XY(p⁻) ↕ XY		
Asymmetric gonadal dysgenesis (MGD)	XO/XY	XY(p⁻)/XY	XY	Male
↕	XO ↕ XY	XY(p⁻) ↕ XY		
Bilateral dysgenetic testes	XO/XY	XY(p⁻)/XY	XY	Pseudohermaphroditism
↕	XO ↕ XY	XY(p⁻) ↕ XY		
Bilateral testes	XY	XY	XY	Normal male

FIGURE 221–5. The abnormalities of testicular differentiation may be thought of as a spectrum of disorders that can be produced by more than one genotype.

external genitalia. Theoretically a delay in testicular differentiation and function in utero could result in delayed secretion of testosterone and müllerian inhibiting factor, completely or partially missing the critically responsive period and resulting in the presence of female or ambiguous genitalia and müllerian structures.

There are subjects with an XO/XY chromosomal complement and bilateral streak gonads as well as XO/XY subjects with bilateral testes. Thus the classic clinical syndrome of mixed gonadal dysgenesis may be one clinical entity in a spectrum ranging from streak gonads and a female phenotype to varied abnormalities of testicular development (symmetric or asymmetric) and genital ambiguity, possibly depending upon the preponderance of a particular cell line, either XO or XY, within the gonad at the time of differentiation (Table 221–1; Fig. 221–5).

Management and Therapy. Owing to the increased incidence of tumor formation, an intra-abdominal testis that cannot be brought into the scrotum should be removed as well as the streak gonad. A scrotal testis should be preserved. In infants, when the testes cannot be brought to the scrotum and must be removed, and the external genitalia are severely ambiguous, the sex of rearing should be female and appropriate genital surgery performed. At the time of puberty, estrogen and progesterone therapy should be given to induce and maintain feminization. If the child is to be raised as a male, testosterone replacement therapy will be needed at the time of puberty.

XY AGONADISM, TESTICULAR REGRESSION, OR VANISHING TESTES SYNDROME. ***Clinical Presentation.***
Typically these subjects are 46 XY phenotypic females with absent gonads and no müllerian or wolffian internal structures. The lack of müllerian structures and gonadal remnants separates this entity from pure XY gonadal dysgenesis. The condition appears to be secondary to regression of the differentiating testis before the onset of androgen secretion, resulting in lack of wolffian differentiation, but after the onset of secretion of müllerian inhibiting factor, resulting in inhibition of female internal structures. There is, however, a phenotypic spectrum of agonadal subjects perhaps related to the time of testicular regression, during or after the critical period of male sexual differentiation. Affected subjects therefore vary widely in phenotypes: from those with total absence of internal sex structures and female external genitalia, to subjects with ambiguous genitalia, to normal males with absent testes.

Pathophysiology. The etiology of the testicular regression is unknown. These subjects are unequivocally 46 XY, and chromosomal abnormalities have never been demonstrated. Familial cases of agonadism in XY subjects occur, however, suggesting that in some cases it may be an inherited condition. Variable phenotypic expression in agonadal siblings from the same kindred also occurs, suggesting that this condition is a clinical spectrum due to the time of regression of the embryonic testes.

Management and Therapy. Sex hormone therapy should be instituted at puberty in accordance with the sex of rearing.

LEYDIG CELL AGENESIS OR DYSGENESIS, GONADOTROPIN UNRESPONSIVENESS. ***Clinical Characteristics.***
Adult subjects with Leydig cell agenesis or dysgenesis have either normal female external genitalia or slight posterior fusion of the labia majora and have been raised as females. An epididymis and vas deferens are present in affected subjects, indicating that little testosterone is needed at a critical period to initiate wolffian differentiation. No müllerian structures are found, confirming that müllerian inhibiting factor is secreted by the Sertoli cells of the seminiferous tubules. In the adults, normal-appearing Sertoli cells with few spermatogonia and few or no Leydig cells are present in the testis.

Pathophysiology. Plasma androgen levels do not significantly change with administration of human chorionic gonadotropin (hCG). Luteinizing hormone (LH) levels are elevated in adulthood.

Theoretically the absence or decrease in Leydig cells can result from (1) an absence of or decrease in precursor cells destined to become functioning Leydig cells under hCG-LH stimulation or (2) a decrease in the hCG-LH receptor or receptor response of the precursor Leydig cells. It can be theorized that the hCG-LH receptor mediates Leydig cell differentiation, and without these receptors, precursor Leydig cells are not formed. A complete phenotypic spectrum of subjects with this disorder can be anticipated, dependent upon the severity of the developmental defect.

Management and Therapy. Affected subjects should be raised in the sex in which they will be more apt to function normally. In most instances because of the severe genital ambiguity this would be female. Thus the testes should be removed and corrective genital surgery performed. At puberty appropriate sex hormone therapy should be instituted concordant with the individual's gender.

DISORDERS OF TESTICULAR FUNCTION

In disorders of testicular function, the testes have differentiated normally, but the secretion of either müllerian inhibiting factor or testosterone is abnormal.

MÜLLERIAN INHIBITING FACTOR DEFICIENCY. *Clinical Presentation.* Males with this condition have a uterus and bilateral fallopian tubes. They have bilateral testes with normal male differentiation of wolffian structures and external genitalia and undergo normal male puberty. This entity most frequently occurs as unilateral cryptorchidism with a contralateral inguinal hernia containing müllerian structures, "uteri inguinale," and a testis. The incidence of testicular tumors is approximately 13 per cent, similar to the incidence in cryptorchidism. An inguinal hernia most often brings affected males to a physician's attention. Although fertility has been described, azoospermia is frequently noted. More than 80 cases have been reported, including at least eight families with two affected sibs. Pedigree analysis suggests an X-linked or autosomal recessive inheritance. In 5 per cent of affected patients, either seminomas or other germ cell tumors occur.

Pathogenesis. Theoretically this entity could be due to a number of abnormalities affecting the synthesis, structure, timing of secretion, or action of müllerian inhibiting factor. Some children with this condition possess no müllerian inhibiting factor and others possess normal amounts, suggesting genetic heterogeneity. Documentation of the precise biochemical abnormalities will have to await further studies of the MIF gene and its receptor. The ultimate effect is lack of suppression of the müllerian anlage, resulting in the presence of a uterus. Androgen secretion is adequate during the critical period of sexual differentiation, and the wolffian ducts and external genitalia differentiate normally.

Management and Therapy. The müllerian structures should be surgically removed if they are in the inguinal canal. Since malignant change in müllerian structures has never been reported, surgical removal is not necessary if they are located in the abdomen. The cryptorchid testes should be brought into the scrotal sac and the patient examined frequently for the development of testicular tumors.

Imperato-McGinley J: Sexual differentiation—Normal and abnormal. Curr Top Exp Endocrinol 5:231, 1983. *Of particular interest in this review is the section on male pseudohermaphroditism, including an extensive bibliography for each clinical entity described.*

DEFICIENCIES OF TESTOSTERONE BIOSYNTHESIS. *Clinical Features.* Five enzymatic steps involving four genes are required to convert cholesterol to testosterone; deficiencies of these enzymatic steps constitute the nonvirilizing forms of the adrenogenital syndrome. The five enzymatic steps are (1) cholesterol 20,22-desmolase, (2) 3β-hydroxysteroid dehydrogenase:Δ$^{5-4}$ isomerase, (3) 17α-hydroxylase, (4) 17,20-desmolase, and (5) 17β-hydroxysteroid dehydrogenase (Fig. 221–6). The enzymatic activities 17α-hydroxylase and 17,20-desmolase reside in the same enzyme. Deficiencies of the enzymes cholesterol 20,22-desmolase and 3β-hydroxysteroid dehydrogenase:Δ$^{5-4}$ isomerase impair production of aldosterone and cortisol. 17α-Hydroxylase deficiency impairs cortisol production, while 17,20-desmolase and 17β-hydroxysteroid dehydrogenase deficiencies affect only androgen biosynthesis. Since androgens are the precursors of estrogens, it follows that estrogen production is also low in all of the enzyme deficiencies except 17β-hydroxysteroid dehydrogenase (Table 221–3). These disorders are inherited as autosomal recessive traits. Genotypic females are phenotypically normal at birth, with the exception of females with 3β-hydroxysteroid dehydrogenase deficiency, who may be mildly virilized.

The testes differentiate normally, and normal amounts of müllerian inhibiting factor are secreted, so müllerian structures

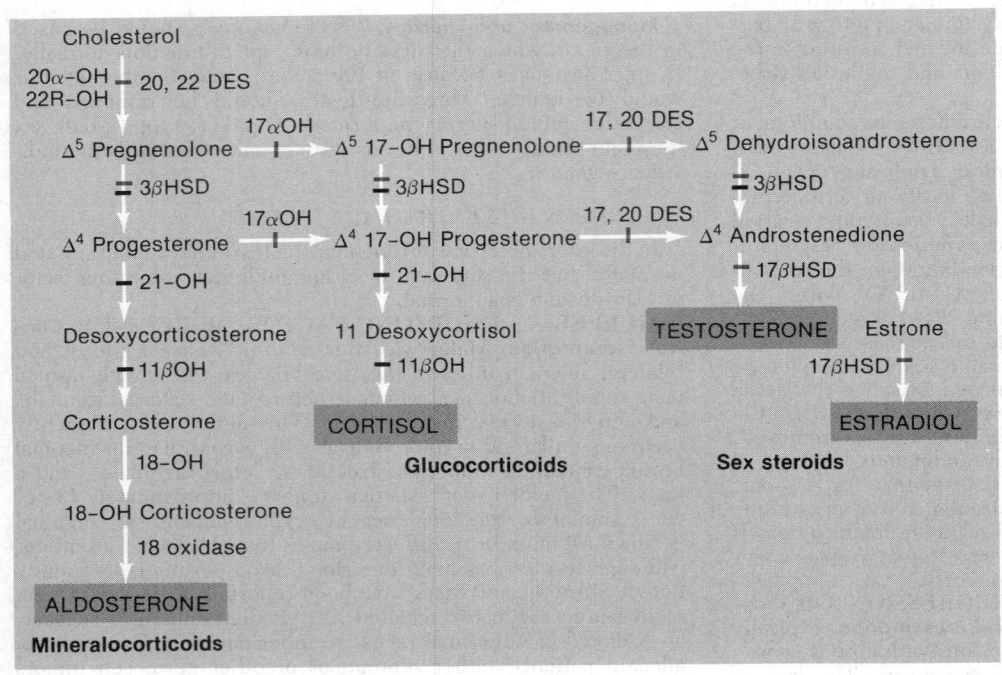

FIGURE 221–6. Congenital adrenal hyperplasia. *Left*, Enzyme deficiencies resulting in male pseudohermaphroditism. Cholesterol 20,22-desmolase, 17α-hydroxylase, 3β-hydroxysteroid dehydrogenase:Δ^{5–4} isomerase, 17,20-desmolase, 17β-hydroxysteroid dehydrogenase. *Center* and *right*, Enzyme deficiencies resulting in female pseudohermaphroditism. 21-Hydroxylase, 11β-hydroxylase, 3β-hydroxysteroid dehydrogenase:Δ^{5–4} isomerase. (DES = desmolase; OH = hydroxylase; HSD = hydroxysteroid dehydrogenase.)

are absent. However, the impaired secretion of testosterone by Leydig cells at the critical period of sexual differentiation in utero causes ambiguity of the external genitalia. Wolffian differentiation is normal. In general, the severity of the enzyme defect is reflected in the degree of external genital ambiguity at birth and the amount of virilization at puberty. Each specific enzyme deficiency, however, may show considerable variation in clinical presentation from totally female external genitalia to males with mild hypospadias and cryptorchidism.

The causes for the enzymatic abnormalities include deletions or mutations at structural gene loci coding for the amino acid sequences of the enzymes. Mutations at sites other than structural loci can be classified as *regulatory*, altering the rate of synthesis or degradation of the enzyme; *architectural*, affecting incorporation of enzyme molecules into active sites in the cell; or *temporal*, affecting the development of the tissue or the time of activation of regulatory systems.

Congenital Lipoid Adrenal Hyperplasia (Cholesterol 20,22-Desmolase Deficiency). A genetic male from a consanguineous marriage exhibited wolffian differentiation but with female external genitalia. The infant died in adrenal crisis at 6 days of age. At autopsy the adrenals were large and yellowish and contained cortical cells with foamy, spongy cytoplasm that stained positively for lipids. Approximately 32 cases have been subsequently described with equal numbers of both sexes affected. Most died in adrenal crisis in infancy, owing to severe deficiencies of glucocorticoid and mineralocorticoid production and with similar pathologic findings.

The affected genotypic males have abdominal or inguinal testes with wolffian differentiation, and no müllerian structures. The external genitalia are either female or severely ambiguous. As would be expected, genotypic females have normal female genitalia.

Pathogenesis. A deficiency in the conversion of cholesterol to pregnenolone results in decreased glucocorticoid, mineralocorticoid, and sex steroid production (Fig. 221–6). All plasma steroid values are low to unmeasurable, and little or no urinary 17-ketosteroids, 17-hydroxysteroids, or aldosterone is found (Table 221–3). cDNA clones that encode the gene responsible for the cleavage of the side chain of cholesterol (P-H50 SCC) have been isolated and the corresponding gene located on chromosome 15. The gene defects in this condition will be forthcoming.

Management and Therapy. Signs of adrenal insufficiency with hyperkalemia and hyponatremia usually occur within the first 2

weeks of life. The condition must be distinguished from 3β-hydroxysteroid dehydrogenase deficiency or congenital adrenal hypoplasia. In a phenotypic female or a patient with ambiguous genitalia and adrenal insufficiency, demonstration of a 46 XY karyotype distinguishes this condition from congenital adrenal hypoplasia. Low urinary 17-ketosteroid and low plasma dehydroepiandrosterone levels distinguish it from 3β-hydroxysteroid dehydrogenase deficiency. Once the diagnosis is established, glucocorticoid and mineralocorticoid therapy should be immediately instituted and is essential for survival. In genotypic males, sex hormone therapy should be instituted at puberty in accordance with the sex of rearing. In most instances, because of the severity of the genital defect, the sex of rearing should be female. Genotypic females also require appropriate female sex hormone therapy at puberty.

3β-Hydroxysteroid Dehydrogenase:Δ^{5–4} Isomerase Deficiency. **Clinical Presentation.** Affected 46 XY subjects with 3β-hydroxysteroid dehydrogenase:Δ^{5–4} isomerase deficiency have genital ambiguity, although mild to moderate hypospadias is more common than severe perineoscrotal hypospadias. Internal male sexual differentiation is normal, with wolffian differentiation and müllerian ductal inhibition. Curiously, genetic males who reach puberty develop gynecomastia, the etiology of which is not known. At birth genotypic females have normal or slightly virilized external genitalia, with clitoral hypertrophy and slight labial fusion.

Severely affected children have adrenal insufficiency and die in infancy as a result of salt-losing crisis if not adequately treated. In the milder cases sufficient cortisol and aldosterone are synthesized to avoid this complication.

Pathogenesis. The enzyme deficiency results in decreased cortisol production, increased ACTH secretion, and increased production of Δ^5,3β-hydroxysteroids (Fig. 221–6). Plasma levels of pregnenolone, 17α-hydroxypregnenolone, and dehydroepiandrosterone and their sulfate conjugates are increased, with decreased levels of aldosterone and cortisol. The slight virilization of the external genitalia in the female is due to the mild androgenic effect of excess plasma dehydroepiandrosterone and its subsequent peripheral conversion to Δ^5-androstenediol and other androgens (Table 221–4). Surprisingly, plasma Δ^4 steroids, i.e., progesterone, 17α-hydroxyprogesterone, androstenedione, and occasionally testosterone, may be normal or even increased. This may reflect intact hepatic and peripheral 3β-hydroxysteroid dehydrogenase:Δ^{5–4} isomerase enzyme activity. Also in some

TABLE 221–3. XY MALE PSEUDOHERMAPHRODITISM WITH AN ENZYMATIC DEFECT IN TESTOSTERONE BIOSYNTHESIS

Enzyme Deficiency	External Genitalia Female or Urogenital Sinus	Ambiguous	Secretion Cortisol	Aldosterone	Androgens	Puberty	Comments
Cholesterol 20,22-desmolase	++++	+	↓	↓	↓	↓	
3β-Hydroxysteroid dehydrogenase:Δ^{5-4} isomerase	+	++++	− ↓	− ↓	↑ DHEA ↑ 17OH preg	Gynecomastia despite low estrogens	Intact peripheral 3βHSD with conversion of Δ^4 to Δ^4 steroids
17α-Hydroxylase	++++	++	− ↓	B ↑ DOC ↑	↓	Gynecomastia despite low estrogens	Hypertension due to ↑ DOC with ↓ renin and aldosterone
17,20-Desmolase	++++	+	−	−	↓		
17β-Hydroxysteroid dehydrogenase	++++	++	−	−	↓ T ↑ Δ^4	Gynecomastia due to increased estrogen and decreased T	Peripheral conversion of androstenedione to E_1

↑ = elevated; ↓ = decreased; − = normal; + = relative frequency of occurrence; B = corticosterone; DOC = desoxycorticosterone; DHEA = dehydroepiandrosterone; 17OH Preg = 17α-hydroxypregnenolone; T = testosterone; Δ^4 = androstenedione; 3βHSD = 3β-hydroxysteroid dehydrogenase; E_1 = estrone.

affected subjects, the gonadal defect is not as severe as the adrenal defect, suggesting that the same enzyme may be under different regulatory control in different areas. The 3-BHSD gene has been cloned and localized to chromosome 1. In both gonadal and adrenal tissue it appears to be encoded by the same structural gene, but under separate regulatory control.

Management and Therapy. In infancy the diagnosis is suggested in a 46 XY male with ambiguous genitalia and adrenal insufficiency. In contrast to an infant with cholesterol 20,22-desmolase deficiency, urinary 17-ketosteroid values are normal to high with increased plasma dehydroepiandrosterone. Treatment involves mineralocorticoid and glucocorticoid replacement therapy. If needed, sex steroid therapy should be instituted at puberty to induce sexual development in accordance with the sex of rearing.

17α-Hydroxylase Deficiency. **Clinical Presentation.** Many cases of 17α-hydroxylase deficiency have been reported in both genetic males and females. In 46 XY subjects the defect of the external genitalia is usually severe, resulting in completely female external genitalia at birth. Müllerian structures are absent, and wolffian structures are either developed or hypoplastic. Often gynecomastia develops at puberty with little or no virilization. Thus, males with this enzyme deficiency can have the same phenotype in adulthood as subjects with the complete androgen insensitivity syndrome. In 46 XX females with this condition secondary sexual development is absent at puberty and there is primary amenorrhea. Classically the affected subjects also have hypertension and hypokalemia.

Pathogenesis. 17α-Hydroxylase activity resides in the same P-450 enzyme as 17,20-desmolase activity (see section below), coded for by a gene located on chromosome 10. 17α-Hydroxylase deficiency can be characterized by partial or complete defects in either or both 17α-hydroxylase/17,20-desmolase activities. Some of the mutations that have been found include (1) a seven base pair (bp) duplication in the N-terminal region XYP17 (P-450 17α), producing a premature stop codon, (2) a triplet deletion of the

TABLE 221–4. CLASSIFICATION OF CAUSES OF FEMALE PSEUDOHERMAPHRODITISM

I. Androgenic influences
  A. Fetal
    1. Congenital adrenogenital syndrome
      a. 21-Hydroxylase deficiency
      b. 11β-Hydroxylase deficiency
      c. 3β-Hydroxysteroid dehydrogenase:Δ^{5-4} isomerase deficiency
  B. Maternal
    1. Excess maternal androgen production
    2. Maternal ingestion of virilizing substances
II. Idiopathic

N-terminal of the CYP-17 gene, (3) a four-base duplication on exon 8, and (4) a stop codon in place of tryptophan at amino acid 17, leading to the formation of a truncated protein.

17α-Hydroxylase activity converts pregnenolone and progesterone to 17α-hydroxypregnenolone and 17α-hydroxyprogesterone, respectively (Fig. 221–6). These steps are necessary for the ultimate formation of cortisol and C19 androgens, including testosterone. Thus a deficiency results in decreased plasma cortisol, an increase in ACTH, and hypersecretion of the plasma precursor 17-deoxysteroids (pregnenolone, progesterone, desoxycorticosterone, corticosterone, 18-hydroxycorticosterone) and their urinary metabolites. Excess circulating desoxycorticosterone increases sodium retention and plasma volume, resulting in hypertension, hypokalemia, and suppression of plasma renin. The plasma aldosterone value is also low secondary to a low level of plasma renin (see Table 221–3). 17α-Hydroxylated steroids are decreased, i.e., plasma 17α-hydroxypregnenolone, 17α-hydroxyprogesterone, 11-deoxycortisol, cortisol, androstenedione, dehydroepiandrosterone, testosterone, and estrogen. Consequently, urinary levels of 17-hydroxysteroids and 17-ketosteroids are low. Despite markedly impaired cortisol production, signs of glucocorticoid deficiency do not generally occur, due to the inherent glucocorticoid activity in the high levels of circulating corticosterone.

In affected adults, gonadotropin values are elevated, sex steroid levels are low, and in the male there is little or no testicular 17α-hydroxyprogesterone and testosterone response to hCG administration. Consanguinity has been documented in some cases, as has an occurrence of the disorder in siblings of both the same and opposite sex.

Management and Therapy. Hypertension associated with hypokalemic alkalosis in an XY individual with female external genitalia or ambiguous genitalia should suggest the diagnosis. It should also be suspected in any XX female with the same symptom complex who has primary amenorrhea and lack of secondary sexual development. Glucocorticoid replacement therapy reverses the metabolic abnormality and lowers the blood pressure. Appropriate sex steroid therapy concordant with the sex of rearing should be administered at puberty.

17,20-Desmolase Deficiency. **Clinical Presentation.** In 1972 a child with male ambiguous genitalia was described with a defect postulated to be secondary to 17,20-desmolase deficiency. A male pseudohermaphroditic cousin and maternal 46 XY "aunt" were included in the report. Since then other cases of the enzyme deficiency in 46 XY males have been reported, all phenotypic females or subjects with severely ambiguous genitalia. A genetic female with primary amenorrhea and lack of secondary sexual development has also been reported.

Pathogenesis. 17,20-Desmolase activity resides in the same P-450 enzyme as 17α-hydroxylase. Partial or complete lack of this activity in the adrenal and gonads results in decreased cleavage of the two-carbon side chain from either 17α-hydroxyprogesterone or 17α-hydroxypregnenolone with a resultant decrease in androstenedione and dehydroepiandrosterone production, respectively (Fig. 221–6). This step is essential for the ultimate formation of testosterone and estrogens. A deficiency in 17,20-desmolase activity can also be associated with a deficiency of 17α-hydroxylase activity (see above).

It is not known why the basal plasma levels of progesterone, pregnenolone, 17α-hydroxyprogesterone, and 17α-hydroxypregnenolone are elevated, particularly in prepubertal subjects with this enzyme deficiency. Since the enzyme 17,20-desmolase is not involved in cortisol biosynthesis, ACTH levels should be normal with subsequent normal amounts of the C21 precursor steroids mentioned above (Fig. 221–6).

Management and Therapy. In genotypic males the sex of rearing depends upon the degree of ambiguity of the external genitalia. In more severe cases, patients should be raised as females, with castration carried out in early childhood. Sex hormone therapy at puberty is invariably necessary. In genotypic females, estrogen and progesterone supplementation is invariably needed at the time of puberty.

17β-Hydroxysteroid Dehydrogenase Deficiency. **Clinical Presentation.** This condition, described only in 46 XY males, is characterized by either female external genitalia or mild ambiguity of the genitalia. With few exceptions, those affected have been raised as girls. In subjects with totally female-appearing external genitalia at birth, the abnormality is not noted until puberty, when virilization frequently occurs with clitoral enlargement. At puberty there are two distinct clinical presentations. Some subjects develop gynecomastia in addition to virilization, while others undergo strong virilization with a male pattern of body hair, deep voice, android build, and no gynecomastia. All subjects raised as females throughout childhood who were castrated prior to or during their teenage years have maintained a female gender identity.

Pathogenesis. 17β-Hydroxysteroid dehydrogenase catalyzes the conversion of androstenedione to testosterone, the final step in the synthesis of testosterone (Fig. 221–6), and the oxidation-reduction of estrone and estradiol, dehydroepiandrosterone, and Δ5-androstenediol. In affected 46 XY subjects, the enzyme deficiency results in increased circulating plasma levels of androstenedione, while plasma levels of testosterone are low to low normal (Table 221–3). Plasma luteinizing hormone (LH) is increased, while plasma follicle-stimulating hormone (FSH) is normal to increased. Approximately 90 per cent of circulating testosterone arises from the extragonadal conversion of androstenedione. Thus in the adult the defect appears to affect the testes while peripheral enzyme activity appears to be intact. However, for masculinization of the external genitalia to be minimal or absent in the fetus, peripheral conversion of androstenedione to testosterone and dihydrotestosterone in the anlage of the external genitalia must be insignificant or absent during early gestation. Thus, peripheral as well as testicular 17β-hydroxysteroid dehydrogenase activity appears deficient in utero, whereas peripheral enzyme activity appears to be intact in the adult. The elevated plasma levels of androstenedione result in increased peripheral conversion to estrone (Table 221–3). In some subjects the conversion of estrone to estradiol also appears to be as severely impaired as the conversion of androstenedione to testosterone, while in others it is impaired to a lesser degree or not at all, suggesting that the 17β-hydroxysteroid dehydrogenase enzyme(s) converting estrone to estradiol and androstenedione to testosterone may be under different regulatory control. The lower the plasma testosterone-estradiol ratio, the greater the likelihood of gynecomastia developing in an affected subject at the time of puberty.

Management and Therapy. 46 XY affected subjects with female external genitalia should be raised as females and castration carried out either before or during early puberty to avoid significant virilization. Female sex hormone therapy should be instituted at puberty. In those subjects with ambiguous genitalia that can be surgically corrected, a male sex of rearing should be considered. If the diagnosis is made peripubertally or postpubertally, careful psychosexual evaluation should be performed to determine the gender identity before any therapy is instituted. If a gender change from female to male has occurred with puberty, corrective male genital surgery is needed.

New MI, White P, Pang S, et al.: The adrenal hyperplasias. *In* Scriver C, Baudet A, Sly W, et al. (eds.): The Metabolic Basis of Inherited Disease, 6th ed. New York, McGraw Hill, 1989, pp 1881–1918. *A review of the biochemical aspects of nonvirilizing and virilizing forms of congenital adrenal hyperplasia.*

Peterson RE, Imperato-McGinley J: Male pseudohermaphroditism due to inherited deficiencies of testosterone biosynthesis. *In* Serio M, Motta M, Zanisi M, et al. (eds.): Sexual Differentiation: Basic and Clinical Aspects. Vol. 2. New York, Raven Press, 1984, pp 301–319. *A detailed study of the clinical characteristics and the biochemistry of male pseudohermaphroditism due to deficiencies in testosterone biosynthesis.*

DISORDERS OF FUNCTION AT ANDROGEN-DEPENDENT TARGET AREAS

COMPLETE ANDROGEN INSENSITIVITY—TESTICULAR FEMINIZATION. *Clinical Presentation.* In this inherited form of male pseudohermaphroditism, genetic and gonadal males have a female phenotype and totally female psychosexual orientation. The testes differentiate and secrete müllerian inhibiting factor, resulting in absent fallopian tubes, uterus, and upper portion of the vagina. Despite normal to high-normal plasma levels of testosterone, wolffian structures are absent or rudimentary, and the external genitalia are totally female. Affected subjects are raised as girls, and the condition is rarely suspected prior to puberty. A prepubertal diagnosis is made when inguinal or labial masses are palpated in a phenotypic female child and are found to be testes.

Adequate breast development occurs at puberty, but pubic and axillary hair is scant to absent. Medical attention is usually sought because of primary amenorrhea. Rarely, patients with 17α-hydroxylase deficiency have the same phenotypic presentation at puberty.

Pathogenesis. In patients with complete androgen insensitivity, absence of high-affinity binding to the androgen receptor (receptor-negative) has been demonstrated in cultured fibroblasts from genital skin. A variety of qualitative abnormalities of the androgen receptor have also been described, suggesting different structural changes of the receptor protein. Deletions and point mutations of the DNA and steroid-binding domains of the androgen receptor have been described in this condition. Postreceptor variants with normal androgen receptor binding have also been demonstrated. In the latter individuals, the mutation may affect the steps in the initiation of androgen action subsequent to nuclear binding, i.e., failure of RNA synthesis or an abnormality in its processing (Fig. 221–7).

The receptor-negative form of complete androgen insensitivity is maternally transmitted with only males expressing the condition, suggesting inheritance as X-linked recessive or autosomal dominant-sex limited (males). The gene for the androgen receptor is on the long arm of the X chromosome near the centromere.

Plasma testosterone levels are normal to high with mild to moderately elevated plasma levels of LH. FSH levels are normal to elevated. Urinary estrogens and plasma estradiol levels are generally in the low female range with increased production rates for estrone and estradiol, which are mainly testicular in origin. The elevated circulating estrogens together with the androgen unresponsiveness result in an unopposed estrogen effect resulting in breast development at puberty.

The histology of the testes resembles that of normal prepubertal males. Postpubertally, Sertoli cells and spermatogonia are present, but no evidence of spermatogenesis exists. The Leydig cells are hyperplastic, correlating with the elevated plasma testosterone levels.

Management and Therapy. Testicular neoplasms occur in approximately 2 to 5 per cent of patients with complete androgen insensitivity, but rarely before the age of 25 to 30 years. For this reason the testes should be removed following puberty to allow complete breast development. Following castration, cyclic estrogen replacement therapy is necessary to maintain adequate breast turgor. In general, the vagina is adequate for normal coital function. Occasionally it is too shallow, but can frequently be enlarged with vaginal dilators, thereby avoiding reconstructive surgery.

PARTIAL ANDROGEN INSENSITIVITY. *Clinical Presentation.* Partial forms of androgen insensitivity occur. Affected subjects range from XY subjects with genital ambiguity and minimal to moderate pubertal virilization and gynecomastia, to normal males with gynecomastia or infertility. Several pedigrees compatible with X linkage have been reported. Studies of genital

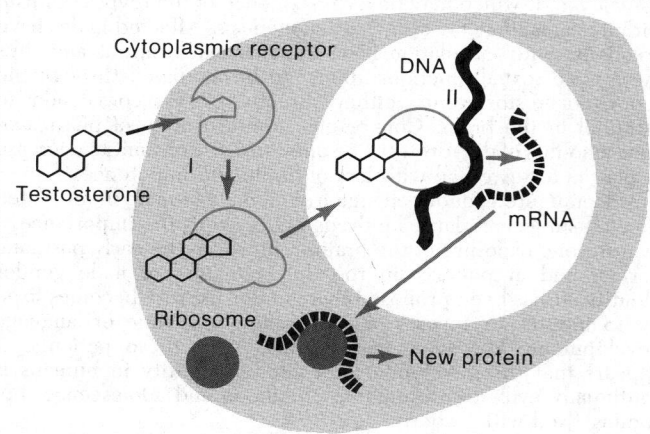

I. Abnormalities affecting binding to the cytosol receptor

  A. Quantitative

    1. Absent binding to cytosol receptor

  B. Qualitative

    1. Thermolability
    2. Failure of stabilization with sodium molybdate
    3. Altered binding affinity
    4. Lability of cytosolic receptor under conditions that normally promote transformation to the DNA–binding state

II. Nuclear or postnuclear receptor binding defect

    1. Impaired nuclear retention
    2. Impaired augmentation of receptor binding following incubation with androgen

FIGURE 221–7. Illustration of the abnormalities of androgen action resulting in androgen insensitivity.

skin fibroblasts from a mother of affected subjects demonstrate two clonal populations, one with normal dihydrotestosterone binding and one with a qualitative abnormality altering binding to the cytosol receptor, confirming X linkage in this form of androgen insensitivity. Affected subjects within the same pedigree may exhibit the variable phenotypes described. Thus these syndromes may represent variable phenotypic expressions of the same gene mutation.

Pathogenesis. In general, the endocrine profile is similar to that demonstrated in subjects with complete androgen insensitivity. Plasma LH and testosterone levels are generally elevated. The total amount of 17β-estradiol produced and the quantity secreted by the testes can be greater than those found in patients with complete androgen insensitivity. However, despite increased estrogen production, the degree of feminization at puberty is not as marked as in complete androgen insensitivity, which may be a consequence of the incomplete androgen resistance with a less severe androgen and estrogen imbalance at the cellular level.

In some affected males with incomplete androgen insensitivity, the binding capacity and affinity of the androgen receptor for dihydrotestosterone are normal. Thus this condition may be a variant of complete androgen insensitivity with normal cytosol-binding activity. Other affected males, however, have a reduced number of binding sites for dihydrotestosterone; this may represent a variant of complete androgen insensitivity with absence of androgen-binding activity. Qualitative defects in the receptor have also been demonstrated.

A form of incomplete androgen insensitivity is infertility in phenotypically normal men with either azoospermia or severe oligospermia. The mean plasma levels of LH and testosterone can be normal or elevated. The most frequent finding in cultured genital skin fibroblasts is a decrease in androgen-binding capacity of the androgen receptor. How frequently this is a cause of infertility is unknown.

Management and Therapy. Subjects with incomplete androgen insensitivity can be distinguished biochemically from male pseu-

dohermaphroditism with defects in testosterone biosynthesis. Following puberty, a normal to elevated plasma testosterone level with a normal androstenedione-testosterone ratio as well as normal plasma progesterone and dehydroepiandrosterone levels distinguishes subjects with this condition from subjects with 17β-hydroxysteroid dehydrogenase deficiency, 17α-hydroxylase deficiency, and 3β-hydroxysteroid dehydrogenase deficiency, who can have the same appearance. True hermaphrodites most commonly have an XX karyotype and can often be distinguished on that basis. Incomplete androgen insensitivity in puberty commonly results in gynecomastia and varying degrees of virilization.

Subjects with moderate to severe defects in masculinization of the external genitalia should be raised as females and castrated before puberty to prevent virilization. Estrogen therapy should be added at puberty. Those with mild hypospadias can be raised as males but require surgery for correction of both the hypospadias and the gynecomastia, if present.

Griffen JD, Wilson JD: The androgen resistance syndromes: 5α reductase deficiency, testicular feminization, and related disorders. *In* Scriver C, Baudet A, Sly W, et al. (eds.): The Metabolic Basis of Inherited Disease, 6th ed. New York, McGraw-Hill, 1989, pp 1919–1944. *A comprehensive review of the biochemical abnormalities in complete and partial androgen insensitivity.*

5α-REDUCTASE DEFICIENCY. *Clinical Presentation.* Most patients with this condition have pseudovaginal perineal hypospadias with separate urethral and vaginal openings within a urogenital sinus. Rarely a blind vaginal pouch opens into the urethra. All patients have epididymides, vas deferens, and seminal vesicles. The incidence of cryptorchidism is significantly higher in childhood than adulthood, suggesting that occasionally the testes descend during puberty.

The pubertal events include deepening of the voice, development of a muscular habitus, growth of the phallus, rugation and hyperpigmentation of the scrotum, and testicular descent. The prostate is small or absent, even in elderly subjects. Subjects have erections with ejaculation from the perineal urethra. Facial hair is decreased or absent and body hair is decreased.

Pathogenesis. The enzyme Δ⁴,5α-reductase catalyzes the reduction of the double bond at the 4–5 position of both C19 steroids, such as testosterone, and C21 steroids. It is present in high quantities in the liver and peripheral tissues, particularly the sebaceous glands, hair follicles, and skin of the external genitalia, where it converts testosterone to dihydrotestosterone (Fig. 221–8). When the enzyme is deficient, plasma testosterone is normal to elevated and dihydrotestosterone is decreased. The urinary 5α-reduced metabolites of testosterone, i.e., androsterone and androstanediol, and of C21 and C19 steroids other than testosterone, i.e., cortisol, corticosterone, 11β-hydroxyandrostenedione, and androstenedione, are decreased. Diminished 5α-reductase activity has been demonstrated both in skin slices and in fibroblasts cultured from genital skin. An autosomal recessive inheritance has been demonstrated.

Male pseudohermaphrodites with 5α-reductase deficiency represent a unique clinical model, defining major actions for testosterone and dihydrotestosterone in male sexual differentiation and development. Since the developmental defect is limited to the external genitalia and prostate, their development appears to be effected through the actions of dihydrotestosterone. In contrast,

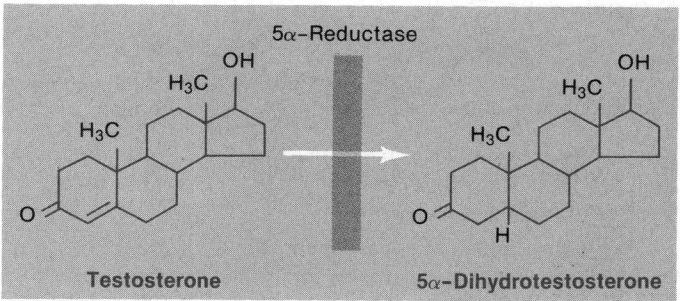

FIGURE 221–8. The conversion of testosterone to dihydrotestosterone by the enzyme 5α-reductase.

wolffian differentiation develops normally and appears to be a testosterone-mediated function (Fig. 221–9). At puberty the affected males develop rugation and hyperpigmentation of the scrotum, growth of the phallus, an increase in muscle mass, and deepening of the voice (Fig. 221–10). Their ultimate height is similar to that of their fathers and normal male sibs. Thus these pubertal events are mainly effected through the actions of testosterone. In contrast, prostatic development or enlargement, acne, normal male facial and body hair, and temporal recession of the hairline do not occur in affected males and appear to be effected mainly through the actions of dihydrotestosterone.

It is puzzling that the effects of dihydrotestosterone in dihydrotestosterone-dependent areas are not mimicked by testosterone, since both androgens share a common cytosol receptor. Two possible explanations can be submitted: (1) the cytosol receptor at certain target sites is modified so that it favors 5α-dihydrotestosterone over testosterone or (2) the 5α-dihydrotestosterone receptor complex has a higher affinity for the acceptor sites in chromatin.

In a few affected subjects with descended testes, testicular biopsy has demonstrated complete spermatogenesis; thus testosterone may be more important than dihydrotestosterone in the process of spermatogenesis. The question of fertility, however, remains unanswered. The cryptorchid testes of most subjects demonstrate seminiferous tubular damage with either Sertoli cells only or aberrant spermatogenesis. Plasma LH is increased despite normal to high plasma levels of testosterone, suggesting a role for dihydrotestosterone in the negative feedback control of LH. The elevated plasma LH levels correlate with the microscopic findings of Leydig cell hyperplasia. Plasma FSH levels are also elevated, which may be a consequence of the cryptorchidism with its damaging effect on spermatogenesis. Affected males have erections, with ejaculation from the perineal urethra, and thus these male sexual functions appear to be mediated through the actions of testosterone, either directly or via conversion to estradiol in the brain. Conversely, administration of pharmacologic amounts of dihydrotestosterone causes a substantial decrease in plasma testosterone with loss of libido and impotence.

A documented gender change from female to male in untreated affected subjects in large kindreds underscores the importance of testosterone exposure of the brain in utero, in the early postnatal period, and at puberty in the determination of male gender identity. It has been proposed that gender identity becomes fixed by 18 months to 4 years of age, around the time of language development. However, from studies with these patients, it appears that the development of gender identity in humans is continually evolving throughout childhood and adolescence, becoming fixed with puberty.

Management and Therapy. Subjects who have been diagnosed in infancy and in early childhood should be raised as males and their sex changed. Dihydrotestosterone cream should be administered to increase phallic size to facilitate surgical correction.

The most serious debate involves how to manage subjects who were raised as females but were diagnosed as having 5α-reductase deficiency in the peripubertal and postpubertal period. After careful psychiatric evaluation some subjects are found to have a male gender identity and should be helped to take their place as males in society. Other subjects who are not able consciously or subconsciously to admit the fact of maleness cannot and should not be encouraged to change gender roles. All these factors must be considered by the physician and a psychiatrist working in concert with the patient and the family before a final decision concerning the sex of rearing is made.

Imperato-McGinley J, Gautier T: Inherited 5α-reductase deficiency. Trends Genet 2(5):130, 1986. *A review of the inheritance and clinical and biochemical findings of this unusual experiment of nature.*
Imperato-McGinley J: 5α Reductase deficiency. *In* Bardin CW (ed.): Current Therapy in Endocrinology and Metabolism—4. Philadelphia, B. C. Decker, 1991. *A review of the condition with a comprehensive discussion of management and therapy.*

XX Males and True Hermaphroditism

XX MALES

Clinical Presentation. Approximately 50 cases of XX males have been reported, including members within the same family. The incidence in newborn males is estimated to be 1 in 20,000. Classically XX adult males have short stature, a normal-sized penis, small firm testes generally less than 2 cm, and infertility. One third have gynecomastia. The phenotypic appearance resembles that of males with Klinefelter's syndrome (XXY) with the notable exception that XX males are shorter in stature than the average male. The histologic features of the testes also resemble those of subjects with Klinefelter's syndrome. The seminiferous tubules are hyalinized and contain only Sertoli cells or a few immature spermatogonia, correlating clinically with azoospermia or oligospermia. The Leydig cells are hyperplastic. Levels of FSH and LH are elevated, with decreased plasma testosterone and increased plasma estradiol levels. XX children with bilateral testes and ambiguous genitalia have been reported, suggesting a phenotypic spectrum of this condition (Table 221–1).

Pathogenesis. Three possible mechanisms for the expression of masculinity in XX individuals have been proposed—(1) translocation of part of the Y chromosome to the X chromosome or to an autosome, (2) undetected mosaicism XX/XY or XXY, and (3) a mutant autosomal gene determining maleness in an XX individual. DNA digests from the nuclei of cells from testes of an XX male have demonstrated Y-specific DNA fragments. Studies using Y-specific DNA probes have demonstrated the presence of Y chromosomal material in the genome of some XX males. Thus, most 46 XX males appear to be a consequence of a paternal X-Y interchange containing the testes-determining gene on the Y chromosome.

TRUE HERMAPHRODITISM

Clinical Presentation. In true hermaphroditism both ovarian and testicular tissue is present with each gonad containing its

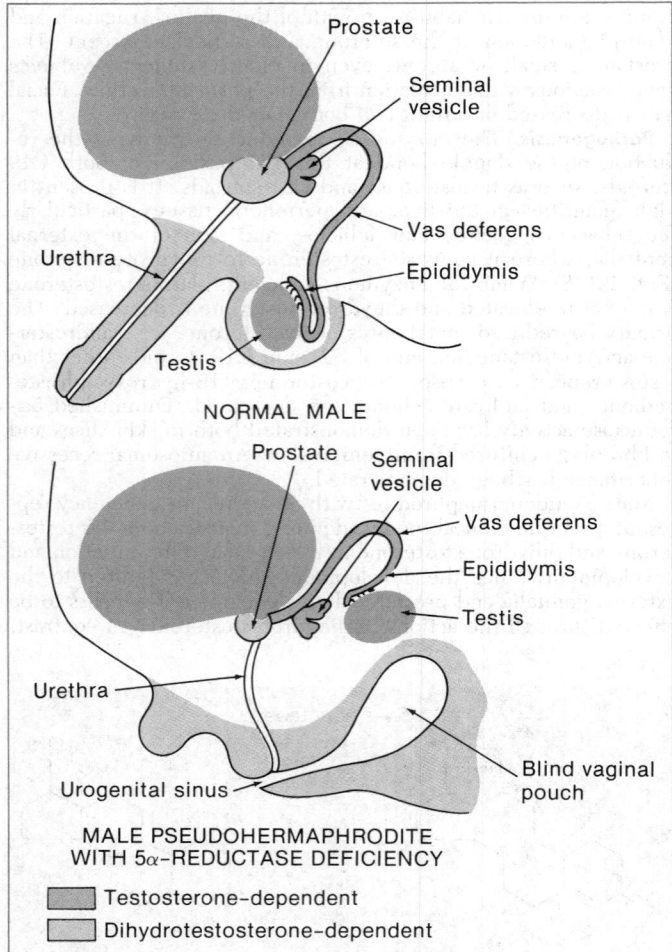

FIGURE 221–9. Illustration of the hypothesis for the specific actions of testosterone and dihydrotestosterone in male sexual differentiation in utero.

corresponding gamete. Most subjects have ambiguous genitalia, although approximately 7 per cent of true hermaphrodites have normal female external genitalia; 75 per cent of affected subjects are raised as males. The most common gonadal associations are an ovary and testis or an ovotestis and ovary. Gonadal tumors occur in approximately 2 per cent.

A fallopian tube is always found adjacent to an ovary and also most commonly adjacent to an ovotestis. An epididymis is present in approximately one third and a uterus in approximately 90 per cent of affected subjects.

With puberty, variable virilization and feminization occur. About half of affected subjects menstruate; in those raised as males with mild or moderate hypospadias or a penile urethra, menstruation can present as cyclic hematuria. Gynecomastia develops in 80 per cent of subjects. Pregnancy and childbirth have been reported in true hermaphrodites following removal of testicular tissue and correction of the external genitalia. A few subjects with functional testicular tissue are fertile (Table 221–1).

Pathogenesis. A 46 XX complement is present in approximately two thirds of cases, XX/XY mosaicism in one third of cases, and 46 XY complement in one tenth of the cases. A reported case of true hermaphroditism in a subject whose brother and paternal uncle were XX males suggests that XX males and XX true hermaphrodites may be variants of the same condition. Interestingly, Y-specific DNA has been found in some XX true hermaphrodites. The pathogenesis of the presence of both ovarian and testicular tissue is unknown.

Management and Therapy. The sex assignment in true hermaphroditism diagnosed in infancy and childhood is best determined by the appearance of the external genitalia, together with the gonadal tissue and internal structures. If an ovary-ovotestis and a uterus are present, the ovotestis and any male internal structures should be removed and feminizing surgery of the external genitalia performed. If bilateral ovotestes are present, and if a good line of demarcation is seen between ovarian and testicular tissue, the testicular portion should be removed, the genitalia surgically feminized, and the child raised as female. If a testis is present on one side and an ovotestis on the contralateral side, the testis should be brought into the scrotum and the child raised as male if the external genitalia can be surgically corrected. If an ovary is present on one side and a testis on the contralateral side, the sex of rearing should be decided by evaluation of the appearance of the external and internal sex structures, and appropriate surgical correction should be performed. Peripubertal

or postpubertal surgical correction of the internal and external sex structures should depend exclusively upon the gender identity of the affected individual. Although testicular tumor formation is rare, if the individual is to be raised as male the testis should be brought into the scrotum, so that periodic examination can be accomplished.

McLaren A: What makes a man a man? Nature 346:216, 1990. *Discussion on the latest development in the quest for the testes determining gene.*

Female Pseudohermaphroditism

Female pseudohermaphroditism can result from either fetal or maternal androgenic influences (Table 221–4). Cases of undetermined etiology have also been described.

CONGENITAL ADRENAL HYPERPLASIA— VIRILIZING FORMS

Three adrenal enzyme defects, 21-hydroxylase deficiency, 11β-hydroxylase deficiency, and 3β-hydroxysteroid dehydrogenase deficiency, can result in increased androgen production in utero with virilization of the female fetus (Table 221–5). They are the virilizing forms of congenital adrenal hyperplasia (Fig. 221–6). 21-Hydroxylase and 11β-hydroxylase deficiency can result in severe virilization of the female fetus. The virilization with 3β-hydroxysteroid dehydrogenase deficiency is mild; it is also a cause of male pseudohermaphroditism, and is discussed in the section Male Pseudohermaphroditism. The adrenal enzyme defects decrease cortisol production; pituitary ACTH secretion therefore increases and drives adrenal androgen overproduction. In the genotypic female, since ovaries and not testes are present, müllerian inhibiting factor is not produced, and the internal structures are female, i.e., uterus and fallopian tubes. Despite the masculinization of the external genitalia, wolffian differentiation does not occur. Affected 46 XY males with either 21-hydroxylase or 11β-hydroxylase deficiency appear phenotypically normal at birth.

21-HYDROXYLASE DEFICIENCY. Clinical Features. 21-Hydroxylase deficiency is the most common cause of ambiguous genitalia in 46 XX infants. Its incidence varies from approximately 1 in 300 births in Alaskan Eskimos to 1 in 15,000 births in Caucasians in Wisconsin. In the classic form of the disease, the spectrum of masculinization varies at birth from female infants with minimal clitoromegaly and fusion of the labioscrotal folds to infants with a penile urethra and the appearance of a cryptorchid

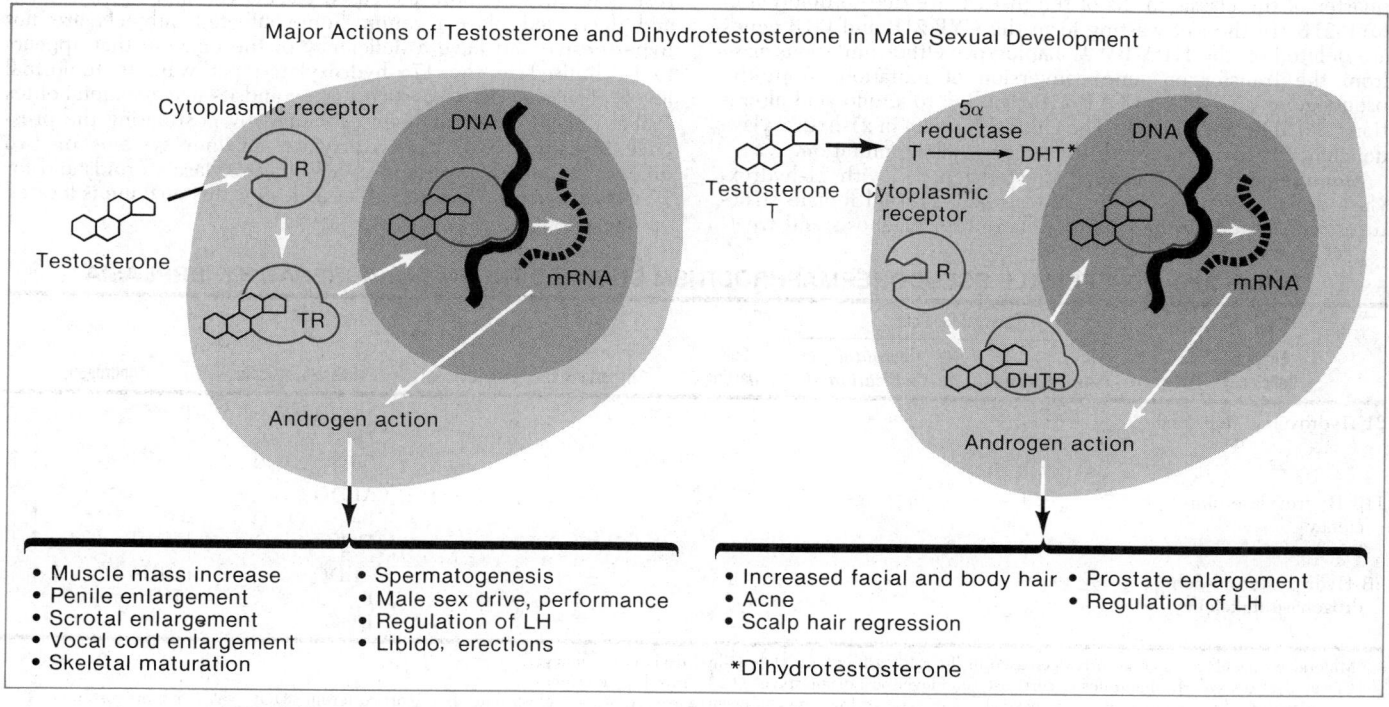

Major Actions of Testosterone and Dihydrotestosterone in Male Sexual Development

- Muscle mass increase
- Penile enlargement
- Scrotal enlargement
- Vocal cord enlargement
- Skeletal maturation

- Spermatogenesis
- Male sex drive, performance
- Regulation of LH
- Libido, erections

- Increased facial and body hair
- Acne
- Scalp hair regression

- Prostate enlargement
- Regulation of LH

*Dihydrotestosterone

FIGURE 221–10. Illustration of the major actions of testosterone and dihydrotestosterone at puberty.

male. Some infants also have salt wasting and may die in infancy. If affected XX children are untreated in infancy, there is rapid acceleration of growth; enlargement of the clitoris; increase in muscle mass; precocious development of pubic, axillary, and body hair; and advancement of bone age. Although they are tall in childhood, premature closure of the epiphyses eventually results in short stature in adulthood. At the time of expected puberty, there is absence of breast development and menstruation. Untreated males with this condition also show precocious maturation with short stature in adulthood. The excessive androgen production can inhibit gonadotropin secretion, so that untreated adult males, although strongly virilized, can have small soft testes and azoospermia. However, because of the adrenal androgen excess, they are capable of having erections. Frequently, however, true puberty occurs in untreated males with normal FSH and LH secretion, testicular enlargement, and spermatogenesis. ACTH-dependent testicular "tumors," most probably of adrenal origin, have been described and can occur either unilaterally or bilaterally.

Females with a nonclassic or late-onset form of the disease are born with normal female genitalia but may develop hirsutism, acne, and menstrual irregularities at puberty.

Pathogenesis. 21-Hydroxylase deficiency results in decreased synthesis of cortisol with consequent increase in ACTH and increase in plasma progesterone, 17α-hydroxyprogesterone, and C19 androgens (dehydroepiandrosterone, androstenedione, and testosterone; Figure 221–6; Table 221–5). In the newborn, determination of plasma 17α-hydroxyprogesterone is the test most diagnostic for this condition. The increased adrenal androgen production in the female fetus in utero virilizes the external genitalia. In the salt-losing form, aldosterone production is deficient, but the salt loss may also be due to increased production of progesterone and 17α-hydroxyprogesterone, which act as aldosterone antagonists. Obligate carrier parents and sibs frequently demonstrate increased 17α-hydroxyprogesterone levels in response to a 1-hour ACTH stimulation test.

The gene for 21-hydroxylase deficiency is closely linked to the HLA locus of chromosome 6. HLA-A3, BW47, DR7, and BW60 are associated with the salt-wasting form, HLA-B5 with the simple virilizing form, and HLA-B14, DR1 with the nonclassic or late-onset form of this condition.

There are two 21-hydroxylase genes, CYP-21A (a pseudogene) and CYP-21B, located adjacent to C4A and C4B genes that encode the fourth component of serum complement. About one quarter of the classic forms of the disease are due to deletion of CYP-21B. In the salt-wasting form the CYP-21B and C4B genes are deleted on the HLA-BW47 haplotype. Other mutations arise from the transfer or gene conversion of mutations from the pseudogene CYP-21A to CYP-21B, leading to amino acid alterations and aberrant splicing. The clinical severity of 21-hydroxylase deficiency is correlated with the severity of the mutation.

Management and Therapy. Affected females with 21-hydroxylase deficiency have ovaries and normal internal female structures with potential for fertility. Therefore, diagnosis and treatment should be carried out early and the child appropriately treated and raised as a female. Surgical correction of the masculinized external genitalia should be performed early so that gender confusion does not occur later on in childhood and adolescence. Medical therapy involves adequate glucocorticoid replacement therapy to lower ACTH secretion and to suppress adrenal androgen excess. Overtreatment should be avoided to prevent the signs and symptoms of glucocorticoid excess, which can lead to growth retardation.

Overt salt losers must be given mineralocorticoid as well as glucocorticoid replacement therapy. Many affected subjects without overt signs of adrenal crisis have impaired mineralocorticoid production, characterized by decreased sodium content and plasma volume with resultant increase in plasma renin, and may benefit from mineralocorticoid supplementation.

The nonclassic or late-onset form of the disease can be treated with a single low dose of a glucocorticoid administered in the late evening. This blunts the rise of ACTH in the morning hours and decreases adrenal androgen production. The treatment results in regulation of menses and improvement in fertility, as well as in hirsutism and acne.

11β-HYDROXYLASE DEFICIENCY. Clinical Features. Females with this disorder can have mild to severe masculinization of the external genitalia. A late-onset form results in mild hirsutism, clitoral hypertrophy, and irregular menses to severe virilization. Males with this condition show precocious male sexual maturation but develop gynecomastia at puberty. The cause of the gynecomastia is unknown, but it has been postulated to be secondary to elevated plasma desoxycorticosterone levels. Patients usually have hyporeninemic hypertension due to elevated desoxycorticosterone levels.

Pathogenesis. 11β-Hydroxylase deficiency results in decreased cortisol production, which causes an increase in ACTH, in C19 androgen secretion, and in desoxycorticosterone production (Fig. 221–6). Elevation of the plasma 11-desoxycortisol level is diagnostic of this enzyme deficiency and distinguishes it from 21-hydroxylase deficiency. Plasma cortisol as well as the urinary cortisol metabolites tetrahydrocortisone and tetrahydrocortisol can be normal to low. Urinary 17-ketosteroids, reflecting adrenal androgen overproduction, and urinary 17-hydroxysteroids, reflecting elevated levels of plasma 11-desoxycortisol, are increased. Excretion of pregnanetriol, a metabolite of 17α-hydroxyprogesterone, is usually normal or slightly increased. Plasma desoxycorticosterone is increased, as is its urinary metabolite tetrahydrodesoxycorticosterone, while corticosterone and aldosterone are decreased. The increased production of desoxycorticosterone results in salt retention, increased plasma volume, hypertension, and decreased plasma renin. Some affected subjects are not hypertensive and have a deficiency of the enzyme that appears to be limited to the 17α-hydroxylated pathway, with normal levels of plasma desoxycorticosterone and its urinary metabolites (Table 221–5). This has been explained by postulating the presence of either two 11β-hydroxylase enzyme systems or two different regulatory systems for 17α-hydroxylase steroids and for 17-desoxysteroids. The gene that codes for this enzyme is located on chromosome 8.

TABLE 221–5. XX FEMALE PSEUDOHERMAPHRODITISM DUE TO CONGENITAL ADRENAL HYPERPLASIA

| Enzyme Deficiency | External Genitalia | | Salt-wasting | Hypertension | Cortisol | Mineralocorticoids | Androgens |
	Ambiguous	Postnatal Virilization					
21-Hydroxylase deficiency	++++	++++	50–80%	−	− ↓	*ALDO ↓ *B ↓ *DOC ↓	T ↑ Δ4 ↑↑↑ 17OHP ↑↑↑↑
11β-Hydroxylase deficiency†	+++	++++	−	++	− ↓	ALDO ↓ B ↓ DOC ↑	T ↑ Δ4 ↑↑ 17OHP ↑↑
3β-Hydroxysteroid dehydrogenase deficiency	++	++	±	−	− ↓	ALDO ↓ − B ↓ − DOC ↓	DHEA ↑↑↑ 17OH preg ↑

*Mineralocorticoids are significantly decreased in the salt-wasting form of 21 O-hydroxylase deficiency.
†Elevated 11-deoxycortisol and desoxycorticosterone levels are diagnostic of 11β-hydroxylase deficiency.
↑ = elevated; ↓ = decreased; − = normal; + = relative frequency of occurrence; ALDO = aldosterone; B = corticosterone; DOC = desoxycorticosterone; T = testosterone; Δ4 = 4-androstenedione; 17OHP = 17-hydroxyprogesterone; DHEA = dehydroepiandrosterone; 17OH preg = 17α-hydroxypregnenolone.

Management and Therapy. Glucocorticoid replacement therapy effects biochemical normalization, decreases blood pressure, and arrests precocious development. In females, surgical correction of the external genitalia should be carried out as in females with 21-hydroxylase deficiency.

VIRILIZATION OF THE FEMALE FETUS SECONDARY TO EXCESS MATERNAL ANDROGEN PRODUCTION OR EXOGENOUS MATERNAL ADMINISTRATION OF VIRILIZING HORMONES

Masculinization of the female infant may occur in mothers with ovarian luteomas, virilizing adrenal tumors, and untreated maternal congenital adrenal hyperplasia. Why virilization of the female fetus does not occur in all states of maternal hyperandrogenicity may be related to the onset and the degree of hyperandrogenicity and the potency of the androgens secreted. The placenta may also offer some protection for the fetus by aromatization of the maternal androgens to estrogens.

Administration of testosterone or its derivatives to pregnant women may virilize a female fetus but with no effect on differentiation of the wolffian ductal system. Paradoxic masculinization of the female fetus associated with maternal administration of diethylstilbestrol early in pregnancy has been reported rarely.

Cutler GB Jr, Laue L: Seminars in Medicine of the Beth Israel Hospital, Boston: Congenital adrenal hyperplasia due to 21-hydroxylase deficiency. N Engl J Med 323:1806, 1990. *A concise, up-to-date review of this most common form of the virilizing forms of congenital adrenal hyperplasia.*

Miller WL: Molecular biology of steroid hormone synthesis. Endocr Rev 9(3):295, 1988. *An inclusive review and bibliography at the molecular level of the enzymes involved in steroid hormone biosynthesis.*

White PC, New MI, Dupont B: Congenital adrenal hyperplasia. N Engl J Med 316:1519, 1580, 1987. *An excellent review and extensive bibliography of the enzyme deficiencies resulting in adrenal hyperplasia, with particular emphasis on 21-hydroxylase deficiency; 107 references.*

222   The Testis and Male Sexual Function

Alvin M. Matsumoto

The testis has three major physiologic functions: (1) During embryogenesis, the testis plays a vital role in normal male sexual differentiation. Production of testosterone by the fetal testis stimulates the development and growth of male internal and external genitalia. The fetal testis also produces müllerian inhibitory factor, which prevents the differentiation of female internal genitalia (see Ch. 221). (2) Beginning at the time of puberty and continuing into adulthood, testosterone produced by the testis is necessary for the development and maintenance of secondary sexual characteristics (virilization) and sexual functioning (libido and potency). (3) Spermatozoa produced by the testis are necessary for fertility.

Disorders of the testis are common and have profound effects on patients. Infertility affects approximately 14 per cent of all married couples in the reproductive age group. Disorders of sperm production cause or contribute to the infertility in 40 per cent of these couples; therefore, 5 to 6 per cent of all men wishing to father children are unable to do so because of a disorder of testicular function. Klinefelter's syndrome, which results in permanent androgen deficiency and infertility, affects approximately one in 400 to 500 males. Impotence and gynecomastia, which often result from testicular dysfunction, are very common complaints for which men seek medical attention. High doses of androgenic steroids are widely used by competitive athletes, often with serious side effects. Finally, cancer of the testis remains one of the most common fatal neoplasms of young men.

Many disorders of the testis can be treated effectively. Testosterone replacement therapy in androgen-deficient men results in the development or restoration of secondary sexual characteristics and normal sexual functioning. Gonadotropin treatment of hypogonadotropic men often stimulates spermatogenesis and induces fertility in addition to restoring androgen secretion. Finally,

seminomas are exquisitely responsive to radiation therapy, and the treatment of nonseminomatous testicular cancers with multidrug chemotherapy has markedly improved survival.

TESTICULAR STRUCTURE AND PHYSIOLOGY

Functional Anatomy

The normal adult testis weighs approximately 20 grams and normally measures 3.5 to 5.5 cm in length and 2.0 to 3.0 cm in width. Normal testis volume is between 15 and 30 ml. About 90 per cent of the volume of the testis is composed of seminiferous tubules, where spermatozoa are produced. Therefore, any significant reduction in testicular size is likely to be reflected in a decrease in total sperm production.

During fetal development, the testes descend from an intra-abdominal position into the scrotum. The scrotal location of the testes allows them to function at a temperature approximately 2°C lower than that of the abdomen. The pampiniform plexus of veins that drains the testes surrounds the testicular artery and cools the arterial blood supply to the testes by a countercurrent heat-exchange mechanism. The lower testicular temperature is necessary for normal spermatogenesis in man. Failure of the testes to descend into the scrotum (cryptorchidism) or an abnormality in the cooling mechanism (varicocele) impairs sperm production.

The testis is composed of two structurally distinct compartments: the *interstitial* or *Leydig cell compartment* and the *seminiferous tubule compartment* (Fig. 222–1). These compartments are responsible for the two major physiologic roles of the testis, namely production of testosterone and spermatozoa, respectively.

The interstitial compartment is composed of *Leydig cells*, which produce sex steroid hormones, primarily testosterone. Leydig cells are nestled between seminiferous tubules, in close proximity to blood vessels. This location is important, since it facilitates delivery of high concentrations of testosterone to the seminiferous tubule compartment (intratesticular testosterone levels being approximately 100 times those found in peripheral blood) and the diffusion of testosterone into the blood vessels, for delivery to the rest of the body. The high intratesticular concentration of testosterone is important in stimulating normal spermatogenesis.

The seminiferous tubule compartment is composed of developing *germ cells* and *Sertoli cells*. Spermatogenesis involves the differentiation and maturation of spermatogonia, the most primitive germ cell, into spermatozoa. In humans, spermatogenesis takes approximately 74 days. Sperm transport through the epi-

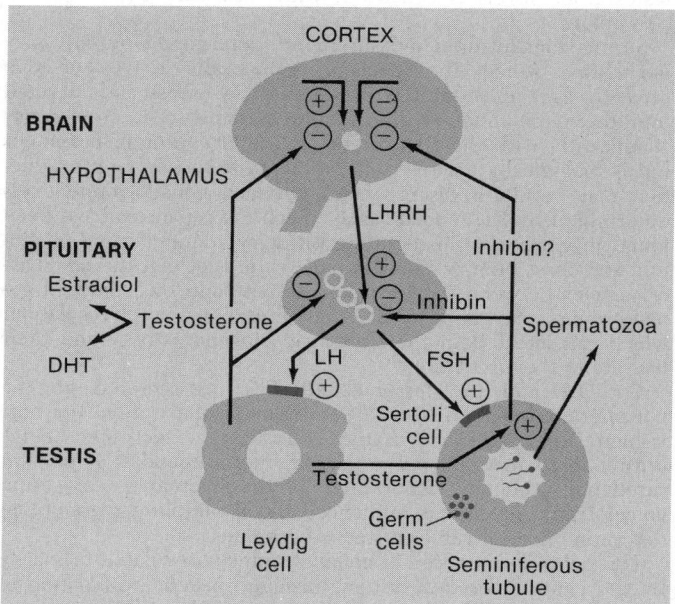

FIGURE 222–1. Diagram of the normal physiology of the hypothalamic-pituitary-testicular axis. (Adapted from Matsumoto AM, Bremner WJ: Bailliere's Clin Endocrinol Metab 1:71, 1987.)

didymis and vas deferens takes another 12 days. Therefore, processes that adversely affect early spermatogenesis may not be manifest by reduced sperm counts in the ejaculate until 2 to 3 months after the insult.

Sertoli cells perform many varied functions. By forming tight junctions at the basal portion of the seminiferous tubules, they maintain a barrier to the passage of macromolecules from the blood and interstitial compartment into the seminiferous tubules (the blood-testis barrier). Sertoli cells support spermatogenesis by synthesizing and secreting androgen-binding protein (ABP) and other protein products, by phagocytosing cellular remnants, and by participating in the movement and release of the maturing sperm and the secretion of fluid into the seminiferous tubule lumen. Sertoli cells produce *inhibin*, a glycoprotein that inhibits follicle-stimulating hormone secretion from the pituitary gland, but whose physiologic role remains unclear. They also produce another glycoprotein, *müllerian inhibitory factor (MIF)*, which is responsible, in the fetus, for causing the regression of the müllerian ducts (which normally develop into the female internal genitalia) during male sexual differentiation (see Ch. 221). Finally, Sertoli cells are capable of aromatizing testosterone to estradiol and producing paracrine factors that modulate Leydig cell function.

Central Nervous System Regulation of Gonadotropin Secretion

Normal testicular function depends on adequate stimulation by the gonadotropins, *luteinizing hormone (LH)*, and *follicle-stimulating hormone (FSH)*, which are secreted by the anterior pituitary gland (Fig. 222–1). Like thyroid-stimulating hormone and human chorionic gonadotropin (hCG), both LH and FSH are glycoprotein hormones composed of an α and a β subunit. These subunits are encoded on different genes, synthesized separately, glycosylated, and noncovalently assembled prior to secretion from the pituitary. The α subunits of all four glycoprotein hormones are identical and biologically inactive, whereas the β subunits are unique for each hormone and determine their biologic activity.

Measurements of serum gonadotropin levels are usually performed by radioimmunoassay (RIA). In normal young men, LH and FSH levels range from 5 to 20 mIU per milliliter (normal ranges vary according to the reference preparations used). Most gonadotropin assays are not sufficiently sensitive to distinguish between low and low-normal gonadotropin levels. Therefore, a hormonal profile of low-normal gonadotropin levels and low testosterone levels is consistent with secondary hypogonadism (see below).

Serum gonadotropin measurements determined by RIA may not always reflect the levels of biologically active hormone present. Free α subunit is synthesized in excess and secreted into the circulation by the pituitary. Because it cross-reacts significantly with the RIA for the intact glycoprotein hormones but is biologically inactive, alterations in free α subunit production may result in discrepancies between gonadotropin levels determined by RIA and bioassay. Such discrepancies have been found in gonadotropin-secreting pituitary adenomas and α subunit-secreting tumors, such as pancreatic islet cell tumors. Discrepancies between the immunoreactivity and bioactivity of gonadotropins may also result from alterations in glycosylation, which can affect both their intrinsic biologic activity and their half-life in the circulation.

Both LH and, to a lesser extent, FSH are secreted into the peripheral circulation from the anterior pituitary in an episodic fashion (Fig. 222–2). Pulsatile gonadotropin secretion begins during sleep in early puberty, and by adulthood it is present throughout the day. Knowledge of the fluctuations of serum gonadotropin levels has influenced blood sampling regimens to determine normal values of these hormones.

The pulsatile secretion of gonadotropins is regulated primarily by the central nervous system through episodic stimulation of the pituitary by *LH-releasing hormone (LHRH)*. LHRH, a decapeptide synthesized by hypothalamic neurons, stimulates release of both LH and FSH from the pituitary gland (see Fig. 222–1). Low-dose pulsatile LHRH administration has been used success-

fully to induce normal testicular function in patients with hypogonadotropic eunuchoidism, who presumably lack endogenous LHRH. By contrast, administration of high-dose, continuous LHRH or potent, long-acting LHRH agonists results in marked suppression of gonadotropin and testicular function. This paradoxic action of superactive LHRH agonists has been used clinically in the treatment of androgen-dependent tumors, such as prostate cancer.

The hypothalamic LHRH neuronal system plays an important integrative role in the regulation of testicular function (see Fig. 222–1). It receives input both from higher neural centers, such as the cerebral cortex and limbic system, through numerous stimulatory and inhibitory neurotransmitter (e.g., catecholamine and serotonin) and neuropeptide (e.g., opioid) systems and from testicular feedback signals, primarily sex steroid hormones. The input from these sources alters LHRH output, which, in turn, regulates pituitary gonadotropin secretion and testicular function. Increasing knowledge of how the central nervous system regulates LHRH secretion has helped to further our understanding of the mechanisms by which stress, malnutrition, and certain pharmacologic agents (such as catecholaminergic and opiate drugs) affect testicular function (Ch. 212).

Gonadotropin Regulation of Testicular Function

LH REGULATION OF TESTOSTERONE PRODUCTION. LH binds to specific membrane receptors on Leydig cells of the interstitial compartment of the testis and stimulates testicular steroidogenesis and secretion of *testosterone*, the major steroid product of the testis (see Fig. 222–1). LH increases the conversion of cholesterol to pregnenolone by the cholesterol side chain cleavage enzyme complex (20,22-desmolase), the rate-limiting step in testosterone biosynthesis.

Testosterone is secreted both locally within the testes and into the peripheral circulation (see Fig. 222–1). Healthy young men secrete approximately 5 to 7 mg of testosterone daily, essentially all from the Leydig cells. Total testosterone concentrations in plasma, as determined by RIA, range from 3 to 10 ng per milliliter (300 to 1000 ng per deciliter). Like gonadotropins, testosterone is secreted in a pulsatile fashion (Fig. 222–2).

In early puberty, testosterone secretion increases from very low to near adult levels during sleep in response to sleep-associated rises in LH levels. In adults, testosterone secretion occurs throughout the entire day. In young healthy men testosterone levels exhibit a circadian variation of about 1.5 ng per milliliter, with maximal levels occurring at 8 A.M. and minimal levels occurring at 9 P.M.

Under the influence of LH stimulation, Leydig cells also convert testosterone to *estradiol*. However, secretion of estradiol by the testis accounts for only about 15 per cent of the daily production of estradiol. The remainder of estradiol in blood is produced from testosterone and androstenedione (an adrenal androgen) by the enzyme aromatase in peripheral tissues, mostly adipose tissue.

TESTOSTERONE TRANSPORT. Like other steroid hormones, the majority of testosterone secreted into the circulation is bound to plasma proteins, primarily albumin and *sex hormone-binding globulin (SHBG)*. Approximately 30 to 40 per cent of total testosterone is bound to SHBG and is not biologically available. Only 1 to 2 per cent is free (i.e., unbound to plasma proteins) and physiologically active. Albumin-bound testosterone seems also to be available to act on many target organs. Therefore, measurement of non-SHBG-bound testosterone may provide the best estimate of biologically available testosterone. In certain clinical situations, alterations in SHBG levels result in total testosterone measurements that do not reflect bioavailable testosterone levels. SHBG (and total testosterone) levels are decreased with obesity, hypothyroidism, androgens, nephrotic syndrome, Cushing's disease, and acromegaly and increased with hepatic cirrhosis, hyperthyroidism, and estrogens. In these situations, free or non-SHBG-bound testosterone levels should be obtained.

PERIPHERAL METABOLISM OF TESTOSTERONE. The metabolism of circulating testosterone plays a very important role in its biologic actions on target tissues. Testosterone may be converted in peripheral tissues to either *dihydrotestosterone (DHT)* or *estradiol*, which mediates many of the physiologic actions of testosterone (see Fig. 222-1). These active metabolites of testosterone can be formed and act locally on androgen target tissues or circulate in blood and act on distant target tissues.

In many androgen-dependent target tissues, testosterone is converted intracellularly to a more potent androgen, DHT, by the enzyme 5 α-reductase. This conversion is required for normal male sexual differentiation. Males with 5 α-reductase deficiency, who cannot form DHT from testosterone in utero, fail to develop normal male external genitalia and as a result are born and raised as phenotypic females (Ch. 221). DHT is also thought to be important in mediating the androgenic effects of testosterone on skin and accessory sexual organs (i.e., prostate, seminal vesicles, and epididymis). In many peripheral tissues, especially in adipose tissue, testosterone is aromatized to estradiol, a potent estrogen. Obesity therefore results in increased peripheral estrogen formation. In men estrogens have diverse physiologic actions that may be agonistic or antagonistic to those of androgens. Therefore, the physiologic effects of testosterone result from the actions of testosterone itself in combination with those of its active metabolites, DHT and estradiol. Finally, 5β-reduced metabolites of androgens may be important mediators of androgen action on bone marrow.

Circulating testosterone and its active metabolites are metabolized to inactive metabolites mostly in the liver, and these inactive metabolites are excreted primarily in the urine. In sexual tissue (including skin and prostate), DHT is efficiently metabolized to 3 α-androstanediol and then to 3 α-*androstanediol glucuronide (3 α-diol G)*. Blood and urine measurements of 3 α-diol G are useful markers of peripheral androgen action. In disorders in which DHT formation is reduced (such as 5 α-reductase deficiency), 3 α-diol G levels are reduced (Ch. 221).

ANDROGEN ACTION AND FUNCTIONS. At the target cell, testosterone and DHT bind to intracellular androgen receptors, which interact with specific chromosomal sites to alter gene transcription and protein synthesis, resulting in expression of androgen action (Ch. 208). Quantitative or qualitative abnormalities of the androgen receptor, resulting in impaired androgen action, cause varying degrees of male pseudohermaphroditism (Ch. 221).

The major functions of androgens are the differentiation of male internal and external genitalia (primary sexual characteristics) during embryogenesis; the development and maintenance of secondary sexual characteristics, sexual functioning (libido and potency), certain behavioral characteristics (such as aggression), and feedback regulation of gonadotropins; and the initiation and maintenance of spermatogenesis.

FSH REGULATION OF SERTOLI CELL FUNCTION. FSH binds to specific membrane receptors on Sertoli cells of the seminiferous tubule compartment of the testis and stimulates the production of seminiferous tubule fluid and a variety of proteins thought to be important in regulating spermatogenesis (e.g., ABP, transferrin, plasminogen activator), in feedback control of pituitary FSH secretion (inhibin and activin), and possibly in intratesticular paracrine modulation of Leydig cell function (see Fig. 222-1). Testosterone produced by adjacent Leydig cells also regulates these Sertoli cell functions through androgen receptors. The relative roles of FSH and testosterone in the regulation of Sertoli cell function are poorly understood. Developing germ cells are enveloped in the cytoplasmic processes of the Sertoli cells, which nurture and coordinate the completion of sperm maturation in the seminiferous tubule.

HORMONAL CONTROL OF SPERMATOGENESIS. Both FSH and LH stimulation are required for the initiation of spermatogenesis at the time of puberty. At this time, LH causes the differentiation of Leydig cells from interstitial connective tissue precursors and stimulates them to produce high intratesticular levels of testosterone, which are essential for the initial phases of sperm production. By stimulating Sertoli cell function, FSH plays an important role in the later stages of spermatid maturation (spermiogenesis) during this initial wave of spermatogenesis.

Normal levels of either FSH or LH do not appear to be absolute requirements for the maintenance of spermatogenesis in adult men. Selective gonadotropin replacement in adult men with experimentally induced gonadotropin deficiency results in stimulation of qualitatively normal sperm production with either FSH or LH treatment alone. However, replacement of both LH and FSH is necessary to maintain quantitatively normal spermatogenesis in these hypogonadotropic men.

Clinically, replacement of both FSH and LH activity is generally required to initiate sperm production in prepubertal hypogonadotropic hypogonadal patients. In contrast, initiation and maintenance of spermatogenesis in postpubertal men with acquired hypogonadotropic hypogonadism can usually be achieved with replacement of LH activity alone.

Seminal fluid analysis is used to evaluate the function of the seminiferous tubules. It is performed on seminal fluid samples obtained by masturbation, usually after 48 hours of abstinence from ejaculation. Normal ejaculate volume ranges from 2 to 6 ml. Although the normal range of sperm concentration is gener-

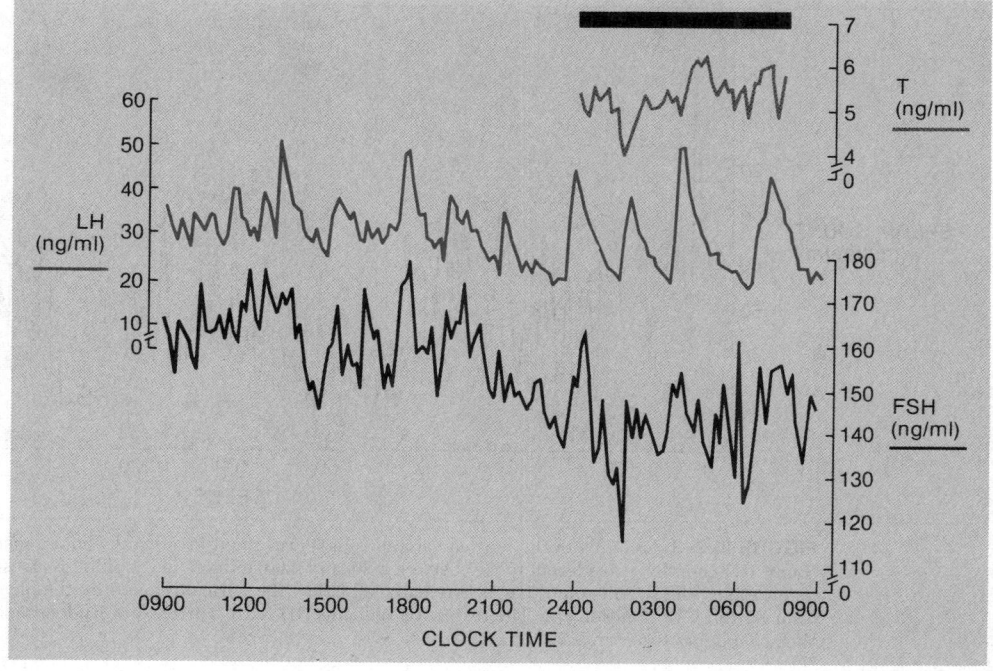

FIGURE 222–2. Example of pulsatile LH and FSH secretion throughout a 24-hour day and episodic testosterone secretion at night in a healthy young man. Blood samples were drawn at 10-minute intervals. Black bar denotes sleep, as documented by electroencephalogram.

ally considered to be 20 to 200 million per milliliter, sperm concentrations below 20 million per milliliter may be sufficient for fertility. In addition to determining sperm count, a careful microscopic examination of the seminal fluid is usually performed to assess sperm motility and morphology. Normally, greater than 60 per cent of sperm examined within 1 hour after ejaculation are motile, and greater than 60 per cent have a normal oval head morphology.

The minimal levels of sperm concentration, per cent motility, and per cent oval forms compatible with fertility are not clearly defined. In any individual, sperm counts normally exhibit extreme variability (Fig. 222-3) and are often temporarily suppressed by factors such as fever. Therefore, a reasonable estimate of mean sperm production requires at least three seminal fluid analyses over a 2-month period. Functional tests of sperm penetration into cervical mucus of various mammalian species or zona pellucida–free hamster ova may be helpful in assessing fertilizing capability of spermatozoa.

Testicular Feedback Regulation of Gonadotropin Secretion

Both steroid and nonsteroidal products of the testis are involved in negative feedback control of pituitary gonadotropin secretion. Increased production of these testicular products results in suppression, whereas decreased production of these factors results in stimulation of gonadotropin secretion (see Fig. 222-1). Testosterone and its active metabolites, DHT and estradiol, exert profound inhibitory effects on both LH and FSH secretion, although the relative roles of these steroids are not clearly defined. Testosterone may affect both the hypothalamic release of LHRH and the pituitary sensitivity to LHRH stimulation. Inhibin, a glycoprotein product of the Sertoli cell, selectively inhibits FSH secretion at the pituitary gland. At present, the physiologic significance of inhibin is unclear.

Knowledge of these negative feedback relationships has proved to be clinically useful in the diagnosis of hypogonadal states (see below). In addition, the potent negative feedback effect of administering exogenous testosterone has been utilized to suppress endogenous gonadotropin and sperm production in the development of male contraceptives.

Matsumoto AM, Bremner WJ: Endocrinology of the hypothalamic-pituitary-testicular axis with particular reference to the hormonal control of spermatogenesis. Bailliere's Clin Endocrinol Metab 1:71, 1987. *This paper reviews the normal physiologic regulation of testicular function, which forms the basis for understanding the pathophysiology and treatment of testicular disorders. An up-to-date discussion of the hormonal regulation of human spermatogenesis is also provided.*

Steiner RA, Cameron JL: Endocrine control of reproduction. *In* Patton HD, Fuchs AF, Hille B, et al. (eds.): Textbook of Physiology: Circulation, Respiration, Body Fluids, Metabolism and Endocrinology, 21st ed. Philadelphia, W. B. Saunders Company, 1989, p 1289. *This chapter contains an excellent, concise, and up-to-date general discussion of the physiology and pathophysiology of the male reproductive axis.*

PHYSIOLOGY OF MALE SEXUAL FUNCTION

Normal male sexual function requires coordinated regulation of the following physiologic events: *libido* or sexual desire, sustained penile tumescence or *erection, ejaculation, orgasm,* and *detumescence.*

Libido

Libido is generated in the central nervous system and stimulated by a variety of visual, tactile, imaginative, auditory, and gustatory stimuli. These stimuli are received in a number of cortical and subcortical regions of the brain, including the limbic system, and relayed via the preoptic–anterior hypothalamic area to spinal cord centers that control penile erection. Therefore, disturbances in libido are nearly always accompanied by disturbed erectile function or impotence.

Libido is regulated primarily by psychic factors and the sex steroid milieu, in particular serum testosterone concentrations. Thus, psychological disturbances of all degrees (from stress to major psychiatric illnesses), central nervous system lesions, drugs that alter brain function, and androgen deficiency may disturb normal libido and potency. Occasionally, castrated males maintain sexual desire and erectile function for long periods, suggesting that the requirement for androgens may be quite variable.

Erection

Erections are generated by two separate but synergistic mechanisms, one involving sensory stimulation of the genitalia, mediated through a spinal reflex arc (reflexogenic erections), and another involving psychogenic stimuli from higher brain centers (psychogenic erections). In reflexogenic erections, afferent sensory fibers from the penis travel in the pudendal nerve to the sacral spinal erection center (S2 to S4). Efferent parasympathetic fibers arising from this center travel in the nervi erigentes and innervate the blood vessels of the corpora cavernosa of the penis; efferent somatic fibers traveling in the pudendal nerve innervate the pelvic floor (ischiocavernosus and bulbocavernosus) muscles. Sympathetic fibers originating in the thoracolumbar spinal erection center (T12 to L1) innervate the muscles of the vas deferens, accessory sex glands, and internal sphincter of the bladder. In psychogenic erections, projections from higher brain centers descend in the lateral spinal columns and regulate both the thoracolumbar and sacral spinal erection centers.

Penile erectile tissue consists of paired corpora cavernosa on

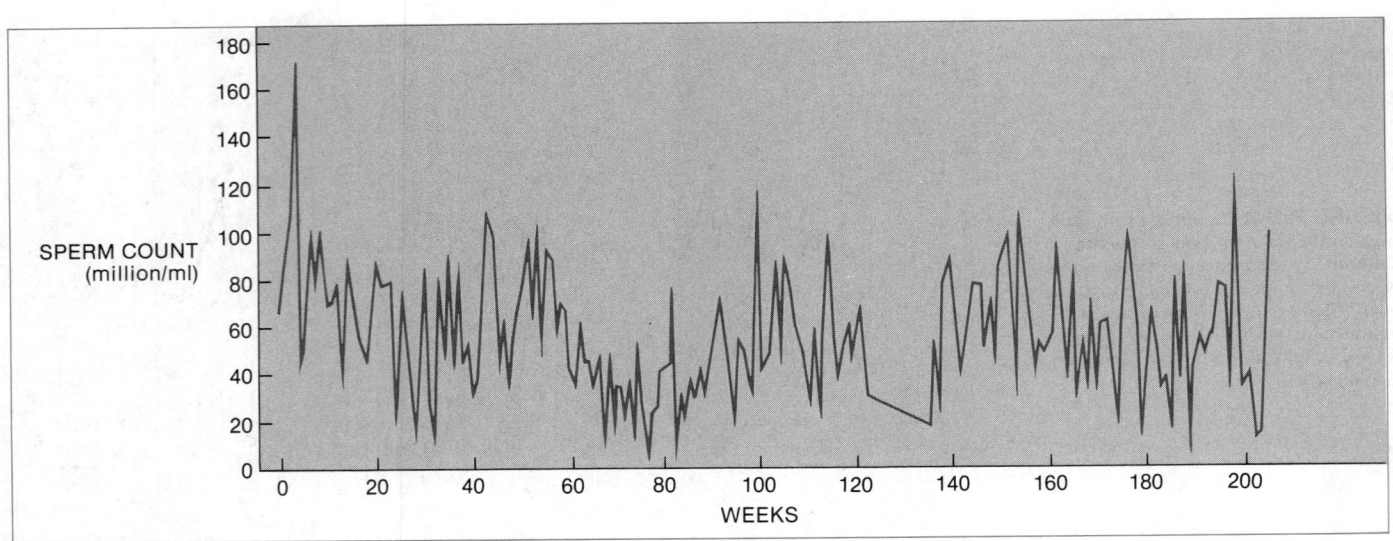

FIGURE 222–3. Example of the normal variations in sperm count in a healthy young man. Normal range of sperm count is generally considered to be between 20 and 200 million per milliliter. Despite good health and no medications, the sperm count may occasionally fall below the normal range, into the oligospermic range. (Adapted from Bardin CW, Paulsen CA: The testes. *In* Williams RH (ed.): Textbook of Endocrinology, 6th ed. Philadelphia, W.B. Saunders Company, 1981.)

the dorsum of the penis and the corpus spongiosum that surrounds the urethra and forms the glans penis. The corpora are composed of spongelike, interconnected trabecular spaces lined by vascular epithelium and smooth muscle and are surrounded by a thick fibrous sheath, the tunica albuginea. Activation of the spinal erection centers results in relaxation of the penile smooth muscle and vasodilation of the cavernosal arteries (branches of the internal pudendal arteries). These actions are mediated by cholinergic, β-adrenergic, and peptidergic (e.g., vasoactive intestinal peptide) receptors. As a result, blood flow into the trabecular spaces of the corpora is increased, causing engorgement of the penis (tumescence). Expansion of the trabecular walls against the tunica albuginea compresses subtunical venules and impedes venous outflow, resulting in sustained tumescence, i.e., an erection.

Failure to achieve an adequate erection or impotence has many potential etiologies, including androgen deficiency, central and peripheral nervous system diseases, vascular disorders, and penile abnormalities. Impotence as it relates to the differential diagnosis of hypogonadism is discussed in a subsequent section of this chapter.

Ejaculation

Ejaculation is stimulated by sympathetic nervous system activation, which results in contractions of the vas deferens and accessory sex glands and emission of seminal fluid into the urethra. Emission is followed by reflex rhythmic contractions of the ischiocavernosus and bulbocavernosus muscles and expulsion of semen from the urethra, i.e., ejaculation. Like erection, the ejaculatory reflex is under considerable control by higher cerebral centers. Sympathetic activation also stimulates closure of the internal urethral sphincter, thereby preventing retrograde ejaculation.

Premature ejaculation is usually due to performance anxiety or an emotional disorder and rarely has an organic etiology. Retrograde ejaculation into the bladder usually occurs in patients with sympathetic neuropathy (e.g., with diabetes) or after bladder neck surgery. Reduced or absent ejaculation may occur with androgen deficiency, sympatholytic drugs, sympathectomy, or extensive retroperitoneal/pelvic surgery.

Orgasm

Orgasm, the pleasurable sensation that usually accompanies ejaculation, is primarily a central nervous system–mediated phenomenon that, under normal circumstances, is influenced by ascending pathways associated with ejaculation. However, orgasm can occur in the absence of erection or ejaculation (e.g., with temporal lobe lesions). Conversely, normal libido, erection, and ejaculation can occur without orgasm; this is nearly always due to a psychological disorder.

Detumescence

Detumescence results from contraction of the penile smooth muscle and α-adrenergic vasoconstriction of the cavernosal arteries, which reduce arterial blood flow into the penis. As a result, the trabecular spaces of the corpora collapse, subtunical venules are decompressed, venous outflow is increased, and the penis becomes flaccid. In many cases, premature detumescence may contribute to the pathophysiology of impotence (e.g., venous leak or incompetence). Failure of detumescence, priapism, is often painful and unrelated to sexual intercourse. It is commonly idiopathic in etiology but may be associated with spinal cord injury, sickle cell disease, chronic myelogenous leukemia, and intracorporal injection of vasodilatory substances used in the treatment of impotence.

Meyer JK: Disorders of sexual function. *In* Wilson JD, Foster DW (eds.): Williams' Textbook of Endocrinology. Philadelphia, WB Saunders Company, 1985, p 476. *This chapter contains a well-organized, clear, and comprehensive discussion of the physiologic and anatomic basis of male sexual function and dysfunction.*

HYPOGONADISM

Hypogonadism is the most common disorder of testicular function encountered in clinical practice. The clinical manifestations of male hypogonadism differ depending on (1) whether there is *impairment of testosterone production*, which is nearly always accompanied by impairment of sperm production, or

isolated impairment of sperm production, with normal testosterone production; (2) whether androgen deficiency occurs *during embryogenesis, before puberty*, or *after puberty;* and (3) whether testicular hypofunction is the result of a *primary* defect in the testis or is *secondary* to hypothalamic-pituitary dysfunction.

Androgen Deficiency

The clinical presentation of androgen deficiency depends on the stage of sexual development in which it occurs.

During early fetal development, testosterone and its active metabolite, DHT, mediate the differentiation of male internal and external genitalia from the wolffian duct system and the indifferent anlage of external genitalia, respectively. Androgen deficiency (e.g., as a result of a genetic androgen biosynthetic enzyme defect) or impaired androgen action (androgen resistance) occurring during this period of development results in varying degrees of ambiguous genital development, or *male pseudohermaphroditism*. These disorders are discussed in greater detail in Ch. 221.

During puberty, testosterone is responsible for the development of male secondary sexual characteristics, such as (1) the growth of the penis and scrotum, (2) the development of accessory sexual organs (prostate and seminal vesicles) necessary to produce an ejaculate, (3) a male pattern of hair growth (face, external ear canals, chest, lower abdomen, pubis, perianal area, legs, and inner thighs) and frontal scalp regression, (4) the enlargement of the larynx and thickening of the vocal cords with consequent deepening of the voice, (5) the development of skeletal musculature and increase in strength (especially in the shoulder and pectoral muscles), (6) a redistribution of body fat, and (7) stimulation of erythropoiesis. Testosterone also stimulates the pubertal spurt of long bone growth and, eventually, the closure of long bone epiphyses, which results in cessation of bone growth. Finally androgens stimulate libido (sexual drive), potency (erectile function), and aggressive behavior and play an important role in initiation of spermatogenesis, which determines the development of fertility.

Patients who develop androgen deficiency before the onset of puberty usually present to physicians as adolescents or young adults with delayed puberty or poor male sexual development. Prepubertal testosterone deficiency results in *eunuchoidism* (Fig. 222–4), which is characterized by infantile development of genital and accessory sexual organs, failure to develop an ejaculate (aspermia), lack of male hair pattern, high-pitched voice, poor muscular development and strength, lower abdominal-pelvic girdle fat distribution, and excessive long bone growth (due to lack of closure of long bone epiphyses). The testes are small, usually less than 2 cm in length or 2 ml in volume. A eunuchoidal body habitus is characterized by excessively long arms and legs in proportion to height. Although there are racial differences in body proportions, eunuchoidal body measurements consist of an arm span that exceeds height by greater than 5 cm or a distance from the floor to the symphysis pubis that is 5 cm greater than that from the symphysis to the crown of the head. Patients with prepubertal androgen deficiency fail to develop normal sexual functioning (libido and potency) and are infertile. Testosterone deficiency before puberty may occasionally result in gynecomastia (benign enlargement of breast tissue).

In the adult, testosterone is responsible for the maintenance of libido, potency, and secondary sexual characteristics and participates in the maintenance of spermatogenesis. The major complaints of men with adult-onset androgen deficiency are poor sexual performance, as a result of diminished libido and/or impotence; infertility, as a result of impaired spermatogenesis; and gynecomastia. Rapid development of severe androgen deficiency (such as surgical castration) may also result in vasomotor instability or hot flushes, similar to those that many women develop at the time of menopause. Androgen deficiency may also result in behavioral changes, such as passivity, lack of motivation, and irritability.

Secondary sexual characteristics do not regress to the prepubertal state in men who develop testosterone deficiency as adults. However, with longstanding androgen deficiency, there may be significant loss of hair in androgen-dependent areas of the body, fine wrinkling of skin (most noticeable around the eyes and mouth), diminished muscle strength and mass, osteoporosis, and altered fat distribution. In hypogonadal men, pubic hair may assume a female type, inverted triangle pattern (female escutcheon), in contrast to the male type, diamond-shaped distribution, with hair extending to the umbilicus (male escutcheon). The amount and distribution of facial and body hair vary considerably, depending on an individual's ethnic and genetic background. The testes are usually small in hypogonadal states that result in androgen deficiency. However, depending on the specific cause and severity of the disorder, testis size may be normal. For example, men with recent onset of gonadotropin deficiency from a destructive pituitary tumor may have normal size testes, despite severe testosterone deficiency.

Serum testosterone levels are low in states of androgen deficiency. Very sensitive and specific RIA's for serum testosterone are generally available and are relatively inexpensive. Routinely available assays measure total testosterone and may give falsely low values in clinical states in which sex hormone–binding globulin is reduced (such as protein deficiency states and obesity). In these instances serum free or non-SHBG-bound testosterone levels should be measured.

Testosterone helps to maintain quantitatively normal spermatogenesis in man; androgen deficiency, therefore, almost always results in abnormalities in sperm production. Impaired spermatogenesis is usually confirmed by a low sperm count on seminal fluid analysis. Sperm counts are highly variable in any individual and are often suppressed by illness (e.g., fever). At least three sperm counts should be obtained over a period of 2 months, while patients are well, before diagnosing low sperm counts (oligospermia).

Isolated Deficiency in Sperm Production

In contrast to patients with androgen deficiency, men with an isolated deficiency of sperm production present postpubertally with infertility as their major complaint, without symptoms of testosterone deficiency. Testis size may be reduced or normal and an undescended testis or *varicocele* (varicose dilatation of the pampiniform venous plexus of the testis) may be found. The remainder of the physical examination is usually unremarkable. Sperm counts are usually low (less than 20 million per milliliter) or zero (*azoospermia*), and there may be isolated or associated abnormalities of sperm motility and/or morphology on seminal fluid analysis. Serum testosterone levels are normal in disorders causing isolated impairment of sperm production.

Differential Diagnosis

The major manifestations of androgen deficiency in adults are impotence, infertility, and gynecomastia. Although hypogonadism resulting in testosterone deficiency is a major cause of these clinical manifestations, there are many other causes.

IMPOTENCE. Impotence is defined as a consistent inability to achieve or maintain penile erection that is adequate for completion of sexual intercourse. It is a commonly encountered complaint in medical practice, occurring in 10 to 35 per cent of adult men with medical problems and increasing in prevalence with advancing age. Impotence is often underdiagnosed because of reluctance of patients and physicians to discuss sexual dysfunction as a medical problem. Although psychogenic impotence is common, the majority of men with impotence who are followed in a general medical clinic have one or more organic causes of erectile dysfunction. Furthermore, organic causes of impotence often result in performance anxiety and secondary psychogenic sexual dysfunction.

Penile erection sufficient to complete intercourse requires (1) normal *central nervous system* and thoracolumbar sympathetic and sacral parasympathetic *spinal cord* outputs to the penis; (2) an intact *arterial supply* and *venous drainage* of the penis; and (3) an *anatomically normal penis*. Dysfunction of any of these components interferes with normal initiation and maintenance of penile erection (Table 222–1).

Normal central nervous system function is necessary to produce adequate penile erections. *Libido* or sexual desire, mediated by the cerebral cortex and limbic system, has a profound influence on erectile function. In most central nervous system disorders that cause sexual dysfunction, reduced libido is usually associated with impotence. All degrees of *psychiatric disturbance*, from minor stress and performance anxiety to major psychiatric illness, such as depression and schizophrenia; *chronic debilitating illness*, such as cardiac, respiratory, renal, or liver disease or malignancy; and *drugs* that affect central nervous system function (sedatives, antipsychotics, antidepressants, centrally acting antihypertensive agents, and alcohol), are central nervous system causes of impotence and generally reduce libido as well as erectile function. *Androgen deficiency, hyperprolactinemia*, and *thyroid dysfunction* (hyperthyroidism and hypothyroidism) also impair libido and potency. Elevated prolactin levels may cause impotence by inducing secondary hypogonadism and androgen deficiency. However, impotence may not resolve with androgen replacement therapy alone and may require, in addition, therapy aimed at reducing the elevated prolactin levels (e.g., bromocriptine). In contrast to these disorders, *destructive or infiltrative diseases* of certain regions of the *brain* (such as tumor or infarction of the

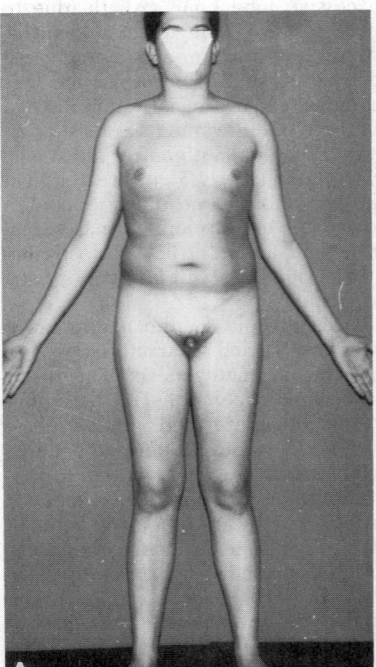
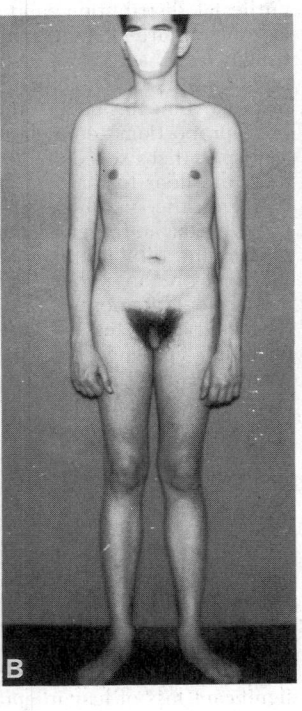
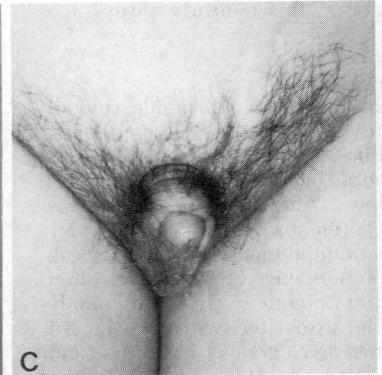
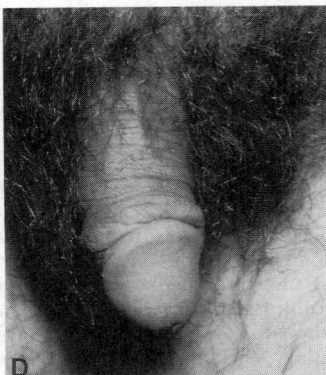

FIGURE 222–4. Example of eunuchoidism as a result of prepubertal androgen deficiency due to functional prepubertal castrate syndrome. *A* and *C*, Before androgen therapy, note the eunuchoidal features of infantile genital development, lack of male hair pattern, poor muscular development, pelvic girdle and lower abdominal fat distribution, and disproportionately long arms and legs. No testicular tissue was identified at the time of surgical exploration. *B* and *D*, After 18 months of testosterone treatment, scalp hair recession, penile development, and pubic hair growth have occurred. A masculine body habitus has developed, with an increase in pectoral and shoulder muscle development and loss of pelvic girdle and lower abdominal fat. (From Bardin CW, Paulsen CA: The testes. *In* Williams RH (ed.): Textbook of Endocrinology, 6th ed. Philadelphia, W.B. Saunders Company, 1981.)

TABLE 222–1. CAUSES OF IMPOTENCE

I. Disorders of Central Nervous System Control	II. Disorders of Peripheral Erectile Response
Psychiatric Illness	Drugs
Stress	Anticholinergic drugs
Performance anxiety	Antidepressants
Depression	Antihistamines
Major psychiatric illness	β-Adrenergic
Chronic Illness	blockers
Cardiac disease	Sympathomimetic
Respiratory disease	drugs
Renal disease	α-Adrenergic agonists
Liver disease	Antihypertensive
Malignancy	agents
Central Nervous System–	Autonomic Neuropathy
Active Drugs	Pelvic surgery
Sedatives	Diabetes
Antipsychotics	Other peripheral
Antidepressants	neuropathies
Central antihypertensives	Vascular Disease
Alcohol	Distal aortoiliac
Endocrine Disorders	atherosclerosis
Hypogonadism (androgen	Diabetes
deficiency)	Trauma
Hyperprolactinemia	Venous incompetence
Thyroid disease	Penile Abnormalities
Central Nervous System	Peyronie's disease
Disease	Chordee
Temporal lobe disorders	Priapism
Limbic system disorders	Trauma
Spinal Cord Disease	Microphallus or
Trauma	micropenis
Multiple sclerosis	
Syphilis	
Other spinal cord lesions	

temporal lobe or limbic system) or *spinal cord diseases* (such as injury, tumor, multiple sclerosis, or syphilis) may cause impotence without associated loss of libido. Patients with high spinal cord lesions (above T11) usually retain the ability to have reflexogenic erections.

In addition to intact central nervous system functioning, normal penile erection requires intact peripheral nervous system function, adequate blood flow to the penis, and normal erectile structures within the penis. *Disorders of peripheral autonomic nerve function* which cause impotence include extensive pelvic surgery, such as aortoiliac bypass, pelvic lymph node dissection, abdominoperineal resection of the rectum, lumbar sympathectomy, and prostatectomy; diabetes; and other conditions causing peripheral autonomic and sensory neuropathy. Atherosclerotic *peripheral vascular disease* involving the distal aortoiliac arteries and *trauma* to these vessels are the most common causes of vascular impotence. These patients usually have diminished or absent femoral pulses and may present with *Leriche's syndrome*, although claudication may be absent in some cases. In addition, autonomic neuropathy and atherosclerotic macro- and microvascular disease are major etiologic factors contributing to erectile dysfunction in the 30 to 50 per cent of diabetic men who develop impotence. Penile venous incompetence (venous leak) resulting in inadequate veno-occlusion to sustain an erection is an uncommon cause of impotence. *Penile abnormalities*, such as Peyronie's disease, chordee, priapism, and microphallus, may also cause erectile dysfunction. *Drugs* may cause erectile dysfunction by inhibiting penile smooth muscle relaxation and arterial vasodilation (anticholinergic drugs, antidepressants, antihistamines, β-adrenergic blockers) or by inducing premature detumescence (sympathomimetic drugs, α-adrenergic agonists). The mechanism of impotence associated with certain antihypertensive agents (e.g., diuretics, vasodilators, sympatholytic agents) is unclear.

Normal testosterone levels are necessary for maintenance of libido and potency. Hypogonadism resulting in androgen deficiency is a cause of impotence in approximately 15 to 20 per cent of men complaining of sexual dysfunction in a general medical clinic. Therefore, all impotent patients should have serum testosterone and gonadotropin levels measured as part of their diagnostic workup.

A thorough history and physical examination provide invaluable clues to the etiology of impotence. Erectile dysfunction that occurs abruptly and is transient, intermittent, or temporally associated with stress is usually psychogenic in origin. Men with psychogenic impotence often have spontaneous nocturnal or morning erections and are able to achieve normal erections with some partners but not with others or with masturbation but not during sexual intercourse. Patients with impotence related to central or peripheral nervous system or vascular disease or penile abnormalities usually demonstrate clinical manifestations of the underlying disorder. A careful drug history may reveal offending medications that cause impotence.

Measurement of nocturnal penile tumescence (NPT) and buckling pressure may be used to differentiate psychogenic from organic impotence. NPT is usually present in psychogenic impotence but absent if there is an organic cause of erectile dysfunction. Formal evaluation is done in a sleep laboratory with EEG monitoring to detect sleep disturbances that may disturb NPT. Resistance of the penis to buckling is also measured; this measurement correlates better than NPT alone with ability to have sexual intercourse. A simpler assessment of NPT can be made by wrapping the penis with perforated paper (e.g., stamps) or a snap gauge; NPT is detected by breaking of the perforations or wires of different tensile strength.

Doppler determination of the ratio of supine penile systolic blood pressure to brachial systolic blood pressure (penile/brachial index) may be useful in diagnosing patients with penile arterial vascular insufficiency. An index greater than 0.75 is normal; one between 0.75 and 0.60 is indeterminate; and one less than 0.6 is suggestive of arteriovascular impotence, which may be confirmed by arteriography. Recently, intracavernosal injection of vasodilatory agents (e.g., papaverine) with and without duplex ultrasonography or direct pressure monitoring has been used in the evaluation of impotence. Development of a sustained erectile response implies normal vascular status, whereas a short-lived, partial, or absent response suggests a hemodynamic abnormality. Corporal veno-occlusion is usually evaluated by cavernosometry and cavernosography following intracavernosal injection of a vasodilating drug. In the absence of neurogenic bladder dysfunction, electromyographic determination of the bulbocavernosus reflex latency and somatosensory evoked response of the dorsal nerve may be useful in detecting peripheral and sacral spinal abnormalities contributing to impotence.

Treatment of impotence is directed at the underlying causes of erectile dysfunction. Psychosexual education, counseling, and therapy are very successful in restoring sexual function in many men with psychogenic impotence. Testosterone therapy should be reserved for hypogonadal men with androgen deficiency in whom libido and potency are restored with adequate androgen replacement. Men with impotence and hypogonadism due to hyperprolactinemia may require agents to lower prolactin levels (e.g., bromocriptine) in addition to testosterone replacement to improve potency. Self-administration of intracavernosal injections of vasodilatory drugs (e.g., papaverine and/or phentolamine) induces penile erections sufficient for sexual intercourse in many patients with impotence. In general, it is very effective and well tolerated. Patients with severe arterial insufficiency or venous leaks are least likely to respond to this therapy. Select patients with vascular impotence are candidates for corrective surgical procedures.

In patients for whom effective therapy is not available, surgical implantation of a penile prosthesis offers rigidity sufficient for sexual intercourse without interfering with ejaculation or orgasm. Recently, vacuum-constriction devices have been introduced as a nonsurgical alternative to penile prostheses for the treatment of impotence. A condom-like cylinder is placed over the flaccid penis; a vacuum is applied to generate negative pressure, drawing blood into the penis and resulting in an erection. A constrictive band is then placed around the base of the penis to prevent the drainage of blood from the penis, maintaining tumescence for the duration of intercourse.

INFERTILITY. Infertility is defined as the inability of a couple to achieve a pregnancy after 1 year of unprotected intercourse. An estimated 5 to 6 per cent of men in the reproductive age group are infertile. Most causes of male infertility result in abnormal sperm count or semen quality, as reflected by an abnormal seminal fluid analysis. About 90 per cent of male infertility is caused by hypogonadism resulting in impaired spermatogenesis; and 80 to 90 per cent of these men have isolated deficiency of sperm production with normal androgen production of unclear etiology, i.e., *idiopathic oligospermia or azoospermia* (see below). Other causes of male infertility include *coital disorders, ductal obstruction, ejaculatory dysfunction,* and *disorders of accessory sexual organs* (Table 222–2). Even if a cause of male infertility is diagnosed, the female partner should undergo diagnostic evaluation, since a concomitant female factor causing infertility is found in 30 per cent of infertile couples.

Although uncommon, *defects* in the *coital technique,* such as timing of intercourse during menses, rather than at the time of ovulation near mid-cycle, premature withdrawal of the penis, prior ejaculation, and infrequent intercourse are causes of male infertility. They are important to remember because they are potentially reversible with proper patient education. Basal body temperature measurements or rapid RIA kits measuring urinary LH levels are commercially available methods often used to estimate the timing of ovulation in the partner's menstrual cycle. *Erectile dysfunction* from any cause may result in unsuccessful intercourse and infertility.

Impediment of sperm transport from the testis to the urethra results in azoospermia and infertility. Causes of *ductal obstruction* include congenital absence of the vas deferens or seminal vesicles; congenital defects of the epididymis or vas, e.g., as a consequence of diethylstilbestrol exposure in utero; fibrosis as a complication of genitourinary infection, especially epididymitis; cystic fibrosis or Young's syndrome, in which thickened, inspissated mucous secretions lead to blockage of the epididymis and vas deferens; and vasectomy.

Obstructive azoospermia must be differentiated from a severe defect in spermatogenesis. Measurement of a serum FSH level is often helpful, since elevated levels generally indicate disordered seminiferous tubular function. Normal FSH levels may occur in either obstructive azoospermia or seminiferous tubule dysfunction. In obstructive azoospermia, radiologic examination, i.e., a vasogram, will demonstrate the ductal obstruction, and a testicular biopsy will reveal normal spermatogenesis. Evaluation of azoospermia is one of the few indications for performing a testicular biopsy. Vasectomy has been used widely and successfully to induce infertility in men who desire fertility control, without any deleterious effects on the hypothalamic-pituitary-testicular axis or general health. Using microsurgical techniques, vasovasostomy has been used successfully to restore fertility in vasectomized men. Despite return of sperm in the ejaculate in 80 to 90 per cent, fertility is restored in only 30 to 50 per cent of men after vasovasostomy.

Ejaculatory dysfunction, such as premature or retrograde ejaculation, can cause infertility by preventing the normal deposition of sperm into the female genital tract. Premature ejaculation is often successfully treated by sex therapy techniques. Retro-

TABLE 222–2. CAUSES OF MALE INFERTILITY

Coital Disorders
  Defects in Technique
    Poor timing with menses
    Premature withdrawal
    Infrequent intercourse
  Impotence

Hypogonadism (Deficiency of Sperm Production)

Ductal Obstruction
  Congenital Defects of Vas Deferens, Epididymides, or Seminal
    Vesicles
  Postinfectious Obstruction
  Cystic Fibrosis/Young's Syndrome
  Vasectomy

Ejaculatory Dysfunction
  Premature Ejaculation
  Retrograde Ejaculation

Disorders of Accessory Glands
  Epididymitis/Seminal Vesiculitis/Prostatitis
  Immunologic

grade ejaculation most commonly results from diabetic autonomic neuropathy, prostatic resection, pelvic surgery, or administration of sympatholytic drugs. It is suspected if orgasm produces little or no ejaculate and is confirmed by the presence of large numbers of sperm in a postejaculation urine sample. Sympathomimetic drugs, imipramine, and harvesting and concentrating of sperm from the urine for artificial insemination have been used to treat retrograde ejaculation.

Disorders of the *accessory sexual organs* result in infertility by a number of mechanisms. Infections of the epididymis, seminal vesicles, and/or prostate have been reported to cause infertility by affecting sperm maturation or function directly or by inducing antisperm antibodies that, in turn, affect sperm function. Offending organisms include *Neisseria gonorrhoea, Chlamydia trachomatis,* coliforms, *Ureaplasma urealyticum,* and *Mycobacterium tuberculosis.* Antisperm antibodies present in the semen may cause sperm agglutination and reduce sperm motility. Induction of these antibodies after vasectomy may be responsible for the discrepancy between the success rate for return of sperm in the ejaculate and restoration of fertility after vasectomy reversal. High-dose glucocorticoid therapy can lower antisperm antibody titers and improve fertility in some patients.

GYNECOMASTIA. Gynecomastia, a benign glandular enlargement of the male breast, is usually asymptomatic, but its rapid development may cause pain and tenderness. It is often very difficult to distinguish between true gynecomastia and an increase in adipose tissue in obese boys or men. The technique used to examine the female breast, namely palpation with the flat of the hand against the chest wall, often misses significant amounts of breast tissue in the male. In order to adequately detect gynecomastia, fingers should be used to grasp the tissue surrounding the areola in a pinching action.

Although usually bilateral, gynecomastia may be markedly asymmetric or rarely unilateral. In these instances, gynecomastia must be distinguished from other benign chest wall tumors (such as lipomas, neurofibromas, and lymphomas) and male breast cancer. In contrast to benign breast conditions, breast carcinoma is usually eccentric in location, hard, and associated with skin or nipple retraction and bloody discharge; lymphadenopathy due to metastatic disease may also be found.

Gynecomastia usually occurs when the breast is exposed to a hormonal milieu of increased estrogen concentration relative to testosterone concentration, i.e., an increased estrogen/testosterone ratio. An increased ratio may result from pathologic conditions or drugs that either increase estrogen or reduce testosterone levels or action of these hormones. Since both of these hormonal alterations commonly result in primary or secondary hypogonadism, hypogonadal states are major causes of gynecomastia. Unless hyperprolactinemia induces androgen deficiency by inhibiting gonadotropin secretion, elevated prolactin levels do not usually cause gynecomastia. Hyperprolactinemia may, however, contribute to the development of *galactorrhea* (milky breast discharge) in patients with gynecomastia. The clinical causes of gynecomastia are summarized in Table 222–3.

Gynecomastia may sometimes be *physiologic* rather than pathologic. Transient gynecomastia is usually seen in neonatal boys, as a result of exposure in utero to high maternal estrogen concentrations. At the time of puberty, gynecomastia is observed in 60 to 70 per cent of boys. This pubertal gynecomastia usually lasts for months to years and does not persist into adulthood. Although there is a transient rise in the estrogen/testosterone ratio during puberty, the pathogenesis of pubertal gynecomastia is unclear. Finally, small amounts of palpable breast tissue (2 to 3 cm in diameter) can be detected by careful examination in 40 per cent of healthy normal adult men, increasing in prevalence with advancing age. This mild gynecomastia is always asymptomatic and generally goes unnoticed.

Most of the pathologic causes of gynecomastia are associated with alterations in the hypothalamic-pituitary-testicular axis, resulting in a hypogonadal hormonal profile. Gynecomastia may occur with any of the causes of hypogonadism that result in *androgen deficiency,* including both primary testicular disorders and those secondary to gonadotropin deficiency.

In addition to androgen deficiency or *disorders of androgen action,* gynecomastia may be caused by a number of *drugs.* Gynecomastia may result from exposure to exogenous estrogen, e.g., from administration of diethylstilbestrol for metastatic pros-

TABLE 222–3. CAUSES OF GYNECOMASTIA

222 THE TESTIS / 1341

I. Physiologic Gynecomastia
  Neonatal
  Pubertal
  Adult

II. Hypogonadism (Deficiency of Androgen Production)

III. Androgen Resistance Syndromes

IV. Drug-Induced Gynecomastia
  Hormones
    Estrogens
    Aromatizable androgens hCG
  Drugs Interacting with Estrogen Receptor
    Marijuana
    Digitalis
  Drugs Altering Androgen Production or Action
    Spironolactone
    Cimetidine
    Ketoconazole
    Cytotoxic agents
  Central Nervous System–Active Drugs
    Antihypertensive agents
    Tranquilizers
    Sedatives
    Antidepressants
    Amphetamines

V. Tumors
  Estrogen-Secreting Tumors
    Adrenal carcinoma
    Leydig cell or Sertoli cell tumor of testis
  Gonadotropin-Secreting Tumors
    Testicular carcinoma
    Lung carcinoma
    Liver carcinoma

VI. Systemic Disorders
  Hepatic Cirrhosis
  Renal Failure
  Thyrotoxicosis

VII. Miscellaneous
  Refeeding Gynecomastia
  Familial
  Increased Peripheral Aromatization
  Local Chest Trauma

tate cancer, ingestion of estrogen-treated animal foodstuffs, use of or contact with estrogen-containing creams, and accidental occupational exposure. Excessive circulating estrogens inhibit endogenous gonadotropin secretion, which results, in turn, in reduced testosterone production. Secondary hypogonadism induced by estrogens may contribute to the development of gynecomastia. Administration of high doses of aromatizable androgens, especially to prepubertal boys or severely hypogonadal men, may induce gynecomastia analogous to that which occurs at puberty. hCG binds to the LH receptor on the Leydig cell of the testis and has biologic activities identical to those of LH. By stimulating relatively greater testicular production of estradiol compared to testosterone, hCG treatment of hypogonadotropic hypogonadal men may cause gynecomastia. Certain drugs result in breast enlargement by interacting with the estrogen receptor (marijuana, digitalis) or by interfering with androgen production or action (spironolactone, cimetidine, ketoconazole, certain chemotherapeutic agents). Finally, many central nervous system–active drugs, such as certain antihypertensives, sedatives, tranquilizers, antidepressants, and amphetamines, are associated with gynecomastia.

Although very uncommon, gynecomastia may be the initial manifestation of an *estrogen-secreting tumor* of the adrenal gland or testis. Feminizing adrenal tumors are usually malignant and present with a palpable abdominal mass. In contrast, estrogen-secreting tumors of the testis are often small and benign. Unlike many exogenous estrogen preparations, which do not cross-react with the RIA for estradiol, these tumors secrete large amounts of estradiol, which are detected in blood by clinically available estrogen assays. *hCG-secreting tumors*, such as testicular, lung, and hepatic carcinoma, may cause gynecomastia by stimulating excessive estrogen relative to testosterone secretion by Leydig cells. hCG cross-reacts with most routinely available LH assays; patients with hCG-secreting tumors may therefore have elevated LH levels. Also, since LH cross-reacts with most intact hCG assays, a specific β-hCG assay should be used to confirm the diagnosis of an hCG-secreting tumor.

Certain *systemic disorders* are associated with gynecomastia. In hepatic cirrhosis, gynecomastia is associated with increased estrogen production, primarily by accelerated peripheral conversion of adrenal androgens (androstenedione) to estrone. In addition, serum SHBG levels are elevated, and total and bioavailable serum testosterone levels are low, which also favor an increased estrogen/testosterone ratio. The gynecomastia observed in patients with renal failure is associated with androgen deficiency resulting from primary testicular failure, and estrogen production is not increased. High estradiol levels and relatively reduced

bioavailable testosterone levels (as a result of increased SHBG levels) are commonly found in patients with thyrotoxicosis and contribute to the development of gynecomastia in this condition.

Gynecomastia is often associated with nutritional repletion and weight gain after a period of starvation and weight loss. This *refeeding gynecomastia* was originally described in former prisoners of World War II who developed tender gynecomastia following their liberation and resumption of a normal diet. A similar condition may occur upon recovery from any prolonged, severe illness associated with malnutrition and weight loss. Refeeding gynecomastia may contribute to the gynecomastia associated with hemodialysis in chronic renal failure patients and to that related to isoniazid treatment in men with tuberculosis. Malnutrition results in severe suppression of the hypothalamic-pituitary-testicular axis. Refeeding and restoration of nutrition and body weight result in resumption of normal gonadal function, a dynamic hormonal situation similar to the onset of puberty. The rapid restoration of gonadal function ("second puberty") may explain the gynecomastia associated with refeeding. *Familial gynecomastia* and *idiopathic increase in peripheral aromatase activity* are very rare causes of gynecomastia.

Treatment of gynecomastia should focus on the correction of the underlying disorder or withdrawal of the offending drug. Prophylactic low-dose irradiation of the breast prior to the institution of diethylstilbestrol treatment in men with prostatic carcinoma prevents gynecomastia. Testosterone treatment of androgen deficiency may occasionally result in resolution of gynecomastia. Experience with the estrogen antagonists (such as tamoxifen), nonaromatizable androgens (such as dihydrotestosterone), and aromatase inhibitors in treating gynecomastia has been limited and variably effective. Severe, longstanding gynecomastia of any cause is usually associated with increased fibrous tissue stroma and requires surgical reduction mammoplasty.

Dial LK (ed.): Geriatric sexuality. Clin Geriatr Med 7:1, 1991. *The entire issue is devoted to sexuality in older adults, with very good chapters on sexuality and impotence in aging men, urologic and endocrine considerations in geriatric sexual dysfunction, and the impact of medications and chronic diseases on sexual function in the elderly.*
Glass AR: Gynecomastia. In Becker KL (ed.): Principles and Practice of Endocrinology and Metabolism. Philadelphia, JB Lippincott Company, 1990, p 1000. *This is a well-organized chapter that provides a very good review of the causes and treatment of gynecomastia.*
Howards SS, Lipshultz LI (eds.): Male infertility. Urol Clin North Am 14:1, 1987. *An excellent, comprehensive discussion of the evaluation and treatment of male infertility by several authors.*
Krane RJ (ed.): Impotence. Urol Clin North Am 15:1, 1988. *The entire issue is devoted to a comprehensive overview of the pathophysiology, evaluation, and treatment of impotence. Chapters on the surgical and nonsurgical treatment of impotence are particularly clear and contain excellent figures.*
Krane RJ, Goldstein I, Saenz de Tejada I: Impotence. N Engl J Med 321:1648, 1989. *An excellent, concise, recent review of the anatomy, physiology, pathophysiology, diagnosis, and treatment of impotence.*
Mahoney CP: Adolescent gynecomastia. Differential diagnosis and management. Pediatr Clin North Am 37:1389, 1990. *An excellent review of pubertal and pathologic gynecomastia in adolescents.*
Stine CC, Collins M: Male sexual dysfunction. Prim Care 16:1031, 1989. *A very good review of the causes and treatment of impotence and premature ejaculation from the standpoint of a primary care physician.*
Swerdloff RS: Infertility in the male. Ann Intern Med 103:906, 1985. *This is an extensive review of the diagnostic evaluation and treatment of male infertility (over 100 references).*

CAUSES OF MALE HYPOGONADISM

Once the diagnosis of male hypogonadism is suspected from the clinical manifestations described above, the diagnosis is confirmed by measurement of serum testosterone level and sperm count. A low serum testosterone concentration confirms androgen deficiency, and reduced sperm counts confirm a deficiency in sperm production.

The majority of hypogonadal men with *androgen deficiency* also have impairment in sperm production. Once androgen deficiency is diagnosed (low serum testosterone and sperm count), an effort should be made to distinguish between disorders that result from primary testicular disease (*primary hypogonadism*) and those that are secondary to inadequate gonadotropin stimulation of the testis (*secondary hypogonadism*), as a result of either pituitary or hypothalamic disease.

In addition to helping to define the specific etiology of androgen deficiency, the distinction between primary and secondary hypogonadism may have practical therapeutic implications. For example, regardless of the specific etiology, primary hypogonadism is usually treated with androgen replacement. In the majority of cases, the infertility in primary hypogonadism is not treatable. However, secondary hypogonadism may result from destruction of pituitary gonadotropin-secreting cells, for example by a pituitary tumor. In this instance, in addition to androgen deficiency, the space-occupying effects of the tumor mass on brain function (such as visual fields and cerebroventricular flow) and alterations (both increase and decrease) in the secretion of other anterior pituitary hormones (such as ACTH, thyroid-stimulating hormone [TSH], growth hormone, and prolactin) need to be considered in formulating a therapeutic plan (Ch. 213). Furthermore, since the testes usually function normally in response to adequate gonadotropin stimulation in patients with secondary hypogonadism, gonadotropins or LHRH may be administered in these patients to stimulate spermatogenesis and induce fertility.

The negative feedback relationship between gonadotropin secretion and circulating testosterone levels (see Fig. 222-1) provides the physiologic basis and rationale for the use of serum gonadotropin levels to distinguish between primary and secondary testicular disorders that result in androgen deficiency. Because the negative feedback effect of testosterone on gonadotropin secretion is reduced, men with *primary hypogonadism* have reduced serum testosterone and elevated serum LH and FSH levels; i.e., they have *hypergonadotropic hypogonadism*. Not uncommonly, serum FSH levels may be disproportionately elevated compared to LH levels, especially with severe seminiferous tubule dysfunction. However, selective elevation of serum LH levels is distinctly unusual and suggests the presence of a substance, such as hCG or α subunit, that cross-reacts in the RIA for LH.

In contrast to primary testicular dysfunction, men with *secondary hypogonadism* are not able to increase gonadotropin secretion appropriately in the presence of reduced testosterone negative feedback and have inadequate gonadotropin stimulation of the testis. These men have a hormonal pattern of reduced serum testosterone and low to low normal serum LH and FSH levels; i.e., they have *hypogonadotropic hypogonadism*. Gonadotropin levels are often in the low normal range in men with secondary hypogonadism because most clinically available gonadotropin assays lack sufficient sensitivity to distinguish low from low normal values.

The majority of hypogonadal patients with *isolated impairment of sperm production* have primary testicular disease. These patients generally present with infertility and have no clinical manifestations of androgen deficiency. Serum testosterone and gonadotropin levels are usually normal. Therefore, hormone determinations are not routinely obtained as part of an infertility workup unless clinical androgen deficiency is also present. Infertile patients who present with no sperm in their ejaculate, i.e., azoospermia, may have either severe seminiferous tubule failure or obstruction of the genital tract. Measurement of serum FSH level may be helpful in evaluation of an azoospermic patient. A selective elevation of serum FSH levels with normal LH levels in a patient with azoospermia implies severe germ cell dysfunction with loss of negative feedback influences (such as inhibin) on the pituitary gland and poor prognosis for fertility. No further workup is usually necessary. A normal serum FSH level in an azoospermic patient leaves open the possibility of a surgically correctable ductal obstruction, and a vasogram and testicular biopsy are usually performed. In addition to severe seminiferous tubule dysfunction, selective elevation in serum FSH levels may be observed in patients with gonadotropin-secreting pituitary adenomas. Uncommonly, isolated deficiency of sperm production results from inadequate gonadotropin stimulation of the testis. In these instances, serum gonadotropin levels are generally reduced, and very rarely selective FSH deficiency may occur.

The vast majority of adults with male hypogonadism have either primary or secondary testicular failure. Very rarely, *disorders of androgen action* may present in adults with a clinical picture of hypogonadism. Unlike the severe androgen resistance syndromes, which present at birth with male pseudohermaphroditism (Ch. 221), these disorders are characterized by mild defects in androgen action, resulting in a nearly normal male phenotype (frequently with varying degrees of hypospadias). Both serum testosterone and gonadotropin levels are usually elevated.

In summary, clinical manifestations combined with measurements of serum testosterone, sperm count, and basal serum gonadotropin levels permit a physiologic classification of the causes of male hypogonadism into *primary* and *secondary hypogonadism* and subclassification into disorders that result in *deficiency of both sperm and androgen production* and those with *isolated deficiency in sperm production* with normal androgen production (Table 222-4).

Primary Hypogonadism

DEFICIENCY OF SPERM AND ANDROGEN PRODUCTION. *Congenital or Developmental Disorders.* *Klinefelter's syndrome* is the most common cause of primary testicular failure resulting in impairment of both spermatogenesis and testosterone production. The syndrome is characterized by small, firm testes, azoospermia, gynecomastia, varying degrees of eunuchoidism and testosterone deficiency, and elevated gonadotropin levels. Klinefelter's syndrome is a very common disorder, affecting 1 in every 400 to 500 men. The incidence of Klinefelter's syndrome increases to 5 per cent when maternal age is over 45 years. The incidence of this syndrome, in particular of its variants, is significantly increased in mentally retarded individuals. The fundamental defect in Klinefelter's syndrome and its variants is the presence of one or a number of extra X chromosomes.

Classically, the karyotype in Klinefelter's syndrome is 47 XXY, resulting from meiotic nondisjunction in either the maternal or paternal gamete. Variants of the syndrome demonstrate a variety of karyotypes, including XXYY, more than two X (poly X) plus Y, and mosaicism. The karyotypes in mosaic Klinefelter's syndrome are a combination of the normal, classic, and variant karyotypes and may vary among different tissues within the same individual. In classic Klinefelter's syndrome (47 XXY), the presence of an extra X chromosome is responsible for the presence of a sex chromatin or Barr body in the nucleus of epithelial cells obtained on buccal smear, a normal finding in females, who carry two X chromosomes. Variant syndromes characterized by more than two X chromosomes may exhibit more than one Barr body per nucleus, the number of sex chromatin bodies always being one less than the number of X chromosomes. Confirmation of the presumptive diagnosis of Klinefelter's syndrome made on buccal smear examination is accomplished by karyotyping of blood lymphocytes or testicular tissue.

Although Klinefelter's disease is a congenital disorder, clinical features are not evident prior to puberty. At the time of puberty, the testes fail to increase in size and become firmer in consistency. This is a result of fibrosis and hyalinization of the seminiferous tubules. The most remarkable clinical feature of Klinefelter's syndrome is the very small size of the testes, rarely exceeding 2 cm in length, in contrast to a lower limit of 3.5 cm in the normal adult. Clinical androgen deficiency is usually present, but the degree of androgen deficiency is variable, resulting in varying degrees of eunuchoidism (Fig. 222-5). In contrast to other conditions that result in prepubertal androgen deficiency and classic eunuchoidism (see above), Klinefelter's syndrome often results in a disproportionate increase in lower extremity compared to upper extremity long bone growth. Careful palpation usually reveals bilateral gynecomastia in about 80 to 90 per cent of patients. Although the incidence of mental retardation is greater, the majority of patients with Klinefelter's syndrome have normal intelligence. Most patients exhibit character and personality disorders, which may be related, in part, to the psychosocial consequences of androgen deficiency. There is a slightly increased incidence of certain systemic diseases in Klinefelter's syndrome. These include diabetes, chronic obstructive pulmonary disease, autoimmune disorders (e.g., systemic lupus erythematosus, Hashimoto's thyroiditis), malignancy (breast cancer, lymphoma, germ cell neoplasms), and varicose veins.

The clinical manifestations of Klinefelter's syndrome variants differ from those of the classic 47 XXY syndrome. In general, the presence of more than two extra X chromosomes results in a much higher incidence of mental retardation and somatic abnormalities, such as hypospadias, cryptorchidism, and bony abnormalities of the radius and ulna. The majority of patients with mosaic Klinefelter's syndrome exhibit less severe clinical manifestations, particularly if a normal XY cell line is present. Indeed, fertility in patients with mosaic Klinefelter's syndrome (XXY/XY) has been documented. Patients with an additional Y chromosome tend to be tall and have extremely aggressive, antisocial behavioral abnormalities. Very rarely, a patient exhibits the classic features of Klinefelter's syndrome with a normal (46 XY) karyotype, a so-called mutant or phenocopy. Finally, phenotypic males with a 46 XX karyotype may demonstrate the typical clinical manifestations of classic Klinefelter's syndrome, except for having shorter stature and a higher incidence of hypospadias. The mechanism by which these individuals develop a male phenotype in the apparent absence of a Y chromosome is unclear (Ch. 221). In some patients with this condition, Y chromosomal material is translocated onto the X chromosome.

Azoospermia is present in over 95 per cent of patients with classic Klinefelter's syndrome. Serum testosterone levels are usually low but may be in the low normal adult range. However, free testosterone levels are reduced in most patients with Klinefelter's syndrome. Serum estradiol levels are often elevated, which results in elevated SHBG concentrations (and total testosterone levels within the normal range) and contributes to the development of gynecomastia. Serum gonadotropin levels, especially serum FSH levels, are uniformly elevated. Occasionally, serum LH levels may fall in the high normal adult range.

Treatment of Klinefelter's syndrome is aimed primarily at correction of the androgen deficiency with testosterone replacement therapy (see below). The infertility is irreversible. Gynecomastia may be a source of great social embarrassment, in which case reduction mammoplasty should be performed.

The *functional prepubertal castrate syndrome (congenital anorchia)* is characterized by bilateral absence of functioning testicular tissue, occasionally associated with absent epididymides, in a genotypic and phenotypic man. The presence of otherwise normal male internal and external genitalia, without müllerian duct derivatives, and descent of the vas and testicular blood vessels into the scrotum imply that a normally functioning testis was present during fetal and prepubertal life. It is hypothesized that testicular damage during the fetal or prepubertal period results in atrophy of the gonads. Patients with this syndrome usually present with delayed puberty, eunuchoidal features with sexual infantilism, absence of palpable testes ("empty scrotum"), and, unlike other conditions associated with eunuchoidism, short stature (see Fig. 222–4). Congenital anorchia must be distinguished from bilateral abdominal cryptorchidism, which also presents with absent scrotal testes. Because of the increased risk of malignancy, intra-abdominal testes require orchiectomy or orchiopexy. The absence of a testosterone response to exogenous hCG (e.g., 2000 IU three times weekly for 3 to 4 weeks) in patients with congenital anorchia may be helpful in distinguishing it from bilateral abdominal testes. However, there have been reports of responses to hCG stimulation in patients with congenital anorchia and absent responses in patients with bilateral cryptorchidism. Laparoscopy or surgical exploration is often necessary to confirm the diagnosis. Treatment of this syndrome consists of androgen replacement therapy to induce full sexual maturation. Insertion of testicular prostheses may be of psychological value.

Noonan (Bonnevie-Ullrich) syndrome, an autosomal recessive disorder, occurs in karyotypically normal males and females. It is characterized by a number of clinical features similar to those of females with Turner's syndrome. Characteristic findings include short stature, typical facies (hypertelorism, antimongoloid eye slant, ptosis, low-set ears, micrognathia, high-arched palate, and dental malocclusions), webbed neck, shield-like chest, pectus excavatum, cubitus valgus, mental retardation, cardiovascular

TABLE 222–4. CAUSES OF MALE HYPOGONADISM

I. Primary Hypogonadism	II. Secondary Hypogonadism
Deficiency of Sperm and Androgen Production	*Deficiency of Sperm and Androgen Production*
Congenital or Developmental Disorders	Congenital or Developmental Disorders
Klinefelter's syndrome and variants	Hypogonadotropic eunuchoidism (Kallmann's syndrome)
Functional prepubertal castrate syndrome	Hemochromatosis
Noonan (Bonnevie-Ullrich) syndrome	Complex genetic syndromes
Myotonic dystrophy	Acquired Disorders
Polyglandular autoimmune disease	Hypopituitarism
Complex genetic disorders	Hyperprolactinemia
? Normal aging	Estrogen excess
Acquired Disorders	Progestins
Orchitis (mumps, leprosy, etc.)	Opiate-like drugs
Surgical or traumatic castration	Systemic Disorders
Drugs (spironolactone, ketoconazole, H_2 receptor blockers, alcohol, marijuana, digitalis, cytotoxic drugs)	Glucocorticoid excess (Cushing's syndrome)
Irradiation	Acute stress or illness
Systemic Disorders	Nutritional deficiency (protein-calorie malnutrition, anorexia nervosa)
Chronic liver disease	Chronic illness
Chronic renal failure	Massive obesity
Malignancy (Hodgkin's, testicular)	*Isolated Deficiency of Sperm Production*
Sickle cell disease	Androgen Excess
Paraplegia	Congenital adrenal hyperplasia (21- and 11β-hydroxylase deficiency)
Vasculitis (periarteritis)	Androgenic anabolic steroids
Infiltrative disease (amyloidosis)	Androgen-secreting tumors
Isolated Deficiency of Sperm Production	Hyperprolactinemia
Congenital or Developmental Disorders	Isolated FSH Deficiency
Germinal cell aplasia (Sertoli cell–only syndrome)	
Cryptorchidism	**Androgen Resistance Syndromes**
Varicocele	*Reifenstein's Syndrome*
Immotile cilia syndrome (Kartagener's syndrome)	*Idiopathic Oligospermia or Azoospermia*
Myotonic dystrophy	*? Celiac Disease*
Acquired Disorders	
Orchitis (mumps, leprosy, etc.)	
Thermal trauma	
Irradiation	
Cytotoxic drugs	
Environmental toxins	
Systemic Disorders	
Acute febrile illness	
Paraplegia	
Idiopathic Oligospermia or Azoospermia	

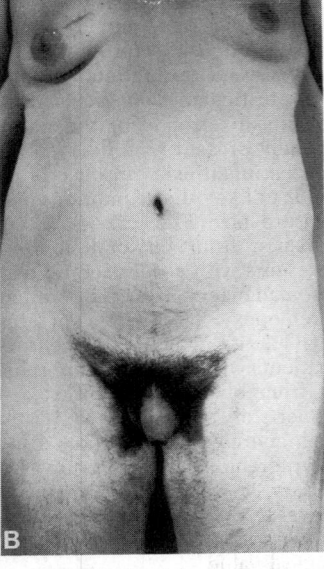

FIGURE 222–5. Two patients with untreated Klinefelter's syndrome, demonstrating the variability in degree of androgenization in this disorder. A, The small penis, diminished pubic hair with a female escutcheon, and sparse body hair indicate severe androgen deficiency. B, Normal penile development and adequate pubic and body hair indicate nearly normal androgen production by the testes. Gynecomastia is present in both patients, although only visible in the patient shown in B. The testes in both subjects were less than 2 cm in length. (From Bardin CW, Paulsen CA: The testes. In Williams RH (ed.): Textbook of Endocrinology, 6th ed. Philadelphia, W.B. Saunders Company, 1981.)

anomalies (pulmonic stenosis and atrial septal defects), and lymphedema. Males with Noonan syndrome (also called male Turner's syndrome) exhibit primary testicular dysfunction with impairment of both sperm and androgen production and elevated serum gonadotropin levels. Cryptorchidism is frequently present. Treatment of this disorder consists of testosterone replacement to correct the androgen deficiency and orchiopexy for associated cryptorchidism, both for psychological reasons and to monitor the testes for malignancy.

Myotonic dystrophy (see also Ch. 504) is an autosomal dominant disorder characterized by progressive weakness and atrophy of muscles, especially those of the face, neck, and distal extremities. An important diagnostic feature in this disorder is the presence of myotonia, or prolonged contraction of muscles. Other characteristic findings include cataracts, cardiac arrhythmias, dysphagia, premature frontal balding, mild intellectual deterioration, and gonadal atrophy. Testicular atrophy, which occurs in middle age, is found in about 80 per cent of men affected by myotonic dystrophy. The majority of these men have isolated impairment of spermatogenesis with normal androgen production. However, approximately 20 per cent of men with myotonic dystrophy have manifestations of androgen deficiency as a result of primary testicular failure. In addition to treating the androgen deficiency, testosterone replacement therapy may help to maintain or improve muscle function in these men.

Polyglandular autoimmune disease (see also Ch. 228) is a disorder in which there is concurrence of organ-specific autoimmune disease involving several endocrine and nonendocrine organs, associated with the presence of circulating autoantibodies to these organs. Specific conditions that occur in association with each other in this disorder are Addison's disease, hypothyroidism, insulin-dependent diabetes, pernicious anemia, ovarian failure, hypoparathyroidism, vitiligo, mucocutaneous candidiasis, Graves' disease, hypopituitarism, and alopecia. Although much less common than primary ovarian failure, primary testicular failure, associated with antitesticular antibodies and resulting in androgen deficiency, may occur in males with polyglandular autoimmune disease.

Normal aging in healthy men significantly reduces levels of total, free, and non-SHBG-bound testosterone and diminishes spermatogenesis compared to that in young men. In addition, the normal circadian variation in testosterone levels is markedly attenuated in old compared to young men. Both LH and FSH levels are significantly elevated in healthy old men, suggesting that the reduction in testosterone levels which occurs with normal aging is mostly the result of primary testicular dysfunction. Indeed, elderly men exhibit reduced testosterone responses to stimulation by exogenous hCG administration. The physiologic significance of reduced testosterone levels in aging men is unknown. Normal aging in men is also accompanied by an increased incidence of sexual dysfunction, as well as decreased muscle and bone mass. Whether these changes in body function with aging are related to the reduction in androgen production remains to be investigated.

Primary hypogonadism may present in a number of *complex genetic disorders,* such as *Alstrom, ataxia telangiectasia, Sohval-Soffer, Weinstein,* and *Werner* syndromes. Rarely, patients with *Prader-Labhart-Willi* and *Laurence-Moon-Biedl* syndromes demonstrate primary, rather than the more commonly associated secondary, hypogonadism.

Acquired Disorders. In general, seminiferous tubule function and spermatogenesis are much more sensitive to external or environmental influences (such as irradiation, cytotoxic agents, or heat) than is Leydig cell production of testosterone. This greater sensitivity is due, in large part, to the fact that spermatogenesis involves active and coordinated cellular division and differentiation, requiring complex regulation. As a result, most acquired primary testicular disorders causing hypogonadism result more commonly in isolated impairment of spermatogenesis with normal androgen production (see below) than in androgen deficiency.

Viral orchitis, most frequently due to *mumps,* is a very common cause of acquired primary testicular failure. Approximately 15 to 25 per cent of males with mumps develop acute orchitis. The few boys who develop mumps orchitis before puberty usually recover completely without subsequent testicular dysfunction. However, acute mumps infection of pubertal or adult testes usually results in permanent seminiferous tubule damage and, in severe cases, Leydig cell dysfunction with androgen deficiency. Although clinical mumps orchitis is unilateral in the majority of cases, degenerative changes have been observed in the clinically uninvolved testis. During the acute phase of orchitis, which usually develops within a few days of parotitis, there is interstitial edema and sloughing of the germinal epithelium. This may be followed by progressive tubular sclerosis and testicular atrophy over the next several months. The availability and use of mumps vaccine have significantly reduced the incidence of mumps orchitis. Orchitis may also complicate infections with viruses such as *echoviruses* and *arboviruses.* Uncommon causes of orchitis include *gonorrhea, leprosy, tuberculosis, brucellosis, glanders, syphilis,* and certain parasitic diseases such as *filariasis* and *bilharziasis.* As in mumps, orchitis complicating these disorders results more commonly in isolated impairment of sperm production, although in severe cases androgen production is also affected.

Bilateral surgical or traumatic castration results in acute androgen deficiency, and castration after puberty often causes hot flushes and irritability, similar to that of women at the time of menopause.

Certain *drugs* may produce androgen deficiency by inhibiting testosterone biosynthesis and/or by blocking androgen action. The aldosterone antagonist *spironolactone* inhibits testosterone synthesis, as well as interfering with androgen action by competitively binding to the androgen receptor. *Ketoconazole,* an antifungal agent, inhibits testosterone synthesis and in high doses may also inhibit adrenal steroidogenesis. *H₂ receptor blockers* (e.g., cimetidine) also block androgen receptors and act as weak androgen antagonists. *Alcohol* has direct toxic effects on both spermatogenesis and steroidogenesis in the testis in the absence of alcoholic cirrhosis. *Marijuana* (tetrahydrocannabinol) has direct inhibitory effects on testicular function in addition to its central nervous system effects. *Digitalis* has been reported to elevate serum estradiol levels and reduce serum testosterone levels, perhaps through its interaction with both the estrogen and androgen receptors. A number of *cytotoxic drugs* used in cancer chemotherapy interfere with spermatogenesis and, more rarely, with androgen production. In some *malignancies,* androgen deficiency may also be present in the absence of exposure to chemotherapeutic agents (e.g., Hodgkin's disease or testicular cancer). Androgen deficiency may be the result of general debilitation and malnutrition associated with some malignancies. *Irradiation* of the testes rarely causes permanent androgen deficiency. However, exposure of the testes to very large doses (over 600 to 800 rads) may compromise Leydig cell function.

Systemic Disorders. A number of systemic diseases cause deficiencies in sperm and androgen production, primarily by affecting testicular function directly, although gonadotropin secretion may also be affected in many of these conditions. In patients with *chronic liver disease* (cirrhosis), gynecomastia and testicular atrophy are commonly present (in 50 to 75 per cent). Total serum testosterone levels are low or low normal. Because SHBG levels are elevated, free or non-SHBG-bound testosterone levels are low. Serum LH levels are usually elevated but may fall in the high normal range. LH secretion may be partially suppressed by the high circulating levels of estrogens found in cirrhotic patients. Increased estrogen concentrations result from impaired hepatic clearance of adrenal androgens (androstenedione), leading to an increased substrate for peripheral aromatization to estrone and estradiol. The increased estrogen/testosterone ratio may contribute to the formation of gynecomastia. Treatment of androgen deficiency in patients with cirrhosis with an aromatizable androgen may result in worsening of gynecomastia.

Chronic renal failure usually causes reductions in both sperm and androgen production. LH and FSH levels are elevated, as a result of increased production as well as reduced renal clearance. The response of testosterone levels to hCG stimulation is impaired. Elevated serum prolactin levels and zinc deficiency may also contribute to testicular dysfunction in uremia. Hemodialysis does not significantly improve testosterone production. However, successful renal transplantation may result in some return of testicular function, which may be tempered by the drugs used for chronic immunosuppressive therapy to prevent graft rejection. In addition to treating androgen deficiency, testosterone replacement therapy may also improve the anemia of renal failure.

Sickle cell disease often results in low serum testosterone and elevated serum gonadotropin levels, implying primary testicular failure. *Paraplegia* may result in a transient reduction in serum testosterone levels that return to normal in the chronic paraplegic state unless chronic malnutrition occurs. *Vasculitis* involving the testis (e.g., periarteritis nodosa) or *infiltrative diseases* (e.g., amyloidosis, leukemia) may also result in primary testicular failure.

ISOLATED DEFICIENCY OF SPERM PRODUCTION.
Congenital or Developmental Disorders. *Germinal cell aplasia, or Sertoli cell–only syndrome,* is an uncommon condition characterized on testicular biopsy by seminiferous tubules of moderately reduced size, lined with Sertoli cells but devoid of germ cells and having little or no tubular fibrosis. Patients with this syndrome are normally androgenized but infertile. They have slightly smaller than normal testes, azoospermia, and elevated serum FSH levels, indicative of severe seminiferous tubule dysfunction. Serum testosterone levels are normal, and LH levels are normal or slightly elevated. Testosterone response to hCG stimulation may be reduced. These findings suggest that mild, subclinical Leydig cell dysfunction may also be present. It is hypothesized that congenital absence of germ cells is the basis for this syndrome. However, in some familial cases of germinal cell aplasia, germ cells have been found on testicular biopsy prior to puberty but are lost during and after puberty. The karyotype is usually 46 XY, although 47 XYY and 47 XXY karyotypes have also been found. Other gonadal disorders causing severe seminiferous tubule damage (such as mumps orchitis, cryptorchidism, irradiation, or cytotoxic drugs) may result in seminiferous tubules lined only with Sertoli cells. In these acquired causes of Sertoli cell–only syndrome, however, the tubules are usually extensively sclerosed and hyalinized and the testes are much smaller. Infertility in congenital germinal cell aplasia is irreversible but may be reversible with time in some acquired cases of severe germ cell damage.

In *cryptorchidism* the testes fail to descend normally into the scrotum. Cryptorchid testes are usually located in the abdomen or inguinal canal. *Ectopic testes* are located outside the normal pathway of testicular descent and may be found in the perineal, femoral, or superficial inguinal areas. To avoid unnecessary treatment, cryptorchid testes must be distinguished from *retractile testes*, which are located in the scrotum, but are withdrawn into the inguinal canal or abdomen with minimal stimulation.

The testes usually descend into the scrotum about the eighth month of fetal life. Undescended testes are found in approximately 3 to 4 per cent of full-term newborn males, but the testes descend during the first year in all but 0.7 to 0.8 per cent. The prevalence of cryptorchidism in adult males is about 0.3 to 0.4 per cent. Inguinal hernia is associated with cryptorchidism in 50 to 80 per cent of cases.

Bilateral cryptorchidism may be the presenting complaint in a number of hypogonadal disorders, such as the functional prepubertal castrate, the Noonan syndrome, and Reifenstein's syndrome. It may also be variably associated with many other causes of hypogonadism, such as Klinefelter's syndrome and hypogonadotropic eunuchoidism. In these disorders, cryptorchidism is usually associated with androgen deficiency. In contrast, when cryptorchidism is not associated with other hypogonadal disorders, it rarely affects Leydig cell function and usually causes isolated impairment of spermatogenesis.

Even when cryptorchidism is unilateral, testicular dysfunction is very common, suggesting that both testes have altered function. Abnormal testicular function may contribute to the failure of the testes to descend properly. In rare instances, normal testicular descent may be impeded by anatomic abnormalities along the pathway of descent, e.g., external inguinal hernias. In these instances, both testes function normally, and orchiopexy before puberty usually results in preservation of normal testicular function.

Careful physical examination of the scrotum should be performed to distinguish cryptorchidism from retractile testes, which is a more common condition. The diagnosis is particularly difficult in obese patients, and repeated examinations may be necessary. Examination should be performed in the standing, squatting, and recumbent positions, and observation in warm water may be helpful. The Valsalva maneuver and applied pressure to the lower abdomen are useful procedures to detect a mobile testis, which does not require therapy. In patients with retractile testes, elicitation of a cremasteric reflex may result in a localized puckering of the scrotal skin. Failure to palpate a testis after repeated examinations suggests that the testis is intra-abdominal, severely atrophic, or absent. Ultrasonography or CT scan may be helpful in localizing nonpalpable testes.

As a result of exposure of the seminiferous tubules to higher extrascrotal temperatures at the time of puberty, the germinal epithelium of cryptorchid testes shows severe degeneration, eventually resulting in tubular fibrosis. Bilateral cryptorchidism causes infertility. Sperm counts are low, and serum FSH levels are usually elevated. Leydig cell function is usually preserved, and serum testosterone and LH concentrations remain normal. The risk of malignancy in undescended testes is five to nine times greater than in scrotal testes, and the risk remains increased even after orchiopexy. Previous reports, based on retrospective studies, markedly overestimated this risk.

Therapy for cryptorchidism should be instituted before puberty, when the degenerative changes of the germinal epithelium occur. The exact age at which treatment should be instituted is controversial. Administration of hCG (1000 IU three times weekly) or LHRH to prepubertal boys with cryptorchidism may cause testicular descent in some patients. When such therapy is successful, it is probable that the testis would have descended spontaneously at puberty. Reports of the efficacy of hormonal therapy are widely discrepant, probably as a result of inclusion of variable proportions of patients with retractile testes. If hormonal therapy is unsuccessful in causing testicular descent, orchiopexy is performed in an attempt to preserve testicular function, to allow easier examination of the testis for malignant degeneration, and for cosmetic reasons. Despite orchiopexy, fertility rates in patients with cryptorchidism are usually reduced, particularly in patients with bilateral undescended testes. Often, bilateral testicular biopsies are performed at the time of orchiopexy to determine the degree of testicular abnormality. If a unilateral cryptorchid testis is atrophic and shows extensive tubular fibrosis, an orchiectomy is usually performed, provided that the contralateral testis is in the scrotum.

A *varicocele* is an abnormal dilatation of the pampiniform plexus of veins surrounding the spermatic cord, caused by retrograde blood flow into the internal spermatic vein. Palpable varicocele occurs in about 10 per cent of the general population and in 30 per cent of men with infertility. Varicocele is clearly associated with infertility. However, approximately 50 per cent of men with varicoceles have normal seminal fluid analyses, and some men with varicocele and abnormal seminal fluid parameters are fertile. About 90 per cent of varicoceles occur on the left side, as a result of valvular incompetence between the left internal spermatic vein and the renal vein. Occurrence of an isolated right-sided varicocele may be an early clue to venous obstruction by malignancy or to situs inversus. Varicoceles may affect testicular function by a variety of mechanisms, including increasing testicular temperature and blood flow. Seminal fluid analysis usually shows low sperm concentration with reduced motility and increased numbers of sperm with abnormal morphology (e.g., increased tapered and amorphous forms). Testicular size and serum testosterone, LH, and FSH levels are usually normal. Surgical repair of varicoceles in infertile men has been reported to improve semen quality and fertility, although well-controlled clinical studies have not been performed.

Immotile cilia syndrome, or *Kartagener's syndrome*, is characterized by sinusitis, bronchiectasis, and situs inversus. Patients usually suffer from chronic respiratory infections because of impaired mucociliary clearance in the respiratory tract. In addition, these patients produce nonmotile spermatozoa. Cilia in the respiratory tract and the sperm tail are immotile in Kartagener's syndrome because of an abnormality in *dynein*, a protein that is important in microtubular filament movement. Other patients have a *deficiency of protein carboxyl methylase*, an enzyme that is important in sperm motility. Infertility in this disorder is not treatable.

The majority of patients with *myotonic dystrophy* (see above) may have isolated impairment of spermatogenesis with normal androgen production.

Acquired Disorders. The majority of adults who develop mumps *orchitis* and orchitis due to other infectious agents sustain severe germ cell damage and isolated impairment of spermatogenesis with normal Leydig cell function (see above). Seminiferous tubule function is much more sensitive to damage from external or environmental agents than is Leydig cell function. Therefore, exposure of the testis to *thermal trauma, irradiation, cytotoxic drugs*, and *environmental toxins* often results in deficiency of sperm production without androgen deficiency. Even relatively minor thermal trauma, such as that induced by tight underwear or hot tubs, may result in suppression of sperm production.

The human testis is very sensitive to irradiation. Only 15 rads of x-irradiation may suppress spermatogenesis temporarily; more than 600 rads usually produces permanent infertility. Doses of radiation used in therapy of malignant lymphoma have been reported to result in permanent germ cell damage and infertility, despite shielding of the testis. Spermatogenesis is also very sensitive to damage by cytotoxic cancer chemotherapeutic agents, especially to alkylating agents. The likelihood of severe seminiferous tubule damage and permanent infertility is greater with combination chemotherapy regimens, such as MOPP for Hodgkin's disease. Despite being very sensitive to radiation and cytotoxic drugs, the germinal epithelium has remarkable regenerative properties, and recovery of spermatogenesis may occur despite very severe germ cell loss associated with high doses of these cytotoxic agents. Both irradiation (over 800 rads) and cytotoxic agents occasionally produce androgen deficiency. Sperm banking offers some hope of fertility for patients who will develop permanent infertility as a result of irradiation or chemotherapy for malignant disease. Sulfasalazine has been associated with oligospermia, reduced sperm motility, and infertility, but these findings may also be related to the underlying inflammatory bowel disease and catabolic state.

Damage to the germinal epithelium has been reported in workers exposed to carbon disulfide, a solvent used in production of rayon, and to dibromochloropropane, an insecticide. A number of other chemical agents used in industry and laboratories have been implicated as direct testicular toxins (e.g., lead, deuterium oxide, cadmium, fluoroacetamide, nitrofurans, dinitropyrroles, diamines, α-chlorhydrin, other insecticides, and rodenticides).

Systemic Disorders. A number of relatively minor *acute febrile illnesses* may result in temporary suppression of sperm production (e.g., minor viral infections). Over 50 per cent of men with spinal cord lesions resulting in *paraplegia* exhibit diminished testicular function, the majority demonstrating impaired sperm production with normal androgen production. Reduced spermatogenesis may be a result of elevated testicular temperature, caused by increased scrotal skin temperature (from loss of lumbar sympathetic innervation) and loss of the cremasteric reflex.

Idiopathic Oligospermia or Azoospermia. In most men who present with infertility and isolated impairment of spermatogenesis, no apparent cause can be found, leading to the diagnosis of *idiopathic oligospermia or azoospermia*. Because of the high prevalence of male infertility (5 to 6 per cent of reproductive age men), idiopathic oligospermia or azoospermia is the most common cause of male hypogonadism. Since the pathogenesis of impaired sperm production is not known, therapy for this disorder has been largely empiric and unsatisfactory. Trials of treatment with large doses of testosterone, gonadotropins, clomiphene citrate, testolactone, cortisone, thyroid hormone, caffeine, and vitamins have generally been unsuccessful in improving fertility rates over those achieved by placebo treatment or untreated patients, who have a 20 per cent fertility rate in 1 year. At present, infertility in these patients should be considered irreversible and couples should be offered artificial insemination, using donor semen, or adoption as alternatives.

Secondary Hypogonadism

Secondary hypogonadism is testicular failure due to inadequate gonadotropin secretion as a result of either hypothalamic or pituitary dysfunction. In the majority of cases, both LH and FSH secretion are diminished, resulting in impairment of both sperm and androgen production. Rarely, there may be isolated deficiency of sperm production.

DEFICIENCY OF SPERM AND ANDROGEN PRODUCTION. Congenital or Developmental Disorders. *Hypogonadotropic eunuchoidism*, or *Kallmann's syndrome*, is a congenital and often familial disorder, characterized by isolated hypogonadotropic hypogonadism (resulting in eunuchoidal features) and anosmia or hyposmia. Gonadotropin deficiency in this disorder is caused by a defect in synthesis and/or release of LHRH from the hypothalamus; chronic exogenous LHRH administration results in stimulation of normal testicular function. A developmental failure of the olfactory lobes is responsible for absent or reduced sense of smell. There is considerable genetic heterogeneity in this disorder. Kallmann's syndrome may be inherited as an autosomal dominant with variable (male-predominant) expression, an autosomal recessive, or an X-linked recessive condition.

Usually, patients with Kallmann's syndrome present with delayed puberty. They exhibit eunuchoidal features and prepubertal size testes. An early prepubertal manifestation of Kallmann's syndrome is micropenis. In addition to anosmia or hyposmia (present in approximately 80 per cent of cases), these patients may also exhibit other mid-line defects (e.g., cleft-lip or -palate, color blindness, renal agenesis, nerve deafness), cryptorchidism, and skeletal abnormalities (e.g., syndactyly, short fourth metacarpals, craniofacial asymmetry). Patients with Kallmann's syndrome are often aspermic (i.e., have no ejaculate). Serum testosterone, LH, and FSH levels are low, while other anterior pituitary functions are normal. The degree of gonadotropin deficiency is highly variable. A single dose LHRH test may not result in stimulation of gonadotropin secretion, but repeated LHRH administration will increase LH and FSH levels. Clomiphene citrate is an antiestrogen that stimulates hypothalamic release of LHRH and as a result increases gonadotropin secretion. In men with Kallmann's syndrome gonadotropins are paradoxically suppressed by clomiphene citrate.

The differentiation between Kallmann's syndrome and constitutional delayed puberty is very difficult (especially in the absence of anosmia or hyposmia) and cannot be reliably made in the prepubertal age range. Usually, androgen therapy is initiated to induce sexual maturation in both of these conditions. It is intermittently stopped to determine whether spontaneous onset of puberty occurs. Patients with Kallmann's syndrome continue to require androgen therapy to achieve and maintain sexual maturation, whereas patients with constitutional delayed puberty do not require treatment after spontaneous endogenous gonadotropin and testosterone secretion begin. When fertility is desired, androgen replacement treatment is discontinued, and spermatogenesis may be induced with gonadotropin or LHRH therapy. Previous androgen therapy does not alter the subsequent testicular response to gonadotropin therapy. However, gonadotropin therapy is much less successful in patients who have associated cryptorchidism, particularly if it is bilateral.

A variant form of Kallmann's syndrome is *isolated LH deficiency*, which is also called the *"fertile" eunuch syndrome*. This syndrome is characterized by a selective deficiency in LH secretion, which results in prepubertal androgen deficiency and eunuchoidism. FSH secretion is preserved, resulting in testes of nearly normal size in which well-advanced spermatogenesis is present. Spermatogenesis is not normal in these patients, however, and they are not fertile, as the name of the syndrome would imply. Treatment with hCG, which contains predominantly LH-like hormonal activity, stimulates Leydig cell production of testosterone, ameliorates androgen deficiency, and increases spermatogenesis.

Hemochromatosis is an autosomal recessive disorder in which there is parenchymal iron deposition in a variety of tissues, most prominently in the liver, skin, pancreas, and heart (Ch. 193). Iron deposition in the pituitary gland selectively inhibits gonadotropin production without significantly affecting other anterior pituitary hormone secretion. The resulting hypogonadotropic hypogonadism and androgen deficiency are responsible for the common complaint of impotence in this disorder. Frequent phlebotomies or treatment with desferrioxamine to decrease iron overload may restore gonadotropin secretion in some patients. Even in the presence of significant iron overload, administration of gonadotropins can stimulate testicular function, including induction of spermatogenesis. Parenchymal iron deposition resulting in hypogonadotropic hypogonadism may also occur in patients with conditions that require frequent blood transfusions, such as thalassemia.

Secondary hypogonadism may be present in a number of *complex genetic syndromes*, such as *Prader-Labhart-Willi, Laurence-Moon-Biedl, Biemond, Carpenter, familial cerebellar ataxia, dyskeratosis congenita, familial ichthyosis, Borjeson, Kraus-Rupert, Lowe, steroid sulfatase deficiency, RUD, CHARGE, LEOPARD, Martsolf, Rothmund-Thompson,* and *Richards-Rundle* syndromes.

Acquired Disorders. Hypopituitarism. Any destructive or infiltrative lesion of the hypothalamus and/or pituitary may cause impairment of gonadotropin secretion, either selectively or in conjunction with deficiency of other anterior pituitary hormones (Ch. 213). Specific pathologic conditions include functioning and nonfunctioning pituitary adenomas; suprasellar tumors, such as craniopharyngioma, meningioma, optic glioma, or astrocytoma; metastatic neoplasms; lymphoma; surgical ablation or irradiation of the pituitary; infarction; vasculitis; apoplexy; hypophysitis; aneurysm; abscess; trauma; granulomatous disease, such as tuberculosis, sarcoidosis, fungal disease, and histiocytosis X; and transfusional iron overload.

Usually, destructive processes involving the pituitary gland result in progressive loss of anterior pituitary function in the following order: Gonadotropin and growth hormone secretion are the first to be affected, followed by TSH production, and finally ACTH secretion. The combination of gonadotropin and growth hormone deficiency is most important to recognize in prepubertal children with growth retardation. In adults, clinical secondary hypogonadism, in the absence of other anterior pituitary dysfunction, may be the initial manifestation of a hypothalamic or pituitary process. Because loss of TSH and ACTH secretion is associated with greater degrees of pituitary destruction, secondary hypothyroidism and hypoadrenalism usually do not occur without concurrent secondary hypogonadism.

Patients with prepubertal gonadotropin deficiency present with delayed puberty and have eunuchoidal features and small testes, usually less than 2 cm. Children with associated growth hormone deficiency also demonstrate short stature (dwarfism). Men with postpubertal gonadotropin deficiency usually present with diminished libido and potency. Initially, testicular size may be normal, but with longstanding gonadotropin deficiency the testes become small. In addition to hypogonadism, patients with hypopituitarism may have findings of deficiency or excess of other anterior pituitary hormones or tumor mass effects.

Serum testosterone levels and sperm counts are low. Serum LH and FSH levels are low or in the low normal adult range. The gonadotropin response to single dose LHRH administration does not reliably differentiate hypothalamic and pituitary causes of gonadotropin deficiency. In many instances, LHRH administration fails to stimulate gonadotropin secretion in patients with hypothalamic disease; alternatively, it may stimulate gonadotropin levels in men with pituitary disease. Clinical evaluation of patients with secondary hypogonadism should include anatomic studies (such as CT scan and visual field examination) to determine the presence and effects of a hypothalamic or pituitary tumor and investigation of other anterior pituitary hormone functions.

Treatment is aimed at the process causing hypopituitarism and correction of androgen deficiency with testosterone replacement therapy. If fertility is desired, androgens are discontinued and gonadotropin therapy is instituted.

Hyperprolactinemia. This condition, resulting from a pituitary adenoma, central nervous system–active drugs (such as phenothiazines and other antipsychotics, opiates, sedatives, antidepressants, stimulants), or adrenergic dopaminergic antagonist drugs (antihypertensives, metoclopramide) may cause secondary testicular failure (Ch. 226). In men, prolactin-secreting adenomas are usually large (macroadenomas), and gonadotropin deficiency may be caused primarily by destruction of pituitary gonadotrophs. Even in the absence of a tumor, prolactin has an inhibitory effect on gonadotropin secretion, resulting in secondary hypogonadism. In some men with hyperprolactinemia, correction of androgen deficiency with testosterone replacement therapy does not correct impotence. The addition of bromocriptine, a dopamine agonist that decreases pituitary prolactin secretion, may be useful in these situations.

The negative feedback effects of *estrogen excess* in men causes inhibition of gonadotropin secretion and secondary hypogonadism. Estrogen excess may result from either exogenous administration of estrogens or estrogenic substances (e.g., diethylstilbestrol administration in men with prostate cancer) or endogenous secretion from an estrogen-producing neoplasm (e.g., feminizing adrenal carcinoma). Patients with estrogen excess usually manifest varying degrees of gynecomastia. *Progestins* (e.g., medroxyprogesterone acetate) and *opiate-like drugs* (e.g., morphine, methadone, and heroin) also inhibit gonadotropin production and may cause secondary hypogonadism.

Systemic Disorders. *Glucocorticoid excess*, as a result of either Cushing's syndrome or high-dosage glucocorticoid administration, suppresses gonadotropin secretion, resulting in secondary testicular failure with loss of libido, impotence, and oligospermia. Activation of the hypothalamic-adrenal axis resulting in stimulation of corticotropin-releasing factor (which is thought to inhibit LHRH secretion) and high circulating levels of endogenous glucocorticoids may contribute to the reduction in serum testosterone, LH, and FSH levels observed with *acute stress or illness*, such as emotional stress, vigorous physical exercise, trauma, myocardial infarction, surgery, burns, sepsis, etc. *Nutritional deficiency*, such as that associated with protein-calorie malnutrition or anorexia nervosa, inhibits gonadotropin production and may cause secondary hypogonadism. Concurrent primary testicular dysfunction may also be associated with inadequate nutrition. Malnutrition may contribute to the secondary testicular failure associated with a number of *chronic illnesses*, such as malignancy and chronic heart, respiratory, liver, and kidney disease. Moderate obesity results in reduction in SHBG and total testosterone levels, with normal free testosterone levels. Some men with *massive obesity* demonstrate clinical androgen deficiency with low free testosterone concentrations and reduced gonadotropin levels.

ISOLATED DEFICIENCY OF SPERM PRODUCTION. *Congenital adrenal hyperplasia* caused by either 21-hydroxylase or 11β-hydroxylase deficiency results in excessive production of adrenal androgens. Androgen excess suppresses gonadotropin secretion, resulting in secondary hypogonadism. Testicular androgen and sperm production are suppressed. Excessive adrenal androgen production causes premature virilization and precocious pseudopuberty, rather than androgen deficiency. Secondary hypogonadism is therefore manifested by isolated impairment of spermatogenesis. Glucocorticoid treatment of some patients with congenital adrenal hyperplasia may result in true precocious puberty, with premature activation of the hypothalamic-pituitary-gonadal axis. These patients demonstrate premature induction of spermatogenesis and normal gonadotropin levels. Androgen excess caused by administration of *testosterone* or *androgenic anabolic steroids* or *androgen-secreting tumors* (e.g., testicular Leydig cell tumors) also result in secondary hypogonadism presenting with isolated deficiency in sperm production with normal androgenization. High doses of testosterone have been used in normal men to suppress sperm production in trials to develop male contraceptives.

Rarely, *hyperprolactinemia* impairs sperm production despite normal gonadotropin and testosterone levels. *Isolated FSH deficiency*, an extremely rare condition, results in normal virilization in males, with normal serum testosterone and LH levels. Spermatogenesis and fertility have not been well characterized in this disorder, although testicular biopsy in one man revealed arrest of sperm maturation at the spermatid stage.

Androgen Resistance Syndromes

Androgen resistance syndromes are caused by defects in androgen action (Ch. 221). The severity of androgen insensitivity determines the clinical presentation of these disorders. Most androgen resistance syndromes result in severely defective androgen action, and patients with these syndromes present at birth as either phenotypic females (testicular feminization) or with ambiguous genitalia (male pseudohermaphroditism). However, some men with mild, incomplete androgen insensitivity or *Reifenstein's syndrome* may present as adults with a clinical picture of mild androgen deficiency with a nearly normal male phenotype. Patients with Reifenstein's syndrome may have hypospadias, gynecomastia, varying degrees of virilization, a small prostate gland, impaired spermatogenesis, and cryptorchidism. They may be distinguished from patients with true hypogonadism by having elevated serum testosterone, LH, and FSH levels. Some men with very mild androgen insensitivity may present with only oligospermia or azoospermia and no other phenotypic abnormalities. Some men with celiac disease are infertile and have elevated serum testosterone and LH levels, suggesting androgen resistance.

Delayed Puberty

Puberty in boys usually begins between the ages of 9 and 14 years. With the maturation of the central nervous system mechanism that regulates LHRH production, pulsatile gonadotropin and testosterone secretions begin, initially during sleep and then throughout the day. The first clinical indications of the onset of puberty are an increase in the testicular size (above 3 cm) and a wrinkling and pigmentation of the scrotal skin. Subsequently, there are increase in penile length and appearance of pubic hair, followed by increasing long bone growth and development of other secondary sexual characteristics, such as hair growth in other androgen-dependent areas, increase in muscle mass, enlargement of the larynx, and growth of the prostate. The increase in testicular size precedes the appearance of pubic hair by about 2 years and the peak velocity in growth of height by 3 years. The onset and duration of puberty and the degree to which secondary sexual characteristics develop vary considerably, largely attributable to the genetic background of an individual.

Delayed puberty is the lack of sexual maturation before the age of 15 years. A number of the disorders discussed above that cause *hypogonadism*, including those causing primary and secondary testicular failure and androgen resistance, may result in delayed sexual maturation. *Severe systemic illnesses* (such as malabsorption, asthma, diabetes, malignancy) that also cause growth retardation and *thyroid hormone deficiency* may also cause delayed puberty. The great majority of boys with delayed puberty, however, have physiologic or *constitutional delayed puberty*. This is a benign form of delayed adolescence which represents a normal variation in the onset of puberty. It is frequently familial. These boys eventually undergo a delayed but normal puberty and attain normal sexual maturation and height.

The diagnosis of constitutional delayed puberty can be strongly suspected in a healthy boy with retardation of growth and bone age, normal growth velocity in relation to bone age, a family history of delayed adolescence, a testicular volume above 2 ml, and a bone age between 12 and 13 years. These clinical features are often not present and the diagnosis can be very difficult. Diagnostic evaluation should be undertaken to exclude organic causes of delayed puberty, i.e., hypogonadism, systemic illness, and hypothyroidism. In the absence of anosmia or other morphologic manifestations, constitutional delayed puberty cannot be distinguished from hypogonadotropic eunuchoidism or Kallmann's syndrome (see above).

Delayed sexual maturation often results in severe psychosocial distress to both the patient and his parents. Therefore, after systemic and endocrine disorders are excluded, patients with delayed puberty are usually treated with androgen replacement therapy to induce sexual maturation. It is generally recommended that patients not be treated with androgens until after 15 years of age. The emotional stress and trauma of delayed puberty often result in treatment beginning at about 13 to 14 years of age, however, so that the onset of sexual maturation coincides with those of his contemporaries. Androgen treatment is intermittently stopped to determine if spontaneous onset of puberty has occurred.

TREATMENT OF HYPOGONADISM
Androgen Therapy

Androgens are principally used to treat testosterone deficiency in hypogonadal men; the therapeutic goal of androgen therapy is to restore the normal physiologic effects of testosterone. In prepubertal androgen-deficient boys, the aim of androgen replacement is to stimulate and maintain male secondary sexual characteristics, somatic development, and sexual function without compromising adult height by premature closure of long bone epiphyses. In adult androgen deficiency, the objective of therapy is to restore and maintain libido, potency, and secondary sexual characteristics. Androgen treatment is very successful in accomplishing these goals. However, testosterone cannot be administered in sufficiently high doses to achieve the high intratesticular levels required to stimulate spermatogenesis.

The long-acting 17β-hydroxyl esters of testosterone, *testosterone enanthate* and *cypionate*, are the most effective, safest, and most practical preparations currently available to treat androgen deficiency. Intramuscular injection of 200 mg of either preparation results in peak serum testosterone levels at the upper limits of the normal adult range in 1 to 2 days. Testosterone levels remain in the normal range for about 2 weeks. Therefore, in adults with androgen deficiency, replacement therapy is usually initiated with either testosterone enanthate or cypionate at a dose of 200 mg intramuscularly every 2 weeks. In these men, testosterone administration generally results in stimulation of libido and potency, improvement in energy level, increase in physical and social drive, and increase in hemoglobin concentration.

In an elderly androgen-deficient man with symptoms of bladder neck obstruction secondary to an enlarged prostate gland, it is wise to begin testosterone therapy gradually with a short-acting testosterone preparation. *Testosterone propionate*, a short-acting 17β-hydroxyl ester of testosterone, given in doses of 25 to 50 mg intramuscularly three times weekly, is useful in this situation. The shorter duration of action of this preparation permits rapid withdrawal if androgen stimulation results in prostatic growth or urinary obstruction.

Androgen replacement therapy is much more complicated in prepubertal boys with delayed puberty. Although testosterone is very effective in inducing secondary sexual characteristics and stimulating long bone growth, overly aggressive androgen therapy can result in premature closure of long bone epiphyses and compromise final adult height. Furthermore, it is often not possible to differentiate patients with constitutional delayed puberty, who require only temporary androgen replacement, from those with permanent hypogonadotropic hypogonadism. Therefore, in boys with delayed puberty whose height is far below the expected adult height, androgen therapy is begun with testosterone enanthate or cypionate, 50 to 100 mg intramuscularly every 2 weeks, and gradually increased to full replacement doses. Androgen therapy is intermittently stopped for 3 to 4 months to determine whether spontaneous pubertal development will occur.

Currently, all oral androgen preparations available in the

United States are 17α-alkylated derivatives of testosterone, which have the potential for serious hepatotoxicity. When used for the treatment of androgen deficiency, parenteral 17β-hydroxyl esters of testosterone do not cause hepatotoxicity. Because of the greater risk of oral androgen preparations, as well as their increased cost and reduced efficacy, they should be avoided in the treatment of androgen deficiency. In the very rare circumstance of a patient who will not or cannot take parenteral androgens, *methyltestosterone*, 25 to 50 mg orally or 10 to 25 mg buccally, or *fluoxymesterone*, 5 to 10 mg orally daily, may be used.

Androgen therapy is absolutely contraindicated in men with androgen-sensitive cancers, i.e., prostatic carcinoma and male breast carcinoma. Full replacement doses of androgens may be inappropriate for hypogonadal men with mental retardation or severe psychopathology and for elderly androgen-deficient men with severe bladder neck obstruction from prostatic hyperplasia, who are not good surgical candidates.

Excessive stimulation of libido and erections by androgens is very uncommon, usually occurring in prepubertal boys or in men with longstanding androgen deficiency given large doses of testosterone. These symptoms usually resolve with time or reduction in dosage. Androgen administration causing acute urinary retention is very uncommon in the absence of underlying prostatic carcinoma. Patients given testosterone to induce puberty may develop acne or gynecomastia, similar to that observed in normal puberty. Adult hypogonadal men less commonly develop acne and rarely develop gynecomastia, except when a predisposing condition such as hepatic cirrhosis exists. Androgens may cause mild weight gain as a result of sodium retention and protein anabolic effects, and patients with underlying edematous states may develop worsening edema during therapy.

Erythropoiesis is stimulated by androgen administration. Occasionally, significant erythrocytosis requiring phlebotomy and reduced testosterone dosage occurs. Testosterone has also been reported to worsen or induce obstructive sleep apnea. All oral 17α-alkylated androgens have been reported to cause hepatic cholestasis and occasionally clinical jaundice. Although rare, more serious and potentially life-threatening complications of oral androgens are the development of peliosis hepatis (blood-filled cysts in the liver), hepatic adenoma, hepatoma, or hepatic angiosarcoma. Hepatotoxicity does not result from replacement dosages of parenteral 17β-hydroxyl esters of testosterone. Depending on the androgen preparation, dose, duration of therapy, and individual susceptibility, androgen administration may induce virilization in women, manifested by acne, hirsutism, and menstrual dysfunction, and in severe cases frontal balding, voice changes, breast atrophy, and clitoral hypertrophy.

Androgens have also been used in the treatment of anemias related to renal and bone marrow failure, micropenis and microphallus, hereditary angioneurotic edema, female breast cancer, lichen sclerosus, endometriosis, and senile osteoporosis. The use of androgenic steroids has not been demonstrated to be of long-term value in promoting protein anabolism in catabolic states associated with a variety of acute and chronic illnesses. However, in many illnesses (such as burns, chronic liver disease, and illnesses requiring chronic glucocorticoid therapy), serum testosterone levels are often low. The efficacy of androgen therapy in this subset of catabolic diseases has not been examined.

Androgenic anabolic steroids are commonly used by competitive athletes with the hope of improving endurance, strength, and performance. Numerous studies have demonstrated that androgens are of dubious value in increasing strength and performance, in the absence of intensive training and high-protein diets. Many athletes often take multiple androgenic anabolic agents (including 17α-alkylated agents) in very high doses, with little regard for potentially serious side effects. Hepatotoxicity (including hepatoma) and impaired spermatogenesis resulting in infertility have been reported in athletes taking these androgenic steroids. Furthermore, the long-term sequelae of taking massive doses of 17β-hydroxyl ester preparations are unknown. The potential risks of high-dose anabolic steroid use far outweigh the potential benefits to athletic performance, and the use of these agents for this purpose should be strongly discouraged.

Gonadotropin and LHRH Therapy

The aim of gonadotropin therapy is to stimulate spermatogenesis and to establish or restore fertility in gonadotropin-deficient hypogonadal patients. The gonadotropin preparations usually used for this purpose are *hCG*, which is purified from the urine of pregnant women and contains LH-like biologic activity almost exclusively; and *human menopausal gonadotropin* (*hMG*, Pergonal), which is purified from the urine of postmenopausal women and contains both FSH and LH activity. A more purified preparation of *human FSH* (*hFSH*, Metrodin) is now available for clinical use; it has been used primarily to induce ovulation so far. Both hCG and hMG are expensive and require multiple injections per week. Therefore, testosterone, rather than gonadotropin therapy, is used to induce and maintain androgenization in patients with hypogonadotropic hypogonadism.

Initiation of spermatogenesis in prepubertal patients with hypogonadotropic hypogonadism usually requires treatment with both hCG and hMG. Because of the relative ineffectiveness of hMG to stimulate the immature testis and the greater expense, treatment is initiated with hCG alone, at a dosage of 2000 IU subcutaneously or intramuscularly two to three times weekly for 6 to 12 months. Clinical evidence of sexual maturation and the increase in serum testosterone levels are monitored to determine the need for adjustments in dose. During hCG treatment, testosterone produced by the Leydig cells causes the Sertoli cells to mature and spermatogenesis to be initiated to varying degrees of completeness. Occasionally, hCG alone stimulates spermatogenesis sufficiently for sperm to appear in the ejaculate. However, the majority of prepubertal patients with hypogonadotropic hypogonadism require FSH activity, in the form of hMG, in addition to hCG to complete spermatogenesis and induce fertility. Therefore, hMG, at a dosage of 75 IU subcutaneously or intramuscularly three times weekly, is usually added to hCG if there is no evidence of sperm in the ejaculate with hCG alone. Gonadotropin induction of sperm production may take as long as 1 year. Even with combined hCG and hMG treatment, sperm output in the ejaculate may not be normal. Despite very low sperm counts, fertility may be induced, however.

Once initiated, spermatogenesis may be maintained with hCG treatment alone. In adults with acquired hypogonadotropic hypogonadism, sperm production may also be restored with hCG treatment alone. Previous androgen treatment does not alter testicular responsiveness to subsequent gonadotropin therapy. The presence of primary testicular disease, such as cryptorchidism, worsens the prognosis for induction of sperm production and fertility by gonadotropin treatment.

In patients with Kallmann's syndrome, pulsatile administration of low doses of LHRH has been used successfully to stimulate endogenous gonadotropin secretion and to initiate and maintain spermatogenesis to induce fertility. Pulsatile administration more closely mimics the normal physiologic situation; however, a portable infusion pump must be used to deliver small doses of LHRH every few hours (e.g., 5 to 20 μg subcutaneously every 2 hours) throughout the day, making LHRH therapy a much more complex management problem than gonadotropin therapy. LHRH and gonadotropin therapy are probably similar in their ability to stimulate spermatogenesis in men with Kallmann's syndrome.

Castro-Magaña M, Bronsther B, Angulo MA: Genetic forms of male hypogonadism. Urology 35:195, 1990. *This is an excellent review article on the pathophysiology, clinical manifestations, and treatment of genetic causes of primary and secondary hypogonadism in men.*

Handelsman DJ, Swerdloff RS: Male gonadal dysfunction. Clin Endocrinol Metab 14:89, 1985. *A very complete review of clinical and laboratory evaluation of male gonadal disorders.*

Hopwood NJ: Pathogenesis and management of abnormal puberty. Spec Topics Endocrinol Metab 7:175, 1985. *An excellent review of pubertal disorders.*

Lee PA, St L O'dea L: Primary and secondary testicular insufficiency. Pediatr Clin North Am 37:1359, 1990. *This is a well-organized and well-written review of the diagnosis and treatment of primary and secondary testicular failure in the pediatric age group.*

Matsumoto AM: Clinical use and abuse of androgens and antiandrogens. In Becker KL (ed.): Principles and Practice of Endocrinology and Metabolism. Philadelphia, JB Lippincott Company, 1990, p 991. *This chapter reviews the pharmacology of androgen preparations, their clinical use in treatment of male hypogonadism and other conditions, the inappropriate use of androgens, and their potential side effects.*

Plymate SR, Paulsen CA: Male hypogonadism. In Becker KL (ed.): Principles and Practice of Endocrinology and Metabolism. Philadelphia, JB Lippincott Company, 1990, p 948. *This chapter contains an excellent comprehensive discussion of disorders causing primary and secondary hypogonadism, with 181 references.*

Rosenfeld RL: Diagnosis and management of delayed puberty. J Clin Endocrinol

Metab 70:559, 1990. *A concise, up-to-date review of the diagnosis and treatment of delayed sexual development.*

PRECOCIOUS PUBERTY

Isosexual precocity is defined as the development of sexual maturation before the age of 9 years. In boys, premature development of secondary sexual characteristics results in virilization. This is accompanied by accelerated skeletal maturation and linear growth and premature closure of long bone epiphyses, resulting in short stature as an adult. *True precocious puberty* is caused by premature secretion of gonadotropins. Testicular androgen and sperm production is stimulated by gonadotropins and results in virilization and increased testis size. *Precocious pseudopuberty* results from secretion of androgens from the adrenal gland or testis. Androgen excess results in virilization, but normal sperm production is not stimulated and the testes remain small. Occasionally, high local testosterone concentrations within the testis can stimulate some degree of spermatogenesis.

True Precocious Puberty

In the majority of cases of true precocious puberty no identifiable cause for premature activation of gonadotropin secretion is found. This condition is called *idiopathic precocious puberty*. It is often inherited as a male-limited autosomal dominant or X-linked recessive trait. Patients have an increased incidence of seizure disorders and abnormal electroencephalograms. The remaining cases of true precocious puberty are primarily caused by *central nervous system lesions* involving the posterior hypothalamus. Lesions include hypothalamic and pineal tumors, craniopharyngioma, hamartomas, hydrocephalus, postencephalitic lesions, congenital brain defects, neurofibromatosis, and tuberous sclerosis. Central nervous system lesions may also result in disturbances of other hypothalamic functions, causing diabetes insipidus, eating disorders, somnolence, emotional lability, and altered temperature regulation, as well as mental and psychomotor retardation and seizures. Precocious puberty may precede the onset of a clinically detectable neurologic lesion. Therefore, a prolonged period of follow-up observation with repeated neurologic evaluation is necessary to exclude central nervous system lesions. Rarely, an *hCG-secreting tumor* (e.g., hepatoblastoma) or *hCG administration* for cryptorchidism (iatrogenic precocious puberty) causes true precocious puberty.

Precocious Pseudopuberty (Ch. 221)

Adrenocortical hyperfunction, either from congenital adrenal hyperplasia (21-hydroxylase or 11β-hydroxylase deficiency) or a virilizing adrenocortical tumor, is the most common condition causing precocious pseudopuberty in boys. Patients with congenital adrenal hyperplasia caused by 21-hydroxylase deficiency usually have markedly elevated serum 17-hydroxyprogesterone and urinary pregnanetriol levels. Rarely, *Leydig cell tumor* of the testis, autonomous Leydig cell function (*testotoxicosis*), and administration of *androgenic steroids* may cause precocious pseudopuberty.

Treatment of these conditions is directed at the underlying cause. For idiopathic precocious puberty, drugs to inhibit pituitary gonadotropin secretion (medroxyprogesterone acetate, LHRH analogues) or androgen synthesis (ketoconazole), or to block androgen action (flutamide, cyproterone acetate) have been used with varying success to prevent further sexual maturation. With the exception of LHRH analogues, these treatments do not usually prevent premature closure of long bone epiphyses.

Kaplan SL, Grumbach MM: Pathophysiology and treatment of sexual precocity. J Clin Endocrinol Metab 71:785, 1990. *A concise and up-to-date review of the pathophysiology and management of precocious pubertal development.*

Wheeler MD, Styne DM: Diagnosis and management of precocious puberty. Pediatr Clin North Am 37:1255, 1990. *This is an excellent, comprehensive review of the diagnosis and treatment of sexual precocity.*

TUMORS OF THE TESTIS

Tumors of the testis are uncommon, representing about 1 per cent of all cancers in men. They occur more commonly in white than in black males. The annual incidence of testicular tumors is 6 per 100,000 males. About 95 per cent of testicular tumors are malignant and derive from the germ cells. The remaining 5 per cent are non–germ cell or stromal tumors derived mostly from Leydig and Sertoli cells of the gonadal stroma and are usually benign. Gonadoblastoma is a rare testicular neoplasm containing both germ cell and stromal elements, arising in dysgenetic testes containing a Y chromosome. The peak age of incidence of testicular cancer is 20 to 35 years. It is the most common malignancy in this age group. Advances in treatment have transformed testicular cancer from the most common cause of cancer death in this age group 20 years ago into one of the most curable of all cancers today. A testicular mass in a patient over 50 years is more likely to be a lymphoma than a germ cell tumor.

The most significant risk factor for developing testicular cancer is cryptorchidism. In unilateral cryptorchidism, the contralateral, normally descended testis also carries an increased risk of malignant degeneration. Orchiopexy at an early age (2 to 3 years) permits easier palpation and detection of testicular cancer and may reduce the risk of neoplasm. Carcinoma in situ has been found in men with oligoazoospermia presenting with infertility and in the contralateral testes of patients with presumed unilateral testicular cancer, suggesting that these conditions may also carry an increased risk for testicular neoplasm.

Germ Cell Tumors

Germ cell cancers may be classified according to their pathologic characteristics into *seminoma* and *nonseminoma*. Nonseminomatous cancers include *embryonal cell carcinomas, choriocarcinomas,* and *teratomas*. Forty per cent of germ cell cancers contain a mixture of seminomatous and nonseminomatous elements. The presence of any nonseminomatous element in a tumor that is predominantly seminoma dictates its classification as a nonseminoma. The distinction between seminoma and nonseminoma is important to plan for staging and subsequent therapy. Seminomas usually metastasize via regional lymph nodes to retroperitoneal, mediastinal, and supraclavicular lymph nodes and are very sensitive to radiation therapy. On the other hand, nonseminomas metastasize by both lymphatic and hematogenous routes (especially to liver and lungs) and are radioresistant.

Most patients with germ cell tumors present with a painless mass in the testis. Rapid onset of a painful testicular mass is usually caused by bleeding into the neoplasm. Back or abdominal pain (from retroperitoneal lymphadenopathy), shortness of breath (from diffuse pulmonary metastases), gynecomastia (from hCG secretion), supraclavicular lymphadenopathy, or ureteral obstruction may also be present.

Germ cell tumors, especially nonseminomatous cancers, often secrete biologic markers (Ch. 160). Embryonal cell cancers may secrete α-*fetoprotein*. Pure seminomas never elaborate α-fetoprotein, and its presence in serum implies the presence of nonseminomatous elements in the tumor or metastases. *hCG* is secreted by nearly all choriocarcinomas, a third of embryonal cell carcinomas and teratocarcinomas and, rarely, by pure seminomas. This marker may be detected and differentiated from crossreacting LH in serum with a specific β-hCG assay. Both of these tumor markers may be used to monitor response to therapy. They may precede clinically detectable disease by weeks to months.

In seminoma, orchiectomy and radiotherapy to the periaortic and iliac lymph nodes have resulted in cure rates of 80 to 95 per cent. In nonseminomatous testicular cancer, the addition of cisplatin to aggressive, multiple-drug chemotherapeutic regimens has resulted in response rates of over 90 per cent and long-term remission in 50 to 90 per cent of patients.

Non–Germ Cell Tumors

Non–germ cell tumors are rare tumors that develop from the two major elements of testicular stroma, the *Leydig* and *Sertoli cells*. They are usually benign, but about 10 per cent are malignant and metastasize via regional lymphatics. Both Leydig and Sertoli cell tumors may secrete a variety of steroid hormones, primarily androgens or estrogens, that may result in virilization or feminization, respectively. These tumors are usually small and difficult to diagnose; selective venous catheterization and sampling to determine the site of increased steroid production are often helpful. Gynecomastia is present in about 30 per cent of patients with non–germ cell tumors. Children may present with either isosexual (virilizing) or heterosexual (feminizing) precocious pseudopuberty. Treatment consists primarily of orchiectomy.

Ozols RF, Williams SD: Testicular cancer. Curr Probl Cancer 13:285, 1989. *An excellent comprehensive review of the classification, epidemiology, staging, treatment, and prognosis of testicular cancer (98 references).*

223 Diseases of the Prostate

Charles B. Brendler

This chapter discusses three common disorders of the prostate: prostatitis, benign prostatic hyperplasia, and adenocarcinoma of the prostate. A brief review of the normal anatomy, physiology, and biochemistry of the prostate is provided first.

THE NORMAL PROSTATE

ANATOMY. The normal adult prostate, a firm, elastic organ weighing about 20 grams, is located caudad to the base of the bladder and is traversed by the first portion of the urethra. It is bordered anteriorly by the symphysis pubis and posteriorly by the rectum. The paired seminal vesicles are attached to the prostate and are located posterior to the bladder (Fig. 223–1).

The human prostate has two concentric anatomic regions: an inner periurethral zone composed of short glands and an outer peripheral zone composed of longer, branched glands. These regions are separated by a thin layer of fibroelastic tissue, the so-called surgical capsule (Fig. 223–2). Benign prostatic hyperplasia (BPH) arises within the inner periurethral zone in a specific region near the verumontanum, called the transition zone. In contrast, prostatic carcinoma usually arises in the outer peripheral zone.

PHYSIOLOGY. The secretions of the prostate and other sex accessory organs presumably protect or enhance the functional properties of the spermatozoa. Of the total average human ejaculate volume of 3.5 ml, the prostate secretes 0.5 ml and the seminal vesicles secrete 2.0 to 2.5 ml.

Two specific components of prostatic secretion, zinc and acid phosphatase, have aroused interest because of their high concentrations in seminal fluid. Zinc is higher in concentration in the prostate than in any other organ in the body, but its function is unknown. The biologic function of acid phosphatase is also unknown. Prostate cancer cells often continue to secrete acid phosphatase after they have metastasized, and the measurement of prostatic acid phosphatase in the serum is used both as a screening test for prostatic carcinoma and to follow the response to therapy in patients with metastatic disease.

BIOCHEMISTRY. The growth and secretory function of the prostate depend on functioning testes; prostatic maturation does not occur in a male castrated before puberty. Testosterone, the major circulating androgen, is converted to dihydrotestosterone (DHT) by the enzyme 5α-reductase in prostatic epithelial cells. DHT, the major active androgenic metabolite within the prostate,

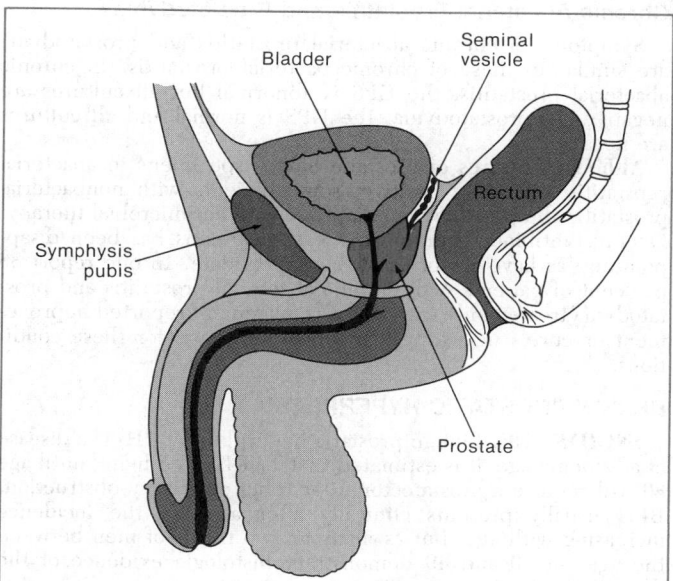

FIGURE 223–1. The anatomic relationship of the prostate to adjacent structures. (After Brendler H. *In* Glenn JF (ed.): Urologic Surgery, 3rd ed. Philadelphia, J. B. Lippincott Company, 1983.)

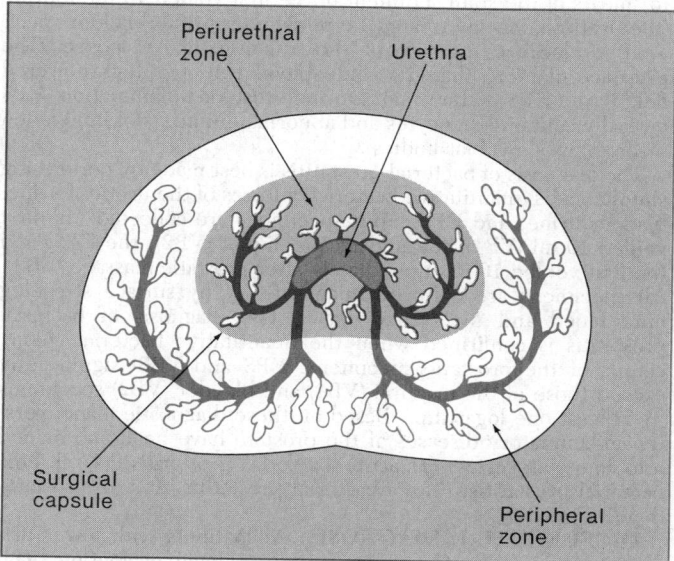

FIGURE 223–2. A coronal section through the prostate demonstrating the anatomic relationships between the urethra, periurethral tissue, surgical capsule, and peripheral tissue. (After Brendler H. *In* Glenn JF (ed.): Urologic Surgery, 3rd ed. Philadelphia, J. B. Lippincott Comany, 1983.)

binds to a cytoplasmic receptor, is transported to the nucleus, and there initiates RNA synthesis, protein synthesis, and cell replication.

Estrogens inhibit prostatic growth, largely by blocking the release of luteinizing hormone from the pituitary, thus inhibiting testicular synthesis of testosterone. If castrated animals are given both estrogens and androgens, normal prostate growth occurs, indicating that estrogens do not block androgen-induced growth in the prostate itself.

PROSTATITIS

INCIDENCE AND ETIOLOGY. About 50 per cent of men experience symptoms of prostatic inflammation during adult life. Only about 5 per cent of these cases are due to bacterial infection of the prostate. The etiology of these symptoms in the remaining 95 per cent of patients is unclear.

Most bacterial infections of the prostate are caused by gram-negative organisms, most commonly *Escherichia coli*. Enterococci, staphylococci, and streptococci are rare causes of prostatic infection. *Chlamydia trachomatis* and *Ureaplasma urealyticum* probably cause prostatitis infrequently, but this topic remains controversial.

PATHOGENESIS. Most episodes of bacterial prostatic infection are due to a previous urethral infection with direct ascent of bacteria from the urethra through the prostatic ducts into the prostate. The organisms that cause bacterial prostatitis are the same as those that produce bacteriuria, and chlamydial and gonococcal infections of the urethra may involve the prostate.

Prostatic infection may also result from impairment of host defense mechanisms. The concentrations of prostatic antibacterial factor and magnesium, zinc, calcium, citric acid, spermine, cholesterol, and lysozyme are decreased in the prostatic fluid of men with chronic bacterial prostatitis. Whether these alterations contribute to or result from prostatic infection is unknown. About 10 per cent of men with chronic bacterial prostatitis have more than one organism, and many after cure develop reinfection of the prostate by a different organism, further suggesting impaired host defense function.

DIAGNOSIS. The diagnosis of prostatitis is based on examination of expressed prostatic secretions (EPS) and quantitative bacterial localization cultures. Although microscopic examination of the EPS is important, it can be misleading. The clinician should always compare the microscopic appearance of the EPS to smears of the spun sediment of the first voided 10 ml of urine (the urethral specimen) and the midstream urine (bladder specimen) to localize the site of the inflammatory response. The presence of more than 20 white blood cells per high-powered field in the EPS is abnormal. During prostatic inflammation, EPS typically contain leukocytes and abnormal numbers of lipid-laden macrophages (oval fat bodies).

The diagnosis of bacterial prostatitis is best made by performing simultaneous quantitative bacterial cultures of the urethral urine, bladder urine, and EPS. Four specimens are collected: the first voided 10 ml (VB1), the midstream aliquot (VB2), the EPS, and the first voided 10 ml immediately after prostatic massage (VB3). All specimens are cultured quantitatively by surface streaking onto blood and MacConkey agar. The diagnosis of bacterial prostatitis is confirmed when the quantitative bacterial colony counts of the prostatic specimens (EPS and VB3) significantly exceed those of the urethral (VB1) and bladder (VB2) specimens by at least one logarithm. Based on these diagnostic maneuvers, the inflammatory diseases of the prostate have been subdivided into four categories: (1) acute bacterial prostatitis, (2) chronic bacterial prostatitis, (3) nonbacterial prostatitis, and (4) prostatodynia.

DIFFERENTIAL DIAGNOSIS. All patients with lower urinary tract complaints require a full urologic evaluation. The differential diagnosis of patients with lower urinary tract irritative symptoms should include upper urinary tract infection with secondary colonization of the bladder, carcinoma of the bladder, neurogenic bladder, prostatic obstruction, and urethral stricture. Because the irritative urinary symptoms in men with prostatitis are identical to those of patients with flat in situ carcinoma of the bladder, a urinary cytology and cystoscopy should be performed in these patients to exclude the presence of bladder malignancy.

Acute Bacterial Prostatitis

Acute bacterial prostatitis is a fulminant condition that occurs mainly between the ages of 20 and 40. Patients present with the acute onset of fever, chills, and malaise associated with marked urinary irritative and obstructive symptoms. Pain may be experienced in the suprapubic region, lumbar spine, and perineum.

On physical examination, patients frequently have a fever as high as 39 to 40°C. Patients may have marked suprapubic tenderness if prostatic infection results in urinary retention. Rectal examination to rule out a prostatic abscess should be done very carefully, as it is extremely uncomfortable for the patient and may result in septicemia or secondary epididymitis if the prostate is massaged too vigorously. The prostate is variably enlarged, markedly tender, and hot to palpation. A prostatic abscess should be suspected if an abnormally fluctuant area is palpated within the prostate.

Patients with acute bacterial prostatitis almost always have associated bacteriuria, and, therefore, a urinalysis and urine culture are helpful in establishing the diagnosis and identifying appropriate antibiotic therapy. With recurrent bacterial prostatitis, intravenous pyelography or abdominal ultrasonography should be done to rule out upper urinary tract pathology. A pelvic ultrasound or computed tomography scan may be helpful in diagnosing a prostatic abscess.

Patients with acute bacterial prostatitis are frequently quite ill and need to be hospitalized for their initial treatment. Urinary retention may necessitate placement of a temporary suprapubic cystostomy or urethral catheter. Intravenous antibiotics are usually given; a combination of gentamicin to cover gram-negative organisms and ampicillin to cover enterococci should be used. Supportive measures include hydration, analgesics, and stool softeners. Following initial intravenous therapy, the patient should be placed on an antibiotic with broad gram-negative coverage that diffuses readily into the prostatic fluid. Trimethoprim, trimethoprim-sulfamethoxazole, and the new quinolone derivatives are the usual choices. Since bacterial infections may be difficult to eradicate, oral antibiotics should be continued for 4 to 6 weeks after the acute episode. It is worthwhile to examine the EPS and VB3 6 to 12 weeks after starting therapy to be sure that the infection has resolved.

Granulomatous lesions of the prostate, observed in about 1 per cent of tissue specimens obtained either by biopsy or by partial prostatectomy, usually result from previous bacterial infection or prior transurethral resection of the prostate. Systemic diseases commonly associated with granuloma formation, such as tuberculosis, account for only a small minority of cases. Granulomatous prostatitis may cause induration that mimics prostatic carcinoma, requiring a biopsy to distinguish the two conditions. Granulomatous prostatitis may result in irritative and obstructive urinary symptoms that usually resolve spontaneously. The value of antibiotics in this condition is controversial.

Chronic Bacterial Prostatitis

Chronic bacterial prostatitis is one of the most common causes of recurrent urinary tract infection in men. The symptoms, similar to but milder than those of acute bacterial prostatitis, include urinary frequency and dysuria along with vague lower abdominal, lumbar, and perineal pain. Fever and urethral discharge are uncommon. The diagnosis is made by examination of the EPS and quantitative bacterial cultures. The EPS should be considered abnormal if there are greater than 10 leukocytes per high power field (hPF) and more than one or two lipid-laden macrophages per hPF. Men with chronic bacterial prostatitis may have a normal EPS while on antibiotic therapy but may continue to have recurrent infections once antibiotics have been discontinued. Furthermore, 5 to 10 per cent of men with no symptoms of prostatic inflammation have more than 10 leukocytes per hPF in their EPS.

An alternative approach to quantitative bacterial cultures, which are expensive and time consuming, is to obtain a quantitative culture of the bladder urine (VB2) and a nonquantitative culture of the EPS on the first office visit. If these cultures are both negative, the prostate is probably not infected. Recovery of gram-negative bacteria from either of these specimens identifies patients who might have chronic bacterial prostatitis and provides a rationale for conventional bacterial localization cultures on the second office visit.

Chronic bacterial prostatitis is frequently difficult to treat. Antibiotic therapy alone eradicates only about 30 to 50 per cent of the infections, but suppressive antimicrobial therapy usually results in complete symptomatic relief and reduces the risks of serious illness. The usual antibiotics used in this condition are trimethoprim-sulfamethoxazole, carbenicillin, or one of the new quinolones, such as ciprofloxacin or norfloxacin, in a 4- to 12-week course of therapy. Suppressive antibiotic therapy with trimethoprim, trimethoprim-sulfamethoxazole, and nitrofurantoin is effective. Experimentally, direct injection of antibiotics, such as thiamphenicol and aminoglycosides, has given promise in patients who failed previous oral antibiotic therapy.

Chronic Abacterial Prostatitis and Prostatodynia

Symptoms of chronic abacterial prostatitis and prostatodynia are similar to those of chronic bacterial prostatitis. In chronic abacterial prostatitis, the EPS is abnormal but all cultures are negative. In prostatodynia, the EPS is normal and all cultures are negative.

Although cultures of prostatic biopsy specimens in abacterial prostatitis are rarely positive, some patients with nonbacterial prostatitis and prostatodynia improve with antimicrobial therapy. Overall, antibiotic therapy in these conditions has been disappointing, as have all forms of therapy to date. In one report 86 per cent of patients with chronic abacterial prostatitis and prostatodynia treated only with stress management reported improvement or cure, suggesting a psychological basis for these conditions.

BENIGN PROSTATIC HYPERPLASIA

INCIDENCE. Benign prostatic hyperplasia (BPH) is a disease of advancing age; it is estimated that 1 in 10 men living until age 80 will require a prostatectomy for relief of urinary obstruction. BPH usually presents clinically after age 50, the incidence increasing with age, but as many as two thirds of men between the ages of 40 and 49 demonstrate histologic evidence of the disease.

ETIOLOGY. BPH is closely related to both aging and age-associated changes in circulating hormones. Circulating androgens clearly play a role; BPH does not develop in men who are castrated or lose testicular function before puberty. Castration causes atrophy of prostatic epithelium.

With aging, serum testosterone levels decline while serum estrogen levels increase, resulting in an increase in the ratio of plasma estrogens to plasma testosterone. It is unclear, however, whether these shifts in circulating hormone levels are directly involved in the pathogenesis of BPH. Androgens and estrogens seem to act synergistically in the development of BPH in the dog, estrogens increasing prostatic androgen receptors by two-fold. Levels of DHT are not actually elevated in BPH tissue, but enzymatic changes occur within the hyperplastic gland that would tend to favor the accumulation of DHT.

PATHOGENESIS. As the hyperplastic prostate enlarges, it compresses the urethra, producing symptoms of urethral obstruction that ultimately may progress to urinary retention. Urethral obstruction may cause incomplete emptying of the bladder, giving rise to urinary stasis, urinary tract infection, and bladder calculi. Furthermore, hypertrophy of the bladder muscle may cause hydronephrosis and bladder diverticula. Bladder neoplasms are more likely to arise in bladder diverticula, especially if the diverticula drain poorly and are chronically infected.

SYMPTOMS. Symptoms due to BPH are either obstructive or irritative. *Obstructive symptoms* include hesitancy to initiate voiding, straining to void, decreased force and caliber of the urinary stream, prolonged dribbling after micturition, a sensation of incomplete bladder emptying, and urinary retention. These symptoms result directly from narrowing of the bladder neck and prostatic urethra by the hyperplastic prostate.

Irritative symptoms include urinary frequency, nocturia, dysuria, urgency, and urge incontinence. These symptoms may result from incomplete emptying of the bladder with voiding or may be due to urinary tract infection secondary to prostatic obstruction. More commonly, irritative symptoms result from reduced bladder compliance as a result of prostatic obstruction. It is important to recognize that irritative symptoms may be caused by other conditions such as bladder carcinoma, neurogenic bladder, and urinary tract infection unrelated to prostatic obstruction. All too frequently, patients with irritative urinary tract symptoms are presumed to have prostatic obstruction without an adequate diagnostic evaluation, resulting in delayed and sometimes inappropriate therapy.

PHYSICAL EXAMINATION. Other than a distended bladder, the usual physical findings in BPH are confined to the prostate. Examination of the prostate should be performed with the patient in either the knee-chest position or bent over the bed with his chest touching his elbows. The examining glove should be well lubricated, and the index finger should be inserted slowly into the rectum to allow the anal sphincter time to relax.

The normal prostate, the size of a walnut, has the consistency of a pencil eraser. The hyperplastic prostate is variably enlarged, usually no more than two or three times normal, but occasionally exceeding the size of a lemon. The consistency remains rubbery but is somewhat more fleshy, particularly in the larger glands. Rectal examination affords only a rough estimate of prostatic size and should never be relied upon to rule out prostatic obstruction. A much more accurate anatomic appraisal of the prostate can be obtained with transrectal ultrasonography and cystourethroscopy. The rectal examination is, however, the single most valuable screening test for prostatic carcinoma. The entire posterior surface of the gland should be examined for areas of induration suggestive of malignancy.

DIAGNOSTIC TESTS. The most valuable test for documenting urinary obstruction is measurement of the urinary flow rate. Inexpensive flowmeters allow an accurate determination of the patient's voided volume and peak urinary flow rate, which can be plotted against the patient's age on a nomogram. A decreased flow rate per se is never an indication for prostatectomy, but, when used and interpreted correctly, uroflowmetry is an excellent physiologic test for prostatic obstruction.

An abdominal ultrasound examination is useful to rule out associated upper tract pathology, such as hydronephrosis, as well as to detect renal masses. Furthermore, ultrasound measurement of postvoid residual urine volumes and prostatic size is extremely accurate.

Cystourethroscopy, although often employed, may be misleading as a screening test for prostatic obstruction. An anatomically small prostate may produce significant obstruction during voiding,

while an anatomically large prostate may produce little or no obstruction at all. The place for cystourethroscopy is in making the decision about whether the prostate is small enough to be resected transurethrally or sufficiently large to require open surgical removal. Before proceeding to prostatectomy, a careful inspection of the bladder is made to rule out bladder diverticula, stones, and, most importantly, tumors.

A retrograde urethrogram may be helpful in evaluating patients with symptoms of BPH when a urethral stricture is suspected. Formal urodynamic testing including a cystometrogram may be indicated in patients with complex voiding symptomatology or a suspected neurogenic bladder.

TREATMENT. The most common treatment for BPH is partial prostatectomy. The indications for prostatectomy are (1) voiding symptoms that are troublesome to the patient; (2) urinary retention; (3) recurrent urinary tract infections caused by postvoid residual urine; (4) compromised renal function due to hydronephrosis from prostatic obstruction; (5) recurrent gross hematuria with no other explanation; and (6) urge incontinence due to prostatic obstruction.

A partial prostatectomy done for BPH attempts to re-establish a wide-open bladder neck and prostatic urethra by selectively removing all of the hyperplastic prostatic tissue down to the so-called surgical capsule, leaving the peripheral prostate intact (Fig. 223–2). This is accomplished either by transurethral resection or by open surgical enucleation of the adenoma, depending usually on the size of the gland. Adenomas less than 70 grams are usually approached transurethrally.

Transurethral prostatectomy (TURP) is generally regarded as a safe and effective procedure, but recent evidence suggests that it may be less effective than open prostatectomy in overcoming urinary obstruction and that TURP may be associated with higher long-term mortality. Alternatives to transurethral prostatectomy include (1) transurethral incision of the bladder neck, (2) balloon dilatation of the prostate, (3) treatment with sympathetic α-adrenergic inhibitors, and (4) antiandrogen therapy.

Transurethral incision is done by making one or two longitudinal incisions with an endoscope through the muscular fibers of the bladder neck and prostatic urethra to spring open the prostate and thus enlarge the caliber of the prostatic urethra. Transurethral incision can be performed as an outpatient procedure under local anesthesia, and operative time and blood loss are greatly reduced. Transurethral incision is probably as effective as transurethral resection in treating small prostates (< 20 grams) but appears less effective for larger, bulkier glands.

Balloon dilatation is done by inflating a balloon endoscopically within the prostatic urethra to a diameter of 90 French for 10 minutes at 4 atm. The pressure from the balloon compresses and may rupture the prostatic tissue, reducing urethral obstruction. Significant hemorrhage may occur infrequently, but morbidity is otherwise minimal. About 70 per cent of patients are improved symptomatically at 6 months; further follow-up is necessary to determine the long-term value of this procedure.

Sympathetic blockade relieves prostatic obstruction by inhibiting α-adrenoceptor–mediated contractions of the prostatic capsule, prostate adenoma, and bladder neck. Selective α_1 blockers, such as terazosin and prazosin, have fewer side effects than nonselective α blockers. Terazosin has the additional advantage of once-daily dosing. The response rate to these agents appears to be about 70 per cent.

Antiandrogen therapy relieves prostatic obstruction by causing atrophy of the prostatic epithelium. Prostate size decreases an average of 30 per cent after 3 to 6 months of therapy, but the prostate quickly regrows after cessation of therapy. Although there is a significant placebo effect on clinical symptoms, urodynamic improvement has been marginal in most studies.

CARCINOMA OF THE PROSTATE

INCIDENCE. Carcinoma of the prostate is rare before age 50, but the incidence subsequently increases steadily with age. Overall, it is the second most common malignancy in American men and the third most common cause of cancer deaths in men over 55 (behind lung and colorectal cancer). Carcinoma of the prostate is more common among black American men (22 deaths per 100,000 men) than white American men (14 deaths per 100,000 men).

ETIOLOGY. The etiology of prostatic carcinoma is unknown. The disease does not occur in men castrated before puberty and regresses following castration or estrogen therapy, but a hormonal etiology has not been established. BPH does not appear to be causally related. Environmental factors may be involved, since men migrating from areas where prostatic cancer is uncommon to areas where it is more common develop the disease with increased frequency. Oncogenic viruses have been detected within prostatic cancer cells, but a direct etiologic relationship has not been established.

PATHOGENESIS. Ninety-five per cent of prostatic cancers are adenocarcinomas, with the remainder being transitional cell carcinomas, squamous cell carcinomas, and sarcomas. Adenocarcinoma of the prostate usually arises in the peripheral region of the prostate (Fig. 223–2), although it commonly invades the periurethral tissue where BPH orginates, subsequently producing urethral obstruction. Prostate cancer may produce ureteral obstruction either by direct extension into the bladder or by spreading behind the bladder through the seminal vesicles. Distant spread occurs through lymphatic and hematogenous routes. Prostatic cancer most commonly metastasizes to the pelvic lymph nodes and skeleton, especially the pelvis and lumbar spine. Visceral metastases, which occur later and less commonly, most frequently involve the lungs, liver, and adrenals.

In its unpredictable natural history, prostatic cancer progresses very slowly in some men, who may do well for many years without treatment. In others the disease exhibits rapid metastatic spread leading to early death. In the absence of the ability to predict which patients can be followed conservatively and which require prompt treatment, we are obliged to treat patients with prostatic cancer aggressively, to the extent that an individual's age and general health permit.

SYMPTOMS. Early carcinoma of the prostate is asymptomatic. As the disease spreads into the urethra, it may cause symptoms of urinary obstruction indistinguishable from those produced by BPH. If the tumor has progressed to obstruct the ureters, the patient may present with uremia. Skeletal pain and pathologic fractures caused by metastatic disease may be the initial symptoms of advanced disease.

PHYSICAL EXAMINATION. The patient may present with lymphadenopathy, signs of uremia, and congestive heart failure, or in urinary retention with a distended bladder. More commonly, the pathologic physical findings are confined to the prostate. On rectal examination the prostate feels harder than the normal or hyperplastic prostate, and the normal boundaries of the gland may be obscured. Approximately 50 per cent of localized indurated areas within the prostate are malignant, with the remainder due to prostatic calculi, inflammation, prostatic infarction, or postsurgical change in a patient having previously undergone a partial prostatectomy for BPH. If induration is detected that is suggestive of carcinoma, the examiner should determine whether it is focal or diffuse in nature and whether it seems to extend beyond the border of the prostate.

DIAGNOSIS. The diagnosis of prostatic cancer is made with an accuracy rate of greater than 90 per cent by a transperineal or transrectal needle biopsy of the prostate. Alternatively, a transrectal fine-needle aspiration of the prostate may be performed for a cytologic diagnosis, although there is less experience with this technique in the United States.

Transrectal ultrasonography is also capable of demonstrating prostate cancers, which typically appear as hypoechoic lesions within the prostate (although some may appear hyperechoic or have mixed echogenicity). Although more sensitive than digital examination, transrectal ultrasonography is not sufficiently specific at present to be used as a screening test for prostate cancer. Overall, only 30 to 40 per cent of the abnormal lesions detected on sonography are malignant. Similarly, measurements of serum prostate specific antigen (PSA) are not sufficiently accurate to diagnose men with early prostate cancer. For example, 15 to 20 per cent of men with BPH have PSA values greater than 10 ng per milliliter (normal, <4.0 ng per milliliter).

STAGING CLASSIFICATION. The treatment of prostatic carcinoma depends primarily on the stage of the disease, as illustrated in the Whitmore staging system (Fig. 223–3).

Stage A prostatic carcinoma refers to tumors that are discovered incidentally on histologic examination of prostatic tissue that has been removed for presumed BPH. Stage A tumors are subdivided into stage A1 lesions, which are well- or moderately well-differentiated tumors involving less than 5 per cent of the removed tissue, and stage A2 lesions, which are either poorly differentiated or involve more than 5 per cent of the removed tissue.

Stage B tumors are palpable on rectal examination and are confined within the boundaries of the prostate. Stage B1 includes tumors involving less than one posterior lobe, and stage B2 includes tumors that involve one whole or both posterior lobes.

Stage C tumors extend beyond the boundaries of the prostate but are confined within the pelvis. These tumors have penetrated the peripheral capsule of the prostate and may extend cephalad into the seminal vesicles or laterally toward the bony pelvic sidewalls.

Stage D tumors are metastatic. Stage D1 tumors have spread to the pelvic lymph nodes, and stage D2 tumors have distant metastases.

STAGING EVALUATION. The treatment of prostatic carcinoma is predicated largely on the stage of the tumor; accurate staging is therefore essential. The digital rectal examination is valuable in assessing the local extent of tumor, but transrectal ultrasonography and magnetic resonance imaging of the prostate may be useful when the findings on physical examination are not definitive.

Enzymatic determination of serum acid phosphatase remains a basic screening test for metastatic prostatic cancer, with an elevated value being about 70 per cent sensitive and virtually 100 per cent specific for metastatic disease. Measurement of serum PSA appears of limited value in the staging of prostate cancer. Ninety per cent of men with prostate cancer have PSA values between 10 and 50 ng per milliliter, but values within this range do not distinguish organ-confined from more advanced disease. Conversely, PSA is extremely helpful in evaluating patients after radical prostatectomy. Since PSA is made only by the prostate, serum levels following surgery should be undetectable. A measurable level of PSA postoperatively is thus highly suggestive of residual disease.

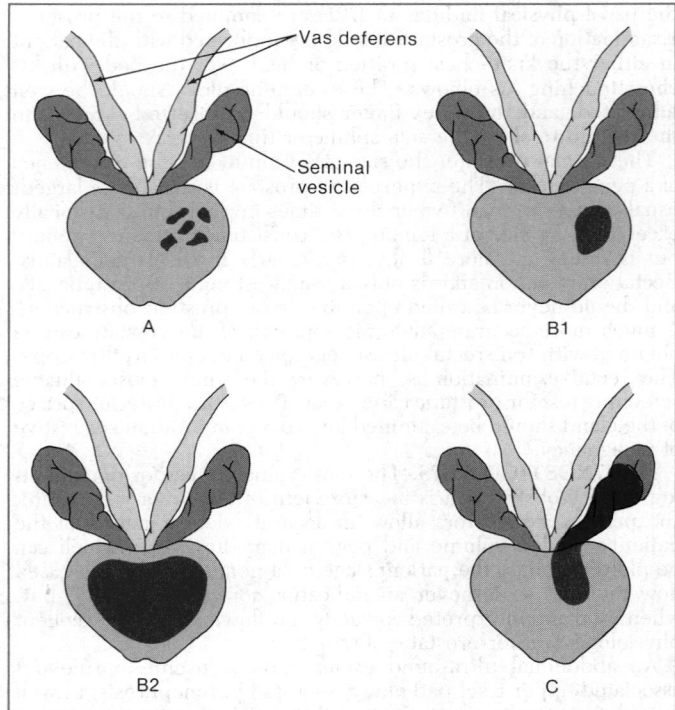

FIGURE 223–3. Whitmore staging classification of prostatic carcinoma. A = Microscopic disease in a clinically benign gland. B1 = Nodule involving less than one posterior lobe. B2 = Nodule involving one entire lobe or both posterior lobes. C = Extension beyond the peripheral capsule of the prostate. D (not pictured) = Metastatic disease.

The radionuclide bone scan is highly accurate and far more sensitive than conventional skeletal radiography in detecting osseous metastases. Pelvic lymph node metastases in prostatic carcinoma are more difficult to detect. Pedal lymphangiography does not consistently demonstrate the primary sites of lymphatic drainage from the prostate, which are the obturator and hypogastric lymphatic chains. Pelvic computed tomography scan has proved similarly unreliable. In patients with otherwise localized disease, a staging pelvic lymphadenectomy is usually done prior to performing a radical prostatectomy, either in conjunction with the operation, relying on a frozen-section evaluation of the lymph nodes, or several days earlier to allow a full histologic evaluation of the nodal tissue. Pelvic lymphadenectomy has a low morbidity and seems justified as a staging procedure to spare those patients with positive lymph nodes from a radical prostatectomy.

TREATMENT. Surgery. Patients with stage A1 disease have traditionally been treated conservatively, since the disease was thought to be latent and of no clinical significance. More recently it has been learned that approximately 16 per cent of untreated patients with A1 disease develop metastatic carcinoma of the prostate within 10 years. Thus, it may be advisable to treat healthy men under age 65 with stage A1 disease aggressively.

Patients with stages A2 and B disease require further therapy, since, untreated, many develop metastatic disease. The treatment options for these clinical stages include radical prostatectomy and radiation therapy. In radical prostatectomy the entire prostate and seminal vesicles are removed through either a perineal or a retropubic approach. The cure rate for patients undergoing radical prostatectomy for localized disease is excellent, with the 15-year survival rate for patients with pathologically confined disease equalling that of age-matched men without prostatic cancer. The major complications of radical prostatectomy are urinary incontinence and impotence. Recent advances in surgical technique, however, have reduced the risk of significant urinary incontinence to less than 5 per cent and have allowed preservation of potency in over 70 per cent of patients.

Radiation. Radiation therapy is administered either via external beam or via interstitial radioactive seeds that are implanted surgically into the prostate. Although the issue remains controversial, radiation therapy seems most appropriate in patients with localized disease who either are unwilling to undergo radical prostatectomy or are not surgical candidates for reasons of age and health. Radiation therapy also is the treatment of choice for patients with clinical stage C disease that has extended beyond the borders of the prostate and is therefore not curable surgically.

Endocrine. Hormonal therapy, the mainstay of treatment for patients with stage D disease, attempts to deprive prostatic tumors of circulating androgens and thereby produce regression of both primary and metastatic lesions. Hormonal ablation can be achieved either by castration or by administration of exogenous estrogens. Diethylstilbestrol (DES), administered at a dose of 3 mg per day, lowers plasma testosterone to castrate levels. Lower doses of DES may produce incomplete suppression of testosterone, whereas doses higher than 3 mg produce no further suppression and are associated with an increased incidence of cardiovascular complications.

Androgen ablation can also be achieved with luteinizing hormone–releasing hormone analogues that inhibit testosterone synthesis, used either alone or in combination with antiandrogens that block androgen action in the prostate itself. In the United States, the most commonly used analogue is leuprolide acetate (Lupron) administered in a depot form intramuscularly, 1 mg monthly. The most commonly used antiandrogen is flutamide (Eulexin), administered in a dose of 250 mg orally three times daily. These agents appear as effective as conventional hormonal therapy with estrogens or orchiectomy, but they seem to provide minimal if any survival advantage. Prostatic cancer is presumably composed of a heterogeneous cell population, some cells being hormone sensitive and others hormone resistant. Relapse following hormonal therapy is due to continued growth of hormone-resistant cells, and further attempts to lower serum testosterone provide no additional palliation.

Patient response to hormonal therapy varies considerably: 10 per cent of patients live less than 6 months, 50 per cent survive less than 3 years, and only 10 per cent live longer than 10 years. The timing of endocrine therapy also appears to make little difference in the course of the disease. Initiation of treatment at

the time of diagnosis may provide a longer symptom-free interval but little in the way of effective palliation once relapse has occurred. For this reason, it may be preferable to delay hormonal therapy until the patient has become symptomatic in the hope of providing increased long-term palliation.

Chemotherapy. Cytotoxic chemotherapy for carcinoma of the prostate has so far yielded discouraging results. A major goal for the future is to develop new forms of therapy that will be effective against the hormone-resistant cell population. The discovery of such agents will represent a major advance in the treatment of this disease.

Blaivas JG: Pathophysiology and differential diagnosis of benign prostatic hypertrophy. Urology 32(6 Suppl):5, 1988. *An excellent review of the physiology and diagnosis of BPH.*
Catalona WJ, Scott WW: Carcinoma of the prostate. *In* Walsh PC, Gittes RF, Perlmutter AD, et al. (eds.): Campbell's Urology, 5th ed. Philadelphia, W. B. Saunders Company, 1986, pp 1463–1543. *This chapter provides a comprehensive review of all aspects relative to the diagnosis and treatment of carcinoma of the prostate.*
Catalona WJ, Smith DS, Ratliff TL, et al.: Measurement of prostate-specific antigen in serum as a screening test for prostate cancer. N Engl J Med 324:1156, 1991. *This large study concluded that measurement of serum PSA levels is a useful addition to screening by rectal examination alone.*
Coffey DS: The biochemistry and physiology of the prostate and seminal vesicles. *In* Walsh PC, Gittes RF, Perlmutter AD, et al. (eds.): Campbell's Urology, 5th ed. Philadelphia, W. B. Saunders Company, 1986, pp 233–274. *An excellent review of prostate biochemistry and physiology.*
Fair WR: Managing prostatitis: Practical aspects of antibiotic therapy. Urology 24:1, 1984. *A symposium on etiology, diagnosis, and treatment of prostatitis.*
Fowler JE Jr: Bacteriuria and associated infections of the reproductive system in men. *In* Urinary Tract Infection and Inflammation. Chicago, Year Book Medical Publishers, 1989, pp 92–123. *An updated review of the etiology, diagnosis, and treatment of male genital tract infections.*
Gittes RF: Medical progress: Carcinoma of the prostate. N Engl J Med 324:236, 1991. *An excellent recent review.*
New approaches in the treatment of benign prostatic hyperplasia. Prostate (Suppl) 3:23, 1990. *A multiauthored review of alternative treatments for BPH.*
Walsh PC: Benign prostatic hyperplasia. *In* Walsh PC, Gittes RF, Perlmutter AD, et al. (eds.): Campbell's Urology, 5th ed. Philadelphia, W. B. Saunders Company, 1986, pp 1248–1265. *A comprehensive review of all aspects relative to the diagnosis and treatment of benign prostatic hyperplasia.*

224 THE OVARIES / 1355

224 THE OVARIES

Robert W. Rebar

The ovaries episodically release female gametes (oocytes or eggs) and secrete sex steroid hormones, principally androstenedione, estradiol, and progesterone. Oocytes are released only during the adult reproductive years when sex steroid secretion is also greatest, but the ovaries are physiologically active throughout life.

Sex steroids affect the growth, differentiation, and function of a variety of tissues and organs throughout the body; therefore abnormalities of the ovaries and of sex steroid secretion should be recognized by all physicians. A rational approach to the diagnosis and treatment of reproductive disorders in women requires an understanding of the functions of the ovaries and of their most important unit, the follicle, throughout life.

EMBRYOLOGY AND ANATOMY OF THE OVARIES

EMBRYOGENESIS AND DIFFERENTIATION. Prior to 6 to 7 weeks of fetal age the gonads are paired, undifferentiated gonadal ridges overlying the mesonephros. By the sixth week of gestation, the primordial germ cells have migrated from their site of origin in the yolk sac to the gonadal ridges. Beginning during the sixth to eighth weeks the ovaries rapidly differentiate, and the number of germ cells, now called oogonia, increases by mitosis to 6 to 7 million. The germ cells next undergo meiosis such that all germ cells (now called oocytes) are arrested in meiotic prophase by the seventh month of gestation. From midgestation onward the number of germ cells progressively decreases until the menopause, by which time virtually no oocytes

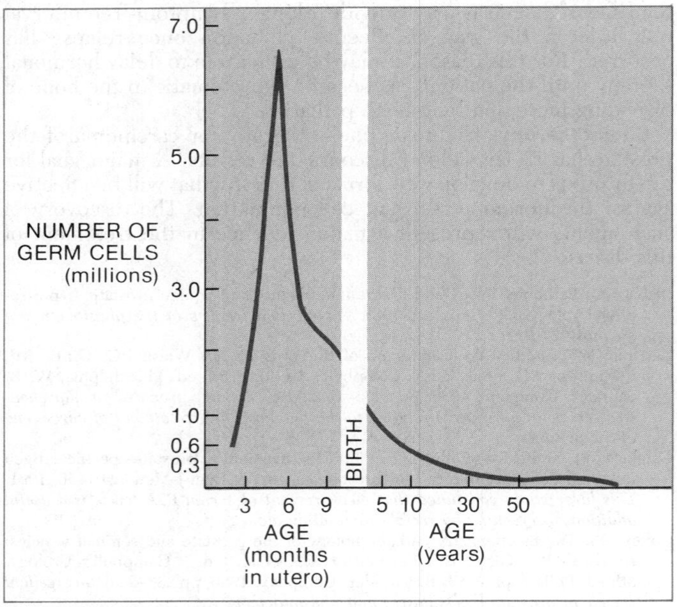

NUMBER OF
GERM CELLS
(millions)

[Graph showing number of germ cells (millions) on y-axis (0.3, 0.6, 1.0, 3.0, 5.0, 7.0) versus age. X-axis shows AGE (months in utero) 3, 6, 9, BIRTH, and AGE (years) 5, 10, 30, 50.]

FIGURE 224–1. The number of oocytes present in both ovaries at different ages. (Adapted from Baker TG: *In* Austin CR, Short RJ (eds.): Reproduction in Mammals. I. Germ Cells and Fertilization. London, Cambridge University Press, 1972, pp 14–45. Reproduced from Rebar RW: Semin Reproduct Endocrinol 1:169–176, 1983.)

remain (Fig. 224–1). Thus the human female is born with a finite and decreasing number of germ cells. The germ cells are eliminated from ovaries by *ovulation* and by *atresia* (degeneration), which accounts for the elimination of 99.9 per cent of all germ cells. The development of the ovaries is described in greater detail in Ch. 221.

THE ADULT OVARY. The adult ovary consists of two principal parts: a central medulla surrounded by the predominant outer cortex (Fig. 224–2). The entire ovary is limited by a single cell layer termed the germinal epithelium. The medulla contains the blood vessels and nerves as well as nests of steroid-secreting hilus or ovarian Leydig cells. The cortex contains the *follicle complexes*, composed of the *oocyte, granulosa cells,* and *theca*

cells. Characteristic changes occur in each component during follicle growth and differentiation. Interactions among the follicular components give rise to the gamete (ovum) and to sex steroid hormones necessary for establishing and maintaining early pregnancy following fertilization of the ovum.

Follicles can be divided into two major classes, nongrowing and growing. The nongrowing or *primordial* follicles comprise 90 to 95 per cent of the ovarian follicles throughout reproductive life of the female. The ability of a woman to menstruate and reproduce depends totally upon the pool of primordial follicles. Each primordial follicle contains a small oocyte arrested in meiotic prophase, surrounded by a layer of squamous cells from which granulosa cells originate. These cells are bounded by the basal lamina, which is selectively permeable to solutes in plasma. This complex is surrounded in turn by stroma, which consists of supporting connective tissue cells, contractile cells, and steroid-secreting thecal interstitial cells. Primordial follicles are recruited sequentially to become growing follicles, which then pass through primary, secondary, and tertiary (or graafian) phases. Atresia may occur in any phase.

Erickson GF, Schreiber JR: Morphology and physiology of the ovary. *In* Becker KL, et al. (ed.): Principles and Practice of Endocrinology and Metabolism. Philadelphia, J. B. Lippincott, 1990, pp 776–788. *A treatise on follicular growth and development.*

OVARIAN FUNCTION IN CHILDHOOD AND PUBERTY

PHYSICAL CHANGES AT PUBERTY. Puberty extends from the earliest signs of sexual maturation until the attainment of physical, mental, and emotional maturity. Pubertal changes in girls result directly or indirectly from maturation of the hypothalamic-pituitary-ovarian unit. Hormonally, human puberty is characterized by a resetting of the negative gonadal steroid feedback loop, the establishment of new circadian and ultradian (frequent) gonadotropin rhythms, and the acquisition in the female of a positive estrogen feedback loop controlling the menstrual cycle as interdependent expressions of the gonadotropins and ovarian steroids. In girls, pubertal development generally occurs between 8 and 14 years of age. The age of onset and the rate of progress through puberty are variable and depend upon genetic, socioeconomic, nutritional, physical, and psychological factors.

Physical changes occur in an orderly sequence over a definite time frame during puberty (Fig. 224–3). Breast budding in girls is usually the first pubertal change, followed shortly by the appearance of pubic hair, with menarche occurring late in pu-

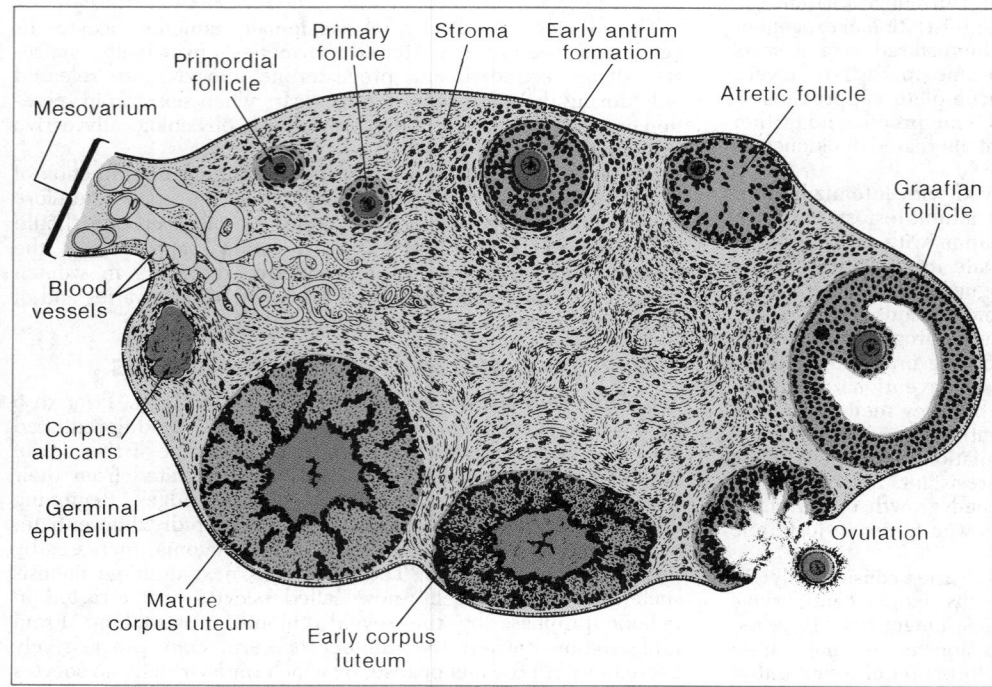

FIGURE 224–2. Diagrammatic illustration of the microscopic anatomy of the ovary. Changes in the components of the follicular complex occurring during atresia and ovulation are shown, progressing clockwise, from a primordial follicle (*upper left*) to a corpus albicans (*lower left*). (Adapted from Ross GT, Schreiber JR: *In* Yen SSC, Jaffe RB (eds.): Reproductive Endocrinology—Physiology, Pathophysiology and Clinical Management, 2nd ed. Philadelphia, W.B. Saunders Company, 1986, pp 115–139.)

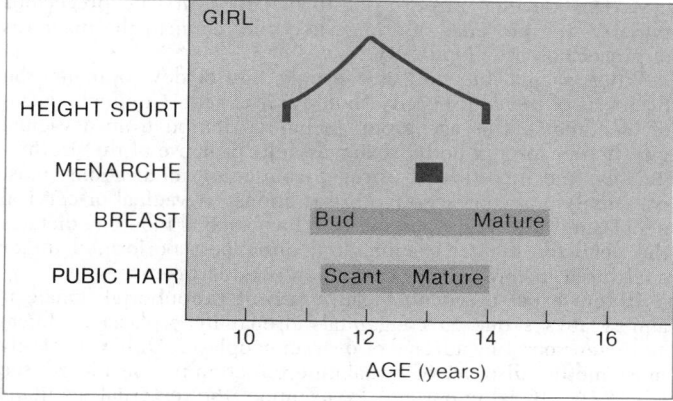

FIGURE 224–3. Temporal sequence of events for the "average" girl during puberty. (Reproduced from Rebar RW: *In* Yen SSC, Jaffe RB (eds.): Reproductive Endocrinology—Physiology, Pathophysiology and Clinical Management, 2nd ed. Philadelphia, W. B. Saunders Company, 1986, pp 683–733.)

bertal development. The time from breast budding (median age of onset 9.8 years) to menarche approximates 2 years. Breast development results from increasing ovarian estrogen production; pubic and axillary hair, from increasing ovarian androgen production. Estrogens are required for growth of pubic hair as well.

The ovarian sex steroids join with growth hormone and adrenal androgens to produce the adolescent growth spurt. Peak growth velocity is achieved relatively early with little growth observed following menarche. Lean body mass, skeletal mass, and body fat are equal in prepubertal boys and girls, but by maturity women have twice as much body fat and less lean body mass and skeletal mass as men, as a result of differences in sex steroid secretion beginning at puberty. Estrogens are necessary for normal formation, mineralization, and maturation of bones. Well-established standards exist for determining radiographically, typically by examining radiographs of the bones of the wrist, whether bone age is appropriate for chronologic age. Estrogen deficiencies retard and excesses advance bone age in relation to chronologic age.

HORMONAL CHANGES. The ovaries function even in early

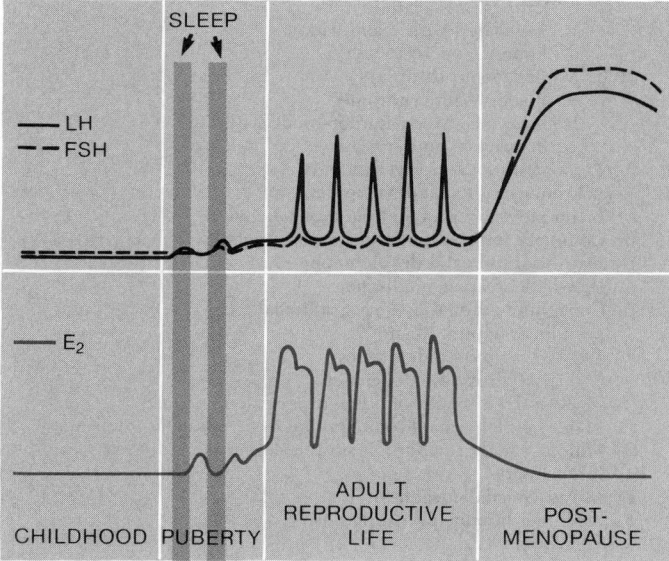

FIGURE 224–4. The changing patterns of LH, FSH, and estradiol (E₂) concentrations in peripheral blood throughout the life of a woman. The elevated levels of LH and FSH present in the first several weeks of life are not shown, nor is the fact that both LH and FSH are secreted in a pulsatile fashion. The pubertal period has been expanded to illustrate the sleep-associated increases in LH and FSH followed by morning increases in E₂ that are observed during puberty. (Reprinted with permission from *Endocrine and Metabolism Continuing Education Quality Control Program*, 1982. Copyright American Association for Clinical Chemistry, Inc.)

childhood. The low levels of luteinizing hormone (LH) and follicle-stimulating hormone (FSH), which are normally present, increase if the ovaries are removed prior to puberty, just as they do later in life, indicating exquisite sensitivity of the hypothalamic-pituitary unit to extremely low circulating sex steroid levels. As puberty nears there is a progressive decrease in sensitivity of the hypothalamic-pituitary unit to sex steroids, leading to increased secretion of pituitary gonadotropins, stimulation of sex steroid output, and the development of secondary sex characteristics. Increased secretion of both LH and FSH initially occurs at night with sleep and is associated with increased estradiol secretion the following morning (Fig. 224–4). As is true for most hormones, both LH and FSH are secreted in an episodic or pulsatile rather than a continuous fashion. It is possible that the sleep-entrained pulsatile secretion of gonadotropins commences in response to increased pulsatile secretion of gonadotropin releasing hormone (GnRH). Later in puberty, secretion of LH and FSH is increased, relative to childhood, throughout the 24-hour period, except during the early follicular phase when nighttime increases still occur. Basal levels of estradiol, the major estrogen secreted by the ovaries, increase throughout puberty. A "critical body mass" may be required for positive estrogen feedback and ovulation. During the first 2 years after menarche, up to 90 per cent of menstrual cycles may be anovulatory because of a delay in the synchronization of the hypothalamic-pituitary-ovarian axis.

ABERRATIONS OF PUBERTAL DEVELOPMENT

DEFINITION. Abnormalities of pubertal development can be divided into four major categories (Table 224–1):

1. *Precocious puberty* represents any pubertal changes before the age of 8 years. The precocious development is *isosexual* when the development is common to the phenotypic sex of the individual and *heterosexual* when the development is characteristic of the opposite sex. *True precocious puberty* is due to premature maturation of the hypothalamic-pituitary axis. In the absence of increased hypothalamic-pituitary activity, *precocious pseudopuberty* exists.

2. *Delayed (or interrupted) puberty* is defined as the absence of any secondary sex characteristics by the age of 13 years or of menarche by age 16 or by passage of 5 or more years from breast budding to menarche.

3. *Asynchronous pubertal development* occurs when there is deviation from the normal pattern of pubertal development.

4. *Heterosexual pubertal development* is development occurring at the appropriate time, but with some features characteristic of the opposite sex.

PRECOCIOUS PUBERTY. Differential Diagnosis. The temporal sequence in which the signs and symptoms of sex steroid hormone excess appear is most important. *Incomplete isosexual precocious puberty* indicates premature development of only a single pubertal feature. If breast budding occurs prior to the age of 8 years in the absence of any other development, the diagnosis may be *premature thelarche*. Premature thelarche is believed due to transient increases in estrogen secretion or increased breast sensitivity to the small quantities of circulating estrogens present prior to puberty. If pubic and/or axillary hair develops alone and persists, *premature pubarche* and *adrenarche* must be considered. These abnormalities are associated with slight increases in adrenal androgen secretion, but not with clitoromegaly or other signs of virilization. These syndromes require no treatment, and affected girls typically begin true puberty at the usual age.

When precocious development is isosexual, the purpose of evaluation is to determine if the cause is central (true precocious puberty) or not. Careful questioning of the patient and her parents may indicate inadvertent ingestion or absorption of sex steroids (iatrogenic or factitious). About 10 per cent of individuals with true precocious puberty have one of several organic brain diseases, including neoplasms, tuberous sclerosis, neurofibromatosis, encephalitis, meningitis, and hydrocephalus. The seriousness of intracranial lesions mandates that girls with precocious puberty have skull films and/or computed tomography (CT) of the brain. In almost 90 per cent of girls with true precocious puberty, however, no cause is identified (idiopathic or constitutional).

The physical examination may also provide critical information about the etiology of the precocious development. Cutaneous café au lait spots, facial asymmetry, polyostotic fibrous dysplasia, and other skeletal abnormalities, cranial nerve deficits, and multiple ovarian follicular cysts suggest *McCune-Albright syndrome* in a girl with precocious puberty. (At present it is uncertain whether the McCune-Albright syndrome produces precocious puberty through a central or a peripheral mechanism stimulating ovarian estrogen secretion.) Precocious development associated with short stature, congenital bodily asymmetry, a triangular facies, and clinodactyly suggests the *Silver-Russell syndrome*. Characteristic signs and symptoms may suggest the coexistence of primary hypothyroidism and precocious puberty, especially if galactorrhea is also present. In these patients, thyroid hormone replacement therapy will halt progression of pubertal development until the expected age of puberty. (Engimatically, primary hypothyroidism may also lead to delayed pubertal development. Thyroid hormone replacement will permit the onset of puberty.)

Abdominal and rectal examination may reveal a mass and suggest an adrenal or ovarian tumor. Because palpable ovarian cysts may develop rarely prior to ovulation in true precocious puberty, the presence of a mass need not confirm the diagnosis of precocious pseudopuberty.

When vaginal bleeding is the only sign of development, the diagnosis of sexual precocity should be suspect. Common causes of bleeding in this age group include irritation from a vaginal infection or foreign body, sexual assault, prolapse of the urethral meatus, and ingestion of estrogen-containing medications (most commonly oral contraceptive preparations). A vaginal or cervical neoplasm is also a rare possibility. Thus, vaginal bleeding dictates the need for vaginal examination, often best performed under anesthesia, before further evaluation is undertaken.

Heterosexual precocity in an apparent prepubertal female is almost always due to congenital adrenal hyperplasia or to an androgen-secreting adrenal or ovarian neoplasm. Only very rarely must another disorder of sexual differentiation be considered (see Ch. 221). It is important to examine the external genitalia carefully because congenital adrenal hyperplasia is usually associated with some degree of sexual ambiguity.

Excessive androgens produced endogenously by abnormal fetal adrenal glands in utero or diffusing across the placenta to the fetus from the mother can virilize the external genitalia and result in female pseudohermaphroditism. The extent of virilization varies from an enlarged clitoris only to sexual ambiguity sufficient to make gender assignment difficult.

Excessive maternal androgen secretion, typically from an ovar-

TABLE 224–1. ABERRATIONS OF PUBERTAL DEVELOPMENT

I. **Precocious development (before age 8)**
  A. Isosexual precocity
    1. Incomplete sexual precocity
      a. Premature thelarche
      b. Premature pubarche
      c. Premature adrenarche
    2. True precocious puberty
      a. Idiopathic (constitutional)
      b. Due to CNS lesions
      c. McCune-Albright syndrome
      d. Primary hypothyroidism
      e. Silver-Russell syndrome
    3. Precocious pseudopuberty
      a. Ovarian neoplasms
      b. Adrenal neoplasms
      c. Iatrogenic (estrogen-containing preparations)
      d. hCG-secreting neoplasms distinct from CNS and ovarian tumors
  B. Heterosexual precocity
    1. Ovarian neoplasms
    2. Adrenal neoplasms
    3. Congenital adrenal hyperplasia
    4. Other rare disorders of sexual differentiation

II. **Delayed pubertal development**
(no development by age 13; absence of menarche by age 16; passage of 5 years or more from breast budding without menarche)
  A. Anatomic abnormalities
    1. Müllerian agenesis or dysgenesis (Rokitansky-Küster-Hauser syndrome)
    2. Distal genital tract obstruction
      a. Transverse vaginal septum
      b. Imperforate hymen
      c. Vaginal agenesis
  B. Hypergonadotropic hypogonadism (FSH > 40 mIU per milliliter)
    1. Gonadal dysgenesis
      a. With stigmata of Turner's syndrome
      b. Pure (46,XX or 46,XY)
      c. Mixed
    2. Ovarian failure with normal ovarian development
      a. Autoimmune disorders
      b. Gonadotropin receptor and/or postreceptor defects (?Resistant ovary or Savage syndrome)
      c. Enzymatic defects (17α-hydroxylase deficiency, galactosemia)
      d. Physical causes
        i. Irradiation
        ii. Chemotherapeutic agents
        iii. Viral agents
      e. Idiopathic

  C. Hypogonadotropic or normogonadotropic hypogonadism (LH and FSH < 10 mIU per milliliter or LH and FSH 6–25 mIU per milliliter with at least one being greater than 10 mIU per milliliter)
    1. Isolated gonadotropin deficiency
      a. In association with midline defects (Kallmann's syndrome)
      b. Independent of associated disorders
    2. Neoplasms of the hypothalamic-pituitary axis
      a. Craniopharyngiomas
      b. Pituitary tumors
      c. Others
    3. Hand-Schüller-Christian disease (eosinophilic granuloma; histiocytosis X)
    4. Idiopathic hypopituitarism
    5. "Hypothalamic" forms of amenorrhea
      a. Psychogenic
      b. Exercise associated
      c. Associated with malnutrition
      d. Anorexia nervosa
    6. Miscellaneous disorders
      a. Prader-Willi syndrome
      b. Lawrence-Moon-Bardot-Biedl syndrome
      c. Primary hypothyroidism
    7. Constitutional delayed puberty

III. **Asynchronous pubertal development**
  A. Incomplete forms of androgen insensitivity
  B. Complete forms of androgen insensitivity

IV. **Heterosexual pubertal development**
  A. Polycystic ovarian syndrome
  B. Congenital adrenal hyperplasia (female pseudohermaphroditism)
    1. 21-Hydroxylase deficiency
    2. 11β-Hydroxylase deficiency
    3. 3β-ol-Hydroxysteroid dehydrogenase deficiency
  C. Male pseudohermaphroditism due to 5α-reductase deficiency
  D. Male pseudohermaphroditism due to partial androgen insensitivity
  E. Mixed gonadal dysgenesis
  F. Androgen-producing neoplasms
    1. Ovarian
    2. Adrenal
  G. Cushing's syndrome

ian or adrenal neoplasm, can lead to virilization of a female fetus. This occurs very rarely, because of the great capacity of the placenta to aromatize naturally occurring androgens to estrogens. Virilization of a female fetus is much more apt to occur if a pregnant woman has ingested a synthetic steroid preparation with androgenic properties, because available synthetic compounds generally cannot be aromatized.

Excessive androgen secretion beginning in utero is usually associated with defective cortisol synthesis. As a consequence, ACTH secretion is increased, resulting in congenital adrenal hyperplasia and excessive androgen secretion. The three different enzyme defects in the steroidogenic pathway that can lead to virilization of the female fetus are described in Ch. 221. 21-Hydroxylase deficiency is the most common form of congenital adrenal hyperplasia, accounting for more than 90 per cent of affected individuals. The defect may vary from partial to complete deficiency of the enzyme.

Diagnostic Tests. MEASUREMENT OF PEPTIDE AND STEROID HORMONES. Increased levels of immunoreactive human chorionic gonadotropin (hCG) may suggest a chorionic gonadotropin (hCG)-secreting neoplasm, most commonly an ovarian teratoma or dysgerminoma. In such cases, the hCG, which is antigenically and biologically similar to LH, stimulates ovarian steroid secretion and pseudopubertal development. Because even specific LH immunoassays show some cross-reactivity with hCG, values for serum LH may be elevated in individuals with hCG-secreting tumors. Immunoreactive hCG is always elevated in the presence of such tumors. Levels and ratios of FSH and LH typical of pubertal as opposed to prepubertal girls help in diagnosing true precocious puberty. Timed urine collections rather than blood samples can be used to measure gonadotropin secretion if necessary. Excessively high circulating levels of estrogen suggest an estrogen-producing neoplasm. High levels of serum testosterone suggest an ovarian source of excess androgen in girls with heterosexual development, while increased levels of dehydroepiandrosterone (DHEA) or its sulfate (DHEA-S) (the principal precursors of 17-ketosteroids) suggest an adrenal source. High levels of serum 17-hydroxyprogesterone imply congenital adrenal hyperplasia (CAH) secondary to 21-hydroxylase deficiency, whereas high levels of serum 11-deoxycortisol imply an 11β-hydroxylase deficiency. In CAH these hormone levels should decrease promptly following oral administration of suppressive doses of dexamethasone. Suppression in response to exogenous corticoids occurs much less consistently in individuals with adrenal cortical adenomas and carcinomas and rarely in those with ovarian androgen-secreting neoplasms (see Ch. 217, 221).

ADDITIONAL STUDIES. Ultrasonic scanning of the adrenals and ovaries and CT of the adrenals may be indicated to confirm clinical suspicions. In girls with ovarian or adrenal neoplasms the tumor can almost always be localized radiographically. Catheterization of the ovarian and adrenal veins and measurements of the effluent steroids from each gland should be pursued only when CT, ultrasonography, or magnetic resonance imaging fails to identify what is suspected to be a neoplasm. Although plain skull films are of use in screening for pituitary and parapituitary tumors, CT or MRI of the skull is indicated in the presence of definite neurologic deficits or if true precocious puberty is suspected. Radiographic estimation of bone age is indicated in all cases and serves as a useful tool to follow the results of treatment.

Treatment. Treatment for precocious puberty should be initiated promptly so that: (1) The patient's ultimate height is not compromised as a result of sex steroid–induced premature epiphyseal closure. (2) Emotional disturbances in the patient and her parents are prevented or attenuated.

Gonadotropin-releasing hormone analogues are now the preferred therapy for suppressing gonadotropin secretion and also may prevent bone maturation. The analogues are not effective in children with McCune-Albright syndrome. Medroxyprogesterone acetate (100 to 200 mg intramuscularly every 2 to 4 weeks) also may be used to suppress gonadotropin secretion. Medroxyprogesterone acetate, however, does not always prevent premature epiphyseal closure and the resultant short stature.

Individuals with CNS or steroid-secreting neoplasms must undergo therapy appropriate for the particular lesion. Girls with congenital adrenal hyperplasia are appropriately managed with glucocorticoids (plus mineralocorticoids when indicated) as outlined in Ch. 221.

DELAYED PUBERTY. Typically girls with delayed puberty present at the age of 16 years or later because of primary amenorrhea, but younger girls may present because of failure to initiate pubertal development. Because of the anxiety generated by delayed puberty, some evaluation is always indicated regardless of the age of the patient.

When pubertal development progresses normally but menstruation does not begin, an abnormality in the genital tract should be considered. Congenital malformations of the müllerian ducts are uncommon, occurring in 0.02 per cent of all women. Most do not cause amenorrhea, and many do not impair reproduction. The anomalies associated with amenorrhea vary in severity from an imperforate hymen to complete aplasia of all müllerian duct derivatives with vaginal atresia. Although aplasia generally involves all of the müllerian duct derivatives, defects may involve only a single part of the distal genital tract.

A müllerian duct anomaly is suggested by (1) normal levels of serum gonadotropins and steroids, (2) an abnormal outflow tract, (3) a history of cyclic abdominal pain with or without a palpable mass, and (4) normal development of secondary sex characteristics. Normal ovarian function still induces endometrial growth and shedding after menarche if the uterus is normal. In the absence of a normal outflow tract, however, the menstrual effluent is retained and may or may not be able to escape into the abdominal cavity. Free in the abdominal cavity, the effluent may cause endometriosis. Constrained to the uterine cavity, the effluent causes hematometra and a large abdominal mass. In the absence of a mass or cyclic pain, a karyotype is indicated in girls with evidence of an abnormal genital tract to rule out any of several disorders of sexual differentiation (see Ch. 221). Such disorders, however, almost never occur together with completely normal pubertal development. In girls with a normal karyotype and a genital tract anomaly, examination under anesthesia and diagnostic laparoscopy should be undertaken to delineate the extent of the defect. When the abnormality consists of an imperforate hymen or transverse vaginal septum only, surgical restoration can be accomplished relatively simply. Attempts to provide an outflow tract for the uterus should not be undertaken if there is no cervix because of the high risk of recurrent pelvic infection. Even with a functional cervix, the creation of an outflow tract that will permit successful pregnancy is unlikely. A functional vagina can be created surgically or by the daily use of ever larger dilators. To prevent shrinkage and scarring, surgery should be deferred until the patient is willing to use dilators postoperatively on a daily basis or she is about to become sexually active.

Other causes of delayed puberty and primary amenorrhea are the same as those that may cause amenorrhea in older women (see below). When no apparent cause for delayed development is found, constitutional delayed puberty must be entertained as a diagnosis of exclusion. A strong family history of delayed maturation adds support to this presumption. Small doses of estrogen may be administered to induce some pubertal development but may obscure a pathologic cause for the delay and may compromise linear growth and ultimate height.

ASYNCHRONOUS PUBERTAL DEVELOPMENT. Asynchronous pubertal development is characteristic of male pseudohermaphroditism due to androgen insensitivity, especially complete testicular feminization. This syndrome of androgen insensitivity is inherited either as an X-linked recessive or as a sex-limited autosomal dominant trait. Despite the presence of intra-abdominal or inguinal testes, there is complete failure of virilization. Affected individuals develop breasts (but only to Tanner stage 3) and a typical female habitus with unambiguous female external genitalia but with absence of internal female structures, generally having only a foreshortened blind-ending vagina. Little or no pubic and axillary hair develops. The karyotype is obviously 46,XY in these individuals. Circulating testosterone levels are equivalent to or higher than those found in normal men, and LH levels are elevated while FSH levels are normal compared to menstruating women. This syndrome is further discussed in Ch. 221.

HETEROSEXUAL PUBERTAL DEVELOPMENT. *Polycystic ovarian (PCO) syndrome,* by far the most common cause of heterosexual pubertal development, is associated with the development of some secondary sex features characteristic of males at the normal age of puberty. Feminization occurs in affected girls, and they develop normal breasts and a typical female habitus, but masculinization also occurs. (In contrast, girls with congenital adrenal hyperplasia generally show little if any female development at puberty.) A heterogeneous syndrome, PCO syndrome most typically begins at or near puberty with hirsutism and irregular menses from the time of menarche. Menarche may be delayed as well, so that young women may present with primary amenorrhea. Basal LH levels tend to be somewhat elevated in perhaps 80 per cent of cases, and circulating levels of all androgens are elevated moderately.

Congenital adrenal hyperplasia is generally diagnosed prior to puberty, and heterosexual precocious pseudopuberty is typical. However, if the defect is mild and changes to the external genitalia are minimal, masculinization may occur at the expected age of puberty. This attenuated or nonclassic form of 21-hydroxylase deficiency seems to occur in families with a strong family history of hirsutism. Affected girls generally have some defeminization with flattening of the breasts, severe hirsutism, relatively short stature, and obesity.

Mixed gonadal dysgenesis designates asymmetric gonadal development, with a germ cell tumor or a testis on one side and an undifferentiated streak, rudimentary gonad, or no gonad on the other. The extent of genital virilization prior to puberty is variable in this rare disorder. The vast majority are reared as girls in whom virilization occurs at puberty; some may note breast development as well. Affected individuals generally have a mosaic karyotype, with 45,X/46,XY being most common. Short stature and other stigmata associated with a 45,X karyotype in Turner's syndrome are less common in patients with tumors than in patients with testes. Gonadectomy is indicated in all individuals with a Y chromosome to eliminate the increased neoplastic potential of such dysgenetic gonads and in all patients in whom virilization occurs at puberty to remove the source of androgen. Estrogen replacement therapy is warranted following gonadectomy. Other causes of male pseudohermaphroditism associated with heterosexual pubertal development are described in Ch. 221.

An androgen-producing neoplasm or Cushing's syndrome may occur rarely during the pubertal years and lead to heterosexual development.

Marshall WA, Tanner JM: Variations in the pattern of pubertal changes in girls. Arch Dis Child 44:291, 1969. *A classic paper that is required reading for all serious students.*

Simpson JL, Rebar RW: Normal and abnormal sexual differentiation and development. *In* Becker KL (ed.): Principles and Practice of Endocrinology and Metabolism. Philadelphia, J. B. Lippincott Company, 1990, pp 710–739. *A detailed discussion of the disorders of sexual differentiation organized similarly to the discussion in this chapter.*

Styne DM, Grumbach MM: Puberty in the male and female. Its physiology and disorders. *In* Yen SSC, Jaffe RB (eds.): Reproductive Endocrinology, 2nd ed. Philadelphia, W. B. Saunders Company, 1986, pp 313–384. *A detailed and excellently referenced discussion of normal and abnormal pubertal development.*

THE NORMAL MENSTRUAL CYCLE

CHARACTERISTICS OF THE MENSTRUAL CYCLE. Between menarche at approximately age 12 years and the menopause at about age 51 years, the reproductive organs of normal women undergo a series of closely coordinated changes at approximately monthly intervals that together comprise the normal menstrual cycle. The menstrual cycle is the expression of the coordinated interaction of the hypothalamic-pituitary-ovarian axis with associated changes in the target tissues (endometrium, cervix, vagina) of the reproductive tract.

A menstrual cycle begins with the first day of genital bleeding (day 1; menses) and ends just prior to the next menstrual period. The median menstrual cycle length is 28 days, but normal ovulatory menstrual cycles may range from about 21 to 40 days in length. Menstrual cycles vary most greatly in length in the years immediately following menarche and in the years immediately preceding menopause, largely because of an increased incidence of anovulatory cycles. Irregularities in menstrual cycle length also may be caused by abrupt changes in diet, exercise, or environment; serious emotional disturbances; and following

parturition or abortion. The menstrual cycle can be divided into three distinct phases: *follicular, ovulatory,* and *luteal.*

The Follicular or Preovulatory Phase. Variable in length, the follicular phase begins with the first day of menstrual bleeding and extends to the day prior to the preovulatory LH surge. A rise in serum FSH begins in the late luteal phase of the previous menstrual cycle, continues into the early follicular phase, and initiates growth and development of a group of follicles (Fig. 224–5). The preovulatory follicle destined for ovulation is selected from this cohort in a manner that is not yet understood. Circulating LH levels rise slowly throughout the follicular phase, but FSH levels fall after the early follicular phase increase. Approximately 7 to 8 days before the preovulatory LH surge, estradiol (E_2) and estrone (E_1) begin to increase, generally reaching a maximum on the day before or the day of the LH surge. The divergence in LH and FSH levels may be related to the follicular secretion of *inhibin* (folliculostatin), a hormone that specifically inhibits the release of FSH. Several days before the LH surge, plasma androgens (androstenedione and testosterone) and some progestins (17α-hydroxyprogesterone and 20α-dihydroprogesterone) begin to increase. They peak on the day of the LH surge. Progesterone itself does not increase until just prior to the onset of the LH surge.

The Ovulatory Phase. During this phase the ovum is released from the mature graafian follicle 16 to 32 hours after the onset of the preovulatory surge of LH by the pituitary gland. The ovulatory phase extends from 1 day prior to the LH surge to 1 day following the LH surge. Some women experience brief (a few minutes to few hours in length), dull, unilateral pelvic pain near the time of ovulation, termed mittelschmerz. The association of this pain to ovulation is unknown, but it may be due to leakage of follicular fluid into the abdominal cavity at ovulation. Mittelschmerz may occur before or after actual ovulation or not at all

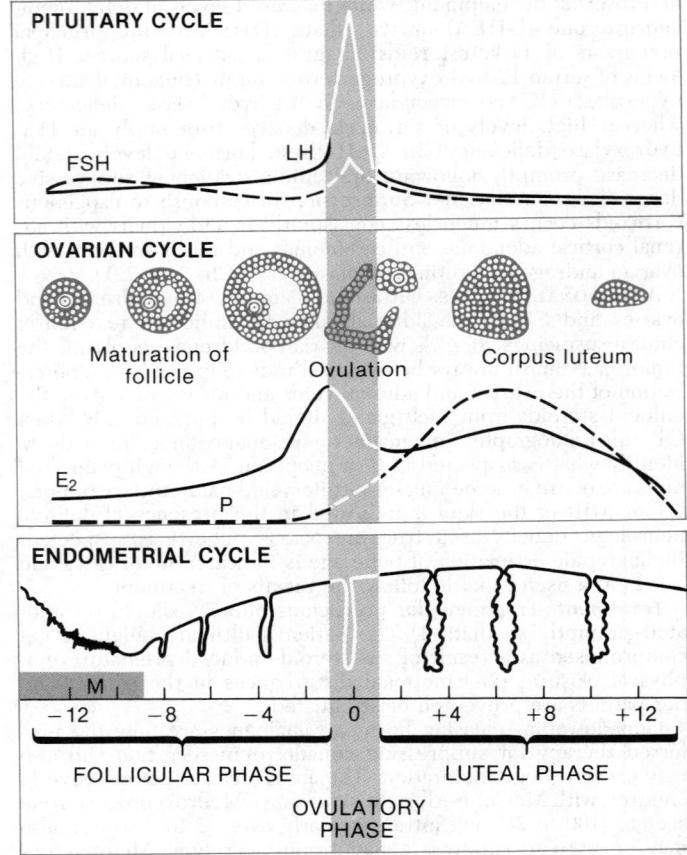

FIGURE 224–5. The idealized cyclic changes observed in gonadotropins, estradiol (E_2), progesterone (P), and uterine endometrium during the normal menstrual cycle. The data are centered about the day of the LH surge (day 0). Days of menstrual bleeding are indicated by M. (Reprinted with permission from *Endocrine and Metabolism Continuing Education Quality Control Program,* 1982. Copyright American Association for Clinical Chemistry, Inc.)

in ovulatory women. During the ovulatory phase a rapid rise in plasma LH results in response to positive estrogen feedback, leading to final maturation of the follicle and to ovulation. As peak LH levels are reached, E_2 levels drop, but progesterone levels continue to increase.

The Luteal or Postovulatory Phase. The more constant half of the menstrual cycle, the luteal phase, is approximately 14 days in length and ends with the onset of menses. This phase represents the functional lifespan of the corpus luteum ("yellow body") of the ovary, which supports the released ovum by secreting progesterone. In the luteal phase, progesterone secretion increases to peak 6 to 8 days after the LH surge. Parallel but smaller increases in 17α-hydroxyprogesterone, E_2, and E_1 levels also occur. Progesterone levels decrease toward menses unless the ovum is fertilized and pregnancy results. The finding of serum progesterone levels greater than 10 ng per milliliter 1 week prior to menses is probably diagnostic of normal ovulation. Progestins increase basal morning body temperature so that a "thermogenic shift" of more than 0.3°C occurring after a nadir is a presumptive sign of ovulation and progesterone secretion. Unfortunately, taking basal temperatures on a daily basis is tedious, subject to error, and not very reliable.

CYCLIC CHANGES IN TARGET ORGANS. Endometrium. During the menstrual cycle the endometrium undergoes remarkable histologic and cytologic changes, which culminate with menstrual bleeding when the corpus luteum ceases to secrete progesterone. The *basal layer of the endometrium*, which is not lost during menses, then regenerates the *superficial layer* of compact epithelial cells lining the uterine cavity and an *intermediate layer of spongiosa*, both of which are shed at each menstruation. Endometrial glands in these layers proliferate under the influence of estrogen in the follicular phase so that the mucosa thickens. In the luteal phase, under the influence of progesterone, the glands become coiled and secretory, with increased vascularity and edema of the stroma. As both E_2 and progesterone decline in the late luteal phase, the stroma becomes increasingly edematous, endometrial and blood vessel necrosis occurs, and endometrial bleeding ensues. Local release of prostaglandins may initiate vasospasm and ischemic necrosis in the endometrium as well as the uterine contractions accompanying menstrual flow. Thus prostaglandin synthetase inhibitors can relieve dysmenorrhea (menstrual cramping). Fibrinolytic activity in the endometrium also peaks at the time of menstruation, accounting for the noncoagulability of menstrual blood. Because the histologic changes during the menstrual cycle are so characteristic, endometrial biopsies are used to date the stage of the cycle and to assess the tissue response to gonadal steroids.

Cervix and Cervical Mucus. During the follicular phase, cervical vascularity, congestion, and edema increase progressively under the influence of estrogen. The external cervical os opens to a diameter of 3 mm at ovulation and then decreases to 1 mm. Cervical mucus increases in quantity (10- to 30-fold) and in elasticity (spinnbarkheit). "Palm leaf" arborization (ferning) becomes prominent just prior to ovulation (if cervical mucus is allowed to dry on a glass slide and examined microscopically). Under the influence of progesterone during the luteal phase, cervical mucus thickens, becomes less watery, and loses its elasticity and ability to fern. The characteristics of cervical mucus are useful clinically to evaluate the stage of the cycle and the amount of estrogen present.

Vagina. When ovarian estrogen secretion is low, as in the early follicular phase, vaginal epithelium is pale and thin. In the follicular phase under the influence of estrogens the epithelium thickens, and the number of mature cornified epithelial cells increases. During the luteal phase, progesterone causes a decrease in the percentage of cornified cells and an increase in the number of precornified intermediate cells and polymorphonuclear leukocytes. There is also increased cellular debris and clumping of shed desquamated cells. Histologic changes in the vaginal epithelium and in the cervical mucus are the most sensitive indicators of estrogen status in the body. However, the reliability of vaginal smears depends upon the absence of infection or exogenously administered steroid hormones that have antiestrogenic effects. Steroid hormones also facilitate progression of spermatozoa toward the ovaries and of ova toward the uterine cavity through effects on the fallopian tubes.

Ovary. A small primordial follicle with a diameter of 50 μm

transforms and grows into a mature graafian follicle 1 to 2 cm in diameter in two distinct phases: (1) The oocyte and follicle grow to form a *primary follicle*, apparently independent of gonadotropin control. The oocyte increases tenfold in diameter (from 15 to 150 μm) and becomes surrounded by a zona pellucida, a translucent "shell" of glycoproteins. In addition, the single layer of cells surrounding the oocyte becomes cuboidal and takes on the characteristics of granulosa cells. (2) In a second phase completely dependent upon gonadotropin and steroid hormones, the follicular unit develops into a *mature graafian follicle*, which is capable of being released in response to the midcycle surge of LH and FSH. Under the influence of FSH, granulosa cells acquire specific receptors for FSH, undergo mitosis, multiply to form secondary follicles consisting of several granulosa cell layers, and also acquire the ability to aromatize androgens to estrogens. Simultaneously, thecal interstitial cells begin to develop around the basement membrane surrounding the granulosa cells, develop specific cell membrane receptors for LH, and synthesize and secrete androgens, primarily Δ4-androstenedione and testosterone, in response to LH. The androgens can diffuse across the basement lamina where they are aromatized to estrogens. The rising E_2 in the follicular phase then feeds back on the hypothalamic-pituitary unit via the systemic circulation (Fig. 224–6). Just described is the so-called *two-cell theory*, which holds that both granulosa and theca are required for estrogen biosynthesis and maturation of the follicle.

A tertiary graafian follicle that contains an antrum or fluid-filled cavity increases from 200 μm to 1 to 2 cm in diameter, primarily because of accumulation of follicular fluid, again under the direct control of FSH. In tertiary follicles, FSH induces the appearance of specific LH receptors on granulosa cell membranes. These LH receptors are responsible for the stimulation of progesterone secretion prior to ovulation (luteinization) and for continued production of progesterone in the luteal phase.

Approximately 2 weeks are required for the presumptive preovulatory follicle to complete its growth and expel a mature oocyte. The oocyte is inhibited from resuming meiotic maturation by granulosa cell–oocyte interaction and an oocyte maturation

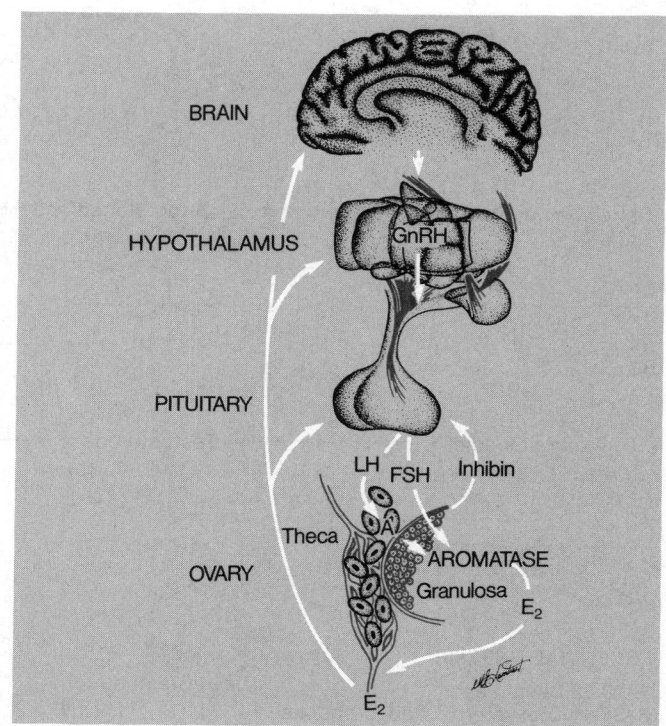

FIGURE 224–6. The hypothalamic-pituitary-ovarian axis in the regulation of follicular maturation and steroidogenesis. A = Androgens; E_2 = estradiol. (Modified from *Endocrine and Metabolism Continuing Education Quality Control Program*, 1982. Copyright American Association for Clinical Chemistry, Inc.)

inhibitor (OMI) until following the LH-FSH surge. Within 36 hours of the onset of the surge the oocyte completes the first meiotic division (reduction to 22 + X chromosomes) and a first polar body is extruded. The second meiotic division is completed only if the oocyte is fertilized by a spermatozoon. During the LH-FSH surge the preovulatory follicle bulges above the surface of the ovary. A stigma or avascular area develops on the follicle surface. Under the influence of local prostaglandins, plasminogen activator, and other hormones, a cluster of granulosa cells surrounding the oocyte and the oocyte itself (together known as the cumulus oophorus) are extruded.

The corpus luteum is formed from the granulosa and theca cells of the former preovulatory follicle following ovulation and secretes progesterone and E₂ for approximately 14 days. It then degenerates unless fertilization occurs. The lifespan of the corpus luteum may depend in part upon prostaglandins and prolactin as well as upon progestin. If fertilization occurs, chorionic gonadotropin (hCG), which is similar to LH, is secreted by the developing blastocyst and helps to support the corpus luteum until the fetoplacental unit can support itself. Pregnancy tests in common use have been developed utilizing antibodies to the specific β subunit of hCG and have little if any cross-reactivity with LH.

OVARIAN STEROIDOGENESIS. The ovaries and the developing follicles synthesize sex steroid hormones (estrogens, androgens, and progestins), which play important roles in ovulation and in preparing the uterus to accept a fertilized ovum via two separate pathways: (1) the so-called Δ^5 pathway, in which 17α-hydroxypregnenolone and DHEA with double bonds between carbons 5 and 6 are intermediates, and (2) the Δ^4 pathway, in which pregnenolone is converted to progesterone and in which 17α-hydroxyprogesterone and androstenedione with double bonds between carbons 4 and 5 are the alternative intermediates (Fig. 224–7).

Although cholesterol as substrate for steroid synthesis is obtained normally from circulating low-density lipoproteins (LDL), it can be synthesized de novo from two-carbon fragments (acetate). Different structures and cells within the ovary synthesize different steroids, in part because of stimulation by the gonadotropins. Gonadotropin binding to its receptor activates adenylate cyclase and stimulates cyclic AMP production. The cAMP in turn activates protein kinases that catalyze phosphorylation of proteins to mediate the cellular effects of each gonadotropin (see Ch. 208). LH also increases phosphatidylinositides within the ovary. LH

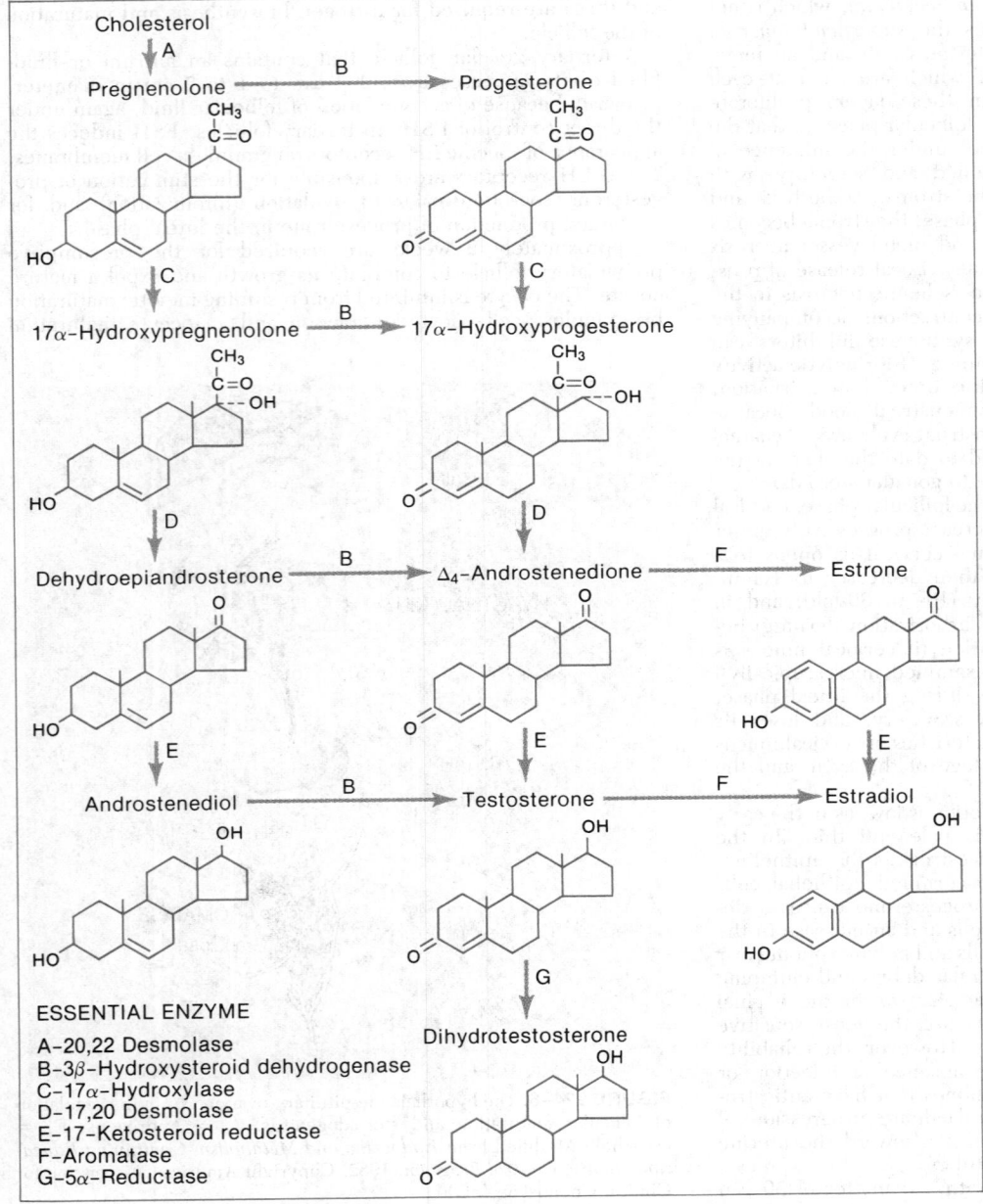

FIGURE 224–7. Steps in ovarian biosynthesis of steroid hormones. (Modified from data of Ross GT: *In* Rudolph AM (ed.): Pediatrics 16:1726, 1977. Copyright American Academy of Pediatrics 1977.)

ESSENTIAL ENZYME

A–20,22 Desmolase
B–3β–Hydroxysteroid dehydrogenase
C–17α–Hydroxylase
D–17,20 Desmolase
E–17–Ketosteroid reductase
F–Aromatase
G–5α–Reductase

acts primarily to regulate the first step in steroid hormone biosynthesis, that is, the conversion of cholesterol to pregnenolone. FSH acts to aromatize androgens to estrogens. Thus, LH acts to enhance substrate flow and the synthesis of androgens and/or progesterone. In the absence of LH, FSH action is reduced because of diminished substrate for aromatization.

Androgens, primarily androstenedione and testosterone, are secreted by interstitial and theca cells and serve as the substrate for the granulosa cell aromatase enzyme for synthesis of estrogens. Androstenedione, the major ovarian androgen, can also be converted to testosterone and estrogens in peripheral tissues. When ovarian androgen synthesis is excessive, as in ovarian androgen-producing tumors, or when conversion of androgen to estrogen in the ovary is reduced, as in PCO syndrome, hirsutism and even virilism can result. Testosterone, the most biologically potent androgen, is bound tightly to sex hormone–binding globulin (SHBG; also known as testosterone-estradiol–binding globulin, TeBG) so that only about 1 per cent of circulating testosterone is biologically free and active. Secretion rates and circulating concentrations in normal adult premenopausal women are given in Table 224–2.

Estrogens are produced predominantly in ovarian follicles by granulosa cell aromatization of the A ring of theca cell androgens. Naturally occurring estrogens are 18-carbon steroids, which by definition stimulate proliferation of the endometrium and bind to specific, saturable cytosolic receptors. The amount of estrogen secretion depends on the phase of the menstrual cycle (Table 224–2). In the early follicular phase the secretion rates of E_2 and E_1 are almost equal (60 to 170 μg per day). As the dominant follicle is selected, E_2 secretion increases to as much as 800 μg per day, with almost all the E_2 synthesized by the dominant follicle. The corpus luteum also produces significant quantities of E_2 (250 μg per day). In the late follicular and luteal phases, E_1 secretion is about one-fourth that of estradiol. The dominant follicle and corpus luteum synthesize about 95 per cent of circulating E_2; E_1 is of little significance in the ovulating woman. In the postmenopausal years, however, E_1 becomes the predominant estrogen in the absence of functioning follicles. E_1 is synthesized by peripheral conversion of adrenal androgens, especially androstenedione. As much estrogen is synthesized during the 9 months of pregnancy as would be synthesized during 100 years of normal menstrual cycles.

Progesterone synthesis is low in the follicular phase, but increases to 10 to 40 mg per day during the luteal phase (Table 224–2). Should pregnancy occur, progesterone production increases to as much as 300 mg per day at term. Why the corpus luteum atrophies at about 14 days is not known, but may be due to the effects of intraovarian estrogen and/or prostaglandins. However, LH stimulation is required for progesterone production by the corpus luteum. Progesterone induces secretory changes in the endometrium in preparation for implantation of the fertilized ovum.

NEUROENDOCRINE REGULATION OF THE OVARIES.

Neurons containing various peptide hormones that can release or inhibit secretion of the gonadotropins are found in the hypothalamus (see Ch. 212). Specifically, cells containing gonadotropin-releasing hormone (GnRH) occur in the area including the arcuate nucleus and median eminence and the preoptic area. Axons from these neurons run in the tuberoinfundibular tract and terminate on capillaries within the median eminence; this allows for delivery of their products through the portal vascular system to the anterior pituitary gland. It appears that classic neurotransmitters, including norepinephrine, dopamine, and serotonin, as well as neuromodulators, such as endogenous opiates and prostaglandins, influence secretion of GnRH by the hypothalamus. In addition, estrogens and androgens bind to cells in the hypothalamus and the anterior pituitary, and progestins bind to cells in the hypothalamus to influence hypothalamic-pituitary regulation of ovarian function.

GnRH is secreted in a pulsatile fashion (perhaps because of an inherent oscillator within the arcuate nucleus) and is responsible for pulsatile release of gonadotropins. Pulsatile gonadotropin release in turn appears to account for the pulsatile secretion of sex steroids from the ovaries. The ovarian sex steroids then feed back on the hypothalamic-pituitary unit to modulate both the frequency and amplitude of the gonadotropin pulse (see Fig. 224–6). Thus, gonadotropin pulses vary throughout the menstrual cycle. Pulses occur at approximately 60- to 90-minute intervals in the follicular phase and at intervals of greater than 180 minutes in the luteal phase.

Gonadal steroids can exert both negative and positive feedback effects on gonadotropin secretion. Among ovarian steroids, 17β-estradiol is the most potent inhibitor of gonadotropin secretion, acting on both the hypothalamus and pituitary. For women to ovulate, E_2 must also elicit a positive feedback effect on gonadotropin release. The feedback effects are both time and dose dependent. In the normal menstrual cycle the positive feedback action of E_2 leading to the LH surge is preceded by a period when lower E_2 levels are present with their negative feedback effects.

It appears that the ovary is the "clock" for the timing of ovulation, with the hypothalamus stimulating pulsatile release of the gonadotropins. The follicle complex and corpus luteum develop in response to gonadotropin stimulation. For appropriate ovarian regulation of reproductive function in women, three biologic characteristics are necessary: (1) an appropriate balance and sequence of negative and positive feedback actions; (2) differential feedback effects on the release of LH and FSH; (3) local intraovarian controls on follicular growth and maturation, separate from but interrelated to the effects of gonadotropins on the ovaries.

di Zerega GS, Hodgen GD: Folliculogenesis in the primate ovarian cycle. Endocr Rev 2:27, 1981. *A detailed discussion of recruitment and selection of the dominant follicle, summarizing a series of elegant studies.*

TABLE 224–2. CONCENTRATIONS, METABOLIC CLEARANCE RATES, PRODUCTION RATES, AND OVARIAN SECRETION RATES OF SEX STEROID HORMONES IN BLOOD

Steroid	Plasma MCR (liters/day)	Binding	Phase of Menstrual Cycle or Stage of Life	Plasma Concentration (ng/dl)	Plasma Production Rate (μg/day)	Ovarian Secretion Rate (μg/day)
Androstenedione	2000	Albumin	Premenopausal	40–240	3200	800–1600
			Postmenopausal	30–120	1600	
Testosterone	700	TeBG, albumin	Premenopausal	19–70	260	
			Postmenopausal	15–70	150	
Estradiol	1350	TeBG, albumin	Early follicular	2.5–6	70–200	60–170
			Late follicular	20–40	445–945	400–800
			Midluteal	15–25	270	250
			Postmenopausal	<1.0–2.5		
Estrone	2200	Albumin	Early follicular	2–6	70–200	60–170
			Late follicular	10–20	300–600	250–500
			Midluteal	10–15	240	160
			Postmenopausal	1.5–5.0	55	
Progesterone	2200	CBG, albumin	Follicular	3–10	700–2500	1500
			Luteal	10–25	3000–30,000	24,000

CBG = Cortisol-binding globulin; MCR = metabolic clearing rate; TeBG = testosterone-estradiol–binding globulin.

Erickson GF, Schreiber JR: Morphology and physiology of the ovary. In Becker KL (ed.): Principles and Practice of Endocrinology and Metabolism. Philadelphia, J. B. Lippincott Company, 1990, pp 776–788. A detailed discussion of ovarian function.

Rebar RW, Kenigsberg D, Hodgen GD: The normal menstrual cycle and the control of ovulation. In Becker KL (ed.): Principles and Practice of Endocrinology and Metabolism. Philadelphia, J. B. Lippincott Company, 1990, pp 788–797. A more detailed discussion of the control of ovulation than is described here.

Richardson GS: Steroidogenesis. In Sciarra JJ (ed.): Gynecology and Obstetrics. Vol. 5. Philadelphia, Harper and Row, 1986 (rev. ed.), pp 1–17. A detailed summary of the steroidogenic pathway.

ABNORMALITIES OF THE REPRODUCTIVE YEARS

DYSMENORRHEA AND ENDOMETRIOSIS. Dysmenorrhea, perhaps the most common of all gynecologic disorders, affects about 50 per cent of postpubertal women. Dysmenorrhea can be classified as primary or secondary.

Primary dysmenorrhea occurs only in ovulatory cycles. Prostaglandins that are released from the endometrium just prior to and during menstruation cause contraction of uterine smooth muscle and produce dysmenorrhea by initiating painful, exaggerated uterine contractions and myometrial ischemia. Associated systemic symptoms include nausea, diarrhea, headache, and emotional changes. Primary dysmenorrhea is much more common than is secondary dysmenorrhea.

In *secondary dysmenorrhea* there is a pathologic cause for the dysmenorrhea. Endometriosis, the ectopic occurrence of endometrial tissue generally within the abdominal cavity, is the most common cause in severe cases. Other possible causes include pelvic inflammatory disease, congenital abnormalities such as atresia of a portion of the distal genital tract and cystic duplication of the paramesonephric ducts, and cervical stenosis.

Prostaglandin synthetase inhibitors such as naproxen, ibuprofen, mefenamic acid, and indomethacin are the mainstays of treatment. If the dysmenorrhea is still severe, addition of an oral contraceptive preparation to inhibit ovulation and limit prostaglandin release is generally effective. In cases in which the pelvic pain still remains intractable, additional evaluation is warranted. If thorough evaluation of the gastrointestinal and urinary tracts fails to reveal a definitive cause, examination under anesthesia and diagnostic laparoscopy may be indicated.

If endometriosis is diagnosed at laparoscopy, treatment varies, depending on the severity of the disease and the goals of the patient regarding fertility. It may be possible to fulgurate implants or lyse adhesions through the laparoscope. In general, endometriosis should be treated medically, with additional surgery deferred until infertility (if present) becomes manifest. Medical therapy can consist of continuous suppression with GnRH analogues, progestins, oral contraceptive agents, or danazol for 3 to 6 months. GnRH analogues are rapidly becoming the most frequent form of medical suppressive therapy. After a course of therapy, use of oral contraceptive agents probably should be continued until fertility is desired. Conservative surgical resection of endometriosis at laparotomy should almost always be deferred until it is established as the cause of infertility. Surgery may be required, however, for continuing severe pain, severe endometriosis, or large ovarian cysts containing endometriosis (endometriomas). If symptoms continue despite adequate treatment or if psychological overlay is suspected, psychiatric evaluation may be indicated. Medical causes of dysmenorrhea, however, should be eliminated first.

PREMENSTRUAL SYNDROME. Premenstrual syndrome (PMS), also known as premenstrual tension (PMT), is a complex of physical and/or emotional symptoms that occur repetitively in a cyclic fashion before menstruation and that diminish or disappear with menstruation. Typically these cyclic symptoms are sufficiently severe to interfere with some aspects of life. Women with definitive psychiatric disturbances probably should not be included among those with PMS. More than 150 different symptoms are now thought to vary with the menstrual cycle (Table 224–3). Estimates of the prevalence of PMS range from 25 to 100 per cent. For most women the syndrome is merely annoying; it is likely that PMS causes serious difficulties for no more than 5 to 10 per cent. The diagnosis is best established by requiring patients to keep prospective daily records of symptoms over a 2- to 3-month period. Less than 50 per cent of women presenting with PMS are found to have the syndrome when such records are examined.

Most women seek help for PMS in their 30's after 10 or more years of symptoms. Many report that their symptoms began at menarche; approximately half state that symptoms began following childbirth. Severity and duration of symptoms are often reported to increase following each successive pregnancy, to become more severe with advancing age. Women with severe longstanding PMS almost always experience secondary psychological reactions, including social difficulties, such as marital discord, difficulty relating to their children, difficulty maintaining friendships, and withdrawal from social activities.

The etiology of PMS is unknown, but theories abound: alterations in the ratio of estrogen to progesterone in the luteal phase, alterations in α-melanocyte stimulating hormone (MSH) or β-endorphin activity, alterations in monoamine neurotransmitters, alterations in prolactin activity, increase in vasopressin secretion, alterations in mineralocorticoid secretion, alterations in prostaglandins, endogenous allergies to steroids (especially progesterone), reactive hypoglycemia, and many others.

Patients should be informed that no one therapy has been effective in all women and that none of the currently popular therapies has proved consistently effective. Still, women with mild premenstrual symptoms often benefit from simple changes in lifestyle, including addition of mild aerobic exercise each day; reduction in intake of xanthine-containing beverages, salt, and refined sugar in the day, particularly in the luteal phase; stress reduction; and adequate rest. Women with more severe PMS may benefit from treating predominant complaints symptomatically. Thus bromocriptine* (generally 2.5 mg twice a day) or danazol (100 to 400 mg daily in two divided doses) may be given continuously for relief of mastalgia, with the understanding that both may have unpleasant side effects. Prostaglandin synthetase inhibitors may help reduce dysmenorrhea and may benefit headaches. Mild sedatives and tranquilizers may help reduce insomnia and anxiety. Mild diuretics (especially spironolactone at doses up to 100 mg each morning) may be of benefit if cyclic edema can be documented by the presence of substantial weight gain in the luteal phase and by signs of dependent edema. The administration of 50 mg of pyridoxine per day has been urged by many as at least a harmless placebo, since it is a required cofactor in several enzymatic reactions, but, rarely, vitamin toxicity can develop when doses as low as 250 mg per day are given for a protracted time.

Since PMS requires the occurrence of cyclic ovulation, oophorectomy is sometimes considered for patients with particularly intractable symptomatology. Because GnRH analogues that induce a "medical castration" appear to have some effectiveness in PMS, the rationale seems valid. However, oophorectomy may create new problems related to estrogen deficiency for women with PMS treated in this permanent fashion.

Natural progesterone, particularly in the form of vaginal suppositories given at doses of up to 800 mg per day, has been used

TABLE 224–3. COMMON SYMPTOMS OF CYCLIC PREMENSTRUAL SYNDROME

Somatic Symptoms

Abdominal bloating	Constipation or diarrhea
Acne	Headache
Alcohol intolerance	Peripheral edema
Breast engorgement and tenderness	Weight gain
Clumsiness	

Emotional and Mental Symptoms

Anxiety	Insomnia
Change in libido	Irritability
Depression	Lethargy
Fatigue	Mood swings
Food cravings (especially salt and sugar)	Panic attacks
	Paranoia
Hostility	Violence toward self and others
Inability to concentrate	Withdrawal from others
Increased appetite	

---

*This use is not listed in the manufacturer's directive.

enthusiastically by many clinicians, but results of double-blind placebo-controlled trials have generally provided no evidence of efficacy. Likewise, the use of large quantities of multiple vitamins or of oil of evening primrose, containing the essential fatty acid γ-linolenic acid, a precursor of prostaglandins, is unsubstantiated.

Keye WR Jr (ed.): The Premenstrual Syndrome. Philadelphia, W. B. Saunders Company, 1988. *A simple multiauthored text detailing what is known about this disorder.*

Stillman R: Endometriosis. *In* Becker KL (ed.): Principles and Practice of Endocrinology and Metabolism. Philadelphia, J. B. Lippincott Company, 1990. *A succinct summary of this enigmatic disorder.*

ABNORMAL UTERINE BLEEDING. *Differential Diagnosis.*

The causes of abnormal uterine bleeding in the reproductive years include complications from the use of oral contraceptive preparations; complications of pregnancy (especially threatened, incomplete, or missed abortion and ectopic pregnancy); coagulation disorders (most commonly idiopathic thrombocytopenic purpura and von Willebrand's disease); and pelvic disease such as intrauterine polyps, leiomyomas, and tumors of the vagina and cervix. Clear-cell adenocarcinoma of the vagina or cervix may occur in women exposed to diethylstilbestrol (DES) during fetal life as a result of maternal ingestion. Affected women also may have congenital abnormalities of the upper vagina, cervix, and uterus. Because a history of DES exposure is not always obtained and because this malignant tumor may be fatal, clinical suspicion should remain high. Women with a history of DES exposure should be reassured, however, that the incidence of malignancy is extremely low. Trauma (postcoital or otherwise), foreign bodies, systemic illnesses including various endocrinopathies (such as diabetes mellitus, hypothyroidism and hyperthyroidism, Cushing's syndrome, and Addison's disease), leukemia, and renal disease may also present with abnormal bleeding.

Dysfunctional uterine bleeding (DUB), abnormal uterine bleeding with no demonstrable organic genital or extragenital cause (75 per cent of cases), is most frequently associated with anovulation. Postmenarchal bleeding in adolescents secondary to immaturity of the hypothalamic-pituitary-ovarian axis accounts for about 20 per cent of all cases, and premenopausal bleeding consequent to incipient ovarian failure constitutes more than half of the cases. Most anovulatory bleeding is due to either estrogen withdrawal or estrogen breakthrough bleeding. In anovulatory women, estrogen stimulates the endometrium unopposed by progesterone. As a consequence, the endometrium proliferates, becomes thicker, and may shed irregularly, especially if estrogen levels drop. Anovulatory bleeding tends to occur at less frequent intervals, while organic lesions tend to cause bleeding more frequently than cyclic menses.

Evaluation and Treatment. All cases of abnormal bleeding should be evaluated, including obtaining a thorough history with special emphasis on the amount and duration of blood loss. Prospective charting of the days that the patient bleeds may be required to evaluate the bleeding pattern. Complications of pregnancy or a bleeding diathesis must always be ruled out.

The physical examination (including the Papanicolaou smear) is normal in dysfunctional bleeding except for signs of anemia in the more severe cases. Laboratory tests should include a complete blood count, platelet count, coagulation studies, thyroid function tests, and fasting blood glucose. DUB must be a diagnosis of exclusion. Management of DUB depends upon the age of the patient and the extent of the bleeding. A sample of the endometrium should be obtained by biopsy or by dilatation and curettage from all women over age 35 and from those at increased risk of developing endometrial carcinoma because of prolonged anovulatory bleeding.

Even profuse bleeding in anovulatory women can almost always be successfully treated by administering one combination oral contraceptive pill every 6 hours for 5 to 7 days. Bleeding should cease within 24 hours, but patients should be warned to expect heavy bleeding 2 to 4 days after stopping therapy. If anemia and signs of acute blood loss are profound, blood transfusion may be necessary. If the bleeding continues despite therapy, curettage can be carried out. Recurrence can be prevented by giving the patient combination oral contraceptive agents cyclically for 3 or more months. If spontaneous cyclic menses do not resume and pregnancy is not desired, the patient can be treated with cyclic progestin (medroxyprogesterone acetate 5 to 10 mg for 10 to 14

days each month) or oral contraceptive agents. If pregnancy is desired, ovulation can be induced, as discussed subsequently.

Acute episodes of anovulatory bleeding also can be treated with conjugated estrogens administered intravenously (25 mg every 4 hours for up to three doses) until bleeding ceases. Progestin therapy (medroxyprogesterone acetate 5 to 10 mg orally for 10 days) should be started simultaneously. Withdrawal bleeding will occur after cessation of therapy, and the patient can then be treated with oral contraceptive agents for at least three cycles.

For individuals with anovulatory bleeding without an episode of profuse bleeding, treatment with cyclic oral contraceptive agents or progestin can be provided unless pregnancy is desired, in which case ovulation must be induced.

Speroff L, Glass RH, Kase NG: Dysfunctional uterine bleeding. *In* Speroff L, Glass RH, Kase NG: Clinical Gynecologic Endocrinology and Infertility, 4th ed. Baltimore, Williams & Wilkins Company, 1989, pp 265–282. *A detailed and logical approach to the treatment of abnormal uterine bleeding.*

AMENORRHEA. *Definition and Etiology.*

Amenorrhea is the absence of menstruation for 3 or more months in women with past menses (*secondary amenorrhea*) or the absence of menarche by the age of 16 years regardless of the absence or presence of secondary sex characteristics (*primary amenorrhea*). If an intact genital outflow tract exists and there is no primary disease of the uterus, amenorrhea is a sign of failure of the hypothalamic-pituitary-ovarian axis to produce cyclically the hormones necessary for menses. Amenorrhea is a sign of any of several disorders involving different organ systems. Amenorrhea is physiologic in the prepubertal girl, during pregnancy and early in lactation, and after the menopause. At any other time it is pathologic and demands evaluation. Use of the term *post-pill amenorrhea* to refer to women who fail to resume menses within 3 months of discontinuing oral contraceptives is inappropriate. Such individuals should be evaluated in the same manner as any woman with amenorrhea. Similarly, individuals with menses occurring at infrequent intervals of greater than 40 days, termed oligomenorrhea, should be evaluated identically to women with amenorrhea.

Clinical Evaluation. The patient with amenorrhea should be viewed as a bioassay subject in whom even subtle hormonal abnormalities may be manifested by obvious signs and symptoms. For example, breast development indicates exposure to estrogens, while the presence of pubic and axillary hair indicates androgenic stimulation.

Patients should be questioned especially closely for evidence of psychological disturbances, dietary and exercise habits, lifestyle, environmental stresses, a family history of genetic anomalies, and abnormal growth and development. Patients should also be asked about and examined for the presence of any signs of hyperandrogenism, including hirsutism, temporal balding, deepening of the voice, increased muscle mass, clitoromegaly, and increased libido, as well as for any signs of defeminization, including decreasing breast size and vaginal atrophy. Any history of galactorrhea, the nonpuerperal secretion of milk from the breasts, should be determined (see Ch. 226). A history of symptoms related to thyroid and adrenal dysfunction should also be sought.

The physical examination should focus on evaluating (1) body dimensions and habitus, (2) the extent and distribution of body hair, (3) breast development and secretions, and (4) the genitalia. In normal adult women the arm span is similar to the height, while in hypogonadal women the span is generally more than 5 cm greater than the height. The general appearance of the patient should be evaluated to determine if the habitus is that of an adult female. The distribution and quantity of body hair should be considered in view of the family history. The extent of any hirsutism (increased sexually stimulated terminal hair; see Ch. 225) should be recorded, preferably by photographs. Other signs of virilization should be sought carefully. Breast development should be graded according to the method of Tanner (Table 224–4). Breast secretion should be sought by applying pressure to the breasts while the patient is seated. Any secretion should be examined microscopically for the presence of perfectly round fat globules of varying size, which are always present in milk and indicate galactorrhea. Finally, the female genitalia should be examined carefully because they are such sensitive indicators of

TABLE 224–4. CRITERIA FOR DISTINGUISHING TANNER STAGES 1 TO 5 DURING PUBERTAL MATURATION

Tanner Stage	Breast	Pubic Hair
1 (Prepubertal)	No palpable glandular tissue or pigmentation of areola; elevation of areola only	No pubic hair; short, fine vellous hair only
2	Glandular tissue palpable with elevation of breast and areola together as a small mound; areolar diameter increased	Sparse, long, pigmented terminal hair chiefly along the labia majora
3	Further enlargement without separation of breast and areola; although more darkly pigmented, areola still pale and immature; nipple generally at or above midplane of breast tissue when individual is seated upright	Dark, coarse, curly hair extending sparsely over mons
4	Secondary mound of areola and papilla above breast	Adult-type hair, abundant but limited to mons and labia
5 (Adult)	Recession of areola to contour of breast; development of Montgomery's glands and ducts on areola; further pigmentation of areola; nipple generally below midplane of breast tissue when individual is seated upright; maturation independent of breast size	Adult-type hair in quantity and distribution; spread to inner aspects of the thighs in most racial groups

Data from Ross GT: Disorders of the ovary and female reproductive tract. *In* Wilson JD, Foster DW (eds.): Textbook of Endocrinology, 7th ed. Philadelphia, W. B. Saunders Company, 1985, pp 206–258; Speroff L, Glass RH, Kase N: Clinical Gynecologic Endocrinology and Infertility, 3rd ed. Baltimore, Williams & Wilkins Company, 1983, p 377; and Kustin J, Rebar RW: Menstrual disorders in the adolescent age group. Primary Care 14:139–166, 1987.

hormonal milieu. The Tanner stage of pubic hair development should be noted (Table 224–4). Since the sensitivity of the genitalia to androgens decreases onward from early in fetal development, the extent of any virilization is important. Fusion of the labia and enlargement of the clitoris with or without formation of a penile urethra are observed in women exposed to androgens during the first 3 months of fetal development (see Ch. 221). Significant clitoromegaly in the absence of other signs of sexual ambiguity and in the presence of other signs of virilization requires marked androgenic stimulation and strongly implicates an androgen-secreting neoplasm in the absence of a history of ingestion of exogenous steroids. The development of the labia minora in postpubertal women indicates the influence of estrogens. Overt anomalies of the distal genital tract and especially any evidence of obstruction to the escape of menstrual blood should be sought in the remainder of the pelvic examination. The vaginal mucosa and the cervical mucus are exquisitely sensitive to estrogen. Under the influence of estrogen the vaginal mucosa changes during sexual maturation from a tissue with a shiny, bright red appearance with sparse, thin secretions to a dull, gray-pink rugated surface with copious, thick secretions.

The history and physical examination quickly differentiate among several causes of amenorrhea, regardless of the age of the patient (Table 224–5). The various disorders of sexual differentiation and the other peripheral causes are often apparent on inspection. Distal genital tract obstruction should be identified at the time of pelvic examination even if the specific abnormality is not obvious. The physical stigmata of Turner's syndrome, discussed subsequently, generally make the diagnosis simple. Any sexual ambiguity indicates the need for chromosomal analysis and the measurement of 17-α-hydroxyprogesterone to rule out congenital adrenal hyperplasia. Pregnancy and gestational trophoblastic disease may be suspected and confirmed by measuring circulating concentrations of hCG. The possibility of intrauterine

TABLE 224–5. CAUSES OF AMENORRHEA

Disorders of sexual differentiation
Distal genital tract obstruction (müllerian agenesis and dysgenesis)
Gonadal dysgenesis
Ambiguity of external genitalia (male and female pseudohermaphroditism)

Other peripheral causes
Pregnancy
Gestational trophoblastic disease
Amenorrhea traumatica (Asherman's syndrome)

Chronic anovulation or ovarian failure
Degree of sexual development
Galactorrhea
Evidence of androgen excess
Evidence suggestive of adrenal or thyroid dysfunction

synechiae or adhesions (Asherman's syndrome) must be considered in individuals developing amenorrhea following curettage or endometritis. Tuberculous endometritis, especially in younger women, may also lead to this disorder. Without hormonal measurements it may be impossible to distinguish among individuals with chronic anovulation, in whom hypothalamic-pituitary-ovarian function is insufficiently coordinated to produce cyclic ovulation, and those with ovarian failure, in whom in most cases the ovaries are devoid of oocytes. Still, it is generally possible to form some strong clinical impressions about the etiology of the amenorrhea. It can be noted if the patient has absence of, incomplete, or complete development of secondary sex characteristics. The presence of excess body hair or galactorrhea may provide clinical evidence of the pathogenesis of the amenorrhea. Signs and symptoms of adrenal or thyroid dysfunction may be important as well.

The administration of a progestin has been advocated to assess the level of endogenous estrogen. This test is of limited value, however, because almost half the young women with premature ovarian failure experience withdrawal bleeding in response to progestin.

To ascertain if the outflow tract is intact, an orally active estrogen, such as 2.5 mg conjugated estrogen daily for 21 days with 5 to 10 mg of oral medroxyprogesterone acetate for the last 5 to 10 days, may be administered. Withdrawal bleeding should occur if the endometrium is normal. Still, hysterosalpingography and hysteroscopy may be required to diagnose Asherman's syndrome because some patients do continue to have some withdrawal bleeding.

Laboratory Evaluation. Basal levels of FSH, prolactin, and TSH should be measured in all amenorrheic and oligomenorrheic women to confirm the clinical impression (Fig. 224–8).

Increased TSH levels with or without increased levels of prolactin imply primary hypothyroidism, and further evaluation for this disorder is indicated (see Ch. 216). Although hypothyroidism commonly results in anovulation, amenorrhea occurs in only some hypothyroid women. Menorrhagia and oligomenorrhea may occur as well. The newly available very sensitive immunoassays for TSH permit identification of women with hyperthyroidism as well because TSH levels are suppressed in those individuals.

If the prolactin concentration is increased (typically greater than 20 to 30 ng per milliliter) and the TSH level is normal (generally less than 5 μU per milliliter), measurement of the prolactin concentration in the basal state should be repeated before more extensive evaluation is undertaken. This is the case because prolactin levels are increased by nonspecific stressful stimuli, sleep, and food ingestion. Prolactin levels may be elevated in as many as one third of women with amenorrhea. Evaluation of galactorrhea and hyperprolactinemia is detailed in Ch. 226.

Increased FSH levels (generally greater than 40 milli International Units [mIU] per milliliter) imply ovarian failure and require further evaluation. Chromosomal evaluation is indicated in all individuals with elevated FSH levels who are under the age of 30 years at the time the amenorrhea begins.

If prolactin and TSH concentrations are within normal ranges and FSH levels are low or normal, the measurement of total testosterone levels is indicated whether or not there is any evidence of hirsutism or virilization. Hyperandrogenic women need not be hirsute because some have relative insensitivity of the hair follicles to androgens. Mildly increased levels of testosterone (and perhaps DHEA-S as well) suggest PCO syndrome. However, total circulating androgen levels are rarely not elevated because of the alterations in metabolic clearance rate and SHBG that are present in PCO syndrome. Circulating levels of LH and FSH may aid in differentiating PCO syndrome from hypothalamic-pituitary dysfunction. LH levels are frequently elevated in PCO syndrome such that the ratio of LH to FSH is increased; however, LH levels may be identical to those observed in normal women in the follicular phase. In contrast, levels of LH and FSH are normal or slightly reduced in hypothalamic-pituitary dysfunction. There is some overlap between women with "PCO-like" disorders and those with hypothalamic-pituitary dysfunction. Radiographic assessment of the sella turcica is indicated in all amenorrheic women in whom both LH and FSH levels are very low (both less than 10 mIU per milliliter) to exclude a pituitary or parapituitary neoplasm. Other pituitary functions should be evaluated in any individual with significantly impaired LH and FSH secretion, as detailed subsequently. Both total testosterone and DHEA-S levels should be measured in hirsute or virilized women. Testosterone levels of greater than 200 ng per deciliter should lead to investigation for an androgen-producing neoplasm, most likely of ovarian origin. DHEA-S levels greater than 7.0 μg per milliliter should lead to evaluation for an adrenal neoplasm, and DHEA-S levels between 5.0 and 7.0 μg per milliliter should lead to evaluation for "adult-onset" congenital adrenal hyperplasia (see Ch. 221).

Hypergonadotropic Amenorrhea (Presumptive Ovarian Failure).

DIFFERENTIAL DIAGNOSIS. Gonadal failure may begin at any time during embryonic or postnatal development and may result from many causes (Table 224–6). Normally the ovaries fail at menopause when virtually no functioning follicles remain. However, premature loss of oocytes prior to age 40 may occur and lead to premature ovarian failure, possibly from abnormalities in the recruitment and selection of oocytes. Since FSH is the principal regulator of folliculogenesis, it would seem that most causes of premature ovarian failure may somehow involve FSH secretion or action. Circulating gonadotropin levels increase whenever ovarian failure occurs, because of decreased negative estrogen feedback to the hypothalamic-pituitary unit.

Genetic Abnormalities. Several pathologic conditions with dys-genetic gonads have elevated gonadotropin levels and amenorrhea. The term *gonadal dysgenesis* refers to individuals with undifferentiated streak gonads without any association with either extragonadal stigmata or sex chromosomal aberrations. Because individuals with gonadal dysgenesis have the normal complement of oocytes at 20 weeks of fetal age but virtually none by birth, this disorder is a form of premature ovarian failure.

Turner's syndrome describes patients with streak gonads composed of fibrous stroma and four cardinal features: (1) a female phenotype, (2) sexual infantilism, (3) short stature, and (4) several physical abnormalities, sometimes including a webbed neck, low-set ears, multiple pigmented nevi, double eyelashes, micrognathia, epicanthal folds, shieldlike chest with microthelia, short fourth metacarpals, an increased carrying angle to the arms, and certain renal and cardiovascular defects (most commonly coarctation of the aorta and aortic stenosis). The diagnosis can sometimes be made at birth because of unexplained lymphedema of the hands and feet. The syndrome is associated with an abnormality of sex chromosome number, morphology, or both. Most commonly the second sex chromosome is absent (45,X). This is the single most common chromosomal disorder in humans, but more than 95 per cent of such fetuses are aborted so that the incidence in newborns is approximately 1 in 3000 to 5000. Chromosomal breakage and mosaicism occur frequently as well. In mosaic individuals with a normal 46,XX cell line, sufficient follicles may persist postnatally to initiate pubertal changes and to cause ovulation so that pregnancy is possible.

Pure gonadal dysgenesis is the term given to phenotypically female individuals with streak gonads who are of normal stature and have none of the physical stigmata associated with Turner's syndrome. Such individuals have either a 46,XX or 46,XY karyotype. The 46,XX defect may be inherited as an autosomal recessive, with 10 per cent having associated nerve deafness. The 46,XY defect may be inherited as an X-linked recessive, with clitoromegaly occurring in 10 to 15 per cent and gonadal tumors developing in 25 per cent if the gonads are not removed.

Trisomy X (46,XXX karyotype) is also associated with premature menopause, while many such individuals actually have normal reproductive lives. Premature menopause can also occur in mosaic individuals with cell lines with excess X chromosomes. When gonadal abnormalities occur in women with excess X chromosomes, they seem to occur after ovarian differentiation so that some ovarian function is possible. Only later in life do such women develop secondary amenorrhea and premature ovarian failure.

OTHER CAUSES. *Physical, Chemical, and Infectious Causes.* Irradiation and chemotherapeutic agents, especially alkylating

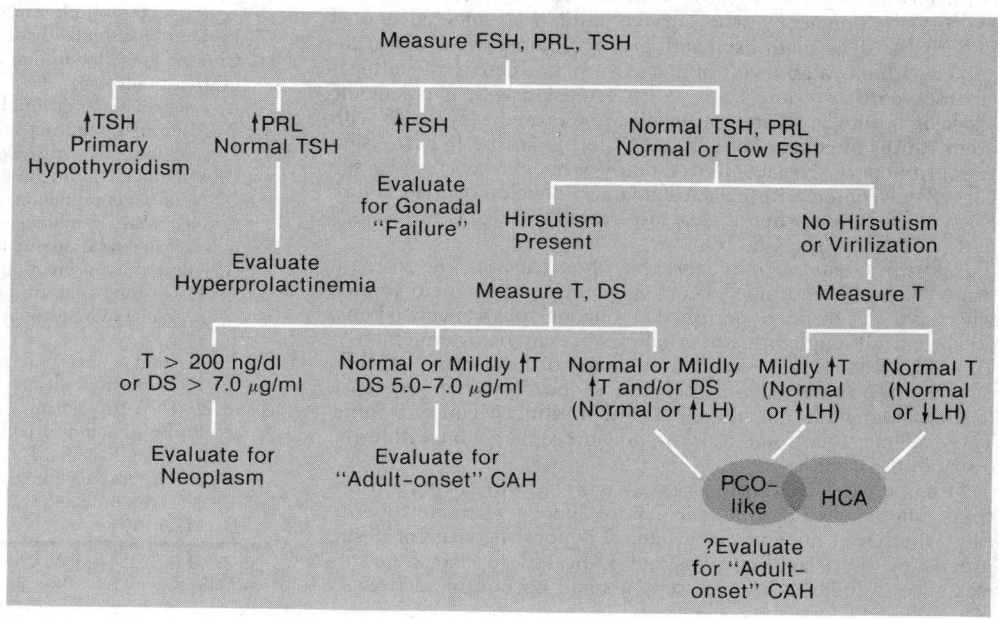

FIGURE 224–8. Biochemical evaluation of amenorrhea. This schema must be considered as an adjunct to the clinical evaluation of the patient. See text for details. **Abbreviations:** FSH = follicle-stimulating hormone; PRL = prolactin; TSH = thyroid-stimulating hormone; T = testosterone; DS = dehydroepiandrosterone sulfate; LH = luteinizing hormone; PCO-like = polycystic ovarian-like; HCA = hypothalamic chronic anovulation; CAH = congenital adrenal hyperplasia.

TABLE 224–6. CLASSIFICATION OF HYPERGONADOTROPIC AMENORRHEA (FSH > 40 mIU PER MILLILITER)

I. Menopause
II. Genetic abnormalities
   A. Genetically reduced cell endowment
   B. Accelerated atresia
   C. Gonadal dysgenesis
      1. With stigmata of Turner's syndrome (45,X)
      2. Pure (46,XX or 46,XY)
      3. Mixed
   D. Trisomy X with or without chromosomal mosaicism
   E. In association with myotonia dystrophica
III. Physical causes
   A. Gonadal irradiation
   B. Chemotherapeutic (especially alkylating) agents
   C. Viral agents
   D. Surgical extirpation
IV. Autoimmune disorders
   A. Polyglandular, involving ovarian failure and any combination of thyroiditis, hypoadrenalism, hypoparathyroidism, diabetes mellitus, myasthenia gravis, vitiligo, mucocutaneous candidiasis, and pernicious anemia
   B. Isolated ovarian failure
V. Enzymatic defects
   A. 17α-Hydroxylase deficiency
   B. Galactosemia
VI. Defective gonadotropin secretion and/or action
   A. Resistant ovary or Savage syndrome
   B. Secretion of biologically inactive forms
   C. α or β subunit defects
VII. Congenital thymic aplasia
VIII. Circulating gonadotropin antibodies
IX. Idiopathic premature ovarian failure

agents, utilized to treat various malignant diseases also may cause premature ovarian failure. Ovulation and cyclic menses return in some of these patients even after prolonged intervals of hypergonadotropic amenorrhea associated with signs and symptoms of profound hypoestrogenism. Rarely, mumps affects the ovaries and causes ovarian failure.

Autoimmune Disorders. Premature ovarian failure may occur in conjunction with a variety of autoimmune disorders. The most well known syndrome involves hypoadrenalism, hypoparathyroidism, and mucocutaneous candidiasis together with ovarian failure (see Ch. 228). Thyroiditis is the most commonly associated abnormality. Antibodies to the FSH receptor have been identified in a very few cases. These associations make it mandatory to rule out other potentially life-threatening endocrinopathies in young women with hypergonadotropic amenorrhea.

Enzymatic Defects. In girls with the rare syndrome of 17α-hydroxylase deficiency who survive until the expected age of puberty, sexual infantilism and primary amenorrhea occur together with elevated levels of gonadotropins. Increased synthesis of desoxycorticosterone leads to hypertension with hypokalemic alkalosis; serum progesterone levels are elevated as well. As with other causes of congenital adrenal hyperplasia, the hypertension is controlled by replacement therapy with glucocorticoids (see Ch. 221). Women with galactosemia also develop ovarian failure early in life, even when a galactose-restricted diet is introduced early in infancy (see Ch. 168).

Defective Gonadotropin Secretion and/or Action. The resistant ovary (Savage) syndrome occurs in young amenorrheic women who have (1) elevated peripheral gonadotropin concentrations, (2) normal (although immature) follicles present on ovarian biopsy, (3) a 46,XX karyotype with no evidence of mosaicism, (4) fully developed secondary sex characteristics, and (5) ovarian resistance to stimulation with human menopausal or pituitary gonadotropins. There seems to be some block to gonadotropin action within the ovary in this syndrome.

THERAPEUTIC CONSIDERATIONS. Women with hypergonadotropic amenorrhea and ovarian failure should be treated identically whether or not they have signs of hypoestrogenism or desire pregnancy. Ovarian biopsy is not indicated to document the existence of follicles because only a small portion of each ovary

can be sampled and because pregnancies have resulted in patients who had biopsies devoid of follicles. Estrogen replacement is warranted to prevent the accelerated bone loss known to occur in affected women (see Ch. 238). The estrogen should be given sequentially with a progestin to prevent endometrial hyperplasia. Young women with ovarian failure may require twice as much estrogen as postmenopausal women for relief of signs and symptoms of hypoestrogenism.

Women with hypergonadotropic amenorrhea are rarely able to become pregnant. Pregnancy is more likely to occur with estrogen replacement therapy than with any other therapy. It is not clear why pregnancy is rarely possible in such women. Even with estrogen replacement the pregnancy rate is less than 10 per cent. The most successful treatment of young women with hypergonadotropic amenorrhea involves hormone replacement to mimic the normal menstrual cycle and embryo transfer utilizing donor oocytes. Pregnancy rates are higher than in other women undergoing in vitro fertilization and typically exceed 30 per cent per cycle.

Differential Diagnosis and Treatment of Chronic Anovulation. Chronic anovulation, the most frequent form of amenorrhea encountered in women of reproductive age, implies that functional ovarian follicles remain and that cyclic ovulation can be induced or reinitiated with appropriate therapy (Table 224–7). Appropriate management requires that the etiology of the anovulation be determined. The pathophysiologic bases for several forms of anovulation are unknown, but the anovulation can be interrupted transiently by nonspecific induction of ovulation in the majority of affected women. It is important to recognize that anovulation can result in either amenorrhea or irregular (generally less frequent) menses.

TABLE 224–7. CAUSES OF CHRONIC ANOVULATION

I. **Chronic anovulation of hypothalamic-pituitary origin**
   A. Hypothalamic chronic anovulation
      1. Psychogenic
      2. Exercise associated
      3. Associated with diet, weight loss, and/or malnutrition
      4. Anorexia nervosa and bulimia
      5. Pseudocyesis
   B. Forms of isolated gonadotropin deficiency (including Kallmann's syndrome)
   C. Due to hypothalamic-pituitary damage
      1. Pituitary and parapituitary tumors
      2. Empty-sella syndrome
      3. Following surgery
      4. Following radiation
      5. Following trauma
      6. Following infection
      7. Following infarction
   D. Idiopathic hypopituitarism
   E. Hypothalamic-pituitary dysfunction or failure with hyperprolactinemia (multiple causes)
   F. Due to systemic diseases
II. **Chronic anovulation due to inappropriate feedback** (i.e., polycystic ovarian syndrome)
   A. Excessive extraglandular estrogen production (i.e., obesity)
   B. Abnormal buffering involving sex hormone–binding globulin (including liver disease)
   C. Functional androgen excess (adrenal or ovarian)
   D. Neoplasms producing androgens or estrogens
   E. Neoplasms producing chorionic gonadotropin
III. **Chronic anovulation due to other endocrine and metabolic disorders**
   A. Adrenal hyperfunction
      1. Cushing's syndrome
      2. Congenital adrenal hyperplasia (female pseudohermaphroditism)
   B. Thyroid dysfunction
      1. Hyperthyroidism
      2. Hypothyroidism
   C. Prolactin and/or growth hormone excess
      1. Hypothalamic dysfunction
      2. Pituitary dysfunction (microadenomas and macroadenomas)
      3. Drug induced
   D. Malnutrition

Modified from Rebar RW: Chronic anovulation. *In* Serra GB (ed.): The Ovary. New York, Raven Press, 1983, pp 217–240.

HYPOTHALAMIC CHRONIC ANOVULATION (HCA). HCA is a heterogeneous group of disorders with similar manifestations. Emotional and physical stress, exercise, diet, weight loss, body composition, malnutrition, environment, and other unrecognized factors may contribute in varying proportions to the anovulation. Abrupt cessation of menses in women under 30 years of age who have no anatomic abnormalities of the hypothalamic-pituitary-ovarian axis and no other endocrine disturbances suggests a diagnosis of HCA. Affected individuals tend to be bright, educated, and engaged in intellectual occupations and may well give a history of psychosexual problems and socioenvironmental trauma. HCA is characterized by low to normal levels of gonadotropins and relative hypoestrogenism. Rarely, however, do affected women present with signs and symptoms of estrogen deficiency. Psychological counseling and/or a change in lifestyle, especially for those women engaged in strenuous exercise programs, may be effective in inducing cyclic ovulation and menses. For women desiring pregnancy, ovulation can also be induced with clomiphene citrate (50 to 100 mg per day for 5 days beginning on the fifth day of withdrawal bleeding). Treatment with human menopausal gonadotropin and human chorionic gonadotropin (hMG-hCG) or with GnRH administered in a pulsatile fashion may be effective in women who do not ovulate in response to clomiphene. Most physicians advocate the use of exogenous steroids to prevent osteoporosis. A regimen can be used consisting of oral conjugated estrogens (0.625 to 1.25 mg), ethinyl estradiol (20 μg), or micronized estradiol-17β (1 to 2 mg) or of transdermal estradiol-17β (0.05 to 0.10 mg) daily with oral medroxyprogesterone acetate (5 to 10 mg) added for the first 12 to 14 days of each month. Sexually active women can be given oral contraceptive agents as an alternative. If steroid therapy is administered, patients must be informed that the amenorrhea probably will be present when therapy is discontinued. Other physicians believe only periodic observation is indicated, with barrier methods of contraception recommended for fertility control. Adequate ingestion of calcium should be ensured regardless of therapy. Contraception is needed for sexually active women with HCA, because the functional defect is mild in these disorders and may resolve spontaneously at any time, with ovulation occurring prior to any episode of menstruation.

Individuals with amenorrhea and significant weight loss should be examined for the possibility of *anorexia nervosa* (see Ch. 202). This disorder may be the most severe form of functional HCA, or it may be a distinct entity.

Kallmann's syndrome (isolated gonadotropin deficiency or familial hypogonadotropic hypogonadism) is a familial disorder consisting of gonadotropin deficiency, anosmia or hyposmia, and color blindness in men or, more rarely, in women. Other midline defects such as cleft lip and palate can occur in the affected individual or in family members. The trait is transmitted as an X-linked recessive or a male-limited autosomal dominant trait, but genetic heterogeneity may occur. Partial or complete agenesis of the olfactory bulb is present on autopsy, accounting for use of the term *olfactogenital dysplasia*. The disorder affects only gonadotropin secretion, and all other pituitary hormones are secreted normally. Isolated gonadotropin deficiency in the absence of anosmia occurs as well. Sexual infantilism with a eunuchoidal habitus is the clinical hallmark of this disorder, but moderate breast development may occur. Circulating LH and FSH levels are quite low, but almost always detectable. Ovulation induction requires use of hMG-hCG or pulsatile GnRH. Estrogen replacement therapy is indicated in these women until such time as pregnancy is desired. It may not be possible to distinguish between partial isolated gonadotropin deficiency and functional HCA in all cases.

Hypopituitarism may be obvious upon cursory inspection or sufficiently subtle to require endocrine testing (see Ch. 213). The clinical presentation depends on the age of onset, the etiology, and the nutritional status of the individual. Failure of development of secondary sex characteristics or for development to progress once puberty is initiated must always raise the question of hypopituitarism. Ovulation can be induced successfully with exogenous gonadotropins when pregnancy is desired and after the hypopituitarism is treated appropriately. Replacement therapy with estrogen is indicated to prevent signs and symptoms of estrogen deficiency.

Galactorrhea associated with hyperprolactinemia, whatever the etiology, almost always occurs together with amenorrhea caused by hypothalamic-pituitary dysfunction or failure. Many conditions can cause excess prolactin secretion (see Ch. 226). It is unclear if all individuals with chronic anovulation associated with hyperprolactinemia and no other cause have pituitary microadenomas, even in the absence of identifiable radiographic changes of the sella turcica. Hirsutism may be observed occasionally in association with amenorrhea-galactorrhea and hyperprolactinemia. Elevated levels of the adrenal androgens DHEA and DHEA-S may be observed and may account for the polycystic-like ovaries present in some hyperprolactinemic women.

The hypothalamic-pituitary unit also may fail to function normally in a number of stressful, debilitating, systemic illnesses that interfere with somatic growth and development. Chronic renal failure, liver disease, and diabetes mellitus are the most prominent examples.

CHRONIC ANOVULATION DUE TO INAPPROPRIATE FEEDBACK. PCO syndrome, which causes anovulation because of inappropriate feedback signals to the hypothalamic-pituitary unit, is a heterogeneous disorder in which there is considerable clinical and biochemical variability among affected individuals. Although patients usually present with amenorrhea, hirsutism, and obesity, affected women may instead complain of irregular and profuse uterine bleeding, may not have hirsutism, and may be of normal weight. Excess androgen from any source or increased extraglandular conversion of androgens to estrogens can lead to the typical findings of PCO syndrome. Included are such diverse disorders as Cushing's syndrome, mild congenital adrenal hyperplasia, virilizing tumors of adrenal or ovarian origin, hyperthyroidism and hypothyroidism, obesity, and primary PCO syndrome with no other recognizable etiology. In the primary syndrome the irregular menses, mild obesity, and hirsutism begin during puberty and typically become more severe with time. Obesity alone can lead to a PCO-like syndrome, with the degree of obesity required to cause anovulation varying widely from individual to individual. All such patients are well estrogenized regardless of whether they present with primary or secondary amenorrhea or dysfunctional bleeding. As noted, LH concentrations tend to be elevated, with relatively low and constant FSH levels, but both may be in the normal range compared to levels in women in the follicular phase of the menstrual cycle. Levels of most circulating androgens, especially testosterone, tend to be mildly elevated. The etiology of PCO syndrome is unknown, but current evidence suggests that the hypothalamic-pituitary unit is intact and that a functional derangement, perhaps involving insulin-like growth factors such as somatomedin C within the ovary, results in abnormal gonadotropin secretion.

The aim of the diagnostic evaluation is to rule out any causes (such as neoplasms) that require definitive therapy. Hirsutism should be evaluated as detailed in Ch. 225. PCO syndrome itself is a benign disorder. Patients generally require therapy for hirsutism, for induction of ovulation if pregnancy is desired, and for prevention of estrogen-induced endometrial hyperplasia and cancer. No ideal therapy exists, but rather the therapeutic approach must be individualized to the needs of each patient.

In the anovulatory woman not desiring pregnancy who is not hirsute, therapy with intermittent progestin administration (such as medroxyprogesterone acetate 5 to 10 mg orally for 10 to 14 days each month) or oral contraceptives can be provided to reduce the increased risk of endometrial carcinoma that is present in such a woman with unopposed estrogen. All women utilizing intermittent progestin administration should be cautioned about the need for effective contraception if they are sexually active, because these agents will not inhibit ovulation when administered intermittently.

The approach to the hirsute anovulatory woman not desiring pregnancy is detailed in Ch. 225. Oral contraceptive agents are the first line of therapy for such women with mild hirsutism and offer protection from endometrial hyperplasia.

In women with PCO syndrome desiring pregnancy, clomiphene citrate is the first approach to inducing ovulation because of its simplicity and high success rate. Approximately 75 to 80 per cent conceive with such therapy. Other possible methods of inducing ovulation include use of hMG-hCG, purified FSH, pulsatile GnRH, wedge resection of the ovaries at laparotomy, and laser or cautery destruction of follicles at laparoscopy. Surgical treatment is warranted only rarely and only in women in whom all other methods fail, in whom there is a question of an ovarian tumor because of ovarian size or circulating androgen levels, and in whom fertility is not an issue (because of the risk of pelvic adhesions from the surgery leading to infertility).

A particularly severe subset of affected women present with marked obesity, anovulation, mild glucose intolerance and high levels of circulating insulin with insulin resistance, acanthosis nigricans, hyperuricemia, and severe hirsutism with markedly elevated circulating androgen levels. These women have *hyperthecosis of the ovaries* in which the androgen-producing cells in the stromal, hilar, and thecal components of the ovaries are increased greatly in number. Although considered a separate entity by some clinicians, hyperthecosis probably should be viewed as a part of the spectrum comprising PCO syndrome.

Chronic Anovulation Due to Other Endocrine and Metabolic Disorders. Adrenal hyperfunction appears to cause chronic anovulation by inducing a PCO-like syndrome secondary to increased adrenal androgen secretion, but other possible mechanisms also exist.

Both hyperthyroidism and hypothyroidism are associated with a variety of menstrual disturbances, including dysfunctional uterine bleeding and amenorrhea as a result of alterations in the metabolism of androgens and estrogens. These metabolic changes in turn result in inappropriate steroid feedback and chronic anovulation.

Rebar RW: Exercise and the menstrual cycle. Exercise-related factors can lead to hypothalamic dysfunction. In Soules MR (ed.): Controversies in Reproductive Endocrinology and Infertility. New York, Elsevier, 1989, pp 41–58. *A detailed discussion of the effects of exercise on reproduction in women.*

Rebar RW: Practical evaluation of hormonal status. In Yen SSC, Jaffe RB (eds.): Reproductive Endocrinology, 2nd ed. Philadelphia, W. B. Saunders Company, 1986, pp 683–733. *A clinician describes a systematic approach to assessing ovarian function and clinical diagnosis. Bibliography is exhaustive.*

Rebar RW, Erickson GF, Coulam CB: Premature ovarian failure. In Gondos B, Riddick D (eds.): Pathology of Infertility. New York, Thieme Medical Publishers, Inc., 1987, pp 123–141. *A detailed discussion of the diagnosis and treatment of premature ovarian failure.*

Yen SSC: Chronic anovulation caused by peripheral endocrine disorders. In Yen SSC, Jaffe RB (eds.): Reproductive Endocrinology, 2nd ed. Philadelphia, W. B. Saunders Company, 1986, pp 441–499. *A detailed discussion of many of the causes of anovulation with an exhaustive bibliography.*

Yen SSC: Chronic anovulation due to CNS-hypothalamic-pituitary dysfunction. In Yen SSC, Jaffe RB (eds.): Reproductive Endocrinology, 2nd ed. Philadelphia, W. B. Saunders Company, 1986, pp 500–545. *A complete discussion of hypothalamic amenorrhea with an extensive bibliography.*

DISORDERS OF FOLLICULOGENESIS.

The recognized disorders of folliculogenesis are not identified until at or following ovulation, but they are believed to be manifestations of abnormalities in follicular development.

Luteinized Unruptured Follicle (LUF) Syndrome. The LUF syndrome describes development of a dominant follicle without its subsequent disruption and release of the ovum. The abnormality can be diagnosed by ultrasonography or by the absence of evidence of ovulation when the ovary is viewed at laparoscopy. The disorder is believed to occur infrequently and sporadically and is probably not a significant cause of infertility. Menstrual cycles in which no ovum is released are characterized by presumptive evidence of ovulation, including biphasic basal body temperatures, secretory endometrium, a normal LH surge, and normal progesterone production in the luteal phase. In fact, although the syndrome is believed to occur, data to substantiate its existence are only circumstantial (although strongly so) at present.

Luteal Phase Dysfunction. Progesterone secretion in the luteal phase may be reduced in duration (termed luteal phase insufficiency) or in amount (termed luteal phase inadequacy). More rarely the endometrium may be unable to respond to secreted progesterone because of the absence of progesterone receptors. These disorders are believed to represent causes for infertility (because of inability of fertilized ova to implant) in approximately 5 per cent of infertile couples. Abnormalities of the follicular phase, especially in the frequency of gonadotropin pulses, may account for most luteal phase dysfunction. Luteal phase defects also may occur sporadically in normally ovulating women approximately once each year.

Luteal phase dysfunction may be associated with several clinical entities, including mild or intermittent hyperprolactinemia (of any etiology), strenuous physical exercise, inadequately treated 21-hydroxylase deficiency, and habitual abortion. Luteal dysfunction occurs more commonly at the extremes of reproductive life and in the first menstrual cycles following full-term delivery, abortion, or discontinuation of oral contraceptives. It also may occur during ovulatory cycles induced with clomiphene citrate or hMG-hCG.

The diagnosis of luteal phase dysfunction can be made either by endometrial biopsy or by serial progesterone determinations. Endometrial biopsies obtained from the uterine fundus in the late luteal phases of two different cycles must be at least 2 days out of phase from the expected date of bleeding, as judged from the subsequent menstrual cycle, for the diagnosis to be made. The absolute concentration that progesterone must achieve and the length of time progesterone must be increased in the luteal phase to exclude luteal dysfunction are unclear. Luteal dysfunction is extremely rare in women with menstrual cycles greater than 25 days in length in whom a single random progesterone determination is greater than 15 ng per milliliter.

Treatment of luteal dysfunction is controversial. Any underlying defect should be treated. If subsequent luteal function depends on prior follicular development, modification of follicular development with either clomiphene citrate (25 to 100 mg daily by mouth for 5 days beginning on cycle day 3 to 5) or FSH (75 to 300 IU intramuscularly for 3 to 5 days beginning on cycle day 3 to 5) is reasonable. hCG (2500 to 5000 IU intramuscularly at 2- to 3-day intervals beginning with the shift in basal body temperature) or progesterone (12.5 mg intramuscularly in oil daily or 25 mg twice a day as rectal or vaginal suppositories) can be utilized as well. Bromocriptine may correct the abnormality in individuals with hyperprolactinemia. Synthetic progestational agents should not be used to treat luteal phase defects because of their possible (although unproven) association with congenital anomalies. Furthermore, the synthetic progestins produce an abnormal endometrium. None of these agents has been shown to increase the pregnancy rate.

Daly DC: Luteal phase defects. In Gondos B, Riddick DH (eds.): Pathology of Infertility. New York, Thieme Medical Publishers, Inc., 1987, pp 169–184. *A complete review of what is known about luteal dysfunction.*

McNeely MJ, Soules MR: The diagnosis of luteal phase deficiency: A critical review. Fertil Steril 50:1, 1988. *A consideration of the difficulties involved in diagnosing luteal dysfunction.*

INFERTILITY. *Infertility* may be defined as involuntary inability to conceive. *Sterility* is total inability to reproduce. In either case the situation may or may not be correctable, especially for each particular couple. Failure to reproduce thwarts a basic human instinct and causes anger, guilt, and depression. More than 10 per cent of couples in the United States seek medical assistance for infertility.

The requirements for pregnancy to occur are several:

1. The male must produce adequate numbers of normal, motile spermatozoa.
2. The male must be capable of ejaculating the sperm through a patent ductal system.
3. The sperm must be able to traverse an unobstructed female reproductive tract.
4. The female must ovulate and release an ovum.
5. The sperm must be able to fertilize the ovum.
6. The fertilized ovum must be capable of developing and implanting in appropriately prepared endometrium.

Infertility is too frequently viewed primarily as a problem of the female. In fact, in approximately 40 per cent of cases, infertility is caused by the male (Table 224–8). In perhaps one third of couples more than one cause contributes to the infertility.

Peak age of fertility in the female is 25 years. For nulliparous women of this age the average time during which unprotected intercourse occurs until conception is 5.3 months. For parous women the average duration of intercourse until conception is 2.7 months. The reproductive performance of couples is influenced by the ages of the female and male partners, the frequency of intercourse, and the length of time the couple has been attempting to conceive. There is a decline in both female and male reproductive performance after age 25.

TABLE 224–8. CAUSES OF INFERTILITY AND THEIR APPROXIMATE INCIDENCE (%)

I. **Male factors (40%)**
  A. Decreased production of spermatozoa
    1. Varicocele
    2. Testicular failure
    3. Endocrine disorders
    4. Cryptorchidism
    5. Stress, smoking, caffeine, nicotine, recreational drugs
  B. Ductal obstruction
    1. Epididymal (postinfection)
    2. Congenital absence of vas deferens
    3. Ejaculatory duct (postinfection)
    4. Postvasectomy
  C. Inability to deliver sperm into vagina
    1. Ejaculatory disturbances
    2. Hypospadias
    3. Sexual problems (i.e., impotence), medical or psychological
  D. Abnormal semen
    1. Infection
    2. Abnormal volume
    3. Abnormal viscosity
  E. Immunologic factors
    1. Sperm-immobilizing antibodies
    2. Sperm-agglutinating antibodies

II. **Female factors**
  A. Fallopian tube pathology (20 to 30%)
    1. Pelvic inflammatory disease or puerperal infection
    2. Congenital anomalies
    3. Endometriosis
    4. Secondary to past peritonitis of nongenital origin
  B. Amenorrhea and anovulation (15%)
  C. Minor ovulatory disturbances (<5%?)
  D. Cervical and uterine factors (10%)
    1. Leiomyomas and polyps
    2. Uterine anomalies
    3. Intrauterine synechiae (Asherman's syndrome)
    4. Destroyed endocervical glands (postsurgery or postinfection)
  E. Vaginal factors (<5%)
    1. Congenital absence of vagina
    2. Imperforate hymen
    3. Vaginismus
    4. Vaginitis
  F. Immunologic factors (<5%)
    1. Sperm-immobilizing antibodies
    2. Sperm-agglutinating antibodies
  G. Nutritional and metabolic factors (5%)
    1. Thyroid disorders
    2. Diabetes mellitus
    3. Severe nutritional disturbances

III. **Idiopathic or unexplained (< 10%)**

Couples who complain of infertility merit evaluation regardless of the length of infertility. If the couple believes there is a problem, it is the physician's responsibility to reassure them by appropriate evaluation and subsequent explanation of all findings and the prognosis.

The evaluation begins with a detailed history obtained from both partners and physical examinations of both individuals. The couple should be seen together for the first visit. Each couple should be questioned together and separately, since separate interviews may uncover information that would not be imparted in the presence of the partner.

Initial evaluation of infertility generally includes (1) assessment of semen, (2) documentation of ovulation by basal body temperature, serum progesterone determination approximately 6 to 8 days before menses, or endometrial biopsy less than 3 days before onset of menses, and (3) evaluation of the female genital tract by hysterosalpingography. Basal serum levels of prolactin and thyroid hormones should be measured. Diagnostic laparoscopy with tubal dye instillation should be performed if all previous tests are normal, since 30 to 50 per cent of women are found to have endometriosis or tubal disease on surgical evaluation. Treatment must be predicated on the findings of the infertility evaluation.

Glass RH: Infertility. *In* Yen SSC, Jaffe RB (eds.): Reproductive Endocrinology, 2nd ed. Philadelphia, W. B. Saunders Company, 1986, pp 571–613. *A summary of the approach to the infertile couple.*

SEXUAL FUNCTION AND DYSFUNCTION. Although sexual responses begin following puberty, they can continue for the duration of a woman's life. Sexual responses generally are divided into four phases: excitement, plateau, orgasm, and resolution.

With sexual arousal and excitement, vasocongestion and muscular tension increase progressively, primarily in the genitals, manifested by vaginal lubrication in the female. The lubrication is due to formation of a transudate in the vagina. Sexual excitement is initiated by any of a variety of psychogenic or somatogenic sexual stimuli and must be reinforced to result in orgasm. With continued stimulation, the excitement phase increases in intensity into a plateau phase during which a high state of sexual interest is maintained. The plateau phase may be short or long, and it is from this phase that an individual can shift to orgasm. The orgasmic phase tends to be brief and is characterized by rapid release from the developed vasocongestion and muscular tension. The orgasmic release is also known as the climax because peak psychological and physical intensity is achieved and there is an attendant feeling of satisfaction. Copious secretions and transudate may flow during orgasm in women. While women may resolve toward sleep following orgasm, many remain responsive to sexual stimulation and may return to plateau and subsequent orgasm.

Characteristic genital and extragenital responses occur during these phases. Estrogens magnify the sexual responses, but responses may occur in estrogen-deficient women. For women these changes occur in the breasts and in the pudendal region and are variable from one response cycle to another. For some women, excitement proceeds quickly through plateau to orgasm, and orgasm is explosive and accompanied by vocalization and involuntary contractions of the pelvic skeletal muscles. For other women, the responses are slow in building, controlled in amplitude, and long lasting. For a few women orgasm never occurs; for many it is intermittently absent.

The somatic sensate focus enabling orgasmic release is variable and may include stimulation of the breast, vagina, or clitoris. The psychological aspect of coitus may involve concentration on the current partner or act or fantasies about other times and persons. While orgasms may vary in physiologic intensity, what is important is psychological satisfaction. Satisfaction for both men and women may be had without orgasm.

Women may seek consultation because of disturbances in normal sexual arousal or orgasm. Such sexual dysfunction may be due to either organic or functional disturbances.

A variety of diseases affecting neurologic function, including diabetes mellitus and multiple sclerosis, may prevent sexual arousal. So, too, may local pelvic disorders, such as endometriosis and vaginitis, which cause dyspareunia and lead to sexual avoidance. Estrogen deficiency causing vaginal atrophy and dyspareunia is a relatively common cause of sexual dysfunction. Debilitating systemic diseases such as malignant disease may also affect sexual function indirectly.

In most cases the cause of sexual dysfunction is psychological. For instance, vaginismus involves involuntary contractions of the muscles surrounding the introitus and leads to dyspareunia. It is a conditioned response engendered by a previous imagined or real traumatic sexual experience. Feelings of guilt, caused by incest or rape as examples; of inadequacy, caused by hysterectomy or mastectomy; or of depression or anxiety may lead to failure to be aroused. Failure to achieve orgasm may be viewed as a dysfunction if the woman is frustrated or dissatisfied.

Treatment of sexual dysfunction is best accomplished by eliminating functional causes and providing the patient, often together with her partner, with appropriate psychological counseling. Behavioral modification is effective in treating many women with psychological sexual dysfunction.

Kaplan HS: The Evaluation of Sexual Disorders: Psychological and Medical Aspects. New York, Brunner-Mazel, 1983. *A good general text detailing sexual disorders.*

Kaplan HS: The Illustrated Manual of Sex Therapy, 2nd ed. New York, Brunner-Mazel, 1987. *A simple text graphically detailing the therapeutic techniques first introduced by Masters and Johnson.*

Kolodny RC, Masters WH, Johnson VE: Textbook of Sexual Medicine. Boston, Little, Brown and Company, 1979. *A widely used text detailing sexual problems and their therapy.*

Masters W, Johnson V: Human Sexual Response. Boston, Little, Brown and

Company, 1966. *The classic work detailing human sexual response. Required reading for all individuals seriously interested in this field.*

Nadelson CC, Marcotte DB (eds.): Treatment Interventions in Human Sexuality. New York, Plenum Press, 1983. *A multiauthored text that considers sexual problems in detail.*

HORMONAL THERAPY DURING THE REPRODUCTIVE YEARS

INDUCTION OF OVULATION. Induction of ovulation should never be attempted until serious disorders precluding pregnancy are ruled out or treated. Furthermore, ovulation induction should be utilized only in women with chronic anovulation, because women with ovarian failure are unresponsive to any form of ovulation induction. In general, the use of pharmaceutical agents does not improve the quality of an ovum, and thus the chance of pregnancy is not improved in women who ovulate regularly.

Clomiphene citrate is the agent that usually induces ovulation most easily. Clomiphene should be utilized in individuals without hyperprolactinemia who have the ability to release LH and FSH. A typical course of clomiphene therapy is begun on the fifth day following either spontaneous or induced uterine bleeding. The initial dosage is 50 mg daily for 5 days. Clomiphene appears to act as an anti-estrogen and stimulates gonadotropin secretion by the pituitary gland to initiate follicular development. If ovulation is not achieved in the very first cycle of treatment, the daily dosage is increased to 100 mg. If ovulation is still not achieved, dosage is increased in a stepwise fashion by 50 mg increments to a maximum of 200 to 250 mg daily for 5 days. The highest dose should be continued for 3 to 6 months before the patient is regarded as a clomiphene failure. The quantity of drug and the length of time that it can be used, as suggested here, are greater than those recommended by the manufacturers, but conform with published series.

The ovulatory surge of LH may occur 5 to 12 days (average, 7 days) after the completion of the last day of clomiphene treatment in each course. Couples are advised to have intercourse every other day during this time interval. Ovulation can be documented by monitoring changes in basal body temperature or preferably by measuring serum progesterone approximately 14 days after the last clomiphene tablet is taken. In addition, menses should occur about 3 weeks after the last day of therapy. Withdrawal bleeding with progestin can be induced if the patient fails to bleed within 4 weeks of therapy and if a serum hCG level documents that the patient is not pregnant.

Some clinicians give 5000 to 10,000 IU of hCG intramuscularly 7 days after the last day of clomiphene therapy to trigger ovulation, but this approach has not been established to increase effectiveness. The administration of hCG, however, does serve to time ovulation and may be helpful in selected couples. Ovulation can be expected to occur approximately 36 hours after hCG administration.

In appropriately selected patients, 75 to 80 per cent will ovulate and 40 to 50 per cent can be expected to become pregnant. About 15 per cent of pregnancies can be expected with each ovulatory cycle. The multiple pregnancy rate is about 8 per cent, with almost all being twins. The incidence of congenital anomalies is not increased.

Side effects of clomiphene are uncommon and very rarely serious. The most serious side effects include vasomotor flushes (10 per cent), abdominal discomfort (5 per cent), breast tenderness (2 per cent), nausea and vomiting (2 per cent), visual symptoms (1.5 per cent), and headache (1 per cent). Significant ovarian enlargement may occur but is rare (5 per cent).

The addition of dexamethasone, 0.5 mg orally at bedtime to blunt the nighttime secretion of ACTH, may be useful in hyperandrogenic women with an adrenal component who fail to ovulate in response to clomiphene. Other individuals failing to respond to clomiphene typically require hMG-hCG or perhaps pulsatile GnRH to induce ovulation.

Bromocriptine, a dopamine agonist, is effective in inducing ovulation in hyperprolactinemic women (see Ch. 226). The drug should be stopped once pregnancy is confirmed. Ovulatory menses and pregnancy are achieved in about 80 per cent of patients with galactorrhea and hyperprolactinemia. The majority of women with prolactin-secreting pituitary tumors remain asymptomatic during pregnancy. It is extremely rare for a patient with either a microadenoma or a macroadenoma to develop a problem related to the tumor that affects either the mother or the fetus during pregnancy. Monitoring during pregnancy need consist only of questioning the patient about the development of visual symptoms and headaches. Formal assessment of visual fields and CT or MRI should be carried out in any patient developing suspicious symptoms. Symptoms generally abate with institution of bromocriptine therapy. No adverse effects of bromocriptine on fetuses or pregnancies have been reported.

hMG, a purified preparation of gonadotropins extracted from the urine of postmenopausal women, must be administered intramuscularly. Each vial contains 75 units of FSH and 75 units of LH. Purified FSH has become available for use recently. Biochemically engineered preparations of both products will become available in the future. hMG is administered at doses of two to four vials for 5 to 12 days to achieve follicular development as monitored by ultrasound and serum or urinary E_2 concentrations. hCG, 5000 to 10,000 IU, is administered as a single intramuscular dose when follicular maturation is apparent. The hCG should be withheld if more than three follicles mature together. GnRH analogues are now being utilized to suppress endogenous follicular activity before initiating therapy with hMG and continued until hCG is given in older women and those with poor responses to hMG alone. Use of the analogues necessitates administration of larger quantities of hMG. Success rates, however, seem to be somewhat improved with this combined therapy.

Because of the expense and the complication rate, thorough evaluation should be carried out to exclude other causes of infertility before hMG-hCG is used. Ovulation can be induced in almost 100 per cent of patients, but pregnancy will occur in only 50 to 70 per cent. There is no increased risk of congenital anomalies with hMG-hCG.

The rate of multiple pregnancies with hMG-hCG may approach 30 per cent, with 5 per cent being triplets or more. Ovarian hyperstimulation is the major side effect and may be life threatening. The ovaries enlarge remarkably in this treatment-induced syndrome, and multiple follicle cysts, stromal edema, and multiple corpora lutea are present. There is a shift of fluid from the intravascular space into the abdominal cavity with resultant hypovolemia and hemoconcentration. The cause of the ascites is unknown. Treatment is conservative, with monitoring of fluid and electrolyte status. Pelvic examinations should not be performed for fear of rupturing the ovaries. The hyperstimulation generally will resolve slowly over about 7 days.

GnRH, administered intravenously or less effectively subcutaneously at doses of 5 to 20 μg every 60 to 120 minutes, also can be used to induce ovulation in women with an intact pituitary gland. It is most effective in individuals with hypothalamic chronic anovulation. hCG can be administered to support the corpus luteum after ovulation at a dose of 1500 IU intramuscularly every 3 days for three to four doses. The advantage of GnRH rests in the fact that hyperstimulation is extremely unlikely. However, reported pregnancy rates have been no greater than those achieved with hMG-hCG. Furthermore, some patients do not tolerate wearing the infusion pump that must be utilized.

Speroff L, Glass RH, Kase NG: Induction of ovulation. *In* Speroff L, Glass RH, Kase NG: Clinical Gynecologic Endocrinology and Infertility, 4th ed. Baltimore, Williams & Wilkins Company, 1989, pp 583–609. *A detailed and practical survey of how to induce ovulation.*

STEROIDAL CONTRACEPTION. *Physiologic Actions and Metabolic Effects.* Oral contraceptive pills are the most widely used contraceptives worldwide, with more than 50 million users. Combination (estrogen-progestin) and progestin only preparations are available. The estrogen may be either mestranol or ethinyl estradiol, while the progestin is usually one of six derivatives of 19-nor-testosterone: norethindrone, norethindrone acetate, norethynodrel, ethynodiol diacetate, norgestrel, and levonorgestrel. New progestins will soon be widely available.

The low-dose combination pills currently in use (containing 30 to 35 μg of estrogen with reduced amounts of progestin) were developed to reduce the biochemical changes produced by contraceptive steroids, but the majority of studies were conducted with the older high-dose preparations. It is known that virtually all biochemical changes are dose related.

Combination oral contraceptives inhibit the midcycle gonadotropin surge by inhibiting GnRH release from the hypothalamus. Cervical mucus becomes thick, viscid, and scanty in amount, thus retarding sperm penetration. Fallopian tube motility and secretion are altered as well, and the endometrial glands produce less glycogen. Efficacy is substantiated by a failure rate of 0.1 per cent during the first year of combination oral contraceptive use, lower than with any other reversible form of contraception.

Oral contraceptives decrease maturation of the vaginal epithelium and somehow render the vagina more susceptible to candidiasis. The endometrium becomes atrophic with variable degrees of decidual change, leading to diminished menstrual flow. Follicular development is arrested with low estrogen and progesterone secretion. Both circulating LH and FSH levels are reduced and constant.

The general metabolic effects of oral contraceptives resemble those of pregnancy. Glucose tolerance is impaired, with an increase in plasma insulin levels. The "mini-pill" containing progestin only in low dosage may cause no changes in glucose metabolism. Levels of circulating triglycerides and of very low density lipoproteins (VLDL) are often increased, almost entirely because of the estrogenic component (see Ch. 172). Only slight changes are seen with the low-dose combination preparations. Only very high estrogenic formulations will increase mean serum cholesterol levels. Because of a direct effect of estrogens on the endoplasmic reticulum in the liver, α_2 globulins, including angiotensinogen, and β globulins are increased, while serum albumin levels are decreased somewhat. A number of blood coagulation factors and carrier proteins (including thyroid-binding globulin, transferrin, ceruloplasmin, SHBG, and corticosteroid-binding globulin) are also increased.

Interactions with Other Drugs. Oral contraceptive steroids interact with several other drugs, leading to reduced effectiveness of the contraceptives or of the other drug. Such interactions occur because of altered drug absorption or metabolism. The majority of these interactions occur only with long-term use of the pharmacologic agent. By inducing hepatic microsomal enzymes, long-term administration of antibiotics may reduce the contraceptive efficacy of the steroids. The short-term use of antibiotics is probably of little concern. Anticonvulsants also sharply reduce the efficacy of contraceptive steroids, as do antacids, which may decrease the absorption of steroids. Conversely, contraceptive steroids oppose the therapeutic effects of anticoagulants, antidiabetic agents, and certain antihypertensive agents, such as guanethidine and α-methyldopa, because of their metabolic effects. Because of the impaired elimination of certain drugs, such as phenothiazines, oral contraceptive users may require lower doses.

Complications, Side Effects, and Benefits. Although the complications and side effects of combination oral contraceptives have been widely reported, the low-dose formulations currently available have minimized the side effects compared to the older, high-dose preparations without sacrificing contraceptive efficacy or reducing the substantial health benefits associated with oral contraceptive use.

The use of oral contraceptives increases the risk of *thromboembolism*, possibly as much as 4- to 13-fold with the doses of estrogens used in early preparations. The estrogen content of oral contraceptives appears to be correlated roughly with the risk of venous thromboembolic disease. Lower dosages of estrogen than were used initially in oral contraceptive preparations may not significantly increase the risk of any cardiovascular complications. Advanced maternal age and smoking seem to be the major risk factors for the use of oral contraceptives. In the absence of smoking and in women under the age of 45 years who do not suffer from obesity, hypertension, diabetes mellitus, or inherited lipoprotein abnormalities, there is little, if any, increased risk to low-dose combination oral contraceptive users for cardiovascular disease, including myocardial infarction. Some clinicians believe that these preparations may be used safely in normal women until the menopause.

In the absence of smoking and hypertension, it appears unlikely that there is an increased risk of fatal and nonfatal stroke from the use of low-dose oral contraceptives, in contrast to the enhanced risk of both thrombotic and hemorrhagic stroke reported earlier from the use of preparations containing larger amounts of estrogens. Some but not all women with migraine headaches may note increasingly frequent headaches with oral contraceptive use. Women with migraine headaches do not seem to be at increased risk of stroke.

Women using oral contraceptives are more likely to become hypertensive, especially if over the age of 35 years. Smoking may contribute to the incidence of hypertension. Increases in blood pressure are generally reversible shortly after oral contraceptives are discontinued. Failure of the blood pressure to return to normal when oral contraceptives are discontinued suggests underlying disease.

Contraceptive steroids do not appear to be teratogenic. Derivatives of 19-nor-testosterone can virilize female fetuses when administered in large doses to women early in pregnancy, but the doses required are far in excess of those contained in oral contraceptives.

Use of oral contraceptives reduces the risk of benign breast neoplasia, including fibrocystic disease and fibroadenoma. Since benign breast disease is a significant risk factor for the subsequent development of breast cancer, oral contraceptives may afford protection against breast cancer in this manner. Indeed, the incidence of breast cancer does not seem to be increased by use of oral contraceptives. Furthermore, oral contraceptives reduce the risk of developing endometrial carcinoma by about half and of developing ovarian carcinoma by about 40 per cent. In the cases of both endometrial and ovarian cancers, the protection is related to duration of use and persists for at least 10 years after stopping oral contraceptives.

Use of combined oral contraceptives may result in an increased risk for the development of *hepatocellular adenoma*, and this risk may increase with increased duration of contraceptive use. Rarely in patients with such adenomas the liver may rupture, and death may even occur because of hemorrhage. There is no evidence of any increased risk of developing liver cancer.

The relationships of oral contraceptive use to cervical carcinoma, pituitary tumors, and melanoma are unclear. Some studies show positive relationships between cervical dysplasia and oral contraceptive use, while other studies do not. Cervical dysplasia is increased in women with first coitus at an early age and those who have multiple sexual partners. Since oral contraceptive use may encourage such sexual behavior, any such relationship is difficult to interpret. In addition, Pap smear screening is much more common among oral contraceptive users so that cervical neoplasia may be detected more frequently in these women. There is some evidence that the incidence of prolactinomas may be increasing in women, but the use of contraceptive steroids has not been shown to increase this risk.

So-called *post-pill amenorrhea* is sometimes regarded as a side effect of oral contraceptive use. The return to ovulation following discontinuation of contraceptive use is variable but occurs within 4 to 8 weeks in most patients. Approximately 1 in 500 patients will have amenorrhea for 6 months or longer, with 15 per cent of these having associated galactorrhea. This prolonged amenorrhea is probably caused by underlying disorders unrelated to oral contraceptive use. In normal women subsequent fertility is unimpaired.

Nausea and vomiting occur occasionally when use begins, but generally abate with continued use. Mastalgia and increased breast size may occur, but also tend to subside in several cycles. Chloasma (hyperpigmentation of the face) is a leading cause of pill discontinuation. Acne is usually improved, but occasionally may be exacerbated. Dizziness, headaches, visual disturbances, depression, and increased or decreased libido have been reported. Easy bruisability due to increased capillary fragility and edema also may occur.

Other therapeutic benefits exist with oral contraceptive use as well. The risk of pelvic inflammatory disease appears reduced by half. Decreased menstrual blood loss results in a lower incidence of iron deficiency anemia. Acne frequently improves and dysmenorrhea decreases in the majority of patients. Symptomatic relief of endometriosis occurs in some patients. The risk of functional ovarian cysts is decreased, as are the incidences of ectopic pregnancies and uterine fibroids. Women with PCO syndrome treated with oral contraceptives are afforded protection from endometrial carcinoma. Oral contraceptives may possibly afford protection against development of rheumatoid arthritis as well.

Absolute contraindications to the use of oral contraceptives include thrombophlebitis, thromboembolic disorders, cardiovascular disease, or a history of these conditions; markedly impaired liver function; known or suspected estrogen-dependent neoplasia; undiagnosed abnormal genital bleeding; known or suspected pregnancy; and congenital hyperlipidemia. Oral contraceptives generally should be administered with caution to smokers, women who are obese, and those with varicose veins. If headaches develop or become more frequent with pill use, oral contraceptives should be discontinued. Because of a possible increase in postsurgical thromboembolic complications in women using oral contraceptives, use of oral contraceptives should be discontinued 2 weeks prior to surgery and begun again 2 weeks postoperatively.

Low-dose combination oral contraceptive pills offer superb protection for sexually active women not desiring pregnancy. For most such individuals the benefits of the low-dose preparations clearly outweigh the adverse effects, but possible side effects and complications must be considered in treating individual patients.

Henzl MR: Contraceptive hormones and their clinical use. In Yen SSC, Jaffe RB (eds.): Reproductive Endocrinology, 2nd ed. Philadelphia, W. B. Saunders Company, 1986, pp 643–682. A detailed discussion of steroidal contraception.

Zatuchni GI: Known and potential complications of steroidal contraception. In Becker KL (ed.): Principles and Practice of Endocrinology and Metabolism. Philadelphia, J. B. Lippincott Company, 1990, pp 868–872. A detailed consideration of the risks of oral contraceptives.

THE MENOPAUSE AND POSTMENOPAUSAL YEARS

DEFINITIONS AND EPIDEMIOLOGY. The *menopause* is the final menstrual period denoting the cessation of cyclic ovarian function as manifested by cyclic menstruation. The *climacteric* is the physiologic period during which regression of ovarian function occurs. Its onset generally is signalled by alterations in the menstrual cycle or vasomotor symptomatology. Menopause occurs at a mean age of approximately 51 years. Today's average woman in the Western world can expect to live one third of her life in the postmenopausal phase.

SYMPTOMATOLOGY AND SIGNS. Most signs and symptoms associated with the postmenopausal years result from decreased circulating estrogen. Common symptoms include hot flushes, paresthesias, palpitations, cold hands and feet, headaches, vertigo, irritability, anxiety, nervousness, depression, fatigue, weight gain, insomnia, night sweats, forgetfulness, and inability to concentrate.

Vasomotor instability is perhaps the most common complaint. Over 75 per cent of women experience hot flushes with decreasing estrogen levels, and these may persist for years. In a typical hot flush, the skin, especially of the head and neck, becomes red and warm for a few seconds to 2 minutes with cold chills thereafter. Accompanying physiologic changes include a rise in skin temperature, peripheral vasodilatation, increased heart rate, decreased skin resistance, and concomitant LH pulses. The mechanism for hot flushes is unknown but must involve thermoregulatory centers in the hypothalamus.

Any increase in bleeding or bleeding after 6 months of amenorrhea demands examination and sampling of the endometrium to exclude carcinoma. Women note relocation of fat deposits, with increased fat in the lower abdomen, hips, and breasts. The genital skin becomes thin and pale, with a decrease in the size of the labia minora, clitoris, uterus, and ovaries, and the women often complain of dyspareunia. Decreased elastic tissue of skin is noted, and osteoporosis may occur in about 25 per cent of postmenopausal women (see Ch. 238).

Menopausal signs and symptoms may begin long before menses have ceased. Symptoms may be difficult to diagnose in women with previous hysterectomies. Following bilateral oophorectomy young women develop identical signs and symptoms.

ENDOCRINOLOGIC CHANGES. During the menopausal transition regular menstrual cycles may continue up to the menopause. The cycles may become shorter, due to shortened follicular phases, with increased FSH, normal LH, and decreased E_2 and progesterone levels in comparison to normal ovulatory cycles. Variable cycles also may occur prior to the menopause, with some being ovulatory and others being anovulatory. Waning ovarian follicular activity with decreasing E_2 production must be central to these changes, and yet some follicles have been found on occasion in ovaries of postmenopausal women.

In postmenopausal women, circulating FSH and LH concentrations are greatly increased. Estrogen levels are decreased markedly, but androgen levels are decreased only slightly. The postmenopausal ovaries continue to secrete substantial amounts of androgen (androstenedione and testosterone), which together with adrenal androgens are converted to estrogens by extraglandular conversion in the periphery. The peripheral conversion of androgens accounts for most circulating estrogen in postmenopausal women.

CLINICAL MANAGEMENT. Treatment of postmenopausal women must be individualized and based on a personal dialogue with each patient. Exogenous estrogen replacement will stop or diminish hot flushes, reverse atrophic genital changes, decrease osteoporotic fractures (see Ch. 238), and may decrease the incidence of atherosclerotic coronary artery disease.

Estrogen replacement therapy is absolutely contraindicated in postmenopausal women with estrogen-dependent tumors of the breast, uterus, or kidney; acute liver disease; cerebrovascular disease; deep-vein thrombosis and embolism; malignant melanoma; and undiagnosed genital bleeding. Replacement therapy must be considered carefully and other therapy may require modification in women with estrogen-associated hypertension, diabetes mellitus, cholecystitis and cholelithiasis, pancreatitis, congestive heart failure, past endometriosis, and neuro-ophthalmologic vascular disease. Individual exceptions to even the absolute contraindications exist.

Many treatment regimens are currently being utilized. Estrogen should be administered together with a progestin in a cyclic fashion to women with a uterus to prevent an increased risk of endometrial hyperplasia and carcinoma. Oral estrone sulfate (0.625 to 1.25 mg), micronized estradiol-17β (1 mg), or transdermal estradiol (0.05 mg) may be given daily. To this should be added a progestin such as medroxyprogesterone acetate (5 to 10 mg orally for 12 to 14 days each month, beginning on the first day of the month). Menstrual bleeding will occur in more than half of the women. As a consequence, continuous daily administration of a combination of an estrogen and a progestin has been advocated. The ratios of estrogen to progestin utilized are empiric. Unfortunately, irregular breakthrough bleeding occurs frequently in the first several months of therapy, even though the majority of women eventually become amenorrheic. Although continuous combined therapy is an option, it cannot be advocated strongly until more data accumulate regarding its safety and efficacy. Still another regimen provides estrogen and progestin Monday through Friday of each week, with no medication given on the weekends. Similar dosages of estrogen alone may be administered continuously to women who have undergone hysterectomy, particularly because progestins may impact negatively on several beneficial metabolic effects of estrogen. Younger women may require twice as much estrogen as older women to alleviate symptoms.

Even the continuous combined replacement therapy differs from oral contraceptive preparations in that the doses of estrogen and progestin are lower. Moreover, the estrogens utilized in replacement therapy have fewer metabolic effects than do the synthetic estrogens used in oral contraceptives. There is no evidence that postmenopausal estrogen administration increases the risk of thromboembolic phenomena.

Before beginning estrogen replacement therapy, patients should have a complete history and physical examination. A pretreatment mammogram is indicated because estrogens stimulate glandular tissue and may make diagnosis of breast masses more difficult. Periodic Papanicolaou smears should be obtained, and patients should undergo endometrial biopsy for any breakthrough bleeding and perhaps at intervals of 1 to 2 years while receiving estrogen replacement therapy. Some clinicians believe endometrial biopsies are not needed so long as there is no abnormal bleeding and withdrawal bleeding does not begin until at least 11 days after beginning progestin.

Side effects of therapy are common and may require modifications of therapy. Breast tenderness occurs frequently if too much estrogen is given. The dose of progestin should be reduced in the woman who complains of depression and/or bloating.

Medroxyprogesterone acetate (20 to 40 mg) or megestrol acetate (40 to 80 mg) orally each day may be utilized to treat hot flushes in women who cannot or will not take estrogens. Clonidine skin patches programmed to deliver 0.1 mg per day may also reduce the intensity and frequency of hot flushes in individuals who cannot take estrogens. Postural hypotension, however, is a common side effect with this therapy. Vaginal lubricants may be used for symptomatic treatment of dyspareunia in such individuals.

EFFECTS OF ESTROGEN ON LIPIDS AND CARCINOMA. Unlike the effects of oral contraceptives in younger women, estrogen replacement in postmenopausal women does not raise blood pressure. This may be true because some estrogens, particularly those synthetic ones used in oral contraceptives, increase hepatic synthesis of renin substrate (angiotensinogen). The naturally occurring estrogens E_2 and E_1, however, do not increase renin substrate.

Estrogen administration tends to lower total cholesterol levels, although the degree of reduction varies with the dose and potency of the estrogen used. More importantly, estrogen decreases the LDL-cholesterol and increases the HDL-cholesterol fraction. Increased levels of the subfraction HDL_2 are most strongly associated with both estrogen ingestion and diminished cardiovascular risk. Thus the net effect of estrogen administration is to shift the HDL-LDL ratio to one associated with a decreased risk of cardiovascular disease. Overall, the risk of cardiovascular disease appears reduced by half in postmenopausal users of estrogen, but this reduced risk has not yet been confirmed by prospective studies. Estrogen administration to postmenopausal women may increase plasma triglycerides slightly, but these increases are generally of no significance except in some individuals with genetic disorders of triglyceride metabolism in whom marked elevations in triglycerides may occur.

Progestins, especially those derived from 19-nor-testosterone (such as norethindrone and norgestrel), oppose the effects of estrogens on plasma lipid and lipoprotein fractions. Even orally administered medroxyprogesterone, which is relatively neutral when given alone, appears to cancel the favorable changes induced by estrogens when given in combination with estrogen.

Estrogen-containing oral contraceptive preparations have not been linked conclusively to increased risks of endometrial or breast cancer. However, as noted, estrogen given alone to postmenopausal women greatly increases the risk of endometrial cancer over those never given estrogen. The risk of endometrial carcinoma is reduced markedly, if not abolished, by the cyclic addition of a progestin. Whether estrogen therapy increases the risk of breast cancer is not clear, but the majority of studies have not shown such a relationship. If there is any increased risk of breast cancer, the increase in risk appears modest. Because the likelihood of death from cardiovascular disease is far greater than that from breast cancer, it appears that the benefits of estrogen replacement therapy outweigh the risks in most postmenopausal women.

Korenman SG (ed.): The Menopause. Norwell, Mass, Serono Symposia, USA, 1990. *A review by leading authorities on the physiologic changes and therapeutic approaches to the menopause.*

Mezrow G, Rebar RW: The Menopause. *In* Sciarra JJ (ed.): Gynecology and Obstetrics, Vol. 4. Revised edition—1990. Philadelphia, J. B. Lippincott Company, pp 1-22. *An up-to-date summary of the management of the menopause.*

OVARIAN TUMORS

Ovarian tumors may cause ovarian dysfunction, either by secreting hormones or by stimulating adjacent non-neoplastic stromal cells. Only perhaps 5 per cent of ovarian tumors, however, show functional activity. Most nonfunctional tumors are asymptomatic until late in their evolution; more than three fourths are diagnosed only in advanced stages. In contrast, women with functioning neoplasms commonly present with altered sexual development or reproductive abnormalities, and thus diagnosis is made much earlier. Ovarian tumors may occur in all age groups but are less common in younger women, especially before puberty.

Ovarian tumors generally are classified as (1) common epithelial tumors derived from coelomic epithelial cells; (2) sex cord stromal tumors composed of granulosa cells, theca cells, Sertoli-Leydig cells, or their progenitors; (3) lipid or lipoid cell tumors; (4) germ cell tumors, including teratomas, dysgerminomas, and choriocarcinomas; (5) gonadoblastomas; (6) soft tissue tumors not specific to the ovary; and (7) secondary metastatic tumors. Each of these major classes of tumors includes several different histologic types. Sex cord stromal tumors are most apt to be functioning.

Ovarian neoplasms must be distinguished from tumor-like conditions of the ovary, which include luteomas of pregnancy (nodular theca-lutein hyperplasia) that may result in virilization of the mother but regress spontaneously post partum; hyperplasia of ovarian stroma (hyperthecosis), frequently associated with severe hirsutism; functional follicle and corpus luteum cysts; germinal inclusion cysts lined by surface epithelium; simple cysts; paraovarian cysts; inflammatory lesions; and endometrial cysts or endometriomas.

Ovarian neoplasms are diagnosed most commonly at the time of routine pelvic examination. Even most functioning neoplasms are palpable; those that are not may be identified by ultrasonography. As an ovarian tumor grows, it distends the abdomen, leading to pressure on the bladder or rectum and a sensation of pelvic fullness and discomfort. Ascites may develop if the neoplasm is malignant or sometimes when it is not (Meigs' syndrome).

TABLE 224–9. CLINICAL FEATURES OF HORMONE-PRODUCING OVARIAN TUMORS

| Tumor | Hormones Produced* | Incidence | | | | Size Range in cm (per cent Palpable) | Miscellaneous |
| | | Age in Years | | | | | |
		Peak	Range	Malignancy	Bilaterality		
Androblastoma (arrhenoblastoma)	*Androgens*, estrogens	20–40	4–69	20%	Rare	<5–>25 (85)	Most common virilizing ovarian neoplasm
Dysgerminoma	Androgens, *chorionic gonadotropin*	10–30	6–76	100%	15%	3–50 (60)	May be "mixed" with other tumors originating from germ cells
Gonadoblastoma	*Androgens*, estrogens	10–30	6–38	50%	40%	<1–>30 (?)	Usually occur in genetic males with female external genitalia
Granulosa-theca cell	*Estrogens*, androgens, progestogens	30–70	<1–92	5–20%	10–15%	<1–>30 (80–90)	Most common functioning ovarian neoplasm
Hilar cell	*Androgens*, estrogens	45–75	4–86	Rare	Rare	1–9 (50)	Hypertension in 50%, diabetes in 50%
Lipoid cell (adrenal-like)	*Androgens*, estrogens	20–50	6–78	20%	Rare	0.5–30	Diabetes associated with lesion in 50%
Teratomas, benign	Serotonin, thyroxine	10–40	<1–78	Rare	10%	2–45 (90)	Carcinoid syndrome only in patients with large carcinoid tumors
Teratomas, malignant	Chorionic gonadotropin	6–15	6–42	100%	Rare	>5 (100)	Not all secrete chorionic gonadotropin

Modified from data of Rose GI, Vande Wiele RL: *In* Williams RH (ed.): Textbook of Endocrinology, 5th ed. Philadelphia, W. B. Saunders Company, 1974, pp 368–422.
*When more than one hormone is secreted, the major one is *italicized*.

Abdominal and pelvic pain may occur with torsion, hemorrhage, or rupture of the tumor.

Functioning ovarian tumors can produce other clinical manifestations as well (Table 224–9). Some tumors are associated with clinical manifestations of decreased hormone production. Intervals of amenorrhea caused by steroid suppression of gonadotropins may alternate with excessive vaginal bleeding produced by steroid stimulation of the endometrium during the reproductive years. In some young girls, steroid-secreting ovarian tumors may cause pseudopubertal development. In postmenopausal women, increased estrogens, secreted by the tumor itself or from peripheral aromatization of androgens secreted by the tumor, may stimulate the endometrium and result in bleeding.

Any pelvic mass identified on examination must be investigated. What constitutes such a "mass" and what evaluation is indicated depend on the age of the individual. Adnexal masses less than 5 cm in diameter may well be due to normal follicular development in women of reproductive age and may resolve with observation over 2 to 8 weeks. Even cystic masses greater than 5 cm in diameter, as documented by ultrasound examination, may resolve over a few weeks. Those that do not resolve require surgical removal. Any palpable adnexal mass in a postmenopausal woman, in whom the ovaries normally atrophy and cannot be detected during examination, should be removed.

Yeh I-T, Zaloudek C, Kurman RJ: Functioning tumors and tumor-like conditions of the ovary. *In* Becker KL (ed): Principles and Practice of Endocrinology and Metabolism. Philadelphia, J. B. Lippincott Company, 1990, pp 848–854. *An excellent discussion of the clinical manifestations of ovarian tumors for any physician who undertakes the medical care of women.*

225 Hirsutism

Roger S. Rittmaster

DEFINITION. *Normal Hair Growth.* Most body hair can be classified as vellus or terminal. Vellus hairs are fine and unpigmented, such as those that cover the face of children. Terminal hairs, pigmented and coarser, may be sex hormone–dependent (such as those over the chin and abdomen of men) or sex hormone–independent (such as eyebrows and eyelashes) (Fig.

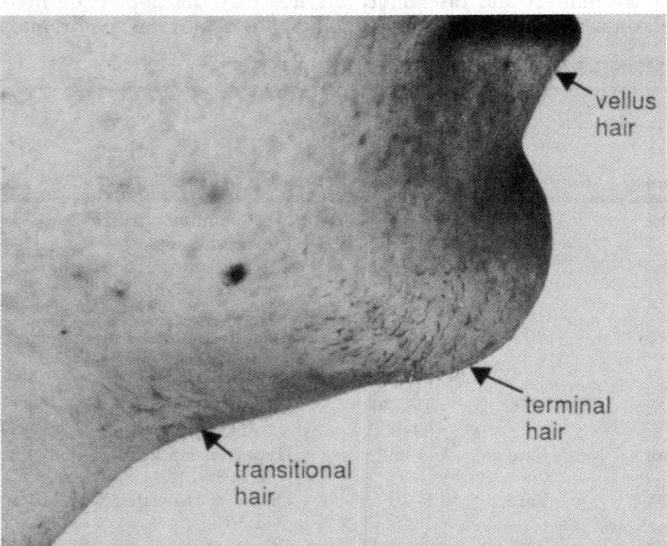

FIGURE 225–1. Facial hair growth in a hirsute woman. Vellus hair is fine, unpigmented hair. Terminal hair is coarse and pigmented. Transitional hair is intermediate between vellus and terminal. This woman also has mild acne, another androgen-dependent process. (Reprinted with permission from Rittmaster RS: Hirsutism. Med North Am 14:2686–2695, 1987.)

225–1). Androgens convert vellus hair to terminal hair in sex hormone–dependent areas.

Hirsutism. Hirsutism is the presence of excess hair in women. This is usually an androgen-dependent process. Twenty-five to thirty-five per cent of young women have terminal hair over the lower abdomen, around the nipples, or over the upper lip. Most women gradually develop more androgen-dependent body hair with age. Nevertheless, "normal" patterns of female hair growth are unacceptable to many women. At the other extreme, severe hirsutism may rarely be the earliest sign of masculinizing diseases. More often, however, severe hirsutism reflects only increased androgen production in women with no serious underlying disorder.

ETIOLOGY. Hirsutism may be divided into androgen-dependent and androgen-independent etiologies. Androgen-dependent hirsutism is restricted to areas where men typically become hirsute and often begins with adolescence. In women, androgens arise from the ovaries, the adrenal glands, or exogenous sources such as anabolic steroids (Table 225–1). Often, no definite abnormality exists; the hirsutism simply results from modestly increased androgen production and/or increased skin sensitivity to androgens.

Androgen-independent hirsutism is caused by drugs (cyclosporine, glucocorticoids, minoxidil, diazoxide, and possibly phenytoin) or starvation (anorexia nervosa); it may be associated with the skin lesions of porphyria; or it may be an inherited condition. Androgen-independent hirsutism is characterized by long, fine hairs occurring over much of the body, including such areas as the forehead and flanks. Androgens may exacerbate androgen-independent hirsutism, giving rise to a clinically confusing presentation. The pathophysiology of androgen-independent hirsutism is unknown.

PATHOPHYSIOLOGY OF ANDROGEN-DEPENDENT HIRSUTISM. To be active in skin, testosterone, the major circulating androgen, must first be converted to dihydrotestosterone by the enzyme 5α-reductase. Hirsute women have elevated skin 5α-reductase compared to nonhirsute women. Nevertheless, increased 5α-reductase alone is usually insufficient to induce hirsutism.

Hirsute women as a group also have increased androgen production from the adrenal glands, the ovaries, or both. Either testosterone itself is secreted, or androgen precursors such as androstenedione are secreted, which are then converted in the liver or skin to active androgens. Most hirsute women do not have an underlying disease, but simply fall at one end of the spectrum of androgen production and skin 5α-reductase activity.

The ovarian and adrenal causes of hirsutism listed in Table 225–1 lead to increased androgen production. Virilizing tumors secrete androgens directly. The pituitary adenomas in Cushing's disease release ACTH, which stimulates the adrenals to secrete both cortisol and androgens (Ch. 217). The virilizing forms of congenital adrenal hyperplasia involve enzyme defects that impair cortisol synthesis, leading to increased ACTH secretion (Ch. 217). The enzyme block causes shunting of cortisol precursors to

TABLE 225–1. CAUSES OF ANDROGEN-DEPENDENT HIRSUTISM

Ovarian causes
   Polycystic ovarian syndrome
   Severe insulin resistance
   Virilizing ovarian tumors
Adrenal causes
   Congenital adrenal hyperplasia
      21-Hydroxylase deficiency
      3β-Hydroxysteroid dehydrogenase deficiency
      11-Hydroxylase deficiency
   Cushing's disease
   Ectopic ACTH-producing tumors
   Virilizing adrenal tumors
Combined ovarian and adrenal causes
   "Idiopathic" hirsutism
Exogenous androgens
   "Anabolic" steroids
   Danazol
   Postmenopausal hormone replacement formulations containing androgens

androgens. The most common form, 21-hydroxylase deficiency, leads to an overproduction of 17-hydroxyprogesterone. While severe forms of 21-hydroxylase deficiency cause ambiguous genitalia in female infants, milder forms may lead only to hirsutism and/or irregular menses. This "attenuated" form of 21-hydroxylase deficiency is present in about 1 per cent of hirsute women.

In the polycystic ovarian syndrome, both the ovaries and adrenals secrete excess androgens, although the majority of the androgens are usually of ovarian origin (Ch. 224). Obesity is an important predisposing factor to the development of polycystic ovarian syndrome and, as such, can indirectly cause hirsutism.

CLINICAL MANIFESTATIONS. Androgen-induced hirsutism of benign origin usually begins in adolescence and becomes gradually worse with time. Family history is often positive. The hirsutism may vary from mild to severe. Usually hair growth begins over the lower abdomen, on the breasts, and over the upper lip. Hirsutism over the chin, above the umbilicus, and over the central chest requires somewhat greater androgenicity. Widespread hirsutism over the upper back, upper abdomen, and upper chest implies severe hyperandrogenism. Some women may have only facial hair or other unusual patterns of hirsutism, probably due to local variation in skin 5α-reductase activity.

Severe, rapidly progressive hirsutism, beginning in childhood or beyond adolescence, suggests an androgen-secreting tumor. Such tumors can cause signs of virilization: deepening of the voice, excess muscle development, and marked clitoral enlargement. Signs of virilization, however, simply imply severe hyperandrogenism and can occasionally be seen with all causes of hirsutism. Androgen-secreting tumors are rare, and most severely hirsute women have either polycystic ovarian syndrome or hirsutism alone.

Attenuated congenital adrenal hyperplasia is clinically indistinguishable from simple hirsutism or polycystic ovarian syndrome, and the diagnosis must be made biochemically. Cushing's disease may be suspected when the patient presents with central obesity, hypertension, diabetes, and/or thinning of the skin (see Ch. 217).

DIAGNOSIS. The diagnostic evaluation of hirsutism is directed at ruling out a significant underlying cause. Important historical points include a drug history (including use of oral contraceptives), age of onset and rate of progression of hirsutism, presence of thinning of scalp hair or deepening of the voice, menstrual history, history of obesity, and family history of hirsutism. The physical examination should include an assessment of the quality and distribution of hair growth, signs of virilization or Cushing's syndrome, and presence of abdominal or pelvic masses.

Laboratory Evaluation. In women with androgen-dependent hirsutism, regular ovulatory menses, and no physical signs of Cushing's syndrome, hormonal evaluation is usually unnecessary. Virilizing tumors have not been reported in such patients, and hirsutism associated with attenuated congenital adrenal hyperplasia need not be treated differently from other benign forms of hirsutism (see Treatment section).

In hirsute women with irregular menses, a reasonable laboratory evaluation includes measurement of serum testosterone, 17-hydroxyprogesterone, prolactin, LH, and FSH. A testosterone level less than 170 mg per deciliter (6 nmol per liter) rules out an androgen-secreting tumor, although re-evaluation may be necessary if the hirsutism continues to progress or signs of virilization appear. Testosterone levels above 170 mg per deciliter may also be seen with polycystic ovarian syndrome. To rule out attenuated 21-hydroxylase deficiency, serum 17-hydroxyprogesterone should be measured between 7 and 9 A.M. during the first week of the menstrual cycle (values may be elevated during the luteal phase). Values less than 200 mg per deciliter (6 nmol per liter) rule out this diagnosis. Mildly elevated values (less than 1000 mg per deciliter) (30 nmol per liter) may be seen in both heterozygous and homozygous 21-hydroxylase deficiency (the heterozygous disorder is not associated with hirsutism) and in polycystic ovarian syndrome. To distinguish between these conditions, 17-hydroxyprogesterone should be measured 30 to 60 minutes after the intravenous administration of 250 μg synthetic ACTH. Levels are greater than 1500 ng per deciliter (45 nmol per liter) in homozygous 21-hydroxylase deficiency. Other forms of attenuated congenital adrenal hyperplasia are too rare to justify routine hormonal screening. Serum prolactin, LH, and FSH are used to evaluate the possibility that a prolactinoma, ovarian failure, or polycystic ovarian syndrome is contributing to the irregular menses. These tests are not directly relevant to the evaluation of hirsutism itself. Measurement of dehydroepiandrosterone sulfate (DHEAS) as an index of adrenal androgen production is generally unhelpful.

TREATMENT. Hirsutism is a cosmetic problem that may have severe psychosocial consequences. Because it is not a disease in itself, the benefits and risks of any therapy should be carefully weighed and the treatment individualized.

Mechanical Hair Removal. For mild hirsutism, bleaching and mechanical hair removal are adequate and safe. Shaving is the easiest method of temporarily removing visible hair. While shaving does not increase hair growth rates, it may leave a stubble and is unacceptable to many women. Plucking and waxing may control mild hirsutism, but they also do not resolve the problem and may lead to scarring. Electrolysis can provide a safe, effective alternative for localized mild to moderate hirsutism and is a useful adjunct to medical therapy in more severe cases. Electrolysis is expensive, however, and long-term treatment may be necessary.

Drug Treatment. Successful medical therapy results in a gradual return of terminal hair to finer, less pigmented vellus hair. Younger women with mild hirsutism of brief duration respond best to medical therapy. More severe hair growth can be prevented, and resolution of the hirsutism is possible. Nevertheless, drug treatment is not a cure, and lifelong therapy may be necessary to prevent recurrence. Generally, 6 months is needed to judge the efficacy of a given therapy, although improvement may continue indefinitely. No drug is currently approved by the Food and Drug Administration for treatment of hirsutism.

Antiandrogens. Antiandrogens (spironolactone, cyproterone acetate), which block the androgen receptor, are the drug treatment of choice for hirsutism. They are effective in reducing hair growth in at least 70 per cent of women, and hirsutism in the remaining women stabilizes. Spironolactone is usually given in a starting dose of 50 mg twice daily. Although higher doses (up to 200 mg daily) may improve efficacy, side effects are dose related. The most common side effect is increased frequency of menses, which can be controlled by combining spironolactone with an oral contraceptive. Spironolactone should not be given to pregnant women or to women with renal insufficiency. Cyproterone acetate, a potent antiandrogen and progestin, is often given as 50 to 100 mg daily on days 5 to 15 of the menstrual cycle, combined with 35 to 50 μg of ethinyl estradiol on days 5 to 26. Alternatively, it may be given with an oral contraceptive, at a starting dose of 50 mg daily from days 1 to 10 of the birth control pill cycle. Side effects are similar to those of the oral contraceptive alone. Although widely used in Europe and Canada, cyproterone acetate has not been approved by the Food and Drug Administration at the time of publication.

Ovarian Suppression. Although oral contraceptives are often used to control menstrual cycles in women given antiandrogens, they are usually ineffective for treating hirsutism when used alone (although they may prevent the hirsutism from becoming worse). Birth control pills differ in the androgenicity of the progestational component, but this difference has never been shown to have clinical significance in the treatment of hirsutism. Gonadotropin-releasing hormone analogues suppress the ovary by suppressing LH and FSH secretion. They are effective in treating hirsutism associated with polycystic ovarian syndrome but are expensive and lead to menopausal symptoms unless estrogens are given concurrently.

Glucocorticoids. Glucocorticoids suppress adrenal cortisol and androgen secretion. They are frequently ineffective in low doses, and higher doses can cause Cushing's syndrome. They also can cause a drug-induced hirsutism in some women and cannot be recommended as a routine treatment. While glucocorticoids have traditionally been used to treat congenital adrenal hyperplasia, antiandrogens are more effective in treating the hirsutism associated with this disorder.

PROGNOSIS. Untreated, hirsutism usually becomes gradually worse with time, and most therapies need to be continued indefinitely. However, worsening hirsutism is easily prevented with antiandrogen therapy, and most women experience a satisfactory improvement with the judicious use of mechanical and medical therapies.

Horton R, Lobo RA (eds.): Androgen metabolism in hirsute and normal females. Clin Endocrinol Metab 15(2):213, 1986. *An excellent collection of reviews on aspects of the pathophysiology and treatment of hirsutism.*

Mahajan DK (ed.): Polycystic ovarian disease. Endocrinol Metab Clin North Am 17(4):621, 1988. *A series of well-written reviews on the pathophysiology and clinical approach to polycystic ovarian syndrome.*

Rittmaster RS: Evaluation and treatment of hirsutism. Fertil Reprod Med Clin North Am 2:511, 1991. *A detailed review of the evaluation and treatment of hirsutism.*

Spritzer P, Billaud L, Thalabard J, et al.: Cyproterone acetate versus hydrocortisone treatment in late-onset adrenal hyperplasia. J Clin Endocrinol Metab 70:642, 1990. *Another example of the excellent clinical results with antiandrogens.*

226 Nonmalignant Diseases of the Breast

Douglas J. Marchant

Approximately one in every four women in the United States requires medical attention for breast symptomatology. More than half of all women have some degree of fibrocystic changes during their lifetime, and most have histologic changes that could be described as "fibrocystic disease." It is recommended, however, that the term *fibrocystic disease* be abandoned and the term *fibrocystic change* or *condition* be substituted because it is more descriptive of the clinical entity.

The physician should be knowledgeable about these common benign conditions and provide treatment or referral when indicated. This chapter discusses growth and development of the breasts, puberty, pregnancy and lactation, and the common benign conditions for which consultation is requested. Diagnostic studies, including examination of the breast, aspiration, and indications for surgical biopsy and referral, are emphasized. Gynecomastia, the main nonmalignant abnormality of the male breast, is described in Ch. 222.

GROWTH AND DEVELOPMENT OF THE BREAST

The functional units of the breast are of ectodermal origin. The epithelial ridge that eventually forms the breast tissue, recognizable by the thirty-fifth day of embryonic life, undergoes a series of alterations to form the lactiferous ducts and alveolae. At 15 weeks, mesenchymal cells differentiate into the smooth muscle of the nipple and the areola. The breast unit is complete at birth, as demonstrated by the occasional appearance of "witch's milk" caused by high levels of maternal hormones. During the third trimester of pregnancy, placental hormones in the fetal circulation stimulate further development of the functional units. This colostral secretion declines within 3 to 4 weeks, the breast tissue involutes, and no additional differentiation occurs until puberty.

Development of the mature breast begins with the onset of puberty and continues for several years. Estrogen levels increase, and the areolae become enlarged and pigmented. Adipose tissue is deposited to form and shape the breast and to provide a steroidogenic milieu for the conversion of hormones directly in the breast. In addition to estrogen and progesterone, insulin, cortisol, thyroxin, growth hormone, and prolactin are required for complete functional development.

The mature breast consists of the functional units—the alveolae, lactiferous ducts, and their supporting tissues. The alveolae are inconspicuous in the nonpregnant, nonlactating breast. The much larger ducts lie embedded in a stromal network consisting of fibrous tissue, fat, blood vessels, and lymphatics.

ABNORMALITIES OF GROWTH AND DEVELOPMENT

A number of congenital anomalies may be referred to the clinician for evaluation and treatment. The most frequently observed is the accessory nipple, or polythelia. This tissue, which may be mistaken for a pigmented nevus, lies along the milk line extending from the axilla to the groin. Rarely, functioning breast tissue is found along this milk line. Most commonly this ectopic breast tissue is located in the axilla, where it may enlarge and become quite painful during pregnancy and lactation.

Patients may be referred for failure of breast development, premature development, and breast hypertrophy. Normal sexual development and puberty are discussed in Ch. 224. Complete absence of the breast is rare and usually is associated with defects in the chest wall and muscles. Premature development is usually associated with the appearance of a mass beneath the nipple-areola complex. Other manifestations of sexual maturation are absent and hormonal studies are normal. A vaginal smear reveals little or no estrogen effect, consistent with the prepubertal state. No treatment is required; in particular to be avoided is surgical removal of the mass in the mistaken belief that it represents a tumor. If this area is removed, breast tissue will not develop on the affected side. Asymmetric breast development is common and requires no further treatment. Breast hypertrophy, on the other hand, is often uncomfortable and disturbing both to the patient and to the parents. These patients require considerable counseling because if reduction mammoplasty is recommended too early, a repeat operation will be necessary. A reduction mammoplasty, if required, should be performed only after completion of breast development, which may take several years.

THE BREAST DURING PREGNANCY AND THE PUERPERIUM

With the completion of breast development during and following puberty, the breasts are quiescent until pregnancy. During pregnancy the breast grows and develops due to lobular alveolar growth, the formation of secretory cells, and changes in the supporting tissues. Insulin responsiveness also is acquired during pregnancy. Further growth requires estrogen, progesterone, prolactin, and human placental lactogen. During pregnancy, serum prolactin increases from a nonpregnant level of approximately 10 ng to 200 ng per milliliter or more at term. Human placental lactogen reaches serum concentrations of approximately 6000 ng per milliliter at term. Lactation is suppressed by estrogen and progesterone, which inhibit prolactin action at the receptor level. With the rapid drop in estrogen and progesterone levels following delivery, this inhibition is removed and milk production begins. A decrease in the prolactin-inhibiting factor (PIF) by suckling increases prolactin and further promotes lactation. In the final event oxytocin is released and acts on the myoepithelial cells to contract the duct system for the delivery of the milk. By the end of the third or fourth month, suckling is the only stimulus required for continued lactation. If breast feeding does not occur, prolactin rapidly returns to nonpregnant levels.

Mastitis occasionally complicates lactation, usually following the first pregnancy. There is a localized area of inflammation and tenderness and slight elevation of temperature. Treatment includes continuation of breast feeding and the use of appropriate antibiotics. Since the most common organism is *Staphylococcus aureus*, penicillin or one of its derivatives is the treatment of choice. If the patient does not respond and if the tenderness and fever persist, a breast abscess should be suspected, for which the treatment is adequate drainage under general anesthesia in an operating room setting. Antibiotics should be continued in full therapeutic doses for 7 to 10 days following adequate drainage. The breast rapidly returns to normal and the cosmetic result is excellent.

The discovery of a dominant mass during pregnancy or lactation requires careful consideration. Early in pregnancy, a dominant mass is easily distinguished from fibrocystic changes. Often the patient gives a history of a mass first discovered many years before and followed in the belief that it represented a benign fibroadenoma. With rare exception, the cause of all dominant masses discovered during pregnancy or the puerperium should be resolved. This requires an open biopsy using a local anesthesia. Biopsy can be safely performed during lactation. The patient is requested to empty the breast early on the day of the operation. The mass is removed with careful approximation of the breast tissues and a pressure dressing temporarily applied. This can be removed later in the day and often the patient can breast feed on the operated side.

FIBROCYSTIC CHANGES

Fibrocystic changes, which represent an exaggerated physiologic response to a changing hormonal environment, include painful lumpy breasts (mastodynia, mastalgia), a dominant mass, and nipple discharge.

The peak incidence of fibrocystic changes occurs between the ages of 30 and 50. Breast tenderness often occurs premenstrually, which suggests that progesterone may play an important role in the development and symptomatology of these changes. In the resting breast there is minimal epithelial proliferation in the proliferative phase of the menstrual cycle and maximal proliferation in the secretory phase, a pattern quite different from that of the endometrium. Whether this dissimilarity between breast and endometrial epithelium reflects receptor content or some more indirect effect on proliferation is unclear. Estrogen is a mitogen for the endometrium but not for the breast, and the idea, derived largely from endometrial studies, that progestins are protective for the breast is difficult to sustain. The relative contributions of estrogen and progesterone to the etiology of benign breast conditions require further investigation.

Most, if not all, women experience these fibrocystic changes, and to label this condition a "disease" is inappropriate. Physical examination usually reveals irregular thickening, particularly in the upper outer quadrants. The changes associated with this process and its symptomatology constitute one of the most difficult challenges in the office practice of the physician.

MASTODYNIA (MASTALGIA)

Breast pain is common; it may occur in as many as 50 per cent of women. Usually the etiology is unclear, and relief of symptoms often is proportional to the time that the physician spends with the patient. The discomfort generally is classified as (1) cyclic mastalgia or mastodynia occurring immediately prior to the menses; (2) fibrocystic changes, including duct ectasia and sclerosing adenosis; or (3) referred pain such as costochondritis.

Almost all women complain of occasional breast discomfort for the first few days preceding the onset of menses, and most do not seek medical attention. It is the discomfort occurring at other times during the menstrual cycle, or throughout the cycle, that brings the patient to the physician.

Perimenopausal patients not infrequently note breast discomfort. The cause is unknown. Postmenopausal patients should be carefully evaluated for referred pain. They often perceive the discomfort to be in the breast when in reality it is related to the pectoral muscles, the chest wall, or even the cardiovascular system. Trauma is not an infrequent cause of breast discomfort. The usual presentation is a tender erythematous or ecchymotic area. In some cases open biopsy must be performed to rule out carcinoma.

NIPPLE DISCHARGE

Nipple discharge may be physiologic or pathologic, provoked or spontaneous. In most cases the patient can be immediately reassured that cancer is unlikely, since 10 per cent or fewer of breast cancers present with nipple discharge. A careful and detailed history is essential. Is the discharge produced only at the time of breast self-examination when the nipple is squeezed? Does it occur only with sexual stimulation? What type of physical exercise does the patient do? Does she wear a sport brassiere? Does she take any medication? Has she ever been pregnant? What is the menstrual history? Most patients can describe the character of the discharge, although not necessarily in a reliable fashion. For example, many patients complain of bloody nipple discharge, but when the secretions are examined on a gauze or by cytology, the color is blackish green and no blood cells are found.

Three types of discharge deserve further comment: galactorrhea, serosanguinous or bloody discharge, and discharge from the postmenopausal breast.

GALACTORRHEA. Galactorrhea is the spontaneous secretion of a milky discharge not immediately associated with a pregnancy. Usually it is persistent and occasionally it is voluminous. Elevated prolactin levels may be associated with galactorrhea. Physiologic causes of hyperprolactinemia include breast stimulation, coitus, eating, exercise, pregnancy, sleep, and stress. Hyperprolactinemia may also be due to pathologic factors, including brain and pituitary disorders, encephalitis, and pituitary microadenomas or macroadenomas. In addition, a number of pharmacologic agents may produce hyperprolactinemia, as noted in Table 226–1.

TABLE 226–1. CAUSES OF NONPUERPERAL GALACTORRHEA

I. **Central origin**
  A. Organic
    1. Suprahypophyseal lesions
      a. Hypothalamic disorders—infiltrative processes (histiocytosis, metastatic diseases); masses (craniopharyngioma, meningioma); infarction; embolism
      b. Pituitary stalk lesions—section; impingement by tumors (all types with suprasellar extension); vascular insult
    2. Hypophyseal tumors
      a. Prolactin secreting* (solitary; part of multiple endocrine adenomatosis syndrome mixed with GH, TSH, ACTH)
  B. Functional
    1. Drug related
      a. Psychotropic (butyrophenones, phenothiazines)*
      b. Antihypertensive (reserpine, α-methyldopa)
      c. Cannabinoids (morphine, heroin)
      d. Contraceptives
      e. Antigastroplegics (metoclopramide)*
    2. Unclassified (idiopathic, stress, empty sella syndrome)
II. **Peripheral origin**
  A. Due to pituitary prolactin
    1. Due to primary failure of target endocrine gland
      a. Hypothyroidism
      b. Addison's disease
    2. Due to excess estrogen formation from target endocrine glands
      a. Feminizing adrenal carcinoma
      b. Polycystic ovarian syndrome
    3. Due to decreased metabolic clearance of prolactin
      a. Renal failure
      b. Liver failure
      c. Hypothyroidism
    4. Due to local breast conditions
      a. Mechanical stimulation or suckling
      b. Thoracic and/or breast trauma, burn
      c. Inflammation, i.e., mastitis, herpes zoster
  B. Due to ectopic prolactin production
    1. Renal neoplasia
    2. Bronchogenic neoplasia

*Most common causes of highest serum prolactin levels.

Prolactin is secreted in a sleep-related circadian rhythm with maximal release between 3:00 A.M. and 5:00 A.M. Serum samples, therefore, should be obtained in a fasting state between 8:00 A.M. and 12:00 noon. Prolactin levels do not change during the menstrual cycle. A serum level of prolactin of greater than 20 ng per milliliter may be abnormal and should be further evaluated. Other diagnostic studies include microscopic evaluation of the breast discharge, which may reveal refractile fat globules, confirming the diagnosis. A thorough history should be taken to rule out physiologic or pharmacologic causes, and the menstrual history should focus on amenorrhea, oligomenorrhea, infertility, or a short luteal phase.

Prolactinomas, or prolactin-secreting pituitary adenomas, are common causes for hyperprolactinemia in women. Prolactinomas may be microadenomas (< 1 cm in diameter) or macroadenomas (> 1 cm). The diagnosis usually is made by computed tomography (CT) scan using contrast media. Modern CT or magnetic resonance imaging has replaced older methods of diagnosing pituitary tumors, such as the cone view tomogram or plain skull film.

SEROUS OR BLOODY BREAST DISCHARGE. This type of nipple discharge must be investigated. Usually it is caused by a benign intraductal papilloma, but carcinoma occurs in 10 to 15 per cent of these patients. Often it is difficult to demonstrate the exact quadrant of the breast from which the discharge appears at the nipple. A microscopic examination of the fluid may identify red blood cells, confirming the clinical impression and the need for open biopsy.

POSTMENOPAUSAL NIPPLE DISCHARGE. Any nipple discharge that occurs during the postmenopausal period must be viewed as suggestive of carcinoma of the breast. Careful examination of the breast may reveal a mass or other findings consistent with carcinoma, which must be followed up, as described in Ch. 227.

DETECTION AND DIAGNOSIS

HISTORY. The diagnostic evaluation begins with a careful history, noting the age of the patient, the date of the last menstrual period, family history of breast disease, use of medication, the date of birth of the first child, and any surgery related to previous breast disease. Inquiry should be made concerning the use of oral contraceptives, including the type of medication and for how long it has been taken. If the patient has received estrogen replacement therapy, the type of medication and the length of time that the medication has been used should be noted. Pelvic surgery, including oophorectomy and a history of pelvic malignancy, particularly ovarian carcinoma and endometrial carcinoma, should be recorded. Did the patient notice the symptom casually or by employing deliberate breast self-examination, or was it first noted by another health care provider? Does the patient wear a brassiere? What type of medication has the patient used to provide relief? Are there any emotional factors that should be considered? The history should be recorded with particular emphasis on the date of onset of the symptom, the exact location in the breast and, finally, the disposition.

PHYSICAL EXAMINATION. For careful evaluation the breasts are first examined in the sitting or standing position. Contour, symmetry, and skin changes are noted. The vascular pattern is observed and the condition of the areola and nipple recorded. These changes may be exaggerated by asking the patient to elevate the arm or to place her hands on the hips, thus contracting the pectoralis major muscles and exaggerating any small change noted on routine observation. While the patient is in this position, the axilla is palpated, being careful to support the arm with the opposite hand. This relaxes the pectoralis muscle and permits careful evaluation of the axilla. While the patient is in the sitting or standing position, the supraclavicular area should be checked for a cervical rib or other unexpected finding. Examination of the neck may reveal thyroid enlargement.

Following these maneuvers, the patient is placed in the supine position. The breast is palpated in a systematic manner with the flat of the hand. The use of Phisohex or talcum powder permits the identification of even minor alterations. Approximately 80 per cent of American women discover their own lesions, often while taking a shower. The use of this so-called "wet technique" permits the identification of very subtle changes in breast texture. Following the careful evaluation of all quadrants, the areola and nipple should be carefully examined and the nipple gently squeezed. Any discharge is evaluated for location, consistency, and color.

The patient often presents with a chief complaint of a lump. This may or may not be confirmed by careful examination. The usual finding is a vague thickening, particularly in the upper outer quadrant.

The physician must carefully evaluate the chief complaint and then, on the basis of a thorough examination, decide whether the findings represent a dominant mass or an exaggeration of normal breast tissue associated with fibrocystic changes. In the obese patient with very large breasts, it is unlikely that any but the most obvious lesion will be discovered by routine examination. The large breast, therefore, is an indication for mammography to augment what in most cases is an inadequate physical examination.

Once a lesion has been characterized as a mass, a lump, or a dominant mass and has been measured or drawn, its cause must be established. There are no obviously benign lesions. The only exception is a mass in the teenager for whom elective treatment of an obvious fibroadenoma may be recommended.

CYST ASPIRATION

A mass may be cystic, solid, benign, or malignant. Attempts should be made to aspirate the mass with a fine (23 or 24) gauge needle. Local anesthesia is not required. The mass is immobilized with the fingers, the needle inserted, and the fluid withdrawn. If the fluid is clear or cloudy and no residual mass is palpated immediately following the aspiration, it is sufficient to arrange a

follow-up examination in 1 month with reassurance and monthly self-examination of the breast. If the mass remains immediately following the aspiration, if the fluid is bloody, or if there is a residual mass on the first follow-up visit, open biopsy is mandatory. If the mass is solid, open biopsy is recommended except for a teenager, for whom excision biopsy can be performed on an elective basis.

Cytologic evaluation of nipple discharge or cyst fluid is seldom rewarding. On the other hand, it is probably advisable to examine spontaneous nipple discharge microscopically, particularly if it is unilateral and serosanguinous or bloody. A positive cytologic examination of cyst fluid in the absence of other indications for biopsy is exceedingly rare. Cytology is not, therefore, recommended as a routine examination.

FINE-NEEDLE ASPIRATION (FNA)

The accurate use of fine-needle aspiration requires an understanding of the techniques involved and a cytopathologist capable of interpreting the smear. A standard disposable syringe can be used with a 23- to 25-gauge needle. Local anesthesia is helpful because several "passes" may be required to obtain an adequate sample of "tissue juice" for appropriate evaluation. The material should not enter the syringe and should be placed directly on the slide and fixed with an appropriate spray. The technique is most useful for the obvious dominant mass. Fine-needle aspiration is useful only if positive; a negative finding is unreliable. Some radiologists prefer that a mammogram be performed prior to fine-needle aspiration because the procedure may distort the anatomy of the breast.

OTHER DIAGNOSTIC STUDIES

Ultrasonography is useful to confirm the presence or absence of macrocysts, particularly when these lesions are discovered by mammography and are nonpalpable. The procedure should not be performed on a routine basis, since it is unsuitable for screening and is an extra expense to the patient. It is much simpler to immediately attempt aspiration with a fine-gauge needle. Thermography and diaphonography are experimental procedures and should not be employed, except with evaluative protocols.

Mammography may be used as a screening examination in the asymptomatic patient or to confirm the findings noted on physical examination. The accuracy of mammography depends upon a number of factors, including the size and density of the breast and the location of the lesion. False-negative results, which occur even in the best institutions, may reach 10 per cent and in some centers approach 25 per cent. The presence of a dominant mass and a negative mammogram clearly do not preclude the recommendation for referral and an open biopsy.

BREAST BIOPSY

Certain features of the breast biopsy are important when discussing such a recommendation with the patient. In the past, open biopsy was performed solely as a diagnostic procedure to determine the presence or absence of cancer. Currently, the biopsy often becomes part of conservative treatment, and therefore it must be executed by surgeons familiar with contemporary treatment for breast cancer (Ch. 227). It is essential that the biopsy be performed in an operating room setting with trained personnel familiar with the biopsy technique and the use of local anesthesia.

MANAGEMENT OF BENIGN BREAST DISORDERS

The medical management of benign breast conditions often challenges even the most well-informed physician. For patients with mild fibrocystic changes and minimal symptomatology, reassurance only is indicated. Occasionally, a well-fitting brassiere, salt restriction, and a mild analgesic to control discomfort are all that is required.

For patients with greater discomfort, a detailed history is often the key to appropriate diagnosis and therapy. Mammography may be helpful in ruling out significant breast pathology and in reassuring the patient. Treatment strategy often depends upon the "complaint threshold of the patient and the safety threshold of the physician." In the absence of highly effective specific therapy, a number of treatment regimens have been proposed:

the topical use of progestational agents, tamoxifen, bromocriptine, various vitamin formulations, and primrose oil. For most patients treatment is directed toward a reasonable and rational explanation rather than any specific medication.

Danazol is effective but for most patients the cost and the side effects are prohibitive. Moderate doses of danazol decrease follicular maturation and increase anovulatory periods. Danazol has intrinsic androgenic activity and also decreases sex hormone–binding globulin, which increases free testosterone levels. Estradiol secretion is reduced because of the lack of follicular maturation. For some patients who have been incapacitated by breast discomfort and nodularity, a short course of danazol (400 to 600 mg daily for 6 months) may provide symptomatic relief and a marked change in the physical examination. The use of danazol should be restricted to those patients who have failed more conservative measures to control their symptomatology.

The treatment of patients with galactorrhea varies according to its etiology and the patient's desires. For patients with a pituitary microadenoma, bromocriptine, 5 mg daily, is usually effective. Unfortunately, if bromocriptine is discontinued, hyperprolactinemia usually returns, leading to galactorrhea and amenorrhea. Therapy therefore must be continued indefinitely.

The objectives for therapy of prolactinomas are to normalize the prolactin levels and menstrual function, to preserve function of the anterior pituitary, and to reduce the tumor mass. Patients with macroadenomas or with extrasellar extension of the tumor should be treated first with bromocriptine, followed by surgery when maximal reduction of the tumor size has been obtained. Surgery should be performed without discontinuing bromocriptine, since the adenoma may rapidly regrow.

Women with no evidence of pituitary adenoma but with unacceptable rates of galactorrhea may benefit from bromocriptine even if the serum prolactin level is normal. If galactorrhea is not symptomatic in such patients, however, treatment is not necessary. It is appropriate to refer most of these patients for further endocrine evaluation and to a reproductive endocrinologist if fertility is desired.

Occasional patients present with nonlactational mastitis, i.e., periodic drainage of purulent material from the nipple-areola complex in spite of previous attempts at drainage. In this condition, known as squamous metaplasia, it is not clear whether infection occurs initially followed by squamous metaplasia and intermittent discharge or whether squamous metaplasia occurs first followed by infection. The treatment, however, is complete excision of the involved duct system. Antibiotics are seldom helpful.

The most common benign neoplasm of the breast is the fibroadenoma, usually first presenting in the teenager but occasionally discovered on routine examination during the early reproductive years. Most of these lesions should be removed. In the occasional young patient with more than one mass, it is appropriate to use ultrasonography to document the actual number of lesions. Most surgeons prefer to remove the palpable lesion, usually as day surgery under local anesthesia, a procedure that is easy to do when the lesion is small. Patients who have discovered these lesions almost invariably request removal. The role of the primary care physician is to document the finding and then arrange for appropriate referral.

SUMMARY

The diagnosis and treatment of nonmalignant diseases of the breast constitute one of the most difficult challenges facing the primary care physician. The symptomatology is extremely subjective, and conclusions based even upon the most careful examination are subject to error.

Even specific complaints, such as nipple discharge, require considerable judgment when recommending treatment or referral. No lesion is obviously benign. Since 80 per cent of women with breast cancer have no identifiable risk factors, careful breast examination must be included as part of every physical examination.

Brookshaw JD: Danazol treatment of benign breast disease: A survey of U.S.A. multi center studies. Postgrad Med J 55:52, 1979. *Danazol has been approved by the FDA for the treatment of fibrocystic changes. It is costly, however, and there are a number of side effects. This article describes the results of a multicenter study in the United States.*
Feig SA: Decreased breast cancer mortality through mammographic screening:

Results of clinical trials. State Art Radiol 167:659, 1988. *Although mammography screening can lead to a remarkable improvement in breast cancer survival, the degree to which any program achieves potential gain depends upon the technical quality of the study, the interpretive expertise of the radiologist, the screening facility, and the number of projections.*
Hindle WH: Fine needle aspiration. *In* Hindle WH (ed.): *Breast Disease for Gynecologists*, Norwalk, CT, Appleton and Lange, 1990, pp 67–118. *This chapter covers the history and evolution of the fine-needle aspiration technique, including recommendations and contraindications for its use.*
Kleinberg DL, Noel GH, Frantz AG: Galactorrhea: A study of 235 cases including 48 with pituitary tumors. N Engl J Med 296:589, 1977. *This classic article is perhaps the most comprehensive report on the clinical entities associated with galactorrhea.*
Leis HP Jr: Management of nipple discharge. World J Surg 13:736, 1989. *This report of a series of over 8000 breast operations discusses the incidence of breast cancer in patients presenting with nipple discharge and the management of significant discharges.*
Love SM, Gelman SR, Silen W: Fibrocystic disease of the breast, a non disease. N Engl J Med 307:1010, 1983. *This article traces the history of fibrocystic "disease." Since most, if not all, women have these changes, the condition should not be called a disease. In most cases there is no relationship between fibrocystic changes and the later development of breast cancer.*
Yen SSC: Prolactin in human reproduction. *In* Yen SSC, Jaffe RB (eds.): *Reproductive Endocrinology.* Philadelphia, W. B. Saunders Company, 1986, pp 237–263. *This chapter describes abnormalities in prolactin secretion and the treatment of the clinical sequelae.*

227 Breast Cancer

Brian J. Lewis

EPIDEMIOLOGY AND PATHOGENESIS

In 1990, 150,000 new cases of female breast cancer and 900 new cases of male breast cancer were projected for the United States. In terms of annual mortality, 49,000 women and 350 men die of breast cancer. These figures and the 1 in 12 lifetime risk that a woman in the United States has for developing breast cancer make this disease a significant health problem.

The cause of breast cancer is unknown, but there are several factors that correlate with its occurrence: age, family history, ethnic influences, and hormonal effects.

AGE. Only about 15 per cent of cases of breast cancer occur before the age of 40. The age-adjusted incidence steadily increases thereafter, with two thirds of cases occurring in postmenopausal women.

FAMILY HISTORY. Daughters or sisters of breast cancer patients have a two- to three-fold greater risk of developing breast cancer than do women without an affected first-degree relative. More specifically, this relative risk can range from 1.5 if the mother or sister was postmenopausal at diagnosis to 8.8 if she was premenopausal and had bilateral disease. Unlike patients in the general population, women with the highest relative risk among those with a positive family history have a greater tendency to have their disease before the age of 40. Careful counseling, screening, and tracking of high-risk patients are essential. Increased monitoring should be given to patients with prior curative treatment for breast cancer, since they have a 10 to 15 per cent lifetime chance of developing a second primary breast cancer.

ETHNIC INFLUENCES. Ninety per cent of breast cancer patients lack a positive family history. While ethnic background has a role, it is necessary to control for the influences of allied cultural and nongenetic factors. Oriental women have a much lower risk of breast cancer than women in western countries. Women of Japanese descent who reside in the United States have a higher risk than women in Japan. Within the United States itself, the probability of developing breast cancer by age 75 shows considerable variation: for white women, it is 8.2 per cent; for black women, 7.0 per cent; for Hispanic women, 4.8 per cent; for native American women, 2.5 per cent; for Japanese-American women, 5.4 per cent; and for Chinese-American women, 6.1 per cent.

HORMONAL EFFECTS. Estrogens have an impact on the development of breast cancer. Early menarche, late menopause, and late or no pregnancy correlate with a higher risk (relative

TABLE 227–1. RISK FACTORS FOR BREAST CANCER IN WOMEN WITH PROLIFERATIVE BREAST DISEASE

Diagnosis	Relative Risk of Breast Cancer (95% Confidence Interval)
Nonproliferative lesions	1.0
Proliferative disease without atypical hyperplasia	1.9 (1.2 to 2.9)
Atypical hyperplasia	5.3 (3.1 to 8.8)
Atypical hyperplasia + family history of breast cancer	11.0 (5.5 to 24)

Data from DuPont WD, Page DL: Risk factors for breast cancer in women with proliferative breast disease. N Engl J Med 312:146, 1985.

risk of 1.3, 1.5 and 2 to 3, respectively). Conversely, premature loss of ovarian function, late menarche, early menopause, and early or more numerous pregnancies correlate with a decreased risk. The chance for developing breast cancer is increased in men with Klinefelter's syndrome or with other disturbances of estrogen metabolism.

Oral contraceptives seem not to increase the risk of breast cancer, and they may ameliorate the symptoms of fibrocystic disease. There is some concern that the use of exogenous estrogens in postmenopausal patients can increase the risk, but this may correlate with higher doses and more prolonged treatment. There is very little evidence that the replacement doses used for the treatment of osteoporosis increase the risk of carcinoma of the breast (Ch. 238).

Historically, there has been a linkage between fibrocystic disease of the breast and an increased risk for breast cancer. A host of terms has been lumped under "fibrocystic disease" (i.e., macrocysts, microcysts, adenosis, apocrine change, fibrosis, fibroadenoma, and ductal hyperplasia). We now know that the majority of women (70 per cent) who have a biopsy for benign disease are not at increased risk for cancer, but the presence of atypical hyperplasia and a family history of breast cancer greatly increase the probability of developing breast carcinoma (Table 227–1).

OTHER RISK FACTORS. Other risk factors include ionizing radiation and possibly diet. Surprisingly, consumption of even moderate amounts of alcohol may increase risk appreciably. Repeated chest fluoroscopy for tuberculosis, therapeutic radiation of mastitis, and exposure of Japanese women to the atomic bomb blast have been linked to increased rates of breast cancer. Animal models and geographic-ethnic differences in incidence suggest that dietary factors, in particular fat (increased in the western diet), may contribute to the development of breast cancer.

DIAGNOSIS

Clinical Presentation

Breast cancer is usually noted as a painless lump and discovered incidentally by the patient, by routine physical examination, or by mammography. Pain and tenderness are nonspecific findings and herald cancer less than 10 per cent of the time. Physical findings suggestive of a malignancy include a hard, irregular mass and skin dimpling or nipple retraction. Nonbloody nipple discharges are rarely associated with cancer. Bloody discharges correlate with intraductal papillomas in about 30 per cent of cases and with invasive cancer in about one third of cases.

Pertinent history includes a family history of breast cancer on the maternal side, especially in first-degree relatives, prior breast biopsies, whether the lump is new or old, and whether it fluctuates in size, consistency, and tenderness with the menstrual cycle. Such cycling is more suggestive of a benign process but by no means rules out cancer. Physical examination should include careful inspection and palpation of both breasts and assessment of the axillary, supraclavicular, and infraclavicular node areas.

Evaluation of a Breast Mass

A suspicious breast mass requires systematic evaluation and follow-up. A negative mammogram or needle aspiration does not ensure that a mass is benign, and if it remains of concern, it must be excised. To avoid distortion of breast anatomy, a mammogram should precede any biopsy procedure. Breast imaging rules out contralateral lesions and multiple foci in the ipsilateral breast, and it is sometimes redone after biopsy to confirm that the area of interest was in fact removed.

Formerly, diagnosis and treatment were a one-step procedure. A woman with a suspicious lesion had an excision under general anesthesia with frozen section analysis of the tumor. If cancer was found, mastectomy immediately followed, and the woman awoke to confront both the diagnosis of cancer and the loss of her breast. A two-step procedure is now used. Fine-needle aspiration cytology or excisional biopsy under local anesthesia allows an outpatient diagnosis. If cancer is found, the patient and surgeon can then review treatment options.

Screening and Detection

Early detection of a tumor improves the chances for cure. Efforts to screen for and detect early breast cancer have centered on self-examination, physician examination, and techniques for imaging the breast.

Self-examination is simple, without cost, and free of risk. It has been shown to result in earlier detection of tumors, and every adult woman should be instructed in its use. Any mass that is new and persists for more than a few weeks, is rapidly enlarging, or changes from a previously stable lump requires a physician's examination.

Examination by a physician as a screening tool is more costly and is applied less frequently than self-examination. Discovery of an unsuspected mass during a periodic examination by a physician leads to detection of tumors at an earlier stage than in patients who do not have periodic breast examinations. The American Cancer Society recommends that every woman have a routine breast examination at least every 3 years.

Breast imaging techniques include thermography, sonography, and radiographic mammography. Thermography has yet to prove sufficiently sensitive for widespread use. Sonography can help distinguish cystic from solid lesions initially found on radiography. Radiographic mammography is a well-studied and standardized methodology. Annual mammography lowers the mortality from breast cancer in screened populations compared with unscreened control groups. It detects smaller lesions with fewer nodal metastases. Current technology allows a lower dose of radiation per examination. Table 227–2 shows guidelines for screening. Annual examinations are also recommended for women with a prior breast cancer regardless of age.

Breast cancer incidence rose gradually over the first half of the century and turned more sharply upward in the 1960's, concomitant with and possibly as a result of increased attention to education and screening. The mortality (deaths per 100,000), however, has remained constant. It may be that tumors are being found earlier and cured more readily, since more of the tumors found are smaller. Alternatively, a proportion of the early asymptomatic (subclinical) cancers being discovered may have a lower malignant potential than tumors that grow faster and more rapidly become clinically apparent. Thus, screening may appear more efficacious than it really is, since some of the patients discovered to have an "early" cancer may represent a subpopulation with indolent disease who would not otherwise have had clinical expression of the tumor. Nonetheless, there has been a definite reduction in mortality from breast cancer in women who are screened with mammography.

TUMOR BIOLOGY

Breast cancer is more than just a local process; local control of tumor is necessary but not by itself sufficient to address the

TABLE 227–2. GUIDELINES FOR MAMMOGRAPHIC SCREENING OF ASYMPTOMATIC WOMEN

1. Baseline mammogram for all women aged 35 to 40
2. Mammography every one to two years from age 40 to 49
3. Mammography annually for women aged 50 or older
4. Mammography annually for women at any age with a personal history of breast cancer
5. Mammography annually for women aged 40 and over who have a family history of breast cancer or who are otherwise at increased risk

TABLE 227–3. STAGING OF CARCINOMA OF THE BREAST

Stage I   Tumor < 2 cm without skin involvement and with no clinically suspicious axillary nodes.

Stage II Tumor < 2 cm with clinically suspicious nodes; any tumor 2 to 5 cm with or without clinically suspicious nodes.

Stage III Any tumor > 5 cm; skin involvement or chest wall attachment; any size tumor with clinically fixed axillary nodes; arm edema; supraclavicular nodes.

Stage IV Metastatic disease.

threat of distant metastases. Breast cancer is also a chronic illness with a potential for recurrence 10 to 15 years after removal of the primary tumor. While one can extirpate apparent disease in the breast and in the axillary nodes in the majority of cases, at least 50 to 80 per cent of women found to have tumor in the axillary nodes and 30 per cent of those without axillary node metastases will have metastatic disease.

STAGING. The system for clinically staging breast cancer reflects the anatomic extent of tumor (Table 227–3). It allows consistent and comparable description and reporting of cases. The stages correlate with survival and are important in planning treatment, but they do not totally predict the clinical behavior of the tumor. A more complete classification scheme would ideally measure the balance between the inherent virulence of the cancer and the intrinsic antitumor defenses of the host. In addition to tumor size and nodal status, hormone receptor content and nuclear grade reproducibly correlate with prognosis. The infrequent histologic subtypes of papillary, colloid (mucinous), and tubular carcinoma are associated with a more favorable outcome. Other variables such as the percentage of cells in S-phase, oncogene expression, epidermal growth factor receptors, cathepsin-D, and stress response (heat shock) proteins may each provide a means for better predicting who will have metastatic disease (Table 227–4).

METHOD OF SPREAD. Breast cancer spreads directly to the bloodstream as well as to the draining lymphatics. Tumor emboli can traverse the lymph nodes and enter the venous system; and tumor cells can presumably reach lymph nodes by way of the bloodstream. In addition, upon discovery, a breast cancer mass usually contains 10^9 or more cells. Given what is known of doubling times, the cell number at diagnosis implies that the cancer may have been growing for a number of years. It seems logical that there will be shedding of the tumor cells into the venous and lymphatic circulation throughout the life of the tumor, especially early, when tumor growth rate is highest.

Accordingly, it is likely that many more patients with breast cancer have micrometastases than we see with clinical recurrence. Negative axillary nodes may not mean that the tumor was never present in the lymphatic system but rather that it had been there and was unable to flourish. Positive lymph nodes do correlate with subsequent metastases and poor survival. This could reflect simple anatomic spread of cancer past the last "line of defense" imposed by the lymph nodes (Halsted). More probably it implies that because the tumor persisted in the nodes, however it arrived there, it will also persist and grow in other organs.

TABLE 227–4. PROGNOSTIC FACTORS IN BREAST CANCER

Factor	Influence on Risk of Metastases
Tumor size	Risk increases with size
Nodal status	Risk increases with presence and number of nodal metastases
Hormone receptor status	Risk increased if receptors not present
Nuclear grade	Risk increased with high grade
Favorable histology	Risk decreases with favorable subtypes
Per cent S-phase	Risk increases with per cent S-phase
Oncogene expression	Risk appears to increase with increased oncogene expression
Cathepsin-D levels	Risk appears to increase with levels
Epidermal growth factor receptor levels	Risk appears to increase with levels
Stress response protein levels	Risk appears to increase with levels

CELL ORIGIN. Most breast tumors derive from mammary epithelium. Eighty per cent of these are infiltrating ductal carcinomas. Less common are infiltrating lobular carcinoma, medullary carcinoma, comedocarcinoma, and tubular, papillary, and colloid carcinoma. Lobular and comedocarcinoma can be bilateral and require increased surveillance of the unaffected breast. Lobular carcinoma in situ poses a special problem. Although it is not an invasive lesion, it is associated with a 1 per cent annual risk for the development of an invasive lesion in either breast. Some surgeons have therefore advocated prophylactic mastectomy. A more conservative approach is to do a "mirror image" biopsy of the contralateral breast to rule out invasive tumor and then to track the patient closely with periodic examinations and prompt biopsy of any suspicious lesions. Ductal carcinoma in situ carries a higher risk for evolving into invasive cancer and requires surgery. Inflammatory breast cancer represents a highly virulent pathologic variant. Clinically, the patient has a red, swollen, warm breast with a characteristic peau d'orange appearance. Microscopically, this is associated with involvement of dermal lymphatics by tumor. It has proven difficult to achieve long-term survival in patients with this diagnosis.

HORMONE RECEPTOR PROTEINS. Estrogen and progesterone receptor proteins (ERP and PRP) are present in normal mammary epithelium and in a proportion of breast cancers. After binding to the steroid, the activated hormone-receptor complex interacts with specific sites on DNA, and this results in the initiation of steroid-specific protein synthesis. One product of estrogen stimulation is PRP, and the presence of PRP signifies functionally intact ERP. A tumor is considered ERP-positive when it contains more than 10 femtomoles of receptor per milligram of protein, as measured using a radioligand binding assay. Monoclonal antibodies against ERP are now available and permit microscopic visualization and enumeration of ERP-positive tumor cells.

ERP is found more frequently and in higher titer in tumors from postmenopausal patients (60 per cent or more versus 30 to 40 per cent positive in premenopausal women). ERP-positive tumors tend to be less virulent and are more likely to respond to hormonal therapy (see below). Tumors that contain both ERP and PRP have the greatest likelihood of regressing after an endocrine maneuver, and the probability of a response increases directly with the titer of the RP. Given the therapeutic and prognostic implications of hormone receptor levels, it is mandatory that all primary breast cancers be submitted for receptor analysis at the time of removal. There is an 80 per cent concordance between the hormone receptor profile of a primary tumor and its metastases, in the absence of intervening hormone treatment. Breast cancers are heterogeneous in the sense that in RP-positive specimens, the majority but not necessarily all of the cells contain RP. When metastatic disease becomes refractory to hormonal therapy after initially responding, the progression reflects the outgrowth of hormone-independent cells that are usually RP-negative.

PRIMARY MANAGEMENT OF BREAST CANCER

Stage I and Stage II Disease

Since Halsted's time, almost three generations ago, the view of breast cancer as a local or regional process has made radical mastectomy or one of its variants the standard approach to the management of resectable tumor confined to the breast and the axillary lymph nodes. Patients often received postoperative radiation therapy to the chest wall and the draining lymph node areas. These treatments have produced a local control rate of 95 per cent, but variations in locoregional therapy have not differed significantly in their impact upon distant recurrence or overall survival. Furthermore, more extensive surgery or surgery followed by radiation increases the risk of arm edema.

These approaches entered general use without the testing of alternative approaches, but recently local tumor excision with breast irradiation has been gaining a wider acceptance. Older, largely uncontrolled studies seemed to indicate similar outcomes either with tumor excision and breast irradiation or with traditional mastectomy. While one cannot refer to the decades of observation on local tumor control and side effects that exist for standard surgical approaches, recent controlled trials show that the techniques are equivalent in terms of tumor recurrence and overall survival.

Public interest in alternatives to mastectomy has increased, and patients are more informed and expect their physicians to provide a comprehensive overview of treatment possibilities, especially ones that would spare them the disfigurement and distress imposed by mastectomy. Likewise, the growing application of plastic surgery for breast reconstruction after mastectomy has lessened the emotional trauma of the operation.

Breast conservation is appropriate therapy for Stage I or Stage II disease. Table 227–5 lists the requirements for its use. Mammography is essential to exclude patients with multifocal disease or with diffuse microcalcifications. (Even if the latter prove benign on biopsy, they will interfere with the subsequent mammographic follow-up used to screen for recurrent cancer.) An adequate surgical resection of the tumor with negative resection margins is essential and is facilitated by inking the margins of the specimen and orienting it for the pathologist. Axillary node dissection determines whether the patient requires adjuvant systemic treatment because of nodal metastasis. Extensive intraductal carcinoma in situ may be a contraindication to breast conservation because of a higher risk of recurrence in the treated breast.

The most common but not necessarily the preferred approach to the primary management of a Stage I or Stage II breast cancer is total mastectomy and axillary lymph node dissection. Postoperative radiotherapy is an individualized rather than "standard" therapy. It is employed when narrow resection margins, extensive nodal disease, the presence of residual tumor, or other high-risk factors for local recurrence are present. With the advent of adjuvant chemotherapy for Stage II disease (see below), there may be even fewer indications for adjuvant radiation therapy, since drug treatment alone may decrease the local failure rate. However, this supposition has yet to be adequately tested in clinical trials.

Clinically suspicious nodes are pathologically negative for tumor 25 to 30 per cent of the time, and, conversely, clinically negative nodes are positive histologically with an equal frequency. With a proper axillary dissection, radiation to the axilla is not usually necessary (and increases the risk for arm edema). While positive axillary nodes increase the likelihood of subclinical supraclavicular and internal mammary node metastases, there is no evidence that adjuvant radiation to those areas will improve survival.

Standard pretreatment evaluation for any of these techniques includes a complete blood count, a profile of serum chemistries with particular reference to studies suggestive of liver or bone

TABLE 227–5. REQUIREMENT FOR LIMITED SURGERY AND RADIOTHERAPY FOR EARLY BREAST CANCER

Patient Selection	Comments
Adequate resection of tumor without major cosmetic deformity	This requires a single discrete tumor, moderate sized breast, tumor diameter < 4–5 cm.
Surgical Criteria	
Wide resection with specimen orientation Hormone receptor analysis Separate axillary incision	Grossly negative surgical margins are essential—re-resection may be required if margins are microscopically involved.
Radiation Therapy	
4500–5000 rad to entire breast + boost to tumor bed	
Treatment of the Axilla	
Level I *and* Level II axillary dissection* (*not* an informal "sampling")	Permits adequate node sampling, controls local tumor, and obviates the need for axillary radiation. Does not impose a major risk for arm edema.

Sources: Harris et al., 1985; Danoff et al., 1985.
*Level I = Complete removal of nodes lateral to the pectoralis minor muscle.
Level II = Removal of nodes beneath the pectoralis minor.

involvement, and a chest radiograph. Many feel that routine bone scans or liver scans are not indicated in patients with clinical Stage I or II disease, although some advocate a baseline bone scan to be used as a reference if the patient should develop skeletal metastases in the future. The yield of positives is extremely low in the absence of symptoms or signs suggesting visceral disease. On the other hand, with locally advanced tumor (Stage III), the yield of screening bone scans is sufficiently high to warrant their use. Likewise, with abnormal blood chemistries suggestive of liver involvement or with symptoms such as bone pain, scans would be required to avoid inappropriate use of a curative procedure in a patient with advanced, incurable disease.

Stage III Disease and Inflammatory Breast Cancer

If a patient's disease is Stage III solely on the basis of tumor size (tumor > 5 cm), but the tumor appears to be as resectable as that of a Stage I or II patient, mastectomy is the primary treatment. For patients with locally advanced but unresectable disease (i.e., invasion of chest wall, fixation of axillary nodes, or positive supraclavicular nodes), control of persistent or recurrent regional disease as well as latent distant metastases is the dominant problem. Inflammatory breast cancer is aggressive locally as well as metastatically. It is properly considered a systemic disease from the outset, even though it appears to be confined to the breast. The treatment plan for the latter two presentations involves an individualized approach using chemotherapy to reduce the tumor volume, followed by radiation therapy and possibly resection of the breast and draining nodes. This strategy requires close consultation from the outset between surgeons, radiation oncologists, and medical oncologists. Prolonged remissions and perhaps cures can be obtained in a fraction of patients.

Metastatic Breast Cancer

CLINICAL FEATURES. Breast cancer most frequently metastasizes to lymph nodes, skin, lung, pleura, bone, liver, brain, and pericardium. In autopsy series, the adrenals are involved in up to half the patients, but adrenal insufficiency is rarely seen. Likewise, the ovaries contain tumor in up to one quarter of patients at autopsy. Rarely metastatic breast cancer may be found incidentally at oophorectomy in a patient whose first sign of breast cancer is an involved ovary presenting as a pelvic mass. Breast cancer is the most common source of metastases to the eye in women.

PATIENT ASSESSMENT. Once a metastatic focus is found, routine studies to map tumor extent include a complete blood count (which can reflect myelophthisis secondary to marrow metastases) and the measurement of serum levels of liver enzymes, bilirubin, and calcium. The carcinoembryonic antigen titer and the CA 15-3 antigen titer can be useful markers for following response to therapy. A chest radiograph is indicated and can reveal lung nodules, mediastinal or hilar node involvement, or a pleural effusion. A bone scan is also mandatory, and positive areas, especially those that are symptomatic or in weight-bearing bones, require follow-up radiographs to determine whether radiation is needed to prevent collapse or pathologic fracture. If physical findings or laboratory studies suggest hepatic involvement, a radionuclide liver scan, a sonogram of the liver, or a liver CT scan confirms the presence of metastatic disease, gauges its extent, and allows comparison with follow-up studies during treatment. "Routine" liver imaging is widely employed, but its yield and cost-effectiveness in the absence of signs suggesting liver metastasis are open to question. The same statement applies to "routine" studies of the brain, although they are clearly indicated in the presence of neurologic symptoms or signs.

COMPLICATIONS. Certain complications occur with some frequency and require urgent attention in patients with metastatic breast cancer: hypercalcemia, metastases to weight-bearing bones, and metastases to the nervous system (the epidural space, the leptomeninges, or the brain).

Hypercalcemia requires standard methods of therapy, such as saline, furosemide, and mithramycin therapy along with treatment of the breast cancer itself (Ch. 235). A positive bone scan, especially in the femur or vertebral column, or bone pain in these areas requires radiographic analysis of the extent of structural damage. Femoral lesions may necessitate orthopedic stabilization and radiation therapy to prevent pathologic fractures.

Vertebral body lesions may require radiation to diminish pain and avoid further collapse.

Patients with persistent back pain are at greater risk for *epidural metastases* and possibly cord compression. Motor or sensory changes in a segmental distribution greatly increase the possibility of an epidural lesion. However, in the presence of back pain, their absence does not exclude an epidural lesion. Pain without a neurologic deficit means that there is still time to treat an epidural lesion with radiation before the cord becomes ischemic and permanently damaged.

Leptomeningeal metastases present with headache and focal sensory or motor changes suggestive of single or multiple nerve root involvement. The diagnosis depends upon the demonstration of breast cancer cells in the cerebrospinal fluid and may require multiple spinal taps to yield a diagnosis (with appropriate studies beforehand, if indicated, to rule out a mass lesion in the brain). Since systemically administered drugs penetrate the blood-brain barrier poorly, intrathecal or intraventricular chemotherapy is necessary.

TREATMENT. The two major types of therapy for disseminated breast cancer are hormonal and cytotoxic. Hormonal therapy is less toxic but can require as long as 8 to 12 weeks to produce maximal benefit. The impact of chemotherapy is more rapid. Responses to all these treatments last a median of 6 to 18 months, and responders have a significantly prolonged survival compared with nonresponders.

The menopausal status of the patient and the hormone receptor profile of the tumor are the major determinants of whether to employ an endocrine maneuver and which particular therapy to use. Other important considerations are the tempo of the disease, the performance status of the patient, and the sites of metastases. A long interval between mastectomy and recurrence suggests indolent disease and would, along with a good performance status, permit the longer observation period needed to gauge response to an endocrine therapy. Bone, soft tissue, and limited pulmonary metastases may respond to hormonal therapy, whereas liver, brain, and extensive lung metastases greatly decrease the probability of a response and therefore require chemotherapy.

Premenopausal Patients. For premenopausal patients with ER-positive tumors, hormonal therapy is first-line treatment in the absence of the contraindications mentioned above. Oophorectomy is the initial choice and causes tumor regression in 30 to 80 per cent of RP-positive patients. If a patient progresses after initial response, then progestins, adrenalectomy (rarely hypophysectomy), and androgens can be used in sequence until there is no longer a response. At that point, the patient should receive chemotherapy.

Some advocate initial endocrine treatment with the antiestrogen tamoxifen, followed later by oophorectomy once the tamoxifen is ineffective. The experience is more limited with this approach. Some women continue to menstruate while receiving tamoxifen, so its exact mechanism of action and the certainty of adequate estrogen blockade are less well established (in premenopausal women). LHRH agonists are being studied and may become the treatment of choice in the next several years.

Adrenal influences can be removed either by surgical adrenalectomy or by use of medical methods to inhibit adrenal function. Surgical ablation requires permanent replacement therapy in addition to the morbidity of surgery. Medical inhibition with aminoglutethimide, by contrast, is reversible once the drug is stopped. Patients receiving aminoglutethimide experience rash and somnolence 10 to 40 per cent of the time, although these side effects wane after several weeks of treatment. The drug blocks adrenal steroidogenesis by inhibiting conversion of cholesterol to pregnenolone. In peripheral tissue, it also blocks the conversion of androstenedione to estrone, a precursor of estradiol. This latter reaction accounts for the bulk of estrogen production in postmenopausal women. In patients who have RP-positive tumors and responded to prior endocrine therapy, responses to aminoglutethimide occur 30 to 60 per cent of the time. Aminoglutethimide therapy requires replacement corticosteroid treatment with hydrocortisone, which also suppresses the increase in pituitary ACTH secretion produced by aminoglutethimide inhibition of cortisol production, an increase that could otherwise override the blockade. A periodic check of plasma dehydroepiandrosterone levels confirms the adequacy of adrenal suppression.

Adrenalectomy is usually chosen over hypophysectomy. The two are roughly equal in therapeutic effect. Hypophysectomy requires a neurosurgeon highly skilled in the transsphenoidal approach (less morbid than the transfrontal route), and complications of the surgery range from incomplete pituitary ablation to cerebrospinal fluid leak and infection. Hypophysectomy also requires permanent thyroid *and* adrenal hormone replacement.

Premenopausal patients with RP-negative tumors, or those originally RP-positive who have become refractory to endocrine treatment, require chemotherapy. Drug classes active against breast cancer include alkylating agents (typically cyclophosphamide), antimetabolites (5-fluorouracil, methotrexate), vinca alkaloids (vincristine, vinblastine), anthracyclines (doxorubicin), and mitomycin-C. In various combinations, these agents effect responses in 60 to 70 per cent of patients, with 10 to 15 per cent achieving a complete remission. These responses have a median duration of only 6 to 9 months, however, and studies are in progress using high-dose chemotherapy and autologous bone marrow rescue to see if selected patients can achieve permanent ablation of metastatic disease.

Postmenopausal Patients. For RP-positive tumors in postmenopausal patients who are candidates for endocrine therapy, the antiestrogen tamoxifen has replaced estrogen therapy (diethylstilbestrol, DES) as initial treatment. Tamoxifen has few side effects, in contrast to DES, which much more frequently produces nausea, anorexia, and salt retention. Both drugs have been associated with a tumor "flare" consisting of increased bone pain and hypercalcemia. This occurs in patients with skeletal metastases during the initial weeks of treatment, more commonly with DES. These reactions usually herald an antitumor effect and do not necessitate cessation of therapy as long as symptoms and calcium levels are controlled by standard supportive treatments. Withdrawal of DES, once the tumor progresses, produces further regression of tumor in 20 to 30 per cent of patients (withdrawal effect is less common with tamoxifen). Once the disease progresses after this initial therapy, serial endocrine maneuvers are employed, as discussed for premenopausal patients, until the tumor becomes refractory to hormonal therapy. Oophorectomy has no role in the treatment of postmenopausal patients. Again, for RP-negative tumors or for tumors resistant to endocrine treatment, chemotherapy becomes the treatment of choice.

Adjuvant Drug Therapy

The goal of prophylactic therapy after mastectomy is to eliminate any micrometastases present. Since eradication of tumor cells is more probable when their number is small, the treatment should be applied as soon after primary treatment as possible. Furthermore, because systemic therapy is quite active against metastatic breast cancer in women who have a high tumor burden, it should be all the more effective against microscopic disease. Table 227–6 summarizes the present indications for adjuvant systemic therapy. Ongoing clinical trials are likely to modify these guidelines in the near future.

The following points should be kept firmly in mind: (1) *optimal* treatment for any subset of patients has yet to be defined; (2) physicians should continue to enroll their patients in controlled trials; and (3) the studies to date in axillary lymph node–negative patients show a statistically significant improvement in relapse-free survival with adjuvant drug therapy. Although not yet demonstrated, there is a strong supposition that overall survival will be increased as well. Since 70 per cent of node-negative

TABLE 227–6. INDICATIONS FOR ADJUVANT SYSTEMIC THERAPY

Axillary lymph node metastases not present
  1. Tumors ≤ 1 cm—no adjuvant therapy (risk of relapse less than 10%)
  2. Tumors >1 cm and especially with adverse prognostic features (see Table 227–4)—consider adjuvant tamoxifen or chemotherapy
Axillary lymph node metastases present
  1. Premenopausal, receptor positive or negative—combination chemotherapy
  2. Postmenopausal, receptor positive—tamoxifen
  3. Postmenopausal, receptor negative—consider chemotherapy, but this cannot be recommended yet as standard practice

women are cured by primary treatment, the challenge remains to identify and treat only the subset at high risk.

The best choice of drugs, dose, schedule, and duration for adjuvant treament is unresolved. To date, no severe long-term sequelae of chemotherapy have appeared in patients who have received adjuvant therapy.

SPECIAL CONSIDERATIONS

Male Breast Cancer

Carcinoma of the male breast occurs with 1 per cent the frequency of female breast cancer. Its clinical presentation and primary therapy are similar to those in women. Abnormalities of estrogen metabolism are cited as a possible causative factor. The vast majority of tumors that have been examined are estrogen RP-positive. Castration is the treatment of choice for the initial management of metastatic disease. Antiestrogen therapy, adrenalectomy, and hypophysectomy may offer some palliation, and the effects of additive hormonal therapy are less certain than in female breast cancer.

Breast Cancer and Pregnancy

Breast cancer complicates approximately one of every 3000 pregnancies. It has been held for some time that pregnancy adversely affects the outcome of breast cancer, with studies citing a high frequency of axillary lymph node metastases and shortened survival when the diagnosis is made during pregnancy. To some extent, these poor results may have related to a delay in diagnosis and in the initiation of treatment rather than inherently different biologic factors. The treatment considerations are the same as for the nonpregnant patients, and a standard surgical approach poses a 1 per cent or less risk to the developing fetus. When patients present with disseminated disease in the first or second trimester, cytotoxic drug treatment is a significant risk to the fetus and usually requires termination of pregnancy. If clinical considerations permit, treatment can be delayed to the third trimester to permit delivery of a viable fetus.

Patients who develop cancer during pregnancy tend to present with more advanced stages of disease than nonpregnant patients. However, when compared stage for stage, pregnant women have only a slightly less favorable prognosis than nonpregnant women. In a woman who has had an apparent cure of a breast cancer, subsequent pregnancy is not associated with an excessive risk of recurrence. Patients with early stage breast cancer who bear children appear to have a survival equal to that of women who do not become pregnant. A 3-year interval between primary treatment of early breast cancer and a subsequent pregnancy has been advocated.

Brinton LA, Hoover R, Fraumeni JF Jr: Interaction of familial and hormonal risk factors for breast cancer. J Natl Cancer Inst 69:817, 1982. *An evaluation of family history of breast cancer as a risk indicator in relation to hormonal factors. A large, case-controlled study.*

Danoff BF, Haller DG, Glick JH, et al.: Conservative surgery and irradiation in the treatment of early breast cancer. Ann Intern Med 102:634, 1985. *A detailed review of the literature on breast conservation in primary breast cancer management.*

Donegan WL: Cancer and pregnancy. CA 33:194, 1983. *An overview of the issues surrounding breast cancer (and other cancers) and pregnancy.*

Dupont WD, Page DL: Menopausal replacement therapy and breast cancer. N Engl J Med 312:146, 1985. *This important, authoritative review of a large number of studies concludes that menopausal therapy consisting of 0.625 mg or less of conjugated estrogens daily does not increase the risk of breast cancer.*

Early Breast Cancer Trialists' Collaborative Group: Systemic treatment of early breast cancer by hormonal, cytotoxic, or immune therapy. Lancet 339:1–15, 71–85, 1992. *A meta analysis of 133 randomized trials involving 31,000 recurrences and 24,000 deaths among 75,000 women. It is a detailed and comprehensive overview of the current status of adjuvant systemic therapy for patients with breast cancer.*

Fisher B: Laboratory and clinical research in breast cancer—a personal adventure. Cancer Res 40:3863, 1980. *This article, plus the following references by Fisher et al. and the reference by Veronesi et al., details a shift in thinking about the biology of breast cancer and update clinical trials of primary management designed to test specific hypotheses about the nature of breast cancer.*

Fisher B, Redmond C, Poisson R, et al.: Eight year results of a randomized clinical trial comparing total mastectomy and lumpectomy with or without irradiation in the treatment of breast cancer. N Engl J Med 320:822, 1989.

Fisher B, Redmond C, Fisher ER, et al.: Ten year results of a randomized clinical trial comparing radical mastectomy and total mastectomy with or without radiation. N Engl J Med 312:674, 1985.

Harris JR, Hellman S, Canellos GP, et al: Cancer of the breast. *In* De Vita VT,

Hellman S, Rosenberg SA (eds.): Cancer. Principles and Practice of Oncology. Philadelphia, J. B. Lippincott, 1985. *A comprehensive treatise detailing areas such as surgical technique, pathology, and chemotherapy.*

Harris JR, Hellman S, Kinne DW: Special report. Limited surgery and radiotherapy for early breast cancer. N Engl J Med 313:1365, 1985. *Summary statement of a workshop held to define surgical procedures, patient selection and criteria, and areas of controversy in the use of more conservative surgery plus radiotherapy for the primary management of breast cancer.*

Kopans DP, Meyer JE, Sadowsky N: Breast imaging. N Engl J Med 310:960, 1984. *A review of mammography and other breast imaging methods which includes a critique of the utility and limitations of each technique.*

McGuire WL, Tandon AK, Allred DC, et al.: How to use prognostic factors in axillary node–negative breast cancer patients. J Natl Cancer Inst 82:1006, 1990. *A summary of the utility of prognostic factors in estimating recurrence risk in node-negative patients.*

Petrakis NL, Ernster VL, King M-C: Breast. *In* Schottenfeld D, Fraumeni JF Jr (eds.): Cancer Epidemiology and Prevention. Philadelphia, W. B. Saunders Company, 1982. *A review of the range of associated risk factors for breast cancer.*

Relman AS: Adjuvant treatment of early breast cancer. N Engl J Med 320:525, 1989. *Two editorials and four articles in this issue show the implications of controlled trials of recent adjuvant treatment in node-negative breast cancer.*

Schatzkin A, Jones DY, Hoover RN, et al.: Alcohol consumption and breast cancer in the epidemiologic follow-up study of the first national health and nutrition examination survey. N Engl J Med 316:1169, 1987. *This article and its accompanying editorial review the increasing evidence that even modest consumption of alcohol increases the risk of breast cancer by 50 to 100 per cent.*

Veronesi U, Del Vecchio M, Greco M, et al.: Results of quadrantectomy, axillary dissection and radiotherapy (QUART) in T₁N₀ patients. *In* Harris JR, Hellman S, Silen W (eds.): Conservative Management of Breast Cancer. Philadelphia, J. B. Lippincott Company, 1983.

Wood WC: National Institutes of Health Consensus Development Conference Statement: Treatment of early stage breast cancer. June 18–21, 1990. *A summary statement of conclusions and recommendations concerning primary treatment of early breast cancer and adjuvant therapy for node-negative patients.*

228 Polyglandular Disorders

John N. Loeb

A number of different syndromes are characterized by autonomous hyperfunction or hypofunction of more than one endocrine gland. Although the majority of these syndromes are clearly of genetic origin, the fundamental mechanisms leading to hyperfunction or hypofunction thus far remain unknown in any instance. The syndromes to be considered in this chapter are those in which dysfunction appears to be autonomous within the affected endocrine glands themselves; multiple glandular abnormalities resulting from primary abnormalities in the hypothalamic-pituitary axis or ascribable to various locally infiltrative processes are discussed elsewhere.

SYNDROMES CHARACTERIZED BY MULTIPLE ENDOCRINE GLAND HYPERFUNCTION OR NEOPLASIA

The major syndromes characterized by multiple endocrine hyperfunction are those of multiple endocrine adenomatosis (MEA) or multiple endocrine neoplasia (MEN). A number of these syndromes are inherited as autosomal dominant traits and are clinically distinct. The term MEN is now generally preferred because it is more inclusive, comprising both hyperplastic and carcinomatous as well as adenomatous abnormalities. Table 228–1 compares the clinical features of some of these syndromes.

MULTIPLE ENDOCRINE NEOPLASIA, TYPE 1 (WERMER'S SYNDROME). In 1954 Wermer reported the familial occurrence of *multiple tumors of the anterior pituitary, parathyroid glands, and pancreatic islet cells* in association with a high incidence of peptic ulcer. This complex of abnormalities is now most commonly referred to as multiple endocrine neoplasia, type 1 (MEN 1). The syndrome may also include tumor or hyperfunction of the adrenal and thyroid glands, but the relation of these latter endocrinopathies to the underlying genetic abnormality is less well defined. Although it has been proposed that the fundamental defect in MEN 1 is an abnormal differentiation of neural crest tissue, current evidence in support of this hypothesis is by no means conclusive (see also below, under MEN 2a). A circu-

TABLE 228–1. COMPARISON OF THE CLINICAL FEATURES OF THE MAJOR SYNDROMES CHARACTERIZED BY MULTIPLE ENDOCRINE GLAND HYPERFUNCTION

Endocrine Abnormality	MEN 1*	MEN 2a*	MEN 2b*
Hyperparathyroidism [Hyperplasia or multiple adenomas]	90–95%, with high incidence of hypercalcemia and nephrolithiasis	20–30%, but only 10% with frank hypercalcemia or nephrolithiasis	Rare
Pancreatic islet cell hyperfunction [Hyperplasia, adenomas, or carcinoma, with hypersecretion (e.g., of gastrin or insulin)]	30–35%	—†	—
Pituitary adenomas ["Nonfunctioning" or with hypersecretion of prolactin (common) or growth hormone (rare)]	20–30%	—	—
Multiple cutaneous lipomas	20%	—	—
Thyroid adenomas, adrenal cortical adenomas, carcinoid tumors	Rare	—	—
Thyroid C-cell hyperplasia with hypersecretion of calcitonin ± medullary carcinoma	—	"100%"‡	"100%"‡
Pheochromocytoma	—	Probably >20%	Probably >20%
Multiple mucosal neuromas; marfanoid habitus	—	—	Characteristic
Inheritance	Autosomal dominant	Autosomal dominant	Autosomal dominant, but frequently "sporadic"
Chromosomal linkage	Chromosome 11	Chromosome 10	—

*Percentages indicate approximate frequencies among affected individuals manifesting hyperfunction of at least one endocrine gland.

†— = *not* part of the syndrome.

‡Generally taken to be an essential component of the syndrome.

lating factor that is mitogenic for parathyroid cells in culture and similar if not identical to basic fibroblast growth factor has recently been found in the plasma of patients with MEN 1 (but not of patients with MEN 2a). The mutant gene for MEN 1 is on chromosome 11.

More than half of patients with MEN 1 have adenomas of two or more different endocrine glands, and involvement of three or more different glands is seen in up to 20 per cent of affected individuals. The approximate frequencies of glandular involvement in patients exhibiting any manifestation of endocrine hyperfunction are, in descending order, parathyroids (90 to 95 per cent), pancreatic islet cells (30 to 35 per cent), and anterior pituitary (20 to 30 per cent). Less commonly there may be hyperfunction (adenomas) of the adrenal cortex and thyroid gland; carcinoid tumors have been reported occasionally. Initial manifestations are most commonly detected in middle age, and many years may elapse between the manifestation of the first endocrine abnormality and ensuing ones. The clinical course is highly variable, depending in part upon which glands are affected and whether the neoplasm results in hypersecretion or instead in compression of surrounding normal glandular tissue with concomitant loss of function. By far the greatest majority of patients

(over 90 per cent) have problems related to hypercalcemia, peptic ulcer, hypoglycemia, or pituitary dysfunction. In patients with pituitary neoplasms symptoms are most commonly attributable to pituitary enlargement, with headache or visual-field abnormalities, or to hypopituitarism. Acromegaly, the galactorrhea-amenorrhea syndrome with hyperprolactinemia, and, considerably more rarely, Cushing's disease, may also be seen.

Parathyroid gland involvement is by far the most common manifestation of MEN 1 but may be clinically "silent" for many years. Patients may have a history of kidney stones or progressive renal failure as the first manifestation of hyperparathyroidism, or, much more commonly, hypercalcemia may be detected incidentally upon routine screening. All four parathyroid glands are usually abnormal, and pathologic study may reveal either hyperplasia or multiple adenomas. Parathyroid carcinoma is rare.

Islet cell tumors of the pancreas can be either adenomas (generally multiple) or carcinomas; they may be preceded by diffuse hyperplasia of islet tissue and most typically secrete excess gastrin. Hypersecretion of gastrin may give rise to the *Zollinger-Ellison syndrome* (see Ch. 98) characterized by marked hypersecretion of hydrochloric acid, peptic ulceration (sometimes involving esophageal, distal duodenal, or jejunal sites), and, often, diarrhea. Abdominal pain, bleeding, and perforation are more common than in ordinary instances of peptic ulcer, and radiographic signs consistent with hypersecretion of gastric acid (e.g., hypertrophied gastric rugae) are frequently seen. Many patients in whom the Zollinger-Ellison syndrome initially appears in isolation represent a subset of individuals with MEN 1 and ultimately develop manifestations of additional endocrine neoplasms. *Duodenal* gastrinomas occur in high incidence in patients with MEN 1 and hypergastrinemia.

Hypersecretion of insulin by islet cell neoplasms (usually nonmetastasizing) may produce hypoglycemia as an initial manifestation, whereas the elaboration of other substances may, considerably more rarely, result in a variety of other syndromes. Vasoactive intestinal peptide and prostaglandins have been proposed as agents possibly responsible for the intractable watery diarrhea that can be seen even in the absence of hypersecretion of gastrin and the Zollinger-Ellison syndrome, and hypersecretion of glucagon with hyperglycemia, weight loss, and a characteristic skin rash ("necrotizing migratory erythema") has been reported. Islet cell tumors may also secrete pancreatic polypeptide or, rarely, ACTH, serotonin, or somatostatin.

Symptoms caused by *pituitary adenomas* in MEN 1 are most commonly due to local encroachment of tumor upon other structures, with headache or visual-field abnormalities, or to deficiency of one or more of the tropic hormones. Many of these tumors secrete prolactin and may give rise to the galactorrhea-amenorrhea syndrome. More rarely there is hypersecretion of growth hormone with resulting acromegaly. Hypersecretion of ACTH in MEN 1 is almost always attributable to an ectopic (pancreatic) site.

Adrenocortical hyperfunction may be due to ectopic production of ACTH or to independently functioning adrenal adenomas or carcinomas. Functioning adenomas most commonly elaborate hydrocortisone, giving rise to signs of glucocorticoid excess, but predominant secretion of aldosterone has been reported in rare instances. Hyperfunction of the *thyroid* gland has been reported least frequently of all, and, in part owing to the high incidence of thyroid abnormalities in the population at large, it is possible that sporadic instances of thyroid hyperfunction in MEN 1 represent incidental occurrences unrelated to the underlying genetic abnormality. Adenomas, thyroiditis, and rarely papillary and follicular cell carcinomas have all been reported in association with MEN 1; medullary carcinomas are *not* a part of this syndrome (cf. MEN 2a and 2b, below). *Other tumors* that can form a part of the clinical picture of MEN 1 include schwannomas, multiple cutaneous lipomas, thymomas, and both bronchial and small intestinal carcinoids.

Management of the various manifestations of MEN 1 is, for the most part, similar to management of the identical manifestations when they occur in sporadic form and hence is considered elsewhere in this textbook. As indicated above, parathyroid involvement, when it occurs, frequently involves more than one gland, and histopathology far more commonly reveals diffuse hyperplasia than a single adenoma. In such instances a number of surgeons now advocate total parathyroidectomy with reimplantation of a glandular fragment in a location conveniently accessible to subsequent exploration if necessary (e.g., the muscle of the forearm). Management of severe peptic ulceration in MEN 1 has usually required either long-term cimetidine or ranitidine therapy or near-total gastrectomy—rather than an attempt to eliminate the source of excess gastrin—since hypersecretion of gastrin by islet-cell tissue in this syndrome is almost always attributable to either multiple tumors or diffuse hyperplasia. A substantial proportion of patients with MEN 1 and the Zollinger-Ellison syndrome have hypergastrinemia on the basis of duodenal rather than pancreatic gastrinomas. The hypergastrinemia can often be cured or markedly ameliorated when these tumors (frequently small) are removed, so the duodenum should be examined first in patients who have MEN 1 and symptomatic hypergastrinemia.

The sporadic nature of the sequential manifestations of this syndrome makes it important to follow affected individuals with particular attention to the development of new abnormalities. Once the diagnosis has been established in a given patient and baseline films of the sella turcica and prolactin levels have proved to be normal, the major requisite is a careful interval history and a periodic (e.g., yearly) determination of the serum calcium and phosphorus.

Because of the high incidence of the syndrome in first-degree relatives, all such family members should be carefully evaluated, as well as any second-degree relatives who have suggestive histories elicited through questioning of the propositus. Determination of fasting blood sugar, serum calcium, and prolactin levels is generally sufficient if menses or sexual potency is present and if the history and physical examination are negative. Films of the sella turcica are usually unrevealing, and CT scanning is too expensive for use as a routine screen.

MULTIPLE ENDOCRINE NEOPLASIA, TYPE 2a (SIPPLE'S SYNDROME). A second and entirely distinct syndrome, multiple endocrine neoplasia, type 2a (MEN 2a), is characterized by *medullary carcinoma of the thyroid, pheochromocytoma, and parathyroid hyperplasia.* First partially described by Sipple in 1961, this syndrome, like MEN 1, is inherited as an autosomal dominant trait. The pheochromocytomas are frequently bilateral, although rarely extra-adrenal, and the medullary carcinoma of the thyroid generally appears to be multifocal in origin. A particularly convenient and virtually constant feature of the medullary thyroid carcinomas is the hypersecretion of calcitonin, which serves as a useful marker for the presence of this neoplasm. Elevated levels of calcitonin, either under basal conditions or in response to the provocative stimuli of calcium and pentagastrin infusions, are an indication of parafollicular C-cell hyperplasia in the thyroid gland and may herald the presence of the genetic abnormality well before pathologic changes appear that are unequivocally malignant. As in the instance of the pancreatic adenomas in MEN 1, the medullary carcinomas of the thyroid in MEN 2a may secrete a variety of hormones and other biologically active substances that are not secreted by the corresponding normal tissue. These include ACTH, prolactin, histaminase, vasoactive intestinal peptide, serotonin, and a number of prostaglandins. Only rarely does medullary carcinoma of the thyroid present as a palpable mass. Pheochromocytoma is observed in about one half of affected individuals, and hyperparathyroidism in about one quarter. Only about 10 per cent of individuals with MEN 2a exhibit hypercalcemia or nephrolithiasis (cf. the much higher incidence of overt hyperparathyroidism in MEN 1). Glial tumors and meningiomas may also be seen in MEN 2a but occur far less frequently.

It has been suggested that MEN 2a represents a form of neuroectodermal dysplasia in which so-called APUD cells (cells capable of *a*mine *p*recursor *u*ptake and *d*ecarboxylation and possessing rather characteristic histologic staining properties)—following their embryonic migration to the foregut and subsequent localization in a variety of endocrine tissues—later become neoplastic and secrete excessive amounts of hormone in response to a specific genetic defect. Although the evidence for a common APUD cell origin is somewhat better in MEN 2a than it is in MEN 1, it is still by no means wholly convincing. In particular, the high incidence of parathyroid involvement is

difficult to reconcile with this theory, since the bulk of present evidence suggests an epithelial rather than a neural crest origin for this tissue. The medullary thyroid carcinomas in MEN 2a may begin as polyclonal hyperplasia followed by clonal carcinomas; that is, these carcinomas may arise as independent clonal "expansions" on a background of initial hyperplasia. The mutant gene for MEN 2a is on the short arm of chromosome 10.

The pheochromocytomas of MEN 2a are generally benign and are treated surgically. Because they are frequently bilateral, an anterior surgical approach is often recommended; CT scanning, multiple-site venous sampling for catecholamines, and angiography can all be helpful in planning surgery. Medullary carcinoma of the thyroid, on the other hand, runs a typically malignant course, and, because of its multifocal nature, requires total thyroidectomy. Elevated levels of calcitonin per se constitute a sufficient indication for total thyroidectomy, even when the tumor is otherwise clinically silent. The tumor is frequently slow growing, and limited node dissection is thus justified; completeness of tumor removal and the possibility of subsequent recurrence are both conveniently monitored by serum calcitonin levels. The isolated finding of medullary carcinoma of the thyroid should prompt a particularly careful inquiry into the family history, since it is likely that at least 10 per cent of such tumors are familial.

Screening of first-degree relatives of patients with MEN 2a is indicated and should include a 24-hour urine collection for vanillylmandelic acid, metanephrines, and catecholamines (even when the blood pressure is normal) as well as calcium and basal calcitonin determinations. If a thyroid mass is present, a fuller workup is indicated, including measurement of calcium-pentagastrin–stimulated calcitonin levels. Restriction-fragment analysis of DNA from peripheral blood lymphocytes can be employed to identify carriers of the MEN 2a gene.

MULTIPLE ENDOCRINE NEOPLASIA, TYPE 2b (MUCOSAL NEUROMA SYNDROME). This syndrome (MEN 2b) resembles MEN 2a but differs in four important respects: (1) The medullary carcinoma of the thyroid and the pheochromocytomas may be accompanied by striking and often disfiguring neuromas of the lips, buccal mucosa, and tongue, as well as by ganglioneuromas of the gastrointestinal tract, thickened corneal nerves visible upon slit-lamp examination, and café-au-lait spots, neuromas, or neurofibromas of the skin; (2) the body habitus may somewhat resemble that seen in patients with the Marfan syndrome; (3) parathyroid hyperplasia sufficient to result in frank hypercalcemia is rare; and (4) mean survival time in MEN 2b is considerably shorter than that in MEN 2a (30 versus 60 years). In contrast to MEN 1 and MEN 2a, MEN 2b is frequently sporadic, a history of affected family members being obtainable in not more than half of the cases.

McCUNE-ALBRIGHT SYNDROME. In 1937 McCune and Albright and their associates both described a syndrome characterized by a triad of *polyostotic fibrous dysplasia, café-au-lait pigmentation of the skin* (typically over the forehead, nuchal or sacral areas, or buttocks), and *precocious puberty in the female.* The precocious puberty, although predominantly seen in the female, may occur in males as well. This syndrome may be accompanied by a variety of other endocrine abnormalities, including pituitary hyperfunction (with Cushing's syndrome, acromegaly, or gigantism), bilateral pheochromocytomas, hyperthyroidism, and hypercorticism resulting from adrenal adenoma. Frank malignant disease has not been described. Although the syndrome was once believed to be hypothalamic in origin, recent evidence suggests that activating mutations of one of the subunits of the G protein that stimulates cyclic AMP production may represent the pathogenetic basis of this disorder.

SYNDROMES CHARACTERIZED BY MULTIPLE ENDOCRINE GLAND HYPOFUNCTION

Syndromes characterized by hypofunction of multiple endocrine organs are discussed under the separate headings of Schmidt's syndrome and the syndrome of polyglandular deficiency associated with mucocutaneous candidiasis. As noted below, however, evidence that the two syndromes actually represent different entities is incomplete. Table 228–2 compares the clinical features of these syndromes.

MULTIPLE ENDOCRINE DEFICIENCY SYNDROME (SCHMIDT'S SYNDROME). In 1926 Schmidt described two

TABLE 228–2. COMPARISON OF THE CLINICAL FEATURES OF THE MAJOR SYNDROMES CHARACTERIZED BY MULTIPLE ENDOCRINE GLAND HYPOFUNCTION

	Multiple Endocrine Deficiency Syndrome (Schmidt's Syndrome)	Polyglandular Deficiency with Mucocutaneous Candidiasis
Hypoadrenalism	Common	Common
Hypothyroidism	Common	Rare
Diabetes mellitus (Type I)	Common	Rare
Gonadal failure	Less common	Less common
Hypoparathyroidism	Rare	Common
Pituitary insufficiency	Rare	Rare
Autoantibodies to endocrine tissues and gastric parietal cells	Often present	Often present
Sex distribution	Strong female predominance	Female preponderance about 4:1
Inheritance	Usually "sporadic," but susceptibility related to HLA haplotype and may be inherited as autosomal dominant	Generally inherited as autosomal recessive; no apparent HLA association; siblings characteristically affected
Time of onset	Usually becomes evident during adult life	Typically becomes evident during childhood preceded by chronic mucocutaneous moniliasis
Other associated "autoimmune" diseases and characteristics	Pernicious anemia; hyperthyroidism; celiac disease; alopecia; vitiligo; myasthenia gravis; isolated red-cell aplasia	Pernicious anemia; malabsorption; alopecia; vitiligo; IgA deficiency; hypergammaglobulinemia; chronic active hepatitis; proliferative glomerulonephritis

patients with biglandular failure characterized by *idiopathic Addison's disease and lymphocytic thyroiditis*. This syndrome has subsequently been expanded to include "primary" failure of other endocrine glands, including the gonads, endocrine pancreas, and rarely the parathyroids, as well as a number of nonendocrine abnormalities of presumed autoimmune origin (see below). Virtually any combination of the foregoing endocrine deficiencies may appear in a single individual. The order of appearance is extremely variable, and a lag of as much as 17 years has been observed in the manifestation of sequential deficiencies. Hypothyroidism and hypoadrenalism are common; diabetes mellitus, (Type 1) and gonadal failure are somewhat less so. The frequencies of the different glandular failures probably vary greatly with ascertainment; if one considers Type 1 diabetes mellitus as part of the syndrome, the association of this with autoimmune thyroid disease may be the most commonly encountered combination.

Characteristic of this syndrome is the presence of autoantibodies to endocrine tissue and at times to gastric parietal cells as well. Such antibodies are often detectable before the appearance of clinical glandular insufficiency and are a hallmark of syndromes of "idiopathic" endocrine failure. Their presence has been implicated in the pathogenesis of the glandular destruction itself rather than merely as reflecting an immune response to tissue antigens released during antecedent glandular degeneration. Thus, for example, approximately two thirds of patients with idiopathic Addison's disease are reported to have autoantibodies to adrenal tissue, whereas such antibodies are generally absent in patients whose adrenal insufficiency is secondary to tuberculous destruction. About twice as many females are affected with idiopathic adrenal insufficiency as males. Although most cases of multiple

deficiency syndromes are sporadic, their occasional appearance in kindreds, as well as the relatively high gene frequency of the HLA-B8 and HLA-DR3 alleles in affected persons, provides strong evidence for a dominantly inherited susceptibility to the development of this type of polyglandular failure. Other "autoimmune" diseases that may accompany the aforementioned endocrine deficiencies include pernicious anemia, celiac disease, myasthenia gravis, alopecia, vitiligo, and isolated red-cell aplasia. Because it occurs in the same families and has the same HLA associations, Graves' disease is considered by many to be another facet of the syndrome.

Although the constellation of adrenal, thyroid, and gonadal failure in a single patient can easily be confused with primary pituitary insufficiency, measurement of the appropriate tropic hormones permits a ready differentiation of the two syndromes. Occasionally the simultaneous presence of hyperpigmentation in such an individual suggests a diagnosis of primary adrenal failure on "clinical" grounds alone. Because of the sporadic appearance and variable sequence of subsequent endocrine deficiencies, patients with a proven idiopathic endocrine deficiency should be periodically screened for evidence of additional endocrine involvement.

POLYGLANDULAR DEFICIENCY ASSOCIATED WITH MUCOCUTANEOUS CANDIDIASIS. A clinical picture somewhat different from that of Schmidt's syndrome is presented by patients with the so-called candidiasis-endocrinopathy syndrome. Characteristically this syndrome is dominated by the presence of extensive mucocutaneous candidiasis that appears in early childhood and is followed by the development of idiopathic adrenal insufficiency or hypoparathyroidism or both. Most typically, but not invariably, the appearance of these endocrinopathies postdates the acquisition of chronic monilial infection (mean age of onset, 13 versus 3 years, respectively). As in Schmidt's syndrome, antibodies against endocrine tissues are frequently demonstrable, and pernicious anemia with antibodies against gastric parietal cells may also be present. Diabetes mellitus, in contrast, is relatively rare. Also contrasting with Schmidt's syndrome, which most typically becomes evident in adult life, is the fact that there is no apparent association with the presence of specific HLA alleles, and the apparent inheritance of the syndrome as an autosomal recessive trait within a single generation of siblings. Chronic active hepatitis and proliferative glomerulonephritis have also been reported. The mucocutaneous candidiasis is associated with hypergammaglobulinemia, IgA deficiency, and anergy to *Candida albicans*. Treatment with oral ketoconazole can produce a striking remission of the mucocutaneous candidiasis, although the latter generally recurs upon discontinuation of therapy. No evidence for disseminated candidiasis has been found in autopsied individuals, nor has *Candida* yet been cultured from an affected endocrine gland.

Albright F, Butler AM, Hampton AO, et al.: Syndrome characterized by osteitis fibrosa disseminata, areas of pigmentation and endocrine dysfunction, with precocious puberty in females. N Engl J Med 216:727, 1937. *One of the two classic descriptions of the McCune-Albright syndrome. Excellent figures.*

Gagel RF, Tashjian AF Jr, Cummings TW, et al.: The clinical outcome of prospective screening for multiple endocrine neoplasia type 2a: An 18-year experience. N Engl J Med 318:478, 1988. *A recent review showing that prospective screening and early treatment of the manifestations of MEN 2a can prevent metastasis of medullary thyroid carcinoma as well as the morbidity and mortality associated with pheochromocytoma.*

Deftos LJ, Catherwood BD, Bone HG III: Multiglandular endocrine disorders. *In* Felig P, Baxter JD, Broadus AE, et al. (eds.): Endocrinology and Metabolism, 2nd ed. New York, McGraw-Hill Book Company, 1987, pp 1662–1691. *Excellent general review with 198 references.*

Pipeleers-Marichal M, Somers G, Willems G, et al.: Gastrinomas in the duodenums of patients with multiple endocrine neoplasia type 1 and the Zollinger-Ellison syndrome. N Engl J Med 322:723, 1990. *Multicenter report of a high incidence of resectable duodenal gastrinomas as a cause of symptomatic hypergastrinemia in patients with MEN 1.*

Rabinowe SL, Eisenbarth GS: Polyglandular autoimmunity. Adv Intern Med 31:293, 1986. *An excellent review of these syndromes with an up-to-date list of 60 references.*

Sobol H, Narod SA, Nakamura Y, et al.: Screening for multiple endocrine neoplasia type 2a with DNA-polymorphism analysis. N Engl J Med 321:996, 1989. *Genetic screening permits identification of individuals at risk for MEN 2a with a high level of certainty.*

Weinstein LE, Shenker A, Gejman PV, et al.: Activating mutations of the stimulatory G protein in the McCune-Albright syndrome. N Engl J Med 325:1688, 1991. *Evidence that activating mutations of the G protein that stimulates cyclic AMP production may be the cause of the McCune-Albright syndrome.*

Wilkin TJ: Mechanisms of disease: Receptor autoimmunity in endocrine disorders. N Engl J Med 323:1318, 1990. *The best recent article on this topic.*

Zimering MB, Brandi ML, deGrange DA, et al.: Circulating fibroblast growth factor–like substance in familial multiple endocrine neoplasia type I. J Clin Endocrinol Metab 70:149, 1990. *Evidence that the parathyroid hyperplasia characteristic of MEN 1 is attributable to a circulating growth factor similar if not identical to basic fibroblast growth factor.*

229 The Adrenal Medullae

Philip E. Cryer

The sympathochromaffin (sympathoadrenal) system consists of two components: (1) the sympathetic nervous system and (2) the chromaffin tissues, including the adrenal medullae. The primary endocrine, neurotransmitter, and perhaps paracrine products of the sympathochromaffin system are the catecholamines—epinephrine (adrenaline), norepinephrine (noradrenaline), and dopamine. Cells of the sympathochromaffin system also contain a variety of peptides of potential biologic importance. Their pathophysiologic roles, if any, are unknown.

Catecholamine excess commonly results in hypertension along with typical symptoms. It has long been suspected, but is still not proven, that increased sympathetic nervous system activity is the cause of primary (essential) hypertension. Catecholamine overproduction from chromaffin cell tumors—pheochromocytomas—is an uncommon, but often curable, cause of hypertension. Deficient sympathetic neuronal norepinephrine release results in postural (orthostatic) hypotension, a sharp decrease in blood pressure when a person stands. Under certain conditions, deficient adrenomedullary epinephrine secretion results in hypoglycemia. Two of these prominent examples of sympathochromaffin pathophysiology are discussed in the paragraphs that follow. Disorders of the sympathetic nervous system are discussed in Ch. 452.

PHYSIOLOGY OF THE SYMPATHOCHROMAFFIN SYSTEM

CATECHOLAMINE BIOSYNTHESIS. The term *catecholamines* is often used to refer to epinephrine and norepinephrine, although dopamine is also a catecholamine, i.e., has the dihydroxyphenyl ("catechol") ring structure and an amine side chain (Fig. 229–1). The catecholamines are synthesized from the amino acid tyrosine, which is derived from the diet or formed by hydroxylation of the essential amino acid phenylalanine. Tyrosine hydroxylase, the enzyme that converts tyrosine to dihydroxyphenylalanine (dopa), is the rate-limiting enzyme in catecholamine biosynthesis. In the presence of a nonspecific decarboxylase, dopa is converted to dopamine, which is the final product in some systems (e.g., interneurons in the sympathetic ganglia). After transport into cytoplasmic vesicles (storage granules), dopamine can be converted to norepinephrine in the presence of dopamine β-hydroxylase. Norepinephrine is the final product in sympathetic postganglionic neurons. Other tissues, such as the adrenal medullae, have cells that also contain phenylethanolamine-N-methyltransferase, the enzyme that converts norepinephrine to epinephrine, the final product of those cells.

Catecholamines are stored in cytoplasmic granules and released from the cell by exocytosis in response to neural stimulation.

CATECHOLAMINE DEGRADATION AND ELIMINATION. Catecholamines are degraded by two principal enzyme systems, catechol-O-methyltransferase (COMT) and monoamine oxidase (MAO) (Fig. 229–1). COMT converts norepinephrine and epinephrine to their respective O-methyl derivatives, the metanephrines (normetanephrine and metanephrine). MAO converts norepinephrine and epinephrine to dihydroxymandelic acid. These intermediates, the metanephrines and dihydroxymandelic acid, can then serve as substrates for MAO and COMT, respectively, resulting in their conversion to the major end product of extra-CNS catecholamine metabolism, vanillylmandelic acid (VMA). Dopamine metabolism (not shown in Figure 229–1) by MAO and COMT leads to the formation of homovanillic acid (HVA).

In general, catecholamine degradation within the sympathochromaffin cells is via MAO, whereas that of released catecholamines is via COMT. Released catecholamines are also conjugated, largely to sulfate in humans, and this may be another important route of inactivation. Sixty to 80 per cent of plasma epinephrine and norepinephrine and roughly half of the catecholamines excreted in the urine are conjugated.

Catecholamines are cleared rapidly from the circulation. Plasma half-times are 1 to 2 minutes. Clearance is largely extrarenal; less than 5 per cent appears in the urine unaltered.

BIOLOGIC ROLES OF THE CATECHOLAMINES. Epinephrine, norepinephrine, and dopamine are neurotransmitters in the CNS. Outside of the CNS, epinephrine is a hormone of the adrenal medulla, and norepinephrine is primarily the neurotransmitter of sympathetic postganglionic neurons. Dopamine is probably also a neurotransmitter, although its physiologic role has not been defined clearly.

Neurally regulated secretion of epinephrine from extra-adrenal chromaffin tissue (not sympathetic neurons) occurs, but in the absence of the adrenal medullae even stimulated plasma epinephrine levels in adults are not high enough to produce measurable biologic effects. Biologic actions of extra-adrenal epinephrine, if any, must be paracrine/neurotransmitter, not hormonal, in nature, at least in adults. Thus, epinephrine functions primarily as a hormone of the adrenal medulla and its plasma concentration is a valid index of its secretion.

Norepinephrine is released from axon terminals of sympathetic postganglionic neurons in direct relation to adrenergic receptors on innervated target cells. Most released norepinephrine is dissipated locally by reuptake into an axon terminal (uptake₁), where it is either stored in vesicles or metabolized, or by uptake into other cells adjacent to the synaptic cleft (uptake₂), where it is metabolized. Only a small fraction escapes into the circulation. The plasma norepinephrine concentration is a reasonable index of sympathetic neural activity under common physiologic conditions, at least in the basal state and during upright activity in humans. However, under some conditions, such as hypoglycemia, substantial amounts of norepinephrine (along with large amounts of epinephrine) are released from chromaffin tissues, specifically the adrenal medulla. Under such conditions the plasma norepinephrine concentration is clearly not an index of sympathetic neural activity. During vigorous physical activity and in a variety of pathologic states such as surgery, acute myocardial infarction, and diabetic ketoacidosis, circulating norepinephrine is probably derived from both the sympathetic nerves and the adrenal medullae, and its concentrations can be high enough to produce measurable effects. Under these conditions norepinephrine may function as a hormone as well as a neurotransmitter.

This physiology is relevant to the clinical use of plasma catecholamine measurements. Norepinephrine release from sympathetic neurons in amounts sufficient to produce biologically active norepinephrine concentrations in the synaptic cleft can be associated with very small, even undetectable, increments in its plasma concentration. On the other hand, if norepinephrine is released directly into the circulation (as from a pheochromocytoma) substantial increments in its plasma concentration are required to produce biologically active synaptic cleft concentrations.

BIOLOGIC ACTIONS OF THE CATECHOLAMINES. Catecholamines produce a variety of hemodynamic and metabolic effects. These are the result of catecholamine occupancy of adrenergic receptors (adrenoceptors) on the surface of target cells and a consequent series of intramembrane and intracellular biochemical events. Adrenergic receptors are divided into α- and β-adrenergic receptors, which are subdivided into α_1- and α_2-adrenergic receptors and β_1- and β_2-adrenergic receptors on the basis of measurements of the responses to various agonists and antagonists and the binding of a variety of ligands (generally antagonists) and competition for binding of these ligands by agonists and antagonists in vitro. In general, β-adrenergic receptors are linked through a stimulatory guanine nucleotide regulatory protein to adenylate cyclase, and α_2- (but not α_1-) adrenergic receptors are linked through an inhibitory protein to adenylate cyclase. A discussion of adrenergic receptors is beyond the scope of this chapter, although selected examples are given.

Catecholamines increase the rate and force of myocardial contraction (β_1) and produce vasoconstriction (α) in most vascular beds, although vasodilatation (β_2) occurs in some vascular beds, e.g., those of skeletal muscle. Norepinephrine produces increased vascular resistance and blood pressure (systolic and diastolic); the increased blood pressure reflexively limits the increase in heart rate. Probably because it has a higher affinity than norepinephrine for β_2-adrenergic receptors, epinephrine normally produces a somewhat different pattern: increased systolic, but not diastolic, blood pressure and increased heart rate.

Catecholamines increase the plasma glucose concentration through complex actions. These involve both stimulation of hepatic glucose production and limitation of glucose utilization and are mediated by both direct and indirect mechanisms. Foremost among the indirect mechanisms is limitation of insulin secretion (α_2). The direct actions are largely β mediated. Catecholamines also stimulate lipolysis, ketogenesis, glycolysis, and mobilization of amino acids such as alanine. They also increase thermogenesis.

Symptoms that occur when the sympathochromaffin system is activated include palpitations, anxiety, headache, and diaphoresis. All but the last are attributable to released catecholamines; diaphoresis has been attributed to a sympathetic cholinergic mechanism.

PHEOCHROMOCYTOMA

Pheochromocytomas are catecholamine-releasing tumors that typically produce hypertension. They are an uncommon cause of hypertension; perhaps 1 in 1000 hypertensive patients harbors a pheochromocytoma. Yet it is important to detect a pheochromocytoma for several reasons: (1) Hypertension due to a pheochromocytoma is usually curable by surgical removal of the tumor. (2) Patients with a pheochromocytoma are at risk for a lethal

hypertensive paroxysm. (3) Some pheochromocytomas are malignant; early detection and removal would be expected to reduce the frequency of metastatic disease. Parenthetically, malignancy is established convincingly only by proven metastases; histologic criteria in the primary tumor are not reliable. (4) The presence of pheochromocytomas can be a clue to the presence of associated endocrine and nonendocrine familial disorders (Ch. 228). Pheochromocytomas are components of the multiple endocrine neoplasia, type 2 (MEN 2a) and type 3 (MEN 2b) syndromes. These familial disorders are inherited as autosomal dominant traits. MEN 2a includes medullary carcinoma of the thyroid, primary hyperparathyroidism, and pheochromocytoma. MEN 2b includes medullary carcinoma of the thyroid, multiple mucosal neuromas, and pheochromocytoma. Pheochromocytomas are not a component of the MEN 1 syndrome (pituitary and pancreatic adenomas and hyperparathyroidism). Familial pheochromocytomas also occur as an isolated disorder, in neurofibromatosis, and in the von Hippel-Lindau syndrome.

PATHOLOGY. Pheochromocytomas arise from chromaffin cells. Chromaffin cells are widespread and associated with sympathetic ganglia during fetal life. Postnatally most chromaffin cells degenerate; the major residual clusters of chromaffin cells comprise the adrenal medullae. Approximately 90 per cent of pheochromocytomas arise from the adrenal medullae. Extra-adrenal pheochromocytomas (paragangliomas) have been found in sites ranging from the carotid body to the pelvic floor. However, the majority are associated with sympathetic ganglia in the abdomen and most of the others with ganglia in the posterior mediastinum. Multiple pheochromocytomas, including bilateral adrenomedullary tumors, occur in up to 10 per cent of apparently sporadic cases. Bilateral adrenomedullary pheochromocytomas, with or without extra-adrenal tumors, are the rule in familial pheochro-

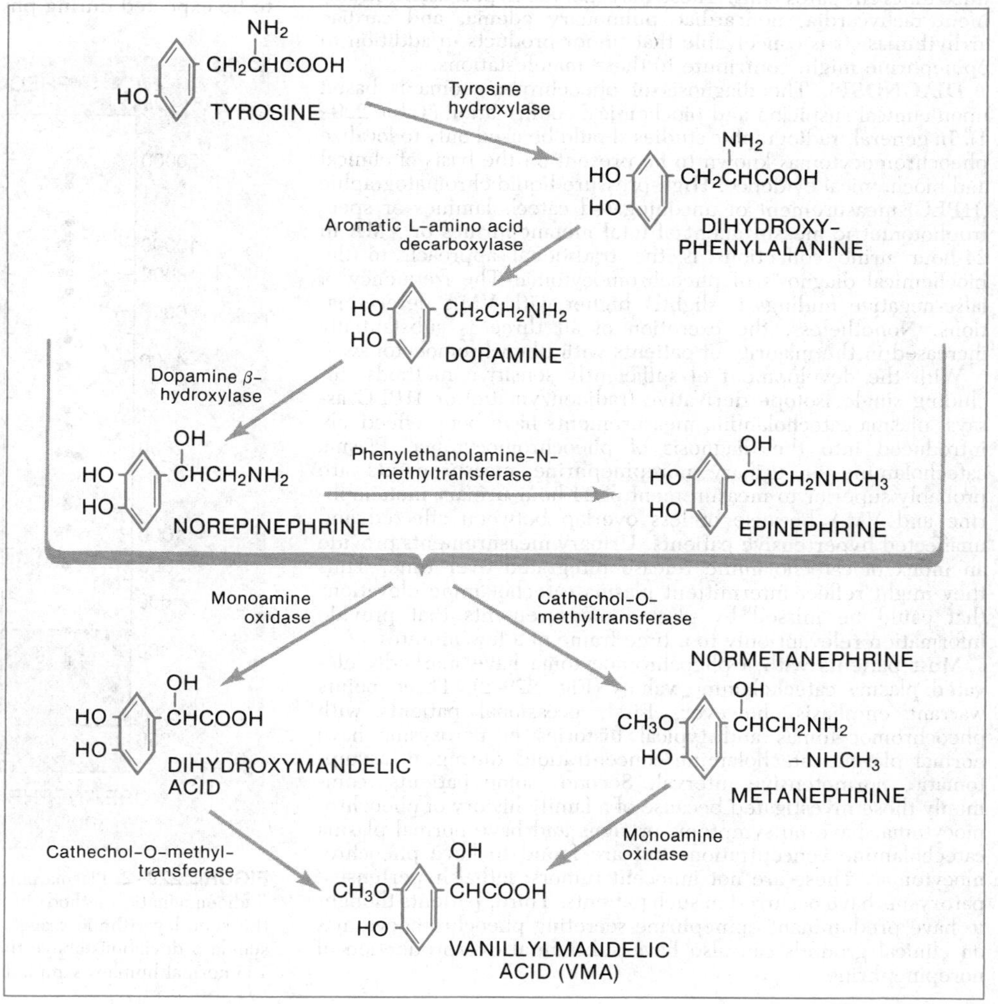

FIGURE 229–1. Catecholamine biosynthesis and metabolic degradation.

mocytoma. Bilateral adrenomedullary hyperplasia, thought to be a precursor to pheochromocytoma, has been found in members of affected families.

The vast majority of pheochromocytomas release norepinephrine, and most also release some epinephrine. Rarely, a pheochromocytoma releases epinephrine predominantly or even exclusively.

CLINICAL MANIFESTATIONS. The clinical manifestations of pheochromocytomas are commonly due to the effects of released catecholamines and only rarely to the mass effect of the tumor. Common symptoms are *headache, palpitations,* and *diaphoresis.* Less common symptoms include abdominal or chest pain, gastrointestinal symptoms, weakness, or visual symptoms. Symptoms are typically paroxysmal and associated with increments in blood pressure. Hypertension is sometimes truly intermittent. In many cases, hypertension is sustained but exhibits marked fluctuations with peak values occurring during symptomatic episodes. In general, plasma catecholamine levels are higher during symptomatic, hypertensive episodes than during asymptomatic, less hypertensive, or even normotensive intervals. The event(s) that precipitates episodic catecholamine release is usually not identifiable. However, the relationship between plasma catecholamine concentrations and blood pressure is not tight. This may reflect contrasting effects of norepinephrine and epinephrine but raises the possibility that hypertension in a patient with a pheochromocytoma may not be exclusively the result of direct effects of circulating norepinephrine on the cardiovascular system. Metabolic features of pheochromocytoma include an increased metabolic rate (some patients complain of heat intolerance, weight loss, or both) and an insulin-resistant state. Glucose intolerance and fasting hyperglycemia occur, but overt diabetes is unusual and probably reflects a coexistent defect in insulin secretion, i.e., genetic diabetes mellitus.

The rare epinephrine-releasing pheochromocytomas can produce different paroxysms. These may include hypotension, prominent tachycardia, noncardiac pulmonary edema, and cardiac arrhythmias. It is conceivable that tumor products in addition to epinephrine might contribute to these manifestations.

DIAGNOSIS. The diagnosis of pheochromocytoma is based upon clinical suspicion and biochemical confirmation (Table 229–1). In general, radiographic studies should be used only to localize pheochromocytomas known to be present on the basis of clinical and biochemical evidence. High-pressure liquid chromatographic (HPLC) measurement of unconjugated catecholamines or spectrophotometric measurement of total metanephrines or VMA in 24-hour urine collections is the traditional approach to the biochemical diagnosis of pheochromocytoma. The frequency of false-negative findings is slightly higher with VMA determinations. Nonetheless, the excretion of all three is substantially increased in the majority of patients with pheochromocytomas.

With the development of sufficiently sensitive methods, including single isotope derivative (radioenzymatic) or HPLC assays, plasma catecholamine measurements have been effectively introduced into the diagnosis of pheochromocytoma. Plasma catecholamine or urinary norepinephrine measurements are probably superior to measurement of 24-hour urinary metanephrine and VMA because of less overlap between affected and unaffected hypertensive patients. Urinary measurements provide an index of catecholamine release integrated over time. Thus they might reflect intermittent plasma catecholamine elevations that could be missed by plasma measurements that provide information relevant only to a time frame of a few minutes.

Most patients with a pheochromocytoma have markedly elevated plasma catecholamine values (Fig. 229–2). Three points warrant emphasis, however. First, occasional patients with pheochromocytomas and typical histories of paroxysms have normal plasma catecholamine concentrations during an asymptomatic, normotensive interval. Second, some patients, commonly those investigated because of a family history of pheochromocytoma, have no symptoms or signs and have normal plasma catecholamine concentrations but are found to have pheochromocytomas. These are not innocent tumors; lethal hypertensive paroxysms have occurred in such patients. Third, patients thought to have predominant epinephrine-secreting pheochromocytomas on clinical grounds can also have substantial overproduction of norepinephrine.

TABLE 229–1. DIAGNOSIS OF PHEOCHROMOCYTOMA

Clinical Suspicion
1. Paroxysmal symptoms (especially headache, palpitations, and diaphoresis)
2. Intermittent or unusually labile hypertension or hypertension refractory to therapy
3. Incidental adrenal mass (rarely a pheochromocytoma in the absence of one or more of the above)
4. Family history of pheochromocytoma, MEN 2, or MEN 3

Biochemical Confirmation
1. Plasma norepinephrine and epinephrine (± dopamine)
   Patient sampled in the basal state (and supine position) and, if possible, during a paroxysm
   Radioenzymatic or HPLC method
   Note blood pressure, heart rate, and any symptoms
2. Urinary catecholamines or metanephrines (or VMA)
   If plasma values are normal or equivocal but clinical suspicion is high, repeated plasma measurements are an alternative
   Can be used as the initial test

Anatomic Localization
1. Computed tomography
   Of the abdomen, including the adrenals, initially; of the pelvis and thorax if the abdomen is negative
   Indicated in the absence of biochemical evidence only if clinical suspicion is very high (e.g., positive family history)
2. Magnetic resonance imaging
3. Iodobenzylguanidine scan

Strict attention to the details of sample collection, handling and storage, the sources of possible biologic variation, and the effects of drugs is critical if diagnostic error is to be avoided in the biochemical assessment of patients with suspected pheochromocytomas. Patients should be studied in the drug-free state if at all possible. Most antihypertensive drugs (other than clonidine) and many other drugs can elevate plasma and/or urine catecholamine levels. Elevated plasma catecholamine concentrations are to be expected during physical or mental stress and in any acute

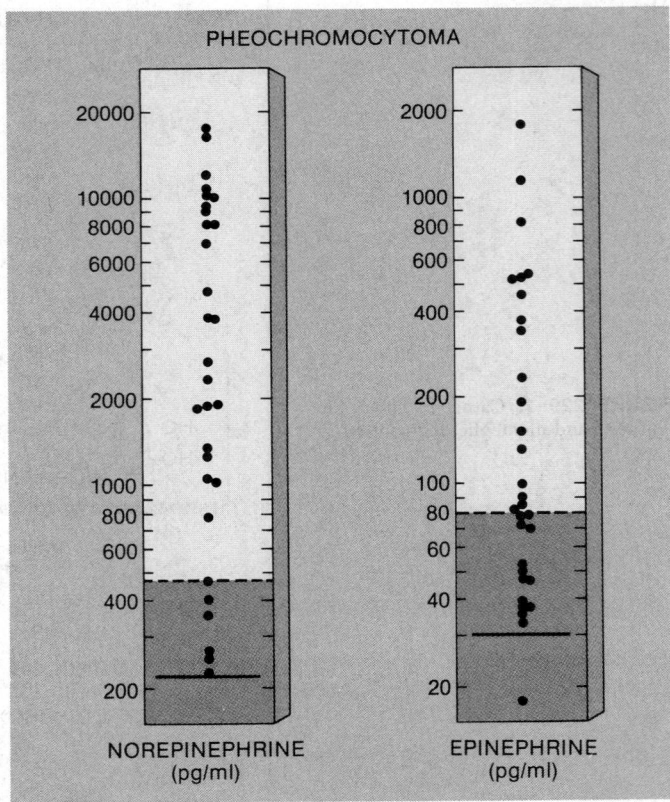

FIGURE 229–2. Plasma norepinephrine and epinephrine concentrations (radioenzymatic method) in 30 patients with pheochromocytomas. Note the semi-logarithmic scales. The interrupted horizontal lines are three standard deviations above the means (solid horizontal lines) of data from 165 normal humans sampled in the supine position.

illness. Elevations, at times marked, have been well documented in patients with acute myocardial infarction, shock, burns, diabetic ketoacidosis, and cerebrovascular accidents, as well as during and immediately after surgery. Stable plasma catecholamine elevations also occur in patients with chronic disorders—for example, hypothyroidism, congestive heart failure, chronic obstructive pulmonary disease, anemia, duodenal ulcer, and depression. Lastly, elevated plasma catecholamine concentrations have been found in some, but certainly not all, patients thought to have essential hypertension.

It is my practice to obtain samples for determination of plasma norepinephrine and epinephrine in the basal state, with the patient supine, when pheochromocytoma is suspected. Substantial elevations over reference values provide strong support for the diagnosis of pheochromocytoma and are commonly found in affected patients. Samples are also obtained during symptomatic paroxysms. However, the interpretation of such values is more judgmental, since reference values cannot be defined precisely. Thus the biochemical diagnosis of pheochromocytoma is more convincingly supported if plasma catecholamine levels are elevated in the basal state and rise further during symptomatic episodes.

It is useful to record the blood pressure and whether or not symptoms are present when plasma samples for catecholamine measurements are drawn from a patient suspected of having a pheochromocytoma. Clearly, normal plasma (or urinary) catecholamine values obtained when the patient is normotensive and free of symptoms do not exclude the presence of a pheochromocytoma. Theoretically, 24-hour urinary catecholamine or metabolite measurements might detect intermittent catecholamine release missed by plasma sampling. These measurements should be obtained if plasma catecholamine levels are normal but clinical suspicion is high.

Substantial plasma norepinephrine elevations are required to produce hypertension in normal humans. Plasma epinephrine elevations within the physiologic range do not raise the diastolic blood pressure. It is reasonable, therefore, to consider normal or even moderately elevated plasma catecholamine levels obtained when the patient is hypertensive to be strong evidence against the diagnosis of pheochromocytoma.

Most patients ultimately found to have pheochromocytomas have distinctly elevated plasma and urinary catecholamine levels. The considerations raised in the preceding paragraphs apply to patients in whom the diagnosis is less clear cut and to the always difficult problem of the degree of certainty of a negative conclusion. Obviously one can never be absolutely certain during life that a given patient does not have a pheochromocytoma. As in many other areas of medicine, clinical judgment must be based upon probability.

Oral clonidine (0.3 mg) suppresses plasma catecholamine levels in hypertensive patients without pheochromocytoma but not in patients with pheochromocytoma. Thus the clonidine suppression test has been suggested to distinguish patients with primary hypertension with elevated basal plasma norepinephrine levels from those with hypertension due to a pheochromocytoma. Definition of the utility of this test awaits further experience. False negatives and false positives have been reported.

LOCALIZATION. Given biochemical confirmation of pheochromocytoma, anatomic localization is desirable. Normal adrenal glands can usually be imaged with modern computed tomography (CT), and the majority of adrenomedullary pheochromocytomas can be seen with this technique. CT is the recommended initial localizing procedure. Magnetic resonance imaging is also useful, and might be more specific. External scanning after the injection of radioactive agents that localize in pheochromocytomas has the conceptual advantage of measuring function rather than anatomy and the practical advantage of permitting scanning of the entire trunk of the body and might, therefore, be expected to localize extra-adrenal pheochromocytomas better than CT scans. The initial experience with [131I]-m-iodobenzylguanidine (MIBG) scans has been encouraging in this regard.

TREATMENT. Treatment is surgical removal of the pheochromocytoma. Patients are usually prepared for surgery by administration of an α-adrenergic antagonist, such as phenoxybenzamine or prazosin, in doses sufficient to produce normal blood pressure and to prevent paroxysms. Treatment for 7 to 10 days prior to surgery is often recommended on the premise that this permits expansion of the blood volume. These drugs can also be used to treat chronic catecholamine excess in patients with metastatic tumor, although they do not influence the growth of a malignant pheochromocytoma. A β-adrenergic antagonist, such as propranolol, can be added to the preoperative regimen if arrhythmias are, or become, a problem.

Most patients are cured by surgery. The differential diagnosis of persistent hypertension includes a missed pheochromocytoma, a surgical complication resulting in renal ischemia, and underlying primary hypertension. Long-term follow-up is important, since late recurrences, including metastatic lesions, are being recognized with increasing frequency.

OTHER NEURAL CREST TUMORS. Pheochromocytomas are tumors of differentiated neural crest cells, the chromaffin cells. Tumors of more primitive cells also occur. These include neuroblastoma, a rather common malignant tumor of infancy and early childhood, usually arising in the adrenal medullae, and ganglioneuroma, a generally benign tumor often arising in sympathetic ganglia. These tumors commonly synthesize catecholamines but usually do not release catecholamines in sufficient quantities to produce clinical manifestations. Presumably the catecholamines are largely inactivated within the tumor. Nonetheless, measurements of catecholamine metabolites such as HVA and VMA are useful, particularly in assessing the response to therapy.

EPINEPHRINE DEFICIENCY

The prevention or correction of hypoglycemia involves both dissipation of insulin and activation of glucose counter-regulatory systems. Whereas insulin is the dominant glucose-lowering factor, there are redundant glucose counter-regulatory factors, and a hierarchy among these. In defense against decrements in plasma glucose, dissipation of insulin is likely most important. Glucagon plays a primary counter-regulatory role. Epinephrine is not normally critical, but it compensates and becomes critical when glucagon is deficient. Hypoglycemia develops or progresses when both glucagon and epinephrine are deficient and insulin is present. Other hormones, neurotransmitters, or substrate effects may be involved, but they are neither critical nor potent.

Selective deficiency of the glucagon response to decrements in plasma glucose is the rule in patients with insulin-dependent diabetes mellitus (IDDM). To the extent that they have deficient glucagon responses, patients with IDDM are largely dependent upon epinephrine to prevent or correct hypoglycemia. Deficient epinephrine responses develop typically later in the course of the disease. Patients with combined deficiencies of the glucagon and epinephrine responses are virtually defenseless against iatrogenic hypoglycemia. They have defective glucose counter-regulation and are at substantially increased risk (25-fold in our experience) for severe hypoglycemia, at least during intensive therapy of IDDM.

Patients with defective glucose counter-regulation often have a history of hypoglycemia unawareness but some do not. They can be identified prospectively with an insulin infusion test. Clearly, euglycemia is not an appropriate therapeutic goal in patients with IDDM and defective glucose counter-regulation, whether the latter is demonstrated with an insulin infusion test or is apparent from recurrent severe hypoglycemia during an attempt at intensive therapy. Administration of a β-adrenergic antagonist such as propranolol impairs recovery from experimental hypoglycemia in most patients with IDDM. Long-term administration of β-adrenergic antagonists has not been shown to increase the frequency of severe hypoglycemia in patients with IDDM, but this has not been examined in the context of intensive therapy.

Bravo EL, Gifford RW Jr: Pheochromocytoma: Diagnosis, localization and management. N Engl J Med 311:1298, 1984. *An extensive experience, including plasma catecholamine data.*

Cryer PE: Pheochromocytoma. West J Med, in press. *A more detailed review of the subject, including discussion of the effects of drugs on catecholamine measurements and other details of diagnostic testing.*

Cryer PE: Diseases of the sympathochromaffin system. *In* Felig P, Baxter JD, Broadus AE, et al. (eds.): Endocrinology and Metabolism, 2nd ed. New York, McGraw-Hill Book Company, 1987, pp 651–692. *A detailed discussion of sympathochromaffin physiology and pathophysiology.*

Cryer PE, Binder C, Bolli GB, et al.: Hypoglycemia in insulin dependent diabetes mellitus. Diabetes 38:1193, 1989. *A review of the physiology and pathophysiology of glucose counter-regulation.*

Duncan MW, Compton P, Lazarus L, et al.: Measurement of norepinephrine and 3,4-dihydroxyphenylglycol in urine and plasma for the diagnosis of pheochromocytoma. N Engl J Med 319:136, 1988. *Includes data comparing plasma and urinary norepinephrine measurements.*

The French MIBG Study Group: Comparison of iodobenzylguanidine imaging with computed tomography in locating pheochromocytoma. J Clin Endocrinol Metab 61:769, 1985. *A large experience demonstrating the strengths and weaknesses of the two approaches.*

230 The Carcinoid Syndrome

Philip E. Cryer

Carcinoid tumors arise from enterochromaffin (Kulchitsky) cells that are located predominantly in the gastrointestinal mucosa. Enterochromaffin cells have the potential to produce a variety of biologically active amines and peptides, including serotonin, bradykinin, histamine, and tachykinins, as well as prostaglandins. Carcinoid tumors are relatively common. Those that release sufficient quantities of mediators into the systemic circulation to produce the clinical carcinoid syndrome—flushing often with diarrhea and sometimes with wheezing or cardiac failure—are rare. Carcinoid tumors are most commonly found in the appendix or rectum, but these rarely produce the carcinoid syndrome. The tumors that produce the syndrome typically arise in the ileum, although the carcinoid syndrome can also result from tumors of the stomach, bile duct, duodenum, pancreas, lung, or even the gonads. Despite the release of a variety of mediators, the biochemical common denominator of the carcinoid syndrome is the overproduction of serotonin and the excretion of its major metabolite, 5-hydroxyindoleacetic acid (5-HIAA).

A variety of ectopic humoral syndromes have been associated with histologic carcinoid tumors. These include Cushing's syndrome (ACTH) and dilutional hyponatremia (vasopressin) with bronchial carcinoids, gynecomastia (chorionic gonadotropin) with gastric carcinoids, acromegaly (growth hormone–releasing hormone) with foregut carcinoids, and hypoglycemia (insulin) with pancreatic carcinoids. Typically, such patients do not have the carcinoid syndrome.

BIOSYNTHESIS AND DEGRADATION OF SEROTONIN. Serotonin is synthesized from dietary tryptophan and later is converted to 5-hydroxyindoleacetic acid through the reactions shown in Figure 230–1.

Approximately 90 per cent of serotonin in the body is normally found in the gut. Serotonin synthesis accounts for only 1 per cent of the metabolism of tryptophan in normal individuals. This may be as high as 60 per cent in patients with the carcinoid syndrome. Indeed, a pellagra-like skin rash has been attributed to diversion of tryptophan from nicotinic acid synthesis in such patients. Normal individuals excrete less than 10 mg of 5-HIAA per 24 hours. Patients with the carcinoid syndrome commonly excrete 50 to 100 mg per 24 hours.

CLINICAL MANIFESTATIONS. Clinical carcinoid syndrome is usually associated with an ileal carcinoid tumor that has metastasized to the liver. Carcinoids in sites, such as those in the lung or ovary, that do not drain into the portal circulation can rarely produce the carcinoid syndrome without evident hepatic metastases. Carcinoid syndrome due to an ileal carcinoid, however, is almost invariably associated with overt hepatic metastases. Presumably the liver clears mediators released from the tumor, and this clearance is impaired by metastatic tumor, resulting in the clinical syndrome.

More than 90 per cent of patients with the carcinoid syndrome have episodes of *cutaneous flushing*. The flush usually begins in the face and may spread to the trunk or even the extremities. It is red initially and then becomes purple; it commonly lasts only a few minutes, but may continue for hours. *Telangiectasias* of the face can result from frequent flushing. The heart rate increases

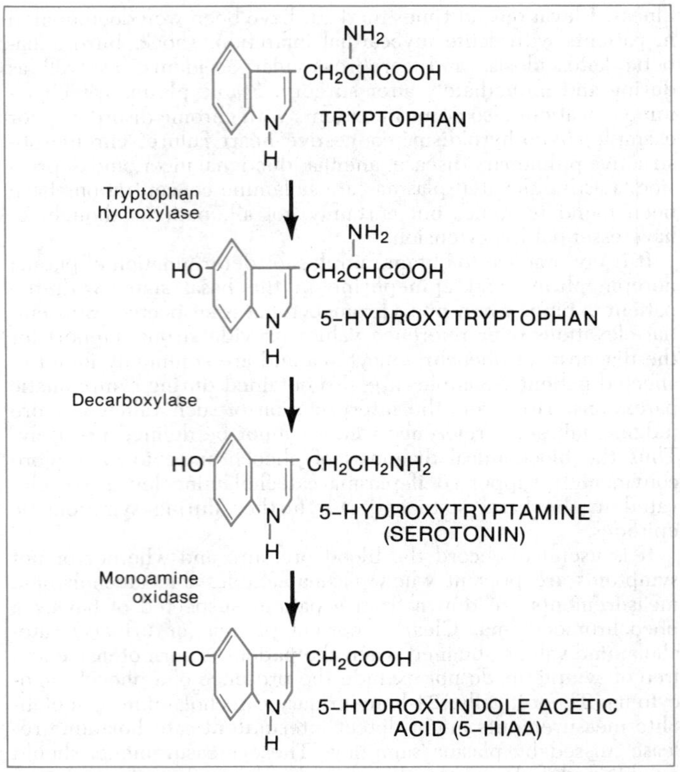

FIGURE 230–1. Synthesis and degradation of serotonin.

and the blood pressure tends to decrease during a flush. This is in contrast to patients with pheochromocytomas who typically have episodes of pallor with hypertension. Bronchial carcinoids may be associated with more intense and long-lasting flushing episodes. In patients with gastric carcinoids, flushing tends to be patchy initially and may be anywhere on the body. Headache commonly follows the flush.

Flushing can be precipitated by alcohol, food, stress, or palpation of the liver, or it may follow the administration of catecholamines, pentagastrin, or reserpine. A single mediator that causes the carcinoid flush has not been identified. It is not serotonin, since inhibition of serotonin synthesis does not prevent flushing. Candidate mediators include bradykinin, histamine, prostaglandins, and tachykinins including substance P.

More than three quarters of patients with the carcinoid syndrome have *diarrhea*, typically exacerbated during episodes of flushing. Serotonin most likely mediates the diarrhea, since it can be reduced by inhibition of serotonin synthesis in most patients. Intestinal symptoms can also result from mesenteric fibrosis. Pleural, peritoneal, and retroperitoneal fibroses also occur. Serotonin may also cause the fibrotic lesions.

Right-sided endocardial fibrosis, perhaps the result of chronic serotonin excess, is found in more than one third of patients with the carcinoid syndrome. Cardiac failure due to pulmonic stenosis or tricuspid insufficiency or both is less common but implies a poor prognosis. Involvement of the left side of the heart is uncommon. It does occur in patients with bronchial carcinoids, which implies that the responsible mediator(s) is ordinarily cleared during passage through pulmonary capillaries.

Bronchoconstriction with wheezing during an episode of flushing is less common, occurring in about 20 per cent of patients. Like flushing, but unlike diarrhea, bronchoconstriction is not prevented by inhibition of serotonin synthesis.

Somatostatin has been reported to decrease flushing, diarrhea, and bronchoconstriction in patients with the carcinoid syndrome. The mechanism(s) of this effect is not known.

DIAGNOSIS. Diagnosis is based upon clinical suspicion—usually a history of flushing and diarrhea—associated with markedly increased urinary 5-hydroxyindoleacetic acid excretion. Metastatic hepatomegaly is common. Since carcinoid tumors produce the carcinoid syndrome rarely, the histologic diagnosis of a carcinoid tumor does not establish the presence of the carcinoid syndrome. Platelet serotonin levels are elevated in most patients with the carcinoid syndrome. Gastric carcinoids appear to have low decarboxylase activity, since 5-hydroxytryptophan, rather than serotonin, is the major product of indole metabolism in some such patients.

Provocative tests, such as the precipitation of episodes with intravenous administration of epinephrine, are seldom necessary and potentially dangerous, since severe hypotension and bronchoconstriction can occur.

False-positive urinary 5-HIAA determinations are common and should be suspected particularly when the values are minimally elevated, e.g., 10 to 20 mg per 24 hours. Increased 5-HIAA excretion can follow the ingestion of chocolate, bananas, tomatoes, pineapples, walnuts, and avocados and the use of drugs, including mephenesin, methamphetamine, methysergide, methocarbamol, reserpine, acetaminophen, and glyceryl guaiacolate (the last in some cough syrups). Increased values have also been reported in Whipple's disease and nontropical sprue.

Computed tomography, radionuclide scans, ultrasonography, and conventional barium-contrast radiographic studies can be used to define tumor anatomy. Despite widespread metastases, the primary tumor can be small and difficult to demonstrate.

TREATMENT. In the presence of documented metastases, resection of a primary ileal carcinoid tumor is not indicated. It may become necessary because of intestinal obstruction or because of intussusception. Rarely, surgical removal of an isolated tumor (e.g., a bronchial or ovarian carcinoid) is curative. Devascularization of metastatic tumor by percutaneous arterial embolization has been reported to produce symptomatic relief in some patients. Resection of localized hepatic metastases and hepatic artery ligation have also been reported to ameliorate symptoms of the carcinoid syndrome temporarily.

Survival of less than 5 years after the onset of the carcinoid syndrome is the rule, but survival for more than 20 years is well documented. Thus, high-risk attempts at curative therapy are generally not indicated. Carcinoid tumors are not radiosensitive. Low-risk chemotherapy has not been very effective.

Symptomatic therapy includes nutritional support plus the provision of nicotinamide to prevent pellagra. Diarrhea has been treated with serotonin antagonists such as methysergide or cyproheptadine as well as with loperamide or even opiates. The drug parachlorophenylalanine, a tryptophan hydroxylase inhibitor, reduces diarrhea. However, allergic reactions and CNS side effects have occurred, and the drug remains experimental. No drug is consistently effective in preventing flushing; H_1 and H_2 histamine antagonists, including cimetidine, are often tried. Phenothiazines and the α-adrenergic antagonist phenoxybenzamine have also been used, as have glucocorticoids. Treatment with leukocyte interferon has been reported to decrease flushing and diarrhea in patients with the carcinoid syndrome. Long-term symptomatic therapy with a somatostatin analogue is promising.

Kvols LK: Metastatic carcinoid tumors and the carcinoid syndrome. Am J Med 81:49, 1986. *A review of chemotherapy and hormonal therapy.*

Norheim I, Theodorsson-Norheim E, Brodin E, et al.: Tachykinins in carcinoid tumors: Their use as a tumor marker and possible role in the carcinoid flush. J Clin Endocrinol Metab 63:605, 1986. *Plasma tachykinin levels often increase during induced flushing and decrease during effective therapy.*

Öberg K, Norheim I, Theodorsson E, et al.: The effects of octreotide on basal and stimulated hormone levels in patients with carcinoid syndrome. J Clin Endocrinol Metab 68:796, 1989. *The somatostatin analogue was shown to block tachykinin release.*

Roberts LJ II: Carcinoid syndrome and disorders of systemic mast-cell activation including systemic mastocytosis. Endocrinol Metab Clin North Am 17:415, 1988. *A more detailed discussion of the carcinoid syndrome.*

231 Ovarian Carcinoma

Howard W. Jones, III

Ovarian carcinoma is the most deadly of the gynecologic malignancies. The age-specific incidence gradually rises, reaching a peak at about age 70, at which time it is 55 per 100,000 among white women. The rate is somewhat lower among black women.

The etiology of ovarian cancer is unknown; except for some relatively rare familial groups, it has not been possible to identify any clinically useful high-risk groups for increased surveillance. Multiple pregnancies and the use of oral contraceptives may be protective because of decreased ovulation and hormonal influences.

Pathology

Four types of ovarian tumors require separate consideration because of their clinical characteristics and prognoses: (1) The common *epithelial tumors* of the ovary include the serous, mucinous, endometrioid, clear cell, and otherwise unspecified adenocarcinomas. These tumors account for almost 90 per cent of ovarian cancers and are most commonly found in postmenopausal women. (2) *Germ cell tumors*, which arise from the totipotent oocytes, are usually benign ("dermoid cysts"). They often occur in young women and are almost always unilateral. When malignant (e.g., dysgerminoma, teratoma), they are highly aggressive but respond very well to combination chemotherapy. (3) *Stromal tumors* are generally low grade, and since they arise from the granulosa, theca, and Sertoli-Leydig cells of the ovary, they may be hormonally functional. They are usually unilateral and may occur in any age group, but most typically in the fourth and fifth decades. Surgical excision alone may be all the therapy required, but combination chemotherapy is effective for metastatic or recurrent disease. (4) Malignancies of other sites that are metastatic to the ovary must always be considered in the evaluation of patients with a pelvic mass. In some cases a pelvic mass is the first indication of a primary gastrointestinal or endometrial carcinoma. Breast cancer also commonly metastasizes to the ovary.

DIAGNOSIS

Clinical Presentation

Early ovarian cancer is usually asymptomatic. Occasionally, ovarian enlargement is found on routine examination and cancer may be discovered incidentally at the time of abdominal or pelvic surgery for other indications. In most cases, however, widespread intra-abdominal metastases are present by the time the diagnosis is made. Symptoms of abdominal swelling, bloating, and pelvic fullness or pressure are common. It is not unusual for the patient to have had vague abdominal complaints or nonspecific gastrointestinal symptoms. Ascites or a palpable abdominopelvic mass may be found on examination. The presence of an irregular mass in the pelvis or cul-de-sac nodularity accompanied by ascites is often diagnostic. Some patients develop malignant pleural effusions and present with shortness of breath.

SCREENING TESTS. Screening tests for ovarian cancer are still controversial. Transvaginal ultrasonography, although quite effective for diagnosing ovarian cysts and tumors, is nonspecific and its use for screening results in surgical exploration of a large number of women with benign ovarian cysts. Even when a cancer is diagnosed by ultrasound screening in an asymptomatic patient, there is still no evidence that survival is improved. Serum levels of the tumor-associated antigen CA-125 above 35 μ per milliliter are highly correlated with serous or endometrioid ovarian cancer in postmenopausal women. Unfortunately, many ovarian tumors (e.g., mucinous, nonepithelial, and about 20 per cent of serous ovarian cancers) do not cause elevated levels of CA-125, while endometriosis, pelvic inflammatory disease, and some benign ovarian tumors may do so. The relative rarity of ovarian cancer, combined with the nonspecific nature of currently available tests, makes ovarian cancer screening unsatisfactory.

DIFFERENTIAL DIAGNOSIS. A pelvic mass can be caused by either a benign or a malignant tumor of the ovary as well as by inflammatory conditions, physiologic cysts, and malignancies of other pelvic organs and structures. Initially, a careful history and physical examination are most helpful in suggesting possible primary sites. Pelvic ultrasonography may allow the dimensions and character of the mass to be determined. Smooth-walled, unilocular ovarian cysts are almost always benign, whereas malignancies are most commonly described as echogenically "complex" with both cystic and solid components. The possibility of ectopic pregnancy must always be considered when a pelvic mass is present. A pregnancy test is, therefore, normally the first laboratory study done in women in the reproductive age group. A careful contraceptive history is important, since functional ovarian cysts, including both follicle cysts and corpus luteum cysts, are common in ovulating women. Inflammatory masses and endometriosis can be confused with ovarian cancer and can cause an elevated CA-125 in addition to a complex adnexal mass. In the older age group, diverticular abscesses and carcinoma of the colon must be considered within the differential diagnosis.

Once a complete history and physical have been done and the size and character of the mass have been confirmed by ultrasonography, several additional studies may be helpful. A barium enema or colonoscopy is almost always indicated prior to surgery to rule out a primary lesion or secondary involvement of the colon. An abdominal and pelvic computerized tomography scan identifies any ureteral obstruction or displacement that may be present and further characterizes the mass. This study may also provide additional information about upper abdominal disease, including aortic lymph node enlargement, omental or liver metastases, and the rare primary carcinoma of the pancreas that mimics ovarian cancer.

Additional studies (e.g., brain scans, bone scans) should generally be reserved for patients whose symptoms or physical findings suggest involvement of the areas to be studied.

TREATMENT

Surgery

In almost all cases of suspected ovarian carcinoma, an exploratory laparotomy is the ultimate diagnostic procedure. If the diagnosis is sustained, tumor debulking, including total abdominal hysterectomy and bilateral salpingo-oophorectomy, if possible, should be done. At this point a definitive diagnosis can be made

TABLE 231–1. DEFINITIONS OF THE STAGES IN PRIMARY CARCINOMA OF THE OVARY*

Stage I	Growth limited to the ovaries
Stage Ia	Growth limited to one ovary; no ascites. No tumor on the external surface; capsule intact.
Stage Ib	Growth limited to both ovaries; no ascites. No tumor on the external surfaces; capsules intact.
Stage Ic	Tumor either Stage Ia or Ib, but with tumor on surface of one or both ovaries; or with capsule ruptured; or with ascites present containing malignant cells or with positive peritoneal washings.
Stage II	Growth involving one or both ovaries with pelvic extension
Stage IIa	Extension and/or metastases to the uterus and/or tubes.
Stage IIb	Extension to other pelvic tissues.
Stage IIc	Tumor either Stage IIa or IIb, but with tumor on surface of one or both ovaries; or with capsule(s) ruptured; or with ascites present containing malignant cells or with positive peritoneal washings.
Stage III	Tumor involving one or both ovaries with peritoneal implants outside the pelvis and/or positive retroperitoneal or inguinal nodes. Superficial liver metastases equal Stage III. Tumor is limited to the true pelvis but with histologically proven malignant extension to small bowel or omentum.
Stage IIIa	Tumor grossly limited to the true pelvis with negative nodes but with histologically confirmed microscopic seeding of abdominal peritoneal surfaces.
Stage IIIb	Tumor involving one or both ovaries with histologically confirmed implants of abdominal peritoneal surfaces, none exceeding 2 cm in diameter. Nodes are negative.
Stage IIIc	Abdominal implants greater than 2 cm in diameter and/or positive retroperitoneal or inguinal nodes.
Stage IV	Growth involving one or both ovaries with distant metastases. If pleural effusion is present, there must be positive cytology to allot a case to Stage IV. Parenchymal liver metastasis equals Stage IV.

*Nomenclature of the International Federation of Gynecology and Obstetrics (FIGO). Staging is based on findings at clinical examination and surgical exploration.

and the extent of the disease accurately staged. Aggressive tumor debulking, even when all cancer cannot be removed, improves the length and quality of survival. If possible, this initial surgery should be done by a gynecologic oncologist whose special training and experience should provide the optimal surgical and postoperative management.

The goal of the initial operation for ovarian cancer is twofold. First, all tumor should be removed if possible to provide the greatest possibility of cure. In approximately two thirds of patients, however, widespread intra-abdominal metastases prevent complete surgical debulking. The second goal of surgery is accurate staging (Table 231–1). In addition to the stage of disease, the volume of residual tumor following initial surgery, the histologic type and grade of the tumor, and the age of the patient have important prognostic significance. Women with minimal residual disease and well-differentiated tumors have the most favorable outcome. Those under age 50 and those with tumors exhibiting mucinous and endometrioid histology also seem to do better.

Careful staging evaluation with peritoneal cytology and multiple biopsies of the upper abdomen (the omentum, diaphragm, and retroperitoneal nodes) is especially important in early stage disease, since microscopic metastases often escape clinical detection. Accurate staging guides the most appropriate postoperative management. Patients with Stage Ia well-differentiated epithelial ovarian cancers do not need additional therapy (Table 231–1).

In patients with advanced disease, aggressive surgical debulking includes bowel resection or colostomy in as many as 25 per cent of patients. Whether such extensive surgical resection actually improves 5- and 10-year survival rates is still controversial. It is agreed, however, that optimal tumor debulking (<1 cm residual) results in prolongation of good-quality survival. This is where the skills and experienced judgment of the gynecologic oncologist are most important.

Chemotherapy

Most patients with ovarian cancer require postoperative chemotherapy. Cisplatin, the cornerstone of most regimens, is usually given in combination with other agents, such as cyclophosphamide, doxorubicin, hexamethylmelamine, or etoposide. Carboplatin, which has fewer renal and neurologic side effects, and ifosfamide are now under investigation. Most patients are treated with intermittent intravenous therapy at 4-week intervals for six monthly cycles, but some centers use intraperitoneal chemotherapy instead. Response rates of 60 to 80 per cent are generally seen, but only about 30 per cent of the treatment group experiences a complete response. Some debilitated patients are still treated with a single alkylating agent, such as oral melphalan, but this therapy is probably not as effective as cisplatin alone or in combination with other cytotoxic drugs. Carboplatin is almost as well tolerated as oral melphalan.

Radiation Therapy

Postoperative external radiation therapy to the whole abdomen is probably as effective as chemotherapy for patients with minimal residual tumor. The toxicity of such therapy, especially that of gastrointestinal obstruction, has usually been greater than that associated with chemotherapy.

Intraperitoneal radioactive colloidal chromic phosphate is also used to treat some women with Stage I or II disease with no gross residual tumor. Only patients with very early disease are good candidates for this therapy, which requires a complete and uniform intraperitoneal distribution of the radioactive suspension.

"Second-look" Surgery

A planned re-exploration in order to evaluate the extent of disease following a course of therapy and to resect any residual malignancy has been called "second-look" surgery. This approach allows an excellent research evaluation of the effect of the primary therapy, but it has not proven to be of significant clinical benefit to patients with ovarian cancer. Measurements of tumor-associated antigens, such as CA-125, used in conjunction with periodic physical examinations and selected radiographic studies, have been helpful in monitoring the disease status of treated patients. Until more effective salvage therapy is available, second-look

TABLE 231–2. CARCINOMA OF THE OVARY: DISTRIBUTION BY STAGE AND 3- AND 5-YEAR SURVIVAL IN THE DIFFERENT STAGES*

| Stage | Patients Treated | | 3-Year Survival (%) | 5-Year Survival (%) |
	Number	(%)		
I	2230	26.1	79.8	72.8
II	1313	15.4	60.5	46.3
III	3339	39.1	27.1	18.6
IV	1391	16.3	10.1	4.8
Unstaged	268	3.1	31.7	21.6
TOTAL	8541	100.0	43.4	34.9

*Data from Carcinoma of the ovary. *In* Pettersson F (ed.): Annual Report on the Results of Treatment in Gynecological Cancer, Vol. 20. Stockholm, Panorama Press AB, 1988. The "Annual Report" is published at regular intervals by the International Federation for Gynecology and Obstetrics and contains vast quantities of statistics generated from institutions which submit their treatment results from throughout the world.

surgery in the asymptomatic patient with a normal physical examination is probably not indicated.

Treatment of Recurrent, Metastatic Disease

The overall survival of patients treated for ovarian cancer is only 30 to 40 per cent; many women develop progressive disease despite appropriate primary therapy. Salvage chemotherapy protocols for recurrent disease lead to only a 10 per cent response rate, which is usually partial and short term. Widespread intra-abdominal metastases with bowel obstruction are frequent, but reoperation with resection, bypass, or enterostomy may provide significant palliation. Pleural effusion may require thoracentesis and pleural sclerosis. With the relative effectiveness of current primary chemotherapy, patients may survive to develop late metastases to the liver, brain, and meninges. Localized radiation has been helpful in some of these patients.

PROGNOSIS

The long-term survival rate of patients treated for epithelial ovarian cancer is still disappointing (Table 231–2). Almost 60 per cent of patients have Stage III or IV disease at the time of diagnosis. Although the majority of women with advanced disease live 2 years with a reasonable quality of life, recurrent cancer eventually becomes symptomatic in most, and by 5 years only about 15 per cent still survive. The results are much better for patients diagnosed at an earlier stage. Almost three fourths of women with Stage I ovarian cancer survive 5 years.

Heintz APM, Hacker NF, Lagasse LD: Epidemiology and etiology of ovarian cancer: A review. Obstet Gynecol 66:127, 1985. *This is an excellent review of the many different factors that might be related to the etiology of ovarian cancer. The authors emphasize the significance of family history.*

Jacobs I, Stabile I, Bridges J, et al.: Multimodal approach to screening for ovarian cancer. Lancet 1:268, 1988. *This study describes the use of pelvic examination, CA-125, and ultrasonography to screen patients for ovarian cancer. There is an excellent discussion with good references.*

Sutton GP, Stehman FB, Einhorn LH, et al.: Ten-year follow-up of patients receiving cisplatin, doxorubicin, and cyclophosphamide chemotherapy for advanced epithelial ovarian carcinoma. J Clin Oncol 7:223, 1989. *This is an excellent review of long-term follow-up of patients treated with platinum-based combination chemotherapy. This group has one of the world's largest experiences, and the discussion and references are superb.*

Williams L, Hoskins WJ: Can cytoreductive surgery aid ovarian cancer survival? Contemp Gynecol Obstet 35:13, 1990. *This recent review examines the role of initial cytoreductive surgery as well as second-look operation for ovarian cancer. An excellent review of the literature.*

Williams SD, Blessing JA, Moore DH, et al.: Cisplatin, vinblastine, and bleomycin in advanced and recurrent ovarian germ-cell tumors. Ann Intern Med 3:22, 1989. *This is a report of a gynecologic oncology group study using new chemotherapy approaches for germ cell tumors of the ovary. The results with platinum-based combination therapy are excellent.*

PART XVII
DISEASES OF BONE AND BONE MINERAL METABOLISM

232 Mineral and Bone Homeostasis

Stephen J. Marx

Calcium, phosphorus, and magnesium, three of the principal body elements, have diverse roles. The calcium ion is particularly versatile. In the crystalline phase, it contributes to the varied structural roles of bone. In a supersaturated solution in blood, it contributes to plasma membrane excitability, plasma enzyme activities, and accretion of all minerals in extracellular matrix of bone. In the cytoplasmic fluid, its extraordinarily low concentrations allow rapid rises of its local concentrations to transmit information among cell compartments via its interactions with high-affinity calcium-binding proteins, such as calmodulin or protein kinase C. Phosphate is the principal intracellular anion, with central roles in cytoplasm as a buffer, energy carrier (mainly via the high-energy phosphate bonds of adenosine triphosphate [ATP]), and molecular switch (through phosphorylation and dephosphorylation). Magnesium is the principal cation in cytoplasm, functioning as a cofactor in many chemical reactions (for example, as an Mg-ATP complex or as a cofactor in many steps of DNA or RNA metabolism).

MINERALS IN BLOOD

The State of Calcium, Phosphate, and Magnesium in Blood

Total calcium concentration is tightly regulated, so that typical diurnal fluctuations are not more than 5 per cent from the mean value. Calcium in blood is divided among protein-bound, complexed, and ionized or free fractions (Table 232–1). Protein binding of calcium in blood is principally to albumin, and this binding is decreased by acid pH. The ionized calcium fraction is the focus for metabolic control by the parathyroid gland, and measurements of ionized calcium in blood give the most valid index of pathologic disruptions of calcium homeostasis.

Phosphate and magnesium in blood are principally unbound (Table 232–1), and the concentration of each is regulated over a broader relative variation from its mean than that for calcium. Neither phosphate nor magnesium has a unique endocrine system dedicated to its control. Rather, their blood concentrations are

sustained indirectly by the hormones directed at calcium control and directly by poorly understood local processes in bone, kidney, and other organs.

Steady-State Flow of Minerals to and from Blood

Only 0.1 per cent of the total body calcium is in blood and extracellular fluid (Table 232–2). This calcium pool is in a rapidly exchanging equilibrium with large calcium pools controlled by three organs (bone, intestine, and kidney), each of which is an important site for the regulation of mineral metabolism. The rate of these daily fluxes (Fig. 232–1) is sufficiently large that disturbance of mineral flux to or from any of these organs can result in abnormally high or low concentrations of one of these minerals in blood.

ORGANS EXCHANGING MUCH MINERAL WITH BLOOD

Bone

BONE FUNCTION AND ARCHITECTURE. Major functions of bone include support, locomotion, encasement of hematopoietic tissue, and reservoir for calcium, phosphate, and magnesium. The architecture of bone responds dynamically to changes in mechanical load. The mechanisms whereby the signals from altered load are transduced are poorly understood. Mature bone adopts one of two macroscopic organizations (Fig. 232–2). The cortices of all bones and the interior of certain bones have a continuous structure termed cortical or lamellar bone. Lamellar bone, which is predominant in the long bones, is characterized by little metabolic activity and few cells. It has a highly organized extracellular matrix of mineral and parallel bundles of type I collagen. During embryonic development or in states with pathologic increase of bone turnover, bone assumes a less organized "woven" architecture. Within the vertebral bodies and in portions of the interior of other bones, bone is organized as a series of thin, interdigitating plates; this is termed trabecular, cancellous, or spongy bone. Its ratio of surface to volume is higher than that found in cortical bone and is thus better suited to rapid turnover.

EXTRACELLULAR MATRIX. Newly deposited osteoid must undergo a poorly understood maturation process for 1 to 3 weeks until it becomes competent for mineral accumulation. The mineral phase of bone extracellular matrix is a mixture of multiple amorphous and crystalline states, the latter principally as hydroxyapatite crystals $(Ca_{10}(PO_4)_6OH_2)$. Ninety to 95 per cent of osteoid, the organic component of the extracellular matrix, is

TABLE 232–1. CONCENTRATIONS AND STATES OF CALCIUM, MAGNESIUM, AND PHOSPHATE IN NORMAL HUMAN PLASMA OR SERUM*

State	Calcium (mM)	Magnesium (mM)	Phosphate (mM)
Protein bound	1.15 (47)	0.26 (31)	0.15 (13)
Filterable or free†			
Complexed	0.25 (10)	0.06 (7)	0.40 (35)
Ionized	1.06 (43)	0.52 (62)	0.60 (52)

*Number in parentheses indicates percentage of total for that mineral.
†Filterable or free = complexed + ionized.

TABLE 232–2. DISTRIBUTION OF CALCIUM, MAGNESIUM, AND PHOSPHATE IN THE BODY OF A 70-KG ADULT*

Compartment	Calcium (g)	Magnesium (g)	Phosphate (g)
Bones and teeth	1300 (99)	14.0 (54)	600.0 (86)
Extracellular fluid	1 (0.1)	0.3 (1)	0.2 (0.03)
Cells	7 (1.0)	12.0 (46)	100.0 (14)

*Most of calcium is in bone; almost half of magnesium is in cells. Phosphate, as the principal counterion to calcium and magnesium in their dominant pools, has an intermediate proportional distribution. Number in parentheses is the percentage of total for that mineral.

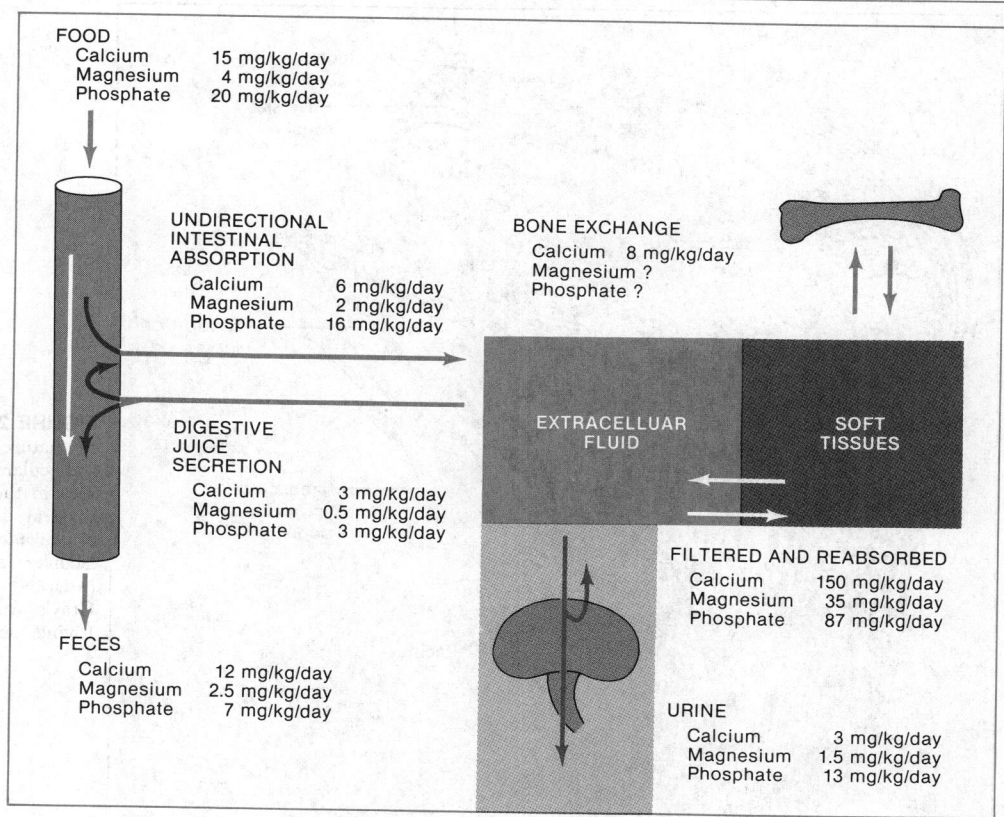

FIGURE 232–1. Typical mineral fluxes in adults. (Modified from Aurbach GD, Marx SJ, Spiegel AM: Parathyroid hormone, calcitonin, and the calciferols. *In* Wilson JD, Foster DW [eds.]: Williams Textbook of Endocrinology. 7th ed. Philadelphia, W.B. Saunders Company, 1985, p 1144.)

composed of bundles of type I collagen, a long triple helix of two alpha₁ (type I) chains and one alpha₂ (type I) chain. The principal collagen of cartilage matrix is type II as a homotrimer of three alpha₁ (type II) chains. Fibrils of collagen play a major role in the strength of bone (type I collagen), cartilage (type II collagen), and elastic tissues (type III collagen). Their disruption results in characteristic disturbances (osteogenesis imperfecta [type I collagen], chondrodysplasia [type II collagen], Ehlers-Danlos syndrome or arterial aneurysms [type III collagen], and even certain variants of familial osteoarthritis [type II collagen]). The second most prominent protein in bone matrix is osteocalcin (or bone gla-protein); it has a molar content of three residues of gamma-carboxyglutamic acid, an unusual amino acid that confers to the molecule high affinity for calcium on bone crystals. The roles of osteocalcin are unknown, but its concentration in blood is a potential index of osteoblast activity. Several other proteins, phosphoproteins, glycoproteins, and so on, in bone matrix have been identified in the search for molecules regulating bone mineral accumulation and bone growth.

BONE CELLS. Several cells are highly characteristic of bone. A flat bone-lining cell (perhaps derived from marrow stroma) with few organelles covers many bone surfaces thought not to be undergoing modification. This cell is perhaps one precursor of the osteoblast. The osteoblast is a cuboidal bone matrix–synthesizing cell. It lines any periosteal, endosteal, or trabecular surface at which bone formation takes place. Its plasma membrane is highly enriched with a bone-specific isoform of the alkaline phosphatase enzyme. This enzyme is believed to promote bone mineralization by catalyzing in supersaturated extracellular fluid of bone the hydrolysis of pyrophosphate and other inhibitors of calcium-phosphate crystallization. The osteocyte is the principal stable cell inside mature bone. It is probably derived from an osteoblast that has encased itself in bone. Osteocytes are interconnected with one another via long processes that traverse bone canaliculi. The role of the osteocyte is unknown, but it is appropriately located to modulate mineral fluxes. The chondrocyte is the dominant cell of cartilage; it releases to the extracellular matrix vesicles that are rich in alkaline phosphatase and that may be a central organelle for calcium accumulation in preparation

for cartilage mineralization. The osteoclast is the main bone-resorbing cell. It is derived from precursors of the premonocyte lineage. It is a highly motile, multinucleated giant cell, with several specialized features for bone. These include organelles that mediate cell attachment to bone surface (podosomes), a strikingly redundant ruffled border at the bone face for ion transport, many enzymes that can function in bone resorption, and a high concentration of carbonic anhydrase II, which participates in acidification of the extracellular pocket between the osteoclast ruffled border and the skeletal resorption surface.

LOCAL REGULATORS OF BONE CELLS. Bone cells are under systemic and local regulation. Known systemic regulators include parathyroid hormone, calcitonin, and calcitriol, which are considered later in this chapter. There is also a highly complex network of local controls. The term "osteoclast-activating factors" was applied in the 1980's to components in incompletely characterized fluids that could activate bone resorption in vitro. Some of their active components have been identified. For example, interleukin 1 and lymphotoxin/tumor necrosis factor–beta are potential stimulators of bone resorption that seem to be released locally by some tumors in bone. They cannot act directly on mature osteoclasts but can act, rather, through nearby cells, such as osteoblasts or marrow stromal cells, that communicate with osteoclasts. Like the activators of bone resorption, the activators of bone formation are poorly understood, particularly since this process involves a complex interplay of osteoblast proliferation and differentiation. Some contributors to this process include type 1 insulin-like growth factor and transforming growth factor–beta; the latter is present selectively and at high concentrations in osteoblasts and osteocytes. In addition, several newly identified proteins (osteogenesis-inducing factor, bone morphogenetic proteins [some of which are homologues of the beta-type transforming growth factor], and so forth) can induce bone formation in soft tissue sites. Prostaglandins can stimulate bone formation or bone resorption, and they may be important mediators in inflammatory processes of the skeletal system.

BONE REMODELING. Bone growth or modeling occurs initially within a membrane or along the edge of cartilage (e.g., periosteum or epiphyseal growth plate). Though it contains few

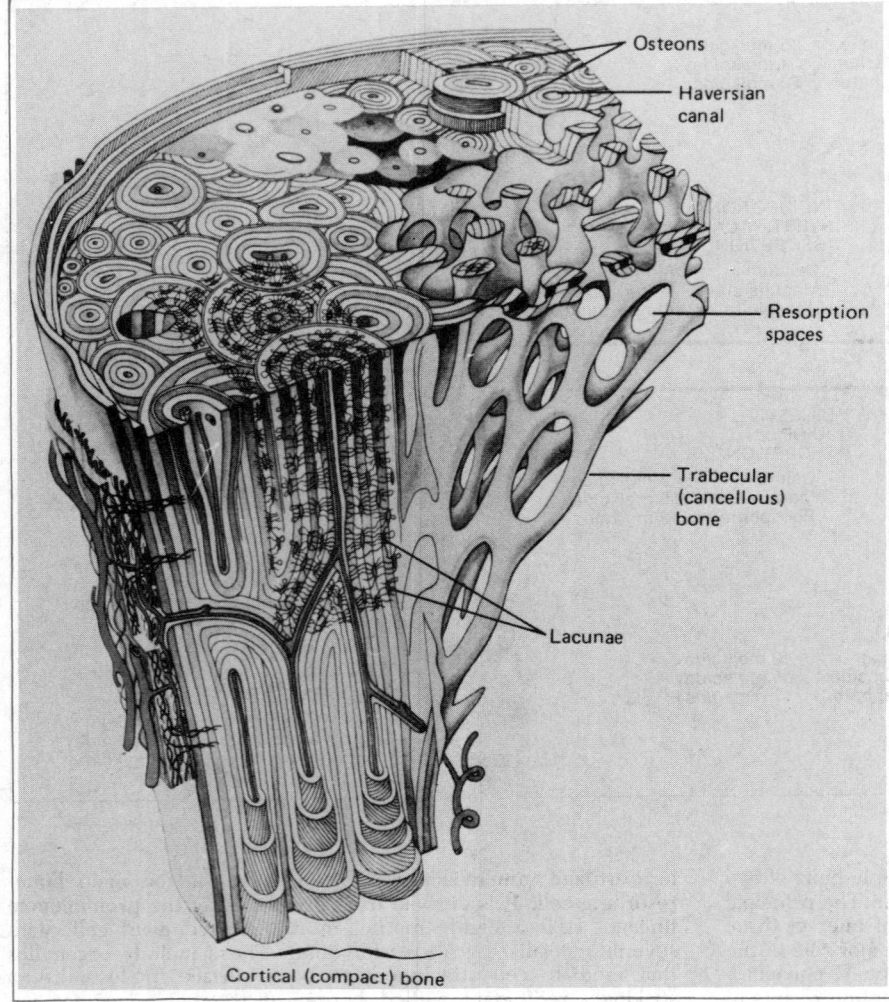

FIGURE 232–2. Bone organization. Microstructure of mature bone; areas of cortical (lamellar) and trabecular (cancellous) bone are shown. The central area in the transverse section shows differences in mineral density as degrees of shading. Note the organization of osteons, the distribution of osteocyte lacunae, and the organization of bone lamellae. (Adapted from Warwick R, Williams PL [eds.]: Gray's Anatomy. 35th ed. Edinburgh, Churchill Livingstone, 1973, p 217.)

cells, cortical bone is constantly going through slow and orderly cycles of localized resorption and then rebuilding. This process is mediated by the local remodeling unit (alternately termed osteon or basic multicellular unit). Remodeling begins with excavation of a cavity by osteoclasts; as the resorption front advances, osteoclasts are replaced by other cells. Over an interval of several months, new bone is deposited in cylindrical lamellae about the rim of the cavity until it is refilled to complete this cycle. This cycle is an important example of the normal, coordinated relation between the bone resorption and bone formation processes. Most perturbations that modify one component of these two processes also modify the other in the same direction. The determinants of this coupling between bone resorption and formation are not known, but they probably include a host of growth factors present at high local concentrations in bone extracellular matrix and exposed or released by the skeletal resorption process.

Intestines

MINERAL ABSORPTION. The intestinal absorption of magnesium and phosphate is not subject to fine regulation and has not been studied intensively. By contrast, intestinal absorption of calcium is tightly regulated, and its quantitation has been analyzed in detail. Most calcium absorption is accomplished in the small bowel. Over a wide range of intakes, approximately one tenth of dietary calcium is absorbed passively; the remainder of net intestinal absorption of calcium is regulated by active vitamin D metabolites, especially $1\alpha,25(OH)_2D$, in blood. With a normal diet, approximately 30 per cent of calcium is absorbed. With low dietary calcium, the secondarily high blood $1\alpha,25(OH)_2D$ level can drive fractional calcium absorption to approach 90 per cent.

Kidney

ION FILTRATION AND REABSORPTION. The non–protein-bound fractions of calcium, magnesium, and phosphate from plasma cross the glomerulus. The distal portions of the nephron have efficient and selective systems capable of completing the reabsorption from tubular fluid of more than 99 per cent of any one of these minerals. Tubular calcium reabsorption is stimulated principally by parathyroid hormone (PTH); thiazides or lithium can also increase tubular calcium reabsorption. Saline loading with or without loop diuretics can inhibit this. Tubular phosphate reabsorption is mainly under negative influence by PTH. The determinants of tubular reabsorption of magnesium are incompletely understood.

Integrated Fluxes: Mineral Balance and Nutrition

Skeletal growth is maximal throughout childhood, nearing completion during adolescence. Until this time, the rate of skeletal calcium accretion is typically 200 to 400 mg (5 to 10 mmole) per day. Fetal mineralization during the last trimester or milk secretion during lactation imposes similar daily increments on calcium efflux from maternal blood. The skeleton remains in a state of approximate zero mineral balance between ages 20 and 35, after which it slowly loses mass. This loss is greatest in the trabecular bone of the vertebrae, attaining peak rates about the menopause (3 to 10 per cent per year during the first 1 to 4 years after surgically induced menopause).

Normal adults can sustain zero calcium balance with daily

TABLE 232–3. EFFECTS OF PRINCIPAL CALCIOTROPIC HORMONES

Hormone	Principal Target Tissues	Action
Parathyroid hormone	Renal proximal convoluted tubule	Increase serum 1,25(OH)$_2$D
	Renal distal convoluted tubule	Increase calcium reabsorption
	Renal proximal and distal convoluted tubules	Decrease phosphate reabsorption
	Bone	Increase calcium and phosphate resorption
Calcitonin	Bone	Decrease calcium and phosphate resorption
1,25(OH)$_2$D	Small bowel	Increase calcium absorption
	Bone	Increase calcium and phosphate resorption
	Parathyroid gland	Decrease release of PTH

calcium intakes between 400 and 1500 mg (10 to 37.5 mmole), mainly as dairy products. Typical daily calcium intakes in the United States are 500 to 800 mg (12.5 to 20 mmole), and there is uncertainty over the minimal level for optimal skeletal health. With a typical daily calcium intake of 700 mg (17.5 mmole), one fourth, or 175 mg (43.7 mmole), is absorbed; during skeletal balance, this amount must equal the amount lost in urinary excretion (disregarding the small amount of calcium lost from skin).

Because of the large mineral fluxes between blood and three principal pools (bone, renal tubular lumen, and intestinal lumen), it is often difficult to assign mild disruptions to one pool. For example, there is uncertainty whether the slow bone losses with idiopathic age-associated osteoporosis reflect primary disturbances of calcium flux in bone, the intestine, or combinations of these.

HORMONAL REGULATORS OF MINERAL HOMEOSTASIS

Parathyroid Hormone

SYNTHESIS, SECRETION, AND METABOLISM. Parathyroid hormone is a rapidly regulated hormone that sustains calcium and 1,25(OH)$_2$D in blood and depresses phosphate in blood (Table 232–3). Parathyroid hormone is stored in the parathyroid cell mainly as a peptide of 84 amino acids. The parathyroid cell secretes PTH as the native molecule or as fragments, only some of which are biologically active. Fragments of PTH are also generated from its metabolism after secretion into blood. The amino-terminus of PTH (residues 1 to 34) contains the requirements for receptor binding and biologic activity. Biologically active forms of PTH are cleared rapidly from blood, perhaps by their receptors, while inactive fragments are cleared more slowly, rendering them likely to be measured in immunoassays not specially designed to measure the intact molecule.

BLOOD CALCIUM EFFECT ON THE PARATHYROID GLAND. The parathyroid gland, as the coordinator of blood levels of PTH and 1,25(OH)$_2$D, is exquisitely sensitive to changes of ionized calcium in extracellular fluid. The parathyroid cell responds to calcium in at least three different ways. First, low calcium concentration is a direct stimulus for the gradual increase in size and numbers of parathyroid cells (secondary hypertrophy and hyperplasia). Second, low calcium stimulates the biosynthesis of PTH over 1 to 2 days. Third, depression of the calcium level stimulates within seconds the secretion of preformed PTH. The parathyroid cell differs strikingly from most other hormone secretory cells, which exhibit accelerated secretion in response to increases of extracellular calcium.

PARATHYROID HORMONE MECHANISMS OF ACTION. Parathyroid hormone binds to a plasma membrane receptor; the PTH receptor then causes a rise of cyclic 3′,5′-adenosine monophosphate (cAMP) and perhaps other second messengers in the cytoplasm of its target cells. The consequence is rapid effects of PTH on the target cells in bone and kidney. A different peptide, termed "parathyroid hormone–related peptide," with homology to PTH at the amino-terminus, is secreted by many cancers, causing hypercalcemia through its interactions with PTH receptors.

PARATHYROID HORMONE ACTION IN BONE. Parathyroid hormone in bone stimulates osteoblasts and osteoclasts. The effects on osteoclasts are indirect, since these cells lack receptors for PTH. Very high PTH levels result in clear excess of bone

resorption over bone formation. Controversy exists over whether mild PTH excess might have a net anabolic effect selectively in trabecular bone.

PARATHYROID HORMONE ACTION IN KIDNEY. Parathyroid hormone acts in the kidney to stimulate the synthesis of 1,25(OH)$_2$D by increasing the activity of 25OHD$_3$ 1α-hydroxylase in the proximal tubules. Parathyroid hormone acts in the distal portions of the nephron to increase tubular reabsorption of calcium. In addition, PTH inhibits phosphate reabsorption in the distal, and perhaps also the proximal, tubules. Parathyroid hormone also inhibits bicarbonate reabsorption.

PARATHYROID HORMONE ACTION ON INTESTINE. Parathyroid hormone has no important direct action on the intestine. However, the direct renal effect of PTH to increase serum 1,25(OH)$_2$D causes highly important secondary effects in the intestine (see Intestinal Actions of Calcitriol, further on).

Calcitonin

CALCITONIN SYNTHESIS AND SECRETION. Calcitonin is a peptide of 32 amino acids that is normally synthesized and secreted by the parafollicular or C cells, which are neuroectodermal cells within the thyroid gland. Its secretion is stimulated by calcium and also by certain intestinal peptides (gastrin and glucagon) (see Ch. 236).

CALCITONIN ACTIONS. Calcitonin, at high concentrations, can directly inhibit osteoclast function. Calcitonin also can act in the kidney to cause mild natriuresis. These calcitonin actions have not been shown to be important in normal physiology. For the present, the principal interests in calcitonin are as a tumor marker, particularly for familial C cell neoplasia, or as a pharmacologic agent to treat bone disorders, such as Paget's disease.

Vitamin D and Its Metabolites

SYNTHESIS OF VITAMIN D. Vitamin D$_3$ is a seco-steroid (i.e., a steroid with one ring opened) synthesized from 7-dehydrocholesterol in the skin (Fig. 232–3), in a reaction catalyzed by ultraviolet light derived from the sun. Vitamin D$_2$, produced synthetically from the plant sterol ergosterol, is a vitamin D$_3$ analogue used as a dietary supplement or drug. The metabolism of vitamin D$_3$ and vitamin D$_2$ is similar in humans (see Ch. 233).

HYDROXYLATIONS OF VITAMIN D METABOLITES. Vitamin D ("D" refers to combinations of the D$_3$ and D$_2$ isoforms) is converted to 25OHD in hepatocytes. This reaction is not under metabolic control and is determined principally by the serum levels of its substrate, vitamin D. 25OHD is normally converted to 1,25(OH)$_2$D only in the renal proximal tubule by an enzyme system stimulated by PTH. A similar PTH-independent 1α-hydroxylation occurs in the normal placenta and abnormally in granuloma tissues, as in sarcoidosis. 25OHD and 1,25(OH)$_2$D can also be hydroxylated at other residues (C-23, C-24, C-26), but these and other conversions probably serve mainly to inactivate vitamin D metabolites.

ABSORPTION AND TRANSPORT OF VITAMIN D METABOLITES. Vitamin D metabolites enter the bloodstream like other sterols, and a small fraction of all vitamin D metabolites undergo an enterohepatic recirculation. When cutaneous synthesis of vitamin D is marginal, any cause of intestinal malabsorption can result in vitamin D deficiency. Vitamin D metabolites are lipid soluble; they circulate in plasma bound to a specific 25OHD binding protein and, to a lesser degree, to other carriers.

MECHANISM OF ACTIONS OF VITAMIN D METABOLITES. Vitamin D is an inactive precursor; 25OHD and

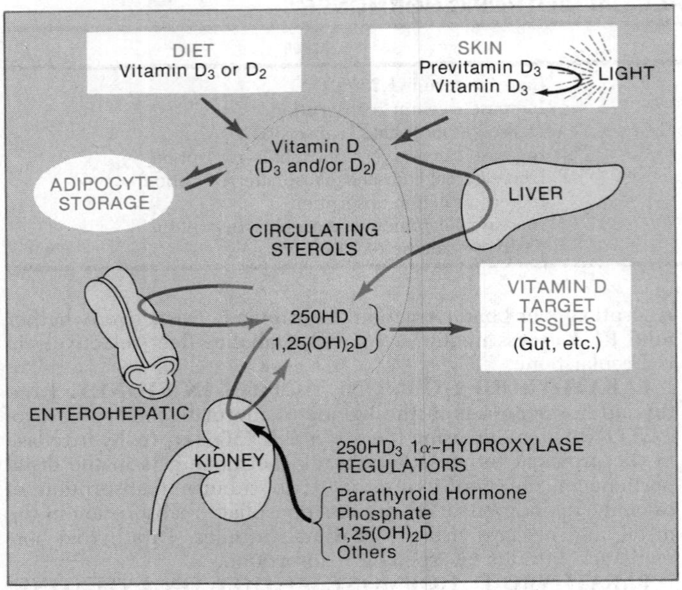

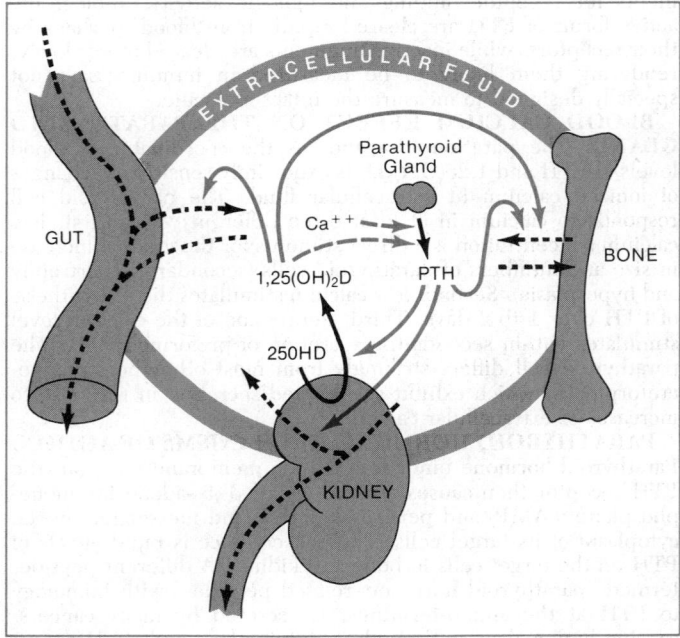

FIGURE 232–3. The vitamin D activation pathway. This involves steps in many different organs. Dysfunction at any step can have clinically important consequences.

1,25(OH)₂D are both active. Though the concentration of 25OHD is about 1000-fold higher than that of 1,25(OH)₂D in blood, the latter has far higher affinity for the vitamin D receptor and normally determines the degree of vitamin D receptor activation. Calcitriol binds to intracellular receptors in target cells and causes gradual changes in the nuclei of those cells. The vitamin D receptor is highly homologous to the receptors for other steroids and to those for thyroid hormone and retinoic acid. Though vitamin D receptors are present in many organs, only those in duodenal mucosa have been established as important in normal physiology.

INTESTINAL ACTIONS OF CALCITRIOL. Calcitriol (1,25(OH)₂D) increases the flux of calcium from the intestinal lumen to blood. Calcitriol, to a much lesser extent, increases the flux of phosphate and magnesium from intestinal lumen to blood. Calcium, magnesium, and phosphate ions have specific processes for their intestinal transport. Calcitriol induces in duodenal mucosa high concentrations of an intracellular calcium-binding protein, termed calbindin. Calbindin belongs to the calmodulin protein family, but its role, if any, in intestinal calcium transport is unknown.

SKELETAL EFFECTS OF CALCITRIOL. The principal effects of calcitriol on bone (antirachitic effects) are indirect results of its action to promote calcium influx from intestinal lumen to blood. The deficient mineralization in vitamin D deficiency states is the consequence of the combination of low calcium in blood and low phosphate in blood, the latter resulting from the renal phosphate-wasting effects from secondary hyperparathyroidism.

The supraphysiologic concentrations of vitamin D metabolites sometimes reached during pharmacotherapy can raise blood calcium in part by increasing osteoclast numbers and activity.

OTHER EFFECTS OF CALCITRIOL. Calcitriol can inhibit PTH biosynthesis and secretion; the direct negative effects of calcitriol might contribute a form of short-loop negative feedback to parathyroid function. Calcitriol exerts direct effects on the renal enzymes that hydroxylate 25OHD; calcitriol inhibits the 25OHD₃ 1α-hydroxylase and stimulates the other hydroxylases that catabolize 25OHD in the renal tubule and in other tissues. Possibly important effects of calcitriol in skin and hair are suggested by its protective effect on psoriatic skin at pharmacologic doses and by the striking association of total alopecia with the rare syndrome of severely defective vitamin D receptors. Vitamin D receptors are present in many additional organs, but no role for them has been identified in normal physiology.

Other Hormones

SEX STEROIDS. Sex steroids, particularly estrogens, have slow but extremely important anabolic effects on bone. The effects are exerted directly on the bone organ, perhaps through receptors in the osteoblast. Estrogen deficiency results in accelerated bone remodeling with disproportionate bone resorption, particularly in trabecular bone.

GLUCOCORTICOIDS. Glucocorticoids affect many of the cells that contribute to mineral metabolism. The most striking effect is bone thinning that results from high glucocorticoid concentrations. This thinning is probably a consequence mainly of inhibition of osteoblasts. In addition, glucocorticoids antagonize the actions of vitamin D metabolites by unknown mechanisms.

THYROID HORMONE. Thyroid hormones also have direct effects on bone cells. Excess of thyroid hormones causes increased release of calcium from bone. The skeletal consequences of deficient thyroid hormone are most evident in the disordered growth of cartilaginous epiphyses associated with congenital hypothyroidism.

GROWTH HORMONE. Growth hormone stimulates the growth of bone and cartilage, in part by stimulating local production of type 1 insulin-like growth factor by osteoblasts and chondrocytes.

ADAPTATIONS TO DISRUPTIONS OF MINERAL METABOLISM

Two principal calciotropic hormones, PTH and 1,25(OH)₂D, interact with each other and with multiple target tissues to control the metabolism of calcium, phosphate, and, to a lesser degree, magnesium (Fig. 232–4 and Table 232–3). These hormones allow for adaptations over time intervals that are short (minutes) or long (months).

Blood levels of ionized calcium are sustained at nearly invariant levels, with minimal diurnal changes reflecting mainly the sudden rises of calcium influx with meals. Serum levels of PTH and 1,25(OH)₂D also show only modest diurnal changes under normal conditions. Serum phosphate typically has broad diurnal fluctuations, with a nadir around 9:00 AM and peaks at around 6:00 PM and 4:00 AM.

Calcium Excess States

States with long-term excess or deficiency of calcium are associated with deviations at multiple steps of the integrated

FIGURE 232–4. Integrated control of secretion and actions of parathyroid hormone (PTH) and calcitriol (1,25(OH)₂ vitamin D = 1,25(OH)₂D) with emphasis on calcium fluxes. Solid black lines show secretion of PTH and calcitriol. Interrupted black lines are calcium fluxes. Solid red lines show stimulatory effects; interrupted red lines show inhibitory effects.

mineral homeostasis system. The most common calcium excess state in adults is primary overfunction of the parathyroid gland. Of course, this has the potential to distort most of the normal calcium regulatory processes. Primary hyperparathyroidism results in high blood levels of PTH and often of 1,25(OH)$_2$D as well. The results are combinations of increased calcium influx to blood dependent upon the evoked dysfunctions in intestinal, skeletal, and renal pools of calcium. A very different integrated metabolic pattern results when calcium excess is caused by dysfunction outside the parathyroid—for example, with osteolytic metastases, skeletal immobilization, or dietary calcium overload (milk-alkali syndrome). In the latter disturbances, the parathyroid gland reacts appropriately and becomes suppressed by the increase of ionized calcium in blood; blood concentrations of PTH and 1,25(OH)$_2$D become low. The abnormally high filtered load of calcium without the anticalciuric effects of PTH results in severe hypercalciuria; irreversible renal damage can occur over a period of only a few weeks.

Calcium Deficiency States

Calcium deficiency states generally result in the parathyroid gland's recognizing the signal of a low ionized calcium level in blood. Increased PTH secretion (within seconds), increased PTH biosynthesis (within days), or parathyroid cell hyperplasia (within weeks) activates the response pathway. The consequences of this secondary hyperparathyroidism are increased renal tubular secretion of 1,25(OH)$_2$D (if there is not underlying deficiency of 25OHD or 1α-hydroxylase) and increased net calcium flux into blood from the intestinal lumen, from bone, and from the renal tubular lumen. The relative contribution of each calcium pool to this integrated response depends in part on the chronic state of that pool and on the relative levels of PTH and calcitriol. Serum calcium typically begins to fall below normal only when the osteolytic response to PTH or 1,25(OH)$_2$D becomes weakened (from depletion of readily exchangeable calcium pools or other types of tachyphylaxis). Secondary hyperparathyroidism has important effects on phosphate homeostasis through direct effects on bone and kidney, increasing phosphate influx from bone and causing a similar increase in phosphate efflux into urine. With forms of hypoparathyroidism, some residual components of mineral homeostasis can be sustained in the face of deficiency of PTH and secondarily of 1,25(OH)$_2$D.

Metabolic Bone Diseases

Certain forms of metabolic bone disease are associated with dramatic imbalances in mineral flux to or from blood; these include increased calcium influx with aggressive osteolytic processes and decreased calcium influx with many forms of osteomalacia. Others, because they do not dramatically compromise the readily exchangeable pools of bone mineral, may have little or no long-term impact on the blood homeostatic system. For example, idiopathic osteoporosis has been categorized into two major forms (perimenopausal and aging associated), but no clearcut changes in blood PTH or 1,25(OH)$_2$D as adaptations to altered serum calcium levels have been identified in either form.

USES OF LABORATORY TESTING

Electrolytes in Blood

CALCIUM IN BLOOD. To stabilize protein concentration, total calcium should be measured in the fasting patient who is seated or recumbent. Most laboratories measure it inexpensively and with high precision. A high or low calcium value during multichannel screening is often the first indication of a treatable disorder. Serum calcium has traditionally been expressed in the United States in units of milligrams per deciliter, with a typical normal range being 8.8 to 10.2 mg per deciliter. Because calcium has a molecular weight of 40 and is divalent, this can be easily converted into milliequivalents per liter (divide milligrams per deciliter by 2.0) or into millimolar units (SI units); divide milligrams per deciliter by 4.0). Simple equations allow measurements of total calcium in serum to be "corrected" for distortions by deviation of albumin concentration (for example, total calcium can be adjusted upward by 1 mg/dl [0.25 mM] for each gram per deciliter that serum albumin is below the normal mean and vice versa). When uncertainty exists with regard to the direction or severity of an abnormality of blood calcium, the ionized calcium

fraction should be evaluated, as it is a more valid and direct reflection of pathophysiology. This is a more demanding laboratory procedure than is total calcium, and the reproducibility is generally worse. An abnormality of blood calcium can arise from an abnormal flux to or from the major sites of calcium turnover—in bone, gut, and renal tubular fluid.

PHOSPHATE IN BLOOD. Phosphate measurements in serum represent only the 30 per cent that is in inorganic compounds. By convention, phosphate is reported in units of elemental phosphorus. These conventions avoid some of the confusion that would result from efforts to consider molar anion content (phosphate in serum is in a variable equilibrium between its monobasic and dibasic states). Its principal determinants are PTH, age, sex, food ingestion, and diurnal rhythm. Serum phosphate is only a weak index of intracellular phosphate stores. Its normal range is far wider than that for calcium.

MAGNESIUM IN BLOOD. Serum magnesium, like phosphate, is determined by its threshold for renal excretion and by total body pools. Primary disturbance of magnesium in blood is unusual, but important abnormalities can occur during major illnesses; for example, in association with chemotherapy or with extensive burns, tissue necrosis may increase blood magnesium levels, or large fluid losses could depress it.

Hormones in Blood

PARATHYROID HORMONE. Parathyroid hormone is often the first regulator that should be examined in an evaluation of a possible disturbance of mineral homeostasis. Two types of immunoassay are in widespread use. Radioimmunoassay (RIA) directed at the mid-region or carboxy-terminus of PTH can provide excellent clinical correlations; this assay is an index equally of PTH secretion rate and of renal clearance of inactive PTH fragments. Therefore, with mild to severe renal failure, the values must be interpreted with caution. A two-site immunoradiometric assay (IRMA) can give a result that is a more valid indicator of intact, biologically active PTH. Clinical correlations are excellent with this assay, and no adjustment is generally needed for renal compromise. Because the intact PTH molecule has a much shorter half-time than do its inactive fragments, normal PTH concentrations with the "intact" IRMA are far lower than with the mid-region or carboxy-terminus RIA (typically, 10 to 60 pg per milliliter versus 100 to 400 pg per milliliter, the latter normal range being especially dependent upon what is selected as the laboratory standard).

CALCITONIN. Calcitonin is measured by RIA. Clinical uses are limited. When the RIA is used in family screening for early stages of C cell neoplasia, it is particularly important that the laboratory provide normal ranges adjusted for the selected C cell challenge protocol and the patient's age.

25-HYDROXYVITAMIN D. Vitamin D itself is rarely measured in clinical settings. Two different vitamin D metabolites can be measured by most laboratories. It is essential to understand that these two metabolites, 25OHD and 1,25(OH)$_2$D, are usually indicators of two entirely different types of process. Serum 25OHD is a useful index of vitamin D nutritional status. It is also a good index of sterol absorption. Low levels can arise from deficiency of sunlight, from deficiency of vitamin D nutritional supplementation, from fat malabsorption, and from accelerated hepatic catabolism of vitamin D metabolites. Since the body easily compensates for concentrations above normal, dangerously high levels occur only during consumption of pharmacologic doses of vitamin D or of 25OHD.

1,25-DIHYDROXYVITAMIN D. 1,25(OH)$_2$D measurement in serum gives an index of the steroid hormone whose renal production is usually finely regulated by blood PTH. Even with vitamin D intoxication, the serum levels of 1,25(OH)$_2$D may be appropriately low because of this regulatory system. Serum 1,25(OH)$_2$D has only limited diagnostic use. However, certain states can be associated with otherwise unexplainable mineral disturbances that reflect high levels of 1,25(OH)$_2$D (sarcoidosis and other granulomas) or low levels (certain renal tubular disorders, such as X-linked hypophosphatemia).

Blood Indices of Bone Disturbance

Alkaline phosphatase enzyme in serum is an index of its sources in bone, liver, and placenta and of its excretion by the biliary tree. With increased osteoblastic activity, the amount of skeletal alkaline phosphatase enzyme in serum can rise dramatically. Skeletal alkaline phosphatase can be measured selectively through its physicochemical properties (it is the heat-labile component of total alkaline phosphatase) or otherwise (e.g., by RIA, a topic for research in several centers). High skeletal alkaline phosphatase levels can point to high bone turnover (hyperparathyroidism, Paget's disease). Other bone-specific proteins are also under investigation as possible specific indicators of skeletal processes. Osteocalcin (sometimes called bone gla-protein) is another osteoblast-specific protein that has been useful in some long-term studies of bone turnover, but its insensitivity to diffuse bone pathology has compromised its broad clinical use.

Measurements on the Skeleton

BONE RADIOGRAPHS AND SCANS. Standard radiography is often the starting point in the evaluation of bone disorders. Images can be specific for numerous conditions or can direct further diagnostic procedures (i.e., bone biopsy) to sites of focal disturbance. A bone scan with technetium-99m diphosphonate may identify a local disturbance that is not accompanied by radiographic change; the label adsorbs to bone mineral, and increased local blood flow without fracture is sufficient to give a positive signal.

BONE MASS INDICES. Bone mass can be measured noninvasively with a wide variety of techniques. These include dual-channel radiographs, single- and dual-channel photon absorptiometry, radiographs with computed tomography (CT), and other methods under development. Selection among these possibilities should depend largely on local expertise. For sequential studies in a patient, these methods are compromised, to varying degrees, by high cost and lack of precision.

BONE BIOPSY. Bone biopsy can be the final diagnostic tool in identifying local or generalized disturbances of bone. It can be particularly useful in distinguishing osteomalacia from osteoporosis. Maximal information about the bone formation process can be obtained by prior administration of two pulses of tetracyclines 14 days apart (tetracyclines selectively adsorb to the mineralization front of osteoid and provide a fluorescent signal in the biopsy). This test should be considered in consultation with persons knowledgeable about its indications and the details of its processing.

Analyses of the Intestines in Mineral Metabolism

Specific tests of intestinal function are rarely used in current clinical practice. Metabolic balance studies are time consuming and expensive. Calcium absorption studies with radioactive or stable isotopes are not applied outside research settings. General indices of intestinal function are considered in other chapters.

Analyses of the Kidney and Urine

Renal biopsy should be done only for the standard indications related to intrinsic or systemic diseases in the kidney. Urinary excretion of hydroxyproline and other collagen metabolites is a useful index of bone resorption rates because 60 per cent of urinary hydroxyproline is normally derived from collagen in bone.

Urinary excretion of calcium, magnesium, or phosphate is useful in screening for total body excess or deficiency of any of these minerals. Urinary excretion of calcium is central in the evaluation of urolithiasis. More detailed discussion of the workup of urolithiasis is presented elsewhere (see Ch. 88).

Aurbach GD, Marx SJ, Spiegel AM: Parathyroid hormone, calcitonin, and the calciferols. Metabolic bone disease. *In* Wilson JD, Foster DW (eds.): Williams Textbook of Endocrinology. 8th ed. Philadelphia, W.B. Saunders Company, 1991. *Detailed review of mineral metabolism with emphasis on calciotropic hormones. Other major textbooks of endocrinology have similar chapters.*

Avioli LV, Krane SM (eds.): Metabolic Bone Diseases and Clinically Related Disorders. 2nd ed. Philadelphia, W.B. Saunders Company, 1990. *A detailed review of the entire field from multiple authors.*

DeGroot LJ, Besser GM, Cahill GF, et al. (eds.): Endocrinology. 2nd ed. Philadelphia, W.B. Saunders Company, 1989. *Volume 2 of this three-volume encyclopedic text contains 22 chapters by many authors covering the field of mineral metabolism. Controversial areas are treated in depth, but coverage of some topics may be outdated.*

Favus MJ (ed.): Primer on Metabolic Bone Diseases and Disorders of Mineral Metabolism. Kelseyville, Calif., American Society for Bone and Mineral Research, 1990. *Concise chapters that quickly advance the reader to the current frontiers of research on a topic.*

Peck WE (ed.): Bone and Mineral Research. Vols. 1–6, 1983–1989. New York, Elsevier. *An annual volume with authoritative reviews of basic and clinical topics in this area.*

233 Vitamin D
Daniel D. Bikle

Vitamin D is a steroid hormone with two molecular forms: vitamin D_3 (cholecalciferol), which is produced in the skin, and vitamin D_2 (ergocalciferol), which is derived from the plant sterol ergosterol. Vitamin D_2 is the usual form of vitamin D available for pharmaceutical use, although both vitamin D_2 and D_3 are used as food supplements. Despite subtle differences in physiology and biochemistry, vitamin D_2 and D_3 have equivalent potency and mechanisms of action in humans. In the ensuing discussion, lack of a subscript after the D implies that both forms of vitamin D are implied.

To achieve biologic potency, vitamin D must be further metabolized. Two of these metabolites, 25-hydroxyvitamin D (25OHD) and 1,25-dihydroxyvitamin D (1,25(OH)$_2$D), are produced by successive hydroxylations; the hepatic enzyme vitamin D 25-hydroxylase catalyzes the formation of 25OHD, and the renal enzyme 25OHD 1-hydroxylase catalyzes the formation of 1,25(OH)$_2$D. Both 25OHD (calcifediol) and 1,25(OH)$_2$D (calcitriol) are available to treat disorders of calcium homeostasis. A third metabolite, 24,25-dihydroxyvitamin D (24,25(OH)$_2$D), also shows promise as a therapeutic agent but as yet is available only for investigational purposes. 24,25(OH)$_2$D, like 1,25(OH)$_2$D, is produced from 25OHD, principally in the kidney.

VITAMIN D ENDOCRINE SYSTEM

The vitamin D endocrine system can be divided into three levels (Fig. 233–1): bioavailability of vitamin D from skin and gut; metabolism of vitamin D to its active forms, principally by the liver and kidney; and the action of these metabolites on target tissues.

BIOAVAILABILITY. Vitamin D_3 is produced in the skin by a multistep process. Irradiation of 7-dehydrocholesterol by ultraviolet (UV) light converts it to previtamin D_3, which then undergoes thermal isomerization to vitamin D_3. No clear regulation of vitamin D_3 production has been observed other than by the amount of UV irradiation that reaches the 7-dehydrocholesterol in the epidermis. Increased melanin in the epidermis reduces the effect of UV irradiation. Aging also appears to result in decreased vitamin D production.

Vitamin D is also available from the diet, as it is commonly used as a food supplement in dairy products. Vitamin D is absorbed principally in the jejunum by a process (chylomicron formation) that is facilitated by bile salts, fatty acids, and monoglycerides. Most of the vitamin D absorbed passes through the lymphatic system before entering the bloodstream. The hydroxylated metabolites of vitamin D (i.e., 25OHD and 1,25(OH)$_2$D) depend less on chylomicron formation for their absorption.

Vitamin D and its metabolites are transported in blood bound mainly to an alpha globulin called vitamin D–binding protein (DBP). This protein has a higher affinity for 25OHD and 24,25(OH)$_2$D than for vitamin D and 1,25(OH)$_2$D. Since the amount of DBP in blood (5×10^{-6} M) far exceeds that of vitamin D and its metabolites (Table 233–1), 1 per cent or less of the total amount of these metabolites is actually free to diffuse into cells. It is unclear whether DBP serves principally as a circulating reservoir for the vitamin D metabolites in blood or facilitates the transport of these metabolites into target tissues. Changes in DBP levels affect total concentrations of vitamin D metabolites without necessarily affecting the free concentrations. Pregnancy and estrogen increase DBP; liver disease and proteinuria decrease DBP. The relative importance of free versus total concentration of the vitamin D metabolites has not been established with certainty, although evidence suggesting that the free concentration is the biologically active concentration is accumulating.

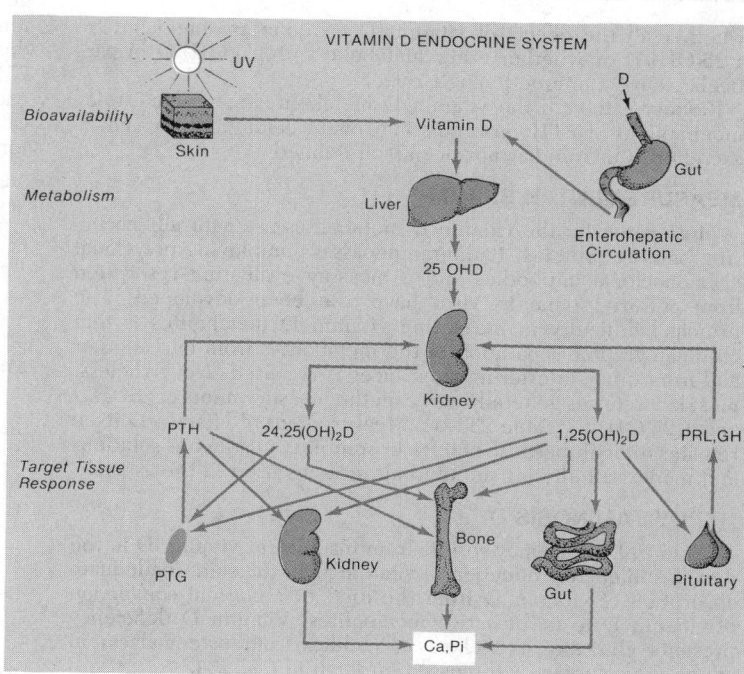

FIGURE 233–1. The vitamin D endocrine system. Vitamin D is made available to the body by photogenesis in the skin and absorption from the intestine. Vitamin D is then hydroxylated in the liver to 25OHD, then in the kidney to 1,25(OH)₂D and 24,25(OH)₂D. The active vitamin D metabolites act on different tissues to produce a variety of responses. The three target tissues principally responsible for calcium (Ca) and phosphate (Pi) homeostasis are kidney, bone, and intestine. Endocrine tissues such as the parathyroid gland (PTG) and anterior pituitary are also target tissues. Their hormones, parathyroid hormone (PTH), prolactin (PRL), and growth hormone (GH), help regulate vitamin D metabolism in the kidney. In addition, PTH has a direct effect on bone and kidney regulation of calcium and phosphate homeostasis. (Reproduced with permission from Bikle DD: The vitamin D endocrine system. *In* Stollerman GH, et al. [eds.]: Advances in Internal Medicine. Vol. 27. Copyright © 1982 by Year Book Medical Publishers, Inc., Chicago.)

METABOLISM. Liver. The first step in the bioactivation of vitamin D occurs in the liver, where vitamin D 25-hydroxylase converts vitamin D to 25OHD. Since 25OHD production by this cytochrome P450 mixed-function oxidase is governed principally by the supply of substrate (i.e., vitamin D), circulating 25OHD levels are a good indicator of vitamin D bioavailability. Hepatic production of 25OHD appears to be well preserved in all but the most severe cases of liver disease unless the vitamin D stores are depleted. Compounds such as phenytoin and phenobarbital, however, which induce drug-metabolizing enzymes in the liver, alter the hepatic metabolism of vitamin D in a manner that may lead to clinical bone disease in subjects with marginal vitamin D stores.

Kidney. The 25OHD produced by the liver is further metabolized to 1,25(OH)₂D and 24,25(OH)₂D, principally in the kidney. Little, if any, 1,25(OH)₂D is produced outside the kidney (except by the placenta) under normal circumstances, although other tissues, such as bone, cartilage, skin, and macrophages may produce 24,25(OH)₂D and 1,25(OH)₂D in limited amounts. Lymphomatous and sarcoid tissue may also contain 1-hydroxylase activity. Both the 1-hydroxylase and the 24-hydroxylase in the kidney are cytochrome P450 mixed-function oxidases located exclusively in the mitochondria of the proximal renal tubule.

TABLE 233–1. VITAMIN D AND ITS METABOLITES

Name	Abbreviation	Generic Name	Serum Concentration*
Vitamin D	D	Calciferol	1.6 ± 0.4 ng/ml
Vitamin D₃	D₃	a. Cholecalciferol	
Vitamin D₂	D₂	b. Ergocalciferol	
25 hydroxy-vitamin D	25OHD	Calcifediol	26.5 ± 5.3 ng/ml
1,25 dihydroxy-vitamin D	1,25(OH)₂D	Calcitriol	34.1 ± 9.8 pg/ml
24,25 dihydroxy-vitamin D	24,25(OH)₂D		1.3 ± 0.4 ng/ml
25,26 dihydroxy-vitamin D	25,26(OH)₂D		0.5 ± 0.1 ng/ml

*Values differ somewhat from laboratory to laboratory, depending on the methodology used and the sunlight exposure and dietary intake of vitamin D in the population studied. Children tend to have higher 1,25(OH)₂D levels than do adults. Data are derived from Lambert PW, Fu IY, Kaetzel DM, et al.: Assay for multiple vitamin D metabolites. *In* Bikle DD (ed.): Assay of Calcium Regulating Hormones. New York, Springer-Verlag, 1983, pp 99–124.

Their activities are closely regulated by a variety of ions and hormones, the most important of which are calcium, phosphate, 1,25(OH)₂D itself, and parathyroid hormone (PTH). Low serum calcium and phosphate levels and elevated PTH levels stimulate 1,25(OH)₂D production. High 1,25(OH)₂D levels inhibit 1,25(OH)₂D production but increase 24,25(OH)₂D production. Other hormones such as prolactin and growth hormone may also stimulate 1,25(OH)₂D production, but whether these hormones are important in the control of 1,25(OH)₂D production under normal physiologic conditions is not known.

TARGET TISSUE RESPONSE. Bone, gut, and kidney are the primary target tissues for vitamin D, but many other tissues, including the pituitary, parathyroid glands, pancreas, brain, activated lymphocytes, thymocytes, skin, and a variety of tumors, contain a specific receptor for 1,25(OH)₂D and respond to it by a change in function. Muscle contains no receptors for 1,25(OH)₂D but appears to be a target tissue for 25OHD. These observations suggest that vitamin D influences a much greater range of biologic phenomena than previously appreciated, such as immunoregulation, cellular differentiation, and neural transmission. Whether all tissues that contain receptors for the vitamin D metabolites have a physiologically important response to normal circulating concentrations of the metabolites has not been established.

Intestine. 1,25(OH)₂D regulates calcium transport across the intestine in a highly integrated sequence of events. First, 1,25(OH)₂D appears to increase the permeability of the brush-border membrane to calcium, permitting calcium to enter from the lumen into the intestinal epithelial cell down a steep electrochemical gradient. The calcium that enters the cell must be accumulated by subcellular organelles, such as the mitochondria, to prevent cytosolic calcium concentrations from reaching toxic levels. 1,25(OH)₂D stimulates this accumulation. The calcium must then be transported through the cell and pumped across the basolateral membrane into the bloodstream. A unique calcium-binding protein (CaBP), induced by 1,25(OH)₂D in the intestine as well as in a number of other target tissues, appears to modulate intracellular calcium concentrations, perhaps by facilitating the removal of calcium from the cell.

Bone. The role of the vitamin D metabolites in calcium movement in and out of bone is less clear. 1,25(OH)₂D is a potent stimulator of bone resorption and inhibitor of collagen production (bone formation) in vitro. On the other hand, 24,25(OH)₂D may stimulate bone and cartilage formation without stimulating bone resorption. These results have engendered a controversy over whether all the effects of vitamin D on bone are mediated by 1,25(OH)₂D or whether other metabolites, 24,25(OH)₂D in particular, have a unique biologic role.

Kidney. Although the vitamin D metabolites may play a role, independent of PTH, in regulating renal calcium and phosphate excretion, this role has not been well defined.

MEASUREMENT IN SERUM

Most assays for the vitamin D metabolites use naturally occurring binding proteins. Radioimmunoassays employing polyclonal or monoclonal antibodies and a bioassay evaluating resorption from cultured bone in vitro have also been developed. The principal difficulty in measuring vitamin D metabolites is that chromatographic separation of the metabolites from one another and from other interfering substances is required. Nevertheless, most laboratories generally agree on the measurements of 25OHD and 1,25(OH)₂D (Table 233–1). Measurement of vitamin D itself remains difficult because of its poor solubility in aqueous solutions and modest affinity for the binding proteins used in the assays.

HYPOVITAMINOSIS D

Vitamin D deficiency results from insufficient vitamin D in the diet, insufficient production of vitamin D in the skin, inadequate absorption of vitamin D from the diet, or abnormal conversion of vitamin D to its bioactive metabolites. Vitamin D deficiency presents clinically as rickets in children and osteomalacia in adults. This subject is discussed in detail in Ch. 234.

HYPERVITAMINOSIS D

Hypervitaminosis D may occur in three general settings: (1) excessive consumption, usually for therapeutic purposes, of vitamin D, vitamin D analogues (such as dihydrotachysterol), or vitamin D metabolites; (2) the abnormal conversion of vitamin D to its biologically active metabolites, as occurs in sarcoidosis and possibly other granulomatous diseases; or (3) a change in the sensitivity of the target tissue to vitamin D, as can occur with the remission of a variety of gastrointestinal diseases associated with calcium malabsorption. The initial signs and symptoms of vitamin D intoxication include weakness, lethargy, headaches, nausea, and polyuria and are attributable to the hypercalcemia and hypercalciuria. Ectopic calcification may occur, particularly in the kidneys, resulting in nephrolithiasis or nephrocalcinosis; other sites include blood vessels, heart, lungs, and skin. Infants appear to be quite susceptible to vitamin D intoxication and may develop disseminated arteriosclerosis, supravalvular aortic stenosis, and renal acidosis.

The dose of vitamin D required to produce toxicity varies among patients, reflecting differences in absorption, storage, and subsequent metabolism of the vitamin as well as in target tissue response to the active metabolites. For example, an elderly patient with senile osteoporosis and a low turnover rate of bone also tends to have a reduced ability to absorb calcium in the intestine and a reduced ability to produce 1,25(OH)₂D in the kidney. Such a patient can usually ingest 50,000 to 100,000 IU of vitamin D per day without developing hypercalcemia or hypercalciuria. In contrast, a patient of similar age with a similar degree of osteoporosis but in whom the osteoporosis develops as a result of primary hyperparathyroidism would almost certainly be harmed by this amount of vitamin D. In the latter patient, the ability of vitamin D to stimulate bone resorption and intestinal calcium absorption is enhanced in part because of the greater rates of 1,25(OH)₂D production and bone turnover observed in primary hyperparathyroidism. Patients with sarcoidosis appear to develop vitamin D intoxication because 1,25(OH)₂D production in the abnormal tissue is not subject to the normal feedback mechanisms that regulate renal production of 1,25(OH)₂D. Analogues of vitamin D, such as dihydrotachysterol, or the renal metabolite of vitamin D, 1,25(OH)₂D, which bypass the normal rate-limiting step of vitamin D bioactivation (the renal 1α-hydroxylase reaction), are more likely than vitamin D or 25OHD to result in hypercalcemia if used in excess.

Hypervitaminosis D is treated by stopping the administration of vitamin D or its analogues or metabolites. If the hypercalcemia is severe, the patient should be placed on a low-calcium diet and

given glucocorticoids (e.g., 60 mg of prednisone every day) and generous amounts of fluids. Acute hypercalcemia, when symptomatic, can be treated with saline and furosemide diuresis, as described under the general management of hypercalcemia (Ch. 235). Hypercalcemia lasts for only a few days when caused by excess 1,25(OH)₂D, but it may persist for weeks or months when caused by excess vitamin D. The hypercalcemia of sarcoidosis tends to respond within days to glucocorticoid therapy.

Adams JS, Singer FR, Gacad MA, et al.: Isolation and structural identification of 1,25-dihydroxyvitamin D₃ produced by cultured alveolar macrophages in sarcoidosis. J Clin Endocrinol Metab 60:960, 1985. *Provides direct evidence that sarcoid macrophages make 1,25(OH)₂D.*

Bikle DD: Regulation of intestinal calcium transport by vitamin D: Role of membrane structure. *In* Aloia RC, Curtain CC, Gordon LM (eds.): Membrane Transport and Information Storage. New York, Wiley-Riss, 1990, pp 191–219. *A comprehensive discussion of the mechanisms by which 1,25(OH)₂D regulates intestinal calcium transport.*

Fraser DR: Regulation of the metabolism of vitamin D. Physiol Rev 60:551, 1980. *A thorough, well-balanced review of vitamin D metabolism in the liver and kidney.*

Holick MF: Capacity of human skin to produce vitamin D₃. *In* Kligman A, Takase Y (eds.): Cutaneous Aging. Tokyo, University of Tokyo Press, 1988, pp 223–246. *A thorough discussion of the biochemistry of vitamin D production in the skin, including the environmental variables that limit this process.*

Lambert PW, Stern PH, Avioli RC, et al.: Evidence for extrarenal production of 1α,25-dihydroxyvitamin D in man. J Clin Invest 69:722, 1982. *The demonstration of 1,25(OH)₂D levels in anephric humans and the suggestion that vitamin D treatment increases these levels.*

Lee DBN, Zawada ET, Kleeman CR: The pathophysiology and clinical aspects of hypercalcemic disorders. West J Med 129:278, 1978. *This article discusses all the major hypercalcemic disorders, including the diagnosis and treatment of hypervitaminosis D.*

Pillai S, Bikle DD, Elias PM: Vitamin D and epidermal differentiation. Evidence for a role of endogenously produced vitamin D metabolites in keratinocytic differentiation. Skin Pharmacol 1:149, 1988. *Describes both the production of 1,25(OH)₂D by epidermal cells and the role of 1,25(OH)₂D in modulating the differentiation of these cells.*

Reichel H, Koeffler HP, Norman AW: The role of the vitamin D endocrine system in health and disease. N Engl J Med 320:980, 1989. *A good overview emphasizing recent concepts regarding the role of 1,25(OH)₂D in cellular growth and differentiation.*

234 Osteomalacia and Rickets
Daniel D. Bikle

DEFINITIONS

Osteomalacia and rickets are caused by the abnormal mineralization of bone and cartilage. Osteomalacia refers to the defect that occurs in bone in which the epiphyseal plates have closed (i.e., in adults), whereas rickets refers to the defect that occurs in growing bone (i.e., in children). Abnormal mineralization in growing bone affects the transformation of cartilage into bone at the zone of provisional calcification. As a result, an enormous profusion of disorganized, nonmineralized, degenerating cartilage appears in this region, leading to widening of the epiphyseal plate (observed radiologically as a widened radiolucent zone) with flaring or cupping and irregularity of the epiphyseal-metaphyseal junctions. This latter problem gives rise to the clinically obvious beaded swellings along the costochondral junctions (rachitic rosary) and the swelling at the ends of the long bones. Growth is retarded by the failure to make new bone. Once bone growth has ceased (i.e., after closure of the epiphyseal plates), the clinical evidence for defective mineralization becomes more subtle, and special diagnostic procedures may be required for its detection.

PATHOGENESIS—OVERVIEW

The best known cause of abnormal bone mineralization is vitamin D deficiency. Vitamin D, through its biologically active metabolites, ensures that the calcium and phosphate concentrations in the extracellular milieu are adequate for mineralization to occur. Vitamin D may also permit osteoblasts to produce a bone matrix that can be mineralized and then allows them to mineralize that matrix in a normal fashion. Phosphate deficiency can also cause defective mineralization. It may act independently or in conjunction with other predisposing abnormalities, since most hypophosphatemic disorders associated with osteomalacia or rickets also affect the vitamin D endocrine system. Dietary calcium deficiency has been implicated as a cause of rickets and may contribute to the osteomalacia and osteoporosis found in elderly patients. Osteomalacia or rickets may develop despite adequate levels of calcium, phosphate, and vitamin D if the bone matrix cannot undergo normal mineralization. For example, the deficiency in alkaline phosphatase in patients with hypophosphatasia can cause a defect in mineralization. This enzyme cleaves pyrophosphate, an inhibitor of bone mineralization, and a deficiency results in reduced removal of this inhibitor. Finally, drugs such as etidronate and heavy metals such as aluminum can interfere with mineralization and lead to osteomalacia or rickets.

Table 234–1 lists diseases associated with osteomalacia and

TABLE 234–1. THE OSTEOMALACIC SYNDROMES*

A. **Disorders in the vitamin D endocrine system**
  1. Decreased bioavailability
      Insufficient sunlight exposure
      Nutritional vitamin D deficiency
      Nephrotic syndrome (urinary loss)
      Malabsorption (fecal loss)
        Billroth type II gastrectomy
        Sprue
        Regional enteritis
        Jejunoileal bypass
        Pancreatic insufficiency
        Cholestatic disorders
        Cholestyramine
  2. Abnormal metabolism
      Liver disease
      Chronic renal failure
      Vitamin D–dependent rickets type I
      Tumoral hypophosphatemic osteomalacia
      X-linked hypophosphatemia
      Hypoparathyroidism (?)
      Chronic acidosis (?)
      Anticonvulsants
  3. Abnormal target tissue response
      Vitamin D–dependent rickets type II
      Gastrointestinal disorders
B. **Disorders of phosphate homeostasis**
  1. Decreased intestinal absorption
      Malnutrition
      Malabsorption
      Antacids containing aluminum hydroxide
  2. Increased renal loss
      X-linked hypophosphatemic rickets
      Tumoral hypophosphatemic osteomalacia
      De Toni-Debré-Fanconi (phosphaturia, aminoaciduria, glycosuria, bicarbonaturia)
      Cystinosis
      Oculocerebrorenal syndrome (Lowe's syndrome)
      Paraproteinemias
      Wilson's disease
      Glycogen storage diseases
      Galactosemia
      Tyrosinemia
      Cadmium poisoning
      Neurofibromatosis
C. **Calcium deficiency**
  1. Dietary insufficiency
  2. Excessive renal loss (?)
  3. Malabsorption of calcium (?)
D. **Primary disorders of bone matrix**
  1. Hypophosphatasia
  2. Fibrogenesis imperfecta ossium
  3. Axial osteomalacia
E. **Inhibitors of mineralization**
  1. Aluminum
      Chronic renal failure
      Total parenteral nutrition
  2. Etidronate
  3. Phenytoin (?)
  4. Fluoride (?)

*This table categorizes diseases that produce osteomalacia according to the presumed mechanism (or mechanisms) by which bone mineralization is inhibited. A question mark indicates that the association of the disease with osteomalacia or the mechanism by which it produces osteomalacia is not established.

rickets according to the presumed mechanism responsible for the mineralization defect. Diseases that appear under multiple headings affect bone mineralization via multiple mechanisms. It is important to understand the mechanism by which a particular disease interferes with bone mineralization in order to choose appropriate diagnostic procedures and therapy.

VITAMIN D DEFICIENCY

Pathogenesis

Vitamin D deficiency results from one, or more often a combination, of the following three causes.

REDUCED SUNLIGHT EXPOSURE. The human skin can generate adequate amounts of vitamin D if exposed to sufficient ultraviolet radiation. In countries with limited sunlight, however, or where the population dresses in a fashion that reduces exposure to sunlight, circulating levels of vitamin D metabolites are often low. These low levels may help explain why the incidence of osteomalacia is higher in Great Britain, the Scandinavian countries, the Middle East, and India than in the United States.

NUTRITIONAL VITAMIN D DEFICIENCY. The fortification of dairy products with vitamin D has made nutritional vitamin D–deficient rickets uncommon in the United States, although it is still prevalent in other parts of the world. Even in the United States, vitamin D deficiency may occur in children of vegetarian mothers who avoid milk products (and presumably have reduced vitamin D stores) and in children who are not weaned to vitamin D–supplemented milk by age 2. The contribution of nutritional vitamin D deficiency to osteomalacia in elderly people is also suspected. Osteomalacia has been observed in 25 to 30 per cent of bone biopsies from elderly patients who have suffered hip fractures in Scandinavia and Great Britain. Most likely, both reduced vitamin D intake and reduced exposure to sunlight contribute to the development of osteomalacia in the elderly.

MALABSORPTION. Fecal loss of vitamin D and its metabolites occurs in patients with malabsorption for several reasons (Fig. 234–1). Ingested vitamin D is absorbed primarily in chylomicrons; disorders that involve the biliary tract, pancreas, or mid to distal portions of the small intestine reduce the efficiency of this process (Ch. 233). Endogenous vitamin D and its metabolites undergo enterohepatic circulation; disorders of the distal small bowel disrupt this circulation. In cholestatic disorders, urinary excretion of vitamin D metabolites is increased, and intestinal absorption is decreased. Drugs, such as cholestyramine, that are used in the treatment of cholestatic disorders may compound the problem by binding to the bile salts required for the absorption of the vitamin D metabolites, thus enhancing their fecal excretion. The resulting bone disease is often a combination of osteomalacia and osteoporosis. The prevalence of osteomalacia in patients with cholestatic and gastrointestinal disorders varies from country to country. It appears to be higher in Great Britain and Northern Europe than in the United States. Fully 25 to 50 per cent of British and European patients who have undergone Billroth type II gastrectomy or jejunoileal bypass or who have cholestatic liver disease or inflammatory bowel disease have osteomalacia when evaluated by bone biopsy.

Diagnosis

In children, the presentation of rickets is generally obvious from a combination of clinical and radiologic evidence. The diagnostic challenge is to determine the etiology. In adults the clinical, radiologic, and biochemical evidence for osteomalacia is often subtle. In situations in which osteomalacia should be suspected (malnutrition, liver disease, malabsorption, and unexplained osteopenia), the clinician must decide whether to obtain a biopsy of bone for histomorphometric examination. This decision must rest on the availability of resources to perform the biopsy and to evaluate the specimen, the index of suspicion coupled with the lack of certainty from other diagnostic procedures, and the degree to which the therapeutic approach will be altered by the additional information.

CLINICAL FEATURES. The clinical presentation of rickets depends on the age of the patient and, to some extent, the etiology of the syndrome (Fig. 234–2). The affected infant or young child may be apathetic, listless, weak, hypotonic, and

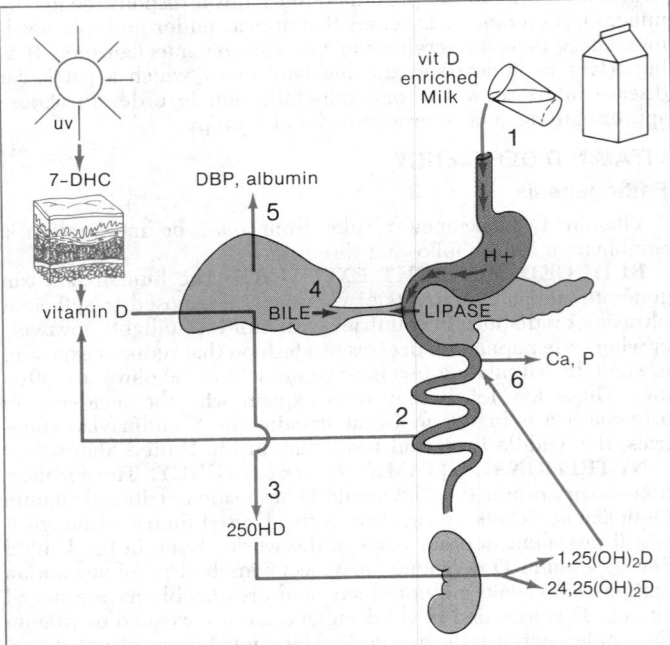

FIGURE 234–1. Six steps in vitamin D absorption and handling that may be altered by hepatogastrointestinal disorders and lead to bone disease. 1, Decreased intake of vitamin D. 2, Decreased absorption of vitamin D secondary to disorders in biliary secretion, pancreatic enzymes, enterocyte function, or intestinal anatomy. 3, Abnormal production of 25OHD by the liver secondary to hepatic parenchymal disease or anticonvulsants. 4, Disruption in the enterohepatic circulation of vitamin D metabolites and conjugates secondary to disorders in biliary secretion. 5, Reduced delivery of vitamin D metabolites to target tissues secondary to decreased vitamin D–binding protein (DBP) and albumin synthesis. 6, Decreased response of the diseased intestine to 1,25(OH)₂D with respect to calcium and phosphorus absorption.

growing poorly. A soft, somewhat misshapen head with widened sutures and frontal bossing may be observed. Eruption of teeth may be delayed, and teeth that do appear may be pitted and poorly mineralized. The enlargement and cupping of the costochondral junctions produce the "rachitic rosary" on the thorax. The tug of the diaphragm against the softened lower ribs may produce an indentation at the point of insertion of the diaphragm (Harrison's groove). Muscle hypotonia can result in a pronounced pot belly and a waddling gait. The limbs may become bowed, and joints may swell because of flaring at the ends of the long bones (including phalanges and metacarpals). Pathologic fractures may occur in patients with florid rickets.

After the epiphyses have closed, the clinical signs of rickets or osteomalacia are subtle and cannot be relied upon to make the diagnosis. Patients with severe osteomalacia complain of bone pain and muscle weakness. Difficulty climbing stairs or rising from chairs may be reported. Such individuals may have a history of multiple fractures. However, osteomalacia is often diagnosed by bone histomorphometry in patients who lack obvious symptoms in their musculoskeletal system.

RADIOLOGIC FEATURES. The radiologic features of rickets, like the clinical manifestations, can be quite striking, especially in the young child. In growing bone, the radiolucent epiphyses are wide and flared, with irregular epiphyseal-metaphyseal junctions. Long bones may be bowed. The cortices of the long bones are often indistinct. Occasionally, evidence of secondary hyperparathyroidism—subperiosteal resorption in the phalanges and metacarpals and erosion of the distal ends of the clavicles—is observed.

Pseudofractures (also known as Looser's zones or Milkman's fractures) are an uncommon but nearly pathognomonic feature of rickets and osteomalacia (Fig. 234–3). These radiolucent lines are most often found along the concave side of the femoral neck, the pubic rami, the ribs, the clavicles, and the lateral aspects of the

scapulae. Pseudofractures may result from unhealed microfractures at points of stress or at the entry point of blood vessels into bone. They may progress to complete fractures that go unrecognized and thereby lead to substantial deformity and disability. Bone density is not a reliable indicator of osteomalacia, since bone density can be decreased in patients with vitamin D deficiency or increased in patients with chronic renal failure. In adults with normal renal function, radiologic evidence of a mineralization defect is often subtle and not readily distinguishable from osteoporosis.

BIOCHEMICAL FEATURES. Vitamin D deficiency results in decreased intestinal absorption of calcium and phosphate. In conjunction with the resulting secondary hyperparathyroidism, vitamin D deficiency leads to an increase in bone resorption, increased excretion of urinary phosphate, and increased renal tubular reabsorption of calcium. The net result tends to be a low normal serum calcium level, low serum phosphorus level, elevated serum alkaline phosphatase level, increased parathyroid hormone (PTH) level, decreased urinary calcium level, and increased urinary phosphate level. Finding a low 25OHD level in combination with these other biochemical alterations strengthens the diagnosis of vitamin D deficiency. The 1,25(OH)₂D level may be normal, making this determination less useful for the diagnosis of osteomalacia. Both 25OHD and 1,25(OH)₂D levels may be reduced in patients with liver disease or nephrotic syndrome, who nevertheless have normal free concentrations of these metabolites and who may not be vitamin D deficient. Other factors, such as age and diet, must be considered. For example, serum phosphorus values are normally lower in adults than in children. Dietary history is important, since urinary phosphate excretion and, to a lesser degree, urinary calcium excretion reflect dietary phosphate and calcium content. Since phosphate excretion depends on the filtered load (the product of the glomerular filtration rate [GFR] and plasma phosphate), urinary phosphate levels may be normal if either the GFR or the plasma phosphate levels are reduced, despite the presence of hyperparathyroidism. Expressions of renal phosphate clearance that account for these variables (e.g., renal threshold for phosphate, or TmP/GFR; TmP = maximal tubular reabsorption of phosphate) are a better indicator of renal phosphate handling than is total phosphate excretion. The TmP/GFR can be calculated from a nomogram using measurements of a fasting serum and urine phosphorus concentration.

HISTOLOGIC FEATURES. Because of the difficulty in di-

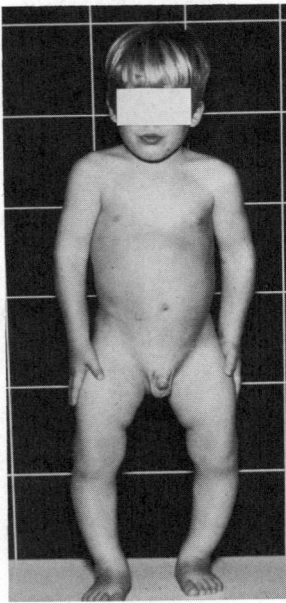 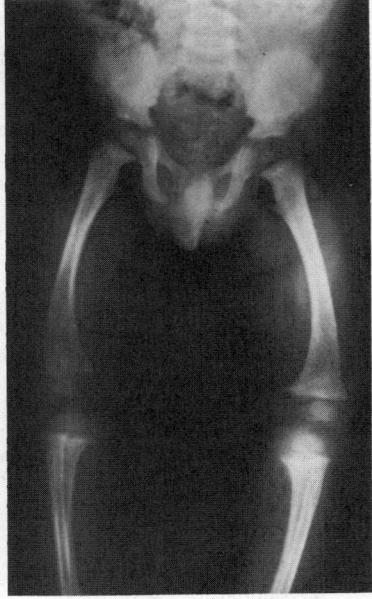

A   **B**

FIGURE 234–2. The clinical (A) and radiologic (B) appearance of a young boy with X-linked hypophosphatemic rickets. The most striking abnormalities are the bowing of the legs, apparent in both femora and tibiae, with flaring of the ends of these bones at the knee. (Photographs courtesy of Dr. Sara B. Arnaud.)

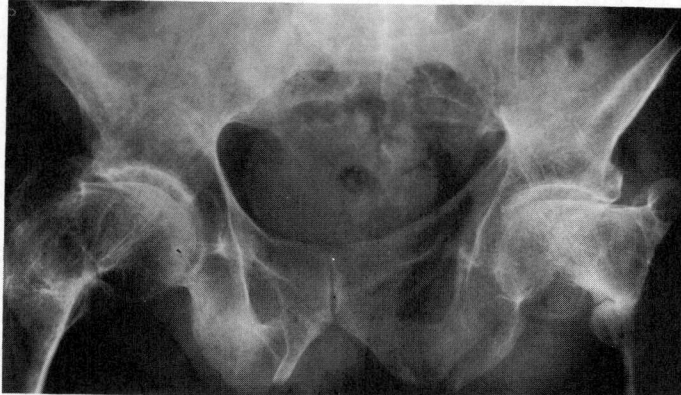

FIGURE 234–3. Roentgenogram of the pelvis of an elderly female with severe osteomalacia. This film reveals marked bowing (varus deformity) of both femoral necks, with pseudofractures of the medial aspect of the femoral necks and the superior aspect of the left pubic ramus. (Photograph courtesy of Dr. Harry K. Genant.)

agnosing osteomalacia in adults by clinical and radiologic means, transcortical bone biopsy may be necessary. A rib or the iliac crest is the site at which a biopsy is generally performed. To assess osteoid content and mineral appositional rate, the bone biopsy specimen is processed without decalcification. This requires special equipment.

In osteomalacia, bone is mineralized poorly and slowly, resulting in wide osteoid seams (>12 μm) and a large fraction of bone covered by unmineralized osteoid. States of high bone turnover (increased bone formation and resorption), such as hyperparathyroidism, can also cause wide osteoid seams and increased osteoid surface, producing a superficial resemblance to osteomalacia. Therefore, the rate of bone turnover should be determined by labeling bone with tetracycline, which provides a fluorescent marker of the calcification front. When two doses of tetracycline are given at different times, the distance between the two labels divided by the time interval between the two doses equals the mineral appositional rate. The normal appositional rate is approximately 0.74 μm per day. Mineralization lag time, the time required for newly formed osteoid to be mineralized, can be calculated by dividing osteoid seam width by the appositional rate corrected by the linear extent of mineralization or calcification front (a measure of the bone surface that is undergoing active mineralization as measured by tetracycline incorporation). It is normally about 20 to 25 days. Depressed appositional rate, increased mineralization lag time, and reduced calcification front clearly distinguish osteomalacia from high turnover states such as hyperparathyroidism. Low turnover states, such as senile osteoporosis, can also have low appositional rates and reduced calcification fronts, but these are distinguished from osteomalacia by normal or reduced osteoid surface and volume.

Treatment

The goal in treating osteomalacia and rickets is to normalize the clinical, biochemical, and radiologic abnormalities without producing hypercalcemia, hyperphosphatemia, hypercalciuria, nephrolithiasis, or ectopic calcification (especially nephrocalcinosis). To realize this goal, patients must be followed carefully, and as the bone lesions heal or the underlying disease improves, the dose of vitamin D, calcium, or phosphate needs to be adjusted to avoid such complications. Table 234–2 lists the available vitamin D metabolites and analogues, including dose range, duration of action, cost, and clinical applications.

Simple nutritional vitamin D deficiency responds to oral doses of 2000 to 4000 IU of vitamin D per day, taken for several months, followed by replacement doses of 200 to 400 IU per day. Radiologic and biochemical evidence of healing requires several months. If the patient fails to respond to treatment, the physician should consider other possible causes of the bone disease.

Patients with malabsorption may respond to large doses of oral vitamin D (25,000 to 100,000 IU per day), or they may require parenteral administration of the vitamin. Since patients with steatorrhea absorb 25OHD (calcifediol) better than they do

vitamin D, 50 to 100 μg of calcifediol per day or every other day should be tried if large doses of vitamin D fail to raise circulating levels of 25OHD into the high normal range. Vitamin D therapy should be supplemented with 1 to 3 grams of calcium per day. Only the osteomalacic component of the bone disease associated with these conditions responds to vitamin D; the osteoporotic component does not. Consequently, patients must be carefully selected for vitamin D treatment and carefully followed. Histomorphometric evaluation of bone biopsies is particularly useful in this regard.

CHRONIC RENAL FAILURE (see also Ch. 77 and 237)
Pathogenesis of Renal Osteodystrophy

Metabolism of 25OHD to 1,25-dihydroxyvitamin D (1,25(OH)$_2$D) and 24,25-dihydroxyvitamin D (24,25(OH)$_2$D) in the kidney is tightly regulated. Renal disease results in reduced circulating levels of both these metabolites. With the reduction in 1,25(OH)$_2$D levels, intestinal calcium absorption falls, and bone resorption appears to become less sensitive to PTH—a result that leads to hypocalcemia. Phosphate excretion by the diseased kidney is decreased, resulting in hyperphosphatemia and aggravation of the hypocalcemia. As a consequence, hyperparathyroidism develops, facilitated by the fact that the levels of the vitamin D metabolites are too low to inhibit PTH secretion. The net effect of deficient 1,25(OH)$_2$D and 24,25(OH)$_2$D and excessive PTH on bone is complex. Patients may have osteitis fibrosa (reflecting excessive PTH), osteomalacia (in part reflecting vitamin D deficiency), or a combination of the two. One particularly debilitating form of renal osteodystrophy is found in a small percentage of patients on hemodialysis in whom only osteomalacia occurs. Such patients have increased aluminum content in their bones, particularly in the zone where mineralization is occurring (calcification front). The aluminum is thought to block mineralization. These patients are particularly debilitated by bone pain, fractures, and muscle weakness.

Diagnosis

Most patients with chronic renal failure and renal osteodystrophy have osteitis fibrosa alone or in combination with osteomalacia (see Ch. 237). If not well controlled, these patients will have a low serum level of calcium and high serum levels of phosphorus, alkaline phosphatase, and PTH. A few patients develop severe secondary hyperparathyroidism in which the PTH level increases dramatically, with restoration of the serum calcium to normal or even elevated levels (sometimes called tertiary hyperparathyroidism). Another small subset of patients with renal osteodystrophy present with normal or low serum levels of PTH and alkaline phosphatase. Their serum calcium levels are often elevated after treatment with small doses of 1,25(OH)$_2$D. These patients have pure osteomalacia on bone biopsy and are thought to suffer from aluminum intoxication (see Ch. 237). Regardless of the type of bone disease, most patients with chronic renal disease have low 1,25(OH)$_2$D and 24,25(OH)$_2$D levels and, unless treated with vitamin D, tend to have low 25OHD levels as well.

Treatment

Patients with renal osteodystrophy generally respond to 1,25(OH)$_2$D (calcitriol, 0.5 to 1.0 μg per day) or dihydrotachysterol (DHT, 0.25 to 0.5 mg per day), calcium supplementation (1 to 3 grams per day), and phosphate restriction (dietary restriction supplemented with phosphate binders such as aluminum hydroxide). The goal is to achieve and maintain normal serum levels of calcium, phosphorus, PTH, and alkaline phosphatase. This regimen treats osteitis fibrosa more effectively than osteomalacia. Some authorities recommend the use of calcifediol rather than calcitriol or DHT, since calcifediol may treat the osteomalacia more effectively. This issue is unresolved. Patients with only osteomalacia usually fail to respond to 1,25(OH)$_2$D alone, but they have responded to 1,25(OH)$_2$D in combination with 24,25(OH)$_2$D, a metabolite not yet available for clinical use. The osteomalacia in renal osteodystrophy also appears to respond to the removal of aluminum with deferoxamine, a drug approved for the treatment of iron overload. Neither 24,25(OH)$_2$D nor deferoxamine has been approved by the United States Food and

TABLE 234–2. AVAILABLE VITAMIN D METABOLITES AND ANALOGUES

	Ergocalciferol	Dihydrotachysterol	Calcifediol	Calcitriol
Abbreviation	D_2	DHT	$25OHD_3$	$1,25(OH)_2D_3$
Physiologic dose	2.5–10 μg (1 μg = 40 units)	25–100 μg	1–5 μg	0.25–0.5 μg
Pharmacologic dose	0.625–5.0 mg	0.2–1.0 mg	20–200 μg	0.25–2.0 μg
Duration of action	1–3 months	1–4 weeks	2–6 weeks	2–5 days
Cost	$0.11/1.25 mg	$0.42/0.4 mg	$0.51/50 μg	$1.50/0.5 μg
Clinical applications	Vitamin D deficiency	Chronic renal failure	Vitamin D malabsorption	Chronic renal failure
	Vitamin D malabsorption	Hypoparathyroidism	Chronic renal failure	Hypoparathyroidism
	Hypoparathyroidism			Hypophosphatemic rickets
	Hypophosphatemic rickets			Acute hypocalcemia
	Anticonvulsant therapy in institutionalized patients			Vitamin D–dependent rickets types I and II

Drug Administration for the treatment of renal osteodystrophy, and both must currently be considered investigational drugs for this purpose.

NEPHROTIC SYNDROME

Even when vitamin D intake is adequate, vitamin D and its metabolites can be lost in the urine. The vitamin D metabolites in serum are tightly bound to an alpha globulin called vitamin D–binding protein (DBP). Patients with the nephrotic syndrome may lose substantial amounts of DBP into their urine and consequently have very low circulating levels of the vitamin D metabolites. Although the total concentration of all the vitamin D metabolites is reduced in this situation, the free (or unbound) concentration may be normal. Thus, the measurement of the total concentration may be misleading as to the severity of the vitamin D deficiency. The incidence of osteomalacia in patients with the nephrotic syndrome is unknown; osteomalacia has only recently been recognized as a complication of this renal disease.

LIVER DISEASE

The hepatic production of 25-hydroxyvitamin D (25OHD) is not tightly controlled. Neither cholestatic nor parenchymal liver disease has much effect on 25OHD production. The low levels of circulating 25OHD found in patients with liver disease can usually be attributed to reduced hepatic synthesis of DBP, poor nutrition, or malabsorption rather than to failure by the liver to metabolize vitamin D. As in patients with the nephrotic syndrome, the low total concentrations of the vitamin D metabolites in patients with liver disease may reflect the low levels of DBP and not a true state of vitamin D deficiency.

ANTICONVULSANTS

Phenytoin and phenobarbital induce drug-metabolizing enzymes in the liver that alter the hepatic metabolism of vitamin D. This effect may account for the lower circulating levels of 25OHD found in patients treated with anticonvulsants. Surprisingly, these drugs do not lead to a reduction in $1,25(OH)_2D$ levels. Chronic anticonvulsant therapy does not seem to lead to clinically significant osteomalacia unless accompanied by other predisposing factors, such as inadequate sunlight exposure or poor nutrition. However, some authorities have raised the possibility that phenytoin may exert a direct inhibitory effect on bone formation. Treatment is generally not required unless serum 25OHD levels are low, in which case modest vitamin D supplementation (400 to 2000 IU per day) may be advised.

HYPOPARATHYROIDISM

Parathyroid hormone is a major stimulator of $1,25(OH)_2D$ production. One would expect osteomalacia to develop when the hormone is absent, because of the reduction in $1,25(OH)_2D$ production. However, osteomalacia appears to be a rare complication of hypoparathyroidism.

VITAMIN D–DEPENDENT RICKETS TYPE I

Vitamin D–dependent rickets type I, or pseudo–vitamin D deficiency, is a rare autosomal recessive disease in which there is a low level of $1,25(OH)_2D$ resulting from a selective deficiency in the renal production of $1,25(OH)_2D$. Although affected patients do not respond to doses of vitamin D that are adequate to treat vitamin D deficiency (i.e., 400 to 4000 IU per day), they do respond to moderate doses (4000 to 40,000 IU per day) of vitamin D or physiologic doses (0.5 to 1.0 μg per day) of $1,25(OH)_2D$.

VITAMIN D–DEPENDENT RICKETS TYPE II

Vitamin D–dependent rickets type II (hereditary $1,25(OH)_2D$–resistant rickets) is a rare condition that occurs in childhood and is not responsive to even huge doses of vitamin D. Many children also present with alopecia. Unlike patients with vitamin D–dependent rickets type I (see above), children with type II disease have high circulating levels of $1,25(OH)_2D$. Their problem involves an abnormality in the number, affinity, or functions of the intracellular $1,25(OH)_2D$ receptor. Recently, the gene for the vitamin D receptor from several affected families has been sequenced, and point mutations in the zinc fingers of the DNA binding domain or in the steroid binding domain (resulting in a premature termination codon) have been identified. Just as the genetic defect in this syndrome varies from family to family, so, too, does the clinical response to $1,25(OH)_2D_3$ (calcitriol), which is generally used in large doses (2 to 6 μg per day).

PHOSPHATE DEFICIENCY

Chronic hypophosphatemia may lead to rickets or osteomalacia independently of other predisposing abnormalities. The principal diseases in which hypophosphatemia is associated with osteomalacia or rickets, however, also include other abnormalities that can interfere with bone mineralization. Chronic phosphate depletion is caused by decreased intestinal absorption or increased renal clearance. Acute hypophosphatemia can result from movement of phosphate into cells (e.g., after infusion of insulin and glucose), but this condition is transient and does not result in bone disease (see Ch. 194).

Seventy to 90 per cent of dietary phosphate is absorbed, primarily in the jejunum. This process is not tightly regulated, although vitamin D, at least in animal models, stimulates phosphate absorption. Meat and dairy products are the principal dietary sources of phosphate, and vegetarian diets that exclude them can cause phosphate deficiency. The incidence of osteomalacia in vegetarians who avoid all meat and dairy products is unknown, but its occurrence has been reported. Since these dietary practices also lead to decreased vitamin D intake, such individuals may be predisposed to bone disease.

Intrinsic small bowel disease and surgical rearrangement of the small bowel interfere with phosphate absorption and, if coupled with diarrhea or steatorrhea, can result in phosphate depletion. The hypophosphatemia may contribute to the osteomalacia seen in such patients, especially when vitamin D levels are reduced.

Eighty-five to 90 per cent of the phosphate filtered by the glomerulus is reabsorbed, primarily in the proximal tubule. This process is regulated by PTH, which reduces renal tubular phosphate reabsorption, and probably also by vitamin D, which appears to increase renal tubular phosphate reabsorption. Many diseases that affect renal handling of phosphate are associated with osteomalacia.

Treatment of phosphate deficiency is generally geared to correction of the primary problem. Oral preparations of phosphate (and the amounts required to provide 1 gram of elemental phosphorus) include Fleet Phospho-Soda (6.12 ml), Neutra-Phos (300 ml), and Phos-Tab (6 tablets). These preparations are usually given in amounts that provide 1 to 3 grams of phosphorus, although diarrhea may limit the dose. Careful attention to both serum calcium and serum phosphate concentrations is required to avoid hypocalcemia or ectopic calcification (should the calcium-phosphate product become too high).

ALUMINUM HYDROXIDE ANTACIDS

A number of widely used antacids (e.g., Mylanta, Maalox, Basaljel, and Amphojel) contain aluminum hydroxide, which binds phosphate and prevents its absorption. Patients who ingest large amounts of these antacids may become depleted in phosphate. This mechanism may contribute to the severity of the osteomalacia observed in patients with chronic renal failure and in those who have undergone partial gastrectomy but who continue to ingest large quantities of antacids (see Ch. 237).

DE TONI-DEBRÉ-FANCONI SYNDROME

The de Toni-Debré-Fanconi syndrome includes a heterogeneous group of disorders characterized by phosphaturia, aminoaciduria, glycosuria, and bicarbonaturia, and frequently mild acidosis and hypercalciuria. In general, the osteomalacia or rickets associated with these proximal tubular disorders responds only to large doses of vitamin D, with correction of the acidosis and hypophosphatemia as needed. The associated bone disease is most likely the result of a combination of systemic acidosis, hypophosphatemia, and abnormal vitamin D metabolism.

X-LINKED HYPOPHOSPHATEMIA

X-linked hypophosphatemia (vitamin D–resistant rickets, or VDRR) is characterized by renal phosphate wasting, hypophosphatemia, and a subtle decrease in $1,25(OH)_2D$ production. Children often present with florid rickets. Although most cases are diagnosed in childhood and have an X-linked dominant form of inheritance, sporadic adult cases and autosomal transmission occur. Most patients have $1,25(OH)_2D$ levels that are inappropriately low for the degree of hypophosphatemia, which ordinarily increases $1,25(OH)_2D$ production. Treatment with oral phosphate and vitamin D suppresses $1,25(OH)_2D$ to even lower levels. The primary abnormality in these patients is thought to be a defect in renal tubular phosphate transport, resulting in renal phosphate wasting. This defect may secondarily alter vitamin D metabolism. X-linked hypophosphatemia is a fairly common form of metabolic bone disease that should be suspected in all individuals who have low levels of serum phosphorus and evidence of bone disease.

The bone disease in patients with X-linked hypophosphatemia responds to the combination of phosphate (1 to 3 grams per day) and either large doses (25,000 to 100,000 IU) of vitamin D or more physiologic doses (0.25 to 1.0 µg per day) of $1,25(OH)_2D$. Neither phosphate nor vitamin D alone is as effective. Unfortunately, oral phosphate preparations also act as laxatives, and tolerance of full doses is sometimes difficult to achieve. A recently recognized complication of such treatment is the development of hyperparathyroidism later in life, thought to be phosphate induced.

TUMOR-INDUCED HYPOPHOSPHATEMIC OSTEOMALACIA

Certain unusual tumors (usually mesenchymal) produce osteomalacia associated with low serum levels of phosphorus and $1,25(OH)_2D$ and increased phosphaturia. The cause of this syndrome is unknown, but it is presumed that a humoral product of the tumor suppresses both $1,25(OH)_2D$ production and phosphate reabsorption in the kidney. Removal of the tumor reverses the abnormalities.

CHRONIC METABOLIC ACIDOSIS

Acute metabolic acidosis results in reduced $1,25(OH)_2D$ production. Although chronic metabolic acidosis is associated with osteomalacia, especially when accompanied by renal loss of phosphate and bicarbonate (as in proximal renal tubular acidosis), it is unclear whether chronic metabolic acidosis has a direct effect on the renal metabolism of vitamin D. Bicarbonate therapy alone is effective in treating the osteomalacia associated with renal tubular acidosis and ureterosigmoidostomy, although the addition of 0.25 to 1 mg of vitamin D per day may facilitate healing.

CALCIUM DEFICIENCY

Calcium deficiency may contribute to the mineralization defect that complicates gastrointestinal disease and proximal tubular disorders, but it is less well established as a cause of osteomalacia than is vitamin D or phosphate deficiency. In one carefully performed study of children who ingested a low-calcium diet, there was clinical, biochemical, and histologic evidence of osteomalacia. The serum phosphorus and 25OHD levels were normal, the serum alkaline phosphatase level was elevated, and the serum and urine calcium levels were low. Since intestinal absorption of calcium decreases with age, the daily requirement for calcium increases from approximately 800 mg in young adults to 1400 mg in the elderly. Calcium deficiency can result not only from inadequate dietary intake but also from excessive fecal and urinary losses. Except in cases in which a renal leak of calcium plays an important role in the etiology of calcium deficiency (certain forms of idiopathic hypercalciuria or following glucorticoid therapy for inflammatory diseases), urinary calcium excretion provides a useful means to determine the appropriate level of oral calcium replacement. Because of its low cost and high percentage of elemental calcium, calcium carbonate is the formulation of choice.

PRIMARY DISORDERS OF THE BONE MATRIX

Intrinsic disorders of bone in which matrix is produced but not normally mineralized are rare. Three diseases appear to fit this category, but none is well understood.

Hypophosphatasia

Hypophosphatasia, transmitted in an autosomal recessive pattern, usually manifests as a severe form of rickets in children, or merely as a predisposition to fractures in adults. The biochemical hallmarks are low serum (and tissue) levels of alkaline phosphatase and increased urinary levels of phosphoethanolamine. The reason these patients develop osteomalacia or rickets is unclear, but the following mechanism has been suggested. Skeletal alkaline phosphatase cleaves pyrophosphate, an inhibitor of bone mineralization; patients deficient in alkaline phosphatase may be unable to hydrolyze this inhibitor and so develop a mineralization defect.

Fibrogenesis Imperfecta Ossium

Fibrogenesis imperfecta ossium is a rare, painful disorder that affects middle-aged men in what appears to be a sporadic fashion. Serum alkaline phosphatase activity is increased. The bones have a dense, amorphous, mottled appearance radiologically and a disorganized arrangement of collagen with decreased birefringence histologically. Presumably, the disorganized collagen matrix retards normal bone mineralization.

Axial Osteomalacia

Unlike fibrogenesis imperfecta ossium, axial osteomalacia is not painful, involves only the axial skeleton, shows no disorganization of collagen on bone biopsy, and is not associated with increased serum alkaline phosphatase activity. The reason for the mineralization disorder in this rare disease is uncertain.

INHIBITORS OF MINERALIZATION

Several drugs are known to cause osteomalacia or rickets by inhibiting mineralization, but in no case is the mechanism fully understood.

Aluminum

Patients on hemodialysis are exposed to aluminum in the dialysate if tap water is used and through the antacid preparations used to control serum phosphorus levels. Most develop bone disease. Bone biopsies show a correlation between the extent of osteomalacia in these patients and the amount of aluminum deposited in bone. It is likely that the aluminum blocks normal mineralization. Severely affected patients respond to a reduction in their exposure to or body stores of the metal.

Many patients who are treated by total parenteral nutrition for extended periods develop bone disease characterized by osteomalacia. In some cases the aluminum content of the casein hydrolysate used to provide amino acids is high. Replacement of casein hydrolysate with purified amino acids may correct or prevent this complication.

Etidronate

Etidronate, the only diphosphonate available for clinical use in the United States, produces osteomalacia at doses greater than 5 to 10 mg per kilogram of body weight. Therefore, the dose must be limited. Etidronate affects osteoblast function and inhibits calcium phosphate crystallization. It is unclear why this drug and not other diphosphonates results in osteomalacia.

Phenytoin

As discussed previously (see Anticonvulsants), phenytoin therapy may cause osteomalacia by inducing enzymes that alter the hepatic metabolism of vitamin D. In addition, phenytoin directly and adversely affects bone mineral metabolism in animals. This effect may also contribute to bone disease.

Fluoride

Fluoride stimulates bone formation, but if it is administered in high doses without adequate calcium supplementation, the bone is poorly mineralized. The mechanism (or mechanisms) by which fluoride alters osteoblast function and bone mineralization is unknown.

Bikle DD: Calcium absorption and vitamin D metabolism. Clin Gastroenterol 12:379, 1983. *A review of the effect of vitamin D on the intestine and the gastrointestinal diseases that lead to osteomalacia.*

Bikle DD, Halloran BP, Gee E, et al.: Free 25-hydroxyvitamin D levels are normal in subjects with liver disease and reduced total 25-hydroxyvitamin D levels. J Clin Invest 78:748, 1986. *This article points out that total vitamin D metabolite concentrations may be reduced in patients with reduced DBP levels without a reduction in the free (and, possibly, the more physiologically relevant) vitamin D metabolite concentrations.*

Brenner RJ, Spring DB, Sebastion A, et al.: Incidence of radiologically evident bone disease, nephrocalcinosis, and nephrolithiasis in various types of renal tubular acidosis. N Engl J Med 307:217, 1982. *The authors point out that bone disease (osteomalacia) is much more common in proximal renal tubular acidosis than in distal renal tubular acidosis.*

Chesney RW, Mazess RB, Rose P, et al.: Long-term influence of calcitriol (1,25-dihydroxyvitamin D) and supplemental phosphate in X-linked hypophosphatemic rickets. Pediatrics 71:559, 1983. *This article discusses the modern therapy for this disease.*

Colussi G, de Ferrari ME, Surian M, et al.: Vitamin D metabolites and osteomalacia in the human Fanconi syndrome. Proc Eur Dial Transplant Assoc 21:756, 1984. *Five patients were evaluated; three had bone disease and low 1,25(OH)₂D levels.*

Curtis JA, Kooh SW, Fraser D, et al.: Nutritional rickets in vegetarian children. Can Med Assoc J 128:150, 1983. *Nutritional vitamin D deficiency continues to be a problem in those who omit milk and dairy products from their diet.*

Dibble JB, Sheridan P, Losowsky MS: A survey of vitamin D deficiency in gastrointestinal and liver disorders. Q J Med 209:119, 1984. *This article reports the results of a survey of 152 patients with gastrointestinal disease and 104 patients with chronic liver disease in whom 25OHD levels were assessed. Low levels of 25OHD were found in many patients, but osteomalacia was detected almost exclusively in patients with 25OHD levels below 2 per milliliter.*

Goldstein DA, Haldimann B, Sherman D, et al.: Vitamin D metabolites and calcium metabolism in patients with nephrotic syndrome and normal renal function. J Clin Endocrinol Metab 52:116, 1981. *This article describes the pathogenesis of osteomalacia in the nephrotic syndrome.*

Hahn TJ, Hendin BA, Scharp CR, et al.: Serum 25 hydroxycalciferol levels and bone mass in children on chronic anticonvulsant therapy. N Engl J Med 292:550, 1975. *The demonstration that chronic anticonvulsant therapy can lead to reduced 25OHD levels and bone mass in children. Vitamin D supplementation increased 25OHD levels.*

Hodsman AB, Iherrard DJ, Wong EGC, et al.: Vitamin D resistant osteomalacia in hemodialysis patients lacking secondary hyperparathyroidism. Ann Intern Med 94:629, 1981. *An early but thorough clinical description of patients with aluminum-associated osteomalacia occurring during hemodialysis.*

Mankin HJ: Rickets, osteomalacia, and renal osteodystrophy. Parts I and II. Am Bone Joint Surg 56A:101, 352, 1974. *A thorough review with an accounting of the history of the subject, a description of the clinical presentation of rickets, and a complete list of the etiologies of bone mineralization disorders.*

Marel GM, McKenna MJ, Frame B: Osteomalacia. Bone Mineral Res 4:335, 1986. *This is an excellent, complete, and up-to-date review of the subject.*

Marie PJ, Pettifor JM, Ross FP, et al.: Histological osteomalacia due to dietary

calcium deficiency in children. N Engl J Med 307:584, 1982. *This study indicates that calcium deficiency alone may be sufficient to cause osteomalacia.*

Parfitt AM, Gallagher JC, Heaney RP, et al.: Vitamin D and bone health in the elderly. Am J Clin Nutr 36:1014, 1982. *A review of the importance of adequate vitamin D intake in adults, discussing, among other issues, the high incidence of osteomalacia found in patients with hip fractures.*

Ritchie HH, Hughes MR, Thompson ET, et al.: An ochre mutation in the vitamin D receptor gene causes hereditary 1,25-dihydroxy vitamin D₃-resistant rickets in three families. Proc Natl Acad Sci USA 86:9783, 1989. *Describes a point mutation leading to a premature termination codon in the steroid binding domain. This same group demonstrated other point mutations in the DNA binding domain of the receptor gene from other families with this syndrome.*

Voights AL, Felsenfeld AJ, Flach F: The effects of calciferol and its metabolites on patients with chronic renal failure. Arch Intern Med 143:960, 1205, 1983. *In this two-part review, the authors evaluate the data concerning the most appropriate vitamin D metabolite (or analogue) to use in the treatment of the various types of renal osteodystrophy.*

Weider N, Cruz DS: Phosphaturic mesenchymal tumors: A polymorphous group causing osteomalacia or rickets. Cancer 59:1442, 1987. *An excellent review of 17 cases of this syndrome of reversible bone disease caused by tumors.*

235 The Parathyroid Glands, Hypercalcemia, and Hypocalcemia
Allen M. Spiegel

THE PARATHYROID GLANDS

EMBRYOLOGY AND ANATOMY. Normally, there are four parathyroids, averaging 120 mg in total weight, but as many as 5 per cent of normal individuals may have more than four glands. The superior parathyroids are derived from the fourth (more caudal) branchial pouches and remain almost stationary during embryologic development. Their typical final location is near the upper poles of the thyroid. Aberrant locations include the tracheoesophageal groove and the retroesophageal space. The inferior parathyroids develop (in association with the thymus) from the third branchial pouches. During normal development, they migrate caudally, assuming a final position near the lower poles of the thyroid. The inferior parathyroids may fail to descend, remaining near the angle of the jaw, or, at the other extreme, may descend into the anterior mediastinum in association with the thymus.

SYNTHESIS AND SECRETION OF PARATHYROID HORMONE (PTH). Parathyroid hormone, together with vitamin D (Ch. 233), is the principal regulator of ionized calcium in extracellular fluid. Parathyroid hormone is synthesized in the parathyroid glands as "preproparathyroid hormone," a precursor composed of 115 amino acids. A hydrophobic "leader" peptide of 25 amino acids is first cleaved from the amino-terminus to yield the prohormone, followed by cleavage of a basic, amino-terminal hexapeptide to yield the mature 84-amino-acid hormone. The latter is the principal secreted form of the hormone. There is no evidence for secretion of either the preprohormone or the prohormone. The prohormone possesses less than 0.2 per cent of the biologic activity of the native, 84-amino-acid hormone. The full biologic activity of the intact hormone resides within the amino-terminal 1–34 fragment, whereas fragments from the midregion and carboxy-terminal regions lack biologic activity (Fig. 235–1).

Secretion of PTH is regulated primarily by the concentration of ionized calcium in the extracellular fluid. Normally, PTH secretion is regulated at a "setpoint" that maintains serum ionized calcium within a relatively narrow range. Deviations below the setpoint stimulate, and deviations above the setpoint inhibit, hormone secretion. Effects of calcium on hormone secretion occur acutely (within minutes); low calcium levels have a slower stimulatory action on hormone synthesis. At high calcium concentrations, there is evidence for intracellular degradation of synthesized hormone and possible release of biologically inactive fragments. High magnesium ion concentrations in extracellular fluid, like high calcium concentrations, inhibit PTH secretion, but hypomagnesemia, unlike hypocalcemia, may inhibit hormone

FIGURE 235–1. Secretion, metabolism, and clearance of parathyroid hormone. *Top,* Parathyroid hormone (PTH) is synthesized as a preprohormone and undergoes successive cleavages within the parathyroid to the mature (1–84), major secreted form of the hormone. Under certain conditions (e.g., hypercalcemia), some of the hormone is cleaved intracellularly into biologically inactive, carboxy-terminal fragments, which are also secreted. *Middle,* The major circulating forms of the hormone are the intact 1–84 species (the shaded region corresponds to the amino-terminal 1–34 portion possessing full biologic activity) and biologically inactive carboxy-terminal fragments. The presence of amino-terminal fragments in the circulation is unclear (indicated by "?"). *Bottom,* Peripheral metabolism of the hormone occurs in liver and kidney. The kidney also clears intact hormone and carboxy-terminal fragments from the circulation. (From Endres DE, Villanueva R, Sharp CF Jr, et al.: Measurement of parathyroid hormone. Endocrinol Metab Clin North Am 18:611, 1989.)

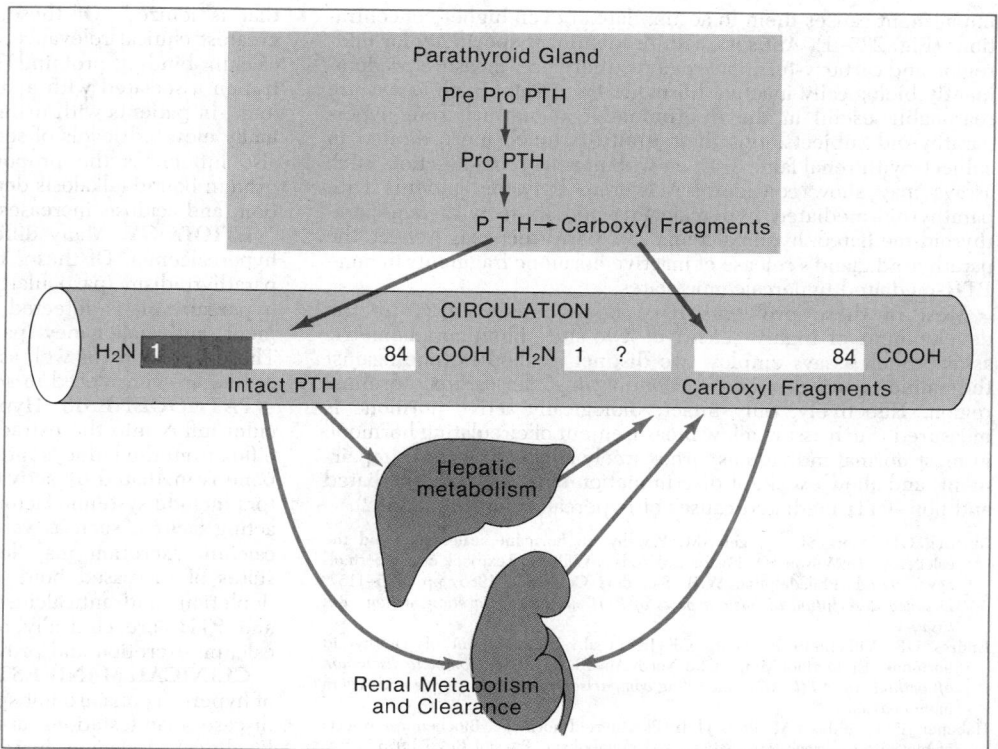

secretion and action. The active metabolite of vitamin D, 1,25(OH)$_2$D (dihydroxycholecalciferol), suppresses both secretion and synthesis of PTH. Reduction in 1,25(OH)$_2$D is a major factor contributing to increased PTH secretion in renal failure.

FORMS OF PARATHYROID HORMONE IN PLASMA. Parathyroid hormone circulates in plasma as the intact hormone secreted from the gland and as fragments derived either from glandular secretion (particularly in hypercalcemic states) or from peripheral metabolism of the intact hormone. Most, if not all, of these fragments lack biologic activity but may, depending on antibody specificity, contribute to immunoreactivity in plasma (Fig. 235–1).

PARATHYROID HORMONE ACTION. Parathyroid hormone acts directly on kidney and bone, and indirectly on the gut, to maintain the normal concentration of serum ionized calcium (see Ch. 232 for a complete discussion of mineral homeostasis). In the kidney, PTH (1) enhances reabsorption of calcium, and also magnesium, from the glomerular filtrate; (2) increases excretion of phosphate and of bicarbonate; (3) activates the enzyme (1-α-hydroxylase) that forms the active metabolite, 1,25(OH)$_2$D, of vitamin D. In bone, PTH causes the release of calcium and phosphate into the extracellular fluid. The hormone acts directly on osteoblasts, which secondarily affect osteoclast activity. The hypercalcemic action on bone and the anticalciuric action on kidney combine to raise the serum calcium level. The phosphatemic action on bone would tend to blunt the hypercalcemic effect of the hormone owing to formation of calcium phosphate complexes, but the phosphaturic action counteracts the tendency to hyperphosphatemia. Stimulation of 1,25(OH)$_2$D formation promotes enhanced intestinal absorption of calcium, which also serves to maintain a normal serum calcium level (see Ch. 233). The clinical consequences of PTH excess (or in the opposite directions, hormone deficiency) follow directly from the actions of the hormone: (1) hypercalcemia; (2) a tendency to hypophosphatemia; (3) a tendency to reduced serum bicarbonate levels and hyperchloremia; (4) increased serum levels of 1,25(OH)$_2$D; and (5) relative reduction in urinary calcium excretion and increase in urinary phosphate excretion for a given filtered load.

MECHANISM OF PARATHYROID HORMONE ACTION. The first step in PTH action is binding to specific plasma membrane–bound receptors on target cells in bone and kidney. Such receptors are coupled to guanosine triphosphate (GTP)–binding proteins—in particular, the Gs protein that links receptors to stimulation of adenylyl cyclase (for a more general description of the mechanism of polypeptide hormone action, see Ch. 208). Adenylyl cyclase catalyzes the formation of the "second messenger," cyclic adenosine monophosphate (AMP), which mediates hormone action by stimulating the phosphorylation of critical intracellular proteins. A clinically useful peculiarity of PTH action on proximal renal tubular cells is that not only are cyclic AMP levels increased intracellularly but, because of overflow into the extracellular fluid, urinary cyclic AMP excretion is also increased. "Second messengers" other than cyclic AMP may also mediate certain actions of PTH.

ASSAY OF PARATHYROID HORMONE IN PLASMA. Normally, the concentration of biologically active PTH circulating in plasma is quite low (<50 pg per milliliter). Bioassays sensitive enough to detect such low levels include a renal cytochemical assay and several assays based on stimulation of cyclic AMP formation in bone or kidney cells. Unfortunately, such assays are too cumbersome for routine clinical use. Total urinary cyclic AMP excretion (normalized to creatinine clearance by simultaneous measurement of serum and urinary creatinine) is an easily measured and sensitive index of circulating PTH bioactivity. It is elevated in primary hyperparathyroidism, is low in hypoparathyroidism, and falls within 1 hour of successful parathyroidectomy in patients with hyperparathyroidism. Increased urinary cyclic AMP excretion, however, is not absolutely specific for PTH hypersecretion; parathyroid hormone–related peptide, secreted by many malignancies, similarly increases urinary cyclic AMP excretion, and this must be taken into account in the interpretation of urinary cyclic AMP measurements in subjects with hypercalcemia (see Hypercalcemia Associated with Malignancy, below).

Radioimmunoassays are sufficiently sensitive and practial for the routine measurement of circulating PTH. Interpretation of assay results requires an understanding of what a particular antiserum is measuring. Immunoreactivity need not correlate with biologic activity. Indeed, the bulk of circulating PTH consists of biologically inactive mid-region and carboxy-terminal fragments. Since such fragments are cleared by the kidney, renal impairment causes them to accumulate at even higher concentrations (Fig. 235–1). Antisera with predominant specificity for mid-region and carboxy-terminal regions, therefore, measure predominantly biologically inactive hormone fragments. Such assays are reasonably useful in the discrimination of normal from hyperparathyroid subjects, but their utility is much more limited in subjects with renal failure. Even with normal renal function, such assays may show considerable overlap between patients with parathyroid-mediated hypercalcemia and those with non–parathyroid-mediated hypercalcemia. In part, this may reflect the parathyroid gland's release of inactive hormone fragments in non–PTH-mediated hypercalcemic states.

Most of these problems have been circumvented by the development of highly sensitive "two-site" immunoradiometric assays. Such assays employ two distinct antibodies, one against the amino-terminal region and one against the carboxy-terminal region. Effectively, only intact, biologically active hormone is measured. Such assays allow measurement of circulating hormone in most normal individuals, are scarcely affected by renal impairment, and allow excellent discrimination between PTH-mediated and non–PTH-mediated causes of hypercalcemia (Fig. 235–2).

Aurbach GD, Marx SJ, Spiegel AM: Parathyroid hormone, calcitonin, and the calciferols. *In* Wilson JD, Foster DW (eds.): Williams Textbook of Endocrinology. 7th ed. Philadelphia, W.B. Saunders Company, 1985, pp 1146–1157. *Detailed description of basic aspects of PTH synthesis, secretion, action, and assay.*

Endres DB, Villanueva R, Sharp CF Jr, et al.: Measurement of parathyroid hormone. Endocrinol Metab Clin North Am 18:611, 1989. *Complete discussion of methods for PTH assay, including comparison of two-site versus mid-region immunoassays.*

Habener JF, Rosenblatt M, Potts JT Jr: Parathyroid hormone: Biochemical aspects of biosynthesis, secretion, action, and metabolism. Physiol Rev 64:985, 1984. *Extensive review of basic aspects of PTH synthesis and action, together with relevant clinical implications.*

Nussbaum SR, Zahradnik RJ, Lavigne RJ, et al.: A highly sensitive two site immunoradiometric assay of parathyrin (PTH) and its clinical utility in evaluating patients with hypercalcemia. Clin Chem 33:1364, 1987. *Description of prototype of most clinically useful assay for PTH.*

HYPERCALCEMIA

DEFINITION. Hypercalcemia is defined as an abnormal elevation in serum ionized calcium concentration.* Since total,

*See Ch. 232 and Part XXVII for calcium and phosphorus reference range values in serum and urine.

rather than ionized, calcium is generally measured, one must be aware of factors that influence the fraction of total serum calcium that is ionized. Of these, serum albumin concentration is of greatest clinical relevance, since albumin is the chief circulating calcium-binding protein. "Normal" total serum calcium concentration associated with a significant reduction in serum albumin (e.g., in patients with malignancy) may actually represent abnormally elevated levels of serum ionized calcium. Acid-base status also influences the proportion of total serum calcium that is protein bound (alkalosis decreases the ionized calcium concentration, and acidosis increases it).

ETIOLOGY. Many different diseases are potential causes of hypercalcemia. Of these, the most common are primary hyperparathyroidism (particularly in asymptomatic individuals whose hypercalcemia is detected by routine serum chemistry measurement) and malignancy (particularly in hospitalized individuals). These disorders, as well as some of the rarer causes of hypercalcemia, are considered in separate sections below.

PATHOGENESIS. Hypercalcemia results from excessive calcium influx into the extracellular fluid from bone and decreased efflux from the kidneys into the urine. Calcium mobilization from bone is mediated by activators of bone resorption. These activators include systemic factors (e.g., PTH, $1,25(OH)_2D$) and locally acting factors, such as various lymphokines. Reduction in renal calcium excretion may lead to hypercalcemia, particularly in states of increased bone turnover. Renal impairment, volume depletion, and anticalciuretic agents, such as thiazide diuretics and PTH, are clinically relevant factors that can reduce renal calcium excretion and provoke hypercalcemia.

CLINICAL MANIFESTATIONS. Many of the manifestations of hypercalcemia are not specific to the underlying cause (specific disease manifestations are discussed under individual disease headings). Extreme hypercalcemia leads to coma and death. Neurologic manifestations in less severe cases may include confusion, lethargy, weakness, and hyporeflexia. Hypercalcemia may be detected by shortening of the QT interval on the electrocardiogram. Arrhythmias are rare, but bradycardia and first-degree heart block have been reported. Acute hypercalcemia may be associated with significant hypertension. Gastrointestinal manifestations include constipation and anorexia; in severe cases, there may be nausea and vomiting. Acute pancreatitis has been reported in association with hypercalcemia of various causes. Hypercalcemia interferes with antidiuretic hormone action, thereby leading to polyuria and polydipsia. Reversible reduction in renal function associated with significant hypercalcemia is

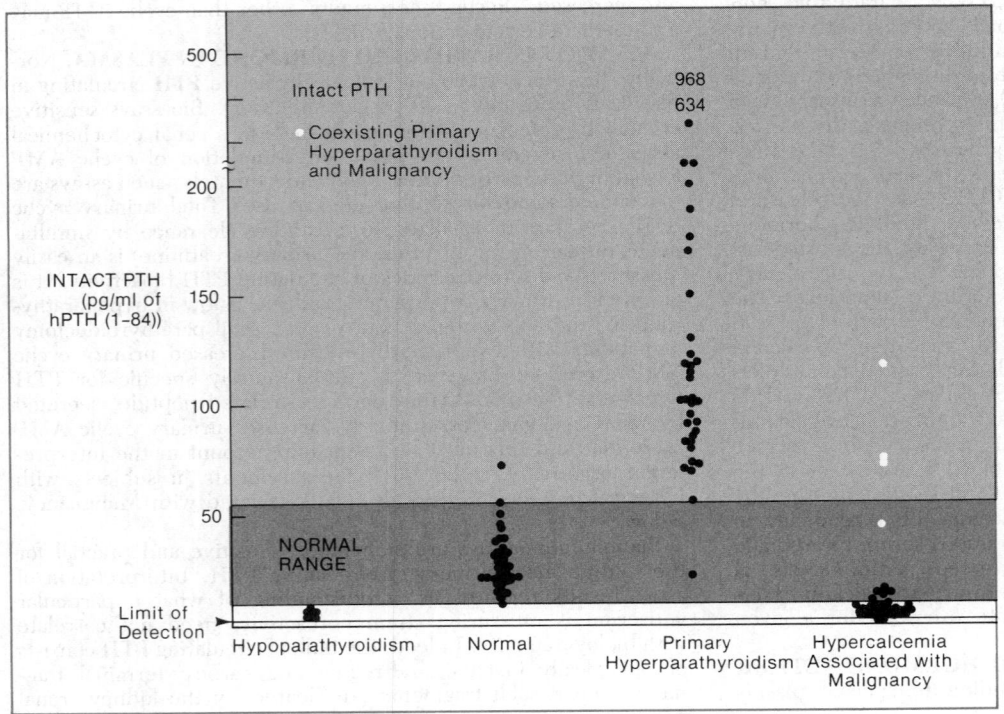

FIGURE 235–2. Two-site immunoassay for PTH in serum. The two-site method measures exclusively intact PTH. The hormone is detectable in the majority of normal subjects and undetectable in patients with various forms of hypoparathyroidism. Almost all patients with primary hyperparathyroidism show values outside the normal range. In contrast, values are low to undetectable in patients with malignancy-associated hypercalcemia, except for four individuals with coexistent primary hyperparathyroidism. (From Endres DB, Villanueva R, Sharp CF Jr, et al.: Measurement of parathyroid hormone. Endocrinol Metab Clin North Am 18:611, 1989.)

TABLE 235–1. CAUSES OF HYPERCALCEMIA

Parathyroid Hormone–Mediated Causes
  Primary hyperparathyroidism
    Sporadic, familial (multiple endocrine neoplasia types I and II)
  Familial hypocalciuric hypercalcemia*
  Ectopic secretion of parathyroid hormone by tumors (very rare)
Non–Parathyroid Hormone–Mediated Causes
  Malignancy associated
    Local osteolytic hypercalcemia
    Humoral hypercalcemia of malignancy
  Vitamin D mediated
    Vitamin D intoxication
    Excessive production of 1,25(OH)$_2$D in granulomatous disorders
  Other endocrinopathies
    Thyrotoxicosis
    Hypoadrenalism
Immobilization with increased bone turnover, e.g., Paget's disease
Acute renal failure with rhabdomyolysis
Calcium carbonate ingestion (milk-alkali syndrome)

*Parathyroid hormone secretion is necessary for hypercalcemia but is not the primary defect.

followed by more permanent damage if hypercalcemia persists. Particularly if serum phosphorus is also increased, hypercalcemia can lead to nephrocalcinosis and interstitial nephritis. Hypercalciuria and nephrolithiasis may also occur. Deposition of calcium in other soft tissues, including skin and cornea, is most likely to occur in patients with associated hyperphosphatemia.

DIFFERENTIAL DIAGNOSIS. Potential causes of hypercalcemia are listed in Table 235–1. These may be divided into PTH-mediated (primary hyperparathyroidism) and non–PTH-mediated diseases (all others). Although ectopic secretion of PTH by tumors was long considered a potential cause of PTH-mediated hypercalcemia, there is now general agreement that ectopic secretion of authentic PTH (as opposed to parathyroid hormone–related peptides; see below) by tumors is extremely rare. The first step in the differential diagnosis of hypercalcemia is to establish whether or not PTH hypersecretion is present, since subsequent diagnostic maneuvers and definitive therapy critically depend on this distinction.

Readily measured blood and urine chemistries may offer some clues to diagnosis. In theory, PTH hypersecretion should be reflected by hypophosphatemia, hyperchloremia, hypobicarbonatemia, increased urinary phosphate excretion, and urinary calcium excretion that is relatively low for the filtered load. Suppression of PTH secretion by hypercalcemia of non-parathyroid etiology should, in theory, change these parameters to the opposite direction. In practice, there is often considerable overlap in each of these parameters between patients with parathyroid-mediated forms of hypercalcemia and those with non–parathyroid–mediated forms. This situation may reflect confounding variables, such as vomiting, diuretic treatment, and renal failure, as well as the ability of certain hypercalcemic agents to mimic many actions of PTH. Most important in this respect is parathyroid hormone–related peptide, first isolated from tumors associated with the syndrome of humoral hypercalcemia. This peptide mimics all of the known actions of PTH on kidney and bone, including increasing urinary cyclic AMP excretion and stimulating renal formation of 1,25(OH)$_2$D. Decreased urinary cyclic AMP excretion (with normal renal function) strongly suggests non–PTH-mediated hypercalcemia, but increased urinary cyclic AMP excretion is compatible with both primary hyperparathyroidism and tumor secretion of parathyroid hormone–related peptide. Serum 1,25(OH)$_2$D concentration also does not allow definitive diagnosis. It may be elevated in primary hyperparathyroidism and vitamin D–related causes of hypercalcemia and may be reduced in other non–parathyroid-mediated causes of hypercalcemia. For reasons that are not entirely clear, the serum 1,25(OH)$_2$D level is often low in patients with malignancies secreting parathyroid hormone–related peptide, despite the ability of the peptide to stimulate 1,25(OH)$_2$D formation.

Definitive distinction between parathyroid- and non–parathyroid-mediated causes of hypercalcemia relies primarily on PTH immunoassay. As discussed earlier, this distinction is best made with the two-site type of assay that measures intact PTH and is unaffected by renal function (Fig. 235–2). An elevated PTH level

secures the diagnosis of primary hyperparathyroidism. In selected cases with coexistent malignancy, the unlikely possibility of ectopic PTH secretion may be excluded by selective venous sampling and assay of PTH, but generally this testing is unnecessary. Hormone levels in the normal range suggest the possibility of familial hypocalciuric hypercalcemia. This entity is discussed further in the section on hyperparathyroidism. Low to undetectable values for PTH place the patient in the non–parathyroid-mediated category. Additional testing is necessary to establish a specific diagnosis within this group. Immunoassays for parathyroid hormone–related peptide have been developed, and these may allow the diagnosis of hypercalcemia caused by tumor secretion of this agent. Complete clinical evaluation, including history (e.g., vitamin ingestion, chronicity of symptoms), physical examination (masses, lymphadenopathy), radiologic studies, and other blood tests (e.g., thyroid and adrenal function), may point to a diagnosis. The diagnostic approach to hypercalcemia is summarized in Table 235–2.

TREATMENT. The definitive treatment of hypercalcemia depends on the specific diagnosis and treatment of the underlying disease, e.g., parathyroidectomy for primary hyperparathyroidism, chemotherapy for a malignancy. The initial treatment of hypercalcemia can be instituted (and in acute hypercalcemic crisis, often *must* be instituted) without a specific diagnosis, but cumulative toxicity and loss of efficacy preclude long-term nonspecific treatment. Measures aimed at reducing the serum calcium level act by increasing urinary calcium excretion and by decreasing bone resorption. General measures applicable to every patient include mobilization as soon as feasible (since immobility increases bone resorption) and hydration (since significant hypercalcemia causes dehydration). Volume depletion, by limiting renal calcium excretion, perpetuates a vicious circle that can lead to acute hypercalcemic crisis. Volume expansion with isotonic saline often significantly reduces the serum calcium level by enhancing renal calcium excretion. Only after volume repletion should diuretics be employed to enhance sodium and thereby calcium excretion. With a vigorous saline diuresis, calcium excretion in the range of 1 to 2 grams per day can be achieved as a temporary measure to reduce the serum calcium level. In patients with renal failure, dialysis can be employed almost as effectively to remove calcium from extracellular fluid. Careful monitoring of cardiac function and serum electrolytes is necessary with both saline diuresis and dialysis treatment.

Since increased bone resorption is the principal factor causing hypercalcemia in most patients, measures aimed at inhibiting bone resorption are generally most effective. Agents that inhibit osteoclast function (the "final common pathway" of bone resorption) are effective irrespective of the specific factor causing

TABLE 235–2. DIAGNOSTIC APPROACH TO HYPERCALCEMIA

1. Distinguish parathyroid hormone–mediated forms of hypercalcemia from non–parathyroid hormone–mediated forms: *Parathyroid hormone immunoassay (preferably two-site type) is the definitive test.*

2. If the parathyroid hormone level is elevated, primary hyperparathyroidism is the most likely diagnosis: *Family history for hypercalcemia should be checked to distinguish sporadic from familial (multiple endocrine neoplasia syndromes and hypocalciuric hypercalcemia) disease. Marginal elevation in parathyroid hormone levels, particularly in young, asymptomatic individuals, should prompt urine calcium measurement to exclude familial hypocalciuric hypercalcemia. In patients with coexisting malignancy, selective venous sampling can be done to exclude ectopic parathyroid hormone secretion, but the latter is extremely rare.*

3. If parathyroid hormone is low or undetectable, further laboratory tests (in addition to complete history, physical, and radiologic studies) are needed to distinguish among the various forms of non–parathyroid hormone–mediated forms of hypercalcemia: *Increased urinary cyclic AMP excretion suggests tumor secretion of parathyroid hormone–related peptide (direct radioimmunoassays for this peptide should shortly become widely available). Increased 1,25(OH)$_2$D suggests granulomatous disease (including some types of lymphoma).*

increased bone resorption. Available agents include calcitonin, plicamycin (mithramycin), and biphosphonates (diphosphonates). Calcitonin should theoretically be the ideal agent, given its low toxicity and specific action in inhibiting osteoclast function. In practice, the effectiveness of calcitonin is often limited and transient. Dosages of up to 32 MRC units per kilogram per day have been given by intravenous infusion. Plicamycin, in doses of 25 μg per kilogram as an intravenous bolus, is generally quite effective in lowering the serum calcium level within 24 to 48 hours. Depending on the underlying process, the effect may last for several days. Unfortunately, repeated treatment causes cumulative liver and renal toxicity, as well as thrombocytopenia. Biphosphonates, effective both orally and parenterally, have been used extensively in Europe but are not available in the United States. Only etidronate is available here, and it must be given intravenously in dosages of 7.5 mg per kilogram per day to treat hypercalcemia effectively.

Inorganic phosphate salts lower the serum calcium level when given intravenously but pose a serious danger of metastatic calcification in the hypercalcemic patient. Sudden hypotension, renal failure, and death have been reported after phosphate infusion treatment. Doses of up to 50 mmole (about 1.5 grams of elemental phosphorus) infused over 6 to 8 hours can be given if the serum calcium level must be lowered and all other measures fail. Oral phosphate is considerably safer. It is useful in patients with significant hypercalcemia who are awaiting definitive treatment and in whom one wishes to prevent development of hypercalcemic crisis. Dosages in the range of 2 grams of elemental phosphorus (10 grams of phosphate salts) per day in divided doses can be given. The serum phosphate level and renal function must be carefully monitored.

Glucocorticoids are highly effective in treating hypercalcemia caused by vitamin D–related mechanisms (vitamin D intoxication, overproduction of $1,25(OH)_2D$ in granulomatous disorders) and by certain malignancies (cytokine release associated with myeloma) but are ineffective in most other forms of hypercalcemia, including hyperparathyroidism and most malignancies. Forty to 100 mg per day of prednisone or the equivalent is the usual dose range. Indomethacin was reported to lower the serum calcium level in prostaglandin-mediated hypercalcemia but has proved generally ineffective. Novel agents under study that may become available in the future include gallium nitrate, shown to be effective in the hypercalcemia of malignancy, and WR-2721, reportedly effective in some cases of parathyroid carcinoma.

PRIMARY HYPERPARATHYROIDISM

DEFINITION. Primary hyperparathyroidism is a disorder in which hypercalcemia is due to hypersecretion of PTH.

ETIOLOGY. In most cases (about 85 per cent), hyperparathyroidism is caused by sporadic, solitary adenomas. Hyperplasia of all four glands occurs in about 10 per cent of cases, and these are most often familial, in the context of three distinct autosomal dominant inherited diseases: multiple endocrine neoplasia types I and II and familial hypocalciuric hypercalcemia. Carcinoma occurs rarely (<5 per cent of cases). The genes for multiple endocrine neoplasia types I and II have been linked to chromosomes 11 (q13) and 10, respectively. In no case has the etiology been clearly defined, but molecular genetic evidence indicates that almost all sporadic adenomas, as well as enlarged glands in multiple endocrine neoplasia type I, are monoclonal tumors. A high percentage of such tumors show loss of alleles at 11q13. This finding suggests that loss of a "tumor suppressor gene" from this locus may be instrumental in tumorigenesis. Epidemiologic evidence demonstrates a higher incidence of parathyroid tumors in subjects receiving neck irradiation in the past. Specific mutations associated with such tumors have not been defined. Finally, it has long been postulated that longstanding secondary hyperparathyroidism (e.g., in response to hypocalcemia of renal failure) may evolve into autonomous hypersecretion, "tertiary hyperparathyroidism." If such a transition occurs, its molecular basis has yet to be identified.

INCIDENCE. The incidence of hyperparathyroidism has increased substantially, largely as a result of routine blood calcium measurement. Age-adjusted incidence rates are between 25 and 50 per 100,000, based on recent surveys. A prevalence between 0.1 and 0.5 per cent has been estimated, with females affected about twice as commonly as males. The incidence rises sharply after age 40.

PATHOLOGY. Microscopic distinction between adenoma and hyperplasia is difficult, if not impossible. The distinction between single-gland and multigland disease relies on gross surgical identification of more than one enlarged gland. In multiple endocrine neoplasia types I and II, there is always multigland involvement, although asymmetric gland enlargement is often present. The chief cell generally predominates in parathyroid tumors; oxyphil cell tumors are much rarer.

PATHOPHYSIOLOGY. The primary disturbance is inappropriate secretion of PTH for the level of serum calcium. Studies in vitro with isolated parathyroid cells show that most adenomas either fail to suppress secretion at high calcium levels or show an altered setpoint, i.e., a higher calcium level is required to suppress secretion than for normal cells. Cells from hyperplastic glands may show a normal calcium setpoint for secretion. Hypersecretion of PTH in such cases may be due to a primary defect causing cellular proliferation and to an inability to suppress hormone secretion completely because of increased cell mass.

Slight increases in PTH secretion act on bone to increase turnover and may cause a reduction in cortical rather than trabecular bone density. At very high levels, PTH causes radiographically detectable subperiosteal bone resorption and, eventually, marrow fibrosis and cystic, reparative bone lesions termed "brown tumors." This is the classic form of the disease called "osteitis fibrosa cystica." Parathyroid hormone increases renal calcium reabsorption, but at high filtered loads of calcium, hypercalciuria, nonetheless, develops. Enhanced $1,25(OH)_2D$ formation by the kidneys is prominent in some patients and is associated with increased intestinal calcium absorption. Such patients may be at particular risk for renal stone formation.

CLINICAL MANIFESTATIONS. Most patients today either are asymptomatic at presentation (discovered through incidental blood calcium measurement) or present with vague, nonspecific symptoms, such as fatigue, weakness, and mental disturbance. Patients with significant hypercalcemia show many of the signs and symptoms of hypercalcemia discussed above. Nephrolithiasis, with or without renal colic, is not specifically associated with hyperparathyroidism but is most commonly seen in this setting. Subperiosteal bone resorption is rarely seen today, and osteitis fibrosa cystica even less commonly. Neuromuscular abnormalities, particularly proximal muscle weakness affecting the lower limbs, may be prominent. Joint manifestations include chondrocalcinosis that may lead to pseudogout. It has been claimed that hypertension, peptic ulcer disease, and osteoporosis are manifestations of hyperparathyroidism, but these are all common, and there is no firm evidence for a causal relationship between hyperparathyroidism and any of these disorders. There are no specific physical findings in hyperparathyroidism. A neck mass, if present, most commonly represents a coincidental thyroid nodule, less commonly a benign or malignant parathyroid tumor. "Band keratopathy," calcification at "3 and 9 o'clock" of the cornea, is best seen by slit-lamp examination and occurs most often when hypercalcemia is accompanied by hyperphosphatemia—thus less commonly in hyperparathyroidism than in other hypercalcemic disorders. Radiologic findings include subperiosteal resorption, which, when present, is best seen at the radial sides of the phalanges, distal phalangeal tufts, and distal clavicles. Lucent bone lesions, representing brown tumors, are seen in rare, severely affected patients. Soft tissue calcification may be evident in the joints, kidneys, and lungs. The calcification is best appreciated on bone scans.

DIAGNOSIS. The differential diagnosis of hypercalcemia is discussed above. Parathyroid hormone immunoassay, preferably one of the newer two-site assays, is the key to diagnosis. In making the distinction between hyperparathyroid and normal states (e.g., in patients presenting with nephrolithiasis), repeated careful serum calcium and PTH (including the mid-region type of assay) measurements are most useful. Hypercalcemic subjects taking lithium or thiazides should be retested for hyperparathyroidism after discontinuation of the drug (this may not be feasible in some patients on lithium), since both drugs may alter serum calcium and parathyroid hormone secretion. In relatively young, asymptomatic individuals, or if the serum PTH level is marginally elevated, hypercalcemia may be due to familial hypocalciuric hypercalcemia rather than hyperparathyroidism (see discussion below under Familial Hypocalciuric Hypercalcemia).

PROGNOSIS AND TREATMENT. Surgical parathyroidectomy is the only definitive treatment for hyperparathyroidism. Oral phosphate treatment can lower the serum calcium level, but the long-term safety and efficacy of this approach are unclear. In mildly affected, older women, estrogen treatment has been advocated, particularly to blunt bone resorption, but, again, long-term efficacy is unknown. Thus, the only alternative to surgery at present is conservative medical follow-up. Most experts recommend surgery for all patients with symptomatic disease and even for asymptomatic patients meeting other, somewhat arbitrary, criteria, such as age below 40 or a serum calcium level higher than 11.5 mg per deciliter. The appropriate management of patients not fitting any of these criteria is controversial, with some advocating surgery for all, and others conservative follow-up. The long-term course of untreated hyperparathyroidism is unknown. Controlled studies comparing surgery versus medical follow-up have not been performed. Small series of patients followed conservatively for several years suggest that mild biochemical disease rarely progresses to severe symptomatic disease, but it is difficult to exclude subtle abnormalities, such as reduced bone density. Since definitive treatment recommendations are not possible, therapy must be individualized. The author personally follows a policy of recommending surgery for all but older patients with only mild, biochemical disease.

If the decision is to perform surgery, the crucial issue is to find a highly experienced parathyroid surgeon. A success rate as high as 95 per cent can be expected for initial neck exploration by a skilled surgeon. The success rate is substantially lower with inexperienced surgeons. Preoperative localization is not needed by the skilled surgeon performing initial exploration. Neither localization studies nor neck exploration itself should serve as *diagnostic* maneuvers. Only after the diagnosis has been established biochemically (by PTH assay) should one recommend surgery. In patients undergoing repeat neck exploration for recurrent or persistent disease, localization studies are extremely helpful. Noninvasive studies include ultrasound, technetium-thallium scanning, computed tomography (CT), and magnetic resonance imaging. Invasive techniques include fine-needle aspiration of imaged lesions for PTH assay, selective arteriography, and selective venous catheterization for hormone assay. The latter techniques are best performed by radiologists with specialized experience.

After successful surgery, hypocalcemia is generally mild and transient and rarely requires treatment. In the rare case of subjects with extensive bone disease, severe, prolonged hypocalcemia secondary to "bone hunger" occurs. Persistent relative hypophosphatemia suggests that bone hunger, rather than hypoparathyroidism, is the cause of hypocalcemia in this setting. Acute treatment with calcium infusions and long-term treatment with vitamin D and oral calcium may be needed. Eventually, treatment can be discontinued if normal parathyroid tissue remains. In patients without residual normal parathyroid tissue, lifelong vitamin D therapy is necessary. Autotransplantation of parathyroid tissue in the forearm is an experimental alternative in such cases. Successful surgery generally halts formation of renal stones in patients with nephrolithiasis and allows skeletal remineralization in patients with bone disease. There is no definitive evidence that surgery corrects hypertension or other nonspecific manifestations of hyperparathyroidism.

FAMILIAL HYPOCALCIURIC HYPERCALCEMIA

DEFINITION. This is an autosomal dominant genetic disease with essentially complete penetrance that causes hypercalcemia and relatively low urinary calcium excretion for the filtered load.

ETIOLOGY. The etiology is unknown, and the chromosomal localization of the "disease gene" has yet to be identified.

INCIDENCE. The disorder is relatively rare, but it is over-represented among patients presenting with unsuccessful neck exploration because of the difficulty in achieving normocalcemia by surgery.

PATHOPHYSIOLOGY. The primary disturbance appears to be in divalent cation transport and/or "sensing" in at least the kidneys and parathyroids. The kidneys show an exaggerated

reabsorption of filtered calcium (and magnesium) that leads to hypercalcemia. The parathyroids, however, fail to suppress fully hormone secretion despite hypercalcemia. The process is PTH dependent, since totally parathyroidectomized subjects become hypocalcemic, but even small amounts of parathyroid tissue are sufficient to maintain hypercalcemia. Parathyroid gland mass is generally only mildly increased.

CLINICAL MANIFESTATIONS. The disease leads to few, if any, clinical manifestations—hence its other name, "familial benign hypercalcemia." Nephrolithiasis and bone disease are, in general, not seen. Pancreatitis has been reported, but the specificity of this association is unclear. Hypercalcemia is present at birth. In some neonates, a clinically severe form of the disease is present. This severe form may be due to inheritance of a double dose of the abnormal gene. Otherwise, the main morbidity is that resulting from unsuccessful neck exploration prompted by failure to distinguish this disorder from conventional hyperparathyroidism. There is no evidence of associated endocrinopathies, as in the multiple endocrine neoplasia syndromes.

DIAGNOSIS. A high index of suspicion is needed to recognize this disease. Hypercalcemia associated with relatively young age, with only slight elevation in the serum PTH level, or with a family history of unsuccessful neck exploration should trigger further evaluation. Hypermagnesemia is suggestive; urinary calcium-creatinine ratios less than 0.01:1 strongly support the diagnosis. Screening of first-degree relatives for hypercalcemia may also be helpful. Until specific genetic probes become available, definitive diagnosis is not possible.

PROGNOSIS AND TREATMENT. Since the disease is compatible with normal life expectancy and is associated with little, if any, morbidity, neck exploration would appear to be contraindicated. Successful surgical treatment, moreover, is quite difficult, with permanent hypoparathyroidism or, more commonly, recurrent hypercalcemia, the usual result.

HYPERCALCEMIA ASSOCIATED WITH MALIGNANCY

ETIOLOGY AND PATHOGENESIS. Malignancies can cause hypercalcemia through two non–mutually exclusive mechanisms. First, local osteolytic hypercalcemia is caused by tumor metastatic to bone. Tumor cells may release bone-resorbing factors or so-called "osteoclast-activating factors," which indirectly lead to bone resorption. Cytokines such as lymphotoxin and interleukin 1 are potent osteoclast-activating factors. Second, humoral hypercalcemia of malignancy is caused by tumor secretion of factors into the circulation that act systemically to increase bone resorption. Such factors may show other PTH-like actions, including increasing urinary cyclic AMP and phosphate excretion and decreasing renal calcium excretion. This condition leads to a syndrome with biochemical features closely resembling those of primary hyperparathyroidism. One such factor commonly associated with many tumors has recently been identified as a polypeptide roughly twice as large as PTH and homologous in amino acid sequence to the biologically active, amino-terminus of PTH. This so-called parathyroid hormone–related peptide may also be secreted by tumors metastatic to bone, so that humoral and local osteolytic mechanisms may combine to cause hypercalcemia. Some tumors cause hypercalcemia through excessive synthesis of $1,25(OH)_2D$, in a manner analogous to that seen in sarcoidosis (see below). A role for additional, as yet unidentified, bone-resorbing agents secreted by tumors has not been excluded.

INCIDENCE. Malignancy-associated hypercalcemia occurs most commonly in patients with bone metastases. Breast carcinoma is one of the most frequent causes. Most subjects with bone metastases are not hypercalcemic because of adequate renal compensatory mechanisms. Slight renal impairment may then provoke hypercalcemia. Treatment of women with breast cancer metastatic to bone with tamoxifen has been associated with acute sharp increases in the serum calcium level. Certain hematogenous neoplasms, such as myeloma and human lymphotropic virus type I–associated leukemia/lymphoma, are frequently associated with hypercalcemia. Humoral hypercalcemia of malignancy is much rarer. It is seen most frequently with squamous carcinomas, but biochemical evidence indicates that almost any tumor type, including breast carcinoma, can produce parathyroid hormone–related peptide.

CLINICAL MANIFESTATIONS. Malignancy-associated hypercalcemia often develops acutely, may be quite severe (hypercalcemic crisis), and is frequently a grave prognostic sign. In most cases, particularly of the local osteolytic hypercalcemia variety, the underlying neoplasm is clinically evident. An otherwise occult neoplasm may occasionally manifest with humoral hypercalcemia of malignancy. Accurate and rapid diagnosis is critical in such cases, since successful tumor removal may be feasible.

DIAGNOSIS. As discussed earlier, PTH radioimmunoassay is the critical test for excluding coexistent primary hyperparathyroidism. Parathyroid hormone–related peptide fails to cross-react in such assays. Recently, specific immunoassays for this peptide have been developed, and these facilitate diagnosis of tumor secretion of the peptide. Increased urinary cyclic AMP excretion (coupled with low or undetectable PTH measurement) also favors tumor secretion of parathyroid hormone–related peptide. If both PTH and urinary cyclic AMP levels are low, one is dealing with a vitamin D–mediated or local osteolytic hypercalcemia.

TREATMENT AND PROGNOSIS. Acute, nonspecific treatment of hypercalcemia is instituted if the diagnosis is unclear (see Ch. 165). Definitive treatment must be directed at the underlying neoplasm, if feasible. When tumor treatment is not possible, vigorous treatment of hypercalcemia may be irrelevant. In those cases mediated by vitamin D or lymphokine release, glucocorticoids are often uniquely effective in lowering the serum calcium level.

HYPERCALCEMIA DUE TO GRANULOMATOUS DISEASES

ETIOLOGY AND PATHOGENESIS. Hypercalcemia is caused by unregulated formation of $1,25(OH)_2D$ in granuloma-associated macrophages. Normally, 1-hydroxylation takes place in the kidney and is sensitive to feedback suppression by high serum calcium levels. Unregulated synthesis of $1,25(OH)_2D$ in patients with granulomatous diseases renders them hypersensitive to vitamin D (from the diet or through sun exposure).

INCIDENCE AND PREVALENCE. This form of hypercalcemia has been observed in almost any disease capable of causing granuloma formation. These diseases include sarcoidosis, tuberculosis and fungal infections, berylliosis, and some lymphomas, such as Hodgkin's disease. Overt hypercalcemia may be seen in only about 10 per cent of patients with sarcoidosis, but hypercalciuria and intestinal hyperabsorption of calcium may occur in almost half of such individuals.

CLINICAL FEATURES. Manifestations are those of the underlying disease, as well as the superimposed effects of hypercalcemia. Because this form of hypercalcemia often coexists with relatively higher serum phosphorus levels than those seen in hyperparathyroidism, soft tissue calcification, nephrocalcinosis, and renal impairment are more common. Patients may present with hypercalcemia and relatively few other findings (e.g., subtle hilar adenopathy in sarcoidosis).

DIAGNOSIS. Parathyroid hormone and urinary cyclic AMP are suppressed. The serum level of $1,25(OH)_2D$ is elevated (in cases of vitamin D intoxication, the serum $1,25(OH)_2D$ level may be normal and only serum $25(OH)D$ is increased).

TREATMENT AND PROGNOSIS. The prognosis depends on that of the underlying disease. Glucocorticoids are extremely effective in lowering the serum calcium level in such cases. Chloroquine has been used effectively in subjects who cannot tolerate glucocorticoid treatment.

Attie MF: Treatment of hypercalcemia. Endocrinol Metab Clin North Am 18:807, 1989. *Complete discussion of treatment options and their pathophysiologic basis.*

Aurbach GD, Marx SJ, Spiegel AM: Parathyroid hormone, calcitonin, and the calciferols, In Wilson JD, Foster DW (eds.): Williams Textbook of Endocrinology. 7th ed. Philadelphia, W.B. Saunders Company, 1985, pp 1170–1198. *Detailed description of primary hyperparathyroidism and malignancy-associated and other forms of hypercalcemia, including differential diagnosis and treatment.*

Broadus AE, Mangin M, Ikeda K, et al.: Humoral hypercalcemia of cancer. N Engl J Med 319:556, 1988. *Review of pathogenesis of this syndrome and discovery of parathyroid hormone–related peptide.*

Brown EM, LeBoff MS, Oetting M, et al.: Secretory control in normal and abnormal parathyroid tissue. Recent Prog Horm Res 43:337, 1987. *Detailed review of control of normal parathyroid hormone secretion and of abnormal secretion in hyperparathyroidism.*

Friedman E, Sakaguchi K, Bale AE, et al.: Clonality of parathyroid tumors in familial endocrine neoplasia type I. N Engl J Med 321:213, 1989. *Description of molecular genetic abnormalities in familial and sporadic forms of parathyroid neoplasia.*

Heath DA: Primary hyperparathyroidism: Clinical presentation and factors influencing clinical management. Endocrinol Metab Clin North Am 18:631, 1989. *Thorough review of clinical features of hyperparathyroidism and arguments for and against surgery.*

Marx SJ, Spiegel AM, Levine MA, et al.: Familial hypocalciuric hypercalcemia. N Engl J Med 307:679, 1982. *Review of clinical and pathophysiologic features of this disease.*

Singer FR, Adams JS: Abnormal calcium homeostasis in sarcoidosis. N Engl J Med 315:755, 1986. *Review of derangements in vitamin D metabolism causing hypercalcemia and hypercalciuria in granulomatous disorders.*

HYPOCALCEMIA

DEFINITION. Hypocalcemia is an abnormal reduction in serum ionized calcium concentration.* Reduction in total serum calcium, as may occur in patients with hypoalbuminemia, does not necessarily reflect a reduction in ionized calcium. Ionized, not total, serum calcium affects neuromuscular function and is therefore the clinically relevant parameter.

ETIOLOGY AND PATHOGENESIS. Normal serum ionized calcium concentration is maintained by the direct actions of PTH on kidney and bone and by the indirect actions (through $1,25(OH)_2D$) on the intestine (see Ch. 232). Hypocalcemic disorders can be divided according to pathogenesis into two broad categories: (1) primary hypoparathyroidism, in which hypocalcemia is due to deficient secretion and/or action of PTH (specific subtypes are discussed under individual headings below); and (2) hypocalcemia due to target organ malfunction (e.g., renal failure, intestinal malabsorption, vitamin D deficiency). Hypocalcemia occurs in this category despite normal or even increased PTH secretion (secondary hyperparathyroidism). In hypoparathyroidism, there is reduced mobilization of calcium from bone, reduced renal reabsorption of calcium, lowered phosphaturia, and reduced $1,25(OH)_2D$ formation with a resultant decrease in intestinal calcium absorption. The end results are hypocalcemia and hyperphosphatemia. Renal failure (see Ch. 237) and acute phosphate loads (as may occur with chemotherapy of certain tumors such as Burkitt's lymphoma) are other causes of hypocalcemia with hyperphosphatemia. With vitamin D deficiency or malabsorption, hypocalcemia occurs with normal or low serum phosphorus levels (the latter reflecting secondary hyperparathyroidism). Hypocalcemia with low or normal serum phosphorus levels is also seen in acute pancreatitis (attributed to calcium soap formation, but this is unproved) and in some patients with osteoblastic tumor metastases. Table 235–3 summarizes the causes of hypocalcemia.

CLINICAL MANIFESTATIONS. Hypocalcemia of any cause is associated with certain typical signs and symptoms. Most prominent among these is increased neuromuscular excitability. Paresthesias of the fingers, toes, and circumoral region are mild manifestations; in more extreme cases there may be muscle cramping, carpopedal spasm, laryngeal stridor, and convulsions.

*See Ch. 232 and Part XXVII for calcium and phosphorus reference range values.

TABLE 235–3. CAUSES OF HYPOCALCEMIA

Hypoparathyroidism
  Deficient parathyroid hormone secretion
    Idiopathic (autoimmune)
    Parathyroid hormone gene mutation
    Surgical
    Infiltrative (iron overload, Wilson's disease)
  Functional
    Hypomagnesemia
    Transient postoperative
  Deficient parathyroid hormone action (hormone resistance)
    Pseudohypoparathyroidism types Ia and Ib
Normal or Increased Parathyroid Hormone Function
  Renal failure
  Intestinal malabsorption
  Acute pancreatitis
  Osteoblastic metastases
  Vitamin D deficiency or resistance

Symptoms reflect not only the degree of hypocalcemia but also the acuteness of the fall in serum calcium concentration. Patients with longstanding severe hypocalcemia may show surprisingly few symptoms. Factors that acutely alter the balance between ionized and protein-bound calcium may precipitate symptoms. For example, alkalosis lowers ionized calcium; thus hyperventilation may provoke symptoms of tetany. Signs of latent tetany include Chvostek's sign (twitching of the upper lip after tapping on the facial nerve below the zygomatic arch) and Trousseau's sign (carpal spasm after inflating a cuff on the upper arm above systolic blood pressure for 2 to 3 minutes).

Various mental disturbances, such as irritability, depression, and even psychosis, have been attributed to hypocalcemia. Papilledema and other signs of increased intracranial pressure have been reported. Intracranial calcifications, particularly of the basal ganglia, may be seen on plain radiographs and even more frequently on CT. Increased sensitivity to the dystonic effects of phenothiazines has been attributed to basal ganglia calcification. Longstanding hypocalcemia may lead to cataract formation. Cardiac effects of hypocalcemia include prolongation of the QT interval and, rarely, congestive heart failure. Dental anomalies depend on age of onset; in children hypocalcemia can cause enamel hypoplasia and failure of the adult teeth to erupt.

DIFFERENTIAL DIAGNOSIS. Measurement of serum calcium, phosphorus, and creatinine levels allows one to categorize the form of hypocalcemia. Hypocalcemia and hyperphosphatemia with normal renal function are pathognomonic of hypoparathyroidism. Low or undetectable PTH by immunoassay despite hypocalcemia confirms the diagnosis. (Rare forms of PTH-resistant hypoparathyroidism show elevated levels of PTH and are discussed further below.) Hypocalcemia and hyperphosphatemia caused by renal failure pose no diagnostic problem. Hypocalcemia with normal or low serum phosphorus levels should prompt measurement of vitamin D metabolites and assessment of gastrointestinal function to check for vitamin D deficiency and malabsorption, respectively. Measurements of PTH should show increased values in such patients, as the normal parathyroids attempt to compensate for hypocalcemia.

TREATMENT. Acute, symptomatic hypocalcemia requires emergency treatment in the form of intravenous calcium infusion. Ten to 20 ml of 10 per cent calcium gluconate solution (contains 10 mg of elemental calcium per milliliter) may be given over 10 to 20 minutes (this may be hazardous in patients taking cardiac glycosides). In less urgent settings, a slow intravenous infusion (over 4 to 8 hours) of 20 mg of elemental calcium per kilogram of body weight may be given. As with hypercalcemic disorders, definitive resolution of hypocalcemia requires treatment of the underlying disease. In patients with hypoparathyroidism, lifelong therapy with vitamin D (with or without oral calcium) is required. This is discussed further under treatment of hypoparathyroidism, below.

HYPOPARATHYROIDISM

DEFINITION. Hypoparathyroidism is defined as deficient PTH secretion and/or action. This condition may lead to overt hypocalcemia and hyperphosphatemia, as discussed above, or may only predispose to hypocalcemia (decreased parathyroid reserve) in times of increased calcium demand, such as pregnancy.

ETIOLOGY AND PATHOGENESIS. *Permanent Deficiency in Parathyroid Hormone Secretion.* This deficiency may result from surgical removal of the parathyroids, from glandular destruction by iron overload (e.g., transfusions in thalassemia) or copper overload (Wilson's disease), and from glandular destruction through a presumed autoimmune mechanism. The latter often has a genetic basis. The parathyroids may fail to develop as part of the DiGeorge syndrome. Some cases termed "idiopathic hypoparathyroidism" may be due to inherited mutations in the PTH gene that prevent synthesis and secretion of PTH.

Transient Deficiency in Parathyroid Hormone Secretion. Reversible hypoparathyroidism can be caused by hypomagnesemia. The latter may compromise both PTH secretion and action. Magnesium replacement corrects the defect. Transient hypoparathyroidism may also result from suppression of normal parathyroids by parathyroid adenomas or other causes of hypercalcemia. This condition rarely lasts more than 1 week. Surgical injury to

the parathyroids is another postulated cause of transiently reduced hormone secretion.

Deficiency in Parathyroid Hormone Action. Secretion of a biologically inactive form of PTH is a theoretical, but unproven, cause of deficient PTH action. Target organ resistance to PTH appears to be the major cause of this form of hypoparathyroidism, which was termed "pseudohypoparathyroidism" by Albright, who described it as the first example of a hormone-resistance disorder. Subsequent studies indicated that the defect in this disease occurs proximal to formation of cyclic AMP (a second messenger of PTH action), since affected subjects lack the normal brisk increase in urinary cyclic AMP excretion observed following infusion of PTH in normal individuals. There are at least two forms of pseudohypoparathyroidism. In type Ia disease, a 50 per cent deficiency has been found in the Gs protein that couples PTH (and many other) receptors to the enzyme that forms cyclic AMP, adenylyl cyclase. This deficiency may limit normal cyclic AMP production in response to PTH as well as to other hormones, such as thyroid-stimulating hormone. As a result, patients with this form of the disease show many abnormalities (e.g., hypothyroidism, hypogonadism) in addition to hypoparathyroidism. In affected subjects from several families with type Ia disease, distinct mutations that prevent synthesis of normal Gs protein have been found in the gene encoding the Gs protein. Inheritance of the mutation is autosomal dominant. In subjects with type Ib disease, the Gs protein is normal, and resistance is limited to PTH. A defective PTH receptor is a likely, but unproven, basis for this disease. In some subjects, hypocalcemia and hyperphosphatemia are associated with radiographically evident osteitis fibrosa cystica. This finding suggests selective renal, as opposed to skeletal, resistance to PTH action. The pathogenesis is unclear.

INCIDENCE. All forms of hypoparathyroidism are relatively rare. The incidence of surgical hypoparathyroidism varies widely as a function of the skill of the surgeon.

CLINICAL MANIFESTATIONS. The manifestations generally associated with hypocalcemia have been discussed above. The clinical features unique to each form of hypoparathyroidism reflect the underlying disease. In autoimmune forms, there may be associated endocrine deficiency, most frequently Addison's disease, as well as a T cell defect predisposing to mucocutaneous candidiasis. Alopecia and vitiligo may also be seen. In pseudohypoparathyroidism type Ib, the appearance is normal, but in type Ia disease, affected individuals show a constellation of abnormal physical findings termed Albright's hereditary osteodystrophy (Fig. 235–3). These findings include obesity; short stature; round face and short neck; metacarpal and metatarsal shortening (most often fourth and fifth), as well as shortening and broadening of the distal phalanges; and subcutaneous calcifications. Such individuals often show slight mental retardation and associated endocrine abnormalities, most commonly hypothyroidism (without goiter) and hypogonadism. First-degree relatives of patients with pseudohypoparathyroidism type Ia may show the physical features of Albright's osteodystrophy without evidence of hormone resistance. This condition has been termed "pseudopseudohypoparathyroidism." Rarely, individuals with pseudohypoparathyroidism (more often of the Ib type) may show radiographic evidence of osteitis fibrosa cystica and elevated serum levels of bone-derived alkaline phosphatase.

DIFFERENTIAL DIAGNOSIS. Low or undetectable serum PTH in the face of hypocalcemia, hyperphosphatemia, and normal renal function establishes the diagnosis of hormone-deficient hypoparathyroidism. Diagnosis of the underlying disease depends on history (e.g., neck surgery), physical findings (e.g., candidiasis, alopecia), and additional laboratory tests (e.g., evidence for hypoadrenalism). Antibodies to parathyroid antigens have been detected in the autoimmune form of the disease, but this test is not available for routine clinical use. If an elevated level of serum PTH is measured by immunoassay in a subject with hypocalcemia, hyperphosphatemia, and normal renal function, this suggests hormone-resistant hypoparathyroidism. Parathyroid hormone infusion (at present with commercially available synthetic 1–34 peptide) and measurement of urinary cyclic AMP excretion can be performed to confirm PTH resistance. Physical appearance can help distinguish type Ia from type Ib pseudohypoparathyroidism, as can testing for other endocrinopathies, such as hy-

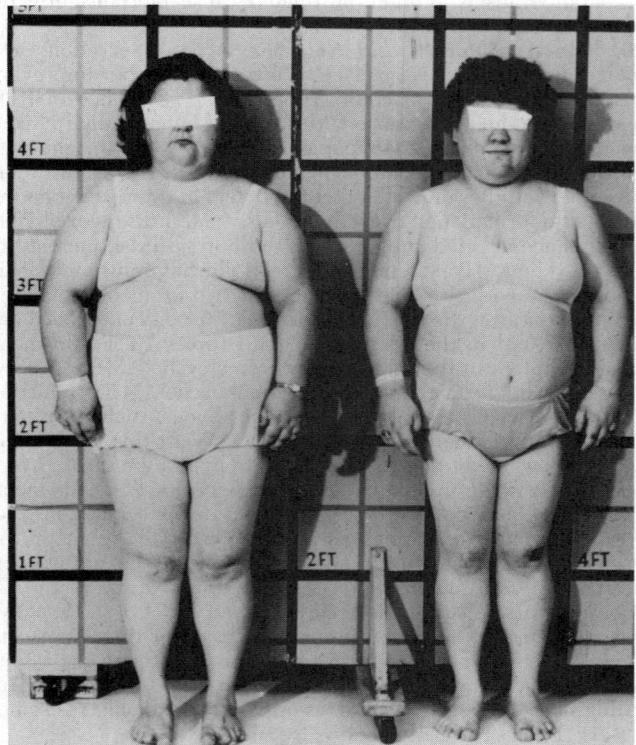

FIGURE 235–3. Phenotypic features of Albright's hereditary osteodystrophy. A mother *(left)* and daughter display many of the features of Albright's osteodystrophy, including obesity, short stature, round face, and short neck. Metacarpal and metatarsal shortening manifest as shortened fourth and fifth fingers (right hands of both subjects) and shortened fourth toes (left feet of both subjects), respectively. Both subjects show resistance to PTH and thyroid-stimulating hormone, as well as deficient Gs protein activity, characteristic of pseudohypoparathyroidism type Ia. (From Spiegel AM: Pseudohypoparathyroidism. *In* Scriver CR, Beaudet AL, Sly WS, Valle D [eds.]: The Metabolic Basis of Inherited Disease. 6th ed. New York, McGraw-Hill, 1989, pp 2013–2027; with permission.)

pothyroidism. Measurement of Gs protein and detection of mutations in the corresponding gene are not routinely available tests.

TREATMENT. Transient forms of hypoparathyroidism may not require treatment. Reversible forms should be treated appropriately, i.e., magnesium replacement for hypomagnesemia. In permanent, hormone-deficient hypoparathyroidism, hormone replacement therapy is not practical. Parathyroid autografting is effective in some patients with surgical hypoparathyroidism. When this is not feasible, and also in subjects with pseudohypoparathyroidism, lifelong treatment with oral vitamin D is required. Vitamin D_2, ergocalciferol (generally 50,000 units per day), is inexpensive by comparison with the active metabolite, $1,25(OH)_2D$ (generally 0.25 µg per day). The latter has the theoretical advantage of more rapid onset (and in case of toxicity, offset) of action, but with appropriate monitoring, vitamin D_2 can be used very effectively. Oral calcium salts (1 to 2 grams of elemental calcium per day in divided doses) may be added for individuals whose dietary calcium intake is highly variable or inadequate. The goal of treatment is the lowest serum calcium concentration compatible with avoidance of symptoms, since without PTH, urinary calcium excretion (and the possibility of nephrolithiasis) will be increased at any filtered load of calcium. Both serum and urine calcium levels, as well as renal function, must be monitored. In forms of hypoparathyroidism that have associated endocrinopathies, appropriate hormone replacement therapy should be instituted.

Ahn TG, Antonorakis SE, Kronenberg HM, et al.: Familial isolated hypoparathyroidism: A molecular genetic analysis of 8 families with 23 affected persons. Medicine 65:73, 1986. *Review of studies of PTH gene as locus of defect in this disease.*

Aurbach GD, Marx SJ, Spiegel AM: Parathyroid hormone, calcitonin, and the calciferols. *In* Wilson JD, Foster DW (eds.): Williams Textbook of Endocrinology. 7th ed. Philadelphia, W.B. Saunders Company, 1985, pp 1199–1207. *Detailed description of clinical and pathophysiologic features of hypocalcemic disorders and the multiple forms of hypoparathyroidism.*

Mallette L: Synthetic human parathyroid hormone 1–34 fragment for diagnostic testing. Ann Intern Med 109:800, 1988. *Description of use of this commercially available peptide in the differential diagnosis of hypoparathyroidism.*

Spiegel AM: Pseudohypoparathyroidism. *In* Scriver CR, Beaudet AL, Sly WS, et al. (eds.): The Metabolic Basis of Inherited Disease. 6th ed. New York, McGraw-Hill, 1989, pp 2013–2027. *Extensive discussion of clinical features and pathogenesis of hormone-resistant forms of hypoparathyroidism.*

236 Calcitonin and Medullary Thyroid Carcinoma

Leonard J. Deftos

Calcitonin (CT) is a 32-residue peptide secreted primarily by the thyroidal C-cells in mammals and by the embryologically related ultimobranchial gland in submammals. The main biologic effect of CT is to decrease bone resorption by inhibiting the osteoclast. This effect results in a decrease in the concentration of blood calcium, with a nadir directly related to bone turnover; thus, the hypocalcemia may be slight in normal adults but considerable when bone resorption is increased pathologically in disease states or physiologically during bone growth. This property of CT makes it an effective drug for hyperresorptive diseases, such as Paget's disease, osteoporosis, and hypercalcemia. The physiologic significance of other reported effects of CT is not well established. The calciuric effect of CT is seen only with pharmacologic doses of the hormone. A variety of gastrointestinal effects are only inconsistently observed. A stimulatory effect on bone formation may be attributable to a CT precursor molecule rather than to CT itself. However, an analgesic effect of CT continues to receive considerable attention and may be related to neuroendocrine features of the hormone. In addition to its role in skeletal physiology and treatment, CT is a serum and tumor marker for medullary thyroid carcinoma (MTC) and is the signal tumor of multiple endocrine neoplasia (MEN) type II.

CALCITONIN

Biochemistry

The 32-residue structure of CT, determined for eight species, reveals a common 1,7 amino-terminal disulfide bridge and carboxy-terminal proline. Seven of the nine amino-terminal residues are identical in all CT molecules. The interspecies structural differences in the rest of the molecule cause the submammalian (ultimobranchial) CT molecules to have a greater potency in mammals than the mammalian CT molecules. Thus, the salmon form of the hormone is widely used for treatment in humans. The greater chemical basicity of these submammalian CT species probably accounts for their increased potency. In contrast to the other major skeletal peptide hormone, parathyroid hormone (PTH), a biologically active fragment of CT has not been identified, and the entire molecule seems to be necessary for biologic activity.

Secretion and Production

The most important secretory regulation of CT is mediated by ambient calcium. An acute increase in blood calcium concentration increases the secretion of CT, and an acute decrease in blood calcium level decreases the secretion of CT. The effects of chronic changes in blood calcium concentration on secretion have not been as well defined. Chronic hypercalcemia may stimulate CT production, but this compensatory response may be limited. Chronic hypocalcemia seems to increase CT storage in C-cells. Although a variety of other factors have been reported to stimulate CT secretion, only pentagastrin and its related peptides are consistent additional secretagogues. The high concentration of pentagastrin necessary to stimulate secretion does not support the presence of a normal entero–C-cell secretory pathway. Nevertheless, pentagastrin and calcium are clinically important agents for the evaluation of CT secretion by both normal and malignant C-cells.

The effect of gonadal steroids and age on CT production remains controversial. It is well established that blood concentrations of CT are higher in males than females and in children than adults. Some studies report a decline in CT secretion during adulthood and a stimulation of CT secretion by estrogens and testosterone. These observations have led to the hypothesis that age- and menopause-related declines in CT production contribute to the corresponding declines in bone mass seen in the elderly, especially postmenopausal women. These observations support the use of CT in the treatment of osteoporosis, but more complex hormonal abnormalities underlie this skeletal disorder.

MEDULLARY THYROID CARCINOMA

Medullary thyroid carcinoma is a tumor of the CT-producing C-cells of the thyroid gland. These cells migrate from the neural crest to the thyroid gland and to other sites of the diffuse neuroendocrine system during embryogenesis in mammals. In submammals, these cells form their own distinct organ, the ultimobranchial gland. The neural crest origin of C-cells accounts for their production of a variety of biologically active substances. This embryologic origin may also explain the common association of MTC with other neuroendocrine tumors. Thus, MTC can occur as part of a multiple endocrine disorder, MEN type II, or sporadically.

Pathology

A palpable tumor is the most common physical finding in the patient with MTC. The tumor is usually firm and located in the middle or upper lobes of the gland. Bilateral tumors are common in MEN. Calcification can be present in the tumor, and this may result in a radiographic pattern that is sufficiently characteristic to assist in clinical diagnosis. Similarly, the presence of amyloid in the tumor can assist in histologic diagnosis. However, cytologic diagnosis is made difficult by the fact that the cells of MTC can be arranged in a variety of patterns. Therefore, the diagnosis of MTC is conclusively made by the demonstration of CT in the tumor by immunohistology. Hyperplasia of the C-cells antedates the frank malignancy of MTC, especially in the familial forms of the tumor. C-cell hyperplasia is often too subtle to be appreciated by light microscopy, and immunohistology for CT is necessary to make this diagnosis.

Tumor Behavior

The clinical behavior of MTC is usually intermediate between that of aggressive anaplastic thyroid cancer and that of indolent papillary and follicular thyroid cancer. Local lymph node spread is common, and metastases to lung and bone can occur. Medullary thyroid carcinoma in which all or most of the cells produce CT may have a better prognosis than a more heterogeneous tumor in which CT production is not uniform. Even in the most aggressive tumors, CT production is usually sufficient to serve as a specific marker for this thyroid cancer. However, there may be rare instances in which CT production has ceased. The 5-year survival of those with MTC approximates 50 per cent. Survival can vary from several months to three decades after diagnosis. Patients under 2 years of age with metastatic disease and over 50 years of age with only localized disease have been reported. C-cell hyperplasia can occur in those as young as 2 years and as old as 45 years of age. Therefore, the tumor can be rapidly aggressive, leading to death within months after diagnosis, or it can be indolent and compatible with survival for decades.

Pathogenesis

Medullary thyroid carcinoma is preceded by C-cell hyperplasia, especially in the familial form of the disease. This progression from hyperplasia to cancer is best documented for MTC in the clinical setting of MEN type II. C-cell adenomas have also been observed. The progression of unregulated growth from hyperplasia to malignancy is similar to that seen in the progression of mucosal cells to a frankly malignant state in colon cancer. In colon cancer, this development is accompanied by a sequential expression of oncogenes. It is thus interesting to speculate that an oncogene cascade is responsible for the progression of normal

C-cells through hyperplasia to cancer in MTC. In the familial form of the tumor, an oncogene abnormality may be related to the chromosome 10 site, to which MEN type IIA has been mapped. Abnormalities in oncogene expression have been observed in MTC, but their role in pathogenesis has not yet been defined. It is notable that this same progression of normal cells to hyperplastic and then neoplastic cells is also observed for the other two endocrine components of heritable MTC, pheochromocytoma and parathyroid neoplasia. Thus, the genetic abnormality on chromosome 10 may result in the overexpression (or undersuppression) of an endocrine cell growth factor.

Diagnosis

Overexpression of the CT gene is the molecular hallmark of MTC. This overexpression results in the increased production of CT by the tumor and increased secretion of the hormone into blood. As a result, most patients with MTC have an increased circulating concentration of CT that can be detected by radioimmunoassay and increased tumor concentrations that can be demonstrated directly by immunohistology or through increased messenger RNA (mRNA) expression by in situ hybridization. Usually, the basal blood concentration of CT is sufficiently elevated to be diagnostic of the presence of the tumor. In the early stages of the diseases, however, the basal concentrations of CT cannot be readily distinguished from normal. In these circumstances, provocative testing of CT secretion can reveal the presence of the abnormal C-cells. Such testing is also clinically indicated for the relative of a patient with familial MTC when early diagnosis is sought. The two most commonly used provocative agents for CT secretion are calcium and the synthetic gastrin analogue pentagastrin, alone or in combination. Most tumors respond to either agent with a diagnostic increase in CT secretion. CT blood measurements can also be used to evaluate therapy and monitor tumor recurrence. Interpretation must be made according to the specific parameters of the procedure utilized.

The primary genetic abnormality in MEN type IIA has been localized to chromosome 10. Molecular genetic techniques allow the assignment of gene carrier status with considerable certainty in a patient at risk and with a well-documented pedigree. However, confounding factors such as mistaken diagnoses and nonpaternity can complicate genetic analysis. The ethical considerations that surround all of genetic screening should be considered in the light of the effective and curative treatment that is available for the components of MEN type IIA.

CT Gene Expression

A wide variety of bioactive substances are overproduced by MTC. Some can be attributed to the neural crest origin of the C-cells and some to deregulated CT gene expression. This gene encodes peptides in addition to CT. The CT gene consists of six exons that generate, through differential mRNA splicing, two distinct mRNA's, one of them the CT precursor and the other a precursor for calcitonin gene–related peptide (CGRP). The CT precursor is processed into three peptides: CT; its amino-terminal flanking peptide, N-pro CT; and its carboxy-terminal flanking peptide, C-pro CT. The CGRP precursor is similarly processed. Thus, the CT gene encodes at least six peptides. The peptides derived from the CT precursor, including CT, act on the skeletal system, and the peptide derived from the CGRP precursor acts as a neurotransmitter. This remarkable genetic economy produces two CT precursor–derived peptides that have opposite skeletal effects, with CT inhibiting bone resorption and N-pro CT, its amino-terminal relative, promoting bone cell mitogenesis. Human CT gene expression is summarized in Figure 236–1.

MULTIPLE ENDOCRINE NEOPLASIA (MEN)

Medullary thyroid carcinoma can occur in association with other endocrine tumors as part of a multiple endocrine neoplasia, designated MEN type II, to distinguish it from MEN type I, which consists of parathyroid, pancreatic, and pituitary tumors. MEN type II is an autosomal dominant syndrome that can be clinically classified into two subtypes, type IIA and IIB (Table 236–1).

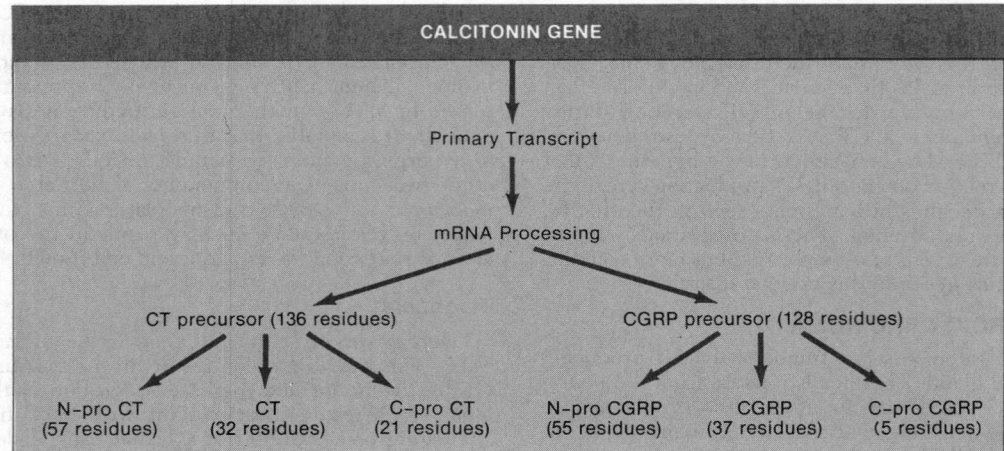

FIGURE 236–1. Summary of human calcitonin (CT) gene expression. The CT pathway occurs primarily in endocrine tissue (e.g., C-cells) and the calcitonin gene–related peptide (CGRP) pathway primarily in neural tissue. The gene has six exons whose primary RNA transcript is differentially spliced into an mRNA for the CT precursor and one for the CGRP precursor. A common 25-residue leader sequence is removed, and these two polypeptide precursors are each processed into their three respective peptide products. (Alternative designations for some of these peptides are as follows: for N-pro CT, PAS-57; for C-pro CT, PDN-21 and katacalcin; for N-pro CGRP, PAS-55). The function of these other peptides is not firmly established.

Pheochromocytoma

Pheochromocytoma is a component of MEN type IIA and IIB. Bilateral and multifocal pheochromocytomas are very common in this clinical setting, with an incidence of over 70 per cent. This figure contrasts with a bilateral incidence of usually less than 10 per cent for sporadic pheochromocytomas and only 20 to 50 per cent for familial pheochromocytomas. Adrenal medullary hyperplasia is a predecessor of the pheochromocytomas seen with MTC. The increase in adrenal medullary mass results from diffuse or multifocal proliferation of adrenal medullary cells, primarily those found within the head and body of the glands. The biochemical as well as clinical manifestations of this tumor may be subtle, so diagnostic tests for pheochromocytoma should be pursued vigorously in MEN type II.

Hyperparathyroidism

Hyperparathyroidism is much more common in MEN type IIA than in MEN type IIB (and it also occurs in MEN type I). The presence of hyperparathyroidism thus should always make one consider the possibility of MEN. Parathyroid hyperplasia is more common than adenoma, an important consideration for surgical treatment. Although a calcium-mediated functional relationship between hyperparathyroidism and MTC has been suggested, the two neoplasias are probably related to the same gene.

Multiple Mucosal Neuromas

The presence of neuromas with a centrofacial distribution is the most consistent component of MEN type IIB. The most common location of neuromas is the oral cavity. The oral lesions are almost invariably present by the first decade and in some cases even at birth. Mucosal neuromas can also be present in the eyelid, conjunctiva, and cornea. The most prominent microscopic feature of neuromas is an increase in the size and number of nerves. These hypertrophied nerve fibers are readily seen with a slit lamp and occasionally by direct ophthalmologic examination.

TABLE 236–1. COMPONENTS OF MULTIPLE ENDOCRINE NEOPLASIA TYPE II AND THEIR FREQUENCY BASED ON AVERAGE FIGURES FROM THE LITERATURE

Component	MEN Type IIA (%)	MEN Type IIB (%)
Medullary thyroid carcinoma	97	90
Pheochromocytoma	30	45
Hyperparathyroidism	50	Rare
Mucosal neuroma syndrome	—	100

Gastrointestinal tract abnormalities are part of the multiple mucosal neuroma syndrome. The most common of these is gastrointestinal ganglioneuromatosis, which usually occurs in the small and large intestines but has also been noted in the esophagus and stomach. The lesions are sometimes associated with swallowing abnormalities, megacolon, diarrhea, and constipation. The diarrhea may also be due to excess production of bioactive substances by the MTC. In any case, diarrhea is the most common symptom of MTC.

Marfanoid Habitus

Patients with this component have a tall, slender body with long arms and legs, an abnormal ratio of upper to lower body segments, and poor muscle development. Other features associated with the marfanoid habitus may include dorsal kyphosis, pectus excavatum or pectus carinatum, pes cavus, and high-arched palate. In contrast to patients with true Marfan's syndrome, these patients do not have aortic arch abnormalities, ectopia lentis, homocystinuria, or mucopolysaccharide abnormalities.

Treatment and Clinical Management

Surgery is the treatment of choice for the three neoplasias in MEN type II. All are potentially lethal—especially MTC and pheochromocytoma—but all can be cured in their early stages by surgery. Aggressive therapy is thus warranted. Management of the individual components of MEN syndromes generally follows the accepted procedures for each of the neoplasias. However, the sequence of treatment is guided by the presence of multiple endocrine tumors. Pheochromocytomas, which are commonly bilateral, should be treated first because they can be life threatening and pose risks for surgery of the other tumors. Thyroid and parathyroid surgery must be aggressive because all glandular tissue may be involved.

An essential feature of appropriate clinical management in MEN type II is evaluation of family members, since these tumors are transmitted in an autosomal dominant pattern. Family members must be re-evaluated periodically because of the varying penetrance of the component tumors. Calcitonin measurement remains the diagnostic procedure of choice. Genetic linkage techniques utilizing restriction fragment length polymorphism (RFLP) are increasingly used to identify individuals at risk for the syndrome.

CALCITONIN AS A DRUG

Calcitonin's primary biologic effect of inhibiting osteoclastic bone resorption makes it useful in treating disorders characterized by increased bone resorption and certain forms of hypercalcemia.

Thus, CT can be prescribed for treating Paget's disease, osteoporosis, and the hypercalcemia associated with malignancy. Both salmon CT and human CT are available, the former being more potent and the latter being less antigenic. Calcitonin is safer than most treatment alternatives, but its effects can be transient. The inconvenience of repeated parenteral administration may be avoided by newer preparations of the peptide.

Burns DM, Birnbaum RS, Roos BA: A neuroendocrine peptide derived from the amino terminal half of rat procalcitonin. Mol Endocrinol 3:140, 1989. *An exposition of the complexities of CT gene expression.*
Deftos LJ: Radioimmunoassay for calcitonin in medullary thyroid carcinoma. JAMA 227:403, 1974. *Early study of the application of CT radioimmunoassay to the diagnosis of MTC.*
Deftos LJ, Roos BA: Medullary thyroid carcinoma and calcitonin gene expression. Bone Miner Res 6:267, 1989. *A detailed exposition of multiple endocrine neoplasia and the regulation of calcitonin-gene products.*
Grauer A, Raue F, Gagel RF: Changing concepts in the management of hereditary and sporadic medullary thyroid carcinoma. Endocrinol Metab Clin North Am 19:613, 1990. *A review of current management approaches.*
Kramer JB, Wells SA Jr: Thyroid carcinoma. Adv Surg 22:195, 1989. *A review of surgical management of medullary thyroid carcinoma.*
Melvin KEW, Tashjian AH Jr, Miller HH: Studies in familial medullary carcinoma. Rec Prog Horm Res 28:399, 1972. *Classic study of MTC.*
Sobol H, Narod SA, Nakamura Y, et al.: Screening for MEN Type IIA with DNA-polymorphism analyses. N Engl J Med 321:996, 1989. *The application of RFLP to genetic analyses in MEN.*

237 Renal Osteodystrophy

Eduardo Slatopolsky

Renal osteodystrophy refers to the complex lesions of bone that are present in the majority of patients with advanced renal failure. The main components of renal osteodystrophy are osteitis fibrosa and osteomalacia (Table 237–1). A lesser role is played by osteosclerosis and osteoporosis. Osteitis fibrosa, a consequence of an increased level of parathyroid hormone (PTH), is characterized by an increase in the number of osteoclasts and an increase in bone resorption and marrow fibrosis. Osteomalacia, a condition secondary in part to alterations in vitamin D metabolism, results from a decreased mineralization of osteoid tissue (shown histologically by an abnormal calcification front in bone). Osteosclerosis is due to localized areas of mineralized woven bone which appear as increased bone density on radiographic studies. Osteoporosis, defined as a decrease in the mass of normally mineralized bone, is an infrequent and minor component of renal osteodystrophy.

OSTEITIS FIBROSA

Secondary hyperparathyroidism occurs universally in chronic renal disease. Chief cell hyperplasia of the parathyroid glands and high levels of immunoreactive parathyroid hormone (i-PTH) are among the earliest findings affecting mineral metabolism in patients with chronic renal failure. Several factors contribute to the development of secondary hyperparathyroidism in renal insufficiency (Table 237–1 and Fig. 237–1).

TABLE 237–1. FOUR COMPONENTS OF RENAL OSTEODYSTROPHY

1. Osteitis fibrosa (secondary hyperparathyroidism)
   a. Phosphate retention
   b. Altered metabolism of vitamin D
   c. Skeletal resistance to PTH
   d. Impaired degradation of PTH
   e. Altered feedback regulation of PTH by Ca^{2+}
2. Osteomalacia
   a. Altered metabolism of vitamin D
   b. Altered synthesis and maturation of collagen
   c. Acidosis
   d. Increased bone magnesium
   e. Increased pyrophosphate
   f. Retention of aluminum
   g. Retention of iron
3. Osteosclerosis ⎫
4. Osteoporosis ⎬ of lesser quantitative importance

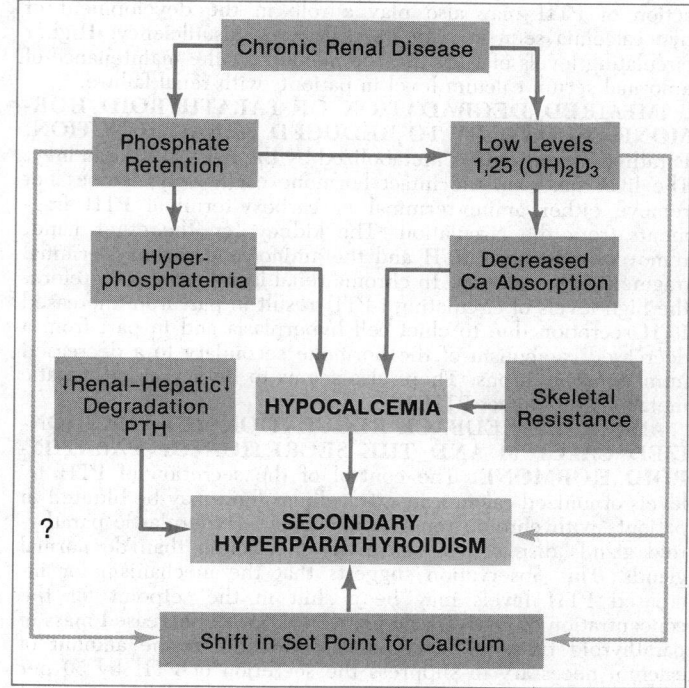

FIGURE 237–1. Diagrammatic representation of the factors involved in the pathogenesis of secondary hyperparathyroidism.

PHOSPHATE RETENTION. An important role of phosphate retention in producing secondary hyperparathyroidism is firmly established. Long-term feeding of a diet high in phosphate to animals with normal renal function can produce secondary hyperparathyroidism. Conversely, restriction of dietary phosphate can prevent the development of secondary hyperparathyroidism in chronic renal failure. The effect of phosphate retention on the parathyroid glands is mediated by lowering the concentration of ionized calcium in extracellular fluid, which in turn results from (1) the complexing of ionized calcium by phosphate; (2) a decreased renal production of calcitriol $(1,25(OH)_2D_3)$, the active metabolite of vitamin D; and (3) a direct effect of phosphate on bone, decreasing calcium mobilization from the skeleton. In patients with far-advanced renal failure (a glomerular filtration rate [GFR] less than 20 ml per minute), correction of hyperphosphatemia alone does not completely reverse secondary hyperparathyroidism, since many other factors also contribute to the increased PTH levels in blood.

ALTERATIONS IN VITAMIN D METABOLISM (see also Ch. 233). Renal osteodystrophy may arise in part because of defective renal production of the active form of vitamin D in advanced renal failure. The liver hydroxylates vitamin D_3 to 25-hydroxycholecalciferol $(25(OH)D_3)$, the predominant form of vitamin D_3 present in plasma. The $25(OH)D_3$ is further hydroxylated to $1,25(OH)_2D_3$, also termed calcitriol, by a specific hydroxylase enzyme found in the mitochondrial fraction of the renal proximal tubular cells. Parathyroid hormone and low-phosphate diets stimulate the activity of this hydroxylase; lack of PTH, hyperphosphatemia, or hypercalcemia decreases the activity of the hydroxylase. Intestinal absorption of calcium is reduced in patients with far-advanced renal insufficiency, and low levels of calcitriol are found in serum as the probable cause. Calcium malabsorption is usually present in patients with GFR's less than 40 ml per minute. In addition, it is now accepted that calcitriol has a direct effect on the synthesis and secretion of PTH. The main action is inhibition of PTH gene transcription and synthesis of Pre-pro PTH messenger RNA (mRNA). Low levels of calcitriol observed in patients with chronic renal failure could potentially play a role in the development of secondary hyperparathyroidism.

SKELETAL RESISTANCE TO THE ACTION OF PARATHYROID HORMONE. Skeletal resistance to the calcemic action of PTH may also play a role in the development of hypocalcemia seen in patients with renal insufficiency. Higher circulating levels of PTH may be needed for the maintenance of a normal serum calcium level in patients with renal failure.

IMPAIRED DEGRADATION OF PARATHYROID HORMONE SECONDARY TO REDUCED RENAL FUNCTION. Parathyroid hormone is metabolized by the liver and the kidney. The liver takes up the intact hormone exclusively; it does not remove either amino-terminal or carboxy-terminal PTH fragments from the circulation. The kidney, on the other hand, removes both intact PTH and the amino- and carboxy-terminal fragments from plasma. In chronic renal insufficiency, therefore, the high levels of circulating i-PTH result in part from increased PTH secretion due to chief cell hyperplasia and in part from a decreased catabolism of the hormone secondary to a decreased number of nephrons. There also seems to be decreased hepatic metabolism of intact PTH.

ALTERED FEEDBACK REGULATION BETWEEN IONIZED CALCIUM AND THE SECRETION OF PARATHYROID HORMONE. The control of the secretion of PTH by levels of ionized calcium in extracellular fluid may be blunted in patients with chronic renal insufficiency. Hyperplastic parathyroid glands display less sensitivity to calcium than do normal glands. This observation suggests that the mechanism for increased PTH levels may be a shift in the setpoint for the concentration of ionized calcium as well as the increased mass of parathyroid tissue. The setpoint is defined as the amount of calcium necessary to suppress the secretion of PTH by 50 per cent. Thus, normal concentrations of ionized calcium may not suffice to suppress the release of PTH by the hyperplastic glands of patients with secondary hyperparathyroidism. Low levels of calcitriol play a role in this abnormal setpoint for calcium-regulated PTH secretion.

OSTEOMALACIA

Osteomalacia is defined as an increase in the osteoid seam width accompanied by a decrease in the mineralization front. The presence of excess osteoid per se does not necessarily indicate osteomalacia. An increase in osteoid tissue may be secondary to the abnormal mineralization of osteomalacia, or it may be due to an increased rate of synthesis of bone collagen that is normally mineralized. The use of double tetracycline labeling of the calcification front in vivo can differentiate between these two possibilities. The use of this technique and quantitative bone histology is critical to the diagnosis of osteomalacia. The mechanisms by which deficiency of vitamin D leads to impaired mineralization of bone are poorly understood. Whether vitamin D or calcitriol can directly stimulate bone mineralization or whether it leads to mineralization only by increasing the levels of calcium and phosphate in the extracellular fluid surrounding bone is uncertain. Although the plasma levels of calcitriol are reduced in patients with far-advanced renal insufficiency, overt osteomalacia is found in only a small fraction of such patients and may be absent even in anephric patients. Thus, other factors could also participate in the pathogenesis of osteomalacia in uremic patients—for example, the plasma level of phosphate. Hypophosphatemia per se can produce severe osteomalacia even in patients with normal renal function. Additional factors include alterations in collagen synthesis and maturation, defective bone crystal maturation, increased bone magnesium concentrations, elevated levels of pyrophosphate, and diminished calcium carbonate levels. The combination of these factors may influence the maturation of bone and potentially contribute to the development of osteomalacia. Acidosis also contributes to the skeletal disease. In chronic renal insufficiency the skeleton assists in buffering the retained acids. Administration of bicarbonate and correction of the acidosis in azotemic patients can reduce fecal calcium excretion.

Another type of osteomalacia in renal insufficiency, one that is resistant to vitamin D therapy, is caused by an excess of aluminum. Patients with osteomalacia secondary to aluminum have pathologic fractures, complain of severe bone pain, and characteristically have low levels of PTH. The source may be a high aluminum content in the water and/or the ingestion of phosphate

binders containing aluminum. The aluminum is deposited in the interface between the osteoid tissue and the calcification front and has a toxic effect on the osteoblast. Severe iron retention can induce a similar form of osteomalacia.

Finally, after total parathyroidectomy the lack of PTH in patients results in low bone turnover and may sometimes precipitate the development of osteomalacia.

CLINICAL MANIFESTATIONS

The symptoms related to renal osteodystrophy usually appear only when renal failure is advanced. On the other hand, certain biochemical alterations may appear early in the course of renal insufficiency. Knowledge of the presence of these alterations may help the physician to introduce treatment early in the course of renal failure and in this way to prevent severe complications in bone and mineral metabolism.

Bone pain can develop and progress slowly to a point where the patient is bedridden, without regard to whether the bone disease is predominantly osteitis fibrosa or osteomalacia. The bone pain is generally vague and commonly located in the lower back, hips, knees, and legs. Low back pain may result from the collapse of a vertebral body, and sharp chest pain may indicate spontaneous rib fracture. Physical findings are frequently lacking.

Muscular weakness, when present, is usually proximal, appears slowly, and progresses with time. Plasma levels of muscle enzymes, creatine phosphokinase, and transaminases are usually normal, and the electron micrographic changes are nonspecific. The pathogenesis of such muscular weakness is uncertain. In patients with myopathy, the myofibrils are disorganized in a patchy fashion and the Z-band material may be dispersed. These changes revert to normal following treatment with $25(OH)D_3$. *Pruritus* due to calcium deposition in skin is a common symptom in uremic patients, particularly with severe secondary hyperparathyroidism.

Vascular calcification and peripheral ischemic necrosis may occur, producing lesions of the tips of the toes and fingers and violaceous discoloration of the skin. Ulcerations and scar formation may occur, with clear demarcation of the lesions from the surrounding skin. Acute pain and swelling around one or more joints may also develop in uremic patients. The syndrome of *calcific periarthritis*, which may be caused by deposition of hydroxyapatite crystals, is accompanied by marked hyperphosphatemia.

Skeletal deformities are common in azotemic children who are growing. Bowing of the tibia and femur and deformities from slipped epiphyses are not uncommon. Children with renal rickets sometimes exhibit typical radiographic findings of vitamin D deficiency. In adults with renal failure, particularly those with osteomalacia, marked skeletal deformities with lumbar scoliosis, thoracic kyphosis, and deformity of the thoracic cage may be observed. Growth retardation is usually seen in young children before and during maintenance hemodialysis. See Chapter 234 for a further discussion of osteomalacia and rickets.

Another clinical manifestation of renal osteodystrophy that occurs in some patients after renal transplantation is aseptic necrosis of the head of the femur. This condition is more frequently seen in patients with severe bone disease (osteitis fibrosa) before renal transplantation and in those who receive very large doses of glucocorticoids.

BIOCHEMICAL FEATURES

Circulating i-PTH is elevated early in the course of renal insufficiency (a GFR of 60 to 80 ml per minute). As the disease progresses (a GFR less than 40 ml per minute), hypocalcemia and low levels of calcitriol appear. With advanced renal insufficiency, however, the serum calcium level may remain close to normal and values below 7.5 mg per deciliter are infrequent. Usually, hypocalcemia is more marked in severe osteomalacia or with profound metabolic acidosis. Occasionally, hypercalcemia may be observed in uremic patients, particularly in those undergoing long-term dialysis. This complication can arise from (1) severe hyperparathyroidism, (2) the ingestion of large amounts of calcium and vitamin D, (3) the presence of unrelated diseases, such as sarcoidosis or malignancies, or (4) a "pure" mineralizing defect, as may occur in osteomalacia secondary to aluminum retention. Hyperphosphatemia is usually present in patients with a GFR less than 25 ml per minute. The degree of hyperphosphatemia depends on the amount of phosphate ingested, the fraction absorbed in the intestine, and that excreted into the urine. If the patient ingests phosphate binders, the serum phosphate level may remain normal despite advanced renal insufficiency. Patients with severe hyperparathyroidism and advanced renal insufficiency usually have higher concentrations of serum phosphate in plasma.

Advanced renal insufficiency (a GFR less than 15 ml per minute) may be associated with hypermagnesemia and an increased content of magnesium in bone. This may adversely affect crystal formation.

Total serum alkaline phosphatase levels are commonly higher in uremic patients with osteitis fibrosa than in those with osteomalacia. Coexistent liver disease should be excluded as a cause of an elevated alkaline phosphatase level.

RADIOGRAPHIC FEATURES

Secondary hyperparathyroidism increases bone resorption, most commonly evident on the subperiosteal surfaces of bone. Erosions that occur in conjunction with formation of new bone may appear as cysts or osteoclastomas (brown tumors). The presence of subperiosteal erosion correlates with serum i-PTH and with the histomorphometric features of osteitis fibrosa on bone biopsy. Subperiosteal resorption of the phalanges may be the most sensitive radiographic sign of secondary hyperparathyroidism. The tuft of the terminal phalanx or the second or third digit commonly shows resorption. With severe tuft erosion there may be a collapse of the soft tissue and change in the contour of the tuft, so that the finger appears to show clubbing. Bone erosions may also occur at the upper end of the tibia, the neck of the femur or the humerus, and the lower surface of the medial end of the clavicle. In the skull, resorption leads to the mottled and granular appearance commonly associated with altering areas of osteosclerosis.

Osteosclerosis is thought to be another feature of osteitis fibrosa arising from an increase in the thickness and number of trabeculae in spongy bone. Osteosclerosis can lead to a typical "rugger jersey" appearance of the spine.

Osteomalacia is far less distinctive radiographically than is secondary hyperparathyroidism. The Looser zone or pseudofracture is the only pathognomonic radiographic finding of osteomalacia in the adult (Fig. 234–2). Rickets, i.e., widening of the epiphyseal growth plate, cannot develop after epiphyseal closure and hence is limited to children. With mechanical stress following severe prolonged deficiency of vitamin D, a Looser zone may extend across the full width of the bone and produce a true fracture with displacement of fragments. In uremia, osteomalacia is commonly associated with secondary hyperparathyroidism, with concomitant radiographic features of both. The diagnosis of osteomalacia rests on histologic examinations and can be established with certainty only by bone biopsy.

Soft tissue calcification is presumed to be influenced by an increase in the calcium phosphate product in plasma, the degree of secondary hyperparathyroidism, the magnitude of alkalosis, and local tissue injury. Three major varieties include (1) calcification of the medium-sized arteries, (2) articular or tumoral calcifications, and (3) visceral calcifications affecting the heart, lung, and kidney.

TREATMENT

The objectives of the treatment of patients with renal osteodystrophy are (1) to return the blood levels of calcium and phosphate to normal; (2) to suppress secondary hyperparathyroidism; (3) to reverse the histologic abnormalities in the skeleton; and (4) to prevent and reverse extraskeletal deposits of calcium and phosphate. Guidelines for the management of renal osteodystrophy are summarized in Table 237–2.

CONTROL OF PHOSPHATE AND CALCIUM. To control phosphate, dietary phosphate intake should be reduced to 700 to 800 mg per day (determined as phosphorus) by restricting the ingestion of dairy products and by decreasing the amount of protein in the diet. In advanced renal failure, in addition to dietary control, phosphate binders are usually required to reduce its intestinal absorption. Phosphate binders should be ingested along with the meal to increase their efficiency. The use of aluminum-containing gels carries the potential of excessive alu-

TABLE 237–2. GUIDELINES FOR MANAGEMENT OF RENAL OSTEODYSTROPHY

Early Treatment
It is important to begin treatment early, i.e., when the GFR is 30 to 40 ml/min, especially for the control of serum phosphate.
Control of Serum Phosphate (P) (3.5 to 4.5 mg/dl)
Restrict phosphorus intake in diet to 600 to 800 mg/day
Phosphate-binding antacids: aluminum carbonate or hydroxide; individualize dosage: Basaljel, Dialume, Alucap, Amphogel, 1–4 capsules with each meal; minimize the use of aluminum binders
Calcium carbonate: 1–3 grams with each meal
Hypophosphatemia should be avoided
Predialysis phosphorus: 4.5–5.5 mg/dl
Adequate Calcium Intake
Oral calcium supplements providing 1–2 grams/day when serum P is controlled: Os-Cal, Titralac
Dialysate calcium, 6.0–6.5 mg per dl (3.0–3.25 mEq/liter)
Use of Vitamin D Sterols
Vitamin D_2 or D_3, 50,000 to 250,000 IU (1.25 to 6.25 mg)/day
Dihydrotachysterol, 0.25–2.0 mg/day
25-Hydroxyvitamin D_3 (calcifediol), 20–100 µg/day (Calderol)
1,25-Dihydroxyvitamin D_3 (calcitriol), 0.5–1.0 µg/day (Rocaltrol)
1,25-Dihydroxyvitamin D_3 (calcitriol) IV, 1.0–3.0 µg 3 times/wk (Calcijex)
Parathyroidectomy: Severe secondary hyperparathyroidism (bone erosions and increased i-PTH) plus any of the following:
Persistent hypercalcemia (serum calcium > 11.5 to 12.0 mg/dl)
Progressive or symptomatic extraskeletal calcification
Persistently elevated serum calcium-phosphorus product
Pruritus not responsive to medical treatment
Calciphylaxis (ischemic ulcers and necrosis)
Symptomatic hypercalcemia after renal transplantation

minum absorption and accumulation. They should, therefore, be used with caution. If the patient develops symptoms and signs suggesting aluminum-induced osteomalacia, this drug should be discounted. If phosphate is not controlled, the patient will develop severe secondary hyperparathyroidism and extraskeletal calcification. Calcium carbonate (1 to 3 grams with each meal) helps to bind phosphate and thereby reduces the amount of aluminum binders needed for the treatment of hyperphosphatemia. During treatment with oral calcium carbonate, it is important to determine the total amount of phosphate ingested during 24 hours and during each meal. In this way the relative amount of calcium carbonate given can be adjusted to the phosphate-binding requirements of specific meals. Calcium carbonate also provides a calcium supplement that helps correct the negative calcium balance secondary to the calcium malabsorption of advanced renal insufficiency. The serum phosphorus level should be maintained at normal or nearly normal levels, between 3.5 and 4.5 mg per deciliter, if the patient is not yet on dialysis. The serum calcium concentration should be maintained in the upper limits of normal. Severe hyperphosphatemia should be corrected before the administration of calcium to reduce the risk of metastatic calcification. Supplemental calcium should be discontinued if the serum calcium level increases above 11.0 mg per deciliter. The concentration of calcium in the dialysate affects serum calcium levels during maintenance hemodialysis. In patients ingesting large amounts of calcium carbonate, the ideal calcium concentration in the dialysate is between 5.0 and 5.5 mg per deciliter.

USE OF VITAMIN D AND ITS METABOLITES. Despite dietary control of phosphate, the use of phosphate binders, an adequate dietary calcium intake, and appropriate levels of calcium in the dialysate, uremic patients may still develop skeletal disease. Thus, vitamin D and its metabolites are important and effective agents in the treatment of renal osteodystrophy. Calcitriol, the most active metabolite of vitamin D, is the drug of choice in the treatment of hypocalcemia and secondary hyperparathyroidism (see Ch. 235). The usual dose is 0.5 to 1 µg per day. Calcitriol, given intravenously during dialysis, at the dosage of 1 to 3 µg three times per week, is the best approach to suppress secondary hyperparathyroidism. If osteomalacia predominates on bone biopsy, excellent results have been obtained with the use of 25(OH)D_3 (20 to 100 µg per day) in addition to calcitriol. With the use of vitamin D or its metabolites, hypercalcemia and, less frequently, hyperphosphatemia may occur as side effects.

PARATHYROIDECTOMY. The regimen outlined above can lead to improved homeostasis of calcium and phosphorus and reverse the symptoms of bone disease and suppression of PTH secretion. Such measures may not be entirely successful, however, and parathyroidectomy may be required. Indications for parathyroid surgery include severe secondary hyperparathyroidism (bone erosions and high levels of i-PTH) in the presence of any of the following: (1) persistent hypercalcemia, particularly when symptomatic; (2) intractable pruritus that does not respond to dialysis or other medical treatment; (3) progressive extraskeletal calcification in conjunction with a high calcium-phosphorus product that is consistently about 75 to 80 despite appropriate phosphate restriction; and (4) the appearance of ischemic lesions of soft tissues. Because of lack of compliance, many patients are unable to control their serum phosphorus levels. In these cases neither calcium supplements nor vitamin D or its metabolites can be recommended safely. Such patients are more likely to develop severe secondary hyperparathyroidism and require parathyroidectomy. Postoperative hypocalcemia may pose a problem if the remaining parathyroid tissue is inadequate and if severe osteitis fibrosa is present preoperatively. Preoperative treatment of such patients with calcitriol (1 to 2 μg per day) may prevent such problems. Serum levels of phosphorus and magnesium sometimes decrease after parathyroidectomy. Aluminum-containing phosphate binders should be withheld if the serum phosphorus level falls below 3.0 mg per deciliter. Rapid remineralization of the skeleton occurs during this period, but once the "hungry bones" have been mineralized, serum calcium levels will rise. A fall in a previously elevated serum alkaline phosphatase toward normal may indicate that rapid skeletal remineralization is nearly complete and that calcium supplements and vitamin D therapy may be reduced or discontinued. In the past, the removal of 3½ parathyroid glands was the procedure of choice. More recently, total parathyroidectomy followed by autotransplantation of some of the parathyroid tissue into the patient's forearm has been utilized. The transplanted tissue is more accessible if subsequent surgical removal is necessary. Total parathyroidectomy without autotransplantation has no place in the management of renal osteodystrophy, since it may predispose to the development of an isolated mineralization defect or osteomalacia in uremic patients. Cryopreservation of removed parathyroid tissue is a useful precaution so that hypoparathyroidism may be treated by reimplantation of parathyroid tissue.

Occasionally after a successful renal transplantation, the patient may develop hypercalcemia. Usually this is due to persistent hyperparathyroidism and increased renal production of calcitriol. In the majority of cases, the hypercalcemia subsides several months after renal transplantation. In some patients, however, severe hypercalcemia (a calcium level of 12 to 13 mg per deciliter) may persist for several months and may affect renal function. In these patients a subtotal parathyroidectomy is recommended.

TREATMENT OF ALUMINUM TOXICITY. If the patient has aluminum-induced osteomalacia, phosphate binders containing aluminum should be discontinued at once. Phosphate should be controlled by using a diet more restrictive in phosphate, and the serum phosphorus level may be allowed to increase to 6 mg per deciliter. Desferoxamine, a drug used for the treatment of iron excess, also chelates aluminum, and its use may relieve aluminum-induced osteomalacia.

Coburn JW, Slatopolsky E: Vitamin D, parathyroid hormone and renal osteodystrophy. *In* Brenner BM, Rector FC (eds.): The Kidney. 4th ed. Philadelphia, W.B. Saunders Company, 1990, pp 2036–2120.

Massry SG: Divalent ion metabolism and renal osteodystrophy. *In* Massry SG, Glassock RJ (eds.): Textbook of Nephrology. Baltimore, The Williams & Wilkins Company, 1983, pp 7.104–7.148.

Slatopolsky E, Weerts C, Norwood K, et al.: Long-term effects of calcium carbonate and 2.5 mEq/liter calcium dialysate on mineral metabolism. Kidney Int 36:897, 1989.

238 Osteoporosis

B. Lawrence Riggs

GENERAL CONSIDERATIONS

Osteoporosis is defined pathologically as an absolute decrease in the amount of bone, leading to fractures after minimal trauma. The disease causes 1.5 million fractures and costs $10 billion in the United States each year. The most common sites of fracture are the vertebrae, distal radius (Colles' fracture), and hip. One third of women over age 65 will have vertebral fractures. By extreme old age, one in every three women and one in every six men will have had a hip fracture; of these, 20 per cent die and another 30 per cent require long-term domiciliary care.

After maximal skeletal mass is achieved in young adulthood, there is a period of stability before bone loss begins. Two distinct phases of bone loss can be recognized: a slow, age-related phase that occurs in both sexes and an accelerated phase that occurs in postmenopausal women. The slow phase begins at about age 35 and continues well into old age, has a similar rate in both sexes, and results in losses of similar amounts of cortical and cancellous bone. Cortical bone predominates in the appendicular skeleton, whereas cancellous bone is concentrated in the axial skeleton, particularly in the vertebrae, and in the ends of the long bones. A transient accelerated postmenopausal phase, caused by estrogen deficiency, is superimposed in women and results in a loss of disproportionately more cancellous than cortical bone. The bone loss declines exponentially with time, and most of the bone is lost during the first 4 to 8 years after menopause.

ETIOLOGY

General

The main underlying cause of fractures in osteoporosis is increased bone fragility as a result of bone loss. Fracture risk is determined by absolute bone density, regardless of age. In the absence of severe trauma, fractures do not occur until bone density has fallen below the values found in young adults (about 1.0 gram per square centimeter for both vertebrae and femur). With further decreases in bone density below the fracture threshold, the incidence of fractures increases. In addition, the increased propensity of the elderly to fall is an independent cause of fractures.

The main factors contributing to osteoporosis are shown in Figure 238–1 and are discussed below.

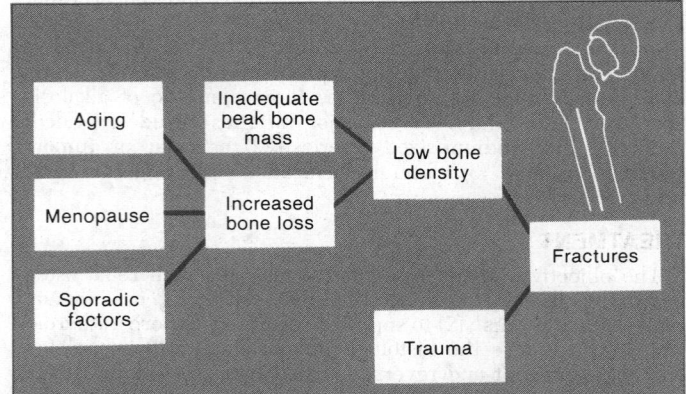

FIGURE 238–1. Model for the pathogenesis of osteoporosis. The major cause of fractures in osteoporosis is a decrease in absolute bone density. In the elderly, trauma due to an increased propensity to fall and an impaired ability to break the fall further increases the incidence of fractures. Low bone density can occur later in life because the amount of bone formed by the completion of growth in young adulthood was inadequate or the rate of bone loss was increased. The latter is a result of the cumulative effect of factors related to aging (that are universally present), of the menopause (in women), and of various sporadic factors (that are present in some but not in other individuals).

Initial Bone Density

Insufficient accumulation of bone mass during skeletal growth predisposes to fractures later in life as age-related bone loss ensues. Differences in bone density at skeletal maturity explain, in part, the racial and sexual differences in the incidence of osteoporosis that have been observed. White women have the lightest skeletons, and black men have the heaviest; white men and black women have skeletons of intermediate density. This rank order corresponds to the rank order for the occurrence of fractures. Women of short stature and of northern European extraction tend to have a more gracile skeleton and also to have an increased incidence of osteoporosis later in life. Moreover, if the rate of bone loss with age is constant, those white women with the lowest bone density values at skeletal maturity are at the greatest risk for fracture in later life. The amount of bone present in young adulthood has been shown to have strong genetic determinants, and the premenopausal daughters of osteoporotic women have lower bone density than do age-matched control women.

Age-Related Factors

Age-related factors are responsible for the slow phase of bone loss. Three age-related factors seem particularly important. First, from the fourth decade onward bone formation is decreased at the cellular level (each osteoblast does less work), and this abnormality becomes more severe with age. Second, as a consequence of impaired calcium absorption, concentrations of serum intact parathyroid hormone increase with aging by about 30 per cent. Impaired calcium absorption is most prominent after age 70 and appears to be caused by impaired metabolism of vitamin D or decreased tissue responsiveness to its active metabolites. The secondary hyperparathyroidism increases overall skeletal turnover (more bone remodeling units are formed), but because of the impairment in osteoblast function, this exacerbates the bone loss. Finally, nutritional vitamin D deficiency may contribute to bone loss in some elderly persons.

Menopause

The excess loss attributable to menopause may be 10 to 15 per cent for the appendicular skeleton and 15 to 20 per cent for the vertebrae. A form of functional hypogonadism associated with decreased vertebral density has been described in female long-distance runners. Postmenopausal administration of estrogen decreases the occurrence of fractures associated with osteoporosis by about one half. Men do not undergo the equivalent of menopause, but gonadal function does decline in some elderly men, and overt hypogonadism is often associated with vertebral fractures.

Sporadic Factors

When present, these sporadic factors increase the rate of bone loss. Smoking and high alcohol consumption increase the risk of developing osteoporosis twofold. Ethanol is toxic to osteoblasts. Obesity is protective, possibly because of increased loading stress to the spine and, in postmenopausal women, because of increased conversion (in fat tissue) of adrenal androgens to estrogens. Nutritional factors may also be important, although this is controversial. Some data suggest that premenopausal women require a calcium intake of 1000 mg per day and postmenopausal women require 1500 mg per day to maintain calcium balance. These levels are well above the average intake—550 mg per day—in middle-aged and elderly women. A high protein intake may decrease retention of dietary calcium, possibly because acid radicals increase urinary calcium excretion.

OSTEOPOROSIS SYNDROMES

Osteoporosis can be classified as primary or secondary, depending on the absence or presence of an associated medical condition known to cause bone loss (Table 238–1). Secondary causes of osteoporosis can be identified in 20 per cent of women and 40 per cent of men presenting with vertebral fractures and should always be sought. Primary osteoporosis may occur, although rarely, in prepubertal boys and girls (juvenile osteoporosis) and characteristically runs an acute clinical course for 2 to 4 years. A spontaneous remission then ensues, followed by resumption of bone growth. An uncommon primary form of

TABLE 238–1. CLASSIFICATION OF CAUSES OF OSTEOPOROSIS

Primary osteoporosis	**Bone marrow disorders**
Juvenile	Multiple myeloma and related
Idiopathic (young adults)	disorders
Involutional osteoporosis	Systemic mastocytosis
Endocrine diseases	Disseminated carcinoma
Hypogonadism	**Connective tissue diseases**
Ovarian agenesis	Osteogenesis imperfecta
Glucocorticoid excess	Homocystinuria
Hyperthyroidism	Ehlers-Danlos syndrome
Hyperparathyroidism	Marfan's syndrome
Diabetes mellitus (?)	**Miscellaneous causes**
Gastrointestinal diseases	Immobilization
Subtotal gastrectomy	Chronic obstructive pulmonary
Malabsorption syndromes	disease
Chronic obstructive jaundice	Chronic alcoholism
Primary biliary cirrhosis	Rheumatoid arthritis (?)
Severe malnutrition	Chronic heparin administration
Alactasia	Chronic administration of
	anticonvulsant drugs (?)

osteoporosis occurs in young adults of either sex (idiopathic osteoporosis) and undoubtedly is heterogeneous etiologically. The main manifestation is vertebral fracture, although fractures of the ribs and appendicular skeleton may also occur. The clinical course may be mild but more often is severe, progressive, and relatively refractory to standard therapy.

The common primary form of osteoporosis, termed "involutional osteoporosis," begins in middle life and becomes increasingly more common with advancing age. Involutional osteoporosis can be separated into two major types based on differences in clinical presentation, in densitometric and hormonal changes, and in the relationship of disease patterns to menopause and aging.

TYPE I ("POSTMENOPAUSAL") OSTEOPOROSIS

This form of the disease typically affects women within 15 to 20 years after menopause. Vertebral fractures and Colles' fractures are the main clinical manifestations. The vertebral fractures are often of the "crush type" and are associated with large deformation and pain. The skeletal sites of these manifestations—vertebral body and the ultradistal radius—contain large amounts of trabecular bone. In patients with type I osteoporosis, the rate of trabecular bone loss is usually two to three times the normal rate, but the rate of cortical bone loss is only slightly above normal. During this accelerated phase, trabecular plate perforation with loss of structural trabeculae weakens the vertebrae and predisposes to acute collapse. Bone turnover is usually high; bone resorption is increased, with inadequate compensatory bone formation. Some osteoporotic women have low bone turnover; these women may have reached a "burned-out" stage and will have little further loss of cancellous bone.

Type I osteoporosis appears to be caused by factors closely related to or exacerbated by menopause. This situation leads to the following cascade: accelerated bone loss, decreased secretion of parathyroid hormone and increased secretion of calcitonin, and functional impairment in 25OHD 1α-hydroxylase activity with decreased production of $1,25(OH)_2D$, therefore leading to decreased calcium absorption. The defect in calcium absorption may further aggravate bone loss. All women are estrogen deficient after menopause, however, and serum levels of sex steroids are similar in postmenopausal women with and without type I osteoporosis. Thus, other factors must augment the rate or duration of the accelerated phase of bone loss; these factors interact with estrogen deficiency to determine individual susceptibility.

TYPE II ("AGE-RELATED") OSTEOPOROSIS

This syndrome occurs in men and women age 70 or older and results from the slow phase of bone loss. It is manifested mainly by hip and vertebral fractures, although fractures of the proximal humerus, proximal tibia, and pelvis are common. The vertebral fractures are often of the multiple-wedge type, leading to dorsal

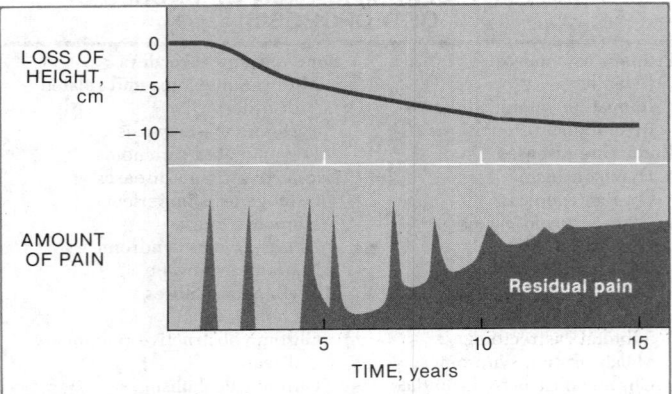

FIGURE 238–2. Clinical course of an untreated or unsuccessfully treated patient with osteoporosis. Upper panel shows continued loss of height. Lower panel shows occurrence of back pain, which is at first acute and intermittent but later chronic.

kyphosis ("dowager's hump"). Thinning of trabeculae associated with the slow phase of bone loss is responsible for gradual and usually painless vertebral deformation. In type II osteoporosis, bone density values for the proximal femur, vertebrae, and sites in the appendicular skeleton are usually in the lower part of the normal range (adjusted for age and sex). This finding suggests proportionate losses of cortical and trabecular bone and a rate of loss that is only slightly higher than the mean for age-matched peers. The age-related processes causing type II osteoporosis affect virtually the entire population of aging men and women, and as the slow phase of bone loss progresses, an increasing number of them have bone density values below the fracture threshold. The two most important of these age-related factors are decreased osteoblast function and secondary hyperparathyroidism. The effects of all risk factors for bone loss encountered over a lifetime, however, are cumulative. Thus, the residual effects of accelerated bone loss after menopause many years before may explain why the incidence of hip fractures is twofold greater in elderly women than in elderly men, although rates of slow bone loss are similar in the two sexes. Conversely, the necessary contribution of age-related slow bone loss accounts for

the absence of an acute increase in the incidence of hip fractures in the immediate postmenopausal period.

CLINICAL CONSIDERATIONS
Clinical Presentation

Osteoporosis is manifested by back pain, loss of height, spinal deformity (especially kyphosis), and fractures of the vertebrae, hips, wrists, and, less frequently, other bones. The most characteristic symptom of osteoporosis is back pain caused by vertebral compression. Typically, a woman within 20 years after menopause develops acute lumbar or thoracic back pain after some ordinary activity, such as raising a window or lifting a sack of groceries. The pain may be mild or severe, and it may be localized or may radiate to the flank. It remits in days or weeks but then recurs with the occurrence of new fractures. After several episodes of acute intermittent pain, a chronic mechanical backache may develop as a result of spinal deformity (Fig. 238–2). In untreated or unsuccessfully treated patients, severe kyphosis may develop, with a loss of 4 to 8 inches of height. In severe cases, the ribcage comes to rest on the pelvic brim. The frequency of occurrence of vertebral fractures and the number of fractures that eventually occur vary widely among patients, but the average is one per year in the initial phase of the disease. In general, progression is slower in elderly women, and substantial dorsal kyphosis and cervical lordosis—the so-called dowager's hump—commonly develop in the absence of significant pain.

Radiologic Findings

Radiographs of the spinal column (Fig. 238–3) show accentuation of the vertebral end-plates, prominence of the weight-bearing vertical trabeculae (caused by disappearance of the horizontal trabeculae), and loss of contrast in radiodensity between the interior of the vertebral body and the adjacent soft tissue. Vertebral deformity may take the form of collapse (reduction of anterior and posterior height), anterior wedging (reduction in anterior height, usually occurring in the thoracic spinal column), or "ballooning" (biconcave compression of the end-plates by pressure of the intervertebral discs, usually occurring in the lumbar spinal column). In addition, the nucleus pulposus may herniate locally into the vertebral body (Schmorl's nodes). Osteoporosis caused by glucocorticoid excess should be considered when there is associated osteoporosis of the skull, fractures of the ribs and pelvic rami, and prominent partially mineralized callus at the site of fracture. In the absence of pseudofractures, osteomalacia may be difficult to distinguish from osteoporosis,

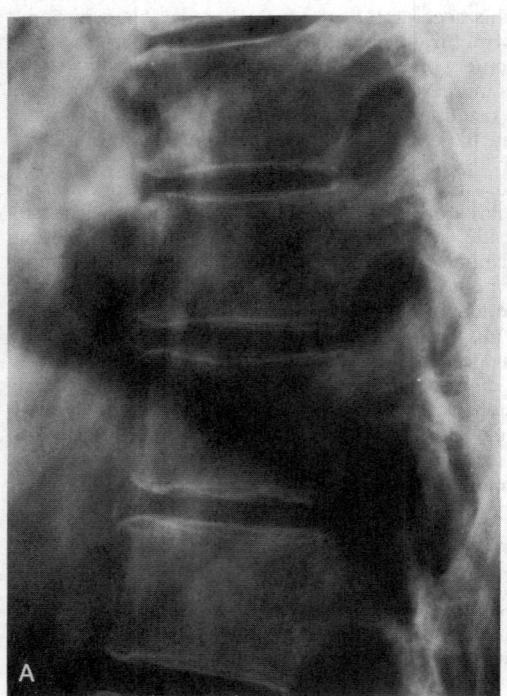
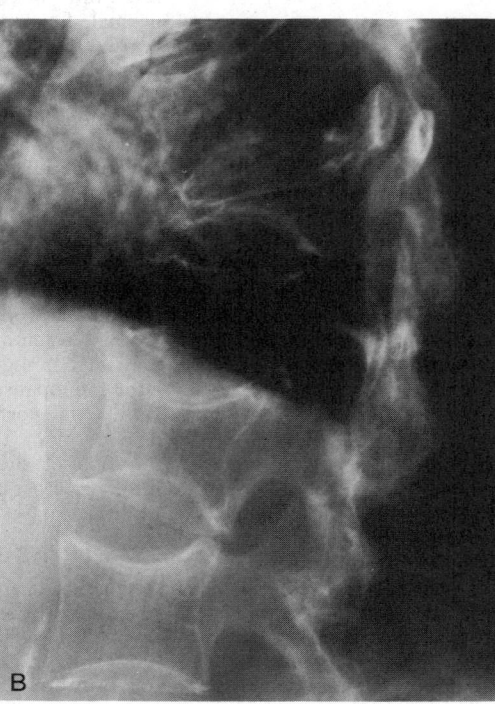

FIGURE 238–3. Radiographs of the spinal column. *A*, Normal bone in a 60-year-old woman. *B*, Vertebral osteoporosis in a 62-year-old woman. There is a decrease in bone density with high-grade collapse fractures of T12 and L1 and ballooning (expansion of the intervertebral discs) of L2 and L3.

but osteomalacia often has a ground glass appearance rather than the characteristic clear glass appearance of osteoporosis. Posterior wedging of a vertebra suggests a destructive lesion rather than osteoporosis.

Diagnostic Evaluation

All patients with newly discovered osteoporosis should have a general medical evaluation to assess severity and exclude secondary diseases that may cause the osteoporosis (Fig. 238–4). Systemic symptoms or abnormal physical findings suggest the presence of an underlying disease. Serum calcium and phosphorus levels are normal in primary osteoporosis. Serum alkaline phosphatase levels also are normal except for transient elevations during healing of vertebral fractures. Sustained elevation of the alkaline phosphatase level, in the absence of liver disease, suggests osteomalacia or skeletal metastasis.

Multiple myeloma may be present without symptoms and with a normal hematogram and erythrocyte sedimentation rate. Although most cases can be diagnosed by serum and urine protein electrophoresis, bone marrow examination may be required to establish its presence (Ch. 151). Sometimes bone marrow examination is also necessary to diagnose disseminated carcinoma.

The severity and the response to treatment can now be assessed directly by measurement of bone density. Three techniques are generally available—dual-photon absorptiometry (DPA), dual-energy x-ray absorptiometry (DEXA), and quantitative computed tomography (QCT)—all of which produce satisfactory clinical results (Table 238–2). Both DPA and DEXA utilize transmission scanning: The photons are generated with a ^{153}Gd source in DPA and an x-ray tube in DEXA. With DPA and DEXA, bone density can be measured at both the lumbar spine and the proximal femur. With QCT, only vertebral density can be assessed. However, unlike the other two methods, QCT can measure cancellous bone in the center of the vertebral body exclusively,

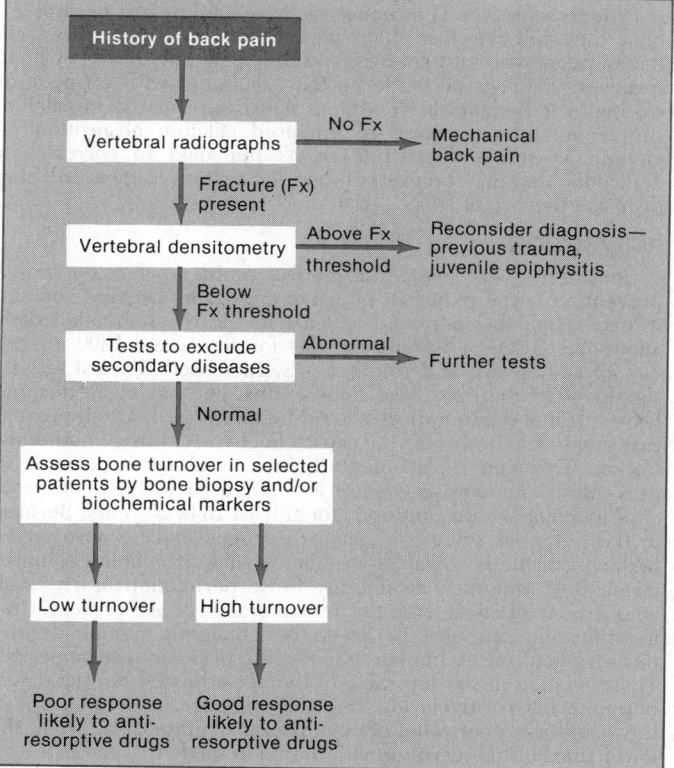

FIGURE 238–4. Diagnostic algorithm for investigation of the patient with osteoporosis. Studies for assessing bone turnover are more important when an effective formation-stimulating regimen becomes available. Nonetheless, it is still important to know whether bone turnover is low, as such patients should be given supplementary calcium and should be saved the expense and side effects of potent antiresorptive drugs, such as estrogen or calcitonin. (Modified from Eastell R, Riggs BL: Diagnostic evaluation of osteoporosis. Endocrinol Metab Clin North Am 17:547, 1988.)

TABLE 238–2. MAJOR METHODS FOR MEASURING BONE MINERAL DENSITY OF THE AXIAL SKELETON

Feature	DPA	DEXA	QCT
Reproducibility (%)	2–4	1–2	3–5
Accuracy (%)	4	4	5–10
Radiation (mrem)	5–10	<5	200–500
Scan time (min)	30	10	10–20

DPA = dual-photon absorptiometry; DEXA = dual-energy x-ray absorptiometry; QCT = quantitative computed tomography.

and it is unaffected by artifacts such as vertebral osteophytes and aortic calcification. In assessing whether therapy has effectively arrested bone loss, measurements should be made at baseline and at yearly intervals during treatment.

Iliac trephine biopsy after double tetracycline labeling may be useful in selected patients to exclude osteomalacia and to assess bone turnover. The biopsy specimen should be processed by an experienced laboratory that will provide quantitative information. Recently, methods have been developed to assess bone turnover noninvasively. Serum osteocalcin, also called bone gla-protein, and serum bone isoenzyme of alkaline phosphatase are specific markers for bone formation. Urine deoxypyridinium reflects the excretion of unique crosslinks of collagen in bone and thus is a specific marker for bone resorption.

TREATMENT

General Therapeutic Measures

Acute back pain responds to analgesics, heat, and gentle massage to alleviate muscle spasm. Sometimes a brief period of bed rest is required. Chronic back pain often is caused by spinal deformity and thus is difficult to relieve completely. Instruction in posture and gait training and institution of regular back extension exercises to strengthen the flabby paravertebral muscles are usually beneficial. Occasionally, use of an orthopedic back brace is required. All patients with osteoporosis should have a diet adequate in calcium, proteins, and vitamins; should be reasonably active physically; and should take precautions to prevent falls.

Drug Therapy

Drugs used in the treatment of osteoporosis can be classified as antiresorptive or formation stimulating (Fig. 238–5). The drugs currently approved by the Food and Drug Administration for the treatment of osteoporosis—calcium, estrogen, and calcitonin—act by decreasing bone resorption. Antiresorptive drugs are most effective when bone turnover is high and have little effect when it is low.

Calcium, which may act by decreasing parathyroid hormone secretion, is safe, well tolerated, and inexpensive. *Vitamin D* or its active metabolite, *1,25-dihydroxyvitamin D*, must be used judiciously, if at all, because the dosage that increases calcium absorption is not much smaller than the dosage that increases bone resorption.

Estrogen effectively reduces bone resorption but has significant untoward effects. These commonly include induction of menstruation, mastodynia, and fluid retention. Less common but more serious side effects are endometrial carcinoma, venous thrombosis and pulmonary embolism, aggravation of hypertension, and cholelithiasis. Some evidence suggests that long-term estrogen therapy increases the risk of breast cancer. Beneficial effects include relief of symptoms due to atrophy of estrogen-sensitive tissues and reduction in the risk of coronary artery disease. Estrogen acts directly on bone cells to decrease bone turnover; estrogen receptors have recently been demonstrated in both osteoblasts and osteoclasts. Androgens and synthetic anabolic agents probably are also antiresorptive but may have weak formation-stimulating activity.

Calcitonin is an effective antiresorptive agent, but calcium supplements must be given concurrently to prevent secondary hyperparathyroidism; disadvantages include the requirement for parenteral administration, a relatively high cost, and the development of neutralizing antibodies in some patients. Preparations

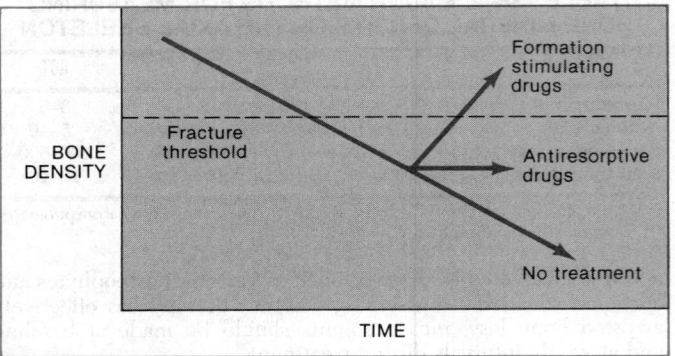

FIGURE 238–5. As bone is lost through the osteoporotic process, the bone density falls below the fracture threshold. As more bone is lost in the untreated patient, progressively more fractures occur. Antiresorptive drug therapy decreases the bone resorption that is responsible for continued bone loss. When a new steady state is attained, after 3 to 6 months of treatment, there is also a decrease in bone formation that approximates the decrease in bone resorption. Thus, the best result that can be obtained with this class of therapeutic agents is maintenance of the existing skeletal mass or slowing of its rate of loss. Regimens that stimulate bone formation have the theoretical potential of increasing bone mass substantially and thus of eliminating the risk of new fractures.

that can be administered transnasally are undergoing clinical trials.

Bisphosphonates are antiresorptive drugs that are adsorbed to bone crystals. When osteoclasts phagocytose bone crystals containing the drug, their metabolic activity is inhibited. The bisphosphonate most widely used in the United States is etidronate. Because this drug also impairs mineralization after long use, it must be administered cyclically. Newer and more potent bisphosphonates are undergoing clinical trials.

Therapy for patients with involutional osteoporosis should be individualized. Calcium supplements (1.0 to 1.5 grams per day) should be given to all patients. Those with more mild disease, especially women within 15 years of menopause, usually receive low-dose estrogen therapy (such as cyclic doses of 0.625 mg of conjugated estrogen or 0.025 mg of ethinyl estradiol daily). Because the risk of endometrial hyperplasia (and therefore carcinoma) is decreased or eliminated by concomitant progestin therapy, 5 mg of medroxyprogesterone acetate should be given daily during the last 10 to 14 days of the cycle. Abnormal menstrual bleeding should be promptly investigated. Continuous estrogen can be given with 2.5 mg of medroxyprogesterone acetate daily without inducing menstrual bleeding in some, but not all, women. The excessive hepatic production of coagulation factors, renin substrate, and bile cholesterol (accounting for an increased risk of venous thrombosis, hypertension, and cholelithiasis) is due to the liver's being exposed to increased estrogen concentration in the first pass after oral administration. These problems can be reduced or eliminated by giving cyclic estrogen as a transdermal patch (0.1 mg of estradiol-17β per day). Annual breast examination and mammograms are mandatory. If bone loss or fractures continue while the patient is receiving hormone treatment, the dosage of both estrogen and progestin should be doubled.

Treatment with vitamin D and its active metabolites should probably be reserved for patients with a documented or suspected impairment in calcium absorption. This impairment can be inferred from a relatively low urinary calcium excretion rate (<75 mg per day), especially if this rate does not increase significantly with calcium supplementation. Calcitonin is an appropriate alternative for women who do not wish to take estrogen or in whom it is contraindicated. The recommended dosage is 50 to 100 units per day accompanied by at least 1.0 gram of supplementary calcium daily.

Regimens that stimulate bone formation have the potential of increasing bone mass substantially and thus of eliminating the risk of new fractures. Sodium fluoride, the synthetic 1–34 fragment of parathyroid hormone in low dosage, and combined therapy with calcitonin and phosphate given orally have been reported to stimulate bone formation, and other regimens are being investigated. Only therapy with sodium fluoride, however, has been widely evaluated. Although fluoride therapy results in large increases in cancellous bone mass, the newly formed bone is qualitatively abnormal. A recent randomized clinical trial showed that it did not decrease the occurrence of vertebral fractures and did increase the occurrence of appendicular fractures.

The same therapeutic approach, with modifications, can be used for other types of osteoporosis. Idiopathic osteoporosis in young adult women often is relatively refractory to therapy. Because the women are premenopausal, there is no reason to prescribe sex steroids. Some of these patients have impaired calcium absorption that is correctable with vitamin D therapy. The mainstay of treatment, therefore, is calcium supplementation with or without pharmacologic doses of vitamin D. Calcitonin can be added to decrease the increased level of bone resorption that may be present.

Although most men with osteoporosis do not have a deficiency of sex steroids, 10 to 20 per cent have partial or complete hypogonadism from various causes. Patients with documented low plasma testosterone levels should receive replacement therapy—for example, with testosterone enanthate in a dose of 200 to 400 mg given intramuscularly every 3 weeks. Calcium supplements with or without pharmacologic doses of vitamin D should also be given.

The most common cause of secondary osteoporosis is chronic use of pharmacologic dosages of glucocorticoids. The single most effective measure is reduction of dosage or, if possible, complete discontinuation of the glucocorticoid. Administering the glucocorticoid once daily or on alternate days may maintain a more favorable balance between its anti-inflammatory and immunosuppressive effects and the osteopenic effect. All patients should be given calcium supplements, and postmenopausal women should be given estrogens. Preliminary data suggest that bisphosphonates may be effective.

Patients with type II osteoporosis have already lost most of the bone they will ever lose, their bone differs little in density from that of peers without fractures, and they generally have low bone turnover. There is no evidence that treatment with estrogen or calcitonin is beneficial. Treatment consists primarily of calcium supplementation (because of impaired calcium absorption), a vitamin D supplement (1000 units per day) to correct any deficiency that may be present, and instruction in measures that decrease the risk of falls.

PREVENTION

Considering the magnitude of the problem of osteoporosis, prevention is the only cost-effective approach. Dietary calcium, if low, should be increased at least to the recommended daily allowance (RDA) of 800 mg per day for adults and 1200 mg per day for adolescents and young adults. Increased physical activity should be encouraged, and bone toxins, such as cigarettes and heavy alcohol consumption, should be eliminated. Of all preventive measures, however, the most effective is estrogen administration. Estrogen replacement therapy is of maximal value in preventing osteoporosis when it is begun at or within a few years after menopause and continued for at least 15 to 20 years. Because of the potential adverse effects of estrogen and because of the high cost of the necessary surveillance while it is being administered, it is important to identify those perimenopausal women who are at greatest risk for future fracture. At present, this identification can best be made by obtaining a bone density measurement of the lumbar spine in the perimenopausal period. Those women in the top third of the age-adjusted normal distribution are at relatively low risk and need not be treated unless this is necessary for relief of menopausal symptoms. Those in the lower third of the distribution are at increased risk, and estrogen replacement therapy should be strongly considered for them. Those in the middle one third of the distribution should have a repeat bone density measurement made after 2 to 3 years and, if substantial bone loss has occurred, should be reconsidered for treatment. In the future, it is possible that bisphosphonate drugs may be substituted for estrogen in some women.

Jackson JA, Kleerekoper M: Osteoporosis in men: Diagnosis, pathophysiology, and prevention. Medicine 69:137, 1990. *Useful review of etiology, presentation, and management of osteoporosis in men.*

Melton LJ III, Eddy DM, Johnston CC: Screening for osteoporosis. Ann Intern Med 112:516, 1990. *Position paper on clinical indications for bone densitometry and the present status of cost-effectiveness of screening. Good discussion on various methods of measurement.*

Riggs BL, Melton LJ III: Medical progress: Involutional osteoporosis. N Engl J Med 314:1676, 1986. *Review of etiology and treatment of osteoporosis and a summary of the evidence that supports the concept of two distinct syndromes of involutional osteoporosis.*

Riggs BL, Hodgson SF, O'Fallon WM, et al.: Effect of fluoride treatment on the fracture rate in postmenopausal women with osteoporosis. N Engl J Med 322:802, 1990. *Results of prospective randomized clinical trial of fluoride therapy in 202 women with type I osteoporosis, using fracture frequency as the end-point. Despite dramatic increases in vertebral bone density, the fracture rate did not change significantly, suggesting that bone strength was decreased.*

Watts NB, Harris ST, Genant HK, et al.: Intermittent cyclical etidronate treatment of postmenopausal osteoporosis. N Engl J Med 323:73, 1990. *Prospective randomized clinical trial in 429 women with type I osteoporosis, showing that this new regimen increases bone mass modestly and reduces the vertebral fracture rate.*

239 Paget's Disease of Bone (Osteitis Deformans)

Frederick R. Singer

INCIDENCE AND EPIDEMIOLOGY

Paget's disease is a common bone disorder second in frequency to osteoporosis. In areas of prevalence, it affects approximately 3 per cent of the population over age 40. The disease is common in the United Kingdom and in the countries to which its inhabitants have migrated, including the United States, Canada, South Africa, Australia, and New Zealand. The disease also is common in France, Germany, and Italy but is rarely found in China, Japan, India, or Scandinavia. There is no major predilection for either sex.

There is evidence of an autosomal dominant transmission that is linked to histocompatibility leukocyte antigens. As many as 25 per cent of patients have been reported to have at least one relative with the disease.

PATHOLOGY

Paget's disease may affect one or many bones, but in the majority of patients most of the skeleton is uninvolved. The earliest phase is characterized by a localized osteolytic process in which proliferation of multinucleated osteoclasts is the dominant lesion. The osteoclasts of Paget's disease may be occasionally quite large and may exhibit more than 100 nuclei in a cross-section of one cell. Adjacent to the advancing osteolytic front, the pathology is characterized by a mixed osteolytic and osteoblastic process of great intensity. Numerous plump osteoblasts line bony trabeculae that have previously been partially resorbed by osteoclasts. The marrow spaces may be devoid of hematopoietic cells and instead are filled with fibroblasts, connective tissue, and blood vessels. The resultant architecture of the bone takes on a "mosaic" pattern in which the cement lines are arranged in a haphazard pattern instead of the normal symmetry of parallel collagen fibers in both cortical and trabecular bone. Occasionally, this abnormal mosaic pattern is present with little or no cellular activity. Osteolytic, mixed osteolytic and osteoblastic, and "burned-out" Paget's disease may be present in a single bone. Paget's disease can usually be readily distinguished from primary hyperparathyroidism, osteomyelitis, and osteomalacia by light microscopy, but electron microscopy studies have provided evidence of a characteristic lesion. The nuclei, and at times the cytoplasm, of the osteoclasts frequently contain abnormal inclusions that resemble the nucleocapsids of viruses of the Paramyxoviridae family. Respiratory syncytial virus and measles virus antigens have been demonstrated in the osteoclasts of Paget's disease by immunohistologic techniques.

ETIOLOGY

Sir James Paget, in his original description of the disease, proposed that the entity was inflammatory in nature. The recent ultrastructural and immunohistologic studies support the concept of a "slow" virus infection, although definitive proof is still to be obtained. No other hypotheses have generated supporting evidence.

CLINICAL FEATURES

In many patients, Paget's disease is not appreciated until an abnormal radiograph or laboratory test is encountered either in the course of a routine evaluation or during assessment of an unrelated complaint. The most common complaints of symptomatic patients are *skeletal deformity* and *musculoskeletal pain*. The bones most likely to be abnormal on physical examination are the cranium, the clavicles, and the long bones, particularly of the lower extremities. The complications associated with skull lesions include hearing loss, vertigo, tinnitus, and, less commonly, headaches. Severe enlargement of the base of the skull may lead to basilar impression and compression of the spinal cord, the brain stem, the cerebellum, and the basilar and vertebral arteries. Slurred speech, impaired swallowing, diplopia, and urinary incontinence may result. Deformity of the facial bones (leontiasis ossea) is much less common in patients with Paget's disease than in patients with fibrous dysplasia, a disease that usually is diagnosed several decades earlier in life. The spine may be involved at any level, but lumbar and thoracic vertebrae are most commonly affected. One or more vertebrae, consecutive or not, can manifest the disease. Back pain may be severe and of complex origin, since degenerative arthritis is common in this age group, and impingement of skeletal tissue on nerve roots or the spinal cord can occur. The sudden onset of intolerable pain suggests that a compression fracture has occurred. Disease affecting the pelvis and proximal femur produces a common severe pain syndrome, weight-bearing pain from degenerative arthritis of the hip. Ambulation may also be impaired when significant lateral or anterior bowing of the femur or tibia develops. These bones are also prone to pathologic fracture. Evidence of disease activity in long bones is manifested by increased skin temperature over the affected bone. This results from the increased cutaneous blood flow associated with the hypervascular bone beneath.

Defects in Bruch's membrane of the retina, termed angioid streaks, may be observed in about 10 per cent of patients and seldom are associated with impaired vision. Cardiac enlargement and frank congestive heart failure may be manifestations of prior increased cardiac output, which is thought to be a consequence of increased vascularity of affected bones. This usually occurs in patients with more than 20 per cent of the skeleton affected by Paget's disease or when the skull is severely involved. Bone tumors such as osteosarcoma and giant cell tumor may develop in lesions of Paget's disease (Ch. 241). A rapid worsening of bone pain or the relatively sudden development of a mass or both are the common modes of presentation.

RADIOLOGY. The radiologic features of Paget's disease are so characteristic that it is seldom necessary to obtain a bone biopsy for diagnosis. The earliest manifestation is a localized osteolytic lesion most readily detected in the skull and at either end of a long bone. In the skull, the circumscribed radiolucent area has been termed osteoporosis circumscripta (Fig. 239–1). The osteolytic lesion in an extremity bone usually progresses with a sharply defined V shape at an average rate of progression of 1 cm per year. Linear cortical radiolucencies may develop in the femur or tibia on the convex surface of a curved bone and may be precursors of fractures. An uncommon variant of the osteolytic lesion may occur at the distal end of the tibia, in which a cystlike expansion of the bone is seen. Osteolytic disease of the vertebral bodies is often associated with sclerotic margins, giving a "picture frame" appearance. These vertebrae are prone to compression fractures.

The radiographic manifestations of osteoblastic activity generally appear years or even decades after the onset of osteolysis. In the skull a "honeycomb" appearance of patchy new bone may fill in the underlying osteoporosis circumscripta, and subsequently the classic "cotton-wool" lesions of exuberant chaotic bone formation appear with a strikingly thickened calvarium (Fig. 239–2). In the long bones, the osteolytic lesions evolve into thickened bone with irregular trabeculation. In the pelvis, thickening of the

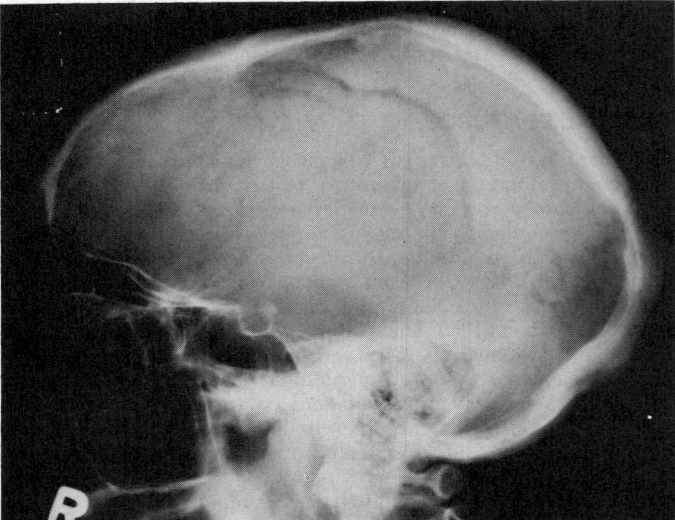

FIGURE 239–1. Osteoporosis circumscripta of the skull, involving the frontal, parietal, and temporal bones.

iliopectineal line, the "brim sign," is nearly pathognomonic of Paget's disease. It is also found in patients with osteopetrosis but rarely in patients with osteoblastic metastases. Enlargement of the ischial and pubic bones is also typical of Paget's disease. Sclerosis of the pagetic vertebral body may be difficult to distinguish from malignant bone involvement, but if the vertebral body is clearly larger than adjacent vertebral bodies, Paget's disease is likely. Computed tomography (CT) of the spine is a useful means of evaluating the detailed anatomy of the spine and is particularly helpful in defining arthritic and neurologic complications in the patient with back pain.

The bone scan is the most sensitive means to detect active lesions of Paget's disease, although it is not a specific diagnostic test. The earliest lesions may not be discernible roentgenographically at the same time an area of increased uptake of the radiolabeled scanning agent is obvious.

BIOCHEMICAL FEATURES

The extent and activity of Paget's disease have been found to correlate reasonably well with serum alkaline phosphatase activity (an index of osteoblastic activity) and urinary hydroxyproline excretion (an index of bone matrix resorption). Patients with very limited active disease have normal biochemical parameters,

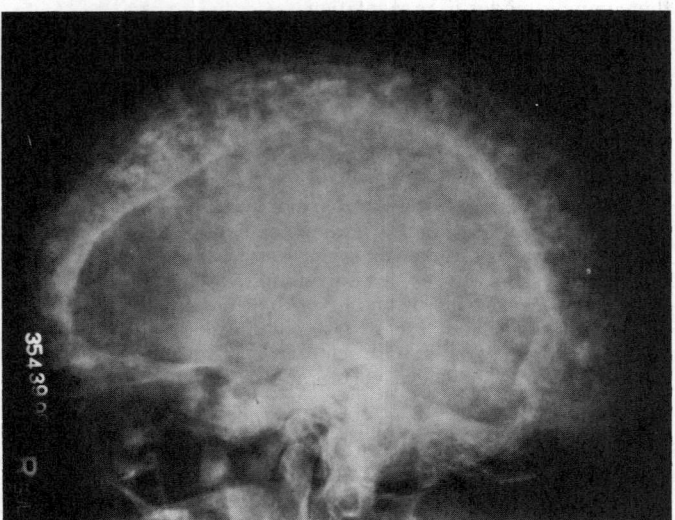

FIGURE 239–2. Advanced involvement of the skull with marked thickening of the entire cranial vault, areas of osteolysis, and patchy new bone formation resulting in a "cotton-wool" appearance.

whereas increases of 50-fold greater than normal sometimes occur in patients with polyostotic disease of greatest extent. The serum calcium concentration is normal except in patients who are immobilized or in whom malignancy or primary hyperparathyroidism develops. Hypercalciuria precedes hypercalcemia in these patients. Hyperuricemia, with or without clinical gout, is sometimes found and may reflect an increased turnover of purines.

MEDICAL AND SURGICAL THERAPY

Most patients with Paget's disease do not require any therapy or may require only analgesic agents, such as aspirin or indomethacin. The leading indications for medical therapy are bone pain and preparation for orthopedic surgery. Prevention of future complications in patients with osteolytic lesions of the skull and weight-bearing bones may be a reasonable objective.

CALCITONIN. Effective and safe therapy of Paget's disease became possible with the availability of salmon calcitonin. Subcutaneous injections of 50 to 100 MRC units daily or on alternate days produce an average decrease of 50 per cent in biochemical parameters and improve many of the manifestations of the disease. Relief of bone pain, healing of osteolytic lesions, reduction of increased cardiac output and elevated skin temperature, stabilization of auditory acuity, and reversal of various neurologic deficits have all been convincingly documented during chronic therapy. Treatment may be necessary for years in patients with active osteolytic lesions. Side effects include nausea, facial flushing, and polyuria, but they seldom require interruption of therapy. Salmon calcitonin elicits an antibody response in more than 50 per cent of patients, since its amino acid sequence differs considerably from that of human calcitonin. Approximately 25 per cent of patients acquire high enough antibody titers to become resistant to hormone action. These patients respond to human calcitonin or to other forms of therapy.

BISPHOSPHONATES. An alternate form of therapy is disodium etidronate, whose main advantage is its oral mode of administration. At a dosage of 5 mg per kilogram of body weight daily for an initial treatment period of 6 months, this drug produces benefits similar to those of calcitonin and can be used in repeated 6-month courses after symptoms return. However, healing of osteolytic lesions has seldom been documented. Long-term use of higher doses should be avoided because of impairment of bone mineralization and resulting susceptibility to fracture. More potent bisphosphonates, which are less likely to impair mineralization, are undergoing clinical trials.

MITHRAMYCIN. Mithramycin is a cytotoxic antibiotic that has not been approved for the treatment of Paget's disease by the Food and Drug Administration (FDA) but has been used in selected patients because of its great potency. The platelet, renal, and hepatic toxicity of this agent warrants great caution in its use. It should be reserved for patients with marked symptomatology in whom other agents fail.

The effectiveness of medical therapy can usually be objectively assessed by measurement of serum alkaline phosphatase activity alone at intervals of 2 to 4 months. Radiographs of osteolytic lesions should be obtained at least annually.

SURGERY. Surgery is an important adjunct to medical therapy in selected patients. Occipital craniectomy may be necessary in patients with basilar impression, and decompression of neurologic structures affected by vertebral lesions is another procedure of critical importance. More commonly, orthopedic procedures are required to enable more normal ambulation in patients with pelvic and lower extremity disease. Degenerative arthritis of the hip is a common complication that can produce severe pain and limit ambulation. Results of total hip replacement are excellent. Deformity of the tibia may also limit ambulation because of knee and ankle pain. Tibial osteotomy leading to restoration of a more normal knee-ankle alignment can also markedly alleviate joint pain and restore a near-normal gait. If possible, 1 to 3 months of medical therapy should be administered prior to surgery to reduce the amount of intraoperative and postoperative bleeding and to prevent immobilization hypercalcemia postoperatively.

Altman RD, Singer FR: Proceedings of the Kroc Foundation conference on Paget's disease of bone. Arthritis Rheum 23:1073, 1980. *A comprehensive coverage of etiologic, metabolic, and therapeutic aspects of the disease.*
Mills BG, Singer FR, Weiner LP, et al.: Evidence for both respiratory syncytial

virus and measles virus antigens in the osteoclasts of patients with Paget's disease of bone. Clin Orthop Rel Res 183:303, 1984. *A study documenting antigens of two Paramyxoviridae viruses in osteoclasts of Paget's disease.*

Rebel A: Symposium: Paget's disease. Clin Orthop Rel Res 217:2, 1987.

Singer FR, Krane SM: Paget's disease of bone. *In* Avioli LV, Krane SM (eds.): Metabolic Bone Disease and Clinically Related Disorders. Philadelphia, W.B. Saunders Company, 1990. *A comprehensive review of clinical features, pathology, biochemistry, and treatment of Paget's disease.*

240 Osteonecrosis, Osteosclerosis, and Other Disorders of Bone

Gordon J. Strewler

OSTEONECROSIS

Osteonecrosis is synonymous with aseptic or avascular necrosis of bone; these terms describe infarction of bone. Bone infarcts may be asymptomatic or associated with self-limited pain if they occur in the shaft, as in sickle cell disease or hyperbaric injury (caisson disease). Syndromes with greater morbidity occur with necrosis of subarticular bone, especially in the femoral head.

ETIOLOGY. The most common cause of osteonecrosis is vascular compromise from fracture or dislocation of the femoral neck. Other bones susceptible to posttraumatic osteonecrosis are the carpal scaphoid, the body of the talus, the humeral head, and the lunate. Nontraumatic vascular compromise, usually of the femoral head, is the likely cause of osteonecrosis in sickle cell disease (sludging of sickled erythrocytes), caisson disease (gas bubble emboli), Gaucher's disease (obstruction by histiocytes), hemophilia, and polycythemia vera. Other important causes are glucocorticoid therapy, cytotoxic chemotherapy, radiation injury, and renal transplantation. The prevalence of osteonecrosis after renal transplantation ranges from 3 to 41 per cent in various reports. In addition to corticosteroid therapy, precedent renal osteodystrophy and persistent secondary hyperparathyroidism may be etiologic factors. Osteonecrosis is associated with alcoholism and diabetes mellitus, but diabetics seem to be relatively protected against its development after renal transplantation. The ossification centers of growing bone in children are susceptible to growth disturbances and sometimes to osteonecrosis; here the relative roles of constitutional factors and trauma are poorly defined. Over 50 eponymic syndromes, collectively called osteochondroses, are associated with growth disturbances at various epiphyseal sites. The most common site of true osteonecrosis is the femoral head (Perthes' disease).

PATHOGENESIS. While in some disorders (e.g., sickle cell disease), osteonecrosis can readily be ascribed to vascular obstruction, in others, such as glucocorticoid excess, its cause is unknown. Better understood are the mechanisms by which infarction of bone leads to its eventual collapse. Dead bone does not lose mechanical stability. Bone resorption occurring as part of the reparative process weakens the infarcted area, predisposing to fractures and fragmentation.

CLINICAL MANIFESTATIONS. Besides the femoral head, common sites of nontraumatic osteonecrosis include the femoral condyles, distal tibia, humeral head, and talus. The presenting symptom is pain, often of acute onset. Radiologic diagnosis may be delayed for weeks or months because dead bone and living bone are radiologically indistinguishable. Magnetic resonance imaging or radionuclide scanning may show abnormalities earlier than the radiograph. It is mostly slow reparative processes that are visualized radiographically. A linear subchondral lucency, the "crescent sign," indicates collapse of subchondral bone. Patchy lucencies reflect resorption; patchy sclerosis indicates growth of new bone over the scaffolding of dead trabeculae. These reparative processes may lead to healing if fragmentation or collapse of weakened bone does not supervene. Initial therapy consists of avoidance of weight bearing, but surgery, such as transpositional osteotomy, arthrotomy with removal of fragments, or arthroplasty, is frequently required.

Kenzora JE (ed.): Symposium on idiopathic osteonecrosis. Orthop Clin North Am 16:593, 1985. *Articles on pathogenesis, diagnosis, and therapy of osteonecrosis.*

DISORDERS OF INCREASED BONE DENSITY

Radiographic evidence of increased bone density (osteosclerosis) usually reflects increased bone mass per unit of volume, rather than increased mineral per unit of bone mass. This increase can result from accelerated synthesis and mineralization of the bone matrix or from decreased bone resorption. The pathogenesis of such disorders is rarely known, and their histologic characteristics are often indistinguishable; hence, they are classified on the basis of their radiographic appearance. Sclerosis of the cortex can produce increased width as the result of new bone formation, and this is sometimes referred to as hyperostosis. Bone shape can also be altered by disorders of modeling, the process by which bones assume their adult shape during development.

Trabecular Osteosclerosis

This form of osteosclerosis is the most frequently encountered. Its causes can be categorized as neoplastic, hematologic, or metabolic.

Neoplastic. Prostatic and breast carcinoma, as well as other neoplasms with osteoblastic metastases, can present on occasion as diffuse osteosclerosis; however, localized blastic or lytic areas are generally also present and permit radiologic diagnosis of malignancy. Generalized osteosclerosis is a rare presentation of myeloma and other hematologic malignancies.

Hematologic. In 40 per cent of cases of agnogenic myeloid metaplasia with myelofibrosis, diffuse skeletal sclerosis is seen. Osteosclerosis is also preceded by myelofibrosis when it occurs in mastocytosis and polycythemia vera. Sickle cell disease is manifested in bone by sclerosis, medullary bone infarcts, and subchondral osteonecrosis.

Metabolic. Renal osteodystrophy characteristically gives rise to sclerosis of the vertebral end-plates—the "rugger-jersey" spine—and to trabecular sclerosis in the metaphyses of long bones and the skull (Ch. 237). Cortical erosions of secondary hyperparathyroidism are also typically present. Diffuse osteosclerosis is an unusual presentation of Paget's disease (Ch. 239) and is rare in primary hyperparathyroidism. Fluorosis occurs endemically in areas of India and Africa where the fluoride content of water is high, following industrial exposure in aluminum and fertilizer plants, and, increasingly, in individuals treated for osteoporosis (see Ch. 238). Uniform sclerosis of bone is accompanied by exostoses and roughened cortical calcifications at muscle and ligamentous insertions, which suggest the diagnosis. Periarticular pain and limitation of motion are common. Histologically, thick trabeculae are covered by wide osteoid seams, which indicate the presence of osteomalacia.

Cortical and Trabecular Osteosclerosis

OSTEOPETROSIS

Osteopetrosis (Albers-Schönberg disease, or marble bone disease), a rare disorder of greatly increased bone density, occurs in several distinct forms. The malignant, autosomal recessive form (osteopetrosis congenita) results in replacement of the marrow space with bone, which causes anemia, infection, and early death. The benign, autosomal dominant form (osteopetrosis tarda) may be asymptomatic and rarely limits survival. A mild form with autosomal recessive rather than dominant inheritance is characterized by renal tubular acidosis and absence of the isozyme carbonic anhydrase II. In obligate heterozygotes for this disorder, carbonic anhydrase II activity is one half of normal. This is undoubtedly an important clue to the nature of osteoclast dysfunction in these individuals.

PATHOLOGY. Osteosclerosis results from defective osteoclast function with a failure of normal bone resorption. The medullary cavity is occupied by thickened bone trabeculae with central zones of entrapped calcified cartilage, which indicates a failure to resorb the primary spongiosa. Osteoclasts are abundant. In some cases, defective osteoclast function is suggested by the absence of a ruffled border, the redundantly invaginated membrane structure normally adjacent to bone in actively resorbing osteoblasts.

MALIGNANT OSTEOPETROSIS. The malignant, autosomal recessive form of osteopetrosis presents in infancy with failure to thrive and delayed development. Proptosis, blindness, and frequently deafness and hydrocephalus ensue before age 2, as bone encroaches upon the cranial foramina. Despite its solid appearance, osteopetrotic bone is fragile, and fractures are frequent. Osteomyelitis is common. Obliteration of the marrow space causes extramedullary hematopoiesis, with hepatosplenomegaly and hypersplenism. Leukoerythroblastic anemia and thrombocytopenia are accompanied by elevated acid and alkaline phosphatase levels and, on occasion, hypocalcemia. Radiologically, the bone is everywhere sclerotic, often with metaphyseal bands of increased density. The long bones are poorly modeled and clublike; ragged metaphyseal-epiphyseal junctions may suggest rickets. Untreated, malignant osteopetrosis results in death from infection, bleeding, or anemia.

BENIGN OSTEOPETROSIS. This autosomal dominant variant is asymptomatic in about half of cases and is usually detected in family studies or as an incidental radiologic finding. The remainder of patients present with fractures of brittle osteopetrotic bone (about 40 per cent) or with osteomyelitis, usually of the mandible. Radiographically, the picture resembles that in the malignant form, but bones are well modeled (Fig. 240–1). The only laboratory abnormality is an increased acid phosphatase level in some patients.

TREATMENT. Bone marrow transplantation from human leukocyte antigen (HLA)–identical sibs has been used successfully for treatment of malignant, autosomal recessive osteopetrosis. Establishment of a chimeric state is accompanied by remarkable regression of osteosclerosis and the reversal of anemia and incomplete nerve deficits. A conceptual by-product of these experiments has been the demonstration that the osteoclast originates from hematopoietic elements.

PYKNODYSOSTOSIS

This disease has only recently been distinguished from osteopetrosis. Inherited as an autosomal recessive trait, it is characterized by short stature and generalized osteosclerosis and is distinguished from osteopetrosis by several additional features: an obtuse mandibular angle with receding chin, multiple wormian bones with persistently open cranial fontanelles, and hypoplasia of terminal phalanges and clavicles. Fractures are common. Toulouse-Lautrec is thought to have suffered from pyknodysostosis.

Cortical Osteosclerosis

HYPERTROPHIC OSTEOARTHROPATHY

The term hypertrophic osteoarthropathy describes subperiosteal formation of new bone in the long bones, secondary to some other condition. It often occurs in conjunction with digital clubbing and arthritis (see Ch. 277). The etiologies include pulmonary, hepatic, and intestinal disease. Bronchogenic carcinoma

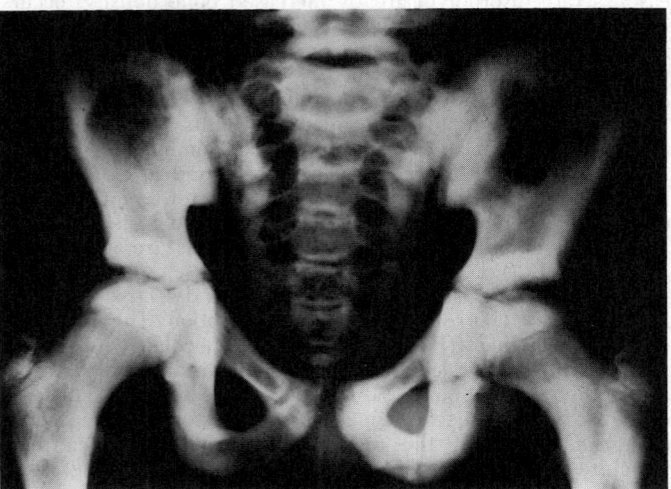

FIGURE 240–1. Roentgenogram of the pelvis of a teenager with the benign, autosomal recessive form of osteopetrosis.

(except small cell carcinoma) is the most common cause of hypertrophic osteoarthropathy and of clubbing; other causes of hypertrophic pulmonary osteoarthropathy are pleural tumors, lung abscesses, and empyema. Hypertrophic osteoarthropathy occurs in as many as 30 per cent of patients with chronic liver disease, often without clubbing. It is occasionally seen in ulcerative colitis and regional enteritis. Hypertrophic osteoarthropathy is unusual in cyanotic congenital heart disease, although clubbing is typically observed.

Hypertrophic osteoarthropathy is usually confined to the distal tibia and fibula and the distal radius and ulna. When advanced, it may involve other bones. However, it rarely involves the distal phalanges, even in the presence of clubbing. Bone pain, tenderness, and soft tissue swelling may be present, but the condition is sometimes asymptomatic. The periosteum is thickened, and subperiosteal formation of new bone is radiographically evident. Initially present as a separate stripe, new bone may eventually fuse with the cortex. The differential diagnosis includes pachydermoperiostosis, thyroid achropachy, hypervitaminosis A, syphilis, and polyarteritis nodosa. The pathogenesis is unknown. However, blood flow to affected extremities is increased, and the condition sometimes responds to vagotomy; these findings suggest that central reflex changes may be operative.

PACHYDERMOPERIOSTOSIS

In pachydermoperiostosis, an autosomal dominant condition, periosteal formation of new bone occurs from puberty in the same distribution as in secondary hypertrophic osteoarthropathy. Also classically present are marked clubbing and thickened, oily skin. Facial features are coarse, and the thickened forehead and scalp are often marked by transverse folds (cutis verticis gyrata). The appearance may superficially resemble that of acromegaly. Pachydermoperiostosis is differentiated from secondary hypertrophic osteoarthropathy by the family history and lack of an antecedent cause.

VITAMIN A INTOXICATION (Ch. 204)

Previously witnessed mostly in abusers of vitamins, this disorder is being seen more often, sometimes with hypercalcemia, in those treated with 13-cis-retinoic acid (isotretinoin) for cystic acne, ichthyosis, or malignancy. The characteristic periosteal new bone is often seen as a fusiform excrescence on the mid-shaft or as anterior spurs on vertebral bodies.

PROGRESSIVE DIAPHYSEAL DYSPLASIA

This rare disorder, also known as Camurati-Engelmann disease, is inherited as an autosomal trait. Classically, it is manifest in childhood by a thin body habitus, muscle wasting and weakness with a waddling gait, and bone pain. The serum biochemistry is usually normal, but the alkaline phosphatase level may be increased; the erythrocyte sedimentation rate is also elevated. Radiographs show characteristic hyperostosis of the diaphyseal cortices with symmetric fusiform enlargement of the long bones. The skull is sometimes involved. These changes progress with time, at a pace that slows in adulthood. Bone pain and muscle weakness sometimes respond to corticosteroids, but the changes in bone do not. Progressive diaphyseal dysplasia exhibits considerable phenotypic variation; asymptomatic individuals and a mild adult variant (Ribbing's disease) are common.

HEREDITARY HYPERPHOSPHATASIA

Hereditary hyperphosphatasia has also been called congenital hyperphosphatasia, osteoectasia with hyperphosphatasia, and juvenile Paget's disease. Children affected by this rare, crippling, autosomal recessive condition present before age 2 with an enlarging skull, bowing of the extremities, bone pain, and fractures. Alkaline and acid phosphatase levels and the urinary hydroxyproline level are greatly increased. The calvaria is thickened, with focal densities that resemble cotton-wool balls. Elsewhere, bones are thickened symmetrically and may be demineralized, sometimes with loss of the normal cortex. Several patients have responded dramatically to calcitonin.

Focal Osteosclerosis

Osteopoikilosis is an asymptomatic, autosomal dominant trait. Pea-sized sclerotic spots, prominent in the metaphyseal area, are accompanied in some kindreds by unique cutaneous lesions (dermatofibrosis lenticularis disseminata). These are yellowish papules or plaques with increased elastin. The combination is known as the Buschke-Ollendorff syndrome. *Osteopathia striata*, another autosomal dominant disorder of the sclerosing type, is usually asymptomatic and is characterized by symmetric, parallel arrays of fine streaks in the long bones and pelvis. *Melorheostosis* is a progressive, painful disorder in which discrete hyperostotic areas appear to flow down the long bones like dripping wax. No hereditary predisposition is evident.

Frame B, Honasoge M, Kottamasu SR: Osteosclerosis, Hyperostosis and Related Disorders. New York, Elsevier, 1987. *A comprehensive, readable, profusely illustrated treatise.*

Hansen-Flaschen J, Nordberg J: Clubbing and hypertrophic osteoarthropathy. Clin Chest Med 8:287, 1987. *A good clinical review.*

Sly WS, Whyte MP, Sundaram V, et al.: Carbonic anhydrase II deficiency in 12 families with the autosomal recessive syndrome of osteopetrosis with renal tubular acidosis and cerebral calcification. N Engl J Med 313:139, 1985.

OTHER DISORDERS OF BONE

Fibrous Dysplasia

Fibrous dysplasia occurs in both monostotic and polyostotic forms. The latter is often associated with cutaneous café au lait spots and precocious pseudopuberty in females, and this triad is called the McCune-Albright syndrome.

The etiology of fibrous dysplasia is unknown. It is not heritable. Individual lesions are composed of dense fibrous tissue in medullary bone, interspersed with thin bone trabeculae (often covered by wide osteoid seams) and sometimes islands of cartilage. Radiographically, the lesions have a multilocular appearance beneath a thinned cortex (Fig. 240–2). Within, they have the appearance of ground glass, owing to their fine trabeculations. Although monostotic and polyostotic forms are histologically indistinguishable, monostotic lesions are not associated with an endocrinopathy. They commonly involve the proximal femur, tibia, or ribs, may occur at any age, and can cause bone pain, fractures, or deformity. Malignant transformation occurs in about 1 per cent of lesions.

Polyostotic fibrous dysplasia usually presents in those between the ages of 3 and 10. It may involve over 50 per cent of the skeleton and frequently produces "shepherd's-crook" deformity of the femur and discrepancies in leg length; skull involvement may cause gross facial disfigurement (leontiasis ossea). Fractures are common. Serum biochemistry is frequently normal except for elevation of the alkaline phosphatase level. The café au lait spots sometimes seen in polyostotic fibrous dysplasia have jagged borders that Albright likened to the coast of Maine, to distinguish them from those in neurofibromatosis, which have smooth borders like the coast of California.

About half of girls with polyostotic fibrous dysplasia undergo precocious puberty, which may precede detection of the bone abnormality. Precocious puberty has also been reported in a few boys with this syndrome. Sexual maturation in both sexes is associated with low gonadotropin levels, and fertility does not occur. Histologically, the ovaries display multiple follicular cysts. Several other endocrinopathies have been described in the McCune-Albright syndrome; these include hyperthyroidism (in about 20 per cent), gigantism with acromegaly, and Cushing's syndrome. Levels of thyroid-stimulating hormone (TSH) are suppressed in hyperthyroidism associated with the McCune-Albright syndrome. In these glands, which thus function autonomously, receptors for the respective tropic hormone–luteinizing hormone (LH), follicle-stimulating hormone (FSH), and TSH—are coupled to adenylate cyclase. However, the nature of the regulatory defect remains to be defined and may be unrelated to the receptor–adenylate cyclase system.

Hereditary Multiple Exostoses

This relatively common disorder (also called diaphyseal aclasis) is inherited as an autosomal dominant trait with high penetrance. Irregular bony excrescences protrude from the expanded metaphyses of the long bones. These osteocartilaginous exostoses arise from the growth plate and grow as the bone does. They may subsequently become isolated from the epiphysis or remain in continuity, but they reproduce normal structure, with an outer cortex and an inner spongiosa continuous with that of the bone of origin. Growth ceases in adulthood. Disability results principally from limb-length discrepancies: Linear bone growth decreases as the bone grows transversely. Less common are syndromes of nerve, spinal cord, and vascular compression. The exostoses undergo sarcomatous degeneration in 3 to 10 per cent of affected individuals, and this must be suspected when a lesion enlarges rapidly, especially during adulthood.

Enchondromatosis (Dyschondroplasia, Ollier's Disease)

A sporadic condition, enchondromatosis becomes symptomatic in childhood as multiple, growing, cartilaginous masses within the trabecular bone, which produce swelling and interfere with linear bone growth. As with cartilaginous exostoses, these arise from the growth plate, growth ceases at puberty, and replacement of cartilage by mature bone may follow. Enchondromas appear radiologically as radiolucent defects in the metaphyseal area of the tubular and flat bones, often with central calcific stippling. Enchondromatosis must be distinguished from hereditary exostoses and from fibrous dysplasia. Malignant degeneration is uncommon. When enchondromatosis is associated with multiple hemangiomas (Maffucci's syndrome), the enchondromas or hemangiomas undergo malignant transformation in 15 per cent of cases.

Achondroplasia

Chondrodystrophies are disorders of cartilaginous growth that typically eventuate in disproportionate short stature. The most common of them is achondroplasia. Affected individuals are easily recognizable: The limbs are short; the trunk is of relatively normal length; and the head is large, with a bulging forehead and scooped-out nose. Achondroplasia is inherited as an autosomal dominant trait. About 80 per cent of cases represent new mutations; the mutation rate increases with paternal age. To account for short bones and a shortened cranial base but a normal cranial vault, the mutation must affect endochondral ossification, as in the limbs and chondrocranium, but not membranous ossification, as in the vault. Surprisingly, the growth plate is not grossly disorganized histologically, and chondrocytes are normal ultrastructurally. The pathogenesis of achondroplasia remains an enigma. Radiographically, the cranial base and foramen magnum are small, lumbar lordosis is greatly exaggerated, and the lumbar spinal canal narrows from the upper to lower lumbar spine, as indicated by a decreasing interpeduncular distance. The long bones appear massive, owing to their disproportionately normal width. Complications can include hydrocephalus, presumably related to the small size of the foramen magnum, and spinal cord and root compression, a potential consequence of even minimal impingement by a disc or osteophyte upon the small spinal canal. Despite its problems, achondroplasia is compatible with good health and a normal lifespan.

Beighton P: Inherited Disorders of the Skeleton. Edinburgh, Churchill Livingstone, 1988. *A comprehensive monograph that includes inherited osteosclerotic disorders as well as bone dysplasias.*

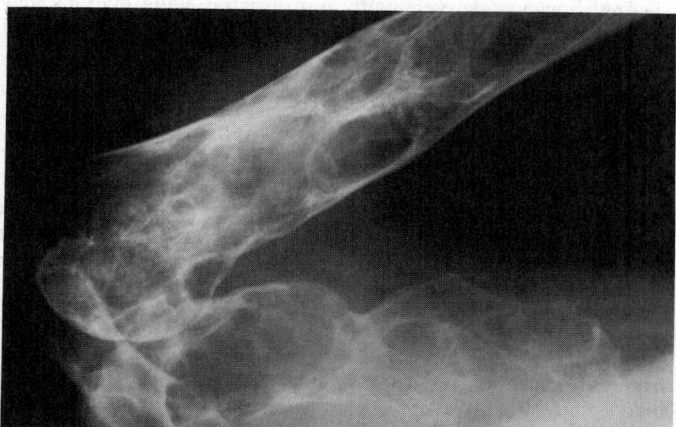

FIGURE 240–2. Roentgenogram of the humerus and scapula of a patient with extensive polyostotic fibrous dysplasia. Both bones are extensively involved with typical lesions.

Nicoletti B, Kopits SE, Ascani E, et al. (eds.): Human Achondroplasia: A Multidisciplinary Approach. New York, Plenum Press, 1988. *Diagnostic, orthopedic, and social aspects.*

241 Bone Tumors

Henry J. Mankin

PRIMARY TUMORS OF BONE

Primary bone tumors are uncommon, but they are important, since they are most frequent in the young (the second to the fourth decades) and they tend to be extraordinarily malignant. Beyond their random occurrence, bone tumors have been associated with (1) genetic disorders of preosseous cartilage (hereditary multiple osteocartilaginous exostoses and enchondromatosis), (2) radiation injury, (3) Paget's disease, (4) bone infarcts, (5) chronic osteomyelitis, and, most recently, (6) specific genetic errors.

CLASSIFICATION AND STAGING

Any connective tissue element that exists in the osseous or preosseous skeleton can be the cell of origin of a neoplastic process; both benign and malignant tumors may be classified according to cell type as osseous, cartilaginous, fibrous, and "other" (including vascular, neural, marrow, lipid, and tumors of unspecified origin). Furthermore, within each broad category, several radiologically, histologically, and biologically distinct types of tumors exist, providing a sometimes puzzling array of diagnoses from which to choose for a patient who presents with an obvious radiographic lesion.

Prior to treatment, all primary bone tumors must be staged to assess the anatomic extent of the lesion (T), the grade of the tumor (G), and the presence or absence of distant metastases (M). The determination of T is best done by physical examination, radiographs, and special imaging studies, including angiography, computed and planar tomography, magnetic resonance imaging, and ^{99m}Tc bone scanning. The grade of the tumor can be determined only by study of biopsy material using both standard and specialized techniques, including, most recently, flow cytometry of DNA kinetics. Since most bone tumors metastasize to the lungs and occasionally other bones, computed tomography of the chest and a bone scan are required to establish "M."

BENIGN BONE TUMORS

Most benign tumors of bone present as a mass or deformity detectable on physical examination, as an incidental finding on a radiograph, or occasionally as a result of a pathologic fracture through a weakened area of the bone. With few exceptions, benign lesions are small and painless. For some, the radiographic features are so characteristic as to be easily recognizable. Benign bone tumors show well-defined cortical margins, absence of a soft tissue mass, and sclerotic bony margination separating the lesion from the normal tissues. Some lesions may require biopsy for definition, and some, particularly those that threaten the integrity of the skeleton, require treatment, which, for most of these lesions, is "intralesional" (such as simple excision or curettage and packing of the defect with methylmethacrylate or autograft or allograft bone), although for some benign lesions the recurrence rate may be high and may necessitate subsequent surgery. An ultimate cure may be anticipated in a high percentage of the cases.

MALIGNANT PRIMARY TUMORS OF BONE

Multiple myeloma, the most common "primary" malignancy of bone, is discussed in Ch. 151. Other primary malignant tumors of bone are considerably less common in frequency than carcinomas or blood element neoplasms. The most frequently encountered bone sarcomas are osteosarcoma and (depending on the age group studied) chondrosarcoma; round cell tumors (Ewing's sarcoma and primary lymphoma of bone), giant cell tumors, and malignant fibrous tumors follow in order of diminishing frequency.

OSTEOSARCOMA. The peak age of incidence for osteosarcoma is in the second decade, with a second, lesser peak occurring in later years (often in association with Paget's disease). The tumor has a predilection for the distal femur or proximal tibia of the rapidly growing child and occurs more frequently in males. Osteosarcoma in later life usually occurs as a complication of Paget's disease, radiation injury of bone, or a bone infarct. Pain, limitation of movement, and swelling are the principal complaints, and even at earliest observation, the radiographic findings show obvious destruction and a soft tissue mass outside the bone. Productive changes within and without the bone suggest the presence of the osteosarcoma. Typically, the serum alkaline phosphatase level is moderately elevated. About 10 per cent of patients have metastases to the lungs at the time of the initial examination or shortly after. If left untreated, the course is fulminant, with a rapid progression of the tumor, widespread metastases, and death in less than a year.

Current treatment consists of preliminary chemotherapy with doxorubicin, methotrexate, and *cis*-platinum, followed by usually limb-sparing surgery using an allograft or metallic implant. Chemotherapy is continued for up to 1 year and has led to survival figures ranging up to 85 to 90 per cent. Even in patients who develop metastases, resection of pulmonary nodules in conjunction with aggressive chemotherapy appears to be successful in effecting cure in over 20 per cent.

ROUND CELL SARCOMA. *Ewing's sarcoma* is a highly malignant tumor of unknown cytogenesis, which primarily affects teenage children and produces a very destructive, lytic tumor often of the pelvis, shaft of the femur, or other long bones. Symptoms and signs include not only local pain, swelling, and a palpable mass, but at times systemic findings, such as fever, malaise, chills, and a rapid erythrocyte sedimentation rate. The prognosis for this tumor is particularly poor without treatment, but the lesions, like the lymphomas of bone, are remarkably chemosensitive and radiosensitive. The combination of chemotherapy and local irradiation or, more recently, of chemotherapy and surgical resection provides a long survival rate exceeding 60 per cent. *Non-Hodgkin's lymphoma* and, less frequently, *Hodgkin's lymphoma* may make their appearance as a bony focus difficult to distinguish radiographically and sometimes histologically from Ewing's sarcoma. Staging of these individuals is essential to be certain that the bone tumor is solitary rather than an osseous focus of diffuse disease. The treatment is similar to that of lymphoma of other sites, depending principally on the radiosensitivity of the primary site and the response of the tumor to chemotherapeutic drugs.

CHONDROSARCOMA. The chondrosarcomas are extraordinarily variable in clinical presentation, degree of malignancy, and biologic behavior. Central chondrosarcomas, most prevalent in middle age, occur most frequently in the pelvis and proximal portions of the appendicular skeleton. Neither radiation nor chemotherapy has proved to be very effective in the treatment of chondrosarcomas, particularly for large tumors. With accurate staging, however, surgery with appropriately wide margins may produce a cure in up to 85 per cent of patients, depending on the stage of the disease.

METASTATIC TUMORS OF BONE

Certain of the malignant neoplasms and tumors of the hematopoietic system have a propensity for metastasis to the skeleton. At times, the presenting complaint for a patient with a primary breast, lung, prostatic, renal, or thyroid carcinoma may be pain in the spine, ribs, or long bones or a pathologic fracture through a metastatic focus. In men, the most frequent source of metastatic carcinoma is carcinoma of the prostate, followed closely by carcinoma of the lung and, with lesser frequency, tumors originating in the genitourinary or gastrointestinal tracts or thyroid gland. In women, carcinoma of the breast is by far the most frequent cause of metastatic bone disease, but the lung is increasingly the primary site in women who smoke. The frequency of metastatic carcinoma far exceeds that of primary tumors of bone, especially in later life, so that staging of any individual with a bone tumor should include a careful clinical, imaging, and laboratory evaluation of the more frequent sites of origin. Conversely, patients who are under treatment for primary tumors of the organs just cited should have frequent bone scans, which are far more sensitive than radiographs in revealing the presence of distant metastases.

Radiographic findings in metastatic bone disease vary with the type of primary tumor and the bony site involved, but almost always the tumorous deposits are in the axial and proximal appendicular skeleton, are centrally placed within the bone, and are quite destructive in appearance. About 90 per cent of prostatic, 50 per cent of breast, and 25 per cent of lung carcinomatous metastases evoke a sclerotic response in the affected bone, producing a mottled increase in osseous density on the radiograph. The treatment of skeletal metastases from a primary carcinoma depends on the patient's general condition, the radiosensitivity of the lesion, the site and extent of involvement, and the proximity of the tumor to vital structures such as the spinal cord. Most skeletal metastases are radiosensitive, and regression and long-term remission can be achieved in some patients with carcinoma of the prostate and breast simply with the use of hormones and radiation (see Ch. 223 and 227). When the integrity of the skeletal system is threatened or a pathologic fracture of a long bone has occurred, prophylactic or therapeutic open reduction and internal fixation are clearly indicated and frequently provide the patient with considerable relief of pain and restoration of function.

Heare TC, Enneking WF, Heare MM: Staging techniques and biopsy of bone tumors. Orthop Clin North Am 20:273, 1989. *Techniques of staging and pitfall of the biopsy.*

Jaffe N: Chemotherapy for malignant bone tumors. Orthop Clin North Am 20: 487, 1989. *A review of current methods of chemotherapy.*

Mankin HJ, Gebhardt MC: Advances in the management of bone tumors. Clin Orthop 200:73, 1985. *An extensive review of this general topic.*

Sweetnam R: Malignant bone tumor management: 30 years of achievement. Clin Orthop 247:67, 1989. *A comprehensive review of progress in the field of bone tumors.*

PART XVIII
DISEASES OF THE IMMUNE SYSTEM

242 Introduction

J. Claude Bennett

The immune system consists of an integrated constellation of various cell types, each with a specifically designated functional role (Fig. 242–1). In addition, secreted molecules (cytokines) are responsible for interactions, modulations, and regulation of the system. Antibody molecules and cells participate in specific interactions with immunogenic epitopes present on foreign materials, i.e., antigens introduced from the exterior world and foreign to the host. Recognition events are the beginning of the physiologic steps identified with the immune response; they initiate a series of processes causing a wide range of effects within the host. These include the pathways through which inflammation takes place, the killing of invading microbial agents, and the disposal of foreign toxic compounds.

Events leading to specific molecular interactions depend upon the differentiation and expansion of the cell clones that are involved. These include production of specific cell-bound receptor molecules (TCR, T-cell receptors) and secreted or cell-bound immunoglobulins (antibodies). The cellular network (Fig. 242–1) results in the elaboration of an enormous array of specific molec-

ular events. Abnormal regulation of the immune system may cause the host to be unable to handle antigenic stimuli, resulting in a state of immune deficiency (see Ch. 244). At the other extreme it may allow the host to react to its own tissues, resulting in an autoimmune process (see Ch. 261).

In an immunocompetent individual, the immune response is initiated by the introduction of an external agent that possesses an immunogenic structural epitope. The appropriate response depends upon the recognition by surface receptors of B and T lymphocytes of the foreignness of the introduced agent. These interactions lead to events that allow proliferation and differentiation of the antigen-stimulated cells. In order to appreciate the exquisite degree of specificity expressed by this remarkable system, one must understand the molecular interactions that result in antigen processing, presentation, and cellular proliferation. B lymphocytes differentiate to produce specifically directed immunoglobulins (antibodies). All such immunoglobulins share an overall structure, but each contains its own antigen-binding area (Fab region) and within any class (e.g., IgG, IgM) a similar constant region (Fc) (Fig. 242–2). Therefore, the product of any given clone of B cells has a unique specificity distinct from that of all other clonal lines of B cells. This provides the enormous diversity in the recognition properties of the immune system. Furthermore, each of the classes of immunoglobulins is imbued with structural elements that set it apart

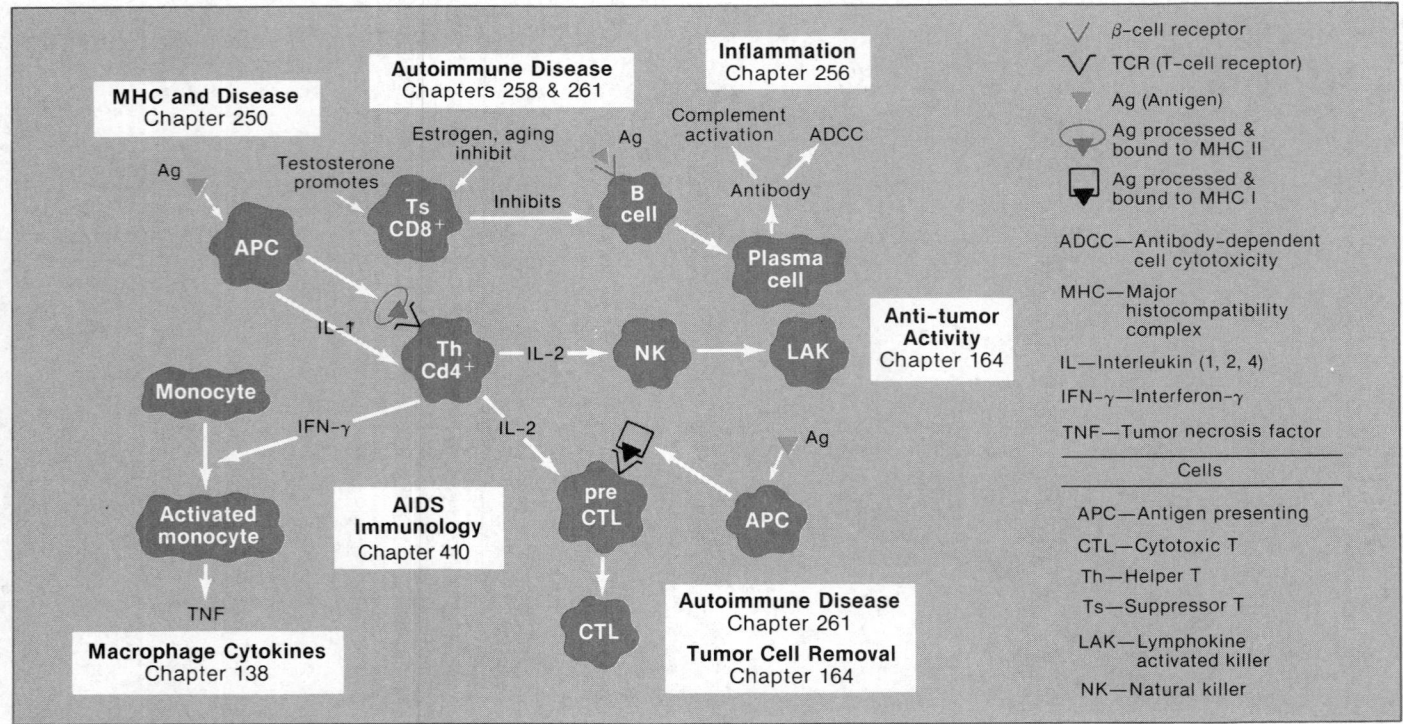

FIGURE 242–1. Schematic diagram of some of the major interactions among the various cell types and secreted molecules of the immune system. Definitions of symbols are given on the right-hand side of the figure. The blocks at various stages in the pathways and at their outcomes indicate their potential significance and refer to chapters elsewhere in this textbook for further reading and in-depth study.

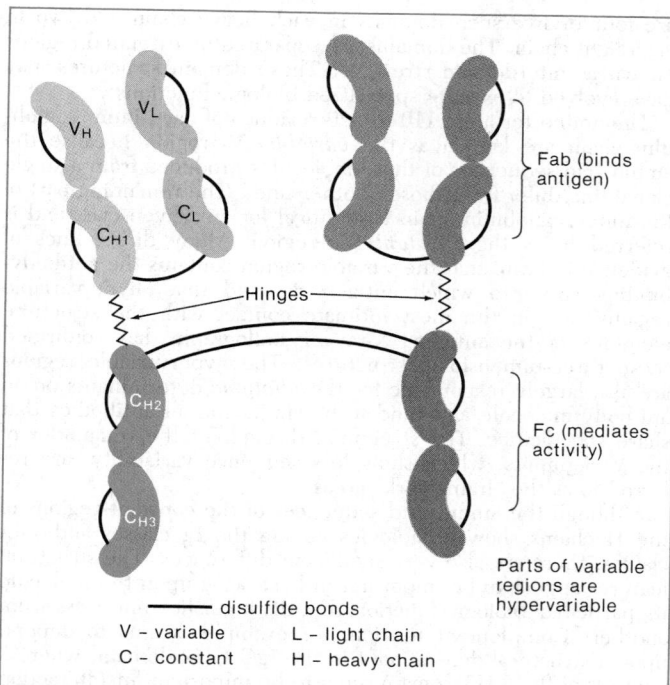

FIGURE 242–2. Diagram of the overall structure of immunoglobulin G, which is the basic structural pattern for all immunoglobulins (see text), drawn to highlight the various reactive areas and to emphasize the globular domain features of the immunoglobulin molecule.

and define its distinct function in biologic effector mechanisms Table 242–1).

During the initiation of the immune process, T lymphocytes respond to antigen on the surface of macrophages or other specialized antigen-presenting cells (APC) (Figs. 242–1 and 242–3). T cells then differentiate as they express various functions, such as cytotoxic potential, enhanced expression of immunity (helper T cells), or down-modulation of the immune response. Therefore, the T lymphocyte becomes pivotal in the development of both *humoral immunity* by way of its stimulation of B lymphocytes and the development of *cellular immunity* and regulation by virtue of its own intrinsic properties and its role in elaboration of cytokines for cellular communication processes.

Reactions of the immune system may stimulate activation of the complement cascade (Ch. 243) and the production of arachidonic acid derivatives such as prostaglandins and leukotrienes (Ch. 256), which play key roles in the expression of inflammation. Both lymphocytes and macrophages secrete a variety of cytokines, which modulate the immune response and the induction of inflammation (Table 242–2).

Immunologic events can be regulated through networks of antibody-forming cells, helper/suppressor mechanisms, and cytokine mediation or through specific mechanisms of immunologic tolerance. Immunodeficiency states and autoimmune diseases represent the endpoints of either a genetically incompetent or a poorly regulated immune system.

B LYMPHOCYTE LINEAGE AND ANTIBODY PRODUCTION

Secreted antibodies are the products of plasma cells, which represent the terminal phase of differentiation of B lymphocytes. The latter are found in all peripheral lymphoid tissues and also in the circulating pool of lymphocytes. Within their surface membranes, B cells have receptors that allow them to recognize foreign antigenic determinants. These receptors are immunoglobulin molecules, and in the initial stages of differentiation are generally of the IgM and IgD classes. Stimulation by a specific antigen in conjunction with appropriate cytokines results in proliferation of these B cells and the production of secreted antibody (see Fig. 242–1).

In the earliest stages of differentiation (Fig. 242–4), B lymphocytes lack membrane immunoglobulin (mIg). However, these cells begin to express in their cytoplasm the μ chain, which is the heavy (H) chain of IgM. Later they produce the light (L) chain (either kappa [κ] or lambda [λ]) which allows IgM molecules to be expressed on the surface. The binding region on the mIg of each cell line is unique in its specificity and is identical to that of the antibody molecule that is to be secreted. This means that at a very early developmental stage, a given cell is locked into its own specificity. This process involves several gene rearrangements (see below).

B-cell activation, proliferation, and differentiation require a variety of cytokines. Perhaps the most important in man is interleukin 2 (IL-2), which seems to play a central role in these events and thus facilitates the production of immunoglobulins of all isotypes. Although other cytokines (e.g., IL-4 and TGF-β) are identified as being able to amplify and modify antibody production, generally they are unable to do this except in the presence of IL-2 (Table 242–2).

IMMUNOGLOBULIN FUNCTION AND STRUCTURE

The basic structure of all immunoglobulin molecules (see Fig. 242–2) is similar among the various classes. Essentially they consist of two types of polypeptide chains—the larger called the heavy (H) chain, the smaller known as the light (L) chain. Each immunoglobulin subunit consists of two identical H and two identical L chains and would therefore have the molecular formula H_2L_2. The heavy and light chains are connected to each other by disulfide bonds, and similarly there are disulfide bridges between the two heavy chains which vary in number for the different classes and subclasses. They are generally located in the center of the heavy chain region, known as the "hinge" region, which

TABLE 242–1. PROPERTIES OF IMMUNOGLOBULINS BY CLASS AND SUBCLASS

Class	IgG				IgA		IgM	IgD	IgE
Molecular weight	160,000				170,000 or polymer		900,000	180,000	190,000
Sedimentation constant	7S				7S (9, 11, 13)		19S	7S	8S
Serum concentration (mg/dl)	1000–1500				250–300		100–150	0.3–30	0.0015–0.2
Valence	2				2 (monomer)		10	2	2
Molecular formula	γ_2L_2				$(\alpha_2L_2)_n$		$(\mu_2L_2)_5$	δ_2L_2	ϵ_2L_2

Subclass	IgG1	IgG2	IgG3	IgG4	IgA1	IgA2	IgM	IgD	IgE
Subclass per cent of class, in serum	65	20	10	5	90	10			
Complement fixation	+ +	+	+ +	–	–	–	+ +	–	–
Alternative complement fixation					+	+		–	–
Placental passage	+	+	+	+	–	–	–	±	±
Fixing to mast cells or basophils	–	–	–	–	–	–	–	–	+
Binding to									
Macrophages	+	±	+	±	–	–	–	–	–
Neutrophils	+	+	+	+	+	+	–	–	–
Platelets	+	+	+	+	–	–	–	–	–
Lymphocytes	+	+	+	+	–	–	+	–	–
Half-life (days)	23	23	8–9	23	6	6	5	3	2.5
Synthesis rate (mg/kg/day)	25	?	3.5	?	44	22	7	0.4	0.02

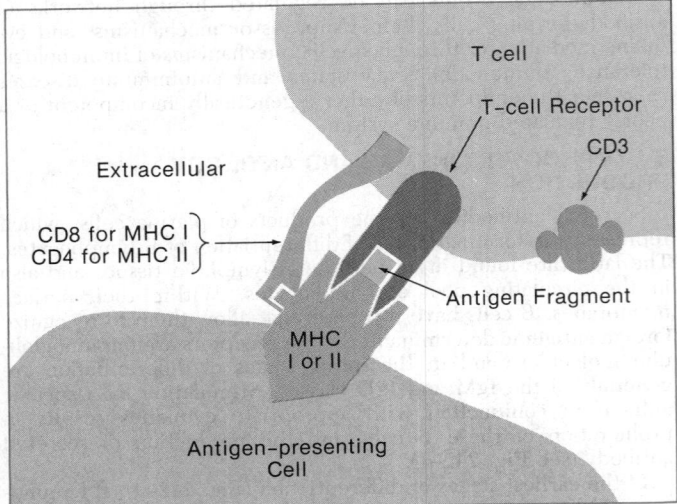

FIGURE 242–3. The molecular events involved in antigen presentation to the T cell. Shown are the interactions among the various molecules, including the major histocompatibility complex (MHC), the T-cell receptor, the CD8 or CD4 molecules, and the CD3 complex. See text for description of the polypeptide chain composition of the various molecules.

is unusually rich in cysteine and proline. Molecular weight of the light chain is about 25,000 daltons, and that of the heavy chain varies between 50,000 and 65,000 daltons. The differences in size of the heavy chains are related to differences in the structure of the hinge region or to the presence of an extra globular domain, as in the case of the μ and ε heavy chains (in IgM and IgE, respectively). Globular domains, formed by intrachain disulfide bonds, each consist of about 110 amino acid residues; and there

are four or five such domains in each heavy chain and two in each light chain. The domains are separated by extended regions known as interdomain stretches. These domain structures may have evolved to execute specialized biologic functions.

The amino terminal 110 to 120 residues of each immunoglobulin chain are known as the *variable* (V) region because the amino acid sequences of those molecules produced from a single clonal line differ from those of other lines. The remaining part of the immunoglobulin chain is identical for any given class and is referred to as the *constant* (C) region. Many direct lines of evidence indicate that the variable region contains the antibody-binding site into which antigen fits and that "hypervariable regions" are in the most intimate contact with the structural elements of the antigen. X-ray crystallography has confirmed these three-dimensional structures. The hypervariable regions are also largely responsible for the *idiotypic* determinants on an antibody molecule and tend to be similar on all antibodies that share specificities. The structures throughout the remainder of the V segments, which show less sequence variability, are referred to as the "framework" areas.

Although the amino acid sequences of the constant regions of the H chains show homologies among the Ig classes and subclasses, there are also very significant differences. The structural features appear to be important in bestowing upon the molecule its particular biologic function that distinguishes one class from another. Complement fixation, for example, seems to depend upon a structural determinant in the IgG CH2 domain, whereas features of the CH3 domain seem to be important for interaction with a variety of cells by way of the Fc receptors. More than one domain in the Fc region of the IgG heavy chain is required for reaction with the binding sites on rheumatoid factors (Ch. 258).

Since Porter's original work on the structure of antibodies, much has been learned about their molecular structure by the use of proteolytic enzymes. For example, papain cleaves IgG into an Fc fragment and two Fab fragments, whereas pepsin degrades the Fc fragment and yields the two Fab fragments still joined by a disulfide bridge (Fab)₂ (see Fig. 242–2). Different enzymes cleave the various classes in different ways, and this approach

TABLE 242–2. CYTOKINES AND THEIR BIOLOGIC ACTIVITIES

Cytokines	T	Macrophages	Other	Major Activities
Interleukin-1α and β (IL-1α and β)		+	+	Fever; bone resorption; prostaglandin release; stimulate cytokine production by macrophages and T cells; proliferation of B and T cells.
Interleukin-2 (IL-2)	+			Activates cytotoxic T cells and NK cells. Stimulates proliferation of T cells and NK cells. Stimulates differentiation of T cells and LAK cells. Costimulates proliferation of B cells and antibody secretion.
Interleukin-3 (IL-3)	+			Supports proliferation of mast cells and pre-B cells. Supports differentiation of stem cells.
Interleukin-4 (IL-4)	+		+	Activates resting B cells and macrophages. Induces IgG and IgE secretion in LPS-activated B cells. Stimulates proliferation of T cells and mast cells. Suppresses TNF-α, IL-1, IL-6 in monocytes.
Interleukin-5 (IL-5)	+			Induces IgA production and IgM secretion from LPS-activated B cells. Proliferation of eosinophils; supports differentiation of cytotoxic T cells.
Interleukin-6 (IL-6)	+	+	+	Induces antibody secretion; differentiation of cytotoxic T cells; proliferation of megakaryocytes. Promotes myeloma cell growth.
Interleukin-7 (IL-7)			Thymic strand cells	Proliferation and differentiation of pre-B cells. Proliferation of thymocytes.
Interleukin-8 (IL-8)		+		Neutrophil and T-cell chemotaxis.
Interleukin-9 (IL-9)	+			Growth of T-helper cell clones.
Interleukin-10 (IL-10)	+			Inhibits production of certain cytokines by selected T-helper cell clones.
Tumor necrosis factor-α (TNF-α) (cachectin)	+	+		Fever; shock; activates macrophages; stimulates PMN chemotoxin; angiogenesis, bone resorption; cytotoxic to many cells.
Tumor necrosis factor-β (TNF-β) (lymphotoxin)	+			Activates endothelial cells, granulocytes, and B cells. Inhibits angiogenesis; cytotoxic to many cells.
Interferon-γ (IFN-γ)	+		NK cells	Activates NK cells, cytotoxic T cells, endothelial cells, and macrophages. Has antitumor activity. Stimulates LAK activity; costimulates B-cell proliferation; inhibits T-cell proliferation.

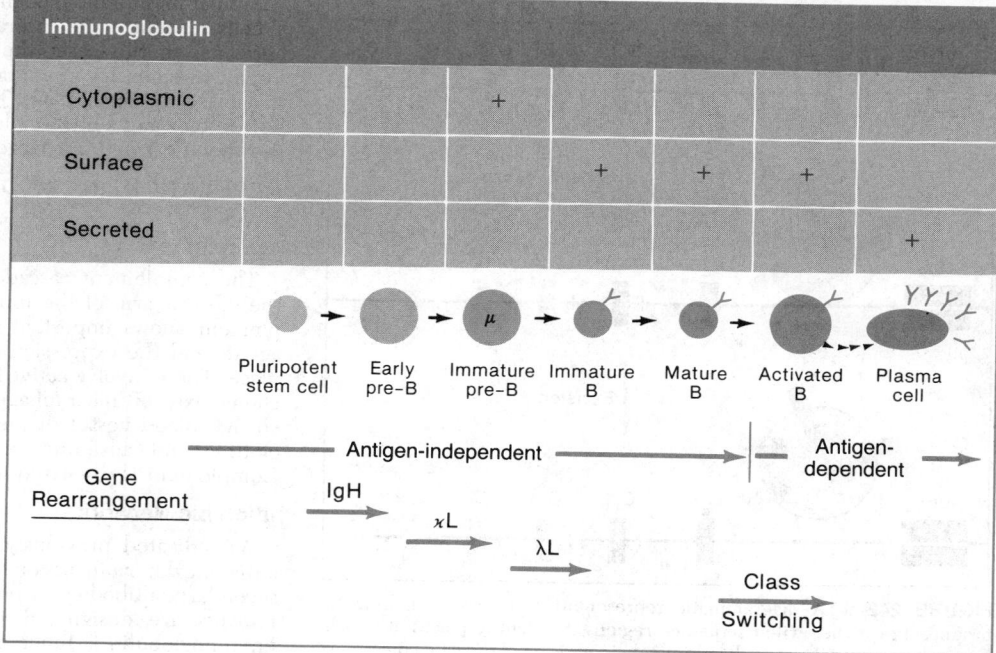

FIGURE 242–4. Presentation of B-cell pathway development in a sequential form showing when immunoglobulin appears in the cytoplasm or on the surface or is secreted. The gene rearrangements that take place at various stages of the differentiation pathway are indicated.

has been important in defining structural corollaries to biologic properties.

Comparisons among the various classes of immunoglobulin are shown in Table 242–1. Certain immunoglobulins appear very different from IgG. For example, IgM is a large molecule but consists of five subunits of the same basic immunoglobulin pattern. It has 10 heavy and 10 light chains and, therefore, 10 antibody-binding sites per molecule. However, because of steric factors, when IgM reacts with large protein antigens, it tends to bind with a valence of five. This can best be seen in the case of IgM rheumatoid factor binding to IgG, which yields a 22 S complex with a formula $(\mu_2 L_2)5\text{-}(IgG)5$.

IMMUNOGLOBULIN GENETICS AND GENE ORGANIZATION

Human immunoglobulin genes are contained on chromosomes 2, 14, and 22 (Table 242–3). Several sequences of events must take place for immunoglobulin genes to be expressed. This requires a random process of gene reorganization. As shown in Figure 242–5, each C region is coded by a single gene, but many gene segments are necessary to form the repertoire of V genes. The latter are formed by rearrangement of DNA to bring one V gene into proximity with a J (junction) gene in the case of the L chains; and in the case of the heavy chains, the V must be brought into proximity with a D (diversity) region and a J region. For any given heavy-chain gene, the total V region is formed from a single V region, a single D, and a single J (Fig. 242–5). Combination with a given constant region would determine the Ig class. Recombination activating genes (RAG) activate the V-D-J recombination, and this suggests that they may encode enzymes that have the properties of being V-D-J recombinases.

TABLE 242–3. CHROMOSOMAL LOCATIONS OF THE HUMAN IMMUNOGLOBULIN AND T-CELL RECEPTOR GENES

Chain	Symbol	Locus
Immunoglobulin		
Heavy chain	H	14q32
Kappa light chain	κ	2p12
Lambda light chain	λ	22q11
T-cell receptor		
Alpha and delta chains	α, δ	14q11–12
Beta chain	β	7q32–35
Gamma chain	γ	7p15

The C region genes are located in tandem, so a switching process must occur in order to allow a given assembled V-D-J region to attach to any constant region. This process results in deletion of all intervening genes from that particular clone (Fig. 242–6). In some B lymphocytes both IgD and IgM are present on the cell membrane at the same time, and this occurs through alternative RNA splicing.

There are several mechanisms for generation of antibody diversity which are inherent in the somatic process of Ig gene formation.

1. *Combinatorial diversity*, which results from the combination of various gene segments as described above
2. *Junctional diversity*, which results at the joining site because of some imprecision in codon formation
3. *Junctional insertion*, by which diversity may arise because of insertion of extra nucleotides
4. *Somatic mutational events*

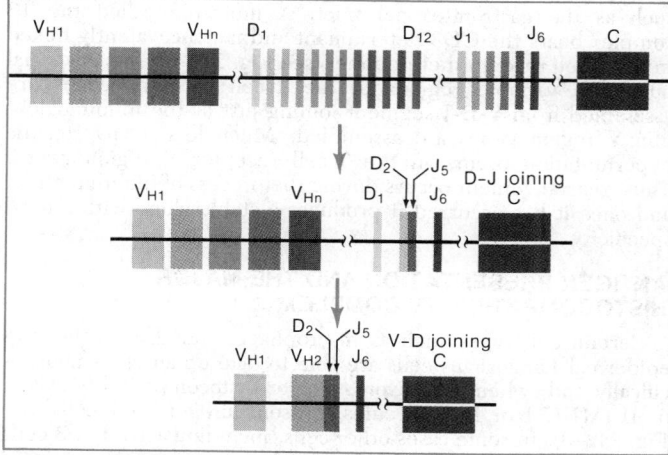

FIGURE 242–5. The mechanisms for DJ and VD joining to form the entire variable region of the heavy chain. Note that intervening gene sequences at each step of joining are deleted, giving rise to the final finished product of an entire V region with the constant region at some distance. This event would be followed by the development of messenger RNA and its splicing to form the entire translatable message sequence (see text for details).

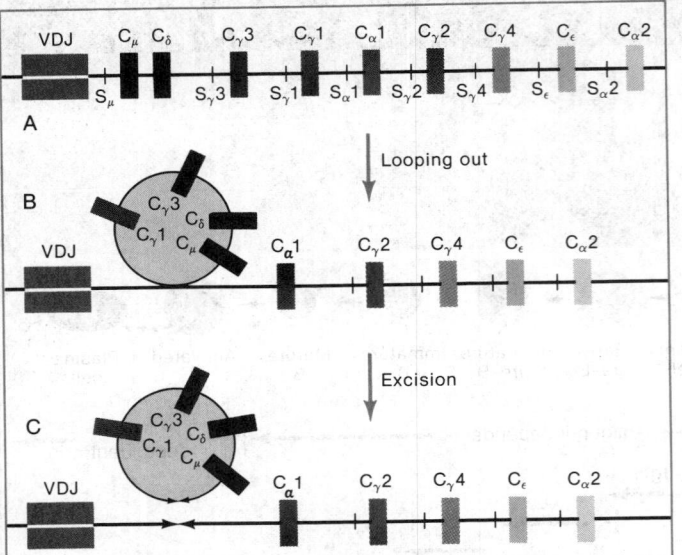

FIGURE 242–6. A diagrammatic representation of class switching to produce IgA₁. The switch sequence regions (S) identify places at which looping can occur. This results ultimately in excision of the loop containing Cμ, Cδ, Cγ₁, and Cγ₃ and brings Cα₁ into close juxtaposition to the rearranged VDJ regions. (Adapted with permission from von Schwedler et al.: Nature 345:452–454, 1990. Copyright © 1990 Macmillan Magazines Limited.)

5. *Exchange rearrangement* of the H segments
6. The *combination of associated heavy and light chains*

This process allows an essentially random extrapolation of combinations into the millions of possibilities; i.e., it *generates* antibody diversity.

T LYMPHOCYTES
T-Cell Receptors

The most common form of T-cell receptor consists of a disulfide-linked heterodimer of α and β chains. Both of these chains contain amino-terminal *variable* regions and carboxy-terminal *constant* regions, just as occur in immunoglobulins. These chains contain carbohydrate and are bound within the surface of the T cell with membrane-spanning regions. A subset of T cells possesses similar receptors made up of γ and δ chains that seem to be highly specialized and located in certain regions of the body, such as the gastrointestinal tract. A molecule called the T3 complex bears the CD3 determinant and is noncovalently linked to the T-cell receptor heterodimer (see Fig. 242–3). It is of special note that variable regions of the T-cell receptor genes are assembled from V-D-J segment joining just as the immunoglobulin V region genes are assembled. Much less if any somatic hypermutation occurs in the T-cell receptor V region genes. Thus, rearrangement occurs during the process of differentiation, and once it has occurred it produces a stable clone with a fixed specificity.

ANTIGEN PRESENTATION AND THE MAJOR HISTOCOMPATIBILITY COMPLEX

Certain cell types such as macrophages, dendritic cells, and epidermal Langerhans cells are able to take up antigens nonspecifically and, when they express major histocompatibility class I or II (MHC I or II) molecules, present antigen to T cells (see Fig. 242–3). In some cases other cells, including activated B cells that may express class II MHC molecules, may also act as antigen-presenting cells. The antigen presented has often been processed so that only a relatively small peptide determinant is bound to the MHC for presentation. The presentation event appears to involve the MHC molecule in conjunction with the processed antigen peptide on the surface of the antigen-presenting cell so that it can react with the T-cell receptor, the T3 complex, and

the CD4 molecule in the case of MHC-II, or with CD8 in the case of MHC-I, on the membrane of the T cell (Ch. 250).

Similar membrane recognition events take place when cytotoxic T cells recognize and interact with cells bearing specific foreign antigens. In this case, the cytotoxic T cell may recognize the foreign antigen in conjunction with a class I MHC molecule, and it does so by virtue of its T-cell receptor in the presence of the T3 complex and a CD8 molecule. Such activated cytotoxic T cells can then destroy their target cells by a lytic process.

REGULATION AND MODULATION OF THE IMMUNE PROCESS
Complement

The complement cascade is important in the modification of the effector arm of the immune system. The activation of complement allows important events such as removal of infectious agents and the expression of the inflammatory response to take place. These involve active fragments of the pathway that enhance chemotaxis of macrophages, alter blood vessel permeability, change blood vessel diameters, cause lysis to cells, alter blood clotting, and cause numerous other subtle points of modification. Complement is discussed in greater detail in Ch. 243.

Idiotypic Networks

As indicated previously, antibody molecules express unique antigenic determinants on their variable regions, thereby allowing secondary antibodies to be produced against them. Such determinants are designated *idiotopes*. Therefore, an idiotope of immunoglobulin is functionally equivalent to the *clonotypic* antigenic determinant of a clonal line of T cells. The idiotypic network concept (Fig. 242–7) holds that the immune system is in a dynamic regulatory equilibrium so that members of each clone within the system are recognized by members of other clones through these anti-idiotype interactions. Conceptually, this interrelated system provides mechanisms for regulation based on recognition of receptors without need for exogenous antigen. This method of regulation may allow certain idiotopes to become dominantly expressed and may be operative with unique *clonal markers*, such as those that are observed due to clonal expansion in malignant lymphoid diseases.

Suppression

Regulation of responses to antigenic stimulation and also control of potential immune responses against self components are essential ingredients of a smoothly operating immune system. Suppressor T cells and the suppressor system represent a series of cell types that act in a highly complex fashion. Several distinct types of suppressor systems have been described, and their sequential action appears to have an amplification effect so that direct and graded regulation can take place. Suppressor effector cells can act on antibody-secreting cells and on T cells to downregulate their expression. Although the mechanism of suppression exists, the T-suppressor cell has yet to be isolated.

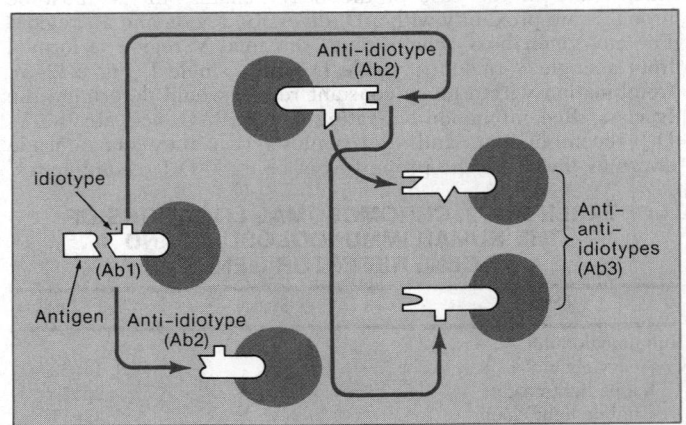

FIGURE 242–7. Diagrammatic representation of the idiotypic network showing the development of anti-idiotypes and anti-anti-idiotypes in sequential processes. This complementary fit mechanism provides the structural basis for the feedback network.

A growing array of molecules have been identified as products of cells that serve to regulate the immune system and to evoke responses in other cells, such as blood vessel endothelial cells and precursor cells in the bone marrow. Cytokines can regulate levels of response or induce differentiation and proliferation of cells. Table 242–2 summarizes the properties of some of these molecules which may be encountered in immune regulation (see also Ch. 256 and 285).

SUMMARY

The immune system is a highly orchestrated and coordinated system that allows a rapid response to foreign substances in a highly specific manner. The organization occurs at the level of the gene, the cell, and the mediator. Therefore, any qualitative or quantitative change in this system can produce profound effects. This is evident as one examines diseases of the immune system, such as those that occur as the result of alteration in immune regulation (see Ch. 258 and 261).

Inflammation, often immunologically mediated and often resulting in tissue damage, is a key feature of diseases of virtually any organ system. Therefore, a knowledge of basic immunology is critical to a clear understanding of the nature of these abnormalities. A student of medicine must be prepared for application of immunology to every branch of internal medicine and for recognizing its importance to an understanding of disease and, hence, the care of the patient.

Balkwill FR, Burke F: The cytokine network. Immunol Today 10:299, 1989. *An excellent integration of cytokine functions.*
Benjamini E, Leskowitz S: Immunology: A Short Course. New York, Alan R. Liss, 1988. *An excellent, manageable general text for the novice.*
Krensky AM, Weiss A, Crabtree G, et al: T-lymphocyte–antigen interactions in transplant rejection. N Engl J Med 322:510, 1990. *Description of T-cell pathways and functional interactions.*
Lai E, Wilson RK, Hood LE: Physical maps of the mouse and human immunoglobulin-like loci. Adv Immunol 46:1, 1989. *Description of the genetic relationships and the methods for generating physical gene maps for this group of structures.*
Maizels N: To understand function, study structure. Cell 60:887, 1990. *A brief discussion of the T-cell receptor structure and its relationship to the structure of immunoglobulins.*
Oettinger MA, Schatz DG, Gorka C, Baltimore D: RAG-1 and RAG-2, adjacent genes that synergistically activate V(D)J recombination. Science 248:1517, 1990. *A detailed description of the mechanisms of Ig class switching.*
Smith KA: Interleukin-2. Sci Am, March 1990, p. 50. *A superb and easy-to-read discussion of the pivotal cytokines in regulation of the immune system.*

243 Complement
John E. Volanakis

Complement is a major effector system of host defense against invading pathogens. It comprises more than 30 proteins that upon activation elaborate protein fragments and protein-protein complexes that interact with specific cellular receptors or directly with cell membranes to mediate acute inflammatory reactions, clearance of foreign cells and molecules, and killing of pathogenic microorganisms. In their native state, complement proteins are either serum soluble or associated with cell membranes (Table 243–1). Most of the serum-soluble proteins are synthesized in the liver. However, a number of other cells—including blood monocytes, tissue macrophages, fibroblasts, epithelial cells of the gastrointestinal and genitourinary tracts, adipocytes, and glial cells—can also produce these proteins. Complement proteins exhibit extensive structural homologies among themselves with remarkable conservation of a small number of repeated structural motifs, indicating that multiple gene duplication events marked the evolution of the system. Functionally, complement proteins are categorized as those participating in the activation sequences, those regulating the activation and activities of the system, and those serving as receptors for biologically active fragments. Some complement proteins overlap these functional categories.

NOMENCLATURE

Eleven of the proteins participating in complement activation are termed complement components and are designated by the letter C and a number from 1 to 9. C1 is a Ca^{2+}-dependent complex of three distinct proteins, C1q, C1r, and C1s. Two additional proteins in this group are designated by the letters B and D. An overbar indicates the enzymatically active form of a complement protein or protein complex, as in $\overline{C1}$. Proteolytic cleavage fragments of complement proteins are symbolized by lower case letters, as in C2a and C2b, and inactive fragments by the letter i, e.g., C2ai. Regulatory proteins are designated by capital letters, as in H and I, or by their abbreviated descriptive names, as in DAF for decay-accelerating factor. Five of the complement receptors are symbolized by the letters CR, for complement receptor, and a number from 1 to 5. The remaining receptors are denoted by the symbol of the protein or protein fragment they bind followed by the letter R, as in C5aR.

COMPLEMENT ACTIVATION

Activation of the complement system is necessary for expression of biologic activity and is characterized by operational simplicity and economy of design. The most important host defense activities are derived from two proteins, C3 and C5, that are structurally homologous and probably represent gene duplication products. Additional biologically active products are derived from C4, another structural homologue of C3. Expression of activity requires cleavage of C3 and C5 by highly specific proteases, termed *convertases* (Fig. 243–1). There are two C3 and two C5 convertases. One of each is assembled during activation of the two pathways of complement, which are termed *classic* and *alternative*. C3 convertases are bimolecular, whereas C5 convertases are trimolecular protein complexes. The two activation pathways utilize different proteins to form these enzymes. In addition, the assembly of the convertases is initiated by different activators in the two pathways. However, the resulting enzymes have identical substrate and peptide bond specificity, giving rise to identical biologically active fragments. Characteristic of the simplicity and economy of design of complement activation is the fact that C5 convertases are derivatives of C3 convertases (Fig. 243–1). In each case, a C3b fragment, produced by the action of C3

TABLE 243–1. PROTEINS OF THE COMPLEMENT SYSTEM*

Prevalent Form in Native State	Functional Group		
	Participating in Activation Sequences	*Regulatory*	*Receptors*
Serum soluble	C1q, C1r, C1s, D C4, C3, C2, B C5, C6, C7, C8, C9	C1 INH C4bp, H, I, P C3a/C5a INA S protein	
Membrane associated		CR1, CR2 DAF, MCP HRF, CD59	C1qR, C3aR, C5aR CR1, CR2, CR3 CR4, CR5

*Established symbols have been used for most complement proteins. In addition, the following generally accepted abbreviations have been used: INH, inhibitor; C4bp, C4b-binding protein; INA, inactivator; R, receptor, e.g., CR1, complement receptor type 1; DAF, decay-accelerating factor; MCP, membrane cofactor protein; HRF, homologous restriction factor.

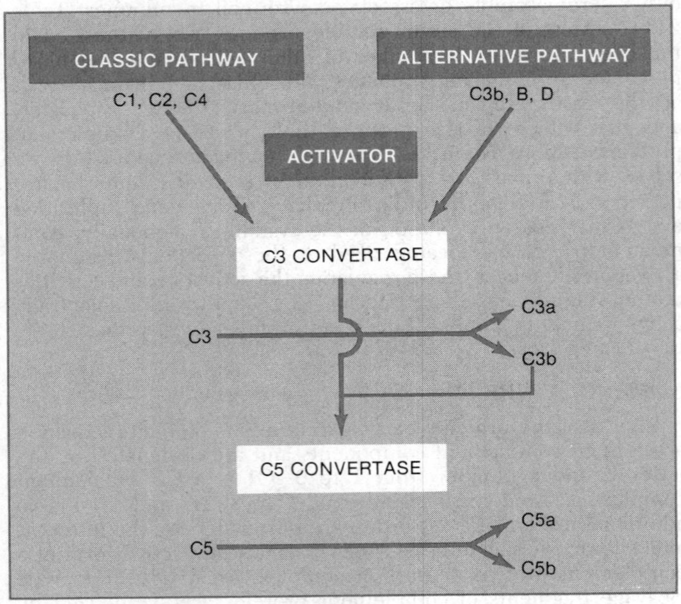

FIGURE 243–1. Activation of the complement system.

completing the assembly of the $\overline{C4b2a}$ complex, which is the C3 convertase of the classic pathway. Cleavage of C3 by the C3 convertase results in the covalent binding of many C3b fragments to the surface of the immune complex and the eventual binding of one C3b to the C4b subunit of the C3 convertase. This leads to the formation of the $\overline{C3b4b2a}$ complex, which is the C5 convertase of the classic pathway.

ALTERNATIVE PATHWAY. Activation of the alternative pathway is initiated by a variety of cellular surfaces, including those of certain bacteria, parasites, viruses, and fungi. Antibodies can also activate this pathway, but they are not usually required. Assembly of the convertases is intimately related to certain structural features of the multifunctional protein C3. C3 is the most abundant complement protein in blood and is characterized by the presence on its α-chain of an unusual, for blood proteins, thioester bond. Under physiologic conditions, this bond is relatively stable, being hydrolyzed at very slow rates to give rise to $C3_{H_2O}$, which is endowed with the ability to initiate the formation of the short-lived *initiation* C3 convertase. This is accomplished by the formation of a complex between $C3_{H_2O}$ and $\underline{B\ and}$ the subsequent cleavage of B by D to generate the $C3_{H_2O}Bb$ complex, the initiation C3 convertase (Fig. 243–3). This series of reactions, starting with the hydrolysis of the thioester bond in native C3 and concluding with the cleavage of C3 into C3a and C3b by the initiation C3 convertase, is considered to occur in the blood continuously at slow rates. Thus, a constant supply of small amounts of freshly generated C3b is available at all times. The initiation C3 convertase is quickly inactivated by the control proteins H and I.

Cleavage of C3 by a C3 convertase induces a pronounced change in the conformation of C3b associated with an extremely labile (metastable) thioester bond that reacts either with water or with hydroxyl or amino groups on the surface of cells or proteins. Thus, C3b becomes covalently attached via an ester or amide bond to surfaces in the immediate vicinity of its generation. The fate of surface-bound C3b depends entirely on the chemical nature of the surface. C3b bound to a nonactivator of the alternative pathway, e.g., host's red cells, is quickly inactivated by the action of control proteins. In contrast, C3b bound to an activator, e.g., *Escherichia coli* cells, preferentially binds B, which is then cleaved by D, generating the $\overline{C3bBb}$ complex, which is the C3 convertase of the alternative pathway. This enzyme is stabilized by the binding of P and is termed the *amplification* C3 convertase because it generates many C3b fragments and thus additional molecules of C3 convertase. Binding of a single C3b molecule to the C3 convertase gives rise to the $\overline{(C3b)_2Bb}$ complex, which is the C5 convertase of the alternative pathway (Fig. 243–3). A biochemical feature determining whether a cell surface can function as an activator of the alternative pathway is the relative amount of sialic acid that is present in membrane-associated glycoproteins and glycolipids. Sialic acid increases the affinity of C3b for the control protein H which prevents the formation of a C3 convertase. Conversely, the absence of cell surface sialic acid favors the binding of B to C3b and the formation of the amplification convertase.

convertase on C3, binds covalently to the C3 convertase and results in the generation of a C5 convertase. Furthermore, C3 and C5 are activated by their respective convertases in similar fashion: A single peptide bond near the NH_2 terminus of the α polypeptide chain of either C3 or C5 is cleaved to generate a small peptide, C3a or C5a, and a large two-polypeptide fragment, C3b or C5b. Each of these four fragments, as well as further cleavage fragments of C3b, express at least one activity important to host defense.

ASSEMBLY OF COMPLEMENT CONVERTASES

CLASSIC PATHWAY. In the classic pathway, assembly of the convertases is initiated by antibodies of the IgG or IgM class complexed with antigen. C1q, one of the three proteins in the C1 complex, binds to two or more Fc regions of antibody molecules within the immune complex. This binding induces a change in the conformation of C1q that causes the autoactivation of C1r, which in turn activates proenzyme C1s to enzymatically active $\overline{C1s}$ (Fig. 243–2). In the next step, $\overline{C1s}$ cleaves C4, resulting in the covalent attachment of its major fragment, C4b, to the surface of the immune complex. Attachment of C4b is accomplished through a transacylation reaction similar to that leading to covalent binding of C3b to activating surfaces (see below). C2 binds to C4b and is also cleaved by $\overline{C1s}$ into two fragments, the larger of which, C2a, remains bound to C4b,

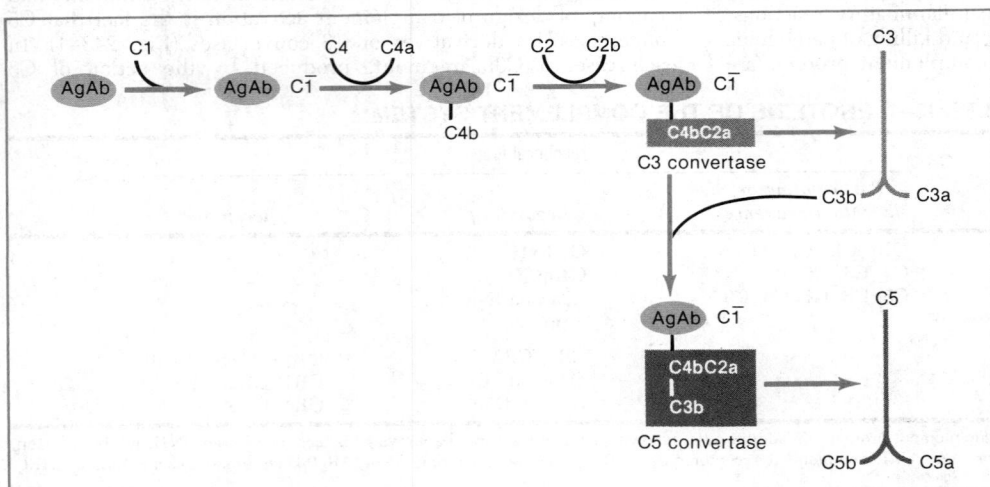

FIGURE 243–2. Formation of complement convertases in the classic pathway of activation.

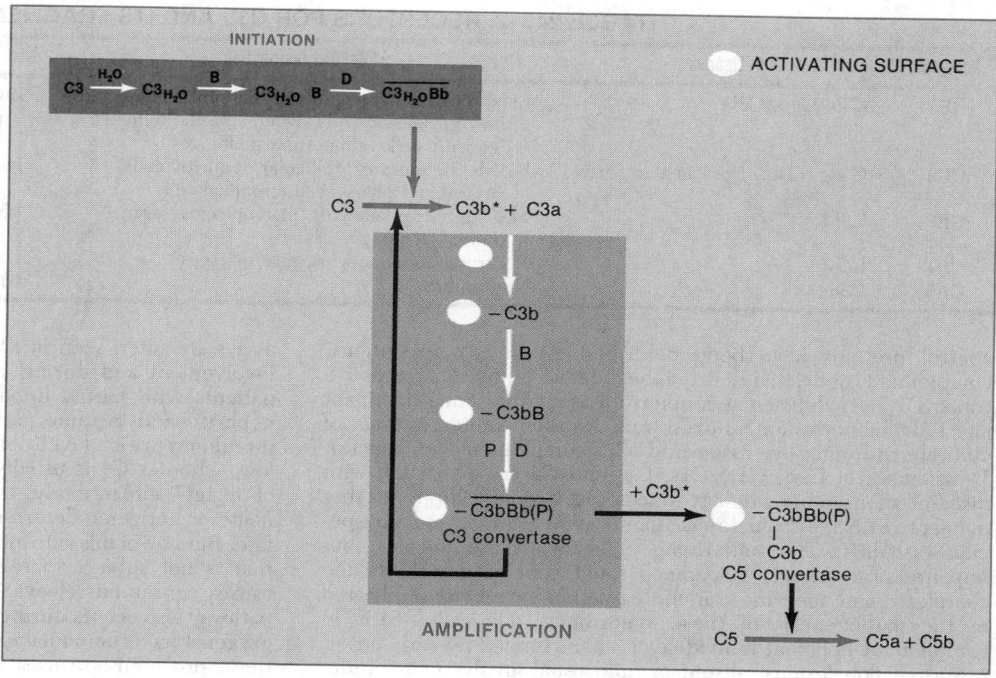

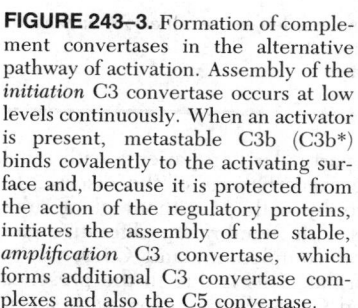

FIGURE 243–3. Formation of complement convertases in the alternative pathway of activation. Assembly of the *initiation* C3 convertase occurs at low levels continuously. When an activator is present, metastable C3b (C3b*) binds covalently to the activating surface and, because it is protected from the action of the regulatory proteins, initiates the assembly of the stable, *amplification* C3 convertase, which forms additional C3 convertase complexes and also the C5 convertase.

BIOLOGIC ACTIVITIES OF COMPLEMENT

With the exception of C5b, the fragments produced by the action of the convertases carry out their biologic functions by interacting with specific cellular receptors (Fig. 243–4). The three complement *anaphylatoxins*, C3a, C5a, and C4a, react with specific receptors to stimulate the release of histamine from mast cells mediating smooth muscle contraction and increased vascular permeability. In addition, C5a evokes neutrophil and monocyte responses, including adherence to vascular endothelia, chemotaxis, release of lysosomal enzymes, and generation of oxygen free radicals. Collectively, the anaphylatoxins allow for the recruitment of host defense molecules and cells to tissue sites invaded by pathogens. C3b and its further cleavage fragments, C3bi and C3dg, react with multiple receptors distributed in a variety of cells (Table 243–2). C3b covalently attached to immune complexes binds to CR1 receptors on erythrocytes, which transport the complexes to the liver, where they are taken up by Kupffer cells and cleared from the circulation. C3b and C3bi interact with CR1 and CR3, respectively, on phagocytic cells to promote ingestion of foreign cells and particles. Reaction of C3bi and C3dg with CR2 on B lymphocytes plays a role in regulating immune responses. C5b initiates the assembly of a large protein-protein complex, termed membrane attack complex (MAC), by interacting sequentially with a single molecule each of C6, C7, and C8 and with 1 to 12 molecules of C9. The MAC interacts directly with the lipid bilayer of biologic membranes through hydrophobic domains of the participating proteins and eventually forms a transmembrane channel that leads to killing of susceptible cells.

CONTROL OF COMPLEMENT ACTIVATION

The multiplicity and potency of the biologic activities generated during complement activation and particularly the ability of complement to mediate acute inflammatory reactions and to produce lethal lesions in cell membranes present a threat not only to invading pathogens but also to the cells and tissues of the host. This self-damaging potential of complement activation is normally kept under effective control by a number of inhibitors and inactivators that act at points of enzymatic amplification and also at the level of effector molecules. C1 INH binds to and inhibits C1̄r and C1̄s, regulating the activation and action of C1̄. A number of plasma and membrane-associated proteins, including C4bp, H, DAF, MCP, CR1, and CR2, control the rate of formation and the activity of complement convertases. Certain of these proteins act as obligatory cofactors for the proteolytic

enzyme I which cleaves C4b and C3b into smaller fragments. The serum S protein, also termed vitronectin, and two cell-associated proteins, HRF and CD59, inhibit the formation of the MAC. HRF and CD59 exhibit species specificity in their action. Finally, C3a/C5a INA, a carboxypeptidase, inactivates the complement anaphylatoxins. Collectively, the complement control proteins perform two important functions: They ensure that complement activation is proportional to the amount and duration of presence of complement activators and protect the cells of the host from the harmful potential of complement activation products.

INHERITED DEFICIENCIES OF COMPLEMENT PROTEINS (Table 243–3)

Hereditary deficiencies of almost all complement proteins participating in the activation sequences and of several of the

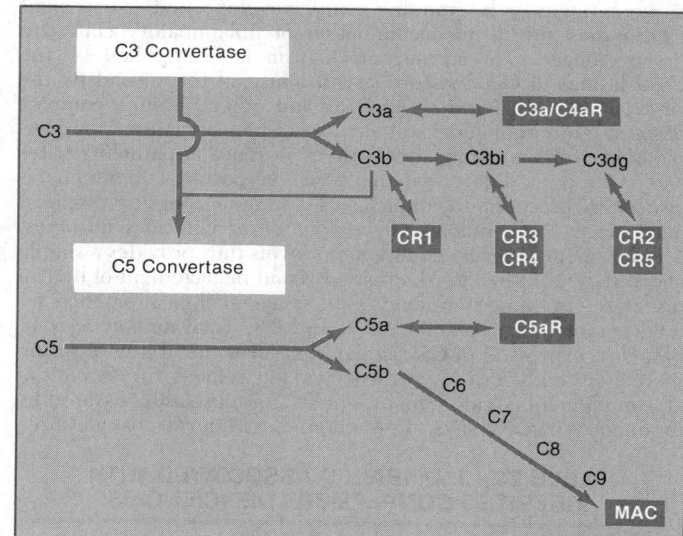

FIGURE 243–4. Interactions of complement fragments with cellular receptors that mediate biologic activities. The complex formed from the binding to C5b of one molecule of C6, C7, and C8 and of 1 to 12 molecules of C9 is termed MAC (membrane attack complex). It forms transmembrane pores by interacting directly with the lipid bilayer of biologic membranes.

TABLE 243–2. RECEPTORS FOR C3b AND ITS FRAGMENTS

Receptor	Ligands	Cellular Distribution	Functions
CR1	C3b, C4b, C3bi	Erythrocytes, neutrophils, eosinophils, monocytes, macrophages, B cells, T-cell subsets, follicular dendritic cells, glomerular podocytes	Immune complex clearance, endocytosis, phagocytosis, immunoregulation
CR2	C3dg, C3bi, Epstein-Barr virus	B cells, thymocytes, follicular dendritic cells, cervical and pharyngeal epithelial cells	Immunoregulation
CR3	C3bi	Neutrophils, monocytes, macrophages, large granular lymphocytes	Phagocytosis, leukocyte adhesion, enhanced cytotoxicity
CR4	C3bi	Neutrophils, monocytes, macrophages	Unknown
CR5	C3dg	Neutrophils	Unknown

control proteins have been described. With two exceptions, complement deficiencies are inherited as autosomal recessive traits. C1 INH deficiency is inherited as an autosomal dominant and P deficiency as an X-linked trait. A rather limited number of clinical syndromes are associated with complement deficiencies. Deficiencies of C1q, C1r, C1s, C4, and C2 are associated with diseases of immune etiology, including systemic lupus erythematosus (SLE), discoid lupus, glomerulonephritis, and nonspecific vasculitis. The underlying mechanisms are unclear, but impaired processing and clearance from the circulation of immune complexes and aberrant immunoregulation have been implicated in the pathogenesis of these syndromes. Clinically, SLE in complement-deficient individuals is characterized by early onset, extensive skin lesions, absent or mild renal involvement, undetectable anti-DNA, and low levels of antinuclear antibodies. Deficiencies of C3, H, I, or P predispose to severe recurrent infections with encapsulated pyogenic bacteria. Lack of or inefficient opsonization of the bacteria by C3b/C3bi apparently causes the susceptibility to infection. Individuals deficient in C5, C6, C7, or C8 are susceptible to disseminated neisserial infections. Direct lysis by complement is probably required for effective defense against gonococci and meningococci. Curiously, individuals with C9 deficiency are usually asymptomatic. Heterozygous deficiency of C1 INH results in hereditary angioedema (Ch. 245), characterized by episodic attacks of circumscribed, nonpruritic edema of the skin or the mucosa of the respiratory or gastrointestinal tract.

Pathophysiology

In certain human diseases, uncontrolled or aberrant activation of complement plays an important pathogenetic role. Activation of the classic pathway at tissue sites by autoantibodies against tissue antigens or by immune complexes deposited at basement membranes results in accumulation of inflammatory cells and tissue damage. The former mechanism is exemplified by the renal lesions of Goodpasture's syndrome and the second by the vascular and renal lesions in SLE and other immune complex diseases. Immunofluorescent staining of biopsy material for complement proteins demonstrates their presence at pathologic sites and is used in differential diagnosis. Hypocomplementemia is also often present in patients with immune complex diseases, particularly SLE, but also in various other clinical syndromes. Measurement of serum complement levels thus provides a simple and widely used tool for the diagnosis and management of human diseases. The most commonly used assays in clinical practice are total hemolytic complement, C4, and C3. Total hemolytic complement, expressed in CH_{50} units, measures the ability of serum to lyse antibody-coated erythrocytes and reflects the activity of all complement components. C4 and C3 are usually measured by immunochemical assays. Low complement levels by all three

TABLE 243–3. DISEASES ASSOCIATED WITH INHERITED COMPLEMENT DEFICIENCIES

Deficient Protein	Diseases
C1q, C1r, C1s, C4, C2	SLE, SLE-like syndrome, discoid lupus, glomerulonephritis, vasculitis
C3, H, I, P	Recurrent pyogenic infections
C5, C6, C7, C8	Recurrent disseminated neisserial infections
C1 INH	Hereditary angioedema

assays are often seen in SLE, particularly in patients with renal involvement and during acute exacerbations of the disease. In patients with partial lipodystrophy with or without glomerulonephritis and in some patients with membranoproliferative glomerulonephritis, levels of total complement and C3 are very low, whereas C4 is usually normal. This is due to the presence of an IgG autoantibody, termed C3 nephritic factor, with specificity for antigenic determinants on the amplification C3 convertase. Binding of this autoantibody to C3bBb creates a stable complex that is not subject to regulation by control proteins and thus causes continuous cleavage of C3. Activation of the alternative pathway also occurs during circulation of the blood through pump oxygenators or hemodialysis machines. The C5a generated during these procedures causes aggregation of neutrophils, leading to their sequestration in the pulmonary vasculature. In some patients this is manifested by symptoms of pulmonary dysfunction and hypoxemia. Complement activation in these cases can best be evaluated by measuring the serum concentration of C3a by radioimmunoassay.

Ahearn JM, Fearon DT: Structure and function of the complement receptors CR1 (CD35) and CR2 (CD21). Adv Immunol 46:183, 1989. *Molecular biology, structure, and function of two important cellular receptors for C3 fragments.*
Campbell RD, Law SKA, Reid KBM, Sim RB: Structure, organization, and regulation of the complement genes. Annu Rev Immunol 6:161, 1988. *An up-to-date review of the genetics and structure of complement proteins.*
Muller-Eberhard HJ: Molecular organization and function of the complement system. Annu Rev Biochem 57:321, 1988. *A comprehensive description of the structure and activation of complement proteins.*
Schifferli JA, Ng YC, Peters DK: The role of complement and its receptor in the elimination of immune complexes. N Engl J Med 325:488, 1986. *Discusses immune complex regulation and disposal.*
Winkelstein JA, Colten HR: Genetically determined disorders of the complement system. In Scriver CR, Beaudet AL, Sly WS, Valle DL (eds.): The Metabolic Basis of Inherited Disease. 6th ed. New York, McGraw-Hill, 1989, pp 2711–2737. *An excellent review of heritable disorders of the complement system.*

244 Primary Immunodeficiency Diseases

Rebecca H. Buckley

Since the first genetic defect in immunity was described in 1952, more than four dozen different primary immunodeficiency syndromes have been reported. Such diseases may involve all components of the immune system, including lymphocytes, phagocytic cells, and the complement proteins. This chapter focuses on abnormalities of lymphocytes. Deficiencies of the complement system (see Ch. 243) are mentioned briefly. A review of neutrophil dysfunction syndromes is presented in Ch. 139 and an overall review of the compromised host is given in Ch. 287. The acquired immunodeficiency syndrome (AIDS) is described in Part XXI.

Despite the large body of knowledge gained regarding functional derangements and cellular abnormalities in the various primary disorders of lymphocytes, the fundamental biologic errors for most of them remain unknown. Exceptions include two defects accompanied by purine salvage pathway enzyme deficiencies—adenosine deaminase (ADA) in some cases of autosomal-recessive severe combined immunodeficiency and purine nucleoside phosphorylase (PNP) in some patients with Nezelof's syndrome. In addition, the absence of three different leukocyte surface glycoproteins due to genetic abnormalities in a common 95 Kd β chain (CD18) is the basis of a condition characterized by defective cytolytic lymphocyte and phagocytic cell functions. The genetic errors in many other immunodeficiencies are known to be on the X chromosome, and the abnormal regions for X-linked agammaglobulinemia, X-linked severe combined immunodeficiency, the Wiskott-Aldrich syndrome, X-linked lymphoproliferative syndrome, properdin deficiency, and chronic granulomatous disease (CGD) have been localized. Immune deficiency can also be associated with broad deficiencies of HLA class I and II antigens and these have been shown to be due to different mutations in transacting factors governing the surface expression of these molecules.

Various classifications of immunodeficiency disorders involving lymphocytes have attempted to postulate the cellular levels at which the defects occur. Cells with mature differentiation markers of both T and B lymphocytes, however, have been found in most of the known defects, despite profound deficiencies of T- and/or B-cell function. Thus, in most cases the suspect cell lineage is not missing but malfunctional. Table 244–1 lists the most prominent functional abnormalities and the presumed cellular level of the defect in 19 primary immunodeficiency syndromes.

In contrast to the acquired immunodeficiency syndrome (AIDS), which has a new case acquisition rate of more than 250 per week, primary immunodeficiency diseases are rare. The incidence of agammaglobulinemia is estimated at 1 in 50,000. Selective absence of serum and secretory IgA, the most common, has a reported prevalence of 1 in 333 to 1 in 700.

APPROACHES TO THE PATIENT WITH SUSPECTED IMMUNODEFICIENCY

The number of patients suspected of having primary immunodeficiency will far exceed the incidences of these diseases. So it is important that the tests selected for immunologic assessment be broadly informative, reliable, and cost effective. Familiarity with certain clinical guidelines aids in the initial selection. Patients with antibody, phagocytic-cell, or complement deficiencies have recurrent infections with high-grade encapsulated bacteria. Therefore, those with only repeated viral respiratory infections are not likely to have any of these disorders. By contrast, patients with deficiencies in T-cell function usually manifest

opportunistic infections. Most defects can be ruled out at little cost to the patient if the proper choice of screening tests is made (Table 244–2). Among the most informative are the complete and differential blood counts and the sedimentation rate. Examination of red cells for Howell-Jolly bodies helps exclude asplenia. A normal platelet count rules out Wiskott-Aldrich syndrome. If the sedimentation rate is normal, chronic bacterial infection is unlikely. If the absolute neutrophil count is normal, congenital and acquired neutropenia and severe chemotactic defects are eliminated. If the absolute lymphocyte count is normal, a severe T-cell defect is unlikely. Beyond this, it is well to keep in mind that tests of immune function are far more informative and cost effective than those measuring immunoglobulin concentrations or enumerating lymphocyte subpopulations.

In assessing B cell function, determinations of antibody titers to protein (such as tetanus and diphtheria toxoids) and polysaccharide (such as pneumococcal and *Haemophilus influenzae*) antigens following immunization are the most useful tests. As a rule, patients with B-cell defects for which there is an effective or indicated treatment do not produce antibodies normally. However, the presence of such antibodies does not exclude IgA deficiency, which would also be missed on a serum electrophoretic analysis. Immunoelectrophoresis is not quantitative and, for that reason, is not useful in evaluating immune competence. The quantification of serum IgA is particularly cost effective. If the IgA concentration is normal, this rules out not only IgA deficiency but all of the permanent types of agammaglobulinemia, since IgA is usually very low or absent in those conditions as well. A particularly uneconomical study is IgG-subclass measurement. It is far more helpful to know the results of the above-mentioned antibody studies, since there are well-documented cases of antibody deficiency despite normal concentrations of all immunoglobulin classes and subclasses.

The most cost-effective test for assessing T-cell function is an intradermal skin test with 0.1 ml of a 1:1000 dilution of a known potent *Candida albicans* extract. If the test is positive, as defined by erythema and induration of 10 mm or more at 48 hours, virtually all primary T-cell defects are excluded and the need for more expensive in vitro tests, such as lymphocyte enumeration on a cell sorter or assessments of responses to mitogens, is obviated. Killing defects of phagocytic cells, which should be suspected if the patient has problems with staphylococcal or gram-negative infections, can be screened for in the office by a

TABLE 244–1. CLASSIFICATION OF PRIMARY IMMUNODEFICIENCY DISORDERS

Disorder	Functional Deficiencies	Presumed Cellular Level of Defect
X-linked agammaglobulinemia	Antibody	Pre–B cell
Common variable ("acquired hypogammaglobulinemia")	Antibody	B lymphocyte
Selective IgA deficiency	IgA antibody	IgA B lymphocyte
Secretory component deficiency	Secretory IgA	Mucosal epithelium
Selective IgM deficiency	IgM antibody	T helper cells
Immunodeficiency with elevated IgM	IgG and IgA antibodies	IgG, IgA B lymphocytes; switch T cell
Transient hypogammaglobulinemia of infancy	None; immunoglobulins low, but antibodies present	Unknown
Antibody deficiency with near-normal immunoglobulins	Antibody	Unknown; ?B cell
X-linked lymphoproliferative disease	Anti-EBV nuclear antigen antibody	B cell; ?also T cell
DiGeorge's syndrome	T cellular; some antibody	Dysmorphogenesis of 3rd and 4th branchial pouches
Nezelof's syndrome (including with PNP deficiency)	T cellular; some antibody	Unknown; ?thymus; ?T cell; metabolic defects
Severe combined immunodeficiency syndromes (autosomal recessive; ADA deficiency; X-linked recessive; defective expression of HLA antigens; reticular dysgenesis)	Antibody and T cellular; phagocytic in reticular dysgenesis	Unknown; metabolic defect(s); ?T cell; ?stem cell; ?thymus
Wiskott-Aldrich syndrome	Antibody; T cellular	Unknown
Ataxia-telangiectasia	Antibody; T cellular	B lymphocyte; helper T lymphocyte
Cartilage-hair hypoplasia	T cellular	G1 cycle of many cells
Immunodeficiency with thymoma	Antibody; some T cellular	B lymphocyte; excessive T suppressor cells
Hyperimmunoglobulinemia E syndrome	Specific immune responses; excessive IgE	Unknown
Chronic mucocutaneous candidiasis	Variable cellular	?Antigen overload
Leukocyte adhesion deficiency	Cytotoxic lymphocytes; phagocytic cells	95 Kd β chain of LFA-1, CR3, and p150, 95

TABLE 244–2. APPROACHES TO THE PATIENT WITH SUSPECTED IMMUNODEFICIENCY

Suspected Deficiency	Tests
All immunodeficiency	Complete and differential blood counts; platelet count; examination of red cells for Howell-Jolly bodies
Antibody deficiency	Immunoglobulin quantification; antibody titers to blood group antigens, protein antigens (tetanus, diphtheria), and polysaccharide antigens (*H. influenzae*, pneumococcal)
T-cell deficiency	Absolute lymphocyte count; intradermal skin test with *Candida albicans* 1:1000
Phagocytic cell deficiency	Absolute neutrophil count; nitroblue tetrazolium assay
Complement deficiency	Freeze serum at −70° C immediately for CH50

nitroblue tetrazolium assay. Complement defects can be most effectively screened for in a CH50 assay, which measures the intactness of the entire complement pathway. If these tests are abnormal, or even if they are normal and clinical features of the patient still strongly suggest a host defect, the patient should be evaluated at a center where more definitive immunologic studies can be done before any type of immunologic treatment is begun.

ANTIBODY DEFICIENCY DISORDERS

Antibody deficiency may occur either as a congenital or an "acquired" abnormality, although in both situations it appears to be genetically determined. Most patients are recognized because they have recurrent infections, but some individuals with selective IgA deficiency or infants with transient hypogammaglobulinemia may have few or no infections. Table 244–3 lists some of the general features of these disorders.

X-LINKED AGAMMAGLOBULINEMIA (XAγ). A majority of boys afflicted with this malady remain well during the first 6 to 9 months of life, presumably by virtue of maternally transmitted immunoglobulin. Thereafter they repeatedly acquire infections with high-grade extracellular pyogenic organisms such as pneumococci, streptococci, and *Haemophilus* unless given prophylactic antibiotics or gammaglobulin therapy. The most common types of infections include sinusitis, pneumonia, otitis, septic arthritis, meningitis, and septicemia. Chronic fungal infections are usually not present, and *Pneumocystis carinii* pneumonia rarely occurs unless there is an associated neutropenia. Viral infections and live virus vaccines are also usually handled normally, with the notable exceptions of hepatitis and enterovirus infections. Several examples of paralysis after polio vaccine administration have occurred, presumably because of mutation of persistent vaccine virus to a more neurotropic form. In addition, a dermatomyositis-like syndrome accompanied by chronic, eventually fatal central nervous system disease caused by various echoviruses has occurred in more than 40 patients. Approximately 20 per cent of patients have an arthritis resembling juvenile rheumatoid arthritis.

TABLE 244–3. CLINICAL CHARACTERISTICS OF ANTIBODY DEFICIENCY DISORDERS

1. Recurrent infections with high-grade extracellular encapsulated pathogens
2. Few problems with fungal or viral (except enterovirus) infections
3. Chronic sinopulmonary disease
4. Growth retardation not striking
5. Antibody deficiency in serum and secretions
6. May or may not lack B lymphocytes with surface immunoglobulins or complement receptors
7. Absence of cortical follicles in lymph node and spleen in X-linked agammaglobulinemia
8. Paucity of palpable lymphoid and nasopharyngeal tissue in X-linked agammaglobulinemia
9. Compatible with survival to adulthood or for several years after onset except for those with persistent enterovirus infections, autoimmune disorders, or malignancy

The diagnosis of XAγ is suspected if serum concentrations of IgG, IgA, and IgM are below the 95-per-cent confidence limits for appropriate age- and race-matched controls (usually there is <100 mg per deciliter total immunoglobulin). The demonstration of antibody deficiency in serum and in external secretions is of great importance in distinguishing this disorder from transient hypogammaglobulinemia of infancy. Tests for natural antibodies to blood group substances, for antibodies to antigens given during standard courses of immunization, and for antibodies to and ability to clear bacteriophage φ × 174 are markedly abnormal. Polymorphonuclear functions are usually normal, but some patients with this condition have had transient, persistent, or cyclic neutropenia.

Lymphopenia is uncommon, and the percentages of T cells and T-cell subsets have been found to be normal or elevated in most instances. In contrast, blood lymphocytes bearing surface immunoglobulin, "Ia-like" antigens, or the EBV receptor, or reacting with a specific anti-B-cell serum, are absent or present in very low numbers. Hypoplasia of adenoids, tonsils, and peripheral lymph nodes is the rule; germinal centers are not present, and plasma cells are rarely found. Conversely, normal numbers of pre–B cells are found in the bone marrow. Mixed lymphocyte responsiveness and lymphocyte responses to antigens and mitogens are normal. Cell-mediated immune responses can be detected in vivo, and the capacity to reject allografts is intact. The thymus has appeared normal in all autopsied cases, and lymphoid cells are abundant in thymus-dependent areas of peripheral lymphoid tissues.

Except in those unfortunate patients who develop polio, persistent echovirus infection, or lymphoreticular malignancy, the overall prognosis is reasonably good if humoral replacement therapy is instituted early. Systemic infection can be prevented by administration of intravenous immune serum globulin (ISG, primarily IgG) at a dose of 400 mg per kilogram every 3 to 4 weeks. Such preparations are known to be free of hepatitis and AIDS viruses. Many patients go on to develop crippling sinopulmonary disease despite this therapy, since no effective means exist for replacing secretory IgA at the mucosal surface. Chronic antibiotic therapy is usually necessary in addition for the management of such patients.

COMMON VARIABLE IMMUNODEFICIENCY (CVID). Patients with this condition (formerly known as acquired hypogammaglobulinemia) may appear similar clinically in many respects to those with XAγ. Although this disorder may occur in infants and young children, most patients present with a history of recurrent infection beginning several years after birth. CVID is distinguished from XAγ by later age of onset, somewhat less severe susceptibility to infections, and almost equal sex distribution. In contrast to patients with the X-linked form, patients with CVID may have normal-sized or enlarged tonsils and lymph nodes, and the latter may have cortical follicles. Additionally, such patients often have normal or nearly normal numbers of circulating immunoglobulin-bearing B lymphocytes. Nevertheless, the serum immunoglobulin and antibody deficiencies are usually just as profound by measurement, and the bacterial etiologic agents are the same as in the X-linked disorder. Echovirus meningoencephalitis is rare in patients with CVID.

This condition has been variably associated with a spruelike syndrome, with or without nodular follicular lymphoid hyperplasia of the intestine; thymoma; alopecia areata; and autoantibody formation leading to hemolytic anemia, gastric atrophy, achlorhydria, and pernicious anemia. Frequent complications include giardiasis (seen far more often here than in XAγ), bronchiectasis, gastric carcinoma, lymphoreticular malignancy, and cholelithiasis. Lymphoid interstitial pneumonia, pseudolymphoma, amyloidosis, and noncaseating granulomas of the lungs, spleen, skin, and liver have also been seen.

Despite normal numbers of circulating immunoglobulin-bearing B lymphocytes and the presence of lymphoid cortical follicles, the lymphocytes do not differentiate in vivo or in vitro into immunoglobulin-producing plasma cells, even in the presence of the polyclonal B-cell activator, pokeweed mitogen. Although the primary biologic error responsible for this defect is unknown, in most patients it appears to be due to abnormal terminal differentiation of the B-cell line. Because this disorder occurs in first-degree relatives of patients with selective IgA deficiency (A Def) and some patients with A Def later become panhypogammaglobulinemic, it is possible that these diseases have a common genetic basis. This concept is supported by the recent finding of rare alleles or deletions of Class III major histocompatibility complex (MHC) genes in individuals with either A Def or CVID, suggesting that the susceptibility gene(s) is in this region on chromosome 6. The treatment of CVID is the same as that for the X-linked disorder.

SELECTIVE IgA DEFICIENCY (A Def). An isolated near-absence (i.e., <10 mg per deciliter) of serum and secretory IgA is the most common primary immunodeficiency disorder, a frequency of 1:333 being reported among some blood donors. Although A Def has been observed in apparently healthy individuals, it is commonly associated with ill health. The kinds of health problems experienced often reflect the type of clinic from which the patients are drawn. Among 75 from an allergy-immunology clinic, there were high frequencies of chronic or recurrent respiratory tract infection and atopic diseases. In contrast, 30 A Def patients drawn from a rheumatology clinic had a high frequency of autoimmune and/or collagen vascular disease.

IgA is the major immunoglobulin of external secretions. As would be expected, its deficiency is associated with infections occurring predominantly in the respiratory, gastrointestinal, and urogenital tracts. Bacterial agents responsible are essentially the same as in other types of antibody deficiency syndromes. A high incidence of viral hepatitis was noted in one group of A Def patients, but there is no clear evidence that patients with this disorder have an undue susceptibility to other viral agents. Children with A Def produce local IgM and IgG antipolio antibodies to killed vaccine given intranasally and IgM and IgG antirubella antibodies during convalescence from natural rubella. Serum concentrations of other immunoglobulins are usually normal in patients with A Def, although an IgG_2 subclass deficiency has been reported in some, and IgM (usually increased) may be of the low-molecular-weight variety.

In addition to limiting the attachment of infectious agents to mucosal surfaces, secretory IgA antibodies probably act to prevent absorption of other foreign antigens, such as those in the diet. There is a high incidence of allergy and of IgG antibodies against cow's milk and ruminant serum proteins in patients with IgA deficiency. The antiruminant antibodies often falsely detect "IgA" in immunoassays which employ goat (but not rabbit) antisera. Intestinal nodular hyperplasia has been seen in a few such patients. A spruelike syndrome may occur in adults with selective IgA deficiency and sometimes responds to a gluten-free diet.

The basic defect leading to A Def is unknown. IgA-bearing blood B cells from most such patients also coexpress surface IgM and IgD, similar to cord blood B cells, suggesting maturation arrest. In addition, the B lymphocytes fail to secrete IgA in vitro. Studies of T-cell function have been normal in most patients. The defect may not always be permanent. The occurrence of IgA deficiency in both males and females and in families suggests autosomal inheritance.

Serum antibodies to IgA are found in as many as 44 per cent of such patients. This observation is of possible etiologic and great clinical significance. At least seven IgA-deficient patients have had severe or fatal anaphylactic reactions after intravenous administration of blood products. For this reason, only multiply washed erythrocytes or blood products from other A Def individuals should be administered to these patients; both intramuscular and intravenous ISG (which contain varying amounts of IgA) are contraindicated.

Currently the only treatment for A Def is vigorous treatment of specific infections with appropriate antimicrobial agents. Even if serum IgA could be replaced (in the face of anti-IgA antibodies), it would not be transported into the external secretions, since the latter is an active process involving only locally produced IgA.

SECRETORY COMPONENT DEFICIENCY. A patient with chronic intestinal candidiasis and diarrhea was found to lack IgA in his external secretions, despite having a normal serum IgA concentration. This was traced to a lack of secretory piece, which prevented the normal secretion of locally produced IgA.

SELECTIVE IgM DEFICIENCY. There are very few well-documented cases of this entity (IgM < 10 mg/ml). Fatal septicemia caused by meningococci and other gram-negative organisms, pneumococcal meningitis, tuberculosis, recurrent staphylococcal pyoderma, periorbital cellulitis, bronchiectasis, and

recurrent otitis have all been reported. There is no specific therapy; early and vigorous treatment with antibiotics is recommended.

IMMUNODEFICIENCY WITH ELEVATED IgM (Hypm). This disorder is characterized by very low serum IgG and IgA but markedly elevated polyclonal IgM. Some patients have low-molecular-weight IgM molecules. Like patients with XAγ, those with this defect commonly become symptomatic during infancy with recurrent pyogenic infections, including otitis media, sinusitis, pneumonia, and tonsillitis. In contrast to patients with XAγ, however, the frequent presence of lymphoid hyperplasia often leads away from a diagnosis of immunodeficiency. There is an increased frequency of autoimmune disorders, such as hemolytic anemia and thrombocytopenia, and transient, persistent, or cyclic neutropenia is common. Thymic-dependent lymphoid tissues and T-cell functions are usually normal, but several patients have had partial T-cell deficiencies. A sex-linked mode of inheritance has been proposed, but several examples of the disorder in females now seem to make this less certain.

Normal or only slightly reduced numbers of Ig-bearing B lymphocytes have been found in the blood; however, cultured B-cell lines from most such patients have shown the capacity to synthesize only IgM, suggesting a B-cell maturation defect. Some patients with this condition have, however, been characterized as having normal B cells but a deficiency of "switch" T cells. Plasma cells in lymph nodes contain only IgM.

Because these patients are unable to make IgG antibodies, the treatment is the same as for agammaglobulinemia.

TRANSIENT HYPOGAMMAGLOBULINEMIA OF INFANCY. Unlike patients with XAγ or common variable agammaglobulinemia, those with this condition can synthesize antibodies to human type A and B erythrocytes and to diphtheria and tetanus toxoids, usually by 6 to 11 months of age, well before immunoglobulin concentrations become normal. The finding of only 11 cases of transient hypogammaglobulinemia of infancy among over 10,000 sera tested by the author over a 12-year period suggests that this is not a common entity.

Gammaglobulin replacement therapy is not indicated in this condition. In addition to the known risks of inducing anti-IgG allotype antibodies, passively administered antibodies could block endogenous primary antibody formation in the same manner that RhoGAM suppresses anti-D antibodies in Rh-negative mothers delivering Rh-positive infants.

ANTIBODY DEFICIENCY WITH NEAR-NORMAL IMMUNOGLOBULINS. The author and her associates have studied the antibody-forming capacities of 12 patients with deficient antibody responses despite apparently normal T-cell function and normal or nearly normal immunoglobulin concentrations. Blood group antibody titers were absent in all but 2, diphtheria titers were low in all, and tetanus titers were low in 10. Geometric mean antibody titers to 13 pneumococcal serotypes were significantly lower than those of normal controls before and after immunization with tridecavalent pneumococcal polysaccharide vaccine. All patients cleared bacteriophage φ × 174 normally, but all primary immune responses were far below the normal range. Secondary responses to φ × 174 were also below the normal range in all but two, but, in both cases, most of the secondary response was IgM rather than IgG. This problem will not be detected unless functional tests of antibody-forming capacity are conducted. It may represent an early stage of "acquired" agammaglobulinemia (or CVID). Patients with this disorder are candidates for immunoglobulin replacement therapy.

X-LINKED LYMPHOPROLIFERATIVE DISEASE. This disorder, also referred to as *Duncan's disease* (after the original kindred in which it was described), is characterized by an impaired immune response to Epstein-Barr virus (EBV). Affected persons are apparently healthy until they experience infectious mononucleosis. Two thirds of the more than 100 patients studied thus far died of overwhelming EBV-induced B-cell proliferation during mononucleosis. A majority of the survivors developed hypogammaglobulinemia or B-cell lymphomas or both. Such individuals have marked impairment in production of antibodies to the EBV nuclear antigen, whereas titers of antibodies to the viral capsid antigen have ranged from zero to markedly elevated. Antibody-dependent cell-mediated cytotoxicity against EBV-infected cells and natural killer function are depressed, and there is a deficiency in long-lived T-cell immunity to EBV. Despite normal numbers of B and T cells, there is an elevated percentage of lymphocytes of the suppressor (CD8) phenotype. In addition, lymphocyte immunoglobulin synthesis in response to polyclonal B-cell mitogen stimulation in vitro is markedly depressed. Thus, both EBV-specific and nonspecific immunologic abnormalities occur in these patients.

CELLULAR IMMUNODEFICIENCY DISORDERS

Some important clinical characteristics of cellular immunodeficiency disorders are listed in Table 244–4. In general, patients with partial or absolute defects in T-cell function have infections or other clinical problems for which there is no effective treatment or which are often of a more severe nature than in those with antibody deficiency disorders. It is therefore rare that such individuals survive beyond infancy or childhood.

THYMIC HYPOPLASIA (DiGEORGE'S SYNDROME). This condition results from dysmorphogenesis of the third and fourth pharyngeal pouches, leading to hypoplasia or aplasia of the thymus and parathyroid glands. Other structures forming at the same age are also frequently affected, resulting in anomalies of the great vessels (right-sided aortic arch), esophageal atresia, bifid uvula, congenital heart disease (atrial and ventricular septal defects), a short philtrum of the upper lip, hypertelorism, an antimongoloid slant to the eyes, mandibular hypoplasia, and low-set (often notched) ears. The diagnosis is usually first suggested by the presence of hypocalcemic seizures during the neonatal period. DiGeorge's syndrome has occurred in both males and females, and chromosomal abnormalities (monosomy 22q11 and 10p13) have been noted in approximately 18 per cent. Familial occurrence is rare.

A variable degree of hypoplasia is more frequent than total aplasia of the thymus and parathyroid glands. Some children with the features of this syndrome have little trouble with infections and show evidence of some cell-mediated immunity. They are often referred to as having partial DiGeorge's syndrome. Those with marked thymic hypoplasia may resemble infants with severe combined immunodeficiency in their susceptibility to infection with low-grade or opportunistic pathogens (i.e., fungi, viruses, and *Pneumocystis carinii*) and to graft-versus-host (GVH) disease from nonirradiated blood transfusions.

Serum immunoglobulins are usually normal for age, but some fractions, particularly IgA, may be diminished and IgE may be elevated. T-cell numbers are decreased, and there is an increased number of B cells. Responses of peripheral blood lymphocytes following mitogen stimulation, like the intradermal delayed hypersensitivity response, have been absent, reduced, or normal. Careful postmortem studies have sometimes revealed tiny nests of thymic tissue containing Hassall's corpuscles and a normal density of thymocytes. Lymphoid follicles usually appear normal, but lymph node paracortical areas and thymus-dependent regions of the spleen show variable degrees of depletion, depending upon the degree of thymic hypoplasia. Because of variability in the severity of the immunodeficiency, it is difficult to evaluate claimed benefits of fetal thymus transplantation.

CELLULAR IMMUNODEFICIENCY WITH IMMUNO-GLOBULINS (NEZELOF'S SYNDROME). This syndrome is characterized by lymphopenia, diminished lymphoid tissue, abnormal thymus architecture, and the presence of normal or increased immunoglobulins. Children with this condition may have recurrent or chronic pulmonary infections, failure to thrive, oral or cutaneous candidiasis, chronic diarrhea, recurrent skin infections, gram-negative sepsis, urinary tract infections, severe varicella, or combinations of these. An autosomal recessive pattern of inheritance has been suggested in some cases, but an X-linked mode seemed more likely in others. Other findings include neutropenia and eosinophilia.

Studies of cellular immune function have shown delayed cutaneous anergy to ubiquitous antigens and low to absent in vitro lymphocyte responses to mitogens and allogeneic cells. Such patients have profound deficiencies of total T cells and T-cell subsets, with usually a normal helper (CD4+) to suppressor (CD8+) cell ratio, in contrast to patients with AIDS, who characteristically have marked inversion of the CD4:CD8 ratio owing to selective deficiency of CD4+ cells. Peripheral lymphoid tissues demonstrate paracortical lymphocyte depletion. The thymuses are very small and have a paucity of thymocytes and usually no Hassall's corpuscles; however, again in contrast to AIDS, thymic epithelium is present. These could all be useful in distinguishing Nezelof's syndrome from pediatric AIDS, since it is the primary immunodeficiency disorder most likely to be confused with it. Fatal or serious infections have included varicella, vaccinia, rubeola, and those due to *Pneumocystis carinii*, cytomegalovirus, *Pseudomonas*, and *Mycobacterium kansasii*. Antibody-forming capacity has been apparently normal in roughly one third of the reported cases. Plasma cells are usually abundant in the lamina propria and lymph nodes. Although very few patients have been reconstituted by bone marrow transplantation, most other forms of therapy have also been unsuccessful.

With Purine Nucleoside Phosphorylase Deficiency. More than 16 patients with Nezelof's syndrome have been found to have purine nucleoside phosphorylase (PNP) deficiency. In contrast to patients with adenosine deaminase (ADA) deficiency, serum and urinary uric acid are markedly deficient, and no characteristic physical or skeletal abnormalities have been noted. Three patients have suffered from a progressive neurologic disorder with spastic tetraplegia, two developed an autoimmune hemolytic anemia, and one, idiopathic thrombocytopenic purpura. Deaths have occurred from generalized vaccinia, varicella, lymphosarcoma, and GVH disease following blood transfusions. In contrast to a majority of patients with Nezelof's syndrome, the thymuses of PNP-deficient patients have had some Hassall's corpuscles, reminiscent of some patients with ADA deficiency. Analyses of lymphocyte subpopulations with monoclonal antibodies in two such patients revealed marked deficiencies of T cells and T-cell subsets but increased numbers of cells with natural killer (NK) phenotype and function. Attempts to correct the immunologic and enzymatic deficiencies of PNP-deficient patients by enzyme replacement or deoxycytidine therapy have not been successful.

SEVERE COMBINED IMMUNODEFICIENCY (SCID) DISORDERS

The syndromes of SCID are characterized by their apparent congenital absence of all adaptive immune function and a great diversity of genetic, enzymatic, hematologic, and immunologic features. Unless immunologic reconstitution can be achieved through immunocompetent tissue transplants or enzyme replacement therapy or unless gnotobiotic isolation can be carried out, death usually occurs before the patient's first birthday. The major subcategories of this disorder are discussed below.

AUTOSOMAL RECESSIVE SEVERE COMBINED IMMU-NODEFICIENCY DISEASE. Within the first few months of life, infants affected with this first-described SCID syndrome have frequent episodes of otitis, pneumonia, sepsis, diarrhea, and cutaneous infections. Growth may appear normal initially, but extreme wasting soon develops. Persistent infections with opportunistic organisms such as *Candida albicans*, *Pneumocystis carinii*, varicella, measles, parainfluenza 3, cytomegalovirus, and BCG frequently lead to death. These infants also lack the ability to reject foreign tissue and are therefore at risk for GVH disease. GVH reactions can result from maternal immunocompetent cells crossing the placenta or from the administration of blood products containing viable histoincompatible lymphocytes.

Immunologic evaluation reveals serum immunoglobulin concentrations to be diminished, and no antibody formation occurs following immunization. There is a lack of cellular immune

TABLE 244–4. CLINICAL CHARACTERISTICS OF CELLULAR IMMUNODEFICIENCY DISORDERS

1. Recurrent infections with low-grade or opportunistic infectious agents such as fungi, viruses, or *Pneumocystis carinii*
2. Delayed cutaneous anergy
3. Accompanied by growth retardation, short life span, wasting, and diarrhea
4. Susceptible to graft-versus-host (GVH) disease if given fresh blood, plasma, or unmatched allogeneic bone marrow
5. Fatal reactions from live virus or BCG vaccination
6. High incidence of malignancy

function, with lymphopenia and absence of lymphocyte responses to mitogens or allogeneic cells, delayed cutaneous anergy, and inability to reject foreign tissues. Marked heterogeneity of lymphocyte subpopulations exists among SCID patients, even among those with similar inheritance patterns. Despite the uniformly profound lack of T- or B-cell function, some patients have had low numbers of both B and T lymphocytes, whereas others have had elevated numbers of B cells. Cytofluorographic studies with monoclonal antibodies to mature T cells and subsets have generally revealed very small numbers of cells reacting with such reagents; however, there is no increase in cells bearing the CD1 antigen present on immature cortical thymocytes. Thus the lymphocytes present appear to have acquired surface markers characteristic of mature T cells. A new phenotype of SCID was characterized in which virtually all of the lymphocytes of some infants with SCID are large granular lymphocytes with NK cell phenotype and function. NK function has been totally lacking in other SCID patients, again illustrating the striking heterogeneity at a cellular level. Typically, these patients have very small thymuses (less than 1 gram), which usually fail to descend from the neck, contain few thymic lymphocytes, lack corticomedullary distinction, and usually lack Hassall's corpuscles (see exception below). Despite the profound thymocyte depletion in SCID patients, thymic epithelium is present—in contrast to the situation in AIDS in which there is marked epithelial atrophy. Both the follicular and paracortical areas of the peripheral lymph nodes are depleted of lymphocytes. Tonsils, adenoids, and Peyer's patches are absent or extremely underdeveloped.

ISG fails to halt the progressively downhill course of SCID. Transplantation of bone marrow cells from HLA genotypically identical or D locus–compatible donors has resulted in apparent complete correction of the immunologic defect in a number of these patients, with some 50 known long-term survivors since 1968. More recently, techniques to deplete all post-thymic T cells from donor marrow have also allowed the use of haploidentical (half-matched) bone marrow cells for correction of SCID. These employ either a combination of soy lectin agglutination and sheep erythrocyte rosetting (the most successful method) or incubation with monoclonal antibodies to human T cells and complement. Both methods leave the stem cells intact. To date, over 100 infants with SCID who would have otherwise died because of lack of an HLA-identical donor have been treated successfully with T-cell–depleted haploidentical bone marrow with few signs of GVH reaction.

With Adenosine Deaminase (ADA) Deficiency. Absence of the enzyme ADA has been observed in approximately 40 per cent of patients with the autosomal recessive form of SCID. Marked accumulations of adenosine, 2'-deoxyadenosine and 2'-O-methyladenosine directly or indirectly lead to lymphocyte toxicity, which causes the immunodeficiency. Adenosine and deoxyadenosine are apparent suicide inactivators of the enzyme S-adenosylhomocysteine (SAH) hydrolase, resulting in the accumulation of SAH. SAH is a potent inhibitor of virtually all cellular methylation reactions. Although most such patients have had profound lymphopenia from the earliest age studied, a few have had early normal or fluctuating lymphocyte counts that declined by 6 weeks to 2 years of life. In marked contrast to "classic" SCID, some ADA–deficient patients have been found to have a few Hassall's corpuscles in their thymuses and changes suggestive of early differentiation. Other distinguishing features of ADA-deficient SCID patients have included the presence of rib cage abnormalities similar to a rachitic rosary and multiple skeletal abnormalities of chondro-osseous dysplasia on radiographic examination.

Both matched sibling and haploidentical post-thymic T cell–depleted bone marrow transplants have resulted in lymphocyte chimerism and partial or complete correction of the immunologic defect in ADA-deficient SCID. Enzyme replacement therapy with irradiated packed normal erythrocytes or polyethylene-glycol–modified bovine adenosine deaminase on a continuing basis has resulted in improvement in some patients. Recently, this condition became the first in which gene insertion therapy was attempted, as the entire ADA gene has been cloned and sequenced.

X-LINKED RECESSIVE SEVERE COMBINED IMMUNODEFICIENCY DISEASE. This is thought to be the most common form of SCID in the United States. Clinically, immu-

nologically, and histopathologically, these patients appear similar to those with the autosomal recessive form.

DEFECTIVE EXPRESSION OF MAJOR HISTOCOMPATIBILITY COMPLEX (MHC) ANTIGENS. There are two main forms: MHC class I antigen deficiency ("bare lymphocyte syndrome") and MHC class I antigen deficiency plus absence of MHC class II antigens. These autosomal recessive conditions are thought to be due to mutations in X-box binding proteins that result in failure of surface membrane expression of the HLA antigens. Sera from affected individuals contain normal quantities of MHC class I antigens and β_2 microglobulin. Patients (usually of North African descent) present with persistent diarrhea in early infancy and have oral candidiasis, bacterial pneumonia, Pneumocystis infection, septicemia, and undue susceptibility to enteroviruses, herpes, and other viral agents. Those with both class I and II antigen deficiencies also have malabsorption. There is variable hypogammaglobulinemia with decreased serum IgM and IgA and poor to absent antibody production. B-cell percentages are usually normal, but plasma cells are absent in tissues. Lymphopenia is only moderate; T-cell functions in vivo and in vitro are decreased but not absent. The thymus and other lymphoid organs are severely hypoplastic. A majority of affected infants die in the first 3 years of life. The associated defects of both B- and T-cell immunity and HLA expression reinforce the important biologic role for HLA determinants in effective immune cell cooperation.

SEVERE COMBINED IMMUNODEFICIENCY WITH LEUKOPENIA (RETICULAR DYSGENESIS). In 1959, identical twin male infants were described who exhibited a total lack of both lymphocytes and granulocytes in their peripheral blood and bone marrow. Seven of eight infants reported died between 3 and 119 days of age from overwhelming infections; the eighth underwent complete immunologic reconstitution from a bone marrow transplant. Autosomal inheritance seems likely from reports of familial occurrences.

PARTIAL COMBINED IMMUNODEFICIENCY DISORDERS

IMMUNODEFICIENCY WITH THROMBOCYTOPENIA AND ECZEMA (WISKOTT-ALDRICH SYNDROME). This X-linked recessive syndrome is characterized clinically by the triad of eczema, thrombocytopenic purpura, and undue susceptibility to infection. Often there is prolonged oozing from the circumcision site or bloody diarrhea during infancy. Atopic dermatitis and recurrent infections usually develop during the first year of life. Infections are caused by pneumococci and other bacteria with polysaccharide capsules, resulting in episodes of otitis media, pneumonia, meningitis, and sepsis. Later, infections with Pneumocystis carinii and the herpesviruses become more frequent. Survival beyond the teens is rare; major causes of death are infections and bleeding, but a 12 per cent incidence of fatal malignancy also occurs in this condition. A papovavirus has been recovered from a reticulum cell sarcoma of the brain and from the urine of patients with this syndrome.

The earliest evidence of immunodeficiency is an impaired humoral immune response to polysaccharide antigens. Absent or markedly diminished isohemagglutinin titers are uniformly found, and poor or no responses are seen following immunization with polysaccharide antigens. Antibody titers to protein antigens also fall with time, and anamnestic responses are often poor or absent. Studies of immunoglobulin metabolism have shown an accelerated rate of synthesis—as well as hypercatabolism—of albumin, IgG, IgA, and IgM, resulting in highly variable immunoglobulin concentrations. The predominant dysgammaglobulinemia is a low IgM, elevated IgA and IgE, and a normal or slightly low IgG concentration. Lymphocyte responses are moderately depressed, and cutaneous anergy is a frequent finding. Analyses of blood lymphocytes with monoclonal reagents have revealed moderately reduced percentages of cells reacting with antibodies to all T cells and to the helper (CD4 +) and suppressor (CD8 +) subsets. In addition, the T lymphocytes have deficient or defective cell surface expressions of the sialoglycoprotein CD43.

The thrombocytopenia appears to be due to an intrinsic platelet abnormality, since antiplatelet antibodies are not usually demonstrated and survival times of allogeneic but not autologous ^{51}Cr-labeled platelets have been normal. Megakaryocytes are present in normal number in the bone marrow, but platelet size is small.

Treatment has been directed primarily toward control of bleeding with platelet transfusions, splenectomy, or both and of infections by intravenous administration of ISG. Several patients have had complete corrections of both the platelet and immunologic abnormalities by HLA-matched sibling bone marrow transplants after being conditioned with irradiation or busulfan and cyclophosphamide.

ATAXIA-TELANGIECTASIA. This is a complex syndrome with neurologic, immunologic, endocrinologic, hepatic, and cutaneous abnormalities. The most prominent clinical features are progressive cerebellar ataxia, oculocutaneous telangiectasias, chronic sinopulmonary disease, a high incidence of malignancy, and variable humoral and cellular immunodeficiency. Ataxia typically becomes evident soon after the child begins to walk. Telangiectasias usually develop by 3 to 6 years of age. Recurrent, usually bacterial, sinopulmonary infections occur in roughly 80 per cent of these patients; common viral exanthems have not usually resulted in untoward sequelae, but varicella was fatal in one of the author's patients.

The malignant tumors reported have usually been of the lymphoreticular type, but others have been seen. Cells from patients and heterozygous carriers have increased sensitivity to ionizing radiation, defective DNA repair, and frequent chromosomal abnormalities. The abnormal gene has been mapped to the long arm of chromosome 11 (11q22-23). An autosomal recessive mode of inheritance seems operative.

The most frequent immunologic abnormality is selective absence of IgA, found in 50 to 80 per cent of these patients. IgG$_2$ or total IgG may also be decreased. IgE concentrations are usually low, and the IgM may be of the low-molecular-weight variety. Specific antibody levels may be decreased or normal. In vivo, there is impaired but not absent cell-mediated immunity, as evidenced by delayed cutaneous anergy and prolonged allograft survival. Death from GVH disease has not been reported. Enumeration of blood T cells and subsets reveals reduced percentages of total T cells and T cells of the helper (CD4) phenotype, with normal or increased percentages of cells of the suppressor (CD8) phenotype. In vitro studies of lymphocyte function have shown moderately depressed proliferative responses to mitogens, decreased T-helper cell function, and an intrinsic defect in B-cell IgA synthesis. The thymus is very hypoplastic and lacks Hassall's corpuscles. No satisfactory treatment has been found.

CARTILAGE-HAIR HYPOPLASIA. An unusual form of short-limbed dwarfism with frequent and severe infections has been reported among the Amish. Features include short and pudgy hands; redundant skin; hyperextensible joints of hands and feet but an inability to completely extend the elbows; and fine, sparse light hair and eyebrows. Severe and often fatal varicella infections appear to be a particular hazard. Progressive vaccinia and vaccine-associated poliomyelitis have also been observed.

The severity of the immunodeficiency varies; in one series, 11 of 77 patients died before age 20, but two were still alive at age 76. Three patterns of immune dysfunction have emerged: defective antibody-mediated immunity, defective cellular immunity, and severe combined immunodeficiency. The most striking abnormality appears to be one of defective cell proliferation due to an intrinsic defect related to the G1 phase, resulting in a longer cell cycle for individual cells. The trait appears to be autosomal recessive with variable penetrance.

IMMUNODEFICIENCY WITH THYMOMA. These patients are adults who almost simultaneously develop hypogammaglobulinemia, deficits in cell-mediated immunity, and benign thymoma (see Ch. 253). The thymomas are predominantly of the spindle cell variety. Eosinophilia or eosinopenia, aregenerative or hemolytic anemia, thrombocytopenia, or pancytopenia may also occur. Antibody formation is poor, although percentages of immunoglobulin-bearing B lymphocytes are normal, and progressive lymphopenia develops. Several patients with this disorder have been shown to have excessive suppressor T-cell activity.

HYPERIMMUNOGLOBULINEMIA E SYNDROME. The hyper-IgE syndrome is a primary immunodeficiency characterized by recurrent staphylococcal abscesses and markedly elevated serum IgE concentrations. The disorder was first reported by the author and her coworkers in two young boys in 1972. These patients all have lifelong histories of severe recurrent staphylococcal abscesses involving the skin, lungs, joints, and other sites. Persistent pneumatoceles develop as a result of their recurrent pneumonias. The pruritic dermatitis that occurs is not typical atopic eczema and does not always persist; respiratory allergic symptoms are usually absent. An autosomal dominant form of inheritance with incomplete penetrance seems possible. Laboratory features include exceptionally high serum IgE concentrations but usually normal IgG, IgA, and IgM concentrations; pronounced blood and sputum eosinophilia; abnormally low anamnestic antibody responses; and poor antibody and cell-mediated responses to neoantigens. In vitro studies have shown normal percentages of CD2-, CD3-, CD4-, and CD8-positive lymphocytes, and there is no increase in the percentage of IgE-bearing B lymphocytes. Lymphocyte responses to mitogens are normal, but responses to antigens or to related allogeneic cells have been absent or very low. Histologic sections of lymph nodes, spleen, and lung cysts show striking eosinophilia.

Phagocytic cell ingestion, metabolism, and killing mechanisms and total hemolytic complement have been normal in all patients. Defects of mononuclear and/or polymorphonuclear chemotaxis are present in some but not most patients and thus are not the basic problem in this syndrome.

The most effective therapy is chronic administration of therapeutic doses of a penicillinase-resistant penicillin, with the addition of other antibiotic or antifungal agents as required for specific infections.

CHRONIC MUCOCUTANEOUS CANDIDIASIS. This clinical syndrome, probably of multiple causes, is associated with chronic candidal infection of the skin and mucous membranes but only rarely life-threatening systemic infections of the types seen in patients with severe T-cell dysfunction. Some patients have endocrinopathies involving the parathyroid, thyroid, adrenal, and/or pancreatic glands (see Ch. 228); however, many have neither associated endocrinopathy nor any demonstrable immunologic abnormality. Ketoconazole (Nizoral) has been found to be the single most effective form of therapy.

LEUKOCYTE ADHESION DEFICIENCY (LAD OR CD11/CD18 DEFICIENCY). This condition is due to an autosomal recessive inherited mutation in the gene encoding the 95 Kd MW β subunit (CD18) shared by three adhesive heterodimers: LFA-1 on B, T, and NK lymphocytes; complement receptor type 3 (CR3) on neutrophils, monocytes, macrophages, eosinophils, and NK cells; and p150,95 (function unknown). Patients have histories of delayed separation of the umbilical cord, omphalitis, gingivitis, recurrent skin infections, repeated otitis media, pneumonia, peritonitis, perianal abscesses, and impaired wound healing. Severe widespread and life-threatening bacterial and fungal infections account for the high mortality. All cytotoxic lymphocyte functions are markedly impaired owing to a lack of the adhesion protein LFA-1; deficiency of LFA-1 also interferes with immune cell interaction and immune recognition. CR3 binds fixed iC3b fragments of C3 and β glucans; its absence causes abnormal phagocytic cell adherence and chemotaxis and a reduced respiratory burst with phagocytosis. Blood neutrophil counts are usually elevated. Deficiencies of these glycoproteins can be screened for by cytofluorography of blood leukocytes with appropriate monoclonal antibodies to CR3 (OKM1, MO1, MAC-1). The disease can be corrected by bone marrow transplantation.

T-CELL ACTIVATION DEFECTS. These conditions are characterized by the presence of T cells that appear phenotypically normal by many criteria but fail to proliferate or produce cytokines in response to stimulation with mitogens, antigens, or other signals delivered to the T-cell antigen receptor (TCR). Recently a number of these have been characterized at the molecular level, including patients who had either (1) defective surface expression of the TCR, (2) defective signal transduction from the TCR to intracellular metabolic pathways, and (3) a pretranslational defect in interleukin-2 (T-cell growth factor) production. These patients have clinical problems similar to those of other severely T-cell–deficient individuals.

PRIMARY DEFICIENCIES OF THE COMPLEMENT SYSTEM

In addition to congenital or hereditary disorders of lymphoid cells, there are several well-defined primary immune defects involving the complement system. Genetically determined deficiencies have been described for all of the components of complement, and undue susceptibility to infection is a characteristic of deficiencies of C2, C3, C5, C6, and C7. The types of infections experienced in C2, C3, and in some with C5 deficiency are with gram-positive encapsulated organisms, whereas those in patients with deficiencies of the terminal components are usually meningococcal or gonococcal. A normal CH50 would exclude all heritable complement deficiencies. The complement system is discussed in detail in Ch. 243.

Alarcon B, Regueiro JR, Arnaiz-Villena A, Terhorst C: Familial defect in the surface expression of the T-cell receptor-CD3 complex. N Engl J Med 319:1203, 1988. *An excellent introduction to the concept of T-cell activation defects.*

Buckley RH: Normal and abnormal development of the immune system. In Joklik WK, Willett HP, Amos DB (eds.): Zinsser Textbook of Microbiology and Immunology. 19th ed. New York, Appleton-Century-Crofts, 1988. *A concise review of ontogeny of the normal human immune system as well as the primary immunodeficiency disorders.*

Buckley RH, Schiff SE, Sampson HA, et al.: Development of immunity in human severe primary T cell deficiency following haploidentical bone marrow stem cell transplantation. J Immunol 136:2398, 1986. *A review of the time course and extent of immune reconstitution in 17 patients with severe T cell defects given haploidentical stem cell transplants.*

Chatila T, Wong R, Young M, et al: An immunodeficiency characterized by defective signal transduction in T lymphocytes. N Engl J Med 320:696, 1989. *An example of a signal transduction defect.*

Fischer A, Lisowska-Grospierre B, Anderson DC, Springer TA: Leukocyte adhesion deficiency: Molecular basis and functional consequences. Immunodef Rev 1:39, 1988. *An excellent review of leukocyte adhesion (CD11/18) deficiency.*

Schaffer FM, Palermos J, Zhu ZB, et al.: Individuals with IgA deficiency and common variable immunodeficiency share polymorphisms of major histocompatibility complex class II genes. Proc Natl Acad Sci USA 86:8015, 1989. *New information concerning the genetic localization of susceptibility genes for selective IgA deficiency and common variable immunodeficiency.*

245 Urticaria and Angioedema

Michael M. Frank

DEFINITION

Urticaria (Table 245–1) is defined as the transient appearance of elevated, erythematous pruritic wheals (hives) or serpiginous exanthem, usually surrounded by an area of erythema. It commonly involves the trunk and extremities, sparing palms and soles, but may involve any epidermal or mucosal surface. The wheals are thought to result from local subcutaneous and intradermal leakage of plasma filtrate from postcapillary venules. In most cases there is associated increased blood flow to the localized area of swelling, resulting in a surrounding erythema. The lesions blanch on pressure, reflecting this pathogenetic process. The appearance of urticaria is thought to reflect an ongoing immediate hypersensitivity reaction.

Angioedema is formed by a similar extravasation of fluid, but in this case the leakage of fluid involves deeper structures, including dermal and subdermal sites. Because of its location in deeper cutaneous structures, it appears as brawny nonpitting edema, usually without well-defined margins. Although urticaria is almost always pruritic, indicating stimulation of nociceptive nerves supplying deeper cutaneous structures, angioedema may be unassociated with itching. Unlike other forms of edema, angioedema is not commonly distributed in dependent areas of the body. Angioedema often involves the lips, tongue, eyelids, genitalia, or dorsum of the hands or feet but also may involve any epidermal or mucosal surface. The transient nature of involvement is important in definition of both urticaria and angioedema; these manifestations appear and peak in minutes to hours and disappear over hours to days.

INCIDENCE AND PREVALENCE

Acute episodes of urticaria/angioedema are arbitrarily defined as those lasting less than 6 weeks. More prolonged episodes are defined as chronic. Acute urticaria and angioedema are very common clinical problems occurring in as many as 20 to 30 per cent of the population at one time or another. They may occur at any age and are the most common form seen in childhood.

TABLE 245–1. CLASSIFICATION OF URTICARIA/ANGIOEDEMA

I. Manifestation of hypersensitivity to a defined agent
  A. Drug reactions
  B. Foods and food additives
  C. Inhaled and contact allergens
II. Presumed immune complex–induced
  A. Collagen disease
  B. Endocrine disease (thyroid disorders)
  C. Serum sickness
  D. Transfusion-induced
  E. Malignancy (tumor antigen–induced)
  F. Infectious agents
III. Physical urticarias
  A. Dermatographism
  B. Familial and acquired cold urticaria
  C. Localized heat urticaria
  D. Cholinergic urticaria
  E. Exercise-induced anaphylaxis/urticaria
  F. Delayed pressure urticaria/angioedema
  G. Familial and acquired vibratory angioedema
  H. Solar urticaria
  I. Aquagenic urticaria
IV. Urticaria pigmentosa and systemic mastocytosis
V. Chronic urticaria and angioedema
VI. Defined complement-related disorders
  A. Hereditary angioedema
  B. Acquired Cl inhibitor deficiency
  C. Complement Factor I deficiency

They occur in persons of all sexes, races, and occupations and at all seasons of the year. Chronic urticaria/angioedema also can occur in individuals of any age, but the peak incidence is noted in young adults. In general, symptoms of urticaria are more striking and are more easily recognized than those of angioedema, and these symptoms are often the presenting complaint. At presentation about 50 per cent of patients are found to have both urticaria and angioedema, approximately 40 per cent have urticaria alone, and about 10 per cent only angioedema. Although the majority of patients clear their lesions spontaneously or respond rapidly to treatment with H_1 antihistamines, a minority of patients continue to have lesions over a period that may last years. It has been reported that of patients with chronic urticaria and angioedema, 75 per cent have symptoms for longer than 1 year, 50 per cent symptoms for longer than 5 years, and 20 per cent symptoms for decades. At times these can be quite debilitating. This clinical syndrome represents a final common pathway of multiple initiating stimuli, and the natural course of disease undoubtedly reflects these multiple initiating factors.

PATHOGENESIS AND PATHOLOGY

Urticaria/angioedema appears to result from dilatation of local small vessels with associated leakage of plasma from local postcapillary venules. Experimentally such leakage can be induced by multiple stimuli. Degranulation of cutaneous mast cells is thought to be the most frequent cause of disease. Mast cells are found in high frequency within the subcutaneous tissues and dermis. Their distribution is particularly rich around blood vessels. These cells stain poorly with the commonly used histopathologic stains and often must be visualized by specific staining techniques. Upon being activated by any of a number of stimuli, these cells degranulate, releasing preformed mediators like histamine present in the granules that can induce capillary permeability and also synthesize various mediators that induce capillary permeability in response to the activation signal, including prostaglandins, HETEs, leukotrienes C, D, and E, and platelet-activating factor (PAF). Recent evidence suggests that with appropriate stimuli, cellular regulatory factors like cytokines can be released without degranulation and release of preformed mediators; these may control the function of other cells within the lesion. Under controlled conditions, the triggering of cutaneous mast cells in normal volunteers induces a typical pruritic hive, lending support to the suggestion that these cells are of critical importance in urticarial reactions in man.

Many stimuli can induce mast cells to degranulate. Probably most important is the interaction of mast cell membrane–bound IgE antibody with specific antigen. Mast cells have on their surface a high-affinity receptor for IgE and in tissues are found coated with IgE antibody derived from plasma or interstitial fluid. Interaction of IgE antibody with its antigen cross-links IgE receptors, a required step in initiating the degranulation process by antigen-mediated cell activation. However, not only IgE meeting its antigen, but also a series of peptides derived from various plasma mediator molecules, can trigger degranulation. For example, peptides derived from activated complement proteins including C3a, C4a, and C5a and small fragments of C2 can induce mast cell degranulation. Similarly, peptides like bradykinin, derived from activation and cleavage of proteins of the kinin-generating system, and neuropeptides like substance P can induce mast cell degranulation. Incompletely defined cellular products derived from circulating mononuclear cells and neutrophils can cause mast cell degranulation as well. Moreover, toxic products from neutrophils and monocytes, whose release is induced by many factors including mast cell products, can on injection induce a typical hive.

Induction of an immediate hypersensitivity response in an allergic individual by the intradermal injection of a sensitizing antigen leads to rapid mast cell degranulation and the immediate appearance of a wheal and flare response that gradually fades. In many individuals 4 to 6 hours later a "late-phase" response is noted with an increase in local inflammation and swelling. Biopsy of such a late-phase reaction reveals the accumulation of neutrophils and eosinophils in the inflamed area and later their gradual replacement by mononuclear cells. The factors that induce the late-phase reaction are not completely defined, but the recent demonstration of the production of chemotactic cytokines some hours after mast cell triggering suggests that these factors may contribute to late-phase inflammation.

An understanding of these experimental findings helps explain biopsy findings in patients with acute and chronic urticaria/angioedema. It should be emphasized that although the disease may be chronic, individual lesions may be quite evanescent, lasting hours to days. On biopsy, subcutaneous edema is prominent with flattened rete pegs, widened dermal papillae, and swollen collagen fibers. There is an increase in the number of cutaneous mast cells noted when compared with normal individuals. Even uninvolved skin from a patient with urticaria shows increased mast cell number when compared with skin of normals. Some mast cell degranulation is seen on biopsy of lesions, and in chronic urticaria a modest mononuclear cell infiltrate containing lymphocytes (predominantly CD4+ helper T cells) and a relatively few monocyte/macrophages is noted. An increase in eosinophils may be seen. Patients with the physical urticaria tend to have more neutrophils and eosinophils on biopsy than are observed in chronic urticaria/angioedema. In a minority of cases with typical urticarial lesions a typical leukocytoclastic vasculitis is observed. This latter finding indicates that the underlying diagnosis is vasculitis and places the patient in a different diagnostic and therapeutic group.

A list of common causes of urticaria/angioedema is provided in Table 245–1. However, it must be emphasized that in most cases the cause of urticaria/angioedema is never found. In one large series 70 per cent of all cases remained in the idiopathic group after all other urticarial syndrome complexes were eliminated. These cutaneous manifestations appear, often are treated, and disappear with no etiologic diagnosis ever made. It is believed that most urticaria/angioedema cases represent hypersensitivity reactions to drugs, foods, or less commonly inhalants, because when a cause is defined it commonly involves one of these sensitizing agents. Penicillin is the drug still most commonly associated with acute urticaria, but aspirin and other nonsteroidal anti-inflammatory agents may exacerbate urticaria, possibly through their inhibition of prostaglandin synthesis, and diuretics, radiocontrast dyes, sulfonamides, and muscle relaxants all are associated with acute urticaria. Opioids can trigger direct mast cell release of histamine and cause urticarial lesions. Among foods, nuts, milk, eggs, chocolate, citrus fruits, tomatoes, fish, shellfish, and food dyes have all been associated with onset of urticaria in some individuals. Nevertheless, so many different antigens, including food additives, drugs, foods, and food contaminants, have been defined as causative in individual cases, and so little antigen may be required to precipitate attacks, that it may be difficult or impossible to define the causative agent. In many patients in whom the disease becomes chronic (defined as lasting longer than 6 weeks) the patient is asked to keep a diary to determine whether a particular food or commercial product is involved with an attack. If it proves impossible to define the precipitating agent by this means, a severely restricted elimination diet, limiting food ingestion to boiled rice and lamb, may be tried to see if elimination of an offending ingested agent will terminate attacks. Too often these attempts are unsuccessful.

There are defined clinical situations in which urticaria and/or angioedema is a common presenting problem: Patients undergoing immune complex–mediated reactions such as occur in active systemic lupus erythematosus and serum sickness may experience waves of urticarial lesions, in this case thought to be due to activation of the various mediatory pathways by circulating immune complexes with generation of kinins and complement-derived anaphylatoxins.

Autoantibodies of various sorts interacting with antigen may induce urticarial reactions. Indeed IgG anti-IgE autoantibodies have been suggested as a major cause of chronic urticaria, and there is some preliminary evidence to suggest that this might be so. Thyroid autoantibodies have been singled out as a cause of urticaria; in one study 90 of 624 patients with chronic urticaria were found to have thyroid autoimmunity, being either hyper- or hypothyroid. Similarly, blood transfusions and infusions of fresh frozen plasma are often associated with hives caused by antibodies in the infused materials encountering host antigen or circulating host antibodies binding antigens in the blood products. One study suggests that as many as 25 per cent of patients receiving fresh frozen plasma (FFP) experience transient urticaria, and some may have anaphylactic symptomatology during the infusion. Similarly, some cancers, for example lymphomas, may be associated with urticarial lesions, thought to be due to an immunologic response to tumor antigens. A similar mechanism is clearly responsible for the hives that may be associated with many infectious agents, particularly viral agents. Here antigens on or released from the infectious agent are bound to antibodies induced in the patient and hives result. Hives are a frequent response to the antibodies formed in the early response to hepatitis A and Epstein-Barr virus infection. Rarely fungal antigens like those derived from Candida albicans may precipitate hives or angioedema. Nevertheless, given the rarity of this observation, it is inappropriate to treat patients with chronic urticaria/angioedema with nystatin unless a clear association with a hypersensitivity response to candidal antigens can be demonstrated. Although rare in the United States, many parasitic diseases can at times be associated with urticaria/angioedema with or without hypereosinophilia. Presumably the presence of the urticaria/angioedema reflects an ongoing immediate hypersensitivity reaction to parasite antigens.

Physical Urticarias and Angioedemas

It is important to consider the physical urticaria/angioedema complex when evaluating patients with chronic recurrent urticaria or angioedema, since in one large series these represent 16 per cent of all chronic urticaria/angioedema patients seen. In some patients a highly specific diagnosis can be made, a clear precipitating factor can be defined, and the patient can learn to avoid attacks. Moreover, specific therapy may be available. When one lists these causes of urticaria/angioedema, they appear to be so easily defined that it appears unlikely that they could be missed. However, in practice this is not the case; a detailed history is required to identify these factors. Indeed it is common for these patients to go years before a correct diagnosis is made. The physical urticarias have in common urticaria/angioedema precipitated by a known physical cause. This response may follow exposure to cold, heat, elevated body temperature, pressure, vibration, specific-wavelength ultraviolet rays, or rarely even application of water to the skin. In some cases these reactions are thought to be IgE mediated, as they can be passively transferred with serum of an affected donor to the skin of an unaffected recipient. In other cases the cause is unknown.

Symptomatic Dermatographism

As many as 2 to 5 per cent of the general population may be dermatographic, with the appearance of blanching followed by a linear streak of edema and erythema within 2 to 5 minutes of stroking of the skin. A small proportion of such individuals have sufficiently severe dermatographism that they become symptomatic. In some cases the symptoms can be transferred to a normal recipient by passive transfer of plasma, suggesting that in some way IgE antibody plays a role. In general these individuals can be treated successfully with H_1 and H_2 antihistamines.

Cold Urticaria

These patients experience urticaria/angioedema on exposure to cold and may become hypotensive on diving into a cold swimming pool. Careful studies have shown that mast cell degranulation with histamine release occurs in these patients on cold exposure. Degranulation may be even more extensive when the patient's tissues are warmed following cold exposure. Placing an ice cube on the skin for 5 minutes and then removing it reveals an area of blanching in the shape of the cube followed by edema formation in the same area surrounded by an erythematous flare caused by local hyperemia. In a percentage of these patients passive transfer to the skin of normals has been demonstrated. It has been suggested that upon cold exposure, certain dermal antigens undergo a conformational change that allows specific IgE autoantibody to bind and initiate mast cell degranulation. These patients are typically treated with cyproheptadine, sometimes with the addition of hydroxyzine. Cold urticaria may occur in some systemic diseases as well. In rare cases this may be associated with the presence of cryoglobulin or cryofibrinogen. The symptom complex, however, is not associated with the presence of cold agglutinins. When cold urticaria is associated with underlying disease, treatment of that disease is an essential part of therapy.

In some patients the disease is atypical in that the patient gives a history of typical urticarial symptoms but the ice cube test is negative. In occasional patients dermatographism is brought out by cold exposure; in others exercise-induced urticaria is noted only in the cold. There is a rare familial type of cold urticaria inherited as an autosomal dominant trait in which patients develop urticarial lesions 9 to 18 hours after cold exposure. This cannot be passively transferred with plasma and the cause is unknown.

In a similar fashion, localized heat urticaria has been described, with a wheal and flare response noted 2 to 5 minutes after application of localized heat to the skin.

Cholinergic or Generalized Heat Urticaria

Typically these patients, representing about 4 per cent of all patients with chronic urticaria, develop small (several millimeters), intensely pruritic wheals on an erythematous base on their upper trunk and arms following exercise with sweating or following hot showers. Essential to the development of lesions is a rise in core body temperature. It is generally believed that the parasympathetic nervous system supply to the neuromuscular junction of cutaneous vessels releases acetylcholine as well as neuropeptide, such as vasoactive intestinal peptide, which in an unknown way causes mediator release. In support of this hypothesis is the fact that a proportion of these patients (30 to 50 per cent) develop typical lesions as well as a series of local satellite lesions upon intracutaneous injection of Mecholyl. Atropine may inhibit the skin test but does not successfully treat the disease. These patients are typically highly responsive to hydroxyzine therapy. There is a subset of patients who respond to heat exposure with the development of large urticarial lesions rather than with the typical lesions of cholinergic urticaria. These patients tend not to develop their hives with exercise and are less responsive to hydroxyzine therapy.

Exercise-Induced Urticaria/Anaphylaxis

These patients note urticarial lesions appearing 5 to 30 minutes after the onset of exercise. They last for 1 to 3 hours. In severe cases anaphylactic reactions may be noted. This is an illness generally of young adults. At times symptoms are difficult to distinguish from those of cholinergic urticaria; however, these patients do not develop urticaria on raising core body temperature as in a hot bath.

Pressure-Induced Urticaria

For unknown reasons, in almost all cases urticarial lesions are common at pressure points on the body, e.g., where clothing is tight. Some patients note the development of marked urticarial lesions 4 to 6 hours after pressure is applied to the body. For example, these individuals may note urticarial lesions on buttocks following a long period of sitting on a hard chair or angioedema or urticaria on their feet after prolonged standing in one place. The lesions may be provoked by placing over the shoulders for 20 minutes a 1-inch strap weighted at the ends with 15-pound weights. A systemic response with malaise and even fever is often noted. The response to antihistamines is often poor. The urticaria but not the systemic toxicity may respond to antihistamine therapy. The most severely affected of these patients may require every-other-day glucocorticoid administration for partial relief. They are reported to be unresponsive to nonsteroidal anti-inflammatory agents.

In a similar way, some patients respond to local vibration with the development of urticarial lesions. Typically symptoms are induced by placing a vibrator or vortex mixer on the arm for 5 minutes. Urticaria appears in 1 to 5 minutes.

Solar Urticaria

In general these patients develop urticarial responses to exposure to sunlight; the patients are divided into groups by the wavelength of light that provokes attacks. Patients whose attacks are provoked by light at 280 to 320 nm (type 1) and 400 to 500 nm (type 4) typically have disease that can be passively transferred with serum to nonaffected recipients. This observation suggests the presence of an IgE-dependent mechanism in these cases. Glass absorbs light with wavelength below 320 nm, and patients with urticaria in response to light wavelengths below 320 nm can be protected easily. The erythema-causing band of the solar spectrum, UVB, is at wavelength 290 to 320 nm, and these patients can sometimes be helped considerably by PABA-containing sunscreens, which absorb light in this range. However, many are not protected by the PABA sunscreens. A newly available sunscreen preparation, butyl methoxydibenzoyl methane, absorbs light in the UVA range and may be more useful for this patient group. There are many types of light sensitivity, and sorting these out may be confusing. They range from metabolic abnormalities (erythrogenic porphyria), in which products of metabolism absorb light energy and undergo chemical alteration with the development of toxic products, to photoallergic reactions, in which skin-sensitizing drugs induce allergic reactions when acted upon by sunlight, to phototoxic reactions, in which drugs localized in cutaneous tissues directly cause tissue-damaging reactions when exposed to light of the proper wavelength. In many of these cases the light energy is absorbed by a complex ring structure in the drug with subsequent release of photons and electrons that lead to local generation of toxic products such as singlet oxygen, hydrogen peroxide, and chloramines. Obviously in each case one attempts to identify the cause of the urticaria and eliminate the offending agent if it can be defined.

Aquagenic Urticaria

These patients respond with urticaria within 2 to 30 minutes to application of water to the skin. Typically this is noted in the course of baths or showers, even with water at tepid temperature. In many cases these individuals are probably exquisitely sensitive to additives in the water, e.g., chlorine, but it is reported that rare individuals develop urticaria in response to distilled water.

Chronic Urticaria/Angioedema

It should be clear from the material presented that chronic urticaria/angioedema can be caused by many agents, and identifying the agent may be difficult or impossible. Often after attempts at identifying the etiology of the urticaria have failed, we are left with a patient who requires treatment. H_1 antihistamines are usually the agents of first choice. Some examples of therapeutic agents are listed earlier in the chapter; in patients with chronic disease, high-dose hydroxyzine and cyproheptadine are often effective. These agents make patients drowsy and may not be well tolerated initially, but drowsiness may pass if the drug is continued. Frequently the dose is increased until drowsiness persists and then the dosage is reduced slightly. It is common to find patients who claim to have been unresponsive to these agents because the drugs have not been used properly. Many more conveniently used and less sedating antihistamines have become available in the last few years and have been shown in controlled studies to be effective in chronic angio-edema/urticaria. These include terfenadine, astemizol, loratidine, and cetirizine. H_2 inhibitory drugs are often added to H_1 inhibitors if the clinical response is not adequate. Other agents have also proven to be beneficial, including doxipen, a tricyclic antide-pressant with anti-H_1 and anti-H_2 properties; nifedipine, a calcium channel blocker; and ketotifin, a drug shown to be efficacious in the physical urticarias. If these agents fail, a course of glucocorticoids may be required. In general one begins with 40 to 60 mg of prednisone per day in divided doses for 1 week. The dosage is then consolidated to a single dose a day, and then the drug is rapidly tapered on an every-other-day schedule until the patient is receiving glucocorticoids once every other day. The dose of glucocorticoids should be tapered to the lowest dose that will maintain the patient with minimal symptoms. Following a course of glucocorticoid therapy, patients often remain in remission for a prolonged time. The illness may recur at a later time or when glucocorticoids are tapered.

DIFFERENTIAL DIAGNOSIS

The etiology of the disorder is multifactorial. Usually the diagnosis of urticaria/angioedema does not present a problem in the patient with clear episodes of pruritic wheals or localized brawny edema. Since many agents can cause these lesions, considerable detective work is required to define these diseases and to develop a suitable specific therapy. During the initial evaluation a number of points must be explored. A history of a fixed rather than evanescent eruption, burning, bruising, or vesiculating lesions must lead one to early biopsy. Similarly, fever or systemic signs and symptoms suggest that further explo-ration is needed. Patients with idiopathic chronic urticaria typi-cally have a normal sedimentation rate, white count, and differ-ential and these should be examined. In appropriate cases, ANA, heterophile, STS, rheumatoid factor level, cryoglobulins and cryofibrinogen, cold hemolysin, C4, and C1 inhibitor levels should be studied for further clues to the underlying diagnosis. In the patient who responds poorly to therapy or who has atypical disease, a biopsy is clearly indicated. Patients with urticarial vasculitis are treated for the underlying vasculitis.

THERAPY

The use of antihistamines is discussed under each of the various entities and in the section on chronic urticaria/angioedema. The use of glucocorticoids has been discussed in that section as well. Epinephrine is of clinical usefulness in acute management of urticaria/angioedema. In this case the drug is administered as a series of injections (0.2 to 0.3 ml) of 1:1000 dilution subcutane-ously, repeated at half-hour intervals two or three times until symptoms are controlled. Obviously the use of epinephrine is contraindicated in certain patient groups such as patients with severe cardiovascular disease. Longer-acting epinephrine prepa-rations such as epinephrine in oil (Sus-Phrine) may be useful.

URTICARIA PIGMENTOSA AND SYSTEMIC MASTOCYTOSIS

Urticaria pigmentosa is characterized by the local accumulation of intradermal masses of infiltrating mast cells (Ch. 252). The lesions may resemble freckles superficially but are raised, as might be expected of infiltrative lesions, and may be somewhat erythematous. They may urticate when stroked (Darier's sign). Systemic mastocytosis is associated with massive accumulation of mast cells in other organs, particularly the bone marrow and gastrointestinal tract. Although some of these patients may pre-sent to the physician with acute or chronic urticaria, that pres-entation is quite rare; systemic signs of histamine toxicity, gas-trointestinal disorders, or disorders consequent to destruction of bone marrow or bone are more common.

HEREDITARY ANGIOEDEMA

Hereditary angioedema (HAE) presents clinically as episodic attacks of brawny nonpitting edema that usually involve the

extremities but may affect any external body surface including the genitalia. Mucosal surfaces are affected as well and patients frequently have attacks of severe abdominal pain due to swelling of the submucosa of the gastrointestinal tract. On rare occasions attacks may affect the airway, where they can cause respiratory obstruction and asphyxiation. Although attacks are sporadic, about half of the patients note that trauma, particularly associated with local pressure, precipitates an attack, and half the patients note a marked increase in attack frequency at times of emotional stress. About one third of patients note an erythema marginatum–like rash at the onset of attacks which they often describe as nonraised, nonpruritic circles on the skin. In general, attacks become progressively more severe over about 1.5 days and then regress over a similar time period. Swelling of the gastrointestinal mucosa may be associated with exquisite abdominal pain.

Although relatively rare (incidence about 1:10,000), this disease has received a great deal of attention because of the high incidence of lethal complications, because its pathophysiologic basis is best understood of all of the angioedemas, and because adequate therapy is available for most patients. Presence of this disease is associated with either low levels or abnormal function of a plasma regulatory protein, the C1 inhibitor (Ch. 243). This protein functions to control activation of the complement, kinin-generating, fibrinolytic, and intrinsic clotting pathways. Although the precise cause of the capillary leakage is unknown, it is believed that a peptide formed during activation of either the complement or the kinin-generating mediator pathway is the responsible factor. HAE has an autosomal dominant inheritance pattern, affecting 50 per cent of the offspring of a patient and occurring with equal frequency in males and females. This autosomal dominant inheritance reflects the presence of one abnormal gene for C1 inhibitor on chromosome 11. This gene may yield no gene product or may code for a nonfunctional protein.

HAE tends to be mild in childhood, becoming more severe at the time of puberty. The factors that initiate attacks are unknown. There is no relationship between the level or activity of C1 inhibitor and the severity of disease. Patients are described who presumably had the defect from birth but whose attacks began at age 70. Diagnosis is established by demonstration of low levels of C1 inhibitor antigen or function and low levels of the comple-ment protein C4 and/or C2. C1 inhibitor inhibits the function of activated C1 of the classic complement pathway. C1 INH acts by binding to the substrate to be inhibited, and the product of one normal gene is insufficient to control mediator activation. C1 when activated cleaves the next two proteins in the cascade, C4 and C2. Since the function of activated C1 is unregulated in the presence of a relative C1 inhibitor deficiency, it continues to cleave C4 and C2. Patients have low levels of circulating C4 and C2 during attacks and usually have low levels between attacks. Interestingly, because of the presence of other control proteins, the levels of C3, the most commonly measured complement protein, are almost always normal. Presumably because of the constant complement activation present in these patients, they have an immune dysregulation, as shown by the higher-than-normal incidence of autoimmune diseases. These include endo-crinopathies, granulomatous bowel disorders, arthritides, and SLE.

Patients' angioedema attacks respond poorly to epinephrine, antihistamines, and glucocorticoids, the mainstays of treatment of urticaria and angioedema caused by immediate hypersensitivity reactions. Nevertheless, acute attacks are treated with epineph-rine, both nebulized racemic epinephrine in the airway (1:1000 given by nebulization) and subcutaneous injections (0.2 to 0.3 ml 1:1000 SQ repeated q 20–30 min × 3). Epinephrine administered very early in an attack often produces some improvement. Patients also receive antihistamines for sedation. Patients often relate that intravenous administration of FFP to supply the missing inhibitor protein terminates attacks. Nevertheless, a rare patient becomes more edematous following FFP, presumably reflecting increased availability of mediator substrates, and FFP therefore is not recommended for treatment of life-threatening laryngeal edema. In this circumstance endotracheal intubation in the operating room under conditions where tracheostomy can be performed is indicated. FFP can be given in nonemergency situations such as in preoperative patients to prevent attacks. The usual dose of FFP is 2 units, an arbitrary amount that has been used extensively and has proven to be effective. Evidence suggests that infusions of purified C1 inhibitor reliably terminate attacks, but this protein has not yet been made available in the United States. Although short-term therapy and therapy of acute attacks of HAE have not been generally satisfactory, long-term therapy has been quite successful. Patients respond to all of the acetylated artificial androgens with increased C1 INH levels that in some cases approach normal values, a correction of serum C4 and C2, and a marked amelioration of symptoms. In the rare patient in whom the drug is ineffective or in whom drug toxicity is a problem, the plasmin inhibitor ε-aminocaproic acid has also been found to be effective. Its mechanism of action is unknown, and there is no change in the amount of C activation reflected in the persistent reduction in the serum level of C4 and C2. With all of these agents there is a high degree of patient-to-patient variation in dosage, and the lowest dose that controls symptoms is chosen. Women are often treated with danazol, an impeded androgen that has few masculinizing side effects. The usual dosage of danazol is 200 to 400 mg per day. Men are often treated with the less expensive but more androgenic agent methyltestosterone in a dose of 10 to 30 mg per day orally.

ACQUIRED C1 INHIBITOR DEFICIENCY

A number of syndromes have been recognized that are associated with a typical hereditary angioedema symptom complex but are a reflection of acquired disease. A decade ago it was recognized that certain patients with malignancies, including lymphosarcoma, leukemia, lymphoma, and paraproteinemia, developed circulating or cellular factors capable of activating C1 and depleting all the C1 inhibitor activity in serum. Later it was noted that rare patients with autoimmune disease also induced massive activation of the complement cascade, with C1 inhibitor utilization and a hereditary angioedema–like clinical picture. More recently, patients have been described with multiple myeloma and anti-idiotypic antibody causing the same symptom complex. Perhaps the most common of these rare individuals are recently described patients who form monoclonal or polyclonal autoantibodies to the C1 inhibitor which destroy its activity. Clinically these patients cannot be distinguished from patients with hereditary angioedema. However, their laboratory tests are unique. All of these patients have profound depressions in functional C1, C4, and C2. Patients with HAE commonly have normal C1 levels. Although their plasma C1 inhibitor antigen level may be normal, these patients have marked depression of C1 INH function. Their treatment involves treating the underlying disease where possible. Some of these patients do respond to danazol or other anabolic steroids. One of the patients with the anti–C1 INH autoantibody has responded to glucocorticoid therapy, and at least one of these patients has responded to cytotoxic therapy.

FACTOR I DEFICIENCY WITH CHRONIC URTICARIA

Factor I is one of the control proteins of the complement activation pathway. The rare individuals with an inherited deficiency of this protein have continuous activation and cleavage of C3 with generation of the anaphylatoxins C3a and perhaps C5a. In vitro these cleavage peptides induce mast cell degranulation and cause chronic urticaria that disappears when the patient is infused with Factor I. In general, this form of urticaria is relatively mild and is treated symptomatically with antihistamines.

Bressler RB, Sowell K, Huston DP: Therapy of chronic idiopathic urticaria with nifedipine: Demonstration of a beneficial effect in a double blinded, placebo controlled, crossover trial. J Allergy Clin Immunol 83:756, 1989. *Seven patients completed this trial. All improved.*

Casale TB, Sampson HA, Harrifin J, et al.: Guide to physical urticarias. J Allergy Clin Immunol 82:758, 1988. *Tables of information on the physical urticarias.*

Champion RH: Urticaria: Then and now. Br J Dermatol 119:427, 1988. *A report of the evaluation of 2300 cases and comments on the literature.*

Champion RH, Greaves MW, Kobza A, et al.: The Urticarias. Edinburgh, Churchill Livingstone, 1985. *The proceedings of a symposium on urticaria-angioedema.*

Frank MM: Hereditary angioedema. *In* Bayless TM, Brain MC, Cherniack RM (eds.): Current Therapy in Internal Medicine 2. Philadelphia, B. C. Decker, 1987, p 42. *Complete discussion of treatment.*

Frank MM, Gelfand JA, Atkinson JP: Hereditary angioedema: The clinical syndrome and its management. Ann Intern Med 84:580, 1976. *Although old, this represents the classic clinical review of this syndrome.*

Leznoff A, Sussman GL: Syndrome of idiopathic chronic urticaria and angioedema with thyroid autoimmunity. A study of 90 patients. J Allergy Clin Immunol 84:66, 1989. *The best review of this patient group.*

Monroe EN: Chronic urticaria. Review of nonsedating H₁ antihistamines in treatment. J Am Acad Dermatol 19:842, 1988. *Comparison of various H₁ agents and review of published studies.*

Wanderer AA: Cold urticaria syndromes. Historical background, diagnostic classification, clinical and laboratory characteristics, pathogenesis and management. J Allergy Clin Immunol 88:965, 1990. *A thorough review of this syndrome.*

246 Allergic Rhinitis

John E. Salvaggio

DEFINITION. Allergic rhinitis is an IgE-mediated inflammatory disease of the nasal mucous membranes characterized by paroxysms of sneezing; itching of the nose, eyes, palate, and pharynx; nasal stuffiness with partial or total obstruction of air flow; and mucous secretion often accompanied by postnasal drainage. The disease is often seasonal, depending on the pollination patterns of inhalant allergens that have direct impact on the respiratory mucosa. The condition may be perennial when due to nonseasonal allergens.

Patients with allergic rhinitis have an increased number of mast cells in nasal secretions. When appropriately sensitized with specific IgE molecules, mucosal mast cells can interact with allergenic airborne particles that initially affect the respiratory mucosa and release water-soluble allergens during inhalation. Mast cells and basophils concentrate IgE on their surface, which fixes to a glycoprotein receptor site on the membrane by its Fc fragment, resulting in an arrangement that permits exposure of the antibody-combining sites (or Fab) to the surrounding milieu. Cross-linking of two IgE antibody molecules by specific antigen aggregates the corresponding receptor sites and results in initiation of a series of cellular biochemical events that culminate in the expulsion of secretory granule contents with release of pharmacologic mediators. The consequences of mediator release may be apparent within minutes or may require hours to develop (late-phase allergic reactions). They are summarized in Figure 246–1. Among the mast cell–derived mediators, either preformed within their granules or generated from precursor molecules, are

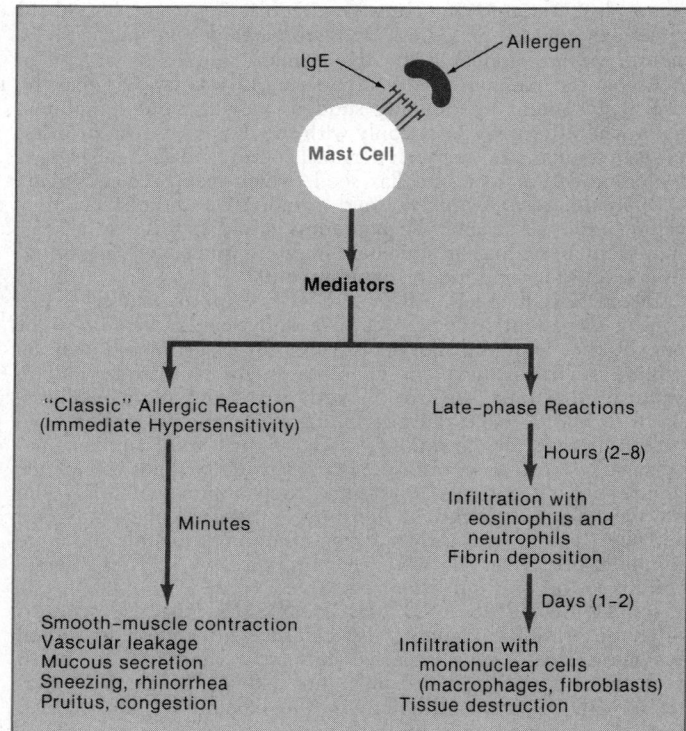

FIGURE 246–1. Mast cell mediator/effector pathways.

histamine; kinins and kininogen; thromboxanes; leukotrienes C_4, D_4, and E_4, which are derived from arachidonic acid released during the allergic reaction; eosinophil chemotactic factors of anaphylaxis (ECF-A), which are derived from the mast cell granule; heparin, which makes up 30 per cent of the dry weight of mast cell granules; superoxide dismutase (SOD), which is formed by the univalent reduction of oxygen; prostaglandins, which are C20 unsaturated fatty acid derivatives of arachidonic acid; platelet-activating factor (PAF), a small phospholipid derivative of phosphoryl choline released from rabbit basophils; neutrophil chemotactic factor of anaphylaxis (NCF-A); inflammatory factors of anaphylaxis, which are constituents of the mast cell granules that can induce a late-phase allergic inflammatory reaction; and a number of enzymes that are found in mast cell granules, such as chymotrypsin, trypsin, and tosyl-arginine-methyl-ester (TAME)-esterase. These enzymes may contribute to the tissue destruction accompanying various late-phase allergic reactions. Both immediate- and late-phase nasal reactions, which occur hours after challenge, have been produced in vivo following nasal challenge with ragweed pollen or other allergens. Histamine; kinins; TAME-esterase; leukotrienes C_4, D_4, and E_4; and prostaglandin D_2 have been directly demonstrated in nasal secretions during the immediate response. With the exception of prostaglandin D_2, these mediators have also been demonstrable in late-phase responses. Since prostaglandin D_2 is released by mast cells but not basophils, this observation suggests an important role for basophils in late-phase reactions. Nasal mucosal biopsy specimens may also reveal increased numbers of ciliated cells, goblet cells, and eosinophils in the epithelium, plus edema and vascular dilation in the submucosa. The inflammation that follows immediate-phase reactions likely results in a primary effect, accounting for much of the hyperreactivity of the allergic nose to a variety of nonspecific stimuli such as strong odors, insecticides, and cigarette smoke.

ETIOLOGY. The most apparent seasonal allergens acting as etiologic agents in allergic rhinitis are pollens such as ragweed. Tree pollens are usually released during the spring, and in most parts of the country the peak of the grass pollen season is late spring to midsummer. Much of the nasal symptoms caused by airborne weed pollens occurs in late summer and early fall. Ragweed pollen is by far the worst offender in the eastern, midwestern, and southern United States. Many individuals with perennial allergic rhinitis have an IgE-mediated response to crude house-dust antigen. In many geographic areas and household situations, mites, including *Dermatophagoides farinae* and *D. petronyssimus*, appear to be the primary sources of antigen in house dusts. Animal danders, particularly cat dander, may be especially potent in inducing sudden, violent nasal symptoms, even when there is contact only with the dander, saliva, or urine of the animal. In certain persons, other inhalant allergens, including cotton seed and flax seed, which may be constituents of animal feeds, fertilizers, and inexpensive upholstery, may cause perennial or sporadic symptoms. Mold spores can be very important perennial or seasonal allergens, since they are found in both outdoor and indoor environments.

INCIDENCE AND PREVALENCE. Approximately 9 per cent of all patients who seek care at a physician's office do so for one of the common allergic diseases. It is estimated that 50 million Americans have allergic diseases: An estimated 9 million suffer from asthma (see Ch. 57) with or without allergic rhinitis; 25 to 30 million have allergic rhinitis alone; and 12 million have other allergic manifestations, such as urticaria, angioedema, eczema, or food, drug, or insect hypersensitivity. These incidence figures are deceptively low, since they approximate only the number of patients who, at the time of the particular study, are actually afflicted with the condition and do not include the large numbers of individuals who have had diseases such as allergic rhinitis in the past but have since "recovered."

PATHOGENESIS AND MECHANISMS. The pathogenesis of allergic rhinitis, including IgE-allergen interaction, mast cell mediator release, sensory nerve stimulation, and CNS-mediated reflex activity, is illustrated in Figure 246–2. The nasal cavity is lined with airways epithelium of the ciliated pseudostratified type. The lamina propria in the anterior part of the nose contains large numbers of seromucous and serous glands. Postganglionic

sympathetic nerves emerge from the stellate ganglion in the neck and reach the nose along arteries. Most of the parasympathetic fibers to the nose travel via the vidian nerve. The parasympathetic fibers are part of a reflex arc with sensory fibers in the trigeminal nerve. The nasal sensory nerves are exposed to stimulation from unconditioned and polluted inhaled air, and there is constant reflex activity in the nerves.

There are immunologic as well as nonimmunologic triggers of this mast cell degranulation process. Histamine sprayed into the nose causes itching, sneezing, discharge, and blockage and directly increases endothelial- and epithelial-cell permeability. This facilitates further allergen penetration into the submucosal areas. Histamine also has a direct effect on vascular H_1 and H_2 receptors, resulting in edema formation. In addition, when released from epithelial basophils, histamine indirectly stimulates sensory nerve H_1 receptors, resulting in a CNS-mediated parasympathetic reflex in the trigeminal and vidian nerves with subsequent itching, sneezing, and increased nasal discharge.

CLINICAL MANIFESTATIONS. Common symptoms include nasal stuffiness, paroxysms of sneezing, profuse mucous secretion, and frequent itching of the nose, eyes, posterior pharynx, or conjunctivae. Soreness or inflammation of the conjunctivae with excessive tearing and mucoid conjunctival discharge may be present in severe cases, and it is not uncommon for patients with recurrent symptoms to note a certain degree of fatigue, malaise, anorexia, and irritability. Many offending plants pollinate during the early morning hours. Thus, morning symptoms may be followed by improvement during the day as exposure lessens. Repeated upward rubbing of the nose to relieve itching may cause a crease to develop across the nose, especially in children. Mouth breathing is common, as are typical dark, discolored infraorbital "shiners" (Fig. 246–3).

Examination of the nasal mucous membranes characteristically reveals bluish, edematous, boggy, pale nasal turbinates, often coated with clear secretion, but many persons with allergic rhinitis have an erythematous, boggy nasal mucosa that can easily be confused with that seen in infectious rhinitis. At times, the nasal airways may be completely obstructed as a result of accumulation of mucus and turbinate swelling. Scleral and conjunctival injection and edema plus periorbital swelling and tearing may be noted. Nasal polyps are relatively uncommonly associated with uncomplicated rhinitis. They may, however, be associated with aspirin intolerance. Since asthmatics with aspirin intolerance often have severe disease, visualization of even small polyps in patients with rhinitis and asthma may provide important diagnostic leads.

In seasonal rhinitis, symptoms recur each year with regularity during the pollination season characteristic for a given area. IgE-mediated perennial rhinitis presents with continuous low-grade symptoms that may improve only if the patient leaves the region of the inciting causes. Perennial rhinitis of unknown cause (also called vasomotor rhinitis) also produces persistent symptoms without correlation to any specific allergen exposure. This type of perennial rhinitis is often worsened by changes in temperature or humidity or with exposure to irritants or other types of air pollutants. It is also often associated with profuse nasal discharge after the patient eats chilled, highly spiced, or very hot foods.

Serous otitis media may be superimposed upon other symptoms of seasonal or perennial allergic rhinitis. In many instances of serous otitis media, however, allergic factors cannot be identified. Serous otitis, which can be an important complication in children, may result from nasal obstruction or obstructive dysfunction of the eustachian tube as a result of mucosal edema and secretions. It can also lead to hearing loss with adverse effects on cognition or speech development in the young child. The tympanic membrane on physical examination is frequently amber colored and retracted and shows decreased motion if there is negative middle-ear pressure or no motion at all if there is a severe effusion.

Chronic sinusitis may be another complication, often manifested by the presence of chronic nasal discharge, nocturnal cough associated with postnasal discharge, pain, fever, headache, and recurrent otitis media. In adults, however, pain, headache, and low-grade fever are the most common signs. Chronic sinusitis as a complication of seasonal allergic rhinitis should be considered whenever symptoms of allergic rhinitis are more protracted than expected, when the patient has severe dull-to-intense throbbing pain over the involved sinus area, or when prolonged or persistent

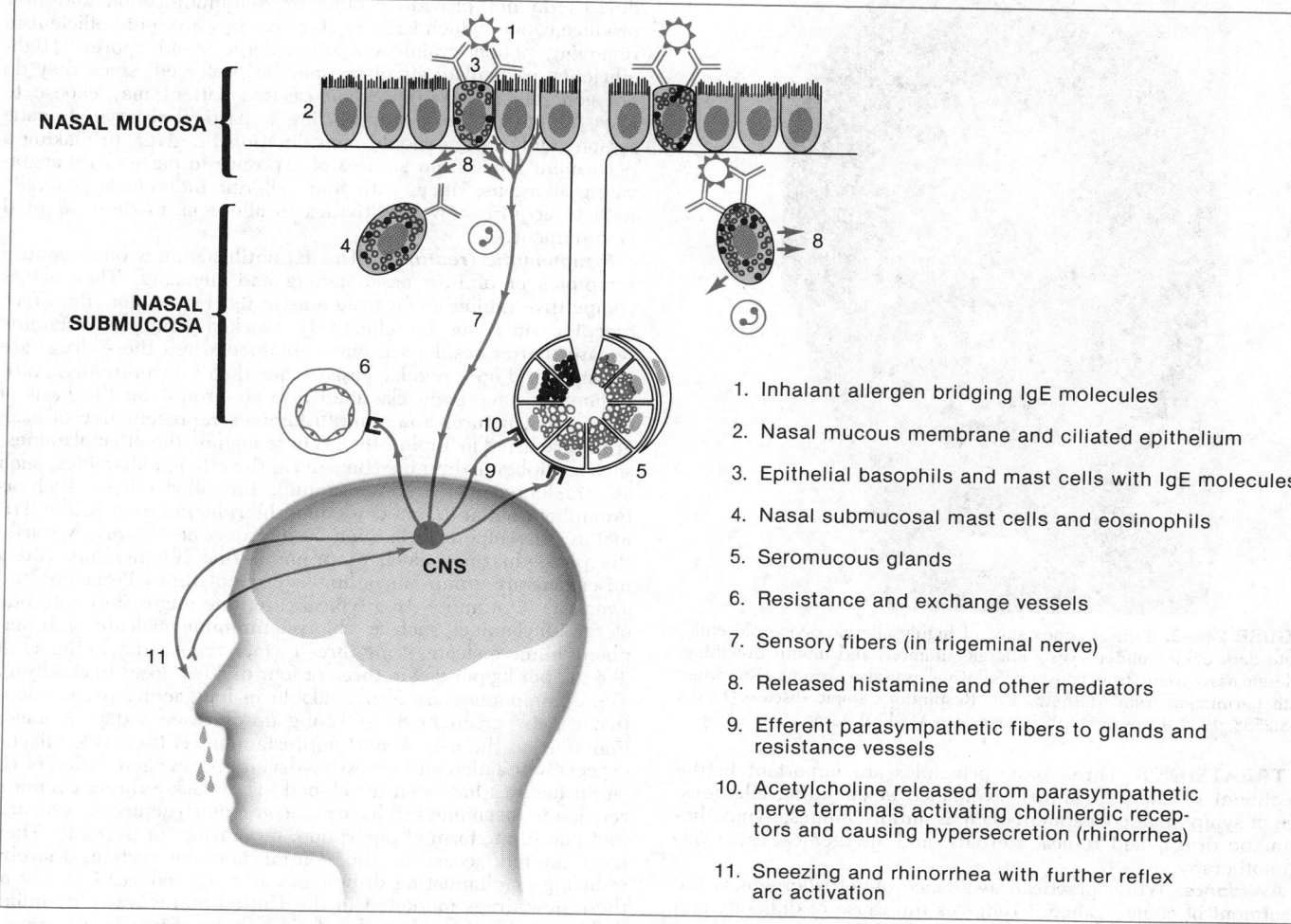

1. Inhalant allergen bridging IgE molecules

2. Nasal mucous membrane and ciliated epithelium

3. Epithelial basophils and mast cells with IgE molecules

4. Nasal submucosal mast cells and eosinophils

5. Seromucous glands

6. Resistance and exchange vessels

7. Sensory fibers (in trigeminal nerve)

8. Released histamine and other mediators

9. Efferent parasympathetic fibers to glands and resistance vessels

10. Acetylcholine released from parasympathetic nerve terminals activating cholinergic receptors and causing hypersecretion (rhinorrhea)

11. Sneezing and rhinorrhea with further reflex arc activation

FIGURE 246–2. Pathogenesis of allergic rhinitis; antigen-antibody interaction and mediator release.

cough develops which is suggestive of bronchitis that has failed to respond to appropriate therapy. Transillumination may be helpful in detecting chronic sinusitis, and equipment for ultrasonic evaluation of the sinuses in the office is also available. Roentgenograms often detect opacification, membrane thickening, or an air-fluid level in one or more sinuses.

DIAGNOSIS (WITH DIFFERENTIAL DIAGNOSIS). A good history is most important in correctly diagnosing rhinitis. In addition to the history of classic symptoms, nasal examination should be performed utilizing a nasal speculum along with high-powered illumination. If nasopharyngeal obstruction is present and its cause has not been detected by simpler means, nasopharyngoscopy should be considered. Careful skin testing with common inhalant preparations together with positive and negative control substances is a mandatory procedure in diagnosing specific allergic factors associated with rhinitis. Direct skin tests of the scratch, prick, and intradermal variety are the least expensive and time consuming. The intradermal test should never be performed without prior performance of negative scratch or prick tests. In general, negative skin test responses with common inhalant allergens indicate that rhinitis is of nonallergic origin. Methods of detecting IgE antibodies in vitro have now been available for several years. In patients who are receiving medications that might prevent skin reactivity or in those with extensive eczema or dermatographia that negates the use of skin tests, these in vitro assays for serum IgE antibodies, such as the radioallergosorbent test (RAST), fluorescent allergosorbent test (FAST), multiple thread allergosorbent test, or enzyme-linked immunosorbent assay (ELISA), may be substituted for direct skin testing. Total serum IgE levels are elevated in only 30 to 40 per cent of patients with allergic rhinitis. They may also be elevated

in many nonallergic conditions. Although frequently elevated in allergic rhinitis, the peripheral blood eosinophil count may be normal. A high peripheral eosinophil count may also be seen in nonallergic perennial rhinitis associated with nasal polyps, hyperplastic sinusitis, and idiopathic asthma. Of more significance is a smear of nasal secretions for eosinophils.

Conditions to be considered in the differential diagnosis of rhinitis are listed in Table 246–1. Clear-cut allergic rhinitis due to inhalant allergens seldom presents a differential diagnostic problem. Symptoms of the common cold may, however, be quite similar, although they usually last less than a week and are often associated with fever, pain, and the presence of considerable numbers of neutrophils in nasal secretions. Symptoms associated with structural abnormalities of the nasal area, such as polyps, deviated nasal septum, enlarged tonsils, or foreign bodies, are often unilateral and relatively constant rather than episodic in classic seasonal allergic rhinitis. A suspected diagnosis of so-called rhinitis medicamentosa due to the rebound effects of nose drops, sprays, ovarian hormonal agents (such as oral contraceptives), reserpine derivatives, or hydralazine can often be confirmed when symptoms gradually improve following avoidance of the suspected agent. Nasal symptoms may accompany metabolic disorders such as hyperthyroidism or emotional states, but the relationship is unclear. During pregnancy and the premenstrual period, hormonally related rhinitis may occur. Eosinophilic nonallergic rhinitis resembles allergic rhinitis but is associated with negative skin test reactions and normal IgE levels and tends to respond well only to topical corticosteroid therapy. A condition known as nasal mastocytosis is associated with symptoms of perennial allergic rhinitis; the diagnosis can be made by nasal mucosal biopsy.

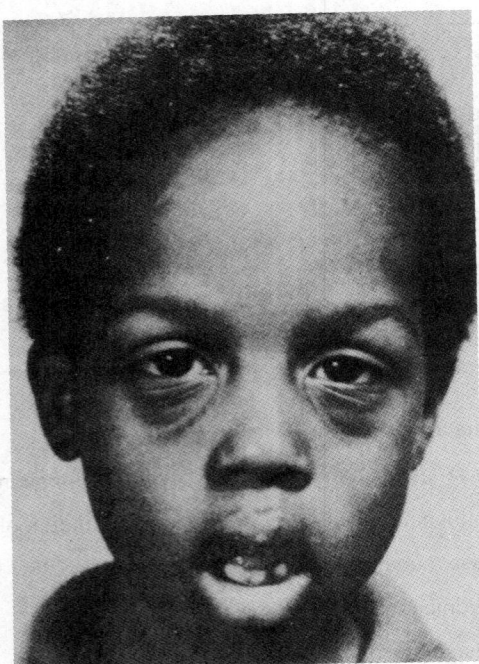

FIGURE 246–3. Typical appearance of highly allergic 6-year-old child. Note dark circles under eyes ("allergic shiners") and mouth breathing. Allergic nasal crease from constant "saluting" was also present. (Reprinted with permission from Mathews KP: Respiratory atopic disease. JAMA 248:2588, 1982. Copyright 1982, American Medical Association.)

TREATMENT. Three basic principles are important in the treatment of allergic rhinitis: avoidance of offending allergens; use of symptomatic treatment such as antihistamines, sympathomimetic drugs, and topical steroids; and allergenic extract immunotherapy.

Avoidance. When practical, avoidance of aeroallergens is the treatment of choice, since it removes the cause of difficulty and prevents symptoms. When a specific food, drug, occupational allergen, or animal dander is involved, avoidance is the only measure that serves both to prevent and to treat disease. All physicians should be familiar, for example, with standard antidust regimens for use in home environments. Although avoidance of outdoor exposure to ubiquitous seasonal and perennial pollens is virtually impossible, common-sense measures to avoid heavy exposure often help to prevent severe exacerbations of symptoms. For example, mold-sensitive patients should avoid barns, working with hay, raking leaves, and mowing grass. Simply keeping doors

TABLE 246–1. DIFFERENTIAL DIAGNOSIS OF RHINITIS

Infections
Allergic
   Seasonal (hay fever)
   Perennial
Eosinophilic nonallergic rhinitis
Rhinitis medicamentosa
Vasomotor rhinitis of pregnancy
"Vasomotor" rhinitis
Disturbed nasal function associated with
   Ciliary dyskinesia
   Hypothyroidism
   Horner's syndrome
   Foreign body
   Nasal polyps
   Nasal septal deviation
   Enlarged tonsils and adenoids
   Nasal mastocytosis
   Sinus disease
   Tumors or granulomas
   Cerebrospinal fluid rhinorrhea
   Aspirin intolerance

and windows closed significantly decreases indoor pollen and mold spore concentrations, and air conditioning makes a closed environment more tolerable. Although electrostatic air-purifying devices do not provide cooling or dehumidification and may produce ozone, which irritates rhinitis, they are quite efficient in removing pollen grains and other large mold spores. High-efficiency particulate air filters may be preferred, since they do not generate ozone. In certain cases a patient may choose to leave an area of exposure during a particularly symptomatic season. Only rarely should consideration be given to making a permanent move from an area of exposure to particularly aggravating allergens, since, with time, allergic individuals generally tend to acquire new sensitivities to allergens in their adopted environment.

Symptomatic Treatment. The H_1 antihistamines often control symptoms of profuse nasal itching and sneezing. They act as competitive inhibitors for histamine at its H_1 receptor site. Since receptor sites can be effectively blocked prior to histamine release, better results are often obtained when these drugs are administered on a regular basis rather than intermittently. Antihistamines have been classified into six groups on the basis of chemical structure. Some antihistamines representative of each group are listed in Table 246–2. These include the ethanolamines, such as diphenhydramine (Benadryl); the ethylenediamines, such as tripelennamine (Pyribenzamine); the alkylamines, such as brompheniramine (Dimetane) and chlorpheniramine (Chlor-Trimeton); the piperazines, such as hydroxyzine (Atarax, Vistaril); the phenothiazines, such as promethazine (Phenergan); and a miscellaneous group, including cyproheptadine (Periactin) and azatadine (Optimine). In a typical case, one might start with one of the alkylamines such as chlorpheniramine maleate or brompheniramine maleate, 4 mg three or four times a day in the adult (0.4 mg per kg per day in three or four divided doses in children). These compounds are also available in long-acting preparations that can be given in 8- to 12-mg doses twice a day. A major limitation to the use of most antihistamines is their side effects, especially sedation and excessive drying. A new generation of H_1 antihistamines has been developed. They lack a direct chemical relation to histamine but have as a common structure an aromatic nitrogen in the form of piperidine, piperazine, or pyridine. They have limited access to the central nervous system, thereby reducing or eliminating drowsiness as a side effect. The first of these new drugs marketed in the United States was terfenidine (Seldane). Another example of these new drugs is astemizole (Hismanil). Several other similar new-generation H_1 antihistamines are under development. Available data have failed to indicate a major enhancement of therapeutic benefit for allergic rhinitis using combined H_1 and H_2 antihistamines.

The most commonly employed sympathomimetic nasal sprays and drops that contain α-adrenergic agonists are phenylephrine hydrochloride, a short-acting agent, and longer-acting preparations such as oxymetazoline hydrochloride. In most cases, use of these compounds for more than a few days results in progressively severe nasal obstruction secondary to rebound swelling of the nasal mucosa that may be a self-perpetuating process (known as rhinitis medicamentosa). Thus these agents are not recommended for long-term use in allergic rhinitis. Sympathomimetic agents administered orally, such as pseudoepinephrine and phenylpropanolamine, may also reduce nasal congestion, although when used alone they may have significant central nervous system effects, often leading to insomnia and nervousness. A 4 per cent solution of cromolyn sodium (Nasalcrom and Opticrom) applied topically can also be beneficial in the treatment and prevention of allergic rhinitis and conjunctivitis if administered frequently. The effect of treatment with Nasalcrom in typical dosage of one spray per nostril four times per day may not be noted until 2 to 4 weeks after initiation of treatment. Thus, there may be an initial need for an antihistamine or decongestant before cromolyn's preventive effect becomes apparent. It is also marketed as a 4 per cent ophthalmic solution that may be employed in treating allergic conjunctivitis. A newer and considerably more potent cromolyn derivative (nedacromil sodium) is currently available in the United Kingdom and Europe but has not yet been approved for marketing in the United States.

Topical corticosteroids are widely used and highly successful in the symptomatic treatment and prevention of allergic rhinitis. These usually include the highly potent and rapidly metabolized

TABLE 246–2. H₁ ANTIHISTAMINE CLASSIFICATIONS

Class (Nonproprietary Name)	Trade Name	Adult	Child
Ethanolamines			
Diphenhydramine hydrochloride	Benadryl	25–50 mg, 3 or 4 times daily	5 mg/kg/day in 3 or 4 divided doses
Carbinoxamine maleate	Clisten	4 mg, 3 or 4 times daily	0.4 mg/kg/day in 3 or 4 divided doses
Ethylenediamine			
Tripelennamine	PBZ	25–50 mg, 3 or 4 times daily	5 mg/kg/day in 3 or 4 divided doses
Methapyrilene hydrochloride	Histadyl	25–50 mg, 4 or 5 times daily	5 mg/kg/day in 3 or 4 divided doses
Alkylamines			
Chlorpheniramine maleate	Chlor-Trimeton, Teldrin, CTM (delayed action), Cosea, Histadur, Rhinihist	4 mg, 3 or 4 times daily; 12 mg, 2 times daily	0.4 mg/kg/day in 3 or 4 divided doses
Brompheniramine maleate	Dimetane; Dimetane (delayed action) Extentabs	4 mg, 3 or 4 times daily; 12 mg, 2 times daily	0.4 mg/kg/day in 3 or 4 divided doses
Piperazines			
Hydroxyzine	Atarax, Vistaril	25–100 mg, 3 or 4 times daily	2 mg/kg/day in 4 divided doses
Phenothiazines			
Promethazine hydrochloride	Phenergan	12.5–25 mg, 2 or 3 times daily	1 mg/kg/day divided into half dose at bedtime and quarter dose every 6 hours in daytime
Trimeprazine tartrate	Temaril	2.5 mg, 4 times daily	2.5 mg in 3 divided doses (3 year olds only); 1.5 mg in 3 divided doses (6 mo to 3 yr)
Miscellaneous			
Terfenadine	Seldane	60 mg, 2 times daily	No recommendation
Astemizole	Hismanil	10 mg, 1 time daily	No recommendation
Cyproheptadine hydrochloride	Periactin	4 mg, 3 or 4 times daily	0.25 mg/kg/day in 3 or 4 divided doses
Azatadine maleate	Optimine	1–2 mg, 2 times daily	No recommendation
Clemastine fumarate	Tavist	2.68 mg, 2 times daily	No recommendation

corticosteroids such as beclomethasone dipropionate (Vancenase and Beconase), flunisolide acetate (Nasilide), budesonide, triamcinolone acetonide, and fluocortin butyl. These agents act primarily topically. Their relatively few side effects may include local burning, irritation, and occasional epistaxis or mild nasopharyngeal candidiasis. Although of substantial value in treating seasonal allergic rhinitis, these may not work well with acute, severe cases associated with considerable nasal mucosal edema and obstruction. They also do not relieve ocular symptoms. If used intermittently on a regular basis, they can help in perennial allergic rhinitis and vasomotor rhinitis. In addition, they may be of some help in weaning patients from excessive use of vasoconstrictor nasal sprays.

Each puff of beclomethasone dipropionate from a nasal inhaler is equal to approximately 42 μg of beclomethasone dipropionate, USP. Seasonal treatment on a daily basis with 400 μg per day is recommended and is considered to be quite harmless. Thus one puff per nostril four times per day from the nasal inhaler would be a typical dosage. In all cases, clinical improvement is usually apparent within several days, but symptomatic relief may not occur in some patients for as long as 2 weeks. There is substantial evidence that no systemic steroid effects occur in adults who use up to 800 μg daily (approximately 16 inhalations). In addition, cushingoid changes probably do not occur until the very large dose of approximately 1 mg* (20 inhalations or more) is reached. When the drug is used, it should be remembered that, in regard to therapeutic potency, eight inhalations is roughly equivalent to 7.5 mg of oral prednisone. These drugs should be used with caution in the presence of viral and fungal nasal diseases such as ocular herpes or related diseases in which there appears to be an associated defect in cell-mediated immunity.

Inhalant Allergen Immunotherapy (Desensitization or Hyposensitization). With this form of therapy, one attempts to alter the immunologic reactivity of an allergic individual so that there is less response upon natural re-exposure to the offending allergen. The clinical decision to use immunotherapy in the patient with allergic rhinitis depends on several factors: (1) the existence of clinically important rhinitis should be confirmed; (2) maximal environmental control procedures should be utilized; and (3) the

response to medication should be well defined. Immunotherapy is usually employed in patients who have substantial allergic components to their illness and who are attaining satisfactory clinical improvement with environmental control and symptomatic treatment. The technique involves injecting increasing amounts of allergen subcutaneously, usually at weekly intervals, starting with a very low dose and gradually increasing (usually a double dose) at each subsequent injection. A satisfactory response to immunotherapy requires achieving an adequate dose with treatment. This can best be achieved using high-quality, well-characterized extracts. The Food and Drug Administration has adopted modern methods of immunologic standardization of allergenic extracts which are significantly improving their quality. After incremental increases in the amount of injected allergen, a maintenance dose is achieved, which is injected at intervals of 2 to 6 weeks, depending upon individual patient activity and requirements. One should always carefully monitor for the development of untoward reactions. In most cases a decrease in nasal symptoms following immunotherapy is obvious during the first 6 months to 1 year and is maximal by 3 years of therapy. Results of a typical controlled clinical study are illustrated in Figure 246–4, which illustrates significant improvement in clinical symptom scores as measured by patient diaries in two groups of patients with ragweed-induced allergic rhinitis who underwent maintenance immunotherapy with aqueous extracts of ragweed prepared by two different methods. There are no universally accepted guidelines for the duration of therapy, and many physicians attempt trials of discontinuation after approximately 4 years of a successful program.

Symptomatic improvement with immunotherapy has been clearly shown in hay fever due to ragweed, grass, mountain cedar pollen, birch pollen, and *Alternaria* sp., and in asthma due to house dust mite, ragweed pollen, grass pollen, and cat dander. Beneficial results depend on a sufficiently high dose of antigen; relapse may occur once continuing maintenance injections are abandoned. Results are specific for particular antigens employed. A variety of immunologic changes have been demonstrated following immunotherapy. Among these changes are a rise in serum IgG-blocking antibodies against the allergens employed; suppression in the usual seasonal rise in IgE antibodies which normally follows environmental seasonal exposure followed by a slow decline in the level of specific IgE antibodies during the

*Exceeds dosage recommended by manufacturer.

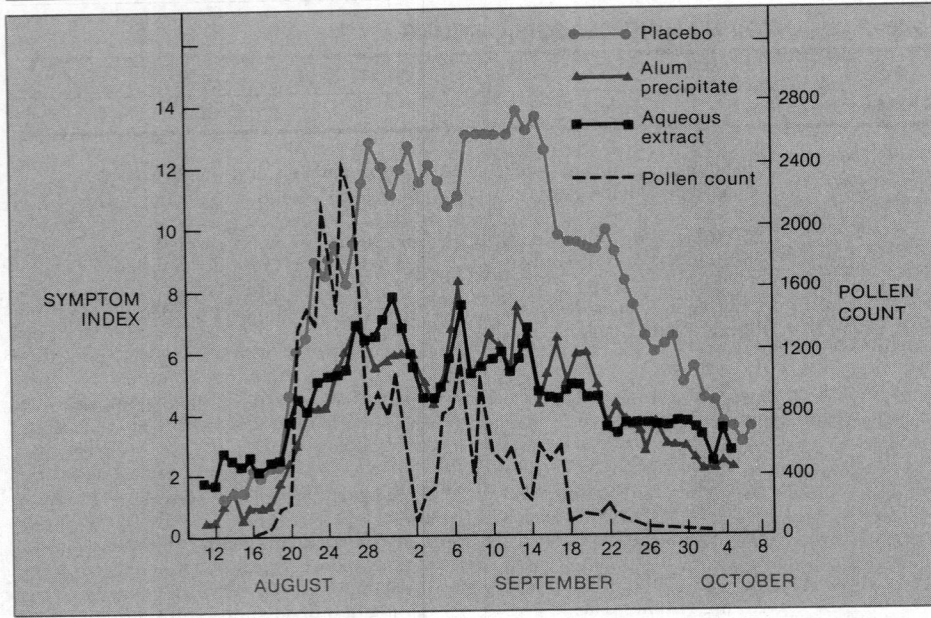

FIGURE 246–4. Daily average symptom scores in three groups of patients. (See text for explanation.) (Reprinted with permission from Norman PS: Trials of alum-precipitated pollen extracts in the treatment of hay fever. J Allergy Clin Immunol 50:31–44, 1972.)

ensuing several years of immunotherapy; increase of blocking IgA and IgG antibodies in secretions; reduced basophil reactivity and sensitivity to allergens; reduced in vitro lymphocyte responsiveness to allergens; and an increase in specific T-suppressor cells following immunotherapy. It is not known which are responsible for clinical improvement, but the serum titer of IgG "blocking" antibodies usually significantly correlates with clinical improvement. In addition, as immunotherapy progresses, the IgG antibodies become largely those of the IgG4 subclass, which are distinguished from antibodies of other IgG subclasses by their inability to cross-link antigen.

New experimental approaches to the therapy of allergic rhinitis include the use of altered antigens (such as allergoids and polymerized forms of antigen) that ultimately result in a heightened degree of immunization, with considerably less chance to trigger sensitized mast cells and produce local or systemic reactions. The use of other routes of antigen administration (e.g., intranasal and oral) has also been attempted, as have efforts to depress specific IgE antibody synthesis, with or without effects on suppressor T cells, by linking allergens to certain agents such as polyethylene glycol, with subsequent production of tolerance. Still other efforts are directed toward such novel ideas as inhibition of IgE receptors on mast cells, basophils, and other IgE receptor–bearing cells.

Therapy of Rhinitis Complications. In treatment of serous otitis media, appropriate medications to keep the nasal airway patent should be used, especially during airplane flights. When fluid and hearing loss persist despite medical treatment, a myringotomy with insertion of a tympanostomy tube usually restores hearing while treatment is continued.

Therapy of chronic sinusitis is based on duration and severity of disease. Since pneumococci, *Haemophilis influenzae*, and β-hemolytic streptococci are frequently offending agents, a broad-spectrum antibiotic such as amoxicillin trihydrate is recommended along with measures to keep the nasal airway patent. Failure to respond to several months of intense therapy may require surgical intervention.

Gershwin ME (ed.): Clinical Reviews in Allergy, Vol. 2, No. 3. New York, Elsevier Scientific Publishing Company, 1984. *A 250-page review of nasal physiology, acute and chronic rhinitis, clinical evaluation, rhinitis therapy, and diagnostic tests.*

Kaplan AP (ed.): Allergy. New York, Churchill Livingstone, 1985. *A comprehensive practical text stressing diagnosis and therapy of common allergic diseases. Diseases based on immediate hypersensitivity are stressed. Chapter on allergic and nonallergic rhinitis by K. P. Mathews is practical and well illustrated.*

Lichtenstein L, Fauci A: Current Therapy in Allergy, Immunology and Rheumatology. Toronto, B. C. Decker, Inc., 1985. *A concise text devoted entirely to the therapy and diagnosis of a wide range of immunologically mediated diseases. Three excellent sections are devoted to allergic rhinitis.*

Lockey RJ, Bukantz SC (eds.): Primer on allergic and immunologic diseases. JAMA 258(20):2581, 1987. *Contains an article by M. Kaliner, P. Eggleston, and K. Mathews on the essentials of respiratory atopic diseases in a setting of other articles that stress the clinical implications of immunology for the medical student and resident.*

Middleton E Jr, Reed CE, Ellis EF: Allergy: Principles and Practice, 3rd ed. St. Louis, C. V. Mosby Company, 1988. *A multiauthored, two-volume reference work, stressing immunologic, pharmacologic, and clinical aspects of the common allergic diseases. A series of pamphlets are sent at intervals to update readers on various chapters as new findings become available.*

Mygind M (ed.): Nasal Allergy. Oxford, Blackwell Scientific Publications, 1978. *A complete text devoted entirely to the structure, function, immunology, diagnosis, and therapy of rhinitis.*

Samter M (ed.): Immunological Diseases. Boston, Little Brown & Co, 1988. *A comprehensive text with in-depth sections on basic immunology, the nonatopic immunologic disorders, the atopic diseases, allergic reaction patterns of the skin, and diseases with prominant immunologic features. The chapter by P. Norman and L. Lichtenstein on allergic rhinitis is particularly thorough in discussing allergenic extract immunotherapy.*

247 Anaphylaxis

Allen P. Kaplan

The term *anaphylaxis* arose from the experiments of Richet and Portier in the early 1900's which showed that dogs who survived a large dose of sea anemone toxin would die within a few minutes after administration of a minute dose a few weeks later. The term meant the opposite of prophylaxis, i.e., a lack of protection rather than the expected immunity. Nevertheless, the reaction is indeed immune in nature and depends upon formation of IgE antibody, the immunoglobulin responsible for typical allergic reactions. The initial sensitization step induces formation of IgE specifically directed to the initiating substance. The IgE binds to high-affinity receptors on basophils and mast cells, and the subsequent combination of antigen with that IgE causes degranulation of basophils and mast cells (see Fig. 246–1). The secretory products of these cells are responsible for the symptoms of allergic reactions (Fig. 247–1). In anaphylaxis, the reaction is systemic in nature, occurs rapidly upon administration of minute concentrations of the offending material, and is potentially fatal. The route of administration of allergen can dictate the manifestations and magnitude of the ensuing allergic reaction; although all routes can lead to anaphylaxis, parenteral administration is more likely than inhaled or ingested allergens to cause elevated circulating levels of unaltered allergen and a systemic reaction. Thus, parenteral administration of medication and insect sting reactions (injected into cutaneous vessels) are among the most common causes of anaphylaxis. Anaphylactoid reactions are de-

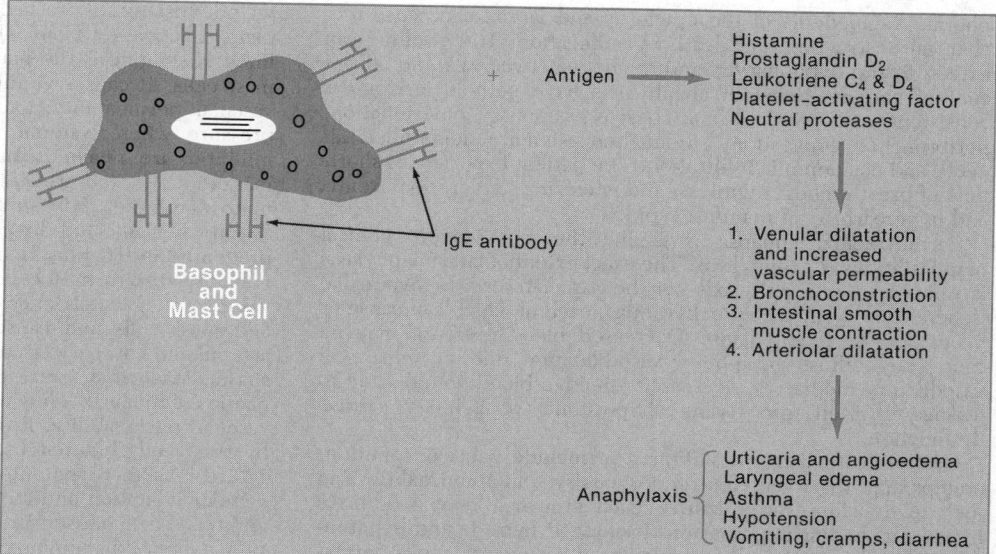

FIGURE 247–1. Acute anaphylaxis.

fined as systemic reactions that have the same symptoms as anaphylaxis but are not due to an IgE-dependent mechanism and are usually not immune. Examples include reactions to radiographic contrast agents and nonsteroidal anti-inflammatory drugs (e.g., acetylsalicylic acid, indomethacin, ibuprofen).

EPIDEMIOLOGY AND ETIOLOGY. The occurrence of anaphylaxis in the early 1900's was largely due to the use of serum from animals immunized with various toxins or bacteria to treat human illness. Between 1895 and 1923, of 41 reported cases of lethal anaphylaxis, 38 were due to serum therapy. Most were due to diphtheria antitoxin injection, and others were due to administration of tetanus antitoxin or antisera to gram-positive bacteria. In the antibiotic era, antibiotics in general and penicillin and sulfa drugs in particular have become the leading causes of fatal anaphylaxis. In recent years, there have been between 100 and 500 deaths per year in the United States due to the administration of penicillin. As new medications and chemicals are produced in a modern society, an ever-expanding number of substances are found capable of causing anaphylaxis. The insect order Hymenoptera is responsible for about 40 deaths each year and is estimated to cause one significant reaction per 10,000 individuals per year, with a mortality of 0.2 per million in the United States. Estimates of penicillin-induced anaphylaxis are 10 to 40 per 100,000 injections.

Although a history of atopy (allergic rhinitis, extrinsic asthma, atopic dermatitis) might be expected to be associated with an increased likelihood of anaphylactic reactions or reactions to antibiotics or insect stings in general, it appears that atopic individuals have, at worst, only a slightly greater risk than nonatopics. Thus, anyone can manifest an IgE response, with clinical symptoms, to the agents responsible for anaphylaxis. There is also no evidence that race, sex, age, occupation, or season intrinsically predisposes an individual to anaphylaxis.

Proteins, polysaccharides, and haptens are capable of eliciting systemic reactions in man (Table 247–1). Proteins are the largest and most diverse group and include antiserum, hormones, seminal plasma, enzymes, Hymenoptera venom (e.g., phospholipase A_2), pollen allergens administered for immunotherapy ("allergy shots"), and foods such as shellfish, eggs, nuts, and wheat products. Polysaccharides such as dextrans are rarer causes. The most common etiologic agents are drugs, low molecular weight substances that are not antigenic themselves but act as haptens and become antigenic upon reaction with host proteins. These include antibiotics, local anesthetics, vitamins, and diagnostic reagents. Although the most common anaphylactic reactions are due to parenteral administration, food-induced anaphylaxis and anaphylactic reactions to an orally administered drug can occur in very sensitive individuals.

CLINICAL MANIFESTATIONS. IgE-mediated reactions can cause symptoms that include the cutaneous, respiratory, cardio-

vascular, gastrointestinal, and hematologic systems (Fig. 247–1). In anaphylaxis, there may be manifestations involving multiple organ systems. The onset and manifestations vary depending on route of administration, dose, the release of and sensitivity to vasoactive substances, and differing sensitivities of the responsive organs. These parameters can vary from person to person, and individuals tend to react in a characteristic pattern. The initial manifestations can begin in seconds or take as long as an hour to develop; in severe reactions the onset is usually within 5 to 10 minutes. Initial manifestations often include skin erythema, pruritus, a generalized feeling of warmth and/or impending doom, light-headedness, shortness of breath, nausea, vomiting, or a lump in the throat. Urticaria is the most common manifestation of anaphylaxis. The rash is generalized and intensely pruritic, and consists of well-circumscribed, erythematous, raised wheals with serpiginous borders and blanched centers. Angioedema may accompany urticaria and typically manifests as swelling of face, eyes, lips, tongue, pharynx, or extremities. The respiratory tract is commonly involved in fatal anaphylaxis. For example, in a study of deaths due to Hymenoptera stings, 70 per cent of victims had involvement of upper or lower airways. The early stages of upper airway edema consist of hoarseness, stridor, and/or dys-

TABLE 247–1. AGENTS CAUSING ANAPHYLAXIS

Type	Common	Rare
Proteins	Venoms (Hymenoptera)	Hormones (insulin, ACTH, vasopressin, parathormone)
	Pollens (ragweed, grass, etc.)	Enzymes (trypsin, penicillinase)
	Foods (eggs, seafood, nuts, grains, beans, cottonseed oil, chocolate)	Human proteins (serum proteins, seminal fluid)
	Horse and rabbit serum (antilymphocyte globulin)	
Haptens and other low molecular weight substances	Antibiotics (penicillins, sulfonamides, cephalosporins, tetracyclines, amphotericin B, nitrofurantoin, aminoglycosides)	Vitamins (thiamine, folic acid)
	Local anesthetics (lidocaine, procaine, etc.)	
Polysaccharides	Dextrans, iron-dextran	

phoria. Angioedema of the epiglottis and larynx can cause mechanical obstruction and death by suffocation. The swelling can extend to the hypopharynx and trachea. Between 25 and 50 per cent of patients dying of anaphylaxis have pathologic changes consistent with severe asthma. There is pulmonary hyperinflation, peribronchial congestion, submucosal edema, edema-filled alveoli, and eosinophilic infiltration. The patient experiences shortness of breath, chest tightness, and wheezing. Severe hypoxemia and hypercarbia can manifest rapidly.

Cardiovascular collapse is among the most severe clinical manifestations of anaphylaxis. The exact extent of fatal anaphylaxis is unknown, as anaphylaxis can be associated with myocardial ischemia and ventricular arrhythmias, each of which can cause or be caused by hypotension. Decreased blood pressure may be caused by diffuse peripheral vasodilatation due to release of vasodilatory mediators, decreased effective blood volume due to leakage of fluid into tissues, hypoxemia, or primary cardiac dysfunction.

Gastrointestinal manifestations can include nausea, vomiting, cramps, and diarrhea. Central nervous system abnormalities can include delirium and seizures, each of which may be due to hypoxemia and/or hypotension. Prolonged hypoxia and hypotension can, of course, lead to a variety of secondary, more permanent changes.

DIFFERENTIAL DIAGNOSIS. The diagnosis of systemic anaphylaxis may be obvious when there is a typical history of antecedent exposure to foreign antigenic material and a sequence of events consistent with the syndrome. Confirmation usually requires demonstration of IgE antibody to the substance by skin testing or by RAST (radioallergosorbent test). When the history is absent or when only a portion of the full syndrome is present, it may be difficult to exclude a vascular, cardiac, or neurologic disorder. Possibilities to be considered include acute myocardial infarction, pulmonary embolism, acute asthma, hereditary angioedema, cold urticaria, a seizure disorder, an anaphylactoid or idiosyncratic reaction, transfusion reaction, or a vasovagal reaction. Vasovagal reactions may occur after an injection (e.g., penicillin, xylocaine) and include symptoms such as pallor, sweating, bradycardia, nausea, and hypotension, which can be confused with anaphylaxis. There is absence of any cutaneous manifestations or evidence of respiratory difficulty, and the diagnosis hinges on the cause of the hypotension. In such instances, skin testing is negative. When positive, an elevated plasma histamine (from basophils or mast cells) or tryptase level (mast cell product) suggests anaphylaxis or anaphylactoid reactions that are mast cell–dependent. Hereditary angioedema is due to absence or dysfunction of C1 inhibitor and is associated with laryngeal edema, peripheral angioedema, and acute abdominal pain. It is typically an autosomal dominant disorder with a family history or prior history of typical episodes. Trauma and infections may precipitate attacks of swelling. Patients with cold urticaria may have systemic symptoms due to water immersion such as while swimming; diffuse urticaria, angioedema, and hypotension may ensue. Anaphylactoid reactions can occur by substances causing direct nonimmune release of mast cell products (opiates, tubocurare, dextrans, sulfobromophthalein), which can cause urticaria, angioedema, chest tightness, wheezing, and hypotension. Aspirin and other nonsteroidal agents can cause upper and lower airway obstruction, urticaria, and/or angioedema with no IgE involvement. These agents have in common the property of inhibition of prostaglandin synthetase (cyclo-oxygenase). IgG–anti-IgA immune complexes may cause anaphylaxis-like symptoms when IgA-deficient patients receive blood. Complement activation appears to have a major role in such instances. Finally, radiocontrast media reactions occur in about 1 per cent of studies that employ them. The mechanism is unknown but may relate to their osmolarity. Newer agents seem to markedly diminish the incidence.

PATHOGENESIS. Antigenic induction of IgE formation requires antigenic processing (see Ch. 242) by dendrite cells or macrophages, T-cell help, and switching of B lymphocytes from IgG synthesis to IgE synthesis. Interleukin 4 may be critical for the latter switch and functions as a T-cell helper factor for IgE formation. Subsequent combination of antigen with IgE bound to high-affinity receptors on mast cells and basophils causes

secretion of a variety of vasoactive substances that may be responsible for the symptoms of anaphylaxis (Fig. 247–1). These include histamine, prostaglandin D_2, leukotrienes C_4 and D_4, and platelet-activating factor (PAF) (1-0-alkyl-2-sn-3 phosphorylcholine). Histamine is the major secretory product of basophils and mast cells. It causes venular and arterial vasodilation, increases vascular permeability, and causes a decrease in diastolic blood pressure when systemic levels of approximately 2.5 ng per milliliter are reached. In studies of insect sting anaphylaxis, markedly elevated arterial levels were documented which lasted up to 90 minutes. Histamine has direct inotropic and chronotropic action when injected directly into cardiac muscle, effects that are prevented by H_1 plus H_2 receptor antagonists. Prostaglandin D_2 is synthesized by mast cells but not by basophils. It is a peripheral vasodilator. Leukotrienes C_4 and D_4 are produced by basophils and mast cells and cause profound constriction of peripheral arterial and coronary circulation and may have a role in bronchospasm, since they cause bronchoconstriction and decreased dynamic compliance. They also cause venular dilation and increase vascular permeability. PAF, like prostaglandin D_2, is synthesized by mast cells but not basophils. On a molar basis, it is about 1000 times more potent than histamine in its ability to cause venular dilatation and an increase in cutaneous vascular permeability. When infused into rabbits, it causes profound hypotension, increased pulmonary resistance, pulmonary hypertension, cardiac arrhythmias, and decreased lung compliance, all manifestations of anaphylaxis. It is also a potent chemotactic factor for eosinophils and may account for much of the eosinophilia seen when allergic reactions persist (see Ch. 246).

Bradykinin is a nine–amino acid peptide that may also contribute to the symptoms of anaphylaxis and is generated by cleavage of kininogen by enzymes known as kallikreins. Kinins are peripheral vasodilators, cause systemic hypotension, and constrict coronary vessels. Basophils and mast cells have a kallikrein-like enzyme; organs containing glands (lung, nasal mucosa) secrete a tissue kallikrein that digests low molecular weight kininogen to release bradykinin. Plasma kinin formation is associated with contact activation of Hageman factor, conversion of plasma prekallikrein to kallikrein, and digestion of high molecular weight (HMW) kininogen.

Anaphylaxis is associated with depletion of clotting factors V, VII, and fibrinogen, activation of complement, and depletion of HMW kininogen consistent with acute intravascular coagulation. Clotting defects such as a prolonged partial thromboplastin time are commonly seen. Activation or depletion of these proteins is likely caused by enzymes released from cells that include not only mast cells and basophils but also monocyte/macrophages, eosinophils, and platelets. The latter group of cells possess low-affinity receptors for IgE (CD23) which may mediate cell secretion upon contact with antigen. The participation of these cells in allergic reactions is an area of current investigation.

PREVENTION AND TREATMENT. Patients who have previously experienced anaphylactic episodes should wear a Medic-Alert bracelet and be instructed regarding the importance of relating details of their specific drug reactions before taking medications. The medical history and medical record must include not only the allergic history but a description of the associated symptoms. The physician must be aware of drugs containing cross-reacting antigens. For example, patients with allergy to sulfa-containing antibiotics should avoid other sulfa-containing substances such as chlorthiazide diuretics, furosemide, sulfonylureas, and dapsone.

There is a 15 per cent incidence of a reaction if a cephalosporin is substituted for penicillin because they share the presence of a β-lactam ring. Reactions with second- and third-generation cephalosporins may also occur, but aztreonam is an exception.

When the patient has a history of drug allergy or of taking a drug suspected of causing a reaction, it is appropriate to substitute another non–crossing-reacting therapeutic agent whenever possible. Penicillin causes more anaphylactic reactions than any other drug, yet the history of "allergy" is unreliable, since close to 80 per cent of patients with such a history have negative skin tests to the major determinant (penicillin polylysine) or a minor determinant mixture (penicillin, penicilloic acid, penicillioylamine) and can tolerate the drug with impunity. Anaphylaxis is highly associated with IgE antibody directed to these minor determinants. Thus, a negative skin test to the commercially available major determinant is insufficient testing to administer the drug given a positive history. The addition of testing for minor determinants with negative results renders anaphylaxis or even any allergic reaction rare indeed. The number of alternative antibiotics that can be used in place of penicillin is ever increasing, and avoidance, in the sensitive patient, is the best approach. Nevertheless, there are circumstances in which administration of penicillin or other agents to a known or suspected sensitive patient is necessary. In this circumstance, the patient can be desensitized by gradual administration of increasing concentration of the drug—first intradermally, then subcutaneously, and finally parenterally. Such a procedure should be carried out by experienced personnel in an intensive care unit setting in which anaphylactic reactions can be effectively treated.

When an anaphylactic reaction is encountered, epinephrine given early quickly reverses most manifestations. Administered at a 1:1000 dilution (0.01 ml per kilogram with a maximum dose of 0.5 ml subcutaneously repeated every 20 minutes as necessary), it is initial treatment once an adequate airway is in place. Further exposure to the inducing substance should be limited. When an anaphylactic reaction is initiated by an injection into the arm or leg, a tourniquet may be applied to limit antigen absorption. In the case of a honeybee sting, care should be taken to remove the stinger without compressing the venom sac. Upper airway obstruction must be differentiated from asthma, since laryngeal and epiglottic edema may require endotracheal intubation or emergency tracheostomy to provide an airway. Asthma can be treated with epinephrine, administration of an inhaled β_2 sympathomimetic, and/or intravenous aminophylline at a 6 mg per kilogram loading dose over 20 to 30 minutes, followed by 0.5 to 1 mg per kilogram per hour.

If any respiratory, vascular, or cardiac complications occur, an intravenous line should be placed promptly and a sample of arterial blood obtained for pH, P_{O_2}, and P_{CO_2} determinations. Supplemental oxygen should be given to reduce hypoxemia. Pulse, blood pressure, and respiratory rate are monitored, and an electrocardiogram is obtained. Hypovolemic shock requires rapid intravenous fluid administration. Additionally, 5 ml of a 1:10,000 solution of epinephrine repeated every 5 to 10 minutes can be given intravenously in severe shock. A vasopressor such as dopamine (2 to 20 µg per kilogram per minute) is indicated to manage hypotension unresponsive to volume expansion. This may increase cardiac output and improve blood flow to coronary, cerebral, renal, and mesenteric vascular beds. Higher doses of dopamine or norepinephrine yield significant α receptor stimulation, which may increase blood pressure but constrict distal vascular beds. In case of significant cardiac dysfunction, an arterial line and a Swan-Ganz catheter should be placed.

Administration of antihistamines at the onset of the acute episode may relieve pruritus, urticaria, and angioedema. Once an intravenous line is placed, 50 to 100 mg of diphenhydramine can be given slowly as a bolus. An H_2-receptor blocker may aid in the therapy of hypotension. Corticosteroids have no value during the acute episode, yet steroids are often also administered intravenously. It takes many hours before their first effect is seen. Thus, administration of steroids helps treat protracted asthma and late reactions that can ensue many hours after the initial episode appears controlled or even 1 to 2 days beyond the initial insult. Thus, observation for at least 24 hours after an anaphylactic event is important.

Dattwyler R, Kaplan AP, Austen KF: Human anaphylaxis. In Kaplan AP (ed.): Allergy. New York, Churchill Livingstone, 1985, pp 559–607. *A textbook review of etiology, pathogenesis, and therapy.*

Peters SP: Systemic anaphylaxis. In Lichtenstein LM, Fauci AS (eds.): Current Therapy in Allergy, Immunology, and Rheumatology, 1985–1986. Toronto, B. C. Decker, Inc., 1985, pp 75–80. *A detailed description of how to treat anaphylaxis.*

Smith PL, Sobotka AK, Blocker ER, et al.: Physiologic manifestations of human anaphylaxis. J Clin Invest 66:1072, 1980. *Physiologic and biochemical changes monitored in human anaphylaxis occurring during a trial of therapy for insect sting allergy. Includes comments and cautions regarding therapy.*

248 Insect Sting Allergy

Lawrence M. Lichtenstein

The stings of insects of the order Hymenoptera have long been recognized as a potential cause of severe, often life-threatening reactions in susceptible individuals. These reactions are unrelated to the toxic chemicals in the venoms, being due to allergic sensitization. Insect sting allergy has recently become the most intensely studied model of anaphylaxis in man, resulting in important advances that have had rapid clinical application.

EPIDEMIOLOGY. The incidence of immediate hypersensitivity to insect stings based on history is 3 per cent; more than 20 per cent of the population, however, has positive skin test reactions to insect venoms without having had a reaction. Other allergies do not seem to predispose to insect sting sensitivity. The frequency varies with exposure and is therefore greater in children and males as well as those inclined to outdoor activities or beekeeping. Systemic reactions to insect stings cause few fatalities, but the morbidity, fear, and change in life style caused by these reactions is significant. A larger number of people suffer prolonged and unusually severe local inflammatory reactions to insect stings, which are allergic in nature. As with other allergies, there appears to be an inherited predisposition, since multiple family members are often affected.

ETIOLOGY. The only insects possessing true stingers are those of the order Hymenoptera. There are two families of importance, the bees (honeybees, bumblebees) and the vespids (yellow jackets, hornets, wasps). The bees have barbed stingers that remain in the skin after a sting. Yellow jackets are the most common culprits, but honeybees are more commonly implicated in the western United States. Wasps are more common in the south central United States (especially Texas). Sensitivity develops to antigens in the insect venom, most of which have enzymatic activity. A major allergen in both insect families is phospholipase A, but they do not cross-react with one another.

PATHOGENESIS. The injection of foreign proteins commonly causes the production of specific antibodies of the IgE and IgG classes. Individuals may develop venom-specific IgE antibodies after any sting, this response sometimes persisting for less than 3 months and in other instances persisting for more than 25 years. Tissue mast cells and circulating basophils bind IgE antibody, thereby becoming sensitized so that a repeat encounter with the offending allergen triggers release of the mediators of anaphylaxis (see Ch. 57). The initiation and persistence of this sensitization are related to inheritable and other unknown determinants. Sensitization may occur at any time in life, even after many uneventful stings. The sensitizing sting itself causes no unusual reaction and is often so remote as to evade recollection.

Generalized mediator release from sensitized basophils and mast cells causes the many manifestations of anaphylaxis (see Table 252–2). Localization of symptoms to specific target tissues is not well understood. The pathology observed in fatal cases includes upper airway edema and obstruction, the visceral consequences of hypotension, or occasionally no discernible abnormality (see Ch. 247 for a discussion of anaphylaxis).

Large local reactions are IgE dependent; their prolonged timecourse is characteristic of the so-called late phase response to antigen which has recently been under intense investigation. These reactions involve a cascade of events beginning with mediator release from mast cells and culminating with local inflammation involving many cell types and numerous mechanisms. The potential roles of eosinophils, neutrophils, basophils, lymphocytes and lymphokines, complement, and mediators with prolonged release or activity are being elucidated.

The venom-specific IgG antibody response to a sting is usually short lived, lasting only a few months. Repeated stings (as in beekeepers) are associated with high titers of IgG antibodies, which protect against allergic reactions. Beekeepers who do not have anaphylactic reactions have high IgG titers, as do affected individuals immunized with venoms. Passive transfer of these IgG antibodies protects sensitive patients from a sting. These protective antibodies are thought to block the allergic reaction by competing with IgE for the allergenic venom proteins and have therefore been termed "blocking" antibodies.

CLINICAL MANIFESTATIONS. Allergic reactions to insect stings are either generalized (systemic) or large local reactions. *Systemic sting reactions* present the classic manifestations of anaphylaxis described in Ch. 247. The observed frequency of the most common symptoms in adult patients is presented in Table 248–1. The risk of a fatal outcome increases, as might be expected, with age and certain drugs, especially antagonists of β-adrenergic receptors. Fatal anaphylaxis may occur without a history of sting allergy.

The onset of systemic symptoms is rapid, within 2 to 3 minutes, and rarely occurs more than 30 minutes after a sting. Symptoms presenting hours later (except large local reactions) are not usually associated with immediate hypersensitivity or IgE antibodies. Unusual reactions such as vasculitis, nephropathies, encephalitis, and other neurologic manifestations have been reported, but no causal relationship has been established. Allergic respiratory symptoms may occur in beekeepers and their families owing to sensitization to the dust in the hives that contain bee body proteins. This sensitivity is unrelated to sting reactions.

Large local reactions are slow in onset and occur with or without concomitant early systemic reaction. The area of induration increases in size progressively for the first 24 to 48 hours and then resolves gradually over several days. These reactions may be so large as to immobilize an entire limb and are a significant cause of morbidity in sensitive individuals. Red streaks resembling lymphangitis may be observed and are often treated with antibiotics despite a lack of evidence for true cellulitis. Some individuals develop large local sting reactions in the absence of allergic sensitivity. These are exaggerated reactions to the toxic and inflammatory venom components and often occur in persons who report similar large swellings after mosquito or fly bites, or who have cutaneous sensitivity to many irritants.

NATURAL HISTORY. The natural history of insect sting allergy has been incompletely documented. The prevalance of venom sensitization in the general population was noted above. It is estimated that about 20 per cent of those at risk by virtue of positive skin tests (but with no history of a systemic reaction) will react on sting. There is considerable variability in the reaction to a sting among those who are clearly allergic as demonstrated by positive skin tests and a history of a previous reaction. In a small study 60 per cent of such adults had a systemic reaction when stung by the appropriate insect. In children, on the other hand, a repeat sting causes a reaction in only 8 per cent. The incidence in adolescents and young adults must lie between these extremes. This variability confounds the prediction of risk associated with sensitization.

Many patients and physicians believe that allergic sting reactions become progressively more severe with every sting. Although some patients progress from large local through mild systemic reactions to life-threatening anaphylaxis, most of those affected maintain a similar pattern of symptoms with every sting. Less than 10 per cent of those experiencing large local reactions subsequently have systemic reactions. Factors favoring a systemic reaction include multiple stings, or stings in close temporal proximity (only weeks apart).

Sensitization generally decreases or disappears in time. This is far more common in children than in adults. However, resensitization has been observed upon re-sting.

DIAGNOSIS. The acute presentation of anaphylaxis is easily diagnosed by the presence of classic symptoms and signs. The insect sting may be inapparent. Differential diagnosis is more

difficult in localized reactions such as acute chest pain and dyspnea or syncope without urticaria.

The diagnosis of insect sting allergy currently rests on a convincing history and positive skin tests. Demonstration in vitro of venom-specific IgE by the radioallergosorbent test (RAST) is less sensitive than skin tests but is equally accurate when positive.

Skin tests are performed intradermally with venoms diluted to concentrations in the range of 1 to 1000 ng per milliliter. Five venoms are used: honeybee (HB), yellow jacket (YJ), yellow hornet (YH), white-faced hornet (WH), and *Polistes* wasp (POL). Positive intradermal skin tests develop, within 20 minutes, a wheal greater than 5 mm in diameter with at least 20 mm of erythema. The degree of skin test sensitivity does not correlate with clinical sensitivity. Within a few months after a systemic sting reaction, skin tests are almost uniformly positive. Stings more remote in time are more commonly associated with an apparent loss of sensitivity (similar to the situation in penicillin-related anaphylaxis).

Honeybee venom sensitivity occurs independent of other venom allergies, but about 10 per cent of patients are sensitive to both bee and vespid venoms. The vespid venoms are highly cross-reactive, so that almost all vespid-sensitive patients have positive YJ, YH, and WH skin tests even though most have been stung only by YJs. Half of these patients are also sensitive to POL venom. Very few individuals are allergic to only one or two of the vespid venoms. In vitro RAST inhibition techniques are useful to distinguish cross-reactivity from specific sensitivity. This is clinically relevant in patients with a positive skin test to *Polistes*. This is usually due to cross-reactivity, and the patient may be spared considerable expense and unnecessary immunization by RAST inhibition analysis.

TREATMENT. The treatment of choice for anaphylactic reactions is subcutaneous epinephrine 1:1000, 0.5 ml initially and repeated twice at 10-minute intervals, if necessary, to reverse the progression of symptoms. Sublingual isoproterenol is probably ineffective. Antihistamines and glucocorticoids do not contribute to the management of life-threatening symptoms but may reduce the duration and severity of cutaneous manifestations. Their use should not be considered until the termination of the acute episode. Intravenous volume expansion or airway maintenance may be necessary. In a few individuals, the process is resistant to epinephrine; in such instances an α-adrenergic agent (i.e., norepinephrine) may be tried. Affected persons not yet protected by immunotherapy are advised to carry, and are instructed in the use of, a kit containing a syringe device preloaded with one or two recommended doses of epinephrine.

Venom immunotherapy is successful in virtually all patients. Less than 2 per cent of those immunized have any systemic symptoms after a challenge sting, and these are uniformly less severe than their previous reactions. The indications for venom immunotherapy are now based on an improved understanding of the natural history of the disease. Those with a history of life-threatening reactions should be treated. The risk of progression from strictly cutaneous to life-threatening respiratory or vascular reactions is uncertain in adults but is rare (<1 per cent) in children. Cutaneous reactors who are more likely to be stung in their daily activities or who for a variety of reasons (location, age, cardiovascular disease) can ill afford a more severe reaction should be treated. The cost and inconvenience of treatment may deter other cutaneous reactors from undergoing immunotherapy. Children, much more commonly than adults, have cutaneous symptoms only. These children may be left untreated. Venom immunotherapy is contraindicated in the absence of positive venom skin tests or RAST. Treatment is currently recommended using all venoms causing a positive skin test (for *Polistes*, see above). While other mechanisms may contribute, the induction of increased serum levels of venom-specific IgG antibodies is the most apparent mechanism of protection for venom immunotherapy; less than 3 μg per milliliter is associated with increased risk of sting anaphylaxis.

Rapid immunization in six to eight weekly visits is recommended, since it is associated with a significantly greater and more rapid immune response and with fewer adverse reactions than a slower (more than 20 weeks) regimen. The maintenance dose of 100 μg of each venom is repeated monthly for at least 6 months, and is then continued at 6- to 8-week intervals for 5 years. If treatment is interrupted for more than 3 months, it is

TABLE 248–1. SYMPTOMS REPORTED BY 245 PATIENTS

Symptom	Per Cent
Cutaneous only	14
Urticaria-angioedema	78
Dizziness-hypotension	61
Dyspnea-wheezing	53
Throat tightness-hoarseness	40
Loss of consciousness	33

likely that protection will diminish to inadequate levels. Loss of venom sensitivity during maintenance immunotherapy occurs in only 10 to 20 per cent of patients during 3 to 5 years of treatment. Skin tests should, therefore, be repeated every 2 years. After 5 years it appears that patients can stop therapy and suffer a sting without serious sequelae. Possible exceptions include patients in whom skin test sensitivity has not diminished in 5 years, those who have had systemic reactions during venom immunotherapy, and those with complicating medical conditions. After stopping venom immunotherapy, venom sensitivity continues to decline and is not increased even after stings.

Adverse reactions to venom immunotherapy may be early or late. Immediate reactions include all the manifestations of anaphylaxis. During the initial course of treatment, 10 to 15 per cent of patients report systemic complaints, only half of which require epinephrine. At maintenance doses, systemic reactions occur rarely. After a systemic reaction, the dose should be reduced by up to 50 per cent on the subsequent visit and then increased gradually toward 100 μg again.

Large local reactions occur frequently. Fifty per cent of treated patients experience at least one such reaction. These occur after 10 of every 100 injections in the induction phase, most commonly in the midrange of doses (10 to 50 μg) and much less often at maintenance doses. Large local reactions do not presage systemic reactions and require a reduction of dose only for the most severe reactions. Long-term side effects have not been observed with venom immunotherapy or in beekeepers stung frequently for over 30 years.

Golden DBK, Addison BI, Gadde J, et al.: Prospective observations on patients who discontinue Hymenoptera venom immunotherapy. J Allerg Clin Immunol 88:162, 1989. *Studies of when and how to discontinue venom immunotherapy.*
Golden DBK, Marsh DG, Kagey-Sobotka A, et al.: Epidemiology of insect sting allergy. JAMA 262:240, 1989. *A review of diagnostic and therapeutic problems in insect allergy.*
Hunt KJ, Valentine MD, Sobotka AK, et al.: A controlled trial of immunotherapy in insect hypersensitivity. N Engl J Med 299:157, 1978. *A comparison of venom immunotherapy with whole body extract and placebo. Demonstrates efficacy of venom therapy and the clinical consequences of challenge stings.*
Valentine MD, Golden DBK: Insect venom allergy. *In* Samter M (ed.): Immunological Diseases. 4th ed. Boston, Little, Brown & Company, 1988, pp 1173–1184. *A general review.*
Valentine MD, Schuberth KC, Kagey-Sobotka A, et al.: The value of immunotherapy with venom in children with allergy to insect stings. N Engl J Med 323:1601, 1990. *A prospective study of the epidemiology and immunotherapy of insect sting allergy in children, indicating that repeat reactions are rare and virtually never of increased severity.*

249 Immune Complex Diseases
Robert R. Rich

DEFINITION. The formation of immune complexes is an invariable consequence of the interaction of antigens with specific antibodies. The inflammatory response that ensues is an important element of normal host defenses, leading to complex clearance and antigen destruction by phagocytic cells. In contrast, immune complex diseases are reflections of excess complex formation or retarded clearance, usually under conditions of exceptional antigen challenge or immunologic dysregulation. Under such circumstances, complexes are deposited or formed at specific tissue sites; the inflammatory response then leads to localized or systemic tissue damage. Clinical manifestations of immune complex disease are protean, with the development of signs and symptoms appropriate to the particular organs involved. This may include virtually any organ, but for reasons described below, sites of predilection include the kidney, lung, skin, joints, and central nervous system. Although immune complex disease may accompany an extraordinary range of pathologic processes, in practice it is encountered most commonly in the course of infectious diseases, in autoimmunity, and as a consequence of therapy for some other primary process.

PATHOGENESIS. Understanding the pathogenesis of immune complex disease requires attention to each of its constituents, i.e., antigen, antibody, the factors that regulate immune complex deposition and clearance, and the inflammatory processes that ensue following their deposition.

Antigens Inducing Immune Complex Diseases. Antigens involved in the development of immune complex diseases can be broadly classified as endogenous, infectious, environmental, and iatrogenic. In many cases the specific antigen is unknown, although the general class can usually be identified. The most familiar example of endogenous immune complexes is the DNA–anti-DNA complexes important to the pathogenesis of systemic lupus erythematosus (SLE). Many other autoimmune diseases are also associated with immune complex formation, but the pathogenetic relevance of the complexes is not always clear. Among autoimmune diseases in which immune complexes are considered important mediators of the inflammatory process are rheumatoid arthritis, cryoglobulinemia, mixed connective tissue disease, polyarteritis nodosa, and other autoimmune vasculitides. Other important sources of endogenous antigens include malignancies in which immune complex formation may contribute to the development of paraneoplastic syndromes.

Infections with organisms of many types, particularly chronic infections, are associated with the development of immune complex disease. Examples among bacterial infections include glomerulonephritis following infection with nephritogenic strains of streptococci, disseminated gonococcal infection, lepromatous leprosy, subacute bacterial endocarditis, allergic bronchopulmonary aspergillosis, secondary syphilis, and chronic *Pseudomonas* infection in patients with cystic fibrosis. Viral diseases in which immune complex deposition may be a prominent feature include hepatitis B infection, dengue, infectious mononucleosis, and subacute sclerosing panencephalitis. Immune complex–mediated disease is also a prominent feature of many parasitic infestations. Particularly noteworthy is the nephrotic syndrome in children with quartan malaria; others include toxoplasmosis, trypanosomiasis, and schistosomiasis.

Extrinsic allergic alveolitis (hypersensitivity pneumonitis) is a frequently encountered immune complex disease associated with exposure to exogenous antigens in the environment. This is usually associated with extraordinary exposure to a particular antigen that is characteristic of certain occupations or hobbies, e.g., the antigens of thermophilic actinomycetes responsible for farmer's lung and bagassosis, and the exposure to avian proteins in patients with pigeon fancier's disease.

A special class of exogenous antigens comprises those encountered as a consequence of medical practice. This includes the prototype of the immune complex diseases, serum sickness, which follows deposition of immune complexes of heterologous serum constituents with autologous antibodies. Serum sickness was regularly seen during the pre-antibiotic decades of the twentieth century when infectious diseases were frequently treated with heterologous antisera. With antibiotic availability, classic serum sickness has been uncommonly encountered. However, as mouse monoclonal antibodies are introduced for treatment of immunologic reactions such as organ transplant rejection, the re-emergence of serum sickness may be anticipated. An iatrogenic disease essentially indistinguishable from classic serum sickness did emerge as a consequence of high-dose antibiotic therapy. The serum sickness–like manifestations of immune responses to drugs reflect the fact that certain drugs, particularly the β-lactam antibiotics and sulfonamides, are effective haptens that are capable of inducing antibody responses upon spontaneous conjugation to autologous proteins. Reactions to tissue allografts following bone marrow or solid organ transplantation are another instance of contemporary practice that may be associated with pathologic immune complex deposition. In the case of solid organ transplants, deposition of complexes within the vasculature of the transplanted organ may contribute importantly to graft rejection.

Factors Affecting Immune Complex Formation and Deposition. Features of both antigen and antibody determine the likelihood of pathologic immune complex formation and deposition. Chief among these are the absolute concentrations of the reactants and their relative molar ration. Most antigens are multivalent for a polyclonal antibody response; antibody molecules are at least bivalent. This theoretically allows for the formation of an extensive antigen-antibody lattice, the size of which is determined largely by the affinity of the antibodies and the molar ration of antigen

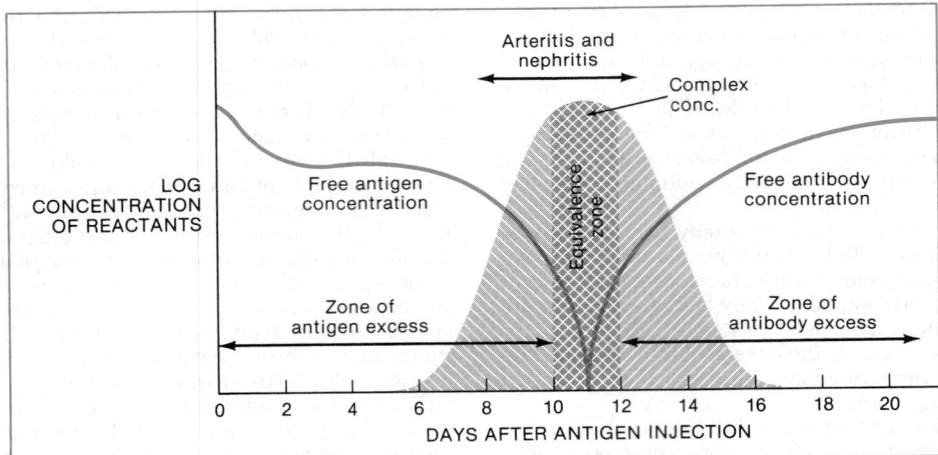

FIGURE 249–1. Development of experimental serum sickness following injection of rabbits with radiolabeled xenogeneic serum. Antibody formation begins after a lag of approximately 5 days. Signs of pathogenic immune complex deposition appear at approximately 8 days and gradually subside with the appearance in the serum of free antibody after the zone of equivalence is passed. Pathogenic complexes are of intermediate size, with a buoyant density of ≥ 19S.

to antibody. As illustrated for an experimental model of serum sickness in Figure 249–1, antibody responses begin under conditions in which antigen is present in excess relative to antibody. After a lag of several days, complexes formed initially are small and exhibit little or no pathogenic activity. In contrast, very large complexes are formed as the amount of antigen becomes limiting late in the course of an antibody response under conditions of antibody excess. Because these large complexes are readily cleared by the reticuloendothelial system, they are also relatively nonpathogenic. Immune complex diseases are usually manifest during conditions of slight antigen excess or near the point of equivalence, where lattice formation is maximal and little if any noncomplexed antigen or antibody is detected in the serum. An additional feature of lattice formation important to rapid precipitation of complexes is interaction between Fc portions of antibody molecules (Fig. 249–2) (see Ch. 242). For example, although the valence of $F(ab')_2$ antibodies does not differ from that of whole immunoglobulins, $F(ab')_2$ antibodies form precipitates more slowly. As noted below, such Fc-Fc interactions are important in complement-mediated regulation of immune complex deposition. Antigen charge also plays a role in determining sites of tissue localization; complexes with a substantial positive charge are preferentially attracted to the strong negative charge of basement membranes, particularly in the renal glomerulus.

Localized presence of antigen may largely account for organ-specific immune complex deposition. Diseases such as Goodpasture's syndrome and myasthenia gravis are generally not classified as immune complex diseases because the complexes are formed in situ rather than being preformed in the circulation and then deposited. Nevertheless, the inflammatory process at the site of antigen-specific antibody deposition is essentially the same as that seen following deposition of preformed complexes. Lupus nephritis is an interesting special case in which the disease develops as a consequence of glomerular deposition of DNA–anti-DNA complexes. It has been demonstrated in experimental animals, however, that single-stranded DNA binds avidly to the glomerular basement membrane, presumably attracted by its cationic nature. Thus, DNA–anti-DNA complexes may be formed at the glomerular basement membrane in addition to the localization of preformed complexes at that site.

Features of blood flow and vascular structure are also important in determining the localization of immune complexes. Chief among these is capillary permeability. Because the capillary endothelium is fenestrated in renal glomeruli, pulmonary alveoli, synovia, the choroid plexus of the brain, and the uveal tract of the eye, complexes preferentially deposit in these sites. Hemodynamic variables enhancing immune complex localization include turbulence of flow and increased blood pressure; both of these conditions promote complex deposition in glomeruli and at artery bifurcations.

Immune Complex–mediated Inflammation. Capillary permeability is markedly increased by the action of vasoactive amines such as histamine and platelet-activating factor, which are elaborated at the site of a nascent inflammatory lesion. Consequently, mast cells, basophils, and platelets are important in the initiation of immune complex–mediated inflammatory responses. Mast cell and basophil degranulation may reflect the effects of IgE antibodies specific for the inducing antigen bound to specific Fcε receptors on their surfaces, as well as the elaboration of the anaphylatoxin components of complement, C3a and C5a, as a consequence of complement activation (Ch. 243). Studies in experimental animals have shown that the deposition of circulating immune complexes is promoted by administration of agents

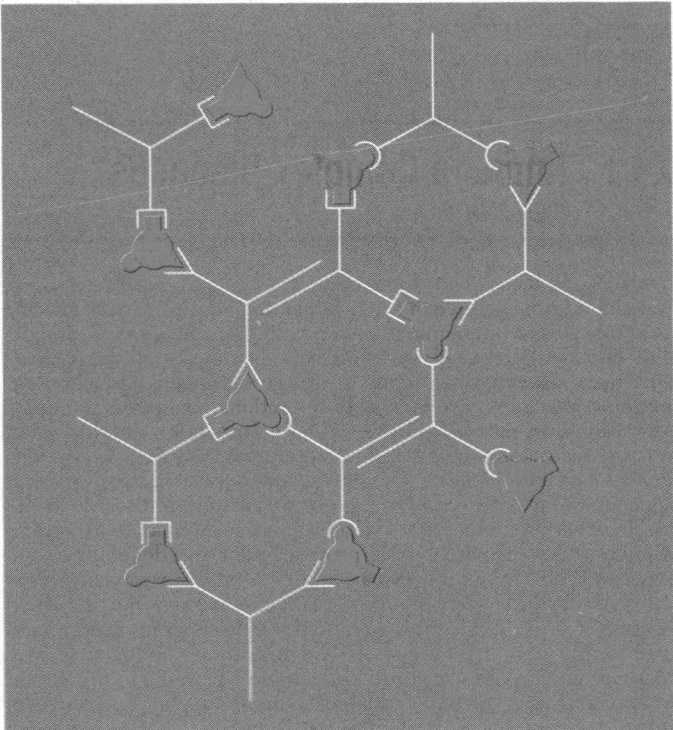

FIGURE 249–2. Immune complex lattice formation near the equivalence point. Neither free antigen nor free antibody is detected. Note that the lattice is formed by noncovalent bonds between antigen and antibody and between Fc portions of adjacent antibody molecules.

that induce mast cell degranulation and is ameliorated by pretreatment with antihistamines. Vascular permeability is also promoted by aggregation of platelets at sites of an inflammatory lesion, with the release of platelet-activating factor and the formation of microthrombi.

The primary cellular effectors of immune complex–mediated inflammation are polymorphonuclear leukocytes in the case of acute immune complex deposition and monocytes and macrophages at sites of chronic deposition. Neutrophils accumulate at the site of immune complex deposition as a consequence of complement activation and production of the chemotactic factor C5a. Their activation and degranulation are promoted by surface binding of complexes to C3b and Fcγ receptors. Tissue damage results from the release of hydrolytic lysosomal enzymes and the formation of toxic oxidants such as superoxide anion (O_2^-) and H_2O_2. Experimental studies of acute immune complex–mediated injury have demonstrated the importance of complement and neutrophils in this process; agents such as cobra venom factor or antineutrophil serum prevent accumulation of neutrophils at the site of complex deposition and consequently prevent injury. Tissue injury at sites of chronic immune complex deposition, for example, in chronic membranous glomerulonephritis and hypersensitivity pneumonitis, is due predominantly to the inflammatory activity of monocytes and macrophages. In experimental models of chronic immune complex deposition, evolution of inflammatory lesions may be inhibited by antimacrophage serum but not by depletion of neutrophils. Mechanisms of monocyte/macrophage-mediated tissue injury are probably similar to those of neutrophils, predominantly the release of hydrolytic enzymes and tissue-reactive oxidants. However, the details of macrophage-mediated inflammation have not been as thoroughly demonstrated experimentally.

Complement and Complement Receptors as Regulators of Immune Complex Deposition. The importance of complement in antibody-mediated inflammation has been appreciated for many years. Consequently, the observation that immune complex diseases, particularly systemic lupus erythematosus, are a prominent feature of genetic deficiencies of complement components presented a difficult paradox. This paradox has been resolved with the more recent realization that complement components can also inhibit immune complex deposition and resolubilize them from sites of deposition. In addition, it is now known that erythrocyte receptors for C3b are important for reticuloendothelial clearance of circulating immune complexes. Analysis of the clinical pattern of immune complex disease in patients with complement deficiencies provides clues to the role of these components in normal prevention of complex deposition. The incidence of immune complex disease in patients with deficiencies of C1q, C1r, C1s, C4, C2, and C3 varies from 60 to 90 per cent, with the majority of these patients exhibiting a lupus-like syndrome. On the other hand, immune complex disease is only occasionally associated with deficiencies of late-acting or alternative pathway components.

The CR1 complement receptors are particularly important to clearance of circulating complexes. Because approximately 90 per cent of blood CR1 molecules are represented on the surfaces of red blood cells, these cells function as efficient scavengers of C3b-containing immune complexes. Studies in baboons revealed that C3b-coated complexes are cleared from erythrocyte surfaces by transfer to the fixed phagocytic cells of the reticuloendothelial system within the liver. Patients with defects in CR1 might be predicted to have deficient complex clearance and an increased predisposition to immune complex disease, a prediction consistent with clinical observations. In patients with SLE but without deficiencies of complement constituents, a significant reduction in the number of erythrocyte CR1 receptors for C3b is frequently observed. The frequent observation of IgA-containing immune complexes and the distinct syndrome of an IgA nephropathy may, at least in part, represent a corollary of these observations. Because IgA does not fix complement via the classic pathway, IgA complexes are less efficiently cleared and are thus more likely to be deposited in capillary beds such as renal glomeruli. At least 60 per cent of patients with focal glomerulonephritis and hematuria following an infectious episode exhibit circulating IgA complexes and complex deposition typical of IgA nephropathy. Whether this represents poor clearance of such complexes, a predisposing defect in IgA regulation, or both requires additional study.

The binding of complement components to immune complexes (Fig. 249–3) prevents the formation of large antigen-antibody lattices and inhibits immune precipitation. This process requires activation via the classic pathway; serum that is deficient in C1q, C4, or C2 does not effectively inhibit lattice formation and complex precipitation. Classic pathway dependence may reflect the initial binding of C1 components, impeding the Fc-Fc interactions between IgG molecules that contribute to immune precipitation. This is followed by covalent bonding of C3b to the complexes, which further inhibits immune precipitation and leads to solubilization of previously deposited complexes. The solubilization process also depends upon activation of components of the alternative pathway, including properdin. Consequently, by promoting clearance of immune complexes and inhibiting their deposition at sites of inflammation, complement components and their receptors should be seen not only as important mediators of immune complex diseases but also as negative regulators that may retard disease development.

EVALUATION OF PATIENTS WITH IMMUNE COMPLEX DISEASES. Because the development of an immune complex disease often represents a secondary immunologic consequence of some other primary process, evaluation of patients with symp-

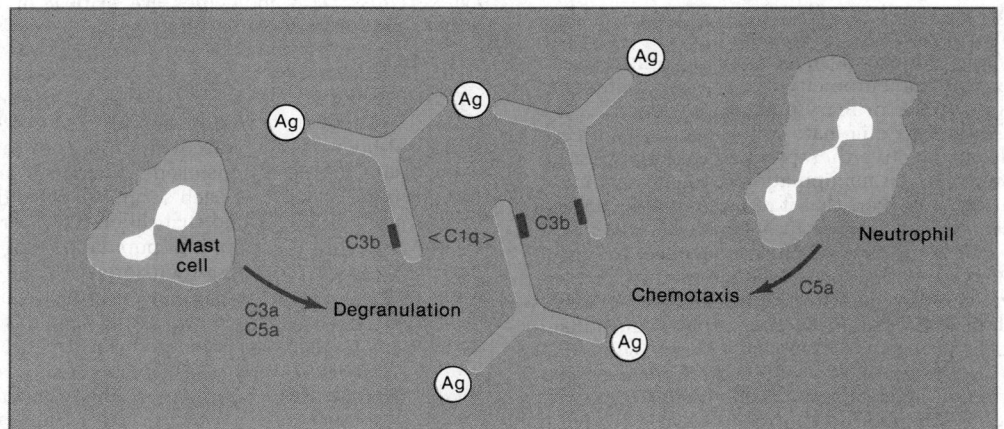

FIGURE 249–3. Positive and negative regulation of immune complex–mediated inflammation by complement components. The anaphylatoxins C3a and C5a, along with antigen binding by surface IgE molecules, promote degranulation of mast cells and basophils and the release of vasoactive amines. C5a also acts as a chemotactic factor attracting polymorphonuclear leukocytes to the site of immune complex deposition. C1q fixation inhibits Fc-Fc interactions between IgG molecules, thereby retarding complex precipitation. Complex formation is inhibited and deposited complexes are solubilized by the covalent attachment of C3b to antibody-antigen complexes; complex solubilization also requires activation of the alternate complement pathway.

toms of immune complex deposition begins with a thorough evaluation of possible sources for high-level antigen exposure. In many instances, such as immune complex disease during a course of antibiotic therapy or as a consequence of chronic infection, the antigen source is obvious. In others, such as hypersensitivity pneumonitis or occasionally in patients with malignancy, an extensive evaluation is required. In cases involving an autoimmune process, the diagnostic process may require extensive serologic investigation. The search for specific antigen within immune complexes is not usually productive. A notable exception is the identification of HBsAg in circulating immune complexes of patients with polyarteritis nodosa, in whom the search provides important insight into the pathogenetic process. More often the actual structure of the antigen is unknown even when its source is identified. A major difficulty is that specific antigen may represent a minor component, particularly with maturation of the antibody response and the development of complexes that form on the basis of immunoglobulin–anti-immunoglobulin interactions.

Many techniques are available for nonspecific detection of immune complexes. The most useful clinically is biopsy with fluorescent or electron microscopic analysis for deposition of various immunoglobulin classes and complement components at the site of a suspected immune complex–mediated inflammatory lesion. Results of such biopsies must be interpreted with caution because complexes may be present at sites not apparently involved in acute inflammation, for example, in apparently normal skin of patients with SLE. Conversely, complexes may have been removed from the site of an ongoing inflammatory process, particularly during its chronic phase. Thus, renal biopsies in acute glomerulonephritis are more likely to reveal immune complex deposition than are biopsies in chronic disease.

Many laboratory methods have been developed for detection of circulating immune complexes based on their physical, chemical, or biologic properties. Among others these include ultracentrifugation, nephelometry, C1q binding, and binding to C3b receptors on a human B-cell line. In all cases, interpretation of the results requires careful attention to conditions of specimen collection and laboratory controls, including appropriate positive and negative standards. Despite the feasibility of quantifying circulating immune complexes, however, the usefulness of such tests has been widely questioned. When appropriately performed, they are often indicative of an ongoing inflammatory process. Nevertheless, a finding of circulating immune complexes is very nonspecific and hence of limited diagnostic usefulness. In addition, the absolute levels do not correlate with disease activity with sufficient predictability to make single determinations helpful in predicting and assessing severity or prognosis. Although serial determinations during the course of disease may correlate roughly with waxing and waning of the inflammatory process, it is only in the unusual patient that such information is particularly helpful in management.

TREATMENT. The therapy of an immune complex disease depends upon its severity and chronicity, the site of inflammatory lesions, and the nature of the primary pathologic process. A first principle when feasible is to eliminate or reduce the source of antigen, for example by effective therapy of an underlying infection, change in an antibiotic, or manipulation of the environment. It should be recognized, however, that if reduction of the antigen load alters the molar ratio of antigen to antibody in complexes, shifting the balance from antigen excess to equivalence, the result may be temporary exacerbation of the inflammatory process. Available alternatives for treatment of the inflammatory process are familiar, including antihistamines, nonsteroidal anti-inflammatory agents, corticosteroids, and cytotoxic agents. When long-term therapy with corticosteroids is anticipated, management with alternate-day therapy is recommended if possible. Cytotoxic agents such as cyclophosphamide have proved to be effective in treatment of systemic vasculitides and severe SLE; a monthly intravenous bolus of cyclophosphamide may prove effective, with reduced toxicity compared to daily therapy. The newer immunosuppressive agents such as cyclosporine are being evaluated for efficacy with chronic immune complex disease developing as a consequence of T-cell dysregulation. Finally, plasmapheresis can dramatically reduce high levels of circulating immune com-

plexes when acute intervention in the inflammatory process is indicated. Such treatment may prove life-saving in patients with severe autoimmune diseases.

Høiby N, Döring G, Schiøtz PO: The role of immune complexes in the pathogenesis of bacterial infections. Annu Rev Microbiol 40:29, 1986.
McDougal JS, McDuffie FC: Immune complexes in man: Detection and clinical significance. Adv Clin Chem 24:1, 1985.
Schifferli JA, Ng YC, Peters DK: The role of complement and its receptor in the elimination of immune complexes. N Engl J Med 315:488, 1986.
Theofilopoulos AN, Dixon FJ: The biology and detection of immune complexes. Adv Immunol 28:89, 1979.
Walport MJ, Lachmann PJ: Erythrocyte complement receptor type I, immune complexes, and rheumatic diseases. Arthritis Rheum 31:153, 1988.
Wilson JG, Fearon DT: Altered expression of complement receptors as a pathogenetic factor in systemic lupus erythematosus. Arthritis Rheum 27:1321, 1984.

250 The Major Histocompatibility Complex and Disease Susceptibility

Benjamin D. Schwartz

The proper functioning of the immune system depends on its ability to distinguish "self" from "nonself." This crucial distinction is achieved via the molecules determined by the major histocompatibility complex, or HLA complex as it is known in humans. It now appears that both foreign and self antigens are recognized by the T lymphocytes of the immune system only in conjunction with HLA molecules. During embryogenesis, a process of T-cell "education" takes place in the thymus whereby T cells recognizing self antigens (in the context of HLA molecules) are normally eliminated and T cells potentially recognizing foreign antigens in the context of self HLA molecules are selected.

For a protein antigen to be recognized by the T lymphocytes of the immune system, it must undergo "processing." During processing, the protein is partially degraded into peptides, some of which are bound by HLA molecules. The peptide and HLA molecule form a complex that is the ligand recognized by the receptor on the T lymphocyte. There appear to be two processing pathways used by the immune system. Intracellular antigens, such as viruses, are processed through the endogenous pathway and are presented by HLA class I molecules to CD8+ (generally cytotoxic) T lymphocytes. In contrast, extracellular antigens are processed through the exogenous pathway and are presented by HLA class II molecules to CD4+ (generally helper) T lymphocytes. Thus, HLA molecules are critical in the recognition of antigen by the immune system.

HISTORY

The existence of a human major histocompatibility complex (MHC) was first suggested in the mid 1950's when leukoagglutinating antibodies were discovered in the sera of multiparous women and multiply transfused leukopenic patients. Analysis of these sera indicated that each serum reacts with the cells of some but not all individuals and that different sera react with the cells of different but overlapping populations of individuals. This pattern suggested that these antisera were detecting alloantigens (i.e., antigens that were present on the cells of some individuals of a given species) which were the products of a polymorphic genetic locus. It was discovered shortly thereafter that these human leukocyte antigens (HLA) had a major role in determining the success of organ transplants, and this finding spurred the initial study of these antigens. Over the ensuing years, the reaction patterns of literally thousands of anti-HLA alloantisera have been codified by computer and have made possible the delineation of the HLA system. In 1973, certain HLA antigens were found to be associated with specific diseases. In addition, at around the same time it was appreciated that the HLA complex regulates several aspects of the human immune response. These findings provided a second impetus for the study of the HLA

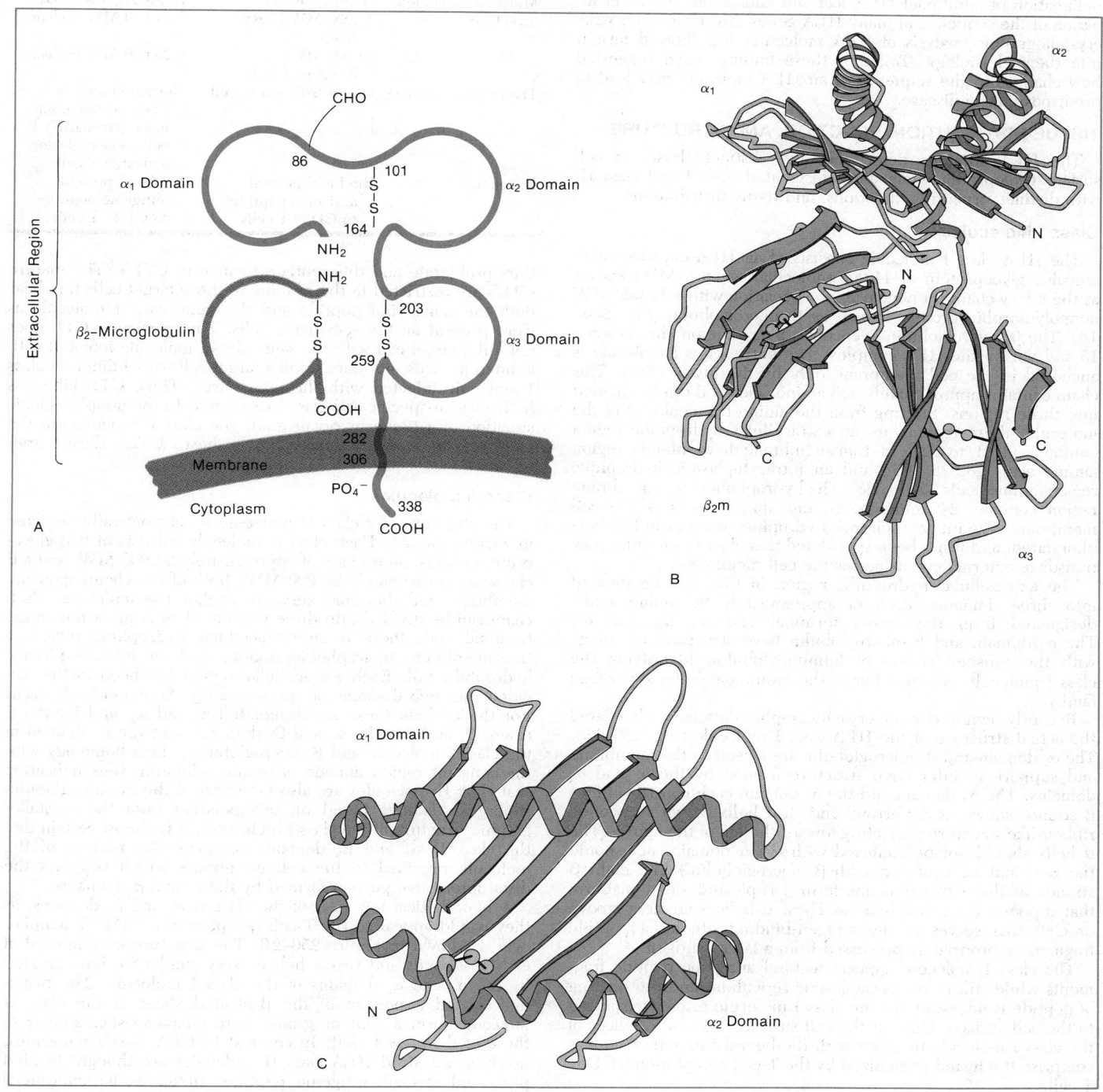

FIGURE 250–1. The HLA class I molecule. *A*, A schematic representation. The molecule consists of a heavy chain, which anchors the molecule in the membrane, noncovalently associated with β$_2$-microglobulin. Numbers indicate amino acid residues where certain features are found. NH$_2$ = amino terminus; COOH = carboxy terminus; CHO = carbohydrate; PO$_4^-$ = phosphate. α$_1$, α$_2$, and α$_3$ are the three extracellular domains. *B* and *C*, The crystallographic structure. β strands are depicted as thick arrows in the amino to carboxy direction, and α helices are represented as helical ribbons. Connecting loops are shown as thin lines. Disulfide bonds are two connected spheres. *B*, Side view. The molecule is shown with the α$_3$ domain and β$_2$-microglobulin at the bottom, and the α$_1$ and α$_2$ domains at the top. The β-pleated sheet is seen edge on. The α helices form the cleft into which peptide can fit. *C*, Top view. The α$_1$ and α$_2$ domains are seen from above. The β-pleated sheet platform and the cleft formed by the α helices are again visible. (*B* and *C* adapted by permission from Nature, Vol. 329, p. 506. Copyright © 1987 Macmillan Magazines Limited.)

complex. The application of molecular biology technology to the study of the HLA complex over the past 10 years has allowed delineation of additional HLA loci and alleles and the determination of the sequence of many HLA genes. Most recently, x-ray crystallographic analysis of HLA molecules has allowed insight into their physiology. Together these findings have suggested how changes in the sequence of an HLA molecule may lead to predisposition to disease.

TISSUE DISTRIBUTION, FUNCTION, AND STRUCTURE

The HLA complex determines two distinct classes of cell surface glycoprotein molecules, designated class I and class II, with distinct structures, functions, and tissue distributions.

Class I Molecules

The HLA class I molecule consists of an HLA-encoded polymorphic glycoprotein of 44,000 molecular weight (MW) known as the heavy chain, in noncovalent association with a 12,000 MW nonpolymorphic protein known as β_2-microglobulin (Fig. 250–1A). The β_2-microglobulin is encoded by a gene on chromosome 15 and not by the HLA complex. The entire class I molecule is anchored in the cell membrane only by the heavy chain. This chain contains approximately 338 amino acids and can be divided into three regions. Starting from the amino terminal end of the molecule, these regions are an extracellular hydrophilic region (amino acids 1 to 281), a transmembrane hydrophobic region (amino acids 282 to 306), and an intracytoplasmic hydrophilic region (amino acids 307 to 338). The hydrophobic transmembrane region contains 24 amino acids, enabling it to span the cell membrane. The intracytoplasmic hydrophilic region can be phosphorylated, and it has been speculated that class I molecules may transduce external events across the cell membrane.

The extracellular hydrophilic region in turn can be divided into three domains, each of approximately 90 amino acids, designated from the amino terminal end α_1, α_2, and α_3. The α_3 domain and β_2-microglobulin have structural homology with the constant region of immunoglobulin, identifying the class I molecule as a member of the immunoglobulin supergene family.

Recently acquired x-ray crystallographic data have elucidated the actual structure of the HLA class I molecule (Fig. 250–1B). The α_3 domain and β_2-microglobulin are closest to the membrane and support an interactive structure formed by the α_1 and α_2 domains. The α_1 domain and the α_2 domain each consists of four β strands shown as flat arrows and an α helix shown as a coiled ribbon-like structure projecting toward the top of the figure. (The α helix should not be confused with the α domain, nor should the β strand be confused with β_2-microglobulin.) The eight β strands of these two domains form a β-pleated sheet platform that supports the two α helices. These α helices create a groove or cleft that serves as the antigen-binding site for a peptide fragment appropriately processed from a larger antigen.

The class I molecule appears to bind antigenic peptide fragments while still in the endoplasmic reticulum, and the binding of peptide is necessary for the class I molecule to be transported to the cell surface. Once at the cell surface, the two α helices of the class I molecule together with the bound antigenic fragment comprise the ligand recognized by the T-cell receptor on a CD8+ T cell.

A top view of the class I molecule as it would appear to the T-cell receptor of a CD8+ T lymphocyte is shown in Figure 250–1C. The β strands of the α_1 and α_2 domains form the floor of the cleft, and the α helices of the same domains form the sides of the cleft. The majority of alloantigenic determinants recognized both by antibodies and by T cells have been shown to be located in the α_1 and α_2 domains.

The class I antigens are found on virtually every human cell (Table 250–1). This tissue distribution is well suited to the physiologic role of the class I antigens to present foreign antigenic peptides such as viral antigenic peptides to cytotoxic T lymphocytes (CTL's). Precursors of CTL's are specific for a particular viral antigenic peptide in the context of a particular class I molecule. When the precursors encounter this particular combination of the viral antigenic peptide and the class I molecule,

TABLE 250–1. COMPARISON OF HLA CLASS I AND CLASS II MOLECULES

	Class I	Class II
Molecules included	HLA-A, -B, -C	HLA-DR, -DQ, -DP
Structure	44,000 MW heavy chain	~34,000 MW α chain
	12,000 MW β_2-microglobulin	~29,000 MW β chain
Tissue distribution	On virtually every cell	Normal limited to immunocompetent cells, particularly B cells, macrophages, activated T cells
Function	Bind and present antigenic peptides to CD8+ T cells	Bind and present antigenic peptides to CD4+ T cells

they proliferate and differentiate to mature CTL's. The mature CTL's are restricted in their killing to those target cells that bear both the same viral peptide and the same class I molecule as were present on the sensitizing cells. That particular CTL does not kill a target cell with the same class I molecule infected with a different virus, nor does it kill a target cell with a different class I molecule infected with the same virus. Thus, CTL killing is both antigen-specific and class I restricted. In the nonphysiologic situation of a tissue or organ graft, the class I antigens are the principal antigens recognized by the host's CTL's during graft rejection.

Class II Molecules

The structure of a class II molecule is schematically depicted in Figure 250–2A. Each class II molecule consists of two glycoprotein chains, an α chain of approximately 34,000 MW, and a β chain of approximately 29,000 MW. Both of the chains span the membrane and therefore serve to anchor the molecule. Each chain can be divided into three regions. Beginning at the amino terminal end, there is an extracellular hydrophilic region, a transmembrane hydrophobic region, and an intracytoplasmic hydrophilic tail. Each extracellular region has been further divided into two domains of approximately 90 amino acids each. For the α chain these are designated α_1 and α_2, and for the β chain, β_1 and β_2. The α_2 and β_2 domains, like the α_3 domain of the class I molecule and β_2-microglobulin, show homology with the constant region domain of immunoglobulin, thus indicating that class II molecules are also members of the immunoglobulin supergene family. Based on extrapolation from the crystallographic structure of the class I molecules, it is almost certain that the class II α_2 and β_2 domains comprise the portion of the molecule proximal to the cell membrane which supports the distal interactive portion formed by the α_1 and β_1 domains.

A hypothetical top view of the class II α_1 and β_1 domains, as they would appear to the T-cell receptor on a CD4+ T lymphocyte, is shown in Figure 250–2B. The structure is composed of eight β strands and two α helices very similar to those created by the α_1 and α_2 domains of the class I molecule. The two α helices and a portion of the β-pleated sheet of the class II molecule form a cleft or groove with characteristics similar to those of the class I cleft. In contrast to HLA class I molecules, newly synthesized HLA class II molecules are thought to bind processed foreign antigenic peptides in an acidic endosomal compartment during their transport to the cell surface. On the cell surface, the α helices of the class II molecule together with the bound peptide constitute the ligand for the receptor on a CD4+ T cell.

In contrast to the HLA class I molecules, the HLA class II molecules have a limited distribution (Table 250–1). They are found predominantly on immunocompetent cells, including B cells, monocytes, dendritic cells, and activated T cells. Interferon-γ can induce increased expression on macrophages and has also been shown to induce expression of class II molecules on cells where they are not normally expressed, e.g., endothelial cells, thyroid cells, epidermal cells, and renal cells.

The physiologic role of the class II molecules parallels that of the class I molecules. Just as CD8+ T cells recognize foreign antigenic peptide in the context of a class I molecule, CD4+

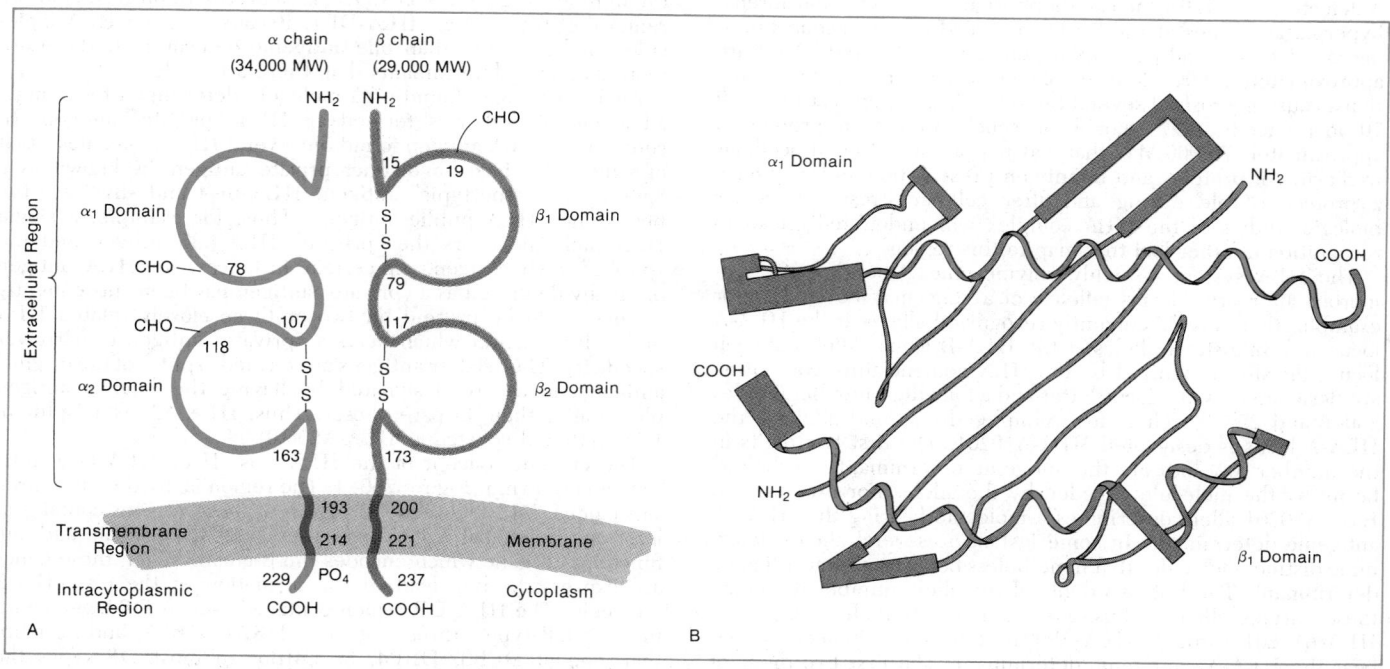

FIGURE 250–2. The HLA class II molecule. *A*, Schematic representation. The molecule consists of an α chain transmembrane glycoprotein noncovalently associated with a β chain transmembrane glycoprotein. The α_1, α_2, β_1, and β_2 domains are indicated. *B*, The postulated crystallographic structure of a class II molecule as seen from above. The antigen-binding cleft is formed by the α_1 and β_1 domains. β strands are depicted as flat thin lines and the α helices as ribbons. The cleft is very similar to that of the class I molecule. For explanation of symbols see Figure 250–1. (*B* adapted by permission from Nature, Vol. 332, p. 845. Copyright © 1988 Macmillan Magazines Limited.)

(generally helper) T cells recognize foreign antigenic peptide in the context of a class II molecule. In nonphysiologic states such as graft transplantation, the class II molecules present on donor cells can initiate an immune response in the host by stimulating the host's helper T cells.

NOMENCLATURE AND GENETIC ORGANIZATION OF THE HLA COMPLEX

The HLA complex is located on the short arm of chromosome 6. Figure 250–3 schematically depicts the genetic loci currently located within the HLA complex. There are three groups or classes of HLA genes and molecules. Genes at the HLA-A, -B,

and -C loci encode the class I or classic histocompatibility molecules, whereas genes at the HLA-DR, -DQ, and -DP loci determine the class II molecules. As noted above, both class I and class II molecules are cell surface bound.

The HLA complex also contains a series of genes that encode soluble proteins. This set of genes is broadly termed the class III genes. Genes at the Bf, C2, C4A, and C4B loci encode properdin factor B and the second and fourth components of the complement system. Genes at the 21-OHA and -OHB loci encode 21-hydroxylase, an enzyme in the adrenal steroid synthetic pathway. The C4B-linked 21-OHB gene is functional, whereas the C4A-linked 21-OHA appears to be a pseudogene; that is, it is not expressed.

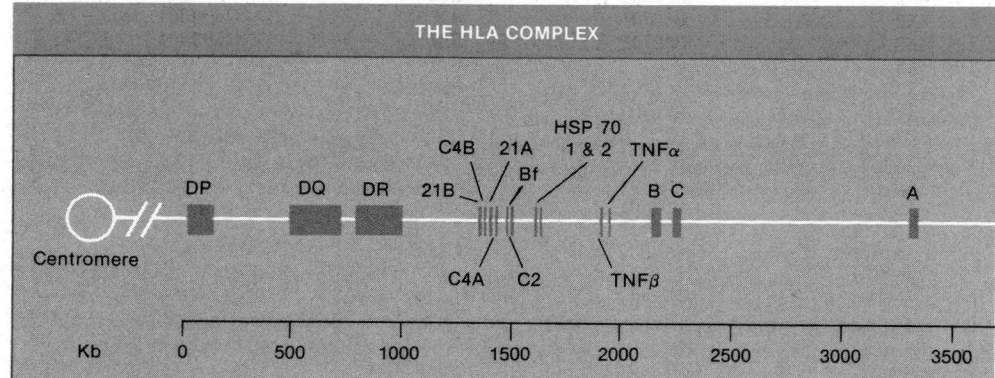

FIGURE 250–3. The current concept of the HLA complex. The class I loci, the class II subregions, and the class III loci are indicated. Distances are given in kilobases (Kb). A, B, and C denote the HLA-A, HLA-B, and HLA-C loci; DP, DQ, and DR designate the HLA-DP, -DQ, and -DR subregions; C2, C4A, C4B, and Bf denote the loci encoding the second, duplicated fourth, and properdin factor B components of the complement system; 21A and 21B designate the 21-hydroxylase A and B loci; TNFα and TNFβ indicate the tumor necrosis factor loci, and HSP 1 and 2 indicate the major heat shock protein 70 loci. Class I loci are shown as thin red blocks, class II loci as thick red blocks, and the complement class III loci as thin vertical bars.

A defective 21-OHB gene can therefore lead to congenital adrenal hyperplasia. Genes at the TNFα and TNFβ loci encode tumor necrosis factor α and β (lymphocytotoxin). TNFα and TNFβ are approximately 20,000 MW cytokines which, among their functions, cause necrosis of several tumors. Finally, genes at the HSP 70 loci encode the major heat shock protein, a protein of approximately 70,000 MW that may play a role in the intracellular trafficking of proteins and in antigen presentation and may have a protective role during and after cellular stress. Molecular biologic studies of the HLA complex will undoubtedly lead to recognition of other loci that map to this region.

The HLA system is highly polymorphic. At each locus, numerous alternative forms (alleles) of a gene may be found. For example, there are 25 currently recognized alleles at the HLA-A locus and 32 distinct alleles at the HLA-B locus. Alleles at each locus officially recognized by the HLA nomenclature committee are designated by the locus letter and a four-digit number (Tables 250–2 and 250–3). Thus, for example, the second allele at the HLA-A locus is designated HLA-A*0201. The first two digits in the number (02) indicate the antigenic determinant (see below) borne by the molecule encoded by the allele. For example the HLA-A*0201 allele determines a molecule bearing the HLA-A2 antigenic determinant. In some instances, several alleles determine distinct molecules that nonetheless bear a common antigenic determinant. The last two digits of the allele number designate these various alleles. Thus, for example, 10 alleles designated HLA-A*0201 through HLA-A*0210 determine molecules that bear the HLA-A2 antigenic determinant. The first two digits of the allele number (02) indicate the HLA-A2 determinant, and the last two digits (01 through 10) designate the 10 distinct alleles, each of which encodes a molecule bearing HLA-A2.

As alluded to above, each functional allele determines a glycoprotein product, the HLA molecule. Each HLA molecule bears antigenic determinants recognized by antibodies. These antigenic determinants are designated by a letter and a number, for example HLA-A1 (Table 250–4). The letter indicates the locus at which the allele encoding the molecule bearing the antigenic determinant is found; the number indicates the number of the antigenic determinant determined by that allele. Antigenic de-

terminants that have been assigned but are not yet officially recognized are signified by a w (for "workshop") placed before the number, e.g., HLA-DRw1. Official recognition results in the removal of the w, e.g., HLA-DR1. Because a given HLA molecule can bear more than one antigenic determinant, there are more antigenic determinants than there are alleles.

An HLA antigen found on a molecule determined by a single allele and no other is termed an HLA "private" antigen. In contrast, an HLA antigen found on several HLA molecules, each of which also bears a distinct private antigen, is known as a "public" or "supertypic" antigen. HLA-Bw4 and -Bw6 are the best-known HLA public antigens. Thus, for example, a single HLA molecule bears the "private" HLA-B35 antigen and the "public" Bw6 antigen. In certain instances, an HLA antigen originally described as a "private" antigen has been subsequently discovered to be present on two or three closely related HLA molecules, each of which bears a "private" antigen of narrower specificity. These latter antigens are termed "splits" of the original antigen and are so designated by having the original antigen placed after them in parentheses. Thus, HLA-A25 is a "split" of HLA-A10 and is listed as HLA-A25(10).

The current concept of the HLA class II or HLA-D genetic region is shown in Figure 250–4. The region is divided into three subregions: DP, DQ, and DR. Each of these regions contains at least one functional A gene which encodes the α chain and one functional B gene which encodes the β chain. When these genes are expressed, they lead to the formation of the class II αβ molecule. The HLA-DR region contains a single DRA gene and, in most DR types, three B genes—DRB1, DRB2, and no more than one of DRB3, DRB4, or DRB5. In most DR types the DRB2 gene is a pseudogene; that is, it is not expressed. However, the DRB1 and one of the DRB3, DRB4, or DRB5 genes are expressed. The DRα chain can combine with either the DRβ1 chain or the DRβ3 (or DRβ4 or DRβ5) chain to produce the DRαβ1 and DRαβ3 (or DRαβ4 or DRαβ5) molecules. The DRαβ1 molecule bears DR antigens 1 through 18, while the DRαβ3 molecule bears DRw52, the DRαβ4 molecule bears DRw53, and the DRαβ5 molecule is associated with DRαβ1 molecules bearing DRw15 and DRw16 and may itself also bear these determinants.

Certain of the HLA-DR B1 allele types have been organized

TABLE 250–2. DESIGNATIONS OF HLA-A, -B, AND -C ALLELES

HLA Alleles	HLA Antigenic Determinant	HLA Alleles	HLA Antigenic Determinant	HLA Alleles	HLA Antigenic Determinant
A*0101	A1	B*0701	B7	Cw*0101	Cw1
A*0201	A2	B*0702	B7	Cw*0201	Cw2
A*0202	A2	B*0801	B8	Cw*0202	Cw2
A*0203	A2	B*1301	B13	Cw*0301	Cw3
A*0204	A2	B*1302	B13	Cw*0501	Cw5
A*0205	A2	B*1401	B14	Cw*0601	Cw6
A*0206	A2	B*1402	Bw65(14)	Cw*0701	Cw7
A*0207	A2	B*1501	Bw62(15)	Cw*1101	Cw11
A*0208	A2	B*1801	B18	Cw*1201	—
A*0209	A2	B*2701	B27	Cw*1301	—
A*0210	A2	B*2702	B27	Cw*1401	—
A*0301	A3	B*2703	B27		
A*0302	A3	B*2704	B27		
A*1101	A11	B*2705	B27		
A*2401	A24(9)	B*2706	B27		
A*2501	A25(10)	B*3501	B35		
A*2601	A26(10)	B*3701	B37		
A*2901	A29(w19)	B*3801	B38(16)		
A*3001	A30(w19)	B*3901	B39(16)		
A*3101	A31(w19)	B*4001	Bw60(40)		
A*3201	A32(w19)	B*4002	B40		
A*3301	Aw33(w19)	B*4101	Bw41		
A*6801	Aw68(28)	B*4201	Bw42		
A*6802	Aw68(28)	B*4401	B44 (12)		
A*6901	Aw69(28)	B*4402	B44 (12)		
		B*4601	Bw46		
		B*4701	Bw47		
		B*4901	B49 (21)		
		B*5101	B51(5)		
		B*5201	Bw52(5)		
		B*5701	Bw57(17)		
		B*5801	Bw58(17)		

into groups based on their occurrence with DRB3, DRB4, or DRB5 alleles. Thus, for example, the DRB1 alleles determining DR3, DR5, DRw6, and DRw8 have been grouped together because they are in linkage disequilibrium (see below) with DRB3 alleles that determine DRw52 (Table 250–5), and are thought to be evolutionarily related. Similarly, the DRB1 alleles encoding DR4, DR7, and DR9 are grouped together because they are in linkage disequilibrium with DRB4, which encodes HLA-DRw53, and are also evolutionarily related. Finally, the DRB1 alleles determining DR2 all are in linkage disequilibrium with DRB5. Linkage disequilibrium is also responsible for the association of particular DR antigens with particular DQ antigens (Table 250–6).

The DQ subregion contains two pairs of A and B genes. One pair, designated DQA2 and DQB2, are pseudogenes and are not expressed. The other pair, designated DQA1 and DQB1, are expressed and result in the formation of the DQαβ molecule. Likewise, the DP subregion contains two pairs of A and B genes. One pair, designated DPA2 and DPB2, contain pseudogenes. The other pair, designated DPA1 and DPB1, encode the DPα and β chains that form the DPαβ molecule.

The polymorphism of the class II molecules (DR, DQ, and DP) varies somewhat for each set. For the DR molecules, the DRα chain is essentially nonpolymorphic between different DR types, while the DRβ chains are highly polymorphic. For the DQ molecules, both the DQα and DQβ chains demonstrate a high degree of polymorphism. For the DP molecules, the DPα chain shows relatively limited polymorphism, while the DPβ chains are again highly polymorphic.

Two additional class II genes have been mapped to the HLA-D region. One has been designated DNA and the second DOB. Neither of these genes has yet been found to be expressed in vivo, although expression has been induced in in vitro systems. The function of these genes is at present unknown.

It should be noted that there is no HLA-D locus or HLA-D molecule per se. The HLA-D antigens are defined and detected solely by a cellular reaction known as the mixed leukocyte reaction (MLR). Responder cells in the MLR appear to be detecting an array of antigenic determinants present on the HLA-DR, -DQ, and/or -DP molecules. In most cases, it is thought that antigenic determinants on HLA-DR molecules contribute most significantly to the MLR. As a result, HLA-D types tend to be most highly correlated with HLA-DR types (see Table 250–3).

The products of the C2, C4, and Bf loci are complement proteins that can be detected serologically and functionally and also display polymorphism (Table 250–7). Alleles determining properdin factor B can be distinguished by their electrophoretic mobility: a common fast form Bf*F, a common slow form Bf*S, a rare fast form Bf*F1, and a rare slow form Bf*SO.7. There are C2 alleles determining two common forms of C2, C2*C and C2*A, and a rare deficiency allele C2*QO. The C4 locus has been duplicated so that there are two distinct C4 loci designated

TABLE 250–3. DESIGNATIONS OF HLA-DR, -DQ, AND -DP ALLELES

HLA-DR Alleles	HLA-DR Determinants	HLA-D–Associated (T-cell–Defined) Determinants	HLA-DQ Alleles	HLA-DQ Determinants	HLA-D–Associated (T-cell–Defined) Determinants	HLA-DP Alleles	Associated HLA-DP Determinants
DRB1*0101	DR1	Dw1	DQA1*0101	—	Dw1,w9	DPA1*0101	—
DRB1*0102	DR1	DW20	DQA1*0102	—	Dw2,w21,w19	DPA1*0102	—
DRB1*0103	DR'BR'	DW'BON'	DQA1*0103	—	Dw18,w12,28,	DPA1*0103	—
DRB1*1501	DRw15(2)	Dw2			Dw'FS'	DPA1*0201	—
DRB1*1502	DRw15(2)	Dw12	DQA1*0201	—	Dw7,w11	DPB1*0101	DPw1
DRB1*1601	DRw16(2)	Dw21	DQA1*0301	—	Dw4,w10,w13,	DPB1*0201	DPw2
DRB1*1602	DRw16(2)	Dw22			w14, w15,w23	DPB1*0202	DPw2
DRB1*0301	DRw17(3)	Dw3	DQA1*0401	—	Dw8,Dw'RSH'	DPB1*0301	DPw3
DRB1*0302	DRw18(3)	DW'RSH'	DQA1*0501	—	Dw3,w5,w22	DPB1*0401	DPw4
DRB1*0401	DR4	Dw4	DQA1*0601	—	Dw8	DPB1*0402	DPw4
DRB1*0402	DR4	Dw10	DQB1*0501	DQw5(w1)	Dw1	DPB1*0501	DPw5
DRB1*0403	DR4	Dw13	DQB1*0502	DQw5(w1)	Dw21	DPB1*0601	DPw6
DRB1*0404	DR4	Dw14	DQB1*0503	DQw5(w1)	Dw9	DPB1*0801	
DRB1*0405	DR4	Dw15	DQB1*0601	DQw6(w1)	Dw12,w8	DPB1*0901	DP'Cp63'
DRB1*0406	DR4	Dw'KT2'	DQB1*0602	DQw6(w1)	Dw2	DPB1*1001	—
DRB1*0407	DR4	Dw13	DQB1*0603	DQw6(w1)	Dw18,Dw'FS'	DPB1*1101	—
DRB1*0408	DR4	Dw14	DQB1*0604	DQw6(w1)	Dw19	DPB1*1301	—
DRB1*1101	DRw11(5)	Dw5	DQB1*0201	DQw2	Dw3,w7	DPB1*1401	—
DRB1*1102	DRw11(5)	Dw'JVM'	DQB1*0301	DQw7(w3)	Dw4,w5,w8,	DPB1*1501	—
DRB1*1103	DRw11(5)	—			w13	DPB1*1601	—
DRB1*1104	DRw11(5)	Dw'FS'	DQB1*0302	DQw8(w3)	Dw4,w10,w13,	DPB1*1701	—
DRB1*1201	DRw12(5)	Dw'DB6'			w14	DPB1*1801	—
DRB1*1301	DRw13(w6)	Dw18	DQB1*0303	DQw9 (w3)	Dw23,w11	DPB1*1901	—
DRB1*1302	DRw13(w6)	Dw19	DQB1*0401	DQw4	Dw15		
DRB1*1303	DRw13(w6)	Dw'HAG'	DQB1*0402	DQw4	Dw8,Dw'RSH'		
DRB1*1401	DRw14(w6)	Dw9					
DRB1*1402	DRw14(w6)	Dw16					
DRB1*0701	DR7	Dw17					
DRB1*0702	DR7	Dw'DB1'					
DRB1*0801	DRw8	Dw8.1					
DRB1*0802	DRw8	Dw8.2					
DRB1*0803	DRw8	Dw8.3					
DRB1*0901	DR9	Dw23					
DRB1*1001	DRw10	—					
DRB3*0101	DRw52a	Dw24					
DRB3*0201	DRw52b	Dw25					
DRB3*0202	DRw52b	Dw25					
DRB3*0301	DRw52c	Dw26					
DRB4*0101	DRw53	Dw4,Dw10,Dw13,Dw14, Dw15,Dw17,Dw23					
DRB5*0101	DRw15(2)	Dw2					
DRB5*0102	DRw15(2)	Dw12					
DRB5*0201	DRw16(2)	Dw21					
DRB5*0202	DRw16(2)	Dw22					

TABLE 250–4. CURRENT LISTING OF RECOGNIZED HLA ANTIGENS

HLA-A	HLA-B		HLA-C	HLA-D	HLA-DR	HLA-DQ	HLA-DP
A1	B5	B51(5)	Cw1	Dw1	DR1	DQw1	DPw1
A2	B7	Bw52(5)	Cw2	Dw2	DR2	DQw2	DPw2
A3	B8	Bw53	Cw3	Dw3	DR3	DQw3	DPw3
A9	B12	Bw54(w22)	Cw4	Dw4	DR4	DQw4	DPw4
A10	B13	Bw55(w22)	Cw5	Dw5	DR5	DQw5(w1)	DPw5
A11	B14	Bw56(w22)	Cw6	Dw6	DRw6	DQw6(w1)	DPw6
Aw19	B15	Bw57(17)	Cw7	Dw7	DR7	DQw7(w3)	
A23(9)	B16	Bw58(17)	Cw8	Dw8	DRw8	DQw8(w3)	
A24(9)	B17	Bw59	Cw9(w3)	Dw9	DR9	DQw9(w3)	
A25(10)	B18	Bw60(40)	Cw10(w3)	Dw10	DRw10		
A26(10)	B21	Bw61(40)	Cw11	Dw11(w7)	DRw11(5)		
A28	Bw22	Bw62(15)		Dw12	DRw12(5)		
A29 (w19)	B27	Bw63(15)		Dw13	DRw13(w6)		
A30 (w19)	B35	Bw64(14)		Dw14	DRw14(w6)		
A31(w19)	B37	Bw65(14)		Dw15	DRw15(2)		
A32(w19)	B38(16)	Bw67		Dw16	DRw16(2)		
Aw33(w19)	B39(16)	Bw71(w70)		Dw17(w7)	DRw17(3)		
Aw34(10)	B40	Bw70		Dw18(w6)	DRw18(3)		
Aw36	Bw41	Bw72(w70)		Dw19(w6)			
Aw43	Bw42	Bw73		Dw20	DRw52		
Aw66(10)	B44(12)	Bw75(15)		Dw21	DRw53		
Aw68(28)	B45(12)	Bw76(15)		Dw22			
Aw69(28)	Bw46	Bw77(15)		Dw23			
Aw74(w19)	Bw47			Dw24			
	Bw48	Bw4		Dw25			
	B49(21)	Bw6		Dw26			
	Bw50(21)						

C4A (formerly Rogers), which determines the electrophoretically more acidic group of C4 components, and C4B (formerly Chido), which determines the electrophoretically more basic group of C4 components. There are four well-defined common structural alleles and one deficiency allele at the C4A locus and three well-defined common structural alleles and one deficiency allele at the C4B locus.

HAPLOTYPE

Because of their close linkage, the alleles at each locus on a single chromosome are usually inherited in combination as a unit. This combination is referred to as the haplotype. Because each individual inherits one set of chromosomes from each parent, each individual has two HLA haplotypes. HLA genes are codominant; therefore, both alleles at a given HLA locus are expressed, and two complete sets of HLA antigens can be detected on cells. By simple mendelian genetics, there is a 25 per cent chance that two siblings will share both haplotypes and be fully HLA compatible, a 50 per cent chance that they will share one haplotype, and a 25 per cent chance that they will share no haplotype and thus will be completely HLA incompatible (Fig. 250–5).

LINKAGE DISEQUILIBRIUM

Because of random matings, the frequency of finding a given allele at one HLA locus associated with a given allele at a second HLA locus should simply be the product of the frequencies of each allele in the population. However, certain combinations of alleles are found with a frequency greater than expected. This phenomenon is termed "linkage disequilibrium" and is quantitated as the difference (Δ) between the observed and expected frequencies. For example, the HLA-A*0101 allele, which determines HLA-A1, and the HLA-B*0801 allele, which determines HLA-B8, are found in the Caucasian population with frequencies of 0.161 and 0.104, respectively. Thus, the expected frequency with which the HLA-A*0101, B*0101 haplotype should be found is 0.161×0.104, or 0.0167. However, this haplotype is found with a frequency of approximately 0.0592, almost four times the expected frequency, for a $\Delta = 0.0592 - 0.0167 = 0.0425$. Table 250–8 lists some common examples of linkage disequilibrium. Several hypotheses have been put forth to explain linkage disequilibrium: (1) a selective advantage of a given haplotype, and (2) recent admixture of two inbred populations.

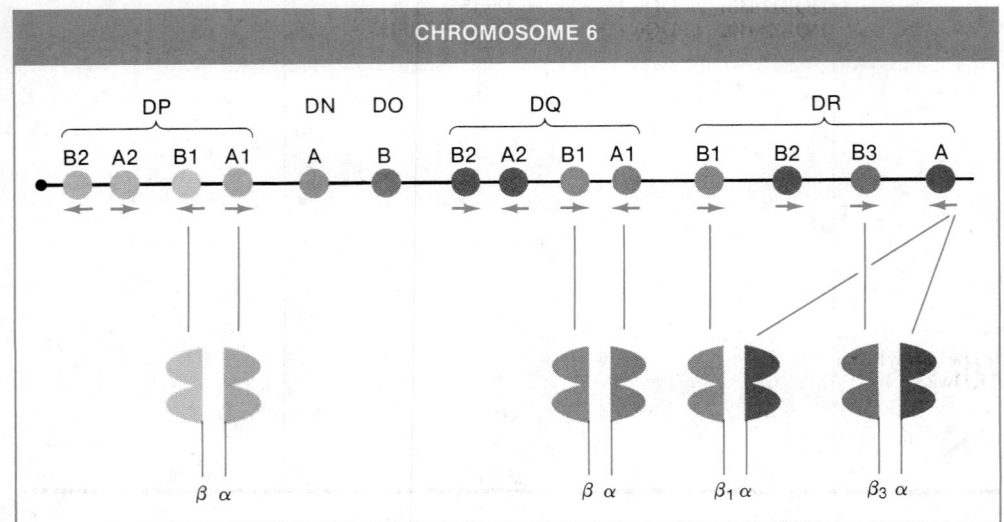

CHROMOSOME 6

FIGURE 250–4. The current concept of the HLA-D region, showing the organization of the three subregions, DP, DQ, and DR. DPA2, DPB2, DQA2, DQB2, and DRB2 are pseudogenes and are not expressed. Pairs of expressed genes (DPA1 and DPB1; DQA1 and DQB1; DRA and DRB1; and DRA and DRB3) which encode class II molecules are indicated. (In other haplotypes, DRA and DRB4 or DRA and DRB5 would be the pair expressed in place of DRA and DRB3.) DNA and DOB are not currently known to be transcribed in vivo. Arrows under genes give the direction of transcription (5' to 3').

TABLE 250–5. ASSOCIATIONS OF DRB1-ENCODED ANTIGENS WITH MOLECULES ENCODED BY DRB3, DRB4, OR DRB5 ALLELES

DRB3	DRB4	DRB5
DR3	DR4	DRw15
DR5	DR7	DRw16
DRw6	DR9	
DRw8		
DRw11 (5)		
DRw12 (5)		
DRw13 (w6)		
DRw14 (w6)		
DRw17 (3)		
DRw18 (3)		

TABLE 250–6. DQ-ASSOCIATED HLA-DR ANTIGENS

HLA-DQ Antigens	Associated HLA-DR Antigens
DQw1	DR1, DRw10, DRw13(w6), DRw14(w6), DRw15(2), DRw16(2)
DQw2	DR3, DR7
DQw3	DR4, DR7, DR9, DRw11(5), DRw12(5)
DQw4	DRw8, DRw15
DQw5	DR1, DRw10, DRw14(w6), DRw16(2)
DQw6	DRw15(2), DRw13(w6)
DQw7	DRw11(5), DRw12(5), DR4
DQw8	DR4
DQw9	DR7, DR9

HLA TYPING

All HLA class I and class II antigens are present on the class I and class II molecules but are defined and detected by different methods. The HLA-A, -B, -C, -DR, and -DQ antigens are defined, detected, and typed serologically by the microlymphocytotoxicity assay. Although some monoclonal antibodies are available for particular HLA antigens, the majority of serologic typing is still done with sera obtained from multiparous women. Typing for the HLA class I antigens is done on purified populations of lymphocytes. Typing of the HLA-DR and -DQ class II antigens is performed on purified populations of B lymphocytes. Alternatively, a two-color dye procedure is used which allows B cells to be distinguished from T cells. HLA-DP antigens are defined and typed by a cellular reaction known as the primed lymphocyte test (PLT), but DP molecules can be detected by monoclonal antibodies. As noted above, HLA-D antigens are defined and typed by the mixed leukocyte reaction (MLR).

The application of molecular biologic techniques to HLA typing has made possible new and more precise methods. The most promising technique is the polymerase chain reaction combined

TABLE 250–7. WELL-DEFINED ALLELES AT THE HLA-LINKED COMPLEMENT LOCI

C2	Bf	C4A	C4B
C2*C	Bf*F	C4A*2	C4B*1
C2*A	Bf*S	C4A*3	C4B*2
C2*Q0	Bf*F1	C4A*4	C4B*3
	Bf*S0.7	C4A*6	C4B*Q0
		C4A*Q0	

with oligonucleotide typing. The polymerase chain reaction is used to amplify the HLA gene(s) to be typed. Because each HLA allele has a unique nucleotide sequence that differentiates it from every other allele, it is possible to synthesize an oligonucleotide (or in some cases, a pair of oligonucleotides) which will hybridize only to this unique sequence. A set of tagged oligonucleotides corresponding to various alleles can therefore be used for HLA typing at the DNA level. Oligonucleotide typing is still in its infancy, and the vast majority of clinical HLA typing is currently done by conventional methodologies.

HLA typing is used primarily for determination of HLA compatibility prior to transplantation and platelet transfusion, for paternity testing, for forensic medicine, and for establishing HLA disease associations.

HLA AND DISEASE

The discovery in 1973 that ankylosing spondylitis (see Ch. 259) is highly associated with HLA-B27 stimulated an intense search for other HLA-disease associations. Well over 100 diseases from virtually all fields of medicine have now been associated with HLA. Despite this broad range of diseases, HLA-associated diseases for the most part share certain common characteristics. In general, these diseases have an hereditary tendency but weak penetrance and do not follow simple mendelian segregation. They lack a known etiologic agent and have an unknown pathophysiology. They are associated with immunologic abnormalities, and many of them are characterized as autoimmune. They follow subacute or chronic courses. Finally, they usually do not affect an individual's ability to bear offspring, thus allowing the HLA-associated diseases to persist in the species.

The association of HLA and disease has been demonstrated by both population and family studies. These two types of studies provide different information. Population studies allow a statistically significant correlation to be established between a particular HLA marker gene and a particular disease state. They do not constitute proof of genetic linkage between a disease susceptibility gene and the HLA marker gene because correlation does not necessarily imply genetic linkage. For example, if a disease susceptibility gene were not linked to HLA but required the presence of a particular HLA antigen for its expression, then an HLA-disease association would be demonstrated in population studies. In contrast, family studies provide an opportunity to determine linkage between a disease susceptibility gene and the HLA marker gene. Because population studies are easier to conduct, the majority of data on HLA and disease derive from this type of study.

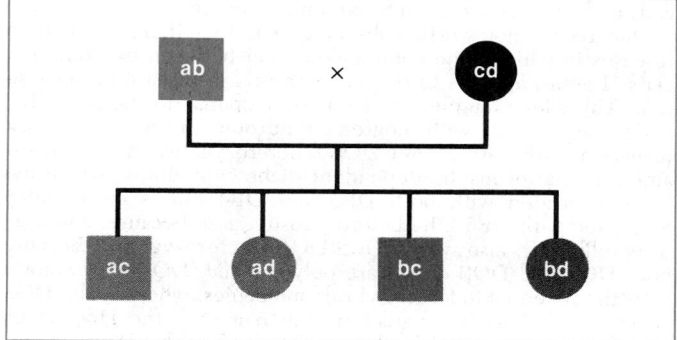

FIGURE 250–5. Inheritance of HLA haplotypes. A haplotype is the combination of alleles at each locus on a single chromosome and is almost always inherited as a unit. Haplotype designations are given by a, b, c, and d. Paternal haplotypes are a and b, and maternal haplotypes are c and d. The mating ab × cd can yield four possible combinations of haplotypes—ac, ad, bc, and bd. Statistically, 25 per cent of the offspring will be HLA identical (e.g., ac and ac), 25 per cent will be total HLA nonidentical (e.g., ac and bd), and 50 per cent will be HLA-haploidentical (e.g., ac and ad).

TABLE 250–8. EXAMPLES OF LINKAGE DISEQUILIBRIUM IN CAUCASIANS

Haplotypes (listed as antigen phenotypes)	Δ ($\times 10^{-3}$)
HLA-A1, B8	53.2
HLA-A2, B44 (12)	14.8
HLA-A3, B7	32.4
HLA-B8, DR3	61.3
HLA-B7, DR2	36.8
HLA-DR2, DQw1	93.6
HLA-DR3, DQw2	37.4
HLA-DR7, DQw2	96.7
HLA-DR4, DQw3	87.5
HLA-A1, B8, DR3	28.0
HLA-A3, B7, DR2	11.5

It should be noted that no HLA-disease association is absolute. The majority of individuals with a given disease-associated HLA antigen do not contract the disease, and a given HLA-associated disease can occur in individuals who lack the usual disease-associated HLA antigen. It is now widely accepted that a combination of a particular HLA antigen, other genetic influences, and environmental agents is necessary for the disease to be manifest.

The strength of the association of a particular disease with a particular HLA antigen is quantitated by calculating the relative risk (Table 250–9). The relative risk (RR) is defined by the formula $RR = (P^+ \times C^-)/(P^- \times C^+)$, where P^+ is the number of patients possessing the disease-associated HLA antigen, C^- is the number of controls lacking that particular HLA antigen, P^- is the number of patients lacking that HLA antigen, and C^+ is the number of controls possessing that HLA antigen. The higher the relative risk above 1, the stronger the association between the HLA antigen and the disease. The relative risk can be stated as the chance of developing the HLA-associated disease for an individual with the disease-associated HLA antigen compared to an individual without that HLA antigen. Because there is usually a significant difference in the frequency of a given antigen among different racial groups, it is mandatory to compare a patient group with a control population of the same race. Thus, for example, HLA-B27 is found in 88 per cent of American white patients with ankylosing spondylitis and approximately 8 per cent of American white controls, yielding a relative risk of approximately 85. In contrast, HLA-B27 is found in 48 per cent of American black patients with ankylosing spondylitis but in only 2 per cent of American black controls, giving a relative risk of 45. Table 250–9 gives the relative risks for selected significant HLA-disease associations.

Because of the phenomenon of linkage disequilibrium and the order in which the HLA class I and class II antigens were defined, a particular disease may have appeared to be associated with a particular antigen at a given HLA locus when in actuality it is more highly associated with a particular antigen at a different HLA locus. Thus, for example, the alleles encoding HLA-DQw2, -DR3, and -B8 are known to be in linkage disequilibrium. Before

TABLE 250–9. SELECTED HLA AND DISEASE ASSOCIATIONS IN WHITE PATIENTS

Disease	Antigen	Approximate Relative Risk
Ankylosing spondylitis	B27	81.8
Reiter's syndrome	B27	40.4
Acute anterior uveitis	B27	7.98
Reactive arthritis (*Yersinia*)	B27	17.6
Rheumatoid arthritis	DR4	6.4
Juvenile rheumatoid arthritis		
Seropositive	DR4	7.2
	Dw4	25.8
	Dw14	47
	Dw4/Dw14	116
Pauciarticular	DR5	2.9
	DPw2	3.9
Systemic lupus erythematosus	DR3	2.7
Behçet's disease	B5	3.3
Sjögren's syndrome	DR3	5.6
High-titer anti-SS-A antibody	DQw1/DQw2	—
Graves' disease	DR3	3.8
Insulin-dependent diabetes mellitus	DR3	3.0
Celiac disease	DR3	13.3
Psoriasis vulgaris	B13	4.5
	B17	3.1
	Cw6	7.2
Pemphigus vulgaris	DR4	21.4
Dermatitis herpetiformis	DR3	18.2
Idiopathic hemochromatosis	A3	6.6
	B14	3.7
Goodpasture's syndrome	DR2	19.8
Multiple sclerosis	DR2	2.8
Myasthenia gravis (without thymoma)	B8	3.3
Narcolepsy	DR2	129

any of the HLA class II antigens were well defined, celiac disease was associated with HLA-B8. The definition of the DR antigens allowed a stronger association to be established between celiac disease and HLA-DR3. The subsequent definition of the HLA-DQ antigens suggested an even more significant association between celiac disease and HLA-DQw2. With the application of molecular biology techniques to the study of HLA and disease associations, restriction endonuclease fragments have been identified in the HLA-DP region which yield even more significant associations. Thus, for example, it has recently been reported that 90 per cent of patients with celiac disease have a genomic DNA fragment that can be detected using a DP β chain cDNA probe. Individuals with this fragment have a relative risk of 46 for contracting celiac disease.

In addition, because of linkage disequilibrium, a number of diseases have been associated with what has been termed extended haplotypes. Two such examples are the association of C2 deficiency with the haplotype A*2501, B*1801, C2*QO, BF*S, C4A*4, C4B*2, DRB1*1501, and systemic lupus with the haplotype A*0101, B*0801, BF*S, C2*C, C4A*QO, C4B*1, DRB1*0301.

Several hypotheses have been suggested to explain HLA-disease associations. Four of these apply to diseases associated with both class I and class II antigens. First, HLA molecules may act as receptors for etiologic agents. If only particular HLA molecules can act as receptors for agents that cause particular diseases, then the HLA-disease association would result. The second hypothesis suggests that the antigen-binding cleft of only a particular HLA molecule can accept the processed antigenic peptide fragment that is ultimately responsible for causing disease. The third hypothesis holds that the actual disease susceptibility genes are not the HLA genes themselves but rather T-cell receptor α and β chain genes. This hypothesis suggests that because a particular T-cell receptor α and β chain combination which predisposes to disease recognizes only a particular antigenic peptide fragment in the context of a particular HLA antigen, an *apparent* association with that HLA antigen is seen. The fourth hypothesis, termed the molecular mimicry hypothesis, states that the disease-associated HLA antigen is immunologically similar to the etiologic agent for the disease and then postulates one of two alternatives. The first alternative suggests that because of the similarity of the etiologic agent and the HLA antigen, no immune response is mounted and therefore the etiologic agent can cause disease unabated. The second alternative suggests that a vigorous immune response is mounted against the etiologic agent, but because of the similarity of the etiologic agent and the HLA antigen, the immune response is turned against the HLA antigen and the resulting autoimmune response produces disease.

The majority of HLA-associated diseases have been associated with the class II antigens. The last hypothesis relates only to class II–associated diseases and suggests that class II molecules aberrantly expressed by cells which normally lack class II molecules may present self-antigenic peptide fragments to CD4+ T cells and thus induce an autoimmune response.

One recent noteworthy observation is that there are certain diseases in which gene complementation between two different class II genes appears to be playing a role in disease predisposition. Thus, for example, the antibody response to the SS-A (Ro) antigen in patients with Sjögren's syndrome and SLE is highest in patients who are DQw1/DQw2 heterozygotes. A second example is that of insulin-dependent diabetes mellitus, which has been associated with both DR3 and DR4 but is most highly associated with DR3/DR4 heterozygosity and, because of linkage disequilibrium, also with DQw2/DQw8 heterozygosity. Because both DQα and DQβ chains are polymorphic, DQ heterozygotes have the potential to form "hybrid" molecules, whereby the DQα chain encoded by one haplotype can pair with the DQβ chain encoded by the second haplotype. Thus, in such heterozygotes, it is possible to form DQw2α/DQw8β and DQw8α/DQw2β molecules. It is postulated that this "hybrid" molecule can present antigenic peptide fragments better than either "parental" molecule to the appropriate CD4+ T cell.

Recently, it has been found that individuals who are predisposed to insulin-dependent diabetes mellitus lack an aspartic acid residue at position 57 of the DQβ chain (i.e., the DQw8 β chain), whereas individuals who are protected from this disease possess an aspartic acid residue at this position (i.e., the DQw7 β chain).

(It should be noted that DQw7 and DQw8 are both splits of DQw3 and have very similar sequences.) Position 57 is found in the α helical portion of the class II peptide-binding cleft. Thus, a single amino acid change in a crucial portion of a class II molecule can dramatically alter disease predisposition.

Finally, it has become apparent that certain regions of the class II molecule, rather than the entire class II molecule, may actually be the elements that confer disease predisposition. These regions have been termed *epitopes*. It has been found that certain DR4 and DR1 class II molecules predispose an individual to rheumatoid arthritis (see Ch. 258). On further analysis, these predisposing DR4 and DR1 molecules were found to share a common amino acid sequence in the α helix of the β chain, and it is thought that this amino acid sequence confers predisposition to rheumatoid arthritis. The fact that two different types of DR molecules share this common disease-predisposing epitope partially explains the lack of absolute HLA-disease associations.

Other mechanisms besides those noted above have also been suggested. It should be emphasized that different mechanisms may be operating to predispose to different diseases and that more than one mechanism may be operating concurrently to produce disease.

McDevitt HO: The HLA system and its relation to disease. Hosp Practice 20:57, 1985. *A clearly written introduction for the neophyte.*
Moller G (ed.): Molecular genetics of class I and II MHC antigens. Parts I and II. Immunol Rev, Vol. 84 & 85. Copenhagen, Munksgaard, 1985. *An in-depth discussion of the organization and basis for polymorphism of the HLA genes.*
Schwartz BD: Infectious agents, immunity, and rheumatic diseases. Arthritis Rheum 33:457, 1990. *A clear discussion of the role of HLA molecules in antigen presentation and the models for HLA-disease associations.*
Tiwari JL, Terasaki PI (eds.): HLA and Disease Associations. New York, Springer-Verlag, 1985. *A comprehensive volume describing virtually all known HLA-disease associations. An excellent referral source.*

251 Drug Allergy
Charles E. Reed

An allergic cause of a drug reaction is suspected when an inflammatory lesion characteristic of those provoked by immunologic mechanisms follows administration of the drug. The variety of drug allergies gives the initial impression that any drug can cause any reaction; in fact, distinct patterns are the rule. Any particular drug tends to cause a similar reaction in different subjects. Typical examples include urticaria after penicillin, lymphocytic pneumonitis after nitrofurantoin, or contact dermatitis from an ointment containing ethylenediamine. Allergic drug reactions need to be distinguished from expected side effects, idiosyncratic reactions of unknown cause, toxic reactions, psychophysiologic reactions, and also from immunologic manifestations of the underlying disease. A further distinction is made between allergic inflammation initiated by a ligand reacting with an antibody or a specifically reacting lymphocyte and similar inflammation initiated by a pharmacologic reaction. Unfortunately these distinctions are not always easily made at the bedside, and there are few reliable clinical or laboratory tests.

Many patients relate a history of allergy to one or more drugs, often without an objective basis. Usually this history can be accepted and serves as a deterrent to excessive drug therapy. Sometimes, however, it is important to evaluate the possibility of allergy to a potentially life-saving drug for which there is no substitute, since many patients with a history of a reaction will tolerate the drug, particularly if several years have passed. If the allergy is still present, taking the drug can be disastrous with fatality from anaphylaxis, Stevens-Johnson syndrome, exfoliative dermatitis, interstitial pneumonitis, or vasculitis. A decision for a particular course of action often rests on judicious weighing of the potential benefits and risks rather than on a definitive diagnosis.

INCIDENCE AND PREDISPOSING FACTORS. Allergic reactions constituted about 6 per cent of all adverse drug reactions in 1968. The frequency is less today because drugs associated with a high frequency of reaction have been displaced by safer ones.

Several predisposing factors exist. Previous drug allergy to the same or a related drug is most important, and the frequency of allergy increases with multiple courses of treatment. Topical administration is the route most likely to sensitize; oral administration, least; and parenteral, intermediate. Parenteral administration provokes more severe reactions, especially anaphylaxis. Children are less likely than adults to react, and men less than women. Persons with history of atopic allergy may be at increased risk of anaphylaxis or urticaria but not of other kinds of allergic drug reactions. Toxic epidermal necrolysis from sulfonamides and several other serious drug allergies are associated with particular HLA phenotypes. The antigenic determinant in drug allergy is often a metabolite rather than the drug itself; genetic differences in drug metabolism therefore influence allergic reactions. For example, persons with reduced acetyltransferase activity were found to be more likely to develop drug-induced systemic lupus erythematosus from procainamide.

MECHANISMS. Foreign macromolecules acting as complete antigens are the most likely to sensitize, eliciting an IgE or IgG antibody response that on a subsequent administration causes anaphylaxis, serum sickness, or vasculitis. Classic serum sickness after injections of large amounts of rabbit or horse serum required large amounts of antigen and relatively high concentrations of circulating immune complexes. Most episodes of urticaria, fever, and arthralgia after relatively small doses involve a combination of IgE- and IgG-initiated events.

Low molecular weight drugs elicit an immune response only after reacting covalently with proteins. This hapten may be the drug itself or a metabolite. The hapten-protein carrier then functions as the complete antigen, both initiating sensitization and eliciting the reaction. An allergic reaction requires a multivalent ligand to cross-link antibody molecules either in fluid phase or bound to cell surface receptors. Univalent haptens actually inhibit cross-linking by occupying the antigen-binding sites. Some chemicals may react with host proteins in such a way that the tertiary structure is altered and the new antigenic determinant is not the hapten itself but the altered structure of the host protein. Drug allergy may take any of the forms of allergic reaction described in Part XVIII. The mechanisms of immune defense and hypersensitivity, like many other biologic functions, exhibit redundancy such that a drug reaction may involve more than one allergic mechanism at the same time. The fact that the hapten often is a drug metabolite may explain the characteristic involvement of some particular organ where the metabolism occurs; alternatively, the hapten may react with a specific organ protein to account for the location of the reaction.

PREVENTION. Avoiding drugs with high sensitizing potential reduces frequency of drug allergy. Interrupted treatment is more likely to sensitize than is continuous treatment, especially with insulin. Beef insulin is more allergenic than pork or human insulin. Recurrence of drug allergy can be reduced by taking a careful history; by exercising a high index of suspicion when fever, rash, or organ damage occurs during treatment; by careful recording of manifestations of drug reactions and diagnosis in the chart when they do occur; and by proper instruction of the patient.

DIAGNOSIS. The history and physical examination provide the essential information for pattern recognition. A key point of the history is the time course of the reaction. Anaphylactic reactions follow within minutes; drug fever, within an hour or two; contact dermatitis, in a day or two; but cholestatic jaundice requires several days or a week. The character of the lesion is also important. Ampicillin characteristically causes a morbilliform rash that may be delayed for 2 days after the drug is stopped. All penicillins may cause urticaria within 10 minutes, but the urticaria may not occur for several days. This distinction is important because the immediate reactions are more likely to be associated with anaphylaxis. A physician observing a drug reaction should record the physical findings for future use. For example, by history alone it is difficult to distinguish between laryngeal edema from anaphylaxis and the hyperventilation syndrome, but the presence of stridor and swelling of pharyngeal or laryngeal

TABLE 251–1. ALLERGIC DRUG REACTIONS

I. Systemic

A. Anaphylaxis
1. Macromolecules
   - Allergenic extracts
   - Dextrans (including iron dextran)
   - Enzymes
     - Asparaginase
     - Chymopapain
     - Trypsin
   - Heparin
   - Hormones (ACTH, insulin, etc.)
   - Human gamma globulin
   - Protamine
   - Vaccines
   - Antisera
2. Diagnostic agents
   - Fluorescein
   - Iodinated contrast media
3. Antimicrobials
   - 5-Aminosalicylic acid
   - Amphotericin B
   - Cephalosporins
   - Cinoxacin
   - Clindamycin
   - Ethambutol
   - Kanamycin
   - Lincomycin
   - Nalidixic acid
   - Penicillins
   - Streptomycin
   - Sulfonamides
   - Tetracyclines
   - Vancomycin
4. Other drugs and other nonsteroidal anti-inflammatory drugs
   - Aspirin
   - Benzyl alcohol
   - Bleomycin
   - Cisplatin
   - Colchicine
   - Cromolyn
   - Cytarabine
   - Dantrolene
   - Ethylenediamine
   - Etoposide
   - Flucytosine
   - Glucocorticoids
   - Indomethacin
   - Local anesthetics
   - Mephyton
   - Meprobamate
   - Niacin
   - Opiates
   - Pentamidine
   - Probenecid
   - Procainamide
   - Sulfite
   - Thiopental
   - Tolmetin
   - Triamterene
   - Tubocurarine and other muscle-relaxing agents
   - Vitamin B_{12}

B. Serum sickness
1. Macromolecules
   - Dextrans
   - Heparin
   - Hormones (insulin, ACTH, etc.)
   - Vaccines
   - Antisera
2. Antimicrobials
   - Cephalosporins
   - Griseofulvin
   - Lincomycin
   - Minocycline
   - Penicillins
   - Streptomycin
   - Sulfonamides
3. Other Drugs
   - Barbiturates
   - Hydantoins
   - Hydralazine
   - Phenylbutazone
   - Procarbazine
   - Propylthiouracil

C. Drug fever
1. Antimicrobials
   - 5-Aminosalicylic acid
   - Cephalosporins
   - Chloramphenicol
   - Erythromycin
   - Isoniazid
   - Kanamycin
   - Nitrofurantoin
   - Norfloxacin
   - Penicillins
   - Pyrazinamide
   - Quinine
   - Streptomycin
   - Sulfonamides
   - Tetracyclines
2. Other drugs
   - Allopurinol
   - Captopril
   - Heparin
   - Hydantoins
   - Hydralazine
   - Hydrochlorothiazide
   - Methyldopa
   - Penicillamine
   - Phenobarbital
   - Pneumococcal vaccine
   - Procainamide
   - Propylthiouracil
   - Quinidine

D. Vasculitis
   - Allopurinol
   - Atenolol
   - Busulfan
   - Carbamazepine
   - Colchicine
   - Diphenhydramine
   - Ethionamide
   - Furosemide
   - Hydantoins
   - Hydroxyurea
   - Ibuprofen
   - Indomethacin
   - Isoniazid
   - Meprobamate
   - Methamphetamine
   - Naproxen
   - Penicillins
   - Phenothiazines
   - Phenylbutazone
   - Propranolol
   - Propylthiouracil
   - Streptokinase
   - Sulfonamides
   - Tetracyclines
   - Thiazide diuretics
   - Vaccines

E. Systemic lupus erythematosus syndrome
   - 5-Aminosalicylic acid
   - Chloroquine
   - Chlorpromazine
   - Ethosuximide
   - Griseofulvin
   - Hydralazine
   - Isoniazid
   - Methyldopa
   - Nitrofurantoin
   - Penicillins
   - Penicillamine
   - Phenytoin
   - Procainamide
   - Propylthiouracil
   - Quinidine
   - Tetracycline
   - Tocainide
   - Trimethadione

II. Skin

A. Urticaria and angioedema
1. Antimicrobials
   - 5-Aminosalicylic acid
   - Aminoglycosides
   - Cephalosporins
   - Ethambutol
   - Isoniazid
   - Metronidazole
   - Miconazole
   - Nalidixic acid
   - Penicillins
   - Quinine
   - Rifampin
   - Spectinomycin
   - Sulfonamides
2. Other drugs
   - Asparaginase
   - Aspirin and other non-steroidal anti-inflammatory drugs
   - Calcitonin
   - Chloral hydrate
   - Chlorambucil
   - Cimetidine
   - Cyclophosphamide
   - Daunorubicin
   - Doxorubicin
   - Ergotamine
   - Ethchlorvynol
   - Ethosuximide
   - Ethylenediamine
   - Glucocorticoids
   - Melphalan
   - Penicillamine
   - Phenothiazines
   - Procainamide
   - Procarbazine
   - Quinidine
   - Tartrazine
   - Thiazide diuretics
   - Thiotepa

B. Morbilliform-maculopapular rash
1. Antimicrobials
   - 5-Aminosalicylic acid
   - Cephalosporins
   - Erythromycin
   - Gentamicin
   - Penicillins
   - Streptomycin
   - Sulfonamides
2. Other drugs
   - Allopurinol
   - Barbiturates
   - Captopril
   - Coumarin
   - Gold salts
   - Hydantoins
   - Thiazide diuretics

C. Toxic epidermal necrolysis and erythroderma and exfoliative dermatitis
   - Allopurinol
   - Amikacin
   - Captopril
   - Carbamazepine
   - Chloral hydrate
   - Chlorambucil
   - Chloroquine
   - Chlorpromazine
   - Cyclosporine
   - Diltiazem
   - Ethambutol
   - Ethylenediamine
   - Glutethimide
   - Gold salts
   - Griseofulvin
   - Hydantoins
   - Hydroxychloroquine
   - Minoxidil
   - Nifedipine
   - Nonsteroidal anti-inflammatory agents
   - Penicillin
   - Phenobarbital
   - Rifampin
   - Spironolactone
   - Streptomycin
   - Sulfonamides
   - Trimethadione
   - Trimethoprim
   - Tocainide
   - Vancomycin
   - Verapamil

D. Erythema multiforme
   - Acetaminophen
   - Barbiturates
   - Carbamazepine
   - Chloroquine
   - Chlorpropamide
   - Clindamycin
   - Ethambutol
   - Ethosuximide
   - Gold salts
   - Hydantoins
   - Hydralazine
   - Hydroxyurea
   - Mechlorethamine
   - Meclofenamate
   - Penicillins
   - Phenolphthalein
   - Phenylbutazone
   - Rifampin
   - Streptomycin
   - Sulfonamides
   - Sulfonylureas
   - Sulindac
   - Vaccines

E. Photosensitive
1. Topical
   - Fluorouracil
   - Hexachlorophene
   - Para-aminobenzoic acid esters
   - Promethazine
   - Sulfanilamide
2. Systemic
   - Carbamazepine
   - Chlorpromazine
   - Griseofulvin
   - Imipramine
   - Lincomycin
   - Nalidixic acid
   - Naproxen
   - Norfloxacin
   - Phenothiazines
   - Piroxicam

TABLE 251–1. ALLERGIC DRUG REACTIONS Continued

2. Systemic *Continued*
- Quinethazone
- Sulfonamides
- Sulfonylureas
- Thiazide diuretics
- Triamterene

F. *Fixed drug eruptions*
- Acetaminophen
- 5-Aminosalicylic acid
- Aspirin
- Barbiturates
- Benzodiazepines
- Chloroquine
- Dapsone
- Dimenhydrinate
- Diphenhydramine
- Gold salts
- Hydralazine
- Hyoscine
- Ibuprofen
- Iodides
- Meprobamate
- Methanamine
- Metronidazole
- Penicillins
- Phenobarbital
- Phenolphthalein
- Phenothiazines
- Phenylbutazone
- Procarbazine
- Pseudoephedrine
- Quinine
- Saccharin
- Streptomycin
- Sulfonamides
- Tetracyclines

G. *Erythema nodosum*
- Bromides
- Oral contraceptives
- Penicillin
- Sulfonamides

H. *Contact dermatitis*
- Ambroxol
- Amikacin
- Antihistamines
- Bacitracin
- Benzalkonium chloride
- Benzocaine
- Benzyl alcohol
- Cetyl alcohol
- Chloramphenicol
- Chlorpromazine
- Clioquinol
- Colophony
- Ethylenediamine
- Fluorouracil
- Formaldehyde
- Gentamycin
- Glucocorticoids
- Glutaraldehyde
- Heparin
- Hexachlorophene
- Iodochlorhydroxyquin
- Lanolin
- Local anesthetics
- Minoxidil
- Naftin
- Neomycin
- Nitrofurazone

- Opiates
- Para-aminobenzoic acid
- Parabens
- Penicillins
- Phenothiazines
- Proflavine
- Propylene glycol
- Streptomycin
- Sulfonamides
- Thimerosal
- Timolol

III. Lung

A. *Asthma*
- Aspirin and other nonsteroidal anti-inflammatory drugs
- Cromolyn
- Sulfite
- Tartrazine
- Occupational exposures to:
  - Cephalosporins
  - Glutaraldehyde
  - Pancreatic enzymes
  - Papain
  - Penicillins
  - Psyllium
  - Thimerosal

B. *Eosinophilic pneumonitis*
- 5-Aminosalicylic acid
- Azathioprine
- Captopril
- Carbamazepine
- Chlorpropamide
- Cromolyn
- Desipramine
- Gold salts
- Imipramine
- Nitrofurantoin
- Penicillins
- Phenytoin
- Sulfonamides
- L-Tryptophan

C. *Fibrotic and pleural reactions*
- Bleomycin
- Busulfan
- Cyclophosphamide
- Gold salts
- Hydralazine
- Hydrochlorothiazide
- Melphalan
- Methotrexate
- Methysergide
- Mitomycin
- Nitrofurantoin
- Procarbazine

IV. Liver

A. *Cholestatic*
- Chlorzoxazone
- Erythromycin estolate
- Ethchlorvynol
- Imipramine
- Nalidixic acid
- Nitrofurantoin
- Phenothiazines
- Sulfamethoxazole

- Sulfonylureas
- Troleandomycin

B. *Hepatocellular*
- 5-Aminosalicylic acid
- Amphotericin B
- Azapropazone
- Ethacrynic acid
- Furosemide
- Gold salts
- Griseofulvin
- Halothane
- Hydantoins
- Isoniazid
- Methyldopa
- Monoamine oxidase inhibitors
- Nitrofurantoin
- Propylthiouracil
- Pyrazinamide
- Quinidine
- Rifampin
- Sulfonamides
- Trimethadione

C. *Chronic active hepatitis*
- Methyldopa
- Nitrofurantoin

V. Kidney

A. *Glomerulitis*
- Allopurinol
- Captopril
- Gold salts
- Nonsteroidal anti-inflammatory agents
- Penicillamine
- Penicillins
- Phenytoin
- Probenecid
- Sulfonamides
- Thiazide diuretics

B. *Interstitial nephritis*
- Allopurinol
- Aztreonam
- Captopril
- Carbamazepine
- Cephalosporins
- Chloramphenicol
- Cimetidine
- Ciprofloxacin
- Colistin
- Furosemide
- Minocycline
- Nonsteroidal anti-inflammatory drugs
- Penicillins, especially methicillin
- Phenytoin
- Polymyxin B
- Rifampin
- Sulfonamides
- Tetracycline
- Thiazide diuretics

VI. Bone Marrow and Blood Cells

A. *Bone marrow aplasia*
- Chloramphenicol
- Gold salts
- Mephenytoin
- Penicillamine
- Phenylbutazone
- Trimethadione

B. *Anemia*
- Acetaminophen
- 5-Aminosalicylic acid
- Captopril
- Cephalosporins
- Chlorpromazine
- Cisplatin
- Hydantoins
- Ibuprofen
- Insulin
- Isoniazid
- Levodopa
- Mefenamic acid
- Melphalan
- Methyldopa
- Methysergide
- Penicillins
- Quinidine
- Quinine
- Rifampin
- Sulfonamides
- Sulfonylureas

C. *Thrombocytopenia*
- Acetaminophen
- Acetazolamide
- Acetylsalicylic acid
- 5-Aminosalicylic acid
- Carbamazepine
- Chloramphenicol
- Chlorpheniramine
- Cimetidine
- Digitoxin
- Diltiazem
- Ethchlorvynol
- Gold salts
- Heparin
- Hydantoins
- Isoniazid
- Levodopa
- Meprobamate
- Methyldopa
- Penicillamine
- Phenylbutazone
- Procainamide
- Quinidine
- Quinine
- Ranitidine
- Rauwolfia alkaloids
- Rifampin
- Sulfonamides
- Sulfonylureas
- Thiazide diuretics

D. *Granulocytopenia*
- Captopril
- Cephalosporins
- Chloral hydrate
- Chlorpropamide
- Penicillins (semisynthetic)
- Phenothiazines
- Phenylbutazone
- Phenytoin
- Procainamide
- Propranolol
- Tolbutamide

E. *Lymphoid hyperplasia*
- Phenytoin
- Mephenytoin

---

mucosa makes the distinction clear. Distinction between a drug reaction and an immunologic event from the underlying disease is important. For instance, many children with viral respiratory infections have transient urticaria that can be mistaken for a penicillin rash. Or, on the first or second day of penicillin treatment a patient with endocarditis may have a macular hem-orrhagic rash and fever, reflecting a reaction to antigens released from the bacteria rather than drug allergy.

Some of the most important patterns of drug reactions are summarized in Table 251–1. For some of the drugs on this list there is no proof that the drug actually caused the reaction. The association is plausible but not certain.

Skin tests may be helpful in predicting anaphylaxis from macromolecules and are usually positive in patients with allergy to foreign serum proteins, insulin, vaccines, and similar materials. With the important exception of penicillin, skin or in vitro allergy tests with low molecular weight drugs are not reliable for detecting anaphylactic (IgE-mediated) drug allergy, although positive skin tests occur after anaphylaxis from muscle-relaxing agents, thiopental, cisplatin, and a few other drugs. Patch tests with single components are useful for identifying contact allergens. Ethylenediamine, one of the ingredients of many creams and ointments, is currently the most frequently encountered contactant. Attempts to adapt lymphocyte transformation tests for diagnosis of drug allergy have been unsuccessful. Eosinophilia, when otherwise unexplained, provides evidence of allergy. Deliberate trial of small doses of the drug strictly for diagnostic purposes is unwise and unnecessary. It may be indicated as a precaution in situations in which the diagnosis of drug allergy is uncertain and no chemically unrelated substitute is available for an urgently needed drug.

MANAGEMENT. In addition to stopping use of the offending drug, symptomatic or supportive treatment of the reaction may be indicated. As a rule it is unwise to attempt to continue using the offending drug under a protective shield of antihistamines or glucocorticoids, although occasional desperate situations may justify an exception. The emergency treatment of anaphylaxis is described in Ch. 247.

SPECIFIC DRUG ALLERGIES. *Penicillin.* Penicillin is one of the most common drugs causing allergy, and being the most fully understood it serves as a model for other drugs. Penicillin reactions include anaphylaxis, urticaria, vasculitis, dermatomyositis, maculopapular rashes, hemolytic anemia, drug fever, interstitial nephritis, pneumonitis, and contact dermatitis. Airborne penicillin can cause asthma in workers who produce or use it. The nature of the reaction is determined not only by the specific metabolite that becomes the hapten but also by the carrier molecule. For example, the penicilloyl determinant commonly evokes IgE antibody in cases of urticaria, but it also evokes IgG, and after complexing with red cell–membrane protein, it may be responsible for hemolytic anemia during intravenous penicillin treatment. Many patients who claim to be allergic to penicillin tolerate it without adverse effect. In such patients, treatment with more expensive or toxic antibiotics would be unnecessary. Reliable tests are available for predicting which patients with a history of penicillin allergy are at risk of immediate allergic reactions. Cautious skin testing with dilute solutions of the antibiotic itself and with commercially available benzylpenicilloyl-polylysine (Pre-Pen) will provide guidance. If skin test reactions are negative to these reagents and to the "minor" determinants (the plain drug, penicilloate, and penilloate), the probability of a mild allergic reaction is about 2 per cent, no higher than in subjects receiving penicillin for the first time. The minor determinants are as yet available only in research settings, but only about 7 per cent of patients react to this reagent alone. Therefore, for patients who give a history of a penicillin reaction and need a penicillin drug for a serious infection, tests with the available reagents interpreted in the light of the history will allow appropriate treatment to proceed. The skin test with penicilloyl-polylysine begins with a prick of the 6.0×10^{-5} M solution, and, if negative in 20 minutes, one proceeds to intradermal testing. Skin testing with the penicillin solution starts with a prick test with a solution containing 6000 units per milliliter of penicillin G or 4 mg per milliliter of other penicillins. Similar testing with cephalosporin is feasible. The frequency of reactions to cephalosporins in patients allergic to penicillin is controversial.

Desensitization can be undertaken when skin test reactions are positive or when there are other reasons for suspecting an appreciable risk of anaphylaxis but the patient has life-threatening infection with an organism for which no alternative antibiotic is available. Oral desensitization is preferred, except in comatose patients when the same principle can be followed parenterally (Table 251–2).

Radiographic Contrast Agents. Iodinated contrast agents injected for radiographic examination are the most common cause of anaphylactic drug reactions. These reactions are not truly anaphylactic, for these materials do not combine with proteins to act as haptens but rather appear to act pharmacologically. As yet these reactions are not fully understood, but it is known that these drugs activate complement and release histamine, probably because they are hyperosmolar. Skin tests or small test doses do not predict reactivity. Persons who have had a previous reaction are at increased risk of a similar reaction from a subsequent injection. When a second examination is necessary, the patient should be given prednisone 50 mg every 6 hours for three doses, ending 1 hour before the procedure, and an antihistamine shortly before. Alternatively, one of the non-ionic agents with low osmolality can be used.

Local Anesthetics. Most adverse reactions to local anesthetics are either toxic or psychophysiologic, but allergic reactions can occur. The most frequent is contact dermatitis; anaphylaxis is more serious although quite rare. It has not yet been determined that skin testing with local anesthetics is useful in predicting anaphylaxis in patients with a history of reactions to local anesthetic. When local anesthesia is needed, an anesthetic as unrelated as possible to the one suspected of causing the reaction should be chosen, and a small test dose should be given first. Lidocaine seems to carry a low risk of allergy.

Aspirin and Other Nonsteroidal Anti-inflammatory Drugs. Shortly after its introduction in the late nineteenth century, aspirin was observed to provoke severe asthma in some asthmatic patients. Such patients react in the same way to other nonsteroidal anti-inflammatory agents. The typical reaction consists of acute bronchospasm, rhinorrhea, and occasionally urticaria. Most of the asthmatic patients who react to these agents also have nasal polyps and lack IgE-mediated allergy to common airborne allergens. In some patients with chronic urticaria but no respiratory disease, urticaria is the only manifestation of the reaction. The mechanism of this adverse response to aspirin is not allergic; extensive search for IgE antibodies has been unrewarding. Rather, it is presumably due to the inhibition of cyclo-oxygenase, but the molecular mechanism is still undefined. Patients who have reacted to aspirin need not avoid other salicylates (except methylsalicylate), and salicylate-free diets are unnecessary. A very few aspirin-reactive subjects react similarly to tartrazine (FD&C yellow No. 5) added to foods or drugs. Skin tests to aspirin and similar agents are not useful and may be dangerous. No biochemical tests are available for diagnosis.

Angiotensin-Converting Enzyme Inhibitors. These drugs may provoke cough and increase the severity and frequency of episodes of angioedema and asthma, presumably by prolonging the action of bradykinin or other vasoactive peptides.

EOSINOPHILIC SYNDROMES. Adulterated cooking oil and contaminated L-tryptophane capsules have been associated with a multisystem systemic inflammatory illness involving skin, muscle, and lung and characterized by eosinophilia of 1000 to 10,000 cells per 10^{-6} liter. Neither the specific causative agent nor the mechanism of the allergic inflammation has yet been identified.

TABLE 251–2. ORAL DESENSITIZATION PROTOCOL FOR PENICILLIN

Dose*	Units	Route†
1	100	P.O.
2	200	P.O.
3	400	P.O.
4	800	P.O.
5	1,600	P.O.
6	3,200	P.O.
7	6,400	P.O.
8	12,800	P.O.
9	25,000	P.O.
10	50,000	P.O.
11	100,000	P.O.
12	200,000	P.O.
13	400,000	P.O.
14	200,000	S.C.
15	400,000	S.C.
16	800,000	S.C.
17	1,000,000	I.M.

*Interval between doses, 15 min.
†P.O. = oral; S.C. = subcutaneous; I.M. = intramuscular.
From Sullivan TJ, Yecies LD, Shaty GS, et al.: Desensitization of patients allergic to penicillin using orally administered β-lactam antibiotics. J Allergy Clin Immunol 69:276, 1982.

American Academy of Pediatrics Committee on Drugs: "Inactive" ingredients in pharmaceutical products. Pediatrics 76:635, 1985. *A useful source of information about allergic reactions to drugs caused by ingredients other than the active drug itself.*

DeSwait RD: Drug allergy. *In* Patterson R (ed.): Allergic Diseases, Diagnosis and Management, 3rd ed. Philadelphia, J. B. Lippincott Company, 1985. *Detailed, well-referenced review of the subject.*

Moscicki RA, Sockin SM, Corsello BF, et al.: Anaphylaxis during induction of general anesthesia: Subsequent evaluation. J Allergy Clin Immunol 86:325–332, 1990. *Description of procedure for diagnosis and management of this life-threatening reaction.*

Rieder MJ, Uetrecht J, Shear NH, et al.: Diagnosis of sulfonamide hypersensitivity reactions by in-vitro "rechallenge" with hydroxylamine metabolites. Ann Intern Med 110(4):286–289, 1989. *An excellent illustration of the direction of contemporary research in drug allergy.*

Sullivan TJ: Drug allergy. *In* Middleton EJ, Ellis EF, Reed CE, et al. (eds.): Allergy Principles and Practice, 3rd ed. St. Louis, C. V. Mosby Company, 1988.

Weist ME, Adkinson NF: Immediate hypersensitivity reactions to penicillins and related antibiotics. Clin Allergy 18:15–40, 1988. *Review of information about the new antibiotics.*

252 Mastocytosis

Dean D. Metcalfe

Mastocytosis is a rare disease characterized by an abnormal increase in mast cells in the bone marrow, liver, spleen, lymph nodes, gastrointestinal tract, and skin. Mastocytosis can present in any age group and demonstrates a slight male predominance (1.5:1.0). The prevalence of the disease is unknown. Familial occurrence is unusual.

The disease is divided into four distinct clinicopathologic entities on the basis of clinical presentation, pathologic findings, and prognosis (Table 252–1). Patients in the first category have a good prognosis, whereas patients in the other three groups do poorly. Indolent mastocytosis is divided into two subgroups: those with isolated skin involvement and those with systemic disease. In most cases such patients gradually accrue more mast cells with progression of symptoms but can be managed successfully for decades using medications that provide symptomatic relief. The second most common form of mastocytosis is that associated with a hematologic disorder. In this group, examination of the bone marrow and peripheral blood reveals the hematologic abnormality. The prognosis in these patients is determined by the prognosis of the associated hematologic disorder. The third category of mast cell disease is mast cell leukemia; it is the rarest form and has the most fulminant behavior. Mast cell leukemia is distinguished from the other categories by its unique pathologic and clinical picture. The peripheral blood smear shows immature mast cells. The fourth category of patients has an aggressive form of mastocytosis; these individuals have poor prognostic features but do not have a distinctive hematologic disorder or mast cell leukemia. A subset of patients with aggressive mastocytosis have a distinct syndrome that has been termed lymphadenopathic mastocytosis with eosinophilia because of the pronounced eosin-

TABLE 252–1. CLASSIFICATION OF MASTOCYTOSIS

I. Indolent mastocytosis
  A. Skin only
    1. Urticaria pigmentosa
    2. Diffuse cutaneous mastocytosis
  B. Systemic
    1. Marrow
    2. Gastrointestinal
    3. ± Urticaria pigmentosa
II. Mastocytosis with associated hematologic disorder (± urticaria pigmentosa)
  A. Dysmyelopoietic syndrome
  B. Myeloproliferative disorders
  C. Acute nonlymphocytic leukemia
  D. Malignant lymphoma
  E. Chronic neutropenia
III. Mast cell leukemia
IV. Aggressive mastocytosis

TABLE 252–2. REPRESENTATIVE MAST CELL PRODUCTS AND THEIR BIOLOGIC EFFECTS

Granule-associated	
Histamine	Pruritus, increased vasopermeability, gastric hypersecretion, bronchoconstriction
Heparin	Local anticoagulation
Tryptase, chymotryptic proteases	Degradation of local connective tissues
Lipid-derived	
Sulfidopeptide leukotrienes	Increased vasopermeability, bronchoconstriction, vasoconstriction (LTC_4); increased vasopermeability, bronchoconstriction, vasodilation (LTD_4 and LTE_4)
Prostaglandin D_2	Vasodilation, bronchoconstriction
Platelet-activating factor	Increased vasopermeability, vasodilation, bronchoconstriction
Cytokines	
Proinflammatory factors	Fibrosis ($TGF\beta$); activation of vascular endothelial cells, cachexia ($TNF\alpha$)
Growth enhancing	Colony-stimulating factor (IL-3); eosinophilia (IL-5)

ophilia, hepatosplenomegaly, and lymphadenopathy. Patients with aggressive disease rapidly increase mast cell numbers and are difficult to manage. Prognosis is less optimistic than in patients with indolent mastocytosis.

ETIOLOGY AND PATHOGENESIS. Mast cells originate from pluripotent bone marrow stem cells and migrate through the blood stream and lymphatics to specific sites within the body, where they mature into a fully granulated cell. The targeting of mast cells to defined locations appears to be determined by the sequential expression of cell surface adhesion molecules, including a laminin-binding protein. Thus, mast cells are often found along endothelial and epithelial basement membrane, along nerves, and around glandular structures rich in laminin. Tissues at interfaces between the external and internal environment, i.e., the skin and gastrointestinal tract, are particularly rich in mast cells. In these sites mast cells are believed to contribute to host defense against parasites.

The regulation of mast cell number and mast cell differentiation is under the control of factors produced both in the hematopoietic marrow and by cells in the tissues in which mast cells finally reside. For example, early mast cell differentiation depends on the colony-stimulating factor interleukin 3 (IL-3) and is inhibited by granulocyte-macrophage colony-stimulating factor (GM-CSF). Final maturation and granule composition may depend upon the production of specific mast cell growth factors by fibroblasts and stromal cells.

Regardless of the etiology of the increased burden of mast cells in patients with mastocytosis, the pathogenesis of the disease is largely the result of the increased production of mast cell mediators, which can have effects either at the site of their production or remote from their origin. Mast cell mediators are of three categories, all of which may distribute through the blood stream and lymphatics and produce biologic effects typical of those observed in patients with mastocytosis (Table 252–2).

CLINICAL FEATURES. The various categories of mastocytosis in general share similar clinical features, which are in turn due to the overproduction of mast cell mediators, although some patterns of disease may predominate in a specific category. The skin, gastrointestinal tract, liver, spleen, lymph nodes, bone marrow, and skeletal system yield the most significant management problems. The respiratory tract and endocrine system are generally spared. Also, although mast cells contain mediators that can inhibit immune responses, patients with mastocytosis do not suffer from recurrent infections.

The most common skin manifestation of mastocytosis is urticaria pigmentosa (Fig. 252–1). It is seen in over 90 per cent of patients with indolent mastocytosis and in less than 50 per cent of patients with mastocytosis with an associated hematologic disorder or those with lymphadenopathic mastocytosis with eosinophilia. The lesions of urticaria pigmentosa appear as small, reddish brown macules or slightly raised papules scattered over the body. Mild trauma, including scratching or rubbing of the lesions, usually

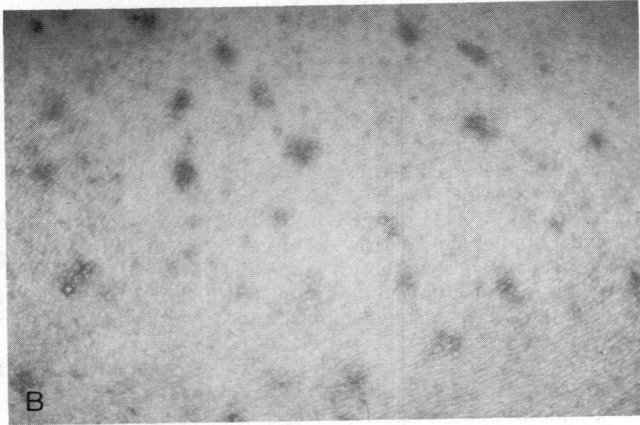

FIGURE 252–1. *A,* Urticaria pigmentosa in a patient with indolent systemic mastocytosis. *B,* Close-up view of urticaria pigmentosa.

causes urtication and erythema around the macules; this is known as Darier's sign. Urticaria pigmentosa is associated with a variable amount of pruritus, which may be exacerbated by changes in climatic temperature, skin friction, ingestion of hot beverages or spicy foods, ethanol, and certain drugs. The diagnosis is confirmed by characteristic skin histopathology. Diffuse cutaneous masto-cytosis consists of a diffuse mast cell infiltration of the skin that can occur without discrete lesions. Solitary lesions called masto-cytomas do occur but are quite rare. Young children with urticaria pigmentosa or diffuse cutaneous mastocytosis may have bullous eruptions.

Gastrointestinal disease often develops in patients with mas-tocytosis. The most common problem is gastric hypersecretion due to elevated plasma histamine with resultant gastritis and peptic ulcer disease. Diarrhea and abdominal pain are common and are followed by the onset of malabsorption in approximately one in three patients. Roentgenographic abnormalities fall into three major categories: peptic ulcers; abnormal mucosal patterns such as mucosal edema, multiple nodular lesions, coarsened mucosal folds, or multiple polyps; and motility disturbances. Histopathology of jejunal biopsies has shown moderate blunting of the villi; however, significant mast cell hyperplasia is uncom-mon.

Hepatic and splenic involvement in indolent systemic masto-cytosis is relatively common, although liver function tests are usually normal. The most common chemical abnormality is an elevated alkaline phosphatase; this must be distinguished from bone-derived alkaline phosphatase, which may also be elevated. The most serious manifestation of hepatic and splenic involvement is portal hypertension and ascites associated with fibrosis of the liver and spleen. These conditions appear most commonly in patients who have mastocytosis with an associated hematologic disorder or in those with aggressive mastocytosis.

Bone marrow lesions consist of focal aggregates of spindle-shaped mast cells, often mixed with eosinophils, lymphocytes, and occasional plasma cells, histiocytes, and fibroblasts (Fig. 252–

2). These lesions are rarely seen in children. Anemia, leukopenia, thrombocytopenia, and eosinophilia may occur in association with systemic disease. Bone marrow infiltration with mast cells may induce bone changes that cause radiographically detectable le-sions in up to 70 per cent of patients. The proximal long bones are most often affected, followed by the pelvis, ribs, and skull. Bone pain is the most common symptom and is present in 19 to 28 per cent of patients. Skeletal scintigraphy (bone scans) is more sensitive than radiographic surveys in detecting and locating active lesions. In severe or advanced disease, pathologic fractures do occur.

Patients in every category of mastocytosis sometimes experi-ence flushing or frank anaphylaxis. In occasional patients, ana-phylaxis may be provoked by alcohol, aspirin, exercise, or infec-tions.

Neuropsychiatric abnormalities have been reported. Problems include a decreased attention span, memory impairment, and irritability. Depression as a consequence of chronic disease or possibly mediated by mast cell products is a possibility.

DIAGNOSIS. The diagnosis of mastocytosis rests on histology, supported by clinical, biochemical, and radiographic data. Mast cells may be overlooked on histologic sections depending on the fixation and/or stain employed. The most useful stains for mast cells include metachromatic stains, such as toluidine blue and Giemsa, and enzymatic stains, such as chloroacetate esterase and aminocaproate esterase. These procedures highlight the granules in the cytoplasm of the mast cell, thereby facilitating identifica-tion. In trephine core bone marrow biopsies, decalcification interferes with subsequent attempts to visualize mast cell gran-ules, making their identification more difficult.

Fortunately, the majority of patients with mastocytosis have either urticaria pigmentosa or diffuse cutaneous mastocytosis, which can be recognized on physical examination. These diag-noses should be confirmed by skin biopsy. Blind skin biopsies are not recommended, as other skin conditions including eczema are associated with an increase in dermal mast cells.

In the absence of skin lesions, mastocytosis may be suspected in patients with one or several of the following: unexplained ulcer disease or malabsorption, radiographic or ^{99m}Tc bone scan abnor-malities, hepatomegaly, splenomegaly, lymphadenopathy, pe-ripheral blood abnormalities, and unexplained flushing or ana-phylaxis. Elevated levels of plasma or urinary histamine or histamine metabolites, prostaglandin D_2 metabolites in the urine, or plasma mast cell tryptase are not diagnostic but do raise the

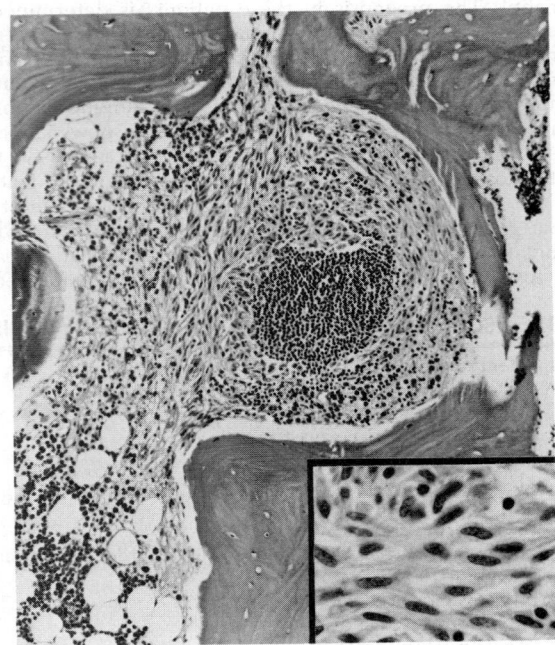

FIGURE 252–2. Bone marrow biopsy shows a characteristic lesion of systemic mastocytosis with nodular, paratrabecular infiltrate of mast cells surrounding a lymphoid aggregate. *Inset:* The mast cells are spindle-shaped, resembling fibroblasts or histiocytes. (Courtesy of W. D. Travis, Bethesda, MD.)

index of suspicion of mastocytosis. Reliable tests for these substances, however, are not generally available except in research laboratories.

Patients suspected of having mastocytosis in the absence of skin lesions should have a bone marrow biopsy and aspirate for diagnosis and categorization of the mastocytosis. Patients with urticaria pigmentosa or diffuse cutaneous mastocytosis should also have this procedure if they have peripheral blood abnormalities, hepatomegaly, splenomegaly, or lymphadenopathy, to determine if they have an associated hematologic disorder. Other tissue specimens, such as lymph nodes, spleen, liver, and gastrointestinal mucosa, define the extent of mast cell involvement but are usually obtained only as dictated by necessity. For example, gastrointestinal biopsies are obtained only if a gastrointestinal workup is indicated, and lymph nodes are biopsied only if lymphoma is considered.

Patients suspected of having mastocytosis should have 24-hour urine 5-hydroxyindoleacetic acid (5-HIAA) and urinary metanephrines measured to help eliminate the possibility of a carcinoid tumor or pheochromocytoma. It should be noted that patients with mastocytosis do not excrete increased amounts of 5-HIAA, suggesting that serotonin, reported in the mast cells of some species, is not synthesized by human mast cells. Idiopathic anaphylaxis and flushing must also be ruled out. Patients with these disorders do not have histologic evidence of significant mast cell proliferation.

TREATMENT. In all categories of mastocytosis, a primary objective of treatment is the control of mast cell mediator–induced signs and symptoms such as anaphylaxis, gastrointestinal cramping, and pruritus. H_1-receptor antagonists such as hydroxyzine and doxepin are helpful in reducing pruritus, flushing, and tachycardia. If insufficient relief occurs, the addition of an H_2 antagonist such as ranitidine or cimetidine may be beneficial. However, many patients continue to complain of bone pain, headaches, and flushing, resulting in part from the inability to block the effects of high levels of histamine with histamine antagonists and the presence of other mast cell mediators. Disodium cromoglycate (cromolyn sodium) is known to inhibit degranulation of mast cells and may have some efficacy in the treatment of mastocytosis. Epinephrine is used to treat episodes of anaphylaxis. Patients should be prepared to self-administer this drug. If subcutaneous epinephrine is insufficient, intensive therapy for anaphylaxis should be instituted. Patients with recurrent episodes of anaphylaxis may be placed on H_1 and H_2 antihistamines to lessen the severity of attacks. Episodes of profound anaphylaxis may be spontaneous but have also been observed following stings from insects.

Methoxsalen with long-wave ultraviolet radiation (PUVA) has been shown to relieve pruritus and whealing after 1 to 2 months of treatment. Relapse of pruritus occurs within 3 to 6 months after stopping treatment. Topical steroids can be used to treat extensive urticaria pigmentosa or diffuse cutaneous mastocytosis, although these lesions eventually recur after discontinuation of therapy.

Treatment of gastrointestinal disease is directed at controlling peptic symptoms, diarrhea, and malabsorption. Gastric acid hypersecretion leading to peptic symptoms and ulcerations is controlled with H_2 antagonists. Diarrhea is difficult to control, and H_2 antagonists are generally not effective. Anticholinergics may give partial relief. Malabsorption, if present, is difficult to manage. In patients with severe malabsorption, systemic steroids have been shown to be effective. Ascites is also difficult to manage. One patient with portal hypertension was successfully managed with a portacaval shunt. Another patient with an exudative ascites was treated successfully with systemic steroid therapy.

Patients with mastocytosis and an associated hematologic disorder are treated as dictated by the specific hematologic abnormality. In mast cell leukemia, chemotherapy has not yet been shown to produce remission or to prolong survival. Chemotherapy has no place in the treatment of indolent mastocytosis. A recent study suggested that splenectomy may improve survival in patients with poor prognostic forms of mastocytosis.

PROGNOSIS. Prognosis must be addressed separately for each category of mastocytosis. One study found seven variables that were strongly associated with poor survival. These included constitutional symptoms, anemia, thrombocytopenia, abnormal liver function tests, lobated mast cell nucleus, a low percentage of fat cells in the bone marrow biopsy, and an associated hematologic disorder. Other poor prognostic variables include absence of urticaria pigmentosa, male sex, absence of skin and bone symptoms, hepatomegaly, splenomegaly, and normal bone radiographic findings.

As a group, patients with indolent mastocytosis and skin involvement alone have the best prognosis. Among children with isolated urticaria pigmentosa, at least 50 per cent of cases resolve by adulthood. Adults with urticaria pigmentosa usually progress gradually to systemic disease and rarely may convert to type II disease. Diffuse cutaneous mastocytosis is usually associated with indolent systemic disease. Patients with mastocytosis with an associated hematologic disorder have a variable course dependent on the prognosis of their hematologic disorder. With mast cell leukemia, mean survival is less than 6 months. Survival with lymphadenopathic mastocytosis with eosinophilia is 1 to 2 years without therapy. The prognosis appears to improve with aggressive symptomatic management.

Cherner JA, Jensen RT, Dubois A, et al.: Gastrointestinal dysfunction in systemic mastocytosis: A prospective study. Gastroenterology 95:657, 1988. *This study describes patterns of gastrointestinal disease in mastocytosis and the implications for clinical management.*

Garriga MM, Friedman MM, Metcalfe DD: A survey of the number and distribution of mast cells in the skin of patients with mast cell disorders. J Allergy Clin Immunol 82:425, 1988. *A study of the value of determination of mast cell numbers in skin biopsies.*

Horny H-P, Kaiserling E, Campbell M, et al.: Liver findings in generalized mastocytosis: A clinicopathologic study. Cancer 63:532, 1989. *A survey of liver histopathology in mastocytosis.*

Schwartz LD, Metcalfe DD, Miller JS, et al.: Tryptase levels as an indicator of mast cell activation in systemic anaphylaxis and mastocytosis. N Engl J Med 316:1622, 1987. *Demonstration of mast cell tryptase in the serum of mastocytosis patients.*

Travis WD, Li C-Y, Bergstralh EJ, et al.: Systemic mast cell disease: Analysis of 58 cases and literature review. Medicine 67:345, 1988. *An excellent review of the histopathologic and clinical features of mastocytosis.*

253 Diseases of the Thymus

Daniel P. Stites

DEVELOPMENT, STRUCTURE, AND FUNCTION. The thymus, a central lymphoid organ, functions in the development and maintenance of immunologic competence. Arising embryologically from the third and fourth branchial clefts, it migrates caudad, as a bilobed organ, to the anterior mediastinum. Ectopic thoracic and cervical thymic rests are present in 30 per cent of normal individuals. The thymus enlarges until late puberty and then involutes, the lymphocytes and epithelial cells being nearly completely replaced with fat by the fifth or sixth decade. The normal thymus varies greatly in size. It is uniquely susceptible to marked involution within hours owing to the stress of serious illness or to treatment with glucocorticoids. The thymus is composed primarily of lymphocytes encased in a lattice of epithelial cells. It also contains a few myoid cells, macrophages, and plasma cells. The thymus is arranged into discrete lobules containing a cortex and medulla. Hassall's corpuscles are specialized aggregates of epithelial cells whose function is unknown.

The thymus begins to function by about 10 to 12 weeks of gestation when immunocompetent T cells can first be detected. Undifferentiated stem cells migrate to the thymus from fetal liver and bone marrow prenatally and from the bone marrow postnatally. Local influences, probably from epithelial cells, induce maturation of thymic lymphocytes, which then divide in the cortex, migrate to the medulla, and emigrate to the peripheral lymphoid tissue as mature T cells. The capacity for self- and nonself-recognition of antigens is conferred upon T cells at this phase within the thymus. The cortex is also the site of intense lymphopoiesis. The thymus secretes a variety of incompletely defined hormones that maintain T-cell competence in peripheral lymphoid organs. The immunosuppressive effects of thymectomy vary with age, being most pronounced at younger ages (see below). The thymus also appears to play an important role in maintenance of tolerance to various antigens, in immune surveillance, and possibly in leukemogenesis (as judged by animal experiments).

THYMIC HYPOPLASIA. Hypoplastic thymus may be either congenital or acquired. In neonates and infants, *congenital thymic hypoplasia* is expressed as marked T-cell and variable B-cell immunodeficiency. Resulting diseases include reticular dysgenesis, severe combined immunodeficiency disease, DiGeorge's and Nezelof's syndromes, and ataxia-telangiectasia (see Ch. 244). Essentially all of these patients are diagnosed in childhood; the severity of the thymic lesion, if untreated, rarely allows survival beyond age 10 or 12 years. Congenital thymic hypoplasia has been treated by thymic or bone marrow transplantation and by thymic hormone injections with variable success. *Acquired hypoplasia* or thymic involution occurs normally with age or results from stress (within hours or days), malnutrition, pregnancy, x-rays, glucocorticoids, or cytotoxic drugs. AIDS and graft-versus-host disease commonly produce severe thymic dysplasia.

THYMIC HYPERPLASIA. An enlarged thymus is very difficult to evaluate accurately because of its large normal variability in size. In the past, so-called status thymolymphaticus, a condition diagnosed with respiratory distress and large thymic shadow on chest roentgenogram, frequently led to unnecessary removal or radiation of normal thymuses. Individuals who received thymic irradiation for "enlarged thymus" have had significant increases in the incidence of thyroid cancer or adenoma. Extrathyroid tumors, particularly breast cancer, also increased slightly but there have been no increases in lymphoreticular malignancy, suggestive of immunodeficiency. The concept of status thymolymphaticus has been abandoned. The thymus may rarely enlarge in thyrotoxicosis, Addison's disease, anencephaly, acromegaly, castration, or tumors (see below). Thymic cysts are usually asymptomatic and the occasional association with neoplasia warrants resection.

THYMUS AND MYASTHENIA GRAVIS. Myasthenia gravis is an autoimmune disease caused by the presence of antiacetylcholine receptor (AchR) antibodies (see Ch. 509). In myasthenia gravis there is a 10 per cent incidence of thymoma. In fact detectable enlargement of the thymus in myasthenia gravis usually heralds the presence of a thymoma. In 65 per cent of cases the thymus is hyperplastic with increased numbers of germinal centers but not clinically enlarged. In the remaining 25 per cent of patients the thymus is normal. In large series of thymomas, 30 to 60 per cent of patients have myasthenia gravis. Rarely myasthenia gravis develops years after total thymectomy for thymoma, which militates against an absolute requirement for thymoma in the pathogenesis of this disorder. Neonatal myasthenia gravis occurs without any thymic abnormality, presumably owing to transplacental transfer of maternal antibody. There is little correlation with serum levels of anti-AchR antibody and clinical improvement in myasthenia following thymectomy. Damage to AchR antigen shared between muscles and thymic epithelial or myoid cells may explain the rather obscure relationship of the thymus to this autoantibody disorder.

EFFECTS OF THYMECTOMY. Total removal of the thymus during the neonatal period in rodents results in severe immunodeficiency, loss of T cells, and a wasting disease, a result of chronic unopposed infection. Thymectomy in adult animals, however, is associated with much subtler changes in T-cell function. What is the effect of thymectomy in humans? Because of the high incidence of extramediastinal thymic rests (30 per cent), thymectomy can rarely be considered total. Total thymectomy intentionally done during cardiothoracic surgery in children does not appear to result in compromised transplantation immunity. In patients with thymoma, a transient decrease in circulating lymphocytes and T-cell functions is noted. Following thymectomy for myasthenia gravis, functional loss in some T-cell populations occurs. However, the long-term effects of thymectomy, either in immunologically normal patients during cardiac surgery or in cancer patients with thymomas, are not known. These individuals should be carefully observed for development of autoimmune disease, infection, certain malignancies, or other signs of T-cell deficiency.

THYMOMA. *Definition.* A thymoma is a neoplasm of thymic epithelial cells. This definition excludes other tumors that may affect the thymus such as lymphoma, germ cell tumors, and carcinoid. Thymomas are rare; fewer than 1000 cases have been reported. Nevertheless, it is the most common tumor of the anterior superior mediastinum (see Ch. 69).

Pathology. Thymomas contain various proportions of epithelial cells and lymphocytes. The latter are T cells and may constitute a large proportion of cellular content of the tumor; hence the term *lymphoepithelioma.* Although their significance is unknown, the activated appearance of these lymphocytes suggests a host reaction to neoplastic epithelial cells. These T cells express surface markers such as CD1a and often such CD4 and CD8 which is characteristic of thymocytes rather than peripheral blood T cells. Various histologic degrees of malignancy from minimal cytologic atypia to undifferentiated carcinoma exist. However, correlation of microscopic appearance with clinical malignancy is notoriously poor. In fact, local invasion of pleura, pericardium, vessels, and nerves is the major criterion for determining clinical malignancy of the tumor.

Clinical Manifestations. Median age of patients with thymoma is about 50 years, and no sex predominance is noted. About 30 per cent of patients present with myasthenia gravis; another 30 per cent are asymptomatic, and the diagnosis is suggested by an anterior mediastinal mass on chest roentgenogram. The remaining 30 to 40 per cent of patients have a variety of symptoms and medical syndromes associated with the tumor (Table 253–1). Symptoms and signs include cough, chest pain, dysphagia, dyspnea, hoarseness, neck mass, and superior vena cava syndrome.

A few patients with spindle cell thymomas have marked *hypogammaglobulinemia.* Whether the relationship is causal is not established. The rare occurrence of red cell aplasia with or without immunodeficiency and thymoma raises the possibility of T cell–mediated suppression of erythropoiesis or immunoglobulin synthesis. Direct evidence to support these notions is only fragmentary.

Diagnosis. The presence of a round or oval anterior mediastinal mass visualized in posteroanterior and lateral chest roentgenograms in the presence of myasthenia gravis or of some other known systemic manifestations is suggestive of thymoma. Computed tomographic (CT) imaging with enhancing contrast media injection is useful in defining the size and location of thymomas and is occasionally useful in differentiating various thymic lesions. Thymic biopsy has no place in evaluation of anterior mediastinal masses, and mediastinoscopy is of little or no value. Some centers claim success with fine needle aspiration and cytology. Thoracotomy with adequate exposure to determine whether capsular invasion has occurred is needed for diagnosis of any thymic tumor. Differential diagnosis includes other primary or secondary thymic tumors (see below), cysts, posttraumatic hemorrhage, aneurysm, or other abnormalities of the anterior mediastinal contents including metastatic tumors, giant lymph node hyperplasia, mesothelioma, thyroid and parathyroid tumors, and paragangliomas (see Ch. 69).

Treatment. Surgical removal of tumor followed by local irradiation if extracapsular extension has occurred is the treatment of choice. Distant metastases are rare; the tumor spreads mainly by local invasion of adjacent structures.

Prognosis. The prognosis is nearly entirely dependent on presence of local invasion and cannot be predicted by histologic appearance of the tumor. Noninvasive thymomas are usually cured by excision. Patients with invasive thymoma have about 50 per cent 5-year survival.

TABLE 253–1. DISEASES ASSOCIATED WITH THYMIC TUMORS

I. Thymoma
    Myasthenia gravis
    Red cell aplasia
    Hemolytic anemia
    Neutrophil agranulocytosis
    Hypogammaglobulinemia (Good's syndrome)
    Systemic lupus erythematosus
    Polymyositis
    Pemphigus vulgaris
    Chronic mucocutaneous candidiasis
II. Carcinoid
    Cushing's syndrome
    Multiple endocrine neoplasia syndromes
    (see Ch. 228)

OTHER TUMORS OF THE THYMUS. *Thymolipoma* probably represents a lipoma arising within normal thymus. This tumor is usually radiolucent and asymptomatic and has not been associated with myasthenia gravis. *Carcinoid tumor* of the thymus arises from neuroendocrine cells within the thymus (see Ch. 230). Fifty per cent produce ACTH-like molecules and cause Cushing's syndrome or hyperparathyroidism, or are associated with multiple endocrine adenomatosis; 30 per cent are malignant and metastasize. Surgery and radiotherapy are indicated. *Carcinomas*, particularly squamous cell types, may rarely occur. *Germ cell tumors* rarely occur: seminoma, teratoma, teratocarcinoma, choriocarcinoma, embryonal cell carcinoma, and yolk sac tumors. The thymus may be involved by *malignant lymphomas*. T-cell lymphomas with acute lymphoblastic leukemia occur in the second decade. Cells from these tumors may have C receptors and are positive for terminal deoxynucleotidyl transferase. Hodgkin's disease usually is of the nodular sclerosing type (see Ch. 147 and 148).

Day DL, Gedgudas E: The thymus. Radiol Clin North Am 22:519, 1984. *A thorough review of thymic anatomy and function. Special emphasis on use of imaging techniques such as CT scans, sonography, and NMR is presented.*

Kornstein MJ, Hoxie JA, Levinson AI: Immunohistology of human thymomas. Arch Pathol Lab Med 109:460, 1985. *Careful phenotypic analysis with monoclonal antibodies of the surface phenotype of various thymomas.*

Namba T, Brunner NG, Grob D: Myasthenia gravis in patients with thymoma with particular reference to onset after thymectomy. Medicine 57:411, 1978. *Excellent review of literature on relationship of thymoma to myasthenia gravis with 72 locally studied cases.*

Salyer W, Eggleston JC: Thymoma. A clinical and pathological study of 65 cases. Cancer 37:229, 1976. *Clinicopathologic description of a large series of thymoma patients, annotating association with other medical syndromes.*

Shore RE, Woodard E, Hildreth N: Thyroid tumor following thymus irradiation. JNCI 74:1177, 1985. *Case control study of 2650 individuals who received thymic irradiation in infancy shows 30 cancers and 59 benign thyroid adenomas in an average of a 29-year follow-up period. No evidence for compromised imune function was detected based on absence of lymphoreticular malignancy.*

PART XIX
MUSCULOSKELETAL AND CONNECTIVE TISSUE DISEASES

254 Approach to the Patient with Musculoskeletal Disease

James F. Fries

The rheumatic diseases present a major challenge to clinical judgment. The chronicity, variability, tendency to exacerbate and remit, biochemical and immunologic complexity, unknown pathogenesis, variable response to specific treatment, and myriad effects upon the patient's lifestyle, family relationships, self-image, and employability combine to complicate the therapeutic equation. Difficult therapeutic decisions must often be made without adequate experimental justification and evaluated against a poorly understood natural history.

In the face of these tremendous uncertainties, contemporary management is relatively straightforward but has recently changed substantially. The therapeutic strategy has shifted from dogma to flexibility. Good management now requires that therapeutic decisions be based upon individual pathophysiology rather than upon diagnosis per se. Further, decisions are never final but are modified in a continuing feedback between application of treatment and observation of response. Decisions change over time as appropriate to the trends, tempo, and previous response of the particular patient. The art of medicine is reborn in the approach to a patient with a chronic disease. The principles underlying contemporary management strategy are set forth in this chapter and are divided into six major topics. The medical history, the physical examination, and the laboratory data, which are discussed in following chapters, are factors in decisions involving these six areas.

DETERMINING THE PATHOPHYSIOLOGY

Diagnosis is *not* the most important factor in selecting management of rheumatic disease. Modern management individualizes therapy within diagnostic categories, based upon subgroups of patients with differing prognoses and different therapeutic requirements. Patients with the same diagnosis often should be managed very differently. Patients with rheumatic disease frequently have features of several diagnostic entities at the same time.

Management in musculoskeletal disease is more closely linked to the underlying pathophysiologic process than to the diagnostic entity. Reversal of the pathophysiologic process (or negation of its impact) requires a clear visualization of that process. Even such a basic pathophysiologic concept as "inflammation" has different therapeutic implications. The inflamed synovial membrane (synovitis) typical of rheumatoid arthritis responds to a different spectrum of anti-inflammatory agents than does the inflammation of ligamentous insertions (enthesitis) typical of ankylosing spondylitis or the inflammation within the joint space induced by microscopic crystals.

Eight specific types of musculoskeletal problems can be readily distinguished by history and physical examination in most patients

and can provide a framework for pathophysiologic categorization. Identification of the predominant pathophysiology in a given patient is usually straightforward. The eight categories are discussed in the following paragraphs and are listed in Table 254–1, together with the prototype disease of the category, examples of the most useful laboratory tests for that category, and the typical treatments required. Management implications for each category are surprisingly distinct and provide guidelines for laboratory investigation and initial treatment. Location of the process is shown in Figure 254–1.

SYNOVITIS. Inflammation of the synovial membrane, with gradual damage to surrounding joint structures, is most strikingly manifested in rheumatoid arthritis. The synovium is tender, thickened, and palpable and may demonstrate warmth and, less often, redness. Joint destruction is caused by the enzymatic products of inflammation and develops slowly over many years. Management is based upon reducing the *rate* of damage to joint structures, and agents directed at retardation of progression (disease-modifying antirheumatic drugs, or DMARD's) should

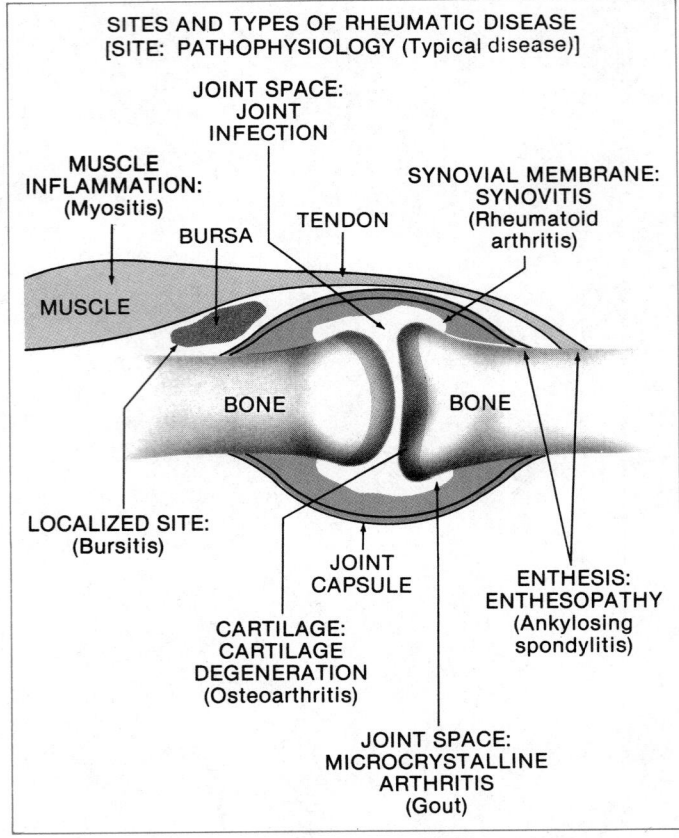

FIGURE 254–1. Location of musculoskeletal disease processes.

usually be employed early in the course and continually throughout. The sedimentation rate is consistently elevated with significant synovitis, and the latex fixation or other tests for rheumatoid arthritis are often useful for further categorization. A wide range of pharmacologic and other treatments may be required, and many patients require sequential trials with a variety of agents. Some useful drugs for synovitis, such as gold, penicillamine, and hydroxychloroquine, have not been proved therapeutically effective in any other category.

ENTHESOPATHY. Inflammation in these diseases is most marked at the enthesis, that transition region where ligament attaches to bone. Such inflammation is the hallmark of a family of rheumatic diseases typified by ankylosing spondylitis and linked to the human leukocyte antigen (HLA)–B27. The distribution of involvement follows the location of regions of enthesis throughout the body. The marked predilection for the sacroiliac joints, heels, and spine identifies a process affecting areas characterized by ligament and tendon attachment. This specific pathophysiology provides a unifying basis for the clinical features of the diseases and their typical response to specific therapy. Rheumatoid factor is predictably absent from the serum. Nonsteroidal anti-inflammatory drugs (NSAID's)—in particular, indomethacin, phenylbutazone, and naproxen—are therapeutically effective and usually are well tolerated over the long term. The spectrum of effective anti-inflammatory drugs used for enthesopathy is different from that in synovitis. Prednisone, for example, is neither indicated nor effective in most patients.

CARTILAGE DEGENERATION. Degenerative and other processes can cause fraying and destruction of the articular cartilage, with subsequent injury to the underlying subchondral bone. This occurrence is usually termed osteoarthritis (or osteoarthrosis), and a group of specific syndromes is recognized within this category. Narrowing of the apparent joint space and development of bone spurs make radiography the most useful investigative procedure; other ancillary tests are usually negative. Few patients have significant inflammation, and it is not surprising that anti-inflammatory treatment is not of great use. The analgesic effects of aspirin or NSAID's may be helpful; doses required for optimal pain relief are often considerably less than doses required for anti-inflammatory effects. Medical treatment is symptomatic and is seldom dramatically effective.

CRYSTAL-INDUCED SYNOVITIS. Microcrystalline arthritis occurs when crystals forming in the synovial fluid (or injected therein) induce an acute inflammatory reaction in the joint fluid and the surrounding synovium. Gout is the prototype disease, with the inflammation induced by crystals of monosodium urate. Similar syndromes may occur with crystals of several other types. The syndrome increases to very intense inflammation within a period of hours and spontaneously resolves without treatment over a period of a few days to a few weeks; this resolution can be markedly accelerated with treatment. The physical factors underlying crystal formation determine that only one or, at most, a few joints are involved at a time. The crucial laboratory observation is inspection of the aspirated joint fluid for crystals under polarized light microscopy. Drugs inhibiting polymorphonuclear leukocytes are particularly effective, as exemplified by colchicine, a drug with little effect in any other rheumatic disease category.

JOINT INFECTION. The synovium encloses a body space that can be the site of direct infection by microorganisms. Critical to investigation of the patient with suspected joint infection is aspiration and culture of the joint fluid and, in many instances, culture of other body fluids as well. Treatment consists principally of prescribing an antibiotic specific for the microorganism involved. Drainage may be required.

MYOSITIS. Inflammation of muscle occurs in two closely related diseases, dermatomyositis and polymyositis, and in an unrelated condition, polymyalgia rheumatica. Determination of muscle enzyme levels and histologic examination of involved muscle may be the critical laboratory observations. In polymyalgia, the sedimentation rate is greatly elevated and is often the sole objective finding. Temporal artery biopsy may be useful when giant cell arteritis is demonstrated. Corticosteroids are almost always required in inflammatory muscle disease and, in contrast to every other rheumatic disease category, are usually required from the outset.

FOCAL CONDITIONS. A wide variety of conditions affecting the musculoskeletal system do not truly warrant the term "disease." Tendinitis, bursitis, low back strain, calcific tendinitis, and other entities can affect almost any area of the body and are the most common of all medical problems. Laboratory aids are few, although radiography may occasionally be useful in locating calcium deposits or spurs or in ruling out fracture. The therapeutic imperative in localized problems (unfortunately often neglected) is to emphasize localized rather than general treatment measures. Treatment of the entire organism for a problem in one local area is seldom rewarding. The use of splints, slings, heat, and local injection is usually the most reasonable initial approach.

GENERALIZED CONDITIONS. A variety of poorly defined entities fall into this category. Terms such as "fibromyalgia" and the "chronic muscle contraction syndrome" are sometimes used to indicate the likelihood of organic disease characterized by sleep disturbance and tender points. The terms "psychogenic rheumatism," "nonarticular rheumatism," and "depressive equivalent" are frequently used to suggest a psychological etiology. These patients are rich in symptoms but poor in objective evidence of pathology. The conditions may be extremely troublesome for the individual but are not progressive and do not result in physical crippling. Laboratory tests, such as the sedimentation rate, give normal results and are employed only to rule out other categories of illness. Treatment is best termed "conservative." The therapeutic approaches to other categories are unlikely to be beneficial, and the physician who attempts pharmacologic intervention rather than reassurance, lifestyle counseling, and support often ends with a drug-dependent patient who gets no better.

These eight categories and the brief descriptions presented are supported by generalizations to which there are some exceptions. However, Table 254–1 summarizes quite specific starting points at which the laboratory investigation and therapeutic approach should begin. The experienced physician soon moves far beyond this table, but it provides a particularly useful framework upon which to place the more detailed clinical knowledge found in the following chapters.

USING THE LABORATORY SELECTIVELY

Laboratory tests in patients with the rheumatic diseases usually provide confirmatory data rather than conclusive evidence. After the three exceptions of (1) the sacroiliac radiograph in ankylosing spondylitis, (2) the identification of specific crystals within the joint fluid, and (3) a positive bacteriologic culture from joint fluid, laboratory tests have varying degrees of lack of sensitivity and lack of specificity and, except in the unusual case, add relatively little to clinical assessment. As a result, the majority of patients presenting with musculoskeletal problems do not require a great amount of laboratory evaluation. The key to appropriate use of the laboratory is selective use. Every test should have a specific indication, and blind "surveys" or "panels" should not be used.

TABLE 254–1. CATEGORIES OF RHEUMATIC DISEASE

Pathology	Prototype	Most Useful Tests	Typical Treatment
Synovitis	Rheumatoid arthritis	Latex, erythrocyte sedimentation rate	Gold
Enthesopathy	Ankylosing spondylitis	Sacroiliac radiographs, HLA-B27	Indomethacin
Cartilage degeneration	Osteoarthritis	Radiographs of affected area	Analgesic
Crystal-induced synovitis	Gout	Joint fluid crystal examination	Colchicine
Joint infection	Staphylococcal	Joint fluid culture	Antibiotics
Myositis	Dermatomyositis	Muscle enzymes, muscle biopsy	Corticosteroids
Focal conditions	Tennis elbow	None, radiographs of affected area	Localized
Generalized conditions	Fibrositis	Erythrocyte sedimentation rate	Conservative

One in six visits by a patient to a health professional is for a musculoskeletal complaint. The great majority of such visits to physicians occur for the common "focal conditions" of life. Low back pain, sprained ankles, tennis elbows, and other common musculoskeletal complaints account for most initial visits. Most such problems are easily identified as self-limited. Optimal management includes ruling out more significant illness, advice about activity or rest, reassurance, occasionally symptomatic medication, and transmission of the expectation that the natural healing process will resolve the difficulty. The usual healing period for local musculoskeletal problems ranges from 2 to 6 weeks, depending upon the magnitude of the often inapparent injury, with the healing process beginning again from the start if there is reinjury during this period. Healing cannot be pharmacologically accelerated. Thus, optimal treatment usually requires "masterly inactivity," with confident reliance upon the natural healing process. Inappropriate vigor with testing or treatment can lead to investigative mishaps, therapeutic side reactions, and an intensity of focus upon the problem inappropriate to its magnitude. The careful clinician uses time to establish the trends and tempo of the condition; time is used to demonstrate the self-limited native condition while avoiding the hazards of inappropriate response.

The critical initial decision, therefore, is whether the problem requires immediate action or whether the decision to investigate or treat can be postponed until the course of the disease and the magnitude of the appropriate response may be better estimated. A 6-week "rule of thumb" is appropriate. In the absence of specific indication or immediate threat, a waiting period of 6 weeks from onset of symptoms serves to minimize inappropriate use of laboratory tests or treatment. Four major exceptions to the 6-week rule obtain. First, a condition that is severe and involves a single joint (or, at most, a few joints) is much more likely, paradoxically, to require immediate attention than is a widespread polyarthritis. Acute gouty arthritis and infections, the usual causes of the "single hot joint," require immediate attention. By contrast, in rheumatoid arthritis, a period of 6 weeks is required even before the criteria for diagnosis can be met, and management in the first days of disease is most appropriately conservative. Many "probable rheumatoid arthritis" patients actually have minor problems that disappear as the viral or minor hypersensitivity reaction subsides. These patients need not be given the emotional burden of a "serious" diagnosis.

Second, a patient who is febrile, systemically ill, and otherwise showing signs of major disease deserves immediate attention. Endocarditis, neoplasm, tuberculosis, and other illnesses are frequently identified through musculoskeletal clues, and a connective tissue disease with systemic manifestations deserves immediate attention.

Third, if the problem is associated with significant trauma, the possible need for immediate orthopedic management should be considered. Fourth, an associated neurologic problem, such as carpal tunnel syndrome, sciatic nerve compression, or cervical nerve root compression may be benefited by immediate attention.

In practice, these four indications for immediate action are relatively unusual. The large majority of patients with initial complaints involving the musculoskeletal system are not found to have conditions requiring either intensive efforts at diagnosis or employment of hazardous therapy.

ESTABLISHING MANAGEMENT GOALS

The impact of disease has too often been defined in terms of numerically expressed test results. The level of autoantibodies, titer of rheumatoid factor, number of radiographic erosions, and sedimentation rate too often become the criteria for therapeutic success. The patient and family are more directly interested in a different list of disease endpoints: in survival, in normal mobility and function, in absence of pain and other symptoms, and in the ability to remain solvent through the duration of a chronic illness. These five "D's" (death, disability, discomfort, drug toxicity, and dollar cost) are the major dimensions of the patient's outcome in the patient's own terms.

In the rheumatic diseases the frequent "trade-offs" among several outcomes must be based upon the values perceived by the particular patient. For example, pain may be reduced by narcotics but disability increased; disability may be reduced by cyclophosphamide but a risk of death incurred; or short-term symptomatic relief by plasmapheresis may be obtained at very high cost.

Establishment of goals must precede development of the individual management strategy. In some instances, a limited goal, such as regaining the ability to walk, may be dramatically useful to the patient and far more valuable than a modest reduction in the general severity of the disease. Some worthy goals may not be achievable in a particular instance, and their pursuit may only increase therapeutic toxicity. The question of what is desirable is subordinate to the question of what is achievable.

PLANNING FOR OPTIMAL LONG-TERM OUTCOME

Hospital-based training tends to focus attention on improving the patient's status by the time of discharge. In chronic illness, such short-term benefits may be desirable but illusory. Corticosteroids, narcotic analgesics, and intra-articular injections often provide obvious short-term benefit. Unfortunately, the agent that provides the best initial response sometimes may lead to iatrogenic disaster over the longer term.

The therapeutic strategy for synovitis has held that simple and less toxic measures should be used first, and hazardous medications withheld unless the simpler approaches fail. Recently, however, it has become recognized that because of severe and prevalent gastric damage, aspirin and NSAID's are more toxic than previously thought and that some DMARD's are relatively well tolerated. As a result, management of synovitis has tended toward earlier and more consistent reliance upon DMARD's, which have a far superior toxic-therapeutic ratio. The old "pyramidal" strategy is being abandoned in favor of a serial DMARD strategy designed to reduce the rate of joint damage.

The inexperienced clinician is often trapped by taking the short view of a chronic illness. A chronic disease cannot be managed by short-term tactics; it requires a long-term strategy, shared and negotiated with the patient.

Such a strategy requires tactical modification at nearly every physician-patient encounter. At each visit, new information is always present, even if only the information about what transpired in response to the last set of decisions. A decision is thus followed by observation, then by further decision, then by another period of observation. The decision strategy is flexible and, in the final analysis, frequently empiric.

USING A COMPLETE CLINICAL REPERTOIRE

Treatment of musculoskeletal disease is frequently discussed in terms of pharmacologic agents. This myopic view neglects the dominant contributions often afforded by reconstructive surgical procedures, by the use of appliances and devices to allow handicapped individuals to function more normally, by exercise to strengthen bones and tissues, or by personal interaction to increase the motivation and improve the self-image of the patient.

A drug-based strategy tends to find its greatest use in early, systemic, inflammatory disease processes. Orthopedic approaches tend to have the greatest utility if the number of joints or regions involved is small, if major problems are concentrated in a single anatomic region, or after an inflammatory process has "burned out." Improvement after occupational therapy is often seen in patients with moderate to major disability who require adaptive devices to render the environment more friendly. Confidence in the ability to live an independent life sometimes can be more important than any specific therapy, and patient confidence (personal efficacy) is a useful therapeutic adjunct. Medical therapy that interferes with mental or emotional adaptation frequently makes things worse.

The novice at managing rheumatic diseases employs only a limited therapeutic repertoire. Typically, the patient requires a diverse program individualized to specific needs and making use of a variety of different disciplines. Development of rational strategies requires intimate knowledge of the strengths and weaknesses of all therapeutic modalities. The physician cannot manage chronic musculoskeletal diseases effectively without knowledge of the techniques of complementary disciplines or a good working relationship with individuals who possess these skills.

ACHIEVING UNDERSTANDING BY THE PATIENT

The informed patient is the physician's greatest single asset in managing chronic illness. Consider even the recommendation that a patient should take aspirin. The lay media describe the hazards of aspirin, colloquialisms associate aspirin with neglect by the physician, and the over-the-counter availability suggests a minor remedy. Yet, for anti-inflammatory treatment with aspirin, the physician may aim for a narrow therapeutic range far above the dose the patient expects. While establishing dosage, the patient is almost certain to encounter one or another side effect, even though the aspirin later may be well tolerated. The informed patient must know that anti-inflammatory and analgesic activities of aspirin are different, that a particular therapeutic range is important, that the drug is active against the inflammatory process itself, and that several weeks may be required to see the full effects of the drug. In the absence of such understanding, it is unusual for a patient to do well on aspirin; education of the patient is a prerequisite for therapeutic success.

Most clinicians believe that patients with positive expectations have better outcomes. While causality is not established by this belief, it is reasonable to assume that restoration of hope and a positive self-image are beneficial parts of treatment. The patient with arthritis is under intense psychological pressures. Self-image is threatened by diseases that may cripple and prevent remunerative employment. The fear of dependence upon others is often present. Yet prognosis is generally better than that anticipated by the patient. The physician who is unaware that every patient with arthritis has significant fears may do great harm by inadvertently increasing those fears.

In addition, the informed patient is more likely to comply with a particular therapeutic regimen. The patient's report of success or failure with previous recommendations is essential for the next clinical decision and must be as accurate as possible, again emphasizing the need for direct patient-physician communication. Unrealistic expectations followed by perceived therapeutic failures are a major cause of a burgeoning business in quack treatment. The patient must be educated to recognize the falsity of overstated claims and the losses in courage, independence, and money that may result. The obscenity of the quack who makes a living by defrauding patients focuses the attention upon the outrage. At the more important level, however, the patient susceptible to the claims of the quack does not have a confident and informed relationship with his or her personal physician.

The management of musculoskeletal disease is directed in large part at maintenance of the independence of the individual. Most persons with arthritis can be independent and healthy individuals despite their musculoskeletal condition. This independence is the final goal of the individualized management strategy.

Fries JF: Toward an understanding of patient outcome measurement. Arthritis Rheum 26:697, 1983. *Review of the concepts and practice of assessment of long-term outcome and the clinical implications thereof.*
Fries JF, Holman HR: Estimating prognosis in systemic lupus erythematosus. Am J Med 57:561, 1974. *Introduction to the concepts of subsets of disease and individualization of prognosis and treatment choice.*
Fries JF, Miller SR, Spitz PW, et al.: Toward an epidemiology of gastropathy associated with non-steroidal anti-inflammatory drug use. Gastroenterology 96:647, 1989. *Review of drug side effect frequency and prevalence, with emphasis upon common, severe, and largely preventable complications.*
Kelley WN, Harris ED, Ruddy S, et al.: Textbook of Rheumatology. 3rd ed. Philadelphia, W.B. Saunders Company, 1989. *Definitive textbook of 2000 pages and many thousand references covering all aspects of rheumatology.*
Schumacher HR (ed.): Primer on the Rheumatic Diseases. 9th ed. Atlanta, Arthritis Foundation, 1988. *Classic, authoritative, current descriptions of all rheumatic diseases and indeed of all rheumatology, available as a public service at nominal cost.*

255 Connective Tissue Structure and Function

Steffen Gay and Renate E. Gay

One of the fundamental characteristics of all connective tissues is the relatively large proportion of extracellular matrix in relation to cells. Until recently, the extracellular matrix was viewed as a passive framework serving mainly as an inert scaffolding for stabilization of the physical structure of tissues. In addition to maintaining this three-dimensional form during morphogenesis and tissue repair, it is now recognized as a dynamic milieu in which cells become organized, exchange signals, and differentiate. Study of these processes has led to discovery of a plethora of new matrix components, matrix receptors, and cell-matrix interactions. The extracellular matrix is composed of multidomain macromolecules that are linked together by covalent and noncovalent bonds to form a highly intricate composite. Two major types of matrices exist: the *interstitium*, which is synthesized by mesenchymal cells and forms the stroma of organs, and the *basement membranes*, which are produced by epithelial and endothelial cells. These matrices comprise four major classes of extracellular macromolecules: (1) the collagens, (2) elastin, (3) noncollagenous glycoproteins, and (4) glycosaminoglycans, which are usually covalently linked to proteins to form proteoglycans.

COLLAGENS. The collagens are the most abundant class of proteins in the human organism, constituting almost 30 per cent of its total protein. The central feature of all collagen molecules is the stiff structure resulting from lengthy domains of triple-helical conformation. Three polypeptide chains, called α chains, are wound around one another to generate a ropelike fold. An absolute requirement for the formation of this triple helix, as well as the most distinctive feature of the α chains, is the presence of lengthy sequences of repeating Gly-X-Y triplets in which the X and Y positions are frequently occupied by prolyl and hydroxyprolyl residues.

Studies based on protein chemistry and complementary DNA (cDNA) sequencing have revealed a genetically determined heterogeneity with as many as 18 homopolymeric or heteropolymeric collagen types. As of this writing, 13 distinct collagen types collectively composed of 25 unique polypeptide chains have been identified. It is of interest that genes coding for the different chains are distributed among several chromosomes in the human genome (Table 255-1). Even simultaneously expressed genes, such as those coding for the two α_1 (I) and one α_2(I) chains of the heteropolymeric type I molecule, are located on different chromosomes. The diversity of the well-defined collagens is reflected by the existence of three distinct forms of general molecular structure. The first of these is represented by the lengthy and essentially linear structure assumed by the triple-helical molecules of the fiber-forming collagens. In contrast, basement membrane collagen type IV molecules contain numerous interruptions of helical conformation within the triple-helical domain, which result in highly flexible molecules. The third molecular form is exemplified by cartilage type IX molecules. These molecules contain three collagenous and four interspersed noncollagenous domains. Most remarkable is the presence of a single chondroitin sulfate chain linked to the noncollagenous domain (NC3) of the $\alpha2$(IX) chain.

Functional diversity of the various collagen types is accomplished by formation of distinct extracellular aggregates. The most obvious are the interstitial linear polymers of fibrils, derived from collagen types I, II, and III. These fibrils with characteristic banding patterns can be readily visualized by electron microscopy. Type I collagen fibers are found in supporting elements of high tensile strength (e.g., tendon and cornea), whereas fibers formed from type II collagen molecules are restricted to cartilaginous structures. The fibrils derived from type III collagen are prevalent in more distensible tissues, such as blood vessels and parenchymal organs. In addition, collagen types V, VI, IX, and XII are also involved in fiber formation, but largely as adducts. This finding is illustrated by the association of collagen types IX, X, and XI with type II collagen in hyaline cartilage. Adaptation for a special function is shown by type VII collagen molecules, which aggregate as antiparallel overlapping dimers to form the anchoring fibrils required to stabilize the dermoepithelial junction of the skin. In contrast to the interstitial types of collagen, type IV molecules form large polygonal aggregates fulfilling the structural and support requirements of basement membranes.

ELASTIN. Elastic fibers are composed of two morphologically and structurally distinct components: elastin and the microfibrils. Elastin, whose gene has now been characterized, is an insoluble protein polymer. The biosynthetic precursor of elastin, tropo-

TABLE 255–1. POLYMORPHISM OF THE COLLAGEN TYPES

Type	Chain(s)	Locus on Chromosome	Major Molecular Species	Major Distribution
I	α1(I)	17q21.3–q22.05	$[\alpha1(I)]_2\alpha2(I)$	Skin, tendon, bone, organ capsules
	α2(I)	7q21.3–q22.1		
II	α1(II)	12q13.1–q13.3	$[\alpha1(II)]_3$	Hyaline cartilage
III	α1(III)	2q31	$[\alpha1(III)]_3$	Blood vessels, parenchymal organs
IV	α1(IV)	13q34	$[\alpha1(IV)]_2\alpha2(IV)$	Basement membranes
	α2(IV)	13q34		
	α3(IV)	—		
	α4(IV)	—		
	α5(IV)	—		
V	α1(V)	—	$[\alpha1(V)]_2\alpha2(V)$	Smooth muscle
	α2(V)	2q31		
	α3(V)	—		
VI	α1(VI)	21q223	$[\alpha1(VI),\alpha2(VI),\alpha3(VI)]$	Minor collagen of stoma matrices
	α2(VI)	21q223		
	α3(VI)	2q37		
VII	α1(VII)	—	$[\alpha1(VII)]_3$	Anchoring fibrils of the dermoepidermal junction
VIII	α1(VIII)	—	$[\alpha1(VIII)]_3$	Descemet's membrane, sclera, dura mater
IX	α1(IX)	6	$[\alpha1(IX),\alpha2(IX),\alpha3(IX)]$	Hyaline cartilage
	α2(IX)	—		
	α3(IX)	—		
X	α1(X)	—	$[\alpha1(X)]_3$	Hypertrophic cartilage
XI	α1(XI)	1p21	$[\alpha1(XI),\alpha2(XI),\alpha3(XI)]$	Hyaline cartilage
	α2(XI)	6p212		
	α1(II)	12q13.1–q13.3		
XII	α1(XII)	—	—	Tendons, ligaments, periosteum
XIII	α1(XIII)	10q11	—	Skin, gut

elastin, is a linear polypeptide composed of about 700 amino acids and is rich in nonpolar amino acids: glycine (>30 per cent), valine, leucine, isoleucine, and alanine. Tropoelastin is synthesized by vascular smooth muscle cells and skin fibroblasts and subsequently incorporated into elastic fibers. Elastic fiber formation involves lysyloxidase-mediated formation of intermolecular crosslinks, called desmosine and isodesmosine. Since these crosslinks do not exist in other proteins and therefore are elastin specific, determination of these two amino acid derivatives in tissue sample reflects the amount of elastin present. The microfibrillar component of interstitial elastic fibers is not fully characterized. However, disulfide-rich glycoproteins, such as *fibrillin*, have been identified and may serve as a scaffold onto which tropoelastin is deposited.

STRUCTURAL GLYCOPROTEINS. The major noncollagenous glycoprotein present in the extracellular matrix is *fibronectin*. Fibronectins are dimeric cell adhesion glycoproteins, composed of two disulfide-bonded subunits and found in rather large quantities in blood plasma (~0.3 mg per milliliter). The diverse functions of fibronectin in cell adhesion are illustrated in Figure 255–1. Some of these functions can be mimicked by synthetic peptides that contain the sequence Arg-Gly-Asp (RGD sequence). Similar sequences are found in other cell adhesion proteins, such as vitronectin, laminin, and collagen type VI. Since fibronectin plays a major role in morphogenesis and tissue remodeling, the regulation of fibronectin biosynthesis by growth factors and cytokines has been a focus of study. For example, it is now established that γ-interferon and transforming growth factor–β

(TGF-β) stimulate fibronectin synthesis, whereas tumor necrosis factor (TNF) and interleukin 1 (IL1) inhibit synthesis.

Vitronectin is a 75-kD protein, which is considerably smaller than the 250-kD fibronectin polypeptide present in plasma and tissue. Vitronectin, also termed serum spreading factor and complement S-protein, promotes cell attachment and spreading, inhibits cytolysis by the complement C5b–9 complex, and modulates antithrombin III–thrombin action in blood coagulation.

Tenascin/hexabrachion is another large glycoprotein of the extracellular matrix. The name hexabrachion refers to the disulfide-linked six-armed structure. Tenascin mediates cell attachment through an RGD-dependent receptor and is expressed in association with mesenchymal-epithelial interactions during morphogenesis and development of undifferentiated tumors. The same protein has also been referred to as myotendinous antigen, GP 250 protein, glial mesenchymal extracellular matrix protein, cytotactin, J1-protein, and brachionectin. As the names suggest, tenascin has been identified in tendons, developing smooth muscle, cartilage, and gut and in neuromuscular and neuronal-glial interactions.

Cartilage Glycoproteins. Several structural glycoproteins have been isolated from various cartilages. They include a 148-kD protein prominent in adult tracheal cartilage, but not present in articular cartilage. On the other hand, articular cartilage contains a 116-kD protein as well as two distinct proteins of 58 kD and 59 kD, which are all localized throughout the interstitial matrix.

PROTEOGLYCANS. Proteoglycans are proteins that carry one or more glycosaminoglycan side chains. Glycosaminoglycans

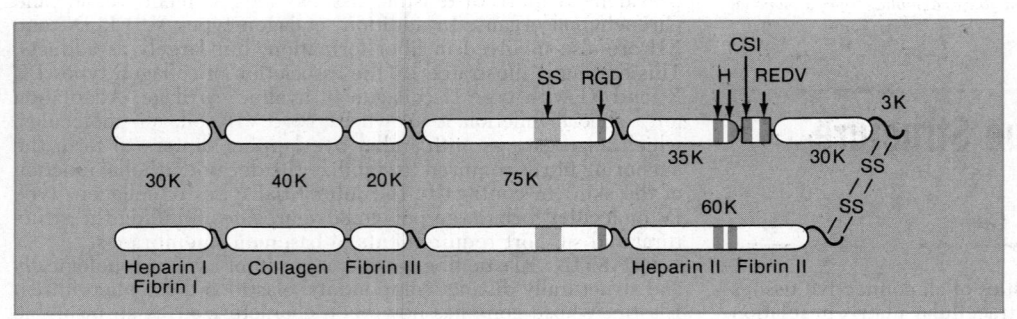

FIGURE 255–1. Multiple cell recognition sites in fibronectin. The fibronectin molecule contains a series of functional domains that bind the indicated ligands. The thick vertical bars indicate cell adhesive recognition sequences. SS = putative synergistic second site; RGD = Gly-Arg-Gly-Asp-Ser site; H = putative sites in the heparin-binding domain; CS1 = the CS1 site in the alternatively spliced IIICS region; REDV = the Arg-Glu-Asp-Val site. (Reprinted with permission from Yamada KM: Fibronectins: Structure, functions and receptors. Curr Opin Cell Biol 1:956–963, 1989. Copyright 1989 by Current Science.)

are long, unbranched polysaccharide chains composed of repeating disaccharide units. One of the two sugar residues in the repeating disaccharide is always an amino sugar (*N*-acetylglucosamine or *N*-acetylgalactosamine). Glycosaminoglycans are highly negatively charged owing to the presence of sulfate and carboxyl groups on multiple sugar residues. In contrast, hyaluronic acid, also called *hyaluronan*, is a polymer of glucuronic acid and glucosamine that is not sulfated and not attached covalently to a protein core connected via a link protein. Proteoglycans of almost all sizes and shapes have been biochemically identified. Nevertheless, since cloning and sequence analysis have often identified the same core proteins, the number of distinct proteoglycans is limited (Table 255–2). With respect to their function, they have been referred to as a "multipurpose glue." Proteoglycans not only bind extracellular matrix components together and mediate cell binding to the matrix but also restrain soluble molecules such as growth factors in the matrix and at cell surfaces. Heparan sulfate proteoglycan, for example, binds basic fibroblast growth factor released from injured endothelial cells. The role of proteoglycans in cell adhesion is best exhibited by a membrane-intercalated proteoglycan termed *syndecan*. This molecule binds to collagen and fibronectin through its heparan sulfate chains and mediates cell adhesion.

BASEMENT MEMBRANES. Basement membranes are thin, sheetlike structures deposited by endothelial and epithelial cells but also found surrounding nerve and muscle cells. They provide mechanical support for resident cells, function as a semipermeable filtration barrier for macromolecules in organs such as the kidney and the placenta, and act as regulators of cell attachment, migration, and differentiation. The major constituents are collagen type IV, laminin, entactin (nidogen), and heparan sulfate proteoglycans. Collagen type IV molecules are $[\alpha1(IV)]_2$ $\alpha2(IV)$ heterotrimers comprising an N-terminal rod 30 μm long (7S), a linear triple helix containing over 20 noncollagenous sequences, and a C-terminal globular domain (NC1). These molecules can spontaneously aggregate into a network consisting of N-terminal tetramers (7S), lateral associations between the triple-helical rods, and C-terminal dimers (NC1). The network is eventually stabilized by disulfide- and lysyloxidase-derived intramolecular and intermolecular crosslinks, which may provide the scaffold for basement membrane formation. Self-assembly has also been observed with *laminin*, a major basement membrane–associated glycoprotein. The typical features of the laminin molecule are a threadlike long arm terminating in a globular domain and three short arms, each consisting of two globular domains separated by short linear segments. Collagen type IV and laminin appear highly integrated in the basement membrane matrix and are closely associated with a 150-kD, sulfated glycoprotein called

TABLE 255–2. PROTEOGLYCANS (PG) CHARACTERIZED BY SEQUENCING OF THE CORE PROTEIN

Proteoglycan	Glycosaminoglycan
Secreted/extracellular matrix PG	
Large aggregating PG	CS/KS*
Versican	CS/DS
Decorin (PG-40, PGII)	CS/DS
Biglycan (PGI)	CS/DS
Basement membrane PG	HS
Type IX collagen	CS
Intracellular granule PG	
Serglycin (PG19)	CS/DS
Membrane-intercalated PG$_S$	
Syndecan	HS/CS
Invariant chain†	CS
Transferrin receptor†	HS
Thrombomodulin†	HS
Lymphocyte-homing receptor†	CS

*CS = chondroitin sulfate; DS = dermatan sulfate; HS = heparan sulfate; KS = karatan sulfate. These glycosaminoglycans are polymers consisting of the repeating disaccharides: glucuronic acid–*N*-acetylgalactosamine (CS), iduronic acid–*N*-acetylgalactosamine (DS), iduronic acid–*N*-acetylglucosamine (HS and heparin), and galactose-*N*-acetylglucosamine (KS). DS, HS, and heparin also contain some disaccharide units in which the uronic acid is glucuronic acid instead of iduronic acid.

†These are so-called "part-time proteoglycans"; only some of the molecules are substituted with glycosaminoglycan, and the rest are free protein molecules.

Reprinted with permission from Ruoslahti J: Proteoglycans in cell regulation. J Biol Chem 264:13369–13372, 1989.

entactin (nidogen) in a stable noncovalent complex. Amino acid sequence data of entactin have revealed epidermal growth factor (EGF)–like cysteine-rich motifs, segments showing homology to the EGF precursor, the low density lipoprotein (LDL) receptor, and thyroglobulin. *Heparan sulfate proteoglycans* occur as an integral component in all basement membranes but play different roles in specific tissues. They control permeability of the glomerular basement membranes and have also been implicated in the anchorage of acetylcholinesterase to the neuromuscular junction.

CONNECTIVE TISSUE MATRIX IN CELL REGULATION

It is now well established that matrix components influence the maintenance of cellular phenotypes mediated through matrix receptors.

RECEPTORS FOR EXTRACELLULAR MATRIX COMPONENTS. Adhesive interactions between cells and their surrounding extracellular matrix are not only important in most developmental events but also essential for maintaining the fundamental life processes. Cell proliferation, polarization, migration, differentiation, and protein synthesis depend on interactions between cells and supporting matrix. Diverse families of structurally similar receptors for matrix components have been identified. They include the transmembrane integrin superfamily, peripheral membrane glycoproteins, glycosyltransferases, and proteoglycans. *Integrins* are a group of α/β heterodimers involved in cell binding, some of which involve recognition of an Arg-Gly-Asp (RGD) sequence present in their ligands. The integrins consist of an α-subunit with a molecular mass of 130 to 210 kD and noncovalently associated β-subunits (95 to 130 kD). The cytoplasmic domain of the β-subunit reveals homologies to the EGF, the insulin receptor, and the *neu* oncogene protein. Both subunits define the integrin subfamilies described in Table 255–3.

Since integrins localize in known junctional regions where actin bundles and myofibrils terminate at the cell surface, the major function of integrin receptors appears to be the linkage of extracellular matrix molecules with the intracellular cytoskeletal network. The connection is thereby mediated through the cytoplasmic domain of the β-subunit. That extracellular matrix components may influence gene expression by signal transduction is shown by the finding that fibronectin degradation products induce, via the fibronectin receptor, collagenase and stromelysin gene expression. The latter pathway may play a major role in inflammatory tissue destruction. The pivotal role of these receptors related to infectious diseases is further illustrated by the observation that bacteria use specific receptors to adhere to host connective tissue. For example, it has been shown that certain strains of *Escherichia coli* express a fibronectin receptor that is involved in colonization.

Nonintegrin peripheral membrane glycoproteins serve as matrix receptors in cell binding to laminin and elastin. Whereas integrin laminin receptors bind to the globular end of the long arm of the molecule, a nonintegrin 67-kD receptor binds to a site in the laminin β1 chain. Other nonintegrin matrix receptors have been shown to be restricted to cells of neural origin or chondrocytes. In this regard, a 34-kD protein that binds to cartilage type II collagen has been isolated and termed *anchorin II*. Anchorin II contains segments that are related to a family of Ca^{2+}- and phospholipid-binding proteins, including calpactin, lipocortin, and endonexin. A 90-kD transmembrane glycoprotein, also known as gp90 Hermes or Hermes antigen, mediates lymphocyte binding to the high endothelium of venules during their movement into lymphoid organs. These observations stress that cell-cell and cell-matrix interactions involve multiple types of receptors.

The most provoking question remains: how do matrix receptors transmit information from the extracellular structure to affect gene expression? Figure 255–2 illustrates a model of "dynamic reciprocity," in which the extracellular matrix is postulated to influence gene expression at all levels, including transcription, messenger RNA (mRNA) processing, and translation, via transmembrane and cytoskeletal components. Elucidating the molec-

TABLE 255–3. THE INTEGRIN FAMILY OF CELL RECEPTORS*

Subunits	Designation	Ligands	Distribution
α1β1	VLA-1; CD-/CD29	Collagens I and IV, laminin	F, BM, aT
α2β1	VLA-2; CD49b/CD29	Collagens I, III, IV, V, and VI	F, En, Ep, aT, Pl
α3β1	VLA-3; CD-/CD29	Collagens I and IV, laminin, fibronectin	F, Ep
α4β1	VLA-4; CD49d/CD29	Fibronectin	F, Nc, T, B, M
α5β1	VLA-5; CD-/CD29	Fibronectin	F, En, Ep, aT, Th
α6β1	VLA-6; CD49f/CD29	Laminin	En
αLβ2	LFA-1; CD11a/CD18	Cell adhesion molecules (ICAM-1, 2)	T, B, M, G
αMβ2	Mac-1; CR3; CD11b/CD18	Fibrinogen, Factor X, C3bi	M, G
αXβ2	p150,95; CD11c/CD18	C3bi	M, G
αIIbβ3	gpIIb, IIIa; CD41/CD61	Fibronectin, fibrinogen, von Willebrand factor	Pl
αVβ3	VNR; CD51/CD61	Fibrinogen, von Willebrand factor, vitronectin (VN)	En
αEβ4	—	—	Ec
αVβ5	CD51/CD-	Fibronectin, vitronectin	Ca

*Cloning of the α- and β-subunits has revealed cell-surface proteins on other cells. These include the very late activation (VLA) antigens and the lymphocyte function–associated antigen 1 (LFA-1)/Mac-1/p 150.95 on leukocytes and the platelet IIb/IIIa glycoprotein.

F = fibroblasts; BM = basement membrane associated; aT = activated T lymphocytes only; En = endothelial cells; Ep = epithelial cells; Pl = platelets; Nc = neural crest melanocytes; T = T lymphocytes; B = B lymphocytes; M = monocytes; Th = thymocytes; G = granulocytes; Ca = UCLA-P3 lung adenocarcinoma cells.

Adapted from Springer TA: Adhesion receptors regulate antigen-specific interactions, localization, and differentiation in the immune system. Prog Immunol Springer 7:121–130, 1989.

ular mechanisms of this message system remains one of the key challenges in cell biology.

PATHOPHYSIOLOGY OF CONNECTIVE TISSUE

Some confusion remains about the role of collagen in a wide variety of diseases involving the connective tissues. Historically, the term "collagen disease"—describing a heterogeneous group of acute and chronic diseases, including rheumatoid arthritis, systemic lupus erythematosus, progressive systemic sclerosis, polymyositis, dermatomyositis, Sjögren's syndrome, arteritis, rheumatic fever, ankylosing spondylitis, and amyloidosis—was based on the erroneous notion that "collagen" was equivalent to "connective tissue." However, as outlined above, the different types of collagen and the macromolecular aggregates derived

from them are now recognized as distinct structural and histologic entities that exist within a meticulously intercalated connective tissue matrix along with structural glycoproteins and proteoglycans. Consequently, no justification exists for use of the anachronistic term "collagen disease" to encompass a group of such diseases initiated by vastly different pathomechanisms and affecting distinct connective tissue entities. The term "collagen diseases" now exclusively pertains to those inherited conditions in which the primary defect has been demonstrated to be at the gene level and to affect collagen biosynthesis, posttranslational modification, or extracellular processing directly. Recent technologies of gene cloning and gene analysis have led to the delineation of mutations in the fibrillar collagen genes. Collagen type I is the target of certain genetic mutations associated with classic clinical variants of dwarfing syndromes, osteogenesis imperfecta, and Ehlers-Danlos syndrome (types IV and VII) (see Ch. 186, 188, and 189). Moreover, polymerase chain reaction amplification of a series of overlapping segments encoding for the entire helical and telepeptide regions of the human α1(I) collagen cDNA is expected to identify potentially all mutations and polymorphisms.

The acquired disorders of connective tissue involving collagen include conditions that result in repair from overt trauma; in diseases characterized by an excessive deposition of collagenous

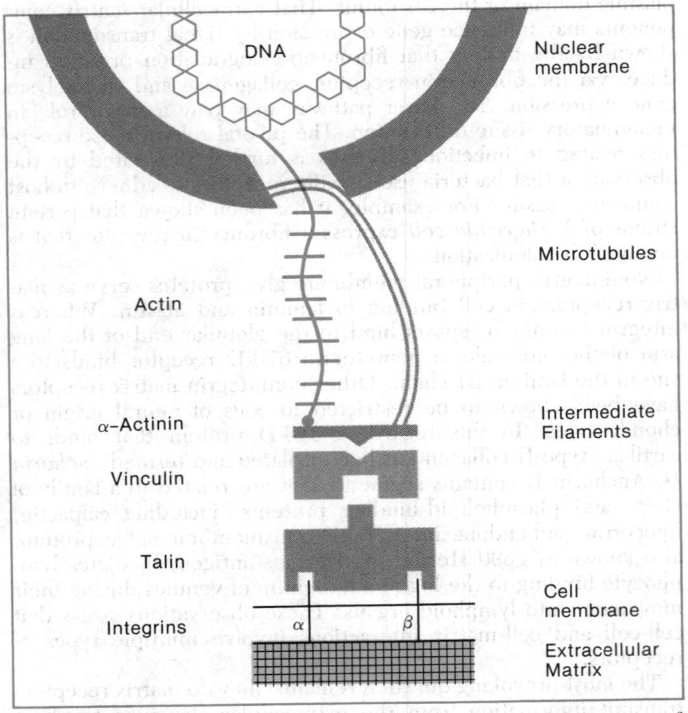

FIGURE 255–2. This refined model for the ultrastructural interaction of cells with extracellular matrix is based on a model of "dynamic reciprocity" whereby the extracellular matrix is postulated to exert an influence on gene expression via transmembrane proteins and cytoskeletal components, proposed originally by Bissell and Carcellos-Hoff (J Cell Sci [Suppl] 8:327, 1987).

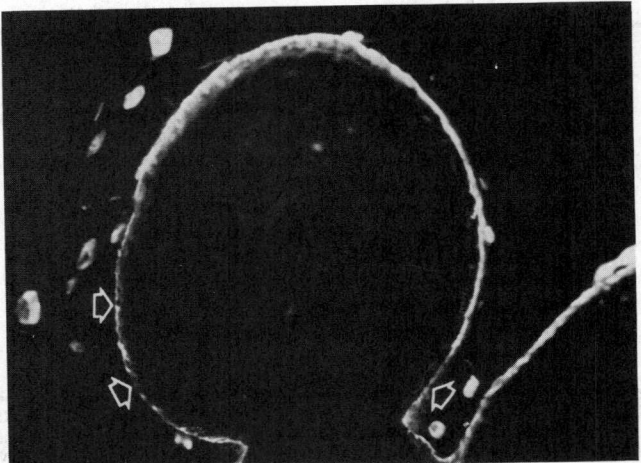

FIGURE 255–3. Frozen section of carcinoma in situ of the breast stained with monoclonal antibodies against human collagen type IV and fluorescence-labeled immunoglobulin antimouse G (IgG). In contrast to other atypical hyperplastic lesions, a thinning and focal loss of basement membrane integrity (arrows) is frequently observed in carcinoma in situ and suggests foci of preceding microinvasion.

FIGURE 255–4. Distribution of collagen types in a normal and rheumatoid joint. The normal synovial lining cell layer is supported by a loose fibrillar network composed of interstitial collagen types I and III, but lacking a continuous basement membrane. Basement membrane collagen type IV is restricted to the vascular endothelium. Vascular smooth muscle cells and pericytes are surrounded with fine, filamentous collagen type V, which is further associated with the interstitial fibers. The vast majority of the interstitial cartilaginous matrix is derived from type II collagen. Collagen types V, IX, and XI are distinctly associated with the hyaline articular interstitium. Synovial fluid normally does not contain collagen. Therefore, detection of collagen in synovial fluid and phagocytes indicates erosive and/or inflammatory joint disease. Detection of type IV collagen suggests endothelial damage and, if found concomitantly with type V collagen, implicates actual necrosis of the vessel walls, i.e., vasculitis. The detection of type I collagen indicates a high level of proteolytic breakdown of synovial stroma and/or bone matrix. Since type II collagen is restricted to the cartilage, the appearance of type II collagen epitopes in synovial fluid and serum represents a sensitive indicator of cartilage destruction and may serve as a tool for monitoring the effects and side effects of antirheumatoid drug therapy. (Reprinted with permission from Gay S, Gay RE: Cellular basis and oncogene expression of rheumatoid joint destruction. Rheumatol Int 9:105–113, 1989.)

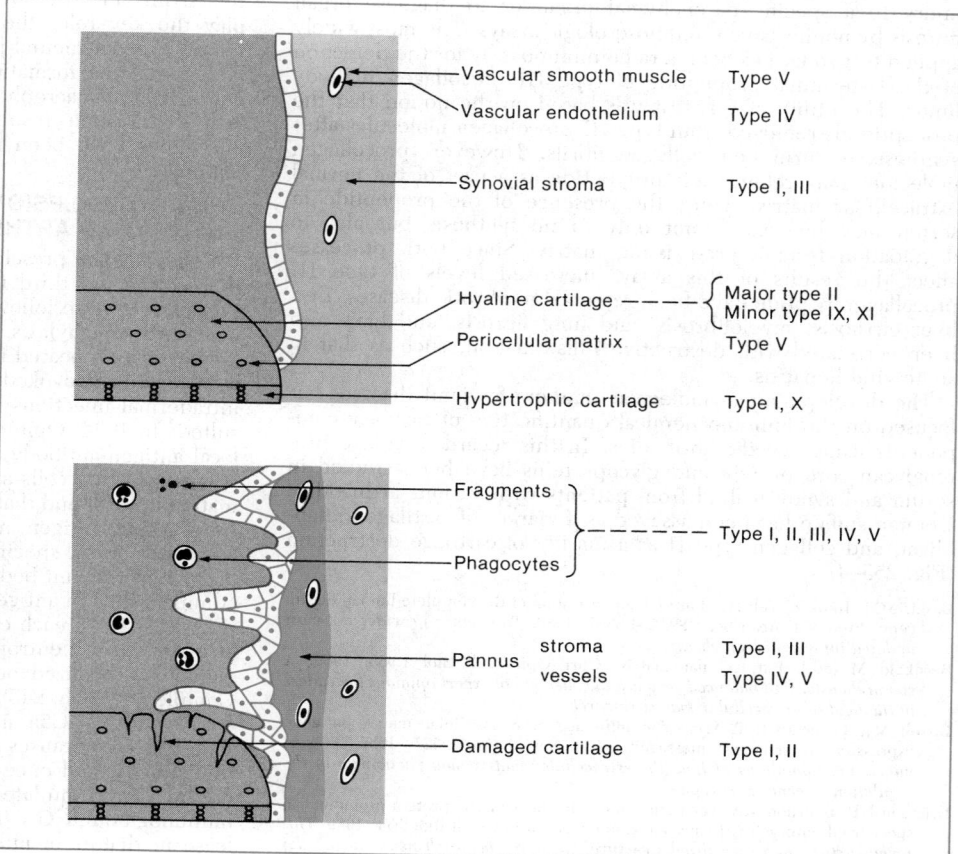

matrix, i.e., fibroproliferative disorders; or in pathologic loss of tissue matrix, including the breakdown of basement membranes in tumor invasion and rheumatoid joint destruction.

Although connective tissue repair after trauma is largely dependent on the type of injury and is, therefore, quite variable, the repair of various connective tissue lesions in wound healing follows a characteristic sequence of events. The initial events involve the synthesis of pericellular and basement membrane collagens in the proliferating epithelial and/or endothelial cells. Subsequently, a loose fibrillar network largely comprising fibronectin and collagen types III and V and single interspersed fibers derived from type I collagen are deposited. Finally, with the formation of scar tissue, the lesions become more fibrous and dense owing to a deposition of collagen fiber bundles derived largely from type I molecules. It is striking that the patterns of collagen deposition in fibroproliferative diseases show certain similarities. For example, damage to the liver is characterized by an initial accumulation of basement membrane collagens in the sinusoidal space of Disse, followed by a fine fibrillar material composed largely of type III collagen and, subsequently, in the case of the development of hepatic fibrosis (cirrhosis, Ch. 122), by an augmented deposition of type I collagen. A similar pattern appears in the development of fibrotic plaques in atherosclerosis (Ch. 47) or the development of cyclosporine-induced myocardial fibrosis in the transplanted human heart.

The major disease affecting almost exclusively the matrix of basement membranes is diabetes mellitus (Ch. 218). The histopathologic hallmark of diabetic microvascular disease is generalized basement membrane thickening. In the kidney, these changes include an increase in glomerular basement membrane permeability followed by decreased glomerular filtration. Evidence exists that accelerated nonenzymatic glycosylation (glycation) plays an important role in the development of diabetic microangiopathy.

The loss of a specialized connective tissue matrix plays a pivotal role in tumor progression and metastasis. With proliferation, malignant tumor cells acquire the capability to invade basement membranes actively and to migrate through the interstitial stroma. Despite the fact that tumor invasion requires a complex sequence of steps, such as the expression of receptors for basement membrane components by the malignant cells, invasion ultimately results in a loss of basement membrane integrity (Fig. 255–3). Severe recessive dystrophic epidermolysis bullosa features a loss of collagen type VII anchoring filaments, which normally connect the epidermal basement membrane to the interstitial matrix of the dermis. In Goodpasture's syndrome, basement membranes are damaged by circulating autoantibodies against basement membrane collagen (Ch. 79). The Goodpasture antigen has been mapped to the C-terminal globular domain of type IV collagen, which explains the high cross-reactivity of the anti–glomerular basement membrane antibodies with alveolar basement membranes.

CONNECTIVE TISSUE MARKERS. The enormous progress in our knowledge of the structure and biology of the connective tissue matrix has caused considerable interest in the development of assays for diagnosis and monitoring therapy in diseases involving connective tissue. Historically, the determination of hydroxyproline as a measure of total collagen content or turnover has been a useful technique in connective tissue research. However, with the discovery of collagen polymorphism and a variety of molecules containing collagenous sequences, the measurement of hydroxyproline now appears to be of only limited value. This observation is based on the fact that there are varying levels of hydroxylation of the different collagens. For example, the type III collagen molecule contains about 30 per cent more hydroxyproline than does type I, and other proteins such as C1q, acetylcholinesterase, and elastin also contain hydroxyproline. Specific immunohistologic and immunoserologic assays have been employed to evaluate the complexity of collagenous proteins in normal and pathologic samples. As illustrated in Figure 255–3, the use of a monoclonal antibody specific for collagen type IV has been advantageous in studies assessing the integrity of basement membranes in neoplastic lesions. Several markers of collagen assembly and turnover have been employed to detect injury to a specific parenchymal organ or to diagnose organ fibrosis by noninvasive immunoserologic assays. The most widely applied test so far has been a radioimmunoassay for the detection of the N-terminal propeptide of type III procollagen in body fluids. The utility of this test was based on the notion that the propeptide is removed from type III procollagen molecules after synthesis to form new collagen fibrils. However, procollagen molecules may retain their propeptide as a part of the normal extracellular matrix. Thus, the presence of the propeptide in serum may be related not only to neosynthesis but also to degradation from a pre-existing matrix. Since both processes affect the results of this assay, increased levels of type III procollagen peptide have been reported in fibrotic diseases, i.e., liver cirrhosis, myelofibrosis, and lung fibrosis, and have also been correlated with destructive inflammation, such as that in acute viral hepatitis.

The development of molecular markers for joint diseases has focused on the immunochemical quantification of cartilage components using specific antibodies. In this regard, cartilage proteoglycan core protein and glycoproteins have been studied in serum and synovial fluid from patients with various arthritides. Keratan sulfate has been assayed as a marker of cartilage metabolism, and collagen type II as a marker of cartilage destruction (Fig. 255–4).

Bashir MM, Indik Z, Yeh H, et al.: Characterization of the complete human elastin gene. Proc Natl Acad Sci USA 264:8887, 1989. *This paper provides the most updated information on elastin.*

Bernfield M (ed.): Extracellular matrix. Curr Opin Cell Biol 1:953, 1989. *A comprehensive and balanced review and collection of expert opinions by leaders in the field of extracellular matrix research.*

Bissell MJ, Carcellos-Hoff MH: The influence of extracellular matrix on gene expression: Is structure message? J Cell Sci (Suppl) 8:327, 1987. *A most interesting hypothesis of how the extracellular matrix may participate in the regulation of gene expression.*

Erickson HP, Bourdon MA: Tenascin: An extracellular matrix protein prominent in specialized embryonic tissues and tumors. Annu Rev Cell Biol 5:71, 1989. *This review article on a specialized structural glycoprotein supplements the articles edited by Bernfield.*

Labhard ME, Hollister DW: Segmental amplification of the entire helical and telopeptide regions of the cDNA for human alpha 1(I) collagen. Matrix 10:124, 1990. *An example of the kind of experimental techniques that are currently applied in hereditary disorders of connective tissue using polymerase chain reaction amplification.*

Lindh E, Thorell JI (eds.): Clinical Impact of Tissue and Connective Tissue Markers. London, Academic Press, 1989. *This book is the proceedings of a recent conference on the use of connective tissue markers.*

McDonald JA: Receptors for extracellular matrix components. Am J Physiol 257:L331, 1989. *A review on how cells interact with matrix via specialized integrin and nonintegrin receptors.*

Miller EJ, Gay S: Collagen structure and function. In Cohen IK, Diegelmann RF (eds.): Wound Healing: Biochemical and Clinical Aspects. Philadelphia, W. B. Saunders, 1991. *A complete review on the biochemistry of collagens.*

Rojkind M: Connective Tissue in Health and Disease. Boca Raton, Fla. CRC Press, 1990. *A review on animal models of human connective tissue diseases and methodologies that are applied in current research of organ fibrosis.*

Ruoslahti J: Proteoglycans in cell regulation. J Biol Chem 264:13369, 1989. *A most concise review of the complex roles different proteoglycans play in cellular regulation.*

Sanderson RD, Lalor P, Bernfield H: B lymphocytes express and lose syndecan at specific stages of differentiation. Cell Regul 1:27, 1989. *An example of the role of a most recent proteoglycan named syndecan in the differentiation of B lymphocytes.*

256 Mechanisms of Tissue Injury in Rheumatic Diseases

Gerald Weissmann

Acute inflammation and tissue injury in the rheumatic diseases are caused by host defense mechanisms that have been designed to attack bacteria or viruses but are instead diverted into an attack on the tissues of the host. The two major inflammatory diseases of rheumatology are rheumatoid arthritis (RA) and systemic lupus erythematosus (SLE), and we understand their pathophysiology thanks to three well-studied models of experimental pathology. Whereas some of their *acute* lesions resemble the Arthus and the Shwartzman reactions, in which neutrophils play the key role, the *chronic* features of RA mimic another model of experimental pathology, the tuberculin reaction and its late granuloma formation, in which cytokines, growth factors, and activated macrophages predominate. Joint injury and cartilage degradation result when synovial cells in which protooncogenes have been activated form an invasive lesion called *pannus*.

THE ARTHUS LESION AS A MODEL FOR RHEUMATOID ARTHRITIS

Following the prescient observation of Magendie in 1839 that the second and third intravenous injections of foreign proteins into rabbits were followed by increasing distress, Richet coined the word anaphylaxis in 1902 to describe acute catastrophes mediated by repeated intravenous injections of antigens. Arthus, in 1903, then provoked "local anaphylaxis" in rabbits by repeated intradermal injections of antigen; inflammation and necrosis resulted. In 1924, Opie confirmed that the lesions of Arthus were local antigen-antibody reactions in which inflammation was mediated by white cells and that proteolysis was critical. In confirmation it was found that the Arthus lesions could also be provoked by planting antigen in the skin followed by the intravenous administration of specific antibody (the "passive Arthus" reaction) or by injecting antibody in the skin followed by the intravenous administration of antigen (the "reversed passive Arthus" reaction) (Fig. 256–1). In each case, one was dealing with the interactions at a surface of neutrophils that had been attracted by immune complexes localized beneath the endothelium of blood vessels. Complement (Ch. 243), activated by immune complexes, releases anaphylatoxins (C5a and C3a), which liberate histamine. Histamine, in turn, causes reversible gaps to appear between endothelial cells, and once breached, the junctions permit egress of neutrophils. Stimulated by discrete receptors for C5a, C3a, and immunoglobulin G's (IgG's) (FcγRII, FcγRIII), neutrophils release mediators of inflammation: reactive oxygen-derived products (O_2^-, H_2O_2), eicosanoids (see below and Ch. 29), and lysosomal enzymes. These products—especially O_2^-, H_2O_2, and proteases—cause irreversible tissue injury. Predictably, Arthus reactions can be abolished by rendering animals deficient in complement or in neutrophils. Antiproteases or antihistamines are somewhat less effective inhibitors of the Arthus lesion; antiplatelet agents or anticoagulants are useless. It is generally agreed that the local Arthus lesion is one model for immune complex vasculitis in humans, which is also due to interactions of neutrophils with immune complexes and complement. In generalized vasculitis of the Arthus type, the *homotypic* clumping of neutrophils to one another and their *heterotypic* sticking to endothelial cells are mediated by receptors for iC3b (CD11b/CD18), whereas the secretory responses of neutrophils are triggered by receptors for C5a and FcγRII.

The central role of neutrophils in this lesion is mirrored by their abundance in the synovial fluid of patients with RA. Their role in *periarteritis nodosa, leukocytoclastic vasculitis*, some of the *vasculitis of SLE*, and *allergic angiitis* is equally important. Although the *raison d'être* for the preponderance of neutrophils in rheumatoid synovial fluid is not yet clear, their sheer number is impressive. Neutrophils constitute more than 90 per cent of cells found in the synovial fluid of patients with RA, and it has been estimated that the turnover of neutrophils in 30 ml of a rheumatoid joint effusion is greater than a billion. The cells take up self-associating complexes of IgG-IgG rheumatoid factor as well as the more common immunoglobulin M (IgM)–IgG complexes; complement is, predictably, activated. *Rheumatoid vasculitis* is another extra-articular problem mediated by neutrophils in seropositive RA patients. Histologic study of the blood vessels of patients with rheumatoid vasculitis associated with hypocomplementemia has shown a predominantly neutrophilic infiltrate, in response to antigen-antibody complexes and depositions of complement in vessel walls.

THE SHWARTZMAN PHENOMENON AS ANOTHER MODEL OF VASCULITIS

Culture filtrates of gram-negative bacteria injected into the skin of rabbits prepare the site for hemorrhagic necrosis when

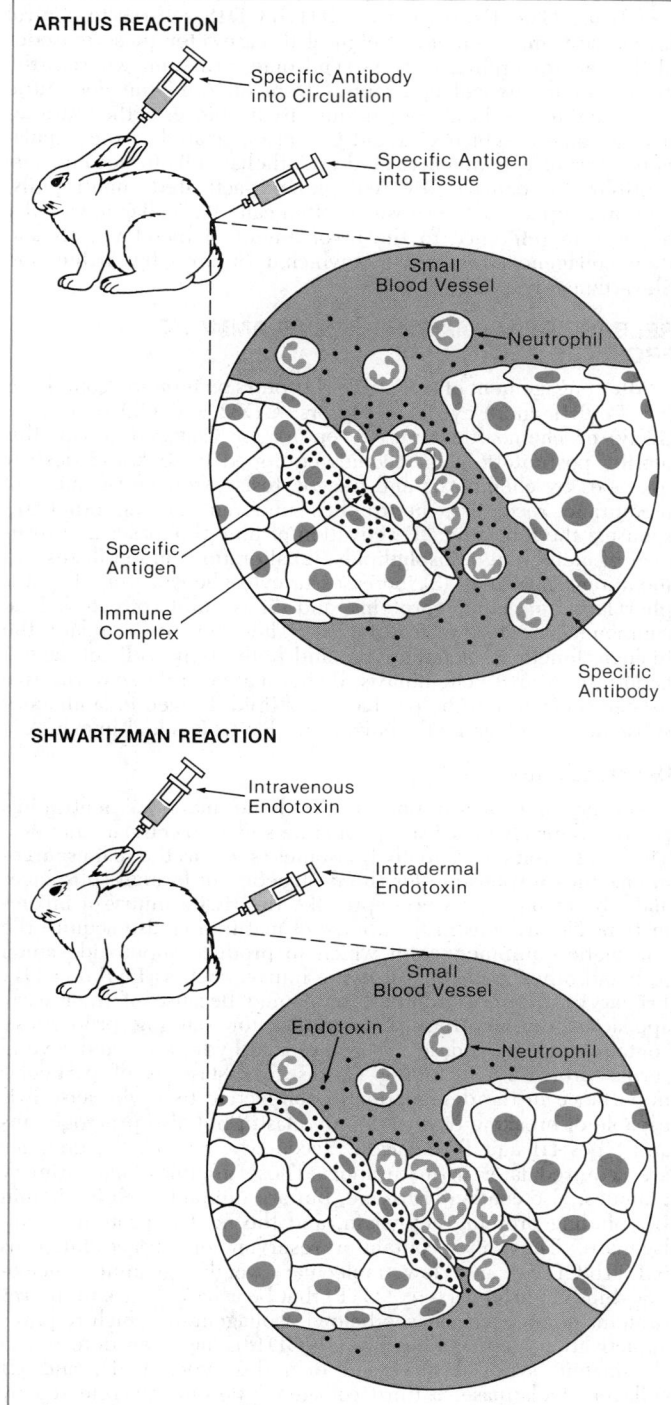

ARTHUS REACTION

Specific Antibody into Circulation

Specific Antigen into Tissue

Small Blood Vessel

Neutrophil

Specific Antigen

Immune Complex

Specific Antibody

SHWARTZMAN REACTION

Intravenous Endotoxin

Intradermal Endotoxin

Small Blood Vessel

Endotoxin

Neutrophil

FIGURE 256–1. In the Arthus model of vascular injury in systemic lupus erythematosus (SLE) *(top)*, intradermal injection of an antigen following intravenous injection of specific antibody leads to immune complex (IC) deposition in vessel walls at the intradermal injection site, which triggers local complement activation, inflammation, neutrophil infiltration, and tissue destruction. In the Shwartzman model *(bottom)*, an intradermal injection of the antigen leads to intravascular alternate pathway complement activation. Antibody is not required, and no IC's are formed. Instead, neutrophils, primed by endotoxin and activated by complement, aggregate within small blood vessels at the intradermal injection, plugging them and causing distal ischemia.

similar filtrates are injected intravenously, a finding first made by Gregory Shwartzman in 1937. The two lesions require a latent, or "preparatory," period of 6 to 24 hours, and the second injection need not be of the same filtrate (Fig. 256–1). The systemic reaction, or "generalized Shwartzman phenomenon," provokes variable degrees of pulmonary or systemic vasculitis and bilateral

renal cortical necrosis as its signature. Like the local lesion, it can be faithfully reproduced by purified endotoxins. Locally or systemically, the *preparatory* injection of endotoxin promotes modest adhesion of neutrophils to postcapillary venules, with escape of some of the white cells from the vessels. The second, or *provocative*, injection leads to microclumps of platelets and leukocytes within the circulation, and these tend to be sequestered in peripheral capillary beds or to attach to the sticky endothelium of venules of the prepared skin site.

The Shwartzman phenomenon can be elicited by second injections not only of endotoxin but also of various polyanions, glycogen, or antigen-antibody complexes, all of which share with endotoxin the capacity to activate complement via the alternate pathway. Moreover, local and systemic Shwartzman reactions can be prevented by rendering animals deficient in complement or neutrophils. In contrast to their inefficacy in the Arthus lesion, anticoagulants and antiplatelet drugs block the local and systemic Shwartzman phenomena. The final Shwartzman lesion is an intravascular insult with secondary damage to endothelial cells. It should be emphasized that the Shwartzman lesion is therefore an exception to the usual circumstances, in which neutrophils fail to injure the endothelial cell layer from which they escape in response to chemoattractants.

Our modern interpretation of the Shwartzman phenomenon is based on recent studies with endotoxin-induced tumor necrosis factor–α (TNF-α) and cellular adhesive molecules displayed by activated endothelial cells and neutrophils. In both the local and the systemic lesions, endotoxin elicits the formation of interleukin 1 (IL1) by Langerhans cells, endothelial cells, or tissue histiocytes and of IL1 and TNF-α from macrophages. These cytokines render venous endothelium sticky—"prepared" in Shwartzman's terms—by inducing the display of adhesive, ligand-like molecules, such as endothelium-leukocyte adhesion molecule 1 (ELAM-1), and by enhancing the procoagulant activity of endothelial surfaces (see below). The enhanced stickiness of endothelial cells induced by endotoxin, TNF, or IL1 leads to *heterotypic* cell-cell adhesion of neutrophils via activation and upregulation of the adhesive integrin CR3 (CD11b/CD18) on the neutrophil surface. The local sites, or small venules in the systemic Shwartzman reaction, have thus been prepared with adherent neutrophils. Some of the neutrophils will already have emigrated to the subendothelium (a noncytotoxic event).

The second, provocative, injection of endotoxin, glycogen, or immune complexes now causes massive *homotypic* neutrophil clumping. With C5a as the major culprit, neutrophils release inflammatory mediators, such as OH_2^-, H_2O_2, eicosanoids, platelet activating factor (PAF), and lysosomal enzymes. As when complement is activated in experimental and clinical examples of the adult respiratory distress syndrome (ARDS; see Ch. 71), leukoaggregates become enmeshed in small capillaries, where the procoagulant effects of endotoxin (via platelets and Factor X) contribute to plugging of the vessels (Fig. 256–2). Tissue injury has been chiefly attributed to H_2O_2 and elastase. Adhesion of neutrophils to endothelial cells—as provoked by TNF, for example—is antagonized by another cytokine: transforming growth factor–β (TGF-β), which in turn is the most potent chemoattractant yet described.

It has now been appreciated that complement-mediated neutrophil aggregation may contribute not only to tissue injury in such diverse conditions as *ARDS, acute pancreatitis, Purtscher's retinopathy, acute thermal injury*, and the *extension of myocardial infarction* but also—especially in SLE—to florid vascular crises. Sera from patients with active SLE contain several factors (among them C5a) that cause normal neutrophils to aggregate. Neutrophil-aggregating activity correlates with the activity of the disease and is most pronounced in patients with central nervous system involvement. The availability of radioimmunoassays specific for complement split products permitted documentation of elevated levels of circulating C3a, C5a, and the C5b–9 membrane attack complex in patients with active SLE. Indeed, elevated C3a levels may predict flares of SLE, rising 2 months before disease becomes clinically apparent. Moreover, complement split products Ba and Bb (generated exclusively by the alternate pathway) are also elevated in active SLE; elevated levels of Ba and Bb are better predictors of clinical disease than are conven-

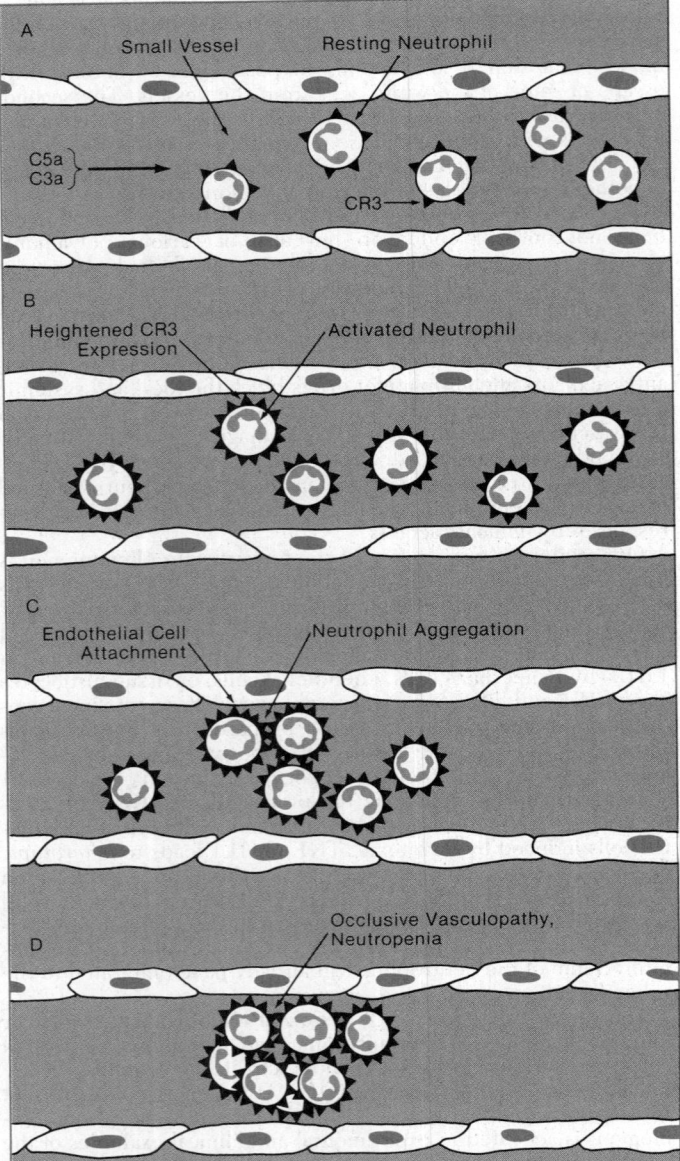

FIGURE 256–2. In active SLE, the process of intravascular complement activation, complement split product (CSP) release, and neutrophil activation may critically involve C5a stimulation of neutrophil CR3 expression (A and B). A hallmark of the activated neutrophil is heightened expression of surface CR3, which makes the cell stickier; that change can be induced in vitro by C5a. Neutrophils with increased numbers of surface CR3 would then aggregate and adhere to the vascular endothelium (C), leading to neutropenia and occlusive vasculopathy (D). The role of cytokines (interleukin 1 and tumor necrosis factor) in the interaction of neutrophils and endothelium in SLE is as yet unclear.

tional assays of total C3 and C4 or CH_{50}. In the course of SLE, microthrombosis without inflammation of the vessel wall (i.e., "vasculitis") has been described in lung, kidney, and brain, and histologic evidence has been found of intravascular leukoaggregation associated with elevated levels of circulating complement split products.

With C5a and C3a active in plasma, it is not surprising that cell receptors for complement become activated and upregulated: CR3 (CD11/CD18; see below) has been best studied. As expected, increases in CD11b/CD18 correlate with increased levels of circulating C5a and C3a. Increased expression of CD11b/CD18 on neutrophils has, again, been demonstrated in patients with active, but not inactive, SLE. The highest levels of neutrophil CD11b/CD18 are found in patients with the most severe disease,

especially *cerebritis*, a group that had the highest levels of circulating C3a. Expression of CD11b/CD18 returns to control levels with improvement of clinical disease after these episodes of the "acute cerebral distress syndrome." In sum, whereas the normal emigration of neutrophils from endothelium does little injury to the vessel wall, the unique circumstances of the Shwartzman lesion—in which C3a and C5a are activated in the circulation—permit cytokine-activated endothelial cells to become susceptible to damage by complement-activated neutrophils. Systemic lupus erythematosus is often called a "collagen vascular disease" in reference to the involvement of blood vessels and their collagenous wickerwork, which is injured by Arthus and Shwartzman reactions.

RELEASE OF MEDIATORS OF INFLAMMATION FROM THE NEUTROPHIL

After engagement of its surface receptors by immune complexes (via FcγRII and FcγRIII receptors; CD32 and CD16, respectively) or chemoattractants (receptors for C5a and so on) this motile, postmitotic cell becomes equipped to seek and destroy microbes by chemotaxis and phagocytosis. After engagement of membrane receptors, neutrophils undergo, among other responses, the following: (1) activation of phospholipases and turnover of membrane phospholipids; (2) alterations in ion fluxes and membrane potential; (3) increases in cytosolic calcium; (4) phosphorylation of cellular proteins; and (5) assembly of cytoskeletal components (actin, microtubules). These events regulate the biologic functions of homotypic and heterotypic cell-cell aggregation (see above), chemotaxis, degranulation, release of reactive oxygen species, and the production of lipid-derived inflammatory substances, such as PAF, leukotriene B_4 (LTB_4), and lipoxin A.

Degranulation

During their maturation in the bone marrow, neutrophils acquire their characteristic populations of intracellular granules. These reservoirs, essentially lysosomes, serve as the main sources of enzymes responsible for the destruction of foreign substances and—by error, as it were—provoke the tissue injury of inflammation. Neutrophils in the course of maturation also acquire the enzymatic equipment with which to produce superoxide anion (O_2^-) and other mediators of tissue injury, such as PAF or LTB_4. Primary (azurophil) granules, so named because of their early appearance in neutrophil maturation (or staining properties), contain myeloperoxidase, lysozyme, acid hydrolases, and several serine proteases, including elastase. Elastase is of particular importance in the degradation of connective tissue because it is capable of breaking down not only elastin but also proteoglycans and types III and IV collagen. Secondary, or specific, granules are acquired later in maturation. These granules, like primary granules, also contain lysozyme, but are uniquely rich in vitamin B_{12}–binding protein, lactoferrin, and the neutral proteinase collagenase. They also contain a reservoir of surface integrins (CD11b/CD18) and low molecular weight guanine nucleotide–binding proteins (e.g., GTP) that bear homologies to the *ras* proteins of oncogenesis (see below). Collagenase, which requires an activation step (as does CD11b/CD18), has been detected in rheumatoid synovial fluid and degrades types I, II, and III collagen. Gelatinase, a third collagenolytic enzyme released by the neutrophil, has been localized to the "C" particle compartment, an additional granule subclass. Gelatinase can degrade types IV, V, and $1\alpha2\alpha3\alpha$ collagen as well as denatured collagen. Thus, neutrophil granules contain three enzymes—elastase, collagenase, and gelatinase—each with different substrate specificity and intracellular origin, which are capable of destroying collagen. These enzymes are differentially released in response to various stimuli.

Neutrophils can discharge the contents of their intracellular granules either *overtly* or *covertly*. During uptake of particles, the neutrophil plasma membrane first invaginates to engulf particles such as immune complexes into a phagocytic vacuole. The vacuole then fuses with lysosomal granules to form a chamber called the phagolysosome, and the granule contents are released into this chamber in the process called *covert degranulation*. Sometimes, however, if the particle is too large, or if the opening of the chamber has not yet closed, lysosomal enzymes are freely discharged into the extracellular milieu, where they may attack host tissues. This *overt degranulation*, a mechanism for extracellular secretion, has been termed "regurgitation during feeding" or, when the material is too large to be ingested (e.g., immune complexes trapped in the matrix of cartilage), has been given the picturesque name of "frustrated phagocytosis" (Fig. 256–3).

Antiproteases, such as alpha$_2$-macroglobulin and alpha$_1$-antitrypsin, may prevent tissue damage caused by degradative proteases released inappropriately during overt degranulation. However, the effect of these antiproteases is readily overcome when they are exposed to hypochlorous acid (HOCl), which inactivates them. Since HOCl is formed in the neutrophil after the interaction of myeloperoxidase, chloride anion, and H$_2$O$_2$ derived from O$_2^-$ via the NADPH (nicotinamide-adenine dinucleotide phosphate, reduced form) oxidase of the cell, HOCl is important in the mediation not only of bacterial killing (see Ch. 138) but also of tissue injury. Indeed, this HOCl inactivates antiproteases, while simultaneously activating latent collagenase and gelatinase. The identification of destructive enzymes such as myeloperoxidase, collagenase, and elastase at extracellular inflammatory sites in RA patients is consistent with this suggestion. Indeed, the unfortunate interaction of granule enzymes and oxygen metabolites released by neutrophils permits proteases to act unopposed and to elicit the inadvertent tissue injury that accompanies brisk phagocytosis.

Release of Toxic Oxygen Products and Lipid Mediators

The H$_2$O$_2$ utilized in the reaction described above is one of several oxygen metabolites, including superoxide anion and hydroxyl radical, that are released during neutrophil activation. The generation of these toxic compounds is governed by the membrane-associated NADPH oxidase system. In addition to contributing to the formation of HClO$^-$, oxygen metabolites can also damage connective tissue directly. For example, superoxide anion is capable of degrading bovine synovial fluid and depolymerizing purified hyaluronic acid.

Neutrophils respond to the engagement of receptors for chemoattractants or immune complexes by mobilizing arachidonate from the sn-2 position of phospholipids. Arachidonate—a fatty acid abbreviated as 20:4 because of its 20 carbons and 4 unsaturated double bonds—is mobilized from membrane stores: directly via a phospholipase A$_2$ (PLA$_2$) or indirectly via a phospholipase C (PLC) and followed by the action of a diacylglycerol lipase on diacylglycerol (DAG). Phospholipases A$_2$, which are associated both with neutrophil granules and with the plasma membrane, have two pH optima (5.5 and 7.5). Purified preparations of PLA$_2$'s require high concentrations of calcium for activity. Neutrophils appear to contain at least two PLC's—one that acts specifically

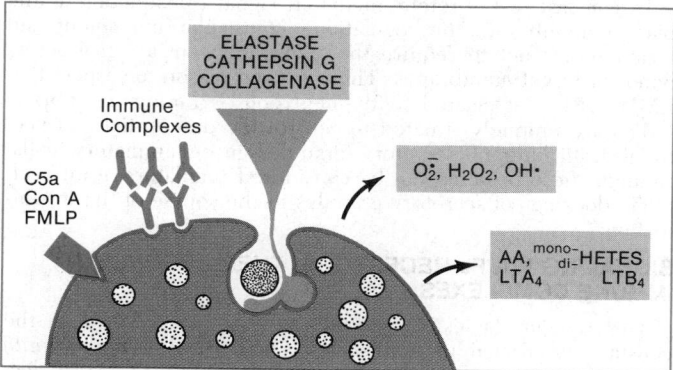

FIGURE 256–3. Release of the mediators of inflammation by the human neutrophil. When neutrophils are engaged by chemoattractants such as formyl-methionyl-leucyl phenylalanine (fMLP), a bacterial peptide analogue), from the complement sequence (C5a), or by lectins (Con A = concanavalin A)—or by immune complexes—they release lysosomal enzymes from intracellular granules to the outside (overt degranulation), assemble and activate the NADPH (nicotinamide-adenine dinucleotide phosphate, reduced form) oxidase that forms toxic oxygen species (O$_2^-$, H$_2$O$_2$, and so on), and turn over membrane phospholipids. These are the precursors for arachidonic acid (AA), which is transformed by an activated 5-lipoxygenase to the intermediate LTA$_4$, which can be used by neutrophils or other cells to form potent mediators: the leukotrienes (e.g., LTB$_4$). HETE = hydroxyeicosatetraenoic acid.

on phosphatidylinositol (PI) and a second that acts on phosphatidylcholine (PC) to yield DAG. Data on the remodeling of lipids show that not only PLA$_2$ activity but also the activity of PLC and phospholipase D (PLD) can explain these changes (see below). After treatment with calcium ionophore or with zymosan particles opsonized by C3b, neutrophils release 20:4 from PI and PC to an almost equivalent extent.

Once released from neutrophil phospholipids, 20:4 is transformed to *eicosanoid* metabolites (eicosa = 20), such as 5-hydroperoxyeicosatetraenoic acid (5-HPETE) by 5-lipoxygenase; the peroxide of 5-HPETE spontaneously forms 5-hydroxyeicosatetraenoic acid (5-HETE) or reacts further with the 5-lipoxygenase to form LTA$_4$, which has an epoxide at the 5,6 position. The 5-lipoxygenase has been purified, sequenced, and cloned. It is a complex enzyme assembly that requires an activation step. Leukotriene A$_4$ is then acted upon by LTA$_4$ hydrolase (LTB$_4$ synthetase) to form 5S, 12R,6, 14-*cis*,8,10-*trans*-dihydroxyeicosatetraenoic acid, or LTB$_4$. Alternatively, LTA$_4$ made by the neutrophil can be processed by other cells as well; transcellular metabolism is a rule with eicosanoids (see Ch. 29). Leukotriene A$_4$ can break down nonenzymatically to 5S,6S or 5S,6R,6,8,10-*trans*,14-*cis*-dihydroxyeicosatetraenoic acid. These nonenzymatic metabolites have, at best, one-tenth the activity of LTB$_4$ in activating neutrophils. In the presence of exogenous arachidonic acid, neutrophils also show 15-lipoxygenase activity, which, in a parallel manner, produces 15-HPETE and 15-HETE. These products, in turn, are acted upon by an LTA$_4$ synthetase–like enzyme to make a 14,15-dihydroxy product and finally, in concert with 5-lipoxygenase, can yield the trihydroxy compounds: lipoxins A and B. Mononuclear cells, in contrast, produce stable prostaglandins (PGE$_2$) and the sulfidopeptides leukotrienes LTC$_4$, LTD$_4$, and LTE$_4$.

Two major candidates for inflammatory mediators made from neutrophils are LTB$_4$ and lipoxin A. Leukotriene B$_4$ is a potent chemoattractant and promotes adhesion of neutrophils to endothelial cells from a variety of arterial and venous sites of several species—an effect not shared with other eicosanoids. Prostacyclin from endothelial cells (PGI$_2$) does not inhibit LTB$_4$-stimulated adhesion. Finally, lipoxin A has potent vasodilating effects in vivo (but not in vitro) and does not mimic the action of endothelium-derived relaxation factor (EDRF) (nitric oxide). Lipoxin A has only modest effects on neutrophil chemokinesis; since its major biologic action appears to be the inhibition of natural killer (NK) cell activity, lipoxin A may chiefly regulate IgG receptor (Fcγ-RIII)–mediated signal transduction.

STIMULUS-RESPONSE COUPLING: THE BASIS OF CELL ACTIVATION IN INFLAMMATION

Phospholipids and Intracellular Calcium

When chemoattractants such as formyl-methionyl-leucyl phenylalanine (fMLP), C5a, C3a, or LTB$_4$ engage their receptors, neutrophils respond by generating inositol trisphosphate (IP$_3$) and DAG. Although signaling via Fc receptors and signaling via receptors for chemoattractants (Fig. 256–4) differ with respect to some details, the general outline of stimulus-response coupling is similar, and neutrophils do not differ in these general pathways from other cells of inflammation.

Cellular IP$_3$ and DAG concentrations substantially increase within seconds after engagement of the fMLP receptor. By 5 seconds, IP$_3$ levels begin to decline. In contrast, both DAG and phosphatidic acid (PA) continue to increase over the course of the next 120 to 300 seconds. Although the exact sequence of enzyme reactions whereby the neutrophil generates these elevated levels of DAG and PA is not yet understood, it is likely that both PA and diglycerides play a critical role in maintaining activation of the neutrophil. Indeed, intracellular signaling in neutrophils or macrophages is more complex than that in "suicide" cells like the platelet. In order for neutrophils or macrophages to respond, over time and in space, two signals must be generated: a short "triggering" signal, with an immediate increase in intracellular messengers (e.g., IP$_3$), and sustained "activation" signals (e.g., DAG or PA) required for the longer processes of chemotaxis and phagocytosis.

But lipid remodeling provides only *some* of the messengers needed for signal transduction. Calcium plays another key role.

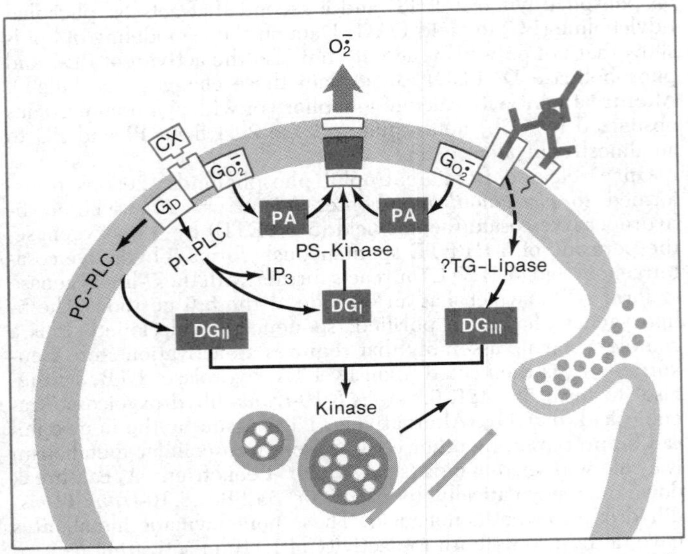

FIGURE 256–4. Stimulus-response coupling in the human neutrophil. Pathways for release of mediators of inflammation by chemoattractants (CX), on the left-hand side of the diagram, differ from those launched by immune complexes (YY), on the right-hand side of the diagram. Three pools of diglyceride (DG) are mobilized, only one of which (DG$_{III}$) is critical for secretion of lysosomal enzymes. Whereas CX-mediated generation of O$_2^-$ is completely inhibited by pertussis toxin–sensitive G-proteins, only some of the O$_2^-$ assembly in response to immune complex requires this intermediate. Phosphatidic acid (PA) seems to be the main intracellular messenger for assembly of the NADPH oxidase. TG = triglyceride; PI-PLC = phosphatidylinositol–phospholipase C; PC-PLC = phosphatidylcholine–phospholipase C; PS = phosphatidylserine; G$_D$ = the G protein of degranulation; G$_{O_2^-}$ = the G protein of superoxide generation.

After treatment with chemoattractants such as C5a or fMLP, neutrophils increase their levels of cytosolic calcium [Ca]$_i$, reaching a peak by 2 to 5 seconds. Over the next 2 minutes, [Ca]$_i$ slowly decreases and then returns *toward*—but not *to*—baseline. The peak levels (300 to 500 nM) are achieved primarily by IP$_3$-induced mobilization from intracellular stores, since similar levels are achieved in the absence of extracellular calcium. The influx of extracellular calcium begins approximately 5 seconds after calcium has been released from intracellular sites and while IP$_3$ levels are still dropping. Although IP$_4$ may in part regulate calcium channels, it is also possible that PA functions in the maintenance of calcium-dependent calcium influx.

Neutrophils break down PI to form DAG and PA within the first 5 seconds of the engagement of receptors by chemoattractants or immune complexes. Suggestions that one or another molecule in the PI-PA cycle mediates these changes in calcium permeability include—among others—the influx via PA-activated "calcium gates" or formation of IP$_4$ from IP$_3$ by specific kinases. However, the turnover of IP$_3$ and IP$_4$ in consequence of specific phosphatases is extremely rapid (5 to 15 seconds), while DAG and PA continue to accumulate (30 to 120 seconds) after treatment of neutrophils with chemoattractants. In contrast, the formation of DAG proceeds in a biphasic fashion. The first peak is at 2 to 5 seconds, consistent with release of the "triggering" messengers, IP$_3$ and DAG, by the hydrolysis of polyphosphoinositides. Before this first wave is completed—by 15 to 30 seconds after treatment with fMLP—a second, more sustained wave of DAG formation commences. In contrast, PA rises throughout the time course of activation. There is general agreement that both PLC and PLD are involved in PA function. The concentrations of DAG and PA remain elevated, compared with those of resting neutrophils, for more than 300 seconds, in what has been called the "activation" phase of neutrophil responses. Although the evidence is by no means complete, it appears likely that the second wave of DAG is important in degranulation, whereas the increased levels of PA are important for assembly of the NADPH oxidase that is responsible for generating O$_2^-$.

GTP-Binding Proteins and Signal Transduction

The superfamily of GTP-binding proteins includes (1) the heterotrimeric proteins which transduce hormonal and sensory signals across the plasma membrane; (2) tubulin (each dimer binds 1 mole of GTP strongly and 1 mole loosely); (3) the elongation and initiation factors of protein synthesis; (4) products of the *ras* oncogene; and (5) putative GTP-binding proteins of cellular secretion. Whereas neutrophils clearly have GTP-binding proteins at their plasmalemma, the protein is neither a classic-G$_s$- or G$_i$-protein and appears instead to be at least one novel G-protein: G$_n$. In turn, at least one function of G$_n$ is to couple receptors for chemoattractants to PLC. Composed of typical β/γ membrane components and an α-subunit of the cytosol, 33 to 50 per cent of the G$_n$-protein is complexed to the β/γ dimer in the membrane, while the remainder is free in the cytosol. Pertussis toxin (PT) binds to the α-subunit at sites distinct from the GTP site; ribosylation by PT of the soluble α-subunit is enhanced 12-fold by the addition of β/γ-subunits, whereas PT ribosylation of membrane G$_n$ is only modestly enhanced. G$_n$ comprises 1 to 3 per cent of membrane proteins; no great excess of these molecules (10^6 per cell) is present over possible receptors (e.g., receptors for IgG and C5a). The neutrophil G-protein (α-subunit) is a substrate for adenosine diphosphate (ADP) ribosylation both by pertussis and by cholera toxins (CT); both toxins inhibit high-affinity fMLP binding, and the protein is antigenically distinct not only from G$_s$- or G$_i$-proteins of other sources, but from the common G$_o$-protein of brain. Predictably, for G-protein–mediated functions, treatment of intact neutrophils with PT inhibits ligand-mediated O$_2^-$ generation, degranulation, chemotaxis, phospholipid turnover, high-affinity fMLP binding, release of eicosanoids, calcium fluxes, and so on.

But the G-proteins of signal transduction are not the only G-proteins of inflammatory cells; a rapidly growing family of low molecular weight GTP-binding proteins (LMW-GBP's), with a molecular weight in the range of 20 to 30 kD are also present. These proteins are characterized by marked sequence homology to the *ras* oncogene product (*ras* p21). In contrast to their high molecular weight counterparts, no clear function has been attributed to any mammalian *ras*-related protein. Microinjection of human *ras* p21, however, causes degranulation of mast cells, suggesting that LMW-GBP's may play a role in exocytosis. Futhermore, recent evidence implicating *ras* p21 in the activation of a PC-specific PLC suggests that this phospholipase is critical for neutrophil secretion. To date, the strongest evidence for the involvement of *ras*-related proteins in the secretory pathway comes from studies of the yeast *Saccharomyces cerevisiae*, in which these proteins regulate vectorial traffic of vesicles within cells.

In contrast to G-protein–mediated signal transduction at the plasma membrane, the regulation of vesicular movement and fusion seems not to require the transduction of a signal across donor or target membranes. There is good reason to suspect that LMW-GBP's associated with neutrophil granule membrane GBP's are uniquely situated to control the differential and vectorial trafficking of secretory granules in inflammatory cells. Indeed, these proteins can be considered regulators of intracellular "docking" of secretory granules in the course of the inflammation.

SIGNALING VIA Fc RECEPTORS: THE RESPONSE TO IMMUNE COMPLEXES

Three major classes of receptors have been described for the constant Fc region of human IgG's. FcγRI is a *high-affinity receptor* for monomeric IgG (K$_a$ = approximately 10^{-8}M, molecular weight = 72 kD) found mainly on mononuclear cells; recognized by monoclonal antibody 32, it is upregulated in response to interferon (IFN). Neutrophils also have two *low-affinity receptors* (K$_a$ = approximately 10^{-6}M), which bind aggregated IgG's or immune complexes much more avidly than monomeric IgG. FcγRII (or CD32), of approximately 40 kD, is present at 15,000 sites per cell (as recognized by monoclonal antibody IV-3) and is also present on B cells, macrophages, and platelets. FcγRII (1) is resistant to elastase, (2) is not linked to the plasmalemma via PI, (3) is present on neutrophils from patients with paroxysmal nocturnal hemoglobinuria (PNH), (4) appears to mediate O$_2^-$ generation and degranulation, and (5) transduces all of the signal for O_2^- generation and some of the signal for degranulation by means of a PT-sensitive G-protein.

FcγRIII (or CD16) also prefers multimeric IgG and is expressed in heterogeneous fashion on neutrophils, macrophages, and NK cells. FcγRIII has a broad range of molecular weight of 50 to 70 kD, is present at approximately 120,000 sites per neutrophil, and is recognized by monoclonal antibody 3G8. The FcγRIII's on neutrophils and NK cells differ with respect to mass and are products of different but very homologous genes. FcγRIII's of the neutrophil are (1) elastase sensitive, (2) linked to the external plasmalemma via PI, (3) reduced to 90 per cent of controls at the plasmalemma—but not the Golgi region—of cells from patients with PNH, (4) an ineffective trigger of cells for O_2^- or enzyme release, and (5) polymorphic with respect to structure and antigenicity because there are two alleles (CNA1 and NA2). FcγRIII's are shed into the supernatant of neutrophils exposed to fMLP, whereas macrophages and NK cells—in which FcγRIII is a transmembrane structure—do not shed this receptor.

Since cells from patients with PNH respond as well as normal cells to IgG-opsonized particles by O_2^- generation, and all O_2^--generating activity in response to IgG is PT sensitive, we must conclude that the FcγRII is linked to GTP-binding proteins, whereas FcγRIII is not (Fig. 256–4). Recent evidence shows that whereas stimulus-response coupling induced by immune complexes in the bulk phase is largely sensitive to PT, degranulation and O_2^- generation induced by immune complexes on a surface are relatively insensitive to PT. From these observations, it appears that FcγRIII may accumulate at the interface between neutrophils and the immune complexes trapped in the subendothelium. Moreover, signaling via Fc receptors differs from signaling via chemoattractant receptors in that the former is dependent on the integrity of cytoplasmic microtubules, whereas chemoattractant-induced signaling is independent of microtubules. *Colchicine therefore inhibits FcγR signaling.* FcγRIII receptors may serve to cluster Fc receptors in the service of "frustrated phagocytosis" when the discharge of neutrophil contents is launched by an IgG-opsonized particulate too large to digest. Therefore, of the two neutrophil Fc receptors for IgG, it appears that FcγRII triggers cells via classic G-protein–mediated signal transduction, as in synovial fluid. In contrast, FcγRIII receptors unlinked to G-proteins mediate neutrophil discharge in vascular lesions where IgG's are trapped at subendothelial sites, as in vasculitis when the release of mediators of inflammation is by "frustrated phagocytosis."

THE INTEGRINS AND INFLAMMATION

The adhesion of formed elements of the blood to endothelium and to one another is mediated by a superfamily of membrane proteins called "integrins." Three major families of mammalian integrins have been described: (1) receptors for extracellular matrix molecules, such as fibronectin and T lymphocyte receptors, known as very late-appearing antigens (VLA); (2) platelet-surface glycoprotein IIb/IIIa and the vitronectin receptor; and (3) the leukocyte function–associated antigen 1 (LFA-1) family of leukocyte adhesion molecules. The most striking characteristic shared by these molecules is their noncovalently linked α/β heterodimer configuration in which the same β-subunit is shared by all members of a family. In addition, many, but not all, integrins contain a domain that recognizes an Arg-Gly-Asp (RGD) sequence present in their respective ligands.

The LFA-1 family of leukocyte adhesion molecules includes three heterodimeric glycoproteins that share a common 95-kD β chain (CD18): LFA-1, Mac-1 (also called Mol, gp165/95, and CR3), and gp 150/90, whose α chains have been designated CD11a, 11b, and 11c, respectively. The expression of these three molecules varies according to lineage and stage of maturation of various hematopoietic cells. In addition to mediating cell-cell adhesion, CD11b/CD18 functions as a receptor for iC3b (CR3) and thereby mediates phagocytosis of opsonized particles.

CD11b/CD18 is probably the major neutrophil adhesion molecule involved in *heterotypic* (neutrophil/endothelium) and *homotypic* (neutrophil-neutrophil) adhesion. Children genetically deficient in all three LFA-1 family adhesion molecules suffer from recurrent bacterial infections, impaired pus formation, delayed wound healing, and poor separation of the umbilical cord. Neutrophils from these patients are defective in functions related

to adhesion, such as aggregation, spreading on surfaces, directed migration, and attachment to endothelial monolayers. Normal human neutrophils treated in vitro with a subset of available anti-CD11b/CD18 monoclonal antibodies exhibit defects indistinguishable from those of neutrophils from patients with deficiency.

Although CD11b/CD18 is clearly implicated in the events of neutrophil adhesion, the molecular mechanisms are unclear. Under normal circumstances, neutrophil sticking must be suppressed to permit cells to circulate. Once neutrophils encounter ligands, cell activation is required to render them sticky. In heterotypic adhesion, the other agonist is the endothelial cell. The endothelial cell plays an active role in adhesion and displays to inflammatory cells an inducible, endothelial surface glycoprotein designated ELAM-1, which partially mediates the adhesion of leukocytes, including neutrophils. Interleukin 1, TNF, lymphotoxin (LT), and endotoxin induce the expression of ELAM-1 on endothelial cells. Intercellular adhesion molecule 1 (ICAM-1), a similar but distinct antigen found on a variety of cells, including endothelial cells, is the ligand for LFA-1 and is therefore one of several molecules that direct lymphocyte binding to high endothelial cells, especially those of the chronically inflamed rheumatoid joint. On the other hand, the endothelial side of the equation can be modified by TGF-β. This factor inhibits the adherence of human neutrophils not only to normal endothelium but also to endothelial cells rendered sticky by ELAM-1 as induced by TNF-α.

In homotypic adhesion (neutrophil-neutrophil), the CD11b/CD18 heterodimer receptor engages an as yet unknown ligand on an adherent neutrophil. The putative ligand is unlikely to be adsorbed iC3b, nor is the adhesive ligand likely to be CD11b/CD18 itself because normal neutrophils are capable of aggregating with neutrophils from CD11b/CD18-deficient patients.

CD11b/CD18 is constitutively expressed on the surface of resting neutrophils at a density of 10,000 to 20,000 molecules per cell. Upon activation by a number of stimuli, including especially chemoattractants, neutrophils "upregulate" their surface expression 5- to 10-fold. Since mature neutrophils synthesize little new protein, it is not surprising that upregulation of CD11b/CD18 is due to the translocation of preformed receptor to the plasma membrane from an intracellular source that cosediments with specific granules.

Because each stimulus that enhances neutrophil adhesion also induces Mac-1 upregulation, it was widely believed that these two phenomena were causally related, but recent studies have dissociated neutrophil-neutrophil aggregation from upregulation of CD11b/CD18. Indeed, whereas the constitutive presence on the cell surface of CD11b/CD18 is *required* for neutrophil adhesion, regulation of cell-cell adhesion appears to involve a structural change in each receptor molecule rather than a quantitative change in the number of receptors.

RHEUMATOID ARTHRITIS AS A FORM OF THE TUBERCULIN REACTION

The histopathology of RA can be divided into two phases: (1) the acute inflammatory lesion, the Arthus-type lesion discussed above; and (2) the more chronic, mononuclear cell–mediated, granulomatous disease proceeding in the deeper layers. This lesion—pannus—is marked by (1) focal collections of β lymphocytes and plasma cells, which synthesize rheumatoid factors locally, (2) various subsets of T lymphocytes, (3) activated macrophages (Fig. 256–5), and (4) the proliferation of other mesenchymal cells of the synovium in which genes for proto-oncogenes have been activated. The two types of activated cells—macrophages and synoviocytes—generate cytokines that cause chondrocytes to participate in their own destruction by releasing proteases and specific collagenase.

The lesions resemble those found in the tuberculin reaction, save for the clusters of B lymphocytes and plasma cells with rheumatoid factor. Indeed, for many years, RA was thought to be a form of tuberculosis, and the gold salts used to treat tuberculosis in the 1920's were first used for RA on the basis of this fuzzy association. We may note that the earliest editions of this text classified RA as a form of "infectious arthritis."

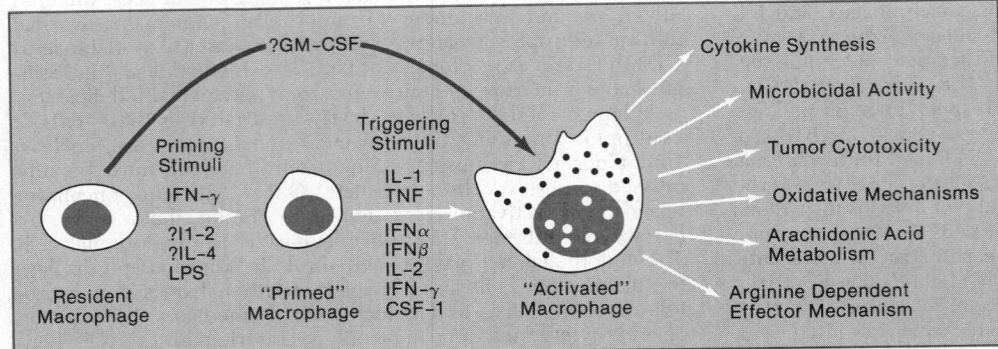

FIGURE 256-5. Schematic depiction of the role of cytokines in the two-stage hypothesis of macrophage activation. Unstimulated cells are primed by treatment with low-dose lipopolysaccharides (LPS), interferon-γ (IFN-γ), and possibly interleukin 2 (IL2). Primed macrophages can be triggered to an activated state by many other cytokines. Activation of the macrophages has classically been defined by demonstrating augmented effector functions as shown.

Although the offending agent of RA is unknown, most modern speculation centers on the likelihood that one or another self-antigen looks very much like the product of a bacterium or virus. The major candidates have been (1) the Epstein-Barr (EB) virus, (2) type II collagen, (3) cartilage proteoglycan, and (4) heat shock (stress) proteins, especially a 65-kD species against which many patients with RA mount a humoral and cellular immune attack. Indeed, there is good evidence that stress proteins are present at the surface of antigen-presenting cells, and recently it was found that a helper T cell clone derived from a patient with tuberculous leprosy reacted with a synthetic peptide found in the third type of variable region of the MLA-DR2 β chain (Ch. 250). The observation that cartilage proteoglycans share epitopes with acetone-extracted fractions of the tubercle bacillus suggests that when humans get RA, they respond to their own tissues as if these were products of the tubercle bacillus or EB virus.

Whatever the offending antigen or antigens prove to be, the mediators released by T and B lymphocytes, by activated macrophages, and by activated synovial cells are the usual battery of cytokines found in chronic inflammation (Table 256-1). These cytokines in turn influence neutrophil function. Indeed, IL1, a proinflammatory cytokine produced chiefly by mononuclear cells, but also by neutrophils, is capable of promoting thymocyte proliferation and synovial fibroblast activation and proliferation. Neutrophils display enhanced adherence to endothelial cells treated with IL1. Among its many other properties, IL1 also induces production of PGE₂ and type II collagenase production by chondrocytes. These actions are regulated by an IL1 inhibitor, which appears to be constitutively present in cartilage cells and in the neutrophil.

Treatment of neutrophils with lymphokine IFN-γ or TNF-β augments neutrophil phagocytic capacity, especially when polymorphonuclear neutrophils are at the surface of cartilage. TNF-β, the most potent chemoattractant, also promotes neutrophil adherence to endothelial cells and stimulates H₂O release and degranulation. Granulocyte-macrophage colony-stimulating factor (GM-CSF), produced largely by fibroblasts, facilitates phagocytosis by neutrophils, possibly by increasing Fc receptor expression. Although many cytokines have no effect on neutrophil chemotaxis, *interleukin 8* (IL8), a macrophage-derived neutrophil chemotactic factor, is one of the most potent neutrophil activators yet found.

Abramson SB, Weissmann G: Complement split products and the pathogenesis of SLE. Hosp Pract 23:45, 1988. *How the Arthus phenomenon and the Shwartzman reaction apply to vasculitis in SLE.*

Bevilaqua MD, Stengelin S, Gimbrone MA, et al.: Endothelial leukocyte adhesion molecule 1: An inducible receptor for neutrophils related to complement regulatory proteins and lectins. Science 243:11, 1989. *Delineation of the critical molecules of endothelial "stickiness."*

Bokoch GM: Signal transduction by GTP-binding proteins during leukocyte activation: Phagocytic cells. *In* Grinstein S, Rotstein OD (eds.): Mechanisms of Leukocyte Activation. New York, Academic Press, 1990, pp 65–101. *A modern discussion of how the molecular biology of G-proteins has permitted an understanding of the control of signal transduction.*

Haines KA, Reibman J, Weissmann G: Triggering and activation of human neutrophils: Two aspects of the response to transmembrane signals. *In* Poste G, Crooke ST (eds.): Cellular and Molecular Aspects of Inflammation. New York, Plenum Press, 1988, pp 31–40. *A detailed analysis of the differences between immediate and prolonged responses to signals at the surface of inflammatory cells.*

Harris ED Jr: Pathogenesis of rheumatoid arthritis: A disorder associated with dysfunctional immunoregulation. *In* Gallin JI, Goldstein IM, Snyderman R (eds.): Inflammation. New York, Raven Press, 1985, pp 751–774. *A review of rheumatoid inflammation with an emphasis on cell-cell interaction in chronic inflammation and cartilage destruction.*

Krane SM, Amento EP, Goldring SR, Stephenson ML: Modulation of matrix synthesis and degradation in joint inflammation. *In* Glauert AM (ed.): The Control of Tissue Damage. Amsterdam, Elsevier, 1990, pp 179–195. *How IL1 appears to be critical for the self-induced destruction in RA as mediated by PGE₂ and collagenase.*

Nathan CF: Secretory products of macrophages. J Clin Invest 79:319, 1987. *The products of macrophages that provoke tissue injury and constitute cell-cell crosstalk are listed here.*

Pike MC: Chemoattractant receptors as regulators of phagocytic cell functions. *In* Grinstein S, Rotstein OD (eds.): Mechanisms of Leukocyte Activators. New York, Academic Press, 1990, pp 19–43. *An overview of how neutrophils escape from the capillaries to produce tissue injury.*

TABLE 256-1. CELLULAR SOURCES AND TARGETS OF MAJOR CYTOKINES

Cytokine	Source	Target
IL1-α	Mφ, EC, fibroblasts	Lymphocytes, EC, HCMφ, fibroblasts, others
IL1-β	Mφ	Lymphocytes, EC, HCMφ, fibroblasts, others
IL2	T cells	Lymphocytes, Mφ, others
IL4	T cells	B cells, T cells, others
IL8	Macrophages	PMN
IFN-α	Lymphocytes	Multiple nucleated cells
IFN-β₁	Mφ	Multiple nucleated cells
IFN-β₂ (IL6)	Fibroblasts, Mφ	HC, lymphocytes, others
IFN-γ	T lymphocytes	Mφ, lymphocytes, others
M-CSF, CSF-1	Mφ	Bone marrow, Mφ fibroblasts
GM-CSF	Fibroblasts	Mφ, PMN
TNF-α	Mφ, fibroblasts	PMN, Mφ, others
TNF-β	Lymphocytes, Mφ	Multiple cells
TGF-β	T lymphocytes	PMN, fibroblasts, Mφ
MDNCF	Mφ	PMN

IFN = interferon; TNF = tumor necrosis factor; IL = interleukin; CSF = colony-stimulating factor; M-CSF = macrophage colony-stimulating factor; GM-CSF = granulocyte-macrophage colony-stimulating factor; TGF-β = transforming growth factor–β; Mφ = macrophage; PMN = polymorphonuclear neutrophil; EC = endothelial cell; HC = hepatocytes.

Ritchlin CT, Winchester RJ: Potential for coordinate gene activation in the rheumatoid synoviocyte: Implications and hypotheses. Springer Semin Immunopathol 11:219, 1989. *A discussion at the molecular level of how proto-oncogenes may mediate the cellular phenotypic changes in synoviocytes from RA.*

Smolen JE: Characteristics and mechanisms of secretion by neutrophils. In Mallett MB (ed.): The Neutrophil: Cellular Biochemistry and Physiology. Boca Raton, Fla., CRC Press, 1989, pp 24–61. *The mechanisms whereby neutrophils release their inflammatory contents.*

Spaethe SM, Needleman P: Biosynthesis and release of lipid mediate of inflammation. In Poste G, Crooke ST (eds.): Cellular and Molecular Aspects of Inflammation. New York, Plenum Press, 1988, pp 153–170. *A review of the cyclo-oxygenase and lipoxygenase pathways in inflammation, with a discussion of the role of essential fatty acid.*

Thomas L: The Youngest Science. New York, Viking Press, 1983, 270 pp. *Read especially Chapters 14 and 15, in which he describes the early days of endotoxin and the Shwartzman reaction.*

Weissmann G: The role of neutrophils in vascular injury. Signal transduction mechanisms in cell/cell interactions. Springer Semin Immunopathol 11:235, 1989. *A review of the Arthus and Shwartzman models and how they relate to the vascular lesions of rheumatic diseases.*

West MA: Role of cytokines in leukocyte activation: Phagocytic cells. In Grinstein S, Rotstein OD (eds.): Mechanisms of Leukocyte Activation. New York, Academic Press, 1990, pp 537–570. *A summary of the effects of cytokines, which are released in rheumatoid inflammation, on the activation of neutrophils and macrophages.*

Winfield JB: Stress proteins and autoimmunity. Arthritis Rheum 32:1497, 1989. *How heat shock proteins may be the link between autoantigens and microbial products in the perpetuation of RA.*

Ziff M: Role of the endothelium in chronic inflammation. Springer Semin Immunopathol 11:199, 1989. *How clusters of lymphocytes arrive in the synovial tissues and what the propulsive and adhesive forces are.*

Zvaifler NJ: Pathogenesis of the joint disease of rheumatoid arthritis. Am J Med 75:3, 1983. *A review of chronic inflammation in the joint, with emphasis on classic pathways of tissue injury.*

257 Specialized Procedures in the Management of Patients with Rheumatic Diseases

William J. Arnold and Robert W. Ike

Since rheumatic diseases may be systemic or localized, patients can present with an array of signs and symptoms reflecting multiorgan involvement or pain with limitation of function in a single anatomic area. Optimal management of these patients relies on a thorough history and physical examination, with appropriate laboratory, imaging, and invasive procedures, to arrive at a correct diagnosis and specific therapy. New, exciting, and highly specialized procedures, such as arthroscopy and magnetic resonance imaging (MRI), provide direct and specific information of particular use in the management of patients with localized rheumatic diseases. New serologic testing for Lyme disease and antiphospholipid antibodies can provide important diagnostic information about puzzling new systemic rheumatic disease. The temptation is to rely heavily on the results of these new tests. However, they and the other procedures discussed below must always be interpreted only in the context of a thorough, comprehensive, multifaceted evaluation.

ASPIRATION OF SYNOVIAL JOINTS AND BURSAE

In any patient with undiagnosed arthritis and an associated joint effusion, examination of the synovial fluid is mandatory. Particularly for patients with infectious and crystal-induced inflammation, aspiration and evaluation of synovial fluid are critical elements in the management. Successful joint or bursal aspiration depends on a thorough familiarity with certain principles.

Successful synovial fluid aspiration begins with a well-informed physician. Although most general internists are able to aspirate the knee or olecranon bursa readily, other commonly inflamed structures, such as the shoulder, ankle, elbow, first metatarsophalangeal joint, and subdeltoid bursa, require special expertise for successful aspiration. If the physician is unsure, the advice of a more experienced physician should be sought. Similarly, a well-informed patient is a prerequisite for success. Before the procedure begins, the physician should inform the patient about the

risks and benefits, and the physician should continue to communicate during the procedure. This is also the time to note possible allergies to lidocaine or iodine.

Next, the appropriate supplies and equipment must be made readily available (Table 257–1). The patient must be comfortably positioned to allow muscle relaxation, which will permit full access through the extensor surface to the joint space. For example, when the knee is being aspirated, the patient should be supine with the knee positioned in 10 degrees of flexion, accomplished by resting it on a pillow. The patient should let the leg fall into external rotation, thereby allowing the quadriceps musculature to relax completely. The best evidence for proper positioning and the patient's comfort is a readily movable patella (side to side). If the patient maintains quadriceps contraction, as evidenced by a relatively immobile patella, aspiration will be difficult and painful, if not impossible.

Following skin preparation with iodine and alcohol, the point of entry is determined with the sterile-gloved, nonaspirating hand. In the case of the knee, this entry is located at the midpoint of the patella on the medial aspect of the knee. Local infiltration of the skin and subcutaneous tissue with 1 per cent lidocaine or topical ethyl chloride to reduce the pain of needle entry is optional. The joint space is then entered with an 18-gauge (1½-inch) needle, with a syringe of up to 20 ml attached, depending on the size of the effusion. Larger syringes are too cumbersome to handle. The knee joint capsule is just below the surface of the skin; however, deeper penetration may be required to access sequestered fluid or to penetrate thickened synovium lining the joint capsule. If fluid is not immediately obtained, the syringe should be rotated while the plunger remains retracted. For diagnostic purposes, a 5-ml sample of synovial fluid is more than adequate for all routine studies, including cultures. However, if additional fluid can be obtained without discomfort to the patient, the Kelly clamp can be used to assist in changing syringes.

Following aspiration, the needle should be removed from the joint with one quick motion and hemostasis ensured by applying pressure at the aspiration site for 1 to 2 minutes. An adhesive bandage dressing is then applied, and the patient can be immediately ambulatory. The synovial fluid specimen can be processed efficiently and accurately by immediately placing a single drop on a clean slide with a coverslip (for microscopy) and then putting one half of the specimen in a heparinized tube (for white blood cell [WBC] count and glucose determination) and transporting the other half in the syringe directly to the bacteriology laboratory for culture.

Analysis of the synovial fluid is undertaken as soon as possible after the aspiration to determine if the fluid is inflammatory or noninflammatory (Table 257–2). Synovial fluid from patients with osteoarthritis is characteristically translucent and noninflammatory, with an average synovial fluid WBC count of 600 per cubic millimeter. In contrast, inflammatory synovial fluid, such as that found in patients with rheumatoid arthritis, has a WBC count of

TABLE 257–1. COMPONENTS OF THE ARTHROCENTESIS TRAY

Skin Preparation
Alcohol sponges, iodine swabs
Sterile gauze (2 × 2)
Adhesive bandages
Sterile disposable gloves
Local Anesthetic
1% Lidocaine
Ethyl chloride spray
Aspirating Equipment
Disposable syringes (5, 10, and 20 ml)
18- and 20-gauge aspirating needles
25-Gauge infiltrating needles
Sterile Kelly clamp
Transporting/Analyzing Equipment
Plain and heparinized test tubes
Clean microscope slides with coverslips
Chocolate agar plates
Aerobic/anaerobic bacteria culture media

TABLE 257–2. SYNOVIAL FLUID ANALYSIS

Diagnosis	Appearance	Total White Cell Count per mm³*	Polymorphonuclear cells	Miscellaneous
Normal	Clear, pale yellow	0–200	Less than 10%	—
Group I (Noninflammatory) Osteoarthritis	Clear to slightly turbid	50–2000 (600)	Less than 30%	Cartilage fragments
Group II (Mildly inflammatory) Systemic lupus erythematosus (SLE) Scleroderma	Clear to slightly turbid	0–9000 (3000)	Less than 20%	—
Group III (Severely inflammatory) Gout	Turbid	100–160,000 (21,000)	Approximately 70%	Monosodium urate crystals
Pseudogout	Turbid	50–75,000 (14,000)	Approximately 70%	Calcium pyrophosphate dihydrate crystals
Rheumatoid arthritis	Turbid	250–80,000 (19,000)	Approximately 70%	—
Group IV (Infectious) Acute bacterial	Very turbid	150–250,000 (80,000)	Approximately 90%	Culture positive
Tuberculosis	Turbid	2500–100,000 (20,000)	Approximately 60%	Culture often negative

*Averages in parentheses.

greater than 2000 per cubic millimeter and may be either translucent or opaque. A rapid determination of opacity can be made by trying to read newsprint placed behind the synovial fluid in a glass tube. Gross tests of inflammation in synovial fluid, such as the mucin clot and string test, can provide additional information about the inflammatory nature of the fluid. Analysis of bursal fluid has shown that bursae react less intensely than synovial joints to specific disease stimuli. A relatively low bursal fluid leukocyte count is often present in patients with septic and gouty bursitis. For instance, in gouty bursitis, an average bursal fluid leukocyte count is 2800 per cubic millimeter, compared with an average of 21,000 per cubic millimeter in synovial fluid.

Every synovial fluid analysis must include a polarizing microscopic evaluation for crystals (see Color Plate 4C). Needle-shaped, intracellular, negatively birefringent crystals of monosodium urate are characteristically seen in patients with gouty arthritis. Rhomboidal, positively birefringent intracellular crystals of calcium pyrophosphate dihydrate are found in patients with the pseudogout syndrome. In both patients with gout and those with pseudogout, a careful, thorough examination of synovial fluid is often necessary to find the pathognomonic crystals. In some patients, both types of crystals may be found. Other crystals found in synovial fluid include calcium oxalate (dialysis-associated arthritis) and calcium hydroxyapatite (Milwaukee shoulder). Occasionally, in patients with chronic effusions accompanied by bleeding (e.g., hemophilia or rheumatoid arthritis), cholesterol crystals may be found. These are platelike and brilliantly birefringent under polarizing microscopy.

The highest synovial fluid WBC counts (15,000 per cubic millimeter or greater) are found in patients with septic arthritis. The most common pathogen is *Staphylococcus aureus*. While a synovial fluid Gram stain revealing gram-positive cocci can be helpful in guiding initial antibiotic therapy, a negative Gram stain does not rule out infection as a cause of the inflammatory arthritis. In these situations, i.e., a negative Gram stain, but with strong suspicion of infectious arthritis, empiric antibiotic therapy must be used until culture results are available.

Neisseria gonorrhoeae is the most frequently found gram-negative organism associated with infectious arthritis. Although gonococcal arthritis may be monoarticular, a polyarticular presentation with fever and skin lesions is characteristic. Gram-negative intracellular diplococci are characteristically seen on a Gram stain of synovial fluid from patients with monoarticular gonococcal arthritis and occasionally (20 per cent) are found in skin lesions of patients with polyarticular gonococcal arthritis.

The clinical course of tuberculous arthritis is usually indolent and monoarticular. The synovial fluid is intensely inflammatory with a high percentage of mononuclear cells. Synovial fluid cultures are usually negative, and signs of active extra-articular disease are minimal. A prompt, accurate diagnosis of tuberculous arthritis requires a high degree of suspicion and culture of synovial biopsy specimens. Often extensive joint destruction is present before a diagnosis of tuberculous arthritis is made.

Determination of the glucose content of synovial fluid is the most valuable chemical assessment performed. When the synovial fluid glucose content is less than 50 per cent of a simultaneously determined serum level, the diagnosis of infectious arthritis should be suspected. In patients with infectious arthritis, serial determinations of synovial fluid glucose level, along with decreasing synovial fluid WBC count and serologic markers of inflammation, such as C-reactive protein level, can be used to follow the efficacy of therapy.

RHEUMATOID FACTOR

Rheumatoid factor is an immunoglobulin M (IgM) antibody directed against normal human immunoglobulin G (IgG). It is usually measured by agglutination tests (agglutination of IgG-coated latex particles) and reported as either negative or positive with a titer. Rheumatoid factor positivity with titers up to 1:320 may be found in otherwise normal people over 70 years old. Rheumatoid factor can be found in 70 to 80 per cent of patients with rheumatoid arthritis but also in patients with other rheumatic diseases (Sjögren's syndrome) and nonrheumatic diseases, such as chronic infections (hepatitis, subacute bacterial endocarditis). In patients with rheumatoid arthritis, the presence of rheumatoid factor is associated with more severe disease, manifested by rheumatoid nodules, rheumatoid vasculitis, and bone erosions. Rheumatoid factor is characteristically absent in patients with the seronegative spondyloarthropathies, such as psoriatic arthritis and ankylosing spondylitis.

ANTINUCLEAR ANTIBODIES

Testing of serum for the presence of antibodies directed against both nuclear and cytoplasmic antigens has contributed greatly to the diagnosis and management of patients with rheumatic diseases. Beginning with Hargraves' description of the LE cell in 1948, subsequent work has refined our knowledge of these antibodies and their clinical associations (Table 257–3).

Routine determination of the presence of antinuclear antibodies is best performed by the indirect immunofluorescent technique

TABLE 257–3. ASSOCIATION BETWEEN RHEUMATIC DISEASES AND ANTINUCLEAR ANTIBODIES

Rheumatic Disease	Antibody Reactive with: (Autoantibody Frequency, %)
Systemic lupus erythematosus	Native DNA (40%), denatured DNA (70%), Sm (30%), nuclear RNP (30%), SSA/Ro (30%), SSB/La (15%)
Drug-induced lupus	Denatured DNA (80%), Histones (> 95%)
Mixed connective tissue disease	Nuclear RNP (> 95%)
Sjögren's syndrome	SSA/Ro (60%), SSB/La (40%)
Dermatopolymyositis	Jo-1 (25%)
Scleroderma	Scl-70 (70% in diffuse scleroderma), centromere (75% in CREST)

Data from Tan EM: Antinuclear antibodies: Diagnostic markers for autoimmune diseases and probes for cell biology. Adv Immunol 44:93–151, 1989.

RNP = ribonucleoprotein; CREST = calcinosis, Raynaud's phenomenon, esophageal dysmotility, sclerodactyly, and telangiectasia.

using Hep-2 cells. The result must be reported as either negative or positive with a titer and pattern. While certain patterns of antinuclear fluorescence correlate loosely with the presence of specific antibodies (e.g., rim pattern with antibodies to native DNA), the presence of specific antibodies can be confirmed only by testing with specific antigens (often referred to as an ANA [antinuclear antibody] profile). Depending on the rheumatic disease, the presence of specific antibodies can be of critical diagnostic significance. For instance, antibody to the Sm antigen is found in only 30 per cent of patients with systemic lupus erythematosus (SLE) but is not found in patients with other rheumatic diseases. The same significance exists for the relationship between antibodies to the Scl-70 antigen and diffuse scleroderma and antibodies to the Jo-1 antigen and polymyositis. Other associations may be of primary therapeutic importance, as in patients with SLE and antibodies to native DNA, in whom there is a higher incidence of renal disease than if these antibodies were absent. There is also a high incidence of complete congenital heart block in infants of normal or SLE mothers who have SSA/anti-Ro antibodies.

SEDIMENTATION RATE

Determination of the sedimentation rate of red blood cells in anticoagulated blood by the Westergren method is a sensitive indicator of the presence of systemic or locally severe inflammation. Characteristically, patients with inflammatory arthritides, such as rheumatoid arthritis and the seronegative spondyloarthropathies, have elevated sedimentation rates, which vary with clinical disease activity. Thus, in this group of patients, determination of the sedimentation rate can assist in following the activity of the disease, but it is of little help diagnostically. In contrast, patients with temporal arteritis and polymyalgia rheumatica frequently have nonspecific symptoms and a negative laboratory serologic evaluation except for an elevated sedimentation rate. In untreated temporal arteritis and polymyalgia rheumatica, a normal Westergren sedimentation rate virtually eliminates the diagnosis. In addition, in these patients, the Westergren sedimentation rate is used together with clinical symptoms to monitor disease activity as a guide to glucocorticoid therapy. Occasionally, as the glucocorticoid dose is tapered, the sedimentation rate rises before symptoms reappear. In patients with the fibromyalgia syndrome, all tests of inflammation are negative or normal, including the sedimentation rate.

C-REACTIVE PROTEIN (CRP)

C-reactive protein is produced in the liver and is normally found in serum in minute amounts (less than 0.6 mg per deciliter). In conditions characterized by inflammation with tissue destruction, particularly bacterial infections, the CRP level may increase 1000-fold in less than 24 hours. Although CRP has been shown to have many effects in the immune system, including complement activation, its specific primary role is still unclear. In the management of patients with rheumatic diseases, serial determinations of the CRP level have certain advantages over following the sedimentation rate. Since numerous serum proteins can influence the sedimentation rate (fibrinogen, haptoglobin, im-

munoglobulin, ceruloplasmin), changes in the sedimentation rate often do not accurately reflect improvement or deterioration in the clinical condition. Owing to its rapid synthesis and degradation, CRP is a sensitive indicator of therapeutic efficacy in situations in which it is elevated. For example, in patients with septic arthritis, serial serum CRP determinations can provide accurate additional information on the efficacy of antibiotic administration.

ANTIPHOSPHOLIPID ANTIBODY SYNDROME

Antiphospholipid antibodies, including the lupus anticoagulant (LA) and anticardiolipin (ACL), have been reported to be associated with thrombosis, central nervous system disease, and multiple spontaneous abortions in patients with SLE. In addition, in patients without SLE or other obvious connective tissue disease, an increased incidence of arterial and venous thrombosis and loss of fetuses has been suggested to be associated with LA and ACL. Determination of ACL levels is done best by enzyme-linked immunosorbent assay (ELISA). However, this method has been shown to have a high degree of variability and often poor reproducibility even in the best laboratories. The LA is determined by prolongation of the partial thromboplastin time (PTT) when normal plasma is mixed with plasma containing LA. Although LA and ACL are distinct antibodies, they are present together in approximately 70 per cent of patients. LA and ACL are found in approximately 34 per cent and 44 per cent of patients with SLE, respectively.

Although this information engenders a great degree of interest, the lack of prospective study of a group of asymptomatic normal or SLE patients with LA or ACL and a matched population without LA or ACL makes uncertain the exact relationship between antiphospholipid antibodies and disease, particularly in normal subjects. However, since the association of LA and ACL with certain syndromes has been so strong, particularly in patients with multiple spontaneous abortions, clinical trials have been instituted. Oral glucocorticoid or heparin and aspirin therapy of LA-positive, clinically normal women with multiple spontaneous abortions has resulted in successful conception and delivery. Glucocorticoid therapy can alter LA levels but has little effect on ACL levels. An increased incidence of thrombosis, fetal loss, thrombocytopenia, and central nervous system disease has been found in ACL-positive patients with SLE, with no relationship to age, duration of disease, disease severity, or other organ involvement.

LYME DISEASE (see Ch. 343)

A virtual epidemic of testing for Lyme antibodies is sweeping the country. In Wisconsin, where the incidence of Lyme disease is 7.5 per 100,000 population, approximately 1200 per 100,000 Lyme antibody titers were performed in 1988. Since Lyme antibody is frequently absent (50 to 70 per cent) early in the disease, when symptoms and signs are characteristically present, an overreliance on such testing can be very misleading. Newer methodologies, including the Western blot analysis for *Borrelia burgdorferi* antigen, are expensive but promise to add specificity and sensitivity. A PCR (polymerase chain reaction) test for *B. burgdorferi* DNA has been devised, but the sensitivity and specificity have yet to be determined.

Particularly in an endemic area, the decision to treat with antibiotics for Lyme disease must be made more on the basis of clinical suspicion than with reliance on serologic results. Patients with fever and erythema chronicum migrans or polyarthritis, with or without Bell's palsy and cardiac abnormalities (particularly congestive heart failure), should receive antibiotic therapy even if the Lyme antibodies are not present. The presence of Lyme antibodies is most useful diagnostically in patients with an atypical clinical presentation or in late disease (monoarticular arthritis or oligoarthritis and isolated central nervous system disease or psychiatric disorder).

BONE DENSITY MEASUREMENTS

The single most important determinant of hip or vertebral fracture in postmenopausal women is bone density. Therefore, detection and treatment of diminished bone density before menopause should reduce the incidence of fracture in later life. There are certain characteristics in perimenopausal women that, when present, have been thought to predict low bone density (Table 257–4). For the most part, when present, these are reliable indicators of low bone density; however, recent studies have shown bone density to be low in some patients without risk factors. While routine screening of every perimenopausal woman for decreased bone density is not recommended, an accurate determination of bone density can be very useful in determining the need for estrogen therapy and in following the efficacy of therapy for established osteoporosis (see Ch. 238).

Noninvasive techniques for assessing bone density include single- and dual-photon analysis, quantitative computed tomography (CT), and dual-energy x-ray absorptiometry (DEXA). The last-named (DEXA) is now the most accurate method, and dual- and single-photon analyses are the most commonly available. Single-photon analysis is used to assess bone density in the distal radius, while dual-photon analysis accurately assesses bone density in the lumbar spine and proximal femur. Changes in bone density of 1 per cent per year can be accurately assessed with dual-photon analysis. With the use of estrogens and salmon calcitonin, the therapy of osteoporosis can be directed at preventing reabsorption of bone, and fluoride and calcium can stimulate calcified matrix formation. Weight-bearing exercise is the only therapy proven to build bone mass; early results of therapy with Didronel (disodium etidronate) to increase bone mass are encouraging.

IMAGING TECHNIQUES

Plain radiographs of the joints are the least expensive and most readily accessible joint imaging technique. They constitute the gold standard for the diagnosis of osteoarthritis and are the most commonly used means to assess the presence and progression of bone erosions in rheumatoid arthritis. Single anteroposterierior radiographs of the hands, feet, pelvis, and knees (weight-bearing joints) are most often used to screen patients with signs or symptoms in these areas. In rheumatoid arthritis, the earliest findings are periarticular osteopenia and soft tissue swelling, particularly evident in the hands. In patients with osteoarthritis, joint space narrowing seen in the medial compartment of the knee on weight-bearing views often precedes the other characteristic features, i.e., subchondral sclerosis, marginal osteophyte formation, subchondral cysts, and varus deformity. A lateral view of the cervical spine in flexion and extension is useful to detect vertebral subluxation (particularly C-1–C-2) in patients with rheumatoid arthritis. A single 20-degree anteroposterior tilt of the pelvis gives excellent visualization of the sacroiliac joints. The limitations of plain radiography in correlating patients' symptoms with intra-articular abnormalities have become evident as more sophisticated imaging techniques have become available. By using both arthroscopic inspection and the newer imaging techniques (MRI), cartilage damage and intra-articular soft tissue abnormalities, such as meniscal tears, have been documented to occur in the presence of normal plain joint radiographs. These observations help to explain the lack of concordance between symptoms and radiographic findings often seen in patients with early osteoarthritis.

Of the new imaging techniques, MRI has had the most dramatic impact on the anatomic assessment of the musculoskeletal system. In a patient with a painful shoulder, the MRI shows rotator cuff inflammation and partial tears with much more sensitivity than does arthography and with more specificity than does ultrasound.

TABLE 257–4. RISK FACTORS FOR OSTEOPOROSIS

Female
Caucasian/Asian
Menopausal
Elderly
Petite female body
Positive family history
Diet deficient in calcium
Alcohol or tobacco consumption
Physical inactivity

In the knee, MRI is extremely sensitive in detecting degenerative changes in menisci and cartilage. Intrameniscal degeneration (grades I and II) unaccompanied by arthroscopically detectable tears is commonly seen on MRI examination in patients with osteoarthritis of the knee. Even meniscal degenerative lesions that appear to be full thickness on MRI (grade III) can occur in the absence of a tear. A similar situation occurs in the lumbosacral spine, where MRI-demonstrable disc degeneration occurs in advance of disc space narrowing on plain radiographs. Thinning and ulceration of hyaline articular cartilage can also be seen before any changes are evident on the plain radiographs. This superior visualization of intra-articular structures holds great promise for the early detection of joint destruction and in guiding specific protective therapy. However, MRI cannot be used to plan or as an indication for arthroscopic interventions in patients with osteoarthritis, since the relationships between the patient's symptoms, the MRI findings, and the response to therapy have not yet been demonstrated.

ARTHROSCOPY

Endoscopic inspection of the joint with therapeutic intra-articular interventions has gone from being "the professor's toy" in the 1970's to being the most commonly performed invasive procedure in the 1990's for patients with arthritis. Fueled by rapid technologic advances, coupled with heightened awareness and expectations on the part of the patient, the dramatic increase in the number of arthroscopies has not yet been accompanied by a clear delineation of the risks and benefits. In addition, the tremendous potential of arthroscopy for research purposes in arthritis to help visually delineate intra-articular abnormalities and obtain synovial biopsy specimens under direct visualization has only just recently begun to be explored.

At present, arthroscopy is performed in an operating room setting, most frequently with the patient under general anesthesia. Sterile conditions are used throughout the procedure. Available instruments include a standard 30-degree rigid operating arthroscope (4 mm in external diameter, fiberoptic light source) in the presence of continuous pressure-controlled saline irrigation. The arthroscope is attached to a television camera, and the image is projected on a screen either in front of or to the side of the arthroscopist. This practice allows accurate visualization as well as the recording of the entire arthroscopic procedure on videotape. Equipment available for arthroscopic intervention includes a variety of motorized and hand-operated instruments. Biopsy forceps and basket forceps for debriding cartilage and menisci come in various sizes and angulations. Motorized equipment includes articular shavers for cartilage and synovial debridement. The basic technique of arthroscopy is triangulation. The arthroscopist must be able to perform diagnostic and therapeutic maneuvers through triangulation while looking at the television screen and not the knee. This is a skill acquired by training on arthroscopic simulators as well as with time and practice. With the use of a standard arthroscope, all compartments of the knee, both weight bearing and non weight bearing, can be inspected, including the posterior compartments and the popliteal space. All intra-articular structures, cruciates, and menisci can be thoroughly inspected and probed to detect defects or laxity. Arthroscopic visualization is now possible for virtually all major joints, including, in order of frequency, the knee, shoulder, ankle, elbow, wrist, and hip. New technologic advances have produced arthroscopes that can be placed in the joint through a 14-gauge needle and now suggest a role for laser therapy in synovial, cartilage, and meniscal debridement.

The most frequent serious complications of arthroscopy at the present time are septic arthritis and hemarthrosis, which occur in fewer than 0.1 per cent of patients. Although no specific series has addressed the complication rate in patients with arthritis, use of local or regional anesthesia rather than general, use of a pressure infusion pump to control bleeding rather than occlusion of blood flow to the leg by thigh tourniquet, and attention to aggressive postoperative rehabilitation should help to lower even further the 1 to 2 per cent overall complication rate for patients with arthritis.

While the role for arthroscopy in the management of patients with arthritis continues to evolve, conceptually, the availability of arthroscopy has already altered the approach to the manage-

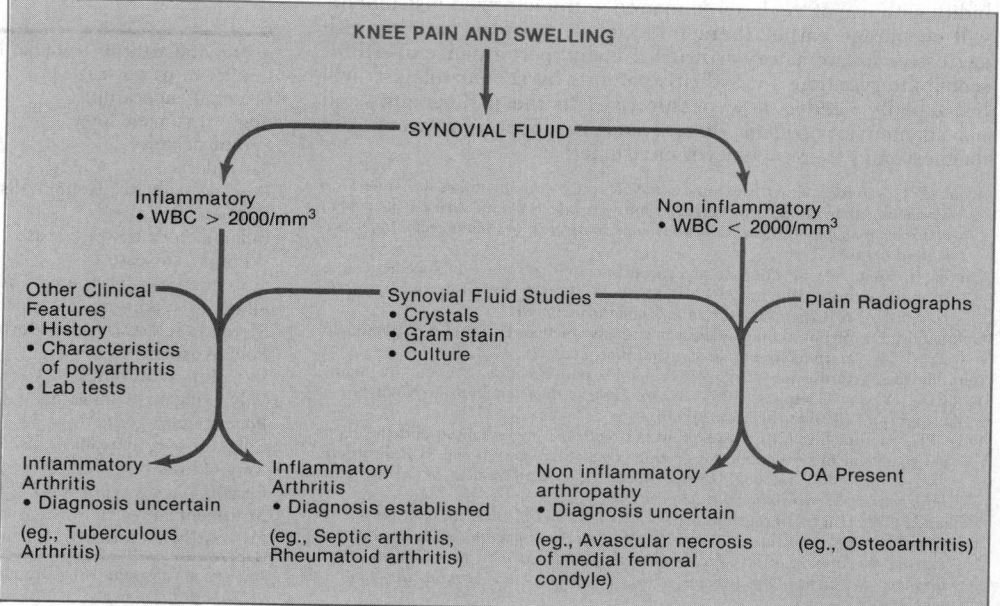

FIGURE 257–1. An arthroscopist's approach to the management of knee arthritis. See text for discussion. WBC = white blood cells; OA = osteoarthritis.

ment of these patients, particularly those with knee arthritis (Fig. 257–1). Clinically, a frequently encountered situation for the rheumatologist is a patient who presents with knee pain and swelling in the absence of trauma. From the arthroscopist's viewpoint, the evaluation of such a patient must be comprehensive and include, in all cases, a complete synovial fluid analysis. If the patient has inflammatory synovial fluid with a positive synovial fluid culture, then immediate management of infectious arthritis will at least involve parenteral administration of antibiotics and repeated needle drainage of the knee. Arthroscopic irrigation and debridement can be used if the infectious arthritis fails to respond. Similarly, if intracellular crystals of monosodium urate are found, then the management should be directed at acute gouty arthritis.

In other patients with knee arthritis and inflammatory synovial fluid, the correct diagnosis of the inflammatory arthritis becomes apparent with time (e.g., rheumatoid arthritis, psoriatic arthritis) and without the need for arthroscopy. More helpful diagnostic information can usually be gained from a thorough history and physical examination that seeks additional articular involvement (e.g., sacroileitis) as well as extra-articular involvement (conjunctivitis, skin rash, digital ulcerations, oral or genital lesions, olecranon nodules, and so on) than from an arthroscopic inspection of an inflamed knee!

However, arthroscopy can be useful at a later time in patients with rheumatoid arthritis, if their comprehensive management program fails to relieve knee pain and disability. These patients usually demonstrate knee inflammation with proliferative synovitis, but at times synovitis can be minimal while the patient notes typical symptoms of internal derangement, such as "locking" and "giving way." Arthroscopic examination might then reveal proliferative synovitis, in which the synovium is capable of being trapped between articular surfaces (synovial impingement syndrome), or actual meniscal tears due to chronic synovitis and loose bodies. These findings can be treated by resection or removal under arthroscopic guidance. Most commonly, a complete, multicompartmental arthroscopic synovectomy will also be performed while addressing any internal derangements present at this time. Patients undergoing complete arthroscopic synovectomy have a much shorter period of rehabilitation and markedly reduced morbidity compared with those who have undergone the previously performed open synovectomy, which is now of historical significance only.

Arthroscopy with synovial biopsy is of greatest value in patients with undiagnosed inflammatory arthritis, particularly if the involvement remains monoarticular. In the past, closed-needle synovial biopsy has been used; however, recent information has documented the dramatic intra-articular variability of synovial inflammation, requiring biopsy under direct visualization for optimal results. Cultures of synovial biopsy specimens may reveal tuberculous or chronic fungal arthritis, such as blastomycosis or sporotrichosis, while noncaseating granulomas are the characteristic synovial histologic finding in patients with chronic sarcoid arthritis. Pigmented villonodular synovitis, ochronosis, and the arthritis of hemochromatosis also have characteristic synovial histologic findings best obtained with arthroscopic guidance.

In patients with a noninflammatory synovial effusion and a negative synovial fluid analysis, plain radiographs and the physical signs of grating of cartilage surfaces with joint motion and varus deformity will allow the diagnosis of osteoarthritis to be made with certainty. Management to reduce pain and disability then follows a standard comprehensive regimen of exercise, use of heat and cold, nonsteroidal anti-inflammatory drugs, intra-articular glucocorticoid injections, gait-assistive devices, orthoses, and special footwear. Only after failure of this program to relieve pain and disability should arthroscopy be considered to document and treat intra-articular abnormalities. Arthroscopic evaluation of patients with early to moderate radiographic changes of osteoarthritis often reveals significant cartilage defects, torn menisci, and localized areas of inflamed synovial tissue. In these patients, arthroscopic debridement of inflamed or damaged tissue, as well as removal of loose intra-articular debris by saline irrigation, has provided pain relief and improved function. In fact, removal of intra-articular debris with closed tidal saline irrigation, even without arthroscopy, has also produced similar improvement in some patients.

It is in those with the noninflammatory synovial fluid and normal radiographs that the most careful evaluation must be performed prior to arthroscopic intervention. Major diagnostic considerations in this group of patients include avascular necrosis of the medial femoral condyle, malignancy, and osteomyelitis in the femur or tibia abutting the joint. In each of these situations, imaging with MRI can identify characteristic abnormalities, thereby avoiding a potentially unnecessary arthroscopic intervention. In the presence of a normal MRI, arthroscopy contributes little and most frequently reveals degenerative cartilage lesions associated with localized synovial inflammation. Classification of these patients as having early osteoarthritis in the absence of characteristic radiographic and physical findings is tempting but clearly beyond the limits of our present understanding of osteoarthritis.

The full promise of arthroscopy as a research tool in patients with arthritis will be realized as technology improves with the development of smaller arthroscopes and the use of lasers. Serial diagnostic arthroscopy with biopsy as an office procedure may be used to document abnormalities and guide therapy. Lower morbidity with use of the laser compared with motorized instruments will encourage earlier therapeutic intervention in patients with aggressive inflammatory arthritis. Finally, performance of arthroscopic interventions for arthritis patients by rheumatologists will bring badly needed new perspectives to the pathogenesis and management of articular disease and may open new avenues of diagnosis and therapy not yet envisioned.

Arnold WJ, Kalunian K: Arthroscopic synovectomy by rheumatologists: Time for a new look. Arthritis Rheum 32:108, 1989. *A modern perspective on the role of arthroscopic synovectomy and the rheumatologist in the management of rheumatoid arthritis.*

Canoso JJ, Yood RA: Reaction of superficial bursae in response to specific disease stimuli. Arthritis Rheum 22:1361, 1979. *First study to delineate clearly the response of superficial bursae to inflammatory stimuli.*

Goldenberg DL: Synovial fluid analysis in current practice. Postgrad Adv Rheumatol 2:3, 1987. *An updated look at synovial fluid analysis.*

Johnson LL: Arthroscopic Surgery—Principles and Practice. 3rd ed. St. Louis, C. V. Mosby Company, 1986. *Arthroscopy is depicted with excellent photographs and clear textual description.*

Love PE, Santoro SA: Antiphospholipid antibodies: Anticardiolipin and the lupus anticoagulant in systemic lupus erythmatosus (SLE) and in non-SLE disorders. Ann Intern Med 112:682, 1990. *Thorough, critical review of all available information on this important association.*

Slemenda CW, Hui SL, Longcope C, et al.: Predictors of bone mass in perimenopausal women. Ann Intern Med 112:96, 1990. *An important study demonstrating the weaknesses of risk factor analysis compared with bone density measurement in identifying women with low bone mass around the time of menopause.*

Sox HC Jr, Liang MH: The erythrocyte sedimentation rate. Guidelines for rational use. Ann Intern Med 104:515, 1986. *Defines the role of the erythrocyte sedimentation rate in the diagnosis and management of patients with rheumatic diseases.*

Steere AC: Lyme disease. N Engl J Med 321:586, 1989. *Complete discussion of clinical, laboratory, and therapeutic aspects of Lyme disease.*

Stoller DW, Genant HK, Helms CA, et al.: Magnetic Resonance Imaging in Orthopedics and Rheumatology. Philadelphia, J. B. Lippincott Company, 1989. *An excellent text devoted to a careful depiction of the MRI findings in the musculoskeletal system.*

Tan EM: Antinuclear antibodies: Diagnostic markers for autoimmune diseases and probes for cell biology. Adv Immunol 44:93, 1989. *Exhaustive, referenced review of the clinical and laboratory significance of antinuclear antibodies.*

258 Rheumatoid Arthritis

Frank C. Arnett

Rheumatoid arthritis (RA) is a chronic systemic inflammatory disease predominantly affecting diarthrodial joints and frequently a variety of other organs. The cause (causes) of RA is (are) unknown, and there is no specific diagnostic test. Therefore, the American College of Rheumatology (ACR) has recently revised classification criteria for RA to guarantee uniformity in investigative and epidemiologic studies (Table 258–1). Although these seven items include the most characteristic clinical features of RA, a variety of other disorders may mimic the disease (see Differential Diagnosis and Table 258–2). It is not recommended that these criteria be relied upon for definitive diagnosis in clinical practice.

Rheumatoid arthritis occurs worldwide in all ethnic groups.

TABLE 258–1. CLASSIFICATION CRITERIA FOR RHEUMATOID ARTHRITIS*

1. Morning stiffness ($\geq$1 hr)
2. Swelling (soft tissue) of three or more joints
3. Swelling (soft tissue) of hand joints (PIP, MCP, or wrist)
4. Symmetric swelling (soft tissue)
5. Subcutaneous nodules
6. Serum rheumatoid factor
7. Erosions and/or periarticular osteopenia, in hand or wrist joints, seen on radiograph

*Criteria 1 to 4 must have been continuous for 6 weeks or longer and must be observed by a physician. A diagnosis of rheumatoid arthritis requires that four of the seven criteria be fulfilled.

PIP = proximal interphalangeal; MCP = metacarpophalangeal.

TABLE 258–2. DIFFERENTIAL DIAGNOSIS OF RA

	Subcutaneous Nodules	Rheumatoid Factor (RF)
Acute viral arthritis (rubella, hepatitis B, parvovirus)	−	−
Bacterial endocarditis	+/−	+
Acute rheumatic fever	+	−
Serum sickness	−	−
Sarcoidosis	+	+
Reactive arthritis (Reiter's disease)	−	−
Psoriatic arthritis	−	−
Inflammatory bowel disease	−	−
Whipple's disease	−	−
Systemic lupus erythematosus	+	+
Sjögren's syndrome	−	+
Systemic sclerosis (scleroderma)	−	+/−
Polymyositis	−	+/−
Vasculitis syndromes	−	+
Polymyalgia rheumatica	−	−
Polyarticular gout	+ (tophi)	−
Calcium pyrophosphate disease	−	−
Amyloidosis	+/−	−
Paraneoplastic syndromes	−	−
Multicentric reticulohistiocytosis	+	−
Osteoarthritis (erosive)	−	−

− = not present; + = frequently present; +/− = occasionally present.

Prevalence rates range from 0.3 to 1.5 per cent in most populations, but frequencies of 3.5 to 5.3 per cent have been found in several Native American tribes (Yakima and Chippewa). The peak incidence of onset is between the fourth and sixth decades, but RA may begin at any time from childhood (see Juvenile Chronic Arthritis) to later life. Females are two to three times more likely to be affected than males.

No definitive description of RA exists before the early nineteenth century, and anthropologic evidence of the disease has been found in New World, but not Old World, skeletons. Thus, it has been proposed, but not proved, that an etiologic agent was carried to Europe by early explorers of the Americas. A.B. Garrod first proposed the term "rheumatoid arthritis" in 1858.

ETIOLOGY

Despite intensive research over many decades, the etiology of RA remains unknown. Three areas of interrelated research are currently most promising: (1) host genetic factors, (2) immunoregulatory abnormalities and autoimmunity, and (3) a triggering or persisting microbial infection.

Genetic susceptibility to RA has been clearly demonstrated. The disease clusters in families and occurs more frequently in monozygotic than in dizygotic twins. The major histocompatibility complex (MHC) allele (and encoded antigen) HLA-DR4 (HLA, human leukocyte antigen) is significantly increased in RA patients in most populations (see Ch. 250). Among Caucasians of western European origin, HLA-DR4 occurs in 60 to 70 per cent of seropositive individuals with RA compared with approximately 30 per cent of normal individuals. The presence of this tissue type correlates even more strongly with rheumatoid factor (RF) titer, severe joint destruction on radiographs, rheumatoid lung disease, and Felty's syndrome. HLA-DR1 is found in the majority of HLA-DR4–negative patients and is most strongly associated with the disease in other ethnic groups (Israelis, Asian Indians). Several subtypes of HLA-DR4 were initially defined by mixed lymphocyte cultures (MLC). The HLA-Dw4, HLA-Dw14, and HLA-Dw15 subtypes predispose to RA, while HLA-Dw10 and HLA-Dw13 do not. Molecular genetic studies have recently demonstrated that these HLA-DR4 subtypes result from only a few amino acid differences in the third hypervariable region of the HLA-DR beta chain. HLA-DR1 shares the same amino acid sequence as the HLA-Dw14 subtype of HLA-DR4. Thus, a "shared epitope" among several MHC class II molecules appears to predispose to RA. The critical region on these molecules appears to be a combining site for the T cell antigen receptor (TCR). Since MHC class II molecules present processed antigen to the TCR on helper (CD4+) T lymphocytes (see Ch. 242), it appears likely that an abnormal antigen-specific cellular and/or humoral immune response is inherent to the etiology of RA. The nature of the antigen, whether self or foreign, remains unknown.

Rheumatoid arthritis appears to be an "autoimmune" disease, similar to other MHC class II–associated disorders (see Ch. 250). Autoantibodies to the Fc portion of immunoglobulin G (IgG) molecules, or RF's, are produced by B lymphocytes in the blood and synovial tissues of 80 per cent of RA patients. Such cases are termed seropositive. High titers of serum RF are associated with more severe joint disease and with extra-articular manifestations, especially subcutaneous nodules. Rheumatoid factor detected by the usual clinical methods (latex fixation or sensitized sheep cell agglutination) are immunoglobulin M (IgM) antibodies. IgG, immunoglobulin A (IgA), immunoglobulin E (IgE), and immunoglobulin D (IgD) RF's have also been described. IgM RF can react with five IgG molecules to produce very large complexes (sedimentation coefficient of 22S), and they appear to participate in the pathogenesis of rheumatoid synovitis. Intermediate-sized complexes (between 7S and 19S) containing only IgG molecules, some of which have RF activity against self, have been found and may occur to a greater extent in individuals with widespread systemic disease and vasculitis.

Despite the extremely strong association of RF's with RA, they clearly do not cause the disease. Production of RF occurs commonly in other diseases or disorders in which there is chronic antigenic stimulation, such as bacterial endocarditis, tuberculosis, syphilis, kala-azar, viral infections, intravenous drug abuse, and cirrhosis. Normal individuals occasionally produce RF, especially with increasing age. In none of these situations is RF associated with HLA-DR4.

An infectious origin for RA has been a continuing hypothesis. Streptococci, diphtheroids, mycoplasmas, and *Clostridium perfringens* have all been proposed and later discarded because of lack of definitive evidence. Viral infections such as rubella, Ross River virus, and, more recently, parvovirus B19 have been shown to produce an acute polyarthritis, but no evidence exists that they initiate chronic RA. The Epstein-Barr virus (EBV) remains a viable but unproven candidate for a pathogenetic role. The EBV is a polyclonal B cell activator capable of stimulating autoantibody production, including RF. Increased numbers of EBV-infected B cells have been found in the blood but not the synovial tissue of RA patients. Antibodies against a nuclear antigen (EBNA) expressed in EBV-infected cells occur in the majority of RA patients, and a variety of other unusual immune responses to EBV are found in RA patients. More recently, an EBV protein has been shown to share the same five amino acids as the HLA-DR4 (Dw4) molecule, which is implicated in susceptibility to RA, thus raising the possibility of "molecular mimicry" as a mechanism. Nonetheless, EBV is highly ubiquitous, and there is no *direct* evidence that this virus initiates the disease.

PATHOLOGY AND PATHOGENESIS

The pathologic hallmark of RA is synovial membrane proliferation and outgrowth associated with erosion of articular cartilage and subchondral bone. Often likened to a malignant tumor, proliferating inflammatory tissue (pannus) may lead subsequently to destruction of intra-articular and periarticular structures and may result in the joint deformities and dysfunction seen clinically.

The events initiating the process are unknown (Fig. 258–1). The earliest findings include microvascular injury and moderate proliferation of synovial cells accompanied by interstitial edema and perivascular infiltration by mononuclear cells, predominantly T lymphocytes. Polymorphonuclear leukocytes and plasma cells are infrequent. With continuation of the process, there is further hyperplasia of lining cells, both DR-positive type A (macrophage-like) and DR-negative type B (fibroblast-like), and the normally acellular subsynovial stroma becomes engorged with mononuclear inflammatory cells, which may collect into aggregates or follicles, especially around postcapillary venules. The composition of cellular infiltrates varies, with some being predominantly T cells, usually CD4+, others being plasma cell rich, and some having a mixed population of lymphocytes (often CD8+), plasma cells, macrophages, and interdigitating (dendritic) cells. Mast cells are also commonly present. Occasionally, germinal centers rich in B lymphocytes can be seen. The proliferating synovium (pannus) becomes villous and is vascularized by arterioles, capillaries, and venules.

Roles for both *cellular* and *humoral* immune mechanisms in the rheumatoid synovium have been proposed, and both are

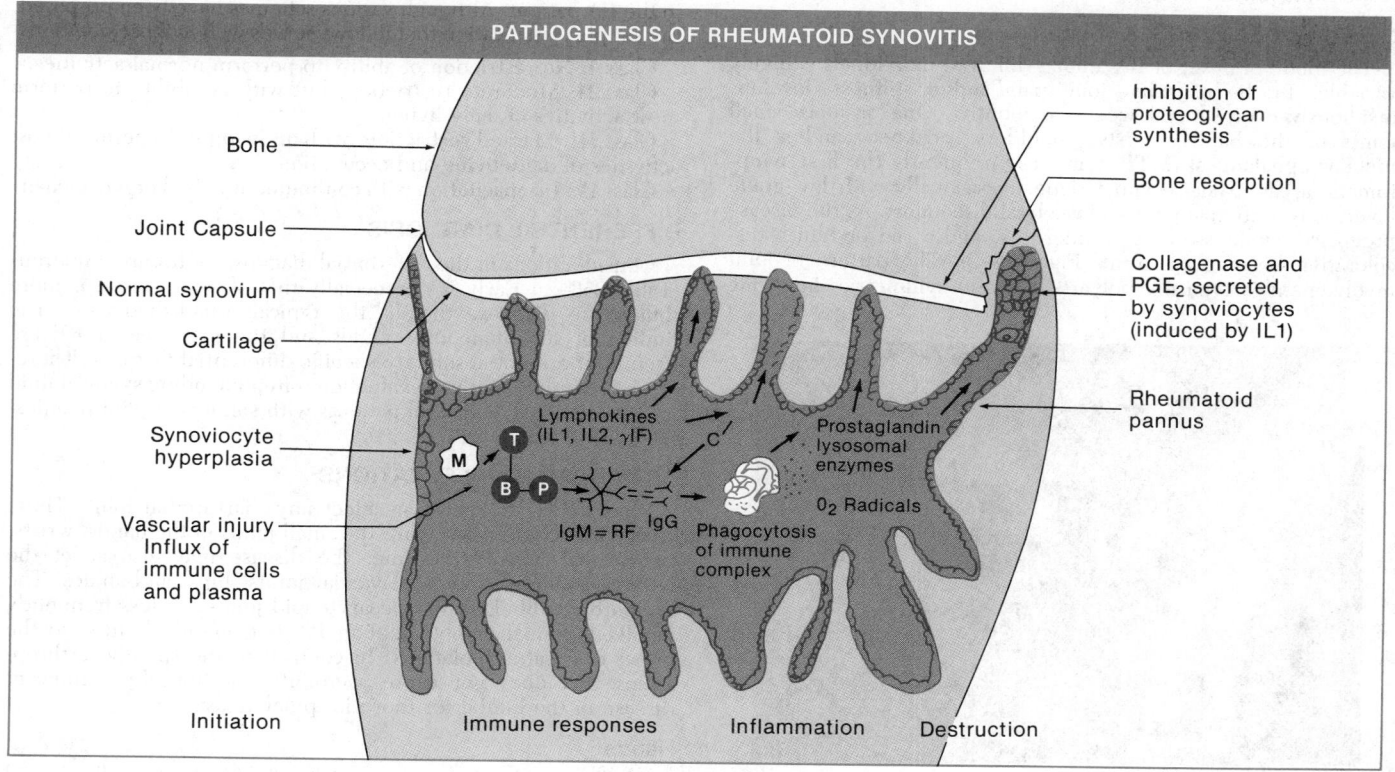

FIGURE 258–1. Events involved in the pathogenesis of rheumatoid synovitis progress from left to right. M = macrophage; T = T lymphocyte; B = B lymphocyte; P = plasma cell; IL1 = interleukin 1; IL2 = interleukin 2; γIF = gamma-interferon; RF = rheumatoid factor; PGE₂ = prostaglandin E₂; IgM = immunoglobulin M; IgG = immunoglobulin G; C = complement.

supported by immunopathologic findings. A cellular mechanism would involve activation of infiltrating T lymphocytes by some unknown antigen (or antigens) presented by DR-positive cells (type A synoviocytes, macrophages, dendritic cells). A release of a variety of soluble mediators would follow, which would then promote further synovial proliferation and inflammation. Indeed, T cells appear to be activated, and T cell–derived lymphokines (such as interleukin 2 and gamma-interferon) probably play important roles in the inflammatory process. Moreover, interleukin 1, produced by the interaction of monocytes and/or macrophages with activated T cells, induces collagenase and prostaglandin E_2 production by synoviocytes. This monokine also promotes degradation and inhibits synthesis of proteoglycan by chondrocytes, as well as enhances resorption of calcium from bone.

Humoral mechanisms are supported by the demonstration of local RF production within the synovium, the formation of IgM-IgG immune complexes, and activation and consumption of complement via the classic pathway. The sequelae of complement activation include increased vascular permeability and phagocytosis of the immune complexes by phagocytic cells. Aggregates of immune complexes within polymorphonuclear leukocytes are often seen in rheumatoid synovial fluid and have been termed "RA cells" or "ragocytes."

Antigen-antibody complexes formed within the joint cavity can become trapped in hyaline cartilage and fibrocartilage, where they cause changes in matrix macromolecules. Within the synovial fluid, immune complexes activate the complement system, kinins, phagocytic cells, and lysosomal enzyme release. Mediators produced in this process stimulate synovial cells to proliferate and to produce proteinases and prostaglandins. These products cause dissolution of the connective tissue macromolecules, as well as articular cartilage. They may also activate fibroblasts to produce a denser connective tissue matrix (fibrosis).

The ultimate destruction of cartilage, bone, tendons, and ligaments probably results from a variety of proteolytic enzymes, metalloproteinases, and soluble mediators. Collagenase, produced at the interface of pannus and cartilage, is probably largely responsible for the typical erosions after its activation by plasmin.

CLINICAL FEATURES

The mode of onset of RA among different individuals is highly variable. In the majority, joint pain and/or stiffness develops insidiously over several weeks to months. One or more small joints of the hands, wrists, shoulders, or knees and/or the metatarsophalangeal (MTP) joints are frequently the first symptomatic areas. Malaise and fatigue, occasionally with low-grade fever, may accompany musculoskeletal discomfort. As the disease progresses, joint swelling, tenderness, and a red or bluish discoloration become apparent (Fig. 258–2). The pattern of joint involvement is typically polyarticular and symmetric, involving

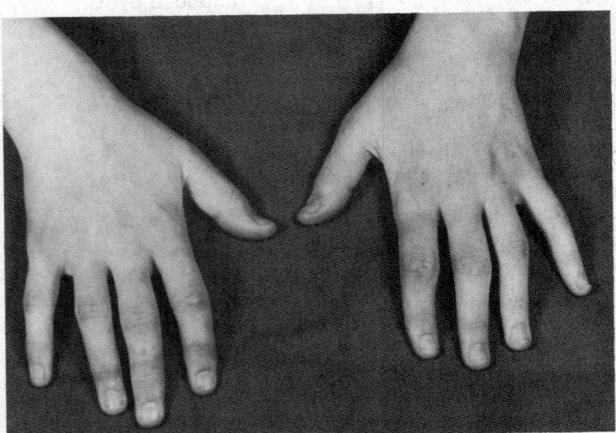

FIGURE 258–2. Early rheumatoid arthritis manifests as symmetric swelling and slight flexion deformities of proximal interphalangeal joints of the hands. Roentgenograms were normal except for evidence of soft tissue swelling.

the proximal interphalangeal (PIP), metacarpophalangeal (MCP), wrist, elbow, shoulder, knee, ankle, and MTP joints. Distal interphalangeal (DIP) joints of the fingers are usually spared. Joint stiffness, especially if lasting more than 1 hour in the morning and after inactivity, is a prominent complaint in RA. So characteristic is this symptom that the duration of morning stiffness is often used as a quantitative guide to the activity of the inflammatory process in both clinical practice and research studies. As the disease process evolves, the patient may experience increasing difficulty with pain and stiffness, as well as impairment of joint function. The simple activities of daily living may be severely compromised, and the ability to continue a productive occupation is threatened. Sleep habits become disturbed, and the patient may experience an associated depression and weight loss.

An "acute" onset occurring over 1 or several days is seen in about 20 per cent of patients. Occasionally, an individual retires in the evening with no symptoms and awakens with acute, generalized RA. Such a rapid onset of pain involving joints, surrounding soft tissues, and muscle can mimic and must be differentiated from acute myositis, viral syndromes, or, if focal, even septic or crystal-induced arthritides. Rare patients experience recurrent (palindromic) episodes of acute monoarthritis, often so severe as to mimic gout, yet lasting only 24 to 48 hours. Such patients, especially if seropositive, eventually develop the typical chronic, symmetric polyarthritis of RA.

The course of RA, like its onset, varies widely. Fluctuating disease activity early in the disease process is usual. Ultimately, joint deformities and variable degrees of disability occur in the majority of patients (Fig. 258–3). Some patients have a relentlessly progressive course leading to early disability or even death, but repeated periods of some degree of remission are the rule. The ACR has proposed criteria for clinical remission in RA. At least five of the following requirements must be fulfilled for at least 2 consecutive months: (1) duration of morning stiffness not exceeding 15 minutes; (2) no fatigue; (3) no joint pain (by history); (4) no joint tenderness or pain on motion; (5) no soft tissue swelling in joints or tendon sheaths; (6) an erythrocyte sedimentation rate (Westergren) less than 30 mm per hour for females or 20 mm per hour for males.

The assessment of functional capacity is frequently necessary in the RA patient. Although various schemes have been proposed, the simple classification that follows serves well in most situations.

Class I: No restriction of ability to perform normal activities.
Class II: Moderate restriction, but with an ability to perform most activities of daily living.
Class III: Marked restriction, with an inability to perform most activities of daily living and occupation.
Class IV: Incapacitation with confinement to bed or wheelchair.

DIFFERENTIAL DIAGNOSIS

Considerations in the differential diagnosis of RA are numerous (Table 258–2). Early RA, especially that of acute onset, is more difficult to diagnose than is the typical established case. The finding of subcutaneous nodules and the presence of RF are useful but are not absolutely specific differential features. Therefore, a complete medical evaluation, often including synovial fluid analysis, is indicated in all patients with significant joint manifestations.

ARTICULAR MANIFESTATIONS

Rheumatoid arthritis can affect any diarthrodial joint. Those most commonly involved are the small joints of the hands, wrists, knees, and feet. With time, the disease may also affect the elbows, shoulders, sternoclavicular joints, hips, and ankles. The temporomandibular and cricoarytenoid joints are less frequently involved. Spinal involvement in RA is generally limited to the upper cervical articulations. In contrast to the spondyloarthropathies, RA does not cause sacroiliitis or clinically significant disease in the lumbar or thoracic spinal areas.

Hands

Swelling of the PIP joints, giving a fusiform or spindle-shaped appearance to the fingers, is one of the most common early signs. Bilateral and symmetric swelling of the MCP joints is also frequent (Fig. 258–2). The DIP joints are usually spared, which

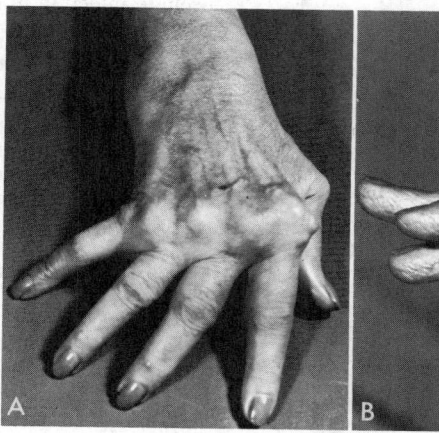
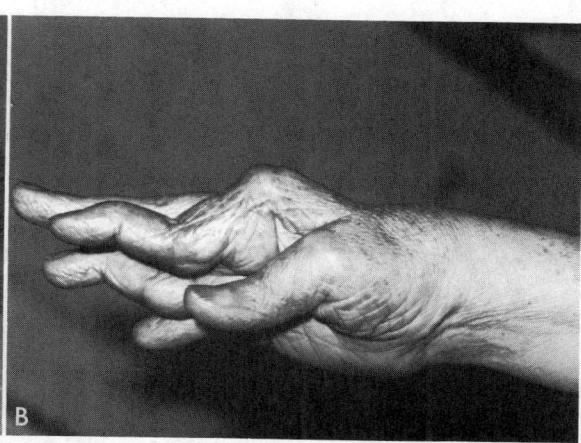

FIGURE 258–3. Hand deformities characteristic of chronic rheumatoid arthritis. *A*, Subluxation of metacarpophalangeal joints with ulnar deviation of digits. *B*, Hyperextension ("swan neck") deformities of proximal interphalangeal joints.

is a useful sign in discriminating RA from osteoarthritis and psoriatic arthritis. Soft tissue laxity gives rise to ulnar deviation of the fingers at the MCP joints (Fig. 258–3A). Swan-neck deformities develop from hypertension of the PIP joints in conjunction with flexion of the DIP joints (Fig. 258–3B). Boutonnière (buttonhole) deformities result from flexion contractures of the PIP joints associated with hyperextension of the DIP joints. These changes result in a loss of strength and dexterity in the hands, as well as the ability to maintain a good pinch. Synovial erosions of extensor tendons, usually at the dorsum of the wrist, may lead to sudden rupture and loss of the ability to extend one or more fingers.

Wrists

The wrists are almost invariably involved in RA and frequently demonstrate easily palpable, boggy synovium, especially over the ulnar styloid. Loss of wrist motion, both flexion and extension,

usually occurs to some degree. The median nerve on the volar side often becomes compressed by proliferating synovium, resulting in a carpal tunnel syndrome (Fig. 258–4). The patient notes paresthesias or pain in the thumb, second and third digits, and radial side of the fourth digit. Symptoms are typically worse at night or with other activities associated with sustained flexion of the wrist. *Tinel's* (Fig. 258–4) and *Phalen's* (Fig. 258–5) signs can usually be elicited, and thenar muscle wasting may be evident.

Knees

Synovial proliferation and effusion are common in these weight-bearing joints. Effusions may be detected by performing ballottement on the patella or by observing a "bulge sign" along the medial aspect of the patella when fluid is pushed into the suprapatellar pouch and then expressed back into the joint. Quadriceps atrophy may occur, and a flexion contracture of the knee may compromise walking. Eventually, destruction of soft tissue around the knee can produce marked joint instability. Popliteal (Baker's) cysts may form owing to effusion or synovial proliferation into the semimembranous bursa (Fig. 258–6). Such synovial cysts may dissect or rupture into the calf, producing symptoms and signs mimicking those of thrombophlebitis. Sonograms are useful in confirming the diagnosis. Venograms may also be necessary because venous occlusion by the cyst can occur.

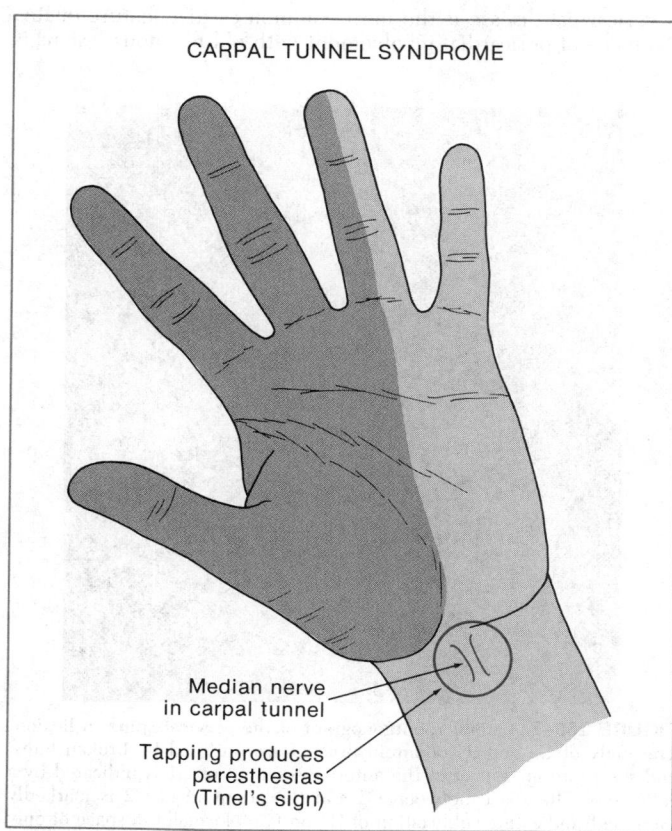

CARPAL TUNNEL SYNDROME

Median nerve in carpal tunnel

Tapping produces paresthesias (Tinel's sign)

FIGURE 258–4. Distribution of pain and/or paresthesias *(shaded area)* when the median nerve is compressed by swelling in the wrist (carpal tunnel).

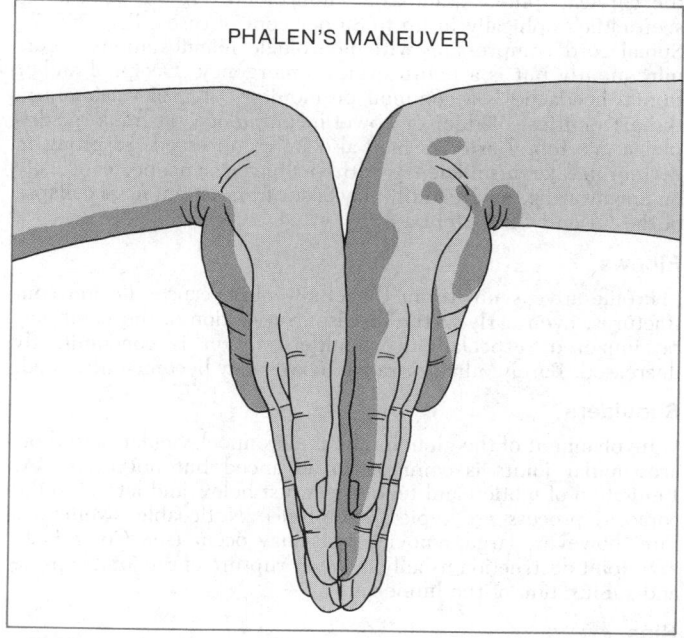

PHALEN'S MANEUVER

FIGURE 258–5. Pain and/or paresthesias are produced in the distribution of the median nerve (Fig. 258–4) when hands are held in forced flexion for 30 to 60 seconds (Phalen's maneuver).

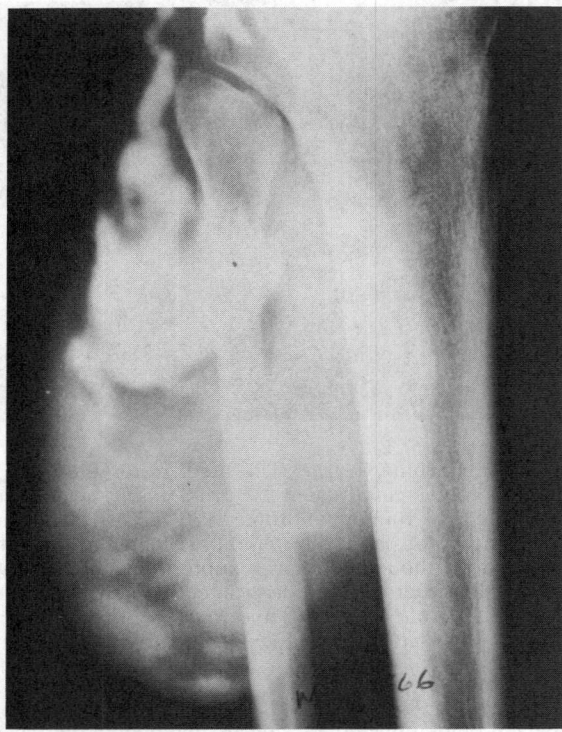

FIGURE 258–6. Arthrogram using a radiocontrast agent injected into the knee. The dye flows into the popliteal space and through a narrow channel into a large synovial cyst (Baker's cyst), which has dissected into the soft tissues of the calf.

Feet and Ankles

The MTP joints are the most commonly involved sites. Subluxation of the metatarsal heads into the soles, often with cock-up and valgus deformities of the toes, results in painful walking and difficulty with footwear.

Neck

Neck pain and stiffness are common. As in other joints, the rheumatoid process can lead to erosion of bone and ligaments in the cervical spine. Atlantoaxial subluxation (C1 on C2) can be seen radiographically in up to 30 per cent of cases (Fig. 258–7). Spinal cord compression with neurologic manifestations occurs infrequently but is a neurosurgical emergency. Occipital and/or frontal headache is a common premonitory sign of weakness in the extremities, bladder or bowel incontinence, or frank quadriplegia. Vertebral arteries may also be compressed, resulting in vertebrobasilar insufficiency with vertigo or syncope, especially on downward gaze. Head tilt may occur from lateral mass collapse of the C1 and C2 vertebrae.

Elbows

Proliferative synovitis in the elbow often causes flexion contractures, even early in the disease. Supination of the hand may be impaired, especially if shoulder motion is concomitantly decreased. Rarely, ulnar or radial nerves may become entrapped.

Shoulders

Involvement of the glenohumeral, acromioclavicular, and thoracoscapular joints is common in advanced but not early RA. Limitation of motion and tenderness just below and lateral to the coracoid process are typical symptoms. Noticeable swelling is rare; however, large synovial cysts may occur (see Color Plate 4D). Joint destruction usually involves rupture of the joint capsule and subluxation of the humerus.

Hips

Pain in the groin, lateral buttock, or lower back may be indicative of hip involvement. Because the hip joint capsule has poor distensibility, severe pain can result if a large effusion occurs. Arthrocentesis should be done to relieve pain and to exclude infection in such cases. Rarely, extreme hip destruction results in protrusion of the femur into the pelvis.

Cricoarytenoid Joints

Synovitis of the cricoarytenoid joints may result in dysphagia, hoarseness, or anterior neck pain. The sudden onset of stridor and dyspnea in a patient with RA is an emergency. Prompt administration of intra-articular or parenteral corticosteroids and/or tracheostomy may be necessary.

EXTRA-ARTICULAR MANIFESTATIONS

Constitutional symptoms, including malaise, fatigue, weakness, low-grade fever and mild lymphadenopathy, are common in RA. All of the extra-articular complications occur almost exclusively in seropositive patients.

Skin

Subcutaneous nodules occur in 20 to 25 per cent of RA patients and are almost always associated with serum RF and more severe articular disease. They occur most commonly in periarticular structures and areas subject to pressure, such as the elbows, extensor and flexor tendons of the hands and feet, Achilles tendons, and, less commonly, occipital and sacral areas. They may occasionally become infected but are usually asymptomatic.

Palmar erythema and fragility of the skin, resulting in easy bruising, are common manifestations. Rheumatoid vasculitis occurs in two major forms. The first is manifested by small, splinter-shaped brown infarcts in the nail folds and digital pulp, often also present over subcutaneous nodules (see Color Plate 4E). Histologic examination may reveal leukocytoclastic vasculitis or a mild venulitis. This is a benign process in most patients and does not indicate serious systemic vasculitis. The second form is a severe necrotizing vasculitis of small and medium arteries indistinguishable from periarteritis nodosa. Digital infarcts, mononeuritis multiplex, fever, and other manifestations of systemic disease should prompt aggressive therapy.

Cardiac Manifestations

Pericardial disease is the most common cardiac feature of RA. Evidence of pericardial involvement with old fibrinous lesions is

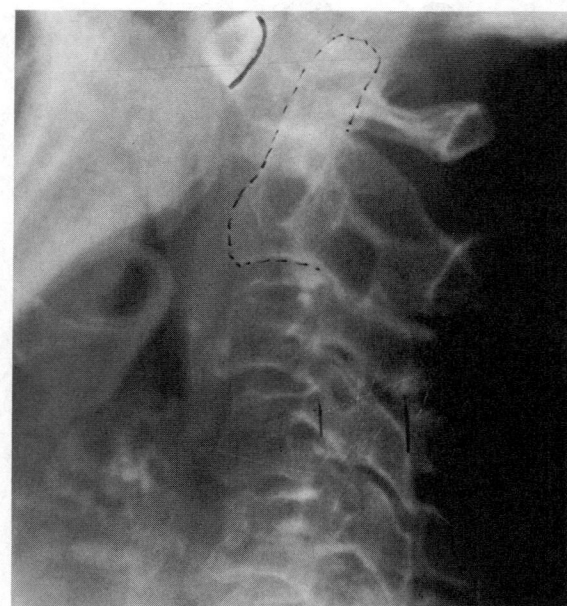

FIGURE 258–7. Lateral roentgenogram of the cervical spine in flexion. The body of C2 and its odontoid process are outlined by broken lines, and the posterior aspect of the anterior segment of C1 is indicated by a solid line. The space between C1 and the odontoid of C2 is markedly increased, indicating subluxation of C1 on C2. Normally, a space of only 2 to 3 mm separates C1 from C2. At a lower level, C3 is also displaced anteriorly owing to rheumatoid erosion of articular and ligamentous structures.

found in approximately 40 per cent of patients at autopsy. A similar frequency of pericardial abnormalities can be detected by echocardiography in asymptomatic RA patients. Clinically evident pericarditis in RA, however, is infrequent. Large pericardial effusions with cardiac tamponade and death are rare. Constrictive pericarditis is somewhat more common and typically presents as dyspnea, right-sided heart failure, and peripheral edema. The pericardial fluid characteristics include a low glucose concentration, increased level of lactate dehydrogenase (LDH), elevated immunoglobulin levels, and low complement activity.

Rheumatoid nodules may develop occasionally in the myocardium or heart valves, and vasculitis may involve the coronary arteries. Conduction abnormalities, valvular incompetence or stenosis, and myocardial infarction are all rare clinical sequelae of rheumatoid heart disease.

Pulmonary Manifestations

Rheumatoid pleural disease, although frequently found at autopsy, is most commonly asymptomatic. Occasionally, a pleural effusion may be of sufficient size to cause respiratory limitation. Neoplasm and infection should be ruled out on the basis of a pleural tap. Typically, the pleural fluid is exudative, and white cell counts vary greatly but generally are less than 5000 per microliter. Glucose levels tend to be low, and the LDH enzyme level is high. Total hemolytic complement, C3, and C4 levels are low. Immune complexes and RF are frequently found in the pleural fluid.

Intrapulmonary nodules may also be seen (Fig. 258–8). Although they are usually asymptomatic, they may become infected and cavitate or rupture into the pleural space, producing a pneumothorax. Malignancy must be excluded in the RA patient, as in any other patient, with a solitary lung nodule. Similar but distinct nodular infiltrates may also be seen in rheumatoid lungs in association with pneumoconiosis (Caplan's syndrome).

Finally, one may see a diffuse interstitial fibrosis with pneumonitis. This may progress to a honeycomb appearance on the roentgenogram, bronchiectasis, chronic cough, and progressive dyspnea. Pulmonary function tests show a diminished compliance and a restrictive ventilatory pattern. Large airways are not involved. An irreversible combination of respiratory insufficiency and resultant right-sided cardiac failure is possible. Rarely, small airway obstruction may develop into a necrotizing bronchiolitis. This complication may also result from therapies with gold and D-penicillamine.

Neurologic Manifestations

Peripheral neuropathies can be produced by proliferating synovium causing compression of nerves. Carpal tunnel syndrome (median neuropathy) (see under Articular Manifestations) is common, and a similar entrapment of the anterior tibial nerve (tarsal

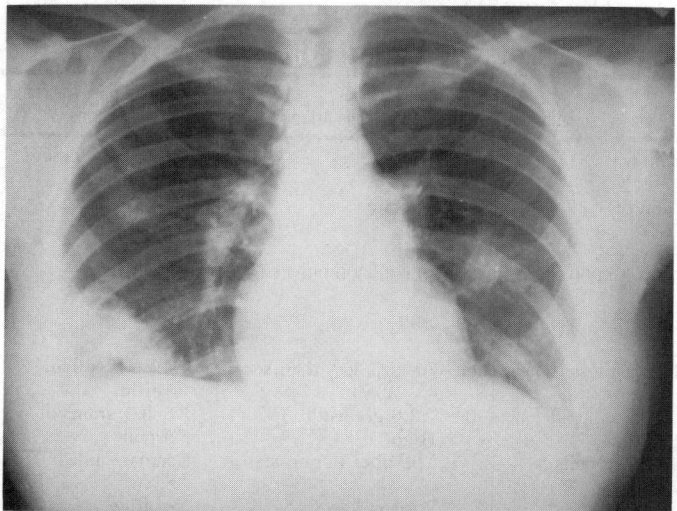

FIGURE 258–8. Chest roentgenogram demonstrating discrete rheumatoid nodules in both right and left lower lobes of the lungs. (Courtesy of Dr. Martin Lidsky, Houston, Texas.)

tunnel syndrome) can result in paresthesias with a foot drop. Rheumatoid vasculitis may cause a mononeuritis multiplex condition with patchy sensory loss in one or more extremities, often in association with a wrist or foot drop. A cervical myelopathy can result from atlantoaxial subluxation (see under Articular Manifestations). The central nervous system is usually spared, although cerebral vasculitis and rheumatoid nodules in the meninges have been described.

Ophthalmologic Manifestations

Sjögren's syndrome is the most frequent ocular complication and may cause corneal damage associated with dryness of the eyes. Xerostomia and/or parotid gland enlargement may accompany ocular dryness. Episcleritis is a self-limited condition associated with redness of the eye and only mild pain. Scleritis is more painful and may result in visual impairment. If this condition progresses to thinning of the tissue, allowing the dark blue color of the choroid below to show through, it is termed scleromalacia perforans. The histologic picture is similar to that of a rheumatoid nodule.

FELTY'S SYNDROME

This triad of chronic RA, splenomegaly, and neutropenia is often accompanied by lymphadenopathy, hepatomegaly, fever, weight loss, anemia, and thrombocytopenia. Hyperpigmentation and leg ulcers may also occur. The syndrome typically appears late in the course of a seropositive, destructive arthritis, often after joint disease is felt to be "burnt out." Recurrent infections with gram-positive organisms constitute the most serious clinical problems and do not correlate with the severity of neutropenia. The bone marrow is typically hyperplastic. Hypersplenism and immune-mediated destruction of white blood cells are believed to cause the neutropenia. Splenectomy may correct the neutropenia and prevent further infections in some patients, but many do not improve. The "large granular lymphocyte syndrome," which is probably a premalignant disorder of T lymphocytes, may mimic Felty's syndrome in RA patients.

LABORATORY FEATURES

A chronic normocytic, normochromic anemia with hematocrit values from 30 to 35 per cent is usual. Typically, both serum iron levels and iron-binding capacity are low. The anemia does not respond to administration of iron, but erythropoietin may be effective when anemia is more severe. The white blood cell count and differential are typically normal, but eosinophilia may occur in severe systemic disease. The platelet count may be moderately elevated owing to chronic inflammation. The erythrocyte sedimentation rate is elevated in most patients but only roughly parallels disease activity. The presence of RF is detected by agglutination methods in more than 80 per cent of cases and is useful in clinical diagnosis. Antinuclear antibodies detected by immunofluorescence, usually in low titer, can be found in 30 to 40 per cent of cases. Although HLA-DR4 can be determined by B cell typing in 60 to 70 per cent of cases, it is not generally useful in diagnosis because it occurs in nearly 30 per cent of normal individuals.

Synovial fluid analysis usually shows a poor mucin clot test and white cell counts in the range of 5000 to 20,000 per cubic millimeter, with 50 to 70 per cent as polymorphonuclear leukocytes (Table 258–3). The synovial fluid glucose concentration is usually normal, but very low values occur occasionally, even in the absence of a superimposed infectious arthritis. Complement levels are typically low.

THERAPEUTIC MANAGEMENT

The prolonged and uncertain course of RA calls for special emphasis on the fact that most patients can continue their accustomed activities, with restrictions tailored to individual cases. Undue or excessive drug therapy, especially adrenocorticosteroids and immunosuppressive agents, can cause greater morbidity than the disease itself. Objectives of management include (1) relief of pain, (2) reduction of inflammation, (3) minimizing undesirable side effects, (4) preservation of muscle strength and joint function, and (5) the return as rapidly as possible to a normal lifestyle. The basic initial program that achieves these objectives for the great majority of patients consists of (1) adequate rest, (2) adequate anti-inflammatory therapy, and (3) physical measures to maintain joint function.

Any confusion arising from the complementary requirements of rest and exercise should be promptly dispelled. As has been noted for many years, it is only a rare patient with RA who does not improve significantly upon being hospitalized. From this we have learned that bed rest tends to decrease the general systemic inflammatory response. Most patients soon learn that their midafternoon fatigue is significantly reduced by a period of rest. During acute attacks, longer rests and perhaps even remaining in bed for the duration of the attack may be required to treat the inflammation.

At the same time, the full range of joint motion should be maintained. This can usually be accomplished by the patient through graded exercise programs. However, during acute attacks, passive range-of-motion exercises by a physical therapist or instructed layperson may be indicated. Physical overexertion increases synovitis and inflammation in the joint affected by RA, but this does not contradict the usefulness of appropriate exercise. Exercise, as well as heat treatments such as showers, baths, warm pools, paraffin baths, or hot packs, should be used to loosen the joints and relieve stiffness. Exercise following the heat treatment maintains the motion of affected joints and prevents muscle atrophy. These goals can generally be achieved without aggressive overactivity and can usually keep a patient fully mobile. Acutely inflamed joints may dictate total body rest or splinting.

NONSTEROIDAL ANTI-INFLAMMATORY DRUGS (NSAID's)

Anti-inflammatory therapy is critical to the basic program. Salicylates are inexpensive, generally well tolerated, and demonstrably effective in controlling RA inflammation. The patient needs to understand that this requires a larger dose than would be used for analgesia alone. A constant blood level of 20 to 30 mg per deciliter is required. For most patients this requires between 3 and 6 grams of aspirin per day. All patients should be monitored for toxic levels by blood tests and should be alerted to report deafness, ringing in the ears, or gastrointestinal intolerance. With the availability of buffered and coated aspirin, a suitable salicylate preparation can be found for almost any patient.

Many other NSAID's that are effective against pain, fever, and inflammation in RA are available. These include derivatives of phenylacetic acid (ibuprofen, ketoprofen, fenoprofen, flurbiprofen), naphthalene acetic acids (naproxen), pyrrolealkanoic acid (tolmetin), indoleacetic acid (indomethacin, sulindac), a halogenated anthranilic acid (meclofenamate sodium), piroxicam, diclofenac, and diflunisal. Most of these drugs are beneficial in RA. They are generally no more effective than aspirin but may be

tolerated in cases in which aspirin is not. Their major problem is high cost. Clinical experience suggests an occasional need to change from one to another of these drugs to minimize side effects and to give maximal benefit to the individual patient.

The NSAID's often cause silent gastrointestinal bleeding. Fortunately, this is usually minimal and tolerable. Overt gastrointestinal tract hemorrhage or ulceration is rare, but if this occurs or gastrointestinal bleeding is contributing to a constant anemia, the therapeutic regimen should be modified. NSAID's should be used cautiously or avoided in patients with impaired renal function.

OTHER THERAPIES

If salicylates and NSAID's fail to control the inflammation or are not tolerated, then one must consider the more slowly acting drugs, including antimalarials, gold, penicillamine, and methotrexate. Antimalarials are usually given as hydroxychloroquine (Plaquenil), 200 mg once or twice daily. This, or chloroquine, may cause retinal lesions and loss of vision; therefore, the patient should be examined by an ophthalmologist at least twice a year.

Gold salts produce remission in many cases. Because of the potential toxicity to kidneys and bone marrow, frequent urinalysis and blood counts must be done, especially during early phases of treatment. An oral gold salt, auranofin, appears to be therapeutically effective and to have less toxicity than do intramuscular injections. A dose of 3 mg two to three times per day is recommended. A therapeutic effect should not be expected before 4 to 6 months. Many patients have been on oral or intramuscular gold therapy for a number of years. Common side effects include pruritic skin rashes and painful mouth ulcers. Severe manifestations include bone marrow suppression, usually leukopenia or thrombocytopenia, renal damage with proteinuria, and rarely a nephrotic syndrome.

Penicillamine may be used in the treatment of RA and is also effective in inducing improvements and sometimes even remissions. Like gold, however, its effects are slow in coming, and it may affect both the bone marrow and the kidneys, so that careful monitoring for toxicity is required. In addition, it may induce other autoimmune diseases, such as myasthenia gravis, Goodpasture's syndrome, or lupus erythematosus.

Immunosuppressive agents such as azathioprine, cyclophosphamide, chlorambucil, and methotrexate have been used to treat especially severe, unremitting RA. Currently, the most widely used and effective form of immunosuppressive therapy for RA appears to be methotrexate. An oral dosage of 7.5 to 15 mg one time per week seems efficacious, and a therapeutic response can be anticipated in several weeks. Side effects include hepatotoxicity and possibly cirrhosis, bone marrow suppression, oral ulcers, and a potential life-threatening pneumonitis. Methotrexate may also cause a leukocytoclastic vasculitis and may promote the formation of rheumatoid nodules.

Because of its side effects, long-term corticosteroid therapy should be reserved for patients with unresponsive and aggressive

TABLE 258–3. SYNOVIAL FLUID FINDINGS IN RHEUMATOID ARTHRITIS AND OTHER FORMS OF ARTHRITIS

Synovial Characteristics	Rheumatoid Arthritis	Gout/Pseudogout	Reiter's/Psoriatic Arthritis	Septic Arthritis	Osteoarthritis, Traumatic Arthritis
Color	Yellow	Yellow-white	Yellow	White	Clear, pale yellow, or bloody
Clarity	Cloudy	Cloudy-opaque	Cloudy	Opaque	Transparent
Viscosity	Poor	Poor	Poor	Poor	Good
Mucin clot	Poor	Poor	Poor	Poor	Good
White blood cell count/mm³	3000–50,000	3000–50,000 or higher	3000–50,000 or higher	50,000–300,000	<3000
% Polymorphonuclear leukocytes	>70	>70	>70	>90	<25
Glucose levels	10–25% less than serum*	10–25% less than serum	10–25% less than serum	70–90% less than serum	5–10% less than serum
Total protein	>3.0 grams/dl	>3.0 grams/dl	>3.0 grams/dl	>3.0 grams/dl	1.8–3.0 grams/dl
Complement	Low	Normal	High	High	Normal
Microscopic features	"RA cells"†	MSU and CPPD crystals	"Reiter's cells"†	Microbes (Gram stain)	Cartilage fibrils†
Culture	Negative	Negative	Negative	Positive	Negative

*Rarely, glucose levels are very low, as in rheumatoid pleural effusions.
†These are not disease specific or diagnostic.
MSU = monosodium urate; CPPD = calcium pyrophosphate dihydrate.

joint disease whose ability to function is threatened. When necessary, the smallest possible dose should be used, i.e., prednisone, 5 mg to 10 mg every other day or daily. Higher doses are necessary for patients with neuropathy, vasculitis, pleuritis, pericarditis, scleritis, and related conditions. Local steroid injections can sometimes be helpful for the relief of persistent effusions and are the treatment of choice for a Baker's cyst of the knee.

Finally, reconstructive orthopedic surgery is of very great importance. Perhaps the greatest contribution of the past two decades to the management of RA has been the development of superb techniques for joint replacement. The use of prosthetic devices for hip and knee joints has given excellent results, and devices for ankle, elbow, and shoulder replacement are improving.

JUVENILE CHRONIC ARTHRITIS

A chronic arthritis beginning in childhood and for which no underlying cause is apparent has been termed *juvenile rheumatoid arthritis*. Because the majority of these cases do not resemble adult RA, the term *juvenile chronic arthritis* (JCA) is a more appropriate designation. Several subgroups of JCA are recognized on the basis of modes of onset, other clinical features, and immunogenetic differences.

Arthritis of systemic onset, or Still's disease, accounts for about 20 per cent of patients. It can begin at any age. Rheumatoid factor and antinuclear antibodies are generally not found. Clinical characteristics include high, spiking daily fevers; an evanescent, salmon-colored rash usually appearing with fever; lymphadenopathy; hepatosplenomegaly; polyserositis; leukocytosis; thrombocytosis; and anemia. Although the disease is rarely life threatening, it can be confused with leukemia or infection. It tends to run a self-limited course in the majority of patients but may recur. Chronic polyarthritis and joint deformities occur in only about 10 per cent of patients.

Disease with a polyarticular onset occurs in approximately 40 per cent of patients. There is a female predominance. The majority of patients are seronegative. Seropositive patients have the worst prognosis, and the disease usually follows a chronic course similar to that in adult RA. HLA-DR4 is strongly associated with seropositive but not seronegative disease. No HLA associations have been found for the seronegative group, except for a small subset with HLA-B27 who develop cervical spine fusion, notably at the C2–C3 apophyseal joints, and, less often, sacroiliitis or ankylosing spondylitis.

Disease with a pauciarticular onset accounts for the remaining 40 per cent of JCA patients. There are at least two subgroups within this group. One is characterized by early age of onset and female predominance. The serum is usually positive for antinuclear antibodies but not RF. Patients in this subgroup are at risk for chronic iridocyclitis, which may progress to blindness. Therefore, frequent ophthalmologic evaluations should be performed. The arthritis usually resolves without deformity. HLA-DR5 and HLA-DRw8 are significantly increased in this subgroup. A second subgroup with pauciarticular onset has a strong male predominance and later age of onset. HLA-B27 occurs in the majority of these patients. The disease in these children follows a course consistent with spondyloarthropathy.

Treatment must be determined on the basis of disease severity. Aspirin is a basic standby, but tolmetin and naproxen can be used safely in children. Physical therapy and psychosocial support are also indicated.

ADULT-ONSET STILL'S DISEASE

Still's disease is one form of juvenile-onset chronic arthritis that may begin in adulthood. Cases have been recognized that span the entire adult age spectrum, including elderly patients. The clinical features are the same as described above. Acute symptoms often respond to salicylates or other NSAID's, but prednisone may be necessary for short periods. The prognosis for complete recovery is good in the majority of patients.

Aptekar RG, Decker JL, Bujak JS, et al.: Adult onset juvenile rheumatoid arthritis. Arthritis Rheum 16:715, 1973. *An excellent clinical discussion of the adult-onset form of Still's disease.*
Arnett FC, Edworthy SM, Bloch DA, et al.: The American Rheumatism Association 1987 revised criteria for the classification of rheumatoid arthritis. Arthritis

Rheum 31:315, 1988. *A more in-depth discussion of the development, recommended uses, and potential pitfalls of criteria for RA.*
Fassbender HG: Normal and pathologic synovial tissue with emphasis on rheumatoid arthritis. *In* Cohen AS, Bennett JC (eds.): Rheumatology and Immunology. 2nd ed. Orlando, Fla., Grune & Stratton, 1986. *Comprehensive discussion with excellent illustrations of the course of synovitis.*
Gregersen PK, Silver J, Winchester RJ: The shared epitope hypothesis. An approach to understanding the molecular genetics of susceptibility to rheumatoid arthritis. Arthritis Rheum 30:1205, 1987. *A discussion of how genetic polymorphism may lead to susceptibility to RA.*
Harris ED Jr: Rheumatoid arthritis: Pathophysiology and implications for therapy. N Engl J Med 322:1277, 1990. *A recent comprehensive review of the pathobiology of RA and theoretical basis for rational therapy.*
Olsen NJ, Callahan LF, Brooks RH, et al.: Associations of HLA-DR4 with rheumatoid factor and radiographic severity in rheumatoid arthritis. Am J Med 84:257, 1988. *A large, well-conducted study of the relation of HLA-DR4 to clinical features of RA.*
Southern P, Oldstone MBA: Medical consequences of persistent viral infection. N Engl J Med 314:359, 1986. *Considerations relating to possible infectious origin of RA.*
Strominger JL: Biology of the human histocompatibility leukocyte antigen (HLA) system and a hypothesis regarding the generation of autoimmune disease. J Clin Invest 77:1411, 1986. *Excellent review of concepts relating to autoimmune features of RA.*
Tugwell P, Bennett K, Gent M: Methotrexate in rheumatoid arthritis. Indications, contraindications, efficacy, and safety. Ann Intern Med 107:358, 1987. *An excellent review of efficacy and safety studies of methotrexate therapy in RA.*
Wees SJ, Sunwoo IN, Oh SJ: Sural nerve biopsy in systemic necrotizing vasculitis. Am J Med 71:525, 1981. *Description of a useful diagnostic procedure for vasculitis and peripheral neuropathy.*
Ziff M: Systemic rheumatoid disease: Immunological aspects. Adv Inflam Res 3:123, 1982. *A comprehensive review of the immunologic mechanisms involving the pathogenesis of RA.*

259 The Spondylarthropathies

Andrei Calin

The seronegative spondylarthritides are characterized by involvement of the sacroiliac joints, by peripheral inflammatory arthropathy, and by the absence of rheumatoid factor. Other features include the following:

1. Pathologic changes concentrated around the enthesis (i.e., the site of ligamentous insertion into bone) rather than the synovium. Nonenthesopathic changes may also develop in the eye, the aortic valve, the lung parenchyma, and the skin.
2. Clinical evidence of overlap among the various seronegative spondylarthritides. Thus, a patient with psoriatic arthropathy may well develop uveitis or sacroiliitis, and a patient with inflammatory bowel disease may develop ankylosing spondylitis or mouth ulcers.
3. A tendency toward familial aggregation, with the suggestion that these entities "breed true" within families.

Types

The spondylarthropathies include ankylosing spondylitis, Reiter's syndrome (both the postvenereal, or endemic, and the postinfective, or epidemic, forms), the reactive arthritides (caused by *Yersinia, Salmonella, Helicobacter, Campylobacter*, and other infections), certain subsets of juvenile arthropathy (juvenile ankylosing spondylitis and the seronegative enthesopathic arthropathy syndrome), enteropathic sacroiliitis (ulcerative colitis and Crohn's disease), psoriatic arthropathy, and perhaps a group of rarer disorders (Whipple's disease, Behçet's syndrome, and pustulotic arthro-osteitis) (Fig. 259–1).

These disorders can be categorized according to the specific periarticular or articular involvement. The various spondylarthropathies can be distinguished from one another according to the particular peripheral joints involved, the associated clinical features (i.e., urethritis, conjunctivitis, skin involvement), and the manner in which the disease progresses (i.e., remission or relapse) (Table 259–1).

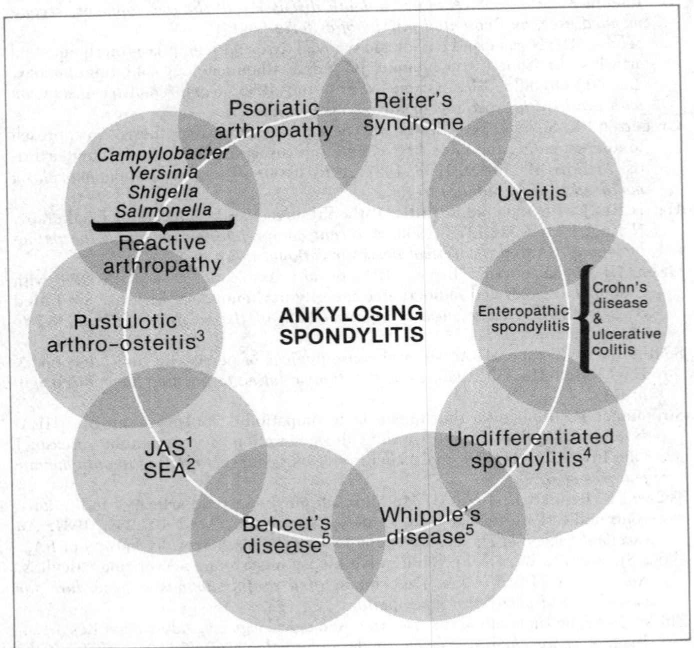

FIGURE 259–1. Individual conditions that overlap to form the spondyl-arthritides. (1) Juvenile ankylosing spondylitis. (2) Seronegative enthesopathic arthropathy syndrome. (3) Considered by Japanese to be part of spondylarthropathy spectrum (rare in United States and Europe). (4) Undifferentiated spondylitis (i.e., subset of patients who have spondylarthropathic features but who fail to meet criteria for ankylosing spondylitis, Reiter's syndrome, or other condition, e.g., dactylitis, uveitis, plus unilateral sacroiliitis). (5) Not universally accepted as members of the spondylarthropathy group.

Hereditary Factors

Hereditary factors play an important role in the development of spondylarthropathies. Some 5 to 20 per cent of individuals positive for HLA-B27 (HLA, human leukocyte antigen) develop ankylosing spondylitis following an unknown environmental event, while 20 per cent develop Reiter's syndrome after exposure to *Shigella* or other environmental trigger.

The explanation for the link between HLA-B27 and the spondylarthropathies remains unknown. Hypotheses include the following: (1) B27 acts as a receptor site for an infective agent; (2) B27 is a marker for an immune response gene that determines susceptibility to an environmental trigger; or (3) B27 may induce tolerance to foreign antigens with which it cross-reacts.

We now know that the risk of developing ankylosing spondylitis for a B27-positive relative of a B27-positive patient is 25 to 50 per cent compared with about 5 per cent for a random B27-positive subject. This argues for genetic differences between the two B27 groups. Splitting of B27 by monoclonal antibodies and cytotoxic T cells has not provided an explanation for these differences, so there must be an additional susceptibility (and perhaps severity) gene or genes (Fig. 259–2). Chromosomes 2, 14, and 19 may also be operative. The extent to which additional environmental triggers modify disease remains unknown. More than 95 per cent of patients with ankylosing spondylitis are HLA-B27 positive, while 80 per cent of those with Reiter's syndrome carry this antigen, as do only 50 per cent of those with psoriatic or enteropathic spondylitis. A new animal model (transgenic B27 + rat) may help elucidate the nature of the link between B27 and disease.

Etiologic Factors

Numerous infective triggers are recognized for the reactive arthropathies (*Shigella, Salmonella, Chlamydia,* and so forth). By contrast, the arthritogenic environmental event in ankylosing spondylitis has not been adequately defined. However, much interest has focused on *Klebsiella,* plasmids, or other extrachromosomal genetic material emanating from gram-negative enteric bacilli, and heat shock or stress protein.

ANKYLOSING SPONDYLITIS

Criteria for Diagnosis

The criteria for diagnosing ankylosing spondylitis have been evolving in recent years. The newly defined European Seronegative Study Group (ESSG) criteria include all spondylarthropathy patients. A simple approach defines ankylosing spondylitis as the presence of symptomatic sacroiliitis. The condition in a patient with back discomfort and radiologic evidence of sacroiliitis would be diagnosed as ankylosing spondylitis.

Prevalence

Once considered a rare disease, the illness is now known to have a prevalence comparable to that of rheumatoid arthritis. The distribution of ankylosing spondylitis follows the population frequency of HLA-B27 and is more common in whites than in blacks.

Ankylosing spondylitis has often gone undiagnosed; inappropriate diagnostic procedures lead to erroneous diagnoses (e.g., mechanical back disease). Such patients often receive incorrect therapy.

Although ankylosing spondylitis was formerly believed to occur predominantly in men, several studies now suggest that there may be a more uniform sex distribution. Most large series report a 2.5:1 ratio in favor of men. The condition in female patients is less frequently diagnosed, perhaps because physicians and radiologists may be reluctant to diagnose a disease that they consider to be rare in women. In women, the disease may be milder and may present with a greater number of peripheral joint manifestations. In the past, many cases of ankylosing spondylitis in women were inappropriately diagnosed as seronegative rheumatoid arthritis.

Clinical Presentation

A history of several of the following five features is suggestive of inflammatory spinal disease: insidious onset of discomfort, age less than 40 years, persistence for more than 3 months, association with morning stiffness, and improvement with exercise.

If this simple screening test is positive, radiologic evidence of sacroiliitis confirms ankylosing spondylitis. Many radiologists have been unfamiliar with rheumatologic joint disease and have diagnosed ankylosing spondylitis only when evidence of major ankylosis of the sacroiliac joints and spine was present. Ankylosing spondylitis can be diagnosed, however, in the presence of only minimal sacroiliitis. What determines whether a patient will have only a mild pelvic disease, ascending spinal disease, extraspinal articular disease, or extra-articular symptoms remains unknown. Presumably, phenotypic expression depends on numerous interrelating genes. The age at onset is of paramount importance. Some 15 per cent of teenagers (at onset) will require a total hip replacement within 20 years, while those with onset in their 20's are much less at risk for major hip or neck involvement.

Early change in the lumbar spine is manifested as squaring of the superior and inferior margins of the vertebral body. This phenomenon is caused by inflammatory disease at the site of insertion of the outer fibers of the annulus fibrosus, i.e., enthesopathy. Later changes result in the classic, though rare, bamboo spine. Comparable spinal changes are seen in primary ankylosing spondylitis and in the spondylitis associated with inflammatory bowel disease. In spondylitis associated with Reiter's syndrome and psoriatic arthropathy, however, the changes tend to be asymmetric and random.

Radionuclide scans, computed tomography, and other advanced radiologic techniques are usually unnecessary. A simple anteroposterior radiograph suffices.

Physical Examination

Examination of the spine may reveal muscle spasm and loss of the normal lordosis. The degree of restriction of forward flexion can be documented by measuring the distraction, on flexion, of two points—the lower point at the level of the lumbosacral junction and the upper point 10 cm above this level. In a normal individual, the distraction of this 10-cm line is 5 to 8 cm, compared with 0 to 6 cm in an untreated patient with spondylitis. Lateral spinal flexion is measured by the distraction, on contralateral flexion, of a 20-cm line drawn in the mid-axillary plane.

THE SPONDYLARTHROPATHIES

THE SPONDYLARTHROPATHIES

TABLE 259–1. COMPARISON OF SERONEGATIVE SPONDYLARTHROPATHIES

	Ankylosing Spondylitis	Reiter's Syndrome	Psoriatic Arthropathy	Enteropathic Spondylitis	Juvenile Arthropathy (JAS* subset)	Reactive Arthropathy
Sex	Male ≥ female	Male ≥ female	Female ≥ male	Female = male	Male > female	Male = female
Age at onset	20	Any age	Any age	Any age	<16	Any age
Uveitis	+ +	+ +	+	+	+	+
Conjunctivitis	−	+	−	−	−	+
Peripheral joints	Lower > upper: often	Lower usually	Upper > lower	Lower > upper	Lower > upper	Lower > upper
Sex differences	Yes	No	No	No	No	No
Sacroiliitis	Always	Often	Often	Often	Often	Often
HLA-B27	95%	80%	20% (50% with sacroiliitis)	50%	90%	80%
Enthesopathy	+	+	+	+	+	+
Aortic regurgitation	+	+	?+	?	?	+
Familial aggregation	+	+	+	+	+	+
Risk for HLA-B27–positive individual	±20%	20%	?	?	?	20%
Onset	Gradual	Sudden	Variable	Gradual	Variable	Sudden
Urethritis	−	+	−	−	−	+/−
Skin involvement	−	+	+ +	−	−	−
Mucous membrane involvement	−	+	−	−	−	−
Symmetry (spinal)	+	−	−	+	−	+
Self-limiting	−	+/−	+/−	+/−	+/−	+/−
Remission, relapses	−	+/−	+/−	−	+/−	+/−

*JAS = Juvenile ankylosing spondylitis.

In this case, normal distraction varies from 5 to 12 cm, compared with 0 to 7 cm in patients with spondylitis.

Peripheral joint involvement, especially in the lower limb, occurs at some stage in approximately 20 to 30 per cent of cases. Inflammatory disease of the hip and shoulder may produce progressive disability. Enthesopathic features include plantar fasciitis, costochondritis, and Achilles tendinitis.

Laboratory Findings

HLA-B27 testing should not be used as a routine screening procedure; it is expensive and usually unnecessary. Elevation of the erythrocyte sedimentation rate occurs in most patients but may be normal despite severe disease. Elevation of immunoglobulin A (IgA) levels and the presence of immune complexes suggest aberrant immunity. Serum creatine kinase and alkaline phosphatase levels may be elevated. Lymphocytes predominate in the synovial fluid, and synovial histologic findings are nonspecific.

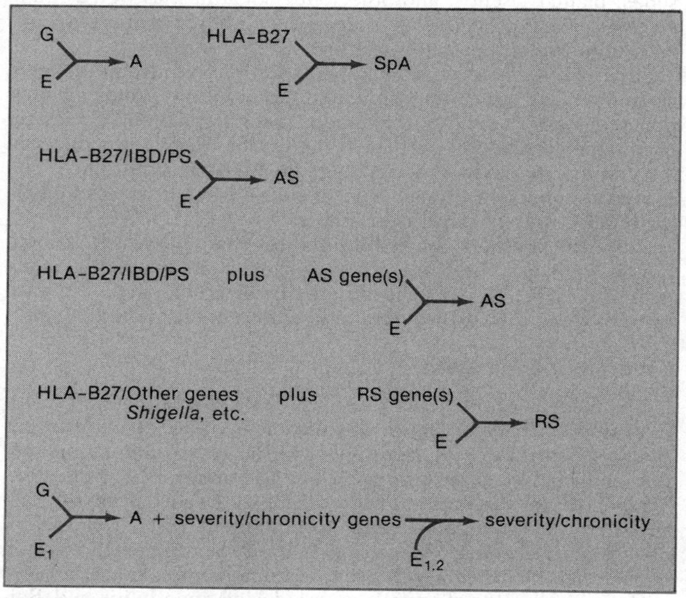

FIGURE 259–2. Relationship between environmental and genetic factors in susceptibility, severity, and natural history of reactive arthropathies and spondylarthritides. G = genetics; E = environment; A = arthritis; SpA = spondylarthropathy; IBD = inflammatory bowel disease; PS = psoriasis; AS = ankylosing spondylitis; E_1 and E_2 = environmental factors; RS = Reiter's syndrome.

Pathology

The synovial lesions of ankylosing spondylitis and rheumatoid arthritis share identical histopathologic characteristics: intimal cell hyperplasia and a diffuse lymphocyte and plasma cell infiltrate. Formation of lymphoid follicles is found less frequently in ankylosing spondylitis than in rheumatoid disease. Synovitis per se, however, does not explain the propensity toward ligamentous ossification and widespread new bone formation observed in ankylosing spondylitis. Inflammation at the enthesis accounts for the unique pathology, or enthesopathy, of ankylosing spondylitis; new bone formation appears to be a specific reparative process occurring at the enthesopathic site. Complications of severe spinal disease include fractures and spondylodiscitis after minimal trauma.

A striking degree of spinal osteoporosis in patients with early and mild disease has been demonstrated, suggesting that bone pathology could be a primary event in disease pathogenesis.

Extraskeletal Involvement

Extra-articular features include fatigue, weight loss, and low-grade fever. Cord compression resulting from spinal fractures or the cauda equina syndrome may cause neurologic symptoms. The negative effects of systemic involvement and of radiotherapy on the survival of patients with ankylosing spondylitis are well recognized.

EYE INVOLVEMENT. Uveitis develops in up to 40 per cent of patients during their illness. It occurs most often in HLA-B27–positive patients. There is no correlation with the severity of the spondylitis, and onset appears to be a random environmental event. The episodes of uveitis are usually self-limited, but may require local steroid therapy.

PULMONARY DISEASE. Patients with severe disease may exhibit chronic infiltrative and fibrotic changes in the upper lung fields that mimic tuberculosis. Pulmonary ventilation is usually well maintained by the diaphragm, despite the chest wall rigidity. The pulmonary fibrosis is occasionally clinically silent, but most affected patients present with cough, sputum, and dyspnea. Cyst formation and subsequent *Aspergillus* invasion may cause hemoptysis.

CARDIOVASCULAR DISEASE. Aortic incompetence, cardiomegaly, and persistent conduction defects occur in 3.5 to 10.0 per cent of patients with severe spondylitic disease. Cardiac involvement may be clinically silent or may dominate the clinical picture. Thickened aortic valve cusps and scar tissue in the root of the aorta represent the major histologic changes.

AMYLOIDOSIS. Amyloid deposition is an occasional complication of ankylosing spondylitis, particularly in Europe.

KIDNEY. In contrast to patients with rheumatoid arthritis, who may show renal impairment as an expression of disease, renal glomerular function is apparently unimpaired in patients with ankylosing spondylitis, despite recognized pathologic changes. An IgA nephropathy, however, has been described in patients with seronegative spondylarthropathy.

Treatment and Prognosis

Ankylosing spondylitis may be a mild or severe disease. As discussed, the younger the age at onset, the more severe the outcome. For example, in an analysis of 1500 cases, 15 per cent of those who were between 15 and 16 years of age at the time of onset needed a total hip replacement within 15 years, compared with 10 per cent of those who were between 19 and 20 years and fewer than 1 per cent of those who were more than 40 years of age (all cohorts were followed for a similar period).

Ankylosing spondylitis is a gratifying condition to recognize and treat early: Much can be accomplished toward ameliorating symptoms and, perhaps, preventing spinal deformity. The primary objectives are to relieve pain, decrease inflammation, begin remedial strengthening exercises, and maintain good posture and function.

Anti-inflammatory agents relieve inflammation, pain, and spasm and permit patients to follow an adequate exercise program. There is some evidence that phenylbutazone decreases the rate of spinal fusion. Nevertheless, indomethacin is the drug of choice. Phenylbutazone, although more efficacious, may be more toxic (in Britain, it can be used only by hospital rheumatologists). Indomethacin, started at a dosage of 25 mg three times a day (or 75 mg slow release at night), may be increased to a maximum of 150 mg daily. The dose should be titrated against response and side effects. Possible side effects include headache, vertigo, and depression, especially in older patients, and nausea, gastric discomfort, and diarrhea in all age groups. Phenylbutazone (100 mg three or four times per day) is remarkably effective but must be used with caution. Dangerous side effects include agranulocytosis and aplastic anemia. Agranulocytosis is an idiosyncratic response, developing chiefly in young individuals within 3 to 6 weeks of the start of therapy. Aplastic anemia appears to be dose-related and occurs primarily in individuals more than 60 years of age.

Nonsteroidal anti-inflammatory drugs (NSAID's) include ibuprofen, naproxen, fenoprofen, tolmetin, sulindac, meclofenamate sodium, piroxicam, diclofenac, and, depending on the country, flurbiprofen, ketoprofen, tiaprofenic acid, etodolac, and others. If indomethacin is efficacious but not tolerated, one of these NSAID's may be given. In general, these agents play a minor role in the management of the spondylarthritides. Phenylbutazone should be tried when indomethacin is ineffective.

Gold and penicillamine have no role to play, but sulfasalazine may be effective. Radiotherapy, once the treatment of choice, is virtually no longer practiced in view of the high risk of inducing leukemia. Azathioprine and methotrexate appear to have no effect on the spinal disease.

The patient also needs remedial strengthening exercises and postural training. A firm mattress and small pillow are ideal when the patient is resting; attention to posture while at work and at rest must be stressed. The best exercise regimen includes extension exercises and hydrotherapy; swimming is highly recommended.

In those few patients who, despite optimal management, develop an irreversible deformity, wedge osteotomy may be indicated. For those with destructive arthropathy of the hip, arthroplasty is a must. The long-term outcome of this procedure is gratifying.

REITER'S SYNDROME

The most common cause of an inflammatory oligoarthropathy in a young man is Reiter's syndrome. This classic triad of urethritis, conjunctivitis, and arthritis represents the one chronic rheumatic disorder related to both a specific genetic background (HLA-B27) and a specific infection. Reiter's syndrome is often not self-limited. Progressive disease may result in major disability. The disease may be defined as an episode of arthropathy within 1 month of urethritis or cervicitis.

Whether a dysenteric (epidemic) or a venereal (endemic) infection is the most common precipitating event is unclear. In young children, the former is the rule. In many cases, the distinction between urethritis as a precipitating factor and urethritis as an integral manifestation of the syndrome remains unclear. In postvenereal Reiter's syndrome, both *Chlamydia* and *Mycoplasma* have been implicated. In a patient with a specific predisposing genetic background, a variety of different organisms may be responsible. *Chlamydia* and *Yersinia* antigenic material has been demonstrated within the synovium, but the "reactive" nature (see below) of Reiter's disease is not in doubt.

Prevalence

Reiter's syndrome develops in at least 1 per cent of patients with nonspecific urethritis. *Shigella* dysentery is followed by Reiter's syndrome in 1 to 2 per cent of cases (i.e., 20 per cent of B27-positive patients). B27 is present in 6 to 14 per cent of whites and 0 to 4 per cent of blacks.

The sex distribution of Reiter's syndrome is difficult to define because the syndrome is diagnosed only with difficulty in women, in whom urethritis and cervicitis are often clinically inapparent. Formes frustes of the syndrome are now being recognized. A woman presenting with or without uveitis and an inflammatory arthropathy of the knee in association with HLA-B27 antigen may have Reiter's syndrome. Similarly, the disorder is difficult to recognize in children; a diagnosis is usually made only if an epidemic of dysentery is present and Reiter's syndrome has been recognized in other family members. Postdysenteric Reiter's syndrome almost certainly has an equal sex distribution.

Clinical Features

Reiter's syndrome should be considered a symptom complex rather than the association of three specific features. The syndrome may manifest as a tetrad (i.e., with the addition of buccal ulceration or balanitis to the classic triad); alternatively, only two of the three cardinal features may be present. Several of the classic features may appear insignificant and be overlooked. For example, the urethritis may be mild, perhaps forgotten; the discharge may be minimal and remembered by the patient only after direct questioning. Balanitis may not be evident unless the prepuce is retracted and the glans penis closely inspected. A red eye may be forgotten or considered irrelevant, and the various skin lesions typified by keratoderma blennorrhagicum may be misdiagnosed.

Rheumatologic features include arthralgias, tenosynovitic episodes, plantar fasciitis, and other enthesopathies, as well as frank arthritis. The typical sausage-shaped digit is a frequent occurrence related to the enthesopathic nature of the disorder.

Some 20 per cent of patients with Reiter's syndrome develop sacroiliitis and ascending spinal disease. Other radiologic evidence of Reiter's syndrome includes plantar spurs and periosteal new bone formation. Cardiac complications similar to those in ankylosing spondylitis occur late in Reiter's syndrome. The hyperkeratotic skin lesions seen in Reiter's syndrome cannot be distinguished from those in psoriasis.

Formerly considered a self-limited process, Reiter's syndrome is now known to be a more or less persistent disease in many patients. About 80 per cent of patients have evidence of disease activity when they are re-examined after a 5-year period.

Laboratory Evaluation

It is unclear whether the presence of HLA-B27 correlates with increased severity of Reiter's syndrome. A patient with severe Reiter's syndrome may have an erythrocyte sedimentation rate in the normal range or one as high as 100 mm per hour or more. Synovial fluid analysis is rarely diagnostic, apart from the fact that it reveals a relatively high complement level (reflecting a nonspecific inflammatory reaction), rather than the low level seen in rheumatoid arthritis (reflecting immune complex disease).

Occasionally, the diagnosis of ankylosing spondylitis and Reiter's syndrome may prove difficult to disentangle. Some patients whose disorder is diagnosed as ankylosing spondylitis may have presented originally with Reiter's syndrome, but the episodes of urethritis have subsequently been forgotten by the physician and patient. Similarly, patients whose disease is diagnosed as Reiter's syndrome may actually have ankylosing spondylitis with peripheral joint disease and a chance of the occurrence of urethritis.

Management

No cure exists for Reiter's syndrome. The patient's feelings of guilt and anxiety about sexual misconduct must be allayed. Although anecdotal evidence suggests that individuals with postvenereal Reiter's syndrome may develop a relapse following sexual activity, many individuals have spontaneous exacerbations. An explanation of allergic response may help the patient: Asthma may develop on exposure to a known or unknown allergen in sensitive individuals; in the same way, Reiter's syndrome may flare up following an unknown allergic event.

Symptomatic management includes the use of indomethacin, phenylbutazone, or other NSAID's. Antibiotic therapy is too late and unnecessary. Patients with severe, recurrent uveitis may require steroid eye drops or subconjunctival preparations. The syndrome may remit, recur, or continue unabated despite steroid or even cytotoxic therapy. For patients with progressive disease, azathioprine or methotrexate may be effective.

THE REACTIVE ARTHROPATHIES

Reactive arthropathy refers to an inflammatory arthritis that follows an infection in which no microbial invasion of the synovial space occurs. The B27-linked arthropathies following *Shigella*, *Salmonella*, *Yersinia*, *Helicobacter*, and *Campylobacter jejuni* infections are in this group. Why some patients develop only an arthropathy whereas others have the full spectrum of Reiter's disease after exposure to one of these agents is unknown.

Yersinia Infection

Yersinia enterocolitica infection may produce the following: fever, mild gastrointestinal illness, and, after a latent period, polyarthropathy and erythema nodosum, especially in B27-positive individuals. The symptom complex may mimic acute rheumatic fever. The arthropathy may last for weeks or months, and in HLA-B27–positive individuals, sacroiliitis may occur.

Salmonellosis

An arthropathy associated with *Salmonella* infections mimics that caused by *Yersinia*. Treatment of these disorders is the same as that of Reiter's syndrome.

JUVENILE CHRONIC ARTHROPATHY

Chronic arthritis in a child or teenager often persists into adulthood; therefore, an awareness of juvenile chronic arthropathy is relevant when attending adult patients. Until recently, the term juvenile rheumatoid arthritis was used, inappropriately, to describe all forms of childhood arthritis. As in adults, arthritis in children may be associated with psoriasis, inflammatory bowel disease, and other conditions. The acute systemic form, Still's disease, manifests with fever, rash, and toxicity in young children who are negative for B27 and rheumatoid factor (IgM anti-IgG). Still's disease is also recognized in adults. Another subset (in the spondylarthropathy group) consists largely of adolescent boys who predominantly exhibit oligoarthropathy affecting the large joints of the lower limbs; such individuals are frequently positive for HLA-B27. This group may develop sacroiliitis or ankylosing spondylitis; the presence of B27 is associated with spinal disease involvement. Another group includes B27-negative individuals (usually girls less than 5 years of age) presenting with an oligoarthropathy characterized by a positive fluorescent antinuclear antibody (FANA) test. These subjects are at risk for developing asymptomatic chronic iridocyclitis, in contrast to FANA-negative and B27-positive patients, who develop clinically obvious acute uveitis. A few older children (preponderantly girls) develop a seropositive, nodular, and erosive disease that resembles adult rheumatoid arthritis. A B27-related syndrome known as seronegative enthesopathy and arthropathy (SEA syndrome) is now also recognized in children. Such individuals often develop sacroiliitis at a later stage.

THE ENTEROPATHIC ARTHROPATHIES

Two major clinical patterns of arthropathy associated with inflammatory bowel disease (ulcerative colitis and Crohn's disease) are peripheral arthropathy and spondylarthropathy.

Peripheral Arthropathy

Approximately 20 per cent of individuals with severe Crohn's disease or ulcerative colitis develop an acute migratory inflammatory polyarthritis, often of abrupt onset and involving the larger joints of the lower extremities. The arthritis resolves in weeks or months. Arthritis flare-ups usually parallel exacerbations of the underlying disorder. The pathogenesis of the joint complication is unknown. The B27 antigen is not present. Treatment is directed at the primary disorder and is more effective in ulcerative colitis than in Crohn's disease.

Spondylarthropathy

About one patient in five with inflammatory bowel disease develops sacroiliitis and, occasionally, severe ankylosing spondylitis. Men and women are equally affected. The spinal disease may precede the bowel disease or follow it. There is no correlation between the severity of the bowel disorder and the spondylitis. Therapy is the same as for classic ankylosing spondylitis. Despite the bowel disease, the NSAID's are usually well tolerated.

A post–intestinal bypass syndrome consisting of arthropathy and occasionally dermatitis is well recognized. Immune alterations appear in these patients, and B27 is occasionally associated with this syndrome.

PSORIATIC ARTHROPATHY

Different subsets of psoriatic arthropathy are recognized, several forms of which appear to be enthesopathic rather than purely synovitic. Uveitis, sacroiliitis, and ascending spinal disease occur in up to 20 per cent of cases. Patients are seronegative for rheumatoid factor and exhibit sausage digits and characteristic radiologic changes. The disease may be markedly destructive.

Psoriasis itself is a genetically determined disease, associated with HLA-B13, HLA-Bw17, and HLA-Cw6. Moreover, HLA-B27 is present in approximately 20 per cent of individuals with psoriatic arthropathy, even in the absence of sacroiliitis. HLA-Bw38, HLA-DR4, and HLA-DR7 appear to be genetic markers for patients with peripheral arthropathy. About 50 per cent of patients with psoriatic spondylitis are B27 negative; thus, as with inflammatory bowel disease, other genetic or environmental factors are relevant.

Psoriatic arthropathy is a common disease, occurring in about 20 per cent of individuals with psoriasis, particularly in those patients with psoriatic nail disease. Women are affected only slightly more commonly than men, in contrast to the more marked sex distribution in rheumatoid disease. Several forms of psoriatic arthropathy, the separation of which is not entirely distinct, have been described.

1. *Asymmetric oligoarthropathy.* In general, little relationship exists between joint and skin activity. Asymmetric involvement of both large and small joints is seen; the sausage-shaped digit is common. Any patient presenting with this form of arthropathy should be carefully examined for signs of psoriasis (scalp, umbilicus, gluteal region, and nails). In the past, many such individuals were considered to have seronegative rheumatoid arthritis.

2. *Symmetric polyarthropathy resembling rheumatoid arthritis.* Rarely, the pattern of arthritis may be indistinguishable from that seen in rheumatoid disease. This form may represent coincidental rheumatoid arthritis in a patient with psoriasis.

3. *Arthritis mutilans.* A resorptive arthropathy, arthritis mutilans is the severest form of destructive arthritis. The telescoping digits appear as the so-called opera-glass hand.

4. *Psoriatic spondylitis.* Approximately 20 per cent of subjects with psoriatic arthropathy have radiologic sacroiliitis (ankylosing spondylitis). Men predominate, with a sex ratio of 3.5:1.

5. *Psoriatic nail disease and distal interphalangeal joint involvement.* Nail pitting, transverse depressions, and subungual hyperkeratosis often occur in association with distal interphalangeal joint disease. The relationship between the psoriasis and the arthritis remains unclear.

Laboratory Features

An elevated erythrocyte sedimentation rate, anemia, and, rarely, hyperuricemia may occur. The frequency of positive tests for rheumatoid factor is the same as that found in the general population. The synovial tissue and fluid changes are nonspecific.

Radiologic Findings

Characteristic changes in this sometimes highly destructive disease include whittling of the distal ends of the phalanges, giving the joints a "pencil-and-cup" appearance; extensive bone resorption can result in an opera-glass hand. Erosions, ankylosis, periostitis, sacroiliitis, and ankylosing spondylitis are other typical radiologic findings.

Therapy

The skin and joints are treated separately. Improvement of the skin disease may be associated with amelioration of the joint inflammation. For mild arthropathy, indomethacin (25 to 50 mg three times per day) is the drug of choice. If this fails, phenylbutazone may be given. Gold and penicillamine may be useful, but few controlled studies have been done. Methotrexate is helpful in resistant cases.

Human Immunodeficiency Virus (HIV) and Spondylarthropathy

It is well recognized that a patient with rheumatoid arthritis who develops HIV disease may enter remission, at least from the point of view of the rheumatologic event. By contrast, patients with Reiter's syndrome or psoriatic arthropathy experience a dramatic exacerbation of the underlying disorder. Presumably, rheumatoid disease requires CD4+ lymphocytes, while the immunologic nature of spondylarthritis is distinct. Any patient who presents with severe Reiter's syndrome or psoriatic arthropathy, particularly when unresponsive to treatment, should be assessed for HIV disease. Methotrexate can have catastrophic effects on the patient with this infection.

Arnett F: The seronegative spondylarthropathies. In McCarty D (ed.): Current Opinion in Rheumatology, Vol. 2, No. 4, 1990. A series of up-to-date review articles on research and clinical subjects in the spondylarthropathy field.
Calin A (ed.): Spondylarthropathy. New York, Grune and Stratton, 1984, pp 1–427. A multiauthored international text on spondylarthropathy, including discussions on immunogenetics, the environment, and ethnic differences.
Feltkamp TEW (ed.): The pathogenetic role of HLA-B27. Scand J Rheumatol Suppl 87:1–163, 1990. An excellent recent review of current understanding of B27.
Will R, Palmer R, Bhalla A, et al.: Marked osteoporosis is present in early ankylosing spondylitis and may be a primary pathological event. Lancet 2:1483, 1989. A study of the spine in early disease, with striking findings.

260 Infectious Arthritis

Stephen E. Malawista

BACTERIAL ARTHRITIS

Bacterial arthritis usually results from bloodborne infection and much less commonly from direct penetration (e.g., needle aspiration) or contiguous osteomyelitis. Acute bacterial joint infections may be divided into two general groups, nongonococcal and gonococcal, based on their typically differing target populations, clinical characteristics, and ease of treatment. Differential features of these two classes of bacterial arthritis are presented in Table 260–1.

Nongonococcal Arthritis

Staphylococcus aureus heads the list of common infecting organisms in this group, followed by other gram-positive cocci (*Streptococcus pyogenes, pneumoniae, viridans*) and gram-negative bacilli (*Escherichia coli, Salmonella* sp., *Pseudomonas*, etc.); *Haemophilus influenzae* is unusual except in children under 4 years of age, before protective immunity develops. Patients are often very young, elderly, immunocompromised, or users of intravenous drugs. Risk factors for bacterial arthritis during septicemia include debilitating chronic disease, immunosuppressive therapy, previous joint damage (e.g., rheumatoid arthritis,

TABLE 260–1. DIFFERENTIAL FEATURES OF DISSEMINATED GONOCOCCAL INFECTION AND NONGONOCOCCAL BACTERIAL ARTHRITIS*

Disseminated Gonococcal Infection	Nongonococcal Bacterial Arthritis
Generally in young, healthy adults	Often in very young, elderly, or immunocompromised persons
Initial migratory polyarthralgias common	Polyarthralgias rare
Tenosynovitis in majority	Tenosynovitis rare
Dermatitis in majority	Dermatitis rare
>50% polyarthritis	>85% monoarthritis
Positive blood culture in <10%	Positive blood culture in 50%
Positive joint-fluid culture in 25%	Positive joint-fluid culture in 85–95%

*From Goldenberg DL, Reed JI: Bacterial arthritis. N Engl J Med 312:764–771, 1985. Reprinted by permission of The New England Journal of Medicine.

neuropathic arthropathy, joint surgery), sickle cell anemia, hypogammaglobulinemia, and intra-articular corticosteroid injections. After prosthetic joint replacement, an increasing problem has been late infection by organisms of low virulence, such as *Staphylococcus epidermidis*.

CLINICAL MANIFESTATIONS. A patient may present typically with the abrupt onset of a single, severely tender, red-hot swollen joint, especially the knee or another weight-bearing joint; shaking chills and fever may occur. However, signs of inflammation may be masked in severely debilitated patients or in those receiving adrenocorticosteroids or immunosuppressive agents. Bacterial arthritis superimposed on a noninfectious inflammatory joint disease may also be easily overlooked. For example, infection in one or a few joints of a patient with rheumatoid arthritis may be mistaken for a flare in the chronic disease. An infected joint in a gouty individual may go unrecognized for too long, even when the patient does not respond to his usual regimen for acute gouty arthritis (a good clue that something else is going on). A high index of suspicion is essential in these circumstances, because delay can lead rapidly to destruction of cartilage and bone and eventual fibrous or bony ankylosis.

DIAGNOSIS. When bacterial arthritis is suspected, prompt joint aspiration and both Gram stain and culture of synovial fluid are imperative; most nongonococcal bacteria will be recovered. Cultures for both aerobic and anaerobic organisms should be made. Synovial fluid leukocyte counts are frequently greater than 50,000 per cubic millimeter, and the glucose level is low and lactate level is high compared with those of serum, but these findings are not specific for infection. Bacteriologic studies should of course be extended to blood and other material (sputum, urine, and so forth) from which the infection may have disseminated. On radiograph, only soft tissue swelling is likely to be seen during the first week, but evidence of loss of articular cartilage and erosion of bone may appear rather soon thereafter in untreated patients.

MANAGEMENT. Successful management of bacterial arthritis depends primarily on early institution of appropriate antimicrobial therapy and effective drainage of the joint space. The selection of antimicrobial agents and recommendations regarding dose and duration of therapy are discussed in other areas of the text (Part XX). Antibiotics are given parenterally, often in high doses, for 2 to 4 weeks or more, depending on the clinical situation and the patient's response. They generally attain adequate levels in joint fluid and need not be given intra-articularly; indeed, the latter procedure may induce a chemical synovitis. For drainage, daily (or even more frequent) closed joint aspiration through a large-bore needle is carried out until fluid no longer accumulates. Open surgical drainage can usually be avoided except when the hip or the shoulder is infected (difficult to evacuate completely by needle); when tissue debris or fibrin interferes with closed aspiration; or when loculations, gross joint destruction, or contiguous osteomyelitis is present. The affected joint should be at rest while inflamed and should be mobilized to prevent atrophy when signs of acute inflammation have subsided.

Gonococcal Arthritis

Gonococcal infection is discussed in Ch. 336. The associated arthritis is by far the most common bacterial joint problem in generally healthy, sexually active teenagers and young adults, especially in urban populations. Gonorrhea is more likely to disseminate in women. The risk of dissemination is particularly high during menses and pregnancy, in the postpartum period, and in individuals with genetic deficiency in the terminal components of serum complement (C5, C6, C7, or C8). Additional features that help to distinguish gonococcal from other bacterial arthritides include a high frequency of associated tenosynovitis and rash and of multiple joint involvement, especially in the wrists and hands. Diagnosis is frequently presumptive because synovial fluid smear and culture are often negative, and corroborating cultural evidence from urethra, cervix, throat, rectum, blood, or skin may be lacking. Highly suggestive diagnostically is a history of fever and migratory polyarthralgias that progress to frank oligoarticular arthritis and are associated with tenosynovitis and skin lesions. The latter are either vesiculopustular on an erythematous base, often with necrotic centers, or hemorrhagic. Similar lesions are seen with arthritis caused by the meningococcus. Response to (even oral) antibiotic therapy (Ch. 336) and drainage is usually dramatic. Resistance to penicillin of gonococci that disseminate is uncommon.

Tuberculous Arthritis

The general decline in the frequency of pulmonary tuberculosis in the Western world is reflected in the relative rarity of tuberculous bone and joint disease. Infection usually reaches the joint from hematogenous dissemination to bone and direct extension from an osteomyelitic focus. Formerly, the classic presentation was chronic low back pain in a child because of involvement of lower thoracic or lumbar vertebrae, leading to collapse and sharp-angle kyphosis (Pott's disease). Currently, the typical target is a tuberculin-positive adult, often without evidence of pulmonary disease, who presents with chronic, insidious pain and swelling, usually in a single joint, especially the hip, knee, or wrist; this presentation is often mistaken for monoarticular rheumatoid arthritis. Tenosynovitis is common. Diagnosis depends upon culture of *Mycobacterium tuberculosis* from synovial fluid (positive in 80 per cent) or synovial biopsy (positive in 90 per cent). Sensitivities to chemotherapeutic agents must be determined; caseating granulomas and acid-fast bacilli are sometimes due to atypical mycobacteria resistant to the usual antituberculous drugs. Usual therapy for uncomplicated infections consists of long-term isoniazid and ethambutol or rifampin.

Goldenberg DL: Infectious arthritis complicating rheumatoid arthritis and other chronic rheumatic disorders. Arthritis Rheum 32:496, 1989. *Problems and recommendations in the diagnosis of infection in joints that have other reasons for being inflamed.*
Goldenberg DL, Reed JI: Bacterial arthritis. N Engl J Med 312:764, 1985. *A compact, well-referenced review of the pathophysiology of bacterial arthritis, clinical and microbiologic characteristics of its common forms, and current approaches to diagnosis and therapy.*

VIRAL ARTHRITIS

Many specific viral infections are associated with polyarthritis, notably hepatitis B, rubella, and parvovirus, but also mumps and vaccinia (and formerly, smallpox) and occasionally adenovirus type 7, Epstein-Barr virus (EBV) (in infectious mononucleosis) and other herpesviruses, and certain enteroviruses. Polyarthritis may dominate the picture of various mosquito-transmitted arbovirus infections, especially epidemic polyarthritis of Australia (Ross River virus) and the denguelike illnesses, chikungunya and o'nyongnyong.

In general, diagnosis is suggested by the exposure history (drug abuse for hepatitis B, immunization for rubella, epidemiologic considerations for arboviruses or enteroviruses); recognition of the associated viral syndrome, which often includes fever, rash, and regional lymphadenopathy; brevity of the joint involvement (days to weeks); and changing antibody titers against specific antigens. Routine laboratory tests are nonspecific, and except for rubella, virus has rarely been recovered from synovial fluid. Little is known about pathogenesis, but studies of hepatitis B and rubella provide some clues.

Transient, often symmetric polyarthritis or arthralgias resembling acute rheumatoid arthritis may be associated with hepatitis B, rubella, or parvovirus infection. In the case of *hepatitis B*, 10 to 30 per cent of patients have arthritis, often accompanied by urticaria, fever, and lymphadenopathy, all occurring days to weeks before the onset of frank hepatitis. This prodromal syndrome typically occurs when hepatitis B surface antigen (HBsAg) is in excess over antibody, hypocomplementemia is present, and serum contains immune complexes composed of HBsAg and anti-HB, other immunoglobulins, and complement components. Similar material has been found in affected dermal blood vessels, and the antigen has been seen in synovial tissue. With the development of antibody excess, complexes disappear, the arthritis and rash resolve, and frank hepatitis may supervene. The process resembles experimental serum sickness and suggests an inflammatory pathogenetic mechanism driven by deposition of immune complexes. Joint symptoms may respond dramatically to salicylates.

Rubella arthritis is primarily a disease of adult women. It usually follows onset of the characteristic rash by a few days, but the rash may be absent and rheumatoid factor present, inviting diagnostic confusion. Arthritis is usually sudden in onset, symmetric and polyarticular in distribution (fingers, knees, wrists), brief in duration (less than a month), and without residua. Salicylates are useful for pain and stiffness.

Arthritis may also occur within a few weeks of vaccination by attenuated rubella virus. Again, attacks are brief but may recur periodically for a few years without permanent joint damage. Rubella virus has been recovered from synovial fluid in both the natural and the vaccine-induced disease and more recently in a few patients with various chronic joint syndromes. It seems capable of replicating in synovium; whether its new association with chronic disease is critical or coincidental remains to be determined.

Human parvovirus B19 causes the highly contagious childhood exanthem fifth disease (*erythema infectiosum;* Ch. 365). In infected adults (especially women), a syndrome of short-lived (weeks) inflammatory joint involvement closely resembles that seen in rubella. As in rubella, the characteristic rash is often absent, and the history (of a sick child) is therefore critical for indicating the correct diagnosis; an elevated titer of specific IgM antibody confirms it. Again, treatment is symptomatic; prognosis, excellent.

Schnitzer TJ: Viral arthritis. *In* Kelley WN, Harris ED, Ruddy S, et al. (eds.): Textbook of Rheumatology. 3rd ed. Philadelphia, W.B. Saunders Company, 1989, pp 1611–1628. *Survey of common and uncommon arthritides associated with specific viral illnesses.*
Wands JR, Mann E, Alpert E, et al.: The pathogenesis of arthritis associated with acute hepatitis B surface antigen–positive hepatitis. Complement activation and characterization of circulating immune complexes. J Clin Invest 55:930, 1975. *Clinical description and characterization of immunologic aspects of the syndrome.*

OTHER FORMS OF INFECTIOUS ARTHRITIS

Lyme Disease (See Ch. 343)

Syphilitic Arthritis

Syphilis is discussed in Ch. 340. Joint disease associated with congenital and acquired syphilitic infections is now rare. In infants with congenital disease, musculoskeletal complaints are related to periostitis and osteochondritis. About the time of puberty, painless knee effusions (Clutton's joints) may be confused with rheumatoid or pyogenic arthritis. With acquired infection, arthralgias, arthritis, or tenosynovitis may accompany classic signs of secondary syphilis: rash, mucous plaques, alopecia, or lymphadenopathy. In tertiary lues, gummatous arthritis or periostitis (tibia, clavicles) may occur. Neuropathic arthropathy (Charcot's joint) is reviewed in Ch. 472.

Fungal Arthritis

Any of the invasive mycoses can affect joints, usually by direct extension from bone. Frequent infectious agents include coccidioidomycosis and histoplasmosis—both of which may also be accompanied by erythema nodosum with joint involvement, sporotrichosis (often by direct penetration: rose thorns), blastomycosis, actinomycosis, and candidiasis. Clinically, the affected joint or joints resemble those in other forms of granulomatous arthritis (e.g., tuberculous). For diagnosis, the causative agent must be seen in appropriately stained synovial biopsy material or grown from synovial tissue or fluid.

261 Systemic Lupus Erythematosus

Alfred D. Steinberg

Systemic lupus erythematosus (SLE) is a disease of unknown etiology characterized by inflammation in many different organ systems associated with the production of antibodies reactive with nuclear, cytoplasmic, and cell membrane antigens. Individual patients may have some, but not necessarily all, of the following: fatigue, anemia, fever, rashes, sun sensitivity, alopecia, arthritis, pericarditis, pleurisy, vasculitis, nephritis, and central nervous system disease. The course is often unpredictable, with variable periods of exacerbations and remissions. There is no one clinical abnormality that definitely establishes the diagnosis, nor is there a single test for the disorder. As a result, criteria have been developed and modified in an attempt to include patients with SLE and to exclude patients with other disorders (Table 261–1). Although these criteria were developed for epidemiologic and research purposes, they are helpful in diagnosis as well. Nevertheless, it is possible to fulfill these criteria and not have SLE, and it is possible to fail to fulfill the criteria and still have SLE. Thus, a teenage girl with a "butterfly" rash of the face, pleurisy, and large amounts of serum antibodies reactive with native DNA undoubtedly has SLE even if she does not yet manifest any other criteria.

INCIDENCE. Although SLE can occur at any age (it has been diagnosed at birth and in individuals in the tenth decade of life), more than 60 per cent of patients experience the onset of disease between ages 13 and 40 years. Among children, SLE occurs three times more commonly in girls than in boys. In patients in their teens, twenties, and thirties, 90 to 95 per cent are female. Thereafter, the female predominance again falls to that observed before puberty.

The disorder is approximately three times more common among American blacks than American caucasians. Certain North American Indian tribes (Sioux, Crow, Arapahoe) have an even greater predisposition toward SLE. Asians are affected to approximately the same extent as American blacks. The overall annual incidence of SLE is about 6 new cases per 100,000 population per year for relatively low-risk populations and approximately 35 per 100,000 for relatively high-risk populations. The chance that a black female will develop SLE in her lifetime is approximately 1 in 250.

These data suggest that both genetic factors and sex hormones may affect the probability of developing SLE. If a family member has SLE, the likelihood of SLE increases (approximately 30 per cent for identical twins and 5 per cent for other first-degree relatives). Although males develop SLE less frequently than do females, their illness is not milder.

ETIOLOGY. The etiology of SLE is unknown. The immune hyperactivity that characterizes SLE appears to derive from abnormal immune activation and loss of self-tolerance (Fig. 261–1). An inherited defect in immune regulation may underlie the disorder in many individuals. Environmental agents that trigger disease include foods, drugs, ultraviolet (UV) light, and micro-organisms (bacteria, viruses, parasites) (Fig. 261–2). Inherited complement deficiency and other deficiencies (see Ch. 243) may predispose to infections that induce disease activity.

The combination of immune stimulation and impaired regulation leads to a loss of self-tolerance and expansion of B cells able to produce a variety of autoantibodies. Androgens protect against both the polyclonal activation and the loss of self-tolerance, whereas estrogens have the opposite effect. Early in life, idiotopes (unique structures expressed on immunoglobulin molecules) stimulate expansion of T cells with receptors that are able to recognize

TABLE 261–1. CRITERIA FOR CLASSIFICATION OF SYSTEMIC LUPUS ERYTHEMATOSUS*

Criterion		Definition
1. Malar rash		Fixed erythema, flat or raised, over the malar eminences, tending to spare the nasolabial folds
2. Discoid rash		Erythematous raised patches with adherent keratotic scaling and follicular plugging; atrophic scarring may occur in older lesions
3. Photosensitivity		Skin rash as a result of unusual reaction to sunlight, by patient history or physician observation
4. Oral ulcers		Oral or nasopharyngeal ulceration, usually painless, observed by a physician
5. Arthritis		Nonerosive arthritis involving two or more peripheral joints, characterized by tenderness, swelling, or effusion
6. Serositis	a.	Pleuritis—convincing history of pleuritic pain or rub heard by a physician or evidence of pleural effusion *OR*
	b.	Pericarditis—documented by electrocardiogram or rub or evidence of pericardial effusion
7. Renal disorder	a.	Persistent proteinuria greater than 0.5 gram per day or greater than 3+ if quantitation not performed *OR*
	b.	Cellular casts—may be red cell, hemoglobin, granular, tubular, or mixed
8. Neurologic disorder	a.	Seizures—in the absence of offending drugs or known metabolic derangements, e.g., uremia, ketoacidosis, or electrolyte imbalance *OR*
	b.	Psychosis—in the absence of offending drugs or known metabolic derangements, e.g., uremia, ketoacidosis, or electrolyte imbalance
9. Hematologic disorder	a.	Hemolytic anemia—with reticulocytosis *OR*
	b.	Leukopenia—less than 4000/mm^3 total on two or more occasions
	c.	Lymphopenia—less than 1500/mm^3 on two or more occasions *OR*
	d.	Thrombocytopenia—less than 100,000/mm^3 in the absence of offending drugs
10. Immunologic disorder	a.	Positive LE cell preparation *OR*
	b.	Anti-DNA: antibody to native DNA in abnormal titer *OR*
	c.	Anti-Sm: presence of antibody to Sm nuclear antigen *OR*
	d.	False-positive serologic test for syphilis known to be positive for at least 6 months and confirmed by *Treponema pallidum* immobilization or fluorescent treponemal antibody absorption test
11. Antinuclear antibody		An abnormal titer of antinuclear antibody by immunofluorescence or an equivalent assay at any point in time and in the absence of drugs known to be associated with "drug-induced lupus" syndrome

*The classification is based on 11 criteria. For the purpose of identifying patients in clinical studies, a person shall be said to have systemic lupus erythematosus if any 4 or more of the 11 criteria are present, serially or simultaneously, during any interval of observation.

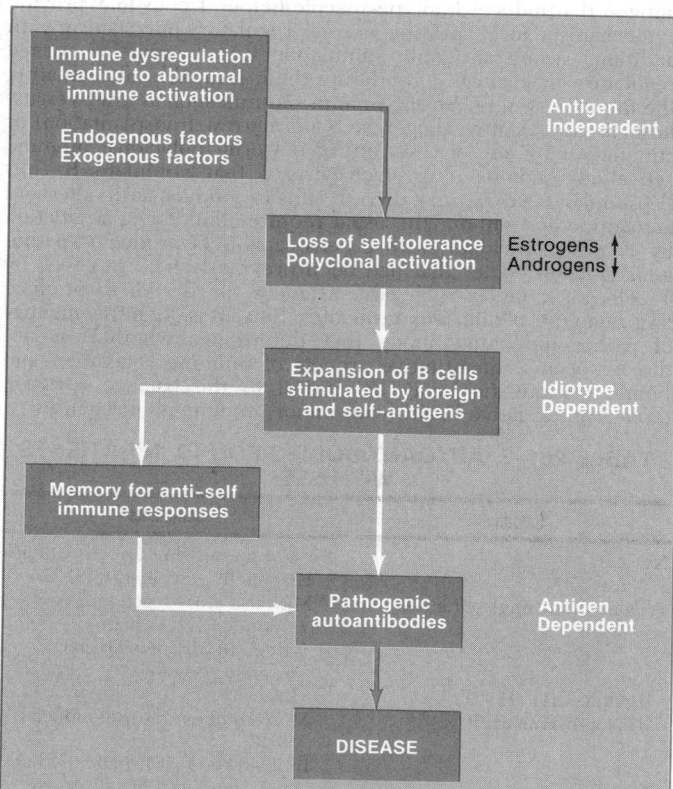

FIGURE 261–1. Flow chart of possible pathogenetic events in systemic lupus erythematosus. A stimulus to humoral immune hyperactivity can result from an endogenous (genetic) predisposition or from environmental triggers, or both. It does not necessarily depend upon stimulation by a specific self-antigen. The immune hyperactivity may lead to a loss of self-tolerance and polyclonal B cell activation. Androgens protect against such effects, whereas estrogens facilitate them. Idiotype stimulation may also contribute to expansion of B cells stimulated by foreign antigens and self-antigens (or antigens cross-reactive with self). Ultimately, selection by self-antigens leads to high-affinity autoantibodies, some of which are pathogenic. Even after the disease is treated, the prior generation of memory B cells allows the autoantibody response to be triggered anew, potentially leading to disease flares.

specific idiotopes but that simultaneously may recognize a self-antigen. In addition, later in life, similar idiotypic stimulation of T cells may provide help for B cells able to produce autoantibodies. For example, an immune complex of antibody and self-antigen (or an antigen cross-reactive with self) may be recognized in such a manner that the idiotype-specific T cell is stimulated by the idiotope on the antibody molecule. This interaction provides help for the B cell, which recognizes the self-antigen and is triggered to produce autoantibodies.

The stimulation of autoreactive B cells leads to both autoantibody-producing cells and memory B cells. The autoreactive B cells are subject to selective pressures by self-antigen, resulting in emergence of clones of B cells able to make antibody of progressively higher affinity for the self-antigen. Some such antibodies are pathogenic and contribute to disease. However, even after treatment, memory B cells may persist. Subsequent stimulation of such B cells may trigger a new disease flare.

Very early in the disease process, autoantibodies may have relatively low affinities for a given self-antigen and may be capable of binding to more than one self-antigen. With time, the selection processes frequently lead to antibodies with high affinity for a given self-determinant and less cross-reactivity with other self-antigens. Therefore, late in disease, the autoantibody "repertoire" becomes relatively fixed.

In some individuals, the inherited predisposition to SLE may be very important, the environmental triggers playing secondary roles. In contrast, other patients may have minimal genetic predispositions and may require very strong environmental triggers for disease expression (Fig. 261–2).

The signs and symptoms are thought to be caused by the

autoantibodies that react with self constituents and initiate inflammatory responses. The more severe the inflammatory response to a given initiator, the more severe the disease. The initiation of this process may be multifactorial and may be different in different individuals. Therefore, several genetic factors may be important in many individuals. These may be genes that allow augmented antibody responses following a variety of stimuli as well as genes that predispose to particular autoantibodies. In addition, hormonal, metabolic, and environmental factors appear to act on the genetically conditioned immune substratum to predispose to or protect against disease expression. Males are protected against SLE by their androgens except in a subgroup of males who inherit a Y chromosome accelerating factor from their fathers. In general, factors that augment humoral immunity favor disease expression, whereas those that retard antibody production tend to protect.

Some patients may have a primary abnormality in the ability of their immune systems to perform normal self-regulatory functions. It is probably best to consider abnormal immune regulation as one of several factors that may contribute to illness. If any one is very abnormal, disease may occur. Under most circumstances, several defects probably combine to incite disease. However, once the process is initiated, impaired self-regulation would favor perpetuation of the disease-inducing abnormalities.

It has long been known that some individuals with SLE have disease exacerbations following exposure to UV light. Several different mechanisms are likely: UV light induces keratinocytes to secrete interleukin 1, which, in turn, stimulates B cells and induces T cells to produce B cell growth and differentiation factors, which stimulate the immune system; UV light impairs processing of antigen and immune complexes, thereby increasing the load of pathogenic complexes on target organs; UV light induces cytosine and thymine dimer formation, which stimulates immune responses.

Certain drugs can cause an SLE-like illness in apparently healthy individuals. The drugs (Table 261–2) do not share common structural or chemical properties. The mechanisms of disease induction probably vary. Even chemicals in foods may induce

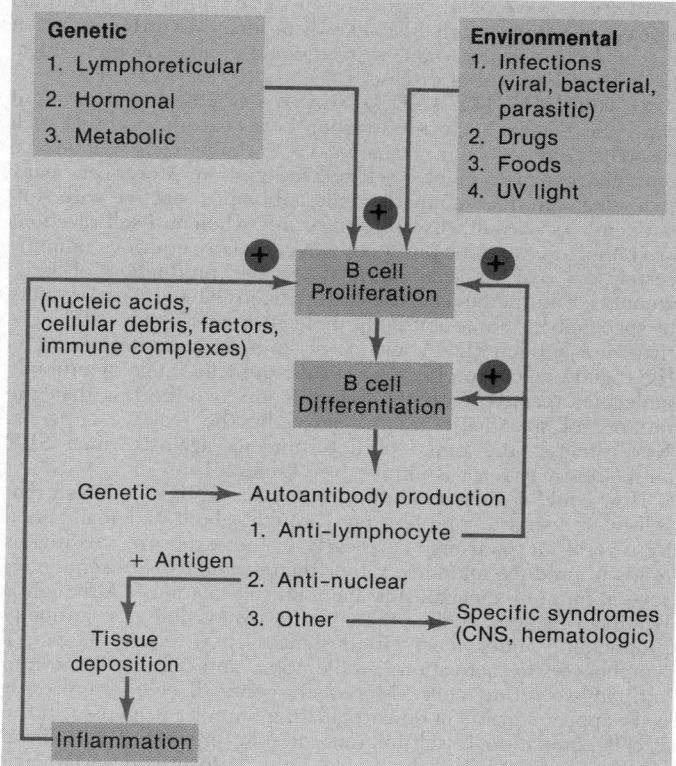

FIGURE 261–2. Initiation and perpetuation of systemic lupus erythematosus.

TABLE 261–2. SOME DRUGS ABLE TO INDUCE FEATURES OF SLE

Related to Dose-Time Administration	More Idiosyncratic
Hydralazine	Aminosalicylic acid
Procainamide	D-Penicillamine
Alpha-methyldopa	Griseofulvin
Isoniazid	Penicillin
Chlorpromazine	Ampicillin
Chlorthalidone	Streptomycin
Phenytoin	Sulfonamides
Mephenytoin	Tetracycline
Trimethadione	Methylthiouracil
Primidone	Propylthiouracil
Ethosuximide	Phenylbutazone
Carbamazepine	Oxyphenisatin
Phenylethylacetylurea	Practolol
	Tolazamide
	Methysergide
	Reserpine
	Quinidine
	Isoquinazepan
	Guanoxan

SLE. For example, alfalfa sprouts contain L-canavanine, which can induce an SLE-like illness. The extent to which "idiopathic" SLE is triggered by such specific environmental factors is unknown.

A variety of complement deficiencies have been associated with SLE. The most common is C2 deficiency. It is not clear whether the association is one of genetic linkage or predisposition because of the deficiency itself. The latter might occur if the deficiency led to increased susceptibility to infections that trigger illness.

For many years it has been thought that there might be a "lupus virus," a particular virus that induces disease. Patients with SLE have, in the endothelial cells of their kidneys and in their lymphocytes, structures that resemble viral nucleocapsids but that are not related to or caused by viruses. In addition, retroviruses have been implicated in the immune complex renal disease of animals with SLE-like disorders. Nevertheless, even if such a virus is important, it is only one of many factors critical to the development of disease.

AUTOIMMUNITY AND DISEASE IN SLE. In past years it was believed that an anti-self response was harmful and that such responses did not occur normally. We now appreciate that normal immune responses involve self-self recognition. Moreover, many individuals produce nonpathogenic antibodies reactive with self-antigens. As a result, disease occurs only when anti-self reactions are either excessive or productive of especially injurious immune responses. SLE is characterized by the production of large amounts of antibodies reactive with antigens having a great variety of specificities. Some antibody molecules cross-react with more than one antigen (DNA and cardiolipin or immunoglobulin G [IgG] and nucleoprotein). As a result, the true range of antibody molecules reactive with self-determinants may be less than the number of specificities as measured by the reactive antigens. Nevertheless, the range of determinants against which SLE antibodies may react is impressive (Table 261–3).

How could such self-reactivity come about? It is believed that self-tolerance is a complex state brought about and maintained by several mechanisms. Very early in life, exposure to antigens tends to produce tolerance rather than immunity. Subsequently, several immune mechanisms maintain self-tolerance. Although B lymphocytes and their progeny are responsible for antibody production, under most circumstances they require helper T lymphocytes for activation, proliferation, and differentiation into antibody-secreting cells. Moreover, some T cells (suppressor cells) appear capable of downregulating immune responses. If the T cell population is self-tolerant, it may prevent B cells from proliferating and differentiating into autoantibody-producing cells. A defect in self-tolerance mechanisms could occur at any of several steps in the immune pathway. Stimulation by a foreign

antigen that induces idiotype-specific helper T cells may provide a mechanism for bypassing normal regulatory mechanisms. In addition, strong antigenic stimulation can overwhelm normal regulatory mechanisms, rendering them incapable of regulating the immune stimuli. Strong immune stimuli such as graft-versus-host disease (as after allogeneic bone marrow transplantation) or stimulation by any of a variety of powerful polyclonal immune activators (endotoxin) or even viruses that stimulate B cells (Epstein-Barr virus), may drive B cells to produce antibodies and autoantibodies without the usual requirements for or regulation by T cells. Individuals with B cells capable of producing pathogenic autoantibodies that had been previously held in check by T cells may, under such circumstances, be driven to produce large amounts of injurious antibodies. Since it is often the quantity of pathogenic autoantibody that determines whether or not disease occurs, quantitative aspects of immune regulation and immune stimulation may be critical to the balance between disease and relative health with minor immune abnormalities.

TABLE 261–3. AUTOANTIBODIES FOUND IN PATIENTS WITH SLE

Specificity	Comments
Nuclear	Present in most but not all patients
Native DNA	Essentially restricted to SLE
Denatured (single-stranded) DNA	May also cross-react with double-stranded DNA; high titers in SLE; lower titers in other diseases
Histones H1, H3-H4	SLE
Histones H2A-H2B	More common in drug-induced SLE
Sm	In 25–60% of SLE patients, but not found in other diseases
Nuclear ribonucleoprotein	Found in SLE, but highest titers in "mixed connective tissue disease"; multiple small proteins and combined RNA have been discovered
Nucleolar antigens	Scleroderma, SLE, Sjögren's syndrome
SS-B (La, Ha)	Sjögren's syndrome, SLE
SS-A (Ro)	Sjögren's syndrome, SLE
Proliferating cell nuclear antigen	SLE
RANA	Especially in rheumatoid arthritis (Epstein-Barr virus)
DNA-RNA hybrids, double-stranded RNA	SLE
Cytoplasmic	Less information available on these
Ribosomal ribonucleoprotein	SLE
Mitochondria	Primary biliary cirrhosis, SLE
Microsomal antigens	Chronic active hepatitis, malignancies
Lysosomes	SLE
Single-stranded RNA, tRNA	SLE
SS-B and SS-A	Sjögren's syndrome, SLE
Cell membrane determinants	Common in SLE
Red cells	May occur without important hemolysis
White cells	Granulocytes, T cells, B cells
Platelets	Common without thrombocytopenia
Lipomodulin	SLE, RA, others ?
Receptors	Insulin, IL2, others
MHC Class II	Interferes with immune functions
Others	
Mitotic spindle and intracellular supporting proteins	SLE and other rheumatic diseases
Immunoglobulins	JRA, RA, SLE, Sjögren's syndrome, others
Clotting factors	SLE and other diseases
Phospholipids (e.g., cardiolipin)	SLE, others, without other disease
Thyroid antigens	Thyroid diseases, SLE, Sjögren's syndrome

RANA = RA nuclear antigen; RA = rheumatoid arthritis; JRA = juvenile rheumatoid arthritis; IL2 = interleukin 2.

PATHOGENESIS. Systemic lupus is often classified as an immune complex type of disorder. This designation is, at best, an oversimplification. SLE is a disease primarily mediated by antibodies; however, the details of pathogenesis are not proved for many of the clinical and pathologic findings. It is clear that patients with SLE produce autoantibodies and that many of these are injurious. This has been well demonstrated for the renal disease associated with SLE. Antibody reacts with antigen either in the circulation or in the glomerulus, and complement is fixed, leading to release of chemotactic factors, attraction of leukocytes, and release of their injurious mediators of inflammation. The degree of pathology is determined, to a large extent, by the magnitude of the antibody deposition and the intensity of the inflammatory process initiated. Continued deposition of antibody and continued induction of inflammation ultimately lead to irreversible renal damage. Similar processes occur in other organs. However, antibody and complement may be deposited in the skin or in the choroid plexus with or without an attendant inflammatory response. The qualitative character of the antibody molecules (affinity, isotype, charge), the nature of the antigen or their combined properties (size, molecular configuration), or additional factors may be critical to pathogenesis.

Antibody plays a role in SLE not only by depositing in vessels but also by binding to the surfaces of cells. Patients with SLE produce antibodies to erythrocytes, granulocytes, lymphocytes, and macrophages. These antibodies can cause such cells to be removed from the circulation by the reticuloendothelial system or to be killed by complement-mediated cytotoxicity or, more likely, by the mechanisms of antibody-dependent cellular cytotoxicity (ADCC). In this non–complement-mediated killing, leukocytes recognize antibody-coated target cells and kill them. ADCC may be responsible for some of the pathology initiated in the kidneys and other organs by other antibody-mediated mechanisms. In addition, antibody directed against renal antigens, e.g., renal tubular or glomerular basement membrane, may be generated as a result of immunization by fragments released from the inflammatory process. Such antibody induces additional renal pathology and may account for much of the disease in some patients.

It appears that many of the inflammatory lesions that occur in SLE are initiated by antibody and that the injury occurs in small vessels. Thus, any organ so affected could be a site of inflammation, with the possibility of scarring, dysfunction, or both. Many of the central nervous system problems of patients (seizures, psychoses), as well as hematologic (anemia, thrombocytopenia, leukopenia), cardiac (coronary artery disease), dermal (alopecia, sun sensitivity), and other clinical and laboratory abnormalities, have additional pathogenetic mechanisms. The hematologic abnormalities could all be explained by antibodies specifically reactive with the formed elements of the blood; however, many relate to suppression at the level of the bone marrow. The central nervous system disorders are multiple, and each may have its own pathogenetic mechanism. Because central nervous system involvement in SLE is not a single entity, individual patients may require different approaches to understanding and therapy.

PATHOLOGY. The pathologic abnormalities of SLE follow directly from the pathogenetic mechanisms; moreover, the same degree of variability is encountered. In organs affected by small vessel vasculitis, the first lesions are usually characterized by granulocytic infiltration and periarteriolar edema. This is usually followed by round cell infiltration and ultimately a relatively acellular eosinophilic material composed of fibrin, immunoglobulins, and complement (fibrinoid) containing scattered hematoxylin bodies. These basophilic-staining bodies are nuclear debris, often associated with antinuclear antibody, and represent a correlate of the LE cell in vivo. Immunofluorescence analysis demonstrates immunoglobulin and complement in the vessels in the affected areas. Arterioles, venules, and sometimes arteries and veins are involved.

Individual organs often have their peculiar abnormalities. The spleen has "onion skin lesions," concentric fibrosis of the walls and surrounding tissues of the central and penicilliary arteries. These lesions are thought to be diagnostic of SLE in patients with "idiopathic" thrombocytopenia. Nonbacterial verrucous endocarditis (Libman-Sacks) consists of vegetations on the heart valves or chordae tendineae; they can extend along the endocardium and become quite large.

The renal pathology varies from mild to severe glomerular inflammation and variable interstitial involvement. Most patients have relatively normal kidneys or a renal lesion consisting of minimal focal hypercellularity, thickening of the capillary basement membrane, and fibrinoid change. In clinically important glomerulonephritis, these lesions are more generalized and are usually a mixture of proliferative and membranous changes, with increases in endothelial, mesangial, epithelial, and inflammatory cells, capsular inflammation leading to crescent formation, and focal thickening of the basement membrane and mesangial hypercellularity. Some kidneys have membranous glomerulonephritis with considerable thickening of the basement membrane. Basement membrane thickening, when associated with fibrinoid changes, results in the so-called wire loop lesions. There may also be hyaline thrombi in glomeruli, focal necrosis, hematoxylin bodies, and sclerosis in healed lesions. Tubular degenerative changes and mixed inflammatory interstitial inflammation are common. Some patients have primarily mesangial disease; this carries a better prognosis than does capillary loop involvement. Extensive crescent formation and substantial glomerular or interstitial scarring are unfavorable prognostic signs.

CLINICAL MANIFESTATIONS. SLE is a highly variable disease in onset and course. A young woman may present with a butterfly rash, a history of recent sun sensitivity, pleuropericarditis, arthritis, fever, extreme fatigue, seizures, and nephrotic syndrome. This "typical" presentation, which is easily recognized as SLE, occurs in only a minority of patients. More commonly, patients may have only one or two signs or symptoms of SLE, such as arthritis and fatigue. Only later do additional features of SLE occur. As a result, the initial presentation may allow neither a definitive diagnosis nor insight into the organ systems that may become involved in the future. Many patients never develop major organ involvement. Some have kidney but not central nervous system involvement or vice versa. Thus, the clinical manifestations of one patient may be very different from those of another. Some associations between serologic findings and clinical features are valid on a statistical basis but may not hold for a given individual. Thus, patients with large amounts of anti-DNA, especially precipitating antibodies, are more likely to have renal disease. Those with antibodies to Ro (SS-A) and La (SS-B, Ha) are most likely to have sicca syndrome, muscle disease, lung disease, and inconsequential or no renal disease. In the paragraphs that follow, individual clinical features of patients with SLE are described (see also Table 261–4). Patients vary greatly in organ system involvement and also in the severity of disease when a given organ system is affected. Thus, most patients do not have many of the abnormalities described. In addition, SLE is characterized by periods of active disease followed by periods of less intense disease or even remission. In rare cases the patient has a rapidly progressive disease, but the majority can look forward to the time when the disease no longer interferes with their lives.

Constitutional Problems. The majority of patients have fatigue, fever, and weight loss at the time of diagnosis. However, before attributing these to SLE, a diligent search is necessary to rule out infection. Later in the illness, the recurrence of one or more of these findings often indicates an increase in disease activity. Fatigue, difficult as it may be to evaluate, often is the first sign that a flare is imminent.

Musculoskeletal Problems. Arthralgias are the single most common manifestation in SLE. They characteristically are much more transitory than in patients with rheumatoid arthritis (RA), lasting minutes to days in a given joint. With more longstanding or more severe disease, the pain may be constant and frank arthritis is observed. It is often symmetric, the proximal interphalangeal joints of the hands, metacarpophalangeal joints, wrists, and knees being most commonly affected. Morning stiffness is reported by many patients with SLE and joint disease. Although the bony erosions characteristic of RA do not occur, deformities similar to those in RA develop in 10 to 15 per cent of patients and are thought to result from tendon disease. Occasionally, patients experience rupture of the Achilles or quadriceps tendon. Myalgias occur in approximately 30 per cent of patients; only a portion of these have muscle tenderness. Many patients with SLE and muscle disease do not have elevations of creatine kinase activity; some of these patients have an elevated aldolase value.

TABLE 261–4. COMMON CLINICAL ABNORMALITIES IN PATIENTS WITH SLE

Abnormality	Approximate Frequency (%)*
Constitutional	90
Fatigue	80
Fever	60
Weight loss, anorexia	
Musculoskeletal	90
Arthritis, arthralgia	30
Myalgia, myositis	
Skin and mucous membranes	60
Butterfly rash	50
Alopecia	50
Photosensitivity	30
Raynaud's phenomenon	30
Mucosal ulcers	20
Discoid lupus	10
Urticaria	10
Edema or bullae	
Eye (conjunctivitis/episcleritis/sicca syndrome)	20
Gastrointestinal	30
Serosal (pleurisy, pericarditis, peritonitis)	50
Lymphoreticular	50
Lymphadenopathy	30
Splenomegaly	
Hepatomegaly	30
Hypertension	30
Bacterial infections	40
Pneumonitis (all)	30
"lupus"	10
Renal (all)	50
severe	20
Central nervous system	
Personality disorders	50
Seizures	20
Psychoses	20
Stroke or long tract signs	10
Migraine headaches	10
Cardiac	
Myocarditis	30
Murmurs and valvular disease	30
Coronary artery disease	20
Hematologic	
Anemia (all)	70
Hemolytic	10
Purpura (all)	50
Thrombocytopenia	10
Peripheral neuropathy	10

*Frequencies are compiled from a number of series and are rounded off to the nearest 10 per cent. There was some variation from series to series depending upon patient population, non-SLE therapy, and therapy for SLE. Some abnormalities are more common in younger patients than in older patients (e.g., splenomegaly and lymphadenopathy) and vice versa (e.g., muscle disease and sicca syndrome).

Skin and Mucous Membranes. The typical butterfly rash varies from a slight blush to a clear-cut and somewhat edematous, nonpapular erythematous covering of both cheeks and the bridge of the nose. Patients with a butterfly rash often look as though they have applied too much rouge. This lesion may occur in the absence of sun exposure but may be exacerbated by the sun. It often precedes other manifestations of disease. A maculopapular erythematous eruption is also common. Indistinguishable from a drug-produced eruption, it is often induced or exacerbated by sunlight and sometimes by a drug (sulfisoxazole [Gantrisin] and ampicillin are common offenders). The palms and soles are not always spared. Healing usually occurs without scarring. Urticaria and angioedema are more common than subepidermal bullae, which occur in only a few per cent of patients. Discoid lupus in

SLE is indistinguishable from discoid lupus without systemic involvement; however, systemic disease may develop in patients with longstanding discoid lesions. In this rash, central atrophy, hyperpigmentation and hypopigmentation, telangiectasia, and follicular plugging accompany the usual stages of erythema followed by hyperkeratosis and then by atrophy. The hypopigmentation may be extensive and particularly disturbing to blacks.

Livedo reticularis occurs commonly in patients with SLE, but only rarely is it severe. Splinter hemorrhages, tender fingertip pulp lesions, and palmar erythema are sometimes remarkable. Purpura is more often secondary to vasculitis or capillary fragility (corticosteroid therapy is often responsible) than to thrombocytopenia.

Lupus profundus (relapsing nodular nonsuppurative panniculitis) occurs rarely in SLE patients. It may be limited to superficial panniculitis or may extend deeply into the thighs or buttocks. The overlying skin may ulcerate, and the deeper lesions often calcify.

One fifth of patients demonstrate vasculitic lesions of the skin. These can occur on the fingertips, forearms, lips, or lower leg (the last-named may ulcerate). Although they are signs of disease activity, they do not usually imply impending disaster. The related mucosal ulcers are often painless and occur on the hard and soft palate, the nasal septum, other parts of the upper respiratory tract, and even the vagina. They are usually harmless, but occasional patients with involvement of the upper airway may require emergency tracheotomy.

Alopecia is usually diffuse; patients report increased hair on comb or brush or pillow. The hair will regrow in areas not scarred by discoid lesions.

Raynaud's phenomenon may be severe enough to cause digital gangrene and spontaneous amputation of the distal parts of the digits. More often it follows a more benign and variable course. Thrombophlebitis occurs in approximately 10 per cent of patients and may be accompanied by pulmonary emboli.

Eyes. Conjunctivitis or episcleritis or both are usually observed in younger patients at times of disease activity. Cytoid bodies (white exudates next to retinal vessels) are associated with active central nervous system involvement. Spasm of the retinal vessels may lead to transient or permanent blindness. Keratoconjunctivitis sicca occurs in 10 per cent of patients and is usually slowly progressive, but it often improves temporarily with therapy for other symptoms.

Gastrointestinal System. Anorexia, nausea, vomiting, and abdominal pain are observed in a minority of patients. Diffuse abdominal pain with or without rebound tenderness may be a manifestation of serositis or mesenteric arteritis. The latter can be complicated by intestinal infarct, which may lead to perforation and death. Corticosteroid therapy often improves symptoms in both situations; however, if perforation has already occurred, the symptoms may be blunted and therapy inappropriately delayed. Pancreatitis is occasionally due to SLE.

Dysphagia may be associated with reduced peristalsis or ulcerations of the esophagus caused by arteritis, or, more commonly Candida albicans infection.

Liver. Liver enlargement is common but usually inconsequential. Fatty infiltration may rarely be associated with hepatic insufficiency. Liver enzyme elevations often occur early in the illness in the absence of therapy. Aspirin treatment may induce such enzyme elevations. Chronic hepatitis is only occasionally observed in patients with SLE.

Heart. Pericarditis is usually symptomatic but without consequence; however, an occasional patient may experience tamponade. The most common electrocardiographic abnormality is nonspecific T wave changes. A prolonged PR interval or evidence of ischemia or infarction may be found. Myocarditis may be manifested by unexplained tachycardia or dyspnea on exertion. More severe involvement is associated with frank heart failure. Coronary artery disease, most often atherosclerotic but occasionally arteritic, can lead to myocardial infarction, even in women in their early twenties.

Lung. Pleuritic chest pain occurs more commonly than does radiographic evidence of effusion; however, massive effusions may occur. Pneumonitis in patients with SLE is often infectious; however, a noninfectious syndrome that varies from fleeting infiltrates (usually hemorrhagic) to marked consolidation and hypoxia occurs in SLE patients. Diffuse interstitial pneumonitis has also been found in SLE.

Hematologic and Lymphoreticular Problems. Lymphadenopathy and splenomegaly with polyclonal immune hyperactivity may be sufficiently marked to suggest a lymphoproliferative disorder. Hematologic abnormalities are almost invariably present in patients with active disease. The most common is a normocytic anemia caused by impaired erythropoiesis. Hemolysis may occur in patients with or without a positive Coombs test result, but significant hemolysis occurs in fewer than 10 per cent of patients. Iron deficiency often contributes to anemia. Many patients with lupus bruise easily; therapy and capillary fragility are more often the cause than is a bleeding disorder. Mild thrombocytopenia occurs in a substantial proportion of patients; however, serious thrombocytopenia occurs in fewer than 10 per cent. Two types of "anticoagulants" occur. In the first, antibodies may react with clotting factors (VIII, IX, XII, and others) and may be responsible for clinically important bleeding. The other is a laboratory finding caused by antibodies reactive with the phospholipids used in the partial thromboplastin time (PTT) test. This abnormality is not associated with prolonged bleeding and is not a cause of concern with regard to surgery or biopsies. However, patients with antibodies reactive with phospholipids often manifest a syndrome characterized by thromboses, repeated abortions, and lung disease. The thromboses may lead to severe central nervous system dysfunction.

Nervous System. Peripheral neuropathies have been observed in about 15 per cent of patients with SLE, sometimes in the absence of other nervous system involvement. In addition to a sensory neuropathy, a mononeuritis multiplex picture (e.g., foot drop) is notable. Central nervous system involvement is quite variable. Psychological problems include personality disorders of every variety and numerous forms of frank psychosis (depression, paranoia, mania, schizophrenia). Differentiating that caused by lupus and that caused by corticosteroids is often a challenge.

Seizures, often grand mal, are common, especially in younger patients. Migraine headaches and cytoid bodies may be indications of disease activity. An organic brain syndrome with impaired mentation can progress to coma. Recovery may be complete, or there may be residual impairment. Movement disorders are more common in younger patients: chorea, athetosis, and hemiballismus are observed. Cerebellar abnormalities may occur independently or with other defects.

Transverse myelitis occurs in patients with SLE. Paralysis may also develop following intracerebral hemorrhage or thrombosis. Sterile meningitis may be observed. Despite the large variety of lupus-related nervous system problems, bacterial and other non-lupus causes must be sought and treated. In addition, the nonsteroidal anti-inflammatory drugs (NSAID's) used in therapy may induce central nervous system signs or symptoms in patients with SLE.

Kidney Disease. The great majority of patients have some degree of renal involvement. In many, the degree of abnormality is mild enough to escape clinical detection. In others, it is clinically detectable but does not progress to functional impairment. Only a minority of patients have renal involvement that is threatening to the function of the organ. Hypertension and lupus renal involvement synergize in bringing about destructive changes. As a result, the presence of untreated hypertension poses a threat in patients with renal abnormalities.

The renal disease of SLE is of several types: rapidly progressive disease (a subacute glomerulonephritis picture), membranous involvement (usually with some mesangial hypertrophy) with nephrotic syndrome, a nephritic picture (mild to severe), and minimal abnormalities. Most patients have mesangial involvement. The progression to capillary loop pathology carries a worse prognosis. The biopsy features can change from one form to another; as a result, the degree of active disease (e.g., necrosis) and scarring (glomerular hyalinization, interstitial) offers a much more useful measure than do precise histologic classifications. The less scarring, the more there is to treat and preserve. Low-grade activity may be associated with slow progression to renal failure. If renal failure occurs, chronic dialysis and renal transplantation are well tolerated. With modern therapy, most patients avoid renal failure. Complete remissions of renal disease occur.

Menses and Pregnancy. Among outpatients with relatively mild SLE, menstruating women tend to be most symptomatic in the period between ovulation and menses. Menses are frequently irregular during active disease. Bleeding may be increased in patients with antibodies to clotting factors or with thrombocytopenia. Repeated spontaneous abortions are common in some women. Others, especially when in remission, carry to term without difficulty. Patients in remission at the time of conception tend to have relatively normal pregnancies. Advanced cardiac, central nervous system, or renal disease is a contraindication to pregnancy. The risk of a disease flare after induced abortion is the same as after delivery. Patients with active renal disease often experience exacerbation during pregnancy and may develop preeclampsia. Patients without renal involvement tend to have calmer pregnancies, but the disease often flares following delivery or abortion. Increased dosage of corticosteroids during the time of delivery and for several weeks thereafter tends to reduce the likelihood of a disease flare. Babies of mothers with antibodies to SS-A may have congenital cardiac problems, including heart block.

LABORATORY FINDINGS. Specific tests for SLE are not available. The presence of large amounts of antibodies to native DNA is the single most useful diagnostic laboratory finding. The LE cell consists of a nucleus that has been phagocytized. The phagocytosis requires antibodies reactive with DNA-histone and complement. In patients with extremely low complement, LE material that has not been phagocytized may be noted. About 80 per cent of patients with SLE are positive for LE cells. A small percentage of patients with related disorders are also positive: rheumatoid arthritis, especially with Felty's syndrome; Sjögren's syndrome; polymyositis-dermatomyositis. The fluorescent antinuclear antibody test (FANA or ANA) has been used as a screening test; however, many patients with related and unrelated diseases may also have positive tests. It is now possible to measure antibodies specifically reactive with various antigens (native DNA, Sm, various low molecular weight RNA species, SS-A, SS-B, and so on). These are much more informative than the FANA despite the improvement in usefulness of the FANA by virtue of analysis of patterns of staining.

Most patients with active SLE have impaired skin tests. Especially important is the common failure to respond to tuberculin in inactive patients as well.

Hematologic. Anemia usually is present in patients with active disease. Although leukopenia occurs in half of the patients, others may manifest leukocytosis. Corticosteroids may increase the white count. Infection in patients with SLE is to be suspected if there is an increase in percentages of granulocytes or immature granulocytes or both, even in the absence of leukocytosis. Thrombocytopenia may precede other features of SLE. Antibodies to coagulation factors may be measured in coagulation abnormalities. Antibodies to phospholipids, which prolong the PTT, do not cause bleeding. A false-positive serologic test for syphilis is also observed in 15 per cent of patients.

Immune. The erythrocyte sedimentation rate (ESR) is usually but not invariably elevated in patients with active disease. Serum albumin levels are usually near normal except in patients with renal disease. Hypergammaglobulinemia may be marked in an untreated patient. Cryoglobulins may be increased. Rheumatoid factor occurs in low titer in patients with SLE. Reduced hemolytic complement levels (CH_{50}) are common in active disease, especially with renal involvement. Some patients have specific congenital complement deficiencies. Immune complexes may be found in the serum or plasma. Antibodies reactive with leukocytes (granulocytes, B cells, T cells) are found in the majority of patients. Platelet-bound immunoglobulin often occurs in the absence of thrombocytopenia, as does a positive Coombs test result in the absence of hemolysis. Antibodies are found that react with DNA, RNA, histones, nuclear ribonucleoprotein, and cytoplasmic antigenic determinants (see Table 261-3). Rarely, antibodies react with heparin (inducing chylomicronemia), insulin receptors (exacerbating difficulties in sugar regulation), and other functional molecules.

Renal. Proteinuria, granular or cellular casts, and cells (red blood cells [RBC], white blood cells [WBC]) are found in the urine of patients with active kidney disease. Elevated serum creatinine levels may be reversible or fixed. Hypertension is common, even in the absence of renal failure. Renal biopsies are best used to determine therapy rather than to confirm the diagnosis.

Cardiac. Abnormal T waves are the most common electrocardiographic abnormality; evidence of coronary artery or hypertensive disease may be noted. Valvular abnormalities and pericardial fluid may be detected with echocardiograms.

Pulmonary. Pleural fluid may be seen on the x-ray film. It is usually an exudate; however, the protein content may not be very high in patients with hypoalbuminemia. The glucose level is usually much higher than that observed in rheumatoid effusions. LE cells may be seen in the fluid. Pleural biopsies can show varying degrees of fibrosis and infiltration. Lung biopsies may show alveolar hemorrhage only, alveolar damage with interstitial edema and hyaline membranes, hypertrophy with or without vasculitis, or acute alveolitis. There is mild to severe hypoxemia. Patients with interstitial fibrosis show decreased vital capacity; others have disproportionately impaired diffusing capacities.

Nervous System. The electroencephalogram most commonly shows diffuse slowing. Seizures often occur in the absence of the typical patterns observed in patients with foci. The cerebrospinal fluid (CSF) may be normal or may have moderately elevated protein levels. The gamma globulin levels usually are not increased. High levels of protein, including high gamma globulins, in the CSF often accompany inflammation of the spinal cord. Granulocytes are indicative of infection; some patients have small numbers of round cells. Aseptic meningitis with numerous lymphocytes in the CSF occurs occasionally. A loss of brain substance may be noted in patients with chronic disease. Isolated loss of cortical or cerebellar neurons occurs.

DIAGNOSIS. SLE should be suspected in any person with a multisystem disease including joint pain. For epidemiologic and study purposes, 4 of the 11 criteria listed in Table 261–1 are required; however, the diagnosis may be made for other purposes with fewer criteria. SLE should be suspected if any of the criteria shown in Table 261–1 are present and unexplained. The disorder should be considered if any of the following are present: unexplained fever, purpura, splenomegaly, adenopathy, pneumonitis, myocarditis, or aseptic meningitis. The presence of a single symptom, such as serositis, along with antibodies to native DNA in a young woman is highly suggestive of SLE.

The condition in children is frequently misdiagnosed as rheumatic fever or juvenile rheumatoid arthritis. The disease in adults is most commonly misdiagnosed as rheumatoid arthritis. Other diagnoses often applied to patients with SLE include Raynaud's disease, hemolytic anemia, idiopathic thrombocytopenia, thrombotic thrombocytopenic purpura, psychosis, vasculitis, progressive systemic sclerosis, lymphoma, autoimmune neutropenia, secondary syphilis, drug reaction, porphyria, multiple sclerosis, myasthenia gravis, polymyositis, glomerulonephritis, Henoch-Schönlein purpura, personality disorder, stroke, and seizure disorder.

In addition to those just listed, other diseases should be considered in patients suspected of having SLE: subacute bacterial endocarditis, bacterial peritonitis, gonococcal septicemia, meningococcal septicemia, tuberculosis, sarcoidosis, serum sickness, leukemia, leprosy, angioimmunoblastic lymphadenopathy, Wegener's granulomatosis, leptospirosis, Lyme arthritis, Rocky Mountain spotted fever, and acquired immunodeficiency syndrome (AIDS).

Overlaps occur between SLE and other diseases such as progressive systemic sclerosis, polymyositis, and Sjögren's syndrome. Some have defined these as "mixed connective tissue disease" or the "overlap syndrome"; others prefer less rigid categorizations.

THERAPY. The management of patients with SLE is often problematic and fraught with difficulties (Table 261–5). The diagnosis of SLE often induces an emotional reaction. In addition, many patients with SLE have psychological problems that may be a result of the disease. Therefore it is necessary to provide effective emotional support. This includes an honest but optimistic assessment. Most patients with SLE can look forward to a normal lifespan, but with the requirement for periodic visits to the physician and treatment with various drugs. Many of the more serious problems do not affect most people. Thus, although the patient must realize the presence of a serious and chronic disease, a dire prognosis usually should not be issued. Early

TABLE 261–5. SOME SUBOPTIMAL PRACTICES FOR PATIENTS WITH SLE

1. All patients*:
   a. Inappropriate view of severity of disease. An excessively pessimistic view that may lead to overtreatment and unnecessary worry on the part of patient and family. On the contrary, an overly optimistic approach may lead to inappropriate reassurance of the patient and inadequate therapy.
   b. Prolonged (>6 weeks) use of high dosages (1 mg/kg/day of prednisone) of daily corticosteroids, which predisposes to toxicities and especially to infections. [If disease becomes controlled, taper dose and move expeditiously to corticosteroid treatment given every other day—aim for 15–20 mg once every 48 hours in the morning. If disease is inadequately controlled, add an antimalarial and/or introduce a cytotoxic drug.]
2. Patients with moderately severe glomerulonephritis:
   a. Treat with daily corticosteroids, and if proteinuria and nephritic sediment persist add azathioprine. [In many individuals this approach may be more likely to lead to renal failure than if the initial therapy were more vigorous.]
   b. Treat a second renal flare with corticosteroids because there was benefit the first time. [The flare usually is more difficult to treat than the initial nephritis.]
   c. Treat either initial disease or a flare with daily corticosteroids, and if the serum creatinine level rises to approximately 2.5 mg/dl give intravenous cyclophosphamide. [It would be desirable to begin cyclophosphamide much earlier. The better the renal function at the initiation of cyclophosphamide therapy, the higher the probability of preventing renal failure.]
   d. Failure to maintain blood pressure control. [Hypertension and nephritis synergize in causing loss of renal function. A blood pressure kept in the middle of the normal range (110–120/70–80 mm Hg) is not as likely to allow progression to renal failure as is one of 140–155/90–100 mm Hg.]
3. Patients with central nervous system involvement:
   a. Failure to distinguish different central nervous system (CNS) syndromes. [Antiphospholipid syndrome with thrombosis may need primarily anticoagulation rather than strong immunosuppression. Guillain-Barré syndrome in a patient with SLE may be due to vasculitis and may require vigorous therapy.]
   b. Failure to utilize diagnostic approaches. [Infection must be ruled out. Magnetic resonance imaging (MRI) and computed tomographic (CT) scan may suggest particular pathologies. A high CSF protein in the absence of infection should suggest vigorous (bolus cyclophosphamide) therapy.]
   c. Use of prolonged high-dose corticosteroid therapy. [This is associated with increased morbidity and mortality because of infections.]
   d. Failure to use intravenous cyclophosphamide early enough. [For many patients with CNS inflammation secondary to SLE, this therapy can be very rapidly effective.]
   e. Inadequate adjunctive therapy. [Repetitive or continuous seizure activity due to SLE may require, on an acute basis, intravenous corticosteroids in addition to anticonvulsant for control. Phenothiazines may be needed in patients with psychiatric manifestations of SLE until immunosuppression is effective.]
   f. Failure to appreciate impending transverse myelitis. [A high CSF protein level and high gamma globulin percentage are suggestive. An MRI study of the spinal cord may be quite helpful.]

*Comments are provided in brackets.

involvement in educational programs and with physical therapists, dieticians, and occupational therapists may be helpful.

Patients with SLE usually need more than normal rest. Ten hours of sleep at night plus an afternoon nap would not be inappropriate. The more active the disease, the more rest needed. Ultraviolet light should be avoided: outdoor swimming should be limited to periods of reduced exposure (not at noon to 1:00 PM ± 4 hours), and sunscreen should be used even for trips to the store. Drugs that augment the effects of UV light, such as tetracyclines and psoralens, should be avoided. The same is true of foods containing large amounts of psoralens (celery, parsnips, figs, and parsley). Exercise should be appropriate to the clinical situation, but exhaustion should be avoided. Stresses, including surgery, infections, childbirth, abortions, and psychological pressures, may exacerbate the process and dictate additional treatment.

Although certain drugs can induce a lupus-like syndrome,

there is little evidence that those drugs are detrimental to patients with SLE. Therefore, such drugs as alpha-methyldopa and phenytoin (Dilantin) may be used without undue concern. However, sulfonamides are often poorly tolerated; patients with active disease often experience a rash. Estrogens may worsen disease. Since hypertension is synergistic with immune complex disease in bringing about pathology, the blood pressure should be kept in the middle of the normal range for age and sex.

Corticosteroids are frequently given. Short-acting drugs such as prednisone or methylprednisolone are preferred so that therapy every other day can be attempted (see Ch. 27) and the hypothalamic-pituitary-adrenal axis not disrupted. The side effects of steroids given every other day are much less than those of daily therapy. Low doses are less than 30 mg per 1.7 square meters per day of prednisone, and every attempt should be made to maintain patients on less than 25 mg per 1.7 square meters every other day. Moderate doses are 30 to 50 mg per 1.7 square meters per day. Higher doses may be necessary for brief periods. Patients with marked multisystem involvement may temporarily require corticosteroids in divided doses. Azathioprine has long been used to treat patients with SLE; its usefulness may be limited to a subset of patients with moderate kidney disease or those with intractable skin disease or arthritis. Vigorous therapy includes boluses of very large doses of corticosteroids (1 gram or more of methylprednisolone) or of cyclophosphamide (0.85 to 2.0 grams per 1.7 square meters) and plasmapheresis.

A major problem in SLE is long-term management. The clinical picture (history plus physical examination) is usually a very good guide to therapy of nonrenal and nonhematologic problems. In the latter two situations, the laboratory measures are helpful. Anemia, fatigue, and hypergammaglobulinemia tend to weigh in favor of more therapy. The long-term toxicities of corticosteroids (cataracts, aseptic necrosis of bone, infections) must always be balanced against the benefits of continued vigorous therapy. The toxicities of immunosuppressive drugs are less than those of prolonged high-dose corticosteroid therapy. Therefore, it is often prudent to initiate immunosuppressive therapy early for serious disease to minimize the toxicities of corticosteroids. In tapering corticosteroids, it is generally advisable to drop rapidly to 30 mg per 1.7 square meters per day and then to reduce dosage more slowly. The lower the dose, the slower the tapering process should be. Rapid tapering can cause a disease flare, which requires re-institution of high doses.

The variable severity and extent of involvement in SLE dictate individualized treatment. It is helpful to divide problems into those of major organs, which therefore are life threatening, and those that are unpleasant but not life threatening (Table 261–6). The major exception to this division is a syndrome of acute toxic

lupus observed primarily in precorticosteroid times: A young woman with high fever, serositis, rash, and arthritis might succumb to SLE in the absence of major organ involvement. This syndrome is usually responsive to therapy with corticosteroids in modest doses.

Non–major organ involvements are best handled with symptomatic therapy: the less medicine the better. Hydroxychloroquine (200 to 600 mg per day) is effective for skin involvement; it also may help treat arthritis and other manifestations. Nonsteroidal anti-inflammatory drugs, such as aspirin and ibuprofen, are useful for arthritis, serositis, and fever. Some patients tolerate one NSAID better than another—bizarre neurologic reactions may occur in SLE patients receiving ibuprofen or other NSAID's; liver enzyme abnormalities may follow aspirin treatment; gastrointestinal tolerance varies. The combination of hydroxychloroquine and NSAID may be sufficient. The addition of low doses of corticosteroids may be necessary. Initial therapy given every other day may not be possible; however, a subsequent switch to alternate-day treatment reduces steroid-induced side effects. In patients with continued disease activity, symptoms may be prominent every other day, necessitating return to daily steroids. Even in the face of corticosteroid therapy, a NSAID and hydroxychloroquine may add substantial benefit and allow a lower steroid dosage. Fevers occurring in spite of daily corticosteroids may respond to NSAID's. Indomethacin may be especially effective in pericarditis.

The management of major organ involvement is usually directed at preservation of function and prevention of organ failure and disability or death. Myocarditis usually responds to the symptomatic treatment of SLE, but occasional patients may require specific treatment; moderate doses of corticosteroids are usually adequate. Thrombocytopenia and hemolytic anemia are treated more or less as they are in the absence of SLE. Both danazol and intravenous gamma globulin have been given for thrombocytopenia in SLE patients. Administration of plasma or plasma exchange may be helpful in patients with features of thrombotic thrombocytopenia (one should look for fragmented RBC's on the peripheral smear). Patients with Factor VIII deficiency caused by specific antibodies are treated with plasmapheresis and immunosuppression. Mild pneumonitis usually responds to moderate doses of corticosteroids; severe disease requires heroic measures. Central nervous system inflammation may require moderate to high corticosteroid dosages; however, since prolonged therapy with high doses of corticosteroids is inappropriate, a switch to cytotoxic therapy should be considered within 2 weeks. In patients with severe involvement, intravenous cyclophosphamide* (0.85 to 2.0 grams per 1.7 square meters) can be life saving. Seizures require treatment with both corticosteroids and anticonvulsants (Table 261–5). The antiphospholipid antibody syndrome is treated with long-term anticoagulation. Warfarin therapy may be effective with minimal toxicity by keeping the prothrombin time at about 15 seconds.

The most studied and controversial area is the treatment of SLE kidney disease. If there is active disease on biopsy and no scarring, high-dose corticosteroids or corticosteroids plus an oral immunosuppressive drug (e.g., azathioprine*) may be sufficient. If there is active disease and any scarring, vigorous therapy must be considered. The currently available data suggest that renal function can be preserved for long periods with cyclophosphamide therapy. Intermittent boluses are safer than daily oral therapy. Despite substantial loss of renal function, a patient with quiescent disease and moderate scarring usually does not benefit from aggressive and potentially toxic therapy (see Table 261–5).

TABLE 261–6. MAJOR VERSUS NON–MAJOR ORGAN INVOLVEMENT IN SLE

Non–Major Organ SLE*	Major Organ SLE†
Alopecia	Glomerulonephritis
Fever	Central nervous system disease
Fatigue	Myocarditis
Anorexia	Pneumonitis
Arthritis	Thrombocytopenic purpura
Myalgia	Hemolytic anemia (marked)
Pleurisy	Severe granulocytopenia (rare)
Pericarditis	Mesenteric vasculitis
Peritonitis	
Rash	
Skin vasculitis	
Raynaud's phenomenon	
Mucosal ulcers	
Splenomegaly	
Lymphadenopathy	
Peripheral neuropathy	
Episcleritis	
Hepatitis	

*Usually does not require high-dose corticosteroids or other vigorous treatment. In all cases, a careful search for infection is carried out.
†Usually requires high-dose corticosteroids or other vigorous treatment. Individual patients vary greatly and some do not require vigorous therapy. Since prolonged high-dose corticosteroid therapy is very toxic, consideration should be given to immunosuppressive drug therapy.

Alarcon-Segovia D: Anti-phospholipid antibodies and the antiphospholipid syndrome in systemic lupus erythematosus. Medicine 68:353, 1989.
Balow JE: Lupus nephritis. Ann Intern Med 106:79, 1987. A symposium devoted to pathogenesis and therapy.
Boey ML (ed.): Proceedings of the Second International Conference on Systemic Lupus Erythematosus, November 26–30, 1989. Singapore, Professional Postgraduate Services International, 1989. Up-to-date coverage of pathogenesis and patient management.
DuBois EL: Lupus Erythematosus. Los Angeles, University of Southern California

*This use is not listed in the manufacturer's directive.

Press, 1978. *A lengthy monograph citing many case reports. Extensively referenced.*

Harris EN, Asherson RA, Hughes GRV: Antiphospholipid antibodies—autoantibodies with a difference. Annu Rev Med 39:261, 1988.

Ropes MW: Systemic Lupus Erythematosus. Cambridge, Mass., Harvard University Press, 1976. *Observations of a physician with over 40 years' experience with SLE patients.*

Sibbitt WL Jr: Magnetic resonance and computed tomographic imaging in the evaluation of acute neuropsychiatric disease in systemic lupus erythematosus. Ann Rheum Dis 48:1014, 1989.

Smith HR, Steinberg AD: Autoimmunity—a perspective. Annu Rev Immunol 1:175, 1983. *Discussion of theoretical aspects of autoimmune diseases as well as their classification and pathogeneses.*

Steinberg AD: Therapy of lupus nephritis. Kidney Int 30:769, 1986. *A completely referenced discussion and thorough analysis of difficult problems.*

262 Systemic Sclerosis (Scleroderma)

E. Carwile LeRoy

Scleroderma (hard skin) is an uncommon disease marked by fibrotic increases in the connective tissue of skin and often of visceral organs as well. It varies widely in extent and severity from isolated hardened skin patches of largely cosmetic importance to a life-threatening, generalized condition that can restrict movement "by an ever-tightening case of steel" (Osler) and lead to insufficiency of the peripheral circulation, the lungs, the gut, the heart, and/or the kidneys. Fortunately, most persons with scleroderma are not at risk for the most severe of its consequences. Since the cause is unknown and no cure is available, the physician must distinguish as early as possible the attendant risks for each patient and manage these prospectively.

Distinctions between localized (skin only) and generalized scleroderma and the conditions that mimic each are shown in Table 262–1. Subsets of generalized scleroderma (systemic sclerosis, SSc) are outlined in Table 262–2. It is on occasion difficult to classify the individual patient in this multisystem, multistage disorder in which each target organ independently progresses through stages of inflammation, induration (fibrosis), and atrophy.

DEFINITION. Systemic sclerosis (SSc) is a generalized disorder of small arteries, microvessels, and the diffuse connective tissue characterized by scarring (fibrosis) and vascular obliteration in the skin, gastrointestinal tract, lungs, heart, and kidneys; hidebound skin is the clinical hallmark and organ compromise the prognostic keystone.

PATHOGENESIS AND PATHOLOGY. The mechanism or mechanisms of fibrosis in SSc is not understood. Mesenchymal cells (fibroblasts, smooth muscle cells, and endothelial cells) become activated by unknown stimuli, resulting in the deposition of increased amounts of the usual components of connective tissue (types I and III collagen, proteoglycan, fibronectin) in the interstitium and in the intima of small arteries. Endothelial cell changes, vasomotor and permeability changes, platelet activation, and perivascular mononuclear cell infiltrates are present in target tissues before fibrosis is prominent.

In SSc scar tissue, lesional fibroblasts produce increased quantities of these connective tissue components on a per cell basis even after removal from the patient and propagation in vitro. These same cells show a growth regulatory abnormality characterized by insensitive responses to growth factors and a persistent state of competence (the state of a cell prepared to divide but not yet triggered to proceed), something of a persistently activated state. Interactions, both autocrine (a factor acting on the cell that produced it) and paracrine (a factor acting on an adjacent cell), between two cytokines, transforming growth factor–beta and platelet-derived growth factor, may begin to explain the state of fibroblast activation in SSc. Gene expression in these cells is unusual and as yet incompletely characterized. Understanding the regulatory defect of fibroblast growth may be a key to understanding the unregulated fibrosis in SSc, and perhaps also

TABLE 262–1. DIFFERENTIAL DIAGNOSIS OF SYSTEMIC SCLEROSIS

Vascular Changes
Peripheral vasospasm
  Idiopathic Raynaud's phenomenon (Raynaud's disease)
  Occupational Raynaud's phenomenon
    Vibration and physical trauma (e.g., jackhammer operator)
  Chemical exposure
    Vinyl chloride (plastics industry)
    Mining exposure (coal, silicates, gold, heavy metals)
    Organic solvents (trichloroethylene, others)
  Environmental and drug-associated Raynaud's phenomenon
    Toxic oil syndrome
    Arsenic
    Bleomycin
    Cisplatin
    Ergotamine
    Beta blockers (high dose)
    5-Hydroxytryptophan and carbidopa
  Reflex sympathetic dystrophy (shoulder-hand, thoracic outlet)
  Other diffuse connective tissue diseases (systemic lupus erythematosus, polyarteritis nodosa, dermatomyositis/polymyositis)
  Intravascular causes (cryoglobulinemia, cold agglutinins, nondistensible RBC's, intravascular coagulation)
  Telangiectasia
    Hereditary telangiectasia (Osler-Weber-Rendu syndrome)
    Hepatic and hormonal spiders (cirrhosis, contraceptives)

Skin Changes
Localized scleroderma
  Morphea (circumscribed, guttate)
  Generalized morphea
  Linear (with hemiatrophy)
  Other localized hamartomas (collagenoma, tuberous sclerosis, keloids, hypertrophic scars)
  En coup de sabre (with or without facial hemiatrophy)
  Tryptophan-eosinophilia-myalgia-fasciitis syndrome
Scleroderma-like skin changes
  Inflammatory-immunologic
    Undifferentiated connective tissue syndromes (mixed)
    Eosinophilic fasciitis
    Overlap syndromes (SSc with SLE, RA, DM/PM, Sjögren's syndrome [sicca complex and its overlaps])
    Chronic graft-vs.-host disease (CGVHD)
  Occupational, environmental, and drug-associated (see Vascular Changes above)
  Metabolic-genetic (pseudosclerodermas)
    Porphyrias
    Phenylketonuria
    Carcinoid syndrome
    Scleredema with or without paraproteinemia
    Scleromyxedema with or without paraproteinemia
    Lichen sclerosus et atrophicus
    Insulin-dependent diabetes mellitus (digital sclerosis)
    Acromegaly
    Amyloidosis
    Heritable premature aging syndromes (Werner's syndrome, progeria, Rothmund's syndrome)

Visceral Disease
Esophageal hypomotility (diabetes mellitus, aging)
Idiopathic pulmonary fibrosis
Sarcoidosis
Amyloidosis
Infiltrative cardiomyopathies
Intestinal hypomotility syndromes
Malignant hypertension (hyperreninemic, accelerated)
Occupational, environmental, and drug-associated interstitial pulmonary disease (see Vascular Changes above)

RBC's = red blood cells; SLE = systemic lupus erythematosus; RA = rheumatoid arthritis; DM = dermatomyositis; PM = polymyositis.

in liver cirrhosis, atherosclerosis, and other examples of unregulated fibrosis.

Prominent vascular and microvascular lesions dominate the early stages of both limited cutaneous and diffuse forms of SSc (Table 262–2). The unusual cyclic vasoconstrictive-vasodilatory features of Raynaud's phenomenon are present in more than 90 per cent of all SSc patients (Table 262–3). Edema is prominent,

TABLE 262–2. SUBSETS OF SYSTEMIC SCLEROSIS (SSc)

Diffuse Cutaneous SSc (dSSc)

Onset of Raynaud's phenomenon within 1 year of onset of skin changes (puffy or hidebound)

Truncal and acral skin involvement

Presence of tendon friction rubs

Early and significant incidence of interstitial lung disease, oliguric renal failure, diffuse gastrointestinal disease, and myocardial involvement

Absence of anticentromere antibodies (ACA)

Presence of anti-topoisomerase I antibodies (variable)

Nailfold capillary dilatation and dropout

Limited Cutaneous SSc (lSSc)*

Isolated Raynaud's phenomenon for years (occasionally decades)

Skin involvement limited to hands, face, feet (acral)

A significant late incidence of pulmonary hypertension, trigeminal neuralgia, skin calcifications, telangiectasia

A high incidence of anticentromere antibodies (ACA, 70–80%)

Dilated nailfold capillary loops without capillary dropout

Systemic Sclerosis *sine* Scleroderma (ssSSc)

Visceral disease without cutaneous involvement

Examples: (1) esophageal hypomotility, duodenal dilatation with malabsorption, wide-mouthed colonic sacculations; (2) Raynaud's phenomenon, dilated nailfold capillary loops, esophageal hypomotility, oliguric renal failure; and (3) Raynaud's phenomenon, dilated nailfold capillary loops, esophageal hypomotility, pulmonary hypertension, and/or interstitial lung disease

*Also termed CREST syndrome, i.e., calcinosis, Raynaud's phenomenon, esophageal hypomotility, sclerodactyly, and telangiectasia.

often occurring episodically, especially in the diffusely involved patient. Circulating evidence of endothelial cell perturbation (elevated plasma levels of Factor VIII–von Willebrand factor) and of platelet activation (elevated serum levels of factors released from platelet alpha-granules) is present in many, but not all, patients. Histologically, vascular lesions are widespread. The small artery lesion in SSc, similar to the lesions seen in chronic homograft rejection, in hemolytic-uremic syndrome, and in thrombotic thrombocytopenic purpura, has three major characteristics: (1) intimal proliferation with smooth muscle cell migration occurring centripetally and the deposition of a mixed mucoid and fibrous connective tissue matrix, (2) medial thinning, and (3) an adventitial cuff of primarily type I collagen, a virtually unique characteristic of the SSc lesion. Cellular proliferation and matrix deposition are prominent in the small arteries of all target organs; when renal involvement, hyperreninemia, and hypertension characterize the clinical course, fibrinoid necrosis is also present. In the nutrient microvascular beds, capillaries are sparse (up to 70 per cent absent), their endothelium is swollen and disrupted, and endothelial basement membranes may be frayed and separated from their cell attachment. Although the endothelial cells bear the brunt of the injury pattern, the basis of this all-out attack on vascular structures in SSc is not known.

Selected immune events point also to the vascular structures. Three of the five defined antigens to which SSc patients show enhanced immune responsiveness are type I collagen, type IV collagen, and laminin (the other two being topoisomerase I and centromere protein), all three components of blood vessels and the second and third being specific for basal lamina, of which the endothelial basement membrane is a prototype. It is possible that a heightened immune response to basement membrane antigens perpetuates the disease in certain immunogenetically selected persons. As in the other rheumatic or diffuse connective tissue disorders that show manifestations of autoimmunity, anti-

nuclear antibodies are prominent in SSc. With the recent introduction of rapidly proliferating human cell substrates (particularly the human laryngeal carcinoma cell line, HEp-2), greater than 90 per cent of SSc patients have circulating antinuclear antibodies in significant titer. The most sensitive and specific of these is the anticentromere antibody (ACA) pattern, a B cell immune response to a major organizing structure of the chromosome called the centromere. ACA patterns are clinically useful in detecting the limited cutaneous type of SSc. Antibodies to a soluble nuclear isomerase, topoisomerase I, are currently emerging as the newest autoimmune serologic "find" in SSc; both clinical and biologic relevance remains to be determined. Recent studies have demonstrated T cell activation in SSC. The data have been interpreted both as increased T helper function and as decreased T suppressor function. One must remember that circulating differences (increases) may indicate reciprocal changes (decreases) in vascular and interstitial lesions. Thus, a T cell component in SSc seems likely; its cause, possibly viral or chemical, remains unclear.

THE PATIENT. *Diffuse SSc.* The usual age of onset is the fourth decade but may range from the first to the eighth. There is no racial or geographic predilection. There are almost as many men as there are women, in contrast to the female preponderance in limited SSc. The onset may be abrupt and may present as swollen hands, face, and feet associated with Raynaud's phenomenon (episodic pallor of the digits, nose, or ears following cold exposure or stress associated with cyanosis and followed by erythema, suffusion, tingling, and pain). Fatigue is common; overt weakness may be present. The skin reveals a nonpitting fullness, an inability to pinch skin folds, and the loss of skin lines and creases in involved areas. These changes may evolve over 12 to 18 months to include the fingers, hands, forearms, arms, face, thorax, and abdomen, as well as the toes, feet, legs, and thighs. The fingers and toes may be dusky or overtly cyanotic and are usually cool to the touch. Blood pressure and pulse may be elevated, and evaluation of swallowing, breathing, urinary excretory, and cardiac functions may reveal abnormalities. Patients with diffuse SSc should be followed closely for visceral involvement (see Table 262–2 and Fig. 262–1). The cumulative survival rate is reduced in diffuse SSc compared with limited SSc (Fig. 262–2).

Limited Cutaneous SSc. The typical patient with limited cutaneous SSc is a female (or a male who has worked with vibrating machines or plastics or in mining), aged 30 to 50, who presents with a 10- to 15-year history of numbness and a "dead" or "wooden" sensation associated with color changes (often pallor only) of, at first, the second and third fingers of the dominant hand. Full-fledged Raynaud's phenomenon usually develops symmetrically in both hands, fingers 2 through 5, with increasing

TABLE 262–3. RAYNAUD'S PHENOMENON IN MUSCULOSKELETAL DISEASE*

Systemic sclerosis	>90%
Overlap, mixed, undifferentiated	80%
Systemic lupus erythematosus	30%
Dermatomyositis, polymyositis	20%
Rheumatoid arthritis	10%

*From Black CM: Scleroderma, dermatomyositis, and polymyositis. *In* Dieppe PA, et al.: Atlas of Clinical Rheumatology. Philadelphia, Lea and Febiger, 1986; with permission.

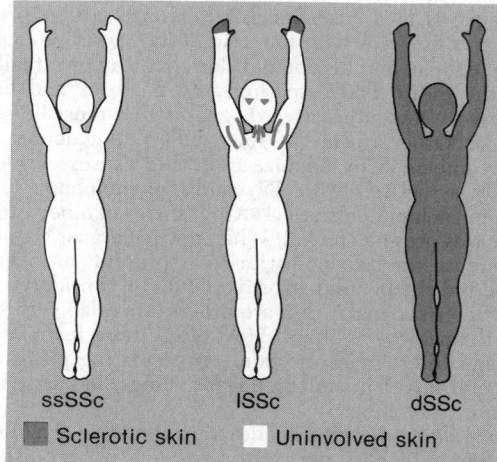

ssSSc	lSSc	dSSc

■ Sclerotic skin □ Uninvolved skin

FIGURE 262–1. A pictorial representation of skin involvement in systemic sclerosis. Note that the limited cutaneous SSc patient (Table 262–2) may have subtle thickening of eyelid, neck fold, and armpit skin. Abbreviations: ssSSc = systemic sclerosis *sine* scleroderma; lSSc = limited cutaneous systemic sclerosis; dSSc = diffuse cutaneous systemic sclerosis. (Adapted from Giordano M, et al.: J Rheumatol 13:911, 1986.)

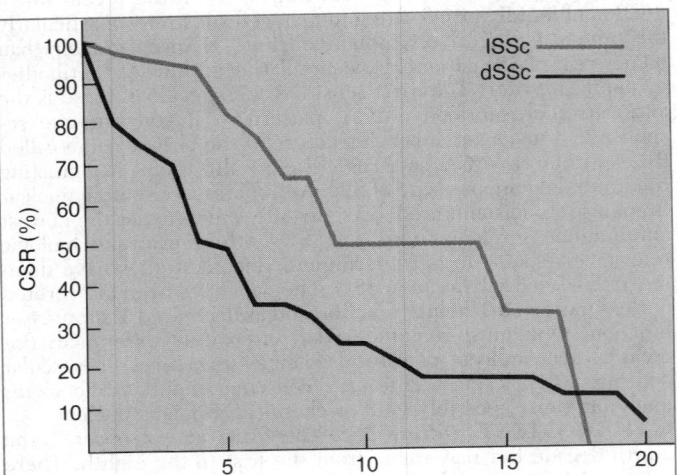

FIGURE 262-2. The cumulative survival rate (CSR, age-adjusted survival) in per cent plotted against time in years for diffuse cutaneous SSc and limited cutaneous SSc (CREST [calcinosis, Raynaud's phenomenon, esophageal dysmotility, sclerodactyly, and telangiectasia] syndrome) patients, showing the substantially reduced survival of diffuse cutaneous SSc patients (Table 262-2). An intermediate group with both intermediate survival and extent of skin involvement has been identified by Giordano et al. Some investigators feel that the intermediate group is not a clearly definable subset as yet. For abbreviations, see Figure 262-1. (Adapted from Giordano M, et al.: J Rheumatol 13:911, 1986.)

frequency, especially in winter; there may be a history of hard, crusting lesions on the fingertips, initially healing in warm weather. General stamina may be decreased, and there may be breathlessness with minimal exertion (see Table 262-2).

DIAGNOSIS. The annual incidence of Raynaud's phenomenon is substantially greater than the incidence of all diffuse connective tissue syndromes combined (Table 262-4). To select those patients with Raynaud's phenomenon who are destined to develop scleroderma and related disorders when a careful history and physical examination reveal no features of connective tissue disease, including no signs of peripheral ischemia, the single best test is wide-field nailfold capillaroscopy—a noninvasive, reproducible, cost-effective, permanent identification of the connective tissue disease–prone patient. Coupled with autoimmune serology and possibly a test of vascular injury or platelet activation/release (such as plasma Factor VIII–von Willebrand factor levels), capillary examination is an important procedure in the early detection of connective tissue disease.

The diagnosis of diffuse SSc is straightforward. A previously well person is now sick with the triad of Raynaud's phenomenon, nonpitting edema, and hidebound skin that may eventually cover virtually the entire body, sparing only the back and buttocks. There are very few alternative diagnoses that must be seriously entertained. Other causes of Raynaud's phenomenon are not usually accompanied by edema, and other causes of edema are not usually associated with Raynaud's phenomenon. The key questions in such patients are (1) Are features of other connective tissue diseases present? and (2) What internal organs are affected?

If symmetric, erosive polyarthritis is present, an overlap between SSc and rheumatoid arthritis should be considered; if fever and a characteristic malar rash are present, overlap with systemic lupus erythematosus is likely. Most often these features are not present, and the second question represents the primary focus. Each visceral target organ (esophagus, lungs, kidneys, heart) of SSc deserves screening.

Abnormal skin texture provides the definitive diagnostic criterion of SSc in over 90 per cent of patients. When distal to the metacarpophalangeal (MCP) joints only, it is called sclerodactyly and is *not* diagnostic of SSc. Firm, taut, hidebound skin proximal to the MCP joints represents the major diagnostic criterion. Skin biopsy is usually *not* more sensitive diagnostically than the experienced touch. Skin changes also distinguish the two prognostically different subsets. If truncal skin changes are present,

TABLE 262-4. POPULATION INCIDENCE OF MUSCULOSKELETAL DISEASE*	
Raynaud's phenomenon	1000†
Rheumatoid arthritis	750
Systemic lupus erythematosus	75
Dermatomyositis, polymyositis	10
Systemic sclerosis	10

*Data from Kammer G: Raynaud's phenomenon. *In* Andreoli TE, et al.: Cecil Essentials of Medicine. Philadelphia, W. B. Saunders Company, 1986; with permission.
†New cases per million adults per year.

the patient has diffuse cutaneous SSc, and close surveillance of visceral function is indicated. If skin changes are limited to the hands, fingers, and face, limited cutaneous SSc is present, yearly evaluation is adequate, and management should focus on the Raynaud's phenomenon. If the skin is of normal texture, two possibilities are suggested: The patient formerly had abnormal skin changes—either diffuse or limited cutaneous—which have subsided; or the patient has visceral disease in the absence of skin changes, which occurs in at least 5 per cent of SSc patients (Table 262-2, SSc *sine* scleroderma).

DIFFERENTIAL DIAGNOSIS. Connective tissue disorders are constellations of organ system involvements (skin, lungs, intestinal tract, serosal surfaces, joints, skeletal muscle, heart, central nervous system); each system involved can show immune-inflammatory, proliferative, or fibrotic-atrophic changes at different stages of the disorder. Virtually none of the systems involved or the stages of involvement of those systems are entirely specific for the particular syndrome or disorder. It is not surprising, therefore, that the nomenclature is confusing. Terms such as mixed connective tissue disease (MCTD), undifferentiated connective tissue syndromes (UCTS), and overlap syndromes have emerged to describe the same patients.

MCTD was introduced to describe anew the already well-known overlap patient with features of myositis, lupus, and scleroderma. The early features of such patients were largely inflammatory and therefore briefly responsive to glucocorticoid therapy; proliferative and fibrotic features were not responsive to treatment. Neither the clinical syndromes, the laboratory tests proposed (extractable nuclear antigen [ENA], antibodies to ribonucleoprotein [RNP]), nor the response to therapy was specific. Therefore, the introduction of MCTD provided no new understanding beyond the time-honored overlap syndrome, which remains the preferred term for established, stable connective tissue disorders with features of more than one traditional disorder (such as rheumatoid arthritis–lupus overlap). In the early patient with inflammatory or edematous features that are insufficient for an established diagnosis, the term undifferentiated connective tissue syndrome (UCTS) is preferred. Some use UCTD here as a hybrid acronym.

Eosinophilic fasciitis is a syndrome that, when acute, is distinct from scleroderma and that blends into the scleroderma spectrum of disorders in its chronic form. Young, vigorous persons note, often after strenuous exertion, the onset of swelling and tautness of the skin of the trunk and proximal extremities with a brawny texture that may be tender. Raynaud's phenomenon is usually absent, and the hands and feet are usually spared. Initially, visceral disease is absent. Deep skin and subcutaneous biopsies show inflammatory changes including the deep fascia, the subcutis, and the dermis. Eosinophilia is present and eosinophils may or may not be present in the skin lesions. Symptoms subside with glucocorticoid therapy and also with no therapy over time. Eosinophilic fasciitis has been associated with aplastic anemia. In a substantial proportion of chronic patients, the visceral involvement of systemic sclerosis has been documented. Several outbreaks of fasciitis-like syndromes, with the added feature of peripheral neuropathy, have recently been documented: the toxic oil syndrome of Spain in 1981–1982 and the L-tryptophan–eosinophilia–myalgia–fasciitis syndrome in the United States in 1989–1990. These events increase the interest in and need for surveillance of environmental triggers in SSc.

CLINICAL MANIFESTATIONS. Peripheral Vascular System. Pallor is the most definitive of the triphasic responses of Raynaud's phenomenon. In the presence of constant or episodic cyanosis alone, the diagnosis should be suspect. The circumstances that provoke pallor and the "dead" sensation of the fingers are usually reproducible in the individual patient (handling cold or frozen items, emotional disturbances). Persistent Raynaud's attacks may lead to a webbing phenomenon (like the frenulum of the tongue) binding the fingernail to the fingertip skin of involved fingers. This is evidence of structural vascular and persistent ischemic disease, as are the more obvious fingertip calluses, digital ulcerations (of fingertips or over dorsal proximal interphalangeal joints), overt ischemic tissue, or calcification; the toes, the nose, and the ears may be affected in Raynaud's attacks as well. The more widespread the areas involved, the more likely is systemic disease.

The Skin. The skin is the most distinctive diagnostic feature of SSc; the diagnosis can be made unequivocally by the texture and location of hidebound skin. In patients with diffuse SSc, skin tautness can limit movement at the wrists, elbows, shoulders, mouth, and thorax (less frequently the hips, knees, and ankles). When fully hidebound, the skin appears to become paper thin over points of bony protrusion, such as the proximal interphalangeal joints, the ulnar styloid process, the olecranon process, the bridge of the nose, and the cheekbones. Gentle pressure over these areas removes all blood from the capillaries; the refilling time can be used as a rough approximation of the degree of ischemia and the propensity to ulcerate.

Gastrointestinal System. If sensitive diagnostic techniques are used, esophageal hypomotility, by far the most common manifestation of gastrointestinal SSc, can be documented in over 90 per cent of patients with both diffuse and limited cutaneous SSc. Many patients do not notice the subtle symptoms of esophageal SSc, which include a vertical substernal burning pain particularly at night, the occasional sense that a pill or large bit of meat "has not gone all the way down," or "heartburn" on lying down soon after a full meal. The single best screening test for esophageal hypomotility is the radionuclide esophageal transit time; it is noninvasive, is safe, and can be relied upon when negative. Because severe esophageal complications, including stricture, can be prevented by early management and because intestinal involvement with SSc does not occur without esophageal involvement, the esophagus of all patients suspected of SSc should be examined for hypomotility. Patients with slow transit times should be further studied both with barium swallow (using light barium and the recumbent position) to detect structural abnormalities (hiatus hernia) and with esophageal motility studies, the definitive procedure for esophageal SSc. The earliest detectable abnormality is a reduction in resting lower esophageal sphincter (LES) pressure, which may be an isolated early finding or may be associated with reduced smooth muscle contraction (secondary and tertiary waves) of the distal two thirds of the esophagus. Upper third, striated muscle dysfunction suggests an overlap syndrome with dermatomyositis. If peptic esophagitis with mucosal ulceration is well established, LES pressure may be increased and the diagnosis of achalasia could be incorrectly entertained. The presence of other features of SSc and reduced LES pressure after treatment are helpful in diagnosis.

Gastric hypomotility may be present but is not often of clinical significance. Small intestinal hypomotility, determined by an upper gastrointestinal (GI) series with small bowel follow-through, occurs in 10 to 20 per cent of patients, all of whom have esophageal hypomotility; this diffuse hypomotility may occur in the absence of cutaneous scleroderma. It need not be searched for in the asymptomatic patient because it consistently declares its presence by postprandial bloating, abdominal distention with diffuse pain, intermittent diarrhea with or without steatorrhea, and weight loss from malabsorption. Abdominal attacks with adynamic ileus may mimic mechanical obstruction and lead to surgical intervention, from which some patients recover poorly and slowly, if at all.

Pulmonary System. Although renal failure was formerly the major threat to life in SSc, the combined impact of several pulmonary abnormalities now seems to be the number one cause of fatal involvement in this disease. Pleurisy and pleural effusions, pulmonary hypertension, interstitial lung disease with fibrosis, and ultimately restrictive pulmonary disease all may be a part of pulmonary SSc. Because the patient is often sedentary from skin or joint restrictions, shortness of breath or dyspnea on exertion is a surprisingly late complaint. Standard chest roentgenography is not a sensitive screening procedure. More than half of SSc patients selected for the absence of pulmonary symptoms and for a normal chest radiograph show reproducible abnormalities on pulmonary function tests. Patients who smoke show a much higher positive proportion. The single-breath diffusion capacity, which measures the balance between ventilation and perfusion, is a sensitive pulmonary screening tool. Mild reductions in vital capacity are common as well. In smokers, there may be evidence of small airway obstruction. The presence of alveolitis, detected by alveolar thickening on thin-section computed tomography (CT) and/or by the presence of inflammatory cells on bronchoalveolar lavage, is predictive of future pulmonary fibrosis and functional insufficiency. Whether therapeutic intervention at the prefibrotic alveolitis stage can prevent pulmonary functional deterioration is currently under study.

Pleural effusions are usually silent and bland. They take on clinical significance primarily in the patient with established restrictive lung disease (decreased vital capacity) in whom the aspiration of an effusion may improve ventilation. They are present in two thirds of patients at postmortem examination. In the immunosuppressed patient, infection may present with "silent" empyema.

Pulmonary hypertension may be sudden in onset and constitutes a medical emergency. All patients with SSc should be followed closely for changes in the second heart sound over the pulmonic area and for the pulmonic valve closure component of that second sound, detected by the splitting of S2 on deep inspiration. The appearance of tricuspid regurgitation or right ventricular enlargement is evidence of established pulmonary hypertension. The chest radiograph may provide evidence of enlarged pulmonary arteries but often does not; the unassisted echocardiogram, while key in detecting cardiac SSc, has been disappointing in detecting pulmonary hypertension. Combined Doppler/echo techniques measuring tricuspid insufficiency (present in most patients with increased right ventricular pressures) are promising in the early detection of pulmonary hypertension. Aggressive attempts to lower pulmonary artery pressure should be instituted (see Ch. 45).

Renal System. At one time, the abrupt onset of accelerated hypertension and oliguria ("scleroderma renal crisis") accounted for the majority of deaths in SSc. Fortunately, with early identification and treatment with inhibitors of angiotensin-converting enzymes (captopril, enalapril, lisinopril), the consequences of renal involvement have been significantly reduced. All patients fulfilling the criteria for diffuse SSc should be suspect for renal involvement and should be followed with 24-hour urine collections for protein excretion and creatinine clearance three to four times a year. Excretion of greater than 750 mg of protein per 24 hours or clearances of less than 60 ml per minute, or distinct changes in either proteinuria or glomerular filtration rate (GFR), should initiate measurements of resting renin levels and, if elevated, treatment. Increases in blood pressure and pulse rate, accelerated increases in edematous skin tightening (rapidly increasing skin score), or the appearance of microangiopathic hemolytic anemia or disseminated intravascular coagulation (see Ch. 155) may also herald the onset of renal involvement.

The sudden appearance of renal SSc when other features of the disease appear more indolent is a characteristic of the kidney's unique ability to autoregulate its own blood flow. The typical small artery lesion of intimal proliferation develops slowly in the kidney of SSc patients, with gradual reduction in renal blood flow, until both renal flow and glomerular flow drop abruptly and renal failure ensues. A rapid acceleration of these changes is associated with the onset of hyperreninemia. It is during this accelerated phase that hypertension, funduscopic vascular changes (hemorrhages and exudates), and microangiopathic hemolytic anemia appear. The key to successful management of renal SSc is to identify the population at risk (those with diffuse SSc), to detect declining GFR early, and to treat expectantly.

One remarkable feature of renal SSc is the ability of some patients to regain renal function after months to years (up to 4 years) of end-stage renal disease and hemodialysis. Very little is known of the mechanisms of this slow reparative process. The aggressive management of renal SSc with captopril and its converting enzyme inhibitor analogues has improved the 1-year survival from 20 per cent to 80 per cent, with current 5-year survival of about 70 per cent, the first dramatic improvement in the natural history of SSc.

Cardiac System. More than 90 per cent of patients with diffuse SSc (truncal skin involvement) have some form of cardiac involvement. Rarely, acute pericarditis with a friction rub is present; more frequently, a silent pericardial effusion appears slowly, with ankle edema and shortness of breath as the presenting features. Echocardiography is the diagnostic procedure of choice. Pericardial effusions may predispose to renal failure by unknown mechanisms. By electrocardiographic monitoring and electrophysiologic studies, 80 per cent of diffuse SSc patients *without* cardiovascular symptoms have evidence of cardiac involvement; in more recent studies, 95 per cent show abnormalities of thallium reperfusion. Intermittent myocardial ischemia with the acute pathologic concomitant of contraction band necrosis seems to precede fibrosis, suggesting that spasm of the intramyocardial vessels plays a role in cardiac SSc. Most, but not all, of these patients have normal coronary arteries by coronary angiography.

Articular and Musculoskeletal System. Approximately 10 per cent of SSc patients present with a symmetric small joint polyarticular synovitis indistinguishable from rheumatoid arthritis. Within a year, the pattern changes abruptly, with subsidence of joint complaints and the appearance of Raynaud's phenomenon, edema, and diffuse cutaneous SSc. The presence of scleroderma-pattern nailfold capillary changes and a positive antinuclear antibody pattern can identify these patients during their polyarticular phase, prior to the development of cutaneous changes, as destined to develop SSc.

About one half of SSc patients develop stiffness and swelling of the fingers, wrists, knees, and ankles, concomitant with cutaneous changes. Morning stiffness may be present. Signs of inflammation are usually mild. Polymorphonuclear leukocytes are usually present in synovial fluid. On biopsy, the synovium is mildly inflamed, with a distinctive deposition of fibrin throughout the synovium. Obliterative microvascular disease and diffuse fibrotic changes occur at a later stage.

Indolent myopathy is common in SSc. It is difficult to distinguish from atrophy caused by taut skin. Most patients show diffuse atrophy of the extremities with slight elevations of muscle enzyme levels (creatine kinase CK and aldolase); these features are refractory to glucocorticoids or to immunosuppressive therapy. Mild myositis of SSc is best left untreated. Less frequently, abrupt proximal muscle weakness develops and is associated with 10- to 50-fold increases in muscle enzymes, electromyographic features of acute myositis, and lymphoid cell infiltration with muscle fiber necrosis on biopsy. These patients generated the initial confusion regarding mixed, overlap, or undifferentiated connective tissue syndromes; they usually respond to glucocorticoid therapy.

Other. In the second and third decades following the onset of Raynaud's phenomenon, a small but significant proportion of patients with limited cutaneous SSc develop unilateral or bilateral trigeminal neuralgia, which can be disabling.

An increasing number of male SSc patients, especially those with diffuse disease, experience impotence after 1 or 2 years of the onset of symptoms. Impotence is thought to have an organic neurovascular cause, because of diminished or absent nocturnal tumescence. It is refractory to treatment.

Dry eyes (keratoconjunctivitis sicca), dry mouth (xerostomia), or both occur in approximately one fourth of SSc patients. Salivary gland biopsies may show mononuclear cell infiltrates or replacement fibrosis. Supportive care with secretion substitution (artificial tears) and stimulation (lemon candy) provides some relief.

TREATMENT. No therapy has been shown to halt the progression of cutaneous or visceral SSc in a controlled, prospective study. A major source of confusion in assessing therapy is the dependence on softening skin as a key outcome measurement and the natural tendency for hidebound skin to soften after several years (dubbed regressive systemic sclerosis). Skin changes should not be taken as indications of the lessening of the vascular and microvascular disease.

The most distinctive change in the natural history of diffuse cutaneous SSc in the past decade has been the reduction in the proportion of patients who develop renal failure. This change has occurred with the advent of more powerful agents to control the accelerated hypertensive phase of renal failure. Indications for immediate treatment are hypertension (an increase of 30 mm Hg systolic or 15 mm Hg diastolic blood pressure, no matter what the absolute level); a reduction in creatinine clearance of 30 ml per minute or to a clearance below 60 ml per minute; and microangiopathic anemia. If the serum creatinine value is less than 4.0 mg per deciliter, the crisis of renal scleroderma can often, but not always, be averted. Continued intensive treatment is indicated even if hemodialysis is instituted, since some patients can regain function sufficient to obviate dialysis after as long as 4 to 5 years.

D-Penicillamine* has been strongly advocated on the basis of retrospective studies that showed skin softening after 2 years. The proportion of patients who develop significant side effects is 30 to 40 per cent. It is a difficult drug to tolerate. Colchicine* has also been proposed as being capable of influencing cutaneous changes in SSc. Brief crossover studies were inconclusive, and longer open studies were promising but uncontrolled. Colchicine is better tolerated than D-penicillamine.

Glucocorticoids in moderate doses (30 to 40 mg per day in divided daily doses) effectively reduce the inflammatory and edematous changes in SSc but have no effect on the fibrotic features. When pulmonary SSc can be shown to have an active inflammatory component by bronchoalveolar lavage, gallium/indium scans, or high-resolution CT, a brief trial of high-dose (60 to 80 mg in divided daily doses) glucocorticoids is indicated. Also, it may help to reduce pulmonary hypertension if used early in the course of its development, usually in conjunction with calcium channel blockers.

The management of Raynaud's phenomenon has improved in recent years (see Ch. 54); nonetheless, even the most successful management of the vasoactive features of SSc does not appear to slow or stop the continuing appearance of new fibrotic or visceral manifestations. Sometimes a change in lifestyle is sufficient. Clothing should protect the trunk to encourage heat dissipation via peripheral vasodilatation. Extremes of cold, exhaustion, or stress should be avoided. Nitroglycerin ointment applied locally along the course of the digital arteries to those fingers showing severe ischemia is helpful. Selective sympathetic blockade, especially postganglionic alpha blockade with prazosin, usually reduces symptoms but may be difficult to tolerate owing to palpitation and orthostatic hypotension. Inhibitors of the slow calcium channels of cell membranes have been a significant advance in the management of Raynaud's phenomenon. At present, nifedipine in gradually increasing doses is popular, but verapamil, diltiazem, and nicardipine have their proponents as well. When tissue necrosis is present (gangrene), prompt hospital admission for stellate ganglion blockade or epidural blocks is indicated.

As an example of how therapeutic trials in SSc must be conducted to provide meaningful results in this indolent, variable disorder, the negative trial of chlorambucil by Furst and colleagues is cited. The agent was not better than placebo. Fifty-two patients, with a mean of 7.2 years of symptoms, were treated for 3 years each. Extensive inpatient evaluation was carried out at 6, 12, 24, and 36 months, looking for skin, skeletal, pulmonary, cardiac (left and right sides of the heart), renal, upper and lower gastrointestinal, muscular, and global involvement. "Slope estimates" for each patient and each organ system were constructed and compared. Never mind that chlorambucil did not change the course of SSc; the study is a prototype of drug trials until we have a much better understanding of the mechanisms involved.

Jimenez SA, Bashley RI, Rosenbloom J: Regulation of macromolecular biosynthesis in cultured dermal fibroblasts of patients with progressive systemic sclerosis. In Black CM, Myers AR (eds.): Current Topics in Rheumatology: Systemic Sclerosis (Scleroderma). New York, Gower Medical Publishing, 1985, pp. 220–225. *A concise review of the data demonstrating that the regulatory defect in the scleroderma fibroblast is at the level of transcription (gene expression).*

Kahaleh MB, LeRoy EC: Vascular factors in the pathogenesis of systemic sclerosis. In Jayson MD, Black CM (eds.): Systemic Sclerosis: Scleroderma. Great Britain, Chichester, John Wiley & Sons, 1988, pp 107–118. *A review of the vascular hypothesis in systemic sclerosis.*

Kahaleh MB, LeRoy EC: Interleukin-2 in scleroderma. Correlation of serum level with extent of skin involvement and disease duration. Ann Intern Med 110:446, 1989. *Clinical-biological correlations between disease progression and exaggerated T helper cell function.*

*This use is not listed in the manufacturer's directive.

Kallenberg CGM: Early detection of connective tissue disease in patients with Raynaud's phenomenon. Rheumatic Dis Clin North Am 16:11, 1990. *A review of the important hypothesis that virtually all future SSc patients can be detected by capillary and serology examinations, when definitive therapy becomes available.*

Korn JH: Immunologic aspects of scleroderma. Curr Opin Rheumatol 2:922, 1990. *A critical appraisal of genetic associations, T cell subsets (lesional and circulatory), in vivo measures of helper T cell function, and the possibility of retroviral molecular mimicry in the immune events of scleroderma.*

LeRoy EC (ed.): Scleroderma. Rheum Dis Clin North Am 16:1–249, 1990. *A multiauthor discussion of the natural history; early detection; cellular, microvascular, and extracellular matrix; immune; and organ-specific characteristics of systemic sclerosis. A useful reference source.*

LeRoy EC, Black C, Fleischmajer R, et al.: Scleroderma (systemic sclerosis). Classification, subsets and pathogenesis. J Rheumatol 15:202, 1988. *The basis for classifying systemic sclerosis into two subsets based on prognosis.*

LeRoy EC, Smith EA, Kahaleh MB, et al.: A strategy for determining the pathogenesis of systemic sclerosis. Is transforming growth factor β the answer? Arthritis Rheum 32:817, 1989. *The hypothesis that wound healing growth factors are involved in the unregulated scarring of systemic sclerosis.*

Silver RM, Heyes MP, Maize JC, et al.: Scleroderma, fasciitis and eosinophilia associated with ingestion of L-tryptophan. N Engl J Med 322:874, 1990. *A newly recognized syndrome in the scleroderma spectrum of disease.*

Steen VD, Shapiro AP, Medsger TA: Outcome of renal crisis in systemic sclerosis. Ann Intern Med 113:352, 1990. *Documentation of the remarkable efficacy of converting enzyme inhibitors in systemic scleroderma renal crisis.*

Tan EM: Antinuclear antibodies: Diagnostic markers for autoimmune diseases and probes for cell biology. Adv Immunol 44:93, 1989. *A thorough review of humoral autoimmunity in scleroderma in the broader context of human autoimmunity in general by an experienced investigator.*

263 Sjögren's Syndrome

Norman Talal

DEFINITION. Sjögren's syndrome (SS) is a chronic inflammatory and autoimmune disease in which the salivary and lacrimal glands undergo progressive destruction by lymphocytes and plasma cells, resulting in decreased production of saliva and tears. The term autoimmune exocrinopathy has been introduced. The spectrum of this illness includes a primary form (sicca complex), a secondary form accompanying rheumatoid arthritis (or occasionally another connective tissue disease), and a form characterized mainly by lymphoproliferation of either a benign infiltrative or a malignant nature. Females are affected 10 times more frequently than males. The typical appearance of a patient with Sjögren's syndrome who has bilateral parotid swelling is shown in Figure 263–1.

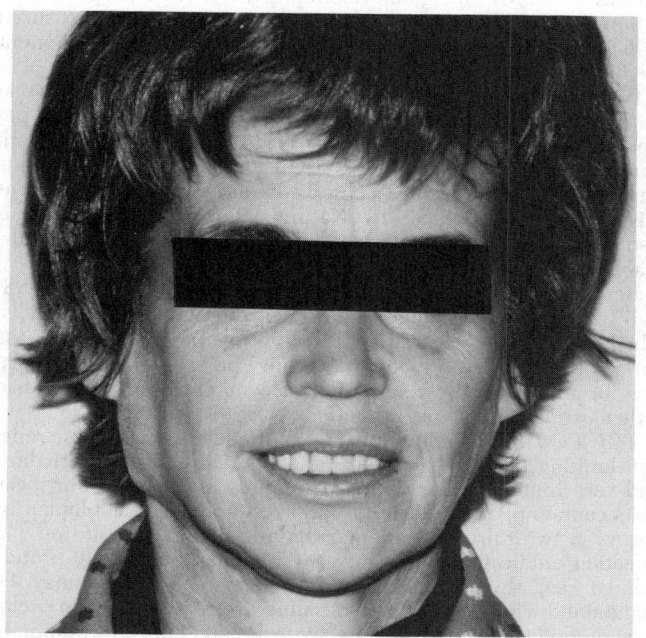

FIGURE 263–1. The characteristic appearance of bilateral parotid swelling has been called the "chipmunk facies" of SS.

A viral etiology for the autoimmune rheumatic diseases has long been suspected but never proved. This possibility has become even more likely because of reports that salivary gland infiltrates and parotid swelling resembling that in SS develop in patients infected with human immunodeficiency virus (HIV). HIV-associated salivary gland disease can occur in adults, children, or after transfusion and may be seen with either AIDS-related complex or AIDS (acquired immunodeficiency syndrome) itself. HIV-related disease must now be added to the differential diagnosis of any patient presenting with parotid swelling. Xerostomia is present in almost all of these patients. Salivary flow rates may be reduced. Dry eyes and arthralgias may also be present. Generalized lymphadenopathy, lymphocytic pulmonary infiltrates, and central nervous system symptoms can occur as well as antinuclear or rheumatoid factor. Anti-Ro/SSA or anti-La/SSB antibodies do not occur. The proper diagnosis can be made by screening for antibodies to HIV with Western blot analysis.

PATHOGENESIS. The several factors involved in the etiology of autoimmune diseases such as SS include genetic, immunologic, hormonal, and probably infectious (? viral) (see also Ch. 261). The discovery of the immune response (IR) genes, which exist in linkage dysequilibrium with other genes in the major histocompatibility complex (see also Ch. 250), has helped distinguish primary from secondary SS. The former is associated with HLA B8, DR3, whereas the latter is associated with DR4 (when rheumatoid arthritis is the accompanying illness). The human leukocyte antigen (HLA) cell-surface antigens, the presumed products of the IR genes, mediate the lymphocyte-lymphocyte and lymphocyte-macrophage interactions necessary for proper immune regulation. Autoimmune diseases probably arise as a consequence of disordered immunologic regulation. Although just how immune regulation becomes disturbed is not yet known, it seems likely that internal factors (such as sex hormones and latent viruses) as well as external factors (drugs or infectious agents) play a role. For example, the predominant female incidence of SS may relate to an ability of androgen to suppress and estrogens to accelerate autoimmune disease, as in the NZB/NZW F_1 mouse model.

CLINICAL MANIFESTATIONS. The symptoms of SS may be subtle and brought out only by careful and persistent questioning.

Ophthalmologic (Keratoconjunctivitis Sicca). The patient may notice accumulation of thick, ropy secretions along the inner canthus caused by a decreased tear film and an abnormal mucous component. Related complaints include erythema, photosensitivity, eye fatigue, decreased visual acuity, and the sensation of a "film" across the field of vision. Desiccation can cause small, superficial erosions of the corneal epithelium. Slit-lamp examination may reveal filamentary keratitis (filaments of corneal epithelium and debris) in severe cases. Conjunctivitis caused by *Staphylococcus aureus* is a complication.

Salivary. Complaints resulting from dryness of the mouth are varied. The "cracker sign" describes the difficulties encountered by trying to eat dry foods without sufficient lubrication. Many subjects require frequent ingestion of liquids. They may resort to carrying water bottles or candy in the purse or pocket. Additional features include oral soreness, adherence of food to buccal surfaces, fissuring of the tongue, and dysphagia. Angular cheilitis resulting from superimposed candidiasis may occur. Patients may lose the ability to discriminate foods on the basis of taste and smell. Dental caries are accelerated. The parotid gland enlarges in many patients (Fig. 263–1) secondary to cellular infiltration and ductal obstruction. Usually asymptomatic and self-limited, the enlargement can be recurrent and associated with pain or erythema. Focal infiltrates of lymphocytes are also found in the minor salivary glands of the lower lip. A biopsy of these lesions provides histologic confirmation and quantification of the degree of infiltration.

Other Symptoms. Dryness may also involve the nasal mucosa, leading to recurrent epistaxis, and may extend throughout the upper respiratory tract, causing hoarseness, recurrent bronchitis, and pneumonitis. Eustachian tube blockage can result in conduction deafness and chronic otitis. Dysphagia may be ascribed to several causes: decreased saliva, infiltration of the glands of the esophageal mucosa, esophageal webbing, and abnormal motility.

Other exocrine gland functions may be affected, leading to loss of pancreatic secretions, hypochlorhydria or achlorhydria, dermal dryness, and lack of vaginal secretions.

Extraglandular Involvement. Extraglandular involvement occurs more frequently in patients with primary than secondary SS. Dependent nonthrombocytopenic purpura is generally associated with hyperglobulinemia. Raynaud's phenomenon is present in 20 per cent of patients. A diffuse interstitial pneumonitis resulting from lymphocytic infiltration may cause dyspnea. Obstructive disease (in the absence of smoking) may result from lymphocytic infiltration surrounding small airways. The most common renal abnormalities involve the tubules, particularly overt or latent renal tubular acidosis and hyposthenuria. The presence of glomerulonephritis should suggest coexisting systemic lupus erythematosus, cryoglobulinemia, or immune complex deposition. Peripheral and cranial neuropathy has been associated with vasculitis involving the vasa nervorum.

Lymphoproliferation and Lymphoma. The incidence of lymphoma is increased 44-fold in SS. Pseudomalignant or malignant lymphoproliferation may be present initially or may develop later in the illness. Most lymphomas belong to the B cell lineage, although the histologic appearance is variable. Many cases previously described as histiocytic lymphoma represent B cell lymphomas and remain sufficiently differentiated to synthesize monoclonal immunoglobulins. Other monoclonal immunoglobulin B cell proliferations in patients with SS include Waldenström's macroglobulinemia, light-chain myeloma, and non–immunoglobulin M (IgM) monoclonal gammopathies (immunoglobulin G [IgG] κ and immunoglobulin A [IgA] λ). A diminution of a previously elevated Ig class may signify malignant transformation. Pseudolymphoma is an intermediate stage in this transition from benign to malignant lymphoproliferation.

Other clinical indications of an increased risk of malignancy include persistent or greatly increased parotid swelling, generalized lymphadenopathy, and splenomegaly. Serial measurement of serum β₂-microglobulin offers another clue to the clinical subset or course. β_2-Microglobulin is elevated in the saliva of patients with SS and in the synovial fluid of patients with rheumatoid arthritis. Salivary levels correspond to the degree of lymphocytic infiltration, and serum levels may be elevated in patients with renal and lymphoproliferative complications.

DIAGNOSIS. *Clinical.* The presence of dry eyes is suggested by a positive Schirmer test (less than 5 mm of wetting per 5 minutes, with the patient unanesthetized), but the frequency of both false-negative and false-positive results is high. The pattern and intensity of staining with rose bengal dye and slit-lamp examination are more reliable in diagnosis. The presence of filamentary keratitis and corneal ulcerations indicates advanced keratoconjunctivitis sicca.

Diminution in stimulated parotid flow rate (PFR) (<5 ml per gland in 10 minutes) is a sensitive indicator of xerostomia. Salivary scintigraphy, which measures the uptake, concentration, and excretion of ^{99m}Tc-pertechnetate by the major salivary glands, is a sensitive index of glandular function. Scintigraphy is expensive, however, and offers no advantage in diagnostic sensitivity over minor salivary gland biopsy. Lip biopsy is a sensitive and specific diagnostic procedure, is well tolerated by the patient, and causes no disfigurement. Further, biopsy offers more information; in addition to confirming the diagnosis, it allows quantification of the degree of lymphocytic infiltration and tissue damage. Aggregates of lymphocytes within the acinar tissue are scored, each aggregate of 50 or more cells representing a focus. The number of foci within 4 sq mm of glandular tissue is determined and constitutes the focus score. A focus score of more than 1 is characteristic of SS and is seen in fewer than 1 per cent of both normal and autopsy controls. Figure 263–2 demonstrates a strongly positive lip biopsy specimen with a focus score of 8. The diagnosis of SS is based upon the presence of two of the following three criteria: (1) focus score of more than 1 in the labial salivary gland biopsy, (2) keratoconjunctivitis sicca, and (3) an associated connective tissue or lymphoproliferative disorder.

Clinically, a "sicca-like" syndrome may be caused by a number of other disease processes, including hyperlipoproteinemias IV and V, hemochromatosis, sarcoidosis, and amyloidosis. Use of anticholinergic drugs as well as a number of other medications

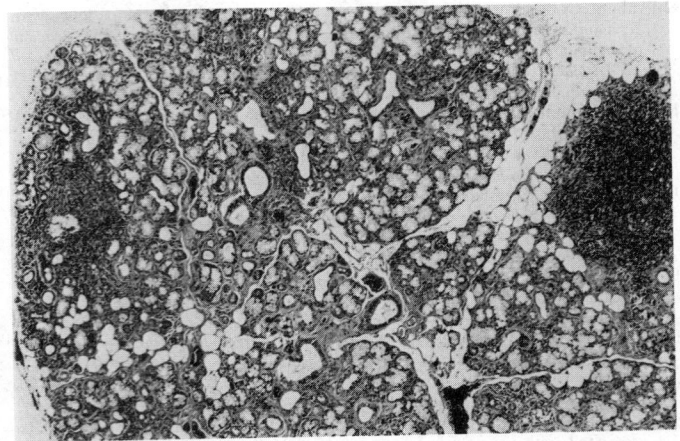

FIGURE 263–2. Several large lymphoid aggregates are seen in this minor salivary gland biopsy from a patient with SS.

may be the single most frequent cause of xerostomia. Thus, it is essential to establish the presence of focal lymphoid infiltrates and autoimmunity in a patient suspected of having SS.

Laboratory. Autoantibodies are common in SS. Rheumatoid factor may be found in 75 to 90 per cent; antinuclear antibodies may be positive in 50 to 80 per cent. Multiple organ-specific antibodies are noted, including antibodies directed against gastric parietal, thyroid microsomal, thyroglobulin, mitochondrial, smooth muscle, and salivary duct antigens.

An autoantibody to a nucleoprotein antigen called SS-B (also termed La) occurs in approximately 50 to 70 per cent of patients with primary SS and, to a lesser extent, in SS accompanied by systemic lupus erythematosus. Antibodies to a related nucleoprotein SS-A (also termed Ro) are less specific for SS, also occur in SLE, and are associated with vasculitis. An antibody (RAP) to an Epstein-Barr (EB) virus–related nuclear antigen (RANA) occurs in secondary SS with rheumatoid arthritis.

Persons with SS manifest B cell hyperactivity. Evidence for this includes the polyclonal hyperglobulinemia seen in more than 50 per cent of patients and the presence of numerous autoantibodies and circulating immune complexes. The lymphoid infiltrates in the salivary glands synthesize immunoglobulins locally. Serum hyperviscosity may result from either macroglobulinemia or polymerizing IgG with rheumatoid factor activity, which forms intermediate complexes. Cryoglobulinemia may be present, as well as vasculitis and glomerulonephritis. A high proportion of patients with SS have circulating immune complexes, as measured by Clq binding and Raji cell assays. Serum levels of complement are only infrequently low.

Peripheral blood T lymphocytes are decreased in about one third of patients. Immunoglobulin-positive lymphocytes in peripheral blood may be increased, particularly in patients with lymphoproliferative or other systemic features. These patients tend to have alterations in T cell subsets and decreased autologous mixed lymphocyte responses. Natural killer (NK) cell activity is also diminished as a consequence of immunoregulatory abnormalities rather than intrinsic deficits.

Reticuloendothelial clearance is defective in patients with SS. In 12 of 19 patients, labeled IgG sensitized autologous red cells, which are usually cleared rapidly by splenic macrophages via surface membrane Fc receptor binding, persisted in the circulation for an abnormally long period. Eleven of the 12 patients had either extraglandular manifestations of SS or secondary SS.

TREATMENT. Treatment of SS is aimed at symptomatic relief and limiting the damaging local effects of chronic xerophthalmia and xerostomia. Ocular dryness responds to the use of artificial tears containing methylcellulose. Since staphylococcal blepharitis occurs in two thirds of patients, the lids should be cultured and infection eradicated. Soft contact lenses may be used to protect the cornea; this practice is controversial. Moisture may be maintained with frequent use of saline drops. Plastic wrap occlusion or diving goggles may be worn at night in an attempt to prevent tear evaporation. Topical steroid use should be avoided unless specifically indicated, because corneal thinning and subsequent perforation may occur. The use of diuretics, many antihypertensive drugs, and antidepressants may further diminish lacrimal and salivary gland function. Xerostomia may respond to an increased fluid intake, use of a 2 per cent solution of methylcellulose, and sour sugar-free candies given as sialagogues. Scrupulous care of teeth is imperative; patients should avoid a high sucrose intake or the frequent use of sugar-containing candies. Vigorous dental plaque control and topical application of fluoride should be used regularly. Oral candidiasis may be treated with nystatin tablets for a prolonged course, with separate treatment of dentures. Vaginal dryness can be treated with propionic acid gels.

Only those patients with severe functional disability or life-threatening complications warrant corticosteroid or immunosuppressive therapy. Prednisone may suppress parotid swelling and improve the restrictive component of pulmonary disease. Immunosuppressive agents have decreased extraglandular lymphoid infiltrates and improved exocrine gland function in some individuals. Their use has been restricted to those patients with severe renal and pulmonary manifestations.

Talal N (ed.): 2nd International Symposium: Sjögren's Syndrome: A Model for Understanding Autoimmunity. London, Academic Press, 1989.
Talal N: Sjögren's syndrome and connective tissue disease with other immunologic disorders. In McCarty D (ed.): Arthritis and Allied Conditions. 11th ed. Philadelphia, Lea & Febiger, pp 1197–1213, 1989.

264 The Vasculitic Syndromes

Sheldon M. Wolff

Vasculitis is a clinicopathologic process characterized by inflammation of the blood vessel wall. Associated with this inflammation may be compromise of the vessel lumen with resulting ischemic changes in the tissues supplied by the vessel. Any size, location, and type of blood vessel may be involved, including large muscular arteries, medium-sized and small arteries, arterioles, capillaries, postcapillary venules, and veins. This heterogeneous category of diseases comprises unique syndromes as well as diseases with overlapping clinical and pathologic features. The vasculitis may be the primary process, or it may be a component of another underlying disease. Furthermore, vasculitis varies considerably in its clinicopathologic manifestations. Certain of the vasculitic disorders are rarely life threatening (e.g., the hypersensitivity vasculitic syndromes in which cutaneous involvement usually predominates). Other vasculitic syndromes may be fulminant and, if untreated, rapidly fatal diseases (e.g., Wegener's granulomatosis and polyarteritis nodosa).

The vasculitic syndromes are generally thought to result from immunopathogenic mechanisms; however, the evidence for this varies among the different syndromes. Among these mechanisms, the deposition of circulating immune complexes with subsequent vessel damage has emerged as the major immunopathologic event associated with most of the vasculitic syndromes. The presence of circulating immune complexes does not prove that the associated vasculitis is caused by them, and complexes per se need not result in vasculitis, even in diseases in which vasculitis is present. In only a few diseases has the actual antigen involved in the immune complex been identified. The most noted of these is the hepatitis B surface antigen that has been demonstrated in the circulating immune complexes, cryoprecipitable serum components, and involved tissues of certain patients with hepatitis B antigenemia–associated vasculitis.

The mechanism of tissue damage from immune complexes is thought to be similar to serum sickness. In this model, soluble immune complexes are formed in antigen excess and deposited in blood vessel walls in areas of increased vascular permeability. The increased permeability is attributed to release of vasoactive amines from platelets or mast cells under the influence of specific immunoglobulin E (IgE). Following deposition of complexes, various components of complement are activated, particularly C5a, which is strongly chemotactic for neutrophils. The neutrophils infiltrate the vessel wall at the site of immune complex

deposition and release intracytoplasmic enzymes such as collagenase and elastase that directly damage the vessel wall. Compromise of the lumen occurs with resulting ischemic changes.

Certain of the vasculitides are characterized by granulomatous inflammation in and around the blood vessels. Although granulomatous responses are generally of the delayed hypersensitivity type, immune complexes themselves can trigger granuloma formation and thereby produce granulomatous vasculitis.

Why certain persons develop vasculitis and others do not is unknown and likely involves a number of host factors, such as genetic predisposition, immunoregulatory mechanisms, and the integrity of the reticuloendothelial system, which clears the complexes from the circulation. In addition, the reasons that certain complexes cause vasculitis and that certain types of vessels and not others are involved probably relate to the size and physicochemical properties of the immune complex and to other physical factors, such as turbulence of blood flow, hydrostatic pressure within vessels, and previously damaged vessel endothelium.

CLASSIFICATION OF THE VASCULITIC SYNDROMES

The heterogeneity and the obvious overlap among the vasculitis syndromes have led to difficulties in classification of this group of diseases. The first report of a vasculitic syndrome was in 1866 by Kussmaul and Maier, who described the clinicopathologic features in a patient with what is now recognized as classic polyarteritis nodosa. It became evident that there were numerous vasculitic syndromes with diverse clinical and pathologic manifestations, but diagnostic criteria were controversial. More precise and accurate classification schemes now have emerged, based upon re-examination of clinical, pathologic, and immunologic features as well as responses to certain therapeutic regimens. Table 264–1 illustrates one such classification scheme.

The first group of vasculitides is the polyarteritis nodosa group. This syndrome is described in detail in Ch. 265. It is the prototype of the serious systemic necrotizing vasculitides and manifests features such as small and medium-sized muscular artery involvement, hypertension, visceral vessel involvement, and a noticeable lack of lung involvement. Eventually physicians recognized a systemic vasculitis that resembled classic polyarteritis nodosa except that lung involvement was a prominent feature and the patients generally manifested eosinophilia, granulomatous reactions, and a strong allergic diathesis, usually severe asthma. Most of these patients had what is now referred to as allergic angiitis and granulomatosis of the Churg-Strauss type. This disease is quite similar to classic polyarteritis nodosa except for the divergent features mentioned above. Many systemic necrotizing vasculitides manifest clinicopathologic characteristics that overlap

TABLE 264–1. THE CLINICAL SPECTRUM OF VASCULITIS

1. Polyarteritis nodosa group
   Classic polyarteritis nodosa
   Allergic angiitis and granulomatosis (Churg-Strauss disease)
   Overlap syndrome
2. Hypersensitivity vasculitis
   Henoch-Schönlein purpura
   Serum sickness and serum sickness–like reactions
   Vasculitis associated with infectious diseases
   Vasculitis associated with neoplasms
   Vasculitis associated with connective tissue diseases
   Vasculitis associated with other underlying diseases
   Congenital deficiencies of the complement system
   Erythema elevatum diutinum
3. Wegener's granulomatosis
4. Giant cell arteritides
   Cranial or temporal arteritis
   Takayasu's arteritis
5. Other vasculitic syndromes
   Angiocentric immunoproliferative lesions
   Mucocutaneous lymph node syndrome (Kawasaki's disease)
   Behçet's disease
   Vasculitis isolated to the central nervous system
   Thromboangiitis obliterans (Buerger's disease)
   Miscellaneous vasculitides

these two syndromes as well as the hypersensitivity group of vasculitides (discussed below). This subgroup has been referred to as the "overlap syndrome" of systemic necrotizing vasculitis.

In addition to the polyarteritis nodosa group of systemic necrotizing vasculitides, certain other vasculitides are systemic and involve multiple organ systems. However, they are referred to by different names, since they possess characteristic clinical and/or pathologic features. This is true of diseases such as Wegener's granulomatosis (see Ch. 266) and the giant cell arteritides. In the latter group, the two major subcategories—cranial or temporal arteritis (see Ch. 267) and Takayasu's arteritis (see Ch. 53)—are systemic diseases involving large muscular arteries with mononuclear cell and often giant cell infiltration within the walls of the involved arteries. Despite the predisposition for certain vessels in these diseases (temporal artery in cranial arteritis and subclavian artery in Takayasu's arteritis), these are systemic diseases that involve multiple arteries. Lymphomatoid granulomatosis (see Ch. 266) is generally considered in the differential diagnosis of systemic necrotizing vasculitis with lung involvement such as Wegener's granulomatosis. However, it is not, strictly speaking, an inflammatory response in vessels but an infiltration of blood vessel walls with atypical and often neoplastic-looking lymphoid cells. Lymphomatoid granulomatosis will often evolve into a lymphoma, and it has been suggested that these patients should be classified as having an "angiocentric immunoproliferative lesion."

The hypersensitivity vasculitides include a broad and heterogeneous group of disorders that have often caused confusion in categorization. These are discussed in detail in this chapter.

Other vasculitic syndromes can be considered under the category of "miscellaneous" for want of a better term. These include Behçet's disease, the major pathologic feature of which is a true vasculitis (see Ch. 269), and thromboangiitis obliterans, which is an inflammatory and occlusive disease of arteries and veins, although its true vasculitic character has been questioned. In addition to the granulomatous vasculitis of the central nervous system, which is seen in association with certain lymphoproliferative malignancies, there is also a rare syndrome of isolated vasculitis of the central nervous system that occurs in the apparent absence of systemic vasculitis or other systemic disease.

HYPERSENSITIVITY VASCULITIS

Hypersensitivity vasculitis is a term applied to a heterogeneous group of disorders that are thought to represent a hypersensitivity reaction to an antigenic stimulus such as a drug or an infectious agent; hence the word "hypersensitivity." Although the antigenic stimuli associated with this group are heterogeneous, these disorders generally share the characteristic of involvement of small vessels. They can be subdivided into two basic groups. The vast majority of the patients manifest involvement of the postcapillary venules, and hence have a venulitis. A smaller group of patients falls into the second category, in which arterioles are predominantly involved (arteriolitis). Most important, there is a predominant and often exclusive involvement of the vessels of the skin. Confusion in the literature generally resulted from grouping this category of vasculitis with the more serious systemic varieties, such as classic polyarteritis nodosa and related diseases. It is true that the hypersensitivity vasculitides may have variable degrees of organ system involvement other than of the skin. However, this is usually less severe than that of typical systemic vasculitis of polyarteritis nodosa and Wegener's granulomatosis. Most frequently, the skin is exclusively involved, or if other organ systems are involved, the cutaneous disease still dominates the clinical picture.

ETIOLOGY. As indicated by the terminology, the etiology is usually a recognizable antigenic stimulus, such as a drug, microbe, toxin, or foreign or endogenous protein. From an etiologic standpoint the hypersensitivity vasculitides segregate into two distinct groups, depending on the source of the sensitizing antigen. In the classic original group, the antigen is foreign to the host. In the second group the antigen is endogenous. For example, certain connective tissue diseases may manifest a typical hypersensitivity small vessel vasculitis. These diseases are generally characterized by circulating immune complexes in which one of the components is an endogenous protein to which antibody is directed. This is true of patients with systemic lupus erythematosus who develop immune complexes composed of endogenous DNA and anti-DNA antibodies; in addition, patients with rheumatoid arthritis may develop immune complexes of rheumatoid factor with antibody activity against endogenous immunoglobulin. Thus, in most of the hypersensitivity vasculitides, the identity of the etiologic agent that triggers the formation of immune complexes is at least strongly suspected.

INCIDENCE AND PREVALENCE. It is difficult to determine an accurate incidence for the hypersensitivity group of vasculitides owing to the marked heterogeneity among these diverse syndromes. However, the hypersensitivity group of vasculitides is much more common than the polyarteritis group and other syndromes such as Wegener's granulomatosis and Takayasu's arteritis. The disease can be seen at any age and in both sexes; however, this varies considerably with the particular subgroup in question.

PATHOLOGY AND PATHOGENESIS. The histopathologic hallmark of the hypersensitivity vasculitides is a leukocytoclastic venulitis. The term leukocytoclasis refers to nuclear debris derived from the neutrophils that have infiltrated in and around the involved vessels. In skin biopsies, this type of involvement is most common in the postcapillary venules just beneath the epidermis. When biopsies are obtained in the acute phase of active disease, the typical pattern of neutrophil infiltration is readily observed. In the subacute or chronic stages, biopsies often reveal mononuclear cell infiltration. In the second and smaller category of hypersensitivity vasculitis, arterioles and capillaries are predominantly involved. In the typical case of hypersensitivity vasculitis with a predominance of cutaneous involvement, the lesions are usually found in the lower extremities or in the dependent areas such as the sacrum in supine patients. This is most likely due to the increase in hydrostatic pressure within the postcapillary venules in these areas.

Although immune complex deposition is widely considered to be the pathogenic mechanism of this group of vasculitis, not every case of hypersensitivity vasculitis has had immune complexes demonstrated, even when carefully sought, as mentioned above.

CLINICAL MANIFESTATIONS. Just as the broad group is etiologically heterogeneous, so too are the clinical manifestations. However, the hallmark of the group is the predominance of cutaneous involvement. The skin lesions may appear as the classic palpable purpura, which results from the extravasation of erythrocytes into the tissue surrounding the involved venules. In addition, one may see macules, papules, vesicles, bullae, subcutaneous nodules, ulcers, and even recurrent or chronic urticaria.

Even though skin lesions generally dominate, various organ system involvements can be seen. Certain constellations of clinicopathologic findings define relatively distinct syndromes. For example, in *Henoch-Schönlein purpura* the typical syndrome consists of palpable purpura (usually over the buttocks), arthralgias, gastrointestinal symptoms, and glomerulonephritis. Henoch-Schönlein purpura is usually seen in children; however, adults of any age may be affected. The disease usually remits spontaneously after 1 week. However, the disease is remarkable for its tendency to recur a number of times over weeks to months before remission is complete. The characteristic skin lesions are present in virtually all patients. The majority of patients also have arthralgias involving multiple joints, but frank arthritis is rare. The gastrointestinal involvement is usually manifested as colicky abdominal pain which may mimic an acute surgical abdomen. Patients may experience nausea, vomiting, diarrhea, constipation, and occasionally the passage of blood and mucus per rectum. In the more severe and rare case, bowel intussusception may occur. Renal disease is a glomerulitis (see Ch. 79), which is usually expressed as microscopic hematuria without significant renal functional impairment. However, in rare cases renal failure can occur. Most frequently, patients recover spontaneously and completely.

Other groups within the hypersensitivity category include *serum sickness and serum sickness–like reactions*. The classic manifestations are fever, urticaria, arthralgias, and lymphadenopathy occurring 7 to 10 days after primary exposure to the antigen in question, which for serum sickness is usually a heterologous serum protein and for serum sickness–like reactions is usually a drug such as penicillin. Most of the manifestations of this disorder are not the result of vasculitis. However, in some cases cutaneous vasculitis typical of the hypersensitivity group is documented. In addition, patients may rarely progress to a typical systemic necrotizing vasculitis involving multiple organ systems.

A number of disorders have vasculitis as a manifestation of an underlying primary disease. Included in these diseases are *systemic lupus erythematosus, rheumatoid arthritis, mixed cryoglobulinemia,* and *other connective tissue diseases.* In these disorders, the manifestations of the underlying disease usually predominate. When vasculitis is observed, it is generally of the small vessel cutaneous type, which is virtually indistinguishable from the vasculitis seen in the hypersensitivity group with recognized exogenous antigens. However, patients with these disorders, particularly systemic lupus erythematosus and rheumatoid arthritis, may also develop a systemic necrotizing vasculitis that closely resembles the polyarteritis nodosa group in manifestations and severity. Nevertheless, in the typical case, the cutaneous vasculitis usually dominates the clinical picture with respect to the vasculitic process.

Other diseases that may fall into this category of small vessel hypersensitivity vasculitis are the *vasculitis associated with congenital deficiencies of various complement components,* such as Clr, Cls, and C2, *erythema elevatum diutinum; hypocomplementemic vasculitis;* the *vasculitis associated with certain neoplasms, particularly of the lymphoid type;* and the *vasculitis associated with other primary disorders such as ulcerative colitis, Crohn's disease, biliary cirrhosis,* and *retroperitoneal fibrosis.*

DIAGNOSIS. The diagnosis of hypersensitivity vasculitis rests on the demonstration of vasculitis on biopsy. Since the predominant organ involved is the skin, histopathologic material is usually readily available. Because cutaneous involvement is often present in severe systemic vasculitides, one should undertake a systematic workup of other organ systems in patients who present with apparently isolated cutaneous vasculitis. Recently, it has been suggested that the presence of antibiotics against the cytoplasm of neutrophils (ANCA) is supportive evidence for a diagnosis of Wegener's granulomatosis (Ch. 266).

TREATMENT AND PROGNOSIS. Therapy of the hypersensitivity group of vasculitides has in general been unsatisfactory. Since most cases resolve spontaneously, the lack of response to therapeutic regimens is of less importance. However, in those patients who go on to develop persistent cutaneous disease or serious organ system involvement, several regimens have been tried with variable results. In cases in which a recognized antigenic stimulus is present, the first order of therapy is to remove the antigen, e.g., to remove sensitizing drugs or responsible organisms by appropriate antibiotic therapy when possible. In situations in which disease appears to be self-limited, no specific therapy is indicated. However, when disease persists or results in organ system dysfunction, a glucocorticosteroid is the drug of choice. Prednisone is usually administered in doses of 1 mg per kilogram per day with rapid tapering when possible, in some instances directly to discontinuation or initially to an alternate-day regimen followed by ultimate discontinuation (see Ch. 27). In cases that prove refractory to corticosteroid therapy, cytotoxic agents such as cyclophosphamide have been used. The efficacy of these regimens has not yet been fully evaluated in hypersensitivity vasculitis. Thus, one should be reluctant to institute cytotoxic agents in persons with disease limited to the skin, particularly since the response of the cutaneous variety of hypersensitivity vasculitis to cytotoxic agents has not been as dramatic as the response of the systemic vasculitides, such as Wegener's granulomatosis (see Ch. 266) and the polyarteritis nodosa group.

The prognosis of most of the diseases in this category is generally excellent, with spontaneous and complete remissions in most patients. However, certain patients may develop persistent and debilitating cutaneous disease, and others may evolve a typical systemic vasculitis with a serious prognosis.

Christian CL, Sergent JS: Vasculitic syndromes: Clinical and experimental models. Am J Med 61:385, 1976. *Excellent review of the vasculitic syndromes with emphasis on the pathophysiologic mechanisms in several of the human diseases as well as in animal models of vasculitis.*

Cupps TR, Fauci AS: The Vasculitides. Philadelphia, W. B. Saunders Company, 1981, pp 1–21. *Comprehensive treatise on the entire spectrum of the vasculitic syndromes. Pathogenesis, clinicopathologic manifestations, and updated therapeutic approaches are discussed in detail.*

Fauci AS, Katz P, Haynes BF, et al.: Cyclophosphamide therapy of severe systemic necrotizing vasculitis. N Engl J Med 301:235, 1979. *One of the first papers to show that aggressive therapy could lead to dramatic and long-term remissions in these diseases.*

Lipford EH Jr, Margolick JB, Longo DL, et al.: Angiocentric immunoproliferative lesions: A clinicopathologic spectrum of post-thymic T-cell proliferations. Blood 72:1674, 1988. *Detailed description of various stages of lymphomatoid granulomatosis.*

Zeek PM: Periarteritis nodosa and other forms of necrotizing angiitis. N Engl J Med 18:764, 1953. *Classic article that represents the first well-organized approach to the rational classification of the vasculitic syndromes. It is still employed as the backbone of most classification schemes.*

265 Polyarteritis Nodosa Group

Sheldon M. Wolff

DEFINITION. In 1866 Kussmaul and Maier described a patient with polyarteritis nodosa. They introduced the term *periarteritis nodosa* to describe segmental nodules of medium-sized muscular arteries. Because the swelling of the arterial walls often led to occlusion, many of the clinical manifestations were secondary to necrosis. Hence, polyarteritis nodosa is often classified as one of the systemic necrotizing vasculitides. Classic polyarteritis does not involve the lung, as do allergic angiitis and granulomatosis of Churg-Strauss.

Polyarteritis associated with hepatitis B antigenemia was described in 1970 by Gocke and colleagues. The association of hepatitis B antigen-antibody complexes and polyarteritis provides strong support for the hypothesis that the vasculitides in general are secondary to the deposition of soluble immune complexes.

In some patients there are manifestations of both classic polyarteritis nodosa and allergic angiitis and granulomatosis of Churg-Strauss. Such patients are classified as being in the group with the so-called overlap syndrome. Their diagnosis, workup, and management are no different from those of other patients in the polyarteritis nodosa group.

Polyarteritis nodosa occurs from infancy to old age, with a peak incidence in the fifth and sixth decades of life, and the male-female ratio has been estimated at 2 to 3:1.

PATHOLOGY. The lesions of polyarteritis involve arteries of medium and small caliber, especially at bifurcations and branchings. The segmental process involves the media, with edema, fibrinous exudation, fibrinoid necrosis, and infiltration of polymorphonuclear neutrophils, and extends to the adventitia and intima. Thrombosis and infarction or hemorrhage occur at this stage. Subsequently, the regions of fibrinoid necrosis are replaced by granulation tissue, and the intima proliferates. Finally the involved segment is replaced by scar tissue with associated intimal thickening and periarterial fibrosis. These changes produce partial occlusion, thrombosis and infarction, and palpable or visible aneurysms with occasional rupture.

In allergic angiitis and granulomatosis the acute fibrinoid necrosis with cellular infiltration involves arterioles and venules as well as medium-sized muscular arteries. It is characteristic of the polyarteritis nodosa group for the vascular lesions to be in different stages of evolution, i.e., acute, subacute, and healed. In allergic angiitis and granulomatosis, the pulmonary granulomatous lesions in vascular and extravascular sites are accompanied by an intense eosinophilic infiltration.

In patients with polyarteritis associated with hepatitis B antigenemia, the specific antigen has been recognized in immune complexes present in the circulation and deposited in affected vessels along with complement proteins. It is presumed that this pathogenetic mechanism prevails in the entire polyarteritis nodosa group, but the basis for arterial deposition is unknown. The deposition of immune complexes in venules and glomeruli is attributed to changes in permeability and to physical trapping.

CLINICAL MANIFESTATIONS AND DIAGNOSIS. The widespread distribution of the arterial lesions produces diverse clinical manifestations, which reflect the particular organ systems in which the arterial supply has been impaired. Among the early symptoms and signs of polyarteritis nodosa are fever, weight loss, and pain in viscera and/or the musculoskeletal system. Striking and specific presenting signs may relate to abdominal pain, acute glomerulitis, polyneuritis, and, on occasion, myocardial infarction. Pulmonary manifestations, especially intractable bronchial asthma, would indicate allergic angiitis and granulomatosis rather than classic polyarteritis nodosa.

Renal. Renal involvement in two forms, renal polyarteritis and a glomerulitis, may occur separately or together. Approximately 70 per cent of patients with polyarteritis nodosa and renal disease have renal vasculitis, whereas the other 30 per cent have glomerulitis. Renal polyarteritis is the most common lesion seen at postmortem examination. Manifestations of the renal involvement include intermittent proteinuria and microscopic hematuria with occasional hyaline and granular casts. The glomerulitis is manifested by microscopic and even macroscopic hematuria, proteinuria, cellular casts, and progressive renal failure. Hypertension is common. Renal involvement is the cause of death in about two thirds of patients with classic polyarteritis nodosa and about one third of those with allergic angiitis and granulomatosis.

Gastrointestinal. Arterial lesions are commonly found in one or more abdominal viscera. The principal manifestation is pain; anorexia, nausea, and vomiting are less prominent. Impaired arterial blood supply to the bowel can produce mucosal ulcerations, perforation, or infarction with melena or bloody diarrhea. Involvement of appendix, gallbladder, or pancreas can simulate appendicitis, cholecystitis, or hemorrhagic pancreatitis. Liver involvement can range from hepatomegaly with or without jaundice to the signs of extensive hepatic necrosis. Splenomegaly is uncommon. There has been no consistent relationship between the development of necrotizing vasculitis and the appearance of liver disease in patients with hepatitis B antigenemia. Some of the observed combinations include necrotizing vasculitis as the initial clinical finding, superimposed upon chronic active hepatitis, or appearing simultaneously with an acute hepatitis.

Central and Peripheral Nervous System. Central nervous system manifestations are generally late occurrences in the course of polyarteritis nodosa, and their particular presentation reflects the specific area of the brain that is compromised. Headache, seizures, and retinal hemorrhages and exudates occur with or without localizing signs referable to the cerebrum, cerebellum, or brain stem; meningeal irritation may occur as a result of subarachnoid hemorrhage. Multiple mononeuropathy, i.e., involvement of several or even many individual nerves at the same or different times, is a common finding and is attributed to arteritis of the vasa nervorum. The peripheral neuropathy is usually asymmetric, with both sensory and motor distribution. The former can be extremely painful, but the latter has attendant muscular degeneration, which can be severe.

Articular and Muscular. Arthralgias and myalgias are frequent in polyarteritis nodosa. Arthralgias are migratory, generally without swelling, and thought to be due to small, localized arterial lesions. Muscle pain or weakness reflects either direct involvement of the arterial supply or a peripheral neuropathy.

Cardiac. Polyarteritis of the coronary arteries and their branches has a frequency approaching that of renal polyarteritis, and heart failure is responsible for or contributes to death in one sixth to one half of the cases. The clinical manifestations of cardiac involvement are those of partial or complete arterial occlusion, as modified by the superimposition of renal hypertension and an appreciable incidence of acute pericarditis without effusion. Whereas the combination of infarction and hypertension commonly leads to left-sided failure, an occasional patient with allergic angiitis and granulomatosis presents with predominantly right-sided decompensation.

Genitourinary. Involvement of the ovaries, testes, and epididymis is frequent, though usually asymptomatic. Mucosal ulceration in the bladder can occasionally precipitate gross hematuria with dysuria.

Cutaneous. Cutaneous involvement of some form is believed to occur in over 25 per cent of those affected with polyarteritis nodosa. The acute cutaneous manifestations include polymorphic exanthemas—purpuric, urticarial, and multiform in character—and severe subcutaneous hemorrhage, resulting from necrotizing arteritis, with secondary gangrene. Ulcerations and a persistent livedo reticularis are associated with the more chronic stage of the disease. A most characteristic but uncommon finding is cutaneous and subcutaneous nodules; these occur at any time in the disease course. The nodules tend to group, appear in crops, are usually movable, may regress in days or persist for months, range in size from a pea to a walnut, and may cause the overlying skin to become reddened or to ulcerate.

Pulmonary. Although the bronchial arteries can be involved in classic polyarteritis, only allergic angiitis and granulomatosis that involves the pulmonary arteries and parenchyma with granulomatous lesions give rise to clinical manifestations. Asthma, when present, is intractable and associated with a marked peripheral eosinophilia. Pneumonic episodes are transient or progressive and may be accompanied by hemoptysis and/or pleuritic pain. Respiratory involvement accounts for about one half of the mortality, with the remainder being attributable to the arteritis of other organs.

COURSE UNTREATED. The course of polyarteritis nodosa is progressive with destruction of vital organs. Intermittent acute episodes resulting from thrombosis of vital or nonvital structures are prominent. Death is most frequently attributed to renal involvement in cases of classic polyarteritis nodosa and to pulmonary lesions in those cases classified as allergic angiitis with granulomatosis. Cardiac failure caused by a combination of infarction and renal hypertension is an additional frequent cause of death in both groups, and acute vascular accidents of the gastrointestinal tract or central nervous system account for much of the remaining mortality. In the retrospective postmortem study of Rose and Spencer, the 5-year survival rate was about 10 per cent in classic polyarteritis nodosa and about 25 per cent in allergic angiitis and granulomatosis if onset was dated from the start of respiratory symptoms. The report of the British Medical Research Council in 1960 placed the 54 months' survival rate in polyarteritis nodosa at nearly 50 per cent. Rare patients with polyarteritis limited to nonvital sites have been reported to experience an unusually long course or even a lasting remission.

LABORATORY FINDINGS. Leukocytosis, predominantly polymorphonuclear, is apparent in over 75 per cent of the cases of polyarteritis nodosa or allergic angiitis and granulomatosis, eosinophilia often being marked in the latter group. Hypocomplementemia, which has not been observed in classic polyarteritis nodosa, has been present in patients with hepatitis B antigenemia. The erythrocyte sedimentation rate is customarily elevated. Abnormalities in the urine sediment, especially hematuria and proteinuria, reflect renal involvement. Abnormalities of the electrocardiogram and electroencephalogram are those expected on the basis of arterial occlusive disease or those secondary to the metabolic disturbances of uremia. Lesions apparent on chest roentgenograms are the rule in patients with allergic angiitis and granulomatosis. The findings range from transient or progressive infiltration to consolidation, cavitation, or scarring; upper and lower lobes are involved with equal frequency. As none of these findings are specific, antemortem diagnosis of polyarteritis depends upon biopsy. Since the arterial involvement is segmental and spotty in distribution, it is advisable to obtain tissue from a symptomatic site, and it is essential to section completely the entire specimen. A deep, open surgical biopsy, including subcutaneous tissue and underlying muscle, should be obtained whenever possible from a skeletal muscle exhibiting pain and tenderness. Involvement of the epididymis and testes is sufficiently common to make this a useful biopsy site if palpation reveals the typical nodularity of segmental vascular lesions. Needle and surgical biopsies of internal organs with clinical involvement, such as liver or kidney, are gaining in favor. As an alternative or additional procedure, angiography to detect aneurysms of medium-sized muscular arteries in renal, hepatic, or intestinal sites may be helpful.

DIFFERENTIAL DIAGNOSIS. The differential diagnosis of the polyarteritis group includes not only the constituent syndromes but also all those conditions associated with systemic necrotizing vasculitis. The key differences between classic polyarteritis nodosa and other causes of necrotizing vasculitis include the absence of extravascular granulomas, sparing of the pulmonary arteries, failure of venous involvement except by contiguous spread, and predilection for medium-sized arteries. For allergic angiitis and granulomatosis the striking granulomatous response excludes all but Wegener's granulomatosis. The prominence of bronchial asthma, peripheral eosinophilia, and the usual absence of necrotizing lesions in the upper respiratory tract permit a tentative clinical distinction between allergic angiitis and granulomatosis and Wegener's granulomatosis. Underlying connective tissue diseases are still recognized by their clinical characteristics even when necrotizing arteritis becomes prominent. For example, cases of rheumatoid arthritis with ulcerating cutaneous lesions and peripheral neuropathy often exhibit prominent rheumatoid nodules and a high titer of rheumatoid factor. The specificities of the immunoglobulins that accompany active systemic lupus erythematosus or mixed cryoglobulinemia are distinctive; in addition, in the presence of active renal disease both entities manifest a reduced serum complement level not generally observed in classic polyarteritis nodosa. The giant cell arteritides (i.e., temporal arteritis, Takayasu's arteritis) lack the glomerulitis, peripheral neuropathy, and cutaneous manifestations notable in polyarteritis nodosa. The combination of progressive nephritis and pulmonary hemorrhage seen in Goodpasture's syndrome is unlike polyarteritis nodosa. The drug-induced hypersensitivity vasculitis group may be difficult to separate on purely clinical grounds, although the history of antecedent drug administration, infrequency of gastrointestinal manifestations, and absence of nodules along arteries are useful points. The clinical presentation in Henoch-Schönlein purpura is distinctive.

TREATMENT. The commonly employed nonsteroidal antiinflammatory agents have no specific therapeutic role in polyarteritis nodosa; thus, corticosteroids have been employed most widely. Large doses, in the range of 40 to 60 mg of prednisone per day, afford symptomatic relief but probably have little effect on the 1-year survival statistics. In our series of 17 patients falling within the polyarteritis group, including 2 with allergic angiitis and granulomatosis and 6 with hepatitis B–associated polyarteritis, 14 experienced dramatic remission with the introduction of cyclophosphamide at a dose of 2 mg per kilogram per day. It was subsequently possible to reduce the cyclophosphamide and to taper the steroids to every other day and yet maintain a remission, and in some instances resolution of microaneurysms on repeat celiac axis angiography was noted.

Churg J, Strauss L: Allergic granulomatosis, allergic angiitis, and periarteritis nodosa. Am J Pathol 27:277, 1951. *This is the classic reference to the polyarteritis nodosa subgroup termed allergic angiitis and granulomatosis; it describes the cardinal clinical and pathologic manifestations.*

Collagen Diseases and Hypersensitivity Panel: Report to Medical Research Council. Br Med J 1:1399, 1960. *This is the classic reference on the natural history of the polyarteritis nodosa group, untreated and with steroid intervention.*

Fauci AS, Katz P, Haynes BF, et al.: Cyclophosphamide therapy of severe systemic necrotizing vasculitis. N Engl J Med 301:235, 1979. *A most important contribution dealing with the effectiveness of cyclophosphamide therapy in the management of a series of patients falling within the polyarteritis group and including such subgroups as allergic angiitis and granulomatosis and hepatitis B–associated polyangiitis.*

Leavitt RY, Fauci AS: Polyangiitis overlap syndrome. Am J Med 81:79, 1986. *Patients are being seen with increasing frequency who do not fit into one of the well-defined vasculitic entities. This is a useful paper that describes 10 such patients.*

Rose GA, Spencer H: Polyarteritis nodosa. Q J Med 26:43, 1957. *This classic article argued most effectively that allergic angiitis and granulomatosis was not a distinct entity from classic polyarteritis nodosa but could most easily be considered polyarteritis nodosa with pulmonary involvement.*

266 Wegener's Granulomatosis and Midline Granuloma

Barton F. Haynes

DEFINITION. Wegener's granulomatosis is a distinct clinical form of systemic necrotizing vasculitis consisting of (1) necrotizing granulomatous vasculitis of the upper and lower respiratory tracts, (2) focal necrotizing glomerulonephritis, and (3) systemic small vessel vasculitis involving numerous organ systems.

ETIOLOGY. The cause of the disease is unknown. It is thought to be a hypersensitivity reaction to unknown inhaled antigen or antigens leading to respiratory tract involvement with granulomatous inflammation, vasculitis, elevated serum immunoglob-

ulin A (IgA) and immunoglobulin G (IgG) levels, and systemic vessel and organ involvement. Although there have been no familial, geographic, or occupational exposure factors associated with the disease, one study has suggested an increased incidence of HLA-B8 antigen in patients with the disease.

INCIDENCE AND PREVALENCE. Originally described in the 1930's, Wegener's granulomatosis is an uncommon, but not rare, disease that is being increasingly recognized in clinical practice. The disease can affect any age group. The mean age at onset is 40 years with a male-female ratio of 3:2.

PATHOLOGY AND PATHOGENESIS. The typical histopathologic lesion seen in the disease is necrotizing vasculitis of small arteries and veins, usually with granuloma formation in the surrounding cellular infiltrates.

In the upper respiratory tract, biopsy of paranasal sinus, nasopharyngeal, or tracheal lesions may show changes of acute or chronic inflammation or may reveal frank vasculitis with or without granulomas. Pansinusitis, nasal crusting with drainage, and serous otitis may result, as well as nasal septal perforation and saddle nose deformity.

Pulmonary lesions are present in 95 per cent of patients, with granulomas and vasculitis the common findings in biopsy material. Lung infiltrates are typically multiple, nodular, bilateral lesions that frequently cavitate. Less frequently, obstructive endobronchial lesions that lead to airway obstruction and atelectasis, or pleural lesions leading to pleural effusions are found. Renal involvement is due to focal segmental glomerulonephritis that can lead to glomerular necrosis, crescent formation, and rapidly progressive renal failure. Any other organ system, most commonly skin and eyes, can be involved with small vessel vasculitis with or without granuloma formation. Although the specific mechanisms that lead to granulomatous vasculitic lesions in Wegener's granulomatosis are poorly understood, considerable evidence suggests that disordered immunity with both antibody- and cell-mediated tissue damage occurs (see Ch. 256). Approximately 50 per cent of patients have elevated levels of circulating immune complexes and test positive for rheumatoid factor, and hypergammaglobulinemia with elevations of serum IgA and IgG levels is common. Deposition of IgG and complement components as well as fibrin can be found in some renal biopsy specimens. Evaluation of pulmonary infiltrates has demonstrated predominantly T cells and macrophages in the granulomatous lesions as well as polymorphonuclear neutrophils (PMN's) in and around inflamed vessels. Some studies have suggested an abnormality of PMN's in this disease, with chemotactic defects, the presence of antineutrophil antibodies, and intravascular lysis of leukocytes reported as early events in the inflammatory process.

It is likely that more than one immunologic mechanism occurs, such that an abnormal or exaggerated antibody response to an inhaled antigen could lead to an immune complex–triggered macrophage–T cell granulomatous response centered in and around vessels.

CLINICAL MANIFESTATIONS. Although Wegener's granulomatosis most commonly presents with upper and lower airway illnesses, it is important to remember that any of the manifestations of the disease can be presenting signs and symptoms (Table 266–1). Organ systems involved during the course of the disease are multiple, with upper and lower respiratory tract, kidney, joint, ear, and eye involvement occurring in 58 to 94 per cent of patients (Table 266–2). Common upper respiratory signs and symptoms include purulent nasal discharge, fever, cough, paranasal sinus pain, nasal mucosal ulceration, and saddle nose deformity. Lung involvement can manifest as cough, hemoptysis, or shortness of breath or can be asymptomatic, with nodular infiltrates seen on routine radiographs.

Renal disease is seen in 85 per cent of patients and is a critical determinant of the clinical outcome. Wegener's granulomatosis of the respiratory tract without renal disease has been termed *limited Wegener's granulomatosis* and was initially thought to be a more benign disease than *generalized Wegener's granulomatosis* with renal and other extrapulmonary system involvement. However, most agree that the limited form constitutes an early form of the generalized disease. Renal manifestations include hematuria, azotemia, proteinuria, and pedal edema. Renal disease can be smoldering but more often, when untreated, rapidly progresses to irreversible renal failure.

TABLE 266–1. PRESENTING SIGNS AND SYMPTOMS IN WEGENER'S GRANULOMATOSIS

Sign or Symptom	%
Pulmonary infiltrates	71
Sinusitis	67
Joint (arthralgia or arthritis)	44
Fever	34
Otitis	25
Cough	34
Rhinitis or nasal symptoms	22
Hemoptysis	18
Ocular inflammation (conjunctivitis, uveitis, episcleritis, and scleritis)	16
Weight loss	16
Skin rash	13
Epistaxis	11
Renal failure	11
Chest discomfort	8
Anorexia or malaise	8
Proptosis	7
Shortness of breath or dyspnea	7
Oral ulcers	6
Hearing loss	6
Pleuritis or effusion	6
Headache	6

Reprinted with permission from Fauci AS, Haynes BF, Katz P, et al.: Wegener's granulomatosis: Prospective clinical and therapeutic experience with 85 patients for 21 years. Ann Intern Med 98:76–85, 1983.

Nearly 70 per cent of patients have some form of joint involvement during the course of the disease. Of those with joint symptoms, one third have an arthritis that is nondeforming and is usually seen in large joints, particularly ankles and knees. The remaining two thirds of patients with joint symptoms have symmetric polyarticular arthralgias without frank arthritis. Eye involvement occurs in 60 per cent of patients and is manifested as proptosis, scleritis, conjunctivitis, uveitis, dacryocystitis, and retinal or optic nerve vasculitis. Scleritis may be in the form of a corneoscleral ring ulcer and in some patients progresses to scleral perforation. Proptosis is usually due to contiguous sinus involvement, with extension of granulomatous inflammation across the lateral wall of the ethmoid sinus into the orbit. Rarely, granulomatous masses can occur in the orbits, causing proptosis in the absence of sinusitis.

Nervous system disease occurs in 20 per cent of patients, involving the peripheral nerves, with mononeuritis multiplex the most common manifestation. Central nervous system involvement can be in the form of cranial nerve dysfunction, diffuse cerebral vasculitis, or hypothalamic granulomas with clinical diabetes insipidus.

Heart involvement is manifested by pericarditis or coronary vasculitis. Less common manifestations of the disease include thyroiditis, mastoiditis, parotid masses, nasolacrimal duct obstruction, pinna and tympanic membrane granulomas, ulcerating breast masses, and anosmia.

Although no laboratory test is diagnostic of the disease, certain laboratory abnormalities are characteristic. These include ele-

TABLE 266–2. ORGAN SYSTEM INVOLVEMENT IN WEGENER'S GRANULOMATOSIS

Organ System	%
Lung	94
Paranasal sinuses	91
Kidney	85
Joints	67
Nose or naospharynx	64
Ear	61
Eye	58
Skin	45
Nervous system	22
Heart	12

Reprinted with permission from Fauci AS, Haynes BF, Katz P, et al.: Ann Intern Med 98:76–85, 1983.

vated erythrocyte sedimentation rate, neutrophilic leukocytosis, anemia, and positive test for serum rheumatoid factor. In addition, the presence of serum antineutrophil antibodies against a cytoplasmic antigen has been reported to be useful for diagnosis.

DIAGNOSIS. The diagnosis of Wegener's granulomatosis should be strongly considered when findings of upper or lower respiratory tract disease, renal disease, and vasculitis involving other organ systems are present. Since early diagnosis and institution of appropriate therapy are essential to preserve renal function and prolong survival, the disease should be considered when any of the typical disease manifestations occurs as an isolated finding (such as proptosis due to granulomatous inflammation and vasculitis) in an otherwise well patient.

To establish a definitive diagnosis of Wegener's granulomatosis, a patient should have evidence of clinical disease in at least two of the following three areas: upper airways, lung, and kidney. Biopsy results should show disease in at least one and preferably two of these organ systems, with lung tissue providing the source of highest diagnostic yield. Open lung biopsy is the procedure of choice to obtain adequate lung tissue for diagnosis. Percutaneous renal biopsy is important early in the evaluation of patients for the disease for both diagnosis and documentation of the extent of renal disease.

Recent studies have shown that serum antibodies against a phorbol myristate acetate–inducible antigen from the cytoplasm of polymorphonuclear leukocytes are specific for Wegener's granulomatosis, and the level of such antibodies correlates with disease activity in Wegener's granulomatosis. Because these antibodies can be found in the serum of patients with vasculitides that do not otherwise fulfill the criteria for Wegener's granulomatosis, at the present time, a positive test for anticytoplasmic antibodies cannot replace a histologic diagnosis.

When the classic triad of Wegener's granulomatosis occurs, the diagnosis, with differentiation from other diseases, is straightforward. However, the diagnosis may be difficult when only isolated features of the disease are present or when less commonly affected organ systems are involved. Thus, the differential diagnosis should include those diseases that can cause pulmonary-renal syndromes, such as Goodpasture's syndrome (see Ch. 79). Idiopathic midline granuloma, also called idiopathic midline destructive disease (see below), is a local disease that destroys facial and palate bones and cartilage, often eroding through maxillary and sphenoidal bones and facial cutaneous tissue. It is not a systemic vasculitis and does not involve lungs or kidneys, but because of the presence of upper airway lesions, it has been confused with Wegener's granulomatosis. Unlike midline granuloma, the lesions of Wegener's granulomatosis do not perforate the palate or erode through major bony structures of the face and upper airway. The only bone commonly destroyed in Wegener's granulomatosis is the medial wall of the orbit, called the *lamina papyracea*.

Another disease frequently confused with Wegener's granulomatosis is *lymphomatoid granulomatosis*. This is a disease characterized by infiltration of various organs with a polymorphic cellular infiltrate consisting of atypical lymphoid and plasmacytoid cells together with granulomatous inflammation in an angiocentric pattern. The disease primarily involves lungs, skin, kidneys, and central nervous system, but not upper airways. Renal involvement is not a glomerulonephritis but rather is an interstitial infiltration with masses of atypical lymphoid cells. Lymphomatoid granulomatosis, unlike Wegener's granulomatosis, is not an inflammatory vasculitis but more likely represents invasion of vessels with premalignant T cells. Up to one half of cases of lymphomatoid granulomatosis evolve into a frank T cell lymphoma that responds poorly even to combined chemotherapy regimens for non-Hodgkin's lymphoma.

TREATMENT AND PROGNOSIS. The treatment of choice for Wegener's granulomatosis is a combination of corticosteroids and a cytotoxic agent. The most efficacious cytotoxic agent in this disease is cyclophosphamide. Irreversible organ system dysfunction can occur if conservative therapy (such as corticosteroids alone) is attempted. In patients with active but stable multisystem disease, oral cyclophosphamide in a dosage of 1 to 2 mg per kilogram per day should be given, with the dosage adjusted to maintain the total leukocyte count above 3000 per cubic millimeter and the PMN count above 1000 to 1500 per cubic millimeter. Close monitoring of the white blood cell count is essential, with weekly assessments necessary to avoid severe leukopenia and infectious complications. In patients with fulminant disease, such as central nervous system vasculitis, severe pulmonary involvement with hypoxemia, rapidly progressive peripheral neuropathy, or rapidly progressive renal failure, cyclophosphamide, in a dosage of 4 mg per kilogram per day, may be given intravenously for 3 days, with a change to the lower oral dosage regimen (1 to 2 mg per kilogram per day) thereafter. Patients should be treated for 1 year after remission has been achieved, and then cytotoxic drug therapy should be stopped and the patient re-evaluated periodically for disease relapse. Complications of cyclophosphamide therapy include hemorrhagic cystitis, bone marrow suppression or failure, opportunistic infections, hair loss, gonadal dysfunction, and rarely bladder carcinoma, leukemia, or lymphoma. Because of the risk of serious complications with cytotoxic therapy, as well as the frequent symptomatic infection of previously damaged upper and lower respiratory tracts with microorganisms such as *Staphylococcus aureus,* the presence of persistent vasculitis should be well documented prior to continuation of long-term cytotoxic therapy (greater than 1 year) for presumed active disease.

Corticosteroids should be administered in an oral daily dose regimen (usually prednisone, 1 mg per kilogram per day) or in divided doses (every 6 hours) for fulminant cases for an initial period (usually 1 to 2 weeks), followed by tapering of the drug to an alternate-day regimen (see Ch. 27). After 3 to 6 months, corticosteroids can usually be discontinued altogether. With this regimen, remissions can be obtained in 90 per cent of patients with Wegener's granulomatosis, once an invariably fatal disease. Those patients who have progressed to end-stage renal failure have had successful renal transplantations while being maintained on this regimen. Patients who relapse while not taking medications or while taking low doses of medication require documentation of disease activity and diagnosis of the disease process present. It is particularly critical in the patient with a new pulmonary infiltrate who has been treated with immunosuppressive therapy to distinguish between a lung infection and a recurrence of pulmonary vasculitis. The use of trimethoprim-sulfamethoxazole oral therapy has been reported to decrease relapses in selected patients with Wegener's granulomatosis, although its use as a first-line drug for the disease remains unproved and cannot be recommended at this time.

Fauci AS, Haynes BF, Katz P, et al.: Wegener's granulomatosis: Prospective clinical and therapeutic experience with 85 patients for 21 years. Ann Intern Med 98:76, 1983. *Long-term follow-up is presented for a large group of patients, detailing presentation, clinical course, and treatment strategy.*

Fauci AS, Haynes BF, Costa, J, et al.: Lymphomatoid granulomatosis. Prospective clinical and therapeutic experience over 10 years. N Engl J Med 306:68, 1982. *Report differentiating lymphomatoid granulomatosis from Wegener's granulomatosis and describing the treatment regimen and outcome for lymphomatoid granulomatosis.*

Haynes BF, Allen NB, Fauci AS: Diagnostic and therapeutic approach to the patient with vasculitis. Med Clin North Am 70:355, 1986. *A concise review that summarizes in detailed tabular form for easy reference the diagnostic and therapeutic approach to patients suspected of having a vasculitic syndrome such as Wegener's granulomatosis.*

Kallenberg CGM, Cohen Tervaert JW, van der Woude FJ, et al.: Autoimmunity to lysosomal enzymes: New clues to vasculitis and glomerulonephritis? Immunol Today 12:61, 1991. *A recent review of the latest theories regarding the pathophysiology of Wegener's granulomatosis.*

Nolle B, Specks U, Ludemann J, et al.: Anticytoplasmic autoantibodies: Their immunodiagnostic value in Wegener granulomatosis. Ann Intern Med 111:28, 1989. *This report shows that if performed using the appropriate techniques, measurement of serum anticytoplasmic antibodies may be an adjunct to the diagnosis of Wegener's granulomatosis and may be of use in monitoring patients with Wegener's granulomatosis for disease activity.*

MIDLINE GRANULOMA

DEFINITION. Idiopathic midline granuloma, also known as idiopathic midline destructive disease, is a progressive, localized destructive process that predominantly involves the nose, paranasal sinuses, and palate, with erosion through bone and soft tissues, frequently involving the face.

ETIOLOGY. The cause of idiopathic midline granuloma is unknown. It has been suggested that the upper respiratory tract and midline facial tissues have an extraordinary capacity to react to antigenic stimulation. In true idiopathic midline granuloma, no primary infectious cause or neoplastic cells are found in involved tissue. Rather, the histologic findings of acute and chronic inflammation with widespread necrosis, with or without granuloma formation, have led to the postulate that this disease is caused by a hypersensitivity reaction to unknown inhaled antigens.

PATHOLOGY. Biopsy of the affected sites demonstrates necrosis and acute and chronic inflammation. Mucosal surfaces of the nose and paranasal sinuses are frequently ulcerated, and inflammation invades and destroys adjacent cartilage and bone. The cellular infiltrate is composed of polymorphonuclear leukocytes, lymphocytes, macrophages, plasma cells, and, less frequently, multinucleated giant cells with well-formed epithelial granulomas. Although perivascular infiltrations and vessel destruction caused by widespread inflammation are common, a primary vasculitis, as a rule, is generally not seen. If foci of atypical lymphocytes or histiocytes are seen, then the presence of an underlying lymphoma or other midline neoplasm should be suspected. Thus, the evaluation of midline granuloma should include a careful search for disseminated lymphoma and other malignancies.

CLINICAL MANIFESTATIONS. Most patients with idiopathic midline granuloma have active sinusitis with superimposed bacterial infections. Symptoms begin with nasal stuffiness and crusting and progress to purulent nasal discharge and nasal bleeding. Ulcerations may appear on the nasal septum, palate, or nose. Progressive perforation and destruction of the nasal septum can occur, resulting in a saddle nose deformity. Destruction of the soft and hard palate can take place, with reflux of food into the upper airway during eating. Paranasal inflammation with swelling is frequently present, resulting in nasolacrimal duct obstruction and dacryocystitis. Relentless midline inflammation

TABLE 266–3. COMPARISON OF CLINICAL FEATURES OF IDIOPATHIC MIDLINE GRANULOMA WITH WEGENER'S GRANULOMATOSIS AND MALIGNANT MIDLINE RETICULOSIS

Feature	Idiopathic Midline Granuloma	Wegener's Granulomatosis	Malignant Midline Reticulosis
Types of upper airway disease	Destructive lesions of sinuses, palate, nose, and facial bones with soft tissue erosions— progesses over months to years	Inflammatory upper airway disease of sinuses and nasal mucosa; palate ulcerations occur without perforation; erosion of medial wall of orbit frequent; otherwise facial bone and soft tissue erosion does not occur	Destructive lesions of sinuses, palate, nose, and facial bones with soft tissue erosion— progresses over weeks to months
Systemic involvment	Disease localized only to upper airway	Systemic involvement of multiple organs characteristic	Destructive lesion local; systemic disease related to disseminated lymphoma
Association with malignancy	None	None	Likely a midline T cell or histiocytic lymphoma
Pathology	Acute and chronic inflammation, with or without granuloma	Necrotizing granulomatous vasculitis	Atypical and pleomorphic cells or frank lymphoma
Treatment	Radiation therapy	Cyclophosphamide and corticosteroids	Radiation therapy and/or combination chemotherapy

Data from Batsakis JG: Ann Otol Rhinol Laryngol 91:541, 1982; Fauci AS, et al.: Ann Intern Med 84:104, 1976.

with necrosis can result in widespread and mutilating destruction of facial bones and tissues, with erosion into the central nervous system, leading to meningitis, or into major blood vessels, leading to life-threatening hemorrhage. Erosion into the orbit can cause retro-orbital masses and lead to orbit destruction and blindness. Loss of smell is common, and recurrent sinus infection with *Staphylococcus aureus* is routine. Most patients are free of systemic signs and symptoms, such as fever, malaise, and arthalgias, except when superimposed bacterial infections are present. There are no characteristic laboratory findings except those related to chronic inflammation and secondary bacterial infections (elevated leukocyte count, erythrocyte sedimentation rate). Computed tomograms and radiographs of the midline structures often show dramatic destruction of facial bones with evidence of widespread sinus inflammation.

DIAGNOSIS. The diagnosis of idiopathic midline granuloma is made by the characteristic clinical presentation of locally destructive lesions restricted exclusively to the upper respiratory tract and the absence of histologic evidence of Wegener's granulomatosis, infections, or lymphoma. Although midline granuloma is a distinct disease, the diagnosis is made by excluding other diseases with similar findings.

While a large number of infectious, collagen vascular, and inflammatory diseases can cause ulcerations of the nose and midline structures, the three entities that are most often confused in the differential diagnosis of idiopathic midline granuloma are presented in Table 266–3. By definition, midline granuloma is a locally destructive disease of the midline facial structures that is relentlessly progressive over months to years. It is not a primary vasculitis and thus is clearly distinct from *Wegener's granulomatosis*. Wegener's granulomatosis is a systemic primary vasculitis that can manifest sinus, nose, and palate lesions. However, the lesions are not progressive; erode only cartilage and thin facial bones, such as the medial wall of the orbit; and frequently heal spontaneously. Erosion of facial bones and tissues in the setting of Wegener's granulomatosis suggests an underlying infection or neoplasm. *Malignant midline reticulosis* is a pleomorphic lymphoma, frequently of the T cell type, that presents with extensive mucosal ulceration, tissue necrosis, bone destruction, and fistula formation in facial midline tissues. Although the clinical picture is similar to that of midline granuloma, the tempo of disease progression is more rapid, and on repeat biopsy, atypical lymphoid cells or frank lymphoma is found. The diagnosis is a difficult one, however, since the clinical picture may suggest an inflammatory process rather than tumor, and on biopsy, the malignant nature of the process may be obscured by an intense inflammatory infiltrate, presumably in response to tumor antigens.

Rarely, other lymphomas, mycosis fungoides, and nonkeratinizing squamous cell carcinomas can produce midfacial destructive lesions. Other less destructive diseases that should be considered in the differential diagnosis of idiopathic midline granuloma are *sarcoidosis* (see Ch. 67), relapsing polychondritis (see Ch. 272), and *necrotizing sialometaplasia*, a self-healing process of 6 to 8 weeks' duration that manifests with large ulcerations of the hard palate and a necrotizing process in minor salivary glands. Infectious diseases that should be ruled out include *chronic bacterial infections, tuberculosis, syphilis, rhinoscleroma* (due to *Klebsiella rhinoscleromatis*), *actinomycosis, leprosy, phycomycosis, blastomycosis, candidiasis, histoplasmosis, coccidioidomycosis,* and *leishmaniasis*. Frequently, there is evidence of secondary bacterial infection in idiopathic midline granuloma. However, for a diagnosis of midline granuloma to be made, there should be no evidence of local or disseminated neoplastic disease.

TREATMENT AND PROGNOSIS. Radiation therapy, approximately 5000 rads, to the midfacial area is the treatment of choice for idiopathic midline granuloma. Prednisone and various types of cytotoxic drug regimens have generally not been successful. Surgical procedures on involved tissues can precipitate acceleration of the destructive process. However, once the disease has been treated with radiation therapy, surgical debridement and aggressive local care measures, such as routine upper airway irrigation and treatment of bacterial superinfections, can aid the healing process. Reconstructive plastic surgery and prosthesis placement for patients with extensive facial disfigurement are often of benefit. In long-term survivors of the disease following radiation therapy, close monitoring for radiation-induced upper airway neoplasia is essential.

Batsakis JG: Midfacial necrotizing diseases. Ann Otol Rhinol Laryngol 91:541, 1982. *A concise paper summarizing the distinguishing features of idiopathic midline granuloma compared with other syndromes.*

Fauci AS, Johnson RE, Wolff SM: Radiation therapy of midline granuloma. Ann Intern Med 84:104, 1976. *Classic paper describing the distinct clinical features of idiopathic midline granuloma and outlining successful management strategies.*

Fechner RE, Lamppier DW: Malignant midline reticulosis. A clinicopathologic entity. Arch Otolaryngol 95:467, 1972. *Detailed report characterizing this midfacial neoplasm and outlining diagnostic and histopathologic criteria.*

Fu YS, Perzin KH: Non-epithelial tumors of the nasal cavity, paranasal sinuses, and nasopharynx: A clinicopathologic study. X. Malignant lymphomas. Cancer 43:611, 1979. *An important study comparing the features of malignant midline reticulosis with other lymphomas of the head and neck.*

Tsokos M, Fauci AS, Costa J: Idiopathic midline destructive disease (IMDD): A subgroup of patients with the midline granuloma syndrome. Am J Clin Pathol 77:162, 1982. *Paper in which clear diagnostic guidelines are emphasized and a more precise term for idiopathic midline granuloma is proposed.*

267 Polymyalgia Rheumatica and Giant Cell Arteritis

Gene Hunder

Polymyalgia rheumatica and giant cell arteritis are common rheumatic diseases of middle-aged and older persons. Although the etiology of these conditions is unknown and their pathogenesis is poorly understood, it is clear that they are closely related. Some believe that a single etiology causes both conditions and that host and other unknown factors determine whether a patient will develop one or both processes. Another theory is that polymyalgia rheumatica and giant cell arteritis are a single disease but that the arteritis is clinically inapparent in many cases of polymyalgia rheumatica.

POLYMYALGIA RHEUMATICA

Polymyalgia rheumatica is characterized by aching and morning stiffness in the shoulder and hip girdles, the proximal extremities, the neck, and the torso. Usually, it is accompanied by evidence of an inflammatory reaction. The mean age at onset is about 70 years, and it nearly always occurs after the age of 50, with women affected twice as commonly as men.

CLINICAL FINDINGS. Polymyalgia rheumatica may begin abruptly but usually develops in a gradual manner over a number of weeks. In mild or early cases, the symptoms may subside 1 to 2 hours after the patient arises in the morning, only to return later after a period of inactivity. Generally, the discomfort becomes severe enough to interfere with usual activities and may confine the patient to bed. Fatigue, sense of weakness, loss of weight, and a low-grade fever may be present. Joint inflammation has been demonstrated in some cases, which supports the contention that polymyalgia rheumatica is a form of synovitis of the proximal joints and periarticular structures. Upon careful testing, muscle strength is found to be normal or nearly normal. Atrophy of the shoulder girdle muscles and restriction of motion compatible with "frozen shoulder" may evolve later. Tenderness of the painful regions is present in half the number of patients or less.

LABORATORY TESTS. A moderate normochromic normocytic anemia is typical. Usually, the erythrocyte sedimentation rate is markedly elevated, averaging 70 mm to 80 mm in 1 hour (Westergren). Other acute phase protein levels may also be elevated. The leukocyte count, the immunoglobulins, and complement all tend to be normal. About one fourth of patients have mild hepatic dysfunction that reverts to normal with treatment. Tests for rheumatoid factor and antinuclear antibodies in the serum are usually negative.

INCIDENCE. Caucasians appear to be affected more frequently than other groups. The highest recorded incidence rates are from northern Europe and the northern United States. In

TABLE 267–1. POLYMYALGIA RHEUMATICA: DIAGNOSTIC CRITERIA

>50 yr of age
Aching and morning stiffness in at least two of the following areas:
 Neck
 Shoulder girdle
 Pelvic girdle
Erythrocyte sedimentation rate (ESR) >40 mm in 1 hr
Duration of symptoms for 1 mo
No other disease present

one population study, 96 patients were identified in a Minnesota community over a 10-year period, producing an average annual incidence rate of 53.7 per 100,000 persons in those 50 years of age and older (the group at risk). The prevalence was approximately 1 in 200 persons in the population 50 years of age or older. Recent reports on incidence rates in Europe show similar findings.

DIAGNOSIS. Several criteria sets for diagnosing polymyalgia rheumatica have been suggested. Most are similar, and that set shown in Table 267–1 is useful. The morning stiffness should last at least one-half hour. The erythrocyte sedimentation rate is an indicator of systemic inflammation. An additional criterion of rapid response to 10 to 20 mg of prednisone per day is suggested by some. These criteria are only guidelines, since patients occasionally have normal sedimentation rates at onset, and a small number may develop symptoms slightly before the age of 50.

DIFFERENTIAL DIAGNOSIS (Table 267–2). A number of other illnesses may manifest similar findings. Some patients with early rheumatoid arthritis lack the more characteristic distal joint involvement and serum rheumatoid factor and have prominent proximal symptoms. A period of observation may be necessary to determine the ultimate course of the patient's illness in such cases.

Polymyositis and polymyalgia rheumatica both limit physical activity. In the former, the limitation is due to a lack of muscle strength without much discomfort on movement; in polymyalgia rheumatica, however, the limitation is associated with pain. Furthermore, in polymyositis, muscle enzymes are elevated, the electromyograms show distinctive changes, and a muscle biopsy shows an inflammatory myopathy; in polymyalgia rheumatica, these tests are normal.

The fibrositis syndrome or fibromyalgia usually affects younger individuals and tends to be associated with more tender spots on physical examination; laboratory tests are normal. When encouraged to do so, patients with fibromyalgia can move the joints through a full range of motion without great difficulty. Both conditions disturb sleep. The wakefulness in polymyalgia rheumatica is due to discomfort caused by movement in bed. In fibromyalgia, however, there is a more generalized, persistent discomfort that is less tangible. In polymyalgia rheumatica, the sounder the sleep at night, the more intense the morning stiffness. In the case of fibromyalgia, the opposite tends to be true.

Other conditions that occasionally need to be distinguished from polymyalgia rheumatica include chronic infections, such as subacute bacterial endocarditis or viral infections, malignancies, hypothyroidism, and other connective tissue diseases.

GIANT CELL ARTERITIS

Giant cell arteritis (temporal arteritis) affects large and medium-sized arteries, especially those branching from the proximal aorta that supply the neck and the extracranial structure of the head and arms. The lesions tend to be scattered irregularly along the involved vessels, but longer, continuously involved segments also occur. Upon histologic examination, a focal or diffuse granulomatous inflammatory infiltration is present with multinucleated histiocytic and foreign body giant cells, histiocytes, lymphocytes, and fibroblasts. Lymphocytes tend to be predominantly helper T cells.

CLINICAL FINDINGS. This disease affects the same population as polymyalgia rheumatica. The manifestations of giant cell arteritis are diverse, and many presentations have been described.

In most patients, symptoms or signs related to the vascular system develop at some time during the course of the disease (Table 267–3). Headache may be focal or generalized, mild or severe, transient or prolonged. Scalp tenderness may be over the arteries of the head or at other sites.

Visual symptoms are present in about one third of patients; half are transient, and half are permanent. The former includes brief visual blurring, amaurosis fugax, or diplopia. Permanent visual loss may be partial or complete and may occur without warning; about half are unilateral, and half are bilateral. The vision loss is due to narrowing or occlusion of the ophthalmic or posterior ciliary arteries. Ocular symptoms become less common a year or more after onset.

Intermittent claudication occurs in about one half of patients, with the jaw muscles most frequently involved. During mastication of firm foods such as meat, fatigue or discomfort is noted. In a small percentage of patients, claudication of the tongue or throat develops with eating and repeated swallowing. Nervous system alterations are found in up to 30 per cent; 14 per cent were found to have either mononeuritis or polyneuropathy, and 7 per cent were found to have transient ischemic attacks or strokes.

Polymyalgia rheumatica occurs in about 40 per cent of patients with giant cell arteritis. It may precede other symptoms or become manifest only during the withdrawal of corticosteroid therapy given for the arteritis. Diffuse or asymmetric myalgias, arthralgias, or joint swelling may be present in other patients with giant cell arteritis.

PHYSICAL EXAMINATION. The temporal, occipital, or other scalp or cervical arteries may be enlarged, tender, and erythematous. Bruits or pulse deficits may be present over the carotid, subclavian, or brachial arteries. Large artery involvement may be present initially or later, as part of an exacerbation. Findings in the eyes of patients with recent visual loss include

TABLE 267–2. DIFFERENTIAL FEATURES IN POLYMYALGIA RHEUMATICA AND SIMILAR DISORDERS

	Polymyalgia Rheumatica	Giant Cell Arteritis	Rheumatoid Arthritis	Dermatomyositis	Fibromyalgia
Morning stiffness > 30 minutes	+	±	+ *	±	Variable
Headache and/or scalp tenderness	0	+	0	0	Variable
Pain with active joint movement	+	0	+ *	0	Inconstant
Tender joints	±	0	+ *	0	Tender spots
Swollen joints	±	±	+	0	0
Muscle weakness	±†	0	+ *	+	0
Normochromic anemia	+	+	+	0	0
Elevated ESR	+	+	+	±	0
Elevated serum creatine kinase	0	0	0	+	0
Serum rheumatoid factor	0	0	70%	0	0
Distinct electromyographic abnormality	0	0	0	+	0
Response to nonsteroidal anti-inflammatory drug (NSAID)	±	0	+	0	0

0 = absent, + = present, ± = present in minority of cases.
* = Associated with affected joints.
† = Pain inhibits movement. Disuse atrophy may occur.

TABLE 267–3. GIANT CELL ARTERITIS: CLINICAL FINDINGS IN 94 PATIENTS*

Clinical Manifestation	Frequency (%)
Headache	77
Abnormal temporal artery	53
Jaw claudication	51
Scalp tenderness	47
Constitutional symptoms	48
Polymyalgia rheumatica	34
Fever	27
Respiratory symptoms	23
Facial pain	14
Diplopia/blurred vision	12
Transient vision loss	5
Blindness (partial or complete)	13
Hemoglobin <11.0 gm/dl	24
Erythrocyte sedimentation rate >40 mm/hr	97

*After Machado EBV, Michet CJ, Ballard DJ, et al.: Trends in incidence and clinical presentation of temporal arteritis in Olmsted County, Minnesota, 1950–1985. Arthritis Rheum 31:745–749, 1988. Adapted from Arthritis and Rheumatism Journal, copyright 1988. Used by permission of the American College of Rheumatology.

papilledema, hemorrhages, and exudates; later, optic atrophy develops.

LABORATORY TESTS. Blood tests are similar to those seen in polymyalgia rheumatica. The platelet count is generally increased. The erythrocyte sedimentation rate averages 80 mm to 100 mm in 1 hour (Westergren), but in 1 to 2 per cent of patients with active arteritis, it is normal or nearly normal. Laboratory tests in patients with visual loss or large artery involvement are not different from tests in patients without these more serious manifestations.

INCIDENCE. Reported incidence rates have varied considerably, from less than 1 per 100,000 persons 50 years of age and older in Israel to about 20 per 100,000 persons 50 years of age and older in northern Europe and the United States. Although the reasons for the variable rates are unknown, ethnic and geographic factors have been suggested. Familial cases of giant cell arteritis and polymyalgia rheumatica have been reported. Giant cell arteritis appears to be one-third as common as polymyalgia rheumatica.

DIAGNOSIS. Giant cell arteritis should be considered in any older person who has developed transient or sudden visual changes, unexplained fever, polymyalgia rheumatica or new headaches, and an elevated erythrocyte sedimentation rate. The arteries of the head, neck, and extremities should be examined carefully. Whereas the significance of slight pulse reductions or minimal degrees of thickness of a temporal artery is difficult to judge, distinct tenderness, redness, and a palpable but nonpulsatile temporal artery are more important clues to the presence of arteritis. In the absence of similar changes in the lower extremities, pulse changes or bruits over the axillary and brachial arteries are more likely to be caused by vasculitis than by arteriosclerosis.

A temporal artery biopsy is recommended for all patients suspected of having giant cell arteritis. A biopsy should be performed on the most clinically abnormal artery segment. When the arteries appear normal on examination, a segment several centimeters long should be removed from one temporal artery, and histologic sections should be examined at multiple levels in an effort to find an involved area. In our experience, if the first temporal artery biopsy is normal, the second site will yield approximately 10 to 15 per cent additional positive cases.

Some patients with polymyalgia rheumatica may be followed carefully without a temporal artery biopsy. If polymyalgia rheumatica is of recurrent onset or has been present for a year or more in the absence of signs or symptoms of vasculitis, biopsy may be deferred and the patient should be followed closely.

DIFFERENTIAL DIAGNOSIS. Conditions that have been confused with giant cell arteritis include systemic infections, amyloidosis with prominent vascular involvement, neoplasms, arteriosclerotic vascular disease in patients with an elevated erythrocyte sedimentation rate that is due to some other cause, arteriovenous fistulas, and other forms of vasculitis.

Follow-up studies of patients who have had a negative temporal artery biopsy have shown that only approximately 10 per cent develop findings of giant cell arteritis and require long-term corticosteroid therapy.

MANAGEMENT

Therapy for polymyalgia rheumatica is aimed at alleviating systemic symptoms and musculoskeletal discomfort. Patients with early or mild polymyalgia rheumatica may try taking nonsteroidal anti-inflammatory drugs. Those not improving with these drugs or those with severe symptoms should be started on 10 mg to 20 mg of prednisone (or the equivalent dose of another corticosteroid). Prednisone acts rapidly, and the patient should notice significant improvement within 24 hours. The corticosteroid dose can be reduced as tolerated after 1 month or earlier. Nonsteroidal anti-inflammatory drugs may be added to control mild discomfort that may occur while corticosteroids are being withdrawn and discontinued.

In giant cell arteritis, the recommended dosage of prednisone is 40 mg to 60 mg per day. Vascular complications seldom occur after corticosteroids have been started. If the response to the initial dose of prednisone is incomplete, the dosage should be increased by 20 mg to 30 mg per day. Usually, if symptoms subside and laboratory values return to normal with a given dose, the disease process is adequately suppressed. Prednisone for both conditions may be administered as a single morning dose or in two to three divided doses per day.

The overall goal of therapy is to administer the lowest dose of corticosteroid that adequately controls the arteritis and prescribe it for the shortest necessary time. The dose needed to achieve control varies among patients and must be determined empirically. There is no evidence that corticosteroid therapy alters the natural course of the disease.

In a small proportion of cases, the corticosteroid dose cannot be reduced without an exacerbation of the disease. Cyclophosphamide, azathioprine, dapsone, and cyclosporine have been reported as steroid-sparing drugs in some instances. However, no controlled studies of these drugs have been done. The average duration of both polymyalgia rheumatica and giant cell arteritis is about 2 years, during which time the intensity of the process may flare up at times but appears to resolve slowly. The course in individual patients, however, varies considerably, and some may continue with active symptoms for several years.

Caselli RJ, Hunder GG, Whisnant JP: Neurologic disease in biopsy-proven giant cell (temporal) arteritis. Neurology 38:352, 1988. *This is a review of the types of neurologic symptoms in 166 consecutive patients with biopsy-proven giant cell arteritis.*

Chuang TY, Hunder GG, Ilstrup DM, et al.: Polymyalgia rheumatica: A 10-year epidemiologic and clinical study. Ann Intern Med 97:672, 1982. *The incidence, manifestations, treatment, course, and outcome of polymyalgia rheumatica in a well-defined population. The relative incidence of giant cell arteritis is also discussed.*

Hunder GG: Giant cell arteritis. Clin Rheum Dis 16:399, 1990. *A discussion on pathogenesis, pathology, diagnosis, and treatment.*

Machado EBV, Michet CJ, Ballard DJ, et al.: Trends in incidence and clinical presentation of temporal arteritis in Olmsted County, Minnesota, 1950–1985. Arthritis Rheum 31:745, 1988. *The incidence and prevalence of giant cell arteritis are determined. Changes in clinical manifestations over a 35-year period are described.*

268 Polymyositis

Robert L. Wortmann

DEFINITION

Polymyositis, an inflammatory disease of skeletal muscle of unknown cause, is characterized by symmetric weakness of limb girdles, neck, and pharynx. The term polymyositis has also been used interchangeably for a group of conditions in which skeletal muscle is damaged by nonsuppurative inflammation; these conditions are more appropriately considered under the classification of idiopathic inflammatory myopathy. These disorders include the traditional diagnosis of adult polymyositis and dermatomyositis (polymyositis with characteristic skin rash) as well as childhood dermatomyositis, cancer-associated myositis, myositis associated with other connective tissue diseases (overlap syndromes), and inclusion body myositis. In this chapter the term idiopathic inflammatory myopathy is used to include all patients with these conditions, and polymyositis is used to denote the adult and prototypic category of inflammatory muscle disease.

INCIDENCE

Idiopathic inflammatory myopathy is a rare condition with an annual incidence ranging between 0.5 and 8.4 cases per million population. The incidence is highest in blacks and lowest in Japanese. Women are more affected than men by a ratio of 2:1. Female predominance is even more pronounced between ages 15 and 44 and in myositis associated with other connective tissue diseases. The sex ratio is equal in older age groups and in myositis associated with malignancy but is reversed in inclusion body myositis. Overall, the age of onset has a bimodal distribution, with peaks in children between 10 and 14 and in adults between 45 and 54. The mean age of onset for the subset of myositis with other connective tissue diseases is similar to that for the associated condition. Individuals with myositis associated with malignancy or inclusion body myositis have a mean age over 60.

PATHOLOGY AND PATHOGENESIS

Abnormalities in skeletal muscle indicative of idiopathic myopathy include muscle fiber degeneration, regeneration, necrosis, phagocytosis, and mononuclear cell infiltration. In polymyositis, necrosis of a single muscle fiber is common, and some nonnecrotic fibers are invaded by T cells and macrophages. Collections of lymphocytes, plasma cells, and histiocytes are found primarily in the endomysium. Inflammatory aggregates contain a high percentage of T cells and few B cells. Over time, fiber diameter variation increases and interstitial fibrosis develops. Although abnormalities in muscle from patients with dermatomyositis may be similar to those in polymyositis, the inflammatory cells tend to be grouped in a perivascular distribution in the perimysium and include a higher percentage of B cells. In the childhood variety of dermatomyositis, vasculopathy, including vascular endothelial hyperplasia, areas of infarction, and perifascicular atrophy, is common, and deposition of immunoglobulin G (IgG), immunoglobulin M (IgM), and C_3 is observed, particularly within the walls of intramuscular arteries and veins. In inclusion body myositis, light microscopy reveals inflammatory changes and characteristic intracellular vacuoles, which are lined with basophilic granules on cryostat sections and eosinophilic material on paraffin sections. Electron microscopy reveals either intracytoplasmic or intranuclear filamentous inclusions. The inclusions are straight and rigid and have periodic striations resembling paramyxoviruses.

The various inflammatory myopathies are believed to be immune-mediated processes that are triggered by environmental factors in genetically susceptible individuals. This theory is in part based on the prevalence of autoantibodies, inflammatory pathology, association with other autoimmune diseases, and response to corticosteroid therapy.

Many patients with polymyositis and dermatomyositis have circulating autoantibodies (Table 268–1). Some are those common in other connective tissue disease (anti-RNP, anti-SSA, anti-SSB), while others occur primarily or exclusively in myositis. The myositis-specific antibodies are directed at cytoplasmic antigens, especially aminoacyl-tRNA (transfer RNA) synthetases. Common antibodies of this type are anti–Jo-1, which is directed at histidyl-tRNA synthetase, and anti-PL7, which is directed at threonyl-tRNA synthetase. These antibodies inhibit the activity of the respective antigenic enzyme protein. Certain picornaviruses can substitute for tRNA and interact with aminoacyl-tRNA synthetase enzymes. It is interesting that some homology exists between amino acid sequences near the active site of histidyl-tRNA synthetase (Jo-1) and some capsid proteins in encephalomyocarditis virus, a *picornavirus* that induces a mouse model of polymyositis. Thus, antibodies initially directed against virus or virus-enzyme complexes could cross-react with homologous areas of host proteins or the enzyme itself. This process is termed molecular mimicry and could explain the autoantibody production.

TABLE 268–1. AUTOANTIBODIES FOUND IN PATIENTS WITH IDIOPATHIC INFLAMMATORY MYOPATHY

Autoantibody	Associated Condition
Anti-SM	SLE
Anti-RNP	SLE, MCTD
Anti-SSA (anti-Ro)	SLE, Sjögren's syndrome
Anti-SSE (anti-La)	SLE, Sjögren's syndrome
Anticentromere	CREST syndrome
Anti-SCL70	Scleroderma
Anti–PM-1	Scleroderma
Anti-Ku	Scleroderma
Anti-Jo-1	PM with interstitial lung disease
Anti–PL-7	PM with interstitial lung disease
Anti–PL-12	PM with interstitial lung disease
Anti–Mi-2	Dermatomyositis

SLE = systemic lupus erythematosus; MCTD = mixed (undifferentiated) connective tissue disease; CREST = calcinosis, Raynaud's phenomenon, esophageal dysmotility, sclerodactyly, telangiectasia; PM = polymyositis.

Several observations emphasize the importance of genetic factors in general and class II antigens (see Ch. 250) in particular in the pathogenesis of inflammatory myopathy. Almost 50 per cent of white patients with polymyositis and dermatomyositis have the HLA-DR3 (HLA, human leukocyte antigen) phenotype. This phenotype is almost always linked with HLA-B8 and is most common in patients with anti–Jo-1 antibodies. HLA-DR52 is found in all patients, black and white, who have myositis and anti-Jo-1 antibodies. The prevalence of the DR1 phenotype is increased threefold in those with inclusion body myositis compared with controls.

Viruses, particularly picornaviruses, are likely causes of myositis. Several viruses, especially coxsackievirus A9, have been associated with myositis in individual cases; elevated titers to coxsackievirus have been found in childhood dermatomyositis; mumps virus antigen has been demonstrated in inclusions in inclusion body myositis; and certain viral infections can induce inflammatory myositis in mice, with inflammation persisting long after virus can be detected. Other infectious agents such as *Toxoplasma gondii* have also been implicated in the pathogenesis of polymyositis.

The pathologic changes in polymyositis and inclusion body myositis appear to result from cell-mediated, antigen-specific cytotoxicity. In these disorders, nonnecrotic muscle fibers are found surrounded by and invaded by CD8+ mononuclear cells, with cytotoxic cells outnumbering suppressor cells by a ratio of 4:1. Studies of circulating mononuclear cells reveal decreased percentages of cells expressing CD8 and increases in those expressing the class II HLA antigen DR, as well as other T cell activation antigens (interleukin 2 receptors; Ta-1, an activation marker also associated with anamnestic responses; and TLiSA-1, a late marker associated with cytotoxic T cell differentiation).

Different immune mechanisms are evident in dermatomyositis. Mononuclear cell invasion of nonnecrotic fibers is rare, cellular infiltration is predominantly perivascular, B cells outnumber T cells, and the CD4-CD8 ratio is higher. In the circulation, DR+ cells and B cells (CD20+ cells) are increased, whereas T cells (CD3+ cells) are decreased. These findings indicate that humoral mechanisms play a significant role in the pathogenesis of dermatomyositis.

Patients with any idiopathic inflammatory myopathy can fulfill the criteria originally developed in 1975 by Bohan and Peter to define polymyositis (Table 268–2).

CLINICAL MANIFESTATIONS

Symptoms usually begin insidiously with no identifiable precipitating event. The cardinal feature of an inflammatory myopathy is symmetric muscle weakness of shoulder and pelvic girdles, at times accompanied by mild pain and tenderness. Weakness of proximal leg and arm muscles, neck flexors, respiratory muscles, and pharyngeal muscles may follow. Early symptoms include difficulty getting up from a chair, climbing stairs, and using hands above the shoulder level. Dysphagia, dysphonia, and dysarthria may develop when the disease affects the pharynx. Morning stiffness, fatigue, and other systemic symptoms are common.

TABLE 268–2. CRITERIA USED TO DEFINE IDIOPATHIC INFLAMMATORY MYOPATHY

1. Symmetric weakness of limb girdle muscles and anterior neck flexors with or without dysphagia
2. Elevation in serum of skeletal muscle enzymes, especially the creatine phosphokinase (CPK)
3. Electromyographic changes consistent with inflammatory myopathy: short, small, polyphasic motor units; fibrillations; positive waves; and bizarre, high-frequency, repetitive discharges
4. Muscle biopsy evidence of fiber necrosis, phagocytosis, and regeneration; variation in fiber size; and inflammatory exudate

Arthralgias are noted with active disease, but frank synovitis is rare. With progression, weakness can become so severe that patients cannot lift their extremities against gravity, involved muscles become atrophic, and contractures develop. An explosive onset with rhabdomyolysis, myoglobinuria, and renal failure is rare. Typically, the neurologic examination is normal except for the motor component of the examination. Deep tendon reflexes are normal or appear slightly decreased because of muscle weakness. Cranial nerve function is normal. Dysphagia is primarily due to weakness of striated musculature in the posterior pharynx and is often associated with a poor prognosis. Patients may have difficulty swallowing liquids, are prone to aspiration, and may have nasal speech. These symptoms may be accentuated by spasm or fibrosis of cricopharyngeal muscles and may require surgical treatment. Esophageal dysfunction may occur but is not often clinically significant.

Pulmonary manifestations develop in some patients because of hypoventilation secondary to muscle weakness, swallowing abnormalities with aspiration, and infection. Approximately 5 to 10 per cent develop interstitial lung disease. Some patients with interstitial pneumonitis have no respiratory symptoms. Others experience nonproductive cough and dyspnea, which may precede the onset of muscle weakness. This restrictive lung disease is associated with bibasilar fine crackles on chest auscultation and reduced diffusing capacity. Symptomatic cardiac problems are unusual, although conduction abnormalities and tachyarrhythmias may be seen on electrocardiograms. Congestive heart failure can result from hypoxemia, pulmonary hypertension, or cardiomyopathy. Raynaud's phenomenon is reported in a small percentage of patients.

Patients with polymyositis may develop periorbital edema. When other cutaneous manifestations are seen, the disease is termed dermatomyositis. Typically, the rash is erythematous and appears on the face, neck, chest, and extensor surfaces of the extremities. The name Gottron's patches is given to raised, red to violet, scaly patches seen over the knuckles, elbows, and knees. A heliotrope rash on the upper eyelids is very characteristic. Capillary nailfold changes are present in some individuals, especially those with Raynaud's phenomenon. These include dilated or distorted capillary loops, sometimes alternating with avascular areas. Childhood dermatomyositis is similar to dermatomyositis in adults except vascular involvement is more prominent. Fever, weight loss, and subcutaneous calcifications are more common, and gastrointestinal tract hemorrhage or perforation may occur.

When myositis occurs in association with another connective tissue or autoimmune disease, the associated conditions may dominate the clinical picture. The most frequently associated disease is systemic lupus erythematosus, but others include scleroderma, rheumatoid arthritis, periarteritis nodosa, giant cell arteritis, autoimmune thyroid disease, insulin-dependent diabetes mellitus, dermatitis herpetiformis, myasthenia gravis, and primary biliary cirrhosis.

Approximately 20 per cent of adults with polymyositis or dermatomyositis also have cancer. Although this may seem higher than expected for the general population, there appears to be no significant difference in the frequency of malignancy when compared with appropriate age-matched control populations. Most often the myositis and malignancy are diagnosed within a year of each other. In general, the location of the neoplasm is as would be expected for the patient's age. Overall, the most commonly associated tumors are of breast and lung. Ovarian and stomach cancers occur more frequently than in the general population; rectal and colon cancers are less frequent. Neoplastic disease is less common in patients with interstitial lung disease or in those with an associated connective tissue disease.

Inclusion body myositis occurs most commonly in older men and can differ from polymyositis by the additional features of distal muscle weakness, asymmetric muscle involvement, and neuropathic findings on physical examination.

CLINICAL COURSE AND PROGNOSIS

The overall 5-year survival rate is approximately 80 per cent, with children having the best prognosis. About half of surviving patients with polymyositis or dermatomyositis essentially recover completely. Older patients, those with associated neoplasms, or those with significant pulmonary, cardiac, and gastrointestinal involvement have a poorer prognosis. Patients with antibodies to aminoacyl-tRNA synthetases (Jo-1) or to signal recognition particles (SRP) do not respond as well to therapy. Patients with inclusion body myositis rarely improve, and they develop fixed or slowly progressive weakness.

LABORATORY DATA

Serum levels of muscle-derived enzymes are elevated at some time during the course of the disease in 99 per cent of patients. Creatine phosphokinase (CPK) levels are the most sensitive, but aldolase, transaminase (serum glutamic-oxaloacetic transaminase [SGOT] and serum glutamic-pyruvic transaminase [SGPT]), and lactate dehydrogenase (LDH) levels are also useful. CPK levels can be used as an index of disease activity or therapeutic response in some but not all patients. When normal CPK values are encountered in the presence of active disease, possible explanations include circulating enzyme inhibitors, a possible associated malignancy, or longstanding disease with severe atrophy. The MB isoenzyme of CPK may be increased in the absence of cardiac involvement owing to its presence in regenerating muscle fibers.

The erythrocyte sedimentation rate remains normal in over half the patients and, when elevated, does not correlate with the degree of weakness. Complete blood count, urinalysis, and other chemistries are usually normal unless an associated connective tissue disease or neoplasm is present.

Antinuclear antibodies are found in low titers in some patients with polymyositis. Certain antibodies (see Table 268–1) may indicate an associated connective tissue disease: anti-SM for systemic lupus erythematosus; anti-SSA and anti-SSB for Sjögren's syndrome; anticentromere for CREST syndrome (calcinosis, Raynaud's phenomenon, esophageal dysmotility, sclerodactyly, and telangiectasia); and anti–PM-1, anti-Ku, and anti-SCL70 for scleroderma. The most common specific autoantibody is to Jo-1. This is found in 10 per cent of patients with dermatomyositis and up to 50 per cent with polymyositis. The majority of patients with anti–Jo-1 antibodies have interstitial lung disease.

The electromyogram (EMG) is abnormal in almost all patients. Classic changes include the triad of (1) small-amplitude, short-duration, polyphasic motor unit potentials; (2) fibrillations, positive waves, and increased insertional irritability; and (3) spontaneous, bizarre, high-frequency discharges. In 10 per cent of patients, the EMG is entirely normal, and in some patients changes are restricted to paraspinal muscles.

DIAGNOSIS AND DIFFERENTIAL DIAGNOSIS

Criteria (see Table 268–2) are useful in establishing the diagnosis of polymyositis. Patients are classified as having definite disease with four, probable disease with three, and possible disease with two. These criteria can be employed only after excluding other causes because no change or test is specific for the diagnosis. Elevation of CPK can occur in a wide number of conditions, as well as with blunt or sharp trauma, aerobic exercise, EMG studies, muscle biopsies, or drugs (such as barbiturate or narcotics) that retard excretion of CPK in the urine. Normal blacks have higher levels of CPK than do whites, frequently with values above the normal ones established for large populations. The EMG changes seen in polymyositis are not specific. Even in the classic case, the change can be considered only myopathic and consistent with inflammation. The EMG is useful in identi-

TABLE 268–3. DIFFERENTIAL DIAGNOSIS OF MUSCLE WEAKNESS

Collagen Vascular
  Polymyositis
  Dermatomyositis
  Polymyalgia rheumatica
  Temporal arteritis
  Rheumatoid arthritis
  Systemic lupus erythematosus
  Polyarteritis nodosa
  Scleroderma

Endocrine
  Hypothyroidism
  Hyperthyroidism
  Hyperparathyroidism
  Hypocalcemia
  Cushing's disease
  Addison's disease
  Hyperaldosteronism

Infectious
  Influenza, coxsackie, human
    immunodeficiency virus
    (HIV), and other viruses
  Infectious mononucleosis
  Rickettsia
  Toxoplasmosis
  Trichinella
  Schistosomiasis
  Bacterial toxins:
    Staphylococcal
    Streptococcal
    Clostridial

Toxic (Drug Related)
  Alcohol
  Clofibrate
  Cocaine
  Colchicine
  Cromolyn
  Cyclosporine
  Emetine
  Gemfibrozil
  Hydroxychloroquine
  L-Tryptophan
  Lovastatin
  Penicillamine
  Zidovudine (AZT)

Psychosomatic
  Hysterical (?)

Idiopathic
  Rhabdomyolysis
  Inclusion body myositis

Neurologic
  Denervating disorders
    Amyotrophic lateral sclerosis
  Neuromuscular junction disor-
    ders
    Myasthenia gravis
    Eaton-Lambert syndrome
  Muscular dystrophies
    Limb-girdle
    Becker's syndrome
  Neuropathies
    Guillain-Barré syndrome
    Diabetes mellitus
    Porphyria

Metabolic-Nutritional
  Uremia
  Hepatic failure
  Malabsorption
  Hypercalcemia
  Hypocalcemia
  Hyperkalemia
  Hypokalemia
  Hypernatremia
  Hyponatremia
  Hypomagnesemia
  Hypophosphatemia
  Periodic paralysis
  Vitamin E deficiency
  Vitamin D deficiency

Carcinomatous
  Neuropathy
  Neuromyopathy
  Myositis
  Microembolization
  Eaton-Lambert syndrome

Storage Diseases
  (enzyme-deficiency states)
  Glycogen
    McArdle's syndrome (myo-
      phosphorylase)
    Phosphofructokinase
    Debrancher enzyme
    Brancher enzyme
    Phosphoglycerate kinase
    Phosphoglycerate mutase
    Lactate dehydrogenase
  Lipid
    Carnitine (primary and
      secondary)
    Carnitine palmitoyltransferase
  Purine
    Myoadenylate deaminase

muscle involvement helps differentiate myasthenia gravis, and EMG changes identify Eaton-Lambert syndrome.

Hyperthyroidism can cause proximal muscle weakness. Hypothyroidism and hyperparathyroidism (or any cause of hypercalcemia) can cause proximal weakness, elevated CPK levels, and myopathic EMG changes. Addison's disease, Cushing's disease, primary aldosteronism, and hypokalemia of any cause may lead to muscle weakness. Steroid myopathy usually begins slowly and is accompanied by other signs of glucocorticoid excess. Other drugs may cause myopathy, including alcohol, chloroquine, cimetidine, clofibrate, colchicine, emetine, heroin, lovastatin, penicillamine, phenytoin, and zidovudine.

Several metabolic myopathies can cause proximal muscle weakness, elevated CPK levels, and myopathic EMG abnormalities. These include carnitine deficiency states, myoadenylate deaminase deficiency, and McArdle's disease in some patients. Other patients with McArdle's disease and those with carnitine palmitoyltransferase deficiency develop rhabdomyolysis and symptoms after strenuous exercise. Muscles become swollen and tender and cramp. Serum CPK and urine myoglobin levels increase dramatically.

Infectious causes of chronic myositis include toxoplasmosis, trichinosis, tropical polymyositis, and several viruses, especially coxsackie and influenza. Polymyositis or a polymyositis-like syndrome can develop in some patients with acquired immunodeficiency syndrome (AIDS). Other causes of myopathic clinical presentations include eosinophilic fasciitis, hypereosinophilic syndromes, sarcoidosis, microembolization of atheromas, diabetic amyotrophy, hepatic failure, and uremia.

TREATMENT

During the active stage of the disease, bed rest is essential, and physical therapy with passive range-of-motion exercise should be performed to maintain function and avoid contractures. Smoking is prohibited, and the head of the bed should be elevated in patients at risk for aspiration. Antacids or H_2 (histamine) antagonists may also be useful to raise the pH of gastric fluids.

Treatment with corticosteroids is empiric but standard. Initially, prednisone is used in single daily doses of 1 to 2 mg per kilogram. In responsive patients, muscle strength usually improves in 1 to 2 months, and the CPK level normalizes in these months. Daily high-dose prednisone should be continued until strength has remained normal for 3 to 6 weeks. Once remission is attained, steroids are tapered very gradually, a process that may require up to 2 years. Alternate-day steroid use is recommended only when the disease is under excellent control.

Steroid failures may be attributed to inadequate initial dosage, tapering too quickly, inaccurate diagnosis, an associated malignancy, refractory disease, or coincident steroid myopathy. An improvement in muscle strength when the steroid dose is raised indicates active disease; improved strength with a lower dose of steroid signifies steroid myopathy. Immunosuppressive agents are used in refractory cases and in patients who continue to require high-dose steroid therapy. Daily oral azathioprine, weekly intravenous or oral methotrexate, or pulses of intravenous cyclophosphamide every 1 to 4 weeks may be used.

Only a small percentage of patients with inclusion body myositis respond to steroid or other immunosuppressive therapy. A therapeutic trial is indicated in this disease, but if improvement is not observed soon, drug therapy should be discontinued to avoid side effects and toxicity.

Bohan A, Peter JB, Bowman RL, et al.: A computer-assisted analysis of 153 patients with polymyositis and dermatomyositis. Medicine 56:255, 1977. *Classic paper in the field that first described the clinical spectrum of inflammatory muscle disease using a rational classification scheme.*
Kagen LJ (ed.): Myositis and myopathies. Curr Opin Rheumatol 1:415, 1989. *Includes up-to-date, expert reviews and annotated bibliographies on topics including immunologic aspects of myositis, treatment, the relationship to malignancy, and inclusion body myositis.*
Plotz PH, Dalakas M, Leff RL, et al.: Current concepts in the idiopathic inflammatory myopathies: Polymyositis, dermatomyositis, and related disorders. Ann Intern Med 111:143, 1989. *Review of present classification scheme as well as clinical features, etiology, pathogenesis, and treatment.*

fying areas of abnormality to undergo biopsy, but biopsy should not include the actual site of EMG needle insertion. Because of the symmetric nature of this disease, it is best to limit the EMG to one side of the body and take the biopsy from the other side. Although the possibility of malignancy should be considered in each patient with myositis, extensive undirected testing is not advised. Clues to the coexistence of neoplastic disease are almost always apparent on history, physical examination, or routine laboratory tests.

A variety of other diseases may cause muscle weakness (Table 268–3), and patients with these may actually fulfill some or all four criteria for polymyositis (see Table 268–2); thus, these disorders must be excluded before the diagnosis can be made. Asymmetric weakness and distal extremity involvement, as well as abnormal reflexes, altered sensation, or cranial nerve abnormalities, should suggest a neurologic disease. Patients with inclusion body myositis may be difficult to distinguish from some patients with muscular dystrophy, but in the latter family history is usually present, symptoms begin earlier in life and progress over years, and the muscles involved vary. Ocular and facial

269 Behçet's Disease

Eugene V. Ball

Although there is no invariable feature of Behçet's disease (BD), certain features occur often enough to constitute a definable syndrome and serve as the basis for diagnostic criteria. One set in common use requires the presence of recurrent oral ulcers and any two of the following: genital ulcers; uveitis; cutaneous or large vessel vasculitis; arthritis; and meningoencephalitis. An "incomplete" form has been defined as recurrent aphthous ulcers and any one of the other features. Although oral ulcers are the linchpin of diagnostic criteria, a diagnosis of probable BD is tenable when several of these features occur together in the absence of aphthous ulcers and other known causes can be excluded. Diagnosis has been possible in some patients only after as many as 20 years of minor symptoms.

CLINICAL MANIFESTATIONS

An ascertainment bias is present in reported frequencies of signs as well as differences in reported frequencies of signs between patients in Europe and America and those of the Middle and Far East. Table 269–1 lists manifestations of the disease in one group of 60 patients. Constitutional signs such as fever and weight loss were noted in 63 per cent. Other significant manifestations include meningoencephalitis and abdominal pain. At least 24 patients from Mediterranean areas have had both BD and secondary (AA) amyloidosis.

Oral ulcers are painful, are round or oval, are usually multiple, and may be the only sign of BD; on the other hand, isolated genital ulcers are seldom indicative of BD. Ulcers occur elsewhere, as in the gut and skin, and there is an assortment of nonulcerative skin lesions, such as erythema, erythema nodosum, photosensitivity, and spontaneous pustules. The pustular reaction of the skin to intradermal needle prick (sometimes referred to as pathergy) was once thought to be pathognomonic of BD, but this reaction occurs in no more than 70 per cent of patients, usually in those with extensive disease. Furthermore, it is nonspecific, occurring in 7 per cent of one group of healthy control subjects.

Ten to 15 per cent of acquired blindness among Japanese is thought to be due to the uveoretinitis of BD. Decreased visual acuity results from inflammation, secondary glaucoma, cataracts, or vitreous hemorrhage; and retinal vein thrombosis leading to sudden blindness is not rare.

Phlebitis or arteritis occur in as many as a quarter of all patients and predisposes to thrombosis or aneurysms. For example, 10 per cent of a group of 450 Tunisians had aneurysms, large artery occlusions, or both. Aneurysms are particularly common in pulmonary arteries and are most often single; as many as 14 have occurred in one patient in less than 1 year. Pulmonary vasculitis produces dyspnea, chest pain, cough, or hemoptysis and is a significant cause of death. Its radiographic signs include scattered infiltrates and pleural effusions.

The arthritis of BD is usually intermittent, self-limited, and localized to the knees and ankles; however, erosive changes have been observed in hip, heel, wrist, knee, ankle, and foot radiographs.

Aseptic meningitis occurs in almost all cases of neurologic BD; other manifestations include encephalopathy, seizures, corticospinal abnormalities, bulbar palsy, ataxia, transient ischemic attacks, strokes, and pseudotumor cerebri. These may be acute or gradual in onset, and they may resolve completely or cause death. Focal intracranial abnormalities are detected by imaging studies.

Small and large ulcers in the gut produce symptoms of inflammatory bowel disease and perforation and are more common in Japanese than in Turkish patients.

PREVALENCE

Behçet's disease is rare in the Americas and Europe. It is more prevalent, as well as virulent, in Turkey and the Middle and Far East. Evidence of BD was found in 19 of 1531 persons aged 10

TABLE 269–1. MAJOR MANIFESTATIONS OF BEHÇET'S DISEASE

Manifestation	Prevalence (%)
Mouth ulcers	97
Genital ulcers	83
Cutaneous lesions	75
Uveitis	48
Joint pain	48
Phlebitis	17

or older in a field survey conducted in rural Turkey; in Hokkaido, Japan, its estimated prevalence was 1 in 1000 persons, but BD is less common in ethnic Japanese living in Hawaii. Its prevalence was estimated at 1 in 25,000 in Olmsted County, Minnesota.

GENETICS AND PATHOLOGY

Although not considered hereditary, BD was present in members of four HLA (human leukocyte antigen)-B51–positive families. HLA-B51 has been detected in 51 per cent of BD patients versus 16 per cent of control subjects in Japan and in 62 per cent with BD versus 29 per cent of control subjects in Iraq. Histopathologic characteristics of BD are nonspecific. Despite its classification as vasculitis, fibrinoid necrosis of vessels is not usually found. Mononuclear cells, found in the epidermis and around small vessels in early lesions, are later replaced by neutrophils and plasma cells. Arteritis, which may be catastrophic, is due to inflammation of the vasa vasorum. Abnormalities of the immune system are inconstant, providing no clues to the cause and pathogenesis of BD, which remain unknown.

TREATMENT

Numerous medications have been tried for symptomatic treatment as well as for prevention. Corticosteroids are given in doses up to 1000 mg per day for serious problems, such as central nervous system disease. Colchicine has been the drug of choice for suppression of uveitis in Japan; however, cyclosporine appears to be superior to colchicine in reducing the frequency and severity of ocular attacks. Other immunosuppressive drugs have been used with variable effectiveness and toxicity. Chlorambucil (0.1 mg per kilogram per day) moderates disease expression; however, long-term use is worrisome with respect to oncogenesis. Azathioprine (2.5 mg per kilogram per day) is superior to placebo in preserving visual acuity in patients with eye disease and in reducing the frequency of oral and genital ulcers and arthritis. Acyclovir has failed to alter the course of BD.

Dilsen N, Konice M, Aral O, et al.: Behçet's disease associated with amyloidosis in Turkey and in the world. Ann Rheum Dis 47:157, 1988. *The features of 8 Turkish and 16 other patients with BD and amyloidosis are described.*

Hamza M: Large artery involvement in Behçet's disease. J Rheumatol 14:554, 1987. *Clinical descriptions of 10 of 450 patients evaluated over a 20-year period who were found to have arterial aneurysms (7) and occlusion (3).*

Lee RG: The colitis of Behçet's syndrome. Am J Surg Pathol 10:888, 1986. *A report of severe colitis requiring colectomy and a review of 29 other published cases.*

Masuda K, Urayama A, Kogure M, et al.: Double-masked trial of cyclosporine versus colchicine and long-term open study of cyclosporin in Behçet's disease. Lancet 1:1093, 1989. *A randomized, 16-week, double-blind study comparing colchicine and cyclosporine in 49 and 47 patients, respectively. Thirty-six patients were enrolled in a long-term study of mean duration of 44 weeks.*

Raz I, Okon E, Chajek-Shaul T: Pulmonary manifestations in Behçet's syndrome. Chest 95:585, 1989. *Seven of 72 patients had pulmonary vascular disease manifested as dyspnea, cough, chest pain, and hemoptysis. The clinical and radiographic data of these and 42 other patients were reviewed.*

Yazici H, Pazarli H, Barnes CG, et al.: A controlled trial of azathioprine in Behçet's syndrome. N Engl J Med 322:281, 1990.

270 Panniculitis and Disorders of the Subcutaneous Fat

Gerald S. Lazarus

The subcutaneous tissue is a fibrofatty layer spread between skin and muscles. It functions not only as a thermal and mechanical insulator but also as an active metabolic organ. The characteristic signet ring lipocytes are organized into lobules by fibrous septa, which are continuous with the dermis and contain the blood and lymph vessels and reticuloendothelial cells.

The diagnosis of panniculitis frequently requires deep skin biopsy. The most important histologic characteristic is the location of the inflammatory process. Inflammation primarily in the septa is designated *septal panniculitis*, whereas inflammatory cells primarily in the fat lobules are called *lobular panniculitis*. The presence or absence of vasculitis further differentiates panniculitis into four major groups.

LOBULAR PANNICULITIS WITHOUT VASCULITIS. Nodular Panniculitis—Weber-Christian Disease. Nodular panniculitis describes a group of syndromes or diseases characterized by subcutaneous nodules and inflammatory cells in the fat lobules. The term Weber-Christian disease is applied when cutaneous lesions are associated with systemic complaints; this eponym should be abandoned because lobular panniculitis includes a variety of distinctive disease entities.

The etiology of this group of diseases is unknown. In the early stages, the fat lobules are infiltrated with polymorphonuclear leukocytes. Later, macrophages appear and ingest fat, producing the characteristic lipophagic granuloma. The lesions heal with lobular fibrosis. Modest septal vasculitis may be observed.

Lobular panniculitis most commonly occurs in women between the ages of 30 and 60, although cases have been reported in all age groups. The lesions begin as red, slightly tender nodules deep in the skin. They appear more or less in symmetric crops on thighs and lower legs, but lesions may also occur on arms, trunk, and face. The number of lesions may vary enormously. The lesions become firmer, less red, and less tender over a period of weeks. They heal, leaving a depressed, hyperpigmented scar. *Liquefying panniculitis* is a variant in which the lesions become necrotic and drain an oily, yellow-brown fluid. A substantial number of patients with this clinical picture may have α_1 proteinase deficiency. Biopsy reveals polymorphonuclear leukocytes in the deep reticular dermis as well as in the fat. *Rothmann-Makai syndrome*, a very rare variant of lobular panniculitis, affects children, in whom numerous large lesions develop; the lesions do not liquefy, and healing usually occurs within 12 months.

Systemic nodular panniculitis is a widespread process affecting cutaneous and visceral fat. Patients usually present with unequivocal cutaneous nodules and arthralgias, malaise, fatigue, weight loss, and abdominal pain. Involvement of the bone marrow may produce anemia, leukocytosis or leukopenia, and bone pain. Hepatomegaly, steatorrhea, and intestinal perforation have also been reported. Inflammation may occur in other internal organs, such as lungs, pleura, pericardium, spleen, kidney, and adrenal glands. Visceral involvement may be confined to the retroperitoneal space, producing abdominal pain, nausea, and vomiting. Mesenteric panniculitis resulting in abdominal pain, diarrhea, constipation, and occasional mass lesions may occur without cutaneous findings. Histiocytic cytophagic panniculitis is a disease characterized by panniculitis, fever, serositis, reticuloendotheliomegaly, and a poor prognosis; it is diagnosed by the presence of T lymphocytes and histiocytosis with phagocytosis of erythrocytes, leukocytes, and platelets.

The prognosis of nodular panniculitis is good in patients with only cutaneous involvement. Remissions and exacerbations of the lesions are frequent. Some patients recover after a few months, and permanent remission is usual after several years. On rare occasions, visceral involvement may be fatal.

No specific therapy exists for this disease. Saturated potassium iodide, increasing from five drops three times per day by one drop per day to 30 drops three times per day, has been suggested. Hydroxychloroquine,* 200 mg two times per day, has also been advocated as treatment. High-dose prednisone, 40 to 60 mg for 1 to 2 weeks, with gradual tapering over 6 to 8 weeks, has also been reported to be of value in patients with severe disease; steroids should be used *only for acute* attacks and for limited periods. There are anecdotal reports that cyclosporine may be of value in patients with severe panniculitis.

Lobular Panniculitis Associated with Pancreatic Disease. The diagnosis is made by skin biopsy, which discloses acute fat necrosis with characteristic ghost cells. These patients often have associated arthritis, ascites, and eosinophilia. Acute pancreatitis, trauma to the pancreas, chronic pancreatitis, pancreatic cysts, and pancreatic carcinoma have been reported to be associated with this syndrome. Diagnosis depends upon the histologic findings at skin biopsy and documentation of a specific pancreatic abnormality. Therapy is directed at the underlying pancreatic disease.

Poststeroid Lobular Panniculitis. Children who receive large doses of steroid for a short period, followed by abrupt discontinuance, may develop lobular panniculitis. Lesions may occur in the viscera, and a fatal case has been reported.

Physical Lobular Panniculitis. Physical trauma of any kind and cold injury, especially in children, can produce lobular panniculitis. A unique traumatic panniculitis occurs in the breasts of obese women in their 50's. Injection of silicones or other foreign materials into female breasts or buttocks and into the male genitalia may induce a granulomatous foreign body nodular panniculitis. Similar inflammatory lesions may be seen following injection of pentazocine (Talwin).

Lobular Panniculitis Associated with Systemic Disease. Lupus erythematosus, sarcoidosis, granuloma annulare, Sweet's disease, acute sudden weight loss from gastrointestinal surgery, and infections, including those caused by deep fungi, mycobacteria, and pyogens, may present as lobular panniculitis. Any patient with acquired immunodeficiency syndrome (AIDS) who has panniculitis must have a biopsy performed and the tissue sent for histologic study and culture to rule out infectious agents. Lymphoma or leukemia may also present as panniculitis; histologically, these lesions demonstrate malignant cells in the fat lobules. Lupus erythematosus confined primarily to the fat is known as lupus profundus. The skin may be exclusively involved, or the panniculitis may be associated with systemic disease.

Lobular Panniculitis with Vasculitis. This category of disease includes *nodular vasculitis* and *erythema induratum*. The eruption consists of recurring, tender, painful nodules on the calves, which often ulcerate and heal with scarring. It is much more common in females than in males. Increased erythrocyte sedimentation rate and hypertension have been associated with this syndrome. Bazin gave the name erythema induratum to this disease when histologic examination revealed caseation necrosis, and the lesions were associated with tuberculosis.

There is no specific therapy. Most patients experience remission of lesions with bed rest. Severe cases have been successfully treated with nonsteroidal anti-inflammatory drugs, dapsone, and prednisone. In the very rare case of nodular vasculitis associated with tuberculosis, appropriate antituberculous therapy is indicated.

SEPTAL PANNICULITIS WITHOUT VASCULITIS. This histologic picture in a patient with nodular, painful, tender lesions, especially on the anterior leg, is diagnostic of *erythema nodosum*, which is discussed in Ch. 525. A chronic disease similar to erythema nodosum clinically and histologically except that the lesions spread peripherally over months, forming rings, is called *subacute migratory panniculitis*. This disease responds to therapy with increasing doses of saturated potassium iodide as described for nodular panniculitis. Septal panniculitis without vasculitis can also be seen in scleroderma, dermatomyositis, and necrobiosis lipoidica diabeticorum. Eosinophilic fasciitis can mimic septal panniculitis. Ingestion of pharmacologic doses of tryptophan for pain or depression has produced a syndrome mimicking acute scleroderma or eosinophilic fasciitis. These diagnostic possibilities should be investigated in all patients.

SEPTAL PANNICULITIS WITH VASCULITIS. *Thrombophlebitis* may present with subcutaneous nodules. Histology reveals inflammation of veins with adjacent panniculitis (see Ch. 54).

Cutaneous polyarteritis is a chronic, recurring, painful nodular eruption, primarily of the legs. An associated mottled livedo vascular pattern is often present. Cutaneous polyarteritis is associated with myalgias, arthralgias, and increased erythrocyte sedimentation rate. Histologic examination demonstrates leukocytoclastic vasculitis of medium-sized arterioles. This disease is not usually associated with systemic involvement. It has a benign course, but lesions may recur for years.

---

* This use is not listed in the manufacturer's directive.

Therapy includes nonsteroidal anti-inflammatory agents and short courses of corticosteroids. Cutaneous polyarteritis associated with granulomatous bowel disease has responded to short courses of cyclophosphamide (Cytoxan).

LIPOATROPHY. Loss of subcutaneous tissue can occur as a consequence of healing in almost any of the panniculitides described previously. The most common diagnosable cause of lipoatrophy is recurrent insulin injection. Insulin lipoatrophy is usually associated with repetitive injections of high doses of insulin in exactly the same location in females. Injections of pentazocine (Talwin) may also produce panniculitis and severe lipoatrophy.

Total lipoatrophy associated with diabetes may occur in children and adults. The clinical picture is dramatic, and there is almost complete loss of subcutaneous fat. Partial lipoatrophy usually begins in children or young adults. It is five times more common in females than in males. Patients often lose the fat in the face and the upper half of the body. In some cases, there is hypertrophy of the fat on the lower half of the body. Patients with partial lipodystrophy often develop progressive mesangio-capillary glomerulonephritis and hypocomplementemia. Diabetes develops in one third of these patients. Retinitis pigmentosum has also been reported with this disease. The prognosis depends upon the severity of the renal disease.

Ackerman AB: Panniculitis. *In* Ackerman AB: Histologic Diagnosis of Inflammatory Skin Diseases. Philadelphia, Lea & Febiger, 1978, pp 779–826. *An outstanding review of the classification and histopathology of panniculitis.*

Alegre VA, Winkelmann RK: Clinical and laboratory studies. Histiocytic cytophagic panniculitis. J Am Acad Dermatol 20:177, 1989.

Bondi EE, Lazarus GS: Panniculitis. *In* Fitzpatrick TB, Eisen AZ, Wolff K, et al. (eds.): Dermatology in General Medicine. 3rd ed. New York, McGraw-Hill Book Company, 1986, pp 1131–1148. *A complete overview of panniculitis, emphasizing clinical description, mechanisms, and treatment.*

Hendrick SJ, Silverman AK, Solomon AR, et al.: Alpha 1–antitrypsin deficiency associated with panniculitis. J Am Acad Dermatol 18:684, 1988.

Panush RS, Yonker RA, Dlesk A, et al.: Weber-Christian disease. Medicine 64:181, 1985. *Excellent review of 15 patients and the world literature.*

Wexner SD, Attiyeh FF: Mesenteric panniculitis of the sigmoid colon. Report of two cases. Dis Colon Rectum 30:812, 1987.

271 Crystal Deposition Arthropathies

H. Ralph Schumacher, Jr.

At least three different calcium-containing crystals are now known to deposit in joints and to be associated with a variety of patterns of arthritis in much the same way as urate crystals cause the various features of gouty arthritis. Calcium pyrophosphate and occasionally calcium oxalate produce linear or punctate calcifications in menisci and articular cartilage that can be readily seen on roentgenograms (Figs. 271–1 and 271–2). These calcifications are termed chondrocalcinosis. Both these crystals and calcium apatite can also deposit diffusely in synovium and peri-articular tissues, giving a soft tissue pattern on roentgenograms. Radiographs may not show obvious calcifications when crystals are relatively few. Definitive diagnosis is made only by aspiration of synovial fluid for identification of the crystal type.

CALCIUM PYROPHOSPHATE DIHYDRATE (CPPD) CRYSTAL DEPOSITION DISEASE (Pseudogout Syndrome)

This disease is defined by the identification of rod- or rhombus-shaped 2- to 20-µm long, weakly birefringent crystals with positive elongation in synovial fluid or articular tissue. This is a common cause of arthritis; it is most frequent in the elderly. Up to 27 per cent of nursing home patients in their 80's have radiographic evidence of chondrocalcinosis on this basis. Familial cases have been described in populations of various ethnic origins. Both sexes are affected.

The cause of CPPD crystal deposition is not established but

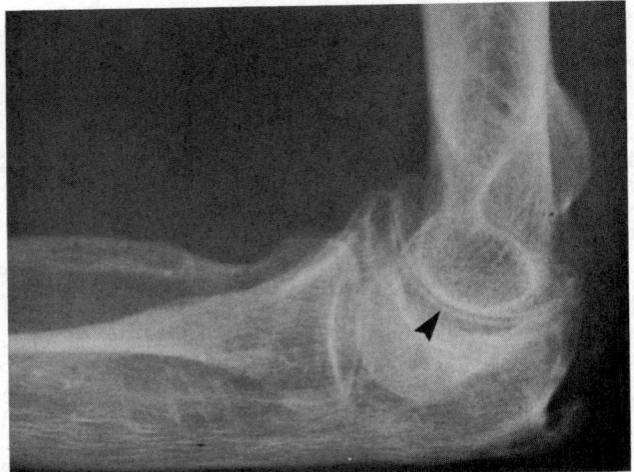

FIGURE 271–1. Chondrocalcinosis (*arrow*) at the elbow joint.

local overproduction of pyrophosphate related to excessive activity of nucleoside triphosphate pyrophosphohydrolase, deficiency of phosphatases, and local changes in proteoglycans are probably important. CPPD crystals deposit only in joints and adjacent tendons or bursae, where they produce hematoxyphilic clumps replacing the normal tissue. Virtually any joint can be involved, but knees, wrists, and second and third metacarpophalangeal joints are most common, so that chronic cases can be confused with rheumatoid arthritis. Acute bouts of crystal-induced arthritis at one or more joints can mimic gout and lead to "pseudogout." Fever with bouts can mimic infection. CPPD crystal deposition often complicates osteoarthritis; this association is more prominent at knees than at hips. Whether crystals contribute to cartilage degeneration in osteoarthritis is not yet clear. Occasional severe arthritis mimics the destruction seen in neuropathic joints. Radiographic evidence of calcification can be present in some cases for years without inducing any symptoms. Others may have crystals in joint fluid with osteoarthritis-like radiographic changes but no visible chondrocalcinosis.

Synovial effusions may have leukocyte counts up to 100,000 per cubic millimeter and with 80 to 90 per cent neutrophils during acute attacks. Between attacks crystals can be seen in clear, noninflammatory joint effusions.

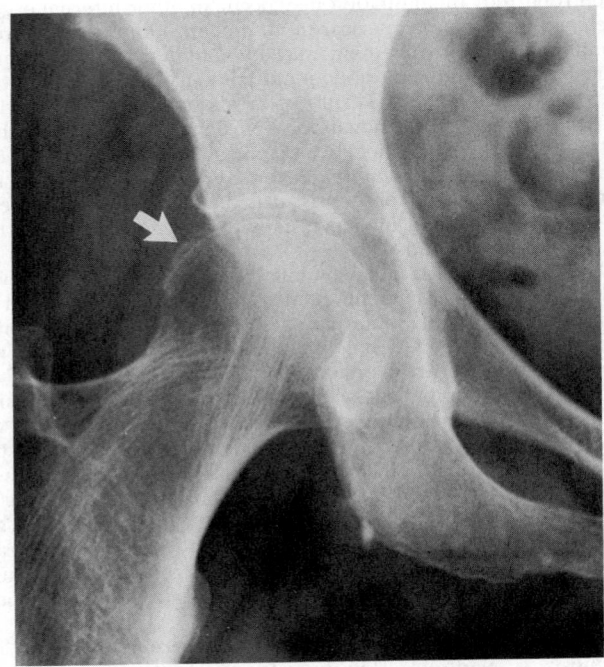

FIGURE 271–2. Chondrocalcinosis in the articular cartilage of the femoral head.

TABLE 271–1. SYSTEMIC CONDITIONS ASSOCIATED WITH CPPD DEPOSITION DISEASE

Hyperparathyroidism
Hemochromatosis
Hypophosphatasia
Hypomagnesemia
Myxedematous hypothyroidism
Ochronosis

CPPD crystal deposition can be an important clue to a number of associated diseases, many of which have specific treatments that can control systemic features if not the arthropathy. Some clearly associated diseases are shown in Table 271–1. CPPD crystal deposition is increased in knees after meniscectomy and may complicate advanced arthritides, such as gout and rheumatoid arthritis.

Treatment of inflammatory episodes with thorough joint aspiration and use of nonsteroidal anti-inflammatory drugs (NSAID's) is generally successful. Intra-articular steroid injections may provide relief in refractory involvement of individual joints. Intravenous colchicine may also be helpful. Chronic therapy with 0.6 to 1.2 mg of colchicine per day can greatly decrease the frequency of acute attacks. Otherwise the prognosis is for slow progression. Joint replacement has been successful when needed.

Alvarellos A, Spilberg I: Colchicine prophylaxis in pseudogout. J Rheum 13:804, 1986. *Colchicine seems well worth trying to prevent acute exacerbations.*

Rachow JW, Ryan LM: Partial characterization of synovial fluid nucleotide pyrophosphohydrolase. Arthritis Rheum 28:1377, 1985. *Overproduction of pyrophosphate by this soluble extracellular enzyme is one possible factor in CPPD crystal deposition.*

Rahman MU, Shenberger KN, Schumacher HR: Initially unrecognized calcium pyrophosphate dihydrate deposition disease as a cause of fever. Am J Med 89:115, 1990. *Even mild crystal-induced joint findings can cause potentially confusing fever.*

Sokoloff L, Varma AA: Chondrocalcinosis in surgically resected joints. Arthritis Rheum 31:750, 1988. *Association of crystals and osteoarthritis is reviewed. CPPD occurs more often in knees than in hips involved with osteoarthritis.*

APATITE CRYSTAL DEPOSITION DISEASE

Individual apatite crystals can be seen only by electron microscopy, but clumps of these crystals appear as 2- to 25-μm shiny (but not generally birefringent) globules that can suggest the diagnosis. Apatite crystal deposition and crystal-induced inflammation are common factors in bursitis and periarthritis. Apatites also occur in some otherwise unexplained acute arthritis, and as with CPPD crystals are common in osteoarthritic joint effusions. Most joints or bursae can be involved, with more common sites including shoulders, hips, knees, and digits. Joint or periarticular inflammation can be acute or chronic. An extremely destructive arthritis has been noted especially at shoulders ("Milwaukee shoulder"), hips, and knees. Radiographs can show soft tissue calcifications with or without bone erosions. Definitive diagnosis of the crystal type is only by electron microscopy with electron probe elemental analysis, x-ray diffraction, or infrared spectroscopy. Other basic calcium phosphates, such as octacalcium phosphate, can be seen along with the apatite. Synovial or bursal effusions can have many or few leukocytes. Serum studies are generally normal except that phosphate levels are often elevated in renal dialysis patients, who are at high risk of apatite deposition.

Apatite deposition can also be associated with scleroderma and the other connective tissue diseases, with repeated depot corticosteroid injections, with tumoral calcinosis due to renal phosphate retention, with central nervous system injury, and with high-dose vitamin D therapy. In most instances the cause of soft tissue apatite deposition is not known. Treatment for acute arthritis or periarthritis is with NSAID's or colchicine. Aspiration of crystals and local injection with depot corticosteroids can also be effective.

Doherty M, Holt M, MacMillan P, et al.: A reappraisal of "analgesic" hip. Ann Rheum Dis 45:272, 1986. *Destructive hip arthritis like the "Milwaukee shoulder" is felt to be related to apatite crystal deposition.*

Paul H, Reginato AJ, Schumacher HR: Alizarin red S staining as a screening test to detect calcium compounds in synovial fluid. Arthritis Rheum 26:191, 1983. *This describes a simple office screening test for apatite and other calcium-containing crystals.*

Pinals RS, Short CL: Calcific periarthritis involving multiple sites. Arthritis Rheum 9:566, 1966. *This recurrent calcific periarthritis is related to apatite crystals.*

Schumacher HR, Somlyo AP, Tse RL, et al.: Arthritis associated with apatite crystals. Ann Intern Med 87:411, 1977. *Clinical picture, diagnostic evaluation, and review.*

OXALATE CRYSTAL DEPOSITION DISEASE

Calcium oxalate deposition can occur in joints along with other tissues of patients with renal failure who are on chronic hemodialysis or peritoneal dialysis, producing radiographic evidence of soft tissue calcification or chondrocalcinosis. Acute or chronic joint effusions with intracellular crystals can be seen. Masses of vertebral oxalates can cause spinal cord compression. Diagnosis is made by identification of typical bipyramidal crystals in joint fluid or biopsy specimens. When less characteristic crystals are seen, other techniques as described under apatite deposition can be used. Vitamin C may potentiate oxalate deposition, so this might be avoided.

Hoffman EC, Schumacher HR, Paul H, et al.: Calcium oxalate microcrystalline-associated arthritis in end stage renal disease. Ann Intern Med 97:36, 1982. *Three cases with oxalosis and arthritis are described. Methods to identify oxalate crystals are included.*

Reginato AJ, Kurnik BRC: Calcium oxalate and other crystals associated with kidney disease and arthritis. Semin Arthritis Rheum 18:198, 1989. *Extensive oxalosis can involve skin, bursae, tendon sheaths, and joints, as well as kidneys and various viscera.*

GOUT

Monosodium urate (MSU) crystal deposition (see Color Plate 4C) in joints and other connective tissues accounts for the most frequent clinical manifestations of gout. The complex genetic, metabolic, and renal factors that interact to produce hyperuricemia and eventually gout are described in detail in Ch. 183. Gouty arthropathy and the gross tophaceous deposits in chronic gout are also described in Ch. 183 but are summarized here, as gout is the most common and prototypical of the crystal deposition diseases.

MSU crystals are rods or needles up to 15 to 20 μm in length and are brightly birefringent with negative elongation when viewed with compensated polarized light. Those from visible tophi or synovial microtophi tend to be more often needle-like. At least some crystals are intracellular during gouty arthritis. Leukocyte counts during attacks usually range from 10,000 to 50,000 per cubic millimeter, with 80 to 90 per cent neutrophils. Gout is most common in middle-aged men but is increasingly seen in women after the menopause and is very rarely noted in premenopausal women but may occur with chronic renal failure. A variety of lower extremity joints are commonly involved, in addition to the classic first metatarsophalangeal joint, but any joint or bursa, including those in the upper extremities, can be affected by either acute or chronic arthritis. Chronic or recurrent acute gout can be polyarticular, can mimic rheumatoid arthritis, and may be misdiagnosed, especially if the typical dramatic early short-lived attacks are not appreciated and synovial fluid is not examined. Tophaceous gout can slowly destroy joints. Crystals are often present in joint fluids even between attacks and may contribute to low-grade inflammation and joint damage.

Radiographs show only soft tissue swelling early in gout but later can reveal cystic erosions with thin, overhanging edges of bone suggestive of gout. Soft tissue tophi are common around joints, in bursae, in Achilles tendons, and at the extensor surface of the forearm; ear tophi appear to be less common than in the past. Gout should be recognized as a syndrome resulting from the many possible causes noted in Ch. 183.

Treatment of acute gouty arthritis can be with NSAID's (although relatively high doses are needed), oral or intravenous colchicine, adrenocorticotropic hormone (ACTH), or prednisone. The last two agents may be needed in complicated patients with renal failure, liver disease, or gastrointestinal disease. Joint aspiration with instillation of depot corticosteroids may also be used if a single joint is involved and infection is excluded. If recurrent attacks develop, chronic low doses of NSAID's or colchicine can suppress inflammation, but crystal accumulation will often continue. Thus, with more frequent attacks or visible tophi, patients should be considered for long-term lowering of urate levels with a uricosuric agent such as probenecid (if renal function is good and the patient is not overexcreting uric acid) or, in other cases, allopurinol, a xanthine oxidase inhibitor.

Lawry GV, Fan PT, Bluestone R: Polyarticular versus monoarticular gout. A prospective, comparative analysis of clinical features. Medicine 67:335, 1988. *Polyarticular gout and other crystal-associated diseases continue to be misdiagnosed without synovial fluid analysis. Fever and other constitutional symptoms are common.*

Wallace SL, Singer JZ: Therapy in gout. Rheum Dis Clin North Am 14:441, 1988. *Some of the complex situations involved in therapy of acute and chronic gout are reviewed. There are risks both from disease progression and from drug toxicities. Colchicine, NSAID'S and allopurinol all require care in appropriate use.*

272 Relapsing Polychondritis
H. Ralph Schumacher, Jr.

This uncommon disease is characterized by recurrent inflammation and destruction of cartilaginous and other connective tissue structures. Frequently involved cartilages are the pinnae of the ears, nasal cartilages, and tracheal rings. Polychondritis occurs nearly equally in both sexes and at any age, but with a peak of onset between the ages of 40 and 60.

The pathologic lesion seen by light microscopy consists of loss of matrix staining, predominantly superficial infiltration with polymorphonuclear neutrophils or lymphocytes, and eventual destruction of normal structures followed by fibrosis. Electron microscopy in addition shows alterations of superficial chondrocytes, matrix, and elastic fibers. The cause of polychondritis is unknown, but the location of lesions and frequency of associated systemic diseases suggest the importance of systemic factors. Antibodies to type II collagen and the presence of cell-mediated immunity to proteoglycan and type II collagen are evidence of immunologic aberrations.

Inflammation of the cartilaginous structures of the ears is the most common initial finding (see Color Plate 10*B*). There may be acute onset of pain and tenderness with erythema and swelling of one or both helices. The lobe is spared. Inner and middle ear involvement can occur, causing hearing loss or vertigo. Nasal cartilage involvement can produce a saddle nose. Laryngeal and tracheal disease can cause hoarseness or life-threatening upper respiratory obstruction. Ocular manifestations are common and include conjunctivitis, episcleritis, iridocyclitis, proptosis, and rarely other problems, such as optic neuritis. Antigens in the eye that are cross reactive with cartilage proteoglycans and their link protein have been identified.

Cardiac involvement, especially of the aortic root with aortic insufficiency, is seen in up to one fourth of cases. There may also be aortic aneurysms. Arthritis is reported in about three fourths of cases. This is generally nondestructive. Fever, rashes, oral or genital ulcers, and neurologic and renal disease can occur. Renal involvement can include glomerulonephritis and immunoglobulin A (IgA) nephropathy.

There are no diagnostic laboratory tests, although the erythrocyte sedimentation rate is often elevated. There may be anemia and leukocytosis. Roentgenograms can detect advanced tracheal narrowing. Cine computed tomographic (CT) scans and pulmonary function tests can detect more subtle airway obstruction.

Relapsing polychondritis is associated with other diseases in one third or more of cases. These include rheumatoid arthritis, systemic lupus erythematosus, Sjögren's syndrome, thyroid disease, ulcerative colitis, psoriasis, spondylarthropathies, Behçet's disease, vasculitis of various types, cryoglobulinemia, diabetes mellitus, biliary cirrhosis, panniculitis, malignancies, sinusitis, and mastoiditis. Lesions of Wegener's granulomatosis can mimic polychondritis.

In mild cases nonsteroidal anti-inflammatory agents can be used for symptomatic treatment, although adrenocorticosteroids in the range of 30 to 60 mg of prednisone per day are generally needed for acute inflammatory episodes and severe respiratory involvement. There is no evidence that steroids alter the long-term course of the disease. Immunosuppressives and cyclosporin A have been used with apparent benefit. Dapsone has been used with variable results in several series.

The course is unpredictable, with about 55 per cent of subjects surviving for 10 years. Infection and systemic vasculitis caused more deaths than did airway obstruction in a recent series. Remissions do occur. Aortic valve disease has required surgery.

Chang-Miller A, Okamura M, Torres VE, et al.: Renal involvement in relapsing polychondritis. Medicine 66:202, 1987. *Glomerulonephritis often responds to corticosteroids or cytotoxic agents.*

Ebringer B, Rook G, Swana T, et al.: Autoantibodies to cartilage and type II collagen in relapsing polychondritis and other rheumatic diseases. Ann Rheum Dis 40:473, 1981. *Immune mechanisms are described and discussed.*

Govet D, Marechaud R, Neu JPH, et al.: Relapsing polychondritis. A critical analysis of the therapeutic effectiveness of dapsone. Presse Med 13:723, 1984. *This interesting agent is not invariably effective.*

Michet CJ, McKenna CH, Luthra HS, et al.: Relapsing polychondritis. Survival and predictive role of early disease manifestations. Ann Intern Med 104:74, 1986. *Anemia, saddle nose deformity, and vasculitis appear to be poor prognostic signs.*

Pazirandeh M, Ziran BH, Khandelwal BK: Relapsing polychondritis and spondylarthropathies. J Rheum 15:630, 1988. *In addition to the many associated autoimmune diseases, one must also consider a possible relationship to psoriasis and spondylarthropathy.*

273 Osteoarthritis *(Degenerative Joint Disease)*
David S. Howell

Osteoarthritis is a complex response of joint tissues to aging and to genetic and environmental factors, characterized by degeneration of cartilage, bone remodeling, and overgrowth of bone. *Idiopathic osteoarthritis* refers to the common variety encountered during aging that is unrelated to known systemic or local diseases and includes certain hereditary and erosive subsets. *Secondary* osteoarthritis refers to the form that is indistinguishable from the idiopathic (primary) type on a pathologic basis but that is clearly provoked by antecedent events, such as an inflammatory, metabolic, endocrine, developmental, or heritable connective tissue disorder (Table 273–1). Effects of a macrotrauma, repeated microtrauma, or prolonged immobilization on normal joints may predispose the joints to secondary osteoarthritis.

When bone hypertrophy estimated by roentgenographic changes is used as a criterion, the majority of the population over 50 years of age is afflicted with osteoarthritis. By the eighth decade there is evidence of disease in 90 per cent of persons. It is the leading cause of joint pain and related disablements in middle-aged and elderly patients.

PATHOLOGY. Minor cartilage softening in non–weight-bearing sites and hypertrophic bone changes may persist a lifetime without producing symptoms. Osteoarthritis depends on development of progressively deepening clefts and erosions, typically in weight-bearing sites. The disease advances over a period of years but rarely reaches the level of severity seen in rheumatoid arthritis; i.e., there is rarely joint fusion or pannus formation, and major subluxations are uncommon.

The earliest histologic changes may be documented in the surface, subsurface, and deep zones of articular cartilage. These changes include loss of staining reactions for proteoglycans, with areas of cell injury, or loss followed by proliferation. Clefts, microcysts, and erosions arise at the site of these changes. Aggressive lesions consist usually of vertical clefts in cartilage, which progress to deep erosions and exposure of subchondral bone. Bone thickening, eburnation, cysts, and bone-on-bone contact across the joint surface typify end-stage disease.

ETIOLOGY. The most accepted premise is that primary changes in articular cartilage underlie development of osteoarthritis. Nevertheless, in a substantial subset of patients, biomechanical deficiencies arising from dysplasias of major or minor nature are causative. Similar biomechanical deficiencies may arise that are related to adolescent and adult remodeling of bones and abnormal distribution of weight-bearing forces (Table 273–1).

Repeated industrial or sports-invoked macrotraumatic and microtraumatic events may produce excessive wear and hypertrophic remodeling responses. Evidence has been obtained for

TABLE 273–1. ETIOLOGIC CLASSIFICATION OF OSTEOARTHRITIS*

Idiopathic (primary)
  Localized
    Hands: Heberden's nodes, erosive interphalangeal
      arthropathy
    Feet: hallux valgus, hammer toes; talonavicular osteoarthritis
    Knees: medial, lateral, patellofemoral compartments
    Hips: sites of cartilage loss—eccentric (superior), concentric (axial,
      medial), diffuse
    Spine: zygoapophyseal joints, osteophytes, intervertebral discs
      (spondylosis); ligaments, e.g., disseminated idiopathic skeletal
      hyperostosis
    Other single sites: shoulder, temporomandibular, carpometacarpal
      joints
  Generalized—Includes three or more areas listed above
  Mineral deposition diseases
    Calcium pyrophosphate deposition disease
    Hydroxyapatite arthropathy
    Destructive disease (e.g., Milwaukee shoulder)

Secondary
  Post-traumatic
  Congenital or developmental
    Legg-Calvé-Perthes hip dislocation
    Epiphyseal dysplasias
    Articular cartilage disorders associated with a gene deficiency (e.g.,
      association with type II procollagen gene mutation)
  Disturbed local tissue structure by primary disease, e.g., ischemic
    necrosis, tophaceous gout, hyperparathyroid cysts, Paget's disease,
    rheumatoid arthritis, osteopetrosis, osteochondritis
  Miscellaneous additional diseases
    Endocrine: diabetes mellitus, acromegaly, hypothyroidism
    Metabolic: hemochromatosis, ochronosis, Gaucher's
      disease
    Neuropathic arthropathies
    Miscellaneous: frostbite, Kashin-Beck disease, caisson
      disease
    Mechanical: obesity, unequal lower extremity length;
      valgus/varus deformities, ligamentous laxity (including
      associations with type I procollagen gene mutations of
      Ehlers-Danlos syndrome).

*Compiled, in part, by Osteoarthritis Diagnostic Criteria Committee. American Rheumatism Association, 1983.

reduced biomaterial properties of cartilage as a function of aging and for possible metabolic disturbances in cartilage metabolism, as in diabetes mellitus, acromegaly, and ochronosis.

The subchondral bone table is disturbed by tissue remodeling early in the disease or by such afflictions as Paget's disease or hyperparathyroidism with subchondral cysts. Hyperlaxity of ligaments per se or as part of certain overt (heritable) disorders of connective tissue can lead to osteoarthritis.

PATHOGENESIS. As a result of a multiplicity of etiologic factors, an apparent final common pathway of disease expression involves breakdown of cartilage both directly by physical injury and by enzymatic degradation resulting from injury to chondrocytes and indirectly by subchondral bone stiffening from remodeling. Most important in this context is injury of the collagen network or framework that holds articular cartilage together. This network retains in a semidehydrated conformed state the abundant, intensely hydrophilic, charged, proteoglycan macromolecules. The latter exert an osmotic pressure of several atmospheres against the network. Ungluing or cleavage of the collagen network by maldistributed or excessive weight-bearing forces or degradation of the network by enzymes elaborated by injured cartilage cells may occur. This response to various precipitating events leads to loss of essential elastic properties.

In early osteoarthritis, repair responses by local chondrocytes are usually of poor quality, leading to almost no replacement of lost tissue. From advanced erosions penetrating the marrow, tissue repair is more effective and consists of mixtures of fibrocartilage and hyaline cartilage. Normal rugged biomaterial properties are never recovered by the repair cartilage. As degeneration proceeds, wear particles and matrix degradation products are released from both original and repair cartilages. These fragments are carried to the synovial lining membrane, where a phagocytic response engenders low-grade inflammation and syn-

ovial effusion, proliferation of synovial cells, and thickening of the synovial membranes. Much evidence has accumulated that membrane-engendered inflammatory factors amplify cartilage breakdown.

Several biochemical abnormalities have been noted in osteoarthritic cartilage: increased water content, decreased aggregation and content of proteoglycans, decreased chain length and altered profiles of glycosaminoglycans, exposure of collagen epitopes indicative of enzymatic cleavage, and increased proteolytic enzyme levels.

CLINICAL MANIFESTATIONS. The clinical presentation may be divided into early and late stages. Throughout these stages, there is deep, aching pain in the afflicted joints, morning stiffness of short duration, and variable joint thickening and effusion. Early stages are dominated by pain on motion with stiffness, night pain, and responsiveness to anti-inflammatory medication. The late stages are dominated by joint instability, predominance of pain at rest that is accentuated on weight bearing, and failure to respond to anti-inflammatory agents. The present description of clinical features is developed largely on an anatomic basis inasmuch as signs and symptoms reflect regional patterns of involvement. Roentgenographic and laboratory workup and treatment are discussed later.

Hands. Heberden's nodes refer to the osteoarthritic disfigurements of distal interphalangeal joints, and Bouchard's nodes signify equivalent lesions of the proximal interphalangeal joints of the hands (Fig. 273–1). Early Heberden's nodes have a soft consistency and may be associated with prominent inflammatory signs. In the chronic stage, they are characterized by bony enlargement and angular deformities with variable symptoms.

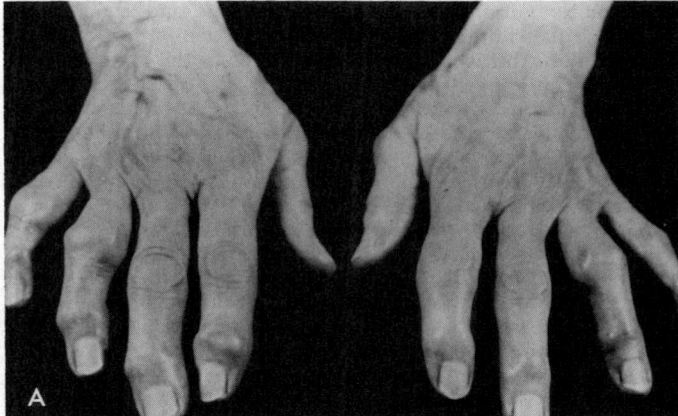
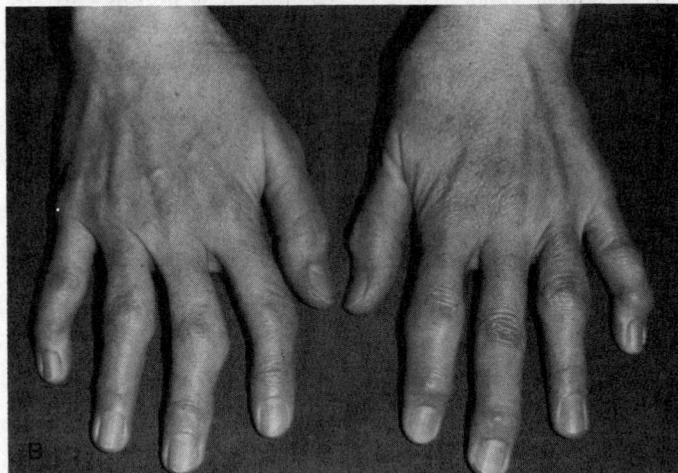

FIGURE 273–1. Typical hand deformities in osteoarthritis. *A,* Typical Heberden's and Bouchard's nodes comprise hypertrophic joint capsular and bony enlargement of the distal and proximal interphalangeal joints, respectively. *B,* Prominent Bouchard's nodes and minor subluxations may cause misdiagnosis of rheumatoid arthritis.

Heredity and sex, in addition to microtrauma, are prominently involved in the development of Heberden's nodes, which are more common in women at menopause or late middle age. The only other common hand lesion involves the first carpometacarpal joint. Such lesions are associated with pain in the radial side of the wrist, pain that is intensified by physical activities such as golf, tennis, and gardening.

Knees. The most common source of major disability in osteoarthritis is knee involvement. At any one time, heat, synovial thickening, or effusions have been documented in at least 50 per cent of cases. Elicitation of crepitus, which persists on repeated flexion and extension of the knee, bony marginal overgrowth, mediolateral instability (in the late stages), and synovial effusion are important diagnostic aids. Degenerative changes are usually more prominent in the medial compartment of the knee, leading to varus (bowleg) deformities. Developmental defects, i.e., knock-knee or bowleg deformity, predispose to osteoarthritis.

Degenerative alteration of the patellofemoral joint is termed chondromalacia patellae. This syndrome of mild effusion and knee pain is usually associated with trauma and occurs predominantly in young adults. It is usually preceded by developmental biomechanical disturbances influencing knee flexion. There is often spontaneous remission of symptoms, but some cases progress to irreversible patellofemoral osteoarthritis.

Hips. Clinical manifestations of primary hip joint disease appear usually in late middle or old age. Perhaps one third or more of cases arise from acetabular dysplasia, as well as growth or maturational disturbances in the femoral neck and head. Altered bone growth as well as developmental thickening at the zenith of the acetabulum may be causative in fewer than 5 per cent of cases. Beyond these factors, there is a background of adult bone remodeling and altered joint incongruity, which may further compromise normal weight-bearing patterns and chondrocyte nutrition. In addition, a variety of acquired disorders, such as rheumatoid arthritis and ischemic necrosis of the femoral head, are important etiologically.

Groin pain on weight bearing or motion is a dominant symptom and is usually referred to the anterior aspect of the thigh above the knee. Over a period of months or a few years, invalidism from severely restricted mobility and pain is a common outcome of untreated disease.

Spinal Osteoarthritis (Including Herniated Disc Syndrome). Throughout the spine, weight-bearing compressive forces are largely supported by one set of articulations—the intervertebral discs. These are elastic organs similar to articular cartilage in respect to the fact that they depend on properties of the semi-dehydrated proteoglycan molecules. A high osmotic pressure at rest results from proteoglycan confinement by cartilage endplates in two dimensions and the annulus fibrosus in the third. An additional important elastic component is provided by the annulus fibrosus. Rotary motions in the back and neck depend upon the zygoapophyseal joints. All of these joints undergo osteoarthritic changes almost identical in nature to those of the peripheral joints (see Ch. 275 for specific clinical features). Ordinarily, the former joints protect the latter against severe torsional trauma; under certain conditions, especially flexion of the lumbosacral spine, the rotary joints are of much less protectional value, and annular tears may occur under these (and several other) conditions. Resultant displacement of discal products into the spinal foramen adjacent to nerve rootlets and/or spinal canal occurs, depending on the conditions of damage. Injury of these structures both by mechanical trauma and by activated inflammatory pathways believed to involve neural peptides constitutes one of several causes of neural dysfunction leading to symptoms. The relationship of the posterior zygoapophyseal joints in the cervical, thoracic, and lumbar spines to their respective nerve roots as they traverse the intervertebral foramina, and the proximity of an additional set of *joints of Luschka* in the cervical spine (segments C2 to C7), have similar importance because of potential damage to nerves by inflammation secondary to mechanical irritation.

Notably, symptoms of osteoarthritis in the cervical spine depend upon the neural segment involved. Pain, aggravated by motion, often radiates into the supraclavicular and upper trapezius regions, as well as the occiput and distal upper extremities.

Overgrowth of bone in either the cervical or the lumbar spine can cause narrowing of the spinal canal and encroachment on the spinal cord rather than the nerve roots. In the neck, a myelopathy of a painless nature may result. Constriction of the spinal cord by surrounding bone, disc, or ligamentous thickening leads to the syndrome of spinal stenosis most common in the lumbosacral spine. Neurogenic claudication pain (resembling vascular claudication) is an important symptom in this condition and must be differentiated from vascular insufficiency (see Ch. 275 for management of discogenic claudication).

Diffuse Idiopathic Skeletal Hyperostosis. This is characterized by a flowing ligamentous calcification along the anterolateral aspects of vertebral bodies. Symptomatology is variable and focused in the spine or multiple tendon osseous junctions (e.g., at the heel); ankylosis of apophyseal and sacroiliac joints is absent. The thoracic spine is most often affected without intervertebral disc narrowing.

LABORATORY FINDINGS. There are no specific clinical tests for osteoarthritis despite recent evidence for the elevation of levels of soluble cartilage-specific breakdown products in synovial fluid and serum. The sedimentation rate is usually within normal limits, synovial fluid is clear and exhibits a normal range of viscosity, and there is a negative mucin clot test result. Leukocyte counts in synovial fluid generally vary from 150 to 1500 per cubic millimeter; wear particles including whole fragments containing proteoglycans and collagen fibers as well as mineral particles are often identified in the fluid.

ROENTGENOGRAPHIC FEATURES. There is usually narrowing of the radiolucent interosseous joint space resulting from destruction of articular cartilage. Bony cysts varying in size may be seen in subchondral or denuded bone, which may be densely sclerotic. Osteophyte formation at the margins of affected joints is the basis for the most striking roentgenographic findings. Degeneration of lumbar and cervical intervertebral discs results in narrowing of the interspaces. A vacuum sign or marked translucency in the disc may be seen. High-resolution computed tomography (CT) and magnetic resonance imaging (MRI) are important steps in the assessment of spinal lesions and occasionally of osteoarthritis in shoulder, hips, and knees. Oblique views are also valuable for defining bony sclerosis and joint space narrowing of the zygoapophyseal joints of the lumbar spine.

DIFFERENTIAL DIAGNOSIS. Osteoarthritis and rheumatoid arthritis are readily distinguished in terms of their usual clinical presentation. The latter is generally associated with prominent signs of joint inflammation, characteristically afflicting the hands and wrists symmetrically, especially the metacarpophalangeal joints. These joints almost never are affected in osteoarthritis.

Differentiation of these disorders is more complicated when seronegative rheumatoid arthritis involves only (or predominantly) the lower extremities. The presence of a normal erythrocyte sedimentation rate, negative serum rheumatoid factor test result, and minimal synovial fluid change supports the diagnosis of osteoarthritis. Despite severe deformities, occasionally seen with Heberden's and Bouchard's nodes, the lack of ulnar drift and metacarpophalangeal and diffuse wrist involvement help to rule out rheumatoid arthritis. Erosive osteoarthritis characteristically shows bone destruction and inflammatory changes in the proximal and distal interphalangeal joints but not in the metacarpophalangeal joints.

Secondary osteoarthritis must be considered in the presence of joint hypermobility, chondrocalcinosis, heritable disorders such as the Ehlers-Danlos syndrome, mechanical derangements of the joints, metabolic bone disorders, ochronosis, neuropathies, and hemochromatosis. Spinal involvement in osteoarthritis is distinctly different from that in ankylosing spondylitis; the latter predominantly afflicts young men and has characteristic and distinctive roentgenographic features involving sacroiliac sclerosis and fusion, calcification and ossification of the annulus fibrosus and adjacent paravertebral ligaments, and formation of bridging syndesmophytes (bamboo spine).

TREATMENT. Although treatment depends in large measure on the site and severity of joint involvement, the outlook with a multidisciplinary long-term management program is relatively optimistic for functional restoration and symptomatic improvement.

Early disease with signs of mild to moderate inflammation but without joint instability can usually be managed successfully with a combination of measures: (1) Pain may be relieved with mild analgesics (e.g., acetaminophen, 500 mg three or four times a day) or nonsteroidal anti-inflammatory drugs (NSAID's) (e.g., aspirin, 2400 to 3600 mg daily) or both. Indomethacin, ibuprofen, naproxen, fenoprofen, piroxicam, sulindac diclofenac, and tolmetin are alternative agents, advantageous as substitutes for aspirin. Where possible, intermittent rather than continuous usage is encouraged to avoid gastrointestinal side effects, especially acid peptic disease. There is a well-documented substantial morbidity in respect to gastrointestinal intolerance to NSAID's, especially during prolonged usage. Use of gastric protective agents is advised almost routinely (e.g., antacids, histamine-2 receptor blockers, and hydrogen ion pump inhibitors (see Ch. 98). (2) Revision of daily schedule of activities, increased joint rest, and selected avoidance of activities unfavorable to the symptomatic joints must be practiced. (3) The joints must be protected with relevant devices, i.e., splints, crutches, walkers, canes, and so on. (4) Weight-reducing diets must be used. (5) Application of moist heat or cold packs may help. (6) Symptomatic response, in refractory cases, to intra-articular or para-articular injections of small amounts of corticosteroid at infrequent intervals is useful. (7) Once pain and muscle spasm have been relieved, a formalized program of physical therapy followed by a prolonged home exercise program is often recommended in the hope of retarding further joint deterioration.

In the case of cervical osteoarthritis, hyperextension and hyperflexion should be avoided. The patient should sleep flat on one pillow. A cervical collar restricts motion and minimizes pain. (See Ch. 275 for treatment of osteoarthritis in the lumbar spine.)

The principal anatomic regions that are most benefited by orthopedic surgery are the knee, hip, and spine. Several surgical procedures are appropriate for patients with severe hip involvement—wedge osteotomy, various arthroplasties, including total joint replacement, and arthrodesis. For the knee, debridement, either through an arthroscope or via open surgery, osteotomy, and a variety of partial or complete arthroplasties are used for treatment. Tibial or femoral osteotomies may be of long-term benefit by realigning weight-bearing forces, but considerable follow-up rehabilitation is required. Otherwise, joint replacement is the treatment of choice for many cases of advanced osteoarthritis of the knees characterized by intractable pain, loss of function, instability, or all three. Some indications for spinal surgery are: (1) advancing intractable nerve deficits, (2) spinal instability, and (3) spinal stenosis affecting bladder or rectal function because of autonomic nerve involvement.

Altman RD (ed): Pain in osteoarthritis (symposium). Semin Arthritis Rheum 18(S2):1, 1989. *A review of recent progress in research on pain production in various forms of osteoarthritis, presented, for the most part, in terms understandable to practicing physicians.*
McCarty DJ (ed.): Arthritis and Allied Disorders. Philadelphia, Lea & Febiger, 1989, pp 1571–1641. *A comprehensive coverage of multiple important topics, well illustrated with radiographs and clarifying tables.*
Moskowitz RW, Howell DS, Goldberg VM, et al. (eds.): Osteoarthritis: Diagnosis and Management. 2nd ed. Philadelphia, W.B. Saunders Company, in press. *Detailed reference emphasizing both medical and surgical approaches of regional and general importance, readily individualized to the patient.*

274 The Painful Shoulder

David S. Howell

Shoulder pain is a common source of incapacitation and can result from numerous causes. Intrathoracic, diaphragmatic, and cervical pathologic lesions all can cause pain referred to the shoulder, a fact that deserves early consideration and strong emphasis. A characteristic of intrinsic painful disorders is that they often originate in periarticular soft structures—synovial membranes, tendons, and associated muscles. These structures have a unique role in joint stabilization. Loading forces are attenuated by the action of muscles across the coordinated bearings—glenohumeral, acromioclavicular, and sternoclavicular joints—as well as across the scapulothoracic surfaces. Multiple bursae and tendons near their attachment sites, particularly the rotator cuff tendons, are subject to microinjury and inflammation. Secondary recurrent pain and muscle spasm occur, followed by atrophic or reflex dystrophic responses or both. The most common disorders afflicting these structures are briefly reviewed in this chapter.

CALCIFIC TENDINITIS. A frequently encountered cause of painful shoulder is focal injury or degeneration of the rotator cuff tendons. Roentgenograms reveal calcium-containing minerals in the tendons of the rotator cuff in roughly 3 per cent of middle-aged persons, usually from prior insults. Mineral deposits in tendinous sites may engender bursal inflammation of variable intensity. Acute shoulder pain with radiation into the upper arm and neck is common. Associated muscle hypertonicity with limitation of shoulder motion and guarding, exquisite local tenderness over the inflamed site, and pain on motion or during prolonged rest are prominent. Most often, roentgenograms show linear densities in the supraspinatus, infraspinatus, or subscapularis tendons. Occasionally, a diffuse calcific pattern in the subacromial bursa is seen. Evidence of acute inflammation usually subsides within 1 week, but subacute rotator cuff tendinitis may persist or recur for months to years.

Management is conditioned by the duration and intensity of attacks. Adequate early pain relief is of paramount importance and is usually attainable by use of moist heat or ice compresses; rest, including arm support; analgesics; and a nonsteroidal anti-inflammatory drug (NSAID). Newer agents are discussed in Ch. 258. In most patients, pain and muscle spasm subside with variable reduction of mineral deposits. Injection of an adrenocorticosteroid derivative commonly hastens symptomatic recovery.

Follow-up evaluation is important to assess completeness of recovery. Residual loss of strength or joint motion or chronic pain deserves a conscientious program of active exercises, including both supervised therapy in a physical medicine facility and a home program of daily exercise. Long-term physical therapy or surgical excision of mineral deposits is seldom necessary.

BICIPITAL TENDINITIS. Inflammation of this tendon and synovial sheath is a frequent cause of shoulder pain. The tendon through attrition may subluxate from the bicipital groove or rupture. Localized tenderness on palpation with accentuation of pain by flexion or extension of the elbow against resistance or by internal rotation and abduction distinguishes the diagnosis clinically.

Treatment includes moist heat or ice compresses, rest, and NSAID's in the acute stages, and frequently the instillation of corticosteroids. Chronic recurrent disease is suggestive of the aforementioned mechanical derangements or an additional rotator cuff tear. Surgical transfer of the tendon may lead to satisfactory recovery.

ROTATOR CUFF TEARS. After heavy work, sports, or accidental injury, degenerative lesions in the rotator cuff often engender breakdown with moderate to major tendinous and ligamentous tears, predominantly in middle-aged persons. Complete rupture of the rotator cuff renders the arm incapable of abduction to 90 degrees. With mild tears, there is pain between 60 and 90 degrees of abduction. Either preceding or following these tears, an impingement syndrome frequently occurs at the coracoacromial arch. Often this is associated radiographically with cysts or sclerosis of the greater tuberosity of the humerus, osteophytes at the anterior margin of the acromion, and narrowing of the distance between the humeral head and acromion. These changes are related to trauma from impingement of the aforementioned bones. Since the rotator cuff forms, in part, the roof of the glenohumeral joint and floor of the subacromial and subdeltoid bursae, tears in the cuff permit synovial joint fluid extrusion into these bursae—demonstrable by arthrogram.

Primary treatment of rotator cuff tears consists of heat and aspirin, 2.4 to 3.6 gm per day, or other NSAID's, such as ibuprofen, 1200 to 2400 mg per day. Partial immobilization and exercise programs are indicated for incomplete tears. When these measures fail, surgical repair is often required.

ADHESIVE CAPSULITIS. This (frozen shoulder) disability of middle-aged persons develops more commonly in women than in men and is of unknown etiology. The diagnosis is suspected when persons with no primary shoulder disease develop active and passive restricted motion of the glenohumeral joint attended by increasing pain in the shoulder over a period of weeks to months, and it is more certain when an arthrogram shows a contracted joint capsule. Fibrosis is seen on pathologic study. Rotator cuff tears, hemarthroses, anterior shoulder capsule tear, psychophysiologic shoulder dysfunction, and shoulder-hand syndrome can all cause immobile painful shoulders and may be confused with adhesive capsulitis.

The key feature of management is prevention of severe pain through early use of heat, analgesics, range-of-motion exercises, and, if these are unsuccessful, the judicious use of intra-articular or systemic corticosteroids.

Manipulation mobilization under general anesthesia followed by a course of intensive physical therapy rarely is required for advanced disease.

SHOULDER-HAND SYNDROME. Shoulder pain and stiffness concurrent with pain, swelling, and vasomotor changes in the hands, wrists, and arms of various intensity and duration characterize this syndrome. Thickening of the skin and edema may follow, resembling Sudeck's atrophy. A small percentage of patients eventually develop adhesive capsulitis and sclerodactyly. This syndrome, which affects patients over age 50 years and follows acute severe illness, such as cerebrovascular accident, myocardial infarction, and trauma to the distal upper extremity, is believed to be caused by reflex sympathetic stimulation. Associated changes of cervical osteoarthritis probably have a minor role if any. When the disease is bilateral, the differentiation from acute rheumatoid arthritis or polymyalgia rheumatica may be difficult. The most important feature of treatment is aggressive physical therapy assisted by analgesics and prednisone in a short, moderate-dosage trial of 20 to 30 mg per day for 3 weeks, tapered at the end of the course. Stellate ganglion blocks and local corticosteroid injections are sometimes employed.

AMYLOID ARTHROPATHY. In two thirds of patients, shoulder involvement is present, usually secondary to myeloma. There is para-articular infiltration with amorphous amyloid fibers, causing the "shoulder pad sign." Acute inflammatory signs are usually absent (see Ch. 197).

ISCHEMIC NECROSIS. This disease is half as common in the humeral head as in the hip. Diffuse shoulder pain precedes conventional radiologic changes, the most helpful of which is an irregular translucent band localized in subchondral bone.

POLYMYALGIA RHEUMATICA. This syndrome is often characterized by severely painful shoulders and upper arms in aged persons with anemia, high sedimentation rates, and a negative rheumatoid factor test, and in a small percentage of cases, temporal arteritis and retinal ischemia threatening to vision (see Ch. 518). The dramatic response of shoulder pain to low-dose corticosteroid administration (prednisone, 10 mg per day) is characteristic.

MILWAUKEE SHOULDER. This syndrome consists of a painful, destructive, bilateral arthropathy in middle-aged and elderly patients with capsular calcification, joint effusions, and a high frequency of eroded rotator cuff tendons. Synovial fluids are virtually free of inflammatory cells despite a reported high collagenase activity.

Kozin F: Painful shoulder and the reflex sympathetic dystrophy syndrome. In McCarty DJ (ed.): Arthritis and Allied Conditions. Philadelphia, Lea & Febiger, 1989, pp 1509–1544. *Detailed coverage of etiopathogenesis, differential diagnosis and management; 301 references.*

Post M: The painful shoulder. Clin Orthop 173:2, 1983. *A symposium by multiple authors on various clinically important syndromes and discussion of current management.*

275 The Painful Back
David S. Howell

The back is a complex structure serving weight-bearing and locomotor functions. It provides for major support of body structures and transmission of loading forces through the sacroiliac joints to the lower limbs. The fundamental functioning unit is an articular triad composed of two zygoapophyseal joints posteriorly and the intervertebral disc anteriorly. The disc is composed of a nucleus pulposus encompassed by the annulus fibrosus. These structures are arranged in a series and stabilized throughout the spine by ligaments. The spinal bones also encase the spinal cord and the cauda equina and through successive foramina rootlets connect the spinal cord with peripheral neural pathways. (See Ch. 273 for detailed discussion of the cervical spine, Ch. 259 for the spondyloarthropathies, and Ch. 490 for intervertebral disc disease.)

ETIOLOGY OF BACK PAIN. In Table 275–1, the numerous causes of back pain are displayed according to disease subgroups. Although all vertebral levels can be affected, pain in the low back is most prevalent. The majority of patients present with problems relating to functional or mechanical disturbances, and these must be distinguished from a wide variety of diseases either of focal origin or referred from multiple organ systems. Among degenerative diseases, low back pain is a leading cause of industrial absenteeism and chronic disablement.

MEDICAL HISTORY. *Sex.* Compression vertebral fractures from osteoporosis have their highest prevalence in postmenopausal women. Gynecologic pathology, such as endometriosis, is the basis for some referred patterns of back pain. Reiter's disease, ankylosing spondylitis, and back injuries are found more commonly in males.

Age. Young people with back pain most commonly suffer from muscle or ligament strains, congenital abnormalities, injury, spondyloarthropathies, and herniated disc syndromes. In middle and old age, osteoporosis, vertebral collapse, degenerative states, including spinal stenosis, and malignant lesions are common.

Family History. Familial patterns of segregation are often detected in respect to spondyloarthropathies and uncommonly in respect to spinal degenerative conditions.

Nature of Pain. Events or conditions that accelerate or retard symptoms should be explored. The chronic inflammatory diseases

TABLE 275–1. ETIOLOGY OF BACK PAIN

Mechanical or Traumatic
Paraspinal ligaments and musculature
  Myofascial syndrome, sacroiliac strain
Spondylogenic
  Osteoarthritis-related lesions—zygoapophyseal joints
  Degenerative lesions—intervertebral discs
  Mechanical insufficiency, congenital and acquired, of ligaments and bones
  Spondylolisthesis
  Spinal stenosis
  Fractures
Metabolic
Vertebral bodies, partial collapse and distortion—osteoporosis; osteomalacia—Paget's disease—often with secondary osteoarthritis
Tumors
Neural tumors, osteosarcoma, metastatic tumors, e.g., from breast, thyroid, kidney
Myeloma, lymphoma, leukemia
Systemic Inflammatory Disease
Spondylitis (ankylosing)—Reiter's disease; psoriatic or enteropathic arthropathy
Disseminated ankylosing skeletal hyperostosis
Infections
Pyogenic, fungal, tuberculous disc infection, herpes zoster infection, paraspinal abscesses
Referred Pain
Vascular—aneurysms, sclerosis of aorta and branches
Tumors or inflammation of pleural, pulmonary, pericardial, cardiac, or neck origin
Viscerogenic disease of gallbladder, pancreas, stomach, intestines, kidneys, ureters, bladder, prostate, uterus
Pelvic or retroperitoneal tumors or inflammation
Nonorganic Components
Hysterical conversion
Learned painful behavior
Psychosis
Litigation neurosis, malingering
Chronic pain syndrome
Substance abuse

(spondyloarthropathies) are associated with increased pain and stiffness on inactivity. Patients with lumbar disc protrusion and radicular pain generally are relieved by lying flat with the knees flexed and are uncomfortable sitting. Sudden or acute onset of symptoms is suggestive of a mechanical or infectious origin of symptoms, respectively. Constitutional symptoms such as fever, weight loss, and fatigue are important clues to infectious, inflammatory, or neoplastic disorders.

In regard to localization, the dorsal segment suggests osteoarthritis, vertebral fracture, neoplasm, herpetic radiculitis, or referred pain from the viscera (see later paragraph). Localization of pain in the low back is usually of little help in regard to differential diagnosis.

Claudication-type pain, with onset after sustained walking, suggests either spinal stenosis or arterial insufficiency. The former condition often refers pain to the thigh and is poorly relieved by standing still. Usually neurogenic claudication is relieved by sitting, whereas vascular claudication is reduced by standing.

Referred Pain. A deep aching pain referred to various sites in the upper and midback may be engendered by lesions in the upper gastrointestinal tract. Pain of malignancy (whether local or referred) is typically severe and unrelieved by change of position or mild analgesics.

In respect to neuropathic symptoms, alteration of the structure of the vertebral foramina may lead to radicular dissemination of pain. In such instances, compression or traction of nerve rootlets or extension of inflammation to them can lead to sensory and motor nerve symptoms and signs, i.e., paresthesias, hypoesthesias, and muscle weakness.

Symptomatology. Discogenic pain is characteristically aggravated by cough or sneeze. Rarely, loss of bowel or urinary sphincter function can result from cord compression or bilateral involvement of sacral nerve roots from spinal stenosis, tumors, or infectious lesions.

PHYSICAL EXAMINATION. General examination of the back is discussed in Ch. 254. Descriptions here are confined to vertebral compression fractures, degenerative disc disease, and lumbosacral strains and sprains.

Lumbosacral Strain. This and related myofascial syndromes are the most common ailments seen in the office practice of rheumatology. A history of injury is often followed by prompt or delayed low back pain. Transient disc prolapse, subluxation of facet joints, and injury to muscles or ligaments are diagnostic considerations. Physical signs are usually limited to paravertebral muscle spasm, tenderness, and restricted lower back motion without evidence of nerve root involvement.

Vertebral Compression Fractures. These are the most common complication of osteoporosis, with the resultant traction or compression of rootlets adjacent to collapsed vertebrae. Severe pain may begin suddenly, associated with the postural strain of lifting heavy objects or hyperflexing the trunk. Major physical findings consist of localized tenderness and muscle spasm related to the level of the nerve roots affected. Poorly localized back pain may be associated with osteoporosis in the absence of vertebral collapse. Metastatic tumor, myeloma, and metabolic bone disease, especially osteopenia of aging, are common underlying conditions.

Discogenic Disease. The most common form of low back pain with radiculitis is associated with prolapse, protrusion, or extrusion of intervertebral disc substance (see Ch. 490). Usually the onset of acute symptoms is preceded by chronic intermittent low back pain, although a discrete injury may precipitate an attack. Ninety per cent of disc herniations are localized at L4–L5 or L5–S1 levels. Discs involving the L4 nerve root may cause pain referred along the course of the femoral nerve upon hip extension and knee flexion. Knee extension may be weak and the patellar reflex reduced or absent. Patients with L5 nerve root disturbance complain of classic sciatic distribution of pain, i.e., radiating to the posterior thigh and the anteromedial leg and foot, in association with weakness of the toe extensors. First sacral radiculopathy is associated with pain over the posterior thigh, calf, and heel, weakness of the ankle and toe flexors, and reduced or absent Achilles tendon reflex. Frequently, loss of neurologic function is subtle and requires repeated testing to document. A positive response to straight-leg raising is most frequently indicative of L4–L5 or L5–S1 disc protrusion. Usually there is pain on hip flexion with the knee extended and absence of pain on

repetition of hip flexion with the knee flexed (Lasègue's sign). The cauda equina syndrome is a form of spinal stenosis and is an uncommon but important complication of massive disc prolapse. In the cauda equina syndrome, central midline disc displacement causes paralysis of the sacral root with bladder and bowel dysfunction. It is characterized by severe bilateral leg pain, urinary retention, weakness of the anal sphincter, and bilateral nerve root abnormalities. Once complete neurologic block has occurred, deceptively pain is often alleviated, and the patient will require a neurologic examination to verify the need for emergency surgery.

Spondylolisthesis. This condition, which refers to forward displacement of one vertebra on another, commonly involves the L4–L5 and L5–S1 levels. Bursts of segmental severe girdle pain are typical, often worse on activity and relieved by rest.

LABORATORY PROCEDURES. These are dictated by the results of medical history and physical examination. Simple radiographs of the back may suffice if a traumatic injury is causative. In instances of suspected metabolic disturbance, appropriate screening tests, such as serum calcium, phosphorus, and alkaline phosphatase measurements, should be obtained. Complete blood counts, sedimentation rate, urinalysis, and automated serum chemical profiles are sometimes justified to clarify the diagnosis. Anemia and an elevated sedimentation rate should prompt a more extensive search for infectious, inflammatory, and neoplastic diseases.

RADIOGRAPHIC STUDIES. *Routine Radiographic Studies.* These include frontal, lateral, and oblique films of the lumbosacral spine, which can demonstrate foraminal encroachment, compression fractures, degenerative changes, and subluxation of zygapophyseal joints, as well as interspace narrowing (see Ch. 272). There may be severe degenerative changes on the radiographs, with few or no relevant symptoms, and severe back pain may occur in the absence of significant radiographic signs and be of discogenic origin.

Additional Imaging Procedures. When surgical intervention is planned or a diagnosis remains questionable and requires an imperative answer and high resolution, computed tomography (CT) and magnetic resonance (MRI) imaging (noninvasive) are increasingly preferred to myelography. It is not usually necessary to perform a discogram (injection of radiopaque dye directly into the disc). When osteomyelitis or neoplastic involvement is likely, radionuclide bone scans are helpful. A percutaneous vertebral biopsy under fluoroscopic guidance may be performed to establish histopathologic diagnosis or bacteriologic diagnosis at highly suspicious sites obvious from scans or radiographs. Electromyography can confirm the presence of nerve root deficits.

MANAGEMENT. Conservative therapy for mechanical disorders of the spine and disc herniation focuses on bed rest, analgesics, and anti-inflammatory medication. Use of long-term anti-inflammatory agents should be accompanied by prophylactic protection against peptic ulceration. Application of moist heat, e.g., hydrocollator packs wrapped with a wet towel, may relieve pain and muscle spasm. The amount of bed rest is dependent on the severity of symptoms. After bed rest, gradual ambulation and a program of exercises, together with back protection including a lumbosacral support, are recommended. Most cases of disc herniation respond to conservative therapy; those unresponsive require further measures, including epidural steroids and nerve root or sleeve infiltrations with steroids. Before surgery is indicated, a psychological assessment and exercises emphasizing back stretching and abdominal strengthening should be attempted.

Progressive muscular weakness and progressive neurologic deficit despite bed rest and other aforementioned measures, as well as the cauda equina syndrome, are indications for surgery. Relative indications for laminectomy are severe pain, unrelieved by bed rest, and recurrent episodes of incapacitating pain. Ninety to 95 per cent improvement following surgery is anticipated, although 70 per cent of patients experience relief of pain whether or not the disc is removed.

Following either conservative therapy or surgery, a program of prophylactic management includes postural education, performance of a daily exercise program to strengthen the lumbar and abdominal muscles, and avoidance of lower spine stress. Besides laminectomy, joint fusion for spondylolisthesis and discogenic disease or unroofing procedures for spinal stenosis are sometimes necessary. Myelography, CT scans, or MRI is indicated preoperatively to establish definitively the nature and extent of disease as well as the level of vertebral involvement.

Acute symptoms from compression fractures require appropriate rest and relief of pain with analgesics. Activities must be selected to avoid additional compression fractures. (See Ch. 238 for management of osteoporosis.)

Brown MD, Rydevik B: Advances in the understanding and treatment of low back pain and sciatica. Orthop Clin North Am 22: April, 1991. *An overview of the present management of low back pain, with emphasis on controlled trials and newer diagnostic techniques.*

Manmiche C, Hessels EG, Bentzen L, et al.: Clinical trials of intensive muscle training for chronic low back pain. Lancet 2:862, 1988. *An appropriate program is described for motivated patients with pain refractory to conventional measures.*

Weber H: Lumbar disc herniation: A controlled prospective study with 10 years of observation. Spine 8:131, 1983. *A classic set of observations on the natural history of the disease and discussion of management.*

276 Systemic Diseases in Which Arthritis Is a Feature

Eugene V. Ball

Eleven per cent of adult Americans interviewed in the National Health Survey claimed to have had one or more episodes of painful joints over a period of 6 weeks. Much of this pain was probably due to soft tissue rheumatism and common rheumatic diseases, such as osteoarthritis and rheumatoid arthritis, that are defined by their own attributes and not by associated signs. The arthralgias of a fraction of these persons might have represented early symptoms of systemic diseases diagnosable only by the later appearance of other clinical signs or by laboratory testing. Table 276–1 illustrates the applicability of general medical laboratory tests to the evaluation of nonspecific joint symptoms. The tests afford significant diagnostic clues for certain systemic diseases in which arthralgias can be the earliest and only symptoms. Brief descriptions of musculoskeletal manifestations of a few systemic disorders follow.

PRIMARY BILIARY CIRRHOSIS (see Ch. 122)

More than half of women with primary biliary cirrhosis (PBC) may have serologic abnormalities, such as rheumatoid factors and antinuclear antibodies, in addition to antimitochondrial antibodies. A large number, primarily in this group, have joint pains or

TABLE 276–1. LABORATORY TESTS IN THE EVALUATION OF NONSPECIFIC JOINT SYMPTOMS

Test	Disease
Liver function tests	Primary biliary cirrhosis; chronic active hepatitis
Calcium and phosphorus	Hyperparathyroidism
Serum protein electrophoresis	Hypogammaglobulinemic arthritis; primary amyloidosis
Serum iron and total iron-binding capacity; ferritin	Hemochromatosis
Lipase or amylase	Pancreatic-arthritis syndrome
Thyroxine (T_4), thyroid-stimulating hormone (TSH)	Thyroid myopathy or arthritis
Complete blood count	Leukemia; sickle cell disease
Lipid analysis	Hyperlipidemia-associated arthritis
Partial thromboplastin time	Vasculopathy; hemophilia
Rapid plasma reagin (RPR) or VDRL	Vasculopathy; syphilis
Anti-HIV (human immunodeficiency virus) antibody	HIV arthritis
Antiparvovirus antibody	Parvovirus arthritis

outright rheumatic disease, mainly rheumatoid arthritis, Sjögren's syndrome, or limited scleroderma (CREST syndrome: calcinosis, Raynaud's phenomenon, esophageal dysmotility, sclerodactyly, and telangiectasia). Other defined causes for bone or joint pains in PBC include osteomalacia and hypertrophic osteoarthropathy.

HEMOCHROMATOSIS (see Ch. 193)

Arthritis is frequently the first sign of hemochromatosis and eventually develops in as many as half of all persons with the disease. Typically occurring between the ages of 40 and 50, the arthritis of hemochromatosis has been reported in persons younger than 30 and is easily overlooked or confused with primary osteoarthritis, even though their distributions often differ. It may also be dismissed as idiopathic tendinitis or bursitis. Pain and stiffness frequently appear first in the metacarpophalangeal joints; other joints involved commonly include the wrists, hips, and knees. Signs of inflammation are negligible except during episodes of pseudogout. Chondrocalcinosis is common on radiographs, as are subchondral cysts, sclerosis, and joint space narrowing. The arthritis is not altered by phlebotomy; treatment is symptomatic and may necessitate arthroplasties, particularly in the hips.

SICKLE CELL DISEASE AND OTHER HEMOGLOBINOPATHIES (see Ch. 136)

Almost all persons with sickle cell disease experience musculoskeletal symptoms. Large joint arthritis lasting a few days to a few weeks results from small vessel occlusion caused by local sickling. The aseptic bone infarcts of SC (or less often SS) disease resemble osteomyelitis, which is far more common in persons with sickle cell disease than in normal persons and is often caused by *Salmonella*. Osteonecrosis occurs in both SS and SC disease, often in the head of the femur; however, multiple areas may be infarcted. Hyperuricemia attributable to SS disease has culminated in gout in older patients. Pain due to microfractures in the lower leg, ankle, or foot, lasting up to 1 to 2 years, has been described in almost one half of a group of 50 patients with beta-thalassemia.

HYPOGAMMAGLOBULINEMIA (see Ch. 244 and 287)

Arthritis as a complication of hypogammaglobulinemia is most typical of the X-linked variety (Bruton's disease) in children; however, it also occurs in other types of primary hypogammaglobulinemia. Septic arthritis is caused by common pathogens or by mycoplasmal organisms such as *Ureaplasma urealyticum*. Nonerosive arthritis, without evidence of infection or other demonstrable cause, often resolves following institution of immunoglobulin therapy. Its resolution with treatment does not necessarily constitute *a priori* evidence of an infectious etiology. Intravenous gamma globulin treatment might suppress arthritis through its complex modulating effect on the immune system (for example, it has been shown to increase suppressor T cell functional activity).

WHIPPLE'S DISEASE (see Ch. 102)

The arthritis of Whipple's disease mimics that of rheumatic fever in some respects. It is painful; there is often warmth, redness, and swelling; it favors large joints; subcutaneous nodules have been noted in a few patients; recurrences are common; and it can be migratory. Less often, small joints of the hands and feet are inflamed, and the arthritis becomes chronic and resembles rheumatoid arthritis. The synovial fluid white cell count is sometimes elevated to 50,000 per cubic millimeter, and rod-shaped bacilli may be identified, usually by electron microscopy, in synovial biopsies. Rheumatoid factors and antinuclear antibody are not features of Whipple's disease. The arthritis may antedate gastrointestinal symptoms by years, making diagnosis difficult.

HYPERLIPOPROTEINEMIA (see Ch. 172)

An association exists between type II familial hypercholesterolemia (both homozygous and heterozygous forms) and musculoskeletal symptoms such as Achilles tendinitis, oligoarthritis, and polyarthritis. Transient pain in the Achilles tendon appears to be more common than frank inflammatory tendinitis, which can last a few days and recur two or three times yearly. A few patients have acute painful monoarthritis or pauciarthritis of the knees, ankles, or small joints that lasts a week or more and recurs frequently. Less common is an incapacitating polyarthritis resembling rheumatic fever, persisting a month or more. In one study, 40 per cent of 73 heterozygous patients were symptomatic; articular manifestations appeared at times before the xanthomas that are the major diagnostic sign of familial hypercholesterolemia. Arthritis may also be a feature of type IV hyperlipoproteinemia.

ENDOCRINE DISORDERS (see Ch. 213, 216, and 235)

Aches and stiffness simulating fibrositis may appear early in hypothyroidism; untreated, this may progress to proximal myopathy with elevated creatine kinase levels, simulating polymyositis, or to a syndrome of synovial thickening and joint effusions, simulating rheumatoid arthritis. There also appears to be an association of hypothyroidism with calcium pyrophosphate deposition disease. Unlike myopathy and arthritis, carpal tunnel syndrome is a common manifestation of hypothyroidism. Hyperthyroidism may cause myopathy without elevations of the creatine kinase level but with muscle wasting, which may be severe. Thyroid acropachy, seen rarely in association with pretibial myxedema and Graves' disease, is characterized by diffuse swelling of the fingers and clubbing.

Hyperparathyroidism is another cause of diffuse, vague musculoskeletal pains resembling those of fibrositis. The other musculoskeletal complications of hyperparathyroidism include back pain due to vertebral body fractures; an erosive arthritis predominantly in the hands and wrists; and chondrocalcinosis (with pseudogout occurring most often after parathyroidectomy).

Carpal tunnel syndrome has been reported in almost one half of persons with acromegaly. Raynaud's phenomenon is rare. The arthritis of acromegaly is clinically indistinguishable from osteoarthritis.

SARCOIDOSIS (see Ch. 67)

Joint or juxta-articular pains are experienced by as many as one third of patients with acute sarcoidosis and may be the only symptom of the disease; however, erythema nodosum often accompanies the arthritis and, together with hilar adenopathy, suggests the diagnosis (one should be aware that arthritis may accompany erythema nodosum of any cause). Arthritis often begins in the ankles and spreads symmetrically. The distal interphalangeal joints are typically spared, but any of the other peripheral joints, as well as the heels, may be painful out of proportion to signs of inflammation, which are meager. Episodes last a few days to a few months, and the arthritis usually resolves completely. The erythrocyte sedimentation rate is often elevated; antinuclear antibodies and rheumatoid factors may be present. Treatment with salicylates, nonsteroidal anti-inflammatory drugs (NSAID's), or prednisone is based on the severity of the arthritis. Progressive, deforming arthritis is a feature of chronic sarcoidosis, as are bone lesions, both lytic and sclerotic. Clinically significant sarcoid myopathy is rare.

FAMILIAL MEDITERRANEAN FEVER (see Ch. 196)

Serositis, fever, and arthritis are the major signs of familial Mediterranean fever (FMF). Arthritis occurs in as many as one half of patients; it is usually monoarticular and confined to large joints in the lower extremities. Although it usually lasts less than 1 week, arthritis has been reported to persist for several months. Synovial fluid contains large numbers of granulocytes, and there is intense infiltration of granulocytes and hyperemia in synovial tissue. Diagnosis is suggested by demographic and other clinical features of the disease. In the absence of these, FMF can be easily confused with juvenile rheumatoid arthritis. Colchicine most often prevents recurrent arthritis as well as amyloidosis.

277 Miscellaneous Forms of Arthritis

Eugene V. Ball

NEUROPATHIC JOINT DISEASE (CHARCOT'S JOINTS)

Recognition of neuropathic joint disease and its association with syphilis preceded reports of its association with diabetes mellitus by 64 years, but syphilis has been superseded by the latter as the leading cause of this disorder. Weakness, decreased pain sensation, and impaired position sense contribute to the massive destruction of the knee (or less often the hip or ankle) seen in syphilis, subacute combined degeneration of the spinal cord, paraplegia, and Charcot-Marie-Tooth disease. In syringomyelia, upper limb involvement is typical. Neuropathic disease of the knee or ankle is suggested by effusions, crepitus, enlargement, and relatively little pain, although pain may be severe late in the disease. Neuropathic joint disease in diabetes mellitus (Fig. 277–1) is more likely to cause painless swelling of one or both feet in a patient with longstanding disease and sensory neuropathy. For mechanical reasons, the joints most frequently involved are the tarsometatarsals and the metatarsophalangeals. Destruction also occurs in the talus, the calcaneus, the ankle joints, and the distal tibia. Radiographs characteristically show loss of joint space, sclerosis, multiple irregular bodies representing chip fractures, and new bone formation; analogous changes are seen in osteomyelitis and malignancy. Less severe, but similar, changes have been reported in calcium pyrophosphate deposition disease. Attempts at stabilizing the involved joint with various orthotic devices are often unsatisfactory, and surgical fusion is difficult.

HEMARTHROSIS

Hemophilia (see Ch. 155) is the major medical cause of hemarthrosis, which (with muscle bleeding) accounts for more than 90 per cent of all bleeding episodes in patients with hemophilia. The severity of hemarthrosis is related directly to the levels of clotting factors. For example, infants with severe factor deficiencies often experience hemarthrosis before the age of 1 year. By the age of 15, virtually all persons with severe, inadequately treated factor deficiencies have some form of chronic joint impairment.

Acute bleeding into a joint (most often the knees, elbows, or ankles) is frequently signified by stiffness or discomfort, followed by pain, swelling, and redness. The joint should be immobilized, and adequate factor replacement should be started as early as possible, preferably during the prodromal phase. The joint changes induced by repeated intra-articular bleeding resemble those of rheumatoid arthritis. Hyperplastic synovium appears to be the source of proteases and other enzymes that destroy cartilage and bone, culminating in the absence of articular carti-

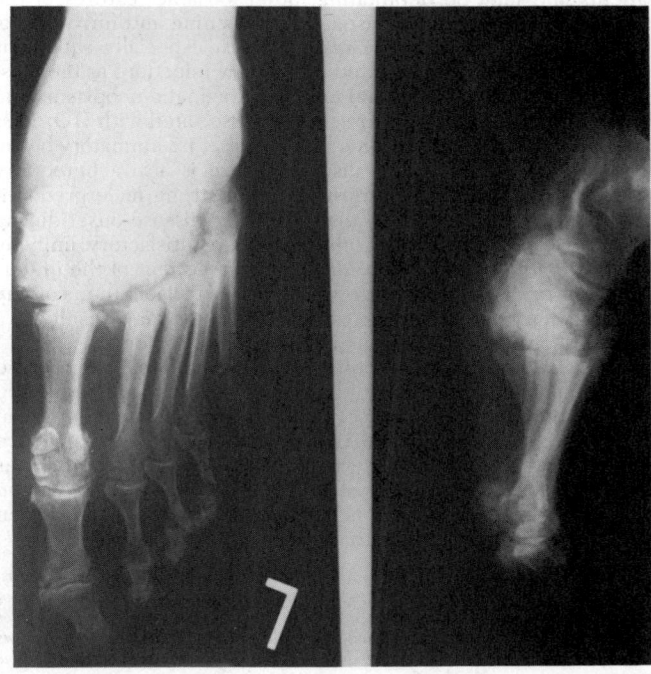

FIGURE 277–1. Diabetes mellitus and neuropathic arthritis. Note lateral displacement of metatarsals (*left*) and fragmentation and osseous debris (*right*).

lage, joint disorganization, and fibrous contractures. Education of the patient and family, as well as home treatment, prevents or attenuates chronic, destructive arthritis. Joint replacements have been done successfully to relieve pain and restore function.

Bleeding into a muscle, which should also be treated with replacement factor, can lead to necrosis and fibrotic scarring. Pseudotumors are cystic bone swellings resulting from intraosseous bleeding and necrosis.

Von Willebrand's disease can produce hemarthrosis and joint destruction comparable to that of hemophilia.

Painful but nondestructive intra-articular bleeding is a common feature of scurvy, and intra-articular tumors such as pigmented villonodular synovitis frequently cause monoarticular bleeding.

MULTICENTRIC RETICULOHISTIOCYTOSIS

The chief manifestations of multicentric reticulohistiocytosis are arthritis and red to purple skin nodules varying in size from 1 to 10 mm. The nodules are found in any part of the skin but tend to concentrate on the face and hands and uncommonly coalesce. The arthritis is most often symmetric and polyarticular. Unlike adult rheumatoid arthritis, it does not spare the distal interphalangeal joints. It can be severely destructive and, in one third of cases, progresses to arthritis mutilans. Systemic signs include fever and weight loss; less often, pericarditis and myositis are present, and it is frequently associated with a malignancy.

The disorder has also been termed lipoid dermatoarthritis because of the lipids contained within the histiocytes and granulomas that constitute the basic lesion. In the absence of a serum or lesional lipid abnormality, lipid deposition is now thought to be nonspecific. Improvement has been reported more consistently with alkylating agents than with prednisone.

HYPERTROPHIC OSTEOARTHROPATHY AND CARCINOMATOUS POLYARTHRITIS

Hypertrophic osteoarthropathy (HO) is a systemic disorder distinguished by periostitis of the distal ends of tubular bones. The lesions presumably begin with increased blood flow and periosteal edema, followed by new bone formation. Isotopic bone scans are positive at an early stage, often preceding radiographic evidence of periosteal new bone. Hypertrophic osteoarthropathy is often manifested as digital clubbing and frequently involves the tibiae, ulnae, radii, femora, metatarsals, and metacarpals. Painful articular swelling appears in approximately 30 per cent of patients and may be debilitating; other variable features of the syndrome include gynecomastia and thickening and furrowing of the facial skin. Intrathoracic malignancies, especially squamous cell carcinoma, have supplanted pulmonary infections as the most common cause of HO. Pleural and diaphragmatic neoplasms and nasopharyngeal carcinomas are strongly associated with HO. Less common causes include chronic liver disease, inflammatory bowel disease, and cyanotic heart disease. There is also a hereditary form termed pachydermoperiostosis, with strong male predominance and a curious bimodal distribution of disease onset during the first year of life or the mid-teens. No satisfactory unifying theory of pathogenesis exists. Successful treatment of the underlying disorder results in regression of HO. In fact, thoracotomy for pulmonary hypertrophic osteoarthropathy may result in a marked decrease in pain and swelling within 24 hours.

The "sudden" onset of polyarthritis resembling rheumatoid arthritis in an older adult should prompt suspicion of an associated malignancy. Carcinomatous polyarthritis may appear months before, or after, detection of malignancy of many types. Its incidence is unknown; in one small series it was almost as common as carcinomatous hypertrophic osteoarthropathy and more common than cancer-related dermatomyositis. Palmar fasciitis has been noted in association with ovarian cancer.

Ginsburg, WW, O'Duffy JD, Morris JL, et al.: Multicentric reticulohistiocytosis: Response to alkylating in six patients. Ann Intern Med 111:384, 1989. *Five of six patients with multicentric reticulohistiocytosis manifesting as skin nodules and polyarthritis were treated with cyclophosphamide. The sixth patient was given chlorambucil. All responded with complete or near-complete remissions lasting as long as 32 months after cessation of treatment.*

Luck JV, Jr, Kasper CKL: General orthopedics: A tribute to J. Vernon Luck Sr.— Symposium: Surgical Management of Advanced Hemophilic Arthropathy: An Overview of 20 Years' Experience. Clin Orthop 242:60, 1989. *A review from a large multidisciplinary hemophilia center of the clinical manifestations of hemophilic arthritis and its management, which included 67 prosthetic arthroplasties.*

Slowman-Kovacs SD, Braunstein EM, Brandt KD: Rapidly progressive Charcot arthropathy following minor joint trauma in patients with diabetic neuropathy. Arthritis Rheum 33:412, 1990. *This report of neuropathic arthropathy progressing rapidly after minor trauma in three patients is based on the authors' research in experimental arthritis.*

278 Nonarticular Rheumatism

Eugene V. Ball

FIBROSITIS

Primary fibrositis has been defined as a chronic pain syndrome with tender points in predictable sites and disturbed sleep. In the absence of diagnostic laboratory tests or objective physical signs, the syndrome is somewhat controversial, and its existence as a distinct entity has been questioned. The pain of fibrositis is often described as muscular or as deep aching or burning. It is generalized but more severe in the trunk and hands and in proximity to tender "trigger" points. These areas are painful to firm palpation in normal persons but are more tender in persons with fibrositis. Some 14 locations have been identified, e.g., in the second costochondral junction and in the periscapular muscles along the medial border of the scapula, and over the medial collateral ligament of the knee.

Patients may have sleep disturbances of possible pathogenetic significance. Fatigue is virtually universal as a component of this syndrome; headaches and heightened anxiety are common. In these respects, the fibrositis syndrome has a close resemblance to the syndrome of mitral valve prolapse, and it too is more common in women past the age of 20 (although it has been diagnosed in children). There are no confirmed biochemical, immunologic, or anatomic abnormalities in patients with fibrositis. Treatment should emphasize its benign nature. The physician should be wary of overuse of drugs to allay anxiety or induce sleep. In limited studies, amitriptyline and cyclobenzaprine have been found to be superior to placebo in decreasing pain and improving sleep.

BURSITIS

Bursae are small, synovial-lined, fluid-filled sacs located between tendons and bones, which serve to reduce friction between opposing muscles or tendons. Most bursae are present from birth; however, others form in response to repeated pressure.

Of the approximately 80 bursae located on each side of the body, only a few are common sources of pain. The subdeltoid is the largest of the bursae around the shoulder; it is located between the deltoid muscle and the shoulder capsule and extends under the acromion. Acute inflammation of this or nearby bursae and tendons is apt to be exceedingly painful, resulting in restriction of the shoulder movement and tenderness over the rotator cuff. Intrabursal injection of lidocaine is diagnostic and often curative; however, recurrences are common. Bursal calcification predisposes to more frequent attacks.

Trochanteric bursitis is thought to occur as a result of chronic strain on weak quadriceps muscles or overuse of hip and thigh muscles. Pain is often perceived in the lateral aspect of the thigh and the low back and is aggravated by abducting the affected leg and by lying on the affected side. Tenderness is present at the edge of the greater trochanter. Injections of lidocaine often abolish the pain.

TENDINOUS LESIONS

Tendinous lesions include tenosynovitis, a lesion of the gliding surfaces of a tendon and its sheath; tendinitis, painful scarring within a tendon; and trigger lesions, which are localized enlargements of the tendon that engage a constricted part of the sheath (as in "trigger finger"). Tendinous lesions are common, occurring in many areas of the musculoskeletal system. An example is de Quervain's disease, which is stenosing tenosynovitis of the abductor pollicis longus and extensor pollicis brevis at the medial

TABLE 278–1. CONDITIONS CAUSING CARPAL TUNNEL SYNDROME

1. Trauma
2. Occupation
3. Infections: for example, Lyme disease and rubella
4. Rheumatoid arthritis and gout
5. Pregnancy
6. Hypothyroidism and acromegaly
7. Amyloidosis
8. Median artery aneurysm
9. Ganglion cyst, increased fat, hypertrophy of abductor pollicis muscle

styloid. Pain can be localized or can radiate into the hand or back to the shoulder. This and carpal tunnel syndrome occur frequently during pregnancy.

CARPAL TUNNEL SYNDROME

The symptoms of carpal tunnel syndrome are paresthesias and pain in the palmar side of the first three fingers and at times the radial half of the fourth finger; the pain may radiate proximally to the shoulder, creating confusion with a cervical disc syndrome. Physical findings include sensory loss, weakness on abduction and opposition of the thumb, and atrophy of the thenar eminence. Carpal tunnel syndrome is caused by an array of conditions that result in pressure on the median nerve as it passes through the bony flexor compartment of the wrist. Some of these causes are listed in Table 278–1.

Diagnosis is confirmed by electrophysiologic nerve tests. (The clinical tests commonly used are of questionable value.) Magnetic resonance imaging may be useful in defining the cause and thus directing treatment, which might include splinting of the wrist, corticosteroid injections, and surgical release of the transverse carpal ligament. Oral pyridoxine is of questionable value.

TENNIS ELBOW

"Tennis elbow" refers to a lesion of the wrist extensor muscles causing pain at the outer elbow, along the back of the forearm or, less commonly, into the shoulder. The burning or aching pain is produced by resisted extension of the wrist, as in grasping and lifting, and rarely is felt as sudden, searing twinges of intensity sufficient to cause momentary grip paralysis. Tennis elbow usually results from repeated forceful extension of the wrist. The tear most often occurs at the origin of the common extensor tendon from the lateral humoral epicondyle; much less frequently, the tear is in the muscle belly. Treatment includes injection of triamcinolone into the painful scar, manipulation, or tenotomy.

Like tennis elbow, "golfer's elbow" is a misnomer in that both conditions occur frequently in people who play neither sport. Golfer's elbow is less painful than tennis elbow; it represents a lesion of the common flexor tendon at the medial epicondyle. Pain is usually localized to the inner side of the elbow and is produced by resisted flexion of the wrist. Treatment includes triamcinolone injection or massage.

TIETZE'S SYNDROME

Tietze's syndrome is a common cause of chest pain that can be mistaken for visceral pain. There is tender, most often unilateral, swelling at one or more costosternal junctions. Biopsy samples of involved areas have revealed chronic inflammatory fibrosis. The syndrome may result from prolonged coughing or hyperventilation, but it is often idiopathic. Injections into the painful area with triamcinolone are sometimes curative.

Goldenberg DL, Simms RW, Geiger A, et al.: High frequency of fibromyalgia in patients with chronic fatigue seen in a primary care practice. Arthritis Rheum 33:381, 1990. *Of 27 patients with chronic fatigue syndrome seen in a primary care practice, 19 had symptoms and signs of fibromyalgia.*

Sheon RP, Moskowitz RW, Goldberg VM: Soft Tissue Rheumatic Pain: Recognition, Management, Prevention. 2nd ed. Philadelphia, Lea & Febiger, 1987.

279 Articular Tumors
Eugene V. Ball

Articular tumors can be classified as those that arise within the synovium; those that arise from cartilage, bone, or contiguous structures; and neoplasms that are nonarticular in origin but that

may metastasize to joints or develop in multiple areas, including joints.

The most common of these are probably synovial chondromatosis and osteochondromatosis, which develop as cartilaginous synovial plaques that sometimes ossify. These cause episodic pain or swelling in a knee, hip, elbow, or shoulder. The joint may lock if the plaques become detached, forming loose bodies. Radiographs reveal multiple opacities if ossification has occurred; arthroscopy may be useful for both diagnosis and treatment.

Pigmented villonodular synovitis (PVNS) is a nonmalignant proliferative disorder of unknown etiology that usually affects the entire synovium of a single joint. This condition occurs most often in early middle age and in the knee in 80 per cent of cases. Uncommonly, two or more joints are involved; similar lesions occur in tendons and bursae. Pain and swelling are characteristic, as is serosanguineous synovial fluid. Radiographic signs include soft tissue swelling, subchondral cysts (particularly in the hip), and pressure erosions. Treatment is synovectomy. Hemangiomas, lipomas, and xanthomas may simulate PVNS.

Synoviomas (synovial sarcomas) are rare, aggressive tumors of young adults. They usually originate in the extremities adjacent to, but not within, a joint. Primary tumors histologically identical to synoviomas have been found in the head and neck, abdominal wall, retroperitoneum, heart, and mediastinum, supporting the view that the tumor originates from mesenchyme rather than synovium. Detection within tumor cells of both cytokeratin (an epithelial intermediate filament) and vimentin (a mesenchymal intermediate filament) has led to the suggestion that the synovioma is a carcinosarcoma. Synoviomas are usually discovered as deep swellings within a tendon sheath, a bursa, or a joint capsule. Pain and tenderness are variable, as are effusions. They metastasize early to lungs, bone, and lymph nodes. Tumor size greater than 4 cm, a high mitotic rate, and local recurrence after excision convey a poor prognosis.

Chondrosarcomas and fibrosarcomas are other malignancies arising within or near joints, and intrasynovial myeloma and lymphoma are rare causes of a swollen or painful joint.

Thorough investigation is required for unexplained pain or swelling within or adjacent to a single joint.

280 Erythromelalgia
Eugene V. Ball

Erythromelalgia (see Ch. 54) is a syndrome of episodic burning pain and redness in the extremities. Attacks may be confined to feet and, if severe and prolonged, may spread to the hands, or they may begin simultaneously in hands and feet. They are most often provoked by increasing environmental temperatures, although a few persons experience attacks only with febrile illnesses. The combination of increasing ambient temperatures and exercise often induces symptoms. Some persons maintain environmental temperatures at levels that are uncomfortably low for themselves, as well as others, to avoid attacks of erythromelalgia. Some sleep bundled up against the cold of an unheated room but with feet protruding uncovered from the blankets. Relief may require immersion of the feet in ice water. The feet appear normal between attacks except in those persons who habitually walk barefoot to avoid attacks provoked by wearing shoes.

Erythromelalgia is sometimes familial. In one remarkable kindred, the disorder is autosomal dominant, afflicting 32 of 66 members. Most often beginning between ages 2 and 8, it has been responsible for severe adjustment problems in youth, engendered in part by an inability to sit comfortably in a heated classroom or to participate in physical activities. In this kindred, the disorder has been frequently misdiagnosed as arthritis, reflex sympathetic dystrophy, or Raynaud's phenomenon; its pathogenesis is unknown, but it is not related to thrombocythemia.

By far the most common recognized cause of nonfamilial erythromelalgia is thrombocythemia, usually a feature of a myeloproliferative disorder. Erythromelalgia was the presenting symptom in 26 of 40 patients with platelet counts in excess of 500×10^9 per liter. Arteriolar inflammation and thrombotic occlusions were found on skin punch biopsy samples. Erythromelalgia disappeared for 3 or 4 days after a single dose of aspirin, which is the duration of its inhibition of platelet aggregation. In the absence of thrombocythemia, aspirins are likely to be ineffective for the treatment or prevention of erythromelalgia.

Other reported associations with erythromelalgia include diabetes mellitus. In addition, nifedipine and bromocriptine can cause an erythromelalgia-like disorder.

Michiels JJ, van Joost T, Vuzevski VD: Idiopathic erythromelalgia: A congenital disorder. J Am Acad Dermatol 21(S Pt. 2): 1128, 1989. *A brief report of idiopathic erythromelalgia in a female whose symptoms began at 2 years of age and increased in severity until age 14, by which time she was sleeping with her feet immersed in ice water.*

Millard FE, Hunter CS, Anderson M, et al.: Clinical manifestations of essential thrombocythemia in young adults. Am J Hematol 33:27, 1990. *Essential thrombocythemia was identified in 13 patients whose median age was 26. Erythromelalgia was the most common complication, occurring in 7 of the 13, of whom 7 were males.*

281 Multifocal Fibrosclerosis

H. Ralph Schumacher, Jr.

In rare instances the delicate fibrous areolar tissue in a certain anatomic region becomes the site of a chronic low-grade inflammatory process, leading to deposition of dense sclerotic plaques, which may obstruct or limit the movement of adjacent viscera. When the process is in the active phase, there are characteristic findings of chronic or granulomatous inflammation, featured by mononuclear cell infiltration, plasma cells, and occasional giant cells. In the end stages the pathologic lesion is simply that of scar tissue, so that by the time this process causes clinical manifestations there may be little evidence of the initial inflammatory reaction. In at least some cases there is an accompanying vasculitis. As a general rule the process tends to originate in the midline, around the great vessels, and then to spread laterally. In most cases a clue to the inciting mechanism is lacking.

Syndromes that have been considered as manifestations of multifocal fibrosclerosis include retroperitoneal fibrosis, mediastinal fibrosis, sclerosing cholangitis (see Ch. 126), Riedel's thyroiditis (see Ch. 216), pseudotumor of the orbit, Peyronie's disease (a sclerotic induration of the corpora cavernosa of the penis), and sclerosing peritonitis. Other sites of a similar fibrosis, such as the testes, vagina, and suprasellar area, have also been reported. Pulmonary and myocardial fibrosis syndromes have generally not been seen as related to multifocal fibrosclerosis, although pleural fibrosis along with retroperitoneal fibrosis can be seen with ergotamine use.

Although most of these syndromes have been described as separate entities, several anatomic areas may become affected in one person. For example, retroperitoneal fibrosis and sclerosing mediastinitis may be present at the same time along with varying combinations of sclerosing cholangitis, Riedel's thyroiditis, and pseudotumor of the orbit. A possible genetic predisposition is suggested by familial cases and by an association between fibrosing syndromes and alpha$_1$-antitrypsin deficiency. Recent reports have also described familial mediastinal or retroperitoneal fibrosis associated with HLA (human leukocyte antigen)-B27 and seronegative spondyloarthropathies; relations to aortic inflammation with a possible element of reaction to atheromatous components has been described.

Comings DE, Skubi KB, Van Eyes J, et al.: Familial multifocal sclerosis. Ann Intern Med 66:884, 1967. *Description of multiple sites of fibrosis in two brothers.*

Goldbach P, Mohsenifar Z, Salick AI: Familial mediastinal fibrosis associated with seronegative spondyloarthropathy. Arthritis Rheum 26:221, 1983. *Two siblings with both diseases.*

RETROPERITONEAL FIBROSIS

In retroperitoneal fibrosis the process usually begins over the promontory of the sacrum and extends laterally across the ureters and as high as the second or third lumbar vertebra. Less commonly, the lesion develops in other extraperitoneal areas, for example, contiguous with the kidneys, duodenum, descending colon, or urinary bladder. In some cases there has been an associated vasculitis in the skin and subcutaneous tissue, manifested by the formation of nodules, erythematous discolorations, and ulcerations. Similarly, inflammatory changes in small vessels at the sites of the sclerosis have been noted. Glomerulonephritis has been seen in a few patients.

The occurrence of retroperitoneal fibrosis in patients taking methysergide for migraine has been reported with greater frequency than could be due to chance. Occasional cases have been reported after use of other drugs such as ergotamine, various beta-adrenergic blocking agents, hydralazine, or methyldopa. Associated diseases in patients with retroperitoneal fibrosis have included systemic lupus erythematosus, vasculitis, scleroderma, eosinophilic fasciitis, biliary cirrhosis, rubella-associated arthritis, and carcinoid. Retroperitoneal tumors, trauma, or surgery may be a factor in some cases. One patient with associated periarticular fibrosis had elevated plasma levels of a platelet-derived growth factor.

The disorder is about twice as common in males as in females, and the peak incidence is in the fifth and sixth decades. Cases have been reported in children. The manifestations are variable, depending on the anatomic location of the process. Pain is the most common symptom; it is vague, tends to be located in the low back, and may be accompanied by symptoms referable to the gastrointestinal tract. The patient is likely to lose weight and have low-grade fever. There may be some anemia and elevation of the erythrocyte sedimentation rate. Although the ureter is the structure most often affected, symptoms referable to the urinary tract are uncommon until obstructive uropathy has led to azotemia and other clinical manifestations of renal insufficiency. The fibrosing process may surround the inferior vena cava, but obstruction of that vessel is uncommon. Thromboembolism and hypertension can be complications. Arterial invasion has been described. Retroperitoneal fibrosis occasionally develops in association with abdominal aortic aneurysm or aortitis.

Diagnosis of retroperitoneal fibrosis has been most often suggested by the findings at intravenous pyelography: displacement of the ureters toward the midline and evidence of obstruction, usually at the level of the pelvic brim. One or both ureters may be affected. In rare instances a mass can be palpated in the pelvis or on the posterior abdominal wall. Ultrasonography, computed tomographic (CT) scanning, and magnetic resonance imaging (MRI) can also identify the fibrosing masses. Once a mass has been disclosed, the main problem in differential diagnosis lies in distinguishing retroperitoneal fibrosis from retroperitoneal tumor. Multiple deep biopsies should be made at the time of laparotomy.

Surgical treatment, if employed before there has been severe renal damage, is often highly successful. Inasmuch as the fibrosing process is seldom invasive, the constricted organ can usually be freed by blunt dissection so that normal movement or flow is restored. Relief of ureteral obstruction is usually achieved by bringing the ureter out on the anterior surface of the sclerotic mass. Occasionally, however, the obstruction recurs months or years after such treatment. Some surgeons wrap the ureters in omentum to try to decrease recurrent obstruction. Steroid therapy may be helpful in the rare case detected early or may be employed as an adjunct to surgical measures. Azathioprine has been used successfully in a few cases. Other drugs such as penicillamine, colchicine, and gamma-interferon, with theoretical ability to limit clinical fibrosis, have not been studied in this disease. Progesterone has been used with some apparent success in Latin America. When the inferior vena cava is obstructed, surgical relief is technically difficult and risky; here it may be preferable to temporize in the hope that development of collateral pathways may alleviate the circulatory block.

The long-term outlook is fairly good if the disease is recognized and if its obstructive consequences can be treated by surgical means. The disease often tends to run its course and subside. Most deaths have been caused by renal failure.

Cohle SD, Leil JT: Inflammatory aneurysm of the aorta, aortitis and coronary arteritis. Arch Pathol Lab Med 112:1121, 1988. *Inflammatory aneurysms of the aorta and other vasculitis may be associated with retroperitoneal fibrosis.*

Ewald EA, Gikas PW, Castor CW: Periarticular fibrosis associated with idiopathic retroperitoneal fibrosis. J Rheum 15: 1443, 1988. *Elevated plasma platelet-derived growth factor is proposed as a possible pathogenetic mechanism.*

MEDIASTINAL FIBROSIS

Taut bundles of collagenous tissue form in the superior and anterior mediastinum, with impingement on the aorta, trachea, bronchi, esophagus, and pericardium, but the predominant manifestations are those caused by obstruction of the superior vena cava: puffy, suffused appearance of the face and conjunctivae; nonpitting edema of the face, neck, and upper extremities; and distended veins in the neck and upper extremities. Rarely the principal vessels affected are the pulmonary arteries, causing pulmonary hypertension. More frequently, the pulmonary veins are involved, and here severe hemoptysis may be the most prominent manifestation. Pericardial fibrosis can lead to constrictive pericarditis. The main task in differential diagnosis is to distinguish this relatively benign condition from obstruction caused by tumor. Roentgenographic examination of the chest may reveal little or no abnormality, but angiographic studies show obstruction of the affected vessels. Thoracotomy may be required for histologic diagnosis.

Histoplasmosis and possibly tuberculosis may cause some mediastinal fibrosis. Mediastinal hemorrhage can lead to fibrosis, and cases have been associated with methysergide use. Some patients with this syndrome have shown gradual improvement over months or years, presumably because of development of collateral circulation. Successful superior vena cava bypass surgery has been described. Steroid and other drug therapy as used with retroperitoneal fibrosis seems reasonable if infection is excluded, but such treatment has not been studied.

Dye TE, Saab SB, Almond MD, et al.: Sclerosing mediastinitis with occlusion of pulmonary veins. J Thorac Cardiovasc Surg 74:137, 1977. *An unusual but serious and treatable cause of hemoptysis.*

Goodwin RA, Nickell JA, Dez Pres RM: Mediastinal fibrosis complicating healed primary histoplasmosis and tuberculosis. Medicine 51:227, 1972. *Excellent review, certainly implicating histoplasmosis.*

SCLEROSING PERITONITIS

A fibrotic syndrome has been observed in patients treated for prolonged periods with the now withdrawn beta-adrenergic blocking drug practolol. Only a few cases have been reported with propranolol or other beta blockers. Some cases have developed a year or longer after cessation of therapy. The peritonitis consists of a thick fibrous encasement of the small intestine, and the symptoms include abdominal fullness, back pain, ascites, weight loss, and signs of subacute obstruction. It has usually been possible to relieve the symptoms by surgery, with blunt dissection to peel away the fibrous tissue. Some improvement occurs with time. A few patients treated with practolol have developed apparently related pericardial or lung disease, conjunctivitis, and dermatitis. Sclerosing peritonitis with many similarities has also been seen in patients treated with chronic ambulatory peritoneal dialysis, in drug abusers, and in an idiopathic form. Silica from talc is a possible factor in some cases. Antibiotics or other agents used in dialysis may also contribute.

Castelli MJ, Armin A-R, Husain A, et al.: Fibrosing peritonitis in a drug abuser. Arch Pathol Lab Med 109:767, 1985. *Perhaps this will become a more common problem.*

Pusateri R, Ross R, Marshall R, et al.: Sclerosing encapsulating peritonitis; report of a case with small bowel obstruction managed by long term hyperalimentation, and a review of the literature. Am J Kidney Dis 8:56, 1986. *This is a serious complication of peritoneal dialysis. Improvement in this patient occurred during parenteral nutrition.*

PART XX
INFECTIOUS DISEASES

SECTION ONE / INTRODUCTION

282 Introduction to Microbial Disease

Gerald L. Mandell

Infectious diseases have profoundly influenced the course of human history. The black plague (caused by *Yersinia pestis*) changed the social structure of medieval Europe. Military campaigns have been profoundly affected by outbreaks of diseases such as dysentery and typhus. Malaria has altered the geographic and racial pattern of distribution of hemogloblins and erythrocyte antigens. The development of *Plasmodium falciparum* is inhibited by the presence of hemoglobin S, and Duffy blood group–negative erythrocytes are resistant to infection with *Plasmodium vivax*. Infections are the major cause of morbidity and mortality in the developing world. AIDS threatens to disrupt the social fabric in some countries of Africa and is severely stressing the health care system in the United States and other parts of the world.

Infection may be defined as multiplication of microbes (viruses, bacteria, fungi, protozoa, or multicellular parasites) in the tissues of the host. The host may or may not be symptomatic. For example, infection with the human immunodeficiency virus may cause no signs or symptoms of illness or tissue damage for years. The definition of infection should also include instances of multiplication of microbes on the surface or in a lumen of the host, causing signs and symptoms of illness or disease. Certain strains of *Escherichia coli* may multiply in the gut and cause a diarrheal illness without invading tissues. This is also considered an infection. Microbes can cause diseases by virtue of toxin production without actually infecting the host. *Clostridium botulinum* can grow in certain improperly processed foods and produce a toxin that can be lethal upon ingestion. At no time does the microbe grow in or on the host. A relatively trivial infection such as that caused by *Clostridium tetani* in a small puncture wound can cause devastating illness because of a toxin released from the organism growing in the tissues.

We live in a virtual sea of microorganisms, and all our body surfaces have an indigenous bacterial flora. This normal flora actually protects us from infection. Reduction of gut colonization increases susceptibility to infection by pathogens such as *Salmonella typhimurium*. The normal flora is thought to exert its protective effect by several mechanisms: (1) utilizing nutrients and occupying an ecologic niche, thus competing with pathogens; (2) production of antibacterial substances that inhibit the growth of pathogens; and (3) induction of host immunity that is cross-reactive and effective against pathogens. In addition to the normal flora, transient colonization may be seen with known or potential pathogens. This may be a special problem in hospitalized patients (see Ch. 289).

Only a very small proportion of microbes may be considered to be principal or professional pathogens, and even among these species only a relatively small number of clones have been shown to cause disease. This supports the concept that pathogenic organisms are highly adapted to the pathogenic state and have developed a set of characteristics which enables them to be transmitted, to attach to surfaces, to invade tissue, and to cause disease. In contrast, opportunistic pathogens cause disease principally in impaired hosts. Organisms that may be harmless members of the normal flora in healthy people may act as virulent invaders in patients with severe defects in host defense mechanisms. Pathogenic organisms may be acquired by several routes. Direct contact has been implicated in the acquisition of staphylococcal disease. Airborne spread, usually by droplet nuclei, is seen in respiratory diseases such as influenza. Contaminated water may be implicated in *Giardia* infection and typhoid fever. Food-borne toxin illnesses may be caused by extracellular toxins produced by *Clostridium perfringens* and *Staphylococcus aureus*. Blood and blood products may be vectors for transmitting hepatitis B virus and the human immunodeficiency virus. Sexual transmission is important for these latter two agents and for a variety of pathogens including *Treponema pallidum* (syphilis), *Neisseria gonorrhoeae*, (gonorrhea), and *Chlamydia trachomatis* (nonspecific urethritis). The fetus may be infected in utero, and this has been seen with rubella virus and cytomegalovirus. Insect vectors may be important, as illustrated by mosquitoes for malaria, ticks for Lyme disease, and lice for typhus.

Pathogens are able to cause disease because of a finely tuned array of adaptations. These include the ability to attach to appropriate cells, often mediated by specialized structures such as the pili on gram-negative rods. Microbes such as *Shigella* species have the ability to invade cells and cause damage in that way. Toxins may act at a distance or may intoxicate infected cells. Pathogens have the ability to thwart host defenses by a variety of ingenious maneuvers. The antiphagocytic capsular coat of the pneumococcus is an example. Organisms may change their surface antigen display so as to outmaneuver the host immune system. This can be seen with influenza virus and trypanosomes. Certain pathogens have the ability to inhibit the respiratory burst of phagocytes (*Toxoplasma gondii*), and others can destroy phagocytic cells that have engulfed them (*Streptococcus pyogenes*). The environment plays an important role in infection, both in transmission and in ability of the host to combat the invader. The humidity and temperature of air may affect the infectivity of airborne pathogens. The sanitary state of food and water is an important factor for the acquisition of enteric pathogens. The "bad air" of swamps associated with malaria turned out to be due to the mosquitoes, but the environmental association was appropriate. The nutritional status of the host clearly is a significant factor in certain infectious diseases. The establishment of infection is a complicated interplay of factors involving the microbe, the host, and the environment.

With rare exceptions, infections are treatable and often curable diseases. Thus it is important to make an accurate etiologic diagnosis and promptly institute appropriate therapy. In acute infections such as pneumonia, meningitis, or gram-negative sepsis, rapid institution of therapy may be life-saving and thus a *presumptive* etiologic diagnosis should be established prior to a *definitive* diagnosis. This presumptive diagnosis can be based on the history, physical examination, epidemiology of illness in the community, and rapid techniques such as microscopic examination of appropriate Gram-stained specimens. Antimicrobial therapy can then be instituted for the presumptive etiologic agents but must be re-evaluated as more definitive diagnostic information becomes available.

283 Introduction to Bacterial Disease

Gerald L. Mandell

Bacteria are classified in the kingdom Procaryotae and contain DNA in a double-stranded loop not bounded by a membrane. The success of bacteria as life forms can be illustrated by the fact that fossils of bacteria 3.5 billion years old have been found. Bacteria are ubiquitous and can grow at temperatures as low as 0°C and as high as 110°C. All bacteria have a bilayered cytoplasmic membrane, and most bacteria (mycoplasma are exceptions) have an outer cell wall containing muramic acid. Morphologic features are often used to categorize bacteria. Bacilli are rods or cylinders with about half the species being motile, while cocci are spherical and nonmotile. It is useful to distinguish bacteria by their ability to retain a basic dye (crystal violet) after iodine fixation and alcohol decolorization (the Gram reaction). Gram-positive organisms retain the dye and contain techoic acids in their cell walls, whereas gram-negative bacteria have an additional outer membrane containing lipopolysaccharide (endotoxin). Capsules may serve as major virulence factors by interfering with the ability of phagocytes to ingest the encapsulated organisms. The capsules of the pneumococcus and *Haemophilus influenzae* are important factors for the virulence of the organisms. Pili or fimbriae are smaller hairlike structures that mediate bacterial attachment to various tissues and body surfaces. Only a very small proportion of species are pathogenic for humans, and new data suggest that even among those pathogenic species only certain clones are true pathogens.

Bacteria may be separated by their ability to reside and replicate intracellularly. Examples of intracellular bacteria include *Salmonella typhi*, *Legionella* species, mycobacteria, and chlamydiae. Extracellular pathogens include streptococci (including pneumococci), staphylococci, and most gram-negative enteric rods such as *Escherichia coli*, *Klebsiella* species, and *Pseudomonas* species. The main technique used for identification of bacteria in patient specimens is culture on artificial media. The ability to grow on the surface of such media in air defines aerobic organisms. Anaerobes cannot grow under such conditions, and facultative organisms can grow either aerobically or anaerobically. Microscopy can be a very useful technique, especially when combined with appropriate staining procedures such as acid-fast stains for mycobacteria or Gram's stain to differentiate gram-positive from gram-negative organisms. Newer techniques utilize direct immunofluorescence (e.g., for *Chlamydia trachomatis*), DNA probes (e.g., for *Legionella* species), and latex agglutination tests to detect antigen (e.g., for pneumococcal capsular antigen in spinal fluid). Assays using the polymerase chain reaction are being studied. Tests for antibodies are less useful but may be helpful in some diseases (e.g., Lyme disease).

284 The Febrile Patient

David C. Dale

Fever or *pyrexia* is an elevation of body temperature to a level above normal, i.e., to more than 37.5°C (99.5°F). It is a useful marker of inflammation; usually the height of the fever reflects the severity of the inflammatory process. Anorexia, malaise, myalgias, headache, and other constitutional symptoms often occur concomitantly. When the body temperature changes rapidly, chills and sweats are also observed. Fever with night sweats is a feature of many chronic inflammatory conditions. *Hyperthermia* is a term for fever due to a disturbance of thermal regulatory control: excessive heat production (e.g., with vigorous exercise or as a reaction to some anesthetics), decreased dissipation (e.g., with dehydration), or loss of regulation (e.g., due to injury to the hypothalamic regulatory center).

Most febrile patients have pain, tenderness, redness, and swelling at the site of inflammation, and the cause of the fever is readily identified. In a general medical practice, the most common causes of fever are respiratory illnesses, urinary tract infections, cellulitis, and superficial abscesses. In hospital patients, pneumonia is the most common cause. In otherwise healthy individuals, fever alone is not a cause for hospitalization unless it is quite high (greater than 39°C, or 102°F) or accompanied by shaking chills, hypotension, a change in the sensorium, or other symptoms suggesting bacteremia. However, in immunosuppressed individuals, the elderly, and patients with recent surgery, greater caution is indicated.

FEVER OF UNKNOWN ORIGIN (FUO)

An FUO is usually defined as an illness lasting more than 3 weeks with temperatures greater than 101°F (38.3°C) in which a diagnosis has not been made despite a good hospital or office evaluation. Ordinarily by this time the workup has included a history, physical examination, routine blood and urine tests and cultures, radiographs, and some specialized serologic tests. With careful further evaluation a diagnosis can be made in 70 to 90 per cent of these cases.

Diagnoses for FUO's fall into six general categories: infections, noninfectious inflammatory conditions, neoplastic diseases, drug fevers, factitious illnesses, and a group of less common causes (Table 284–1). The pattern of fever is only occasionally helpful in pointing to a specific diagnosis, e.g., the alternate-day fever in established *Plasmodium vivax* infections, the sustained fever in untreated *Salmonella typhi* infections and other continuous bacteremias, and the relapsing (Pel-Ebstein) fever in Hodgkin's disease and other lymphomas.

Evaluation of the FUO Patient

In patients with persisting fevers, it is important first to carefully review the medical history and repeat the physical examination. New clues may be found in the social, occupational, travel, and medication history. Previous medical and surgical

TABLE 284–1. CAUSES OF FEVER OF UNKNOWN ORIGIN

Infections
  Abscesses—hepatic, subhepatic, gallbladder, subphrenic, splenic, periappendiceal, perinephric, pelvic, and other sites
  Granulomatous—extrapulmonary and miliary tuberculosis, atypical *Mycobacteria*, fungal infection
  Intravascular—endocarditis, meningococcemia, gonococcemia, *Listeria*, *Brucella*, rat-bite fever, relapsing fever
  Viral, rickettsial, and chlamydial—infectious mononucleosis, cytomegalovirus (CMV), human immunodeficiency virus (HIV), hepatitis, Q fever, psittacosis
  Parasitic—extraintestinal amebiasis, malaria, toxoplasmosis

Noninfectious inflammatory disorders
  Collagen-vascular diseases—rheumatic fever, systemic lupus erythematosus, rheumatoid arthritis (particularly Still's disease), vasculitis (all types)
  Granulomatous—sarcoidosis, granulomatous hepatitis, Crohn's disease
  Tissue injury—pulmonary emboli, sickle cell disease, hemolytic anemia

Neoplastic diseases
  Lymphoma/leukemia—Hodgkin's and non-Hodgkin's lymphoma, acute leukemias
  Carcinoma—kidney, pancreas, liver, gastrointestinal tract, lung, especially when metastatic
  Atrial myxomas

Drug fevers
  Sulfonamides, penicillins, thiouracils, barbiturates, quinidine, laxatives (especially with phenolphthalein)

Factitious illnesses
  Injections of toxic materials, manipulation or exchange of thermometers

Other causes
  Familial Mediterranean fever, Fabry's disease, cyclic neutropenia

illnesses, alcohol intake, and animal contacts are important. On physical examination, special attention should be given to the skin, lymph nodes (including epitrochlear, postauricular, axillary), mucous membranes (including the conjunctivae), and abdominal region (masses, tenderness, and size of the liver and spleen). Usually the basic laboratory tests—CBC, differential, sedimentation rate, urinalysis, liver function tests, skin tests for delayed hypersensitivity (e.g., PPD, mumps), and stool for occult blood—should be repeated. Most patients with active inflammation are anemic, and the leukocyte differential can provide valuable clues. Neutrophilia suggests an occult bacterial infection. Monocytosis suggests tuberculosis, brucellosis, inflammatory bowel disease, or other chronic inflammatory conditions. Severe lymphopenia suggests immunodeficiency or a malignancy. A very elevated sedimentation rate suggests giant cell/temporal arteritis, polymyalgia rheumatica, Still's disease, bacterial endocarditis, or other occult infections, and a normal test rarely occurs with any of these illnesses. If the alkaline phosphatase is elevated, obstructive or infiltrative disease of the liver is the most likely cause, although nonspecific elevation is not uncommon. Other tests, e.g., antinuclear antibodies, febrile agglutinins, complement assays, may be positive but are rarely helpful in the FUO evaluation.

A definitive diagnosis is usually made through a combination of imaging studies, microbiologic tests, and/or biopsies. Previous radiographs should be reviewed carefully for evidence of sinusitis, apical inflammation or small nodules in the lungs, hilar adenopathy, or an intra-abdominal mass. Abdominal ultrasonography, computed tomography (CT), or magnetic resonance imaging (MRI) is very helpful to examine the liver, gallbladder, spleen, and pelvic areas for tumors and abscesses. These tests have reduced, but not completely eliminated, the need for exploratory laparotomies.

Cultures of blood (including for *Mycobacterium avium* in HIV patients), urine (including mycobacterial cultures if tuberculosis is suspected), and other bodily fluids (e.g., cerebrospinal, peritoneal, pleural) should be obtained if at all suggested by the clinical examination. It is useful to do anaerobic cultures of materials from suspected abscess cavities and to examine blood cultures for fastidious bacteria, yeast, and fungi in difficult cases. A tissue diagnosis often can be made from a biopsy of abnormal skin or lymph nodes or the bone marrow. Biopsies or needle aspirations of liver, lung, bone, or other deep tissue sites are also valuable when abscesses or tumors are suspected.

THERAPY

Therapeutic trials with antibiotics, corticosteroids, or antipyretics before the diagnosis is clear can confuse the evaluation. In some instances a trial may be justified but should be time limited, i.e., about 2 weeks. In patients with deep tissue abscesses, fever usually persists despite antibiotics. In patients with noninfectious inflammatory diseases, e.g., sarcoidosis, Still's disease, or vasculitis, a good clinical diagnosis usually can be made before such therapies are begun. In patients with malignancies, rational therapy depends upon a tissue diagnosis. Patients with factitious illness often have serious underlying psychiatric disorders. Care in confrontation is essential to prevent desperate acts including suicide.

Extensive workups of FUO's can be very expensive. In every patient the need for hospital care and testing should be continuously reassessed. When the patient is not severely ill, it is frequently worthwhile to use observation alone as a diagnostic tool. Sometimes even a short period of observation allows an obscure diagnosis to become obvious. In other cases, the fever disappears without the necessity for further diagnostic tests.

Aduan RP, Fauci AS, Dale DC, et al.: Factitious fever and self-induced infection: A report of 32 cases and a review of the literature. Ann Intern Med 90:230, 1979. *A comprehensive review of a large series of patients.*

Bor DH, Makadon HJ, Friedland G, et al.: Fever in hospitalized medical patients: Characteristics and significance. J Gen Intern Med 3:119, 1988. *A careful review of the frequency and outcome of illnesses with fever in an acute care hospital.*

Dinarello CA, Wolff SM: Fever of unknown origin. *In* Principles and Practice of Infectious Diseases. New York, Churchill, Livingstone, 1990, pp 468–478. *A comprehensive discussion of the diagnosis of FUO.*

Larson EB, Featherstone HJ, Petersdorf RG: Fever of undetermined origin: Diagnosis and follow-up of 105 cases 1970–1980. Medicine 61:269, 1982. *A comparison of a series of cases from the 1970's with the series studied by Petersdorf and Beeson in the 1950's.*

Mackowiak PA, LeMaistre CF: Drug fever: A critical appraisal of conventional concepts: An analysis of 51 episodes in two Dallas hospitals and 97 episodes reported in the English literature. Ann Intern Med 106:728, 1987. *Illustrates the causes and courses of drug fevers in 51 cases, with a review of the literature.*

Rowland MD, Del Bene VE: Use of body computed tomography to evaluate fever of unknown origin. J Infect Dis 156:408, 1987. *Outlines the usefulness of CT for FUO patients.*

285 The Pathogenesis of Fever

Bruce Beutler and Steven M. Beutler

FEVER: DEFINITION

Fever (pyrexia) entails an elevation of core body temperature above the level that is normally maintained by the individual. Under normal circumstances, core body temperature (the temperature of blood in the right atrium) is tightly regulated, exhibiting circadian variations over a range that usually does not exceed 0.6°C (1°F), with a mean value of 37°C (98.6°F) (the normal "set point"). An array of thermoregulatory mechanisms, described in detail below, ensures that this temperature is maintained. During episodes of fever, the thermoregulatory set point is shifted, such that the same thermoregulatory mechanisms are employed to maintain an abnormally elevated temperature.

It is important to realize that fever is not equivalent to an elevated core temperature, but to an elevated set point. Under many circumstances, ranging from intense physical exertion to immersion in hot liquids, core temperature may be elevated yet fever does not exist, since an attempt to cope with the departure from homeostasis is in progress. Failure of thermoregulation may also be associated with elevated core temperature; this problem (which obtains in malignant hyperthermia) is also distinct from fever.

THERMOREGULATORY MECHANISMS

Central to any consideration of fever is an understanding of the larger issue of thermoregulation. Core body temperature is determined by two opposing processes, each of which is regulated by the central nervous system. On the one hand, energy in the form of heat is generated by living tissues through a process termed *thermogenesis*. Energy may be passively absorbed from the environment as well. On the other hand, energy is inevitably lost to the environment, chiefly through the emission of infrared radiation and through transfer of energy to a surrounding medium, or to water, which is then volatilized. The temperature at which tissues are maintained is related to heat capacity (i.e., to the amount of energy required to elevate temperature by a defined increment) and to the quantity of energy lost or gained by the system.

Heat is liberated as a product of exothermic chemical reactions, which occur in both anabolic and catabolic pathways. Several "futile cycles" have been defined in which the energy stored in phosphate bonds is liberated in the absence of other net chemical transformation. Such cycles may supply a substantial fraction of the heat produced in thermogenesis. A second thermogenic mechanism consists in the utilization of ATP for the directional transport of ions across biologic membranes. Uncoupling agents, which disrupt the proton gradient so generated in mitochondria, stimulate thermogenesis by increasing the number of chemical transformations performed to achieve a given quantity of work. In humans, liver and muscle tissue are capable of liberating the major portion of energy in the form of heat, although all cells participate to some degree. In other species and in human infants, brown adipose tissue is also an important source of heat.

Metabolic reactions proceed more rapidly at an elevated temperature. Therefore, the passive warming effect of a febrile state leads to accelerated production of energy in the form of heat: For each temperature increment of 0.6°C (1°F), basal metabolic rate increases by approximately 10 per cent. This may, at times, be quite significant from a nutritional point of view. While the resting energy output of an average 70-kg man might approximate 60 watts, it would be expected that the same individual would exhibit an energy output of at least 100 watts when febrile to a temperature of 40.6°C (105°F), based solely upon the accelerated rate of exothermic reactions. Of course, a still greater expenditure of energy might be required to maintain the fever itself.

Muscle is a particularly flexible transducer of chemical energy, since its metabolic activity is largely controlled by the central nervous system. *Shivering thermogenesis* refers to the involuntary process whereby muscles are recruited to produce energy through the exercise of activity, leading to an enhanced metabolic demand. This is one mechanism responsible for the rise in body temperature witnessed in fever. Hence, a sharp "chill" often heralds the onset of fever.

Conservation of energy is effected through piloerection in mammals other than humans. In humans, the development of "gooseflesh" is the equivalent response. Other dermal reactions are also involved: "Flushing" represents a redistribution of circulation to dermal vessels and facilitates heat loss; a blanched appearance of the skin indicates an attempt to conserve heat. Fever is frequently accompanied by a perception of "coldness," prompting efforts to seek warmth.

INITIATION OF FEVER

The neural pathways responsible for thermoregulation originate in the hypothalamus. The exact location of thermoregulatory centers in man remains unknown, although preoptic, supraoptic, anterior, ventromedial, paraventricular, and suprachiasmatic areas have been implicated in animals. A local sensing mechanism exists, wherein the temperature of blood is coupled to the development of autonomic discharge. Elevation of body temperature depends primarily upon sympathetic outflow, leading to shivering thermogenesis and dermal vasoconstriction, whereas cooling mechanisms (sweating and dermal vasodilation) involve a mixture of sympathetic and parasympathetic pathways.

Certain neurotropic drugs are capable of disrupting the hypothalamic thermosensory mechanism or blunting the hypothalamic response and so may interfere with the development of fever. Among these, phenothiazines are the best known for their "poikilothermic" effect. These agents are not specifically active in febrile states; rather, they act to disable thermoregulatory mechanisms at all times following their administration.

CLINICAL ASPECTS OF FEVER

Although fever patterns tend to be nonspecific, they may sometimes provide diagnostic clues. Well known is the alternate-day fever pattern often seen with *Plasmodium vivax* and *Plasmodium ovale* infection. *Plasmodium malariae*, on the other hand, results in fever occurring every third day. A relapsing fever pattern is seen with *Borrelia* infection. Fevers occur daily for 3 to 6 days; a fever-free interval of about 1 week's duration then supervenes. A similar phenomenon is seen in rat-bite fever. Cases of brucellosis and typhoid may be characterized by a continuous "undulating fever." Hodgkin's disease is sometimes accompanied by periodic pyrexia (Pel-Ebstein phenomenon) with cycles lasting variable periods.

Intermittent fevers are seen in many conditions and are therefore of little help in discriminating between various disorders. Intermittent fever may also be caused by the interruption of a continuous fever with antipyretics or cooling measures; such interventions must be taken into account when attempting to analyze a temperature curve.

In addition to considering patterns of pyrexia, it is worthwhile to note the relationship between core temperature and other vital signs. For example, a dissociation between temperature and pulse is sometimes seen in cases of typhoid fever, Legionnaires' disease, psittacosis, and brucellosis. Factitious fever is also accompanied by an inappropriately low pulse. In addition, the respiratory rate may remain unchanged, and normal superimposed diurnal variations in temperature may be absent in factitious fever.

Drug fever may occur in association with nearly any medication. Antibiotics, particularly β-lactam agents, sulfonamides, and nitrofurantoin, are most frequently responsible. Drug fever usually develops within 5 to 10 days following initiation of therapy but can develop after a single dose or after months of administration. Drug fever may persist for several days after withdrawal of the offending agent and occasionally begins after the drug has been withdrawn. There is no characteristic fever pattern. Fevers due to drug allergy tend to be well tolerated but may be accompanied by other allergic phenomena such as nephritis or neutropenia. These, along with rash, may occur in 20 to 60 per cent of patients with drug fever. In the remaining cases, fever may be the sole manifestation. On occasion, drugs appear to induce fever by behaving as exogenous pyrogens (see below).

The response to antipyretics or antibiotics may shed light on the etiology of the fever. For example, fever due to malignancy uncomplicated by infection sometimes responds dramatically to low doses of nonsteroidal anti-inflammatory drugs. Such therapy usually proves ineffective in eliminating fever due to an unremitting infection. Fever caused by pneumococcal pneumonia characteristically resolves promptly upon administration of penicillin; similarly, administration of appropriate antimalarial drugs may result in rapid cessation of fever caused by malaria. Resolution of fever following withdrawal of a medication is characteristic of a drug fever.

Extreme pyrexia (characterized by a core temperature exceeding 41°C, or 106°F) often indicates failure of a distal mechanism of thermoregulation, occurring alone or in combination with infection. Examples of noninfectious causes of such extreme pyrexia include heat stroke, neuroleptic malignant syndrome, and malignant hyperthermia associated with succinylcholine.

CYTOKINES AND FEVER

Hypothalamic dysregulation and fever are triggered by proteins released from cells of the immune system (Fig. 285–1). This communication between the immune system and the nervous system is perhaps the most thoroughly studied "neuroimmunoendocrine" link. In response to invasive stimuli, including components of various microorganisms (e.g., lipoteichoic acid, lipopolysaccharides, and other constituents [collectively termed *exogenous pyrogens*]) or certain chemical agents (e.g., amphotericin and perhaps other drugs), cells of the immune system (principally macrophages and, to a lesser extent, lymphocytes) produce proteins that behave as *endogenous pyrogens*. These proteins are designated "monokines" and "lymphokines," respectively, and are often denoted under the more general heading of "cytokines." During the past decade, several of the cytokines active in the pathogenesis of fever have been isolated, and their structures have been determined by molecular cloning. At present, 11 proteins with pyrogenic activity have been identified (Table 285–1), and it is likely that many others exist. Although mononuclear phagocytes are the principal source of pyrogenic cytokines, the same proteins may sometimes originate from nonimmune cells of neoplastic tissue, in which autonomous production and secretion may occur.

The pyrogenic cytokines are structurally diverse proteins with well-established effects in hematopoiesis, inflammation, and the regulation of cell metabolism. Individual agents are often markedly pleiotropic in their actions. In addition to their involvement in the mediation of fever, cytokines mediate the "acute phase response," which is characterized by increased production of "acute phase reactants" in the liver (fibrinogen, C-reactive protein, complement proteins B, C3, C4, α_2-acid glycoprotein, serum amyloid A, and a variety of proteinase inhibitors among them), decreased production of albumin and transferrin, hypoferremia, hypertriglyceridemia, and other metabolic changes.

Pyrogenic cytokines are presumed to bind to receptors present on vascular endothelial cells that lie within the hypothalamus. They act to reset the hypothalamic thermoregulatory center, prompting an elevation of core body temperature. The resetting is believed to depend largely upon endothelial cell production of prostaglandins (PGE_2 and perhaps $PGF_{2\alpha}$). Thromboxanes and lipoxygenase products may also affect the set point. Cytokines may also interact directly with neural tissues; there is evidence to suggest that the release of corticotropin-releasing factor (CRF) may trigger thermogenesis in response to at least one cytokine (interleukin 1β).

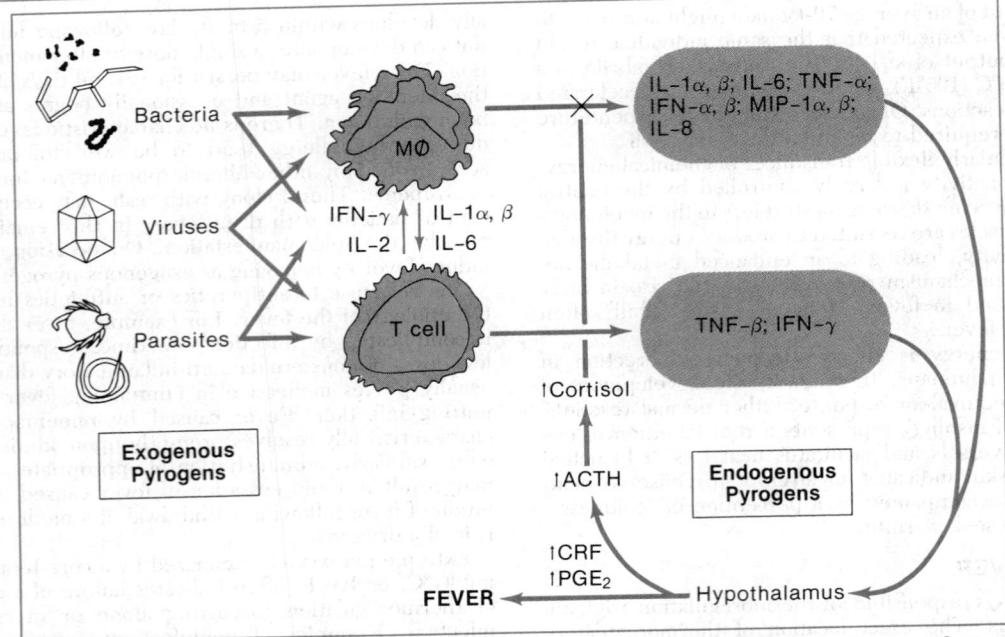

FIGURE 285–1. Production of endogenous pyrogens by macrophages and T lymphocytes. A variety of microbial pathogens produce molecules that function as exogenous pyrogens, triggering the release of endogenous pyrogens from mononuclear cells. ACTH = Adrenocorticotropic hormone; CRF = corticotropin-releasing factor; PGE₂ = prostaglandin E₂; other abbreviations are defined in the text and Table 285–1.

TABLE 285–1. PROTEINS WITH PYROGENIC ACTIVITY

Endogenous Pyrogen	Other Names/ Abbreviations	Principal Source	Induced by	Principal Effects in Addition to Pyrogenesis	Physical Characteristics
Cachectin/tumor necrosis factor-α	TNF-α	Macrophages	LPS, other microbial products	Fever, shock, anorexia, wasting, tumor necrosis, bone resorption, ↓ adipocyte lipoprotein lipase, neutrophil activation, ↑ endothelial cell adhesiveness/procoagulant effect	Homotrimer; 17 kDa subunit size (nonglycosylated)
					↕ 26% identity
Lymphotoxin/tumor necrosis factor-β	TNF-β; LT	Lymphocytes (T & B)	Antigenic/mitogenic stimulation		Homotrimer; 20–25 KDa subunit size (glycosylated)
Interleukin-1α (IL-1α)	Leukocyte ativity factor (LAF), leukocyte endogenous mediator (LEM), mononuclear cell factor (MCF), endogeneous pyrogen (EP)	Macrophages and many other cell types	LPS, other microbial products, TNF	Fever, IL-2 production, bone resorption, pannus formation, neutrophil activation, ↑ endothelial cell adhesiveness/procoagulant effect	Monomer; 17 KDa (glycosylated)
					↕ 26% identity
Interleukin-1β (IL-1β)					Monomer; 17 KDa (glycosylated)
Interferon-α	IFN-α; leukocyte interferon	Leukocytes (esp. monocyte-macrophages)		Induction of antiviral state	22 KDa (glycosylated)
					↕ 23% identity
Interferon-β	IFN-β; fibroblast interferon	Fibroblasts	LPS, viral infection, double-stranded RNA		22 KDa (glycosylated)
Interferon-γ	IFN-γ; immune interferon; type 2 interferon	T lymphocytes		Macrophage activation Upregulation of Class I and Class II MHC molecules	20–25 KDa (glycosylated)
Interleukin-6 (IL-6)	Interferon-β₂, hepatocyte-stimulating factor (HSF), B-cell stimulating factor-2 (BSF-2), B-cell differentiation factor (BCDF)	Many cell types	LPS, TNF	↑ Synthesis of acute phase reactants Weak antiviral effect Terminal differentiation of B cells; T-cell activation	21–26 KDa (glycosylated)
Macrophage inflammatory protein 1α	MIP 1α		LPS		7.9 KDa (nonglycosylated)
					↕ 57% identity
Macrophage inflammatory protein 1β	MIP 1β	Macrophages		Neutrophil chemotaxis	7.8 KDa (nonglycosylated)
Interleukin-8 (IL-8)	Monocyte-derived neutrophil chemotactic factor (MDNCF)		LPS, TNF, IL-1		8.0 KDa (nonglycosylated)

No single cytokine is capable of provoking fever of a magnitude equivalent to that elicited by endotoxin, for example. However, it is probable that combined production of several cytokines, as may occur in an inflammatory state, is sufficient to explain most fevers.

One monokine known as cachectin (also referred to as tumor necrosis factor-α) seems capable of reproducing many of the physiologic derangements observed in septic shock and thus appears to mediate most of the deleterious effects of bacterial endotoxin, including fever. A lymphokine known as lymphotoxin (also referred to as tumor necrosis factor-β) is homologous to cachectin, binds to the same receptor as cachectin, and elicits many of the same effects. Two other cytokines (interleukin 1α and interleukin 1β), while incapable of causing shock by themselves, produce many effects similar to those of cachectin, and in some instances synergistic responses have been noted.

Many of the cytokines are mutually inducing, and the concept of a "cytokine cascade" has been offered to describe the production of several factors occurring in response to the elaboration of one member of the group. The temporal sequence of induction may be reflected in the course of fever in vivo. For example, injection of a bolus of cachectin into a rabbit causes an immediate rise in body temperature, as well as a delayed rise, apparently related to secondary production of interleukin 1.

The production of certain cytokines is augmented by the presence of others: For example, cachectin biosynthesis is enhanced by interferon-γ, which also potentiates many of the effects of cachectin. Inhibitory feedback, from the production of glucocorticoid hormones, for example, may block further cytokine synthesis (see below). Thus, a complex relationship exists through which the release of one cytokine may augment (or at times inhibit) the production and effects of a second agent.

MECHANISMS OF ANTIPYRESIS

Nonsteroidal antipyretic agents inhibit fever by blocking the synthesis of prostaglandins within the endothelium of the hypothalamic vasculature, which is accomplished through inhibition of cyclo-oxygenase. However, they do not diminish the elaboration of endogenous pyrogens and may actually increase the production of some of these proteins (notably cachectin). Nonsteroidal antipyretics do not produce poikilothermic effects: They are capable of reducing fever but cannot lower body temperature beneath its normal set point.

Glucocorticoid hormones directly impede the production of endogenous pyrogens by mononuclear phagocytic cells. This is their mechanism of antipyresis and likely explains much of the total anti-inflammatory effect that they exhibit. Inhibition of cytokine synthesis is achieved at more than one level and has been studied most thoroughly in the case of cachectin biosynthesis. Both transcription of the cachectin gene and translation of the cachectin mRNA are downregulated by glucocorticoid agonists. The latter effect seems to depend upon the presence of a sequence motif that is commonly observed in the 3′-untranslated region of mRNA molecules specifying inflammatory mediators; however, the exact means by which glucocorticoid hormones prevent effective translation have not yet been elucidated.

The cyclic (often circadian) course followed in many febrile illnesses has not been fully explained. In some instances (e.g., in malaria), a clear relationship to the life cycle of the pathogen has been demonstrated. Cyclicity may, in other cases, follow from the fact that cells comprising the chief source of endogenous pyrogens are rendered refractory by continued exposure to the stimulatory agent and must recover or be replaced.

THE EVOLUTIONARY BENEFITS OF FEVER

It has been argued that the febrile response would not exist if it did not promote survival. By inference, it has been suggested that antipyretic therapy is best avoided in all but life-threatening circumstances. Modulation of various immune functions has been reported at elevated temperatures in vitro. Moreover, in specific instances, elevation of core temperature has been correlated with a beneficial effect on the course of disease. Most notably, the progression of tertiary syphilis in man is retarded by fever. In an experiment involving rabbits, spirochetal lesions of the skin have been shown to develop more rapidly in those regions of the skin that have been shaved of fur to allow for local cooling.

Failure to develop a fever in the course of a severe infection foretells a poor outcome. A causal effect has been suggested by studies performed with the lizard Dipsosaurus dorsalis. Poikilotherms that are capable of elevating their body temperature only by passive absorption of heat, these animals have been shown to resist lethal infection more effectively at warm temperatures than at cool temperatures.

Contrary to these arguments in support of a beneficial effect, it may be noted that tertiary syphilis is not characterized by fever; hence the causative agent appears to have evolved so as to avoid triggering a febrile response. Indeed, by virtue of their short generation time, microorganisms are generally capable of evading defense mechanisms of the host when compelled to do so in an evolutionary context. Thus, those pathogens that elicit fever may well be impervious to the effects that fever produces. The absence of a pyrogenic response during sepsis could, of course, simply reflect failure of thermoregulatory systems as a result of overwhelming infection.

Ultimately, it must be acknowledged that the immune response is imperfect in that many aspects of immune function may actually injure the host. Fever, like many phenomena associated with inflammation, might sometimes serve no useful function.

TREATMENT OF FEVER

In the absence of specific knowledge concerning the benefits of fever, a conservative approach to the treatment of fever is advisable. Core temperatures beneath 40.6°C (105°F) are well tolerated by most individuals. Moreover, when its source has been defined, fever often serves as an important indicator of therapeutic effect.

Under certain circumstances, aggressive treatment of fever is warranted. Patients with myocardial ischemia, patients predisposed to seizures, and pregnant women may require treatment with antipyretics, since elevation of core temperature increases cardiac output and myocardial oxygen demand, increases the likelihood of seizures, and may exert a teratogenic effect. Acetaminophen or nonsteroidal anti-inflammatory agents are adequate for this purpose in the majority of cases. Physical methods for increasing heat dissipation may also be employed.

Temperatures that exceed 41.1°C (106°F) are life-threatening and must be lowered immediately. Antipyretics are often ineffective in such instances, since pyrexia of this degree does not result from an aberrant hypothalamic set point. It is advisable, in such cases, to lower temperature by any means possible; the most effective action is to immerse the patient in ice water while monitoring core temperature to be certain that a state of hypothermia is not induced.

286 The Acute Phase Response
Charles A. Dinarello

ACUTE PHASE CHANGES. Infections, trauma, inflammatory processes, and some malignant diseases induce a constellation of host responses that are collectively referred to as the "acute phase response." The response is associated with characteristic metabolic changes in liver protein synthesis, but, on closer examination, changes also occur in several other systems that include hematologic, endocrinologic, neurologic, and immunologic dysfunctions. These changes are called acute because most are observed within hours or days following the onset of infection or injury, although some acute phase changes also indicate chronic disease. The full spectrum of the response includes dramatic increases in the synthesis of several unique hepatic proteins that are not produced in health. One of these, C-reactive protein, is a marker of the acute phase response and can be used as an indicator of disease. The increased plasma concentrations of acute phase hepatic proteins, glycoproteins, and globulins are responsible for elevated erythrocyte sedimentation rates. Although the liver is producing increasing amounts of a variety of proteins, hepatic albumin synthesis is decreased. Increases in gluconeogenesis, energy expenditure, and muscle proteolysis occur and contribute to weight loss. However, anorexia is often present and may account for most of the weight loss. Fever may be present, and increased sleep and lethargy are frequent clinical complaints. Leukocytosis with increased numbers of circulating immature neutrophils is common, and serum iron and zinc levels are depressed while increased ceruloplasmin levels result in elevated serum copper. Thyroid dysfunction can be present, and there is often abnormal glucose tolerance and lipid metabolism. In addition, anemia develops despite adequate stores of iron, and hypergammaglobulinemia often occurs.

Although the most florid presentation of the acute phase response is observed in patients with bacterial infections, burns, or multiple injuries, clinicians also encounter acute phase changes in patients with occult infections or chronic illnesses such as rheumatoid arthritis, Crohn's disease, and several autoimmune diseases. The presence of acute phase changes can also serve as an indicator of silent disease and some cancers, particularly renal cell carcinoma and Hodgkin's disease. The acute phase response has the outstanding characteristic of being a generalized host reaction irrespective of the localized or systemic nature of the inciting disease. The various components of the response are remarkably consistent despite the considerable variety of pathologic processes that induce it. For example, plasma levels of several acute phase proteins are elevated following myocardial infarction, fracture of a bone, or bacterial pneumonia.

INDUCTION OF ACUTE PHASE CHANGES. How are infections, injuries, and immunologic and inflammatory reactions able to elicit acute phase changes in the host? Moreover, does the acute phase response serve any purpose, and can its presence be used for diagnosing or monitoring the progression of disease? The initiation of the acute phase response is linked to the production of hormone-like polypeptide mediators, now called cytokines. Several cytokines induce acute phase changes: interleukin 1, tumor necrosis factor, interferon-γ, interleukin 6, and leukemia inhibitory factor. Interleukin 1 and tumor necrosis factor induce the production of interleukin 6 from a variety of cells. Interleukin 1 and tumor necrosis factor are produced from phagocytic mononuclear cells, enter the circulation, and affect distant organ systems. Although the primary sources of interleukin 1 and tumor necrosis factor are blood monocytes, phagocytic lining cells of the liver and spleen, and other tissue macrophages, specialized cells such as keratinocytes, gingival and corneal epithelial cells, renal mesangial cells, and brain microglial and astroglial cells also produce these molecules. Interleukin 1 and tumor necrosis factor produced by these latter cell types exert their primary effects within these tissues. In fact, the ability of microbial and inflammatory substances to stimulate the production of these mediators in these strategically located, specialized cells appears to be part of local pathologic changes in many diseases.

Interferon is produced primarily during viral infections. Although it shares with interleukin 1 and tumor necrosis factor the ability to produce fever, sleep, and lethargy, interferon does not induce certain other acute phase changes, and, hence, elevated erythrocyte sedimentation rates and neutrophilia are not commonly observed during viral infections.

The patient with a localized bacterial infection represents an excellent example of the development of the acute phase response. At the onset of the infection, blood monocytes and tissue macrophages become activated either by phagocytosis of the invading microbe or by exposure to its products or toxins; the process results in the synthesis and release of various cytokines within 1 to 2 hours. These mediators enter the circulation and reach the brain where they initiate fever. Fever is the result of prostaglandin E_2 synthesis induced by pyrogenic cytokines in the thermoregulatory center of the brain. Whereas fever is clearly one of the most obvious signs of the acute phase response, other components of the response can be present without apparent clinical manifestations. One of the most sensitive measures of the acute phase response is an increase in the number and immaturity of circulating neutrophils. The release of neutrophils is due to

the direct action of interleukin 1 on the bone marrow. In human subjects injected with small doses of endotoxin or interleukin 1, marked neutrophilia can be measured in the absence of fever. Although not routinely measured, serum zinc and iron levels are depressed. Low serum iron associated with anemia in the face of adequate iron stores is characteristic of the acute phase response. There is a large body of evidence that decreased serum iron probably plays an important role in protecting the host against various bacteria. For example, the reduction in serum iron can suppress the growth rate of several microorganisms and certain tumor cells that have a strict requirement for iron as a growth factor.

Within 8 to 12 hours after the onset of infection or trauma, the liver increases the synthetic rate of the so-called acute phase proteins. The response includes increases in proteins normally found in health as well as the appearance of new proteins that serve as markers of a pathologic event. Several normal plasma proteins increase several-fold during the acute phase response. These include haptoglobin, certain protease inhibitors, complement components, ceruloplasmin, and fibrinogen. However, true acute phase reactants increase several hundredfold. These include serum amyloid A protein, a precursor of the amyloid fibril in secondary amyloidosis, and C-reactive protein. C-reactive protein was named for its ability to interact with the C-polysaccharide of pneumococci and was the first acute phase protein described. Table 286–1 lists the characteristic pattern of increased plasma proteins observed during the acute phase response. Note one exception: The plasma concentration of albumin is decreased.

Of all the acute phase proteins, C-reactive protein and serum amyloid A protein are clinically the most important because their presence serves as an indicator of disease. These proteins are structurally related. C-reactive protein is particularly useful as a marker of the hepatic acute phase protein response and can be measured easily in most hospital clinical laboratories.

Despite the anabolic processes of the liver, the acute phase response is accompanied by a pronounced catabolism of muscle protein associated with loss of body weight and overall negative nitrogen balance. Fever increases oxygen and caloric demands (usually 7 per cent per degree F), and most of the negative nitrogen balance results from oxidation of amino acids from skeletal muscle, which contributes to wasting. These amino acids are largely used for gluconeogenesis. In addition, there can be demineralization of bone. Although the metabolic demands of elevated temperature contribute to the increased need for energy substrates, the host also requires a large supply of amino acids for synthesis of new protein at a time when food intake may be severely impaired or appetite reduced. Amino acids are required for immunologic and reparative processes such as the clonal expansion of lymphocytes and the proliferation of fibroblasts. Also, they are needed for synthesis of hepatic acute phase proteins, immunoglobulins, and collagen. The mechanism of providing ample amino acids for these cellular functions seems to be well orchestrated during the acute phase response. The catabolism during infection and inflammation differs from that of starvation. Unlike starvation, in which large amounts of ketones

TABLE 286–1. PLASMA PROTEINS THAT INCREASE DURING THE ACUTE PHASE RESPONSE

C-reactive protein
Serum amyloid A protein
Alpha-1-acid glycoprotein
Ceruloplasmin
Alpha-macroglobulins

Complement components (C1-C4, factor B, C9, C11)

Alpha-1-antitrypsin
Alpha-1-antichymotrypsin

Fibrinogen
Prothrombin
Factor VIII
Plasminogen

Haptoglobin
Ferritin
Immunoglobulins

Lipoproteins

are spilled into the urine, a septic individual excretes protein with small amounts of ketones. Interleukin 1 and tumor necrosis factor, the primary mediators of acute phase changes, inhibit lipoprotein lipase and hence interfere with lipid metabolism. In addition, these cytokines directly stimulate hepatic lipogenesis, and this mechanism likely accounts for the hypertriglyceridemia observed in patients with acute phase responses, in association with either acute or chronic disease.

MEASUREMENT OF ACUTE PHASE CHANGES IN CLINICAL MEDICINE. The acute phase response is nonspecific. However, the presence of certain acute phase changes in an otherwise healthy individual can alert the physician to hidden disease. Measuring the levels of ACTH, cortisol, growth hormone, and vasopressin is not particularly useful, although they are elevated during acute phase responses. Increased peripheral neutrophils and erythrocyte sedimentation rate are often used to detect an acute phase response. Measurement of C-reactive protein can assist the physician in determining the presence of disease in patients with vague, constitutional complaints. C-reactive protein levels are usually less than 100 µg per liter but increase within hours 10- to 1000-fold. In severe bacterial infections, the serum level can rise from undetectable to over 100 mg per liter in 48 hours. The presence of elevated levels of C-reactive protein or serum amyloid A protein, even in the absence of fever or neutrophilia, may indicate occult infection or malignant change. Increases in C-reactive protein and serum amyloid A protein occur in patients of any age and also in immunocompromised patients with opportunistic infections.

Not all inflammatory diseases are associated with elevated C-reactive protein. A refractory state can develop in certain diseases such as scleroderma, ulcerative colitis, and lupus erythematosus. Failure to develop hepatic protein changes and the neutrophilia of the acute phase response seems to be related to the presence of circulating inhibitors of cytokines.

TREATMENT OF ACUTE PHASE RESPONSES. Measurements of fever, acute phase plasma proteins, and peripheral leukocyte numbers are well-established procedures for monitoring many disease states. Although nonsteroidal anti-inflammatory agents are used to treat the fever and associated myalgias of acute phase responses, these drugs do not affect other acute phase changes in the liver, various endocrinologic parameters, or the bone marrow response. Antipyretic blood levels of aspirin and therapeutic concentrations of drugs such as indomethacin or ibuprofen do not reduce production of interleukin 1, tumor necrosis factor, or interleukin 6. On the other hand, corticosteroids are highly effective in reducing cytokine synthesis as well as the effect of these mediators on various tissue targets. Patients receiving therapeutic doses of corticosteroids have blunted acute phase responses with ongoing infections, inflammatory processes, or immunologic reactions.

Most clinicians would agree that alleviation of fever is indicated in many situations, such as in patients with seizure or cardiovascular disorders, in patients with joint destruction, and in patients with debilitating muscle wasting. Treating fever with antipyretics reduces the metabolic and caloric demands of elevated temperature and at the same time ameliorates many of the symptoms of the acute phase response such as headache and myalgias.

The role of acute phase proteins in host defense and repair is not entirely clear. Studies suggest that the major role of C-reactive protein is to bind serum lipids or opsonize pneumococci, whereas serum amyloid A is thought to be immunosuppressive. Ceruloplasmin scavenges toxic free oxygen radicals that are injurious to many tissues. What is clear, however, is that the production and physical structure of these acute phase proteins have been conserved through 400 million years of evolution, and therefore they have presumably been useful to the host. The Limulus crab and fish make C-reactive protein that is nearly identical to human C-reactive protein. This argues that the acute phase response plays a role in survival.

Beisel WR: Magnitude of the host nutritional responses to infection. Am J Clin Nutr 30:1236–1247, 1977. *Discussion of the metabolic imbalances seen in patients with infection and injury.*

Dinarello CA: Interleukin-1 and its biologically related cytokines. Adv Immunol. 44:153–205, 1989. *A comprehensive review of the biologic activities of interleukin 1, interleukin 6, and tumor necrosis factor.*

Feingold KR, Soued M, Serio MK: Multiple cytokines stimulate hepatic lipid synthesis in vivo. Endocrinology 125:267–274, 1989. *Evidence that interleukin*

1, tumor necrosis factor, and interferon may account for the hyperlipidemias observed in patients with acute or chronic inflammatory disease.

Kushner I, Gewurz H, Benson MD: C-reactive protein and the acute-phase response. J Lab Clin Med 97:739–749, 1981. *A brief discussion of the usefulness of measuring C-reactive protein levels in clinical practice.*

Pepys MB, Baltz ML: Acute phase proteins with special reference to C-reactive protein and related proteins (pentaxins) and serum amyloid A protein. *In* Dixon FJ, Kunkel HG (eds.): Advances in Immunology, Vol 34. New York, Academic Press, 1983, pp 141–211. *A comprehensive discussion of the hepatic acute phase protein pattern observed during the acute phase response, with special attention to the acute phase response in various autoimmune diseases.*

287 The Compromised Host

Philip A. Pizzo

Compromised host is a term used to describe patients who have an increased risk for infectious complications as a consequence of a congenital or acquired qualitative or quantitative abnormality of one or more components of the host defense matrix (Table 287–1). Until the early 1980's, this term was largely restricted to patients with congenital immunodeficiencies (Ch. 244) or to those who became immunocompromised as a consequence of cancer or its treatment, bone marrow failure, or treatment with immunosuppressive therapy. The advent of the acquired immunodeficiency syndrome (AIDS) has given the term *compromised host* a new meaning and relevance. The compromised host with AIDS is discussed in detail in Part XXI. In this chapter, the focus is on non-AIDS patients with altered immune defenses. However, many of the complications and approaches to diagnosis and management are generic.

PHYSICAL DEFENSE BARRIERS

The skin and mucosal surfaces represent the primary defense against both endogenous and exogenous sources of infection. Disruption of skin and mucosa may result from trauma, tumor invasion, the cytotoxic effects of chemotherapy or radiotherapy, the use of invasive diagnostic or therapeutic procedures (e.g., intravenous catheters), and effects of locally destructive infections such as oral herpes simplex. Such mucosal alterations provide a nidus for microbial colonization, a focus for localized infection, and a portal of entry for systemic invasion.

The skin and various mucosal surfaces are normally colonized by aerobic and anaerobic bacteria. However, in patients who have been hospitalized, who are neutropenic, or who have received prior broad-spectrum antibiotics, the normal gram-positive flora of the skin can be replaced by other gram-positive organisms such as CDC group JK *Corynebacterium* or *Bacillus* species or by gram-negative organisms (e.g., pseudomonads, enteric gram-negative rods), fungi (e.g., *Candida albicans* or *Aspergillus* species), and atypical *Mycobacterium* species such as *M. chelonei* or *M. fortuitum*.

Similarly, the gastrointestinal tract is normally colonized by an array of aerobic and anaerobic bacteria as well as some fungi, and disruption of its mucosa may lead to infections by a variety of pathogens including polymicrobial infections. A common cause for disruption of the gastrointestinal mucosal integrity is cytotoxic chemotherapy to patients with malignancy, particularly cytarabine (ara-C), the anthracyclines (daunorubicin and doxorubicin), methotrexate, 6-mercaptopurine, and 5-fluorouracil. Although stomatitis is usually the most clinically recognizable manifestation of gastrointestinal toxicity, diffuse gastrointestinal involvement is also likely. Frequently, the differentiation between chemotherapy-induced stomatotoxicity and localized infection (e.g., necrotizing gingivitis due to anaerobic bacteria or mucosal lesions due to herpes simplex virus) can be difficult, particularly in the neutropenic patient.

In addition to mucosal breakdown, mechanical obstruction of body passages can also increase the risk of serious localized infection due to stasis of local body fluids and resultant overgrowth of potentially pathogenic colonizing organisms. Common sites of secondary infection due to obstruction include the lung, urinary tract, biliary tract, or eustachian tube. One should consider an obstructive process when infection at any of these sites fails to respond to appropriate antibiotics.

Anatomic changes can also contribute to the risk of infection. For example, in patients with sickle cell disease, macrophage and splenic dysfunction predisposes to the development of certain bacteremias, especially by *Streptococcus pneumoniae* and *Salmonella* species. Anatomic abnormalities of bones and joints as a result of vaso-occlusive crises caused by infarction of bone marrow, bony cortex, or synovium in patients with sickle cell disease

can also predispose to development of infections such as osteomyelitis or arthritis caused by these organisms.

PHAGOCYTE DEFECTS

The polymorphonuclear leukocyte (PMN) and the monocyte are the two most important components of cellular host defense that protect against invasive bacteria and fungi. Both quantitative and qualitative defects affecting PMN and monocytes may occur in compromised patients.

Quantitative Abnormalities of Phagocytes

Granulocytopenia is among the most important risk factors for serious infection in the compromised host. However, it is impor-

TABLE 287–1. PREDOMINANT PATHOGENS IN COMPROMISED PATIENTS: ASSOCIATION WITH SELECTED DEFECTS IN HOST DEFENSE

Host Defense Impairment	Bacteria	Fungi	Viruses	Other

Neutropenia	Gram-negative
	  Enteric organisms
	    (*E. coli, K. pneumoniae, Enterobacter* spp., *Citrobacter* spp.)
	  Pseudomonas aeruginosa
	Gram-positive
	  Staphylococci
	    (coagulase negative, coagulase positive)
	  Streptococci
	    (enterococci α-hemolytic)
	  Anaerobes
	    (anaerobic streptococci, *Clostridia* spp., *Bacteroides* spp.)
		Candida species
		  (*C. albicans* > *C. tropicalis* > other species)
		Aspergillus species
		  (*A. fumigatus, A. flavus*)		

Abnormal cell-mediated immunity	*Legionella* *Nocardia asteroides* *Salmonella* spp. Mycobacteria (*M. tuberculosis* and atypical mycobacteria) Disseminated infection from live bacteria vaccine (BCG)	*Cryptococcus neoformans* *Histoplasma capsulatum* *Coccidioides immitis* *Candida*	Varicella-zoster virus Herpes simplex virus Cytomegalovirus Epstein-Barr virus Herpes virus 6 Disseminated infection from live virus vaccines (vaccinia, measles, rubella, mumps, yellow fever, live polio)	*Pneumocystis carinii* *Toxoplasma gondii* *Cryptosporidium* *Strongyloides stercoralis*

Immunoglobulin abnormalities	Gram-positive
	  Streptococcus pneumoniae, S. aureus
	Gram-negative
	  Haemophilus influenzae
	  Neisseria spp., enteric organisms
			Enteroviruses
			Disseminated infection from live virus vaccines (vaccinia, measles, rubella, mumps, yellow fever, polio)
				Giardia lamblia

Complement abnormalities
C3, C5
	Gram-positive
	  S. pneumoniae, staphylococci
	Gram-negative
	  H. influenzae, Neisseria spp., Enteric organisms			

C5-C9	*Neisseria* species (*N. gonorrhoeae, N. meningitidis*)			
Anatomic disruption Oral cavity	α-Hemolytic streptococci, oral anaerobes (*Peptococcus, Peptostreptococcus*)	*Candida*	Herpes simplex virus	
Esophagus	Staphylococci, other colonizing organisms	*Candida*	Herpes simplex virus Cytomegalovirus	

Lower gastrointestinal tract	Gram-positive
	  Enterococci
	Gram-negative
	  Enteric organisms
	Anaerobes (*B. fragilis, C. perfringens*)
		Candida		*Strongyloides stercoralis*

Skin (IV catheter)	Gram-positive
	  Staphylococci, streptococci
	  Corynebacterium, Bacillus spp.
	Gram-negative
	  P. aeruginosa, enteric organisms
	Mycobacteria
	  M. fortuitum, M. chelonei
		Candida
		Aspergillus		

Urinary tract	Gram-positive
	  Group D streptococci
	Gram-negative
	  Enteric organisms
	  P. aeruginosa
		Candida		

Splenectomy	Gram-positive
	  S. pneumoniae
	Gram-negative
	  DFZ bacillus
	  H. influenzae
	  Salmonella (sickle cell disease)
				Babesiosis

Modified from Rubin M, Walsh TJ, Pizzo PA: Clinical approach to infections in the compromised host. *In* Hoffman R, Benz EJ Jr, Shattil SJ, et al. (eds.): Hematology: Basic Principles and Practice. New York, Churchill Livingstone, 1991.

tant to keep in mind that except for congenital neutropenias, there are often other alterations of the host defense matrix that occur in concert with granulocytopenia and can further alter the risk for infection as well as the types of infectious complications that occur.

Granulocytopenia is most commonly associated with malignant disease and its treatment with cytotoxic therapy. This includes patients with hematologic malignancies and lymphomas as well as the increasing number of patients with solid tumors who receive cytotoxic chemotherapy. Patients with primary or secondary bone marrow failure also have neutropenia as their predominant risk for infection. In addition to the neutropenia per se, the patterns of infection are also influenced by the other disease- or treatment-related immune abnormalities. For example, despite equivalent degrees of granulocytopenia, the patient with acute myelogenous leukemia (AML) may present with a different pattern of infection than the patient with aplastic anemia. The disruption of a mucosal defense barrier which occurs in the patient with AML who is receiving cytotoxic therapy appears to increase the risk for infection with enteric gram-negative bacteria, α-streptococci, or anaerobes. In contrast, the patient with aplastic anemia who does not have impaired mucosal integrity may be able to sustain longer periods of granulocytopenia without developing a systemic bacterial infection. On the other hand, if the patient with aplastic anemia is treated with steroids or cyclosporine, the risk for viral or fungal infection may be increased.

Regardless of these modifying factors, the relationship between granulocytopenia and serious infection has been established unequivocally by the classic study of Bodey and colleagues (Table 287–2). This study demonstrated that the risk of infection begins to increase significantly when granulocyte counts fall below 1000 per microliter and is most marked when the counts are 100 per microliter or less. In addition to the absolute granulocyte count, the duration of granulocytopenia is also directly related to the direction of granulocytopenia as well as to whether the counts are rising or falling.

For practical purposes, granulocytopenia is usually defined as a count of 500 or fewer PMN's and band forms per microliter. However, a patient with an absolute granulocyte count of 500 to 1000 per microliter that is rapidly falling is probably at greater risk for infection than a patient with a count of 200 per microliter that is rising. Thus, the absolute granulocyte count, the duration of granulocytopenia, and whether the neutrophil count is falling or rising must all be considered when assessing the risk to any individual patient. Some clinicians also include the monocyte count in this equation to generate an absolute phagocyte index.

Granulocytopenia primarily predisposes patients to bacterial and fungal infection and does not of itself appear to increase the incidence of severity of viral and parasitic infections. In the 1950's and 1960's, when cytotoxic therapy was first being developed, gram-positive bacteria (especially *Staphylococcus aureus*) predominated. In the early 1970's, with the availability of antibiotics to control gram-positive bacteria (e.g., methicillin), gram-negative organisms (e.g., *Escherichia coli, Klebsiella, Pseudomonas aeruginosa*) emerged as the predominant pathogens in neutropenic patients, perhaps because of the increasing use of more aggressive chemotherapy regimens for the treatment of patients and the use of broader-spectrum antibiotics. During the 1980's, gram-positive organisms re-emerged as common bacterial isolates, and at many centers they now represent the most frequently encountered organisms.

TABLE 287–2. ASSOCIATION OF GRANULOCYTE LEVEL AND CHANCE OF DEVELOPING SIGNIFICANT INFECTION

Granulocyte Level (per cu mm)		Percentage of Serious Infections (Duration of Granulocytopenia in Weeks)							
Initial	*Change*	*1*	*2*	*3*	*4*	*6*	*10*	*12*	*14*
Any level	Any fall	12							
Any level	Fall to 2000	2							
Any level	Fall to 1500	5							
Any level	Fall to 1000	10	30	45	50	65	70	85	100
Any level	Fall to 500	19							
Any level	Fall to <100	28	50	72	85	100			

Adapted from Bodey GP, Buckley M, Sathe YS, et al.: Quantitative relationships between circulatory leukocytes and infection in patients with acute leukemia. Ann Intern Med 61:328–340, 1966.

In addition to these changes in the pattern of infection, institutional variations in the causes of infection and the antibiotic sensitivity patterns of isolates cannot be overemphasized, making it imperative for the physician to have a working knowledge of the specific isolates encountered at his or her own clinical setting.

The gram-negative organisms encountered most commonly in granulocytopenic patients are *E. coli, K. pneumoniae,* and *P. aeruginosa.* Together, these have generally accounted for approximately 90 per cent of the gram-negative isolates at most centers. A precise source for gram-negative bacteremia is identified in only a minority of cases, but the gastrointestinal tract, respiratory tract soft tissue, and urinary tract are the most probable sources for infection. Of these three organisms, *P. aeruginosa* is often the most virulent in neutropenic hosts, although in most developed countries the incidence of infection due to *Pseudomonas* declined in neutropenic patients during the 1980's. But as a general rule, virtually any organism can be pathogenic if the host defenses are severely impaired. *Enterobacter* species, *Citrobacter* species, and *Serratia marcescens* are less frequently encountered but are notable because they rapidly become resistant to β-lactam antibiotics through the induction of chromosomally mediated β-lactamases. Other less common gram-negative isolates include *Acinetobacter* species, *Haemophilus* species (usually nontypable *H. influenzae*), and non-*aeruginosa* pseudomonads (often catheter-related and antibiotic-resistant).

The gram-positive organisms most frequently encountered are the coagulase-negative staphylococci (most commonly *S. epidermidis*), coagulase-positive staphylococci (*S. aureus*), enterococci, and α-hemolytic streptococci (e.g., *S. mutans* or viridans group streptococci). Both coagulase-positive and -negative staphylococci are most commonly isolated from the blood, often from patients with indwelling intravenous catheters, or from foreign bodies such as prosthetic heart valves or orthopedic implants. *S. aureus* tends to be significantly more virulent and its sensitivity to β-lactam antibiotics (e.g., methicillin, oxacillin, or nafcillin) can vary from center to center, making it imperative for the physician to be aware of the frequency of methicillin-resistant *S. aureus* (MRSA) at his or her institution. In contrast, the coagulase-negative staphylococci tend to be relatively indolent. During the last decade, the coagulase-negative staphylococci have become increasingly resistant to β-lactam antibiotics, and the majority (50 to 80 per cent) are methicillin-resistant and generally require treatment with vancomycin. Notable are the recent reports of α-hemolytic viridans streptococci that have been associated with septic shock and the adult respiratory distress syndrome (ARDS) in patients who are receiving high-dose cytosine arabinoside and who develop oral mucosal disruption. Other gram-positive bacteria that may be encountered in neutropenic patients include *Bacillus* species (often catheter-related), group CDC-JK *Corynebacterium* (often catheter-related and relatively antibiotic-resistant), *Enterococcus faecium* (may be resistant to vancomycin), and *Lactobacillus* (may also be resistant to vancomycin).

Infections due solely to anaerobic bacteria are less common and are usually associated with a concomitant abnormality in gastrointestinal mucosal integrity. While *Bacillus fragilis* and *Clostridium perfringens* are the most common organisms, other *Bacteroides* species, as well as other *Clostridium* species (e.g., *C. tertium, C. septicum*), which are often clindamycin-resistant, can be clinically important. Anaerobes are frequent components of intra-abdominal infections, including peritonitis, intra-abdominal abscesses, and perirectal cellulitis or abscesses. *C. difficile* is a common cause of colitis in neutropenic patients who are treated with antibiotics or cytotoxic agents.

Infections due to *Mycobacterium* species are not increased in frequency in neutropenic patients, although patients with hairy cell leukemia (HCL), who have profound monocytopenia in addition to neutropenia, appear to have an increased risk for developing atypical mycobacterial infection (e.g., *M. kansasii, M. fortuitum, M. chelonei,* and *M. avium-intracellulare* complex). Rapidly growing mycobacteria (*M. fortuitum* and *M. chelonei*) may also cause exit site infections in patients with indwelling intravenous catheters, or wound infections following surgery.

In contrast to the bacterial infections, which are often associated with the onset of fever in neutropenic patients, fungal infections only rarely cause primary infection (i.e., initial infection in patients not yet receiving antibiotics). More commonly, fungal infections occur as a secondary process in patients receiving antibacterial agents. Although a variety of fungal infections may be encountered in the neutropenic host, *Candida* and *Aspergillus* species predominate.

The vast majority of infections due to *Candida* species are caused by *C. albicans*, with other potential pathogens including *C. tropicalis*, *C. parapsilosis*, *C. krusei*, and *C. glabrata* (also known as *Torulopsis glabrata*). In neutropenic patients, *Candida* infections may include candidemia, catheter-related infections, invasive mucosal infections (e.g., oral, esophageal, or lower gastrointestinal), and disseminated disease, in which the most commonly affected organs are the liver and spleen (so called hepatosplenic candidiasis), the eye (endophthalmitis), and the skin.

Aspergillosis is usually due to *A. fumigatus* and *A. flavus*, although *A. niger* and *A. terreus* can also result in infection. The upper airways (e.g., oral cavity, nasal cavity, or sinuses) and lung are the primary sites involved with *Aspergillus*, and spread is usually by direct invasion into contiguous areas, although widespread dissemination has been described to sites including brain, liver and spleen, gastrointestinal tract, heart, and kidneys. However, positive blood cultures virtually never occur.

Other fungal pathogens that may occur in neutropenic patients include the Mucoraceae species (*Mucor, Rhizopus, Absidia*, and *Cunninghamella*—often clinically resembling *Aspergillus* species infections), *Trichosporon beigelii* (which may cause disseminated visceral and cutaneous disease), *Fusarium* species, *Drechslera, Pseudallescheria boydii*, and *Malassezia furfur*.

Qualitative Abnormalities of Phagocytes

The microbicidal activity of granulocytes and monocytes involves complex interactions between the cell and the organism or inflammatory site. Some of the major functions important for microbicidal activity include migration of the cell to the inflammatory site (or chemotaxis), cell activation, phagocytosis, and intra- and extracellular killing via both oxygen-dependent and -independent pathways. These qualitative abnormalities can be operationally divided into the following categories: (1) those associated with malignant or myeloproliferative disease itself, (2) those associated with diseases that do not primarily affect the leukocytes, (3) iatrogenic causes (such as administration of pharmacologic agents or radiation), and (4) primary disorders of phagocytes.

PATIENTS WITH MALIGNANT DISORDERS AND MYELODYSPLASIA. Significant functional defects in mature PMN's can occur in patients with AML and acute lymphoblastic leukemia prior to therapy. Although it has been largely assumed that granulocytes from patients with chronic myelogenous leukemia (CML) have normal microbicidal activity, some studies have documented significant impairment in neutrophil function of morphologically mature PMN's from patients with CML, including abnormalities in phagocytosis, random migration, chemotaxis, and bactericidal activity. Nevertheless, during the stable chronic phase of the disease, infectious complications are rarely seen in these patients.

In addition to immunoglobulin deficiencies that impair opsonization, patients with chronic lymphocytic leukemia (CLL) and multiple myeloma may also have such abnormalities as defective granulocyte adherence, decreased granulocyte migration, a decrease in the number of granulocyte receptors for C3b and IgG, and decreased chemotaxis of monocytes.

Significant defects in granulocyte function have also been found in PMN's from patients with myelodysplastic syndromes and preleukemic states. The clinician should probably assume that neutrophils from patients with myelodysplastic syndromes or preleukemia are functionally defective, and thus patients with "borderline" granulocyte counts should be approached as if they had an absolute neutropenia.

NONMALIGNANT HEMATOLOGIC DISEASE. Although the predominant defect in host defense in most patients with aplastic anemia is neutropenia, followed by immune suppression as a result of therapy (e.g., steroids, antithymocyte globulin, or cyclosporine), deficient production of superoxide and a deficiency of myeloperoxidase can sometimes be observed. Patients with

paroxysmal nocturnal hemoglobinuria (PNH) appear to have an increased susceptibility to bacterial infection. Impaired chemotaxis despite normal phagocytosis and bacterial killing has been described in PNH, and the Fc receptor type III (the major Fc receptor in blood and on neutrophils) has also been shown to be deficient in PNH.

In addition to splenic dysfunction, abnormal complement activation, and defective serum opsonizing capacity, defective phagocytic function has been described in patients with sickle cell anemia, although the significance of this is unclear. Neutrophils from infection-prone children with sickle cell disease have been shown to have defective bactericidal activity, perhaps secondary to zinc deficiency.

Some patients with severe G6PD deficiency appear to have an increased susceptibility to infections caused by catalase-positive bacteria. The clinical picture resembles that of chronic granulomatous disease of childhood, although only rarely are infections reported in the first decade of life. The granulocytes show normal phagocytosis and chemotaxis but defective bactericidal activity.

Although most studies address disseminated intravascular coagulation (DIC) secondary to overwhelming bacterial infection, the potential role of fibrinogen degradation products (FDP's) in modifying PMN function has been suggested by the finding that two FDP's (FDP D and FDP E) can cause substantial in vitro inhibition of PMN chemotaxis, oxidative metabolism, and killing of *E. coli*. DIC associated with infection, then, may represent a vicious circle in which the organism triggers the coagulation abnormalities, which in turn may result in neutropenia and defective PMN function, thus worsening the infection.

PHARMACOLOGIC AGENTS AND RADIOTHERAPY. Most cytotoxic drugs used for treatment of malignant and autoimmune diseases or transplantation have antiproliferative effects, resulting in neutropenia and monocytopenia. Among the antineoplastics, the most commonly implicated agents include methotrexate, 6-mercaptopurine, vincristine, vinblastine, anthracyclines, cyclophosphamide, carmustine, and platinum compounds.

Glucocorticoids are associated with increased susceptibility to infection. As a general rule, the signs and symptoms of even severe infections may be masked or greatly reduced in patients receiving steroids. Steroids impair neutrophil chemotaxis, and at high dosages PMN phagocytosis, microbicidal activity, and antibody-dependent cytotoxicity may also be altered. In addition, steroids may cause monocytopenia as well as defects in monocyte chemotaxis, phagocytosis, and killing of bacteria and fungi. In addition to their action on granulocytes and monocytes, steroids may enhance susceptibility to infection by impairing wound healing, increasing skin fragility, and depressing lymphocyte function, the production of cytokines, and humoral immune responses.

Biologic agents (e.g., colony-stimulating factors [CSF], interleukins, interferons) are being employed increasingly in clinical medicine, and their impact on the host defense matrix must be assessed. Studies to date suggest that granulocyte-macrophage (GM)-CSF or granulocyte (G)-CSF not only may increase cell number but also may enhance a number of neutrophil functions, including oxidative metabolism, phagocytosis, microbicidal activity, and antibody-dependent cytotoxicity. At the same time, in adults undergoing autologous bone marrow transplantation, there appears to be the unanticipated finding of a marked decrease in migration of PMN's toward a sterile, artificially created inflammatory site on the skin during periods of GM-CSF administration. Although the clinical significance of any of these effects has not yet been established, these data underscore the importance of carefully evaluating biologics as they are introduced into the therapeutic armamentarium. For example, although interleukin 2 (IL2) appears promising in mediating tumor lysis (with either lymphokine-activated killer [LAK] cells, tumor infiltrating lymphocytes [TIL], or interferon-α), impaired granulocyte function, decreased chemotaxis, and decreased Fc receptor γ-III expression have been noted in some patients receiving high doses of IL2 and may be associated with an increased incidence of significant infections due to *S. aureus*. In contrast, other biologic agents such as interferon-γ may increase phagocyte function and decrease the risk for infection (e.g., in patients with chronic granulomatous disease).

PRIMARY DISORDERS OF PHAGOCYTE FUNCTION. Chronic granulomatous disease (CGD) has served as a prototype for diseases characterized by defective oxidative metabolism of phagocytes. Although CGD represents a heterogeneous group of disorders from a molecular and genetic perspective, the common denominator is that phagocytes lack essential components of oxidative metabolism and fail to generate the respiratory burst in response to various stimuli, including certain pathogenic organisms. The organisms that cause serious infections in patients with CGD are most often those that contain the enzyme catalase. In the absence of cellular production of H_2O_2, the peroxide generated by non–catalase-containing organisms is enough to ameliorate the neutrophil deficiency and allow microbicidal activity. However, if the organism also contains catalase, the H_2O_2 it produces is rapidly degraded and is not available for participation in oxidative-based killing. The majority of infections in patients with CGD are caused by *S. aureus*, although serious infections can also result from enteric gram-negative bacilli (e.g., *E. coli*, *K. pneumoniae*, or *Serratia* species), *P. cepacia*, *Nocardia asteroides*, and *Aspergillus* species.

Serious recurrent infections usually begin in the first year of life in children with CGD. The lung is the most common site of infection (pneumonias and abscesses), with other common infections including skin and soft tissue abscesses, visceral abscesses (particularly hepatic), osteomyelitis (especially of the small bones in the hands and feet), and suppurative lymphadenopathy. Uncommonly, CGD can present in adolescence or adulthood, although with careful history, infectious complications often date back to childhood.

Prophylactic antibiotics, with trimethoprim-sulfamethoxazole, have been advocated by many investigators. Recently, interferon-γ has been shown to reduce the incidence of serious infection and hospital days for patients with CGD.

Myeloperoxidase (MPO) deficiency is perhaps the most common of all granulocyte disorders, with an estimated frequency ranging from 1 in 2000 to 1 in 4000. MPO is a lysosomal enzyme that catalyzes the formation of hypochlorous acid from H_2O_2 produced in the respiratory burst. Interestingly, the majority of individuals identified with MPO deficiency are healthy, and infectious complications are exceedingly rare. Systemic *Candida* infections have occurred in a small number of MPO-deficient patients who also had diabetes mellitus.

Chédiak-Higashi syndrome (CHS) is a rare disorder characterized by autosomal recessive inheritance, recurrent infections, partial oculocutaneous albinism, central and peripheral neuropathy, and increased bleeding time. Neutropenia can also be present. Infections result from combined effects of neutropenia and functional defects in phagocytes, which include impaired degranulation and defective chemotaxis. Infections frequently involve the skin, respiratory tract, and mucous membranes and are most commonly caused by *S. aureus* or gram-negative bacilli. Deficiency of the iC3b receptor (also known as CR3, Mo1, and MAC-1), which is important for adherence and phagocytosis, is a rare disorder. Accordingly, neutrophils demonstrate defects in aggregation, margination, chemotaxis, and phagocytosis. The most common infections are skin and subcutaneous tissue infections, otitis, mucositis, gingivitis, and periodontitis.

A number of disorders have been described which are characterized by defects in chemotaxis of granulocytes and/or monocytes. Infections in these patients tend to be cutaneous, and the most common pathogens are *S. aureus*, streptococci, *C. albicans*, *E. coli*, and *Trichophyton rubrum*. Depending on the specific syndrome, deep-seated infections may also occur. The "lazy leukocyte" syndrome may also be associated with neutropenia and is characterized by gingivitis, recurrent otitis media, rhinitis, and stomatitis. Hyperimmunoglobulin E syndrome (Job's syndrome) is usually associated with multiple cutaneous abscesses caused by staphylococci, but deep-seated infections and infections due to other organisms such as pseudomonads and *Candida* have also been reported. Wound healing does not appear to be a problem, as it is in CGD. Chemotaxis defects have been reported in patients with congenital ichthyosis and recurrent *T. rubrum* infections.

DEFECTS IN CELL-MEDIATED IMMUNITY (CMI)

Cellular immune dysfunction either may be primary, as in a number of congenital immunodeficiency states, or may occur secondary to other disorders of therapeutic interventions. Defec-

tive CMI may lead to infections caused by bacteria, fungi, viruses, and protozoa. The predominant pathogens are intracellular organisms (those microbes that survive inside of macrophages) and include mycobacteria (both *M. tuberculosis* and atypical mycobacteria), *Legionella*, *N. asteroides*, *Salmonella* species, *Cryptococcus neoformans*, *Histoplasma capsulatum*, *Coccidioides immitis*, varicella-zoster virus (VZV), herpes simplex virus (HSV), cytomegalovirus (CMV), Epstein-Barr virus (EBV), *Pneumocystis carinii*, *T. gondii*, *Cryptosporidium*, and *Strongyloides stercoralis*.

Patients with Malignant Disorders

Hodgkin's disease and the non-Hodgkin's lymphomas are associated with altered CMI not only when the malignancy is active, but in some instances even when the malignancy is in remission.

CMI defects have been postulated to help explain the incidence of atypical mycobacterial infections in patients with hairy cell leukemia and also occur in relatively rare T-cell malignancies such as mycosis fungoides and T-cell CLL. CMI defects exist in children with ALL, as evidenced by their increased susceptibility to infections due to *P. carinii* or disseminated VZV, but it is likely that concurrent therapy plays a major role. Clinically significant impairment of CMI has not been well established for other malignancies.

Patients with Nonmalignant Hematologic Disorders

Impaired CMI is not a prominent feature of nonmalignant hematologic disorders unless associated with therapy or acquisition of HIV-1 infection. Abnormalities in CMI have been best described in patients with hemophilia who have received Factor VIII concentrates even in the absence of apparent HIV-1 infection. Patients with sickle cell anemia have been found to be anergic in association with zinc deficiency and decreased nucleoside phosphorylase activity.

A number of infections may produce impaired CMI either directly (e.g., by infecting key cellular components such as T lymphocytes or macrophages) or by affecting other immunoregulatory mechanisms. The most notable viral infection associated with impaired CMI is HIV-1. Other viral infections that also are associated with CMI defects include CMV, EBV, RSV, hepatitis B, and influenza. Other nonviral infections that have been variably associated with impaired CMI by in vitro testing have included tuberculosis, leprosy, bacterial pneumonia, brucellosis, typhoid fever, coccidioidomycosis, syphilis, and a variety of parasitic diseases.

Noninfectious disorders that have been linked to abnormal CMI include chronic protein-calorie malnutrition, uremia, diabetes mellitus, surgery, anesthesia, sarcoidosis, and cystic fibrosis.

Pharmacologic Agents

Corticosteroids are the pharmacologic agents most often associated with CMI abnormalities, although they may also cause immune suppression owing to effects on other host defense mechanisms. The degree of immunosuppression and the relative risk of infection depend on the dose and duration of corticosteroids as well as the underlying disease. Patients receiving pharmacologic doses of steroids (e.g., brain tumor patients, patients with inflammatory bowel disease, patients with autoimmune disorders) may have impaired CMI and should be considered at risk for mycobacterial, viral, and parasitic infections. Patients who are to be treated with corticosteroids and who have a known history of tuberculosis or a positive PPD skin test should be placed on prophylactic INH to prevent reactivation and potential dissemination of disease.

A number of cytotoxic agents are also associated with impaired CMI, including methotrexate, cyclophosphamide, 6-mercaptopurine, and azathioprine. Cyclosporine is an immunosuppressant used to suppress transplant rejection and is associated with alterations in helper T cells, effector T cells, and NK cells. It has not been established, however, that the use of cyclosporine per se is associated with an increased risk of infection.

Radiotherapy may also result in impaired CMI, especially when used in combination with other immunosuppressive agents or for treatment of patients with underlying diseases associated with intrinsic CMI defects (e.g., as a component of the preparatory regimen for bone marrow transplantation or for treatment of Hodgkin's disease).

Primary Disorders of Cell-mediated Immunity
(see Ch. 244)

Defects in CMI are found as components of mixed primary B- and T-cell abnormalities, including severe combined immunodeficiency disease (SCID), Wiskott-Aldrich syndrome, ataxia-telangiectasia, and certain purine pathway enzyme deficiencies. Infections in patients with these disorders tend to begin early in life and may be caused not only by pathogens associated with CMI abnormalities but also by those seen with humoral defects, such as the encapsulated bacteria.

SCID is associated with a marked decrease in both B- and T-cell numbers and extremely low levels of immunoglobulins. Patients fail to react to skin tests and have a negligible antibody response following immunizations. Failure to thrive and recurrent infections are seen within the first few months of life. Infections are due to S. aureus, S. pneumoniae, H. influenzae, P. carinii, Candida, and herpes group viruses. Affected infants usually die by 2 years of age. A variant of SCID has been described that is associated with chronic skin eruption, hepatosplenomegaly, eosinophilia, and histiocytic infiltration of the lymph nodes (Omenn's disease). P. carinii pneumonia may be a common presenting symptom in this disorder.

In patients with Wiskott-Aldrich syndrome, the major abnormality is an inability to respond to polysaccharide antigens. Infections are caused by polysaccharide-encapsulated bacterial pathogens such as S. pneumoniae and H. influenzae. However, patients may also lose T-cell functions and may have increased susceptibility to pathogens such as HSV and certain fungi and protozoa.

Ataxia-telangiectasia is associated with absent serum and secretory IgA. The thymus is hypoplastic, and thymus-dependent zones in lymph nodes are empty. Infection with encapsulated bacteria predominates, especially recurrent sinopulmonary infections. Many patients have progressive loss of T-cell function over time and may become susceptible to associated pathogens.

Purine pathway enzyme deficiencies (adenosine deaminase deficiency or nucleoside phosphorylase deficiency) may be associated with either combined B- and T-cell defects or isolated B- or T-cell abnormalities. The type of infection depends on the predominant immune defect. Infections may not appear until 6 to 12 months of age.

The primary cellular immunodeficiencies associated with T-cell abnormalities include thymic hypoplasia (DiGeorge's syndrome), combined immunodeficiency with predominant T-cell defect (Nezelof's syndrome), purine nucleoside phosphorylase deficiency, and chronic mucocutaneous candidiasis.

DiGeorge's syndrome develops when the third and part of the fourth pharyngeal pouches fail to develop during embryogenesis, resulting in absence of the thymus and parathyroid glands. Children with DiGeorge's syndrome lack T lymphocytes and have severe depression of CMI, making them susceptible to overwhelming infections due to a variety of organisms, including HSV, VZV, C. albicans, and P. carinii. Nezelof's syndrome can be differentiated from DiGeorge's syndrome by the absence of parathyroid and cardiac involvement.

Cartilage-hair hypoplasia is a form of short-limbed dwarfism associated with a virtual absence of T-cell function. Interestingly, susceptibility to infection is not as pronounced as in other T-cell deficiencies. Overwhelming viral infections due to vaccinia or varicella viruses may occur.

Chronic mucocutaneous candidiasis involves impairment in CMI, and infection is almost always limited to the skin and mucous membranes.

ABNORMALITIES OF HUMORAL DEFENSE MECHANISMS—IMMUNOGLOBULINS AND COMPLEMENT

Immunoglobulins and complement are among the most important components of the humoral immune system, and defects or deficiencies in either may be associated with serious infections. Other proteins that have been classified as part of the humoral defense system include lysozyme, lactoferrin, tuftsin, and fibronectin. Immunoglobulins may be opsonic (enhance phagocytosis) or neutralizing (inhibits replication of viruses) or with complement may lyse microbes or cells. The humoral system functions predominantly against bacterial infections. Patients with either primary or secondary defects or deficiencies in these proteins are at highest risk for developing serious infections due to the encapsulated bacteria and to a lesser extent the enteroviruses and Giardia lamblia.

Patients with Malignant Disorders

The degree of humoral impairment in multiple myeloma appears to be related to the stage of the disease, primarily due to malignant plasma cell induction of a protein that is synthesized by macrophages and that selectively suppresses B-cell function. Myeloma patients are most susceptible to recurrent infections from encapsulated bacteria such as S. pneumoniae or H. influenzae early in the course of the disease. Infections due to enteric gram-negative rods and staphylococci are also encountered, especially in patients with refractory or advanced disease. Sites of recurrent infection are most often the upper respiratory tract, urinary tract, or skin.

Patients with B-cell CLL appear to have an unbalanced immunoglobulin chain synthesis and resultant hypogammaglobulinemia. The incidence of infection correlates with the duration and stage of the disease as well as the serum levels of immunoglobulins (particularly IgG). Encapsulated bacteria predominate, although infections due to staphylococci and enteric gram-negative bacilli also occur. Upper and lower respiratory tract infections are encountered most commonly, although other sites such as urinary tract and skin are frequently involved.

Nonmalignant states (e.g., nephrotic syndrome, burns, protein-losing enteropathy) can be associated with increased immunoglobulin catabolism or loss and may lead to decreased antibody levels and enhanced susceptibility to infection. Clinically significant acquired complement defects are unusual.

Primary Deficiencies

Isolated B-cell immunodeficiency states and their associated risks for infection in children include transient hypogammaglobulinemia of infancy, which is not usually associated with serious infections; sex-linked hypogammaglobulinemia, which is associated with recurrent pyogenic infections and septicemia due to S. pneumoniae, H. influenzae, S. aureus, N. meningitidis, and P. aeruginosa; hypogammaglobulinemia associated with hyperimmunoglobulin M, in which patients have recurrent respiratory, soft tissue, and gastrointestinal infections; selective IgM deficiency, in which patients have severe recurrent infections due to pyogenic bacteria; and selective IgA deficiency, in which certain patients may have increased numbers of upper respiratory tract infections whereas others appear not to be at increased risk. Chronic diarrhea due to G. lamblia is also associated with IgA deficiency. Common variable hypogammaglobulinemia is associated with respiratory tract infections due to S. pneumoniae, H. influenzae, and S. aureus. Diarrhea due to G. lamblia also occurs.

Many patients with B-cell deficiencies, particularly those with congenital hypogammaglobulinemia, appear to be at risk for the development of chronic central nervous system infections due to enteroviruses.

A number of primary defects in complement components have also been described. Although deficiencies of the early classic pathway components (C1, C2, C4) have been reported, associated infection is rare, probably because the alternative pathway remains functional and is able to compensate. Deficiencies of C3 or C5, on the other hand, often lead to severe infections due to encapsulated organisms, enteric gram-negative bacteria, and staphylococci. Absence of the later components (C5b, C6, C7, C8, C9) leads to an increase in infections, primarily due to Neisseria species, both N. gonorrhoeae and N. meningitidis. Although the defects in these later components may be present from birth, infectious episodes do not typically begin until the teenage years. Indeed, any patient with recurrent infections due to Neisseria species should be investigated for the possibility of complement deficiency.

SPLENECTOMY AND SPLENIC DYSFUNCTION

Splenectomy may be performed either as a part of staging or as a therapeutic intervention in a number of disorders, including Hodgkin's disease, agnogenic myeloid metaplasia, paroxysmal nocturnal hemoglobinuria, hereditary spherocytosis, thalassemia, and a variety of autoimmune disorders.

The spleen probably plays an adjunctive role in host defense by removing organisms from the blood that have been ineffectively opsonized by complement. In addition, it participates in the primary immunoglobulin response and is involved in the regulation of the alternative complement pathway, with low levels of immunoglobulins and properdin reported in patients following splenectomy. A decrease in the opsonic peptide tuftsin has also been reported following splenectomy, and alternative pathway defects may be important in patients with sickle cell disease and splenic dysfunction.

The risk of developing serious infection, as well as the types of infections may vary depending on the reason for abnormal splenic function and the presence or absence of other immune abnormalities. Patients who undergo post-traumatic splenectomy appear to be at a lower risk for infection. An increased risk of *Salmonella* infections appears to be unique for the sickle cell population. Most asplenic patients or patients who have undergone splenectomy are at increased risk for serious bacterial infections primarily due to *S. pneumoniae* and *H. influenzae*, as well as *Neisseria* species and the DF2 bacillus. The initial presentation of even overwhelming infection may be deceptively subtle, with fever often being the only sign of infection. Asplenic patients with an underlying hematologic disease who present with fever should be managed initially as potentially septic.

EVALUATION AND MANAGEMENT OF THE FEBRILE GRANULOCYTOPENIC PATIENT: A PARADIGM FOR THE COMPROMISED HOST

A classic tenet of infectious disease is that antibiotic therapy is based on the isolation and identification of a specific organism or on a reliable prediction of a specific organism from a clinically involved site of infection. The overall management of neutropenic patients is based on the use of empiric antibiotics directed against a wider array of potential pathogens. Indeed, it is well accepted that when a neutropenic patient develops a new fever (usually defined as one oral temperature $\geq 38.5°C$, or more than two successive readings of $\geq 38°C$ in a 12-hour period), an empiric broad-spectrum antibacterial regimen should be started expeditiously. The rationale for this approach evolved from the observation that bacteremias in neutropenic patients were rapidly lethal, especially those due to gram-negative organisms, if antibiotic therapy was delayed until an organism was isolated or a site of infection identified. Although the goal of the pre-antibiotic evaluation of a newly febrile neutropenic patient is to identify potential sources, the majority of patients will not have a source of infection identified to explain the fever.

The standard initial evaluation should include a careful physical examination with particular attention to areas that may "hide" an infection, notably the oral cavity and the perianal area. Examination of the perirectal area, including deep palpation, should be performed, and only if there are findings suggestive of a localized inflammatory site (e.g., pain or fluctuance) should a judicious digital examination be performed. At a minimum, two sets of blood samples for culture should be obtained. If the patient has an indwelling intravenous catheter, then at least one set should be drawn through the catheter and another from a peripheral vein. For patients with multilumen intravenous catheters, a culture should be obtained through *each* lumen and the specific lumen clearly identified on the culture bottle. This is important, because catheter infection may be limited to a single lumen. Because of the absence of granulocytes, microscopic examination of the urine may be normal even in the presence of a urinary tract infection. A chest radiograph can serve as a valuable baseline, although some investigators have questioned the use of this procedure in patients without pulmonary symptoms. In addition, accessible sites of potential infection should be aspirated or biopsied, with appropriate material sent for Gram's stain, culture, and histologic examination.

Even with a comprehensive evaluation, an infectious etiology for the fever is found in only 30 to 50 per cent of patients.

Nonetheless, even subtle indications of inflammation must be considered as sites of potential infection in the presence of granulocytopenia. For example, minimal perirectal erythema and tenderness may be harbingers of a perirectal cellulitis. Minimal erythema or serous discharge at the exit site of an indwelling intravenous catheter may herald a tunnel or exit-site infection.

Colonization with microorganisms often precedes development of significant infection. However, routine "surveillance" cultures are not of practical benefit in a neutropenic patient, since colonization of no single body site is consistently predictive and multiple potential pathogens are usually isolated from any single site, making it difficult to predict the organism responsible for infection. Moreover, since empiric broad-spectrum antibiotics are administered under any circumstance, the expense of routine surveillance cannot be justified.

Tests such as nuclear scanning have also been used to define occult sites of infection. Although gallium citrate accumulates in inflammatory lesions because of its avid binding to lactoferrin, this test has not been shown to be useful in granulocytopenic patients. Autologous or allogeneic leukocytes labeled in vitro with indium-111 have been used with some success in the evaluation of febrile granulocytopenic patients.

Because of these diagnostic difficulties, even fevers that are temporally associated with the administration of blood products or with fever-producing antineoplastic agents should be considered potentially infectious in etiology and treated as such. In sum, virtually all new fevers in the neutropenic population warrant careful clinical and microbiologic evaluation, followed by prompt initiation of empiric antibiotic therapy. Conversely, any clinically evident site of potential infection mandates expeditious broad-spectrum therapy, even in the absence of fever.

Since the goal of empiric antibiotic therapy is to protect against the early morbidity and mortality that result from untreated bacterial infections, regimens have been formulated to maximize activity against organisms that are commonly encountered and are particularly virulent. However, empiric regimens cannot realistically be designed to cover every potential bacterial pathogen. Moreover, no regimen is capable of completely eliminating the risk of development of subsequent infections in persistently neutropenic patients.

Management of Indwelling Intravenous Catheters

Although gram-positive bacterial infections (especially staphylococcal) are the most frequent causes of catheter-related infections, other bacterial and nonbacterial species can be encountered, particularly in the neutropenic patient. These include resistant *Corynebacterium*, *Bacillus* species, gram-negative organisms, and fungi. In approaching the patient with a catheter-related infection, it is important to consider the specific type of infection, the location of the infection (i.e., bacteremia versus exit site versus tunnel), the type of access device (e.g., Hickman versus implantable subcutaneous reservoir), and the duration of symptoms.

In general, the vast majority of simple catheter-related bacteremias and exit-site infections can be cleared using appropriate antibiotics and do not necessitate catheter removal. This applies to both neutropenic and non-neutropenic patients. If multilumen devices are used, the antibiotic infusion should be rotated among the ports, since infection may be limited to one lumen (failure to do so can be a cause of persistent infection despite antibiotics). Diagnostic cultures should also be drawn through all ports of any multilumen device. If there is persistent bacteremia after 48 hours of appropriate therapy, the catheter should be removed. Failures of therapy are more common when the infections are due to certain organisms, such as *Bacillus* species or *Candida albicans*, and when these are isolated, the catheter usually should be removed.

Infections extending to involve the tunnel of a Hickman catheter also mandate prompt removal of the device, as antibiotics alone rarely cure this "closed-space" infection, particularly in the granulocytopenic host. Likewise, infections around the reservoir of an implantable subcutaneous device may be difficult to eradicate without catheter removal. Patients with recurrent catheter infections (despite a history of appropriate therapy) are also candidates for prompt catheter removal.

It is unresolved whether a non-neutropenic patient with an indwelling catheter who becomes newly febrile should receive antibiotics empirically. The safest policy is to begin antibiotics (using a third-generation cephalosporin like ceftriaxone or an aminoglycoside plus vancomycin) and continue them pending culture results and clinical response. This approach protects against rapid progression of undetected yet virulent infections (such as *S. aureus*) and may minimize the need for ultimate catheter removal. If by 72 hours the cultures are negative and the patient is stable, antibiotics can be discontinued.

Initial Management of the Neutropenic Patient Who Becomes Febrile

Traditionally, gram-negative bacteria have been the most frequently isolated pathogens in the neutropenic population. Of the gram-negative bacteria, *E. coli*, *K. pneumoniae*, and *P. aeruginosa* have been the most common. While gram-negative bacteria still predominate at some institutions, there has been a trend in recent years toward more gram-positive infections, and these now comprise the majority of isolates at many centers. In general, the gram-negative infections tend to be more virulent, and early empiric regimens have been formulated to provide protection primarily against these organisms while maintaining a broad spectrum of activity against other potential pathogens. Indeed, adequate coverage of these gram-negative organisms is still an essential property of any empiric regimen.

Although there is no single best regimen or recipe, there are a number of appropriate options. The selection of a specific antibiotic regimen depends on many factors, including institutional sensitivity patterns, individual and institutional experience, and clinical parameters.

The standard approach to the empiric management of the febrile neutropenic patient has been to use combination antibiotic regimens. Until recently, this has been the only way to provide coverage broad enough to encompass the predominant gram-positive and gram-negative organisms. Moreover, some combinations have been considered to provide synergy and to have the potential for decreasing the emergence of resistant isolates. Aminoglycoside–β-lactam combinations were the first empiric regimens with acceptable efficacy in the setting of fever and neutropenia. Such combination regimens are still widely used and represent a standard against which newer regimens are tested. Many variations have been studied and include aminoglycosides combined with either an extended-spectrum penicillin, a cephalosporin, or as a component of a triple-drug regimen. If an aminoglycoside-containing combination regimen is to be employed, the choice of specific antibiotics should be based primarily on the institutional antibiotic sensitivity patterns and secondarily on toxicity and cost differences.

Non–aminoglycoside-containing combination regimens have also been studied. These have consisted of combinations of two β-lactam antibiotics, or so-called double β-lactam regimens, usually consisting of an expanded-spectrum carboxy- or ureido-penicillin plus a third-generation cephalosporin (e.g., piperacillin and ceftazidime).

New or Novel Antibiotics for Neutropenic Patients

The advent of β-lactam antibiotics with broad-spectrum activity which achieve high serum bactericidal levels has made monotherapy another option for the initial empiric therapy of the febrile neutropenic patient (Table 287–3). The third-generation cephalosporins and the carbapenems are the two classes that include potential candidates for empiric single-agent therapy. Ceftazidime has been the most extensively studied of the third-generation cephalosporins as monotherapy because of its superior activity against *P. aeruginosa*.

A large, randomized study evaluating 550 consecutive episodes of fever and neutropenia was conducted at the National Cancer Institute (NCI). In this study, patients with fever and granulocytopenia underwent a standard initial evaluation and then were randomized to receive either a combination of antibiotics (cephalothin, gentamicin, and carbenicillin) or ceftazidime as a single agent. The overall results show that monotherapy compared favorably with a standard combination regimen. Approximately two thirds of the episodes in both groups were successfully treated for the entire duration of their granulocytopenia, without requiring *any* changes in their initial regimen. Another one third of the episodes required some change or modification (such as addition of an antibacterial, antifungal, or antiviral drug) to ensure a successful outcome (see indications for modifications below), and an equally low number in both groups (about 5 per cent) died of infection. None of the deaths was attributable to a specific deficiency in one regimen that was not present in the other.

Two subgroups of patients were identified who required more frequent modifications of the initial regimen in order to achieve a successful outcome: (1) those presenting with a documented source of infection to account for the initial fever, and (2) those having relatively protracted periods of granulocytopenia (> 1 week). The need for modification in these subgroups was identical for those episodes treated with monotherapy and those treated with combination therapy. In this study, these modifications did not represent a failure of either regimen per se but instead were reflective of the limitations of any regimen in treating patients who are at high risk for development of subsequent infections.

Concerns regarding the use of ceftazidime as a single agent for fever and neutropenia include the lack of synergy against documented gram-negative infections, lack of activity against certain gram-positive isolates, poor antianaerobic activity, and the potential for development of resistance.

In addition to the third-generation cephalosporins, other anti-

TABLE 287–3. ACTIVITY OF NEWER ANTIBIOTICS AGAINST BACTERIAL PATHOGENS COMMONLY ENCOUNTERED IN IMPAIRED HOSTS

Antibiotic	Enteric Gram-negative	P. aeruginosa	Coagulase-positive Staphylococci	Coagulase-negative Staphylococci	Enterococci	Non-Group D Streptococci	Anaerobes
Ceftazidime	Good	Good	Moderate (poor against methicillin-resistant strains)	Poor against the majority (most are methicillin-resistant)	Poor	Good	Poor
Cefoperazone	Good	Moderate	Moderate (poor against methicillin-resistant strains)	Poor against the majority	Poor	Good	Poor
Other third-generation cephalosporins	Good	Poor	Moderate (poor against methicillin-resistant strains)	Poor against the majority	Poor	Good	Poor to moderate (moxalactam and ceftizoxime have some activity)
Imipenem	Good	Good	Good (poor against methicillin-resistant strains	Poor against the majority	Good	Good	Good
Quinolones	Good	Good	Good (including most methicillin-resistant strains)	Good (limited clinical experience)	Poor to moderate	Poor to moderate	Poor
Aztreonam	Good	Good	Poor	Poor	Poor	Poor	Poor

Modified from Rubin M, Walsh TJ, Pizzo PA: Clinical approaches to infections in the compromised host. *In* Hoffman R, Benz EJ, Shattil SJ, et al. (eds.): Hematology: Basic Principles and Practice. New York, Churchill Livingstone, 1991.

biotics are also being evaluated in neutropenic patients. Imipenem, for example, is a member of the carbapenem class of antibiotics. It is formulated in fixed combination with cilastatin, which inhibits a renal enzyme that can degrade imipenem. Overall, it has the broadest spectrum of activity of any available antibiotic. Of note is its excellent in vitro activity against enterococci as well as many anaerobes.

Early results of two randomized studies appear to corroborate its efficacy in this setting—one comparing it with an aminoglycoside-containing combination and another being performed at the NCI comparing it with monotherapy with ceftazidime. Interestingly, neither of these studies appears to demonstrate superior efficacy for imipenem. Two potential drawbacks to its use include a relatively high incidence of the development of resistant *P. aeruginosa* and its potential to decrease the seizure threshold in patients with central nervous system pathology. In addition, in the ongoing NCI trial, a higher than expected frequency of nausea has been found with imipenem.

Because of the increasing incidence of gram-positive infections in cancer patients during the 1980's and their increased resistance to β-lactam antibiotics, some authorities have recommended that vancomycin be added to empiric regimens. Conversely, it has been argued that since many of these organisms are of relatively low virulence, vancomycin may be safely withheld until the gram-positive isolate has been identified microbiologically.

Although two randomized studies demonstrated a reduction in gram-positive infections in patients receiving a vancomycin regimen, there were no significant differences in outcome or survival when vancomycin was added in a pathogen-directed manner. A retrospective analysis from the NCI also indicated that there was no excess morbidity in delaying the institution of vancomycin by waiting for either a microbiologic or clinical indication for its use (i.e., a positive culture for a resistant gram-positive organism or a clinical infection developing with other antibiotics).

At the present time, it seems reasonable not to routinely include vancomycin in all empiric antibiotic regimens. Its use, however, should be guided by institutional experience and sensitivity patterns. For example, in a center with a high incidence of methicillin-resistant *S. aureus,* routine use of vancomycin is clearly warranted, since this may be a particularly virulent organism if not treated. In addition, fluctuations in patterns of infecting microorganisms may occur over time. For example, penicillin-resistant α-hemolytic streptococci have recently been identified as particularly virulent pathogens in some centers (perhaps related to the use of high-dose cytosine arabinoside). Clearly, the emergence of new pathogens or pathogens with altered sensitivity profiles may force dramatic changes in our use of antibiotics in the future.

The appropriate role for the quinolones in the neutropenic patient has yet to be defined. Because of their relatively poor activity against certain gram-positive organisms, they should not be used for empiric therapy alone. They may, however, be useful for completion of therapy in patients who initially respond to intravenous antibiotics and who have had either a fever of undetermined origin or a susceptible bacterial isolate.

A particularly useful feature of aztreonam is its apparent lack of cross-reactivity with the other β-lactams in patients who have penicillin or β-lactam allergies. In this group of patients empiric therapy might begin with a combination of vancomycin, aztreonam, and an aminoglycoside.

Also recently introduced are combinations of β-lactams with β-lactamase inhibitors (i.e., clavulanic acid and sulbactam). Three preparations are now available, including amoxicillin + clavulanic acid (oral formulation only), ticarcillin + clavulanic acid, and ampicillin + sulbactam. A number of studies have documented the efficacy of ticarcillin + clavulanic acid combined with aminoglycoside for initial empiric therapy of fever in neutropenic patients. The expanded gram-positive coverage may obviate additional anti–gram-positive agents.

APPROACH TO THE PATIENT WITH PROLONGED GRANULOCYTOPENIA

How Long Should Antibiotics Be Continued?

A question of practical importance is how long empiric antibiotics should be continued in persistently neutropenic patients.

Should they always be continued until the granulocyte count recovers, or can they be safely discontinued prior to that time?

The question of duration of therapy can be approached by placing patients in two categories: those whose initial workup (at the time of presentation with fever and neutropenia) did not reveal a source of infection (i.e., a fever of undetermined origin, or FUO) and those whose initial workup revealed an infection to account for the fever (i.e., a positive culture, clinically infected site, or both). The majority of patients (approximately 60 per cent) fall into the FUO category, although this varies with the institution, the therapy, and the patient population (Fig. 287–1).

FUO PATIENTS. There are only limited data that specifically address the issue of duration of empiric therapy in neutropenic patients presenting with an FUO. For patients with an expected short duration of granulocytopenia (e.g., < 1 week), waiting to stop antibiotics until recovery of the counts is practical and effective. However, the real dilemma arises in the population with more prolonged granulocytopenia.

In a study from the NCI, patients with FUO and persistent granulocytopenia were randomized either to discontinue antibiotics on day 7 of therapy or to continue them until the resolution of the neutropenia. Nearly 40 per cent of afebrile patients in whom antibiotics were stopped developed recurrent fever, and 38 per cent of febrile patients whose antibiotics were discontinued developed hypotensive episodes. It was concluded that day 7 was too early to discontinue antibiotics in this group.

A subsequent study randomized persistently neutropenic, afebrile patients to continue or discontinue antibiotics on day 14. Preliminary analysis showed no difference between the two groups: Approximately one third of patients became febrile again regardless of whether they stopped or continued antibiotics. However, those whose fevers recurred following discontinuation of antibiotics responded to a reinstitution of their initial regimens, whereas those remaining on antibiotics required addition of amphotericin B. On this basis, it seems reasonable to discontinue antibiotics and carefully observe FUO patients who are predicted to have a long duration of neutropenia and who have remained afebrile after 14 days of therapy.

PATIENTS PRESENTING WITH DOCUMENTED INFECTIONS. There are even fewer data that address the issue of duration of antibiotics in patients with defined sites of infection. For persistently neutropenic patients who have had clinical and microbiologic resoluton of their infection and who are afebrile at day 14 (for a minimum of 7 days), antibiotics should be discontinued. The ultimate decision of whether to continue or discontinue rests on a number of clinical parameters, such as the degree of or potential for antibiotic toxicity, the predicted duration of neutropenia, the seriousness of the initial infection, and the presence or absence of a continued site of infection or other factors predisposing to subsequent infection. It should be emphasized that any neutropenic patient whose antibiotics are discontinued requires careful, meticulous follow-up in order to quickly detect new fevers or infection.

Modifications of Antibiotic Therapy During the Course of Granulocytopenia

Empiric antibiotics have their greatest impact early in the course of neutropenia. However, it is during a prolonged granulocytopenic episode when the patient is at highest risk for the development of multiple types of secondary infections or superinfections. Many of these dictate specific modifications of the initial regimen (Table 287–4).

Bacterial isolates that are resistant to the initial empiric regimen are invariably encountered when managing neutropenic patients. For example, at most centers, the majority of coagulase-negative staphylococci are resistant to β-lactams, and breakthrough infections might be anticipated. Fortunately, coagulase-negative staphylococci are relatively indolent, and the risk for secondary infection can be balanced accordingly. Thus, for the patient who develops evidence of gram-positive infection while receiving β-lactam or who has evidence of a catheter site infection, vancomycin is an appropriate addition to the initial antibiotic regimen. Similarly, if the coverage of the initial regimen has limited antianaerobic activity, secondary infection with anaerobics might be anticipated.

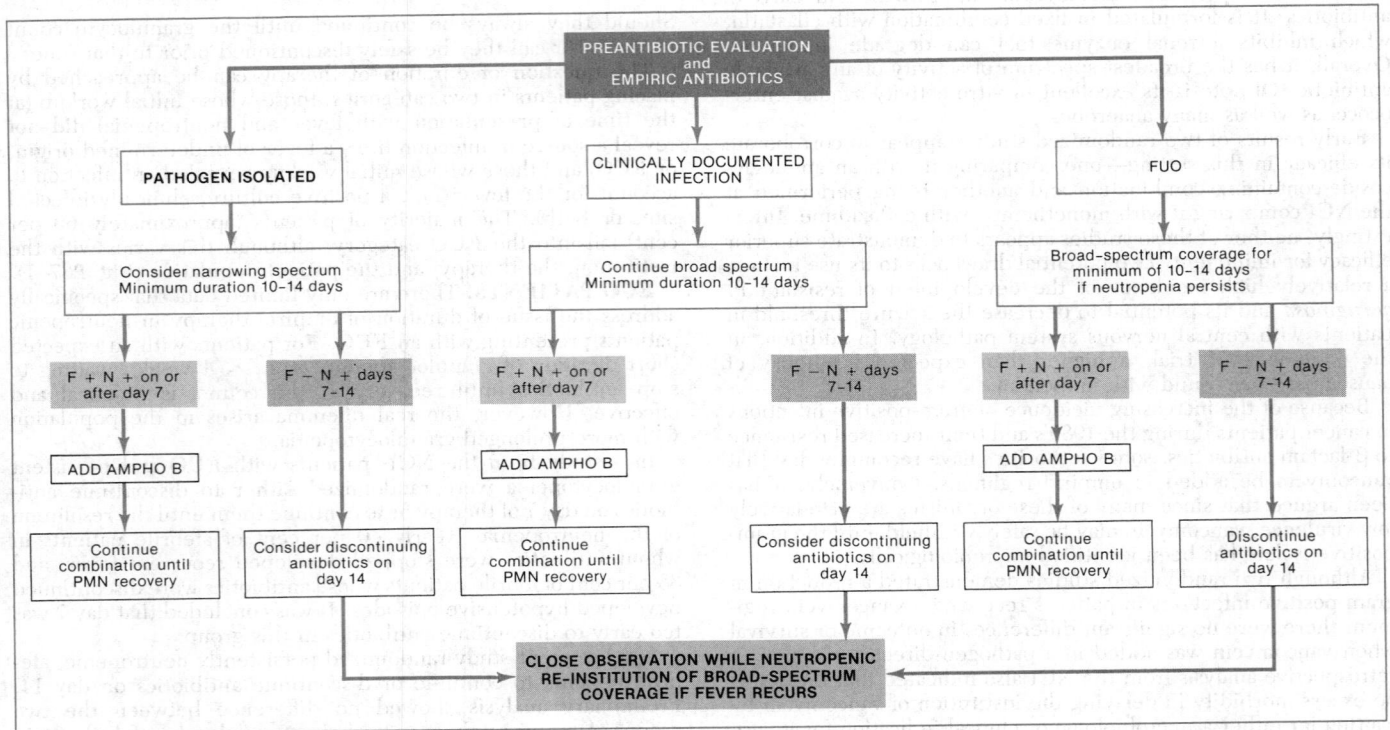

FIGURE 287-1. Management of fever and neutropenia. F + N + = Febrile, neutropenic. F − N + = Afebrile, neutropenic. FUO = No source for fever on preantibiotic evaluation. AMPHO B = Amphotericin B. (From Rubin M, Walsh TJ, Pizzo PA: Clinical approach to infections in the compromised host. *In* Hoffman R, Benz EJ, Shattil SJ, et al. (eds.): Hematology: Basic Principles and Practice. New York, Churchill Livingstone, 1991.)

The appearance of "secondary" resistance is seen more frequently with certain organisms. For example, *Enterobacter* species, *Citrobacter* species, and *Serratia* have inducible β-lactamases, and the appearance of a clinically significant clustering of resistant *Enterobacter* in a neutropenic population has been recently observed. Accordingly, when these organisms are isolated from a patient, careful observation for emergence of resistance is warranted, and for patients receiving monotherapy with a broad-spectrum β-lactam an aminoglycoside should be added. *P. aeruginosa* may develop resistance to imipenem through a relatively novel mechanism involving a change in the porins. Hence, patients receiving single-agent therapy for *P. aeruginosa* infection should also have an aminoglycoside added to their regimens. Secondary development of resistance by gram-positive organisms is somewhat rarer, although it has been described. Of

note, recent studies have documented the emergence of vancomycin-resistant coagulase-negative staphylococci and enterococci in patients receiving vancomycin.

The appearance of a new site of infection (e.g., cellulitis or pneumonia) or the progression of a previously documented site of infection is an additional reason for changes or modifications of the antimicrobial regimen. For example, the development of marginal or necrotizing gingivitis is relatively common in patients who have received intensive cytotoxic therapy. Anaerobic organisms contribute to this process, and an antianaerobic agent such as clindamycin or metronidazole should be added to the empiric regimen if gingivitis is diagnosed.

The most common pathogens contributing to perianal cellulitis are the aerobic gram-negative bacilli, enterococci, and bowel anaerobes. Therefore, when it occurs in a patient already receiv-

TABLE 287-4. MODIFICATION OF THERAPY

Clinical Event	Possible Modifications of Therapy
Breakthrough bacteremia	If gram-positive isolate (e.g., *S. epidermidis*), add vancomycin If gram-negative isolate (i.e., presumably resistant), switch to new regimen
Catheter-associated infection	Add vancomycin (as well as gram-negative coverage if not already being given)
Severe oral mucositis or necrotizing gingivitis	Add specific antianaerobic agent (e.g., metronidazole)
Esophagitis	Oral clotrimazole, fluconazole, or IV amphotericin B

Pneumonitis
  Diffuse or interstitial
  New infiltrate in a granulocytopenic patient also receiving antibiotics
	Trimethoprim-sulfamethoxazole and erythromycin (plus broad-spectrum antibiotics if the patient is granulocytopenic)
	If granulocyte count is rising, watch and wait
	If granulocyte count is not recovering, biopsy to establish diagnosis; if biopsy cannot be done, add amphotericin B empirically

Perianal tenderness	If patient is already receiving broad-spectrum antibiotics, add a specific antianaerobic agent If patient is not on antibiotics, begin broad-spectrum therapy with anaerobic coverage
Persistent fever and neutropenia	Continue antibiotics and after 1 week of persistent fever and neutropenia, add systemic antifungal therapy

ing broad-spectrum antibiotics, the addition of an antianaerobic agent as well as a change in the broad-spectrum coverage may be necessary. Similarly, any suspected intra-abdominal site of infection should prompt addition or inclusion of antibiotics active against aerobic gram-negative bacilli, enterococci, and bowel anaerobes.

The development of a new site of infection may also warrant the addition of antimicrobial agents directed at fungi, viruses, or parasites. The appearance of burning retrosternal pain is frequently an indicator of esophagitis, most often caused by cytotoxic therapy, *Candida*, or herpes simplex. The development of pulmonary infiltrates might raise suspicion not only of resistant bacteria, but also of *P. carinii*, fungi, or a viral pneumonia. A new localized infiltrate in a neutropenic patient whose white blood count is rising while receiving broad-spectrum antibiotics with the "new" infiltrate may simply represent an inflammatory reaction at a previous unrecognized site of infection. Close observation without any modification may be appropriate. If, however, the granulocyte count is not rising and the patient has been neutropenic for only a short period of time ($\leq$ 1 week), then a bacterial process is most likely. If the patient has been persistently neutropenic for a more prolonged period, then a fungal pneumonia should also be strongly considered and amphotericin B added while a diagnostic workup is initiated.

Patients who develop hypotension while receiving broad-spectrum antibiotics should be presumed septic with a resistant organism or breakthrough infection. In such patients, changes in the empiric regimen should be made expeditiously and continued for the duration of treatment if an organism is not recovered. So-called culture-negative sepsis may occur when the growth of resistant organisms is suppressed by marginally effective antibiotics or when samples for culture are not drawn during the bacteremic episode.

Empiric Antifungal Therapy

The diagnosis of a disseminated fungal infection is difficult in an immunocompromised patient. Neutropenic patients who remain persistently febrile despite a 4- to 7-day trial of broad-spectrum antibacterial therapy are particularly likely to have a fungal infection. Empiric antifungal therapy might be expected to have a dual effect: the prevention of a fungal overgrowth in patients with prolonged neutropenia and the early treatment of "subclinical" fungal disease.

To date, the only proven agent for empiric therapy has been amphotericin B. Amphotericin B should be begun at 0.5 mg per kilogram per day and administered along with antibiotics until the resolution of neutropenia. A number of new azole and triazole antifungal agents are being evaluated and offer the promise of less toxic alternatives to amphotericin B.

Patients who remain febrile after the resolution of neutropenia should be evaluated for hepatosplenic candidiasis. The diagnosis is suggested by "bull's-eye" lesions on CT scan or ultrasonography of the liver and spleen. MRI scanning of the liver may be even more sensitive. Biopsy and histologic examination are essential. Patients with hepatosplenic candidiasis may require extended courses of antifungal therapy. The average amount of amphotericin B required for resolution of these lesions is approximately 5 grams, often in conjunction with 5-flucytosine (100 mg per kilogram per day).

PREVENTION OF INFECTIONS

Because bacteria account for the majority of infections in compromised patients, prophylactic strategies have focused on these pathogens. The strategies that have been explored include mechanical techniques to prevent acquisition of new pathogens; absorbable or nonabsorbable oral antibiotic regimens to either prevent acquisition or decrease the number of potentially pathogenic colonizing organisms; and methods to improve the host defense matrix, including immunization, and more recently, biologic agents (e.g., the colony-stimulating factors) (Table 287–5).

Perhaps the most important infection prevention strategy of all, however, is hand washing. Although taken for granted, this simple procedure is frequently overlooked to the detriment of the patient.

TABLE 287–5. METHODS FOR PREVENTING INFECTION IN HIGH-RISK PATIENTS

Prevent Acquisition and/or Suppress or Eliminate Microbial Flora	Improve or Modify Host Defenses
Isolation	Immunization
Simple or reverse isolation	Active
Isolation with HEPA air fil-	*Pseudomonas*
tration	Pneumococcus
Prophylactic antibiotics	VZV
Nonabsorbable antibiotics	Passive
Trimethoprim-sulfamethoxa-	J-5 core glycolipid
zole erythromycin	Pooled immunoglobulins
Selective decontamination	Hyperimmune globulins
Quinolones	Monoclonal antibodies
Prophylactic antivirals	Cell-component replacement
Acyclovir	Leukocyte transfusions
Amantadine	Accelerate granulocyte recovery
Prophylactic antifungals	Lithium
Nystatin	G-CSF
Imidazoles	GM-CSF
Triazoles	Immunomodulations
Amphotericin B	Interferons
Prophylactic antiparasitics	Interleukins
Thiabendazole	
Trimethoprim-sulfamethoxa-	
zole	
Combination-comprehensive	
Total protective isolation	

Modified, with permission of the University of Chicago Press, from Pizzo PA: Considerations for the prevention of infectious complications in patients with cancer. Rev Infect Dis 11:S1551–1563, 1989.

Neutropenic Patients

MECHANICAL TECHNIQUES. Reverse isolation (i.e., single room with gowns, masks, and gloves) following the onset of neutropenia does not prevent infection. This is because most of the infections arise from the patient's endogenous microbial flora. In addition, having a patient wear a surgical mask outside of his or her room does little to protect against subsequent infection. Although some authorities have recommended that all foods be thoroughly cooked and that fresh fruits and vegetables be avoided to decrease the acquisition of gram-negative bacteria, the value of these measures in preventing infection remains unproven.

The total protective environment (TPE) is a comprehensive regimen designed to reduce the patient's endogenous microbial burden as well as the acquisition of new organisms. The TPE includes a HEPA-filtered laminar airflow room together with an aggressive program of surface decontamination, including the sterilization of all objects that enter the room, and an intensive regimen to disinfect the microbial diet. A number of studies have documented that TPE can reduce infections in profoundly granulocytopenic individuals. However, TPE is expensive, and because of the improvement in treating established infections, it does not offer a current survival advantage to most patients. Thus TPE is not necessary for the routine care of the majority of granulocytopenic patients.

ORAL ANTIBIOTIC REGIMENS. Numerous studies have evaluated both nonabsorbable antibiotics (such as gentamicin, vancomycin, polymyxin, or colistin) and antibiotics that are absorbed from the gastrointestinal tract (e.g., trimethoprim-sulfamethoxazole, erythromycin, or quinolones). The goal of antibiotics has ranged from "total decontamination" of the alimentary tract with oral nonabsorbable antibiotics to "selective decontamination," in which the goal is to eliminate the potentially pathogenic aerobic flora (mostly the enteric gram-negative bacteria) while preserving the majority of anaerobic organisms and thus preserving "colonization resistance." Although the introduction of each new prophylactic regimen has been met with enthusiasm, over time these strategies have failed because of the emergence of resistant organisms.

The fluoroquinolones (mostly norfloxacin and ciprofloxacin) have been used in recent years for prophylaxis in neutropenic patients. These agents are well absorbed and their use may really represent "early treatment" rather than prophylaxis. Although studies evaluating quinolones have demonstrated a reduction in gram-negative infections in the patients who receive them, caution about the widespread use of quinolones for prophylaxis should be underscored. Organisms resistant to the quinolones have already been described, and the indiscriminate use of these agents only accelerates this process. Since the quinolones are useful for the treatment of both immunocompromised and immunocompetent individuals, the use of these antibiotics for prophylaxis should be discouraged.

PATIENTS WITH SICKLE CELL ANEMIA. Since patients with sickle cell anemia are prone to infections with encapsulated organisms (e.g., *S. pneumoniae*, *H. influenzae*), especially in young children, the pneumococcal vaccine and prophylactic penicillin have been used to prevent these infections. Unfortunately, the vaccination has not resulted in an effective antibody response. Prophylactic penicillin can, however, significantly reduce the incidence of infection, and it is recommended that penicillin prophylaxis be begun by 4 months of age in children with sickle cell anemia and that it be continued beyond the third birthday.

Prevention of Fungal Infections

Although the increasing incidence of fungal infection makes a preventive strategy desirable, to date no clear evidence of benefit has been demonstrated. It is hoped that newer azole and triazole antifungal agents may improve the ability to control these opportunistic pathogens.

Prevention of Viral Infections

HERPES SIMPLEX. Herpes simplex is a frequent cause of morbidity in compromised patients, particularly in association with bone marrow or renal transplantation or intensive chemotherapy regimens. Several studies have demonstrated that acyclovir administered either orally or intravenously at dosages of 250 mg per square meter every 8 hours can reduce the incidence of herpetic gingivostomatitis. Accordingly, it seems reasonable to administer prophylactic oral or intravenous acyclovir in patients who are HSV seropositive (titers ≥1:16) or who have a prior history of infection and are undergoing bone marrow transplantation or intensive therapy for acute leukemia.

VARICELLA-ZOSTER VIRUS. One of the most important ways to prevent VZV transmission is to prevent contact of immunosuppressed individuals with infected individuals. This includes patients with either primary VZV (chicken pox) or secondary VZV (zoster). If a seronegative individual has had contact with an infected individual, passive immunization with ZIG (zoster immune globulin) has been shown to reduce the incidence of pneumonitis and encephalitis. Administration of ZIG (1 vial per 15 kg) must occur within 72 hours after exposure.

A varicella vaccine has been shown to reduce infection in children with leukemia. The live vaccine may be released soon for administration in normal healthy children and if effective should reduce the overall population of infected individuals.

CYTOMEGALOVIRUS. Strategies aimed at prevention of CMV infection have included use of seronegative blood products in seronegative patients, passive immunization, and chemoprophylaxis with acyclovir.

Prevention of Parasitic Infections

The clearest benefit of prophylaxis has been demonstrated in preventing *P. carinii* pneumonia with trimethoprim-sulfamethoxazole. The decision to administer prophylaxis for *P. carinii* should be influenced by the patient's underlying disease, the intensity or immunosuppression of the therapy being delivered, and the center where treatment is being administered. Recent studies have demonstrated that trimethoprim-sulfamethoxazole can be effective and safe at a dosage of 75 mg per square meter twice a day given on 3 consecutive days each week. Alternatives include aerosolized pentamidine and dapsone.

Improving Host Defense

Immunization against bacterial and viral pathogens has played an extremely important role in decreasing the incidence and/or severity of many infectious diseases. Unfortunately, active immunization is generally unsuccessful in immunocompromised hosts, since they are unable to mount or to sustain an antibody response to most vaccines.

Passive immunization, on the other hand, involves administration of preformed antibodies to high-risk patients. ZIG, for example, is effective in preventing infection and decreasing the incidence of morbidity and mortality associated with primary chicken pox in susceptible hosts. Another "hyperimmune" preparation that has been investigated in high-risk patients is the so-called J-5 antisera, collected from patients with high titers of antibody directed against the core glycolipid of Enterobacteriaceae. The results of early clinical trials with the J-5 antisera appeared encouraging, although confirmatory studies have not been consistent. Monoclonal antibodies have been developed and suggest that they may reduce morbidity in some patients with gram-negative sepsis. Pooled immunoglobulin preparations do not appear to offer benefit for neutropenic hosts but are of benefit to patients who have either congenital or acquired (e.g., CLL, multiple myeloma) hypogammaglobulinemia.

Perhaps the most exciting new developments will be the therapeutic use of cytokines and lymphokines to enforce the host defense repertoire. Clearly, as new factors become defined, the prospect for restoring function in the compromised host stands as the opportunity for the 1990's.

Graybill JR: Systemic fungal agents—diagnosis and treatment I: Therapeutic agents. Infect Dis Clin North Am 3:805–825, 1988. *Comprehensive review of diagnostic and therapeutic advances in the management of patients with systemic mycoses.*
Hill HR: Infections complicating congenital immunodeficiency syndromes. In Rubin RH, Young LS (eds.): Clinical Approach to Infection in the Compromised Host. New York, Plenum Medical Book Company, 1988, pp 407–438. *Practical overview of the serious infectious complications that occur in children with congenital immune deficiency diseases.*
Hirsch MS: Herpes group virus infections in the compromised host. In Rubin RH, Young LS (eds.): Clinical Approach to Infections in the Compromised Host. New York, Plenum Medical Book Company, 1988, pp 347–366. *Details the important issues related to the serious infections caused by herpes simplex, varicella-zoster, and cytomegalovirus in immunocompromised hosts.*
Immunization Practices Advisory Committee, CDC. General recommendations on immunization. Guidelines from the Immunization Practices Committee. Ann Intern Med 111:133–142, 1989. *Offers recommendations for immunization practices for adults.*
Leher RJ, Ganz T, Selsted ME, et al.: Neutrophils and host defense. Ann Intern Med 109:127–142, 1988. *Comprehensive review of phagocyte function and its relevance to host defense.*
Mandell GL, Douglas RG, Bennett JE (eds.): Principles and Practice of Infectious Diseases, 3rd ed. New York, Churchill Livingstone, 1990.
Pizzo PA: Considerations for the prevention of infectious complications in patients with cancer. Rev Infect Dis 11:S1551–S1563, 1989. *Provides a critical overview of preventive strategies aimed at suppressing or eliminating the host's microbial burden or at augmenting altered host defenses.*
Pizzo PA, Hathorn JW, et al.: A randomized trial comparing combination antibiotic therapy to monotherapy in cancer patients with fever and neutropenia. N Engl J Med 315:552, 1986. *A large prospective randomized clinical trial that provides a basis for the evaluation of empiric antibiotics for adults and children who become febrile while neutropenic.*
Pizzo PA, Robichaud KJ, Wesley R, et al.: Fever in the pediatric and young adult patient with cancer. A prospective study of 1001 episodes. Medicine 61:153–165, 1982. *Reviews the clinical presentation and outcome of children, adolescents, and young adults with cancer who develop fever.*
Rubin RH, Young LS (eds.): Clinical Approach to Infection in the Compromised Host. New York, Plenum Medical Book Company, 1988.
Rubin M, Walsh, TJ, Pizzo PA: Clinical approaches to infections in the compromised host. In Hoffman R, Benz EJ Jr, Shattil SJ, et al. (eds.): Hematology: Basic Principles and Practice. New York, Churchill Livingstone, 1991, pp 1063–1114. *Detailed review of infections in compromised hosts.*
The International Chronic Granulomatous Disease Cooperative Study Group: A controlled trial of interferon gamma to prevent infection in chronic granulomatous disease. N Engl J Med 324:509, 1991. *Demonstrates the clinical benefits of reduced infection frequency when interferon gamma was administered to children with chronic granulomatous disease.*
Walsh T, Pizzo PA: Nosocomial fungal infections: A classification for hospital-acquired fungal infections and mycoses arising from endogenous flora or reactivation. Annu Rev Microbiol 42:517–545, 1988. *Reviews the major fungal pathogens that contribute to infectious complications in cancer patients and provides a system for their classification.*

288 Shock Syndromes Related to Sepsis

John N. Sheagren

Sepsis is defined as the presence of various pus-forming and other pathogenic organisms or their toxins in the blood or tissues. A presumptive diagnosis of sepsis is often made on the basis of historical, physical, and laboratory data even in the absence of proof. The most serious complications are produced when infection spreads from the original focus to the bloodstream. Bacteremia can produce two different types of complications: microbiologic and inflammatory. The microbiologic complications result from the local and systemic proliferation and seeding of the causative organism, which cause direct tissue or organ damage. The inflammatory complications are produced locally and can result in tissue or organ destruction independent of toxic factors produced by the causative organism. Bacteremia triggers intravascular activation of the same inflammatory systems that are protective within tissues but which, during severe sepsis, combine with stress-generated endocrine responses to produce a deleterious sequence of metabolic events. The end stage of these events is systemic vascular collapse, traditionally termed *septic shock,* and/or the constellation of symptoms referred to as the "multiple system organ failure" (MSOF) syndrome. The clinical definition of septic shock is a systolic blood pressure less than 90 mm Hg which has become unresponsive to adequate volume replacement.

Morbidity and mortality associated with septic shock are high: Approximately two thirds of such patients die, and the cause of death is usually progressive failure of one or more vital organs. Prevention of septic shock should be the primary goal. It is possible to recognize clinically the changes that occur in patients in the early stages of septic shock. Intervention at early stages can reduce morbidity and mortality.

INCIDENCE AND EPIDEMIOLOGY. Infections most commonly occur in the hospital setting. Many infected patients become bacteremic. It is estimated that of 100 randomly chosen patients who appear to be infected (septic) in a hospital setting, approximately 90 per cent actually are infected. Of these, about 20 per cent develop some evidence of hemodynamic instability and appear, at least temporarily, "shocky." About half of shocky patients (or about 10 per cent of all septic-appearing patients) go on to frank septic shock and/or manifest serious end-organ malfunction related to the septic episode (MSOF) such as adult respiratory distress syndrome (ARDS), renal failure, or disseminated intravascular coagulation (DIC). Since about 5 per cent of all hospital patients either are admitted with or develop an infection during hospitalization, the number of patients at risk of developing septic shock is large. The clinician must be familiar with the manifestations and differential diagnosis of the septic-appearing patient and have in mind rapid comprehensive diagnostic and therapeutic plans of action.

Shock Related to Gram-Negative as Opposed to Gram-Positive Organisms. Septic shock more commonly follows gram-negative than gram-positive septic episodes, and many textbooks refer to generic septic shock as gram-negative sepsis or endotoxic shock because endotoxin is found only in gram-negative bacterial cell walls. In patients who are bacteremic with gram-negative microbes, the incidence of metabolic complications and shock is high (about 25 per cent). However, about 10 per cent of patients with gram-positive bacteremia, especially those infected with *Staphylococcus aureus,* develop shock. The incidence of suppurative complications (metastatic seeding to bones, joints, viscera, and so on), on the other hand, is much higher with gram-positive microorganisms. Gram-positive bacteria have the capability of adhering to endothelial cells and subendothelial matrix substances (such as fibronectin, laminin, fibrinogen, and endothelial cell proteins) to a much greater degree than do gram-negative organisms, so that seeding to heart valves, to other organs, and especially to foci of trauma and/or pre-existing inflammation is much more common.

PATHOGENESIS. Sepsis can cause shock in many ways, either related to the primary focus of infection or to the systemic effects of bacteremia. These mechanisms of shock are listed in Table 288–1.

The classic *septic shock syndrome* results primarily from the sequence of events triggered by bacteremia during which cell wall bacterial substances (endotoxin in gram-negative organisms, the peptidoglycan/teichoic acid complex in gram-positive organisms, and polysaccharide substances in yeast cell walls) activate the monokine, complement, coagulation, kinin, and ACTH/endorphin systems. Endotoxin (and probably other toxic microbial cell wall substances) is the strongest stimulus known to produce tumor necrosis factor-α (also known as TNF-α and cachectin) (see

TABLE 288–1. MECHANISMS OF SHOCK CAUSED BY SEPSIS

1. Shock related to a localized primary focus of infection
   Hypovolemic shock: severe local infection may
   —cause sufficient local fluid accumulation to produce systemic hypovolemia.
   —produce severe diarrhea with gastrointestinal fluid loss.
   —erode into a local vessel with mycotic aneurysm formation and rupture.
   Cardiogenic shock: extension of a pericardiac infection (usually pneumonia) into the pericardium
   —may cause purulent pericarditis and tamponade.
   Toxigenic shock (the toxic shock syndrome): a toxin is produced locally, causing
   —endothelial cell damage with capillary leakage.
   —cardiodepression.
2. Shock related to bacteremic infections
   Cardiogenic shock: seeding of the organism through the bloodstream may cause
   —valvular malfunction (endocarditis).
   —myocarditis secondary to multiple metastatic myocardial abscesses.
   —purulent pericarditis (metastatic).
   Inflammatory-system–mediated shock: bacterial cell wall substances activate the complement, coagulation, kinin, and ACTH/endorphin systems and thus cause
   —vasodilation (roles of endorphins, kinins, and complement).
   —capillary leakage (primarily due to the intracapillary adherence and aggregation of activated polymorphonuclear leukocytes).
   —disseminated intravascular coagulation.
   —cardiodepression (encephalins, vasopressin, monokines, possibly other substances).

Ch. 286) by macrophages. TNF-α, in high enough concentration, impairs functioning of surrounding cells in multiple ways, and data are now firmly in hand to indicate that TNF-α plays a central role in mediating the toxic effects of endotoxin and other microbial products. All these mediators initiate a series of metabolic events that ultimately may progress to a state of shock.

Severe sepsis produces hemodynamic changes in two phases. Septic patients initially have hemodynamic changes primarily reflecting vasodilation. Systemic vascular resistance is decreased, pulse rate increases to compensate, and cardiac output is dramatically increased. Paradoxically, a state of cardiodepression exists during severe sepsis, and a circulating myocardial depressant factor (MDF) has recently been rediscovered. This MDF turns out probably to be TNF-α. Septic patients develop a fall in cardiac ejection fractions down to 20 to 25 per cent despite the markedly increased cardiac output.

As this hyperdynamic state develops, complement-mediated leukoagglutination combines with other inflammatory mediators (such as bradykinin, histamine, and the endorphins) to cause a severe capillary leak, intravascular volume decreases, blood pressure falls, and cardiac output now further declines. Several additional factors contribute to the decline in cardiac output: Peripheral resistance increases in late septic shock and other cardiodepressants participate such as vasopressin and encephalin. Individual organs may be damaged independently of the hypotensive events; for example, direct pulmonary damage by the activated leukocytes may result in ARDS, or the patient may develop renal malfunction. Presumably these end-organ manifestations are related to localized direct inflammatory damage. It is in this stage that DIC associated with severe hypoperfusion may occur, resulting in extremely high morbidity and mortality.

An important pathophysiologic concept in understanding the damage that occurs during bacteremia or fungemia is that of the syndrome of multiple system organ failure (MSOF). Septicemia is the most important of a number of precipitating causes. Other causes include severe trauma, burns, pancreatitis, and all other causes of shock. Once the syndrome of MSOF is triggered, by whatever cause, the patient becomes febrile and hypermetabolic, exhibits hyperactive hemodynamic measurements, and develops progressive failure of one or more organs. Mortality approaches 90 per cent despite all modern therapeutic measures.

Figure 288–1 outlines the sequence of early events initiated from the localized focus of infection. From these events are derived the various complications of bacteremia, which include metastatic abscess formation and the metabolic complications described earlier. Antibiotics limit metastatic abscess formation (the microbiologic complications of bacteremia). However, the other metabolic events, when initiated and independent of bacterial proliferation, still produce substantial morbidity and mortality. Therefore, therapy in addition to antibiotics is being sought to counter these deleterious metabolic sequelae.

The ACTH/Endorphin System. During systemic stress, increased ACTH release occurs. For each molecule of ACTH produced, a molecule of one of the endorphins or encephalins is also produced. The endorphins provide pain and anxiety relief during severe stress, but high levels of circulating endorphins may contribute to hypotension, changes in vascular permeability, and alterations in mentation.

Coagulation/Kinin System Activation. Bacterial endotoxins and other cell wall materials directly activate the coagulation system both by initiating platelet aggregation and by activating Hageman factor. Subsequently, kinin system activation (see Ch. 256) results in the production of bradykinin, a powerful vasodilator.

Complement System Activation. The complement system is also directly activated by high molecular weight bacterial and fungal polysaccharides, primarily by means of the alternative pathway. A sequence of intravascular events ensues, resulting in histamine release (contributing, to vasodilation), microvascular instability, and activation of circulating polymorphonuclear leukocytes (PMN's). The activated PMN has enhanced bactericidal capabilities but also an enhanced capability of damaging host tissues. The activated PMN possesses increased amounts of lysosomal enzymes and produces a variety of toxic metabolites of molecular oxygen, all of which are both bactericidal and cytocidal. Furthermore, the activated PMN produces both inflammatory prostaglandins and several products of the lipoxygenase system, many of which enhance inflammation by also producing vasodi-

lation, capillary leakage, chemotaxis, and PMN activation. The activated PMN's adhere to each other (the *leukopenic phase* of sepsis during which PMN aggregates form in capillaries) and to endothelial cells to cause severe damage and capillary leakage.

CLINICAL MANIFESTATIONS. *The Septic Patient.* The clinical situation in which a patient is considered septic (highly likely to be infected) is common. High fever and a chill strongly indicate that bacterial sepsis is occurring. In this setting, the physician must be alert for signs of septic shock. When a clinical diagnosis of septic shock can be made, the mortality rate is high. Therefore, it is important to develop the concept of a "preshock phase of septic shock" predicated on identifying a subgroup of infected patients more likely than others to develop shock. Treatment before shock develops undoubtedly prevents some of the morbidity and mortality associated with sepsis.

Table 288–2 lists several systemic signs and a variety of physical findings likely to be predictive of septic shock. Extremes of body temperature are often associated with shock. Specifically, fever in excess of 40.6° C and hypothermia associated with sepsis should be alerting signs that hypotension may soon follow. Also, in the febrile patient with a distinct change in mentation the mortality rate is higher. In association with such a finding, primary central nervous system infection may be present, and lumbar puncture is often indicated. Febrile patients who have hemodynamic instability (who are orthostatic with a blood pressure decrease of 30 mm Hg or greater) should be considered on the verge of septic shock.

While it is not possible to distinguish between simple dehydration and early septic shock solely on the basis of orthostatic blood pressure changes, hemodynamic monitoring shows an increase in peripheral vascular resistance in the former case and a reduction in the latter. Also, fluid challenge alone rapidly stabilizes the purely hypovolemic patient. Sepsis is associated in the early stages with a state of "warm shock" in which there is an orthostatic decrease in blood pressure but good perfusion in the extremities (they are warm and pink rather than cool and cyanotic). Tachypnea with hypoxemia or metabolic acidosis or both may be predictive of impending ARDS. The development of peripheral edema, often with a suddenly decreased serum albumin concentration, as in toxigenic shock (see Toxic Shock Syndrome in Ch. 300), may be caused by an unrecognized bacteremic event.

Laboratory Data Suggesting Bacteremia or Toxemia. Several laboratory tests are often helpful in the evaluation of a potentially septic patient (Table 288–2). The blood may show hypoxemia and a metabolic acidosis. Serum lactate elevation is highly predictive of deterioration leading to septic shock. Decreasing urine output, often associated with rising blood urea nitrogen and creatinine, may be seen early in sepsis as renal failure occurs. Serum albumin measurements may show decreases in excess of that calculated by catabolism alone. Often such patients show signs of progressive peripheral edema. In early sepsis, the total white count may be low, with most of the decrease in the PMN count, owing to complement-induced leukoaggregation. As white cells aggregate, platelets become caught up in the process. Thrombocytopenia is predictive of high risk of septic shock and ARDS.

In the future, assistance in clinical decision making may be provided by rapid laboratory measurements of the levels of

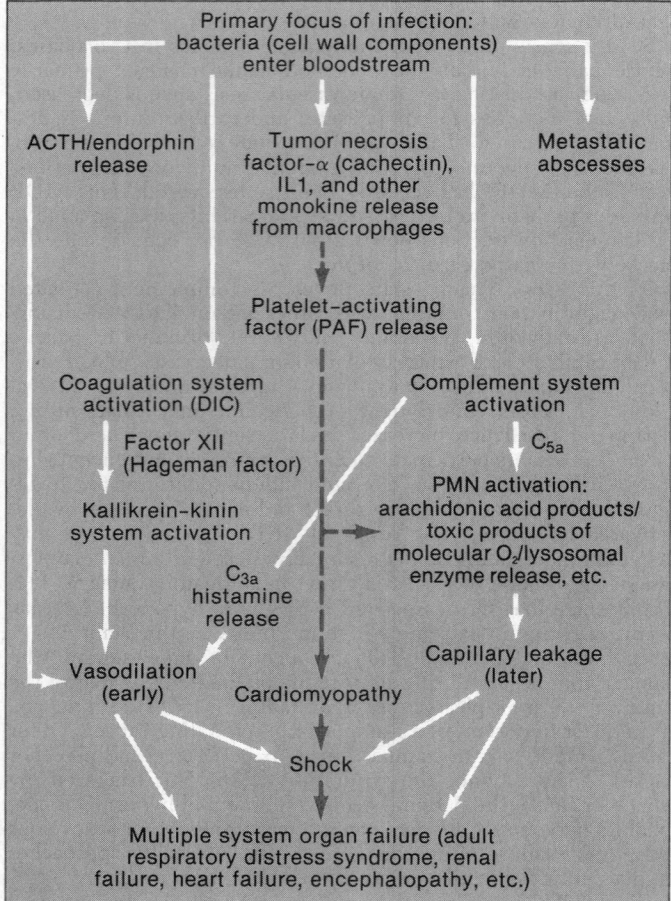

FIGURE 288–1. The complications of severe sepsis.

TABLE 288–2. PHYSICAL SIGNS AND LABORATORY DATA LIKELY TO BE PREDICTIVE OF THE DEVELOPMENT OF SEPTIC SHOCK

1. Extremes of body temperature (fever > 40.6°C or hypothermia)
2. Altered mental status
3. Orthostatic blood pressure decrease (>30 mm Hg) or sustained unexplained hypotension.
4. Decreasing urine output
5. Unexplained edema, usually associated with a falling serum albumin concentration
6. Tachypnea with hypoxemia and/or the development of a metabolic acidosis
7. Elevated serum lactate concentration
8. Development of leukopenia (predominantly neutropenia)
9. Development of thrombocytopenia with or without petechial skin rash
10. Unexplained end-organ failure (e.g., renal, hepatic)

activating bacterial products (e.g., endotoxin) and/or products of the mediator systems shown in Figure 288–1. For example, the rapid identification of an elevated level of TNF-α, a falling total complement level, and elevated levels of C5a, prostaglandins, or endorphins might predict subgroups of septic patients at higher risk of developing shock.

DIAGNOSIS. The presumptive diagnosis of sepsis must be made when the setting and attendant clinical signs are suggestive. In general, patients with fever should be considered septic until proven otherwise. Therapy should always be initiated for high-risk febrile patients in advance of microbiologic confirmation of sepsis.

Evaluation of the Septic Patient. The setting in which the episode is occurring should be evaluated promptly. Crucial to appropriate initial decision making are the background history, which may help to define the type of host defense defect present, and prior cultural data, which might predict the infecting organism. The physical examination should be directed at quickly but thoroughly searching for the septic source as well as signs of end-organ failure that might indicate progression to shock such as altered mental status, progressive edema, hypotension, and so on (Table 288–2). All potentially infected foci should be appropriately sampled, and the material obtained should be Gram-stained and cultured.

Differential Diagnosis of Severe Sepsis. Having done a thorough preliminary evaluation and initiated therapy (see below), one can reassess the clinical situation on subsequent days and stop antibiotic therapy if the episode later turns out not to be infectious. Many nonseptic events can cause high fever with or without hemodynamic instability. For example, a variety of hypersensitivity reactions (often caused by drugs) may mimic sepsis. Vasculitic disease may present with high fever, unstable blood pressure, and altered mentation. Pulmonary emboli occur frequently in the hospital setting, and especially if the patient develops fever, the embolic event initially may be confused with sepsis. Myocardial infarction may result in hemodynamic instability, and in the subset of patients who develop higher than average fever may lead to initial confusion with sepsis.

There are infectious syndromes against which antimicrobials are of no use and in which bacterial sepsis may be suspected. For example, viral syndromes such as those caused by influenza viruses, enteroviruses, adenoviruses, cytomegalovirus, and hepatitis viruses may all produce high fever and be difficult to diagnose. Malaria can be difficult to identify unless the parasite is detected on the peripheral blood smear.

TREATMENT. Possible therapeutic modalities for the septic patient are outlined in Figure 288–2.

Antibacterial Therapy. Broad coverage is required in patients with severe sepsis. It is best to initiate therapy with a combination of antibiotics when the infecting organism is unknown. An aminoglycoside should always be used, and gentamicin remains the aminoglycoside of choice unless other considerations (such as abnormal renal function and known microbial resistance) dictate the use of tobramycin or amikacin. In the granulocytopenic patient, the aminoglycoside should be combined with high doses of piperacillin. In the patient likely to have an anaerobic focus of infection in which *Bacteroides fragilis* is likely to be present, such as an intra-abdominal or gynecologic infection, or decubitus and lower extremity vascular and neuropathic ulcers, clindamycin or cefotetan or cefoxitin is combined with gentamicin. For all other patients, gentamicin plus cefazolin or ceftriaxone is the combination of choice. If β-lactam antibiotic–resistant (methicillin-resistant) staphylococci are possible, then vancomycin must be added to the above combinations. When cultures define the causative microbe(s) or other data point to a specific organism, therapy can be tailored to the most appropriate, most specific, least toxic, and least expensive single antibiotic.

Antishock Therapy. The most important component of the therapy of shock associated with sepsis is volume replacement. Sufficient quantities of an appropriate solute (or, where indicated, a colloid such as albumin or whole blood) should be administered in an attempt to provide adequate volume support. Evidence is accumulating, especially in the surgical literature, that colloid-containing solutions are more efficacious than solute solutions once capillary leakage has developed or after approximately 4 liters of a solute have been administered. Hemodynamic monitoring is mandatory and is preferably carried out in the intensive

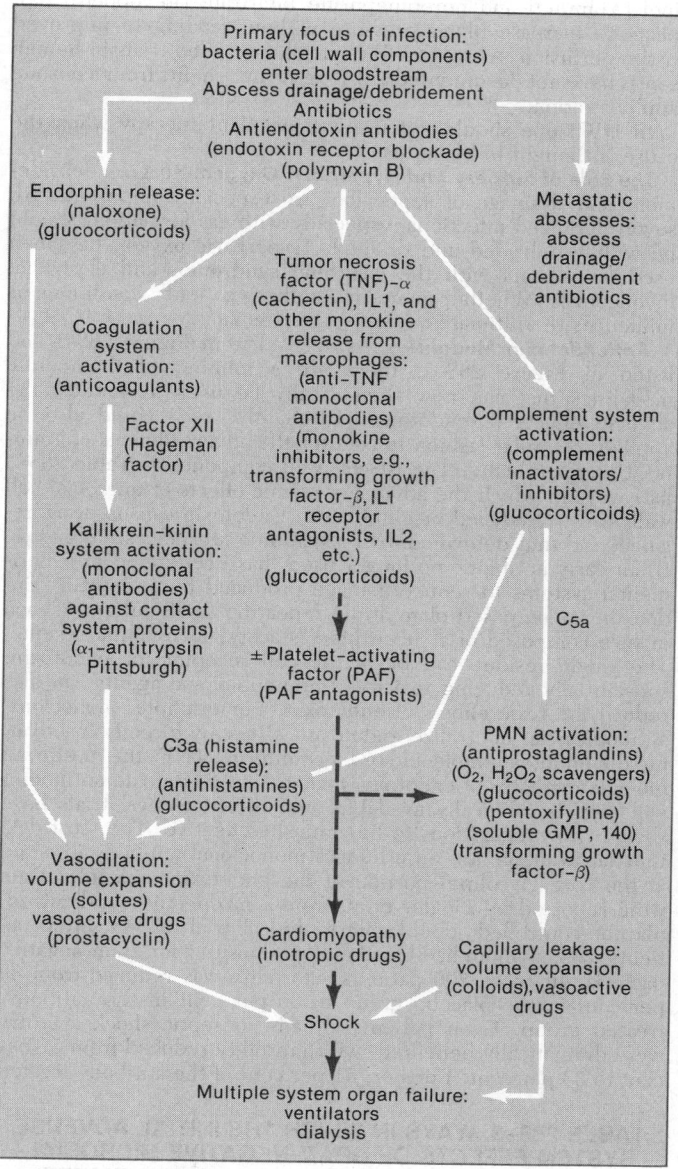

FIGURE 288–2. Therapy for the complications of severe sepsis. Theoretically efficacious but unproven or ineffective therapeutic modalities are in parentheses.

care unit (see Ch. 71). Fluid administration should be just sufficient to bring the pulmonary capillary wedge pressure to the high normal range.

Recently two multicenter studies prospectively compared high doses of methylprednisolone sodium succinate (MPSS) with placebo in a blinded protocol in over 600 severely septic patients. Glucocorticoids were administered within 4 hours of recognition of the septic event. Both studies showed *no* efficacy of MPSS and one study showed *increased* mortality in patients who have mild degrees of renal malfunction (creatinines of 2 mg per deciliter or greater) or who have developed ARDS. Thus, glucocorticoid therapy has no proven role in the treatment of human sepsis.

The use of other anti-inflammatory drugs such as the antiprostaglandins is under active investigation. These agents may selectively suppress inflammatory damage caused by the activated PMN without interfering with the antibacterial capabilities of these important host defense cells.

Some clinicians have tried to use naloxone in severe sepsis on the basis of the contribution of the endorphin system to hemodynamic instability in experimental models of septic shock.

However, in primate models naloxone, like α-agonists (metaraminol [Aramine] and norepinephrine bitartrate [Levophed]), appears to increase blood pressure without leading to improved tissue perfusion. Also, data from small controlled trials in human sepsis have not documented any long-term benefits from naloxone administration.

In DIC, one should not use anticoagulant therapy when the cause is thought to be sepsis.

The Role of Surgery and Hyperbaric Oxygen. Surgical debridement and drainage of septic foci are especially important. All severe localized infections, especially with gas formation, should be widely debrided and drained. Hyperbaric oxygen has been used in patients with the gangrene syndromes and clostridial myonecrosis. Whether or not it stabilizes patients' conditions or influences the ultimate outcome is unknown.

Antiendotoxin Modalities. As derived from Figure 288–1 and listed in Figure 288–2, there are a number of therapeutic modalities that can now theoretically be used to counter the adverse effects of endotoxin. Ultimately, each could also be applied in similar fashion to counter the adverse effects of gram-positive microbial and yeast cell wall components. Table 288–3 lists ways in which the adverse systemic effects of microbial cell walls can be reduced or eliminated. Endotoxin can be disaggregated, and thus detoxified, by polycationic substances. Polymyxin B, an early antibiotic no longer used, has been found in experimental systems to reduce damage produced by endotoxin. Endotoxin is composed of multiple repeating small subunits, each in turn composed of a substituted N-acetylglucosamine residue. The single residue can block the cell receptor for endotoxin, substantially reducing toxicity. Immunobiologic agents can also reduce the toxic effects of endotoxin. For example, monoclonal antibodies can neutralize endotoxin, either by directly inactivating the endotoxin molecule or by countering TNF, the most toxic biologic mediator of endotoxin toxicity. Antiendotoxin antibodies will soon be clinically available, and recent clinical trials have shown two preparations to be clinically effective. The most data thus far available are on a human monoclonal antibody directed at the core glycolipid portion of the endotoxin molecule. Data were reported by Ziegler et al. from a prospective randomized, placebo-controlled, double-blind clinical trial of 543 septic patients, 200 of whom had blood cultures positive for gram-negative bacteria. In those 200 patients, mortality was reduced from 49 per cent in the placebo group to 30 per cent in the antibody-treated group. Even patients already in septic shock at entry were dramatically benefited, with mortality reduced from 57 per cent to 33 per cent. Further, 51 per cent of the antibody-treated

TABLE 288–3. WAYS IN WHICH THE INITIAL ADVERSE SYSTEM EFFECTS OF GRAM-NEGATIVE MICROBIAL CELL WALLS CAN BE REDUCED OR ELIMINATED

1. **Endotoxin "dissolution":** By administering polymyxin B (a polycationic antibiotic) or other detergents; probably causes disaggregation of the organized complexes or endotoxin, reducing toxicity.
2. **Endotoxin receptor blockade:** Small subunits of disaggregated endotoxin bind to endotoxin receptors on macrophages and, while not causing toxicity themselves, block toxic monokine (TNF-α, IL1, etc.) release.
3. **Antiendotoxin antibodies:** Antibodies can be directed either (1) against the "core endotoxin" moiety, resulting in "detoxification," or (2) against the antigenic polysaccharide side chains ("O-antigens"), resulting in enhanced opsonization and/or antibody-mediated killing of the bacterium.
4. **Monokine neutralization:** Specific monoclonal antibodies directed against TNF-α decrease the systemic effects either of purified endotoxin or of live, whole microbes.
5. **Monokine antagonists:** The effects of TNF-α are inhibited by transforming growth factor-β and IL2. IL1 synergizes with TNF-α, and an inhibitor of IL1 (known as IL1 receptor antagonist) ameliorates the effects of bacteremia. Many other biologic inhibitors of the monokines undoubtedly exist.
6. **Platelet-activating factor (PAF) antagonists:** In some experimental systems, PAF seems to play an important role in the damage produced by monokines. Thus, PAF antagonists may play potential therapeutic roles.

patients survived to be discharged from the hospital, compared with only 29 per cent of the placebo-treated group. Another product, a mouse monoclonal preparation, has also shown efficacy in a randomized, double-blind clinical trial reported in abstract form; mortality in patients with gram-negative sepsis was reduced if the patient was not yet in septic shock. Thus, when released for clinical use (possibly by the time of publication of this text), a dose of one or another of these preparations will be indicated at the point where initial stabilization measures have failed in the course of severely septic patients who are at high risk of being infected with gram-negative microbes.

Finally, as noted above, there may be a therapeutic benefit in neutralizing or in other ways countering the effects of TNF and/or other monokines (especially IL1). A monoclonal antibody preparation that neutralizes TNF can increase survival in animal models of septic shock. There are also a number of biologic antagonists of TNF, such as transforming growth factor-β, IL2, and an IL1 receptor antagonist (see Table 288–3) that could prove useful. Inhibiting any or all of the other mediators generated by the septic event is being explored. For example, the kallikrein-kinin system may play a very important role, and new ways of inhibiting contact system proteins or in other ways impairing bradykinin generation may become clinically feasible (Fig. 288–2).

PROGNOSIS. Most febrile patients lacking other signs of severe sepsis (as described in Table 288–2) will usually do well even when bacteremic. Such patients usually respond quickly to fluid administration, antibacterial therapy, and drainage of the primary focus of infection. However, the presence of shock and/or progressive dysfunction in any organ system dramatically increases morbidity and mortality. Even when the inciting infection is localized, shock (with the exception of the toxic shock syndrome) is associated with a 30 to 50 per cent mortality. Full-blown, bacteremia-associated septic shock has greater than a 50 per cent mortality. A favorable outcome in a patient in frank shock depends on the skill of management in the intensive care unit. Early diagnosis and therapy of severely septic patients decrease morbidity and mortality.

PREVENTION. Prevention of infection, especially in the hospital, is the key to reducing morbidity and mortality associated with septic shock. Strict adherence to the hospital infection control program with avoidance of Foley catheters and meticulous attention to the placement and maintenance of intravascular lines dramatically reduces the incidence of bacteremic infections. The concept of the preshock approach to the therapy of septic shock is useful; in all such patients fluids should be administered and broad antibiotic coverage started early. Controlled studies of anti-inflammatory therapy in severe sepsis are under way, and better guidelines should be forthcoming.

Abraham E, Shoemaker WC, Bland RD, et al.: Sequential cardiorespiratory patterns in septic shock. Crit Care Med 11:799, 1983. *Describes the hemodynamic patterns occurring in patients as they develop septic shock.*

Beutler B: The tumor necrosis factors: Cachectin and lymphotoxin. Hosp Pract 25:45, 1990. *Describes roles of cachectin (TNF-α) and lymphotoxin (TNF-β) in tissue damage during infection.*

Beutler B, Cerami A: Cachectin: More than a tumor necrosis factor. N Engl J Med 316:379, 1987. *Excellent review of the role of cachectin in inflammation, sepsis, and septic shock.*

Bone RC, Fisher CJ, Clemmer TP, et al.: Sepsis syndrome: A valid clinical entity. Crit Care Med 17:389, 1989. *Describes clinical criteria for prospectively identifying a patient population at risk of severe septic complications.*

Cerami A, Beutler B: The role of cachectin/TNF in endotoxic shock and cachexia. Immunol Today 9:28–31, 1989. *Reviews history, structure, mechanism of production and biologic effects of TNF.*

Parillo JE, Parker MM, Natanson C, et al.: Septic shock in humans: Advances in the understanding of pathogenesis, cardiovascular dysfunction and therapy. Ann Intern Med 113:227, 1990. *An excellent review of cardiovascular patterns, pathogenesis, and therapy of septic shock.*

Sibbald WJ, Sprung CL: New Horizons—Perspectives on Sepsis and Septic Shock. Fullerton, CA, Society of Critical Care Medicine, 1986. *A complete review of all basic and clinical aspects of the sepsis and multiple organ system failure syndromes.*

Tracey KJ, Beutler B, Lowry SF, et al.: Shock and tissue injury induced by recombinant human cachectin. Science 234:470, 1986. *Cachectin (tumor necrosis factor) is capable of producing most of the deleterious effects of endotoxin.*

Zeigler EJ, Fisher CJ, Sprung CL, et al.: Treatment of Gram-negative bacteremia and septic shock with HA-1A human monoclonal antibody against endotoxin. N Engl J Med 324:429, 1991. *Conclusively demonstrates that a human monoclonal IgM antibody that binds to the lipid A domain of endotoxin is safe and effective treatment of patients with severe sepsis caused by gram-negative bacteria.*

289 Prevention and Control of Hospital-Acquired Infections

William Schaffner

HISTORY. Hospitals are viewed today as institutions where scientific advances are used to provide the most up-to-date diagnostic and therapeutic services for patients. This optimistic view is tempered, however, by the realization that the hospital also can be a dangerous place for patients. The application of technology is not without hazards, and among these hospital-acquired infection has the longest history. When hospitals first were established in Europe during the Middle Ages, they were primarily places where the gravely ill were taken to die. Because facilities were primitive, infections that prompted the admission of some patients were readily spread to others. Hospital typhus and typhoid were commonplace, for example, and hospitals acquired the reputation of pest houses.

These circumstances remained basically unchanged until the mid-nineteenth century, when a Hungarian physician, Ignaz P. Semmelweis, was appointed to direct the obstetric service of the prestigious Allgemeines Krankenhaus (General Hospital) in Vienna. Semmelweis encountered a puzzling situation concerning the hospital's two obstetric wards. They were ostensibly similar and admitted patients on alternate days. Yet the mortality rates on the two wards were strikingly different. Semmelweis performed a seemingly elementary exercise but one that was unique in his time. He tabulated the monthly mortality rates on the two wards and documented that on Ward I the rates regularly were 8 to 10 per cent or even higher, whereas on Ward II they rarely rose above 2 per cent. The cause of this extraordinary mortality was puerperal sepsis (childbed fever), a rapidly fatal septic illness. Semmelweis worked before the formulation of the germ theory of disease, but we now know puerperal sepsis to be caused by the group A β-hemolytic streptococcus. He systematically examined a series of hypotheses attempting to explain the disparate mortality rates, but none proved valid. Among the more far-fetched notions was that the disease was psychosomatic and that intense anxiety was provoked when monks made their rounds, tolling hand-bells in mourning for those recently dead. Semmelweis persuaded the monks not to ring the bells and, of course, the occurrence of puerperal sepsis continued unaffected.

At that point a pathologist cut his finger while performing an autopsy of a woman who had died of puerperal sepsis. He soon developed a fatal illness with a clinical course that was entirely similar to puerperal sepsis. Because the pathologist had been inoculated with trace amounts of material during the autopsy, Semmelweis drew an insightful analogy: Perhaps the obstetric patients also were being inoculated with infectious material. It was then that a seemingly trivial difference between the two obstetric wards became important. The deliveries on the low-mortality ward were performed by midwives; on the high-risk ward they were performed by medical students and physicians. Furthermore, the autopsy room was directly adjacent to the ward and Semmelweis deduced that the unwashed contaminated hands of students and physicians going from autopsies to the delivery room were the vehicles for transmitting infection to patients. Despite protestations from the medical staff, Semmelweis then insisted upon hand washing after autopsies and before the examination of each patient. The mortality rate on Ward I promptly fell to levels even lower than those on the other ward.

Semmelweis is honored as the originator of hospital infection control efforts. His process of systematically gathering data, performing an analysis, and instituting control measures still is followed today. Furthermore, his emphasis on the hands of caregivers as the means for carrying pathogens from patient to patient remains valid. Unfortunately, as in the last century, contemporary physicians still require constant reminders to wash their hands during their patient care duties.

After the acceptance of the germ theory of disease, rapid advances in microbiology, disinfection, and aseptic technique around the turn of the century substantially enhanced the safety of patient care in hospitals. Starting in the 1930's, the introduction of antimicrobials made possible the development of progressively more elaborate surgery. However, predictions that hospital infections soon would become inconsequential have not come true. Rather, the types of hospital infection have changed in response to advancing medical science.

Most recently, the 1950's and 1960's witnessed a global pandemic of hospital infections caused by *Staphylococcus aureus*. Previously very susceptible to penicillin, the new penicillin-resistant epidemic strain (phage type 80/81) became the scourge of hospitals worldwide. It stimulated research into all aspects of hospital-acquired infection and persuaded authorities that every hospital should have a formal infection control program. For reasons that still are not clear, the staphylococcal pandemic waned in the 1970's and gram-negative bacilli, often antibiotic-resistant, became the dominant nosocomial pathogens. In the 1980's there again was a shift; staphylococci returned (now methicillin-resistant), enterococci rose in importance, and *Candida* and other yeast infections caused a larger proportion of nosocomial infections in seriously ill patients. Predictions for the 1990's suggest that antibiotic-resistant organisms of all kinds will assume even greater importance in hospitals. Thus, it seems that there will be no infection-free utopia; each era presents infection control challenges anew as yesterday's saprophyte becomes tomorrow's pathogen.

INTRODUCTION. Infections that are acquired during hospitalization and are neither present nor incubating at the time of hospitalization are defined as *nosocomial** infections. The occurrence of a nosocomial infection does not per se indicate that the hospital or its personnel were at fault or committed an error in caring for the patient. Current preventive measures still cannot prevent many nosocomial infections. Medicolegal liability regarding a nosocomial infection occurs when it can be demonstrated that physicians or hospital personnel have been negligent in not adhering to appropriate standards of care and that an infection resulted from the failure to perform consistent with the standard.

It is estimated that five to eight nosocomial infections occur for every 100 admissions to acute-care hospitals in the United States, resulting in 2 to 4 million such infections annually. Some nosocomial infections are more serious than others, but taken together they are estimated to require over 6 million days of excess hospital stay a year and contribute to the deaths of a substantial number of patients (Table 289–1).

Most studies of nosocomial infections have been performed in the high-technology hospitals of the developed countries. Although less attention has been given to delineating nosocomial infections in developing countries, it is clear that they are an important problem there as well. Hospital outbreaks of measles and shigellosis as well as infections related to a lack of disinfectants and other supplies occur regularly. Because developing countries have only modest resources, it is especially unfortunate that their efforts to provide medical care are so often thwarted by nosocomial infections. The World Health Organization recently has acknowledged that nosocomial infections are a substantial international public health issue.

PREDISPOSING FACTORS. All patients do not have an equal risk of developing a nosocomial infection. The inherent resistance of the patient to infection is probably the most important determinant of risk. The extremes of age, poor nutritional status, the severity of underlying diseases, and breaks in the integrity of the skin and mucous membranes all increase a patient's risk of nosocomial infection.

The second strong influence on risk of nosocomial infection is the array of diagnostic and therapeutic manipulations undertaken for the patient's benefit. Every invasive procedure carries some risk of infection because it violates either a cutaneous or mucosal barrier to microbial invasion. The risk varies with the degree of invasiveness. For example, an intramuscular injection usually has virtually no risk of infection, whereas 15 to 20 per cent of colorectal operations are complicated by wound infections despite meticulous surgical technique, preoperative bowel preparation, and appropriate antibiotic prophylaxis. Thus, physicians should

---

Nosocomial has a derivation from the Greek word for hospital or infirmary.

subject every invasive procedure to an assessment of potential benefits weighed against potential risks. Medical therapy also can make patients extremely susceptible to nosocomial infections. Cancer chemotherapy eliminates virtually all of a patient's circulating neutrophils, and the immunosuppressive regimens used in organ transplantation ablate the normal immune response to invading microorganisms (see Ch. 287). Infection control measures are designed to protect the patient until periods of such exquisite vulnerability have passed and the patient again has normal or nearly normal phagocytic and immune functions. In addition, the antibiotics used to combat infection can be considered a two-edged sword. Although their use does not generally confer an increased risk of complicating infection, when new infections occur in the face of antibiotic therapy, the pathogens often are resistant to the antibiotics being used (so-called suprainfections). Lastly, it follows that the longer a patient remains in the hospital, the more likely it is that a nosocomial infection will occur.

MODES OF TRANSMISSION. Nosocomial pathogens can be found in both the animate and inanimate environment of the hospital. It is not generally appreciated how clean the hospital's inanimate environment has become. The furniture, bedclothes, curtains, and other inanimate surfaces in the hospital only very rarely harbor microorganisms that cause infections in patients. Nevertheless, reservoirs of nosocomial pathogens still can be established in inanimate areas of the hospital occasionally, especially in specialty care areas. For example, if the countertop in the intensive care unit where urine specific gravity determinations are performed remains wet, it may harbor multiresistant gram-negative bacilli. Nurses' hands then become contaminated and the organisms can be carried back to patients in the unit. Although similar infection hazards in the inanimate environment are detected periodically and need to be remedied, we cannot look to enhanced housekeeping of the general hospital environment to reduce nosocomial infection rates further.

Whereas the hospital's general inanimate environment has receded as a source of nosocomial infections, the role of contaminated medical devices has increased substantially; over 100,000 device-related infections are estimated to occur each year. Medical devices are examples of imaginative medical technology that offer new benefits to patients. However, manufacturers often do not consider the potential infection risks of new devices fully and physicians often employ devices in ways that were not initially anticipated. For example, when intravascular pressure transducers first were introduced, their use was associated with outbreaks of bacteremia. Investigations revealed that instruments were being inadequately disinfected because the instruments were very fragile. When appropriate disinfection protocols were developed, this new infection risk associated with technologic innovation was virtually eliminated.

The animate hospital environment consists of the patients and their caregivers. These humans are the sources of most nosocomial pathogens, and the intimacies of patient care often result in their sharing their microbial flora.

A familiar scenario involves *Staphylococcus aureus*, a classic hospital pathogen. Hospital personnel have a higher rate of asymptomatic carriage of *S. aureus* (often over 30 per cent) than does the general population. Staphylococci may be transmitted from hospital workers to patients, where they later can produce, for example, postoperative wound infections. Such "hospital staph" often are more antibiotic-resistant than community-acquired *S. aureus*, providing a distinctive marker that enables their movement to be readily traced. However, hospital personnel are not the only source of resistant microbial flora. Recent investigations have demonstrated that on admission to the hospital, some patients already may be colonized with small numbers of resistant bacterial strains. After antibiotic treatment, these resistant strains have a survival advantage and multiply to emerge as potential causes of nosocomial infection. Indeed, the endogenous flora is the major source of both the bacterial and viral pathogens that cause nosocomial infections in patients who receive organ transplants and are immunosuppressed for long periods.

Over 100 years have passed since Semmelweis implicated the hands of the students and physicians as the means of spreading pathogens to patients. Nevertheless, such direct contact continues to be the most common way patients are colonized with microorganisms of exogenous origin. At times the microorganisms may be from the caregiver's own flora. Usually, however, the hands of nurses or doctors are contaminated transiently while caring for one patient, and the pathogens then are carried over to the next patient (this process is aptly called "cross-infection" in Britain). Gram-positive skin flora (*S. aureus* and *S. epidermidis*), many gram-negative bacilli (*Enterobacter* and *Serratia,* for example), and even viruses (respiratory syncytial virus, rotavirus) are spread by this means. Over a century ago Semmelweis introduced the most effective way to interrupt transmission by contaminated hands: hand washing. In order to promote hand washing after every patient contact, modern hospitals have located sinks conveniently and have provided disinfectant soap wherever patient examinations and manipulations take place, with special attention to intensive care areas, treatment rooms, and the like. However, persuading medical staff, especially physicians, to routinely wash their hands remains a challenge, especially in the hectic environment of the intensive care unit.

Airborne transmission once was thought to have an important role in the spread of pathogens in the hospital. Today this seems not to be the case, although occasional explosive outbreaks of tuberculosis and chickenpox strongly suggest airborne transmission from a source patient. *Aspergillus* infections have occurred in immunosuppressed patients whose rooms drew air from the vicinity of major construction sites in or adjacent to the hospital. Likewise *Legionella* infections have been produced by the contaminated water spray from an air conditioning cooling tower. Concern about the role of airborne infection in the operating room continues to influence the design and construction of these areas. Most studies indicate that the bacteria causing wound infections originate from the resident flora of either the patients themselves or the operating team. This suggests that transmission likely occurs by direct contact or droplet spread. Nevertheless, because only a few bacteria can infect in certain elaborate procedures that implant foreign bodies (such as total joint replacements), such procedures are performed in laminar air flow facilities where the air stream is designed to flow away from the operative field.

ANTIMICROBIAL RESISTANCE. Since the pandemic of the 1950's and 1960's caused by staphylococcal strains newly resistant to penicillin, it has become axiomatic that antibiotic resistance has been a major feature of nosocomial infections. Although antibiotic-resistant bacteria are not inherently more virulent than their susceptible counterparts, they reduce the physician's therapeutic options and often require the use of more expensive antibiotics.

Currently, both gram-positive and gram-negative hospital pathogens have developed patterns of antimicrobial resistance. *S. aureus* infections are resurgent, and many strains now have developed resistance to methicillin and other similar β-lactam antibiotics that have been mainstays of therapy until recently. Many physicians turned to the quinoline antibiotics as alternate therapy, but quinoline-resistant strains were recovered with

TABLE 289–1. IMPACT OF HOSPITAL-ACQUIRED INFECTIONS IN ACUTE CARE HOSPITALS

Anatomic Site	Number of Infections per 100 Admissions	Proportion of All Hospital-Acquired Infections	Estimated Direct Mortality	Estimated Number of Excess Hospital Days per Infection	Proportion of All Excess Hospital Days
Urinary tract	2.5	30–40%	<1%	2	19%
Postoperative wound	1.5	20–25%	1–2%	7	33%
Pulmonary	1	10–20%	5–10%	8	21%
Bloodstream	0.5–1	5–15%	25%	14	16%
Others	1	20–25%	Varies with site	2	12%

extraordinary rapidity in hospitals where these drugs were used widely. *S. epidermidis* has become a notable nosocomial pathogen in some intensive care units; these organisms have a very diverse pattern of antibiotic resistance. Likewise, gram-negative bacilli have developed distinctive resistance profiles in some hospitals; *Enterobacter cloacae, Pseudomonas aeruginosa,* and *Acinetobacter calcoaceticus* particularly have been involved. It has become clear that genes determining antibiotic resistance are often carried on extrachromosomal plasmids that can be transferred among bacterial species. Thus, some medical centers have been subjected to outbreaks of resistant gram-negative bacillary infections that have extended over years. The distinctive antibiotic resistance pattern first was detected in one bacterial species (among *Serratia,* for example) and then over time also was found among other gram-negative nosocomial pathogens (among *Enterobacter* and *Klebsiella* sequentially). Investigations that combine studies of infections in hospital populations with molecular biologic studies of the pathogens have been called "molecular epidemiology."

During the early 1950's bacterial pathogens isolated from infections virtually anywhere in the United States had essentially identical antibiotic susceptibility patterns. Shortly after antimicrobial resistance was recognized, however, it became apparent that different hospitals began to develop antibiotic resistance patterns among their hospital pathogens that were distinctive and different from each other. Thus, one hospital might have a problem with multiresistant *Serratia,* whereas another hospital directly across the street might encounter almost no such isolates. Although never precisely explained, these differences have been attributed to differences in patient populations, severity of illness, length of stay, and, most importantly, patterns and intensity of antibiotic use. Physicians needed to be aware of these differences, so clinical microbiology laboratories maintained surveillance of resistance patterns and reported them periodically to the medical staff. The more sophisticated surveillance systems were able to distinguish resistance patterns between community-acquired and hospital-acquired infections. Just recently it has become clear that such hospital-wide surveillance is insufficient in large, complex medical centers. Rather than a uniform hospital-wide nosocomial flora, there are a number of independent subpatterns that are specific to each special care area. Thus, the burn unit, neonatal intensive care unit (NICU), and surgical intensive care unit each may have a distinctive nosocomial flora, each with its own localized resistance problem. Laboratories have started to adapt their computerized data management systems so that specialty unit–specific surveillance data can be provided to the physicians who practice in each unit.

COMMON NOSOCOMIAL INFECTIONS, BY ANATOMIC SITE (see Table 289–1)

URINARY TRACT INFECTIONS. Urinary tract infections continue to be the most common nosocomial infection, accounting for 30 to 40 per cent of all hospital-acquired infections. They occur so frequently because almost all are linked to prior urinary tract instrumentation, most often with the seemingly innocuous bladder catheter. Even single in-and-out catheterization is associated with 2 to 3 per cent bacteriuria in otherwise healthy persons. The urethral meatus is colonized with bacteria and even after appropriate cleansing, some are inoculated into the bladder during the catheterization process. The healthy bladder almost always rids itself of small numbers of introduced bacteria. If the bladder and urethra are traumatized, however, an infection is more likely to be established. After complicated labor with its associated urethral and bladder trauma, 23 per cent of postpartum women develop a urinary tract infection after only a single catheterization.

Given these risks, the use of indwelling Foley catheters is preferred, and 10 to 20 per cent of hospitalized patients are treated with these devices. Because of their frequent use, Foley catheters are the leading factor predisposing to nosocomial urinary tract infections. The longer the catheter is in place, the more likely it is that an infection will occur; approximately 5 per cent of patients with a catheter develop bacteriuria per day. The infecting strains colonize the urethral meatus. Through movement of the catheter as well as their own motility they gain entrance to the bladder. Contemporary urinary drainage systems are well designed so that ascending infection from the reservoir bag now is quite uncommon.

Most nosocomial urinary tract infections are asymptomatic or mild, clear with little or no therapy after catheter removal, and do not prolong hospital stay very much (an average of 1 to 2 days only). They are important, however, for two reasons. They are occasionally severe, and 1 of every 200 nosocomial urinary tract infections results in bacteremia. In addition, many nosocomial urinary tract infections are caused by antibiotic-resistant bacterial strains. Thus, the infected catheter systems become reservoirs of resistant gram-negative bacilli, especially in intensive care units where they can be spread easily to other very ill patients. The most common organisms producing nosocomial urinary tract infections include *E. coli* (30 per cent), enterococci (16 per cent), *Pseudomonas* (12 per cent), and *Klebsiella* (6 per cent). Pseudomonas and other multiresistant gram-negative bacteria account for a gradually increasing proportion of these infections as the hospitalized population becomes older, is more severely ill, and receives more intensive antibiotic treatment.

The prevention of nosocomial urinary tract infections has received sustained attention and considerable success. Of course, assuring that catheters are used only for patients who genuinely require continuous bladder drainage is the first guiding principle. It follows that catheters should be removed as soon as possible when patients no longer need them. Industry has been very responsive by producing reliable, sturdy, closed drainage systems. In the past, catheters were disconnected from drainage bags to empty the bags, obtain diagnostic urine specimens, and the like. Every such interruption was an opportunity to introduce bacteria into the catheter system. Contemporary designs facilitate maintenance of the system's integrity by allowing the catheter to be aspirated with a needle and syringe.

These systems work so well that catheters need not be changed routinely, nor is catheter irrigation required unless the catheter becomes obstructed. The use of triple-lumen catheters with a closed prophylactic antibiotic irrigation system has been proposed, but these systems offer no great advantage in preventing infection and are difficult to manage by ward nurses. They may be useful in some patients after urologic surgery in order to prevent obstruction by blood clots and proteinaceous debris. There is no need to culture the urine routinely at the time of catheter removal; the practice of cutting off the catheter tip and culturing it has no value.

Regular perineal hygiene and antibiotic-containing creams have not proven to be of value in reducing infection. Likewise, catheters impregnated with a variety of antibacterial materials have offered no substantial advantage. The use of prophylactic systemic antibiotics to "cover" an indwelling catheter has been decried for 30 years, yet some data suggest they may be efficacious for the first 4 days of catheterization. A serious prospective trial has not been undertaken, perhaps because of the fear of selecting antibiotic-resistant strains.

BACTEREMIA. If urinary tract infections are the most frequent nosocomial infections, nosocomial bacteremias are the most serious. Bacteremias may be secondary to recognized infection at some site, or they may be primary and cannot be attributed to an obvious infection in another anatomic location. Identifying the source of a secondary bacteremia permits one to treat it as well as the bacteremia and prevent recurrences.

The occurrence of a primary bacteremia should always prompt a thorough review of all the patient's intravenous infusions as well as other intravascular devices, as they are frequent sources of bloodstream infections. More than 25 per cent of hospitalized patients receive intravenous fluids. Other diagnostic and therapeutic procedures require access to the venous or arterial systems for either brief or prolonged periods. An intravenous pyelogram and cardiac catheterization are examples of abbreviated procedures, whereas intra-arterial pressure monitoring may continue for days. Although all these procedures create an access for bacteria to enter the bloodstream, they are remarkably safe. Nevertheless, the history of intravascular technology is punctuated with many studies of endemic and epidemic bloodstream infections. The procedures that offer an assurance of reasonable safety today were hard won, and any lapse in appropriate care can result in a device-related bacteremia. As more patients have required admission to intensive care units, the rate of nosocomial bacteremia has gradually risen during the 1980's.

Intrinsic contamination of intravenous fluid by the manufacturer is fortunately a rare event. Most episodes of infusion-related sepsis are caused by microorganisms that enter the system during its use (extrinsic contamination). The major locus of contamination is the cannulation site. The longer the catheter is left in place, the more likely it is that infection will occur. The catheter site may be purulent and phlebitis may be evident, but these overt clinical manifestations frequently are not present. Suppurative thrombophlebitis is an unusual event in which a substantial segment of vein becomes a linear abscess, the entire lumen being filled with pus. S. aureus and S. epidermidis are the most frequently isolated pathogens, but an array of gram-negative bacilli and Candida species also regularly are associated with catheter sepsis.

Any indwelling vascular access device can be associated with infection. Hickman-Broviac catheters that are tunneled under the skin of the anterior chest wall before they enter the subclavian vein were developed to provide long-term vascular access (as for cancer chemotherapy) and minimize the risk of infection. They have been largely successful. When infection does occur, it often is possible to treat the infection, leaving the catheter in place. Although such catheters have an enhanced risk for developing another infection, enough time is often gained to complete a course of chemotherapy.

The essentials of prevention begin with meticulous aseptic catheter insertion technique. Because the risk of infection increases with increasing duration of use, strict nursing protocols exist to ensure that all catheters are discontinued on a regular rotation and that new catheters are inserted at different sites. As a reminder, the dressings at the insertion site are dated; peripheral catheters should be left in place no longer than 72 hours unless there is no alternative. If a catheter must remain in place, a note providing the reasons should be written in the chart. Likewise, the infusions themselves also must be changed regularly; infusions should hang no longer than 24 hours. Because most infections originate at the insertion site, in-line filters have not reduced infection rates; they add expense without increasing safety. The catheter insertion site is protected by a single dressing for the duration of the catheter's routine use; daily dressings and antibiotic ointments are no longer considered useful.

NOSOCOMIAL PNEUMONIA. Hospital-acquired lower respiratory tract infections (including pneumonia and bronchitis) account for 10 to 15 per cent of nosocomial infections. Almost 1 per cent of patients admitted to the hospital develop pneumonia. Elderly patients with serious underlying illnesses are at risk, as are all patients receiving mechanical ventilation. These infections usually extend a patient's hospital stay for 7 days or more, produce substantial morbidity, and contribute to the deaths of already seriously ill patients.

In contrast to community-acquired pneumonia in younger patients, nosocomial pneumonia usually is a mixed infection involving more than one organism. Although a hospital's intensive care unit may develop a dominant bacterial respiratory tract pathogen, the list of bacteria associated with nosocomial pneumonia is large. Aerobic gram-negative bacilli are associated with more than half the cases, including P. aeruginosa, Enterobacter, Klebsiella, E. coli, and Acinetobacter, among others. Acinetobacter particularly is associated with ventilated patients in busy intensive care units. Among gram-positive organisms, S. aureus is isolated with regularity but may not always have a major pathogenic role. Pneumococci contribute to about 3 per cent of nosocomial pneumonias, usually in elderly patients with predisposing lung disease. Most clinical laboratory routines do not process respiratory tract specimens anaerobically, and even research methods have limitations in ascribing a role for anaerobes in lower respiratory tract infections. Although aerobic pathogens clearly are dominant, most authorities believe that anaerobes are involved in about one third of nosocomial pneumonias. Legionella pneumophila can be a vexing problem in some hospitals, where it can be isolated from the water supply. Viral respiratory infections are increasingly recognized as causes of nosocomial pneumonia and as infections predisposing to subsequent bacterial invasion. Respiratory syncytial virus, influenza, and cytomegalovirus are the viruses most commonly identified.

Endotracheal tubes and tracheostomies bypass the upper respiratory tract defense mechanisms and can traumatize mucous membranes. When managed improperly, these devices can provide direct access for the introduction of hospital pathogens on the hands of personnel or by contaminated suction tubing. Ventilator machines often produced contaminated aerosols in past years, but current maintenance protocols have made nosocomial pneumonia due to the machine itself an unusual event.

Aspiration of oropharyngeal secretions is the principal initiating event in nosocomial pneumonia. Patients who have an impaired gag reflex, are sedated, or have altered consciousness are more likely to aspirate. The volume and pH of the aspirate as well as its bacterial population contribute to the likelihood of lung injury. The bacterial population is determined by the organisms colonizing the oropharynx. The flora of the normal pharynx is largely gram-positive. Gram-negative bacillary colonization occurs in older persons with a variety of underlying diseases, after antibiotic therapy, and in patients who are leukopenic.

Gastric alkalinization can permit the multiplication of gram-negative bacteria in the stomach. These bacteria can then become the source of oropharyngeal colonization. Antacids and histamine type-2 (H_2) blockers are often given to patients in ICU's who are being ventilated in order to prevent stress ulcers. Because they raise gastric pH, these drugs promote the growth of bacteria in the stomach and increase the risk of nosocomial pneumonia. Because it does not neutralize gastric acidity, sucralfate is preferred for stress ulcer prophylaxis.

The prevention of nosocomial pneumonia is a daunting challenge. Positioning patients with their heads raised may reduce somewhat the occurrence of aspiration. Scrupulous hand washing inhibits the transmission of nosocomial pathogens. Meticulous maintenance of ventilatory equipment and assiduous pulmonary toilet by nurses reduce risks. The role of selective decontamination of the gastrointestinal tract with combinations of oral and systemic antibiotics currently is being studied.

SURGICAL WOUND INFECTIONS. Postoperative wound infections account for 20 per cent of nosocomial infections. These infections account for a substantial amount of morbidity, increase hospital stay considerably, and are costly. Some postoperative infections extend down from the skin incision to the depths of the surgical field where they can destroy vascular anastomoses or disrupt an implanted prosthetic device. Bacteremia may accompany such infections. The extent of the surgical procedure and its anatomic location, the severity of the patient's underlying illness, and the surgeon's skill are all important determinants of risk. When surgery involves tissues that normally are not subjected to a large microbial population during the procedure ("clean" operations), wound infection rates often are less than 2 per cent. Such operations include inguinal herniorrhaphy and vascular surgery in the neck, for example. When procedures transect mucosal surfaces, such as in a colectomy ("contaminated" operations), up to 20 per cent of patients have a postoperative wound infection. If patients are malnourished, at the extremes of age, or have serious underlying diseases, wound infections are more likely to occur. The longer the duration of the operation, the more likely that a postoperative infection will occur. A surgeon's skill is critical. If tissues are traumatized, the vascular supply is unnecessarily interrupted, devitalized tissue or blood clots are left in the wound, or wound layers are not realigned properly, the risk of wound infection increases.

S. aureus and S. epidermidis are the most commonly isolated pathogens from wound infections, reflecting their common residence on human skin. A wide variety of other organisms contribute to these infections, including enterococci, E. coli, P. aeruginosa, and Bacteroides, largely determined by the organ undergoing surgery. The infecting bacteria most often originate in the patient's own endogenous microbial flora, whether on the skin or on a mucosal surface. A smaller contribution comes from the bacterial flora of the surgeon and other members of the operating team. Even clean wounds are not truly sterile; small numbers of bacteria can be recovered from virtually all wounds at the time of wound closure. Thus, for the most part, the infecting bacteria are in the wound when the patient leaves the operating room, unless there is a drain or packing in the incision. Occasionally bacteremia originating from another infected site implant at the operative site; there have been a few well-described instances in which a wound was infected during postoperative care.

A whole array of techniques are employed to minimize the occurrence of wound infection. The architecture, air handling, and housekeeping in the operating room have made the physical environment very clean. Special laminar flow rooms are used for some procedures, such as implantation of an artificial joint. An elaborate ritual of aseptic practice involves both the patient (shaving the surgical area, baths with disinfectant soap, skin preparation just before surgery, among others) and the surgeon (precise hand scrubbing, operating room gowns and masks, use of sterile gloves, and the like). The importance of the appropriate use of antibiotic prophylaxis cannot be overemphasized. Indeed, some medical historians suggest that the most important consequence of the discovery of antibiotics was that their use permitted the development of the technologically adventurous procedures that characterize contemporary surgery. In recent years it has been amply confirmed that for antibiotics to be effective in preventing wound infection they need to be given only briefly, chosen to be effective against the most commonly expected pathogens at the surgical site, and given in amounts sufficient to provide killing concentrations in the tissues. The brevity of their use (often no longer than 24 hours) results in very little drug toxicity or development of bacterial resistance.

MISCELLANEOUS SITES. In addition to the most commonly occurring infections discussed above, nosocomial infections also occur in numerous other sites and circumstances. The extent of nosocomial infectious diarrhea is only now being recognized. Among children, the most common pathogen is rotavirus; among adults, *Clostridium difficile* colitis is a complication of antibiotic therapy. Epidemics of keratoconjunctivitis due to adenoviruses can be propagated by the contaminated hands of ophthalmologists as well as contaminated tonometers. Meningitis, usually caused by *S. epidermidis*, can follow the placement of shunts in the cerebral ventricles. Meningitis also can occur in immunocompromised organ transplant recipients. In renal transplant patients *Cryptococcus* and *Listeria* are the most frequent pathogens. Transfusions of blood and blood products have resulted in the transmission of hepatitis B virus and human immunodeficiency virus as well as other viruses and bacteria.

INFECTION CONTROL PROGRAMS

Although many efforts were being made to prevent infections in hospitals, most institutions did not have a formal organized program until the 1960's. At that time it became apparent that the previous focus by hospitals on environmental hygiene was insufficient. Strongly influenced by the Centers for Disease Control, the American Hospital Association, and the Joint Commission on Accreditation of Health Care Organizations, every hospital now must have an active infection control program in order to secure accreditation. Central to the program is an Infection Control Committee whose members are broadly representative of hospital administration and the professional disciplines. A physician knowledgeable about infection control is designated the Hospital Epidemiologist. It is recommended that the hospital employ one infection control practitioner (usually a nurse with special infection control training) for every 250 beds. These practitioners organize a wide variety of infection control activities, but all who work in hospitals must realize that the practitioners alone cannot produce the safest milieu for patients. Rather, all who work in hospitals must assume responsibility: Infection control is everyone's business.

A critical element of the program is a system of surveillance for detecting nosocomial infections, analyzing the data, and reporting on distinctive events. Surveillance may involve reviewing microbiology laboratory reports, visiting wards, inspecting surgical wounds, and the like. It now has been well demonstrated that such surveillance provides more pertinent information than routinely culturing features of the environment, a practice that has largely ceased.

The infection control practitioners also orchestrate the institution's control measures, ranging from appropriate isolation systems to responses when an epidemic is detected. Each unit in the hospital contributes its own section of procedures to a hospital-wide infection control manual. Its procedures are reviewed on 1- to 2-year cycles and as needed when new developments occur.

Sophisticated support from the clinical microbiology laboratory

is necessary for a successful infection control program. The laboratory provides its routine data for surveillance purposes, may be asked to process extra cultures when an outbreak is under investigation, and may undertake special studies with nosocomial pathogens.

Other hospital service units also provide critical support for the infection control program. Although the role of the inanimate environment has been de-emphasized, the housekeeping department must maintain a high level of cleanliness throughout the institution. They also are responsible for managing and disposing of the hospital's solid waste. Heavily contaminated wastes (such as from the microbiology laboratory) must be incinerated. Solid waste disposal has become a major political issue over the last several years and has become very expensive, so this function has grown in importance.

The central supply operation cleans and either disinfects or sterilizes reusable materials that are employed in the diagnosis and therapy of patients. The laundry collects and launders soiled linen. Linen need be sterilized only for use in operative procedures. The hospital kitchen or outside food service must adhere to strict hygiene standards in preparing the many and varied diets for patients. Fortunately, foodborne outbreaks in hospitals are not common.

The occupational health service has special responsibilities to protect hospital personnel from acquiring an infection from patients while performing their patient-care duties, and, in turn, also to prevent employees from transmitting their own infections to patients. In this regard, several diseases have assumed particular importance.

AIDS (see Part XXI). Although the risk of acquiring HIV infection from occupational exposure is very low, this disease has received great attention from hospital infection control programs over the past several years. AIDS has raised a number of scientific, ethical, social, and legal issues that have had an impact on the ability of the infection control team to devise solutions. Not every issue has as yet been adequately addressed, largely because certain essential data are lacking.

Because HIV is not transmitted through casual contact, routine interactions with patients are not hazardous. Exposures that are associated with a risk of acquiring HIV infection are injuries by "sharps" (needles and scalpels, primarily) contaminated with the body fluid (blood, most commonly) or tissue of an HIV-infected patient. A number of studies have indicated that approximately 1 of every 250 such exposures results in transmission of HIV infection to the health care worker. Transmission is more likely to occur when the exposures are multiple and deep and when a substantial volume of blood is inoculated during the injury. The prospective studies of exposures on skin or mucous membranes have not shown any seroconversions, but there have been anecdotal reports suggesting that such exposures rarely might result in transmission. Much remains to be learned in this regard.

Standard protocols have been developed to manage the hospital worker who sustains an occupational injury involving a patient's blood or other body fluid. These include testing the source patient for HIV infection (if the patient can be identified), counseling the hospital worker, and possibly offering zidovudine prophylaxis. Such injuries often are major anxiety-provoking events, and the cooperation of the occupational health service and the infection control team in the supportive counseling of the hospital worker is extremely important. See Ch. 413 for additional discussion of AIDS prevention and control.

TUBERCULOSIS. Health care workers have always been at greater risk than the general population for acquiring tuberculosis. The patient who is diagnosed with tuberculosis is only a modest hazard. Respiratory isolation techniques and antituberculosis therapy quickly reduce the hazard of nosocomial transmission. Rather, the risk is from the cryptic case, the patient with as yet undiagnosed tuberculosis. After a steady decline for years, tuberculosis is again resurgent because of the recent wave of immigrants from Southeast Asia and Central America and the frequency with which tuberculosis complicates HIV infection.

All hospitals are obliged to have a tuberculosis control program. All personnel receive a tuberculin skin test on employment. Those who are skin test–negative are followed by periodic skin testing, usually at yearly intervals, although high-risk persons may be tested at shorter intervals. Those who convert to a positive skin test are evaluated for active disease and are candidates for isoniazid (INH) preventive therapy. There is no place for annual chest roentgenograms, a now discarded practice.

HEPATITIS B. Like HIV infection, hepatitis B is transmitted in the hospital by exposure to blood and other body fluids that contain the virus. Hospital personnel who are exposed to blood and use needles, scalpels, and other sharp objects are at increased risk of hepatitis B infection. Programs to prevent hepatitis B infection are two-pronged. First, strong attempts must be made to reduce injuries through education, designing safer devices, and providing for the secure disposal of sharps in impervious containers. These precautions help avert not only hepatitis B infections, but all other blood-borne pathogens including retroviruses and other viral hepatitis agents. Secondly, hepatitis B vaccine must be offered to all workers at potential risk. Ideally, all students of the health care professions should be immunized early in their training. In addition, insistent attempts to immunize current health care workers, including physicians and nurses, must continue. After an injury, standard protocols are used by the occupational health service to evaluate the health worker and the source patient and to offer appropriate prophylaxis.

In addition to providing hepatitis B vaccine, hospitals should provide other vaccines for the protection of personnel. Measles, mumps, and rubella have produced outbreaks in hospitals resulting in a great deal of unnecessary illness, turbulence, and expense. In these outbreaks, hospital workers have both acquired these viral infections and transmitted them to patients. It now is recommended that hospital workers born since 1957 receive a second dose of measles vaccine. If this is provided as the combined measles-mumps-rubella (MMR) vaccine, protection is achieved against all three diseases.

Finally, as the United States population ages, as hospitals care for increasingly sicker patients, and as medical technology continues its aggressive advances in organ transplantation and other invasive therapies, the importance of nosocomial infections will likely continue to increase. Infection control programs must be alert to these changes and be prepared to respond to them with equally new and innovative preventive measures.

American Hospital Association: Management of HIV Infection in the Hospital, 3rd ed. Recommendations of the Technical Panel on Infections Within Hospitals. Chicago, American Hospital Association, 1988. *A booklet available from the AHA that discusses aspects of caring for HIV-infected patients in hospitals. Not a clinical text.*
Bennett JV, Brachman PS: Hospital Infections. Boston, Little Brown & Company, 1986. *A comprehensive treatment of hospital infection issues.*
Centers for Disease Control: Guidelines for prevention of transmission of human immunodeficiency virus and hepatitis B virus to health care and public safety workers. MMWR 37(No. S-6):3–37, 1989. *The official recommendations.*
Kaiser AB: Antimicrobial prophylaxis in surgery. N Engl J Med 315:1129–1138, 1986. *A comprehensive review.*
Pugliese G, Lynch P, Jackson MM: Universal Precautions. Policies, Procedures, and Resources. Chicago, American Hospital Publishing Company, 1991. *An excellent resource for practical suggestions.*
Weber DJ, Rutala WA: Nosocomial infections: New issues and strategies for prevention. Infect Dis Clin North Am 3(4):671–929, 1989. *A collection of papers discussing a wide variety of current infection control issues.*
Wenzel RP: Prevention and Control of Nosocomial Infections. Baltimore, Williams & Wilkins, 1987. *A scholarly text on nosocomial infections.*

290 Advice to Travelers

Bruce M. Greene

Overseas travel by U.S. citizens is steadily increasing, including travel to developing countries. Approximately 15 million people from the United States travel overseas each year, including an estimated 7 million to developing countries. It is the latter group, who are exposed to a variety of health hazards as a consequence of overseas travel, that this chapter addresses. Importantly, most of such health problems are entirely or partially preventable.

The precautions that one can recommend to travelers to developing countries include general preventive health measures, vaccinations, and medications. What is recommended depends greatly on the specific itinerary and living conditions. It is incumbent upon the physician making such recommendations to be cognizant of the most recent epidemiologic information pertinent to the situation.

GENERAL PREVENTIVE HEALTH MEASURES

TRAVELER'S DIARRHEA. Travelers to developing countries frequently experience gastroenteritis. The risk of this problem can be minimized by avoiding indiscriminate consumption of high-risk foods, such as lettuce salads, unpeeled fruits, raw vegetables, local water and milk, ice cubes made from local water, creamy sauces and other obvious rich foods that serve as a good culture medium, and food prepared and served by sidewalk vendors. Eating food that is prepared in a reputable restaurant, cooked well and served hot, and drinking bottled water, carbonated drinks, or hot tea or coffee reduce the risk of gastroenteritis. Finally, it is important to recall that airline food is usually prepared locally.

Boiling water for 10 minutes at usual elevations (longer at high elevations with low atmospheric pressure) is the most reliable way to purify water. Purification tablets and filtration devices are less effective. Bottled mineral water in which the seal is unbroken is usually safe. For further details of the clinical aspects of this syndrome, see Ch. 319.

MALARIA. Minimizing exposure to mosquito bites is an important precaution for malaria prevention. No prophylactic agent is completely effective, and wearing protective clothing and utilizing appropriate insect repellent (containing DEET) are essential. Mosquito exposure is usually worst in the evening and early morning. In areas with high-intensity exposure to infected mosquitoes, mosquito bed nets and knockdown sprays should be used for sleeping.

Large urban areas usually are malaria transmission–free; however, many urban areas of Africa are exceptions. Travel to a game park even for a day or overnight travel through rural areas is sufficient to create a significant risk of malaria.

Most important, travelers to malaria-endemic areas should be advised that, even though all preventive measures are taken and observed carefully, acquisition of malaria is still a possibility. Therefore, because of the risk of rapidly fatal falciparum malaria, such individuals should be advised to report promptly to an emergency room for unexplained fever that occurs within 6 months of returning. It is imperative to note that the fever associated with falciparum malaria frequently does *not* demonstrate a regular pattern and can even be unremitting.

ACUTE MOUNTAIN SICKNESS. An individual whose travel results in an increase in altitude of greater than approximately 2500 to 3000 meters within a 48- to 72-hour period has a risk of developing acute mountain sickness. This syndrome, associated with headache, nausea, vomiting, diarrhea, and fever, can be extremely debilitating and is preventable. Treatment with acetazolamide, 250 mg three times a day starting 24 hours before travel and continuing for 5 days after arrival, minimizes symptoms. The individual should be questioned regarding sulfa allergy and warned of the mild diuretic effect of acetazolamide.

ADVICE TO INDIVIDUALS WITH UNDERLYING CARDIOPULMONARY DISEASE. Persons with severe angina pectoris should be advised against air travel. On the other hand, persons with well-compensated, stable ischemic heart disease should be able to travel without undue risk, although it is apparent that access to medical care will be suboptimal during travel.

Individuals with underlying respiratory insufficiency may be able to travel by air, although supplemental oxygen may be required during travel. Guidelines have recently been proposed to assist in making these determinations (see references).

MOTOR VEHICLE ACCIDENTS. One of the most serious threats to visitors to developing countries is motor vehicle accidents. The traveler must exert special vigilance and a high level of individual responsibility in safeguarding against this possibility. In this regard, knowing and having a record of one's blood type may be important.

SPECIAL RISKS. Schistosomiasis can be acquired by even transient exposure to fresh water lakes and ponds. Rabies is quite

PLATE 9   INFECTIOUS DISEASES

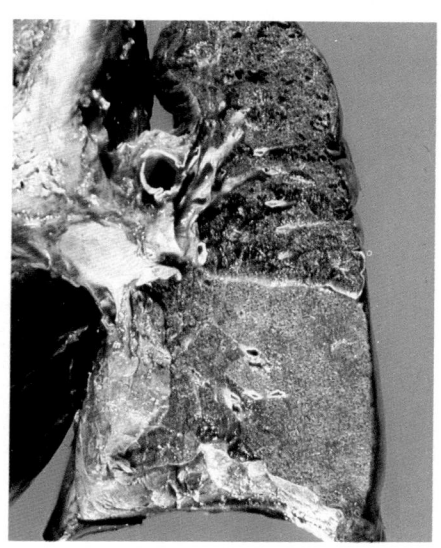

A, Autopsy specimen revealing lobar consolidation (gray and red hepatization) of the left lower lobe due to *Streptococcus pneumoniae*. Note the absence of abscess formation and the presence of dense consolidation extending from the hilum to the pleural surface.

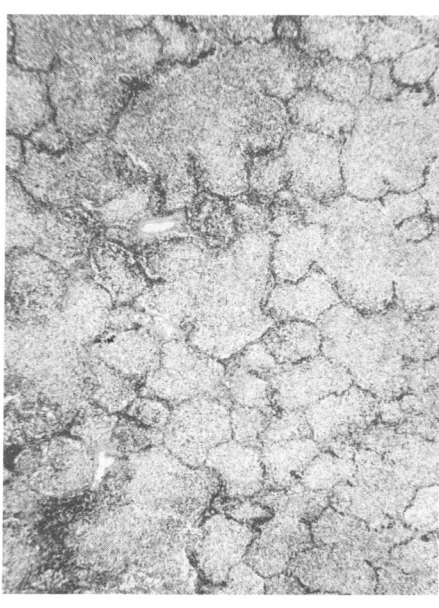

B, Low-powered magnification (×100) of hematoxylin and eosin (H & E) stain of tissue section from left lower lobar pneumonia pictured in A. Note intact alveolar walls and alveoli filled with edema and thick cellular exudate.

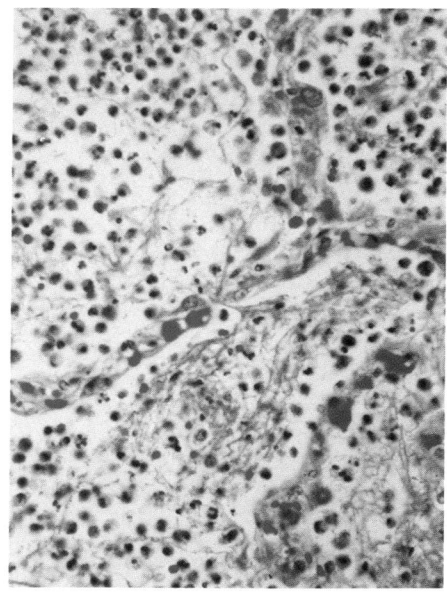

C, Higher magnification (×500) of H & E stain depicted in B. Note heavy infiltrate of polymorphonuclear cells and intact alveolar walls.

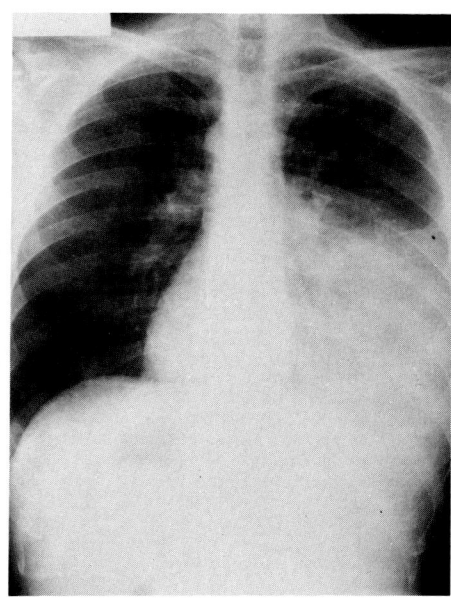

D, Roentgenogram (posteroanterior view) of the chest of a patient with left lower lobar pneumonia due to *S. pneumoniae,* with concomitant pleural effusion. Note obliteration of the left diaphragmatic shadow and the air bronchogram effect seen near the hilum, consistent with air space or alveolar exudative disease.

E, Fluid removed from the pleural space in a patient with early pneumococcal pneumonia and pleural effusion. The fluid may be serous, serosanguineous, green, or thick and white.

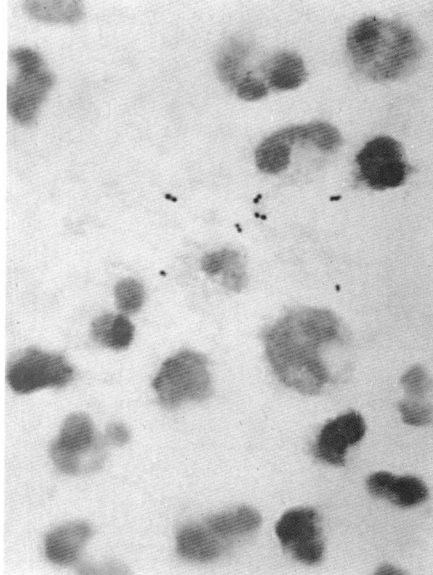

F, Gram's stain of pleural fluid shown in E, revealing the presence of polymorphonuclear cells and typical gram-positive diplococci in pairs, consistent with pneumococci.

G, Erysipeloid. Characteristic indolent, violaceous, nonpurulent lesion on a finger.

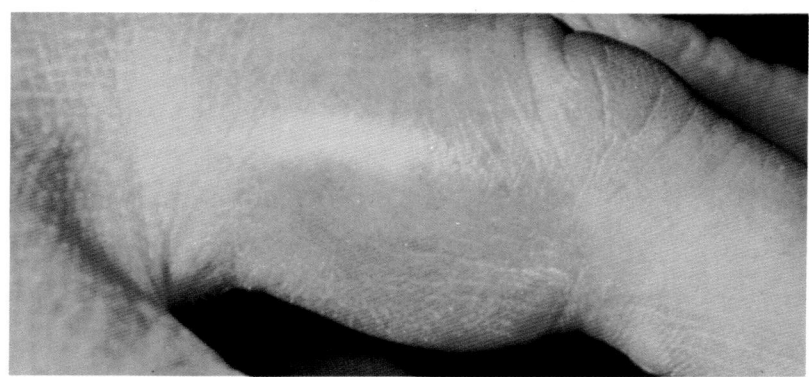

PLATE 10   LYME DISEASE, POLYCHONDRITIS, AND LEISHMANIASIS

A, Erythema chronicum migrans (ECM), the major dermatologic manifestation of Lyme disease. Four days after onset of ECM, this patient has developed secondary annular lesions; some of their borders have merged. (From Steere AC, Bartenhagen NH, Craft JE, et al.: The early clinical manifestations of Lyme disease. Ann Intern Med 99:76–82, 1983; with permission.)

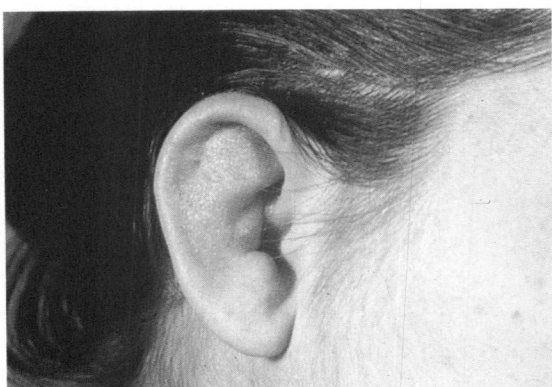

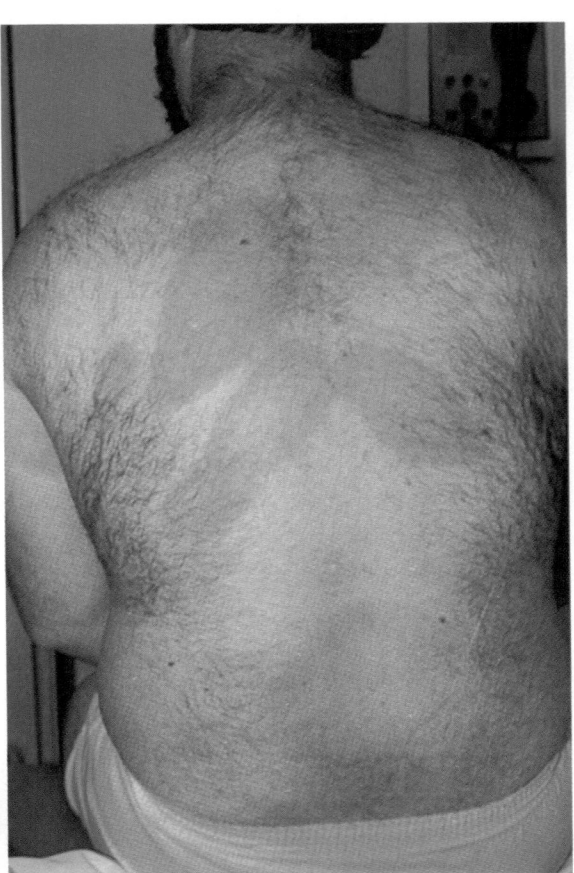

B, Polychondritis. Note nodularity of ear.

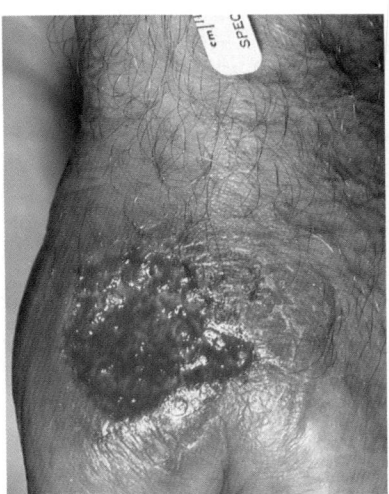

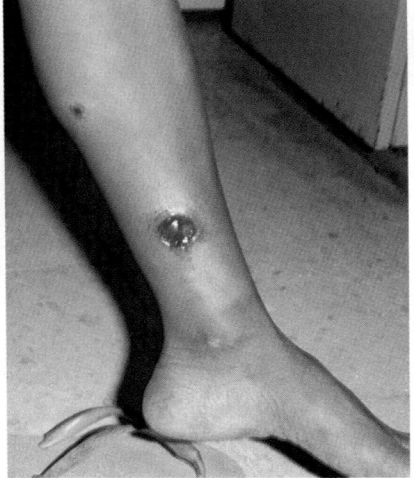

C, Left, Exudative cutaneous leishmanial lesion on the dorsum of the hand *(L. braziliensis)* acquired in the jungle of southeastern Peru. *Right,* Cutaneous leishmanial lesion on the lower leg *(L. mexicana)* of an inhabitant of southern Mexico.

PLATE 11.   *See figure on the opposite page*

Protozoan diseases. *A* to *D* show various erythrocyte forms of falciparum or vivax malaria (× 1500).

A, "Ring forms" of *Plasmodium falciparum.* Note the delicate rings and an erythrocyte containing two organisms.

B, Trophozoite of *Plasmodium vivax.* The red cell is enlarged, Schüffner's dots are seen, and the parasite is large and ameboid.

C, Schizont of *Plasmodium vivax* with at least 18 merozoite nuclei.

D, Gametocyte of *Plasmodium falciparum.* The crescent or banana shape is characteristic.

E, Trypanosoma rhodesiense in the peripheral blood. It has a nucleus, posterior kinetoplast, undulating membrane, and flagellum (× 1500).

F, Spleen smear showing a cell filled with *Leishmania donovani.* The rod-shaped kinetoplast and large, round nucleus appear as two adjacent red dots.

G, Methenamine silver nitrate stain of clump of *Pneumocystis* cysts. They appear as black circles against the blue background (× 800). It should be noted that *Pneumocystis* is no longer considered a protozoan.

H, Stool sample observed by light microscopy, showing a motile *Entamoeba histolytica* moving in a straight line across the field. The ameba contains lucent vacuoles and shows a pseudopod directed to the upper right (× 500).

(A, C, D, and *F* are photographs taken by T. C. Jones from the Cornell Parasitology teaching slides; *B* is from the collection of H. Zaiman, originally photographed by M. Wittner; *E* and *G* were provided by R. B. Roberts; *H* is a photograph of fresh material provided by T. C. Jones.)

PLATE 11 PROTOZOAN DISEASES

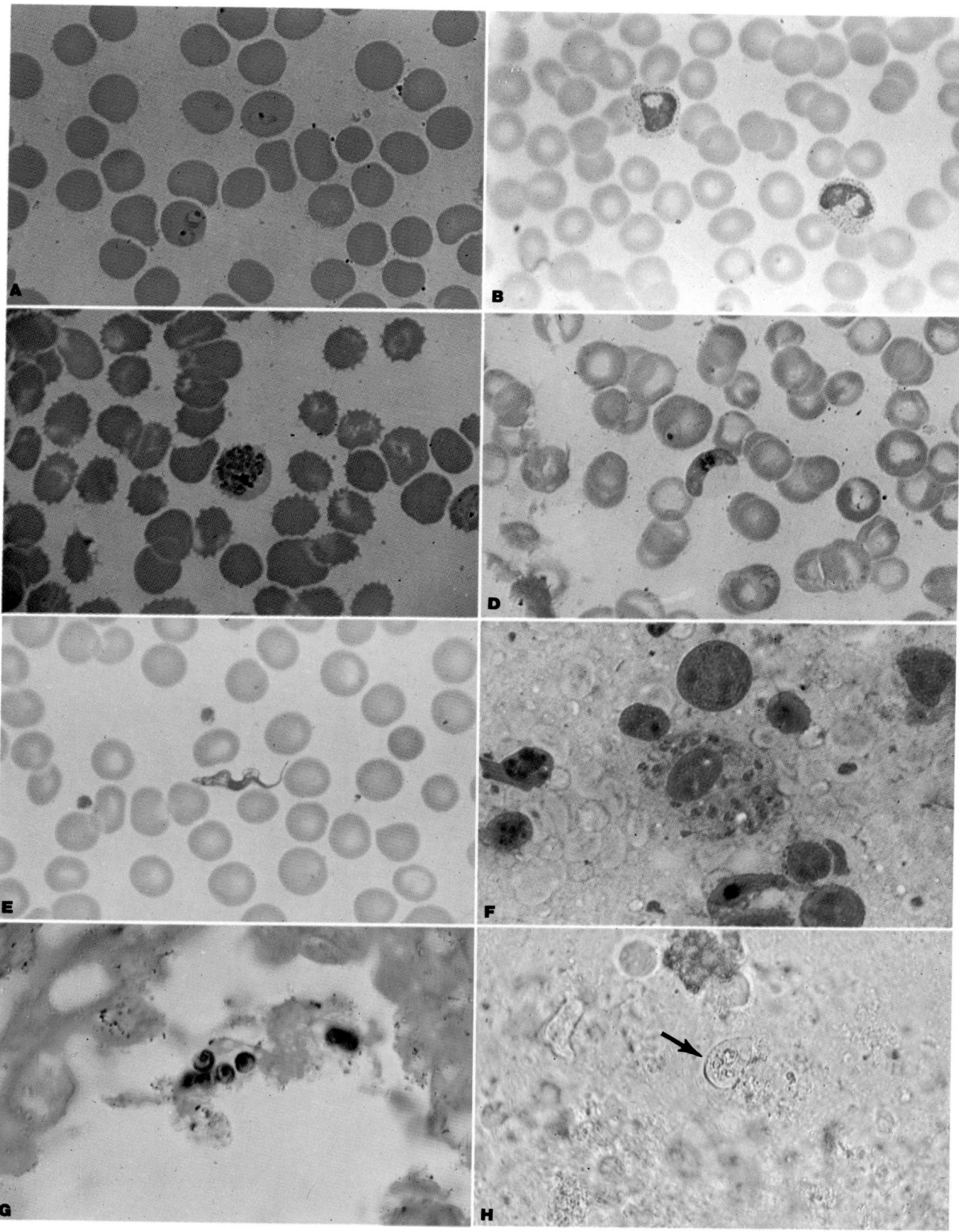

See legend on the opposite page

PLATE 12   HIV AND ASSOCIATED DISORDERS

A to E show dermatologic abnormalities in AIDS.

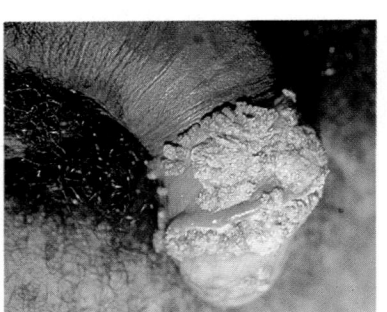

A, Prominent condyloma surrounding the corona and the shaft of the penis.

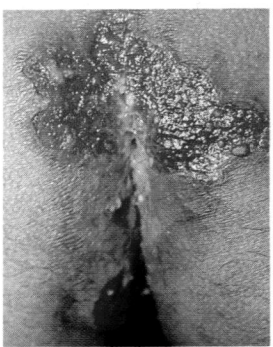

B, Chronic ulcerative herpetic infection is commonly seen in the intergluteal fold.

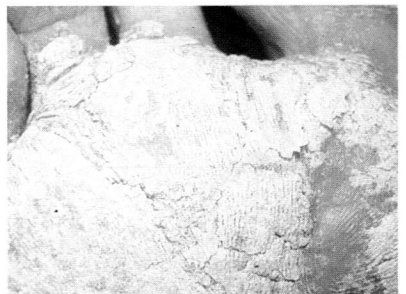

C, Marked hyperkeratosis characterizes keratoderma blennorrhagicum of Reiter's syndrome in HIV-seropositive patients.

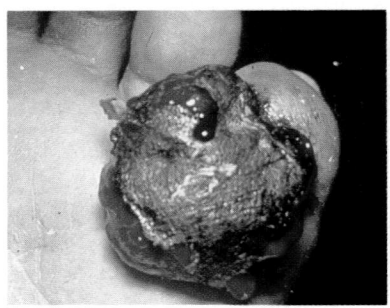 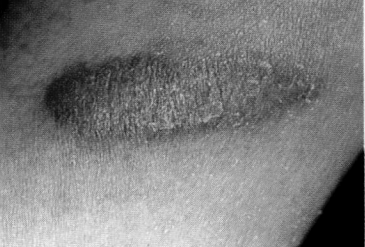

D, Left, An exophytic tumor of Kaposi's sarcoma on the sole. Right, Lesion demonstrating the linear configuration frequently noted in Kaposi's sarcoma of the skin in patients with AIDS.

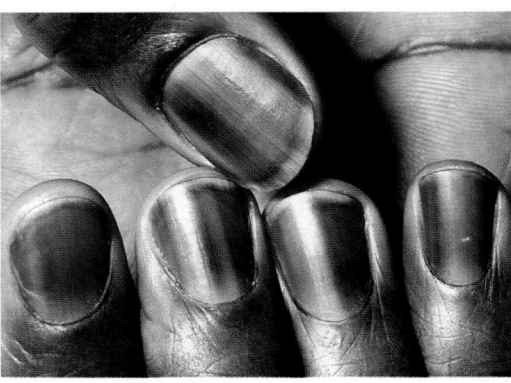

E, Vertical bands in the nail plates developed during treatment with AZT.

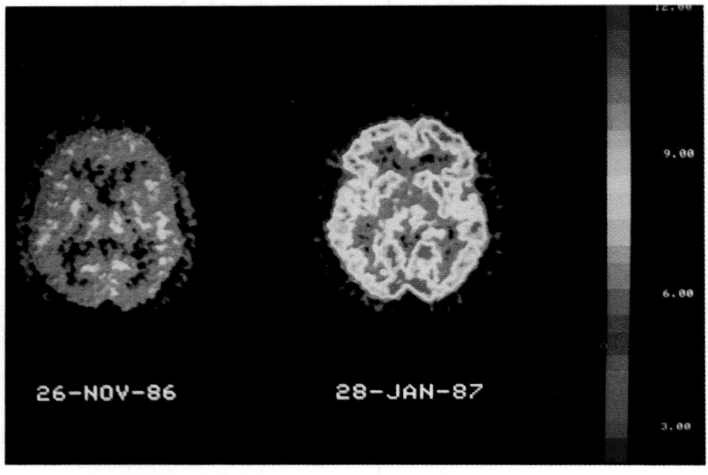

F, Positron emission tomography (PET) scan showing glucose metabolism in the brain of a patient with AIDS dementia before (left) and during (right) therapy with AZT. This patient had marked improvement in his cognitive function that was associated with a relative normalization of glucose metabolism in the brain. (Reproduced with permission from Brunetti A, Berg G, Di Chiro G, et al.: Reversal of brain metabolic abnormalities following treatment of AIDS dementia complex with 3' - azido - 2', 3' - dideoxythymidine (AZT, zidovudine): A PET - FDG study. J Nucl Med 30:581–590, 1989.)

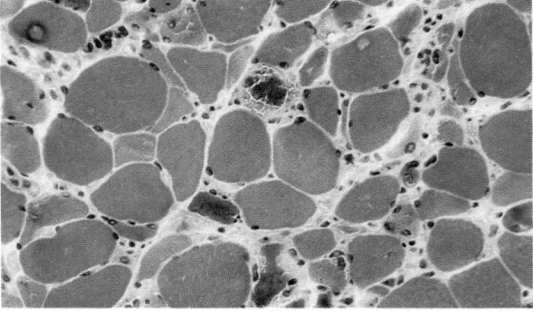

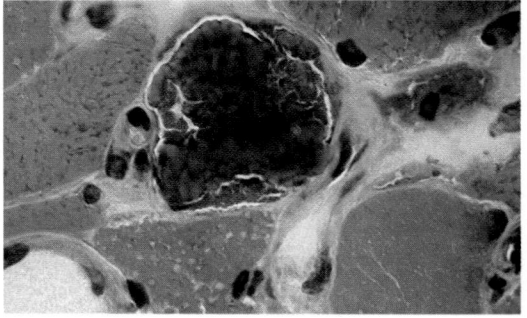

G, Pathologic findings in a patient with AZT-induced myopathy. Top, Destructive changes with variation in fiber size and a "ragged-red" fiber. Inflammatory changes can be seen in both AZT-induced myopathy and the myopathy of HIV infection. However, ragged-red fibers are seen only in patients receiving AZT. Transverse section, stained with the modified Gomori trichrome stain (× 320). Bottom, Detail showing a ragged-red fiber (× 900). (Photographs courtesy of Dr. M.C. Dalakos.)

common in developing countries, and dogs and other vertebrate animals should be avoided. Cysticercosis is a particular threat in some countries, e.g., Mexico, and the usual source is not under-cooked meat, but rather a food handler harboring an adult *T. solium* worm. Similarly, trichinosis is a risk in many countries, and pork may be used as a substitute for other meats in some dishes. In West and West Central Africa, loa loa is a risk and can be prevented with weekly diethylcarbamazine. Finally, individuals who are medication-dependent should pack an extra supply of critical medications and ensure their safe passage by packing strategically.

JET LAG. Individuals traveling to a time zone that is more than 3 hours different from that to which they are accustomed frequently experience extreme fatigue, somnolence, and disordered sleeping patterns. This results in part from lack of adequate sleep in transit and in part from the necessary resetting of the individual's biologic clock. To counter the first problem, short-acting benzodiazepines are helpful and can ensure adequate sleep. Upon arrival in the new time zone, resetting of the biologic clock is facilitated by forcing oneself to live according to the new time schedule. This frequently necessitates increased consumption of coffee or tea and sometimes further use of short-acting hypnotics. There is no clear evidence that more extensive and elaborate programs to avoid jet lag are of value.

PRETRAVEL VACCINATIONS AND OTHER INJECTIONS

It is important to review the individual patient's overall immunization status, including those vaccines addressed below as well as others such as pneumococcal and influenza vaccines that may be indicated for some persons. Prior to administration, full details concerning the injectable reagent, available in the manufacturer's package insert, should be consulted.

IMMUNE SERUM GLOBULIN (GAMMA GLOBULIN). For travel to most developing countries, individuals who have not had hepatitis A infection should receive 0.06 ml per kilogram for a stay of greater than 3 months' duration, to be repeated every 5 months; for travel with a total duration of less than 3 months, a single injection of 0.02 ml per kilogram is adequate. Following deep intramuscular injection, the site usually remains sore for 1 to 3 days. Immune serum globulin has been found to have some efficacy in preventing food-borne non-A, non-B hepatitis.

YELLOW FEVER. This is recommended for travelers to endemic areas in South and Central America and Africa. Although it is a live virus vaccine, yellow fever immunization is not affected by concurrent administration of immune serum globulin preparations in the United States. Occasionally (in 2 to 5 per cent of vaccinees), fever, headache, and myalgias develop 6 to 10 days after injection during the phase of virus replication. Because of the time required for virus replication, yellow fever vaccine must be given at least 10 days prior to travel to an endemic area. Administration once every 10 years is required. As with all live virus vaccines, except oral polio vaccine, it is not recommended that yellow fever vaccine be given with known or possible pregnancy. Egg allergy is a contraindication. Further, infants less than 4 months of age and some persons with altered immune status should not receive yellow fever vaccine.

TETANUS. Travelers to developing countries should receive a tetanus booster if they have not been immunized within the previous 5 years. This is because of the risk of hepatitis B and HIV infection associated with needle injection in the event that a tetanus-prone injury is sustained in a developing country. In adults, tetanus-diphtheria (Td) is recommended.

POLIO. Adults who are traveling to developing countries where polio is a risk should receive a polio booster if none has been given since childhood. Those who previously received a primary course of immunization with oral polio vaccine should receive trivalent OPV on one occasion. Those who are uncertain of what they received previously, or who received inactivated polio vaccine, should receive a booster dose of enhanced efficacy inactivated polio vaccine (eIPV). Adults who have no prior history of polio immunization should receive a primary series with eIPV. Refer to the first reference below for further details.

Oral polio vaccine is a live virus and can lead to paralytic polio in nonimmunized adult contacts of those who receive OPV. Further, individuals with immunodeficiency (IgA deficiency, common variable immunodeficiency, acquired immunodeficiency syndrome, and others) *should not* receive OPV.

MEASLES. Because of the recent outbreaks of measles in previously immunized populations, the Immunization Practices Advisory Committee on Measles Prevention has recently changed policy to recommend that every person receive a two-dose vaccination regimen. For adults, it is recommended that, irrespective of any travel plans, every person born after 1956 receive a second dose of measles vaccine. Revised recommendations for children are also available.

For full effect, measles immunization should precede administration of immune serum globulin by at least 2 weeks. As the time interval between measles immunization and administration of immune serum globulin decreases from 4 weeks, measles vaccination efficacy may decrease, and one must consider giving a second dose of measles vaccine 3 months after the last administration of immune serum globulin (or 6 months later if the larger dose of immune serum globulin has been administered). Live measles vaccine, when given as a component of combined measles/rubella or measles/mumps/rubella vaccine should not be given to women known to be pregnant or who are considering becoming pregnant within the subsequent 3 months. Women who are given measles vaccines should not become pregnant for at least 30 days after vaccination. Individuals with severe alterations of immune competence should not be given measles vaccine.

MENINGOCOCCAL MENINGITIS. Outbreaks of meningo-coccal meningitis occur in epidemic form across sub-Saharan Africa. In addition, recent major outbreaks have occurred in Nepal, northern India, and Saudi Arabia and may occur unpredictably across much of Africa and in Brazil. Meningococcal vaccine is available that protects against the A, C, Y, and W-135 capsular strains. Although the risk to casual visitors to endemic areas is extremely small, it is recommended that meningococcal vaccine be given to individuals who will spend more than simple in-transit time in areas with a risk of major outbreaks.

TYPHOID. Avoiding intake of potentially contaminated food and drink is the most effective means of prevention of typhoid infection. The overall risk to American travelers is less than 1 case in 10,000 trips, but travelers to higher-risk countries such as India have about a fourfold increased incidence. For primary immunization, the newly licensed oral live-attenuated Ty21a vaccine is recommended. One capsule is taken every other day for a total of four doses. Concurrent antibiotic use is contraindicated. For booster immunization, either oral vaccine (as for primary immunization) or heat-phenol–inactivated vaccine, 0.5 cc subcutaneously in adults, can be used. Booster is necessary after 5 years following oral immunization or after 3 years when parenteral immunization has been used. The available typhoid vaccines provide approximately 50 to 90 per cent protection.

CHOLERA. This vaccine, because of its short duration of effect and lack of efficacy (approximately 50 per cent protection), as well as the lack of substantial risk of disease for most U.S. travelers, is no longer recommended. Concomitant administration with yellow fever vaccine may result in a reduced vaccine response to yellow fever virus.

MUMPS. This live vaccine should be given to susceptible persons unless there is a contraindication, such as immune defects and pregnancy or possible pregnancy.

JAPANESE ENCEPHALITIS. This mosquito-borne viral encephalitis occurs in epidemics, primarily in late summer and autumn, in the temperate regions and the northern part of tropical zones in Bangladesh, Burma, China, India, Japan, Kampuchea, Korea, Laos, Nepal, Thailand, Vietnam, and the eastern areas of the USSR. There is a lower risk to visitors to endemic areas, which include the tropical zones of southern India, Indonesia, Malaysia, Philippines, Singapore, Sri Lanka, Taiwan, and southern Thailand. Persons who intend to live for prolonged periods of time in an endemic or epidemic area are at greater risk. Because of fear of litigation, the manufacturer of the vaccine no longer makes it available in the United States, but the American Consulate in many cities in China and in various clinics in other capitals in endemic and epidemic areas can administer the Japanese encephalitis vaccine.

HEPATITIS B. This is indicated for travelers to developing countries who may have blood or other significant body fluid exposure. HIV infection risk must, of course, also be considered.

PLAGUE. This vaccine is rarely indicated and should be reserved primarily for travelers to known endemic areas, particularly Vietnam. Individuals who are at extreme risk of developing plague should be given antibiotic chemoprophylaxis with tetracycline, 500 mg 4 times per day during periods of exposure.

RABIES. Rabies occurs commonly in many developing countries, and travelers should be forewarned about the risk associated with even seemingly totally healthy dogs and other animals. Preexposure vaccination with human diploid cell vaccine (HDCV) is recommended for individuals who will be living or visiting for more than 30 days in countries where rabies is a constant threat. In addition, veterinarians, animal handlers, spelunkers, and some laboratory workers should receive rabies vaccine. Chloroquine phosphate may interfere with developing an antibody response to HDCV, but intramuscular injection can overcome this problem.

RUBELLA. Rubella vaccine is recommended for susceptible, unvaccinated adolescents and adults, particularly females. Even though thought to be safe during pregnancy, this vaccine is not recommended for women known to be pregnant or those who may become pregnant within 3 months of vaccination. In addition, individuals with immunodeficiency should not be given this live vaccine.

SMALLPOX. This vaccine is no longer available and should not be administered, since the last human case in nature occurred in 1977.

TYPHUS. This vaccine is not available in the United States and is only very rarely indicated.

MEDICATIONS

MALARIA PROPHYLAXIS. Because of the explosive spread of chloroquine-resistant strains of *Plasmodium falciparum* and the emergence of resistance to alternative drugs in Asia, East and West Africa, and South America, recommendations regarding chemotherapeutic approaches to prevent malaria are changing rapidly.* In rural Thailand, where chloroquine and dihydrofolate reductase inhibitor resistance is ubiquitous, doxycycline, 100 mg per day orally, has given good results. Mefloquine is the recommended agent for most other areas with drug-resistant *P. falciparum*. Unfortunately, significant central nervous system side effects can be associated with mefloquine. The recommended dosage for prophylaxis is 250 mg per week starting 1 week prior to travel and for 4 weeks after departure from the malarious area. With intensive exposure that may include *P. vivax* and *P. ovale*, chloroquine prophylaxis is recommended, followed by primaquine to eliminate liver stage parasites. See Ch. 424 for further details regarding antimalarial prophylaxis and treatment.

TRAVELERS' DIARRHEA PREVENTION. For short-term (less than 5 days) visitors to developing countries, norfloxacin, 400 mg taken once a day, provides considerable protection. Two tablets of bismuth subsalicylate taken four times per day provide similar results.

Treatment of mild diarrhea consists of restricting intake to fluids (Coca-Cola or hot tea with sugar), soups, and toast. Loperamide is recommended as an effective antiperistaltic agent. Norfloxacin, 400 mg orally twice a day for 5 days, is useful in more severe cases. High fever with diarrhea or bloody diarrhea indicates the need for medical consultation. See Ch. 319 for further details regarding possible etiologies and treatment of travel-associated diarrheal diseases.

ANTIBIOTICS FOR INFECTED WOUNDS AND OTHER SKIN INFECTIONS. It is recommended that antibiotic ointment (e.g., bacitracin–polymyxin B) and bandages be taken to treat minor cuts and scrapes. For prolonged treks away from civilization, cephalexin tablets may be recommended for pyogenic infections. Because of the frequency of fungal infections in tropical climates, it is advisable for travelers to take antifungal powder and, in the case of females, vaginal antifungal cream or suppositories.

---

*For up-to-date information on malaria prevention from the Centers for Disease Control, U.S. Public Health Service, telephone (404) 639-1610. For other information, telephone (404) 639-3311 (main switchboard).

Centers for Disease Control, Department of Health and Human Services: Health Information for International Travel. Washington, D.C., U.S. Government Printing Office, 1991. *Excellent concise source of current information on health risks in overseas locations, as well as key information on vaccines and drugs. Obtainable from the Superintendent of Documents, U.S. Government Printing Office, Washington, D.C. 20402, telephone (202) 783-3238. Updated yearly.*

Conrad ME, Lemon SM: Prevention of endemic icteric viral hepatitis by administration of immune serum gamma globulin. J Infect Dis 156:84–91, 1987.

Gong H: Advising patients with pulmonary diseases on air travel. Ann Intern Med 111:349–351, 1989.

Hill DR, Pearson RD: Health advice for international travel. Ann Intern Med 108:829–852, 1988. *Authoritative recent review.*

Johnson TS, Rock PB: Current concepts: Acute mountain sickness. N Engl J Med 319:841–845, 1988.

Steffen R, Rickenbach M, Wihelm U, et al.: Health problems after travel to developing countries. J Infect Dis 156:84–91, 1988. *Most detailed study available providing follow-up data on cohorts of travelers to developing countries.*

---

291 Antimicrobial Therapy

Lowell S. Young

The advent of antimicrobial therapy represented an historic milestone in the cure and control of many infectious diseases. Invariably fatal infections, like bacterial endocarditis, became treatable for the first time. Subsequently, abundant evidence has accumulated that early treatment of localized bacterial infections may obviate further complications. The greatest progress during the modern era of antimicrobial therapy has been in the treatment of acute bacterial infections, although a few chronic diseases such as tuberculosis are usually successfully treated. New developments offer promise in controlling viral diseases and parasitic infections that are a major burden on much of humankind. There have been some modest developments in the antifungal area as well. Nonetheless, the initial enthusiasm that greeted the introduction of new agents with antibacterial activity has been tempered by a more sobering perspective. Antimicrobial agents are not always innocuous to the host, and their widespread usage appears to have fostered increasing drug resistance throughout the world. The growing complexities of antimicrobial therapy appear to be related to the rapid proliferation of agents of several classes, increasing drug resistance, and a greater recognition of interactions between pharmacologic agents.

SOME DEFINITIONS

The terms *antibiotic*, *antimicrobic*, and *chemotherapeutic agent* have often been used interchangeably to designate defined chemical substances that possess activity against specific microorganisms. Indeed, antibiotic was first defined as a substance produced in nature by living microbes that inhibited the growth of other microbial organisms at low concentrations. Viewed in this light, antibiotics seem to be a product of evolution and may confer a selective advantage on the producer in a specific ecosystem. Technically, antibiotics differ from chemotherapeutic agents in that the latter represent the products of chemical synthesis, such as the sulfonamide dyes that were subsequently found to have antibacterial activity. Antibiotics in common use, such as penicillins and aminoglycosides, are derived from natural products but from a functional point of view may be considered interchangeable with chemotherapeutic agents. As the development of new antibacterial agents has proliferated, restrictive technical terms have become outdated. For instance, new penicillins, cephalosporins, and aminoglycosides contain synthetic or semisynthetic modifications of existing structures that confer potent new biologic activity. The term "antimicrobic" has been proposed to describe all substances with antimicrobial activity, whether of natural or synthetic origin, but its acceptance has been variable.

GENERAL PRINCIPLES

The goal of antimicrobial therapy is to kill or inhibit the growth of an infecting pathogen without causing harm to the host. Thus, the basis for such an effect is *selectivity*, whereby the parasite is specifically targeted by virtue of some difference between it and mammalian cells. The first widely used antimicrobial compounds, sulfonamides and penicillins, illustrate this principle very clearly. Sulfonamides are inhibitors of para-aminobenzoic acid, an essential requirement for nucleic acid synthesis in many bacteria but not in humans. Penicillins and related agents that contain a beta-lactam ring act to disrupt the synthesis of peptidoglycan, which gives the bacterial cell wall its shape and strength. Mammalian cells have no cell wall, making penicillin-type drugs the ideal antibacterial agent in terms of selectivity.

Table 291–1 summarizes the mechanism of action of some of the major groups of antibacterial agents. Unfortunately, the selective action of some important compounds on the infecting microbe is not as specific as with penicillin, and important toxic effects on host cells may be encountered. Some drugs like the sulfonamides merely inhibit the growth of organisms and are *bacteriostatic*. When these agents are used, eradication of an infecting agent depends on host defenses such as phagocytic cells and antibodies. Others, like penicillins and the aminoglycosides, inhibit bacteria at relatively low concentration and at higher (but still usually therapeutic) concentrations can kill them; these are *bactericidal* agents. These designations of a bacteriostatic or bactericidal agent may vary, depending on the type of organism: Penicillin G is usually bactericidal for gram-positive cocci but is only static against the enterococcus (*Streptococcus faecalis*), while chloramphenicol is usually bacteriostatic even at very high concentrations but can be bactericidal against *Haemophilus influenzae*. Spectrum refers to range of microorganisms affected by a particular agent, which varies from relatively narrow for low doses of penicillin G to quite broad for large doses of the new cephalosporins. Breadth of spectrum is not necessarily related to mechanism of action.

The interaction between a microbe and therapeutic agent can be complex, and many important variables affect outcome. Intrinsic virulence differs considerably among infecting agents, so that the progression of infection ranges from a very indolent tempo to a fulminating course. Host factors should influence selection of bactericidal versus bacteriostatic agents and the breadth of spectrum of therapy. The site of infection influences dose and duration of treatment. The proliferation of therapeutic choices compels the physician to obtain in-depth knowledge of any agent prescribed. Treatment can be guided by laboratory studies, but therapeutic choices must be based on knowledge of antimicrobial spectrum, mode of action, pharmacology, toxicity, and all major factors that affect drug activity.

IDENTIFICATION OF THE INFECTING AGENT

It is highly desirable to have the infecting agent identified prior to initiation of treatment, but in most circumstances culture confirmation and tests in vitro of antimicrobial susceptibility will not be available for at least a day. Clinical decision making is usually based on a perception of probabilities and on simple tests, the most important of which is the Gram stain. Even the latter

is not necessary in the case of exudative pharyngitis, because the only treatable bacterial causes of the syndrome are hemolytic streptococci and now, rarely, *Corynebacterium diphtheriae*. Other isolates can usually be ignored and therapy with a penicillin initiated. When only a single infecting organism seems likely, therapy with a narrow-spectrum agent is preferable.

In reality, many infectious processes initially begin as mixed infections: The aspiration of secretions into the lung usually results in the deposition of many types of oral microbes that can lead to pneumonia or lung abscess, or the perforation of an abdominal viscus leads to release of millions of aerobic and anaerobic bacteria into the abdominal cavity. What may survive to be cultured in respiratory secretions or from abdominal drainage may well be the hardiest of bacteria, and not necessarily all of those that were associated with initial infectious morbidity. Not all mixed infectious processes require treatment with broad-spectrum agents, but the presence of multiple pathogens might explain clinical failure when a mixed infection is being treated and only one component of that infection is being affected by a particular drug regimen.

Initiation of antibiotic therapy prior to obtaining appropriate cultures is perhaps the leading explanation for the failure to document infecting pathogens. On the other hand, the Gram stain or immunofluorescent staining of secretions can identify the cause of infection after treatment is started. Irrespective of when it is done, the Gram stain can provide valuable semiquantitative information about predominant pathogens and can help the clinician decide whether a subsequent culture result can actually be relied upon. For instance, the validity of a sample of respiratory secretions is greatly enhanced by the detection of phagocytic cells, such as neutrophils or alveolar macrophages. In contrast, the presence of squamous epithelial cells should be the basis for rejecting the validity of expectorated sputum, since they reflect oropharyngeal contamination. With regard to quantitative evaluation of a potentially infected body fluid, isolation of greater than 10^5 organisms per milliliter has been accepted as establishing the validity of a urine culture result. However, microscopic examination of uncentrifuged urine may still yield an approximate idea of the degree of infection (any organism seen corresponds with 10^5 bacteria per milliliter), as well as the nature of the infection that is taking place in the urinary tract. Isolation of organisms in pure culture from blood or normally sterile body fluids (like spinal fluid) is an unambiguous laboratory result that establishes an infectious etiology. Occasionally, some bloodstream infections are polymicrobial. Some blood culture isolates may be rejected as contaminants. The latter are usually skin flora like corynebacteria or coagulase-negative staphylococci. However, repeated isolation of such organisms from blood culture in association with signs of infection calls for careful clinical assessment. Coagulase-negative staphylococci and corynebacteria can be valid pathogens in immunosuppressed subjects and patients with prosthetic devices.

TABLE 291–1. MECHANISM OF ACTION OF ANTIMICROBIAL AGENTS

Agent	Site of Action	Effect	Cidal	Static
Penicillins, cephalosporins	Cell wall	Inhibit crosslinking of peptidoglycan, resulting in spheroplast formation	+	Occasionally
Vancomycin	Cell wall	Block transfer of pentapeptide from cytoplasm to cell membrane	+	Occasionally
Polymyxin B, colistin	Cytoplasmic membrane	Bind phospholipid and disrupt membrane	+	
Aminoglycosides	Ribosome	Bind to 30S ribosomal subunit, thereby inhibiting attachment of messenger RNA; also affect transfer RNA	+	
Tetracyclines	Ribosome	Bind to 30S subunit and inhibit binding of transfer RNA		+
Chloramphenicol	Ribosome	Bind to 50S subunit and inhibit messenger RNA translation	Occasionally	+
Erythromycin, clindamycin	Ribosome	Inhibit messenger RNA translation	Occasionally	+
Rifampin	Nucleic acid synthesis	Impaired RNA formation by inhibiting DNA-dependent RNA polymerase	+	Occasionally
Metronidazole	Nucleic acid synthesis	Damages nucleic acid structure	+	
Quinolones	Nucleic acid synthesis	Inhibit DNA gyrase	+	
Sulfonamides	Nucleic acid synthesis	Competes with para-aminobenzoic acid, thereby blocking formation of thymidine and purines		+

SUSCEPTIBILITY, RESISTANCE, AND ANTIBACTERIAL SPECTRA

Appropriate antimicrobial therapy is based on the results of laboratory tests and validated by the clinical effect of treatment. Test results and treatment are not always consistent: Patients who have excellent or intact host defenses may recover from infection irrespective of whether the antibiotic they receive has an effect on the infecting agent. Nevertheless, in a serious deep-seated or bloodstream infection, laboratory tests do provide an invaluable guide to the selection or adjustment of therapy. Usually a microbe is considered susceptible to an antibacterial agent if it can be inhibited or killed by a concentration of the drug that is realistically achievable at the site of the infection. The levels of drug that must be achieved in the host vary, depending on the site of infection, and could be limited by toxic side effects. A common practice is to set the range of susceptibility at or above realistically achievable blood levels, but there are some notable exceptions. For instance, some agents like nalidixic acid or nitrofurantoin are rapidly excreted in the urine, and only very low blood levels are achieved. Low doses of drugs that are effective for some infections are totally inadequate for deep-seated infections. The best example is the relatively low dose of benzyl penicillin G that is required to cure pneumococcal pneumonia, sometimes less than 100,000 units of penicillin per day, which contrasts with the dose of approximately 20 million units per day that may be necessary to treat pneumococcal endocarditis or meningitis. With aminoglycosides the levels for effective therapy of bloodstream infections have been projected to be in the range of 4 to 6 μg per milliliter of gentamicin or tobramycin, and such concentrations are usually accepted as the upper boundary for susceptibility in vitro. However, it is clear that the peak levels of aminoglycosides like gentamicin and tobramycin are sustained for less than an hour. Nonetheless, that period seems sufficient to achieve rapid killing of many bacterial strains.

Many methods have been introduced to determine the susceptibility of bacteria to antimicrobials in vitro. They have been best standardized for rapidly growing organisms. The most common involve measuring inhibition of growth in a broth medium or around an antibiotic-impregnated disc placed on the surface of agar containing the test strain (disc diffusion test). By varying drug concentrations in a series of test tubes or wells, the broth dilution test yields quantitative data on the drug concentration required to inhibit the organism, the minimum inhibitory concentration, or MIC (usually expressed in micrograms per milliliter). Subcultures of broth media make it possible to determine the concentration of drug that kills the test strain—the minimum bactericidal concentration, or MBC. In the disc diffusion test, only growth inhibition can be determined, but the diameter of the zone of inhibition usually correlates inversely with the MIC. The two methods give generally similar results (with the disc test being perhaps somewhat easier to perform), and for most infections susceptibility results based on inhibitory measurements are satisfactory. In treating endocarditis, meningitis, and septicemias occurring in immunocompromised hosts, MBC data on infecting isolates are desirable. Bactericidal activity appears to be a requisite for cure of enterococcal endocarditis, as penicillin G or ampicillin inhibits but does not kill this group of organisms. The phenomenon of "tolerance" has also been observed: a wide discrepancy, 32-fold or more, between MIC and MBC. Some investigators believe that strains of staphylococci isolated from patients with endocarditis or osteomyelitis that prove to be tolerant to penicillins or vancomycin should be treated with the addition of gentamicin or rifampin, but this policy remains controversial.

Table 291–2 summarizes the susceptibilities of clinically important gram-positive and gram-negative bacteria in vitro and indicates agents of choice and alternative therapies. The darkened squares (resistant or not indicated) may include drug-pathogen combinations for which clinical evidence fails to support an effect in vitro. Susceptibility testing in vitro is needed because no one agent is predictably effective against all categories of bacteria and because of the increasing incidence and changes in patterns of resistance. There are a few exceptions to this dogma, such as the uniform susceptibility of group A streptococci to penicillin. On the other hand, relative resistance (intermediate susceptibility) of pneumococci to penicillin G may be increasing, and it is advisable to test blood and cerebrospinal fluid (CSF) isolates.

Antimicrobial resistance may be absolute, in which case increasing the concentration of the agent has no effect, and relative, in which case it may be overcome by dose augmentation. The basis and mechanisms of resistance have become complex, and the simplest approach is to consider (a) the genetic basis for resistance and (b) the actual mechanisms involved. Chromosomal alterations or mutations were the first basis for resistance recognized. These occurred at a relatively predictable rate. Subsequently, a much more common genetic basis has emerged: Plasmids or extrachromosomal DNA elements include R-factors or genetic elements that encode for synthesis of enzymes that functionally inactivate or modify antibiotics. The rapid spread of resistance in some hospital and community settings has been related to acquisition of plasmids by the process of conjugation among gram-negative bacilli and transduction by phages among gram-positive cocci. The mechanisms of resistance are summarized in Table 291–3. The most familiar are the beta-lactamases that hydrolyze to varying degrees agents possessing the beta-lactam ring (penicillins, cephalosporins, monobactams). A great variety of these have been described, occurring in both cocci and bacilli and having both a constitutive and an inducible nature. The latter poses real problems in laboratory diagnosis, as organisms that are initially thought to be susceptible (like *Enterobacter* species) may harbor inducible enzymes. Beta-lactamases may be of either chromosomal or plasmid origin and are usually responsible for high-level resistance that cannot be overcome by dosage escalation. Inactivation can destroy the usefulness of drugs outside the beta-lactam class. A growing number of R-factor–encoded enzymes have been identified that can modify aminoglycosides by the addition of an adenyl, acetyl, or phosphorylating group to hydroxyl or amino groups on the drug structure. These additions create a sterically altered molecule with ablated or reduced antibacterial activity. Conversely, the design of innovative new antimicrobial agents that prove invulnerable to inactivating enzymes involves further modifications of antibiotic structures that can block the access of inactivating enzymes to target sites. In this sense, the development of new aminoglycosides is analogous to the substitutions that protect the beta-lactam ring from hydrolysis and yield the antistaphylococcal penicillins.

One of the most worrisome mechanisms of resistance involves the ability of bacteria to exclude antimicrobial agents from the cell. Aminoglycosides are actively transported into bacteria, but high-level, multiresistant strains seem to be impermeable to all aminoglycosides. These appear to arise from chromosomal mutation and are selected by aminoglycoside use. The active transport system for aminoglycosides is oxygen dependent. This probably explains the lack of effect of aminoglycosides on anaerobic bacteria, since anaerobic conditions impair the activation of the transport system.

Another type of enzymatic resistance is illustrated by organisms that have acquired a plasmid-encoded "bypass" enzyme that subverts the metabolic block of the sulfonamides.

To have an effect, antibiotics that resist hydrolysis or modification must enter the bacterial cell and reach their target site. Target site alteration explains sudden high-level streptomycin resistance (30S ribosomal subunit) or erythromycin resistance (50S ribosomal subunit). The basis for these changes appears to be chromosomal mutations. A similar basis is postulated for alterations in penicillin-binding proteins, which can result in both low- and high-level resistance.

The indiscriminate use of antimicrobial agents generally favors the emergence of resistance. Antibiotics are not mutagens and do not "create" resistant bacteria. Rather, usage selects for strains that are resistant by virtue of chromosomal mutations or spread of plasmids among the bacterial population. Emergence of resistance during treatment is common with some gram-negative rods such as *Serratia* and *Pseudomonas*. This phenomenon must be distinguished from superinfection, in which a new and usually resistant pathogen becomes a secondary invader. Superinfection may be a consequence of prolonged high-dose therapy and may be avoided by use of narrow-spectrum agents in doses that are not excessive.

PHARMACOLOGIC FACTORS

Laboratory conditions for testing antibacterial agents may differ strikingly from conditions in vivo. In clinical situations the rates of growth of bacteria may be slow, thus affecting the rapidity with which cell wall–active drugs can work. More important, blood and tissue concentrations fluctuate with frequency and method of dosing, and the concentration of drug at the active site of infection may differ from that in body fluids that are more easily sampled. The distribution of agents even within the same class can vary considerably, as they may be metabolized, inactivated, and eliminated by different pathways. Such factors have a crucial effect on the size of doses, the interval between dosing, and possible drug toxicity. Also, the properties of the infecting agent may affect dosing. After exposure of bacteria to an antibiotic, a certain proportion of the population is killed or inhibited, and there may be a significant lag time before multiplication of bacteria resumes after the drug concentration falls. This time interval for regrowth has been called the "postantibiotic effect." For different organisms and with different antibiotics, there may be varying postantibiotic effects. Thus, intermittent dosing of agents may be quite feasible if there is rapid killing and a long postantibiotic effect. Some of the more recalcitrant organisms like *Pseudomonas* regrow rapidly after exposure to antipseudomonal penicillins, and there is very little postantibiotic effect. This argues for more frequent or even continuous dosing, but for the great majority of clinical situations the latter has proved impractical, and the clinical superiority of continuous dosing has not been established.

Table 291–4 summarizes the recommended doses and some pharmacologic data on most of the commonly used agents. Tissue penetration is linked to serum protein binding. The quantity of drug that diffuses into a site of infection is related to the "peak" or maximum serum concentration of free or unbound drug and the duration that the maximum level is maintained. On the other hand, therapeutic outcome does not always correlate with protein-binding affinity, probably because protein binding is usually easily reversible. Lipid solubility of an antibiotic is another factor affecting tissue penetration and influences the ability of an agent

TABLE 291–2. SUSCEPTIBILITIES OF CERTAIN BACTERIA TO SELECTED ANTIBIOTICS

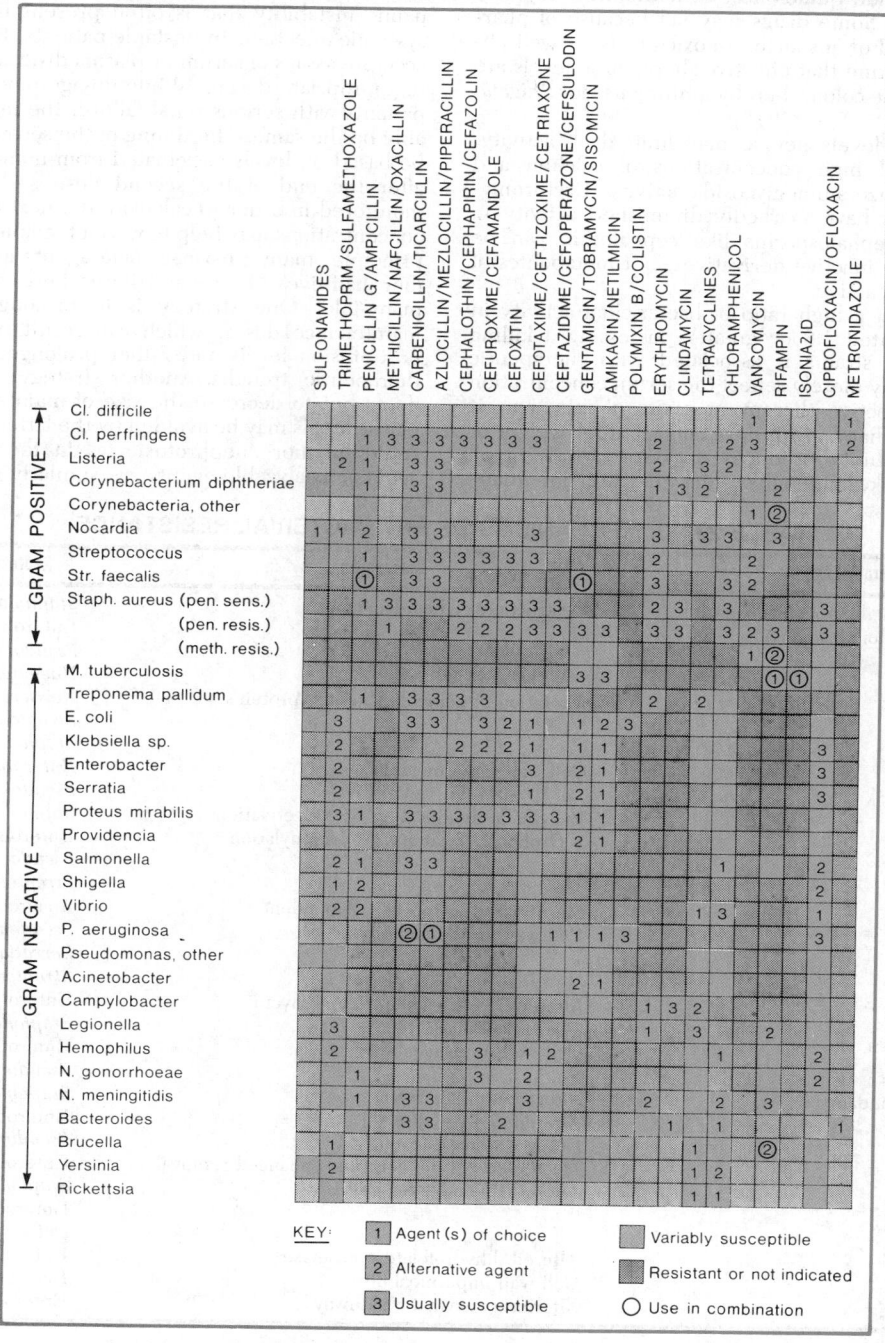

	SULFONAMIDES	TRIMETHOPRIM/SULFAMETHOXAZOLE	PENICILLIN G/AMPICILLIN	METHICILLIN/NAFCILLIN/OXACILLIN	CARBENICILLIN/TICARCILLIN	AZLOCILLIN/MEZLOCILLIN/PIPERACILLIN	CEPHALOTHIN/CEPHAPIRIN/CEFAZOLIN	CEFUROXIME/CEFAMANDOLE	CEFOXITIN	CEFOTAXIME/CEFTIZOXIME/CETRIAXONE	CEFTAZIDIME/CEFOPERAZONE/CEFSULODIN	GENTAMICIN/TOBRAMYCIN/SISOMICIN	AMIKACIN/NETILMICIN	POLYMIXIN B/COLISTIN	ERYTHROMYCIN	CLINDAMYCIN	TETRACYCLINES	CHLORAMPHENICOL	VANCOMYCIN	RIFAMPIN	ISONIAZID	CIPROFLOXACIN/OFLOXACIN	METRONIDAZOLE
Cl. difficile																			1				1
Cl. perfringens			1	3	3	3	3	3	3	3						2		2	3				2
Listeria		2	1	3	3										2		3	2					
Corynebacterium diphtheriae			1	3	3										1	3	2			2			
Corynebacteria, other																			1	②			
Nocardia	1	1	2	3	3					3			3				3	3		3			
Streptococcus			1	3	3	3	3	3	3						2				2				
Str. faecalis			①	3	3						①				3			3	2				
Staph. aureus (pen. sens.)			1	3	3	3	3	3	3	3	3				2	3		3				3	
(pen. resis.)				1			2	2	2	3	3	3	3		3	3		3	2	3		3	
(meth. resis.)																			1	②			
M. tuberculosis												3	3							①	①		
Treponema pallidum			1	3	3	3									2		2						
E. coli		3			3	3		3	2	1		1	2	3									
Klebsiella sp.		2				2	2	2		1		1	1									3	
Enterobacter		2								3		2	1									3	
Serratia		2								1		2	1									3	
Proteus mirabilis		3	1		3	3	3	3	3	3		1	1										
Providencia												2	1										
Salmonella		2	1	3	3													1				2	
Shigella	1	2																1				2	
Vibrio	2	2															1	3				1	
P. aeruginosa					②	①					1	1	1	3								3	
Pseudomonas, other																							
Acinetobacter												2	1										
Campylobacter															1		3	2					
Legionella		3													1	3				2			
Hemophilus		2						3		1	2							1				2	
N. gonorrhoeae			1						3	2												2	
N. meningitidis			1	3	3					3					2			2		3			
Bacteroides				3	3											1	1	1					1
Brucella		1															1			②			
Yersinia		2															1	2				1	
Rickettsia																	1	1					

KEY:
- 1 Agent(s) of choice
- 2 Alternative agent
- 3 Usually susceptible
- Variably susceptible
- Resistant or not indicated
- ○ Use in combination

(GRAM POSITIVE: Cl. difficile through M. tuberculosis; GRAM NEGATIVE: Treponema pallidum through Rickettsia)

to pass through membranes by nonionic diffusion. Penetration of drug into the spinal fluid is related not only to the drug itself but also to the degree of inflammation in the meninges. Lipid-soluble agents such as chloramphenicol, isoniazid, rifampin, sulfonamides, and metronidazole penetrate spinal fluid well. Aminoglycosides, amphotericin B, and polymyxins do not penetrate well even in the face of inflammation. Penicillins and vancomycin generally penetrate CSF when inflammation is present. Most antibiotics commonly used are excreted primarily through the kidney, but notable exceptions include erythromycin and chloramphenicol. Thus, it may be possible to treat infections of the urinary tract with doses smaller than are required for serious systemic disease, because high urine levels are achieved with most agents. Urine and bile regularly contain higher concentrations of antibiotics than does serum. Penicillins and tetracyclines are concentrated in bile, but aminoglycosides enter bile less well, particularly when liver disease or obstruction is present. Drugs like tetracyclines and clindamycin diffuse readily into bone and have been used successfully in osteomyelitis. Agents that enter prostate tissue well include quinolones, trimethoprim, erythromycin, and doxycycline. Some drugs may fail because of pharmacokinetic properties. For instance, amoxicillin is so well absorbed in the small intestine that effective therapeutic levels are usually not achieved in the colon, thereby limiting use for *Shigella* infections.

Factors besides drug levels per se may limit drug activity. Purulent secretions and high concentrations of calcium and magnesium ions antagonize aminoglycoside activity. Erythromycin and aminoglycosides have markedly diminished activity in acidic environments. Cephalosporins like cephalothin can be metabolized to relatively inactive derivatives, but metabolites of cefotaxime are still quite active.

There is evidence that a high ratio of bactericidal activity in serum (e.g., serum diluted 1:8 or greater possessing a killing effect) against infecting strains is associated with therapeutic success. Such activity may merely reflect the serum concentration required to achieve effective therapy at a site of infection. It should not be assumed that a given dose corrected for weight or body surface area reliability produces the same levels in all patients. With agents like aminoglycosides that are potentially

toxic, therapeutic monitoring is clearly indicated during serious systemic infection. For example, gentamicin peak (postinfusion) levels should exceed 4 μg per milliliter, and trough (or "valley") levels should be less than 2 μg per milliliter. Route of administration is important, since orally administered drugs may be poorly absorbed in serious systemic infections. For patients who are in shock, intramuscular or subcutaneous injections should clearly be avoided, and all medications should be given intravenously.

MODIFICATION OF DRUG DOSES IN RENAL AND HEPATIC FAILURE

Since the majority of antibiotics are excreted via the kidney, dosage adjustment must be considered in moderate to severe renal failure. Many studies have related serum creatinine level or creatinine clearance to degree of dosage modification, and useful nomograms have been derived that may aid in the calculation of dosage. Table 291–4 indicates the agents affected by renal failure and dialysis. Many of these guidelines have been derived by study of patients who are in the "steady state," i.e., patients in renal failure who are on dialysis programs but who may not be infected. Thus, they may not manifest the hemodynamic instability that is often present in patients with serious systemic infection. In unstable patients, there is no substitute for accurate assays of serum or plasma drug concentrations as a guide to appropriate dosing. While dosage modification is indicated in patients with serious renal failure, the initial doses should probably be the same. The timing of the second dose should probably be based on levels anticipated from nomograms, but peak levels after the end of the second dose and third dose should be monitored in order to calculate the next doses. Increased trough concentrations may help to warn of incipient toxicity. As a general principle, many pharmacologic agents are given every three to four half-lives. In renal failure these half-lives are prolonged many-fold. One strategy is to prolong the interval between maintenance doses, which can result in fairly high "peak" or postinfusion levels and rather prolonged (and occasionally subtherapeutic) troughs. Another strategy is to give more frequent doses but to decrease the size of maintenance doses. Subtherapeutic levels may be avoided by the latter tactic, but the approach could be more nephrotoxic (as in the case of aminoglycoside agents). Dialyzable agents are similarly cleared by peritoneal or

TABLE 291–3. MECHANISMS OF ANTIBACTERIAL RESISTANCE

Antimicrobial Agent	Mechanisms	Representative Organisms
Beta-lactams (penicillins, cephalosporins, carbapenems, monobactams)	Destruction by beta-lactamase	*Staphylococcus aureus* Enterobacteriaceae *Pseudomonas aeruginosa* *Haemophilus influenzae*
	Alteration of penicillin-binding proteins	*Neisseria gonorrhoeae* *Streptococcus pneumoniae* *Staphylococcus aureus*
	Cell wall impermeability	*Enterobacter* species *Pseudomonas aeruginosa*
Aminoglycosides	Enzymatic modification by *N*-acetylation, *O*-phosphorylation, or *N*-adenylation	*Staphylococcus aureus* Enterobacteriaceae *Pseudomonas aeruginosa* *Streptococcus faecalis*
	Membrane transport O₂ dependent Cell wall impermeability	Anaerobes *Pseudomonas aeruginosa* *Serratia* species *Streptococcus faecalis*
	Altered 30S ribosome (streptomycin)	Enterobacteriaceae
Chloramphenicol	*O*-acetylation Cell wall impermeability	*Staphylococcus aureus* Enterobacteriaceae *Pseudomonas aeruginosa*
Erythromycin, clindamycin	Alteration of 23S RNA	*Staphylococcus aureus*
Quinolones	Altered DNA gyrase Cell wall impermeability	Enterobacteriaceae *Pseudomonas aeruginosa*
Tetracyclines	Decreased permeation plus enhanced removal	Enterobacteriaceae
Sulfonamides	Altered thymidylate synthetase	*Staphylococcus aureus* Enterobacteriaceae *Neisseria gonorrhoeae*
Trimethoprim	Altered dihydrofolate synthetase Cell wall impermeability Alternate enzymatic pathway	Enterobacteriaceae *Pseudomonas aeruginosa* Enterococci

TABLE 291–4. DOSAGE, PHARMACOLOGIC FACTORS, AND ADJUSTMENT IN RENAL AND HEPATIC FAILURE

Class/Agent	Dose Systemic Infection	Oral	Protein Binding (%)	Normal Serum Half-Life (hr)	Dose Adjustment Hepatic Failure	Dose Adjustment Renal Failure	Serum Levels Affected by Dialysis
Aminoglycosides							
Amikacin	5–7 mg/kg/q8	—	0	2–3	No	Major	Yes
Gentamicin	1.7 mg/kg/q8	—	0	2–3	No	Major	Yes
Netilmicin	1.7 mg/kg/q8	—	0	2–3	No	Major	Yes
Tobramycin	1.7 mg/kg/q8	—	0	2–3	No	Major	Yes
Antifungal Agents							
Amphotericin B	0.7–1 mg/kg/d	—	90	24	No	No	No
Flucytosine	40 mg/kg/q6	Yes	10	3	No	Major	Yes
Ketoconazole	6 mg/kg/d	Yes	98	8	Avoid	No	No
Miconazole	5 mg/kg/q6–8	—	92	2.2	Avoid	No	No
Antituberculous Agents							
Ethambutol	15 mg/kg/d	Yes	10	1.5	No	Major	Yes
Isoniazid	5 mg/kg/d	Yes	10	3	Yes	Minor	Yes
Rifampin	10 mg/kg/d	Yes	70	3	Yes	Minor	No
Cephalosporins							
Cefaclor	7 mg/kg/q6	Yes	20	1	No	Yes	Yes
Cefamandole	30 mg/kg/q6	—	70	1	No	Yes	Yes
Cefazolin	15 mg/kg/q6	—	80	2	No	Major	Yes
Cefotetan	30 mg/kg/q12	—	85	3	No	Major	Yes
Cefoxitin	30 mg/kg/q6	—	70	0.7	No	Yes	Yes
Cephalothin	30 mg/kg/q6	—	70	0.7	Minor	Yes	Yes
Cephalexin	7 mg/kg/q6	Yes	15	1	No	Yes	Yes
Cefoperazone	30 mg/kg/q8–12	—	90	2	Some	Minor	Yes
Cefotaxime	30 mg/kg/q6	—	50	1.2	Some	Minor	Yes
Cefsulodin†	30 mg/kg/q6–8	—	20	1.6	No	Major	Yes
Ceftizoxime	30 mg/kg/q6–8	—	50	1.3	No	Minor	Yes
Ceftriaxone	30 mg/kg/q12–24	—	90	8	No	Yes	Yes
Ceftazidime	30 mg/kg/q8	—	60	2	No	Major	Yes
Moxalactam	30 mg/kg/q8–12	—	50	2	No	Major	Yes
Penicillins							
Amoxicillin	7 mg/kg/q6	Yes	20	1	No	Yes	Yes
Ampicillin	30 mg/kg/q6	Yes	20	1	No	Yes	Yes
Azlocillin	50 mg/kg/q6	—	50	1	Minor	Major	Yes
Carbenicillin	70 mg/kg/q4	—	50	1	Minor	Major	Yes
Cloxacillin	7 mg/kg/q6	Yes	95	0.5	Minor	Minor	Yes
Dicloxacillin	7 mg/kg/q6	Yes	97	0.5	Minor	Minor	No
Methicillin	30 mg/kg/q4–6	—	30	0.5	No	Minor	No
Mezlocillin	50 mg/kg/q6	—	50	1	No	Major	Yes
Nafcillin	30 mg/kg/q4–6	—	90	0.5	Yes	Minor	No
Oxacillin	30 mg/kg/q4–6	—	90	0.5	Yes	Minor	Yes
Penicillin G	0.3–4 million U q4–6	Yes	60	0.5	No	Yes	Yes
Penicillin V	7 mg/kg/q6	Yes	80	1	No	Minor	Yes
Piperacillin	40 mg/kg/q6	—	50	1	Minor	Major	Yes
Ticarcillin	40 mg/kg/q4–6	—	50	1	Minor	Major	Yes
Quinolones							
Ciprofloxacin	10 mg/kg/q12	Yes	30	3	No	Major	Yes
Nalidixic acid	15 mg/kg/q6	Yes	90	1.5	No	Avoid	No
Norfloxacin	6 mg/kg/q12	Yes	15	3	No	Major	Yes
Tetracyclines							
Chlortetracycline	7 mg/kg/q6	Yes	50	5	Avoid	Avoid	No
Demeclocycline	7 mg/kg/q12	Yes	50	10	Avoid	Avoid	Yes
Doxycycline	1.5 mg/kg/q12–24	Yes	90	15–20	No	No	No
Minocycline	3 mg/kg/q12–24	Yes	90	15	Avoid	Avoid	No
Oxytetracycline	7 mg/kg/q6–12	Yes	35	8	Avoid	Avoid	No
Tetracycline HCL	7 mg/kg/q6	Yes	50	7	Avoid	Avoid	No
Sulfonamides							
Sulfadiazine	15 mg/kg/q6	Yes	50	3	Avoid	Major	Yes
Sulfamethoxazole	12 mg/kg/q8	Yes	50	6	Avoid	Major	Yes
Trimethoprim (used with above)	2.3 mg/kg/q8–12	Yes	60	10	No	Major	Yes
Sulfisoxazole	15 mg/kg/q6	Yes	50	6	Avoid	Major	Yes
Other Agents							
Aztreonam	30 mg/kg/q8	—	60	2.0	No	Major	Yes
Chloramphenicol	7–15 mg/kg/q6	Yes	30	1.5	Some	Minor	Yes
Clindamycin	7 mg/kg/q6	Yes	90	2.5	Some	Minor	No
Colistin	2 mg/kg/q12	—	0	5	No	Avoid	No
Erythromycin	7 mg/kg/q6	Yes	20	1.5	Some	No	No
Imipenem	7.5 mg/kg/q6	—	15	1	No	Avoid	Yes
Metronidazole	15 mg/kg/q6	Yes	20	8	No	No	Yes
Nitrofurantoin	1 mg/kg/q6	Yes	60	0.3	No	Avoid	No
Polymyxin B	1.5 U/kg/q12	—	0	5	No	Avoid	No
Spectinomycin	30 mg/kg	—	0	2	No	Avoid	No
Vancomycin	7 mg/kg/q6	Yes*	10	6	No	No	No

*Not systemically absorbed.
†Not available in the United States.

extracorporeal hemodialysis. Following dialysis, a dose approximately two thirds to three quarters of a maintenance dose should be given, depending upon the degree of removal of the antibiotic by dialysis and the timing of the previous maintenance dose.

Several important antibiotics are metabolized in the liver and are partially excreted in the bile. Agents primarily metabolized by the liver include the sulfonamides, chloramphenicol, and tetracycline. There is usually little reason to alter the dose of penicillin, cephalosporins, and aminoglycosides in patients with liver disease. Even with erythromycin, ethambutol, and clindamycin, there is little evidence that dosage reduction is necessary except in severe hepatic failure. For instance, clindamycin should probably be reduced to half-normal doses after 2 to 3 days of treatment. Chloramphenicol total dosage should be restricted to 1.5 to 2.0 grams per day (adult), and erythromycin should be reduced to perhaps one-half the normal dose after 2 to 3 days of treatment. Drugs to be avoided in hepatic failure include sulfonamides and tetracyclines.

COMBINATION ANTIMICROBIAL THERAPY

Use of combinations of antibacterial agents is exceedingly common. The rationale for their use may be summarized as follows: (1) Prior to the identification of pathogens infecting critically ill subjects, combinations offer a broader, more comprehensive antibacterial spectrum than does a single agent. (2) Use of a drug combination may eradicate an infection that cannot be cured by a single agent, such as the effect of penicillin on enterococci. Addition of an aminoglycoside or a potentiating agent such as rifampin may result in bactericidal activity at a deep-seated focus of infection, as in endocarditis. (3) Combinations are indicated in the treatment of mixed infections, since not all of the pathogens may be susceptible to a single agent. (4) Combinations may decrease the opportunity for emergence of resistance. This has been best documented in tuberculosis. (5) Combinations may interact additively or synergistically against infecting organisms. As a result, there may be an enhancement of antibacterial activity and/or enhanced rate of killing. The latter may lead to more rapid clearing of infection with reduction in duration of therapy. Combinations may permit the use of a lower dosage of one or more components of the regimen, particularly the more toxic component, thereby avoiding undesirable side effects. More rapid killing or greater potency in vivo may be more directly beneficial in patients with impaired host defenses. Some clinical studies suggest an improved clinical response not only when drugs used to treat endocarditis interact synergistically but also in sepsis occurring in immunocompromised patients.

The converse of synergism is antagonism between antimicrobial agents. This is best described for combinations of bactericidal plus bacteriostatic agents. Penicillin-type drugs require cell growth to exert their lethal effect. When penicillins are combined with static drugs like tetracycline, only growth inhibition may result. Clinical studies in humans indicate poorer results in treatment of pneumococcal meningitis with penicillin plus tetracycline than with penicillin alone.

Empiric therapy is presumptive or "blind" therapy given when the clinical severity of a likely infection dictates that treatment be started. It is not necessarily combination therapy, as some single agents can still be quite effective. Intelligent choices in the absence of microbiologic information can be made based on the clinical syndrome and the likely infecting pathogen. Epidemiologic factors as well as host factors enter into the decision. The setting in which the patient develops infection or a prior exposure or travel history can be of considerable value. Pneumonias contracted outside the hospital are usually due to streptococci (and pneumococci) and penicillin-sensitive anaerobes. An "atypical" or diffuse pattern raises the likelihood that community-acquired pneumonia will be better treated with erythromycin than penicillin. Infections that occur in the nosocomial setting or in markedly neutropenic patients should always be initially treated with therapy directed against gram-negative bacilli.

Table 291-5 summarizes recommendations for initial empiric therapy by clinical syndrome.

SPECIFIC ANTIMICROBIAL AGENTS

Table 291-2 summarizes recommended choices of antimicrobial agents for specific infecting agents. The organisms are divided into gram-positive and gram-negative isolates, and antimicrobial agents that are similar are grouped together. Clearly, such a table oversimplifies the appropriate choices for various agents. In some situations, there is no clear-cut agent of first choice, and any member of a class may be appropriate. Differences in pharmacology, cost, and side effects might lead to a selection of one agent in preference to another. There is an increasing divergence in antibacterial spectrum among the newer beta-lactam agents, such as the antipseudomonal penicillins and the third-generation cephalosporins. Among the aminoglycosides, anticipated efficacy may be expressed as follows: While gentamicin and tobramycin remain the most widely prescribed, gram-negative bacilli that are resistant to these agents are more likely to be inhibited by netilmicin and amikacin.

Few oral agents are listed in Table 291-2, but it may be inferred that any of the oral antistaphylococcal agents, such as cloxacillin or dicloxacillin, could be used to treat mild infections due to penicillinase-producing staphylococci. The spectrum of oral cephalosporins such as cephalexin or cephradine mimics that of cephalothin or cefazolin. In the case of group A hemolytic streptococci, it would not be necessary to test for susceptibility of these organisms against penicillin G and related penicillins in vitro, since all would be expected to be susceptible. It would, however, be highly desirable if one were to use a penicillin against the Klebsiella species to test that penicillin for susceptibility in vitro; it should probably not be presumed that antibiotics such as piperacillin or mezlocillin will be effective in vitro and in vivo without specific testing. Some agents should always be used in combination to treat serious bloodstream or systemic infections, such as antituberculous therapy (isoniazid plus at least one other agent) or enterococcal sepsis with or without endocarditis (the combination of either a penicillin or a vancomycin with an aminoglycoside). Older agents of the aminoglycoside class, such as streptomycin or kanamycin, are no longer widely used because their activity is more comprehensively covered by newer drugs (gentamicin and amikacin). The exception to this might be in the conventional treatment of disease caused by Mycobacterium tuberculosis, for which streptomycin is still indicated.

Sulfonamides and Sulfa-Containing Combinations

Sulfonamides were the first chemotherapeutic agents to be introduced into wide clinical use. They are bacteriostatic and previously were quite active against many gram-positive and gram-negative organisms. They are, however, no longer among the first choices for serious systemic infections, the exception being Nocardia asteroides infections. Sulfonamides remain effective therapy for coliform organisms causing community-acquired urinary tract infections, but they are unreliable against hospital-acquired microorganisms. More commonly used to treat a wide variety of more serious bacterial infections is the fixed combination (1:5) of trimethoprim and sulfamethoxazole. Synergism in vitro against many enteric bacteria can be demonstrated with this combination, yet trimethoprim is a highly active agent itself. A major argument in favor of continued use of the fixed combination is that it may reduce the likelihood of the development of resistance to one component in the pair. Trimethoprim-sulfamethoxazole is usually active against enteric bacteria and H. influenzae (including most penicillinase-producing strains), and it has been effective against Pneumocystis carinii. The diffusion of trimethoprim into prostate fluid makes it a useful agent in prostatic infections. Central nervous system penetration is good. The oral preparation is well absorbed, although a parenteral form is available for patients in whom gastrointestinal absorption may be erratic. Occasional side effects include neutropenia and all of the dermal and systemic hypersensitivity reactions that have been well associated with sulfonamides.

Penicillin G and Related Agents

The primary spectrum of penicillin G (benzyl penicillin) is gram positive, with such organisms as Streptococcus pyogenes, Streptococcus pneumoniae, and Streptococcus viridans remaining exquisitely susceptible. Procaine penicillin is readily administered intramuscularly, and because of slow absorption, dosing of 600,000 units every 12 hours remains effective therapy for pneumococcal pneumonia. Benzathine penicillin is a long-acting (2 to 3 weeks) agent that is slowly released after intramuscular injection and provides therapeutic levels for streptococcal pharyngitis and some forms of syphilis and prophylactic effect against acute rheumatic fever. For oral use in mild respiratory infections, phenoxymethyl penicillin (V) is acid stable and preferable to penicillin G. In large doses penicillin G is still effective against *Neisseria meningitidis*, most *N. gonorrhoeae,* and anaerobic organisms, including *Clostridium* species, but usually not against strains of *Bacteroides fragilis*. Against enterococci, penicillin G or ampicillin should be used in combination with an aminoglycoside such as streptomycin or gentamicin. Ampicillin may be effective in the treatment of *Salmonella* infections, central nervous system infections due to *Haemophilus* strains, and *Listeria monocytogenes* infections. When used in large doses, penicillin G or ampicillin is effective against a few gram-negative organisms, most notably *Proteus mirabilis* (but not other *Proteus* species). Penicillin G and related penicillins should not be used against the great majority of coagulase-producing staphylococci, most of which now produce beta-lactamases.

Antistaphylococcal Penicillins

The antistaphylococcal penicillins are beta-lactamase–stable and relatively narrow in spectrum. Parenteral preparations include methicillin, nafcillin, and oxacillin. There is little choice among this category of agents in terms of antistaphylococcal activity. There may be some differences in side effects, with methicillin possibly associated with more hypersensitivity nephritis and oxacillin with a greater incidence of abnormal serum elevations of hepatic enzymes. When used in appropriate doses, the central nervous system penetration is probably adequate to treat meningitis. The oral antistaphylococcal agents should not be used to treat serious infections, but mild or moderately severe infections may respond to dicloxacillin or cloxacillin. Combination of antistaphylococcal penicillins with an aminoglycoside or rifampin has been recommended for refractory staphylococcal infections or when the isolates demonstrate tolerance. Coagulase-negative staphylococci may produce beta-lactamase like most coagulase-positive *Staphylococcus aureus* organisms. However, serious infections like prosthetic valve endocarditis are better treated with vancomycin plus rifampin or vancomycin plus an aminoglycoside.

Broad-Spectrum Penicillins and Related Compounds

Although ampicillin and amoxicillin are technically classified as broad-spectrum penicillins, the extended spectrum really only includes *Escherichia coli, H. influenzae, Salmonella,* and *Shigella* species. Even then, amoxicillin should not be used orally for *Shigella* infections because excellent absorption from the upper gastrointestinal tract results in subtherapeutic levels in the lower gut. Other penicillins like carbenicillin, ticarcillin, mezlocillin, azlocillin, or piperacillin are notable for their activity against *Pseudomonas aeruginosa,* most *Proteus* species, and anaerobic pathogens such as *Bacteroides fragilis*. On a weight basis, car-

benicillin and ticarcillin have relatively weak antipseudomonal activity and so must be used in considerably larger doses than most penicillins, in the range of 18 to 30 grams a day for adults (200 to 400 mg per kilogram). The large sodium load given with such doses may aggravate congestive failure and cause electrolyte abnormalities. While these antipseudomonal penicillins are important agents for serious infections, emergence of resistance and variable stability to beta-lactamases has led to the tendency to combine these agents with an aminoglycoside. They are quite active against the coccal organisms that ampicillin usually inhibits, but none of these agents should be used against coagulase-positive staphylococci. The combination of a beta-lactamase inhibitor (clavulanate) with amoxicillin or ticarcillin confers stability on staphylococcal penicillinase and broadens coverage of some gram-negative bacilli. Other potential uses of extended-spectrum penicillins include treatment of infection caused by *Acinetobacter* species, *Listeria,* and a variety of anaerobes. Like the antistaphylococcal penicillins, their half-life is relatively short, but protein binding is low. Thus, frequent dosing at 4- to 6-hour intervals is usually necessary. Newer antipseudomonal penicillins, such as mezlocillin, azlocillin, or piperacillin, are augmented in their antipseudomonal activity, in the case of the last two approximately six- to eight-fold by weight in comparison to carbenicillin when organisms are tested at low inoculum concentrations. On the other hand, the tendency has been to use smaller doses of these more potent penicillins to avoid the side effects associated with large doses of carbenicillin. The result is that no clear-cut clinical differences have been found between these agents when they are used in combination with aminoglycosides. Some of these newer penicillins, such as mezlocillin and piperacillin, have variable activity against *Klebsiella* species and must be tested prior to use.

Newer compounds that possess a beta-lactam nucleus (and thus are related to the penicillins) include (1) imipenem, an agent with very broad activity against gram-positive and gram-negative bacteria; and (2) monobactams, such as aztreonam. The latter compound is devoid of activity against gram-positive bacteria, but like the third-generation cephalosporins, they are potent agents for treatment of gram-negative bacillary infections.

Cephalosporins

Cephalosporins are structurally related to penicillins, yet there are major differences in activity between these agents in vitro and in vivo. The first cephalosporins, such as cephalothin, cephaloridine, and cefazolin, were effective against penicillinase-producing staphylococci as well as pneumococci and streptococci (except enterococci). Additionally, they offered good activity against several important gram-negative pathogens, such as *E. coli, Klebsiella,* and *Proteus mirabilis*. Despite activity in vitro, they are not effective against *Salmonella* and *Shigella* and do not

TABLE 291–5. INITIAL EMPIRIC THERAPY FOR SERIOUS INFECTION

Syndrome	Qualifying Factors	Recommended Treatment
Septicemia	Immunocompromised host	
	Neutrophil count >500 μl	Third-generation cephalosporin or
		Cephalosporin (cefalozin) + aminoglycoside (gentamicin, tobramycin)
	Neutrophil count <500 μl	Piperacillin or ceftazidime + aminoglycoside (amikacin, tobramycin)
	Normal host	
	Urinary source	Ampicillin + gentamicin or third-generation cephalosporin
	Biliary source	Ampicillin + gentamicin or imipenem
	Abdominal or pelvic source	Aminoglycoside + clindamycin or cefoxitin, or broad-spectrum penicillin
	No source	Oxacillin + gentamicin or third-generation cephalosporin
	Neonate or child	
	<48 hr old	Ampicillin + either cefotaxime or ceftriaxone
	>48 hr old	Ampicillin + oxacillin + aminoglycoside
Meningitis	<6 yr	Ampicillin + cefotaxime or ceftriaxone
	>6 yr	Ampicillin, penicillin G, or ceftriaxone
Brain abscess		Penicillin G + cefotaxime or ceftriaxone + metronidazole
Pneumonia	Community acquired	Ampicillin or penicillin G ± erythromycin
	Postinfluenzal	Antistaphylococcal penicillin or cephalosporin
	Postaspiration	Ampicillin or clindamycin
	Nosocomial	Azlocillin or piperacillin + aminoglycoside, or third-generation cephalosporin + aminoglycoside

penetrate the blood-brain barrier. The enormous popularity of these agents appears related to a low incidence of side effects, fairly broad coverage against community-acquired respiratory and urinary tract pathogens, and the availability of both oral and parenteral dosing. Nevertheless, these compounds have not been considered the agents of choice for any serious systemic infections. They have been successfully used to treat patients with a history of mild penicillin-type reactions, such as rash, but not urticaria or anaphylaxis. With the development of newer cephalosporins, the principal advantages of these older compounds (often referred to as "the first generation") have been in prophylactic surgical usage and relatively greater activity against penicillinase-producing Staphylococcus aureus.

The so-called "second-generation" cephalosporins offer a few improvements over cephalothin and cefazolin. Cefoxitin is a compound with fairly consistent activity against B. fragilis. Cefamandole and cefuroxime lack the anaerobic spectrum of cefoxitin but have modestly improved activity against some gram-negative organisms not inhibited by the first generation, such as H. influenzae and Enterobacter species. Oral agents include cefaclor, which has greater activity against penicillinase-producing H. influenzae than does cephalexin.

The newest cephalosporins (often referred to as "third generation") or structurally related compounds such as moxalactam, a 1-oxy-beta-lactam, have markedly enhanced activity against enteric bacteria as well as variable coverage of P. aeruginosa. These compounds are stable against the beta-lactamases of H. influenzae and N. gonorrhoeae and cross the blood-brain barrier in sufficient concentrations to offer effective therapy for gram-negative meningitis (with perhaps the exception of P. aeruginosa infection). Among the agents shown to be effective in gram-negative central nervous system infections are cefotaxime, moxalactam, ceftazidime, and ceftriaxone. Several of these agents have a much longer half-life than first-generation cephalosporins, permitting dosing intervals of 8 to 12 hours. In the case of one agent, ceftriaxone, once-a-day dosing has been possible in some infections because of an 8-hour half-life. The antipseudomonal activity of these compounds is variable; nonetheless, newer antipseudomonal cephalosporins like cefsulodin* and ceftazidime represent some of the most potent antipseudomonal agents introduced into clinical practice, and these compounds appear to be significantly safer than aminoglycosides. Table 291–6 summarizes the relative properties of these agents, as well as selected comments. As a general rule, the increased activity against gram-negative pathogens is also coupled with relatively diminished activity against gram-positive cocci. While the gram-positive, particularly antistaphylococcal, coverage of these agents may be satisfactory for initial therapy, serious staphylococcal disease as well as pneumococcal infection is better and certainly more economically

treated with older beta-lactam agents (e.g., oxacillin, penicillin G, respectively). These agents are also not without serious untoward effects, including the triggering of disulfiram reactions, inhibition of platelet adhesiveness, and hypoprothrombinemia. In many patients with community-acquired and mild to moderately severe nosocomial infections, third-generation cephalosporins offer the potential of effective single-agent therapy. The results in immunocompromised hosts suggest that these compounds may still be more efficacious when combined with aminoglycosides.

Chloramphenicol

Chloramphenicol is an oral or parenterally administered drug whose spectrum makes it useful for a wide variety of bacterial and rickettsial infections. The antibacterial spectrum includes gram-positive organisms such as streptococci and staphylococci, but the agent has not been considered to be one of the more potent antistaphylococcal compounds. It is usually bacteriostatic except against H. influenzae, against which it is bactericidal. Many enteric organisms are inhibited by chloramphenicol, but Pseudomonas strains are usually resistant. Important therapeutic uses include typhoid fever, central nervous system infections, anaerobic infections, intraocular infections, and serious rickettsial infections. Against B. fragilis, it remains one of the most useful agents. On the other hand, chloramphenicol can cause severe hematologic toxicity. In the great majority of individuals receiving courses in excess of 1 week of chloramphenicol, there is a dose-dependent inhibition of erythropoiesis. Some patients, estimated at 1 in 50,000, have developed irreversible aplastic anemia following oral or parenteral dosing. While it remains a highly effective agent in selected situations, there are now a number of very reasonable alternatives to chloramphenicol. The unpredictability of the hematologic toxicity should lead physicians to reserve this agent for serious infections in which there are major indications for avoiding alternative drugs.

The Tetracyclines

Tetracyclines inhibit a wide range of gram-positive and gram-negative bacteria as well as Mycoplasma species, but they are not agents of choice for any serious bacterial infections. Their activity against gram-positive organisms is static, and the results do not appear to approach those obtained with bactericidal agents. Gram-negative coverage includes E. coli and Klebsiella species, but there are major gaps in their spectrum, including Pseudomonas, Serratia species, and other serious nosocomial pathogens. Tetracycline may be useful in urinary tract infections, rickettsial infections, mycoplasmal infections, and the prophylaxis or treatment of traveler's diarrhea (caused by toxigenic E. coli). Older preparations such as chlortetracycline or oxytetracycline have been supplanted by tetracycline HCl, minocycline, or doxycycline. The last-named two preparations have certain pharmacologic advantages, including less frequent dosing, and doxycycline may be used in renal failure.

---

*Investigational drug in the United States.

TABLE 291–6. THIRD-GENERATION CEPHALOSPORINS AND RELATED COMPOUNDS

Agent	Protein Binding (%)	Peak Serum Levels (μg/ml) After 1 gm IV	Half-Life (hr)	Comments
Aztreonam	60	50	2.0	No activity vs. gram-positive organisms
Cefmenoxime*	77	40	1.0	Weak antipseudomonal activity
Cefoperazone	90	125	2.1	Primary excretion is biliary with little dose adjustment in renal failure
Cefotaxime	38	40	1.1	Good CNS penetration but weak antipseudomonal activity
Cefsulodin*	30	65	1.5	Primarily antipseudomonal activity; not much else
Ceftazidime	20	70	1.9	Potent antipseudomonal activity
Ceftizoxime	30	75	1.4	Potent gram-negative activity except for Pseudomonas
Ceftriaxone	85	140	8.0	Very long half-life, good CNS penetration, but poor antipseudomonal activity
Imipenem	15	50	0.9	Broad gram-positive and gram-negative activity
Moxalactam	50	60	2.3	Good anaerobe coverage but associated with coagulopathy

*Not available in United States.
CNS = central nervous system.

Erythromycin

This is the most commonly available member of the class of macrolide antibiotics. Traditionally, erythromycin has been regarded as an agent of second choice for streptococcal and staphylococcal infections, to be used in those patients with history of serious penicillin allergy. In this regard, erythromycin remains a useful agent, but its primary appeal in recent years has been its clinical efficacy against several important new causes of infection, such as *Mycoplasma*, *Legionella*, *Chlamydia*, and *Campylobacter* species. Against all of these pathogens, erythromycin can be considered the agent of choice. In serious respiratory infections, erythromycin should be administered parenterally, but this use is associated with a high incidence of phlebitis. The compound is one of the safest of all antimicrobials, but mild gastrointestinal disturbances are common. Several oral preparations are available, but none seems clinically superior.

Clindamycin and Lincomycin

Clindamycin and lincomycin mimic some of the spectrum of erythromycin. Their major advantage over erythromycin is greater activity against anaerobes, particularly *B. fragilis*. Nonetheless, the antianaerobic spectrum of these compounds is not complete. In the treatment of intra-abdominal infections, these agents are usually combined with aminoglycosides for gram-negative coverage. A major problem with clindamycin therapy has been antibiotic-associated diarrhea and pseudomembranous colitis. The incidence and severity of this complication vary, and the problem is not always associated with clindamycin. The development of gastrointestinal symptoms on treatment should be a warning to discontinue use of these agents.

Metronidazole

Metronidazole has long been used for the therapy of trichomoniasis, amebiasis, and giardiasis. Subsequently, it has been found to be a highly effective and bactericidal agent against many anaerobic pathogens, including *B. fragilis*. It is available in both oral and parenteral forms and must be considered the therapy of choice for *B. fragilis* infections involving deep-seated foci, such as heart valves and the central nervous system. Many infections involving anaerobes are mixed processes that also involve aerobic organisms. Because it is almost exclusively active against anaerobic pathogens, metronidazole is usually combined with other antimicrobials. The drug must be metabolized to its active form. Its excellent distribution, rapid bactericidal activity, and penetration in "closed spaces" are appealing characteristics, but it also has the potential of inducing disulfiram reactions and potentiating the effects of warfarin (Coumadin). Metronidazole's carcinogenicity in animals and mutagenicity in bacteria have not been demonstrated in humans, but it seems wise to restrict this agent to use in severe infections.

Rifampin

Rifampin is a semisynthetic derivative of rifamycin B and has been used principally for the therapy of tuberculosis. It is one of the most potent and effective antituberculous agents available, with a spectrum that includes both *M. tuberculosis* and atypical organisms. It has been found to be very active against the wide variety of gram-positive and gram-negative organisms, including staphylococci (both coagulase-positive and coagulase-negative types) and *Legionella* species. The compound is one of the few that have been effective in terminating meningococcal carrier state, and it inhibits methicillin-resistant staphylococci. The principal drawback to the use of rifampin is that almost all microorganisms have the ability to develop resistance rapidly. Therefore, even in tuberculosis this drug must be combined with another active agent. It seems useful as an adjunct to other antibacterial agents, such as in combination with antistaphylococcal penicillins to treat "tolerant" strains in endocarditis and meningitis. It inhibits methicillin-resistant staphylococci but is best used with vancomycin. Another potential advantage has been excellent penetration into phagocytic cells. A disadvantage, however, is its potent ability to induce enzymes that decrease the half-life of a number of other pharmacologic agents, including steroids, sulfonylureas, and digitoxin.

Vancomycin

Initially developed during an intense search for agents active against coagulase-producing staphylococci, this agent acquired a reputation for efficacy as well as toxicity to the eighth cranial nerve and to renal function. More modern preparations of vancomycin do not appear to be strongly associated with these side effects. Indeed, the compound has been used effectively to treat serious infections in patients with renal failure because it is not significantly excreted by the kidneys; prolonged bactericidal activity results from widely spaced doses. The spectrum includes not only *Staphylococcus aureus* but also coagulase-negative staphylococci, *Staphylococcus faecalis* (enterococci), and *Corynebacterium* species. Vancomycin has not been considered an agent of primary choice for *Staphylococcus aureus* but is an effective alternative in the penicillin-allergic patient. In prosthetic valve endocarditis caused by coagulase-negative staphylococci, it is often considered the agent of choice in combination with rifampin or gentamicin or both.

Aminoglycosides

Aminoglycosides are rapidly bactericidal against most of the clinically important gram-negative bacilli, including enteric bacteria and *P. aeruginosa*. Most isolates of *Staphylococcus aureus* are also inhibited by aminoglycosides. The initial compounds of this series, like streptomycin, were also shown to be effective against *M. tuberculosis*, and in combination with a penicillin, either streptomycin or gentamicin offers the best available therapy for deep-seated enterococcal infections. Older agents like streptomycin, neomycin, and kanamycin are considerably less useful today because they appear to be relatively more toxic or have been supplanted by agents with greater activity against *P. aeruginosa*. The contemporary aminoglycosides include gentamicin, tobramycin, netilmicin, and amikacin. The last two compounds offer some advantages in that they are stable to inactivation by some of the plasmid-encoded enzymes that acetylate, adenylate, or phosphorylate the older agents. Thus, amikacin or netilmicin may be preferred to treat infections caused by gentamicin- or tobramycin-resistant strains, but susceptibility testing in vitro is necessary because some isolates may be resistant to all agents within this class. Rapid bactericidal effect and good distribution except for the central nervous system make these highly desirable compounds for the treatment of serious systemic gram-negative infections. Unfortunately, aminoglycosides are toxic to renal function, can cause eighth cranial nerve (both cochlear and vestibular function) and renal damage, and occasionally manifest curare-like effects. Pharmacologically, there is a narrow range between the therapeutic levels achievable by dosing every 8 to 12 hours and levels that are associated with toxicity. Aminoglycoside therapy should be closely monitored by frequent blood level determinations in treating serious infections when large doses are used for prolonged courses. These agents are either additive or often synergistic with beta-lactam compounds against pathogens such as *P. aeruginosa*, *Serratia* species, and other gram-negative rods. For immunocompromised hosts, aminoglycosides remain an important component of therapy, usually as part of a combination with a beta-lactam agent. Aminoglycosides do not adequately penetrate the central nervous system or bone and are not absorbed via the oral route. They are perhaps overused as topical agents, and in that setting the rapid emergence of resistance has been documented. For prophylaxis in colonic surgery, older aminoglycosides like neomycin or kanamycin may suffice in regimens that transiently suppress the growth of aerobic bowel flora.

Spectinomycin also belongs to the aminoglycoside class and is used exclusively for the treatment of gonorrhea when penicillin-type agents have failed. Such antigonococcal activity is shared by other members of the class.

Polymyxin, Colistin (*Polymyxin E*)

Polymyxin B and colistin (polymyxin E) are closely related cationic polypeptide detergents that bind to the lipoproteins of many gram-negative outer cell membranes. They are rapidly bactericidal in vitro, particularly against *P. aeruginosa* and enteric rods except *Proteus* species and *Serratia*. These agents are without effect against gram-positive organisms. Resistance has rarely emerged on therapy. Because of poor clinical results and nephrotoxic potential, the use of these compounds has decreased markedly. Lack of clinical efficacy could be due to properties of poor diffusion and rapid binding to tissues.

Quinolones

The quinolone group of agents includes older compounds like nalidixic acid and newer, more active agents such as ciprofloxacin, norfloxacin, and ofloxacin. Nalidixic acid has few modern uses and may be regarded as a urinary antiseptic for suppression of chronic infection. The newer quinolones have very broad activity against both gram-positive and gram-negative organisms (including *Mycoplasma* and *Legionella*) and can be administered orally. Their use is best defined for urinary tract infection and gastrointestinal infection. Quinolone therapy for serious systemic infections is justified following defervescence achieved with intravenous antibiotics.

Urinary Antiseptics

Mandelamine, nitrofurantoin, and nalidixic acid are agents that are effective only in urinary tract infections and usually as suppressive therapy in chronic infections. Resistance to some of these compounds may emerge rapidly. They may be useful in situations where the goal is suppression rather than a cure because of unremediable anatomic abnormalities. Gastrointestinal side effects have been commonly associated with each of these preparations. Additionally, the optimum antibacterial effect of mandelamine is at urine pH of less than 5.0, so that additional acidification of the urine with acidic substances is required for efficacy.

DURATION OF THERAPY

There are no easy formulas for determining duration of therapy, although a practical guide is treating for 2 to 4 days after defervescence and resolution of signs of infection. The site of infection, host factors, the nature and antimicrobial susceptibility of infecting organisms, the severity of infections, and the response to treatment should be taken into consideration. For bloodstream infections not accompanied by endocarditis or bone involvement, 10 to 14 days is a usual course of treatment. Most respiratory infections are adequately treated in the same interval. Uncom-

plicated meningitis caused by the meningococcus or pneumococcus is probably adequately treated by 7 to 10 days of high-dose parenteral penicillin G. Endocarditis, deep-seated bone infections, and infections involving prostheses require a minimum 4- to 6-week course of treatment but in some cases more. It is important to remember that signs of inflammation, particularly pulmonary infiltration, may persist long after infecting organisms are killed or contained by host defenses, and delayed resolution of lung infiltrates is not uncommon. On the other hand, deep-seated infections like endocarditis and osteomyelitis may have to be treated for periods long after subsidence of signs of infection. Thus, the decision to continue or stop treatment at the end of an appropriate interval must be based on thorough clinical examination and careful reasoning. Patients with impaired host defenses may require longer therapy than those individuals who are basically healthy. A single dose of an effective antimicrobial agent may be adequate to cure lower urinary tract infection involving the bladder, but a much longer duration, on the order of several weeks, is required to ensure therapeutic success in treatment of intrarenal infection.

FAILURE TO RESPOND TO TREATMENT

One of the most important clinical dilemmas is the persistence of fever and other manifestations of infection after a course of costly and potentially toxic therapy has been started. At the same time that every component in antimicrobial therapy is being reassessed, an alternative explanation for fever, pain, and inflammation must also be sought. For instance, tumors or hypersensitivity reactions can incite febrile reactions. Usually, an interval of 2 to 5 days is necessary to judge the efficacy of treatment. At that point, the following are indicated: (1) assessing the accuracy of the diagnosis of infection; (2) determining if the drug selection is appropriate, and particularly if the dose and mode of administration are responsible for the lack of success of therapy; and (3) searching for (a) presence of anatomic abnormalities, (b) foreign body, (c) undrained abscess, (d) infarction of tissue, (e) development of superinfection, (f) emergence of resistance, or (g) presence of a simultaneous infectious process that is not being treated by antibacterial therapy. If these are unrevealing, a noninfectious origin of fever or drug reaction should be considered.

In the severely immunosuppressed host, fever and signs of infection may persist despite appropriate therapy. In these patients clinical failure of drug treatment is more realistically regarded as host failure; if any improvement is possible in this

TABLE 291–7. UNTOWARD EFFECTS OF SOME ANTIMICROBIAL AGENTS

Target	Agent	Mechanism	Manifestation
Endocrine	Ketoconazole	Altered steroid synthesis	Gynecomastia
	Sulfonamides	Block iodine uptake	Goiter
Gastrointestinal	All agents, especially ampicillin, clindamycin	(1) Altered bowel flora	Diarrhea
		(2) Exotoxin of *Clostridium difficile*	Pseudomembranous colitis
	Isoniazid, rifampin, tetracyclines	Hepatocellular necrosis	Hepatitis
	Neomycin	Villous damage	Malabsorption
Hematologic	Chloramphenicol	(1) Protein synthesis inhibition	Reversible anemia, leukopenia
		(2) Idiosyncratic	Aplastic anemia
	Carbenicillin, others	Inhibition of platelet aggregation	Bleeding
	Moxalactam	Impaired prothrombin synthesis	Bleeding
	Penicillins, many others	Impaired leukopoiesis, thrombopoiesis	Neutropenia, thrombocytopenia
	Sulfonamides	Glucose-6-phosphate dehydrogenase (G6PD) deficiency	Hemolytic anemia
Kidney	Aminoglycosides, polymyxins	Tubular damage	Renal failure
	Amphotericin	Tubular damage	Hypokalemia, renal failure
	Carbenicillin	Na-K exchange	Hypokalemia
	Penicillins	Interstitial nephritis	Renal failure
	Sulfonamides	Tubular crystallization	Renal failure
Nervous	Aminoglycosides	(1) Damage to hair cells of Corti	Deafness
		(2) Vestibular damage	Vertigo
		(3) Neuromuscular blockade	Respiratory arrest
	Isoniazid	Pyridoxine antagonism	Neuropathy
	Penicillins, cephalosporins	Cortical irritation	Seizures
	Polymyxins	Neuromuscular blockade	Respiratory arrest
Pulmonary	Nitrofurantoin	Interstitial inflammation	Fibrosis
Skin	Tetracyclines	Bind to dermal structures	Photosensitivity
	Penicillins, sulfonamides, tetracyclines, others	Allergic reactions	Rash, serum sickness, erythema multiforme

difficult situation, it usually correlates with improvement in underlying disease or the immunologic status of the host. If an infection is documented and responds poorly to initially prescribed treatment, then a change to an alternate regimen is indicated. If signs and symptoms progress or new complications appear in spite of seemingly appropriate treatment, a change in therapy is indicated as well as a search for superinfection or an undiagnosed process such as a viral or fungal infection. One of the greatest clinical dilemmas is presented by the patient in whom drug fever or a hypersensitivity reaction is suspected but in whom discontinuing treatment could be dangerous. In such individuals, it is usually prudent to give alternative medication rather than to stop antibacterial therapy completely.

ANTIBIOTIC TOXICITY AND UNTOWARD REACTIONS

A large proportion of drug reactions are related to antimicrobial agents. As many as 10 per cent of patients receiving penicillins and sulfonamides experience some type of toxic or hypersensitivity reaction. These reactions can be fatal, as in the anaphylaxis associated with penicillin or the aplastic anemia due to chloramphenicol. Table 291–7 summarizes some of the major untoward reactions to antibiotics. The majority of toxic reactions are, however, short lived and reversible. Nephrotoxicity secondary to aminoglycosides may be averted by careful therapeutic drug monitoring. A commonly recognized complication of antibiotic therapy is diarrhea and/or pseudomembranous colitis. This is due to bowel overgrowth by C. difficile, which elaborates an exotoxin that is responsible for symptoms. Discontinuation of antibiotic therapy will usually lead to resolution of treatment, but some patients require vancomycin or metronidazole.

Besides anaphylaxis, other hypersensitivity reactions include fever, hemolytic anemia, serum sickness, and a wide variety of dermal reactions that include rash and exfoliation. When serious infection is being treated, mild hypersensitivity reactions may be suppressed by a variety of symptomatic medications. Manifestations of hypersensitivity such as rash may fade despite continued treatment, as is common with ampicillin. The decision to continue therapy in the face of such reactions must be based on severity

of infection and the lack of reasonable alternatives. Another issue of great clinical importance that is not fully resolved is the potential cross-reactivity between penicillins and cephalosporins. However, the great majority of patients who have only rash following exposure to penicillin, ampicillin, or related penicillins can be safely treated with cephalosporin compounds. The immediate hypersensitivity-type reactions, such as anaphylaxis, wheezing, and urticaria, should be carefully noted. Patients with a history of immediate reactions to penicillin should not be rechallenged with cephalosporins unless they have life-threatening infections and can be observed under close medical supervision.

MAJOR ANTIBIOTIC DRUG INTERACTIONS

An increasing number of interactions have been reported between antimicrobials, or antimicrobials and other pharmacologic agents that seriously ill patients may be receiving. Some of these are summarized in Table 291–8. Some noteworthy examples include the induction of hepatic enzymes by rifampin, which may hasten the metabolism of other antibiotics or drugs. An unexplored area of drug interactions is that which may involve more than two agents. Penicillins like ampicillin or carbenicillin gradually inactivate aminoglycosides like gentamicin in renal failure, when a long half-life for both types of drugs provides opportunity for complexing between the two classes of agents. While this effect is not apparent when patients have normal renal function, the net effect in patients in renal failure is effectively to lower the levels of circulating aminoglycosides and penicillin.

USE OF TOPICAL ANTIBIOTICS

Topical antibiotics or antiseptics have been commonly applied to burns and open wounds, and they are often incorporated into irrigants. A few studies suggest that topical agents can suppress bacteria in burn wounds and reduce sepsis originating from this source. Some topical antiseptics, such as those that contain iodine, are probably too toxic to inflamed tissues, and their local appli-

TABLE 291–8. IMPORTANT ANTIBIOTIC DRUG INTERACTIONS

Antimicrobial Agent	Interacting Drug	Result
Amphotericin B	Curariform drugs	Increased curare-like effect
Aminoglycosides	Neuromuscular blockers (i.e., tubocurarine, pancuronium)	Additive blockade
	Diuretics: ethacrynic acid, furosemide	Increased ototoxicity
	Antibiotics: amphotericin B	Increased nephrotoxicity
	Carbenicillin/ticarcillin (other penicillins)	Inactivation, resulting in reduced activity
Ampicillin/amoxicillin	Allopurinol	Rash
Cephalosporins (cefamandole, cefoperazone, moxalactam)	Alcohol	Disulfiram reaction
Chloramphenicol	Warfarin	Decreased warfarin metabolism and inhibition of vitamin K–producing gut bacteria, thus increasing prothrombin time
	Phenytoin	Decreased phenytoin metabolism levels
	Oral hypoglycemic agents	Increased hypoglycemia
Isoniazid	Warfarin, phenytoin	Increased risk of toxicity by decreased drug metabolism
	Disulfiram	Psychosis
	Rifampin, para-aminosalicylic acid	Additive hepatotoxicity
	Oral contraceptives	Decreased contraceptive effect
Metronidazole	Alcohol	Disulfiram-like reaction (nausea)
	Disulfiram	Psychosis
Nalidixic acid	Warfarin	Increased prothrombin time
Polymyxins	Curariform drugs	Increased curare-like effect
Quinolones	Theophylline	Increased theophylline blood levels
Rifampin	Warfarin, phenytoin	Decreased warfarin, phenytoin effect
	Isoniazid	Additive hepatotoxicity
	Methadone	Withdrawal symptoms
	Oral contraceptives	Decreased contraceptive effect
	Steroids	Decreased steroid effect
Sulfonamides	Procaine	Decreased sulfonamide effect
	Hypoglycemic agents	Hypoglycemia
	Warfarin, phenytoin	Displace drugs from protein-binding sites, causing increased warfarin and phenytoin effects
Tetracyclines	Antacids, oral iron	Decreased tetracycline absorption

cation should be discouraged. Topically applied antibiotics can provide only surface suppression of microbial flora. They also provide ample opportunity for development of resistance, since large numbers of organisms may be present on injured skin. Antibiotics in irrigants may be irritating, may be absorbed in large quantities so as to cause increased toxicity, and may offer little advantage over irrigation per se.

Bennett WM, Aronoff GR, Morrison G, et al.: Drug prescribing in renal failure: Dosing guidelines for adults. Am J Kidney Dis 3:155, 1983. *A highly practical guide to antibiotic dose reduction in renal failure.*

Hooper DC, Wolfson JS: Drug therapy: Fluoroquinolone antimicrobial agents. N Engl J Med 324:384, 1991. *Succinct review of the most important "new" group of antibiotics.*

Krogstad DJ, Moellering RC Jr: Antimicrobial combinations. *In* Lorian V (ed.): Antibiotics in Laboratory Medicine. 2nd ed. Baltimore, The Williams and Wilkins Company, 1986, pp 537–595. *A laboratory-oriented review with practical guidelines for clinicians.*

Lupski JR: Molecular mechanisms for transposition of drug-resistance genes and other movable genetic elements. Rev Infect Dis 9:357, 1987. *An up-to-date summary of a rapidly changing field.*

Neu HC: β-Lactam antibiotics: Structural relationships affecting *in vitro* activity and pharmacologic properties. Rev Infect Dis 8(Suppl 3):237, 1986. *An important and well-written overview of the single most important group of antibiotics.*

Peterson PK, Verhoef J (eds.): The Antimicrobial Agents Annual. Vol 3. Amsterdam, Elsevier, 1988. *One of the most comprehensive reviews of all major categories of antimicrobial agents.*

Siegenthaler WE, Bonetti A, Luthy R: Aminoglycoside antibiotics in infectious diseases. Am J Med 80(Suppl 6B):2, 1986. *Succinct summary of this group of agents, which remain important in modern antimicrobial chemotherapy.*

Young LS: Empirical antimicrobial therapy in the neutropenic host. N Engl J Med 315:580, 1986. *Summarizes, with relevant references, the debate over the merits of combination antimicrobial therapy versus the use of a single agent for empiric treatment of immunocompromised hosts.*

SECTION TWO / BACTERIAL DISEASES

292 Pneumococcal Pneumonia

Richard J. Duma

DEFINITION. Pneumococcal pneumonia is an acute, suppurative infection of the lungs produced by an encapsulated bacterium, *Streptococcus pneumoniae* (pneumococcus). It is the most commonly occurring bacterial pneumonia in the world; in the United States, an estimated 150,000 to 500,000 cases occur annually.

MICROBIOLOGY. Virulent S. *pneumoniae* organisms are encapsulated, gram-positive cocci about 0.8 μm in diameter that occur in chains (streptococci) or pairs (diplococci) (see Color Plate 9*F*). When in pairs, cocci are characteristically described as lancet shaped; i.e., each coccus is pointed at the end like the tip of a lance, and the bases are in juxtaposition. The capsule, which is a polysaccharide and which varies in thickness from strain to strain, is not seen with Gram stain but may be recognized by negative staining (e.g., with India ink or methylene blue). In purulent clinical specimens, some pneumococci stain negatively rather than positively on the Gram stain, as aging, exposure of the cell wall to a variety of destructive host enzymes (e.g., lysozyme), and/or inhibition of cell wall synthesis by antibiotics (e.g., penicillin) result in incomplete or abnormal bacterial cell walls that no longer retain the iodine-fixed crystal violet stain.

Pneumococci are fastidious, facultative bacteria that grow best in the presence of blood or serum and in air supplemented with 10 per cent carbon dioxide. Since they are fermentative and since lactic acid is the usual end-product, concentrations of glucose must be controlled in the culture media and should not exceed 1 per cent. In addition, since they produce hydrogen peroxide (H_2O_2) but not catalase, the addition of a catalase source (e.g., red blood cells) enhances growth. Viability is reduced by drying, a low pH (<6.5), and prolonged incubation.

On blood agar plates after overnight incubation at 37°C, colonies generally appear mucoid, glistening, and dome shaped and are surrounded by an area of greening (α-hemolysis) within the blood agar. With continued incubation, as aged bacteria undergo autolysis, the colony domes of highly encapsulated strains collapse centrally and appear umbilicated. An important biologic feature that distinguishes S. *pneumoniae* from other streptococci is its bile solubility or susceptibility to surface-active agents, such as sodium deoxycholate and ethyl hydrocuprein chloride (optochin). The latter agent (optochin) is incorporated into a standardized 5-μg disc and is utilized worldwide to identify pneumococci rapidly. However, since optochin-resistant pneumococci occur and since some nonpneumococcal, α-hemolytic streptococci are optochin sensitive, for purposes of species determination, the usefulness of this biologic property may be questioned.

Pneumococcal virulence and pneumococcal pneumonia are often studied in the mouse, since this animal is highly sensitive to encapsulated pneumococci (with the exception of type 14). Indeed, the sensitivity of mice to encapsulated pneumococci may be utilized for rapidly and selectively isolating virulent pneumococci from sputum specimens or from clinical materials containing mixtures of other bacteria. If the specimen in question contains pneumococci and is injected into the peritoneal cavity of the mouse, a peritoneal exudate containing pneumococci may be harvested in 24 hours.

Unlike many other streptococci, particularly those belonging to Lancefield group A, and unlike other pyogenic bacteria that may produce pneumonia, S. *pneumoniae* organisms do not possess or produce any clinically important toxins, and particularly none that are tissue destructive. Some strains may elaborate hyaluronidase, and all contain a hemolysin (pneumolysin O) that produces α- or β-hemolysis on blood agar under aerobic or anaerobic conditions, respectively; however, no clinical importance is assigned to any of these substances, and their values are principally for strain identification purposes.

The most important factor defining virulent S. *pneumoniae* is the presence of a high molecular weight, complex polysaccharide capsule, which is a potent inhibitor of neutrophil phagocytosis. At least 84 different immunogenic types of capsules exist, and two different nomenclatures (Danish and American) are used to number them (which is often a source of confusion). Antigenically distinct capsules are easily identified with polyvalent antisera in an agglutination or precipitin test or by the Neufeld quellung reaction, a rapid test based on visualization of refractile swelling of the capsule after application of a polyvalent or monovalent type-specific antiserum to the bacterium in question. Rough or nonencapsulated pneumococci, which are generally avirulent, do not react with antipolysaccharide antisera. Although the identification of pneumococcal capsular antigen in certain body fluids or secretions may suggest active pneumococcal infection (see below), immunologic tests to detect such antigens must be interpreted with caution, since antibodies against some pneumococcal capsular serotypes cross-react with polysaccharides of other streptococci (particularly group B), *Haemophilus influenzae* type B, *Escherichia coli*, *Klebsiella pneumoniae*, *Salmonella* species, and even human ABO blood group isoantigens.

TABLE 292–1. MIC$_{90}$ OF SOME COMMONLY USED BETA-LACTAM ANTIBIOTICS AGAINST PENICILLIN-RESISTANT PNEUMOCOCCI

Antibiotic	MIC$_{90}$ (µg/ml)*	
	Intermediate Penicillin Resistance	High-Level Penicillin Resistance
Ampicillin	0.5	8
Oxacillin	4.0	31
Methicillin	—	64
Carbenicillin	32.0	64
Ticarcillin	64.0	128
Piperacillin	1.0	8–16
Mezlocillin	1.0–2.0	8–15
Azlocillin	1.0	16
Cephalothin	1.0	8–31
Cefaclor	4.0–16.0	16
Cefonicid	16.0	16
Cefoxitin	4.0–8.0	32–125
Cefamandole	0.5–2.0	8–31
Cefuroxime	0.25–0.44	—
Cefotaxime	0.125–1.0	1–4
Ceftriaxone	0.12–0.5	1
Ceftazidime	3.2–32.0	64
Cefoperazone	1.0–2.0	2–16
Moxalactam	2.0–4.0	128
Imipenem	0.06–1.0	1–2

*MIC$_{90}$ = Minimal inhibitory concentration at which 90 per cent of strains are susceptible.

Adapted with permission from Klugman KP: Pneumococcal resistance to antibiotics. Clin Microbiol Rev 3:171–196, 1990.

The susceptibility of pneumococci to most chemotherapeutic antibacterials is generally excellent. Noteworthy among antipneumococcal drugs are the beta-lactams, especially penicillins, cephalosporins, cefamycins, and carbapenems (but *not* monobactams). In addition, erythromycins, lincosines (e.g., clindamycin), vancomycin, chloramphenicol, and teicoplanins are effective. For penicillin G, the antibiotic against which all other antipneumococcal agents are compared, *susceptibility* is defined as inhibiting the growth of pneumococci at a concentration of less than 0.1 µg per milliliter (referred to as the *minimal inhibitory concentration*, or MIC). Indeed, the MIC of penicillin G worldwide for the vast majority of pneumococcal strains is predictably 0.1 µg per milliliter or less. However, since 1968, when penicillin-resistant strains were first identified in Australia, a significant per cent (in some studies as high as 10 per cent) of isolates may be moderately or intermediately resistant (i.e., the MIC is 0.1 to <2.0 µg per milliliter), and a small per cent may be highly resistant (i.e., the MIC is ≥ 2.0 µg per milliliter). Isolates that are highly resistant to penicillin G are also usually resistant to a wide array of other antibacterials (Table 292–1), although such bacteria are uniformly susceptible to vancomycin and occasionally to third-generation cephalosporins or carbapenems. The resistance of pneumococci to beta-lactams is *not* due to bacterial production of a beta-lactamase and is *not* plasmid mediated, as is so often the case with most other bacteria (especially gram-negative bacilli), but rather it is chromosomally mediated and appears to result from point mutations that dictate the production of target membrane penicillin-binding proteins (PBP's) with an affinity for penicillin G that differs from that of the PBP's of penicillin-susceptible strains.

Pneumococci are relatively resistant to aminoglycosides; in fact, gentamicin is frequently incorporated into primary culture media for selective isolation of pneumococci from sputum, since it suppresses the growth of concurrent or contaminating bacteria. Similarly, quinolones at low or clinically achievable concentrations are generally ineffective in inhibiting the growth of most pneumococci; further, in some studies, more than 50 per cent of pneumococcal isolates are resistant to tetracyclines.

EPIDEMIOLOGY. Pneumococcal pneumonia is a sporadic disease that occurs most often during the coldest months of the year. The vast majority of such pneumonias occur after aspiration of "normal" oropharyngeal secretions that contain encapsulated pneumococci, followed by an inability to clear such bacteria-containing secretions adequately; thus, oropharyngeal carrier rates of pneumococci are important in understanding the dynamics of acquiring pneumococcal pneumonia, its spread, and its frequency of occurrence within a population.

Since most data referable to oropharyngeal carrier rates come from studies performed prior to the development and distribution of a commercially available pneumococcal vaccine, the prevalence of colonization with (or carriage of) certain serotypes and the relative importance of factors that have an impact on carriage must be interpreted with caution. Nevertheless, since most estimates suggest that only 10 per cent of people at increased risk for pneumococcal pneumonia receive pneumococcal vaccine, and since some studies suggest that the presence of pre-existing, type-specific, circulating serum antibody does not prevent oropharyngeal colonization, prevaccine data on carriage rates are probably applicable and useful.

In longitudinal, prevaccine studies of pneumococcal oropharyngeal carriage by people living in temperate zones, serotypes with USA numbers of 23 or less are most frequently encountered, further suggesting that humans are infected by their own endogenous flora, since more than half the cases of pneumococcal pneumonia and bacteremia are caused by these strains. Clustering of one serotype within a family commonly occurs, and the prevalence of carriage does not appear to be affected by sex. Rates of carriage are higher in children, particularly those of a preschool age, than in adults; and among adults, rates are highest in those intimately exposed to preschool children. Oropharyngeal carriage appears to be highest during the coolest months of the year (fall, winter, and early spring), when respiratory infections are common. Although some studies suggest that respiratory infections do not affect pneumococcal carriage rates, others indicate that the spread of carriage within families occurs in association with the appearance of respiratory tract infections due either to the pneumococcus or to certain respiratory viruses, such as the rhinovirus. Although the prevalence of oropharyngeal carriage in the surrounding community or within households affects the risk of individual acquisition, crowding does not appear to be critical or even important, as is the case with infections by group A streptococci. The duration of oropharyngeal carriage of a particular serotype ranges from 2 weeks to years, the mean being 6 to 8 weeks. Reacquisition of the same serotype with no change in risk factors for acquisition commonly occurs. In children, initial acquisition within a family setting is frequently associated with rises in homotypic serum antibody and occasionally with illness, but in adults, both of these phenomena are observed infrequently.

Although epidemics of pneumococcal pneumonia may occur, they are *rare* and generally appear in special populations known to be at high risk for pneumococcal disease, such as domiciliary populations of alcoholics, institutionalized elderly, Navajo Indians, New Guinea highlanders, Alaskan natives, and South African gold miners.

In studies of ambulatory adult populations, a variety of conditions or specific risk factors appear to predispose to the development of pneumococcal pneumonia (Table 292–2): extremes of age, dementia, seizure disorders (aspiration), cigarette smoking, congestive heart failure, cerebrovascular occlusions or severe neurologic impairments (especially those associated with chronic aspiration and paralysis of respiratory muscles or impaired cough reflex), chronic obstructive pulmonary disease, chronic bronchitis, bronchiectasis, malignancies (particularly solid tumors of the lung), institutionalization, immunologic deficiencies (e.g., of immunoglobulins G [IgG] or A [IgA]), recent viral infections (particularly those caused by myxoviruses, such as influenza), and splenic dysfunction (e.g., sickle cell anemia).

IMMUNOLOGY. In nonimmunized, untreated patients, specific anticapsular humoral antibody (immunoglobulin M [IgM] and immunoglobulin G [IgG]) can be detected in the blood 5 to 10 days after infection and correlates with the clearance of pneumococci and eventual recovery. Complement (C3) and type-specific, opsonizing antibody, principally IgG, enhance phagocytosis by polymorphonuclear leukocytes, the major host defense mechanism for eradicating pneumococci. Patients with deficiencies of biologically active IgM, IgG, and, to a lesser degree, IgA (particularly secretory) are more susceptible to developing pneumococcal pneumonia and other pneumococcal infections than are normal persons without such deficiencies. In normal persons,

TABLE 292-2. RISK FACTORS OR UNDERLYING CONDITIONS PREDISPOSING TO THE DEVELOPMENT OF PNEUMOCOCCAL PNEUMONIA OR SERIOUS PNEUMOCOCCAL INFECTIONS

Age (extremes)
Alcoholism
Bone marrow transplantation
Bronchiectasis
Cerebrovascular occlusions or severe neurologic impairment
Chronic bronchitis
Chronic lymphocytic leukemia
Chronic obstructive pulmonary disease (COPD)
Cirrhosis or chronic liver disease
Complement deficiency (particularly C3)
Conditions associated with aspiration (e.g., seizures)
Congestive heart failure
Dementia
Diabetes mellitus
Immunologic deficiencies (acquired, hereditary, or iatrogenic)—humoral (IgG or IgA) or cellular (e.g., acquired immunodeficiency syndrome [AIDS])
Institutionalization
Malignancy (particularly solid tumors of the lung)
Multiple myeloma
Nephrotic syndrome
Neutropenia
Smoking
Splenic dysfunction (e.g., in sickle cell disease) or asplenia
Viral diseases, especially influenza

once specific anticapsular antibodies form, they generally persist for life.

PATHOGENESIS AND PATHOLOGY. Most cases of pneumococcal pneumonia result from the aspiration of oropharyngeal material containing indigenous, virulent pneumococci into terminal bronchioles and alveoli and then the inability to clear such bacteria adequately from these sites. Although microaspiration is a natural, common event that occurs during sleep, pneumonia seldom results, because pulmonary bacterial clearance and/or local host defense mechanisms are adequate and intact and are not defective or suppressed. These important defense mechanisms, which serve as either a barrier against or a clearance for bacteria, are the epiglottic reflex, ciliary escalator and mucous blanket, secretory and humoral immunoglobulins, surfactant, alveolar macrophage and polymorphonuclear leukocyte activity, and lymphatic drainage. When these mechanisms are blunted or overwhelmed by large volumes of aspirated noxious material, by large inocula of pneumococci, by a highly virulent strain, and/or by material containing additional virulent pathogens, pneumonia may result. After aspiration, atelectasis or bronchiole obstruction (which predisposes to or abets infection) may occur, and infection may follow; once infection follows, further atelectasis from inspissated material may result. These events may be modified by the level of type-specific humoral and/or secretory immunity present in the host.

Once virulent pneumococci establish a base in the lung, the first visible evidence of an inflammatory response is localized capillary dilatation and hyperemia, the appearance of serous edema within alveoli, and margination, diapedesis, and chemotaxis of polymorphonuclear cells induced by immunoglobulins and/or activated complement. Fluid-filled alveoli enhance the passage of bacteria through the pores of Kohn and into terminal bronchioles, with spread to contiguous, uninfected alveoli, forming the advancing margins of the disease. If clearance and host immune mechanisms are adequate at this stage, the infection may resolve. However, if not, the disease may spread further until the pleura and interlobar fissures are reached and consolidation with dense infiltrates of polymorphonuclear leukocytes and extravasated red blood cells occurs (see Color Plates 9A to C).

Pneumococcal pneumonia may involve an entire lobe (lobar pneumonia), multiple lobes (multilobar pneumonia), or just segments of a lobe, producing a patchy area (or areas) of pneumonia (pneumonitis). At times, infection spreads concentrically from bronchi (bronchopneumonia), a pattern occasionally seen in infants and in the elderly. In the central and oldest portions of infection, consolidation with massive numbers of polymorphonuclear leukocytes predominates, while peripheral to this are new areas of hemorrhage, infiltrating polymorphonuclear cells, and edema. Early pathologists referred to these areas in the lung as "gray hepatization" and "red hepatization," respectively, because of the gross resemblance of involved lung to liver tissue (see Color Plate 9A). In fully developed, untreated pneumococcal pneumonia, all stages of the cellular inflammatory process may be present.

In 5 to 10 per cent of patients, infection may extend into the pleural space, resulting in an *empyema*, or in 15 to 25 per cent of patients, bacteria may enter the bloodstream (*bacteremia*) via the lymphatics and thoracic duct. Invasion of the bloodstream by pneumococci may lead to serious metastatic or secondary infections at a number of extrapulmonary sites (Table 292-3), the most important and most frequent of which is the subarachnoid space *(meningitis)*. Other infections that may occur from bacteremic spread are *septic arthritis, pericarditis, endocarditis* (infection of the heart valves), and, in patients with ascites, *peritonitis (spontaneous bacterial peritonitis,* or SBP). In addition, organs of the sinopulmonary system may be concomitantly and acutely infected by pneumococci; involved structures include the air sinuses *(sinusitis)*, mastoids *(mastoiditis)*, ears *(otitis media)*, conjunctivae (pyogenic *conjunctivitis)*, epiglottis *(epiglottitis,* particularly in infants), or rarely the soft tissues of the neck or retropharyngeal area *(Ludwig's angina)*.

CLINICAL FINDINGS. The presentation of acute bacterial pneumonia due to *S. pneumoniae* may be highly variable, depending on when the patient presents to the physician in the course of the disease, the patient's age, whether or not effective antibiotics were previously administered, the presence or absence of satisfactory host defenses, and the existence of risk factors for dissemination of pneumococci (e.g., asplenia, neutropenia, and agammaglobulinemia). The presentation may be mild or explosive and rapidly lethal. Classically, the onset of acute pneumococcal pneumonia is sudden and is characterized by an abrupt occurrence of cough, chills, high fever (up to 40°C), myalgias, tachypnea, shallow respirations, tachycardia, weakness, and often frank rigors. Initially, the cough may be productive of scant mucopurulent or blood-streaked sputum; later (after 24 to 48 hours), it may be thick, purulent, frankly bloody or rust-colored, and consistent with an alveolar, hemorrhagic, exudative process. If the infecting pneumococcus is highly encapsulated, a gelatinous, blood-tinged sputum may be seen. The presence of pleuritic pain is specific clinical evidence that the pneumonia is probably bacterial and, in the presence of most of the above findings, pneumococcal.

The patient with pneumococcal pneumonia is generally diaphoretic and, in addition, may be dehydrated and hypotensive. Anorexia, nausea, and vomiting are common. If allowed to continue untreated, single-lobe disease may progress to multilobe involvement, and the patient may become dusky, cyanotic, and confused. If bacteremia occurs, chills and rigors may persist, and rarely shock, a disseminated intravascular coagulopathy (DIC), and/or an adult respiratory distress syndrome (ARDS) may supervene and ultimately lead to the patient's death.

A history is frequently elicited of a recent upper respiratory or viral-like illness that has occurred prior to the appearance of

TABLE 292-3. CONCURRENT OR COMPLICATING PNEUMOCOCCAL INFECTIONS OCCURRING IN PNEUMOCOCCAL PNEUMONIA

Otitis media
Sinusitis/mastoiditis
Conjunctivitis (suppurative)
Epiglottitis
Tracheobronchitis
Pleuritis (empyema)
Soft tissue cellulitis (e.g., Ludwig's angina)
Pericarditis*
Endocarditis*
Meningitis*
Arthritis (septic)*
Peritonitis (in presence of ascites)*

*Usually blood borne.

clinical pneumonia, especially during the winter months, when influenza is common. Risk factors for aspiration, such as alcoholism, seizures, or vomiting, or for acquiring pneumococcal pneumonia, may be present (see above).

On physical examination, the acutely ill patient is tachypneic and may be observed to use accessory muscles for respiration (intercostal, abdominal, and sternocleidomastoid) and even to exhibit nasal flaring. If pleuritic pain is severe, reflex splinting of the ipsilateral thorax is observed. Fever and tachycardia are present, and although hypotension may occur, frank shock is unusual, except in the later stages of infection or if DIC occurs.

Auscultation of the chest reveals bronchovesicular or tubular breath sounds and wet rales over the involved lung. As consolidation occurs, vocal and tactile fremitus is increased; however, if a concurrent pleural effusion is present, breath sounds and fremitus may be diminished or absent. A localized, grating pleural friction rub may occasionally be heard.

Examination of the upper respiratory passages may be helpful in suggesting a diagnosis of pneumococcal pneumonia. For example, in children the absence of an exudative pharyngitis and the presence of otitis media might suggest pneumococcal involvement. In older children and adults, the air sinuses and/or mastoids may be acutely infected. (But this infection can also occur in streptococcal, staphylococcal, and *H. influenzae* pneumonia.)

Evidence of extrapulmonary infections may be present, particularly in untreated disease lasting more than 48 hours; for example, signs of meningeal irritation (stiff neck, Kernig's or Brudzinski's signs) with abnormalities in mentation may suggest meningitis; the appearance of pathologic heart murmurs, splenomegaly, and heart failure may be evidence of endocarditis; or the presence of pain, swelling, tenderness, heat, and possibly redness of one or more joints may point toward a septic arthritis of hematogenous origin.

Additional findings unrelated to pneumonia per se, but related, rather, to sepsis and/or toxicity, may be noted: a paralytic ileus with abdominal pain, distention, and loss of bowel sounds; mild jaundice due to a reactive hepatitis or to intrapulmonary hemorrhage associated with the pathology of the disease; frank shock; purpuric lesions resulting from DIC; or symmetric gangrene and purpura of the fingers and/or toes (*purpura fulminans*) associated with bacteremia.

LABORATORY FINDINGS. The peripheral white blood cell (WBC) count is often two to three times the normal value; however, in alcoholics or immunosuppressed patients, it may be normal or low. Of more value is the WBC differential, which consists predominantly of bands and polymorphonuclear leukocytes (left shift). If DIC is suspected, then thrombocytopenia and pleomorphism of red blood cells (schistocytes and helmet cells) are present and may be seen on the peripheral blood smear, prothrombin and partial thromboplastin times are prolonged, and hypofibrinogenemia and circulating fibrin-split products may be detected.

In some patients, the total bilirubin and hepatic cellular enzyme levels may be slightly elevated. Since dehydration and hypovolemia commonly occur (owing to fever, diaphoresis, nausea, and vomiting), the hemoglobin, hematocrit, and serum sodium level may be elevated. When pneumonia is the dominant clinical event, arterial blood gas studies, which reflect pulmonary function and compensatory events, usually reveal hypoxemia (low Po_2), hypocarbia (low Pco_2), and alkalosis (blood pH above 7.4) resulting from hyperventilation and shunting. However, if frank shock intervenes, a metabolic acidosis may result (blood pH less than 7.4); if it is not corrected, death may follow.

Good posteroanterior and lateral chest roentgenograms are important to obtain (see Color Plate 9D), first to confirm the presence and to ascertain the extent and radiographic character of the pneumonia and second to determine if underlying predisposing pulmonary diseases are present, such as bronchiectasis, bronchial obstruction, emphysema, tumor, or tuberculosis. In severely dehydrated or profoundly neutropenic or immunodeficient patients, early inflammatory infiltrates may not be seen radiographically or may be patchy and irregular in appearance; but after hydration or restoration of circulating levels of inflammatory cells, patterns of lobar consolidation may become apparent.

Characteristically, in immunocompetent patients with untreated, frank pneumococcal pneumonia, chest roentgenograms reveal a lobar distribution and an air space (or alveolar exudative) pattern of disease with an air bronchogram effect. However, if prior, partially effective antibiotic usage has occurred, the pattern may be atypical, and a lobar distribution may be the exception rather than the rule. Interlobar fissures may bulge, owing to considerable fluid content within the involved lung associated with large amounts of capsular material. In severe cases, more than one lobe may be involved (multilobar pneumonia). In 30 per cent of cases, a pleural effusion may be present and may be readily detected by a lateral decubitus film. Such effusions may be sterile and represent parapneumonic collections of fluid, or occasionally they may be infected with pneumococci, in which case they are called *empyemas*.

If blunting of the costophrenic angle is noted radiographically, and the finding is believed to represent an effusion, then at least 300 to 500 ml of fluid is probably present, and a thoracentesis is indicated. Unless contraindicated, *every pleural effusion associated with an acute bacterial pneumonia in which the etiology of the pneumonia is unclear should be tapped and the fluid studied for microorganisms* (see Color Plate 9E). Ordinarily, fluid removed from the pleural space is sterile, so that any bacteria seen on a Gram stain or cultured from the fluid represent pathogens until proved otherwise.

Other important laboratory studies *that must be obtained early in the patient's workup* are routine cultures of the blood, a microscopic examination of a Gram stain and a culture *of purulent material from the site of infection* (alveoli, bronchi, or lung), and an examination of any infected material that can be removed from a secondarily infected extrapulmonary focus. In pneumococcal pneumonia, 15 to 25 per cent of blood cultures may be positive for *S. pneumoniae*. However, the results of blood cultures are generally not available for 18 to 24 hours and thus cannot assist the physician in making a presumptive diagnosis or in initially selecting appropriate chemotherapy. Often, in asplenic patients, a high-grade bacteremia occurs, so that examination of the peripheral WBC smear or of the buffy coat for pneumococci may be useful.

Microscopic examination and cultures of expectorated purulent sputum from a patient with acute bacterial pneumonia are essential if a correct presumptive etiologic diagnosis is to be made and an appropriate antibiotic is to be given. Ideally, these tests should be done before therapy is initiated; however, a significant delay in instituting therapy should not be permitted. Attention must also be given to obtaining a diagnostically useful sputum sample; that is, material must be purulent and thus presumed to be from the site of infection. Ideally, saliva or oropharyngeal contamination of the sample should be avoided.

In a patient with the clinical picture of acute bacterial pneumonia, the finding of gram-positive diplococci in expectorated sputum that contains many ($\geq$50 bacterial cells per $100\times$ field) polymorphonuclear cells (purulent sputum) and few (<10 squamous cells per $100\times$ field) or no squamous epithelial cells (which indicates little or no oropharyngeal contamination of the specimen) is strong presumptive evidence of pneumococcal pneumonia.

Cultures of expectorated sputum are also important but are not without problems; for example, since *S. pneumoniae* is fastidious, it may fail to grow in culture, but this does not exclude its presence. In addition, pneumococci may be overlooked, since they may be overgrown by other organisms or mixed with similar-appearing, nonpneumococcal, α-hemolytic streptococci, which are normally present in oropharyngeal secretions. On the other hand, since *S. pneumoniae* is often present normally in the oropharynx, its growth from sputum, especially from that which is expectorated, may not be indicative of pneumococcal disease. Perhaps the main value of securing a sputum culture is to confirm or question observations made from the Gram stain and, if pneumococci (and/or other bacteria) are ultimately isolated, to perform antibiotic susceptibility testing.

If the patient is unable to expectorate purulent sputum for microscopic examination and culture, and if other infected materials (e.g., pleural or joint fluid) either are not available or are negative for pneumococci, various procedures for obtaining pus from the infected lung must be considered. Cough can be induced by having the patient inhale an aerosol of warm 3 per cent NaCl;

a plastic catheter can be inserted into the trachea via the nose or throat and suction applied; a direct transtracheal needle and catheter aspiration may be performed (a procedure not without complications); the patient may undergo endoscopy (provided the arterial Po_2 is ≥ 50 mm Hg), and alveolar washings or bronchial brushings may be obtained; or rarely, direct aspiration of the pneumonic infiltrate through the chest wall with a long, "skinny" needle (22 gauge) may be employed (a procedure also not without risks). Open lung biopsies for pneumococcal pneumonia are not indicated, although they may be for certain complications, ill-defined superinfections, or underlying diseases. In any acute bacterial pneumonia, the guiding principles for deciding what procedure, if any, to use for obtaining purulent sputum from the involved lung are as follows: (1) If expectorated sputum is satisfactory (i.e., purulent and relatively free of contaminating oropharyngeal material), further efforts to obtain pus from the deeper recesses of the lung are probably not necessary or indicated; (2) if additional procedures are necessary, one should select first the procedure that is least traumatic and invasive and is risk free and then proceed, if necessary, in a stepwise fashion to the next least invasive, risk-free procedure until satisfactory material is obtained; (3) one should not delay more than several hours before beginning chemotherapy, and if the patient is extremely ill, one must rely on clinical judgment and not delay treatment at all; and (4) one must make every effort to identify the etiologic agent (or agents) responsible for the pneumonia early in the course of the illness, since once this goal is realized, the chances of managing the patient successfully are markedly enhanced.

A variety of other tests may be applied to sputum specimens to identify pneumococci in acute bacterial pneumonia; but in skilled hands, few, if any, are better, less costly, easier to do, and more informative than the Gram stain. All tests done on sputum possess a similar problem in interpretation, namely, determining whether or not bacteria present in the sample are responsible for the pneumonia observed. If blood or pleural fluid cultures are subsequently positive for S. pneumoniae, the etiologic agent is confirmed, although the presence of additional pathogenic bacteria within the lung may not be entirely excluded, as, rarely, blood or pleural fluid cultures may yield other bacteria (polymicrobial infection) in addition to pneumococci.

Detection of pneumococcal capsular antigen generally requires the presence of approximately 10^5 bacteria per milliliter, about the same concentration as required to observe an average of one bacterium per $1000\times$ (or an oil immersion field on a standard light microscope) on a Gram stain. Cross-reactions with other antigens of other bacteria are frequent, and with certain serotypes, false-negative results are common. Perhaps the greatest value of capsular antigen detection is to confirm the presence of pneumococci in those patients who have been partially treated and in whom sputum cultures may be negative and a Gram stain may reveal few, if any, intact bacteria.

Colony counts of bacteria from bronchoalveolar lavage (BAL) washings obtained during endoscopy are seldom available early in the course of illness. Specimens must be obtained with a special cuffed endoscope so that oropharyngeal contamination does not occur with insertion of the scope. Generally, counts of colony-forming units (CFU) of bacteria higher than 10^3 to 10^5 per milliliter of fluid removed are considered significant, but this is not invariably so.

DNA hybridization studies may be performed, but as with capsular antigen detection, adequate numbers of bacteria must be present for the test to be positive. Utilization of the polymerase chain reaction (PCR) may amplify pneumococcal DNA and improve the potential for detection; however, such enhanced sensitivity may lead to false-positive tests caused by very small numbers of contaminating pneumococci.

Elastase or elastin fibers in sputum may suggest the presence of a gram-negative bacillary necrotizing pneumonia, particularly that due to Pseudomonas, but this test is of little value in the diagnosis of pneumococcal pneumonia (other than the test should be negative), since necrosis of the lung is not produced by pneumococci.

DIFFERENTIAL DIAGNOSIS (see also Ch. 61 and chapters dealing with specific organisms). The clinical picture and many of the routine laboratory and roentgenographic features associated with pneumococcal pneumonia are often indistinguishable from those of other acute bacterial pneumonias. Thus, collecting appropriate microbiologic data is essential if the correct etiologic diagnosis is to be made.

In adults, the second most common community-acquired, acute bacterial pneumonia is that caused by H. influenzae. The Gram stain of purulent sputum from such patients often reveals myriads of tiny gram-negative coccobacilli, with the observation of an occasional filamentous form. Such an infection often occurs in a patient with chronic bronchitis or chronic obstructive pulmonary disease and usually is due to nonencapsulated H. influenzae (as opposed to highly encapsulated, serotype B strains commonly infecting young children).

Staphylococcus aureus is another bacterium occasionally producing acute pneumonia, but when this kind of pneumonia is community acquired, it usually occurs during or just after an epidemic of viral influenza. In the hospital setting, S. aureus may be seen year round, as it is a commonly occurring nosocomial infection. If a highly virulent, toxin-producing strain is responsible, the "toxic shock syndrome" may be observed. On a Gram stain of purulent sputum, clusters of gram-positive cocci and characteristic tetrads of cocci are seen. Late in the clinical course, abscess formation or destruction of the lung occurs.

Group A streptococci (S. pyogenes) also produce acute pneumonia, and in such instances, the patient may be more toxic appearing than the extent of involvement of the lung might suggest. Classically, a small, peripherally located, wedge-shaped infiltrate is commonly seen, and a thin, watery, serosanguineous pleural effusion is often present. A roentgenogram of the chest may suggest a pulmonary infarction. An upper respiratory tract infection, particularly an exudative or erythematous pharyngitis or tonsillitis (especially in children), may be present; and an erythematous rash produced by streptococcal erythrogenic toxin (scarlet fever) may be seen. A Gram stain of purulent sputum usually reveals numerous short chains of gram-positive cocci or diplococci. Thus, the Gram stain may not differentiate group A streptococcal from pneumococcal pneumonia.

Moraxella catarrhalis, which in the recent past was referred to as Neisseria or Branhamella catarrhalis, may produce acute pneumonia, but usually in the elderly and particularly in those with chronic bronchitis or obstructive lung disease. It is a relatively benign infection, compared with those produced by other pyogenic bacteria, and is rarely, if ever, associated with bacteremia. A Gram stain of purulent sputum is again important, and the diagnosis should probably be made only when numerous gram-negative diplococci, in the absence of other potentially pathogenic bacteria, are seen. N. meningitidis (meningococci) are morphologically similar to M. catarrhalis organisms and must also be included in the differential diagnosis. However, in such instances patients are generally young adults, and the infection is associated with significant toxicity.

Gram-negative bacilli, particularly those belonging to the family Enterobacteriaceae (e.g., E. coli, Klebsiella, Enterobacter, Serratia, and Proteus) must also be considered as causative agents in the differential diagnosis of pneumococcal pneumonia, particularly if the patient is debilitated and is residing in a nursing home or similar institution, and certainly if the patient is hospitalized. Aerobic gram-negative bacilli are often responsible for nosocomial but infrequently for community-acquired pneumonias. This is because gram-negative bacilli rarely colonize the oropharynx of otherwise healthy people in the community, but they are common oropharyngeal residents in debilitated, hospitalized, or institutionalized patients. In addition, the patient in question may exhibit certain risk factors associated with invasion by gram-negative bacilli, such as the receipt of prior antibiotics, corticosteroids, inhalation therapy, or tracheostomy and the existence of profound neutropenia or severe debilitation. The pneumonic process is usually necrotizing, and gas formation may be detected on roentgenograms. A Gram stain of purulent sputum usually reveals many large, bipolar-staining gram-negative rods. Elastin fibrils may also be seen on a KOH preparation of sputum from the site of infection.

Anaerobic bacteria may also produce acute suppurative pneumonia. The anaerobes most frequently involved are Bacteroides species (usually B. melanogenicus), Peptostreptococcus, and Fusobacterium. Frequently, anaerobic infections are polymicrobial and may include bacteria other than strict anaerobes (e.g., *S. aureus*). The occurrence of anaerobic infection is usually preceded by gross aspiration and is enhanced if the individual has anaerobic oral infections or solid tumors of the oropharyngeal structures or tracheobronchial tree (tumors that may outstrip their blood supply, necrose, and provide an ideal anaerobic environment). The clinical presentation of anaerobic pleuropneumonic disease may be indolent rather than abrupt, and it may be accompanied by expectorated sputum or empyemas that have fetid and nauseating odors. (However, the absence of such an odor does not exclude the presence of anaerobes.) As with gram-negative bacillary pneumonias, necrosis of the lung with gas formation may be noted.

Mycoplasma pneumoniae, *Chlamydia*, and *Legionella* may also produce acute pneumonias, which are usually best described as atypical. With mycoplasmal pneumonia, patients are ordinarily young, and prolonged communicability, especially within households, may often be documented. The clinical, radiographic, and pathologic features are usually those of an interstitial pneumonia, rather than lobar consolidation and an alveolar exudative process. Serum cold agglutinin levels may be elevated, and the disease is rarely, if ever, fatal. Chlamydial pneumonia, especially that due to *C. psittaci*, is contracted from infected psittacine birds; or in the case of *C. pneumoniae* or TWAR agent (derived from the designation of the first two isolates, TW-183 and AR-39), infection is acquired from other infected humans. *C. pneumoniae* is the most common species producing chlamydial pneumonia in humans, and the clinical picture is usually that of pharyngitis, often with laryngitis, and segmental pneumonia of a single lobe without pleural effusion. Seroepidemiologic studies reveal a higher prevalence of antibodies in males than females and in older adults than children. Legionnaires' disease, which may be produced by a variety of *Legionella* species but principally by *L. pneumophila*, is associated with considerable systemic toxicity (nausea, vomiting, and diarrhea) and may be very difficult to differentiate from pneumococcal pneumonia. However, in the temperate zones, community-acquired legionnaires' disease is usually seasonal, occurring in the warmer months or summer; patients are typically male construction workers and smokers in their fifties whose clinical manifestations include fever, chills, myalgias, headache, dry cough, and nonspecific pulmonary infiltrates. Anti-*Legionella* fluorescein-labeled antibodies, which may be employed to examine sputum for *Legionella*, as well as antigen detection techniques applied to the urine, may be helpful in the early diagnosis of this disease.

Patients with the acquired immunodeficiency syndrome (AIDS) and acute pneumonia present considerable diagnostic problems. Although pneumococcal pneumonia and infections from encapsulated bacteria occur with greater frequency in patients with AIDS than in normal individuals, pneumocystosis and cytomegalovirus pneumonia occur more frequently than pneumococcal pneumonia in these patients and thus must also be excluded.

Finally, not only does pneumonia due to microbes other than the pneumococcus have to be considered in a differential diagnosis, but also a variety of noninfectious conditions may mimic the clinical picture of pneumococcal pneumonia. Pulmonary infarction, with emboli (e.g., in right-sided endocarditis) or without emboli (e.g., in sickle cell anemia), may present a considerable diagnostic challenge, even after differential lung scanning and pulmonary angiography. Chemical pneumonitis, localized or diffuse (Mendelson's syndrome), often caused by aspiration of gastric juice of low pH, may also be difficult to differentiate from pneumococcal or other bacterial pneumonias; however, in the absence of antibiotic therapy, a Gram stain of purulent sputum consistently reveals a paucity of bacteria.

TREATMENT. All patients with suspected pneumococcal pneumonia should be treated as promptly as possible with an effective antimicrobial agent. One should not wait for cultural confirmation of the diagnosis to initiate therapy. Although many patients may recover without antibacterial therapy, effective antimicrobial agents reduce morbidity, mortality, and complications.

At present, *penicillin G* is the therapy of choice, and it is the standard against which all other antipneumococcal agents are compared. Susceptible strains exhibit an MIC of less than 0.1 μg per milliliter, levels that are easily achieved in a variety of tissues with therapeutic dosing of 1.2 to 2.4 million units per day. If

complicating pneumococcal bacteremia occurs, only 10 to 15 per cent of untreated patients may be expected to survive; this figure may be increased to 85 to 90 per cent with penicillin G treatment. A variety of other penicillins or related beta-lactam antibiotics are also effective and may be used in special circumstances, as when bacteria other than or in addition to pneumococci are seriously considered in the differential diagnosis or when penicillin-resistant pneumococci are present. Ideally, initial therapy should be parenteral to ensure delivery and adequate serum and tissue levels. If the patient is in shock or has heart failure, the route of delivery should be intravenous. Later in the course of therapy, if the patient's progress is good, the route of administration may be changed to oral. Treatment with any effective agent should be for at least 5 to 7 days.

For patients who are believed to be allergic to penicillin, a variety of other antibacterial agents may be used. Usually, a first-generation cephalosporin is selected, since its molecular configuration is slightly different from that of penicillin G (a six-membered thiazole ring rather than a five-membered one) and since the frequency of serious reactions due to cross-allergenicity appears to be low. However, careful observation of the penicillin-allergic patient during the initial use of a cephalosporin must still be made, since the threat of a serious side effect exists. If the patient has a clear history of a type I (immediate) hypersensitivity reaction, all beta-lactams should be avoided. For such patients, erythromycin is an excellent choice, even though an increasing frequency of resistance (MIC $\geq$ 1.0 μg per millileter) to erythromycin is being observed worldwide. Tetracyclines should be avoided because the frequency of resistant strains is often widespread and high (up to 80 per cent of isolates in some parts of the world). Similarly, quinolones should also not be used because concentrations at which most strains are susceptible are too high to predict a satisfactory outcome.

With the advent of penicillin-resistant pneumococci (see above), different strategies of therapy may have to be devised on the basis of susceptibility or resistance to other agents (Table 292–4). At present, in the United States, such strains are infrequent, sporadic, localized to certain geographic areas, and generally of intermediate resistance (MIC between 0.1 and 2.0 μg per milliliter). Nevertheless, each locale or hospital needs to monitor its own isolates, and therapeutic strategies should be based on these results. If strains are intermediate in resistance, simply increasing the dose of penicillin G to 6 million units per day will suffice (unless the complication of meningitis or endocarditis exists). However, if strains highly resistant to penicillin G (MIC $\geq$ 2.0 μg per milliliter) are repeatedly or frequently isolated, then penicillin G should not be routinely employed as initial therapy. In fact, such highly resistant isolates are generally resistant to most other beta-lactam antibiotics (see Table 292–1), as well as many other antimicrobials, so that agents such as vancomycin, teicoplanin, or rifampin may have to be used (with or without empiric penicillin) until the results of susceptibility data are available. Among currently available beta-lactams, cefotaxime, ceftriaxone, and imipenem appear to be most active against highly resistant pneumococci (see Table 292–1).

If effective antibacterial therapy is employed, the patient's temperature usually falls to or below normal by crisis within 24

TABLE 292–4. CRITERIA FOR RESISTANCE OF *S. PNEUMONIAE* TO SOME COMMONLY USED ANTIBIOTICS*

Antibacterial Agent	MIC (μg/ml)†
Penicillin G	
Intermediate	$\geq$0.1
High level	$\geq$2.0
Erythromycin	$\geq$1.0
Trimethoprim/sulfamethoxazole	$\geq$1/19
Tetracycline	$\geq$8.0
Rifampin	$\geq$2.0
Chloramphenicol	$\geq$8.0

*Based on criteria established by the National Committee for Clinical Laboratory Standards (NCCLS).
†MIC = Minimal inhibitory concentration.

hours. However, in some instances, perhaps because of the nature of the pathology or complications that occur (e.g., pleural effusion), the patient's temperature may fall by lysis over 2 to 3 days. Resolution and recovery from pneumococcal pneumonia generally result in restoration of normal pulmonary architecture. Occasionally, healing may be via fibrosis, in which instance persistence of pulmonary infiltrates on roentgenograms may be evident for months after clinical recovery.

In addition to effective antibacterial therapy, a variety of supportive measures are generally employed in the initial management of acute pneumococcal pneumonia; these include bed rest, monitoring of vital signs and urine output, insertion of a Swan-Ganz catheter to monitor cardiac output, administration of an occasional analgesic to relieve pleuritic pain to permit more effective breathing and coughing, fluid replacement if the patient is dehydrated, electrolyte correction, oxygen therapy, and relief of an ileus with nasal gastric suctioning. In relieving pleuritic pain or in providing sedation in situations requiring it (e.g., delirium tremens), care should be taken not to use excessively high doses that would depress the respiratory center. Intercostal nerve blocks, which do not interfere with respiratory drive, may be employed. In patients with neuromuscular disorders, particularly those involving defective conduction at the myoneural junction, aminoglycosides should be avoided. If possible, antipyretics should also be avoided, since the use of these agents interferes with the evaluation of fever as a measurement of the patient's progress (or lack of).

COMPLICATIONS. Approximately 5 per cent of patients with pneumococcal pneumonia develop an empyema, although a larger per cent (up to 30 per cent) commonly develop sterile pleural effusions. Most effusions resolve with or after successful antibacterial therapy, although empyemas often require drainage. Empyemas usually consist of thick pus composed of fibrin, serous proteins, large numbers of leukocytes and/or their products, and pneumococci. Initially, such collections may be drained by needle aspiration; however, later, as loculations occur, drainage via chest tubes is usually necessary. Chest roentgenograms with lateral decubitus films are often useful in the early recognition of pleural effusions; however, at a later time and in the course of removal and follow-up, ultrasonography and/or computed tomography (CT) may be necessary. In any acute bacterial pneumonia, pleural fluid that has been removed should be subject to a Gram stain, aerobic and anaerobic cultures, pH determination, cell count and differential, protein and sugar analysis, and a lactate dehydrogenase determination.

If pneumococcal bacteremia occurs, extrapulmonary complications, such as *meningitis, septic arthritis,* and *endocarditis,* must be excluded, since their therapy generally requires higher dosages of penicillin G and, in the case of septic arthritis, may require drainage. A spinal tap with examination of cerebrospinal fluid should be done if meningitis is suspected, and multiple pretreatment blood cultures and echocardiography of the heart valves should be obtained if endocarditis is suspected. Other complications that might occur are *pyogenic pericarditis,* which may produce tamponade and require drainage, and *peritonitis* in those with ascites (e.g., cirrhosis or nephrotic syndrome).

PROGNOSIS. The case fatality rate for untreated pneumococcal pneumonia is about 25 per cent, whereas in those treated promptly with penicillin G, it may be less than 5 per cent. Fatality rates differ considerably among patient groups, depending on such factors as presence or absence of bacteremia, multilobe involvement, neutropenia, asplenism, underlying diseases (particularly of the heart or lung), age of the patient (the prognosis being poor at the extremes), complicating extrapulmonary pneumococcal infections (e.g., meningitis), the occurrence of shock, the serotype of pneumococcus responsible (type 3 being highly virulent), delayed therapy, penicillin susceptibility or resistance, and prior immunization with polyvalent pneumococcal vaccine. However, it is noteworthy that since the advent of penicillin G in the 1940's (but prior to widespread use of the pneumococcal vaccine) the case fatality rate of pneumococcal pneumonia and bacteremia remains essentially unchanged.

PREVENTION. At present, the single most important preventive measure that is readily available is polyvalent pneumococcal vaccine. This vaccine contains 23 antigenic capsular poly-

saccharide types, which in the United States account for up to 90 per cent of bacteremic infections. In immunocompetent populations, it is estimated to be 80 per cent protective, inducing antibodies of the IgG2 subclass, which enhance opsonization, phagocytosis, and killing of pneumococci by polymorphonuclear leukocytes and fixed macrophages. It is virtually free of life-threatening side effects, and obviously it cannot produce a pneumococcal infection in itself, since it contains no viable, intact pneumococci. About 15 to 30 per cent of patients who receive the vaccine may develop fever, localized swelling, and/or pain at the injection site. As with all polysaccharide vaccines, it is poorly immunogenic in infants and may be less immunogenic in the very elderly and in those with a variety of conditions generally associated with poor vaccine responsiveness (e.g., those having uremia, hemodialysis, previously treated Hodgkin's disease, multiple myeloma, AIDS, and splenic dysfunction syndromes, as well as immunosuppressed transplant recipients, to name a few). Nevertheless, the vaccine should probably be given to immunodeficient patients, as mortality may still be reduced in a significant number of vaccine recipients. In normal individuals, if antibodies result from vaccination, they usually persist for more than 5 years and possibly for life. At present, new vaccines in which the capsular antigens are conjugated to proteins are under development and may prove more immunogenic.

The U.S. Public Health Service specifically recommends the currently available pneumococcal vaccine for patients with underlying conditions that are associated with increased susceptibility to pneumococcal infections or increased risk of mortality from such infections, namely, healthy adults 65 years or older and those with chronic cardiac or pulmonary diseases, anatomic or functional asplenia, chronic liver disease, alcoholism, diabetes mellitus, and cerebrospinal fluid leaks. In addition, although antibody responsiveness may be less than desirable, recommendations for receipt of the vaccine also are made for those with chronic renal failure or those on hemodialysis, for those with Hodgkin's disease, chronic lymphocytic leukemia, multiple myeloma, and AIDS; or for those receiving or about to receive chemotherapy for cancer, organ transplantation, or splenectomy.

Antibiotic prophylaxis with penicillin G or similar agents in otherwise healthy patients with viral upper respiratory infections is not routinely indicated, is not cost effective, and may only lead to superinfections with antibiotic-resistant bacteria or to adverse side effects from the antibiotic itself. However, in individuals with seriously compromised pulmonary, cardiac, or immune function, a narrow-spectrum agent, such as penicillin G, may be given in low dosages during a viral syndrome for a limited time to reduce the risk of morbidity and mortality from potentially invasive pneumococci. Such prophylaxis may especially apply to those in households where pneumococcal infections recently occurred.

Finally, it should be appreciated that pneumococcal infections, including pneumonia, are generally not acquired by otherwise normal people from exposure to other patients with pneumococcal pneumonia; thus patients with pneumococcal pneumonia do not require isolation, and prophylaxis for medical staff exposed to such infections is not indicated.

Austrian R: Prevention of pneumococcal infection by immunization with capsular polysaccharides of *Streptococcus pneumoniae*: Current status of polysaccharide vaccines. J Infect Dis 136(Suppl):S38, 1977. *A review of early and more recent studies of successes and difficulties with pneumococcal vaccines by a real authority.*

Austrian R: Life with the Pneumococcus. Notes from the Bedside, Laboratory, and Library. Philadelphia, University of Pennsylvania Press, 1985. *An array of interesting observations, both clinical and laboratory, on pneumococcal infections by an outstanding authority and the father of the modern capsular polysaccharide pneumococcal vaccine.*

Austrian R, Gold J: Pneumococcal bacteremia with especial reference to bacteremic pneumococcal pneumonia. Ann Intern Med 60:759, 1964. *A landmark clinical study that clearly points out the major risk factors involved in pneumococcal pneumonia and bacteremia.*

Burman LA, Norrby R, Trollfors B: Invasive pneumococcal infections: Incidence, predisposing factors, and prognosis. Rev Infect Dis 7:133, 1985. *An analysis of 494 Swedish patients with 508 culturally confirmed pneumococcal infections.*

Coonrod JD: Pneumococcal pneumonia. Semin Respir Infect 4:4, 1989.

Finland M, Barnes MW: Changes in occurrence of capsular serotypes of *Streptococcus pneumoniae* at Boston City Hospital during selected years between 1935 and 1974. J Clin Microbiol 5:154, 1977. *A thorough study of the distribution of pneumococcal serotypes in bacteremia, empyema, and meningitis useful for a complete understanding of vaccine efficacy by world-renowned investigators in the field of pneumococcal disease.*

Heffron R: Pneumonia, with Special Reference to Pneumococcal Lobar Pneumonia. New York, Commonwealth Fund, 1939. *Complete descriptions of the natural history of patients with pneumococcal pneumonia during the preantibiotic era.*

Hook EW III, Horton CA, Schaberg DR: Failure of intensive care unit support to influence mortality from pneumococcal bacteremia. JAMA 249:1055, 1983. *A clinical study that reveals that even intensive care and special units have not influenced the survival rate in pneumococcal pneumonia and bacteremia since the advent of penicillin, thus further emphasizing the need for prevention.*

Jabes D, Nachman S, Tomaz A: Penicillin-binding protein families: Evidence for the clonal nature of penicillin resistance in clinical isolates of pneumococci. J Infect Dis 159:16, 1989. *A study of the molecular abnormalities and mechanisms involved in penicillin-resistant pneumococci by some of the leading investigators in this field.*

Klugman KP: Pneumococcal resistance to antibiotics. Clin Microbiol Rev 3:171, 1990. *A complete, in-depth microbiologic, epidemiologic, and clinical review, evaluation, and update of the problem of penicillin resistance by an authority with considerable experience with such isolates.*

Palmer DL, Jones CC: Diagnosis of pneumococcal pneumonia. Semin Respir Infect 3:131, 1988. *A thorough review of the issues complicating the diagnosis of pneumococcal pneumonia and an update on tests that might be helpful in the future.*

293 Mycoplasmal Infections

Stephen G. Baum

In the late 1930's, a group of pneumonias was delineated that did not resemble typical bacterial lobar pneumonia. Because the cause of the pneumonias was unknown, and because the radiographic appearance and low mortality distinguished these cases from pneumococcal and other bacterial respiratory infections, these were called *primary atypical pneumonias.* In the 1950's, the organism responsible for many cases of so-called atypical pneumonia was isolated by Eaton and was shown to be similar to one causing pleuropneumonia in cattle; hence the names Eaton agent and pleuropneumonia-like organisms (PPLO). In 1962, this agent was reclassified as *Mycoplasma pneumoniae.*

The most significant human infections caused by mycoplasmas are diseases of the respiratory tract, including pharyngitis, tracheobronchitis, and pneumonia. Also, one species of mycoplasmas, *Mycoplasma hominis,* and a closely related organism, *Ureaplasma,* have been etiologically implicated in some diseases of the human urogenital tract and in respiratory disease of the neonate.

The high incidence of mycoplasmal infection is not generally appreciated. Factors responsible for this include lack of familiarity with mycoplasmal syndromes; the absence of specific, rapid tests for diagnosis in the early phases of these diseases; and the relative difficulty of growing the organisms in the diagnostic laboratory.

Accurate etiologic diagnosis of mycoplasmal diseases, however, is of considerable clinical importance. Mycoplasmal infections do not respond to the antimicrobial therapies usually used for respiratory or genital infections, but treatment with erythromycins or tetracyclines leads to amelioration of symptoms, decrease in the likelihood of spread, and eventually, true microbiologic cure.

DESCRIPTION OF THE ORGANISM AND RELATIONSHIP TO PATHOGENESIS. The mycoplasmas, members of the class Mollicutes, represent the smallest free-living forms, i.e., they do not require host cells for replication. For many years the question of whether these organisms were viruses or bacteria was debated. However, it appears that they are neither, and there is no significant DNA similarity between mycoplasmas and any known bacterium or virus.

The average diameter of mycoplasmas (125 to 150 nm) is in the size range of large viruses. They have no cell wall but are bounded by a limiting membrane containing lipid. Absence of a cell wall renders them susceptible to lysis by hypotonic solutions but insensitive to cell wall–active antibiotics, such as the penicillins. Mycoplasmas and *Ureaplasma* can be grown on agar supplemented with serum proteins and sterols. Most *Mycoplasma* species form 200- to 300-μm colonies, which look much like a fried egg. They have a peripheral halo and a thicker central portion lying just below the surface of the agar. *M. pneumoniae* colonies, however, lack the halo and resemble a mulberry. When

M. pneumoniae is grown on agar containing mammalian erythrocytes, it rapidly produces a clear zone of hemolysis similar to β-hemolysis of some bacteria. *M. pneumoniae* also differs from many other mycoplasmas in that it grows more slowly, ferments glucose to produce acid, adsorbs red cells to growing colonies, and reduces the dye tetrazolium under aerobic conditions. All of these characteristics have been exploited to establish a rapid microbiologic diagnosis.

When mycoplasmas contaminate tissue culture systems, as they often do, they are found intracellularly. This fact has led to speculation about the mechanisms of persistence of these organisms in vivo. However, electron microscopic studies using tracheal organ culture systems have demonstrated most of the infecting organisms extracellularly at the base of the cilia of epithelial cells.

Two properties of *M. pneumoniae* seem to correlate extremely well with its pathogenicity in humans. *M. pneumoniae* has a selective affinity for respiratory epithelial cells and produces hydrogen peroxide. The H_2O_2 is thought to be responsible for much of the initial cell disruption in the respiratory tract. H_2O_2 also causes damage to erythrocyte membranes. In the laboratory, this damage results in hemolysis and, in the patient, may alter erythrocyte antigens, thereby stimulating cold agglutinins. These agglutinins appear in the serum of over 50 per cent of patients who develop mycoplasmal pneumonia and are capable of clumping red blood cells in vitro at 4°C. They are different from cold precipitins or cryoglobulins occurring in other diseases. Cold agglutinins are immunoglobulin M (IgM) antibodies directed at the I antigen on the surface of normal erythrocytes. There is increasing evidence that cold agglutinins are antibodies to a glycolipid in the membrane of *M. pneumoniae,* which happens to cross-react with a similar erythrocyte antigen. Cold agglutinins occur rarely in other diseases, including influenza and adenoviral pneumonia.

RESPIRATORY DISEASES CAUSED BY *M. pneumoniae*

DEFINITION. Respiratory infection by *M. pneumoniae* may be asymptomatic or may lead to inflammation of the upper airways (pharyngitis or tracheitis) or lower respiratory tract (bronchitis or pneumonia). In the vast majority of cases, disease is self-limited, but proper antibiotic therapy can shorten the duration of symptoms.

EPIDEMIOLOGY. Each year about one of every thousand people in the United States experiences mycoplasmal pneumonia. The incidence of all other mycoplasmal upper and lower respiratory infections is probably 10 times that of mycoplasmal pneumonia. One quarter to three quarters of all pneumonias occurring in "closed" populations (military recruit camps, boarding schools, and colleges) are caused by *M. pneumoniae.* Patients with hypogammaglobulinemia may have increased susceptibility, and *M. pneumoniae* infection may often exacerbate bronchial asthma.

Mycoplasmal respiratory infection is most common in children and young adults, with a peak incidence in the age range of 5 to 20 years; however, infants and elderly patients are also infected. Distribution is worldwide. Although documented epidemics have occurred primarily in the fall months, this disease does not have the marked seasonal predominance that is found with influenza.

Infection is spread from person to person by respiratory secretions expelled during bouts of coughing. The organism is present in these secretions for several days prior to the onset of symptoms and peaks in titer in the sputum during the first week of clinical illness. *M. pneumoniae* organisms persist in the sputum, albeit in reduced numbers, for weeks after the cessation of appropriate antimicrobial therapy.

In open populations under nonepidemic conditions, the infection seems to be spread most easily among playmates and within the household. The index case is usually a child. The majority of households having an index case will experience secondary infections, and the majority of susceptible family members become infected, with resultant symptomatic disease or asymptomatic seroconversion.

In comparison with viral respiratory disease, the incubation period for mycoplasmal infection is relatively long, averaging 2 to 3 weeks. Therefore, unless two or more people from a household are simultaneously infected from an index case, it is unusual for several family members to be ill at the same time, and the disease may take several months to run its course through a household.

CLINICAL PRESENTATIONS. Mycoplasmal infection of the upper airways is impossible to distinguish clinically from infection by other agents. On the other hand, mycoplasmal pneumonia has several characteristics that may help the physician to diagnose this disease (Fig. 293–1). The onset of mycoplasmal pneumonia is usually insidious, in contrast to the abrupt onset of adenoviral or influenzal pneumonia. Mild fever is usually the first sign of infection. The hallmark of the disease is severe, disabling, paroxysmal cough, which usually becomes prominent 2 or 3 days after the onset of fever and often requires narcotic medication for suppression. Although usually nonproductive, the cough may yield small amounts of whitish sputum. Occasionally, the sputum may contain flecks of blood, but grossly purulent sputum and marked hemoptysis are rare. Production of purulent or bloody sputum is actually more prevalent in tracheobronchitis than in pneumonia.

Headache occurs commonly in conjunction with the cough. During the first week of illness, many patients complain of burning soreness in the chest, though true pleuritic pain is uncommon. Fever rarely exceeds 39.5° C (102 to 103° F), and mild myalgias and malaise occur early in the disease. A history of shaking chills, severe myalgias, or gastrointestinal complaints is unusual.

On physical examination, the pharynx may be slightly injected or inflamed. Much diagnostic emphasis has been placed on the presence of bullous myringitis in patients with mycoplasmal respiratory disease. This finding was noted in fewer than 25 per cent of volunteers experimentally infected with M. pneumoniae and is very rare in naturally occurring mycoplasmal infection. Bacteria are much more commonly cultured than are M. pneumoniae from patients with bullous myringitis, and the relationship between M. pneumoniae infection and bullous myringitis or otitis remains tenuous.

Examination of the chest usually fails to show signs of dense consolidation or fluid accumulation. Auscultation reveals fine rales either unilaterally or bilaterally, which are often not very impressive. Findings from the remainder of the physical examination are usually normal.

The radiographic appearance of the lungs frequently presents a surprise. There is marked patchy infiltration of the lungs consistent with extensive interstitial pneumonia; bilateral involvement is evident in about one quarter of the patients. Infiltration is most prominent at the base of the lungs, although mycoplasmal pneumonia can be seen in any pulmonary segment. There may be slight blunting of the costovertebral angle on the affected side (or sides) in 10 to 20 per cent of patients, but large pleural effusions are rare. If thoracentesis is performed, it yields a serous or serosanguineous transudative fluid.

COMPLICATIONS. Spread of infection within the lung and pleural effusions are the most common pulmonary complications. Involvement of a number of extrapulmonary sites has been attributed to infection with M. pneumoniae, usually occurring as complications of pulmonary disease. Occasionally, they have been seen without pneumonia, and mycoplasmal causation has been substantiated on the basis of culture of the organism from involved organs, fourfold or greater rises in mycoplasma-specific antibodies, or demonstration (described later) of less specific cold hemagglutinins.

Three extrapulmonary complications are relatively common (occurring in 2 to 10 per cent of seriously ill patients). These deserve comment because, when present, they help to confirm the diagnosis of mycoplasmal pneumonia.

Erythema Multiforme Major (Stevens-Johnson Syndrome). Some patients with mycoplasmal pneumonia develop blistering lesions involving the mouth, eyes, and skin. Usually, although the lesions look quite severe, they heal with minimal scarring. However, when the cornea is involved, blindness may ensue, and local and systemic steroid therapy is often recommended in these instances. This dermatologic syndrome has many causes, including adverse reaction to drugs. When, however, it occurs in conjunction with interstitial pneumonia in a child or young adult, its presence helps confirm the clinical diagnosis of mycoplasmal pneumonia.

The pathogenesis of this syndrome is unknown. There is one report of isolation of M. pneumoniae from skin lesions, but most authorities consider Stevens-Johnson syndrome an allergic reaction. A great variety of other skin rashes in mycoplasmal pneumonia have been described, but these are not diagnostically helpful.

Raynaud's Phenomenon. A second syndrome, occurring in fewer than 5 per cent of mycoplasmal pneumonia patients, is Raynaud's phenomenon. This consists of painful blanching of the distal parts of fingers and toes upon exposure to cold and may occur whether or not the patient has a history of Raynaud's phenomenon unrelated to mycoplasmal infection. The pathogenesis of this complication in M. pneumoniae infection is unknown. However, it is tempting to hypothesize that high titers of cold hemagglutinins could play a role by creating minute thrombi in

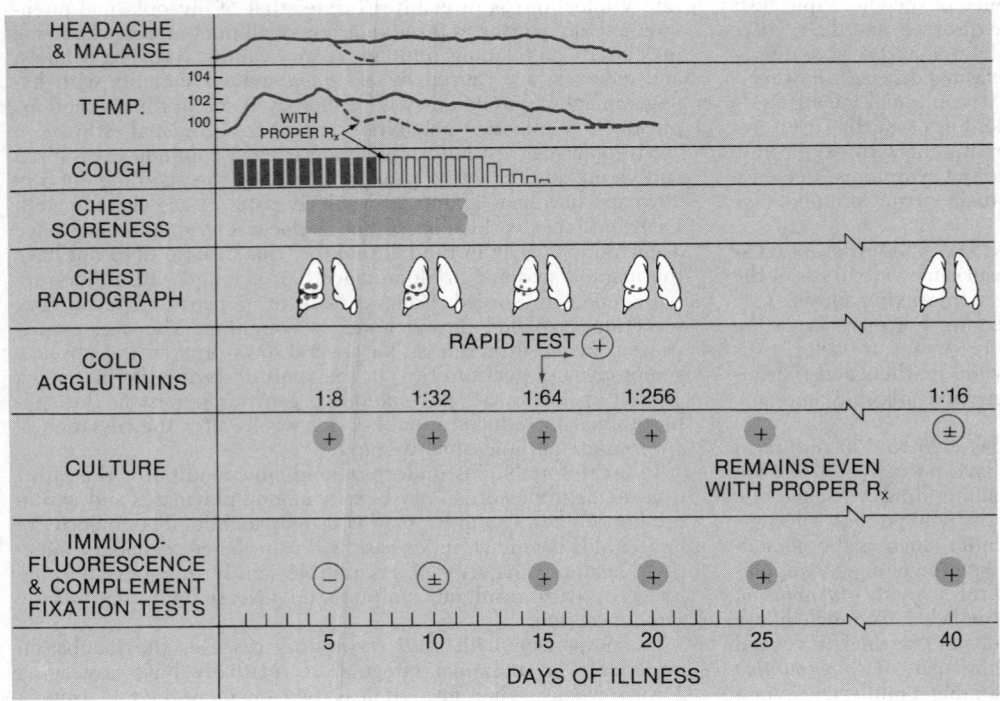

FIGURE 293–1. Major clinical manifestations of mycoplasmal pneumonia.

the microcirculation of the distal extremities when exposed to cold. Patients with sickle cell disease may have particularly severe symptoms when they contract mycoplasmal pneumonia. In the presence of extremely high titers of cold agglutinins (1:20,000), gangrene of the distal parts of fingers and toes in these patients has been reported.

Hemolysis. Patients with cold agglutinin titers of greater than 1:500 may experience rapid and severe hemolysis with decreases of 50 per cent in hematocrit. This complication occurs in fewer than 5 per cent of patients in the second or third week of illness.

LESS COMMON COMPLICATIONS. Among the organ systems reported to be rarely involved in mycoplasmal infection are the cardiovascular, skeletal, and central nervous systems. In a very few cases involving each of these systems, the organism has been cultured directly from the affected organ.

NEUROLOGIC COMPLICATIONS. Aseptic meningitis, meningoencephalitis, cranial nerve neuritis, peripheral neuritis, Guillain-Barré syndrome, transverse myelitis, and psychosis all have been reported as complications of *M. pneumoniae* infection. Most often, etiologic diagnosis is made on the basis of exclusion of other agents and antibody response to *M. pneumoniae*. Spinal fluid cell counts and glucose and protein levels are extremely variable in these cases, ranging from normal to patterns consistent with aseptic meningitis. In some cases, elevated cerebrospinal fluid proteins were found to contain antibodies to *M. pneumoniae*, but these often paralleled serum antibody levels, and it was unclear whether or not cerebrospinal fluid antibody represented diffusion from the serum. There are only two or three reports of isolation of *M. pneumoniae* from cerebrospinal fluid or neural tissue, and the prevailing hypothesis is that mycoplasmal central nervous system disease occurs on the basis of allergic reaction.

Patients with neurologic complications seem to have greater mortality than is commonly associated with mycoplasmal disease. This could either signify a group of patients at increased risk of death from mycoplasmal infection or, alternatively, support the hypothesis that these patients had a second (concurrent) undiagnosed disease with greater inherent mortality.

CARDIOVASCULAR COMPLICATIONS. Pericarditis and myocarditis are the most commonly reported cardiovascular complications of mycoplasmal infection. In general, the major criteria of heart disease have been congestive failure and abnormal electrocardiographic results. Large pericardial effusions have not occurred. There have been a few deaths during the acute phase of the disease, but recovery without sequelae is the rule. In most cases documentation of *M. pneumoniae* infection has been made by noting seroconversion. In one retrospective study based on seroconversion, 8 per cent of patients with *M. pneumoniae* infection had evidence of pericarditis or myocarditis. The average age of these patients was 46 years, considerably greater than the mean for patients with *M. pneumoniae* infection.

MUSCULOSKELETAL COMPLICATIONS. Arthralgias are common in association with mycoplasmal pneumonia, but frank arthritis is rare. When it does occur, arthritis may continue long after the other manifestations of mycoplasmal infection are gone. Large joints seem to be preferentially affected, and the arthritis may be migratory. *Mycoplasma* has not been cultured from joint fluid of immunocompetent patients.

M. pneumoniae and other mycoplasmas have been implicated as the causative agents of a number of other connective tissue diseases, including rheumatoid arthritis, juvenile rheumatoid arthritis, and Reiter's syndrome. Nonhuman mycoplasmas have been shown to cause arthritis in the animals they infect, and *M. pneumoniae* has been cultured on several occasions from the joints of immunocompromised patients. To date, however, there is no evidence that human mycoplasmas cause joint disease, except perhaps as an acute complication of pneumonia.

CLINICAL COURSE. Mycoplasmal respiratory disease is almost invariably self-limited and very rarely results in death. In the absence of treatment, upper respiratory infection usually lasts 1 to 3 weeks, and pneumonia may persist from 4 to 6 weeks. Recovery is gradual, with clinical improvement preceding roentgenographic clearing. Development of any of the severe cardiovascular, dermatologic, hematologic, or neurologic complications described earlier may prolong resolution. Proper treatment, which is often not begun until other antibiotics have failed, would appear to shorten the duration of symptoms by about one half. Results might be even better if treatment were begun earlier.

Relapse occurs in 5 to 10 per cent of patients. In most cases, these patients have received courses of therapy less than 2 weeks in duration.

Two groups of patients commonly appear to develop severe disease. The first group consists of infants who, until recently, were thought not to be particularly susceptible to *M. pneumoniae* infection. Many infants develop severe respiratory distress requiring intubation and supported respiration. Fortunately, despite severe illness the prognosis for these children is excellent. The second group comprises patients with sickle cell disease. In addition to digital gangrene, these patients are prone to develop large multilobar pneumonias and pleural effusions. The possibility of mycoplasmal infection should be considered in a patient with sickle cell crisis and interstitial pneumonia.

PATHOLOGY. Since death is rare in patients with mycoplasmal pneumonia, descriptions of pathologic changes in this disease rest on a very small number of specimens. The tracheobronchial tree and lungs are generally hyperemic. There is evidence of interstitial pneumonia with engorged lungs consistent with the findings on radiographs. Cellular infiltrate, usually minimal, consists mostly of mononuclear elements. Tracheal organ culture systems have been used to demonstrate that infection with *M. pneumoniae* causes a marked decrease of ciliary action, followed by complete loss of cilia and sloughing of epithelial cells.

IMMUNITY. There are varied antibody responses to infection with *M. pneumoniae*. It is unclear what role these immune responses play in the pathogenesis of, and recovery from, infection. Secretory immunoglobulin A (IgA) antibody is thought to be the most protective immunoglobulin in this disease. Individual immunity may be relatively short lived, and there are well-documented instances of recurrent disease within 2 to 10 years following primary infection.

DIAGNOSIS. A clinical diagnosis of mycoplasmal pneumonia should be seriously entertained whenever interstitial pneumonia occurs in a young adult. Examination of the Gram-stained sputum is helpful in that it reveals inflammation but no bacterial organisms. The peripheral leukocyte count may be normal or slightly elevated. There is minimal shift toward immature forms, and mild lymphopenia may exist. The diagnosis is substantiated by finding a cold agglutinin titer greater than 1:32 in the serum.

Hospital bacteriology or serology laboratories titrate cold agglutinins in the patient's serum using Rh-positive, type O erythrocytes to avoid reactions due to major blood group isoantibodies present in the patient's serum. However, a simple, rapid bedside procedure for finding cold agglutinins can be performed using only the patient's blood. One milliliter of freshly drawn blood is placed in a tube containing anticoagulant. The tube used for prothrombin determinations is suitable. The tube is chilled on ice for 2 or 3 minutes and then gently rotated in a horizontal position. Development of small clumps of erythrocytes, similar to those seen when typing blood, which disappear on warming the tube between the hands, indicates the presence of cold agglutinins. The agglutination-dissociation cycle can be repeated many times with the same blood sample. This differentiates the reaction from direct hemagglutination by viruses—a process that generally cannot be recycled. A positive test result correlates with a cold agglutinin titer of 1:64 or greater. When the cold agglutinin titer is extremely high, an easily dissociable clot may form in the tube. Blood from a patient with an unrelated disease should be used as a control. Cold agglutinins are usually found during the second and third weeks of illness and may peak 1 month or more after the onset of symptoms.

Diagnosis of mycoplasmal pneumonia should be further supported by finding rising titers of specific antibodies to the *Mycoplasma* organism. These can be measured by complement fixation, inhibition of metabolism, indirect hemagglutination, or immunofluorescence techniques. In addition, patients with mycoplasmal pneumonia may develop a false-positive test result for syphilis.

Definitive diagnosis of mycoplasmal pneumonia rests, however, on coupling an antibody rise with culturing *M. pneumoniae* from sputum. Although growth on agar may take 2 to 3 weeks, rendering results useless for initiating drug therapy, a more rapid (3 to 4 days) presumptive diagnosis can be based on the use of a diphasic medium available in some diagnostic laboratories.

DIFFERENTIAL DIAGNOSIS. The most common respiratory infections mimicking mycoplasmal pneumonia are influenza and adenoviral and *Legionella* pneumonia. These tend to be more fulminant in onset and are associated with more severe systemic symptoms and greater respiratory insufficiency. Patients with legionnaires' disease are likely to be older men with a history of smoking. Confusion and gastrointestinal disturbance are common in *Legionella* pneumonia. Often one cannot definitively distinguish between these diseases, and a therapeutic trial with erythromycin (which also is used to treat *Legionella pneumophila*) may be warranted. Psittacosis and ornithosis (chlamydial diseases) and Q fever (a rickettsial disease) should also be considered in the diagnosis. In such cases, history of exposure to birds on the one hand and to cattle on the other may prove diagnostically helpful.

THERAPY. Treatment with appropriate antibiotics can terminate symptoms abruptly and usually must be begun on the basis of clinical diagnosis. Penicillins, cephalosporins, and aminoglycosides, such as streptomycin, kanamycin, and gentamicin, have little or no effect against these organisms.

M. pneumoniae is sensitive in vitro and in vivo to erythromycin and to the tetracyclines. These agents appear to be equally effective in diminishing the symptoms of the disease. Because there are fewer adverse effects, especially in children under age 10 years, erythromycin is preferred. The dosage for either drug is 250 to 500 mg four times daily for 2 to 3 weeks. Although erythromycin and the tetracyclines are effective in ending symptoms, *M. pneumoniae* can be isolated from the sputum of patients for several weeks after the onset of therapy. The mechanism of persistence is unknown but does not depend on the emergence of drug-resistant organisms.

PREVENTION. The frequency of mycoplasmal infection makes the development of a vaccine an attractive objective. Inactivated vaccines, while producing rises in serum antibody levels, give little protection.

The possible role of IgA antibodies in combating disease has prompted the trial of intranasally administered vaccines using live temperature-sensitive (ts) mutants of *M. pneumoniae*. The rationale was that these mutants would induce a localized nasopharyngeal immune response but would not replicate in the warmer lower respiratory tree and cause disease. The results of initial trials of these vaccines have been variable.

GENITAL AND NEONATAL INFECTION BY MYCOPLASMA AND UREAPLASMA

INTRODUCTION. One strain of human mycoplasmas, *M. hominis*, and a closely related organism, *Ureaplasma urealyticum*, frequently colonize the male and female genital tracts. During the past decade, there has been increasing interest in discovering the role these organisms might play in causing disease of the genitourinary system in adults and pulmonary and central nervous system disease in infants.

EPIDEMIOLOGY. *M. hominis* and ureaplasmas can be included in the group of venereally transmitted infectious agents. Infants are colonized during birth, but carriage of the organism is lost during the first year of life. After this, the prevalence of colonization increases with age and sexual experience, as it does for other sexually transmitted organisms. At all ages, females seem to be more readily colonized than males, and colonization is found most frequently in patients from lower socioeconomic groups. *U. urealyticum* carriage may decrease with increasing age over 40 and with hypoestrogenism.

CLINICAL PRESENTATIONS. *M. hominis, U. urealyticum*, or both organisms have been implicated in nongonococcal urethritis (NGU) and inflammatory disease of the prostate, vagina, cervix, upper urinary tract, and female pelvic organs. In addition, colonization by one or both of these organisms has been associated with male and female infertility, habitual abortion, and recurrent production of premature and underweight infants.

INFECTION OF THE LOWER URINARY TRACT. Chlamydia are responsible for a large percentage of cases of NGU. *U. urealyticum* is probably the cause of many of the remaining cases of NGU. Evidence for this stems from the many patients with NGU from whom ureaplasmas are cultured and from these patients' poor clinical response to treatment with sulfa drugs, to which chlamydia are susceptible and to which *Ureaplasma* is not. *M. hominis* probably does not cause urethritis.

INFECTION OF THE UPPER URINARY TRACT. *M. hominis* has been isolated from the kidneys and ureters of patients with clinical pyelonephritis. Antibody to the organism was detected in serum and urine from some of these patients, providing moderately strong evidence that *M. hominis* causes some cases of pyelonephritis. *U. urealyticum* infection may infrequently play a role in urinary calculus formation.

INFECTION OF THE FEMALE GENITAL TRACT. *M. hominis* probably causes a small proportion of the cases of vaginitis and cervicitis. Infection of the uterus and fallopian tubes with this organism has also been documented. *Ureaplasma* rarely, if ever, causes infection in the female pelvis.

MYCOPLASMAS AND REPRODUCTIVE ABNORMALITIES. *U. urealyticum* has been cultured from the sperm of males with fertility disorders. Treatment to eradicate *Ureaplasma* has resulted in increased motility and number of sperm as well as improved morphology. However, recent studies do not indicate a causal role for ureaplasmas in infertility.

Ureaplasma has also been isolated from the internal organs of the products of conception of patients with repeated spontaneous abortions. In addition, in some studies *U. urealyticum* was more often isolated from the genital tracts of women with this syndrome than from control populations. Finally, treatment with tetracycline prior to conception in women with a history of habitual abortion has been reported to increase fetal salvage rate. Unfortunately, few if any of these studies took into account the presence of chlamydia, which might have been responsible for the reproductive disorders.

LOW BIRTH WEIGHT. Prior to the realization that tetracycline is contraindicated in pregnancy, it was shown that tetracycline treatment of mothers who habitually gave birth to underweight fetuses would increase birth weight. In addition, vaginal colonization by ureaplasmas was correlated with decreased birth weight. However, these studies did not take into account the presence or absence of chlamydia. Despite numerous studies, the relationship of genital mycoplasmal colonization to prematurity and abortion remains controversial.

INFECTION OF NEONATES AND INFANTS. *U. urealyticum* has been the most commonly isolated organism from the upper and lower respiratory tract of premature and low birth weight infants with respiratory disease. Infants colonized or infected with this organism at birth, whether or not they manifested respiratory distress at that time, were significantly more likely to develop chronic lung disease than were noncolonized infants. Infection appeared to occur in utero and was also related to neonatal death. The requirement for oxygen therapy in these neonates may have played a role in the pathogenesis of the chronic lung disease. *M. hominis* was the second most commonly isolated organism in preterm infants, but the relationship to disease appears more tenuous.

U. urealyticum and *M. hominis* have also commonly been cultured from the cerebrospinal fluid of premature infants with meningitis, hydrocephalus, and intraventricular hemorrhage.

PUERPERAL INFECTION. *M. hominis* infection and septicemia have been associated with some cases of postpartum fever. This organism has been found in the blood of up to 10 per cent of women with fever after delivery, and antibody response indicating true infection has been noted in many cases.

THERAPY. Mycoplasmas and *Ureaplasma* are all susceptible to the tetracyclines. *U. urealyticum* is sensitive to erythromycin, but *M. hominis* is not. Spectinomycin, an antimicrobial agent used in cases of penicillin-resistant gonococcal disease, appears to be effective against both *M. hominis* and *U. urealyticum*. Since both *U. urealyticum* and *C. trachomatis* are sensitive to tetracycline, it is recommended that patients with NGU be treated with a tetracycline at a dose of 1 to 2 grams daily for 1 to 2 weeks. The patient should abstain from sexual intercourse during this period, and sexual partners should be evaluated for therapy.

In addition, tetracycline therapy prior to conception and erythromycin therapy during pregnancy should be considered for couples with gestational problems who are shown to harbor *U. urealyticum* in the genitourinary tract.

Episodes of postabortal and puerperal fever are usually self-limited and do not require antimicrobial therapy directed at mycoplasmas. Should such therapy be deemed necessary, tetracycline is the drug of choice.

Couch RB: Mycoplasma diseases. *In* Mandell G, Douglas RG, Bennett JE (eds.): Principles and Practice of Infectious Diseases. 3rd ed. New York, Churchill Livingstone, Inc., 1990, pp 1445–1458. *An up-to-date chapter dealing with both clinical and microbiologic aspects.*

Sanchez PJ, Regan JA: *Ureaplasma urealyticum* colonization and chronic lung disease in low birth weight infants. Pediatr Infect Dis J 7:542, 1988. *A prospective study of the relationship of genital mycoplasmas and neonatal lung diseases.*

Taylor-Robinson D, McCormack WM: The genital mycoplasmas. N Engl J Med 302:1003, 1980; 302:1063, 1980. *A comprehensive two-part article on epidemiology, microbiology, clinical presentation, and therapy.*

Waites KB, Rudd PT, Crouse DT, et al: Chronic *Ureaplasma urealyticum* and *Mycoplasma hominis* infections of central nervous system in preterm infants. Lancet 1:17, 1988. *A study showing the high incidence of congenital mycoplasmal central nervous system infection in the newborn.*

294 Pneumonia Caused by Aerobic Gram-Negative Bacilli

Waldemar G. Johanson, Jr.

Over the past 30 years, the group of organisms known collectively as aerobic gram-negative bacilli (GNB) has assumed an increasing importance in clinical respiratory infections. There is no evidence that this phenomenon is due to a change in the virulence of these organisms. Rather, it is due to changes in the human hosts they infect and, to some degree, to changes in the environment induced by antibiotics and other factors, especially in hospitals. Each of the GNB has its place (or places) in nature. Many are regular inhabitants of the human gastrointestinal tract, while others are found in water or other sites in the environment. None is especially virulent for the respiratory tract of healthy mammalian hosts; all are distinctly inferior to the pneumococcus, for example, in that regard. A careful review of the preantibiotic literature reveals that the presence of these organisms in the respiratory tracts of seriously ill patients is not a recent occurrence; rather, the presence of these organisms was disregarded for many years, an approach that was not unjustified, considering the preeminence of the pneumococcus as a cause of fatal pneumonia prior to the availability of highly efficacious antibiotics. The emergence of GNB as respiratory pathogens in recent years is the result of suppression of more aggressive organisms by effective therapy and the long-term survival of people who would have succumbed to other infections or other processes in an earlier era.

PATHOGENESIS. Pneumonias due to GNB are caused by one of three mechanisms: inhalation of contaminated aerosols, hematogenous infection of the lungs from another primary source of infection, or aspiration of oropharyngeal secretions that are colonized by these organisms.

Contamination of respiratory therapy equipment by GNB, usually *Pseudomonas aeruginosa*, was recognized as a major cause of nosocomial pneumonias in the 1960's. With the advent of disposable nebulizers and other control strategies, this problem has been largely eliminated, although sporadic outbreaks remind us that continued vigilance is required. However, as a practical matter, pneumonias due to GNB are rarely caused by inhalation of contaminated aerosols today.

The incidence of pneumonia caused by bacteremic spread to the lungs has probably been overestimated in the literature. *P. aeruginosa* causes a distinctive vasculitis involving pulmonary arteries and veins, and pneumonia in adjacent lung units associated with bacteremia, but this is uncommon with other organisms. It is likely that most instances of bacteremia from a nonpulmonary source, such as the gastrointestinal or urinary tract, associated with pulmonary infiltrates, fever, and hypoxemia, represent noncardiogenic pulmonary edema, or the "adult respiratory distress syndrome," and not actual pneumonia. In fact, pneumonia due to this cause is sufficiently uncommon that the presence of gram-negative bacteremia in association with new pulmonary infiltrates should initiate a vigorous search for a primary site of infection outside the lungs before it is concluded that pneumonia is responsible.

Aspiration of oropharyngeal secretions that contain GNB is the usual event leading to pneumonia caused by these organisms. Colonization of the upper respiratory tract with GNB occurs in 10 per cent or fewer of normal people, but the prevalence of such colonization is markedly increased among patients with acute or chronic diseases. Colonization rates are similar among populations with chronic disease, such as alcoholics and residents of skilled nursing facilities, and previously healthy individuals with acute but severe illnesses or trauma; in both types of patient groups, colonization rates approach 50 per cent. Similarly, colonization of the oropharynx by GNB among healthy persons undergoing elective surgical procedures rises from essentially zero to 35 to 50 per cent within 24 hours following surgery. The organisms responsible for colonization vary from one study to another, but only rarely can this sudden acquisition of GNB be attributed to demonstrable environmental sources. Instead, colonization appears to be caused by a translocation of the patient's fecal flora or the transfer of organisms from one patient to another on the hands of personnel. However, the root cause of this colonization is the great susceptibility of ill patients to the acquisition of GNB from the immediate environment.

Healthy people are resistant to the implantation of GNB in the oropharynx; even gargling a broth culture of GNB fails to produce colonization. This difference between healthy and ill people is related to the ability of GNB to adhere to epithelial cells of the oropharynx. Buccal epithelial cells obtained from healthy subjects adhere few GNB during incubation in vitro, while cells obtained from either acutely or chronically ill patients adhere large numbers. The ability of cells to resist adherence by GNB is directly related to the concentration of fibronectin on the cell surface; loss of cell surface fibronectin, whether removed by proteolytic enzymes experimentally in vitro or by endogenous enzymes in vivo, appears to expose binding sites on the cells to which GNB can adhere and thus achieve colonization.

Once established in the oropharynx, GNB multiply, achieve high concentrations in secretions, and are aspirated in small liquid boluses into the lungs (see Ch. 61). Since lung defenses are often impaired by the same underlying conditions that promote changes in cell resistance to adherence and colonization, the ability of the lungs to handle this bacterial inoculum is insufficient and pneumonia results. The specific lung defense mechanism that might be impaired in a given patient varies with the nature of the underlying illness. For example, patients with chronic airway obstruction have impaired mucociliary transport and alveolar hypoxia that hinders the effectiveness of phagocytic cells. Some data suggest that the bronchial abnormalities in these patients allow persistent colonization of the distal airways by potentially pathogenic bacteria, a factor that affords the bacteria the advantage of access to the distal lung. Patients who are neutropenic are remarkably predisposed to develop pneumonias with GNB, a clinical observation that correlates nicely with the experimental finding that swift recruitment of circulating neutrophils into the lungs is a crucial aspect of host defense against *Pseudomonas* infection. Alcoholism seems to predispose to GNB pneumonias in several ways. Malnutrition promotes colonization of the upper tract by GNB, aspiration is facilitated by episodes of impaired consciousness, and acute alcohol intoxication hinders the ability of phagocytes to migrate to the site of inflammation.

Of the many species of gram-negative aerobic bacilli that colonize human hosts, only *Haemophilus influenzae* can be classified as a true respiratory pathogen, if the ability of the organism to produce infections in previously normal individuals is accepted as a reasonable criterion of pathogenicity. All of the others together, including Enterobacteriaceae (*Escherichia coli, Klebsiella, Enterobacter, Serratia,* and *Proteus*), *Pseudomonas,* and *Acinetobacter,* account for 10 to 20 per cent of community-acquired pneumonias, and these occur almost exclusively in patients with serious underlying disease. The genus *Klebsiella* contains four species, of which only *K. pneumoniae* and *K. oxytoca* cause pneumonia; infections due to *K. pneumoniae* are by far the most common.

Pneumonia caused by *Klebsiella* has been held separate from that caused by other gram-negative bacilli largely for historical reasons. It was the first such organism to be recognized as a pulmonary pathogen, and the pneumonia it caused was distinct from that caused by the pneumococcus, especially in its lack of response to early forms of treatment and its predilection to cause upper lobe pneumonias in alcoholic men. However, the classic features of *Klebsiella* pneumonia as described in the earlier literature, such as "currant jelly" sputum (a mixture of blood and mucus), the bulging fissure associated with upper lobe consolidation, and the syndrome of "chronic cavitary pneumonia," are rarely observed today. While *Klebsiella* remains an important pulmonary pathogen, the illness it causes cannot be clinically differentiated from that caused by other aerobic gram-negative bacilli, and its treatment is similar.

CLINICAL MANIFESTATIONS. Pneumonias caused by GNB may be community acquired or hospital acquired (nosocomial). Virtually all patients with community-acquired pneumonias caused by GNB have serious underlying chronic illnesses, especially chronic obstructive lung disease, alcoholism, or malignancy. Nosocomial pneumonias resulting from GNB occur principally in patients with severe, acute illnesses whether or not they have underlying chronic disease as well. Thus, these infections are most likely to be found in postoperative patients or patients who require intensive care for other reasons. The clinical manifestations of infection are influenced by the nature of the associated processes.

Community-acquired gram-negative bacillary pneumonias share the common features of all bacterial pneumonias—fever, cough productive of purulent sputum, chest pain, and shortness of breath. The illness tends to be abrupt and associated with prominent systemic signs and symptoms, such as mental confusion, vomiting, and hypotension. Physical examination reveals rales in most patients, but the classic findings of dense consolidation are uncommon. Pleural effusion is present in 15 to 20 per cent of patients. Radiographic infiltrates may involve any lobe and are bilateral in about one third of patients. Although cavitation is most likely to occur in pneumonia caused by *Klebsiella*, it also occurs commonly with *Pseudomonas* infections and occasionally with other organisms. Laboratory features include leukocytosis or leukopenia, either of which is characteristically associated with a marked left shift. Leukopenia is a poor prognostic sign.

Nosocomial pneumonia produced by GNB can be an explosive illness similar to the community-acquired form but frequently proceeds with a more indolent but seemingly inexorable course. Often the patient is in respiratory failure, intubated, and receiving mechanical ventilation. GNB are initially found colonizing the oropharynx, and over the subsequent few days appear in tracheal secretions, followed by increasing numbers of neutrophils. Finally, the patient becomes febrile and develops new radiographic infiltrates and worsening hypoxemia. Another common presentation is fever on the second or third postoperative day. Postoperative pneumonias are most common after lateral thoracotomies (especially combined thoracoabdominal procedures) and upper abdominal incisions. When nosocomial GNB pneumonia complicates the course of an already seriously ill patient, it is frequently associated with evidence of impaired function of other organs, commonly the liver, kidneys, hematopoietic system, and central nervous system. Upper gastrointestinal bleeding and impaired coagulation are also common. This phenomenon is referred to as the syndrome of multiple organ failure and is the most common cause of death in patients with protracted serious illness. The occurrence of any of these complications should alert the clinician to the probable presence of bacterial infection. If no apparent site is found elsewhere in the patient, the lungs must be highly suspect even in the absence of strong clinical signs, since such pulmonary infections are often difficult to detect in the setting of serious disease.

DIAGNOSIS. Confirmation that GNB are responsible for pneumonia is a difficult clinical problem created largely by colonization of proximal airways by these organisms. Thus, GNB are often present in the secretions of ill patients whether they have pneumonia or not and whether or not the GNB are the cause of pneumonia. Blood cultures are positive in 20 to 30 per cent of patients with community-acquired infections but in as few as 8 per cent of those with nosocomial pneumonias. Nevertheless, because the information gained from a positive blood culture regarding the causative organism and its antimicrobial susceptibility is so important in patient management, blood cultures

should always be obtained when GNB pneumonia is suspected. Similarly, while pleural effusion is usually not present, the yield of positive cultures from such fluid when it is present is about 30 per cent, and a diagnostic thoracentesis should be performed if a sufficient volume of fluid is identified radiographically.

Invasive sampling via the fiberoptic bronchoscope adds significantly to the accuracy of diagnosis, especially among mechanically ventilated patients. The best technique appears to be the "protected specimen brush" (PSB), in which samples are collected from the peripheral lung without contamination by proximal secretions. The PSB sample should be cultured quantitatively. Samples containing more than 10^3 organisms are indicative of pneumonia. This technique may be especially useful in ruling out significant infections. Fewer than one half of mechanically ventilated patients who meet the clinical criteria of pneumonia have positive PSB cultures; those who do not may be safely managed without antimicrobial treatment for pneumonia.

TREATMENT. Recommendations for the antimicrobial treatment of pneumonia due to GNB are changing rapidly as new drugs aimed at this group of organisms are entering clinical practice. It must be remembered that GNB are relatively poor respiratory pathogens and that patients susceptible to infection by them are at even greater risk of pulmonary infection by more virulent organisms, such as the pneumococcus, *Haemophilus*, and *Staphylococcus aureus*. Thus, despite the presence of GNB in sputum, initial treatment of these pneumonias—particularly those acquired outside the hospital or in the absence of concomitant antibiotic therapy—should include coverage of the usual respiratory pathogens. The use of multiple agents is advisable for initial therapy for several reasons: The susceptibility of the infecting organisms is not known, and two agents provide broader coverage; emergence of antibiotic resistance may be retarded by the use of multiple agents; and antibacterial synergism may result from the use of multiple agents. The agents chosen must be given parenterally and in adequate dosage. Metabolic clearance rates of the aminoglycosides in particular vary widely, and standard dosages based on body weight and renal function may result in either excessively high or low plasma concentrations in the individual patient. Improved clinical outcomes in the treatment of pneumonia caused by GNB have been associated with peak plasma levels of 6 μg per milliliter for gentamicin or tobramycin and 28 μg per milliliter for amikacin.

On the basis of the foregoing, a reasonable therapeutic approach to the patient with a community-acquired pneumonia suspected to be of gram-negative bacillary etiology would be to initiate treatment with a beta-lactam agent plus an aminoglycoside, for example, cefuroxime or cephalothin plus gentamicin or tobramycin. This combination provides coverage for the usual respiratory pathogens as well as the most common GNB (*K. pneumoniae* and *E. coli*) in this setting. If the patient has recently received antimicrobial therapy or has been recently hospitalized, a third-generation cephalosporin, such as cefotaxime or ceftazidime, can be substituted for the other beta-lactam agents.

Treatment of nosocomial infection is often made more difficult by previous antimicrobial therapy, and drug susceptibility studies are critically important. However, empiric therapy must usually be initiated before the results of such studies are available. Agents should be chosen on the basis of several factors, including knowledge of local resistance patterns, previous cultures, and prior treatment. For example, resistance of *P. aeruginosa* to gentamicin varies from 5 to 50 per cent in different hospitals, and knowledge of resistance patterns in one's hospital can be very helpful in selecting empiric therapy. Most clinicians choose an aminoglycoside, usually amikacin because of the less frequent resistance to this agent, and a third-generation cephalosporin such as ceftazidime. If *P. aeruginosa* is strongly suspected on the basis of previous cultures or the clinical setting (respiratory failure, neutropenia), an agent with greater antipseudomonas activity, such as piperacillin or ticarcillin, can be substituted for the cephalosporin. Because new beta-lactam agents with good activity against gram-negative bacilli are less active than earlier generation agents against a number of important respiratory pathogens, great care needs to be given to the spectrum of organisms covered until the results of cultures are available.

PROGNOSIS. The mortality of GNB pneumonias remains high—in the range of 30 to 50 per cent. It has been argued that this is the result of the underlying disease usually present in patients who develop these pneumonias. This notion could lead to therapeutic nihilism. Other data clearly indicate that GNB pneumonias increase hospital mortality among patients who have nonlethal disease processes, a finding that would support an aggressive diagnostic and treatment approach. It is probable that both conclusions could be correct, depending on the population of patients studied. There is little doubt that GNB pneumonias represent the terminal event for a number of patients with irreversible and lethal diseases and that such patients form a large fraction of all hospital patients. On the other hand, there is reason to expect recovery rates of 80 per cent or more among patients who develop GNB pneumonias in the context of acute, severe, but nonlethal disease processes, and in these patients aggressive diagnostic maneuvers and intensive therapy are clearly indicated.

COMPLICATIONS. Pneumonias caused by GNB are more likely than other pneumonias to be complicated by one or another adverse event. Important complications include empyema, lung necrosis, superinfections, and multiple organ failure; metastatic seeding of infection to other sites is an uncommon complication.

Empyema occurs in perhaps as many as 30 per cent of patients with GNB pneumonias. Criteria for the diagnosis of empyema, besides the presence of gross pus, include the presence of bacteria on Gram stain, a pleural fluid pH of 7.2 or less, or a pleural fluid white cell count exceeding 30,000 per deciliter. Each of these criteria indicates a condition that is unlikely to respond to antimicrobials alone but that usually requires drainage of the pleural space as well. Thus, the term "complicated effusion" has gained favor over "empyema" to identify pleural fluid collections for which drainage needs to be considered. The occurrence of a complicated effusion generally prevents the recovery of the patient until it is recognized and effectively treated. Signs and symptoms of continuing illness, such as fever, persistent leukocytosis, and the onset of multiple organ failure, in a patient undergoing treatment for a GNB pneumonia should raise suspicion of a complicated effusion. If pleural fluid is identified on upright posteroanterior and lateral chest radiographs, thoracentesis should be performed; useful studies of the fluid obtained include measurements of pH and glucose, white cell count, Gram stain, and cultures for aerobic and anaerobic organisms.

If the fluid qualifies as a complicated effusion, most authorities recommend prompt placement of a thoracostomy tube and drainage. Alternative approaches, principally repeated thoracentesis, are less successful owing to loculation of the pleural space. Surgical drainage of the pleural space, using localized resection of an overlying rib with creation of a larger drainage tract, is reserved for patients who do not respond to tube drainage. Decortication of the pleura may be necessary if the clinical signs of uncontrolled infection are not ameliorated by simple drainage plus antimicrobial therapy. In such patients, radiographic evidence of effusion persists, along with continued fever and leukocytosis. At surgery, the pleural space is found to contain numerous loculated pockets of pus. The timing of intervention with these techniques requires excellent clinical judgment, because the patients are usually seriously ill and poor candidates for surgical treatment of any kind; on the other hand, they will not recover unless the pleural space is adequately drained.

Extensive lung necrosis has been termed "lung gangrene" because of the rapid occurrence of pulmonary cavitation associated with marked systemic toxicity and the appearance of extensive devitalization of lung tissue at necropsy. Occasionally, an entire lung appears to dissolve within a few days, leaving multiple cavities with air-fluid levels. This complication occurs with all of the common GNB, although perhaps more commonly in infections produced by *K. pneumoniae* and *P. aeruginosa*. Lung necrosis may be caused by the extracellular products of these organisms. *P. aeruginosa* makes a number of "virulence factors," including exotoxin A, exoenzyme S, elastase, and a neutral protease. However, *K. pneumoniae* makes none of these, and the propensity of this organism to cause lung necrosis remains unexplained.

Extensive lung necrosis may be followed by massive hemoptysis, continued suppuration because of inadequate drainage of the massively disrupted lung parenchyma, or bronchopleural fistula caused by extension of the necrotizing process through the pleura. The last must be promptly treated with placement of a chest tube because of the attendant pneumothorax. However,

the definitive treatment of extensive lung necrosis is surgical resection of the involved lobe or lobes. As with management of complicated effusion, the timing of such an intervention must be carefully considered in light of the control of the underlying infection, the severity of complicating problems (hemoptysis, air leak, and so on), and the patient's general condition.

Assessment of the patient with multiple organ failure in the context of a serious illness complicated by a GNB pneumonia is always difficult. The major question is usually whether a new complication such as oliguria is due to the underlying disease, to the current treatment, or to the infection. Each of the common manifestations of multiple organ dysfunction—altered liver function, acute renal failure, hematopoietic abnormalities, upper gastrointestinal bleeding, and altered mental state—may be multifactorial in etiology, and the antimicrobial agents used to treat GNB pneumonia may cause most of them. The guiding principles are to treat the infection aggressively and to correct life-threatening complications as they occur.

Superinfections may develop during the treatment of GNB pneumonia, just as GNB pneumonia may occur as a superinfection of a previous pneumonia. Unfortunately, treatment of the patient's pneumonia does not prevent colonization of the oropharynx and tracheobronchial tree by additional GNB or fungi. Thus, the clinician is often faced with evaluating a new set of microorganisms recovered from the patient's secretions. The guiding principle here is to treat patients, not culture results. If the patient is responding well and appears to be improving, the new cultures can be disregarded for the time being. On the other hand, if the new cultural data correspond to a worsening clinical course, the process of evaluation and revision of treatment must be begun again.

Fagon JY, Chastre J, Hance AJ, et al.: Detection of nosocomial lung infection in ventilated patients. Am Rev Respir Dis 138:110, 1988. *A study that documents the usefulness of invasive sampling with the protected specimen brush (PSB) technique in diagnosing or excluding pneumonia.*

Karnad A, Alvarez S, Berk SL: Pneumonia caused by gram-negative bacilli. Am J Med 79(Suppl 1A):61, 1985. *Many well-documented cases are described that indicate clearly the variable clinical presentation of these infections and the generally poor response to treatment.*

Levison ME, Kaye D: Pneumonia caused by gram-negative bacilli: An overview. Rev Infect Dis 7(Suppl 4):S656, 1985. *A thorough review from the standpoint of microbiology and antimicrobial therapy.*

Nolan PE, Bass JB: New drugs for treating lung infection. Chest 94:1076, 1988. *A review of the role of new antimicrobial agents in the treatment of lung infections.*

295 Recurrent Aspiration Pneumonia

Waldemar G. Johanson, Jr.

Categorization of the various syndromes associated with aspiration of liquids into the tracheobronchial tree is not an area distinguished by precise terminology or even consistency in the use of terms. Most of the important syndromes are dealt with elsewhere in this volume: gastric acid aspiration (Ch. 528), anaerobic pneumonias and lung abscess (Ch. 62), lipoid pneumonia (Ch. 66), and hydrocarbon aspiration (Ch. 528). In this chapter, we concentrate on an infrequent but difficult problem: that of recurrent bacterial pneumonias associated with aspiration. Such pneumonias are defined as recurring clinical illnesses characterized by fever, purulent sputum, and new radiographic infiltrates in the lungs in a patient with known or suspected chronic aspiration of oropharyngeal contents.

ETIOLOGY. Most patients afflicted with this problem have serious problems with swallowing for one or another reason. Common predisposing conditions are carcinoma of the esophagus with obstruction, tracheobronchial fistula (usually following treatment for cancer), and neurologic diseases affecting deglutition. Strokes are certainly the most common cause of the latter but amyotrophic lateral sclerosis (including bulbar palsy), multiple sclerosis, and the myopathies may be responsible. Recurrent nocturnal aspiration of gastric contents by patients with esophageal reflux represents the one situation in which the swallowing mechanism may be intact in this syndrome.

Impaired swallowing having neural or myopathic causes is most pronounced when the patient attempts to swallow liquids. By contrast, dysphagia caused by obstruction is always worse with solid foods. Thus, it is not surprising that the patient with myoneural deficits of the pharyngeal musculature repeatedly aspirates oropharyngeal secretions. In patients with esophageal obstruction, secretions accumulate proximal to the obstruction, especially at night, and are aspirated. Gastric contents are normally sterile. However, as the patient with reflux aspirates gastric contents, a certain volume of oropharyngeal secretions is necessarily carried along.

Oropharyngeal secretions are massively contaminated, containing 10^6 to 10^8 aerobic bacteria per milliliter and about 10 times as many anaerobic organisms. Although the majority of organisms composing the normal flora of this region have little invasiveness for the normal host, highly pathogenic organisms, including *Streptococcus pneumoniae*, *Staphylococcus aureus*, and *Haemophilus influenzae*, may be present in the secretions of normal people. Since most of the patients susceptible to recurrent aspiration have serious underlying diseases, their upper respiratory tracts are likely to be colonized by enteric gram-negative bacilli and *Pseudomonas* as well.

Normal individuals aspirate small volumes of oropharyngeal secretions during sleep but do not develop recurrent pneumonias. The difference between normal people and those who do develop recurrent pneumonias is probably the volume of material aspirated and the underlying chronic illnesses of the latter patients; differences in the bacterial flora of secretions may play a role as well.

CLINICAL MANIFESTATIONS. Episodes of recurrent pneumonia associated with aspiration tend not to be acute, fulminant illnesses but rather are characterized by progressive fever, purulent sputum production, shortness of breath, and systemic symptoms (such as loss of appetite and malaise) over a period of days. The frequency of such episodes in an individual prone to recurrent aspiration varies widely. In patients with tracheobronchial fistulas, the episodes are essentially continuous until an effective preventive measure can be implemented or the patient dies. By contrast, patients with esophageal reflux may go years between episodes. The frequency of episodes is usually directly related to the frequency and volume of material aspirated and thus is increased in conditions in which aspiration is a daily event, especially if coupled with a decreased level of awareness, as occurs in some patients following strokes.

Physical findings include those related to the underlying illness and the presence of coarse rhonchi over dependent lung zones. Rales and signs of consolidation may or may not be present. Fever and leukocytosis are regularly present. Radiographs of the chest reveal infiltrates of varying intensity, with a preponderance of change in the dependent zones, i.e., posterior aspects of the lower lobes and posterior segments of the upper lobes. Pleural effusion is uncommon unless anaerobic infection is present.

DIAGNOSIS. Examination of expectorated sputum is helpful in confirming the suspicion of aspiration pneumonia but of little help in defining a specific bacterial etiology. Typically, the sputum of such patients is intensely purulent, with a wide spectrum of bacterial forms present on Gram stain. Culture of this material yields the same flora as in upper respiratory secretions, and the clinical problem consists of trying to discern which of several pathogenic organisms should be treated. Cultures should be obtained, however, since knowledge of the sensitivity of the organisms present may be needed to guide therapy. Blood cultures are rarely positive. The presence of food particles in tracheal secretions is clear evidence of aspiration. In patients receiving enteral feedings, the presence of glucose in secretions may be demonstrable by bedside tests. Since normal secretions contain an undetectable level of glucose, a positive result is highly specific for aspiration. Dietary lipids form large intracellular deposits when ingested by phagocytic cells, and examination of sputum with a lipid stain may confirm the clinical impression of chronic aspiration. The microscopic appearance of the large lipid

deposits is important in differentiating this type of lipid inclusion from the foamy deposit that occurs in macrophages owing to the accumulation of endogenous lipid distal to an obstructing lesion in the airways.

When the diagnosis of recurrent aspiration is in doubt, cineradiographic studies of the patient swallowing a thin, water-soluble contrast material is usually definitive. Thick barium should be avoided, as aspiration of this material compounds the patient's problems and the use of a thick solution is less likely to identify the swallowing difficulty. The procedure may need to be repeated with the patient in the supine position in questionable cases. Follow-up films of the chest reveal the presence of contrast material in the airways.

Patients with infrequent episodes of recurrent pneumonia caused by esophageal reflux and nocturnal aspiration represent a somewhat different problem. The presence of a hiatal hernia or the demonstration of reflux during an upper gastrointestinal contrast study does not necessarily prove that pneumonia was caused by this mechanism, although that would be a reasonable presumption if other aspects of the patient's presentation were compatible with the diagnosis. Probably the best diagnostic test in uncertain circumstances is to monitor the pH in the upper esophagus during sleep. Reflux into the upper esophagus is marked by a sudden fall in pH, an event that is easily captured on a long-term strip chart recorder for review the next morning. Attempts to document aspiration by placing contrast material or radioisotopes in the stomach prior to sleep are of limited value, since such patients do not aspirate every night.

TREATMENT. Initial antibiotic therapy should provide broad coverage. Pending the results of culture and sensitivity studies, therapy with intravenous penicillin and an aminoglycoside is reasonable. Alternatively, a second- or third-generation cephalosporin can be used as long as coverage for gram-positive, gram-negative, and anaerobic organisms is provided. Supportive care, including aggressive tracheobronchial toilet, is required. Nutrition must not be overlooked despite the difficulties encountered in many of these patients. If swallowing is impossible and a small feeding tube cannot be placed in the intestinal tract via the nose or mouth, parenteral nutrition should be provided while a long-term solution to the patient's problem is sought. Failure to address the nutritional deficits of these patients is a common cause of protracted and often lethal complications.

Surgical intervention to prevent esophageal reflux is indicated for the patient in whom recurrent pneumonia can be reasonably attributed to this mechanism. Long-term solutions for the other patients with this syndrome often involve difficult choices. Bypassing the mouth to facilitate feeding can be accomplished with a feeding gastrostomy or enterostomy. The former can be performed noninvasively via fiberoptic gastroscopy, with the feeding tube being passed percutaneously into the stomach. In some patients, cessation of swallowing food diminishes the frequency and severity of aspiration and successfully ameliorates the clinical problem. However, in many it does not because patients must still handle their own secretions. Drug therapy aimed at reducing the volume of secretions in this situation is usually not successful. The only certain preventive measure is tracheostomy with all of the complications attendant to this procedure. Even tracheostomy does not negate the possibility of aspiration around the tube unless the larynx is removed or the vocal cords are sewn together. The latter can be undone at a later date if the patient's condition improves. These procedures should not be contemplated in all patients with the syndrome of recurrent aspiration, since many patients have underlying conditions that will be lethal in a short time. However, if the patient has a reasonable chance of long-term survival in the absence of recurrent episodes of pneumonia, these steps should be considered.

Bartlett JG: The triple threat of aspiration pneumonia. Chest 68:560, 1975. *A useful classification and review of the bacteriology of aspiration pneumonias.*

Lorber B, Swenson RM: Bacteriology of aspiration pneumonia. A prospective study of community and hospitalized cases. Ann Intern Med 81:329, 1974. *Emphasizes the differences in bacteriology among these two groups of patients.*

Shike M, Berner YN, Gerdes H, et al.: Percutaneous endoscopic gastrostomy and jejunostomy for long-term feeding in patients with cancer of the head and neck. Otolaryngol Head Neck Surg 101:549, 1989. *This study documents the safety and benefit of percutaneous endoscopic gastrostomy in patients at risk of aspiration due to cancer.*

Winterbauer R, Durning R Jr, Baron E, et al.: Aspirated nasogastric feeding solution detected by glucose strips. Ann Intern Med 95:67, 1981. *Provides insight into the problem and a simple approach to diagnosis.*

296 Legionellosis

Paul H. Edelstein

DEFINITION. Legionellosis is the term used to describe infections caused by bacteria of the genus *Legionella*. The most important of these diseases is pneumonia, called legionnaires' disease. Either as part of legionnaires' disease or distinct from it, the legionellae may cause infections elsewhere in the body, usually in the form of abscesses. Finally, a type of transient and mild febrile illness, called Pontiac fever, is assumed to be caused by legionellae, though this is unproved.

HISTORY. Legionnaires' disease was first recognized as a distinct entity when it caused epidemic pneumonia among members of the American Legion attending a convention in Philadelphia in 1976; this resulted in 29 deaths and in 182 cases of pneumonia. Despite evidence that people who were not legionnaires became ill during the same epidemic, the disease earned the name "legionnaires' disease." Charles McDade and William Shepard, of the United States Centers for Disease Control, determined that this disease was caused by an ostensibly newly discovered bacterium. The bacterium was named *Legionella pneumophila* to honor the legionnaires who had the disease, as well as to denote the organ that the bacterium infects. It has been subsequently determined that neither the disease nor the bacterium is new. The first documented epidemic of legionnaires' disease occurred in a meat packing plant in Minnesota in 1957, and the first recorded isolation of the bacterium was in 1943. In fact, three different *Legionella* species had been isolated from humans prior to 1976, although they were thought to be rickettsia-like agents. Several unsolved epidemics of pneumonia, including one in Philadelphia in 1974, were recognized to have been due to legionnaires' disease.

BACTERIOLOGY. Twenty-nine *Legionella* species have been recognized to date. About half of these have been isolated from patients with legionnaires' disease, and about half have been isolated only from the environment. The species that most commonly cause disease are *L. pneumophila, L. micdadei, L. bozemanii, L. dumoffii,* and *L. longbeachae.* Fourteen serogroups are recognized for *L. pneumophila,* while several other species contain up to two serogroups. *L. pneumophila* causes up to 90 per cent of cases of legionnaires' disease in nonimmunocompromised individuals, and about 90 per cent of these cases are caused by *L. pneumophila* serogroup 1. *Legionella micdadei* is probably the second most common cause of legionnaires' disease and is a very common cause of legionnaires' disease in immunocompromised patients.

The legionellae are small, gram-negative, obligately aerobic, asaccharolytic, and usually motile bacilli. *Legionella* requires complex growth media, having an absolute nutritional requirement for L-cysteine. Optimal growth occurs on a buffered charcoal yeast extract medium supplemented with iron, L-cysteine, and α-ketoglutarate (BCYEα). These bacteria do not grow on conventional bacteriologic media, such as tryptic soy blood agar, MacConkey's agar, or unsupplemented chocolate agar. Their usual habitat is natural and treated waters, such as lakes, ponds, and tap water. Legionellae are found in highest concentration in warm water, especially in hot water heaters, hot water plumbing fixtures, and cooling towers. They appear to be obligate or facultative parasites of fresh water amoebae, such as *Hartmannella* and *Acanthamoeba.* Humans are very likely accidental hosts of these bacteria.

Virulence factors have been examined for relatively few strains each of *L. pneumophila* and *L. micdadei* and are not well understood. The bacteria produce endotoxins and exotoxins, which may cause tissue damage independently or in concert with the host immune system.

PATHOGENESIS. Legionnaires' disease is acquired by inhalation of aerosolized water containing *Legionella* organisms. It is also possible that some patients acquire disease by pulmonary aspiration of contaminated water. The contaminated aerosols are derived from humidifiers, shower heads, respiratory therapy equipment, industrial cooling water, and cooling towers. Aerosols formed by contaminated water in plumbing systems and in cooling towers are the most common sources of infection. Inhaled organisms are phagocytosed by pulmonary alveolar macrophages, which are unable to kill the bacteria. The bacteria inhibit phagolysosomal fusion and multiply within the phagosome. Eventually, the multiplying bacteria, which produce cytotoxins, kill the macrophage and are released extracellularly. The intracellular infection cycle is reinitiated in another macrophage. Continuing bacterial multiplication and consequent lung damage produce symptoms 2 to 14 days after the initiation of infection. Bacterial uptake and multiplication are curtailed by the action of cytokines (e.g., gamma-interferon), which are produced by macrophages and lymphocytes. Natural killer and lymphokine-activated killer cells probably lyse infected macrophages, aborting the intracellular infection cycle. The role of polymorphonuclear phagocytes is unclear, although they probably have some part in eliminating bacteria, especially after activation by interleukin 2 and tumor necrosis factor. Antibody appears to have little function in host immunity or defense, whereas T lymphocytes play a major role in the immune process. The actual mechanism of pulmonary damage is not well understood and could be due to bacterial toxins, immune reactions to infection, or both. The bacteria may spread to extrapulmonary sites via the lymphatic system and bloodstream; they are likely transported in the blood by infected blood mononuclear cells. The mechanism whereby the pneumonia exerts systemic effects is unknown but could be the result of disseminated bacterial infection, the effect of toxin, or the production of host factors such as tumor necrosis factor.

The pathogenesis of Pontiac fever is still a mystery. On the basis of epidemiologic and microbiologic findings, inhalation of water contaminated with many different types of bacteria, including *Legionella* species, produces the disease. The incubation period of the disease, 12 to 36 hours, is too short to allow for bacterial infection and multiplication. Therefore, it is possible that bacterial or fungal toxins present in the water produce this illness, as has been hypothesized for a closely related disease, humidifier fever. Another possibility is an immune response to one or more of the multiple microorganisms found in the water. Antibody to *Legionella* species found in the contaminated water is present in most disease victims, but it is unclear what this means.

EPIDEMIOLOGY. Legionnaires' disease occurs worldwide but is primarily a disease found in technically advanced countries. Case reports from underdeveloped countries are rare, perhaps because of limited diagnostic facilities and also perhaps because of the infrequent use of air conditioning and complex plumbing systems. Normal children have this disease very rarely. Elderly adults are at increased risk, as are cigarette smokers and those with chronic pulmonary or cardiac disease. Glucocorticosteroid administration, or its endogenous production, is the major risk factor for legionnaires' disease. OKT3 administration may also predispose to this illness, but cyclosporine administration probably does not. Administration of cytotoxic agents does not appear to be a risk factor, nor are hematologic malignancies (except hairy cell leukemia), neutropenia, or acquired immunodeficiency syndrome (AIDS), in the absence of glucocorticoid administration. Patients in the immediate postoperative period appear to be at increased risk of acquiring legionnaires' disease, perhaps because of inhalation of contaminated water aerosols during anesthesia, transient paralysis of local lung defenses, or both. Males get legionnaires' disease about twice as often as females, although this does not hold true for several epidemics of legionnaires' disease. No good evidence exists for person-to-person spread of legionnaires' disease.

Legionnaires' disease may occur in epidemics originating in a single building or area. Outbreaks of the disease have occurred among hotel guests, hospital inpatients and outpatients, office building workers, and factory workers. There appears to be little, if any, increased risk of disease acquisition among people with occupational water exposure.

It is estimated that from 1 to 5 per cent of all pneumonias in adults are due to legionnaires' disease. In some geographic regions, community-acquired legionnaires' disease is more common, with average prevalence rates of 10 to 20 per cent of all pneumonias. When the disease occurs in endemic or epidemic nosocomial form, 1 per cent to as many as 20 per cent of hospitalized patients with pneumonia have this disease.

Pontiac fever has been recognized primarily as an epidemic illness, with attack rates in excess of 90 per cent. It has been noted to occur in office and factory workers and in recreational bathers using spa or Jacuzzi-type baths. The disease very likely has a sporadic form, but the lack of specific diagnostic tests makes diagnosing this form very difficult.

PATHOLOGY. Specific pathologic changes are found only in the lung in the vast majority of fatal cases of legionnaires' disease. Intense inflammation is present in the alveolus, alveolar ducts, respiratory bronchioles, and alveolar septa. The inflammatory process consists of bacteria, polymorphonuclear leukocytes, and macrophages. On occasion, pleuritis, pleural empyema, pericarditis, and cavitary lung disease are found. Very rarely, abscess formation occurs outside the chest cavity; this is characterized by the presence of polymorphonuclear leukocytes.

CLINICAL PRESENTATION. Legionnaires' disease manifests as a febrile systemic illness with pneumonia. Several prospective and retrospective studies of patients with different types of pneumonia have shown that legionnaires' disease has few, if any, characteristic clinical features and that it cannot be distinguished clinically from pneumococcal pneumonia. However, clinical observations during epidemics of legionnaires' disease have often documented characteristic clinical findings. It is probable that the spectrum of clinical presentations is wide, ranging from a "typical" form of legionnaires' disease to one indistinguishable from other causes of pneumonia. This chapter describes the "typical" form of legionnaires' disease, which in reality may be present in the minority of patients. A prodromal illness consisting of malaise, low-grade fever, and anorexia may develop several days before the onset of more severe symptoms. Myalgia, extreme fatigue, and high fever then develop. Gastrointestinal complaints are common, such as generalized or localized abdominal pain, nausea, vomiting, and diarrhea; the diarrhea is generally watery and not dehydrating. Recurrent rigors and prostration may occur. Symptoms referable to the respiratory tract may not develop until later. It is this paucity of respiratory tract symptoms, despite evidence of a systemic febrile illness, that can either be a clue to diagnosis or mislead clinicians. When the patient is pressed for details regarding symptoms, a history of a nonproductive cough, or one productive of nonpurulent, sometimes bloody, secretions, is usually obtained. Production of large amounts of grossly purulent sputum is unusual. Pleuritic chest pain, sometimes in concert with hemoptysis, may be present and may mislead the clinician into considering pulmonary infarction. Mental confusion is reported commonly in some series; obtundation, seizures, and focal neurologic findings may also occur less frequently.

Fever is almost uniformly present in cases of legionnaires' disease, although there are reports of short (days) afebrile periods in some immunosuppressed patients with *L. micdadei* pneumonia. Some patients have pulse-temperature dissociation. Chest examination early in the disease may reveal only scattered rales or evidence of pleural effusion. However, later in the course, most patients have classic findings of consolidating pneumonia. Abdominal examination may reveal generalized or local tenderness and, in rare cases, evidence of peritonitis. Splenomegaly is uncommon. Findings of pericarditis, myocarditis, and focal abscesses are rare. No rash is associated with this disease, except that caused by other factors, such as drug therapy.

The fatality rate of untreated legionnaires' disease is about 10

TABLE 296–1. EXTRAPULMONARY INFECTIONS CAUSED BY *LEGIONELLA*

Dialysis shunt infection
Sinusitis
Pericarditis
Prosthetic valve endocarditis
Peritonitis
Abscesses
  Skin
  Brain
  Bowel
  Rectum
  Kidney
  Myocardium

to 30 per cent in nonimmunosuppressed patients and up to 80 per cent in immunocompromised ones. Thus, the majority of previously healthy people recover from untreated legionnaires' disease after 7 to 10 days of severe illness; those who do not recover die of progressive respiratory and multisystem failure.

Clinically significant extrapulmonary infection in patients with legionnaires' disease is quite rare (Table 296–1).

Pontiac fever is a nonfatal influenza-like disease, with symptoms of myalgia, fever, headache, and malaise occurring in 60 to 90 per cent of patients. Arthralgia occurs with variable frequency, as do cough, anorexia, and abdominal pain. The illness is generally not severe enough, nor long enough in duration, to cause most patients to seek medical attention. Not much is known about physical findings early in the disease; findings after 3 to 5 days of illness are generally normal except for fever and possibly tachypnea. Pneumonia does not occur. The illness lasts about 3 to 5 days, although some patients may have persistent fatigue or nonfocal neurologic complaints for weeks to months afterward.

CHEST ROENTGENOGRAPHIC FINDINGS. Legionnaires' disease causes alveolar filling infiltrates that usually eventuate in consolidation. Interstitial infiltrates are rare, although they may occur early in the course of disease and then progress to consolidating infiltrates. The infiltrates may be unilateral or bilateral and can spread very quickly to involve the entire lung. Pleural effusion, usually small in volume, occurs commonly and may be the sole abnormal radiographic finding in early disease.

DIAGNOSIS. The results of multiple nonspecific laboratory tests may be abnormal in patients with legionnaires' disease. These abnormal findings include proteinuria, pyuria, hematuria, leukocytosis, leukopenia, and thrombocytopenia. Disseminated intravascular coagulation may be seen in patients with respiratory failure caused by legionnaires' disease. Hyponatremia, hypophosphatemia, hyperbilirubinemia, and elevated serum alanine transaminase (ALT), serum aspartate transaminase (AST), and alkaline phosphatase concentrations may also be found. Elevation of creatine kinase (MM isoenzyme) is common, and some patients develop myoglobinuria and renal failure. The cerebrospinal fluid is usually normal, although rare patients may have 25 to 100 white blood cells per microliter of cerebrospinal fluid.

Legionnaires' disease can be diagnosed using specific laboratory tests (Table 296–2). The most sensitive and specific test is culture of respiratory tract secretions, such as sputum. Sputum culture for *Legionella* should be performed on every patient suspected of having this disease. Serologic testing is more useful to epidemiologists than to clinicians, because of cross-reactions with antibodies to unrelated organisms. No laboratory test currently available is 100 per cent accurate for the diagnosis of legionnaires' disease. Thus empiric therapy must be considered in appropriate clinical settings.

The diagnosis of Pontiac fever is based on demonstration of legionellae in water to which the patient was exposed, significant increases in antibody to the isolated *Legionella* species, and a clinical course compatible with this diagnosis. To be certain about the diagnosis of Pontiac fever, it is almost always necessary to perform extensive studies of unaffected people and their environments. This is because recovery of legionellae from water and the elevation of antibodies to *Legionella* are relatively common events. Thus, it is nearly impossible to diagnose nonepidemic cases of Pontiac fever specifically.

The differential diagnosis of legionnaires' disease is especially broad, especially in immunosuppressed hosts. Mycoplasmal pneumonia is generally much less severe and causes significant respiratory system complaints. Pneumococcal pneumonia, in contrast to legionnaires' disease, is usually penicillin-responsive. Psittacosis and Q fever can have clinical presentations quite similar to that of legionnaires' disease.

THERAPY. Erythromycin is considered the drug of choice for this disease, on the basis of retrospective studies, which show that the case fatality rate is lowered about fivefold by prompt administration of erythromycin. The drug is given every 6 hours in a dosage of 0.5 to 1.0 gram intravenously until there is clinical improvement, which usually occurs in 2 to 4 days. Therapy can then be changed to oral erythromycin, 0.5 gram every 6 hours for 3 weeks. Possible alternative drugs include doxycycline (100 mg twice daily), sulfamethoxazole-trimethoprim (15 mg per kilogram per day of the trimethoprim component, three times daily), or ciprofloxacin (750 mg twice daily); clinical experience is not

TABLE 296–2. SPECIFIC DIAGNOSTIC TESTS FOR *LEGIONELLA*

Type	Suitable Specimens	Sensitivity (%)*	Specificity (%)	Notes
Culture	Sputum, lung, pleural fluid, blood, abscess contents	—	100	Use of special and selective media required; 3 to 5 days required for growth
Immunofluorescent microscopy	Sputum, lung, pleural fluid, abscess contents	25–75	95–99.9	Species-specific monoclonal antibody available; not helpful for diagnosis of all species; highest specificity for *L. pneumophila*; relatively low specificity for other species; 2 to 3 hours required for testing
DNA probe	Sputum, lung	50–60	99.1–99.9	Genus specific; may have lower sensitivity for detection of some species and for detection of organism in pleural fluid and transtracheal aspirates; 2 to 3 hours required for testing
Urine enzyme-linked immunosorbent assay (ELISA)	Urine	90–95	>99.9	Useful only for detection of *L. pneumophila* serogroup 1, the most common cause of legionnaires' disease; 2 to 3 hours required for testing
Antibody	Serum	60–70	90–99	Requires testing of paired specimens; seroconversion may not occur until 2 to 3 months after infection; most specific for *L. pneumophila* serogroup 1; cross-reactions with antibodies to many other bacteria

*Sensitivity versus culture. Culture is the most sensitive diagnostic technique, but its absolute sensitivity is unknown; reasonable estimates are 80 to 90 per cent.

substantial with any of these alternative drugs and they should not be used unless erythromycin cannot be tolerated, so they remain second choices. Quinolone antimicrobials (ciprofloxacin, pefloxacin) are much more effective than erythromycin in experimental laboratory studies; with further clinical experience, they may become the drugs of choice. Because of its potent in vitro activity and efficacy in experimental models, many clinicians would add rifampin (600 mg twice daily) to erythromycin for the treatment of severe cases of legionnaires' disease. There are no clinical data indicating the superiority of this combination. Penicillins, cephalosporins (first, second, and third generation), and aminoglycosides are ineffective for the therapy of legionnaires' disease. In fact, the failure of pneumonia to respond to these agents should prompt consideration of legionnaires' disease, and perhaps initiation of erythromycin therapy. No effective therapy for Pontiac fever is known.

Most patients with legionnaires' disease respond within 1 to 4 days to specific antimicrobial therapy. The symptoms clearing most rapidly are rigors, mental confusion, myalgia, anorexia, fatigue, and abdominal complaints. Fever may persist for a week after initiation of therapy but starts a downward trend within a few days. Despite this clinical evidence of improvement, other findings may falsely imply disease progression, such as evidence of increased pulmonary consolidation on physical examination and on roentgenography. Weeks to months are required for the resolution of pulmonary infiltrates. Patients with respiratory failure have a relatively poor prognosis and tend to have a much slower response to therapy.

Doebbeling BN, Wenzel RP: The epidemiology of *Legionella pneumophila* infections. Semin Respir Infect 2:206, 1987. *A recent comprehensive review.*

Edelstein PH: The laboratory diagnosis of legionnaires' disease. Semin Respir Infect 2:235, 1987. *Expands on laboratory diagnosis.*

Kirby BD, Snyder KM, Meyer RD, et al.: Legionnaires' disease: Report of sixty-five nosocomially acquired cases and review of the literature. Medicine (Baltimore) 59:188, 1980. *Classic description of the disease.*

Winn WC Jr: Legionnaires' disease: Historical perspective. Clin Microbiol Rev 1:60, 1988. *Good review of most aspects, extensively referenced.*

Streptococcal Diseases

297 Streptococcal Diseases

Richard M. Krause

Streptococci are ubiquitous, gram-positive globular bacteria that grow in chains. They were first described by Billroth in 1874 in purulent exudates from erysipelas lesions and infected wounds. Subsequently they were shown to cause different forms of streptococcal disease, including streptococcal sore throat, scarlet fever, streptococcal skin infections (impetigo or pyoderma), suppurative infections (including abscesses and pneumonia), food poisoning, septicemia, bacterial endocarditis, and urinary tract infections. A single streptococcal species may be responsible for a variety of diseases, and many different kinds of streptococci may be cultured from humans and animals.

The first classification of these organisms was based on their capacity to lyse red blood cells. When streptococci are cultured on blood agar plates, three types of hemolytic reactions are observed. Streptococcal colonies surrounded by a clear zone of hemolysis are termed beta (β), colonies surrounded by green partial hemolysis are termed alpha (α), and the nonhemolytic colonies are termed gamma (γ).

Primarily through the efforts of Lancefield, the β-hemolytic streptococci were further differentiated into a number of serologic categories, designated groups A to H and K to T, on the basis of specific polysaccharide antigens. Most streptococci causing pharyngitis and impetigo belong to group A. Rheumatic fever occurs only after group A pharyngitis. Streptococci belonging to certain other Lancefield groups are now recognized as important causes of infection. α-Hemolytic and gamma streptococci can cause endocarditis and other forms of sepsis with systemic illness.

Group A streptococcal pharyngitis has been intensely studied over the years because it may give rise to the delayed, nonsuppurative sequelae acute rheumatic fever (ARF) and acute glomerulonephritis (AGN). While ARF is less common in the United States today than 30 years ago, it still persists as a common cause of heart disease in the developing world. Pyoderma due to group A streptococci may lead to AGN but not to ARF.

CLASSIFICATION OF STREPTOCOCCI OF CLINICAL IMPORTANCE

The classification of streptococci on the basis of hemolysis patterns on blood agar plates and antigenic composition was a major advance. Nevertheless, it is frequently necessary to employ a combination of features, including growth characteristics and biochemical reactions, to characterize fully these organisms because they are such a heterogeneous group. A classification of streptococci with a clinical orientation for the most important streptococcal infections is presented in Table 297–1. While group A streptococci remain important human pathogens, β-hemolytic non–group A, α-hemolytic, and nonhemolytic streptococci are of increasing importance as the cause of suppurative infections in all regions of the body.

GROUP A INFECTIONS. Group A streptococci are the most common cause of streptococcal pharyngitis. They are recognized by the characteristic group A carbohydrate cell wall antigen, which is identified by serologic reactions to specific rabbit antiserum. In this way they can be distinguished from other β-hemolytic streptococci that are also frequently isolated from the human pharynx, vagina, or skin.

GROUP B INFECTIONS. Group B streptococci are identified serologically by their characteristic cell wall polysaccharide. First recognized as a cause of bovine mastitis, since the 1960's they have emerged as a major cause of neonatal sepsis with or without meningitis. Carriage of group B streptococci in the female genital tract is a major source of these infections.

GROUP D INFECTIONS. Group D streptococci consist of two major categories: enterococci (such as *S. faecalis*) and non-enterococci (such as *S. bovis*). Strains isolated from clinical cultures are usually nonhemolytic or α-hemolytic, but β-hemolytic strains are seen.

Enterococci are present in the normal intestinal flora and are a significant cause of community-acquired and hospital-acquired sepsis and septicemia. Enterococci are a frequent cause of urinary tract infections, particularly in patients with structural abnormalities of the urinary tract. They are also a frequent cause of endocarditis. Enterococci are frequently resistant to many antibiotics, which complicates treatment. For the treatment of enterococcal endocarditis, combined therapy should be employed, including intravenously administered penicillin in high doses plus an aminoglycoside antibiotic. In combination, these drugs have a synergistic killing effect on enterococci.

In contrast to enterococci, nonenterococcal group D streptococci isolated from patients with endocarditis are extremely sensitive to penicillin. Because of these differences in antibiotic sensitivity, it may be necessary to perform additional biochemical tests to differentiate enterococci from nonenterococcal group D organisms. One simple culture procedure employs broth containing 6.5 per cent sodium chloride. Enterococci usually grow under these conditions, whereas other streptococci do not.

OTHER STREPTOCOCCAL INFECTIONS. Not infrequently, the β-hemolytic streptococci cultured from the throat or other sites are identified as groups C or G organisms. Most commonly when they colonize the pharynx, these organisms produce no symptoms or illness. But on occasion pharyngitis occurs, which may be exudative. A rise in the convalescent antistreptolysin O titer indicates that these groups actually can cause an infection of the pharynx and other sites and are not just passively carried. An unexpected event was the occurrence of 10 cases of group C streptococcal sepsis, including meningitis, in New Mexico in the summer of 1983. In addition to groups C and G, case reports indicate that streptococci belonging to most of the other groups can cause sporadic infections, including meningitis, infected heart valves, visceral abscesses, and soft tissue infections following surgical procedures. Furthermore, these less common organisms are now known to cause opportunistic infections in individuals with diminished resistance due to other diseases or treatments.

The predominant aerobic flora of the oral pharynx normally consists of a large variety of streptococci. These are classified as *viridans*, α-hemolytic, or green streptococci. They may play some useful role by maintaining a favorable ecologic balance. However, they can produce disease in abnormal circumstances. They are a common cause of subacute bacterial endocarditis and enter the bloodstream most often from diseased teeth and gums.

Special interest has now centered on a species of these organisms identified as *S. mutans*. These bacteria colonize the oral cavity and have been implicated in the development of dental caries. They produce a mucoid substance that becomes part of the plaque adhering to the tooth enamel. The bacteria remain embedded in the plaque and excrete metabolic products that are a factor in the production of caries. Currently there is evidence that dental caries can be prevented by decreasing sugar in the diet to diminish the growth of these bacteria as well as by practicing proper oral hygiene to remove the plaque containing the *S. mutans* organisms.

Anaerobic streptococci are also a prominent part of the normal flora in the mouth, intestine, and vagina. It is suspected that they maintain an ecologic balance on the surface of these tissues, but the mechanism is unknown. The presence of this normal flora appears to be important, however, because when the ecologic balance is disturbed by the use of antibiotics, pathogens such as *Candida albicans* may cause infections of these sites.

Anaerobic streptococci may cause abscesses in many different regions of the body, including retropharyngeal spaces, paranasal sinuses, dental structures, and the brain. Visceral infections include lung abscesses and empyema fluids, abscesses of the liver and other intra-abdominal viscera, and perirectal and pelvic abscesses. Anaerobic streptococci are especially prone to thrive in dead or devitalized muscle, skin, or subcutaneous tissue. A rapidly progressing necrotizing fasciitis or *progressive synergistic gangrene* is usually produced by these anaerobic streptococci along with *Staphylococcus aureus*. While these anaerobic organisms are frequently sensitive to penicillin, debridement and drainage of abscesses are important aspects of treatment.

GROUP A STREPTOCOCCAL INFECTIONS

BACKGROUND AND PATHOGENESIS. Although streptococci were identified as the cause of scarlet fever and tonsillitis in 1895, it was not until later that a major advance was made in classification, when these organisms were classified serologically into groups by Lancefield and into types by Lancefield and Griffith. With these developments it was possible to identify

TABLE 297–1. CLINICAL CLASSES OF STREPTOCOCCAL INFECTIONS

Lancified Groups	Hemolysis on Blood Agar	Representative Species	Major Clinical Syndromes	Colonization (Carriage)
A	β	*S. pyogenes*	Pharyngitis (scarlet fever), pyoderma, wound infection, sepsis, rheumatic fever, acute glomerulonephritis	Pharynx
B	β	*S. agalactiae*	Perinatal sepsis, newborn meningitis, subacute bacterial endocarditis, urinary tract infection, adult sepsis	Adult urogenital tract, gastrointestinal tract, throat, rectum, pharynx
C and G	β		Mild pharyngitis	Pharynx
D	Variable (usually nonhemolytic)	Enterococci (*S. faecalis*)	Subacute bacterial endocarditis, urinary tract infection	Bowel
		Nonenterococci (*S. bovis*)	Subacute bacterial endocarditis	
Nongroupable: viridans streptococci	α (green)	*S. salivarius, S. sanguis, S. mutans*	Subacute bacterial endocarditis, caries	Oropharynx, saliva
Anaerobic (microaerophilic streptococci)	γ (nonhemolytic) or variable	*Peptostreptococcus*	Abscesses, gangrene, necrotizing fasciitis, peritonsillar abscess	Mouth, intestine, vagina

group A streptococci as the most common cause of streptococcal pharyngitis. The ability to measure serologic responses was another important advance. Most widely used has been the antistreptolysin O (ASO) test developed by Todd in 1932. This was a major achievement because a rise in an ASO titer or a markedly elevated titer was found to be indicative of a prior streptococcal infection. These immunologic and bacteriologic developments led to the firm conclusion that ARF and AGN are nonsuppurative sequelae to group A streptococcal infections and that infections by *any* of the other streptococcal groups do not result in such sequelae. The rare exception to this rule is that, on occasion, group C streptococcal infections appear to cause AGN. ARF is observed *only* after group A pharyngitis, but AGN is seen after pharyngitis and pyoderma.

Epidemics of streptococcal disease in the armed forces have been known since the Civil War. The epidemics in World War I, World War II, and the Korean War were studied in detail, and much of the current knowledge concerning the epidemiology of group A streptococcal disease rests on this research. A major advance was the primary prevention of rheumatic fever by penicillin treatment of streptococcal pharyngitis and the use of penicillin prophylaxis to prevent recurrences of ARF. Epidemics of streptococcal sore throat and scarlet fever were once commonly observed among school children, and this resulted in extensive programs for the early detection and treatment of pharyngitis to prevent rheumatic fever. While epidemics of streptococcal pharyngitis are now less common, sporadic outbreaks in schools or other closed populations still occur as minor epidemics. Indeed, during the past several years there has been an unexpected increase in the occurrence of rheumatic fever in school children and military recruits.

Group A streptococci are subdivided into M types on the basis of an antigen known as *M protein*. More than 80 antigenically distinct M types have been identified. This substance plays a very important role in the pathogenesis of group A streptococcal infections. The M protein is a surface component of the streptococcus and is correlated with its ability to resist phagocytosis. Streptococci that have large amounts of M protein are highly resistant to phagocytosis, whereas those with no or a sparse amount of M protein are susceptible to phagocytosis. Following an infection with streptococci of a particular M type, homologous type-specific immunity develops, so that the individual is resistant to infection by organisms of the same M type; this immunity persists for many years. Reinfection with the same M type is rare. Because there are numerous M types of streptococci, repeated streptococcal infections caused by different M types are common, particularly in childhood and early adult life. Penicillin or other antibiotic therapy can suppress the type-specific immune response. For this reason, reinfection with the same M type has been seen since the use of antibiotics.

Because of the importance of M type–specific immunity in resistance to group A streptococcal infections, intensive research has centered on the immunochemistry of the M protein and the immune response to it. The complete chemical structure of several different M proteins is now known, and with the use of recombinant DNA technology, pure type 6 M protein has been produced by *Escherichia coli*. It should now be possible to examine at the molecular level the chemical basis for the antiphagocytic properties of M protein and to explore the molecular interactions that occur when specific antibody promotes phagocytosis of group A streptococci. While these recent developments on the chemistry of M protein have raised again the possibility of a multivalent streptococcal vaccine for use in regions where streptococcal disease still flourishes, a number of theoretical and practical impediments to the development of such a vaccine have to be overcome.

The T antigen is another streptococcal surface protein that has assisted in the classification of streptococci isolated from clinical material. As with M proteins, there are multiple serotypes of T antigens. While T antigens (unlike M proteins) play no part in virulence, they have become very useful antigenic markers, particularly in the recognition of less virulent strains that have lost their M protein. The T antigen classification also has been useful in identifying strains isolated from patients with pyoderma for which an M protein has not yet been identified.

Group A streptococci grown in vivo and in vitro produce a great variety of antigenic extracellular products, such as the two hemolysins—streptolysin O and streptolysin S—streptokinase, hyaluronidase, nicotinamide adenine dinucleotidase (NADase), and several deoxyribonucleases (DNases). The antibody responses to several of these substances are useful in clinical diagnosis. Streptolysin O is reversibly inhibited by oxygen. Because anaerobic conditions prevail beneath the surface of the blood agar, hemolysis in this region is due to streptolysin O. Streptolysin O is produced by almost all group A strains as well as by many group C and G organisms. Since streptolysin O is a good antigen, titration of ASO antibodies in human sera is the most widely used serologic procedure in clinical practice to detect a prior group A streptococcal infection. In recent years, a test to measure anti-DNase B antibodies has been used in the evaluation of streptococcal pyoderma as well as upper respiratory tract infections. A rise in ASO antibodies is not observed in pyoderma.

The erythrogenic toxins cause the typical erythema of scarlet fever. There are three serologically distinct toxins, each neutralized by its respective antibody. For this reason scarlet fever may occur more than once. Not all strains of streptococci produce an erythrogenic toxin. In the past several years, there have been numerous reports of the occurrence of a toxic shock–like syndrome associated with group A streptococcal infections, but there is still uncertainty if this is due to erythrogenic toxin or some other streptococcal product.

Group A streptococci most commonly infect the tonsils, nasopharynx, and skin. A number of features of streptococcal skin infections set them apart from streptococcal tonsillitis, and for this reason, the clinical features of skin infections are considered separately.

EPIDEMIOLOGY. Streptococcal pharyngitis and tonsillitis are the most common group A streptococcal infections. Their most frequent occurrence is in children between 5 and 15 years of age, but both younger and older persons are still highly susceptible to infection. This is particularly true when special environmental circumstances enhance transmission. For example, mobilization of troops during wartime results in an increased incidence of streptococcal infections in individuals 18 to 25 years of age. The high attack rate in children and military recruits is related to the close contact between susceptible individuals and either infected persons or healthy carriers who carry contagious streptococci in the pharynx. Organisms are transmitted from one person to another on saliva droplets produced by sneezing or coughing.

Untreated patients are the primary source of the spread of streptococcal disease, especially during the period of acute pharyngitis and for the first several weeks of convalescence. Studies of kindergarten and school-age children indicate that an untreated child is often the source of the disease in the classroom as well as in the home. It is therefore important to identify and treat patients as soon as possible to prevent secondary spread of the disease.

Throat cultures of untreated patients obtained during the illness and early convalescence (1 to 3 weeks) usually reveal large numbers of streptococci, and therefore the source of spread. Small numbers of streptococci may be detected in the throat cultures for many weeks or months after an untreated infection. However, individual carriers in whom small numbers of streptococci persist for long periods are an unusual source of secondary spread.

Nasal or throat carriage (or both) of virulent streptococci is also a source of infection of open wounds and skin abrasions as well as of puerperal sepsis. Secondary infection of the lungs may occur, particularly after a respiratory infection such as influenza. Indeed, streptococcal pneumonia may be seen with greater frequency during an influenza epidemic.

A confusing aspect of streptococcal pharyngitis is that a significant number of individuals have "silent" infections that are detected by positive throat cultures *and* a rise in the ASO titer. In early studies it was learned that at least 25 to 30 per cent of all patients who developed ARF had had a preceding silent throat infection. Such silent infections complicate the control of spread of streptococcal disease in a family or community. Epidemiologic studies have shown that patients with subclinical or silent infection are capable of disseminating the streptococci to other individuals, who then may develop overt disease.

Currently there is debate concerning reasons for the declining frequency of severe acute pharyngitis with exudate. Certainly the number of such patients with severe disease is much smaller than it was 30 years ago, while the mild form appears more common. It is unknown whether this change in the clinical picture is due to a decline in the virulence of the streptococci, to host factors, or to the widespread use of antibiotics to treat patients who have been infected with the more virulent forms of streptococci, thus eliminating these organisms from the reservoir of potential pathogens.

A number of epidemiologic factors influence the spread of streptococcal disease. Clearly, socioeconomic factors that promote crowding will result in close contact between individuals and therefore in the spread of streptococci. Climate, season, and geography also can enhance the spread of streptococci because of their influence in bringing people into close contact. It has already been mentioned that military recruits are susceptible because they are clustered in large camps under crowded conditions. Similarly, streptococcal disease is common in civilian populations where poverty and poor housing promote crowding and therefore the spread from one individual to another. It is probable that these factors continue to influence the widespread occurrence of streptococcal disease, and therefore ARF and rheumatic heart disease, in developing countries.

Scarlet fever is now uncommon in the United States. The reasons for this are not clear, because the decline began before the widespread use of antibiotics. Streptococcal strains that produce scarlet fever are the same as those that produce group A infections except that they are lysogenized by a bacteriophage that induces the production of erythrogenic toxin.

Although streptococcal pharyngitis is most common in the winter months, when close contact between individuals is greatest, streptococcal pyoderma occurs in the late summer and early fall. Presumably this is due to exposure of uncovered skin, during the warmer months, to minor trauma and insect bites, which favor skin infections. Although streptococcal pharyngitis and streptococcal pyoderma occur worldwide, geography clearly influences the occurrence of these diseases. Pharyngitis is more common in temperate and cold climates, and pyoderma is more frequent in hot or tropical climates.

The attack rate of ARF after streptococcal infections may vary widely. During the major epidemics of World War II and the Korean War, the attack rate was 3 per cent or more in military recruits with untreated group A streptococcal infections. Since that time, studies of children and other civilian populations, particularly those experiencing the sporadic infections that occur today, have suggested that the attack rate may be as low as 0.3 per cent or less.

The epidemiology and bacteriology of the streptococcal infections that precede ARF differ in important respects from those of the streptococcal infections that precede AGN. In the early years of streptococcal bacteriology, ARF was seen as a complication of epidemic pharyngitis due to nearly all of the different types of group A streptococci. For example, certain M types, such as 1, 3, 5, 6, 14, 18, 19, and 24, have all produced epidemics of pharyngitis in the United States that have resulted in ARF. In contrast, AGN was not a constant complication of these epidemics. The occurrence of AGN has been associated with epidemics of pharyngitis caused by a limited number of M types, such as type 12. Such differences in the bacteriology of ARF and AGN have raised speculation concerning "rheumatogenic" and "nephritogenic" strains of streptococci. However, such designations become blurred on the basis of epidemiologic information. Sporadic outbreaks of AGN caused by types 1, 3, and 6 have been seen, all of which have been associated with ARF. There is no doubt that certain outbreaks of type 12 pharyngitis have resulted in an unusually high incidence of AGN, but type 12 strains in the general population have not consistently resulted in outbreaks of AGN. Therefore, no single M type can be arbitrarily designated "nephritogenic." Clearly the *antecedent* streptococcal infection that results in AGN must be due to an organism that has acquired some special characteristic other than a particular M protein. Despite intensive study, there is no certainty about the nature of this special characteristic. Efforts are under way to identify streptococcal antigens in the immune complexes of patients with AGN that are associated with "nephritogenic" streptococci. It is tempting to speculate that strains acquire the "nephritogenic" property by some form of gene transfer from those streptococci that already possess the capacity to produce AGN.

As attention was focused on the epidemiology of streptococcal infections and AGN, additional M serotypes that had not been associated with pharyngitis were identified, primarily from skin infections. AGN has been associated with skin infections due to several of these types, such as M types 49, 55, and 57.

Streptococcal Sore Throat

The usual incubation period of streptococcal pharyngitis is between 2 and 4 days. Typically, in both children and adults there is a rather abrupt onset of sore throat. A particular characteristic is pain on swallowing. Hoarseness is rare. Other symptoms include headache, malaise, feverishness, and anorexia. Chilliness is common, but not rigor. Nausea, vomiting, and abdominal pain are common in children. The patient appears mildly to moderately ill, but signs and symptoms depend upon the severity of the illness. Temperature frequently exceeds 38.5°C. In the moderately severe case, examination of the throat reveals diffuse erythema, edema, and lymphoid hyperplasia of the posterior pharynx. The uvula may be edematous. The tonsils are enlarged and reddened. A yellow-gray exudate, when present, may be punctate or confluent. There may be discrete areas of exudate about 1 to 2 mm in diameter on the posterior pharynx. The anterior cervical nodes are usually enlarged and tender. The white blood cell count is usually greater than 12,000 per cubic millimeter. When properly taken, the throat culture usually reveals large numbers of group A β-hemolytic streptococci. Not uncommonly, group A streptococci are the predominant organisms observed on the culture plate. The course of streptococcal pharyngitis is usually self-limited, and the fever and other symptoms abate within 3 to 4 days.

A pharyngitis of the severity just described is typical of the infections seen in earlier years in civilian populations and during military epidemics, but such infections occur less commonly today. Many patients do not have all of the signs and symptoms just described. For example, in mild pharyngitis, there may be no exudate and the throat culture may reveal modest numbers of group A streptococci.

If antimicrobial therapy has not been used, group A streptococci may persist in the pharynx for weeks or months following acute pharyngitis. Some patients who are treated with penicillin will carry the streptococci for several weeks. If the course of antibiotics has been adequate, these patients need not be retreated, since they are unlikely to be a source of spread to other individuals.

The diagnosis of streptococcal pharyngitis in infants and small children presents a special challenge. The disease lacks a well-defined onset. Often rhinorrhea is a dominant manifestation. Fever is low grade. Usually the physical signs in the throat are not helpful in the differential diagnosis. A throat culture is positive when properly taken, as is the culture of the anterior nares. Despite the mildness of the pharyngitis in infants, suppurative complications such as otitis media can occur.

Scarlet Fever

Scarlet fever occurs in those patients with streptococcal pharyngitis in whom the infected organism produces an erythrogenic toxin and who are not immune to the toxin because they have had no prior exposure. The enanthem of scarlet fever includes a tongue that may be bright red with large papillae (raspberry tongue) or coated, with the red papillae protruding (strawberry tongue). These manifestations of the disease are rarely seen in adults. The rash appears shortly after the onset of the sore throat, usually within 2 days, and involves the neck, upper chest, and back and then spreads to the remainder of the trunk and the extremities. The palms and the soles are spared. The rash consists of a diffuse erythema that blanches on pressure, with numerous 1-mm punctate elevations that give a sandpaper texture to the skin. There is a generalized facial flush with a pale area often seen around the mouth, the *circumoral pallor*. The distribution of the rash is variable. The trunk and inner aspects of the arms and thighs are most often affected, but in milder cases the rash is seen only in the axilla or groin. Linear striations of confluent petechiae are known as *Pastia's lines*. A tourniquet applied to the arm for 5 minutes results in large numbers of petechiae distal to the obstruction in nearly all cases (the *Rumpel-Leede sign*). The erythema usually disappears by the sixth to ninth day after the onset of infection. Desquamation of the skin is a characteristic of scarlet fever. It begins with a fine scaling of the face and body and is usually completed during the second week. There then occurs an extensive and characteristic desquamation of the palms and soles. Eosinophilia has been observed, particularly during the period of desquamation.

SUPPURATIVE COMPLICATIONS. The most frequent suppurative complications of streptococcal pharyngitis are perinasal sinusitis, otitis media, and mastoiditis. Suppurative cervical adenitis may occur. Bacteremia was seen more commonly in earlier times prior to the use of antibiotics; this resulted in metastatic lesions in joints, bones, and other sites. Group A streptococcal meningitis is now uncommon.

Recent reports have called attention to unusually severe group A streptococcal infections of skin or wounds, which then extended to soft tissue infection and septicemia, associated with a toxic shock–like syndrome. Cellulitis and fasciitis were common. Most patients developed shock and acute respiratory distress syndrome. The constellation of renal failure, shock, hypocalcemia, and thrombocytopenia is similar to that seen in staphylococcal toxic shock syndrome. In one series, 6 of 20 patients died. The severe complications of these patients are listed in Table 297–2.

An unusual and infrequent complication of streptococcal tonsillitis is *peritonsillar abscess*, or *quinsy*. While it is probable that the streptococcal infection leads to the formation of the abscess, the abscesses themselves do not contain group A streptococci but a variety of oropharyngeal flora, including anaerobic bacteria. This complication should be suspected if there is an abrupt increase in (1) soreness in the throat, (2) swelling in the neck, and (3) fever during or shortly after streptococcal pharyngitis. Inspection of the throat reveals the displacement of the tonsil on the affected side toward the midline. A fluctuant mass may be felt in the affected area with a gloved finger; it should be treated promptly because complications arise when the infection extends farther into the neck and surrounding tissues.

NONSUPPURATIVE COMPLICATIONS. The nonsuppurative complications of streptococcal disease are ARF and AGN. These are discussed in Ch. 298 and 79, respectively.

DIAGNOSIS. Group A streptococcal pharyngitis must be differentiated from pharyngitis due to other bacterial and viral agents. Gonococcal tonsillopharyngitis should be suspected if there is a history of homosexuality or fellatio. *Vincent's angina* usually has an insidious onset without the constitutional symptoms characteristic of a streptococcal sore throat. Signs of this infection, including an exudate, are commonly unilateral, whereas streptococcal pharyngitis is not. *Diphtheria* is now rare, although it should be recognized by the presence of the characteristic diphtheritic membrane as well as the other signs and symptoms of the disease.

TABLE 297–2. COMPLICATIONS OF GROUP A STREPTOCOCCAL SOFT TISSUE INFECTION*

Complication	No. of Patients (%)
Shock	19 (95)
Acute respiratory distress syndrome	11† (55)
Renal impairment	16 (80)
Irreversible	2 (10)
Reversible	14 (70)
Amputation	2 (10)
Desquamation of the skin	4 (20)
Fasciotomy	9‡ (45)
Sepsis	12 (60)
Death	6 (30)

*In a total of 20 patients.

†Diffuse pulmonary edema and hypoxia developed in one patient; both complications were resolved with diuresis and supplemental oxygen.

‡Amputation of a limb was ultimately required in two patients who underwent fasciotomies.

From Stevens DL, Tanner M, Winship J, et al.: Severe group A streptococcal infections associated with a toxic shock–like syndrome and scarlet fever toxin A. N Engl J Med 321:1–7, 1989. Modified by permission of the New England Journal of Medicine.

The major confusion in the differential diagnosis stems from viral respiratory infections, which not only occur more frequently than do streptococcal infections but which also may cause pharyngeal and tonsillar exudate. While many upper respiratory infections have a "common cold–like" quality, the symptoms may overlap considerably with those of streptococcal disease. Adenoviruses can cause an exudative pharyngitis clinically indistinguishable from that due to group A streptococci. A severe exudative pharyngitis with fever and toxicity is seen in infectious mononucleosis. The generalized symptoms and signs associated with infectious mononucleosis, however, should assist in the differential diagnosis. Pharyngitis due to group A coxsackieviruses (herpangina) or to herpes simplex results in the formation of vesicles. When these rupture, they may leave shallow ulcers that can often be differentiated from streptococcal disease by inspection. Because it is frequently not possible to distinguish streptococcal from nonstreptococcal sore throat on clinical grounds, precise diagnosis requires a throat culture.

Before any antimicrobial therapy is administered, swabs should be passed through the mouth under direct vision and a good light and rubbed over the tonsils and posterior pharynx. The swabs should be streaked directly, with a minimum of delay, on a sheep blood agar plate of low dextrose content. After incubation overnight, the number of hemolytic streptococci present should be recorded in a roughly quantitative manner. The organisms are very numerous in most cases if they are the cause of the infection, but in some instances as few as 10 to 20 colonies are observed. The presence of a few colonies does not provide convincing evidence that they are responsible for the illness, because 5 to 10 per cent of the general population (and a higher percentage of children) may be nasopharyngeal carriers of these organisms, so growth of a few colonies is not by itself an indication of infection. Serologic grouping and typing of the isolated organisms are usually not necessary for routine clinical diagnosis. Because the growth of group A streptococci is inhibited in vitro by paper discs containing less than 0.02 unit of bacitracin, some laboratories routinely determine the bacitracin susceptibility of hemolytic streptococci. Hemolytic bacteria resistant to such low concentrations of bacitracin are unlikely to be group A streptococci. On the other hand, approximately 5 per cent of non–group A hemolytic streptococci are also susceptible to this low concentration. New rapid antigen detection systems have been developed to identify group A streptococci directly from the cotton swab, including latex agglutination of throat swab extracts. The specificity of these tests is reasonably good, but when small numbers of streptococci are present, the test is less sensitive than the culture methods. If the test is negative and pharyngitis is suspected on clinical grounds, a throat culture should be done.

If the pharyngitis persists with adequate penicillin therapy, it is unlikely to be due to group A streptococci. However, viral pharyngitis is often of brief duration, and if such patients are treated with penicillin, it may appear that there has been a therapeutic response when in fact the disease has abated spontaneously.

The ASO test is not useful in the diagnosis of streptococcal pharyngitis. An elevation in titer is evidence of a recent infection and is employed in the diagnosis of patients with rheumatic fever and rheumatic heart disease.

TREATMENT. There are four reasons for treating streptococcal pharyngitis: (1) the prevention of suppurative complications; (2) the prevention of the nonsuppurative complications ARF and AGN; (3) the prevention of spread of the disease to family contacts or to persons in small social units, such as school rooms and army barracks, and (4) the relief of symptoms. The recent occurrence of streptococcal pharyngitis followed by rapid onset of a toxic shock–like syndrome that may be fatal is now a compelling reason for early diagnosis and treatment. Prevention of ARF depends upon the eradication of the organism from the pharynx, and this requires treatment for at least 10 days. Because signs and symptoms frequently subside in a few days, there is a tendency to shorten the time antibiotics are given. Brief periods of antibiotic therapy do not eliminate the streptococci from the pharynx. Patients treated briefly have a greater risk of developing ARF than do those who are adequately treated for at least 10 days.

Penicillin is the drug of choice. Group A streptococci are highly susceptible in the action of penicillin. Despite its use for over 40 years, no penicillin-resistant strains have developed. A single intramuscular injection of 1.2 million units of benzathine penicillin G provides a sufficiently prolonged level of penicillin in the blood to eradicate the organism. For children weighing less than 60 pounds, the dose is 600,000 units. If oral therapy is used, 250,000 units of penicillin G or 250 mg of penicillin V, three or four times daily, is the treatment of choice. If penicillin allergy is suspected or known to exist, erythromycin is the drug of choice, 20 mg per pound per day (not to exceed 1 gram per day) for a period of 10 days. Erythromycin resistance is not yet a serious problem in the United States. Many group A streptococci have developed resistance to tetracycline, and it is no longer recommended for treatment of group A infections. Sulfonamides, when used to treat streptococcal pharyngitis, are ineffective in preventing rheumatic fever. They do not suppress the immune response, do not terminate pharyngeal carriage of streptococci, and thus do not reduce the attack rate of subsequent rheumatic fever. They may be used, however, as continuous prophylaxis to prevent new infections in patients who have had an initial attack of rheumatic fever.

Treatment of streptococcal sore throat should be started as soon as a definite diagnosis of streptococcal infection is made. Because of the occurrence of toxic shock–like syndrome with streptococcal infections, if the clinical picture suggests streptococcal pharyngitis, a throat culture should be done and the treatment begun without delay. It has been shown, however, that a short delay while awaiting throat culture results (even for several days) in initiating antimicrobial therapy does not significantly interfere with rheumatic fever prevention. One exception to this statement involves the patient with a history of rheumatic fever. In such a patient, the prevention of rheumatic occurrence is not always possible unless treatment is instituted at the first clinical sign of streptococcal infection. For such a patient, any delay of therapy entails the risk of reactivation of the disease.

If severe suppurative streptococcal infections such as mastoiditis, pneumonia, wound infections, or other forms of sepsis are present, patients should receive 600,000 units of procaine penicillin G twice a day intramuscularly for several days until the illness is under control. Then a shift can be made to benzathine penicillin or oral penicillin. It may be necessary to prolong therapy for several weeks whenever pus or necrosis is present, particularly when adequate debridement is not possible.

STREPTOCOCCAL PNEUMONIA

Streptococcal pneumonia is now uncommon. It can be seen, however, as a complication of influenza, measles, pertussis, or varicella. It is characterized by abrupt onset of fever, chills, myalgia, dyspnea, cough, pleuritic chest pain, and hemoptysis. Patients are severely ill. Radiologically, there is usually bronchopneumonia. Lobar consolidation is less common. One characteristic feature of streptococcal pneumonia is the early and rapid accumulation of a large volume of thin empyema fluid. The pneumonic infection can extend to the mediastinum and pericardium. Bacteremia occurs in 10 to 15 per cent of the cases. Bacteriologic diagnosis depends on recovering group A streptococci from the sputum, empyema fluid, and blood. Because the patient is very ill, treatment should be started promptly. Therapy consists of 4 to 6 million units of parenteral procaine penicillin G given daily; this total daily dose is given in two to four intramuscular injections. There must also be adequate drainage of the empyema fluid. This may require insertion of a chest tube.

STREPTOCOCCAL SKIN INFECTIONS

PYODERMA. Group A streptococci can produce localized purulent skin infections known as pyoderma. While some of the lesions represent secondary infections of wounds or burns, most commonly the infection is primary and is usually referred to as *streptococcal impetigo* or *impetigo contagiosa*. Intensive studies over the past 20 years have revealed a number of important bacteriologic and epidemiologic differences between streptococcal impetigo and streptococcal pharyngitis (Table 297–3). Impetigo occurs in the summer and fall, but pharyngitis is seen in the winter and spring. Children between the ages of 2 and 5 years

TABLE 297–3. COMPARISON OF THE FEATURES OF STREPTOCOCCAL PHARYNGITIS AND PYODERMA*

Features	Pharyngitis	Pyoderma
Clinical illness	Acute	Indolent
Laboratory		
Leukocytosis	Usually present	Often absent
Antistreptolysin O response	Common	Uncommon
Epidemiology		
Seasonal occurrence	Winter and spring	Late summer and early fall
Geographic distribution	More common in temperature or cold climates	Common in hot or tropical climates
Age	School-aged children	Children of preschool age
Transmission	Direct spread from human reservoirs	Unknown; insects may be mechanical vectors
Carrier state	Common in pharynx of many populations	Unusual on skin
Preceding trauma	Not present	May predispose to infection
Complications		
Acute nephritis	Occurs; partially preventable (50%)	Occurs; preventability unknown
Acute rheumatic fever	Occurs; preventable	Does not occur
Treatment		
Local	Not important	Removal of crusts and scrubbing with hexachlorophene soap
Systemic	Single intramuscular injection of benzathine penicillin or oral penicillin for 10 days	May not be necessary; extensive lesions may require intramuscular benzathine penicillin

From Wannamaker LW: N Engl J Med 282:23, 78, 1970. Modified by permission of the New England Journal of Medicine.

are more commonly infected. They are usually from underprivileged families residing in the southern United States or the tropics. Nevertheless, outbreaks can be seen among children of similar circumstances in other areas of the United States, such as those on American Indian reservations.

Epidemiologic studies have not clarified the mode of spread of streptococcal pyoderma, but it is reasonable to assume that personal contact with those infected, and perhaps insect vectors, may be important. Despite the uncertainty about the mode of spread, a number of important epidemiologic and clinical facts have emerged from recent studies. In general, the streptococci that cause pyoderma are the higher numbered M types, whereas pharyngitis is usually due to M types 1 through 40. Children who develop streptococcal impetigo and who carry the higher types on the skin may then develop pharyngeal carriage of these skin strains, which are unlikely to cause pharyngitis. Such pharyngeal carriage must be taken into consideration in the diagnosis of respiratory disease in these children, because carriage of these strains alone is not indicative of streptococcal pharyngitis.

Differences have been seen also in the immune response, depending on the site of the streptococcal infection. While the ASO response is usually brisk following streptococcal pharyngitis, it is weak or absent in patients with impetigo. It has been suggested that inactivation of streptolysin O by the lipids present in the skin accounts for this feeble antibody response. Brisk antibody responses do occur, however, to DNase B in patients with impetigo. M type–specific protective antibodies are almost always produced after streptococcal pharyngitis, but the response to the M type–specific antigens is variable in the case of impetigo. It is not surprising, therefore, that lesions due to the same serotype may persist for months if untreated.

The lesions of streptococcal impetigo occur over the exposed areas of the body. They are more common on the lower extremities, undoubtedly because abrasions of the skin are more common in these areas. The lesions begin as papules but rapidly evolve into vesicles surrounded by erythema. They may be localized but are often multiple. As the papules enlarge, they break down over 5 or 6 days to form a thick crust. The lesions heal slowly, leaving a depigmented area. While there may be some regional lymphadenitis, systemic symptoms are not usually present.

While streptococcal impetigo can be suspected from the history as well as the examination, definite diagnosis requires bacteriologic culture. The crust must be removed to obtain specimens from the base of the lesion after washing the infected area of the skin with sterile water. Soap or other detergents can kill or reduce the number of group A streptococci. Culturing the surface of the lesion itself usually gives a negative result. Culture results may show both group A streptococci and *Staphylococcus aureus*, but it is generally believed that the streptococcus is the primary pathogen. In many instances mild impetigo responds to local treatment. The crusts should be removed and the skin washed with soap and water. Topical antibiotics and other antiseptics have little or no value in treatment or prevention. When the lesions are more extensive, parenteral use of benzathine penicillin G is indicated. The lesions respond well to penicillin therapy. The antibiotic regimen is the same as that used for the treatment of pharyngitis. Even though the *S. aureus* present may produce penicillinase, this does not interfere with penicillin treatment. Prevention of impetigo is achieved with good personal hygiene and liberal use of soap and water.

The importance of streptococcal impetigo beyond the inconvenience and some disfiguration of the skin relates to its association with AGN. Not all strains of group A streptococci that cause impetigo and other forms of pyoderma result in AGN; nevertheless, certain M types, such as 49, 55, and 57, have been associated with sporadic cases as well as large epidemics of pyoderma-associated AGN. These have occurred in many different geographic regions. Although there is evidence to suggest that treatment of streptococcal pharyngitis prevents AGN 50 per cent of the time, there is no conclusive evidence that treatment of an individual case of pyoderma prevents subsequent occurrence of AGN. Nevertheless, treatment of the individual is important, particularly in a setting in which AGN is occurring or has occurred in the past, because this eradicates the streptococcus from the environment. The individual is therefore less of a risk to siblings and other school children.

A more severe ulcerated form of pyoderma is known as *ecthyma*. During the Vietnam conflict, this was seen in combat troops serving in the jungle. The ulcers, located on the ankle or dorsum of the foot, are circular, have a punched-out appearance, and are 0.5 to 3 cm in diameter. They contain purulent material and may be covered with a yellowish-gray crust. They are surrounded by a zone of erythema, and in more severe cases there may be cellulitis and lymphadenitis.

ERYSIPELAS. Erysipelas (St. Anthony's fire) is an acute infection of the skin and subcutaneous tissues caused by group A streptococci. The disease is more common in infants, young children, and elderly people. It is most commonly seen on the face and has a "butterfly" distribution when the bridge of the nose and the cheeks are involved. Eyelids are edematous and often swollen shut. The source of the infection is the patient's nasopharynx. Erysipelas may also develop from streptococcal infections elsewhere on the body, including surgical incisions and wounds. In some cases, the disease has been seen in association with dermatophytosis.

As with streptococcal pharyngitis, the onset is usually abrupt, and similar systemic symptoms are frequently present. The lesion initially begins with an area of mild discomfort at the site of infection. Erythema follows and enlarges rapidly, reaching a maximum in 3 to 6 days. The lesion, pink to deep red in color, has an advancing irregular margin. It is warm to the touch. Vesicles and bullae may appear, which then rupture and become crusted. As the margin advances, the central area begins to clear and the skin returns to a normal appearance, usually with some residual pigmentation.

While recovery is usually seen in a week or 10 days, this varies with the severity of the infection. High fever and bacteremia were often present before antibiotics were available, and mortality was not uncommon, particularly in patients who had bacteremia. Death is rare when the disease is adequately treated with penicillin or another appropriate antibiotic. Early diagnosis and treatment are important in infants and in elderly, debilitated, or immunosuppressed individuals. Death can occur in these cases if treatment is not prompt. Not uncommonly the disease will recur in the same site, particularly if there are areas of lymphatic obstruction.

Large numbers of group A streptococci can usually be cultured from the nasopharynx of patients with early erysipelas. Efforts to culture the streptococci from the edema fluid of the lesion are not always successful. Diagnosis is primarily made on the basis of clinical findings.

PREVENTION AND PROPHYLAXIS OF GROUP A STREPTOCOCCAL DISEASES AND THEIR NONSUPPURATIVE SEQUELAE

Views on the antibiotic treatment of streptococcal pharyngitis to prevent ARF and AGN are undergoing re-evaluation because of the decrease in the severity of streptococcal pharyngitis in recent years and the dramatic decline in the occurrence of ARF. Do the low attack rates of ARF (1 to 2 per 100,000 people per year for the age group 5 to 17 years) justify intensive efforts to detect streptococcal infections by bacteriologic cultures? Do they justify a prolonged course of antibiotic therapy for all patients in whom streptococcal infection is suspected, however mild it may be? There has been some discussion about possible relaxation of the vigorous efforts used in the past to diagnose and treat streptococcal pharyngitis. Any relaxation of efforts to diagnose and treat even mild infections shoud be tempered by consideration of the recent outbreaks of rheumatic fever and severe, even fatal, infection associated with a toxic shock–like syndrome.

From this debate several principles are emerging. While direct proof is lacking, it is probable that the decline in the incidence of ARF and the clinical severity of streptococcal pharyngitis is due at least in part to the widespread use of penicillin to treat this infection during the past 50 years. It is difficult to believe that this decline in disease has occurred as a result of genetic changes in the streptococci. This would have required the simultaneous occurrence of similar genetic events in a large number of different streptococci during this interval, which seems unlikely. Certainly the decline in both diseases has been too precipitous to have been the result of changes in the genetic background of the population that would have enhanced natural immunity. These considerations suggest that the treatment of pharyngitis with penicillin has been a major factor in reducing the incidence of this infection; it follows that penicillin treatment has also influenced the decline in ARF. It seems likely that continuation of treatment in the future will maintain this low incidence. It is known that virulent group A streptococci lurk in the shadows and are the cause of occasional outbreaks of streptococcal pharyngitis and ARF. It is certainly conceivable that such outbreaks would become more common if penicillin treatment were no longer used. Therefore, arguments to discontinue the use of throat cultures for diagnosis and of penicillin to treat streptococcal pharyngitis, even though the disease is generally less virulent today than in previous times, are reminiscent of the arguments to discontinue the use of pertussis or poliomyelitis vaccines now that these diseases are rare. We know that failure to vaccinate will result in the re-emergence of these diseases. It is likely that the failure to treat streptococcal infections will have the same consequences.

Until there is more evidence concerning the benign nature of most streptococcal diseases that are occurring today, it is prudent to maintain vigilance concerning streptococcal infections.

The occurrence of an index case of either ARF or AGN should alert the physician to the possibility that an outbreak of streptococcal disease is occurring in a family or school.

It is apparent from this discussion concerning the infrequency of ARF and the milder nature of most streptococcal disease that there is probably much less risk today of the recurrence of rheumatic fever in patients with prior history of the disease following an untreated streptococcal infection. Continuous antibiotic prophylaxis has been employed in the past to prevent recurrences of rheumatic fever in such patients, and while discussions are under way concerning modification of the recommendations, the three regimens listed below are still recommended at this time, particularly since there has been an unexpected resurgence of rheumatic fever in recent years.

1. Benzathine penicillin G given in a single injection of 1.2 million units every 4 weeks usually provides protection for about 30 days. The disadvantages and discomfort of this regimen should be weighed against the individual patient's susceptibility to

rheumatic occurrences. Those with rheumatic heart disease, those who have had a recent attack of rheumatic fever, and those exposed to an environment in which the incidence of streptococcal infection is frequent deserve the most effective protection. For such patients, benzathine penicillin by monthly injection is recommended.

2. Sulfonamide given daily by mouth in the form of 1.0 gram of sulfadiazine or one of the other sulfapyramidines provides satisfactory prophylaxis, but failures do occur. Toxic reactions may be observed during the first 60 days of continuous treatment. These have been rare, however, with the small doses of sulfadiazine that have been employed extensively.

3. Oral penicillin V is the preferred form because it is relatively resistant to gastric acid. The dose is 125 or 150 mg twice a day. This regimen has not been any more effective, however, than the daily dose of 1.0 gram of sulfadiazine. Indeed, 200,000 units of penicillin twice daily has not proved as yet to be clearly superior to the single dose. It is possible that the oral dose of penicillin may have to be increased to nearly therapeutic proportions to be more effective than sulfonamides, and this would increase further its expense and impracticality.

GROUP B STREPTOCOCCAL INFECTIONS

In the past, group B streptococci were primarily of interest to veterinarians because they were the cause of bovine mastitis. However, in recent years human strains of group B streptococci that appear to be distinct from the bovine strains have received considerable attention because they frequently produce neonatal sepsis. Group B streptococci are subdivided by means of surface polysaccharides into five serotypes: Ia, Ib, Ic, II, and III. Recent evidence suggests that group B streptococci normally colonize the intestine, and it is speculated that there is then secondary spread from the rectum to the vagina. This raises the possibility of sexual transmission of these organisms. Vaginal carriage is asymptomatic in postpubertal women. The incidence of carriage and of neonatal infection varies widely, depending on socioeconomic status and geographic residence.

Infections due to group B streptococci are associated with perinatal events. Maternal infections include chorioamnionitis, septic abortion, and puerperal sepsis. Group B streptococci are now recognized as one of the most frequent causes of neonatal sepsis and meningitis. Extensive clinical and epidemiologic studies have delineated two forms of the disease. "Early-onset disease" primarily involves infection of the lungs. The disease usually occurs within the first 10 days of life, but cases after this period have been reported. The organisms are usually acquired from the maternal genital tract. This infection may be secondary to aspiration of infected amniotic fluid. Septicemia usually is present. Early-onset disease occurs as frequently as 5 in every 1000 live births, although this varies, depending upon the region of the country and the specific hospital reporting. Early-onset disease tends to occur in infants of certain high-risk pregnancies, such as those involving prematurity, prolonged rupture of membranes, and maternal infection. The other form of group B streptococcal neonatal infection has been referred to as "late-onset disease." Affected infants develop meningitis and bacteremia. The infant is usually over 10 days old, but cases have occurred at 4 or 5 days of age. Infection may be due to nosocomial transmission. The disease has a much lower mortality than does early-onset disease. Type III organisms predominate as the cause of early- and late-onset disease.

Because all the evidence suggests that early-onset disease in the newborn infant is acquired by vertical transmission from the mother who has vaginal colonization by group B streptococci, intravenous administration of ampicillin sodium has been used to treat such women during labor in an effort to prevent transmission. While recent reports suggest that the disease in newborns is prevented by selective chemoprophylaxis of the mother, more research remains to be done in this important area.

While group B streptococci frequently may be cultured from the throat, they rarely, if ever, cause pharyngitis. Group B streptococci infection can, however, cause urinary tract infections in both sexes. Infected men are likely to be elderly. Group B streptococci may produce suppurative gangrenous lesions in

adults with insulin-dependent diabetes mellitus who have peripheral vascular insufficiency. Any large series of infectious diseases reveals group B streptococci as a cause of endocarditis, pneumonia, empyema, meningitis, peritonitis, and terminal bacteremia in patients with malignancy.

All group B streptococci are susceptible to penicillin. It is the drug of choice for these infections. Thus far, most strains are susceptible to erythromycin. Tetracycline should not be used because the organisms have developed resistance to this antibiotic.

Anthony B: Group B streptococcal infections. In Feigin R, Cherry J (eds.): Textbook of Pediatric Infectious Diseases. 2nd ed. Philadelphia, W.B. Saunders Company, 1987, pp 1322–1336. A thorough review of the epidemiology, microbiology, and clinical aspects of group B neonatal infections, including medical management.
Bass JW: Treatment of streptococcal pharyngitis revisited. JAMA 256:740, 1986. An excellent recent review of current indications for treatment and the choice of therapy.
Fischetti A: Streptococcal M protein: Molecular design and biologic behavior. Clin Microbiol Rev 21:285, 1989. A thorough review of the molecular biology of M protein, including the identification of the antigenic epitopes that stimulate type-specific immunity, with a commentary on the biologic and medical implications.
Kaplan L, Markowitz M: The fall and rise of rheumatic fever in the United States: A commentary. Int J Cardiol 21:3, 1988. A thoughtful review of the recent "resurgence" of rheumatic fever in the United States, which calls attention to the need for continued vigilance in the diagnosis and treatment of streptococcal pharyngitis.
Kimura Y, Kotami S, Shiokawa Y: Recent Advances in Streptococci and Streptococcal Diseases. IX Lancefield International Symposium. Bracknell, United Kingdom, Reedbooky, 1985. Brief reports by international scientists on most aspects of steptococcal bacteriology, immunology, epidemiology, and clinical research on streptococcal disease and pathogenesis.
McCarty M: Streptococci. In Davis BD, Dulbecco R, Eisen HN, et al. (eds.): Microbiology. 4th ed. New York, Harper & Row, 1990, pp 525–538. A good brief review of all aspects of streptococcal bacteriology and streptococcal disease.
Rheumatic Fever Committee, American Heart Association: Prevention of rheumatic fever. Circulation 70:1118A, 1984. Standard recommendations for the prevention of rheumatic fever, which should be basic knowledge for all physicians.
Shulman ST (ed.): Management of Pharyngitis in an Era of Declining Rheumatic Fever. Columbus, Ohio, Ross Laboratories, 1984. A collection of papers that thoroughly reviews the changing patterns of streptococcal diseases and the implications of these changes for treatment.
Stevens D, Tanner M, Winship J, et al.: Severe group A streptococcal infections associated with a toxic shock–like syndrome and scarlet fever toxin A. N Engl J Med 321:1, 1989. An excellent recent review of the recent occurrence of this syndrome, which may be lethal and is seen in association with group A streptococcal infections in various sites, accompanied by septicemia and toxic shock.
Wood HF, Feinstein AR, Taranta A, et al.: Rheumatic fever in children and adolescents. III. Comparative effectiveness of three prophylaxis regimens in preventing streptococcal infections and rheumatic recurrences. Ann Intern Med 60 (S5):31, 1964. A classic controlled long-term study of the prevention of rheumatic recurrences and the relative effectiveness of the three regimens commonly in use for secondary prophylaxis.

298 Rheumatic Fever

Alan L. Bisno

DEFINITION. Rheumatic fever is a delayed, nonsuppurative sequel of upper respiratory infection with group A streptococci. The disease is characterized by inflammatory lesions involving primarily the joints, heart, and subcutaneous tissues; its pathogenesis remains obscure. The clinical manifestations include polyarthritis, carditis, subcutaneous nodules, erythema marginatum, and chorea in varying combinations. In its classic form, the disorder is acute, febrile, and largely self-limited. However, damage to heart valves may be chronic and progressive, causing cardiac disability or death many years after the initial episode.

ETIOLOGY. The development of acute rheumatic fever (ARF) requires antecedent infection with a specific organism, the group A *Streptococcus*, at a specific body site, the upper respiratory tract. Cutaneous streptococcal infection, a precursor of poststreptococcal acute glomerulonephritis, has never been shown to cause rheumatic fever.

Strains representing a number of the more than 80 M protein serotypes of group A streptococci are capable of causing ARF.

There is a substantial body of evidence to indicate, however, that group A streptococci vary in their rheumatogenic potential. Analysis of epidemics of ARF caused by a variety of serotypes shows a striking absence of certain highly prevalent types (e.g., type 12) and an overrepresentation of types 5 and 18 and a number of others. Reports from the preantibiotic era document epidemics of streptococcal tonsillitis, even among rheumatic subjects, in which ARF failed to appear. Prospective studies in which poststreptococcal acute glomerulonephritis and ARF occur simultaneously in the same indigent population suggest that the streptococcal strains responsible for each sequel are serotypically distinct.

Streptococci epidemiologically associated with recent ARF outbreaks in the United States belong to the classic "rheumatogenic" serotypes and often exhibit mucoid colonial morphology.

PATHOGENESIS. The mechanism by which group A streptococci elicit the connective tissue inflammatory response that constitutes ARF remains unknown. Various theories have been advanced, including (1) toxic effects of streptococcal products, particularly streptolysins S and O, both of which are capable of initiating tissue injury; (2) inflammation mediated by antigen-antibody complexes, perhaps localized to sites of tissue injury; and (3) "autoimmune" phenomena induced by the similarity of certain streptococcal and human tissue antigens.

Efforts to discriminate among these potential pathogenetic mechanisms have been hampered by the lack of an animal model of rheumatic fever. Most authorities currently favor the theory that ARF is an "autoimmune" disorder, in which tissue damage is mediated by the host's own immunologic responses to the antecedent streptococcal infection. This theory is rendered more credible by the relatively long latent period between the onset of pharyngitis and ARF and by the demonstration of numerous examples of antigenic similarity between somatic constituents of the group A *Streptococcus* and human tissues. The most intensively studied of these antigenic cross-reactions is that between streptococci and human heart. Many patients with ARF (as well as patients with uncomplicated streptococcal infections) have in their sera antistreptococcal antibodies that cross-react with heart tissue in a variety of test systems. Components of the streptococcal cell wall (including group A carbohydrate and M protein) and of the cell membrane contain epitopes that share antigenic determinants with certain constituents of the human heart.

Patients with ARF have, on the average, higher titers of antibodies to streptococcal extracellular and somatic antigens than do patients with uncomplicated streptococcal infections. Data relating to cellular immunity are more limited. ARF patients exhibit an exaggerated cellular reactivity to streptococcal cell membrane antigens, as demonstrated by inhibition in vitro of migration of peripheral blood lymphocytes.

Chronic remittent nodular lesions have been produced in dermal connective tissue following injection into experimental animals of a streptococcal mucopeptide-polysaccharide cell wall complex. Antibodies to the cytoplasm of neurons located in the caudate and subthalamic nuclei of the brain have been identified in sera of patients with Sydenham's chorea, and such antibodies cross-react with group A streptococcal membranes. Streptococcal extracellular products appear to be present in immune complexes circulating in the blood of ARF patients. Taken together, these and other reported immunologic cross-reactions and toxic phenomena could theoretically account for most of the manifestations of ARF. As yet, however, there is no direct evidence that any of them is of pathogenetic significance.

Several observations suggest that development of rheumatic fever may be modulated, at least in part, by the specific genetic constitution of the host. These include (1) the tendency of rheumatic fever to affect more than one member of a given family; (2) the fact that only a small percentage of all individuals experiencing an immunologically significant streptococcal infection develop ARF; (3) the tendency of rheumatic individuals to experience recurrent attacks; (4) the propensity of rheumatic subjects to exhibit exaggerated immunologic responses to streptococcal antigens; and (5) the fact that certain class II histocompatibility antigens are encountered significantly more frequently in ARF patients than in controls. Recently, a unique antigen has been found to be strongly expressed on the B cells of virtually all ARF patients but in fewer than 20 per cent of controls.

EPIDEMIOLOGY. The epidemiology of ARF mirrors that of streptococcal pharyngitis. The peak age of incidence is 5 to 15 years, but both primary and recurrent cases occur in adults. ARF is rare in children less than 4 years of age, a fact that has led some observers to speculate that repetitive streptococcal infections are necessary to "prime" the host for the disease. There is no clear-cut sex predilection, although females are more likely to develop certain manifestations such as Sydenham's chorea and mitral stenosis.

The frequency with which ARF develops following untreated group A streptococcal upper respiratory infection differs with the epidemiologic circumstances. In the years following World War II, careful prospective studies were conducted among personnel in military recruit camps suffering from exudative tonsillitis or pharyngitis caused by M-typable group A streptococci. Under such circumstances, in which cases of streptococcal pharyngitis tend to be clinically severe and to appear in epidemics, approximately 3 per cent of untreated patients developed ARF. Studies of endemically occurring streptococcal infection among open populations of children are complicated by the difficulties of differentiating cases of streptococcal pharyngitis from viral pharyngitis occurring in streptococcal carriers; nevertheless, the ARF attack rate in such circumstances is clearly lower than in the military experience, with an overall attack rate of less than 1 per cent.

Certain features of the antecedent streptococcal infection are associated with an increased risk of ARF. Among these are the magnitude of the antistreptolysin O (ASO) titer rise and the persistence of the infecting organism in the pharynx. Prospective civilian studies indicate that ARF is more likely to occur following clinically severe exudative pharyngitis than following mild, nonexudative illness. On the other hand, one third or more of cases of ARF occur after streptococcal infections that are asymptomatic or so mild as to have been forgotten by the patient.

Patients with a history of ARF are at greatly increased risk of recurrent disease following an immunologically significant streptococcal infection. In long-term prospective studies of rheumatic subjects carried out at Irvington House, a rheumatic fever sanitarium outside New York City, one of every five documented streptococcal infections gave rise to a recurrence of ARF. The risk of recurrence is greater in patients with pre-existing rheumatic heart disease and in those experiencing symptomatic throat infections; the risk declines with advancing age and with increasing interval since the most recent rheumatic attack. Nevertheless, rheumatic patients remain at increased risk well into adult life, perhaps indefinitely.

Rheumatic fever occurs in all parts of the world; there is no known racial predisposition. In temperate climates, ARF peaks in the cooler months of the year, in the winter and early spring or shortly after schools open in the fall. The major environmental factor favoring occurrence appears to be crowding, as in military barracks or similar closed institutions and in large households. Crowding favors interpersonal spread of group A streptococci and perhaps enhances streptococcal virulence by frequent human passage.

ARF remains rampant in developing areas such as the Middle East, the Indian subcontinent, and many nations of Africa and South America. It has been estimated that rheumatic heart disease causes 25 to 40 per cent of all cardiovascular disease in the Third World. In striking contrast, the incidence of ARF and the prevalence of rheumatic heart disease have declined dramatically both in North America and in Western Europe over the past four to five decades. During this time, the disease has become extremely uncommon in the affluent suburbs of many United States cities, while persisting among lower socioeconomic groups, particularly those massed in the densely populated core areas of major urban centers.

The mid-1980's, however, witnessed some startling developments in the epidemiology of ARF in the United States. Outbreaks of the disease were reported in Salt Lake City, Utah; Columbus and Akron, Ohio; Pittsburgh, Pennsylvania; Nashville and Memphis, Tennessee; and a number of other communities. Equally surprising was the fact that, in many of these outbreaks, the victims were predominantly white, middle-class children dwelling in the suburbs. Moreover, ARF epidemics occurred in military training bases in Missouri and California, a phenomenon that had not been observed for two decades. There is as yet no evidence that these events presage a major national resurgence of ARF.

PATHOLOGY. ARF is characterized by exudative and proliferative inflammatory lesions in the connective tissues, especially those of heart, joints, and subcutaneous tissues. The early lesions consist of edema of the ground substance, fragmentation of collagen fibers, cellular infiltration, and fibrinoid degeneration. In the heart, diffuse degeneration and even necrosis of muscle cells may be observed. At a slightly later stage, focal perivascular inflammatory lesions develop. These so-called *Aschoff nodules* (Fig. 298–1), considered virtually pathognomonic of rheumatic fever, consist of a central area of fibrinoid surrounded by lymphocytes, plasma cells, and large basophilic cells, some of them multinucleate. Many of these cells have elongated nuclei with a distinctive chromatin pattern, sometimes called "caterpillar" or "owl-eye" nuclei, depending on their orientation in microscopic cross-section. Cells containing these nuclei are called "Anitschkow myocytes," despite the fact that most authorities believe them to be of mesenchymal origin.

Cardiac findings may include pericarditis, myocarditis, and endocarditis. Foci of coronary arteritis may also be observed. A thickened and roughened area ("MacCallum's patch") is frequently present in the left atrium above the posterior leaflet of the mitral valve. Valvular lesions appear early as small verrucae along the line of closure. Later, as healing occurs, the valves may become thickened and deformed, the chordae shortened, and the commissures fused. These changes result in valvular stenosis or insufficiency. The mitral valve is most commonly involved, followed by the aortic, the tricuspid, and, rarely, the pulmonic.

Pathologically, the *arthritis* of ARF is characterized by a fibrinous exudate and sterile effusion without erosion of the joint surfaces or pannus formation. *Subcutaneous nodules* have many histologic features in common with the Aschoff nodules. These consist of central zones of fibrinoid necrosis surrounded by histiocytes, fibroblasts, occasional lymphocytes, and rare polymorphonuclear cells. Inflammation of the smaller arteries and arterioles may occur throughout the body. Despite pathologic evidence of diffuse vasculitis, aneurysms and thrombosis are not typical features of ARF.

CLINICAL MANIFESTATIONS. Rheumatic fever may involve a number of different organ systems, most notably the heart, joints, skin, and central nervous system. The clinical picture of the disease may thus be quite variable (Table 298–1), depending upon which systems are attacked, whether they are involved singly or in combination, the order in which they are affected, and the severity of the involvement. Five clinical

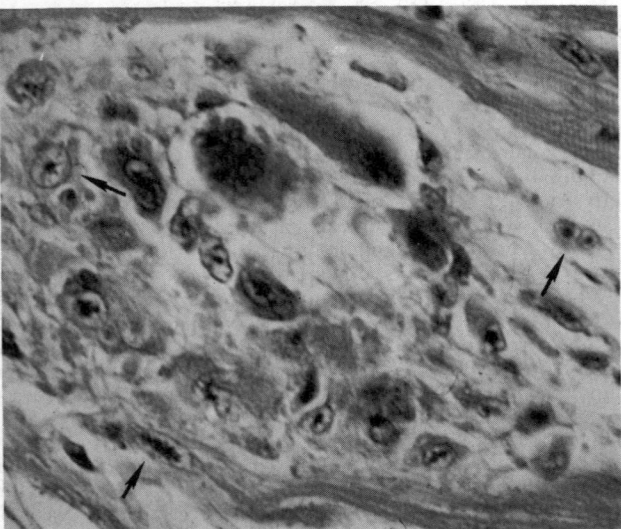

FIGURE 298–1. Myocardial Aschoff nodule demonstrates areas of fibrinoid degeneration and numerous large cells with polymorphous nuclei; several of the nuclei have "owl-eye" or "caterpillar" configurations (*arrows*). × 630. (Courtesy of Robert Peace, M.D.)

TABLE 298–1. THE MANY FACES OF ACUTE RHEUMATIC FEVER: POSSIBLE PRESENTATIONS

High fever, prostration, crippling polyarthritis
Lassitude, tachycardia, new cardiac murmurs
Acute pericarditis
Fulminant heart failure
Sydenham's chorea, without fever or toxicity
Acute abdominal pain, mimicking appendicitis
Varying combinations of the above

features of the disease are so characteristic that they are recognized as "major manifestations" according to the revised Jones criteria (see below) for diagnosis of ARF: carditis, polyarthritis, chorea, subcutaneous nodules, and erythema marginatum. Certain other findings, frequently present but nonspecific, have been designated "minor manifestations." These include arthralgia, fever, history of previous rheumatic fever or evidence of pre-existing rheumatic heart disease, and certain laboratory findings (see below).

In cases in which it can be determined, the *latent period* between the antecedent streptococcal infection and the onset of symptoms of ARF ranges between 1 and 5 weeks. The average latent period is 19 days for both primary and recurrent attacks. When acute polyarthritis is the presenting complaint, the onset is often rather abrupt and may be marked by high fever and toxicity. If isolated carditis is the initial manifestation, the onset may be insidious or even subclinical. Between these two extremes, a wide variety of gradations exist in the initial presentation of ARF (Table 298–1). In most attacks, fever and joint involvement are the earliest clinical manifestations, although they may occasionally be preceded by abdominal pain localized to the periumbilical or infraumbilical areas. At times the location and severity of the pain, as well as fleeting signs of peritoneal inflammation, may lead to a misdiagnosis of acute appendicitis. Carditis, if it is to appear, usually does so within the first 3 weeks of the illness. In contrast, chorea tends to occur later in the course of the disease, sometimes after all other manifestations have subsided. Fortunately, chorea and polyarthritis almost never occur simultaneously. Epistaxis may be a feature of ARF, occurring both at the onset and throughout the acute phase of the illness; it may be quite severe.

Overall, arthritis occurs in approximately 75 per cent of first attacks of ARF, carditis in 40 to 50 per cent, chorea in 15 per cent, and subcutaneous nodules and erythema marginatum in fewer than 10 per cent. The incidence of individual manifestations, however, varies with age. Carditis is more frequent in the youngest age groups and is relatively uncommon in first attacks occurring in adults. Chorea occurs primarily in persons between age 5 years and puberty. It is seen more frequently in females and virtually never occurs in adult males. Thus, the majority of ARF attacks occurring in adults are manifested primarily by arthritis.

Arthritis. Joint involvement ranges from arthralgia alone to acute, disabling arthritis characterized by swelling, warmth, erythema, severe limitation of motion, and exquisite tenderness to pressure. The larger joints of the extremities are usually involved—most frequently the knees and ankles, but also the wrists and elbows. The hips and small joints of the hands and feet are affected occasionally. Involvement of shoulders and lumbosacral, cervical, sternoclavicular, and temporomandibular joints occurs in a relatively small percentage of cases. The synovial fluid contains thousands of white blood cells, with a marked preponderance of polymorphonuclear leukocytes; bacterial cultures are sterile.

Characteristically, the articular involvement in ARF assumes a pattern of *migratory polyarthritis*. This does not mean that inflammation in one joint disappears before the next is attacked. Rather, a number of joints are affected in succession, and the periods of involvement overlap. Inflammation in one joint may subside while another is becoming symptomatic, so that the process seems to migrate from joint to joint. In untreated cases, as many as 16 joints may be affected, and about half the patients develop arthritis in more than six joints. When effective anti-inflammatory therapy is administered early in the course of the disease, the involvement not infrequently remains monoarticular or pauciarticular.

In most instances, inflammation in any one joint begins to subside spontaneously within a week, and the total duration of involvement is no more than 2 or 3 weeks. The entire bout of polyarthritis rarely lasts more than 4 weeks and resolves completely, leaving no residual joint damage. Some authors have described the rare occurrence of *Jaccoud's arthritis*, so-called chronic post-rheumatic fever arthropathy of the metacarpophalangeal joints, following repetitive bouts of rheumatic polyarthritis. This entity is not a true arthritis but a form of periarticular fibrosis; its relationship to rheumatic fever remains unresolved.

Carditis. Rheumatic fever may involve the endocardium, myocardium, and pericardium (Table 298–2), and thus the disease is capable of inducing a true *pancarditis.* Carditis is the most important manifestation of ARF because it is the only one capable of causing significant permanent organ damage or death. Although the clinical picture may at times be fulminant, it is more frequently mild or even asymptomatic and may escape notice in the absence of more obvious associated findings, such as arthritis or chorea. The diagnosis of carditis requires the presence of one of the following four manifestations: (1) organic cardiac murmurs not previously present, (2) cardiomegaly, (3) pericarditis, or (4) congestive heart failure. In practice, the characteristic murmurs of ARF are almost always present in cases of rheumatic carditis, unless the ability to hear them is obscured (e.g., loud pericardial friction rub, large pericardial effusion, low cardiac output, severe tachycardia). The diagnosis of carditis should be made with caution in the absence of one of the following three murmurs: apical systolic, apical mid-diastolic, and basal diastolic. Such murmurs, if they are destined to develop, do so usually within the first week and almost always within the first 3 weeks of illness. (An exception to this rule may occur in the patient with "pure" chorea; see later discussion.) The *apical systolic murmur* of relative or actual mitral regurgitation encompasses most of systole. It is blowing, relatively high pitched, and heard best at the apex; it radiates to the axilla and at times to the base of the heart or the back. It must be distinguished carefully by quality, location, and radiation from a variety of functional precordial systolic murmurs heard in normal individuals, especially in children. The *apical mid-diastolic* (Carey-Coombs) murmur is a low-pitched sound replacing or immediately following the third heart sound and ending distinctly before the first heart sound. It may be heard in a variety of conditions associated with increased flow across the mitral valve and is thus not pathognomonic of ARF. It may be differentiated from the diastolic rumble of mitral stenosis by the absence of an opening snap, presystolic accentuation, or accentuated first sound at the mitral area. The high-pitched, descrescendo *basal diastolic murmur* of aortic regurgitation is best heard along the upper left sternal border or over the aortic area. It may be brief and faint, best heard after expiration with the patient leaning forward. The prognostic significance, if any, of echocardiographically recorded valvular regurgitation in the absence of audible murmurs remains to be determined.

Other prominent auscultatory findings in patients with active rheumatic carditis include tachycardia, which persists during sleep; protodiastolic, presystolic, or summation gallops; an indistinct or "mushy" quality to the first heart sound (resulting in some cases from first-degree heart block); pericardial friction rub; or muffling of heart tones caused by pericardial effusion. In the early stages of congestive heart failure, rapid distention of the hepatic capsule may lead to right upper quadrant aching and tenderness over the liver. All the usual clinical findings of pericarditis or congestive failure may be observed.

A number of different rhythm disturbances may occur during

TABLE 298–2. CLINICAL MANIFESTATIONS OF CARDITIS IN ACUTE RHEUMATIC FEVER

Murmurs*
   Apical systolic
   Apical mid-diastolic (Carey-Coombs murmur)
   Basal diastolic
Pericarditis
Cardiomegaly
Congestive heart failure

*At least one of the characteristic murmurs is almost always present in acute rheumatic carditis (see text for details).

the course of ARF. By far the most common is first-degree atrioventricular block. Second- and third-degree heart block, nodal rhythm, and premature contractions may also be observed; atrial fibrillation, on the other hand, is usually a feature of chronic rather than acute rheumatic involvement. Conduction disturbances do not in themselves indicate acute carditis, and their presence or absence is unrelated to the subsequent development of rheumatic heart disease.

In cases of ARF with severe carditis, areas of patchy pneumonitis are sometimes seen. Many observers feel that these pulmonary infiltrates represent a specific *rheumatic pneumonia.* The case is difficult to prove, however, because of the confusion induced by such confounding clinical entities as pulmonary edema, pulmonary embolization, superimposed bacterial pneumonia, and the acute respiratory distress syndrome in these severely ill and toxic patients.

Sydenham's Chorea (Chorea Minor, "St. Vitus' Dance"). This neurologic syndrome occurs after a latent period that is variable but on the average longer than that associated with the other manifestations of ARF. It frequently occurs in "pure" form, either unaccompanied by other major manifestations or, after a latent period of several months, at a time when all other evidence of acute rheumatic activity has subsided. Chorea is characterized by rapid, purposeless, involuntary movements, most noticeable in the extremities and face. The arms and legs flail about in erratic, jerky, incoordinated movements that may sometimes be unilateral (hemichorea). Facial tics, grimaces, grins, and contortions are evident. The speech is usually slurred or jerky. The tongue, when protruded, retracts involuntarily, while asynchronous contractions of lingual muscles produce a "bag of worms" appearance. The involuntary motions disappear during sleep and may be partially suppressed by rest, sedation, or volition.

Patients with chorea display generalized muscle weakness and an inability to maintain a tetanic muscle contraction. Thus, when the patient is asked to squeeze the examiner's fingers, a squeezing and relaxing motion occurs that has been described as "milkmaid's grip." The knee jerk may have a pendular quality. There is no cranial nerve or pyramidal involvement, and sensory modalities are unaffected. The electroencephalogram may display abnormal slow wave activity.

Emotional lability is characteristic of Sydenham's chorea and often may precede other neurologic manifestations, leaving teachers and parents puzzled over apparently inexplicable personality changes.

Subcutaneous Nodules. These are firm, painless subcutaneous lesions that vary in size from a few millimeters to approximately 2 cm. The skin overlying them is freely movable and is not inflamed. The lesions tend to occur in crops over bony surfaces or prominences and over tendons. Sites of predilection include the extensor surfaces of elbows, knees, and wrists; the occiput; and spinous processes of the thoracic and lumbar vertebrae (Fig. 298–2). Nodules are virtually never the sole major manifestation of ARF; they almost always appear in association with carditis, and the cardiac involvement in such cases tends to be clinically severe. Nodules ordinarily do not appear until at least 3 weeks after the onset of an attack, usually lasting 1 to 2 weeks. They may appear in repeated crops in patients with protracted carditis. Similar nodules may be seen in systemic lupus erythematosus and in rheumatoid arthritis. Subcutaneous nodules in the latter disease are larger and more persistent than those in rheumatic fever.

Erythema Marginatum. The rash begins as an erythematous macule or papule, which then extends outward, while the skin in the center returns to normal. Adjacent lesions coalesce, forming circinate or serpiginous patterns. The lesions are neither pruritic nor indurated, and they blanch on pressure. They vary greatly in size and appear mostly upon the trunk and proximal extremities, sparing the face. Erythema marginatum may be raised or flat; the latter was termed *erythema annulare* in the older literature. The lesions are evanescent, migrating from place to place, at times changing before the observer's eyes, and leaving no residual scarring. The erythema may be brought out by the application of heat. Individual lesions may come and go in minutes to hours, but the process may go on intermittently for weeks to

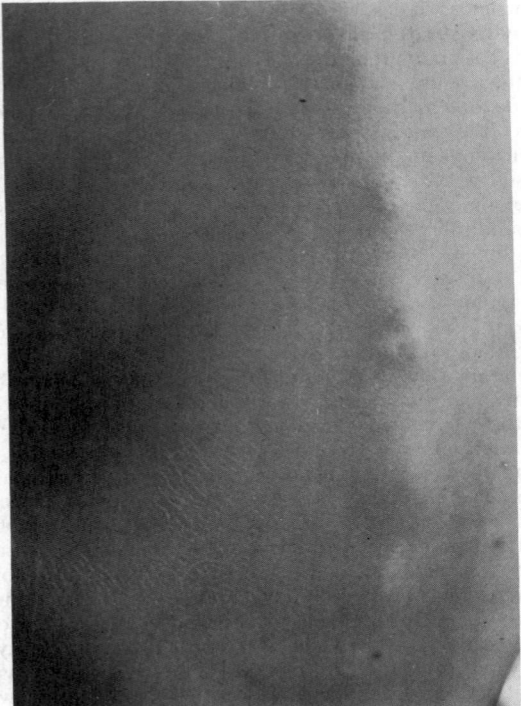

FIGURE 298–2. Subcutaneous nodules over spinous processes on the back of a patient with acute rheumatic carditis. (Courtesy of S. Levine, M.D.)

months uninfluenced by anti-inflammatory therapy; its persistence is not necessarily an adverse prognostic sign. In the great majority of cases, erythema marginatum is accompanied by carditis; it also tends to be associated with subcutaneous nodules.

LABORATORY FINDINGS. No specific laboratory test is diagnostic of ARF. Usually there is a leukocytosis with an increase in the proportion of polymorphonuclear leukocytes. A mild to moderate normocytic normochromic anemia is the rule. In some patients the serum aspartate aminotransferase (AST) level is elevated. Evidence of acute inflammation is prominent, including readily detectable quantities of C-reactive protein in the blood and elevation of the erythrocyte sedimentation rate. An exception is "pure" chorea, which may appear long after indices of inflammation have returned to normal.

The urine may contain protein, white cells, and red cells. Biopsy studies have revealed a variety of renal abnormalities, but the classic proliferative glomerular abnormalities that characterize poststreptococcal acute glomerulonephritis occur quite rarely in ARF. Electrocardiographic and radiographic studies may reveal evidence of rhythm disturbances, pericarditis, or congestive heart failure. Echocardiography may document myocardial and valvular dysfunction and pericardial effusion.

The major laboratory contribution to the workup of ARF is the documentation of recent group A streptococcal infection. Throat culture should always be performed but is positive in only a minority of cases. This is perhaps due to the time lapse of several weeks between the onset of the pharyngeal infection and the throat culture. The serum titer of ASO is elevated in 80 per cent or more of ARF patients. If two streptococcal antibody tests, e.g., ASO plus either anti-DNase B or antihyaluronidase, are performed, an elevated titer of at least one will be found in 90 per cent of ARF patients. A battery of three tests establishes the presence of recent, immunologically significant streptococcal infection in more than 95 per cent of individuals experiencing an acute rheumatic attack. The definition of an "elevated" titer varies, depending upon the test employed, age of the patient, and geographic locale. ASO titers greater than 200 to 250 Todd units per milliliter are generally considered elevated. At times, serial sampling may detect a rising titer of streptococcal antibodies in patients seen early in the course of a rheumatic attack.

COURSE AND PROGNOSIS. The average duration of an untreated attack of ARF is approximately 3 months. The duration tends to be longer, up to 6 months, in patients with severe carditis. Fewer than 5 per cent of patients have continuing rheumatic activity for longer than 6 months. In a few of these the disease is limited to chorea and is otherwise benign. Other patients exhibit evidence of persistent inflammatory activity, including arthritis, carditis, and subcutaneous nodules. "Chronic rheumatic fever" occurs more frequently in patients who have had one or more previous attacks; cardiac involvement in chronic rheumatic fever tends to be frequent and severe.

Death from intractable myocarditis during the acute phase of ARF is now very rare. Once the acute attack has subsided, the only long-term sequel is that of rheumatic heart disease, manifested primarily by insufficiency and/or stenosis of the mitral and aortic valves. The prognosis from a cardiac standpoint is very much dependent upon the clinical findings at the time the patient is first seen. In one large study, for example, 347 patients were examined during an acute rheumatic attack and again 10 years later. Among patients who had been free of carditis during their acute attack, only 6 per cent had residual heart disease on follow-up. Patients with no pre-existing heart disease and with mild carditis during their acute attack (i.e., apical systolic murmur without pericarditis or heart failure) had a relatively good prognosis in that only approximately 30 per cent had heart murmurs 10 years later. About 40 per cent of subjects with apical or basal diastolic murmurs and 70 per cent of subjects with failure and/or pericarditis during their acute attacks had residual rheumatic heart disease. The prognosis was worse in patients with pre-existing heart disease and in those who had experienced recurrent attacks of ARF in the 10-year interval.

The data cited above indicate that patients who do not develop carditis during an acute attack and are protected from ARF recurrences are most unlikely to suffer from rheumatic heart disease. The patient with "pure" chorea represents an exception to this rule. A significant proportion of such patients who have no evidence of carditis when first examined may develop rheumatic valvular disease on prolonged follow-up. Although the explanation for this phenomenon is unknown, it is conceivable that in view of the long latent period associated with chorea, signs of carditis might have been present earlier but subsided by the time the neurologic abnormality became evident.

DIAGNOSIS. Although ARF is readily recognized in the individual who presents with multiple major manifestations or in epidemic circumstances, at other times the disease may be extraordinarily difficult to diagnose with confidence. This is because of the variability of its clinical presentation, the frequency with which only a single major manifestation is detected, and the fact that there is no definitive diagnostic laboratory test. Nevertheless, precise diagnosis is especially important in this disease because of the necessity to advise the patient regarding prolonged antimicrobial prophylaxis (see below).

The diagnostic criteria of T. Duckett Jones, as subsequently modified by a committee of the American Heart Association, attempt to minimize overdiagnosis and underdiagnosis (Table 298–3). Two major manifestations, or one major and two minor manifestations, indicate a high probability of ARF, *provided that there is supporting evidence of recent streptococcal infection.* Although a positive throat culture for group A streptococci technically satisfies this requirement, streptococcal carriage rates of 15 per cent are not uncommon among school-aged children during the fall and winter. Elevated titers of antibodies to streptococcal extracellular products, although not diagnostic of ARF, do indicate a recent, *immunologically significant* streptococcal infection. Conversely, if a battery of streptococcal antibody tests fails to reveal any evidence of recent infection, the diagnosis of ARF must be considered unlikely. This statement does *not* necessarily hold true in patients whose only rheumatic manifestation is Sydenham's chorea. Because of the long latent period associated with chorea, previously elevated antibody titers may have declined to normal.

The modified Jones criteria are, of course, only guidelines. They are most difficult to apply confidently when polyarthritis is the single major manifestation. Under such circumstances, serious consideration must be given to various other entities, including rheumatoid arthritis, Still's disease, viral arthritides (e.g., rubella, hepatitis B), the early prepurpuric phase of Henoch-Schönlein purpura, and septic arthritis, including gonococcal arthritis.

TABLE 298–3. JONES CRITERIA (REVISED) FOR GUIDANCE IN THE DIAGNOSIS OF RHEUMATIC FEVER*

Major Manifestations	Minor Manifestations
Carditis	*Clinical*
Polyarthritis	Previous rheumatic fever or rheumatic
Chorea	heart disease
Erythema marginatum	Arthralgia
Subcutaneous nodules	Fever
	Laboratory
	Acute phase reactions
	Erythrocyte sedimentation rate,
	C-reactive protein, leukocytosis
	Prolonged PR interval
	Plus

Supporting evidence of preceding streptococcal infection (increased ASO or other streptococcal antibodies; positive throat culture for group A *Streptococcus;* recent scarlet fever).

The presence of two major criteria, or of one major and two minor criteria, indicates a high probability of the presence of rheumatic fever if supported by evidence of a preceding streptococcal infection.

*Reprinted from Jones criteria (revised) for guidance in the diagnosis of rheumatic fever. Circulation 69:204A, 1984, by permission of the American Heart Association, Inc.

Serum sickness is frequently a serious consideration, particularly if the patient has received penicillin or other antibiotics for a preceding respiratory infection. Systemic lupus erythematosus, sickle cell hemoglobinopathies, and infective endocarditis may involve the joints and the heart. Other differential diagnostic considerations include congenital heart lesions, viral and idiopathic forms of myocarditis and pericarditis, and functional heart murmurs. Nonfamilial forms of chorea have been described in systemic lupus erythematosus and rarely in association with the use of birth control pills. It remains uncertain how often episodes of chorea occurring during pregnancy ("chorea gravidarum") represent attacks of rheumatic fever. Other disorders that may at times be confused with ARF are gout, sarcoidosis, Hodgkin's disease, and acute leukemia.

Following an episode of acute streptococcal pharyngitis, a small proportion of patients may experience persistent symptoms of malaise, arthralgia, low-grade fever, and lymphadenopathy plus laboratory evidence of mild inflammation. It is difficult to classify such cases, but the affected individuals do not meet the criteria for diagnosis of ARF and, moreover, do not appear to be at risk for the delayed cardiac sequelae of ARF.

TREATMENT. Antibiotics neither modify the course of a rheumatic attack nor influence the subsequent development of carditis. Nevertheless, it is conventional to give a course of antibiotics designed to eradicate any rheumatogenic group A streptococci remaining in the tonsils and pharynx, at least in part to prevent spread of the organism to close contacts. The recommended regimens are those conventionally used for treatment of acute streptococcal pharyngitis (Ch. 297). Benzathine penicillin G is preferred in the non–penicillin-allergic patient. Following completion of this therapy, continuous antistreptococcal prophylaxis should commence (see below).

Treatment with anti-inflammatory agents is effective in suppressing many of the signs and symptoms of ARF. These agents do not "cure" the disease, nor do they prevent the subsequent evolution of rheumatic heart disease. They should be avoided in very mild or equivocal cases because, by suppressing the clinical manifestations, they may obscure the diagnosis. The two drugs most widely used are aspirin and corticosteroids. The former is used in patients with acute polyarthritis, provided that carditis is either absent or mild and there is no evidence of congestive heart failure. Aspirin is very effective in decreasing fever, toxicity, and joint inflammation. It should be given in a dosage of 90 to 100 mg per kilogram per day in children and 6 to 8 grams per day in adults. This is administered in equally divided doses, every 4 hours for the first 24 to 36 hours; thereafter it may be given in four doses during waking hours. A salicylate level of 25 mg per deciliter is usually satisfactory. The incidence of nausea

and vomiting may be minimized by starting somewhat below the optimal dosage level and gradually increasing over a few days. The patient should be observed for evidence of significant gastrointestinal bleeding and for signs and symptoms of salicylism. After 2 weeks, the dosage is reduced to 60 to 70 mg per kilogram per day for an additional 6 weeks. These dosage schedules represent general guidelines only. The precise aspirin dose must be determined by the patient's clinical response, blood salicylate levels, and tolerance of the drug.

Corticosteroids are generally reserved for patients who have severe carditis manifested by congestive heart failure, who are unable to tolerate large doses of salicylates, or whose signs and symptoms are inadequately suppressed by aspirin. As with aspirin, the dosage must be individualized. Prednisone, 40 to 60 mg per day in divided doses, may be used initially; after 2 to 3 weeks it should be withdrawn slowly over an additional 3-week period. In cases of fulminating carditis with profound heart failure, intravenous corticosteroids may be employed. Aspirin should be administered for a month after discontinuation of prednisone. As is the case for other patients receiving corticosteroids, the physician should be alert to problems such as gastrointestinal bleeding, sodium and water retention, and impairment of glucose tolerance. Suppression of the pituitary-adrenal axis or of the host immune system is a potential problem but not ordinarily a major one during this relatively short course of treatment. The role of nonsteroidal anti-inflammatory agents in management of ARF remains to be defined.

Following cessation of anti-inflammatory therapy, clinical or laboratory evidence of ARF may reappear. Such therapeutic "rebounds" occur more frequently after corticosteroid therapy than after treatment with aspirin. They may be minimized by prolonging salicylate therapy for 9 to 12 weeks and, when corticosteroids have been required, by continuing aspirin use for a month after corticosteroids have been discontinued.

Congestive heart failure is managed by the usual measures of bed rest, sodium restriction, diuretics, and, if necessary, oxygen and digitalis. The potential risk of digitalis-induced arrhythmias in the patient with active myocarditis must be borne in mind.

All patients should be kept at bed-chair rest for the first 3 weeks of illness, during which time carditis will usually manifest itself if it is destined to appear. Bathroom privileges may be allowed unless arthritis or chorea makes this infeasible or unless frank heart failure supervenes. Subsequently the level of physical activity should be guided by the patient's clinical status, primarily by the presence and activity of rheumatic carditis. Patients with congestive heart failure should be kept at rest until compensation has been achieved. Patients with Sydenham's chorea require a quiet environment, and sedatives such as phenobarbital may be helpful.

Once the acute attack has subsided completely, the patient's subsequent level of physical activity is dependent upon cardiac status. Patients without residual heart disease may resume full and unrestricted activity. It is important that the patient not be subjected to unwarranted invalidism, either because of his or her own inaccurate perceptions of the nature of the rheumatic process or because of those of parents, teachers, or employers.

PREVENTION. "Primary prevention" of ARF consists of accurate diagnosis and appropriate treatment of streptococcal sore throat (Ch. 297). Although straightforward in theory, primary prevention is often frustratingly difficult to achieve. In many of the densely populated, indigent communities in which the risk of ARF is greatest, children with self-limited illnesses such as sore throats may never come to medical attention, and throat culture services are usually unavailable to aid in diagnosis. Moreover, in one third or more of cases, ARF may arise after a clinically inapparent streptococcal infection.

Perhaps the most effective strategy for avoiding the mortality and chronic cardiac disability associated with ARF is that of "secondary prevention." This strategy focuses upon the group of persons who have already suffered a rheumatic attack and who are inordinately susceptible to a recurrence following an immunologically significant streptococcal upper respiratory infection. Recurrent attacks tend to be mimetic in nature, so that patients who have suffered carditis with their previous attack are likely to have repetitive cardiac involvement and progressive cardiac damage. Because even patients who experienced only arthritis or chorea may develop carditis with recurrent attacks of ARF, *all* patients who have experienced a documented attack of ARF should receive continuous antimicrobial prophylaxis to prevent either symptomatic or asymptomatic streptococcal infections. The specific regimens to be used are indicated in Ch. 297. By far the most effective of these is intramuscular benzathine penicillin G every 4 weeks. Rheumatic recurrences are very unusual in patients faithfully adhering to this regimen.

The total duration of intramuscular or oral rheumatic prophylaxis remains unresolved. Some authorities recommend lifelong prophylaxis. On the other hand, the risk of rheumatic recurrence is known to diminish with increasing age and increasing interval since the most recent rheumatic attack. Patients who escape carditis during their initial attack are less likely to experience rheumatic recurrences and less likely to develop carditis if a recurrence does ensue. These facts suggest that prophylaxis need not be perpetual for all rheumatic subjects. Continuous prophylaxis should be maintained indefinitely for those with clinically significant rheumatic heart disease. Other rheumatic subjects should be protected until reaching adulthood, for at least 5 years after their most recent attack, and if they are in an epidemiologic circumstance that places them at high risk of streptococcal acquisition (e.g., parents of small children, school teachers, military recruits, nurses, pediatricians, or residents of areas with a high incidence of ARF). The decision to remove a rheumatic subject from continuous prophylaxis should be an individualized one, based upon the physician's assessment of the risk and likely consequences of recurrence, and taken with the patient's informed consent. Patients taken off prophylaxis must be instructed to return immediately for medical follow-up whenever symptoms of pharyngitis occur.

Patients with rheumatic valvular heart disease must receive prophylaxis designed to avoid bacterial endocarditis whenever they undergo dental or surgical procedures likely to evoke bacteremia. This is not necessary in the rheumatic subject who is free of residual heart disease. The regimens for prevention of endocarditis (see Ch. 299) are different from those prescribed for prevention of ARF, and the fact that a patient is receiving rheumatic fever prophylaxis does not exempt him or her from endocarditis prophylaxis. This is a frequent point of confusion not only among patients but among physicians and dentists as well.

Bisno AL: The resurgence of acute rheumatic fever in the United States. Annu Rev Med 41:319, 1990. *A review that places in historical perspective the epidemiologic and bacteriologic features of the recent outbreaks of ARF in the United States.*

Committee on Rheumatic Fever, Infective Endocarditis, and Kawasaki Disease, American Heart Association: Prevention of rheumatic fever. Circulation 78:1082, 1988. *Official recommendations of the American Heart Association for primary and secondary prevention of rheumatic fever. Includes specific antimicrobial regimens.*

Stollerman GH: Rheumatic Fever and Streptococcal Infection. New York, Grune & Stratton, 1975. *A comprehensive, extremely readable summary of all aspects of rheumatic fever.*

Endocarditis

299 Infective Endocarditis

David T. Durack

When microbes colonize the endocardium, they cause the disease termed *infective endocarditis*. The organism is usually a common bacterium, the site affected is usually one of the heart valves, and the characteristic lesion is a vegetation. For general use, the term infective endocarditis is more appropriate than *bacterial endocarditis*, because this disease also can be caused by fungi and chlamydia. Serviceable terms in general use include *subacute* and *acute bacterial endocarditis* (SBE and ABE), *native valve endocarditis* (NVE), *prosthetic valve endocarditis* (PVE), and *nonbacterial thrombotic endocarditis* (NBTE).

MICROBIOLOGY. Most of the species of bacteria that can colonize or infect humans have been reported to cause endocarditis. However, a few common gram-positive species account for the great majority of infections. Streptococci and staphylococci dominate the list; together these organisms cause more than 80 per cent of infections on native valves. Table 299–1 shows representative figures for the reported frequency of the main etiologic microbes on native valves, on prosthetic valves, and in drug addicts. Individual and local experience may differ widely.

The Gram-Positive Cocci. The various α-hemolytic (viridans) streptococci together cause more cases of endocarditis than any other bacteria. These relatively avirulent streptococci are found in large numbers in the oropharyngeal and gastrointestinal flora. In order of frequency, the species that cause SBE most often are *Streptococcus sanguis*, *S. mutans*, *S. intermedius*, and *S. mitis*. Next in frequency among the streptococci causing endocarditis are the group D streptococci, *S. bovis* and *Enterococcus faecalis*. *S. bovis* bacteremia and endocarditis are associated with the presence of lower gastrointestinal lesions, including polyps and colonic cancer. Therefore, recovery of this species from blood cultures should be followed up by investigation for colonic tumors, whether or not the patient has any symptoms. *E. faecalis* (the enterococcus) causes endocarditis in association with infections of the genital and urinary tract in women of childbearing age and of the urinary tract in elderly men with prostatic disease.

S. pneumoniae occasionally causes acute endocarditis. The triad of coexisting pneumococcal pneumonia, meningitis, and endocar-

TABLE 299–1. APPROXIMATE FREQUENCY OF VARIOUS ORGANISMS CAUSING INFECTIVE ENDOCARDITIS ON NATIVE VALVES, IN DRUG ABUSERS, AND ON PROSTHETIC VALVES*

	NVE (%)	Intravenous Drug Abusers (%)	Early PVE (%)	Late PVE (%)
Streptococci	65	15	10	35
Viridans, alpha-hemolytic	35	5	<5	25
S. bovis (group D)	15	<5	<5	<5
E. faecalis (group D)	10	8	<5	<5
Other streptococci	<5	<5	<5	<5
Staphylococci	25	50	50	30
Coagulase-positive	23	50	20	10
Coagulase-negative	<5	<5	30	20
Gram-negative aerobic bacilli	<5	15	15	10
HACEK group	5	<5	<1	<5
Fungi	<5	5	10	5
Miscellaneous bacteria	<5	5	5	5
Diphtheroids, propionibacteria	<1	<5	5	<5
Other anaerobes	<1	<1	<1	<1
Legionella	0	0	0	<1
Rickettsia	<1	<1	<1	<1
Chlamydia	<1	<1	<1	<1
Polymicrobial infection	<1	5	5	5
Culture-negative endocarditis	5	<5	<5	<5

*These are representative figures collated from the literature; wide local variations in frequency are to be expected.

Adapted from Durack DT: Infective and non-infective endocarditis. *In* Hurst JW (ed.): The Heart, 6th ed., pp 1130–1157. Copyright © 1986 by McGraw-Hill, Inc. Used by permission of McGraw-Hill Book Company.

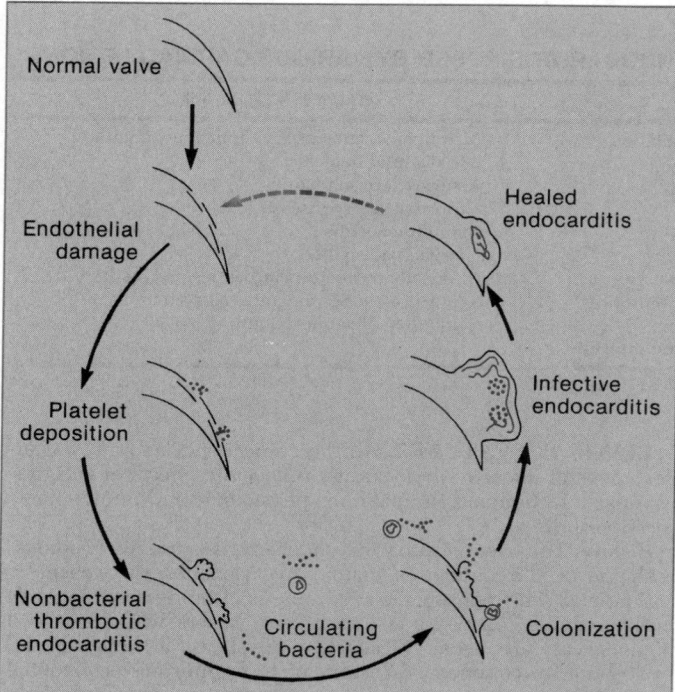

FIGURE 299–1. A diagram to illustrate the main events in pathogenesis of subacute bacterial endocarditis. (Adapted from Durack DT: Infective and non-infective endocarditis. *In* Hurst JW (ed.): The Heart, 5th ed. Copyright © 1982 by McGraw-Hill, Inc. Used by permission of McGraw-Hill Book Company.)

ditis is known as *Austrian's syndrome*. It often occurs in debilitated alcoholics and carries a very poor prognosis.

A few cases of endocarditis are caused by nutritionally dependent streptococci that require media supplemented with L-cysteine or pyridoxine for growth. These fastidious organisms can be difficult to isolate from blood cultures, and the infections they cause are more difficult to cure than infections caused by other streptococci.

Staphylococcus aureus is the leading cause of acute bacterial endocarditis, is the predominant species in narcotic addicts with endocarditis, and is an important cause of PVE (Table 299–1). *Staphylococcus epidermidis* rarely causes NVE, but it is a leading cause of PVE.

Other Etiologic Organisms. Gram-negative and fungal infections are described later. Endocarditis caused by *Haemophilus* species is usually caused by *H. aphrophilus, H. paraphrophilus,* or *H. parainfluenzae,* rarely *H. influenzae. Neisseria gonorrhoeae* causes acute endocarditis; this complication of gonorrhea has become rare since the introduction of penicillin. Cases of endocarditis caused by anaerobic bacteria or by more than one species (polymicrobial infection) also are rare, accounting for less than 1 per cent of cases.

PATHOGENESIS AND PATHOLOGY. Figure 299–1 illustrates the sequence of events in pathogenesis of SBE, which usually develops on previously abnormal heart valves. Forty years ago, the underlying cardiac condition was most often chronic rheumatic valvular heart disease. Today, the leading pre-existing condition for SBE in the United States is congenital heart disease in its

various forms, including mitral valve prolapse. The number of cases engrafted upon rheumatic valvular disease will decline even further in the United States and other developed countries as the prevalence of chronic rheumatic heart disease in the general population continues to fall. Other important predisposing conditions are cardiac surgery (especially if a prosthetic valve has been implanted) and previous episodes of infective endocarditis. ABE can attack previously normal as well as damaged valves and prosthetic valves. Estimates of the frequency of the main underlying heart conditions for patients of various ages with acute or subacute endocarditis are shown in Table 299–2. Table 299–3 ranks the relative risks for endocarditis posed by various cardiac lesions.

The pathogenetic sequence leading to SBE begins with endothelial damage. When subendothelial connective tissue containing collagen fibers is denuded of endothelium, platelets aggregate at the site. These aggregates have been found occasionally on normal valves, but they occur more frequently on the surfaces of valves damaged by congenital or rheumatic disease or by a previous episode of infective endocarditis. These microscopic platelet thrombi may form and resolve harmlessly, but sometimes they are stabilized by deposition of fibrin and grow to form nodular sterile vegetations that are referred to as NBTE. Microscopic examination shows bundles of degenerating platelets held together by strands of fibrin, with few other cells present. This process can be induced in experimental animals by passing a catheter into the heart; NBTE forms at sites where the catheter damages the endothelium. Intracardiac pressure-monitoring catheters produce NBTE in humans in the same way. For unknown reasons, patients with cachexia caused by advanced malignancy or other wasting diseases are prone to form NBTE, which in this setting is usually termed *marantic endocarditis*. The sterile vegetations found in a few patients with systemic lupus erythematosus (Libman-Sacks endocarditis) are another form of NBTE.

The vegetations of NBTE are irregular friable white or tan masses of variable size that are usually found along the lines where valves touch upon closing. They may be so small as to be easily missed on inspection but are frequently rather large. Because there is no inflammatory reaction at the site of attachment, the vegetations of NBTE can often be picked off easily with forceps at necropsy, leaving a normal-looking valve surface. These easily dislodged vegetations embolize frequently, often blocking peripheral arteries and causing infarction in myocardium, spleen, kidney, brain, gut, or extremities.

When NBTE is colonized by circulating bacteria, infective endocarditis results. Two important factors that determine which organisms are most likely to cause endocarditis are (1) the frequency with which they are found in the blood and (2) their ability to adhere to fibrin and platelet thrombi. Viridans streptococci enter the blood from the oral cavity frequently (probably daily) and adhere well to platelets and fibrin. Therefore, it is not surprising that they are the leading cause of SBE (Table 299–1). In contrast, *Escherichia coli* adheres poorly and rarely causes infective endocarditis, even though it is a very frequent cause of bacteremia.

Once lodged upon the surface of NBTE, bacteria multiply rapidly and attain high numbers within the vegetation, after which many enter the stationary or resting phase. The presence of bacteria is a powerful stimulus for further localized thrombosis, which causes vegetations to enlarge by accretion of new layers of fibrin. Because these layers protect bacteria from phagocytes, the

TABLE 299–2. APPROXIMATE FREQUENCY OF THE MAJOR CATEGORIES OF PRE-EXISTING CARDIAC LESIONS IN PATIENTS WITH INFECTIVE ENDOCARDITIS IN THE UNITED STATES

	Children Under 2 Years Old (%)	Children 2 to 15 Years Old (%)	Adults 15 to 50 Years Old (%)	Adults > 50 Years Old (%)	Adults, Intravenous Drug Abusers
No known heart disease	50–70	10–15	10	10	50
Congenital heart disease	30–50	70–80	20–30	10	10
Mitral valve prolapse	Rare	Rare	30	30	10
Rheumatic heart disease	Rare	<10	10	10	<10
Degenerative heart disease	0	0	Rare	10–20	Rare
Prosthetic valve	Rare	<10	10–20	10–20	20
Previous endocarditis	Rare	<5	5	5–10	20

Adapted from Durack DT: Infective and non-infective endocarditis. *In* Hurst JW (ed.): The Heart, 6th ed., pp 1130–1157. Copyright © 1986 by McGraw-Hill, Inc. Used by permission of McGraw-Hill Book Company.

TABLE 299–3. ESTIMATED RELATIVE RISK FOR INFECTIVE ENDOCARDITIS POSED BY VARIOUS CARDIAC LESIONS

Relatively High Risk	Intermediate Risk	Very Low or Negligible Risk
Prosthetic heart valves	Mitral valve prolapse with regurgitation	Mitral valve prolapse without regurgitation
Aortic valve disease	Pure mitral stenosis	Atrial septal defects
Mitral insufficiency	Tricuspid valve disease	Arteriosclerotic plaques
Patent ductus arteriosus	Pulmonary valve disease	Coronary artery disease
Ventricular septal defect	Previous infective endocarditis	Syphilitic aortitis
Coarctation of the aorta	Asymmetric septal hypertrophy	Cardiac pacemakers
Marfan's syndrome	Calcific aortic sclerosis	Surgically corrected cardiac lesions (without prosthetic implants, more than 6 months after operation)
	Hyperalimentation or pressure-monitoring lines that reach the right atrium	
	Nonvalvular intracardiac prosthetic implants	

Adapted from Durack DT: Infective and non-infective endocarditis. *In* Hurst JW (ed.): The Heart, 6th ed., pp 1130–1157. Copyright © 1986 by McGraw-Hill, Inc. Used by permission of McGraw-Hill Book Company.

vegetation provides a sanctuary in which even avirulent bacteria can flourish.

Approximate figures for the frequency with which vegetations are found at various locations in the heart are given in Table 299–4. The frequency with which a cardiac valve is involved by endocarditis is related to the mean blood pressure acting upon it. Accordingly, the aortic and mitral valves are infected far more often than the tricuspid and pulmonary valves. This rule does not hold for acute endocarditis in intravenous drug abusers, in whom tricuspid valve infection is common (Table 299–4).

Endocarditis usually develops at sites where blood flows from a high-pressure source (e.g., the left ventricle) through an orifice (e.g., a ventricular septal defect) into a low-pressure sink (e.g., the right ventricle). Examples of cardiovascular conditions subject to infection that fit these criteria include mitral regurgitation, aortic stenosis, ventricular septal defect, patent ductus arteriosus, and coarctation of the aorta. Vegetations are usually located on the "downstream" side of these anatomic abnormalities, where pressure effects and turbulence favor deposition of bacteria from the swift stream of blood. Vegetations also may develop at sites where a turbulent regurgitant jet of blood strikes the wall of a cardiac chamber, causing endothelial roughening and reactive endocardial fibrosis. These are called *jet lesions*.

The vegetations of infective endocarditis are variable in appearance. Some are small warty nodules, whereas others have the cauliflower-like polypoid appearance that gave rise to the descriptive term *vegetation*. Some are less than 1 sq mm in size, whereas others are so large as to block valve orifices and cause functional stenosis. They may be white, red, tan, or gray. Vegetations on the tricuspid valve are often larger than those on left-sided valves. Microscopic examination shows colonies of bacteria or masses of fungal hyphae embedded in fibrin and platelets. Infected vegetations usually contain surprisingly few leukocytes. Inflammatory cells may accumulate at the base of the vegetation, where it attaches to the valve. This distorts the valve, superimposing new damage on any pre-existing pathology. If this reaction is severe, the valve may perforate, or an abscess may develop in adjacent tissues. Abscess formation is common in ABE and PVE but not in SBE.

Antibodies to many of the commensal organisms that cause SBE are present in low titer before infection occurs, increase in titer during the course of SBE, and decrease after successful treatment. These antibodies do not arrest the progress of SBE and do not provide immunity to future endocardial infection.

The healing process begins even in untreated endocarditis but reaches completion only if antibiotic treatment kills the bacteria. Host cells move in to organize the vegetation; macrophages ingest bacterial and cellular debris; and fibroblasts lay down new collagen. The vegetations gradually shrink over a period of weeks or months and become endothelialized. Recognizable but nonviable bacteria can sometimes be found in sections of valves resected at operation or necropsy, months after infection has been eradicated. The healed valve is often scarred, thickened by fibrosis, and calcified. It may be perforated, and the supporting structures may be damaged. Residual hemodynamic dysfunction, mild or severe, is therefore likely. This condition may worsen over time, even though the bacteria had been eradicated long before by antibiotic treatment. The scarred valve remains susceptible to reinfection for life.

CLINICAL FEATURES. All the clinical and laboratory manifestations of infective endocarditis reflect the effects of an intravascular infection and the patient's physiologic and immunologic reaction to it.

History. The onset of subacute endocarditis is usually insidious, with nonspecific complaints, general malaise, anorexia, weakness, and fatigue. This nonspecific syndrome is often described as a "a flu-like illness." Low-grade intermittent fevers with chills and night sweats are usual. Headaches, myalgias, arthralgias, and back pain are common. A history of heart murmur, congenital heart disease, rheumatic fever, or cardiac surgery may help identify the underlying lesion. The patient may conceal intravenous drug abuse, which should be kept in mind during both interview and examination as a likely mode of infection.

Symptoms of heart failure must be carefully sought because their presence is of great prognostic significance. Embolization and infarction can cause sudden onset of neurologic syndromes, such as hemiparesis, or abdominal pain due to infarction of spleen, kidney, or gut. Embolization of a coronary artery can cause silent or symptomatic myocardial infarction. Perforation of a valve or rupture of chordae tendineae can cause sudden onset of severe heart failure.

Physical Examination. Patients with subacute endocarditis may have nonspecific symptoms of subacute systemic infection including pallor, asthenia, and sweating. A variety of interesting peripheral signs may be found on further examination, including petechiae, splinter hemorrhages, Roth's spots, Osler's nodes, Janeway lesions, and clubbing of the fingers. Some of the characteristics of these signs are summarized in Table 299–5.

Examination of the spleen often shows moderate enlargement, usually without notable tenderness unless there is a splenic abscess or recent embolic infarction.

On examination of the cardiovascular system, the peripheral pulse is often rapid because of fever, heart failure, or both. A collapsing pulse may be present, indicating aortic incompetence

TABLE 299–4. FREQUENCY WITH WHICH ANATOMIC SITES ARE INVOLVED IN SUBACUTE ENDOCARDITIS, ACUTE ENDOCARDITIS, AND ENDOCARDITIS IN INTRAVENOUS DRUG ABUSERS

	SBE (%)	ABE (%)	Endocarditis in Intravenous Drug Abusers (%)
Left-sided valves	85	65	40
Aortic	15–26	18–25	25–30
Mitral	38–45	30–35	15–20
Aortic *and* mitral	23–30	15–20	15–20
Right-sided valves	5	20	50
Tricuspid	1–5	15	45–50
Pulmonary	1	Rare	2
Tricuspid *and* pulmonary	Rare	Rare	3
Left- *and* right-sided sites	Rare	5–10	5–10
Other sites (patent ductus, VSD, coarctation, jet lesions)	10	5	5

Adapted from Durack DT: Infective and non-infective endocarditis. *In* Hurst JW (ed.): The Heart, 6th ed., pp 1130–1157. Copyright © 1986 by McGraw-Hill, Inc. Used by permission of McGraw-Hill Book Company.

associated with pre-existing aortic valve disease, or new aortic insufficiency associated with endocarditis. Individual peripheral arteries may be occluded by emboli, or they may be the site of a mycotic aneurysm.

One or more cardiac murmurs are present in virtually all patients with endocarditis. Murmurs may be caused by pre-existing heart disease, by endocarditis itself, or by both. Up to 15 per cent of patients do not have a heart murmur when first examined, but nearly all develop a murmur before the disease has run its course. New murmurs and changing murmurs are more likely to occur in acute endocarditis than in subacute disease. Development of a new murmur of aortic insufficiency during a febrile illness of unknown origin strongly suggests the diagnosis of infective endocarditis.

COMPLICATIONS. Heart failure is by far the most important complication of infective endocarditis; it exerts more influence on prognosis and treatment than any other. In one representative series, some degree of heart failure was present in 75 per cent of patients with aortic valve disease and endocarditis, in 50 per cent with mitral valve involvement, and in 19 per cent with tricuspid disease.

Arterial embolization is diagnosed in about one third of patients with subacute endocarditis and in up to two thirds of patients with acute endocarditis. Many small or large arterial emboli go undetected. Any artery may be affected. In order of frequency, arteries supplying the brain, lung, myocardium, spleen, and extremities are involved.

Neurologic manifestations of endocarditis are common and clinically important. These include toxic confusional states, stroke, meningoencephalitis, cranial or peripheral nerve lesions, and psychiatric symptoms. About 10 per cent of patients with endocarditis have complaints involving the central nervous system at presentation, and 30 to 50 per cent have nervous system involvement at some point during the course of the disease. Cerebral infarction is usually caused by embolism, while cerebral hemorrhage, which is less common than infarction, may be associated with emboli or rupture of a mycotic aneurysm. Heparin therapy increases the risk that an intracranial hemorrhage will occur during the course of infective endocarditis.

Cerebritis secondary to impaction of infected emboli or hematogenous spread of bacteria is quite common, especially in acute bacterial endocarditis caused by *S. aureus*. Cerebritis may progress to form a frank cerebral abscess, which is found in 1 to 5 per cent of cases of acute endocarditis. However, brain abscesses rarely complicate subacute endocarditis.

In up to 15 per cent of patients, examination of the cerebrospinal fluid may show reactive changes consisting of the presence of polymorphonuclear leukocytes and moderately elevated protein concentration. Such reactions are particularly common in acute staphylococcal endocarditis. In most cases cerebrospinal glucose concentrations do not decrease, cultures are negative, and true bacterial meningitis does not develop, except in a few patients with acute pneumococcal or staphylococcal endocarditis.

Mycotic aneurysm is an unusual but important complication that is diagnosed in 3 to 5 per cent of patients. The true incidence is probably higher, but a number pass undetected, especially small aneurysms in the brain. Mycotic aneurysms are caused by an inflammatory reaction in the arterial wall associated with septic microemboli to vasa vasorum or with impaction of an infected embolus in the arterial lumen. The site most often involved is the proximal aorta, including the sinuses of Valsalva, followed by arteries to the viscera, extremities, and brain. Living organisms are seldom found in the wall of these aneurysms, even when the underlying endocardial infection is still active. Presumably, the damage that weakened the arterial wall was caused by an inflammatory reaction to infected emboli. If an aneurysm enlarges to a certain critical size (probably about 1 cm in diameter), it is likely to continue to enlarge and eventually rupture as a result of the physical forces exerted by the arterial pressure, despite eradication of the infecting organisms by antimicrobial therapy.

Many patients with subacute endocarditis show abnormalities in the urinary sediment. In some cases this is due to glomerulonephritis, a relatively common complication that occasionally causes significant renal failure. Glomerulonephritis is caused by deposition of immune complexes on the glomerular basement membrane. Other inflammatory manifestations of subacute infective endocarditis that may be mediated by immune complexes include arthritis, tenosynovitis, and possibly pericarditis, Osler's nodes, and Roth's spots. In a few patients with long-term SBE, glomerulonephritis is severe enough to necessitate dialysis. Renal function usually recovers steadily within a few weeks after the start of effective treatment.

TABLE 299–5. CHARACTERISTICS OF SOME PERIPHERAL SIGNS OF INFECTIVE ENDOCARDITIS

	Petechiae	Splinter Hemorrhages	Roth's Spots	Osler's Nodes	Janeway's Lesions	Clubbing
Appearance	Tiny red hemorrhagic spots	"Splinters" under nails; red when fresh, then brown or black	Small bright red patches with white centers	Pea-sized red or purplish nodules	Red macules	Curvature of the nails in two planes, with swelling of the terminal phalanges
Distribution	Anywhere, especially above clavicles, in mouth and in conjunctivae	Distal third of nails	Retinae	Fingers and toes; occasionally hands and feet	Palms and soles; occasionally on flanks, forearms, ankles, feet, ears	Fingers and/or toes
Incidence	Common, in both SBE and ABE	Common, in both SBE and ABE	Infrequent; usually in SBE	Infrequent; usually in SBE	Infrequent; usually in ABE	Rare; in SBE only
Pathology	Increased capillary permeability; microemboli	Blood in avascular squamous epithelium under nail; due to microemboli or increased capillary fragility	Inflammation and hemorrhage	Intracutaneous local vasculitis; bacteria rarely found; occasional abscess formation; probably embolic in origin	Origin uncertain; possibly embolic or allergic in origin	Soft tissue proliferation, occasionally periosteal new bone formation
Pain	None	None	None	Mild to moderately severe	None	Usually none; sometimes painful
Duration	Days	Weeks	Days	Days	Several hours to days	Weeks to months
Diagnostic significance	Nonspecific; also found in septicemia, after cardiac surgery, and in many other disorders	Nonspecific; found in up to 10% of normal people and up to 40% of patients with mitral stenosis	Strongly suggestive of endocarditis but not diagnostic	Almost pathognomonic for endocarditis	Unusual in bacteremia without endocarditis	Nonspecific; found in many cardiopulmonary disorders; can be congenital

Adapted from Durack DT: Infective and non-infective endocarditis. *In* Hurst JW (ed.): The Heart, 5th ed., pp 1250–1277. Copyright © 1982 by McGraw-Hill, Inc. Used by permission of McGraw-Hill Book Company.

SPECIAL FORMS OF INFECTIVE ENDOCARDITIS

ACUTE BACTERIAL ENDOCARDITIS. Several important features distinguish acute from subacute bacterial endocarditis. The clinical course is usually measured in days rather than in weeks or months. The associated systemic illness is more severe, and early mortality is higher than in subacute endocarditis. The diagnosis is usually made within 7 days from onset of symptoms.

Acute endocardial infection is usually caused by primary pathogens capable of producing invasive infection at other sites. S. aureus is the most common cause of acute endocarditis. This species alone accounts for 50 to 70 per cent of cases. The patient is more likely to suffer rapid destruction of the valve, including perforation, so the likelihood that valve replacement will be required is greater. Patients with acute bacterial endocarditis are also more likely to have one or more focal infections outside the heart—in brain, bone, lungs, or other sites. Such foci could be either primary infections (that is, the portal of entry for the organism causing endocarditis) or secondary hematogenous infections. In contrast, the organisms that cause subacute bacterial endocarditis rarely cause localized hematogenous infection elsewhere in the body.

Abscesses in the fibrous cardiac skeleton or myocardium are much more likely to form in acute than in subacute endocarditis. If such abscesses are adjacent to the fibers of the conduction system, they may cause conduction defects. Abscesses may be responsible for antibiotic treatment failure.

Because acute bacterial endocarditis is caused by invasive organisms and progresses rapidly, treatment should not be delayed until blood culture results are available. It is important to clear the bloodstream of circulating organisms as soon as possible, both to reduce the risk of death from septicemia and to lessen the chances that metastatic infection will develop elsewhere. When acute endocarditis is strongly suspected, empiric antibiotic therapy should be started immediately after three blood samples have been drawn for culture.

ENDOCARDITIS IN DRUG ADDICTS. Endocarditis is the most important of the many bacterial infections experienced by intravenous drug abusers. Salient features that distinguish endocarditis in this subgroup from the disease in general include a younger age of onset, a higher proportion of acute cases, a correspondingly higher proportion of cases involving normal cardiac valves, and a high frequency of tricuspid valve infection. The etiologic organisms can gain entry into the bloodstream in various ways: directly, by injection of contaminated drugs; or indirectly, from the patient's skin flora, from cellulitis caused by subcutaneous injection of drugs, or from suppurative thrombophlebitis or drug-related infections in other sites such as the lungs. S. aureus is the leading etiologic organism. Addicts also have an increased incidence of endocardial infection with gram-negative bacilli, especially Pseudomonas species, and fungi.

Drug addicts with acute endocarditis usually experience a brief, severe illness, with heavily positive blood cultures. Because the etiologic organisms are often primary pathogens, hematogenous infections at other sites in the body are common. A frequent finding on admission is multiple patches of pneumonitis visible on chest radiography. These are caused by septic pulmonary emboli arising from vegetations on the tricuspid or occasionally the pulmonary valve. Although acute disease is typical, subacute endocarditis also is common in addicts, especially in those who have had previous episodes of endocarditis.

The prognosis for young drug addicts with right-sided S. aureus infection is good, with mortality rates being less than 5 per cent. Factors that worsen the prognosis include left-sided involvement, particularly aortic, and infection with gram-negative bacilli or fungi. Recurrent episodes of endocarditis are common in addicts who continue to use drugs after their first episode of endocarditis, especially if a prosthetic valve has been inserted.

PROSTHETIC VALVE INFECTION. Prosthetic valve endocarditis should be regarded as a special category, because it differs in many ways from other forms of endocarditis. By arbitrary definition, early PVE occurs within 60 days of valve placement and late PVE more than 60 days postoperatively. Early PVE occurs at a rate of about 0.5 per cent, although this figure varies between hospitals. Late PVE is estimated to occur at an overall rate of about 1 per cent per year. The rate for infection of aortic valve prostheses is three to five times higher than for mitral prostheses.

The progress of PVE may be either acute or subacute, but this cannot be predicted reliably from the infecting organism. For example, even S. epidermidis, a "nonpathogen" that causes indolent chronic disease on native valves, can cause an acute syndrome in early PVE.

The spectrum of organisms causing PVE is quite distinct. S. epidermidis, which rarely infects native valves, is a leading cause of both early and late prosthetic valve infection. Gram-negative bacilli and fungi infect prosthetic valves notably more often than they do native valves, especially in early onset cases. The later the onset of PVE after operation, the more nearly the spectrum of etiologic organisms resembles that of native valve endocarditis.

In addition to forming vegetations, infection may spread around the circumference of the sewing ring of the prosthesis, often causing partial dehiscence and paravalvular leaks. Abscess formation in fibrous tissue or myocardium adjacent to the sewing ring is common. Despite these adverse factors, when a prosthetic valve is replaced because of infection, early reinfection with the same organism is uncommon.

In general, PVE is harder to cure than most other forms of endocarditis (Table 299–6). This is due partly to the increased frequency of antibiotic-resistant organisms in PVE, partly to the fact that a foreign body is present at the site of infection, and partly to the high frequency of perivalvular abscesses. Not surprisingly, the risk of relapse after antibiotic therapy is much higher for PVE than for native valve infection. Valve replacement is often necessary to achieve cure. Antibiotic treatment usually must be continued for a minimum of 4 to 6 weeks, sometimes for many months. In some cases in which repeated valve replacement is contraindicated, cure cannot be achieved but suppressive antibiotic therapy is continued indefinitely.

GRAM-NEGATIVE BACTERIAL ENDOCARDITIS. This term usually refers to infection with enteric or environmental gram-negative aerobic bacilli such as Klebsiella, Pseudomonas, Serratia, Enterobacter, and E. coli. (Haemophilus species are not considered in this group.) Gram-negative endocarditis is a rare disease except in two settings: early prosthetic valve infection and intravenous drug addiction. In these two groups, gram-negative bacilli can account for up to 15 per cent of cases.

TABLE 299–6. ESTIMATED BACTERIOLOGIC CURE RATES FOR ETIOLOGIC ORGANISMS TREATED WITH ANTIMICROBIAL THERAPY ALONE OR ANTIMICROBIALS PLUS SURGERY*

Native Valve Endocarditis	Antimicrobial Therapy Alone	Antimicrobial Therapy Plus Surgery
Viridans streptococci, group A streptococci, S. bovis, pneumococci, gonococci	98	98
E. faecalis	90	>90
S. aureus (in young drug addicts)	90	>90
S. aureus (in elderly patients with chronic underlying diseases)	50	70
Gram-negative aerobic bacilli†	40	65
Fungi	<5	50

Prosthetic Valve Endocarditis	Early PVE (No Surgery)	Late PVE	Early PVE (With Surgery)	Late PVE
Viridans streptococci, group A streptococci, S. bovis, pneumococci, gonococci	‡	80	‡	90
E. faecalis	‡	60	‡	75
S. aureus	25	40	50	60
S. epidermidis	20	40	60	70
Gram-negative aerobic bacilli†	<10	20	40	50
Fungi	<1	<1	30	40

*Morbidity and mortality will be significantly greater than these figures for *bacteriologic* cure indicate.
†Excluding *Haemophilus* species, which carry a better prognosis.
‡Insufficient data to estimate rate.
Adapted from Durack DT: Infective and non-infective endocarditis. In Hurst JW (ed.): The Heart, 5th ed., pp 1250–1277. Copyright © 1982 by McGraw-Hill, Inc. Used by permission of McGraw-Hill Book Company.

Gram-negative endocarditis often progresses acutely. Patients may develop septic shock. The mortality rate is higher than for gram-positive infections, approaching that of fungal endocarditis. Antibiotic treatment alone is often unsuccessful, so valve replacement is frequently necessary. Treatment with combinations of two or more antibiotics for 6 weeks or more is often necessary. Relapse after antibiotic treatment is much more common than for gram-positive infection.

HACEK ENDOCARDITIS. The acronym HACEK refers to a group of unusual organisms that share some characteristics and, taken together, cause a significant number of cases of infective endocarditis. They are *Haemophilus* species (but usually not *H. influenzae*), *Actinobacillus actinomycetemcomitans*, *Cardiobacterium hominis*, *Eikenella corrodens*, and *Kingella* species. These are fastidious gram-negative bacteria that have a tendency to cause subacute endocarditis with large vegetations. They are more likely to be sensitive to β-lactam antibiotics, especially ampicillin and ceftriaxone, than other aerobic gram-negative bacilli. Endocarditis caused by these organisms has a fairly good prognosis and often can be cured without valve replacement, even in some cases of prosthetic valve infection.

FUNGAL ENDOCARDITIS. Like gram-negative endocarditis, fungal infection of the endocardium is rare except in two groups of patients: those with prosthetic valves and intravenous drug addicts. Although a wide variety of fungal species have been recovered from patients with endocarditis over the years, only two predominate: *Candida* and *Aspergillus* species. *C. albicans* endocarditis occurs in patients with central intravascular lines, especially hyperalimentation lines that are allowed to reach the level of the tricuspid valve. Therefore, these infections often involve the right side. *C. parapsilosis* and *C. tropicalis* are more likely to occur in drug addicts and can infect valves on either side of the heart. Fungal vegetations tend to be bulky and often cause infarctions as a result of embolization of peripheral arteries. Because blood cultures are commonly negative in fungal endocarditis (see earlier discussion), surgical removal of a large embolus from an artery to one of the limbs may be diagnostic as well as therapeutic. Histologic examination may show hyphae of the infecting fungus in tissue sections.

Few drugs are available for treatment of fungal endocarditis. Amphotericin B is generally used, but the chance of achieving cure with drug therapy alone is extremely low. Cure rates can be increased by surgical removal of vegetations and valve replacement, but mortality remains relatively high compared with that for other forms of endocarditis (Table 299–6).

ENDOCARDITIS IN INFANTS AND CHILDREN. Infective endocarditis is an unusual occurrence in infants. When it does occur, it is most often only one component of systemic bacterial infection caused by an invasive organism such as *S. aureus*. The endocardial infection is likely to follow an acute course, being discovered unexpectedly at necropsy in an infant who has died with bacterial infection. Often a normal cardiac valve is involved, as in other forms of acute endocarditis. The remaining cases are associated with congenital cardiac defects. Because the diagnosis is often delayed or missed, endocarditis in infants has a higher mortality than in other age groups.

In children more than 1 year old, infective endocarditis is not rare. Most affected children have subacute disease involving congenital cardiac defects. The spectrum of etiologic organisms and the approach to diagnosis and treatment are similar to those in adults with infective endocarditis. However, the age and physical size of children must be carefully considered when choosing the best time for cardiac surgery, especially when prostheses must be implanted.

ENDOCARDITIS IN OBSTETRIC AND GYNECOLOGIC PRACTICE. Pregnancy itself poses little increased risk for infective endocarditis. Septic abortion or pelvic infection related to intrauterine contraceptive devices can lead to endocarditis in susceptible patients. Occasionally, infective endocarditis develops during delivery or in the puerperium. If the mother has pre-existing valvular disease, bacteremias associated with perinatal infective complications such as amnionitis, endometritis, parametritis, septic thrombophlebitis, or urinary tract infection can seed the endocardium. The leading etiologic organisms in this setting are *E. faecalis*, *S. agalactiae* (group B), *S. aureus*, and only occasionally *Bacteroides* or gram-negative enteric bacilli.

NOSOCOMIAL ENDOCARDITIS. Intensive medical care can predispose to endocarditis in many ways. Endothelial damage can be caused by intracardiac surgery, pressure-monitoring catheters, ventriculoatrial shunts, and hyperalimentation lines if they reach into the right atrium. Portals of entry for microorganisms are provided by wounds, burns, biopsy sites, intravenous and arterial catheters and pacemakers, hemodialysis access sites, urinary catheters, and intratracheal airways. Nosocomial bacteremias are common in seriously ill patients. Therefore, it is not surprising that hospital-acquired infective endocarditis has become increasingly common in the past two decades, as intensive care units have proliferated. Perhaps the highest risk is found in severely burned patients, who may sustain repeated episodes of bacteremia while pressure-monitoring catheters are kept in the right side of the heart for long periods. In contrast, diagnostic right heart catheterization over brief periods in patients in a coronary care unit, who seldom develop bacteremia, presents a very low risk for infective endocarditis.

The microbes likely to cause nosocomial endocarditis are staphylococci, *Candida* species, and gram-negative bacilli. The prognosis is worse than for most other forms of infective endocarditis. This is because the patients have serious pre-existing diseases that may obscure the symptoms and signs, thus delaying diagnosis. Also, nosocomially acquired organisms are more likely to be resistant to antibiotics.

CULTURE-NEGATIVE ENDOCARDITIS. This term refers to the situation in which the endocardium is infected, but blood cultures remain persistently negative. Possible causes include antibiotic therapy, and infection by slow-growing or fastidious microorganisms that are missed because of suboptimal blood culture technique. Culture-negative endocarditis is an uncommon disease. Therefore, when blood cultures from a patient not receiving antibiotics remain *persistently* negative in the absence of antibiotic therapy, that patient probably does not have endocarditis. Fungal endocarditis is an exception. Blood cultures are positive in only about half of patients with *Candida* endocarditis and in less than one fifth of those with *Aspergillus* infection. When culture-negative disease does occur, it is much more likely to follow a subacute than an acute course.

If the clinical findings strongly support the diagnosis of culture-negative endocarditis, a therapeutic trial of antibiotic therapy may be given. This usually consists of a penicillin plus an aminoglycoside for subacute infection, a combination that covers viridans streptococci, enterococci, HACEK organisms (see above), and diphtheroids. If the disease is acute, treatment for *S. aureus* must be included. To be of any diagnostic value, a proper therapeutic trial must be continued for at least 2 weeks, unless new diagnostic information changes the clinical situation.

INFECTIVE ENDARTERITIS. An infection located within an artery can mimic infective endocarditis. Possible sites of vegetations include patent ductus arteriosus, coarctation of the aorta, arteriovenous fistulas, and prosthetic vascular grafts. In the past, about one quarter of all patients with an uncorrected patent ductus arteriosus eventually developed bacterial endarteritis. Because many of the underlying lesions are surgically correctable, infective endarteritis is now uncommon in developed countries, with the exception of infections in arteriovenous shunts constructed for the purpose of hemodialysis. When bacterial endarteritis occurs in an aneurysm, the etiologic organisms are usually found within a multilayered thrombus in the lumen of the aneurysm rather than in vegetations.

RECURRENT ENDOCARDITIS. The term *recurrent endocarditis* includes both *relapses* and *reinfections*. Recurrent endocarditis has been reported in 2 to 30 per cent of cases. This wide variation is partly explained by variable duration of follow-up. Intravenous drug abusers are at higher risk than any other group for recurrent endocarditis. A few patients with more than four separate episodes of infective endocarditis have been reported.

The likelihood of relapse after treatment of different forms of infective endocarditis can be predicted from published experience (Table 299–6). Because occasional relapses occur even after optimal treatment, careful follow-up for several months after treatment is mandatory. Most relapses occur within a few days or weeks of ending treatment, but occasional late relapses occur as a result of a few organisms surviving in a metabolically inactive state deep within vegetations.

Reinfection means that a new episode of endocarditis has developed after a cure of a previous episode. Reinfections have become more common in recent years, as more patients are followed for longer periods after a first episode. Usually a different species or strain of etiologic organism is involved, but if the second organism is a common viridans streptococcus that appears identical to the first, one cannot be certain, without special tests, whether an episode of recurrent endocarditis represents reinfection or relapse.

DIFFERENTIAL DIAGNOSIS. The differential diagnosis of endocarditis is very wide because its manifestations are numerous and often nonspecific. SBE must be considered in the evaluation of every patient with fever of unknown origin. It can be confused with rheumatic fever, osteomyelitis, tuberculosis, meningitis, intra-abdominal infections, salmonellosis, brucellosis, glomerulonephritis, myocardial infarction, stroke, endocardial thrombi, atrial myxoma, connective tissue diseases, vasculitis, occult malignancy (especially lymphomas), congestive heart failure, pericarditis, and even psychoneurosis. ABE shares many manifestations with septicemias caused by *S. aureus, Neisseria,* pneumococci, and gram-negative bacilli in patients who do not have endocarditis. ABE may mimic pneumonia, meningitis, brain abscess, stroke, malaria, acute pericarditis, vasculitis, and disseminated intravascular coagulation.

INVESTIGATIONS. *Routine Tests.* Results of urinalysis are abnormal in about 50 per cent of cases, showing microscopic hematuria or slight proteinuria or both. Gross hematuria suggests that renal infarction may have occurred. Red cell casts and heavy proteinuria indicate that immune complex glomerulonephritis may be present.

The automated blood count shows only nonspecific abnormalities. Anemia is usual in SBE and fairly common in ABE. Anemia is most often of the hypoproliferative type, with a normochromic normocytic smear. ABE may cause acute hemolysis.

A moderate leukocytosis with some immature forms apparent on smear is often found in SBE, but in many cases the leukocyte count is normal. Patients with ABE often show neutrophilia with band forms, vacuoles, Döhle bodies, and toxic granulation. In a few cases, careful examination of a Gram-stained smear of the buffy coat reveals organisms within neutrophils.

The erythrocyte sedimentation rate is usually elevated, except in a few acute cases of brief duration.

Blood Culture. This is the single most important investigation in diagnosis of endocarditis. Blood cultures should be drawn from all patients with fever and heart murmur unless their illness is clearly due to another diagnosed disease or the fever resolves quickly without recurrence. Blood cultures should also be taken if a patient with a heart lesion susceptible to endocarditis has other symptoms or signs consistent with infection.

The bacteremia of infective endocarditis is usually continuous, with between 1 and 100 organisms per milliliter of blood in subacute cases. Therefore, it is seldom necessary to draw a large number of blood cultures. The causative organism can be recovered from culture samples taken on the first day of admission in over 90 per cent of patients with culture-positive endocarditis. No more than three separate venous blood cultures should be drawn on the first day. If these show no growth by the second day, two or three further culture samples may be drawn. If the patient has received prior antibiotic therapy, further blood samples may be taken over the following week in a search for recrudescence of bacteremia after antibiotic effect has passed. Otherwise, repeated blood cultures are likely to be uninformative and wasteful.

After careful skin cleansing, 10 to 20 ml of blood should be drawn for each culture. Skin preparation is especially important because common skin flora (*S. epidermidis* and diphtheroids) can cause endocarditis, and their isolation from blood cultures can cause diagnostic confusion. Pour plates can help to distinguish contaminants from true positive cultures. The culture medium should be adequately supplemented to allow growth of fastidious, nutritionally variant bacteria. When endocarditis is suspected, cultures should be incubated for at least 3 weeks and stains made at intervals even if no growth is apparent on inspection.

Subacute endocarditis stimulates the humoral immune system to produce both nonspecific and specific antibodies. A positive test for rheumatoid factor is found in 40 to 50 per cent of subacute cases, but rarely in ABE. This can provide a useful diagnostic clue in culture-negative cases. A polyclonal increase in gamma globulins is characteristic. Occasional false-positive serologic test results for syphilis occur. Hemolytic complement levels may be moderately elevated, normal, or low. The lowest levels are found in patients with immune complex glomerulonephritis. Circulating immune complexes are present in more than 80 per cent of patients with either ABE or SBE. All these immunologic findings revert to normal after eradication of the organisms.

Electrocardiography. Electrocardiography may reveal evidence of myocardial infarction due to embolization of a vegetation to a coronary artery. When a disturbance of conduction develops during the course of endocarditis, extension of infection into the myocardium may have occurred. This could be focal myocarditis or an abscess located close to the conduction system.

Echocardiography. Modern echocardiographic imaging is essential for optimal management of infective endocarditis. Serial two-dimensional studies with color flow Doppler can detect most vegetations and provide valuable additional data on underlying heart conditions and cardiac function. Introduction of transesophageal imaging has greatly improved sensitivity for detection of small vegetations, prosthetic valve infections, and abscesses. Echocardiography, valuable though it is, does have some limitations in this application. Because the sensitivity for small vegetations is not perfect, a negative echocardiogram cannot rule out endocarditis, especially when a prosthetic valve is present. Occasional false-positive readings for vegetations occur, particularly in cases with myxomatous changes affecting a valve. Finally, the echocardiographic appearance of vegetations during and after therapy is not a reliable criterion for success or failure of antibiotic therapy.

Radiography. The chest radiograph is most useful as a means of providing evidence of congestive heart failure. Multiple small patchy infiltrates in the lungs of an intravenous drug abuser with fever strongly suggest the diagnosis of septic emboli arising from right-sided infective endocarditis. Valvular calcification may identify a valve affected by chronic rheumatic or congenital disease. A mycotic aneurysm could cause widening of the aorta.

Abnormal motion of a prosthetic valve can be detected by fluoroscopy, indicating presence of a vegetation or partial dehiscence of the valve from the aortic root. This information can indicate that valve replacement is needed during management of PVE.

Computerized axial tomography can be very useful to define the cause of focal neurologic lesions in patients with endocarditis. Such lesions could be caused by various complications, including cerebritis, infarction, hemorrhage from a mycotic aneurysm, or brain abscess. Angiography is occasionally necessary to demonstrate mycotic aneurysms in the brain or elsewhere.

Cardiac catheterization and cineangiography are not necessary for most patients who respond well to antimicrobial therapy without developing cardiac failure. When treatment seems to be failing and/or operation is considered, cardiac catheterization can provide vital information. In one study of 35 patients who underwent cardiac catheterization during active endocarditis, the precatheterization assessment was significantly modified for 23, the diagnosis of site of valve involvement was altered for 14, and six valve ring abscesses were revealed. Surgery was postponed or cancelled for six patients when catheterization indicated only mild hemodynamic abnormalities. There were no serious complications. This study suggests that catheterization for selected patients with endocarditis provides such important information that it should not be avoided for fear of dislodging emboli.

TREATMENT. *General Measures.* The patient should be informed of the diagnosis and treatment plan and comforted. Heart failure, if present, should be managed with bed rest, salt restriction, and drug treatment as necessary. High temperatures and headaches can be treated symptomatically.

Antibiotic Therapy. For optimal antibiotic therapy, certain microbiologic information on the infecting organism is necessary. For most bacteria, both the minimal inhibitory concentration (MIC) and minimal bactericidal concentration (MBC) of the antibiotics likely to be used should be determined. This forms the basis for choice of curative therapy.

The serum bactericidal titer (SBT or Schlichter test) is frequently used and is sometimes useful in the management of endocarditis. The infecting organism is exposed in vitro to the patient's serum, which is drawn while antibiotic therapy is being administered, to determine the maximum dilution of serum that will inhibit and kill the organism. The SBT provides assurance that the antibiotic(s) present in the patient's serum is actually capable of killing the infecting organism. Clinical experience indicates that the SBT should be 1:8 or higher at intervals during each day of treatment. For gram-positive organisms the serum usually can kill the organism without difficulty, and SBT's are often very high (1:128 to 1:1024). In such cases, SBT's need not be measured repeatedly. SBT's for gram-negative bacilli are usually rather low (1:2 to 1:16). The SBT is most likely to be clinically helpful when the physician is treating an unusual organism, using unusual antibiotics, using an unusual regimen (such as oral treatment), or encountering treatment failure. If treatment with unusual combinations of antibiotics is needed, further laboratory tests should be performed to find out whether they are synergistic, indifferent, or antagonistic in combination.

Bactericidal antibiotics should be used for treatment of endocarditis whenever possible. Some patients have been cured with bacteriostatic drugs, but results of treatment with these agents are usually poor, presumably because host defense mechanisms are inadequate in the vegetations. With respect to treatment, the vegetations of infective endocarditis provide a contrast to bacterial pneumonia, in which phagocytes are plentiful and bacteriostatic antibiotics are usually effective. Curative antibiotic therapy for endocarditis must eradicate organisms completely, without the help of phagocytes to eliminate microbes that are relatively resistant to antibiotics because they are in the resting phase.

Clinical experience with treatment of the common forms of bacterial endocarditis caused by gram-positive cocci is so extensive that specific therapeutic regimens can be recommended with confidence. Standard regimens for streptococcal and staphylococcal endocarditis are listed in Table 299–7. Regimens for treatment of endocarditis caused by less common organisms are not listed. For these, treatment must be chosen on the basis of more limited published experience, together with the results of tests performed upon the infecting organism in the microbiology laboratory. One of the β-lactam antibiotics should be included in the regimen whenever possible.

Empiric Therapy. When the causative organism is unknown, the choice of empiric therapy depends upon whether the patient has acute or subacute disease. For ABE, broad-spectrum therapy that will cover *S. aureus* as well as many species of streptococci and gram-negative bacilli is required. For SBE, a regimen that will treat most streptococci including *E. faecalis* is appropriate. To meet these requirements, the following regimens are suggested:

1. For ABE, a combination of nafcillin, 2 grams intravenously every 4 hours, plus ampicillin, 2 grams intravenously every 4 hours, plus gentamicin, 1.0 mg per kilogram intravenously every 8 hours.
2. For SBE, a combination of ampicillin, 2 grams intravenously every 4 hours, plus gentamicin, 1.0 mg per kilogram intravenously every 8 hours.

These regimens should be adjusted if and when the causative organism is identified.

Duration of Therapy. Because infective endocarditis carries significant mortality even when well managed, it is important that treatment be continued long enough to ensure that relapse will not occur. On the other hand, patients with the most easily treated forms of endocarditis should not be subjected to unnecessarily long and expensive treatment in hospital. Extensive experience with treatment of the streptococci provides sufficient grounds for firm recommendations on duration of therapy for these organisms (Table 299–7).

In contrast, the natural history of *S. aureus* endocarditis is more variable. Some patients recover swiftly without complications, whereas others remain febrile for several weeks, sometimes owing to manifestations of disseminated staphylococcal disease such as osteomyelitis. While 4 weeks of therapy is adequate for most cases, this must not be regarded as a rigid rule because some patients require treatment for 6 to 8 weeks or longer to achieve cure. In general, the less extensive the published experience with a particular infective agent, the more one should lean

toward prolonging treatment in order to provide a reasonable margin of safety. Guidelines on duration of treatment for other organisms are not listed because the duration required varies greatly according to individual circumstances.

Anticoagulants. Although the infected vegetation is essentially a thrombotic lesion, there is no evidence that anticoagulants provide any useful therapeutic effect in endocarditis. In fact, simultaneous treatment with antibiotics plus heparin carries a higher risk of serious or fatal intracerebral hemorrhage from mycotic aneurysm or infarction than treatment with penicillin alone. However, Coumadin can be given to most patients with endocarditis without excessive risk.

It is therefore best to avoid use of heparin entirely in endocarditis and to discontinue or avoid anticoagulation therapy if possible. However, Coumadin may be given if there is a clear-cut indication, taking care not to allow the prothrombin time to rise above 1.5 times normal values. An antibiotic treatment regimen that does not require intramuscular injections should be used if the patient is receiving anticoagulant therapy.

Surgical Treatment. Modern operative treatment constitutes the greatest advance in management of endocarditis since the advent of antibiotics. Surgical consultation should be obtained early, so that prompt operative intervention is available if needed.

Aortic or mitral valvular incompetence with consequent acute left ventricular failure can occur without warning, even in the most favorable forms of endocarditis. These patients need valve replacement in order to reverse cardiac failure resulting from new or worsening valvular dysfunction. Replacement of an infected prosthesis is often necessary for cure because prosthetic valve infection is more difficult to eradicate with antibiotics than is native valve infection. Repeated major emboli constitute a relative indication for valve replacement. Occasionally, a patient remains septic despite antibiotic therapy. Operation may then be required for infection control rather than for the hemodynamic consequences of infection. Operation to close a patent ductus arteriosus or septal defect, to excise a coarctation of the aorta, or to relieve asymmetric septal hypertrophy may be required as part of treatment of endocarditis engrafted upon these lesions.

Good surgical management for endocarditis depends on correct timing for valve replacement. If operation is undertaken too soon, unnecessary operative mortality and early and late morbidity of valve replacement may result. Some patients respond quickly to medical therapy, so that operation can be postponed indefinitely. If time is available for treatment of septicemia, renal failure, pneumonia, myocarditis, conduction defects, or other complications before valve replacement, ventricular function will improve and operative risk will be correspondingly lower. Given for a few days, antibiotic therapy should eradicate or at least greatly reduce the population of organisms on the valve, thus increasing the chance that an artificial valve can be inserted without itself becoming infected. However, if surgery is delayed too long patients may die suddenly, or their hemodynamic status may deteriorate so that operation is no longer feasible. This is a tragic error, because some of these patients could have been saved by earlier operation.

Frequent re-examination of the patient, together with echocardiography and/or cardiac catheterization to extend the clinical findings, is indicated in every case in which operation may be needed. The natural history of the type of endocarditis being treated should be taken into account. Penicillin-sensitive streptococcal endocarditis can almost always be bacteriologically cured (see Table 299–6), and the prognosis is good if cardiac failure does not occur. Thus, operation should usually be considered only for patients with cardiac failure who do not respond to medical treatment. Similarly, narcotic addicts with acute staphylococcal endocarditis have a relatively good prognosis, so operation should be reserved for those who develop serious heart failure. At the other end of the spectrum, the likelihood that fungal prosthetic valve endocarditis can be eradicated with antifungal drugs alone is negligible, even in the absence of heart failure (see Table 299–6). Such patients usually should undergo valve replacement early, without waiting to test the remote possibility that antifungal treatment could eradicate the infection. Aortic valve involvement, staphylococcal infection in patients other than drug addicts, gram-negative infection, prosthetic valve infection, and extension of infection into the myocardium should be regarded as other relative indications favoring early valve replacement.

For selected cases, excision of vegetations with valve repair is a desirable option that can avoid the morbidity associated with a prosthetic valve.

PROGNOSIS. Infective endocarditis is unusual among infectious diseases in that it is always fatal if untreated. Most of the rare cases of apparent recovery reported in the preantibiotic era probably did not have infective endocarditis, which can be diagnosed with absolute certainty only at operation or necropsy. The median interval between onset of symptoms and death in patients with untreated subacute endocarditis was about 6 months, with wide individual variation. Almost all patients with acute infective endocarditis died in less than 4 weeks.

Favorable prognostic factors include infection with penicillin-sensitive streptococci, a youthful patient, absence of serious pre-existing diseases, and early diagnosis and treatment. The rate of recovery for many young drug addicts with *S. aureus* infection of the tricuspid valve is excellent—greater than 95 per cent.

Heart failure is by far the most important adverse prognostic factor. Other adverse factors include aortic valve involvement, renal failure, culture-negative disease, gram-negative or fungal

infection, prosthetic valve infection, and presence of an abscess in the valve ring or myocardium.

Today, bacteriologic cure can be achieved in most patients with bacterial endocarditis (see Table 299–6). This is not true for infection with resistant gram-negative bacilli and fungi, but fortunately these are uncommon. Despite the ability to eradicate most organisms, both early and long-term mortality and morbidity of infective endocarditis remain significant because of damage already done before treatment. Follow-up of patients cured of infective endocarditis shows a 5-year survival of only 60 to 70 per cent.

PREVENTION. Because endocarditis is a serious disease, antibiotics are usually given to susceptible patients during medical and dental procedures known to cause bacteremia, in an attempt to prevent this infection. Unfortunately, there is no proof that this practice is effective. Meaningful cost-benefit ratios cannot be calculated, and any recommendations are therefore necessarily empiric.

One approach is to consider two factors in each situation: (1) the relative risk for endocarditis posed by the patient's heart condition and (2) the relative risk for endocarditis posed by the procedure. If both risks are judged to be significant, prophylactic antibiotics should be given. If one or both of these risk factors are judged to be negligible, prophylaxis should be omitted. The first of these two questions can be approached by using a ranking like that shown in Table 299–3. The second can be approached

TABLE 299–7. TREATMENT REGIMENS

Organism	Antibiotic Regimen	Duration (Weeks)	Comments
Alpha-hemolytic (viridans) streptococci, *S. bovis*	1. Penicillin G, 10–20 million U/day IV in six equal doses, plus gentamicin, 1 mg/kg IV or IM q 8 h	2	For patients <65 years old without renal failure, eighth-nerve defects, or serious complications
	2. Penicillin G, 10–20 million U/day IV in six equal doses, plus gentamicin, 1 mg/kg IV or IM q 8 h (for first 2 weeks only), *or*	4	For patients with complicated disease, e.g., CNS involvement, shock, moderately penicillin-resistant organism, failed previous treatment
	3. Penicillin G, 10–20 million U/day IV in six equal doses, *or*	4	For patients >65 years old or with renal failure or eighth-nerve defect
	4. Ceftriaxone, 2 grams IV or IM once daily, *or*	4	For patients allergic to penicillin
	5. Vancomycin, 15 mg per kilogram (not to exceed 1 gram) q 12 h IV	4	For patients allergic to penicillin
Group A streptococci, *S. pneumoniae*	1. Penicillin G, 2 million U q 6 h IV, *or*	2–4	These organisms are usually highly sensitive to penicillin; 2–3 weeks will be adequate for most cases
	2. Cefazolin, 2 grams q 8 h IV	2–4	
E. faecalis, other penicillin-resistant streptococci	1. Ampicillin, 2 grams q 4 h IV, *plus* gentamicin, 1 mg per kilogram q 8 h IV, *or*	4–6	Four weeks will be adequate for most cases; serum levels must be checked and dose adjusted accordingly
	2. Vancomycin, 15 mg per kilogram (not to exceed 1 gram) q 12 h IV, *plus* gentamicin, 1 mg/kg IV or IM q 8 h	4–6	Four weeks will be adequate for most cases; the dose of streptomycin may have to be reduced as treatment progresses, to avoid toxicity
S. aureus	1. Nafcillin, 2 grams q 4 h IV, *or*	4 or longer	Standard regimen
	2. Nafcillin as above *plus* gentamicin, 1.0 mg per kilogram q 8 h IV for the first 3–5 days, *or*	4 or longer	For patients with severe disseminated staphylococcal disease, gentamicin synergy may be advantageous during early stages of treatment
	3. Cephalothin, 2 grams q 4 h IV, *or*	4 or longer	For patients allergic to penicillin
	4. Vancomycin, 15 mg per kilogram (not to exceed 1 gram) q 12 h IV	4 or longer	For patients allergic to penicillin and cephalosporin; for resistant organisms
HACEK group	1. Ampicillin, 2 grams q 4 h IV, *plus* gentamicin, 1 mg/kg q 8 h IV or IM, *or*	4	Standard regimen
	2. Ceftriaxone, 2 grams IV or IM once daily	4	For patients allergic to penicillin, or for outpatient therapy

TABLE 299–8. AUTHOR'S RECOMMENDATIONS FOR PROPHYLAXIS OF ENDOCARDITIS*

	Indications	Drug and Dosage
Standard regimen	For dental procedures and oral or upper respiratory tract surgery	Amoxicillin, 3 grams orally 1 hour before, then 1.5 grams 6 hours later†
Special regimens	Parenteral regimen for high-risk patients; also for gastrointestinal or genitourinary tract procedures	Ampicillin, 2 grams IM or IV, *plus* gentamicin, 1.5 mg per kilogram IM or IV, 0.5 hour before†, then 1.5 grams amoxicillin orally 6 hours later
	Parenteral regimen for penicillin-allergic patients	Vancomycin, 1 gram IV *slowly* over 1 hour, starting 1 hour before; *add* gentamicin, 1.5 mg per kilogram IM or IV, if gastrointestinal or genitourinary tract is involved†
	Oral regimen for penicillin-allergic patients (oral and respiratory tract procedures)	Erythromycin, 1 gram orally 2 hours before, then 0.5 gram 6 hours later,† *or* clindamycin, 300 mg orally 1 hour before, then 150 mg 6 hours later
	Oral regimen for minor gastrointestinal or genitourinary tract procedures	Amoxicillin, 3 grams orally 1 hour before, then 1.5 grams 6 hours later†
	Parenteral regimen for cardiac surgery including prosthetic valve placement	Cefazolin, 2 grams IV on induction of anesthesia, repeated 8 and 16 hours later,‡ *or* Vancomycin, 1 gram IV *slowly* over 1 hour, starting on induction of anesthesia, then 0.5 gram IV 8 and 16 hours later‡

*These are empiric suggestions. No regimen has been proven effective, and prevention failures may occur with any regimen. These recommendations are not intended to cover all clinical situations; practitioners should use their own judgment on safety and cost-benefit issues in each individual case. Several additional doses may be given if the period of risk for bacteremia is prolonged, but prophylaxis should not be extended for days.

†Pediatric dosages: ampicillin, 50 mg per kilogram; erythromycin, 20 mg per kilogram for first dose, then 10 mg per kilogram; gentamicin, 2 mg per kilogram; vancomycin, 20 mg per kilogram; penicillin V, cefazolin, and amoxicillin for children weighing more than 60 pounds, use same dose as for adults; for children weighing less than 60 pounds, use half the adult dose.

‡Gentamicin, 1.5 mg per kilogram IV, may be given with each dose only if postoperative gram-negative infections have occurred with significant frequency.

Adapted from Durack DT: Nine controversies in the management of endocarditis. *In* Petersdorf RG, et al. (eds.): Update V. Harrison's Principles of Internal Medicine, pp 35–46. Copyright © 1984 by McGraw-Hill, Inc. Used by permission of McGraw-Hill Book Company.

by knowing something of the frequency of bacteremia after the procedure in question and the number of cases of endocarditis attributed to it. For example, if a patient with aortic stenosis were to have dental extraction or urologic surgery, attempted prevention with antibiotics would be appropriate. If the same patient were to undergo gastroscopy, antibiotics would not be indicated because that procedure poses very little risk for endocarditis.

Prophylaxis for endocarditis is not required to cover the most common gastrointestinal diagnostic procedures such as endoscopy or radiocontrast studies, nor for normal delivery, therapeutic abortion, dilation and curettage, insertion or removal of intrauterine contraceptive devices in the absence of local infection, cardiac catheterization, insertion of pacemakers, endotracheal intubation, or bronchoscopy. However, some physicians choose to cover even these low-risk procedures in patients with prosthetic valves because they are at higher risk for endocarditis.

The indication for prophylactic antibiotics in patients with mitral valve prolapse remains controversial. MVP increases an individual's risk for endocarditis by five to eight times and underlies a significant proportion of cases of subacute bacterial endocarditis. However, mitral valve prolapse is very common in the general population, while endocarditis is relatively uncommon, so prolapse should be regarded as a low-risk lesion for endocarditis. Many authorities currently recommend prophylaxis for patients with prolapse, especially those with mitral regurgitation, but an estimate of benefits in relation to costs has indicated that parenteral prophylaxis for prolapse is probably not cost-effective. In the author's opinion, it is reasonable to give oral antibiotic prophylaxis to MVP patients undergoing procedures that cause significant bacteremia because the costs and risks of oral penicillin therapy for an individual are very low, and a serious disease may occasionally be prevented. However, use of antibiotics in this setting should be considered optional rather than mandatory. Parenteral prophylaxis for MVP patients probably should be avoided to reduce the risk of anaphylaxis.

Specific recommendations for prophylaxis of endocarditis are listed in Table 299–8.

Bisno AL: Treatment of Infective Endocarditis. New York, Grune & Stratton, 1982. *This book deals with many aspects of endocarditis besides treatment. It provides a good source for references.*

Bisno AL, Dismukes WE, Durack DT, et al.: Antimicrobial treatment of infective endocarditis due to viridans streptococci, enterococci, and staphylococci. JAMA 261:1471–1477, 1989. *A resource paper from the American Heart Association Committee appointed to review and recommend therapy for the common forms of endocarditis caused by gram-positive cocci. This is a detailed publication with seven large tables that list definitive recommendations for most situations involving infective endocarditis caused by gram-positive cocci.*

Durack DT: Infective and non-infective endocarditis. *In* Hurst JW (ed.): The Heart, 7th ed. New York, McGraw-Hill Book Company, 1990, pp 1230–1225. *A general review of infective and noninfective endocarditis in a leading cardiology textbook (204 references).*

Durack DT: Prophylaxis of endocarditis. *In* Mandell GL, Douglas RG, Bennett JE (eds.): Principles and Practice of Infectious Diseases, 3rd ed. New York, John Wiley & Sons, 1990, pp 716–721. *This chapter analyzes the problems of endocarditis prophylaxis in detail and reviews current recommendations (74 references).*

Karchmer AW, Dismukes WE, Buckley MJ, et al.: Late prosthetic valve endocarditis: Clinical features influencing therapy. Am J Med 64:199, 1978. *This paper reports on patients with late prosthetic valve endocarditis, comparing survival according to etiologic organisms and medical as opposed to surgical treatment. Various features that carry a poor prognosis are identified, and relative indications for surgery are discussed.*

Rahimtoola SH: Infective Endocarditis. New York, Grune & Stratton, 1978. *A heavily referenced book, with good material on pathogenesis, pathology, and endocarditis in addicts and fungal endocarditis.*

Reisberg BE: Infective endocarditis in the narcotic addict. Prog Cardiovasc Dis 22:193, 1979. *A useful review of infective endocarditis in narcotic addicts. The importance of tricuspid valve infection and the effect of different infecting organisms and the sites involved on prognosis are analyzed.*

Reller LB: The serum bactericidal test. Rev Infect Dis 8:803, 1986. *A concise analysis of the strengths and weaknesses of the SBT as a means to monitor therapy.*

Weinstein L: Infective endocarditis. *In* Braunwald E (ed.): Heart Disease. A Textbook of Cardiovascular Medicine. Philadelphia, W. B. Saunders Company, 1988. *A long, detailed chapter in a major cardiology textbook (approximately 400 references).*

Staphylococcal Infections

300 Staphylococcal Infections

John N. Sheagren

Staphylococci are ubiquitous in nature. All humans are colonized by "nonpathogenic" staphylococci. In addition the "pathogenic" coagulase-producing *Staphylococcus aureus* is present transiently in a high percentage of people and is chronically carried by about 15 per cent of the normal population.

S. aureus itself is one of the most important bacterial pathogens of man. It can be aggressively invasive, spreading rapidly through soft tissues, directly invading bones and other support structures, and ultimately, under conducive circumstances, seeding the bloodstream to produce septic shock and disseminated intravascular coagulation. Conversely, *S. aureus* can lie dormant deep within tissues for years without causing disease. The balance between host and parasite that results in infection with a given strain of staphylococci is not known and continues to be the subject of active research.

Staphylococci rank only behind *Escherichia coli* in overall incidence of infections in the hospital setting. In the community, staphylococci, particularly *S. aureus*, are the leading cause of acute, serious, and progressive skin, soft tissue, and post-traumatic infections. A thorough understanding of the pathogenetic mechanisms and clinical manifestations of staphylococcal infections is crucial to the care of septic patients in every medical environment.

BACTERIOLOGY. Staphylococci are members of the family Micrococcaceae, of which there are two genera of major clinical importance, the micrococci and the staphylococci. These two genera are both catalase positive, but only staphylococci can anaerobically ferment glucose to produce acid. The staphylococci in turn have three clinically important species: *S. aureus*, *S. epidermidis*, and *S. saprophyticus*. *S. aureus* alone has the capacity to produce coagulase. Most laboratories label all coagulase-negative organisms as "*S. epidermidis*," which results in the failure to differentiate at least one clinically important subspecies, *S. saprophyticus*. *S. saprophyticus* ferments mannitol and can also be identified by resistance to novobiocin. *S. saprophyticus* is a frequent cause of urinary tract infections, almost always in young women; these organisms are sensitive to all generally prescribed urinary tract antibiotics.

The word *aureus* comes from the Latin word meaning gold and refers to the fact that most *S. aureus* colonies develop a bright golden-yellow color on blood agar media. However, *S. aureus* speciation is now assigned to all strains producing coagulase, whether or not they are golden in color. In addition, almost all strains of *S. aureus* ferment mannitol and contain deoxyribonuclease (DNAase). Staphylococci grow well both anaerobically and aerobically: thus, both aerobic and anaerobic bottles in a blood culture set from a truly bacteremic patient are usually positive.

The name *staphylococcus* comes from the Greek word "staphyle" (literally, "a bunch of grapes") for these organisms grow in "grape-like" clusters in liquid or semisolid media or within tissues when causing infection. However, in material obtained from abscesses, the organisms can sometimes be confusing in morphology, being quite variable in size, shape, and tendency toward clustering. Occasionally the organisms may grow in pairs or even chains, and confusion with streptococci is possible. Nonetheless, to the trained eye the size and general characteristics of the organism usually permit an accurate diagnosis of a pure staphylococcal lesion when the stained smear is carefully examined.

No reproducible serologic typing schemes are available to classify staphylococci. However, bacteriophage typing has been extremely useful in identifying strain characteristics of *S. aureus* and in providing epidemiologic data. Recently, bacteriophage typing has begun to be applied to *S. epidermidis*, and over 50 per cent of recovered strains can now be typed by this system. Recent techniques of plasmid profile analysis have been very useful in studying the epidemiology of hospital-associated *S. aureus* and *S. epidermidis* infections. Plasmid (the extrachromosomal DNA in staphylococci) analysis using electrophoretic techniques provides distinctive patterns for individual strains of staphylococci.

EPIDEMIOLOGY. Staphylococci may colonize almost all animal species, and *S. epidermidis* is universally present on the human skin. The carrier state of *S. aureus* is clinically important. Humans carry *S. aureus* predominantly in the nasopharynx, although some individuals can be heavily colonized in the axillae, groin, and perineal region. The heavily colonized individual may become a source of recurrent infections both to himself and to surrounding contacts. Most humans probably carry a few *S. aureus* organisms among the normal flora of every body site but at such a low level that routine cultures rarely reveal the organism. About 15 per cent of normal, non–hospital-associated persons more or less chronically carry a heavy growth of *S. aureus* in their noses.

The definition of the carrier state is a simple one: from swab culture of the anterior nares of a carrier, multiple colonies of *S. aureus* are visually identified on a blood agar culture plate. Clearly this definition is imprecise, because the more intensely one focuses attention on the organism the higher will be the percentage of normal individuals found to carry it. Nonetheless, colony counts of the nasopharyngeal flora consistently indicate a small group of persons who harbor relatively large numbers of the organism.

The factors that result in high growth rates and numbers of *S. aureus* in the nares of certain individuals and not in others are unknown. There is no evidence that the immune response to the organism (for example, secretory immunoglobulins or other inhibitory substances) plays a major role in the acquisition and loss of the organism from the nose and throat, as is the case for the meningococcus. Data indicate that the teichoic acid moiety in the cell wall of *S. aureus* mediates the adherence of the organism to nasal mucosal cells, a phenomenon of major import in mucous membrane colonization. Also, it is highly probable that the carrier state is influenced by the ability of other members of the normal bacterial flora of the nose, throat, and skin to suppress growth of a given strain of *Staphylococcus*. Most probably, other staphylococci or micrococci (or both) will turn out to be instrumental in controlling the growth of a newly introduced staphylococcal strain. In fact, clinical use of this concept has already been attempted via the process termed *bacterial interference*. Bacterial interference is the concept that a nonpathogenic strain of *Staphylococcus*, once established, seems to reduce the likelihood of acquisition of another, more pathogenic strain (see later section).

There is an interesting association between the nasal carriage of *S. aureus* and any condition associated with small breaks in the skin and mucous membranes. It has been known for a long time that patients with a variety of dermatoses, especially atopic dermatitis, are very likely to be heavily colonized with *S. aureus*. In fact, patients with eczematous skin diseases may be heavily colonized in the lesions but have few organisms on the intervening normal skin. Possibly related to these observations is the fact that patients who regularly use needles have an increased rate of carriage of *S. aureus*. Drug addicts, diabetics injecting insulin, patients on hemodialysis, and even patients receiving brief courses of allergy shots all have an increased rate of nasal carriage of *S. aureus*. Recently, AIDS patients have been identified as frequent carriers of *S. aureus* (probably because of the frequency of chronic dermatologic conditions), and serious *S. aureus* infections are being increasingly recognized in AIDS patients. Another group of patients recently described as having a high risk of

S. *aureus* bacterium are those treated with interleukin 2 (IL2, an immunotherapeutic agent now available for melanoma, renal cell carcinoma, lymphoma, and some other solid tumor therapy). About 20 per cent of IL2-treated patients develop bacteremia, the vast majority of which (approx. 70 per cent) are caused by S. *aureus*. Probably, dermal IL2 toxicity leads to increased colonization followed by invasion and dissemination. In addition, IL2 produces an acute defect in polymorphonuclear leukocyte (PMN) chemotaxis which undoubtedly contributes to its propensity to cause bacterial infections, especially with S. *aureus*.

The carrier state, especially of S. *aureus*, is clinically important, because the organism carried in the nose and throat is often identical to that in the bloodstream of drug-abusing patients with endocarditis. Similarly, studies done years ago demonstrated that patients who entered hospitals for surgical procedures and who were carriers of S. *aureus* had increased rates of wound infections with the carried organism. The same phenomenon has recently been shown for hemodialysis patients, 60 to 80 per cent of whom are colonized in the nose with S. *aureus*. The colonizing organism often causes recurrent infections. Prophylaxis of the nasal carrier state in hemodialysis patients with rifampin significantly reduces the subsequent incidence of infections (see later section on Treatment of Chronic Carriers).

Thus, the sequence of events leading to infection with S. *aureus* seems to be the following: Persons who for whatever reason begin to carry the organism in the nose are at risk of seeding the organism to other bodily sites and to breaks in the skin (for example, wounds or points of insertion of intravascular catheters). From such colonized peripheral sites, the organism may invade and cause destructive and rapidly progressive local and systemic septic complications.

Carriage of staphylococci within the gastrointestinal tract has not been extensively studied. However, normally a few staphylococci can usually be isolated. S. *epidermidis* is not uncommonly isolated from the stool but probably represents contamination from the perianal skin. Staphylococci, especially S. *aureus*, may grow to very high titers in the gastrointestinal tract in the presence of antibiotic therapy and cause gastrointestinal symptoms; the presumption is that antibiotics suppress the more sensitive normal floral components that are responsible for inhibiting the growth of S. *aureus*. This rationale is similar to that for the emergence of C. *difficile* in the syndrome of antibiotic-associated colitis (see Ch. 308).

Newborn infants rapidly experience an increasing rate of colonization following birth. It is not uncommon within nurseries to note infant colonization rates of 25 to 30 per cent. Most infants remain asymptomatic; on occasion, however, outbreaks of disease within nurseries may occur, sometimes traceable to a common carrier. Adult patients become increasingly colonized with S. *aureus* the longer they remain in the hospital. Once a hospitalized individual becomes a carrier (especially individuals with open, actively infected lesions), the nasally carried organisms may spread to other anatomic sites, to clothing and other items within the room, and to individuals with whom the patient has contact. The most effective technique for stopping transmission of staphylococci from person to person, especially in a hospital setting, is to wash one's hands meticulously immediately before and after examining each patient. This process is particularly important when examining a patient with a gross, obviously staphylococcal lesion or with a chronic exudative dermatosis. Such patients should always be appropriately isolated while they are hospitalized.

PATHOGENESIS. Whether or not an infection develops with any microorganism depends on the balance between the aggressiveness of the organism and the level of defense provided by the host. Thus, organisms that are highly virulent may regularly infect normal hosts and, conversely, nonpathogenic (saprophytic) organisms usually cause infection only in the face of a significant impairment of host defense. The following paragraphs first describe those microbial characteristics that lead to the presence or absence of virulence and then the primary mechanisms by which the host attempts containment.

Microbial Virulence. The factor that makes certain strains of staphylococci virulent and others nonpathogenic is unknown. Several extracellular enzymes are produced by S. *aureus*, many probably participating in the pathogenic capabilities of the organism. For example, as in the case of streptococci, hyaluronidase probably assists the organism in its rapid spread through tissues. A variety of other enzymes may also degrade other tissue elements, may lyse inflammation-associated coagulation (coagulase), and may be directly toxic to either white cells (leukocidins) or platelets. Studies in experimental models have shown a high correlation between coagulase production and organism virulence.

The ability of S. *aureus* to adhere to damaged endothelial surfaces explains why the organism has a high likelihood of seeding to traumatized or inflamed tissues. Adherence is mediated by receptors on the surface of S. *aureus* for laminin and fibronectin (components of the subendothelial matrix), fibrin and fibrinogen (coagulation factors), and endothelial cell surface protein components.

Numerous toxins are produced by S. *aureus*. Some have endotoxic capabilities when injected into tissues (for example, the α and β toxins). S. *aureus* frequently produces an enterotoxin, and at present six enterotoxins (A through F) have been described. Enterotoxin F is identical to pyrogenic exotoxin C, the toxin found to be involved in the toxic shock syndrome and now called "toxic shock syndrome toxin-1" (abbreviated TSST-1). Another well-described toxin is the exfoliative toxin responsible for the staphylococcal scalded skin syndrome.

The capsular and cell wall components of S. *aureus* clearly participate in the pathogenesis of certain clinical syndromes produced by the organism. Many S. *aureus* strains have a polysaccharide capsule covering the complex rigid cell wall matrix that consists of peptidoglycan and teichoic acid (ribitol in S. *aureus* and predominantly glycerol in S. *epidermidis*), and recent data suggest that the encapsulated strains of staphylococci are major causes of bacteremic episodes. In most strains of S. *aureus*, a unique substance, *protein A*, is also part of the cell wall. Protein A is an immunologically active substance having high affinity for the Fc fragment of immunoglobulins, particularly subgroups of IgG. Thus, protein A binds to and aggregates IgG molecules and, interestingly, fixes complement in the process. Protein A has emerged as an extremely useful immunochemical substance for extraction and quantitation of IgG molecules from biologic specimens. Whether protein A plays a role in any of the clinical syndromes produced by S. *aureus* is unknown.

The presence of a capsule varies greatly from strain to strain and may explain some of the biologic differences between organisms as they invade tissues or the bloodstream. The capsule inhibits phagocytosis by interfering with the interaction between the underlying teichoic acid–peptidoglycan complex and complement, which is activated primarily via the alternative pathway. Thus, encapsulated strains are protected in tissues from the complement-mediated attack by PMN leukocytes. Along with the enzymes described above, the capsule undoubtedly increases the ability of S. *aureus* to protect itself as it spreads through tissues and therefore is an important virulence factor for tissue infections. Paradoxically, while unencapsulated organisms are more likely to be contained in tissues, should the bloodstream be reached (for example in a narcotics addict directly injecting carried organisms into the blood stream), the syndrome of septic shock and disseminated intravascular coagulation (DIC) may result. The syndrome of septic shock follows massive intravascular activation of monokines (especially tumor necrosis factor-α [TNF-α] and the complement, coagulation, and kinin systems (Ch. 243 and 285). In such a situation, unencapsulated strains of S. *aureus* produce septic shock exactly like gram-negative bacteria wherein the cell wall lipopolysaccharide (endotoxin) activates the responsible inflammatory systems.

Host Defense Aspects. The primary mechanism by which the host defends against staphylococci, especially S. *aureus*, is via the nonspecific defense system. The specific antibody and T cell–mediated host defenses appear to participate very little, if at all, in defense against S. *aureus*. Thus, antibodies are of theoretical value against encapsulated strains of S. *aureus*, and at present, attempts to induce anticapsular antibodies as therapeutic modalities are being revived. Previous attempts to develop vaccines against the organism, however, have not yielded documented clinical benefits.

The nonspecific host defense system consists of the barrier systems (skin and mucous membranes) plus the complement-mediated PMN leukocyte assault on invading organisms. Patients with defects in intracellular killing of bacteria by the PMN (for example, as in the chronic granulomatous disease of childhood or the Chédiak-Higashi syndrome) are particularly prone to develop serious infections with *S. aureus*. AIDS patients probably also have a subtle bactericidal defect in their PMN's as well as frank neutropenia in the end stage of the disease.

Certain pathologic states with highly elevated levels of IgE predispose the patient to recurrent, chronic infections with *S. aureus*. *Job's syndrome* is a condition wherein an elevated IgE level associated with eczematous skin changes somehow predisposes the patient to recurrent soft tissue infections. No one knows how or why staphylococcal infections are enhanced by highly elevated levels of IgE. The theory is that mast cell activation in the neighborhood of a focus of *S. aureus* infection somehow impairs normal PMN-mediated defense mechanisms. Some recent studies have shown that antihistamines may at least partially correct the defect demonstrated in these patients. Interestingly some AIDS patients have increased IgE production associated with a chronic, diffuse dermatitis, a combination of events strongly predisposing to infection with *S. aureus*.

The presence of a foreign body has a dramatic effect on the development of staphylococcal infections. For example, infections with *S. epidermidis* strains are particularly common in patients harboring foreign bodies such as prosthetic heart valves, cerebrospinal fluid shunts, and artificial joints. As for *S. aureus*, the inoculum required experimentally to produce a skin infection in a healthy individual is very large (10^6 to 10^7 organisms); however, the presence of even a small foreign body such as a suture reduces the dose required to produce an infection to less than 100 organisms. Thus, foreign bodies must provide a nidus of chronic inflammation in which leukocyte accumulation and function are impaired.

CLINICAL MANIFESTATIONS

This section reviews two broad categories of human diseases produced by staphylococci: first, diseases related to the production of toxins by staphylococci (exclusively *S. aureus*) and, second, diseases related to direct organism invasion.

TOXIN-PRODUCED DISEASES. Clinically, the most important toxins produced by *S. aureus* are the enterotoxins and exfoliative toxin. The distinction between the different types of toxins is becoming less clear: For example, the toxin involved in the toxic shock syndrome (pyrogenic exotoxin C) has recently been shown to be identical to enterotoxin F; furthermore, that toxin clearly has exfoliative properties.

Staphylococcal Gastroenteritis. Most cases of gastroenteritis caused by *S. aureus* follow the ingestion of foods containing a preformed toxin. The toxin itself is not produced within the gastrointestinal tract. A number of extracellular toxins are produced in large amounts when the culture media contain high amounts of carbohydrate (as in sugary and starchy foods contaminated by *S. aureus*) and when such a mixture is incubated at appropriate conditions of temperature and acidity. Toxin ingestion results in increased intestinal peristalsis, profuse nausea, vomiting, diarrhea, and in some cases fever. The organism and its preformed toxin can usually be identified in point source outbreaks from the epidemiologically implicated foodstuff. Toxin-mediated staphylococcal gastroenteritis is usually self-limited, lasting anywhere from 12 to 24 hours; however, supportive therapy (fluid and electrolyte maintenance) may on occasion be required. Antibiotics are not useful.

The Toxic Shock Syndrome (TSS). TSS is almost certainly caused by the production of one or more toxins at the site of a localized, often relatively asymptomatic or unnoticed infection with any strain of *S. aureus* capable of toxin production. The most common site of infection is still the vagina, usually in association with tampon usage. About 25 per cent of TSS cases reported to the CDC in 1989 were not associated with infection of the female genital tract; most of those were associated with infected foreign bodies (such as sutures) in surgical wounds, or other sites, often relatively asymptomatic, of *S. aureus* colonization and/or infection. As stated earlier, the toxin responsible for TSS is now named TSST-1, although recent data also implicate staphylococcal

enterotoxin-A (SEA) in some cases of TSS. TSST-1 production by strains of *S. aureus* isolated from cases of TSS has been shown to be related to lysogeny, the presence of a temperate bacteriophage. Presumably, the clinical manifestations of the syndrome are produced when the toxin is absorbed either through mucous membranes or from a subcutaneous tissue site of colonization or infection. TSST-1 production by toxigenic strains of *S. aureus* is markedly enhanced in Mg^{++}-depleted media; further, superabsorbent tampon materials chelate Mg^{++} and/or in other ways result in ideal conditions for toxin production, explaining the relationship between superabsorbent tampon introduction and the TSS. The toxin probably produces its systemic effects both by directly damaging cell membranes in peripheral tissues and by stimulating production of monokine mediators, especially TNF-α. Interestingly, TNF-α production by mononuclear cells is triggered because TSST and SEA bind specifically to MHC class II molecules.

The clinical syndrome that results is dramatic. The patient, almost always unaware of the focus of toxin production, experiences the abrupt onset of high fever, myalgias, and profuse nausea, vomiting, and watery diarrhea. Within the first several days, a sunburn-like rash appears, and the conjunctivae become injected. On biopsy of the skin lesions, the epidermis exhibits cleavage in the basilar layers, differentiating it from the staphylococcal scalded skin syndrome (discussed later) and from viral and drug eruptions. The patient often becomes progressively more ill and is frequently in frank shock when presenting for care. A diffuse capillary leak syndrome rapidly develops, and the serum albumin concentration often plummets to less than 2 grams per 100 ml. Hypotension and frank shock are common and are often associated with the adult respiratory distress syndrome (ARDS), acute renal failure, and abnormalities in literally every organ system evaluated. For example, almost all patients exhibit an altered state of mentation, hepatocellular malfunction, elevated levels of muscle enzymes, thrombocytopenia, and a low serum calcium concentration (far out of proportion to the hypoalbuminemia). Highly elevated levels of calcitonin are present for which no explanation currently exists.

Therapy is both supportive and specific. Identification of site of infection, drainage thereof (most frequently consisting of removal of contaminated tampons), and antibiotic therapy with β-lactamase–resistant antistaphylococcal agents are all indicated. Antibiotics do not change the course of the initial illness but seem to prevent relapse, at least in tampon-associated cases. Patients with TSS are rarely bacteremic, and therefore this type of shock syndrome is different from bacteremic, inflammatory system-mediated shock (see Ch. 286), wherein complement, coagulation, and kinin system activation seem to be primary events.

The prognosis in TSS is favorable despite the fact that most patients are critically ill for a period of time in the hospital. In the early 1980's, between 5 and 10 per cent of patients studied died; in 1989, no deaths were reported to the CDC among women with menstrual TSS. Since recurrences, generally milder, are relatively common following tampon-associated TSS (up to 10 per cent over the subsequent three menstrual cycles), women who have recovered from TSS should avoid tampon use for at least 6 months following the illness.

The Staphylococcal Scalded Skin Syndrome (SSSS). SSSS is another toxin-mediated disease produced by certain strains of *S. aureus*, usually of phage group II. These organisms produce an exfoliative toxin that when injected experimentally into infant mice produces dramatic skin desquamation and mimics in every way the clinical syndrome seen in human infants. The human disease is produced by a toxin originating in a distant focus of infection. The exfoliative toxin is absorbed and disseminated systemically and causes cleavage of the middle layers of the epidermis, bulla formation, and ultimately slippage of the superficial layer of the epithelium on gentle pressure (a positive *Nikolsky's sign*). The skin is often tender and very erythematous, producing a sunburn-like rash during the initial phase. Infants are most commonly involved, and outbreaks of this syndrome have occurred in nurseries after introduction of a toxin-producing strain. Often mild or asymptomatic omphalitis is the source. In older children, the portal of infection can be any minor skin abrasion, furuncle, or some other infected local site. The conjunctival sac may be the source as a result of mild conjunctivitis, and this source often goes undetected. The syndrome has occasionally been reported in adults. The rash proceeds rapidly to desquamation, but healing is rapid and is related to how promptly the peripheral site has been treated. Mortality of SSSS is very low.

Differentiation of SSSS from viral exanthems and drug allergies is very important. The most important disease with which SSSS can be confused is *toxic epidermal necrolysis (TEN)*, an often fatal variant of erythema multiforme usually caused by a drug allergy (see Ch. 525). The two illnesses can be differentiated on skin biopsy, and therapy is very different for each: Local care and antibiotics suffice to cure SSSS, whereas high-dose systemic glucocorticoids are indicated in TEN, with mortality still remaining high.

DISEASES RELATED TO DIRECT INVASION AND SYSTEMIC SPREAD OF STAPHYLOCOCCI. In the following subsections, the classic clinical manifestations of invasive staphylococcal infection, bacteremia, and endocarditis are described.

Dermal Infections. Most minor skin infections in man are caused by either *S. aureus* or group A β-hemolytic streptococci. There is no way clinically to differentiate between diseases produced by the penicillin-sensitive streptococci and *S. aureus*; obviously, this is an important point, for all skin infections in which antibiotic therapy seems indicated therefore require the use of a β-lactamase–resistant antibiotic. Direct invasion through minor breaks in skin and mucous membranes is the hallmark of disease produced by *S. aureus*. A wide variety of dermal and soft tissue infections may result, including cellulitis, local abscess formation (furuncles and carbuncles), lymphangiitis, and lymphadenitis. Direct extension can occur to deep support structures such as bones and joints and result in primary osteomyelitis and septic arthritis. Even dermal staphylococcal infections that appear minor are important to recognize because they may become a source of bacteremia. When a patient with a localized *S. aureus* skin infection manifests fever and chills, bacteremia must be assumed to be present, and prompt diagnosis and therapy should be initiated.

Diagnosis of dermal infections is usually relatively easy. The aspirate of a large, well-developed abscess (furuncle or carbuncle) almost always reveals typical, creamy, yellow pus; and on Gram's stain the clustered cocci are mixed with inflammatory debris. One should perform Gram's stains of materials from every dermal infection because occasionally gram-negative organisms may cause a clinical picture similar to that of gram-positive infections, especially in immunocompromised hosts, and obviously the initial therapeutic approach will be very different.

Therapy must always be initiated with a β-lactamase–resistant antibiotic if antimicrobial therapy is indicated at all. In fact, the backbone of therapy of dermal staphylococcal infections continues to be debridement and drainage. Only large lesions associated with signs of surrounding cutaneous spread or systemic clinical symptoms need be treated with antibiotics. It is usually wise, however, before incising a large staphylococcal abscess (even when localized) to treat the patient with an oral dose of a penicillinase-resistant antibiotic (e.g., 250 mg of dicloxacillin). Such a dose should be administered 30 minutes to 1 hour before incision and drainage are carried out.

The prognosis for most localized infections is excellent, but infections due to *S. aureus* often recur. Population surveys have found that each year most persons develop one to several isolated local lesions, most probably caused by *S. aureus*. However, not infrequently an individual may suffer from recurrent crops of extremely debilitating local skin lesions. In this situation the patient is usually found to be carrying the causative organism in the anterior nares, axilla, groin, or perirectal region. Most such individuals are nasal carriers, and an attempt to eradicate nasal carriage is worth making (see later section on Treatment of Chronic Carriers).

Bone and Joint Infections. Through a variety of mechanisms *S. aureus* commonly involves bone (osteomyelitis, see Ch. 304) and joints (see Ch. 260 on septic arthritis). Direct inoculation by *S. aureus* can occur in trauma or penetrating wounds. Bone and joint infections can also result from bacteremia. In children and young adults it is assumed that bacteremia originates from a minor dermal source (such as folliculitis) or from heavily colonized mucous membranes. Seeding of *S. aureus* from the blood tends to occur to areas previously traumatized or harboring foreign bodies. In young children, the organism tends to seed into the diaphyseal plates of the long bone, areas of greatest vascularity. The affected area (usually on the ankle, knee, or shin) becomes acutely warm and swollen and may appear at first to be a primary cellulitis. Fever and shaking chills are common. Blood cultures are usually positive. In adults, the syndrome of hematogenous osteomyelitis is usually less acute, often involving the lumbar vertebrae. The individual begins to develop low-grade fever, night sweats, and back pain that gradually becomes localized to an area of point tenderness. In such cases, *S. aureus* may be grown from the blood, but more commonly the organism is isolated from an aspirate of the bone or intervertebral space obtained by an orthopedic surgical consultant.

Staphylococcal septic arthritis usually involves a joint afflicted by pre-existing chronic arthritis (such as rheumatoid arthritis or osteoarthritis). Again, an episode of bacteremia causes seeding to a previously inflamed joint. The only indication in some patients is the development of increasing symptoms in one joint, usually accompanied by fever. Joint aspiration reveals a purulent effusion; Gram's stains may be negative, but the organism can usually be cultured. *S. epidermidis* increasingly is being described as a cause of chronic osteomyelitis, especially in debilitated patients such as those on hemodialysis or with underlying neoplastic diseases.

The diagnosis of staphylococcal bone and joint infections depends on recovering the organism from an aspirate of the involved site; every effort should be made, with the assistance of an orthopedic surgeon, to aspirate or biopsy the involved area *before* antibiotics are started. Newer techniques permit core biopsies to be obtained from deep tissues and may in the future permit more frequent definitive bacteriologic diagnosis of low-grade, chronic bone and joint infections. The diagnosis becomes especially difficult if patients have been treated with antibiotics before appropriate culture material has been obtained. In such cases a rising or significantly elevated teichoic acid antibody titer may assist in diagnosing deep infections due to *S. aureus* (see later section on The Teichoic Acid Antibody Assay).

Treatment of osteomyelitis in adults must be prolonged. While it is becoming customary to treat children with a brief course of parenteral antibiotics, adults on oral antibiotics tend to relapse if a prolonged parenteral course of antibiotics is not administered. Four weeks of parenteral therapy is the minimum acceptable course, and most clinicians prefer to treat for 6 to 8 weeks. Much of such a course of prolonged parenteral therapy can be administered at home. An oral antistaphylococcal agent (for example, dicloxacillin 2 grams daily) should be continued for several weeks following completion of the parenteral course. Gradual reduction of the dose of oral antibiotic over a 3- to 6-month period may leave the patient symptom-free for an extended period of time. Some clinicians treat isolated septic arthritis for only 2 weeks; however, it is extremely difficult to differentiate septic arthritis *without* bone involvement from that with osteomyelitis. Therefore, a 4-week course of therapy with appropriate parenteral antibiotics is recommended. Staphylococcal osteomyelitis tends to relapse even after years of quiescence, and one can never be sure of complete eradication of the disease. Once a relapse has occurred, chronic recurrence will be the rule. In such situations carefully planned surgical debridement and drainage under the cover of a prolonged parenteral and oral course of antibiotics may result in extended quiescence or even apparent cure. The availability of microsurgical techniques to apply muscle grafts over areas of chronic osteomyelitis now permits healing to occur even in some extraordinarily recalcitrant cases. Some of the newer β-lactam antibiotics have favorable pharmacokinetics, permitting once-daily parenteral therapy to be administered long term to outpatients. The most widely used such antibiotic is ceftriaxone.

Staphylococcal Pneumonia and Empyema. Although most cases of *S. aureus* pneumonia follow acute viral infections of the lower respiratory tract (especially influenza), the disease occasionally occurs de novo in elderly and debilitated individuals. *S. aureus* pneumonia is most often acquired in the hospital. Primary staphylococcal pneumonia is most common in children and usually evolves radiologically from patchy pulmonary infiltrates into harder nodules and then pneumatoceles. Rapid development of pleural effusions and empyema often accompanied by pneumothorax may occur. Staphylococcal bronchitis and recurrent pneumonias are also seen in children and young adults with cystic fibrosis, and a young adult suffering from recurrent bronchitis from which *S. aureus* and/or *Pseudomonas aeruginosa* (usually with mucoid colonial morphology) are isolated should have a sweat test evaluation.

Adult patients with influenza have an increased incidence of *S. aureus* pneumonia. The patient is usually recovering from typical symptoms of influenza when the rapid onset of fever, chills, and chest pain supervenes. Gram's stain of the sputum in such cases reveals large clumps of gram-positive cocci. Therapy must be intense with appropriate antibiotics. Nonetheless, such patients often do poorly and frequently develop secondary infections with gram-negative organisms, chronic respiratory failure, and progressive debility. Mortality rates remain high. Even in young people, morbidity is substantial, related to serious, rapidly progressive pulmonary disease often with empyema as well as the sequelae of the accompanying bacteremia.

In particular, pleural effusions accompanying *S. aureus* pneumonia require early drainage to prevent empyema formation. If thorough drainage cannot be accomplished by needle aspiration, a chest tube must be inserted. Every effort should be made to avoid the debilitating, prolonged sequelae that result from an extensive, multiloculated *S. aureus* infection of the pleural space.

Staphylococcal Meningitis, Cerebritis, and Brain Abscess. Meningitis due to *S. aureus* most commonly develops as a complication of a central nervous system diagnostic or neurosurgical procedure. Occasionally, however, meningitis may develop during an episode of bacteremia from a peripheral site. Many patients with staphylococcal bacteremia, with or without endocarditis, develop transient but sometimes focal central nervous system symptoms. On lumbar puncture, such patients commonly have a PMN pleocytosis with elevated protein but a normal to low normal glucose concentration and a *negative* Gram's stain. These individuals probably have begun to develop multiple perimeningeal foci or areas of cerebritis (or both) and not yet frank meningitis. Almost certainly, if left untreated such patients would develop frank brain abscesses or fulminant staphylococcal meningitis. On occasion, such a patient may also exhibit purpura, disseminated intravascular coagulation, and shock in which the differentiation from *meningococcal meningitis* (see Ch. 302) is difficult. Treatment of such patients is particularly difficult, for the initial inclination is to use penicillin, an inappropriate antibiotic choice. Thus, for any patient whose Gram's stain of the spinal fluid does not reveal identifiable organisms (such as meningococci or pneumococci), a β-lactamase–resistant antibiotic must be included in the initial antibiotic coverage.

Brain abscesses in general are usually caused by anaerobes, but not infrequently *S. aureus* is found to accompany them. Therefore, antistaphylococcal drugs should be included with antianaerobic antibiotics in the initial coverage of such individuals. For example, nafcillin plus metronidazole is an excellent combination for the patient who has a brain abscess with the source and causative organisms not yet defined. Surgical drainage is required only if the abscess is large and encapsulated.

Therapy of staphylococcal meningitis and cerebritis is usually that of the underlying syndrome (for example, endocarditis). However, even in the rare patient with an uncomplicated case of pure meningitis, therapy should be prolonged, at least 4 weeks parenterally, in contrast to the customary 10 to 14 days of therapy for patients with uncomplicated meningitis caused by *S. pneumoniae* or *N. meningitides*.

Staphylococcus epidermidis may cause meningeal signs and symptoms, almost always in a patient with a central nervous system shunt in place. In such instances, the infection has originated in the shunt, and the organism has proliferated and seeded back into the spinal fluid. In many such cases, the individual known to have a shunt in place simply has fever with few if any central nervous system signs. Only an aspirate of the shunt itself reveals the organism. Therapy may result in suppression of symptoms, but removal of the infected shunt is almost always required before cure can be accomplished.

Staphylococcal Urinary Tract Infections. Here the species spectrum changes, and coagulase-negative staphylococci become the more common infecting organisms. *S. epidermidis* may occasionally cause urinary tract infections, especially in elderly hospitalized men with obstructive urinary tract pathology or indwelling Foley catheters.

Staphylococcus saprophyticus accounts for between 5 and 10 per cent of urinary tract infections in otherwise healthy young women. Presumably the organism colonizes the genitalia and for reasons not yet ascertained may ascend the urethra to involve the bladder and cause symptomatic cystitis. *S. saprophyticus* is easily treated, being sensitive to essentially all commonly used antibiotics, including penicillin, ampicillin, sulfonamides, and cephalosporins.

S. aureus may involve the urinary tract by either of two mechanisms: First, the organism may seed to the renal cortex during an episode of staphylococcal bacteremia; second, usually in patients with lower urinary tract pathology or indwelling Foley catheters, the organism may ascend to cause a primary lower urinary tract infection. Approximately 10 per cent of patients with staphylococcal bacteremia eventually excrete the organism in the urine; other studies have found that about 25 per cent of patients with a defined urinary tract infection caused by *S. aureus* had had a preceding bacteremic episode. Thus, small cortical abscesses must occur frequently during bacteremia and ultimately rupture in some patients into the tubules and the urine. Most such patients respond promptly to therapy for the underlying disease, and renal carbuncles are now rare.

Conversely, about 5 per cent of patients with a primary staphylococcal urinary tract infection may develop secondary bacteremia. In some patients, the renal infection may seed to the perinephric and retroperitoneal structures, with resultant chronic infection and fibrosis. Frank perinephric abscess is a complication associated with high morbidity and mortality. This condition occurs most frequently in patients with chronic underlying renal diseases who are also often diabetic. Aggressive drainage along with prolonged antibiotic therapy is required for cure.

Staphylococcal Endocarditis. This condition follows staphylococcal bacteremia during which a nidus of infection becomes established on one or more heart valves. Endocarditis consists of two clinical syndromes (see Ch. 299): The first is "subacute" bacterial endocarditis, and the second is "acute" bacterial endocarditis.

Subacute Bacterial Endocarditis. The patient presents with a history of days to weeks of low-grade fever with or without chills, myalgias, night sweats, and weight loss. The word *subacute* refers to the clinical manifestations: The clinical course is one of a chronic, febrile illness. The patient almost always has a history of pre-existing organic valvular heart disease, and the species of *Staphylococcus* involved is usually *S. epidermidis*. *S. epidermidis* accounts for approximately 5 per cent of all cases of subacute endocarditis, the vast majority being caused by streptococcal species. *S. epidermidis* is the most common cause, however, of endocarditis occurring in association with prosthetic heart valves (see Ch. 299). The organism, being a contaminant from the patient's or surgeon's skin flora, is inoculated at the time of the surgical valve replacement. Most such infections occur within the initial 2 months after surgery. In such instances, the outlook for therapy with antibiotics alone is poor, and reoperation with removal of the infected valve or valve ring is often required. More than half of such patients die.

Acute Bacterial Endocarditis. The word *acute* refers to the clinical presentation of the patient who experiences the rapid onset of fever, chills, and myalgias, often with back pain or some gastrointestinal symptoms. The fever is often quite high (103 to 105° F), and the individual at first has the feeling of developing a very bad case of the flu. In the majority of cases, the individual has not had a history of pre-existing valvular heart disease, although it is assumed that many of these individuals have had asymptomatic organic valvular lesions (such as a fenestrated or bicuspid aortic valve, mitral valve prolapse, and so forth). Frequently, therapy for such individuals, who previously had been well, is delayed because the patient and the physician do not realize the gravity of the situation.

S. aureus is almost always the cause of the syndrome of acute endocarditis, and recent data suggest that this syndrome is *increasing* in frequency. At the time of presentation, the patient may not have an obvious heart murmur or show evidence of embolic phenomenon. Thus, the differentiation between primary staphylococcal bacteremia, which may remain uncomplicated, and acute staphylococcal bacterial endocarditis is clinically difficult. The physician must closely follow every patient whose blood samples grow *S. aureus* and must examine carefully each day for the presence of a new murmur, the signs of embolic phenomena, or the observable development of vegetation(s) by echocardiography. Valve destruction, especially of the aortic valve, may progress quite rapidly, and surgery may be necessary even within the first few days of presentation.

S. aureus endocarditis in the drug addict is almost always on one of the right-sided heart valves, usually the tricuspid valve. Therefore, pleuritic chest pain and pulmonary infiltrates are common occurrences due to embolization. In drug-abusing patients who have surreptitiously taken antibiotics, the syndrome may be of a much lower grade and may mimic that of subacute bacterial endocarditis.

The treatment of bacterial endocarditis must be prolonged (see Ch. 299). Four weeks of parenteral therapy is the minimum for staphylococcal endocarditis, although some authors have reported that 2 weeks may suffice for the drug addict, usually a young, otherwise healthy individual with right-sided endocarditis. All staphylococcal infections should be treated with a "cidal" antibiotic, and serum bactericidal levels must be monitored to guide effective therapy. For infections caused by β-lactam antibiotic–resistant staphylococci, whether *aureus* or *epidermidis* species, a cephalosporin is not adequate therapy (see later discussion of treatment), although data may indicate sensitivity to the cephalosporins in vitro. As noted earlier, patients with prosthetic valve endocarditis often require surgery to eradicate the infection. Even those patients with prosthetic valve infections who respond to antibiotics alone probably should be treated with a prolonged course of an appropriate oral antistaphylococcal drug following the 6-week course of parenteral therapy in the hospital.

The prognosis for patients with staphylococcal endocarditis is guarded. Patients with prosthetic valve endocarditis have about a 50 per cent mortality rate. Patients with acute bacterial endocarditis caused by *S. aureus* on native valves do well if they are young and otherwise healthy and especially if the vegetations are on the right-sided valves. The older the patient with left-sided valvular involvement, the higher the mortality (approaching 60 to 80 per cent). Pre-existing symptomatic heart disease is a particularly ominous prognostic sign. The patients who have the subacute syndrome due to *S. epidermidis* not on prosthetic valves, in which the organism is susceptible to the usual antibiotics, usually do quite well: Survival rates are comparable to those of patients with streptococcal endocarditis (in the range of 90 per cent).

Staphylococcal Bacteremia. Sustained true bacteremia due to *S. epidermidis* is uncommon: Although blood cultures frequently yield the organism, 80 to 90 per cent of the time it is a contaminant. True, sustained *S. epidermidis* bacteremia is usually caused by infection of an intravascular line or a prosthetic valve. The most common species causing true bacteremia, especially in the hospital, is *S. aureus*.

There are two varieties of *S. aureus* bacteremia: primary and secondary. Primary bacteremia exists when a patient presenting with fever and chills grows *S. aureus* out of multiple blood cultures but does *not* have an identifiable primary focus of infection. The patient usually has unrecognized endocarditis and should be treated accordingly. Secondary bacteremia is that associated with an obvious, peripheral focus of infection, for example, an intravascular line. Many such patients have a benign clinical course after line removal and a brief course of antibiotic treatment. The problem is to select from the overall group of such patients those who have not developed metastatic septic complications. Patients without metastatic sequelae usually do well with a short (14-day) course of therapy. The typical patient who develops *S. aureus* bacteremia has usually been hospitalized for some other medical problem and has had a neglected peripheral or central venous or arterial access line in place. The patient suddenly develops fever and chills with or without signs of local infection at the site of the line. Other common sources are hemodialysis access shunts, postsurgical or traumatic wounds, and decubitus ulcers. The diagnosis of staphylococcal bacteremia is made when *S. aureus* grows from several blood cultures obtained before an empiric course of antibiotics is begun. Some patients already have an obvious metastatic complication of the bacteremic episode when first examined.

TABLE 300–1. CRITERIA FOR ANTIBIOTIC THERAPY FOLLOWING *STAPHYLOCOCCUS AUREUS* BACTEREMIA

1. Host defenses are normal.
2. The patient has no seedable sites (pre-existing valvular heart lesions, implanted prostheses, chronic arthritis).
3. The primary focus of infection is obvious and easily managed.
4. There is a prompt, complete response to the initial course of antimicrobial therapy.
5. The *S. aureus* recovered is fully sensitive to the antibiotics initially chosen.
6. No clinical evidence of a metastatic, suppurative complication is found during 10–14 days of careful follow-up examinations.

The complications of an episode of *S. aureus* bacteremia are of two varieties: The first type is *nonsuppurative*, i.e., patients who exhibit the septic shock syndrome, some also developing disseminated intravascular coagulation; the second type is *suppurative*, involving the metastatic spread of the organism via the bloodstream to heart valves or other organs. The development of endocarditis in this setting is distinctly uncommon; most suppurative spread occurs to bones, joints, and kidneys, occasionally to other deep viscera, and rarely to the meninges. Following the episode of bacteremia, the patient is placed first on broad, empiric and later on specific antistaphylococcal antibiotic therapy. Throughout this period, the patient must be examined carefully each day for metastatic suppurative sites. Laboratory evaluation may also be helpful, yielding pyuria and the organism from the urine, abnormalities of liver function, and other data. Vegetations may become demonstrable by echocardiography. Radionuclide scans may reveal infectious foci within bones, joints, or soft tissues.

Those patients who develop a clinically evident metastatic focus are treated as dictated by the type of complication that has evolved. Approximately 20 per cent of previously healthy persons who acquire *S. aureus* bacteremia develop some type of complication. Administration of an oral antistaphylococcal drug (dicloxacillin) should be continued for several weeks if there is any doubt about the possibility of residual metastatic abscesses.

If the criteria listed in Table 300–1 are present, such patients usually do well with a short course (14 days) of antibiotic therapy following an episode of *S. aureus* bacteremia.

Septic Shock Syndromes Due to Staphylococci. Staphylococci can produce shock by five mechanisms (Table 300–2). Massive local infection due to staphylococci is uncommon, and such infections usually involve several organisms, usually anaerobes coinfecting with *S. aureus*. *S. epidermidis* may be a part of the flora in these infections but is probably not pathogenic. Specifically, patients with one of the gangrene syndromes (for example, necrotizing fasciitis or synergistic gangrene) may develop shock not caused by bacteremia but by fluid accumulation in the infected area. Such individuals require massive fluid and albumin replacement, extensive local debridement, and broad antibiotic coverage, including effective antianaerobic drugs.

Diarrhea, nausea, and vomiting may be so severe in some patients with staphylococcal food poisoning that shock may develop from hypovolemia secondary to gastrointestinal fluid loss. Hospitalization with fluid replacement may be required.

TABLE 300–2. MECHANISMS OF SHOCK CAUSED BY STAPHYLOCOCCI

1. The local infection can generate a massive inflammatory reaction resulting in sufficient "third spacing" (i.e., fluid accumulation into the area of infection) to lead to hypovolemic shock.
2. Enterotoxin-producing *S. aureus* occasionally causes diarrhea severe enough to cause hypovolemia and shock.
3. Cardiogenic shock can be produced by staphylococci by causing either valve malfunction (usually aortic), multiple myocardial abscesses, or purulent pericarditis.
4. Endotoxic-like shock can be produced via inflammatory mediator activation (see Ch. 288).
5. Toxigenic shock—the toxic shock syndrome—can produce shock, probably both by activating inflammatory mediators and by direct capillary endothelial and end-organ damage.

Cardiogenic shock is self-explanatory (see Ch. 41).

During acute sepsis S. aureus may produce shock that mimics that produced by endotoxin during gram-negative organism septicemia (see Ch. 288). Briefly, the primary event in endotoxic shock is the following: On entering the bloodstream, endotoxin activates a sequence of endocrine and inflammatory events leading first to vasodilation and subsequently to a monokine (especially TNF-α)-, complement-, and PMN-mediated capillary leak syndrome resulting in full-blown septic shock. The coagulation and kinin systems also become activated, and such patients may suffer frank DIC. The presence or absence of a capsule seems to be a major factor determining whether or not a particular strain of S. aureus in the bloodstream will cause an endotoxic shock–like syndrome. Encapsulated organisms are virulent in tissues and are *more* likely to reach the bloodstream in the course of a peripheral infection. However, once there they are *less* likely to produce the septic shock syndrome. Unencapsulated strains activate inflammatory mediators readily in tissues and therefore are *more* likely to be contained and are least likely to reach the bloodstream and to cause bacteremia. Yet, these are the organisms that can cause shock when directly inoculated into the bloodstream, as by a parenteral drug user or when having colonized an intravascular line.

For a discussion of the toxigenic shock caused by S. aureus, refer to the earlier section on the toxic shock syndrome.

Miscellaneous Staphylococcal Infections. This section focuses on several relatively unusual infections that require special diagnostic and therapeutic considerations.

Staphylococcal Pyomyositis. This malady is primarily a tropical disease of malnourished persons, rare enough to be reportable in the United States. The patient develops pain, warmth, and swelling over a muscle region, usually of the lower extremities and buttocks. The overlying skin may appear quite normal or may look like a mild cellulitis; however, when drainage is attempted, the surgeon discovers that the infection extends into muscle, often with extensive destruction.

S. Aureus Epidural Abscess. This infection is often related to the presence of vertebral osteomyelitis wherein periosseus inflammation extends into the epidural space. The inflammation causes localized tenderness over the spine at point of infection followed by weakness and progressive neurologic signs of paraplegia. Effective therapy depends on early diagnosis and *prompt* surgical intervention and drainage.

DIAGNOSIS. Knowledgeable interpretation of the Gram's stain of an adequately obtained specimen usually suggests the presence of staphylococci. Culture of such a specimen almost always yields the responsible staphylococcus, and confirmation is provided by positive blood cultures. Some judgment is required in deciding whether S. epidermidis in blood cultures is a contaminant or a true infection. The presence of the organism in *more than two* consecutive blood cultures and associated with proper clinical circumstances (the presence of an indwelling intravascular catheter or a prosthetic device) strongly suggests true bacteremia. The vast majority (80 to 90 per cent) of S. epidermidis isolated from blood culture bottles are single organisms, usually in only one of the two bottles in a set, and are contaminants. While S. aureus may on occasion contaminate blood cultures, the clinician must consider the isolation of S. aureus from the blood under any condition to be significant until proven otherwise. In most cases multiple blood cultures are positive, and there is no question about the diagnosis of the true bacteremic state. If there is any doubt as to the origin of S. aureus either in blood, urine, or other fluid specimens, appropriate therapy should be continued.

The Teichoic Acid Antibody (TA-AB) Assay. This assay measures the presence (and titer) or absence of antibodies to staphylococcal cell wall teichoic acids. It is of no use in diagnosing infections with S. epidermidis because it only identifies antibodies to the ribitol teichoic acid moiety in the wall of S. aureus. Approximately 90 per cent of patients with S. aureus endocarditis develop a significant titer of teichoic acid antibodies. The test is fairly sensitive but only moderately specific for other types of serious, deep-seated S. aureus infections. The major role of the TA-AB assay is not primarily to diagnose S. aureus infections, most of which are diagnosed on clinical grounds, but to assist the clinician in deciding how long to treat bacteremic patients. Patients with S. aureus bacteremia who develop disseminated or metastatic abscesses usually develop an increase in the titer of TA-AB acid antibodies as opposed to those with benign, self-limited bacteremias. The predictive value of a negative assay in someone who has experienced an episode of S. aureus bacteremia is high; therefore, the test may be useful in *ruling out* metastatic infections in such patients. In general, however, clinical parameters suffice in such clinical decision-making, and the TA-AB assay rarely provides additional, helpful information.

TREATMENT. Effective therapy of staphylococcal infections depends on early, effective debridement and drainage of the primary focus of infection along with the selection of antibiotics to which the organisms are susceptible. At present, more than 90 per cent of all organisms, whether nosocomial or community-acquired, are resistant to penicillin. Therefore, no patient suspected of having an infection with S. aureus should be started on any penicillinase-susceptible penicillin. Most staphylococci are still susceptible to nafcillin and oxacillin; methicillin is an antiquated drug, more toxic than either of the aforementioned parenteral alternatives. Usual doses of nafcillin and oxacillin are in the range of 6 to 12 grams daily, and patients with endocarditis should receive between 9 and 12 grams daily. In the penicillin-allergic individual, the cephalosporins can be used in the absence of a history of an anaphylactic type of penicillin hypersensitivity; however, the most effective alternative continues to be vancomycin. Vancomycin is used in a dose of 2 to 4 grams per day parenterally and has been considered equal to the penicillins and cephalosporins in terms of therapeutic efficacy. Recently, however, some studies have shown relatively poorer clinical responses to vancomycin than to the β-lactam antibiotics, and a switch to nafcillin or oxacillin in patients not infected by a β-lactam–resistant strain of staphylococcus is probably indicated.

β-Lactam Antibiotic–Resistant Staphylococci (BLARS). These organisms are usually referred to as "methicillin-resistant staphylococci." However, methicillin is simply the drug used to determine resistance of these organisms and many methicillin-resistant organisms remain sensitive to the cephalosporins in vitro. However, the clinical responses to the cephalosporins of cephalosporin-sensitive but methicillin-resistant organisms have not been good. Thus, when any species of staphylococcus has been identified as being methicillin-resistant (or, therefore, nafcillin- or oxacillin-resistant) it should be considered resistant to *all* β-lactam antibiotics regardless of contrary data in vitro. The drug of choice in the treatment of BLARS continues to be vancomycin. Alternative drugs include rifampin and trimethoprim-sulfamethoxazole (TMS). Some BLARS remain sensitive to the aminoglycosides, and aminoglycosides may provide a synergistic effect with whatever other antibiotic is used. Newer antibiotics that will be effective against BLARS are teichoplanin* and the quinolones, although recent data indicate increasing quinolone resistance. A new β-lactam–like antibiotic, imipenem (a carbapenem), should probably not be used against BLARS, despite sensitivity in vitro. These recommendations hold true both for S. aureus and S. epidermidis. Fusidic acid, an antibiotic which inhibits ribosomal GTPase (elongation factor), has been used for many years in England and Canada. It should be thought of when one encounters a serious, resistant S. aureus infection in a patient who is intolerant of the glycopeptide antibiotics or who requires an oral agent to treat such infections.

Treatment of Chronic Carriers. Certain individuals may suffer recurrent staphylococcal infections of the skin (furunculosis), and eradication of the nasal carrier state may be required to terminate the series of infections. Nasal carriage termination may be difficult by local, topical measures. Traditionally, individuals so afflicted have been advised to observe meticulous personal hygienic measures such as frequent bathing or showering, using pHisoHex or other bactericidal soap preparations, and the application of an antibacterial ointment such as bacitracin to the anterior nares. While such a treatment program clears a portion of chronic carriers, many relapse and continue to develop recurrent crops of boils. One drug very helpful in this situation is rifampin, known to be excreted in bactericidal concentrations in external (nasal) secretions. Rifampin should always be used with another

---

*Investigational drug.

oral antistaphylococcal drug that, even though present in low concentrations, will delay the emergence of rifampin resistance. Thus, a 5-day course of rifampin* (600 mg twice daily) plus, for example, dicloxacillin (125 mg four times a day) or in the penicillin-allergic patient cephalexin or TMS is very effective in eliminating nasal carriage of S. aureus and the associated dermal infections. A percentage of individuals reacquire the organism and the course of therapy may have to be repeated; the physician should be sure to ascertain that the carried organism is still sensitive to rifampin. As discussed earlier, 5 days of rifampin treatment administered every 3 months to colonized hemodialysis patients significantly reduced the incidence of subsequent infections with S. aureus. Another agent recently introduced for topical use is mupirocin (Bactroban). Application of mupirocin ointment to the anterior nares 3 times a day for 5 days rapidly eliminates nasal carriage; however, 10 per cent relapse occurs in 3 weeks and 40 per cent by 14 weeks. Some mupirocin resistance may be developing. Other antibiotics that may help clear nasal carriage include the oral quinolones and clindamycin.

Bacterial Interference. Bacterial interference is the process of recolonizing an individual with an organism in order to displace a more pathogenic microbe. Initially, investigators found that patients heavily colonized with an aggressive strain of S. aureus that was associated with recurrent infections (boils, omphalitis, or conjunctivitis) could be helped by being recolonized with a nonpathogenic strain (designated strain 502A) of the organism. Reports in the 1960's and 1970's attested to the efficacy of bacterial interference. However, from time to time, there were reports of a serious infection caused by the 502A strain of S. aureus. The use of bacterial interference to treat recurrent infections due to a carried strain of S. aureus therefore has declined. The potential usefulness of this process should be kept in mind as one considers therapeutic approaches to patients with recurrent furunculosis recalcitrant to repeated courses of therapy.

PREVENTION. Prevention of nosocomial staphylococcal infections depends on breaking the chain of transmission between a carrier and a susceptible noncarrier. Transmission from person to person is effectively interrupted by thorough handwashing before and after examination of each patient. Certain other hospital infection control recommendations and procedures apply in particular to staphylococcal infections. For example, hospitals are required to have specific recommendations about the placement and maintenance of intravascular catheters; such instructions should be followed *meticulously.* Staphylococci are among the leading causes of infection of indwelling intravascular catheters, and proper catheter maintenance substantially reduces the incidence of nosocomial infections with these organisms.

While in theory vaccines containing capsular polysaccharides might enhance host defenses against the encapsulated strains of staphylococci, vaccines developed in the past were not shown to be of major clinical benefit. It is probable that some acquired immunity does develop against staphylococci, since the incidence of S. aureus infections decreases with increasing age. Also, recent data have shown that anticapsular antibodies facilitate opsonization of encapsulated strains. New monoclonal antibody technology will revitalize attempts to develop passive and possibly active immunization of patients at high risk of S. aureus bacteremia.

Bergdoll MS, Chesney PJ: Toxic Shock Syndrome. Boca Raton, Fla., CRC Press, in press. *New volume addressing all aspects of the toxic shock syndrome.*

Brumfitt W, Hamilton-Miller J: Methicillin-resistant *Staphylococcus aureus.* N Engl J Med 320:1188–1196, 1989. *Up-to-date review of all aspects of infections with β-lactam antibiotic–resistant staphylococci.*

Chambers HF, Korzeniowski OM, Sande MA: *Staphylococcus aureus* endocarditis. Clinical manifestations in addicts and nonaddicts. Medicine 62:170–177, 1983. *Data from a prospective, multicenter study describe and contrast the clinical presentation of the syndromes in addicts and nonaddicts.*

Esperson F, Frimodt-Møller N: *Staphylococcus aureus* endocarditis: A review of 119 cases. Arch Intern Med 146:1118–1121, 1986. *Excellent review of the syndrome of acute bacterial endocarditis with emphasis on community-acquired cases.*

Haley RW: Methicillin-resistant *Staphylococcus aureus:* Do we just have to live with it? Ann Intern Med 114:162–164, 1991. *Succinct review of the problem of nosocomial MRSA infections.*

Musher DM, McKenzie SO: Infections due to *Staphylococcus aureus.* Medicine 56:383–409, 1977. *A nice review of most clinical aspects of* S. aureus *infections; still relevant today.*

Sheagren JN: *Staphylococcus aureus*—the persistent pathogen. N Engl J Med 310:1368–1372, 1437–1442, 1984. *A complete review of all aspects of infections with* S. aureus.

Yu VL, Goetz A, Wagener M, et al.: *Staphylococcus aureus* nasal carriage and infection in patients on hemodialysis. Efficacy of antibiotic prophylaxis. N Engl J Med 315:91–96, 1986. *The rate of infection in hemodialysis patients can be decreased by treating the nasal carrier state.*

*This use of rifampin is not listed in the manufacturer's directive.

Bacterial Meningitis

Morton N. Swartz

301 Bacterial Meningitis

Meningitis is an inflammation of the arachnoid, the pia mater, and the intervening cerebrospinal fluid. The inflammatory process extends throughout the subarachnoid space about the brain and spinal cord and regularly involves the ventricles. Pyogenic meningitis, considered in this chapter, is usually an acute infection with bacteria that evoke a polymorphonuclear response in the cerebrospinal fluid (CSF). One of its major forms, that caused by meningococci, is considered in Ch. 302; less acute forms of bacterial meningitis, characterized by a mononuclear cell response in the CSF, are discussed in Ch. 332 and 456.

ETIOLOGY AND INCIDENCE. Approximately 20,000 to 25,000 cases of bacterial meningitis occur annually in the United States. If all cases are included regardless of the age of patients, data from the Centers for Disease Control indicate that *Haemophilus influenzae* type b is the most frequent bacterial cause (48 per cent), followed by *Neisseria meningitidis* (19 per cent) and *Streptococcus pneumoniae* (13 per cent). About 70 per cent of all cases occur in children under 5 years of age. The relative frequencies with which the different bacterial species cause meningitis are age related (Table 301–1). In the newborn, gram-negative bacilli (most frequently *Escherichia coli*, but also other enteric bacilli and *Pseudomonas*) and group B streptococci are the principal causes. In the past 25 years the group B *Streptococcus* has increased in importance in neonatal meningitis; in some hospitals it is the single most frequent etiology, surpassing *E. coli.* Beyond the first month of life and extending through childhood, *H. influenzae* and *N. meningitidis* are the most fre-

TABLE 301–1. BACTERIAL CAUSES OF MENINGITIS

	Neonates (≤1 month) (%)	Children (1 month– 15 years) (%)	Adults (>15 years) (%)
S. pneumoniae	0–5	10–20	20–40
N. meningitidis	0–1	25–40	10–20
H. influenzae	0–3	40–60	2–4
Streptococci	20–40*	2–4	5–10
Staphylococci	5	1–2	5–15
Listeria	2–10	1–2	5–10
Gram-negative bacilli	50–60†	1–2	10–20

*Almost all isolates from neonatal meningitis are group B streptococci.
†Of all cases of neonatal meningitis, *E. coli* accounts for about 40 per cent and *Klebsiella-Enterobacter* for about 8 per cent.

quent causes of bacterial meningitis. In adults *S. pneumoniae*, *N. meningitidis*, and gram-negative bacilli are responsible for most cases. Meningococcal meningitis is the only type that occurs in outbreaks; its relative frequency among the meningitides depends on whether statistics have been gathered in a hyperendemic area or during an epidemic period. In about 10 per cent of patients with pyogenic meningitis the bacterial cause cannot be defined. Simultaneous mixed meningitis is rare, occurring in the setting of neurosurgical procedures, penetrating head injury, erosion of the skull or vertebrae by adjacent neoplasm, or intraventricular rupture of a cerebral abscess; the isolation of anaerobes should strongly suggest the latter two of these.

Important changes have occurred in the frequencies of several types of bacterial meningitis over the past 25 years. Gram-negative bacillary meningitis has doubled in frequency in adults, probably reflecting more frequent and extensive neurosurgical procedures as well as other nosocomial factors. *Listeria monocytogenes* has increased eight- to tenfold as a cause of bacterial meningitis in urban general hospitals, reflecting the enlarging immunosuppressed population at particular risk. *Listeria* infections appear to be food borne (dairy products, uncooked vegetables) and involve particularly organ transplant recipients, other patients receiving corticosteroids and cytotoxic drugs, patients with liver disease, pregnant women, and neonates. Meningitis due to *Staphylococcus epidermidis*, essentially unheard of 30 years ago, now represents about 3 per cent of cases in large urban hospitals. It occurs as a complication of neurosurgical procedures and may present a particular therapeutic problem due to methicillin resistance of many of the *S. epidermidis* strains.

CLINICAL SETTINGS. The clinical setting in which meningitis develops may provide a clue to the specific bacterial cause. Meningococcal disease, including meningitis, may occur sporadically and in cyclic outbreaks. In the past, military recruits were particularly susceptible, but now meningococcal vaccine (polysaccharides of groups A, C, Y and W135) is employed for protection. Large urban outbreaks can occur.

Certain predisposing factors are frequently associated with the development of *pneumococcal meningitis. Acute otitis media* (± *mastoiditis*) occurs in about 30 per cent of patients. *Pneumonia* is present in about 15 per cent of patients with pneumococcal meningitis, a much higher frequency than in meningitis caused by *H. influenzae* or *N. meningitidis. Acute pneumococcal sinusitis* is occasionally the initial focus from which infection spreads to the meninges. A significant head injury (recent or remote) has occurred in about 10 per cent of patients with pneumococcal meningitis. CSF rhinorrhea (usually caused by a defect or fracture in the cribriform plate) is present in about 5 per cent of patients with pneumococcal meningitis. Meningitis occurring in young children with sickle cell anemia is most likely to be caused by *S. pneumoniae*. A variety of defects in host defenses (primary or acquired immunoglobulin deficiencies, the asplenic state) may predispose to severe pneumococcal disease, particularly bacteremia and meningitis. Alcoholism is an underlying problem in 10 to 25 per cent of adults with pneumococcal meningitis in urban hospitals.

S. aureus meningitis is seen most commonly as a complication of a neurosurgical procedure, following penetrating skull trauma, or occasionally secondary to staphylococcal bacteremia and endocarditis. Meningitis caused by *gram-negative bacilli* takes one of three forms: neonatal meningitis, meningitis following trauma or neurosurgery, or spontaneous meningitis in adults (e.g., bacteremic *Klebsiella* meningitis in a patient with diabetes mellitus). The most common causes of gram-negative bacillary meningitis in the adult are *E. coli* (about 30 per cent) and *Klebsiella-Enterobacter* (about 40 per cent). The most frequent causes of bacterial meningitis in patients with neoplastic disease are gram-negative bacilli (particularly *Pseudomonas aeruginosa* and *E. coli*), *Listeria monocytogenes, S. pneumoniae*, and *S. aureus*. Meningitis caused by *group A streptococci* is uncommon but occasionally occurs following acute otitis media.

The age-related incidence (children under 5 years) of *H. influenzae* type b meningitis is so striking that the occurrence of this disease in an adult should raise the question of the presence of an underlying anatomic or immunologic defect, circumventing the usual barrier interposed by serum bactericidal mechanisms.

Neonatal Meningitis. The incidence of meningitis is higher in the first month of life than in any other single month. The principal cause, *E. coli* strains containing the K1 capsular antigen, is usually acquired by the neonates from their mothers who carry the organism in their stool. In the newborn the group B *Streptococcus* can produce either an "early onset" (occurring within 8 days of delivery and characterized by a fulminant illness with septicemia, severe respiratory distress, and sometimes meningitis) or a "late onset" (occurring 10 days to 2 months after delivery and presenting a more insidious, slowly progressive illness which usually includes meningitis) infection.

The clinical signs in neonatal meningitis suggest sepsis but not necessarily central nervous system involvement: fever (in only 60 per cent), jaundice, diarrhea, lethargy, poor feeding or vomiting, respiratory distress (including apnea), seizures, irritability, bulging fontanel (in only 30 per cent), and nuchal rigidity (15 per cent). Frequently, only by examination of the CSF can the presence of meningitis be ruled in or out.

PATHOLOGY. The purulent exudate is distributed widely in the subarachnoid space, most abundant in the basal cisterns and about the cerebellum initially, but also extending into the sulci over the cerebrum. There is no direct invasion of cerebral tissue by the infecting organism or the inflammatory exudate, but the subjacent brain becomes congested and edematous. The effectiveness of the pial barrier accounts for the fact that cerebral abscess does not complicate bacterial meningitis. Indeed, when these two processes coexist, the sequence usually has been that of an initial abscess subsequently leaking its contents into the ventricular system, producing meningitis. There are two possible exceptions to the aforementioned generalization: (1) neonatal meningitis due to *Citrobacter*, in which the organisms appear to invade the brain after producing a necrotizing vasculitis of small penetrating blood vessels; (2) *Listeria* rhombencephalitis, a very rare process in which brain stem infection can occur simultaneously with *Listeria* meningitis (or alone). Structures adjacent to the meninges may show a variety of pathologic changes secondary to bacterial meningitis. *Cortical thrombophlebitis* results from venous stasis and adjacent meningeal inflammation. Infarction of cerebral tissue may follow. *Involvement of cortical and pial arteries* with peripheral aneurysm formation and vascular occlusion occurs occasionally in bacterial meningitis. Rarely, narrowing of the supraclinoid portion of the internal carotid artery at the base of the brain occurs as a result of arteritis and arterial spasm. In fulminating cases (particularly meningococcal meningitis), *cerebral edema* may be marked even though the CSF pleocytosis is only moderate. Rarely such patients develop temporal lobe and cerebellar herniation, resulting in compression of the midbrain and medulla. *Damage to cranial nerves* occurs in areas where dense exudate accumulates; the third and sixth cranial nerves are also vulnerable to damage by increased intracranial pressure. *Ventriculitis* probably occurs in most cases of bacterial meningitis; rarely this progresses to the accumulation of pus, *ventricular empyema. Hydrocephalus* can develop during meningitis from obstruction to CSF flow within the ventricular system (obstructive hydrocephalus) or extraventricularly (communicating hydrocephalus). *Subdural effusions* are sterile transudates that develop over the cerebral cortex in about 15 per cent of infants with bacterial meningitis. Rarely such effusions become infected, producing a subdural empyema. In the past the diagnosis has been made almost exclusively in infants, in whom abnormal transillumination or increasing head size can be detected. Now, sterile or infected (showing peripheral contrast enhancement) subdural collections can be demonstrated readily by CT scan as low-density areas about the cerebrum.

PATHOGENESIS. Bacteria may reach the meninges by several routes: (1) systemic bacteremia, (2) direct ingress from the upper respiratory tract or skin through an anatomic defect (e.g., skull fracture, eroding sequestrum, meningocele), (3) passage intracranially via venules in the nasopharynx, or (4) spread from a contiguous focus of infection (infection of the paranasal sinuses, leakage of a brain abscess). Bacteremic spread to the meninges is probably the most frequent path of infection. However, not all bacteremic organisms have the same likelihood of causing meningitis. Most bacterial species causing meningitis (*H. influenzae* b, *N. meningitidis, S. pneumoniae, E. coli* K1, group B *Streptococcus*) have definable capsules which are antiphagocytic. Whether the capsular polysaccharide confers some special meningeal tropism, possibly through surface receptors, is not known. The primary focus initiating the bacteremia is usually in the upper respiratory tract or lung (pneumonia) but may be in the heart (endocarditis) or the gastrointestinal or urinary tracts. Experiments in infant primates infected with *H. influenzae* suggest that the initial site of inflammation in the central nervous system may be the choroid plexus. Once established in any part of the meninges, infection quickly extends throughout the subarachnoid space. Bacterial replication proceeds relatively unhindered, since CSF levels of complement are low early in meningeal inflammation, resulting in minimal opsonic and bactericidal activity (or none), and since surface phagocytosis of unopsonized organisms is meager in such a fluid environment. A secondary bacteremia may follow meningeal infection and itself contribute to continuing further inoculation of the cerebrospinal fluid.

Acute meningeal inflammation can be induced in animal models by intracisternal inoculation of pneumococcal cell wall components or of *H. influenzae* type b lipopolysaccharide, probably through the release of inflammatory cytokines such as interleukin 1, tumor necrosis factor (TNF), or prostaglandins. Increased CSF levels of TNF have been found in bacterial, but not viral, meningitis.

CLINICAL MANIFESTATIONS. History. An acute onset of fever, generalized headache, vomiting, and stiff neck are common to many types of meningitis. The majority of patients with pyogenic meningitis of the three common causes have had an antecedent or accompanying upper respiratory tract infection, acute otitis (or mastoiditis), or pneumonia. Myalgias (particularly in meningococcal disease), backache, and generalized weakness are common symptoms. The illness usually progresses rapidly with development of confusion, obtundation, and loss of consciousness. Occasionally the onset may be less acute, with meningeal signs present for several days to a week.

General Physical Findings. Evidences of meningeal irritation (drowsiness and decreased mentation, stiff neck, Kernig's and Brudzinski's signs) are usually present. In certain patients the findings of meningitis may be easily overlooked; infants, obtunded patients, or elderly patients with congestive failure or pneumonia may develop meningitis without prominent meningeal signs. Their lethargy should be investigated carefully and meningeal signs should be sought; if any doubt exists, examination of the CSF is indicated.

The presence of a petechial, purpuric, or ecchymotic rash in a patient with meningeal findings almost always indicates meningococcal infection and requires prompt treatment because of the rapidity with which this infection can progress (see Ch. 302). Rarely, extensive petechial and purpuric lesions occur in meningitis caused by *S. pneumoniae* or *H. influenzae*. Very rarely skin lesions almost indistinguishable from those of meningococcal bacteremia occur in patients with acute *S. aureus* endocarditis who also have meningeal signs and a CSF pleocytosis (secondary either to staphylococcal meningitis or to embolic cerebral infarction). Usually one or two of the lesions in such a patient are those of purulent purpura; aspiration of material reveals staphylococci on Gram's stain. In the summer months viral aseptic meningitis may produce meningeal signs, macular and petechial skin lesions, and a CSF pleocytosis of several hundred cells, sometimes with neutrophils predominating initially.

Neurologic Findings and Complications. *Cranial nerve abnormalities,* involving principally the third, fourth, sixth, or seventh nerves, occur in 10 to 20 per cent of patients with bacterial meningitis. These usually disappear shortly after recovery. Persistent sensorineural hearing loss occurs in 10 per cent of children with bacterial meningitis. In another 16 per cent a transient conductive hearing loss develops. The most likely sites of involvement in persistent sensorineural deafness appear to be the inner ear (infection or toxic products possibly spreading from the subarachnoid space along the cochlear aqueduct) and the acoustic nerve. In children permanent hearing impairment is more common following meningitis due to *S. pneumoniae* than to *H. influenzae* or *N. meningitidis*.

Seizures (focal or generalized) occur in 20 to 30 per cent of patients and may result from readily reversible causes (high fever in infants; penicillin neurotoxicity when large doses are administered intravenously in the presence of renal failure) or from focal cerebral injury. Seizures can occur during the first few days or can appear with associated focal neurologic deficits caused by

cortical vein phlebitis 7 to 10 days after the onset of the meningitis. In adults with seizures accompanying meningitis, *S. pneumoniae* is more commonly the cause, but alcoholism is a confounding factor.

Brain swelling and increased CSF pressure are associated with seizures, third nerve dysfunction, abnormal reflexes, coma, hypertension, and bradycardia. Two anatomic features of brain capillaries account for the functioning of the blood-brain barrier in controlling the concentration of substances in brain interstitium. They are the presence of tight junctions fusing brain capillary endothelial cells together and the paucity of pinocytotic vacuoles in the same cells. With bacterial meningitis, separation of intercellular junctions occurs, and pinocytotic vacuoles increase, probably accounting for the development of complicating cerebral edema. In approximately one quarter of fatal cases of community-acquired meningitis in adults, cerebral edema accompanied by temporal lobe herniation is observed at autopsy.

Papilledema is rare in bacterial meningitis even with high CSF pressures. Its presence should indicate the possibility of some other associated or independent suppurative intracranial process (subdural empyema, brain abscess). Marked central hyperpnea sometimes occurs in patients with severe bacterial meningitis; CSF acidosis (principally caused by increased lactic acid levels) provides much of the respiratory stimulus.

Focal cerebral signs (principally hemiparesis, dysphasia, visual field defects, and gaze preference) occur in about 25 per cent of adults with community-acquired bacterial meningitis. They may develop during early meningitis secondary to occlusive vascular processes or some days later. Also, cerebral blood flow velocity may be decreased in the presence of increased intracranial pressure and lead to temporary or lasting neurologic dysfunction. It is important to distinguish lateralizing findings resulting from postictal changes (Todd's paralysis), which usually persist for no more than several hours.

Prompt treatment of bacterial meningitis usually results in rapid recovery of neurologic function. Persistent or late-onset obtundation and coma without focal findings suggest development of brain swelling, subdural effusion (in the infant), hydrocephalus, loculated ventriculitis, cortical thrombophlebitis, or sagittal sinus thrombosis. The last three are commonly associated with fever and continuing CSF pleocytosis.

Residual neurologic damage remains in 10 to 20 per cent of patients who recover from bacterial meningitis. Developmental delay and speech defects are each observed in about 5 per cent of children. In infants surviving neonatal meningitis, significant sequelae are much more frequent (30 to 50 per cent).

LABORATORY DIAGNOSIS. Cerebrospinal Fluid Examination. Initial CSF pressure is usually moderately elevated (200 to 300 mm H_2O). Striking elevations (over 450 mm) occur in occasional patients with acute brain swelling complicating meningitis in the absence of an associated mass lesion.

Gram-Stained Smear. By the time of hospitalization, most patients with pyogenic meningitis have large numbers (at least 10^5 per milliliter) of bacteria in the cerebrospinal fluid. Careful examination of the Gram-stained smear of the spun sediment of CSF reveals the etiologic agent in 70 to 80 per cent of cases. In most instances when gram-positive diplococci (or short chaining cocci) are observed on stained CSF smear they are pneumococci. In certain clinical settings it is important to distinguish this organism from the relatively penicillin-resistant *Enterococcus*, which would require the addition of an aminoglycoside to penicillin in treatment. This can be done by identifying pneumococcal polysaccharide in the CSF by latex particle agglutination (or by employing the quellung reaction). Culture of the cerebrospinal fluid reveals the etiologic agent in 80 to 90 per cent of patients with bacterial meningitis.

Special Immunologic and Serologic Procedures. In patients in whom the etiologic agent is not identified on Gram-stained smear of the CSF, rapid diagnosis may often be made by detection of specific bacterial antigens by latex agglutination (LA) or countercurrent immunoelectrophoresis (CIE). These techniques have been employed most extensively in the rapid diagnosis of meningitis caused by *H. influenzae* type b, but have also been used in the diagnosis of meningococcal (groups A,B,C, and Y) and pneumococcal meningitis, and meningitis due to group B streptococci. Antigen detection by LA is more sensitive and provides results more rapidly than CIE. Since *E. coli* K1 and *N. meningitidis* serogroup B share a common antigenic determinant, immunologic cross-reactivity may cause a false-positive reaction with the group B meningococcal reagent. Since the bacterial cause can be found on Gram-stained smear in most cases of bacterial meningitis, the role of latex agglutination appears to be as an adjunct in rapid diagnosis when no organisms are observed or in providing a specific rather than a morphologic (Gram's stain) diagnosis.

The limulus gelation assay for endotoxin is positive in the CSF of patients with meningitis caused by gram-negative but not by gram-positive bacteria.

Cell Count. The cell count in untreated meningitis usually ranges between 100 and 10,000 per cubic millimeter, with polymorphonuclear leukocytes predominating initially (80 per cent or more) and lymphocytes appearing subsequently. Extremely high cell counts (>50,000 per cubic millimeter) may occur rarely in primary bacterial meningitis but should also raise the possibility of intraventricular rupture of a cerebral abscess. Cell counts as low as 10 to 20 may be observed early in bacterial meningitis (particularly that caused by *N. meningitidis* and *H. influenzae*). Occasionally, in granulocytopenic patients or in the elderly with overwhelming pneumococcal meningitis, the CSF may contain very few leukocytes and yet may appear grossly turbid because of the presence of myriads of organisms. Meningitis caused by several bacterial species (*M. tuberculosis*, *B. burgdorferi*, *T. pallidum*) characteristically produces a lymphocytic pleocytosis. *Listeria monocytogenes* meningitis in infants may produce a primarily lymphocytic response in the CSF; in the adult there is usually a polymorphonuclear response, but rarely lymphocytes predominate.

Glucose. The CSF glucose is reduced to values of 40 mg per deciliter or below (or less than 50 per cent of the simultaneous blood level) in 50 per cent of patients with bacterial meningitis; this finding can be very valuable in distinguishing bacterial meningitis from most viral meningitides or parameningeal infections. A normal CSF glucose does not exclude the diagnosis of bacterial meningitis. The simultaneous blood glucose level should be determined, because patients with diabetes mellitus (or who are receiving intravenous glucose infusions) have an elevated level of glucose in the CSF, and its significance can be appreciated only on comparison with the simultaneous blood level. However, it may take 90 to 120 minutes for equilibration to occur after major shifts in the level of glucose in the circulation. The hypoglycorrhachia characteristic of pyogenic meningitis appears to be due to interference with normal carrier-facilitated diffusion of glucose.

Protein. The level of protein in the CSF is usually elevated above 100 mg per deciliter, and the higher values are more commonly observed in pneumococcal meningitis. Extreme elevations, 1000 mg per deciliter or more, indicate subarachnoid block secondary to the meningitis.

Other Abnormalities in the CSF. Elevated levels of lactic acid occur in pyogenic meningitis. Although lactic dehydrogenase levels are higher in patients with bacterial meningitis than in those with viral infections of the central nervous system, these alterations are not of help in determining the specific etiologic agent involved. C-reactive protein is increased in about 95 per cent of patients with bacterial meningitis and is not increased in most patients with viral meningitis. However, it does not seem to provide more information than the CSF cell count, is not helpful in diagnosing bacterial meningitis in newborns, and does not provide clues to the bacterial species involved.

Other Laboratory Tests. Blood and Respiratory Tract Cultures. Bacteremia is demonstrable in about 80 per cent of patients with *H. influenzae* meningitis, 50 per cent of those with pneumococcal meningitis, and 30 to 40 per cent of those with meningococcal meningitis. Cultures of the upper respiratory tract are not helpful in establishing an etiologic diagnosis. Determination of serum creatinine and electrolytes is important in view of the gravity of the illness, the occurrence of specific abnormalities secondary to the meningitis (syndrome of inappropriate secretion of antidiuretic hormone), and problems in therapy in the presence of renal dysfunction (seizures and hyperkalemia with high-dose

penicillin therapy). In patients with extensive petechial and purpuric skin lesions, evaluation for coagulopathy is indicated.

Radiologic Studies. In view of the frequency with which pyogenic meningitis is associated with primary foci of infection in the chest, nasal sinuses, or mastoid, roentgenograms of these areas should be taken at the appropriate time after institution of antimicrobial therapy. Computerized tomography (CT) scans are not indicated in most patients with bacterial meningitis. If a mass lesion (cerebral abscess, subdural empyema) is suspected by history, clinical setting, or physical findings (papilledema, focal cerebral signs), then CT scans should be performed. *Bacterial meningitis is a medical emergency requiring immediate diagnosis and rapid institution of antimicrobial therapy.* Delay in performing a diagnostic lumbar puncture in order to obtain a CT scan should be avoided except on the basis of findings indicative of a parameningeal collection or other intracranial mass lesion. Changes may be observed on CT scan during meningitis itself: cerebral edema, enlargement of the subarachnoid spaces; contrast enhancement of the leptomeninges and the ependyma; or patchy areas of diminished density caused by associated cerebritis and necrosis. Patients with meningitis rarely have significant CT abnormalities in the absence of focal neurologic findings. In the patient with meningitis whose clinical status deteriorates or fails to improve, the CT scan may be helpful in demonstrating suspected complications: sterile subdural collections or empyema; ventricular enlargement secondary to communicating or obstructive hydrocephalus; prominent persisting basilar meningitis; extensive areas of cerebral infarction resulting from occlusion of major cerebral arteries or veins; or marked ventricular wall enhancement, suggesting ventriculitis or ventricular empyema.

DIAGNOSIS. Diagnosis of bacterial meningitis is not difficult in a febrile patient with meningeal symptoms and signs developing in the setting of a predisposing illness. The diagnosis may be less obvious in the elderly, obtunded patient with pneumonia or the confused alcoholic patient in impending delirium tremens. Examination of the CSF should be carried out promptly whenever there is any question of meningitis.

Headache, fever, vomiting, stiff neck, and CSF pleocytosis are features of meningeal inflammation and are common to many types of meningitis (e.g., bacterial, fungal, viral) and also to some parameningeal processes. The CSF findings are most helpful in distinguishing among these processes (see Ch. 471). In the patient with meningitis whose CSF does not reveal the etiologic agent on examination of Gram-stained smear, particularly when the CSF glucose is normal and the polymorphonuclear pleocytosis is atypical, certain treatable processes which can mimic bacterial meningitis should be considered in differential diagnosis: (1) *Parameningeal infections.* The presence of infections (chronic ear or nasal accessory sinus infections, lung abscess) predisposing to brain abscess, epidural (cerebral or spinal) abscess, subdural empyema, or pyogenic venous sinus phlebitis should be sought. Neurologic findings may appear in the course of primary bacterial meningitis, but their presence should alert the physician to the need for close scrutiny for the presence of a space-occupying infectious process in the central nervous system. Neurologic symptoms or findings antedating the onset of meningeal symptoms should suggest the possibility of a parameningeal infection. The isolation of an anaerobic organism should suggest the possibility of intraventricular leakage of a cerebral abscess. (2) *Bacterial endocarditis.* Bacterial meningitis may occur during bacterial endocarditis caused by pyogenic organisms such as *S. aureus* and enterococci. In subacute bacterial endocarditis sterile embolic infarctions of the brain may occur and produce meningeal signs and a CSF pleocytosis containing several hundred cells, including polymorphonuclear leukocytes. A history of dental manipulation, fever, and anorexia antedating the meningitis should be sought; careful examination for heart murmurs and peripheral stigmata of endocarditis is indicated. (3) *"Chemical" meningitis.* The clinical and CSF findings (polymorphonuclear pleocytosis and even reduced glucose level) of bacterial meningitis may be produced by chemically induced inflammation. Acute meningitis following a diagnostic lumbar puncture or spinal anesthesia may be due to bacterial or chemical contamination of equipment or anesthetic agent. Endogenous chemical meningitis resulting from leakage into the subarachnoid space of material from an epidermoid tumor or a craniopharyngioma can produce a polymorphonuclear pleocytosis and hypoglycorrhachia. Birefringent material may be seen on polarizing microscopy of the CSF sediment.

Rarely, a patient develops meningitis characterized by subacute onset and persistent neutrophilic CSF pleocytosis lasting weeks or months without ready bacteriologic diagnosis. The etiologic agent in such cases of *chronic neutrophilic meningitis* has usually been either a fungus (*Aspergillus, Candida, Blastomyces*, etc.) or a bacterium such as *Nocardia* or *Actinomyces* species.

NON-NEUROLOGIC COMPLICATIONS. Shock. When shock occurs in pyogenic meningitis it is usually a manifestation of an accompanying intense bacteremia, as in fulminant meningococcemia, rather than of the meningitis itself. Management is guided by the principles of septic shock therapy with appropriate modifications for myocardial failure (see Ch. 302).

Coagulation Disorders. Coagulopathies are frequently associated with the intense bacteremias (usually meningococcal, occasionally pneumococcal) and hypotension which can accompany meningitis. The changes may be mild such as thrombocytopenia (with or without prolongation of prothrombin and partial thromboplastin times) or more marked with clinical evidences of disseminated intravascular coagulation (see Ch. 302).

Septic Complications. **Endocarditis.** Previously, 5 to 10 per cent of patients with pneumococcal meningitis, particularly those with bacteremia and pneumonia as well, developed acute endocarditis, most commonly on the aortic valve. The incidence is currently much lower, as a result of earlier treatment of the initiating infection. In such patients, febrile relapse and a new murmur may appear shortly after completion of antimicrobial therapy for meningitis.

Pyogenic Arthritis. Septic arthritis may result from the bacteremia associated with meningitis caused by *S. pneumoniae, N. meningitidis,* or *H. influenzae.*

Prolonged Fever. With appropriate antimicrobial treatment of meningitis of the three most common bacterial causes, patients become afebrile within 2 to 5 days. Sometimes fever persists beyond this or recurs after an afebrile period. In the patient with persisting headache, obtundation, and cerebral findings, inadequate drug therapy or neurologic sequelae (cortical venous thrombophlebitis, ventriculitis, subdural collections) are important considerations. Re-evaluation of the CSF, particularly Gram-stained smear and culture, is essential under these circumstances. Drug fever may be responsible in the patient who continues to show clinical improvement in all other respects. Metastatic infection (septic arthritis, purulent pericarditis, thoracic empyema, endocarditis) may be the cause of continuing or recurrent fever.

A syndrome consisting of fever, arthritis, and pericarditis 3 to 6 days after initiation of effective antimicrobial therapy of meningococcal meningitis occurs in about 10 per cent of patients (see Ch. 302).

RECURRENT MENINGITIS. Repeated episodes of bacterial meningitis generally indicate a host defect, either in local anatomy or in antibacterial and immunologic defenses (e.g., recurrent *N. meningitidis* infections in patients with congenital or acquired deficiencies of complement, particularly late-acting components). Eleven per cent of patients with pneumococcal meningitis have had more than one episode, whereas 0.5 per cent of patients with meningitis caused by other organisms have had recurrent attacks. *S. pneumoniae* is the cause of one third of episodes of community-acquired recurrent meningitis; various streptococci, *H. influenzae,* and *N. meningitidis* are the causes of another one third of episodes. In contrast, in nosocomial recurrent meningitis, gram-negative bacilli and *S. aureus* are the causes of about 60 per cent of episodes. A history of head trauma is much more frequent in patients with recurrent meningitis. Organisms may directly enter the subarachnoid space, through a defect in the cribriform plate (the most common site), in association with the empty sella syndrome, via a basilar skull fracture, through an erosive sequestrum of the mastoid, through congenital dermal defects along the craniospinal axis (usually evident before adult life), or as a consequence of penetrating cranial trauma or neurosurgical procedures. The anatomic defect may produce a frank CSF leak (rhinorrhea or, less commonly, otorrhea) or may entrap a vascular cuff of meninges which might subsequently serve as a direct route for organisms to reach the meninges. CSF rhinorrhea may be intermittent, and meningitis may occur months or years after head injury.

Any patient with bacterial meningitis, particularly if meningitis is recurrent, should be evaluated carefully for any congenital or post-traumatic defects. The presence of CSF rhinorrhea should be sought at admission and subsequently (rhinorrhea may clear during active meningitis only to recur when inflammation has resolved). Clinical clues suggesting the presence of a CSF fistula through the cribriform plate, pericranial air sinuses, or temporal bone include (1) salty taste in the throat, (2) positionally dependent rhinorrhea (rhinorrhea only in the lateral recumbent or prone position suggests an otic or sphenoid origin), (3) anosmia (cribriform plate leak), and (4) hearing loss or full feeling in the ear, often with a finding of fluid or bubbles behind the tympanic membrane (leakage into the middle ear). Demonstration of glucose in nasal secretions with glucose oxidase "sticks" (Dextrostix) suggests the presence of CSF. Quantitative determination of glucose and chloride content of nasal secretions can definitively establish the presence of CSF rhinorrhea.

Recurrent pneumococcal meningitis may occur without apparent predisposing circumstances, and cryptic CSF leaks should be sought actively in such patients by polytomography of the frontal and mastoid regions and by radioisotope techniques. (Radioiodine-labeled albumin is introduced intrathecally, and pledgets of cotton placed in the nares are subsequently examined for the radionuclide. Radioisotopic cisternography has been used successfully recently.) Intrathecal introduction of fluorescein as a visual tracer (under ultraviolet light) can be employed similarly in detecting active leaks. Surgical closure of CSF fistulas should be carried out to prevent further episodes of meningitis. Newer extracranial approaches via the ethmoid sinuses for repair of cribriform plate or sphenoid sinus dural defects are successful and avoid the higher morbidity associated with craniotomy.

In most patients with CSF otorrhea and rhinorrhea following an acute head injury, the leak ceases in 1 or 2 weeks. *Persistent rhinorrhea for more than 4 to 6 weeks is an indication for surgical repair.* Prolonged administration of penicillin does not prevent pneumococcal meningitis and may encourage infection with more drug-resistant species.

Rarely, recurrent meningitis of nonbacterial etiology may mimic bacterial meningitis. *Mollaret's meningitis* consists of repeated febrile episodes of mild meningeal symptomatology, usually without neurologic abnormalities. Initially, large "endothelial" cells may be seen in the CSF along with polymorphonuclear leukocytes, which subsequently are replaced by lymphocytes. *Behçet's syndrome,* characterized by relapsing oral and genital ulcers and ocular lesions (hypopyon), may exhibit a variety of neurologic abnormalities, including recurrent meningitis.

PROGNOSIS. The introduction of antimicrobial agents has converted bacterial meningitis from a disease that was almost always fatal to one in which the majority of patients survive without significant neurologic residua. The mortality rate for community-acquired bacterial meningitis varies with the etiologic agent and the clinical circumstances. With current antimicrobial therapy the mortality rate for *H. influenzae* meningitis is below 5 per cent and that for meningococcal meningitis is about 10 per cent. The highest mortality is with pneumococcal meningitis, in which the rate is about 25 per cent. The mortality rate for gram-negative bacillary meningitis in adults has been 20 to 30 per cent, but it appears to be decreasing in the past 5 to 10 years. The mortality rate for recurrent community-acquired meningitis in adults (about 5 per cent) is strikingly lower than the 20 per cent rate for nonrecurrent episodes. Poor prognostic factors include advanced age, presence of other foci of infection, underlying diseases (leukemia, alcoholism), coma, and delay in instituting appropriate therapy.

TREATMENT. Antimicrobial Agents. Antimicrobial therapy should be begun promptly in this life-threatening emergency. Treatment should be aimed at the most likely causes based on clinical clues (age of the patient, presence of a purpuric rash, a recent neurosurgical procedure, CSF rhinorrhea). If the infecting organism is observed on examination of the Gram-stained smear of the CSF sediment, specific therapy is initiated. If the etiologic agent is not seen on smear (or not detected by latex agglutination), treatment for bacterial meningitis of unknown etiology should be carried out (see below).

With the exception of chloramphenicol, the commonly employed antimicrobial agents do not readily penetrate the normal blood-brain barrier; but the passage of penicillin and other antimicrobials is enhanced in the presence of meningeal inflammation. Antimicrobial drugs should be administered intravenously throughout the treatment period; reduction in dosage as the patient improves should be avoided, because normalization of the blood-brain barrier during recovery reduces the CSF levels of drug that are achievable. Bactericidal drugs (penicillin, ampicillin, third-generation cephalosporins) are preferred whenever possible in the treatment of meningitis caused by susceptible bacteria. In animal models of bacterial meningitis CSF levels of antibiotics at least 10 to 20 times the minimal bactericidal concentration appear to be needed for optimal therapy. Several antimicrobial drugs (first- or second-generation cephalosporins, clindamycin) do not provide effective levels in the cerebrospinal fluid and should not be used.

Meningitis of Specific Bacterial Cause. The treatment of choice for pneumococcal meningitis in the adult is penicillin (24 million units daily in divided doses every 2 to 3 hours) or ampicillin (12 grams daily in divided doses every 2 to 3 hours). In the patient with a major penicillin allergy, chloramphenicol (4 to 6 grams intravenously daily in the adult) is a reasonable alternative. However, several points of caution should be made: (1) resistance to chloramphenicol has been reported from Spain in 45 per cent of pneumococcal strains, (2) the response to chloramphenicol of granulocytopenic patients may be suboptimal, and (3) recently, isolates of S. pneumoniae that are relatively resistant (minimum inhibitory concentration [MIC] of 0.1 to 1.0 µg per milliliter) or highly resistant (South African strains with MIC of 2 to 8 µg per milliliter) to penicillin have been identified. In the United States, relative pneumococcal resistance to penicillin, not due to β-lactamase production but rather to alterations in penicillin-binding proteins, occurs in 0 to 2 per cent of clinical isolates (in a few geographic areas the figures are as high as 6 to 8 per cent). (In one area of Spain 50 per cent of pneumococcal isolates have been reported to be penicillin resistant.) In addition to cases of meningitis due to highly penicillin-resistant S. pneumoniae that occurred during the outbreak in South Africa in the late 1970's, seven cases of meningitis due to moderately penicillin-resistant strains (including two that were multiply resistant) have been described in the United States and abroad. Thus, antimicrobial susceptibilities should be determined for all pneumococcal isolates from cerebrospinal fluid, blood, or sterile body fluids. If the isolate is, or is suspected to be, relatively penicillin resistant, a third-generation cephalosporin (e.g., cefotaxime or ceftriaxone) or chloramphenicol (provided the strain is not multiply resistant) is a reasonable alternative to penicillin G. If the isolate should prove to be highly penicillin resistant, vancomycin is the antimicrobial of choice.

The treatment of meningococcal meningitis is the same as for pneumococcal meningitis (see Ch. 302).

At present 30 per cent of isolates of H. influenzae b in the United States are ampicillin resistant. Thus, cefotaxime (200 mg per kilogram intravenously daily in divided doses every 4 to 6 hours for children; 12 grams daily in adults) or ceftriaxone (loading dose of 75 mg per kilogram intravenously followed by 50 mg per kilogram intravenously every 12 hours in children; not to exceed a total of 4 grams daily) is appropriate therapy for H. influenzae b meningitis. The combination of chloramphenicol (100 mg per kilogram intravenously daily for a child; 4 grams intravenously daily for an adult) and ampicillin (300 to 400 mg per kilogram intravenously per day for a child; 12 grams intravenously per day for an adult) is an acceptable alternative. If the isolate proves susceptible to ampicillin, the chloramphenicol may be discontinued. Although in Spain over 50 per cent of isolates are chloramphenicol resistant, less than 1 per cent have been resistant in the United States. Cefuroxime, a second-generation cephalosporin, has been used extensively the past half-dozen years, but the third-generation cephalosporins are preferable because of reports indicating slower sterilization of CSF and a higher incidence of sensorineural hearing loss with cefuroxime.

Adult meningitis caused by methicillin-sensitive S. aureus should be treated with a penicillinase-resistant penicillin (nafcillin, 10 to 12 grams intravenously per day). Rifampin (600 mg orally or intravenously daily), because adequate CSF levels can be achieved and because of its capacity to penetrate leukocytes and kill intracellular organisms, may be added as a second antimicrobial in difficult cases. In the penicillin-allergic patient,

vancomycin (2.0 grams intravenously in divided doses every 6 hours) is the alternative of choice. Since penetration of vancomycin into the CSF is limited, adjunctive intrathecal therapy (5 to 20 mg of vancomycin in 10 ml of 5 per cent dextrose–0.85 per cent NaCl slowly in the adult)* has been used when CSF cultures have remained positive after 48 hours of intravenous therapy alone. For adult meningitis due to methicillin-resistant S. aureus, intravenous vancomycin (with adjunctive intrathecal vancomycin as needed) is the treatment of choice. In refractory cases the addition of another drug for systemic therapy (rifampin or gentamicin) may be warranted.

Treatment of enterococcal meningitis in the adult involves the use of intravenous penicillin (24 million units daily) or ampicillin (12 grams daily), supplemented with parenterally administered gentamicin (3 to 5 mg per kilogram daily in divided doses every 8 hours). In the patient who fails to respond promptly to parenteral therapy, adjunctive intrathecal therapy with gentamicin (3 to 5 mg per day) should be considered.

Cefotaxime (12 grams daily intravenously in divided doses every 4 hours in adults) or ceftriaxone is now being used extensively in the treatment of meningitis known to be due to susceptible gram-negative bacilli (E. coli, Klebsiella, Proteus, etc.). It should not be used in the treatment of meningitis due to less susceptible species such as Pseudomonas aeruginosa and Acinetobacter. Initial treatment (on the basis only of findings on Gram-stained smear of CSF) of adults with gram-negative bacillary meningitis involves the combination of cefotaxime (or ceftazidime) with an aminoglycoside (e.g., gentamicin, 5 mg per kilogram daily in divided doses every 8 hours). Adjunctive intrathecal therapy with gentamicin (3 to 5 mg administered at intervals of 24 hours for the first few days) may be indicated as well if there is no response to initial systemic therapy. Following identification of the specific pathogen and determination of its drug susceptibilities, alterations in antimicrobial therapy may be indicated. If the organism is Pseudomonas aeruginosa, a third-generation cephalosporin with antipseudomonal activity, ceftazidime (2 grams intravenously every 6 or 8 hours in an adult), is combined with parenteral (and intrathecal, if needed) aminoglycoside in treatment. If necessary, alternative therapy would be a combination of an antipseudomonal penicillin (e.g., piperacillin or azlocillin, 3 to 4 grams intravenously every 4 to 6 hours in an adult) with an aminoglycoside.

Bacterial Meningitis of Unknown Etiology. Initial treatment of meningitis when the etiologic agent cannot be identified on Gram-stained smear of cerebrospinal fluid is based on available clinical clues. *In the neonate,* a wide range of gram-positive (group B streptococci, Listeria) and gram-negative organisms (E. coli, Klebsiella, H. influenzae) may be the cause, indicating the intravenous use of combined therapy with drugs such as ampicillin with gentamicin (or amikacin), or ampicillin with cefotaxime (or ceftriaxone), until results of cultures become available. *In children,* therapy is directed at the three most frequent pathogens: H. influenzae, S. pneumoniae, and N. meningitidis. The appearance of ampicillin resistance among strains of H. influenzae almost two decades ago necessitated the shift from single-drug therapy (ampicillin) to a two-drug approach (ampicillin-chloramphenicol) in the treatment of meningitis of unknown cause in this age group, pending results of culture. Now, ceftriaxone (same dosage as for H. influenzae meningitis) or cefotaxime is most commonly employed in many pediatric centers. *In adults,* therapy with ampicillin or penicillin is directed at the most common community-acquired pathogens (S. pneumoniae and N. meningitidis; L. monocytogenes in older adults and in the previously mentioned high-risk groups). In the highly penicillin-allergic individual, trimethoprim-sulfamethoxazole is a suitable alternative in the treatment of Listeria meningitis. Because H. influenzae type b infections appear to be increasing in adults, and because of the increased incidence of gram-negative bacillary and staphylococcal meningitis in certain clinical settings, broader initial therapy may be indicated if clinical features suggest unusual organisms.

Duration of Therapy. The frequency of cerebrospinal fluid examinations depends on the clinical course, but a repeat exam-

---

*Intrathecal use is not mentioned in the manufacturer's package insert approved by the U.S. Food and Drug Administration. Therefore its use in these circumstances must be considered investigational.

ination should be done in 24 to 48 hours if there has not been satisfactory improvement. Routine "end-of-treatment" CSF examination is unnecessary in most patients with the common types of community-acquired bacterial meningitis. Meningococci are rapidly eliminated from the circulation and CSF with appropriate antimicrobial therapy, which should be continued for 5 to 7 days after the patient becomes afebrile. If the patient has responded well, a follow-up lumbar puncture is not necessary. *H. influenzae* meningitis should be treated for 10 days (at least 7 days after the patient becomes afebrile). Follow-up CSF examination may be omitted in those patients who have responded with rapid clinical resolution of the meningitis. In pneumococcal meningitis antimicrobial treatment should be continued for 10 to 14 days and follow-up examination of the CSF should be done. More prolonged therapy is indicated with concomitant parameningeal infection. Treatment of gram-negative bacillary meningitis with parenteral antimicrobials is prolonged, usually for a minimum of 3 weeks (particularly in patients with a recent neurosurgical procedure) in order to prevent relapse. Repeated examinations of the CSF are necessary both during and at the conclusion of treatment to determine whether bacteriologic cure has been achieved.

Other Aspects of Treatment. Occasional patients with acute bacterial meningitis develop marked brain swelling (CSF pressure exceeding 450 mm H_2O), which may lead to temporal lobe or cerebellar herniation following lumbar puncture. To reduce this increased pressure, an intravenous infusion of 20 per cent mannitol solution (0.25 to 0.5 gram per kilogram) is administered over 20 to 30 minutes. Continued control of increased intracranial pressure, if needed thereafter, may be effected with mannitol, dexamethasone (10 mg intravenously, followed by 4 mg every 6 hours), or both. Brain swelling is about the only current indication for the use of corticosteroids in the treatment of pyogenic meningitis in adults; they should be employed only when the appropriate antimicrobial drugs are administered. Fluid restriction (1200 to 1500 ml daily in adults) is advisable during the first 24 to 48 hours to minimize brain swelling.

In a recent placebo-controlled trial of adjunctive dexamethasone therapy in community-acquired childhood bacterial meningitis, those treated with the corticosteroid became afebrile earlier and were less likely to have complicating bilateral sensorineural hearing loss. However, complicating gastrointestinal bleeding occurred in several patients, dictating caution if this approach is considered in the treatment of severe childhood meningitis. In mild cases of bacterial meningitis use of dexamethasone to reduce the incidence of sensorineural hearing loss should await results of confirmatory studies. There is no evidence in adults, as yet, of a similar reduction in the incidence of sensorineural hearing loss with adjunctive corticosteroids.

Patients with acute bacterial meningitis should receive constant nursing attention to ensure prompt recognition of seizures and to prevent aspiration. If seizures occur, they should be treated acutely with diazepam (Valium) administered slowly intravenously in a dose of 5 to 10 mg in the adult. Maintenance anticonvulsant therapy can be continued thereafter with intravenous phenytoin (Dilantin) until the medication can be administered orally. Sedation should be avoided because of the danger of respiratory depression and aspiration.

Surgical treatment of an accompanying pyogenic focus such as mastoiditis should be carried out when complete recovery from the meningitis has occurred, but under continuing antibiotic administration. Rarely, the mastoid infection (e.g., Bezold abscess) is so hyperacute that early drainage may be required after 48 hours or so of antibiotic therapy when the acute meningeal process has subsided somewhat.

Berk SL, McCabe WR: Meningitis caused by gram-negative bacilli. Ann Intern Med 93:253, 1980. *Good descriptions of gram-negative bacillary meningitis occurring spontaneously and after surgery.*

Del Rio M, Skelton S, Chrane D, et al.: Ceftriaxone versus ampicillin and chloramphenicol for treatment of bacterial meningitis in children. Lancet 1:1241, 1983. *A clinical and bacteriologic study of meningitis in 78 children showing the equivalence of ceftriaxone treatment to that of the heretofore conventional regimen.*

Dodge PR, Davis H, Feigin RD, et al.: Prospective evaluation of hearing impairment as a sequela of acute bacterial meningitis. N Engl J Med 311:869, 1984. *An excellent detailed prospective study of deafness as a complication of childhood meningitis. A model study of this sort.*

Durack DT, Spanos A: End-of-treatment spinal tap in bacterial meningitis. Is it worthwhile? JAMA 248:75, 1982. *Places in perspective the role of end-of-treatment CSF examination.*

Geiseler PJ, Nelson KE, Levin S, et al.: Community-acquired purulent meningitis: A review of 1316 cases during the antibiotic era, 1954–1976. Rev Infect Dis 2:725, 1980. *Extensive experience at one of the last contagious disease hospitals in the United States is recounted. Effects of prior antibiotic therapy on culture results are particularly well studied.*

Hyslop NE Jr, Montgomery WW: Diagnosis and management of meningitis associated with cerebrospinal leaks. In Remington JS, Swartz MN (eds.): Current Clinical Topics in Infectious Diseases, 3. New York, McGraw-Hill Book Company, 1982, pp 254–285. *Most complete review of the bacteriology, anatomy, diagnostic approach, and surgical repair of CSF leaks associated with meningitis.*

Lebel MH, Freij BJ, Syrogiannopoulos GA, et al.: Dexamethasone therapy for bacterial meningitis. Results of two double-blind, placebo-controlled trials. N Engl J Med 319:964, 1988. *Results from a controlled trial involving 200 infants and children with bacterial meningitis indicate that dexamethasone as adjunctive therapy with antibiotics (ceftriaxone or cefuroxime) reduced the incidence of moderate or severe bilateral sensorineural hearing loss.*

New PFJ, Davis KR: The role of CT scanning in diagnosis of infections of the central nervous system. In Remington JS, Swartz MN (eds.): Current Clinical Topics in Infectious Diseases, 1. New York, McGraw-Hill Book Company, 1980, pp 1–33. *Comprehensive review of the changes on CT scan in a wide variety of CNS infections. Large number of illustrative scans with good descriptions.*

Saez-Llorens X, Ramilo O, Mustafa MM, et al.: Molecular pathophysiology of bacterial meningitis: Current concepts and therapeutic implications. J Pediatr 116:671, 1990. *A thorough review of the bacterial components implicated in initiating toxic effects in the central nervous system, the cytokines involved in enhancing the inflammatory response in the subarachnoid space, and potential therapeutic interventions.*

Sande MA, Smith AL, Root RL (eds.): Bacterial Meningitis. New York, Churchill–Livingstone, 1985. *A collection of articles reviewing current issues and recent progress in understanding bacterial meningitis. Provides valuable insights in pathogenesis and pathophysiology.*

Schaad UB, Suter S, Gianella-Borradori A, et al.: A comparison of ceftriaxone and cefuroxime for the treatment of bacterial meningitis in children. N Engl J Med 322:141, 1990. *This study of 106 infants and children with bacterial meningitis indicates that in a direct comparison ceftriaxone produces more rapid sterilization of CSF and is less frequently complicated by sensorineural hearing loss than is cefuroxime.*

Swartz MN, Dodge PR: Bacterial meningitis—a review of selected aspects. N Engl J Med 272:725, 779, 842, 898, 954, 1003, 1965. *Detailed account of experience at the Massachusetts General Hospital. Particularly good on clinical aspects, neurologic complications, and differential diagnosis.*

Tunkel AR, Wispelwey B, Scheld WM: Bacterial meningitis: Recent advances in pathophysiology and treatment. Ann Intern Med 112:610, 1990. *An up-to-date and comprehensive review of the pathogenesis, pathophysiology, and treatment of bacterial meningitis. Practical therapeutic guidelines are presented.*

302 Meningococcal Disease

DEFINITION. Meningococcal infections are caused by *Neisseria meningitidis*. The best known syndromes are *meningococcal meningitis* ("epidemic cerebrospinal meningitis") and *fulminant meningococcemia*. Infections also occur in the upper and lower respiratory tracts, joints, pericardium, eyes, and genitourinary tract.

ETIOLOGY. *N. meningitidis* is a gram-negative coccus that appears on smears of infected fluids as biscuit-shaped diplococci, located either extracellularly or within polymorphonuclear leukocytes. Colonies are best isolated on blood, "chocolate," or enriched Mueller-Hinton agar in an atmosphere of 3 to 10 per cent CO_2. Modified Thayer-Martin selective medium is useful in detection of meningococcal carriers or in initial isolation of *N. meningitidis* from areas with an extensive indigenous flora. The organism is susceptible to drying or chilling, and specimens should be inoculated and incubated promptly. Sodium polyetholesulfonate, frequently included in commercial blood culture media as an anticoagulant and to neutralize inhibitory factors in human blood, may inhibit isolation of occasional strains of *Neisseria* species.

Since other *Neisseria* species and related organisms (*Moraxella catarrhalis*), as well as morphologically similar gram-negative coccobacilli (e.g., other *Moraxella* species, *Acinetobacter*, *Kingella*), may be isolated from clinical specimens, biochemical and immunologic methods are needed for identification. *Neisseria* species are oxidase positive. Whereas *N. gonorrhoeae* ferments only glucose (but not maltose or lactose) to acid, *N. meningitidis* ferments both glucose and maltose (but not lactose). *N. lactamica*, a species sometimes present in throat cultures, may be mistaken for the meningococcus, since it too ferments both glucose and maltose; however, it also utilizes lactose. Occasional maltose-negative strains of *N. meningitidis* have been noted; fluorescent antibody or coagglutination tests or electrophoretic analysis of hexokinase isoenzymes may be helpful in distinguishing such strains from *N. gonorrhoeae*, particularly when isolated from atypical locations.

N. meningitidis are classified by serogroup and further defined by serotype. There are 13 serogroups, including groups A, B, C, D, X, Y, Z, 29E, and W135; they differ in the structures of their capsular polysaccharides and can be identified by agglutination reactions with specific antisera. Most meningococcal disease is due to strains belonging to groups A, B, C, and Y. Twenty to 50 per cent of isolates from carriers are nongroupable (unencapsulated). Subcapsular protein antigens located in the outer bacterial membrane have been used to identify 20 serotypes among the various serogroups, providing a classification useful in epidemiologic studies. Serotype 2 (2a, 2b) strains are responsible for most cases of meningococcal disease due to group B (50 per cent) and group C (80 per cent) organisms (and also are associated with groups Y and W135), but they are rarely isolated from carriers not in direct contact with clinical cases. In contrast, other serotypes are commonly isolated, but primarily from carriers. More detailed differentiation between strains can be carried out by including lipopolysaccharide typing in addition. Group A meningococcal strains show no variation in their outer membrane proteins and are unrelated serologically to the serotypes of other groups.

Strains of *N. meningitidis* produce extracellular proteases that cleave the IgA1 heavy chain in the hinge region. Although the role of this protease in infection is unknown, its elaboration also by the other principal causes of bacterial meningitis (*H. influenzae, S. pneumoniae*) and the importance of IgA in mucosal immunity at the pharyngeal portal for these organisms suggest a possible role in pathogenicity.

Fresh isolates of *N. meningitidis* from the pharynx of carriers and from patients with meningococcal disease contain pili, which appear to have an important role in attachment to nonciliated columnar human nasopharyngeal cells.

Meningococci contain endotoxins, and these lipopolysaccharides may play a role in the purpura and other clinical features of meningococcemia.

INCIDENCE. *N. meningitidis* is second only to *H. influenzae* as a cause of bacterial meningitis in this country. In the period 1984 to 1990, 2400 to 2700 cases of meningococcal infection were reported annually in the United States.

EPIDEMIOLOGY. The natural reservoir of *N. meningitidis* is the human nasopharynx, and transmission occurs principally through airborne droplets or close contact. Infection may occur as the *asymptomatic carrier state* (the most common form), *endemic disease* (sporadic cases occurring at a relatively stable rate), *hyperendemic disease* (cyclic waves of increased incidence), or *epidemic disease* (major outbreaks involving large portions of the population or focal outbreaks involving particularly lower socioeconomic groups).

Carrier State. Nasopharyngeal carrier rates may fluctuate widely. The rate varies with age: 0.5 to 1.0 per cent in children 3 to 48 months of age, 5 per cent in those 14 to 17 years of age, and 20 to 40 per cent in young adults. In the nonepidemic setting carriage usually lasts weeks to months. The carrier rate in close family contacts of a case of meningococcal disease is increased and may reach 40 per cent. In crowded populations (e.g., military training camps) the carrier rate has ranged between 20 and 60 per cent and has reached 90 per cent during epidemics. Although it has often been stated that meningococcal outbreaks occur when the rate of nasopharyngeal carriage exceeds 20 per cent in a military camp, there is in reality no clear relation between the overall carriage rate in a community and the occurrence of meningococcal disease. The strain (serotype)-specific acquisition rate appears to be a more reliable indicator of an outbreak than the group-specific carriage rate.

Spread of disease appears to be mediated by carriers rather than by direct case-to-case transmission. An adult family member generally is the one who brings *N. meningitidis* into a household, where it spreads to others and often colonizes younger children and infants last. As yet unknown host and environmental factors are of decisive importance in determining whether the organism will be confined to the nasopharynx or dissemination will take place.

Meningococcal Disease. The annual attack rate for meningococcal disease in the United States in recent years has been about 1.2 cases per 100,000 population. The highest incidence is in the first year of life (17.1 per 100,000), declining in the 1- to 4-year age group (5.2 per 100,000), and ultimately reaching the level of 0.3 per 100,000 in adults. During epidemics of meningococcal disease, overall annual attack rates of 5 to 24 cases per 100,000 are observed (as high as 370 per 100,000 in Sao Paulo, Brazil, in 1974), and the age incidence tends to shift to older children and young adults. The peak incidence is in the winter and early spring.

During a nonepidemic period the risk of meningococcal illness for household contacts of an initial case is about 3 per 1000 (500- to 1000-fold higher than the overall endemic rate for meningococcal disease) and stems from the higher carriage rate in this setting. The secondary attack rate appears to be age related, with most cases occurring in younger children.

Major meningococcal epidemics, caused primarily by group A strains, tend to recur at 20- to 30-year intervals (e.g., as occurred during World Wars I and II). More circumscribed outbreaks have taken place in interepidemic periods, as in Detroit in 1929, when about 750 cases occurred. Aside from several minor urban outbreaks, particularly among alcoholics, group A strains have only rarely been implicated in meningococcal disease in North America during the past decade. However, serious epidemics caused by group A meningococci have occurred in Finland in 1973, in Brazil in 1974, and in northern Nigeria in 1977. The outbreak in Nigeria is but one of many that have occurred about once every 10 years in the "meningitis belt" in sub-Saharan Africa. In the 1948–49 epidemic, about 93,000 cases were reported, with over 14,000 deaths. Although group A meningococci had been susceptible to sulfonamides in the past, resistant strains first appeared in the epidemics in Africa in the late 1960's and subsequently in Brazil and Finland.

Although group A meningococci have been involved in the most extensive epidemics of meningococcal disease, groups B and C have been responsible for focal outbreaks and for *endemic disease* both in this country and abroad. In the United States in 1963 and 1964, outbreaks caused by group B meningococci (noteworthy for their frequent resistance to sulfonamides) occurred in military camps. By 1967 serogroup B was responsible for the majority of infections occurring in military and civilian populations. By the early 1970's serogroup C strains were those most frequently isolated, only to be supplanted by group B in the mid 1970's. Currently, serogroup B accounts for 50 to 55 per cent of cases; serogroup C, for 20 to 25 per cent; serogroup W135, for 15 per cent; serogroup Y, for 10 per cent; and serogroup A, for 1 to 2 per cent.

Just as serogrouping of meningococcal strains has been invaluable in the study of major epidemics and in the development and use of polysaccharide vaccines, serotyping can be helpful in evaluating changes in ambient strains. Between epidemics sporadic cases are caused by heterogeneous strains belonging to many serogroups and a variety of serotypes. In military recruit populations, the serogroup carried is not a valid indicator of epidemic potential. At intervals of 5 to 10 years a single serotype (e.g., serotype 2, present in most disease-related strains of groups B and C and in some strains of groups Y and W135 during this past decade) becomes pre-eminent, producing *hyperendemic disease*, sometimes accompanied by scattered small outbreaks.

Meningococci can be further subdivided by clonal analysis based on the electrophoretic mobilities of a series of cytoplasmic isoenzymes and outer membrane proteins. In an analysis of over 400 serogroup A strains of diverse epidemiologic origins isolated from around the world from 1915 to 1983 (including 23 outbreaks or epidemics since 1960), seven clones have been identified as responsible for sets of epidemics. At least two of these sets represent mutually exclusive pandemics, involving numerous epidemics between 1967–75 and 1973–83, respectively. Case strains showed little clonal diversity during individual epidemics, indicating that such a typing scheme can be useful in defining the etiology of outbreaks.

Similarly, several serogroup B epidemics have involved changes in serotypes from 2a to 2b. This change did not result from antigenic drift or genetic recombination among strains, but rather represented clonal replacement, since these serotypes are linked to distinctive groups of clones.

Nosocomial transmission of infection occasionally occurs. Meningococcal meningitis has developed in several physicians who gave mouth-to-mouth resuscitation to infected patients. Group Y meningococci particularly have been implicated in meningococcal pneumonia, and such patients, if not isolated, may be responsible for nosocomial spread of infection.

Immunity. The age-specific incidence of meningococcal disease is inversely proportional to the prevalence of antimeningococcal bactericidal antibodies (against serogroups A, B, C). At birth, over 50 per cent of infants have bactericidal antibody as a result of transplacental transfer. Group B organisms present a special problem that accounts for the occurrence of group B meningococcal disease in neonates. Because the capsular polysaccharide of group B meningococci is a polymer of α 2–8–linked sialic acid and is immunologically identical to oligosaccharides of several human glycoproteins (including brain gangliosides), immunologic tolerance for this molecule exists in humans. IgM antibody can be induced but without the usual switch to IgG. As a result, maternal antibody to group B capsular antigen is entirely IgM and cannot be passed transplacentally. All infants are born lacking antibody to group B (but not to other common serogroup) capsular antigens. Because the capsular polysaccharide of E. coli K1 is the same, infants are born also lacking antibody to this organism, the major cause of neonatal sepsis and meningitis.

From 6 to 24 months of age, the prevalence of antibodies is lowest, and thereafter it increases to early adulthood, when over 70 per cent of individuals have bactericidal activity. The protective role of bactericidal antibodies against N. meningitidis was demonstrated during an outbreak of group C meningitis among army recruits in 1968. Eleven per cent of recruits lacked serum antibody against the outbreak-associated strain, and one quarter of these susceptibles acquired this strain during their training period. Of the susceptibles exposed, 38 per cent developed systemic meningococcal disease; in contrast, only 1 per cent of the entire trainee group developed disease.

IgA antibody to meningococcal polysaccharide may have a paradoxic effect. When a large part of an individual's antibodies to a meningococcal serogroup is of this class, serum complement-mediated immune lysis by IgM is blocked, enhancing susceptibility to meningococcal disease. This was demonstrated in several outbreaks. Sera drawn from susceptibles at the time of acute meningococcal infection lacked bactericidal activity for the infecting strain; removal of IgA restored this activity which was in the IgM class. This odd phenomenon is observed for a short time following the induction of IgA by asymptomatic carriage of N. meningitidis or an immunologically related organism.

Following meningococcal meningitis serum bactericidal antibody develops, and the patient is immune to clinical reinfection with the same serogroup. However, this is not the usual means of acquiring immunity. Nasopharyngeal carriage of N. meningitidis is an effective immunizing process, producing rises in bactericidal antibody within 5 to 12 days of acquisition of the organism. About 90 per cent of carriers of group B, C, or Y meningococci develop increased serum bactericidal titers, primarily to the colonizing strain but also to heterologous strains. Similarly, nasopharyngeal carriage of nongroupable meningococci, strains rarely causing human disease, can induce antibodies against various groupable pathogenic isolates.

The group-specific capsular polysaccharides of group A and group C meningococci are good immunogens and have been used in successful vaccines. The capsular polysaccharide of group B meningococci is a very poor immunogen because of its immunologic identity with oligosaccharides of several human glycoproteins, and this likely contributes to the failure to develop an effective group B vaccine.

In young children, colonization with N. lactamica may induce cross-reactive antibodies to N. meningitidis and thus contribute to natural immunity. N. lactamica is relatively avirulent and has only rarely been involved in systemic infections. During the first

8 years of life the age-related prevalence of meningococcal carriage is between 0.5 and 2 per cent, whereas that of N. lactamica is considerably higher (4 to 20 per cent).

In addition to antibody, complement is an important component of serum bactericidal activity. Isolated congenital deficiency of one of the late complement components (C5–C8) is rare and has been associated with recurrent or, occasionally, chronic (chronic meningococcemia) infections with N. meningitidis. Repeated episodes of meningococcal meningitis have occurred in patients with late complement component deficiencies in the absence of enhanced susceptibility to organisms other than N. meningitidis. Measurement of total hemolytic complement is helpful for screening purposes in a patient with recurrent systemic Neisseria infections. The course of infection, whether meningitis or meningococcemia, is not unusual, and the response to antimicrobial treatment is satisfactory. Complement deficiency may be an important risk factor, as well, for the occurrence of first episodes of endemic meningococcal disease. Although the latter occur in persons with deficiencies of early-acting components (C2–C4), which are often due to complement-depleting underlying diseases (systemic lupus, multiple myeloma, C3 nephritic factor, hepatic failure), their frequencies are similar to those of infections caused by other encapsulated bacteria. In contrast, essentially the only clinical features of deficiency of late components are meningococcal infections. Fulminant meningococcal disease has also occurred in several members of a family with properdin deficiency. Preliminary evidence suggests that immunization with meningococcal vaccine can correct the bactericidal defect in sera of affected male members with familial properdin deficiency.

PATHOGENESIS AND PATHOLOGY. The factors that determine whether initial exposure to N. meningitidis will result in benign nasopharyngeal carriage or serious invasive infection are unclear. Binding by pili to microvilli of nonciliated columnar mucosal cells of the nasopharynx may allow surface multiplication and colonization by N. meningitidis. Transport across these specialized mucosal cells appears to occur within phagocytic vacuoles and provides a potential mechanism for invasive meningococcal disease. About one third of patients with invasive infection have had antecedent symptoms referable to the upper respiratory tract. Whether these prodromal symptoms are produced by N. meningitidis or a predisposing viral respiratory infection is difficult to determine, particularly since many cases of meningococcal disease occur in winter when viral respiratory infections are frequent. A simultaneous outbreak of meningococcal disease and influenza A2 infection has occurred in a closed institutional setting. The predisposing role of influenza for meningococcal lower respiratory infections may be clearer (e.g., numerous cases of meningococcal pneumonia complicating influenza during the 1918–19 pandemic).

The incubation period from initiation of nasopharyngeal infection to bloodstream dissemination is probably under 10 days. The incubation period may be quite short, judging by the fact that the interval between primary and secondary cases in the same household is often only 1 to 4 days. Also, among prospectively studied military recruits cultured within 7 days preceding hospitalization for meningococcal disease, only about 20 per cent were carriers of the implicated strain. Once the organism has entered the circulation, the predominant (over 90 per cent) clinical expression is meningitis or meningococcemia.

The pathologic findings in acute meningococcemia are observed when shock and disseminated intravascular coagulation have occurred. The skin lesions show evidence of fibrin thrombi and vasculitis in small blood vessels. N. meningitidis can be seen in endothelial cells and in neutrophils surrounding damaged vessels. The prominent purpura has been attributed to the enhanced capacity to elicit the dermal Shwartzman reaction of its endotoxin compared to endotoxin from enteric gram-negative bacilli. Hemorrhagic adrenal infarction is often observed in patients with fulminant meningococcemia (Waterhouse-Friderichsen syndrome). Shock in this disease is a consequence of bacteremia and not of adrenal failure, since (1) fulminant meningococcemia can occur without adrenal hemorrhage, (2) serum cortisol levels are normal or elevated, and (3) patients who have recovered have not developed Addison's disease. It has been suggested that the shock, purpura, and widespread microvascular thrombi are consequences of an endotoxin-initiated generalized Shwartzman-like reaction or endotoxin-activated disseminated intravascular coagulation. Increased levels of circulating endotoxin are associated with the development of severe septic shock and death in systemic meningococcal disease. Serum levels of tumor necrosis factor, a cytokine induced in macrophages by endotoxin, correlate with the severity of meningococcemia. Depressed levels of complement components are found in some patients with acute meningococcemia and may reflect complement activation by circulating endotoxin. Interstitial myocarditis is observed in about 70 per cent of cases of fatal meningococcal disease.

CLINICAL MANIFESTATIONS. Overt illness develops when the initial, often minimally symptomatic nasopharyngeal infection has progressed to bloodstream invasion. The subsequent clinical picture may be mild, or sudden in onset and fulminant, and may reflect principally the bacteremia or features referable to metastatic localization of infection. The most common clinical syndromes are acute meningococcemia, acute purulent meningitis, and a combination of the two (meningococcemia-meningitis).

Meningitis. Most cases occur in children between 3 months of age and adolescence. Isolated meningitis is less common than meningococcemia-meningitis. The clinical picture may be dominated by manifestations of either meningococcemia or meningitis. In the latter instance the findings are similar to those of meningitis caused by any of the common pyogens (see Ch. 301). Predisposing acute otitis media or pneumonia is unusual in contrast to *H. influenzae* or pneumococcal meningitis. The onset of meningeal symptomatology (1) may be rapid (less than 24 hours) without premonitory symptomatology, (2) may follow an upper respiratory infection of 1 or 2 weeks' duration, or (3) may evolve gradually over several days of upper respiratory or nonlocalizing symptoms. Rarely, the clinical course with fever and meningismus may be indolent and persist unchanged for a week or longer, suggesting the diagnosis of "aseptic" meningitis. In the last-named instance CSF examination during this period may reveal minimal or no increase in cell count and no organisms on Gram-stained smear, but *N. meningitidis* may be isolated, indicating early meningeal involvement. A "clear" CSF in this setting should *not* preclude careful culture. The rapid onset of delirium is seen occasionally in bacterial meningitis (more frequently meningococcal), but it also may occur with a temporal lobe abscess or encephalitis. The neurologic features and complications of meningococcal meningitis are generally the same as for other bacterial meningitides.

The course of meningococcal meningitis may differ from that of other pyogenic meningitides in the occasional occurrence during convalescence of a nonseptic arthritis-pericarditis syndrome.

Meningococcemia. About 20 per cent of patients with meningococcal disease have meningococcemia without meningitis. The clinical expression of meningococcemia varies from an acute process (mild systemic illness or rapidly lethal course) to a chronic, indolent, relapsing disease that may go on for months.

Mild Acute Meningococcemia. This is the most common form of meningococcemia, characterized by the rapid development of malaise, fever, chills, myalgias, and arthralgias, often following a minor upper respiratory infection. In a few patients diarrhea has been an early symptom. The subsequent course may follow one of several paths: (1) Symptoms may abate in 2 or 3 days, and the diagnosis is made in retrospect when *N. meningitidis* is isolated from a blood culture. (2) Initial symptomatology is followed over 24 to 48 hours by recurrent chills and the appearance of erythematous macular lesions, particularly on the extremities, often accompanied by petechiae. In more severe infections, purpura and ecchymotic areas with gunmetal gray necrotic centers appear. Tachycardia and tachypnea are prominent. Mild hypotension may be present, and shock is a feature if fulminant meningococcemia ensues. In some patients headache may appear and confusion and stiff neck develop; the syndrome then becomes one of combined *meningococcemia-meningitis.* A meningoencephalopathic picture has been described in up to 15 per cent of patients. This probably represents a heterogeneous group (some with meningitis and others with fulminant meningococcemia and central nervous system changes secondary to shock), in whom confusion, delirium, or coma is striking. (3) Occasionally, initial malaise, fever, and arthralgias (accompanied by a few macular and petechial skin lesions) may persist for about a week, during which one or more joint effusions may develop. Blood cultures reveal *N. meningitidis*, and all manifestations promptly subside on treatment with penicillin.

Fulminant Meningococcemia. This is the most dramatic form of infection, with an abrupt onset and extraordinarily rapid progression (occasionally less than 10 hours from onset to fatal termination). It occurs in about 10 per cent of patients with meningococcal disease. Violent chills, high fever, dizziness, headache, and profound weakness develop over a few hours. Petechiae appear initially on the extremities; they rapidly increase in number and coalesce as new ones appear in the conjunctivae and buccal mucosa. Hypotension with peripheral vasoconstriction quickly appears. Purpura soon develops (Fig. 302–1). At this point the patient may still be febrile or may have become hypothermic. As shock supervenes, restlessness, mental obtundation, and coma may follow in rapid succession. Disseminated intravascular coagulation (DIC) is commonly present, with enlarging hemorrhagic areas in the skin and sometimes mucosal and gastrointestinal bleeding. Cardiac (myocarditis) and respiratory ("shock lung") failure may be terminal events. *The relentless course, once shock develops, makes mandatory early diagnosis*

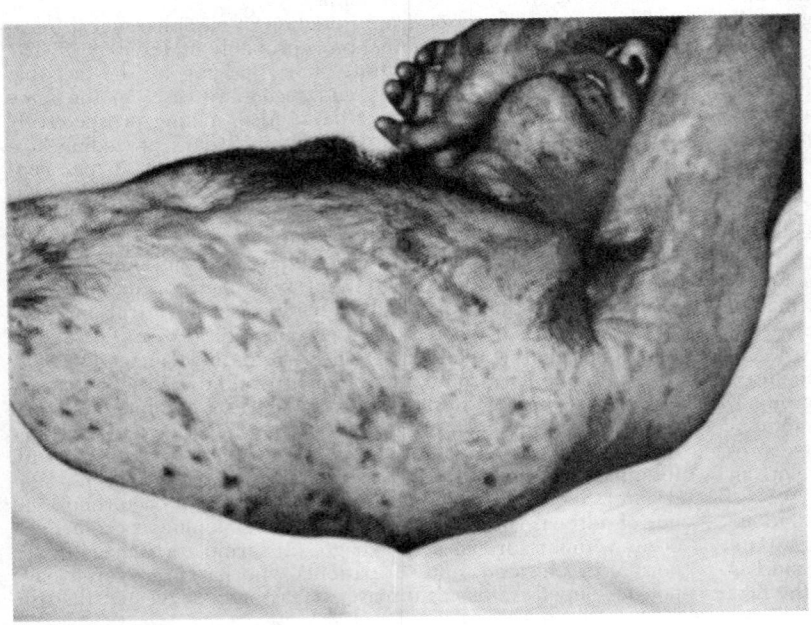

FIGURE 302–1. Skin lesions in fulminating meningococcemia. (Courtesy of Dr. Worth B. Daniels.)

and immediate institution of antibiotic treatment even while parts of the initial examination are being performed.

Chronic Meningococcemia. This uncommon form of meningococcemia is characterized by intermittent febrile episodes lasting 1 to 6 days, or, rarely, by sustained fevers for several weeks. It begins with chills, migratory arthralgias (or occasionally mild arthritis), and headache, but minimal toxicity. A transient polymorphous (erythematous macules and papules, rare petechiae, and purpuric nodules) nonpruritic rash appears with each febrile episode. The total number of skin lesions is small, and Gram's stain and culture only rarely reveal the etiologic agent. Biopsy reveals a leukocytoclastic angiitis, which may be mistaken for a collagen disease or allergic vasculitis. Splenomegaly is observed in 20 per cent of patients. Blood cultures are not positive during apyrexial periods and may not yield the organism until the second or third febrile episode.

Untreated, about 20 per cent of patients ultimately develop meningitis. Rarer complications include endocarditis and epididymitis.

Where the organism resides between episodes is unclear. Throat cultures frequently have not revealed meningococci. The occurrence of chronic meningococcemia in several patients with congenital late complement component deficiencies suggests a possible factor in pathogenesis.

Upper Respiratory Tract Infection. How frequently nasopharyngeal infection is symptomatic is unclear. Nasopharyngeal symptoms preceding some systemic meningococcal infections may be due to this organism or to ambient viral respiratory infections.

Pneumonia. Meningococcal pneumonia is much more often of bronchogenic than of hematogenous origin. Other than during the 1918 influenza pandemic, it has been reported only rarely until this past decade. Primary meningococcal pneumonia is most often due to group Y; 15 years ago among recruits pneumonia caused by group Y was the most common form of meningococcal disease. Primary meningococcal pneumonia may be segmental, lobar, or bronchopneumonic in pattern. It sometimes follows antecedent influenza or adenoviral infection. Clinical features are similar to those of community-acquired pneumonias. The onset may be gradual or abrupt. Lower lobes are usually involved. Bacteremia occurs in about 15 per cent of cases. In some patients purulent sputum is produced, containing numerous gram-negative diplococci; in others sputum is scanty, and diagnosis is made on a transtracheal aspirate or by blood culture. Response to treatment with penicillin is prompt.

Meningococcal pneumonia occasionally develops in the course of clinical meningococcemia or meningitis, but the clinical picture is dominated by the extrapulmonary aspects.

To be distinguished from meningococcal pneumonia are pulmonary infections due to *Moraxella catarrhalis* (gram-negative biscuit-shaped diplococci) or rarely to other usually noninvasive *Neisseria* species (e.g., *N. sicca*). Such infections usually take the form of acute exacerbations of chronic bronchitis or of pneumonia, occurring particularly in immunodeficient individuals, patients with chronic pulmonary disease, or as a nosocomial infection. *M. catarrhalis* can also be the cause of acute sinusitis, bacteremia, and, rarely, meningitis. In children this organism, after *S. pneumoniae* and *H. influenzae*, is the third most common cause of acute otitis media. β-Lactamase production occurs in 75 per cent of strains isolated currently from children. Alternatives to ampicillin or penicillin for therapy, based on in vitro susceptibilities, include trimethoprim-sulfamethoxazole, amoxicillin-clavulanic acid, chloramphenicol, tetracycline, and cefuroxime.

Arthritis. Arthritis complicates 2 to 16 per cent of acute meningococcal illness and may take several forms: (1) *Isolated, acute suppurative meningococcal arthritis* is a rare type occurring in the absence of meningitis or clinical meningococcemia. The joint fluid has the characteristics of septic arthritis. (2) *Early onset (first 2 to 3 days) arthritis* during meningococcal meningitis or meningococcemia is the most common form. It is a polyarthritis with acutely inflamed joints; effusions are small or absent. It responds promptly to penicillin. (3) *Late onset (fourth to tenth day, when meningitis is subsiding) arthritis* is commonly a subacute mono- or oligoarthritis accompanied by joint effusions. It is associated with recrudescence of fever, pleuropericarditis, and, occasionally, new papulobullous skin lesions. Synovial and pericardial fluids are characteristically serosanguineous (but sometimes purulent) and sterile. Immunopathologic study of synovial lesions implicates immune complex formation in their genesis. Treatment involves joint aspiration and the use of anti-inflammatory agents.

Pericarditis. Pericarditis complicates 2 to 20 per cent of meningococcal disease. It may take several forms: (1) *Early onset pericarditis*, appearing in the first several days of clinical meningococcemia or meningitis, may be purulent and may be due to invasion by *N. meningitidis*. (2) *Late onset pericarditis*, developing 4 to 10 days after onset of meningitis, may cause large sterile, serosanguineous effusions. The favorable response to anti-inflammatory agents and adrenal corticosteroids supports the proposed role of hypersensitivity in pathogenesis. (3) *Isolated purulent pericarditis*, occurring in the absence of meningitis or clinical meningococcemia, is the least common form of meningococcal pericarditis and usually presents with a purulent effusion and tamponade requiring surgical intervention.

Other Meningococcal Infections. Ocular involvement (panophthalmitis, conjunctivitis) occurs in less than 1 per cent of patients with meningococcal disease. Primary conjunctivitis, an acute purulent process, is even less common. Since dissemination develops in 10 per cent of children with primary meningococcal conjunctivitis, systemic therapy with penicillin should be employed along with topical antimicrobials.

Genital tract and anal infections with *N. meningitidis* occasionally occur, the latter in homosexual males. In the female symptomatic or asymptomatic infections of the cervix and vagina may be associated with salpingitis or subsequent clinical meningococcemia. Urethral infection is less common than anal infection but is usually symptomatic. Treatment, as for gonococcal infection, is warranted to eliminate symptomatic disease and to prevent the rare instance of disseminated infection.

COURSE AND COMPLICATIONS. Acute meningococcemia may run a varied course, from that of mild disease to that of fulminant illness with death in a day or less. Certain features (particularly if present simultaneously) indicate a poor prognosis: (1) petechiae for less than 12 hours prior to hospitalization (rapid development of crops of new petechiae and purpura from one hour to the next is ominous); (2) shock; (3) fever above 40° C; (4) absence of meningitis; (5) leukopenia; (6) thrombocytopenia or evidence of DIC; and (7) extremes of age.

Extensive purpura, acral cyanosis, hemorrhagic bullae, and peripheral gangrene are features of fulminant meningococcemia, usually occurring in the presence of shock and DIC. DIC may be evident on hospitalization or may develop precipitously in some patients who are stable initially. In acute DIC platelets, fibrinogen, prothrombin, and Factors V, VII, and VIII are reduced. Abnormalities in three screening tests (prothrombin time prolongation, platelet count reduction, hypofibrinogenemia) aid in detection of DIC, which occurs to some extent in about one quarter of patients with meningococcemia. The partial thromboplastin time may also be prolonged. Confirmation is provided by demonstration of circulating fibrin degradation products in concentrations greater than 40 μg per milliliter. These coagulation defects can result in upper gastrointestinal bleeding, hematuria, and bleeding from the respiratory tract. Despite all therapeutic interventions, some patients show progressive deterioration with marked tachycardia, hyperventilation, refractory shock, metabolic acidosis, deepening coma, and "shock lung." Myocardial involvement may be manifest as either transient electrocardiographic changes or left ventricular failure.

In those who recover, resolution of the hemorrhagic or gangrenous lesions is slow and may require skin grafting. Areas of the hands and feet may remain edematous, cold, and cyanotic and may show demarcation after some weeks.

DIAGNOSIS. Laboratory Findings. Bacteriologic diagnosis is established by the finding of organisms on stained smears from an infected area (in an appropriate clinical setting), by isolation of *N. meningitidis* from blood or infected body fluids, or by demonstration by latex agglutination of group A, B, C, or Y polysaccharide antigen in blood or CSF. Blood cultures reveal *N. meningitidis* in about one third of patients with meningococcal meningitis and in 50 to 75 per cent with clinical meningococcemia or meningococcemia-meningitis. In rare patients with fulminant meningococcemia, diplococci can be seen on Gram-stained smears of blood or buffy coat. Demonstration of organisms on scrapings from skin lesions in acute meningococcemia has been variable: 70 per cent in one study, but much lower in more recent experience.

Since *N. gonorrhoeae* can be isolated from the pharynx and *N. meningitidis* can occasionally be found in the anogenital area, since both species may invade the bloodstream, and since gonococci and *N. lactamica* have on rare occasions been implicated in meningitis, accurate bacteriologic identification is important. However, 0.5 to 5 per cent of meningococci are maltose negative and may thus resemble gonococci and cause confusion.

Meningococcal polysaccharide antigen is demonstrated in the CSF of about 70 per cent of patients with meningococcal meningitis. Antigen is detected in the blood of 10 to 25 per cent of patients with meningococcemia, and its presence is associated with a poorer prognosis and higher incidence of late onset arthritis.

The CSF findings in meningococcal meningitis are those of pyogenic meningitis.

Differential Diagnosis. The differential diagnosis of meningococcal meningitis in the absence of clinical meningococcemia is that of acute meningitis with a purulent CSF formula. With the meningococcemia-meningitis syndrome it should be remembered that very rare instances of meningitis caused by *H. influenzae* and *S. pneumoniae* may be accompanied by petechial skin lesions. Occasional patients with enteroviral meningitis may have a brisk CSF pleocytosis (up to several thousand cells, with as many as 50 to 80 per cent neutrophils and a maculopetechial rash). Rarely, acute bacterial endocarditis caused by *Staphylococcus aureus* can produce a clinical picture almost indistinguishable from that of meningococcemia-meningitis, with a polymorphonuclear CSF pleocytosis and petechial and purpuric skin lesions. In *S. aureus* endocarditis there are a few skin lesions of purulent purpura which show the etiologic agent on Gram-stained smear. Occasionally measles or other viral exanthems may resemble early meningococcemia. Rocky Mountain spotted fever may mimic meningococcemia, but the absence of meningitis in the former, epidemiologic considerations, and demonstration of the etiologic agent aid in distinguishing between these processes.

Chronic meningococcemia, because of its protean manifestations, may be mistaken for Henoch-Schönlein purpura, acute vasculitis, gonococcemia, rheumatic fever, and subacute bacterial endocarditis.

TREATMENT. Antibiotic Management. As soon as the diagnosis is made, the patient should be put on respiratory isolation to minimize nosocomial spread of infection. Whereas practically all meningococci isolated prior to 1963 were susceptible to sulfadiazine (formerly the treatment of choice), since that time isolates resistant to sulfonamides have become common. Sulfonamide resistance in this country peaked in 1970, when 67 per cent of strains were resistant, and has since decreased (1980) to 12 per cent (8 per cent of group B, 30 per cent of group C, 4 per cent of group W135; all group Y strains susceptible). Should resistance to sulfonamides decline to less than 10 per cent, sulfonamides may again become appropriate drugs for prophylaxis.

Antimicrobial therapy should be initiated *immediately* in patients with suspected meningococcal meningitis or clinical meningococcemia because of the rapidity with which the illness may progress. Intravenous penicillin G is the drug of choice (24 million units daily in the adult in divided doses every 2 to 3 hours) for meningococcal meningitis. Alternatively, intravenous ampicillin can be employed in the adult (12 grams daily in divided doses every 2 to 3 hours). In patients allergic to penicillin, intravenous chloramphenicol (4 to 6 grams daily in the adult) is the recommended alternative, with appropriate monitoring of the hematopoietic system. Third-generation cephalosporins such as cefotaxime and ceftriaxone are active in vitro against *N. meningitidis* and have been used successfully in treatment of meningococcal meningitis. They may now provide an alternative when the use of chloramphenicol is considered. The duration of treatment of meningococcal meningitis and the management of complications are considered in Ch. 301.

Until the mid 1980's clinical isolates were uniformly susceptible to penicillin and ampicillin. However, in the past 5 years penicillin-resistant *N. meningitidis* (Groups B and C) have been

isolated from blood and CSF of patients in Spain (up to 5 per cent of isolates), England, Ireland, and South Africa. Almost all of these isolates have been relatively penicillin resistant (non–β-lactamase–producing) strains, with minimum inhibitory concentrations of 0.25 to 0.7 μg per milliliter due at least in part to altered forms of penicillin-binding protein 2. Three isolates (β-lactamase–producing) have been highly penicillin resistant, and at least one of these contained a β-lactamase plasmid. Although high doses of penicillin have been effective in treatment of meningococcemia due to relatively resistant strains, this treatment might not be effective for meningitis due to similar strains or for invasive infections due to β-lactamase–producing strains. Alternative antimicrobial agents in such situations include cefotaxime and chloramphenicol.

Intravenous penicillin G is the treatment for acute clinical meningococcemia without meningitis. Although 8 to 10 million units daily is usually adequate to sterilize the blood and most areas of metastatic infection, it may not provide therapeutic CSF levels in the patient with incipient meningitis. For this reason, initial therapy with "meningitis" doses is often employed. Treatment is continued until the patient has been afebrile for 5 days. Penicillin (5 to 8 million units daily intravenously in the adult) is effective treatment for chronic meningococcemia.

Other Aspects of Treatment. Treatment of severe meningococcemia requires supportive measures to deal with shock and other complications (DIC, congestive failure, metabolic acidosis, "shock lung"). These include cardiovascular monitoring in an intensive care setting, initial volume expansion, use of vasoactive agents, attention to fluid balances, maintenance of adequate oxygenation, and possible use of digoxin. A central venous pressure (CVP) catheter is placed (a flow-directed pulmonary catheter for evaluation of left atrial and ventricular filling pressures may be necessary if cardiac decompensation develops). Volume expansion (dextrose-saline infused rapidly) is necessary initially to assure that intravascular volume is optimal. If there is no sudden or progressive rise in CVP, then volume expansion (utilizing both crystalloid and colloid) is continued until shock is corrected or fluid overload (increased CVP, rales) develops. Urine output should be monitored and maintained at 40 to 50 ml per hour.

If rapid improvement does not follow volume expansion or if the CVP exceeds appropriate limits, a catecholamine should be added to enhance cardiac output and raise arterial pressure to the range of 90 to 100 mm Hg. Dopamine has been widely used because of its ability to increase renal blood flow (at dosage below 6 μg per kilogram per minute) while increasing cardiac contractility. It is administered by continuous intravenous (initial rate of 2 to 5 μg per kilogram per minute) infusion at a rate sufficient to maintain an adequate arterial pressure and urine volume.

Controlled multicenter clinical trials have not shown a beneficial effect of adrenal corticosteroids in high dosage (30 mg per kilogram of methylprednisolone or 6 mg per kilogram of dexamethasone) as adjunctive therapy in sepsis or septic shock. One or two pharmacologic doses (3 mg per kilogram of dexamethasone or 30 mg per kilogram of methylprednisolone intravenously) have been used in patients not responding to the aforementioned initial measures. Smaller maintenance doses do not appear beneficial, and continued administration predisposes to superinfection. If adrenal insufficiency is suspected, replacement doses of corticosteroids are indicated.

Adequate oxygenation is essential in a patient with shock, particularly if meningitis is also a feature (in which hypoxia can aggravate cerebral edema). Oxygen administration, and intubation with ventilatory assistance if needed, should be an integral part of therapy aiming at restoring the arterial Po_2 to appropriate levels (80 to 120 mm Hg). Acidosis should be corrected by intravenous administration of sodium bicarbonate (45 mEq) as needed. Digoxin is not of value in meningococcemic shock but may have a role if fluid overload complicates volume expansion or secondary myocarditis. Generally, diuretics such as furosemide have been of more value in this acute situation.

The initial enthusiasm for heparin treatment of DIC in meningococcemia and septic shock has waned, since evidence of efficacy in reducing mortality has been conflicting despite improvement in coagulation factors. Heparin treatment on the basis of laboratory abnormalities alone is inadvisable. Reversal of hypotension is often associated with improvement in laboratory evidences of

DIC and a halt in further clinical progression of the coagulopathy. Only if bleeding into deep tissues or thrombotic manifestations occur in the presence of DIC might heparinization be considered. After initiation of heparin therapy coagulation factor deficiencies can be repaired by administration of fresh frozen plasma. Once heparin is started, prothrombin time and partial thromboplastin time determinations are no longer helpful in following laboratory evidences of DIC; levels of fibrin degradation products, fibrinogen, and platelets are of greatest assistance.

PREVENTION. Chemoprophylaxis. Close contacts (e.g., same household or daycare center, medical personnel exposed by intimate contact prior to institution of proper isolation precautions) of a patient with meningococcal disease are at increased risk of developing systemic disease and should receive chemoprophylaxis. Since secondary (or coprimary) cases usually occur within 4 days of the initial case, prophylactic treatment should begin as soon as the initial case is identified. Rifampin has been shown to be 80 to 90 per cent effective in eliminating meningococci from the nasopharynx of asymptomatic carriers, and minocycline has been almost as effective. Because of reports of vestibular side effects with minocycline, rifampin is the recommended drug for chemoprophylaxis. It is administered for 2 days: to adults at a dosage of 600 mg orally every 12 hours; to children (1 month of age or older) at a dosage of 10 mg per kilogram every 12 hours; and to children under 1 month of age, at a dosage of 5 mg per kilogram every 12 hours. Since even the high doses of penicillin used to treat meningococcal meningitis or meningococcemia may not eradicate nasopharyngeal carriage, rifampin should be administered also to the index patient prior to discharge from hospital. Rifampin-resistant strains appear readily and would be selected if use of the drug for prophylaxis were widespread. Preliminary evidence indicates that ciprofloxacin also is effective in eradicating pharyngeal carriage of *N. meningitidis*.

Meningococcal Vaccine. A quadrivalent (groups A, C, Y, W135) vaccine is now commercially available. A previous serogroup A vaccine showed efficacy of 85 to 95 per cent and was helpful in controlling epidemics; similar clinical efficacy has been demonstrated for a serogroup C vaccine in military recruits and in an epidemic. The polysaccharide vaccines are immunogenic in adults but do not induce a good antibody response in children under 2 years of age. A vaccine against serogroup B, the major cause of meningococcal disease in the United States, is not available.

The principal indication for use of meningococcal vaccines is the presence of outbreaks of meningococcal disease caused by *N. meningitidis* belonging to serogroup A or C (or more recently Y and W135).

The routine immunization of individuals against meningococcal disease is not recommended because of the low risk of disease in the absence of outbreaks. However, immunization would be advisable for high-risk groups such as those with complement deficiencies or with anatomic or functional asplenia. Also, vaccination should be considered for travelers to countries in which there is epidemic meningococcal disease. Since about 50 per cent of secondary cases among close contacts occur more than 5 days following the primary case, consideration should be given to the use of immunization as an adjunct to chemoprophylaxis to extend protection if the latter has been unsuccessful.

PROGNOSIS. The mortality from meningococcal meningitis before any treatment was available was about 75 per cent, and residual neurologic damage in the survivors was extensive. The advent of the sulfonamides brought a dramatic reduction in mortality to 5 to 15 per cent. Despite the emergence of sulfonamide-resistant *N. meningitidis*, mortality has been kept at the same low level through the use of high doses of penicillin G or ampicillin. The case-fatality ratio for patients with meningococcemia without accompanying meningitis is higher (25 per cent) than for meningococcal meningitis and reflects the fulminant course in some patients. The case-fatality ratio is highest in children under 2 years of age and in adults over 50.

Band JD, Chamberland ME, Platt T, et al.: Trends in meningococcal disease in the United States, 1975–1980. J Infect Dis 148:754, 1983. *Review of incidence of meningococcal disease in the United States, with emphasis on the role of various serogroups and the prevalence of sulfonamide resistance.*

Benoit FL: Chronic meningococcemia. Case report and review of the literature. Am J Med 35:103, 1963. *The best review of the clinical features of this fascinating entity.*

DeVoe IW: The meningococcus and mechanisms of pathogenicity. Microbiol Rev

46:162, 1982. *Comprehensive review of the biologic properties of N. meningitidis and of the epidemiologic and immunologic aspects of meningococcal disease.*

Duerden BI (ed.): Meningococcal infection. J Med Microbiol 26:161, 1988. *A series of papers reviewing newer aspects of the epidemiology, pathogenesis, and immunology of meningococcal infections based on the recent European experience.*

Feldman HA: Meningococcal infections. Adv Intern Med 18:117, 1972. *The best overview of the major aspects of meningococcal disease, including epidemiology, clinical aspects, treatment, and prevention. Authoritative; very well referenced.*

Goldschneider I, Gotschlich EC, Artenstein MS: Human immunity to the meningococcus. I. The role of humoral antibodies. J Exp Med 129:1307, 1969. *A most important paper, relating susceptibility to meningococcal infection to the lack of serum bactericidal activity against N. meningitidis. A lucid presentation of the basic facts necessary to understand the epidemiology of meningococcal disease.*

Goldschneider I, Gotschlich EC, Artenstein MS: Human immunity to the meningococcus. II. Development of natural immunity. J Exp Med 129:1327, 1969. *A second landmark paper by these authors on immunity to meningococcal infection. The role of the carrier state as an immunizing process is clearly demonstrated.*

Griffiss JM, Brandt BL: Nonepidemic (endemic) meningococcal disease: Pathogenetic factors and clinical features. In Remington JS, Swartz MN (eds.): Current Clinical Topics in Infectious Disease, 7. New York, McGraw-Hill Book Company, 1986, pp 27–50. *Provides important insights into the endemic and hyperendemic forms of meningococcal disease in the United States. The role of host-parasite interactions is emphasized.*

Koppes GM, Ellenbogen C, Gebhart RJ: Group Y meningococcal disease in United States Air Force recruits. Am J Med 62:661, 1977. *A very good description of the spectrum of disease produced by group Y meningococci. The importance of pneumonia in a recruit population is emphasized.*

Olyhoek T, Crowe BA, Achtman M: Clonal population structure of Neisseria meningitidis serogroup A isolated from epidemics and pandemics between 1915 and 1983. Rev Infect Dis 9:665, 1987. *An extensive and thorough study of serogroup A isolates from around the world over a period of about 70 years, indicating that most epidemics have been associated with a single or predominant clone. Seven predominant clones have been identified as causing groups of epidemics worldwide since 1915.*

Peltola H: Meningococcal disease: Still with us. Rev Infect Dis 5:71, 1983. *Authoritative evaluation of the status of meningococcal disease around the world.*

303 Infections Caused by *Haemophilus* Species

DEFINITION. *Haemophilus* infections involve primarily the upper respiratory tract and the bronchopulmonary system. Invasive infections (bacteremia, meningitis, pericarditis, septic arthritis, cellulitis) may sometimes ensue; they occur predominantly in young children and are almost aways due to one species, *H. influenzae* type b. Endocarditis is occasionally caused by *Haemophilus* species other than *H. influenzae* b. One *Haemophilus* species (*H. ducreyi*) is the cause of chancroid (see Ch. 339).

GENERAL MICROBIOLOGIC FEATURES. The various *Haemophilus* species (Table 303–1) are similar in morphology (small, pleomorphic, gram-negative bacilli) and growth requirements (facultatively aerobic, media supplemented with blood). *H. influenzae* requires for aerobic growth both the X factor (hematin) and the V factor (NAD, NADP, or nicotinamide nucleoside) present in erythrocytes. Since some strains of *H. influenzae* grow best in 5 to 10 per cent carbon dioxide and other *Haemophilus* species have a CO_2 dependence, clinical specimens

TABLE 303–1. DIFFERENTIAL PROPERTIES OF *HAEMOPHILUS* SPECIES

| Species | Growth Factor Requirement | | | |
	X	V	CO_2 Dependence	Hemolysis
H. influenzae	+	+	−	−
H. parainfluenzae	−	+	−	−
H. aphrophilus	−, +	−	+	−
H. paraphrophilus	−	+	+	−
H. hemolyticus	+	+	−	+
H. ducreyi	+	−	−	−

should be incubated in a CO_2 incubator. Media for isolation of *Haemophilus* species include chocolate agar, agar containing horse (*not* sheep) blood, or enrichment agar (Levinthal).

H. hemolyticus rarely is isolated from sites outside the upper respiratory tract and is of dubious pathogenicity.

INFECTIONS DUE TO *HAEMOPHILUS INFLUENZAE.*

Etiology. *H. influenzae* strains are either encapsulated (typable) or unencapsulated (nontypable). The former consist of six distinguishable types, designated a to f. Type b capsular polysaccharide contains both ribose and ribitol phosphate (PRP). In children 95 per cent of *H. influenzae* strains causing meningitis and bacteremia belong to type b, and the remaining strains are mainly nontypable. However, encapsulated strains make up only a small percentage of all clinical isolates of *H. influenzae*. Nontypable strains are more likely to be implicated in localized or surface infections such as otitis media in children and lower respiratory tract infections (exacerbations of chronic bronchitis and pneumonia) in adults. *H. influenzae* bacteremia is uncommon in adults, but when it occurs only about 30 per cent of isolates are type b strains and the remainder are mostly nontypable. Encapsulated strains can be identified by a variety of methods employing antisera to their capsular antigens (immunofluorescence; production of immunoprecipitin halos ringing colonies on agar plates containing antiserum; demonstration by counterimmunoelectrophoresis or latex particle agglutination of capsular antigen in culture supernatants). The outer membrane of *H. influenzae* strains contains a lipopolysaccharide with the properties of endotoxin. A classification of *H. influenzae* b into 21 subtypes based on differences in outer membrane proteins has been developed and is of use in epidemiologic studies.

H. aegyptius (Koch-Weeks bacillus) is a cause of sporadic or epidemic summer conjunctivitis. It has the same growth factor requirements as *H. influenzae*, and, since it shares over 70 per cent nucleotide sequence homology with *H. influenzae*, it is now designated *H. influenzae* biogroup *aegyptius*. It is nonencapsulated. Strains of this biogroup have been responsible for an invasive bacteremic illness, Brazilian purpuric fever (BPF), which resembles meningococcemia and occurs in Brazil, often following conjunctivitis. Strains of biogroup *aegyptius* from BPF appear to be more virulent in animal models than strains of this biogroup isolated from patients with only conjunctivitis.

Genetic relationships (clonality) between strains of *H. influenzae* differing both geographically and temporally in isolation can be identified by electrophoretic studies of cytoplasmic enzymes and outer membrane proteins. Examination by such multilocus enzyme electrophoresis of numerous isolates from around the world suggests certain conclusions: (1) most invasive disease caused by *H. influenzae* type b is caused by a limited number (about nine) of clones; (2) some geographic variation in clonal composition of serotype b *H. influenzae* populations exists on a continental or regional basis; (3) nontypable strains belong to distinctive clone clusters (much more diverse as a group than clones of type b) rather than represent variants that have simply lost the capacity to elaborate polysaccharide capsule; (4) no clear associations of clone groups with clinical manifestations have been defined with the possible exceptions of certain clones of nontypable *H. influenzae* involved in meningitis and bacteremia in neonates and in urogenital disease in women.

Smears of clinical specimens usually show pleomorphic gram-negative coccobacilli. Occasionally, in underdecolorized Gram-stained smears of spinal fluid, bipolar concentration of stain may incorrectly suggest gram-positive diplococci.

Incidence and Prevalence. Nontypable *H. influenzae* are commonly carried in the nasopharynx of asymptomatic individuals. Rates of carriage for encapsulated strains (usually type b) are much lower (less than 5 per cent of children and less than 1 per cent of adults). However, the carriage rate of household contacts, at the time of hospitalization of a child with invasive *H. influenzae* b, is much higher, 20 to 25 per cent (50 per cent in children under 5 years). Nasopharyngeal carriage of *H. influenzae* b may develop in some persons in the presence of circulating antibody to PRP, and successful antibiotic treatment of *H. influenzae* meningitis may not eliminate it from the upper respiratory tract. The carrier state may persist for weeks to months.

H. influenzae b is the principal (estimated 8000 to 11,000 cases annually) cause of bacterial meningitis in the United States. It is estimated to cause an additional 6000 cases per year of other invasive diseases such as bacteremia, epiglottitis, pneumonia, and cellulitis. By 5 years of age, one in every 200 children has had a systemic infection from *H. influenzae* b. In the past decade many clinicians have had the impression that systemic disease caused by *H. influenzae* b has become more frequent in adults. Systemic infection with *H. influenzae* probably should be considered in the adult in the proper setting more frequently than was formerly the case. *H. influenzae* type f is probably the second most frequent encapsulated *H. influenzae* pathogen in adults.

Epidemiology. Infections in the first 2 months of life are rare, probably because of transplacental transfer of maternal antibody. Most cases (about 80 per cent) of meningitis and invasive infections caused by *H. influenzae* in the United States occur in children under 2 years of age. The mean age of children with epiglottitis is 3 to 5 years. Host factors appearing to contribute to increased susceptibility include immune globulin deficiencies, sickle cell disease, CSF fistulas, splenectomized states, and chronic pulmonary infections. Alcoholism appears to be a risk factor in adults. In certain racial groups (Eskimos, American Indians, blacks) children are at higher risk of invasive *H. influenzae* infection; socioeconomic factors undoubtedly play a role.

Unlike *Neisseria meningitidis*, *H. influenzae* b does not cause epidemics in the community, but it is responsible for an increased incidence of secondary cases among susceptibles in families or possibly in daycare centers exposed to an index case. The risk of serious *H. influenzae* illness among exposed household contacts of a child with *H. influenzae* meningitis is age dependent: 4 per cent among children under 2 years of age, 2 per cent among children 2 to 3 years of age, and 0.1 per cent among children 4 to 5 years of age. The risk of infection in household contacts represents a 600-fold increase over the age-adjusted risk in the population at large.

Pathogenesis and Immunity. Most nasopharyngeal infections with *H. influenzae* are unrecognized and occur by age 5 years. Type b strains may occasionally invade locally, producing epiglottitis, pneumonia, or buccal cellulitis, or may be disseminated directly from the nasopharynx via the bloodstream, producing meningitis. Intense ($>10^3$ organisms per milliliter of blood) sustained bacteremia resulting from intravascular bacterial replication (rather than growth at a focal site of initial infection) appears to be a prerequisite for the development of meningitis. Pathogenicity of type b strains owes principally to the antiphagocytic activity of its PRP capsule. Nonencapsulated strains rarely produce bacteremic infection but can produce disease involving the upper (otitis media, sinusitis) and lower (pneumonia, exacerbations of chronic bronchitis) respiratory tracts.

In Finland, studies of anti-PRP antibodies by radioimmunoassay indicate an inverse correlation between age-related antibody levels and incidence of bacteremic *H. influenzae* disease (confirming Fothergill and Wright); 90 per cent of children (3 to 12 months of age) had antibody levels below 150 ng per milliliter, whereas all adults had higher levels. In the presence of complement, IgG class antibodies to PRP are not only bactericidal (bacteriolytic) but are also opsonic. Such antibodies are protective in vivo. Antibodies to outer membrane proteins also play a role in immunity, but they appear to be protective primarily against strains of the same subtype.

The antibody response to *H. influenzae* b meningitis is age related (infants responding poorly and older children and adults developing high titers) and related to PRP load and clearance rate. Antigenemia may persist for as long as several weeks in younger children; an antibody response may be delayed until antigenemia has cleared. Anti-PRP antibody responses are observed within about 3 months in about 80 per cent of children with meningitis.

Failure of specific anti-PRP antibody response occurs in individuals with agammaglobulinemia and with IgG_2 subclass deficiency. In addition, during the first 1 or 2 years of life polysaccharide antigens such as PRP vaccine are not efficient immunogens. The rare recurrence of *H. influenzae* b meningitis in the first 24 months of life may reflect failure even of invasive infection to elicit a protective antibody response.

It has been suggested that the age-related acquisition of anti-PRP antibodies is too rapid and extensive to be accounted for by the low incidence of *H. influenzae* b carriage or disease, and that cross-reacting *E. coli* strains in the intestine may serve as the primary immunogen.

Clinical Manifestations. In one survey of children with serious *H. influenzae* infections, meningitis was the most common manifestation (about 50 per cent), followed by pneumonia (15 per cent), bacteremia without definable portal (10 per cent), cellulitis (10 per cent), epiglottitis (10 per cent), and pericarditis (4 per cent).

Among adults with *H. influenzae* bacteremia, pneumonia is the most common cause. Other sources of *H. influenzae* bacteremia in adults include obstetric infections (nontypable strains), meningitis, occult bacteremias, cellulitis, acute sinusitis, and epiglottitis. Metastatic *H. influenzae* infections in the adult include septic arthritis and purulent pericarditis.

Meningitis (See Ch. 301). *H. influenzae* type b is the preeminent cause of bacterial meningitis in childhood, most cases occurring between age 4 months and 2 years. The clinical features are not distinctive except as they relate to pyogenic meningitis occurring at that age. The manifestations may be nonspecific (fever, irritability, listlessness, poor feeding, vomiting) initially, especially in the younger child, and there may be only minimal nuchal rigidity. If the fontanel is still open, it may not be tense, particularly if the infant is dehydrated. Subdural effusions occur more frequently (20 to 30 per cent) with *H. influenzae* meningitis, but this is related to age and ease of detection by transillumination.

Anemia is more frequent in children with *H. influenzae* b meningitis and invasive infections than in those with comparable meningococcal or pneumococcal illnesses. It appears, in patients with prolonged antigenemia coinciding with production of antibody to PRP, to be a consequence of splenic removal of PRP-coated erythrocytes to which antibody and complement have been bound, or of intravascular hemolysis.

In adults *H. influenzae* b causes only about 4 per cent of cases of bacterial meningitis, and a CSF leak is a predisposing factor in about half of such cases.

Epiglottitis. This pediatric otolaryngologic emergency begins abruptly with a severe sore throat, fever, and dysphagia; progression is swift, usually requiring hospitalization (and intubation) within 12 hours of onset. In the adult the onset of epiglottitis may be more prolonged and respiratory difficulty less pronounced initially despite severe pharyngitis and dysphagia; occasionally, the clinical picture may be mistaken for that of asthma. Airway obstruction in the child develops early with a sensation of choking, inspiratory (but not expiratory) distress, drooling, and anxiety. Speech is muffled, but the barking cough observed in croup is uncommon. The patient sits leaning forward with arms, back, and neck hyperextended to provide maximal airway. Pneumonia occurs in 15 to 25 per cent of patients, but simultaneous meningitis is uncommon. *Intraoral examination of the child (particularly in the supine position) may precipitate a cardiorespiratory arrest and should be performed only with the means of establishing an airway immediately at hand.* The pharynx is reddened; the epiglottis is bright red and markedly swollen. Lateral radiographs of the neck can demonstrate swelling of the epiglottis, but are of less value in acute cases (the procedure may delay establishment of an adequate airway) than in subacute ones.

Viral croup may resemble epiglottitis but occurs in younger children (3 to 36 months), has a more gradual onset, and frequently is preceded by an upper respiratory infection; the airway obstruction is subglottic.

Pneumonia. Most cases occur in children, are caused by type b, and are accompanied by bacteremia. Lobar consolidation occurs more commonly than bronchopneumonia, and pleural effusions (or empyema) are present in 75 per cent of cases. Lung abscess is rare. Meningitis occurs in about 15 per cent of patients. In the adult, *H. influenzae* pneumonia occurs more frequently in the setting of chronic lung disease, alcoholism, immunologic deficiency, or following viral respiratory tract infection, but it may develop in previously healthy individuals. The majority of sputum isolates are nontypable, as are most blood isolates from the approximately 20 per cent of patients in whom bacteremia occurs. The radiologic pattern is usually that of bronchopneumonia. Small sterile parapneumonic effusions are common. The diagnosis can be suspected on the basis of findings on Gram-stained smears of sputum, but confirmation requires isolation of the organism from blood, pleural fluid, or lower respiratory tract.

Bronchitis. *H. influenzae* (nontypable) has been associated with purulent sputum and clinical exacerbations (dyspnea, wheezing, low-grade fever) of chronic bronchitis. Gram-stained smears of sputum show numerous neutrophils and small pleomorphic gram-negative bacilli. A direct etiologic role may be difficult to establish because of the frequent (20 to 80 per cent) carriage of these organisms in the upper respiratory tract of normal adults.

Bacterial Tracheitis. This acute upper airway infection particularly of children is characterized by fever, stridor, subglottic edema without epiglottal involvement, and abundant purulent tracheal secretions. Inspissation of the latter may lead to pseudomembrane formation requiring removal. This bacterial infection, often due to *H. influenzae* but even more often due to *Staphylococcus aureus*, is usually secondary to a primary parainfluenza virus respiratory infection.

Cellulitis. *H. influenzae* b causes cellulitis in children below 2 years of age, but may also cause cellulitis on rare occasions in older adults. The cheek, periorbital area, head, and neck are the most common sites. An associated ipsilateral otitis media or upper respiratory infection is a frequent precursor. It begins with fever, local pain, and increasing toxicity. The lesion develops within a few hours and progresses rapidly; it is poorly demarcated, tender, and edematous. Although usually described as having a distinctive bluish purple color, the lesion is commonly erythematous like other types of cellulitis. Bacteremia occurs in 80 per cent of cases. Diagnosis is made on the basis of the appearance and location of the lesion, the patient's age, Gram-stained smears and culture of an aspirate, and blood cultures.

Bacteremia Without Obvious Portal. *H. influenzae* b is responsible for about 20 per cent of cryptogenic bacteremias occurring in febrile children with mild nonspecific illnesses. Such patients are at considerable risk for subsequent serious localized infection (meningitis, pneumonia, epiglottitis). Unsuspected *H. influenzae* bacteremia also occurs in patients with neoplastic disease undergoing chemotherapy. Fulminant *H. influenzae* bacteremia with fatal shock and disseminated intravascular coagulation can develop in splenectomized patients.

Skeletal Infections. Septic arthritis accounts for 1 to 8 per cent of cases of invasive *H. influenzae* b infection in children. It is the cause of pyogenic arthritis in about one half of cases in children under 2 years of age. Weight-bearing joints are most often involved. Most commonly pyarthrosis is secondary to bacteremic spread from an upper respiratory tract infection, but joint involvement may result from direct spread of adjacent osteomyelitis in the first year of life.

A "reactive" arthritis has recently been described in children in association with *H. influenzae* b meningitis. Whereas the articular manifestations of pyogenic arthritis are usually present within the first day of admission with meningitis, the joint findings in the "reactive" form usually appear about a week following institution of appropriate antimicrobial therapy. Gram's stains and cultures of repeated synovial fluid aspirates are negative. Whether this process is comparable to the reactive arthritis of meningococcal meningitis, in which immune complexes are present in blood and synovial fluid, is not known. Joint effusions with a neutrophilic pleocytosis occurring in this setting should be considered to be those of pyogenic arthritis until results of repeated bacteriologic studies are available.

H. influenzae is a rare cause of osteomyelitis in children, usually occurring in the first year of life.

Pericarditis. *H. influenzae* b is the cause of 10 to 15 per cent of cases of purulent pericarditis in children. It is a rare cause of pericarditis in adults. Over one half of the children have an associated pneumonia. The hemodynamic manifestations of cardiac tamponade are commonly present. Treatment involves pericardiocentesis for diagnosis followed by surgical drainage (closed catheter drainage or anterior pericardectomy), along with antimicrobial therapy. With treatment 85 to 95 per cent of patients recover.

Otitis Media and Sinusitis. *H. influenzae* is second in frequency to *Streptococcus pneumoniae* as the cause of acute otitis media in children. In most instances the *H. influenzae* strains are not typable, but type b strains can be isolated in 10 per cent of cases. Serous middle ear fluid in children with chronic low-grade otitis media with effusion may be colonized by *H. influenzae*, which may contribute to its persistence. *H. influenzae* also appears to be a significant cause of otitis media in older children and adults. The manifestations of acute otitis media caused by *H. influenzae* are indistinguishable from those caused by other pyogens: otalgia, fever, hyperemia of the tympanic membrane, and middle ear fluid. Tinnitus, vertigo, and nystagmus may develop.

Acute sinusitis is more common in adults than in children. In about 25 per cent of cases *H. influenzae* (nontypable) is the cause. Facial pain, frontal headache, purulent nasal discharge or nasal obstruction, anosmia, and nasal speech are common features. Sinus tenderness and opacity on transillumination are helpful findings.

Conjunctivitis. *H. influenzae* biogroup *aegyptius* mucopurulent conjunctivitis occurs principally in children, particularly in the summer. The findings of acute catarrhal conjunctivitis are present, but petechial hemorrhages on the tarsal and epibulbar conjunctivae are suggestive of *H. influenzae* or a pneumococcal cause. Diagnosis is made on the basis of Gram-stained smears of conjunctival scrapings and culture of the outer eye.

H. influenzae biogroup *aegyptius* conjunctivitis is often self-limited, clearing in 7 to 14 days. Treatment consists of moist soaks to keep the eyelids clean and topical antimicrobials (e.g., 10 to 30 per cent sulfacetamide eyedrops).

Brazilian Purpuric Fever (BPF). This recently recognized, frequently fatal infection of young children in Brazil usually follows recovery from purulent conjunctivitis that began 1 or 2 weeks earlier. Clinical features include acute onset with fever and toxicity, abdominal pain and vomiting, rapidly followed by the appearance of petechiae, purpura, hypotension, and shock. *H. influenzae* biogroup *aegyptius*, previously identified only with cases of purulent conjunctivitis worldwide, is responsible for this bacteremic illness resembling meningococcemia. The fulminant clinical picture associated with BPF is consistent with the lack of close genetic relatedness of BPF strains with other isolates of the same biogroup and with the greater pathogenicity of BPF strains of biogroup *aegyptius* in infant rats compared with control conjunctival isolates of the same biogroup.

Other Infections. *H. influenzae* is a very rare cause of endocarditis and brain abscess. *H. influenzae* may occasionally be the cause of nonexudative pharyngitis (with prominent pain and dysphagia), but its presence in the pharynx often merely represents colonization. Rare cases of genital tract infections (salpingitis, endometritis, puerperal sepsis) and urinary infections have occurred.

Diagnosis. Certain serious infections (purulent meningitis, epiglottitis, facial and orbital cellulitis) in young children should suggest the possibility of *H. influenzae* b as the cause. In meningitis the presence of gram-negative pleomorphic coccobacillary forms in smears of CSF is highly suggestive of *H. influenzae*, but other organisms (*Pasteurella multocida, Acinetobacter*) which only rarely cause meningitis may have a similar appearance. Rapid and sensitive methods of antigen (PRP) detection such as latex particle agglutination (LPA), coagglutination (CoA), countercurrent immunoelectrophoresis (CIE), and enzyme-linked immunosorbent assay (ELISA) have detected *H. influenzae* b antigen in initial CSF specimens of 60 to 90 per cent of cases of *H. influenzae* meningitis; they are particularly helpful in early diagnosis and in the diagnosis of patients whose cultures may be negative because of prior antibiotic therapy. LPA is positive in 90 to 95 per cent of culture-confirmed cases of *H. influenzae* b meningitis and has the advantages over CIE and ELISA of being easier to perform and more rapid. Antigenemia can be demonstrated in 60 to 100 per cent of patients with *H. influenzae* b meningitis but much less frequently in children with epiglottitis and cellulitis. False-positive reactions may occur owing to cross-reactive antigens in other bacteria such as *E. coli*, but these are infrequent.

Bacteremia is commonly demonstrable in patients with invasive infections (at least 80 per cent of children with meningitis, epiglottitis, or cellulitis) caused by *H. influenzae* b. *H. influenzae* is generally isolated on cultures of the epiglottis, joint fluid, and empyema fluid when it is the cause of infection in those areas.

Treatment. Currently, about 30 per cent of strains of *H. influenzae* b isolated in this country from systemic infections are ampicillin resistant. Resistance to chloramphenicol is found in less than 1 per cent of strains. Regional variations in resistance patterns exist. In a pediatric hospital in Barcelona, Spain, 60 per cent of meningeal isolates are ampicillin resistant; 66 per cent are resistant to chloramphenicol; and 57 per cent are resistant to both drugs. Most ampicillin-resistant *H. influenzae* strains are resistant by virtue of plasmid-encoded β-lactamase production. Detection of β-lactamase production is commonly employed to determine ampicillin resistance. Recently rare isolates of ampicillin-resistant *H. influenzae* that are resistant because of alterations in penicillin-binding proteins rather than β-lactamase production have been detected. Since routine testing for β-lactamase would indicate incorrectly such strains to be ampicillin susceptible, special disc or agar-dilution testing would be required if this were suspected. About 15 per cent of strains (usually nontypable) associated with childhood otitis media are ampicillin resistant, as are 8 to 20 per cent of strains (mostly nontypable) isolated from adults with invasive infections or chronic bronchitis.

Because of the prevalence of ampicillin resistance, ampicillin should not be used as single-drug therapy of systemic illnesses caused by *H. influenzae* b unless it has been established that the organism is ampicillin susceptible (a non–β-lactamase producer). Several forms of initial therapy are currently being employed (see Ch. 301). These include a third-generation cephalosporin such as ceftriaxone or cefotaxime; chloramphenicol (alone, or in combination with ampicillin until testing for ampicillin resistance has been performed); and, for nonmeningeal infections, cefuroxime (a second-generation cephalosporin resistant to many β-lactamases). Ceftriaxone or cefotaxime would be the drug of choice, particularly in areas where resistance to both chloramphenicol and ampicillin exists or when such resistance is suspected on the basis of clinical response to other therapy.

Amoxicillin (20 to 40 mg per kilogram per day in three divided doses) or ampicillin (50 to 100 mg per kilogram per day in four divided doses), because each is active against *S. pneumoniae* and most strains of *H. influenzae*, is still the drug of choice for initial treatment of otitis media in children. Alternatives include amoxicillin-clavulanate, trimethoprim (TMP)-sulfamethoxazole (SMX) (8 mg per kilogram of TMP and 40 mg per kilogram of SMX per 24 hours, given in two divided doses every 12 hours), the combination of penicillin (or erythromycin) with a sulfonamide, cefaclor or cefuroxime-axetil. Treatment should be continued for 10 to 14 days. Initial treatment of *H. influenzae* pneumonia in the adult should be with ampicillin or amoxicillin, since these infections are infrequently caused by ampicillin-resistant strains, and there is sufficient time to shift therapy (cefuroxime, amoxicillin-clavulanate, chloramphenicol) if the response is unsatisfactory. Based on the bacteriology (*S. pneumoniae* and *H. influenzae* are frequently identified) of acute sinusitis, ampicillin is a reasonable initial antibiotic choice. (In the patient with rapidly progressive frontal sinusitis, *S. aureus* must be considered as a cause as well, and a penicillinase-resistant penicillin should be included in the initial therapeutic program.)

Prevention. A vaccine (*Haemophilus* b polysaccharide vaccine) against invasive infection with *H. influenzae* b was licensed in 1985 for use in the United States in children who are 24 months or older. This vaccine was demonstrated in Finland to have 90 per cent efficacy among children 18 to 71 months of age. It was not possible statistically to demonstrate efficacy in children immunized at 18 to 23 months of age. The vaccine was ineffective in children under 18 months of age. Subsequent case-control studies in the United States of children of 24 months and older indicate that this vaccine is somewhat less effective in this country than would have been anticipated from results of the Finnish trial, suggesting possible regional differences in vaccine efficacy. Consideration may be given to immunization of children in high-risk groups (sickle cell disease, asplenic states, malignancies associated with immunosuppression) at 18 months of age even though efficacy has not been established in this age group. If this is done, a booster dose within 18 months may be necessary.

Since the majority of cases of *H. influenzae* meningitis occur in the first 18 to 24 months of life, when the current polysaccharide vaccine is not efficacious, other vaccines have been developed. Since there appears to be an age-specific defect in the response of infants to polysaccharide antigen (thymus-independent), attempts have been made to overcome this limitation by linking the PRP antigen to a protein (e.g., diphtheria toxoid), thus invoking T cell participation and establishing immunologic memory. A large-scale Finnish field trial of *H. influenzae* type b polysaccharide–diphtheria toxoid conjugate vaccine in infancy (administered at 3, 4, 6, and 14 months of age) indicated that the vaccine afforded 83 per cent protection. A recent comparable study of the same vaccine in Alaskan native infants showed only very limited protective efficacy, suggesting again unexplained possible regional variation in vaccine efficacy. This conjugate vaccine is currently approved for immunization of children as young as 15 to 18 months of age. Other *H. influenzae* polysaccharide–protein conjugate vaccines, employing as the protein moiety either *N. meningitidis* outer membrane protein or a nontoxic antigenically identical mutant diphtheria toxin, are being developed for immunization of younger infants.

The rate of secondary cases among young children who are close household contacts of a patient with invasive *H. influenzae* b infection indicates the need for an effective prophylactic antibiotic program. Since rifampin has efficacy in eliminating nasopharyngeal carriage of *H. influenzae* b, the following management of household contacts has been recommended: (1) if another child less than 4 years of age resides in the household of an index case, all household members (including adults) should receive rifampin (20 mg per kilogram orally once daily for 4 days, with a maximal daily dose of 600 mg); (2) rifampin in the same dosage should also be administered to the index patient prior to discharge from the hospital, since nasopharyngeal carriage may reappear after discontinuation of antimicrobial therapy for systemic infection; (3) rifampin prophylaxis is probably not indicated if over 2 weeks have elapsed since illness began in the index patient or if the youngest child in the household is 4 years of age or older.

Whether the risk of subsequent invasive *H. influenzae* infection is increased in contacts of patients in daycare facilities is controversial; the risk may vary from region to region. If 2 or more cases occur in a daycare center within 60 days, rifampin prophylaxis should be given to all contacts in the facility, including adults. Whether to do likewise if only one case has occurred is controversial. However, if any of the exposed classroom contacts is under 2 years of age, institution of chemoprophylaxis seems warranted.

INFECTIONS CAUSED BY OTHER *HAEMOPHILUS* SPECIES. *Haemophilus parainfluenzae.* This *Haemophilus* species is part of the normal flora of the nasopharynx and is found in dental plaque. It is very uncommonly responsible for human disease. It has been a rare cause of meningitis, epiglottitis, otitis media, puerperal bacteremia, brain abscess, and pneumonia in adults. Ampicillin is the drug of choice, except when ampicillin resistance is present (6 per cent of isolates), in which case a third-generation cephalosporin or chloramphenicol is an alternative. The most common association of *H. parainfluenzae* with disease has been with infective endocarditis. It may take as long as 14 to 18 days to grow out of blood cultures. The only distinctive clinical feature (also observed with *H. aphrophilus* endocarditis) appears to be the frequent occurrence of embolic occlusion of large arteries. For endocarditis in the adult, treatment with ampicillin (12 grams daily intravenously) alone or in combination with gentamicin (4 mg per kilogram per day in divided doses every 8 hours intravenously) for 4 to 6 weeks has been employed successfully.

Haemophilus aphrophilus. This organism is part of the normal gingival flora and is a rare cause of disease, generally acting as an "opportunist." The infections it produces, often following oropharyngeal foci of infection or trauma, include abscesses (particularly brain abscess), bacteremia, and endocarditis. Most strains are susceptible to penicillin, ampicillin, third-generation cephalosporins, chloramphenicol, and gentamicin. Successful treatment of endocarditis has involved the use of ampicillin or penicillin, alone or in combination with streptomycin, for 4 to 6 weeks.

Haemophilus ducreyi. See Ch. 339.

Haemophilus influenzae

Campos J, Garcia-Tornel S, Gairi JM, Fabregues I: Multiply resistant *Haemophilus influenzae* type b causing meningitis: Comparative clinical and laboratory study.
J Pediatr 108:897, 1986. *Summarizes the extent of a major endemic problem in Spain of resistance to ampicillin and chloramphenicol in* H. influenzae *strains. Alternative therapeutic approaches are suggested.*

Cherry JD: Acute epiglottitis, laryngitis, and croup. *In* Remington JS, Swartz MN (eds.): Current Clinical Topics in Infectious Disease, 2. New York, McGraw-Hill Book Company, 1981, pp 1–30. *Provides a particularly vivid clinical picture of acute* H. influenzae *epiglottitis. Valuable points on differential diagnosis and treatment are emphasized. A very well organized and thoroughly referenced presentation.*

Dajani AS, Asmar BI, Thirumoorthi MC: Systemic *Haemophilus influenzae* disease. J Pediatr 94:355, 1979. *This is a thorough review of an extensive pediatric experience with systemic* H. influenzae *b infections. It provides helpful data on the relative frequencies of the various clinical syndromes and an extensive bibliography.*

Eskola J, Peltola H, Takola AK, et al.: Efficacy of *Haemophilus influenzae* type b polysaccharide–diphtheria toxoid conjugate vaccine in infancy. N Engl J Med 317:717, 1987. *This article describes a 5-month follow-up of a very large trial in Finland of the type b capsular polysaccharide–diphtheria toxoid vaccine, which protected children from 7 to 14 months of age against invasive* H. influenzae *infection.*

Fothergill LD, Wright J: Influenzal meningitis: Relation of age incidence to bactericidal power of blood against causal organism. J Immunol 24:273, 1933. *This is the original and "classic" study demonstrating an inverse relationship between the presence of serum bactericidal antibody and the incidence of* H. influenzae *meningitis at various ages.*

Granoff DM, Ward JI: Current status of prophylaxis for *Hemophilus influenzae* infections. *In* Remington JS, Swartz MN (eds.): Current Clinical Topics in Infectious Disease, 5. New York, McGraw-Hill Book Company, 1984. *Provides excellent background regarding secondary spread of* H. influenzae *infections and concrete recommendations for chemoprophylaxis of close family and daycare center contacts.*

Mayo-Smith MF, Hirsch PJ, Wodzinski SF, et al.: Acute epiglottitis in adults. An eight year experience in the state of Rhode Island. N Engl J Med 314:1133, 1986. *A clinical and bacteriologic review of 56 cases of acute epiglottitis (supraglottitis) in adults, indicating that* H. influenzae *is an important cause in this age group (28 per cent of published cases in which blood cultures were obtained). Practical management issues are considered.*

Murphy TF, Apicella MA: Nontypable *Haemophilus influenzae*: A review of clinical aspects, surface antigens, and the human immune response to infection. Rev Infect Dis 9:1, 1987. *A detailed review of the antigenic nature and biologic properties of nonencapsulated* H. influenzae. *The role of such strains in clinical infections in adults and children is very thoroughly covered.*

Musser JM, Kroll JS, Granoff DM, et al.: Global genetic structure and molecular epidemiology of encapsulated *Haemophilus influenzae*. Rev Infect Dis 12:75, 1990. *This represents an enormous study by multilocus electrophoresis of over 2200 isolates of encapsulated* H. influenzae *from around the world. It provides insights into the clonal population structure of this species and indicates patterns of intercontinental and regional geographic distribution.*

Peltola H, Kayhty H, Virtanen M, et al.: Prevention of *Haemophilus influenzae* type B bacteremic infections with the capsular polysaccharide vaccine. N Engl J Med 310:1561, 1984. *This article describes a long-term follow-up of a very well conducted, large scale trial of the type b capsular polysaccharide vaccine, which protected against bacteremic* H. influenzae *b disease in children older than 24 months of age.*

Shurin SB, Anderson P, Zollinger J, et al.: Pathophysiology of hemolysis in infections with *Hemophilus influenzae* type b. J Clin Invest 77:1340, 1986. *In a careful laboratory study the authors demonstrate that the anemia observed in invasive* H. influenzae *b infections is hemolytic in origin and may be due to coating of PRP on erythrocytes and their subsequent immune destruction.*

Spagnuolo PJ, Ellner JJ, Lerner PL, et al.: *Haemophilus influenzae* meningitis: The spectrum of disease in adults. Medicine 61:74, 1982. *These 15 cases represent the largest series of cases of* H. influenzae *meningitis reported in the past 20 years. Particular emphasis is on predisposing factors in this unusual form of meningitis in adults.*

Wallace RJ Jr, Musher DM, Septimus EJ, et al.: *Haemophilus influenzae* infections in adults: Characterization of strains by serotypes, biotypes, and β-lactamase production. J Infect Dis 144:101, 1981. *This is a detailed review of 103 cases of* H. influenzae *bacteremia or meningitis. Noteworthy is the frequency of nontypable strains among blood isolates in adults and the infrequency of ampicillin resistance in the same group.*

Haemophilus parainfluenzae and Haemophilus aphrophilus

Bieger RC, Brewer NS, Washington JA II: *Haemophilus aphrophilus*: A microbiologic and clinical review and report of 42 cases. Medicine 57:345, 1978. *A comprehensive review of the bacteriologic features, ecologic niche, and clinical impact of this uncommon cause of human disease.*

Oill PA, Chow AW, Guze LB: Adult bacteremic *Haemophilus parainfluenzae* infections: Seven reports of cases and a review of the literature. Arch Intern Med 139:985, 1979. *The type of infection (exclusive of endocarditis) caused by* H. parainfluenzae *and the antibiotic susceptibilities of this organism are summarized concisely.*

Osteomyelitis

304 Osteomyelitis

Francis A. Waldvogel

DEFINITION. Osteomyelitis is an infection by microorganisms that invade and destroy bone. Osteomyelitis is a well-known, albeit rare, consequence of bacteremia. In most situations nowadays, open fractures, wounds, and orthopedic procedures allow the microorganism to gain access to bone from a contaminated or infected contiguous structure. Peripheral bones can also be invaded by contiguity in cases of severe vascular insufficiency. In the latter case, metabolic and neurologic factors often play an important contributory role.

ETIOLOGY. Most cases of osteomyelitis are of bacterial origin. Of all pathogenic organisms, *Staphylococcus aureus* is still the most common offending agent, whatever the mechanism of the infection. However, *S. epidermidis* has emerged in recent years as a frequent offender as well, for instance, in hematogenous spread to a vertebral body from an infected intravenous line. *S. epidermidis* is also responsible for many bone infections secondary to implantation of prosthetic material, such as total hip prosthesis, where it can account for up to 30 per cent of the cases.

Other etiologic agents include gram-negative enteric organisms, which are often responsible for hematogenous vertebral osteomyelitis, certain *Salmonella* species that cause hematogenous disease in patients with sickle cell anemia, and often *Pseudomonas aeruginosa*, which can involve the spine in heroin addicts. Anaerobic organisms, most often in mixed cultures, have been isolated from infected bone in the vicinity of an anaerobic reservoir (mandible, sinuses, sacrum), after human or animal bites, or from infected extremities in diabetic patients. *Mycobacterium tuberculosis* should always be considered a diagnostic possibility in osteomyelitis of the spine, especially in patients presenting with limited periosteal reactions, and in nonhealing bone infections. Various fungi can cause osteomyelitis under exceptional conditions, such as hematogenous spread from a chronically infected intravenous device or in connection with prosthetic material. Finally, exceptional cases of viral osteomyelitis have been described after chickenpox.

All causes of osteomyelitis have not yet been discovered. Thus, multifocal hematogenous osteomyelitis is a syndrome occurring in children and young adults characterized by multiple, lytic inflammatory bone lesions in patients with various skin conditions such as pustulosis palmoplantaris and acne fulminans. Bacterial cultures of biopsy specimens are negative, and the disease usually evolves toward cure without specific antibacterial therapy.

INCIDENCE, PREVALENCE, AND EPIDEMIOLOGY. Hematogenous osteomyelitis has a biphasic incidence, occurring mainly in children, in whom it shows a predilection for the metaphysis of long bones, and in adults beyond the age of 50 years, in whom it most often involves the spine. Any factor favoring bacteremia (urinary tract infection, prostatitis, various skin infections, prolonged intravenous therapy, or repeated injections) can occasionally lead to hematogenous osteomyelitis of the spine. Osteomyelitis secondary to a contiguous focus varies in frequency acccording to the primary trauma, the invasive procedure performed, the type of material inserted, the underlying disease, and the degree of contamination of the wound. For instance, in well-planned aseptic interventions such as total hip replacement, the risk of infection is usually around 0.4 per cent; insertions of total knee prostheses, on the other hand, are associated with a higher risk of infection, particularly in patients with rheumatoid arthritis; at the other end of the spectrum, the prevalence of postoperative osteomyelitis can reach 15 per cent after comminuted fracture.

PATHOGENESIS AND PATHOLOGY. The development of

experimental models and the collection of better morphologic data have shed some new light on the mechanisms leading to bone destruction in osteomyelitis. The porous structure of bone, its canaliculi filled with capillaries and/or osteoblast cytoplasmic extensions, and the space between these organic structures and the mineral constituents, account for a nonnegligible fluid volume in bone, in the range of 5 per cent. In hematogenous osteomyelitis, microorganisms settle probably first in this fluid phase, where they stimulate an active inflammatory reaction. Whether microorganisms have to adhere on the hydroxyapatite surface or on collagen to escape host defense mechanisms, as suggested by other infection models, is currently suggested by some experimental data. Since microorganisms per se are unable to destroy bone tissue, one has to postulate that the inflammatory reaction, the metabolic alterations, and the vascular changes triggered by the bacterial invasion play predominant roles in the development of an osteomyelitic focus, i.e., in bone destruction and regeneration. From a morphologic point of view, the following major alterations can be identified: (1) bone necrosis, with death of the cellular constituents and disappearance of bone mass. Sometimes devitalized bone persists as a dead fragment called a sequestrum; (2) a heavy inflammatory reaction, in which granulocytes predominate initially but are replaced over time by a mononuclear infiltrate; (3) new bone apposition, originating from periosteal activation. In some cases, this bone apposition can be exuberant and lead to bridging of two adjacent bone structures, as in vertebral osteomyelitis. In other cases, bone apposition is very modest, and radiographic examination may show only an intraosseous, punched-out radiolucent lesion, as in subacute hematogenous osteomyelitis (Brodie's abscess) (Fig. 304–1).

CLINICAL MANIFESTATIONS. Acute hematogenous osteomyelitis involving long bones usually does not pose any major diagnostic problems: It starts as an acute episode with chills and fever, the young patient usually complaining of severe pain in the affected bone, most often the tibia or femur, more rarely the humerus. Clinical examination of the affected limb is usually unremarkable, except for pain on palpation of the affected area, usually the metaphysis. Characteristically, the adjacent joint is freely mobile and painless. If the infection is caused by an organism less virulent than *S. aureus*, however, the onset can be protracted, the pain less severe, and the fever moderate.

In hematogenous osteomyelitis of the spine, the clinical pres-

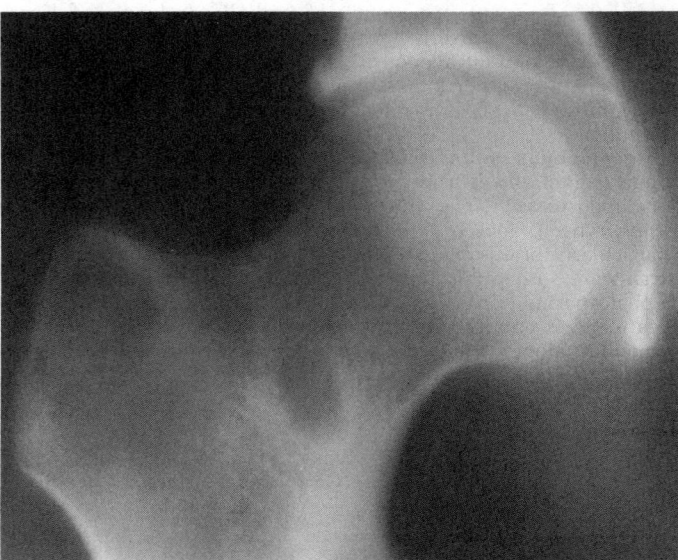

FIGURE 304–1. Subacute osteomyelitis (Brodie's abscess), hematogenous, in the right femur of a 31-year-old male.

entation is often characterized by progressive, ill-defined pain with low fever, following, for instance, an episode of urinary tract infection, bacteremia, or skin infection. The dull pain is usually located in the lower dorsal or lumbar segments of the spine ("febrile lumbago"). Any vertebral body can occasionally become involved by the disease, even the cervical spine ("febrile torticollis"). On physical examination, the mildly febrile patient usually has vertebral and paravertebral tenderness, but the overlying skin is normal. At this stage, there is no radicular pain and no sign of pyramidal tract involvement. Either of the two latter findings suggests a spinal epidural abscess, a dreaded complication of vertebral osteomyelitis calling for immediate neuroradiologic evaluation, surgical decompression, and appropriate antibiotic therapy (see Spinal Epidural Abscess in Ch. 471).

Under exceptional circumstances, a patient with hematogenous osteomyelitis—usually of long bones—will present only with pain in the affected area, without fever. Radiographs show a punched-out lesion, without expansion beyond cortical bone. Without biopsy, it is difficult to differentiate such a lesion (Brodie's abscess) from benign or even malignant tumors.

Osteomyelitis secondary to a contiguous focus of infection after open trauma or secondary to orthopedic reconstructive surgery is a diagnostic challenge, since pain, low-grade fever, local signs of low-grade inflammation, and radiographic findings are compatible with both postoperative repair and infection. Recurrence of mild fever 1 week after surgery or trauma, increasing pain on weight bearing after total joint prosthetic replacement (Fig. 304–2), poor healing of the incision, and drainage of increased amounts of serosanguineous fluid should alert the physician to the possibility of ongoing infection.

DIAGNOSIS AND DIFFERENTIAL DIAGNOSIS. In hematogenous osteomyelitis, blood cultures are positive in about 25 to 30 per cent of cases, yielding most frequently *S. aureus*. Positive cultures for *S. epidermidis* should not be discarded as

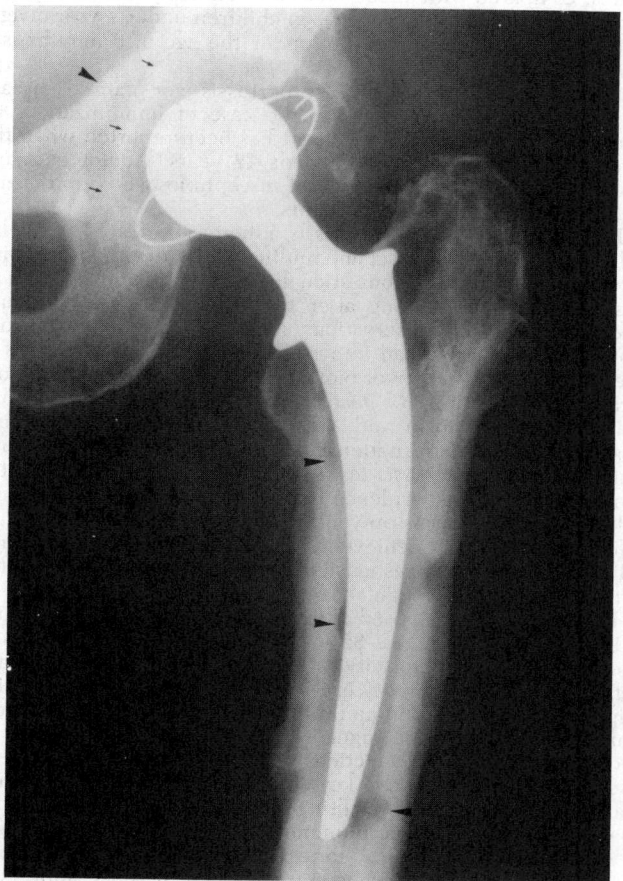

FIGURE 304–2. Osteomyelitis secondary to a contiguous focus of infection (*arrows*): infection after placement of a total hip prosthesis in a 63-year-old patient.

contaminants, but the organism should be further characterized as to sensitivity patterns, biotype, even plasmid contents, since this organism—often nosocomial—has become a common pathogen in bone infection. If the blood cultures remain negative, a direct aspiration and/or bone biopsy should be done for full microbiologic diagnosis. This is particularly true for vertebral osteomyelitis, which can be due to a great variety of microorganisms.

In osteomyelitis secondary to a focus of infection, the clinician is often tempted to perform a local superficial aspiration or to culture the fistulous tract for microbiologic diagnosis. Such cultures often yield multiple organisms, and it is often difficult to differentiate the pathogenic organisms from contaminants. Deep bone aspiration and/or biopsy is of greater value under these circumstances, and usually yields the offending organism in pure culture. For all cases of osteomyelitis, other laboratory tests are noncontributory: Erythrocyte sedimentation rate is usually increased; the white blood cell count is normal or high; and blood chemistry values are normal.

Radiologic changes are delayed, appearing several weeks after the onset of the disease. In hematogenous osteomyelitis of long bones, periosteal elevation and subsequent bone destruction are the first changes to be observed. In vertebral osteomyelitis, progressive piecemeal destruction of two adjacent vertebral plateaus, narrowing of the intervertebral space, and progressive anterior periosteal bridging are the hallmarks of the disease, bone sclerosis being a late event. All of these changes occur over several weeks. In tuberculous osteomyelitis of the spine, the changes just mentioned are delayed and occur over several months, periosteal reaction usually being absent.

In most cases of hematogenous osteomyelitis, ^{99m}Tc-pyrophosphate uptake, although nonspecific, can be of great diagnostic help by identifying the suspected areas of infection for appropriate tomograms at a stage when conventional radiographic results are still normal. In osteomyelitis secondary to a contiguous focus of infection, radiologic techniques and bone scanning are less helpful, since they cannot distinguish between normal bone reaction and infection. When detailed radiologic information is mandatory, such as in identifying an abscess in acute osteomyelitis, demonstrating sequestra in chronic osteomyelitis, or searching for a possible paraspinal abscess in vertebral body infection, CT scanning can offer additional diagnostic help. However, besides identifying such complications, this procedure has not been helpful in decreasing the delay in early diagnosis of osteomyelitis. In vertebral osteomyelitis, magnetic resonance imaging studies (MRI) have been particularly helpful in identifying infection and assessing its extension within and beyond osseous structures.

Acute hematogenous osteomyelitis of long bones must be differentiated clinically from septic arthritis, bursitis, and cellulitis. These more superficial infections are accompanied by local skin changes, and radiographic results remain normal. Osteomyelitis of the spine is a diagnostic challenge and has to be differentiated from bone tumors such as myeloma and metastases, which usually do not involve two adjacent vertebral plateaus. In case of doubt, bone biopsy is usually indicated.

TREATMENT. The therapeutic approach to osteomyelitis is both surgical and medical. For instance, although acute hematogenous osteomyelitis is usually treated medically, an orthopedic surgeon should be ready to intervene in case of abscess or sequestrum formation, pathologic fracture, etc. Conversely, osteomyelitis after total hip replacement will need surgical intervention for debridement, and possibly prosthetic replacement, under coverage of antibiotic therapy.

Appropriate medical treatment of osteomyelitis presupposes isolation of the offending organism and a complete assessment of its antibiotic sensitivities. In case of *S. aureus* sensitive to oxacillin, nafcillin should be used at a dosage of 1.5 grams to 2 grams every 4 hours parenterally. In case of an *S. aureus* or *S. epidermidis* resistant to oxacillin, vancomycin at a dosage of 1 gram given every 12 hours as a slow infusion is the treatment of choice. Dose adjustment is required for patients with renal dysfunction. For all other organisms, a similar rule can be applied: Those parenteral antibiotics usually effective for the treatment of septicemia due to a particular organism are also appropriate for osteomyelitis, provided that they are administered over a 4- to

6-week period. Thus, osteomyelitis of the spine caused by a gram-negative organism will be cured by a 4- to 6-week course of ampicillin, a first- or second-generation cephalosporin, an aminoglycoside, or a fluoroquinolone, depending on the sensitivity patterns. Bed rest is usually recommended until all signs of inflammation have abated, pain has subsided, and radiographs show signs of improvement. This is particularly true for osteomyelitis of the spine. Surgery is generally unnecessary in hematogenous infection, except for drainage of intramedullary abscesses, removal of sequestra, and decompression if neurologic signs supervene in vertebral osteomyelitis. In osteomyelitis secondary to a contiguous focus of infection, however, careful evaluation of the situation by a skilled orthopedic surgeon is mandatory. In case of infected fractures or prostheses, stable union is a prerequisite for bacteriologic cure. Union should be achieved first despite sepsis, and infection is controlled subsequently by antibiotic therapy after removal of the foreign material. In case of nonunion of a fracture or loosening of the prosthesis, the foreign material should be removed and, if possible, replaced by an external fixation device. Infected prostheses should also be removed and the infected focus cleaned out, with reinsertion of new material in a one-step or two-step procedure.

PREVENTION. At present, there is no preventive treatment available for hematogenous osteomyelitis, since the occurrence

of the disease after bacteremia is unpredictable. Infection rates after insertion of hip prostheses have been shown to be markedly decreased by short-term coverage (1 to 2 days) with parenteral antistaphylococcal antibiotics. Such coverage should also be considered in high-risk operations, such as reduction of comminuted fractures, open fractures, and insertion of joint prostheses in high-risk patients.

Kido D, Bryan D, Halpern M: Hematogenous osteomyelitis in drug addicts. Ther Nucl Med 118:356, 1973. *A concise study of 32 cases, most of them due to Pseudomonas species. Discusses their clinical and radiologic manifestations.*

Larde D, Mathieu D, Frija J, et al.: Vertebral osteomyelitis: Disk hypodensity on CT. AJR 139:963, 1982. *Thirty-six cases of vertebral osteomyelitis, investigated by CT scan for early diagnosis of complications.*

Norden CW (ed.): Osteomyelitis. Infect Dis Clin North Am 4:361, 1990. *A comprehensive, up-to-date monograph that focuses on epidemiologic, clinical, diagnostic, and therapeutic aspects of osteomyelitis (12 chapters).*

Waldvogel FA: Use of quinolones for the treatment of osteomyelitis and septic arthritis. Rev Infect Dis 11 (Suppl 5):S1259–1263, 1989.

Waldvogel FA, Medoff G, Swartz MN: Osteomyelitis: A review of clinical features, therapeutic considerations and unusual aspects I. II. III. N Engl J Med 282:198, 260, 316, 1970. *A retrospective review of 247 cases of osteomyelitis, their clinical and radiologic presentations, and their treatment.*

Waldvogel FA, Vasey H: Osteomyelitis: The past decade. N Engl J Med 303:360, 1980. *A review update of newer approaches in diagnosis and treatment of osteomyelitis, with emphasis on a combined surgical and medical approach.*

Wing VW, Jeffrey RB, Federle MP, et al.: Chronic osteomyelitis examined by CT. Radiology 154:171, 1985. *The additional information obtained by CT scanning in case of sequestra is well illustrated in 14 out of 25 patients with chronic osteomyelitis.*

Whooping Cough

305 Whooping Cough (Pertussis)

Richard B. Johnston, Jr.

DEFINITION. Whooping cough (synonym, pertussis) is a noninvasive, highly communicable bacterial respiratory illness. It occurs at all ages but is most common and most severe in infants and young children. The etiologic agent of the syndrome is usually *Bordetella pertussis*. The descriptive name derives from a distressing, prolonged inspiratory effort that follows paroxysmal coughing. Whooping cough is estimated to cause 600,000 to 1 million deaths yearly in infants from areas where pertussis immunization is not practiced.

ETIOLOGY. When first isolated, *Bordetella pertussis* is a small, nonmotile, weakly staining, gram-negative coccobacillus, 0.5 to 1.0 μm in length. Capsules can be demonstrated by special procedures, and bipolar metachromatic granules are present. The complex medium containing blood originally employed by Bordet and Gengou is still used (in modified form) for cultivation. *Primary isolates do not grow on conventional laboratory media.*

An estimated 5 to 10 per cent of clinical whooping cough is caused by *B. parapertussis*. The animal pathogen *B. bronchiseptica* is responsible for a minor percentage of cases. These organisms can be differentiated from *B. pertussis* by growth requirements, enzyme production, and presence of species-specific antigens. It has been suggested that adenoviruses, alone or in concert with *B. pertussis*, and *Chlamydia trachomatis* may play an etiologic role in some cases of whooping cough.

EPIDEMIOLOGY. In nonimmune households the attack rate is 80 to 90 per cent. Transmission is by droplet infection. Carriers of *B. pertussis* are found infrequently, but persons previously immunized have been shown during outbreaks of disease to excrete the organism in the absence of clinical symptoms or in the presence of mild or atypical illness.

The mortality rate from whooping cough has fallen since the beginning of the twentieth century owing to improved supportive therapy. The incidence of whooping cough, however, did not change until after the 1940's, when immunization of young children became standard practice. In the 1940's, approximately

200,000 cases of pertussis were reported annually in the United States, compared with about 4000 cases annually in recent years. Over 70 per cent of deaths occur in children under 1 year of age. The case fatality rate in infants under the age of 6 months is 1 per cent.

Neither immunization against pertussis nor natural disease provides lifelong protection. In the case of immunization, an attack rate greater than 50 per cent has been reported when the interval after immunization exceeds 12 years. Adolescents and adults represent a large reservoir of susceptibles who can transmit the disease to unimmunized infants.

PATHOGENESIS. *B. pertussis* adheres to ciliated epithelial cells of the respiratory tract and multiplies there without invading the tissues. Yet this colonization leads to profound changes in tissues which persist long after the responsible bacteria have been cleared. Such observations suggest that a toxin or toxins from the bacteria play an important part in the pathogenesis of the syndrome. A variety of biologic activities have been demonstrated by injecting *B. pertussis* products into experimental animals. An endotoxin and a heat-labile toxin that can cause tissue necrosis have been identified among these bacterial factors, but the exotoxin *pertussis toxin* (PT) is the best candidate at the moment for a major virulence factor. Immunization with chemically detoxified PT can prevent severe whooping cough with an efficacy similar to that achieved with the standard cellular vaccine. PT is believed to be responsible for the characteristic lymphocytosis of whooping cough.

PT is a protein composed of five noncovalently linked subunits (S1–S5). The subunits S2–S5 form a nontoxic unit that binds to the cell membrane; toxicity is mediated by the enzymatically active subunit, S1. Activity of S1 inhibits a subclass of guanosine triphosphate (GTP)–binding proteins (G proteins) that are essential for transmembrane signaling and, thus, certain types of receptor-mediated cell functions. Genetic engineering has been used to replace one or two key amino acids within the enzymatically active S1 subunit, resulting in a stable nontoxic form of PT that can be used as a safe immunogen.

Adherence of *B. pertussis* to respiratory epithelium is required for the pathogenesis of whooping cough. Adherence appears to involve a bacterial outer membrane protein with a molecular weight of 69 kilodaltons, termed 69kD outer membrane protein (OMP), P69, or pertactin. An antigenically similar protein exists on *B. parapertussis* and *B. bronchiseptica*. Injection of this protein into mice or humans elicits agglutinating antibody to *B. pertussis* and protects the mice against lethal *B. pertussis* respiratory challenge. Synthesis of 69kD OMP is controlled by a regulatory gene at the *vir* (virulence) locus, which modulates synthesis of PT and additional factors that may contribute to pathogenesis, including filamentous hemagglutinin.

PATHOLOGY. Lesions caused by *B. pertussis* are found principally in the bronchi and bronchioles, but changes are also seen in the nasopharynx, larynx, and trachea. Masses of bacteria and mucopurulent exudate are intertwined with the cilia of the columnar epithelium. There is necrosis of the midzonal and basilar epithelium with infiltration of polymorphonuclear leukocytes and macrophages. The most frequent findings in the lung are bronchopneumonia, interstitial pneumonitis, and numerous small areas of atelectasis. The brain can show edema and scattered petechiae at autopsy.

CLINICAL MANIFESTATIONS. The incubation period lasts 7 to 14 days (rarely over 2 weeks). It is customary to divide the clinical course into three stages.

Catarrhal Stage. Whooping cough begins with symptoms indistinguishable from those of a mild viral upper respiratory infection. Sneezing is frequent, conjunctivae are injected, and a nocturnal cough appears. The temperature may be slightly elevated. Infectivity is greatest at this stage.

Paroxysmal Stage. Seven to 14 days after onset, the cough becomes more frequent, then paroxysmal. In a typical paroxysm there is a series of 15 to 20 short coughs of increasing intensity, and then a deep inspiration, making the "whoop." A tenacious mucous plug is usually expelled, and vomiting frequently follows. Paroxysms may occur as often as every half hour and are accompanied by signs of increased venous pressure, including deeply engorged conjunctivae, periorbital edema, petechial hemorrhages, particularly about the forehead, and epistaxis. During the attack the infant may be cyanotic until the crowing whoop occurs. Between paroxysms the child usually feels well, although justifiably apprehensive. This phase lasts 2 to 4 weeks.

Physical examination of the chest is often unremarkable except for scattered rhonchi. The chest roentgenogram sometimes reveals hilar and mediastinal nodal enlargement. The presence of fever should immediately suggest the development of a secondary infectious process.

Convalescent Stage. The paroxysms gradually become less frequent and less intense; vomiting ceases, and slow recovery ensues. Convalescence requires 4 to 12 weeks. For many months even a mild, unrelated respiratory infection can induce a return of paroxysmal cough and whoop.

In infants less than 6 months old the paroxysms and the whoop are often absent; choking spells and apneic episodes may be the major manifestations. Second attacks of whooping cough as well as disease occurring in previously immunized individuals often present simply as an upper respiratory illness or bronchitis.

Complications. Recurrent vomiting can lead to metabolic alkalosis or malnutrition. Central nervous system changes can result from cerebral anoxia or hemorrhages consequent to the elevated venous pressure. Rarely, cortical degeneration occurs, but the exact pathogenesis of the encephalopathy is unknown. A serous meningitis with lymphocytosis of the cerebrospinal fluid has been described. Pneumothorax and interstitial emphysema are infrequently seen. Secondary bacterial otitis media occurs frequently. The major cause of death in whooping cough is pneumonia, either primary or caused by other bacteria or viruses.

DIAGNOSIS. There is little difficulty in making the clinical diagnosis of whooping cough in a patient who, after a period of coryzal symptoms, develops paroxysmal coughing with a terminal inspiratory whoop. Lymphocytosis often occurs toward the end of the catarrhal stage or early in the spasmodic phase. Characteristically the leukocyte count ranges from 15,000 to 30,000 per microliter or higher, and 80 per cent of the cells are small lymphocytes. Polymorphonuclear leukocytosis suggests a secondary bacterial complication.

Microbiologic identification of the organisms may be required to make the diagnosis in abortive or mild cases or in young infants. During the early stages *B. pertussis* can be isolated from approximately 90 per cent of patients. By the third or fourth week the organism can be recovered in only 50 per cent of cases, and in the convalescent stage it is unusual to obtain a positive culture.

Specimens for culture are best obtained by pernasal swab rather than by the cough plate method. A sterile cotton swab wrapped about a flexible copper wire is passed through the nares, and mucus is obtained from the posterior pharynx. *B. pertussis* is readily killed by desiccation, so the specimen should be quickly plated onto fresh medium, to which penicillin has been added to prevent overgrowth of adventitious organisms.

A fluorescent antibody staining procedure can be applied directly to clinical specimens or organisms grown in culture. It greatly accelerates the identification of cultured organisms after isolation but is less reliable with nasopharyngeal swabs or other clinical material.

Serologic procedures are of little help in the diagnosis of whooping cough because a rise in titer of most antibodies does not occur until at least the third week of illness. Tests are not well standardized, and few laboratories perform them.

TREATMENT. *Supportive Therapy.* Young infants, particularly those under 6 months of age, should be hospitalized. Supportive measures combined with careful nursing care are of paramount importance. Specific attention must be devoted to the maintenance of proper water and electrolyte balance, adequate nutrition, and sufficient oxygenation. Constant alertness for the presence of secondary infectious complications such as pneumonia is required. Mild cases require only supportive treatment.

Antimicrobials. Specific therapy of severe whooping cough has been disappointing despite the in vitro susceptibility of *B. pertussis* to various antimicrobial agents. Antimicrobials given in the catarrhal stage may ameliorate the disease. In the established paroxysmal stage the organisms can be readily eliminated by antimicrobials, but the course of the illness is unaltered. Antibiotics may be justified in order to render the patient noninfectious. Erythromycin is the drug of choice. The daily dose is 50 mg per kilogram of body weight given in four divided doses. The organism is eliminated after a few days of therapy, but because bacteriologic relapse may occur, treatment should be continued for 14 to 21 days. Trimethoprim-sulfamethoxazole (8 mg per kilogram and 40 mg per kilogram per day in two doses) is a possible alternative for patients who do not tolerate erythromycin.

PREVENTION. Unfortunately, the diagnosis is usually not made until the end of the catarrhal stage, and by then spread of the disease has already occurred. Exposed susceptibles should receive erythromycin prophylaxis, and close (household, daycare, classroom) contacts under 7 years of age who have been previously immunized should receive a booster dose of vaccine in addition to erythromycin. Booster doses of vaccine have been used to protect adults, such as hospital staff, but side effects tend to be frequent, and erythromycin chemoprophylaxis may be preferable.

Active Immunization. Women of childbearing age generally do not have significant levels of protective antibody in their sera, and most newborns have received no passive protection. Consequently, active immunization is begun as early as is practicable. At present, it is recommended that the infant receive three injections of pertussis vaccine (inactive *B. pertussis* organisms) at 8-week intervals commencing at age 2 months. The pertussis suspension is mixed with alum-precipitated diphtheria and tetanus toxoids (DTP). A fourth injection is given 6 to 12 months after the third dose (15 to 18 months of age), and a booster is given before entering kindergarten. Administration of pertussis vaccine to those over 6 years of age is not generally recommended because of an apparent increased incidence of untoward reactions and the diminished risk of the illness itself in the older child. However, low doses have been administered to adults without incident.

As previously noted, immunization does not confer lifelong protection. Approximately 80 per cent of those vaccinated within 4 years of exposure are protected, whereas 80 to 90 per cent of a matched unimmunized group with similar exposure contract pertussis. The prophylactic efficacy of pertussis vaccine was clearly demonstrated when epidemics occurred in the United Kingdom in 1977–79 and 1982 following a 3- to 5-year period during which vaccine acceptance had declined to very low levels. More than 170,000 cases of whooping cough were reported, including 42 deaths, principally among children under 5 years of age. Similar outbreaks have followed diminished vaccine utilization in Japan and Sweden.

Reactions at the injection site as well as fever and hyperirritability occur commonly after injection of pertussis vaccine. The incidence of postinjection encephalopathy is uncertain, and it is not clear whether the vaccine can cause permanent neurologic damage. A recent British study suggests a risk of 1 in 140,000 immunizations for previously normal infants, with residual neurologic damage in 1 in 330,000 immunizations. This estimated risk of neurologic complications from pertussis immunization is far less than the hazards of whooping cough in the young child. Nevertheless, in infants with a personal history of convulsions or other neurologic disorders, pertussis immunization should be deferred until the condition has stabilized. Acellular vaccines containing various combinations of pertussis toxin, 69kD OMP, filamentous hemagglutinin, or other *B. pertussis* products are being studied. Acellular vaccines cause far fewer reactions than does the whole bacterial cell vaccine. If tests currently under way of their immunogenicity and prophylactic efficacy are convincing in field use, acellular vaccines should replace the killed whole-cell vaccine.

Geller RJ: The pertussis syndrome: A persistent problem. Pediatr Infect Dis J 3:182, 1984. *A succinct state-of-the-art presentation of diagnosis, clinical picture, and management.*

Griffin MR, Ray WA, Mortimer EA, et al.: Risk of seizures and encephalopathy after immunization with the diphtheria-tetanus-pertussis vaccine. JAMA 263:1641, 1990. *A careful (and unrevealing) search for neurologic sequelae associated with DTP immunization. Accompanying editorial, p. 1679.*

Manclark CR (ed.): Proceedings of the Sixth International Symposium on Pertussis. Department of Health and Human Services, United States Public Health Service, Bethesda, Md. DHHS Publication No. (FDA) 90-1164, 1990. *Comprises a review of recent research on virulence factors, surface proteins, host-parasite interactions, genetic regulation of virulence factors, epidemiology, diagnosis, and clinical aspects.*

Pittman M: The concept of pertussis as a toxin-mediated disease. Pediatr Infect Dis J 3:467, 1984. *A thorough review of pathogenesis, immunity, and immunization.*

Wardlaw AC, Parton R (eds.): Pathogenesis and Immunity in Pertussis. New York, John Wiley and Sons, 1988. *A superb source of current information on clinical and microbiologic aspects of whooping cough and on pertussis vaccines.*

Diphtheria

306 Diphtheria

Erik L. Hewlett

Diphtheria is an acute, toxin-mediated infectious disease caused by toxigenic *Corynebacterium diphtheriae*. Classically, the infection usually localizes to the pharynx, larynx, and nostrils, with skin infection representing an increasing proportion of cases in developed nations. Severe systemic disease and mortality occur most frequently in patients with pharyngeal infection and are largely attributable to an exotoxin released by the bacteria at the site of localized infection. The disease, but not necessarily the local infection, is preventable by immunization with diphtheria toxoid.

ETIOLOGY. *C. diphtheriae* is a pleomorphic, non–spore-forming, non–acid-fast, nonmotile gram-positive rod that on smears is often seen in palisades or configurations resembling Chinese characters. Its club-end appearance is the origin of the name *Corynebacterium*, from the Greek "korynee," meaning club. The heterogeneous morphology of corynebacteria makes diagnosis on the basis of stained smear unreliable. *C. diphtheriae* grows well on tellurite agar or Loeffler's serum slants under aerobic conditions and is distinguished from related corynebacteria by fermentation of glucose and maltose but not sucrose. Although the organisms are killed by mild heating (56°C for 10 minutes), they are strikingly resistant to damage from drying and can be cultured from floor dust for 5 weeks or longer.

The species is divided into three stable biotypes, named *gravis*, *intermedius*, and *mitis*, to indicate their relative virulence in epidemics during the early twentieth century. Although biotypes are still used to characterize strains, there is not a direct correlation between biotype and severity of disease. In fact, the *intermedius* biotype is most frequently toxigenic (98.9 per cent), followed by *gravis* (84.0 per cent) and *mitis* (34.1 per cent). Recently, DNA hybridization, using an insertion sequence probe, has enabled identification and epidemiologic tracking of strains in a population.

The major virulence determinant is an exotoxin that is produced by organisms infected by a lysogenic β-phage. The toxin structural gene is carried in the genome of the phage, and toxin is produced by lysogenized *C. diphtheriae* only after depletion of the iron in the medium. Toxigenicity of an isolate can be determined in vitro by ELISA or by the Elek test, in which the clinical isolate is streaked at right angles to an antitoxin-impregnated strip of filter paper on a plate. If the strain is toxigenic, a precipitin line of toxin-antitoxin complex forms during culture. Toxigenicity testing in vivo involves intraperitoneal injection of a suspension of organisms into naive and antitoxin-treated guinea pigs. Death of the test animal, but not the antitoxin recipient, in 1 to 4 days indicates toxin production.

EPIDEMIOLOGY. Diphtheria is a highly contagious infection that is spread most easily under socioeconomic conditions in which there is poor personal hygiene, crowding, and limited access to medical care. The primary route of transmission has been by aerosol or other transfer of respiratory secretions from an infected individual. As illustrated by several outbreaks among adults in the United States, however, spread from cutaneous lesions of subjects with little or no systemic disease by direct contact or by fomites (such as unclean blankets) is of increasing importance epidemiologically. The skin infections of these carriers may occur in many different forms, such as purulent punched-out ulcers, impetiginous lesions, and wound infections. As a result, it is often difficult to make the diagnosis of diphtheria without classic symptoms in their contacts. Furthermore, the diagnosis may be missed because of the presence of a mixed infection with staphylococci or streptococci. Such localized infections with limited toxin absorption are postulated to be the source of acquired immunity among nonimmunized children in the tropics. Although infections of animals, especially cattle, can be the source of human disease, this is an uncommon mechanism of transmission and there are no known reservoirs in nature. Molecular epidemiologic studies indicate that among toxigenic strains, some may be more virulent than others, and severe disease results from transmission of more virulent strains in a population.

Immunization status influences susceptibility to infection and severity of disease in the individual patient. When disease does occur in immunized or partially immunized patients, mortality (1.3 per cent) is 10-fold lower than in nonimmunized individuals (13.4 per cent). Herd immunity has a major impact on patterns of transmission and carriage of *C. diphtheriae*. Although it was expected by some that immunization with diphtheria toxoid would increase the rate of carriage of *C. diphtheriae* in a population, the opposite is true. The selective advantage of toxigenicity is lost, and fewer toxigenic strains are found in an immunized population. Serologic surveys indicate a high proportion of susceptible adults in many populations. Although clinical diphtheria is at its lowest level ever, with no cases reported in the United States in 1986, the potential exists for disease in the setting of unrecognized exposure.

PATHOGENESIS. Following arrival of *C. diphtheriae* at the site of infection, organisms proliferate and elaborate toxin. As with other bacterial diseases that are mediated in large part by exotoxins, the rapidity of onset, severity of disease, and ultimate outcome are determined by the rate of production, absorption, and dissemination of the toxin. The determinants of these variables include the site of infection, the virulence of the strain (quantity of toxin produced and availability of ancillary factors to facilitate toxin absorption), and the status of host immunity. For example, individuals with *C. diphtheriae* infection of the skin, middle ear, or anterior nares—sites from which toxin absorption is less than across the pharyngeal mucosa—may have little or no systemic disease. Prior immunity, by virtue of immunization or prior infection, may prevent systemic manifestations of disease without affecting the localized carriage of the organism.

Diphtheria toxin, among the best studied of all bacterial toxins, is synthesized as an inactive single polypeptide of 61,000 molecular weight. It is activated by proteolytic cleavage and reduction of the interchain disulfide bonds, yielding two subunits (A or active subunit and B or binding subunit). Upon reaching the host cell, the B subunit attaches to a specific glycoprotein receptor, a step that is required for internalization by receptor-mediated endocytosis. Within mammalian cells, the A subunit catalyzes the transfer of the adenosine diphosphate ribose (ADPR) portion of nicotinamide adenine dinucleotide (NAD) to a specific target amino acid (modified histidine named diphthamide because of this reaction) on a single protein, elongation factor 2, which is required for protein synthesis. The consequence to the cell is interruption of protein synthesis, disruption of cell processes requiring new proteins, and, ultimately, cell death. The consequences to the infected host depend upon the types of cells intoxicated and the extent of intoxication.

CLINICAL MANIFESTATIONS. The manifestations of infection with *C. diphtheriae* can range from a single, localized lesion without systemic signs or symptoms to a rapidly progressive, fatal illness. In general, the severity of the disease is correlated with the magnitude and site of the local lesion, and, in fact, the different clinical presentations have been classified on the basis of the primary site of infection.

Symptoms begin after an incubation period of less than 1 week. Patients with cutaneous, anterior nasal, or middle ear infection with *C. diphtheriae* are generally well, with little or no local pain and often only purulent drainage from the involved site. Occasionally, a thin membrane with associated crusting can be seen. Because of the infrequent occurrence of systemic toxicity, these lesions can become chronic, providing a source for transmission to contacts. This presentation is now the predominant one in developed countries.

Tonsillar or faucial diphtheria, although not frequently life-threatening, can be associated with severe complications. At the time of presentation, patients are moderately ill, with complaints of low-grade fever, fatigue, headache, and sore throat. The typical adherent, grayish green membrane may be localized to one tonsil or may extend across the midline and anteriorly. Such patients have the potential for abrupt deterioration and warrant close observation.

Pharyngeal diphtheria, especially associated with laryngeal and bronchial extension, represents an extreme in the spectrum of clinical presentations. The patient is gravely ill with weak pulse, restlessness, and confusion, but at the same time may be afebrile. The diphtheritic membrane may be extensive, covering the posterior pharynx and extending upward into the nasopharynx, forward onto the hard palate, and downward through the larynx. The thick, partially necrotic membrane is difficult to remove and is the source of the classic, but not diagnostic, foul odor associated with this disease. Development of anterior cervical warmth and edema resulting in the "bull neck" appearance is not uncommon in extensive pharyngeal disease. Patients in whom the membrane extends to the larynx and beyond experience airway obstruction with stridor and cyanosis.

Clinical diphtheria may be associated with dysfunction of a variety of tissues, especially heart and nerve, and these complications are the major cause of morbidity and mortality. Myocarditis, for example, occurs in 50 per cent of patients with moderately severe disease, apparently as a result of direct toxin action on myocardial cells and perhaps subsequent inflammation and fibrosis. The onset may be slow, with manifestations after the local pharyngeal lesion is improving. There are concurrent abnormalities of the cardiac conducting system, as indicated by electrocardiographic (ECG) abnormalities such as ST-T wave changes, arrhythmias, and heart block. The rapid onset of ECG changes, circulatory collapse, and congestive heart failure indi-

cates a high level of systemic intoxication and a very poor prognosis.

Functionally significant intoxication of neural tissue occurs in 10 to 20 per cent of patients and is manifested by cranial nerve palsies, peripheral neuropathies, and frank paralysis. Patients may experience difficulty swallowing, with regurgitation and aspiration of liquids, extremity weakness, and even respiratory failure. These deficits may be first recognized 4 or more weeks after onset of the illness, but, if the patient survives, are generally slowly reversible.

DIAGNOSIS. Although bacteriologic identification is a critical feature of diphtheria diagnosis, therapy for this life-threatening illness must not await culture confirmation. Gram-stained or fluorescent antibody–stained material can be used to increase the index of suspicion but is not adequate for definitive diagnosis. Swabs from nose and pharynx or other sites should be cultured on Loeffler's slants and the more selective tellurite agar as well as blood agar. All clinical isolates of *C. diphtheriae* should be tested for toxigenicity by ELISA or Elek test. Since coinfection with staphylococci and streptococci can occur, the presence of these organisms does not rule out diphtheria.

In milder cases, the diphtheritic membrane may not be striking and other physical findings are not distinguishing. Although the sore throat is generally less than with a streptococcal infection, the differential diagnosis should include streptococcal pharyngitis, oral candidiasis, infectious mononucleosis, and Vincent's angina.

TREATMENT AND PREVENTION. The goals of therapy in a patient with presumed or documented diphtheria are neutralization of free toxin, elimination of further toxin production, control of the local infection, support during the course of the systemic intoxication phase, and prevention of transmission. The mainstays of treatment, therefore, are (1) equine diphtheria antitoxin (human diphtheria immune globulin is not available in the United States), (2) antibiotics, (3) supportive intervention directed at complications such as respiratory compromise, congestive heart failure, cardiac arrhythmias, neuropathies, renal failure, and bleeding diatheses, and (4) strict isolation.

Presumptive diagnosis of diphtheria is adequate justification for use of diphtheria antitoxin, since the severe life-threatening complications are the result of toxin action at distal sites and immediate neutralization of circulating toxin is essential. The dose of antitoxin is based upon the site and extent of local infection and the severity and duration of symptoms at the time of presentation. Patients with cutaneous infection generally do not experience toxicity, but a low dose of antitoxin (20,000 units) is sometimes given. A dose of 20,000 to 40,000 units of antitoxin is recommended for patients with limited pharyngeal disease of 2 days' or less duration. Patients with more extensive nasopharyngeal involvement, especially of greater than 3 days' duration and associated with bull neck and other complications, require 80,000 to 100,000 units of antitoxin. The antitoxin is most effective when given intravenously, but because it is of equine origin, patients must be tested for hypersensitivity before administration and desensitized as necessary.

Antibiotics are required for prevention of further toxin production, control of local infection, and reduction of transmission, as untreated convalescent carriage can persist for weeks. Treatment with penicillin or erythromycin should be followed by repeat culture to document elimination of the organism because resistance to erythromycin has been observed. Since the consequences of toxin action within target cells cannot be reversed pharmacologically, patients with life-threatening complications need intensive monitoring and specific supportive therapy as indicated. For example, myocarditis with arrhythmias and congestive heart failure may necessitate salt restriction, digitalis, antiarrhythmics, and even temporary pacing during the height of illness. As with other toxin-mediated diseases, there may not be a sufficient immune response to provide future protection, and convalescent individuals should receive diphtheria toxoid immunization.

All contacts should be cultured. Those immunized 5 or more years previously should receive a booster, and those never immunized should be treated prophylactically with antibiotics. All asymptomatic carriers should be treated with antibiotics to eliminate the organism and immunized with either a primary series or booster as indicated.

The only effective measure for prevention of clinical diphtheria is immunization with diphtheria toxoid. The primary series is three doses given in conjunction with tetanus toxoid and pertussis vaccine during the first 6 months of life. Boosters are given at 15 months and 4 to 6 years of age. In order to maintain immunity during adolescence and adulthood, boosters are needed at 10-year intervals using a preparation containing a reduced amount of the diphtheria toxoid, owing to adverse reactions related to some prior immunity. The reduced dose for adults is available alone or in combination with tetanus toxoid (Td).

Although not commonly determined at the present time except as an epidemiologic research tool, susceptibility of an individual to clinical diphtheria can be assessed by quantitation in vitro of toxin-neutralizing antibody in the serum or by the Schick test, which involves injection of a low dose of native diphtheria toxin intradermally and observation for evidence of local toxin damage (redness, edema at 48 to 96 hours). A positive reaction indicates lack of neutralizing antibody and susceptibility to disease.

Björkholm B, Böttiger M, Christenson B, et al.: Antitoxin antibody levels and the outcome of illness during an outbreak of diphtheria among alcoholics. Scand J Infect Dis 18:235, 1986. *Illustration of the reduced level of immunity in adult population and significance of "protective" antibody levels.*

Dixon JMS, Noble WC, Smith GR: Diphtheria; other corynebacterial and coryneform infections. In Smith GR, Easmon CSF (eds.): Topley and Wilson's Principles of Bacteriology, Virology and Immunity. 8th ed. Vol. 3. London, Edward Arnold, 1990, pp 55–79. *Useful compilation of microbiologic and epidemiologic data.*

Harnisch JP, Tronca E, Nolan CM, et al.: Diphtheria among alcoholic urban adults. A decade of experience in Seattle. Ann Intern Med 111:71, 1989. *Extensive summary of diphtheria in the United States in the last 20 years.*

Hewlett EL: Selective primary health care: Strategies for control of disease in the developing world. XVIII. Pertussis and diphtheria. Rev Infect Dis 7:426, 1985. *Review of approaches to control of diphtheria, compared and contrasted with pertussis.*

Pappenheimer AM: Diphtheria: Studies on the biology of an infectious disease. The Harvey Lectures, Series 76. New York, Academic Press, 1982, pp 45–73. *Detailed description of the cellular and molecular biology of toxin structure and function.*

Rappuoli R, Perugini M, Falson E: Molecular epidemiology of the 1984–1986 outbreak of diphtheria in Sweden. N Engl J Med 318:12–14, 1988. *Demonstration of the utility of a molecular probe and the concept of alternative virulence factors it raises.*

Clostridial Diseases

John G. Bartlett

307 Clostridial Myonecrosis and Other Clostridial Diseases

Clostridia are gram-positive, spore-forming anaerobic bacteria that are widely distributed in soil and in the normal intestinal microflora of humans and animals. Sporulation permits survival in adverse conditions so that these organisms can be isolated with ease from almost any environmental source. Concentrations vary considerably, but any fertile loam is expected to contain at least 10^3 clostridia per gram. Clostridia have been found in the intestinal tract of almost all animals examined. Most humans harbor 10^9 to 10^{10} clostridia per gram of stool; these organisms are less commonly found in the normal flora of the skin, oral cavity, and female genital tract. *Clostridium perfringens*, the most frequent clinical isolate, is found in virtually all soil samples and, along with *C. ramosum*, is the most frequent clostridial species found in the intestinal flora of humans. Nevertheless, there are over 60 recognized species, and about 30 species have been found in human infections. Most clinical laboratories do not perform the extensive biochemical testing necessary to speciate clostridial isolates, and even when this is done, many organisms do not fit current taxonomic schema.

Clostridia cause diverse disease processes including bacteremia, localized infections at various anatomic sites, and the histotoxic clostridial syndromes. The latter refer to diseases caused by toxins elaborated under appropriate cultural conditions by specific clostridial species (Table 307–1). The most commonly encountered histotoxic species is *C. perfringens*, which is divided into five types designated A to E on the basis of the production of the four major lethal toxins designated alpha, beta, epsilon, and iota. All *C. perfringens*, and many other species of clostridia (Table 307–1), produce alpha toxin, a phospholipase that splits lecithin to phosphoryl choline and a diglyceride. Intravenous administration of alpha toxin in experimental animals causes massive hemolysis, platelet destruction, and widespread capillary damage. Other clostridial toxins cause diseases of the intestine (enteric toxins) or of the nervous system (neurotoxins). The toxins of *C. botulinum* and *C. tetanus* are lethal to mice in doses of 1 ng. By extrapolation, the lethal dose in the bloodstream of humans is approximately 10^{-9} mg per kilogram body weight, making these toxins the most potent microbial poisons known. The toxins of

C. difficile and the alpha toxin of *C. perfringens* are about 100 to 1000 times less potent in mouse lethality testing.

Smith LDS: The Pathogenic Anaerobic Bacteria, 2nd ed. Springfield, IL, Charles C Thomas, 1975, pp 109–324. *The author, a noted authority in the field, provides a scholarly review of clostridia, including a description of the species, their natural habitat, their toxins, and their role in disease.*

CLOSTRIDIAL MYONECROSIS

DEFINITION. Clostridial myonecrosis, or gas gangrene, is a life-threatening infection involving muscle caused by toxins produced by clostridia, usually *C. perfringens*.

ETIOLOGY. Clostridial myonecrosis usually follows wounding from trauma or surgery, contamination with histotoxic clostridia, and toxin elaboration. It is estimated that 30 to 80 per cent of serious, traumatic, open wounds are contaminated by clostridia, although gas gangrene remains a relatively rare infection. This experience emphasizes the decisive role of local conditions that promote toxin production primarily by decreasing the oxidation-reduction potential. Contributing factors to tissue hypoxia include vascular insufficiency, the presence of foreign bodies, tissue necrosis, and concurrent infection involving other microbes.

The most frequent pathogen, *C. perfringens*, is found in approximately 80 per cent of cases with positive cultures. Other clostridial species implicated include *C. novyi*, *C. septicum*, *C. histolyticum*, *C. bifermentans*, and *C. fallax*. In many instances, there are several clostridial species isolated from the infected site. Species causing gas gangrene produce over 20 exotoxins,

TABLE 307–1. HISTOTOXIC CLOSTRIDIAL SYNDROMES

Disease	Agent	Toxin
Enteric diseases		
Food poisoning	*C. perfringens*, type A	Enterotoxin
Antibiotic-induced diarrhea or colitis	*C. difficile*	Toxins A and B
Enteritis necroticans	*C. perfringens*, type C	Beta toxin
Neurologic syndromes		
Botulism	*C. botulinum*	Botulinal toxins A, B, E, F, and G
Tetanus	*C. tetanus*	Tetanospasmin
Myonecrosis (gas gangrene)	*C. perfringens*, *C. novyi*, *C. septicum*, *C. histolyticum*, *C. bifermentans*, *C. fallax*	Multiple toxins, especially alpha toxin

including seven that are lethal to experimental animals. In appropriate environmental conditions, vegetative forms of the histotoxic clostridia replicate and elaborate toxins that diffuse into adjacent soft tisssue to promote local spread as well as extensive systemic effects.

CLINICAL MANIFESTATIONS. Gas gangrene is a devastating infection characterized by prominent findings at the site of injury and profound systemic toxicity. Most cases occur in association with wounding from trauma or surgery. The usual clinical settings are (1) traumatic injury or penetrating wound; (2) surgery, especially intestinal or biliary tract operations; (3) uterine gas gangrene, which most frequently follows delivery or septic abortions; (4) soft tissue lesions associated with vascular insufficiency; (5) intestinal gas gangrene, which is most commonly found in compromised hosts, especially patients with leukemia or colonic carcinoma; and (6) "spontaneous gas gangrene," a rare form of the disease in which there is no readily identifiable predisposing condition. During peacetime in the United States approximately 50 per cent of cases follow severe traumatic injury and 40 per cent follow surgery. The most frequent traumatic injuries are car accidents, crush injuries, industrial accidents, and gunshot wounds. The most frequent antecedent surgical procedures are colon resection and biliary tract surgery. About two thirds of cases involve extremities, and one third involve the abdominal wall.

The usual incubation period from the time of wounding to the onset of symptoms is 1 to 4 days, with a range of 8 hours to several weeks. The first symptom is usually sudden and severe pain at the site of injury. Observations at this time typically show tense edema and tenderness. Gas may be noted in the soft tissues by palpation, radiography, computed tomography, or ultrasound studies. The skin is initially pale and then progresses to a magenta or bronze discoloration, and there is often cutaneous necrosis with hemorrhagic bullae. As the lesion evolves, there may be a thin, serosanguineous discharge with characteristic sweet odor. The systemic findings that accompany the evolving changes at

the wound are profound. These include diaphoresis, low-grade fever, and tachycardia. Common complications include hemolytic anemia, hypotension, and renal failure. The patient is typically anxious throughout the disease but remains alert despite profound systemic toxicity.

DIAGNOSIS. The diagnosis of clostridial myonecrosis is based on a constellation of clinical findings and supporting microbiologic data. Roentgenographic studies often show gas bubbles in the soft tissue, computed tomography shows gas and myonecrosis, and Gram's stains of discharge typically show large, gram-positive or gram-variable bacilli with blunt ends and a paucity of polymorphonuclear leukocytes. Approximately 15 per cent of patients have clostridial bacteremia. Nevertheless, the findings of Gram's stain and the detection of gas in the soft tissue cannot be considered specific, and most patients with clostridial bacteremia do not have myonecrosis. The definitive diagnostic procedure is surgical incision to expose muscle that may appear pale and edematous, beefy-red, or, in the most advanced stages, black and friable. The muscle is nonviable, it fails to contract with stimulation, and the cut surface does not bleed.

The differential diagnosis includes a number of soft tissue infections that may also involve clostridia, or occur in association with severe systemic toxicity, tissue necrosis, a fulminant course, or gas formation. Important findings in the differential diagnosis are summarized in Table 307–2. This classification includes two anatomic patterns: infections involving the enveloping fascia and infections within the fascial compartment. The latter category includes infections associated with myonecrosis which are classified by microbiologic pattern as streptococcal myonecrosis, synergistic necrotizing cellulitis due to mixtures of aerobic and anaerobic bacteria, and gas gangrene. None of these infections is common, but all require aggressive treatment including early surgical intervention. Clinical clues suggesting these devastating conditions include severe systemic toxicity, severe pain that is

TABLE 307–2. DEEP AND SERIOUS SOFT TISSUE INFECTIONS

	Gas-Forming Cellulitis	Synergistic Necrotizing Cellulitis	Gas Gangrene	"Streptococcal" Myonecrosis	Necrotizing Fasciitis	Infected Vascular Gangrene	Streptococcal Gangrene
Predisposing conditions	Traumatic	Diabetes, prior local lesion, perirectal lesion	Traumatic or surgical wound	Trauma, surgery	Diabetes, trauma, surgery, perineal infection	Arterial insufficiency	Traumatic or surgical wound
Incubation period	>3 days	3–14 days	1–4 days	3–4 days	1–4 days	>5 days	6 hours–2 days
Etiologic organism(s)	Clostridia, others	Mixed aerobic-anaerobic flora	Clostridia, esp. *C. perfringens*	Anaerobic streptococci	Mixed aerobic-anaerobic flora	Mixed aerobic-anaerobic flora	*S. pyogenes*
Systemic toxicity	Minimal	Moderate to severe	Severe	Minimal until late in course	Moderate to severe	Minimal	Severe
Course	Gradual	Acute	Acute	Subacute	Acute or subacute	Subacute	Acute
Wound findings							
Local pain	Minimal	Moderate to severe	Severe	Late only	Minimal to moderate	Variable	Severe
Skin appearance	Swollen, minimal discoloration	Erythematous or gangrenous	Tense and blanched, yellow-bronze, necrosis with hemorrhagic bullae	Erythema or yellow-bronze	Blanched, erythema, necrosis with hemorrhagic bullae	Erythema or necrosis	Erythema, necrosis
Gas	Abundant	Variable	Usually present	Variable	Variable	Variable	No
Muscle involvement	No	Variable	Myonecrosis	Myonecrosis	No	Myonecrosis limited to area of vascular insufficiency	No
Discharge	Thin, dark, sweetish or foul odor	Dark pus or "dishwater," putrid	Serosanguineous, sweet or foul odor	Seropurulent	Seropurulent or "dishwater," putrid	Minimal	None or serosanguineous, no odor
Gram stain	PMN's, gram-positive bacilli	PMN's, mixed flora	Sparse PMN's, gram-positive bacilli	PMN's, gram-positive cocci	PMN's, mixed flora	PMN's, mixed flora	PMN's, gram-positive cocci in chains
Surgical therapy	Debridement	Wide filleting incisions	Extensive excision, amputation	Excision of necrotic muscle	Wide filleting incisions	Amputation	Debridement of necrotic tissue

spontaneous (tenderness suggests a more superficial infection such as cellulitis), bullae, gas in the soft tissue, and rapid extension. Computed tomography or magnetic resonance imaging often demonstrates the tissue plane of involvement, and deep aspirates and blood cultures may reveal microbiologic patterns. However, surgery provides a definitive diagnosis.

TREATMENT. The most important facet of treatment is extensive surgical debridement with wide excision of involved muscle, amputation when an extremity is involved, or hysterectomy with uterine gas gangrene. The preferred antibiotic is aqueous penicillin G given intravenously in doses of 10 to 40 million units daily for adults. Alternative antimicrobial agents include intravenous metronidazole (2 grams per day), chloramphenicol (2 grams per day), or clindamycin (1800 mg per day). Cephalosporins are generally less active against clostridia. The therapeutic value of hyperbaric oxygen is controversial. Advocates claim that this clearly demarcates the necrotic tissue to simplify surgery and improve survival rates. Nevertheless, controlled studies to document efficacy are not available, and there may be major problems in transferring critically ill patients to centers with this type of facility. Surgery should not be delayed. Supportive measures include fluid and electrolyte replacement, control of acidosis, transfusions for severe anemia, and appropriate measures for renal failure.

PROGNOSIS. Clostridial myonecrosis is a devastating infection that often requires mutilating surgery and prolonged hospital courses. The overall mortality rate in 116 reports summarizing over 1200 cases is 25 per cent. However, many reported cases actually represent other types of soft tissue infections involving clostridial species, and the mortality rate for true gas gangrene is probably far higher.

PREVENTION. The inoculum of *C. perfringens* required to produce gas gangrene is reduced by 10^6 organisms in experimental animals if the organism is delivered into devitalized muscle containing dirt instead of normal tissue. As noted earlier, contamination of wounds by clostridia either from soil sources or from the endogenous fecal flora is common with both traumatic injuries and surgical incisions. The incidence of clostridial myonecrosis following battlefield injury was 10 per cent in World War I, 1 per cent in World War II, and 0.01 per cent (22 cases in 139,000 battle injuries) in the Vietnam War. These figures reflect improvements in the management of battlefield injuries with major emphasis on prompt and thorough debridement. There should also be care in preserving the vascular supply, particularly with the use of tourniquets and casts. Judicious decisions regarding closure of traumatic wounds and the prophylactic use of antibiotics are also important. There is no effective means of active immunization.

Baxter CR: Surgical management of soft tissue infections. Surg Clin North Am 52:1483, 1972. *Soft tissue infections are reviewed using three categories: infections requiring incision and drainage, infections requiring excision of tissue, and infections not requiring extensive surgery.*

Dellinger EP: Severe necrotizing soft tissue infections. JAMA 246:1717–1721, 1981. *The author reviews management principles for severe soft tissue infections and enphasizes the differential diagnosis based on clinical presentation, Gram's stain, and operative inspection.*

Heimbach RD: Gas gangrene: Review and update. HBO Review 1:41, 1980. *The author reviews gas gangrene and presents an endorsement for hyperbaric oxygen treatment which may be overly enthusiastic.*

Stevens DL, Maier KA, Laine BM, et al.: Comparison of clindamycin, rifampin, tetracycline, metronidazole, and penicillin for efficacy in prevention of experimental gas gangrene due to Clostridium perfringens. J Infect Dis 155:220, 1987. *A provocative report showing multiple antimicrobial agents to be superior to penicillin in an animal model of gas gangrene.*

Weinstein L, Barza M: Gas gangrene. N Engl J Med 289:1129, 1972. *A review of clinical features and management recommendations for gas gangrene.*

OTHER CLOSTRIDIAL DISEASES

SEPTICEMIA. Clostridia account for up to 3 per cent of all positive blood cultures in most clinical microbiologic laboratories. The most frequent species is *C. perfringens*, which accounts for 50 to 60 per cent. Most patients have other conditions and the significance of the clostridia is enigmatic. Less frequently there is an associated mixed infection, such as an intra-abdominal abscess, that represents the presumed portal of entry. Gas gangrene is rare and this diagnosis should be based on compatible

clinical features. Special notation must be made for bacteremia with *C. septicum*. Many of these patients have leukemia in relapse, neutropenia, or colonic carcinoma. The usual portal of entry is the distal ileum or cecum ("neutropenic enterocolitis"), most patients are acutely ill, the mortality rate is high, and aggressive resectional surgery combined with intravenous penicillin is indicated. *Clostridium tertium* may cause a similar syndrome, but the mortality rate is low and most patients respond to antibiotics without surgery.

MISCELLANEOUS INFECTIONS. Clostridia are frequently isolated from infections involving the host's normal flora. This situation especially applies to cases in which the infecting flora originates in the colon, such as in intra-abdominal sepsis, wound infections after intestinal surgery, and wounds such as ischemic ulcers, diabetic ulcers, or decubitus ulcers located on the lower trunk or lower extremities. These organisms are especially common in infections associated with gas formation such as emphysematous cholecystitis, emphysematous cystitis, and crepitant cellulitis. Clostridia are also found in 5 to 10 per cent of anaerobic pulmonary infections and with similar frequency in nonvenereal infections of the female genital tract. Such infections usually involve a mixture of aerobic and anaerobic bacteria so that the role of clostridia is uncertain. Penicillin G is generally considered the preferred antibiotic for clostridial infections, although increasing resistance is noted with some species other than *C. perifringens*. Alternative agents include imipenem, metronidazole, chloramphenicol, or a β-lactam–β-lactamase inhibitor.

CLOSTRIDIA ENTEROTOXEMIAS. Clostridia cause three different types of enteric disease, each of which is ascribed to a unique toxin (Table 307–1). *C. difficile*, the major cause of antibiotic-associated colitis, is discussed in Ch. 308.

C. perfringens is commonly responsible for foodborne outbreaks of a self-limited enteric disease. More recent studies show that this organism may also cause diarrhea in other settings such as sporadic diarrhea, antibiotic-associated diarrhea, and diarrhea in chronic care facilities. The mechanism is an enterotoxin produced by some type A strains during sporulation. Requirements for the foodborne form are (1) ingestion of at least 10^8 viable vegetative cells; (2) enterotoxigenic potential of the ingested strain; and (3) sporulation with toxin production in the alkaline medium of the small bowel. The usual symptoms are diarrhea and abdominal cramps ascribed to fluid secretion, morphologic damage to the intestinal mucosa, and altered motility in the small bowel. Less frequent symptoms are nausea, vomiting, and fever. The usual vehicle in outbreaks is meat or food made with meat, such as stews, meat pies, gravies, or casseroles. The attack rate among exposed persons is usually 30 to 60 per cent, and the incubation period ranges from 7 to 15 hours. The diagnosis is suspected in any outbreak of gastrointestinal disease associated with typical symptoms and incubation period among persons sharing a common and likely food source. Confirmation requires the recovery of *C. perfringens* in concentrations of at least 10^5 per gram of epidemiologically implicated food, recovery of at least 10^6 spores per gram of stool obtained within 48 hours after onset of symptoms from victims, or, preferably, detection of enterotoxin in stool. Nearly all patients have spontaneous resolution of symptoms within 6 to 24 hours and do not require any specific form of therapy.

Enteritis necroticans is a serious gastrointestinal disease caused by the beta toxin of *C. perfringens*, type C. This disease, once called "darmbrand," occurred in epidemic form in malnourished individuals from Norway and Germany at the end of World War II. More recently, the same condition, known locally as "pigbel," has been found to be endemic in the highlands of New Guinea. Sporadic cases have been reported in Africa, Southeast Asia, China, and western countries. In New Guinea, most victims are children who have participated in pig feasts. The toxin is susceptible to proteolytic enzymes including trypsin. However, toxin inactivation in the small bowel fails because of enzyme deficiency ascribed to protein malnutrition, excessive consumption of sweet potatoes, which contain trypsin inhibitors, or colonization with *Ascaris lumbricoides*, which secretes trypsin inhibitors. The predilection for children presumably reflects antigenic naiveté. Pathologically, enteritis necroticans is a segmental disease of the small bowel which is characterized by mucosal infarction, edema, hemorrhage, and infiltration with polymorphonuclear cells. In advanced stages the bowel is thinned, friable, and subject to perforation. Medical therapy consists of intestinal decompression, penicillin or chloramphenicol, and intravenous fluid support. About half of the patients require resectional surgery, and the overall mortality rate is 15 to 40 per cent. Prevention is achieved with a beta-toxoid vaccine that is currently recommended for children in the endemic area.

Editorial: Clostridium septicum and neutropenic enterocolitis. Lancet 2:608, 1987. *The authors review "typhlitis" with C. septicum bacteremia.*

Gorbach SL, Thadepalli H: Isolation of Clostridia in human infections: Evaluation of 114 cases. J Infect Dis 131:S81–S85, 1975. *The authors review their experience with 152 strains of clostridia recovered from 144 patients at Cook County Hospital. Sixty-five patients had soft tissue infections or intra-abdominal sepsis, and 84 per cent of these had polymicrobial infections. Clostridia bacteremia in 49 patients usually occurred with no apparent relation to the clinical setting.*

Larson HE, Borriello SP: Infectious diarrhea due to Clostridium perfringens. J Infect Dis 157:390, 1988. *The authors review diarrhea due to enterotoxin-producing strains of C. perfringens, calling attention to some unique clinical features such as a prolonged clinical course and the potential utility of stool analysis for enterotoxin.*

Lawrence G, Walker PD: Pathogenesis of enteritis necroticans in Papua New Guinea. Lancet 1:125–126, 1976. *The authors, noted authorities in the field, provide a postulate for the pathophysiology of pigbel.*

Ramsay AM: The significance of Clostridium welchii in the cervical swab and blood stream in postpartum and postabortum sepsis. J Obstet Gynecol Br Commonwealth 56:247–258, 1949. *The author refers to C. perfringens (welchii) as a "harmless saprophyte" in a discussion of 28 women with bacteremia, since most had minimal clinical disturbance despite the fact that the majority were studied before antibiotics were available.*

Shaudera WX, Tacket CO, Blake PA: Food poisoning due to Clostridium perfringens in the US. J Infect Dis 147:167–170, 1983. *The authors review the Centers for Disease Control's experience with C. perfringens food poisoning.*

Van Damme–Jongsten M, Rodhouse J, Gilbert RJ, et al.: Synthetic DNA probes for detection of enterotoxigenic Clostridium perfringens strains isolated from outbreaks of food poisoning. J Clin Microbiol 28:131, 1990. *The DNA probes described proved useful in identifying enterotoxin-producing strains of C. perfringens.*

308 Pseudomembranous Colitis

DESCRIPTION. Pseudomembranous colitis is a severe gastrointestinal disease characterized by exudative plaques on the colonic mucosa.

ETIOLOGY. Pseudomembranous colitis is usually found in association with other conditions, although occasional cases occur in healthy persons with no identifiable risk factors. The great majority of cases represent a complication of antimicrobial use, and the etiologic agent in nearly all cases of antibiotic-associated pseudomembranous colitis is *Clostridium difficile*. The pathophysiologic mechanism is elaboration of toxins during replication of vegetative forms of *C. difficile*, a process that is presumably promoted by suppression of the competitive flora.

INCIDENCE. The incidence of antibiotic-associated pseudomembranous colitis depends on the frequency with which endoscopy is performed to establish the diagnosis, antimicrobial use patterns, and epidemiologic patterns. Nearly all antimicrobials with an antibacterial spectrum of activity have been implicated. The most frequent are ampicillin, clindamycin, and cephalosporins. Less frequent are penicillins other than ampicillin, erythromycin, and sulfamethoxazole-trimethoprim. Drugs rarely implicated include tetracyclines, chloramphenicol, sulfonamides, quinolones, and parenterally administered aminoglycosides. *C. difficile*–induced diarrhea or colitis may occur sporadically or in clusters within institutions. Epidemiologic studies indicate that *C. difficile* may be found in the colonic flora of about 3 per cent of healthy adults, is widely distributed in the environment, and is especially common in areas subject to fecal contamination from patients who have *C. difficile*–induced diarrheal complications. This last observation provides an explanation for focal outbreaks of the disease in hospitals and nursing homes where there is clustering of vulnerable patients, mainly the elderly and antibiotic recipients.

MECHANISM. *C. difficile*–induced colitis is a toxin-mediated enteric disease in which there is no microbial invasion of the intestinal mucosa. Toxin A appears to be responsible for the clinical features of the intestinal disease; toxin B is strongly

cytopathic and accounts for positive results in the tissue culture assay. Most strains of *C. difficile* produce both toxins, although there is substantial strain variation in the quantities of toxins produced.

CLINICAL MANIFESTATIONS. Virtually all patients are at risk for antibiotic-associated pseudomembranous colitis, although there appears to be an increased risk with increasing age. The most common symptom is diarrhea consisting of watery or semiliquid stools without visible blood. Stool examination may show fecal leukocytes, but this is inconsistent and nonspecific. Many patients also have fever, which is usually moderate but may reach 40° C. Other common findings are abdominal cramps, lower quadrant tenderness, leukocytosis, and hypoalbuminemia. Systemic symptoms and abdominal findings are not invariably present, and some patients simply have annoying diarrhea. Complications in severe cases include dehydration, hypoalbuminemia with anasarca, electrolyte disturbances, toxic megacolon, and colonic perforation. Symptoms may begin at any time during the course of antimicrobial treatment or up to 6 weeks after antimicrobials have been discontinued. The differential diagnosis includes acute and chronic diarrhea caused by enteric pathogens other than *C. difficile*, an adverse reaction to drugs other than antibiotics, intra-abdominal sepsis, and idiopathic inflammatory bowel disease.

DIAGNOSIS. The preferred method to establish the anatomic diagnosis is colonoscopy to demonstrate typical punctate, raised, yellowish-white plaques with "skip areas" of a normal mucosa or a mucosa showing erythema or edema. The plaques are usually 2 to 10 mm wide but may enlarge and coalesce over extensive segments of the colon in the late stages. Microscopic examination of colonic biopsies shows epithelial necrosis, goblet cells distended with mucus, and infiltration of the lamina propria with polymorphonuclear cells and eosinophilic exudate. The pseudomembrane is attached to the surface epithelium and is composed of fibrin, mucin, and polymorphonuclear cells.

The preferred diagnostic test to implicate *C. difficile* is a tissue culture assay of stool to demonstrate a cytopathic toxin that is neutralized by antitoxin to *C. difficile* or *C. sordellii*. Antitoxin neutralization with antisera to *C. sordellii* reflects antigenic cross-reactivity. Toxin titers may also be performed using serial dilutions of stool specimens, although there is little correlation between the toxin titer and the severity of the disease. Alternative methods to detect *C. difficile* toxins, including the latex agglutination assay, are considered less reliable. Stool cultures for *C. difficile* often show high rates of false-positive results due to carrier rates of 10 to 30 per cent among hospitalized patients and persons receiving antibiotics without diarrheal complications. However, cultures of stool or rectal swabs are appropriate for evaluating epidemics of *C. difficile*–associated enteric disease.

Anatomic changes in the colonic mucosa noted in patients with the diarrheal complications of antibiotic use include an entirely normal colonic mucosa; erythema or edema; colitis with friability, ulceration, or hemorrhage; and pseudomembranous colitis. The toxin of *C. difficile* has been implicated in the entire spectrum of anatomic changes, but the frequency of this toxin correlates to a large extent with the severity of the disease process. Tissue culture assays for *C. difficile* toxin are positive in over 90 per cent of patients with pseudomembranous colitis and in approximately 20 per cent of those with antibiotic-associated diarrhea and an entirely normal colonic mucosa. Thus, the tissue culture assay defines the etiologic agent and does not establish the anatomic diagnosis. There is no identifiable pathogen in most patients with antibiotic-associated diarrhea or colitis in whom the assay for *C. difficile* toxin is negative, except for occasional cases that may involve *S. aureus*, Salmonella, or *C. perfringens*.

TREATMENT. Most important is discontinuation of the implicated antibiotic. This often results in resolution of symptoms with no necessity for further diagnostic tests or therapy. Patients with severe or persistent symptoms should have stool examination to detect *C. difficile* cytotoxin. Patients with severe fluid, albumin, or electrolyte depletion often require intravenous replacement and may require hyperalimentation. The role of corticosteroids and attempts to manipulate the flora, as with oral lactobacilli or fecal enemas, is not established. Antiperistaltic drugs are contraindicated.

Specific therapy is available for diarrhea caused by *C. difficile*, using cholestyramine to bind the toxin or antibiotics to inhibit the pathogen. The preferred agent for seriously ill patients is orally administered vancomycin, 125 to 500 mg four times daily for 7 to 14 days. Vancomycin is active against virtually all strains of *C. difficile*, the levels in the colon with oral administration are extremely high, and systemic toxicity is nil owing to poor absorption. The major problems with vancomycin are high cost, noxious taste, and relapses in 15 to 35 per cent of patients when vancomycin is discontinued. Relapses are characterized by the recurrence of typical symptoms, positive tissue culture assays for *C. difficile* cytotoxin, and stool cultures that yield vancomycin-sensitive strains of *C. difficile*. The frequency of relapses is not influenced by the dose of vancomycin, the duration of treatment, or the selection of vancomycin versus metronidazole.

Alternative and less expensive treatments are anion exchange resins that bind *C. difficile* toxins, such as cholestyramine (4 gm packet orally three times daily for 5 to 10 days) and metronidazole (500 mg orally 3 or 4 times daily for 7 to 14 days). These drugs should be reserved for less seriously ill patients. Patients with relapses may be treated with metronidazole or vancomycin for 10 to 14 days, followed by cholestyramine (above doses) or low dose vancomycin (125 mg on alternate days) for 3 weeks.

PROGNOSIS. *C. difficile* causes a disease spectrum ranging from asymptomatic carriers of the toxin to patients with life-threatening pseudomembranous colitis. The most common clinical expression is "simple diarrhea" that resolves when the implicated antibiotic is discontinued. Even patients with PMC usually recover without specific forms of therapy. However, symptoms may be prolonged and debilitating, with persistent diarrhea for several weeks or months. Reports that focus on more seriously ill patients indicate mortality rates of 10 to 30 per cent. With early institution of vancomycin therapy there is a prompt symptomatic response, and virtually all patients recover. The incidence of relapse following vancomycin or metronidazole treatment is 15 to 35 per cent, and some patients suffer multiple relapses following each course of treatment.

PREVENTION. The most important preventive measure is judicious use of antimicrobial agents. Patients with *C. difficile*–induced diarrhea or colitis should be isolated and placed on enteric precautions to limit spread to susceptible hosts within institutions. Additional maneuvers sometimes suggested in facilities where this complication is endemic or epidemic include sequestering *C. difficile* carriers, restriction of afflicted patients to rooms with private bathrooms, antibiotic control programs, and treatment of carriers with oral vancomycin.

Bartlett JG, Gorbach SL: Pseudomembranous colitis. Adv Intern Med 22:455, 1977. *Review of the topic with extensive reference list for publications prior to evidence implicating* C. difficile.

Bartlett JG: Treatment of *Clostridium difficile* colitis. Gastroenterology 89:1192, 1985. *Editorial review of treatment strategies.*

Bartlett JG: Clostridium difficile: Clinical considerations. Rev Infect Dis 12(Suppl 2):S243, 1990. *Review of the topic including clinical features, diagnostic tests, and therapy.*

Fekety R, Kim K-H, Brown D, et al.: Epidemiology of antibiotic-associated colitis. Am J Med 70:906, 1981. *A survey of the epidemiology of* C. difficile.

McFarland LV, Mulligan ME, Kwok RYY, Stamm WE. Nosocomial acquisition of *Clostridium difficile* infection. N Engl J Med 320:210, 1989. *The authors document the frequency of* C. difficile *as a nosocomial pathogen, although most of the colonized patients remained asymptomatic.*

Price AB, Davis DR: Pseudomembranous colitis. J Clin Pathol 30:1, 1977. *A review of histopathologic changes.*

309 Botulism

DEFINITION. Botulism is a severe neuroparalytic disease caused by botulinal toxin produced by clostridial species, usually *C. botulinum*. There are four recognized disease categories: (1) foodborne botulism, (2) infant botulism, (3) wound botulism, and (4) unclassified cases.

ETIOLOGY. *C. botulinum* is a gram-positive, spore-forming obligate anaerobe that is widely distributed in nature and frequently found in soil, marine environments, and agricultural products. Adults regularly ingest *C. botulinum* spores from fresh agricultural products without deleterious consequences, and this organism is not recognized as a component of the normal fecal flora. Each strain produces one of eight antigenically distinct toxins of approximately 150,000 daltons, designated A through H. Human disease is caused by types A, B, E, and rarely by F and G. *C. barati* and *C. butyricum* have been implicated in infant botulism with production of type F and E toxins, respectively. Botulinal toxins are hematogenously disseminated to peripheral cholinergic synapses where they bind irreversibly and block acetylcholine release. The result is hypotonia with a descending symmetric flaccid paralysis. Botulinal toxin is the most potent poison of man; it has an estimated lethal dose in the bloodstream of 10^{-9} mg per kilogram. Type A botulinum toxin is now available for injection as treatment for ocular muscle disorders, such as strabismus and blepharospasm, and dystonias, such as torticollis and hemifacial spasm.

FOOD POISONING. Foodborne botulism results from the ingestion of preformed toxin in inadequately prepared food, although *C. botulinum* in the intestine may be responsible or may serve as a continuing source of toxin. There are an average of 15 "outbreaks" annually in the United States, most of which involve a single case. The most frequently implicated vehicle in the United States is home-canned foods, which usually have a putrefactive odor. Meat and meat products are more commonly responsible in Europe, and preserved fish is most frequent in Japan, Scandinavia, and Russia. Type A and B organisms predominate in the United States, type A west of the Mississippi River and type B in eastern states. Type E organisms are usually, but not exclusively, associated with an aquatic source in northern latitudes, where they are found in coastal waters, lakes, and intestines of fish that inhabit these areas.

CLINICAL MANIFESTATIONS. The incubation period is usually 18 to 36 hours but may be as short as 2 hours or as long as 8 days. Persons with the shortest incubation period usually have the most severe disease. The bulbar musculature is affected first, with resultant diplopia, difficulty in focusing to a near point, dysphonia, dysarthria, and dysphagia. Involvement of the cholinergic autonomic nervous system may cause decreased salivation with a dry mouth and sore throat, ileus, or urinary retention. Common gastrointestinal symptoms include nausea, vomiting, and abdominal pain. Neurologic examination shows lateral rectus muscle weakness (cranial nerve VI), ptosis, dilated pupils with sluggish reaction, decreased gag reflex, or medial rectus paresis. This is followed by descending involvement of the motor neurons to peripheral muscles, including the muscles of respiration. Some patients have only mild illness, whereas others have severe paralysis that may require intensive supportive care for weeks. Mentation remains clear, there is no fever, and neurologic dysfunction is bilateral but not necessarily symmetric. The principal causes of death are respiratory or bulbar paralysis and infectious complications during the period of supportive care.

DIAGNOSIS. The usual laboratory test in suspected cases is analysis of serum, stool, gastric contents, and/or food for botulinum toxin and analysis of stool and/or food for *C. botulinum*. The classic toxin test is a mouse assay in which specimens are injected intraperitoneally to demonstrate a lethal toxin that is neutralized by type-specific antitoxin. Alternative antigen assays, such as the enzyme-linked immunoassay, have been developed, but are not widely available. Among patients with clinical evidence of botulism, the toxin is detected in sera from one third, the toxin is found in the stool from one third, and the organism is recovered in stool from 60 per cent.

Botulism should be suspected in patients with acute flaccid paralysis, especially when there is bilateral sixth cranial nerve dysfunction, associated gastrointestinal symptoms, prior ingestion of possibly contaminated food, and typical symptoms in other persons who shared this food. The differential diagnosis includes myasthenia gravis, Guillain-Barré syndrome, tick paralysis, cerebrovascular accident involving branches of the basilar artery, trichinosis, the Eaton-Lambert syndrome, hypocalcemia, hypermagnesemia, organophosphate poisoning, atropine poisoning, paralytic poisoning caused by shellfish or puffer fish, and psychiatric syndromes. Electromyography using repetitive stimulation at 40 Hz or greater is useful in differentiating botulism from other neurologic syndromes. This shows a diminished amplitude of muscle action potentials with a single supramaximal stimulus and facilitation of action potentials using paired or repetitive stimuli. These findings do not appear until the patient develops peripheral muscle weakness and are most likely to be positive in an affected limb.

TREATMENT. Sudden respiratory arrest is the most important serious complication, so that patients must be carefully observed with monitoring of vital capacity and liberal use of ventilatory support. Elimination of the toxin from the gastrointestinal tract may be facilitated using gastric lavage, cathartics, and enemas early in the course. Antitoxin is usually given irrespective of the duration of illness, since the toxin may persist in the blood for extended periods. Treatment is initiated using two vials of the trivalent antitoxin, each containing 7500 IU type A, 5500 IU type B, and 8500 IU type E antitoxin; one vial is given intravenously, one is given intramuscularly, and the two-vial treatment is then repeated at 2 to 4 hours. The antitoxin is horse serum and is associated with a 20 per cent incidence of hypersensitivity reactions, the most serious being anaphylaxis in 3 to 5 per cent. Efficacy of the antitoxin is most clearly established with type B and type E botulism. Other therapeutic considerations include guanidine hydrochloride (15 to 50 mg per kilogram daily) to enhance acetylcholine release, but efficacy has not been established. Some advocate penicillin to help eradicate *C. botulinum* from the intestine, since this represents a potential source of additional toxin.

PROGNOSIS. The case fatality rate for foodborne botulism was formerly 60 to 70 per cent. Improved methods of management, especially support of respiratory function, have reduced the fatality rate to less than 10 per cent. Patients who survive generally have complete recovery.

PREVENTION. Foodborne botulism is caused by germination of spores in food with toxin produced by vegetative forms, although the toxin may also be produced in vivo by simultaneous ingestion of spores. The disease may be prevented by destruction of spores in the original food source, inhibition of germination, or destruction of preformed toxin. Specific measures are as follows:

1. Destruction of spores with heat or irradiation. Spores of types A and B may survive boiling for several hours, especially at high altitudes (such as in Colorado) where the boiling point may be substantially lower. These spores may be destroyed if kept at 120°C for 30 minutes using pressure cookers. Spores of type E are most heat-labile and are killed with heating at 80°C for 30 minutes.

2. Germination may be inhibited by a reduction in pH, refrigeration, freezing, drying, or addition of salt, sugar, or other inhibitory substances such as sodium nitrite.

3. Inactivation of preformed toxin is accomplished by terminal heating for 20 minutes at 80°C or 10 minutes at 90°C.

INFANT BOTULISM. Infant botulism results from production of botulinal neurotoxin in vivo following colonization of the gastrointestinal tract in children ages 1 to 9 months. This is the most common form of botulism in the United States, where 30 to 80 cases are documented annually. Spores of *C. botulinum* (but not the toxin) have been found in about 10 per cent of honey supplies, which presumably account for one third of cases. The disease spectrum varies considerably, ranging from "failure to thrive" or mild changes in bowel habits to the sudden infant death syndrome or "crib death." The most commonly recognized form of the disease is the "floppy baby syndrome." Initial symptoms are lethargy, diminished suck, constipation, weakness, feeble cry, and diminished spontaneous activity with loss of head control. This is followed by extensive flaccid paralysis. The diagnosis is established with the recovery of *C. botulinum* or its toxin in stool. The toxin has rarely been detected in the serum. Fecal carriage of the organism and the toxin may persist for weeks to months following clinical improvement and hospital discharge. The major therapeutic need is supportive care with special attention to nutrition and maintenance of respiratory function. The role of antitoxin, guanidine, and antibiotics in this form of botulism has not been established, and generally their use is not advised. The mortality rate for hospitalized patients given supportive care is only 2 per cent.

WOUND BOTULISM. This is a rare form of botulism in which a traumatic wound is infected by *C. botulinum* with toxin

production in vivo. Types A and B have been implicated, reflecting their presence in soil. Clinical features are identical to those of foodborne botulism except that the incubation period from the time of injury is 4 to 14 days and there is a paucity of gastrointestinal symptoms. The diagnosis is established by recovering *C. botulinum* from the wound or by detection of the toxin in serum. Management includes wound debridement and other treatments described for foodborne botulism except for bowel cleansing.

UNCLASSIFIED BOTULISM. This category includes persons over the age of 12 months who have typical symptoms and signs of botulism with no identifiable vehicle. It is possible that some cases result from production of toxin in vivo by organisms colonizing the intestine in a fashion comparable to the mechanism described for infant botulism.

SPECIAL NOTE. Physicians who suspect foodborne botulism or wish to receive botulinal antitoxin should contact the state health department (daytime and 24-hour numbers listed in JAMA 256:1105, 1986) or contact the CDC 24-hour number (404-329-2888).

Arnon SS: Infant botulism: Anticipating the second decade. J Infect Dis 154:201, 1986. *An authoritative review of infant botulism based on the 10-year experience following its original report in 1976.*

Botulinum toxin for ocular muscle disorders. The Medical Letter 32:100, 1990. Medical Letter *consultants review the uses of botulinum toxin (Oculinum) for occular muscle disorders and other dystonias, a growing role of this potent toxin.*

Chia JK, Clark JB, Ryan CA, et al.: Botulism in an adult associated with food-borne intestinal infection with *Clostridium botulinum*. N Engl J Med 315:239, 1986. *This is a case report of an adult with the infant form of botulism and an accompanying editorial that places this observation in perspective.*

Dowell VR Jr, McCroskey LM, Hathaway CL, et al.: Coproexamination for botulinal toxin and *Clostridium botulinum*. JAMA 238:1829, 1977. *Reviews methods to establish the diagnosis in foodborne botulism.*

Merson MH, Hughes JM, Dowell VR, et al.: Current trends in botulism in the United States. JAMA 229:1305, 1974. *Summary of the CDC experience with foodborne botulism.*

Tacket CO, Shandera WX, Mann JM, et al.: Equine antitoxin use and other factors that predict outcome in type A foodborne botulism. Am J Med 76:794, 1984. *A review supporting the previously controversial role of antitoxin in type A botulism in adults.*

310 Tetanus

DEFINITION. Tetanus is a neurologic syndrome caused by a neurotoxin elaborated at the site of injury by *Clostridium tetani*.

ETIOLOGY. *C. tetani* is an anaerobic, gram-positive, slender, motile bacillus. The sporulated form has a characteristic drumstick or tennis racket shape with a terminal spore. The vegetative form produces tetanospasmin, a protein neurotoxin with a molecular weight of approximately 150,000. Tetanospasmin ranks with botulism toxin as the most potent known microbial toxin; 1 mg is capable of killing 50 to 70 million mice. The vegetative forms of *C. tetani* are highly susceptible to heat, disinfectants, and other adverse environmental conditions, but the spores are highly resistant and can survive in soil for months to years. Killing of spores requires boiling for at least 4 hours or autoclaving for 12 minutes at 121°C.

EPIDEMIOLOGY. *C. tetani* can be found in 20 to 65 per cent of soil samples, the highest yields being in cultivated land and the lowest yields, in virgin soil. The organism can also be found in stool from a variety of animals, house dust, operating rooms, and contaminated heroin. Approximately 10 per cent of humans harbor *C. tetani* in the colon.

Tetanus is most common in warm climates and in highly cultivated rural areas. The greatest problem is in economically deprived countries, owing to poor immunization standards and unhygienic practices. An example is the practice of dressing the umbilical stump with animal dung or "dusting powder," a local dried clay sold for cosmetic purposes, after childbirth by unimmunized mothers. It is estimated that the annual toll from neonatal tetanus in developing countries is 1 million. In the United States, there are 40 to 60 reported cases annually, and almost all occur in unimmunized or inadequately immunized persons. Of these cases 60 to 80 per cent are associated with acute wounds, 15 to 20 per cent represent complications of chronic wounds, 3 to 10 per cent are complications of parenteral drug abuse, and 5 to 10 per cent have no clearly identified source. Over 70 per cent of these patients are 50 years of age or older, and less than 4 per cent are under 20 years; there is only about one case of neonatal tetanus per year. This predilection for the disease in the elderly appears to reflect waning immunity associated with aging.

PATHOGENESIS. Clinical tetanus requires a source of the organism, local tissue conditions that promote toxin production, and immunologic naiveté. The usual portals of entry are traumatic wounds, surgical wounds, subcutaneous injection sites, burns, skin ulcers, infected umbilical cords, and otitis media with tympanic membrane perforation. The spores are ubiquitous in the environment, and most cases reflect contamination from exogenous sources, although endogenous infection is conceivable in occasional cases that follow intestinal surgery. Important factors at the site of injury are necrotic tissue, suppuration, and the presence of a foreign body. These are responsible for a reduction in the local oxidation-reduction potential (eH), thus promoting reversion of spores to the vegetative forms that produce tetanospasmin. Tetanospasmin is taken up by the peripheral nerve terminals and carried intra-axonally within membrane-bound vesicles to spinal neurons at a transport rate of approximately 250 mm per day. Upon reaching the perikarya of the motor neurons the toxin passes to the presynaptic terminals where it blocks release of neurotransmitters, including glycine, which is the neurotransmitter used by group 1A inhibitory afferent motor neurons. Loss of the inhibitory influence results in unrestrained firing with sustained muscular contraction. The result with spinal cord neurons is rigidity. In severe cases there is also involvement of the sympathetic chain causing autonomic dysfunction.

CLINICAL FEATURES. Forms of tetanus include generalized, localized, cephalic, and neonatal.

Generalized tetanus is the most common. The extent of the associated trauma varies from a rather trivial injury that may be forgotten by the patient to a severe, contaminated crush injury. The usual incubation period is 7 to 21 days, depending largely on the distance of the site of injury from the central nervous system. The "onset period" refers to the time from the first clinical symptoms of tetanus to the first generalized spasm. An incubation period of less than 9 days and an onset period of less than 48 hours appear to be associated with more severe symptomatology. Trismus is the presenting complaint in 75 per cent of cases, so the patient is often initially seen by a dentist or oral surgeon. Other early features include irritability, restlessness, diaphoresis, and dysphagia with hydrophobia and drooling. Sustained trismus may result in a characterisic sardonic smile, or "risus sardonicus," and persistent spasm of the back musculature may cause opisthotonos. These early manifestations reflect involvement of the bulbar muscles and paraspinous muscles, possibly because they are innervated by the shortest axons. Waves of opisthotonos are highly characteristic of the disease. With progression, the extremities become involved in episodes characterized by painful flexion and adduction of the arms, clenched fists, and extension of the legs. Noise or tactile stimuli may precipitate spasms and generalized convulsions, although they occur spontaneously as well. Involvement of the autonomic nervous system may result in severe arrhythmias, oscillation in the blood pressure, profound diaphoresis, hyperthermia, rhabdomyolysis, laryngeal spasm, and urinary retention. In most cases the patient remains lucid. Complications include fractures from sustained contractions and convulsions, pulmonary emboli, bacterial infections, and dehydration.

Localized tetanus refers to involvement of the extremity with a contaminated wound and shows considerable variation in severity. In the more severe cases there are intense, painful spasms that usually progress to generalized tetanus. Cases that remain localized tend to be less severe. This is a relatively unusual form of tetanus, and the prognosis for survival is excellent.

Cephalic tetanus generally follows a head injury or occurs with *C. tetani* infection of the middle ear. The clinical symptoms consist of isolated or combined dysfunction of the cranial motor nerves, most frequently the seventh cranial nerve. This may remain localized or progress to generalized tetanus. Again, this is a relatively unusual form of tetanus, but the incubation period is only 1 or 2 days, and the prognosis for survival is extremely poor.

Tetanus neonatorum refers to generalized tetanus resulting from *C. tetani* infection in neonates. This occurs primarily in underdeveloped countries where various contaminated materials are used to sever or dress the umbilical cord in newborn infants of unimmunized mothers. The usual incubation period following birth is 3 to 10 days, and it is sometimes referred to as "the disease of the seventh day," reflecting the average incubation period. The child typically shows irritability, facial grimacing, and severe spasms with touch. The mortality rate exceeds 70 per cent.

DIAGNOSIS. The diagnosis of tetanus is usually made on the basis of clinical observations. The putative agent, *C. tetani*, is infrequently recovered with cultures of the wound. A confirmed history of immunization or a serum antitoxin level of 0.01 units per deciliter or higher makes tetanus very unlikely. Spinal fluid analysis is entirely normal, and the electroencephalogram generally shows a sleep pattern. The differential diagnosis depends on the dominant clinical features and includes oculogyric crisis secondary to phenothiazine toxicity, meningitis, dental abscess, seizure disorder, subarachnoid hemorrhage, hypocalcemic or alkalotic tetany, alcohol withdrawal, and strychnine poisoning. Strychnine poisoning produces very similar symptoms but differs from tetanus in that patients usually recover rapidly following supportive care.

TREATMENT. *Surgery.* Debridement of any associated wound. (This may pose a problem in "skin poppers," who often have multiple possibly infected sites.)

Antibiotics. Penicillin G should be given parenterally in doses of 1 to 10 million units daily for 10 days; tetracycline, erythromycin, and chloramphenicol are alternative agents for penicillin-allergic patients.

Antitoxin. Human tetanus immunoglobulin (TIG) should be given as soon as possible to neutralize toxin that has not entered neurons. The dose is arbitrary, ranging from 500 to 6000 units, and the route of administration may be intramuscular or as split doses intramuscularly and by infiltration into the wound. Some authorities advocate intrathecal administration of 250 units of TIG. Equine tetanus immune globulin (10,000 to 100,000 units intravenously or intramuscularly) is equally effective, but the rate of reactions is high owing to the equine source. Epinephrine 1:1000 should be readily available for severe reactions. This preparation is far less expensive and is consequently used most extensively in underdeveloped countries.

Active Immunization. Natural infection does not result in detectable levels of circulating antibody, so a full course of immunization with tetanus toxoid in three doses should be given.

Muscle Spasms. Chlorpromazine (50 to 150 mg every 4 to 8 hours in adults), meprobamate (400 mg every 3 to 4 hours in adults*), or diazepam (2 to 20 mg intravenously every 2 to 8 hours) are given to control spasms and convulsions, and short-acting barbiturates are useful for sedation. Overuse of these agents may lead to hypoventilation. When muscle spasms are severe or interfere with ventilation, therapeutic paralysis should be introduced using pancuronium bromide or metocurine combined with mechanical ventilation.

Supportive Care. Trismus, dysphagia, laryngeal spasm, respiratory muscle spasm, and sedatives all contribute to the high frequency of pulmonary complications. Maintenance of a patent airway is imperative, often with intubation followed by a tracheostomy. The patient may then be maintained with mechanical ventilation in conjunction with diazepam in intravenous doses titrated to relieve rigidity without excessive sedation.

Patients with dysphagia should be fed via a nasogastric tube. Fluid balance needs to be followed assiduously, since large losses may occur and may be difficult to measure owing to profuse sweating. Autonomic nervous system involvement may result in tachycardia and hypertension with high cardiac output and cardiac arrhythmias. Alpha- and beta-adrenergic blocking agents were used formerly, but beta blockade was sometimes complicated by cardiac arrest. Other considerations with autonomic instability include morphine, epidural blockade, or magnesium sulfate in-

---

*May exceed manufacturer's recommended dosage.

TABLE 310–1. GUIDELINES FOR TETANUS PROPHYLAXIS IN WOUND MANAGEMENT

History of Adsorbed Tetanus Toxoid	Clean and Minor Wounds		Other Wounds*	
Number of Doses	Td†	TIG‡	Td†	TIG‡
Unknown or less than three	Yes§	No	Yes§	Yes
Three or more	Yes if over 10 years since last dose	No	Yes if over 5 years since last dose	No

*Included but not limited to wounds contaminated with dirt, feces, soil, saliva, puncture wounds; avulsions; and wounds resulting from missiles, crushing, burns, and frostbite.

†Td: Tetanus and diphtheria toxoids adsorbed. Children under 7 should receive DPT (diphtheria and tetanus toxoids and pertussis vaccine adsorbed). Too frequent booster doses of tetanus toxoid have been associated with hypersensitivity reactions.

‡TIG: Tetanus immune globulin in a dose of 250 to 500 units intramuscularly. The usual dose is 250 units. The usual prophylactic dose of equine tetanus immune globulin is 1500 to 5000 units intramuscularly. When tetanus toxoid is given concurrently there should be separate syringes and injection sites.

§Unimmunized or incompletely immunized persons (1 or 2 doses of toxoid) should receive complete immunization with Td at time 0, 4–8 weeks later, and 6–12 months later.

fusions. Additional concerns are pulmonary emboli requiring anticoagulation, gastrointestinal bleeding that may be prevented with sucralfate, rhabdomyolysis with myoglobinuria and renal failure that may require dialysis, superimposed infections requiring judicious use of antibiotics, hyperthermia requiring a cooling blanket, and hypotension requiring pressor agents.

PROGNOSIS. The overall mortality rate for generalized tetanus is 25 to 50 per cent even in modern medical facilities with extensive resources. Important prognostic features are the form of tetanus, as described above, the incubation period, the onset period, patient's age, and severity of symptoms. Patients with mild disease have only trismus with or without minor and brief muscle spasms. Moderate disease is characterized by trismus, dysphagia, rigidity, and intermittent muscle spasms. With severe tetanus there are generalized convulsions. Patients with moderate or severe generalized tetanus generally require 3 to 6 weeks for recovery. They may require intensive care during most of this time, but if they survive their recovery is usually complete. The highest mortality rates are at the extremes of age. The most frequent cause of death is pneumonia, but many patients have no obvious findings at autopsy, suggesting that death was directly due to the neurotoxin.

PREVENTION. Nearly all cases of tetanus occur in unimmunized or inadequately immunized individuals. The Immunization Practices Advisory Committee recommends active immunization of infants and children with DPT (diphtheria and tetanus toxoids and pertussis adsorbed) at 2 months, 4 months, 6 months, 15 months, and 4 to 6 years. Tetanus toxoid is a highly effective antigen and protective levels of serum antitoxin in persons who complete the primary series persist for at least 10 years. Td (tetanus and diphtheria toxoids adsorbed for adult use) is rec-

ommended every 10 years at mid-decade ages (15 years, 25 years, 35 years, etc.). This is commonly neglected as disclosed by serosurveys showing that 40 per cent of persons over 60 years in the United States lack protective levels of tetanus antitoxin. The recommended primary immunization series for unimmunized persons over 7 years is Td at time 0, 4 to 8 weeks, 6 to 12 months after the second dose, and then every 10 years. Nearly all states now require DPT immunization for school enrollment. About 95 per cent of tetanus cases in the United States occur in persons who have not received the primary series of tetanus toxoid. Immunized childbearing women confer protection on their infants through transplacental maternal antibody.

Prevention of tetanus after injury requires appropriate wound management, assurance of adequate immunity, and consideration of antibiotic prophylaxis. The aim of surgery is to eliminate necrotic tissue, purulent collections, and foreign bodies that promote the environmental conditions necessary for spore germination. Guidelines for immunoprophylaxis based on immunization status and wound characteristics are summarized in Table 310–1. Passive immunization is recommended only for "tetanus prone" wounds, preferably with TIG prepared from plasma of adults hyperimmunized with tetanus toxoid. The alternative is tetanus antitoxin equine prepared from hyperimmunized horses. The horse serum is associated with a high reaction rate including pain at the injection site, serum sickness, and anaphylactic shock. Equine antitoxin also generates immune complexes that are rapidly excreted so that larger doses are required to produce sustained blood levels. The definition of *tetanus-prone* depends on the interval between injury and treatment, the degree of contamination, the extent of devitalized tissue or foreign bodies within the site of injury, and the depth of the injury. Antimicrobial agents such as penicillin, erythromycin, or metronidazole may be given to inhibit replication of the vegetative forms of *C. tetani*, but immunization and wound cleansing are considered more important, so the use of antibiotics is generally dictated by other considerations.

Armitage P, Clifford R: Prognosis in tetanus: Use of data from therapeutic trials. J Infect Dis 138:1–8, 1978. *Data for 1385 patients with tetanus in India are reviewed to propose a prognostic classification.*

Bizzini B: Tetanus toxin. Microbiol Rev 43:224, 1979. *An extensive discussion of tetanus toxin.*

Centers for Disease Control: Tetanus—United States 1987 and 1988. MMWR 39:37–41, 1990. *A review of the clinical experience with tetanus in the United States and the revised guidelines for tetanus prophylaxis.*

Dowell VR Jr: Botulism and tetanus: Selected epidemiologic and microbiologic aspects. Rev Infect Dis 6(Suppl 1):202, 1984. *A review of the reported experience in the United States for these neurologic syndromes.*

Faust RA, Vickers OR, Cohn L Jr: Tetanus: 2,449 cases in 68 years at Charity Hospital. J Trauma 16:704–712, 1976. *The authors review a large clinical experience with tetanus in a United States hospital.*

Griffin JW: Local tetanus. Johns Hopkins Med J 149:84–88, 1981. *A good review of local tetanus and the pathophysiology of tetanospasmin.*

Olsen KM, Hiller FC: Management of tetanus. Clin Pharm 6:570, 1987. *A review of management guidelines with emphasis on the important role of benzodiazepines.*

Schofield F: Selective primary health care: Strategies for control of disease in the developing world XXII. Tetanus: A preventable problem. Rev Infect Dis 8:144, 1986. *The author reviews the tetanus problem in the developing world.*

Anaerobic Bacteria

311 Diseases Caused by Non–Spore-forming Anaerobic Bacteria

Sherwood L. Gorbach

DEFINITIONS. Anaerobic bacteria are the major constituents of the microflora that colonizes the gastrointestinal tract, upper respiratory tract, skin, and vagina. Under normal circumstances these organisms exist in a *commensal* (literal meaning "dining at the same table") relationship with their host. Anaerobic bacteria require reduced oxygen tension for growth; the more fastidious strains cannot survive exposure to atmospheric oxygen for more than 5 minutes. As a general rule, anaerobes associated with infectious processes are relatively aerotolerant. Teleologically, aerotolerance provides anaerobic bacteria with a survival advantage in mammalian tissues, since the extremely oxygen-sensitive forms perish almost immediately upon escape from their natural ecologic niche, whereas aerotolerant forms can establish a septic focus.

Regardless of the organ site, anaerobic infections have three characteristics in common. First, such infections are truly endogenous, since the pathogens originate from the normal flora of the host. Second, certain pathogenic conditions predispose to anaerobic infections by initiating spread of the normal flora beyond the confines of mucosal barriers. These inciting events also produce a low *oxidation-reduction potential* (Eh) in the tissues, thereby favoring the growth of anaerobic organisms. Compromised vascular supply, trauma, tissue destruction, and antecedent infections caused by aerobic bacteria or viruses that result in necrosis are among the situations that precede anaerobic infection. Third, the infecting flora is highly complex. Abdominal infections, for example, harbor an average of five different bacterial species, usually three anaerobes and two aerobic or facultative strains.

ANAEROBIC GRAM-NEGATIVE BACILLI. *Bacteroides.* *B. fragilis* is the pre-eminent anaerobic pathogen in humans. This distinction is based on its virulence, its ubiquity in various organ sites, and its resistance to many conventional antimicrobial drugs. The organism frequently produces abscesses and causes tissue destruction. The *B. fragilis* group has been divided into five distinct species, based on biochemical differences and DNA homology: *B. fragilis*, *B. distasonis*, *B. vulgatus*, *B. ovatus*, and *B. thetaiotaomicron*. Although these organisms are recognized pathogens, they all lack one of the prime virulence factors of other gram-negative organisms, endotoxin. *Bacteroides* strains do possess a surface *lipopolysaccharide* (LPS), but this substance differs in chemical composition from LPS of other gram-negative organisms. In addition, *B. fragilis* LPS lacks the biologic activities of classic endotoxin, such as production of septic shock and vascular collapse in experimental animals. On the other hand, *B. fragilis* contains on its outer cell membrane a specific, large molecular weight capsule composed of polysaccharide. In a purified form the capsular material is highly antigenic, and it can produce abscesses when it is injected into experimental animals.

B. fragilis causes infections in the abdominal cavity that are associated with contamination by the intestinal flora. These organisms also are found in female pelvic infections and in mixed infections of skin and soft tissue such as decubitus ulcer, diabetic foot ulcer, and gangrene of the perineum.

B. bivius and *B. disieus* are frequent isolates in female pelvic infections. These organisms often are resistant to conventional penicillins and cephalosporins.

The *Bacteroides oralis*/*B. melaninogenicus* group and the asaccharolytic *Bacteroides* are found in the normal flora but may be associated with various infections. The major distinguishing feature of the asaccharolytic *Bacteroides* is the production of a brown-black pigment, formed in the colony after 5 to 7 days of growth on blood agar. Many strains require blood and vitamin K or its analogues for growth. Infections caused by these organisms are most commonly found in the respiratory tract, head and neck region, and female pelvic area.

Fusobacterium. The major species found in clinical specimens are *F. nucleatum* and *F. necrophorum*. In Gram-stained preparations, these organisms take up stain poorly and appear as slender spear-shaped bacilli with parallel sides and tapered ends. The LPS of *F. nucleatum* causes septic shock and vascular collapse when injected intravenously into rabbits, in contrast with the material found in *B. fragilis*, which is biologically inactive in this model. *Fusobacterium* species are regular constituents of the normal flora of the oral cavity, gastrointestinal tract, and female genital tract. Among the infectious processes, these organisms are major causes of pleuropulmonary infections and various abscesses of the head and neck region. They are also responsible for bacteremia. The most common sites of origin are the female genital tract, orofacial region, and lower respiratory tract.

ANAEROBIC GRAM-POSITIVE COCCI. This diverse group of organisms ranks second in importance to *Bacteroides* in frequency of isolation from infected sites. The major genera are *Peptostreptococcus*, which includes strains formerly classified as *Peptococcus*. Anaerobic streptococci, a disease group of aerotolerant and anaerobic organisms, are distinguished by producing mainly lactic acid. (There are also gram-negative cocci known as *Veillonella*, that are only rarely involved as pathogens.) Anaerobic gram-positive cocci are important components of the

normal flora of humans. Within the oral cavity these organisms represent a significant percentage of the anaerobic isolates in saliva and dental plaque. They are also among the leading components of the fecal flora and the vaginal flora. As pathogenic organisms these anaerobic cocci are found in virtually all sites where anaerobes have been identified. Approximately 50 per cent of such isolates in a clinical bacteriology laboratory are from surgical wounds, mostly associated with abdominal operations and hysterectomies. The gram-positive cocci are also found in skin and soft tissue infections and in blood cultures. About one third of anaerobic pleuropulmonary infections are associated with these gram-positive cocci. In the female genital tract they are probably the most important cause of salpingitis and are frequently isolated in cases of pelvic abscess.

GRAM-POSITIVE NON–SPORE-FORMING BACILLI. The two leading isolates are *Propionibacterium acnes* and various species of *Eubacterium*. *P. acnes* is the most frequent anaerobe found on normal skin. This organism is commonly recovered from blood cultures, most often as a contaminant, or from wound infections as part of a mixed flora. Although these organisms have little intrinsic pathogenicity, they are important causes of infection in patients with artificial heart valves, vascular grafts, orthopedic prostheses, or ventricular shunts. *Eubacterium* is isolated from wound infections, particularly in association with *Bacteroides*. Insofar as can be determined, *Eubacterium* plays no pathogenic role in the infective process. A newly described genus, *Mobiluncus*, consists of gram-variable or gram-negative curved rods that are implicated in vaginal infections.

PATHOGENESIS OF ANAEROBIC INFECTIONS. *Unitarian Compared with Synergistic Infections.* Our theoretical models of infections are based on concepts of microbial monoetiology. Pasteur established that certain microorganisms are responsible for a specific disease state. His theory was formalized by Robert Koch in his famous postulates. Finally, Erhlich created the concept of a single drug, the "magic bullet," designed for a specific infection. Thus, the principle states: one microbe, one disease, one drug. This concept applies to classic infections such as typhoid fever, diphtheria, and cholera. However, the classic design does not fit most infections associated with anaerobic bacteria, since these processes harbor multiple strains of organisms with varying oxygen sensitivities and undefined pathogenic potentials. Anaerobic infections follow the model of bacterial synergy, in which several bacteria behave in a cooperative fashion to produce infection. In experimental model systems of mixed infection, various microbial components contribute virulence factors or growth substances that permit other more pathogenic forms to invade the tissues. Most clinical anaerobic infections are mixed, containing several species of bacteria. Because it is not clear which are the primary pathogens and which are the symbionts and commensals, it is often necessary to treat all of the potential pathogens.

Virulence Factors. The microenvironment of an anaerobic abscess has features that ensure its own survival. An abscess has an Eh of −250 mv, with an extremely low concentration of oxygen. Anaerobiosis is a hostile condition for host-defense mechanisms. Within this oxygen-free zone, neutrophils are unable to kill bacteria by their oxidative metabolic pathway. Low oxygen tension also inhibits the activity of aminoglycoside antibiotics, since they require an oxidative transport system to cross the bacterial cell envelope. The abscess itself contains a large concentration of microorganisms, approximately 10^8 to 10^9 per milliliter. A high inoculum and a relatively low growth rate are adverse conditions for the activity of β-lactam antibiotics. Thus, host defenses and antibiotic interventions are hindered in an anaerobic abscess.

Individual anaerobic microorganisms possess virulence factors that promote their survival in the host's tissues. *B. fragilis* elaborates a polysaccharide capsule that provides protection against phagocytosis by neutrophils. Membrane-associated enzymes are found in many virulent anaerobes, including β-lactamases and superoxide dismutase (SOD). The β-lactamases destroy antibiotics such as penicillin and cephalosporin. SOD, an enzyme present in virtually all pathogenic anaerobes studied thus far, seems to protect the organism in its initial exposure to oxygenated tissues.

Immunologic factors are affected by anaerobic bacteria. Several species of anaerobes are more resistant to phagocytosis than coliforms and other facultative organisms. Anaerobic bacteria can also interfere with phagocytosis of aerobes when both organisms are present in a mixed infection. Infection with *B. fragilis* induces T cells of CD4$^+$8$^+$ phenotype, leading to abscess formation. Thus, abscess is related to cellular, rather than humoral immune mechanisms.

Role of Facultative Organisms. Facultative or aerobic organisms are frequent partners in anaerobic infections. In some settings these organisms seem to initiate the infective process, perhaps by promoting early tissue necrosis or by consuming oxygen in the tissues. In abdominal infections coliforms and *Bacteroides* are often isolated together.

An animal model of intra-abdominal infection has delineated the role of these pathogens in the septic process. Following intestinal perforation, the initial phase consists of peritonitis, bacteremia, and septic shock. This phase is caused, at least in the animal model, by coliforms such as *E. coli* and *Proteus*. The later abscess formation is associated with anaerobes, particularly *Bacteroides*. Antimicrobial drugs active only against coliforms suppress the initial septicemic and shock phase but have no effect on abscess formation. Similarly, antianaerobic drugs do not protect against coliform bacteremia, but they do suppress formation of abscess. The clinical picture is complex, with overlapping of the septic shock stage and the abscess stage. However, the therapeutic implications are clear: Both components of abdominal sepsis should receive appropriate antimicrobial attention.

ANAEROBIC BACTERIA IN VARIOUS INFECTIONS. Aerobic and facultative microorganisms have been traditionally considered the major pathogens in infectious diseases. Recent improvements in laboratory techniques have facilitated the identification of anaerobic bacteria, and it has become clear that these oxygen-sensitive organisms share responsibility for a significant number of infections seen in clinical practice (Table 311–1).

Intra-abdominal Infections. Infections within the peritoneal cavity usually are related to contamination by the intestinal flora. The microflora of the upper intestine, from the stomach to the upper ileum, consists of sparse numbers of facultative gram-positive organisms derived from the oropharynx. Relatively few coliforms and obligate anaerobes are encountered. The lower bowel, on the other hand, harbors a luxuriant flora in which anaerobes outnumber facultative organisms such as coliforms by a factor of 1000 to 1. Hence, injuries to the upper intestinal tract, such as perforated ulcer or trauma, result in a small inoculum of microorganisms and a low risk of infection. But colonic perforations release a large inoculum of bacteria, causing a high rate of infection.

TABLE 311–1. PRINCIPAL TYPES OF ANAEROBIC INFECTIONS

Location	Type of Infection
Head and neck	Brain abscess
	Gingivitis
	Chronic sinusitis
	Chronic otitis media
	Odontogenic and oropharyngeal-space infections
Respiratory tract	Aspiration pneumonia
	Necrotizing pneumonia
	Lung abscess
	Empyema (adults)
Gastrointestinal tract	Peritonitis
	Intra-abdominal abscess
	Liver abscess
Female genital tract	Tubo-ovarian abscess
	Salpingitis (30–50% of cases)
	Septic abortion and endometritis
	Bartholin's gland abscess
	Bacterial vaginosis
Skin and soft tissue	Crepitant cellulitis
	Necrotizing fasciitis
	Myonecrosis (gas gangrene)
	Decubitus ulcer
	Diabetic foot ulcer
	Bite wounds

From Styrt B, Gorbach SL: Recent developments in the understanding of the pathogenesis and treatment of anaerobic infections. N Engl J Med 321:240–246, 1989. Reprinted by permission of the New England Journal of Medicine.

Peritonitis and intra-abdominal abscess are associated with anaerobic bacteria in 95 per cent of cases. The most frequent finding is a mixture of aerobes and anaerobes. (Infection by a single facultative organism such as *E. coli* is uncommon and usually is seen in *primary peritonitis* associated with cirrhosis of the liver.) In a large series of intra-abdominal infections, an average of five different organisms were isolated from each patient, including three types of anaerobes and two aerobes. Of the anaerobes, *Bacteroides, Clostridium,* anaerobic cocci, and *Fusobacterium* are the major pathogens. The specific site of infection does not determine the flora, since the same pathogens are found in peritonitis, appendicitis, subphrenic abscess, and diverticular abscess.

Anaerobic Pleuropulmonary Infections. Anaerobic infections of the lower respiratory tract produce four clinical conditions: *aspiration pneumonia, lung abscess, necrotizing pneumonia,* and *empyema.* The pathogenesis of these conditions is aspiration of oropharyngeal contents, a situation associated with compromised state of consciousness, obstruction of the esophagus, and neurologic deficits. The oral flora is permitted admission to normally sterile regions of the lower respiratory tract. Approximately 90 per cent of patients with aspiration pneumonia have anaerobes as the major infecting flora. The situation applies to patients who have aspirated outside the hospital or shortly after admission, since they harbor normal oral flora. When the aspiration event occurs after hospitalization or after treatment with antibiotics, at which time the oral flora becomes colonized by gram-negative facultative organisms, the aspirated flora assumes a different character consisting of coliforms and *Pseudomonas.* Lung abscess is associated with anaerobic bacteria in over 90 per cent of cases. The aerobes that occasionally cause a solitary lung abscess include *Klebsiella* and *S. aureus.* Necrotizing pneumonia is actually an earlier stage of lung abscess in which a specific segment or lobe of the lung is extensively damaged with multiple small abscesses. In the more advanced stage these abscesses coalesce to form a single large cavity, leaving in its wake a large area of destroyed lung. Necrotizing pneumonia is a more aggressive condition than lung abscess, with higher mortality. Anaerobes are responsible for the vast majority of cases. Empyema is an infection usually associated with underlying pneumonitis or lung abscess. Nearly 75 per cent of the cases of empyema are associated with anaerobes, most frequently in patients with chronic infection. The remaining cases are caused by the classic aerobic pathogens such as staphylococci, group A streptococci, and pneumococci; these organisms produce an acute onset and a more virulent course. Formerly, most cases of empyema were caused by these aerobic gram-positive organisms, but the situation has been reversed with the advent of antimicrobial agents.

Anaerobic pleuropulmonary infections involve multiple bacterial species including *B. melaninogenicus, F. nucleatum,* and anaerobic gram-positive cocci. *B. fragilis* is found in 15 per cent of cases. The fact that these organisms are found in the same relative concentrations in the various clinical cases suggests that the inoculum of oral contents is similar in each setting.

Obstetric and Gynecologic Infections. The source of infections of the female upper genital tract is the vaginal flora, which has aerobic and anaerobic bacteria as normal constituents. The clinical conditions in which anaerobes are frequently encountered include tubo-ovarian abscess, pelvic abscess, septic abortion, endomyometritis, and postoperative wound infection (following hysterectomy). Polymicrobial bacteremia is a frequent occurrence in patients with severe pelvic infections. The major anaerobic pathogens are *Bacteroides, Peptostreptococcus, Fusobacterium,* and *Clostridium.* Pelvic inflammatory disease, also known as salpingitis, is a milder condition that is caused by an array of organisms, including gonococci, *Chlamydia,* and anaerobes, particularly *Peptostreptococcus.*

Head and Neck Infections. Because the anaerobic bacteria in the normal flora of the upper airways have limited invasive properties, they require an antecedent event that permits their movement into deeper structures. Dental manipulation, trauma, prior bacterial or viral infections, and operative interventions can provide the initiating circumstance. Necrotizing infections of the gingiva and endodontal infections are usually associated with oral strains of *Bacteroides* and *Fusobacterium.* Spirochetes have been found at the advancing border of inflammation in histologic sections of acute ulcerative gingivitis, noma, and lung abscess. Since these organisms cannot be grown in subculture, their role in pathogenesis cannot be assessed. In patients with *sinusitis*, anaerobes are recovered from 50 per cent of patients with chronic processes. However, acute or subacute sinusitis, lasting 3 months or less, is rarely associated with anaerobes. *Otitis media* may be either acute or chronic. As in sinusitis, anaerobes may be present in the chronic forms but are rarely present in the more acute cases. *Space infections*, occurring in the potential spaces formed by fascial planes of the head and neck, are usually associated with three types of organisms: either *S. aureus, Streptococcus pyogenes*, or anaerobic bacteria. The first two organisms occur in space infections related to overlying skin processes such as boils or impetigo. Anaerobes are associated with space infections that arise from diseases of the mucous membrane, dental manipulations, or in those cases that occur spontaneously. *Ludwig's angina* is an example of a space infection associated with anaerobes.

Of the central nervous system infections, *brain abscess* is the one most frequently associated with anaerobic bacteria. These organisms are isolated from 85 per cent of suppurative brain abscesses unrelated to trauma or operative procedures. Gram-positive cocci, followed in frequency by *Fusobacterium* and *Bacteroides*, are the most common strains, often in association with facultative streptococci and coliforms. *Subdural empyema* may also be caused by anaerobes, particularly when it occurs in association with a parameningeal focus in an ear or nasal sinus. Classic pyogenic meningitis, however, is rarely caused by anaerobes.

Skin, Bone, and Soft Tissue Infections. The predisposing factors in anaerobic skin and soft tissue infections are trauma, ischemia, and surgery. The organisms often derive from the fecal or oral flora, particularly in wounds associated with intestinal surgery, decubitus ulcer, and human bites. The clinical presentations are *crepitant cellulitis, synergistic gangrene* or *cellulitis*, and *necrotizing fasciitis*. Anaerobes are also regularly encountered in *diabetic foot ulcers;* 75 per cent of such lesions are associated with *Bacteroides*, anaerobic cocci, and *Clostridium*, usually in mixed culture. Anaerobic *osteomyelitis* is associated with trauma or prior surgery, although some cases arise from hematogenous spread.

CLUES TO PRESUMPTIVE DIAGNOSIS OF ANAEROBIC INFECTION. Clinicians should suspect the diagnosis of an anaerobic infection before the bacteriologic results are available on the basis of the following features: (1) Any infection that is contiguous or in proximity to a mucosal surface normally harboring an anaerobic flora—the gastrointestinal tract, female genital tract, and oropharynx. (2) A foul-smelling discharge; this odor is pathognomonic evidence of anaerobic infection. The absence of odor, however, is not helpful, because 50 per cent of anaerobic infections lack the characteristic odor. (3) The presence of severe tissue necrosis, abscess formation, fasciitis, or gangrene. (4) Gas in the tissue, which is highly suggestive, although not absolutely diagnostic. (5) A mixed infection, indicated by a Gram's stain of exudate showing a polymorphic array of organisms. Certain anaerobes have a characteristic appearance under the microscope, especially *Clostridium, Fusobacterium, Actinomyces*, and certain strains of *Bacteroides*. (6) The failure to recover organisms by conventional aerobic culture in the presence of clinical infection. (7) Failure to respond to antibiotics that have poor anaerobic activity, such as aminoglycosides and certain penicillins and cephalosporins.

TREATMENT STRATEGIES FOR ANAEROBIC INFECTIONS. Successful therapy for anaerobic infections involves rational antibiotic selection in conjunction with judicious surgical resection and drainage. The operative approach may be ultimately decisive, but it should be emphasized that surgical intervention alone may be inadequate. Anaerobic infection can continue to simmer with intermittent sepsis and insidious extension of the process unless appropriate antimicrobial agents are employed. Selection of initial antibiotic therapy should be based on knowledge of the pathogens likely to be present in a specific clinical setting. Because many anaerobic infections tend to be mixed with coliforms and other facultative organisms, it is advisable to use antimicrobial drugs active against both components. With regard

to the anaerobic components, important differences are seen in infections above and below the diaphragm. Anaerobic infections above the diaphragm, including those in the central nervous system, head and neck region, and pleuropulmonary area, tend to involve organisms sensitive to penicillin. This observation is not invariably true, since certain organisms, especially *Bacteroides*, can elaborate β-lactamases, which inactivate penicillins and cephalosporins. Anaerobic infections below the diaphragm, such as those in the abdominal cavity and female genital tract, commonly involve the *B. fragilis* group as a major pathogen. Because these organisms are commonly resistant to several antimicrobial agents, infections in these sites require special consideration for choice of antimicrobial drugs.

TREATMENT. The range of choice among antimicrobial drugs is somewhat limited with regard to anaerobic bacteria in general and even more so with members of the *B. fragilis* group. A United States survey of antibiotic susceptibility among strains of *B. fragilis* from eight medical centers was conducted from 1981 to 1986. Among the β-lactam antibiotics, imipenem and ticarcillin–clavulanic acid were the most active, followed by piperacillin, cefoxitin, and moxalactam. Since high blood levels can be achieved with these drugs, they can be used to treat clinical infections caused by this organism. Disappointing results were seen with penicillin, carbenicillin, ticarcillin, cephalothin, cefamandole, cefotetan, and certain third-generation cephalosporins such as cefotaxime and cefoperazone. The drugs in this grouping are not considered good choices for infections associated with *B. fragilis*. Clostridia, fusobacteria, and gram-positive cocci are usually sensitive to several drugs, including penicillins, cephalosporins, clindamycin, and metronidazole.

The explanation for variations in activity of the β-lactam drugs against anaerobes is the presence in certain strains of constitutive β-lactamases. This enzyme is found in most strains of *Bacteroides* and in occasional strains of *Fusobacterium* isolated from clinical sources. The increased activity of cefoxitin, imipenem, and ticarcillin–clavulanate against *Bacteroides* is based on their resistance to hydrolysis by β-lactamase elaborated by anaerobic organisms.

Metronidazole, a bactericidal drug, has excellent activity against *Bacteroides, Fusobacterium, Clostridium*, and most strains of anaerobic cocci. Resistance to metronidazole among *Bacteroides* is extremely rare. Since the drug has a spectrum limited almost exclusively to anaerobes, another agent such as an aminoglycoside or a cephalosporin should be included for facultative organisms. In clinical trials metronidazole has produced excellent results in intra-abdominal infections, female pelvic infections, brain abscess, and anaerobic osteomyelitis. Many failures, however, have been noted in anaerobic pleuropulmonary infections, probably related to the relatively poor activity against microaerophilic organisms that may accompany this infectious process.

Clindamycin is highly active against most anaerobic isolates with resistance rates among *Bacteroides* running at about 5 per cent. Some resistant isolates of *Clostridium* and *Fusobacterium* have been encountered, but they have been relatively uncommon in clinical practice. The drug is also active against streptococci, both aerobic and anaerobic, and most strains of *S. aureus*. Because it has very little activity against coliforms and other facultative gram-negative organisms, a second drug is used in mixed anaerobic infections. Clindamycin has produced excellent results in intra-abdominal infections, female pelvic infections, and skin and soft tissue infections. Some authorities consider it the drug of choice for anaerobic pleuropulmonary infections, preferring it to penicillin because of apparent failures associated with penicillin treatment. Erythromycin is less active than clindamycin, although resistance patterns commonly overlap. The problem with erythromycin is the difficulty in administering it parenterally. By the oral route only low serum levels of erythromycin are obtained, often below the amount needed to inhibit many anaerobic bacteria.

Tetracyclines were once touted as drugs of choice for anaerobic infections, but their performance against *Bacteroides* and many gram-negative cocci has considerably altered this view. Widespread tetracycline resistance has been noted. As a result, this class of compounds is not recommended for treatment of anaerobic infections. Chloramphenicol shows excellent activity in vitro against *Bacteroides* and most other anaerobic pathogens. It also has activity against coliforms, staphylococci, and streptococci.

Whereas some clinical trials have shown good results with chloramphenicol, others have encountered therapeutic failures. In addition, animal models of anaerobic infection have shown poor results with chloramphenicol treatment.

Aminoglycoside and quinilone antimicrobial drugs, as well as aztreonam and ceftazidime, are inactive against most anaerobic bacteria. These drugs are included in antimicrobial regimens for therapy of mixed infections, although their role is clearly to suppress the facultative gram-negative components.

PROGNOSIS. Prognosis of anaerobic infections is related to the site of infection, the type of pathogen, the underlying condition of the patient, and the choice of antimicrobial therapy. In general, anaerobic pleuropulmonary infections have a good outcome, especially when adequate drainage can be achieved. Penicillin G has been successful in treating these infections in the past, curing up to 95 per cent of patients with aspiration pneumonia or lung abscess, for example. Some failures have been noted with penicillin, and in such instances clindamycin has been used to advantage. Metronidazole treatment has been associated with failures in lung abscess.

Severe intra-abdominal infections have a failure rate of 10 to 20 per cent even with optimal surgery and antimicrobial therapy. Higher failure rates in controlled clinical trials have been associated with treatment regimens using antimicrobial agents with poor activity against *B. fragilis* such as cephalothin, doxycycline, cefamandole, and cefoperazone. Infections of the female genital tract generally have a good prognosis, since most patients tend to be rather healthy prior to the onset of the septic process. Good results have been reported with cefoxitin, clindamycin,

and metronidazole, usually in association with another antibiotic. In one clinical trial penicillin combined with gentamicin produced a poor result in endomyometritis when compared with the alternative regimen of clindamycin and gentamicin.

In general, clinical trials with new antimicrobial agents have corroborated the findings in animal models and susceptibility testing in vitro. Because of the vast array of anaerobic organisms and their varying patterns of susceptibility, it is best to base empiric therapy on known sensitivity patterns and performance of the specific drugs in controlled clinical trials.

Bartlett JG, Louie TJ, Gorbach SL, et al.: Therapeutic efficacy of 29 antimicrobial regimens in experimental intra-abdominal sepsis. Rev Infect Dis 3:535, 1981. *An experimental model of intra-abdominal infections that explains the pathophysiologic events and the rationale for antimicrobial treatments.*

Cuchural GJ, Tally FP, Jacobus NV, et al.: Comparative activities of newer β-lactam agents against members of the *Bacteroides fragilis* group. Antimicrob Agents Chemother 34:479, 1990. *Seven medical centers in the United States collaborated on this survey of antibiotic efficacy against the pre-eminent anerobic pathogens.*

Finegold SM, George WL (eds.): Anaerobic Infections in Humans. New York, Academic Press, 1989. *A collection of authoritative articles by the "Who's Who" in anaerobic bacteriology.*

Kasper DL, Onderdonk AB (eds.): International Symposium on Anaerobic Bacteria and Bacterial Infections. Rev Infect Dis 12:S2, 1990. *Complete clinical, laboratory, and therapeutic aspects, presented by foremost experts in the field.*

Styrt B, Gorbach SL: Recent developments in the understanding of the pathogenesis and treatment of anaerobic infections. N Engl J Med 321:240–246, 298–302, 1989. *An update of advances, with an extensive bibliography.*

Enteric Infections

312 Introduction

Bruce M. Greene

Included in this section are bacteria that are pathogenic in humans as a consequence of their intraintestinal localization and multiplication, and biologic properties that lead to disease through toxin production and its physiologic effects, direct damage to intestinal epithelial cells, or invasion across the mucosa into lymphoid tissues with subsequent multiplication and dissemination. Although the major global impact of most of these pathogens is in developing countries, in the aggregate they represent a major and poorly controlled threat to human health in many developed countries, including the United States. Furthermore, diarrhea in travelers to developing countries, most commonly due to strains of *Escherichia coli*, is a major health problem, affecting one third to one half of those who spend significant time abroad.

The clinical manifestations associated with this group of pathogens are quite diverse. Typhoid fever is dominated by systemic manifestations in the majority of cases, particularly early in the infection, and in only approximately one third of cases is diarrhea a significant manifestation. Intestinal perforation and hemorrhage are frequent. Conversely, at the other end of the spectrum, cholera is manifest almost exclusively as a secretory diarrhea, with systemic manifestations reflecting fluid loss. Shigellosis shows a combination of febrile and toxic manifestations as well as fluid loss reflecting damage to colonic epithelium. Nontyphoidal salmonellae may cause classic enteric fever as well as severe diarrheal syndromes. Strains of diarrheogenic *E. coli* vary considerably in their mode of pathogenesis and consequently in the associated clinical manifestations. Campylobacter enteritis is a febrile illness associated with diarrhea that is frequently bloody.

Differential diagnostic features of this group of infections are indicated in Table 312–1. Importantly, in addition to these agents it may be difficult to exclude amebic dysentery from consideration, as well as rotavirus enteritis, giardiasis, yersinia infection, and food poisoning due to other bacterial pathogens such as *Bacillus cereus*, clostridia, *Vibrio parahemolyticus*, and *Staphylococcus aureus*. Therefore, specific epidemiologic features in an individual case may be crucial in establishing the correct diagnosis and in instituting proper therapy. Furthermore, the presence of

TABLE 312–1. DIAGNOSTIC FEATURES OF COMMON ENTERIC INFECTIONS

Causative Agent(s)	Typical Clinical Manifestations	Signs and Laboratory Manifestations	Epidemiologic Features
Salmonella typhi	Fever, intestinal perforation, or hemorrhage	Rose spots, relative leukopenia	Travel to or residence in endemic areas
Vibrio cholera	Severe watery diarrhea; dehydration	Fecal leukocytes absent	Residence in endemic areas
Shigella species	Fever, cramps, explosive diarrhea	Abundant fecal leukocytes	Travel to developing countries; residence in a custodial institution
Nontyphoidal salmonellae	a. Fever, diarrhea b. Typhoidal fever	a. Fecal leukocytes (moderate) b. Relative leukopenia	Consumption of undercooked poultry, eggs, processed meats; nursing homes
Diarrheogenic *E. coli*	a. Fever, diarrhea b. Hemorrhagic diarrhea	Fecal leukocytes prominent in enteroinvasive forms	Travel to developing countries; consumption of inadequately cooked processed food
Campylobacter jejuni	Fever, diarrhea	Fecal leukocytes present	Consumption of undercooked poultry, unpasteurized milk, contaminated water

immunodeficiency, especially AIDS, necessitates consideration of multiple additional pathogens and reordering of the likelihood of causative agents (see Ch. 416 for gastrointestinal manifestations of AIDS).

313 Typhoid Fever

Thomas Butler

DEFINITION. Typhoid fever is a bacterial disease caused by *Salmonella typhi.* It is characterized by prolonged fever, abdominal pain, diarrhea, delirium, rose spots, and splenomegaly and complicated sometimes by intestinal bleeding and perforation. Enteric fever is synonymous with typhoid fever, which is occasionally caused also by *S. enteritidis* bioserotype paratyphi A or B.

ETIOLOGY. The typhoid bacillus is a motile gram-negative rod in the family Enterobacteriaceae. It possesses a flagellar (H) antigen, a cell wall (O) lipopolysaccharide antigen, and a polysaccharide virulence (Vi) antigen located in the cell capsule. The polysaccharide side chain of the O antigen confers serologic specificity to the organism and is essential in virulence because salmonellae other than *S. typhi* and *S. enteritidis* bioserotype paratyphi A or B do not produce enteric fever in humans. These antigens play critical roles in permitting the organisms to invade lymphoid tissue from the gut lumen and to multiply within macrophages.

INCIDENCE AND PREVALENCE. Typhoid fever has been almost eliminated from developed countries because of sewage and water treatment facilities but remains a common disease in developing countries. In 1980, the number of cases occurring yearly was estimated as about 7 million in Asia, over 4 million in Africa, and 0.5 million in Latin America. About 500 cases are diagnosed each year in the United States, and over half of these are in recently arrived travelers who contracted their infections abroad.

EPIDEMIOLOGY. Adults and childen of all ages and both sexes appear equally susceptible to infection. In developing countries, most cases occur in school-age children and young adults. Although acquired immunity provides some protection, reinfections have been documented. Typhoid fever occurs during all seasons.

Transmission is by the fecal-oral route through contaminated water or food. The main human sources of infection in the community are asymptomatic fecal carriers and cases during either disease or convalescence. Females and older males are prone to become chronic fecal carriers because underlying cholecystitis enables them to harbor chronic infection in the gallbladder. *S. typhi* is resistant to drying and cooling, thus allowing bacteria to survive prolonged periods in dried sewage, water, food, and ice.

Vi-phage typing of *S. typhi* is a useful epidemiologic tool to trace cases of typhoid fever to a carrier or food source. Single-source outbreaks of typhoid fever are rare. In endemic situations, multiple phage types are present, and several phage types may be responsible for an epidemic.

PATHOGENESIS AND PATHOLOGY. After ingestion of *S. typhi*, the part of the inoculum that survives the acidity of the stomach enters the small intestine, where bacteria penetrate the mucosa and enter mononuclear phagocytes of ileal Peyer's patches and mesenteric lymph nodes. Inocula of at least 10^5 bacteria are necessary to initiate disease, and inocula of 10^7 and more cause disease regularly. The incubation period ranges from 8 to 28 days, depending on inoculum size and immune status of the host. Bacteria proliferate in mononuclear phagocytes and spread by way of the blood to the spleen, liver, and bone marrow, where further proliferation in macrophages occurs. The earliest symptoms of fever and chills (Table 313–1) are associated with bacteremia. Inflammatory reactions occur in the spleen, liver, bone marrow, Peyer's patches mainly in the terminal ileum, and skin, consisting of mononuclear cell infiltration, hyperplasia, and focal necrosis. Focal collections of mononuclear leukocytes are called "typhoid nodules." Fever and other constitutional symptoms are probably caused by the release of interleukin 1 (endogenous pyrogen) from infected mononuclear phagocytes. Endotoxemia does not occur in typhoid fever. Intestinal manifestations are caused by hyperplasia of Peyer's patches with ulcerations of overlying mucosa, resulting in pain, diarrhea, bleeding, or perforation.

CLINICAL MANIFESTATIONS. In the first days of illness the nonspecific symptoms of fever, chills, and headache are mild and in the typical case build up in intensity during the first week, resulting in prostration. The evolution of disease syndromes occurs stepwise over 1 to 3 weeks (Table 313–1) but may be variable in the time of appearance. The early symptoms of fever, abdominal pain, and prostration tend to persist throughout the illness, which in untreated cases lasts a month or longer. Abdominal pain occurs in more than half of patients and is frequently diffuse or located in the right lower quadrant over the terminal ileum. Diarrhea occurs in about a third of patients and consists of either watery stools or semisolid stools described as "pea soup." Melena occurs less commonly. Rose spots occur in more than half of light-skinned individuals but are often not visible in dark-skinned patients. The rash is seen most commonly on the shoulders, thorax, and abdomen and rarely affects the extremities. The lesions are erythematous macules or papules about 1 to 5 mm in diameter which typically blanch with pressure but may become hemorrhagic. They fade quickly after a few days of treatment. Many patients display abnormal behavior or altered mental status that may be out of proportion to the severity of the systemic illness. Among the common presentations are "toxic" staring, delirium, aphonia, and coma. Seizures are common in children. Patients are rarely jaundiced.

In about 5 per cent of patients, intestinal bleeding or intestinal perforation occurs, usually after the second week of illness. Bleeding occurs from ileal ulcers and may present as melena or bright red blood in stools. Brisk bleeding develops rarely but is an occasional cause of death. Intestinal perforation presents as the sudden onset of more severe abdominal pain, distention, and tenderness. Bowel sounds are diminished and the abdominal radiograph usually reveals free air. Perforation most often occurs unexpectedly after a few days of treatment when a patient has started to improve. Other complications of typhoid fever include pneumonia, which develops as a superinfection due to other bacteria, myocarditis, acute cholecystitis, and acute meningitis.

Relapses occur in about 10 to 20 per cent of patients treated with chloramphenicol. Patients with relapses experience the reappearance of typical symptoms about 7 to 14 days after the

TABLE 313–1. EVOLUTION OF TYPICAL SYMPTOMS AND SIGNS OF TYPHOID FEVER

Disease Period	Symptoms	Signs	Pathology
First week	Fever, chills gradually increasing and persisting; headache	Abdominal tenderness	Bacteremia
Second week	Rash, abdominal pain, diarrhea or constipation, delirium, prostration	Rose spots, splenomegaly, hepatomegaly	Mononuclear cell vasculitis of skin, hyperplasia of ileal Peyer's patches, typhoid nodules in spleen and liver
Third week	Complications of intestinal bleeding and perforation, shock	Melena, ileus, rigid abdomen, coma	Ulcerations over Peyer's patches, perforation with peritonitis
Fourth week and later	Resolution of symptoms, relapse, weight loss	Reappearance of acute disease, cachexia	Cholecystitis, chronic fecal carriage of bacteria

end of treatment. Relapses tend to be less severe than the initial episode.

DIAGNOSIS. The preferred method of diagnosis is isolation of *S. typhi* from a blood culture, which is positive in most patients during the first 2 weeks of illness. Urine and stool cultures are positive less frequently but should be taken to increase the diagnostic yield. The bone marrow culture is the most sensitive test, positive in nearly 90 per cent of cases, and can be used when a bacteriologic diagnosis is crucially needed or in patients who have been pretreated with antibiotics. The duodenal string test to culture bile has also been used with success in typhoid fever.

The Widal test for agglutinating antibodies against the somatic (O) and flagellar (H) antigens of *S. typhi* is widely used for serodiagnosis. An O agglutinin titer of ≥1:80 or a fourfold rise supports a diagnosis of typhoid fever, whereas the H agglutinins are more often nonspecifically elevated by immunization or previous infections with other bacteria. Serodiagnosis is of limited value because false-positive results are often obtained in endemic areas and false-negative results occur in some cases of bacteriologically proven typhoid fever.

Other laboratory findings are anemia of variable severity and a white blood cell count that is normal or decreased with an increased percentage of band forms. Platelets are often diminished, and signs of disseminated intravascular coagulation are present. Liver function tests frequently show elevated aminotransferases and bilirubin concentrations. Renal failure is an infrequent complication. In patients with diarrhea, the stool shows fecal leukocytes.

The differential diagnosis depends on infections that are endemic in the area where an individual contracted the infection. For returned travelers from developing countries, the common possibilities are malaria, hepatitis, typhus, amebic liver abscess, shigellosis, nontyphoid salmonellosis, and leptospirosis. In the United States one must consider septicemias originating from the urinary tract, GI tract, or gallbladder as well as influenza, infectious mononucleosis, meningococcemia, miliary tuberculosis, and bacterial endocarditis.

TREATMENT. Chloramphenicol has remained the drug of choice since its introduction in 1948 because no other drug has been demonstrated to cause more rapid or consistent improvement of disease. Resistance to chloramphenicol mediated by plasmid R factors has been reported only occasionally in patients who acquired infections in Mexico, India, and Thailand. Chloramphenicol is given orally in a dose of 50 to 60 mg per kilogram of body weight per day in four equal portions every 6 hours. After defervescence and clinical improvement the dosage can be reduced to 30 mg per kilogram per day to complete a 14-day course. In patients unable to take oral medication the same dosage should be given intravenously until the patient can take capsules.

Alternative drugs should be considered when *S. typhi* resistant to chloramphenicol is isolated or strongly suspected. Several are nearly equal to chloramphenicol in efficacy. Trimethoprim-sulfamethoxazole is effective in a standard adult dose of 160 mg trimethoprim and 800 mg sulfamethoxazole given orally or intravenously twice a day for 14 days. Other drugs that are effective include ampicillin (intravenously), amoxicillin, cefoperazone, and ceftriaxone.

Patients who are dehydrated, anorectic, or suffering from diarrhea should receive intravenous saline with attention to electrolyte and acid-base disturbances. Patients with brisk intestinal bleeding require blood transfusion. Patients with suspected perforation should have an abdominal radiograph to look for free air and peritoneal fluid. Laparotomy should be undertaken as early as possible to suture the perforation, and gentamicin should be added to broaden coverage for polymicrobial peritonitis.

In some high-risk patients with delirium, coma, or shock, high-dose dexamethasone in addition to antibiotics reduces mortality. The dose should be 3 mg per kilogram initially, followed by 1 mg per kilogram every 6 hours for 48 hours. One must be cautious with this therapy because signs and symptoms of perforation are masked by steroids. Antipyretic drugs such as aspirin should be administered with caution because they occasionally cause marked reductions in blood pressure.

Patients with relapses of typhoid fever should be treated the same as patients with a first attack. Chronic fecal carriers (asymp-

tomatic excretion for a year or longer) should be given high doses of ampicillin or amoxicillin, 100 mg per kilogram per day, plus probenecid 30 mg per kilogram per day for 4 to 6 weeks. Trimethoprim-sulfamethoxazole is also effective. Patients with gallstones or cholecystitis may require cholecystectomy for eradication of the carrier state. Chloramphenicol neither prevents nor effectively treats the chronic carrier state.

PROGNOSIS. Typhoid fever carried a case fatality rate of about 12 per cent in the preantibiotic era which was reduced to about 4 per cent after chloramphenicol became available. Case fatality rates over 10 per cent continue to be reported in developing countries despite availability of antibiotics, whereas developed countries show case fatality rates less than 1 per cent. After treatment with chloramphenicol or other effective drug, most patients become afebrile in 4 to 7 days. In the preantibiotic era about 10 per cent of recovered patients had relapses, and chloramphenicol treatment has not reduced this rate. Intestinal bleeding or perforation occurs in about 5 per cent of patients and may not be prevented by antibiotic treatment. Thus, bleeding or perforation is occasionally detected after patients have defervesced during treatment. About 1 to 3 per cent of patients become chronic fecal carriers after recovery.

PREVENTION. Travelers to developing countries should avoid consuming untreated water, drinks served with ice, peeled fruits, and other food that is not served hot. American international travelers face an overall risk of developing typhoid fever of less than 1 case in 10,000 trips, but travelers to high-risk countries like India and Pakistan have a probability of about 4 in 10,000 trips of getting typhoid fever. Travelers wishing immune protection should receive either live oral vaccine Ty21a (Berna Products [1-800-533-5899]) given as one capsule every other day for a total of four capsules or typhoid vaccine, U.S.P., administered as two subcutaneous injections of 0.5 ml each at intervals of 4 weeks, with booster doses given every 3 years if needed. These vaccines give only partial protection, and thus vaccinated persons should still exercise dietary precautions. The traditional method of controlling typhoid is to follow stool cultures of convalescent cases and report positive cultures to the Health Department. The Health Department investigates nonimported typhoid cases to identify possible food sources or contact with a chronic carrier.

Butler T, Islam A, Kabir I, et al.: Patterns of morbidity and mortality in typhoid fever dependent on age and gender: Review of 552 hospitalized patients with diarrhea. Rev Infect Dis 13:85, 1991. *Severe and fatal disease in Bangladesh was more common in young children and adults and was correlated with high incidences of seizures, delirium or coma, intestinal perforation, and pneumonia.*

Hornick RB: Selective primary health care: Strategies for control of disease in the developing world. XX. Typhoid fever. Rev Infect Dis 7:536, 1985. *A useful review of pathogenesis, epidemiology, and prevention of this infection.*

Islam A, Butler T, Nath SK, et al.: Randomized treatment of patients with typhoid fever by using ceftriaxone or chloramphenicol. J Infect Dis 158:742, 1988. *Study of treatment in Bangladesh showed that chloramphenicol remains the treatment of choice because of low cost and rapid defervescence, but newer cephalosporins are good alternatives.*

Klotz SA, Jorgensen JH, Buckwold FJ, et al.: Typhoid fever: An epidemic with remarkably few clinical signs and symptoms. Arch Intern Med 144:533, 1984. *In 34 patients in Texas who were infected after eating Mexican food at a restaurant, illness was characterized by fever without localizing signs and symptoms; there were no deaths or complications.*

Levine MM, Ferreccio C, Black RE, et al.: Large-scale field trial of Ty21a live oral typhoid vaccine in enteric-coated capsule formulation. Lancet 1:1049, 1987. *In Chilean school children, three capsules given every other day conferred 67 per cent protection during 3 years; oral vaccination is preferred to parenteral vaccine because of absence of toxic reactions.*

---

314 Salmonella Infections Other Than Typhoid Fever

Donald Kaye

DEFINITION. *Salmonella*, a genus of the family Enterobacteriaceae, can cause an asymptomatic intestinal carrier state or clinical disease in both humans and animals. In humans the most common clinical manifestation is enterocolitis with diarrhea as the major symptom. Some patients develop bacteremia without gastrointestinal manifestations. Localization from bacteremia may result in osteomyelitis, a mycotic aneurysm, or other localized infection. *S. typhi*, a pathogen of humans only, causes enteric fever. Enteric fever produced by *S. typhi* is called typhoid fever, whereas enteric fever caused by other salmonellae is named paratyphoid fever.

An asymptomatic intestinal carrier state of variable duration may follow inapparent or symptomatic infection. Most carriers are transient carriers. A chronic carrier state, defined as lasting more than 1 year, is usually permanent and is most often related to persistent infection in the gallbladder. With the exception of *S. typhi*, in which a human carrier is always implicated, most salmonella infections are acquired from food products derived from infected animals (e.g., eggs, poultry, meat, milk).

ETIOLOGY. Salmonellae are motile, gram-negative, non–spore-forming members of the family Enterobacteriaceae. They are differentiated from other Enterobacteriaceae by biochemical tests. They ferment glucose, maltose, and mannitol but not lactose or sucrose. Almost all salmonellae produce acid and gas with fermentation and are ornithine- and trehalose-positive. Exceptions to the rules which are helpful in identification are the following: *S. typhi* does not produce gas and is ornithine-negative; *S. choleraesuis* is trehalose-negative; and *S. gallinarum-pullorum* is nonmotile. As another confounding exception, lactose-fermenting strains of salmonellae have been isolated.

Salmonellae can be differentiated into over 2000 serotypes by their somatic (O) antigens, which are composed of lipopolysaccharides and are part of the cell wall, and flagellar (H) antigens. Proper nomenclature has divided the salmonellae into three species: *S. typhi*, *S. choleraesuis*, and *S. enteritidis*. The first two consist of only one serotype each, whereas the third contains all the rest of the serotypes. These latter serotypes are recognized as *S. enteritidis* serotype _____(e.g., *S. enteritidis* serotype typhimurium). However, in a less confusing and cumbersome system, each serotype is commonly referred to as a separate species and is so indicated in this chapter. In this system, using common O antigens, salmonellae have been divided into five major groups, A through E. Some of the important serotypes and their groups are *S. typhi* (group D), *S. choleraesuis* (Group C₁), *S. typhimurium* (group B), and *S. enteritidis* (group D).

S. typhimurium is the most common cause of human disease and represents about 25 per cent of *Salmonella* isolates in the United States reported to the Centers for Disease Control (CDC). Other common isolates are *S. enteritidis*, *S. heidelberg*, *S. newport*, *S. hadar*, *S. infantis*, *S. agona*, *S. montevideo*, *S. thompson*, and *S. braenderup*. In 1987, these 10 serotypes accounted for 73 per cent of the human isolates reported to the CDC. Recently, *S. enteritidis* outbreaks related to eggs have been increasing.

EPIDEMIOLOGY. *S. typhi*, *S. paratyphi* A, *S. schottmuelleri* (*S. paratyphi* B), *S. hirschfeldii* (*S. paratyphi* C), and *S. sendai* are either solely or almost always pathogens in man only, and human-to-human transmission is important.

The remaining serotypes of salmonellae are widely spread in the animal kingdom, and salmonellae have been isolated from virtually all species, including birds, poultry, mammals, reptiles, amphibians, and insects. Salmonella infection in man usually occurs from ingestion of contaminated animal food products, most often eggs, poultry, and meat. Eggs usually become contaminated from feces on the surface of the egg, with small cracks allowing entry into the egg. However, infection of the ovary allows primary incorporation of salmonellae into the egg. Meat and poultry become widely contaminated at the slaughterhouse with salmonellae spread from carcass to carcass, usually on the surface. *S. choleraesuis* is associated with pig products and *S. dublin* with cattle and consumption of unpasteurized milk from cattle. Salmonellae may survive cooking at relatively low temperatures in the center of eggs or turkeys, or food may be contaminated after cooking from kitchen utensils or from the hands of food preparers who handle raw food.

Salmonella infections have been acquired following contamination of food or water with feces of pet turtles, chicks, birds, dogs, cats, and many other species. These pets become infected from their food.

Salmonella infection can also be acquired by eating food or less commonly drinking water contaminated by a human carrier who has not washed his hands adequately. Infection has been spread by the fecal-oral route in children, by contaminated enema and fiberoptic instruments, and by diagnostic and therapeutic preparations made from animal or insect products (e.g., pancreatic extract, carmine dye).

Outbreaks of salmonellosis occur in institutionalized patients, who are probably more prone to develop salmonella infections for three reasons. First, there are more underlying diseases which decrease host defense mechanisms against salmonellae such as disorders of gastric acidity and intestinal motility; second, use of antimicrobial agents reduces the normal, protective intestinal flora; and third, institutional food prepared in bulk is more likely to be contaminated than individually prepared meals. Outbreaks in nurseries and in the elderly in nursing homes have the highest mortality rates (i.e., over 5 per cent).

Most cases of salmonella infection occurring in the United States are sporadic rather than related to outbreaks. However, when an infection occurs in a family, other members of the household also tend to have positive stool cultures. About 40,000 cases of salmonella infection have been reported to the CDC in recent years, a marked increase over the past 30 years. However, this undoubtedly represents only a fraction of actual cases. It has been estimated that over 1 million cases actually occur each year. A disproportionate number of infections occur in July through October, probably related to the warm weather. Salmonella infections are most common in infants and children under 5 years of age.

Salmonellae have become increasingly resistant to antibiotics, with many strains now resistant to ampicillin. Resistance to ampicillin and other antibiotics is usually by means of bacterial acquisition of resistance transfer factors. It is believed that much of the resistance has been related to widespread use of antimicrobial agents in farm animals.

PATHOGENESIS. Following ingestion of organisms, the determinants of whether or not infection results, as well as the severity of infection, are the dose and virulence of the *Salmonella* strain and the status of host defense mechanisms. Large inocula such as 10⁷ bacteria are usually required to produce clinical infection in the normal host. Smaller inocula are more likely to result in no infection or to produce a transient intestinal carrier state. Gastric acid serves as a host defense mechanism by killing many of the ingested organisms, and intestinal motility is also probably a host defense mechanism. In the absence or decrease of gastric acidity (as in the elderly, following gastrectomy, vagotomy or gastroenterostomy, with H₂-receptor antagonists, and with antacids) and with decreased intestinal motility (as with antimotility drugs), much smaller inocula can produce infection and the infection tends to be more severe.

Administration of antimicrobial agents prior to ingestion of salmonellae can markedly reduce the size of inoculum needed to produce infection, presumably by reducing the protective bowel flora.

While any *Salmonella* serotype can produce any of the salmonella syndromes (transient asymptomatic carrier state, enterocolitis, bacteremia, enteric fever, and chronic carrier state), each serotype tends to produce certain syndromes much more often than others. For example, *S. anatum* usually causes asymptomatic intestinal infection, whereas *S. typhimurium* usually causes enterocolitis. *S. choleraesuis* is more likely to produce bacteremia (often with metastatic infection) than asymptomatic infection or enterocolitis, and some serotypes such as *S. typhi* are most likely to cause enteric fever as well as the chronic carrier state. Fortunately, most *Salmonella* serotypes are of relatively low pathogenicity for man, and therefore, although food products are commonly contaminated, large outbreaks occur only when more virulent serotypes are involved.

In order to produce infection (even asymptomatic intestinal infection), enteric pathogens (including salmonellae) must first adhere to intestinal mucosal epithelial cells. Pili on the surface of salmonellae adhere to specific receptor sites on the epithelial cells. Following adherence, invasion of the mucosal cell may result, or multiplication may occur without invasion, resulting in asymptomatic infection. When the organisms reach the lamina propria, polymorphonuclear leukocytes serve as a defense mechanism to prevent invasion of lymphatics. Certain serotypes seem more able than others to invade lymphatics and subsequently produce bacteremia. For example, *S. dublin*, which has been isolated from unpasteurized milk, commonly produces bacteremia following intestinal infection. Both the small intestine and colon are involved in the inflammatory process. The diarrhea in salmonella enterocolitis results from the inflammation. In addition, watery stools may occur, apparently the result of secretion of water and electrolytes by small intestinal epithelial cells in response to an enterotoxin secreted by some of the *Salmonella* strains or in response to tissue mediators of inflammation.

Patients with diseases that impair host defense mechanisms seem to have an increased frequency of severe salmonella infection. For many years, a striking association has been recognized between diseases producing hemolysis and salmonella bacteremia. Specifically, salmonella bacteremia is common in patients with sickle cell disorders, malaria, and bartonellosis. In fact, because of the frequency of salmonella bacteremia in sickle cell diseases and the underlying bone disease in these patients to which salmonellae localize, these organisms are the most common cause of osteomyelitis in patients with sickle cell disorders. Prolonged salmonella bacteremia occurs in patients with hepatosplenic schistosomiasis, probably related to localization on and in the intravascular schistosomes. Patients with lymphoma and leukemia also are more prone to develop salmonella bacteremia. Recently, prolonged and recurrent refractory salmonella bacteremia has been observed in patients with AIDS.

CLINICAL SYNDROMES. *Asymptomatic Intestinal Carrier State.* The asymptomatic intestinal carrier state may result from inapparent infection, which is the most common form of salmonella infection, or may follow clinical disease (convalescent carrier). The carrier state is usually self-limited to several weeks to months, with the incidence of positive stool cultures rapidly decreasing. By 1 year far less than 1 per cent still have positive stools. The major exception is with *S. typhi*: About 3 per cent of those infected excrete the organism for life. A patient who has had *Salmonella* in his or her stool for 1 year (chronic carrier) is likely to become a lifelong carrier. Patients with *Schistosoma haematobium* infections are predisposed to become chronic urinary carriers of *Salmonella*.

Enterocolitis. After an incubation period, which is usually 12 to 48 hours, the illness starts suddenly with crampy abdominal pain and diarrhea. A chill is common. Although occasional patients have nausea and vomit once or twice, vomiting is not persistent. The diarrhea may be watery and of large volume or small volume. The stools may contain mucus and occasionally blood. Polymorphonuclear leukocytes are present in the stool. Diarrhea may be mild or may be severe with up to 20 to 30 stools a day. Fever is present in most patients and may reach 40°C (104°F) or higher. The abdomen is tender to palpation. Transient bacteremia may occur and is most likely in infants, the elderly, and patients with impaired host defense mechanisms.

Symptoms usually improve over a period of days, with fever lasting no more than 2 to 3 days and diarrhea no more than 5 to 7 days. However, these symptoms may occasionally persist for up to 14 days.

Enteric Fever. Paratyphoid fever is an enteric fever syndrome identical to typhoid fever but produced by a serotype other than *S. typhi* (most often *S. paratyphi* A, *S. schottmuelleri*, or *S. hirschfeldii*). On occasion, it may immediately follow classic enterocolitis caused by the same organism. The syndrome, characterized by prolonged sustained fever, relative bradycardia, splenomegaly, rose spots, and leukopenia, is described in Ch. 313. Enteric fever produced by serotypes of *Salmonella* other than *S. typhi* is usually milder than typhoid fever, and the chronic carrier state follows less commonly than after typhoid fever.

Bacteremia. Patients with the syndrome of salmonella bacteremia usually complain of fever and chills for a period of days to weeks. Gastrointestinal symptoms are unusual, but in some patients the syndrome of salmonella bacteremia follows classic enterocolitis. Other symptoms are nonspecific such as malaise, anorexia, and weight loss. Metastatic infection of bones, joints, mycotic aneurysm (particularly of the abdominal aorta), meninges (mainly in infants), pericardium, pleural space, lungs, heart valves, cysts, uterine myomas, malignancies, and other sites is common, and symptoms may be related to the site of metastatic infection. Stool cultures are usually negative for *Salmonella*, but blood cultures are positive.

Although any *Salmonella* serotype can produce the syndrome of bacteremia, *S. choleraesuis* is most likely to cause this syndrome; over 50 per cent of *S. choleraesuis* infections are bacteremic. *S. choleraesuis* infection also has the highest mortality rate of infection caused by any *Salmonella*.

Salmonella bacteremia occurs with increased frequency in infants and the elderly and in patients with diseases associated with hemolysis (such as sickle cell diseases, malaria, and bartonellosis), with lymphoma, and with leukemia. Localization to bone is common in patients with sickle cell diseases.

Prolonged salmonella bacteremia lasting for months occurs in patients with hepatosplenic schistosomiasis. Patients with AIDS develop recurrent, relapsing salmonella bacteremia that is difficult to cure with antibiotics.

DIAGNOSIS. The diagnosis of salmonella infection is made by isolation of the organism from the stool in enterocolitis, from the blood in bacteremia, from blood and stool in enteric fever, and from the local site in localized infection. Serologic studies are of little clinical value in salmonella infections other than typhoid fever, but they may be of use in epidemiologic studies. The white blood cell count is usually normal in enterocolitis, normal or low in enteric fever, and normal in bacteremia. A stained smear of the stool usually demonstrates polymorphonuclear leukocytes in patients with salmonella enterocolitis.

The differential diagnosis of salmonella enterocolitis includes all causes of acute diarrhea, including invasive bacteria such as *Campylobacter jejuni*, *Shigella* species, invasive *E. coli*, *Yersinia enterocolitica*, and *Vibrio parahaemolyticus*; toxigenic bacteria such as *Vibrio cholerae*, enterotoxigenic *E. coli*, *S. aureus*, *B. cereus*, *C. perfringens*, and *C. difficile*; viruses; and protozoa such as *E. histolytica*, *G. lamblia*, and *Cryptosporidium* species. Invasive bacterial causes of diarrhea and *C. difficile* infection are also associated with polymorphonuclear leukocytes in the stool, whereas bacterial toxigenic causes (other than *C. difficile*), viruses, and protozoa generally are not. The bacterial toxigenic causes of diarrhea other than *C. difficile* do not produce fever.

Stool culture is definitive for the diagnosis of salmonella enterocolitis, but by the time the results of the stool culture are available, most patients are recovering.

The differential diagnosis of salmonella bacteremia includes all acute infectious and noninfectious causes of fever, including bacteremia caused by other organisms.

The differential diagnosis of enteric fever is the same as discussed in Ch. 313.

TREATMENT. *Enterocolitis.* The primary approach to treatment of salmonella enterocolitis is fluid and electrolyte replacement. Oral fruit juices and carbonated sodas are useful for those who can take fluids orally. Intravenous fluids are necessary in those who are unable to take oral fluids or who are severely dehydrated, most often the very young and the elderly.

Drugs with antiperistaltic effects such as loperamide or diphenoxylate with atropine can relieve cramps but should be used sparingly, as they can prolong the diarrhea.

Salmonella enterocolitis is self-limited, and the large majority of cases do not require antimicrobial therapy. However, infants, the elderly, and those with sickle cell disease, lymphoma, leukemia, or other serious underlying diseases who are severely ill and may have bacteremia may benefit from antimicrobial therapy. Amoxicillin, 1 gram every 6 hours orally, or trimethoprim-sulfamethoxazole, one double-strength tablet every 12 hours orally in adults, can be used in those who are able to take oral drugs. Ampicillin, 1 to 2 grams IV every 6 hours, and trimethoprim-sulfamethoxazole, 10 mg per kilogram per day IV of the trimethoprim component, have been used in those who are more severely ill. Antibiotic susceptibility studies should be performed on the isolates, as many strains are now resistant to ampicillin. Therapy is continued for 5 days.

There has been a reluctance to treat salmonella enterocolitis, as antibiotic therapy has been reported to have no effect on the clinical course and furthermore to prolong the period of time that salmonellae are excreted in the stool. In addition, most patients are improving by the time that salmonellae or other bacterial pathogens are isolated from the stool. Perhaps most important, effective, single-drug therapy active against *Salmonella*, *Shigella*, *Campylobacter*, and other bacterial causes of diarrhea has been lacking until recently, and early empiric antimicrobial therapy for diarrhea suspected to be of bacterial origin has therefore been problematic.

In the past few years, the availability of norfloxacin and ciprofloxacin has changed some of these factors. These agents are active against virtually all bacterial pathogens that cause diarrhea except for *C. difficile* and can be used empirically in the early therapy of severe diarrhea of presumed bacterial etiology. Furthermore, several preliminary studies indicate that these agents decrease the duration of the clinical course of salmonella enterocolitis but may increase the duration of fecal excretion. These observations of efficacy must be confirmed and extended before routine use of these agents can be advocated for suspected salmonella enterocolitis.

Bacteremia and Enteric Fever. The major therapeutic agents are chloramphenicol, 50 mg per kilogram per day in four equally divided doses orally or IV, or ampicillin, 2 grams IV every 6 hours. With resistant organisms or when these agents cannot be used for other reasons, trimethoprim-sulfamethoxazole IV may be substituted at a dose of 10 mg per kilogram per day of the trimethoprim component. Ampicillin is preferred when localized infection (especially intravascular) is present. After response, oral amoxicillin or oral trimethoprim-sulfamethoxazole can be given in the doses described under enterocolitis. In patients infected with salmonellae resistant to these agents, third-generation cephalosporins such as cefotaxime, ceftizoxime, ceftriaxone, and ceftazidime may be useful. First- and second-generation cephalosporins such as cephalothin and cefamandole do not seem to be acceptably effective. With further experience, ciprofloxacin may also prove to be a very useful agent. Therapy is continued for 2 weeks for enteric fever and bacteremia without localization of organisms and for much longer periods of time with localization to bone, aneurysms, heart valves, and various other sites. Surgical drainage or removal of foreign bodies is often necessary for cure of localized infection.

Cure of the schistosomiasis in patients with salmonella bacteremia may cure the bacteremia. Patients with AIDS tend to relapse repeatedly after treatment courses for salmonella bacteremia. Long-term suppressive therapy has been recommended by some.

Carriers. Chronic carriers (i.e., over 1 year) of salmonellae other than *S. typhi* are rare. Stools of convalescent carriers spontaneously become negative over a period of weeks to months, and no therapy should be given. The rare chronic carrier of non–*S. typhi* serotypes (usually infected with *S. paratyphi* A, *S. schottmuelleri*, or *S. hirschfeldii*) may be treated with 4 to 6 grams of ampicillin plus 2 grams of probenecid orally each day in four divided doses for 6 weeks. Strains resistant to ampicillin may respond to ciprofloxacin. Patients who relapse usually will have gallbladder disease (most often calculi) and will not be cured with antimicrobial therapy. Cholecystectomy plus antimicrobial therapy may cure these patients, but it is doubtful that the carrier state per se is a sufficient indication for cholecystectomy.

PROGNOSIS. Mortality in salmonella enterocolitis is rare; infants and the elderly are at greatest risk, with death occurring from dehydration and electrolyte imbalance. Mortality from salmonella bacteremia or enteric fever is not uncommon and is most likely to occur in the very young and the very old. *S. choleraesuis* bacteremia has the highest mortality rate of any *Salmonella* serotype, as high as 20 to 30 per cent.

PREVENTION. Salmonella infection is best prevented by proper management of the water supply and sewage disposal, cooking and refrigeration of foods made from animal products, pasteurization of milk and milk products, and handwashing before preparing foods and after handling animals and uncooked animal products. Despite these precautions, because of the widespread presence of salmonellae in the animal kingdom, it is unlikely that the frequency of salmonella infections will be significantly diminished.

There is no vaccine for any salmonellae other than *S. typhi*.

Asperilla MO, Smego RA Jr, Scott LK: Quinolone antibiotics in the treatment of salmonella infections. Rev Infect Dis 12:873–889, 1990. *A review of the effectiveness of the newer quinolones in salmonella infections.*

Centers for Disease Control Salmonella Surveillance. Annual Survey 1987. U.S.

Public Health Service, 1988, pp 1–90. *A compilation of the serotypes of* Salmonella *isolated from human and nonhuman sources in the United States.*

Fischl MA, Dickinson GM, Sinave C, et al: Salmonella bacteremia as manifestation of acquired immunodeficiency syndrome. Arch Intern Med 146:113–115, 1986. *A paper illustrating the refractoriness of salmonella bacteremia in patients with AIDS.*

Neill MA, Opal SM, Heelan J, et al.: Failure of ciprofloxacin to eradicate convalescent fecal excretion after acute salmonellosis: Experience during an outbreak in health care workers. Ann Intern Med 114:195–199, 1991. *A study demonstrating a high relapse rate of fecal excretion of salmonella with a prolonged carriage state after ciprofloxacin treatment of convalescent carriers.*

Soe GB, Overturf GD: Treatment of typhoid fever and other systemic salmonelloses with cefotaxime, ceftriaxone, cefoperazone and other new cephalosporins. Rev Infect Dis 9:719–736, 1987. *A review of use of third-generation cephalosporins in systemic salmonella infections.*

315 Shigellosis

Thomas Butler

DEFINITION. Shigellosis is an acute bacterial infection caused by the genus *Shigella* resulting in colitis affecting predominantly the rectosigmoid colon. Bacillary dysentery is synonymous with shigellosis. The disease is characterized by diarrhea, dysentery, fever, abdominal pain, and tenesmus. Shigellosis is usually limited to a few days. Early treatment with antimicrobial drugs results in more rapid recovery.

ETIOLOGY. Shigellae are nonmotile gram-negative bacilli belonging to the family Enterobacteriaceae. Four species of shigellae are recognized on the basis of antigenic and biochemical properties: *S. dysenteriae* (group A), *S. flexneri* (group B), *S. boydii* (group C), and *S. sonnei* (group D). Among these species there are over 40 serotypes, each of which is designated by the species name followed by a specific Arabic number. *S. dysenteriae* 1 is called the Shiga bacillus and causes epidemics with higher mortality than other serotypes. With the exception of *S. flexneri* 6, they do not ferment lactose.

Serotypes are determined by the O polysaccharide side chain of the lipopolysaccharide (endotoxin) in the cell wall. Endotoxin is detectable in the blood of severely ill patients and may be responsible for the complication of the hemolytic-uremic syndrome. To be virulent, shigellae must be able to invade epithelial cells, as tested in the laboratory by keratoconjunctivitis in the guinea pig (Sereney test) or HeLa cell invasion. Bacterial invasion of cells is genetically governed by three chromosomal regions and a 140 Mdal plasmid. Shiga toxin is produced by *S. dysenteriae* 1 and in lesser amounts by other serotypes. It inhibits protein synthesis and has enterotoxic activity in animal models, but its role in human disease is uncertain.

INCIDENCE AND PREVALENCE. In the United States in 1988, there were over 30,000 reported cases of shigellosis. The predominant species in the 1980's was *S. sonnei* (64 per cent), followed by *S. flexneri* (31 per cent), *S. boydii* (3 per cent), and *S. dysenteriae* (2 per cent). Most cases were in young children, and a large proportion occurred in population groups living in homes for the mentally ill or in nursing homes. A large outbreak occurred in 1987 in Tennessee affecting more than 1000 persons camping under unsanitary conditions at a mass gathering.

Worldwide most cases of shigellosis occur in children of developing countries, where *S. flexneri* is the predominant species. During the past 20 years, major epidemics due to *S. dysenteriae* 1 have occurred in Central America, Central Africa, India, and Bangladesh.

EPIDEMIOLOGY. Shigellosis is transmitted by the fecal-oral route. Crowded living conditions, low standards of personal hygiene, poor water supply, and inadequate sewage facilities all contribute to an increased risk of infection. Transmission most often occurs by close person-to-person contact through contaminated hands. During clinical illness and for up to 6 weeks after recovery, organisms are excreted in the feces. Although the organisms are sensitive to desiccation, they may survive several months in food or water, which are occasional vehicles of transmission.

Children between 1 and 4 years of age have the greatest risk of developing shigellosis. Inhabitants of custodial institutions, such as homes for retarded children, are at highest risk. Intrafamilial spread follows often when the initial case has occurred in a pre-school child. In young adults the incidence is higher in women than men, which probably reflects closer contact of women with children. The male homosexual population in the United States is at increased risk for shigellosis, which is one of the causes of the "gay bowel syndrome."

Humans and higher primates are the only known natural reservoirs of shigellosis. Transmission shows variable seasonal patterns in different regions. In the United States, the peak incidence is in late summer and early autumn.

PATHOGENESIS AND PATHOLOGY. Since the microorganisms are relatively resistant to acid, shigellae pass the gastric barrier more readily than other enteric pathogens. In volunteer studies, as few as 200 ingested bacilli regularly initiate disease in 25 per cent of healthy adults. This contrasts strikingly with the much larger numbers of typhoid or cholera bacilli required to produce disease in normal individuals. During the incubation period, usually 12 to 72 hours, the organisms traverse the small bowel, penetrate colonic epithelial cells, and multiply intracellularly. An acute inflammatory response ensues in the colonic mucosa attended by prodromal symptoms (Table 315–1). Epithelial cells containing bacteria are lysed, resulting in superficial ulcerations and shedding of shigella organisms into stools. The mucosa is friable and covered with a layer of polymorphonuclear leukocytes. Advancing inflammation causes the formation of crypt abscesses. Initially the inflammation is confined to the rectosigmoid colon but after about 4 days of illness may advance to involve the proximal colon also. In severe cases, there may be pancolitis with extension of inflammation into the terminal ileum; a pseudomembranous type of colitis may develop. Diarrhea results because of impaired absorption of water and electrolytes by the inflamed colon.

Although the colonic inflammation is superficial, bacteremia occurs occasionally, especially in *S. dysenteriae* 1 infections. Susceptibility of organisms to serum complement–mediated bacteriolysis may explain the infrequency of bacteremia and disseminated infection. Colonic perforation is a rare complication during toxic megacolon. Children with severe colitis due to *S. dysenteriae* 1 are prone to develop the hemolytic-uremic syndrome. In this complication fibrin thrombi are deposited in the renal glomeruli, causing cortical necrosis and fragmentation of red cells.

CLINICAL MANIFESTATIONS. Most patients with shigellosis begin their illness with a nonspecific prodrome (Table 315–1). The height of the temperature varies, and children may have febrile convulsions. The initial intestinal symptoms soon follow as cramps, loose stools, and watery diarrhea, which usually precede the onset of dysentery by 1 or more days. The average fecal output is about 600 grams a day for adults. The dysentery consists typically of flecks and small clots of bright red blood and mucus in stools that are small in volume. Frequency of passage is often as high as 20 to 40 times a day, with excruciating rectal pain and tenesmus during defecation. Some patients develop rectal prolapse during severe straining. The amount of blood in stools varies widely but usually is small because of the superficial colonic ulcerations. Abdominal tenderness is often most marked in the left lower quadrant over the sigmoid colon but may also be generalized. The fever is likely to abate after a few days of

dysentery, making afebrile bloody diarrhea an occasional clinical presentation. After 1 to 2 weeks of untreated disease, spontaneous improvement occurs in most patients. Some patients with mild disease develop only the prodrome or experience only watery diarrhea without dysentery.

Complications include dehydration, which can be a cause of death, especially in children and the elderly. Shigella septicemia occurs mainly in malnourished children with *S. dysenteriae* 1 infections. The leukemoid reaction and hemolytic-uremic syndrome may develop in children late in the course after antimicrobial treatment when the dysentery has started to improve. Neurologic manifestations can be striking and include delirium, seizures, and nuchal rigidity.

The important postdysenteric syndromes are arthritis and Reiter's triad of arthritis, urethritis, and conjunctivitis (see Ch. 259). These are nonsuppurative phenomena that occur in the absence of viable *Shigella* organisms about 1 to 3 weeks after resolution of dysentery.

DIAGNOSIS. Shigellosis should be considered in any patient with acute onset of fever and diarrhea. Examination of the stool is essential. Blood and pus are grossly apparent in severe bacillary dysentery; even in milder forms of the disease, microscopic examination of the stool often reveals numerous leukocytes and erythrocytes. The fecal leukocyte examination should be performed with a portion of liquid stool, preferably containing mucus. A drop of stool is placed on a microscopic slide, mixed thoroughly with two drops of methylene blue, and overlaid with a coverslip. The presence of abundant polymorphonuclear leukocytes helps in distinguishing shigellosis from diarrheal syndromes caused by viruses and enterotoxigenic bacteria. The fecal leukocyte examination is not helpful in distinguishing shigellosis from diarrheal illnesses caused by other invasive enteric pathogens (nontyphoidal *Salmonella*, *Campylobacter*, and *Yersinia*). Amebic dysentery is excluded by the absence of trophozoites on a microscopic examination of fresh stool under a cover slip. The peripheral white cell count is of little diagnostic value, since it may range from less than 3,000 to more than 30,000. Sigmoidoscopic examination reveals diffuse erythema with a mucopurulent layer and friable areas of mucosa with shallow ulcers 3 to 7 mm in diameter.

Definitive diagnosis depends upon isolating shigellae by selective media. A rectal swab, a swab of a colonic ulcer obtained by sigmoidoscopic examination, or a freshly passed stool specimen should be inoculated immediately on culture plates or into carrying media. Since isolation rates of shigellae from freshly passed stools of patients with shigellosis may be as low as 67 per cent, culturing for 3 successive days is recommended. Stool cultures are generally positive within 24 hours after onset of symptoms and may remain positive for several weeks in the absence of antimicrobial therapy. Appropriate culture media include blood, desoxycholate, and Salmonella-Shigella (S-S) agars. Selected colonies should be diagnosed by agglutination with polyvalent *Shigella* antisera. S-S agar is inhibitory for *S. dysenteriae* 1.

Definitive bacteriologic diagnosis becomes of critical importance in distinguishing the more severe and prolonged cases of shigellosis from ulcerative colitis, with which it may be confused both clinically and on sigmoidoscopic examination. Patients with

TABLE 315–1. EVOLUTION OF CLINICAL SYNDROMES IN SHIGELLOSIS

Stage	Time of Appearance After Onset of Illness	Symptoms and Signs	Pathology
Prodrome	Earliest	Fever, chills, myalgias, anorexia, nausea, vomiting	None or early colitis
Nonspecific diarrhea	0–3 days	Abdominal cramps, loose stools, watery diarrhea	Rectosigmoid colitis with superficial ulceration, fecal leukocytes
Dysentery	1–8 days	Frequent passage of blood and mucus, tenesmus, rectal prolapse, abdominal tenderness	Colitis extending sometimes to proximal colon, crypt abscesses, inflammation in lamina propria
Complications	3–10 days	Dehydration, seizures, septicemia, leukemoid reaction, hemolytic-uremic syndrome, ileus, peritonitis	Severe colitis, terminal ileitis, endotoxemia, intravascular coagulation, toxic megacolon, colonic perforation
Postdysenteric syndromes	1–3 weeks	Arthritis, Reiter's syndrome	Reactive inflammation in HLA-B27 haplotype

shigellosis have been subjected to colectomy because of a mistaken diagnosis of ulcerative colitis; a positive culture should prevent such a misadventure.

TREATMENT. The effectiveness of antimicrobial agents in treating shigellosis has been well established. Appropriate antimicrobial therapy instituted early may decrease the duration of symptoms by 50 per cent and decrease the duration of excretion of shigellae (an important epidemiologic factor) by a far greater percentage. Because of the increasing frequency of plasmid-mediated antimicrobial resistance to *Shigella* infections, drug susceptibility testing is important. Trimethoprim-sulfamethoxazole administered in standard doses twice daily for 5 days is now the treatment of choice for *Shigella* strains of unknown antibiotic sensitivity in both adults and children. Alternative drugs include ampicillin, tetracycline, nalidixic acid, norfloxacin, and ciprofloxacin.

Fluid losses in shigellosis are qualitatively similar to those in other infectious diarrheal diseases, and the patient should be treated with appropriate intravenous or oral electrolyte repletion fluids in quantities adequate to correct clinical signs of saline depletion. The requirement for fluids is generally small, but fluid repletion is lifesaving in exceptional cases.

Agents that decrease intestinal motility should not be used. Such preparations as diphenoxylate and paregoric may exacerbate symptoms, presumably by retarding intestinal clearance of the microorganisms. There is no convincing evidence that pectin- or bismuth-containing preparations are helpful.

PROGNOSIS. The mortality rate in untreated shigellosis is dependent upon the infectious strain and ranges from 10 to 30 per cent in certain outbreaks caused by *S. dysenteriae* 1 to less than 1 per cent in most *S. sonnei* infections. Even with infection caused by *S. dysenteriae* 1, mortality rates should approach zero if appropriate fluid replacement and antimicrobial therapy are initiated early.

About 2 per cent of patients may develop arthritis or Reiter's syndrome weeks or months after recovery from shigellosis.

PREVENTION. Individuals excreting shigellae should be excluded from all phases of food handling until negative cultures have been obtained from three successive stool specimens collected after completion of antimicrobial therapy. In institutional outbreaks, strict and early isolation of infected individuals is mandatory. Targeted antimicrobial chemoprophylaxis has been disappointing. The most important control measure is scrupulous handwashing by all individuals involved in handling of food. Reporting of shigellosis cases to health authorities should be mandatory.

For the traveler to countries with major *Shigella* problems, no chemoprophylactic agent is an adequate substitute for good personal hygiene and the avoidance of contaminated food and water. A variety of vaccines has been developed and tested, but no vaccine is now commercially available.

Bennish ML, Harris JR, Wojtyniak BJ, et al.: Death in shigellosis: Incidence and risk factors in hospitalized patients. J Infect Dis 161:500, 1990. *Among more than 9000 infected inpatients, 9 per cent died, with death more likely in infants, the malnourished, and patients with low serum protein concentrations and thrombocytopenia.*

Butler T, Islam MR, Azad MAK, et al.: Risk factors for development of hemolytic uremic syndrome during shigellosis. J Pediatr 110:894, 1987. *In children with S. dysenteriae 1 infection, hemolytic-uremic syndrome developed after antibiotic therapy, which was usually inappropriate for the susceptibilities of the isolated bacterial strains.*

Butler T, Speelman P, Kabir I, et al.: Colonic dysfunction during shigellosis. J Infect Dis 154:817, 1986. *Studies perfusing the human colon showed diminished colonic water absorption, increased potassium secretion, and normal ileocecal flow rates.*

Haltalin KC, Kusmiesz HT, Hinton LV, et al.: Treatment of acute diarrhea in outpatients. Am J Dis Child 124:554, 1972. *An unequivocal demonstration of the value of appropriate antimicrobial therapy in the management of shigellosis.*

Levine MM: Bacillary dysentery. Mechanisms and treatment. Med Clin North Am 66:623, 1982. *A good review of microbiologic and clinical aspects of shigellosis.*

Wharton M, Spiegel RA, Horan JM, et al.: A large outbreak of antibiotic-resistant shigellosis at a mass gathering. J Infect Dis 162:1324, 1990. *Poor sanitation at a campsite in Tennessee led to an attack rate of more than 50 per cent in several thousand attendees; the Shigellosis was caused by multiresistant S. sonnei.*

316 *Campylobacter* Enteritis

Richard L. Guerrant

Enteric infection with a member of the genus *Campylobacter* usually results in an inflammatory, occasionally bloody diarrhea or dysentery syndrome. In industrialized, temperate areas, *Campylobacter jejuni* is often the most commonly recognized cause of inflammatory enteritis. The diarrhea may also be watery, especially in developing, tropical areas. An enterocolitis or proctocolitis syndrome similar to that seen with *C. jejuni* is also increasingly appreciated in homosexual males with several "*Campylobacter*-like organisms." The other major *Campylobacter* species that infects humans is *C. fetus*, a relatively uncommon cause of bacteremia and occasional intravascular infection in immunocompromised hosts. Finally, *Helicobacter pylori* (previously called *Campylobacter pylori*) has been increasingly associated with histologic gastritis and peptic ulcer disease.

ETIOLOGY. *Campylobacter* (meaning curved rod) is a curved or spiral, motile, non–spore-forming, gram-negative rod measuring 1.5 by 3.5 μ which is distinguished from Enterobacteriaceae by its inability to ferment or oxidize carbohydrates. It was formerly called a vibrio, but is now recognized as a separate genus, on the basis of its distinctive DNA content. It is both oxidase- and catalase-positive and is a microaerophilic organism that requires reduced oxygen (5 to 10 per cent) and increased carbon dioxide (3 to 10 per cent). The organism does not grow at either aerobic or strictly anaerobic conditions. Perhaps reflecting its avian reservoir, *C. jejuni* also requires an increased temperature to 42°C for optimal growth. *C. jejuni* is distinguished from *C. fetus* by its higher growth temperatures, cephalothin resistance, and nalidixic acid sensitivity. As shown in Table 316–1, the additional *Campylobacter* species that infect humans include *C. laridis*, a thermophilic organism commonly found in healthy sea gulls which has been reported in children with mild recurrent diarrhea and in an elderly patient with sepsis and terminal multiple myeloma. The weak or non–catalase-producing *C. upsaliensis* may cause diarrhea or bacteremia and *C. hyointestinalis*, like *C. fetus*, causes occasional bacteremia in compromised hosts. These organisms are also inhibited by cephalothin that is in some selective culture media. Up to three distinct species of "*Campylobacter*-like organisms" (including proposed species names *C. fennelliae* and *C. cinaedi*) are associated with proctocolitis in homosexual males and occasionally with bacteremia or diarrhea in women and children. Like *C. fetus*, these *Campylobacter*-like organisms do not grow at 42°C or in the presence of cephalosporin antibiotics and may require several days to a week or more to

TABLE 316–1. HUMAN *CAMPYLOBACTER* INFECTIONS

Species	Growth Temperature	Reservoir	Clinical Manifestations
C. jejuni/coli	37–42°C	Poultry, mammals	Common cause of dysentery/diarrhea
C. fetus (sub sp. *fetus*, old sub sp. *intestinalis*)	25–37°C	Cattle, sheep	Uncommon, bacteremia; intravascular infections in debilitated hosts
C. laridis	30–42°C	Sea gulls	Uncommon, childhood diarrhea, one case of sepsis
C. upsaliensis	37–42°C	Dogs	Occasional diarrhea
C. hyointestinalis	37°C	Swine	Occasional bacteremia in compromised hosts
"Campylobacter-like organisms": (including *C. cinaedi*, *C. fennelliae*)	37°C	?	Proctocolitis, rarely sepsis, in homosexual males
Helicobacter pylori (formerly *C. pylori*)	37°C	?	Histologic gastritis, peptic ulcer disease

grow in culture. *C. jejuni* is further subdivided into over 90 serotypes on the basis of heat-stable O antigens or over 50 serotypes on the basis of heat-labile capsular and flagellar antigens, markers that are helpful in tracing the epidemiology of this common enteric pathogen.

EPIDEMIOLOGY. Although the frequency of other *Campylobacter* infections is either low or unclear, *C. jejuni* infections are extremely common throughout the world. In many studies, the frequency of *Campylobacter* enteritis exceeds that of *Salmonella* or *Shigella* infections, and it has been estimated that as many as 2 million *Campylobacter* enteritis cases occur annually in the United States. The reservoirs of *C. jejuni/coli* include a wide range of mammalian species. Thirty to 100 per cent of chickens, turkeys, and water fowl may be infected asymptomatically in their intestinal tracts, and commercially prepared poultry in supermarkets can often be shown to be culture positive. In addition, swine, cattle, sheep, horses, and even household pets and rodents may carry *Campylobacter jejuni*, *C. coli*, or *C. fetus*. Enteric symptoms may be found, particularly in puppies, kittens, calves, or lambs, which may have diarrhea when infected. Furthermore, the organisms survive days to weeks in fresh or salt water and in milk and are killed most effectively by pasteurization, chlorination, drying, or freezing.

The transmission of *Campylobacter* infections is likely via the fecal-oral route. Fecal-oral spread may occur by contact among animals, homosexual males, and those in day care centers. However, secondary transmission is relatively infrequent and the infectious dose appears to vary from 500 to over 1 million organisms. The majority of infections, however, are probably acquired via ingestion of contaminated food, water, or milk vehicles. Many cases and outbreaks are associated with ingestion of inadequately cooked poultry, unpasteurized milk, inadequately treated water, and even cake icing, salads, beef, and clams.

The majority of those infected in well-described outbreaks are symptomatic. Asymptomatic infection appears to be relatively infrequent in temperate climates and in adults. An exception is among young children in certain tropical developing areas such as Bangladesh, where as many as 39 per cent of children under the age of 2 years may be infected asymptomatically (Table 316–2). These frequent asymptomatic infections in tropical areas raise important questions about possible strain differences in virulence, host susceptibility, and protective immunity against disease that might be acquired very early in developing areas.

Throughout the world, *Campylobacter* infections appear to predominate during the warmer or wet season. As with diarrheal illnesses in general, the highest age-specific attack rate is in young children. However, the greatest proportion of positive fecal cultures occurs in older children and young adults. There is little if any sexual predominance of recognized *C. jejuni* infections.

PATHOGENESIS AND PATHOLOGY. *C. jejuni* and *C. coli* are reasonably susceptible to gastric acidity. However, the reported variation in infectious dose suggests considerable host or strain variability. After an incubation period of 1 to 7 (median 4) days, symptoms of the enteric infection begin. *C. jejuni* organisms are attracted toward mucus and fucose in bile, and the flagellae may be important in both chemotaxis and adherence to epithelial cells or mucus. Adherence may also involve lipopolysaccharide or other outer membrane components. Several laboratories around the world have documented the production by *C. jejuni* of a cholera-like, heat-labile enterotoxin that binds to ganglioside and is neutralized by anticholera toxin antiserum. However, the genetic code and role of this toxin in disease remain elusive to date. Studies from Mexico have shown that antitoxic immunity

TABLE 316–2. CLINICAL PRESENTATIONS OF CAMPYLOBACTER JEJUNI INFECTION

	Industrialized Countries	Developing Countries
Per cent of all diarrhea with *C. jejuni*	5–13	2–35
Per cent of *C. jejuni* diarrhea with:		
Fecal PMN	78–93	22–46
Blood in stool	60–65	5–17
Asymptomatic infection rates (%)	<2	0–39*

*Depending on age—39% if less than 2 years old.

develops after infection, often with watery diarrhea, suggesting that this toxin is significant in those infections.

However, more characteristic in temperate areas is a diffuse, often bloody exudative enteritis involving the ileum and colon. These pathologic changes may include nonspecific crypt abscesses that on colonoscopy and histopathology may mimic the changes seen with inflammatory bowel disease. Such invasive pathology is also seen in rabbit, chick, mouse, dog, and monkey models of infection. Although *C. jejuni* is negative in the Sereny test for guinea pig conjunctivitis, some have reported the production of cytotoxins by certain strains of *C. jejuni* that may be involved in the pathogenesis of the invasive colitis. The relative infrequency of bloodstream invasion by *C. jejuni*, compared with *C. fetus*, likely relates to the relative serum sensitivity of most *C. jejuni* strains and to the rapid development of bactericidal antibody with infection in normal individuals. Volunteer studies suggest that effective immunity develops to rechallenge with the homologous strain, and animal studies suggest that protective immunity may be transferred in immune milk to suckling offspring. Additional evidence of effective immunity comes with the decreasing illness:infection ratio among children in endemic areas as well as among regular consumers of raw milk.

Once patients are infected, they shed 10^7 to 10^9 organisms per gram of stool for a median duration of 2 to 3 weeks, if not treated with effective antibiotics. Although some may continue to excrete the organism for 2 to 3 months, chronic asymptomatic intestinal carriage is rare.

CLINICAL MANIFESTATIONS. As noted in Table 316–1, the major recognized disease with human *Campylobacter* infections is the characteristic diarrheal illness seen with *C. jejuni* or *C. coli* infections. Although asymptomatic infections and watery, noninflammatory diarrhea are seen with *C. jejuni* infections in tropical, developing areas as shown in Table 316–2, *C. jejuni* is characteristically associated with an inflammatory, febrile enteritis in industrialized countries throughout the world. After an incubation period of 1 to 7 days, a brief prodrome of fever, headache, and myalgias lasting for 12 to 24 hours is promptly followed in a case of *C. jejuni* enteritis in a child or young adult with the symptoms of acute enteritis. These characteristically include crampy abdominal pain, fever to 39 or 40°C, and diarrhea with up to 10 or more loose, often bloody bowel movements per day. Occasionally the crampy abdominal pain may predominate as an appendicitis-like syndrome, with mesenteric adenitis or terminal ileitis being the predominant pathology. On physical examination the abdomen is diffusely tender and may mimic appendicitis. Although the acute febrile enteritis is usually self-limited to 5 to 7 days, 10 to 20 per cent of cases may last longer than 1 week and 5 to 20 per cent of untreated cases may relapse with a similar illness.

Complications, particularly if antimotility agents are used, include toxic megacolon, pseudomembranous colitis, and colonic hemorrhage. In addition hemolytic-uremic syndrome, postinfectious polyneuritis, or Guillain-Barré syndrome may follow *C. jejuni* enteritis. As with many inflammatory colitis syndromes, reactive arthritis and full-blown Reiter's syndrome may follow weeks after *Campylobacter* enteritis. Bacteremia may occur relatively rarely (< 1 per cent of cases), particularly in the very young or the elderly, in whom meningitis, endocarditis, cholecystitis, urinary tract infections, and pancreatitis have been described. In patients with hypogammaglobulinemia or HIV infection, *C. jejuni* infections may be prolonged or severe despite appropriate antimicrobial therapy.

In striking contrast to *C. jejuni*, the slow-growing *C. fetus* is primarily an uncommon cause of bacteremia, often in immunocompromised hosts. Although *C. fetus* would be missed on most routine stool cultures for *C. jejuni*, studies with filtration methods suggest that it is a relatively infrequent cause of diarrhea. Instead, *C. fetus* tends to cause intravascular, meningeal, or localized infections such as arthritis, cellulitis, abscesses, cholecystitis, and urinary, placental, or pleural infections, often in elderly or debilitated hosts. As it does in animals, *C. fetus* may cause stillbirth or septic abortions more often than generally recognized in humans. *C. fetus* infections are often recognized only by astute clinical microbiology technicians who methodically examine or subculture specimens of blood or other body fluids after 1 week in the laboratory. The clinical course of *C. fetus* bacteremia is often related to its recognition and appropriate treatment as well as to the underlying disease.

DIAGNOSIS. The diagnosis of *Campylobacter* infections is related to a careful history for exposure or characteristic clinical syndromes, direct stool examination, and selective culture methods. *C. jejuni* enteritis should be suspected in anyone presenting with a febrile enteritis, especially if there is a history of recent ingestion of inadequately cooked poultry, unpasteurized milk, or untreated water. As suggested in Figure 316–1, such a history should prompt the obtaining of a fecal specimen in a cup if at all possible and direct microscopic examination using methylene blue or Gram's stain for leukocytes as well as gross and/or occult blood. In many industrialized areas, the presence of blood or fecal leukocytes with fever strongly suggests the presence of a cultivable enteric pathogen such as *C. jejuni*, *Salmonella*, or *Shigella*, with *C. jejuni* being most common. Additional imme-

diate clues to *C. jejuni* infection may be seen on darkfield or phase microscopy for characteristic darting motility or on a carbolfuchsin Gram's stain of stool for characteristic curved rods or sea gull morphology. However, darkfield and Gram's stains, while reasonably specific with trained observers, are each only 50 to 66 per cent sensitive. Patients with febrile enteritis, particularly with blood and leukocytes in the stool, should be cultured for *C. jejuni*.

Additional differential diagnostic possibilities for febrile inflammatory enteritis include *Salmonella* and *Shigella* infections, for which one should seek a history of an outbreak or contact exposure (such as in day care centers or among homosexual males, respectively). If the patient has recently taken antibiotics, *C. difficile* colitis or *Salmonella* enteritis should be considered. Recent ingestion of raw seafood should prompt investigation for *Vibrio* infection that may present with either inflammatory or noninflammatory diarrhea. A history of sick pet exposure, persisting abdominal pain, or unexplained inflammatory diarrhea should also prompt consideration of *Yersinia enterocolitica* infections, and

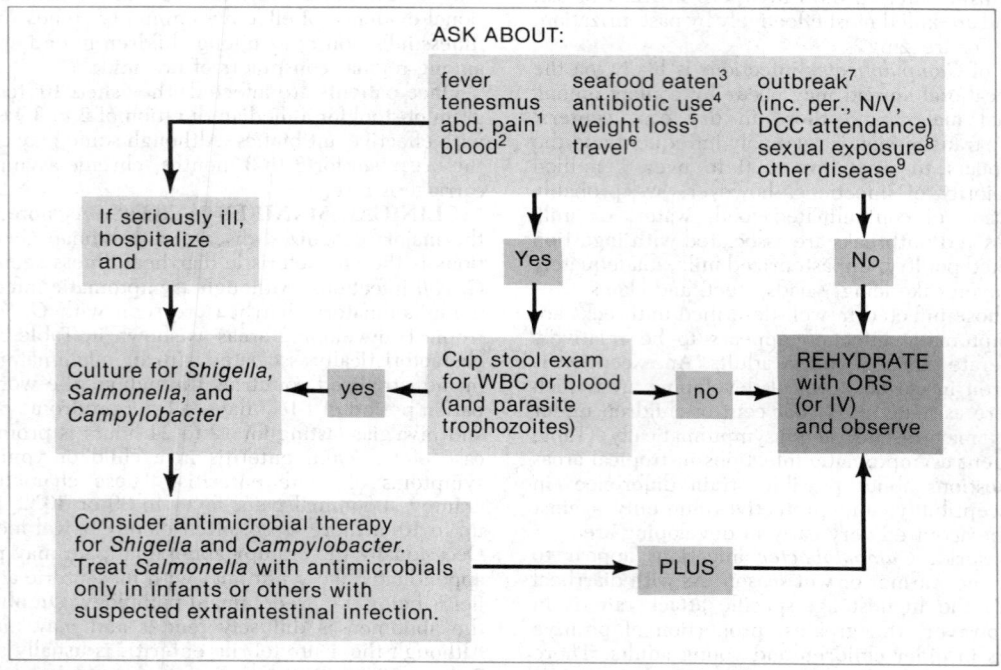

FIGURE 316–1. Approach to the diagnosis and management of acute infectious diarrhea.

1. If unexpected abdominal pain and fever persist or suggest an appendicitis-like syndrome, culture for *Yersinia enterocolitica*.

2. Bloody diarrhea, especially if without fecal leukocytes, suggests enterohemorrhagic (Shiga toxin–producing) *E. coli* 0157 or amebiasis (where leukocytes are destroyed by the parasite).

3. Ingestion of inadequately cooked seafood should prompt consideration of *Vibrio* infections or Norwalk-like viruses.

4. Associated antibiotics should be stopped if possible and cytotoxigenic *C. difficile* considered.

5. Persistence (> 10 days) with weight loss should prompt consideration of giardiasis or cryptosporidiosis.

6. Travel to tropical areas increases the chance of enterotoxigenic *E. coli* as well as viral (ex. Norwalk-like or rotaviral), parasitic (ex. *Giardia; Entamoeba, Strongyloides, Cryptosporidium*), and, if fecal leukocytes are present, invasive bacterial pathogens as noted in the algorithm.

7. Outbreaks should prompt consideration of *S. aureus, B. cereus, Anisakis* (incubation period < 6 hours), *C. perfringens,* ETEC, *Vibrio, Salmonella, Campylobacter, Shigella* or EIEC infection. If unexplained, consider saving *E. coli* for LT, ST, invasiveness, adherence testing, and serotyping, and save stool for rotavirus and stool + paired sera for Norwalk-like virus testing.

8. Sigmoidoscopy in symptomatic homosexual males should distinguish proctitis in the distal 15 cm only (caused by herpesvirus, gonococcal, chlamydial, or syphilitic infection) from colitis [*Campylobacter, Shigella, C. difficile,* or chlamydial (LGV serotypes) infections] or noninflammatory diarrhea (due to giardiasis).

9. Immunocompromised hosts should have a wide range of viral (ex. CMV, HSV, coxsackie, rotavirus), bacterial (ex. *Salmonella, Mycobacterium avium-intracellulare, Listeria*), fungal (ex. *Candida*), and parasitic (ex. *Cryptosporidium, Strongyloides, Entamoeba,* and *Giardia*) agents considered.

(Adapted from Guerrant RL, Shields DS, Thorson SM, et al.: Evaluation and diagnosis of acute infectious diarrhea. Am J Med 78:91–98, 1985.)

travel exposure to tropical areas or residence in an institution where careful hygiene is difficult should prompt an examination of stool and possibly rectal biopsy specimens for *E. histolytica* (which often destroys fecal leukocytes). Another frequent diagnosis that is considered, especially if *Campylobacter* enteritis has relapsed once or twice, is inflammatory bowel disease. However, it is imperative that anyone who is being considered for that diagnosis have treatable causes such as *Campylobacter* enteritis or amebiasis excluded by appropriate cultures or stains, as treatment with steroids may worsen *Campylobacter* or amebic enteritis with potentially devastating consequences. Additional noninfectious causes of bloody diarrhea with abdominal pain include intussusception and vascular insufficiency.

The diagnosis of *H. pylori* infections is best made by documenting the organism by culture and histology of gastric biopsies. Additional clues may be provided by urease tests of biopsies, breath tests for urease degradation of ingested urea, or serologic tests for anti–*H. pylori* antibody.

THERAPY. The most important treatment for *Campylobacter* enteritis, as with all diarrheal illnesses, is adequate rehydration and maintenance fluid therapy, which can often be accomplished with oral glucose-electrolyte solutions. The effectiveness of specific antimicrobial therapy remains debated. Although most *C. jejuni* strains are sensitive to erythromycin as well as to tetracyclines, chloramphenicol, clindamycin, quinolones, and aminoglycosides, they are characteristically resistant to penicillin, ampicillin, cephalosporins, and sulfamethoxazole-trimethoprim. Indications for antibiotic treatment remain controversial. Several studies have failed to show a significant reduction in the duration of illness with erythromycin treatment despite its prompt eradication of the organism from the stool. Some reserve antimicrobial treatment for those with particularly severe symptoms of high fever, bloody or severe diarrhea, young children in day care centers, or prolonged or relapsing illnesses. Antimotility agents should be avoided in *Campylobacter* enteritis, as with any inflammatory diarrhea.

It should be remembered that erythromycin orally may not be adequate for systemic *C. jejuni* or *C. fetus* endovascular infections, which probably warrant 2 to 4 weeks of parenteral bactericidal antimicrobial therapy.

H. pylori infections, although difficult to eradicate with a single agent, may be eradicated by combinations of agents such as bismuth compounds plus metronidazole, provided that the organism is susceptible.

PROGNOSIS. The prognosis of *C. jejuni* enteritis is generally quite good, and the disease is usually self-limited with or without specific therapy.

PREVENTION. As most *Campylobacter* infections arise from fecal contamination, often from animal reservoirs, many if not most *Campylobacter* infections are potentially preventable by education. The most common recognized vehicles of spread are inadequately cooked food, unpasteurized milk, and inadequately treated water. Consequently, thorough cooking of meats, careful handwashing after food preparation, pasteurization of milk, and adequate chlorination of drinking water should greatly reduce the frequency of *Campylobacter* infections. Parents should be warned that sick pet kittens or puppies may harbor potential human pathogens such as *C. jejuni* and keep them away from small children and practice careful hygienic measures in their care.

Blaser MJ: *Helicobacter pylori* and the pathogenesis of gastroduodenal inflammation. J Infect Dis 161:626–633, 1990. *Excellent overview of the rapidly emerging work on this important, newly recognized pathogen.*

Blaser MJ, Wells JG, Feldman RA, et al.: *Campylobacter* enteritis in the United States. Ann Intern Med 98:360–365, 1983. *Critical analysis of the presentation of* C. jejuni *and other enteritides in the United States.*

Butzler JP, Skirrow MB: *Campylobacter* enteritis. Clin Gastroenterol 8:737–765, 1979. *Good review of cultivation methods, epidemiology, clinical presentation, and models of* C. jejuni *infections.*

Guerrant RL, Lahita RG, Winn WC, et al.: Campylobacteriosis in man: Pathogenic mechanisms and review of 91 bloodstream infections. Am J Med 65:584–592, 1978. *Review of both* C. fetus *and* C. jejuni *infections and their presentations as bacteremic illnesses.*

Guerrant RL, Shields DS, Thorson SM, et al.: Evaluation and diagnosis of acute infectious diarrhea. Am J Med 78:91–98, 1985. *Review of a more cost-effective approach to selecting patients for stool culture who are likely to have an identifiable bacterial pathogen, such as* C. jejuni.

Perlman DM, Ampel NM, Schiffman RB, et al.: Persistent *Campylobacter-jejuni* infections in patients infected with the human immunodeficiency virus: Asso-
ciation with abnormal serological response to *C. jejuni* and emergence of erythromycin resistance during therapy. Ann Intern Med 108:540–546, 1988. *Report of persistent, severe* C. jejuni *enteritis and occasional bacteremia in patients with HIV infection who fail to mount a serum antibody response.*

Quinn TC, Corey L, Chaffee RG, et al.: The etiology of anorectal infections in homosexual men. Am J Med 71:395–406, 1981. *Review of the clinical manifestations and diagnostic approach to the wide range of enteric infections commonly seen in promiscuous homosexual males.*

Ruiz Palacios GM, Torres J, Torres NI, et al.: Cholera-like enterotoxin produced by *Campylobacter jejuni*. Lancet 2:250–252, 1982. *Original report of evidence for production of a cholera-like enterotoxin by* C. jejuni *in a developing area.*

Walker RI, Caldwell MB, Lee EC, et al.: Pathophysiology of *Campylobacter* enteritis. Microbiol Rev 50:81–94, 1986. *Excellent recent review of the virulence traits, pathogenic mechanisms, and animal models of* C. jejuni *infections.*

317 Cholera

William B. Greenough, III

DEFINITION. Cholera is an acute watery diarrheal disease caused by *Vibrio cholerae*, serogroup 1, which occurs both sporadically and as large outbreaks. Fluid loss may be extreme, exceeding 1 liter per hour. In such cases loss of solute-rich body fluids in stools rapidly depletes circulating plasma volume, producing vascular collapse and death in hours. Without treatment, mortality approaches 60 per cent of those affected; however, mild cases and carriers also occur and participate in the spread of disease.

ETIOLOGY. *V. cholerae* are short, slightly curved, rapidly motile, uniflagellate gram-negative bacteria that grow aerobically at 37°C on relatively simple media. They are currently classified as Enterobacteriaceae and are members of a very large group of surface water organisms distributed in all parts of the world, especially favoring brackish or salt-fresh water interfaces. There are many O serogroups of *V. cholerae*, but only serogroup 1 causes epidemic human disease. It occurs as two major serotypes, Ogawa and Inaba, with a less common Hikojima variant occasionally observed. There are also two main biotypes, "classic" and "eltor." The eltor biotype is recognized by its resistance to polymyxin B and by characteristic vibriophage susceptibility. These markers are of use epidemiologically. *V. cholerae* produces a potent exotoxin (choleragen) that binds to intestinal epithelium, producing a chloride ion–driven secretion and malabsorption of sodium ion and water. Other vibrios can produce exotoxins but do not have other biologic characteristics that lead to spreading epidemic disease.

EPIDEMIOLOGY. Cholera is thought to be a disease of antiquity, with clear written descriptions dating before 500 BC. The present global spread (seventh pandemic) has been due to an eltor biotype first recognized in 1911 at the El Tor quarantine station in the Persian Gulf. Epidemics due to this organism first appeared in the Celebes in the 1930's, spreading westward through Southeast Asia and reaching the Mediterranean and Africa in the 1970's. In 1991, for the first time in a century, a large epidemic struck the Western Hemisphere, involving more than 20,000 people in Peru and Ecuador in less than 6 weeks. However, in the Ganges delta, epidemics of classic *V. cholera* were replaced by eltor late in the 1960's. There have been small but regular outbreaks of cholera in the United States in the Mississippi delta regions since 1973. The eltor strains isolated have not been the same as the global epidemic strain. If special methods are applied, *V. cholerae* serogroup 1 can be isolated from many waters and may be associated in an altered state with phytoplankton. The main puzzle of where the interepidemic reservoir of *V. cholerae* is in nature has yet to be solved.

Mode of Spread. During epidemics cholera is mainly waterborne. Large numbers of vibrios enter many water sources from the voluminous liquid stools that soak clothing and linens and contaminate the environment. The setting for epidemics is often extreme poverty with lack of safe water supplies. However, an outbreak in Portugal affected the most careful travelers who used only bottled water, which unfortunately had been supplied from a spring contaminated with *V. cholerae*. Occasionally, contaminated foods spread disease. Most often raw or undercooked shellfish or fresh vegetables washed with contaminated water are responsible. There is a high risk of secondary spread in families or institutions in which water and food are shared. Contamination of household food and water sources is the rule. It is easy to understand how this occurs when an adult patient may produce 30 to 50 liters of stool in 2 to 3 days and is usually too weak to use a commode or toilet. Mild cases and rare convalescent carriers probably spread the disease between communities. True long-term carriers are rare enough to be reportable.

Susceptibility to Cholera. In areas where cholera occurs each year, children under 5 years are the main victims. Older children and adults in such endemic areas have acquired a lasting and strongly protective local intestinal immunity. Breast-fed infants in such circumstances do not get cholera and are solidly protected by antibodies from their mother's milk. When cholera attacks a population that has not experienced it for many years, as was true in recent spread to the Philippines and Africa, all ages are attacked equally, but morbidity and mortality are greatest among the very young and very old. Individuals with low gastric acid production, who are on acid-suppressing medications, or who have had gastrectomies are especially vulnerable, since *V. cholerae* is quite sensitive to acid. Cholera tends to attack persons of blood group O with greater severity, whereas individuals with AB blood group have less severe disease. People with a safe, piped water supply and effective disinfected waste disposal are at least risk regardless of host susceptibility.

PATHOGENESIS. After ingesting *V. cholerae*, vomiting and diarrhea may begin as early as 12 hours or not appear for more than a week. Illness occurs when viable organisms reach the duodenum and jejunum where favorable conditions, such as alkaline pH, nutrients, and bile salts, exist for growth. Multiplication occurs rapidly, with a doubling time of 20 to 30 minutes. Actively motile vibrios penetrate mucous layers and attach to the brush border of the intestinal epithelium where they secrete a potent exotoxin. This toxin is a protein of 84,000 daltons consisting of five B subunits that bind irreversibly to a specific chemical receptor on the cell surfaces (GM1-ganglioside). The toxic moiety or A subunit is linked to the B aggregate and gains entry once binding has occurred. It catalyzes an ADP ribosylation reaction that results in increased adenylate cyclase activity and consequent raised cyclic AMP levels in the enterocytes or any other affected cells. The most visible result in the small intestine is the profuse watery diarrhea resulting from abolition at the villous tips of the normal absorption of sodium ion and with it anions and water, and stimulation of crypt cells to secrete chloride, drawing with them cations and water from the bloodstream into the gut lumen. The resulting solute-rich stream originating in the duodenum and jejunum is profuse, eliciting vomiting as it progresses cephalad and diarrhea as it flushes through the colon. The fluid lost in cholera is a slightly fishy-smelling nonfecal whitish mucous-flecked liquid ("rice water stool"). There is no cellular damage and no inflammation or loss of plasma proteins or formed elements of the blood. There is also increased secretion of hepatic and pancreatic fluids, prostaglandin, and other intestinal hormones. All signs and symptoms of cholera derive from the fluid losses, which approach in composition an ultrafiltrate of plasma enriched in potassium and bicarbonate (Table 317–1). There is no evidence

TABLE 317–1. TYPICAL CHEMICAL VALUES IN STOOL AND PLASMA FROM PATIENTS WITH SEVERE CHOLERA

| | Stool | Plasma | |
		Untreated	Treated†
Sodium*	138 (105)	141	142
Chloride*	102 (90)	107	106
Potassium*	18 (25)	4.5	3.6
Bicarbonate*	45 (30)	9	21
Arterial pH	—	7.21	7.43
Plasma specific gravity	—	1.040	1.026

*Milliequivalents per liter. Stool values in parentheses are for children less than 10 years old.

†Four hours after water and electrolyte replacement.

for systemic effects by cholera toxin itself, since *V. cholerae* does not invade the body. It exerts all of its effects topically by adhering to the intestinal lining and producing toxin that is bound at cell surfaces.

CLINICAL MANIFESTATIONS. In its most dramatic presentation cholera can reduce a perfectly healthy robust adult to shock and death in 4 to 6 hours. More usually death ensues in 18 or more hours. In rare instances "cholera sicca" shock and death occur before diarrhea appears, the voluminous secretions pooling in distended loops of bowel and not escaping as either diarrhea or vomiting. Despite the capacity of cholera to cause severe illness, many of the infected patients have only a mild diarrhea indistinguishable from that of ordinary gastroenteritis. In epidemics about half of those infected have either no symptoms or very mild illness.

Without fluid replacement cholera patients demonstrate signs of severe volume depletion—sunken eyes, poor skin turgor, hoarse voice, extreme thirst, faint heart sounds, weak or absent peripheral pulses, and severe muscle cramps. Patients are oriented but appear apathetic except for thirst. If patients survive and have not received adequate hydration, fever secondary to sepsis and pneumonia is common and pulmonary edema can ensue with even modest fluid replacement.

In children, unconsciousness and/or convulsions may signal hypoglycemia. In both children and adults, adequate early volume replacement with a correctly formulated oral hydration solution can prevent all signs and symptoms except diarrhea. Initial laboratory values from depleted cholera patients (Table 317–1) reflect the loss of isotonic fluid without larger molecules such as albumen. This results in increased concentrations of plasma proteins and blood cells. Loss of bicarbonate leads to acidosis with a low arterial pH and bicarbonate. Potassium depletion is not reflected by low plasma values until acidosis has been corrected.

DIAGNOSIS. Cholera should be ruled out in any patient with acute watery diarrhea. Travel or residence in a cholera-endemic area should raise the index of suspicion. In clusters of acute watery diarrhea, particularly where sanitation is poor, it is especially important to recognize cholera early to permit advance actions to prevent deaths of large numbers of people.

Treatment does not depend on an etiologic diagnosis. Fluid replacement should be started without delay as soon as diarrhea begins. After initiating treatment, stool should be examined directly for red and white blood cells. Except in mixed infections with invasive organisms, which do occur in cholera outbreaks, fecal red and white cells are not a feature of cholera. If phase or darkfield microscopy is available, the characteristic darting motility of vibrios can be recognized in fresh wet preparations. To be certain that these motile bacteria are *V. cholerae*, serogroup 1 antisera can be applied to wet preparations, immobilizing the organisms in a rapid and specific diagnostic test. For greater sensitivity of this test, a stool sample or rectal swab can be incubated in an enrichment medium for vibrios, such as alkaline peptone water, for 12 to 18 hours. Stool culture is best done on a selective medium, since colonies of *V. cholerae* may be overgrown or are easily missed on standard enteric media. A simple method uses thiosulfate-citrate-bile salt-sucrose (TCBS) agar, which is very stable and selective for vibrios. Opaque flat yellow colonies form on TCBS agar in 18 hours at 37°C. Confirmation of serogroup and serotype can be done by direct slide agglutination with specific antisera. Biotyping requires more elaborate procedures, but resistance to polymyxin B is a quick way to recognize the eltor biotype.

Although the first line of immune defense is local at the intestinal epithelium, circulating antibodies occur to the specific O antigens. Testing for these is of use only as an epidemiologic tool to judge prevalence of disease in a specific population.

TREATMENT. Early and complete replacement of fluid losses averts death and all complications. It does not decrease diarrhea, however, unless an advanced oral hydration solution based on food polymers is used. In all except the most severe cases, oral rehydration therapy is sufficient to treat cholera, especially if started as soon as diarrhea begins. All varieties of watery diarrhea lose fluid of similar composition, depending principally on the rate of loss. Oral hydration therapy is the treatment of choice in all situations except when a patient has been permitted to become depleted and is in vascular collapse or is comatose. It is as

TABLE 317–2. CHOLERA AND ACUTE DIARRHEA TREATMENT SOLUTIONS (ORAL AND INTRAVENOUS)

	Substrate (g/L)	Na+	K+ (millimoles/L)	*Base	Cl⁻	Osmolarity
Oral						
WHO/UNICEF	20 (glucose)	90	20	30	80	330
Pedialyte	25 (glucose)	45	20	30	35	300
Rice solution	80 (rice)	90	20	30	80	240
Ricelyte	30 (rice digest)	50	25	30	45	200
Intravenous						
Dhaka solution	0	134	13	48 (bicarbonate)	99	294
Ringer's†	0	130	4	28 (lactate)	109	271

*Citrate is generally used but bicarbonate is equally effective, and lactate or acetate are used in intravenous solutions.
†Also contains calcium, 3.0 mEq per liter.

appropriate to use oral rehydration therapy in hospitals as at home or in the field, as it entails fewer risks, is much less costly, does not require trained medical personnel for administration, and is equally effective. The discovery that absorption of sodium by cotransport pathways of intestinal mucosa is spared during cholera and other diarrheal diseases opened the way for a safe, inexpensive, and effective oral replacement solution. Glucose, amino acids, and small peptides, when absorbed by separate cotransport pathways of the intestine, carry with them sodium ions. Water and anions follow down the osmotic and electochemical gradients from the gut lumen to the bloodstream. Originally oral rehydration solutions were based only on glucose, and these were and remain very effective but do not diminish diarrheal fluid losses. Recent use of complex carbohydrates and proteins in foods, such as rice and other starchy foods, as the source for cotransporting substances has resulted in oral rehydration solutions that not only replace losses but also markedly reduce diarrhea. The composition of available oral rehydration solutions is listed in Table 317–2, together with some standard intravenous solutions.

Intravenous fluid replacement should be reserved for neglected patients who have not received oral replacement and are in shock or close to it. In a cholera epidemic it is essential that all individuals at risk be thoroughly familiar with oral rehydration therapy and use it early to minimize deaths and the need of intravenous fluids. Thirst and urination are adequate guides to oral replacement therapy even in small children. This eliminates the need for accurate intake and output measurements and weighings, which even in excellent hospitals are difficult and are out of the question under epidemic conditions. Intravenous replacement for patients who are depleted and in shock should be given rapidly through a large-bore needle to ensure infusion rates of 50 to 100 ml per minute until a strong radial pulse has been achieved. Remaining fluid deficits may then be replaced less rapidly over 2 hours. The fluid deficit in a severely depleted patient is about 10 per cent of body weight (for a 50-kg patient— 5 liters). As soon as patients are strong enough to drink, oral rehydration therapy should begin, preferably with a rice- or other cereal-based solution of the proper solute composition. If this is done adequately, no further intravenous fluids are needed. In semicomatose patients who are unable to cooperate, nasogastric intubation permits adequate enteral replacement. For both intravenous and oral solutions the composition is of critical concern and should be within a range to properly replace losses of solutes and water (Table 317–2). It should be noted that many drinks ordinarily given to diarrhea patients are not adequate, although they may be allowed as a complement to intravenous or oral rehydration therapy. Vomiting is not a contraindication for use of oral rehydration therapy.

If a commercial preparation of oral rehydration salts is not available, a home solution can be prepared. The safest and most effective of these is a thick but drinkable suspension prepared from rice or other suitable ground starchy foods. If precooked products are available, these are very convenient but not essential. To a quart of water with cereal thickly suspended, a half level teaspoon (two three-finger pinches of salt) are added and the mixture cooked only long enough to soften the ground cereal powder. The mixture should be used within 6 hours and may be taken warm or cold. In cholera it may be necessary to drink a

great deal of fluid every hour for the first day. The patient must be offered a small cup every few minutes to minimize overloading the stomach and consequent vomiting. This is labor intensive but does not require medical skills. Especially in epidemics, family members are essential and effective participants in the treatment program.

In treating either children or adults, fluid therapy should be guided by thirst, observations on the circulation, urine output, and presence of edema or rales at the lung bases. Feeding is important and should be initiated immediately. Breast feeding is especially useful in affected infants, although few breast-fed babies contract cholera except in nonendemic areas where maternal milk lacks protective antibodies. Feeding should be with appetizing complex carbohydrates and proteins culturally adapted to the taste of the patient.

Adjunctive antibiotic therapy shortens diarrhea. This varies with the epidemic strain, but tetracycline and doxycycline have been effective when resistance is not present.

PREVENTION. Safe water supplies and appropriate disposal of human waste prevent spread of cholera but may not be achievable. *V. cholerae* is a fragile organism and cannot withstand drying, mild oxidation, or acid conditions. Thus a wide variety of disinfectants are effective for soiled articles. Bleaching powder is frequently used. Handwashing with soap before food handling is important.

There are no effective vaccines currently available, but several oral vaccines are in experimental use and have proven effective. Antibiotic prophylaxis has not been useful and encourages the emergence of resistant strains.

Barua D, Greenough WB III: Cholera. New York, Plenum Scientific Publishing Co., 1991. *A broad review of all aspects of cholera.*
Carpenter CCJ, Mitra PP, Sack RB: Clinical studies in Asiatic cholera. Parts I–VI. Bull Johns Hopkins Hosp 118:165, 1966. *This is an excellent series of reports concerning the pathophysiology of cholera, rational fluid replacement, and the value of antibiotic therapy.*
Hirschhorn N: The treatment of acute diarrhea in children. An historical and physiologic perspective. Am J Clin Nutr 33:637, 1980. *A thorough review of the special concerns that surround treatment of acute diarrhea, including cholera, in children. The review serves to "bridge" the traditional pediatric literature and the recent literature on cholera and related diarrheal diseases.*
Johnston JM, Martin DL, Perdue J, et al.: Cholera on a Gulf Coast oil rig. N Engl J Med 309:523, 1983. *Describes outbreaks of cholera along the coast of the Gulf of Mexico.*
Layseca CV: Cholera—Peru 1991. MMWR 40:108–110, 1991.
Rabbani GH, Greenough WB III: Cholera. *In* Lebenthal E, Duffey H (eds.): Textbook of Secretory Diarrhea. New York, Raven Press Ltd., 1990. *An up-to-date review of current knowledge about cholera.*

318 Enteric *Escherichia coli* Infections

Richard L. Guerrant

Escherichia coli is the predominant aerobic, coliform species in the normal colon. However, *E. coli* can also be an enteric pathogen and cause intestinal disease, usually diarrhea. Diarrhea caused by *E. coli* may be watery, inflammatory, or bloody, depending on which genetic codes for virulence traits the organism happens to possess. Consequently, diarrheogenic *E. coli* must be defined more specifically according to its virulence traits. Specific virulence traits determine the type of disease the organism causes, such as enterotoxigenic, enteroinvasive, enterohemorrhagic, enteropathogenic, or enteroadherent *E. coli* diarrhea. Each of these categories is being further resolved by the type of enterotoxin (such as the cholera-like, heat-labile toxin, LT, or the heat-stable toxin, ST) or adherence (such as close, focal, epithelial cell effacing, or diffuse) it causes. Taken separately, organisms such as enterotoxigenic *E. coli* constitute major bacterial causes of diarrhea morbidity and mortality on a global scale, particularly among children in tropical, developing areas and in travelers. Taken together, the varied types of *E. coli* diarrhea not only constitute the major category of bacterial enteric pathogens, but illustrate the wide array of ways that enteric pathogens can cause disease.

As noted in Table 318–1, at least three different types of *E. coli* enterotoxins may cause intestinal secretion (ETEC), others are enteroinvasive (EIEC), still others cause food-borne hemorrhagic colitis (EHEC) and produce large amounts of Shiga-like toxin (EHEC), while the classically recognized enteropathogenic *E. coli* (EPEC) serotypes are neither enterotoxigenic nor invasive but may focally attach and efface the epithelium. Further information is emerging on additional types of enteroadherent *E. coli* (EAEC) that exhibit autoaggregating (EAggEC) or diffuse adherence (DAEC) traits and may be associated with prolonged diarrhea among children in tropical developing areas.

ETIOLOGY. *Escherichia coli* is a small, catalase-positive, oxidase-negative, gram-negative bacillus in the family Enterobacteriaceae. It characteristically reduces nitrates, ferments glucose and usually lactose, and is either motile (with peritrichate flagella) or nonmotile. It gives a positive methyl red reaction and negative reactions with Voges-Proskauer, urease, phenylalanine deaminase, and citrate agents. *E. coli* constitutes the predominant facultative gram-negative bacillus in the intestinal tract of humans and other mammals. As with other gram-negative organisms, the lipopolysaccharide cell wall contains lipid A and 2-keto-3-deoxyoctanate (KDO), a core glycolipid that has been used in vaccine

development to provide cross-protection against systemic infections with other gram-negative organisms. Smooth (S) forms of *E. coli* have O specific carbohydrate chains attached to this core glycolipid to provide 169 O serogroups as well as at least 60 heat-labile protein flagellar (H) antigens by which strains are currently serotyped. Historically some 80 variably heat-labile capsular (K) antigens have also been described (L, B, and A), not to mention the more recently appreciated numerous adherence, enterotoxin, cytotoxin, and invasiveness factors that may be gained or lost by a particular serotype, as they are characteristically encoded on transmissible genetic elements such as plasmids or bacteriophages. Consequently, this common inhabitant of the normal human intestinal tract becomes a pathogen when it houses one or more specific traits that contribute to its colonization and virulence in the intestinal tract. Other traits such as O and H serogroup appear also to be important for certain enteropathogenic and enteroinvasive organisms. For reasons that remain obscure, only a few O serogroups tend to predominate in the normal human colon (O groups 1, 2, 4, 6, 7, 8, 18, 25, 45, 75, and 81), while others noted in Table 318–1 tend (albeit not absolutely) to be associated with specific virulence traits and thus different types of pathogenesis in the intestine. The O antigens of invasive *E. coli* often cross-react with various *Shigella* species, suggesting further that, in addition to the 140 Mdal plasmid, serotype also has a role in pathogenesis.

EPIDEMIOLOGY. Enteric *E. coli* infections are essentially acquired by the fecal-oral route, reflecting primarily a human reservoir for most recognized types of *E. coli* enteropathogens. Enterotoxigenic *E. coli* is also an important veterinary pathogen, especially in calves and piglets. However, the attachment traits of animal strains are different from those that infect humans and likely substantially influence their epidemiology.

The infectious doses of enterotoxigenic *E. coli* and enteroinvasive *E. coli* have been determined in volunteers to be 10^6 to 10^8, numbers that usually require multiplication in contaminated food or water vehicles for their transmission. Heavy contamination with enterotoxigenic *E. coli* has been documented in foods prepared in homes, restaurants, and at street vendors as well as in drinking water in many tropical areas, and contaminated water and foods likely represent the major sources of their acquisition, primarily in the warm or wet season. In the United States, major outbreaks of water- or food-borne *E. coli* diarrhea of different

TABLE 318–1. DIFFERENT TYPES OF ENTERIC E. COLI INFECTIONS

Type	Mechanism	Predominant O Serogroups	Genetic Code	Detection	Clinical Syndromes
Enterotoxigenic E. coli (ETEC):					
1. Cholera-like, heat-labile toxin (LT)	Activates intestinal adenylate cyclase & adhesin fimbriae	6, 8, 11, 15, 20, 25, 27, 63, 80, 85, 139	Plasmid	ELISA, RIA, PIH, CHO, Y1 cells, 18 h loops, gene probe	Watery diarrhea, Travelers' diarrhea
2. Heat-stable toxin (STa: STh or STp)	Activates intestinal guanylate cyclase & adhesin fimbriae	12, 78, 115, 148, 149, 153, 159, 166, 167	Plasmid (transposon)	ELISA, RIA, suckling mice, 6 h loops, gene probes	Watery diarrhea, Travelers' diarrhea
3. Heat-stable toxin (STb)	?; Not cAMP or cGMP		Plasmid	Piglet loops, gene probe	?
Enteroinvasive E. coli (EIEC):					
4. Enteroinvasive E. coli (EIEC)	Invasive	11, 28ac, 29, 124, 136, 144, 147, 152, 164, 167	Plasmid (140 Mdal, pWR110)	Sereny test, gene probe, (lys⁻, NM, oft. lactose⁻)	Inflammatory dysentery
Enterohemorrhagic E. coli (EHEC):					
5. Enterohemorrhagic E. coli (EHEC)	Shiga-like toxin(s) & adhesin fimbriae	26, 39, 113, 121, 128, 139, 145, 157, occ 55, 111	Phage(s) & adhesin plasmid(s)	Serotype, HeLa, Vero cells, sorbitol	Bloody noninflammatory diarrhea; hemolytic-uremic syndrome
Enteropathogenic E. coli (EPEC):					
6. Focal attaching and effacing EPEC	Attach, then efface the mucosa	55, 111, 119, 125, 126, 127, 128, 142, 158	Plasmid (50 Mdal, pMAR2)	Serotype, focal HEp2 adhesion, gene probes for EAF or eae	Infantile diarrhea
7. Other EPEC	?	44, 86, 114	?	Serotype	?
Enteroadherent E. coli (EAEC):					
8. Enteroadherent-aggregating E. coli (EAggEC)	Colonize; ? toxin(s)		? Plasmid	HEp2 cell adherence; AA or DA probes	? Prolonged diarrhea
9. Diffusely adherent E. coli (DAEC)			? Plasmid		

types have been documented in the last 10 to 15 years. A large water-borne outbreak of diarrhea at a popular national park was found to be caused by enterotoxigenic *E. coli* (ETEC), and a widespread outbreak of enteroinvasive *E. coli* (EIEC) enteritis was traced to consumption of French Camembert cheese. More recently, bloody, noninflammatory diarrhea was noted in two states in association with enterohemorrhagic *E. coli* (EHEC) (O157) in specialty hamburgers in a fast-food chain. Occasional nosocomial outbreaks of enterotoxigenic *E. coli* and enteropathogenic *E. coli* serotypes (EPEC) have also occurred in hospitalized infants in the United States and other industrialized countries.

As with most diarrheal illnesses, the highest age-specific attack rates of enterotoxigenic *E. coli* infections are in young children, especially at the time of weaning, when enterotoxigenic *E. coli* account for 15 to 50 per cent of illnesses. Like immunologically inexperienced young children, the traveler visiting tropical areas has a 30 to 50 per cent chance of acquiring travelers' diarrhea over a 2- to 3-week stay unless untreated water or ice and uncooked foods such as salads are strictly avoided. The most commonly recognized pathogen associated with travelers' diarrhea around the world is enterotoxigenic *E. coli* that produces either the STa, LT, or both enterotoxins (see Ch. 319).

Of potential immunologic significance is the continued occurrence of symptomatic infections with *E. coli* which produce the less immunogenic STa in adult residents of tropical or other areas endemic for enterotoxigenic *E. coli* infections. In contrast, adult residents in endemic areas often carry LT-producing *E. coli* asymptomatically, suggesting that they may be protected from symptoms, if not from colonization.

Limited data on invasive *E. coli* suggest that the infectious doses are relatively high. As with enterotoxigenic *E. coli* infections, such large numbers have been readily spread in food with high attack rates. Enteropathogenic *E. coli* have been recognized primarily in urban areas, especially among hospitalized infants in their first year of life, with apparent cross-infection in hospital nurseries. While sporadic cases still occur, nosocomial outbreaks of EPEC diarrhea during summer months appear to have become less common and less severe in industrialized countries in the last decade or two.

PATHOGENESIS AND PATHOLOGY. The pathogenesis of enteric *E. coli* infections begins with the ingestion of the organism in contaminated food or water, which then faces the normal gastric acid barrier. Both enterotoxigenic *E. coli* and enteroinvasive *E. coli* appear to be sensitive to gastric acid; neutralization by gastric acid reduces the infectious dose by 100- to 1000-fold. This is followed by an incubation period of 2 to 7 days, during which colonization of the involved part of the intestinal tract and enterotoxin production or invasion takes place. Best characterized is the colonization by enterotoxigenic *E. coli* in the upper small bowel which involves one of at least three major colonization factor antigen groups (which are fimbriate or fibrillar protein structures on the surface of the organism). The colonization fimbriae bind the organism to cell surface receptors in the upper small bowel where the enterotoxin is delivered to reduce normal absorption and cause net electrolyte and water secretion. The heat-labile toxin (LT) with a molecular weight of about 86,000 has a binding and active subunit that, like choleratoxin, binds to a monosialoganglioside (Gml) receptor. Also like choleratoxin, the active subunit ADP-ribosylates the regulatory subunit of adenylate cyclase to activate adenylate cyclase. The consequently increased chloride secretion and reduced sodium absorption combine to cause net isotonic electrolyte loss that must be replaced to prevent severe dehydration and hypotension and its potential consequences. Other strains produce the heat-stable toxin (STa), a much smaller molecule of 18-19 amino acids (molecular weight less than 2000) which activates intestinal particulate guanylate cyclase. Like cyclic AMP, the cyclic GMP thus formed also causes net secretion. A third type of *E. coli* enterotoxin (STb) causes secretion in porcine intestine without activating adenylate or guanylate cyclase; STb has no known role in human disease. Both the colonization traits and enterotoxin production are encoded on transmissible plasmids. Besides the complications of dehydration, the only significant pathologic change is depletion of mucus from intestinal goblet cells.

Other *E. coli*, often of certain serogroups noted in Table 318–1, have the capacity, analogous to *Shigella*, to invade and multiply in epithelial cells, cause conjunctivitis in guinea pigs (Sereny

test), and cause inflammatory colitis and dysenteric or bloody diarrhea. As seen with shigellosis, there is a striking inflammatory response with sheets of polymorphonuclear leukocytes in the stool. The colon shows patchy, acute inflammation in the mucosa and submucosa with focal denuding of the surface epithelium but usually without deeper invasion or systemic spread. While epithelial cell invasiveness in both enteroinvasive *E. coli* and *Shigella* appears to be encoded on a large 120-140 Mdal plasmid, several chromosomal determinants, including the O antigen, are critical for full invasive virulence.

Classically recognized enteropathogenic *E. coli* serotypes often fail to produce known enterotoxins or to be invasive. Nevertheless, they are well established causes of infantile diarrhea. Recent studies document at least two separate mechanisms by which different EPEC serotypes may cause diarrhea. The first, demonstrable with the majority of classically recognized EPEC serotypes such as O55 and O111, is a plasmid-encoded adherence to epithelial cells. This close adherence is associated with dissolution of the glycocalyx, disruption and effacement of the microvilli, villus atrophy, mucosal thinning, inflammation in the lamina propria, and variable crypt cell hyperplasia. These morphologic changes are associated with a reduction in the mucosal brush border enzymes and may contribute to the impaired absorptive function and diarrhea.

Other *E. coli*, notably of serogroups O26, 39, and 157, have been associated with food-borne outbreaks of bloody, noninflammatory diarrhea and with the hemolytic-uremic syndrome. These organisms produce large amounts of Shiga-like toxin that may be responsible for the characteristic colonic mucosal inflammation, edema, and hemorrhage. Sigmoidoscopy usually reveals only moderately hyperemic mucosa, and barium enema may reveal a thumb-print pattern of submucosal edema in the ascending and transverse colon. Some patients have superficial ulceration with mild neutrophil infiltration in the edematous submucosa.

Still other EPEC serotypes have historically been associated with diarrhea and have caused diarrhea in volunteers without recognized attachment, enteroadherence, enterotoxin, or enteroinvasiveness traits to date, suggesting that still other mechanisms remain to be unraveled for *E. coli* strains that cause diarrhea. The roles of a recently recognized LT-like toxin (which activates adenylate cyclase but is immunologically distinct from LT), of STb (a unique large heat-stable toxin that causes secretion without altering cyclic AMP or cyclic GMP in porcine intestine), or of colonization alone offer three additional potential types of enteric *E. coli* infections for which roles in human disease remain unclear at present.

CLINICAL MANIFESTATIONS. The most common clinical manifestation of enteric *E. coli* infections is the watery diarrhea that characterizes enterotoxigenic *E. coli* infections, particularly in young children and travelers to tropical or developing areas. This may range from mild to severe, cholera-like diarrhea that may be life-threatening, especially in small children and elderly patients who are particularly prone to suffer the most severe consequences of dehydration, undernutrition, and electrolyte imbalance (especially hypokalemia and acidosis).

The incubation period (2 to 7 days) varies with the size of the inoculum. Characteristic symptoms include malaise, abdominal cramping, anorexia, and watery diarrhea, occasionally associated with nausea, vomiting, or low-grade fever. The illness is usually self-limited to 1 to 5 days and rarely extends beyond 10 days or 2 weeks. Infections with *E. coli* which produce both ST and LT or ST alone may be more severe than those with only LT-producing *E. coli*. The persistence of impaired mucosal absorptive capacity for 1 to 3 weeks may further compound the cycle of malnutrition that complicates diarrheal illnesses in children in developing, tropical areas.

Infection with enteroinvasive *E. coli* is characterized by inflammatory colitis, often with abdominal pain, high fever, tenesmus, and bloody or dysenteric diarrhea essentially like that seen with *Shigella*, to which this organism is closely related. The incubation period is usually 1 to 3 days with the duration usually self-limited to 7 to 10 days.

Outbreaks of enteropathogenic *E. coli* infections in newborn nurseries have ranged from mild transient diarrhea to severe and rapidly fatal diarrheal illnesses, especially in premature or otherwise compromised infants. The more severe illnesses appear to have been more common in industrialized countries prior to 1950. However, more recent outbreaks and sporadic cases are well documented.

Recently recognized outbreaks of hemorrhagic colitis associated with the Shiga-like toxin producing *E. coli* (EHEC) O157:H7 and O26:H11 have been characterized by grossly bloody diarrhea with remarkably little fever or inflammatory exudate in the stool. Although the diarrheal illnesses have been self-limited, a significant number of children have subsequently developed a hemolytic-uremic syndrome. In addition, outbreaks of hemorrhagic colitis due to EHEC in nursing homes may be quite severe and more common than previously appreciated. The incubation period in two outbreaks has been 3 to 4 days (range 1 to 7 days), and the illness is characteristically self-limited to 5 to 12 days (mean 7.8).

DIAGNOSIS. A definitive etiologic diagnosis of *E. coli* diarrhea requires the documentation of a specific virulence trait such as enterotoxin, invasiveness, enteroadherence, or serotype, which usually requires specialized immunologic, tissue culture, animal bioassay, or gene probes that are available only in research and reference laboratories. Such tests are rarely cost effective or clinically indicated, except in outbreak or research situations. Fortunately, a likely diagnosis can often be suspected by the clinical and epidemiologic setting. For example, self-limited, noninflammatory diarrhea in tropical, developing areas is most likely due to enterotoxigenic *E. coli*, rotaviruses (young children), or Norwalk-like viruses (older children and adults). Noninflammatory diarrhea in winter months in temperate areas in older children or younger adults is more likely to be due to Norwalk-like viruses. Specific tests for the respective virulence traits of different types of *E. coli* are noted in Table 318–1. One should also consider *Vibrio* infections in areas endemic for cholera or in any coastal area where inadequately cooked seafood may be eaten. If noninflammatory diarrhea persists, especially with weight loss, one should also consider *Giardia lamblia* or *Cryptosporidium* infection. In outbreaks of food poisoning, *S. aureus*, *Clostridium perfringens*, and *Bacillus cereus* should be considered.

Inflammatory colitis with high fever, tenesmus, and leukocytes, mucus, and blood in the stool may well be due to enteroinvasive *E. coli* but should prompt a stool culture for more common invasive pathogens such as *Campylobacter jejuni*, *Shigella*, and *Salmonella* or even *Clostridium difficile*, *Yersinia enterocolitica*, or non-cholera *Vibrio* (see Ch. 316). On the other hand, bloody diarrhea without high fever or fecal leukocytes should prompt consideration of the Shiga-like toxin producing enterohemorrhagic *E. coli* (EHEC) such as strain O157:H7. This organism is often suspected as a sorbitol-negative *E. coli*, which may require further study for serotype or Shiga-like toxin production.

THERAPY. As with all diarrheal illnesses, the primary treatment is replacement and maintenance of water and electrolytes. Losses of water and electrolytes may be particularly severe and even life-threatening with enterotoxigenic *E. coli* and can usually be replaced with a simple oral rehydration solution that employs the intact, sodium-coupled glucose, and/or amino acid absorption to replace fluid losses, as described in Ch. 317. This oral rehydration solution should be given ad libitum with free water and, in breast-fed infants, continued breast feeding and early refeeding to compensate for the nutritional losses.

Because most *E. coli* diarrhea is self-limited, the role of antimicrobial agents is debated and remains of secondary importance to rehydration. In areas where the enterotoxigenic *E. coli* remains sensitive, early initiation of sulfamethoxazole-trimethoprim, tetracycline, or new quinolone derivatives may reduce a 3- to 5-day illness to a 1- to 2-day illness if started with the first loose stool in travelers to endemic, tropical areas (see Ch. 319). The use of antimotility agents should be tempered by the potential added risk of worsening or prolonging inflammatory diarrheas and by their lack of effectiveness in reducing fluid loss even though abdominal cramping and overt diarrhea may be temporarily reduced. Because of the potential severity of the disease in infants, some pediatricians use neomycin, 100 mg per kilogram per day P.O., divided into three daily doses for 5 days, for documented enteropathogenic *E. coli* infections in neonates.

Bismuth subsalicylate may reduce symptoms in travelers' diarrhea but should be used with caution to avoid toxic doses of salicylate. A number of pharmacologic agents have been shown to enhance absorption or reduce secretion with experimental diarrhea but remain inadequately studied or too toxic for recommended use to date.

PROGNOSIS. The overall prognosis in *E. coli* diarrheas of the various types noted, if fully and adequately treated, is generally excellent. However, the impact of *E. coli* and other common diarrheas on mortality and morbidity (particularly with repeated infections compounding malnutrition in developing young children) remains one of the major health problems on a global scale; this problem may actually be worsening in some transitional areas.

PREVENTION. The prevention of *E. coli* enteric infections is ultimately related to basic economic development and adequate sanitary facilities and wide availability of sufficient quality and quantity of water. In the interim, especially in areas where adequate water supplies and sanitary facilities are not available, such measures as breast feeding for at least 6 to 12 months and hygienic measures like handwashing should reduce the likelihood of acquiring *E. coli* enteric infections. Travelers to developing or tropical areas should avoid drinking untreated or unboiled water or ice and eating uncooked fruits or vegetables that may have been "freshened" with highly contaminated water. Although a number of antimicrobial agents have been documented to be effective over short periods of time when taken prophylactically, their effectiveness is sharply limited by the rapidly emerging resistance to antimicrobial drugs as well as by the potential side effects of their indiscriminate, widespread use. For example, tetracycline resistance among enterotoxigenic *E. coli* is common, and combined sulfamethoxazole-trimethroprim resistance is rapidly emerging around the world. Finally, currently developing toxoid or colonization factor vaccines hold considerable promise for the prevention of enterotoxigenic *E. coli* diarrhea.

Bhan MK, Raj P, Levine MM, et al.: Enteroaggregative *Escherichia coli* associated with persistent diarrhea in a cohort of rural children in India. J Infect Dis 159:1060–1064, 1989. *A first report of a clinical role for new types of enteroadherent* E. coli.

Black RE, Merson MH, Hug I, et al.: Incidence and severity of rotavirus and *Escherichia coli* diarrhoea in rural Bangladesh. Implications for vaccine development. Lancet 1:141–143, 1981. *Concise report of community-based studies of enterotoxigenic* E. coli *and rotaviral diarrhea in a rural area of Bangladesh.*

Carter AO, Borczyk AA, Carlson AK, et al.: A severe outbreak of *E. coli* O157:H7 associated hemorrhagic colitis in a nursing home. N Engl J Med 317:1496–1500, 1987. *A common source outbreak with secondary, probable person-to-person spread, of this serious cause of bloody diarrhea and hemolytic-uremic syndrome in the institutionalized elderly.*

DuPont HL, Formal SB, Hornick RB, et al.: Pathogenesis of *Escherichia coli* diarrhea. N Engl J Med 285:1–9, 1971. *Classic early clinical, pathologic, and pathogenetic studies of enterotoxigenic and enteroinvasive* E. coli *diarrhea in human volunteers.*

Guerrant RL, Kirchhoff LV, Shields DS, et al.: Prospective study of diarrheal illnesses in northeastern Brazil: Patterns of disease, nutritional impact, etiologies and risk factors. J Infect Dis 148:986–997, 1983. *A detailed study of endemic diarrhea in a tropical area, including seasonality, risk after weaning, and nutritional impact, as well as relationship of enterotoxigenic* E. coli *to other pathogens.*

Guerrant, RL, Hughes JM, Lima NL, Crane JK: Diarrhea in developed and developing countries: Magnitude, special settings and etiologies. Rev Infect Dis 12:S41–S50, 1990. *Overview of community-based and hospital-based studies of diarrhea that reviews the relative importance of* E. coli *among other pathogens in developing and developed countries.*

Levine MM, Edelman R: Enteropathogenic *Escherichia coli* of classic serotypes associated with infant diarrhea: Epidemiology and pathogenesis. Epidemiol Rev 6:31–51, 1984. *A thorough historical review of classic enteropathogenic* E. coli *diarrhea as well as an update on recent volunteer studies and pathogenesis.*

Levine MM: *Escherichia coli* that cause diarrhea: Enterotoxigenic, Enteropathogenic, Enterohemorrhagic, and Enteroadherent. J Infect Dis 155:377–389, 1989. *A good overview of major pathogenic mechanisms of* E. coli *diarrhea.*

Microbial Toxins and Diarrheal Diseases. CIBA Foundation Symposium No. 112, 1985. *Thorough review of the mechanisms of enterotoxin action, relating the pharmacology of* E. coli *toxins (LT, STa, STb, Shiga) to those of other enteric pathogens like* V. cholerae, Shigella, *and* C. difficile.

NIH Consensus Development Conference on Traveler's Diarrhea. JAMA 253:2700–2704, 1985. *A balanced critical appraisal of the epidemiology, etiologies, presentation, and treatment of concise travelers' diarrhea.*

Sansonetti PJ, Hale TL, Oaks EV: Genetics of virulence in enteroinvasive *Escherichia coli*. Microbiology, 1985, pp 67–82. *One of a series of three brief reviews that offer a considerable amount of new information on the pathogenesis of the major types of* E. coli *enteric infection including ETEC, EIEC, EPEC, and EHEC.*

319 The Diarrhea of Travelers

R. Bradley Sack

Travelers from the developed world who visit the developing world are highly susceptible to an acute diarrheal illness known as "travelers' diarrhea" or by more colorful names that fit the locale in which the travelers find themselves incapacitated. Although at one time this condition was blamed on a change in diet, minerals in the water, and travel fatigue, it is now known to be an acute infection, caused by enteric pathogens that are endemic throughout the areas of the world where sanitation is less than optimal. In those areas the diarrhea produced by these pathogens is primarily a childhood disease that decreases markedly in incidence after the first few years of life, because of the development of protective immunity. Travelers are, in a sense, immunologically naive "children" who are suddenly placed in an endemic area of infection and therefore are highly susceptible to the disease. The predictable, high attack rates of diarrhea in travelers make this syndrome one that can be conveniently and intensively studied by investigators attempting to prevent and treat it. Perhaps other than a common source outbreak of diarrheal disease, the attack rates among travelers are the highest known in any identifiable population. Among travelers from the United States to the developing world, attack rates vary from about 25 to 75 per cent during the first 3 weeks of stay, with rates decreasing markedly as immunity develops.

By way of contrast, travelers from developing countries who visit other developing countries usually have a considerably lower attack rate, based on their prior exposure to these organisms. However, they are still susceptible to "new" agents that they may not have encountered previously. Visitors from the developing countries who visit the developed world, on the other hand, have a very low attack rate of diarrhea, as would be expected.

ETIOLOGY. Multiple studies have now been done on the etiology of this syndrome throughout the world, and it is clear that enterotoxigenic *Escherichia coli* (Ch. 318) is the predominant organism. Other bacteria, viruses, and protozoa are also involved, but with lesser frequency (Table 319–1). In different geographic areas, the rank order of these pathogens varies, but *E. coli* heads the list; because of this observation, studies of treatment and prophylaxis have been possible by focusing on this single group of organisms. However, a considerable percentage of episodes is undiagnosed etiologically, in spite of the best available laboratory techniques; evidence from studies employing antimicrobials suggests that a large number of these are also bacterial in origin. Contrary to "popular" notions about travelers' diarrhea, relatively few cases are caused by protozoa, particularly *Entamoeba histolytica*.

PATHOGENESIS AND CLINICAL PICTURE. The clinical syndrome of travelers' diarrhea is typically that of a secretory watery diarrhea caused by the enterotoxins of *E. coli* (see Ch. 318). The entire process is analogous to the pathogenesis of cholera (Ch. 317). The watery diarrhea usually lasts 3 to 4 days, and when most severe, may result in watery stools as frequent as 15 to 20 times per day, with significant water and electrolyte loss, leading to clinical signs of dehydration. Although deaths due to this illness are extremely rare, definitive replacement of fluid

TABLE 319–1. ETIOLOGIC AGENTS OF TRAVELERS' DIARRHEA

Agent	Percentage
Enterotoxigenic *E. coli*	30–70
Shigella	5–10
Salmonella	<5
Campylobacter	<5
Enteroadherent *E. coli*	5–10
Rotavirus	<5
Giardia lamblia	<5
Entamoeba histolytica	<3
Cryptosporidium	<5
Unknown agents	30–40

and electrolytes lost in the stool may be necessary, and hospitalization may be required. The vast majority of illnesses are much milder, however, consisting of only three to five diarrheal stools per day, and are of importance primarily because of limitation of activities.

Those episodes due to *Shigella* organisms are usually typical of a dysentery-like illness, with abdominal pain, fever, and blood and inflammatory cells in the stool.

Nearly all episodes are self-limited, but a few (less than 1 per cent) may become persistent and require evaluation following return home.

Although the clinical syndrome in children traveling to the developing world has been less well studied, there are a number of reports of severe, persistent diarrhea and marked nutritional wasting following visits to high-risk areas.

TRANSMISSION. The transmission of the enteric pathogens occurs almost exclusively through fecally contaminated food and water. Of highest risk to the traveler are foods that are not cooked or peeled and are consumed raw. Foods obtained from road-side vendors or foods kept unrefrigerated for long periods of time are also in the highest risk category.

PREVENTION. Since the mode of transmission is known, prudent attention to the ingestion of uncontaminated food and water should entirely prevent the disease. This has been shown in the military and on board cruise ships, where all food is hygienically prepared and packaged. For the usual traveler, however, food must be obtained from local sources, and contamination cannot be entirely prevented. Even the "best" hotels in the developing world may have unsanitary kitchens, and "first class" travelers are therefore not exempt.

A number of studies have been carried out in an attempt to prevent the disease with drugs, and many agents have been shown to be highly protective. The most protective are antimicrobials directed against the most common etiologic agents, the enterotoxigenic *E. coli*. Either doxycycline (100 mg), trimethoprim-sulfamethoxazole (160 + 800 mg), norfloxacin (400 mg), or ciprofloxacin (500 mg), taken once daily for a period of up to 3 weeks, has provided a high degree of protection against travelers' diarrhea, in the neighborhood of 75 to 90 per cent. Because the antibacterial spectrum of norfloxacin and ciprofloxacin includes *Campylobacter jejuni*, these drugs may theoretically provide a broader spectrum of coverage against the known etiologic agents of travelers' diarrhea. A nonantimicrobial drug, bismuth subsalicylate taken four times a day, has also given a significant degree of protection (approximately 60 per cent). Other antimicrobial drugs have also been used successfully (erythromycin, mecillinam, trimethoprim alone) but have not been tested as extensively. Drugs that have been tested and found to be of little or no benefit include neomycin, streptotriad, hydroxyquinolines, and *Lactobacillus* preparations.

The main questions relating to the use of prophylactic medications are not the efficacy, but rather the side effects; this issue will be further discussed later.

THERAPY. Therapy is based on recognition of clinical disease and a general knowledge of the causative organisms, since identity of specific etiologic agents will usually not be known (Table 319–1). The therapy of travelers' diarrhea falls under three general categories: (1) replacement of fluid and electrolytes lost to prevent and treat the resulting dehydration, (2) symptomatic therapy directed at relieving the frequency of stooling or the attendant abdominal cramps, and (3) specific antimicrobial therapy directed at the causative agent, in order to decrease the severity and shorten the duration of the illness.

Replacement therapy is done best with the oral glucose-electrolyte solutions developed for therapy of all dehydrating diarrheas, regardless of etiologic agent or age of the patient. These are now available commercially in packets, which can be carried by the traveler and used as required by mixing the contents with the appropriate volumes of potable water.

Symptomatic therapy may be useful for travelers with a typical secretory diarrhea who need to participate in certain vital events, such as long bus rides or important business or social occasions. The drugs used (loperamide, diphenoxylate) primarily interfere with intestinal motility and therefore can decrease the rate of stooling in persons with mild disease. However, because of this action, there is the possibility of actually intensifying the clinical illness due to invasive bacteria, since they are more slowly cleared from the bowel.

Preparations of bismuth subsalicylate have also been shown to give mild symptomatic relief, although the mechanism of action is unknown. Kaolin/pectin preparations are of no significant effect in treatment.

Specific antimicrobial therapy has been shown to be highly effective for this illness. The same drugs used for prophylaxis—trimethoprim-sulfamethoxazole (160–180 mg), norfloxacin (400 mg), ciprofloxacin (500 mg), and doxycycline (100 mg) in twice-daily doses—are also effective in shortening the duration of the disease to 24 to 36 hours. A 3-day course of therapy is sufficient.

THE STRATEGY OF MANAGING THE PROBLEM OF TRAVELERS' DIARRHEA. The questions relating to the prevention and treatment of travelers' diarrhea were reviewed at an NIH Consensus Conference, which should be consulted for further details. The most difficult issue is who, if anyone, should receive prophylactic antimicrobials. Since antimicrobials are widely available as over-the-counter medications throughout the developing world, the small addition to the antimicrobial pool by tourists is thought to be inconsequential to the larger issue of antibiotic pressure on a worldwide basis. Of more importance is the issue of adverse reactions to the drugs being taken for prophylaxis. Although none of the published controlled studies demonstrated any significant side effects, all were done using primarily young healthy adults. Since these drugs have significant side effects, although at low frequency, they are not recom-

mended for routine prophylaxis. For the short-term individual traveler, however, who is advised of the possible side effects and who wishes to avail him/herself of the protection, these drugs can be considered for use.

Since the same drugs can be taken as treatment, the preferred strategy in most cases would be to have the traveler carry along sufficient medication, so that he or she can administer appropriate treatment when indicated. Oral rehydration therapy should be given simultaneously for the prevention of dehydration. For milder episodes of diarrhea, drugs like bismuth subsalicylate or antimotility drugs can be taken for symptomatic relief.

The problem of travelers' diarrhea will continue until the general sanitation of the developing world approaches that of the industrialized countries or until effective vaccines against the major diarrheal pathogens are available. Neither of these occurrences is expected soon, and therefore this common syndrome will need to be addressed for some time; this can now be done rationally and effectively based on our knowledge of etiologies and modes of transmission.

Consensus Conference: Travelers' Diarrhea. JAMA 253:2700, 1985. *A summary of the NIH conference in which all aspects of the problem were reviewed; a complete publication of the conference is given in Rev Infect Dis 8:(Suppl 2), 1986.*

DuPont HL, Reves RR, Galindo E, et al.: Treatment of travelers' diarrhea with trimethoprim/sulfamethoxazole and with trimethoprim alone. N Engl J Med 307:841, 1982. *A controlled therapeutic study showing marked efficacy of these drugs.*

Sack RB: Treatment and prevention of travelers' diarrhea. *In* Holmgren J, Lindberg A, Mollby R (eds.): Development of Vaccines against Diarrhea, 11th Nobel Conf., Stockholm 1985, pp 289–301. Lund, Sweden, Studentlitteratur, 1986. *A comprehensive review of all controlled studies of prophylaxis and treatment.*

Other Bacterial Infections

320 Extraintestinal Infections Caused by Enteric Bacteria

Elizabeth J. Ziegler

Bacteria constitute over half the dry weight of stool. *Bacteroides* species far outnumber other genera, at 10^{12} organisms per gram. Other anaerobes such as *Fusobacterium*, *Clostridium*, and peptostreptococci also are abundant. Among the facultative bacteria, members of the family Enterobacteriaceae predominate, at about 10^9 organisms per gram. Pseudomonads, enterococci, other non-hemolytic streptococci, and yeasts are present as well.

These bacteria that normally inhabit the human gastrointestinal tract perform important functions beneficial to the host. *Bacteroides fragilis*, *Clostridium*, and enterococci deconjugate bile acids for participation in fat metabolism. Some intestinal bacteria synthesize menaquinone, or vitamin K, a cofactor for blood coagulation. Normal gut flora discourage colonization of the bowel with primary pathogens and overgrowth of bacteria usually present in small numbers. Colonization resistance is not understood completely, but it must involve bacteriocins, regulation of local oxidation-reduction potential, and balance of nutrients as well as unknown factors. Breakdown of colonization resistance is illustrated by the increase in susceptibility of antibiotic-treated animals to *Salmonella* and by the emergence of fecal *Pseudomonas aeruginosa* and *Candida* in patients receiving antimicrobial agents.

PATHOGENESIS OF INFECTIONS

Enteric bacteria are not primary pathogens but cause disease when they escape from their usual gastrointestinal habitat. Direct penetration of the bowel wall by surgical, traumatic, or spontaneous rupture spills fecal contents into the peritoneal cavity and

into open wounds. Gut bacteria on the perineal skin gain access to the urinary tract and proliferate there, especially when the flushing action of urine flow is disrupted by mechanical obstruction or neurologic dysfunction. When the biliary tract is obstructed by gallstones or tumor, the upper small bowel, which normally is sterile, becomes colonized with facultative bacteria (*Escherichia coli*, *Klebsiella*, enterococci) or, less often, with *Bacteroides* and *Clostridium*, which then infect the gallbladder and bile ducts. Intestinal flora can be introduced into the respiratory tract from contaminated skin or the environment; they proliferate there under the influence of antibiotics and in the presence of underlying pulmonary disease and tracheal instrumentation. Penetrating foreign bodies, such as intravenous catheters and intraventricular cerebral pressure monitors, become colonized by gut flora on the skin and in respiratory secretions and then induce infection in adjacent tissues. In burns, destruction of the skin barrier, the rich culture medium of oozing tissue fluid, and a shift of surface flora by application of local and systemic antibacterial agents result in local necrotizing infection of the burn wound with gut flora and frequent secondary gram-negative bacteremia.

In the absence of mechanical and surface abnormalities such as those outlined above, systemic resistance to enteric bacteria is very strong. The mainstay of this resistance is the polymorphonuclear neutrophil, destruction or malfunction of which leads almost inevitably to bloodstream invasion by bowel bacteria. Serum complement must be protective against invasion of some organisms, since very few of the gram-negative bacilli isolated from blood are sensitive to complement-mediated bacteriolysis, whereas many enteric rods in feces are susceptible. Newborn infants, whose neutrophils and complement activity have not fully matured, are at high risk of disseminated infections with facultative enteric rods. Microbial factors are important, too. Although anaerobes predominate over facultative bacteria and aerobes in the gut, these anaerobes rarely cause bacteremia or metastatic infection even in neutropenia. The presence of certain bacterial polysaccharide capsules (e.g., *E. coli* K1) or production of large amounts of capsule (e.g., by *Klebsiella pneumoniae* in hyperglycemic or glycosuric diabetics) predisposes to systemic invasion by these organisms.

Infections with enteric bacteria have increased dramatically during the past four decades. The reasons should be apparent from the discussion above. Advances in surgical and intensive care, trauma and burn management, blood transfusion, antimicrobial and cancer chemotherapy, transplantation, and immunosuppression all create opportunities for these infections. The average lifespan has lengthened, so that those receiving medical attention carry the added risks of advanced age. The majority of extraintestinal infections with enteric bacteria now arise in the hospital, and they exact a high toll in mortality and increased hospital costs. Furthermore, they jeopardize the success of the advanced treatments we have worked so hard to develop. For these reasons, physicians should understand the pathogenesis of each infection so that they can effect a cure and prevent recurrence if possible.

SPECIFIC LOCAL INFECTIONS WITH ENTERIC BACTERIA

The diagnosis and management of each of the following gram-negative infections are discussed in depth in the appropriate section elsewhere in the textbook. A few points are emphasized here.

PERITONITIS (see Ch. 110). It can be difficult to recover bacteria from patients with spontaneous bacterial peritonitis; large volumes of fluid should be submitted for culture. Patients undergoing chronic peritoneal dialysis frequently develop peritonitis. If the same organism is isolated from repeated episodes and especially if it is an enteric rod or *Pseudomonas*, infection of the subcutaneous catheter tunnel should be suspected. A radiolabeled white blood cell scan can be helpful in detecting such infections so that the infected catheter can be removed.

PYELONEPHRITIS (see Ch. 84). Urinary tract infections localized to the bladder or kidneys can have important implications for therapy. Symptoms may be misleading, selective ureteral catheterization carries considerable risk, and examination of urine for antibody-coated bacteria is not practical in routine laboratories. A simple culture technique can differentiate between upper and lower urinary tract infections in difficult cases in which parenteral antibiotics would be required for kidney infection. In brief, the test (Fairley, 1967) employs a newly placed three-way bladder catheter through which a combination antibiotic and enzyme mixture (fibrinolysin and DNase) is instilled to sterilize the bladder. Neomycin is employed for most organisms; polymyxin can be used for *Pseudomonas* and amphotericin for yeast. Bladder instillation is followed by a large-volume sterile water wash. Then the catheter is clamped, and three 10-minute specimens are collected. Increasing bacterial counts after the wash point to pyelonephritis. If infection is limited to the bladder, the Fairley procedure can cure it. The test is unreliable in patients with low urinary output, and it should not be performed in patients with neutropenia.

PROSTATITIS (see Ch. 223). Most antibiotics available for treatment of infections with enteric bacilli do not penetrate the prostate well. For this reason, chronic prostatitis rarely is cured. However, the role of chronic prostatitis as a nidus of recurrent acute urinary tract infection in males can be curbed by low levels of suppressive antibiotics in bladder urine, achieved by a single tablet of an oral antibiotic given daily.

MENINGITIS (see Ch. 301). Enteric rods, especially *E. coli* and *Klebsiella*, are a frequent cause of neonatal meningitis. In adults, meningitis with enteric bacilli is exceedingly rare except in cases of head trauma or neurosurgery. Bacteria may be infrequent and difficult to see on stained smears of spinal or ventricular fluid. Treatment with a third-generation cephalosporin that penetrates the blood-brain barrier at high dose may be sufficient, but infections with organisms resistant to such drugs may require chloramphenicol or a combination of intravenous and intrathecal aminoglycosides. Infected foreign bodies must be removed.

PNEUMONIA (see Ch. 61, 294, 295). Seeing gram-negative rods in respiratory secretions or growing them from the secretions does not necessarily imply infection. Susceptible patients often have severe chronic lung disease with abnormal chest radio-

graphs. Many are on respirators with inflammation around endotracheal tubes and have abnormal gram-negative nasopharyngeal flora. Evidence of increasing infiltrates, fever, increasing leukocytosis, and/or worsening respiratory function should be sought before the diagnosis of gram-negative pneumonia is made in such cases.

INFECTIONS OF INTRAVENOUS CATHETERS. Patients who are critically ill may have limited numbers of sites for placement of intravenous catheters. If catheter infection is suspected, it may be impractical or impossible to remove all the lines. Comparison of quantitative blood cultures drawn through each catheter and from one peripheral vein can identify the infected site and preserve the uninfected catheters in place.

INFECTIONS IN NEUTROPENIA (see Ch. 287). The most common bowel infection in neutropenia is perirectal abscess. Inflammation may be modest, but patients complain of severe pain. Examination can cause bacteremia. Surgical drainage may not be required unless neutropenia resolves and fluctuance develops. A less common but much more serious condition is typhlitis, an infection of the cecum associated with gas in the bowel wall, peritonitis, perforation, and bacteremia. This condition can be fatal within hours. Surgical resection has been helpful in a few cases, but surgical mortality is very high. Aggressive antibiotic therapy should be directed against *E. coli* and *P. aeruginosa*, the most common etiologic agents.

Necrotic skin lesions can accompany gram-negative bacteremia in neutropenic patients. These lesions are called ecthyma gangrenosum, and they are seen most frequently in *Pseudomonas* bacteremia. Cases have been reported with other gram-negative rods and with *Candida* and *Aspergillus* septicemia as well. The lesions can be scraped to search for the organism on smear. If nothing is seen, a punch biopsy for culture and histologic section can be done safely even in severe thrombocytopenia. In fungemia, the histologic section may be the only premortem diagnostic specimen obtained.

GRAM-NEGATIVE BACTEREMIA AND ENDOTOXIC SHOCK

Gram-negative bacteria gain access to the bloodstream from foci of tissue infection or, when host resistance is depressed, from sites of heavy colonization and minor trauma. Although bacteremia creates the opportunity for metastatic infections, a more immediate and serious consequence of gram-negative bacteremia is septic shock. The incidence of gram-negative bacteremia has risen steadily during the past three decades. It is estimated that at least 200,000 episodes occur in the United States each year, of which 20 to 60 per cent are fatal. Mortality varies with the severity and nature of underlying disease, the source of bacteremia, and the incidence of serious sequelae of sepsis, such as the adult respiratory distress syndrome (ARDS) and disseminated intravascular coagulation (DIC). Death is caused by either irreversible hypotension or damage to vital organs such as lung or kidney, which cannot be salvaged despite recovery from circulatory collapse.

Rates of shock vary in different series from less than 20 per cent to more than 50 per cent. In comparable groups, shock is somewhat more frequent in gram-negative bacteremia than in gram-positive bacteremia or fungemia. However, gram-negative bacteremia is distinguished from the other septicemias by the fact that very small numbers of circulating bacteria are associated with hypotension. It is generally agreed that the principal trigger of gram-negative shock is endotoxin, a major structural component of the gram-negative bacterial cell wall, for the abnormalities seen in endotoxic shock can be duplicated with intravenous infusions of pure endotoxin in experimental animals. Endotoxin is a lipopolysaccharide (LPS) consisting of a long chain of strain-specific repeating sugar subunits at one end, some connecting core sugars in the middle, and lipid A, a fatty acid– and phosphate-substituted diglucosamine, at the other end, embedded in the cell wall. Lipid A, the biologically active portion of the molecule, is highly conserved with little variation among gram-negative bacteria. An exception is *Bacteroides fragilis*, which makes an unusual lipid A; its LPS is virtually nontoxic and pure *B. fragilis* bacteremia is infrequently associated with shock.

Endotoxin has been detected in the plasma of patients with gram-negative bacteremia who are sick enough to exhibit signs of peripheral hypoperfusion. There is evidence that antibiotics, especially those directed at the cell wall, release substantial amounts of LPS from bacteria while killing them; this may explain the transient worsening of hypotension occasionally seen after the first dose of antibiotics.

The human is one of the species most sensitive to endotoxin. Subnanogram quantities of LPS stimulate beneficial host responses, such as lymphocyte activation and fever (interleukin 1). However, nanogram quantities given intravenously can elicit a panoply of toxic reactions, including complement activation, production of procoagulant factors with DIC, neutrophil aggregation, lung capillary damage, and perturbation of circulatory control with splanchnic pooling of blood, hypotension, and metabolic acidosis. Many mediators are involved in these toxic reactions; recent work suggests that tumor necrosis factor, a small protein produced by endotoxin-stimulated macrophages, may be responsible for many of the phenomena leading to death from endotoxin (see Ch. 285, 286). High levels of interleukin 6, another cytokine, have been correlated with a fatal outcome in septic shock. It has not yet been determined whether interleukin 6 mediates some of the toxic reactions or whether it is an "alarm hormone" that merely reflects the severity of cell injury in sepsis.

CLINICAL MANIFESTATIONS (see also Ch. 288). Since focal infections usually precede bloodstream invasion, patients are likely to have had fever and leukocytosis for several days before the sudden deterioration that marks the onset of gram-negative bacteremia. The temperature may suddenly increase or it may fall to subnormal levels, especially in elderly patients or those who are debilitated. Rarely, fever is obliterated by chronically administered high-dose steroids. There may be frank shaking chills. Patients may exhibit new anxiety, agitation, or confusion. The first clue to sepsis in an already critically ill patient may be an increase in cardiac output or an inability to absorb enteral nutrition. For some reason, patients with burns often develop unexplained ileus as one of the few signs of bacteremia on a background of fever, leukocytosis, and vascular instability associated with the burn itself. Even though blood pressure still may be normal, orthostatic pulse and blood pressure changes may be seen. Resting tachycardia and/or increased respiratory rate is helpful (unless the patient has a pacemaker, is on drugs that affect heart rate, or is on a respirator at controlled rate). In patients under less strict surveillance, the first symptom of hypotension may be a significant decrease in urine output. When the blood pressure is obtained, it is important to consult the medical record for the patient's normal reading. Formerly hypertensive patients will suffer poor perfusion at levels of blood pressure that are normal for most individuals. In general, the traditional distinction between "warm" and "cold" shock has not been helpful in separating gram-positive from gram-negative shock, and no reliance should be placed on it. When measured, cardiac output generally is high and systemic resistance is low in cases of endotoxic shock uncomplicated by other diseases. In late stages of untreated or irreversible shock, patients exhibit intense vasoconstriction, then cyanosis. Symptoms of shock-induced organ failure—bleeding, ARDS, azotemia, and infarcts of brain, heart, and bowel—will appear and may dominate the picture.

DIAGNOSIS. The term "sepsis" has come to denote a syndrome in which there is a systemic response to infection in the form of fever or hypothermia, tachycardia, tachypnea, and either hypotension (in 50 per cent of cases) or evidence of hypoperfusion of one or more organ systems. Analysis of clinical series suggests that 30 to 50 per cent of patients with the sepsis syndrome have gram-negative bacteremia documented by blood culture. Many of those without gram-negative bacteremia have gram-negative focal infections. Most patients with measurable endotoxin in the blood have gram-negative bacteremia, but a few do not. Figure 320–1 is a schematic representation of these relationships. Other considerations in the differential diagnosis of sepsis include infection of the bloodstream by gram-positive bacteria and fungi, staphylococcal toxic shock syndrome, clostridial shock, pulmonary embolus, acute allergic reactions, myocardial infarction, and a long list of less common conditions.

For therapeutic purposes, the diagnosis of gram-negative bac-

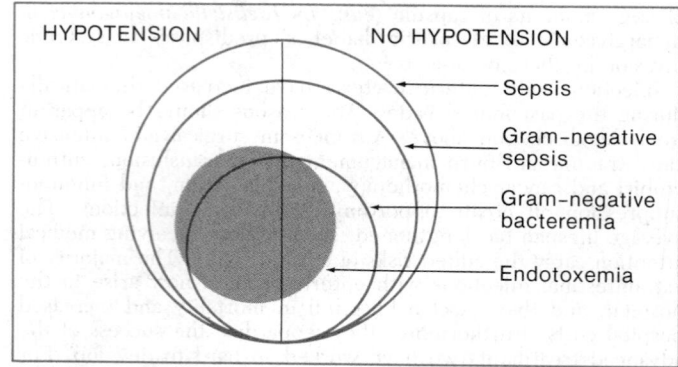

FIGURE 320–1. Schematic representation of etiologies of the sepsis syndrome. (Courtesy of Craig R. Smith.)

teremia cannot await the results of blood cultures but must be made on clinical grounds alone. The clinical setting is very helpful. A diagnosis of gram-negative bacteremia should be considered when sudden deterioration occurs in patients with focal infections usually caused by gram-negative bacteria (e.g., pyelonephritis, cholecystitis), in patients with significant focal infections from which gram-negative bacteria already have been isolated, and in patients with compromise in host defenses (e.g., neutropenia, burn injury), rendering them susceptible to their own bacterial flora. Neutropenic patients rarely have physical signs to localize the source of their bacteremia, but careful conversation often reveals a history of minor trauma, slight pain, or diarrhea.

Gram-negative bacteremia and endotoxin infusion both cause transient neutropenia followed by neutrophilic leukocytosis. Large "toxic" vacuoles are seen. The first leukocyte count often is obtained after the leukopenic phase, but patients recovering from chemotherapy may have limited leukocyte reserves and thus exhibit only an apparent reversal of marrow recovery. Isolated thrombocytopenia or full-blown disseminated intravascular coagulopathy is not diagnostic of gram-negative bacteremia but, if present, is good supporting evidence. Arterial blood gas determinations may reveal unexplained hypoxemia without overt pulmonary disease, followed by metabolic acidosis.

TREATMENT. Three elements are essential in the management of gram-negative bacteremia: physiologic support, antibiotics, and identification of the source so that it can be eradicated. These are listed in the order in which they should be addressed, but all three should be considered urgently, generally within 1 hour. If the patient is in shock or impending shock, physiologic monitoring in an intensive care unit should be applied if available. Good intravenous access should be obtained and a bladder catheter placed for hourly measurement of urine flow.

The aim of physiologic support is to restore adequate tissue perfusion. This is judged most easily by urine flow and mental status; perfusion of vital organs may be adequate when systolic blood pressure remains low and there is marked peripheral vasoconstriction. The principles of management of septic shock are the same as those used for other kinds of shock. If urine flow is less than 0.5 ml per kilogram per hour, fluids should be infused at the maximum rate tolerated by the patient. The composition, infusion rate, and total amount of fluid must be tailored to individual cardiovascular capacity. If urine flow is not restored with the pulmonary artery wedge pressure at the upper limits of normal or if the wedge pressure cannot be raised by fluids, a sympathomimetic amine, such as dopamine or dobutamine, should be administered without delay. If excessive quantities of fluid are used, severe pulmonary edema may develop just as the patient is recovering from septic shock. Dopamine is diluted to a concentration of 0.8 to 1.6 mg per milliliter and is given intravenously at an initial rate of 1 to 5 μg per kilogram per minute. At the lowest dose, dopamine acts only on dopaminergic receptors to cause vasodilation in renal, mesenteric, and other peripheral vascular beds. In patients with severe hypotension, the infusion may be started at 5 μg per kilogram per minute and gradually increased by 5 to 10 μg per kilogram per minute up to 20 to 50 μg per kilogram per minute as needed. At higher doses, dopamine acts on β-adrenergic and then α-adrenergic receptors to raise blood pressure. Dobutamine may be preferable in patients with congestive heart failure because it does not increase the pulmonary artery wedge pressure; however, in contrast to dopamine, it does not produce renal vasodilation. Therefore, dopamine is preferable in profound, prolonged shock. If shock is not responsive to dopamine, isoproterenol and then norepinephrine should be tried. If pressors are used for many days, patients may require very slow weaning; continued hypotension does not necessarily imply continuing infection.

The correct choice of antibiotics is crucial to successful treatment of gram-negative bacteremia. When inappropriate drugs are used or the doses are too low, outcome is poor. It is never wise to give a single antibiotic to a patient at the onset of a bacteremic episode, even if the diagnosis and etiology seem certain. Many other infections can mimic gram-negative bacteremia, as discussed. Sometimes more than one bacterial species is involved. In neutropenia, the outcome of *Pseudomonas* bacteremia is much better if more than one effective antibiotic is used. The choice of empiric antibiotics should be made on the basis of the site of the focal infection (or infections) present, the known antimicrobial sensitivities of previous isolates from the patient and of agents of recent nosocomial infections in the hospital, and the patient's underlying diseases. At the present time the best regimen seems to be a combination of an aminoglycoside with a third-generation cephalosporin. An antistaphylococcal drug should be added if *S. aureus* infection is likely. If bowel perforation or infarction has occurred, *Bacteroides fragilis* must be covered. If *Clostridium perfringens* is suspected to be part of a mixed infection, concomitant high-dose penicillin should be used. (*C. perfringens* decolorizes easily in the Gram stain and may be distinguishable from gram-negative rods only by its boxlike rectangular shape.) A common mistake in the use of aminoglycosides is to tailor the initial regimen to the first renal function tests. If azotemia is acute and attributable to poor perfusion, initial low doses will give inadequate levels as soon as hypotension is reversed. Renal toxicity from these drugs rarely occurs early; it is far more important to treat infection effectively in the first 24 hours than to avoid aminoglycoside toxicity.

Gram-negative bacteremia cannot be cured without eradication of the source of bacteremia. In cases of infection associated with ureteral or biliary obstruction, bacteremia and shock may persist in the face of adequate antibiotics until the obstruction is relieved. All likely sites of infection should be cultured, if possible, before antibiotics are given. However, antibiotic treatment should not be delayed for this reason. Wound cultures often remain positive after blood and urine have been sterilized. The physician should not be content until he or she has found a satisfactory explanation for bacteremia. New fever or clinical deterioration can signal a new infection in a susceptible patient, the emergence of resistant bacteria, spread of the original focal infection, inadequate antibiotic levels, or a drug reaction. Such an episode requires complete re-evaluation with physical examination and repeat cultures.

Several modes of adjunctive treatment for endotoxic shock are being evaluated at the present time. High-dose corticosteroids were used empirically for many years because of beneficial effects seen in experimental animal models of septic shock, but two recent large clinical trials have demonstrated no benefit and a possible deleterious effect on resolution of secondary infections. Nonsteroidal anti-inflammatory drugs also are being studied in endotoxic shock. Because endotoxin seems to play a central role in the evolution of gram-negative shock, several groups have raised antibodies to LPS determinants common to most gram-negative bacteria and have found these anti-endotoxin antisera effective in preventing LPS toxicity and bacteremic death in experimental gram-negative infections. A controlled clinical trial of human anti-LPS antiserum to treat established bacteremia showed a lower bacteremic death rate in patients given antiserum than in those given preimmunization control serum; the protective effect extended to patients in profound endotoxic shock. In an extension of this work, two double-blind, placebo-controlled trials of monoclonal antibodies to lipid A in patients with gram-negative sepsis have recently been completed. In one study, a therapeutic effect of a murine monoclonal antibody has been reported in some patients with gram-negative sepsis. In the other study, treatment with a human monoclonal antibody resulted in a 39 per cent decrease in mortality among patients with gram-

negative bacteremia, compared with placebo treatment, and the antibody was effective in patients who were in septic shock. Adjunctive immunotherapy with antiendotoxin monoclonal antibody may soon become part of the standard regimen for treating patients in sepsis who have gram-negative bacteremia.

Bone RC, Fisher CJ Jr, Clemmer TP, et al.: Sepsis syndrome: A valid clinical entity. Crit Care Med 17:389, 1989. *A description of the clinical presentation of patients in sepsis, many of whom have gram-negative bacteremia.*

Fairley KF, Bond AG, Brown RB, et al.: Simple test to determine the site of urinary tract infection. Lancet 1:427, 1967. *A brief description of the details of the Fairley test.*

Hack CE, DeGroote ER, Felt-Bersma RJF, et al.: Increased plasma levels of interleukin 6 in sepsis. Blood 74:1704, 1989. *A good analysis of cytokine dynamics in sepsis.*

Kreger BE, Craven DE, Carling PC, et al.: Gram-negative bacteremia. III. Reassessment of etiology, epidemiology and ecology in 612 patients. Am J Med 68:332, 1980. *A recent classic clinical description of gram-negative bacteremia in an academic hospital setting, with emphasis on the pathogenesis and the influence of the underlying condition on outcome.*

Tracey KJ, Beutler B, Lowry SF, et al.: Shock and tissue injury induced by recombinant human cachetin. Science 234:470, 1986. *An excellent review of tumor necrosis factor and experimental evidence of its role in the shock of gram-negative bacteremia.*

Van Deventer SJH, Buller HR, ten Cate JW, et al.: Endotoxemia: An early predictor of septicemia in febrile patients. Lancet 1:606, 1988. *Use of the Limulus lysate test to show endotoxin in the circulation of septic patients, most of whom had gram-negative bacteremia.*

Ziegler EJ, Fisher CJ Jr, Sprung CL, et al.: Treatment of gram-negative bacteremia and septic shock with HA-1A human monoclonal antibody against endotoxin. N Engl J Med 324:429, 1991. *Description of the randomized, double-blind, placebo-controlled trial of human monoclonal IgM anti–lipid A antibody in gram-negative bacteremia, with a review of previous work.*

321 *Yersinia* Infections

Thomas Butler

PLAGUE

DEFINITION. Plague is a bacterial infection of animals and humans caused by *Yersinia pestis*. The most common clinical form is *acute regional lymphadenitis*, called *bubonic plague*. Less common forms include *septicemic, pneumonic, cutaneous,* and *meningeal plague*. Mortality is high in untreated cases, but antibiotic treatment administered early in the course of the disease markedly reduces fatalities.

HISTORY. *Y. pestis* has caused devastating pandemics with high mortality rates throughout history. The fourth great pandemic in the world is currently under way. The first three are believed to have occurred in the following times: the first originated in Egypt in 542 A.D. and spread to Turkey and Europe. The second started in the 14th century in Asia Minor and Africa; after spreading to Europe the black death killed about a fourth of the continent's people. The third occurred in Europe during the 15th to 18th centuries. The present fourth pandemic began around 1860 in the Chinese province of Yunnan. It spread to the southern coast of China, reaching Hong Kong in 1894. Subsequently plague was carried by ship to India, other countries of Asia, Brazil, and California. An estimated 10 million deaths were caused by this disease in India during this century. The plague bacillus was discovered by Alexandre Yersin in 1894 in Hong Kong and was called *Pasteurella pestis* until 1970. Transmission by flea bites was suggested by Ogata in 1897.

ETIOLOGY. The causative agent, *Y. pestis*, belongs to the family of bacteria Enterobacteriaceae. It is virulent by virtue of plasmid-mediated V and W antigens, which confer calcium dependency and are believed to enable the plague bacillus to proliferate inside mammalian mononuclear phagocytic cells. In the capsular envelope there is an antiphagocytic protein called Fraction 1 antigen. In the cell walls there is a potent lipopolysaccharide endotoxin, which produces fever, disseminated intravascular coagulation, and complement activation. In addition, *Y. pestis* elaborates *murine toxin*, which produces β-adrenergic blockade, but the role of this exotoxin in human disease is unclear.

DISTRIBUTION AND EPIDEMIOLOGY. During 1980 to

1986, 4522 cases of human plague were reported to the World Health Organization. Countries reporting the most cases were Vietnam, Brazil, Peru, Tanzania, Burma, Madagascar, and United States. In the United States, plague is limited almost entirely to the Southwestern states of New Mexico, Arizona, Colorado, Nevada, and California.

Plague is a zoonotic infection that is transmitted among animal reservoirs by flea bites or by ingestion of contaminated animal tissues. Throughout the world domestic and urban rats are the most important reservoirs. In sylvatic foci of plague, however, as occur in the United States, reservoirs are the ground squirrel, rock squirrel, and prairie dog. Humans are an accidental host in the natural cycle of plague, when rodent fleas bite people, and appear to play no role in the maintenance of plague in nature. Only rarely, during epidemics of pneumonic plague, is the infection passed directly from person to person. Occasionally, the infection develops in humans by the direct handling of contaminated animal tissues, as when hunters skin dead rabbits.

The incidence of plague in humans for any particular locality is a function of both the frequency of infection in local rodent populations and the intimacy with which the people live with the infected rodents and their fleas. In the United States, the season for plague is April to September, when people are out of doors. Off-season cases often involve hunters who handle their prey.

PATHOGENESIS AND CLINICAL FEATURES. The most common clinical form is bubonic plague, which presents a distinctive clinical picture (Table 321–1). During an incubation period of 2 to 8 days following a bite by an infected flea, bacteria proliferate in the regional lymph nodes. Patients are typically affected by the sudden onset of fever, chills, weakness, and headache. Usually at the same time, or after a few hours or the next day, patients notice the *bubo*, which is signaled by intense pain in one anatomic region of lymph nodes, usually the groin, axilla, or neck. A swelling evolves that is so tender that the patient typically avoids any motion that would provoke tenderness of the affected nodes. The bubo contains acute inflammatory cells, a high density of bacteria, and hemorrhagic necrosis.

The buboes of patients with plague are oval swellings varying from about 1 to 10 cm in length and elevating the overlying skin, which may appear stretched or erythematous. They appear either as a smooth, uniform, egg-shaped mass or as an irregular cluster of several nodes. There is warmth of the overlying skin and an underlying, firm, tender, nonfluctuant mass. Usually around the lymph nodes there is considerable edema, which can be gelatinous or pitting in nature. Occasionally, edema extends into the skin region drained by the affected lymph nodes. Although infections other than plague can produce acute lymphadenitis, plague is unique for the suddenness of onset of the fever and the bubo, the rapid development of intense inflammation in the bubo, and the fulminant clinical course that can produce death as quickly as 2 to 4 days after the onset of symptoms. The bubo of plague is also distinctive for the usual absence of a detectable skin lesion and likewise for the absence of an ascending lymphangitis nearby.

In uncomplicated *bubonic plague*, the patients are typically prostrate and lethargic and often exhibit restlessness or agitation. Occasionally, they are delirious with high fever, and seizures are common in children. Temperature is usually in the range of 38.5 to 40.0°C, and the pulse rate is increased. Blood pressure is characteristically low, in the range of 100/60 mm Hg. Pressure determinations may be unobtainable if shock ensues. The liver and spleen are often palpable and tender. Abdominal pain, vomiting, and diarrhea are common.

The majority of patients with bubonic plague do not have skin

TABLE 321–1. PLAGUE SYNDROMES

Syndrome	Features
Bubonic	Fever, painful lymphadenopathy (bubo)
Septicemic	Fever, hypotension without bubo
Pneumonic	Cough, hemoptysis with or without bubo
Cutaneous	Pustule, eschar, carbuncle, or ecthyma gangrenosum usually with bubo
Meningitis	Fever, nuchal rigidity usually with bubo

lesions. About a fourth of patients in Vietnam, however, did show pustules, vesicles, eschars, or papules near the bubo or in the anatomic region of skin that is lymphatically drained by the affected lymph nodes. These presumably represent sites of flea bite inoculations. When these lesions are opened, they usually contain white cells and plague bacilli. These skin lesions rarely progress to extensive cellulitis or abscesses. Ulceration may lead, however, to a larger plague carbuncle. Another kind of skin lesion in plague is purpura, which may become necrotic, resulting in gangrene of distal extremities that is the probable basis of the term "black death." These purpuric lesions result from vasculitis and thrombosis.

A distinctive feature of plague is the propensity for massive growth of bacteria in the blood. In the early acute stages of bubonic plague, all patients probably have intermittent bacteremia. Single blood cultures obtained at the time of hospital admission from Vietnamese patients were positive in 27 per cent of cases. A hallmark of moribund patients with plague is high-density bacteremia, so that a blood smear revealing characteristic bacilli has been used as a prognostic indicator in this disease. Occasionally in the pathogenesis of plague infection, bacteria are inoculated and proliferate in the body, producing bacteremia without a bubo. This syndrome has been termed *septicemic plague*.

One of the feared complications of bubonic plague is secondary pneumonia. The infection reaches the lungs by hematogenous spread from the bubo. In addition to the high mortality, plague pneumonia is highly contagious by airborne transmission. It is characterized by fever and lymphadenopathy with cough, chest pain, and often hemoptysis. Radiographically, there is patchy bronchopneumonia or confluent consolidation. The sputum is usually purulent and contains plague bacilli. *Primary inhalation pneumonia* is rare now but is a potential threat to the individual exposed to a patient with plague who has a cough.

Plague meningitis is a rarer complication and typically occurs more than a week after inadequately treated bubonic plague. Less commonly, plague meningitis appears as a primary infection without antecedent lymphadenitis. Bacteria are frequently demonstrable with a Gram stain of spinal fluid sediment.

LABORATORY FEATURES. The white blood cell count is typically elevated in the range of 10,000 to 20,000 cells per cubic millimeter, with a predominance of immature and mature neutrophils. Blood platelet counts may be normal or low in the early stages of bubonic plague. Although a generalized bleeding tendency from profound thrombocytopenia is rare, disseminated intravascular coagulation (DIC) is common. Fibrinogen-fibrin degradation products in the serum that are indicative of DIC were detected in elevated titers in most patients tested in Vietnam.

DIAGNOSIS. Plague should be suspected in febrile patients who have been in known endemic areas. A bacteriologic diagnosis is readily made in most patients by smear and culture of a bubo aspirate. The aspirate is obtained by inserting a 20-gauge needle on a 10-ml syringe containing 1 ml of sterile saline solution into the bubo and aspirating several times until the saline solution has become blood tinged. It may be necessary to inject some of the saline solution and to reaspirate it immediately. Drops of the aspirate should be placed on microscope slides. The Gram stain reveals polymorphonuclear leukocytes and gram-negative coccobacilli and bacilli. Smears of blood, sputum, or spinal fluid can be handled similarly.

The aspirate, blood, and other appropriate fluids should be inoculated onto blood and MacConkey's agar plates and into infusion broth. For definitive identification, cultures can be mailed in double containers to the Centers for Disease Control, Plague Branch, P.O. Box 2087, Fort Collins, Colorado 80422 (telephone no.: 303–221–6450). At this same laboratory, a serologic test, the passive hemagglutination test utilizing Fraction 1 of *Y. pestis*, can be performed on acute and convalescent phase serum. For patients with negative cultures, a fourfold or greater increase in titer or a single titer of greater than or equal to 1:16 is presumptive evidence for plague infection.

The differential diagnosis of bubonic plague includes tularemia, streptococcal and staphylococcal lymphadenitis, secondary syphilis, and lymphogranuloma venereum. For pneumonia, the physician should also consider common forms of bacterial and viral pneumonia. For meningitis and septicemia, the common bacterial causes need to be assessed by age groups.

TREATMENT AND PROGNOSIS. Untreated plague has an estimated mortality of greater than 50 per cent. Therefore, the early institution of effective antibiotic therapy is mandatory. In 1948, streptomycin was identified as the drug of choice for the treatment of plague by reducing mortality to less than 5 per cent. No other drug has been demonstrated to be more efficacious or less toxic. Streptomycin should be administered intramuscularly in two divided doses daily, totaling 30 mg per kilogram of body weight per day for 10 days. Most patients improve rapidly and become afebrile in about 3 days. If the serum creatinine concentration rises significantly, the dose of streptomycin should be reduced. In mild renal failure, the recommended dose is about 20 mg per kilogram per day and in advanced renal failure, 8 mg per kilogram every 3 days.

For patients allergic to streptomycin or for whom an oral drug is strongly preferred, tetracycline is a satisfactory alternative. It is administered orally in a dose of 2 to 4 grams per day in four divided doses for 10 days. For patients with meningitis who require a drug that penetrates the cerebrospinal fluid effectively and for patients with profound hypotension in whom an intramuscular injection may not be well absorbed, chloramphenicol should be administered intravenously with a loading dose of 25 mg per kilogram of body weight followed by 60 mg per kilogram per day in four divided doses. After clinical improvement, oral chloramphenicol administration should be continued to complete a total course of 10 days; the dosage may be reduced to 30 mg per kilogram per day to reduce the magnitude of bone marrow suppression. The three antibiotics streptomycin, tetracycline, and chloramphenicol given alone are clinically very effective, and relapses are exceedingly rare. Therefore, there is no rationale for using multiple antibiotics to treat plague.

Because patients are febrile and often have nausea or vomiting, hypotension, and dehydration, intravenous 0.9 per cent saline solution should be given to most patients for the first few days of the illness or until improvement occurs. Patients in shock require additional quantities of fluid, with hemodynamic monitoring.

The buboes usually recede without need of local therapy. Occasionally, however, they may enlarge or become fluctuant during the first week of treatment and require incision and drainage. The aspirated fluid should be cultured for evidence of superinfection, but this material is usually sterile.

PREVENTION. All patients with suspected plague should be reported to the local health department. Those with cough or other signs of pneumonia must be placed in strict respiratory isolation for at least 48 hours after the start of antibiotic therapy or until the sputum culture is negative. The bubo aspirate and blood must be handled with gloves. Standard bacteriologic techniques that safeguard against skin contact with and aerosolization of infected fluids and cultures should be adequate to protect laboratory personnel.

Persons living in endemic areas should protect themselves against rodents and fleas. Measures include living in ratproof houses, reducing opportunities for rodent harborage near homes, wearing shoes and garments to cover the legs, and application of insecticide dusts to houses and household pets. A formalin-killed vaccine, plague vaccine U.S.P. (Cutter Laboratories, Berkeley, California 94710) is available for travelers to epidemic areas, for individuals who must live and work in close contact with wild rodents, and for laboratory workers who must handle live *Y. pestis* cultures. A primary series of two injections is recommended, with a 1- to 3-month interval between them. Booster injections are given every 6 months for as long as exposure continues.

Butler T: Plague and other *Yersinia* infections. New York, Plenum Publishing, 1983. *This monograph gives full clinical description and contemporary literature citations.*

Hull HF, Montes JM, Mann JM: Septicemic plague in New Mexico. J Infect Dis 155:113, 1987. *One fourth of 71 recent cases of plague in New Mexico were septicemic without a bubo. To prevent the observed 33 per cent mortality rate, earlier empiric antibiotic treatment is advised.*

Welty TK, Grabman J, Kompare E, et al.: Nineteen cases of plague in Arizona. West J Med 142:641, 1985. *This paper describes clinical features of recent cases in Arizona.*

OTHER *YERSINIA* INFECTIONS

DEFINITION. The nonplague yersinioses are caused by *Yersinia enterocolitica* and *Y. pseudotuberculosis*. These gram-negative rod bacteria produce fever, diarrhea, and abdominal pain that can mimic acute appendicitis. The common pathologic lesions in yersiniosis are acute enteritis and mesenteric lymphadenitis. Extraintestinal disease may result from septicemia or may appear as arthritis and erythema nodosum.

ETIOLOGY. Of the 34 different O serotypes of *Y. enterocolitica* that have been identified, the ones most commonly associated with human disease are types 3, 8, and 9. All virulent strains possess a plasmid that encodes the V and W antigens, which confer calcium dependency on the bacteria. Like other gram-negative bacteria, the yersiniae contain a lipopolysaccharide endotoxin in the cell wall that may be responsible, in part, for the fever and inflammation.

EPIDEMIOLOGY. The yersinioses are distributed worldwide. Large numbers of confirmed cases have been reported in Europe, Canada, the United States, and Japan. In the United States, infection with *Y. enterocolitica* appears to be rare when compared with infection with *Salmonella* and *Shigella* species. Both adults and children are susceptible to infection. Males acquire the infection more commonly than do females. The natural reservoirs of *Y. enterocolitica* are farm animals, especially pigs and goats, and other domestic animals, including dogs and cats. The natural reservoirs of *Y. pseudotuberculosis* include birds and other diverse domestic and farm animals. These animals harbor the bacteria in their intestines and excrete them in feces. Humans become infected by ingesting food or water contaminated by animal feces or directly by the ingestion of certain fomites. Person-to-person transmission seems to be rare. Blood transfusion has transmitted infections. Well-defined outbreaks of *Y. enterocolitica* infection have occurred in children in Georgia whose caregivers handled raw pork intestines, in a New York school at which chocolate milk was the source of infection, in members of a Brownie scout troop in Pennsylvania who ate infected bean sprouts, and in persons who drank milk from a dairy in Tennessee. There are no clear seasonal patterns of infection.

PATHOGENESIS OF CLINICAL SYNDROMES. An inoculum with as many as 10^9 organisms may be required to produce infection. During the incubation period, estimated at 4 to 10 days, bacteria proliferate in the small bowel; invade the mucosa, especially that of the ileum; and elicit an acute inflammatory response. Ulcerations may occur, and polymorphonuclear leukocytes appear in the stool. Some bacteria migrate via the lymphatics to the mesenteric lymph nodes, where inflammation occurs. The initial symptoms include fever and either diarrhea or abdominal pain. In these instances, the corresponding pathologic finding is terminal ileitis or mesenteric lymphadenitis or both. The colon is less frequently affected, but aphthoid ulcers and hemorrhagic colitis have been described in yersiniosis. The tissues are affected by acute inflammation, thrombosis of blood vessels, hemorrhage, and necrosis. The diarrhea results from the mucosal invasion by bacteria or the action of an enterotoxin. Diarrhea varies from semisolid or watery to grossly bloody. In some patients the abdominal pain is severe and located in the right lower quadrant and may be mistaken for appendicitis; the appendix is usually normal. A few days later, some patients may develop extraintestinal complications of arthralgias, arthritis, and erythema nodosum. Synovial fluid contains bacterial antigen, and an immunologic reaction has been postulated to explain the pathogenesis of these complications. Arthritis, including sacroileitis, is more likely to occur in individuals of haplotype HLA-B27, and erythema nodosum occurs more commonly in women. Septicemia is a rare complication that occurs in the setting of prior liver disease, malignancies, immunosuppressive therapy, or after blood transfusion. Rarer clinical forms of yersiniosis include pneumonia, pharyngitis, and meningitis. Antibodies appear in the blood against the O and other antigens of *Y. enterocolitica*, and nearly all infections are self-limited. However, fatalities have occurred from extensive ulceration and necrosis of the intestine and septicemia.

DIAGNOSIS. The diagnosis requires the isolation of yersiniae from stool, blood, or surgical specimens. The number of bacteria in stool may be small, and a cold-enrichment technique has been used. A rectal swab or piece of stool is placed into 0.067M phosphate-buffered saline solution at a pH of 7.6 and incubated at 4°C for 4 weeks. Most other stool bacteria die, whereas *Y.*

enterocolitica grows. At weekly intervals, subcultures should be made on MacConkey's agar. A presumptive diagnosis can be made from serologic test results by showing a rise in agglutinin titer in paired serum specimens. The existence of cross-reacting antigens in the genera *Brucella*, *Vibrio*, and *Salmonella* indicates that false-positive serologic results sometimes occur.

TREATMENT AND PROGNOSIS. Yersiniosis is usually self-limited and so rarely diagnosed that it is impossible to assess the possible benefits of antibiotic treatment. Most isolates of Y. *enterocolitica* are susceptible to streptomycin, gentamicin, tetracycline, chloramphenicol, and sulfamethoxazole-trimethoprim and resistant to the penicillins and cephalosporin antibiotics. Y. *pseudotuberculosis* isolates usually have been susceptible to penicillin. It is important to suspect the diagnosis in patients with severe abdominal pain to avoid unnecessary surgery for appendicitis. The recognition that early fever accompanies yersiniosis may be helpful, as is epidemiologic information pertaining to outbreaks in the community.

PREVENTION AND CONTROL. The presumed origin of Y. *enterocolitica* infection in farm and domestic animals suggests that transmission may be similar to that of *Salmonella*. Meat and dairy products and other farm produce should periodically be examined for Y. *enterocolitica* content. During outbreaks, public health authorities should identify sources of infection in food (especially milk and pork), water, or persons.

Cover TL, Aber RC: *Yersinia enterocolitica*. N Engl J Med 321:16, 1989. *This comprehensive review covers epidemiology, clinical features, diagnosis, and treatment and has 201 references.*

Lee LA, Taylor J, Carter GP, et al.: *Yersinia enterocolitica* 0:3: An emerging cause of pediatric gastroenteritis. J Infect Dis 163:660, 1991. *Outbreaks of diarrhea are being recognized, and some involve black children whose caregivers are exposed to raw pork intestines during holiday seasons.*

Tertti R, Vuento R, Mikkola P, et al.: Clinical manifestations of *Yersinia pseudotuberculosis* infection in children. Eur J Clin Microbiol Infect Dis 8:587, 1989. *In an outbreak affecting 34 Finnish school children, fever and abdominal pain led to unnecessary laparotomies in 3 cases.*

322 Tularemia

Richard B. Hornick

DEFINITION. Tularemia is a rare infectious disease caused by a small gram-negative pleomorphic rod, *Francisella tularensis*. This organism is acquired from an animal reservoir, frequently cottontail rabbits, by direct contact with diseased animal tissues, the bite of an infected tick or deer fly, ingestion of contaminated food or water, and inhalation of aerosolized bacteria. Clinical manifestations usually include a cutaneous ulcer with enlargement of regional lymph nodes. Rarely, a pneumonitis results from inhalation of *F. tularensis* or secondary spread from the skin ulcer and lymph nodes. Confirmation of the diagnosis by cultural technique is not advocated because of the high contagion risk to personnel handling this organism. The therapeutic response to effective antibiotic therapy is rapid.

The typhoidal form of tularemia was first described in Japan in 1818. A clear description of the organism occurred in 1906 when McCoy uncovered a "plaguelike" disease among ground squirrels in Tulare County, California. In Japan, tularemia may be referred to as Ohara's disease or Yato-byo (wild hare disease).

ETIOLOGY, SPECIFIC LABORATORY DIAGNOSIS, AND EPIDEMIOLOGY. *F. tularensis* is a small gram-negative pleomorphic rod-shaped bacterium. Organisms are not seen in smears of infected tissue unless special staining techniques are used. Fluorescent antibody conjugate staining and modified Dieterle staining are the best methods for demonstrating them. All tularemia strains are serologically identical, but there are biochemical and virulence differences for mammals that have allowed differentiation of two strains. These are called Jellison A and B; the former, found only in North America, is lethal for domestic rabbits (*Oryctolagus*) and causes severe disease in humans. The unique biochemical capabilities of this strain—e.g., it ferments

glycerol and contains citrulline ureidase—do not explain its increased virulence. Strain B lacks these biochemical features, is not lethal for cottontails, causes milder disease in humans, usually is isolated from rodents or from water, and is distributed over Europe, Asia, and North America. Reasons for the differences in virulence are unknown.

Culture Methods. The direct isolation of *F. tularensis* from blood (rarely), pus from ulcers or buboes, sputum, or pharyngeal or gastric aspirations in a patient with pneumonitis can be achieved by two methods. This is a class 4 organism requiring an effective hood or an adequate isolation laboratory to prevent human disease or epizootics. The two methods for isolation are intraperitoneal inoculation of guinea pigs and direct plating of a specimen onto glucose cysteine blood agar, cystine heart agar, or eugon agar. As few as one to five viable organisms will cause the death of guinea pigs in 5 to 10 days. Appropriate facilities are needed to prevent spread of the disease to other animals. The media employed to isolate the organism usually contain drugs to suppress other flora and allow the tularemia colonies to be visible. Useful additions are 0.1 mg of cycloheximide and 20 units of penicillin per milliliter of media. The colonies are small on these media; they appear in 48 to 72 hours of incubation at 37°C.

Serologic Diagnosis. The measurement of serum agglutinating antibodies is a useful and safer method of diagnosing tularemia. Titers begin to rise in about 7 to 10 days and peak in 3 to 4 weeks. Paired serum specimens obtained 2 weeks apart and demonstrating a fourfold or greater rise are diagnostic of tularemia. However, a single specimen with a titer of 1:160 or greater in a patient thought to have tularemia on clinical grounds is diagnostic. Antibiotic therapy does not appear to dampen the antibody response. Titers remain elevated for 6 to 8 months and then decline in the subsequent 1 to 1.5 years to low or undetectable levels. There is a cross-reaction with brucella antigen during the early phase of the antibody response. The brucella titer falls off faster than and is never so high as the tularemia titer.

Skin Testing. A skin test antigen has proved to be reliable for diagnostic and epidemiologic purposes. A positive test result, similar in appearance to a tuberculin test response, is present during the first week of illness, frequently before the agglutinins are detectable, and remains positive for years. There is no known cross-reacting skin test antigen. The antigen is derived from *F. tularensis* by ether extraction; however, it is not commonly available. It can be obtained from the Centers for Disease Control, Atlanta. In 10 per cent of patients, the skin test antigen may boost pre-existing agglutinating antibody titers. Skin test reactivity can be shown to be associated with sensitized lymphocytes.

Epidemiology. Tularemia is a sporadic disease; humans acquire it when bitten by an infected tick or deer fly or when handling an infected animal. In the process of dressing a rabbit or skinning a muskrat, the hands may become contaminated with infected blood, subcutaneous abscesses, or liver and spleen that contain millions of organisms. The act of eviscerating the animal can create an aerosol that can be inhaled. The ingestion of contaminated water or food is the least likely method of acquiring tularemia. Many carnivores such as dogs, cats, bull snakes, and others may feed on diseased rabbits. This results in contamination of the teeth and saliva. These animals are relatively resistant to tularemia. Contact with the teeth of a pet dog or cat has resulted in ulceroglandular tularemia. Studies in volunteers have quantified the susceptibility of humans to infection and disease and the virulence of *F. tularensis* for humans. As few as 50 type A organisms injected subcutaneously cause ulceroglandular disease. Pneumonic tularemia can be induced by a similar inoculum size if the aerosolized and inhaled particles are small (less than 5 μm). Type B organisms require an inoculum about 1000 times larger to induce ulceroglandular or respiratory disease in humans.

The incidence of tularemia is low, 150 to 300 cases a year having been reported in each of the past 20 years. The peak incidence was in 1939, when almost 2300 cases were reported. Laws passed at that time prohibited the sale of wild rabbits, especially cottontails, and this legislation plus increased public awareness of the danger of handling sick or dying wild animals has contributed to the decline. Most cases occur in the Midwest, but the disease is not restricted to any one geographic location in the United States. Cottontail rabbits in urban and suburban areas throughout the country provide the reservoir from which tularemia can occur. Epizootics among these or other animals can cause epidemics in humans. Tularemia has been reported only north of the 30th parallel. The cottontail rabbit is not found in Europe; various rodents such as voles, muskrats, and hares carry *F. tularensis* (Jellison B type) in that part of the world. Diseased jackrabbits, found west of the Mississippi River, may be an important source of contamination of ticks and deer flies.

In the summer months, most cases of tularemia are caused by tick or deer fly bites. Ulceroglandular disease begins with an ulcer at the site of the bite, e.g., groin, axilla, or scalp. In the fall, during hunting season, sporadic cases, usually ulceroglandular, occur among hunters and trappers. In the Scandinavian countries, epidemics have occurred in the winter months when farmers handling stored hay contaminated by diseased voles inhaled *F. tularensis* and developed pneumonic tularemia.

MECHANISMS OF INFECTION AND PATHOLOGY. The most common form of tularemia results from the penetration of *F. tularensis* into the skin. This penetration may be through hair follicles or minute areas of trauma. The development of the subsequent disease takes 2 to 6 days, depending upon the number of bacteria and their virulence. The organisms multiply in the dermis and induce a marked inflammatory process consisting primarily of mononuclear cells with a perivascular distribution. This process produces an erythematous tender papule. The inflamed area continues to swell until the induced ischemia causes the skin to ulcerate. The base of the ulcer becomes black and depressed. The edges are sharply demarcated. At the time of penetration, some organisms may be phagocytized and transported in the lymph to regional nodes. There is no clinically apparent lymphangitis. The nodes enlarge and become painful when caseation occurs. Histologic sections reveal geographic necrosis and disruption of the capsule. Fluctuation of the node is a late and rare event. It may then rupture. The necrotic, purulent, painful lymph node is termed a bubo. Healing of a bubo takes months even with appropriate antibiotic treatment. Aspiration of an unruptured node may lead to an indolent draining sinus tract. *F. tularensis* may remain in the necrotic tissue and purulent drainage for many weeks. The ulcer heals slowly and usually leaves a depigmented, rounded area in the skin.

Oculoglandular tularemia may occur when the conjunctival sac is infected from an ulcer or contaminated finger. Small yellowish granulomatous lesions develop on the palpebral conjunctivae, accompanied by enlargement of the preauricular lymph nodes. In untreated patients the cornea may perforate.

Inhaled small particle aerosols (<5 μm in diameter) containing *F. tularensis* (usually type A) are ultimately deposited in the terminal bronchioles and alveoli, although infection of the trachea and large bronchi also occurs. A peribronchial inflammation develops, with infiltration by neutrophils and mononuclear cells. This produces necrosis of alveolar walls and results in localized pneumonitis. In humans, small areas of pneumonitis represent the most common findings on chest roentgenograms. Often these are ill defined and difficult to interpret. Lobar consolidation or lung abscesses represent extensive spread and necrosis. These are infrequent in humans. Mediastinal and peritracheal lymph nodes enlarge and may be apparent on chest x-ray films. They may be partially responsible, along with the bronchitis, for the substernal burning that is common in patients with tularemic pneumonia. The incubation period for this form of tularemia varies inversely with the size and virulence of the inhaled inoculum. Following an inoculum of 10 to 50 organisms, disease appears in about 4 to 7 days in volunteers.

Typhoidal tularemia follows systemic spread of *F. tularensis* from the oropharynx and probably the gastrointestinal tract when a huge inoculum is swallowed. Enlargement of cervical lymph nodes, and presumably nodes in the mesentery, occurs. This latter process causes abdominal pain and is associated with an ileus. This is the most unusual form of tularemia in this country.

CLINICAL MANIFESTATIONS. Disease initiated by a tick bite is manifested by an ulcer at the site or adjacent to it. The tick defecates after feeding, and the infected feces may be scratched into the epidermis. Usually the lesion is in the inguinal, axillary, or scalp skin. If contact with tularemia organisms results from the handling of an infected animal, an ulcerative lesion evolves in the skin of the hands, frequently around a fingernail. This lesion may be so trivial that it is ignored by the patient.

The ulcer is depressed into the dermis, has sharply demarcated edges, and gradually develops a black base. In the initial stage of development the lesion produces a thick, yellowish exudate. Regional lymph nodes enlarge and are tender to palpation. Fever and chills are common. The temperature curve is usually remittent or continuous in character. Without antibiotic therapy, most patients remain febrile for several weeks, the ulcer heals slowly over weeks to months, and the enlarged lymph nodes persist for months. Untreated patients may occasionally develop a secondary necrotizing pneumonia as a consequence of bacteremia. These patients may be acutely ill.

Primary tularemia pneumonia presents with the sudden development of substernal burning and a nonproductive paroxysmal cough associated with fever and chills. Headache, myalgia, photophobia, malaise, and prostration are common findings. The temperature elevates quickly to 39.4 to 40°C and remains at that level (continuous fever curve) until antibiotic treatment is given. Sixty to 70 per cent of patients survive without specific therapy, and in these a slow defervescence occurs over several months. Radiographs of the lungs may reveal ill-defined, scattered oval areas of infiltration, with enlarged peritracheal lymph nodes. Pleural effusions, lobar consolidation, and lung abscess are other manifestations of this form of tularemia. Cervical lymph nodes are palpable and tender.

DIAGNOSIS AND DIFFERENTIAL DIAGNOSIS. The diagnosis of ulceroglandular tularemia is made on the basis of the clinical manifestations and serologic studies. Paired serum specimens collected over a 2- to 3-week period are required to demonstrate a fourfold rise in titer. A baseline agglutinin titer of 1:160 in a patient with a history of an indolent ulcer for 2 or more weeks is diagnostic of tularemia. Culture of an ulcer and blood should be performed only if the hospital laboratory has appropriate protective isolation hoods. Patients with sporotrichosis or *Mycobacterium marinum* infections may have ulcers suggestive of tularemia but are usually afebrile. Enlarged lymph nodes extending centripetally as a beaded chain are a characteristic finding in sporotrichosis. Lesions of the fingers infected with staphylococci or β streptococci usually produce more pus and may be associated with lymphangitis. *Bacillus anthracis* can produce an ulcer (anthrax) with black-based, sharply demarcated edges similar to that initiated by *F. tularensis*. A careful history and serologic data help in the differential diagnosis. In patients in whom any form of tularemia is suspected, the use of the skin test antigen is helpful. The test result is usually positive prior to the development of agglutinating antibodies.

Tularemia pneumonia must be differentiated from the more common bacterial, viral, and mycoplasmal pneumonias. The history and the presence of ulceroglandular disease are helpful. Skin testing and serologic studies are diagnostic. The chest radiographs may yield suggestive findings consisting of ill-defined, small, oval, multiple infiltrates but is not diagnostic.

Patients infected with *F. tularensis* usually have a normal leukocyte count with an elevation of the sedimentation rate. The white count is elevated when a bubo or a lung abscess is present.

COMPLICATIONS. Pericarditis and meningitis are rare events that usually occur in patients who have been misdiagnosed and have received inappropriate treatment. Pericarditis results from direct extension of the infection from the purulent, necrotic mediastinal lymph nodes or the involved lung. Constrictive pericarditis has been reported. Meningitis develops rarely, represents a seeding of the meninges during bacteremia, and is characterized by a lymphocytic pleocytosis in the cerebrospinal fluid.

TREATMENT. Patients with all forms of tularemia respond to the following antibiotics: streptomycin, gentamicin, tetracycline, and chloramphenicol. The aminoglycoside antibiotics are recommended, since they produce a prompt cure of patients with the most severe form of tularemia. Patients with pneumonitis are afebrile within 24 to 48 hours and do not relapse. Ulcers and tender lymph nodes heal in 7 to 10 days. Gentamicin, 5 mg per kilogram per day in divided doses, is given for 10 days. Streptomycin was the principal drug for treating tularemia before gentamicin; 1 gram is given every 12 hours for 10 days. Treatment with tetracycline or chloramphenicol may produce an equally rapid response, but relapses occur in 15 to 20 per cent of the patients. These drugs are not recommended unless gentamicin and streptomycin are contraindicated. Doses of 3 to 4 grams of tetracycline or 3 grams of chloramphenicol daily for 10 days can be employed. Naturally acquired resistance to any of these antibiotics has not been found.

Patients with ulceroglandular tularemia respond well to these antibiotics. Fluctuant lymph nodes should not be aspirated until the patient has finished the course of the antibiotic treatment. Isolation of patients with any form of tularemia is not required; there is no evidence of person-to-person spread.

PROGNOSIS. The mortality for untreated ulceroglandular disease is about 5 per cent. Patients infected with type B strains and untreated probably have a mortality less than 1 per cent. Many of these patients probably go undiagnosed, as the disease is mild and self-limiting. Treatment with antibiotics prevents death and promotes healing in a week to 10 days.

The mortality for pneumonic tularemia in the preantibiotic period was 30 to 40 per cent. Treatment with streptomycin or tetracycline has lowered this figure to less than 1 per cent. Healing occurs without residual lung damage or deficits in pulmonary function.

PREVENTION. Patients who recover from tularemia have a high degree of resistance to reinfection. If *F. tularensis* is reintroduced into the skin, a positive skin test reaction ensues without ulceration. Resistance to pulmonary disease may be associated with sensitized lymphocytes and alveolar macrophages.

A live attenuated strain of *F. tularensis* has been prepared as a vaccine. This can be administered by the acupuncture route, and it produces excellent immunity. The vaccine can be obtained from the Commander, U.S. Army Medical Research Institute of Infectious Diseases, Frederick, Maryland 21701. Its use is limited to persons considered at high risk, such as selected laboratory workers, forest rangers, game wardens, and perhaps others known to be exposed during an outbreak. The vaccine exerts its effect through the stimulation of cellular immune mechanisms. Circulating agglutinins are not associated with resistance to disease.

Buchanan TM, Brooks GF, Brachman PS: The tularemia skin test; 325 skin tests in 210 persons: Serologic correlation and review of the literature. Ann Intern Med 74:336, 1971. *This study is an extension of the study reported by Young et al. (see below). It clearly presents proof of the efficacy of the skin test as a diagnostic test for tularemia. In addition, it shows the amount of antigen stimulation needed to cause a conversion to a positive reactor.*

Evans ME, Gregory DW, Schaffner W, et al.: Tularemia: A 30-year experience with 88 cases. Medicine 64:251, 1985. *An excellent summary of the clinical presentations of* F. tularensis *disease.*

Penn RL, Kinasewitz GT: Factors associated with a poor outcome in tularemia. Arch Intern Med 147:265, 1987. *A retrospective study of the factors leading to poor outcomes. One significant factor was delay in diagnosis and treatment.*

Young LS, Bicknell DS, Archer BG, et al.: Tularemia epidemic: Vermont, 1968. Forty-seven cases linked to contact with muskrats. N Engl J Med 280:1253, 1969. *This represents one of the largest outbreaks occurring in the United States in the past 20 years. It is one of the best described epidemiologic studies of infection caused by the Jellison type B organism.*

323 Anthrax

Jonas A. Shulman

DEFINITION. Anthrax is a zoonotic disease caused by *Bacillus anthracis*, a large gram-positive, spore-forming bacillus that is transmitted to humans by contact with infected animals or contaminated animal products. Other names for anthrax include woolsorter's disease, Siberian ulcer, malignant pustule, charbon, malignant edema, and ragsorter's disease. In 1877, Koch described *B. anthracis* as one of the first microbes identified as a cause of a specific disease, thereby making anthrax the prototype for Koch's postulates and the first disease to satisfy them. Anthrax has all but disappeared from North America, Western Europe, and Australia since being nearly eradicated in livestock following extensive veterinary programs, including vaccination. The disease is still prevalent in many developing countries, however, especially Asia, Africa, and Central America, where livestock are only marginally subjected to veterinary control and where environmental conditions are favorable for an animal-to-soil-to-animal cycle.

Anthrax occurs primarily in herbivorous animals, especially cattle, goats, and sheep, but many other animals, including pigs, buffalo, and elephants, have also been infected with the disease. Cattle are particularly susceptible to the systemic form of anthrax and clinically progress to death in 24 to 48 hours. The large numbers of organisms found in infected cattle may contaminate not only the animal but also its products and environs, thereby allowing infection to occur in animals more resistant to anthrax, such as humans.

The primary forms of anthrax in humans are cutaneous, inhalation, gastrointestinal, and oropharyngeal. Septicemia and meningitis may occur from any of these primary foci. By far, the most common form of the disease in the United States is the cutaneous lesion, which accounts for more than 95 per cent of clinical cases. Inhalation anthrax has occurred only rarely in the United States in the past 25 years, and gastrointestinal anthrax has never been reported in this country.

ETIOLOGY. *Bacillus anthracis* is a large gram-positive, nonmotile, spore-forming bacillus (1 to 1.3 × 3 to 8 μm). Although spores of *B. anthracis* do not form in living tissue, they are induced by aerobic conditions in the external environment and may persist for years in the soil, in animal products, or in an appropriate industrial setting. The organism grows well aerobically on ordinary laboratory media at 35° to 37°C. The colonies produced are especially sticky (positive tenacity test, positive string of pearls test) and have a tendency to stand up in stalagmite fashion when lifted with a bacteriologic loop. The colonies are nonhemolytic, rough, and flat, with many comma-shaped outgrowths on blood agar. Microscopic examination of organisms growing on artificial media shows long, parallel chains of organisms frequently described as having a rather characteristic "boxcar" appearance. Spores are oval and occur either centrally or paracentrally but cause no swelling of the bacillus. Material from fresh lesions reveals single or short chains of two or three bacilli, which may appear encapsulated, the ends of which are slightly rounded.

Anthrax organisms can be differentiated from the saprophytic *Bacillus* species by fluorescent antibody staining, lysis with a specific γ bacteriophage, and virulence for mice, guinea pigs, and rabbits. Parenteral inoculation into these species results in death in 1 to 3 days.

INCIDENCE AND PREVALENCE. *Bacillus anthracis* is a soil organism that has a worldwide distribution. Animal anthrax is endemic in some areas of Asia, Africa, and Latin America, especially in the less socioeconomically developed regions that have inadequate animal vaccination programs and poor animal husbandry. These countries are more likely to have a number of human cases as well. Certain areas within the United States and other parts of the world may provide a particularly favorable environment for large numbers of resistant spores to survive in the soil for many years. In fact, a number of epizootics related to focal regions of heavily contaminated soil have occurred.

Since no reliable reporting of anthrax exists, and in many instances the diagnosis may never be made, the actual worldwide incidence of anthrax is not known. Estimates in the past have ranged between 20,000 and 100,000 human cases per year, but these figures have more recently been estimated at 2000 to 20,000 cases per annum. In the United States, approximately one case of human anthrax per year was reported between 1970 and 1985, but only two cases have been documented since 1984. Reports of human anthrax have been especially frequent in areas of the world such as Turkey, Pakistan, Iran, Haiti, and several Asian and African countries. There are probably many parts of the world with significant endemic problems but from which data are not available.

The potential for large outbreaks in animals and humans continues to exist, especially when economic or political upheaval is present. One of the largest epidemics of anthrax was reported in Zimbabwe between 1978 and 1980, when nearly 10,000 human cases of cutaneous anthrax and a few cases of gastrointestinal anthrax occurred, resulting in approximately 100 deaths. This outbreak was related to an extensive epizootic infection in cattle. Another major outbreak of anthrax occurred in Siberia in 1979. It was initially thought by some to be related to inhalation, but more recently the route of infection has been identified as the ingestion and handling of infected "black market" meat. The source of anthrax in the cattle in this epidemic appeared to be a single 29-ton lot of bone meal used as animal feed that likely was made from the bones of animals that had died of anthrax the previous year.

Very rare cases of inhalation anthrax have developed in workers exposed to aerosolized anthrax spores generated during the processing of contaminated materials such as woolens, hides, or bone meal, and even more rarely in people who have simply been in the vicinity of a wool-processing mill or tannery but who were not directly involved in the processing of the product. Cases have even been reported in home weavers, such as those using contaminated goat yarn, or in individuals working with contaminated bone meal fertilizer.

In the United States, the average annual occurrence has diminished. From 1977 to 1988, the number of cases was only 0.8, as opposed to 127 cases reported to occur annually between 1916 and 1925. The case fatality rate of the 221 U.S. cases of cutaneous anthrax from 1955 to 1986 was approximately 5.0 per cent (11 of 221), whereas the case fatality rate was 82 per cent in the patients with inhalation anthrax (9 of 11). The overall mortality rate in these 232 American cases of anthrax was 8.6 per cent.

EPIDEMIOLOGY. Cases of anthrax are classified generally as either agricultural or industrial. Most of the agricultural cases of human anthrax result from direct contact with contaminated discharges from infected animals. Occasional human cases have been transmitted by bites of flies that have fed on the carcasses of animals that have died of anthrax. Industrial cases usually result from contact with anthrax spores contaminating animal products, such as goat hair, wool, hides, and skin, and animal bones, especially those imported from areas of high endemicity. Transmission usually occurs during the processing of these animal products, either by direct contact with the contaminated raw material or by indirect contact with a contaminated environment; rarely, transmission may occur via airborne particles produced during the manufacturing process. Because the B. anthracis spores can survive for long periods, a wide variety of unusual products have been associated with human infection, such as imported bongo drums made with goat skins, shaving brushes, various leather or woolen blankets, and ivory piano keys. Laboratory-acquired infections have been reported; however, human-to-human transmission of anthrax is not thought to occur.

Most cases of anthrax in the United States are sporadic, but occasional epidemics have been reported. In 1957, the largest and most serious of these occurred in New Hampshire, where nine employees of a textile mill acquired anthrax while processing a batch of contaminated goat hair imported from Asia. This outbreak included four cutaneous cases and five inhalation cases, with four fatalities reported in the latter group.

PATHOGENESIS. The virulence of B. anthracis is determined by both a plasmid-mediated group of exotoxins and another plasmid-mediated antiphagocytic polydiglutamic acid capsule. Three toxic proteins (exotoxins) have been identified and cloned, including a protective antigen (PA), an edema factor (EF), and a lethal factor (LF). A combination of two of these proteins (PA and EF) has been demonstrated to decrease polymorphonuclear neutrophil function, suggesting that in this way host susceptibility to infection with B. anthracis may be increased.

In cutaneous anthrax, the organism is introduced either through a wound or by means of infected animal fibers that disrupt the skin. The organism is not known to penetrate intact skin. Once in the subcutaneous tissue, the anthrax spore is thought to germinate, multiply, and produce both its exotoxin and the antiphagocytic capsular material. The toxins are capable of provoking a marked edematous response and tissue necrosis with a paucity of neutrophil invasion. Phagocytosis of the organisms by local macrophages occurs, and these bacilli are then spread to regional lymph nodes, where further production of toxins produces a hemorrhagic, necrotic, and edematous lymphadenitis. Bacilli may enter the circulation, at times producing meningitis, pneumonia, and systemic toxicity.

Inhalation anthrax is fortunately a very uncommon clinical presentation of anthrax, as it is associated with close to 100 per cent mortality. In the United States, inhalation anthrax is now essentially obsolete, with only two cases reported during the past 20 years; however, this is still a cause of significant disease in

many parts of the world. Inhalation anthrax, commonly known as "woolsorter's disease," occurs not as a result of direct contact with infected animals but rather by inhalation of an aerosol of spores in particle sizes less than 5 μm. These aerosols have usually occurred during the processing of contaminated material. In humans, spores are inhaled, reach the alveoli, and may then eventually be phagocytized by macrophages and carried by these cells to the mediastinal lymph nodes. Germination, growth, and toxin formation at this site can produce a severe, massive hemorrhagic lymphadenitis and mediastinitis. B. anthracis may also directly affect the pulmonary capillary endothelium, causing thrombosis and respiratory failure. Pleural effusion is common. Anthrax is not thought to cause a primary pneumonia, but secondary bacterial pneumonia may complicate inhalation anthrax. Bacillus anthracis may also enter the bloodstream from this site, with the evolution of an intense bacteremia. The number of organisms per milliliter of blood may be so great that the organism may be seen on smears of the peripheral blood. In some instances, a hemorrhagic meningitis ensues. Respiratory failure, shock, and pulmonary edema are frequent causes of death.

Ingestion of markedly contaminated, poorly cooked meat may result in either the oropharyngeal or the gastrointestinal form of infection. When oropharyngeal anthrax occurs, there is localized swelling of the pharynx, sometimes causing tracheal obstruction, and marked cervical adenopathy with overlying brawny edema. Similarly, the organism may reach the small and large intestines and cause a gastrointestinal syndrome. In this case, the spores that are deposited in the submucosa of the intestinal tract may germinate, multiply, and produce toxin, again resulting in marked edema, hemorrhage, and necrosis. Regional mesenteric lymphadenopathy is common, and findings associated with the syndrome include fever, vomiting, abdominal pain and distention, massive bloody diarrhea, mesenteric adenitis, hemorrhagic ascites, and septicemia. Gastrointestinal anthrax is a very severe form of the disease, has a high mortality rate (25 to 75 per cent), and is rarely diagnosed during life except in the setting of an epidemic.

It is important to note that although antimicrobial agents may rapidly eradicate the organism, the persistence of the toxin that has been produced may result in continued development of the disease process until the toxin is metabolized. Thus, although the mortality rate may be diminished by appropriate antibiotic therapy, especially in the cutaneous form of the disease, the clinical process may continue to progress even after the institution of antimicrobial therapy. Antitoxins have been tried by some in the past, but such antitoxins are not currently available.

CLINICAL MANIFESTATIONS. Cutaneous anthrax is the most common form of the disease in humans, accounting for more than 95 per cent of cases. After an incubation period of 1 to 5 days, the infection generally begins with a small, somewhat pruritic papule at the site of an abrasion, which over the next several days develops into a vesicle containing serosanguineous fluid teeming with organisms. The lesion generally occurs on the upper extremities, especially the arms and hands, or on the face, neck, or other areas that are likely to be exposed to the contaminated animal product or infected soil. As the lesion progresses, ulceration occurs, with formation of a necrotic ulcer base that is frequently surrounded by smaller vesicles. The characteristic black eschar evolves over several weeks to a size of several centimeters, gradually separating and leaving a scar. This black eschar accounts for the name "anthrax," which comes from the Greek word for coal. The edema is frequently nonpitting, gelatinous, and brawny and is very striking. It may be quite extensive, spreading over a wide area in severe cases. With involvement near the eye, periorbital swelling may be especially intense. The edema may be so dramatic that hypotension occurs in part owing to the loss of intravascular volume as fluid enters the subcutaneous tissues. This edema, in combination with the vesicle progressing to the necrotic black eschar, forms the lesion that is highly characteristic of anthrax. Despite the dramatic appearance of the lesion, it is frequently painless.

In association with the localized cutaneous lesion, most patients present with minimal constitutional findings, such as fever, malaise, myalgias, and headaches. In those with extensive edema, the systemic symptoms may be more severe. Localized lymphadenopathy may occur at times and may be complicated by bacteremia and even meningitis. Death is rare if appropriate antimicrobial therapy is instituted; in untreated cases of cutaneous anthrax, however, the mortality rate remains about 25 per cent.

Bacterial adenitis due to staphylococci and streptococci, tularemia, plague, orf, cat scratch disease, localized herpes, and ecthyma gangrenosum are diagnostic considerations, and lesions seen in these diseases may be confused with those of anthrax. The diagnosis of cutaneous anthrax will rarely be missed if the disease is considered in any patient who has had exposure to an appropriate animal or animal product and who develops a painless ulcer surrounded by small vesicles, along with marked edema and eschar formation. Gram stains of the vesicular fluid and lesion usually readily demonstrate the characteristic gram-positive bacilli, as the organisms are present in large numbers in these lesions and are readily isolated by culture. Informing the bacteriology laboratory of the possibility of the diagnosis of anthrax is important to prevent the organism from being discarded as merely a probable contaminant of *Bacillus* species, which is frequently not fully characterized. At times, secondary bacterial infection may occur in these ulcers. Rarely, more than one lesion may be present, resulting from co-primary infections.

Inhalation anthrax is very rare, usually fatal, and extremely difficult to diagnose. The incubation period in this syndrome is generally 1 to 6 days, and the illness is generally biphasic. Initially, a brief, nonspecific "influenza-like" illness occurs, manifested by high fever, fatigue, myalgias, malaise, a nonproductive cough, and at times some chest discomfort. Few physical findings are noted at this time; however, within several days after a short period of clinical improvement, the patient becomes much more ill. This second phase is manifested by severe dyspnea, cyanosis, hypoxia, hemoptysis, stridor, chest pain, and diaphoresis. Physical examination may reveal some crepitant rales and evidence of pleural effusions. Some subcutaneous brawny edema of the chest wall and neck may be noted. The chest radiograph in these patients shows a rather distinctive clinical finding, namely, a widened mediastinum. Bacteremia, shock, and meningitis are frequently present, and death generally follows within 1 to 2 days of the onset of the respiratory distress. The mortality rate is 80 to 100 per cent, even with appropriate therapy.

Inhalation anthrax should be considered in patients with an appropriate exposure to an animal product, such as in a weaver using imported goat hair or a textile mill worker. The most important clue is the presence of an appropriate epidemiologic history in a patient developing severe respiratory distress and a rapidly enlarging mediastinum.

Gastrointestinal anthrax is an extremely rare disease and has an incubation period of 2 to 5 days, although there are some cases in which a more prolonged incubation period has been postulated. The diagnosis is rarely suspected before death except in areas where anthrax is highly endemic and in which multiple human cases are occurring. The symptoms include severe abdominal pain, hematemesis, melena, rapid onset of ascites, and at times marked diarrhea. Paracentesis may reveal hemorrhagic ascites, and sometimes these cases may simulate acute surgical abdomens. The disease usually progresses to bacteremia, toxemia, shock, and eventually death in many patients. No cases of intestinal anthrax have been reported in the United States.

Oropharyngeal anthrax presents as severe sore throat with neck swelling, adenopathy, dysphagia, and at times tracheal compression and dyspnea. Cervical and submandibular lymphadenopathy is common. Again, bacteremia and its complications may ensue.

The meningitis caused by anthrax is a complication of any of the forms of anthrax and almost never is found without a primary focus of infection. It is frequently hemorrhagic and most often fatal.

DIAGNOSIS. The clinician who elicits a careful epidemiologic history and who has a high index of suspicion of anthrax will not have problems establishing the diagnosis in cutaneous anthrax and will even be alert to the rarer and more difficult to recognize cases of inhalation, gastrointestinal, or oropharyngeal anthrax.

Inhalation anthrax is rarely suspected before death and only if an epidemiologic history of aerosol exposure is obtained or if an epidemic is recognized. The major finding in the clinical evaluation, other than epidemiologic history, is the presence of a widened mediastinum or at times hemorrhagic pleural effusions or an associated hemorrhagic meningitis. Ordinarily, Gram stains of sputum and cultures do not demonstrate *B. anthracis*. These patients frequently do develop bacteremia, however, and in these cases the organism can be readily isolated and sometimes seen on stains of the peripheral blood.

A number of serologic tests are available to diagnose anthrax retrospectively, but many of these very ill patients die so quickly that the initial serologic studies may not be especially helpful to the clinician. In some cases, however, serology has been a helpful diagnostic tool, especially when prior antibiotics have eradicated the bacteria before cultures or smears were obtained. Current serologic tests considered to be of value include an enzyme-linked immunosorbent assay (ELISA), which detects antibodies to the capsular antigen, and an electrophoretic immunotransblot test, which detects antibodies to the PA exotoxin. Both of these serologic tests are quite sensitive and specific enough to be useful, but the test for antibody to the PA exotoxin may be more specific.

TREATMENT. Penicillin G is the drug of choice for treatment of anthrax. Only a few isolates of *B. anthracis* have been identified as resistant to penicillin G. In cutaneous anthrax, cultures of the infected blisters have become negative for the organism within 5 hours of receiving 2 million units of penicillin G. As previously mentioned, however, the presence of the toxin may persist, and the cutaneous lesion frequently goes through its various phases of evolution, even though the organism has been eradicated and the mortality rate reduced.

For cutaneous anthrax, intravenous penicillin G is given, 2 million units every 6 hours for several days, followed by a 7- to 10-day course of oral penicillin G. In patients presenting with severe, overwhelming edema, corticosteroids have been thought by some to be helpful, although no controlled studies of its use have been performed. Severe neck swelling may require intubation or tracheostomy. In patients who are allergic to penicillin, effective alternatives include streptomycin, erythromycin, tetracycline, and chloramphenicol. No local surgery should be performed on these patients, since no pus requiring drainage is usually present and since excision of the lesion has been reported to increase the severity of symptoms and the spread of the organism. The lesion should be covered with a sterile dressing. There have been no definite cases of spread of anthrax from human to human.

In inhalation, gastrointestinal, or oropharyngeal anthrax or in anthrax meningitis, high dosages of intravenous penicillin G, in the range of 24 million units per day, are recommended, along with excellent supportive care for the problems of hypotension and respiratory distress. Some authors encourage the addition of parenteral streptomycin in a dosage of 1 to 2 grams per day to the penicillin G therapy in these cases. When the patient is hospitalized, good infection control practices are required. Soiled dressings must be incinerated or autoclaved.

PROGNOSIS. Inhalation anthrax is considered to be fatal in 80 to 100 per cent of cases, and gastrointestinal anthrax has a case fatality rate of 25 to 75 per cent. The case fatality rate for cutaneous anthrax is about 20 to 25 per cent without treatment but generally is less than 1 per cent with appropriate treatment.

PREVENTION. Control of anthrax in animals is essential to control of the disease in humans. All cases of animal anthrax, as well as human anthrax, should be reported to the state health department or the appropriate veterinary agency. Live avirulent animal vaccines are effective and may help control anthrax in endemic areas. Animals dying of anthrax should be cremated or buried, and care must be taken at autopsy to avoid additional contamination of the environment by infected blood and tissues. Prevention of human anthrax can be partially accomplished through proper disposal of the infected animals. In addition, formaldehyde has been used successfully to decontaminate raw wool and hair. A cell-free filtrate vaccine has been shown to protect humans from anthrax and is available from the Michigan State Department of Health. This vaccine should be offered to workers likely to be exposed to contaminated animal products in high-risk industries. Newer vaccines are being evaluated, such as a protective antigen (PA) toxoid vaccine and a protective antigen (PA)–producing live vaccine. In the Soviet Union, in addition to the chemical vaccine, a live anthrax spore vaccine has been widely used for prophylaxis against anthrax in both humans and animals. Good personal hygiene, as well as the use of protective clothing and respirators when contaminated aerosols are likely to be encountered, may also prove to be helpful preventive measures. Gastrointestinal anthrax can be prevented by proper cooking of meat and by avoiding ingestion of potentially contaminated meat.

Care must be taken in the laboratory when working with *B. anthracis*, since cases of anthrax have been acquired in this setting.

Brachman PS: Anthrax. *In* Evans A, Feldman H (eds.): Bacterial Infections of Humans: Epidemiology and Control. New York, Ms. Hilary Evans Publishing Company, 1982, pp 63–74. *Comprehensive summary of all aspects of anthrax, with emphasis on the epidemiology.*

Brachman PS: Inhalation anthrax. Ann NY Acad Sci 353:83, 1980. *A review of all aspects of inhalation anthrax.*

Gold H: Anthrax. Arch Intern Med 96:387, 1955. *Excellent clinical summary.*

Harrison LH, Ezzell JW, Abshire TG, et al.: Evaluation of serologic tests for diagnosis of anthrax after an outbreak of cutaneous anthrax in Paraguay. J Infect Dis 160:706, 1989. *Newer serologic methods for diagnosis and detection of immunity.*

Ivins BE, Welkos SL: Recent advances in the development of an improved human anthrax vaccine. Eur J Epidemiol 4:12, 1988. *New approach to vaccines for anthrax.*

Knudson GB: Treatment of anthrax in man: History and current concepts. Milit Med 151:71, 1986. *Reviews the history of anthrax with emphasis on treatment.*

Little SF, Knudson GB: Comparative efficacy of *Bacillus anthracis* live spore vaccine against anthrax in guinea pigs. Infect Immun 52:509, 1986. *Compares two different anthrax vaccines and discusses ELISA testing.*

Plotkin SA, Brachman PS, Utell M, et al.: An epidemic of inhalation anthrax, the first in the twentieth century. I. Clinical features. Am J Med 29:992, 1960. *Summarizes the clinical features of an epidemic of inhalation anthrax in the United States.*

324 Diseases Caused by Pseudomonads

Stephen C. Schimpff

PSEUDOMONADS

Pseudomonads are gram-negative aerobic bacilli that prefer moist environments and are relatively noninvasive, yet can cause serious and often fatal infection when the host defense mechanism is damaged or deficient. Each species is different in its pathogenic properties, each causes somewhat different types of infection, and each invades as a result of different host defense defects, but with each pseudomonad, the environmental source is usually water, moist soil, or a contaminated medical device, infusion, or injection.

Pseudomonads are divided into five major groups based upon RNA/DNA homology (Table 324–1). For purposes of discussion,

TABLE 324–1. CLASSIFICATION OF PSEUDOMONADS THAT HAVE BEEN ISOLATED FROM CLINICAL SPECIMENS

Group/Subgroup	Genus and Species
RNA group I	
Fluorescent group	*P. aeruginosa*
	P. fluorescens
	P. putida
Nonfluorescent group	*P. stutzeri*
	P. alcaligenes
	P. pseudoalcaligenes
RNA group II	*P. mallei*
	P. pseudomallei
	P. cepacia
	P. pickettii
RNA group III	*P. acidovorans*
	P. testosteroni
RNA group IV	*P. diminuta*
	P. vesicularis
RNA group V	*Xanthomonas maltophilia*

this chapter considers *Pseudomonas mallei* (the cause of melioidosis), *Pseudomonas pseudomallei* (the cause of glanders), *Pseudomonas aeruginosa* (which principally causes bacteremia, endocarditis, pneumonia, keratitis, and urinary tract infections), and *Pseudomonas cepacia* and *Pseudomonas (Xanthomonas) maltophilia* (which cause bacteremia, pseudobacteremia, endocarditis, and urinary tract infections).

Pseudomonas pseudomallei. This organism causes melioidosis, which is often characterized as a glanders-like infectious disease. It was first described in Rangoon among debilitated morphine addicts. The term "melioidosis" means "a similarity to distemper of asses." Despite the clinical resemblance to glanders, it has a totally different epidemiology. Melioidosis occurs in animals and humans in endemic areas of southeast Asia and northern Australia and has now been recognized to occur in epidemic-like form in specific areas, given the combination of the environment (an appropriate rainy season with water-covered rice paddies) and a susceptible host (abraded skin in barefoot farmers who have a high prevalence of diabetes mellitus and renal calculi).

P. pseudomallei is a gram-negative, motile, aerobic bacillus that is small and may grow in filamentous chains. Staining with methylene blue or Wright's stain shows a bipolar "safety pin" pattern. *P. pseudomallei* has a characteristic wrinkling appearance of the colonies on agar if held long enough. The organism, like most pseudomonads, can be isolated from soil and water and particularly streams, rice paddies, and ponds of the endemic areas and on plants, including commonly consumed vegetables. Most human infection probably occurs through skin abrasions. However, laboratory animals have been found to become infected by the respiratory route, so inhalation may be a possible human route of acquisition, which would explain the occurrence of primary pneumonia.

At the conclusion of American involvement in the Vietnam War, 343 cases were reported, with 36 deaths among the American military; however, serologic surveys suggest that either mild or inapparent infection may be fairly common, with positive serologies found in 1 to 2 per cent of healthy, nonwounded U.S. Army troops returning to the United States. This would suggest that as many as 225,000 Americans may have had subclinical infection with *P. pseudomallei*. The importance of this observation is that recrudescence of disease has been observed many years after primary infection.

In addition to inapparent infection or asymptomatic pulmonary infection, the frequently observed forms of melioidosis are an acute, localized, suppurative soft tissue infection, an acute pulmonary infection, and an acute septicemic presentation. The localized infections are probably related to skin abrasion, with the development of a nodule with secondary lymphangitis and regional lymphadenitis. It is likely that this is the form of infection that progresses to the acute septicemic phase. An apparent primary pulmonary infection ranges from bronchitis to necrotizing pneumonia. For the patient with pneumonia, there is usually high fever and signs and symptoms of consolidation, ordinarily in an upper lobe. It is an acute pyogenic process, frequently leading to early cavitation and giving a pulmonary appearance consistent with tuberculosis. Progression to bacteremia is rare.

Patients with the acute septic form characteristically present with a short history of fever and no clinical evidence of focal infection. Most are profoundly ill, with signs of sepsis, such as tachypnea or Kussmaul's breathing, and occasional evidence of septic shock. Clinical and radiologic evidence frequently demonstrates progression to diffuse bilateral and patchy pulmonary infiltrate, which progresses to abscess and cavity formation if the patient survives. Subcutaneous abscesses are relatively uncommon but can occur at multiple sites, as can visceral abscesses, such as in the liver or spleen.

The diagnosis should be considered in any patient living in an endemic area who has a febrile illness and especially one who is occupationally at risk and, perhaps, who is at further risk of sepsis because of diabetes or renal disease. The diagnosis should be highly suspected in such an individual who presents with a rapidly progressive, extensive pulmonary process if there are subcutaneous lesions or in one whose condition progresses to a cavitary form indistinguishable from tuberculosis. A Gram stain of pulmonary or abscess exudate shows small gram-negative bacilli, and methylene blue staining shows the bipolar "safety pin" characteristic. The organism grows on standard media and is usually detected in blood cultures within 48 hours.

In northeast Thailand, a report from a hospital that serves a population of nearly 2 million rural rice farming families determined that about 20 per cent of all community-acquired bacteremias were caused by *P. pseudomallei* and that during the rainy season, when the paddy fields are under water (from June to September), *P. pseudomallei* was the single most common organism isolated from blood culture, representing nearly one half of all documented cases of community-acquired bacteremia in the month of August (Fig. 324–1). An interesting observation was the higher than expected frequency of both diabetes mellitus and renal calculi in patients with sepsis who are from this region, where both diabetes and calculi are common.

Treatment of pulmonary or suspected septic forms should probably begin with a combination of agents. The standard recommended treatment has been a combination of chloramphenicol, doxycycline, and trimethoprim-sulfamethoxazole. These agents, however, are bacteriostatic rather than bactericidal and do not represent a regimen one would wish to use for suspected community-acquired bacteremia. Although clinical data remain limited, the third-generation cephalosporin ceftazidime is now likely the drug of choice, with carbapenem, imipenem, piperacillin, or amoxicillin–clavulanic acid as reasonable alternatives. The addition of an aminoglycoside during empiric therapy might be appropriate until culture results are known. Treatment apparently needs to be prolonged, including intravenous therapy (ceftazidime, imipenem, or piperacillin) for 2 to 4 weeks, followed by oral therapy (perhaps amoxicillin–clavulanic acid) for 6 months or longer to prevent recrudescence.

The prognosis for patients with localized disease should be excellent with appropriate therapy. However, those with the septicemic form are often gravely ill at the time of admission, and the mortality rate reported in 1989 was 68 per cent. Some groups of patients with the highest mortality were those who were hypothermic, azotemic, or unable to produce a leukocytosis. It should be pointed out that in the reported survey only 27 per cent of the patients with septicemic melioidosis were given an antibiotic active against *P. pseudomallei* as part of the initial empiric regimen. Thus, it remains unclear what the survival rate would be in patients treated promptly with an appropriate agent, especially ceftazidime, imipenem, or amoxicillin–clavulanic acid.

Evidence also exists that melioidosis may be more frequent

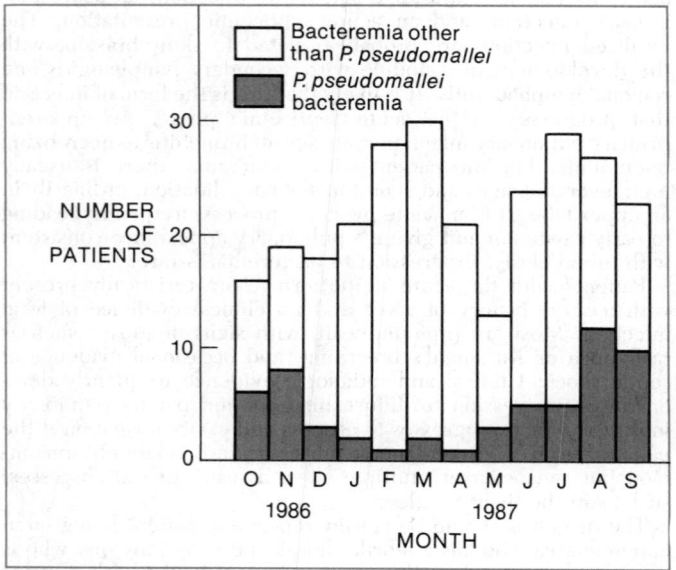

FIGURE 324–1. Number of persons with community-acquired bacteremia caused by *P. pseudomallei* and other organisms, in northeast Thailand from October 1986 to September 1987. (From Chaowagul W, White NJ, Dance DAB, et al.: Melioidosis: A major cause of community-acquired septicemia in northeastern Thailand. J Infect Dis 159:890–899, 1989; by permission of the University of Chicago Press, 1989.)

among immunocompromised individuals. In a report from Bangkok, Thailand, 49 cases of melioidosis seen over a 12-year period occurred exclusively among patients with diabetes mellitus, collagen vascular disorders, leukemia, lymphoma, or aplastic anemia. Twenty-nine of the 49 had the disseminated, or septic, form of the infection. Some associated infections included tuberculosis, candidiasis, aspergillosis, cytomegalovirus infection, and Epstein-Barr virus infection, all being infections associated with depressed cellular immunity. Among these patients, the mortality in those with localized melioidosis was low, whereas it was high in those with disseminated disease. An interesting finding among a subgroup of these patients demonstrated that the four patients with localized melioidosis who were evaluated had normal numbers of lymphocytes, including T-helper and T-suppressor lymphocytes, whereas the seven evaluated patients with disseminated melioidosis had a marked reduction in total lymphocytes and one third of the lower limit of normal for T-helper lymphocytes. This finding suggests that dissemination of *P. pseudomallei* is at least in part a function of an effective cellular arm of the immune system.

Pseudomonas mallei. *P. mallei* can cause an infection in horses, mules, and donkeys that occasionally has been transmitted to humans. The name "glanders" comes from the prominent pulmonary involvement, although the infection can, instead, be characterized by subcutaneous ulcerative lesions or lymphatic thickening with nodules (known as farcy).

Glanders was never a common human infection, and with the decline in the use of horses for day-to-day activities and with improved sanitation, glanders has become a very rare disease. Apparently, there have been no naturally acquired infections in the United States since 1938, although the occasional case occurs in other countries.

Like melioidosis, glanders tends to occur as an acute localized suppurative infection, an acute pulmonary infection, an acute septicemic infection, or a chronic suppurative infection. An abraded area of skin may lead to a local nodule with acute lymphangitis. Inoculation into an abraded mucous membrane can lead to extensive ulcerating granulomatous lesions. These forms of infection seem to have an incubation period of 1 to 5 days; in contrast, after inhalation, a primary pneumonia tends to develop 10 to 14 days later. Symptoms are relatively nonspecific and include fever, occasional rigors, malaise, fatigue, and headache. Examination findings depend upon the form of infection. Leukocytosis is common. Chest radiographs of the acute pulmonary form usually show densities consistent with early lung abscess; however, lobar or bronchopneumonia-type infiltrates are common. Chronic suppurative disease involves multiple subcutaneous and intramuscular abscesses, especially on the extremities, with lymphatic involvement and, in many, a nasal discharge with or without ulceration.

The organism is usually difficult to find in exudates, but, when seen with a Gram stain or methylene blue, appears similar to *P. pseudomallei*. The organism is reasonably easy to cultivate.

The treatment of glanders is uncertain because of the rarity of the disease and therefore the inability to carry out clinical trials. A reasonable recommendation is to initiate therapy with regimens found effective for melioidosis, recognizing that the acute septicemic form has been uniformly fatal in the past and suggesting that the full dosage of intravenous combinations of agents be given initially.

Pseudomonas aeruginosa. The name "aeruginosa" comes from the flourescent blue-green pigment pyocyanin, produced by many, but not all, strains. Other pigments produced by *P. aeruginosa* include pyoverdin (green) and, occasionally, pyorubin (deep red) and pyomelanin (black). Like other pseudomonads, *P. aeruginosa* grows well in multiple moist settings with limited nutrients. Found in soil, in water, and on plants, it can also be a normal commensal in animals and humans. Colonization in humans usually takes place in moist areas, such as perineum, auditory canal, axillae, and the lower alimentary canal. It is commonly found in sink traps, ice machines, and kitchen settings in the hospital; it can become a particular problem when it contaminates medications or medical devices with a moist environment, such as ventilators, endoscopes, pressure monitors, and the like. It can withstand many disinfectants and is resistant to a broad variety of antimicrobial agents. In the nonhospital setting, infections have been related to growth in swimming pools, contact lens solutions, and hot tubs.

Infection with *P. aeruginosa* has become, to a large degree, a by-product of medical advances in technology. In the 20 years prior to 1960 at the Johns Hopkins Hospital, only 91 cases of *P. aeruginosa* bacteremia occurred. Today, *P. aeruginosa* is the fourth most common cause of primary nosocomial gram-negative bacteremia and is the fourth most frequently isolated nosocomial pathogen, causing about 10 per cent of all hospital-acquired infections, 13 per cent of all nosocomial pneumonias, 12 per cent of urinary tract infections, and 7 per cent of surgical wound infections.

The most common infections caused by *P. aeruginosa* include nosocomial bacteremia; nosocomial pneumonia; nosocomial urinary tract infection; surgical wound infection; endocarditis related to intravenous drug abuse or placement of artificial heart valves; respiratory infection associated with cystic fibrosis; external otitis, including "malignant" external otitis (see Ch. 471); corneal keratitis; and uncommon occurrences of spinal osteomyelitis in heroin addicts (see Ch. 304) and rare cases of meningitis or brain abscess. A common origin of bacteremia in the granulocytopenic patient is infection along the alimentary canal, especially perianal cellulitis, colonic lesions, and, occasionally, pharyngitis or esophagitis. Finally, extensive burns are commonly colonized by *P. aeruginosa*, with progression to sepsis and death.

P. aeruginosa almost never causes infection in the absence of (1) damage to a normal host defense mechanism (e.g., cancer chemotherapy–induced mucosal damage to the alimentary canal or extensive third-degree burns); (2) deficiency or alteration in a defense mechanism (e.g., the progressive respiratory tract changes of cystic fibrosis); or (3) bypass of a normal defense mechanism (e.g., respiratory assist device directly inoculating organisms into the bronchial tree while concurrently limiting or damaging the mucociliary mechanism, or insertion of an indwelling urinary catheter, circumventing the normal bladder clearance mechanism). Thus, infections with *P. aeruginosa* are most commonly seen in patients with a urinary catheter; those neutropenic from disease, chemotherapy, or both; those with cystic fibrosis; those with extensive thermal injuries; those in the intensive care unit who are subjected to any number of invasive procedures; those with head trauma, allowing entry either directly or via a pressure monitoring device; those with artificial heart valves or damaged endocardium from contaminants in illicit drugs; and those who have had extensive surgery, particularly when there is consequent need for open drainage.

Pollack has pointed out three distinct stages of *Pseudomonas* infection: stage I—bacterial attachment and colonization; stage II—local invasion; and stage III—bloodstream dissemination and systemic disease. Stage I is a prerequisite to stage II, which, in turn, is a prerequisite to stage III, although obviously not all colonized individuals have local invasion and not all those with local invasion progress to dissemination or systemic disease. The three stages relate to the fact that this organism is both invasive and toxigenic. Colonization in a normal person is relatively uncommon at most sites, although over time, a fair proportion of the population will have transient colonization of the colon. However, hospitalized patients have a much higher frequency of colonization, related, in part, to changes in host defenses, as discussed above, and, in part, to the frequency of hospital reservoirs of this organism. In addition, broad-spectrum antimicrobial therapy suppresses other normal microbial flora, especially along the alimentary canal. This suppression reduces the body's normal mechanism of colonization resistance, so that an organism such as *P. aeruginosa* or other species resistant to the antibiotics used can more readily colonize multiple locations in high concentration. Additional specific factors further predispose to colonization by *P. aeruginosa*. These include the presence of pili for attachment, flagella for motility, and exoproducts, especially proteinases. Also involved is the secretory protease-induced loss of fibronectin from epithelial cells during serious illness (among patients hospitalized or not), which, in turn, allows the pili or fimbriae to adhere to the oral, pharyngeal, and respiratory epithelium. Thus, the illness determinants of protease production are major modulators of the oral flora. This colonization, in turn, can be accentuated by local damage caused by an endotracheal tube, by viral infection (such as influenza), by thermal injury, or by cancer chemotherapy and is exacerbated by antibiotics. *P. aeruginosa*, in some settings, can help protect itself from defense mechanisms by the production of a glycocalyx, a carbohydrate produced by many bacteria, which, by surrounding the cell and anchoring it to epithelial cells or invasive devices, such as an intravascular or urinary catheter, protects the bacterium from antibody, complement, and polymorphonuclear leukocytes or macrophages.

After colonization, *P. aeruginosa* can invade in the appropriate setting through the effect of extracellular enzymes (toxins). These include elastase, alkaline protease, and perhaps also cytotoxin and hemolysins. Elastase and protease have been demonstrated to cause necrotizing lesions in the skin, lung, and cornea, along with small vessel necrotizing lesions, which cause the characteristic skin finding known as ecthyma gangrenosum. It is this combination of local necrosis and blood vessel destruction that is the essence of the initial invasive characteristic of *P. aeruginosa*.

The third stage of *Pseudomonas* infection, dissemination and systemic disease, is due, in the first case, to these same extracellular enzymes and, in the second case, to *Pseudomonas* liposaccharide (endotoxin) and exotoxin A. As with other septicemias caused by gram-negative bacilli, endotoxin is thought to be a critical factor in the activation of the clotting, fibrinolytic, kinin, and complement systems, along with the production of prostaglandins and leukotrienes, the release of β-endorphins, and the release of cytokines, including tumor necrosis factor. By some interaction of many or all of these factors come fever, shock, disseminated intravascular coagulation (which is relatively uncommon with *Pseudomonas* bacteremia), and the adult respiratory distress syndrome. The other factor, exotoxin A, is similar to diphtheria toxin in that it inhibits protein synthesis. It causes local necrosis and encourages bacterial dissemination to the systemic circulation and, in itself, has been shown to produce shock in animal models.

Pseudomonas bacteremia occurs most commonly in cancer patients who are receiving intensive chemotherapy that produces granulocytopenia in patients with extensive third-degree burns, and, occasionally, in patients with immunoglobulin or hypocomplementemia states. It is also a common cause of bacteremia in the patient with urinary catheterization. It is the fourth most frequent cause of primary hospital-acquired gram-negative bacteremia. Sepsis in burn patients arises from the thermally damaged skin. Bacteremia in neutropenic patients arises principally from the lower intestinal tract and occasionally from primary pneumonia. Surveillance cultures have documented that granulocytopenic patients frequently become colonized, and nearly all colonized patients will develop bacteremia if profound (<100 per microliter) granulocytopenia persists for more than a few days. Ecthyma gangrenosum, usually a sign of fairly advanced systemic infection, is not pathognomonic but is most frequently associated with *P. aeruginosa* bacteremia. These skin lesions at first are small and indurated, and then they rapidly enlarge, become necrotic, and may ulcerate. Bacteria, on histologic section, are seen to be invading small arteries and veins, with remarkably minimal evidence of inflammation. A histologically similar lesion can be found in the lungs as a secondary consequence of bacteremia. The mortality of *Pseudomonas* sepsis is high, with the underlying status of the patient's host defenses and the promptness of institution of empiric antibiotic therapy being the two critical factors affecting survival. The presence of septic shock, the evidence of septic metastases, or both, at the initiation of antibiotic administration are usually considered adverse prognostic signs but, in reality, represent another measure of late institution of therapy.

The standard approach to suspected gram-negative sepsis, including that caused by *P. aeruginosa*, is a combination employing an antipseudomonal β-lactam (penicillin or cephalosporin) with an aminoglycoside. Two newer drugs, imipenem or the antipseudomonal quinolones—again, in combination with an aminoglycoside—are also effective. Although in some cases, such as in the febrile, neutropenic patient, monotherapy has been recommended with agents such as ceftazidime or imipenem, a two-drug regimen is advised for initial empiric therapy. A number of studies suggest that survival is improved when two antibiotics to which the organism is susceptible are administered immediately and that survival is further improved if the two agents prove to be synergistic in activity. For the future, we must look also to immunologic approaches to bacteremia prevention and treatment, such as monoclonal antibodies to lipopolysaccharide.

Respiratory tract infections (see also Ch. 294) can take the form of a primary pneumonia, a secondary pneumonia due to bacteremia, or a chronic infection with intermittent exacerbations. Primary pneumonia occurs almost exclusively in hospitalized patients whose oropharynx or tracheobronchial tree is colonized by *P. aeruginosa* as a result of intubation. Frequently, *Pseudomonas* pneumonia occurs in the setting of additional pulmonary damage, such as blunt trauma, substantial atelectasis, or hemothorax. Atelectasis appears to be a key contributing pathogenic factor. Early, aggressive physiotherapy for the chest sometimes clears what appears to be a pneumonia but, in fact, is atelectasis that has resulted in fever, purulent sputum production, and a positive chest radiograph. However, once actual pneumonia has begun, the prognosis is poor, and early empiric therapy is critical.

The pneumonia that follows bacteremia is usually fulminant, with multiple areas of hemorrhage around small and medium-sized pulmonary arteries and lesions caused by necrosis of the small muscular arteries and veins in a fashion similar to ecthyma gangrenosum. Survival is limited even with prompt, aggressive therapy.

Chronic *Pseudomonas* respiratory infections are largely limited to patients with cystic fibrosis (see also Ch. 64), with the frequency of this infection increasing with age, so that, ultimately, almost all patients will have significant *Pseudomonas* pulmonary infection. The age differential is probably related to the progressive development of airway obstruction, which seems to be a critical factor in the development of *Pseudomonas* infection. This chronic infection is associated with chronic cough, nutritional losses, and progressive loss of pulmonary function. The standard treatment has been an antipseudomonal penicillin plus an aminoglycoside. The development of resistance is common, so therapy must therefore be based on susceptibility patterns. Ceftazidime, imipenem, or a quinolone may also be considered. Acute exacerbations may be reduced or even prevented with intermittent therapy a number of times each year, irrespective of whether the infection is currently quiescent.

OTHER PSEUDOMONADS

Pseudomonas cepacia. This species of *Pseudomonas* can grow as well in distilled water as it can in trypticase soy broth; it is resistant to many of the commonly used hospital disinfectants; it can use penicillin as a carbon source; and it is resistant to many of the commonly used antimicrobials. Its virulence properties are not understood.

Community-acquired infections are, without doubt, rare. However, certain hosts are at substantially increased risk. Endocarditis has occurred among intravenous drug abusers; skin infections related to extensive burns have occurred; a necrotizing, occasionally recurrent pneumonia has occurred among patients with the phagocytic dysfunction of chronic granulomatous disease; and an emerging problem for cystic fibrosis patients has been a relentless, often fulminating pneumonia caused by *P. cepacia*.

Nosocomial infections and pseudoinfections are considered together because of a common origin and because it is sometimes difficult to distinguish between the two. The source of *P. cepacia* in the hospital setting is usually a moist or water-based reservoir, which, given the technologic advances of medicine in recent decades, suggests that *P. cepacia* has the potential to become a not infrequent cause of infection and pseudoinfection in the high-technology or intensive care setting. *P. cepacia* has been found to cause pneumonitis, endocarditis, wound infections, and urinary tract infections, along with primary bacteremia. The origins of iatrogenic bacteremia can be conveniently divided into those related to contaminated solutions, injectables, and medical devices. Among the contaminated solutions that have been implicated in bacteremia or pseudobacteremia have been disinfectant solutions, heparinized flushing solutions, distilled water, topical anesthetics, and intravenous infusates, including human serum albumin and cryoprecipitate. Contaminated injectables have included saline, methylprednisolone, and fentanyl. The implicated devices all have the common property of including a moist environment where the organism can multiply; pressure monitoring devices, respiratory assist devices, peritoneal dialysis machines, reusable hemodialysis coils, and blood gas analyzers have been documented as point sources.

Figure 324–2 shows an epidemic of *P. cepacia* bacteremia among patients at the Clinical Center of the National Institutes of Health. The figure indicates that *P. cepacia*–positive blood cultures were uncommon in the years preceding this outbreak and that the majority during the epidemic occurred within the medical intensive care unit. A blood gas analyzer in an adjoining laboratory was found to be contaminated, and this served as the point source for this series of bacteremias. Although some were apparently pseudobacteremias, (i.e., the blood culture became positive owing to contamination by skin or other sources), others were true bacteremias with significant morbidity. Indeed, among those highly compromised patients, many with cancer and significant immune suppression, the mortality resulting from the *P. cepacia* infection itself was 38 per cent.

P. cepacia is resistant to many of the commonly used broad-spectrum antibiotics but does usually tend to be susceptible to trimethoprim-sulfamethoxazole.

Pseudomonas maltophilia (Xanthomonas maltophilia). *X. maltophilia* is atypical of the other pseudomonads in that the oxidase test is negative or equivocal. It is probably a fairly common commensal and a part of the transient flora, especially of hospitalized patients. In the hospital environment, it is not infrequently found in moist or wet settings. The organism is resistant to most of the first- and second-generation cephalosporins, semisynthetic penicillins, and aminoglycosides, although it has variable susceptibility to the antipseudomonal penicillins. It is generally susceptible to many of the third-generation cephalosporins, trimethoprim-sulfamethoxazole, and rifampin. Synergy has been noted with trimethoprim-sulfamethoxazole plus carbenicillin and with the triple regimen of trimethoprim-sulfamethoxazole plus carbenicillin and rifampin.

X. maltophilia is an uncommon cause of a wide spectrum of diseases that, in general, are less severe than infections caused

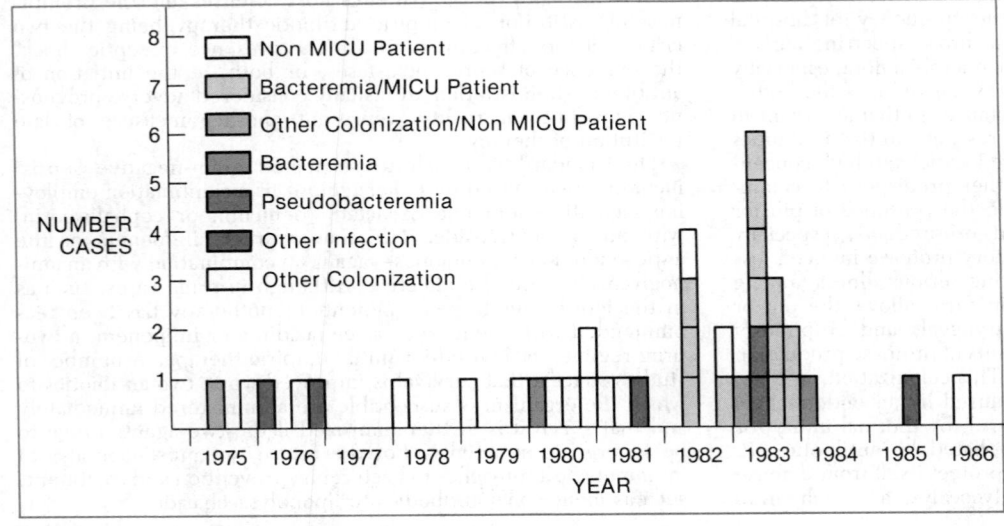

FIGURE 324–2. An epidemic of *Pseudomonas cepacia* bacteremia among patients at the Clinical Center of the National Institutes of Health. MICU = medical intensive care unit. (Reprinted with permission from Henderson DK, Baptiste R, Parillo J, et al.: Indolent epidemic of *Pseudomonas cepacia* bacteremia and pseudobacteremia in an intensive care unit traced to a contaminated blood gas analyzer. Am J Med 84:75–81, 1988.)

by other gram-negative bacilli in similar locations. Currently, *X. maltophilia* infections are relatively responsive to antimicrobial therapy. The most common types of infection are pneumonia, endocarditis, urinary tract infection, and iatrogenic bacteremia or pseudobacteremia. Cholangitis and meningitis have been reported but are quite unusual, and wounds, although a common site for *X. maltophilia* isolation, are rarely infected by this organism. Pneumonias tend to occur in debilitated patients with prior antibiotic therapy in a nosocomial setting, but they are very uncommon, and the organism should be questioned as causative in the absence of a pure culture via bronchoscopy, thoracentesis, or blood. Endocarditis in the community occurs among intravenous drug abusers and in the hospital as a complication of open heart surgery, usually among those with abnormal valves.

X. maltophilia bacteriuria is found somewhat often in patients with indwelling long-term catheters; however, only rarely has the organism been shown to cause clinical infection. When infection has occurred, it has usually been in association with significant instrumentation, genitourinary surgery, or both. The morbidity has tended to be low, and therapy, especially with trimethoprim-sulfamethoxazole, has frequently been effective.

Iatrogenic bacteremia and pseudobacteremia caused by this organism have been reported often. In one epidemic of 25 patients with positive blood cultures, it was determined that these cases were pseudobacteremias due to contaminated blood collection tubes. In another setting, eight children were found to have bacteremia after open heart surgery, apparently as a result of contamination of the monitoring transducers in the intensive care unit. *X. maltophilia* has been found to contaminate the deionized water used for diluting disinfectants, and the organism can even survive in the diluted disinfectant. It is important to emphasize that not all of these bacteremias have been "pseudobacteremias"; for example, two fatal cases of endocarditis have been noted as a result of bacteremia caused by a contaminated device or solution.

Bodey GP, Jadeja L, Elting L: *Pseudomonas* bacteremia: Retrospective analysis of 410 episodes. Arch Intern Med 145:1621, 1985. *A review of* P. aeruginosa *bacteremia.*

Curtin JA, Petersdorf RG, Bennett IL: Pseudomonas bacteremia: Review of ninety-one cases. Ann Intern Med 54:1077, 1961. *A classic paper describing* P. aeruginosa *bacteremia.*

Dance DAB, Wuthiekanun V, Chaowagul W, et al.: The antimicrobial susceptibility of *Pseudomonas pseudomallei.* Emergence of resistance *in vitro* and during treatment. J Antimicrob Chemother 24:295, 1989. *New data on the antimicrobial susceptibility of* P. pseudomallei *to the newer antibiotics, with reference to clinical trials.*

Henderson DK, Baptiste R, Parillo J, et al.: Indolent epidemic of *Pseudomonas cepacia* bacteremia and pseudobacteremia in an intensive care unit traced to a contaminated blood gas analyzer. Am J Med 84:75, 1988. *A nice review of bacteremia and pseudobacteremia due to* P. cepacia.

Marshall WF, Keating MR, Anhalt JP, Steckelberg JM: *Xanthomonas maltophilia:* An emerging nosocomial pathogen. Mayo Clin Proc 64:1097, 1989. *A thorough review of infection due to* Pseudomonas (Xanthomonas) maltophilia.

Palleroni NJ: Family Pseudomonadaceae. *In* Kreig NR, Holt JG (eds.): Bergey's Manual of Systematic Bacteriology. Vol. 1. Baltimore, The Williams and Wilkins Company, 1984, pp 141–219. *Basic reference manual for taxonomy of bacteria.*

Pollack M: *Pseudomonas aeruginosa. In* Mandell GL, Douglas RG Jr, Bennett JE (eds.): Principles and Practice of Infectious Diseases. 3rd ed. New York, Churchill Livingstone, 1990, pp 1673–1691. *A very thorough discussion of the microbiology, epidemiology, pathogenic factors, and clinical syndromes of* P. aeruginosa.

Sanford JP: Pseudomonas species (including melioidosis and glanders). *In* Mandell GL, Douglas RG Jr, Bennett JE (eds.): Principles and Practice of Infectious Diseases. 3rd ed. New York, Churchill Livingstone, 1990, pp 1692–1696. *Broad discussion of melioidosis and glanders by an expert in infections of importance to the U.S. military.*

325 Listeriosis

Alan M. Stamm

DEFINITION. Listeriosis is an infectious disease caused by the bacterium *Listeria monocytogenes*. The majority of afflicted patients are immunocompromised and present with meningoencephalitis.

ETIOLOGY. *Listeria monocytogenes* is a gram-positive bacillus but may stain unevenly and/or appear coccoid. It is facultatively anaerobic, non–spore forming, and β-hemolytic on blood agar. It grows optimally at 35 to 37°C, grows less well at temperatures as low as 4°C, and exhibits tumbling motility at 20 to 25°C.

Although at least 16 serotypes of *L. monocytogenes* are identified, each of the types 1/2a, 1/2b, and 4b accounts for about 30 per cent of human disease in the United States. These serotypes are uniformly distributed throughout this country. Six other species of *Listeria* exist, but they are rarely pathogenic for humans.

EPIDEMIOLOGY. *Listeria monocytogenes* is distributed widely in nature throughout the world. It is recovered from water, soil, decaying vegetation, silage, sewage, insects, crustaceans, fish, birds, and wild and domestic mammals. Sporadic as well as epizootic disease, manifest as meningitis, encephalitis, or spontaneous abortion, occurs in sheep, cattle, and goats. Asymptomatic human intestinal carriage is present in 1 to 5 per cent of normal adults and in 20 to 25 per cent of case contacts.

Neonates and the elderly have the highest attack rates of listeriosis. The sexes are equally represented. The incidence of disease is not significantly different across the United States or from one continent to another. Consistent seasonal patterns are noted, with disease occurring most commonly in domestic animals in late winter to early spring and in humans in late summer to early fall. However, the correlation between the number and location of animal cases and human cases is poor in any one region, and direct animal-to-human transmission of disease is rarely documented.

Epidemiologic investigations of outbreaks of listeriosis have demonstrated their frequent foodborne etiology. Manure from infected sheep was used to fertilize cabbage plants in the Maritime Provinces of Canada; 41 cases of human disease in 1980–1981 were linked to the ingestion of cole slaw prepared from these cabbages. Milk from cows was pasteurized but nonetheless implicated in 49 cases of listeriosis in Massachusetts in 1983; whether the microorganism survived pasteurization or contaminated the product afterward remains controversial. The largest epidemic occurred in southern California in 1985; 142 cases were associated with the consumption of soft, Mexican-style cheese made with unpasteurized milk. Similarly, an outbreak of 122 cases in Switzerland during 1983–1987 was attributed to a soft cheese. During periods of increased disease activity, the organism causing an epidemic is differentiated from those causing sporadic disease by serotyping, phage typing, or electrophoretic enzyme typing. All four of these outbreaks were due to *L. monocytogenes* serotype 4b.

Further evidence for foodborne acquisition of *L. monocytogenes* is provided by recent microbiologic investigations. The microorganism has been identified as a fairly common contaminant of raw and pasteurized milk; ice cream; raw beef, pork, and lamb; ready-to-eat meat products, including salami, sausages, and hot dogs; retail poultry; cooked shrimp and crab; raw vegetables such as cabbage, cucumbers, potatoes, and radishes; and packaged salads. Studies to date have not shown contamination of eggs or fruits. Although commercial food production methods may effectively kill the microorganism, products may become contaminated during subsequent processing and packaging before leaving the production facility.

PATHOGENESIS. The majority of adults with listeriosis have impaired cell-mediated immunity caused by cytotoxic chemotherapy for malignancy, immunosuppressive therapy for organ transplantation, or pregnancy. Both helper and suppressor T cells are centrally involved, whereas immunoglobulin and complement play lesser roles as opsonins. The gastrointestinal tract is the usual portal of entry. Bacteria are taken up from the lumen by endocytosis of epithelial cells covering intestinal villi. The inoculum required to cause disease may depend on the immunologic health and gastric acidity of the host as well as the virulence characteristics of the microorganism.

Dissemination occurs via simple bacteremia and/or circulation of infected monocytes. *Listeria monocytogenes* is a facultative intracellular parasite capable of multiplying within the nonimmune monocyte-macrophage. Listeriolysin O, a hemolysin structurally similar to streptolysin O, may be an important virulence factor in this process. Phagocytosis of the bacterium stimulates its production; it binds to cholesterol in cell membranes, leading to their disruption. This feature may allow the microorganism to escape from phagolysosomes but to persist and multiply within macrophages, ultimately leading to their destruction.

Factors external to the human host and the bacterium may also be important. Investigation of an outbreak of 36 cases of listeriosis in Philadelphia in 1986–1987 identified no predominant serotype. It is hypothesized that an epidemic co-infection may have triggered disease through an effect on the mucosal barrier or on intestinal motility in those previously merely colonized by *L. monocytogenes*.

Transmission from the pregnant woman to the fetus may occur either transplacentally or at the time of vaginal delivery. Listeriolysin O may increase uterine contractility and contribute to fetal loss.

CLINICAL MANIFESTATIONS. The incubation period between acquisition of infection and onset of disease varies from days to weeks. The clinical presentation of listeriosis is as meningitis in 50 to 60 per cent of cases; bacteremia without evident localized disease in 25 to 30 per cent; parenchymal disease of the central nervous system (CNS), with or without meningitis, in 10 per cent; and endocarditis in 5 per cent. Infrequent manifestations due to hematogenous dissemination include anterior uveitis, endophthalmitis, cervical lymphadenitis, pneumonia, empyema, pericarditis, peritonitis, hepatitis, liver abscess, cholecystitis, mycotic aneurysm, osteomyelitis, and arthritis.

Listeria monocytogenes is the etiologic agent in about 1 per cent of cases of acute bacterial meningitis. However, among patients with cancer, it is responsible for more than one fifth of episodes. Conversely, among patients with *Listeria* meningitis, 25 per cent have a malignancy; 25 per cent are transplant recipients; 20 per cent have another underlying disorder, such as diabetes mellitus or cirrhosis, or are receiving glucocorticosteroids; and 30 per cent have no predisposing condition. Two thirds of patients experience a fairly sudden onset of symptoms, but one third note an insidious progression over several days. No features distinguish *Listeria* meningitis. High fever is almost always reported. Headache, meningismus, and a decreased level of consciousness are present in more than one half of patients. Focal neurologic deficits and seizures are found in about one fourth. Most patients have 100 to 10,000 white blood cells per cubic millimeter of cerebrospinal fluid (CSF), with two thirds of them being polymorphonuclear cells. The CSF glucose level is less than 50 mg per deciliter in one half of cases, and the protein level is usually 50 to 300 mg per deciliter. The Gram stain of CSF is interpreted as revealing gram-positive bacilli in only 25 per cent of cases. Cultures of blood are positive in 60 to 75 per cent. The differential diagnosis includes disease due to *Streptococcus pneumoniae*, a gram-negative bacillus, or *Cryptococcus neoformans*.

Parenchymal disease of the CNS is associated with clinical and CSF findings of meningitis in only 50 per cent of cases. Anatomically, the spectrum of disease includes diffuse and localized cerebritis, brain stem meningoencephalitis (rhombencephalitis), and macroscopic abscess formation in the brain or spine. All patients are febrile; other common symptoms and signs are decreased consciousness in two thirds of patients, headache and hemiparesis in one half, and seizures and cranial nerve palsies in one third. *Listeria* rhombencephalitis merits special mention. Eight of the first 11 reported victims have been previously healthy. The illness has a biphasic course: A 3- to 10-day prodrome of fever, headache, and vomiting is terminated by the abrupt onset of palsies of cranial nerves V, VI, VII, IX, and/or X. In patients without concurrent meningitis, the analysis of CSF is usually normal or reveals only a mild pleocytosis and increased protein; Gram stain and culture are rarely positive. Blood cultures are positive in most patients with parenchymal CNS disease. The differential diagnosis includes tuberculosis, toxoplasmosis, nocardiosis, mycoses, and stroke.

Bacteremia without evident localized disease (primary bacteremia) occurs in patients with hematologic malignancies (33 per cent of cases), organ transplant recipients (25 per cent), pregnant women (13 per cent), and individuals suffering from alcoholism or cirrhosis (11 per cent). *Listeria* bacteremia has no distinguishing features. Up to one fourth have premonitory gastrointestinal symptoms: nausea, vomiting, abdominal pain, and/or diarrhea. Less frequently, upper respiratory symptoms may precede the onset of fever, chills, hypotension, tachycardia, and malaise.

Endocarditis occurs not in immunocompromised hosts but usually in those with underlying valvular heart disease. The aortic valve is involved in two thirds of cases and the mitral valve in one third, and prosthetic valve disease is well described. The onset of illness is subacute, with a median duration of symptoms prior to hospitalization of 5 weeks. Fever is cited in 75 per cent of reported cases, a new or changing murmur in 40 per cent, splenomegaly in 35 per cent, and hepatomegaly, CNS emboli, and pulmonary emboli each in 25 per cent.

One third of all cases of listeriosis are associated with pregnancy. Most commonly, in the third trimester, the mother develops a "flulike" illness with fever, sore throat, myalgias, crampy abdominal pain, and diarrhea. After 3 to 7 days, premature labor or abortion ensues. Transplacental transmission of disease becomes clinically evident in the newborn within hours of delivery; this severe septicemic illness is known as granulomatosis infantisepticum. Babies may also acquire infection in the birth canal or nosocomially in the nursery; at a mean of 14 days of life, disease presents as anorexia, fever, or meningismus. *Listeria monocytogenes* is the third most common cause of neonatal sepsis and meningitis after *Escherichia coli* and group B streptococci.

The complete spectrum of listeriosis is seen among patients with acquired immunodeficiency syndrome (AIDS), but the cumulative prevalence is much less than 1 per cent. Chemoprophylaxis of pneumocystosis with trimethoprim-sulfamethoxazole may prevent listeriosis.

TREATMENT. Ampicillin is the antimicrobial agent of choice for listeriosis. Although no comparative trials have been conducted, it has an established record of efficacy and can be administered safely even during pregnancy and infancy. The standard dosage in patients with meningitis is 200 mg per kilogram per day in six divided doses given intravenously. The duration of therapy necessary to effect a cure consistently is 3 weeks. Seriously ill and immunocompromised patients are treated with ampicillin plus gentamicin; the latter drug is administered intravenously in doses sufficient to yield peak serum concentrations of 5 to 8 μg per milliliter and predictable CSF concentrations of 1 to 2 μg per milliliter. The majority of the data from in vitro studies and animal model trials suggest that these two drugs act synergistically against *L. monocytogenes*.

Trimethoprim-sulfamethoxazole has emerged as the preferred therapy for patients allergic to penicillins. The combination is bactericidal at achievable serum and CSF concentrations. Ten case reports have appeared in the literature, including those of immunocompromised patients with CNS disease, and all 10 were cured. Experience to date suggests an initial dosage of 160 mg of trimethoprim plus 800 mg of sulfamethoxazole given intravenously every 12 hours in adults with normal renal function. Erythromycin and tetracycline are alternative therapies.

The inordinate number of treatment failures and relapses among patients treated with cephalosporins or chloramphenicol indicates that these agents are not to be used. Newer β-lactams, including imipenem, are not as active as ampicillin against *L. monocytogenes*. The quinolones do not appear to be sufficiently active at achievable concentrations to be useful clinically. There has been no significant change in the antimicrobial susceptibility profile of *L. monocytogenes* over the past two decades.

DIAGNOSIS. The microbiologic diagnosis of listeriosis is established by culture of blood, CSF, or tissue. In cases of granulomatosis infantisepticum, meconium, amniotic fluid, and lochia are cultured. Initial growth in the laboratory may be slow and may require several days. Unwary technicians may misinterpret these gram-positive bacilli as diphtheroids and label them contaminants.

PROGNOSIS. The overall mortality rate of *Listeria* meningitis is 30 per cent, being higher in patients with cancer, hypoglycorrhachia, or bacteremia and lower in previously healthy individuals. Parenchymal CNS disease and endocarditis are fatal in 50 per cent of cases.

PREVENTION. Individuals at increased risk should avoid raw milk, wash raw vegetables carefully, and cook meats thoroughly. In the hospital, patients with listeriosis should be isolated from immunocompromised hosts.

Carvajal A, Frederiksen W: Fatal endocarditis due to *Listeria monocytogenes*. Rev Infect Dis 10:616, 1988. *A detailed survey of 44 cases.*

Gellin BG, Broome CV: Listeriosis. JAMA 261:1313, 1989. *An excellent analysis focusing on pathogenesis and epidemiology.*

Nieman RE, Lorber B: Listeriosis in adults: A changing pattern. Report of eight cases and review of the literature, 1968–1978. Rev Infect Dis 2:207, 1980. *A comprehensive review of the clinical aspects of disease in 186 patients.*

Schlech WF III: Virulence characteristics of *Listeria monocytogenes*. Food Technol 42:176, 1988. *A concise discussion relating virulence factors to epidemiology.*

Schwartz B, Hexter D, Broome CV, et al.: Investigation of an outbreak of listeriosis: New hypotheses for the etiology of epidemic *Listeria monocytogenes* infections. J Infect Dis 159:680, 1989. *Description of an outbreak that may have been precipitated by a co-infecting organism.*

Stamm AM, Dismukes WE, Simmons BP, et al.: Listeriosis in renal transplant recipients: Report of an outbreak and review of 102 cases. Rev Infect Dis 4:665, 1982. *An extensive review of disease in an immunocompromised population.*

WHO Working Group: Foodborne listeriosis. Bull WHO 66:421, 1988. *An in-depth analysis of this problem.*

326 Erysipeloid

W. Edmund Farrar

DEFINITION. Erysipeloid is a localized skin infection that is almost always limited to the fingers and hands and is caused by *Erysipelothrix rhusiopathiae*. The term "erysipeloid" was coined by Rosenbach to distinguish the lesion from that of human erysipelas. Usually, only a single lesion is present, but diffuse skin involvement and endocarditis occur rarely.

ETIOLOGY. *E. rhusiopathiae* is a straight or slightly curved, thin, non–spore-forming gram-positive rod that grows readily on most ordinary laboratory media. It is nonmotile, catalase negative, nonhemolytic, or α-hemolytic on blood agar and able to form hydrogen sulfide on triple sugar iron (TSI) slants; these properties help to distinguish it from corynebacteria (diphtheroids) and *Listeria monocytogenes*.

EPIDEMIOLOGY. Human infection with *E. rhusiopathiae* almost always results from exposure to infected animals. Infection occurs worldwide in many species of wild and domestic animals, including, especially, swine, sheep, rodents, and birds. Disease in swine, sheep, turkeys, and ducks is of substantial economic importance. Although the organism appears not to cause disease in fish, it can grow and persist for long periods in the mucoid exterior slime of these animals. It can survive for months in soil after initial contamination and may remain viable in foods after salting, pickling, and smoking, but it is killed within 15 minutes by moist heat at 55°C. Most human cases are related to occupational exposure; individuals at greatest risk include butchers, fishermen, fish handlers, abattoir workers, veterinarians, and homemakers.

CLINICAL MANIFESTATIONS. Most human cases probably occur via scratches or puncture wounds of the skin. Within a few days after inoculation, itching, pain, and a characteristic violaceous erythema appear (see Color Plate 9G). The lesion may spread slowly to involve other fingers but rarely progresses beyond the wrist. Systemic effects are uncommon. Low-grade fever and arthralgias or arthritis occur in approximately one tenth of cases, and lymphangitis and lymphadenopathy occur in about a third. The absence of suppuration, along with the violaceous color, lack of pitting edema, and disproportionate pain, helps to distinguish erysipeloid from staphylococcal or streptococcal infection. Erysipeloid is a self-limited disease, and the lesions usually resolve within 3 or 4 weeks without therapy.

Approximately 50 cases of systemic infection with *E. rhusiopathiae* have been reported; 90 per cent of the patients had endocarditis. All but one involved native valves. Compared with endocarditis due to other microorganisms, infection with *E. rhusiopathiae* is more likely to occur in males (probably reflecting occupational exposure), is more likely to involve the aortic valve, and results in a higher mortality rate (38 per cent). In nearly 60 per cent of patients, endocarditis due to *E. rhusiopathiae* develops on previously normal heart valves. The clinical picture with respect to fever, peripheral skin stigmata of endocarditis, emboli, splenomegaly, hematuria, and mycotic aneurysm is similar to

that produced by other bacterial organisms. Antecedent or concurrent skin infection has been noted in only about a third of cases of endocarditis.

TREATMENT. Most strains of *E. rhusiopathiae* are highly susceptible to penicillins, cephalosporins, erythromycin, and clindamycin; most strains are resistant to sulfonamides, trimethoprim-sulfamethoxazole, aminoglycosides, and vancomycin. Although skin lesions usually heal spontaneously within 4 weeks, healing is hastened by antibiotic therapy. Oral penicillin V is probably the best choice for therapy.

Endocarditis or septicemia due to *E. rhusiopathiae* should be treated with large dosages of penicillin G (12 to 20 million units per day), given by the intravenous route, for 4 to 6 weeks. Cephalosporins may be used in patients who are allergic to penicillins. The resistance of *E. rhusiopathiae* to vancomycin is noteworthy because this agent is often used in empiric therapy for prosthetic valve endocarditis and in the treatment of native valve endocarditis caused by gram-positive organisms in individuals who are allergic to penicillins.

Barnett KJ, Estes SA, Wirman JA, et al.: Erysipeloid. J Am Acad Dermatol 9:116, 1983. *A good review of the clinical features and appearance of the lesions on electron microscopy and enunciation of the hypothesis that L-forms may play a role in the pathogenesis of the infection.*

Gorby GL, Peacock JE: *Erysipelothrix rhusiopathiae* endocarditis: Microbiologic, epidemiologic and clinical features of an occupational disease. Rev Infect Dis 10:317, 1988. *An up-to-date review that compares this infection with endocarditis due to other bacteria.*

Klauder JV: Erysipeloid as an occupational disease. JAMA 111:1345, 1938. *An account of the epidemiology of the infection in 100 patients, together with a vivid, illustrated clinical description.*

Reboli AC, Farrar WE: *Erysipelothrix rhusiopathiae*: An occupational pathogen. Clin Microbiol Rev 4:354, 1989. *A concise review of epidemiology, clinical features, and bacteriology.*

327 Actinomycosis

Ward E. Bullock

DEFINITION. Actinomycosis is a chronic bacterial infection that induces both a suppurative and a granulomatous inflammatory response. It spreads contiguously through anatomic barriers and frequently forms external sinuses, from which may extrude "sulfur granules" that are characteristic but not pathognomonic. The most common clinical forms are cervicofacial, thoracic, abdominal, and, in females, genital.

ETIOLOGY. Members of the genus *Actinomyces* are prokaryotes with cell walls that contain both muramic acid and diaminopimelic acid. Unlike the cell walls of fungi, the cell walls of these organisms do not contain sterols and are insensitive to polyene antibiotics. *Actinomyces israelii* is the species most often recovered from human cases of actinomycosis. However, *A. naeslundii*, *A. odontolyticus*, *A. viscosus*, *A. meyeri*, and a related genus, *Arachnia propionica*, cause identical clinical infections and bear close resemblance in primary culture. *Actinomyces bovis* produces "lumpy jaw" in cattle but is not a human pathogen. These gram-positive bacteria are filamentous (0.5 to 1.0 μm in diameter) with branching and are non–acid fast, with a tendency to break up into coccobacilli. They require anaerobic to microaerophilic conditions for growth, which is quite slow; usually, 3 to 10 or more days are required before these organisms can be macroscopically detected in culture.

EPIDEMIOLOGY. Actinomycosis is observed throughout the world, and its prevalence is unrelated to climate, occupation, race, or age. The disease has been reported more commonly in men than in women (3:1). However, since the recognition of pelvic actinomycosis in association with the use of intrauterine contraceptive devices (IUCD's), the male prevalence ratio may be decreasing. The number of cases of actinomycosis reported annually to the Centers for Disease Control is fewer than 100. These infections are not easily recognized by clinicians, and the organisms are fastidious; therefore, it is likely that the true incidence is substantially greater. Although many animal species are susceptible to actinomycosis, infection is neither transmissible from animal to human nor transmissible from person to person. *Actinomyces* species are part of the indigenous microbiota colonizing the teeth and oral cavity. They may also be found in the tonsillar crypts of asymptomatic individuals, in the fecal flora, and within the female reproductive tract.

PATHOGENESIS AND PATHOLOGY. The *Actinomyces* maintain their niche within the microbial community of the mouth by adherence to oral surfaces, especially to dental plaque, a thin film of salivary proteins and glycoproteins that coats the enamel surface. Adherence is achieved by complex protein-protein stereochemical interactions and by lectin-carbohydrate interactions, the latter of which also mediate cellular coaggregation of oral *Actinomyces* with *Streptococcus milleri*, *Streptococcus sanguis*, and other mouth flora. This propensity for coaggregation may explain, in part, why actinomycotic infections often are polymicrobic, with "associate" mouth flora frequently isolated from cervicofacial, thoracic, and central nervous system abscesses. The associate flora may play a synergistic role in infection by maintaining the low oxygen tension necessary for growth of the *Actinomyces*. To cause disease, these organisms must be introduced into tissue through a break in the mucous membrane resulting from dental infections and manipulations or from aspiration of infected dental debris. They may enter the abdominal cavity by perforation of the lower gastrointestinal tract or by ascending infection of the genital tract in women.

Actinomycotic infection evokes a combination of suppurative and granulomatous inflammatory responses that are accompanied by intense fibrosis. Plasma cells and multinucleated giant cells often are observed within lesions, as may be large macrophages with foamy cytoplasm around purulent centers. The infection spreads through fascial planes and ultimately may produce draining sinus tracts, especially in infections of the pelvis and abdomen. Sulfur granules within lesions and sinus drainage are a typical feature, though not always present. These granules are gritty aggregates of organisms measuring 1 to 2 mm in diameter; the centers have a basophilic staining property, with eosinophilic rays terminating in pear-shaped "clubs" on the surface. They contain calcium phosphate, probably as a result of phosphatase activity of both the host and the organisms.

CLINICAL MANIFESTATIONS. Cervicofacial actinomycosis comprises 50 to 60 per cent of reported cases. Infection is usually observed in a setting of poor oral hygiene with tooth decay, periodontal disease, or gingivitis, in which mucosal integrity is disrupted by dental manipulations or other injury. The infection generally evolves as a chronic or subacute soft tissue swelling or mass involving the submandibular or paramandibular region. The swelling may have a ligneous consistency that is caused by tissue fibrosis. More rapidly developing lesions often simulate pyogenic infections. Trismus may be present, and advanced lesions may discharge odorless pus containing "sulfur granules" through one or more sinuses. Fever, pain, and leukocytosis may be present. The infection can extend to the tongue, salivary glands, pharynx, and larynx. Bone (most commonly the mandible) may be invaded from the adjacent soft tissue. Cervical spine or cranial bone infection may lead to subdural empyema and invasion of the central nervous system. The differential diagnosis includes tuberculosis (scrofula), fungal infections, nocardiosis, suppurative infections by other organisms, and neoplasms.

Thoracic actinomycosis comprises 15 to 30 per cent of the disease spectrum and usually results from aspiration of infective material from the oropharynx. Less commonly, thoracic infection may be introduced by esophageal perforation, by extension into the mediastinum from the neck, or by spread from an abdominal site; hematogenous spread to the lung is rare. Pulmonary actinomycosis commonly spreads from an early pneumonic focus across lung fissures to involve the pleura and the chest wall, with eventual fistula formation and drainage containing sulfur granules (Fig. 327–1). Granules rarely are present in the sputum. The incidence of this complication, as well as the destruction of thoracic vertebrae and adjacent ribs, has declined in the antibiotic era.

The complaints of patients with thoracic actinomycosis are nonspecific. The most common of these are a productive cough,

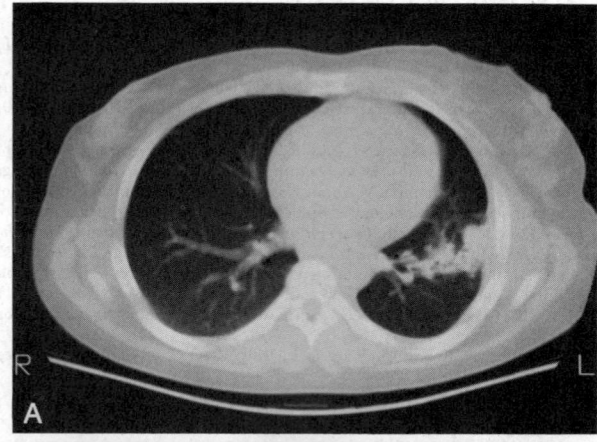
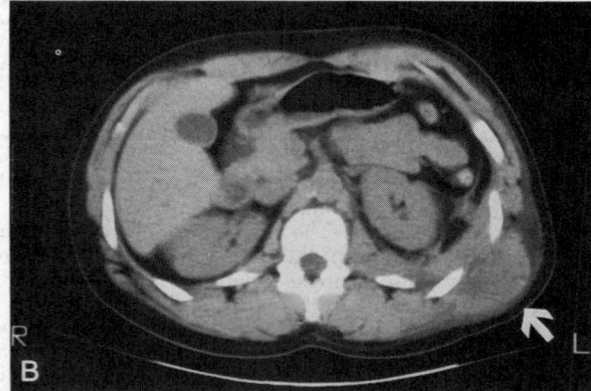

FIGURE 327–1. Thoracic computed tomographic (CT) scan of a 43-year-old woman with pulmonary actinomycosis. There is consolidation within the left lung and pleural thickening adjacent to the parenchymal disease (*A*). Abscess extended into the left breast and inferiorly to the costophrenic sulcus, to the retroperitoneum, and into the lateral abdominal wall (*arrow*) (*B*).

dyspnea, weight loss, fever, and chest pain. Anemia, mild leukocytosis, and an elevated sedimentation rate are relatively common. There often is a history of underlying lung disease, and patients rarely present in an early stage of infection. The pulmonary lesions may resemble tuberculosis, especially when cavity formation occurs, and blastomycosis, which may destroy ribs posteriorly but rarely form sinuses. Nocardiosis, bronchogenic carcinoma, and lymphoma can also mimic thoracic actinomycosis.

ABDOMINAL-PELVIC ACTINOMYCOSIS. Actinomycosis of the abdomen and pelvis is a chronic, localized inflammatory process that often is preceded weeks or months by surgery for acute appendicitis with perforation or for perforated colonic diverticulitis, or by emergency surgery upon the lower intestinal tract after trauma. Occasionally, abdominal actinomycosis may manifest without identifiable predisposing factors. The ileocecal region is involved most frequently, with the formation of a mass lesion. The infection extends slowly to contiguous organs, especially the liver, and may involve retroperitoneal tissues, the spine, or the abdominal wall. Persistent draining sinuses may form, and those involving the perianal region can simulate Crohn's disease or tuberculosis. The extensive fibrosis of actinomycotic lesions, presenting to the examiner as a mass, often suggests tumor. Constitutional symptoms and signs are nonspecific; the most common are fever, weight loss, nausea, vomiting, and pain.

An association has been recognized between long-term use of IUCD's and actinomycosis of the genital tract. Manifestations of infection may range from a chronic vaginal discharge to pelvic inflammatory disease with tubo-ovarian abscesses or pseudomalignant masses. No association exists between actinomycotic infection and the type of IUCD employed. Accurate data on the prevalence and incidence of infection among IUCD users are sparse, since cytologic criteria and fluorescent antibody staining techniques are the principal means of detecting *Actinomyces* in vaginal smears and other genital tract specimens. Anaerobic cultures of the female genital tract generally are unsuccessful.

Currently, it is generally agreed that *Actinomyces* species may be part of the indigenous genital tract flora of females and that demonstration of their presence by morphologic criteria and fluorescent antibody stains does not predict disease. However, colonization of the endometrium appears to require the presence of an IUCD. Although many cases of genital-pelvic actinomycosis associated with IUCD use have been reported, the actual incidence of disease appears to be low relative to the millions of those who use IUCD's.

Central nervous system (CNS) and disseminated actinomycosis are very uncommon. Most infections of the CNS manifest as encapsulated brain abscesses that are indistinguishable from those caused by other organisms. Most actinomycotic infections of the CNS are thought to be seeded hematogenously from a distant primary site; however, direct extension of cervicofacial disease is well recognized. Sinus formation is not a characteristic of CNS disease. The rare meningitis caused by *Actinomyces* is chronic and basilar in location, and the pleocytosis usually is lymphocytic. Thus, it may be misdiagnosed as tuberculous meningitis.

Unlike *Nocardia* species, *Actinomyces* usually are not opportunistic in the immunocompromised host. To date, few systemic actinomycotic infections have been reported among patients with the acquired immunodeficiency syndrome (AIDS).

DIAGNOSIS. Critical to the diagnosis of actinomycosis is a high index of suspicion that is communicated to the microbiology diagnostic laboratory, along with material from draining sinuses, from deep needle aspiration, or from biopsy specimens. Anaerobic culture is required, and no selective media are available to restrict overgrowth of the slow-growing *Actinomyces* by associated microflora. The presence in pus or tissue specimens of non–acid-fast, gram-positive organisms with filamentous branching is very suggestive of the diagnosis. The characteristic morphology of "sulfur granules" and the presence of gram-positive organisms within are helpful. However, the granules must be distinguished from similar structures that are sometimes produced in infections and that are caused by *Nocardia, Monosporium, Cephalosporium, Staphylococcus* (botryomycosis), and others. *Actinomyces* and *Arachnia* generally can be differentiated from other gram-positive anaerobes by means of growth rate (slow), by catalase production (negative, except *A. viscosus*), and by gas-liquid chromatographic detection of acetic, lactic, and succinic acids produced in peptone-yeast-glucose broth. Direct fluorescent antibody conjugates can be employed to detect *Actinomyces* in clinical material or culture but are not readily available to clinical microbiology laboratories. There are no reliable serologic tests or skin tests.

TREATMENT. Penicillin G is the drug of choice for treatment of infection caused by any of the *Actinomyces*. It is given in high dosage over a prolonged period, since the infection has a tendency to recur, presumably because antibiotic penetration to areas of fibrosis and necrosis and into "sulfur granules" may be poor. Most deep-seated infections can be expected to respond to intravenous penicillin G, 10 to 20 million units per day given for 2 to 6 weeks, followed by an oral phenoxypenicillin in a dosage of 2 to 4 grams per day. A few additional weeks of oral penicillin therapy may suffice for uncomplicated cervicofacial disease; complicated cases and extensive pulmonary or abdominal disease may require treatment for 12 to 18 months. To date, little evidence exists of acquired resistance to penicillin G by *Actinomyces* during prolonged therapy. Radical excision of large sinus tracts should be considered in some cases. Alternative first-line antibiotics for treatment of infection caused by *Actinomyces* include tetracycline, erythromycin, and clindamycin. First-generation cephalosporins and imipenem also are highly effective. Antifungal drugs are not active against these organisms. In vitro antibiotic sensitivity testing of *Actinomyces* is difficult, and the results may not be predictive of antibiotic activity in vivo.

The need to employ combination antibiotic therapy to attack microorganisms that are isolated in association with *Actinomyces* has not been established. The generally good results obtained with penicillin G alone over nearly three decades indicate that monotherapy is effective in most cases. In complicated infections of the lower abdomen, where anaerobic gram-negative organisms, among others, may be the "associates," combination antibiotic therapy is appropriate.

The presence of organisms presumed to be *Actinomyces* on a Papanicolaou smear, obtained from an asymptomatic female with or without an IUCD in place, is not an indication for therapy. When patients experience well-defined IUCD-related symptoms and Papanicolaou smears demonstrate *Actinomyces* by specific fluorescent-labeled antibody, the device should be removed. Antibiotic administration for a 2-week period may be indicated. More serious infections require prolonged therapy as recommended above.

PROGNOSIS. The advent of antibiotics has greatly improved the prognosis for all forms of actinomycosis. At present, cure rates are high, and neither deformity nor death is common.

Bennhoff DF: Actinomycosis: Diagnostic and therapeutic considerations and a review of 32 cases. Laryngoscope 94:1198, 1984. *A helpful general review.*

Bernardi RS: Abdominal actinomycosis. Surg Gynecol Obstet 149:257, 1979. *A thorough review of all aspects of actinomycosis, with emphasis on the abdominal form.*

Cisar JO, Sandberg AL, Clark WB: Actinomycosis of the central nervous system. Rev Infect Dis 9:855, 1987. *A good review of 70 cases of CNS actinomycosis.*

Flynn MW, Felson B: The roentgen manifestations of thoracic actinomycosis. AJR 110:707, 1970. *An outstanding guide to roentgenographic diagnosis of pulmonary actinomycosis.*

Nayar M, Chandra M, Chitraratha K, et al.: Incidence of actinomycetes infection in women using intrauterine contraceptive devices. Acta Cytol 29:111, 1985. *Ten of 350 women using intrauterine contraceptive devices (IUD's) had Actinomyces-like organisms in Papanicolaou-stained smears; 8 of the 10 were symptomatic. Seven of the 10 patients had been using an IUD for more than 2 years.*

Richtsmeier WJ, Johns ME: Actinomycosis of the head and neck. CRC Crit Rev Clin Lab Sci 11:175, 1979. *An excellent review, with an emphasis on infection of the head and neck.*

Smego RA Jr: Molecular aspects of adherence of Actinomyces viscosus and Actinomyces naeslundii to oral surfaces. J Dent Res 68:1558, 1989. *A brief summary for those wishing to know more about adherence mechanisms.*

328 Nocardiosis
Ward E. Bullock

DEFINITION. Nocardiosis is a subacute or chronic bacterial infection that evokes a suppurative response. The most common sites of primary infection are, first, the lung and then the skin, from which bacteria may disseminate hematogenously to the central nervous system and other tissues. The infection often pursues a more acute and aggressive course in immunosuppressed patients.

ETIOLOGY. *Nocardia* species are gram-positive, aerobic actinomycetes, many of which are weakly acid fast in tissue or on initial isolation. They reproduce by filamentous branching, with fragmentation into bacillary and coccoid forms. *Nocardia* species are distributed widely in nature and commonly are found in soil, grasses, and rotting vegetation. Of the three species that cause most infections in humans, *N. asteroides* is by far the predominant pathogen. *N. caviae, N. farcinica,* and *N. brasiliensis* also produce pulmonary and disseminated infections, but much less frequently. *N. brasiliensis* is the most common cause of actinomycetoma in Latin and South America.

INCIDENCE AND PREVALENCE. A 1976 survey estimated the incidence of nocardiosis in the United States to be 500 to 1000 new cases per year. At present, the incidence undoubtedly is higher as a consequence of an expanding population of individuals who are immunosuppressed iatrogenically or by underlying diseases. Nocardiosis has been reported worldwide in all ages and races, and is two to three times more common in men than in women. No occupation-related risks have been found. Thus, possible hormonal effects on bacterial growth or virulence have been postulated.

EPIDEMIOLOGY. The majority of infections caused by *N. asteroides* are encountered in patients with impairment of cell-mediated immunity (CMI). However, the organism clearly is capable of infecting apparently normal persons. Nocardiosis presumably is acquired by inhalation of airborne bacteria, since the primary site of infection is the lung in the majority of cases. Other mammals can be infected. However, no well-established evidence exists for animal-to-person transmission or for person-to-person transmission. Occasional clusters of nocardial infection have been reported among immunosuppressed hospital patients, suggesting possible nosocomial acquisition. *Nocardia asteroides* has been recovered from the sputum, skin, and other body regions of patients who do not have apparent disease. Nevertheless, repeated isolation of *Nocardia* species from any immunocompromised person should be considered evidence of infection rather than colonization, and treatment should be initiated. Nocardiosis can manifest as a primary cutaneous infection (especially *N. brasiliensis*) after inoculation through local injury and may disseminate to other organs.

PATHOGENESIS AND PATHOLOGY. The typical nocardial lesion within the lung and other tissues is one of liquefactive necrosis with abscess formation. Polymorphonuclear leukocytes predominate in association with varying proportions of macrophages and lymphocytes. Granuloma formation is infrequent, and in contrast with actinomycotic lesions, fibrosis is rare. Confluent daughter abscesses are common. Sulfur granules are not present in visceral lesions, as they are in actinomycosis. However, they may be seen in nocardial lesions of the skin.

That CMI plays a major role in host defense against nocardiosis is suggested by the fact that immunocompromised patients are prone to this infection. The importance of antigen-specific T lymphocyte immune function is illustrated by the increased susceptibility of athymic nude mice to *Nocardia* infection and by the capacity of T lymphocytes from rabbits immunized with *N. asteroides* to augment phagocytosis and growth inhibition of these organisms by macrophages. Neutrophils exhibit poor nocardicidal activity in vitro but may inhibit growth of organisms during an early phase of infection prior to maturation of cellular immune responses.

Among the mechanisms that may be employed by *N. asteroides* to counter host defenses are inhibition of lysosome-phagosome fusion that enables phagocytic cells to kill ingested bacteria, production of superoxide dismutase and catalase, and the capacity to block the acidification of parasitized phagosomes.

Nocardia species are not visible in tissue specimens stained by hematoxylin and eosin or by the periodic acid–Schiff procedure. They can be visualized by a tissue Gram stain or after slight overstaining by the Gomori methenamine silver method, which demonstrates the filamentous structure of the organisms. Many *Nocardia* are weakly acid fast and can be seen on a modified Ziehl-Neelsen stain.

CLINICAL MANIFESTATIONS. Pulmonary infection is the most frequent manifestation of nocardiosis (about 75 per cent of the reported cases). The clinical manifestations are nonspecific and include fever, cough, weight loss, and dyspnea. The range of pulmonary involvement extends from transient or inapparent infection to confluent bronchopneumonia with complete consolidation. Radiographic examination of the chest may reveal one or more of the following: fluffy infiltrates, multiple abscess formation with cavitation in 10 to 20 per cent of cases, bulging fissures, masses, nodules, and empyema. Hilar involvement and calcification are infrequent. *Nocardia* can disseminate to other organs from pulmonary lesions, especially in patients who are immunosuppressed following organ transplantation. Patients who have received extensive x-irradiation and chemotherapy for malignancies and those who are treated with steroids in high dosage also are prone to metastatic infection, and evidence thereof should be sought aggressively.

In 20 to 40 per cent of patients with pulmonary nocardiosis, dissemination to the central nervous system occurs, and therefore, computed tomography (CT) scanning of the head should be considered. Loculated brain abscesses, either singular or multiple, are common and are often accompanied by headache and focal neurologic findings; meningitis is infrequent. Other common sites of dissemination include the skin and subcutaneous tissues, kidneys, eyes, liver, and lymph nodes. In cases of apparently localized nocardial lesions of skin, it is important to distinguish between the possibilities of primary inoculation and hematogenous dissemination to the skin from another site.

DIAGNOSIS. The clinical and radiographic findings in pulmonary nocardiosis are nonspecific. Consequently, it may be confused with a variety of other bacterial infections of the lung,

including actinomycosis and tuberculosis, as well as fungal infections and malignancies. Alertness to the possibility of nocardiosis can expedite the diagnostic workup, especially in immunosuppressed patients, in whom the disease may coexist with other opportunistic infections. Cultures and stains should be done on specimens of sputum, pleural fluid, and bronchial lavage fluid, as well as on percutaneous lung aspirates or open lung biopsy specimens. Needle biopsy of cerebral mass lesions should be considered strongly in patients with the acquired immunodeficiency syndrome (AIDS) who have pulmonary nocardiosis because of the multiplicity of infections and tumors that can manifest in a similar manner.

Skin lesions should be aspirated if fluctuant, or biopsied, and specimens should be submitted for culture and the smear preparations or histologic sections examined for organisms. Nocardiosis can often be diagnosed with a high degree of confidence by direct examination of sputum or purulent material. The presence of gram-positive, filamentous branching rods that stain unevenly with crystal violet to give a beaded appearance is highly suggestive of either *Actinomyces* or *Nocardia*. If the organisms are acid fast on a modified Ziehl-Neelsen stain, the probability of *Nocardia* is high. However, lack of acid-fast staining does not exclude *Nocardia*.

Nocardia species are not fastidious and grow aerobically, though slowly, on routinely used media. Characteristic heaped, waxy colonies, often colored tan, orange, or even purple, may be seen after 2 to 7 days of culture. Longer times may be required. Thus, the microbiology laboratory should be advised of possible nocardiosis to ensure that plates are held for 10 to 14 days and that steps are taken to limit overgrowth by microbial contaminants, particularly in sputum samples. The use of defined carbon-free medium to which paraffin is added may enhance the chances of isolating *N. asteroides* from sputum because it can utilize paraffin as a sole source of carbon, in contrast to most other organisms. Several simple tests can assist in the presumptive differentiation of *Nocardia* from other aerobic actinomycetes and from rapidly growing *Mycobacteria*, as, for example, the decomposition of casein, xanthine, tyrosine, and 1 per cent ethylene glycol. However, most clinical laboratories should rely on reference facilities for definitive taxonomic designations.

TREATMENT. The sulfonamides are equally efficacious and are first-line agents for treatment, as is the combination of trimethoprim-sulfamethoxazole (TMP-SMX). Typically, sulfadiazine should be given in a dosage of 6 to 10 grams per day, with adjustment as needed to achieve peak serum levels of 12 to 15 mg per deciliter. These antimicrobials penetrate the central nervous system and other body compartments well. A high percentage of *Nocardia* isolates are sensitive to sulfonamides and to TMP-SMX by in vitro testing. However, the techniques of in vitro sensitivity testing with *Nocardia* have not been standardized, in part because of technical difficulties created by slow growth in culture and problems in obtaining a homogeneous suspension of cells for standardization of the inoculum. Thus, the results of in vitro tests frequently are poor predictors of in vivo efficacy and should be interpreted with caution.

Not all patients respond to sulfonamide or TMP-SMX therapy. Acquisition of resistance to the sulfonamides during therapy has been documented, and metastatic lesions can appear during the course of apparently successful treatment. Hypersensitivity reactions or hemopoietic toxicity induced by these drugs may force discontinuation of treatment, especially in patients with AIDS. The alternative antibiotics that have proved to be most efficacious, both in vitro and clinically, are minocycline, amikacin, and imipenem. Ceftriaxone, cefuroxime, and cefotaxime display in vitro activity against many strains of *Nocardia*. However, it remains to be determined if the last-named three antibiotics will prove valuable for treatment of nocardiosis. Although some in vitro studies indicate that certain combinations of antibiotics may exert synergistic activity against *Nocardia*, no good clinical evidence exists that combination antibiotic regimens are superior to single-agent therapy.

Treatment should be prolonged, since relapse of nocardiosis is common. In patients with intact host defenses, treatment should be continued for 6 weeks after clinical recovery. In those who have AIDS or who are otherwise immunocompromised, treatment should be continued for a year or more. As a rule, it is necessary to perform surgical drainage of brain abscesses, empyema, and subcutaneous abscesses. Patients with cerebral nocardiosis or other deep abscesses should be monitored by serial CT scans. If patients are receiving immunosuppressive drugs, the dosage should be reduced if at all possible.

PROGNOSIS. The prognosis for clinical cure of nocardiosis is influenced by the location of the infection, by pre-existing impairment of cellular immunity from underlying disease or drug therapy, and by the aggressiveness of the patient's management. Mortality rates range from near 0 per cent in patients with isolated skin lesions to more than 40 per cent in cases of central nervous system involvement. The overall mortality rate in patients with pulmonary disease is in the range of 15 to 30 per cent, even in those who are immunocompromised.

Barnicoat MJ, Wierzbicki AS, Norman PM: Cerebral nocardiosis in immunosuppressed patients: Five cases. Q J Med 268:689, 1989. *Presentation of five cases with a good bibliography on the topic.*

Feigin DS: Nocardiosis of the lung: Chest radiographic findings in 21 cases. Radiology 159:9, 1986. *A good descriptive study.*

McNeil MM, Brown JM, Jarvis WR, et al.: Comparison of species distribution and antimicrobial susceptibility of aerobic actinomycetes from clinical specimens. Rev Infect Dis 12:778, 1990.

Palmer DL, Harvey RL, Wheeler JK: Diagnostic and therapeutic considerations in *Nocardia asteroides* infection. Medicine 53:391, 1974. *A comprehensive literature review of 243 cases of nocardiosis (including 13 patients in the authors' own experience).*

Smego RA Jr, Moeller MB, Gallis HA: Trimethoprim-sulfamethoxazole therapy for *Nocardia* infections. Arch Intern Med 143:711, 1983. *This article provides an extensive literature review and discusses TMP-SMX in depth.*

Wallace RJ Jr, Steele LC, Sumter G, et al.: Antimicrobial susceptibility patterns of *Nocardia asteroides*. Antimicrob Agents Chemother 32:1776, 1988. *An examination of antibiotic sensitivity patterns among 78 clinical isolates of N. asteroides by a group experienced in the complexities of in vitro sensitivity testing with these organisms.*

Wilson JP, Turner HR, Kirchner KA, et al.: Nocardial infections in renal transplant recipients. Medicine 68:38, 1989. *A current and well-written review of nocardiosis, with emphasis upon disease manifestations in renal transplant patients.*

329 Brucellosis

Robert A. Salata

DEFINITION. Bacteria of the genus *Brucella* cause disease with protean manifestations. Transmission of infection to humans from animals occurs as a consequence of occupational exposure or ingestion of contaminated milk products. Despite the attempt to institute effective control measures, brucellosis remains a significant health and economic burden in many countries.

ETIOLOGY. Brucellae are slow-growing, small, aerobic, nonmotile, nonencapsulated, non–spore-forming, gram-negative coccobacilli. *B. abortus*, *B. suis*, *B. melitensis*, and *B. canis* are known to infect humans and are typed on the basis of biochemical, metabolic, and immunologic criteria. There are differences in virulence among these four species. *B. abortus*, with a reservoir in cattle, usually is associated with mild sporadic disease; suppurative or disabling complications are rare. *B. suis* infection, resulting from swine contact, is often associated with destructive, suppurative lesions and may have a prolonged course. *B. melitensis*, with a reservoir in sheep and goats, may cause severe, acute disease and disabling complications. *B. canis*, spread to humans from infected dogs, causes disease with an insidious onset, frequent relapse, and a chronic course that is indistinguishable from infection related to *B. abortus*.

EPIDEMIOLOGY. Over 500,000 cases of brucellosis are reported yearly to the World Health Organization. *B. melitensis* infection, distributed primarily in the Mediterranean region, Latin America, and Asia, accounts for the majority of cases. *B. abortus* infection occurs worldwide but has been effectively eradicated in several European countries, Japan, and Israel. *B. suis* occurs mainly in the midwestern United States, South America, and Southeast Asia, whereas *B. canis* infection is most common in North and South America, Japan, and Central Europe.

In association with effective control programs in animals, human brucellosis has decreased dramatically in the United States, from over 6000 cases in 1947 to fewer than 200 cases

since 1980 (Fig. 329–1). States reporting the greatest number of cases include Texas, California, Virginia, and Florida. In North America, brucellosis occurs mainly in spring and summer and is most common in adult males, usually related to occupational exposure.

Brucella infection in the United States most frequently occurs in high-risk groups, including slaughterhouse workers, farmers and dairymen, veterinarians, travelers to endemic areas, and laboratory workers handling the organisms. Over one half of reported cases occur in the meat-processing industry, particularly in the kill areas, where infection is spread through abraded or lacerated skin and the conjunctiva, possibly by aerosolization, and rarely by ingestion of infected tissue. Many cases of *B. abortus* infection in veterinarians have accidentally occurred from the strain 19 vaccine used to immunize cattle. In American travelers or immigrants, Mexico has been the most frequent source of *B. melitensis* infection, transmitted through the ingestion of goat's milk cheese. *Brucella* infections associated with unpasteurized milk and accidental strain vaccine injections may account for an increasing proportion of cases reported in the United States.

Brucellosis in children accounts for only 3 to 10 per cent of all reported cases, is most common in endemic areas, and is often a mild, self-limited process. There is no convincing evidence to associate *Brucella* infection with abortion in humans.

PATHOGENESIS AND IMMUNITY. After penetrating the epithelial cells of human skin, conjunctiva, pharynx, or lung, *Brucella* organisms initially induce an exuberant polymorphonuclear neutrophil response in the submucosa. Following ingestion of organisms by neutrophils and tissue macrophages, spread to regional lymph nodes occurs. If host defenses within the lymph nodes are overwhelmed, bacteremia follows. The usual incubation period between infection and bacteremia is 1½ to 3 weeks. Bacteremia is accompanied by phagocytosis of free *Brucella* organisms by neutrophils and localization of bacteria primarily to the spleen, liver, and bone marrow, with the formation of granulomas.

If the inoculum is large and the patient is untreated, large granulomas may form, suppurate, and serve as a source of persistent bacteremia with the potential for multiorgan spread.

Both virulent and attenuated strains of *Brucella* are readily phagocytized by neutrophils after opsonization with normal human serum. Whole bacteria and extracts of *Brucella* species may inhibit neutrophil oxidative burst activity and degranulation. Intracellular killing of ingested bacteria has been demonstrated

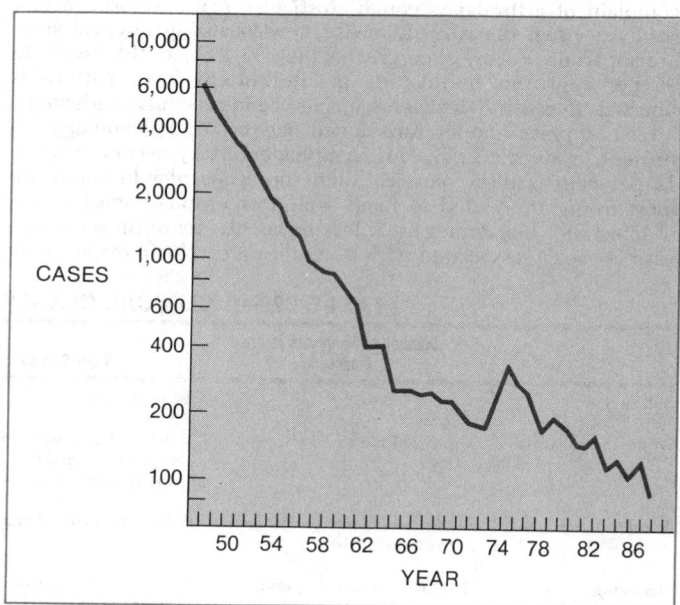

FIGURE 329–1. Incidence of human brucellosis, United States, 1947 to 1988. Following the implementation of eradication programs in cattle, the incidence of human brucellosis in the United States has steadily declined from 6321 cases in 1947 to fewer than 100 cases in 1988.

with *B. abortus* but not *B. melitensis*; this may explain differences in pathogenicity between these species.

Humoral factors may be important in the host defense against *Brucella*. Even in the absence of specific agglutinating antibody, normal human serum is bactericidal for *Brucella* organisms; *B. abortus* is more susceptible to serum lysis than is *B. melitensis*. The intracellular location of the organism may provide a means for the bacteria to escape the lethal effects of serum. Specific serum agglutinating antibody has opsonic activity but does not correlate with the development of protective immunity.

A role for mononuclear phagocytes and cell-mediated immunity in brucellosis has been demonstrated. Protection against *Brucella* infection in animals is associated with preceding infection with *Listeria monocytogenes* or *Mycobacterium tuberculosis*, both of which stimulate cell-mediated immune mechanisms. Skin testing with *Brucella* proteins elicits a typical delayed hypersensitivity response in infected individuals. Macrophages, activated with lymphokines, kill *Brucella* in vitro. In some cases of chronic brucellosis, depressed proliferative responses to classic T cell mitogens or to *Brucella* antigen occur. An increased incidence of *Brucella* infection has been seen in patients with Hodgkin's disease and other lymphomas.

CLINICAL MANIFESTATIONS. Clinically, human brucellosis may be conveniently divided into subclinical illness, acute/subacute disease, localized disease and complications, relapsing infection, and chronic disease (Table 329–1).

Subclinical Illness. Detected only by serologic testing, asymptomatic or clinically unrecognized human brucellosis often occurs in high-risk groups, including slaughterhouse workers, farmers, and veterinarians. Greater than 50 per cent of abattoir workers and up to 33 per cent of veterinarians have high anti-*Brucella* antibody titers but no history of recognized clinical infection. Children in endemic areas frequently have subclinical illness. Subclinical cases outnumber clinically evident cases of brucellosis by 12 to 1.

Acute and Subacute Disease. After an incubation period of several weeks or months, acute brucellosis may occur as a mild, transient illness (with *B. abortus* or *B. canis*) or as an explosive, toxic illness with the potential for multiple complications (with *B. melitensis*). Approximately 50 per cent of patients have an abrupt onset over days, while the remainder have an insidious onset over weeks. Symptoms in brucellosis are protean and nonspecific. Over 90 per cent of patients experience malaise, chills, sweats, fatigue, and weakness. More than 50 per cent of patients have myalgias, anorexia, and weight loss. Fewer patients complain of arthralgias, cough, testicular pain, dysuria, ocular pain, or visual blurring. Likewise, few localizing physical signs are apparent. Fever, often greater than 39.4°C (103°F), occurs in 95 per cent. An undulating or intermittent fever pattern is unusual. Because *Brucella* organisms are intracellular pathogens, a relative pulse-temperature deficit may occur. Splenomegaly is present in 10 to 15 per cent, lymphadenopathy occurs in up to 14 per cent (axillary, cervical, and supraclavicular locations are most frequent, related to hand-wound or oropharyngeal routes of infection); hepatomegaly is less frequent. Acute/subacute disease is usually associated with a significant serologic response by the standard tube agglutination assay. Other laboratory findings in acute or subacute disease may include mild anemia, lymphopenia or neutropenia (especially with bacteremia), lymphocytosis, thrombocytopenia, or (rarely) pancytopenia. The majority of infected individuals recover completely without sequelae if the diagnosis is appropriately made and prompt therapy is initiated.

Localized Disease and Complications. *Brucella* organisms may localize in almost any organ, most commonly in bone, central nervous system, heart, lung, spleen, testes, liver, gallbladder, kidney, prostate, and skin. Localized disease may occur simultaneously at multiple sites. Localized complications most often appear in association with a more chronic course of illness, although complications may occur with acute disease due to *B. melitensis* or *B. suis*. In the United States, localized disease is most frequently related to *B. suis*.

Relapsing Infection. Up to 10 per cent of patients with brucellosis relapse after antimicrobial therapy. This probably results from the intracellular location of the organisms, which protects the bacteria from certain antibiotics and host defense mechanisms. Relapses occur most frequently within months after initial infection but may occur as long as 2 years after apparently successful treatment. Relapsing infection is difficult to distinguish from reinfection in high-risk groups with continued exposure. Nearly all relapsed cases respond to a repeated course of antimicrobial agents.

Chronic Disease. Disease with a duration greater than 1 year has been called chronic brucellosis. A majority of patients classified as having chronic brucellosis really have persistent disease caused by inadequate treatment of the initial episode, or they have focal disease in bone, liver, or spleen. About 20 per cent of patients diagnosed as having chronic brucellosis complain of persistent fatigue, malaise, and depression. These symptoms frequently are not associated with clinical, microbiologic, or serologic evidence of active infection.

DIAGNOSIS. Many more common illnesses mimic the clinical presentation of brucellosis. The most conclusive means of establishing the diagnosis of brucellosis is by positive cultures from normally sterile body fluids or tissues. Special media are necessary because of the unusual metabolic requirements and slow growth of *Brucella*. The culture of *Brucella* organisms is potentially hazardous to laboratory personnel; a laboratory should not undertake isolation and identification of *Brucella* unless Biosafety Level 3 facilities are available. Therefore, most cases of brucellosis are diagnosed by serologic testing.

In acute brucellosis, positive blood cultures are obtained in 10 to 30 per cent of cases (as high as 85 per cent with *B. melitensis*). Blood culture positivity decreases with increasing duration of illness. With *B. melitensis* infection, bone marrow cultures are of higher yield than are blood cultures. Blood cultures processed in radiometric detection systems may yield positive cultures in less than 10 days. With localized brucellosis (e.g., lymph nodes, spleen, liver, or skeletal system), cultures of purulent material or tissues usually yield *Brucella* organisms. Culture of cerebrospinal fluid is positive in 45 per cent of patients with meningitis. Antibody against *Brucella* may be demonstrated in cerebrospinal fluid by enzyme-linked immunosorbent assay (ELISA).

Most patients mount significant serologic responses to *Brucella* infections. The most frequently utilized test is the standard tube

TABLE 329–1. CLINICAL CLASSIFICATION OF HUMAN BRUCELLOSIS

	Duration of Symptoms Before Diagnosis	Major Symptoms and Signs	Diagnosis	Comments
Subclinical	—	Asymptomatic	Positive (low titer) serology, negative cultures	Occurs in abattoir workers, farmers, and veterinarians
Acute and subacute	Up to 2–3 mo and 3 mo to 1 yr	Malaise, chills, sweats, fatigue, headache, anorexia, arthralgias, fever, splenomegaly, lymphadenopathy, hepatomegaly	Positive serology, positive blood or bone marrow cultures	Presentation can be mild, self-limited (*B. abortus*), or fulminant with severe complications (*B. melitensis*)
Localized	Occurs with acute or chronic untreated disease	Related to involved organs	Positive serology, positive cultures in specific tissues	Bone/joint, genitourinary, hepatosplenic involvement most common
Relapsing	2–3 mo after initial episode	Same as acute illness but may have higher fever, more fatigue, weakness, chills, and sweats	Positive serology, positive cultures	May be extremely difficult to distinguish relapse from reinfection
Chronic	Greater than 1 yr	Nonspecific presentation but neuropsychiatric symptoms and low-grade fever most common	Low titer or negative serology, cultures negative	Most controversial classification; localized disease may be associated

agglutination (STA) test, measuring antibody to *B. abortus* antigen. A fourfold or greater rise in titer to 1:160 or higher is considered significant. A presumptive case is one in which the agglutination titer is positive (≥1:160) in single or serial specimens, with symptoms consistent with brucellosis. By 3 weeks of illness, over 97 per cent of patients demonstrate serologic evidence of infection. Several problems exist, however, with the STA test. This test equally detects antibodies to *B. abortus*, *B. suis*, and *B. melitensis*, but not to *B. canis*. Serologic confirmation of *B. canis* infection requires *B. canis* or *B. ovis* antigen. Despite adequate antibiotic treatment, significant STA titers can persist for up to 2 years in 5 to 7 per cent of cases. As the STA titer may remain elevated, it is not useful in differentiating relapsing infection from other febrile illnesses in patients with past *Brucella* infections. Individuals with subclinical infection may demonstrate significant STA titers. In chronic localized brucellosis, STA titers may appear absent or low owing to a prozone phenomenon. This prozone effect appears to be related to the presence of immunoglobulin G (IgG) or immunoglobulin A (IgA) blocking antibodies; it can be eliminated if dilutions are carried out to at least 1:1280. False-positive STA titers due to immunologic cross-reactivity have been associated with *Brucella* skin testing, cholera vaccination, or infections due to *Vibrio cholerae*, *Francisella tularensis*, or *Yersinia enterocolitica*.

Immunoglobulin M (IgM) is the major agglutinating antibody formed in the first few weeks following infection with *Brucella* organisms. Thereafter, IgG levels also rise. The STA test measures both IgM and IgG. With prompt and adequate therapy, IgG antibody levels usually become undetectable after 6 to 12 months. If therapy is given, those patients who develop persistent *Brucella* infection usually maintain elevated IgG agglutinins. The addition of 2-mercaptoethanol (2-ME) to the STA test results in the detection of only IgG antibodies. In the absence of rising STA titers, a single elevated 2-ME *Brucella* agglutination titer (≥1:160) suggests either current or recent infection. Since a substantial number of patients maintain elevated IgM antibodies for years after treatment, the 2-ME agglutination test helps to identify those patients who have been cured, as IgG titers usually disappear within 6 months of adequate treatment. Certain newer antibody tests, including an ELISA and radioimmunoassay (RIA), are more sensitive than the STA; these methods have not been widely employed, and agglutination tests remain the standard for serologic diagnosis.

TREATMENT. Antibiotic treatment of *Brucella* infections is complicated by a number of complex issues, including the requirement for antibiotics that penetrate intracellularly, for prolonged therapy to prevent relapse, and for bactericidal antibiotics in treating central nervous system infection and endocarditis, as well as the lack of controlled, randomized, double-blind studies comparing different antimicrobial regimens. Debate is still considerable regarding which antibiotic regimens are clearly superior.

Patients treated with single agents such as tetracycline, streptomycin, chloramphenicol, rifampin, or trimethoprim-sulfamethoxazole have a 10 to 40 per cent chance of failure or relapse. Therefore, most authorities consider that combination antibiotic therapy for brucellosis is indicated. In acute brucellosis, without evidence of endocarditis or central nervous system involvement, the antibiotic regimen of tetracycline (2 grams per day) for 6 weeks plus streptomycin (1 gram per day) for 3 weeks has been used widely and has a low rate of relapse. Intramuscular administration of streptomycin makes this therapy difficult in some circumstances. Currently, doxycycline (200 mg per day) plus rifampin (600 to 900 mg per day) for 6 weeks is considered the antibiotic regimen of choice by the World Health Organization. Acute brucellosis in children can be treated with trimethoprim-sulfamethoxazole.

In central nervous system brucellosis, the combination of a third-generation cephalosporin with rifampin should be considered. In localized brucellosis, surgical drainage of abscesses should be pursued in conjunction with antimicrobial therapy for 6 or more weeks. *Brucella* endocarditis, which accounts for the highest mortality rates among *Brucella* infections, requires bactericidal drugs; early valve replacement is often necessary because of aortic valve destruction and/or major arterial emboli.

PROGNOSIS. Brucellosis appropriately treated within the first month of symptom onset is curable. Acute brucellosis often produces severe weakness and fatigue, and patients are frequently unable to work for up to 2 months. Immunity to reinfection follows initial *Brucella* infection in the majority of individuals. With early antimicrobial therapy, cases of chronic brucellosis or localized disease and complications are rare. Of patients who die of brucellosis, 84 per cent have endocarditis involving a previously abnormal aortic valve, often associated with severe congestive heart failure.

PREVENTION. The control of human brucellosis relates directly to prevention programs in domestic animals and avoidance of unpasteurized milk and milk products. With control in animals and the resultant marked decrease in human cases, the need for a vaccination program in humans has been less pressing. In other countries, the experience with human vaccination has shown a narrow range between efficacy and toxicity. In slaughterhouses, important means of prevention include careful wound dressing, protective glasses and clothing, prohibition of raw meat ingestion, and the use of previously infected (immune) individuals in high-risk areas. Eradication of human cases requires elimination of disease in animals and a greater awareness by the physician of the epidemiology, nuances of clinical presentation, and available diagnostic and treatment strategies in *Brucella* infections.

Ariza J, Gudiol F, Valverde J, et al.: Brucella spondylitis: A detailed analysis based on current findings. Rev Infect Dis 7:656, 1985. *The epidemiologic, clinical, diagnostic, and therapeutic features of spondylitis due to B. melitensis are detailed in 20 patients included in a 10-year prospective study from Barcelona, Spain.*

Arnow PM, Smaron M, Ormiste V: Brucellosis in a group of travelers to Spain. JAMA 251:505, 1984. *Describes the risk of brucellosis in travelers to endemic areas and the value of epidemiologic investigation to detect unrecognized cases.*

Bouza E, Garcia de la Torre M, Parris F, et al.: Brucella meningitis. Rev Infect Dis 9:810, 1987. *An excellent review about the variable clinical manifestations and approaches to the diagnosis and treatment of meningitis due to Brucella.*

Buchanan TM, Faber LC, Feldman RA: Brucellosis in the United States, 1960–1972: An abattoir-associated disease. I. Clinical features and therapy. Buchanan TM, Sulzer CR, Frix MK, et al.: II. Diagnostic aspects. Buchanan TM, Hendricks SL, Patton CM, et al.: III. Epidemiology and evidence for acquired immunity. Medicine 53:403, 415, 427, 1974. *A very complete description of all aspects of brucellosis derived from a study of 160 patients in a large Iowa slaughterhouse.*

Fernandez-Guerrero ML, Martinell J, Aguado JM, et al.: Prosthetic valve endocarditis. Arch Intern Med 147:1141, 1987. *Highlights the expanding spectrum of brucellosis to include prosthetic valve infections and issues regarding management.*

Gazapo E, Gonzalez Lahoz J, Subiza JL, et al.: Changes in IgM and IgG antibody concentrations in brucellosis over time: Importance for diagnosis and follow-up. J Infect Dis 159:219, 1989. *Patterns of antibody responses correlating with successful treatment, chronic disease, or drug relapses and failures were followed prospectively and proved clinically useful.*

Gotuzzo E, Carrillo C, Guerra J, et al.: An evaluation of diagnostic methods for brucellosis—the value of bone marrow culture. J Infect Dis 153:122, 1986. *The high yield of bone marrow culture in patients with B. melitensis infection is emphasized.*

Hall WH: Modern chemotherapy for brucellosis in humans. Rev Infect Dis 12:1060, 1990. *A comprehensive analysis of the world's literature related to therapy of brucellosis that stresses that prolonged combined chemotherapy in conjunction with surgery, where indicated, is the key to successful treatment.*

Jacobs F, Abramowicz D, Vereerstraeten P, et al.: *Brucella* endocarditis: The role for combined medical and surgical treatment. Rev Infect Dis 12:740, 1990. *A review of 39 cases of cured Brucella endocarditis.*

330 Cat Scratch Disease

Andrew M. Margileth

DEFINITION. Cat scratch disease is characterized by tender regional chronic lymphadenopathy that is frequently preceded by a primary skin lesion related to cat contact or scratches. The disease is usually benign, and the adenopathy resolves spontaneously in 3 weeks to several months. In about 3 per cent of patients, severe systemic disease (pulmonary hilar adenopathy, hepatosplenomegaly with granuloma, neuroretinitis, encephalopathy, angiomatoid papules) has occurred.

ETIOLOGY. Since 1983, studies by Wear et al. have continued to identify a pleomorphic gram-negative rod-shaped bacterium in tissue from patients with clinical and histopathologic criteria of cat scratch disease. These specimens include about 900 lymph nodes, 10 primary inoculation skin lesions, and over 12 from patients with ocular granulomas. Recently, a gram-negative pleomorphic bacillus was cultured from over 20 patients with subacute cat scratch disease. Further identification of this organism is pending.

EPIDEMIOLOGY. Since the initial description by Debré (1950), over 3000 patients with cat scratch disease have been reported. Cat scratch disease may occur in preschool children and in adults, but over 60 per cent of cases present between ages 5 and 21 years. An estimated 2000 unreported cases occur annually in the United States. The disease is worldwide, occurring in all races, with a predominance in males (55 per cent). In temperate zones, most cases have occurred during fall and winter. Seasonal variation is minimal in warmer climates. There is a familial clustering in 5 per cent of cases.

TRANSMISSION AND COMMUNICABILITY. The mode of transmission is presumably by direct contact, since the bubo usually follows a scratch, bite, or lick from a young cat. Cat contact occurs in 94 per cent of patients. The disease has also developed after a dog bite or scratch and rarely after a scratch from a thorn, wood splinter, or fish bone or after insect bites. Person-to-person transmission has not been reported. Attempts to isolate an infectious agent from cat saliva or claws have been unsuccessful. The healthy cat—often a kitten—apparently acts as a mechanical vector for the infective agent, for skin tests with cat scratch antigen on the implicated cats have been nonreactive. Studies in family outbreaks have shown that the family cat usually transmits the causative agent no longer than 2 to 3 weeks.

PATHOGENESIS AND PATHOLOGY. No serologic test is available to measure antibodies to the causative agent. Fortunately, the cat scratch skin test is reliable and has a high degree of specificity; the reaction is a delayed hypersensitivity type. A positive reaction is usually detected at the time the clinical diagnosis is suspected; however, conversion may be delayed up to 4 weeks thereafter. Cutaneous reactivity lasts up to 10 years. Recurrent lymphadenopathy has been reported recently in three adults.

Histopathologic findings of biopsied lymph nodes may show a broad spectrum of reactions: arteriolar proliferation and widening of arteriolar walls, reticulum cell hyperplasia, multiple microabscesses, frank abscess formation, and round or stellate granulomas. Other than the vascular changes, similar histopathologic findings may be found in tularemia, brucellosis, tuberculosis, lymphogranuloma venereum, and the solid granulomas in sarcoidosis. One presentation, reticulum cell hyperplasia and granulomas, is suggestive of Hodgkin's disease. Cat scratch bacilli were best demonstrated by the Warthin-Starry silver impregnation stain in nodes removed during the first 3 to 4 weeks of the illness. In early lesions these bacteria were abundant in clumps or filaments and were most readily found in vessel walls, collagen fibers, and microabscesses. The bacilli ranged in size from 0.2 to 0.3 µm in diameter and 0.5 to 1.5 µm in length.

CLINICAL MANIFESTATIONS. The patient usually is not ill in spite of impressive lymphadenopathy; however, malaise, fever, fatigue, headache, and anorexia may be present. Three to 10 days elapse from the time of the scratch or contact until a primary skin papule or pustule forms. One or more erythematous papules may be observed. Unilateral conjunctival granuloma or conjunctivitis occurred in 6 per cent of the author's 1237 patients. An inoculation site (a scratch or a primary lesion, or both) may be detected in 64 to 96 per cent of patients, depending on the thoroughness of the examination and the duration of the bubo. Most primary lesions persist for 1 to 3 weeks, rarely for months, and heal without scar formation. Regional lymphadenopathy usually develops about 2 weeks after the scratch (range, 5 to 50 days). Lymphangitis has not been observed. Tender nodes, present in 80 per cent of patients for the first 1 or 2 weeks, are commonly found in the head, neck, or axilla. Epitrochlear, inguinal, femoral, or occipital areas are involved less frequently. Multiple site involvement occurred in one third of the author's cases. Node size varies from 1 to 8 cm. Enlargement persists for 2 to 4 months, rarely for 6 to 24 months. Suppuration occurs in

TABLE 330–1. CLINICAL FEATURES IN 1237 PATIENTS WITH CAT SCRATCH ADENOPATHY AND A POSITIVE SKIN TEST (APRIL 1975 TO JANUARY 1990)

Category	Percentage of Patients
Animal contact	
Cat	94
Dog	5
None	1
Animal scratch	
Cat	75
Dog	2
None	23
Primary lesion	
Skin papule or pustule	54
Eye granuloma	6
Mucous membrane	4
Symptoms and signs	
None except adenopathy	48
Fever (38.3–41.2°C)	32
Malaise/fatigue	30
Headache	14
Anorexia/emesis/weight loss	15
Splenomegaly	11
Sore throat	8
Exanthem	5
Parotid swelling	1.3

about 10 per cent of patients seen in office practice and in about 25 per cent of those admitted to hospitals.

About one half of patients have no clinical signs other than lymphadenopathy. About one third have fever (38.3 to 41.2°C) lasting for 5 to 9 (range, 1 to 60) days; 30 per cent have malaise or an influenza-like syndrome lasting about 4 (range, 1 to 21) days. Less common manifestations include splenomegaly (11 per cent), the oculoglandular syndrome of Parinaud (6 per cent), central nervous system involvement (2 per cent), and severe chronic systemic disease (2 per cent) (see Tables 330–1 and 330–2). Rarely, thrombocytopenic purpura, hepatosplenomegaly, breast tumor, and osteomyelitis have been reported.

Central or peripheral nervous system involvement may develop in all age groups. Encephalopathy, meningitis, neuroretinitis, radiculitis, polyneuritis, or myelitis with paraplegia has been observed in over 110 patients. Onset of neurologic symptoms is sudden, usually with fever, and occurs within 1 to 6 weeks of the

TABLE 330–2. CAT SCRATCH LYMPHADENOPATHY IN 1237 PATIENTS: CLINICAL CHARACTERISTICS OF INVOLVED NODES AND DURATION OF ADENOPATHY (APRIL 1875 TO JANUARY 1990)

Adenopathy (N = 1237)	Per Cent	Size (cm) (N = 1237)	Per Cent
Single node	42.5	1.0 to <3.0	41.4
Multiple nodes	24	3.0 to <5.0	39
Multiple sites	33	≥5.0	19.6
Tender nodes	79		
Suppuration	16		

Location (N = 1636*)	Per Cent	Duration of Node (N = 818)	Per Cent
Head: total (N = 286†)	17.5	Prior to diagnosis‡	
Submandibular	12	1 to <4 weeks	45
Preauricular	5	1 to <2 months	31
Neck: total (N = 634)	39	2 to <4 months	15
Posterior	14	4 to <6 months	3
Anterior	21	6 to <12 months	3
Supraclavicular	3	Regression (months, <1.0 cm)§ (N = 1235)	
Extremities: total (N = 712)	43.5	1 to <2	15
Axillary	25	2 to <6	63
Epitrochlear/brachial	7.3	6 to <12	14
Inguinal	7	12 to <24	5
Femoral	4.3	≥24	0.8

*Mediastinal = 3, breast = 2, pancreas = 1, mesenteric = 1: N = 7 (0.5%).
†Occipital = 16 (1%).
‡Duration ≥12 months = 22 (3%).
§2 to 4 weeks = 27 (2.2%).

onset of adenopathy. There may be cerebrospinal fluid pleocytosis, elevated protein levels, or both. Electroencephalograms are abnormal in most patients. Severe manifestations last for 1 to 2 weeks, with complete recovery in 1 to 12 months.

Cat scratch disease in individuals with acquired immunodeficiency syndrome (AIDS) is less well recognized and is often confused with other clinical manifestations related to AIDS. Although cat scratch disease in children with AIDS has not been reported, the syndrome in adults has unusual manifestations and responds to antibiotic therapy. Recently, the first case of culture-proven cat scratch disease in an AIDS patient was reported. The patient with AIDS often presents with numerous lesions ranging from pink to deep reddish-purple papules to sessile nodules or pedunculated nodules on any part of the body. The skin lesions occur most frequently on the head, trunk, or extremities but may also occur on the conjunctival, oral, or nasal mucosa. The nodules are firm, indurated, and usually nontender and range in size from 1 mm to 6 cm in diameter. Clinically, the lesions are indistinguishable from Kaposi's sarcoma, histiocytoid hemangioma, epithelioid hemangioma, or pyogenic granuloma. Radiographs of lesions over bone may show increased bone loss and periostosis and a marked increase in soft tissue mass.

DIAGNOSIS. Regional lymphadenopathy developing 2 weeks after cat contact, and especially if a primary inoculation papule or pustule followed a scratch, suggests cat scratch disease. Three of the four following manifestations would confirm the diagnosis in a typical case, whereas all four would be necessary in an atypical case: (1) a history of animal (usually cat) contact, with the presence of a scratch or a primary dermal, eye, or mucous membrane lesion; (2) negative laboratory studies (serology, cultures of aspirated pus or lymph node, PPD-T, and PPD-Battey) for other causes of lymphadenopathy; (3) a positive skin test result to one or two cat scratch antigens; (4) node biopsy revealing typical histopathology, especially if pleomorphic rod-shaped bacilli can be demonstrated with the Warthin-Starry silver stain.

If a negative skin test result is found to one or two different cat scratch antigens applied simultaneously and again 4 weeks later, and if results of other studies are negative, a biopsy must be considered to rule out a benign tumor or lymphoma. The presence of tenderness favors cat scratch or a pyogenic or mycobacterial adenopathy rather than a neoplasm. Ultrasonography has been very useful in deciding whether or not to aspirate nontender or nonfluctuant cervical masses. It may also aid needle placement for cyst or abscess aspiration.

Skin Tests. A skin test using cat scratch antigen is positive in 98 per cent of patients who are clinically suspected of having cat scratch disease. A negative result often occurs if the duration of illness is less than 3 or 4 weeks, and 1 to 2 per cent of patients with typical cat scratch disease have negative test results with one or two different antigens. The positive reaction consists of a wheal or papule with 5 mm or more of induration, with or without erythema, occurring 48 to 72 hours after intradermal inoculation of 0.1 ml of antigen. Induration may persist for 5 to 6 days or longer. A positive test result may be obtained for years (10 to 28) after the initial episode.

Positive reactions have been reported in veterinarians (12 to 29 per cent), healthy persons (5 per cent), and family contacts (18 per cent); the overall incidence is 5 per cent. Thus the limit of confidence for a positive reaction in a person suspected of having cat scratch disease is about 95 per cent. If the reaction is negative at 4-week intervals, the disease can be excluded with reasonable certainty, especially if two different antigens are used. Repeated skin testing with cat scratch antigen in the same patients has not produced positive reactions.

Since cat scratch antigen is not available commercially, aspirated pus from affected nodes should be saved to prepare test antigen. Cat scratch antigen for medical diagnosis is usually available from the author upon written request.

Laboratory Data. Laboratory tests are not diagnostic. Eosinophilia has been reported. At the onset there may be a mild leukocytosis. The erythrocyte sedimentation rate is usually elevated during the first few weeks of adenopathy.

DIFFERENTIAL DIAGNOSIS. Cat scratch disease should be considered in all patients with persistent lymphadenopathy (over 3 weeks), because it is the most common cause of chronic regional lymphadenitis in children or adolescents. The presence of an inoculation (dermal or ocular) lesion strongly suggests cat scratch

disease. Other less common causes are sporotrichosis, primary syphilis, lymphogranuloma venereum, typical or atypical tuberculosis, other bacterial adenitis, tularemia, brucellosis, histoplasmosis, coccidioidomycosis, sarcoidosis, toxoplasmosis, infectious mononucleosis, and benign or malignant tumors. In atypical forms of cat scratch disease, one may observe benign parotid lymphosialadenopathy, Parinaud's oculoglandular disease, encephalitis, pneumonia, thrombocytopenic purpura with or without anemia, erythema nodosum, angiomatoid papules, and osteomyelitis, as well as fluctuant lymphadenopathy simulating cystic hygroma or a thyroglossal duct cyst. If cat scratch skin test reactions, appropriate cultures, and serologic and PPD-T and PPD-Battey skin tests are negative, a node biopsy will usually determine the cause.

TREATMENT. The best therapy is reassurance that the adenopathy is benign and in most cases will subside spontaneously within 2 or 3 months. Management consists of appropriate follow-up examination, analgesics for pain, and aspiration if suppuration occurs. Commonly used antimicrobials are usually ineffective. Gentamicin or trimethoprim-sulfamethoxazole (TMP-SMX) may be effective. Gentamicin sulfate is given intramuscularly, 5 mg per kilogram per 24 hours in divided doses. TMP-SMX is given orally, 6 to 12 mg of TMP and 30 to 60 mg of SMX per kilogram twice daily for 7 days. In the child whose node suppurates, needle aspiration on an ambulatory basis is preferred to incision and drainage. After washing with povidone-iodine (Betadine) cleanser, a needle (18 or 20 gauge) is inserted through normal unanesthetized skin at the base of the mass to avoid a chronic sinus tract in the event that a tuberculous lesion is present. Aspiration provides material for skin test antigen, relieves painful adenopathy, and usually allows the patient to become symptom free within 24 to 48 hours. If fluid recurs, reaspiration may be necessary. Application of moist soaks to the primary lesion may facilitate drainage and shorten the duration of lymphadenopathy. The efficacy of steroid therapy is questionable, and it is not recommended. Excisional biopsy of the node may be necessary in selected patients because of persistent pain or for diagnostic purposes.

Paradoxically, patients with human immunodeficiency virus (HIV) infection and associated skin, bone, liver, or spleen lesions, lymphadenopathy, and associated systemic illness due to cat scratch disease have responded promptly to common antibiotics (erythromycin, doxycycline, antimycobacterial drugs). In vitro studies have shown the English-Wear bacillus to have microbial susceptibility to aminoglycosides, cefoxitin sodium, cefotaxime sodium, netilmicin sulfate, and mezlocillin sodium.

PROGNOSIS. The prognosis is excellent; lymphadenopathy usually regresses spontaneously in 2 to 4 months. One attack appears to confer lifelong immunity. Three adults had a recurrence of cat scratch disease. Complications and sequelae are almost nonexistent. Rarely, patients have been observed to have chronic adenopathy for 2 to 3 years.

PREVENTION. Because of the number of household pets (50 million cats in the United States), cat scratch disease is difficult to prevent. Disposal of the suspect cat is not recommended, because the cat involved is invariably well. Four to 9 per cent of family members scratched by the same cat may develop cat scratch disease. The patient with the disease does not require isolation or quarantine. Active or passive protection is not available.

Bogue CW, Wise JD, Gray GF, et al.: Antibiotic therapy for cat-scratch disease? JAMA 262:813, 1989. *Three patients with cat scratch disease were treated successfully with intramuscular gentamicin sulfate. Two patients had extensive hepatic involvement, and one had marked inguinal lymphadenitis.*

Carithers HA, Margileth AM: Cat scratch disease: Acute encephalopathy and other neurologic manifestations. AJDC 145:98, 1991. *Sixty-one patients developed encephalopathy within one-half to 6 weeks of the onset of cat scratch disease. The average age of the patients was 10.6 years (1 to 66 years). Convulsions occurred in 46 per cent and combative behavior in 40 per cent. Lethargy with or without coma was accompanied by variable neurologic signs. The "English-Wear" bacillus was demonstrated in 10 of 14 biopsy specimens. All 61 patients recovered within ½ to 12 months.*

Collipp PJ: Cat scratch disease therapy. AJDC 143:1261, 1989. *Eleven patients with proven CSD responded to oral TMP-SMX therapy within 1 week.*

English CK, Wear DJ, Margileth AM, et al.: Cat scratch disease: Isolation and culture of the bacterial agent. JAMA 259:1347, 1988. *A gram-negative bacterium or its cell wall defective variants were isolated from lymph nodes of 10 patients with cat scratch disease. Vegetative bacteria produced lesions in the skin of an armadillo identical to early lesions in human skin. These vegetative bacteria were recovered from the lesions in the armadillo.*

Kemper CA, Lombard CM, Deresinski SC, et al.: Visceral bacillary epithelioid angiomatosis. Am J Med 89:216, 1990. *Two adults, one HIV infected and one not HIV infected, are reported. The HIV-infected patient had bacillary epithelioid angiomatosis of liver and bone marrow, causing hepatic failure. The cardiac transplant recipient had fever of unknown origin with hepatic and splenic bacillary epithelioid angiomatosis, with positive Warthin-Starry cat scratch–like organisms.*

Koehler JE, LeBoit PE, Egbert BM, et al.: Cutaneous vascular lesions and disseminated cat-scratch disease in patients with the acquired immunodeficiency syndrome (AIDS) and AIDS-related complex. Ann Intern Med 109:449, 1988. *Four patients with AIDS developed angiomatous nodules involving skin and bone, two of whom were scratched by a cat. Numerous bacteria were noted in these nodules by the Warthin-Starry stain and electron microscopy. Rapid resolution of skin and osseous lesions occurred after treatment with erythromycin, doxycycline, or antimycobacterial antibiotics.*

Relman DA, Loutit JS, Schmidt TM, et al.: The agent of bacillary angiomatosis. N Engl J Med 323:1573, 1990. *Tissue from three unrelated patients with bacillary angiomatosis yielded a unique 16S gene sequence. These 16S sequences belong to a previously uncharacterized microorganism, most closely related to Rochalimgea quintana, a rickettsia-like organism.*

Schlossberg D, Morad Y, Krouse TB, et al.: Culture-proved disseminated cat-scratch disease in acquired immunodeficiency syndrome. Arch Intern Med 149:1437, 1989. *An HIV-positive adult with cat scratch disease developed papillitis and retinitis that responded to TMP-SMX and dexamethasone. Subsequently, epithelioid hemangioma, liver abscesses, pleural effusion, and gingival Kaposi's sarcoma developed. Cultures of lymph node, pleural fluid, and liver yielded gram-negative bacilli believed to be the causative agent of cat scratch disease.*

331 Bartonellosis

C. Glenn Cobbs

DEFINITION. Bartonellosis (Carrión's disease) is an insect-borne bacterial disorder characterized by two well-defined clinical stages. It has a striking geographic restriction, occurring only on the western coast of South America at altitude. The first stage, Oroya fever, was recognized in the nineteenth century when it caused an outbreak of febrile hemolytic anemia among railway workers in Peru. Even before that time, the cutaneous stage, verruga peruana, had been described. The common bacterial etiology of the two forms of the disease was established in 1885 by Daniel Carrión, a Peruvian medical student, when he died of acute hemolytic anemia 39 days after inoculation with material from a verruga lesion.

ETIOLOGY. In 1909, Barton described the causative microorganism, *Bartonella bacilliformis*, a small, motile, pleomorphic bacillus that can be grown on various enriched media.

EPIDEMIOLOGY. Bartonellosis is generally restricted to the habitat of its main vector, the sandfly, *Phlebotomus verrucarum*. Other *Phlebotomus* species have rarely been associated with transmission. The sandfly breeds and transmits the infection in river valleys of the Andes Mountains at an altitude between 2500 and 9000 feet. Humans provide the only known reservoir of the microorganism. Convalescent individuals may have low-grade bacteremia for months to years after infection, and *B. bacilliformis* may be recovered from 5 to 10 per cent of apparently healthy persons in an endemic area. These carriers present the greatest epidemiologic threat.

Similar hemotropic bacterial species have occasionally been described in other geographic locales, but these microorganisms are distinguishable from *B. bacilliformis*.

PATHOLOGY. After inoculation by the vector, the bacteria replicate in the human host and invade erythrocytes and endothelial cells. Red cell parasitization results in increased fragility of red cells and increased phagocytosis by the reticuloendothelial system. In severe cases, as many as 90 per cent of the circulating erythrocytes may be parasitized. The hemolytic anemia that ensues results in fever, anemia, and weakness. Peripheral blood smears reveal a normochromic macrocytosis, striking polychromasia, Howell-Jolly bodies, Cabot rings, and nucleated erythrocytes. The Coombs test and other assays for red cell agglutinins and hemolysins are usually negative. Cells of the reticuloendothelial system may demonstrate intracellular organisms, presumably as a result of erythrophagocytosis, and reactive hyperplasia of lymphatic tissue is common.

Most untreated patients who survive the acute hemolytic anemia go on to develop the chronic cutaneous lesions of verruga peruana. These hemangiomatous nodules consist of proliferating small vessels infiltrated by lymphocytes and macrophages. Verrugas may also occur in the viscera, bone, and central nervous system.

CLINICAL MANIFESTATIONS. Within 2 to 6 weeks after the sandfly bite, the nonimmune host develops Oroya fever, characterized by the insidious onset of myalgias and low-grade fever, followed by high fever, headache, and painful muscles and joints. Tender lymphadenopathy is common, but splenomegaly should suggest some other disorder. Erythrocyte counts decrease rapidly within a few days and many fall as low as 1 million per cubic millimeter. The combination of anemia and jaundice results in a lemon color in light-skinned individuals. In some patients, the disease is characterized by a febrile crisis, followed by rapid resolution of symptoms and signs, increased erythropoiesis, and gradual reduction in fever. Recurrence of fever after initial improvement suggests secondary infection. *Salmonella* disease is an especially important complication of bartonellosis, as it is in other disorders associated with hemolysis, such as sickle cell anemia.

After resolution of the febrile hemolytic anemia, immunity develops, and relapses or reinfections are distinctly unusual. After a latent period, which ranges in untreated patients from weeks to months, many patients manifest the second stage of bartonellosis, verruga peruana. This disorder is characterized by hemangiomatous nodules that are reddish-purple, are 1 to 2 cm in diameter, and typically evolve over 1 to 2 months in crops on exposed skin but also on mucous membranes and internal organs. The lesions are usually nontender and morphologically may vary, appearing as ulcers or secondarily infected pustules. In some instances, these may be mistaken for Kaposi's sarcoma or other malignant disorders of skin. The verrugas may persist for months to years in untreated patients.

DIAGNOSIS. The diagnosis is made by examining the peripheral blood film. There bacilli may be seen within red cells, either singly or in pairs or clusters. With a Giemsa stain, the bacilli appear as 0.3- to 1.5-µm red or reddish-purple rods with some pleomorphism. The microorganism may be cultured from blood if appropriate media are utilized. Identification of the microorganisms in the verrucal lesion is possible but more difficult.

TREATMENT AND PROGNOSIS. The mortality in untreated Oroya fever approaches 50 per cent and is a result of both acute hemolytic anemia and secondary infectious disorders, such as *Salmonella* disease, as noted above. Malaria, amebiasis, and tuberculosis also appear to be more common in these patients. Penicillin, chloramphenicol, and possibly tetracycline or streptomycin all seem to be clinically effective. Chloramphenicol, at a dose of 2 to 4 grams daily for 7 or more days, is the therapy of choice because of the frequent association of *Salmonella* infection. In patients so treated, fever generally disappears within 2 to 3 days, although blood smears may remain positive for some time longer.

PREVENTION. Insecticides, particularly those with dichlorodiphenyl trichloroethane (DDT), are of use in eradicating the vector.

Schultz MG: A history of bartonellosis (Carrión's disease). Am J Trop Med Hyg 17:503, 1980. *A fascinating summary of the initial historical accounts, medical descriptions, and investigations into the etiology and epidemiology of the disease.*

Diseases Due to Mycobacteria

332 Tuberculosis

Emanuel Wolinsky

DEFINITION. Tuberculosis is a chronic infectious disease caused by mycobacteria of the "tuberculosis complex," mainly *Mycobacterium tuberculosis*.

INCIDENCE. During the Industrial Revolution of the eighteenth and ninteenth centuries, the disease was known as the *white plague*. It was the leading cause of death in young people all over the world. Today, despite great progress in its treatment and control, it remains an important medical problem in many developing countries. There are still 4 to 10 million new cases and about 1 million deaths each year from tuberculosis. In the United States tuberculosis mortality decreased from a rate of 202 per 100,000 in 1900 to less than 1 in 1982. The new case rate has also declined from about 60 per 100,000 in 1950 to 9 in 1985. During the last few years, however, there has been little decline, and even an upsurge in 1986, in the number of new cases reported, thought to be primarily related to the association of tuberculosis with the acquired immunodeficiency syndrome (AIDS).

The rate of infection as determined by skin test surveys remains high in many developing countries. In the United States the rate has become increasingly difficult to estimate because of the abandonment of large-scale testing in cities. Information obtained in 1977 from selected urban areas of the country indicated that the rate of infection varied from less than 3 per cent in young children to 14 to 40 per cent in adults over the age of 65. Tuberculosis is becoming more and more a disease of middle-aged and older nonwhite men in residual urban pockets of disease associated with poverty and overcrowding.

ETIOLOGY. The microorganism that causes tuberculosis belongs to the genus *Mycobacterium*, which is classified in the family Mycobacteriaceae of the order Actinomycetales. Taxonomists do not agree on the further classification of the genus, but a useful concept is that of the tuberculosis complex to include *M. tuberculosis*, *M. bovis*, and probably *M. africanum*. Some taxonomists would subdivide *M. bovis* into European, Afro-Asian, and African variants. A few suggest that there should be just one species, *M. tuberculosis*, with subclassifications of bovine type, African type, and so forth.

M. tuberculosis is an obligate intracellular parasite that shares with other mycobacteria a characteristic staining quality. The popular abbreviation *AFB* for *acid-fast bacilli* is based on this quality. Acid-fastness is the result of retention of carbol fuchsin (or certain fluorochrome dyes) after washing with acid, alcohol, or both. It is not unique to mycobacteria, since *Nocardia* and certain *Corynebacterium* strains may also be acid fast. Mycobacterial cell walls are rich in lipids, existing mainly as complexes with peptides and polysaccharides. Certain stains can form a stable complex with one of these lipid compounds, mycolic acid, provided that the latter is contained within an intact cell wall structure.

In addition to the members of the tuberculosis complex, the genus *Mycobacterium* may be divided into about 30 species. Again, there is disagreement among the taxonomists on the definition of some of these species (see Ch. 333).

PATHOLOGY AND PATHOGENESIS. Tuberculosis is derived from the word *tubercle*, meaning a small lump or nodule. Histopathologically, the tubercle is a more or less discrete focus of granulomatous inflammation consisting of lymphocytes, epithelioid cells, macrophages, and giant cells. The granulomas seen in tuberculosis are characterized by a form of tissue necrosis known as *caseation*, so called because the caseum has the consistency of soft cheese. Prior to the time of necrosis the lesion may heal completely by resolution, but once necrosis and caseation have occurred it heals by fibrosis, encapsulation, calcification, and scar formation. Breakdown of the pulmonary lesion occurs when the caseum softens and liquefies and is expelled through the bronchial system. This process results in the formation of a cavity in the lung. Spread of disease may occur by local extension, by an intrabronchial route, or through the lymphohematogenous pathway. Early in the primary infection the organisms are transported to the draining lymph nodes and may be widely disseminated throughout the body. In the apical posterior areas of the upper lobes the seeded organisms may remain dormant in inactive lesions for many years only to reactivate during a period of lowered host immunity. The processes of healing and breakdown may occur sequentially and repeatedly so that various stages of the inflammatory reaction are seen in different areas.

The primary lesion in a nonsensitized individual consists of an area of nonspecific pneumonitis in a middle or lower lung zone at the site of deposition of the inhaled droplet nuclei carrying tubercle bacilli. The initial inflammatory response is the same as that seen in any bacterial pneumonia and consists mainly of fibrin, edema, and polymorphonuclear leukocytes. The extent of this primary exudative response varies with the number and virulence of the bacilli inhaled, the native resistance of the host, and the effectiveness of the immune response. The change to a granulomatous type of reaction occurs coincidentally with the development of delayed hypersensitivity after 2 or 3 weeks. The mechanisms of cellular immunity may allow the host to wall off the lesion and to halt the lymphohematogenous spread. It is the softening and liquefaction of the caseous focus that leads to further trouble and the provision of a favorable environment for the rapid multiplication of the mycobacteria. In the encapsulated lesion that does not soften, the bacilli slowly lose their viability.

Stages in the natural history of untreated pulmonary tuberculosis, especially as it occurs in childhood, may be described as follows:

1. During the primary phase and throughout the development of the lesions there are usually no symptoms. Even in the so-called manifest primary stage, symptoms may be mild or absent despite parenchymal lesions and enlarged hilar or mediastinal lymph nodes. Pleurisy with effusion may occur. Life-threatening complications at this stage are meningitis and miliary disease.

2. The primary disease usually heals, leaving evidence of its presence in the form of a calcified pulmonary scar along with calcifications in the draining lymph nodes, which together are known as a *Ghon's complex*.

3. The third stage is one of latency, during which the bacilli remain dormant but still viable within inactive lesions. This situation may exist for the remainder of the patient's life.

4. Reactivation may occur in a relatively small proportion of infected individuals. This is the mechanism by which tuberculosis in the adult usually develops, either in the lung or in an extrapulmonary site.

5. Exogenous reinfection occasionally may be documented by the demonstration of bacilli with a different phage type or drug sensitivity pattern from those of the primary infection.

EPIDEMIOLOGY. Infection is usually transmitted from person to person by the inhalation of infective droplet nuclei that result from the aerosolization of respiratory secretions. The source of the infected material usually is an adult with cavitary pulmonary tuberculosis. The most important determinants of infectivity are the concentration of organisms in the sputum and the closeness and duration of contact with the index case. Other factors of importance are the cough frequency and the personal habits of the index case, the efficiency with which aerosols are produced by such activities as singing, loud talking, and laughing, and the air circulation and ventilation in the area of contact. A situation favorable to acquisition of infection would be an overcrowded and poorly ventilated house in which there were several young children and an adult with highly positive sputum.

Ingestion is no longer a common pathway for infection, although in the days of unpasteurized milk and widespread tuberculosis in cattle this was a common route of infection for *M. bovis*, especially for the production of tuberculosis of the tonsils and subsequent involvement of the submandibular lymph nodes. Another route of infection that still may be observed, however, is primary inoculation through the skin. Laboratory workers may inoculate themselves with actively growing cultures via needle puncture or broken glass, and pathologists may sustain a penetrating injury while doing a postmortem examination.

Many localized outbreaks or miniepidemics have been reported in the past and continue to be observed today (Lincoln, 1967; Stead, 1979). The pattern of airborne transmission in a closed environment is well described in these accounts of infections aboard ships, in day care centers, nursing homes, prisons, industrial school dormitories, and school buses, and among members of a choir.

Tuberculosis Control. Tuberculosis is perpetuated by the repeated cycle of new infections that result from the inhalation of infected droplet nuclei coughed into the air by adults with cavitary pulmonary disease. This cycle may be attacked at several points. Case-finding efforts are needed to recognize individuals with active disease so that they may be placed under treatment to terminate the infectivity. Large-scale roentgenographic surveys have been abandoned in favor of contact investigation, recognition of symptomatic cases at entry points to the medical care system, and surveillance of high-risk groups such as hospital personnel, prisoners, and nursing home patients.

Protection from the complications of primary disease may be afforded by vaccination with bacille Calmette-Guérin (BCG). This was a strain of *M. bovis* attenuated by many passages on artificial media. There are now many different strains, each unique, maintained in laboratories across the world. Vaccination has been utilized mainly in areas that have a high rate of tuberculosis infection. Although vaccination may protect the individual, it does not reduce the overall rate of infection in the community, since it does not prevent the transmission of infection. Its effectiveness depends on an enhancement of the immune response, which enables the host to eliminate most of the bacilli before tissue destruction and dissemination occur. The efficacy of BCG is controversial. It has not been used extensively in the United States because it interferes with the subsequent use of the tuberculin test in recognizing tuberculosis infection and because the major source of morbidity is people already infected. Nevertheless, a case could be made for BCG in certain special circumstances such as to protect the infant whose noncompliant mother has active disease and to prevent infection in close contacts of an index case with drug-resistant bacilli.

Chemoprophylaxis may prevent infection in close contacts with negative skin tests, prevent disease in those already infected, and prevent subsequent recurrences in individuals with inactive pulmonary disease. The recommended drug for prophylaxis is isoniazid, once daily, in a dosage of 300 mg for adults and 10 mg per kilogram (not to exceed 300 mg) for children. When taken for 1 year, such treatment results in a reduction of at least 70 per cent in the appearance of primary disease in household contacts. Protection is about 90 per cent in those who actually take the drug as prescribed, and it continues for many years. There is some evidence that isoniazid for only 9 months is almost equally effective, and even shorter two-drug courses are being investigated. The two principal drawbacks to this method of control are isoniazid-related hepatitis and the failure of about 30 per cent of patients to take the prescribed medication.

The risk of developing active disease in recent tuberculin converters of any age is about 3 to 5 per cent in the first year after infection. From 5 to 15 per cent may progress to active disease within 5 years. The risk is greater in infants. Chemoprophylaxis is recommended for close contacts of patients with recently diagnosed active disease; for persons with recent infection documented by skin test conversion within the past 2 years; for individuals with positive skin test results, radiographic findings consistent with inactive tuberculous disease, and neither positive bacteriologic findings nor a history of adequate chemotherapy;

and for individuals with positive skin test results who have additional risk factors (such as malignancy or severe diabetes) or who are undergoing prolonged immunosuppressive or corticosteroid therapy. Although chemoprophylaxis is one of the important methods of tuberculosis control in this country, it has not been accepted in many other parts of the world. Isoniazid does not prevent disease resulting from infection with isoniazid-resistant bacilli. Rifampin alone, or combined with pyrazinamide for a few months, has been suggested as an alternative.

IMMUNOLOGY. Tuberculosis is the classic example of disease caused by an intracellular parasite. Protection is afforded by the mechanisms of cell-mediated immunity rather than by those associated with antibodies. Immunity may be natural or acquired, but in either case it is the macrophage that assumes the major burden of protection. Polymorphonuclear leukocytes have the ability to phagocytize but not to destroy mycobacteria. Although the results of some experiments are contradictory, most researchers have been able to demonstrate that macrophages from an immunized animal kill the bacilli more efficiently and at a more rapid rate than do control cells. Macrophages may be activated by immunologically specific mechanisms as well as by nonspecific stimulation. Specific stimulation occurs when sensitized T lymphocytes contact mycobacterial antigens that have been properly processed by macrophages. The lymphocytes then release a number of active chemical substances known as *lymphokines*, one variety of which activates macrophages.

Native immunity certainly has played a role in the global aspects of tuberculosis. Good examples exist in the animal kingdom; the rat and the cat are quite resistant to infection with *M. tuberculosis*, in contrast to the guinea pig and the monkey, which are highly susceptible. Lurie was able to breed two races of rabbits, one susceptible and one resistant to infection. Although it is difficult to separate the factors of social and economic conditions from those of race, the Eskimo peoples and blacks are considered by some researchers to be more susceptible. The forces of natural selection probably contributed to the decline of tuberculosis prior to the introduction of chemotherapy, although improved socioeconomic conditions played an important role. Acquired immunity may occur as a result of natural infection or by vaccination. Recovery from tuberculosis confers protection against reinfection with a new inoculum, even though the original bacilli may remain latent for many years and be capable of producing recrudescent disease. Whether acquired by natural infection or vaccination, the protection is only relative and may be overwhelmed by a sufficiently large infecting dose.

The relationship between delayed hypersensitivity and immunity is still controversial. The two functions appear at about the same time after infection and are intimately related thereafter. Nevertheless, it has been shown in experimental animals that immunity may remain despite abolition of a positive skin test result by desensitization and that immunity may be induced by ribosome preparations that do not induce a positive skin reaction.

The balance between the reactions of delayed hypersensitivity and those of the humoral antibody response is very important in determining the clinical presentation and prognosis in leprosy. A similar but less dramatic situation exists in tuberculosis. A more favorable prognosis may be expected for patients who have strong reactivity in their cell-mediated immune functions than for those who are hypoergic and have abundant antibody production. Patients with nonreactive tuberculosis tend to have disseminated disease with almost unopposed multiplication of the organisms in reticuloendothelial cells and a lack of granulomatous response. The question of whether the anergic state is the cause or the result of severe tuberculosis is moot. Recovery of the compromised cell-mediated immune functions, including delayed hypersensitivity, usually accompanies clinical improvement. A patient's location in the immune spectrum usually is dynamic and changeable rather than fixed.

The Tuberculin Skin Test. The biologically active material in the liquid medium after growth of *M. tuberculosis* was named *tuberculin* by Robert Koch. This crude material was later called *Old Tuberculin (OT)*. A purified protein derivative of tuberculin *(PPD)* was made by Siebert in 1924 by precipitation with saturated ammonium sulfate. The World Health Organization adopted a large batch, designated *PPD-S*, as the international standard tuberculin. Five tuberculin units *(TU)* was defined as the biologic activity contained in a specified weight of PPD-S. Solutions with much greater stability were achieved by the addition of a wetting agent. All preparations of PPD commercially available in this country must be bioequivalent to 5 TU of PPD-S as demonstrated by comparative testing in humans.

The intracutaneous, or Mantoux, test is performed by injecting 5 TU contained in 0.1 ml of solution intracutaneously with needle and syringe. This is known as the intermediate-strength test. It corresponds to 0.1 µg of the standard preparation. A more dilute solution containing 1 TU is available to test those who may be expected to have a very strong reaction, especially children. This preparation is known as first-strength PPD and is essentially a fivefold dilution of the 5 TU material. Second-strength PPD contains what is calculated to be 250 TU.

In the sensitized individual a reaction of redness, swelling, and induration begins at about 6 hours, reaches a maximum intensity at 36 to 60 hours, and then fades over the next several days. A positive result usually is defined as 10 mm or more of induration at 48 hours. This arbitrary definition is based on results of large-scale testing that showed that a reaction of 10 mm best separated those with from those without tuberculosis. The reading of the test is a subjective evaluation, with wide observer variation. It is only by averaging multiple readings made blindly by at least two expert readers that an accuracy within 3 mm may be approached.

It is unwise to have an arbitrary definition of a positive reaction in the diagnostic evaluation of a sick patient. Many factors may diminish the response in a nonspecific manner. They include virus infections or live virus vaccination; immunosuppression by disease, drugs, or steroids; malnutrition; overwhelming infection of any kind; and old age. It is best to measure the induration as accurately as possible and, in addition, to describe the intensity of both the erythema and the induration. Well-defined erythema that persists for 72 hours is usually indicative of a positive reaction. In case of doubt, it is often useful to repeat the test using 250 TU. If there is no reaction to the second-strength material, the odds against the diagnosis of nondisseminated tuberculosis are overwhelming. It is helpful to determine the reaction to other antigens utilizing the so-called *anergy panel*. The most useful are mumps, *Candida*, trichophytin, tetanus toxoid, and a streptococcal antigen such as streptokinase. Failure to react to the panel indicates a generalized state of cutaneous anergy, which may be expected to include tuberculin. Several multiple puncture devices are available for performing a tuberculin test. They should all be regarded as screening tests, and any doubtful or positive reactions should be tested with the Mantoux technique.

Intradermal administration of tuberculin in the recommended dosage does not induce an immunologic response even after repeated injections. However, a second injection from 2 weeks to 12 months after an original negative reaction may produce a booster response from recall of waning delayed hypersensitivity. To avoid the assumption that the positive reaction represents a new infection, it has been suggested that negative reactors be retested up to a week later in surveillance programs such as those for hospital personnel. Infection with any mycobacterium and probably with organisms of related genera, such as *Nocardia* and *Corynebacterium*, may give cross-reactions with the tuberculin test materials available today. Tuberculin reactivity is a quantitative function that may vary in intensity from time to time in a given person.

Factors Modifying the Course of Tuberculosis. Before chemotherapy, tuberculosis patients were considered to be at risk for recrudescent disease for the rest of their lives. Mitchell was able to follow over 2000 patients for 15 to 25 years after their moderately or far advanced disease had become inactive. He found a relapse rate of 28 per cent. Even with modern drug therapy relapse occasionally may occur, depending mainly on whether or not the patient was cooperative in taking medication. A study of 20,000 cases reported to the Centers for Disease Control in 1980 revealed that 7 to 8 per cent represented recurrent disease.

Many conditions are known to increase the risk for the recurrence of tuberculosis. Among these are emotional stress, malnutrition, drug addiction, alcoholism, immunosuppression by diseases that interfere with cell-mediated immunity, and the use of drugs such as corticosteroids. Gastric resection is a risk factor, presumably in relation to malnutrition. A risk over 10 times that of suitable controls has been documented for patients with chronic

renal failure on maintenance dialysis or for those with renal transplants. Influenza, pneumonia, and cancer of the lung may cause local reactivation of dormant lesions. Another local factor is pneumoconiosis, especially silicosis and coal worker's pneumoconiosis.

CLINICAL DESCRIPTION. **Pulmonary Tuberculosis.** Tuberculosis may involve any organ system, but the lung is the usual site of the primary lesion and the principal organ involved. In roughly one half of patients with extrapulmonary disease, however, the original pulmonary lesions may not be discernible clinically or radiographically.

Primary Tuberculosis. Primary tuberculosis refers to disease in a person not previously infected with a virulent mycobacterium of the tuberculosis complex. Primary tuberculosis formerly was seen almost exclusively in children and was known as the childhood type. At present it is not uncommon in adults of all ages. Most primary infections are subclinical and not detectable by ordinary radiographic procedures. They may be recognized, however, by a documented tuberculin skin test conversion. When accompanied by symptoms or radiographic evidence, or both, the disease is called manifest or overt primary tuberculosis. Enlarged hilar lymph nodes are almost always seen. Complications of the primary infection include pleurisy with effusion, miliary disease, meningitis, bone and joint disease, and progressive primary infection. In progressive primary disease the lesions enlarge, caseate, liquefy, and cavitate. Primary disease in adults is especially prone to progression and cavity formation.

The morbidity and mortality associated with primary infection are related to age. Although usually benign in older children and adults, it is life threatening when it occurs in infants. In a New York City study before the development of chemotherapy, tuberculosis in children less than 6 months of age had a mortality rate of 50 per cent. Congenital tuberculosis, often fatal, may be acquired from a mother with active disease by the hematogenous route or by the aspiration or ingestion of contaminated amniotic fluid. A unique finding in primary tuberculosis of young children is the development of consolidated and collapsed segmental lesions resulting from a combination of bronchial compression from enlarged hilar lymph nodes and extrusion of caseous contents into the bronchial lumen. This situation usually is clinically benign despite the alarmingly unhealthy appearance of the chest roentgenogram. The spectrum of primary tuberculosis in adults was documented by Stead and colleagues in 1968. In almost half of 37 adults the disease progressed without interruption into chronic pulmonary tuberculosis.

Reactivation Tuberculosis. This term refers to the pattern of disease in adults. It usually results from the reactivation of dormant foci in the posterior portions of the upper lobes that had been seeded by the bloodstream during the early primary infection. Occasionally adult disease is the result of a new inoculum of tubercle bacilli in a person already sensitized by a previous infection *(exogenous reinfection)*. Adult disease is characterized by chronicity, caseation, sloughing of liquefied caseous material, cavity formation, and the simultaneous occurrence of healing and progression in different areas of the lung. Lymph node involvement is usually minimal or absent, at least in those nodes that directly drain the pulmonary foci. Phage typing of strains recovered from different areas of the body and correlation between antimicrobial susceptibility patterns and the history of drug intake have been used to document both recrudescence of an old infection and exogenous reinfection.

The onset of disease may be *insidious, catarrhal, hemoptoic,* or *acute.* With insidious onset there is gradual development of fatigue, anorexia, weight loss, and other vague complaints. Later, a low-grade intermittent fever may develop that is commonly associated with excessive sweating at night. The temperature elevation tends to occur in the late afternoon. The catarrhal onset is characterized by an increasingly productive cough and occasional blood streaking of the sputum. Fever and night sweats may also be noted. In the hemoptoic variety, the presenting symptom is hemoptysis either with or without other symptoms already mentioned. Occasionally, the onset is acute and influenza-like with high fever, chills, myalgia, and productive cough. Pleuritic pain may be the presenting complaint, often without pleural fluid but sometimes ushering in the appearance of an effusion. Many cases of adult-type pulmonary tuberculosis in the past were discovered by routine chest films in asymptomatic persons. Some individuals might recall minor symptoms, such as slight pleurisy, night sweats, or tiredness, but others would deny all warning signs despite the presence of advanced disease. Before the advent of chemotherapy it was not unusual for the patient to have hoarseness or perirectal abscess—both conditions being secondary to the long-term presence of highly positive sputum.

Diagnosis. A careful history and physical examination often suggest the diagnosis of pulmonary tuberculosis before any laboratory test is ordered. The most characteristic physical findings of adult-type disease are rales heard posteriorly near the apex of one or both lungs. The chest radiographs then confirm the presence of disease in the posterior portion of the upper lobes. Visualization of one or more cavities strengthens the diagnosis. In primary tuberculosis the initial pneumonic area may be anywhere in the lung, especially in the middle or lower lobes, with enlargement of the draining lymph nodes at the lung root. These characteristic patterns are not always seen, however. In a report from a large teaching hospital, the diagnosis of tuberculosis was not suggested by the radiologist in 26 per cent of 100 consecutive cases. A wide variety of unusual patterns may be encountered, from mass lesions resembling malignancy to widespread interstitial disease of a nonspecific nature. Diabetics are more likely than nondiabetics to have lower lobe disease, which may also be noted as a bronchogenic spread from apical cavities. Nonapical, noncavitary, and thoracic lymph node disease is common in AIDS patients with tuberculosis.

Confirmation of the diagnosis should be sought by bacteriologic examination of the sputum. It may be necessary to obtain specimens by the inhalation of nebulized distilled water or saline solution or by gastric lavage. In addition to properly stained smears and cultures for acid-fast bacilli, it is useful to search for elastic fibers by unstained potassium hydroxide wet mounts. The presence of these fibers indicates destruction of lung tissue and should be accompanied by smears positive for AFB. Occasionally, it may be necessary to resort to bronchoscopy and even to lung biopsy to establish the diagnosis.

The tuberculin skin test is very useful in diagnosis, despite the fact that 5 to 20 per cent of those with newly diagnosed cases may have a negative response to the initial test. Transient depression of cell-mediated immune reactions either may be specific for tuberculin or may take the form of a generalized anergy to all skin test antigens. For immediate diagnostic purposes in such cases, it is useful to apply a second-strength PPD containing 250 TU, which will give a false-negative reaction in no more than 2 or 3 per cent of patients without disseminated disease or severe debility.

Recent innovations in laboratory tests include automated radiometric culture methods that allow for more rapid results and simultaneous differentiation of M. tuberculosis from other mycobacteria; immunoassays and polymerase chain reaction for specific antigens in sputum and body fluids; DNA probes specific for organisms of the tuberculosis complex applied to growing cultures (available now) and to sputum (investigational); and serodiagnosis by enzyme-linked immunosorbent assay to detect antibodies against specific M. tuberculosis antigens.

Differential Diagnosis. Many subacute and chronic pulmonary conditions, both infectious and noninfectious, may be confused with tuberculosis. Some pulmonary mycoses, especially histoplasmosis, may present with a similar clinical and radiologic picture. Pyogenic lung abscess as well as pneumonia with a delayed resolution may be confused with tuberculosis. A pyogenic lung abscess is likely to have more fluid within it, hence a higher air-fluid level, and more dense consolidation around it. When repeated examinations of the sputum are negative for AFB, one should increase efforts at establishing another diagnosis. Tuberculomas may be confused with similar lesions arising from several different fungal infections and with pulmonary neoplasms. Sarcoidosis and tuberculosis may have similar manifestations. One third of cases of fever of unknown origin are due to infection, and extrapulmonary tuberculosis is still prominent among these cases.

TREATMENT. Historical Perspective. For many decades the physician relied upon nonspecific measures to treat tuberculosis.

These measures included fresh air, good food, bed rest, and graded exercise, among others. The idea of the cottage sanatorium was started in this country in 1884 to accommodate these feeble attempts at treatment. Measures designated to collapse cavities and to put diseased portions of the lungs "at rest" included artificial pneumothorax, pneumoperitoneum, phrenic nerve crush, and various forms of thoracoplasty. Resectional surgery became popular after the introduction of effective drug therapy.

The era of chemotherapy began in 1945 with Waksman's discovery of streptomycin. In 1949 it was shown that treatment with the combination of streptomycin and para-aminosalicylic acid (PAS) delayed the emergence of streptomycin-resistant tubercle bacilli. With the introduction of isoniazid in 1952 it became possible to treat the disease with two drugs given by mouth. A course of 18 to 24 months was recommended by studies of relapse rates and the bacteriology of lesions removed at lung resection as related to duration of treatment. Ethambutol, marketed in 1961, replaced PAS because of its relative lack of annoying side effects. These drugs rendered all previous modes of therapy obsolete, and most sanatoriums in this country were closed by 1960. A study done in India in 1960 demonstrated that home treatment was not risky for the patient or his or her family. It was documented in 1973 that supervised intermittent treatment twice a week was just as beneficial as daily treatment, especially for the ambulatory continuation phase after a period of daily drug therapy. Such intermittent treatment is especially suited for uncooperative patients. The introduction of rifampin in 1966 provided not only another very powerful antituberculosis agent, but also the opportunity to shorten the duration of therapy by at least one half. Published reports on short-course chemotherapy began to appear in 1972. With proper combinations and rhythm of administration it is now possible to achieve excellent results with 6 months of treatment, provided that all doses are consumed as prescribed.

The Antituberculosis Drugs. *Isoniazid (INH)* is the most important drug in original treatment regimens. It is easily synthesized, highly stable, inexpensive, and well tolerated. The drug is well absorbed when given by mouth and also may be administered parenterally. It is widely distributed throughout the body, including the central nervous system, and it reaches bacilli within cells. The drug exerts a bactericidal effect on actively multiplying bacilli. Adverse reactions may occur in approximately 5 per cent of cases with a dose of 5 mg per kilogram per day, usually given as 300 mg once daily for adults. A common toxicity is peripheral neuropathy, based on interference with the metabolism of pyridoxine. It is directly related to the dose and blood level and is more likely to be seen in genetically constituted slow acetylators and in malnourished individuals. Neuropathy can be prevented by the administration of 25 mg of pyridoxine daily and is not likely to occur when ordinary doses of INH are used in nonalcoholic, nondiabetic, well-nourished, and relatively young patients. The most important adverse reaction is hepatitis of the hepatocellular variety. Although approximately 10 per cent of healthy individuals may have asymptomatic elevations of aminotransferases within the first 2 months of treatment, the enzyme levels usually return to normal despite the continued administration of the drug. The risk of hepatitis is related to age, being less than 1 per cent in those under 35 and increasing with age to 2.3 per cent at age 60. Hepatitis usually occurs within the first few months of treatment but occasionally appears in later stages. Heavy alcohol intake is associated with a greater risk of hepatitis. Several fatalities from INH hepatitis have been reported, mainly in patients whose reaction occurred late and in those who continued to take the drug despite progressive symptoms.

Some rare untoward effects include encephalopathy, loss of memory, optic atrophy, convulsions, hemolytic anemia, and purpura. The usual hypersensitivity reactions such as drug fever and skin rash occasionally may be seen. Isoniazid is one of several drugs that can produce a lupus-like syndrome. Although INH is excreted promptly and mainly by the kidneys, the half-life is prolonged only slightly in patients with renal failure.

Rifampin (RMP) is comparable to INH in its bactericidal effect on metabolically active bacilli. It is an antibiotic of the rifamycin family and is much more expensive than INH. Well absorbed when taken orally in a fasting state, the drug is widely distributed and penetrates well into cells and into the central nervous system when the meninges are inflamed. It differs from most of the antituberculosis drugs in that it has good activity against a variety of gram-positive and gram-negative bacteria. Its activity depends upon inhibition of DNA-dependent RNA polymerase activity. Rifampin is well tolerated by most patients in a dosage of 10 mg per kilogram per day, usually given to adults as 600 mg once daily by mouth. An intravenous preparation recently has become available. Hepatitis is the most important adverse effect, occurring in about 1 per cent of patients. There are conflicting reports on the risk of hepatitis when INH and RMP are given together. Most studies now indicate no excessive risk. An exception occurs in the treatment of children, for whom a dosage of greater than 10 mg per kilogram per day of INH given with RMP is associated with a high risk of hepatitis.

Allergic reactions occasionally occur, especially in those individuals who take the drug irregularly or in those who are given intermittent treatment twice weekly in a dosage greater than 600 mg. These reactions include chills and fever and more rarely acute renal failure, thrombocytopenia, and massive hemolysis. Rifampin may induce enzymes in the liver that increase metabolic degradation of several other drugs, such as oral contraceptive agents and anticoagulants. The drug is excreted mainly by the liver and biliary tract and therefore must be given with caution to patients with liver failure.

Ethambutol (EMB) is a synthetic chemical compound that is well absorbed when given by mouth and is excreted mainly in the urine. Thus, the drug should be given with great care to patients with poor renal function, for whom dosage must be reduced and blood levels followed carefully. Aside from its principal toxicity, optic neuritis, there are very few adverse effects. Optic nerve toxicity is directly related to dosage and blood levels. At the recommended dosage of 15 mg per kilogram per day, optic neuritis is very rare, but some physicians administer 25 mg per kilogram per day for the first 2 or 3 months, at which dosage approximately 3 per cent of patients may have impaired visual acuity. When the higher dose is used, periodic examinations for visual acuity are indicated. The toxicity usually is reversible if administration of the drug is discontinued promptly.

Pyrazinamide (PZA) is an important drug because of its excellent tissue-sterilizing ability when used in combination with other bactericidal drugs. It is well absorbed from the gastrointestinal tract, is widely distributed throughout the body water, and penetrates well into the central nervous system. The drug is active against only one species of *Mycobacterium, M. tuberculosis*, and then only at the low pH of 5.0 to 5.5. It is especially useful to kill tubercle bacilli within macrophages, into whose acidic environment it penetrates well. It is excreted mainly by way of the kidneys. Allergic reactions are rare, but joint pains and occasionally gout may occur as the result of a hyperuricemic effect. Hepatitis may occur in about 1 per cent of patients receiving the recommended daily dose of 20 to 30 mg per kilogram, usually 1.5 grams for small and 2.0 grams for large adults, given by mouth once daily.

Streptomycin (SM) is an aminoglycoside antibiotic that has been chemically defined and synthesized. It is not absorbed when given by mouth. The principal method of elimination is through the kidneys, so that dosage adjustment is necessary when renal function is reduced. It is distributed largely in the extracellular fluid and does not enter appreciably into the central nervous system or into macrophages. The dosage is 10 to 15 mg per kilogram per day, given intramuscularly, usually as 0.75 to 1.0 gram once daily in adults with normal renal function. As with other aminoglycosides, damage to the renal tubules is common, as manifested by cylindruria, but renal function is not compromised unless blood levels of the drug are excessive. The major toxicity is exerted against the eighth nerve, of which the vestibular division is more likely to be affected, although deafness may also be produced. The seriousness of these reactions makes periodic testing of renal and eighth nerve function advisable, especially in the elderly. Measurements of blood levels should be obtained whenever renal function is in question. Allergic reactions are fairly common, as are paresthesias of the lips and extremities immediately after injection. The drug is bactericidal against tubercle bacilli. The maximum effect is exerted at a pH of 7.7.

Kanamycin and *capreomycin* are used as substitutes for SM when the organisms are resistant to that drug or on the rare occasions when the patient cannot tolerate SM. Dosages, methods

of administration, and adverse reactions are similar to those of SM. More care is needed with kanamycin, since it is slightly more ototoxic and nephrotoxic than SM, especially on the cochlear division of the eighth nerve.

Ethionamide and *cycloserine* are not used for initial therapy but are reserved for retreatment cases and for special situations of drug intolerance and bacillary resistance. Both drugs are given by mouth in dosages of 10 to 15 mg per kilogram per day. The administration of ethionamide is accompanied by rather severe gastrointestinal upset and occasionally by hepatitis, and allergic reactions are common. Allergic reactions with cycloserine are rare, but aberrations of mental function and seizures are quite common. Other drugs under investigation include the quinolones ciprofloxacin and ofloxacin, rifabutin, and several long-acting rifamycins (rifapentine is one that has a name).

Drug Regimens. Until the landmark short-course chemotherapy studies of the British Medical Research Council and its cooperative investigators, the conventional drug regimens for initial treatment consisted mainly of INH and EMB for 1.5 to 2 years, supplemented by RMP or SM for the first month or two in patients with far-advanced disease. An intermittent schedule of supervised twice-weekly drug administration often was used after the initial 2 or 3 months of daily treatment for noncompliant patients. The main problems were those related to compliance with and cost of the long-term administration of two or more drugs. The conventional regimen has been all but abandoned in favor of short-course treatment.

Short-Course Treatment. The first report of successful short-course treatment was published in 1968 and involved experience in East Africa. From the results of many other trials conducted since then, it appears that the minimum requirements include therapy with INH and RMP for at least 9 months. The addition of a third drug—EMB, SM, or PZA—for the first 1 to 3 months of intensive treatment guards against the eventuality of infection with INH- or RMP-resistant bacilli. To shorten the course to 6 months, a third drug is necessary. That drug should be PZA for the initial 2 months. Treatment may then be continued with daily INH plus RMP for the remaining 4 months. When the patient is in a high-risk group for infection with INH-resistant or RMP-resistant organisms, use of a four-drug regimen has been suggested for the first 2 months (INH/RMP/PZA/SM), followed by administration of two or three drugs, depending on drug susceptibility, for 4 months. Even shorter regimens consisting of INH/RMP/PZA/SM daily for 4 months may be advisable for problem patients for whom ambulatory treatment of any kind is unsuitable, with expected success rates of 70 to 80 per cent.

Short-course treatment has the obvious advantages of smaller amounts of drugs used and less time needed at the ambulatory health facility for supervision of treatment. Another benefit is more rapid sputum conversion. In addition, if relapse occurs following short-course treatment, it is usually caused by drug-susceptible organisms. The main disadvantage of intensive three- and four-drug regimens, drug toxicity, has proved to be less troublesome than was predicted. Many experts believe that the 6-month INH/RMP regimen supplemented with PZA for the first 2 months should be the standard initial treatment for tuberculosis. Directly observed, twice-weekly therapy for the last 4 months should be utilized for poorly cooperative individuals.

The remarkable success of short-course treatment has been attributed to special characteristics of certain drugs, e.g., the ability of INH, RMP, and PZA to penetrate macrophages and to kill rapidly growing bacilli; the effectiveness of PZA in the acid environment of the phagolysosome; and the more rapid bactericidal activity of RMP during periods of intermittent growth of otherwise dormant bacilli.

Results of Treatment. The success of treatment may be judged by clinical assessment, decreased bacillary count of the sputum, and clearing of the lungs as shown on radiographs. The temperature usually returns to normal within a week or two, but in some patients who are highly febrile, defervescence may not occur for many weeks. The speed of radiographic improvement depends upon the nature and extent of pulmonary disease and the age of the patient. Chronic, cavitary, and fibrotic lesions do not clear rapidly. The sputum should be examined at frequent intervals during the first few months of treatment, since a decreasing number of acid-fast bacilli is the surest indication of successful treatment. The best of regimens in patients with far-advanced disease takes 4 to 6 weeks to convert sputum cultures to negative in 50 per cent of cases; to convert 75 per cent of cases usually requires about 10 weeks. The rate of conversion depends on the same factors that determine the rate of radiographic clearing. Failure of the sputum to convert to negative or a rise in the bacillary count after an initial decrease represents a treatment failure. Such failures are usually the result of poor compliance on the part of the patient but occasionally are related to bacillary drug resistance or an inappropriate drug regimen. The aim of chemotherapy is an initial success rate of 100 per cent without relapses. When relapse occurs, it is usually within a year of the completion of therapy. Rarely, relapses may occur with decreasing frequency up to 5 to 10 years after completion of therapy. This is so infrequent after adequate drug therapy that it is no longer necessary for the local health department to carry out periodic follow-up examinations.

Corticosteroids. Corticosteroids may be a useful adjunct to chemotherapy for selected patients. They usually produce a dramatic reversal of overwhelming sepsis and prompt defervescence in those patients who remain febrile, anorectic, and debilitated despite apparently adequate drug treatment. Absorption of the fluid may be hastened in tuberculous pleurisy and pericarditis, although there is no evidence that late complications in the pleural and pericardial spaces are prevented. Steroids should be given for as short a time as possible, preferably for no longer than 3 or 4 weeks. A more controversial issue is whether or not to use INH prophylaxis to cover the administration of steroids in the patient with a history of tuberculosis or with a positive tuberculin skin test result. This situation is most likely to occur in patients receiving steroids to prevent rejection of transplanted organs, to help control lymphoma or leukemia, or to control severe asthma. One year of INH preventive therapy is recommended when steroids are used on a long-term basis.

Reversal of Infectiousness. Some experts believe that it takes only about 2 weeks of effective chemotherapy to render patients noninfectious to others, even when large numbers of viable acid-fast bacilli are still present in the sputum. The evidence for this is inconclusive, and it is more reasonable to consider a patient with smear-positive sputum to represent a gradually diminishing risk until the smears are negative.

Drug Resistance. The phenomenon of clinical bacillary resistance was recognized soon after SM was tried as single drug therapy. The emergence of drug-resistant strains was at least delayed, if not prevented, by the use of two or more drugs in combination. Resistant populations emerge by a selective process in which resistant cells are favored which have arisen by spontaneous random mutation at the rate of about 1×10^{-8} to 1×10^{-10} per bacterium per generation.

Modern drug regimens are designed to prevent the emergence of drug resistance unless the patient is noncompliant or infection occurs with strains already resistant to one or more drugs—a situation known as *primary drug resistance*. The rate of primary drug resistance in a community influences the choice of drug regimens for initial treatment. In this country the overall rate is 7 per cent and varies in different locations from 3 to 15 per cent, depending mainly on the relative numbers of Asian and Hispanic individuals in the population. Age is another important factor; the highest rate is seen in young children. The highest single drug rate is for INH, with SM second. In a 1980 study from the Centers for Disease Control, 41 per cent of unsuccessfully treated patients harbored strains resistant to at least one drug. In the face of known or suspected drug-resistant bacilli, it is preferable to use at least three drugs until susceptibility test results are available.

Retreatment. The choice of proper therapy for initial treatment failures and disease that relapses after apparently successful treatment requires special expertise. Accurate drug susceptibility testing is a prerequisite for devising the best drug regimen, but while awaiting test results the following guidelines may be followed: A single new drug should not be added to a regimen that has failed, since rapid emergence of resistance to the new drug may occur. Instead, the new regimen should contain at least two drugs that the patient has never received previously.

In selecting the proper drugs, all available information should be gathered from the patient, the patient's family and former physicians, and health departments. It may be necessary to use combinations of four or more drugs, some of which have high rates of adverse reactions. After two or three relapses, especially when the infecting strain is resistant to INH, RMP, and SM, the chances of success are slim. The best approach to retreatment of patients with multiply resistant strains is to prevent this unfortunate turn of events by proper supervision of the initial course of drug therapy.

Patients with Impaired Renal and Hepatic Function. Isoniazid is excreted mainly in the urine, and it has been reported that the drug will accumulate in patients with markedly impaired renal function. However, the drug is dialyzable, and others have reported that the half-life is prolonged only slightly in patients with renal failure. It is probably not necessary to reduce the dosage, but pyridoxine supplementation should be given and patients should be monitored for hepatitis and peripheral neuropathy. It may also be advisable to assay INH serum concentrations from time to time. Rifampin is metabolized in the liver and excreted mainly in the bile. When hepatic function is impaired, the drug may accumulate to toxic levels. It is only slightly, if at all, dialyzable. Both EMB and SM are cleared by dialysis and are excreted mainly through the urine. The dosage of SM must be reduced in proportion to the renal function; serum levels should be checked frequently, and the patient should be monitored for signs of eighth nerve toxicity. In a similar fashion, the dosage of EMB must be reduced, serum levels checked, and the visual acuity monitored. Since about 20 per cent of EMB is metabolized in the liver, it would be wise to check serum levels when there is hepatic failure. There is insufficient information upon which to base recommendations for use of PZA, ethionamide, and cycloserine in patients with impaired renal or hepatic function. Since PZA and cycloserine are excreted mainly by the kidneys, the dosage should be reduced and blood levels monitored when these drugs are used in patients with poor kidney function. It is not known how ethionamide is metabolized; only a very small amount may be found unchanged in the urine. Drug levels should be monitored to avoid accumulation.

Treatment of Pregnant Women. Ethionamide and SM should be avoided, the first because of teratogenic potential and the second because eighth nerve damage has been reported in the offspring. Cycloserine and PZA should also be avoided because of a lack of information on possible adverse effects. Although rifampin crosses the placental barrier readily and inhibits ribonucleic acid (RNA) polymerase, there is no evidence of its association with fetal damage. Recommended treatment for pregnant women with active tuberculosis is INH/RMP for 9 months, supplemented with EMB if necessary.

Treatment of Children. There are conflicting recommendations for drug regimens and dosages of individual drugs for treatment of children with tuberculosis. The most suitable combination is INH 10 mg per kilogram daily (maximum of 300 mg daily) and RMP 15 mg per kilogram daily (maximum of 600 mg daily). A third drug should be added if there is risk of infection with drug-resistant organisms. The third drug, given for the first 2 or 3 months of therapy, may be SM, EMB,* or PZA. All three drugs have drawbacks: SM has a high rate of adverse effects and must be given by injection; young children cannot be monitored for the major toxicity of EMB, optic neuritis; and experience with PZA is limited. Directly observed, twice-weekly therapy should be considered for a poorly cooperative family. Nine months has been suggested for duration of treatment, perhaps reduced to 6 months when PZA is used as a third drug.

Surgical and Collapse Procedures. The need for collapse procedures such as pneumothorax, pneumoperitoneum, and phrenic nerve crush and for excisional surgery with or without thoracoplasty has been virtually eliminated by the success of chemotherapy. The surgeon may still be called upon to correct late complications of previous attempts at treatment such as bronchopleural fistula, persistent empyema, and hemoptysis from bronchiectasis or aspergilloma.

EXTRAPULMONARY DISEASE. In contrast to the declining incidence of pulmonary tuberculosis, there has been little change

---

*Not recommended for use in children under 13 years of age.

in the number of extrapulmonary cases reported in the United States since 1964, about 4000 per year. This may be partially explained by the higher rate of infection in the immunocompromised states associated with old age, renal failure (including dialysis and transplant patients), cirrhosis, malnutrition, hematologic malignancies, and AIDS. In England, extrapulmonary disease is reported mainly in recent immigrants from the Asian subcontinent.

Thoracic Cavity and Chest Wall. Tuberculosis of the pleura is almost always associated with disease of the lung, arising by contiguous spread or rupture of a subpleural tubercle. It usually begins as a localized fibrinous inflammation, which produces pleuritic chest pain. Pleurisy with effusion is often associated with primary infection. When this occurs in young adults who are untreated, approximately 75 per cent may be expected to develop overt pulmonary tuberculosis within 5 years. The onset may be either abrupt or insidious, with cough and fever accompanying the chest pain. Pain and friction rub often disappear as pleural fluid accumulates. Most primary tuberculous pleural effusions resorb spontaneously, sometimes within a week or two, but the diagnosis can be made on the basis of a positive tuberculin skin test result, the exudative characteristics of the fluid, and the preponderance of lymphocytes. Tubercle bacilli are usually very scarce in the fluid so that stained smears may be negative and cultures only weakly positive. Imprints and cultures made from pleural tissue removed by closed needle biopsy are more likely than the fluid to be positive. Histologic examination also may be helpful. Pleural effusions in young adults who have positive tuberculin skin test results are best treated as tuberculosis unless some other cause can be identified. The fluid should be aspirated for diagnosis and perhaps once or twice more if it accumulates rapidly. Chest tube drainage should be avoided. Corticosteroids should not be used routinely but may be given in selected cases to hasten symptomatic improvement and absorption of the fluid. Pleural effusion may also occur in disseminated tuberculosis with multiple organ and serous membrane involvement. Tuberculous empyema may be secondary to involvement of the vertebral column or result from a bronchopleural fistula.

Endobronchial tuberculosis commonly accompanies pulmonary disease but now rarely results in identifiable symptoms and signs. In primary tuberculosis of children it is the pressure of enlarged lymph nodes together with ulceration and rupture through the bronchial wall that produces endobronchial disease. Endobronchial disease in adults usually starts as inflammatory lesions from repeated implantations of tubercle bacilli originating in lung parenchyma. These lesions may progress to ulceration and narrowing of the bronchi and eventually to cicatricial stenosis. Secondary changes include atelectasis and obstructive pneumonitis, tension cavity from involvement of the distal small bronchi or bronchioles, and accumulation of fluid within cavities. The symptoms of endobronchial disease are spasmodic coughing and a localized wheeze. Bronchial ulceration or erosion of a caseating lymph node may cause positive sputum in the absence of recognizable pulmonary disease. Bronchoscopy usually serves to identify the lesions.

Although tuberculosis of the endocardium and myocardium has been described, the most common involvement of the heart is *pericarditis.* Rupture into the pericardium of nearby caseous lymph nodes is the common route of infection, although lymphohematogenous dissemination may occur. The serofibrinous pericardial effusion usually is associated with substernal pain, fever, pericardial friction rub, and left-sided pleural effusion. Cardiac tamponade occasionally develops in the acute stage. A search for tuberculosis elsewhere and a tuberculin skin test should be performed. A thorough examination of the pericardial fluid obtained by needle aspiration or surgical drainage also may be helpful. Obtaining a pericardial biopsy sample in the operating room may be justified in obscure cases because of the importance of early drug treatment. The differential diagnosis includes benign or viral pericarditis, pyogenic infection, other granulomatous inflammations, connective tissue disease, and malignant effusion. The diagnosis is made more difficult by the facts that the skin test reaction is negative in a sizable minority; the fluid rarely contains enough organisms to be positive by smear and often not even by culture; the characteristics of the fluid are nonspecific; and about half of the individuals have no other obvious sites of tuberculosis. The administration of corticosteroids may be beneficial, but antituberculosis drugs should be used in addition even when tuberculosis is only suspected.

The most important sequela is constrictive pericarditis, which usually occurs 2 to 4 years after the acute disease. At this stage the heart is small and relatively immobile and there is a paradoxical pulse and obstruction of venous return to the heart, with congestion of the liver, peripheral edema, and later ascites. Calcification of the pericardium may be seen on x-ray films. Treatment consists of removal of the pericardium, although it is preferable to perform the operation at an earlier stage.

The chest wall may be the site of one or more subcutaneous abscesses as a result of hematogenous dissemination or sometimes as the peripheral manifestation of an empyema necessitatis as it burrows through the chest wall. Chest wall abscesses may also result from drainage of underlying caseous lymph nodes along the intercostal lymphatics.

Extrathoracic. Lymphatic. Tuberculous lymphadenitis is the most common manifestation of extrathoracic disease throughout the world, and the most frequently involved nodes are cervical. The disease in this location was known as *scrofula,* or the *King's Evil.* The latter name was used because the condition was supposedly amenable to cure by the royal touch. Although it was once thought that infection with *M. bovis* was responsible for most cases of scrofula, a recent study from England emphasized that *M. tuberculosis* accounted for more cases than did the bovine organism, although the latter is relatively more common in lymphatic tuberculosis than in other forms of the disease. Infection of the tonsils through the ingestion of contaminated milk was the usual route of infection for the tonsillar node high in the neck, near the angle of the jaw. At present, scrofula in young children is mainly due to infection with mycobacteria other than *M. tuberculosis* and *M. bovis* (see Ch. 333). Supraclavicular node involvement usually arises by lymphatic spread from mediastinal disease. Affected nodes elsewhere in the neck, as well as those in the axilla and inguinal area, the other common sites of involvement, may be the result of drainage from a primary site or from hematogenous spread. Both intra- and extrathoracic node involvement is common in tuberculosis of AIDS patients.

The infected nodes are usually detectable by sight and palpation. Although the nodes usually are not painful, they may be tender during the phase of rapid enlargement early in the infection. Later they become matted together and eventually soften, slough, and drain. Draining sinuses may persist for many months, sometimes for years, with intermittent healing and breakdown. The diagnosis may be made by bacteriologic study of the pus from draining sinuses or by biopsy together with bacteriologic studies. The presence of calcific densities in the neck and axilla as seen in the chest radiograph may provide evidence of healed tuberculous adenitis.

Lymphatic tuberculosis tends to heal but often not completely, so that relapse is common even many years after the primary infection. Treatment with antituberculosis drugs is usually successful, although the tendency to late relapse may still be seen. Good results have been reported with short-course regimens. Excision of large caseous nodes in accessible sites sometimes is advisable.

Genitourinary. The second most common site of infection is the genitourinary tract. Disease is usually centered in the kidney, which becomes seeded either during the primary infection or later. These foci may remain dormant for many years. When reactivation occurs, one or more renal abscesses are produced, followed by spread to the remainder of the urinary tract. Extensive scarring of the ureters eventually occurs. This scarring produces obstructive hydronephrosis, which together with renal caseation may destroy the kidney completely. Specific symptoms may be lacking until the hydronephrotic kidney becomes secondarily infected or until the development of tuberculous cystitis manifested by frequency and dysuria. Long before the onset of symptoms, the examination of the urine may show hematuria, pyuria, and albuminuria, along with cultures negative for pyogens. The diagnosis is made by radiographic examination of the urinary tract, cystoscopy, and demonstration of tubercle bacilli by cultures of first morning voided urines. It was found that approximately 10 per cent of a general tuberculosis patient population had positive urine cultures, and in 7 per cent of these patients the urinary tract disease was completely unanticipated. Renal tuberculosis responds well to drug treatment. According to recent recommendations, conventional long-term regimens may be replaced by 6- to 9-month courses of INH, RMP, and a third drug (either EMB or PZA). The role of surgery remains controversial. Some urologists would remove destroyed kidneys and repair strictures of the ureter, while others claim that surgery is almost never indicated.

Genital tuberculosis in the male may involve the prostate, seminal vesicles, and epididymis. The acute inflammation is later replaced by induration and hard nodules, sometimes followed by obstruction, calcification, and chronic draining sinuses of the scrotum. The diagnosis is made by finding tubercle bacilli in the urine, sinus drainage, or biopsied tissues. In the female, tuberculous salpingitis is the common manifestation, followed by disease of the uterus and ovaries. Sterility almost always results, and peritonitis may occur secondarily. The symptoms are those of chronic pelvic inflammatory disease. Diagnosis should be based on examination of tissue from the endometrium and from lesions visible through the laparoscope and cultures of the menstrual fluid or vaginal discharge. As with renal tuberculosis, drug therapy usually is successful, but excisional surgery may be indicated for residual lesions or persistently draining sinuses.

Skeletal Tuberculosis. The presence of a gibbus or hunchback deformity of the thoracic spine (Pott's disease) has served as a marker of tuberculosis since prehistoric times. *Tuberculous spondylitis* is still the most common manifestation of bone and joint infection. At present, it is mainly a disease of adults that arises by reactivation of dormant foci. The common areas of involvement are thoracic and lumbar; the cervical spine may be involved in 2 to 3 per cent of cases. The destructive process usually begins in the intervertebral discs, where it first produces narrowing of the disc space, then destruction of the two adjacent vertebral bodies through the bony end-plates. Sometimes, however, the anterior portion of the vertebral body is destroyed first. Inflammation often extends into the soft tissues surrounding the spine, either in the form of a spreading, phlegmonous reaction or as a cold abscess that may be paravertebral, in and around the psoas muscle, or retropharyngeal, depending upon the site of disease. The symptoms are usually dominated by back pain, sometimes followed by the neurologic manifestations of compression of the spinal cord and nerve roots. There may be fever. Active tuberculosis of the lungs may be absent, although some evidence of past disease usually is seen.

Radiographic examination of the spine shows destructive lesions in the commonly involved sites. The paraspinal involvement appears as widening of the mediastinum or an oval-shaped density behind the heart. It may be manifested as a psoas abscess, a retropharyngeal abscess, or a mass in the groin or in the supraclavicular area. A similar radiographic appearance may occur in pyogenic infection of the spine. A needle biopsy sample usually is necessary to establish the proper diagnosis. Occasionally open biopsy of the vertebral body may be necessary. Imaging of the spine by magnetic resonance and computed tomography is valuable in the differential diagnosis and to delineate the extent of disease.

The disease has a natural tendency to heal by spontaneous fusion of the vertebral bodies. Treatment consists of antituberculosis chemotherapy according to the modern regimens described under Treatment. Preliminary results with short-course treatment are encouraging, but they cannot be recommended for routine use until further experience has accumulated. Prolonged bed rest, immobilization of the spine, and spinal fusion usually are not necessary, although some indications still exist for surgical procedures: evidence of cord compression and other major neurologic deficits, instability of the spine, and involvement of the upper and midthoracic spine.

Tuberculous arthritis occurs mainly in hips and knees but also may involve many other joints, including elbows, shoulders, and the joints of the hands and feet. The patient usually has chronic monoarticular arthritis. Diagnosis is made by synovial biopsy and bacteriologic study of tissues and pus. The process usually responds to antituberculosis chemotherapy without the necessity for operative procedures, but occasionally excision of extensively destroyed synovium and temporary immobilization may be beneficial.

Tuberculous tenosynovitis is usually secondary to involvement of adjacent bone. At least two distinctive processes may result from involvement of the hand: carpal tunnel syndrome, and compound palmar ganglion, a distinctive bilobed swelling on either side of the volar carpal ligament. Chemotherapy often needs to be supplemented by debridement and evacuation of fibrinous material.

Abdominal Tuberculosis. *Intestinal tuberculosis* secondary to chronic pulmonary disease once was so common that patients were routinely screened by radiography of the small bowel upon admission to the sanatorium. This situation continued long after the ingestion of *M. bovis* was brought under control by the pasteurization of milk. Lately, the emphasis has been on primary intestinal disease in the absence of recognizable pulmonary lesions. The route of infection in these cases remains unknown. Tuberculosis may involve all parts of the alimentary canal from top to bottom, but by far the most common location is in the ileocecal area. The predominant tissue reaction may be either ulcerative or hyperplastic, with accompanying bleeding, perforation, fistula formation, obstruction, or combinations of two or more of these processes. The early symptoms are nonspecific, consisting mainly of anorexia, loss of weight, abdominal pain, and alternating periods of diarrhea and constipation. The clinical picture is not unlike that of Crohn's disease, especially since a fibrogranulomatous tissue reaction is characteristic of both. Tuberculosis of the colon also may occur and needs to be distinguished from carcinoma, diverticulitis, and inflammatory bowel disease of nonspecific nature. Perirectal abscess and fistula formation may result from lower colon lesions. The disease usually responds well to antituberculosis chemotherapy, but surgical correction may be necessary for the complications described earlier. The diagnosis often is made unexpectedly at surgery or autopsy.

Tuberculous peritonitis may result from bloodborne infection or by extension of disease from the intestine, mesenteric lymph nodes, or fallopian tubes. The classic form is that of a chronic adhesive peritonitis that produces a doughy, tender abdomen, abdominal masses, low-grade fever, anorexia, and weight loss. A much more common manifestation is painless ascites. When this occurs in adults with alcoholic cirrhosis and ascites, it makes for a difficult differential diagnosis. Tuberculosis should be suspected when the combination of fever, ascites, and a positive tuberculin skin test reaction is found. Examination of the fluid is helpful. A high total protein concentration with a moderate number of leukocytes, mostly lymphocytes, is suggestive of tuberculosis. A more definitive diagnosis may be obtained by laparoscopy or laparotomy. Usually the entire peritoneal surface is studded with tubercles that are easily differentiated from carcinomatosis histologically. The fluid is rarely positive for AFB by stained smear and even by culture is positive in somewhat less than 50 per cent of cases. Response to antituberculosis chemotherapy is good.

Isolated tuberculosis of the liver or spleen occasionally has been described. These organs are usually involved in disseminated or miliary tuberculosis, but occasionally a liver biopsy done in an attempt to explain enlargement of the liver, jaundice, or abnormal liver function studies leads to a diagnosis of tuberculosis when there is apparently no disease elsewhere.

Central Nervous System. In the past, *tuberculous meningitis* was one of the most dreaded complications of primary tuberculosis in young children, appearing in about one in a thousand cases and almost always resulting in fatality. It usually occurred 2 to 6 months after the primary infection in infants and was commonly associated with miliary tuberculosis. In this country it is now more likely to be seen in adults than in children. Invasion of the meninges occurs by direct extension from subjacent caseous foci in the cerebral cortex, cerebellum, choroid plexus, middle ear, or spine. Brain infarcts secondary to tuberculous arteritis sometimes occur. The syndrome of inappropriate secretion of antidiuretic hormone may accompany the meningitis.

The inflammatory reaction is concentrated around the base of the brain, where the thick exudate may eventually obstruct the basal foramina to produce hydrocephalus. Examination of the spinal fluid reveals a characteristic pattern of high protein, low sugar, and a moderate number (up to a few hundred) of leukocytes, most of which are lymphocytes. However, early in the course of the disease neutrophils may predominate; rarely the shift to a lymphocytic exudate does not occur; the sugar level may be normal or only slightly decreased; and the number of leukocytes may reach several thousand. Occasionally the protein content is high enough that a thin web or pellicle appears in undisturbed refrigerated fluid. Acid-fast bacilli may be seen in this web, although they are not visible in the sedimented fluid. Stained smears of the fluid are usually positive in no more than 25 per cent of samples, but there are a few colonies of tubercle bacilli in cultures in about 75 per cent of cases. The larger the sample of spinal fluid submitted, the greater the chance of finding the organism. The tuberculin skin test should be positive in approximately 75 per cent of cases, provided that those nonreactive to 5 TU are retested with 250 TU. A careful search reveals evidence of tuberculosis elsewhere in the majority of cases, although the disease in the lungs may appear to be inactive.

The onset is usually insidious, extending over a period of many weeks. Occasionally, however, there is a much more acute onset that resembles pyogenic or aseptic meningitis. The most common symptoms are headache, fever, lethargy, and confusion. Later, focal neurologic signs appear in the form of ocular palsies, other cranial nerve palsies, and increasing stupor progressing to coma. Stiffness of the neck is common. The outcome of therapy depends mainly on the stage of disease at the time treatment is instituted. Treatment should start immediately when tuberculous meningitis is suspected, without waiting for confirmation of diagnosis. A triple-drug regimen including INH and RMP is recommended. Ethionamide and PZA achieve therapeutic concentrations in spinal fluid even in the absence of an inflammatory reaction. Ethambutol penetrates reasonably well through inflamed meninges. It should be remembered that SM does not appear in therapeutic concentrations and that infections with INH-resistant organisms occur more often in children than in adults. Treatment should be continued for at least 1 year, although administration of the third drug may be discontinued after 2 or 3 months once it has been determined that drug resistance is not a problem. The use of corticosteroids is controversial, but should be considered in the presence of coma or spinal fluid block. Intrathecal treatment is usually not necessary.

Tuberculomas of the brain may be seen at any age. Cases involving children still predominate in the developing countries, while in the United States they occur mainly in adults. The clinical presentation is that of a brain tumor with signs and symptoms of increased intracranial pressure, focal seizures, and focal neurologic defects. Indications of infection, such as fever, often are absent. Lesions may be single or multiple and must be differentiated from tumor and abscess. The spinal fluid may show slight lymphocytosis and elevated protein concentration, but often it is normal. The correct diagnosis may be suggested by radiographic or magnetic resonance scanning techniques, a positive tuberculin skin test reaction, and the presence of tuberculosis elsewhere, but the definitive procedures are needle aspiration through a burr hole and craniotomy for open biopsy. Drug treatment similar to that used for tuberculous meningitis should be used.

Miscellaneous. Almost every organ and tissue of the body can be involved in tuberculosis. In the upper respiratory tract and oral cavity, the larynx and the middle ear are most prone to infection. *Tuberculous laryngitis* used to be a rather common complication that was considered to be secondary to longstanding highly positive sputum associated with chronic cavitary disease. It was extremely painful and resulted in such difficulty in swallowing that severe inanition resulted. Response to drug treatment, even to administration of SM alone, was rapid and dramatic. The new face of tuberculous laryngitis is that of a primary laryngeal lesion that must be distinguished from carcinoma. Tuberculous middle ear disease, formerly common, is now rare. It was usually associated with advanced pulmonary or disseminated disease. Involvement of the eye is in the form of chronic uveitis, such as chorioretinitis, iridocyclitis, or iritis. Phlyctenular conjunctivitis produces small, yellowish vesicles. Direct inoculation into the eye may produce conjunctivitis or keratitis. The specific origin of eye disease is difficult to prove. Cutaneous tuberculosis has all but disappeared, except for lesions associated with direct inoculation in laboratory workers and pathologists. Other manifestations include lesions like lupus vulgaris, in which tubercle bacilli may be located, and the tuberculids that are considered to be hypersensitivity reactions, in which the organisms usually are not found. The larger blood vessels may harbor

infections in their walls. Tuberculosis is a rare cause of aortic aneurysm. At one time tuberculosis of the adrenal gland was a common cause of adrenal insufficiency. Occasional cases of tuberculosis of the thyroid, breast, and soft tissues elsewhere than in the chest wall are still being reported.

DISSEMINATED AND MILIARY TUBERCULOSIS. These terms are used synonymously, although miliary tuberculosis is but one form of disseminated tuberculosis in which the widely dispersed small tubercles resemble millet seeds. During life these lesions usually are first recognized in the chest roentgenogram as very small nodules of uniform size that are evenly distributed throughout both lungs. The acute form was predominantly an early complication of untreated primary tuberculosis, occurring mainly in young children and often associated with meningitis. During the past three decades the predominant age group has changed to the elderly, and the disease has become more subacute in its progression.

The diagnosis often is missed because it is difficult to distinguish the tuberculosis symptoms from those of the many underlying conditions that could be responsible for the weight loss, increasing fatigue, and low-grade fever. Skin test anergy and frequent absence of chronic pulmonary tuberculosis may compound the difficulty. This sort of subacute disseminated tuberculosis has been called *cryptic* or *nonreactive tuberculosis*. In a series of autopsied cases analyzed by Slavin and colleagues in 1980, only 15 per cent of patients admitted during the antibiotic era had the correct diagnosis made ante mortem. A composite of such a case would be an elderly anergic patient without previously recognized tuberculosis who presented to the hospital with malignancy, renal failure, a renal transplant, or chronic alcoholism. Constitutional symptoms would be nonspecific, mainly fever, loss of weight, and increasing fatigue. Examinations would reveal no obvious tuberculosis in lungs or other organs, no hepatosplenomegaly, and no enlarged peripheral lymph nodes. There would be moderate anemia, a slight elevation of alkaline phosphatase, and a negative initial bacteriologic workup. The correct diagnosis depends upon a high index of suspicion and the demonstration of characteristic microscopic lesions and mycobacteria by biopsy. The most productive tissue is the liver, usually sampled by needle biopsy, with bone marrow next in line. Blood cultures should be obtained, since they are sometimes positive at this stage of disease. At a later stage choroidal tubercles may be seen and radiographs of the lungs may show the typical miliary pattern.

Miliary tuberculosis almost always results from the discharge of infected caseous material into the bloodstream, usually from a well-hidden lymph node in the mediastinum or the abdomen. When multiple bacteremic episodes occur, the process may be protracted. The patient may have serositis manifested by pleural effusion, pericardial effusion, or ascites. Hematologic abnormalities may be so prominent that a primary blood disease is suspected. The most common abnormality is a leukemoid reaction, although leukopenia, thrombocytopenia, and hemolytic anemia may occur. More commonly the primary disease is hematologic, complicated by a secondary tuberculosis dissemination, especially when large doses of corticosteroids have been given.

Treatment should consist of an intensive antituberculosis drug regimen using at least three drugs. After a few months, when a good response has occurred and after the drug susceptibility pattern of the infecting strain is known, the third drug can be discontinued. The total duration of therapy has not been established, but it probably should be at least 1 year.

TUBERCULOSIS AND AIDS. The pandemic of AIDS has had a major impact on the worldwide tuberculosis problem. The incidence of tuberculosis in AIDS patients has been reported to be 5 to 21 per cent in New York, Newark, and Florida, and 3.8 per cent nationwide. Those at highest risk are intravenous drug users. In addition, analysis of patients with active tuberculosis revealed an HIV seropositivity rate of 40 per cent in Zaire and 30 per cent in Florida. The association of the two infections accounts for the failure of the tuberculosis case rate curve to move downward since 1984.

Tuberculosis usually occurs early in the course of AIDS and may even be the sentinel infection. Diagnosis is difficult because the characteristic pulmonary symptoms, signs, and radiographic appearance often are absent. Disease tends to be extrapulmonary, disseminated, and lymphatic. Pulmonary lesions, when present, often are noncavitary and nonapical. Skin test reactions are not dependable. Diagnosis may depend upon biopsies of lymph node, liver, and bone marrow, blood cultures, and bronchoscopy. Modern chemotherapy regimens usually are successful but probably should be continued for a year. All patients with risk factors for HIV infection or with ARC should be skin tested and, if positive, given a course of the best preventive chemotherapy available. See also Part XXI.

NEW DIAGNOSTIC TESTS. Several innovative techniques have been proposed for the rapid diagnosis of tuberculosis. The most promising are (1) specific antigen detection by enzyme-linked immunosorbent assay (ELISA) or antibody-sensitized latex particles, (2) detection of DNA sequences by probes and polymerase chain reaction, and (3) demonstration of tuberculostearic acid by chromatography and mass spectrometry, which is especially useful for body fluids such as cerebrospinal fluid (CSF).

Abernathy RS: Tuberculosis in children and its management. Sem Respir Infect 4:232, 1989. *The latest thorough review of this subject.*

Anonymous: Tuberculosis in chronic renal failure. Lancet 1:909, 1980. *A short leading article documenting an incidence 10 times as high as in a control population.*

Ben-Dov I, Mason GR: Drug resistant tuberculosis in a southern California hospital; trends from 1969 to 1984. Am Rev Respir Dis 135:1307, 1987. *Resistance to at least one drug was found in 35 per cent of 281 hospitalized patients. Resistance was primary in 23 per cent, acquired in 59 per cent.*

Centers for Disease Control: Primary resistance to antituberculosis drugs—United States. MMWR 32:521, 1983. *The final report of a 7-year study in which 20 selected laboratories throughout the country submitted over 12,000 cultures to the CDC laboratory to be tested for drug susceptibility in a uniform manner.*

Chapman M, Murray RO, Stoker DJ: Tuberculosis of the bones and joints. Semin Roentgenol 14:266, 1979. *This is a thorough clinical review, replete with excellent pictures, from the Royal National Orthopaedic Hospital in London.*

Daniel TM, Debanne SM: The serodiagnosis of tuberculosis and other mycobacterial diseases by enzyme-linked immunosorbent assay. Am Rev Respir Dis 135:1137, 1987. *This state-of-the-art review takes us from the early work of Arloing in 1898 through many decades of failures up to the present, when we can look forward to having soon a useful clinical diagnostic test.*

Dannenberg AM Jr: Macrophages in inflammation and infection. N Engl J Med 293:489, 1975. *This study utilizing skin lesions in rabbits demonstrates the dynamic nature of mycobacterial lesions. Macrophages enter the arena as novices, become activated locally by interaction with immune lymphocytes, ingest bacilli, die, and are replaced by fresh cells recruited from the circulation.*

DeWit D, Steyn L, Shoemaker S, et al: Direct detection of Mycobacterium tuberculosis in clinical specimens by DNA amplification. J Clin Microbiol 28:2437, 1990. *Specific DNA was detected in specimens of CSF, pleural and pericardial fluid, and tissue. The test was "at least as sensitive as conventional culture techniques."*

Edwards D, Kirkpatrick CH: The immunology of mycobacterial disease. Am Rev Respir Dis 134:1062, 1986. *A relatively brief state-of-the-art review that brings this subject up to date.*

Elias J, DeConing JP, Vorster SA, et al.: The rapid and sensitive diagnosis of tuberculous meningitis by the detection of tuberculostearic acid in cerebrospinal fluid using gas chromatography–mass spectrometry with selective ion monitoring. Clin Biochem 22:463, 1989. *In this study from South Africa, the authors document a satisfactory 5-hour test using 35 samples of spinal fluid.*

Fertel J, Pitchenik AE: Tuberculosis in acquired immune deficiency syndrome. Semin Respir Infec 4:198, 1989. *An excellent review of tuberculosis in AIDS from a well-informed Miami team.*

Fine PEM: BCG vaccination against tuberculosis and leprosy. Br Med Bull 44:691, 1988. *The author reviews the history and the public health impact of BCG vaccines. He concludes that they have had a substantial impact.*

Fox W: The chemotherapy of tuberculosis: A review. Chest 76S:785, 1979. *An excellent review of antituberculosis drug treatment up to 1979.*

Jacobs RF, Abernathy RS: Management of tuberculosis in pregnancy and the newborn. Clin Perinatol 15:305, 1988. *A valuable review for coverage of clinical management as well as drug therapy.*

Kallo JR, Pulliam L: The BACTEC radiometric system for detection and rapid identification of mycobacteria. Lab Med 20:692, 1989. *The automated system compared favorably with culture controls in over 1,000 specimens, confirming several previously reported large-scale studies.*

Lichtenstein IH, MacGregor RR: Mycobacterial infections in renal transplant recipients: Report of 5 cases and review of the literature. Rev Infect Dis 5:216, 1983. *Among the cases were two that probably represented reactivation tuberculosis in the transplanted kidney. A survey of 26 transplantation centers revealed a tuberculosis rate of 480 cases per 100,000.*

Lifeso RM, Weaver P, Harder EH: Tuberculous spondylitis in adults. J Bone Joint Surg 67A:1405, 1985. *Experience with 107 cases from Saudi Arabia allows the authors to reach valid conclusions regarding the role of surgery. They report good results with chemotherapy and selected anterior decompression and fusion.*

Lincoln EM: Epidemics of tuberculosis. Arch Environ Health 14:473, 1967. *A review of 109 epidemics in 12 countries, the majority of them occurring in schools.*

Mackay AD, Cole RB: The problems of tuberculosis in the elderly. QJ Med 53:497, 1984. *The case rate of tuberculosis is increasing among the elderly, and physicians should understand the special problems of diagnosis and management so well presented in this report.*

O'Brien RJ: Present chemotherapy of tuberculosis. Semin Respir Infect 4:216, 1989. *An excellent presentation from the Division of Tuberculosis Control, CDC.*

Omari B, Robertson JM, Nelson RJ, Chiu LC: Pott's disease, a resurgent challenge to the thoracic surgeon. Chest 95:145, 1989. *Recounts good results with combined medical and surgical treatment of 19 patients from Los Angeles.*

Rieder HL, Snider DE Jr, Cauthen GM: Extrapulmonary tuberculosis in the United States. Am Rev Respir Dis 141:347, 1990. *The latest statistics on all varieties of extrapulmonary disease from the Division of Tuberculosis Control, CDC.*

Sahn SA, Lakshminarayan S: Tuberculosis after corticosteroid therapy. Br J Dis Chest 70:195, 1976. *This review emphasizes the usefulness of preventive therapy with isoniazid in patients already infected with M. tuberculosis.*

Schofield PF: Abdominal tuberculosis (leading article). Gut 26:1275, 1985. *The author gives a good discussion of all aspects of abdominal disease as it is seen today.*

Slavin RE, Walsh TJ, Pollack AD: Late generalized tuberculosis: A clinical pathologic analysis and comparison of 100 cases in the preantibiotic and antibiotic eras. Medicine 59:352, 1980. *This study, from the Department of Pathology at Johns Hopkins University, consists of an analysis of 200 autopsied cases. It contains a wealth of useful information on one form of disseminated tuberculosis.*

Stead WW: Control of tuberculosis in institutions. Chest 76 (suppl):797, 1979. *Reviews recent outbreaks in nursing homes, prisons, schools, and hospitals and suggests common-sense methods of control.*

Stead WW, Kerby GR, Schlueter DP, et al.: The clinical spectrum of primary tuberculosis in adults. Ann Intern Med 68:333, 1968. *Primary pulmonary disease was documented in 37 adults, of whom 9 had only minor symptoms, 11 developed pleural effusion, and 16 showed progression to adult-type chronic pulmonary disease.*

Stead WW, Senner JW, Reddick WT, Lofgren JP: Racial differences in susceptibility to infection by Mycobacterium tuberculosis. N Engl J Med 322:422, 1990. *The authors provide convincing epidemiologic evidence that blacks are more readily infected than whites, at least in the nursing home setting. Once infected, the progression to clinical disease was not different.*

333 Other Mycobacterioses

Emanuel Wolinsky

Organisms of the tuberculosis complex are not the only mycobacteria associated with human disease. The most popular label at present for these other mycobacteria is "nontuberculous." They have become more prominent in the total picture of mycobacterial disease because of the declining incidence of tuberculosis and a greater awareness and recognition of the other mycobacterioses. Indeed, there is evidence that the frequency of nontuberculous pulmonary disease may be increasing in certain areas of the country. In addition, disseminated mycobacterial infection is now recognized much more frequently as an opportunistic infection in immunosuppressed individuals, especially in those with the acquired immunodeficiency syndrome (AIDS). Infection with other mycobacteria has been blamed, perhaps unfairly, for the apparent failure of bacille Calmette-Guérin (BCG) vaccination to protect adults in South India from subsequent tuberculosis. Leprosy, also a mycobacterial disease, is discussed in Ch. 334.

Although the existence of nontuberculous mycobacteria was recognized in the late 1800's, they were first identified as causes of human disease in the mid 1950's.

MYCOBACTERIA. *Mycobacterium avium-intracellulare (MAI).* Mycobacteria of this species or complex constitute the most important agents of nontuberculous mycobacteriosis throughout the world. The organism known as the avian tubercle bacillus was described in 1890, although tuberculosis of chickens had been recognized for 22 years before that time. Supposedly quite resistant to infection with *M. avium*, people with documented *M. avium* disease were the subjects of occasional literature reports. Recognition of the expanded role of these mycobacteria in pulmonary and disseminated disease occurred in the 1950's, when the organism was misnamed *Nocardia intracellularis* and given the common name of Battey bacillus. The official name of *Mycobacterium intracellulare* was assigned in the 1960's. The realization that *M. intracellulare* could not be distinguished from *M. avium* in most laboratories dictated another change to the term MAI or *M. avium complex*. In this complex one can recognize 28 types by seroagglutination, of which types 1 to 3 represent the classic *M. avium* strains. By using DNA probes, one can differentiate *M. avium* (serotypes 1–6, 8–11, 21) from *M. intracellulare* (types 7, 12–20). Strains of MAI grow slowly; usually are nonpigmented or slightly yellow, becoming more highly pigmented with age but independently of light; are resistant to most antituberculosis drugs; and often produce colony variants of two or three types, including smooth translucent, smooth domed, and rough opaque. Of the three variants, the translucent colonies are usually most drug resistant and most virulent for experimental animals. Strains of MAI may be associated with all varieties of mycobacterial disease, especially pulmonary disease, childhood lymphadenitis, and disseminated infection in patients who have AIDS. AIDS-associated strains tend to be deeply pigmented and, in the United States, are mainly serotypes 1, 4, and 8.

Mycobacterium scrofulaceum. This is a scotochromogenic mycobacterium similar in many ways to MAI. The pigmentation varies from light yellow to dark orange. In some publications these organisms are lumped together with MAI, and the combination is called the *MAIS complex*. The name derives from the fact that the organism was recognized as the cause of scrofula in young children. Rarely, *M. scrofulaceum* may be associated with pulmonary disease in adults. Most of the disease-associated strains belong to one of three seroagglutination types, but it is not uncommon to see a strain of *M. scrofulaceum* agglutinate in one of the MAI serotypes.

Mycobacterium kansasii. The "yellow bacillus" was described in 1953 in Kansas City and was later given the official name of *M. kansasii*. It is responsible for a large number of pulmonary mycobacteriosis cases in some areas of the world. The organisms may be recognized in the initial sputum smears as large cross-barred acid-fast bacilli. Positive cultures may be identified by their distinctive photochromogenicity. The yellow color is light dependent, developing within hours after the colonies have been exposed to light. Most strains are fully susceptible to rifampin and only slightly resistant to isoniazid, ethambutol, and streptomycin. *M. kansasii* is not found in nature except occasionally in samples of water.

Mycobacterium fortuitum-chelonae. Strains of this group grow rapidly, even on ordinary laboratory media. They are sometimes spoken of as the *M. fortuitum complex*, but it is better to retain at least two separate species because they can be distinguished from each other readily in the laboratory, and *M. chelonae* tends to be much more drug resistant than *M. fortuitum*. Both species are pathogenic for mice and resistant to the usual antituberculosis drugs. Long known for their ability to produce injection site abscesses and severe infections of traumatic wounds, strains of this group recently have become prominent as the cause of sternal osteomyelitis after cardiac surgery, of wound infection after implantation of silicone breast prostheses, of disseminated and localized infection in dialysis patients, of prosthetic valve endocarditis, and of disseminated infections with skin lesions in the immunosuppressed host.

Mycobacterium marinum. This organism is distinctive by virtue of its photochromogenicity and an optimal growth temperature of 30 to 33° C. It was named and recognized as a pathogen of fish in 1926. It is a common contaminant in fresh and salt water, accounting for the frequent occurrence of skin infection in individuals who work or play in a marine environment, including those with home aquariums. Deep infections of the hand may also occur. Almost all strains are resistant to isoniazid but susceptible to rifampin and ethambutol. The organisms are also susceptible to tetracycline and sulfonamides.

Other Slow-Growing Species. *Mycobacterium xenopi* has an optimal growth temperature of 43° C and has been found as a contaminant in hot water generators and storage tanks. From these sites several outbreaks have occurred of respiratory tract colonization and pulmonary disease in the hospital environment. Other species that may cause disease are *M. simiae*, *M. szulgai*, and *M. malmoense*. Two species that may be associated with superficial soft tissue disease but not with pulmonary disease are *M. ulcerans* and *M. hemophilum*.

Species of Low Pathogenic Potential. A few cases have been reported in which strains of the *M. terrae* complex (including *M. triviale)* were the cause of pulmonary disease, arthritis, or tenosynovitis. Strains of this complex may be found in the soil. An organism long associated with water and considered to be saprophytic is *M. gordonae*. Documented infections with this organism now range from bursitis to widely disseminated disease. Cases of pulmonary disease and synovitis also have been ascribed to *M. flavescens*, an organism with an intermediate growth rate that was previously considered to be nonpathogenic for humans.

EPIDEMIOLOGY. In contrast to tuberculosis, the other mycobacterioses are not transmitted from person to person but are acquired from the environment by mechanisms that are not well understood. For *M. xenopi* and *M. kansasii* the evidence points to the inhalation of aerosols of infected water. Strains of MAI may be found in domestic animals, soil, dust, and water. There is evidence that infected droplet nuclei may be produced along coastlines. Still largely unexplained is the geographic variability in the incidence of other mycobacterioses and the relative proportion of these infections attributable to each of the two most important agents of disease, MAI and *M. kansasii*. In this country the highest rates of *M. kansasii* disease have been reported from New Orleans, Dallas, Houston, Kansas City, and Chicago, while Milwaukee and the states of Georgia and Florida have reported a predominance of MAI disease. From one institution in St. Louis, 27 per cent of newly diagnosed cases of mycobacterial pulmonary disease were associated with an equal proportion of MAI and *M. kansasii*. Australia, Israel, and Japan have reported an overwhelming predominance of MAI infections over those caused by *M. kansasii*. In the Scandinavian countries, southeast England, and the Canadian province of Ontario, *M. xenopi* is an important pathogen. These figures refer to pulmonary disease; they do not reflect the distribution of disseminated infections. A recent increase in MAI and a concomitant decrease in *M. kansasii* pulmonary disease have been reported from Virginia and have been noted elsewhere, as well.

PATHOGENESIS. The localization of disease in the lungs suggests that the inhalation of infectious aerosols represents the primary route of infection. In many cases infection occurs by inoculation as a result of surgery, puncture wounds, lacerations, and foreign bodies. The question of whether the disease in adults usually represents primary infection or recrudescence of dormant foci cannot be answered at this time. The alimentary tract may be the route of infection in AIDS, since the intestinal tract is so often involved.

CLINICAL DESCRIPTION. *Pulmonary Disease.* The classic description is that of chronic cavitary disease resembling tuberculosis that occurs in a middle-aged rural man who has one or more of the following predisposing conditions: pneumoconiosis, healed tuberculosis, chronic bronchitis and emphysema, bullous disease, bronchiectasis, and malignant disease. However, there are many exceptions: The disease may be seen in all age groups except rarely in children, in either sex, and in some individuals without any apparent predisposing factor. It sometimes appears as an acute condition in which there is an infected bulla or cyst or in a case resembling pneumonia. Solitary pulmonary nodules also have been described.

The diagnosis may be suspected from the clinical appearance and the x-ray film, but it is the laboratory that must supply the correct identification of the mycobacterial agent. Skin tests are not helpful owing to a lack of adequately standardized antigens and the poor specificity of the currently available reagents. Pulmonary changes are characterized by one or more thin-walled cavities with little or no pleural disease or spread to the basal segments of the lungs. The sputum usually contains many acid-fast bacilli visible on smear and yields a heavy growth of the infecting agent. It may be possible to recognize the large banded forms of *M. kansasii* in the direct smear. A single positive culture result in which there are only a few colonies usually represents environmental contamination. Repeatedly positive specimens may be indicative of transient or long-term colonization of the respiratory tract when they are not associated with new or enlarging cavities and a compatible clinical picture.

Treatment for *M. kansasii* disease usually is highly successful, provided that rifampin is included in the regimen. It is recommended that isoniazid, rifampin, and ethambutol be given for 1 year after the sputum becomes negative for the organism. Results of preliminary trials of short-course treatment have not been encouraging.

Therapy for MAI disease, on the other hand, has proved to be difficult. Most strains are resistant to the available antituberculosis drugs as well as the other anti-infectives, and the drug regimens recommended up to now have been chosen empirically. The necessity for treatment must first be established by an observation period to determine the stability of disease and the rate of progression if it is advancing. During this period the sputum should be examined at frequent intervals, and the patient should receive a comprehensive course of bronchial hygiene, including cessation of smoking, bronchodilator therapy, chest physiotherapy, and antibiotics if there are purulent secretions. These maneuvers have served to eliminate the organism from the sputum of some patients with chronic pulmonary disease. It may be necessary to initiate therapy immediately in certain cases of severe acute disease with a new cavitary lesion and no other apparent cause. Drug treatment may be considered at three levels. Level 1 is a triple-drug regimen consisting of isoniazid, rifampin, and ethambutol for a duration of at least 2 years provided there is some response within the first few months. This level would be suitable for a patient who had chronic stable disease with consistently positive sputum test results and in whom the mycobacterial infection was adding to the burden of pulmonary disease. Level 2 treatment consists of the same three drugs plus daily streptomycin administration for at least 2 years. Administration of streptomycin may be reduced to two or three times a week after an initial response has been demonstrated. This treatment level would be suitable for a patient who had slowly progressive disease, who had a poor response to level 1 treatment, or who had a relapse after discontinuation of level 1 drug therapy. Drug treatment at level 3 may be empiric combinations of five or six drugs or, more reasonably, a regimen based on drug susceptibility studies: drugs used for level 2 with the addition of ethionamide, cycloserine, ciprofloxacin, or clofazimine (available); and rifabutin and other rifamycin derivatives or new macrolides (investigational).

The response to drug treatment depends to a large extent on the underlying chronic lung disease and on the rate of progression of the mycobacterial infection. For those patients who have rapidly progressive infection in lungs that are already severely damaged, the prognosis is poor even with level 3 treatment. Some of these individuals have defects in cellular immune functions, especially those associated with T cells. Resectional surgery should be considered after a few months of treatment for those patients who have adequate pulmonary function and sufficiently localized mycobacterial disease. Treatment is not necessary for solitary pulmonary nodules that result from MAI infection, usually recognized after resection.

Disease caused by *M. xenopi* and *M. szulgai* usually is amenable to drug therapy. The exact combinations of drugs to be used depend on the drug susceptibility patterns in vitro. Suggested for *M. xenopi* disease is a regimen consisting of isoniazid, rifampin, and streptomycin and for *M. szulgai*, rifampin, ethambutol, and either ethionamide or streptomycin.

Infections associated with *M. scrofulaceum*, *M. simiae*, and *M. fortuitum-chelonae* are more difficult to control because of natural drug resistance. Strains of *M. simiae* usually are resistant to all of the antituberculosis drugs except cycloserine and ethionamide. Limited information on susceptibility of *M. scrofulaceum* suggests that ethionamide, rifampin, and ethambutol are most likely to be active in vitro. The same considerations as those described for MAI infection are applicable to these resistant infections. Although pulmonary infections with *M. fortuitum-chelonae* are quite rare, there is some information about the response to drug treatment from cases of extrapulmonary disease. Before sensitivity test results are available, full doses of amikacin should be given intramuscularly, together with one or more of the following drugs: doxycycline, erythromycin, ciprofloxacin, cefoxitin, and a sulfonamide.

Lymphadenitis. Mycobacterial lymphadenitis is almost exclusively a disease of children of preschool age. Data from British Columbia published in 1974 indicated that the case rate for this new kind of scrofula was 0.37 per 100,000 persons per year, about 10 times higher than for that caused by *M. tuberculosis*. Involved nodes may be found in the femoral, inguinal, epitrochlear, and axillary areas, although the most common location is around the angle of the jaw. The route of infection to the groin area is a penetrating injury or splinter entry into an extremity. The cervical nodes probably become infected by mucous membrane penetration in the mouth or pharynx. Examination shows a child who has had a painless localized swelling for several weeks and who is otherwise healthy. An unknown proportion of cases goes on to suppuration and breakdown. Draining sinuses, whether spontaneous or following incision and drainage, may persist for many months. *M. scrofulaceum* was the most common cause of this infection, with MAI the second. However, there has been a recent reversal of this ratio so that strains of MAI now are the most common isolates from these infected nodes. Rare cases caused by several other species have been reported.

Correct diagnosis depends on the physician's familiarity with the disease, a positive tuberculin skin test result (sometimes requiring the use of second-strength purified protein derivative), the absence of a history of contact with tuberculosis, absence of thoracic disease, and the location as well as the appearance of the involved nodes. Other conditions that need to be differentiated are tuberculosis, pyogenic lymphadenitis, cat scratch disease, congenital cyst, and lymphoma. The treatment of choice is excision of the involved nodes. In about 10 per cent of cases there is a recurrence of the infection in another group of nodes near the original site, occasionally on the other side. Rarely there may be a third episode. Recurrences should be treated in the same manner as the original infection. There is no convincing evidence that drug treatment is beneficial. It should be remembered that as a result of this infection a child may have a positive tuberculin skin test reaction for many years.

Skin and Soft Tissue Infections. **Cutaneous Granuloma.** Localized groups of papules have been called swimming pool granuloma or fish tank granuloma, depending on the source of infection. In another form of the disease there is a local abscess at the inoculation site, usually on the hand, followed by a series of secondary nodules that progress centrally along the lymphatics in a manner not unlike that seen in sporotrichosis. A few deep hand infections have also been described; such cases should be referred to a hand surgeon. The infection is not uncommon as an occupational or recreational illness in people who work or play in a marine environment. With few exceptions, the etiologic agent is *M. marinum*. Most superficial infections are self-limited. When treatment is deemed necessary, the physician may use a combination of rifampin and ethambutol, rifampin alone, one of the tetracyclines, or trimethoprim-sulfamethoxazole. All of these regimens have been reported to be successful.

Local Abscess. Many cases of local abscess following subcutaneous or intramuscular injection have been reported, some in outbreaks. The trouble usually is traced to a contaminated multiple injection vial, and the etiologic agent usually is *M. fortuitum-chelonae*. Incision and drainage usually will suffice to control the infection.

Local Trauma. Most of these infections caused by *M. fortuitum-chelonae* occur as a result of penetrating or lacerating wounds contaminated with soil. Expert surgical handling is necessary, along with appropriate drug therapy as outlined under Pulmonary Disease.

Disseminated Nodules. Multiple nodules and abscesses may be associated with widely disseminated mycobacterial disease, almost always in an immunocompromised host. The species most often isolated is *M. fortuitum-chelonae*. In addition, such nodules have been described in renal transplant patients as a result of infection with *M. hemophilum*.

Buruli Ulcer. This deeply penetrating ulcer caused by *M. ulcerans* is confined mainly to Africa, Papua New Guinea, Malaysia, and Australia. The treatment is difficult and controversial.

Skeletal Infections. The synovia, tendon sheaths, and bursae are involved more often than other parts of the skeletal system in nontuberculous mycobacterial infections. A wide variety of species may be associated, including environmental strains with little pathogenicity for humans, such as *M. terrae*, *M. gordonae*, and *M. flavescens*. Leading the list of etiologic agents is *M. kansasii*, with *M. fortuitum-chelonae* and MAI following in that order. Many of these infections follow trauma in which the wound is contaminated with soil or water. Others have occurred after injections of corticosteroids into arthritic joints; in these cases it is difficult to determine which condition was primary. The most common site is the hand, where the infection produces an indolent but persistent tenosynovitis, including the carpal tunnel syndrome. Osteomyelitis may occur in the form of multifocal lesions from hematogenous dissemination, often as a slowly progressive rather than a fulminant infection. The principal etiologic agent in these cases is MAI.

Treatment for skeletal infection usually demands close cooperation between a skilled surgeon and a physician specializing in infectious disease. Drug therapy depends on the etiologic agent (refer to earlier discussion).

Postsurgical Infections. Infections following surgery mainly are caused by *M. fortuitum-chelonae*. They include prosthetic valve endocarditis, sternal wound infection and osteomyelitis after open heart surgery, wound infection after augmentation mammoplasty, and infections associated with hemodialysis and peritoneal dialysis.

Disseminated Disease. Patients who develop disseminated disease usually are severely immunocompromised from the standpoint of cellular immune functions. The arrival of AIDS has been associated with a dramatic increase in disseminated mycobacterial infections, since up to 50 per cent of such patients coming to autopsy in several cities have been found to have disseminated MAI infections. Prior to 1980 there were relatively few cases of disseminated mycobacterial disease reported throughout the world. They usually involved patients who had underlying hematologic malignancies or who were under treatment with corticosteroids, or both. Both children and adults were affected, and the most common etiologic agents were *M. kansasii* and MAI. The case fatality rate was very high, even with the most intensive multiple-drug treatment. Diagnosis is most commonly made by biopsy and culture of liver, bone marrow, or lymph nodes. Cultures of the blood are often positive. Skin lesions or subcutaneous nodules or abscesses should be biopsied and examined for acid-fast bacilli. Strains of *M. fortuitum-chelonae* often are associated with these superficial lesions. The tissues may show a nonspecific necrotizing reaction in which macrophages are loaded with acid-fast bacilli, rather than a granulomatous reaction. In AIDS patients, disseminated infection usually occurs in the late stages of the disease, and the diagnosis may be made quickly by finding AFB in the stool or in the buffy coat.

Treatment for disseminated disease is based on the same principles as those outlined for pulmonary disease. Infections caused by drug-sensitive organisms such as *M. kansasii* can usually be brought under at least temporary control provided that the human host is able to provide an adequate immune response. For infections related to MAI a multiple-drug regimen is usually chosen as outlined earlier, with the realization that, for the AIDS patient, the response usually is poor and the side effects may be severe.

Chester AC, Winn WC Jr: Unusual and newly recognized patterns of nontuberculous mycobacterial infection with emphasis on the immunocompromised host. Pathol Ann 21:251, 1986. *This is an extensive review, well referenced, and presented from the standpoint of the pathologist.*

Davidson PT: The diagnosis and management of disease caused by *M. avium* complex, *M. kansasii*, and other mycobacteria. Clin Chest Med 10:431, 1989. *An excellent contribution from an established leader in the clinical mycobacterial arena.*

Grange JM, Yates MD: Infections caused by opportunist mycobacteria: A review. J R Soc Med 79:226, 1986. *A succinct, informative account of mycobacteriosis as seen in England.*

Grange JM, Yates MD, Boughton E: The avian tubercle bacillus and its relatives. J Appl Bacteriol 68:411, 1990. *The important historical, ecological, and microbiological facts are presented admirably.*

Horsburgh CR Jr, Mason UG III, Farhi DC, et al.: Disseminated infection with *Mycobacterium avium-intracellulare*: A report of 13 cases and a review of the literature. Medicine 64:36, 1985. *A thorough analysis of 13 cases from the National Jewish Hospital and 24 cases from the literature, with emphasis on response to treatment. Patients with AIDS were excluded.*

Lichtenstein IH, MacGregor RR: Mycobacterial infections in renal transplant recipients: Report of five cases and review of the literature. Rev Infect Dis 5:216, 1983. *Renal transplant recipients have a high risk of disseminated mycobacteriosis, and 34 per cent of reported cases have been attributed to nontuberculous species.*

Marchevsky AM, Damsker B, Green S, et al.: The clinicopathological spectrum of nontuberculous mycobacterial osteoarticular infections. J Bone Joint Surg 67A:925, 1985. *A report of eight cases, attributed to five different species, with a good literature review. Infection of bone, synovium, and tendon sheaths may be seen.*

Margileth AM, Chandra R, Altman RP: Chronic lymphadenopathy due to mycobacterial infection: Clinical features, diagnosis, histopathology, and management. Am J Dis Child 138:917, 1984. *From Washington and New York comes this informative report of 153 cases, of which 86 per cent were due to*

nontuberculous mycobacteria. Unfortunately, no speciation of the positive cultures is presented.

Moran JF, Alexander LG, Staub EW, et al.: Long-term results of pulmonary resection for atypical mycobacterial disease. Ann Thorac Surg 35:597, 1983. *This report documents the good results of resectional surgery in 37 patients seen by the surgical group at Duke University from 1967 to 1981. All disease was attributed to M. avium-intracellulare.*

O'Brien RJ: The epidemiology of nontuberculous mycobacterial disease. Clin Chest Med 10:407, 1989. *This is a unique review dealing with such features as ecology of the organisms, mechanisms of transmission, and prevalence of disease (roughly 2 per 100,000 in the United States).*

Roth RI, Owen RL, Keren DF, et al.: Intestinal infection with *Mycobacterium avium* in AIDS: Histological and clinical comparison with Whipple's disease. Dig Dis Sci 30:497,1985. *A good account of the fascinating similarity of some MAI intestinal infections to Whipple's disease.*

Wallace RJ Jr: The clinical presentation, diagnosis, and therapy of cutaneous and pulmonary infections due to the rapidly growing mycobacteria, *M. fortuitum* and *M. chelonae*. Clin Chest Med 10:419, 1989. *Dr. Wallace has been at the forefront of clinical research in diseases associated with rapidly growing mycobacteria. This review is excellent.*

Wallace RJ Jr, O'Brien R, Glassroth J, et al.: Diagnosis and treatment of disease caused by nontuberculous mycobacteria. Am Rev Respir Dis 142:940, 1990. *This is an authoritative review and an official statement of the American Thoracic Society.*

Wolinsky E: Nontuberculous mycobacteria and associated diseases. Am Rev Respir Dis 119:107, 1979. *A state-of-the-art review of the entire subject.*

Woodring JH, Vandiviere HM, Melvin IG, Dillon ML: Roentgenographic features of pulmonary disease caused by atypical mycobacteria. South Med J 80:1488, 1987. *A retrospective study of 40 cases, with good radiographic pictures.*

Woods GL, Washington JA: Mycobacteria other than *Mycobacterium tuberculosis*: Review of microbiologic and clinical aspects. Rev Infect Dis 9:275, 1987. *From the Cleveland Clinic comes this helpful review of the epidemiologic, pathologic, and clinical features of each species.*

Young LS, Inderlied CB, Berlin OG, Gottlieb MS: Mycobacterial infections in AIDS patients, with an emphasis on the *Mycobacterium avium* complex. Rev Infect Dis 8:1024, 1986. *A good exposition of the subject from Los Angeles, which includes a section on the authors' laboratory studies of potentially useful combination drug regimens.*

334 Leprosy—Hansen's Disease

Zanvil A. Cohn and Gilla Kaplan

DEFINITION. Leprosy is a bacterial disease of great chronicity and low infectivity which occurs worldwide. The primary host is the human, in whom the causative agent *Mycobacterium leprae* accumulates largely in the skin and peripheral nerves, leading to a variety of cutaneous lesions and loss of nerve conduction. Serious disfigurement and loss of digits and extremities may result and represent the stigmata of this biblical disease. The clinical manifestations are largely governed by the ability of the host to mount a cell-mediated immune (CMI) response to the organism and its antigens. Patients unable to generate an immune attack develop widely distributed skin lesions of the *lepromatous* state and allow unrestricted growth of bacilli. In contrast, a moderate to vigorous immune response leads to the local cutaneous lesions of the *tuberculoid* form. In addition to these polar states there are intermediate forms that demonstrate gradations in reactivity. Modulation of the disease toward more polar forms can occur and may lead to tissue damage via humoral (immune complex) and cellular (CMI) mechanisms. Therapy with multiple drugs leads to a prompt reduction in viable organisms and transmissibility but must be maintained for long periods for the disappearance of skin lesions and a reduction in bacterial load.

TRANSMISSION. Little detailed information is available about how the bacillus is transmitted from one individual to another. This deficit in our understanding is related to the long incubation period (>3 years) and the absence of adequate techniques to identify the organism in the environment. Other than in humans the disease has been discovered in feral armadillos studied in Louisiana and Texas. These animals contain large numbers of acid-fast bacilli in parenchymatous organs which by DNA hybridization and restriction fragment length polymorphism analysis techniques are identical to bacilli obtained from humans. The sooty mangabey, a new world monkey, can become infected naturally in the wild or when injected with human bacilli. In both armadillos and monkeys it takes 18 to 24 months for the injected bacilli to reach high numbers. These infections are quite unlike the spectrum of human disease.

The localized lesions of tuberculoid leprosy and the generalized distribution of lepromatous disease are in keeping with suggested pathways for the introduction of bacilli. Direct inoculation via such means as trauma and puncture wounds might lead to an initial focus with environmental bacilli. Some suggest that the initial route may be through the respiratory or gastrointestinal tract. Biting insects have been considered, but no clear evidence exists regarding them as an intermediate vector. It seems reasonable, however, that at some point during the infection in lepromatous leprosy patients, hematogenous spread occurs with wide seeding of the body.

It is likely that the number of environmental bacilli is correlated with transmission. The incidence of the disease within a household containing an infected tuberculoid or lepromatous index patient may be four to eight times that of the general population. In particular, lepromatous patients with lesions in the nasal mucosa discharge large numbers of organisms. Bacilli recovered from dry nasal discharges retain some viability for up to 7 to 10 days, with somewhat greater viability under conditions of higher humidity. Transmission of the disease from an untreated, infected mother to an infant is not uncommon and should always be considered. In general, clinical wisdom indicates that disease transmission takes place only after years of exposure. Little likelihood of transmission is present in a ward or hospital setting and patients are now cared for on an ambulatory basis with a minimum of precautions.

SUSCEPTIBILITY. Leprosy occurs worldwide and in individuals of all ages. It appears more frequently in young adults, but this may be related to a parental index case and the long period of incubation. The incidence of the disease is greater in males than in females. However, it is unlikely that this represents differences in gender but possibly reflects the greater likelihood that males seek and obtain medical attention in the Third World.

A large number of studies suggest, but do not prove, that the overall susceptibility to leprosy is not controlled by immune response genes and their expressed major histocompatibility class II antigens. Early analysis of the disease incidence and susceptibility in identical twins has not been conclusive. More recent studies suggest that the type of leprosy rather than overall disease susceptibility may be controlled by HLA determinants. No clear-cut conclusions on the genetic basis of susceptibility can therefore be accepted at this time. In this context, environmental factors such as nutrition and coincident microbial and parasitic infections must be considered as alternatives.

The physiologic immunodeficiency of the newborn may lead to an early colonization with the bacillus. The AIDS pandemic has been associated with a rise in the incidence of other mycobacterial diseases, and this association may become more apparent in leprosy in the future.

EPIDEMIOLOGY. The worldwide number of leprosy cases has been estimated to be between 12 and 15 million. In many countries valid statistics are not available, and the incidence in outlying, rural areas is poorly documented. The highest prevalence rates are in Asia and Africa, followed by Central and South America and Oceania. The highest rates do not usually exceed 55 per 1000 but may be as high as 200 per 1000 in selected villages. Many accept the fact that with effective chemotherapy the worldwide incidence is dropping and will continue to do so with advanced diagnostic and public health methods.

The majority of leprosy cases are found in tropical areas. Socioeconomic condition, availability of health care, and body exposure to the environment may all contribute. The disease also occurs in the colder climates of Tibet, Nepal, Korea, and Siberia. In the previous centuries the disease occurred more commonly in Scandinavia and those countries bordering the North Sea. Small numbers (300 to 500 per year) of cases currently occur in the United States. The majority of these are in immigrant groups from Asia and South America, although occasional cases are seen in the southern states and those bordering Mexico.

The nature of the disease varies considerably with geographic distribution. African and Asian countries have a predominance of tuberculoid leprosy, and 20 per cent or fewer of the cases are of the lepromatous type. In contrast, larger numbers of lepromatous cases are reported in Brazil and Venezuela. Early infection and/or sensitization with cross-reacting antigens of other mycobacteria has been considered as an explanation for the variation in type of leprosy with which an individual presents.

ETIOLOGIC AGENT. *Mycobacterium leprae* is the causative agent of human leprosy, and no evidence of strain variation has been noted by DNA–DNA hybridization or restriction fragment length polymorphism. The organism is acid-alcohol fast when stained by the Ziehl-Neelsen method. *M. leprae* is an obligate intracellular parasite and has never been cultivated extracellularly in laboratory media. It is a resident of the phagolysosomes of macrophages, Schwann cells, and endothelial cells. *M. leprae* is classified as a mycobacterium and contains mycolic acid, arabinogalactan, and phenolic glycolipid. The latter molecule is the only *M. leprae*–specific component. Most other carbohydrates, peptidoglycans, and proteins share antigenic determinants with other mycobacterial species, making serologic diagnosis especially difficult.

The absence of a culture system for *M. leprae* has complicated any investigations of the physiology and pathogenicity of the organism. Many advances in this field have resulted from the ability of the armadillo to support the growth of the mycobacteria. Eighteen to 24 months after inoculation, large numbers of bacilli (10^9 per gram) can be purified from liver and spleen and serve as a source for antigenic and chemical analysis. *M. leprae* is one of the few pathogenic mycobacteria which lacks the enzyme catalase and is susceptible to killing by oxygen metabolites such as hydrogen peroxide. Many of the metabolic activities of *M. leprae* appear to be low compared with other mycobacteria, and de novo purine biosynthesis appears to be missing. *M. leprae* replicates very slowly within host cells and has a doubling time of approximately 13 days. It prefers ambient temperatures below 37°C and grows selectively in cooler portions of the body such as skin, testes, and nasal mucosa.

Within the vacuolar apparatus, the bacillus is surrounded by a loose matrix of secreted phenolic glycolipid which also serves as a scavenger of oxygen intermediates. Specific *M. leprae* proteins have been identified by direct chemical analysis and through recombinant DNA technology. Other polypeptides are cross-reactive with those of *M. tuberculosis* and other mycobacteria.

The determination of bacillary viability and resistance to chemotherapeutic agents depends upon its slow growth in the foot pads of mice—a bioassay taking about 12 months. Accelerated growth occurs in the athymic nude mouse but still requires 6 or more months. These properties impose severe restrictions on rapid diagnosis. Application of the polymerase chain reaction, in which selected DNA sequences are amplified a millionfold, may lead to the specific identification of as few as 10 bacilli within a few days.

IMMUNOLOGIC CONSIDERATION. A major immunologic defect occurs in patients with lepromatous leprosy. This is expressed as a selective unresponsiveness of T cells to *M. leprae* and is evident in skin test anergy and the in vitro lymphocyte transformation test to *M. leprae* antigens (Table 334–1). Patients

TABLE 334–1. IMMUNOLOGIC FEATURES OF LEPROSY PATIENTS

	Tuberculoid	Borderline Tuberculoid	Mid Borderline	Borderline Lepromatous	Lepromatous
Acid-fast bacilli in skin lesion	−	−/+	+	+++	+++
Lepromin (Mitsuda) reaction	+++	++	−	−	−
Lymphocyte transformation test	15%	5.7%	2%	0.4%	0.3%
Anti–*M. leprae* antibodies	−/+	−/++	++	+++	+++
CD4+/CD8+ T-cell ratio in skin	1.35	1.11	NT	0.48	0.20

with the tuberculoid form of the disease respond normally, and in neither form of the disease are there abnormalities in humoral immunity. The association between cell-mediated, T cell–directed immunity and the number of *M. leprae* in the tissues is shown in Figure 334–1. These two parameters are inversely related. In the absence of *M. leprae*–specific T-cell reactivity, lymphokine formation is depressed or absent and tissue macrophages fail to be activated into an antimicrobial state. Normally, macrophage activation occurs largely through the local release of interferon-γ (IFN-γ), a lymphokine that enhances the production of toxic oxygen intermediates in these cells. Bacilli taken up by "resting" and "aged" macrophages of the skin are able to multiply intracellularly, leading in the case of lepromatous disease to multibacillary vacuoles. In tuberculoid forms, the bacilli are largely destroyed and only small numbers survive to perpetuate the cell-mediated immune reactions.

Lepromatous patients, although unresponsive to *M. leprae* antigen, develop adequate reactions to other antigens to which they have been sensitized. These include skin test antigens such as PPD, mumps, *Candida*, trichophytin, and tetanus toxoid. The highly selective anergy of leprosy may be related to the loss of T cells with surface recognition receptors rather than suppressor cell phenomena.

CLINICAL DIAGNOSIS. Patients with leprosy are first seen and followed by dermatologists because the cutaneous lesions are often the presenting complaint. The range in immunity to *M. leprae* is reflected clinically by a wide variation of skin lesions and peripheral nerve involvement. In this section we review the characteristics of the major polar forms.

Polar Tuberculoid Leprosy (TT). This form presents as one to three plaques or macules defined by a sharp, raised border. In dark-skinned patients they are often hypopigmented centrally with a more erythematous border. The central area is scaly, lacks hair, and is anesthetic. Nerves may be palpably enlarged in and adjacent to the plaque, and these are commonly found leading to the area of the ear, elbow, and knee. Almost any area of the skin may be affected except for the warmer regions of the scalp, axilla, and perineum.

Borderline Tuberculoid Leprosy (BT). As the body burden of antigen increases, in association with a partial reduction in immunity, the number, distribution, and nature of the cutaneous lesions increase in complexity and the sequelae of peripheral nerve damage increase in severity. The skin exhibits a polymorphic array of macular, erythematous, hypopigmented lesions involving the trunk, extremities, and face. These vary in number and distribution in a seemingly random fashion. Larger nerve trunks are involved with a granulomatous reaction, leading to foot drop, flexion contractions of the digits, and corneal abrasions.

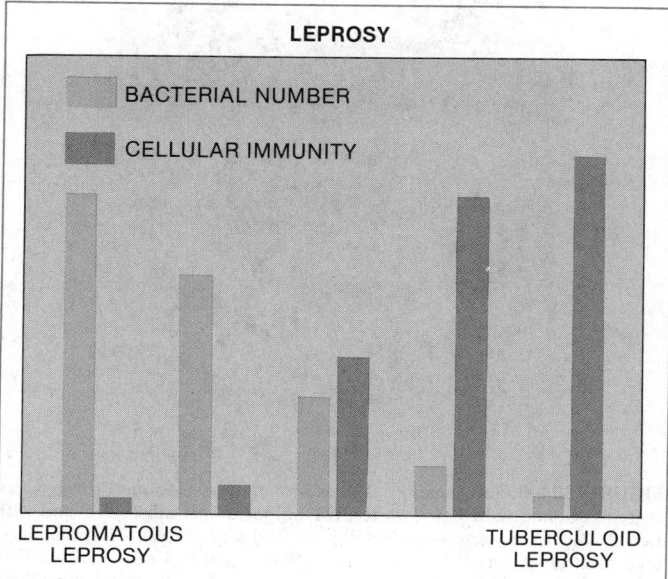

FIGURE 334–1. Cellular immunity and bacterial numbers across the clinical spectrum of leprosy.

The anesthesia of hands and feet and the resulting damage from burns, trauma, and secondary infection leads to loss of digits, plantar ulcerations, and blindness. These widely dispersed lesions suggest hematogenous spread and a cell-mediated reaction that is not capable of fully controlling bacillary growth.

Lepromatous Leprosy (LL). Here there is little or no CMI, and tremendous numbers of organisms are dispersed throughout the body. Again the lesions are pleomorphic but often are less "angry" or erythematous than in borderline disease. Macules, papules, and nodules may cover wide areas of the trunk and extremities, and lesion distribution is often symmetric. Almost any area of affected or "normal" looking skin contains bacilli. Often there are no obvious lesions but the skin looks shiny and "full," as the dermis is expanded with macrophages containing bacilli. This is particularly prominent on the ears, eyebrows, and face, giving rise to an appearance called leonine facies. Eyebrow loss is frequent; a saddle nose deformity may result from cartilage destruction; gynecomastia from reduced testosterone levels secondary to testicular damage may be present; and blindness and iridocyclitis, laryngeal stenosis, loss of incisor teeth, and loss of digits may occur. These results of long-term untreated lepromatous leprosy are the stigmata that ostracized the leper from his community and necessitated custodial care. This is almost never the case today, and patients undergoing chemotherapy remain members of their households. Nerve damage in lepromatous leprosy is more slowly progressive but is eventually severe and diffuse and leads to a sensory polyneuropathy. Rigid, swollen nerves are palpable in many locations.

REACTIONAL STATES. *Erythema Nodosum Leprosum (ENL).* The release of *M. leprae* antigen, often following the initiation of therapy in multibacillary patients with or without the formation of immune complexes, results in an acute reactional state that may lead to death. Suddenly, painful, erythematous nodules and papules arise diffusely and may eventually lead to necrosis and suppuration. These symptoms, accompanied by fever and malaise, can continue for months, are extremely debilitating, and are often accompanied by acute inflammation of the eyes, testes, nerves, lymph nodes, and joints. Some patients develop glomerulonephritis with the deposition of complement and immune complexes in the glomeruli. This serious complication requires prompt diagnosis and therapy.

Reversal Reactions. This reactional state may also occur after chemotherapy but differs from ENL in that tissues are infiltrated with newly recruited T lymphocytes. The acceleration of the local cell-mediated reaction, observed mostly in borderline patients of the tuberculoid as well as the lepromatous type, is accompanied by widespread erythema and induration of pre-existing lesions as well as systemic symptoms, e.g., pyrexia. The onset of this state is slower, takes weeks to months, and may persist for many months if not properly treated. Rapid progression of pre-existing peripheral nerve damage may take place. These irreversible changes in nerve conduction should be considered a medical emergency and treated accordingly.

LABORATORY DIAGNOSIS. In addition to clinical manifestations the primary method for the diagnosis of leprosy is the identification of acid-fast bacilli in the skin. The slit smear technique is used throughout the world. Skin is incised with a scalpel, squeezing the area to maintain a bloodless field. The edges of the slit are scraped with the edge of the scalpel, smeared on a slide, fixed, and stained by the Ziehl-Neelsen method. A microscopic logarithmic score (1^+ to 6^+), (5^+ equals 100 to 1000 acid-fast bacilli per high-power field), is used to quantitate the bacterial load. Usually six sites on the ear lobes, eyebrows, elbow, knee, and a lesion are prepared. This simple method when skillfully applied is as sensitive as any diagnostic procedure.

A more definitive estimate of bacillary numbers in the skin comes from biopsy material. Biopsies are fixed, sectioned, and stained for acid-fast organisms as well as the background host cells. A logarithmic score is made by counting the number of bacilli in high-power fields. This ranges from 1^+ to 6^+ and is a useful index in following the response of patients to therapy in terms of bacillary numbers and histopathologic classification. (Bacterial Index: 0—no bacilli in 100 microscopic fields ($\times 100$); $1+ = 1$ to 10 bacilli in 100 fields; $2+ = 1$ to 10 bacilli in 10 fields; $3+ = 1$ to 10 bacilli per field; $4+ = 10$ to 100 bacilli per

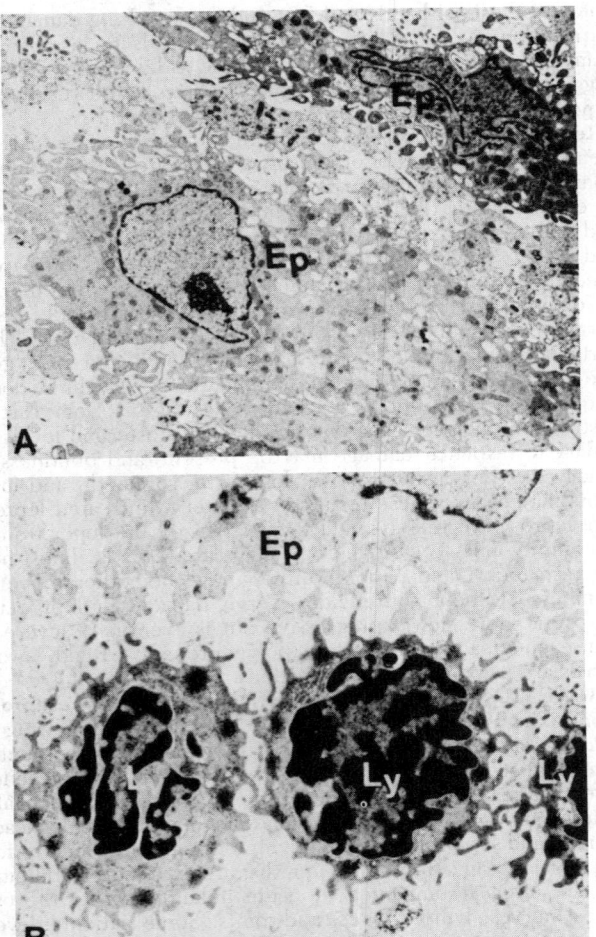

FIGURE 334–2. Transmission electron photomicrographs of cutaneous granulomas from a patient with tuberculoid leprosy. *A,* The granuloma contains large epithelioid cells (Ep) with multiple cytoplasmic organelles (× 4500). *B,* Three T lymphocytes (Ly) and an epithelioid cell are observed (× 9000).

field; 5+ = 100 to 1000 bacilli per field; and 6+ = many 1000s per field.)

A skin test may be employed which distinguishes the immunologically reactive (tuberculoid) and nonreactive (lepromatous) poles of the disease. A crude antigen consisting of heat-killed bacilli from lepromatous skin nodules is injected and induces local induration and the formation of granulomas in 3 to 4 weeks in most tuberculoid patients. Patients with lepromatous leprosy fail to react to the antigen and may remain unresponsive long after effective chemotherapy.

Serologic tests are useful in assaying the level of anti–*M. leprae* antibodies in multibacillary lepromatous but not in the paucibacillary tuberculoid forms. However, the many cross-reactive antigenic epitopes shared with other mycobacteria complicate interpretation and differential diagnosis. ELISA tests, which recognize antibodies against the carbohydrate moieties of the phenolic glycolipids, the only molecule that is *M. leprae*–specific, are positive in patients with lepromatous but not tuberculoid disease and decline after the initiation of chemotherapy. Patients with lepromatous leprosy have a polyclonal hypergammaglobulinemia, acute phase reactants such as C-reactive protein, and immune complexes in the circulation. Ten per cent give false-positive tests for syphilis and 30 per cent have cryoglobulinemia.

HISTOPATHOLOGY AND IMMUNOPATHOLOGY. Microscopic analysis of tissue plays a primary role in diagnosing and classifying the various clinical forms of leprosy and employs the standardized classification described by Ridley and Jopling. Five groups have been defined spanning the spectrum from polar tuberculoid (TT) to polar lepromatous (LL) and include borderline

(BB) as well as borderline tuberculoid (BT) and borderline lepromatous (BL). Our discussion focuses on the polar forms, and the details pertaining to the intermediate manifestations can be found in more specialized texts.

Lesions of the Skin. **Tuberculoid Leprosy.** Microscopic examination of H & E–stained sections of biopsies obtained from a TT macular plaque reveals heavy infiltration of the dermis by mononuclear leukocytes organized in well-developed granulomas. These contain large numbers of lymphocytes scattered between and surrounding other components of the granulomatous response, including macrophage-derived epithelioid cells and Langhans-type multinucleated giant cells (Fig. 334–2). Occasional plasma cells but no granulocytes are found. Langhans cells are found within the dermal infiltrate in significant numbers. Staining with monoclonal antibodies shows that the majority of lymphocytes are T cells and that the CD4+ "helper type" phenotype predominates over CD8+ "suppressor/cytotoxic" cells.

The epidermis overlying the dermal infiltrate is thickened (two- to threefold), and individual keratinocytes are enlarged. The keratinocytes display large amounts of MHC class II determinants on their surface. This is a response to the local production of IFN-γ in the dermis and is accompanied by the expression of other IFN-γ–induced molecules by keratinocytes and other cell types.

Acid-fast staining of sections reveals an occasional bacillus or bacillary remnants within macrophages. Borderline tuberculoid (BT) lesions are similar except that acid-fast bacilli are more readily seen.

Lepromatous Leprosy. In contrast to TT lesions, the lepromatous lesion contains only small numbers of lymphocytes, predominantly of the CD8+ phenotype, scattered through a background of loosely organized dermal macrophages and collagen (Fig. 334–3). The macrophages often have a pale, foamy cytoplasm and may contain large clumps of *M. leprae* called globi (Fig. 334–4). By electron microscopy these organisms are seen to reside within large cytoplasmic vacuoles, embedded in a lucent matrix that contains a phenolic glycolipid. Remnants of the osmiophilic bacilli are always present along with structurally intact organisms (Fig. 334–4B and C). A gram of skin may contain 10^9 bacilli. The small proportion of lymphocytes is predominantly

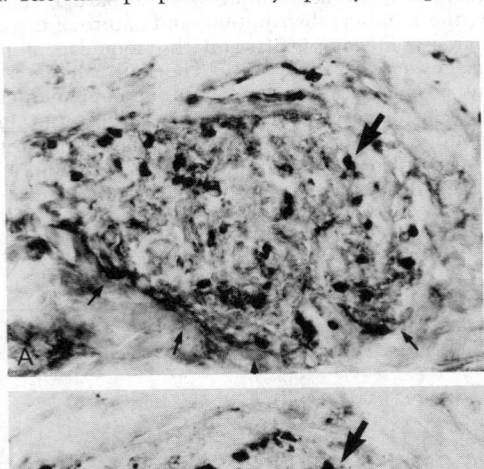

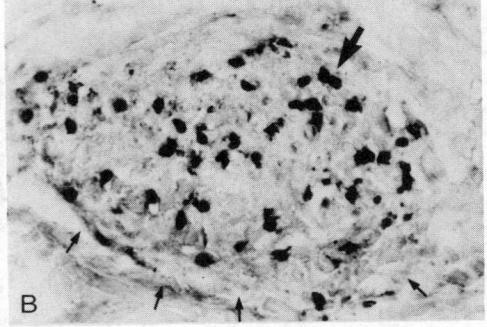

FIGURE 334–3. Lepromatous leprosy—cutaneous lesion. Frozen serial sections stained with Leu 3 (anti CD4–helper T-cell subset) *(A)* and with Leu 2 (anti CD8–suppressor/cytotoxic T-cell subset) *(B).* The inflammatory infiltrates *(small arrows)* contain few T cells. Cells of the CD4+ subset *(large arrow* in *A)* are less numerous than those of the CD8+ subset *(large arrows* in *B).* Immunoperoxidase, counterstained with hematoxylin (× 200).

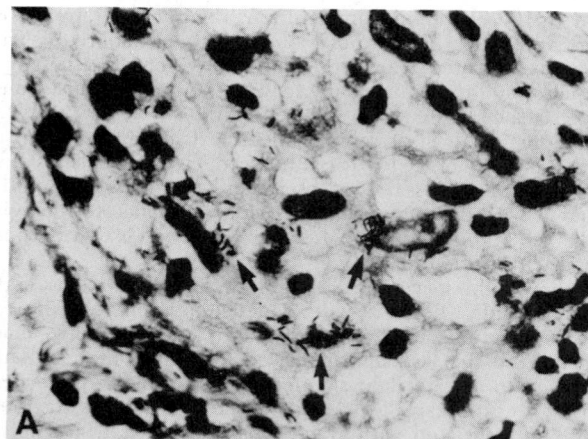

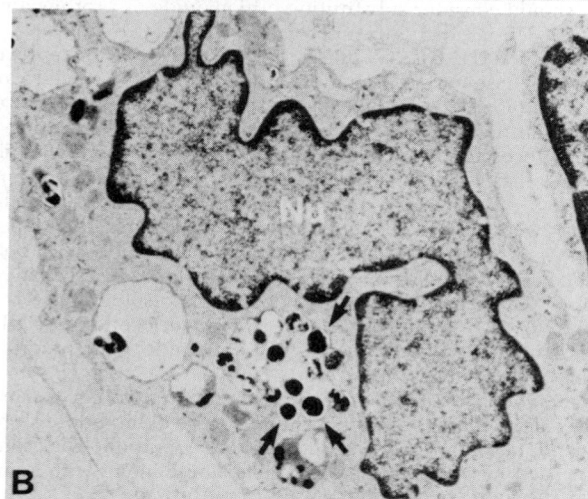

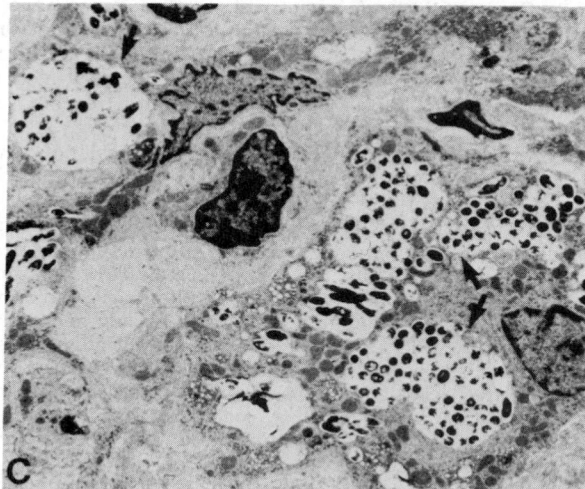

FIGURE 334–4. Lepromatous leprosy—cutaneous lesions. Acid-fast staining of histologic section *(A)* and transmission electron photomicrographs *(B and C)* of *M. leprae*–parasitized foamy macrophages *(arrows)*. The phagocytes have large nuclei and many light and electron lucent vacuoles containing darkly staining bacteria (*A,* × 500; *B,* × 9000; *C,* × 3000).

of the CD8+ subset, and very small numbers of CD4+ helper cells are present. Langhans cells are rarely seen in the dermis; the overlying epidermis is thin and atrophic and fails to show surface MHC class II antigens usually associated with local IFN-γ production.

The loose infiltrates of LL and its bacilli are present in almost every area of the skin examined and individual infected macrophages may be observed surrounded by collagen bundles.

***Lesions of Peripheral Nerve.* Tuberculoid Leprosy.** The pau-

cibacillary granulomatous response is associated with significant destruction of peripheral nerve fascicles and late in the disease may lead to caseous necrosis of nerve trunks. Large numbers of T cells and mononuclear phagocytes breach the perineurium and lead to destruction of Schwann cells and axons alike. By the time the skin lesion is apparent, nerve damage and sensory loss have occurred. The mechanism of the nerve damage in TT is unclear but is related to the granulomatous response.

Lepromatous Leprosy. Many bacilli are observed within Schwann cells and macrophages surrounding and within the perineural sheath in a reaction involving the majority of subcutaneously placed nerve trunks (Fig. 334–5). Nerve damage is relatively slow as compared to TT but more extensive and insidious. Few if any lymphocytes are part of the lesion. Eventually more enlargement and displacement by connective tissue result. Schwann cells are particularly capable of taking up *M. leprae* and serve as permissive hosts for their replication (Fig. 334–5).

Other Organs. Granulomatous lesions can be seen in the lymph nodes, liver, spleen, bone marrow, endocrine organs, and eye. These contain bacilli but are not considered to be an important source of infection. Patients with untreated multibacillary disease can have a constant bacteremia of 10^5 AFB per milliliter, all of which are present within monocytes. The total body burden of *M. leprae* can reach 10^{12}.

***Lesions of Reactional States.* Erythema Nodosum Leprosum (ENL).** Patients with BL and LL disease maintain high levels of circulating anti–*M. leprae* antibodies as well as high antigen levels in tissue depots. Following effective chemotherapy a prompt and extensive kill of bacilli takes place, and large amounts of soluble antigens are liberated extracellularly. More than 50 per cent of such patients develop ENL and present with painful erythematous skin nodules, fever, iridocyclitis, neuritis, glomerulonephritis, and other systemic manifestations. Examination of the skin nodules shows extensive infiltration of neutrophils, mononuclear cells, and tissue necrosis. Immune complexes are evident and there is a panvasculitis of dermal arteries and veins. These are all hallmarks of an extensive acute inflammatory response resulting in tissue damage.

Reversal Reactions. Patients with BT, BB, or BL leprosy, who are partially responsive to *M. leprae* antigens, occasionally undergo an upgrading reaction after several months of therapy. This differs from ENL in the migration of a predominantly T-cell infiltrate into pre-existing inflammatory sites. Many of the T cells are of the helper phenotype and are secreting lymphokines into

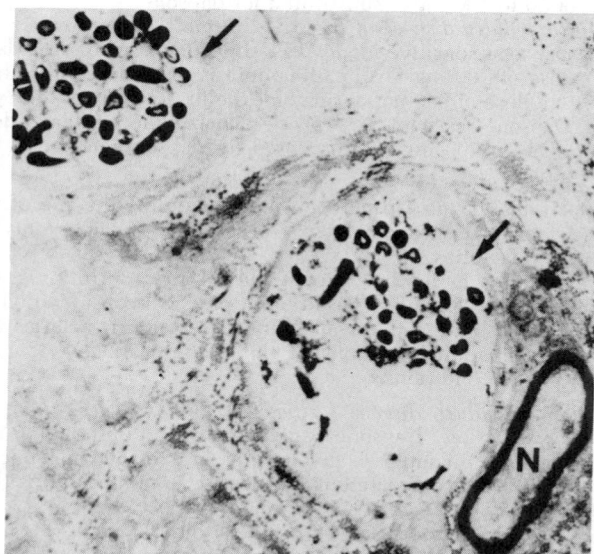

FIGURE 334–5. Transmission electron micrograph of an infiltrated peripheral nerve of a cutaneous lesion from a lepromatous leprosy patient. The myelinated neuron (N) and two *M. leprae*–infected Schwann cells *(arrows)* are observed (× 9000).

their environment. T-cell migration into skin lesions is associated with mononuclear phagocyte differentiation into organized granuloma and is often associated with the rapid progression of peripheral nerve damage. This enhancement of CMI leads to limited bacillary destruction. Such reactions may continue for weeks or months and are associated with severe morbidity leading to serious sequelae.

PATHOGENESIS. Recovery from infections with obligate intracellular parasites such as *M. leprae* requires the host to mount an effective CMI response. For this purpose, antigen-presenting dendritic cells must recognize and cluster with appropriate T cells, leading to T-cell stimulation, differentiation, and replication. T cells then follow two distinct pathways. In the first, helper cells synthesize and secrete a variety of hormone-like lymphokines which seem to enhance the microbicidal activity of monocytes and macrophages as well as stimulate other cells in the environment, e.g., keratinocytes, endothelial cells, and fibroblasts. A second pathway leads to the development of T cells which are of the CD4$^+$ phenotype and are antigen specific and MHC class II restricted. Along with NK (natural killer) and LAK (lymphokine-activated killer) cells, they serve as potent specific and nonspecific cytotoxic effector cells.

In lepromatous leprosy and in the absence of local lymphokine production, bacilli multiply in macrophages that have neither the capacity to kill the organism nor to be activated by lymphokines. To modify this fertile intracellular culture environment, the host must destroy the heavily parasitized macrophage, liberating its contents into the extracellular milieu. Here newly emigrated monocytes ingest, kill, and degrade *M. leprae* with the help of a lymphokine stimulus. This is the situation which applies in the tuberculoid form of the disease and is lacking in the lepromatous state. The immunomodulation necessary to mobilize host defense in lepromatous disease is discussed in a later section.

RECOMMENDED TREATMENT SCHEDULES. The most commonly used drug in the therapy of leprosy is 4,4'-diaminodiphenylsulfone (dapsone, DDS). Because of the widespread emergence of dapsone-resistant strains of *M. leprae*, all patients now receive multidrug therapy. The components and schedules vary depending upon the presence of dapsone-sensitive strains and the part of the world in which the patient resides. In the United States the following regimens are employed:

1. *Paucibacillary disease of the TT and BT categories.*
   a. Dapsone-sensitive *M. leprae*—Dapsone is given in a daily dose of 100 mg for 4 to 7 years and rifampin at a daily dose of 600 mg for 6 months.
   b. Dapsone-resistant *M. leprae*—Clofazimine at a daily dose of 50 to 100 mg is substituted for dapsone.
2. *Multibacillary disease of the BB, BL, and LL categories.*
   a. Dapsone-sensitive *M. leprae*—Dapsone is given in a daily dose of 100 mg for life. Rifampin is given in combination in a dose of 600 mg per day for the first 3 years of therapy.
   b. Dapsone-resistant *M. leprae*—Clofazimine at a daily dose of 50 to 100 mg is substituted for dapsone and given for life.

The evaluation of dapsone sensitivity requires the use of the mouse foot pad assay and is a procedure available only in specialized facilities.

A modified schedule for third world country control programs was issued in 1982 and is based upon practical consideration by the WHO, including the availability of slit smear facilities and financial constraints. Portions of the therapy are given under unsupervised conditions.

   1. *Paucibacillary disease*—a bacillary index of less than 2+ at all six skin sites. Dapsone is given daily at a dose of 100 mg, unsupervised. Rifampin is given at a dose of 600 mg once a month, supervised. Treatment is given for 6 months and is then discontinued.
   2. *Multibacillary disease*—a bacillary index of more than 2+ at any one of six skin sites. Dapsone is given daily at 100 mg with clofazimine 50 mg daily, unsupervised. Rifampin 600 mg and clofazimine 300 mg are given once monthly, supervised. This therapy is continued for 2 years or preferably until slit smears are negative.

The WHO schedule for intermittent rifampin therapy is based in part upon its expense and upon clinical and laboratory trials. It should be noted, however, that many leprologists employ rifampin at 450 to 600 mg daily for 2 to 3 years. Relapses under the WHO schedule occur not infrequently.

Rifampin is the most rapidly effective bactericidal agent and kills the majority of *M. leprae* within 2 to 3 weeks. This is evident by mouse foot pad assays and occurs only after 2 to 6 months of treatment with dapsone or clofazimine. Resistance to rifampin is well known in the therapy of *M. tuberculosis* and is now becoming evident with *M. leprae*.

Therapy with clofazimine, a phenazine derivative, has certain unpleasant side effects based upon its lipophilicity. The compound is a red-purple dye taken up and concentrated by macrophages of the skin, causing increased skin pigmentation. This is distressing to certain light-skinned patients. Clofazimine is also deposited in the small intestine, where it causes segmental thickening associated with crampy pain and diarrhea. The physician should consider substituting ethionamide or prothionamide at 250 to 375 mg daily, unsupervised.

THERAPY OF REACTIONS. *Erythema Nodosum Leprosum.* The acute onset of ENL may be mild enough to require only salicylates or other cyclo-oxygenase inhibitors. With severe episodes, high doses of corticosteroids (prednisone 60 to 80 mg per day) are necessitated and should be tapered off as soon as feasible. However, exacerbations occur frequently and repeated dosing is necessary. A particularly useful drug in severe ENL is thalidomide. It is given initially at 200 mg twice a day and then tapered to levels of 50 to 100 mg per day. Thalidomide is a potent teratogen and should be assiduously avoided if pregnancy is possible. Clofazimine has also been found useful in ENL but requires 4 to 6 weeks to achieve therapeutic effects. ENL in some patients responds poorly to thalidomide, and prednisone and/or clofazimine is employed.

Reversal Reactions. The chronicity and potential nerve damage of this cell-mediated reaction require the use of high-dose steroids and careful evaluation of peripheral nerve condition. Thalidomide is not used in this condition but clofazimine along with steroids allows the more rapid withdrawal of prednisone.

Other Complications. A variety of surgical procedures are available at specialized leprosy hospitals to help correct foot drop, hand deformities, madarosis, and lagophthalmos. Plastic surgical procedures can replace nasal septa and aid in the closure of large plantar ulcerations. On occasion patients request the removal of glandular tissue for gynecomastia.

The presence of a cold abscess of a peripheral nerve with sudden increase in pain and functional loss requires immediate decompression by surgical drainage.

IMMUNOMODULATION. The availability of recombinant lymphokines that can enhance the microbicidal properties of macrophages and stimulate the expression of CMI may find a place in the care of leprosy patients. Preliminary studies with the T-cell mitogen interleukin 2 (IL2) have already been carried out in patients with lepromatous leprosy. The intradermal injection of IL2 leads to a local cell-mediated reaction associated with induration, the destruction of parasitized macrophages, and a marked reduction in the bacillary load. Trials with more prolonged administration have demonstrated that a systemic response can be achieved.

PROGNOSIS. Tuberculoid leprosy is usually self-limited and responds well to chemotherapy. Nerve damage is, however, irreversible. In lepromatous disease, prolonged courses of multiple drugs arrest the progression of the illness when compliance is good. It is the ability of the public health infrastructure to monitor compliance that is central to effective therapy. Recurrences due to poor maintenance therapy are not infrequent.

PREVENTION AND PROPHYLAXIS. Education of the general public plays an important role in sensitizing individuals to the nature of leprosy lesions and the ability to cure the illness with medication. Once a case has been identified in a household, careful physical examination of all contacts with the biopsy of suspicious lesions should be carried out. The threat of contagion is much higher in children under 16 years of age. In this adolescent category the prophylactic use of dapsone should be considered.

A number of vaccine trials are currently underway, many sponsored by the World Health Organization. These are employ-

mycobacteria in highly endemic areas of Africa, Asia, and India. There is suggestive evidence that BCG alone may reduce the incidence of disease.

Guinto RS, Abalos RM, Cellona RV, Fajardo TT: An Atlas of Leprosy. Sasakawa Memorial Health Foundation, 1983. *Excellent pictorial presentation of diagnostic signs.*
Hansen GA: Causes of leprosy. Norsk Laegevidensk 4:76–79, 1874. *The classic work on leprosy.*
Hastings EC: Leprosy. New York, Churchill Livingstone, 1985.
Hastings RC, Franzblau SG: Chemotherapy of leprosy. Annu Rev Pharmacol Toxicol 28:231–245, 1988. *Current update of therapy and complications thereof.*

Job CK: Nerve damage in leprosy. XIII Leprosy Congress State of the Art Lectures. Int J Leprosy 57:532–539, 1989. *Good discussion of mechanisms of nerve damage.*
Kaplan G, Britton WJ, Hancock GE, et al.: The systemic influence of recombinant interleukin 2 on the manifestations of lepromatous leprosy. J Exp Med, in press. *Systemic modulation of CMI with IL-2.*
Kaplan G, Kiessling R, Teklemariam S, et al.: The reconstitution of cell-mediated immunity in the cutaneous lesions of lepromatous leprosy by recombinant interleukin 2. J Exp Med 169:893–907, 1989. *Discussion of our current understanding of the immunopathology of leprosy.*

Sexually Transmitted Diseases

P. Frederick Sparling

335 Introduction and Common Syndromes

Sexually transmitted diseases (STD's) are a diverse group of infections, caused by biologically dissimilar microbial agents, which are grouped together because of certain common clinical and epidemiologic features. In recent years there has been a remarkable accumulation of information about venereal infections. Advent of the acquired immunodeficiency syndrome (AIDS) has heightened public awareness of the importance of STD's and the dangers of unsafe sexual practices. New knowledge has accumulated rapidly about old diseases; for instance, it is now clear that cervical carcinoma is a complication of certain human papillomavirus (genital wart virus) infections. Some relatively less severe infections, such as chlamydial ones, are known to be alarmingly prevalent in young persons. This chapter discusses certain common features of some of these infections, as well as the differential diagnosis and management of several of the common syndromes of genital infections.

DEFINITIONS. Those infectious agents that are frequently transmitted by sexual contact, and for which sexual transmission is epidemiologically important, are considered sexually transmitted diseases. In some cases, such as gonorrhea and genital herpes simplex virus infection, sexual transmission is the only important mode of transmission, at least between adults. In others, such as the hepatitis viruses, giardiasis, shigellosis, and amebiasis, there are also important nonsexual means of acquiring infection. Table 335–1 lists the important infectious agents that are commonly transmitted sexually, as well as their known or probable disease syndromes. "Sexual" includes the full range of heterosexual or homosexual behavior, including genital, oral-genital, oral-anal, and genital-anal contact.

EPIDEMIOLOGIC CONSIDERATIONS. Sexually transmitted infections are prevalent in many segments of society, but, for obvious reasons, are most prevalent in the groups with the most promiscuous sexual activity. It is not sexual activity per se but the number and type of different sexual partners that determine the risk of acquiring STD. The highest rates of gonorrhea are found in the young (15 to 30) and unmarried and in groups of low educational and socioeconomic status. Rates of gonococcal infection may be 50-fold higher in young, single inner-city persons than in married middle- to upper-middle-class persons. Decisions regarding the cost-effectiveness of screening for STD should be governed by these considerations; screening is most effective in high-risk groups.

Multiple infections are frequent in patients with sexually transmitted infection. In venereal disease clinics, about 20 per cent of men with gonorrhea also have urethral chlamydial infection, and 30 to 50 per cent of women with gonorrhea also have cervical chlamydial infection. In women with vaginitis, one study showed that 16 per cent of cases were caused by mixed infection with various combinations of *Candida, Trichomonas,* and *Gardnerella vaginalis.* However, there is no convincing evidence that one sexually transmitted infection directly increases the risk of acquiring others. Rather, the frequent coexistence of multiple sexually acquired infections probably reflects the frequency of these organisms and the multiplicity of sexual partners among patients who were the subjects of these studies.

Control of sexually transmitted infections is complicated by the frequent lack of significant symptoms. The majority of gonococcal and chlamydial infections in women probably are associated with few symptoms. From 10 to 50 per cent of urethral gonococcal infections in men are oligo- or asymptomatic. Urethral chlamydial infections of men are more common than gonococcal infections and frequently are asymptomatic. The importance of the asymptomatic male is underscored by the repeated observation that women with gonococcal pelvic inflammatory disease have male partners whose infection is asymptomatic. Thus, one of the crucial issues in management is proper diagnosis and treatment of the asymptomatically infected partner.

STD IN HOMOSEXUAL MALES. Homosexual males are recognized as a group at particularly high risk of acquiring sexually transmitted disease, including human immunodeficiency virus (HIV) infection. HIV is but one of many STD-related problems in homosexual males, however. Syphilis remains a serious problem in homosexual males, although it also is a problem in drug-abusing heterosexuals. Some homosexual males are exceptionally promiscuous and are at high risk of acquiring not only syphilis but also gonococcal urethritis, proctitis, and pharyngitis; herpes genitalis and proctitis; hepatitis A and B; and a variety of enteric infections that are rarely transmitted in heterosexual sex, including giardiasis, amebiasis, and shigellosis. These enteric infections are probably transmitted by oral-anal or anal-penile-oral contact. In recent years, however, the incidence of some STD's, such as gonorrhea, has declined in homosexual males owing to adoption of changed and safer sex practices (fewer partners, condoms) resulting from the fear of acquiring AIDS. Homosexual women apparently do not have increased rates of STD.

INCIDENCE OF STD's. The true incidence of the STD's is not known in the United States because of serious problems of under-reporting. Gonorrhea is the most common of the reported infectious diseases in the United States, with over 1,000,000 reported infections annually. Although genital chlamydial infections generally are not reported, their prevalence certainly exceeds that of gonorrhea. Herpes simplex virus (HSV) and human papillomavirus (HPV) infections also are more prevalent than gonorrhea. The relative incidence of STD is quite variable in different areas of the world. For instance, chancroid is currently uncommon in the United States but is about as common as gonorrhea in certain areas of the Far East.

COMMON SYNDROMES. *Urethritis in Males.* Urethritis in males is a very common syndrome. It is ordinarily classified as either gonococcal or nongonococcal urethritis (NGU), depending on whether the presence of gonococci can be demonstrated by

TABLE 335–1. SEXUALLY TRANSMITTED AGENTS AND THEIR SYNDROMES*

Microorganism	Syndromes
Bacteria	
Neisseria gonorrhoeae	Urethritis, cervicitis, bartholinitis, proctitis, pharyngitis, salpingitis, epididymitis, conjunctivitis, perihepatitis, arthritis, dermatitis, endocarditis, meningitis, amniotic infection syndrome
Mobiluncus species and *Gardnerella vaginalis*	"Nonspecific" vaginosis
Treponema pallidum	Syphilis (multiple clinical syndromes)
Haemophilus ducreyi	Chancroid
Calymmatobacterium granulomatis	Granuloma inguinale
Shigella species	Enteritis in homosexual men
Campylobacter species	Enteritis in homosexual men
Group B *Streptococcus*	Neonatal sepsis and meningitis
Chlamydiae	
Chlamydia trachomatis	Nongonococcal urethritis, purulent hypertrophic cervicitis, epididymitis, salpingitis, conjunctivitis, trachoma, pneumonia, perihepatitis, lymphogranuloma venereum, Reiter's syndrome
Mycoplasmas	
Ureaplasma urealyticum	Nongonococcal urethritis, ? premature rupture of membranes and abortion
Mycoplasma hominis	Postpartum fever, pelvic inflammatory disease
Viruses	
Herpes simplex virus (HSV)	Genital herpes, proctitis, meningitis, disseminated infection in neonates
Hepatitis A virus	Hepatitis in homosexual men
Hepatitis B virus	Hepatitis, ? periarteritis nodosa, hepatoma; especially prevalent in homosexual men
Cytomegalovirus	Congenital infection (birth defects, infant mortality, mental deficiency, hearing loss); mononucleosis syndrome
Human papillomavirus (HPV)	Condyloma acuminatum; cervical carcinoma
Molluscum contagiosum virus	Molluscum contagiosum
Human immunodeficiency virus (HIV)	Acquired immunodeficiency syndrome and related illnesses
Protozoa	
Trichomonas vaginalis	Trichomonal vaginitis, occasional urethritis
Entamoeba histolytica	Enteritis in homosexual men
Giardia lamblia	Enteritis in homosexual men
Fungi	
Candida albicans	Vaginitis, balanitis
Ectoparasites	
Phthirus pubis	Pubic lice infestation
Sarcoptes scabei	Scabies

*The relative importance of sexual transmission in the epidemiology of several of these agents remains to be defined; these include Group B streptococci, hepatitis A virus, cytomegalovirus, *Candida albicans*, and others.

Gram's stain or culture. In venereal disease clinics, the prevalence of gonococcal and nongonococcal urethritis is similar, but NGU is considerably more common in private practice and in college infirmaries. Several recent studies of asymptomatic sexually active young persons found a prevalence of up to 15 per cent of genital chlamydial infection.

A large number of studies have established *Chlamydia trachomatis* as a cause of approximately 40 per cent of cases of NGU. Case-control studies have provided suggestive evidence that *Ureaplasma urealyticum* (formerly "T-strain" mycoplasma) is a

significant factor in chlamydia-negative NGU. In addition, urethral inoculation of volunteers with pure cultures of *U. urealyticum* produced rather typical NGU. In practice, however, it is difficult to define the importance of *Ureaplasma* infection in patients with urethritis, because up to 70 per cent of asymptomatic sexually active persons are colonized by these organisms. A very small proportion of cases of NGU in men is due to *Trichomonas vaginalis* or herpes simplex virus infection.

Diagnosis of urethritis requires demonstration of an inflammatory urethral exudate. A discharge may not be evident if the patient has recently voided, and patients preferably should be examined several hours after their last urination. The discharge may be present only in the morning, prior to urination. Demonstration of discharge often requires urethral "milking" and may require insertion of a small calcium alginate or similar swab into the anterior urethra, with examination of a direct Gram-stained smear of the swab for leukocytes. Presence of an average of at least five polymorphonuclear leukocytes per high power (100×) field suggests the diagnosis of urethritis.

The patient should be questioned for past history of urethritis and for symptoms suggestive of systemic diseases such as Reiter's syndrome or disseminated gonococcal infection. Examination should be made for signs of conjunctivitis, arthritis, dermatitis, and epididymitis. Prostatitis is rarely present unless there are symptoms of perineal, suprapubic, or rectal discomfort, and rectal examination is not routinely indicated. Rectal examination and urine culture are indicated in men with dysuria but without signs of anterior urethral discharge.

Laboratory studies are ordinarily limited to a Gram's stain of urethral exudate. Demonstration of typical gram-negative diplococci, many of which are inside neutrophils, establishes the diagnosis of gonococcal urethritis. At least 90 per cent of men with symptomatic culture-proven urethral gonorrhea have a positive Gram's stain. In occasional patients, especially those with equivocal Gram's stain, it may be necessary to culture the anterior urethra or freshly voided urine sediment for gonococci. This is particularly important in asymptomatic male contacts of patients with disseminated gonococcal infection or gonococcal salpingitis, since Gram's stain of urethral contents is positive in only about 60 per cent of men with asymptomatic urethral gonorrhea.

Diagnosis of NGU usually is made by exclusion of gonorrhea. Monoclonal antibodies are available for diagnosis of chlamydiae in secretions; results indicate a sensitivity of over 90 per cent compared with culture, with nearly 100 per cent specificity. This test requires use of a fluorescence microscope, and cost considerations preclude widespread use. Other immunoassays are available, with comparable efficacy. A DNA hybridization test recently was introduced. Culture for *Chlamydia* is now more widely available than in the past and is the best (but expensive) test. There is no serologic test that is clinically useful. Tests for *Ureaplasma* are not readily available and rarely are indicated. Examination of a saline suspension of urethral exudate occasionally may reveal motile trichomonads in patients with recurrent urethritis who fail to respond to appropriate therapy. A serologic test for syphilis should be obtained, but the diagnostic yield is low.

Management is outlined in Figure 335–1 and is discussed further in Ch. 336. Sexual partners of men with gonococcal or nongonococcal urethritis should be treated both to prevent reinfection of the patient and to prevent development of complications in the partners.

The syndrome of *postgonococcal urethritis* (persistence or crudescence of urethritis after administration of therapy that has eradicated gonococcal infection) is usually due to concomitant urethral chlamydial infection that was not eradicated by the original treatment. This syndrome is more common after therapy with a β-lactam antibiotic than after a regimen of tetracycline, undoubtedly because of the greater efficacy of tetracycline for treating chlamydial infections. Accordingly, there is considerable merit to use of oral tetracycline to follow up ceftriaxone therapy for genital gonorrhea.

Genital Ulcer Syndrome. Genital skin lesions may be either ulcerative or nonulcerative. In patients seen in a venereal disease clinic, the most common sexually transmitted nonulcerative genital lesions are due to scabies, genital warts, molluscum contagiosum, or *Candida* species, but differential diagnosis includes a long list of dermatologic conditions.

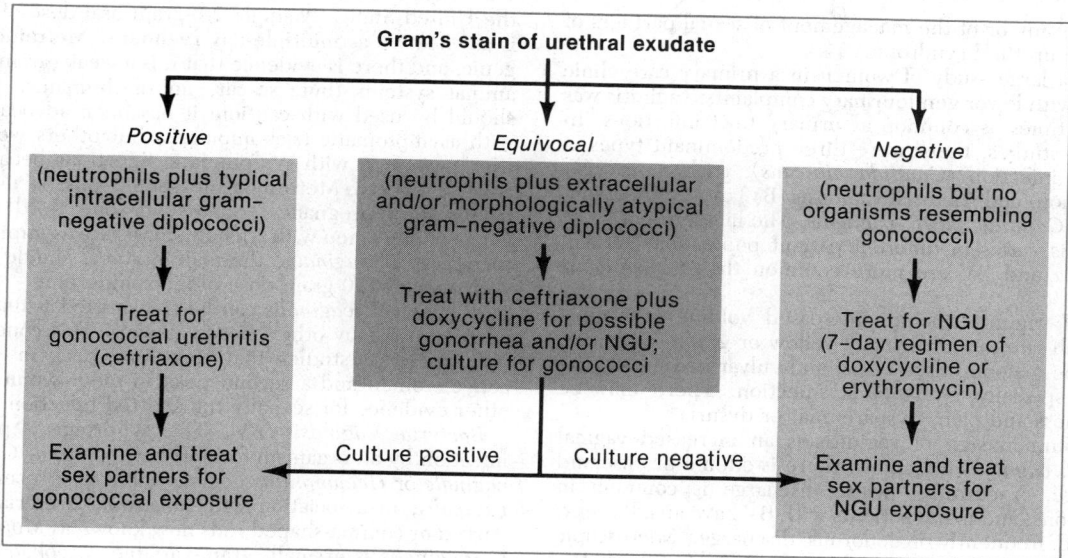

FIGURE 335–1. Management of male patients with urethritis.

The most common cause of ulcerative genital lesions in patients in the United States is herpes simplex virus, but differential diagnosis includes syphilis, chancroid, lymphogranuloma venereum (LGV), granuloma inguinale (GI), and trauma. Chancroid is becoming more common in certain cities in the United States; LGV and GI are rare. The most important distinction is between syphilis, genital herpes, and chancroid. Sometimes, the appearance is virtually diagnostic: Grouped, painful, superficial vesicles are nearly diagnostic of herpes, whereas a single, clean-based, nonpainful ulcer with indurated margins suggests primary syphilis. In recent studies, only about 60 per cent of penile syphilitic chancres had this classic appearance. Painful ulcers suggest herpes or chancroid. Genital herpes may present as a single ulcer, particularly in patients with recurrent herpes, and syphilis may present with multiple ulcers. Secondarily infected lesions of primary syphilis may be painful.

It is a useful rule to obtain a serologic test for syphilis on all patients with genital ulcers, and, if the initial serology is negative and if the diagnosis remains uncertain, to obtain a second serology about 2 weeks later. A darkfield examination for syphilis should also be done, and it should be repeated twice on successive days if syphilis is seriously suspected and the initial examination is negative.

Infection by herpes simplex virus may be efficiently diagnosed by viral culture or by immunofluorescent methods, but these are frequently unavailable in practice. Papanicolaou's smear is suggestive of herpes in about two thirds of culture-positive cases. Giemsa's or Wright's stain of cells scraped from the base of a vesicle may reveal multinucleate giant cells (Tzanck's test), but this test is particularly insensitive in herpetic lesions that have become ulcerated. Serologic tests for herpesvirus are not helpful in management but may indicate persons with latent infection. Referral of patients to centers with capability of viral culture may be indicated in diagnostically difficult patients.

In addition to herpesvirus infection, chancroid should be suspected in patients with painful genital ulcers. Chancroid is occurring in epidemics in certain United States cities, particularly among crack house clients. Attempts should be made to isolate the causative agent, *Haemophilus ducreyi;* selective culture media are an improvement over previously available methods. No serologic tests are available.

Therapy clearly depends on the correct diagnosis. Topical antibiotics are never indicated. Initial genital herpes (first infection) is best treated with topical or oral administration of acyclovir or intravenous administration for severe infections. Therapy of chancroid is with co-trimoxazole, erythromycin, or ceftriaxone. Occasional empiric trials of oral co-trimoxazole or erythromycin are warranted in patients with persistent genital ulcers not readily attributable to herpesvirus or syphilis, but repeated attempts to isolate *H. ducreyi* should be made in such instances. It is not possible to arrive at an unequivocal diagnosis of the cause of genital ulcers in all patients.

Lower Genital Tract Infections in Women. Infections of the female genitourinary tract produce a variety of syndromes, often with overlapping symptoms (dysuria, vaginal discharge, vulvar irritation). These infections are very common, relatively poorly understood by most physicians, sometimes difficult to treat, and often frustrating for both doctor and patient. However, the various syndromes usually can be distinguished on relatively simple clinical and laboratory grounds, and a precise microbial etiology often can be established.

It is most helpful first to determine the primary anatomic site of infection: urethra or bladder, endocervix, or vagina. This can sometimes be accomplished by history; women with urinary tract infection (UTI) usually experience "internal" dysuria, whereas women with dysuria associated with vaginitis usually experience "external" dysuria owing to passage of urine over inflamed labia. Cervicitis is diagnosed by physical examination; there are mucopurulent secretions emanating from the endocervical canal, and there is often a hypertrophic, mucoid, reddened "cobblestone" appearance to the cervical mucosa. Patients with cervicitis may also have urethritis or vaginitis. Vaginitis is associated with increased vaginal discharge of several types, as discussed below, and frequently there are associated signs and symptoms of vaginal, vulvar, and perineal irritation (dyspareunia, external dysuria, itching, pain). In patients with lower genitourinary infection, it is important to determine whether there is involvement of the upper genitourinary tract (pyelonephritis, salpingitis).

The Urethral Syndrome. Bacterial cystitis with or without pyelonephritis is usually diagnosed in women with dysuria, urinary frequency, and pyuria if they have colony counts of at least 10^5 bacteria per milliliter of urine. If similar symptoms are present but routine cultures grow less than 10^4 bacteria per milliliter of voided urine, the "urethral syndrome" is likely.

In a study of sexually active young women who presented to walk-in clinics with dysuria and urinary frequency, and who did not have vaginitis or active herpes simplex infection, 43 per cent had the urethral syndrome (urethritis). Among women with urethritis, 25 per cent had positive urethral cultures for *Chlamydia trachomatis.* Isolation of chlamydiae from the urethra was uncommon in women without urethritis. In other studies, gonococci also were shown to cause this syndrome. Thus, women as well as men may present with urethritis caused by gonococci and chlamydiae.

Management of patients with the urethral syndrome has not been carefully evaluated. Patients with symptoms of urinary tract infection who do not have bacteriuria should have urethral and cervical cultures for *Neisseria gonorrhoeae.* If these cultures are also negative, a therapeutic trial may be made with a tetracycline or a sulfonamide for approximately 7 days. There are no controlled trials of such therapy or of the management of sexual partners of women with the urethral syndrome.

Vaginitis. In a large study of women in a primary care clinic who presented with lower genitourinary complaints, vaginitis was more than five times as common as urinary tract infections. In this and similar studies, there were three predominant types of vaginitis: yeast infection (*Candida albicans*), trichomonas (*T. vaginalis*) infection, and bacterial vaginosis (BV) caused by organisms other than *Candida* and *T. vaginalis*. The incidence of these types of vaginitis varies in different patient populations, but in general *Candida* and BV are more common than *T. vaginalis* vaginitis.

Symptoms of vaginitis include increased volume of vaginal discharge, which is often abnormally yellow or green in appearance and may be malodorous. Vaginal and vulvar itching may be troublesome, especially in *Candida* infection. There may be vaginal tenderness and pain, dyspareunia, or dysuria.

The most common sign of vaginitis is an increased vaginal discharge. In *T. vaginalis* infections, there is often a profuse and frothy discharge. A curdlike, white discharge is common in *Candida* infections, and many patients with BV have an adherent, often gray, and frequently malodorous discharge. Microscopic examination shows many polymorphonuclear leukocytes in the discharge in all but BV. Speculum examination may show signs of endocervicitis as well, with purulent discharge issuing from the cervical os. In occasional patients, no objective signs of vaginal inflammation are found despite the presence of troublesome symptoms. See Table 335–2.

Candida Vaginitis. Most vaginal yeast infections are due to *C. albicans*. Diagnosis is usually made by visualizing yeasts or pseudohyphae by microscopic examination of vaginal secretions suspended in normal saline or 10 per cent KOH. Microscopic examination is less sensitive than culture. However, many asymptomatic women have positive vaginal cultures for *C. albicans*, and therefore some authorities advocate using microscopy in preference to culture. The discharge in *Candida* vaginitis is not malodorous and has a pH of less than 4.5 when a drop is applied to pH paper with a range of 4.0 to 5.5.

Therapy of *Candida* vaginitis is with one of the imidazole compounds (e.g., clotrimazole, miconazole, butaconazole, or teraconazole) once each night for 3 to 7 days intravaginally. There is no convincing evidence that attempts to eradicate yeast from the gastrointestinal tract have a significant effect on rates of cure or relapse of *Candida* vaginitis. There is no evidence to warrant therapy of sexual partners. Attempts should be made to correct ancillary conditions that increase susceptibility to vaginal candidiasis: antibiotic therapy, diabetes, or oral anovulatory steroids. Relapse is a significant problem in some patients. No therapy is indicated for asymptomatic vaginal carriers of *C. albicans*.

T. vaginalis Vaginitis. Diagnosis is made ordinarily by visualizing motile trichomonads in a normal saline suspension of vaginal secretions. The organisms are easily seen at high-dry (100×) magnification, and may usually be seen under low-power magnification. The saline suspension should be examined promptly. Culture is more sensitive, but about 80 to 90 per cent of culture-positive cases are detected by microscopy. Addition of a drop of 10 per cent KOH to vaginal secretions usually results in liberation of a detectable fishlike odor, attributed to release of volatile amines. The pH of vaginal secretions is usually greater than 5.0. In these latter two respects, *T. vaginalis* vaginitis is similar to BV.

Therapy of trichomoniasis is with one of the nitroimidazoles,

either metronidazole or newer compounds such as tinidazole. The latter is extensively used in Europe but is not approved in the United States. A single 2.0-gram oral dose of metronidazole is as effective as multiple-day regimens. Metronidazole is mutagenic, and there is evidence that it is a weak carcinogen in certain animal systems (but, so far, not in humans). Accordingly, it should be used with caution; it has been advocated for women with asymptomatic trichomoniasis, but others would reserve its use for women with symptomatic infections because of possible adverse effects. Metronidazole should not be used in the first trimester of pregnancy. Since over one third of male sexual partners of women with trichomoniasis are asymptomatic urethral carriers of *T. vaginalis*, the male partners should also be treated with a single 2.0-gram dose of metronidazole.

Although *T. vaginalis* can be transmitted sexually, it probably is transmitted by other means as well. This conclusion is based on prevalence studies that show one peak in young, sexually active women and a second peak in older women who have no other evidence for sexually transmitted infection.

Bacterial Vaginosis (BV). This syndrome is probably due to infection by an organism formerly called either *Corynebacterium vaginale* or *Haemophilus vaginalis*, but now termed *Gardnerella vaginalis*, in association with anaerobic bacteria, including the curved or comma-shaped rods now known as *Mobiluncus* species. *G. vaginalis* is a small, gram-variable coccobacillus that can be grown quite successfully on partially selective enriched media. Among women with abnormal vaginal discharge who do not have yeast infection or trichomoniasis, over 90 per cent grow *G. vaginalis*, whereas fewer than 10 per cent of matched controls grow the same organism. There usually are increased numbers of anaerobic vaginal bacteria as well, and decreased numbers of the normal vaginal lactobacilli. Development of full symptoms may require both *G. vaginalis* and vaginal anaerobes, although the precise pathophysiology of this syndrome is still under investigation.

Diagnosis of bacterial vaginosis is by exclusion of trichomoniasis, candidiasis, and purulent cervicitis. Abnormal cells termed "clue cells" are often seen in a wet mount of vaginal secretions in normal saline; these are stippled, granular-appearing vaginal epithelial cells that contain large numbers of adherent *G. vaginalis*. Few polymorphonuclear leukocytes are present. Addition of a drop of 10 per cent KOH usually results in production of an unpleasant fishy odor. The pH of the vaginal secretions is nearly always greater than 5.0.

Optimal therapy is being investigated. Metronidazole has only borderline activity in vitro against *G. vaginalis*, but in a dose of 500 mg by mouth twice daily for 7 days it was effective in eradicating both *G. vaginalis* and the symptoms of vaginitis from 80 of 81 patients in one trial; similar results have been obtained in other trials. This suggests that the principal cause of this syndrome is an anaerobe, since metronidazole is principally effective against anaerobes. Clindamycin (300 mg orally twice daily for 7 days) also is effective. Over 90 per cent of male partners are urethral carriers of *G. vaginalis* and therefore probably should be treated with the same regimen as the patient, although data to support this are lacking at present.

Mixed Vaginitis. In 2 to 16 per cent of patients, vaginitis may be due to polymicrobial infection with two or three organisms. Such mixed infection may account for some instances of treatment failure. Particular care should be given to identification of all causative organisms in patients who have recurrent or relapsing vaginitis.

Cervicitis. Two organisms are recognized as probable causes of mucopurulent endocervicitis: *N. gonorrhoeae* and *C. trachomatis*. Women who are sexual partners of men with chlamydia-positive NGU have a much higher rate of isolation of chlamydiae from the cervix than do women who are partners of men with chlamydia-negative NGU, and they also have significantly higher rates of mucopurulent cervicitis. Herpes simplex virus can also cause cervicitis, especially in primary infection. However, the clinical appearance in herpetic cervicitis is different, with cervical vesicles and ulcers rather than mucopurulent cervicitis.

True cervicitis should not be confused with cervical ectopy, which is merely the appearance of endocervical columnar epithelium on the exposed, visible exocervix. This results in a red-appearing cervix and may result in increased production of a mucoid vaginal discharge but does not require therapy.

TABLE 335–2. DIFFERENTIAL DIAGNOSIS OF VAGINITIS

Characteristics of Vaginal Discharge	Organism Causing Vaginitis		
	C. albicans	*T. vaginalis*	BV
pH	4.5	>5.0	>5.0
White curd	Usually	No	No
Odor with KOH	No	Yes	Yes
Clue cells	No	No	Usually
Motile trichomonads	No	Usually	No
Yeast cells	Yes	No	No

Diagnosis of mucopurulent endocervicitis requires visualization of purulent discharge from the cervical os. There often is a roughened "cobblestone" appearance to the cervix. Gram's stain is about 60 per cent sensitive and over 90 per cent specific for gonorrhea if typical intracellular gonococci are seen, but cultures for *N. gonorrhoeae* should be taken. Tissue culture for isolation of *C. trachomatis* may be employed if available. Cytology is not sufficiently sensitive to warrant widespread use. New immunoassays for *C. trachomatis* allow rapid, sensitive, specific diagnosis from patient secretions and undoubtedly should be more widely employed to document etiology and to initiate proper treatment for cervicitis due to chlamydiae.

Antibiotic therapy appears to result in clinical improvement in mucopurulent cervicitis. Patients with negative cultures for the gonococcus probably should be treated with doxycycline (100 mg twice daily for 7 days) or erythromycin in a dose of 500 mg four times daily for at least 7 days; their sexual partners probably should be treated similarly. One should recognize that only modest data support these recommendations. No other form of cervicitis has been shown to respond to antimicrobial therapy.

Upper Genital Tract Disease in Women: Salpingitis. Full coverage of this important topic is precluded by space considerations. This is a very important clinical problem, resulting in considerable morbidity in the estimated 250,000 to 500,000 women who are affected yearly in the United States.

Etiology. The gonococcus may account for as many as 50 per cent of cases in the United States, particularly among women with relatively severe and first-episode salpingitis. About 15 to 20 per cent of women with gonococcal cervicitis probably subsequently develop salpingitis. Strong evidence now implicates genital chlamydial infections as another significant cause of salpingitis; in Sweden, more cases of salpingitis are due to *C. trachomatis* than to *N. gonorrhoeae.* Salpingitis due to genital chlamydial infections may be mild, and patients may not seek medical care. Nevertheless, complications may follow, particularly tubal scarring and infertility. There is less convincing evidence that *Mycoplasma hominis* may occasionally cause a similar syndrome. Many cases of salpingitis are caused by mixed infection with microaerophilic streptococci and enteric bacilli, often including *Bacteroides* species. These polymicrobial infections appear to be more common in recurrent attacks of salpingitis.

Diagnosis. Clinical diagnosis of salpingitis is inexact. Perhaps only 20 per cent of patients have the classic syndrome of lower abdominal pain and tenderness, cervical tenderness, fever, leukocytosis, and elevated sedimentation rate. The most common findings are lower abdominal tenderness, which is usually bilateral, and adnexal and cervical tenderness. Patients with gonococcal salpingitis are more likely to present with fever, and more commonly have onset near the menses, whereas patients with nongonococcal salpingitis more commonly present with adnexal masses. Laparoscopy is commonly used to diagnose salpingitis in certain countries but is invasive and requires general anesthesia. In the United States, laparoscopy is usually used only in selected patients whose differential diagnosis includes ectopic pregnancy, appendicitis, ruptured abscess, or other potential emergencies.

Complications. Complications are primarily infertility and ectopic pregnancies. Rates of involuntary infertility are about 15 per cent after one attack of salpingitis and about 75 per cent after three or more attacks. Total hysterectomy may eventually be necessitated by symptoms of chronic salpingitis.

Therapy. Recommendations from the Centers for Disease Control suggest initial therapy of outpatients with cefoxitin 2.0 grams intramuscularly along with probenecid 1.0 gram orally, followed by doxycycline 100 mg orally twice daily for 10 to 14 days. There are no controlled data on efficacy of various regimens used for hospitalized patients. Current recommendations call for doxycycline 100 mg twice daily plus cefoxitin 2.0 grams intravenously four times daily; or clindamycin 900 mg intravenously three times daily plus gentamicin 1.5 mg per kilogram three times daily. After discharge, doxycycline should be given in a dose of 100 mg twice daily to complete 10 to 14 days of therapy. Patients should usually be hospitalized if they are very ill, are pregnant, have significant adnexal masses, or have failed previous therapy, or if the differential diagnosis includes surgical emergencies such as appendicitis or ectopic pregnancy.

Prevention. Sexual partners of women with gonococcal salpingitis must be identified, examined, and treated to prevent subsequent reinfection of the patient. About one half of the infected male partners of women with gonococcal salpingitis are asymptomatic. Treatment of women with tetracycline (as compared with penicillin) to eradicate chlamydiae from the cervix reduces the incidence of post-therapy salpingitis (Rees, 1980), which suggests that increased emphasis on treatment of chlamydiae in the male and female genital tract might reduce the incidence of salpingitis.

Bowie WR, Wang S-P, Alexander ER, et al.: Etiology of nongonococcal urethritis: Evidence for *Chlamydia trachomatis* and *Ureaplasma urealyticum.* J Clin Invest 59:735, 1977. *An excellent epidemiologic and clinical study of the etiology and therapy of nongonococcal urethritis in males.*

Brunham RC, Paavonen J, Stevens CE, et al.: Mucopurulent cervicitis—the ignored counterpart in women of urethritis in men. N Engl J Med 311:1, 1984. *Genital chlamydial infection causes mucopurulent cervicitis, and proper diagnosis leads to effective treatment.*

Holmes KK, Mårdh P-A, Sparling PF, et al. (eds.): Sexually Transmitted Diseases, 2nd ed. New York, McGraw-Hill, 1990. *The definitive textbook on STD's, heavily referenced.*

Mårdh P-A, Møller BR, Paavonen J: Chlamydial infection of the female genital tract with emphasis on pelvic inflammatory disease. A review of Scandinavian studies. Sex Transm Dis 8(Suppl):140, 1981. *Review of the role of chlamydiae in pelvic inflammatory disease.*

Nettleman MD, Jones RB, Roberts SD, et al.: Cost-effectiveness of culturing for *Chlamydia trachomatis*: A study in a clinic for sexually transmitted diseases. Ann Intern Med 105:189, 1986. *Cultures were most cost effective in low-risk women. In high-risk groups, empiric therapy is suggested.*

Pheifer TA, Forsyth PS, Durfee MA, et al.: Nonspecific vaginitis: Role of *Haemophilus vaginalis* and treatment with metronidazole. N Engl J Med 298:1429, 1978. *A clinical and therapeutic study of nonspecific vaginitis, showing that both G. vaginalis and vaginal anaerobes are probably important in causation of the syndrome and also that metronidazole is effective therapy.*

Rees E: The treatment of pelvic inflammatory disease. Am J Obstet Gynecol 138:1042, 1980. *Treatment of women with chlamydial infection of the cervix with tetracycline compared with penicillin reduced the incidence of subsequent salpingitis.*

Stamm WE, Harrison HR, Alexander ER, et al.: Diagnosis of *Chlamydia trachomatis* infections by direct immunofluorescence staining of genital secretions: A multicenter trial. Ann Intern Med 101:638, 1984. *Immunofluorescence was reasonably sensitive (89 to 92 per cent) and specific (96 to 99 per cent) in the diagnosis of genital chlamydial infection in symptomatic men and women, compared with culture. Other reports show less sensitivity in asymptomatic screening.*

Stamm WE, Koutsky LA, Benedetti JK, et al.: *Chlamydia trachomatis* urethral infections in men: Prevalence, risk factors, and clinical manifestations. Ann Intern Med 100:47, 1984. *Asymptomatic male urethral carriers of chlamydiae are very common.*

Stamm WE, Wagner KF, Amsel R, et al.: Causes of the acute urethral syndrome in women. N Engl J Med 303:409, 1980. *Females may also develop a form of nongonococcal urethritis resulting from infection with Chlamydia trachomatis.*

Tait IA, Rees E, Hobson D, et al.: Chlamydial infection of the cervix in contacts of men with nongonococcal urethritis. Br J Vener Dis 56:37, 1980. *Chlamydia trachomatis is shown to cause mucopurulent cervicitis, and appropriate antibiotic therapy results in clinical improvement.*

Taylor-Robinson D, Csonka GW, Prentice MJ: Human intraurethral inoculation of ureaplasmas. Q J Med 46:309, 1977. *Inoculation of the investigator's urethra with ureaplasmas resulted in nonspecific urethritis.*

336 Gonococcal Infections

INTRODUCTION. *Neisseria gonorrhoeae* is a common sexually transmitted organism that causes anterior urethritis in males and endocervicitis and urethritis in females. Other types of primary infection include pharyngitis, proctitis, conjunctivitis, and vulvovaginitis; the last-named disorder occurs principally in prepubescent females. Complications may occur by direct extension of infection, including epididymitis, prostatitis, Bartholin gland abscess, salpingitis, and perihepatitis. Bacteremia may occur, with production of characteristic cutaneous lesions, arthritis, and tenosynovitis; rare complications include endocarditis and meningitis. Conjunctival infection formerly was a common cause of blindness in neonates.

Gonorrhea is the most common reportable infectious disease in the United States, with about 1 million reported cases annually. The true incidence is probably at least 2 million cases annually.

EPIDEMIOLOGY. The only natural hosts for *N. gonorrhoeae* are humans. The organism normally resides on the columnar epithelium of mucosal surfaces and is usually transmitted by intimate sexual contact.

The prevalence of gonorrhea varies greatly in different groups. As many as 5 per cent of persons in high-risk populations may be infected at any time. Surveys of private practices in the United States in the 1970's showed that about 2 per cent of sexually active young women had positive endocervical cultures for the gonococcus. Highest prevalence was found in young (15 to 30) single persons of low socioeconomic and educational status, probably because these factors correlate positively with sexual promiscuity.

The risk of acquiring infection depends on the type of contact with an infected person. About 60 to 80 per cent of females in contact with a male with urethral gonorrhea develop gonococcal cervicitis. By contrast, it is estimated that only 20 to 30 per cent of males having sex with an infected female develop gonorrhea. This difference may be due to exposure of females to a larger inoculum of gonococci. A person having oral sex with a male with gonococcal urethritis has considerable risk of acquiring pharyngeal gonorrhea. Transmission of infection by oral contact with the genitals of an infected female is rare. Infection is apparently efficiently spread by penile-rectal contact.

Gonococci die rapidly upon drying, and transmission by fomites is rare. Epidemics were reported in prepubertal females living in close proximity in orphanages, but such episodes are now very uncommon.

Control of gonorrhea is difficult because of the frequency of asymptomatic infection. Perhaps 50 per cent of infections in females are asymptomatic or only minimally symptomatic, and at least 10 per cent of infected males are asymptomatic.

In past years there was considerable emphasis on case finding by endocervical culture of young, sexually active females. The merit of this strategy depends on the prevalence of infection in the community and the lifestyle of the patient. A more cost-effective method for finding infected patients is to culture patients about 6 weeks after treatment for gonorrhea; as many as 15 to 20 per cent of such persons are culture positive, usually because of reinfection.

THE ORGANISM. *N. gonorrhoeae* is a gram-negative, aerobic diplococcus. Many strains require 3 to 10 per cent CO_2 for optimal growth. They are highly autolytic and die rapidly when outside their normal human environment. They are sensitive to fatty acids and grow best on media with added starch to inhibit fatty acids present in agar. Several partially selective media are available; most employ antibiotics such as trimethoprim, vancomycin, colistin, and nystatin to inhibit growth of other microorganisms. Replacement of vancomycin with lincomycin seems to improve the rate of isolation of gonococci.

Presumptive identification in vitro is made by colonial morphology, Gram's stain, and a positive oxidase test. Differentiation from the closely related meningococcus and the various nonpathogenic *Neisseria* is ordinarily by patterns of utilization of various simple carbohydrates; gonococci use glucose but not maltose or sucrose.

Gonococci are highly variable and occur in a number of different colonial forms. Small colonial types are piliated and more virulent in humans than the larger, nonpiliated variants. Variation is also found in certain outer membrane proteins. Gonococci undergo rapid variation in the antigenic type of pilus expressed, which probably contributes to prolonged infections without treatment and to the ability of persons to acquire repeat infections after treatment. The importance of surface components of the gonococcus in the pathogenesis of infection is under intense investigation.

Gonococci can be serotyped on the basis of antigenic differences in pili, outer membrane proteins, and other antigens. They also can be reliably biotyped by definition of their nutritional requirements on defined agar media ("auxotypes"). These tests are not routinely available at present.

PATHOGENESIS. The minimal infective dose of gonococci for establishment of urethritis in male volunteers is between 100 and 1000 colony-forming units. Surface pili undoubtedly help to attach the bacteria to the mucosal surface, and they also help prevent ingestion and killing by polymorphonuclear leukocytes. Typical urethral infections result in a moderately severe inflammatory response, which is probably due to release of toxic lipopolysaccharide from gonococci and to production of chemotactic factors that attract neutrophilic leukocytes. Certain strains are likely to cause asymptomatic urethral infection for reasons not completely understood. These strains are usually penicillin sensitive, resistant to the bactericidal effects of normal human serum, and particularly likely to cause bacteremia and septic arthritis.

In the preantibiotic era, symptoms usually persisted for 2 to 3 months before host defenses finally succeeded in eradicating the infection. Host defenses include serum opsonic and bactericidal antibodies, as well as local (mucosal) antibodies of the IgG and IgA classes. All gonococci produce an enzyme, IgA protease, which cleaves the major class of secretory IgA, perhaps contributing to persistence of local gonococcal infections.

Serum bactericidal antibodies are undoubtedly important in prevention of bacteremic infection. The best evidence for this has been provided by patients who suffer from homozygous deficiency of one of the complement components C6, C7, C8, or C9. This results in deficiency of serum bactericidal activity but no alteration of serum opsonic activity. Such individuals are particularly prone to recurrent bacteremic gonococcal infection or to recurrent meningococcal meningitis or meningococcemia.

CLINICAL PATTERNS OF DISEASE. *Gonorrhea in Males.* Gonococcal urethritis in males ("the clap" or "the strain") is characterized by a yellowish, purulent urethral discharge and dysuria. The usual incubation period is 2 to 6 days. The discharge of gonorrhea is slightly more copious and purulent than in nongonococcal urethritis (NGU). Symptoms are probably produced by 90 per cent of infections, although asymptomatic infections do occur and may persist for many months. Males with asymptomatic infection do not seek treatment, whereas those with symptomatic infection are usually promptly treated and cured. This is the probable explanation for prevalence studies that show that up to 50 per cent of infected males are asymptomatic. Asymptomatic infection in males and females is of great epidemiologic importance, since such carriers may continue to spread infection to new sexual partners for months if they are not properly diagnosed and treated.

Complications of gonococcal urethritis in males are now rare. Urethral stricture was formerly a common complication but was probably due in part to the use of caustic treatment regimens. Epididymitis and prostatitis, relatively common complications in the past, are seen only occasionally today. The principal complication is disseminated gonococcal infection, which is estimated to affect about 1 per cent of men with gonorrhea. This entity is discussed below.

The differential diagnosis of gonococcal urethritis is discussed in Ch. 335.

Gonococcal infections of the pharynx and rectum are common problems in homosexual males. Most patients with pharyngeal infection are asymptomatic, but occasional patients have exudative pharyngitis with cervical adenopathy. Gonococcal infection of the rectum causes a wide spectrum of symptoms, ranging from asymptomatic carriers to severe proctitis with tenesmus and bloody, mucopurulent discharge. Although approximately 40 per cent of females with cervical gonorrhea also have positive rectal cultures, symptoms of proctitis in females are unusual. This has suggested that the trauma of rectal intercourse may contribute to the proctitis observed in males. Sigmoidoscopy may be indicated to exclude ulcerative colitis, Crohn's colitis, rectal lacerations, or other infections such as shigellosis, amebiasis, or syphilis, all of which are common in male homosexuals.

Gonococcal epididymitis is usually unilateral. Both *Chlamydia trachomatis* and the gonococcus are significant causes of epididymitis in men under 35 years, whereas coliform bacteria are the usual cause in older males. The differential diagnosis includes trauma, tumor, and torsion of the testicle, the last of which is suggested by sudden onset and elevation of the testicle. If there is question of testicular torsion, consultation with a urologist is necessary. In epididymitis there is often a urethral exudate, which should be cultured for gonococci and other bacteria. Treatment of gonococcal epididymitis includes scrotal elevation and 7 to 10 days of appropriate antibiotics, as indicated in Table 336–1.

Gonorrhea in Females. In prevalence studies, approximately one half of women infected with the gonococcus are asymptomatic or have so few symptoms that they do not seek medical care. The most commonly involved site is the endocervix (80 to 90 per cent), followed by the urethra (80 per cent), rectum (40 per cent), and pharynx (10 to 20 per cent). Most pharyngeal, urethral, and rectal infections cause few or no symptoms. Cervical infection may result in vaginal discharge or abnormal menstrual bleeding. Neither of these symptoms is specific for gonococcal infection. Gonococcal urethritis may mimic cystitis caused by enteric bacilli, although standard urine cultures are negative because gonococci do not grow on culture media ordinarily used to diagnose urinary tract infection. Culture methods are discussed below under Laboratory Diagnosis. The differential diagnosis of cervicitis, vaginitis, and the urethral syndrome is discussed in Ch. 335.

The most important complication of gonorrhea is salpingitis. The less precise term "pelvic inflammatory disease" (PID) is often used synonymously. Although many other organisms can cause a similar syndrome, the gonococcus accounts for about half of the estimated 500,000 annual cases of PID in the United States. About 15 per cent of women with gonococcal cervicitis develop PID, often in close proximity to a menstrual period. Symptoms usually include abdominal pain, and often there is fever. Physical examination usually discloses cervical motion tenderness and bilateral adnexal tenderness; in a small proportion of cases the disease may be unilateral, causing confusion with appendicitis or ectopic pregnancy. There may be signs of generalized peritonitis. Laboratory studies often show an elevation of the white blood cell count and sedimentation rate. The diagnosis of PID is inexact, as shown by laparoscopic examination; many patients with PID are missed if undue reliance is placed on presence of fever or elevation of white blood cell count or sedimentation rate.

Although PID is uncommon in pregnancy, it may be particularly severe, and pregnant patients with PID should probably be hospitalized. The incidence of gonococcal PID is increased about threefold in women using an intrauterine device (IUD) for contraception.

A single attack of gonococcal PID seems to increase twofold the risk of developing another bout of PID with subsequent gonococcal cervicitis. About half of the male sexual partners of women with gonococcal PID are infected, and half of these infections are asymptomatic. Failure to diagnose and treat properly the male partners exposes the patient to the risk of further attacks of PID. After the patient has been effectively treated, it often is wise to refer her and her sexual partners to a public health clinic for follow-up.

The major complication of gonococcal PID is tubal scarring and infertility. The incidence of involuntary infertility is estimated as 15 per cent after one attack of PID and about 50 per cent after three attacks. The incidence of ectopic pregnancy is increased from seven- to tenfold in women with previous salpingitis, with resultant increased fetal and maternal mortality. Treatment is indicated in Table 336–1.

Gonococci may spread upward to the liver, causing perihepatitis (Fitz-Hugh-Curtis syndrome). Gonococcal perihepatitis causes tenderness and pain in the region of the liver, mimicking acute cholecystitis. However, it resolves promptly with appropriate antibiotic therapy. Peritoneoscopy may be indicated rarely for diagnostic purposes; "violin-string" adhesions between the liver capsule and the peritoneum are seen.

Gonorrhea in Children. Infants born to a mother with cervicovaginal gonorrhea may develop a gonococcal conjunctivitis, although routine use of prophylactic 1 per cent silver nitrate eye drops (or, in some hospitals, topical erythromycin or tetracycline) has markedly reduced the incidence of this problem. Neonates may also acquire pharyngeal, respiratory, or rectal infection and may develop gonococcal sepsis. Older children up to 1 year of age usually acquire conjunctival or vaginal infection by accidental contamination from an adult, whereas from 1 year to puberty most childhood gonorrhea is the result of purposeful sexual abuse by an adult.

Gonococcal Bacteremia. Approximately 1 per cent of adults with gonorrhea develop the syndrome of gonococcal bacteremia, dermatitis, and arthritis, or disseminated gonococcal infection (DGI). In most series, the majority of patients with DGI are women. The regional incidence of DGI probably varies because of geographic differences in prevalence of the usually antibiotic-sensitive, serum-bactericidal-resistant strains of *N. gonorrhoeae* that cause this syndrome. The severity of the syndrome is variable, from a slowly evolving mild illness with little or no fever, mild arthralgias, and few skin lesions to a fulminant illness with high fever and prostration. Most episodes of DGI are relatively mild in comparison with meningococcemia.

Many patients with DGI have no local symptoms of gonococcal infection. Initial manifestations are usually migratory asymmetric polyarthralgias and skin lesions that are often accompanied by fever. Many patients have tenosynovitis, typically involving the flexor tendon sheaths of the wrist or the Achilles tendon (colloquially known as "lover's heels"). Skin lesions are few in number (fewer than 30 usually), are acral in distribution (fingers, toes, extremities), and may be painful before they are visible. The individual lesions may be papules, pustules, or bullae on an erythematous base; less commonly seen are petechiae or necrotic lesions. The rash is not pathognomonic but is sufficiently typical that it should strongly suggest DGI when seen in young patients with polyarthralgia. Blood cultures are often positive at this stage, and circulating immune complexes may be present. Gram's stain of the skin lesions is positive in only about 5 per cent of patients, but gonococcal antigens can be detected in these lesions in about two thirds of patients by use of immunofluorescent-labeled antigonococcal antibody.

The early stage of gonococcemia may subside spontaneously or may merge indistinctly after about 1 week into a second stage of septic arthritis. Skin lesions have usually disappeared by this time, and blood cultures are nearly always negative. Septic

TABLE 336–1. ANTIBIOTIC REGIMENS RECOMMENDED FOR GONOCOCCAL INFECTION

Diagnosis	Treatment
Uncomplicated genital, rectal, or pharyngeal infection of men and women	Ceftriaxone, 250 mg IM once, plus doxycycline, 100 mg orally twice daily for 7 days *or* Spectinomycin, 2.0 grams IM once, plus doxycycline, 100 mg orally twice daily for 7 days
Treatment failure (patients should be recultured and isolates tested for production of β-lactamase)	Spectinomycin, 2.0 grams IM *or* Ceftriaxone, 250 mg IM
Gonorrhea in pregnancy	Ceftriaxone, 250 mg IM once, plus erythromycin base, 500 mg orally four times daily for 7 days *or* Spectinomycin, 2.0 grams IM plus erythromycin (as in ceftriaxone regimen)
Salpingitis—outpatient	Cefoxitin, 2.0 grams IM, plus doxycycline, 100 mg orally twice daily for 10–14 days (see text)
Salpingitis—inpatient	Doxycycline, 100 mg IV twice daily, plus cefoxitin, 2.0 grams IV four times daily until improved, followed by doxycycline, 100 mg PO twice daily to complete 14 days of therapy; alternative regimens include clindamycin plus an aminoglycoside (see text)
Disseminated gonococcal infection	Ceftriaxone, 1 gram IM every 24 hours *or* Spectinomycin, 2 grams IM every 12 hours (see text)

arthritis may occur without preceding skin lesions or polyarthralgia. One large joint (elbow, wrist, hip, knee, ankle) is usually involved, although some series report involvement of two joints in a significant minority of patients. On infrequent occasions symmetric involvement of the fingers may mimic acute rheumatoid arthritis. Physical examination typically discloses a swollen, warm joint with evident intra-articular fluid. Aspiration of the joint often reveals a marked neutrophilic leukocytosis (50,000 to 100,000 leukocytes per cubic millimeter), although early in the development of the septic joint the synovial leukocyte count may be much lower. Cultures of joint fluid are often positive if the leukocyte count is 80,000 or greater but are often negative when leukocyte counts are 20,000 or less.

Other complications of gonococcal bacteremia include mild hepatitis, myocarditis, the Fitz-Hugh-Curtis syndrome, meningitis, and endocarditis. In the preantibiotic era gonococcal infection accounted for up to 10 per cent of all endocarditis, but it is now rare. Gonococcal endocarditis is often a rapidly progressive infection with severe valvular damage; it should be suspected in patients with a new murmur, severe prostrating illness, severe myocarditis, or evidence of renal failure, or in the presence of stigmata of peripheral embolization.

The differential diagnosis of the gonococcal bacteremia arthritis syndrome includes Reiter's syndrome, rheumatic fever, rheumatoid arthritis, systemic lupus erythematosus, other infectious or postinfectious arthritis, subacute bacterial endocarditis, meningococcemia, and viral hepatitis. In young males, Reiter's syndrome is the principal consideration. Conjunctivitis is rarely seen in gonococcemia but is common in Reiter's syndrome. In the absence of typical skin lesions, DGI may not be suspected until culture results are known.

Diagnosis of DGI is secure when gonococci are recovered from the blood, skin lesions, or synovial fluid. The diagnosis of DGI is probably correct in patients in whom the only positive cultures are from local mucosal surfaces but in whom there are both typical skin lesions and a prompt response to antigonococcal therapy.

LABORATORY DIAGNOSIS. Gram's stain of urethral exudate in symptomatic males has a sensitivity of 90 to 98 per cent and a specificity of 95 to 98 per cent. Accordingly, urethral cultures are not ordinarily indicated in untreated symptomatic males. Since the sensitivity of the Gram stain is only about 60 per cent in asymptomatic male urethral infection, cultures of the anterior urethra or fresh urine sediment are recommended when epidemiologic evidence suggests possible asymptomatic urethral infection. Gram's stain of the endocervix is about 50 to 60 per cent sensitive and about 82 to 97 per cent specific in women with positive cervical cultures for N. gonorrhoeae. Care must be taken to avoid mistaking normal endocervical flora and neutrophils for gonorrhea; only smears showing several neutrophils with multiple, typical intracellular gram-negative diplococci should be read as presumptively positive for gonorrhea. All women should be cultured for N. gonorrhoeae, even if the Gram's stain appears positive.

Cultures should be plated immediately if possible onto chocolate agar or chocolate agar containing selective antibiotics (e.g., modified Thayer-Martin medium, MTM). Holding media such as Amies' or Stuart's transport media may be used if necessary, but viability of gonococci drops after 12 to 24 hours in such media. In infected women, a single endocervical culture on MTM is about 80 to 90 per cent sensitive, as judged by yields obtained with multiple cultures from multiple sites. About 3 to 5 per cent of women have their only positive culture at the pharyngeal, urethral, or rectal site. The yield from these sites is too low to warrant routine pharyngeal, urethral, or rectal cultures. Urethral cultures are indicated in women with the urethral syndrome. Both cervical and rectal cultures should be obtained as part of the test of cure in women after treatment, since inclusion of the rectal culture increases the diagnostic yield of treatment failures by as much as 50 per cent. Pharyngeal cultures should be obtained from patients with symptomatic pharyngitis or from persons exposed by fellatio to infected males. Patients with possible disseminated gonococcal infection should have culture samples taken from all possible mucosal sites (pharynx, urethra, cervix, rectum), as well as blood and synovial fluid.

Cultures of the cervix should be taken under direct visualization during speculum examination, using a cotton-tipped swab. Lubricant jellies may be deleterious to gonococci and should be avoided. Cultures of tampons can be used if speculum examination is not possible. Cultures of the anterior urethra of males should be taken with calcium alginate swabs or a sterile wire loop.

Positive cultures from the pharynx or rectum should be carefully evaluated by the microbiology laboratory to avoid confusion between gonococci and meningococci. Meningococci are more common than gonococci in throat cultures. Male homosexuals apparently transmit meningococci sexually, and positive rectal cultures for meningococci are relatively common in this group.

A variety of inexpensive office kits are available for culturing gonococci. These offer the advantages of media with long shelf life. They are approximately equal to standard cultures when their use is limited to urethral or cervical samples; the currently available systems should not be used for pharyngeal or rectal cultures.

A variety of serologic tests for gonorrhea have been developed in the past, and more are being tested currently. No test available in 1991 is sufficiently sensitive and specific to merit use for screening purposes. Patients with complications of gonorrhea usually have detectable serum antibodies against crude or purified gonococcal antigens, but none of the tests is routinely available at present.

TREATMENT. Gonococci frequently have chromosomal mutations that result in relative resistance to penicillin, tetracycline, and other antibiotics. The resistance in these strains is relatively low and usually can be overcome by appropriate doses of penicillin. Recently, strains with slightly higher levels of chromosomally mediated resistance (CMRNG strains) have become prevalent in certain areas of the United States and are more common in parts of Asia. These strains do not respond to penicillin but do respond to spectinomycin or ceftriaxone. As many as 5 to 10 per cent of all gonococci in the United States now are CMRNG.

Gonococci that carry a β-lactamase (penicillinase) plasmid recently emerged in the Far East and elsewhere in 1975 and have spread to much of the world. Penicillinase-producing gonococci (PPNG) account for about 30 per cent of all gonorrhea in certain cities in the Africa and the Far East but are less common in the United States. The prevalence of PPNG is about 1 to 5 per cent in the United States and seems to be rising. There are two closely related gonococcal penicillinase plasmids of either 3.2 or 4.4 × 10^6 daltons; each encodes a typical enteric-type TEM β-lactamase. The gonococcal plasmids are similar to penicillinase plasmids found in Haemophilus species. PPNG are resistant to clinically attainable doses of penicillins but are sensitive to spectinomycin and to certain cephalosporins (cefuroxime, cefoxitin, ceftriaxone). PPNG are known to cause DGI and salpingitis.

Quite recently, a new problem has arisen: plasmid-encoded tetracycline resistance, Tc^r. These strains do not respond to tetracycline but do respond to spectinomycin or ceftriaxone and may respond to penicillin. Prevalance of Tc^r gonococci is increasing and approximates 5 to 15 per cent in various cities in the United States.

The antibiotic regimens recommended for gonorrhea in the United States are summarized in Table 336–1. Ceftriaxone now has replaced penicillin and ampicillin, because of the prevalence of CMRNG and Pc^r strains. Tetracyclines no longer are acceptable therapy for gonorrhea because of the prevalence of Tc^r strains. Because gonococcal infections commonly are associated with genital chlamydial infection, most authorities now recommend a 7-day course of a tetracycline (usually doxycycline) for all patients with gonorrhea as follow-up to initial ceftriaxone therapy.

Each of the recommended regimens is highly effective for genital gonorrhea. If patients fail to respond to therapy, they should be cultured so that their isolates can be tested for production of penicillinase, and spectinomycin should be used for retreatment. However, most apparent failures are really reinfections. Some studies show that 15 per cent of patients are reinfected within 6 weeks of successful therapy. On this basis, many authorities recommend that patients should be recultured 6 weeks after treatment.

In the absence of an effective vaccine, control of this disease depends on proper diagnosis and treatment of patients' sexual contacts. If patients are given simple instructions, many bring their contacts to the physician for examination. There are sound epidemiologic reasons for treating contacts immediately. Local health departments are not utilized sufficiently for help in examination and treatment of contacts.

Treatment of salpingitis (PID) has not been studied adequately (see Table 336–1). Most authorities recommend removal of intrauterine devices in women with PID. It is crucial to examine and treat all sexual partners of women with gonococcal PID.

Therapy of gonococcal arthritis is ordinarily highly successful with each of the recommended regimens (Table 336–1). Failure to improve in 3 days suggests that the patient does not have DGI. Septic joints should be aspirated, both to make the initial diagnosis and to remove inflammatory exudate. Open drainage is rarely indicated, except in infection of the hip in childhood. Repeat closed aspiration may be necessary if joint fluid rapidly reaccumulates, but most patients require only one or a few joint aspirations. Antibiotics should not be injected into the joint space. Most patients with DGI should be hospitalized initially, but outpatient therapy may be used occasionally in carefully selected, compliant patients with a definite diagnosis and only mild infection. Antibiotics indicated in this situation include cefuroxime, 500 mg orally twice daily, or ciprofloxacin, 500 mg orally twice daily. Therapy should be continued for 7 days.

Gonococcal conjunctivitis should be treated by immediate saline irrigation and intravenous ceftriaxone.

PREVENTION. Although vaccines are currently under intense study, an effective gonococcal vaccine is still only a hope. Condoms prevent most infection, but those who need them most often do not use them. Certain contraceptive foams have antigonococcal activity but are of unproven efficacy clinically.

Barlow D, Phillips I: Gonorrhoea in women: Diagnostic, clinical, and laboratory aspects. Lancet 1:761, 1978. *A concise description of the clinical and laboratory findings in a large group of women.*

Collier AC, Judson FN, Murphy VL, et al.: Comparative study of ceftriaxone and spectinomycin in the treatment of uncomplicated gonorrhea in women. Am J Med 77:68, 1984. *Ceftriaxone was effective in a single dose of 125 mg intramuscularly without probenecid for oropharyngeal and genital infections. Spectinomycin resulted in a 50 per cent failure rate in oropharyngeal infection, in agreement with earlier reports.*

Dans PE, Judson F: The establishment of a venereal disease clinic. II. An appraisal of current diagnostic methods in uncomplicated urogenital and rectal gonorrhea. J Am Vener Dis Assoc 1:107, 1975. *A critical examination of the utility of various diagnostic methods, including multiple cultures and Gram's stains.*

Eisenstein BI, Sox T, Biswas G, et al.: Conjugal transfer of the gonococcal penicillinase plasmid. Science 195:998, 1977. *Gonococci contain a conjugal plasmid that enables them to transfer sexually their penicillinase plasmid with efficiency.*

Faruki H, Kohmescher RN, McKinney WP, et al.: A community-based outbreak of infection with penicillin-resistant *Neisseria gonorrhoeae* not producing penicillinase (chromosomally mediated resistance). N Engl J Med 313:607, 1985. *Drug resistance among gonococci is an increasing problem everywhere.*

Handsfield HH, Lipman TO, Harnisch JP, et al.: Asymptomatic gonorrhea in men: Diagnosis, natural course, prevalence and significance. N Engl J Med 290:117, 1974. *Asymptomatic infection of the male urethra by gonococci is carefully described and is shown to be much more common than previously recognized.*

Handsfield HH, Murphy VL: Comparative study of ceftriaxone and spectinomycin for treatment of uncomplicated gonorrhoea in men. Lancet 2:67, 1983. *Among newer antibiotics, ceftriaxone appears most promising for single-dose therapy of penicillin-resistant gonorrhea.*

Handsfield HH, Wiesner PJ, Holmes KK: Treatment of the gonococcal arthritis-dermatitis syndrome. Ann Intern Med 84:661, 1976. *This is probably the best evaluation of the efficacy of various regimens for therapy of disseminated gonococcal infection.*

Hook EW, Holmes KK: Gonococcal infections. Ann Intern Med 102:229, 1985. *An excellent, clinically relevant review.*

Lebedeff DA, Hochman EB: Rectal gonorrhea in men: Diagnosis and treatment. Ann Intern Med 92:463, 1980. *This paper briefly reviews the clinical findings, diagnostic methods, and efficacy of various methods of treatment for gonococcal proctitis in men.*

Luciano AA, Grubin L: Gonorrhea screening: Comparison of three techniques. JAMA 243:680, 1980. *Culture of the first-voided urine in asymptomatic males is shown to be a highly reliable method for diagnosis.*

337 Lymphogranuloma Venereum

Lymphogranuloma venereum (LGV) is an acute to chronic sexually transmitted disease caused by strains of *Chlamydia trachomatis*. LGV typically produces transient genital lesions followed by significant regional lymphadenopathy, which may progress to late fibrosis and tissue destruction in untreated cases.

ETIOLOGY. The organisms causing LGV are closely related to the *C. trachomatis* strains that cause trachoma (serotypes A–C) or nongonococcal urethritis (serotypes D–K). By use of a microimmunofluorescent procedure the LGV strains have been grouped into three serotypes (L1, L2, and L3), of which L2 is apparently the most common. On one occasion the related organism *Chlamydia psittaci* caused a similar syndrome. All chlamydiae contain a common group antigen, but an LGV-specific protein antigen has been partially characterized. As is the case with all chlamydiae, the LGV strains can be isolated only in tissue culture or in yolk sac culture.

EPIDEMIOLOGY. LGV is more common in tropical and subtropical climates but does occur in relatively low incidence throughout the Western world. The true incidence is unknown. Screening of patients in venereal disease clinics with the LGV complement fixation test has sometimes shown 10 per cent with positive serologies; however, this may merely reflect cross-reactions between antibodies directed against the *Chlamydia trachomatis* serotypes D–K (the causes of nongonococcal urethritis and related syndromes) and the LGV serotypes L1, L2, and L3.

The disease is almost always transmitted by sexual contact. The site of primary infection is usually around the genitals but may be anal or oral, depending on the mode of sexual practice.

PATHOGENESIS AND PATHOLOGY. The incubation period is uncertain but has been estimated to be anywhere from a few days to several weeks. In approximately one fourth of patients a small, evanescent primary lesion develops at the site of inoculation, but in the other three fourths of patients no primary lesion is clinically evident. Occasional patients may have symptoms of nonspecific urethritis, presumably owing to intraurethral infection. Approximately 2 to 6 weeks after sexual contact most patients develop significant regional lymphadenopathy. Primary infection of the anterior vulva or penis results in inguinal adenopathy, whereas primary infection of the vagina or posterior vulva or rectum results in primary perirectal or pelvic adenopathy. Most patients seen in venereal disease clinics are males with inguinal adenopathy. In about one third of patients the adenopathy is bilateral. Involvement of lymphatic tissue may result in significant lymphedema and, if untreated, may lead to elephantiasis of the external genitalia. Chronic infection of the perirectal tissues may lead to rectal strictures. The histologic appearance of involved tissues is nonspecific with acute and chronic inflammation.

CLINICAL MANIFESTATIONS. The transient primary lesion usually appears as an infiltrated papule or small erosion. It may mimic herpes but is frequently unnoticed or not present. In its earlier stages the adenopathy syndrome is manifested by discrete, tender, movable nodes. After several days the nodes become matted, with an ovoid, firm, lobulated swelling with adherent, erythematous overlying skin. In about 10 to 20 per cent of patients, nodes are involved above and below the inguinal ligament, and fibrosis may result in the so-called "groove sign" (linear depressions parallel to the inguinal ligament). The nodes may undergo necrosis, and, if not aspirated, spontaneous fistula tracts may develop. Lymphatic obstruction may result in vulvar edema or polypoid masses around the anal orifice. In early stages anal masses may resemble hemorrhoids. There may be fever, chills, and headache, associated with other nonspecific systemic symptoms such as nausea and weight loss. Infrequently, there is generalized rash, polyarthralgia, splenomegaly, generalized lymphadenopathy, or meningismus. Cutaneous manifestations may include erythema nodosum, erythema multiforme, urticaria, or a scarlatiniform eruption.

Late complications are usually limited to strictures or scarring of the rectum. This complication is more common in women but is now fortunately rare. There is often no preceding adenopathy syndrome. The strictures may be bandlike or may involve extensive areas of the lower large bowel.

DIAGNOSIS. LGV must be considered in patients with enlarged inguinal lymph nodes, draining inguinal fistulas, and rectal strictures. Differential diagnosis includes reactive nodes secondary to distal sites of pyogenic infection on the extremities (which may be small and not noticed unless careful examination is performed), chancroid, granuloma inguinale, syphilis, and a variety of other diseases associated with adenopathy or adenitis. Diagnosis is made by one of two methods: either by direct demonstration of LGV organisms in lesion material or by appropriate serologic tests. Material may be obtained for culture from affected lymph nodes by inserting a needle into the area of fluctuance, being careful to insert the needle through normal skin. The aspirated pus is characteristically extremely viscous. Organisms may sometimes be directly demonstrated in this material by immunofluorescence, although this test is not routinely available. Culture may be performed in yolk sacs or in tissue cell culture. A complement fixation test, using group-specific antigen, is widely available for serologic diagnosis. In the presence of a compatible clinical syndrome, a titer greater than or equal to 1:16 is strongly suggestive of LGV. Serial samples frequently show a fourfold or greater rise in titer in the acute stage of the disease. Most patients with LGV develop peak titers of at least 1:64. Other serologic tests are under development, including indirect immunofluorescence and counterimmunoelectrophoresis; each of these tests uses antigens specific for LGV, but neither is widely available at present. A direct immunofluorescence test employing monoclonal antibodies against *C. trachomatis* serotypes L1, L2, and L3 offers promise for rapid specific diagnosis, but it is not yet widely available.

Other laboratory tests are of little help. Many patients have a modest elevation in total leukocyte count with predominance of lymphocytes. There may be a reversal of the albumin globulin ratio, and some patients have elevated cryoglobulins or rheumatoid factor.

TREATMENT. Both tetracycline and sulfonamide drugs are effective. Usual therapy for adults is tetracycline, 500 mg four times daily for at least 3 weeks. When tetracycline is contraindicated, as in pregnancy, sulfisoxazole may be given in a dose of 500 mg four times daily for at least 3 weeks. Tense nodes should be aspirated through normal skin to prevent formation of fistulous tracts. Patients with early stages of the disease respond well to therapy, but those with late complications, including chronic lymphatic obstruction and rectal stricture, respond poorly or not at all to antibiotic therapy. Surgery may be needed to correct rectal stricture. After an initial course of treatment, patients should be seen at least every 3 months for 1 year, and the titer of the LGV complement fixation test should be followed. Retreatment should be given if there is a fourfold increase in serologic titer or if there is clinical evidence of relapse. Sexual contacts should be treated similarly.

PREVENTION. There are no specific data regarding modes of prevention. Presumably, use of condoms would help to prevent transmission. An effective vaccine is not available.

Klotz SA, Drutz DJ, Tam MR, et al.: Hemorrhagic proctitis due to lymphogranuloma venereum serogroup L2: Diagnosis by fluorescent monoclonal antibody. N Engl J Med 308:1563, 1983. *LGV may cause hemorrhagic proctitis that mimics ulcerative colitis in homosexual males; monoclonal antibodies provide rapid diagnosis.*

Schachter J: Lymphogranuloma venereum and other nonocular *Chlamydia trachomatis* infections. *In* Hobson D, Holmes KK (eds.): Nongonococcal Urethritis and Related Infections. Washington, D.C., American Society for Microbiology, 1977, pp 91–97. *An excellent short review of the biology of the organism and the clinical manifestations of the disease.*

Sowmini CN, Gopalan KN, Chandrasekhara RG: Minocycline in the treatment of lymphogranuloma venereum. J Am Vener Dis Assoc 2:19, 1976. *Tetracyclines were effective in infected military personnel in Vietnam.*

338 Granuloma Inguinale (Donovanosis)

Granuloma inguinale, also known as donovanosis, is a slowly progressive ulcerative disease involving principally the skin and subcutaneous tissues of the genital, inguinal, and anal regions. It is primarily transmitted sexually, but probably can be transmitted by nonsexual contact as well. Multiple sexual contacts with an infected partner seem necessary for transmission of infection.

The disease is uncommon in the United States, with less than 100 recorded cases annually. It is quite common, however, in certain other areas of the world, especially Papua New Guinea.

ETIOLOGY. The causative organism is *Calymmatobacterium granulomatis*, a gram-negative bacterium which is immunologically related to certain *Klebsiella* strains. Current evidence suggests that *C. granulomatis* is not a member of the *Klebsiella-Enterobacter-Serratia* family; its exact taxonomic status is uncertain. The organism can be grown in yolk sacs, but only with great difficulty on artificial medium. It is apparently a facultative intracellular parasite, since in infected lesions it is found primarily in histiocytes or other mononuclear cells.

CLINICAL MANIFESTATIONS. The initial lesion usually appears as a subcutaneous nodule that erodes through the surface and develops into a beefy, elevated granulomatous lesion. This usually is painless and unassociated with systemic symptoms. Secondary bacterial infection may cause a necrotic painful ulcerative lesion that may be rapidly destructive. A cicatricial form may also occur with a depigmented elevated area of keloid-like scar containing scattered islands of granulomatous tissue. Lesions in the genital area are commonly associated with pseudobuboes in the inguinal region; these swellings are usually not due to involvement of the inguinal lymph nodes but rather to granulomatous involvement of the subcutaneous tissues. Metastatic infection of bones or other viscera is occasionally seen. Clinical experience suggests that secondary carcinomas may be a complication of granuloma inguinale.

DIFFERENTIAL DIAGNOSIS. The differential diagnosis includes tumor, lymphogranuloma venereum, chancroid, syphilis, and other ulcerative granulomatous diseases. Chancroid is usually differentiated by its irregular undermined borders, which are not seen in the usual cases of granuloma inguinale. Darkfield examination and serologic tests should help to distinguish syphilis. Biopsies may be necessary to distinguish granuloma inguinale from certain tumors.

DIAGNOSIS. Diagnosis is made by demonstrating intracellular "Donovan bodies" in histiocytes or other mononuclear cells from lesion scrapings or biopsies. Wright's stain and Giemsa's stain of fresh impression smears or unfixed biopsies usually demonstrate the bacilli relatively easily, although multiple biopsies may be necessary in chronic cases. Culture is not practical at present. A serologic test has been devised but is not clinically available. Histologic examination of biopsies shows mononuclear cells with some infiltration by polymorphonuclear leukocytes but no giant cells.

TREATMENT. Treatment consists of tetracycline or sulfisoxazole in a dose of 0.5 gram four times daily for at least 3 weeks. Other regimens that have proved effective include ampicillin, chloramphenicol, gentamicin, or co-trimoxazole. Limited experience suggests that lincomycin may be used successfully. Patients should be followed for at least several weeks after discontinuation of treatment because of the possibility of relapse. Although the risk of communicability appears to be low, sexual contacts should also be examined; at present, treatment of contacts is not indicated in the absence of clinically evident disease.

PREVENTION. No effective prevention is known.

Breschi LC, Goldman G, Shapiro SR: Granuloma inguinale in Vietnam: Successful therapy with ampicillin and lincomycin. J Am Vener Dis Assoc 1:118, 1975. *Ampicillin was frequently effective in patients previously unresponsive to tetracycline.*

Garg BR, Lal S, Sivamani S: Efficacy of co-trimoxazole in donovanosis. A preliminary report. Br J Vener Dis 54:348, 1978. *Trimethoprim and sulfamethoxazole were effective.*

Kuberski T: Granuloma inguinale (donovanosis). Sex Trans Dis 7:29, 1980. *An excellent short review.*

Maddocks I, Anders EM, Dennis E: Donovanosis in Papua New Guinea. Br J Vener Dis 52:190, 1976. *A description of the epidemiology and clinical manifestations in an endemic area of granuloma inguinale.*

Rosen T, Tschen JA, Ramsdell W, et al.: Granuloma inguinale. J Am Acad Dermatol 11:433, 1984. *An American epidemic of this relatively rare disease is described.*

339 Chancroid

Chancroid is a sexually transmitted infection caused by the gram-negative bacillus *Haemophilus ducreyi*.

EPIDEMIOLOGY. On a worldwide basis chancroid is considerably more common than syphilis, and in parts of Africa and in Southeast Asia is nearly as great a problem as gonorrhea. In the United States it is an uncommon disease, but the incidence is rising. Epidemics have been documented in several cities in North America in recent years. The majority of reported cases occur in males. An outbreak in Greenland was exceptional in that about 40 per cent of cases were noted in women. It is quite likely that there has been significant underdiagnosis in women in the past.

CLINICAL MANIFESTATIONS. The usual incubation period is 2 to 5 days but may be up to 14 days. In the Greenland outbreak the incubation period averaged nearly 2 weeks in women. The initial clinical manifestation is an inflammatory macule that then becomes a vesicle-pustule and finally a sharply circumscribed, somewhat ragged, and undermined painful ulcer. The base is moist and may be covered with a grayish necrotic exudate. Removal of the exudate reveals purulent granulation tissue. There is usually surrounding cutaneous erythema. Lesions typically are single but may be multiple, possibly owing to autoinoculation of nearby tissues. There are rarely systemic symptoms. Inguinal adenopathy is noted in one half of patients, approximately two thirds of whom have unilateral adenopathy. Lesions are usually noted on the shaft or glans of the penis or around the anal orifice in males. In females lesions may occur on the cervix, vagina, vulva, or perianal area. Lesions may occasionally occur primarily on or spread to the abdomen, thigh, breast, fingers, or lips. Intraoral lesions are uncommon.

There are reports of a transient genital ulcer, followed by significant inguinal adenopathy. This may be difficult to distinguish from lymphogranuloma venereum. Other uncommon clinical variants include the *phagedenic type* of ulcer with secondary suprainfection and rapid tissue destruction; *giant chancroid,* which is characterized by a very large single ulcer; *serpiginous ulcer,* which is characterized by rapidly spreading, indolent, shallow ulcers on the groin or the thigh; and a *follicular* type with multiple small ulcers in a perifollicular distribution.

DIFFERENTIAL DIAGNOSIS. The differential diagnosis includes syphilis, herpes genitalis, lymphogranuloma venereum, traumatic ulcers, and granuloma inguinale. Of these the most commonly confused are syphilis and herpes genitalis. Multiple infections are relatively common. Outpatients with suspected chancroid should have a serologic test for syphilis and preferably a darkfield examination as well.

DIAGNOSIS. The diagnosis of chancroid is made on the basis of the clinical appearance of the lesions plus either morphologic demonstration of typical organisms in the lesions or recovery of *H. ducreyi* by culture. Culture is the preferred method. Positive cultures can be obtained in over 80 per cent of cases. Best culture results seem to be obtained with a chocolate agar medium containing 3 µg per milliliter of vancomycin. Necrotic debris should be removed from the ulcer with physiologic saline. The base and edges of the ulcer should be swabbed with a cotton-tipped swab and inoculated directly onto the culture plate if possible; swabs may be put into Amies transport medium if culture plates are not immediately available. Smears obtained from the undermined edges should be gently rolled onto a slide. *H. ducreyi* is a small gram-negative bacillus with rounded ends, which typically forms chains or parallel aggregates in lesions. Typical organisms are seen in 50 to 80 per cent of cases. Organisms may also be obtained by aspiration of inguinal nodes. Nodes should be aspirated by placing the needle through normal skin to avoid formation of fistulous tracts. Nodes should not be incised. There is no serologic test for chancroid.

TREATMENT. The drug of choice is probably erythromycin, in a dose of 500 mg orally four times daily for 7 to 10 days. A single intramuscular dose of ceftriaxone (250 mg) is curative. Combinations of trimethoprim and sulfamethoxazole (co-trimoxazole) usually are effective. Ciprofloxacin, 500 mg orally twice daily for 3 days, is highly effective. Ampicillin should not be used, since some strains of *H. ducreyi* produce a typical TEM-type β-lactamase and are quite ampicillin resistant. Interestingly, the plasmids containing the gene for production of β-lactamase are very closely related to the penicillinase plasmids found recently in *H. influenzae* and *Neisseria gonorrhoeae.* Tetracycline resistance is common. All regular sexual partners should be examined and epidemiologically treated with a similar regimen.

PREVENTION. No vaccine is available. Use of a condom is presumably helpful. There are no data regarding efficacy of antibiotic prophylaxis.

Blackmore CA, Limpakarnjanarat K, Rigau-Perez JG, et al.: An outbreak of chancroid in Orange County, California: Descriptive epidemiology and disease-control measures. J Infect Dis 151:840, 1985. *A very large continental United States outbreak is described. Sulfa and tetracycline resistance was common, but erythromycin and co-trimoxazole were effective.*

Hammond GW, Slutchuk M, Scatliff J, et al.: Epidemiologic, clinical, laboratory, and therapeutic features of an urban outbreak of chancroid in North America. Rev Infect Dis 2:867, 1980. *An excellent summary of a recent epidemic in Winnipeg.*

Lykke-Olesen L, Larsen L, Pedersen TG, et al.: Epidemic of chancroid in Greenland 1977–78. Lancet 1:654, 1979. *A remarkable epidemic, affecting 3 per cent of the adult population. Tropical climates are not necessary for disease transmission or expression.*

Plummer FA, D'Costa LJ, Nsanze H, et al.: Antimicrobial therapy of chancroid: Effectiveness of erythromycin. J Infect Dis 148:726, 1983. *Documents the efficacy of erythromycin.*

Taylor DN, Pitarangsi C, Echeverria P, et al.: Comparative study of ceftriaxone and trimethoprim-sulfamethoxazole for the treatment of chancroid in Thailand. J Infect Dis 152:1002, 1985. *Ceftriaxone appears to be effective for this infection as well, in a single intramuscularly administered dose of 250 mg.*

340 Syphilis

DEFINITION. Syphilis is a subacute to chronic infectious disease caused by the bacterium *Treponema pallidum.* It is usually acquired by sexual contact with another infected individual. Syphilis is remarkable among infectious diseases in its large variety of clinical presentations. It progresses, if untreated, through primary, secondary, and tertiary stages. The early stages (primary and secondary) are infectious. Spontaneous healing of early lesions occurs, followed by a long latent period. In about 30 per cent of untreated patients, late disease of the heart, central nervous system, or other organs ultimately develops. At one time this disease was termed "the great imitator." Although the disease is less common now than previously, it remains a great challenge to the clinician because of its protean manifestations and is of great interest to biologists as well because of the long and tenuous balance between the host and the invading spirochete.

ETIOLOGY. The etiology of syphilis was discovered in 1905 by Schaudinn and Hoffman when they visualized spirochetal organisms in early infectious lesions. The causative agent of syphilis, *Treponema pallidum,* is closely related to other pathogenic spirochetes, including those causing yaws (*Treponema pertenue*) and pinta (*Treponema carateum*).

T. pallidum is a thin, helical cell approximately 0.15 µ wide and 6 to 50 µ long. Ordinarily there are approximately 6 to 14 spirals. The organism is tapered on either end. It is too thin to be seen by ordinary Gram's stain but can be visualized in wet mounts by darkfield microscopy (see below) or by silver stains or fluorescent antibody methods.

The organism bears considerable structural resemblance to gram-negative bacteria. A superficial hyaluronic acid slime layer is formed around the organism and may contribute to virulence. Beneath the slime layer is the outer membrane, or outer envelope, which is structurally similar to the outer membrane of gram-negative bacteria. Between the outer membrane and the peptidoglycan cell wall are six axial fibrils. The axial fibrils are attached three at each end and overlap in the center of the organism. They are structurally and biochemically similar to flagella and may be in part responsible for the motility of the organism.

It is possible to culture *T. pallidum* in vitro, but yields are very low; culture is of limited use in research but of no use in clinical practice. *T. pallidum* can be maintained by serial passage in rabbits without loss of virulence. Only a few strains have been isolated in rabbits and carefully studied, and little evidence is available regarding the genetic diversity of the organism. All studied isolates have been susceptible to penicillin and are similar antigenically. Immunity to the homologous strain develops after prolonged infection in rabbits. The only known natural hosts for *T. pallidum* are humans and certain monkeys and higher apes.

PATHOGENESIS AND HOST RESPONSE. *T. pallidum* may penetrate through normal mucosal membranes and also through minor abrasions of epithelial surfaces. In experimental rabbit syphilis, spirochetes can be found in the lymphatic system within 30 minutes of inoculation and are found in blood shortly thereafter. There have been occasional instances in humans of transfusion syphilis resulting from use of blood from a donor who was in the incubation stage of the disease. Therefore it seems clear that syphilis is a systemic disease from the onset in humans as well. However, the first lesions appear at the site of primary inoculation, presumably because of the large numbers of treponemes implanted at this site. In laboratory animals, there is an inverse relationship between numbers of treponemes inoculated and time required for development of the primary cutaneous lesion. The minimal number of treponemes required to establish infection is not known but may be as low as one treponeme. Multiplication of organisms is very slow, with a division time in rabbits of approximately 33 hours. Similarly slow growth of treponemes in humans probably accounts in part for the protracted nature of the illness and for the relatively long incubation period.

T. pallidum is not known to produce any toxins. Although the outer membrane structurally resembles those of gram-negative bacteria, there is no biologically active endotoxin in *T. pallidum*. Treponemes are capable of specific attachment to host cells, but it is not known whether attachment results in damage to host cells. Most treponemes are found in intercellular spaces, but occasional treponemes can be seen within phagocytic cells. However, there is no evidence for intracellular survival of treponemes.

The primary pathologic lesion of syphilis is a focal endarteritis. There is an increase in adventitial cells, endothelial proliferation, and presence of an inflammatory cuff around affected vessels. Lymphocytes, plasma cells, and monocytes predominate in the inflammatory lesion, and in some cases polymorphonuclear cells are seen as well. The vessel lumen is frequently obliterated. With healing there is considerable fibrosis. Treponemes may be seen in most early lesions of syphilis and in some of the late lesions such as the meningoencephalitis of general paresis.

Granulomatous reaction is also frequent in secondary syphilis and in late syphilis. The granuloma is histologically nonspecific, and cases of syphilis have been incorrectly diagnosed as sarcoidosis or other granulomatous diseases. Human inoculation studies suggest that the pathogenesis of the gumma, which is a granulomatous lesion, involves hypersensitivity to small numbers of virulent treponemes introduced into a previously sensitized host.

Intracutaneous inoculation of patients with syphilis in various stages with partially purified antigens of *T. pallidum* showed that delayed cellular hypersensitivity developed only in late secondary syphilis but was uniformly present in latent syphilis. There may be temporary hyporesponsiveness of lymphocytes from patients with primary and secondary syphilis to treponemal antigens. It is possible but not proved that the unusual waxing and waning of lesions in early syphilis depend on the balance between development of effective cellular immunity and suppression of thymus-derived lymphocyte function.

The host also responds to infection with production of numerous antibodies, and in some instances circulating immune complexes may be formed. The nephrotic syndrome has been recognized occasionally in secondary syphilis, and renal biopsies from such cases have shown membranous glomerulonephritis characterized by focal subepithelial basement membrane deposits. The deposits contain both IgG and C3, and treponemal antibody.

Rarely patients may develop paroxysmal cold hemoglobinuria. This is due to production of an IgG antibody that binds to the red cell at 4°C and, upon rewarming of the blood in the presence of complement, results in hemolysis. Thus patients may develop massive hemolysis and hemoglobinuria after cold exposure. This was formerly usually due to congenital syphilis but is now almost always due to other infections. Treatment with penicillin usually stops the attacks.

Antibodies useful in diagnosis are discussed under Serologic Tests, below.

EPIDEMIOLOGY. Syphilis, with the exception of congenital syphilis, is acquired almost exclusively by intimate contact with the infectious lesions of primary or secondary syphilis (chancre, mucous patches, condylomata lata). This is usually through sexual intercourse, including anogenital and orogenital intercourse. Health workers have sometimes been infected during unsuspecting examination of patients with infectious lesions. Infection by contact with fomites is extremely uncommon.

Syphilis is most common in large cities and in young, sexually active individuals. The highest rate in both men and women occurs at ages 20 to 24, followed by ages 25 to 29 and 15 to 19 years. Among predominantly rural areas in the United States the disease is most prevalent in the southeast.

Syphilis spares no class, race, or group but is more prevalent in the United States among the poorly educated and economically deprived than among more prosperous groups. Increased numbers of different sexual partners and perhaps indiscriminate choice of partner increase the risk of acquiring sexually transmitted disease. Patients with primary and secondary syphilis name on the average nearly three different sexual contacts within the previous 90 days. A cornerstone of syphilis control is epidemiologic investigation of sexual contacts of patients with primary or secondary lesions, and of patients with early latent disease. Recent evidence suggests that syphilis is strongly correlated with drug use and anonymous sex, and epidemiologic investigations are less efficacious in this situation.

In recent years male homosexuals have accounted for an increasing proportion of the total cases of infectious syphilis. The ratio of male:female cases of primary and secondary syphilis in the United States rose from 1.6:1.0 in 1965 to 2.5:1.0 in 1975 and about 3:1 in the mid 1980's. Currently, more than half of all white males with infectious syphilis name at least one male sexual partner during the recent past. In contrast, only 2 per cent of primary and secondary syphilis in females occurs in women who name a female sexual contact. Similar trends have been noted in other countries. Unfortunately, syphilis increased dramatically in 1989–1990 in many parts of the United States, particularly among nonwhite heterosexuals, many of whom probably exchanged sex for drugs. In many cities, incidence of infectious syphilis increased 50 to 100 per cent in 1990, which is worrisome both because syphilis is a serious disease and because it is a cofactor for acquisition of HIV.

The annual incidence of syphilis has generally declined worldwide for approximately 100 years with the exception of periods of extensive war. With the introduction of penicillin there was a rapid decline in primary and secondary syphilis after World War II, to annual rates of approximately 4 cases per 100,000 in 1957. This resulted in declining federal expenditure for syphilis control, however, and there was a subsequent resurgence in infectious primary and secondary syphilis in the United States, reaching peaks of over 12 cases per 100,000 several times in the period 1965–1983. Since many cases of syphilis are not reported, the true incidence is much higher, perhaps 75,000 to 100,000 annually.

Reported deaths from syphilis declined from 2434 in 1965 to 200 in 1976. Infant deaths from syphilis fell by 98 to 99 per cent by 1980, but rose sharply in 1988–1990. Patients with clinically manifest late syphilis, particularly those with gummas, are becoming less common, perhaps as a result of the effectiveness of penicillin therapy for early syphilis. However, surveys indicate that there still are significant numbers of patients with untreated cardiovascular and neurologic syphilis, especially among older age groups. There is suggestive evidence that neurosyphilis may be presenting with atypical clinical manifestations and therefore may not be easily recognized. There is considerable clinical evidence that early syphilis is more severe and more difficult to treat in patients with HIV infection.

NATURAL COURSE OF UNTREATED SYPHILIS. The incubation period from time of exposure to development of the primary lesion at the place of initial inoculation of treponemes averages approximately 21 days but ranges from 10 to 90 days. A painless papule develops and gradually breaks down to form a clean-based ulcer with raised, indurated margins. This persists for 2 to 6 weeks and then heals spontaneously. Several weeks later the patient characteristically develops a secondary stage characterized by low-grade fever, headache, malaise, generalized lymphadenopathy, and a mucocutaneous rash. There may be involvement of visceral organs. The secondary eruption may occur while the primary chancre is still healing or several months after the disappearance of the chancre. The secondary lesions heal spontaneously within 2 to 6 weeks, and the infection then enters latency. Some patients may later develop relapsing lesions similar to those of the secondary stage; rarely the relapse takes the form of recurrence of the primary chancre. About one third of untreated patients eventually develop late destructive tertiary lesions involving one or more of the eyes, central nervous system, heart, or other organs, including skin. These may occur at any time from a few years to as late as 25 years following infection.

The incidence of late complications of untreated syphilis is currently unknown but seems less than noted previously. Cases of gumma are at present so rare as to be reportable.

CLINICAL MANIFESTATIONS. _Primary Syphilis._ The typical lesion of primary syphilis is the chancre, a painless, clean-based, indurated ulcer. The chancre starts as a papule, but then superficial erosion occurs, resulting in the typical ulcer. The borders of the ulcer are raised, firm, and indurated. Occasionally, secondary infections change the appearance, resulting in a painful lesion. Most chancres are single, but multiple ulcers are sometimes seen, particularly when skin folds are opposed ("kissing chancres"). The untreated chancre heals in several weeks, leaving a faint scar. The chancre is usually associated with regional adenopathy, which may be either unilateral or bilateral. The regional nodes are movable, discrete, and rubbery. If the chancre occurs in the cervix or in the rectum, the affected regional iliac nodes are not palpable. See Figure 340–1.

It was formerly taught that 90 per cent of chancres occurred in the genital region. Currently, a much higher proportion of nongenital chancres is observed, particularly among male homosexuals, in whom chancres in or near the rectum are common. Rectal chancres may have an atypical appearance, mimicking rectal fissures or other more benign lesions, and are frequently overlooked. Conversely, they have also been mistaken for malignant disease. In general it is reasonable to assume that any ulcer occurring in the genital area or, in male homosexuals, around the rectum is syphilitic until proved otherwise. Chancres may also be seen in the pharynx, on the tongue, around the lips, on the fingers, on the nipples, or in diverse other areas. The morphology depends in part on the area of the body in which they occur and also on the host immune response. Chancres in previously infected individuals may be small and may remain papular. Chancres of the finger may appear more erosive and may be quite painful.

The _differential diagnosis_ of a genital ulcer should include genital herpes. Herpetic ulcers can usually be distinguished because they are multiple, superficial, and, if seen early, vesicular. They are often painful. Herpetic ulcers, unlike syphilitic ulcers, may yield positive findings on Tzanck's test—multinucleated giant cells in the base of the ulcer. The ulcers of chancroid are usually painful, often multiple, and frequently exudative and nonindurated. Lymphogranuloma venereum may produce a small papular lesion associated with a regional adenopathy. Other conditions that must be distinguished include granuloma inguinale, drug eruptions, carcinoma, superficial fungal infections, traumatic lesions, and lichen planus. Final distinction in most cases is made on the basis of darkfield examination, which is positive only in syphilis.

Secondary Syphilis. Approximately 4 to 8 weeks following the appearance of the primary chancre, patients typically develop lesions of secondary syphilis. They may complain of _malaise, fever, headache, sore throat,_ and other systemic symptoms. Most patients have generalized lymphadenopathy, including the epitrochlear nodes. Approximately 30 per cent of patients have evidence of the healing chancre, although many patients, including male homosexuals and women, give no history of a primary lesion.

At least 80 per cent of patients with secondary syphilis have cutaneous lesions or lesions of the mucocutaneous junctions at some point in their illness. The diagnosis is usually first suspected on the basis of the cutaneous eruption. The rash is often minimally symptomatic, however, and many patients with late syphilis do not recall either primary or secondary lesions. The rashes are quite varied in their appearance but have certain characterisitc features. The lesions are usually widespread and are symmetric in distribution. They often are pink, coppery, or dusky red, particularly the earliest macular lesions. They usually are nonpruritic, although occasional exceptions have been noted, and are almost never vesicular or bullous in adults. They are indurated except for the very earliest macular lesions and frequently have a superficial scale (papulosquamous lesions). They tend to be polymorphic and rounded, and on healing they may leave residual pigmentation or depigmentation. The lesions may be quite faint and difficult to visualize, particularly on dark-skinned individuals.

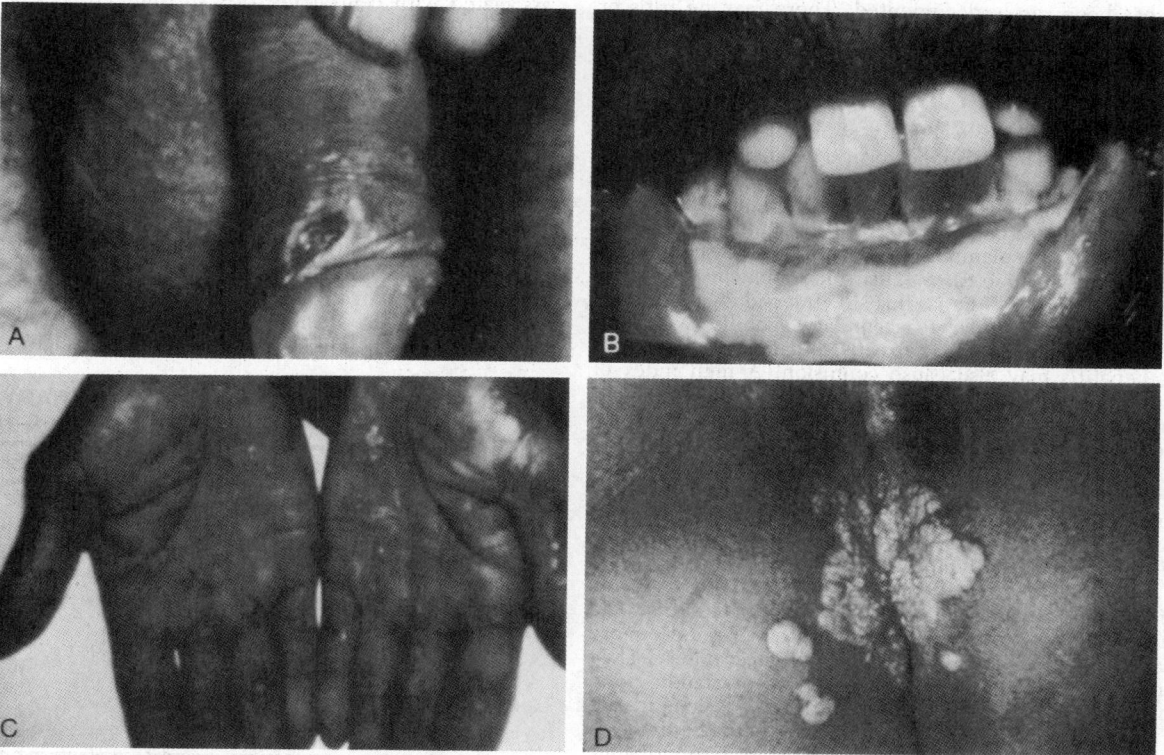

FIGURE 340–1. _A,_ Primary syphilis, chancre. _B,_ Secondary syphilis, mucous patch. _C,_ Secondary syphilis, papulosquamous rash. _D,_ Secondary syphilis, condylomata lata.

The earliest pink macular lesions are frequently seen on the margins of the ribs or the sides of the trunk with later spread to the rest of the body. The face is often spared except around the mouth. Subsequently a papular rash appears, which is usually generalized but is *quite marked on the palms and soles*. These rashes frequently are associated with a superficial scale and may be hyperpigmented. When the rash occurs on the face, it may be pustular, resembling acne vulgaris. On occasion the scale may be so great as to resemble psoriasis. Deep nodular lesions may cause confusion. Ulceration may occur, producing lesions resembling ecthyma. In malnourished or debilitated patients extensive destructive ulcerative lesions with a heaped-up crust may occur, the so-called rupial lesion. Lesions around the hair follicles may result in patchy alopecia of the beard or of the scalp.

Ringed or annular lesions may occur, especially around the face, particularly on black individuals. Lesions at the angle of the mouth or the corner of the nose may have a central linear erosion (the so-called "split papule").

In warm, moist areas such as the perineum, large, pale, flat-topped papules may coalesce to form condylomata lata. These may also be seen in the axilla and rarely in a generalized form. They are extremely infectious. They are not to be confused with the common venereal warts (condylomata acuminata), which are small, often multiple, and more sharply raised than condylomata lata.

Other lesions of the mucous membranes are common. The palate and pharynx may be inflamed. Approximately 30 per cent of patients develop the so-called mucous patch. This is a slightly raised oval area covered by a grayish-white membrane, which when raised reveals a pink base that does not bleed. These may be seen on the genitalia, in the mouth, or on the tongue and, like condylomata lata, are highly infectious.

Other manifestations of secondary syphilis include hepatitis, which has been reported in up to 10 per cent of patients in some series. Jaundice is rare, but an elevated alkaline phosphatase is common. Liver biopsy reveals small areas of focal necrosis and mononuclear infiltrate or periportal vasculitis. Spirochetes can often be visualized with silver stains. Periostitis with widespread lytic lesions of bone has been reported occasionally; use of bone scans appears to be a sensitive test for early syphilitic osteitis. An immune complex type of nephropathy with transient nephrotic syndrome has been rarely documented. There may be iritis or an anterior uveitis. From 10 to 30 per cent of patients have pleocytosis in the cerebrospinal fluid, but symptomatic meningitis is seen in less than 1 per cent of patients. Symptomatic gastritis may be present.

Differential diagnosis of secondary syphilis includes a large number of diseases. The cutaneous eruptions may be mimicked by pityriasis rosea, which can be differentiated by the occurrence of lesions along lines of skin cleavage and frequently by the presence of a herald patch. Drug eruptions, acute febrile exanthems, psoriasis, lichen planus, scabies, and other diseases must also be considered in some cases. The mucous patch may superficially resemble oral candidiasis (thrush). Infectious mononucleosis may appear very similar to secondary syphilis, with sore throat, generalized adenopathy, hepatitis, and a generalized rash. Infectious hepatitis may also cause confusion. A high index of suspicion is required to make the diagnosis of syphilis in some cases. Unfortunately even classic cases with widespread, hyperpigmented, papulosquamous lesions involving the palms and the soles are not infrequently misdiagnosed in the current era. Fortunately, if the serologic tests for syphilis are obtained, they are positive in 99 per cent of patients. The condylomata lata and mucous patches contain large numbers of treponemes on darkfield examination. Aspiration of lymph nodes may occasionally reveal motile *T. pallidum*.

Relapsing Syphilis. Condylomata lata are likely to recur. The skin manifestations tend to be unilateral, the eruptions more dense, marked, with fewer lesions, and sometimes solitary. They are also more infiltrated and of somewhat longer standing and have some characteristics that resemble the skin lesions in late syphilis. This reflects the increasing immunity with the duration of the early disease. Neurorecurrences, as well as ophthalmic and other relapsing manifestations, may occur. If the patient has been inadequately treated, relapses may be delayed.

Latent Syphilis. By definition latent syphilis is that stage in which there are no clinical signs of syphilis and the cerebrospinal fluid is normal. Latency begins with the passing of the first attack of secondary syphilis and may last for a lifetime thereafter. It is usually detected by positive specific treponemal antibody tests for syphilis. The test must be shown to be reactive on more than one occasion to rule out technical errors. Diseases known to cause occasional false-positive treponemal reactions for syphilis, such as systemic lupus erythematosus, must be excluded. In addition, congenital syphilis must be excluded before the diagnosis of latent syphilis can be made. Patients may or may not have a history of earlier primary or secondary syphilis, although such history is obviously helpful in making a firm diagnosis of latent syphilis.

Latency has been divided into two stages: *early* and *late latency*. Evidence suggests that most relapses occur in the first year, and epidemiologic evidence shows that the most infectious spread of syphilis occurs during the first year of infection. *Therefore early latency in the United States is defined as the first year after infection.* Late latent syphilis is ordinarily not infectious except for the case of the pregnant woman, who may transmit infection to her fetus after many years.

Late Syphilis. Late, or tertiary, syphilis is the destructive stage of the disease and can be crippling. Late syphilitic complications are still important medical problems, but newly recognized cases of late syphilis have been declining steadily in the United States since World War II. Although the incidence of late syphilis is unknown, the prevalence of various types of late syphilis has been approximated (Table 340–1).

Late syphilis is usually very slowly progressive, although certain neurologic syndromes may have sudden onset owing to endarteritis and thrombosis in the central nervous system. Late syphilis is noninfectious. Any organ of the body may be involved, but three main types of disease may be distinguished: late benign (gummatous), cardiovascular, and neurosyphilis.

Late Benign Syphilis. Late benign syphilis, or gumma, was the most common complication of late syphilis in the Oslo Study of untreated patients (1891–1951). In the penicillin era gummas are rare. They typically develop from 1 to 10 years after the initial infection and may involve any part of the body. Although they may be very destructive, they respond rapidly to treatment and therefore are relatively benign. Histologically the gumma is a granuloma. The histologic findings are nonspecific and may be associated with central necrosis surrounded by epithelioid and fibroblastic cells and occasionally giant cells. There is sometimes vasculitis. *T. pallidum* is ordinarily not demonstrable by silver stains but can sometimes be recovered by inoculation of rabbits.

Gummas may be solitary or multiple. They are usually asymmetric and are often grouped. They may start as a superficial nodule or as a deeper lesion that breaks down to form punched-out ulcers. They are ordinarily indolent and slowly progressive with curving or polycyclic borders. They are indurated on palpation. There often is central healing with an atrophic scar surrounded by hyperpigmented borders. Cutaneous gummas may resemble other chronic granulomatous ulcerative lesions caused by tuberculosis, sarcoidosis, leprosy, and other deep fungal infections. Precise histologic diagnosis may not be possible. However, the syphilitic gumma is the only such lesion to heal

TABLE 340–1. NEWLY DIAGNOSED TERTIARY SYPHILIS IN 105 PATIENTS IN DENMARK, 1961–1970

Type of Tertiary Syphilis	Number Observed*
Neurosyphilis	72
Asymptomatic	45
Tabes dorsalis	11
General paresis	13
Meningovascular	1
Optic atrophy	2
Cardiovascular syphilis	44
Aortic insufficiency	16
Aortic aneurysm	13
Uncomplicated aortitis†	15
Late benign syphilis (gumma)	4

*Some patients had more than one form of late syphilis.
†Autopsy diagnoses only.

dramatically with penicillin therapy. Another form of gumma is papulosquamous and may mimic psoriasis.

Gummas may also involve deep visceral organs, of which the most common are the respiratory tract, the gastrointestinal tract, and bones. In earlier centuries gummas of the nose and palate commonly resulted in septal perforations and disfiguring facial lesions. Gummas may also involve the larynx or the pulmonary parenchyma. Gumma of the stomach may masquerade as carcinoma of the stomach or lymphoma. Gummas of the liver were once the most common form of visceral syphilis, presenting often with hepatosplenomegaly and anemia, occasionally with fever and jaundice. Skeletal gummas typically produce lesions in the long bones, skull, and clavicle. A characteristic symptom is nocturnal pain. Radiologic abnormalities, when present, include periostitis and either lytic or sclerotic destructive osteitis.

Cardiovascular Syphilis. The primary cardiovascular complications of syphilis are aortic insufficiency and aortic aneurysm, usually of the ascending aorta. Less commonly other large arteries may be involved, and rarely involvement of the coronary ostia results in coronary insufficiency. These complications in all cases are due to obliterative endarteritis of the vasa vasorum with resultant damage to the intima and media of the great vessels. This results in dilatation of the ascending aorta and eventually in stretching of the ring of the aortic valve, producing aortic insufficiency. The valve cusps remain normal. Death may eventually result from congestive heart failure. There has been some success with placing prosthetic heart valves in patients with syphilitic aortic insufficiency. Aneurysms occasionally present as a pulsating mass bulging through the anterior chest wall. Syphilitic aortitis may involve the descending aorta, but this is almost always proximal to the renal arteries, unlike atherosclerotic aneurysms, which typically involve the descending aorta below the renal arteries.

The disease usually begins within 5 to 10 years after initial infection but may not become clinically manifest until 20 to 30 years after infection. Cardiovascular syphilis is thought to be more common in men than in women and possibly in blacks than in whites. Cardiovascular syphilis does not occur after congenital infection—a phenomenon that remains unexplained.

Asymptomatic aortitis is best diagnosed by visualizing linear calcifications in the wall of the ascending aorta by radiography. The signs of syphilitic aortic insufficiency are the same as for aortic insufficiency of other causes. In aortic insufficiency resulting from dilatation of the aortic ring, the decrescendo murmur is often loudest along the *right* sternal margin. Syphilitic aneurysms may be fusiform but are more typically saccular and do not lead to aortic dissection. Approximately 10 to 25 per cent of patients with cardiovascular syphilis have coexistent neurosyphilis, and it is therefore mandatory to do a lumbar puncture in all patients with cardiovascular syphilis.

At present, syphilis is a relatively more common cause of aortic insufficiency among the elderly than among younger patients; this is due to the progressively decreasing incidence of new cases of late cardiovascular syphilis.

Neurosyphilis. Neurosyphilis may be divided into four groups: asymptomatic, meningovascular, tabes dorsalis, and general paresis. These are more fully described in Ch. 472. Division is not absolute, and there may be considerable overlap between syndromes. Current cases of neurosyphilis are more likely than heretofore to be variants of the classic syndromes, possibly as a result of use of antimicrobials for other diseases.

Asymptomatic Neurosyphilis. Asymptomatic neurosyphilis is diagnosed when there is a positive VDRL* in the cerebrospinal fluid (CSF) in the absence of signs and symptoms of neurologic disease. False-positive VDRL test results are very rare in CSF in the absence of a traumatic tap. The CSF usually shows an increased total protein and a lymphocytic pleocytosis. If the CSF is normal 2 or more years after the initial infection, the patient is not likely to develop a positive CSF later. Although up to 30 per cent of patients with untreated secondary syphilis have an abnormal CSF, penicillin therapy apparently prevents progression to late symptomatic neurosyphilis. Because of this, routine lumbar punctures for examination of CSF are not indicated in early syphilis unless the patient is known to have HIV infection.

Unfortunately, it has become common practice to avoid lumbar punctures in later stages of syphilis as well. Instead, patients are treated with doses of penicillin thought to be effective for neurosyphilis, if present. As a result, there are few data on the present frequency and course of asymptomatic neurosyphilis.

Some laboratories perform an FTA-ABS* test on spinal fluid. Interest in tests such as this has been prompted by good evidence that patients with untreated neurosyphilis may have a negative CSF-VDRL. There are published reports of positive FTA-ABS test results in the CSF of patients with otherwise normal spinal fluid, in whom there were clinical signs and symptoms compatible with neurosyphilis. However, the CSF FTA-ABS test has not been standardized, and there is some evidence that positive CSF test results are caused by passive transfer of serum antibody into spinal fluid. At present no diagnosis of asymptomatic (or symptomatic) neurosyphilis should be based solely on the CSF FTA-ABS* test.

Meningovascular Syphilis. An acute to subacute aseptic meningitis may occur at any time after the primary stage but usually within the first year of infection. It frequently involves the base of the brain and may result in unilateral or bilateral cranial nerve palsies. In about 10 per cent of cases, the onset of meningitis coincides with the rash of secondary syphilis. The spinal fluid shows a lymphocytic pleocytosis with increased protein and usually normal glucose concentration. The CSF-VDRL is nearly always positive. Rarely CSF glucose concentration is decreased. This syndrome can mimic tuberculous or fungal meningitis or nonpurulent meningitis of various causes.

In other patients, the meningeal involvement may be less prominent, but there is sufficient endarteritis and perivascular inflammation to result in cerebrovascular thrombosis and infarction. This usually occurs 5 to 10 years after the initial infection and is more common in males. There often is an associated aseptic meningitis as well. Most cerebrovascular accidents are not due to syphilitic arteritis even in patients with a positive serologic test for syphilis. However, syphilis should be considered as the cause in young patients with a history of syphilis and without other causes for cerebrovascular accidents.

Tabes Dorsalis. Tabes dorsalis is a slowly progressive degenerative disease involving the posterior columns and posterior roots of the spinal cord, resulting in progressive loss of peripheral reflexes, impairment of vibration and position sense, and progressive ataxia. There may be chronic destructive changes in the large joints of the affected limbs in far-advanced cases (Charcot's joints). Incontinence of the bladder and impotence are common. Sudden and severe painful crises of uncertain cause are a characteristic part of the syndrome. These may involve the larynx, vagina, rectum, or other organs. Not infrequently severe, sharp abdominal pains lead to exploratory surgery. Lightning pains in the extremities may require opiates for relief. These may be triggered by exposure to cold or other stresses or may arise with no obvious precipitating cause.

Optic atrophy is seen in 20 per cent of cases. The pupils are abnormal in 90 per cent of cases, with bilaterally small pupils that fail to constrict further in response to light but that do constrict normally to accommodation (Argyll Robertson pupils).

The cause of tabes dorsalis is unclear. Spirochetes cannot be demonstrated in the posterior column or dorsal root.

Onset of the disease is usually delayed, often 20 to 30 years after initial onset of infection. It is thought to be more common in whites and in males. Typical cases of patients presenting with lightning pains, ataxia, Argyll Robertson pupils, absent deep tendon reflexes, and loss of posterior column function are easy to diagnose. Atypical cases may be more troublesome, particularly because the VDRL test result in the serum is normal in as many as 30 to 40 per cent of patients, and 10 to 20 per cent of patients (even before the advent of penicillin) have normal CSF-VDRL results as well. The FTA-ABS test in serum is nearly always positive.

Treatment is unsatisfactory. Penicillin does not reverse the symptoms, although it does usually result in clearing of the abnormal spinal fluid. Carbamazepine in doses of 400 to 800 mg per day has been reported to be effective in treatment of the lightning pains.

Tabes dorsalis is now thought to be uncommon, although a

---

*See Serologic Tests, below. Also refer to Table 340–2.

survey of newly diagnosed late syphilis in Denmark in the decade 1961 to 1970 showed that in approximately 10 per cent of all persons with late syphilis and 40 per cent of all with clinical neurosyphilis there was evidence of tabes dorsalis.

General Paresis. This form of neurosyphilis is a chronic meningoencephalitis resulting in gradually progressive loss of cortical function. It typically occurs 10 to 20 years after the initial infection. Pathologically there is a perivascular and meningeal chronic inflammatory reaction with thickening of the meninges, a granular ependymitis, degeneration of the cortical parenchyma, and abundant spirochetes in the tissues.

The most devastating effect of general paresis is on the mind. With effective penicillin therapy this disease has become much less common; in the United States, first admissions to mental hospitals because of syphilitic psychosis declined from 7694 in 1940 to 154 in 1968, the last year for which definite figures are available.

In its early stages general paresis results in nonspecific symptoms such as irritability, fatigability, headaches, forgetfulness, and personality changes. Later there is impaired memory, defective judgment, lack of insight, confusion, and often depression or marked elation. The patients may be delusional, and seizures are sometimes seen. There may also be loss of other cortical functions, including paralysis or aphasia.

Physical signs are primarily those of the altered mental status. Cranial nerve palsies are uncommon. Optic atrophy is rare. The complete Argyll Robertson pupil is also uncommon, but irregular or otherwise abnormal pupils are not infrequent. Peripheral reflexes are often somewhat increased.

The CSF is nearly always abnormal with lymphocytic pleocytosis and increased total protein. The VDRL is usually reactive in both spinal fluid and serum. The disease responds well to penicillin therapy if administered early, although as many as a third of treated patients may develop progressive neurologic decline in later years. Fever therapy induced with malaria was formerly an effective adjunct to treatment with arsenicals but has now been abandoned.

Even though classic general paresis is now infrequent, it remains reasonable to suspect syphilis as the cause of undiagnosed neurologic illness. Since the VDRL may be negative in patients with late neurologic syphilis, the FTA-ABS test on serum must be performed before syphilis can be excluded.

Congenital Syphilis. Congenital syphilis results from transplacental hematogenous spread of syphilis from the mother to the fetus. The incidence of congenital syphilis among newborns or infants under 1 year of age in the United States rose from 180 cases in 1957 to 422 cases in 1972 but declined to about 100 cases annually thereafter. Unfortunately, the recent rise in heterosexually acquired syphilis has been accompanied by a rise in congenital syphilis as well. Each case of congenital syphilis represents a tragedy that could have been prevented by better case reporting and by proper prenatal care. A VDRL should be obtained in all expectant mothers at the beginning and near the end of pregnancy.

Spirochetes can be found in abortuses of as little as 9 to 10 weeks' gestation. The risk of fetal infection is greatest in the early stages of untreated maternal syphilis and declines slowly thereafter, but the mother may infect her fetus during at least the first 5 years of her infection. Adequate treatment of the mother prior to the sixteenth week usually prevents manifest clinical illness in the neonate. Later treatment may not prevent late sequelae of the disease in the child. Untreated maternal infection may result in stillbirth, neonatal death, prematurity, or syndromes of early or late congenital syphilis among surviving infants.

Manifestations of early congenital syphilis are often seen in the perinatal period but may not develop until the infant has been discharged from the hospital. The disease resembles secondary syphilis of the adult except that the rash may be vesicular or bullous, which is extremely rare in adults. There often is rhinitis, hepatosplenomegaly, hemolytic anemia, jaundice, and pseudoparalysis (immobility of one or more extremities) resulting from painful osteochondritis. There may be thrombocytopenia and leukocytosis. The early stages of congenital syphilis must be differentiated from rubella, cytomegalovirus infection, toxoplasmosis, bacterial sepsis, and other diseases.

Late congenital syphilis is defined as congenital syphilis of more than 2 years' duration. The disease may remain latent with no manifest late damage. Cardiovascular alterations have not been observed in congenital syphilis. Neurologic manifestations are common, and there may be eighth cranial nerve deafness and interstitial keratitis. The latter occurs in over 10 per cent of patients but may not be manifest until the tenth year of life or later. Periostitis may result in prominent frontal bones, depression of the bridge of the nose ("saddle nose"), poor development of the maxilla, and anterior bowing of the tibias ("saber shins"). There may be late-onset arthritis of the knees (Clutton's joints). The permanent dentition may show characteristic abnormalities known as Hutchinson's teeth; the upper central incisors are widely spaced, centrally notched, and tapered in the manner of a screwdriver. The molars may show multiple poorly developed cusps (mulberry molars). Some of the late manifestations such as interstitial keratitis and Clutton's joints may be due to hypersensitivity responses and are benefited by corticosteroids in some cases.

DIAGNOSIS. *Darkfield Examination.* The most definitive means of making a diagnosis is finding spirochetes of typical morphology and motility in lesions of early acquired or congenital syphilis. The darkfield examination is almost always positive in primary syphilis and in the moist mucosal lesions of secondary and congenital syphilis. It may occasionally be positive in aspirates of lymph nodes in secondary syphilis. Problems arise, however, because of false-negative results in primary syphilis owing to application by the patient of soaps or other toxic compounds to the lesions. A single negative result is therefore insufficient to exclude syphilis. Patients with suspicious lesions but with an initially negative darkfield examination should be instructed to avoid washing the lesion and to return daily for two successive examinations. Confusion may also arise because of the presence of spirochetes that are morphologically indistinguishable from *T. pallidum* in the mouth, particularly around the gingival margins. For lesions in these areas, therefore, diagnosis often depends upon clinical appearance, history, and serologic testing.

To perform the darkfield examination, the surface of the suspected ulcerative lesion should be cleaned with saline solution and gauze without production of bleeding. The presence of red cells in the specimen makes it difficult to visualize small numbers of *T. pallidum*. Squeezing of the lesion (with gloves on) may help produce serous fluid, which is picked up on a glass slide, covered with a coverslip, and examined with the darkfield microscope. Living *T. pallidum* organisms demonstrate gradual motion to and fro, rotational movement around the long axis, and rather sudden 90-degree bending near the center of the organism. Since most physicians do not have the proper equipment and are not familiar with the techniques of darkfield microscopy, the state public health authorities can be called for assistance.

T. pallidum may also be demonstrated in biopsies or pathologic specimens by fluorescent antibody stains or by silver stains.

Serologic Tests. Two basic types of humoral antibody are stimulated by infection with *T. pallidum*: nonspecific antibody directed against diphosphatidylglycerol (cardiolipin), which is a normal component of many tissues; and specific treponemal antibodies. Nonspecific antibodies against cardiolipin were formerly designated "reagin," a term that should be discarded to avoid confusion with another "reagin," IgE. The kinds of tests used in syphilis are summarized in Table 340–2.

Nonspecific Tests. Anticardiolipin antibodies were first discovered by Wassermann in 1907, using extracts of congenitally syphilitic livers as the antigen for a complement fixation test. Subsequently it was shown that normal livers contained the same antigen as do many other tissues; the antigen for this class of test is now extracted from beef heart. As yet there is no convincing explanation for why patients infected with *T. pallidum* develop increasing titers of antibody against a normal tissue component. The Wassermann test has now been replaced by related tests. The standard test in use today for detection of anticardiolipin antibody is the Venereal Disease Research Laboratories (VDRL) test, which is an easily quantified slide flocculation test. Many similar tests, including the rapid plasma reagin (RPR) test and the unheated serum reagin (USR) test, are frequently used for screening for syphilis.

The VDRL and related tests are simple, well standardized, cheap, and the screening tests of choice. The VDRL is the test

TABLE 340–2. SEROLOGIC TESTS FOR SYPHILIS

Type	Use
Nonspecific (anticardiolipin) antibodies:	
VDRL (slide flocculation)	Screening, quantitation, following response to treatment
RPR (circle-card) (agglutination)	Screening
Specific treponemal antibodies:	
FTA-ABS (immunofluorescence with absorbed serum)	Confirmatory, diagnostic, not for routine screening
MHA-TP (microhemagglutination)	Similar to FTA-ABS but can be quantified and automated

VDRL = Venereal Disease Research Laboratories test.
RPR = Rapid plasma reagin test.
FTA-ABS = Fluorescent treponemal antibody absorption test.
MHA-TP = Microhemagglutination assay for *T. pallidum*.

of choice for following the response of patients to treatment. Since the VDRL detects antibody against a normal tissue component, it may be falsely positive in a significant number of patients. The relative proportion of patients with a false-positive VDRL depends on the prevalence of syphilis in the community; the lower the prevalence of syphilis, the higher the proportion of positive VDRL tests that are due to nonsyphilitic causes.

The VDRL test begins to turn positive 1 to 2 weeks after the onset of the chancre. In large series of patients with primary syphilis, approximately two thirds have had a positive VDRL test result. Obviously, then, a negative VDRL test does not exclude primary syphilis, particularly if the lesion is less than 2 weeks old. The VDRL is positive in 99 per cent of patients with secondary syphilis, the only exceptions being patients with such high titers of antibody that they are in antibody excess; dilution of the serum will then paradoxically result in conversion of a negative test to positive. There is some evidence that AIDS delays or diminishes the serologic response in early (primary and secondary) syphilis. VDRL reactivity tends to diminish in later stages of the disease, and only about 70 per cent of patients with cardiovascular or neurosyphilis have a positive VDRL test result.

The *quantitative titer* of the VDRL test is somewhat useful in diagnosis and quite useful in following therapeutic response. The titer is reported as the highest dilution that gives a positive response. Most patients with secondary syphilis have titers of at least 1:16. Most patients with false-positive VDRL tests have titers of less than 1:8. No single titer is in itself diagnostic. Significant rises (fourfold or greater) in paired sera, however, are strongly indicative of acute syphilis.

Treponemal Tests. There are many varieties of specific treponemal antibody tests. The most widely used is the fluorescent treponemal antibody absorption (FTA-ABS) test. Patient serum is absorbed with extracts of nonpathogenic cultivable treponemes to remove cross-reacting group treponemal antibody. Agglutination of red cells to which *T. pallidum* antigens have been fixed is the basis of the microhemagglutination assay for *T. pallidum* (MHA-TP).

The precise nature of the antigens involved in these tests is not known. Characterization of the antigens of *T. pallidum* has been greatly hindered by inability to grow the organism in cell-free culture. Recent success in cloning *T. pallidum* antigens into *Escherichia coli* may circumvent this problem. Antibodies reactive in the various tests are found in all major immunoglobulin classes (IgG, IgM, IgA). A modification of the FTA-ABS test has been developed using fluorescein-labeled anti–human IgM (IgM FTA-ABS). The IgM FTA-ABS test is of some use in the diagnosis of early congenital syphilis but is of no use in distinguishing acute disease from old infections in adults.

The FTA-ABS test is best used as a confirmatory test. It is somewhat more difficult to perform than the VDRL test and cannot be easily quantified. It is sensitive and has a high degree of specificity, being positive in only approximately 1 per cent of normal individuals. It is positive in 85 per cent of patients with primary syphilis, 99 per cent with secondary syphilis, and at least 95 per cent with late syphilis. It may therefore be the only test positive in patients with cardiovascular or neurologic syphilis. In late syphilis the FTA-ABS test usually remains positive for life despite adequate therapy. It (as well as the MHA-TP) is positive in other treponemal diseases, such as pinta, yaws, and bejel.

The FTA-ABS test is reported in terms of relative brilliance of fluorescence, from borderline to 4+. Borderline reactivity has the same meaning as nonreactive for clinical purposes. Most laboratories report 1+ positive tests as reactive, but some studies have shown that such tests may be difficult to reproduce. Occasional laboratories therefore report only as positive tests with 2+ or greater reactivity. In patients lacking historical or clinical evidence of syphilis but with a reactive FTA-ABS test, one should repeat the FTA-ABS test. Use of another treponemal test such as the MHA-TP may be helpful in problem cases.

The MHA-TP test is less sensitive than either the VDRL or the FTA-ABS test in primary syphilis. Its sensitivity and specificity otherwise are nearly identical to those of the FTA-ABS test, being positive in nearly all patients with secondary syphilis and in 95 per cent or more of patients with late syphilis. The reactivity of serologic tests for syphilis in various stages of disease is shown in Table 340–3.

False-Positive Serologic Test Results for Syphilis. The VDRL or RPR test may be positive in a variety of diseases other than syphilis. A false-positive result is defined as a reproducible positive test in a patient with no clinical or historical evidence of syphilis and whose serum FTA-ABS or MHA-TP test is negative.

"Acute" (less than 6 months) false-positive VDRL test results occur with low frequency in atypical pneumonia, malaria, and other bacterial or viral infections and may occur after smallpox or other vaccinations as well. *Chronic false-positive VDRL tests* (lasting longer than 6 months) are relatively common in autoimmune disorders such as systemic lupus erythematosus (SLE), in narcotic addicts, in leprosy, and in aged persons. From 8 to 20 per cent of patients with SLE have been reported as having a false-positive VDRL test, and the false-positive result may develop many years prior to the onset of other manifestations of the disease. A chronic false-positive VDRL test in females age 20 or younger carries a significant risk of future development of SLE, thyroiditis, or other autoimmune disorders, and such patients should be followed carefully for a considerable period of time. As many as one third of patients with narcotic addiction have a false-positive VDRL test. Over 1 per cent of patients aged 70 and 10 per cent of patients over age 80 have a low-titer false-positive VDRL test. Most false-positive VDRL tests have a titer of 1:8 or less, although occasional patients with lymphoma and other diseases have been described with very high-titer false-positive VDRL tests.

A positive FTA-ABS result is usually indicative of recent or past syphilis. However, there is an increased incidence of false-positive FTA-ABS results in SLE and in other chronic diseases associated with hyperglobulinemia, including rheumatoid arthritis, biliary cirrhosis, and others. False-positive results are of two kinds in SLE: The most common is one with a beaded pattern of fluorescence, which has been shown to be due to anti-DNA antibodies; there also may be homogeneous fluorescence of the treponeme indistinguishable from a true positive result in syphilis. Patients with SLE who have a false-positive FTA-ABS result almost always have a negative VDRL result (and conversely, patients with SLE with a positive VDRL usually have a negative FTA-ABS).

Occasionally one encounters reproducible positive FTA-ABS results in patients with no clinical or historical evidence of syphilis and in whom there is no evidence of diseases associated with false-positive FTA-ABS results. It may be wise to obtain CSF for examination of total protein, cells, and VDRL reactivity in order to rule out neurosyphilis. If in doubt and if the patient is not allergic to penicillin, it is often wisest to treat such patients for possible syphilis.

IgM FTA-ABS Test for Congenital Syphilis. Mothers with a positive VDRL or FTA-ABS deliver infants with a positive VDRL

TABLE 340–3. FREQUENCY OF POSITIVE SEROLOGIC TESTS IN UNTREATED SYPHILIS

Stage	VDRL (%)	FTA-ABS (%)	MHA-TP (%)
Primary	70	85	50–60
Secondary	99	100	100
Latent or late	70	98	98

and FTA-ABS because of passive transfer of the IgG antibodies reactive in these tests. Since many infants with congenital syphilis are clinically normal at birth but develop serious symptomatic disease some weeks later, it is important to determine whether a newborn with a positive VDRL or FTA-ABS test has passively transferred maternal antibody or is actively infected. Since maternal IgM antibodies are not passively transferred to the fetus, an IgM FTA-ABS test has been developed to detect syphilis in the newborn. Unfortunately there is approximately a 35 per cent incidence of false-negative IgM FTA-ABS test results in delayed-onset congenital syphilis. There also is a false-positive rate of approximately 10 per cent. For these reasons the IgM FTA-ABS test is of limited use in the diagnosis of neonatal syphilis.

If the mother has been adequately treated for syphilis during pregnancy and the infant is clinically normal at birth, one may elect to follow the infant carefully by serial examination and VDRL titers. If the positive VDRL in the infant is due to passively transferred maternal antibody, the titer of reactivity falls markedly in the first 2 months of life. A rising titer indicates active disease and the need for treatment. Many physicians are unwilling to risk failure of proper follow-up of VDRL-positive but clinically normal neonates and instead administer effective therapy immediately. The risk of penicillin allergy in neonates is very low.

TREATMENT. *T. pallidum* is highly susceptible to penicillin, being inhibited by less than 0.01 µg of penicillin G. Since treponemes divide slowly, and since penicillin acts only on dividing cells, it is necessary to maintain serum levels of penicillin for many days. Studies in animals and in humans show that more therapy is required as the length of infection increases. Current recommendations for treatment of syphilis are summarized in Table 340–4.

Early (Less Than 1 Year) Infectious Syphilis. Early syphilis may be treated with a single injection of 2.4 million units of *benzathine penicillin G*, which provides low but effective serum levels for over 2 weeks. Extensive studies in the 1940's and 1950's with regimens that provided similar serum levels and duration of therapy showed that approximately 95 per cent of patients were cured by such treatment. Many of the remaining 5 per cent who had clinical or serologic evidence of relapse may actually have been reinfected. It is not necessary to examine the CSF at this stage because penicillin prevents development of later neurosyphilis. Motile treponemes disappear from primary lesions in 24 hours.

A single injection of 2.4 million units of *aqueous procaine penicillin*, which provides relatively high serum levels for a brief period, is ineffective in established early syphilis but is curative if the disease is still in the incubating stage. The ceftriaxone regimen currently useful for gonorrhea probably is curative for incubating syphilis, but data are few, and careful follow-up is indicated if there is reason to suspect exposure to syphilis in a patient treated for gonorrhea with ceftriaxone. The incidence of incubating syphilis in gonorrhea patients is 2 per cent or more in several series.

For patients allergic to penicillin, tetracycline hydrochloride may be given in a total dose of 30 grams over 15 days, or doxycycline 100 mg twice daily for 14 days. Particularly careful follow-up is necessary in patients treated with drugs other than penicillin, because patients may not be fully compliant with these prolonged courses of oral therapy and these regimens have been less fully evaluated clinically. Ceftriaxone, 2 gram IM daily for 10 days, may be effective but has not been well studied. Chloramphenicol is of equivocal efficacy and for this reason, as well as because of the risk of toxicity, should not be used. Spectinomycin has essentially no effect on syphilis. Erythromycin is of questionable efficacy.

Syphilis of More Than 1 Year's Duration. Larger doses of penicillin are needed for *neurosyphilis* (see Ch. 472) than for syphilis of less than 1 year's duration. In general, patients with general paresis respond better to treatment than do patients with tabes dorsalis, although patients with paresis should be expected to show residual effects of the infection. This is particularly true in advanced cases. Meningovascular syphilis usually responds well, except for residual damage to cranial nerves or cortical function resulting from ischemic infarcts. Published studies show that a total of 6.0 to 9.0 million units of penicillin G results in a

TABLE 340–4. PENICILLIN TREATMENT PRACTICE IN SYPHILIS AS RECOMMENDED BY UNITED STATES PUBLIC HEALTH SERVICE

Indications for Syphilis Therapy†	Dosage and Administration*	
	Benzathine Penicillin G	Aqueous Benzyl Penicillin G or Procaine Penicillin G
Primary, secondary, and early latent syphilis (<1 year); epidemiologic treatment	Total of 2.4 million units; single IM dose of two injections of 1.2 million units in one session	Total of 4.8 million units IM in doses of 600,000 units daily for 8 consecutive days
Late latent (>1 year) or when CSF was not examined in "latency"; asymptomatic neurosyphilis (HIV negative), cardiovascular syphilis, late benign (cutaneous, osseous, visceral gumma)	Total of 7.2 million units IM in doses of 2.4 million units at 7-day intervals, over 21 days	Total of 9 million units IM in doses of 600,000 units daily over 15 days
Symptomatic neurosyphilis or asymptomatic neurosyphilis in an HIV-positive patient	2 to 4 million units of aqueous (crystalline) penicillin G intravenously every 4 hours for at least 10 days	2 to 4 million units procaine penicillin IM daily and probenecid, 500 mg orally 4 times daily for 10–14 days
Congenital Infants	CSF normal: Total of 50,000 units per kilogram IM in a single or divided dose at one session	CSF abnormal: Total of 50,000 units per kilogram IM per day for 10 consecutive days‡
Older children	CSF normal: Same as for early congenital syphilis, up to 2.4 million units	CSF abnormal: 200,000–300,000 units/kg/day IV aqueous crystalline penicillin for 10–14 days

*Individual doses can be divided for injection in each buttock to minimize discomfort.

†In *pregnancy*, treatment is dependent on the stage of syphilis.

‡For aqueous penicillin, give in two divided IV doses per day; for procaine penicillin, give as one daily dose IM.

satisfactory clinical response in approximately 90 per cent of patients with neurosyphilis, in the absence of HIV infection.

Currently used benzathine penicillin regimens have received relatively little study in neurosyphilis. Benzathine penicillin G in a total dose of 7.2 million units given as 2.4 million units weekly for 3 successive weeks is effective in most patients. However, there are reports of patients who have failed standard penicillin therapy for neurosyphilis but who responded to intensive intravenous therapy that provided high serum levels of penicillin. Benzathine penicillin does not provide measurable levels of penicillin in the spinal fluid or aqueous humor of the eye. There are anecdotal reports of increased treatment failures in patients with concomitant HIV infection. *Therefore in cases of symptomatic central nervous system syphilis, which is a serious disease, or in asymptomatic neurosyphilis in HIV-positive patients there is considerable rationale to treatment with intravenous penicillin G (20 million units per day for at least 10 days in hospital).* Therapy of neurosyphilis not infrequently results in increased CSF pleocytosis for 7 to 10 days after starting treatment and may transiently convert a normal CSF to abnormal.

Limited evidence suggests that treating *latent syphilis* with 7.2 million units total dose of benzathine penicillin is curative even if the patient has asymptomatic neurosyphilis. However, because of the possible lack of the efficacy of benzathine penicillin in some patients with central nervous system syphilis, it is desirable to examine CSF in all patients with latent syphilis to exclude asymptomatic neurosyphilis. This is particularly important in

HIV-positive patients. Alternatively, one may reasonably elect to perform a lumbar puncture at the conclusion of the follow-up period (2 years); if the CSF is normal, the patient can be reassured that neurosyphilis will not develop.

There is no evidence that therapy with antimicrobial drugs is clinically beneficial to patients with *cardiovascular syphilis*. Nevertheless, treatment of cardiovascular syphilis is recommended in order to prevent further progression of disease and because approximately 15 per cent of patients with cardiovascular syphilis have associated neurosyphilis.

There is no evidence regarding the efficacy of other antimicrobials in the treatment of later syphilis. Therefore if patients are allergic to penicillin, it is mandatory that the CSF be examined before therapy is undertaken. Either tetracycline or doxycycline taken for 4 weeks is probably effective.

Syphilis in Pregnancy. All pregnant women should be examined with a VDRL or RPR test during pregnancy; if they are at high risk for syphilis, a second test should be obtained before delivery. Because of the risk to the fetus, evaluation and treatment of the VDRL-positive patient should be done as rapidly as possible, particularly for patients first seen in the later stages of pregnancy. If a confirmatory FTA-ABS is positive and the patient has not been treated, penicillin should be administered in doses appropriate for early or late syphilis as outlined above. Penicillin-allergic patients should not be treated with tetracycline or erythromycin because of toxicity (tetracycline) or lack of efficacy (erythromycin). Penicillin desensitization may be considered but also carries risks. For patients who are VDRL positive but FTA-ABS negative and who have no clinical signs of syphilis, treatment may be withheld. In such patients a quantitative VDRL test and another FTA-ABS test should be repeated in 4 weeks. If the VDRL titer has risen by fourfold or more, or if clinical signs of syphilis have developed, the patient should be treated. If after repeat examination the diagnosis remains equivocal, the patient should be treated to prevent possible disease in the neonate. After treatment a quantitative VDRL titer should be followed monthly; if it rises fourfold, the patient should be treated a second time.

Congenital Syphilis. Proper treatment of the mother usually prevents active congenital syphilis in the neonate. However, infected infants may be clinically normal at birth, and the infant may be seronegative if the mother's infection was acquired late in pregnancy. The infant should be treated at birth if the mother has received no or inadequate treatment, or has been treated with drugs other than penicillin, or if the infant cannot be carefully followed up for several months after birth. The CSF should be examined before treatment of the infant. If the CSF is normal, treatment may be with a single injection of 50,000 units per kilogram of benzathine penicillin G. If the CSF is abnormal, treatment should be with aqueous penicillin G, 50,000 units per kilogram intramuscularly or intravenously daily, given in two divided doses, for a minimum of 10 days. Alternatively, a single daily intramuscular injection of procaine penicillin G, 50,000 units per kilogram, may be given for 10 days. These recommendations are based upon the failure of benzathine penicillin to provide adequate treponemicidal levels in spinal fluid and on evidence that aqueous or procaine penicillin does provide adequate CSF levels of penicillin. Many experts believe that all syphilis in infected infants should be treated with either procaine or aqueous penicillin to ensure adequate CSF levels. Tetracycline should not be used to treat children of less than 8 years of age. Antimicrobial agents other than penicillin are not recommended for treatment of congenital syphilis.

Follow-up Examinations. All patients with early syphilis or congenital syphilis should return for quantitative VDRL titers and clinical examination 3, 6, and 12 months after treatment. Patients with late latent syphilis should be examined also at 24 months after therapy; if CSF was not examined prior to therapy, a lumbar puncture should be done prior to discharge to rule out inadequately treated asymptomatic neurosyphilis.

The quantitative VDRL titer should return to normal within 12 months after therapy of primary syphilis or 24 months after therapy of secondary syphilis. In a small percentage of patients with early syphilis, the VDRL remains reactive in low titer for long periods of time. Chronic low-titer VDRL reactivity after therapy is much more common in late syphilis and should not be viewed with alarm. The FTA-ABS test usually remains positive

for years, despite adequate therapy. The influence of therapy on serologic tests is shown in Table 340–5. A fourfold or greater rise of VDRL titer after therapy is sufficient evidence for retreatment. Patients with treated early syphilis are fully susceptible to reinfection, and many clinical and serologic relapses after therapy are probably reinfections. As such they represent failures of proper epidemiologic case finding and of preventive therapy of the patient's sexual contacts.

Patients with neurosyphilis should be followed with serologic tests for at least 3 years and with repeat examination of CSF at 6-month intervals. The CSF pleocytosis is the first abnormality to disappear, but cell counts may not be normal for 1 to 2 years. The elevated CSF protein level falls more slowly, followed by the positive CSF-VDRL test, which may take years to become negative. It is not known whether use of high-dose intravenous penicillin therapy accelerates the return of CSF to normal. Rising CSF cell counts, protein, and VDRL titer obtained at follow-up are an indication for retreatment.

Epidemiologic Investigation and Treatment. All patients with syphilis should be reported to public health authorities. In the absence of an effective vaccine, control of syphilis depends on finding and treating persons with infectious lesions of primary and secondary syphilis before they can further transmit the disease and on finding and treating persons with incubating syphilis before they develop infectious lesions. All patients with early syphilis (less than 1 year) should be carefully interviewed by qualified persons to determine the nature of their recent sex contacts. Approximately 16 per cent of the named recent contacts of patients with early syphilis are found to have active untreated syphilis on examination, and a similar proportion of individuals named as suspects or associates also have active syphilis.

Most authorities, particularly in the United States, recommend treatment of sexual contacts of patients with early syphilis even if the contacts are clinically and serologically normal on examination. This is justifiable, because 30 per cent of clinically normal individuals named as contacts of persons with infectious lesions of syphilis within the previous 30 days go on to develop syphilis if untreated. In general, preventive treatment is given to all sexual contacts of the past 90 days, although nearly all cases of syphilis in contacts develop within 60 days of exposure.

Jarisch-Herxheimer Reactions. Up to 60 per cent of patients with early syphilis, and a significant proportion of patients with later stages of syphilis, experience a transient febrile reaction after therapy for syphilis. This usually occurs in the first few hours after therapy, peaks at 6 to 8 hours, and disappears within 12 to 24 hours of therapy. Temperature elevation is usually low grade, and there is often associated myalgia, headache, and malaise. The skin lesions of secondary syphilis are often exacerbated during the Herxheimer reaction, and cutaneous lesions that were not visible may become visible. It is usually of no clinical significance and may be treated with salicylates in most cases. In patients with syphilis of the coronary ostia or of the optic nerve, there is a theoretic risk that local inflammation coincident with the Herxheimer reaction could precipitate serious damage. This is the subject of much discussion in the old literature, but there is little current evidence that "local Herxheimer rections" constitute a significant risk to the patient. Corticosteroids have been used to prevent adverse effects of the Herxheimer reaction, but there is no evidence that they are

TABLE 340–5. EFFECT OF RECOMMENDED TREATMENT SCHEDULES ON SEROLOGIC TESTS FOR SYPHILIS

Stage of Disease When Treated	Time to Follow-up (years)	Frequency of Positive Serologic Tests (%)	
		VDRL†	FTA-ABS
Primary (seropositive)*	2	0–3‡	>80
Secondary	2	0–24	>80
Late latent or tertiary	5–13	56–70	98

*Patients with primary syphilis and a positive VDRL test.
†Positive VDRL tests after treatment are almost always *low titer* unless reinfection or relapse has occurred.
‡The range of results reflects inclusion of data from several series, using different patient selection and treatment regimens.

clinically beneficial (other than reducing fever) or necessary. Institution of treatment with small doses of penicillin does not prevent the Herxheimer reaction.

The pathogenesis of the Herxheimer reaction is unclear. It may be due to liberation of antigens from the spirochetes. There is evidence of activation of the complement cascade, including transient consumption of C3, C4, C6, and C7, and of transient decrease in treponemal antibodies coincident with the Herxheimer reaction. There is also evidence for endotoxemia, obtained by positive limulus amebocyte gelatin tests, at the time of the Herxheimer reaction, although *T. pallidum* does not contain biologically active endotoxin. These seemingly contradictory observations could be explained if the reaction resulted in release of endogenous endotoxin from the gut.

Persistence of Treponemes After Treatment. Studies in humans and in rabbits have shown that spiral forms may be visualized by silver stains in lymph nodes after effective treatment. Living virulent treponemes have occasionally been recovered by rabbit inoculation from lymph nodes, CSF, or ocular fluids after effective treatment has been given. These documented cases of treponemal persistence are very rare, however. At present there is little reason to worry about persistence of virulent treponemes after therapy with penicillin, with the possible exception of central nervous system syphilis, which needs further evaluation. There is no evidence for selection of penicillin-resistant mutants of *T. pallidum* to date.

PROSPECTS FOR PREVENTION. Solid immunity develops in rabbits following prolonged infection with virulent *T. pallidum*. It has not yet been possible to transfer immunity passively in laboratory animals by either immune serum or immune lymphocytes alone, suggesting that both cellular and humoral systems are necessary for immunity. Rabbits have been effectively immunized with multiple injections of treponemes that have been rendered avirulent by irradiation or by exposure to cold. However, a very large number of injections and a large mass of treponemes are necessary to effect immunity in the laboratory animal. For this reason and since *T. pallidum* cannot yet be grown in a virulent state in cell-free medium, there is no immediate prospect for a vaccine. However, significant immunity does develop in humans after prolonged infection. For the present, control depends entirely on clinical awareness on the part of physicians, adequate reporting to public health authorities, and vigorous application of epidemiologic investigation and preventive treatment of sexual contacts.

Drusin LM, Singer C, Valenti AJ, et al.: Infectious syphilis mimicking neoplastic disease. Arch Intern Med 137:156, 1977. *A fascinating and frightening account of diagnostic problems caused by oral, rectal, or lymphatic syphilis, nearly leading to cancer surgery.*

Feher J, Somogyi T, Timmer M, et al.: Early syphilitic hepatitis. Lancet 2:896, 1975. *A description of the frequency and histology of early syphilitic hepatitis.*

Fischer A, Kristensen JK, Husfelt V: Tertiary syphilis in Denmark 1961–1970. A description of 105 cases not previously diagnosed or specifically treated. Acta Dermatovener 56:485, 1975. *One of few studies of the prevalence of newly diagnosed late syphilis in the antibiotic era.*

Gamble CN, Reardan JB: Immunopathogenesis of syphilitic glomerulonephritis: Elution of antitreponemal antibody from glomerular immune-complex deposits. N Engl J Med 292:449, 1975. *Clear evidence for an immune-complex etiology of syphilitic nephrosis.*

Gjestland T: The Oslo study of untreated syphilis: An epidemiologic investigation of the natural course of the syphilitic infection based upon a re-study of the Boeck-Bruusgaard material. Acta Derm Venereol 35:Suppl 34, 1955. *A medical classic, in which the long-term course of untreated syphilis is evaluated.*

Holmes KK, Märdh P-A, Sparling PF, et al.: Sexually Transmitted Diseases, 2nd ed. New York, McGraw-Hill Book Company, 1990. *The definitive text on sexually transmitted diseases.*

Lee TJ, Sparling PF: Syphilis. An algorithm. JAMA 242:1187, 1979. *An algorithm for management of patients who present with a positive VDRL or similar test.*

Lugar A, Schmidt B, Spendlingwimmer I, et al.: Recent observations on the serology of syphilis. Br J Vener Dis 56:12, 1980. *A current evaluation of the merits of serologic tests for syphilis.*

Magnuson HJ, Thomas EW, Olansky S, et al.: Inoculation syphilis in human volunteers. Medicine 35:33, 1956. *A classic paper, in which prison volunteers were inoculated with virulent T. pallidum. Immunity to inoculation syphilis was observed only in individuals who had congenital or late syphilis.*

Raskind MA, Eisdorfer C: Screening for syphilis in an aged psychiatrically impaired population. West J Med 125:361, 1976. *Syphilitic disease of the central nervous system may be more prevalent than hospital surveys suggest.*

Tramont EC: Persistence of *Treponema pallidum* following penicillin G therapy: Report of two cases. JAMA 236:2206. *At least one of the cases of neurosyphilis probably was a true penicillin treatment failure.*

Wilner E, Brody JA: Prognosis of general paresis after treatment. Lancet 2:1370, 1968. *Neurosyphilis frequently shows clinical progression despite what is probably adequate therapy.*

Spirochetal Diseases Other Than Syphilis

341 Nonsyphilitic Treponematoses*

Thomas Butler

DEFINITION. The nonsyphilitic treponematoses are the skin diseases called *yaws, bejel,* and *pinta.* They occur predominantly in tropical regions and are transmitted by skin contact with infected persons. Disfiguring ulcerations of the skin may be produced, and invasion of bone and other tissues has been described. Treatment with benzathine penicillin G is effective, and the World Health Organization has carried out extensive treatment campaigns in endemic areas.

ETIOLOGY. Yaws is caused by *Treponema pertenue;* pinta is caused by *T. carateum;* and bejel is caused by a treponeme that is indistinguishable from other species. Like *T. pallidum,* these treponemes are spirochetal bacteria with helical structures and measure about 0.2 μ in diameter and 10 μ in length. They are visible by darkfield microscopy but cannot be cultivated in vitro.

DISTRIBUTION AND EPIDEMIOLOGY. Yaws is prevalent in rural areas of tropical Africa, the Americas, Southeast Asia, and Oceania. The highest incidence is in children between ages 2 and 5 years. Bejel occurs in Africa, in Eastern Mediterranean countries, on the Arabian peninsula, in Central Asia, and in Australia. It is most prevalent in arid regions. Pinta occurs in rural areas of tropical Central and South America. Pinta affects mostly older children and adolescents. Humans are the only known carriers of the nonsyphilitic treponematoses. The portal of entry is the skin, which must be broken, as by a scratch or insect bite, before the spirochete can enter. Transmission is believed to occur by contacting the skin directly or indirectly by contaminated hands or fomites and is facilitated by conditions of poor personal hygiene and crowding.

CLINICAL FEATURES. *Yaws* produces a skin papule at the site of inoculation after an incubation period of 3 to 4 weeks. The most common sites are the legs and buttocks. The papule enlarges, ulcerates, and develops a serous crust from which treponemes can be recovered. Regional lymphadenitis may accompany the papule, which will heal spontaneously within 6 months. A generalized secondary rash will occur before or after healing of the initial lesion, and these rashes are also papular and often covered with brown crusts. Relapsing crops of lesions can occur. Papillomas may result, and the plantar surfaces of the feet are involved with hyperkeratotic lesions. Periostitis of long bones leads to tender bones, and fever may be present. Relapsing lesions may occur over several years, resulting in chronic ulcerations and destructive gummatous lesions affecting the skin and bones.

Bejel produces patches on the mucous membranes of the oral cavity and pharynx and can cause split papules at the mucocutaneous junction of the oral angles. Anal, genital, and other

---

*The author acknowledges the contribution of Dr. Thorstein Guthe on this subject in the 16th edition of the *Cecil Textbook of Medicine*, pages 1584–1589, and refers the interested reader to this more complete treatment of the subject, which includes photographs of skin lesions.

intertriginous skin areas can be affected by lesions that resemble secondary syphilis. Regional lymphadenitis is common, and generalized rashes are rare. Healing of these early lesions is followed by latency manifested by seropositivity or by late lesions that resemble tertiary syphilis. These include nodular ulcers of skin, deformities of bones, and gummatous lesions that can perforate the palate.

Pinta starts similarly as a cutaneous papule with regional lymphadenitis that is followed by a generalized maculopapular eruption. One to 3 years after healing of the initial lesion, large hyperpigmented macules that are brown or blue develop and subsequently lose their pigment and become white. The time required for lesions to pass through these stages varies, so that the same patient may have coexisting areas of increased pigment and loss of pigment.

DIAGNOSIS. By darkfield microscopy, the causative spirochetes from early skin lesions can be observed directly. Spirochetes have been demonstrated also in lymph node aspirates. Serologic tests for syphilis detect cross-reacting antibodies in these diseases. The VDRL test, the serologic test for syphilis, and the fluorescent treponemal antibody absorption test all give positive results if serum is taken at least 2 weeks after the appearance of initial lesions.

TREATMENT AND PROGNOSIS. Long-acting benzathine penicillin G given as 1.2 million units intramuscularly is the preferred treatment for patients with early lesions. For patients with late manifestations, this therapy should be repeated twice at approximately 7-day intervals. The early lesions heal rapidly, and most seropositive patients convert to seronegative status. Late destructive lesions take longer to show improvement.

PREVENTION. The prevalence of these diseases has been reduced in several areas of the world by mass treatment campaigns using penicillin. The World Health Organization has treated about 53 million cases of yaws and 350,000 cases of pinta in the field with good results. These campaigns, however, are not adequate to eradicate the disease. It has been suggested that reduction in transmission requires improvements in the sanitation and economic standards of people living in endemic areas.

Guthe T: Clinical serological and epidemiological features of framboesia tropica (yaws) and its control in rural communities. Acta Dermatovener 49:343, 1969.

Hackett CJ, Lowenthal LJA: Differential Diagnosis of Yaws. WHO Monograph Series No. 45. Geneva, WHO, 1960.

Kantor I, Wilentz JM, Berger BB: Yaws. Arch Dermatol 103:546, 1971.

Vorst FA: Clinical diagnosis and changing manifestations of treponemal infection. Rev Infect Dis 7(Suppl 2):S327, 1985. *This paper shows that yaws in populations after mass treatment with penicillin assumes attenuated forms characterized by shorter duration of papillomas and lower antibody titers.*

342 Relapsing Fever

Thomas Butler

DEFINITION. Relapsing fever is an acute febrile illness caused by blood spirochetes belonging to *Borrelia* species. The two major kinds of relapsing fever are *louse-borne relapsing fever*, for which the human is the reservoir and the body louse is the vector, and *tick-borne relapsing fever*, for which rodents and other animals are the predominant reservoirs and ticks are the vectors. The clinical course consists of one or more phases of fever and spirochetemia, which last for several days and are separated by afebrile intervals of several days without spirochetemia. The relapsing fevers are effectively treated with antibiotics, but after treatment patients often experience a Jarisch-Herxheimer–like reaction.

ETIOLOGY. Relapsing fevers are caused by spirochetes of *Borrelia* species, which belong to the order of bacteria Spirochaetales. *Borrelia* species differ from the other two genera of pathogenic spirochetes, *Leptospira* and *Treponema*, by structure, biochemical characteristics, and antigenic determinants. *Borrelia* spirochetes are spiral organisms that measure 5 to 40 μ in length and about 0.5 μ in diameter. They are too thin to be seen reliably by light microscopy of wet preparations, but they are visible by darkfield or phase contrast microscopy and display corkscrew-like

motility. They are stainable with aniline dyes, such as Wright's or Giemsa's stains, and can be visualized well in tissue by the application of silver stains. Between the cell wall and the cytoplasmic membrane there are 15 to 20 flagella, which are anchored to the ends of the spirochete and wrap around its body until they meet at the middle region. *Borrelia* spirochetes are microaerophilic and fermentative in their growth characteristics. They require long-chain fatty acids for growth and are cultivable in Kelly's medium.

The species names of the tick-borne *Borrelia* are derived from the species names of *Ornithodorus* tick vectors that carry them. The more common ones in North America are *B. turicatae, B. hermsii,* and *B. parkeri* and in Africa *B. duttonii.* Louse-borne disease is caused solely by *B. recurrentis. Borrelia* spirochetes produce fever when injected into rabbits but do not possess endotoxin.

The relapsing feature of *Borrelia* infection has been attributed to antigenic variation in the infecting population of spirochetes. In experimental infections of rats with *B. hermsii,* three separate serotypes emerged sequentially during relapses, and specific antibody appeared in response to each of the antigenic variants.

DISTRIBUTION AND EPIDEMIOLOGY. The two types of relapsing fever, louse-borne and tick-borne, differ so much in their epidemiology that they must be considered separately. *Epidemic relapsing fever* refers to the louse-borne kind and *endemic* or *sporadic relapsing fever* to the tick-borne variety. For louse-borne relapsing fever, the cycle of infection is from person to person via the louse. Body lice acquire the infection by feeding on a spirochetemic person, and they remain infected for their entire lifespan, which is 10 to 61 days under laboratory conditions. Spirochetes do not reach the salivary glands or ovaries of the lice. Therefore, infection is not transmitted to humans by bites of lice. Infection is believed to be transmitted to humans by the crushing of lice on the skin, which allows liberated spirochetes to penetrate through a bite site or through intact skin.

The persons at greatest risk for acquiring louse-borne relapsing fever are those living under crowded, unhygienic conditions that favor infestation with body lice. Migrant workers and soldiers in war are particularly prone to develop this infection. Males are at much greater risk than females. A strain-specific, short-lived acquired immunity develops following infection. This immunity helps to explain why migrant workers coming into an endemic area are more susceptible to infection than are the permanent inhabitants. In some endemic areas, such as Addis Ababa, Ethiopia, there is an increased incidence during the cool winter season when people wear heavier clothing that becomes louse infested.

The vectors for tick-borne relapsing fever are argasid soft ticks of the genus *Ornithodorus.* The major reservoirs of tick-borne relapsing fever are wild rodents, including squirrels, deer mice, rats, chipmunks, and rabbits. The infection is passed between the reservoir animals by tick bites, and humans are accidental hosts when they come into contact with infected animal ticks.

Ticks acquire the infection by biting and sucking blood from a spirochetemic animal. Transmission of the infection to animals or to humans follows injection of infected saliva through the bite site or intact skin. Ticks are more durable vectors than body lice, being able to survive as long as 15 years between blood meals and to harbor viable spirochetes for years. In addition, female ticks can pass *Borrelia* spirochetes transovarially to their offspring, thus permitting ticks to be infective without having previously bitten an infected host.

Persons at greatest risk of infection are those who come in contact with infected ticks from wild rodents. The largest outbreak of tick-borne relapsing fever occurred in 62 campers and employees in the National Park at the Northern Rim of the Grand Canyon, Arizona, in 1973. They had all slept in log cabins that were inhabited by wild rodents. Another outbreak in Washington State affected 42 boy scouts who also camped in a log cabin.

CLINICAL SYNDROMES AND PATHOGENESIS. Following an incubation period of 4 to 18 days after exposure to ticks or lice, illness begins abruptly with shaking chills, fever, headache, and fatigue. Most patients have these symptoms almost continuously throughout the day, whereas some patients report intermittent symptoms several times a day. Patients complain frequently of myalgias, arthralgia, anorexia, dry cough, and abdominal pains. These symptoms are usually mild on the first day of illness and increase in intensity over a few days, until they result in prostration and a visit to a physician. The nonspecific nature of the symptoms leads the patient or the physician to believe the illness is flulike.

The temperature is elevated in the range of 38.5° to 40°C, and the pulse rate is increased. The blood pressure is lowered to about 105/70 mm Hg. Patients appear lethargic or may be delirious. Common physical signs are conjunctival injection, petechial skin rash that is more apparent on the trunk than on the extremities, and palpable liver and spleen. Jaundice is occasionally present. Generalized muscle weakness is common. Some patients have nuchal rigidity.

The white blood cell count is usually normal, with increased band forms and decreased eosinophils. The platelet counts are often less than 50,000 per cubic millimeter, and there may be prolongation of prothrombin and partial thromboplastin times. Liver function test results are frequently abnormal, with elevations in concentrations of serum alanine aminotransferase and bilirubin that are evenly divided between the conjugated and unconjugated fractions. Renal function studies often show mild abnormalities of the serum urea nitrogen and creatinine values, and patients may have proteinuria and microscopic hematuria.

DIAGNOSIS. The diagnosis of relapsing fever depends on the demonstration of spirochetemia. In most patients, this is readily accomplished by obtaining peripheral blood by either fingerstick or venipuncture methods and preparing a thin film on a microscope slide. *Borrelia* spirochetes are stained blue by aniline dyes. Thus a routine blood smear stained with Wright's or Giemsa's stain is adequate. Blood smears, thin or thick, prepared for examination for malaria parasites, are also satisfactory. Spirochetes lie in the plasma spaces between blood cells or may overlie the blood cells. Febrile patients with relapsing fever typically have large numbers of spirochetes in the blood, approximately 10^6 to 10^8 per milliliter, or several per high-power field. Patients who are afebrile in the interval between relapses have smears negative for *Borrelia* and should be re-examined when the fever reappears. Spirochetemia also may be detected by darkfield or phase contrast microscopy. A drop of fresh blood is diluted with another drop of 0.9 per cent NaCl and overlaid with a coverslip. Spirochetes are readily identified by their characteristic rotational motility.

TREATMENT AND PROGNOSIS. The relapsing fevers are effectively treated with tetracycline and erythromycin. Tetracycline is the treatment of choice except in children less than 7 years old and in pregnant women, in whom tetracycline may stain developing fetal teeth. Recent studies in Ethiopia indicate that a single oral dose of tetracycline, 500 mg, is as effective in clearing spirochetemia and preventing relapse as a longer course of treatment. Erythromycin, 500 mg given orally as a single dose, is equally effective and is a satisfactory alternative to tetracycline. For patients unable to take oral medication, intravenous injections of 250 mg of tetracycline or erythromycin are curative. For children weighing less than 30 kg, the dosage of tetracycline or erythromycin should be reduced to approximately 10 mg per kilogram. Penicillin G has been used to treat relapsing fever, but its use has been associated with slow clearance of spirochetes and relapses following treatment.

In most patients with louse-borne relapsing fever and in some with tick-borne relapsing fever, a distressing Jarisch-Herxheimer–like reaction occurs within 4 hours after antibiotic treatment. During the reaction, the patient is extremely uncomfortable, feeling very cold with severe headache and myalgia. The blood leukocyte and platelet counts sharply decrease, and spirochetes disappear from the plasma. The patient may require intravenous infusions of 0.9 per cent NaCl to maintain adequate blood pressure. Over several hours, the temperature declines and the patient's condition improves. Attempts to ameliorate the severity of the reaction by giving antipyretic or anti-inflammatory drugs have not been entirely successful. The best approach is to anticipate the reaction and to provide intensive nursing care and intravenous fluid support during the first day of treatment.

The prognosis is favorable for complete recovery in 95 per cent or more of treated cases of relapsing fever. Bad prognostic signs are the presence of jaundice, high spirochete counts in the blood,

and hypotension. The prognosis of untreated disease is grave in the case of louse-borne relapsing fever, for which mortality rates of 40 per cent have been reported during recent epidemics. Causes of death include liver failure, cerebral hemorrhage, and cardiac arrhythmia due to myocarditis. Untreated patients experience relapses. In louse-borne relapsing fever, the first attack lasts about 6 days and is followed by an afebrile period of about 9 days. There usually is one relapse, which lasts only about 2 days. In tick-borne relapsing fever, the first attack lasts about 3 days and is followed by an interval of about 7 days, after which an average of three relapses occur, each lasting about 2 days. Relapses are usually milder in intensity than the first attacks.

PREVENTION. Available approaches for the control of relapsing fevers include the detection and treatment of human cases, vector control, rodent control, and public health education. Delousing of clothing and bodies with insecticides such as DDT (chlorophenothane) can be employed, as can the application of insect repellents. In known epidemic situations, prophylactic antibiotics are a temporary measure to contain spread of infection to persons at high risk. For tick-borne relapsing fever, campers and hikers going into endemic areas should be advised to avoid cabins that are inhabited by rodents and ticks and to apply topical tick repellents to the skin.

Barbour AG, Hayes SF: Biology of *Borrelia* species. Microbiol Rev 50:381, 1986. *Review of recent knowledge about this genus of spirochetes and similarity of relapsing fever and Lyme disease.*
Butler T: Relapsing fever: New lessons about antibiotic action. Ann Intern Med 102:397, 1985. *Reviews clinical research in Ethiopia relating to mechanisms of Jarisch-Herxheimer reaction.*
Horton JM, Blaser MJ: The spectrum of relapsing fever in the Rocky Mountains. Arch Intern Med 145:871, 1985. *This report of 23 recent cases indicated an increased incidence of the disease in Colorado. Severe Jarisch-Herxheimer reactions occurred in four patients.*

343 Lyme Disease

Stephen E. Malawista

Lyme disease is a tick-borne inflammatory disorder caused by a newly recognized spirochete, *Borrelia burgdorferi*. Its clinical hallmark is an early expanding skin lesion, *erythema chronicum migrans* (ECM), which may be followed weeks to months later by neurologic, cardiac, or joint abnormalities. Symptoms may refer to any one of these four systems alone or in combination. All stages of Lyme disease may respond to antibiotics, but treatment of early disease is the most successful. Although cases of the illness are concentrated in certain endemic areas, foci of Lyme disease are widely distributed within the United States and Europe.

"Lyme arthritis" was recognized in November 1975 because of unusual geographic clustering of children with inflammatory arthropathy in the region of Lyme, Connecticut. It soon became clear that this was a multisystem disorder (Lyme *disease*) occurring at any age, in both sexes, and often preceded by a characteristic expanding skin lesion, *erythema chronicum migrans* (ECM). In Europe ECM had been associated with the bite of the sheep tick, *Ixodes ricinus*, and with tick-borne meningo-polyneuritis. In the Lyme region, a closely related deer tick, *Ixodes dammini*, was implicated as the principal disease vector on epidemiologic grounds. In 1982, Burgdorfer and associates isolated a spirochete, now called *Borrelia burgdorferi*, from *Ixodes dammini* and linked it serologically to patients with Lyme disease. It was soon recovered from patient specimens.

DISTRIBUTION AND EPIDEMIOLOGY. Lyme disease is widespread. In the United States there are three distinct foci: the Northeast from Massachusetts to Maryland, the Midwest in Wisconsin and Minnesota, and the West in California, southern Oregon, and western Nevada. However, the illness has been reported in 43 states, as well as throughout Europe and Asia. The earliest known cases in the United States occurred on Cape Cod in 1962 and in Lyme, Connecticut, in 1965; annual cases now number in the thousands. Disease can occur at any age and in either sex. Onset of illness is generally between May 1 and November 30, with the peak in June and July.

The primary vectors of Lyme disease are tiny ixodid ticks. Major foci of disease correspond to the distribution of *I. dammini* (Northeast, Midwest), *I. pacificus* (West), *I. ricinus* (Europe, western USSR), and *I. persulcatus* (Asian USSR, China, Japan), but other vectors, including the Lone Star tick, *Amblyomma americanum*, are likely in some areas. In one United States study, 31 per cent of 314 patients recalled a tick bite at the skin site where ECM developed days to weeks later. The six ticks that were saved were invariably nymphal *I. dammini*, whose peak questing period is May through July; the nymphal stage is primarily responsible for transmission of disease. Preferred hosts for *I. dammini* nymphs are white-footed mice and, for adults, white-tailed deer, in whose fur they mate.

The rising incidence of Lyme disease in recent years in the United States may be explained by multiple factors including an increase in the numbers of ixodid ticks, the outward migration of residential areas into previously rural woodlands (habitats favored by ixodid ticks and their hosts), an exploding deer population, and increased recognition.

In areas endemic for Lyme disease, the prevalence of *B. burgdorferi* in nymphal *I. dammini* ranges from about 20 per cent to over 60 per cent (cf. *I. pacificus*, 1 to 3 per cent). The organism has been isolated, or specific antibody found, in blood and tissues of a wide variety of large and small animals, including domestic dogs and birds. Indiscriminate feeding on a variety of animals by immature *I. dammini* may favor the spread of infection.

PATHOGENESIS. Recovery of *B. burgdorferi* is straightforward from the tick but difficult from patients, in part because of a relative paucity of organisms in specimens of tissue and fluids from the latter. Nevertheless, rare positive cultures are reported at all stages of the illness—from blood (early), *erythema chronicum migrans*, secondary annular lesions, meningitic cerebrospinal fluid, heart, joint fluid, and even a late skin lesion, *acrodermatitis chronica atrophicans*, that had been present for 10 years. Spirochetes have been identified by silver stain or by immunofluorescence in some histologic sections of ECM and rarely of secondary annular lesions, synovium, brain, eye, heart, striated muscle, liver, spleen, kidney, and bone marrow.

From these data, combined with clinical (see below) and epidemiologic features of Lyme disease, the following pathogenetic sequence is likely. *B. burgdorferi* is transmitted to the skin of the host via the tick vector. After an incubation period of 3 to 32 days, the organism migrates outward in the skin (ECM), spreads in lymph (regional adenopathy), or disseminates in blood to organs (e.g., central nervous system, joints, heart, and presumably liver and spleen) or other skin sites (secondary annular lesions; see below). Maternal-fetal transmission is distinctly uncommon. Although organisms are hard to find in later stages of Lyme disease, it is likely that persistent live spirochetes are driving the illness throughout its course. Evidence for this interpretation includes the responsiveness of many patients to antibiotics, the rare sightings of spirochetes in affected tissues, and an expansion of the antibody response to additional spirochetal antigens over time.

Lyme disease is associated with characteristic immune abnormalities. At disease onset (ECM), almost all patients have evidence of circulating immune complexes. At that time, the findings of elevated serum immunoglobulin M (IgM) levels and cryoglobulins containing IgM predict subsequent nervous system, heart, or joint involvement—i.e., early humoral findings have prognostic significance. Serial determinations of serum IgM are often the single most helpful laboratory indicator of disease activity. These abnormalities tend to persist during neurologic or cardiac involvement. Later in the illness, when arthritis is present, serum IgM levels are more often normal. By then, immune complexes are usually lacking in serum but are present uniformly in joint fluid, where their titers correlate positively with the local concentration of polymorphonuclear leukocytes. Mononuclear cells from peripheral blood increase their antigen-specific proliferative response as the disease progresses, but the greatest reactivity to antigen is seen in cells from inflamed joints. Adjacent to that joint fluid, one sees on biopsy a proliferative synovium often replete with lymphocytes and plasma cells that are presumably capable of producing immunoglobulin locally. Thus, an initially disseminated, immune-mediated inflammatory disorder becomes in some patients localized and propagated in joints.

In addition to factors related to the pathogenicity of specific isolates of *B. burgdorferi*, immunogenetic make-up may play a role in whether an infected individual is able to rid himself of spirochetes. Patients with chronic arthritis have been reported to have an increased frequency of the B-cell alloantigen HLA DR4 or DR2, and individuals with another late manifestation, *acrodermatitis chronica atrophicans*, have an increased frequency of DR2.

CLINICAL CHARACTERISTICS. Lyme disease is conveniently divided into three clinical stages, but the stages may overlap, most patients do not exhibit all of them, and, in fact, seroconversion can occur in asymptomatic individuals. The illness usually begins with ECM and associated symptoms (stage 1), sometimes followed weeks to months later by neurologic or cardiac abnormalities (stage 2) and weeks to years later by arthritis (stage 3). Chronic neurologic and skin involvement may also occur years after onset.

Early Manifestations. Erythema chronicum migrans, the unique clinical marker for Lyme disease, begins as a red macule or papule at the site where the tick vector, usually long gone, had engorged. As the area of redness expands to 15 cm or so (range, 3 to 68 cm), there is usually partial central clearing. The outer borders are red, generally flat, and without scaling. The centers are occasionally red and indurated, even vesicular or necrotic. Variations may occur—multiple rings, for example. The thigh, groin, and axilla are particularly common sites. The lesion is warm to touch, but not often sore, and is easily missed if out of sight. Routine histologic findings are nonspecific: a heavy dermal infiltrate of mononuclear cells, without epidermal change except at the site of the tick bite.

Within days of onset of ECM, one half of United States patients develop multiple annular secondary lesions (see Color Plate 10A; Table 343–1). They resemble ECM itself but are generally smaller, migrate less, and lack indurated centers; they are not associated with the sites of previous tick bites. Individual lesions may come and go, and their borders sometimes merge. Other occasional skin lesions are noted in Table 343–1. In addition, benign lymphocytoma cutis has been reported in Europe. *Erythema chronicum migrans* and secondary lesions fade in 3 to 4 weeks (range, 1 day to 14 months). They may recur.

Skin involvement is often accompanied by flulike symptoms—malaise and fatigue, headache, fever and chills, myalgia, and arthralgia (Table 343–2). Some patients have evidence of meningeal irritation or mild encephalopathy—for example, episodic attacks of excruciating headache and neck pain, stiffness, or pressure—but typically lasting only for hours at this stage of the illness, and without spinal fluid pleocytosis or objective neurologic deficit. Except for fatigue and lethargy, which are often constant, the early signs and symptoms are typically intermittent and

TABLE 343–1. EARLY SIGNS OF LYME DISEASE

Signs	No. of Patients	
	N = 314	(%)
Erythema chronicum migrans	314	(100)*
Multiple annular lesions	150	(48)
Lymphadenopathy		
Regional	128	(41)
Generalized	63	(20)
Pain on neck flexion	52	(17)
Malar rash	41	(13)
Erythematous throat	38	(12)
Conjunctivitis	35	(11)
Right upper quadrant tenderness	24	(8)
Splenomegaly	18	(6)
Hepatomegaly	16	(5)
Muscle tenderness	12	(4)
Periorbital edema	10	(3)
Evanescent skin lesions	8	(3)
Abdominal tenderness	6	(2)
Testicular swelling	2	(1)

Erythema chronicum migrans was required for inclusion in this study.
From Steere AC, Bartenhagen NH, Craft JE, et al.: The early clinical manifestations of Lyme disease. Ann Intern Med 99:76, 1983.

TABLE 343–2. EARLY SYMPTOMS OF LYME DISEASE

Symptoms	No. of Patients N = 314	(%)
Malaise, fatigue, and lethargy	251	(80)
Headache	200	(64)
Fever and chills	185	(59)
Stiff neck	151	(48)
Arthralgias	150	(48)
Myalgias	135	(43)
Backache	81	(26)
Anorexia	73	(23)
Sore throat	53	(17)
Nausea	53	(17)
Dysesthesia	35	(11)
Vomiting	32	(10)
Abdominal pain	24	(8)
Photophobia	19	(6)
Hand stiffness	16	(5)
Dizziness	15	(5)
Cough	15	(5)
Chest pain	12	(4)
Ear pain	12	(4)
Diarrhea	6	(2)

From Steere AC, Bartenhagen NH, Craft JE, et al.: The early clinical manifestations of Lyme disease. Ann Intern Med 99:76, 1983.

changing. For example, a patient may have meningitic attacks for several days, a few days of improvement, and then the onset of migratory musculoskeletal pain. This last may involve joints (generally without swelling), tendons, bursa, muscle, and bone. The pain tends to affect only one or two sites at a time and to last a few hours to several days in a given location. The various associated symptoms may occur several days before ECM (or without it) and last for months (especially fatigue and lethargy) after the skin lesions have disappeared.

Later Manifestations. **Neurologic Involvement.** Within several weeks to months of the onset of illness, about 15 per cent of patients develop frank neurologic abnormalities, including meningitis, encephalitis, chorea, cranial neuritis (including bilateral facial palsy), motor and sensory radiculoneuritis, or mononeuritis multiplex, in various combinations. The usual pattern is fluctuating meningoencephalitis with superimposed cranial nerve (particularly facial) palsy and peripheral radiculoneuropathy, but Bell's palsy may occur *alone*. By now, patients with meningitic symptoms have a lymphocytic pleocytosis (about 100 cells per cubic millimeter) in cerebrospinal fluid and sometimes diffuse slowing on electroencephalogram. However, the neck is rarely stiff except on extreme flexion; Kernig's and Brudzinski's signs are absent. Neurologic abnormalities typically last for months but usually resolve completely (late neurologic complications are noted below).

Cardiac Involvement. Also within weeks to months of onset, about 8 per cent of patients develop cardiac involvement. The most common abnormality is fluctuating degrees of atrioventricular block (first-degree, Wenckebach, or complete heart block). Some patients have evidence of more diffuse cardiac involvement, including electrocardiographic changes compatible with acute myopericarditis, radionuclide evidence of mild left ventricular dysfunction, or, rarely, cardiomegaly, None has had heart murmurs. Cardiac involvement is usually brief (3 days to 6 weeks), but it may recur.

Arthritis. From weeks to as long as 2 years after the onset of illness, about 60 per cent of patients develop frank arthritis, usually characterized by intermittent attacks of asymmetric joint swelling and pain primarily in large joints, especially the knee, one or two joints at a time. Affected knees are commonly more swollen than painful, often hot, and rarely red; Baker's cysts may form and rupture early. However, both large and small joints may be affected, and a few patients have had symmetric polyarthritis. Attacks of arthritis, which generally last from weeks to months, typically recur for several years, decreasing in frequency with time. Fatigue is common with active joint involvement, but fever or other systemic symptoms at this stage are unusual. Joint fluid white cell counts vary from 500 to 110,000 cells per cubic

millimeter, with an average of about 25,000 cells per cubic millimeter, mostly polymorphonuclear leukocytes. Total protein ranges from 3 to 8 grams per deciliter. The C3 and C4 levels are generally greater than one-third, and glucose levels usually greater than two-thirds, that of serum. Rheumatoid factor and antinuclear antibody are absent.

In about 10 per cent of patients with arthritis, involvement in large joints may become chronic, with pannus formation and erosion of cartilage and bone. Synovial biopsy findings may mimic those of rheumatoid arthritis: surface deposits of fibrin, villous hypertrophy, vascular proliferation, and a heavy infiltration of mononuclear cells. In addition, there may be an obliterative endarteritis and (rarely) demonstrable spirochetes. In vitro, *B. burgdorferi* stimulates mononuclear cells to produce interleukin 1, and concentrations of this cytokine have been elevated in synovial fluid. In one patient with chronic Lyme arthritis, synovium grown in tissue culture produced large amounts of collagenase and prostaglandin E_2. Thus, in Lyme disease the joint fluid cell counts, the immune reactants (except for rheumatoid factor), the synovial histology, the amounts of synovial enzymes released, and the resulting destruction of cartilage and bone may be similar to those in rheumatoid arthritis.

Other late findings (years) associated with this infection include a chronic skin lesion—*acrodermatitis chronica atrophicans*—well known in Europe but still rare in the United States. One sees violaceous infiltrated plaques or nodules, especially on extensor surfaces, that eventually become atrophic. Uncommon late chronic neurologic disease includes transverse myelitis, diffuse sensory axonal neuropathy, and demyelinating lesions of the central nervous system. Mild memory impairment, subtle mood changes, and chronic fatigue states may also occur.

LABORATORY TEST RESULTS. The diagnosis of Lyme disease is based on the recognition of clinical features of the illness in a patient with a history of possible exposure to the causative organism. Culture of *B. burgdorferi* from patients is definitive but has rarely been successful except from skin biopsy specimens. Recently, the organism was isolated from blood in a significant minority of patients with systemic manifestations of early disease (it grows very slowly). Special tissue staining techniques generally have a low yield and are not readily available. Determination of specific antibody titers is currently the most helpful adjunctive test for Lyme disease. In serum, specific IgM antibody titers against *B. burgdorferi* usually reach a peak between the third and sixth weeks after the onset of disease; specific immunoglobulin G (IgG) antibody titers rise more slowly and are generally highest months later when arthritis is present (Fig. 343–1). Individuals with Lyme disease of more than 6 weeks' duration can be expected to have elevated levels of specific antibodies. However, the tests employed are not yet standardized, and results from different commercial laboratories may vary, especially for boderline elevations. The vast majority of individuals with established Lyme arthritis have elevated specific IgG titers. This finding makes antibody titers against *B. burgdorferi* particularly useful in differentiating Lyme disease from other rheumatic syndromes, especially when ECM is missed, forgotten, or absent. This antibody cross-reacts with other spirochetes, including *Treponema pallidum*, but patients with Lyme disease do not have positive VDRL test results.

Other tests under development seek to identify spirochetal material in host fluids or tissues. They include a test for spirochetal protein in urine and use of the polymerase chain reaction to detect spirochetal DNA in host material; neither has been perfected for clinical use as of this writing.

The most common nonspecific laboratory abnormalities, particularly early in the illness, are a high erythrocyte sedimentation rate, an elevated serum IgM level, or an increased serum glutamic-oxaloacetic transaminase (SGOT) level. The enzyme levels generally return to normal within several weeks. Patients may be mildly anemic early in the illness and occasionally have elevated white cell counts with shifts to the left in the differential count. A few patients have had microscopic hematuria, sometimes with mild proteinuria (dipstick); values for creatinine and blood urea nitrogen have been normal. Throughout the illness, serum C3 and C4 levels are generally normal or elevated. Rheumatoid factor and antinuclear antibodies are usually absent.

DIFFERENTIAL DIAGNOSIS. *Erythema chronicum migrans* is the unique herald lesion of Lyme disease (see Color Plate

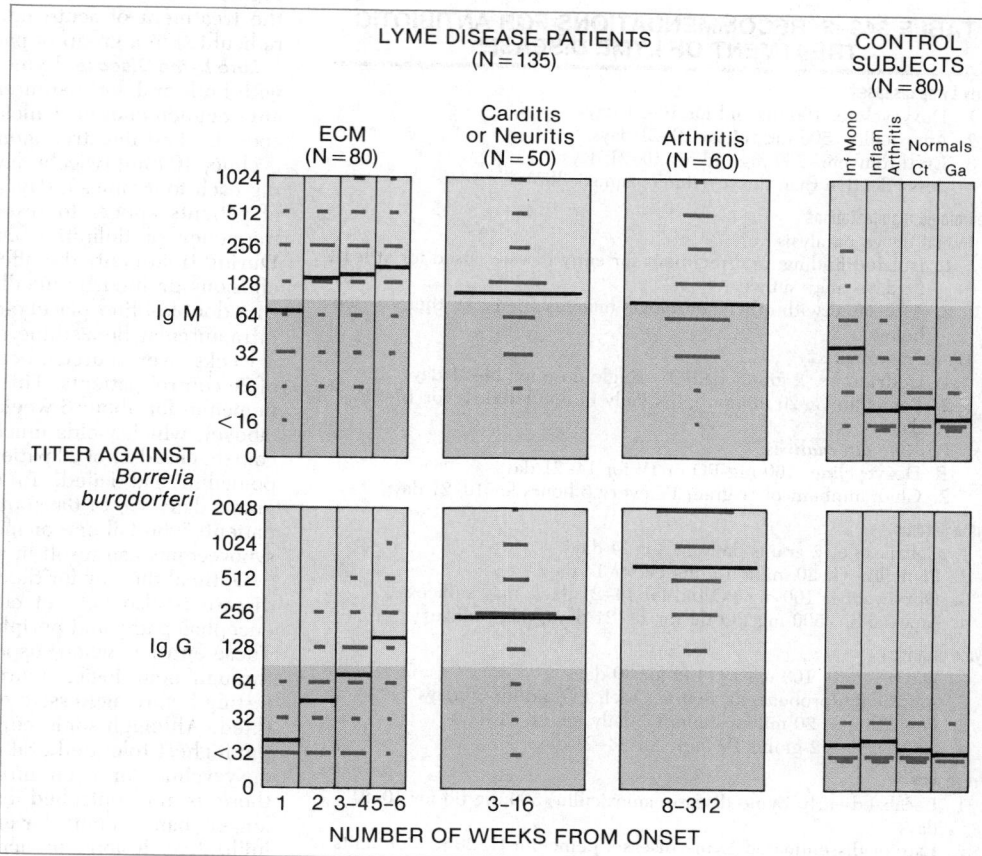

FIGURE 343–1. Antibody titers against *Borrelia burgdorferi* are shown in serum samples from 135 patients with different clinical manifestations of Lyme disease, and from 80 control subjects with infectious mononucleosis, inflammatory arthritis, or no disease (titers determined by indirect immunofluorescence). The black bar shows the geometric mean titer for each group; the pink shaded areas indicate the range of values generally observed in control subjects. Note that all patients with Lyme arthritis have elevated IgG antibody titers. (Adapted from Steere AC, Grodzicki RL, Kornblatt AN, et al: The spirochetal etiology of Lyme disease. N Engl J Med 308:733–740, 1983. Reprinted by permission of the New England Journal of Medicine.)

10A). When present in its classic form, there is little else that might be confused with it. However, some patients are not aware of having had ECM, and in others, its appearance is not always characteristic. Secondary lesions might suggest *erythema multiforme*, but blistering, mucosal lesions, and involvement of the palms and soles are not features of Lyme disease. Malar rash may suggest systemic lupus erythematosus; an urticarial rash, hepatitis B infection or serum sickness. Evanescent blotches and circles may resemble *erythema marginatum*, but those of Lyme disease do not expand.

Early flulike symptoms may be misleading, especially when *erythema chronicum migrans* is absent or missed or is not the first manifestation. Severe headache and stiff neck may suggest aseptic meningitis; abdominal symptoms, hepatitis; and generalized tender lymphadenopathy and splenomegaly, infectious mononucleosis. As in the last infection, profound fatigue in Lyme disease may be a major and persistent complaint.

In later stages, Lyme disease may mimic other immune-mediated disorders. Like rheumatic fever, Lyme disease may be associated with sore throat followed by migratory polyarthritis and carditis, but without evidence of valvular involvement or of a preceding streptococcal infection. Migratory pain in tendons and joints may also suggest disseminated gonococcal disease. An isolated facial weakness may mimic Bell's palsy of other causes. Late neurologic involvement may suggest multiple sclerosis (transverse myelitis), Guillain-Barré syndrome (symmetric peripheral neuropathy), primary psychosis, or brain tumor. In adults with Lyme arthritis, the large knee effusions can resemble those in Reiter's syndrome, and the occasional symmetric polyarthritis, that of rheumatoid arthritis. In children, the attacks of arthritis, although generally shorter, may be identical to those seen in the oligoarticular form of juvenile rheumatoid arthritis, but without iridocyclitis.

TREATMENT. The major goal of therapy in Lyme disease is to eradicate the causative organism. Like other spirochetal diseases, Lyme disease is most responsive to antibiotics early in its course. Treatment regimens have evolved over time based on both controlled clinical data and on clinical experience. Because of the difficulty in proving that bacteria have been eradicated and the common persistence of some symptoms long after treatment, the endpoint of antibiotic therapy is not always clear. The treatment regimens presented here represent guidelines that will no doubt be refined in time (Table 343–3).

Early Lyme Disease. If patients are treated early with oral antibiotics, *erythema chronicum migrans* typically resolves promptly, and major later sequelae (myocarditis, meningoencephalitis, or recurrent arthritis) usually do not occur. Prompt treatment is therefore important, even though such patients may be susceptible to reinfection. For adults, antibiotic choices in order of preference include oral doxycycline, 100 mg twice a day; amoxicillin, 500 mg three times a day; and erythromycin, 250 mg four times a day, each for 10 to 21 days depending on the rapidity of clinical response. Failures are more common with erythromycin than the other two agents. In children younger than 9 years, amoxicillin, 30 mg per kilogram per day (not less than 1 gram or more than 2 grams per day), is given in divided doses for the same period or, in cases of penicillin allergy, erythromycin, 30 mg per kilogram per day, in divided doses for 10 to 21 days.

About 10 per cent of patients with early Lyme disease experience a Jarisch-Herxheimer–like reaction (higher fever, redder rash, or greater pain) during the first 24 hours of antibiotic therapy. Whichever drug is given, 30 to 50 per cent of patients have brief (hours to days) recurrent episodes of headache, musculoskeletal pain, and fatigue which may continue for extended periods. The etiology of these symptoms is unclear at present; they may result from undegraded spirochetal antigen(s) rather than persistence of live spirochetes. It is clear, however, that the risk of delayed resolution is greatest in individuals with disseminated manifestations of disease (multiple skin lesions, headache, fever, lymphadenopathy, or Bell's palsy) prior to the institution of antibiotics.

Later Lyme Disease. For Lyme meningitis, with or without other neurologic manifestations (cranial neuropathy or radiculoneuropathy), intravenous ceftriaxone, 2 grams daily in a single dose, or intravenous penicillin G, 20 million units a day in six divided doses, each for 10 to 21 days, is effective therapy.

TABLE 343-3. RECOMMENDATIONS FOR ANTIBIOTIC TREATMENT OF LYME DISEASE*

Early Lyme disease†
1. Doxycycline, 100 mg bid for 10–21 days
2. Amoxicillin, 500 mg tid for 10–21 days
3. Erythromycin, 250 mg qid for 10–21 days
   (less effective than doxycycline or amoxicillin)

Neurologic manifestations
Facial nerve paralysis
  1. Isolated finding: oral regimens for early disease, used for at least 21 days, may suffice.
  2. Associated with other neurologic manifestations: IV therapy (see below)
Lyme meningitis‡
  1. Ceftriaxone, 2 grams daily by single dose for 14–21 days
  2. Penicillin G, 20 million units daily in divided dose for 10–21 days
  Possible alternatives
  1. Doxycycline, 100 mg PO or IV for 14–21 days
  2. Chloramphenicol, 1 gram IV every 6 hours for 10–21 days

Lyme carditis
1. Ceftriaxone, 2 grams daily IV for 14 days
2. Penicillin G, 20 million units IV for 14 days
3. Doxycycline, 100 mg PO bid for 14–21 days, may suffice§
4. Amoxicillin, 500 mg PO tid for 14–21 days, may suffice§

Lyme arthritis
1. Doxycycline, 100 mg PO bid for 30 days
2. Amoxicillin/probenecid, 500 mg each PO qid for 30 days
3. Penicillin G, 20 million units IV daily for 14–21 days
4. Ceftriaxone, 2 grams IV daily for 14–21 days

Pregnancy
1. Localized early Lyme disease: amoxicillin, 500 mg tid for 10–21 days
2. Late or disseminated Lyme disease: penicillin G, 20 million units daily for 14–21 days
3. Asymptomatic seropositivity: no treatment necessary

*These are guidelines, to be modified by new findings and to be applied always with close attention to the clinical context of individual patients.

†Shorter courses are reserved for disease that is limited to a single skin lesion only.

‡Regimens for radiculoneuropathy, peripheral neuropathy, and encephalitis are the same as those for meningitis.

§Oral regimens have been reserved for mild cardiac involvement (first-degree heart block, normal ventricular function), but there is no substantiation that more severe degrees of heart involvement require more aggressive antibiotic therapy.

Reprinted with permission from Rahn DW, Malawista SE: Lyme disease: Recommendations for diagnosis and treatment. Ann Intern Med 114:472, 1991.

Headache and stiff neck usually begin to subside by the second day of therapy and disappear by 7 to 10 days; motor deficits and radicular pain frequently require 7 to 8 weeks for complete recovery but do not require longer antibiotic courses. Possible alternative oral regimens are listed in Table 343–3. For Bell's palsy alone, oral regimens may suffice, but these patients may be at higher risk of later sequelae than are individuals with early disease without neurologic dissemination.

Despite the generally benign course of Lyme carditis in most patients, intravenous antibiotics are commonly employed for all but the mildest forms of cardiac involvement (first-degree atrioventricular block of less than 0.4 second; Table 343–3). This practice is warranted by the knowledge that B. burgdorferi can invade myocardium directly and by the frequency of other manifestations of dissemination in these patients. Prednisone, 40 to 60 mg a day in divided doses, has, in the past, seemed to hasten resolution of high-grade heart block, but one should hesitate to institute glucocorticoids during antibiotic administration, as they may impede eradication of infecting organisms. If second- or third-degree heart block is present, patients should be admitted to hospital for cardiac monitoring; temporary pacing is occasionally required for complete heart block.

In clinical practice, ceftriaxone (2 grams daily for 14 to 21 days) has largely replaced penicillin for the therapy of disseminated Lyme disease. Arguments in favor of this practice are a once-daily administration schedule which is amenable to outpatient intravenous antibiotic programs, and improved penetration of the cerebrospinal fluid in comparison with that noted with penicillin. Penicillin and cefotaxime have been found equally effective for the treatment of acute neurologic Lyme disease (meningitis or radiculitis) in a group of patients studied in Germany.

Late Lyme Disease. Lyme arthritis has been successfully treated with both oral and parenteral antibiotics, but failures occur with any regimen chosen. Unless central nervous system involvement coexists, first-line treatment with a month-long course of doxycycline, 100 mg twice a day, or amoxicillin plus probenecid, 500 mg each four times a day, is recommended. Roughly two thirds of patients appear to respond to these oral regimens, but the frequency of definitive cures will await long-term follow-up. During treatment, the affected joint should be kept at rest and effusions drained by needle aspiration as for any infected joint. In a double-blind placebo-controlled trial, 7 of 20 patients given intramuscular benzathine penicillin, 2.4 million units weekly for 3 weeks, were cured (mean follow-up 33 months), versus none of 20 control patients. This regimen provides low serum levels of penicillin for about 6 weeks. High-dose intravenous penicillin G (above), which yields much higher serum levels over its 10-day course, cured 11 of 20 patients, including two in whom benzathine penicillin had failed. In one comparative trial, ceftriaxone (2 grams daily for 14 days) outperformed intravenous penicillin. In patients who fail one or more courses of antibiotics, arthroscopic synovectomy can result in a long-term response and perhaps cure.

Optimal therapy for the later neurologic complications of Lyme disease is also not yet clear. The frequency of subtle chronic encephalopathy and peripheral neuropathy is debated at present. These entities, when suspected, should be carefully documented through neurologic, neuropsychological, and electrophysiologic testing before aggressive or prolonged antibiotic therapy is instituted. Although some current thinking favors longer periods of the highest tolerated oral doses of amoxicillin (with probenecid), doxycycline, or even intravenous antibiotics in difficult cases, there is no controlled experience with courses of antibiotics longer than 1 month for any manifestation of Lyme disease. The infiltrative lesions of acrodermatitis chronica atrophicans are usually cured by 3 weeks of oral phenoxymethyl penicillin, 2 to 3 grams daily in divided doses.

Pregnancy. Because the spirochetes that cause relapsing fever and syphilis can cross the placenta, there has been concern regarding this possibility in Lyme disease. Maternal-fetal transmission of B. burgdorferi resulting in either neonatal death or stillbirth has been reported in rare instances in which symptomatic early Lyme disease occurred early in pregnancy and was either untreated or inadequately treated. In follow-up studies conducted by the Centers for Disease Control, maternal Lyme disease was not directly implicated as a cause of fetal malformations. There have been no cases of fetal infection occurring when currently recommended antibiotic regimens for Lyme disease have been used during pregnancy. A lower threshold for initiating therapy for suspected Lyme disease in pregnancy is understandable, but women acquiring the illness during pregnancy should be reassured that the vast majority of infants born to women in these circumstances have been entirely well.

Tick Bites. A final treatment issue regards the advisability of administering antibiotics prophylactically to individuals sustaining ixodid tick bites in endemic areas. The single study completed to date has not supported this common practice. Because nymphal ixodid ticks must, in general, feed for a day or more before transmitting spirochetes (at least in mice), ticks removed prior to this time are unlikely to have transmitted B. burgdorferi even if infected. Tick bite sites should be observed for development of ECM and patients cautioned regarding the common associated symptoms of early Lyme disease.

Malawista SE, Steere AC, Hardin JA: Lyme disease: A unique human model for an infectious etiology of rheumatic disease. Yale J Biol Med 57:473, 1984. *The larger significance of Lyme disease, a disorder that is infectious in origin but inflammatory or "rheumatic" in expression.*

Rahn DW, Malawista SE: Lyme disease: Recommendations for diagnosis and treatment. Ann Intern Med 114:472, 1991. *Critical review of the literature supplemented by 15 years of clinical experience with this illness.*

Steere AC, Green J, Schoen RT, et al.: Successful parenteral penicillin therapy of established Lyme arthritis. N Engl J Med 312:869, 1985. *Cure by antibiotics of a rheumatoid "look-alike."*

Steere AC, Grodzicki RL, Kornblatt AN, et al.: The spirochetal etiology of Lyme disease. N Engl J Med 308:733, 1983. *Borrelia recovered from blood, ECM, and cerebrospinal fluid of patients.*

Steere AC, Malawista SE, Syndman DR, et al.: Lyme arthritis: An epidemic of oligoarticular arthritis in childen and adults in three Connecticut communities. Arthritis Rheum 20:7, 1977. *The first description of a new nosologic entity, recognized because it clusters geographically; rheumatoid arthritis does not.*

Steere AC, Pachner AR, Malawista SE: Neurologic abnormalities of Lyme disease: Successful treatment with high-dose intravenous penicillin. Ann Intern Med 99:767, 1983. *Meningitis, formerly treated with high-dose prednisone tapered over months, responds to penicillin in days.*

344 Leptospirosis

J. Bruce McClain

The term *leptospirosis* designates an infection with any serovar of *Leptospira interrogans,* regardless of the syndrome. Old names such as canicola fever, Fort Bragg fever, Weil's disease, or peapicker's disease are potentially confusing and should be avoided.

ETIOLOGY. *Leptospira* consists of three species: *interrogans,* which is pathogenic, and *biflexa* and *parva,* which are saprophytic. Serotyping and serogrouping have established over 170 serovars in the species *L. interrogans.* The proper designation of a serovar is *L. interrogans* serovar Pomona, not *L. pomona.* The latter usage, although widespread, represents serovars as species and is incorrect. The organism is a tightly coiled spirochete with one axial filament. It is gram-negative but with a diameter of 0.15 μm it is difficult to see on light microscopy and so is usually visualized by phase contrast or darkfield techniques. It is easily cultured on Fletcher's medium and is an obligate aerobe.

EPIDEMIOLOGY. Leptospirosis is a ubiquitous enzootic disease. Reservoirs of infection include rodents, skunks, foxes, domestic livestock, dogs, and frogs. Many animals exhibit a prolonged urinary shedding of the organism without clinical illness. When humans contact infected tissues, fluids, or contaminated waters they contract the illness. Transmission may occur through cuts, mucous membranes, and possibly unabraded skin. In earlier series, illness was reported associated with occupational exposure such as among sanitation, dairy, slaughterhouse, and fishing workers. The epidemiology has changed over the last 15 years owing to the advent of multiuse land development, with farmlands draining into recreational bodies of water. More recent reports indicate that at least one half of cases result from nonvocational exposure. There has been a corresponding decrease in the age of persons infected, although males still comprise 80 per cent of cases. In the United States between 50 and 150 cases are reported annually.

The national attack rate is 0.05 per 100,000, although rates as high as 1 per 100,000 occur in Hawaii. The disease is probably substantially under-reported. Leptospirosis peaks annually in the summer months and displays a 4- to 5-year periodicity in attack rate over the last 25 years.

PATHOLOGY AND PATHOGENESIS. Gross anatomic findings in patients dying from leptospirosis are (1) widespread hemorrhage in skin, mucosa, serosa, heart, lungs, spleen, liver, and kidneys; (2) hepatomegaly without prominent splenomegaly; (3) bile staining and enlargement of the heart and kidneys. Histologic examination of the liver in autopsy material shows nonspecific inflammatory changes, bile stasis, and disruption of the limiting plate. Biopsy material under light and electron microscopic examination shows similar features with less destruction of architecture.

Kidneys in autopsy series show a spectrum of changes that reflect an initial tubular injury that is acellular. As the disease progresses and antibodies appear, inflammatory changes occur that represent an overt interstitial nephritis with disruption of the tubular architecture. Biopsy series show similar changes to a lesser degree. The glomeruli have foot process fusion and mesangial hypertrophy but are otherwise spared. Leptospiras are seen in most of the renal material. Hemorrhagic manifestations are associated with areas of capillary wall damage and necrosis with perivascular round cell infiltration. Striated muscle is frequently involved with degeneration of individual fibrils and loss of architecture associated with inflammation. This pattern is considered specific for leptospirosis. The myocardium is affected with similar changes. In one fourth of autopsy cases myocarditis is listed as serious enough to be a contributing cause of death.

The mechanism by which *Leptospira* organisms cause damage to tissues is obscure. Toxic factors have been identified in culture supernatants, but organisms that do not produce some of these factors may cause serious disease. Early in the illness the evidence favors direct toxicity to certain tissues, while late in the illness damage secondary to inflammation is more pronounced.

CLINICAL FEATURES. Most natural infections appear 7 to 14 days after the exposure, although the incubation period ranges from 2 to 20 days. The length of the incubation period has no prognostic significance. Clinical findings vary among reported series, but a general description includes fever and headache, 95 per cent; myalgia and conjunctival suffusion, 80 per cent (in nonmilitary series suffusion is reported less often); gastrointestinal symptoms (nausea, vomiting, or abdominal pain), 60 per cent; cough or pharyngitis, 40 per cent; lymphadenopathy, 25 per cent; hepatomegaly, 15 per cent; rash, 10 per cent; and jaundice and gastrointestinal hemorrhage, 5 per cent each. Less commonly reported symptoms are splenomegaly, uveitis, and diarrhea. About one half of patients exhibit a "brutal beginning," with an abrupt onset of symptoms over a 1- to 2-hour period. The clinical picture that should bring leptospirosis to mind is a febrile patient with severe muscle aches and pain who is nauseated or vomiting. The presence of conjunctival suffusion may be helpful in detecting the illness in military populations. It is not conjunctivitis as seen in allergic or viral conjunctivitis but rather a *pericorneal reddening or hyperemia.* The fever is high, usually above 38°C and frequently up to 40°C, and is accompanied by chills. Headache is severe and is characterized as retro-orbital or occipital. The presence of headache, high fever, and neck stiffness or pain due to profound myalgia suggests meningitis and may necessitate a lumbar puncture. Spinal fluid is usually acellular in the first 5 to 7 days of illness, although leptospiras may be seen. With the onset of antibody in the serum, an aseptic meningitis may occur in up to 90 per cent of patients, but only one half have meningeal symptoms. Other neurologic manifestations such as changes in the level of consciousness, encephalitis, and cranial nerve palsies have been reported less often. The muscle pains and tenderness are truly remarkable. The severity of myalgia may even prevent the patient from standing. The presence of nausea, vomiting, and anorexia with abdominal tenderness caused by muscle involvement can mimic pancreatitis. Acute dilatation of the gallbladder and cholecystitis can occur in leptospirosis and make the clinical evaluation of an ill patient very difficult, especially since there is already laboratory evidence of inflammation.

The illness usually lasts 4 to 9 days. During that period all clinical findings resolve simultaneously, and both doctor and patient are surprised at how quickly the recovery has taken place and at how well the patient feels. In about 15 per cent of patients the illness persists beyond the ninth day. It rarely may last 6 to 7 weeks.

Leptospirosis is generally a monophasic illness. In a minority of patients after an initial illness there is a period of apparent recovery, after which symptoms worsen. This second phase is termed the immune phase. It lasts 2 to 4 days in most patients. It differs from initial illness in being more variable. Fever is not so high, myalgia and gastrointestinal symptoms are not so severe, but meningitis and abnormal spinal fluid and iridocyclitis are more common. The immune phase is so named because of its correlation with the onset of antibodies to leptospirosis in the blood, the disappearance of leptospiremia, and the increased positivity of urine cultures for the germ.

The term *Weil's syndrome* is applied to one pole of a continuum of illness. It is not a specific subgroup of leptospirosis; it is simply severe leptospirosis. Any of the several manifestations of Weil's syndrome may occur alone. The clinical findings of intense jaundice, mental status changes, hemorrhage, purpura or petechiae, and renal insufficiency occurring in a previously normal patient are so memorable that this syndrome stimulated the search for leptospiras. The first manifestation of severe illness is usually jaundice that develops between the fifth and ninth days. The intensity of jaundice has no prognostic significance. Renal insufficiency may develop concomitantly with jaundice. Oliguria is a grave prognostic sign. Hemorrhagic manifestations may develop: Purpura and petechiae may appear on the oral, vaginal, or conjunctival mucosa. A biphasic pattern may be seen, although the stages tend to merge into a single severe illness. Convalescence is rapid in most patients but has taken up to 10 weeks. Several reports in the Far Eastern literature describe a distinctive presentation of severe leptospirosis seen in China and Korea, where the dominant syndrome is an influenzal illness. These pneumonias may be frankly hemorrhagic.

Childhood Disease. A recent report of nine pediatric cases reiterated the close contact of children to a common reservoir such as dogs. The pediatric syndrome shares many features of adult disease but is more intense, with several atypical features such as shock, hydrops of the gallbladder, skin desquamation, and chest radiographic abnormality.

LABORATORY FEATURES. Leukocyte counts are usually below 15,000 per cubic millimeter but may be as high as 50,000 per cubic millimeter. There is almost always neutrophilia. Hematocrit is normal in anicteric illness, but in prolonged illness anemia is common. The causes of anemia are many, with blood loss, microangiopathy, and leptospiral hemolysin all implicated in clinical cases. Thrombocytopenia is seen in severe cases. Coagulation studies occasionally demonstrate a vitamin K–reversible prolongation of prothrombin time. However, this is not responsible for the hemorrhagic diathesis of severe leptospirosis. The sedimentation rate is elevated in one half of the cases.

Liver function tests reveal a mean serum glutamic-oxaloacetic transaminase/serum glutamic-pyruvate transaminase (SGOT/SGPT) elevation of 5 times normal, with occasional patients having elevations up to 20 times normal. The direct bilirubin concentration may rise as a manifestation of severe disease and may reach 64 mg per deciliter, but in most icteric cases it is below 20 mg per deciliter. The pattern is one of intrahepatic cholestasis.

Early in the illness 80 per cent of patients have abnormal urine findings, the most common of which are microscopic hematuria, pyuria, and 2+ proteinuria. Gross hematuria rarely has been reported. One fourth of patients demonstrate elevations of the blood urea nitrogen between 20 and 100 mg per deciliter. The most common electrolyte abnormality is hyperkalemia, primarily in patients with renal failure.

The chest radiograph appears abnormal in one fourth to two thirds of patients, including anicteric cases. The most common abnormality is patchy bronchopneumonia. A small pleural effusion is seen in 10 per cent of patients. Recent reports from the Far East indicate a distinctive pulmonary presentation with radiographic abnormalities in 64 per cent of cases.

Electrocardiographic abnormalities occur in 10 to 40 per cent of patients, with bradycardia and low voltage accounting for one half of abnormalities. The remainder consist of nonspecific ST-T wave changes.

Cerebrospinal fluid may be abnormal in up to 90 per cent of patients. In 70 per cent of specimens the total cell count is below 500 per cubic millimeter, with frequent presence of neutrophils. Protein ranges from 50 to 110 mg per deciliter in 80 per cent of cases. The glucose concentration is usually normal. IgM antibodies may be detected in blood by day four or five of illness in most patients.

DIAGNOSIS. A diagnosis of leptospirosis must be suspected in any patient with fever, myalgia, headache, and nausea or vomiting. The presence of conjunctival suffusion is an early and helpful sign. The most common misdiagnosis of a patient with leptospirosis is aseptic meningitis followed by viral hepatitis, viral syndrome, fever of unknown origin, bronchitis, influenza, nephritis, and rickettsiosis. The following differential points aid the clinician: (1) The myalgias of leptospirosis are not a prominent feature of viral hepatitis; (2) creatine kinase is frequently elevated in leptospirosis, and this seldom occurs in viral hepatitis; (3) liver enzyme values in viral hepatitis may average 10 to 15 times higher than normal, but the average is 5 times higher in leptospirosis; (4) conjunctival suffusion is very helpful in separating leptospirosis from other processes; (5) in the first 3 days of leptospirosis, although spirochetes are present in the cerebrospinal fluid, the cytology is usually normal; early in the course of aseptic meningitis the cytology is usually abnormal.

The diagnosis may be confirmed by culture (on Fletcher's semisolid medium) of the blood in the first week of illness or of the urine thereafter. Cultures are usually positive in 2 weeks but may take up to 8 weeks to become positive. Since leptospiras may be excreted in the urine for prolonged periods, the diagnosis may be established by urine culture in untreated patients even after clinical illness is over. Direct examination of the urine and blood is not sufficient to establish the diagnosis. Some artifacts may be mistaken for leptospiras as well as nonpathogenic spirochetes. When cultures are performed three or four times, organisms are recovered with regularity. The diagnosis may be established serologically by two methods. The macroagglutination method is a screening test that uses pooled antigens from all of the serogroups of leptospirosis. Diagnosis is made by a fourfold rise in titer. This test is broadly available but does not detect infecting serovars that are not included in the pooled test antigens. Microagglutination requires a live pathogenic leptospiral culture and therefore is performed mainly in reference laboratories. Techniques for detecting genus-specific antibody or antigen using hemolytic assays and counterimmunoelectrophoresis have been published and are available as research tools. The most promising test for early diagnosis is a genus-specific antibody detection system.

PROGNOSIS. In most untreated cases this is a nonfatal, self-limited illness. The reported mortality of leptospirosis varies greatly among series. In military populations it is around 0.1 per cent. In civilian series it ranges from 5 to 10 per cent. In both military and civilian series mortality is related to age and the presence of jaundice. Thirty per cent of patients over age 60 die. Jaundiced patients have a 15 per cent mortality. The differences in mortality may have to do with the underlying health of the host and the bias toward reporting more serious cases. In the military series, involving large groups of well men, high attack rates have been documented and physicians are sensitive to the diagnosis. If the patient lives, sequelae are uncommon even in severe cases. When sequelae occur, they consist of focal cerebral or peripheral nerve deficits or ocular problems caused by persistent uveitis. Several patients have been reported with persistent renal abnormalities.

THERAPY AND PREVENTION. Antibiotics are effective in the therapy of leptospirosis, although patients have died despite therapy. Tetracycline and doxycycline (in controlled trials) are both effective in shortening the course of anicteric leptospirosis when they are given in the first 2 to 4 days of illness. Penicillin G, even given late in the course of severe leptospirosis in a blinded controlled trial, has been shown to be effective in shortening illness. Both doxycycline and penicillin prevent leptospiruria in infected patients. Chloramphenicol is not effective therapy. Although in vitro activities within the achievable levels have been demonstrated for penicillin, cephalosporins, erythromycin, gentamicin, and quinolones, they have not been studied in a controlled trial. Vancomycin and daptomycin lack activity. Ceftriaxone is effective in animal studies. The balance of therapy in leptospirosis consists of careful attention to the details of care in patients with renal, hepatic, hematologic, and central nervous system complications.

Doxycycline, 100 mg once a week, prevents leptospirosis in high-risk groups for 3 weeks. Efficacy in longer periods of exposure has not been studied. There are no licensed human vaccines, although effective animal vaccinations are available.

Feigin RD, Anderson DC: Human leptospirosis. CRC Crit Rev Clin Lab Sci 5:413, 1975. *The most comprehensive review of leptospirosis, including history, microbiology, pathogenesis, clinical findings, and therapy.*

Im J, Yeon KM, Han MC, et al.: Leptospirosis of the lung: Radiographic findings in 58 patients. AJR 152:955, 1989. *A description of radiographic findings seen in the Far Eastern pulmonary presentation of leptospirosis.*

McClain JBL, Ballou WR, Harrison SH, et al.: Doxycycline therapy of leptospirosis. Ann Intern Med 100:696, 1984. *A placebo-controlled trial of oral doxycycline in the therapy of anicteric leptospirosis.*

Takafuji ET, Kirkpatrick JW, Miller RN, et al.: An efficacy trial of doxycycline chemoprophylaxis against leptospirosis. N Engl J Med 310:497, 1984. *A placebo-controlled trial of oral doxycycline demonstrated efficacy in preventing illness in American soldiers.*

Watt G, Padre LP, Tuazon ML, et al.: Placebo-controlled trial of intravenous penicillin for severe and late leptospirosis. Lancet 1:433, 1988. *A placebo-controlled blinded trial demonstrating the effectiveness of penicillin G in patients who were ill for over 5 days with renal and hepatic impairment.*

Watt G, Padre LP, Tuazon M, et al.: Limulus lysate positivity and Herxheimer-like reactions in leptospirosis: A placebo controlled study. J Infect Dis 162:564, 1990. *A description of these reactions in treated patients.*

Diseases Caused by Chlamydiae

Walter E. Stamm

345 Introduction

Because of their obligate intracellular growth cycle, chlamydiae were originally considered large viruses and were variously called *Bedsonia* or *TRIC* (for *trachoma-inclusion conjunctivitis*) agents. These terms have been discarded, and chlamydiae now constitute a separate order (Chlamydiales), family (Chlamydiaceae), and genus (*Chlamydia*). All members of the genus are obligate intracellular pathogens, but they more closely resemble bacteria than viruses in that they possess both deoxyribonucleic acid (DNA) and ribonucleic acid (RNA), divide by binary fission, have bacterial ribosomes and a cell wall not unlike that of Enterobacteriaceae, and can be inhibited by antibiotics. Compared with other bacteria, they have a small genome of 6 to 8 × 10^5 base pairs. They also lack adenosine triphosphate (ATP)–generating enzymes and hence depend entirely upon host cell metabolism for energy production.

The genus *Chlamydia* originally contained two species, *C. psittaci* and *C. trachomatis*. The former is a ubiquitous cause of infection in birds and lower mammals, with humans being occasional accidental hosts, while *C. trachomatis* infects humans and has no apparent natural animal hosts. Characteristically, *C. psittaci* produces long-lived, persistent infections of birds and mammals. Transmission to humans occurs via exposure to infected animal tissues or secretions. Persistent infections caused by *C. trachomatis* in humans may also be common but have been less well documented. In most of the developed world, *C. trachomatis* is transmitted sexually and from mother to infant at the time of birth. Trachoma, still endemic in arid parts of the developing world but rare in industrialized countries, spreads within families via close nonsexual contact. Recently, Grayston and colleagues described a fastidious new strain of chlamydia that was originally called the TWAR agent. Subsequent genetic studies have identified this organism as a new chlamydial species, *Chlamydia pneumoniae*. *C. pneumoniae* appears to be a common cause of both upper respiratory tract infections and pneumonia worldwide and often occurs episodically in community-wide epidemics. No animal reservoirs have been identified, and the mode of transmission is presumed to be from person to person via respiratory droplets and secretions.

All three chlamydia species possess a genus-specific, heat-stable lipopolysaccharide antigen that serves as the basis for the widely available complement fixation serologic test. Species- and immunotype-specific antigens have also been described, and the latter serve as the basis for subdividing *C. trachomatis* into 15 immunotypes using the microimmunofluorescence test of Wang and Grayston. Specific immunotypes tend to cause particular clinical syndromes. Types A, B, Ba, and C produce endemic trachoma (see Ch. 346). Types D, E, F, G, H, I, J, and K cause oculogenital infections in adults (see Ch. 335) and ocular, respiratory, and genital infections in infants. Types L1, L2, and L3 produce lymphogranuloma venereum (LGV) (see Ch. 337) and proctocolitis, primarily in homosexual men (see Ch. 103). LGV strains of *C. trachomatis* possess properties that distinguish them from non-LGV strains biologically, including more efficient cell entry and cell-to-cell infectivity in tissue culture, as well as increased mouse lethality upon intracerebral injection. Only one serovar of the new species, *C. pneumoniae*, has been identified to date.

Chlamydiae replicate by means of a unique life cycle unlike that of other bacteria. The 300-nm elementary body (the infective and extracellular form of chlamydia) initiates infection by attachment to receptors in the susceptible host cell's outer membrane. Subsequently, the elementary body enters the host cell by endocytosis. Within the resulting phagosome, the elementary body reorganizes within 6 hours into the larger 800- to 1000-nm and more metabolically active reticulate body. These reticulate bodies undergo repeated binary division until a large inclusion occupying much of the cell's cytoplasm and containing many reticulate bodies is formed. Reticulate bodies possess many ribosomes and synthesize deoxyribonucleic acid (DNA), ribonucleic acid (RNA), proteins, and other molecules but cannot generate ATP. After 24 hours, some of the reticulate bodies condense to form compact elementary bodies in the mature inclusion, and the latter are released into the extracellular environment to begin the cycle anew by infecting adjacent cells.

C. trachomatis preferentially infects columnar epithelial cells. In most patients, *C. trachomatis* infections remain superficial, involving mucosal surfaces of the eye, nasopharynx, cervix, urethra, and rectum (Table 345–1). Many of these infections produce few or no symptoms and tend to be subacute in nature and mild in terms of the signs they produce. Ascending infections of the endometrium, fallopian tube, liver capsule, epididymis, or lung produce more severe symptoms and signs and can be regarded as more extensive or invasive infections. Infection of the upper genital tract in women is of particular importance, often leading to tubal scarring with resultant complications of infertility and ectopic pregnancy. LGV strains of *C. trachomatis* infect lymphoid cells and macrophages as well as epithelial cells and cause the most invasive disease, manifested either by proctocolitis or by painful inguinal adenopathy and fever. *C. trachomatis* occasionally causes nongenital systemic infection, including culture-negative endocarditis, peritonitis, and pneumonia in adults. Both *C. pneumoniae* and *C. psittaci* preferentially infect respiratory epithelial cells, but the latter has a broader host range that includes macrophages (see Ch. 348). *C. psittaci* also causes culture-negative endocarditis.

Since many chlamydial infections produce either no symptoms or nonspecific symptoms and signs, laboratory confirmation of infection should be sought. Available techniques include direct microscopic examination of tissue scrapings or secretions for typical inclusions or for elementary bodies; isolation of the

TABLE 345–1. CLINICAL SPECTRUM OF C. TRACHOMATIS INFECTIONS*

Males	Females	Infants
Uncomplicated Infections		
Urethritis (NGU, PGU)	Cervicitis	Conjunctivitis
Proctitis	Urethritis	Pharyngitis
Conjunctivitis	Proctitis	Asymptomatic rectal and vaginal carriage
Pharyngitis	Conjunctivitis	
	Pharyngitis	
	Bartholinitis	
Invasive Infections		
Proctocolitis	Endometritis	Pneumonia
Lymphogranuloma venereum	Salpingitis	? Otitis media
Epididymitis	Perihepatitis	
? Prostatitis	Postpartum endometritis	
Complications	Infertility	? Chronic pulmonary impairment
Reiter's syndrome	Ectopic pregnancy	
Rectal strictures	Chronic salpingitis	
? Urethral strictures	Complications of pregnancy (? prematurity, stillbirth)	
? Sterility		

*Excludes trachoma.
NGU = nongonococcal urethritis; PGU = postgonococcal urethritis.

organism in cell culture; and assessment of antichlamydial antibody in serum or secretions. Adoption of cell culture techniques for isolation of *C. trachomatis* from patients' secretions or biopsies (replacing the more cumbersome embryonated yolk sac method) has been a major factor contributing to recognition of the wide spectrum of infections caused by *C. trachomatis*. Inclusions formed in cell culture monolayers can be visualized using iodine, Giemsa's, or immunofluorescent staining procedures. Despite widespread use in research laboratories, cell culture procedures for isolation of *C. trachomatis* have not been generally available to clinicians because of their expense and technical difficulty. Lack of an available confirmatory diagnostic test and the inability to screen high-risk populations for infection have been major factors contributing to the increasing incidence of genital and neonatal *C. trachomatis* infections in this country. Newer immunodiagnostic procedures that detect chlamydial antigen in patients' secretions have recently been developed and can be used for diagnostic confirmation and for screening where cultures are not available. These tests utilize monoclonal or polyclonal antichlamydial antibodies to demonstrate the presence of chlamydial antigens in infected secretions by either enzyme-linked immunosorbent assay (ELISA) or immunofluorescence techniques, and have approximate sensitivities of 80 to 90 per cent and specificities of 97 to 99 per cent compared with culture in high-risk populations. Nucleic acid hybridization tests using chlamydia-specific DNA and RNA probes have also been developed and have similar sensitivity and specificity. Neither cultures, specific antigen detection, nor nucleic acid probes are routinely available for the diagnosis of *C. pneumoniae* and *C. psittaci* infections; hence, these infections must be diagnosed serologically.

Chlamydial infection stimulates both a humoral and a cellular immune response, but neither appears to be completely protective against subsequent infection with either homologous or heterologous strains. Both local and systemic antibody can be demonstrated after acute infection, and immunoglobulin G (IgG) antibody neutralizes infective elementary bodies. Some have advocated that the immune response actually participates in the disease process by producing continued inflammation. Serodiagnosis of chlamydial infections has limited applicability except in specific circumstances. The complement fixation test, available in most health department laboratories, should be used for confirmation of suspected psittacosis or LGV. A titer of 1:64 or greater in a patient with a clinical syndrome compatible with LGV can be regarded as diagnostic. In patients with pneumonia, however, the complement fixation test does not distinguish between *C. psittaci* and *C. pneumoniae* infection (see Ch. 348). The microimmunofluorescence test is useful in the diagnosis of infant pneumonia, pelvic inflammatory disease, or Fitz-Hugh-Curtis syndrome as well as suspected LGV or *C. pneumoniae* infection but is available only in research laboratories. Uncomplicated genital infections evoke only low titer-antibody responses, and acute infections cannot be easily distinguished from pre-existing antibody in many patients.

C. trachomatis infections can be treated with a variety of antimicrobial agents. Those with greatest activity in cell culture assays and in clinical studies include the tetracyclines (tetracyline HCl, doxycycline, and minocycline), erythromycin, sulfonamides, sulfamethoxazole-trimethoprim, and rifampin. Ofloxacin, a new fluoroquinolone antibiotic, has in vitro activity against chlamydia and has been effective in clinical trials of uncomplicated infection. The β-lactam antibiotics produce abnormal inclusions in cell culture and inhibit replication but have been largely ineffective in clinical treatment trials. The aminoglycosides, vancomycin, and spectinomycin have no activity against chlamydiae. In general, chlamydial infections require 7 to 21 days of antibiotic treatment; single-day regimens have been largely ineffective. Treatment failure usually indicates noncompliance, reinfection, or inadequate duration of drug therapy. Clinically significant resistance to tetracycline or erythromycin has not been described.

Bowie WR, Caldwell HD, Jones RP, et al. (eds.): Chlamydial Infections. Cambridge, Cambridge University Press, 1990, pp 1–601. *Excellent source of most recent knowledge on all aspects of chlamydial infection, including 13 comprehensive review articles.*

Grayston JT: *Chlamydia pneumoniae*, Strain TWAR. Chest 95:664–669, 1989. *Excellent overview of knowledge regarding this new pathogen.*
Stamm WE: Diagnosis of *Chlamydia trachomatis* genitourinary infections. Ann Intern Med 108:710–717, 1988. *Review of clinical criteria and new diagnostic tests for common chlamydial infections.*

---

346 Trachoma

Chlamydia trachomatis causes two epidemiologically distinct patterns of ocular infection. In trachoma-endemic parts of the world, *C. trachomatis* immunotypes A, B, Ba, and C cause trachoma, a chronic eye disease that may lead to severe visual impairment or blindness. In nonendemic areas, immunotypes D through K produce a milder, self-limited conjunctivitis in infants born to mothers with cervical infection or in adults who acquire ocular infection after secondary spread from genital sites.

Since antiquity, trachomatous infection has been recognized in the Mediterranean basin and in the Orient, and it remains prevalent in Africa and Asia. Although the incidence has been decreasing over the last 30 years, millions have eye infections with chlamydiae, with millions blinded as a result. Trachoma flourishes in hot, dry areas that have a shortage of available water and poor hygienic customs. Initial infection usually occurs in early childhood, and in certain parts of the world virtually the entire population is infected with chlamydiae before reaching adulthood. Specific chlamydia antigens may stimulate a local immune response resulting in a hypersensitivity reaction. Repeated exposure to chlamydiae and the high prevalence of bacterial superinfection with *Haemophilus* spp., pneumococci, staphylococci, and Enterobacteriaceae in these populations contribute to the severity of the resulting eye disease. In the United States, trachoma is occasionally seen on Indian reservations in the Southwest, in Mexican-Americans, and in immigrants from endemic areas, but such cases rarely result in major visual impairment.

Persons with active trachoma shed chlamydiae in desquamated conjunctival cells, in conjunctival exudate, and in tears, which then may be transmitted by fingers, fomites, and perhaps flies. In endemic areas, transmission by these routes occurs through close personal contact, especially within family units and in groups of young children. Patients with early active infection shed more infective chlamydiae than those with chronic infection. However, even patients with long-term eye disease unaccompanied by signs of current activity may shed chlamydiae and thus serve as a source of infection.

Typically, trachoma in children begins insidiously at about age 2 as a follicular conjunctivitis, most noticeable in the conjunctiva of the upper lid and the tarsal plate. Histologically, inclusion bodies appear within the conjunctival epithelial cells, polymorphonuclear leukocytes infiltrate the epithelium, and subepithelial lymphoid follicles develop. Reinfection is common during this period. Next the cornea becomes involved, with epithelial keratitis and subepithelial corneal infiltration resulting in opacities. Blood vessels from the limbus, accompanied by fibroblasts, invade the cornea to form a pannus. Progression of the inflammatory response leads to necrosis and scarring of the conjunctiva and gradual corneal vascularization from the upper limbus downward. Eventually a dense fibrovascular pannus extends over part or all of the cornea to grossly impair vision. Linear or stellate scars appear on the conjunctiva. Progressive scarring of the subepithelial tissues leads to deformation of the tarsal plate and results in entropion, trichiasis, and further corneal damage. Destruction of the conjunctival goblet cells and lacrimal ducts and gland produces xerosis. The latter changes often follow secondary bacterial infection, which may also produce corneal ulceration and accelerate loss of vision. Typically there are no systemic symptoms or signs of infection. Active infection with chlamydia is common between the ages of 2 and 5, but then resolves. The disease process may evolve over about 10 years in hyperendemic areas, but is milder and more slowly progressive in most cases, evolving over 20 to 40 years.

The traditional diagnostic criteria for trachoma include lymphoid follicles on the upper tarsal plate, limbal follicles, typical conjunctival scars, and vascular pannus. Early in the disease the last two can be detected only by slit-lamp examination. The presence of any two of these features confirms the diagnosis. Laboratory confirmation of trachoma is based on (1) identification of typical inclusions in epithelial cells from a conjunctival swab or scraping (usually done by Giemsa's or immunofluorescence staining); (2) cultivation of chlamydiae from a conjunctival specimen in cell culture; (3) microimmunofluorescent antibody in high titer in tears; or (4) demonstration of chlamydia using noncultural tests such as antigen detection or nucleic acid hybridization. Approximately 20 to 60 per cent of children with early inflammatory trachoma have Giemsa-positive scrapings; higher yields result from cultures of chlamydiae.

In the differential diagnosis of ocular chlamydial infection, epidemic keratoconjunctivitis (usually caused by adenovirus type 8 or type 19), herpetic keratoconjunctivitis, Newcastle disease virus conjunctivitis, acute hemorrhagic conjunctivitis caused by enterovirus type 70 or coxsackievirus, reactions to allergens and irritating chemicals, and other bacterial causes of conjunctivitis must be considered. Some of these entities may coexist with chlamydial infections, and repeated ophthalmologic examinations and extensive laboratory evaluation may be required to establish a correct diagnosis.

Adult inclusion conjunctivitis caused by *C. trachomatis* usually presents as an acute follicular conjunctivitis with preauricular lymphadenopathy. Untreated, it regresses slowly, but keratitis with marginal infiltrates, subepithelial opacities, and corneal neovascularization may develop in the conjunctiva. Unlike trachoma, adult inclusion conjunctivitis rarely impairs vision permanently.

Control of chronic trachoma in endemic areas has been attempted using tetracycline or erythromycin ointment in the eyes of all affected children in the community for 21 to 60 days. Oral administration of erythromycin has been used as an alternative. Antibiotic therapy usually suppresses clinical activity and chlamydiae as well as bacterial growth but may not eradicate chlamydiae permanently. However, in endemic areas, repeated courses of drug treatment are beneficial because they reduce severity of eye disease and thus avoid progression toward blindness. Even one dose per month of doxycycline, 300 mg (2.5 to 4 mg per kilogram), can provide clinical benefit by converting severe to mild eye disease. Drug therapy has no influence on scars or pannus. Surgical correction is required for serious entropion or trichiasis. Topical corticosteroids and caustic substances have no place in therapy. For acute adult inclusion conjunctivitis, tetracycline HCl, 2.0 grams given orally daily in divided doses, or erythromycin, 2.0 grams given orally daily in divided doses for 1 to 2 weeks, successfully treats genital tract as well as ocular involvement. Sulfisoxazole, 4 grams daily, may also be effective. Sexual partners must be treated simultaneously in order to avoid reinfection.

The potential measures to prevent trachoma include efforts to increase the supply of water; practices to maintain cleanliness, such as frequent handwashing and avoidance of use of common towels; and measures to reduce flies. The disease has disappeared in many areas coincident with improved hygienic conditions. It is important to detect mild early infection in young children in endemic areas and to apply effective drug treatment repeatedly to prevent the blinding progression of the disease. Detection and treatment of adults who already have visual impairment probably can reduce the source of infection for children. Entire family groups or communities should be treated simultaneously. Efforts to prevent trachoma with a vaccine have been unsuccessful.

Dawson CR: Eye disease with chlamydial infection. *In* Oriel D, Ridgway G, Schachter J, et al. (eds.): Chlamydial Infections. Cambridge, Cambridge University Press, 1986, pp 135–144. *Excellent overview of all aspects of trachoma.*

Schachter J, Dawson CR: Epidemiology of trachoma predicts more blindness in the future. Scand J Infect Dis Suppl 69:55–62, 1990. *Reviews trends in the epidemiology and control of trachoma.*

347 Neonatal Chlamydial Infections

Between 5 and 22 per cent of pregnant women have *Chlamydia trachomatis* infection of the cervix, with neonatal infection occurring when the infant passes through the infected birth canal. Ascending intrauterine infection of the fetus has not been demonstrated. After birth, 30 to 50 per cent of infants born to infected mothers have cultural evidence of infection, 25 per cent manifest clinically apparent conjunctivitis, and 10 to 15 per cent acquire nasopharyngeal infection, which in some cases progresses to chlamydial neonatal pneumonia. Otitis media and symptomatic nasopharyngitis may be caused by *C. trachomatis* in some infants. Untreated neonatal infections may become chronic and persist over many months.

Neonatal *C. trachomatis* inclusion conjunctivitis typically begins 5 to 14 days after birth. In infants given ocular prophylaxis, however, onset may be delayed for weeks or months. The infection must be differentiated from gonococcal ophthalmia (which has a shorter incubation period of 1 to 3 days) and from other common causes of neonatal conjunctivitis (*Streptococcus pneumoniae, Haemophilus influenzae, Staphylococcus aureus,* and group D streptococci). Typical manifestations include lid and conjunctival swelling, mucopurulent ocular discharge, conjunctival hyperemia, and membrane formation. Untreated, the disease persists 3 to 12 months but usually heals without sequelae. Rarely, conjunctival scarring and corneal neovascularization occur. Neonates with inclusion conjunctivitis frequently have concomitant chlamydial infection of the nasopharynx, rectum, urethra, and vagina, usually without associated clinical manifestations at these sites.

The diagnosis can be rapidly established by demonstration of chlamydial inclusions or elementary bodies in conjunctival scrapings stained by Giemsa's stain or immunofluorescence. Alternatively, demonstration of chlamydial antigen in ocular secretions by ELISA or cultures for *C. trachomatis* can be used if available.

The relative effectiveness of topical ocular prophylaxis for chlamydial eye infection using silver nitrate, erythromycin ointment, or tetracycline ointment has become increasingly unclear. Early studies suggested that topical erythromycin was most effective and silver nitrate least effective, but more recent studies have found little difference among these three regimens. Many health departments currently recommend the use of topical erythromycin. However, topical erythromycin prophylaxis does not cure concomitant nasopharyngeal or rectal infection. Thus, a better preventive approach would be screening and treatment of pregnant women for *C. trachomatis* infection before term. This approach essentially eliminates *C. trachomatis* infections in neonates and should be the strategy of choice in high-risk women.

Since many infants with inclusion conjunctivitis have concomitant nasopharyngeal, rectal, and vaginal *C. trachomatis* infection, systemic rather than topical therapy should be used. In addition, relapses often follow topical therapy. Erythromycin, 40 to 50 mg per kilogram per day in four divided doses for 14 to 21 days, cures more than 80 per cent of cases. Both parents should be examined for *C. trachomatis* infection and should be treated with tetracycline or erythromycin (for nursing mothers) if cultures or immunodiagnostic tests are not available.

Approximately 10 per cent of infants born to infected mothers develop a distinctive subacute chlamydial pneumonia between the first and fourth months of life. Typically, tachypnea, a staccato cough, inspiratory rales, elevated serum globulin concentrations, and eosinophilia are seen, but fever is absent. Hyperinflated lungs with scattered interstitial infiltrates are evident on chest radiographic examination. The disease lasts for weeks to months but is mild in most infants and resolves without specific therapy. However, marked hypoxemia and apnea have been reported in some cases. Lung biopsies have demonstrated chlamydial inclusions, alveoli with inflammatory exudate, and a lymphocytic interstitial infiltration of the bronchial submucosa. In some cases, *C. trachomatis* has been recovered from lung tissue. Diagnosis in most instances can be suspected on clinical grounds and confirmed by the demonstration of chlamydial inclusions or elementary bodies on Giemsa- or immunofluorescent-stained smears of the conjunctivae or nasopharynx. *C. trachomatis* should be sought by cell culture of eye scrapings, nasopharyngeal swabs, or rectal swabs if they are available. Rising high-titer immunoglobulin M (IgM) microimmunofluorescent antibody to *C. trachomatis* can be demonstrated in the majority of infants with pneumonia. Erythromycin, 50 mg per kilogram per day in four divided doses for 14 to 21 days, has been recommended for treatment of pneumonia in infants, although there are no control trials demonstrating the benefits of this regimen. Chronic respiratory impairment and persistent pulmonary symptoms may develop in some patients.

Hammerschlag MR, Cummings C, Roblin PM, et al.: Efficacy of neonatal ocular prophylaxis for the prevention of chlamydial and gonococcal conjunctivitis. N Engl J Med 320:769–772, 1989.

Harrison HR: Chlamydial infection in neonates and children. *In* Oriel D, Ridgway G, Schachter J, et al. (eds.): Chlamydial Infections. Cambridge, Cambridge University Press, 1986, pp 283–292. *Excellent review.*

Laga M, Plummer FA, Piot P, et al.: Prophylaxis of gonococcal and chlamydial ophthalmia neonatorum: A comparison of silver nitrate and tetracycline. N Engl J Med 318:653–657, 1988. *Good discussion of the issues of ocular prophylaxis.*

348 Infections Due to *Chlamydia psittaci* and *Chlamydia pneumoniae**

PSITTACOSIS

Psittacosis (ornithosis), an infection of birds caused by *Chlamydia psittaci*, can produce asymptomatic infection, a transient influenza-like illness, or serious pneumonic disease when transmitted to humans.

Parrots and parakeets are common carriers and until recently were the major source of human infection. With better control of psittacine disease in aviaries, other birds now cause more human infections, including turkeys, pigeons, ducks, and other fowl. Persons working with birds are at greatest risk, notably pet shop employees, pigeon handlers, and poultry workers. There is no risk associated with eating poultry products.

The agent is present in the blood, tissue, feathers, and discharges of infected birds. Although avian disease can be fatal, infected birds frequently show only minimal evidence of illness. Birds having active infections are most likely to transmit the disease, but asymptomatic carriers are common, and birds can transmit the agent for months.

Psittacosis is generally acquired by the respiratory route through inhalation of infected dried bird excreta or by handling of infected birds. Cases have been reported after only brief exposure to birds, and 20 per cent of patients can recall no history of exposure to birds. Person-to-person transmission of psittacosis is rare.

PATHOLOGY. In birds, the principal sites of disease are the liver, spleen, and pericardium. In humans, the lung is most commonly involved. *C. psittaci* gains access to the human body via the respiratory route, rapidly enters the blood, and reaches the reticuloendothelial cells of the liver and spleen. After replication in these sites, invasion of the lung occurs via hematogenous spread. Lobar pneumonitis results from inflammation and progressive edema of the alveoli, often accompanied by small hemorrhages. Thick, gelatinous plugs of mucus may fill major and minor bronchi and account for the severe cyanosis and progressive anoxia seen in fatal cases. Foci of necrosis may occur in more severely affected parts of the lung and are sometimes associated with capillary thrombi. The process is generally most severe in

dependent bronchopulmonary segments. Monocytes and macrophages containing cytoplasmic inclusion bodies, which represent the agent (LCL bodies), are characteristic. Hyperplasia and monocytic infiltration of pulmonary and hilar lymph nodes and splenic enlargement with occasional areas of focal necrosis occur. Rarely the liver shows intralobular focal necrosis and swollen Kupffer's cells containing psittacosis elementary bodies. Pathologic changes in the myocardium, heart valves, pericardium, meninges, brain, adrenal glands, pancreas, and kidneys have been reported.

CLINICAL MANIFESTATIONS. Wide variations can occur in the clinical picture. The incubation period ranges from 7 to 15 days but may be longer. Asymptomatic or mild influenza-like infections probably are the rule. Moderate or severe infections, although less frequent, are more commonly diagnosed. The onset of illness may be insidious, but it often starts with chills and a fever that rises slowly to 39 to 40.5°C during the first week of illness. The pulse may be slow relative to the level of the fever. Headache is severe. Malaise, anorexia, nausea, vomiting, severe myalgias, particularly in the neck and back, and arthralgias are common. Cough is generally prominent but may be delayed until late in the first week. Small amounts of mucoid sputum with occasional blood streaking are the rule. Changes in mentation are often seen. Delirium or stupor may occur in severe cases toward the end of the first week and usually are associated with severe pulmonary involvement, cyanosis, and anoxia. Other neurologic manifestations are uncommon. A macular rash (Horder's spots) resembling that seen in typhoid has occasionally been described. Jaundice and progressive renal failure have been reported in severe cases. Severe dyspnea, tachypnea, tachycardia, cyanosis, jaundice, delirium, and stupor are all poor prognostic signs.

The physical findings of pneumonia are usually sparse. Chest roentgenograms often reveal infiltrates not detected at the bedside. Examination may reveal only fever, painful muscle groups, an elevated respiratory rate, and a relative bradycardia. Fine, crepitant rales may be heard in localized areas over the lungs, but true consolidation is less common. Pleurisy with effusion occurs but is unusual. Mild hepatomegaly is frequent. A palpable spleen has been noted in a substantial number of patients. Splenomegaly in a patient with undiagnosed acute pneumonitis should raise the consideration of psittacosis. An erythematous pharynx may be noted. In rare instances there may be signs of pericarditis or myocarditis. In prolonged, severe illness, thrombophlebitis and pulmonary infarction have been reported as late complications.

Patients with mild cases may recover in 7 days. More severe infections may last 12 to 21 days without specific treatment. Defervescence is generally slow, and a prolonged convalescence is common. Relapses have been reported even after appropriate treatment. Reinfections have been described. Occasional cases of endocarditis caused by *C. psittaci* in patients with sterile blood cultures have been described.

LABORATORY FINDINGS. The leukocyte count is usually normal or slightly elevated. The erythrocyte sedimentation rate is generally elevated. Chest roentgenograms show soft, patchy infiltrates radiating outward from the hilum, which tend to be more prominent in dependent lobes or segments. Occasionally diffuse miliary, nodular, or frank lobar distribution of infiltrates is seen.

A specific diagnosis can be made only by isolation of the agent or by serologic studies. The agent is present in the blood and sputum during the first 2 to 3 weeks, but owing to the high risk of laboratory-acquired infection, isolation is hazardous and should not be attempted except in special laboratories. Diagnosis is generally made by a fourfold rise in complement-fixing antibodies. A significant change in antibody titers is generally present by the twelfth to fourteenth day of disease; the titers are usually maximal by 30 days, then slowly wane. Treatment can delay or suppress antibody response. A serum complement-fixation titer of 1:32 during the acute illness is presumptive evidence of psittacosis. However, the complement fixation test is also positive in infections with LGV strains of *C. trachomatis* and with *C. pneumoniae* infections (see below). False-positive complement-fixation tests have been reported with Q fever, brucellosis, and legionnaires' disease.

DIFFERENTIAL DIAGNOSIS. Establishing a specific diag-

---

*Portions of this chapter are based upon "Psittacosis (Ornithosis, Parrot Fever)" by William Schaffner, in the 17th edition of the *Cecil Textbook of Medicine*.

nosis of psittacosis is of importance because of its potential severity, its response to antimicrobials, and the public health significance of psittacosis. All cases should be reported to the local health department. The syndrome of idiopathic pneumonia accompanied by protracted high fever, usually severe headache, and relative bradycardia should suggest psittacosis. Often a history of contact with birds is the only clue to diagnosis and may be elicited only by repeated questioning of the patient and family. When pneumonic symptoms are prominent, psittacosis must be differentiated from legionnaires' disease, viral pneumonias, mycoplasmal pneumonia, influenza, Q fever, tularemia, tuberculosis, fungal infection, and other bacterial pneumonias. If pneumonic symptoms are not prominent, psittacosis can be confused with other systemic febrile illnesses such as typhoid fever, brucellosis, infectious mononucleosis, infectious hepatitis, miliary tuberculosis, or the viral meningoencephalitides.

TREATMENT. The tetracyclines are the drugs of choice, and early diagnosis and initiation of treatment may be lifesaving. After institution of therapy with 2 to 3 grams daily, both fever and symptoms are generally controlled within 48 to 72 hours, although the response may be indolent. Although the disease apparently responds to penicillin in doses above 2 million units daily and to erythromycin, tetracycline remains the drug of choice. Treatment should be continued for at least 10 days after defervescence to prevent relapse. With treatment, mortality rates as low as 1 to 5 per cent can be achieved.

CHLAMYDIA PNEUMONIAE (Strain TWAR)

A new species of chlamydia, *Chlamydia pneumoniae*, has recently been established. Current evidence indicates that *C. pneumoniae* (formerly called the TWAR organism) is a frequent cause of upper and lower respiratory tract infection in both children and adults. Seroprevalence studies show that about 40 per cent of most adult populations tested worldwide have evidence of prior infection with this agent. Infections are uncommon in children under the age of 5 but are frequent in children between the ages of 8 and 15 and in young adults. *C. pneumoniae* has been identified as a cause of epidemics of respiratory infection in closed populations such as military recruits. The organism may be transmitted in communities in a cyclic fashion. Thus, in some years many infections occur, whereas in other years very few are noted. Studies to date have failed to identify an animal reservoir for *C. pneumoniae*. It is believed to be an exclusively human pathogen that is transmitted from person to person via respiratory secretions in much the same way as many viral respiratory infections and *M. pneumoniae*. Transmission has been demonstrated within households, schools, and military barracks.

Chlamydia pneumoniae is an obligate intracellular pathogen with 10 per cent or less DNA relatedness to *C. psittaci* or *C. trachomatis*. Like other chlamydiae, it produces cytoplasmic inclusions in infected cells. *C. pneumoniae* has unique pear-shaped elementary bodies and forms dense oval inclusions that do not contain glycogen. Only a single serovar of *C. pneumoniae* has been recognized to date. The organism can be cultured in HeLa 229 and McCoy cells but has been difficult to isolate from patients with suspected infection. More recently, HL cells have been identified as a more sensitive cell line for isolation of *C. pneumoniae*.

Clinically, *C. pneumoniae* produces a spectrum of respiratory infections that differ somewhat in manifestations by age. In children, teenagers, and young adults, the most common manifestations are bronchitis, sinusitis, and mild pneumonia. Occasionally, pharyngitis is seen. It is thought that many infections are asymptomatic or produce mild nonfebrile upper respiratory tract infections. *C. pneumoniae* infection, however, may frequently be prolonged, lasting for several weeks. Clinically, the pneumonia produced by *C. pneumoniae* generally resembles that seen with mycoplasma infection. Chest radiographs most commonly show small, single, subsegmental infiltrates, and more extensive consolidation is rarely seen. In adults, pneumonia may be more severe and bronchitis and sinusitis more prolonged. With most infections due to *C. pneumoniae*, the white blood cell count is normal.

Specific diagnosis of infection due to *C. pneumoniae* is difficult. Although the organism can be cultivated in HL cells and other cell lines, it is not easily grown and most laboratories are not equipped to undertake cultures. Similarly, specific serologic testing is not widely available. The complement fixation test for chlamydiae can be utilized and is available to most clinicians. A fourfold titer rise or a single titer of 1:64 or greater suggests the diagnosis. However, antibodies to *C. psittaci* or *C. trachomatis* infection are also measured by this test, and hence it is not specific for *C. pneumoniae*. The microimmunofluorescence test for *C. pneumoniae* provides a specific means of diagnosis but is not widely available. Using this test, a fourfold titer rise, an IgM of 1:16 or greater, or a single IgG titer of 1:512 or greater supports the diagnosis. More sensitive and easily performed methods for diagnosis of *C. pneumoniae* infection are clearly needed.

In vitro, tetracyclines and erythromycin are the most effective drugs against *C. pneumoniae*. Sulfonamides are not effective. Although no controlled trials have been conducted, it is currently recommended that therapy with tetracycline or erythromycin, 2 grams per day, be provided for 10 to 14 days.

Grayston JT: *Chlamydia pneumoniae*, strain TWAR. Chest 95:664–669, 1989.

Grayston JT, Wang SP, Kuo CC, Campbell LA: Current knowledge of *Chlamydia pneumoniae* strain TWAR, an important cause of pneumonia and other acute respiratory diseases. Eur J Clin Microbiol Infect Dis 8:191–202, 1989. *Reviews current knowledge of* C. pneumoniae.

Jariwalla AG, Davies BH, White J: Infective endocarditis complicating psittacosis: Response to rifampicin. Br Med J 1:155, 1980. *Endocarditis caused by psittacosis is reviewed concisely.*

Macfarlane JT, Macrae AD: Psittacosis. Br Med Bull 39:163, 1983. *A well-written review.*

Schaffner W, Drutz DJ, Duncan GW, et al.: The clinical spectrum of endemic psittacosis. Arch Intern Med 119:433, 1967. *Good descriptions of clinical presentations.*

Rickettsial Diseases

Richard B. Hornick

349 Introduction

The rickettsiae are small obligate intracellular, gram-negative pathogens. They do not have a symbiotic relationship with human host cells and therefore cause metabolic derangements that result in cell death. Infections with the typhus and spotted fever groups of rickettsiae involve endothelial cells. This host-pathogen interaction results in a perivasculitis. Q fever induces granulomas in the liver plus interstitial pneumonia. Ehrlichiosis is a new human disease caused by a rickettsial organism that has long been associated with disease in dogs. *Ehrlichia canis* appears to be transmitted by ticks, can be demonstrated rarely inside leukocytes, and induces antibodies. Fortunately, these small, gram-negative organisms are susceptible to tetracycline and chloramphenicol antibiotics so that patients recover quickly once the drugs are administered.

Each of the rickettsiae is transmitted to humans by ticks, mites, lice, fleas, or aerosols originating from animal products (placentas, Q fever) or from feces of the aforementioned insects. In the United States, there are relatively few cases of rickettsial infections. Rocky Mountain spotted fever is the most prevalent, 600

TABLE 349–1. SUMMARY OF SOME EPIDEMIOLOGIC FEATURES OF SELECTED RICKETTSIAL DISEASES OF HUMANS

Disease	Organism	Natural Cycle Arthropod Vector	Natural Cycle Reservoir/ Mammalian Host	Usual Mode of Transmission to Humans	Common Occupational or Environmental Association	Geographic Distribution
Typhus group Murine typhus	*Rickettsia mooseri* (*R. typhi*)	Flea	Rodents	Infected flea feces into broken skin or aerosol to mucous membranes	Rat-infected premises (shops, warehouses, grain elevators)	Scattered foci, worldwide
Epidemic typhus	*R. prowazekii*	Body louse	Humans*	Infected crushed louse of feces into broken skin or aerosol to mucous membranes	Lousy human population with louse transfer	Worldwide
Brill-Zinsser disease	*R. prowazekii*	Recrudescence months to years after primary attack of louse-borne typhus			Unknown; ?stress	Worldwide
Spotted fever group (selected examples) Rocky Mountain spotted fever	*R. rickettsii*	Ixodid ticks	Ticks/small mammals	Tick bite, mechanical transfer to mucous membranes, ?airborne	Tick-infested terrain, houses, dogs	Western hemisphere
Ehrlichiosis	*Ehrlichia canis*	Ticks	?Dogs	Tick bite	Tick-infested areas	At least 12 states in US, primarily southern states
Boutonneuse fever	*R. conorii*	Ixodid ticks	Ticks/rodents, dogs	Tick bite	Tick-infested terrain, houses, dogs	Mediterranean littoral, Africa, ?Indian subcontinent
Rickettsialpox	*R. akari*	Mouse mite	Mite/mice	Mouse mite bite	Unique mouse- and mite-infested premises (incinerators)	United States, U.S.S.R., Korea, ?Central Africa
Scrub typhus Tsutsugamushi disease	*R. tsutsugamushi* (multiple serotypes)	Chigger	Chigger/?rodents	Chigger bite	Chigger-infested terrain; secondary scrub, grass airfields, golf courses	Asia, Australia, New Guinea, Pacific Islands
Q fever	*Coxiella burnetii*	?Ticks	Ticks/mammals	Inhalation of dried airborne infective material; ?tick bite	Domestic animals or products, dairies, lambing pens, slaughterhouses	Worldwide
Trench fever	*Rochalimaea quintana*	Body louse	Humans	Infected crushed louse or feces into broken skin; ?aerosol to mucous membranes	Lousy human population with louse transfer	Africa, Mexico, ?South America, ?Eastern Europe

*Recent isolations of putative *R. prowazekii* from flying squirrels in the eastern United States have not been evaluated as reservoirs for human infection. Previous claims of involvement of domestic animals are now largely discounted.

to 700 cases having been reported annually from 1985 to 1989. Fewer cases of Q fever and murine typhus are identified each year. Certain other rickettsial infections are major public health problems in developing countries but are not found in the United States, e.g., scrub typhus. The potential for tourists to return to the United States with an emerging rickettsial infection is increasing. Because of the rarity of rickettsial infections in the United States, diagnosis may be delayed. Delays in diagnosing these illnesses can adversely affect the potential for recovery.

In this introductory chapter, three tables are included that summarize, first, the epidemiologic features of rickettsial infections; second, the host cells involved in the pathogenesis of the disease; and third, those clinical manifestations of the clinical features that will assist in differentiating the various forms of rickettsial infections. The following chapters provide additional details on the major rickettsial infections that are found in this country or that represent potential threats to persons traveling abroad.

TABLE 349–2. RICKETTSIA TARGET CELL RELATIONSHIPS, PATHOLOGIC LESIONS, AND CLINICAL MANIFESTATIONS OF HUMAN RICKETTSIOSES*

Disease	Target Cell	Host-Cell Association	Basic Lesion	Clinical Manifestations
Typhus-like fevers Typhus group	Endothelial	Free intracytoplasmic	Vasculitis	Acute self-limited fever
Scrub typhus	Endothelial	Free intracytoplasmic	Vasculitis	Acute self-limited fever
Spotted fever group	Endothelial, smooth muscle	Free intracytoplasmic and intranuclear	Vasculitis	Acute self-limited fever
Ehrlichiosis	Leukocytes	Intracytoplasmic inclusion body	Leukopenia, thrombocytopenia, liver cell damage	Acute self-limited fever
Q fever	Reticuloendothelial	Intracytoplasmic vacuole	Granulomas	Acute self-limited fever, "atypical pneumonia," subacute hepatitis, subacute endocarditis
Trench fever	Unknown	Pericellular (in louse and cell culture)	Unknown	Recurring febrile episodes

*Adapted from Stickland (ed.): Hunter's Tropical Medicine. Philadelphia, W. B. Saunders Company, 1984.

TABLE 349–3. SOME CLINICAL FEATURES OF SELECTED RICKETTSIAL DISEASES

Disease	Usual Incubation Period (Days)	Eschar	Rash Onset, Day of Disease	Distribution	Type	Usual Duration of Disease* (Days)	Usual Severity†	Fever After Chemotherapy (Hours)
Typhus group								
Murine typhus	12 (8–16)	None	5–7	Trunk → extremities	Macular, maculopapular	12 (8–16)	Moderate	48–72
Epidemic typhus	12 (10–14)	None	5–7	Trunk → extremities	Macular, maculopapular, petechial	14 (10–18)	Severe	48–72
Brill-Zinsser disease	—	None		Trunk → extremities	Macular	7–11	Relatively mild	48–72
Spotted fever group								
Rocky Mountain spotted fever	7 (3–12)	None	3–5	Extremities → trunk, face	Macular, maculopapular, petechial	16 (10–20)	Severe	72
Ehrlichiosis	7–21	None	Rare?	Unknown	Petechial	7 (3–19)	Mild	72
Boutonneuse fever	5–7	Often present	3–4	Trunk, extremities, face, palms, soles	Macular, maculopapular, petechial	10 (7–14) 7	Moderate	—
Rickettsialpox	?9–17	Often present	1–3	Trunk → face, extremities	Papulovesicular	7 (3–11)	Relatively mild	—
Scrub typhus (tsutsugamushi disease)	1–12 (9–18)	Often present	4–6	Trunk → extremities	Macular, maculopapular	14 (10–20)	Mild to severe	24–36
Q fever	10–19	None		None		7 (2–21)	Relatively mild‡	48 (occasionally slow)

*Untreated disease.
†Severity can vary greatly.
‡Occasionally subacute infections occur (e.g., hepatitis, endocarditis).

350   The Typhus Group

This group of conditions includes three established clinical and epidemiologic entities: epidemic louse-borne typhus fever, the oldest disease known to be caused by rickettsiae; Brill-Zinsser disease, a classic example of reactivation of a latent infection; and flea-borne murine typhus. The first two conditions are induced by *Rickettsia prowazekii*, a pathogen transferred from person to person by the bite of body lice. Persons who have recovered from epidemic typhus have persistent rickettsiae in various host cells, presumably in the reticuloendothelial cells; stresses that cause a defect in the suppressive lymphocytes will, years later, permit these rickettsiae to be reactivated, resulting in a mild typhus-like illness, called Brill-Zinsser disease. In 1975, *R. prowazekii* was isolated from flying squirrels in the southeastern United States. A number of persons acquired typhus fever from squirrels living in their attics and probably harboring infected fleas or lice or both.

Flea-borne murine typhus, caused by *R. typhi*, is a mild form of typhus fever occurring in this country and elsewhere. It is transmitted by fleas from rodents (Fig. 350–1). *R. canada* is a tick-borne (mouse-rabbit reservoirs), rickettsial organism, formerly classified with the typhus group. It is distinct from the typhus, as well as the spotted fever group. Whether it is a significant human pathogen requires more study. It has been implicated by serologic means as the cause of acute febrile cerebrovasculitis in one patient.

EPIDEMIC LOUSE-BORNE TYPHUS

INTRODUCTION. Synonyms include classic, historic, and European typhus; jail, war, camp, and ship fever; *Flichfieber* (German); *typhus exanthematique* (French); and *tifus exantematico* and *tabardillo* (Spanish). Many of these names indicate the

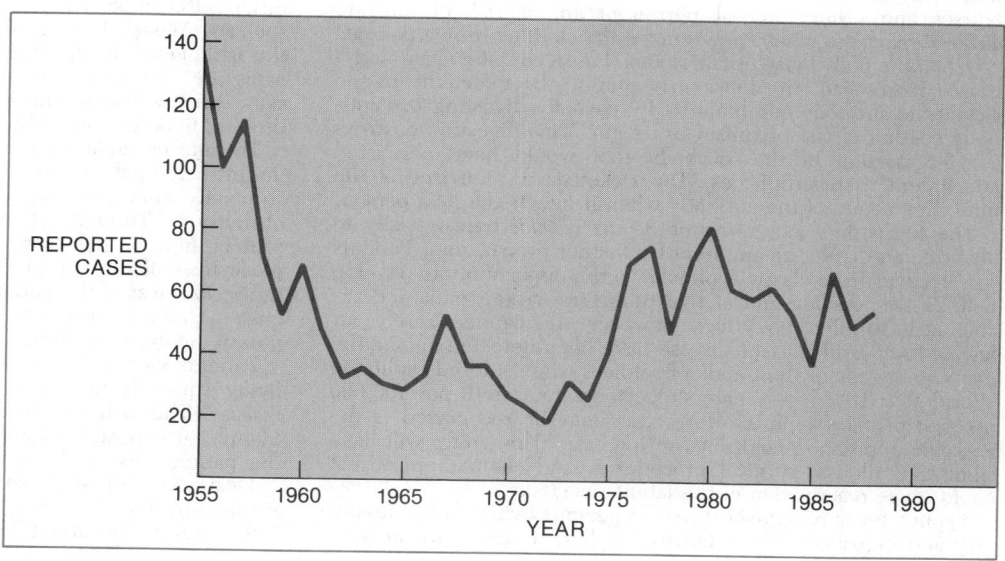

FIGURE 350–1. Flea-borne (endemic, murine) typhus fever: cases, by year in the United States from 1955 to 1988. For 1988, 54 cases of murine typhus were reported from 10 states. Thirty of the cases were reported from Texas, 10 from California, and 7 from Hawaii.

location of the outbreaks—military and concentration camps, crowded ships with poor and starved immigrants, outbreaks in persons living in occupied countries during wartime, and so forth. Each implies crowded, unsanitary living conditions where bathing and laundry facilities are inadequate. These conditions allow for the breeding and propagation of body lice. The impact of typhus fever on military campaigns and immigration patterns is a fascinating and provocative story. The reader is referred to Woodward for an introduction to the effects of this disease on history.

DEFINITION. Classic typhus fever is manifested by the sudden onset of headache, fever, rash, and an altered mental state. (Typhus is derived from the Greek word meaning cloudy or misty. Applied to typhus, it describes the obtunded, lethargic state of mind.) *R. prowazekii* is transmitted by human body lice (*Pediculus humanus humanus*).

ETIOLOGY. *R. prowazekii* is a small obligate intracellular, gram-negative bacillus. In cells it stains red when exposed to Gimenez's stain. Viable rickettsiae stimulate the endothelial cell to act like a phagocyte to engulf the rickettsiae in a phagosome and internalize it. If rickettsiae do not break out of the phagosome promptly, they begin to disintegrate, perhaps owing to enzymatic activities. The rickettsiae have an enzyme, phospholipase A, that enables them to lyse the phagosome wall and to multiply freely in the cytoplasm. *R. prowazekii* escape from the cell by destroying it. The necrotic cell stimulates an inflammatory response that leads to the vasculitis and subsequent clotting abnormalities.

TRANSMISSION AND EPIDEMIOLOGY. The unique feature of infection with *R. prowazekii* is that no animal reservoir has been implicated, at least until its isolation from the flying squirrel (*Glaucomys volans*). It is still uncertain how significant the flying squirrel will be in amplifying the incidence of this disease. Very few, if any, cases of classic typhus occur each year in this country (Centers for Disease Control does not have an active surveillance for it). Fifteen cases were reported in 1980 and 1981, all in persons having contact with flying squirrels.

Classic typhus is a disease of humans. An individual with rickettsemia can infect body lice. The lice acquire the organisms in their blood meal. These ectoparasites may then find another person to whom they transmit the rickettsiae via infected feces. Body lice do not survive the ingestion of rickettsiae. The organisms multiply in the gut of the louse, destroy the epithelial cells, and the louse dies (usually in 1 to 3 weeks). However, during the period of infection, the louse passes feces heavily laden with rickettsiae. Either the human host scratches the site of the bite and thereby self-inoculates the rickettsiae, or the feces and rickettsiae can contaminate minute apertures in the epidermis, allowing the organisms to find cells in which to multiply. Dried, contaminated feces can also become airborne, e.g., by shaking out one's clothes loaded with lice and feces and thereby creating an infectious aerosol. When inhaled, the rickettsiae can penetrate the mucosal cells and enter endothelial cells. Laboratory accidents frequently generate aerosols that induce infection in technicians. Nurses and other medical personnel are at risk of inhaling airborne particles when they remove the clothing from a patient.

When the body louse obtains a blood meal containing antibody-coated rickettsiae, the louse may modify the infectivity of the rickettsiae-antibody combination by partially digesting the antibody coating of the organism in its gut. This digestion destroys the Fc portion of the antibody that would have permitted attachment to macrophages. The rickettsia is then free of the inhibiting action of the antibody when it infects the next person.

The louse does not transmit *R. prowazekii* transovarially to offspring and is not an amplifier for further propagation. Patients who recover from classic typhus have the opportunity to develop Brill-Zinsser disease and at that time have rickettsemia and are able again to infect body lice. However, this happens rarely, for few cases of Brill-Zinsser disease have been detected among the many hundreds of thousands of soldiers who acquired typhus in World War II; one estimate suggested a rate of 10 per 100,000 cases of primary typhus. More cases may be recognized as the geriatric population continues to increase. This group will have significant illness, surgical procedures, and chemotherapy that could cause reactivation of the latent rickettsiae.

Typhus fever remains a threat to persons living under unsanitary and deprived circumstances. As long as there are persons who are latent reservoirs for *R. prowazekii*, an epidemic can erupt. One country with persistent typhus is Ethiopia. There, prolonged drought, poverty, and malnutrition contribute to the perpetuation of the disease.

PATHOLOGY. The rickettsiae invade only endothelial cells, as described in Ch. 351. This leads to vasculitis, with differing pathologic changes in various organs. There is no eschar in this disease. The rash appears to have its origin in the leakage of blood and fluid from the damaged capillaries. The damage to the endothelial cells results in cell death, and at these sites platelet-fibrin thrombi form, platelet-active substances are released, and vasoconstriction and occlusion of small vessels occur. These changes can lead to infarcts in various organs, edema of tissue, leakage of inflammatory cells around small blood vessels ("typhus nodules" of the brain, for instance), stimulation of clotting mechanisms, and the development of shock. Almost all organs are involved in patients with untreated disease. The inflammatory exudate consists of mononuclear cells, plasma cells, histiocytes, and polymorphonuclear leukocytes. Gangrene of skin and limbs occurs in the presence of extensive thrombotic activity.

CLINICAL MANIFESTATIONS AND COURSE. The incubation period is about 7 days on the average but can range from 6 to 15 days. The onset is abrupt with intense headache, chills, fever, and myalgia. There is back or leg pain—presumably due to the muscle damage secondary to the vasculitis. Bites of lice may cause pruritus, and persons infested with lice may have numerous scratches in the skin. Sometimes the skin has a yellow-gold hue because of frequent louse bites. The headache is described as the "worst ever," and the pain is unremitting unless treated with narcotic analgesics. The temperature rises quickly during the first 2 days and persists for about 2 weeks, maintaining a continuous fever pattern if not altered by antibiotics or antipyretic medications. During the first week, there is a bradycardia relative to the temperature elevations of 39° to 41°C. Conjunctivae are injected, and photophobia is present. Deafness, tinnitus, and sometimes vertigo are prominent features. The patient appears to be in a toxic state, with a flushed face, obtundation, and profound weakness. There may be a cough, but no rales are apparent on auscultation of the lungs. The pharyngeal mucous lining is dry and inflamed.

The rash, characteristic of the typhus group, appears on the fourth to seventh day of disease. The lesions appear first on the trunk and axillary folds (areas of skin stress) and spread to the extremities but spare the palms and soles of the feet. The lesions are reddish-pink macules that fade on pressure. With treatment or in mild cases, the rash disappears within several days. In untreated patients, it can spread and coalesce, leading to gangrene of portions of the skin, especially over regions of bony prominences. In 5 to 10 per cent of patients, the rash may not be present.

These and other manifestations of the disease occur because of the initial unchecked multiplication and spread of the rickettsiae, involving ever-enlarging segments of the endothelial surface. The resulting damage to the organs evolves because of the compromised circulation and the associated acute inflammatory responses. Whether rickettsial toxin or endotoxin contributes to the pathologic changes is still a debated point. Whatever processes are involved, certain organs are regularly involved: the skin, heart, kidneys, and skeletal muscle. In patients with severe disease, hypotension and renal failure portend a fatal outcome.

The altered mental status that occurs as the disease progresses (in untreated patients) is striking. The patient may progress from stupor to coma. The stupor may be interrupted by brief periods of delirium. The patient may have to be restrained in order to protect him or her from trauma. At this stage, lymphocytic pleocytosis of the cerebrospinal fluid may be present. Despite the seriousness of the patient's condition, complete recovery can ensue. Cranial nerve lesions are common. There are also temporary mental aberrations.

Patients who have acquired typhus fever in this country from flying squirrels have had signs and symptoms of the classic disease. The rash was noted in 8 of 15, and it was evanescent. Significant central nervous system involvement was reported in five patients; two had coma and three had confusion or delirium.

Death in untreated patients occurs between the ninth and eighteenth days. Recovery from the disease begins with a rapid lysis of fever after about 2 weeks of disease. With the disappearance of fever, mental function returns quickly. Recovery of a sense of well-being is protracted owing to the need to counter the stresses of prolonged negative nitrogen balance, inanition, and loss of muscle mass.

Brill-Zinsser disease is manifested in a manner similar to classic typhus. All signs and symptoms are milder, presumably because the host has well-developed immune mechanisms that can regain control in a short time. Serologic studies in these patients demonstrate immunoglobulin G (IgG) rather than immunoglobulin M (IgM) antibodies. Occasionally, patients with unrecognized Brill-Zinsser disease die. An underlying disease or procedure may permit activation of the latent rickettsiae, and this combination can culminate in death. Reactivation has been noted following surgical procedures and the use of immunosuppressive drugs. In experimental animals that have recovered from the primary disease, isolation of rickettsiae at a future date is facilitated by the administration of steroids.

PROGNOSIS. The fatality rate in untreated groups of patients with classic typhus is 10 to 60 per cent. Children usually have a mild illness with minimal risk of death. Patients over 60 years of age have the highest mortality rate. Recovery is the rule with appropriate antibiotic treatment.

TREATMENT. R. prowazekii responds well to tetracycline and chloramphenicol antibiotics. Doxycycline, 200 mg as a single oral dose, is the treatment of choice. Tetracycline, 25 mg per kilogram daily in four doses, or chloramphenicol, 50 mg per kilogram daily in four doses, is an effective alternative. Therapy should be continued for 2 to 3 days after the fever has defervesced. Most patients are afebrile within 48 to 72 hours and improve quickly from the debilitating headache or mental aberrations or both. Relapses occur in persons who are treated early, on day 1 or 2 of illness. Such patients do not develop the required immune mechanisms to contain the proliferation of the residual rickettsiae. Furthermore, both antibiotics are rickettsiostatic and do not eradicate all of these intracellular parasites even with the introduction of specific immune mechanisms. Recovery from disease without the assistance of antibiotic therapy also allows rickettsiae to remain in cells, later to be activated and cause Brill-Zinsser disease. In the severely ill patient, fluid therapy and proper nutrition are mandatory. Fortunately, antibiotic therapy has simplified the need for supportive care.

PREVENTION AND CONTROL. To prevent and control the spread of classic typhus, the body lice (and feces) associated with patients and their clothes must be destroyed. The clothing should be carefully placed in plastic bags and sealed and carefully removed only in the area where they are to be treated. Clothes that can sustain boiling are boiled, and the rest should be subjected to steam and dry heat. It is also possible to kill the lice (also the eggs present in seams and elsewhere—these eggs will hatch in a week) with insecticides. Formerly, 10 per cent DDT (chlorophenothane) was used, but lice are now generally resistant to it. Resistance has also become a problem with 1 per cent lindane dust. Malathion (1 per cent) and 2 per cent temefos (Abate) are effective in most areas. These dusts are applied to the fully clothed individual. This approach controls the acute outbreaks of disease when applied to all persons in the community. Long-time use of insecticides is not effective because of the development of resistance, because long-term compliance is difficult, and because the insecticides may have a deleterious effect on the ecology of the region. Control requires improvement of sanitary conditions and standards of living as well as health education.

Health personnel who encounter patients with classic typhus are at risk for acquiring the disease from lice picked up from the patient or his or her clothes. There is no risk of direct human-to-human transfer of the rickettsiae other than by aerosolized, dried, contaminated feces. Once the patient has been deloused, no isolation barriers are required.

No vaccine is currently available for preventing classic typhus.

Travelers to endemic areas are rarely at risk unless, for example, they work in camps for displaced persons or carry out relief work that brings them in contact with persons with lice. Decontaminating the clothing overnight with insecticides or wearing insect repellent–treated clothes provides some protection. Prophylactic doxycycline has been effective when given weekly to prevent scrub typhus and would be expected to be effective in preventing R. prowazekii infections. This drug should

be used only for short periods, 2 to 4 weeks. It is important under these circumstances to monitor the temperature for 2 weeks at least, as the drug may have masked the initial infection and delayed the onset of symptoms. Retreatment with doxycycline at the onset of the fever is curative.

MURINE TYPHUS

DEFINITION. Murine typhus, a milder form of classic typhus, is caused by *Rickettsia typhi* and is transmitted from rodents to humans by means of the rat flea (*Xenopsylla cheopis*). It is the only disease of the typhus group that occurs regularly in the United States, albeit in small numbers.

ETIOLOGY. *R. typhi* is a small, gram-negative, obligate, intracellular pathogen. Like *R. prowazekii*, it can penetrate into endothelial cells by induced phagocytosis. Its disease potential resides in its ability to multiply in these cells, destroy them, and initiate a vasculitis. *R. typhi* is catalogued with the typhus group because it shares common antigens with *R. prowazekii* and *R. canada*. In addition, there is cross-immunity between *R. prowazekii* and *R. typhi* induced by infections. Despite these similarities, it is clear from deoxyribonucleic acid (DNA) homology studies that the two are not closely related.

TRANSMISSION AND EPIDEMIOLOGY. *R. typhi* causes disease worldwide. Wherever there are large rodent populations, there is the potential for outbreaks. The rat and other small animals serve as reservoirs of this disease. *Rattus rattus* and *Rattus norvegicus* are two species of rats that can sustain the *R. typhi*, serve as a source of rickettsiae for the rat flea, and have no obvious illness from carrying this human pathogen. The rat flea disseminates the infection not through its bite but by placing contaminated feces on the skin. These may be rubbed or scratched into the skin; they can be carried to the conjunctival sac or mucous membranes on the fingers, where the rickettsiae can invade; or they can be aerosolized after drying and cause infection if inhaled. In the flea, the rickettsiae multiply in the enterocytes in the gut, do not kill the flea, and continue to be shed in the feces for the life of the flea. The rickettsiae are not transmitted by fleas to their offspring.

The numbers of cases reported to the Centers for Disease Control (CDC) from 1955 to 1988 are shown in Figure 350–1. Fifty-four cases were reported in 1988, most from Texas and California. These numbers probably represent an under-reporting of the true incidence. There was a dramatic drop in the number of reported cases after the mid 1940's. In 1944 there were over 5400 cases. By 1954 there were 163. This decline was due to intensive efforts at rodent control. Most of the cases occur in the warmer months, when rat fleas are plentiful.

PATHOLOGY. Descriptions of the pathologic lesions in this disease are few because of the rarity of fatal cases. Since the rickettsiae are known to invade endothelial cells, the pathologic consequences should mimic those seen in other rickettsial infections. The reasons for the differences in virulence of these rickettsiae and the varying severity of illnesses produced are unknown.

CLINICAL MANIFESTATIONS AND COURSE. Headache, fever, and myalgia are the principal symptoms and signs associated with illness produced by *R. typhi*. These appear after an incubation period of about 1 to 2 weeks. A faint macular-papular pink-colored rash appears in about 80 per cent of patients after 4 to 5 days of illness. It may be difficult to see in poor light. When present, it may be visible for 4 to 8 days before it gradually fades.

Rarely are there any significant complications of this infection, but as it is an infection of the endothelial cells, there is a vasculitis that can cause widespread organ derangement. The patients, especially if older, are debilitated by the infection when not treated. They may remain febrile, with a temperature of 39 to 40°C for 2 weeks. This metabolic stress necessitates prolonged convalescence. Antibiotic therapy brings about a prompt recovery.

DIAGNOSIS. This disease has no distinguishing characteristics during the early days of symptoms. The rash appearing on the fourth or fifth day of illness should alert the physician to the possibility of a rickettsial infection. The history of a possible exposure to areas where rats are known to exist, e.g., grain elevators, port facilities, and farm buildings, provides useful information. Flea bites, if seen early, are discrete and may have a central hemorrhagic punctum. The location and grouping of flea bites are important diagnostic features. They occur in covered parts of the body, in irregular groups of several to a dozen or more. They may be in the region of the belt, shoulders, and hips or on the legs.

Differentiating this disease from Rocky Mountain spotted fever (RMSF) may be difficult. The rash of RMSF usually begins on the wrists and palms and on the soles of the feet and then extends to the skin of the thorax and abdomen. In murine typhus the lesions are on the skin of the chest and abdomen and rarely on the extremities. The history of a tick bite or exposure provides evidence for a clinical diagnosis of RMSF.

Serologic studies confirm the rickettsial infection. Weil-Felix OX-19 reaction is positive in most patients who have not received antibiotic treatment. This test, however, does not distinguish murine typhus from the spotted fever group of infections. The indirect immunofluorescent test can be used to identify *R. typhi* infections. However, because of the common antigens shared with *R. prowazekii*, the serum requires cross-absorption with special antigens from these two rickettsia strains. Isolation of the organism is possible but should be done only in special laboratories where containment facilities are available.

PROGNOSIS. The mortality rate is less than 5 per cent in untreated patients. Appropriate antibiotic treatment results in prompt cure, and the mortality rate is reduced almost to zero. One death was reported between 1977 and 1986.

TREATMENT. Tetracycline and chloramphenicol are effective drugs for treating this rickettsial infection. A 5- to 7-day course of either is effective. The usual dosage of 25 mg per kilogram of tetracycline per day in four doses or chloramphenicol, 50 mg per kilogram per day in four doses, effects a prompt cure. The organisms are sensitive to these antibiotics. No resistant strains have been identified. Relapses do occur when antibiotics are administered early in the course of the illness. Retreatment with the antibiotic of choice provides prompt response.

PREVENTION AND CONTROL. There is no vaccine to prevent this disease. Control of rats has been shown to be very effective. When rat control programs are instituted, appropriate insecticides should be simultaneously used to prevent the fleas from seeking humans for feeding as the rat population is decreased.

Bozeman FM, Maisello SA, Williams MG, et al.: Epidemic typhus rickettsia isolated from flying squirrels. Nature 225:545, 1975.
Duma RJ, Sonenshine DE, Bozeman FM, et al.: Epidemic typhus in the United States associated with flying squirrels. JAMA 245:2318, 1981. *These two papers provide a good background on the discovery of the flying squirrel as a reservoir of* R. prowazekii *and the disease associated with exposure to these animals and their ectoparasites.*
Gaon JA, Murray ES: The natural history of recrudescent typhus (Brill-Zinsser disease) in Bosnia. Bull WHO 35:133, 1966. *Classic paper describing the studies conducted to prove that Brill-Zinsser disease is truly a recrudescence of classic typhus fever.*
Linneman CC, Pretzman CI, Peterson ED: Acute febrile cerebrovasculitis. A nonspotted fever group rickettsial disease. Arch Intern Med 149:1689, 1989. *An intriguing case report and discussion of the probable role of* R. canada *in causing this clinical entity.*
Walker TS: Rickettsial interactions with human endothelial cells in vitro: Adherence and entry. Infect Immun 44:205, 1984.
Wohlbach SB, Todd JI, Palfrey FW: The Etiology and Pathology of Typhus. Cambridge, Mass., Harvard Press, 1922. *This book provides the reader with an excellent description of the natural course of classic typhus fever.*
Woodward TE: A historical account of the rickettsial diseases with a discussion of unsolved problems. J Infect Dis 127:5, 1973.

351 Rocky Mountain Spotted Fever

SYNONYMS. Rocky Mountain spotted fever (RMSF) is also known as typhus fever, tick-borne, by the Centers for Disease Control (CDC), *fiebre manchada* (Mexico), *fiebre petequial* (Colombia), and *febre maculosa* or Sao Paulo typhus (Brazil).

DEFINITION. Rocky Mountain spotted fever is a sometimes fatal systemic infection manifested by fever, severe headache, rash, and other organ disease caused by the vasculitis induced by *Rickettsia rickettsii*. The organism is usually transmitted to humans from animal reservoirs by a tick bite.

ETIOLOGY. *R. rickettsii* organisms are small, gram-negative, coccobacillary bacteria that can grow only inside eukaryotic host cells. They cannot be isolated on cell-free culture media. In human infections the rickettsiae invade and multiply within endothelial cells of arteries and veins. Different strains of *R. rickettsii* vary in virulence in human as well as animal hosts. Mortality rates appear to be higher in Montana than on the Eastern seaboard. Attempts to correlate virulence with structural components in the polysaccharide portion of the cell wall have been unsuccessful. However, two surface proteins, with molecular weights of 120,000 and 155,000, have been identified as possible virulence factors (protective antigens), and the latter has been produced from cloned genes in *Escherichia coli*. The antigenic material protects mice from lethal infection and will be studied as a potential vaccine.

DISTRIBUTION AND INCIDENCE. This disease was named for the geographic site of its original discovery; the causative agent was named for the discoverer, Howard T. Ricketts. By the 1940's the disease had become more common on the East Coast than in the West. The incidence rose sharply beginning in 1971 and peaked at 1.91/100,000 population in 1980 in the eight South Atlantic states. Subsequently, it has fallen to a value similar to that of 1970. A total of 603 cases of RMSF were reported in 1989 in the United States (Fig. 351–1).

Serologic surveys in children and adults in North Carolina, the state with the highest number of reported cases, demonstrate that subclinical infections occur. Almost 20 per cent of the children had OX-19 agglutination titers in the diagnostic range, and a smaller number had positive indirect fluorescent antibody titers, a more specific test. None of these children was previously diagnosed as having had Rocky Mountain spotted fever.

TRANSMISSION AND EPIDEMIOLOGY. Ninety-five per cent of reported cases occur between April 1 and September 30, with two thirds in May, June, and July. Children and young adults account for about 40 per cent of cases. Ninety per cent of patients give a history of a tick bite or attachment or of having been in a tick-infested area 14 days prior to onset of illness. Infected ticks are found in urban as well as rural areas. A park in New York City was the source of ticks that transmitted *R. rickettsia* to four children, one of whom died.

Rocky Mountain spotted fever occurs in humans when an infected tick bites and injects *R. rickettsii* into the skin. Probably fewer than 10 organisms injected intradermally are sufficient to induce disease.

Several species of ticks are commonly involved in transmission of disease: *Dermacentor andersoni*, the wood tick, in the Rocky Mountain states; *Dermacentor variabilis*, the dog tick, in the East and Oklahoma; *Amblyomma americanum* in Texas and Oklahoma; and *Rhipicephalus sanguineus* in Texas and Mexico. These ticks feed on small mammals such as ground squirrels and rabbits as well as on larger animals such as bear and deer. Dogs serve as a reservoir to infect ticks and then other animals or humans. Figure 351–2 shows the distribution of cases of Rocky Mountain spotted fever by state in the United States in 1989.

Laboratory-acquired infections have occurred in persons exposed to droplets from accidental generation of aerosols from solutions of the organism. However, even in circumstances conducive to airborne transmission, person-to-person transmission does not occur. Rocky Mountain spotted fever can also be acquired by the transfusion of contaminated blood.

PATHOLOGY. The basis of the pathologic changes in this disease, as in other rickettsial infections, is the inflammatory response stimulated by the irreparable damage of the endothelial cells. In patients dying within 3 to 5 days of onset of disease, significant coagulation abnormalities are present. Causes may include damage to the endothelial cells with release of Factor VIII; and stimulation of the release of platelet factors by damage to the endothelium or by activation of the kallikrein-kinin system by the Hageman factor. Microinfarcts result from occlusions of small vessels, and edema and hemorrhages occur secondary to increased permeability of the vasculature. Such lesions can be found in the heart, kidneys, adrenals, lungs, brain, skin, spleen, and subcutaneous tissues.

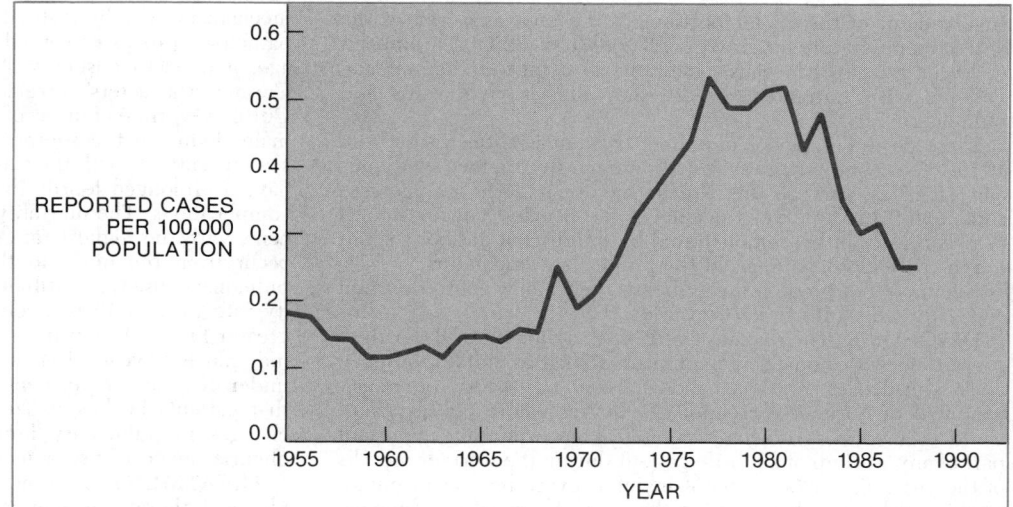

FIGURE 351–1. Rates of reported Rocky Mountain spotted fever cases, by year, in the South Atlantic states and all other states, from 1955 to 1988.

The rash is thought to result from the vasculitis and the associated permeability changes. Petechial lesions are caused by microhemorrhages secondary to the vasculitis and thrombocytopenia.

Patients with glucose-6-phosphate dehydrogenase (G6PD) deficiency appear to be prone to severe infections caused by *R. rickettsii* and other rickettsial agents. These patients have severe hemolytic reactions and significant thrombotic lesions in the glomeruli, resulting in oliguria.

CLINICAL MANIFESTATIONS. The incubation period of naturally acquired disease has a range of 2 to 14 days with an average of 7 days. The onset of disease in the typical case is sudden, with a severe headache, often retrobulbar in location, chills, fever, myalgia, malaise, nausea and vomiting, conjunctival injection, and photophobia. Tenderness may be present in large muscle groups. The duration of fever in untreated cases is about 2 weeks, but recovery from the debilitating effects of the disease requires several additional weeks.

Rash appears in 80 to 90 per cent of patients—usually on the third or fourth day of fever, rarely after 5 or more days. It consists of pink macules, 2 to 5 mm, often noted first about the wrists and ankles. Lesions then spread to arms, chest, face, feet, and abdomen. Rarely does the rash involve the mucous membranes. Initially, these lesions blanch with pressure, but after 2 to 3 days they become fixed and turn dark red or purple and then slowly disappear during convalescence. The latter lesions represent microhemorrhages. Lesions on the palms and soles of the feet, in conjunction with the rash elsewhere, and petechial lesions in the skin folds of the axillae and around the ankles, constitute the classic distribution of the rash. Biopsy of the rash reveals perivascular round cell infiltration. Staining of the specimens of skin with fluorescent tagged antibodies to *R. rickettsii* reveals the intracellular organisms.

In patients with unrecognized and inappropriately treated disease, the rash coalesces as the spread of the infectious process involves additional and larger vessels. This can result in large ischemic and gangrenous lesions. Especially susceptible is the skin of the tip of the nose, ear lobes, digits, and scrotum.

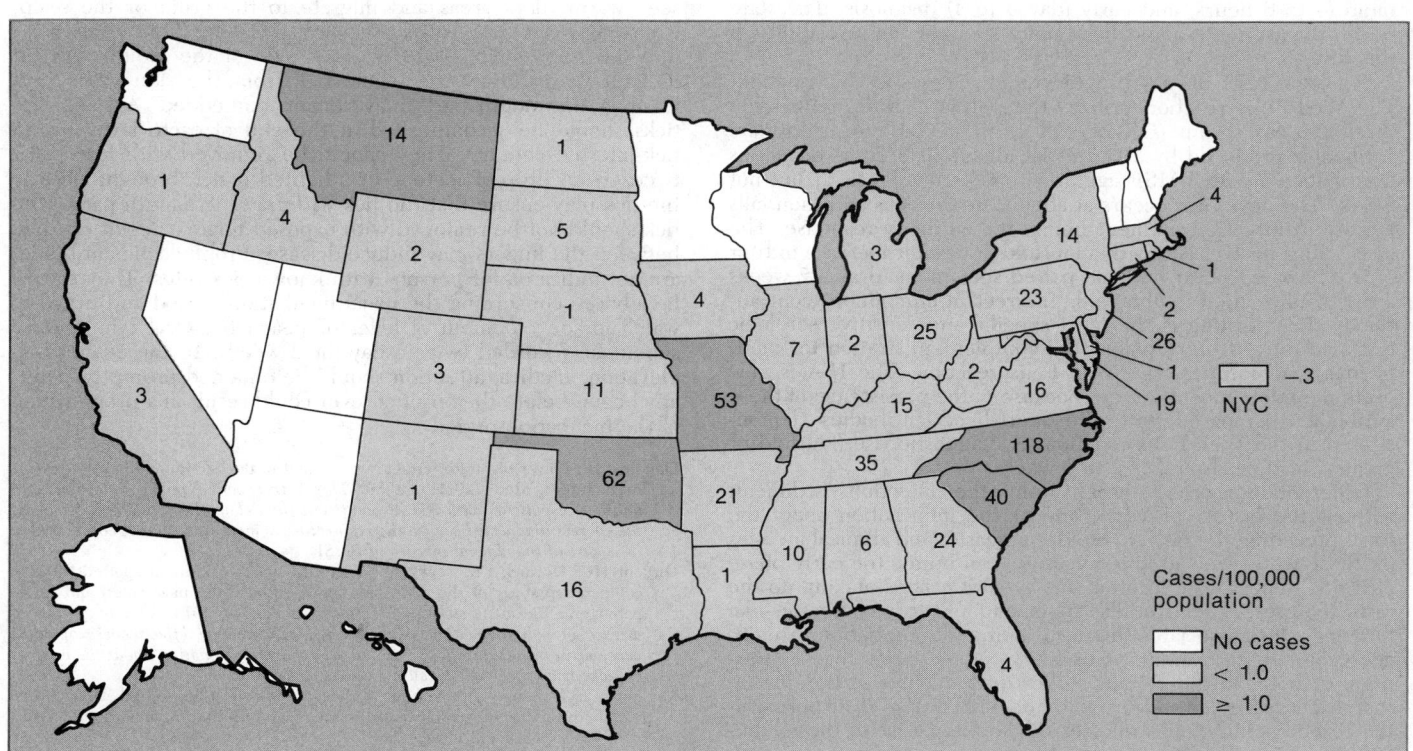

FIGURE 351–2. Rocky Mountain spotted fever: Cases, by state, in the United States in 1989.

Involvement of the cooler portions of the body may reflect the optimal temperature for growth of *R. rickettsii* (32°C). Thrombosis of larger arteries can cause gangrene of a limb or hemiplegia. Patients with untreated disease may die of myocarditis and pulmonary edema.

The reported incidence of pulmonary abnormalities varies from 10 to 40 per cent in large series of patients. Respiratory symptoms and signs as part of this illness have not been emphasized sufficiently. In fact, after the spleen, the heaviest concentrations of rickettsiae can be demonstrated by fluorescent antibody staining in the endothelial cells of the pulmonary vasculature.

Edema of the brain and ring hemorrhages may cause delirium and stupor and ultimately lead to death.

DIAGNOSIS. The diagnosis of RMSF is difficult in the patient presenting with nonspecific complaints such as sudden onset of fever, headache, myalgia, and malaise. A history of travel, camping, or outdoor recreational activities where tick exposure could occur and of recent tick bites is an especially important part of any workup of a febrile patient during the warmer months of the year. The patient complains of a severe headache, photophobia, and pain when moving the eyes. There is no meningismus. Lumbar puncture usually reveals normal cerebrospinal fluid (CSF). Patients with stupor or coma may demonstrate elevated CSF protein and a few mononuclear cells. The presence of a faint, pink-colored rash on wrists and ankles should raise a suspicion of RMSF. Helpful in making the diagnosis is the knowledge that the rash appeared after the fever.

A search for an attached tick should concentrate on the scalp and groin. Hard body ticks such as *D. andersoni* tend to remain attached for long periods. The finding of an engorged tick should provide the needed information for a clinical diagnosis. There usually is no ulceration or scar from the tick bite.

Most patients have thrombocytopenia but not significant clotting abnormalities. In severe cases, disseminated intravascular coagulopathy (DIC) occurs with hypofibrinogenemia and prolonged prothrombin and partial thromboplastin times. Other laboratory studies are not helpful in making a diagnosis. The white blood cell count is usually normal.

Confirmation of RMSF is achieved by immunofluorescence staining of tissue specimens and by serologic analyses. The detection by immunofluorescence of rickettsiae in tissues, such as skin or rash biopsies, is the one test that can provide the most rapid (4 to 6 hours) and early (day 3 to 4) diagnosis. The state health department should be contacted about the availability of this test.

Serologic tests do not provide rapid diagnostic confirmation. The Weil-Felix reaction utilizes the polysaccharide antigens of three *Proteus* strains (OX-19, OX-2, and OX-K) to agglutinate antibodies produced by a rickettsial infection. Serum specimens from patients with RMSF agglutinate OX-19 and OX-2, but not OX-K. The peak titer occurs at about 2 to 3 weeks and then falls rapidly. Antibiotic treatment blunts the antibody response. The test is inexpensive, and with a fourfold or greater increase in titer of OX-19 or OX-2, or both, in paired specimens (drawn 2 weeks apart) confirmation is obtained. Indirect immunofluorescent antibody (IFA) testing is the most specific and sensitive serologic test available. It has replaced the complement fixation test and, in many laboratories, the Weil-Felix reaction. The IFA is now used in epidemiologic surveys because of the persistence of these antibodies compared with the short-lived antibodies demonstrated in the Weil-Felix reaction. A diagnostic rise (fourfold or greater) in titer also takes 2 to 3 weeks.

Differentiation of this disease from other infections is difficult without the history of a tick bite or the information about the fever preceding the rash. In children measles and atypical measles (in those who received killed vaccine) can mimic the early phase of RMSF illness. The location and type of lesions making up the rash, the presence of Koplik's spots, and a history of measles-like illness in close associates should permit a differentiation. Meningococcemia with meningitis usually produces petechiae or purpura, or both, in the patient earlier in the course of the disease than expected in all but rare patients with RMSF. Furthermore, the cerebrospinal fluid indicates the septic nature of the meningitis caused by the meningococci.

PROGNOSIS. Patients with RMSF have a serious infectious disease that involves endothelial cells throughout the host. Prompt antibiotic therapy is necessary to assist cellular immune mechanisms to eliminate the pathogen. In some patients, the pathologic processes spread rapidly and cause irreversible damage, and death ensues within 3 to 5 days (fulminant disease). Certain risk factors correlate with severe diseases: presence of G6PD/A−, time of onset of specific antibiotic therapy, and black males living in the southeastern United States during the tick season. Patients with the classic form of RMSF who are untreated have a prolonged febrile illness lasting 2 to 3 weeks with many complications. The mortality rate in such patients is 20 to 30 per cent, with the highest rate occurring in the elderly. Death may occur from the ninth to the fifteenth day, often from severe pulmonary disease. Antibiotic treatment has lowered the mortality rate to 3 to 10 per cent. The 1985 case fatality rates were greater for blacks (16 per cent) than whites (3 per cent) and for individuals 40 years of age or older (9 per cent) than for individuals under 40 years (2 per cent). This is a serious disease requiring that patients be hospitalized and carefully monitored to detect changes in pulmonary findings and evidence of hypotension, oliguria, myocarditis, or increasing intracranial pressure.

TREATMENT. Prompt initiation of tetracycline or chloramphenicol therapy is mandatory to ensure optimal chances for recovery. Tetracycline (25 to 50 mg per kilogram per day), doxycycline (100 mg every 12 hours in adults), and chloramphenicol (50 mg per kilogram per day) are the drugs of choice. Usually the fever abates in 2 to 3 days, and concurrently a sense of well-being is restored. Antibiotic treatment can be discontinued 2 to 3 days thereafter. No instances of strains resistant to the tetracyclines or chloramphenicol have been reported. The newer third-generation cephalosporins or the aminoglycoside antibiotics have not been evaluated in RMSF. Evaluation of four aminoquinolone antibiotics in various infected tissue culture cell lines have revealed antibacterial activity equal to that of tetracyclines. Clinical evaluations are not available. Relapses after tetracycline or chloramphenicol treatment are uncommon.

PREVENTION AND CONTROL. Immunity to reinfection after recovery from RMSF appears to be complete. No naturally acquired second cases have been reported. There is no effective vaccine.

The best method for preventing disease is to avoid contact with ticks. Ticks are brushed off leaves or blades of grass onto clothes or skin as one comes in contact with such vegetation. Ticks usually remain stationary until the host is quiet. They then seek warm, dark areas and migrate to the groin or the scalp, where they can grasp hair shafts while inserting their mouth parts into the skin. Small barbs on each side of the mouth make it difficult to withdraw the whole tick from the skin while it is feeding; the mouth parts may remain embedded. A search for ticks should be accomplished at the end of each day spent in tick-infested country. They should be removed with forceps or tweezers. A drop of acetone or a lighted match brought close to the tick may ensure that the tick withdraws its mouth parts. The tick should not be removed with exposed fingers. A tick crushed between the fingers may induce disease. Prophylactic antibiotics are not indicated for persons with known tick bites. They should be advised concerning the usual incubation period and urged to watch for development of fever or headache. Oral temperature should be recorded twice a day for 2 weeks. In the event of an elevation, medical attention should be obtained promptly. Therapy begun before the onset of fever could result in a prolongation of the incubation period.

Donohue JF: Lower respiratory tract involvement in Rocky Mountain spotted fever. Arch Intern Med 140:223, 1980. *This retrospective review of pulmonary findings in patients with RMSF points out the delays that occurred in making the correct diagnosis because the respiratory symptoms were not considered to be a part of the clinical picture of RMSF.*

DuPont HL, Hornick RB, Dawkins AT, et al.: Rocky Mountain spotted fever: A comparative study of the active immunity induced by inactivated and viable pathogenic *Rickettsia rickettsii*. J Infect Dis 128:340, 1973. *A study of induced disease in volunteers that demonstrated the minimal effectiveness of killed vaccines in preventing RMSF. In addition, new information about the number of rickettsiae required to cause diseases was obtained.*

Kaplowitz LG, Lange JV, Fischer JJ, et al.: Correlation of rickettsial titers, circulating endotoxin, and clinical features in Rocky Mountain spotted fever. Arch Intern Med 143:1149, 1983.

Marx RS, McCall CE, Abramson JS, et al.: Rocky Mountain spotted fever: Serological evidence of previous subclinical infection in children. Am J Dis

Child 136:16, 1982. Wilfert CM, MacCormack JN, Kleeman K, et al.: The prevalence of antibodies to *Rickettsia rickettsii* in an area endemic for Rocky Mountain spotted fever. J Infect Dis 151:823, 1985. *Two good studies attempting to assess the specificity and sensitivity of various serologic tests in measuring antibodies as an indicator of subclinical infections.*

Rao AK, Schapira M, Clements ML, et al.: A prospective study of platelets and plasma proteolytic systems during the early stages of Rocky Mountain spotted fever. N Engl J Med 318:1021, 1988. *An excellent presentation of the events that lead to the pathologic changes in patients with RMSF.*

Silverman D: *Rickettsia rickettsii*—induced cellular injury of human vascular endothelium in vitro. Infect Immun 44:545, 1984. *Electron microscopic study of cellular derangements caused by* R. rickettsii.

352 Other Tick-Borne Rickettsioses

DEFINITIONS. *Mediterranean spotted fever,* also known as North African tick typhus, Kenya tick-bite fever, Indian tick typhus, and boutonneuse fever, is caused by *Rickettsia conorii.* A second disease, called North Asian tick-borne rickettsiosis, is induced by *Rickettsia siberica.* A third tick-borne rickettsial infection, called Queensland tick typhus, is caused by *Rickettsia australis.* The disease produced by these agents consists of headache, fever, rash, myalgia, and malaise. The rickettsiae induce disease by invading endothelial cells and producing a vasculitis. The outcome of disease is usually favorable. The illnesses are mild compared with Rocky Mountain spotted fever (RMSF). One other difference is the usual presence of a depressed, black ulcer—the site of the tick bite. This is the *tache noire,* or eschar, and has been likened to a cigarette burn.

ETIOLOGY, DISTRIBUTION, AND EPIDEMIOLOGY. Mediterranean spotted fever (MSF) occurs in countries bordering the Mediterranean Sea, but also in the Middle East, India, and Pakistan. Several species of ticks are involved. The brown dog tick, *Rhipicephalus sanguineus,* is the main vector, but ticks common to wild animals transmit *R. conorii* in African countries. Italian epidemiologists have demonstrated a dramatic increase in the incidence of this disease in Italy, Spain, and Israel. The assumption is that the suburbanization of cities and towns resulted in increased opportunities for humans to contact ticks.

The distribution of *R. siberica* extends from European Russia through Siberia to the Soviet Far East and south into the Indo-Pakistan subcontinent. Several species of hard, or ixodid, body ticks appear to be the vectors: *Haemaphysalis concinna, Dermacentor sylvarum,* and *Dermacentor nuttallii.* Transovarian transmission occurs in these three naturally infected ticks.

Queensland tick typhus is one of several rickettsial infections found in Australia. The *R. australis* is carried by the tick *Ixodes holocyclus,* and marsupial animals are among known animal reservoirs.

PATHOLOGY. These three rickettsiae are very similar to *R. rickettsii.* There is greater than 90 per cent homology by DNA hybridization between the latter strain and *R. conorii.* All share group-specific antigens but have species-specific antigens as well that allow for their identification. These strains invade endothelial cells and cause cell death, resulting in a vasculitis (see Ch. 351). Each of these three strains produces an eschar (*tache noire*) at the site of the tick bite.

SYMPTOMS, LABORATORY FINDINGS, AND DIAGNOSIS. The onset of disease caused by each of these three rickettsiae is sudden and characterized by fever, headache, malaise, myalgia, and conjunctival injection. These symptoms and signs appear about 5 to 7 days after the tick bite. The eschar is the distinguishing sign that confirms the diagnosis. It should be looked for in the scalp, axillae, and groin area, regions of the body favored by ticks. Because of the necrotic nature of the eschar, lymph nodes draining the region of the eschar are enlarged. The lesion has been appropriately likened to a cigarette burn, about 2 to 5 mm in diameter with a black center and a raised, erythematous rim. The lesion is only mildly tender.

As with RMSF, a rash appears on the fourth to fifth day. The faint pink macular-papular lesions represent small hemorrhages into the skin. The rash is generalized, including the palms and soles of the feet. The duration of the disease is about 2 weeks. Mortality is unusual.

The Weil-Felix reaction demonstrates agglutinating antibodies to OX-19 antigen in most patients; these appear in the second to third week of disease. The microimmunofluorescence test for detection of antibodies to *R. conorii* is the serologic test of choice, if available.

A skin biopsy stained with immunofluorescent antibody stain is the most rapid and earliest diagnostic procedure. This approach is indicated only when the diagnosis of spotted fever is suspected and a *tache noire* eschar is not present.

TREATMENT. Tetracycline and chloramphenicol are the drugs of choice. Defervescence occurs within 2 days. Therapy (see Ch. 351) should be continued for at least 2 days after the patient becomes afebrile.

PROPHYLAXIS. Prevention of human disease requires avoidance of tick bites. Travelers into wild game country of Africa should check their clothes and skin carefully for ticks. Tourists traveling to southern European countries should search for ticks if they go on hiking tours through suburban and rural areas during the spring and summer months.

Recovery from these rickettsial infections imparts solid immunity. In experimental animals *R. conorii* is relatively avirulent compared with most strains of *R. rickettsii.* However, animals recovered from infections with the former strain are protected against challenge with virulent *R. rickettsii.* This protection is mediated by T lymphocytes that recognize antigens on other species of rickettsial agents of the spotted fever group.

HUMAN EHRLICHIOSIS (SPOTLESS ROCKY MOUNTAIN SPOTTED FEVER). The first recognized case occurred in 1986. The organism *Ehrlichia canis* is catalogued in the family Rickettsiaceae. As the species name indicates, it causes disease in canines and is known to be transmitted by ticks (*R. sanguineus*—brown dog tick). The reservoir of *E. canis* is unknown. Much of what is known of this disease has been acquired through retrospective serologic studies and prospective studies of hospital admissions who present with signs and symptoms suggestive of the disease, as well as comparisons of human illness with induced and acquired disease in dogs.

Serologic surveys of febrile hospitalized patients have demonstrated an equal or greater incidence than RMSF. Oklahoma and Georgia surveys in 1987 and 1988 revealed an estimated incidence of 3.3 and 5.3 cases, respectively, per 100,000 persons per year. The Centers for Disease Control reported an informal, laboratory-based survey from 1989 in which 38 cases were detected. Only 4 cases were from Oklahoma and 2 from Georgia. Each state had many more cases of RMSF (see Fig. 351–1). The other 32 cases were from Missouri (14), Virginia (10), Washington (2), Arkansas (1), Illinois (1), Louisiana (1), and Texas (1). Serologic surveys have revealed low titers (1:40 or less) of antibodies in 96 per cent of normal persons. The significance of these low titers is uncertain but may suggest that the infection is more common than RMSF and that many infections must be asymptomatic. As with RMSF, peak incidence is in spring and early summer months.

E. canis has not yet been isolated from patients who have been diagnosed by serologic tests and/or visualization of the organism in leukocytes. Although this does not satisfy Koch's postulates, the serologic evidence is compelling, and the electron microscopic pictures of the organisms in white blood cells are morphologically compatible with *E. canis.* The demonstration of the organisms in inclusion bodies in leukocytes (most likely in lymphocytes, but also in monocytes and neutrophils) is rare. These bodies are round or ovoid, purple to dark blue (Leishman stain), and 2 to 5 μm in diameter. One to four bodies have been seen per infected cell. The electron microscope reveals these bodies to contain a few to as many as 40 microorganisms. Their size of 0.2 to 0.8 μm is consistent with that of rickettsiae and of *E. canis.*

Infected humans (and dogs) present with fever, thrombocytopenia, leukopenia (lymphopenia), and anemia. Bone marrow biopsies reveal hypocellularity and occasional noncaseating granulomas. Evidence of liver cell damage appears subsequently; in dogs this is thought to be due to enlargement of cells of the reticuloendothelial system with compression of adjacent parenchyma. Many patients are asymptomatic and are diagnosed only by serologic surveys. A few hospitalized patients have had significant disease; the manifestations may have been due to hemorrhage into various part of the body, perhaps a vasculitis (seen in dogs) or secondary infections. Fever is usually short-lived (3 to 7 days), but one untreated patient was febrile for 19 days. Rash is unusual, but petechial lesions are likely with thrombocytopenia. Myalgia, headache, asthenia, nausea, or vomiting are common complaints. Physical findings are minimal; the presence of fever, petechial rash, and history of tick bite plus leukopenia is very suggestive of RMSF and of ehrlichiosis. The absence of a rash, but with the other characteristics, should suggest *E. canis* infections. Therapy is the same—tetracycline or chloramphenicol. This treatment for patients thought to have RMSF, but with minimal or no rash and subsequently no serologic response, probably cured many patients with ehrlichiosis. Diagnosis is made by demonstrating a fourfold rise in antibody titer. Single titers of 1:160 or greater have been interpreted as indicative of recent infection. An indirect fluorescent antibody (IFA) test using *E. canis* grown in primary canine monocyte blood cultures has been the discriminating serologic standard.

De Micco C, Raoult D, Toga M: Diagnosis of Mediterraneam spotted fever by using an immunofluorescence technique. J Infect Dis 153:137, 1986.

Raoult D, De Micco C, Gallais H, et al.: Laboratory diagnosis of Mediterranean spotted fever by immunofluorescent demonstration of *Rickettsia conorii* in cutaneous lesions. J Infect Dis 150:145, 1984. *These investigators studied two groups of patients to demonstrate the usefulness of the technique and then to establish the sensitivity and specificity of the procedure.*

Fishbein D, Kemp A, Dawson JE, et al.: Human ehrlichiosis: Prospective active surveillance in febrile hospitalized patients. J Infect Dis 160:803–810, 1989.

Harkess JR, Ewing SA, Crutcher JM, et al.: Human ehrlichiosis in Oklahoma. J Infect Dis 159:576–579, 1989. *These two papers provide important epidemiologic evidence about the incidence of E. canis infections in Georgia and Oklahoma. They also compare the incidence to that of RMSF in those states.*

Harris RL, Kaplan SL, Bradshaw MW, et al.: Boutonneuse fever in American travelers. J Infect Dis 153:126, 1986. *Excellent color print of eschar. Provides warning to American physicians to be alert to the tick-borne rickettsial disease that tourists can acquire overseas.*

Maeda K, Markowitz N, Hawley RC, et al.: Human infection with *Ehrlichia canis*, a leukocytic rickettsia. N Engl J Med 316:851–856, 1987. *The first reported case of ehrlichiosis. This patient had intracytoplasmic inclusion bodies in leukocytes that led eventually to the correct diagnosis.*

Mansueto S, Tringali G, Walker DH: Widespread simultaneous increase in the incidence of spotted fever group rickettsiosis. J Infect Dis 154:539, 1986.

Vicente V, Alegre A, Ruiz R, et al.: Kinin-prekallikrein system in Mediterranean spotted fever. J Infect Dis 154:541, 1986. *These authors carefully studied the kinin system and found that unlike in RMSF, it was not activated in MSF; additional laboratory evidence confirmed the lesser virulence of R. conorii.*

353 Rickettsialpox

DEFINITION. Rickettsialpox is a rare mite-borne infectious disease caused by *Rickettsia akari*. This mild, self-limited illness consists of headache, fever, an eschar at the site of the mite bite, and a papulovesicular rash.

ETIOLOGY. *R. akari* is classified with the spotted fever group of rickettsia. It is a small, gram-negative, coccobacillus-shaped, obligate intracellular organism.

DISTRIBUTION AND INCIDENCE. Rickettsialpox was first described in 1946. In the subsequent few years, more than 500 cases were diagnosed, primarily in New York City. Since the early 1950's, only one outbreak has occurred, again in New York City. The disease is virtually unknown throughout the rest of the United States.

TRANSMISSION AND EPIDEMIOLOGY. The original description of this disease included the isolation of *R. akari* from persons with the disease, from mites (*Allodermanyssus sanguineus*) that feed on rodents, and from house mice (*Mus musculus*). Engorged mites were occasionally found on the mice; attachment was usually around the rump. The mites remain in the nest, where access to mice is readily available. Intrusion into this animal-ectoparasite cycle by humans can result in an infected mite's biting and inducing disease. The ecologic range of *A. sanguineus* covers most of the United States, and mice are

ubiquitous animals. Thus the elements for potential epidemics exist. Isolated cases may develop from unusual exposure to mice, as in persons working in land fills or in homeless persons sleeping in abandoned buildings.

Rickettsialpox is fairly common in some urban areas of the Ukraine, where rats appear to be the animal reservoir. In Korea small field mice are infected.

PATHOLOGY. The known pathologic changes are limited to the skin, since this is a nonfatal infection. Histologic examination of the eschar (site of mite bite) reveals intense inflammation with necrosis. Other findings are similar to those in Rocky Mountain spotted fever: thrombosis and necrosis of capillaries, edema, and a monocytic perivascular infiltrate. The characteristic rash in this disease is papulovesicular. The lesions contain fluid that may yield *R. akari* on culture.

CLINICAL MANIFESTATIONS AND COURSE. The bite of the mite is not painful and goes unnoticed. This site undergoes a localized inflammatory reaction over the next week to 10 days. During this time the edema and cellular components of the reaction create a slowly enlarging, firm, erythematous papule, which may reach 1 to 1.5 cm in diameter. The involved skin separates gradually, creating a vesicle that finally breaks down to form an ulcer. The base of the ulcer is usually black and is surrounded by a rim of erythematous skin. This progression occurs over a 3- to 7-day period, at the end of which there is the sudden onset of fever, chills, sweats, headache, backache, and malaise. The lymph nodes draining the area of the eschar enlarge but are nontender. These symptoms and signs may be present for a week if no specific antibiotic treatment is administered.

As with other members of the spotted fever group, a rash appears after 2 to 3 days of illness. Initially the lesions are maculopapular, few in number, and distributed mostly on the trunk and abdomen, rarely involving the palms or soles. The lesions evolve quickly and uniformly into vesicular lesions; the vesicle appears to sit on top of an erythematous papule. These lesions persist for about a week; the fluid in the vesicle is slowly absorbed, and a scab forms, which leaves a brownish discoloration in the skin after it falls off. This gradually clears without leaving a scar. There is no significant internal organ involvement.

DIAGNOSIS. The diagnosis is made by clinical observation; the unique lesions of the rash, the presence of the eschar, and a history that suggests contact with rodents in the past 2 weeks provide sufficient evidence to make the diagnosis. Serologic studies confirm the diagnosis; complement-fixing antibody titers have been the standard, but indirect immunofluorescent antibodies are more specific, when available. Confusion exists regarding whether the Weil-Felix reaction can be used to diagnose rickettsialpox. In about 10 per cent of patients in small series, significant titer rises to OX-19 and OX-2 have been observed. The test lacks sensitivity for confirming the diagnosis. The organism can be isolated from the vesicular fluid or from clotted blood specimens. These materials must be injected into animals or embryonated eggs. Laboratory tests are of no diagnostic help, although leukopenia is common.

The rash may be confused with the lesions of chickenpox, but no eschar is present in chickenpox. In addition, the lesions of chickenpox are usually in various stages of maturity, whereas the character of those in rickettsialpox is more uniform. Finally, the vesicle of rickettsialpox appears to sit on a papule, whereas those of chickenpox lack such a base.

PROGNOSIS. Rickettsialpox is a benign illness, and recovery occurs without therapy.

TREATMENT. Treatment with tetracycline or doxycycline shortens the febrile period and hastens recovery. Antibiotic treatment need only be administered for 3 to 4 days to ensure a cure. No relapse will occur.

PREVENTION AND CONTROL. Rickettsialpox is a zoonosis involving a common house pest, the mouse. Control of this reservoir through elimination of mouse harborages and the application of residual acaricides to walls adjacent to mice-infested areas should control mite populations. There is no available vaccine.

Brettman LR, Lewin S, Holzman RS: Rickettsialpox: Report of an outbreak and a contemporary review. Medicine 60:363, 1981. *Good summary of clinical features of recent outbreak.*

Dolgopol VB: Histologic changes in rickettsialpox. Am J Pathol 24:119, 1948.

Greenberg M, Pelliteri O, Klein IF, et al.: Rickettsialpox—a newly recognized rickettsial disease. II. Clinical observations. JAMA 133:901, 1947. *Original clinical description of a newly recognized spotted fever group infection.*

Huebner RJ, Stamps P, Armstrong C: Rickettsialpox—a newly recognized rickettsial disease. I. Isolation of the etiological agent. Public Health Rep 61:1605, 1946. *Excellent description of the discovery of rickettsialpox.*

Lackman DH: A review of information on rickettsialpox in the United States. Clin Pediatr 2:296, 1963. *A resource for information on rickettsialpox in the United States.*

354 Scrub Typhus

DEFINITION. Scrub typhus is an acute febrile illness caused by *Rickettsia tsutsugamushi* (from the Japanese: *tsutsuga*, "dangerous"; *mushi*, "bug"). This rickettsia is inoculated into humans during the bite by a chigger. The site of the bite develops into an eschar.

ETIOLOGY. *R. tsutsugamushi* (*R. orientalis*) is a small, gram-negative, obligate intracellular organism. Unlike other rickettsial infections, infection with *R. tsutsugamushi* does not induce solid protection against additional bouts of scrub typhus. This results from the variable antigenic compositions of the strains.

This is the only rickettsia whose polysaccharides bear an antigenic relationship to *Proteus* OX-K. This *Proteus* strain is used in serologic tests to confirm scrub typhus.

DISTRIBUTION. This disease occurs almost exclusively in the large triangular region extending from the northern islands of Japan southwest to Australia and southeast to the South Pacific Islands. This region contains the larval form of mites that are both vector and reservoir of rickettsiae.

TRANSMISSION AND EPIDEMIOLOGY. *R. tsutsugamushi* is transmitted to humans by the bite of the larva of trombiculid mites (chiggers). Chiggers are the only stage in the life cycle of these mites (*Leptotrombidium deliensis* and others) that can feed on humans. Chiggers are almost microscopic, often brilliantly colored (red bugs). The chiggers feed on rats and other small rodents. The word "scrub" was applied because of the type of vegetation—transitional between forests and clearings—that maintains the chigger-mammal relationship. But other regions (semiarid, sandy beaches, and so on) also support rodents and mites. Humans encounter scrub typhus when they enter such areas to build roads, to clear fields or forests, or on military expeditions. Circumscribed regions are highly endemic, a reflection of the lack of mobility of the chiggers and their rodent hosts. Mites transmit the rickettsiae to their offspring via the ova. In this fashion they can serve as vector and reservoir of the etiologic agent.

This disease has been called river or flood fever because of the increased incidence during the rainy seasons. Chiggers and mites proliferate in warm, wet environments.

PATHOLOGY. *R. tsutsugamushi* invades endothelial cells to produce a vasculitis (see Ch. 351). The serious pathologic manifestations in untreated patients are predominantly myocarditis, meningoencephalitis, and pneumonitis. Coagulopathy develops but is less severe than in Rocky Mountain spotted fever or typhus.

The site of the chigger bite develops into a papular lesion that ulcerates to form an eschar. This is associated with regional and later generalized lymphadenopathy.

CLINICAL MANIFESTATIONS AND COURSE. The incubation period for development of the primary papular lesion ranges from 6 to 18 days. This lesion can occur anywhere on the body. It enlarges, undergoes central necrosis, and crusts to form the eschar. As the eschar matures, the patient has the sudden onset of headache, fever, chills, and malaise. Over the next several days, these symptoms increase in severity with further elevation of the temperature. The patient, if untreated, may become stuporous as meningoencephalitis develops. Signs of cardiac dysfunction, including minor electrocardiographic abnormalities such as first-degree heart block and inverted T waves, can appear. The rash of scrub typhus appears at the end of the first week of disease. This is a faint, pink maculopapular rash appearing first on the trunk and spreading to the extremities.

Physical findings late in the first week of illness include generalized lymphadenopathy and palpable spleen and occasionally liver. Pulmonary findings are often absent despite radiographic evidence of interstitial pneumonia. In those patients with myocarditis, there may be a gallop rhythm, poor-quality heart sounds, and systolic murmurs.

Various cranial nerve deficits have been noted in untreated patients. Deafness, dysarthria, and dysphagia may occur but are usually transient, although deafness can last for several months.

All of 87 (nonimmune) soldiers in Vietnam who developed scrub typhus had fever and headache, 46 per cent had an eschar, and 35 per cent had a rash. Eighty-five per cent had generalized lymph node enlargement. It is not surprising that many were misdiagnosed as having infectious mononucleosis.

Laboratory studies reveal leukopenia early in the disease with subsequent increase of white blood cell counts to normal levels. Coagulopathies can be demonstrated, but only rare patients develop the disseminated intravascular clotting syndrome. Liver enzyme values may be elevated, indicating hepatocellular damage. Proteinuria is common.

Patients with untreated disease remain febrile for about 2 weeks and have a long convalescence of 4 to 6 weeks thereafter.

DIAGNOSIS. The variable presentations in this disease make the clinical diagnosis difficult. The eschar and rash should suggest a rickettsial infection, but these may be found in fewer than one half of patients. Furthermore, the eschar and rash may suggest other rickettsial infections, such as tick-borne typhus. A knowledge of the endemic foci of scrub typhus and determination of whether the patient has traveled or worked in such areas constitute important epidemiologic information. A therapeutic trial of tetracycline or chloramphenicol is indicated in patients in whom the diagnosis of scrub typhus is suspected. Defervescence should occur within 24 hours.

The specific serologic test is the detection of significant increases (greater than fourfold) of indirect immunofluorescent antibodies in paired serum specimens obtained 2 weeks apart. The *Proteus* OX-K antigen test is readily available and inexpensive, so that it is frequently employed in endemic areas. About 50 per cent of patients have diagnostic titers. In Malaya, the sensitivity and specificity of both tests were found to be about the same, but their usefulness was enhanced when they were used concurrently.

R. tsutsugamushi can be isolated from a patient's blood by inoculating it, intraperitoneally, into white mice. The rickettsiae can be demonstrated in the tissues of the mice.

PROGNOSIS. Without treatment, the mortality rate ranges from 0 to 30 per cent depending upon virulence and resistance factors; with treatment, survival is the expected outcome. Second or third attacks of scrub typhus, caused by different serotypes, usually result in a mild illness, usually with no eschar or rash.

Persistence of *R. tsutsugamushi* in lymph node tissues has been demonstrated 1 year after recovery. This finding raises the possibility of reactivation of disease during immunosuppression.

TREATMENT. Tetracycline, doxycycline, and chloramphenicol are all effective. The drug should be continued for at least 2 days after the patient has become afebrile.

PREVENTION AND CONTROL. Vaccines were developed and tested during and after World War II. Some were effective against homologous strains. However, no single antigen has been identified that induces protection against all of the antigenically diverse strains of *R. tsutsugamushi*. In military populations in endemic areas, weekly doses of doxycycline protect against scrub typhus.

Avoidance of chigger attachment can be accomplished by insect repellents applied to the skin and by wearing protective clothing impregnated with benzyl benzoate. Diethyltoluamide preparations such as OFF and DEET are also effective if sprayed on clothing and exposed skin but are removed rapidly by water. Application of this chemical to socks is especially important in preventing chigger bites.

Berman SJ, Kunidin WD: Scrub typhus in South Vietnam: A study of 87 cases. Ann Intern Med 79:26, 1973. *A good analysis of the clinical features of scrub typhus appearing in United States troops. Helpful in assessing potential for disease in tourists returning from endemic areas.*

Brown GW, Saunders JP, Singh S: Single dose doxycycline therapy for scrub typhus. Trans R Soc Trop Med Hyg 72:412, 1978. *Clinical investigation on the feasibility of a single dose of drug to treat scrub typhus.*

Traub R, Wisseman CL Jr: The ecology of chigger-borne rickettsiosis (scrub typhus) (review article). J Med Entomol 11:237, 1974. *Excellent summary by two experts who have clarified much of what is now known about the ecology of this disease.*

355 Trench Fever

DEFINITION. Trench fever is caused by a louse-borne rickettsial organism *Rochalimaea quintana*. Patients have a self-limited but relapsing illness characterized by headache, fever, and severe pain in bones, joints, and muscles. Because of these latter complaints, the disease has been called shin-bone fever. Other synonyms include Volhymia fever and 5-day or quintan fever.

ETIOLOGY AND EPIDEMIOLOGY. *R. quintana* is distinct from other rickettsia because it can be grown extracellularly and can be cultivated on cell-free blood agar. It is transmitted to humans by the body louse *Pediculus humanus humanus*. The organism lives in the digestive tract of lice, a permanent carrier state, and is excreted in the feces. It is the deposition of the feces on scratched or abraded skin that allows the organisms to penetrate into the human host. Once in the bloodstream, *R. quintana* may persist for months to years. This rickettsemia serves as a source of infection for other lice and may be associated with relapses of disease, or the host may remain asymptomatic despite it. Late relapses may be precipitated by stresses to the immune system such as other infections, malignancies, or vaccine administration.

Trench fever is rarely diagnosed in the United States. Epidemics occurred during World Wars I and II in Europe. Cases have been reported from Mexico and Bolivia and in Africa and Asia. Diagnosis of the disease is usually made during epidemics.

PATHOLOGY AND CLINICAL MANIFESTATIONS. Little is known of the pathologic changes associated with this disease. The rash that occurs has been biopsied and these specimens revealed perivascular infiltrates consisting of lymphocytes, but no endothelial damage has been seen. It is not known where the organism resides in the human host.

The clinical manifestations are variable and nonspecific. The incubation period ranges from 14 to 35 days (average 22 days). Most patients have the sudden onset of fever with chills, headache, retro-orbital pain, especially on moving the eyes, and pain in joints, bones, and muscles. Bone pain is often severe in the shin, thighs, and back. The temperature may rise to 39.5° to 40°C and persists for several days to a week. There may be an evanescent erythematous macular rash; the lesions blanch with pressure. Only a few lesions are present on the chest, back, and abdomen, and they disappear within 24 hours.

On physical examination, the spleen and liver may be enlarged and the conjunctivae are injected. Laboratory findings are of no diagnostic help; white blood cell count is variable, and proteinuria and polyuria are common.

Relapses of disease occur in 50 per cent of patients. These are associated with a short, variable, febrile course. Multiple relapses are not unusual.

DIAGNOSIS. Isolated cases in immigrants or travelers are difficult to diagnose. The finding of body lice in clothing or on the patient should alert the physician to the diagnosis. Blood cultivated on agar containing 10 per cent fresh defibrinated horse blood yields *R. quintana*. Serologic tests are available in some state laboratories or at the Centers for Disease Control. The disease can be confused with influenza, relapsing fever, louse-borne typhus, malaria, dengue, leptospirosis, and typhoid fever.

TREATMENT AND PROGNOSIS. No therapeutic regimen has been proven in clinical trials. Tetracycline and chloramphenical are antibacterial in in vitro testing. Tetracycline therapy appears to control the acute phase of the disease. Relapses, however, do occur despite this treatment. Mortality, even without antibiotic treatment, is very rare. Eventual recovery does occur in most patients; the remainder continue to have recurrences for months or years.

PREVENTION. Control of body lice is the key. Obviously, preventing the acquisition of lice through bathing and clean clothing would be effective, but not practical in times of war. Dusting of clothing, especially the seams, with DDT 10 per cent, Allethrin, or Abate 2 per cent, may be done. The lice that may be present on the patient should be removed with Kwell Shampoo and/or lotion or cream.

Hurst A: Trench fever. Br Med J 2:318, 1942. *A good resource document outlining the variety of clinical manifestations of trench fever.*

Vinson JW: *In vitro* cultivation of the rickettsial agent of trench fever. Bull WHO 35:155, 1966.

356 Q Fever

DEFINITION. Q fever is a systemic infection caused by the inhalation of small numbers of *Coxiella burnetii*. Domestic animals and pets are the usual sources of infection for humans. This highly infectious rickettsial agent induces mild febrile illness, occasionally associated with pneumonitis, but in a few patients causes chronic hepatitis and life-threatening endocarditis.

ETIOLOGY. *C. burnetii* is unique among the rickettsiae in the following ways: It is not transmitted to humans by arthropod vectors; rather, it is readily disseminated by aerosols. No rash ensues despite the similarity of the infection of endothelial cells (vasculitis) as occurs with *Rickettsia rickettsii*. The organism resides uniquely inside the phagolysosome in the cytoplasm of the infected cell. *C. burnetii* does not have cross-reacting antigens with *Proteus vulgaris,* and, therefore, antibodies developed during infection do not agglutinate in the Weil-Felix test. These rickettsiae are resistant to destruction by environmental stresses, e.g., sunlight, humidity.

Isolation of *C. burnetii* from pulmonary secretions, liver biopsies, and surgical cardiac valve specimens is possible but not recommended unless appropriate laboratory facilities are available. This is a highly infectious agent that can readily cause laboratory-acquired infections. These materials are injected into eggs and/or guinea pigs. In the latter, the production of agglutinating antibodies confirms the presence of the organism. *C. burnetii* can exist in two phases. Phase I organisms are usually associated with chronic, severe clinical illnesses, such as endocarditis. Phase II organisms evolve (through the loss of mono- and polysaccharide chains of the lipopolysaccharide surface antigens) following multiple transfers in eggs. Phase II is equivalent to the rough and Phase I to the smooth form of gram-negative bacteria. Antibodies to Phase II organisms are predominant in the majority of patients with Q fever. However, patients with endocarditis have higher titers of antibodies to Phase I organisms, specifically IgA and IgG; the latter two types of antibodies are diagnostic for this entity.

Three different types of plasmids have been found in *C. burnetii*. These may account for the variations in virulence of strains but do not account for the phase variation, since plasmids are found in organisms in either phase. Persons with mild infections have isolates that contain different plasmids from those isolated from patients with endocarditis. These plasmids control the production of proteins that may be involved in the infectious process. Another virulence factor appears to be the lipopolysaccharide antigens. These antigens are variable, but are strain-specific and thus are unique for those strains associated with chronic disease, such as endocarditis. Similarly, other specific antigens are on strains that cause mild disease.

EPIDEMIOLOGY. Human disease is acquired by inhalation of aerosols containing *C. burnetii*. The organisms are disseminated from domestic and pet animals (cats). The placentas from these animals contain huge concentrations of rickettsiae. During delivery of the placenta, aerosols are generated which may be wind borne to contaminate soil, clothing, and the wool or fur of other animals or may be transmitted hundreds of yards to susceptible persons. Trucks carrying sheep appear to disseminate organisms to persons passed on the streets. Sheep regularly transported to research laboratories through hallways in a medical center caused an epidemic that persisted for 6 months. Organisms are also found in the mammary glands and milk of sheep and cows, amniotic fluid, and feces. The ability of *C. burnetii* to form sporelike structures that resist environmental destruction allows these organisms to cause disease long after the initial contamination occurs and at sites distant from the original source.

The animals are infected by ticks. There are ticks that transmit the organisms among wild animals, such as the kangaroo in Australia. Spread to domestic animals occurs when the two populations of animals intermingle. Ticks have not been implicated in the transmission from animals to humans. Q fever is a mild and inapparent infection in animals. It may be responsible for placental deficiencies that lead to stillbirth of kittens and lambs.

Various volunteer studies, designed to evaluate vaccine effectiveness, have demonstrated that very few organisms, probably less than 10, are sufficient to induce disease. For this reason, as well as the ability to survive in most environments, *C. burnetii* is a hazardous organism with which to work. In one laboratory 21 of 50 cases diagnosed over a 15-year period occurred in persons working in laboratories (or offices) not directly involved in Q fever research. Presumably, these persons were infected by widely disseminated aerosols from laboratory accidents or from contaminated clothing of workers socializing outside their laboratory. Despite the infectious nature of the organism and its presence in sputum, human-to-human transmission does not occur and respiratory isolation for infected patients is not needed.

In the United States and Canada, *C. burnetii* (and antibodies) have been found in milk from numerous herds of cattle. Despite this evidence, documented cases of Q fever occurring after the ingestion of unpasteurized milk from such cows have not been identified. The ingestion of 10^5 organisms by mouth by volunteers failed to induce disease. If disease occurs, it could originate from aerosols created in the act of pouring the milk into a glass.

The incubation period varies indirectly with inoculum size. Large doses result in disease at about 7 days. Most persons develop symptoms at 13 to 18 days.

PATHOLOGY. Knowledge of the pathologic changes is greatest for the more severe form of this disease. For example, microscopic examinations of liver biopsies and autopsy material from patients dying of chronic hepatitis and from heart valves infected with *C. burnetii* are available. Patients with pneumonitis usually have a mild illness so tissue specimens are scarce. Animal studies have provided complementary pathohistologic data.

Hepatitis. Granulomas with fatty necrosis are typical microscopic findings. These granulomas are doughnut-shaped. While they are common in Q fever, they also are seen in patients with tuberculosis. Fatty metamorphosis is also seen. Patients with mild forms of Q fever may have elevated liver enzyme values indicative of minimal liver cell damage.

Subacute and Chronic Endocarditis. This is a life-threatening disease because of the difficulty in eradicating the infection. These patients may have large vegetations on the aortic valve and less likely on the mitral valve. They have negative blood cultures and frequently have a history of a febrile illness with or without pneumonitis months previously. The vegetations have a histologic picture similar to that in other forms of endocarditis, an avascular collection of fibrin and platelets. These patients also have enlarged livers and spleens, plus signs of vasculitis associated with endocarditis, e.g., splinter hemorrhages, Roth spots, and petechiae.

Pneumonitis. In the few autopsies performed, consolidation similar to that of other bacterial pneumonias was the gross finding. The microscopic examination revealed an exudate loaded with histocytes and no polymorphonuclear leukocytes. This inflammatory response is compatible with a nonbacterial process. The histologic features have been described as those of a "severe intra-alveolar, focally necrotizing, hemorrhagic pneumonia with associated necrotizing bronchitis and bronchiolitis."

The portal of entry of *C. burnetii* is the respiratory tract; small particles less than 3 to 5 μ in diameter can reach the terminal bronchioles. The pneumonia does not appear until the third or fourth day of fever. In a mouse model, the rickettsia enter

pneumatocytes, histiocytes, and fibroblasts. The self-limiting nature of this infection is probably related to the destruction of the organisms in the macrophages. However, *C. burnetii* can persist for 2 months inside those cells. Some of the macrophages can be damaged by *C. burnetii*, leading to an inflammatory response. Cellular immune mechanisms attack these damaged cells. Numerous factors are involved in the pathogenesis of pneumonia—the number and virulence of the rickettsiae, particle size, and the functional status of the macrophages and parenchymal cells of the lung.

CLINICAL MANIFESTATIONS. The onset of Q fever is very abrupt; the manifestations are not specific. The patient develops a high fever that is associated with headache, chills, myalgia, and malaise. This flulike syndrome differs from influenza disease because of the height of the temperature, frequently 39.4° to 40°C. The fever also persists for 10 to 14 days. No rash occurs. Retro-orbital pain, common in other rickettsial infections, is reported in 10 to 15 per cent of patients.

Patients may have a dry, nonproductive cough indicative of the bronchiolitis and the minimal pneumonitis produced by the invading *C. burnetii*. Physical findings of consolidated lung are lacking early in the course of the pneumonia. There may be decreased breath sounds, but rales are unlikely until resolution of the lesion(s) begins. The chest films reveal patchy infiltrates that frequently are multiple round, segmental opacities. These are discrete lesions. Larger areas of the lung may show consolidation, and linear atelectatic lesions occur in about half the patients with pneumonia. Resolution of the lesions is slow. The incidence of pneumonitis varies from 4 to 97 per cent in series of cases reported from the United States (28 per cent), Australia (4 to 75 per cent), and Switzerland (97 per cent). The reasons for these variations are unknown.

Most patients (85 per cent) with Q fever have hepatic involvement as measured by abnormal liver cell enzymes. Hepatomegaly is noted in about 65 per cent of patients, but few patients (10 per cent) have liver tenderness. Jaundice is unlikely (about 5 per cent of cases) unless chronic hepatitis ensues, a very rare manifestation. Liver biopsies have demonstrated, by direct immunofluorescent studies, rickettsia residing in hepatic cells. Q fever may account for a few cases of acute hepatitis. Patients with a strong exposure history should be evaluated for infection by *C. burnetii*.

The clinical manifestations of Q fever endocarditis are characteristic of those associated with the syndrome of endocarditis, e.g., splenomegaly, splinter hemorrhages, and heart murmurs. In the United States, endocarditis caused by *C. burnetii* is an extremely rare condition. Evidence of endocarditis in a patient occurs years after the acute infection. This fact, plus the lack of positive blood cultures, leads to a delay in diagnosis. The diagnosis is made by serologic means, demonstrating a high titer or a rising titer of Phase I antibodies, especially IgA and IgG classes. The level of Phase I antibodies is higher than that of Phase II, a reversal of what is seen in the common forms of Q fever. Presumably, the polysaccharide nature of the Phase I antigens is the reason they are poor immunogens, but their chronic presence leads finally to high antibody production.

DIAGNOSIS. The key to making a diagnosis of Q fever in a patient with a debilitating febrile illness is obtaining a history of contact with sheep, cattle, goats, or cats or the skins or wool from these animals. This history should be compelling enough to initiate antibiotic treatment and to obtain acute and convalescent serum for serologic studies. These latter studies are the practical and definitive diagnostic aids. Phase II antibodies (complement fixing [CF] or indirect fluorescent antibody [IFA]) are present in two thirds of patients at the end of 2 weeks of illness and in 90 per cent at 1 month. Phase I antibodies, if present, are found in titers lower than Phase II antibodies. IFA is more sensitive than CF in detecting early antibody formation (IgM) and also in demonstrating persistence of antibody at 1 year or longer. The presence of Phase I antibodies in excess of Phase II, and specifically Phase I IgA, is diagnostic of Q fever endocarditis.

The nonspecific clinical manifestations of early symptoms and signs of Q fever, e.g., headache, fever, myalgia, suggest numerous infectious diseases. Influenza infections are seasonal, the temperature is less than that of Q fever, and liver function tests are normal. The white blood cell count is not helpful, as it is normal in both infections. Other diseases such as typhoid fever and brucellosis can be diagnosed by bacterial cultures. Viral hepatitis can be mistaken for Q fever. Appropriate serologic studies and liver biopsy provide diagnostic evidence. In those patients with pneumonitis, the differential diagnosis includes viral or mycoplasmal etiologies, tularemia, psittacosis, and *Legionella pneumophila*. Serologic and culture results identify these organisms.

TREATMENT AND PROGNOSIS. *C. burnetii* is known to be susceptible to a number of antibiotics. Sensitivity studies have been conducted in eggs, guinea pigs, and recently in acute and chronically infected tissue culture cells. Tetracycline and doxycycline or chloramphenicol have been effective in vitro as well as in clinical studies. Early institution of tetracycline (within 3 days of onset) reduces the febrile course by half. Tetracycline, 500 mg four times a day, or doxycycline, 100 mg twice a day, should be continued for at least 1 week after the patient becomes afebrile (usually 2 to 3 days). The prognosis with such therapy is excellent, with no mortality expected. Those patients who receive no antibiotics also do well, with a recovery rate of over 99 per cent. If a febrile relapse occurs, retreatment with the same antibiotic is effective.

The recommended treatment of patients with Q fever endocarditis is not settled. Long-term therapy (1 year or more) with combinations of antibiotics has been effective in small numbers of patients. Tetracycline plus trimethoprim-sulfamethoxazole and rifampin plus doxycycline are two such combinations. Evidence from tissue culture studies indicates that the quinoline antibiotics in combination with rifampin may offer a therapeutic advance. Surgical resection of infected valves is usually required because the large vegetations cause hemodynamic deficiencies in cardiac function.

PREVENTION. There is no commercially available vaccine for Q fever. Experimental vaccines using either Phase I or Phase II organisms have been effective in preventing disease in volunteers and in several field trials. For those persons at high risk, such as researchers working with sheep, veterinarians, or exposed laboratory workers, vaccine can be obtained under an investigational new drug (IND) application.

Focusing on controlling disease in the workplace is more effective than attempting to control the disease in animals. Three recommended measures include knowledge of the serologic status of the employees, not permitting pregnant women or persons with valvar heart disease to be in the high-risk jobs, and confining the research on sheep to a building dedicated solely to that purpose. Vaccination of employees should also be attempted.

Derrick EH: "Q" fever, a new fever entity: Clinical features, diagnosis and investigation. Med J Aust 2:281, 1937. *The original description of Q fever.*

Khavin T, Tabibzadeh S: Histologic, immunofluorescence, and electron microscopic study of infectious process in mouse lung after intranasal challenge with *Coxiella burnetii*. Infect Immun 56:1792, 1988.

Meikeljohn G, Reimer EG, Graves PS, et al: Cryptic epidemic of Q fever in a medical school. J Infect Dis 144:107, 1981. *A good epidemiologic study of Q fever originating in a research laboratory.*

Millar JK: The chest film findings in "Q" fever—a series of 35 cases. Clin Radiol 29:371, 1978.

Sawyer LA, Fishbein DB, McDade JE: Q Fever: Current concepts. Rev Infect Dis 9:935, 1987. *An excellent review of recent investigations concerning Q fever.*

Urso FP: The pathologic findings in rickettsial pneumonia. Am J Clin Pathol 64:335, 1975.

Yeaman MR, Roman MJ, Baca OG: Antibiotic susceptibilities of two *Coxiella burnetii* isolates implicated in distinct clinical syndromes. Antimicrob Agents Chemother 33:2053, 1989. *A new method to evaluate sensitivities of Q fever isolates to antibiotics.*

Zoonoses

357 Zoonoses

J. Bruce McClain

Many infectious diseases are zoonoses with which we come into contact by way of occupation, avocation, or bad luck. Since the manifestations of disease change with each species, a mild infection for one species can be lethal for another. Many zoonoses are treated fully elsewhere in this book. This chapter is an attempt to inform practitioners of diseases contracted from animals which may deserve mention although not extensive description and are treated more fully and properly in subspecialty textbooks.

There are still three main venues where zoonotic illness is contracted: agriculture, laboratory work, and pets. Laboratory-acquired disease depends on the agents in the laboratory as well as agents proper to the species. A review summarizing the experience from several large research institutions dealing in biomedical research indicated that the most common occupational illnesses are, in decreasing order, brucellosis, Q fever, typhoid, infectious hepatitis, tularemia, tuberculosis, dermatomycoses, Venezuelan equine encephalitis, typhus, and psittacosis. Common pet-acquired illnesses are toxoplasmosis, toxocariasis, dermatomycoses, psittacosis, salmonellosis, cat scratch disease, campylobacteriosis, and lymphocytic choriomeningitis. Common agricultural illnesses are brucellosis, hydatid disease, leptospirosis, Q fever, yersinosis, cryptosporidiosis, campylobacteriosis, and anthrax. Brief descriptions of zoonoses not covered elsewhere in this text are found in Table 357–1.

Donham KJ: Zoonotic diseases of occupational significance in agriculture: A review. Int J Zoon 12:163, 1985. *An extensive description of 40 of the most important zoonoses.*

Miller CD, Songer JR, Sullivan JF: A twenty-five year review of laboratory-acquired human infection at the National Animal Disease Center. Am Ind Hyg Assoc J 48:271, 1987. *A summary of all major reports from large research institutions on occupational zoonoses.*

Stehr-Green JK, Schantz PM: The impact of zoonotic diseases transmitted by pets on human health and the economy. Vet Clin North Am: Small Anim Pract 17:1, 1987. *A description of the number of cases and fatality of pet-transmitted disease.*

TABLE 357–1. CHARACTERISTICS OF SELECTED ZOONOSES

Microorganism	Common Name(s)	Epidemiology	Syndrome	Mode of Transmission	Reservoir	Diagnosis	Treatment	Prevention
Corynebacterium ovis	Pseudotuberculosis	12 cases in agricultural workers of sheep and goats	Lymphadenitis	Mechanical inoculation from infected animals	Sheep and goats, 10–80% of herds	BI blood agar 10% CO_2	Penicillin, erythromycin, resistant to TMX	B
Pasteurella multocida	—	14,000 cases/year in pet owners and laboratory workers	Cellulitis, respiratory infection, bacteremia, similar to *H. influenzae*	Animal bites, contact with oral secretion	Dogs, cats, other domestic and wild mammals	BI	Oral AMP, TCN, IM/IV PEN G, CEF	B
Rhodococcus equi	*Corynebacterium equi*	19 cases in immunosuppressed patients	F, Mal, C, L, lung abscess	Aerosol	Cattle, pigs, sheep, cats	BI	CHL, VAN, GEN	None
Streptobacillus moniliformis	Rat-bite fever, Haverhill fever	1–2 cases/year; 12% mortality untreated	HA, N&V, My, R, arthritis 70%, endocarditis	Rat bite, trauma, food contamination	Rats, mice, weasels, dogs, pigs	Isolation on special medium, SC	PEN G, AMP, TCN, CHL × 10 days	B
Spirillum minus	Rate-bite fever, sodoku	<1 case/year; 7% mortality untreated	Local eschar, F, HA, N&V, R	Subcutaneous inoculation of infected mammals	Rodents and other mammals	Animal passage, darkfield of peripheral blood	PEN × 25 days	B
Herpesvirus simiae	Virus W	Laboratory workers, 24 cases reported, 18/24 fatal	Encephalitis, preceded by local itching or numbness	Skin defect in contact with infected saliva or animal tissues. Human-to-human transmission has occurred.	*Macaca mulatta*; lethal epizootics have occurred in bonnet macaques, pata, and colobus monkeys	SC, VI	Hyperimmune globulin not useful. ACY used in 2 human cases; ACY effective in animal model	?ACY, B
Parapoxvirus infections	Orf, milker's nodule, bovine papular stomatitis[a]	Agricultural workers	Granulomatous ulcerative lesions with regional adenopathy	Contact with infected secretions or trauma from virus-contaminated objects	Goats, cows	Histopathology, VI, electron microscopy	None	B
Paramyxovirus	Newcastle disease	Poultry workers	Follicular conjunctivitis, F, C, Mal	Direct contact with infected birds or environmental aerosols	Poultry and other birds	SC, VI	None	B, mask
Orthopox virus	Monkeypox (mouse pox, cow pox, buffalo pox[b])	Agricultural, laboratory workers, pets	L, F, R, skin pox, fever, HA, Mal, like smallpox	Direct contact	Multiple species	SC to specific virus, VI	None	B
Rhabdovirus	Vesicular stomatitis virus	Agricultural and veterinary workers	F, My, N&V, Mal, oral vesicles	Direct contact with infected animal	Horses, cattle, wild and domestic swine, plus others	SC, VI from blood	None	B
Animal herpes virus	Pseudorabies, mad itch	7 cases with animal contact	Dysphagia, altered taste and smell, cutaneous dysesthesia, paresthesia, pruritus, cranial nerve palsy	Skin and mucous membrane contact	Pigs, cats, livestock	SC, VI	None; cases resolved	B
Arenavirus	Lymphocytic choriomeningitis virus	Outbreaks from pets and labs	Aseptic meningitis	Aerosols and direct contact	Mice, hamsters	SC, VI	None	Extermination

[a]There are subtle differences between isolates from the above three diseases, but the lesions and virions are morphologically indistinguishable and serology is not useful, so the name depends on the epidemiologic setting.

[b]These are distinct viruses and the syndromes differ, but the histopathology of the lesions is similar.

Abbreviations

ACY	= acyclovir	CEF	= cephalosporin	N&V	= nausea and vomiting
AMP	= ampicillin	CHL	= chloramphenicol	PEN	= penicillin
B	= barrier techniques taken to mean physical separation and or quarantine for affected animals	F	= fever	R	= rash
		GEN	= gentamicin	SC	= seroconversion
		HA	= headache	TCN	= tetracycline
BI	= bacterial isolation	L	= lymphadenopathy	TMX	= sulfa/trimethoprim
C	= cough	Mal	= malaise	VAN	= vancomycin
		My	= myalgia	VI	= virus isolation

SECTION THREE / VIRAL DISEASES

358 Introduction to Viral Diseases

R. Gordon Douglas, Jr.

Viruses are among the simplest and smallest of all forms of life. They are obligate intracellular parasites that require host cell structural and metabolic components for replication. They infect bacteria as well as plants and animals. More than 400 distinct viruses infect humans. They produce diseases ranging from subclinical infections and mild, self-limited, localized infections to common systemic infections and overwhelming, highly lethal infections such as meningoencephalitis or hemorrhagic fever with shock.

CHARACTERISTICS OF VIRUSES

Essentially, virus particles, or virions, consist of nucleic acid enclosed in a protein coat. They lack metabolic activity and do not possess ribosomes or most enzymes necessary for replication. In addition, some possess a lipid envelope. Both the lipid and the protein coats protect the nucleic acid from enzymatic degradation. The nucleic acid may be either deoxyribonucleic acid (DNA) or ribonucleic acid (RNA). It may code for only a few or, in some cases, several hundred proteins. The protein coat, or capsid, consists of repeating, identical subunits called capsomeres. The capsid and nucleic acid together are called the nucleocapsid. The smallest (parvoviruses) are only 18 nm in diameter, whereas some poxviruses may be as large as 450 nm in diameter.

There are two major types of structure of virus particles. In the first type, capsomeres are arranged as a regular polyhedron with 20 triangular faces and 12 corners. Such a virus exhibits icosahedral symmetry. Many nonenveloped viruses are of this type. Other viruses exhibit helical symmetry in which a helix is formed of ribonucleoprotein and nucleic acid. Helical viruses are always enveloped, whereas icosahedral viruses may be enveloped

or nonenveloped. The envelope is derived from host cell membranes and modified by insertion of one or more spike-like glycoproteins. These and other proteins on the surface of enveloped or nonenveloped viruses are important for two reasons: They provide specific interaction with receptors on host cells, and they serve as the major antigens of the virus.

Figure 358–1 demonstrates schematically the marked variety in size, shape, and structure of human viruses. In addition, there is great diversity in the structure of the viral genome: Either RNA or DNA may be single stranded or double stranded. The genome may be linear or circular and may exist as single or multiple segments.

Viruses are classified by the International Committee on Taxonomy of Viruses according to the scheme presented in Table 358–1. The following order of virion characteristics is used: nucleic acid type, presence or absence of envelope, genome replication strategy, positive- or negative-sense genome, and genome segmentation.

As a result of the variety of structures of viruses and the complexities of genomes, mechanisms of replication are diverse and dependent upon the structure of the virus and its genome. Following a random collision between a virus particle and a cell surface, attachment occurs by binding of a surface protein of a virus to a host cell virus receptor. Penetration of the plasma membrane of the cell occurs by endocytosis, a process similar to receptor-mediated endocytosis of nonviral ligands, or by nonendocytic pathways such as direct translocation across the plasma membrane. Following acidification of the endosome, fusion of the viral membrane with that of the vesicle occurs, releasing the nucleocapsid. After uncoating of the viral nucleic acid, macromolecular synthesis of nucleic acid and protein occurs. The strategy for genome replication is dependent on the type of nucleic acid. Assembly of virus components then occurs, with release of mature viruses by budding, in the case of enveloped viruses, or by lysis of the cell, in the case of some nonenveloped viruses. Such released virions are infectious for other cells.

Viruses cause cell injury by a number of mechanisms: directly by lysis resulting from viral replication, by lysis induced by

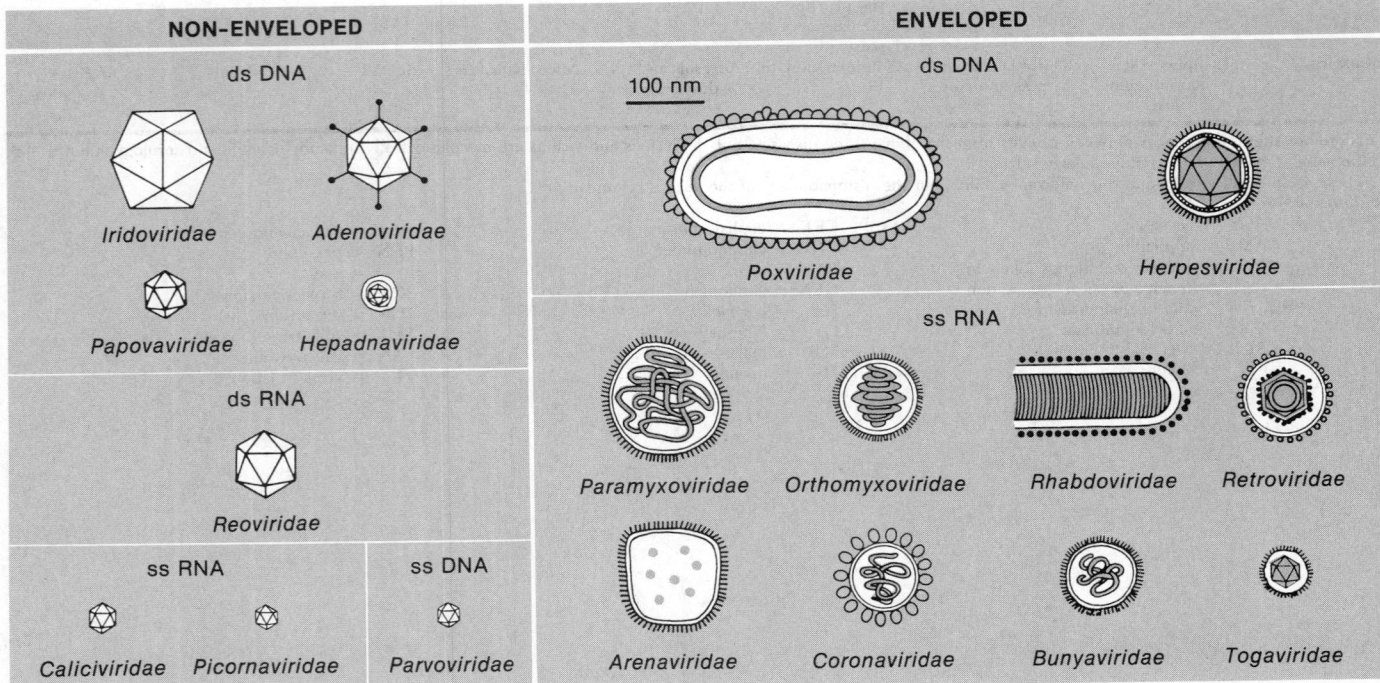

FIGURE 358–1. Structure and relative size of human virus families. (Modified from Matthews REF: Intervirology 12:158, 1979.)

TABLE 358–1. CLASSIFICATION OF HUMAN VIRUSES

Dividing Characteristics	Virus Families	Important Human Viruses
DNA Viruses		
dsDNA, enveloped	Poxviridae	Variola (smallpox) virus
		Vaccinia virus
	Herpesviridae	Herpes simplex virus types 1 and 2
		Varicella-zoster virus
		Human cytomegalovirus
		EB virus
		Human herpesvirus type 6
dsDNA, nonenveloped	Adenoviridae	Human adenovirus
	Papovaviridae	Papillomavirus
	Hepadnaviridae	Hepatitis B virus
ssDNA, nonenveloped	Parvoviridae	Parvovirus B19
RNA Viruses		
dsRNA, nonenveloped	Reoviridae	Colorado tick fever virus
		Human rotaviruses
ssRNA, enveloped		
No DNA step in replication		
Positive-sense genome	Togaviridae	Alphavirus: Eastern equine encephalitis, Western equine encephalitis
		Rubivirus: Rubella virus
	Flaviviridae	Yellow fever virus
		Dengue viruses
		St. Louis encephalitis
	Coronaviridae	Human coronaviruses
Negative-sense genome		
Nonsegmented genome	Paramyxoviridae	Parainfluenza virus
		Measles virus
		Respiratory syncytial virus
	Rhabdoviridae	Rabies virus
	Filoviridae	Marburg and Ebola viruses
Segmented genome	Orthomyxoviridae	Influenza A and B virus
	Bunyaviridae	California encephalitis virus
	Arenaviridae	LCM virus
		Lassa virus
DNA step in replication	Retroviridae	HTLV I, II
		HIV I, II
ssRNA, nonenveloped	Picornaviridae	Polioviruses, coxsackieviruses, echoviruses, rhinoviruses
	Caliciviridae	Norwalk virus

EB = Epstein-Barr; LCM = lymphocytic choriomeningitis; ss = single stranded; ds = double stranded.

From Murphy FA: Virus taxonomy. *In* Fields BN: Virology. New York, Raven Press, 1985. With permission.

antiviral antibody and complement, or by cell-mediated immune mechanisms recognizing infected host cells. As virus infection spreads and sufficient numbers of cells are injured, disease results. A role for viral toxins has never been established, and such enzymes that are virus coded have a role in viral replication, but not directly in cellular injury, and they do not affect host tissues at distant sites. However, release of products of inflammation from sites of cell injury and circulating interferon and other lymphokines may contribute to the signs and symptoms of viral infection.

In addition to lytic effects on cells, viral infection may transform cells so that they proliferate continuously, and in vertebrates, mammals, and humans, may produce tumors, sometimes as a result of the occurrence of viral oncogenes in such viruses.

HOST DEFENSE MECHANISMS

In addition to nonspecific barriers such as skin, respiratory epithelium, gastric acidity, and so on, three main host defense mechanisms against viral infections have been described: (1) production of specific antiviral antibody; (2) development of specific cell-mediated immunity involving cytotoxic T cells and nonspecific effector cells such as natural killer (NK) cells; and (3)

proliferation of macrophages that restrict virus replication and dissemination and can also destroy infected cells.

Antiviral antibodies develop in response to viral infection and to immunization with attenuated or inactivated virus or viral components. In the serum, antibodies of all classes and subclasses of immunoglobulins are found; in addition, secretory antibodies consisting predominantly of immunoglobulin A (IgA) molecules develop on mucosal surfaces in response to infection of their surfaces. They are of critical importance in diseases in which the primary site of inoculation is a mucosal surface.

The immune system may interact with extracellular (free) virus or cell-associated virus. Specific antibody inactivates (neutralizes) extracellular virus, and this activity may be enhanced by complement. Thus, it can prevent initial infection or restrict cell-to-cell spread of virus through extracellular fluids. It cannot, however, penetrate into cells and neutralize intracellular virus. Thus, virus may escape the effects of antibody by direct cell-to-cell transfer. Virus-infected cells possess viral antigens on their surface and may be lysed by specific antibody and complement, by specific cytotoxic T cells, or by nonspecific cells such as NK cells or macrophages. Virus released in the process may be neutralized by antiviral antibody.

Cytotoxic T cells (Tc), which are HLA class I antigen restricted, also develop in response to infection or immunization (Ch. 242). They are important in limiting the growth of certain viruses in the infected host. This has been most clearly shown for influenza infections in mice, and Tc are undoubtedly important in a number of viral infections in humans.

Natural killer cells are another important host defense mechanism against viral infections. During early stages of viral infection, the numbers of natural killer cells and their activity are greatly augmented by virus-induced interferon. Mice deficient in NK cells are more sensitive to cytomegalovirus infection, and NK activity has been demonstrated in a number of human infections.

Virus-induced interferons (α and β) have important roles in protection against virus infection through their ability to prevent viral replication in many cells throughout the body and by means of their regulatory function in the immune system. In experimental infections in animals in which interferon activity is neutralized by specific antibody, potentiation of viral infection occurs. In humans, in a number of infections, development of endogenous

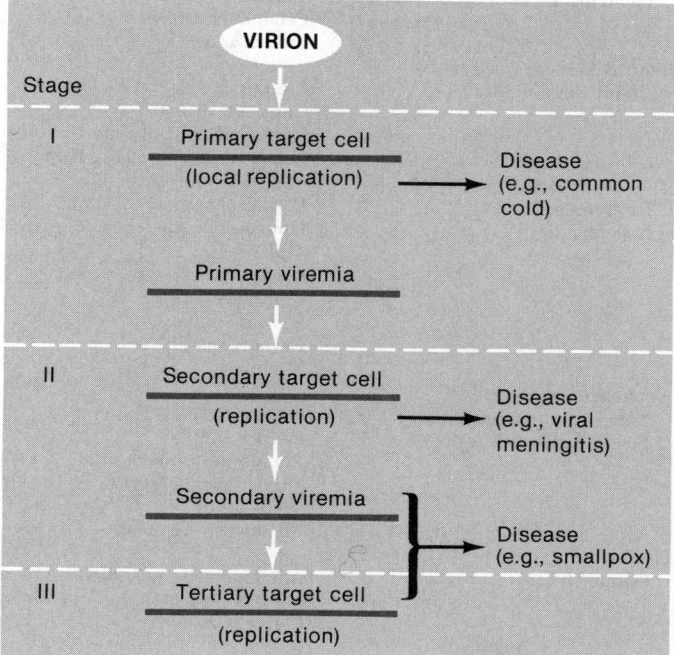

FIGURE 358–2. Stages of viral pathogenesis. Initial invasion may involve only primary target cells or may lead to secondary or tertiary target cell invasion, which results in the characteristic disease. (Courtesy of ED Kilbourne.)

interferon in serum or secretions correlates with recovery: decreasing virus titers and amelioration of symptoms. Since administration of interferon to humans produces a number of side effects, such as fever, leukopenia, and myalgias, interferon may also account, in part, for some of the systemic signs and symptoms that accompany viral infections.

Interferon-γ is induced as a result of immune stimulation. It also has antiviral effects and is a major immune regulatory protein that induces Tc, activates macrophages and NK cells, and regulates antibody production by B cells.

MECHANISMS OF PATHOGENESIS

Infection is initiated, often when one or a very few virus particles are deposited in the respiratory tract, gastrointestinal tract, or genitourinary tract or are injected percutaneously or pass transplacentally. As shown in Figure 358–2, human viral infections may be classified according to mechanisms of pathogenesis. Many infections are limited to cells at the portal of entry, and dissemination does not occur. Conjunctivitis due to adenovirus type 8 and common colds due to rhinoviruses and to other respiratory viruses are excellent examples of this type of pathogenesis.

Other virus infections spread hematogenously to distal sites. Infection at the primary site may or may not result in symptoms, but viral replication in the distal site usually results in the characteristic illness associated with such a virus infection. Enteroviruses such as coxsackievirus and echovirus infect the gastrointestinal tract as their primary site, and this infection is usually clinically silent but produces a primary viremia, following which encephalitis, meningitis, or other central nervous system disease may occur as these tissues are infected.

In other infections, viral replication in the secondary site produces a viremia that results in replication in still other sites. Such was the case with smallpox and may be the case with measles. Rash may be a manifestation of either primary or secondary viremia.

Many virus infections have clinical characteristics that permit diagnosis: measles, mumps, chicken pox, and poliomyelitis. However, many others do not, and many syndromes have multiple etiologies, as is shown in Table 358–2. In fact, as many as 200 serologically distinct viruses may cause the common cold and related disorders. In the case of some syndromes—for example, atypical pneumonia—the etiology may be shared with other infectious organisms: *Mycoplasma pneumoniae*, *Chlamydia pneumoniae*, and *Legionella pneumophila*. Others, however, are exclusively viral in etiology.

TABLE 358–2. VIRUSES COMMONLY ASSOCIATED WITH DIFFERENT SYNDROMES

Disease Category	Common Associated Virus	Disease Category	Common Associated Virus
Respiratory Tract		*Immune System*	
Upper respiratory infection (including common cold and pharyngitis)	Rhinoviruses Coronaviruses Parainfluenza 1–3 Influenza A, B Herpes simplex Adenoviruses Echoviruses Coxsackieviruses Epstein-Barr virus Respiratory syncytial	Acquired immunodeficiency syndrome	Human immunodeficiency virus I
		Gastrointestinal Tract	
		Gastroenteritis	Rotavirus Norwalk-like agents Adenovirus
		Hepatitis	Hepatitis A Hepatitis B Hepatitis C Delta virus Hepatitis E Epstein-Barr virus Cytomegalovirus
Croup	Parainfluenza 1–3 Influenza A, B Respiratory syncytial		
Bronchiolitis	Respiratory syncytial Parainfluenza 1–3	*Skin*	
Pneumonia (adults)	Influenza A	Maculopapular rash	Measles Rubella Parvovirus B19 Echoviruses Coxsackievirus A16 Enterovirus 71
Pneumonia (children)	Respiratory syncytial Parainfluenza 1–3 Influenza A		
Central Nervous System		Hemorrhagic rash	Herpesvirus G Alphavirus Bunyavirus Flaviviruses
Aseptic meningitis	Mumps Coxsackievirus B1–5 Coxsackievirus A9 Echovirus 4, 6, 9, 11, 14, 18, 30, 31		
		Localized lesions	Herpes simplex Human papillomavirus 1, 2, 4, 41 Molluscum contagiosum
Paralysis	Polio 1–3		
Encephalitis	Human immunodeficiency virus I Alphaviruses Flaviviruses Bunyaviruses Herpes simplex 1 Enterovirus 71 Mumps	*Neonatal*	
		Teratogenic effects	Rubella Cytomegalovirus
		Disseminated disease	Coxsackievirus B1–5 Echoviruses Hepatitis B Parvovirus B19 Cytomegalovirus Herpes simplex
Genitourinary Tract			
Vulvovaginitis, cervicitis	Herpes simplex 2		
Penile and vulvar lesions	Herpes simplex 2 Molluscum contagiosum Human papillomavirus 6, 10, 11, 40–45, 51	Lower respiratory disease	Respiratory syncytial Influenza
		Enteritis	Rotavirus
Acute hemorrhagic cystitis	Adenovirus 11	*Other*	
Ocular		Arthritis	Rubella Parvovirus B19 Hepatitis B
Conjunctivitis	Adenovirus 3, 4, 7, 8, 19 Herpes simplex Varicella-zoster Measles	Myositis	Togaviruses Influenza B
Acute hemorrhagic conjunctivitis	Enterovirus 70 Coxsackievirus A 24	Carditis	Coxsackievirus B
		Parotitis, pancreatitis, and orchitis	Mumps

Modified from Menegus MA, Douglas RG Jr: Viruses, rickettsia, chlamydiae, and mycoplasmas. *In* Mandell GL, Douglas RG, Jr, Bennett JE: Principles and Practice of Infectious Diseases, 3rd ed. New York, Churchill Livingstone, 1990.

Recent advances in antiviral chemotherapy have produced a number of specific antivirals that are available and effective for prophylaxis or treatment, or both, of certain viral diseases. Drugs such as trifluridine, amantadine, ribavirin, acyclovir, vidarabine, zidovudine, and ganciclovir are available in the United States. For many other viral infections, however, no specific therapy exists. Proper use of antivirals requires specific viral diagnosis. Fortunately, in the case of herpes zoster, the diagnosis can usually be made clinically, and in influenza, the diagnosis can often be made on clinical and epidemiologic grounds; however, for many infections, viral diagnosis is required. Viral diagnostic laboratories are more common than in the past, and rapid techniques are gaining acceptance.

Vaccines are available for a number of viral infections, and many have greatly affected morbidity and mortality due to specific infections. Antibodies induced by vaccination may block initiation of infection in a primary site, as in the case in influenza. Others, such as inactivated poliomyelitis vaccine, are designed to prevent primary viremia after initial infection has occurred. Live attenuated viruses induce cell-mediated as well as humoral immune response.

Fields BN (ed.): Virology, 2nd ed. New York, Raven Press, 1990. *Excellent recent definitive textbook of basic virology.*
Mandell GL, Douglas RG Jr, Bennett JE (eds.): Principles and Practice of Infectious Diseases, 3rd ed. New York, John Wiley & Sons, 1990. *Excellent reference work about clinical aspects of viral infections; both syndromes and specific viruses are discussed, as well as vaccines, antivirals, and diagnostic virology.*

359 Antiviral Therapy

Mark Middlebrooks and Richard J. Whitley

Compared with the progress made in the treatment of bacterial infections over the past four decades, advances in the chemotherapy of viral diseases have come much more slowly. In the United States, only a few antiviral agents of proven clinical value are available and for a limited number of indications. The problems associated with the development of antiviral agents can be summarized as follows: (1) viruses are obligate intracellular parasites that utilize biochemical pathways of the infected host cell, so that it is difficult to achieve clinically useful antiviral activity without also adversely affecting host cell metabolism; (2) early diagnosis of viral infection is crucial for effective antiviral therapy, yet by the time symptoms appear several cycles of viral multiplication may have occurred and replication has begun to wane; (3) precise diagnosis is difficult for many viral infections because of the lack of specificity of symptoms; and (4) since many of the disease syndromes caused by viruses are common, relatively benign, and self-limiting, the therapeutic index (ratio of efficacy to toxicity) must be extremely high for therapy to be acceptable.

As with all infectious diseases, the effectiveness of therapy is related to host defenses. Not only is the incidence of reactivation of certain viral diseases high in the immunocompromised host, but these infections are often much more severe. These patients require high doses of antiviral agents for long periods of time and have a high morbidity and mortality with currently approved antiviral therapy.

ANTIVIRALS FOR HERPESVIRUS INFECTIONS
Vidarabine

MECHANISM OF ACTION. Also known as vira-A or adenine arabinoside (9-β-D arabinofuranosyl adenine), vidarabine is a purine nucleoside analogue that is phosphorylated intracellularly to its active triphosphate derivative. This compound competitively inhibits DNA-dependent DNA polymerases of some DNA viruses approximately 40 times more than those of host cells. In addition, it is incorporated into DNA, thus inhibiting elongation. Although viral DNA synthesis is blocked at lower doses of drug than is host cell DNA synthesis, large doses of vidarabine are cytotoxic to dividing host cells.

LICENSED USES. Vidarabine is licensed currently for intravenous treatment of herpes simplex encephalitis (HSE), neonatal herpes simplex virus (HSV) infections, and varicella-zoster virus (VZV) infections in immunocompromised patients. In addition, vidarabine 3 per cent ophthalmic ointment is approved for the treatment of HSV keratoconjunctivitis and recurrent epithelial keratitis.

TOXICITY AND ADVERSE CLINICAL EFFECTS. When therapeutic doses are given intravenously, vidarabine causes few adverse effects in most patients. The most common side effects (10 to 15 per cent incidence) are gastrointestinal disturbances (e.g., anorexia, nausea, vomiting, diarrhea), which are usually mild. Central nervous system disturbances occasionally include tremors, dizziness, confusion, hallucinations, ataxia, and psychoses. An elevated aspartate aminotransferase level and blood urea nitrogen may also be seen. Doses of 20 mg per kilogram per day may cause more pronounced central nervous system effects as well as leukopenia and thrombocytopenia. Vidarabine is a relatively insoluble drug that requires continuous administration in large volumes of fluid given over 12 hours. This relative difficulty in administration as compared with acyclovir, as well as acyclovir's more favorable safety profile, has resulted in the latter becoming the drug of choice for virtually all HSV and VZV infections.

Vidarabine should be recognized historically as the first drug licensed for systemic use in the treatment of a viral infection. Although it is efficacious for a number of herpesvirus infections, for the most part it has been replaced by acyclovir.

Acyclovir

MECHANISM OF ACTION. Acyclovir, 9-((2-hydroxyethoxy)methyl) guanine, is an acyclic analogue of guanosine. Virus-specified thymidine kinase phosphorylates acyclovir to its monophosphate derivative, an event that does not occur in uninfected cells to a significant extent. Acyclovir is then further phosphorylated by cellular enzymes to its triphosphate derivative. Acyclovir triphosphate binds viral DNA polymerase, acting as a DNA chain terminator. Because acyclovir is taken up selectively by virus-infected cells, the concentration of acyclovir triphosphate is 40 to 100 times higher in infected than in uninfected cells. Furthermore, viral DNA polymerase exhibits a 10- to 30-fold greater affinity for acyclovir triphosphate than do cellular DNA polymerases. The higher concentration in infected cells plus the affinity for viral polymerases results in the very low toxicity of acyclovir for normal host cells. Although Epstein-Barr virus (EBV) and cytomegalovirus (CMV) do not have virus-specific thymidine kinases, acyclovir does have minimal activity against these viruses.

LICENSED USES. Acyclovir is available in ointment, capsule, and intravenous formulations. In the topical form, acyclovir is licensed for the management of primary herpes genitalis in both immunocompetent and immunocompromised hosts as well as in limited, non–life-threatening mucocutaneous HSV infections in immunocompromised hosts. It is less active topically than when delivered by other routes.

Oral acyclovir is indicated in the management of most cases of primary or initial genital herpes in all patient populations and as suppressive therapy in normal hosts with frequently recurrent genital herpes (six or more recurrences a year). Oral acyclovir is also used as prophylaxis and treatment in immunocompromised patients with a history of HSV infections, e.g., herpes labialis or genital herpes. High-dose oral acyclovir (i.e., 800 mg five times per day) has recently been approved for use in immunocompetent patients with localized herpes zoster. However, there has been no conclusive demonstration of a decrease in the incidence of postherpetic neuralgia after treatment with acyclovir.

Intravenous acyclovir is indicated in severe initial herpes genitalis of immunocompetent patients and in the treatment of some initial and recurrent mucocutaneous infections in immunocompromised patients, as well as in the treatment of HSE (licensure pending). Recently, intravenous acyclovir was approved for treatment of VZV infections in immunocompromised hosts. Oral high-dose administration for the treatment of VZV infections in immunocompromised patients is currently under investigation.

TABLE 359–1. DOSAGE ADJUSTMENT FOR INTRAVENOUS ACYCLOVIR IN PATIENTS WITH IMPAIRED RENAL FUNCTION

Creatinine Clearance (ml/min/1.73 M²)	Percentage of Standard Dose	Dosing Interval (Hours)
>50	100	8
25–50	100	12
10–25	100	24
0–10*	50	24

*Administered after hemodialysis.

TOXICITY. Acyclovir has an excellent safety profile and is well tolerated. The major adverse effect of acyclovir is alteration of renal function. High-dose bolus injection of acyclovir can cause crystallization in renal tubules and subsequent acute tubular necrosis, or simply a reversible elevation of serum creatinine. Dehydration, pre-existing renal insufficiency, and higher doses of acyclovir are risk factors for renal toxicity. Dosage alterations are required with renal impairment (Table 359–1). In addition, there have been a few brief reports suggesting CNS toxicity after intravenous administration of acyclovir. Oral acyclovir has not been associated with renal toxicity, even when given in high doses (800 mg five times a day).

Because acyclovir is a nucleoside analogue that can be incorporated into both viral and host-cell DNA, it has been studied extensively for its potential as a carcinogen, teratogen, and mutagen. There is no significant evidence that acyclovir is a carcinogen in humans, and animal studies indicate that acyclovir is not a significant teratogen in clinically used doses. Acyclovir is not a significant mutagen in vitro but seems to be able to induce chromosomal events in a manner similar to that of caffeine. Because of the many possible indications for acyclovir during pregnancy, as well as the likelihood of frequent first-trimester exposures to drug before pregnancy is established, it is extremely important to define the risk of acyclovir in pregnancy. An "Acyclovir in Pregnancy Registry" has been established to gather data on all reported prenatal exposures to oral acyclovir. Although no significant risk to the mother or fetus has been documented, the total number of monitored pregnancies remains too small to detect any risk that is not overwhelming. The safety of acyclovir in pregnancy, therefore, has not been unequivocally established. Since acyclovir crosses the placenta and can concentrate in amniotic fluid, there is valid concern about the potential for renal toxicity in the fetus.

RESISTANCE TO ACYCLOVIR. Resistance to acyclovir develops through mutations in one of two HSV genes, namely those specifying viral thymidine kinase (TK) or DNA polymerase. Clinical isolates resistant to acyclovir are almost uniformly deficient in TK. Until recently such resistance has been rare; all such mutants had reduced neurovirulence and did not readily establish latency. However, acyclovir-resistant HSV mutants are being reported more frequently in the immunocompromised patient population. These mutants are deficient in viral TK and sensitive to vidarabine and foscarnet, drugs that do not require viral TK for activation. Importantly, a small number of isolates are fully neurovirulent and able to establish latency in a murine model, a finding somewhat unusual for TK-deficient viruses. With the growing population of immunocompromised patients (due to both HIV infection and therapeutic immunosuppression) who suffer from frequent and severe herpesvirus infections, it is expected that acyclovir resistance will become more prevalent.

Ganciclovir

MECHANISM OF ACTION. Ganciclovir, also known as DHPG, is an acyclic nucleoside analogue of acyclovir that has increased in vitro activity against all herpesviruses as compared with acyclovir, including an 8 to 20 times greater antiviral activity against CMV. Like acyclovir, the activity of ganciclovir in HSV-infected cells depends upon phosphorylation by virus-specific TK. Also like acyclovir, ganciclovir monophosphate is further converted to its di- and triphosphate derivatives by cellular kinases. In cells infected by HSV-1 or HSV-2, the triphosphate (DHPG-TP) competitively inhibits the incorporation of guano-sine-TP into viral DNA and terminates chain synthesis. The mode of action of ganciclovir against CMV and EBV (which do not produce virus-specific TK) is not entirely known, but it has been suggested that these viruses may induce a cellular TK or other kinase that efficiently promotes the obligatory initial phosphorylation of ganciclovir to its monophosphate.

LICENSED USES. Ganciclovir has been licensed by the United States Food and Drug Administration for the treatment of CMV retinitis and life-threatening CMV diseases in AIDS and other immunocompromised patients.

TOXICITY. The most important side effects of ganciclovir are the development of neutropenia and thrombocytopenia. Neutropenia occurs in approximately 35 per cent of patients and is usually (but not always) reversible with dose adjustment or discontinuation. Thrombocytopenia occurs in about 20 per cent of patients. Numerous other side effects possibly related to ganciclovir, such as nausea, vomiting, dizziness, and headache, are usually not of clinical significance. Agents with significant myelotoxicity, such as antimetabolites or alkylating agents, cannot be used concomitantly with ganciclovir. Zidovudine (azidothymidine, or AZT) may be used cautiously in low doses in patients receiving ganciclovir, but hematologic parameters must be monitored closely.

Ganciclovir also has significant gonadal toxicity in animal screening systems, most notably as a potent inhibitor of spermatogenesis. As an agent affecting DNA synthesis, ganciclovir has carcinogenic potential.

CLINICAL USE. Ganciclovir has been the most widely tested drug for the treatment of CMV infections. There is support for clinical benefit in immunocompromised patients with CMV retinitis and gastrointestinal infection. Benefit is suggested but has been less dramatic for CMV pneumonia in AIDS patients and organ transplant recipients. There are many issues requiring further study to determine the optimal use of ganciclovir, including the indications, dose, duration of maintenance therapy, prophylactic use, usefulness of other modalities in combination (e.g., immunoglobulin therapy), and use in treatment of other life-threatening herpesvirus infections.

Idoxuridine and Trifluorothymidine

Idoxuridine and trifluorothymidine are analogues of thymidine. When administered systemically, these nucleosides are phosphorylated by both viral and cellular TK to active triphosphorylate derivatives that inhibit both viral and cellular DNA synthesis. The result is antiviral activity but also sufficient host cytotoxicity to prevent the systemic use of these drugs. Toxicity of these compounds is not significant, however, when applied topically to the eye in the treatment of HSV keratitis. Both idoxuridine and trifluorothymidine, as well as vidarabine, ophthalmic ointments are effective and licensed for such treatment. Acyclovir as an ophthalmic preparation also appears to be effective but is not yet licensed. Trifluorothymidine appears to be the most efficacious of these compounds. Although these agents are not of proven value in the treatment of stromal keratitis and uveitis, trifluorothymidine is more likely to penetrate the cornea. Some forms of stromal keratitis and uveitis are thought to be caused by immune mechanisms and thus would not respond to antiviral drugs. The ophthalmic preparations of idoxuridine, vidarabine, and trifluorothymidine may cause local irritation, photophobia, edema of the eyelids and cornea, punctual occlusion, and superficial punctate keratopathy.

ANTIVIRALS FOR RESPIRATORY VIRAL INFECTIONS

It is difficult to overestimate the impact of respiratory viral illnesses on human health. Almost 90 per cent of the population experiences one of these illnesses each year, resulting in a staggering number of days lost from work and school, as well as significant potential for serious morbidity and even death. Nonetheless, since these conditions in most patient populations are self-limited and rarely fatal, the requirements for new drugs are stringent: an extreme degree of safety, moderate to high effectiveness, ease of administration, and low cost. Accordingly, only two such antivirals are approved for use in the United States, each with fairly limited indications. Because of the number of developmental programs identifying new antivirals for treatment of respiratory viruses, it seems likely that an expanded armamentarium will be forthcoming.

Amantadine and Rimantadine

MECHANISM OF ACTION. Amantadine has a narrow spectrum of activity, and at concentrations achievable in humans it is useful only against influenza A infections. Although amantadine was the first antiviral to be approved in the United States, its mechanism of action is not yet completely understood. Influenza A viruses differ in their susceptibility to amantadine, and the drug may have different actions depending upon the concentration and virus strain. Early studies indicated that amantadine acted by preventing the penetration of the virus and/or by uncoating it. In more recent studies, low concentrations of the drug were shown to inhibit virus assembly by interacting with hemagglutinin; high concentrations appear to inhibit an early stage of the infection involving fusion between the virus envelope and the membrane of secondary lysosomes.

LICENSED USES. As an antiviral agent, amantadine is licensed for both the chemoprophylaxis and the treatment of influenza A infections. Amantadine can be used for any unimmunized member of the general population who wishes to avoid influenza A, but prophylaxis with amantadine is especially recommended for control of presumed influenza outbreaks in institutions housing high-risk persons. High-risk individuals include adults and children with chronic disorders of the cardiovascular or pulmonary systems requiring regular follow-up or hospitalization during the preceding year, as well as residents of nursing homes and other chronic-care facilities. In these instances, amantadine should be administered to all residents of the institution, whether or not they received influenza vaccination the previous fall. To reduce spread of virus and to minimize disruption of patient care, it is also recommended that amantadine prophylaxis be offered to unvaccinated staff who care for high-risk patients. Amantadine prophylaxis is also recommended in the following situations:

1. As an adjunct to late immunization of high-risk individuals. Amantadine does not interfere with antibody response to the vaccine.

2. For persons who have not been immunized and who care for high-risk persons in home settings, both to reduce spread of virus and to allow persons to maintain care for high-risk persons in the home setting.

3. For immunodeficient persons, who may be expected to have a poor antibody response to vaccine.

4. For persons for whom influenza vaccine is contraindicated, e.g., for persons hypersensitive to egg protein.

Amantadine is also indicated in the treatment of uncomplicated respiratory illness caused by influenza A. Studies have shown a beneficial effect on the signs and symptoms of acute influenza, as well as a significant reduction in quantity of virus in respiratory secretions. Because of the short duration of disease, amantadine must be administered within 48 hours of symptom onset to show benefit. The effect of amantadine on the prevention of complications in high-risk groups is under evaluation.

Rimantadine is a structural analogue of amantadine, with the same spectrum of activity, mechanism of action, and clinical indications. Rimantadine is used extensively in the Soviet Union and has been widely tested in the United States. It is anticipated that this drug will be licensed soon in the United States. Rimantadine is somewhat more effective than amantadine against influenza type A viruses at equal concentrations. Absorption of rimantadine is delayed when compared with amantadine, and, furthermore, equivalent doses of rimantadine produce lower plasma levels than does amantadine. The lower plasma levels may explain the lower incidence of side effects at similar doses. Rimantadine has similar CNS side effects even though, unlike amantadine, this drug does not affect CNS catecholamine release and is not effective in the treatment of Parkinson's disease. The efficacy of rimantadine in both the prophylaxis and treatment of influenza A infections is similar to that of amantadine. There has been a recent report of rimantadine-resistant strains of influenza isolated from patients treated for acute influenza A.

TOXICITY. Amantadine is reported to cause side effects in 5 to 10 per cent of healthy young adults taking the standard adult

TABLE 359–2. DOSAGE ADJUSTMENT FOR ORAL AMANTADINE IN PATIENTS WITH IMPAIRED RENAL FUNCTION

Creatinine Clearance (ml/min/1.73 M²)	Suggested Oral Maintenance Regimen After 200 mg (100 mg bid) on the First Day
≥ 80	100 mg bid
60–80	100 mg bid alternating with 100 mg daily
40–60	100 mg daily
30–40	200 mg (100 mg bid) twice weekly
20–30	100 mg 3 times each week
10–20	200 mg (100 mg bid) alternating with 100 mg every 7 days
<10	100 mg every 7 days

dose of 200 mg per day. These side effects are usually mild, cease soon after amantadine is discontinued, and often disappear even with continued use of the drug. Central nervous system side effects are most common and include difficulty in thinking, confusion, lightheadedness, hallucinations, anxiety, and insomnia. Activities requiring mental alertness (e.g., driving) should be avoided until it is reasonable to assume that these symptoms will not occur. More severe adverse effects, e.g., mental depression and psychosis, are usually associated with doses exceeding 200 mg daily. About 5 per cent of patients complain of nausea, vomiting, or anorexia. Older individuals are more likely to experience side effects. Rimantidine appears to be somewhat better tolerated.

Patients with renal disease should receive doses based on their creatinine clearance (Table 359–2). Doses for older people and children are usually lower as well. Persons with an active seizure disorder may be at increased risk for seizures when amantadine is given at standard doses.

Ribavirin

MECHANISM OF ACTION. Ribavirin is a nucleoside analogue whose mechanisms of action are poorly understood and probably not the same for all viruses; however, its ability to alter nucleotide pools and the packaging of mRNA appears to be important. This process is not totally virus specific, but there is a certain selectivity in that infected cells produce more mRNA than noninfected cells. The capacity of viral mRNA to support protein synthesis is markedly reduced by ribavirin. High concentrations also inhibit cellular protein synthesis.

LICENSED USES. The development of a mechanism to deliver ribavirin via a small-particle aerosol greatly enhanced the potential usefulness of this drug for respiratory viral infections. At this time ribavirin is licensed for the treatment, by aerosol administration, of carefully selected hospitalized infants and young children with severe lower respiratory tract infections caused by respiratory syncytial virus (RSV). The vast majority of infants and children with RSV infection have disease that is mild and self-limited and do not require ribavirin.

TOXICITY AND CLINICAL PROBLEMS. No adverse effect has been clearly attributable to aerosol therapy with ribavirin, although reports of adverse effects during or following therapy of infants with RSV have included bronchospasm, pulmonary function test changes, pneumothorax in ventilated patients, apnea, cardiac arrest, hypotension, and concomitant digitalis toxicity. Precipitation of drug within the ventilatory apparatus of patients on mechanical ventilation can be a serious problem. When proper precautions are taken, such as frequent changes in ventilator tubing, safe delivery of ribavirin to ventilated patients can be accomplished. Reticulocytosis, rash, and conjunctivitis have been associated with the use of ribavirin aerosol. Although there are no pertinent human data, ribavirin has been found to be teratogenic and mutagenic in nearly all species in which it has been tested. This drug is, therefore, contraindicated in women who are or may become pregnant. Some concern has been expressed about the risk to persons in the room with infants being treated with ribavirin aerosol, particularly females of childbearing age. Although this risk seems to be minimal with limited exposure, awareness and caution are warranted.

FUTURE ANTIVIRALS

Advances in molecular virology continue to define those sites of viral replication which may be vulnerable to attack without harm to the host cell. Further characterization of the viral DNA polymerase, required for replication but not utilized by the host cell, is a major research focus. In addition, classes of compounds, many of them nucleoside analogues, are being systematically evaluated in order to identify more efficacious and less toxic antivirals. A description of some of the most promising drugs follows.

Several compounds have activity against the herpesviruses, including foscarnet sodium (trisodium phosphonoformate, PFA), 1-β-D-arabinofuranosyl-E-5-(2-bromovinyl) arabinosyluracil (BV-araU), fluoroidoarabinosyl cytosine (FIAC), and (S)-1-((3-hydroxy-2-phosphonylmethoxy)propyl) adenine (HPMPA).

Foscarnet, a pyrophosphate analogue of phosphonoacetic acid (PAA), has potent in vitro and in vivo activity against herpesviruses. Unacceptable toxicity was demonstrated with PAA (deposition in bone), but foscarnet has been less toxic. These drugs inhibit the DNA polymerase of all human herpesviruses by blocking the pyrophosphate binding site and preventing chain elongation. Unlike acyclovir, which requires activation by a virus-specific thymidine kinase, foscarnet acts directly on the virus DNA polymerase. Thymidine kinase–deficient, acyclovir-resistant herpesviruses remain sensitive to foscarnet. Foscarnet has recently attracted attention as an inhibitor of HIV replication and is undergoing evaluation in patients with AIDS. It is in clinical trials as a treatment for CMV infection. The lack of marrow toxicity of foscarnet offers an advantage over ganciclovir. Renal toxicity, however, has been demonstrated.

Bromovinyl arabinosyl uracil, BV-araU, is a potent inhibitor of HSV-1 and EBV. More importantly, it is exquisitely active against VZV, being over 1000 times more potent than acyclovir. Like acyclovir, the mechanism of action of BV-araU is based upon the phosphorylation of the parent compound by herpesvirus TK, which restricts its action to virus-infected cells. BV-araU appears to have a favorable toxicity profile and will soon begin clinical trials in the United States.

Fluoroiodoarabinosyl cytosine (FIAC) and fluoroiodoarabinosyl uracil (FIAU), its principal metabolite, are both potent selective inhibitors of herpesviruses. Like acyclovir and BV-araU, their activity depends on phosphorylation by herpesvirus TK. The parent compound is converted rapidly to the triphosphate in infected cells, selectively utilized by virus DNA polymerase, and incorporated into viral DNA, resulting in the formation of very short DNA chains. In vitro, FIAC has greater activity than acyclovir against HSV-1; it is also active against HSV-2, VZV, and CMV. Because of its oral bioavailability, FIAC is thought to have potential usefulness in the treatment of CMV retinitis in patients with AIDS.

HPMPA is a potent, broad-spectrum antiviral agent that is one of a new class of nucleotide analogues structurally characterized as phosphonylmethyl ethers of acyclic nucleoside derivatives. The associated guanine and cytosine analogues are designated HPMPG and HPMPC. HPMPA has in vitro activity against HSV-1, HSV-2, CMV, VZV, EBV, adenovirus, and a retrovirus. The mechanism of action of HPMPA is thought to be similar to that of acyclovir, i.e., the triphosphate analogue inhibiting viral DNA polymerase. The difference, however, is that HPMPA is a monophosphate equivalent and does not require phosphorylation by a virus-specific TK, allowing HPMPA to have an expanded spectrum of activity. Of all these compounds, HPMPC is emerging with the most clinical potential. Although its in vitro potency is only moderate, HPMPC exhibits impressive potency in vivo.

INTERFERONS

HISTORY AND INTRODUCTION. Interferons (IFN) are glycoprotein cytokines (intracellular messengers) with a complex array of immunomodulating, antineoplastic, and antiviral properties. The name *interferon* was derived from landmark experiments by Isaacs and Lindemann in 1957, demonstrating the existence of a biologic substance that "interfered" with viral replication in infected cells. Interferons are currently classified as α, β, or γ, with natural sources of these classes, in general, being leukocytes, fibroblasts, and lymphocytes, respectively. Each type of IFN can now be produced via recombinant DNA technology. The complexity of the response to IFN, including the variability of dose response, duration of therapy, and combination with other treatments, creates enormous challenges to determine appropriate clinical scenarios in which IFN might be a worthwhile therapeutic agent.

MECHANISM OF ACTION. Binding of IFN to the intact cell membrane is the first step in establishing an antiviral effect. Interferon binds to specific cell surface receptors; IFN-γ appears to have a different receptor from either IFN-α or -β, which may explain the purported synergistic antiviral and antitumor effects sometimes observed when IFN-γ is given with either of the other two IFN species.

A prevalent view of IFN action is that, following binding, there is synthesis of new cellular RNA's and proteins, which mediate the antiviral effect. The antiviral state is not fully expressed until these primed cells are infected with virus. In addition to their antiviral effect, IFN's have a number of other biologic activities, including inhibition of cell proliferation and enhancement of the cytotoxic activities of lymphocytes, the expression of cell surface antigens, and the phagocytic and tumoricidal activities of macrophages. These properties may play an important role in the in vivo antiviral and antitumor effects of the IFN's.

LICENSED USES. Although promising for a number of viral infections and HIV-associated conditions, the only licensed use of IFN as an antiviral is its intralesional administration in the treatment of condyloma acuminatum, or genital warts, which are caused by human papillomaviruses. Only IFN-α is licensed.

TOXICITY AND CLINICAL PROBLEMS. Side effects are frequent with IFN administration and are usually dose-limiting. Influenza-like symptoms, i.e., fever, chills, headache, and malaise, commonly occur, but these symptoms usually become less severe with repeated treatments. At doses used in the treatment of condyloma acuminatum, these side effects rarely cause termination of treatment and may be reduced in severity by pretreatment with acetaminophen. For local treatment (intralesional injection) pain at the injection site does not differ significantly from that in placebo-treated patients and is short-lived. Leukopenia is the most common hematologic abnormality, occurring in up to 26 per cent of patients treated for condyloma. Leukopenia is usually modest, not clinically relevant, and reversible upon discontinuation of therapy. Increased alanine aminotransferase levels may also occur, as well as nausea, vomiting, and diarrhea.

At higher doses of IFN, neurotoxicity is encountered, as manifested by personality changes, confusion, loss of attention, disorientation, and paranoid ideation. Early studies with IFN-γ show similar side effects as treatment with IFN-α and -β but with the additional side effects of dose-limiting hypotension and a marked increase in triglyceride levels.

CLINICAL TRIALS. Interferon has potential use against virtually all viral infections. Its ultimate utility depends on a number of factors, including the acceptability of side effects, cost, and the availability of other antivirals. Of the many viral infections in which IFN has been tested, treatment of condyloma acuminatum, chronic hepatitis B, chronic hepatitis C, and recurrent respiratory papillomatosis and prophylaxis of rhinovirus and coronavirus upper respiratory infection have been promising.

Condyloma Acuminatum. Several large controlled trials have demonstrated the clinical benefit of IFN-α therapy of condyloma acuminatum. These studies have demonstrated clearance rates of treated lesions from 36 to 62 per cent. Up to one third of lesions treated with IFN recur. Much research remains to be done to examine the effects of different routes of administration, prolonged therapy, repeated courses of treatment, and combined treatment with other therapeutic modalities (i.e., cryotherapy, podophyllin, and laser ablation).

Respiratory Papillomatosis. Recurrent respiratory papillomatosis is a disease in which squamous papillomata relentlessly recur within the larynx and trachea of both children and young adults. Standard management consists of careful microendoscopic excision, usually with a CO_2 laser. In recent years, there have been numerous case reports and uncontrolled studies supporting benefit from IFN as an adjunct to surgical treatment. Results of placebo-controlled trials have suggested benefit.

Hepatitis. The inhibitory effect of human leukocyte IFN-α on hepatitis B virus (HBV) replication was first reported more than

TABLE 359–3. INDICATIONS FOR THE USE OF AVAILABLE ANTIVIRAL AGENTS

Indication	Antiviral Agent	Route	Dose	Comments
Respiratory syncytial virus infection (infants)	Ribavirin	Aerosol	Diluted in sterile water to a concentration of 20 mg/ml, then delivered via aerosol for 12–18 hrs/day for 3–7 days	Only for infants at high risk
Life- or sight-threatening CMV infections in immunocompromised hosts	Ganciclovir	IV	5.0 mg/kg q12h × 14 days	Maintenance therapy of 5.0 mg/kg/day recommended for AIDS patients. Leukopenia is a frequent complication; in bone marrow transplant patients with CMV pneumonia, CMV immune globulin may be a useful adjunct
Condyloma acuminatum	Interferon-α	Intralesional	1.0 million units injected into the base of each lesion, up to 3 times per week for 3 weeks	Flu-type symptoms may occur with administrations
Influenza A infection	Amantadine	Oral	Adults: 100–200 mg/day for 5–7 days Children ≤ 9 years: 4.4–8.8 mg/kg/day for 5–7 days not to exceed 150 mg/day	Normal person >65 years of age should receive 100 mg/day
Prophylaxis against influenza A virus infection	Amantadine	Oral	Adults: 100–200 mg/day Children ≤ 9 years: 4.4–8.8 mg/kg/day (not to exceed 150 mg/day)	Continued for the duration of the epidemic or for 2 weeks in conjunction with influenza vaccination (until vaccine-induced immunity develops); normal persons >65 years of age should receive 100 mg/day
Herpes simplex virus (HSV) encephalitis	Acyclovir	IV	10 mg/kg (1 hour infusion) every 8 hours for 10–14 days	Morbidity and mortality are significantly lower in patients treated with acyclovir than with vidarabine
Neonatal herpes	Vidarabine or Acyclovir	IV IV	30 mg/kg/day (continuous infusion over 12 hours) for 10 days 10 mg/kg (1 hour infusion) every 8 hours for 10 days	Efficacy of vidarabine is established; vidarabine and acyclovir show equal efficacy
Mucocutaneous HSV in immunocompromised hosts	Acyclovir or Acyclovir or Acyclovir	IV Oral Topical	250 mg/M² or 6.2 mg/kg (1 hour infusion) every 8 hours for 7 days 400 mg 5 times/day for 10 days 5% ointment; 4–6 applications/day for 7 days or until healed	Choice of topical, oral, or intravenous preparation depends upon clinical severity and setting; topical acyclovir is appropriate only when it can be applied to all lesions; it does not affect untreated lesions or systemic symptoms Least desirable
Prophylaxis against mucocutaneous HSV during intense immunosuppression	Acyclovir or Acyclovir	Oral IV	200 mg 3–4 times/day 250 mg/M² every 8 hours or 5 mg/kg every 12 hours (1 hour infusion)	Oral therapy most convenient; lesions recur when therapy stops Lesions recur when therapy stops
Treatment of initial genital HSV infections	Acyclovir or Acyclovir	Oral IV	200 mg 5 times/day for 10 days 5 mg/kg (1 hour infusion) every 8 hours for 5–7 days	Drug of choice in most clinical settings; treatment has no effect on subsequent recurrence rates For patients requiring hospitalization or with neurologic or other visceral complications
Recurrent genital herpes	Acyclovir	Oral	200 mg 5 times/day for 5 days	No effect on subsequent recurrence rates; efficacy greater if used early in attack
Prophylaxis against frequently recurring genital herpes	Acyclovir	Oral	200 mg 3–5 times/day	Occasional "breaking through" attacks and/or asymptomatic virus shedding during treatment; re-evaluation every 6 months recommended
Treatment of HSV keratitis	Trifluorothymidine or Vidarabine or Idoxuridine	Topical Topical Topical	One drop of 0.1% ophthalmic solution every 2 hours while awake (up to 9 drops/day) One-half-inch ribbon of 3% ophthalmic ointment 5 times/day One-half-inch ribbon of 0.5% ophthalmic ointment 5 times/day	3% acyclovir ointment (ophthalmic) is equal or superior to idoxuridine, vidarabine, and trifluridine for treatment of HSV keratitis but is not available in the United States
Localized herpes zoster in immunocompetent hosts	Acyclovir	Oral	800 mg 5 times/day for 7–10 days	Shortens time to lesion healing, but not shown to decrease the incidence of postherpetic neuralgia
Chickenpox in immunocompromised hosts	Acyclovir or Vidarabine	IV IV	500 mg/M² (1 hour infusion) every 8 hours for 7 days 10 mg/kg/day (continuous infusion over 12 hours) for 5 days	In the absence of comparative data, acyclovir is preferred because of its ease of administration and lower toxicity.
Treatment of severe localized or disseminated herpes zoster in immunocompromised hosts	Acyclovir or Vidarabine	IV IV	500 mg/M² or 12.4 mg/kg (1 hour infusion) every 8 hours for 5–7 days 10 mg/kg/day (continuous infusion over 12 hours) for 5–7 days	Comparative trials in severe localized and disseminated herpes zoster are under way; pending results, acyclovir is preferred because of its ease of administration and lower toxicity

10 years ago. Treatment with IFN-α in chronic hepatitis B subsequently has been investigated in several large, randomized, controlled trials. The earlier studies were encouraging, but the response rate was low at approximately 30 per cent.

In an attempt to enhance the efficacy of antiviral therapy, combinations of IFN with other agents have also been studied. Vidarabine and acyclovir have been used in such studies with little success. It has been observed, however, that the use of a short course of corticosteroids before treatment with IFN-α results in "immunologic rebound" after prednisone withdrawal. This phenomenon, which seems to be directed at virus-infected hepatocytes, is characterized by an acute hepatitis-like elevation of serum aminotransferases and a transient decline in levels of HBV DNA polymerase and HBV DNA. The results of a large multicenter trial comparing patients randomly assigned to receive one of two doses of IFN-α versus prednisone followed by IFN-α, or no treatment, were recently published. The authors found that a 4-month treatment regimen of subcutaneous IFN-α in a dose of 5 million units daily resulted in a complete response (loss of serum HBeAg and HBV DNA) in nearly 40 per cent of patients, and that reactivation of infection within 6 months after treatment was no greater than 2 per cent. The beneficial effect of pretreatment with a tapering dose of prednisone was limited to patients with low baseline levels of alanine aminotransferase (less than 100 units per liter). The best predictor of response in this study was the HBV DNA level before treatment, with approximately half of the patients having levels less than 100 pg per milliliter experiencing a complete response. Long-term follow-up studies are required to determine the duration of antiviral effect and the impact on survival.

The efficacy of IFN for treatment of chronic hepatitis C (non-A, non-B hepatitis) has also recently been investigated. Both acyclovir and corticosteroids have been ineffective, but preliminary reports suggest benefit with the use of IFN. The first large, randomized, placebo-controlled study of IFN-α therapy in patients with chronic hepatitis C showed that the serum alanine aminotransferase levels declined to normal in 38 per cent of patients treated with 3 million units of IFN-α for 6 months, compared with 4 per cent of untreated patients. However, only 52 per cent of the patients who initially responded to treatment remained in remission during 6 months of follow-up.

Respiratory Infections. The upper respiratory infection known as the "common cold" has a multitude of possible viral causes (see Ch. 360). It has been demonstrated that nasal spray or drops of IFN-α provide prophylaxis against the common cold caused by rhinovirus or coronavirus infection. Although clinical benefit was demonstrated in these studies, administration of IFN-α for 2 to 3 weeks led to hemorrhage of nasal mucosa.

IMMUNOGLOBULIN THERAPY

Efficacy has been established for prophylactic immunoglobulin administration for several viral infections, but the use of immunoglobulin alone for therapy of established disease has not been proven unequivocally beneficial for any viral infection. Benefit has been shown for the administration of intravenous immunoglobulin or CMV hyperimmune globulin when combined with ganciclovir in the treatment of CMV pneumonia in bone marrow transplant recipients. Survival was increased to 52 to 79 per cent, which is significantly better than that of historical controls treated with either agent alone. Currently active areas of research include the efficacy of CMV hyperimmune globulin for prevention and treatment of disease in bone marrow, kidney, and heart transplant patients, and that of CMV monoclonal antibody in the treatment of established CMV disease in AIDS patients.

CONCLUSION

Although relatively few antiviral drugs are licensed for use at this time, there is significant interest in the development of antiviral compounds. Table 359–3 summarizes the use of currently available antivirals for indications other than therapy of HIV infections. Systematic approaches have revealed a number of promising new drugs and biologic agents that are in various stages of evaluation. A better understanding of the molecular biology of virus replication and pathogenesis should elucidate agents with enhanced virus-specific activity.

Buhles WC, Mastre BJ, Tinker AJ, et al.: Ganciclovir treatment of life- or sight-threatening cytomegalovirus infection: Experience in 314 immunocompromised patients. Rev Infect Dis 10:495–503, 1988. *Describes the clinical efficacy of ganciclovir when used to treat infections of the retina, gastrointestinal tract, and lungs.*
Couch R: Respiratory diseases. In Galasso G, Whitley R, Merigan T (eds.): Antiviral Agents and Viral Diseases of Man, 3rd ed. New York, Raven Press, 1990, pp 327–372. *This chapter contains a summary of the published work regarding the efficacy and toxicity of amantadine, rimantadine, and ribavirin for influenza and respiratory syncytial virus infections.*
Davis GL, Balart LA, Schiff ER, et al.: Treatment of chronic hepatitis C with recombinant interferon alfa. N Engl J Med. 321:1501–1506, 1989. *The first large, randomized, placebo-controlled trial of interferon therapy of chronic hepatitis C.*
Dorsky DI, Crumpacker CS: Drugs five years later: Acyclovir. Ann Intern Med 107:859–874, 1987. *A detailed analysis of the chemistry, antiviral activity, and clinical efficacy of acyclovir.*
Hayden FG, Belshe RB, Clover RD, et al.: Emergence and apparent transmission of rimantadine-resistant influenza A virus in families. N Engl J Med 321:1696–1702, 1989. *Postexposure prophylaxis with rimantadine in families was not as effective as pre-exposure prophylaxis during community outbreaks.*
Hirsch MS, Kaplan JC: Antiviral Agents. In Fields BN, Knipe DM, Chanock E (eds.): Virology, 2nd ed. New York, Raven Press, 1990, pp 441–468. *A comprehensive text which includes a detailed analysis of antiviral therapy.*
Matthews T, Boehme R: Antiviral activity and mechanism of action of ganciclovir. Rev Infect Dis 10:490–494, 1988. *A concise description of the antiviral activity and mechanism of action of ganciclovir.*
Perrillo RP, Schiff ER, Davis GL, et al.: A randomized, controlled trial of interferon alfa-2b alone and after prednisone withdrawal for the treatment of chronic hepatitis B. N Engl J Med 323:295–301, 1990. *A multicenter study of combination therapy for chronic hepatitis B.*
Reichman RC, Oakes D, Bonnez W, et al.: Treatment of condyloma acuminatum with three different interferons administered intralesionally. Ann Intern Med 108:675–679, 1988. *Intralesional injections of three different interferon preparations were found to be efficacious in the treatment of condyloma acuminatum.*
Reines ED, Gross PA: Antiviral agents. Med Clin North Am 72:691–721, 1988. *An excellent review of the principles and applications of antiviral chemotherapy.*

Viral Infections of the Respiratory Tract

360 The Common Cold

Albert Z. Kapikian

DEFINITION. Although the term "common cold" does not denote a precisely defined disease, it has an almost universally comprehended meaning of an acute, self-limited, common illness of all age groups, in which the major clinical manifestations involve the upper respiratory tract, with nasal discharge (coryza) or nasal obstruction as the predominant symptom.

ETIOLOGY. Although it was known since 1914 that bacteria-free filtrates of nasal secretions from patients with a common cold could induce a similar illness in volunteers inoculated intranasally, the discovery of etiologic agents from common colds eluded scientists for many years. Despite the isolation of numerous viruses that were associated etiologically with acute respiratory illnesses, such as influenza virus in 1933, and the adeno-, parainfluenza, and respiratory syncytial viruses in the 1950's, it was clear that the major etiologic agent or agents of the common cold had not yet been discovered. However, beginning gradually in the 1950's and escalating rapidly in the 1960's, about 100 distinct common cold viruses were discovered and shown to be the major causative agents of the common cold. These heretofore fastidious agents were named rhinoviruses (rhin- is Greek for nose), because they caused predominantly nasal symptoms. Shortly thereafter, another group of fastidious viruses, the coronaviruses, were discovered and shown to be the second most important etiologic agents of the common cold and related diseases.

Rhinoviruses have emerged as the major known etiologic agents of adult upper respiratory illnesses such as common colds. They have been isolated from approximately 15 to 40 per cent of adults with these illnesses (Table 360–1). The isolation rate is lower in children with upper respiratory tract illnesses, as only about 5 per cent are rhinovirus positive. Rhinoviruses are classified as a genus in the picornavirus family and possess certain common characteristics, including small size (approximately 27 nm), ribonucleic acid (RNA) core, ether resistance, and complete or almost complete inactivation at pH 3. The last property is a major characteristic distinguishing rhinoviruses from another genus of the picornaviruses, the enteroviruses (poliovirus, coxsackievirus, and echovirus), which are stable at pH 3. There are now 100 officially designated rhinovirus serotypes and a single subtype, and it appears that this number includes most circulating strains.

The second most important etiologic agents of common colds are the coronaviruses, which are associated with 10 to 20 per cent of common colds in adults. Their importance as etiologic agents of common colds in infants and young children has not been determined. The human coronaviruses possess certain common characteristics, including (1) a unique electron microscopic appearance characterized by pleomorphic 100- to 150-nm enveloped particles possessing relatively widely spaced club- or pear-shaped surface projections (reminiscent of the solar corona, from which the name coronavirus is derived); (2) an RNA genome; and (3) ether and acid lability. There are at least three distinct human coronavirus serotypes, designated B814, 229E, and OC43. As a result of difficulties in propagating these fastidious agents, fewer than 50 isolates have been recovered since their discovery; most epidemiologic studies have thus relied on serologic studies with the 229E and OC43 viruses, for which suitable antigens could be prepared. As shown in Table 360–1, many other viruses, such as influenza, parainfluenza, respiratory syncytial, adeno-, echo-, and coxsackieviruses, can also cause common cold–like symptoms. These other agents are described in other sections of this text. A determination of the etiology of a common cold cannot be made clinically, since the agents causing the syndrome are so numerous. In addition, about one third to one half of common colds have yet to be associated with an etiologic agent.

INCIDENCE AND PREVALENCE. The common cold is probably the most frequently occurring illness in humans worldwide. The National Center for Health Statistics estimated that in the United States in 1988 the population experienced more than 68 million common colds for an incidence of 28.5 per 100 persons per year. Common colds represented 16.3 per cent of all acute conditions and were estimated to cause over 175 million days of restricted activity. The incidence of common colds was estimated to be 70.8 per 100 infants and young children under 5 years of age.

TABLE 360–1. PERCENTAGE OF COMMON COLDS ASSOCIATED WITH SPECIFIC ETIOLOGIC AGENTS IN ADULTS*

Rhinoviruses (100 serotypes)	15–40%
Coronaviruses (at least 3 serotypes)	10–20%
Influenza viruses A, B, C Parainfluenza viruses (4 serotypes) Respiratory syncytial virus (1 serotype) Adenoviruses (various serotypes)	5–10%
Coxsackieviruses (various serotypes) Echoviruses (various serotypes)	1–2%
Group A β-hemolytic streptococci	2–10%
No specific agent known but presumed to be viral	30–50%

*Each of these agents can also cause common colds in the pediatric age group, but their relative roles are not clearly defined. Viruses associated with specific syndromes such as rubeola, rubella, and varicella have also been associated with common cold–like symptoms in the pediatric age group.

In the Cleveland Family Study, which spanned a period of about 10 years and included close surveillance of over 25,000 illnesses, common respiratory diseases accounted for 60 per cent of all illnesses. The overall incidence of common respiratory diseases (which included illnesses diagnosed as the common cold, rhinitis, laryngitis, bronchitis, and other undifferentiated acute respiratory illnesses) was 5.6 per person per year. Children under 1 year of age experienced about seven respiratory illnesses per year; the highest incidence occurred in the 1-year age group (8.3 cases per year) and the incidence remained rather high through age 5 (7.4 cases per year). A progressive decrease was observed beginning at age 6. As expected, adults had relatively fewer common respiratory illnesses than children (adults averaged over four per year). The average incidence was slightly greater in boys than in girls, whereas in adults, mothers experienced higher rates than fathers. In addition, the incidence of common respiratory diseases was greater in young children attending school than in those of the same age who were not in school; also, preschool siblings of school children had more respiratory illnesses than preschool siblings without brothers or sisters attending school. The incidence of common respiratory diseases increased progressively as family size increased from three to seven members. Such illnesses were introduced into the home most frequently by school children under 6 years of age, followed in order of decreasing frequency by preschool children, school children 6 years of age and over, mothers, and fathers. Analysis of secondary attack rates in families revealed that on the average 25 per cent of all exposures in the home were followed by illness; 1- and 2-year-olds experienced the highest secondary attack rates (about twice the average).

In a more recent survey of acute respiratory illnesses over a 6-year period in Tecumseh, Michigan, the mean incidence of respiratory illnesses per person per year was 3. The highest incidence was in the 1-year age group (6.1) and the next highest in the 1- to 2-year age group (5.7). A viral or potentially pathogenic bacterial agent was isolated from about 25 per cent of the specimens collected, with rhinoviruses accounting for 38.5 per cent of the total number of isolates, a figure representing more than twice the number of isolates of the next most frequently detected group, the parainfluenza viruses.

Studies of the prevalence of neutralizing antibodies in serum against various rhinovirus serotypes have revealed a gradual acquisition of antibody beginning early in childhood and reaching a maximum of at least 50 per cent in the fifth decade. The prevalence of serum antibody to specific serotypes was not consistent. Although all individuals studied had neutralizing antibodies to each of the 55 serotypes tested, the prevalence of antibody to each serotype varied from about 10 to 80 per cent. Limited surveys of the prevalence of neutralizing antibody to rhinoviruses in various developed and developing countries, including several tropical areas, indicated a generally worldwide presence of rhinovirus antibody.

The prevalence of coronavirus serum antibody has been difficult to determine, because only two serotypes, 229E and OC43, can be cultivated with consistency in cell cultures and, in addition, results have been variable in different locations with these two viruses. For example, in one study in the United States, 29 per cent of children and 69 per cent of adults had serum complement-fixing (CF) antibody to OC43 virus. Such antibody to 229E virus was present very infrequently in children, whereas about one third of adults were antibody positive. However, in the United Kingdom, about 25 per cent of children and 41 per cent of adults had neutralizing antibody to 229E virus. In United States marine recruits, over 80 per cent had serum hemagglutination inhibition antibody to OC43 virus and 12 per cent had CF antibody to 229E virus. By recently developed enzyme- or radio-immunoassays, the prevalence of serum antibody to 229E and OC43 or related coronaviruses was over 80 per cent in adults in different geographic areas. A true evaluation of the prevalence of antibody to the coronavirus group must await the development of serologic assays for other members of this fastidious group of agents.

EPIDEMIOLOGY. In the temperate climates common colds occur most frequently in the colder months of the year. For example, in the Cleveland Family Study a consistent pattern of a low summer and high winter incidence of common respiratory diseases was documented. In September, a rise in respiratory illnesses to about six cases per person-year from a summer low of three cases per person-year was observed. After a slight dip in October an average rate of about seven cases per person-year was observed for each month from November through March.

Rhinoviruses are spread from person to person by aerosol, direct contact, or indirect contact involving environmental objects (fomites) via virus-contaminated respiratory secretions. In early volunteer studies, rhinoviruses induced common colds when administered in nasal drops or by swabbing the nasal mucosa or conjunctiva but not by swabbing the throat. More recent volunteer studies have yielded conflicting views on the most efficient mode of transmission of rhinovirus-induced common colds. One view highlights a mode of transmission that involves self-inoculation of the nasal mucosa or conjunctiva with a rhinovirus-contaminated finger. Virus was recovered in 15 of 16 trials from fingers that were rubbed on plastic surfaces contaminated with rhinovirus 1 to 3 hours previously. In addition, rhinovirus dried on volunteers' fingers could be transferred to uncontaminated fingers of other volunteers following skin contact, in three of five trials. The efficiency of transmission of infection from experimentally infected volunteers to susceptible volunteers by hand-to-hand contact followed by self-inoculation was compared with that of transmission by large- and small-particle aerosols. It was striking that 11 of 15 hand-to-hand exposures initiated infection, whereas only 1 of 12 large-particle exposures (donor and contact in social setting) and none of 10 small-particle exposures (donor and contact separated by double mesh barrier) induced such infection. In contrast, another view stresses the major role of aerosol transmission since following exposure to rhinovirus-infected "donors," 10 of 18 restrained volunteers (i.e., they could not touch their faces) and a similar number (12 of 18) of unrestrained volunteers developed common colds. However, none of 12 unrestrained individuals exposed to presumably rhinovirus-contaminated fomites (playing cards, etc.) developed illness. Thus, under the conditions of these separate volunteer studies, aerosol, direct contact, and indirect contact with fomites were capable of inducing common colds. However, the relative importance of each mode of transmission is still a matter of controversy.

In another study, rhinovirus communicability was evaluated in childless married couples who lacked serum neutralizing antibody to the challenge viruses. The overall transmission of a rhinovirus-related cold between partners was 38 per cent, which is similar to the secondary attack rate in the Cleveland Family Study or to those in epidemiologic studies of naturally occurring rhinovirus infections. Transmission rarely occurred unless (1) at least 1000 TCID$_{50}$ (50 per cent tissue culture infective doses) of virus were present in the donor's nasal washing, (2) the donor's hands and anterior nares were rhinovirus positive, (3) the donor had at least moderate symptoms, and (4) the partners spent many hours together (at least 122 hours during a 7-day period). Virus in saliva was not strongly associated with transmission.

The effect of exposure to cold temperatures on the course of common colds was evaluated in volunteers who were challenged with rhinovirus by small-particle aerosol or intranasal instillation. Exposure to the cold environment did not have a significant effect on host resistance to rhinovirus infection and illness. Exposure to cold temperature did not induce a common cold in uninoculated volunteers. This finding is consistent with results of early studies on the epidemiology of common colds on the island of Spitzbergen. These studies demonstrated that very few colds occurred during the bitter Arctic winter, but sharp outbreaks began shortly after the first ship arrived at the end of May. Thus, cold weather by itself did not induce common colds; the ingredient needed to initiate the outbreak was exposure to infected individuals. In early volunteer studies using common cold virus–like agents for challenge, fatigue and sleep deprivation caused an insignificant increase in the frequency with which colds occurred; however, in females, susceptibility was related to the menstrual cycle, with attempts to induce colds during menstruation being relatively unsuccessful.

The incubation period of rhinovirus-related common colds is quite short, ranging from 1 to 5 days with a mean of 2 days. Virus shedding generally begins with the onset of symptoms and continues for 1 week or even longer. Although there are 100 distinct rhinovirus serotypes, no one serotype has assumed special importance because numerous serotypes usually circulate at the same time. Rhinoviruses can be detected during most months of the year but reach peak prevalence during the fall and spring seasons. They are least prevalent during the cold winter months of December, January, and February, when common colds still occur frequently. However, coronavirus infections have been found to be prevalent during the late fall, winter, and early spring, when rhinovirus infections occur less frequently. Thus, coronaviruses can be considered to be the major known etiologic agents of the common cold in the winter.

A cyclic pattern in infection rates of coronaviruses 229E and OC43 has been described. With the 229E virus, infections appear to occur in the same years in various locations, including Chicago, Maryland, Virginia, and Michigan; a 2-year cycle of activity has been suggested. For OC43 virus, a 2- to 4-year cycle was found that did not coincide in all locations. The 229E virus was shed in nasal washings of volunteers for 1 to at least 4 days after challenge; the peak frequency of virus excretion generally coincided with the peak of clinical symptoms. Virus shedding was also detected in certain volunteers who did not develop colds after challenge. Reinfections have also been observed frequently with coronaviruses under natural conditions; however, volunteers inoculated with the same coronavirus strain 8 to 12 months after initial challenge failed to develop illness on rechallenge.

It appears that serum antibody to a specific rhinovirus serotype correlates with protection against natural or experimental challenge with that serotype. However, serum antibody may not in itself be responsible for protection but may be a reflection of the level of specific nasal secretory antibodies. In one volunteer study in which the protective effects of neutralizing antibody in serum and in nasal secretions were compared, it was found that only nasal secretory antibody was associated with resistance to rhinovirus infection and illness.

PATHOLOGY. The pathologic mechanisms whereby a common cold is induced by a virus are not known. However, the pathology of viral rhinitis in general has been described. In the initial acute period of viral rhinitis the nasal mucosa is thickened and edematous and, depending on the degree of hyperemia, is pale gray to red in color and covered by a thin, watery mucoid discharge. The nasal cavities are narrowed by the enlargement of the turbinates. Histologically, there is extreme edema of the mucosal tissue, which is also infiltrated sparsely with neutrophils, lymphocytes, plasma cells, and eosinophils. Secretory hyperactivity of the mucus-secreting submucosal glands is also observed. The edematous nasal mucosa can cause obstruction of the orifices of the accessory air sinuses and lead to sinusitis. Extension of bacterial superinfections can result in serious sequelae, including osteomyelitis, cavernous sinus thrombophlebitis, epidural or subdural abscess, meningitis, or brain abscess. However, such complications are exceedingly rare.

Information on the pathologic findings in acute rhinovirus infections is extremely limited. Biopsies of nasal epithelium obtained from volunteers with experimentally induced rhinovirus colds failed to demonstrate consistent histologic changes. However, sloughed ciliated epithelial cells are found in nasal secretions.

CLINICAL MANIFESTATIONS. The major clinical manifestation of common colds occurring under natural or experimental conditions is coryza or nasal congestion. The most common complaints in naturally occurring rhinovirus-positive respiratory illnesses in 139 civilian adults were rhinorrhea and sneezing, which were recorded in one half to two thirds of the cases. The next most frequent complaint was sore throat, which occurred in nearly one half, whereas hoarseness and cough were less common, being present in one quarter to one half of the cases. Temperature elevation was unusual. An oral temperature of 99.6°F (37.6°C) or greater at the time of study was documented in less than 1 per cent of the cases. Nonrespiratory complaints were not common except for headache, which occurred in approximately one quarter of the cases. The mean duration of symptoms was about 9 days with a median of 7.4 days and a mode of 4 days.

The clinical manifestations of coronavirus 229E–like infections under natural conditions in adults are quite similar. Of nine patients who shed this agent, all had coryza, eight had nasal congestion, seven had sneezing, and five had sore throat at the time of study. Less common manifestations were headache (in four), cough (in three), muscular or general aches (in three), and chills and fever (in two). Coryza or nasal congestion was the chief complaint in eight of the nine patients.

Administration of rhinoviruses or coronaviruses to volunteers has provided an opportunity to define the clinical manifestations associated with these agents under carefully controlled conditions (Table 360–2). The mean incubation period of colds induced by coronaviruses was significantly longer (about 1 day), the duration of the illness somewhat shorter, and the mean maximum number of paper tissues used per day (for nasal discharge) greater than in rhinovirus-induced illnesses. In later studies, each of six other coronavirus strains was also administered by the nasal route to volunteers: cumulatively, 35 of 49 volunteers developed common cold–like illnesses. Thus, the ability to induce common colds in adults under experimental conditions is now as firmly established for the coronaviruses as for the rhinoviruses.

Rhinoviruses also cause common colds in children. The role of rhinoviruses as etiologic agents of bronchitis, bronchiolitis, bronchopneumonia, pneumonia, and croup in the pediatric age group is unclear. However, it appears certain that rhinoviruses are not important causes of these syndromes, even though nasal inhalation of a rhinovirus by small-particle aerosol induces a tracheobronchitis in volunteers. Rhinoviral respiratory illness has also been implicated as an important precipitant of asthmatic attacks in children with a history of asthma. Rhinoviruses have been recovered from certain hospitalized pediatric patients with lower respiratory tract disease; most of these patients had significant underlying disease involving the immune or cardiopulmonary system. In addition, rhinoviruses were recovered from patients with cyanosis and apnea in an intensive care nursery. Coronaviruses can also cause common cold–like illnesses in children. In one study, coronavirus 229E was recovered from two infants with pneumonia, and serologic evidence of coronavirus infection was demonstrated in 8.2 per cent of pediatric patients hospitalized with lower respiratory tract disease. However, in other studies such an association was not found. Coronavirus infection has been associated with exacerbations of wheezing in young children with asthma. Coronavirus OC43 and rhinovirus infections also were observed in several military trainees with pneumonia with pleural reaction and with atypical pneumonia, respectively. The etiologic significance of such associations is not known. Rhinovirus and coronavirus infections have been associated with exacerbations of chronic bronchitis in adults. A transient decrease in pulmonary function has also been observed in volunteers infected with rhinovirus. Rhinovirus has also been recovered from the lung of an adult patient with a fatal pulmonary infection and other underlying disease involving the immune system. Other complications of common colds include sinusitis, otitis media, and extension of infection into the central nervous or vascular system, as noted in the pathology section. Rhinovirus has been recovered from sinus and middle ear fluids. The role of bacteria acting in concert with the virus infection in certain of these complications must be kept in mind in establishing therapeutic regimens.

DIAGNOSIS. Since most respiratory viruses can induce common colds, an etiologic diagnosis cannot be made on clinical grounds. Specific viral diagnosis of the common cold is essentially a research procedure that requires tissue or organ cultures for virus isolation or antigens for certain serologic studies. Serologic evidence of rhinovirus infection is demonstrated by an antibody rise to a specific serotype by neutralization assay in tissue culture. Complement fixation (229E, OC43), hemagglutination-inhibition (OC43), enzyme-linked immunosorbent assay (229E), or radioimmunoassay (OC43) can be performed in order to detect serologic evidence of infection with certain coronaviruses. However, antigens for such tests are not generally available. Molecular biologic techniques are being introduced for the diagnosis of rhinovirus or coronavirus infection. The most important test for a patient with a common cold–like illness is a throat culture for group A β-hemolytic streptococci because symptoms of illnesses associated with the common cold viruses and the streptococcus may overlap. Appropriate antibiotic therapy is available for treatment of this bacterial infection.

TREATMENT AND PREVENTION. There is no specific treatment for patients with the common cold. Only symptomatic treatment measures should be employed. At this time, it appears that acetylsalicylic acid (aspirin) should not be used in children with colds because of the epidemiologic association of this drug with Reye's syndrome (see Ch. 480) when the drug is administered during a viral illness, usually influenza or varicella, both of which can cause symptoms resembling those of the common cold (Table 360–1).

Antibiotics have no value in the therapy of the uncomplicated common cold. Clinical trials evaluating the efficacy of antihistamines for treatment of common colds have yielded inconsistent, inconclusive results. Thus, it appears from currently available evidence that the routine use of antihistamines for treatment of the common cold is not indicated. Previous tonsillectomy did not significantly affect the number of common respiratory illnesses or the induction of experimental colds in volunteers in the Cleveland Family Study. Available evidence indicates that vitamin C does not reduce the number of episodes of respiratory illness but does decrease somewhat the total number of days of disability. The routine use of large doses of vitamin C for preventive treatment of common colds does not appear to be warranted from evidence available at this time. The efficacy of steam (heated, humidified air) inhalation for the treatment of common colds has yielded variable results and needs further evaluation.

Currently 100 serotypes of rhinovirus are known to exist, and no one serotype or group of serotypes appears to be consistently more important than others. Experimental rhinovirus vaccines against single serotypes have been made and shown to be effective in preventing or modifying illnesses induced by the serotype present in the vaccine. Although some heterotypic antibody responses have been observed with experimental decavalent rhinovirus vaccines, the production of a rhinovirus vaccine appears to be impractical because of the multiplicity of serotypes. Until the number of serotypes of coronaviruses can be elucidated and the role of antibody in preventing or modifying illnesses can be established, consideration of a coronavirus vaccine is premature.

Since the three-dimensional structure and the cellular recep-

TABLE 360–2. COMPARISON OF THE CLINICAL FEATURES OF COMMON COLDS PRODUCED BY INTRANASAL ADMINISTRATION OF CORONAVIRUSES OR RHINOVIRUSES

	Coronaviruses		Rhinoviruses	
	229E	**B814**	**Type 2 (HGP or PK)**	**DC**
Number of volunteers inoculated	26	75	213	251
Number getting common colds	13 (50%)	34 (45%)	78 (37%)	77 (31%)
Incubation period (days)				
Mean	3.3	3.2	2.1	2.1
Range	2–4	2–5	1–5	1–4
Duration (days)				
Mean	7	6	9	10
Range	3–18	2–17	3–19	2–26
Maximum number of tissues used daily				
Mean	23	21	14	18
Range	8–105	8–120	3–38	3–60
Malaise	46%	47%	28%	25%
Headache	85%	53%	56%	56%
Chill	31%	18%	28%	15%
Pyrexia	23%*	21%	14%	18%
Mucopurulent nasal discharge	0	62%	83%	80%
Sore throat	54%	79%	87%	73%
Cough	31%	44%	68%	56%
Number of volunteers with common colds of indicated severity				
Mild	10 (77%)	24 (71%)	63 (80%)	36 (47%)
Moderate	2 (15%)	7 (20%)	12 (15%)	28 (36%)
Severe	1 (8%)	3 (9%)	4 (5%)	13 (17%)

*Between 99.2°F (37.3°C) and 100.4°F (38°C) (oral). After Bradburne, Bynoe, Tyrrell: Br Med J 3:767, 1967.

tors of rhinovirus have been determined recently, it may be possible to design effective and practical antiviral compounds based on these findings. In addition, there has been renewed interest in the use of interferon to prevent common colds, since interferon can now be produced by recombinant deoxyribonucleic acid (DNA) techniques. Interferon applied topically by nasal spray was effective in reducing the number of symptomatic illnesses when given prophylactically to volunteers challenged with rhinovirus or following natural exposure to a rhinovirus cold in a family setting. Nasal irritation from interferon was minimized by short-term application. However, in a recent study, another interferon preparation was not effective for prophylaxis of naturally occurring common colds when administered as a nasal spray. Interferon nasal sprays are not effective as treatment for common colds caused by rhinovirus after symptoms have begun. Prophylactic interferon nasal spray has also been shown to shorten the duration and reduce the severity of coronavirus (229E)–induced cold symptoms. The use of interferon for prophylaxis of common colds does not appear practical for general usage but may be beneficial under special circumstances.

One method available for preventing rhinovirus-induced colds may be the application of rigid personal hygienic measures when a family member has a common cold. This would entail handwashing and avoidance of finger-eye and finger-nose contact.

Recently, the use of virucidal paper handkerchiefs has been shown to interrupt the transmission of rhinovirus-induced colds. This intervention awaits further evaluation in various settings.

Committee on Infectious Diseases of the American Academy of Pediatrics (Fulginiti VA, Brunell PA, Cherry JD, Ector WL, Gershon AA, Gotoff SP, Hughes WT, Mortimer EA Jr, Peter G): Special Report: Aspirin and Reye syndrome. Pediatrics 69:810, 1982. *After weighing the available evidence, this Committee has made a strong recommendation against the use of aspirin under usual circumstances in children with varicella or influenza (both of which can cause common cold–like symptoms).*

Couch RB: Rhinoviruses. *In* Fields BN, et al. (eds.): Virology, 2nd ed. New York, Raven Press, 1990, pp 607–629. *An up-to-date review of the rhinoviruses (196 references).*

Dick EC, Jennings LC, Mink KA, et al.: Aerosol transmission of rhinovirus colds. J Infect Dis 156:442–448, 1987. *Presents evidence of the importance of aerosol transmission of rhinovirus-induced common colds in a volunteer setting.*

Fox JP, Cooney MK, Hall EC, et al.: Rhinoviruses in Seattle families, 1975–1979. Am J Epidemiol 122:830, 1985. *A comprehensive epidemiologic study of rhinovirus infections in families in Seattle, Washington.*

Gaffey MJ, Kaiser DL, Hayden FG: Ineffectiveness of oral terfenadine in natural colds: Evidence against histamine as a mediator of common cold symptoms. Pediatr Infect Dis J 7:215–220, 1988. *A study demonstrating the lack of effect of an antihistamine on the treatment of naturally occurring common colds. Describes the inconsistent results in the evaluation of antihistamines in the treatment of common colds.*

Greve JM, Davis G, Meyer AM, et al: The major human rhinovirus receptor is ICAM-1. Cell 56:839–847, 1989. *Describes continued progress in the elucidation of cellular receptors of rhinoviruses, which may lead to the development of antiviral compounds.*

Hendley JO, Gwaltney JM Jr: Mechanism of transmission of rhinovirus infections. Epidemiol Rev 10:242–258, 1988. *Reviews the various modes of transmission of rhinovirus common colds (60 references).*

Kim S, Smith TJ, Chapman MS, et al.: Crystal structure of human rotavirus serotype 1A (HRV1A). J Mol Biol 210:91–111, 1989. *A basic paper describing further advances in determining the structure of rhinoviruses and the application of this information to the development of antiviral compounds.*

Lowenstein SR, Parrino TA: Management of the common cold. Adv Intern Med 32:207–233, 1987. *A balanced, careful description of the management of common colds (121 references).*

Macknin ML, Mathew S, Medendorp SV: Effect of inhaling heated vapor on symptoms of the common cold. JAMA 264:989–991, 1990. *A recent study describing the ineffectiveness of steam (heated, humidified air) inhalation on common cold symptoms. Includes a review and references which demonstrate the variable results with this therapy.*

McIntosh K: Coronaviruses. *In* Fields BN, et al. (eds.): Virology, 2nd ed. New York, Raven Press, 1990, pp 857–864. *An up-to-date review of the coronaviruses (74 references).*

Remington PL, Rowley D, McGee H, et al.: Decreasing trends in Reye syndrome and aspirin use in Michigan, 1979 to 1984. Pediatrics 77:93, 1986. *The decreasing use of aspirin in children with colds or influenza and the decrease in Reye syndrome in Tecumseh, Michigan, is evaluated.*

Sperber SJ, Hayden FG: Chemotherapy of rhinovirus colds. Antimicrob Agents Chemother 32:409–419, 1988. *A review of various approaches—experimental and available—for treating the rhinovirus common cold (119 references).*

Sperber SJ, Levine PA, Sorrentino JV, et al.: Ineffectiveness of recombinant interferon-β serine nasal drops for prophylaxis of natural colds. J Infect Dis 160:700–705, 1989. *Demonstrates the variability of results of efficacy of interferon in prophylaxis of common colds.*

Tyrrell DAJ: Common colds. Intervirology 25:177–189, 1986. *A review of common colds from a historical perspective by a pioneer in this field.*

361 Viral Pharyngitis, Laryngitis, Croup, and Bronchitis

Maurice A. Mufson

DEFINITION. Viral infections that localize to the upper and middle respiratory passages produce an acute inflammatory response and, depending upon the anatomic site involved, evoke the clinical manifestations of pharyngitis, laryngitis, croup (laryngotracheobronchitis), and bronchitis. These infections do not ordinarily involve the pulmonary alveoli. Pharyngitis, laryngitis, and bronchitis can occur in persons of any age. Croup occurs exclusively in children and mainly during the second year of life. These illnesses usually begin abruptly with predominant upper respiratory tract signs and symptoms and limited systemic findings, and the uncomplicated illness abates after 5 to 10 days. Croup can be a life-threatening illness; the most common complications include respiratory failure and pneumonia.

ETIOLOGY. The major viral pathogens of the respiratory tract that can cause pharyngitis, laryngitis, croup, and bronchitis include members of the myxoviruses (influenza, parainfluenza, and respiratory syncytial viruses), adenoviruses, coronaviruses, picornaviruses (rhinoviruses and enteroviruses), and herpesviruses (Table 361–1). However, they differ in their propensity to cause these illnesses (Table 361–2). An etiologic diagnosis requires either isolation of virus or visualization of viral antigen in respiratory secretions by immunofluorescence, detection of antigen by enzyme immunoassay, or demonstration of a rise in antibody during convalescence.

Pharyngitis also can occur as part of systemic viral illnesses associated with *Epstein-Barr virus* (see Ch. 373) or *cytomegalovirus* (see Ch. 372) infection, and laryngitis and bronchitis occur in *measles* virus infection (see Ch. 367). When coryza represents the main feature of an upper respiratory infection, the term *common cold* (see Ch. 360) prevails. When the infecting virus is an influenza virus, the designation *influenza* describes an acute respiratory tract infection with fever and prostration (see Ch. 364).

INCIDENCE AND PREVALENCE. Most children and adults experience three to five viral infections of the upper respiratory tract each year. Croup is a serious illness of infants and children; the incidence of croup peaks in the second year of life, as high as 47 cases per 1000 children per year, and by age 4 to 5 it declines to under 15 cases per 1000 children per year (Denny, 1983).

EPIDEMIOLOGY. Viral pharyngitis, laryngitis, croup, and bronchitis occur during all months of the year, with peaks of occurrence paralleling epidemics of individual viruses. Respiratory syncytial virus, influenza A and B viruses, and parainfluenza virus type 1 occur in epidemics, mainly in the late fall, winter, and spring (see Table 361–3). The other viral pathogens occur endemically or sporadically. Virus infections of the respiratory tract spread by direct person-to-person contact, by infectious aerosols, or by fomites.

CLINICAL MANIFESTATIONS. *Viral Pharyngitis.* Acute viral pharyngitis is characterized by a scratchy and sore throat, but pain upon swallowing is not a prominent or constant feature. Dysphagia occurs infrequently in viral pharyngitis. Cough is not a feature of acute viral pharyngitis. Fever and malaise accompany influenza and adenovirus infections, but these findings are infrequent with the other respiratory viral pathogens. Pharyngeal erythema and edema and enlarged and tender lymph nodes may

TABLE 361—1. VIRUSES THAT CAUSE PHARYNGITIS, LARYNGITIS, CROUP, AND BRONCHITIS

Virus	Serotype
Influenza	Types A, B
Parainfluenza	Types 1, 2, 3
Respiratory syncytial	Subgroups A, B1, B2
Adenovirus	Types 1, 2, 3, 4, 5, 6, 7 (also others)
Coronavirus	Types 229E, OC43 (also others)
Rhinovirus	Most or all of more than 100 serotypes
Enterovirus	At least some of more than 75 serotypes
Herpes simplex	Type 1

TABLE 361–2. RELATIVE IMPORTANCE OF VIRUSES CAUSING PHARYNGITIS, LARYNGITIS, CROUP, AND BRONCHITIS

Virus	Occurrence in Indicated Illness*			
	Pharyngitis	*Laryngitis*	*Croup*	*Bronchitis*
Influenza A	+ + + +	+ + + +	+	+ + + +
B	+ +	+ +		+ +
Parainfluenza 1	+ +	+ +	+ + + +	+ +
2	+	+	+ + +	+
3	+ +	+ +	+ + + +	+ +
Respiratory syncytial	+		+	+ + +
Adenovirus	+ + + +	+ +		+ +
Coronavirus	+	+		+ + +
Rhinovirus	+ + + +	+		+
Enterovirus	+			
Herpes simplex	+ +			+

*Graded from minimal (+) to major (+ + + +) importance; blank means unlikely occurrence.

be the only physical findings. Adenovirus pharyngitis may be associated with conjunctivitis. Exudative tonsillitis occurs in adenovirus infections, infectious mononucleosis associated with Epstein-Barr virus infection, herpetic pharyngitis (with or without vesicles or small ulcers), as well as streptococcal pharyngitis. Exudative tonsillitis alone does not distinguish these infections. Bronchospasm occurs as a feature of herpes tracheobronchitis in elderly persons.

Viral Laryngitis. In acute viral laryngitis, hoarseness predominates, associated with difficulty in talking, pain on clearing respiratory secretions, and often fever, depending upon the infecting virus. Cough and pharyngitis may be present. The larynx is erythematous and edematous, and the regional lymph nodes are slightly enlarged and tender. Wheezes may be audible upon auscultation.

Viral Croup. The clinical picture of croup characteristically includes inspiratory stridor, hoarseness, and a brassy cough. This distinctive triad of symptoms reflects the acute and intense edema and mucoid exudative secretions of the larynx and associated obstruction of the subglottic portion of the upper airway. These symptoms develop acutely, accompanied by fever, cough, tachypnea, and wheezing. Retractions of the chest wall occur. Hemoptysis does not occur. Rhonchi, rales, or wheezes, alone or in combination, may be audible upon auscultation of the lungs. Radiographic examination of the neck can demonstrate subglottic narrowing, and a chest roentgenogram may show hyperinflation of the lungs. In the uncomplicated case, the findings resolve in several days, but some children develop respiratory failure and pneumonia. Children who perviously experienced multiple episodes of croup manifest hyperreactive airways several years later.

Viral Bronchitis. In acute viral bronchitis, cough, with or without sputum production, and fever are the main features. The sputum is slightly mucoid or watery and white. Other common symptoms include hoarseness, nonpleuritic substernal chest pain, and malaise. Rhonchi or rales may be heard upon auscultation of the chest. The chest roentgenogram may show increased intensity of the vascular pattern, but pulmonary infiltrates do not occur. Acute bronchitis associated with influenza or coronavirus infection occurs often as an exacerbation of chronic bronchitis.

TREATMENT AND PROGNOSIS. Viral pharyngitis, laryngitis, and bronchitis are self-limited illnesses, and not severe, except for herpes tracheobronchitis infections. The symptoms of these illnesses should be treated with analgesics, fluids, and rest.

TABLE 361–3. EPIDEMIOLOGY OF VIRUSES THAT CAUSE PHARYNGITIS, LARYNGITIS, CROUP, AND BRONCHITIS

Epidemic	Endemic	Sporadic
Parainfluenza 1*	Parainfluenza 3	Parainfluenza 2
Influenza A†	Adenovirus	Herpes simplex
Influenza B	Coronavirus	
Respiratory syncytial‡	Rhinovirus	
	Enterovirus	

*Alternate years, usually.
†Epidemic and pandemic.
‡Annual epidemics.

Persistent cough can be treated with suppressant preparations. Antibiotics are not indicated, except when secondary bacterial infection occurs; it is likely to develop mainly with influenza virus infections. In pharyngitis, pharyngeal pain or dysphagia should be treated with analgesics and fluids.

The less serious cases of croup can be managed by having the child rest in bed at home. Vaporizers that produce a mist of moist air may be beneficial. Children with severe croup require hospitalization, supportive treatment, and constant monitoring for the development of respiratory distress. If hypoxemia develops, oxygen therapy is essential; hypoxemia requiring oxygen can develop even before cyanosis becomes evident. Subglottic edema may be reduced by the administration of racemic epinephrine. Administration of corticosteroids in the treatment of croup may have limited benefit. Antiviral drug therapy is available for influenza A, respiratory syncytial, and herpes simplex viruses (Table 361–4). Ribavirin lessens the severity of serious respiratory syncytial virus infection in the infant and child. Herpes tracheobronchitis can be successfully treated with acyclovir. Influenza virus vaccine must be administered to persons in the high-risk group (unless contraindicated) to diminish the chance of infection (see Ch. 16).

Avila MM, Carballal G, Rovaletti H, et al.: Viral etiology in acute lower respiratory tract infections in children from a closed community. Am Rev Respir Dis 140:634, 1989. *One fifth of 94 children with bronchitis had virus infections; respiratory syncytial virus and adenoviruses were the most common.*
Houvinen P, Lahtonen R, Ziegler T, et al.: Pharyngitis in adults: The presence of coexistence of viruses and bacterial organisms. Ann Intern Med 110:612, 1989. *About one fourth of 106 adults with pharyngitis had virus infections; respiratory syncytial and influenza A viruses were most common.*
Mufson MA, Örvell C, Rafnar B, et al.: Two distinct subtypes of human respiratory syncytial virus. J Gen Virol 66:2111, 1985. *New description of two subtypes (or subgroups) of respiratory syncytial virus recognized by their pattern of reaction with monoclonal antibodies generated against the major proteins of the virus.*
Sherry MK, Klainer AS, Wolff M, et al.: Herpetic tracheobronchitis. Ann Intern Med 109:229, 1988. *Successful treatment of adults with severe herpes infection of trachea and bronchi with intravenous acyclovir.*
Thom DH, Grayston JT, Wang SP, et al.: Chlamydia pneumoniae strain TWAR, Mycoplasma pneumoniae, and viral infections in acute respiratory disease in a university student health clinic population. Am J Epidemiol 132:248, 1990. *One tenth of college students with either bronchitis or pharyngitis had virus infections; influenza A and B viruses predominated.*

TABLE 361–4. ANTIVIRAL DRUG THERAPY OF VIRUSES THAT CAUSE PHARYNGITIS, LARYNGITIS, CROUP, AND BRONCHITIS

Virus	Drug	Dose (Duration)	Route
Influenza A	Amantadine*	200 mg daily (10 days)	Oral
	Rimantidine*	200–300 mg daily (10 days)	Oral
Respiratory syncytial	Ribavirin	20 mg/ml solution (12–18 hours)	Aerosol
Herpes simplex†	Acyclovir	8 mg/kg q8hr (7–10 days)	IV

*More commonly used for prophylaxis at same daily dose over longer periods of time until the virus leaves the community.
†Herpes simplex tracheobronchitis treated with IV acyclovir.

362 Respiratory Syncytial Virus

Robert M. Chanock

DEFINITION. Respiratory syncytial virus (RSV) is the most important cause of viral lower respiratory tract disease in infants and children. This ubiquitous virus causes an extensive epidemic every year during fall, winter, or early spring. During these epidemics there is a dramatic increase in admission to hospitals of infants and young children with severe lower respiratory tract disease. Older children and adults commonly undergo reinfection, but disease is usually milder than that experienced during infancy and early childhood.

ETIOLOGY. RSV, an enveloped virus that belongs to the family Paramyxoviridae, genus *Pneumovirus*, resembles the parainfluenza viruses of the genus *Paramyxovirus* but differs from them in morphology of its nucleocapsid, in failure to agglutinate erythrocytes (hemagglutination), and in absence of a neuraminidase enzyme. The RSV negative (−) strand RNA genome, approximately 15,000 bases in length, is transcribed as a series of 10 separate messenger ribonucleic acids (mRNAs), each of which is translated into a separate viral protein. One of these proteins, nucleocapsid protein, coats the viral RNA to form a helical nucleocapsid. This structure is enclosed within a bilayer lipid membrane that is studded with two different viral glycoproteins. One of these, the fusion protein, lyses the host cell membrane, permitting entry of virus into the cell. This protein is also responsible for fusion of infected cells to neighboring cells, a process that results in syncytium formation, a prominent feature of the virus during its growth in tissue culture.

Although antigenic variation among strains has been noted, it does not appear to have major epidemiologic significance. A related RSV is a common cause of respiratory disease in calves, but this virus does not appear to infect humans.

EPIDEMIOLOGY. Whenever appropriate studies have been performed, RSV has been found to be the major pediatric respiratory tract viral pathogen. The highest incidence of severe lower respiratory tract disease is observed in infants between 1 and 6 months of age, with a peak incidence at 2 months. Serious lower respiratory tract disease occurs more commonly in males than in females and in nonblack than in black infants. Approximately 50 per cent of infants who live through a single RSV epidemic become infected. In certain settings, such as day care centers, the attack rate approaches 100 per cent during an outbreak.

Reinfection occurs with high frequency during childhood. Adults are also reinfected frequently, particularly when there is exposure to a large amount of virus. For example, in families into which virus is introduced, spread of RSV among older siblings and parents occurs with high frequency (40 per cent). In individuals of all ages, reinfection is usually symptomatic, and adults exposed to a large amount of virus may develop an influenza-like disease.

Most individuals infected with RSV have upper respiratory illness. However, a surprisingly large proportion of infants (25 to 40 per cent) also develop lower respiratory tract disease. Hospitalization of infants for RSV disease varies with environmental and socioeconomic conditions. Overall, 1 in 120 to 1 in 200 infants requires hospital care for RSV pneumonia or bronchiolitis during the first year of life. RSV is responsible for approximately 50 to 75 per cent of bronchiolitis and for 20 to 25 per cent of pneumonias that necessitate admission of infants and young children to hospital.

In developed countries, severe RSV lower respiratory tract disease is rarely fatal (0.5 to 2.5 per cent). Fatal RSV disease occurs most often in infants with other underlying illnesses, particularly congenital heart disease (37 per cent), bronchopulmonary dysplasia, serious renal disease, and diseases such as cancer that are treated with immunosuppressive drugs. In a British study of 46 infants and children who died with lower respiratory tract disease, 13 were infected with RSV. In addition, a number of babies dying of sudden infant death syndrome are infected with RSV.

RSV has a clear seasonality in temperate zones of the world. In urban centers, epidemics occur yearly in the late fall, winter, or spring but not during the summer. In the northern hemisphere, the virus is rarely isolated during August or September. Each RSV epidemic lasts approximately 5 months, with 40 per cent of infections occurring during the peak month in the temporal center of the outbreak. In the northern hemisphere, most outbreaks peak in February or March, but the peak may occur as early as December or as late as June. RSV is spread by infected respiratory secretions in the form of large droplets or through fomite contamination.

During epidemic intervals, RSV is one of the most common causes of hospital-acquired infection on pediatric wards. The risk of infection increases as the hospital stay is extended beyond 1 week. The mortality in such hospital-acquired infections is considerably higher than in community-acquired infections because the patients involved are frequently at high risk from other diseases, malnourishment, or immunosuppressive drugs.

Since reinfection with RSV is common and often associated with disease, it is clear that immunity is neither permanent nor complete. However, multiple reinfections induce temporary immunity to infection and a more long-term resistance to severe RSV lower respiratory tract disease. Studies in adult volunteers indicate that immunity to induced upper respiratory tract infection correlates better with the level of nasal neutralizing immunoglobulin A (IgA) antibodies than with serum antibodies. On the other hand, there is some epidemiologic evidence that the high levels of maternally derived RSV antibodies possessed by many small infants provide protection from serious lower respiratory tract disease. However, lower levels of such antibodies present in the serum of older infants are not protective.

CLINICAL MANIFESTATIONS. During infancy, RSV infection usually causes upper respiratory symptoms. In 25 to 40 per cent of infections the respiratory tract below the larynx is also involved. Lower respiratory tract signs are preceded by a prodromal phase of rhinorrhea that is sometimes accompanied by a decrease in appetite. Low-grade fever is common. Cough is often accompanied by wheezing, and if disease is mild, symptoms may not progress beyond this stage. Examination usually reveals moderate tachypnea, diffuse rhonchi, fine rales and wheezes, as well as profuse rhinorrhea and intermittent fever. Otitis media is also common. The chest radiograph usually appears normal. In most instances, uneventful recovery occurs after 7 to 12 days.

In more severe cases, coughing and wheezing progress and the child becomes dyspneic and refuses feedings. Hyperexpansion of the chest is evident, and there may be intercostal and subcostal retractions. Severe tachypnea is common even in the absence of visible cyanosis, and in advanced disease, as the child tires and hypoxia becomes more extreme, listlessness and apnea occur. The chest may appear normal on radiographic examination, but often there is a combination of air trapping (hyperexpansion) and peribronchial thickening or interstitial pneumonia. Segmental or lobar consolidation is also occasionally seen, usually involving the right upper lobe. Pleural effusion is rare. In infants with underlying cardiac or respiratory disease, the progression of symptoms may be rapid. In these instances, respiratory failure requiring intubation and ventilation may appear on the second or third day of illness.

Almost all infants who require hospitalization are hypoxemic on admission and remain so for a prolonged period—up to several weeks—although recovery has ensued. The hypoxemia reflects an abnormally low ventilation-perfusion ratio. Hypercarbia may also be present.

In infants who were born prematurely, and sometimes in normal infants under 6 weeks of age, apneic spells may develop during RSV infection. These often occur in the absence of significant respiratory signs and may be the predominant symptom bringing the infant to medical attention. Such apneic spells, while often recurrent during acute infection, are usually self-limited and rarely cause neurologic or systemic damage. However, exceptions to this pattern occur, and such episodes are an indication for hospitalization and careful medical supervision. Apnea at the peak of severe illness is a poor prognostic sign.

In the newborn infant, most RSV infections produce only upper respiratory symptoms. Bronchiolitis is rare, and severe infection is more often characterized by lethargy, irritability, and fever or unstable body temperature than by specific respiratory signs.

Children who have apparently recovered completely from RSV bronchiolitis or pneumonia may still retain both measurable and symptomatic respiratory abnormalities for many years. A study of 23 children examined 10 years after an episode of bronchiolitis found that although all were symptom free (a criterion for admission to the study), 20 had some measurable physiologic abnormality of lung function or arterial blood gases.

Acute RSV infections are common in adults, particularly in medical personnel or in those caring for small children. These reinfections are occasionally asymptomatic but usually are associated with rhinorrhea, pharyngitis, cough, constitutional symptoms of headache and fatigue, and fever. Disease usually lasts about 5 days but may be more prolonged, particularly in hospital staff. Alterations in pulmonary function, such as elevated total respiratory resistance and increased airway reactivity, often last for 8 weeks. There is some evidence that RSV infection in the elderly is a cause of febrile bronchitis and severe or even fatal pneumonia.

DIAGNOSIS. Presumptive diagnosis of RSV infection can often be made on the basis of the clinical syndrome in relation to the time of year and other epidemiologic features. Definitive diagnosis depends upon the laboratory. In older children and adults, an increase in serum RSV antibody concentration, either complement fixing (CF) or neutralizing, is a fairly sensitive index of reinfection with RSV. Serologic tests in infants are less sensitive, particularly in patients under 4 months of age. In young infants, only 2 to 15 per cent of RSV infections are detectable by CF and 2 to 20 per cent by neutralization assay. Antibody measurement by solid-phase immunoassay (enzyme-linked immunosorbent assay, or ELISA) recently has been shown to be a more sensitive indicator of infection in small infants than CF or neutralization. At all ages, however, isolation of virus or detection of antigen in respiratory secretions is the procedure of choice. Specimens are best obtained by aspiration or gentle washing out of nasopharyngeal secretions. These may be examined by inoculation of tissue culture, immunofluorescence, or ELISA. Infectivity of RSV in secretions is labile; hence samples should be placed on wet ice while being transported to a tissue culture laboratory.

TREATMENT AND PREVENTION. Treatment of RSV infections of the lower respiratory tract consists primarily of supportive care: mechanical removal of secretions, proper positioning of the infant, administration of humidified oxygen, and in severe cases respiratory assistance. When wheezing is an important symptom, some patients, particularly those over a year of age, benefit from the use of theophylline or adrenergic drugs.

Ribavirin (1β D-ribofuranosyl-1,2,4-triazole-3-carboxamide), delivered by small-particle aerosol, is now licensed for treatment of severe RSV disease in young infants. The drug has a beneficial effect on illness and diminishes virus shedding. Recently, intravenous inoculation of 2 grams per kilogram of human IgG containing a high titer of RSV neutralizing antibodies was shown to decrease virus shedding and improve oxygenation. In the case of both ribavirin and human IgG it remains to be shown that treatment decreases duration of hospitalization.

Because immunity to RSV is neither permanent nor complete, the goal of immunoprophylaxis is prevention of severe lower respiratory tract disease. It should be possible to achieve this through the cumulative effect of repeated vaccination. Efforts to develop an effective vaccine have been frustrated by the ineffectiveness of formalin-inactivated virus and by the genetic instability of satisfactorily attenuated temperature-sensitive mutants that initially showed promise as live virus vaccine strains. Perhaps recent success in preparing purified RSV surface glycoproteins and in constructing vaccinia virus or adenovirus recombinants that express RSV surface glycoproteins may open the way to effective immunoprophylaxis for this virus because each of these experimental vaccines induces significant resistance to RSV infection in experimental animals.

Groothuis JR, Woodin KA, Katz R, et al.: Early ribavirin treatment of respiratory syncytial viral infection in high-risk children. J Pediatr 117:792, 1990. *Early administration of ribavirin by small-particle aerosol to high-risk infants and children with RSV lower respiratory tract disease had a beneficial effect on severity of clinical illness and oxygenation but did not reduce duration of hospitalization.*

Hall CBH, Geiman JM, Biggar R, et al.: Respiratory syncytial virus infections within families. N Engl J Med 294:414, 1976. *Longitudinal surveillance of RSV infections in families. During an epidemic, infection occurred in 44 per cent of families; within these families the infection rate was 62 per cent in infants and 43 per cent in adults, the latter rate representing reinfection.*

Hemming VG, Rodriguez W, Kim HW, et al.: Intravenous immunoglobulin treatment of respiratory syncytial virus infections in infants and young children. Antimicrob Agents Chemother 31:1882–1886, 1987. *Intravenous inoculation of 2 grams per kilogram of human IgG with a high titer of RSV neutralizing antibodies effected a significant reduction in virus shedding and an improvement in oxygenation.*

Henderson FW, Collier AM, Clyde WA Jr, et al.: Respiratory-syncytial-virus infections, reinfections and immunity. N Engl J Med 300:530, 1979. *Longitudinal surveillance of children in a day care center demonstrated high frequency of reinfection; also, after several reinfections partial immunity developed to RSV.*

McIntosh K, Chanock RM: Respiratory syncytial virus. In Fields B, Knipe D (eds.): Virology. New York, Raven Press, 1990, pp 1045–1072. *A summary of biologic properties of RSV as well as its epidemiology and the pathogenesis of the disease.*

Olmsted RA, Elango N, Prince GA, et al.: Expression of the F glycoprotein of respiratory syncytial virus by a recombinant vaccinia virus: Comparison of the individual contributions of the F and G glycoproteins to host immunity. Proc Natl Acad Sci USA 83:7462, 1986. *Immunization of cotton rats with a vaccinia virus—RSV surface glycoprotein gene recombinant induces resistance to RSV infection in the lungs.*

363 Parainfluenza Viral Diseases

Robert M. Chanock

DEFINITION. Infection with parainfluenza viruses occurs early in life and is an important cause of *pediatric respiratory tract disease*. The spectrum of illness varies from mild upper respiratory disease to severe croup, pneumonia, or bronchiolitis. Reinfection is common in later life and is associated with mild respiratory tract disease.

ETIOLOGY. The parainfluenza viruses are enveloped viruses that belong to the family Paramyxoviridae, genus *Paramyxovirus*. The single-stranded ribonucleic acid (RNA) viral genome has negative polarity (antimessenger sense) and is approximately 15,000 bases in length. Its genetic information is expressed as a series of messenger RNA's (mRNA's) transcribed from the viral genome that codes for eight or nine viral-specific proteins. One of these proteins, nucleocapsid protein, coats the viral RNA to form a helical nucleocapsid. This structure is enclosed within a lipid bilayer envelope that is studded with the two viral glycoprotein surface antigens, the hemagglutinin-neuraminidase, and the fusion protein. Parainfluenza viruses share many properties with the influenza viruses, but they differ from these agents in their wider RNA nucleocapsid (18 nm as compared with 9 nm) and in the distribution of hemagglutination and neuraminidase functions on their surface glycoproteins. Both parainfluenza hemagglutinin and neuraminidase are located on the same surface glycoprotein, whereas these functions reside on separate surface glycoproteins of the influenza viruses. The parainfluenza viruses have common antigens that are not shared by the influenza viruses. Mumps virus shares the foregoing properties, as well as related antigens, with the parainfluenza viruses.

There are four antigenically distinct serotypes of human parainfluenza virus. Related parainfluenza viruses cause respiratory disease in mice (Sendai virus, a subtype of type 1), dogs (SV5, a subtype of type 2), calves (bovine shipping fever virus, a subtype of type 3), and birds (seven distinct serotypes not closely related to human parainfluenza viruses). Animal and avian parainfluenza viruses are distinct antigenically from human parainfluenza viruses and do not appear to infect humans.

EPIDEMIOLOGY. The four parainfluenza virus types have wide geographic distribution. The first three types have been identified in most areas where appropriate tissue culture and hemadsorption techniques have been applied to the study of childhood respiratory tract diseases. So far, type 4 viruses (subtypes 4A and 4B), which are more difficult to recover in tissue culture, have been isolated in fewer areas, but serologic studies suggest that they are also relatively ubiquitous.

The parainfluenza viruses are exceeded only by *respiratory syncytial virus (RSV)* as an important cause of lower respiratory tract disease in young children. These viruses, particularly type 3, commonly reinfect older children and adults to produce upper respiratory tract disease. Illness usually occurs less often and is less severe during reinfection than during primary infection.

There is considerable diversity in both epidemiologic and clinical manifestations of infections caused by the parainfluenza viruses. Parainfluenza virus type 1 is the principal cause of croup (laryngotracheobronchitis) in children, and parainfluenza virus type 3 is second only to RSV as a cause of pneumonia and bronchiolitis in infants less than 6 months of age. Parainfluenza virus type 2 resembles type 1 virus in clinical manifestations but causes serious illness less frequently. Infections with parainfluenza virus type 4 are detected infrequently, and associated illnesses are usually mild.

The parainfluenza viruses are most important as respiratory tract pathogens during infancy and childhood, when they (types 1 through 3) cause a spectrum of effects ranging from inapparent infection to life-threatening lower respiratory tract disease. Studies in different parts of the world indicate that types 1, 2, and 3 are associated with approximately 40 to 70 per cent of severe croup. In addition to croup, these three viruses are also responsible for a smaller but appreciable percentage of other acute respiratory tract diseases of infancy and early childhood. Eighty per cent of individuals undergoing primary infection with type 3 virus develop a febrile illness, and in one third there is involvement of the lower respiratory tract. Approximately one half of initial type 1 virus infections and two thirds of initial type 2 virus infections produce a febrile illness. Severe croup, although the most dramatic and serious manifestation of initial parainfluenza virus infection, is noted in only 2 to 3 per cent of primary type 1 or type 2 virus infections.

Primary parainfluenza virus infection generally occurs early in life. Type 3 virus often causes illness during the first months of life while infants still possess circulating neutralizing antibodies derived from their mothers. In contrast, in young infants, maternally derived antibodies appear to prevent both infection and severe disease caused by type 1 and type 2 viruses. After age 4 months, there is an increase in the incidence of croup and other lower respiratory tract diseases caused by type 1 and type 2 viruses. This high incidence continues until approximately 6 years of age, after which there is a much lower incidence. It is unusual for type 1 or type 2 virus to cause lower respiratory tract illness during adolescence or adult life, although this does occur on occasion.

At present, type 1 and type 2 virus epidemics are synchronous, occurring during the autumn of odd-numbered years. For many years, type 3 virus exhibited an endemic pattern, with infection occurring during all seasons of the year. Within this endemic pattern, small outbreaks occurred, but there was no predictable periodicity. Within the past 10 years, there has been a shift toward yearly spring epidemics of type 3 virus infection. Nosocomial infection of infants and young children with the parainfluenza viruses, particularly type 3 virus, is common and often leads to serious lower respiratory tract disease.

Transmission of parainfluenza viruses is by direct person-to-person contact or large droplet spread. The high rate of infection early in life, coupled with the high frequency of reinfection, suggests that these viruses spread readily from person to person. Reinfected individuals appear to be infectious, and a relatively small inoculum is able to initiate infection. Type 3 virus appears to be the most transmissible of the parainfluenza viruses.

In experimental infection of adult volunteers, the interval between administration of type 1, 2, or 3 virus and onset of upper respiratory tract symptoms ranged from 3 to 6 days. The incubation period in pediatric infections has not been defined; however, the interval between exposure to type 3 virus and the subsequent initial shedding of this virus is 2 to 4 days. Resistance to type 1 or type 2 parainfluenza virus infection and associated upper respiratory disease appears to be a function of local respiratory tract, secretory, immunoglobulin A (IgA)–neutralizing antibodies. Infants may also be partially protected from infection and lower respiratory tract disease by serum antibodies. This

protective relationship is suggested by the relative sparing of young infants from type 1 and type 2 virus infection and associated disease at a time when they possess serum antibodies passively acquired from their mother. Also, the risk of infection with type 3 virus during the first 4 months of life is inversely related to the level of neutralizing antibodies present in cord serum at birth. However, the protective effect of passive immunity is less than that observed for type 1 and type 2 viruses, since a significant number of infants with moderately high levels of maternally derived serum antibody become infected with type 3 virus and develop severe illness.

CLINICAL MANIFESTATIONS. In children, the most common type of illness consists of rhinitis, pharyngitis, and bronchitis, usually with fever. The most common initial symptoms are cough, hoarseness, and fever. The cough may be croupy, but respiratory distress is not present. Approximately three fourths of such ill children have a temperature above 37.8°C; fever usually lasts 2 to 3 days. Coarse breath sounds, rhonchi, erythema of the pharyngeal mucous membranes, and rhinitis are characteristic physical findings. Cervical adenopathy is uncommon.

When croup develops, the initial symptoms of rhinitis, pharyngitis, fever, and cough progress. After several days, the cough worsens and becomes brassy, seal-like, or barking, and stridor ensues. At this stage, most children recover uneventfully after 24 to 48 hours, but in some air hunger develops, with cyanosis, sternal and intercostal retractions, and progressive airway obstruction. The lateral radiograph of the neck (which should be obtained only under carefully controlled medical supervision, if at all) shows glottic and subglottic narrowing (the "steeple sign") and differentiates this disease from epiglottitis.

When bronchiolitis or pneumonia develops, fever persists and the cough progresses and becomes somewhat productive. It is accompanied by wheezing, tachypnea, and retractions and in severe cases by cyanosis. The x-ray film shows interstitial or perihilar infiltrates and air trapping. In some patients a combined bronchopneumonia-croup syndrome occurs.

DIAGNOSIS. Presumptive diagnosis of parainfluenza virus infection can be made on the basis of age, history, clinical findings, and relation to known or characteristic prevalence of virus in the community. Definitive diagnosis, however, requires recovery of the virus from appropriate specimens taken from the respiratory tract or identification of viral antigens in respiratory tract secretions by immunofluorescence or another form of immunoassay. Serodiagnosis by hemagglutination inhibition, complement fixation, or neutralization can establish that infection with a member of the parainfluenza virus group has occurred, but frequent heterotypic responses make type-specific diagnosis by serology extremely difficult.

TREATMENT. Symptomatic treatment of croup usually includes humidification of air by ultrasonic nebulizer and periodic inhalation of racemic epinephrine. Antibiotics are usually contraindicated. The use of corticosteroids is controversial, but many physicians prescribe high doses of dexamethasone if croup is severe. Specific antiviral treatment or effective vaccines for prevention of parainfluenza virus disease are not available.

Chanock RM, McIntosh K: Parainfluenza viruses. *In* Fields B (ed.): Virology. New York, Raven Press, 1990, pp 963–988. *Summary of natural history of parainfluenza virus infection and pathogenesis of disease.*

Chanock RM, Parrott RH, Johnson KM, et al.: Myxoviruses: Parainfluenza. Am Rev Respir Dis 88:152, 1963. *A discussion of the importance of parainfluenza viruses in pediatric respiratory tract disease and the first description of pattern of spread and reinfection.*

Denny FW, Murphy TF, Clyde WA, Jr, et al.: Croup: An 11-year study in a pediatric practice. Pediatrics 71:871, 1983. *Eleven-year evaluation of the role of parainfluenza viruses in croup. These viruses accounted for 74 per cent of all virus isolates from croup patients.*

Fox JP, Hall CE: Infections with other respiratory pathogens: Influenza, mumps, and respiratory syncytial viruses; *Mycoplasma pneumoniae.* In Fox JP (ed.): Viruses in Families. Littleton, MA, John Wright/PSG Inc, 1980, pp 335–381. *Longitudinal surveillance of families for parainfluenza virus infection and illness. Infection rate was 44 per 100 person-years for all ages, while attack rate for illness associated with parainfluenza virus infection was 76 per cent for babies under age 2 years and 25 per cent for adults.*

Glenzen WP, Denny FW: Epidemiology of acute lower respiratory disease in children. N Engl J Med 288:498, 1973. *Excellent summary of contribution of parainfluenza viruses to pediatric respiratory disease.*

364 Influenza

R. Gordon Douglas, Jr.

DEFINITION. Influenza is an acute, usually self-limited febrile illness that occurs in outbreaks of varying severity almost every winter. The causative virus is transmitted by the respiratory route; however, systemic symptoms are out of proportion to those in the respiratory tract. Infection with influenza virus can produce several other clinical syndromes common with infection with respiratory viruses, such as common colds, pharyngitis, croup, tracheobronchitis, bronchiolitis, or pneumonia. Conversely, infections with other respiratory viruses, such as respiratory syncytial virus, rhinovirus, or adenovirus, may produce sporadic cases indistinguishable from those of typical influenza. In addition to enormous morbidity and loss of time from school and work, influenza epidemics are associated with substantial mortality caused in large part by pulmonary complications.

Since the year 1510, 31 pandemics of respiratory disease similar to modern influenza have been described, 5 of which have occurred in the twentieth century (1900, 1918, 1957, 1968, and 1977). Of these, the pandemic of 1918 was the most severe, accounting for at least 21 million deaths. Over 500,000 deaths have occurred in the United States from epidemic influenza in the past 20 years.

ETIOLOGY. Influenza viruses belong to the family Orthomyxoviridae. Influenza A virus constitutes one genus and influenza B virus another. The virion is a medium-sized (80 to 100 nm in diameter) enveloped spherical or elongated particle covered with surface projections that are glycoproteins possessing either hemagglutinin (H) or neuraminidase (N) activity (Fig. 364–1). The envelope is composed of a lipid bilayer, on the inner surface of which is the matrix (M) protein. Within the envelope are eight segmented pieces of nucleocapsid, formed by a single species of protein, the nucleoprotein (NP), and single-stranded ribonucleic acid (RNA). Three polymerase (P) proteins and three nonstructural (NS_1, NS_2, and M2) proteins of unknown function are found within the envelope. The H is responsible for binding of the virus to the cell. Antibody to this protein neutralizes viral infectivity and thus is the major determinant of immunity. The viral N is instrumental in release of virus from cells. Antineuraminidase antibody is not neutralizing but limits viral replication and therefore the severity of infection. The M protein plays a role in stability of the membrane and in organization of the virion

during assembly. The three polymerases are important in viral replication. The internal M, NP, and P proteins are antigenically indistinguishable in all influenza A viruses but vary from those found in influenza B and C viruses. Thus, type-specific (A, B, or C) distinction of influenza viruses depends on serologic reactions mediated by these internal antigens. However, the surface proteins (H and N) do vary, not only among influenza virus types but also among subtypes of influenza A.

The viral *genome* comprises eight segments of RNA, each of which codes for one or two viral proteins. Reassortment of gene segments occurs frequently during coinfection of cells with two influenza A viruses. Influenza B and C viruses have been studied much less but appear to be structurally similar to influenza A virus. Antigenic variation is much less frequent with influenza B, and it may not occur with influenza C.

EPIDEMIOLOGY. *Antigenic Variation.* One of the unique and most remarkable features of influenza virus is the frequency with which changes in antigenicity occur. Such changes help explain why influenza continues to be a major epidemic disease in humans. As noted previously, antigenic variation involves only the H and N proteins among the proteins of influenza virus. The H is the more important, since it is more frequently involved in antigenic variation than the N protein and since antibody to this protein neutralizes infection. Antigenic variation is referred to as *antigenic drift* or *antigenic shift*, depending on whether the variation is small or great.

Antigenic Drift. Antigenic drift refers to relatively minor changes that occur frequently (every year or every few years) within an influenza A subtype. Each subtype is named by its hemagglutinin and neuraminidase. To date, three hemagglutinins (H1, H2, and H3) and two neuraminidases (N1 and N2) have been recognized in humans. The former designations, HO and HSW, are now classified as variants of H1. Each strain within the subtype is identified by site and year of isolation. Thus, influenza A/Bangkok/79/H3N2 indicates an influenza virus of type A and subtype H3N2 that was isolated in 1979 in Bangkok. The original H3N2 variant, A/Aichi/68/H3N2, was isolated in Aichi, Japan, in 1968. All isolates worldwide for the next 3 years were serologically identical. Subsequent antigenic drifts resulted in recovery of variants possessing minor differences: A/England/72/H3N2, A/Port Chalmers/73/H3N2, A/Scotland/74/H3N2, A/Georgia/74/H3N2, A/Victoria/75/H3N2, A/Texas/77/H3N2, A/Bangkok/79/H3N2, A/Philippines/2/82/H3N2, A/Mississippi/1/85/H3N2, A/Shanghai/11/87/H3N2, and so on. Antigenic drift results from point mutations that usually affect the RNA segment coding for the hemagglutinin, resulting in an alteration in protein structure that involves one or a few amino acids. Four antigenic sites have been described and complete nucleotide sequencing of hemagglutinins of several H3 strains has been determined, in support of this hypothesis. There is immunologic selection in which a new virus is favored over the old for person-to-person transmission because of the less frequent presence of antibody in the population to the new virus.

Antigenic Shift. Major antigenic shifts result from genetic reassortment when two influenza viruses simultaneously infect a single cell. Such an event results in a hemagglutinin or neuraminidase, or both, that is completely new in comparison with the previously circulating strain. Because of the high level of immunity to the old strain and lack of immunity to the new strain within the human population, the new strain, provided that it possesses intrinsic viral properties such as virulence and transmissibility, can readily cause a major outbreak of influenza.

Epidemic Influenza. An epidemic is an outbreak of influenza confined to one location such as a city, town, or country. In a given community, epidemics of influenza A virus infection have a characteristic pattern. A graphic description of an epidemic due to an A/Victoria/75/H3N2–like virus, which occurred in 1976 in Houston, Texas, is shown in Figure 364–2. Such localized epidemics begin rather abruptly, reach a sharp peak in 2 to 3 weeks, and last 5 to 6 weeks. Reports of increased numbers of children with febrile respiratory illness are often the first indication of influenza in a community. This is soon followed by the occurrence of influenza-like illnesses among adults. The next event is increased hospital admissions of patients with pneumonia, exacerbation of chronic obstructive pulmonary disease, croup, and

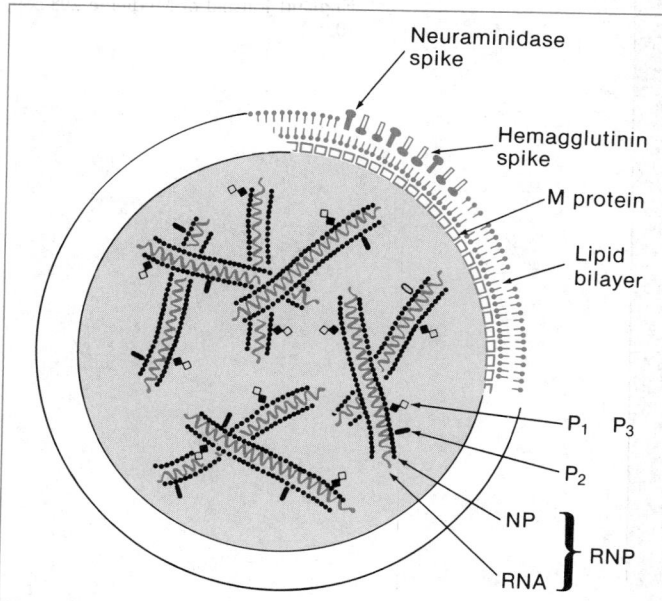

FIGURE 364–1. Schematic model for influenza virus virions. (Modified from Ginsberg HS: Orthomyxoviruses. *In* Davis BD, Dulbecco R, Eisen HN, Ginsburg HS [eds.]: Microbiology, 3rd ed. Hagerstown, MD, Harper & Row, Publishers, 1980, p 1119.)

Neuraminidase spike

Hemagglutinin spike

M protein

Lipid bilayer

P_1 P_3

P_2

NP

RNA

RNP

congestive heart failure. There are increases in school and industrial absenteeism and in the number of deaths caused by pneumonia and influenza. Although the latter finding is a highly specific indicator of influenza, it invariably lags behind the others. Viral isolation studies show a peak that parallels that of acute febrile respiratory illness. Year-round studies indicate that almost all isolates are obtained during the epidemic period. It is rare to recover influenza virus during other periods of the year, although occasionally there is serologic evidence of infection during other months.

Epidemics occur almost exclusively during the winter months—October through April in the northern hemisphere and May through September in the southern hemisphere. When observed in large countries such as the United States or Australia, regional differences in the time of occurrence of influenza outbreaks are apparent. It is not uncommon to have major outbreaks occurring in some communities or regions while others are experiencing no activity whatsoever. Often those so spared experience similar outbreaks at a later time, particularly if the prevalent virus demonstrates significant antigenic variation compared with previously prevalent viruses. During epidemics, the average overall attack rates are estimated to be 10 to 20 per cent;

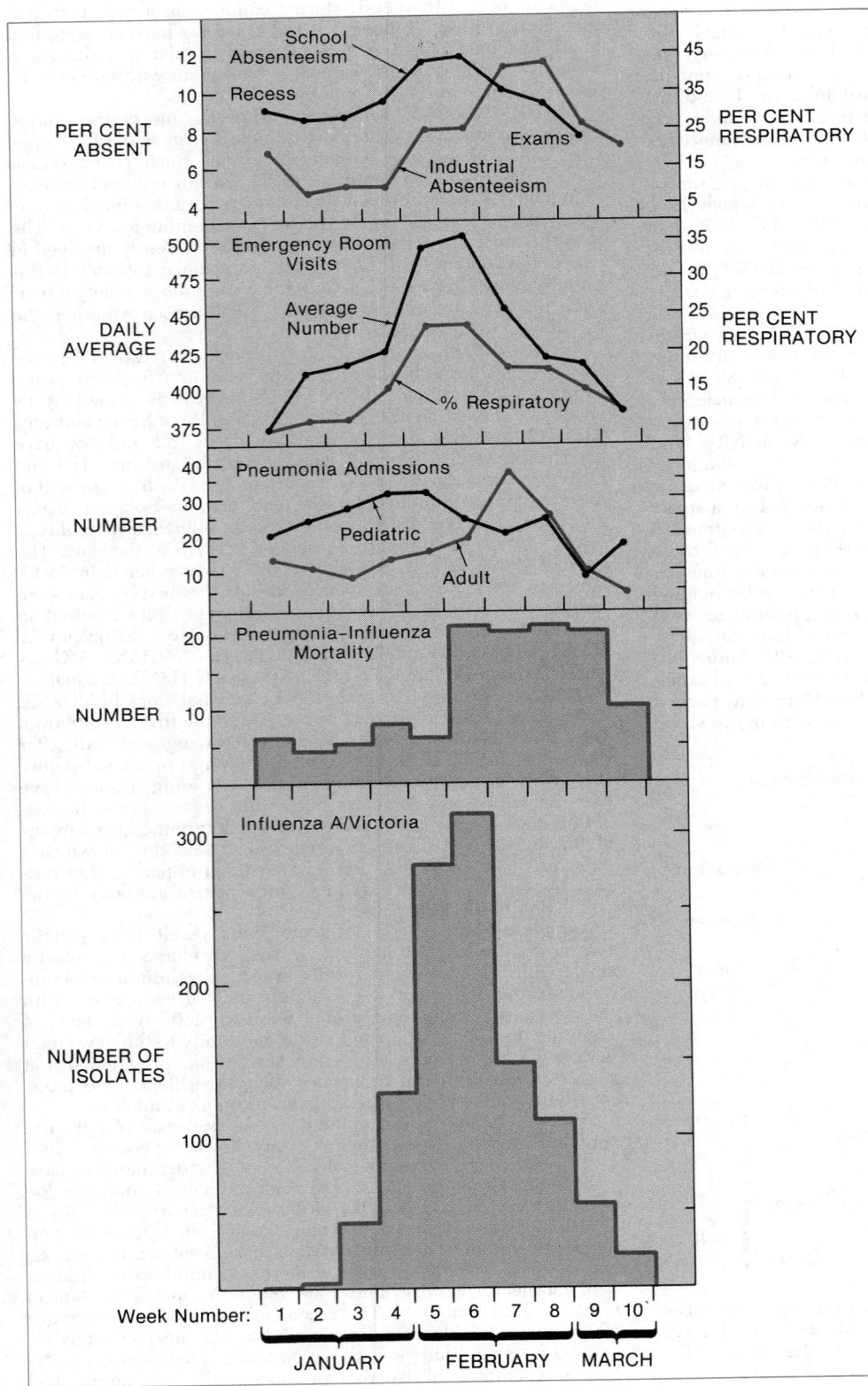

FIGURE 364–2. Correlation of the nonvirologic indexes of epidemiologic influenza with the number of isolates of influenza A/Victoria virus according to week, Houston, 1976 (industrial absenteeism is indicated by percentage with respiratory complaints). (Modified, by permission, from the New England Journal of Medicine 298:589, 1978.)

however, in selected populations of age groups, attack rates of 40 to 50 per cent are not uncommon. For many years it had been thought that during an epidemic of influenza a single strain of influenza virus prevailed and that other respiratory viruses were diminished or disappeared. However, we now know that two different strains within a single subtype, for example, A/Victoria/3/75/H3N2 and A/Texas/1/77/H3N2, or two different influenza virus subtypes, H1N1 and H3N2, may cocirculate. Furthermore, outbreaks of influenza A and B or simultaneous outbreaks of influenza A and respiratory syncytial virus infection have been demonstrated. Studies indicate that strains circulating at the end of one season's epidemic are most likely to be responsible for the next season's outbreak (the so-called *herald wave phenomenon*).

Pandemic Influenza. Pandemics of influenza result from the emergence of a new virus to which the overall population contains no immunity, so that epidemics of influenza progress to involve all parts of the world. The association of different subtypes of influenza A virus with pandemic influenza for the past 80 years is shown in Table 364–1. The pandemics of 1957, 1968, and 1977 all began in mainland China and then spread east and west, but primarily to the USSR and Western Europe before reaching the American continent. The interval between pandemics is variable and unpredictable, and this fact, in part, led to the national immunization program against swine influenza, when a small outbreak of A/H1N1 infection was detected at Fort Dix, New Jersey. This virus, A/New Jersey/76/H1N1, was very similar to the virus responsible for the 1988 outbreak. The most severe pandemics have resulted when there were major antigenic alterations in both of the major surface antigens. A striking exception to this occurred when A/USSR/77/H1N1 did not cause a severe pandemic in 1977 to 1978, despite major shifts in both surface glycoproteins. This discrepancy may reflect that much of the world's population in 1977 had been alive during the previous H1N1 era and thus possessed partial protective immunity. Furthermore, it appears that transmissibility from person to person and intrinsic virulence are virus-coded functions that vary much as does antigenicity. Intrinsic virulence with H1N1 viruses appears to be milder than with H3N2 viruses.

Proposed Mechanism of Epidemic Behavior. When a new virus with appropriate characteristics of virulence and transmissibility is introduced into a population lacking appropriate antibody, pandemic influenza results. After one or more waves of pandemic influenza, the level of immunity in the population increases. Such a chain of events provides a setting for emergence of a variant showing antigenic drift, since the level of immunity to it is less than that to the original strain. Repeated epidemics caused by strains showing antigenic drift within the subtype occur in subsequent years. After 10 to 40 years of circulation of variants within this given subtype, the population's immunity to all variants within the subtype is very high, and the conditions for the spread of a new virus are favorable. Such a virus originates by genetic reassortment. It possesses an H or N, or both, that is markedly different from the prior subtype. When such a virus circulates, the next pandemic occurs. Antigenic variation does not provide the entire explanation. Virus factors also contribute to virulence and transmissibility. Furthermore, other than the association of influenza outbreaks with colder seasons, the factors that allow an epidemic to develop or those responsible for the tapering off of an epidemic after 5 or 6 weeks, when only a

TABLE 364–1. ANTIGENIC SUBTYPES OF INFLUENZA A VIRUS ASSOCIATED WITH PANDEMIC INFLUENZA

Year	Interval (Years)	Designation	Extent of Antigenic Change in Indicated Surface Protein*	Severity of Pandemic
1870	—	H2N?	?	Moderate
1889	19	H3N8	H + + + N?	Severe
1918	29	H1N1†	H + + + N + + +	Severe
1957	39	H2N2	H + + + N + + +	Severe
1968	11	H3N2	H + + + N −	Moderate
1977	9	H1N1	H + + + N + + +	Mild

*+ = Minor change; + + = moderate change; + + + = major change; − = no change.

†Former designation was Hsw1N1 (35).

portion of susceptible persons is infected, are unknown. Finally, where the virus resides between epidemics is not understood.

Mortality. Pneumonia and influenza deaths fluctuate annually in predictable fashion, with peaks in the winter and troughs in the summer. When pneumonia and influenza deaths exceed the predicted number, this is due to influenza A or occasionally to influenza B virus activity. Although mortality is greatest during pandemics, substantial mortality occurs with epidemics, and the cumulative mortality from epidemics may exceed that of pandemics. Excess deaths due to influenza in the United States average 30,000 per epidemic (Fig. 364–3).

PATHOGENESIS AND PATHOLOGY. Influenza virus infection is acquired by transfer of virus-containing respiratory secretions from an infected to a susceptible person. Small-particle aerosols (less than 10 μ mass medium diameter) may be most significant in such person-to-person transmission. Once the virus has been deposited in the respiratory tract epithelium, unless it is prevented by specific secretory antibody, nonspecific mucoproteins, or mechanical actions of the mucociliary blanket, it attaches to and penetrates columnar epithelial cells by pinocytosis. Viral replication lasts 4 to 6 hours, and virus release continues for several hours before cell death ensues. Infection of adjacent and nearby cells follows, so that within a few replication cycles large numbers of cells in the respiratory tract are infected. The duration of the incubation period until onset of illness and virus shedding, which occur in close proximity, varies from 18 to 72 hours, depending in part on the inoculum size. Quantitation of virus in respiratory tract specimens reveals a characteristic pattern that correlates with severity of illness, suggesting that a major mechanism in the production of illness is cell death resulting from viral replication. Serum or secretory antibody or cell-mediated immune mechanisms are not detectable at this time, indicating that immunologic mechanisms are probably not involved in production of illness, with the exception of circulating interferon, which may contribute to systemic symptoms and fever. Viremia is rare.

Interferon is frequently detected in respiratory tract and serum specimens. Shedding of virus precedes by 1 to 2 days the appearance of interferon, which is correlated with improvements of signs and symptoms and decrease of virus titer, suggesting that interferon is active in the recovery process.

Neutralizing, hemagglutination-inhibiting (HAI), antineuraminidase, complement-fixing, enzyme-linked immunosorbent assay (ELISA), and immunofluorescent antibodies begin to develop in the sera of persons with primary influenza virus infection during the second week after exposure to antigen and reach a peak by 4 weeks. Secretory antibodies develop in the respiratory tract after influenza infection and consist predominantly of immunoglobulin A (IgA) antibodies that reach peak titers in 14 days. Protection against infection is afforded by serum HAI titers of 1:40 or greater, serum-neutralizing titers of 1:8 or greater, or nasal-neutralizing antibody titers of 1:4 or greater.

Nasal and bronchial biopsy specimens from persons with uncomplicated influenza reveal desquamation of the ciliated columnar epithelium. Individual cells show shrinkage, pyknotic nuclei, and loss of cilia. In addition, the lungs in fatal influenza show extensive hemorrhage, hyaline membrane formation, and paucity of polymorphonuclear cell infiltration. Patients with secondary bacterial pneumonia have the changes characteristic of bacterial pneumonia in addition to the tracheobronchial findings of influenza in the tracheobronchial tree.

CLINICAL FINDINGS. Many patients can pinpoint the hour of onset. Initially, systemic symptoms predominate and include feverishness, chilliness or frank shaking chills, headache, myalgias, malaise, and anorexia. In more severe cases, prostration is observed. Usually myalgias or headaches are the most troublesome symptoms, and their severity is related to the level of the fever. Arthralgias are commonly observed. Ocular symptoms, although less commonly present, are helpful diagnostically and include photophobia, tearing, burning, and pain on moving the eyes. Respiratory symptoms, particularly dry cough and nasal discharge, are usually also present at the onset but are overshadowed by the systemic symptoms. Nasal obstruction, hoarseness, and dry sore throat may also be present.

Fever is the most important physical finding. The temperature usually rises rapidly to a peak of 38 to 40°C and occasionally to 41°C within 12 hours of onset, concurrently with the development of systemic symptoms. Fever is usually continuous but may be intermittent, especially if antipyretics are administered. On the second and third days of illness, the temperature elevation is usually less than on the first day. As fever subsides, the systemic symptoms diminish. Typically, the duration of fever is 3 days, but it may last from 1 to 5 or more days. In a few cases, a second fluctuation in fever occurs on the third or fourth day, resulting in a biphasic fever curve. Early in the course of illness, the patient appears toxic, the face is flushed, and the skin is hot and moist. The eyes are watery and reddened. Clear nasal discharge is common, but nasal obstruction is uncommon. The mucous membranes of the nose and throat are hyperemic, but exudate is not observed. Small, tender cervical lymph nodes are often present, and transient, scattered rhonchi or localized areas of rales are found in less than 20 per cent of cases.

As systemic signs and symptoms diminish, respiratory complaints and findings become more apparent. Cough is the most frequent and troublesome of these symptoms and may be accompanied by substernal discomfort or burning. Nasal obstruction, discharge, pharyngeal pain, and injection are also common. Such symptoms and signs usually persist 3 to 4 days after fever subsides; however, cough, lassitude, and malaise may persist for 1, 2, or more weeks before full recovery.

This pattern of illness just described occurs with any type or subtype of influenza A or B virus. Attack rates are higher in children than in adults, although the incidence of pulmonary complications is lower in children. Maximum temperatures are higher in children, cervical adenopathy may be more frequent, and croup occurs only among children.

PULMONARY COMPLICATIONS. Three kinds of pulmonary complications are well recognized: *primary influenza viral pneumonia, secondary bacterial pneumonia,* and *mixed viral and bacterial pneumonia.* In addition, during an outbreak of influenza, less distinct and milder pulmonic syndromes often occur that may represent viral tracheobronchitis, localized viral pneumonia, or possibly mixed viral and bacterial infection.

Primary Influenza Viral Pneumonia. This syndrome first became well documented in the pandemic of 1957 to 1958. However, it is clear that many of the deaths in the 1918 to 1919 outbreak were due to this syndrome in healthy young adults. Primary influenza viral pneumonia has occurred predominantly among persons with cardiovascular disease, especially rheumatic heart disease with mitral stenosis. Although this syndrome occurs in healthy young adults in every large outbreak, other chronic disorders and pregnancy have been implicated as risk factors in some epidemics. Following a typical onset of influenza, there is rapid progression to fever, cough, dyspnea, and cyanosis. Physical examination and chest roentgenograms reveal bilateral findings consistent with the adult respiratory distress syndrome. Blood gas studies show marked hypoxia. Gram's stain of the sputum fails to reveal significant bacteria, and bacterial culture yields sparse growth of normal flora. Viral cultures of sputum or tracheal aspirates yield high titers of influenza virus. Such patients do not respond to antibiotics, and mortality is high.

Secondary Bacterial Pneumonia. Bacterial superinfection is often clinically distinguishable from primary viral pneumonia. The patients are most often elderly or have chronic pulmonary, cardiac, metabolic, or other diseases. Following a typical influenza illness, a period of improvement lasting from 1 to 4 days may occur. Recrudescence of fever is associated with symptoms and signs of bacterial pneumonia, such as cough, sputum production, and a localized area of consolidation apparent on physical and chest roentgenogram examination. Gram's stain and sputum culture reveal predominance of a bacterial pathogen, most often *Streptococcus pneumoniae, Staphylococcus aureus,* or *Haemophilus influenzae.* Such patients usually respond to specific antibiotic therapy.

Mixed Viral and Bacterial Pneumonia. During an outbreak of influenza, many cases are observed that do not clearly fit into either of the categories just described. The disease is not relentlessly progressive, and yet the fever pattern may be persistent and not biphasic. These patients may have a milder form of primary viral, secondary bacterial, or mixed viral and bacterial infection. Many respond to antibiotics. Milder forms of primary viral pneumonia involving only one lobe or segment have been described that do not invariably lead to death. Such cases are more likely to be confused with a pneumonia due to *Mycoplasma pneumoniae* than to that produced by bacterial infection. Pneumonia may occur in children, but it is less common than in adults. In addition, bronchiolitis and croup may be caused by influenza A or B virus infection.

Exacerbation of Chronic Obstructive Pulmonary Disease. In

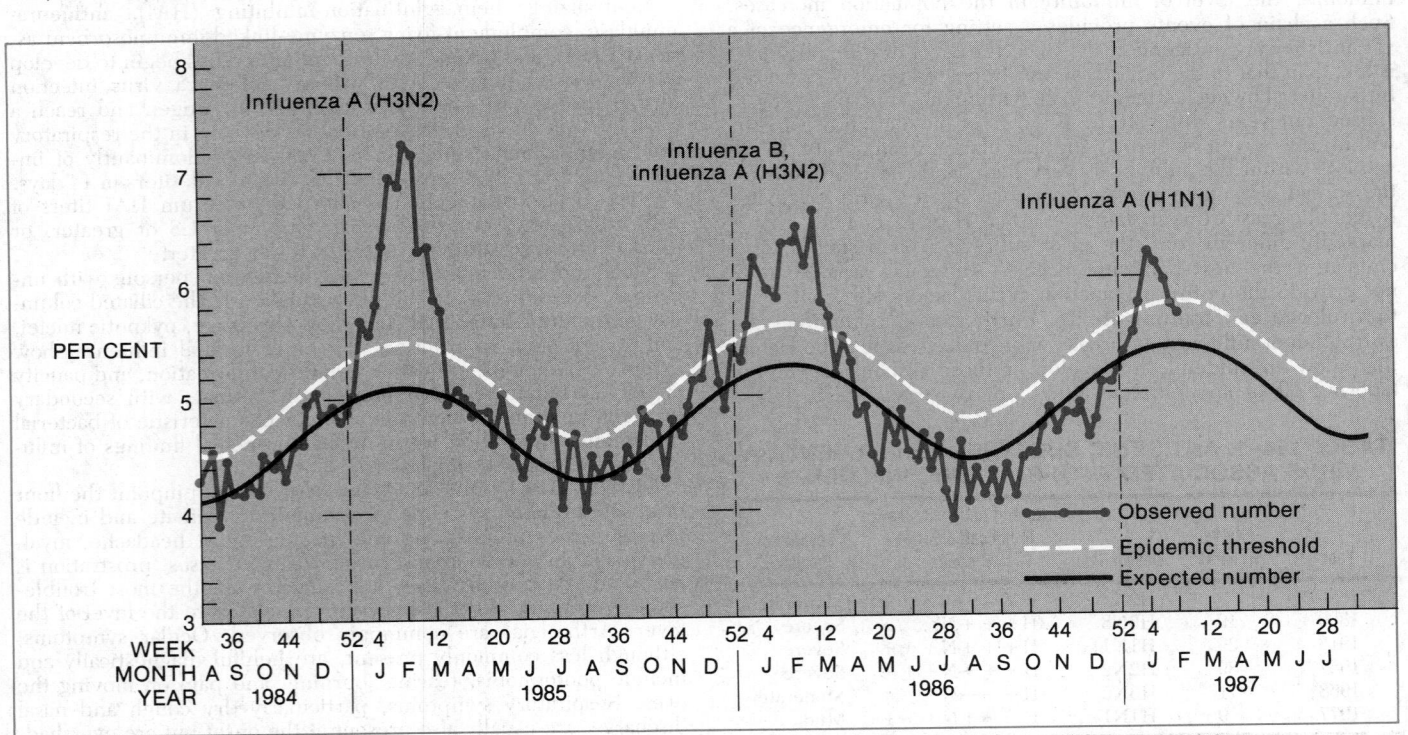

FIGURE 364–3. Pneumonia and influenza deaths as a percentage of total deaths in 121 cities from August 1984 through February 1987. (From Centers for Disease Control: Update: Influenza activity—United States. MMWR 36:116, 1987.)

adults with chronic obstructive pulmonary disease, influenza A or B virus infection may lead not only to pneumonia but also to acute exacerbation of chronic bronchitis, a syndrome that is associated with other respiratory viruses and bacteria as well.

NONPULMONIC COMPLICATIONS. *Reye's Syndrome.* Reye's syndrome is a frequently recognized hepatic and central nervous system complication of influenza A and B infection. Reye's syndrome is discussed in Ch. 480.

Other Complications. Myositis and myoglobinuria with tender leg muscles and elevated serum creatine kinase (CK) levels have been reported, mostly occurring in children. Myocarditis, pericarditis, and myocardial infarction rarely have been associated with influenza A and B virus infection. Gullain-Barré syndrome has been reported to occur after influenza A, but no definite causal relationship has been established. Transverse myelitis and encephalitis have also been reported rarely. Toxic shock syndrome due to infection of the respiratory tract with toxin-bearing *S. aureus* has been reported.

DIAGNOSIS. In an individual case, influenza often cannot be distinguished from infection with a number of other viruses and bacteria that produce headache, muscle aches, fever, and cough. On occasion, other respiratory viruses can produce an influenza-like illness, as can streptococcal pharyngitis. In the summer months, enteroviruses produce a clinically indistinguishable picture, and the acute manifestations of many other infections, such as dengue, may mimic influenza. On the other hand, in the context of an epidemic, influenza may be readily distinguished from other acute infections. When local, state, or national health authorities report an epidemic of influenza A or B virus infection in a given community, and a patient is seen with the acute onset of fever, headache, muscle aches, and cough, it is highly likely that these symptoms are caused by an influenza virus infection.

Definitive diagnosis depends on detection of infectious virus or viral antigen in secretions from patients or the detection of a serum antibody response. Influenza virus is readily isolated from throat or nasal specimens, sputum, or tracheal secretion specimens in the first 2 or 3 days of illness. Usually infectivity is detected within 48 to 72 hours in cell cultures. Viral antigen may be detected more rapidly in such specimens by use of immunofluorescence or ELISA. Serologic methods are less useful clinically because they require a convalescent serum obtained 10 to 14 days after the onset of infection. However, they are of great use in epidemiologic studies and to document the occurrence of an outbreak. A fourfold increase in antibody titer, comparing an acute with a convalescent phase, is diagnostic. The complement fixation antibody test is most useful for diagnosis because it is not dependent on strain or subtype variation, as is hemagglutination inhibition.

TREATMENT. Amantadine shortens the duration of fever and of systemic and respiratory symptoms by about 50 per cent. The dose is 100 to 200 mg per day orally for 3 to 5 days. Rimantadine, although not yet licensed, has a similar effect and reduces the likelihood of the mild, transient central nervous system side effects that occur with amantadine. Other symptomatic measures include antipyretics and cough suppressants. Many authorities consider that aspirin should not be used, especially for persons under 16 years of age, because of its association with the occurrence of Reye's syndrome. There is no evidence that amantadine or rimantadine is effective in treatment of pulmonary complications of influenza.

Currently, primary influenza viral pneumonia in its severe stages is best managed in an intensive care unit with supportive measures such as respiratory therapy, supplemental oxygen, and fluids. Secondary bacterial pneumonia should be treated with appropriate antibiotics. When studies of the sputum do not clearly indicate which bacterium may be infecting the patient, coverage should include antibiotics that are effective against *S. aureus*, *S. pneumoniae*, and *H. influenzae*.

PREVENTION. The mainstay of prevention is the use of inactivated influenza virus vaccines. These vaccines provide about 80 per cent protective efficacy. The antigenic composition is reviewed annually so that the vaccine contains the most recently circulating strains. Usually the vaccine is a trivalent product containing one or more subtypes of influenza A and influenza B virus. The recent vaccines have been purified by density gradient centrifugation or chromatography and have very low reaction rates. One to two per cent of persons vaccinated have fever and systemic symptoms peaking at 8 to 12 hours after vaccination, and up to 25 per cent may have mild local reactions at the site of vaccination. "Split" virus (subvirion) vaccines contain antigens with disrupted virus and may be less reactigenic than "whole" virus vaccines. The highest priority for vaccination should be given to persons with cardiac or pulmonary conditions requiring ongoing medical care and to residents of nursing homes and other chronic care facilities. Physicians, nurses, and other personnel including home health-care providers who have extensive contact with high-risk patients constitute the next priority for vaccination. Finally, persons over age 65 and persons with other chronic disease of any age should be vaccinated. Vaccine may also be given to well persons under age 65 who wish to reduce the likelihood of acquiring influenza. Vaccine should be administered each year in the fall prior to the influenza season.

Amantadine and rimantadine are also effective in preventing influenza A and should be used to supplement vaccine programs. Persons who are not vaccinated in the fall should be placed on amantadine when an outbreak occurs or throughout the influenza season for the highest risk group. If vaccine is available, persons may be vaccinated simultaneously, and amantadine therapy should be stopped after 14 days. Alternatively, if vaccine is not available, amantadine administration may be continued for the duration of the outbreak, the dose being 100 to 200 mg per day orally. In the family setting, prophylaxis may fail owing to emergence of resistant viruses. Amantadine, administered to patients and staff alike, is very helpful in managing nosocomial outbreaks.

Arden NH, Patriarca PA, Fasano MB, et al.: The roles of vaccination and amantadine prophylaxis in controlling an outbreak of influenza A (H3N2) in a nursing home. Arch Intern Med 148:865–868, 1988. *Useful data to manage a common problem.*

Barker WH, Mullooly JP: Pneumonia and influenza deaths during epidemics: Implications for prevention. Arch Intern Med 142:85–89, 1982. *Best study of the devastating effects of an influenza epidemic.*

Centers for Disease Control: Prevention and Control of Influenza. Part I. Vaccines. MMWR 38:297–298, 303–311, 1989. *Details of extensive revisions of recommendations for use of influenza vaccine as well as a summary of recent epidemiology.*

Dolin R, Reichman RC, Madore HP, et al.: A controlled trial of amantadine and rimantadine in the prophylaxis of influenza A infection. N Engl J Med 307:580, 1982. *Definitive study comparing prophylactic efficacy of amantadine and rimantadine.*

Douglas RG Jr.: Prophylaxis and treatment of influenza. N Engl J Med 322:443–450, 1990. *Recent review of vaccines and antivirals for influenza.*

Hayden FG, Belshe RB, Clover RD, et al.: Emergence and apparent transmission of rimantidine resistant influenza A virus in families. N Engl J Med 321:1696–1702, 1989. *A problem possibly limiting usefulness of antiviral prophylaxis.*

Kendel AP, Patriarca PA (eds.): Options for the Control of Influenza. New York, Alan R. Liss, 1986. *Excellent recent review of rationale for vaccine and amantadine use. In addition, an up-to-date summary of epidemiology.*

Younkin SW, Betts RF, Roth FK, et al.: Reduction in fever and symptoms in young adults with aspirin or amantadine. Antimicrob Agents Chemother 23:577, 1983. *Study comparing therapeutic effects of amantadine and aspirin.*

365 Adenovirus Diseases

Stephen G. Baum

The most clinically significant diseases caused by adenoviruses are infections of the respiratory system and the eye. Recently, adenoviruses have been shown to play a significant role in causing diarrheal disease in children and respiratory infections in immunocompromised patients. Adenoviruses are the object of intensive research efforts because they possess several fascinating and important biologic capabilities, including oncogenesis and latency. Today they are perhaps the best characterized human virus group.

ETIOLOGIC AGENT. Adenoviruses are double-stranded DNA viruses that average 70 nm in diameter and have a unique outer structure, which permits their morphologic identification by electron microscopic examination. The virus is icosahedral with 20 equilateral triangular faces and 12 vertices. The faces are made up of hexon subunits, and the vertices each contain a penton subunit. From each vertex, an antenna-like structure, the fiber, projects with a knob at the end. Each class of these surface subunits differs antigenically from the others. The hexon contains group-specific and type-specific antigens. Forty-seven serotypes of human adenovirus have been identified (types 1 to 47). Many of the serotypes have been associated with specific syndromes, but over half the adenovirus types have not been shown to cause disease. The 47 serotypes have been divided into six groups by DNA homology and four groups according to ability to agglutinate different erythrocytes. The latter grouping correlates well with the ability of different serotypes to cause specific syndromes and to induce tumors in animals.

In acute infections, adenoviruses cause cell death and lysis with release of new progeny virions. The mechanisms of latency and animal oncogenesis are not completely understood, although many of the functions of adenovirus have been accurately mapped on the deoxyribonucleic acid (DNA) genome. Adenoviruses can form a family of hybrid viruses with an unrelated DNA virus, SV40. Portions of the DNA of adenovirus and SV40 are covalently linked within an adenovirus outer coat. The hybrid virus has unique biologic and oncogenic capabilities in vitro and in animals in vivo. Neither adenovirus alone nor the hybrid viruses have been shown to cause cancer in humans.

A small defective DNA parvovirus has been isolated from some adenovirus preparations and from some patients with adenovirus infection. This *adeno-associated virus (AAV)* requires adenovirus for its replication. It is not known to cause disease by itself and does not appear to contribute to adenovirus pathogenesis. A related parvovirus (B19) has recently been implicated as the cause of erythema infectiosum (fifth disease), aplastic crisis in patients with hemoglobinopathies, and arthropathy in adults.

EPIDEMIOLOGY. Most people experience an adenovirus infection during the first decade of life. The initial infecting serotype and the syndrome it causes are a function of the age of the patient and the route of infection. Studies of large populations show that adenoviruses cause 3 to 5 per cent of all clinically apparent infections in children. Adenoviruses are the most common viral isolates in this age group, and at least half of these isolations are associated with subclinical infections. Respiratory infection is transmitted by person-to-person contact or through contaminated swimming water.

Conjunctival infection may be transmitted directly, through water, or by fomites such as towels or ophthalmologic equipment and solutions. Pneumonia and urinary tract infection in immunocompromised patients may be acquired exogenously or may represent reactivation of latent infection. There are many adenoviruses that infect other animals and birds, but these play no known role in human disease.

CLINICAL PRESENTATIONS OCCURRING MOSTLY IN CHILDREN. Respiratory Infection. Infants most commonly manifest adenovirus infections as coryzal symptoms, but occasionally adenovirus type 7 causes fulminant bronchiolitis and pneumonia in this age group. Recently, Reye's syndrome has been reported as a complication of severe adenovirus infection in infants. In older children, pharyngitis and tracheobronchitis are most prevalent. Adenoviruses are the most common viral isolate from children with the whooping cough syndrome. It is not known whether this virus contributes to the pathogenesis of *Bordetella pertussis* infection or whether adenovirus alone can cause the syndrome.

Pharyngoconjunctival Fever. This syndrome occurs in small epidemics in summer camps where it is probably spread in swimming water. Adenovirus type 3 has been the most common isolate. The onset of symptoms is acute and includes pharyngitis, rhinitis, conjunctivitis, cervical adenitis, and elevation in temperature to about 38°C. The bulbar and palpebral conjunctivae have a granular appearance. The symptoms last 3 to 5 days. Permanent sequelae are rare, and there is no specific therapy.

Intestinal Disease. Immunoelectron microscopy has revealed viruses in the stool in many cases of infantile diarrhea. The most common viruses visualized are rotaviruses and adenoviruses. These adenoviruses appear to be defective in their replication and require special cells for isolation in tissue culture. Serotypes 40 and 41 have been found most often in this situation. Intussusception in children has also been linked to adenovirus types 1,

2, 3, and 5, although a causal role is unproven. Many of the children with this syndrome have intercurrent adenoviral respiratory infection.

Hemorrhagic Cystitis. Adenovirus types 11 and 21 have been associated with hemorrhagic cystitis in as many as 20 to 50 per cent of American and Japanese children with this syndrome. Boys are affected more often than girls, in contrast to the situation with bacterial cystitis. Gross and microscopic hematuria may persist for 1 to 2 weeks.

CLINICAL PRESENTATIONS OCCURRING MOSTLY IN ADULTS. Respiratory Infection. The first isolation of adenoviruses directly from sick patients occurred during an epidemic of acute respiratory disease in military recruits. This population seems extremely susceptible to infection with types 4 and 7, as it is to infection with *Mycoplasma pneumoniae* and the meningococci. In general, the manifestations are those of atypical pneumonia, of which up to 40 per cent of cases are caused by adenovirus. Fever to 39°C, cough, pharyngitis, rhinorrhea, and pulmonary rales are the most common signs and symptoms. Radiographic examination of the chest shows patchy interstitial infiltrates that are unilateral in most cases. Small pleural effusions can occur.

In nonepidemic situations, it is impossible to make a definitive clinical diagnosis of adenoviral pneumonia. Some factors useful in comparing adenoviral with mycoplasmal pneumonia are lower incidence of cold agglutinins, shorter incubation period, and better correlation of radiographic and physical findings in the chest in adenovirus infection. Influenza and parainfluenza viruses produce similar syndromes. Adenoviral pneumonia usually lasts about 1 week. There is no specific therapy, and bacterial superinfection and death are rare.

Adenoviruses have been isolated from the lungs and urine of immunocompromised patients including renal transplant recipients and patients with acquired immunodeficiency syndrome (AIDS). Several of the higher serotypes were first isolated from such patients. In these instances, adenovirus operates as an opportunistic agent.

Neurologic Disease. Central nervous system infection, most often appearing as meningoencephalitis, has been attributed to adenovirus. It sometimes occurs in minor epidemic form and is frequently associated with recent respiratory infection. The clinical presentation is that of encephalitis or aseptic meningitis. There are no pathognomonic findings.

Epidemic Keratoconjunctivitis. The initial epidemic of adenoviral keratoconjunctivitis involved shipyard workers who sustained minor eye trauma from paint and rust fragments. Adenovirus type 8 was isolated in this and many other epidemics. Serotypes 19 and 37 have caused keratoconjunctivitis that was spread by fomites such as roller towels. Contaminated ophthalmic solutions have also transmitted infection. The incubation period is from 3 to 24 days. The onset is insidious, and both eyes often are affected. Eye irritation and exudation may last 1 to 4 weeks. Preauricular adenopathy often occurs early. Corneal involvement is a late complication and may persist for a month or more with blurring of vision. Residual blindness is unusual. There is no specific antiviral therapy as there is for herpes keratitis. Secondary spread to household contacts occurs in about 10 per cent of cases, varying with the duration of the index case.

DIAGNOSIS. Diagnosis is usually made on clinical grounds alone. In the case of diarrheal illness, immunoelectronmicroscopy and DNA hybridization assays have proved useful, but these are not at present generally available. Antibody and nucleic acid probes have also been developed for diagnosis of adenovirus keratoconjunctivitis. Virus culture is, of course, the definitive assay.

TREATMENT AND PREVENTION. There is no effective antiviral chemotherapy for human adenoviral infections. Live, enteric-coated oral adenovirus vaccines of types 4 and 7 have been effective in immunizing military populations. In epidemic situations, mass immunization with the live virus vaccine promptly interrupts the epidemic. The vaccine is not recommended or available for civilians because of the low incidence and sporadic occurrence of infection with adenovirus types 4 and 7.

Baum SG: Adenovirus. *In* Mandell A, Douglas RA, Bennet JE (eds.): Principles and Practice of Infectious Diseases. 3rd ed. New York, Churchill Livingstone

Inc., 1990, pp 1185–1191. *An expanded version of the material in this chapter, containing correlative tables, fully referenced.*

Horwitz MS: Adenoviridae and their replication. *In* Fields BN, Knipe DM (eds.): Virology, 2nd ed. New York, Raven Press, 1989, pp 1679–1721. *An encyclopedic chapter on the molecular biology of the adenoviruses.*

366 Viral Gastroenteritis

Albert Z. Kapikian

DEFINITION

Viral gastroenteritis (acute infectious nonbacterial gastroenteritis, epidemic diarrhea, winter vomiting disease, sporadic infantile gastroenteritis) is a common acute infectious disease of all age groups, characterized by vomiting or watery diarrhea, or both, that may be accompanied by fever, nausea, anorexia, and malaise. It ranges from a mild, self-limited illness of short duration to life-threatening dehydration, especially in infants and young children.

The importance of this disease in a developed country was highlighted in the Cleveland Family Study, in which infectious gastroenteritis, presumably nonbacterial, was the second most common disease experience, accounting for 16 per cent of some 25,000 illnesses in a period of almost 10 years. In developing countries the impact of diarrheal illnesses is staggering: In Asia, Africa, and Latin America, 3 to 5 billion cases of diarrhea and 5 to 10 million diarrhea-associated deaths occur annually, with the major impact in infants and young children. In addition, diarrheal illness was ranked first among infectious diseases in incidence and mortality in these developing areas.

In spite of major discoveries in bacteriology and parasitology in the past century, the etiology of most acute diarrheal illnesses remained elusive for many years. In the 1940's and 1950's, oral administration of bacteria-free stool filtrates from patients with acute diarrhea induced illness in volunteers, but the suspected viral etiologic agent could not be identified. In 1972, Kapikian and colleagues, employing immune electron microscopy (IEM), discovered virus-like particles in a stool suspension derived from a gastroenteritis outbreak in Norwalk, Ohio. In 1973, Bishop and associates, employing electron microscopy (EM), discovered rotavirus particles in duodenal biopsies from infants and young children hospitalized with acute gastroenteritis.

ETIOLOGY

NORWALK VIRUS GROUP. The Norwalk virus is the prototype strain of a group of fastidious, nonenveloped particles usually named after the geographic location of the gastroenteritis outbreak from which they are recovered. They share these common characteristics: (1) a diameter of approximately 27 nm; (2) indistinct morphology; (3) presence in feces; (4) noncultivable in vitro; (5) unknown nucleic acid content; and (6) a characteristic buoyant density of 1.36 to 1.41 grams per cubic centimeter in cesium chloride. The group includes at least four serotypes —Norwalk, Hawaii, Ditchling, and Snow Mountain agents—and several other strains (Montgomery County, "W," cockle, Taunton, and Parramatta) that share an antigenic relationship with one of the known serotypes or have not been characterized. Classification of these fastidious viruses into a virus family has not been feasible. However, the protein composition of Norwalk and Snow Mountain viruses resembles that of the caliciviruses, since they each possess a single primary virion-associated protein with an approximate molecular weight of 60,000. The Norwalk virus was recently cloned and found to contain a positive sense single-stranded ribonucleic acid (RNA) genome.

ROTAVIRUS. Rotaviruses are classified as a genus in the family Reoviridae and are etiologic agents of diarrhea in humans and in numerous animal and a few avian species. They are 70 nm in diameter, with a genome consisting of 11 segments of double-stranded RNA, and possess a distinctive double-layered capsid. The name rotavirus (rota = wheel) was adopted because the sharply defined circular outline of the outer capsid was reminiscent of the rim of a wheel placed on short spokes radiating from a wide hub (the inner capsid). The virions (see Fig. 366–1)

have a density of 1.36 grams per cubic centimeter in cesium chloride and are antigenically distinct from the three reovirus serotypes. Rotaviruses possess three important antigenic specificities—group, subgroup, and serotype—which are mediated by different proteins: group specificity prominently by VP6 and subgroup by VP6 alone (encoded by RNA segment 6). Serotype specificity has been defined by VP7, a glycoprotein that is one of the two major neutralization antigens located on the outer capsid (encoded by RNA segment 7, 8, or 9). The other outer capsid protein VP4 (formerly designated VP3), which is encoded by RNA segment 4 and which protrudes from the smooth outer surface as a spike of about 12 nm in length, also induces neutralizing antibodies. VP4 is the hemagglutinin in certain strains. Antibodies to both VP4 and VP7 are associated with protection against rotavirus illness. There are seven human rotavirus serotypes as defined by VP7, of which those numbered 1 to 4 are of epidemiologic importance. Several human and animal rotavirus strains share VP7 serotype specificity. Most animal and human rotaviruses share the common group antigen and are thus classified as group A rotaviruses, and these are further divided into subgroups. The human rotaviruses have only recently been grown efficiently in cell culture. Several human and animal rotavirus strains have been discovered that do not share the common group antigen and are classified as non–group A rotaviruses (groups B to G). They were formerly designated "pararotaviruses." In this chapter, when the term rotavirus is used, it is meant to describe only those rotaviruses belonging to group A, unless specified otherwise.

OTHER AGENTS. Other viral agents have been associated with gastroenteritis and include enteric adenoviruses belonging to types 40 and 41 (70 to 80 nm in diameter); caliciviruses (30 to 40 nm); astroviruses (28 to 30 nm); small, round viruses other than the Norwalk virus group (20 to 30 nm); putative coronavirus–like particles (100 to 150 nm); the Otofuke, Sapporo, and Osaka agents (33 to 40 nm); the "minireoviruses" (30 nm); the pleomorphic, fringed, Breda or Berne virus-like particles (toroviruses) (100 to 140 nm); 35 nm "picobirnavirus"; and a pestivirus antigen. The role of these viruses as etiologic agents of severe infantile diarrhea appears to be minor, with the exception of the enteric adenoviruses, which are associated with approximately 5 to 10 per cent of the diarrheal illnesses of infants and young children requiring hospitalization. In addition, the role of these other agents in epidemic viral gastroenteritis appears to be minor. Additional studies are needed to assess the role of these other agents in gastroenteritis. It should be noted that about one third to one half of gastroenteritis episodes have yet to be associated with an etiologic agent.

EPIDEMIOLOGY

NORWALK VIRUS GROUP. The Norwalk group of viruses comprises major etiologic agents of acute nonbacterial gastroenteritis, which typically occurs as a sharp outbreak affecting adults, school-age children, and family contacts. The location or source of contamination responsible for these outbreaks includes various settings such as schools, camps and recreational areas, nursing homes, swimming facilities, cruise ships, and restaurants. For example, the Norwalk virus was derived from an outbreak in an elementary school in Norwalk, Ohio, in which 50 per cent of the students and teachers developed gastroenteritis within a 2-day period. Norwalk virus has been linked with 42 per cent of 74 nonbacterial gastroenteritis outbreaks investigated from 1976 to 1980 and approximately 10 per cent of all acute gastroenteritis outbreaks. In the United States, antibody to the Norwalk virus is usually acquired gradually in childhood and somewhat more rapidly in the adult years, so that by age 50 at least 50 per cent of individuals have serum antibody. In developing countries, infants and young children acquire Norwalk antibody at an earlier age, and the virus is associated with mild gastroenteritis in this age group.

Norwalk virus is most likely transmitted via the fecal-oral route; however, it has also been detected in vomitus. Although sporadic cases attributed to person-to-person transmission may occur, the explosive nature of outbreaks associated with the Norwalk virus group often suggests a common source of infection, such as water or food. Common-source outbreaks have been attributed to contamination of community and noncommunity public water systems, stored water on cruise ships, or recreational swimming water and to ingestion of tainted oysters, cockles, lettuce, or cake frosting. Secondary person-to-person transmission to contacts is relatively common. The incubation period ranges from 10 to 51 hours, with a mean of 24 hours, and symptoms usually last 24 to 60 hours. Norwalk virus outbreaks occur throughout the year without a peak season.

Norwalk virus infections have been detected in individuals with travelers' diarrhea. However, this agent is not considered to be an important cause of this disease.

ROTAVIRUS. Rotaviruses are the major known etiologic agents of severe diarrhea in infants and young children in most areas of the world and are usually associated with sporadic infantile gastroenteritis, which differs from epidemic viral gastroenteritis associated with the Norwalk virus group in the following characteristics: (1) it usually does not occur in sharp outbreaks; (2) it is associated with a severe diarrheal illness in infants and young children; (3) it does not usually cause illness in adults; and (4) the attack rate among family contacts of index cases is low, although subclinical infections occur frequently in contacts.

The most compelling evidence for the importance of rotaviruses in severe infantile gastroenteritis has emerged from numerous cross-sectional studies in developed and developing countries. In developed countries, including the United States, rotaviruses are associated with approximately 35 to 52 per cent of acute diarrheal illness requiring hospitalization of infants and young children. The contribution of other enteric pathogens is consistently relatively minor. A similar pattern is also usually observed in developing countries, where rotaviruses are the most frequently detected pathogens in children less than 2 years of age who have severe gastroenteritis; however, bacterial agents also play an important role in such areas. It is estimated that in developing countries 873,000 infants and young children under 5 years of age die from rotavirus diarrhea each year. It should be noted that during longitudinal studies in a community setting where all diarrheal episodes are monitored, the incidence of rotavirus diarrhea is lower than that of diarrhea caused by other pathogens, but dehydration is more often associated with rotavirus disease than with illness caused by other agents.

In temperate climates, rotavirus gastroenteritis has a characteristic seasonal occurrence during the cooler months of the year with peak prevalence in the winter months. In tropical countries it occurs throughout the year, with less pronounced peaks. Rotavirus diarrhea occurs most frequently in children between 6 months and 24 months of age. Infants less than 6 months of age have the next highest frequency, although in certain studies the highest frequency is observed in this age group. The low frequency of clinical illness in neonates who undergo rotavirus infection is an unusual paradox that has not been explained.

Rotavirus gastroenteritis occurs infrequently in adults, but subclinical infections are common.

Rotaviruses are likely transmitted by the fecal-oral route, although respiratory transmission remains a possibility, since there is such a rapid acquisition of serum antibody during the first 2 years of life regardless of hygienic conditions. Nosocomial rotavirus infections occur frequently. The incubation period of rotavirus illness is approximately 2 to 4 days. There are seven recognized human rotavirus serotypes of which those numbered 1 to 4 appear to be of clinical importance. Group B rotavirus is responsible for widespread outbreaks of gastroenteritis in adults in China, and a relatively small number of group C rotaviruses have been recovered from individuals with gastroenteritis in various countries. With the exception of the group B rotaviruses in China, the role of the non–group A rotaviruses in other regions of the world appears to be relatively minor at this time.

Rotavirus infections have been observed in individuals with travelers' diarrhea. However, rotaviruses are not considered to be an important cause of this illness.

PATHOLOGY AND PATHOGENESIS

NORWALK VIRUS GROUP. Histopathologic lesions following Norwalk or Hawaii virus infections are characterized by a reversible involvement of the upper jejunum. The jejunal mucosa remains intact with marked broadening and blunting of the villi and shortening of the microvilli, along with mononuclear cell infiltration and cytoplasmic vacuolization. Functional alterations may include a transient malabsorption of fat, D-xylose, and lactose and a significant decrease in levels of small intestinal brush border enzymes (alkaline phosphatase and trehalase). Adenylate cyclase activity in the jejunum is not elevated. Delay in gastric emptying may be responsible for the nausea and vomiting associated with these agents.

The nature of immunity to Norwalk virus is perplexing, because a high percentage (~50 per cent) of adults are susceptible to both natural and experimental illness. In addition, although immunity has been observed in approximately 50 per cent of adults, it appears to correlate inversely with the level of serum or local jejunal antibody.

ROTAVIRUS. The major histopathologic lesions are characterized by reversible involvement of the proximal small intestine. The mucosa remains intact, with shortening of the villi, mononuclear cell infiltration in the lamina propria, distended cisternae of the endoplasmic reticulum, mitochondrial swelling, and sparse, irregular microvilli. Functional alterations may include impaired D-xylose absorption and depressed levels of disaccharidases (maltase, sucrase, and lactase).

The mechanism of immunity to human rotaviruses is not completely clear. Although serum antibodies correlate with resistance to illness, the role of local intestinal immunity has not been elucidated. Animal studies indicate that antibody in the small intestine is the major determinant of resistance to illness. A high rate of subclinical infection in neonates is well documented and may be related to passively acquired maternal antibody, host

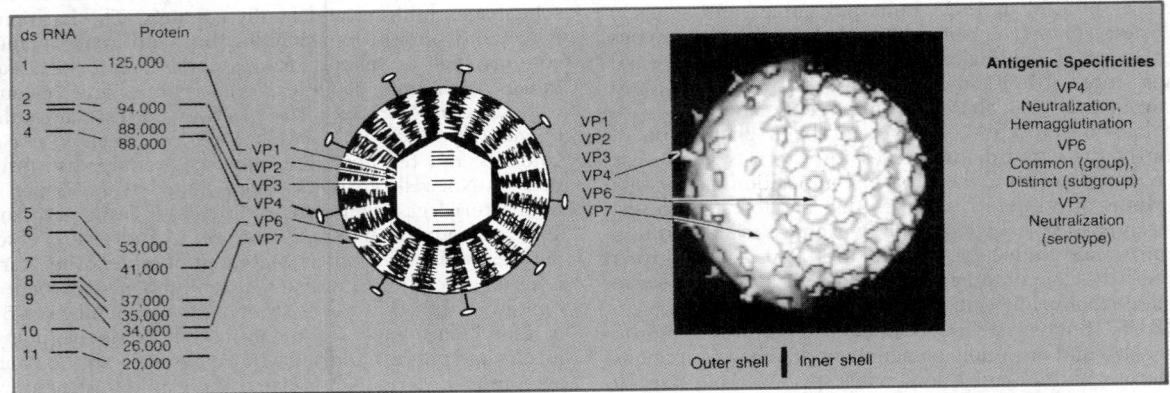

FIGURE 366–1. *Left,* Schematic representation of the rotavirus double-shelled particle. *Right,* Surface representations of the three-dimensional structures of a double-shelled particle (on the left half) and a particle (on the right half) in which most, if not all, of the outer shell and a small portion of the inner shell mass have been removed. (From Kapikian AZ, Chanock RM: Rotaviruses. *In* Fields BN, et al. (eds.): Virology, 2nd ed. New York, Raven Press, 1990; with permission. Figure on right from Prasad BV, Wang GJ, Clerx JP, et al.: Three-dimensional structure of rotavirus. J Mol Biol 199:269–275, 1988; with permission.)

factors, or naturally attenuated rotaviruses that are able to persist in newborn nurseries.

CLINICAL MANIFESTATIONS

NORWALK VIRUS GROUP. Clinical characteristics of illness induced by the Norwalk group of viruses include nausea, vomiting, diarrhea, anorexia, or abdominal discomfort, or any combination. Accompanying clinical manifestations may also include myalgias, low-grade fever, headache, and chills. In children, vomiting occurs more often than diarrhea, whereas in adults the opposite is observed. The onset of illness may be abrupt, marked by vomiting, diarrhea, or both. The illness is usually mild and lasts about 24 to 60 hours. However, severe gastroenteritis has been observed in middle-aged patients and has contributed to the death of elderly, debilitated individuals. The stools are characteristically loose and watery; blood, mucus, and leukocytes are not typically present. A transient decrease in the T, B, and null cell lymphocyte subpopulations has been observed.

ROTAVIRUS. Rotavirus infection can produce a variety of responses in infants and young children, ranging from subclinical infection and mild diarrhea to a severe and occasionally fatal dehydrating illness. Clinical characteristics include vomiting, diarrhea, abdominal discomfort, or fever, or any combination. Fever and vomiting often develop before the diarrhea. Accompanying clinical manifestations may include dehydration, irritability, and pharyngeal or tympanic membrane erythema. In hospitalized patients, the mean duration of confinement is 4 days, with a range of 2 to 14 days. The stools are characteristically loose and watery and only infrequently contain blood or leukocytes.

Although rotaviruses can cause severe or fatal dehydrating illnesses in developing countries, deaths have also been documented in developed countries. In a study in Canada, rotavirus gastroenteritis was implicated in the deaths of 21 children 4 to 30 months of age (mean 11 months) over a period of about 5 years. Twenty children were dead or moribund upon arrival at hospital, and one child was infected nosocomially. With the exception of the latter patient and one other, each child was considered healthy prior to the rotaviral illness. Death occurred within 1 to 3 days of onset of symptoms. Dehydration and electrolyte imbalance leading to cardiac arrest were believed to be the major cause of death in 16 patients; aspiration of vomitus was the cause of death in 3 patients, and seizures were a contributing factor in the remaining 2 patients.

Rotavirus can also induce chronic symptomatic diarrhea with prolonged fecal shedding of the virus and antigenemia in patients with primary immunodeficiency diseases. Infections with rotaviruses or other viral and bacterial enteric pathogens may be especially severe in individuals who are immunosuppressed for bone marrow transplantation. In one study, 8 of 78 such patients (average age of entire group, 20.5 years) shed rotavirus in stools and 5 of the 8 died. In addition, a non–group A rotavirus was associated with severe gastroenteritis in an 8-year-old bone marrow transplant patient. Rotavirus infections have also been persistent and severe in children with severe combined immunodeficiency. Rotavirus infections have also been associated with necrotizing enterocolitis and hemorrhagic gastroenteritis in neonates.

Outbreaks of rotavirus gastroenteritis have occurred in elderly individuals in nursing homes with several fatalities.

DIAGNOSIS

NORWALK VIRUS GROUP. Since a specific diagnosis of infection with this group cannot be made by clinical observation, the diagnosis must be made in the laboratory and relies on the detection of virus in the stool or a serologic response to a viral-specific antigen. These tests include IEM (for the entire group), radioimmunoassay (Norwalk and Snow Mountain agents), and enzyme-linked immunosorbent assay (ELISA) (Norwalk, Snow Mountain, and Hawaii viruses). These are still research procedures, because reagents are not generally available. Virus shedding is maximal at or shortly after onset of illness and minimal at 72 hours following onset. The characteristic absence of fecal leukocytes in Norwalk infection may be helpful for differentiation from *Shigella* or *Salmonella* enteritis.

Although a specific clinical diagnosis of infection with Norwalk virus cannot be made in the individual patient, a tentative diagnosis of infection can be made during an outbreak if certain criteria are met: (1) bacterial or parasitic pathogens are not detected; (2) vomiting is present in at least 50 per cent of cases; (3) incubation period is 24 to 48 hours; and (4) mean or median duration of illness is 12 to 60 hours.

ROTAVIRUS. The clinical manifestations of rotavirus gastroenteritis are not distinctive enough to enable diagnosis. Thus, diagnosis requires either detection of the virus or demonstration of a significant serologic response to rotavirus in paired acute and convalescent sera. The epidemiologic pattern relating to the age of the patient, the temporal occurrence of illness, and the signs and symptoms of illness, however, may suggest the diagnosis. In addition, the usual absence of fecal leukocytes in rotavirus diarrhea may help in early differentiation from *Shigella* or *Salmonella* enteritis.

Stools obtained from the first to fourth day of illness are optimal for rotavirus detection, but virus shedding may continue up to 21 days. Virus is characteristically present in stools during the early phase of diarrhea, but diarrhea may continue for 2 to 3 days after the cessation of virus shedding.

Over 25 assays have been developed for the detection of rotavirus in stools. The most rapid method is still direct EM because in negatively stained preparations these agents have a distinctive morphologic appearance and are present in large amounts. The non–group A rotaviruses, which do not share the common group antigen, can also be detected by EM. However, an electron microscope may not be readily available, and its use may be impractical when evaluating a large number of specimens. Thus, other rapid and highly effective methods for virus detection have been developed, including ELISA, counterimmunoelectro-osmophoresis (CIEOP), radioimmunoassay (RIA), reverse passive hemagglutination assay (RPHA), latex agglutination (LA), RNA electrophoresis, dot hybridization, and recently by utilizing the polymerase chain reaction. Commercial kits are now available for the ELISA, LA, RPHA, and RNA electrophoresis assays. A popular method is the confirmatory ELISA because it is simple to perform, is sensitive, does not require specialized equipment, and has a negative serum antibody control for detecting nonspecific reactions. An ELISA using monoclonal anti-VP7 antibody is also available. The non–group A rotaviruses cannot be detected by these assays, because they lack the common group antigen; however, an ELISA for group B rotaviruses has recently been developed. Diagnosis of group A rotavirus infection by growth in cell cultures is not practical.

There are many methods for measuring a serologic response to rotavirus infection, including IEM, complement fixation (CF), immunofluorescence, immune adherence hemagglutination assay, ELISA, neutralization, hemagglutination-inhibition (HI), and inhibition of RPHA. Complement fixation is an efficient assay for detecting a serologic response to rotavirus in patients 6 to 24 months of age but is not as effective in adults or infants below 6 months of age.

Detection of rotavirus or demonstration of a serologic response does not necessarily establish an etiologic association with the patient's illness, especially in newborns and adults, who frequently undergo subclinical infection.

TREATMENT

NORWALK VIRUS GROUP. Since the Norwalk group of viruses characteristically causes a mild, self-limited gastroenteritis, replacement of fluid and electrolyte loss with orally administered isotonic fluids is usually sufficient. However, if severe vomiting or diarrhea occurs, parenteral fluid replacement may be necessary. Oral administration of bismuth subsalicylate significantly reduces the severity of abdominal cramps, with a decrease in the median duration of gastrointestinal symptoms from 20 hours to 14 hours. However, the number, weight, and water content of stools and the level of virus excretion are not affected significantly.

ROTAVIRUS. Because rotavirus gastroenteritis may lead to severe dehydration in infants and young children, the early replacement of fluids and electrolytes is essential. Intravenous fluids have been used effectively in the treatment of dehydration.

However, in many parts of the world where such treatment is not feasible, efforts have been made to evaluate the effectiveness of an oral rehydration salts (ORS) solution. In a double-blind study comparing ORS with intravenous fluids in children with rotavirus gastroenteritis, ORS solution containing either glucose (20 grams per liter) or sucrose (40 grams per liter) plus electrolytes was found to be as effective as intravenous therapy for rehydration. Glucose electrolyte solutions are recommended for optimal results. The recommended World Health Organization (WHO) ORS solution is made by adding the following to 1 liter of water: sodium chloride, 3.5 grams; trisodium citrate, dihydrate, 2.9 grams; potassium chloride, 1.5 grams; and glucose, anhydrous, 20 grams. Sodium bicarbonate, 2.5 grams, may be substituted for the trisodium citrate, dihydrate. The efficacy of oral glucose-electrolyte solutions that contained either 90 mmol of sodium per liter (as in the WHO formula above) or 50 mmol of sodium per liter, plus additional electrolytes, was examined in well-nourished ambulatory or hospitalized children with mild or moderate dehydrating diarrheal illnesses of varied etiology (including rotavirus but excluding cholera), and each was found to be safe and effective. After the initial calculated fluid deficit is corrected by the ORS, water or fluids without added electrolytes, such as breast milk or some other form of low-solute feeding, should be given orally in addition to the ORS solution, to replace both continued diarrheal fluid and electrolyte losses and to provide normal daily fluid requirements. If oral rehydration fails to correct the fluid and electrolyte loss or if the patient is severely dehydrated or in shock, intravenous therapy must be given.

In a recent study, rice-based ORS solution was found to be effective in the rehydration of infants and young children hospitalized with mild to moderate dehydration caused by diarrhea associated with various pathogens, including rotavirus. Although either a glucose-based or a rice-based ORS solution was effective in rehydration, the latter was associated with decreased stool output and greater absorption and retention of fluid and electrolytes when compared with the glucose-based solution.

In a limited study, chronic rotavirus illness in immunodeficient children has been treated effectively by oral feeding of pooled human milk that contained rotavirus antibody. However, oral administration of preparations containing rotavirus antibody is not effective for treatment of normal children during episodes of rotavirus gastroenteritis.

PREVENTION

NORWALK VIRUS GROUP. There are no specific methods for the prevention of illness by the Norwalk virus group. However, because of the extremely infectious nature of these agents, careful handwashing and proper disposal of contaminated material should minimize transmission. In addition, hygienic preparation of food and measures to decrease contamination of drinking water or swimming facilities should limit the frequency of Norwalk virus outbreaks. Active immunization against this group of viruses is not yet feasible.

ROTAVIRUS. Epidemiologic studies indicate the global need for a rotavirus vaccine to prevent rotavirus diarrhea in the first 2 years of life, when illness is most severe. Current efforts are focused on developing a live, attenuated oral vaccine that is effective against all serotypes. A promising initial strategy involved the "Jennerian" approach, in which a related rotavirus from a nonhuman host (a bovine or rhesus rotavirus strain) was used as the immunizing agent. Efficacy trials of several such candidate rotavirus vaccines gave variable results and it soon became clear that these vaccines did not induce satisfactory heterotypic immunity in infants not primed by previous rotavirus infection. The rhesus rotavirus vaccine (a VP7 serotype 3 strain) induced protection against rotavirus diarrhea in the 1- to 4-month age group in a study in which VP7 serotype 3 was predominant, but it failed in other studies to protect unprimed infants against illnesses caused by other than serotype 3 rotaviruses. Thus, the "Jennerian" approach has been modified with the goal being a quadrivalent vaccine composed of rhesus rotavirus (serotype 3) and three reassortant rotaviruses each containing 10 rhesus rotavirus genes and a single human rotavirus gene that encodes VP7 serotype 1, 2, or 4 specificity. Efficacy trials of this vaccine are underway.

Finally, a non-Jennerian approach to rotavirus vaccination is also being evaluated. It involves the use of a neonatal rotavirus strain, M37, that appears to be naturally attenuated. The feasibility of this approach is based on the observation in an Australian study that neonates who developed a subclinical rotavirus infection in the first 14 days of life were protected against severe rotavirus diarrhea during a 3-year follow-up.

Breast milk is generally considered to confer some degree of protection against clinically significant rotavirus diarrhea during infancy. The prophylactic oral administration of human serum globulin containing rotavirus antibody to low birth weight neonates provides significant protection against rotavirus diarrhea. In addition, passive oral immunization of infants and young children with bovine colostrum that contained antibodies to human rotavirus was effective in preventing rotavirus illness when compared with a control group.

Chiba S, Yokohama T, Nakata S, et al.: Protective effect of naturally acquired homotypic and heterotypic rotavirus antibodies. Lancet 2:417, 1986. *An important study that examines the relationship of serotype-specific and heterotypic rotavirus neutralizing antibodies to immunity against rotavirus gastroenteritis.*

Ciba Foundation Symposium 128: Novel Diarrhea Viruses. Chichester, John Wiley and Sons, 1987. *An entire volume by various contributors, with special emphasis on non–group A rotaviruses, enteric adenoviruses, caliciviruses, astroviruses, Berne and Breda or Breda-like viruses, the Norwalk virus and rotavirus vaccines.*

Estes MK, Cohen J: Rotavirus gene structure and function. Microbial Rev 53:410–449, 1989. *A review of the molecular biology of rotaviruses with application to an understanding of the natural history of rotavirus infection. Has extensive bibliography of 358 references.*

Green KY, Taniguchi K, Mackow ER, Kapikian AZ: Homotypic and heterotypic epitope specific antibody responses in adult and infant rotavirus vaccines. J Infect Dis 161:667–679, 1990. *An analysis of serologic responses to various rotavirus vaccines by an epitope blocking assay and by neutralization. Demonstrates the influence of prior rotavirus infection on the response to vaccination and the role this might have on vaccination strategy.*

Jiang X, Graham DY, Wang K, Estes MK: Norwalk virus genome cloning and characterization. Science 250:1580–1583, 1990. *A study describing the cloning of the fastidious Norwalk virus.*

Kapikian AZ, Chanock RM: Norwalk group of viruses. In Fields BN, et al. (eds.): Virology, 2nd ed. New York, Raven Press, 1990, pp 671–693. *A detailed current review of the Norwalk group of viruses from a virologic, epidemiologic, and clinical point of view. Has extensive bibliography with 219 references.*

Kapikian AZ, Chanock RM: Rotaviruses. In Fields BN, et al. (eds.): Virology, 2nd ed. New York, Raven Press, 1990, pp 1353–1404. *A detailed current review of rotaviruses from a virologic, epidemiologic, and clinical point of view. Has extensive bibliography with 780 references.*

Kapikian AZ, Flores J, Midthun K, et al.: Strategies for the development of a rotavirus vaccine against infantile diarrhea with an update on clinical trials of rotavirus vaccines. Adv Exp Biol Med 257:67–89, 1989. *A perspective on various approaches to rotavirus vaccination with a description of several field trials.*

Kaplan JE, Gary WG, Barron RC, et al.: Epidemiology of Norwalk gastroenteritis and the role of Norwalk virus in outbreaks of acute nonbacterial gastroenteritis. Ann Intern Med 96:756, 1982. *A review of outbreaks of viral gastroenteritis associated with the Norwalk virus from 1976 to 1980.*

Matsui SM, Kim JP, Greenberg HB, et al.: The isolation and characterization of a Norwalk virus specific cDNA. J Clin Invest 87:1456–1461, 1991. *A study describing the cloning of the fastidious Norwalk virus.*

Matsui SM, Machow ER, Greenberg HB: Molecular determinant of rotavirus neutralization and protection. Adv Virus Res 36:181–214, 1989. *A review of the rotavirus proteins involved in neutralization and protection (116 references).*

Perez-Schael I, Garcia D, Gonzalez M, et al.: Prospective study of diarrheal diseases in Venezuelan children to evaluate the efficacy of rhesus rotavirus vaccine. J Med Virol 30:219–229, 1990. *A detailed description of a field trial with a rotavirus vaccine candidate.*

Pizarro D, Posada G, Sandi L, Moran JB: Rice-based oral electrolytic solutions for the management of infantile diarrhea. N Engl J Med 324:517–521, 1991. *A study evaluating the efficacy of two rice-based rehydration solutions and a conventional glucose-based solution.*

Prasad BUV, Burns JW, Marietta E, et al.: Localization of VP4 neutralization sites in rotavirus by three-dimensional structure of a rotavirus and Fab fragments. Nature 343:476–479, 1990. *Demonstrates the three-dimensional structure of a rotavirus and Fab fragments of a rotavirus-neutralizing monoclonal antibody directed at VP4. Identifies the spikes as VP4.*

Rodriguez WJ, Kim HW, Arrobio JO, et al.: Clinical features of acute gastroenteritis associated with human reovirus-like agent in infants and young children. J Pediatr 91:188, 1977. *A comprehensive description of the clinical features of rotavirus gastroenteritis from a clinical, epidemiologic, and laboratory point of view.*

Santosham M, Burns B, Nadkarni V, et al.: Oral rehydration therapy for acute diarrhea in ambulatory children in the United States: A double-blind-comparison of four different solutions. Pediatrics 76:159, 1985. *A evaluation of various oral rehydration solutions in infants and young children with diarrhea and mild dehydration. Of special interest to the clinician.*

Santosham M, Daum RS, Dillman L, et al.: Oral rehydration therapy of infantile diarrhea. A controlled study of well-nourished children hospitalized in the United States and Panama. N Engl J Med 306:1070, 1982. *An evaluation of oral glucose-electrolyte rehydration solutions containing different sodium con-*

centrations in children hospitalized with diarrhea. An important study for the clinician.

Tyrrell DAJ, Kapikian AZ (eds.): Virus Infections of the Gastrointestinal Tract. New York, Marcel Dekker, Inc., 1982. *An entire volume on viral infections of the gastrointestinal tract by numerous contributors. Includes relevant data on viral agents associated with gastroenteritis with extensive references.*

367 Measles *(Morbilli, Rubeola)*

Philip A. Brunell

DEFINITION. Measles is an acute, highly contagious disease characterized by fever, coryza, cough, conjunctivitis, and both an enanthem and an exanthem.

ETIOLOGY. The virus is an enveloped, negative-stranded RNA paramyxovirus (genus *Morbillivirus*) measuring 120 to 250 mm in diameter, similar to other members of the Paramyxovirus family but lacking neuraminidase. Its single antigenic serotype has been remarkably stable throughout the world for many years with no variation noted. The virus contains six major polypeptides, which are responsible for a number of structural and functional properties, including hemagglutination (of primate erythrocytes), hemolysis, cell fusion, and others. Isolation of virus from clinical specimens is most successful with primary kidney cell cultures of human or simian origin. Selected laboratory strains grow well in other continuous cell lines of mammalian origin.

EPIDEMIOLOGY. With the introduction of routine immunization against measles in the United States in 1963, the incidence of measles fell by about 99 per cent. Smaller outbreaks have occurred at increasing intervals in 1971, 1976, and 1986. A somewhat larger outbreak started in 1989. Prior to the advent of measles vaccine, almost every child got measles, most before school entry. The frequency increased every other year. This pattern still is seen in developing countries where measles in the very young is common. It is estimated that there are from 1 to 2 million deaths annually worldwide. Many developed countries have a less stringent policy toward measles immunization than does the United States.

During the 1989 epidemic in the United States, the highest attack rate was in preschool children, which was more than twice that of 15- to 19-year-olds, the group with the second highest incidence. Most of the former were immunized, whereas the majority of the older group had received measles vaccine. There were more than 400 cases in those born prior to 1957. About 30 per cent of the deaths occurred in the latter group; most occurred in those who were immunocompetent. Almost all of the remaining deaths occurred in those under 5 years of age, most of whom were unimmunized and otherwise normal.

Communicability. Measles is one of the most highly contagious infections. Almost all unprotected household contacts are infected. Demonstration of virus in nasopharyngeal secretions during the prodromal, pre-eruptive phase and in the first days of rash is in accord with epidemiologic evidence of contagiousness. Close physical proximity or direct person-to-person respiratory droplet contact is the usual requisite for infection, although airborne transmission has been documented.

Immunity. An unmodified attack of measles is followed by lifelong immunity. Passively transferred maternal antibody protects the young infant during the early months of life.

PATHOLOGY AND PHYSIOLOGIC RESPONSES. Pathologic changes in fatal measles usually represent the compound effect of viral and secondary bacterial infection. Pneumonia is almost invariably present; it is most frequently interstitial. More representative are changes of the uncomplicated viral diseases within the tonsillar, nasopharyngeal, and appendiceal tissue removed during the prodrome. These changes consist of round cell infiltration and the presence of multinucleated giant cells. Giant cells also are observed in tissue cultures infected with measles virus. The skin and mucous membranes contain perivascular round cell infiltrates with congestion and edema. Koplik's spots are inflammatory lesions of the submucous glands with similar microscopic features.

Simultaneous with the onset of rash, measles-specific antibodies are detectable in serum. Leukopenia is observed on the first day of rash mainly owing to a decrease in lymphocytes; subsequently, granulocytopenia ensues as well. Measles virus replicates in lymphoid tissues (spleen, thymus, lymph nodes), can multiply in vitro in peripheral blood T and B lymphocytes and monocytes, and can be isolated from blood leukocytes during the course of the disease. The virus is propagable in a suspension of leukocytes in vitro.

Immunosuppressive Effects of Measles. It has long been known that cell-mediated immunity is impaired during measles. There is transient suppression of the tuberculin reaction (observed also with measles vaccines); improvement in eczema and allergic asthma and the induction of remissions in nephrosis have been described. Infection of activated lymphocytes may explain the depression of cell-mediated immunity during the acute disease. In severe disease, the magnitude of depression of the total lymphocytes has been positively correlated with a lessened chance of recovery.

CLINICAL MANIFESTATIONS. After an incubation period that averages 11 days, measles becomes clinically manifest with symptoms of fever, malaise, myalgia, and headache. Within hours *ocular symptoms* of photophobia and conjunctival injection occur. The palpebral and, to a lesser extent, the bulbar conjunctivae are involved. There is usually no exudate. Sneezing, coughing, and nasal discharge occur almost simultaneously. Less commonly, hoarseness and aphonia may reflect laryngeal involvement. In this prodromal stage of 1 to 4 days' duration, tiny white spots on the buccal mucosa may herald the appearance of skin rash. The white lesions described by Koplik characteristically occur lateral to the molar teeth and typically are mounted on a bluish-red areola of injected mucosa, superimposed on a diffuse red background. They generally appear a day or so prior to rash and disappear within 2 days after its appearance. They constitute a pathognomonic diagnostic sign. The enanthem may involve other mucous membranes such as the palpebral conjunctiva and vaginal lining.

The *rash* of measles follows the prodromal symptoms by 2 to 4 days, occasionally as late as 7 days. It first appears behind the ears or on the face and neck as a blotchy erythema, spreads downward to cover the trunk, and finally is manifest on the extremities. The hands and feet may escape involvement. Initially, the eruption consists of discrete red macules that blanch with pressure. Subsequently, these lesions become papular, tend to coalesce, and may develop a red, nonblanching component. In adults the rash generally is more extensive, with a greater tendency to become confluent and slightly raised and redder than in children. This is particularly true on the face. The rash fades in the order of its appearance; its disappearance about 5 days after onset may be attended by a fine, powdery desquamation that spares the hands and feet. In adults malaise may continue for 1 to 2 weeks.

The *fever* of measles may persist for about 6 days and frequently reaches 40 or 41°C. Throughout the febrile period, productive cough and auscultatory evidence of bronchitis may be evident. These manifestations may persist after defervescence, and cough is often the last symptom to disappear. Bronchopulmonary symptomatology is an integral part of the primary viral infection; roentgenographic evidence of pulmonary involvement is frequently seen in the uncomplicated disease in the absence of leukocytosis and obvious bacterial infection. Generalized lymphadenopathy accompanies the acute febrile illness and may persist for several weeks thereafter. Nausea and, less commonly, emesis appear to be more common in adults. Diarrhea may also be present.

COMPLICATIONS. The persistence or recurrence of fever and development of leukocytosis are presumptive evidence of the common bacterial sequela of otitis media or pneumonia. Pneumococcus and Group A streptococcus are the most common secondary invaders.

Serious complications directly related to the measles virus are rare. Laryngitis of sufficient severity to embarrass respiration has been observed and may warrant tracheostomy. Keratoconjunctivitis is part of the acute phase but rarely progresses to actual corneal ulceration. Electrocardiographic abnormalities may be found in as many as 30 per cent of children, but clinical evidence of cardiac disease is absent. Abdominal pain or diarrhea may be related to invasion of lymphoid tissue of the appendix or Peyer's patches. These symptoms may lead to unnecessary surgery before the appearance of the typical rash.

Encephalomyelitis. A rare (0.1 per cent) but serious consequence of measles is a demyelinating encephalomyelitis that may appear from 1 to 14 days after the onset of infection. This complication is associated with recurrence of fever and headache, vomiting, and stiff neck. Stupor and convulsions usually follow. Localizing neurologic symptoms may be present. Death ensues in about 10 per cent of patients; more than half of survivors suffer permanent residuals of varying severity. Abnormal electroencephalograms were recorded in about half of children with measles without clinical signs of encephalitis. In some of the children the abnormal encephalographic findings were persistent. Infection of brain cells results in an incomplete viral replicative cycle with production of defective virions lacking the matrix (M) measles virus protein. Studies of patients with acute measles encephalomyelitis and those with late-onset subacute sclerosing panencephalitis show high titers in serum and cerebrospinal fluid of antibodies to all the measles virus proteins except M.

Other late sequelae of measles are thrombocytopenic purpura and exacerbation or activation of pre-existing pulmonary tuberculosis. The late complication of subacute sclerosing panencephalitis is discussed in Ch. 478.4.

Giant-Cell Pneumonia. In patients who are immunocompromised, e.g., those with AIDS, measles virus may induce an interstitial pneumonia characterized by giant cells and intracellular inclusion bodies. The disease is usually fatal.

Measles Modified by Antibody Administration. Attenuation of the natural disease by antibody prophylaxis may result in an illness of lessened severity comparable to the milder infection as seen in infants with illness modified by maternally acquired antibody. Fever alone may be observed, but some degree of exanthem is usually apparent. Koplik's spots may not appear. In general, the course is truncated and relatively uncomplicated. Lasting immunity is uncertain. Later routine immunization of these individuals is probably indicated.

Atypical Measles. From 1963 to 1967, two types of measles vaccine, one live attenuated, the other inactivated or "killed," were available in the United States. The live attenuated vaccine has been the sole product licensed and used in this country since 1967. A severe illness was reported in killed vaccine recipients after exposure to natural measles. These patients had high fever, pneumonia with pleural effusion, obtundation, and an unusual rash. The exanthem was hemorrhagic and was most marked on the extremities. In some instances vesicular, macular, or maculopapular phases have been observed. The rash is sometimes accompanied by edema of hands and feet. Concomitantly these patients' sera revealed extraordinarily high titers of measles-specific antibodies.

Subsequent investigations showed that patients who had received inactivated measles vaccines failed to develop antibodies to the fusion (F) protein of the virus. Lack of antibodies to the cell fusion factor is believed to have permitted these patients to support measles infection. Thus, the atypical measles syndrome

is believed to be due to an anamnestic antibody response in the face of an abundance of measles antigens.

In addition to the rash and pulmonary findings, these patients may have elevated liver enzymes, disseminated intravascular coagulation, and marked myalgia. Nodular pulmonary changes have persisted in some patients. Some cases of pneumonia are reported to have occurred in the absence of rash. Initial diagnoses on presentation have included Rocky Mountain spotted fever and meningococcemia because of the similarities of rash and toxicity. Since inactivated vaccines were available only from 1963 through 1967, the past recipients are now young adults. This atypical measles syndrome is of increasing importance to the internist. Atypical measles has been reported in some patients who received live vaccine alone or after killed vaccine. Recipients of killed vaccine who later received live vaccine may have severe local and systemic reactions to reimmunization.

DIAGNOSIS. The diagnosis should be suspected during an epidemic or following history of exposure. Prior to the appearance of rash, the diagnosis may be difficult unless Koplik's spots are present. Finding in a darkened room an uncomfortable patient who has conjunctivitis, coryza, and cough should make one suspect measles. The rash in adults may be more violaceous, confluent, slightly raised, and more extensive than in children. A history of having received measles vaccine does not preclude the diagnosis, as most individuals with measles of school age have had the vaccine.

Differential diagnosis (Table 367–1) includes consideration of rubella, scarlet fever, infectious mononucleosis, secondary syphilis, drug eruptions, toxic shock syndrome, and Kawasaki's disease. Of value in excluding these possibilities are the milder course, postauricular nodes, and pinker rash of rubella; the sore throat, eventual desquamation, strawberry tongue, and leukocytosis of scarlet fever; and serologic tests for infectious mononucleosis. Fever, enanthem, and catarrh are uncommon with the cutaneous manifestations of drug hypersensitivity. Erythema infectiosum is usually an afebrile illness with rash on the cheeks, arms, and legs. There is no prodrome or accompanying respiratory tract involvement. Kawasaki's disease is rare in adults.

Specific Diagnosis. Virus isolation is technically difficult. Increase in specific antibody may be detected as early as the first or second day of rash. Generally, acute and convalescent sera are required. Demonstration of measles IgM is available in some laboratories.

Presumptive diagnosis may be made if giant cells are detected in stained smears of nasal exudate in the pre-eruptive period.

PROGNOSIS. Uncomplicated measles is rarely fatal, and complete recovery is the rule. Fatalities are almost always the result of pneumonia, occurring in adults or in children below the age of 2 years. Congestive cardiac failure is a common cause of death in patients over 50 years old. The prognosis is particularly poor in patients with AIDS or other immunocompromised patients (see Ch. 410).

Antimicrobial drugs effective against the usual secondary invaders have reduced the case fatality rate of measles sharply. They have proved effective in therapy of bacterial complications, but not in prophylaxis.

Encephalitis occurs as frequently in mild as in severe measles (i.e., about one in 1000 cases); subacute sclerosing panencephalitis

TABLE 367–1. A GUIDE TO THE DIFFERENTIAL DIAGNOSIS OF MEASLES

	Conjunctivitis	Rhinitis	Sore Throat	Enanthem	Leukocytosis	Specific Laboratory Tests Available
Measles	+ +	+ +	0	+	0	+
Rubella	±	±	±	±	0	+
Exanthem subitum	±	±	0	0	0	0
Enterovirus infection	0	±	±	0	0	+
Adenovirus infection	+	+	+	0	0	+
Scarlet fever	±	±	+ +	0	+	+
Infectious mononucleosis	0	0	+ +	±	±	+
Drug rash	0	0	0	0	0	0

0 Not usually present; no test available.
± Variable in occurrence.
+ Present; test available (virus or bacterial culture, serology).
+ + Present and severe.

occurs about 7 years after measles and has essentially disappeared with widespread vaccine use.

TREATMENT. There is no specific antiviral therapy for measles with demonstrated efficacy.

Symptomatic Therapy. In the absence of complications, bed rest is the essence of treatment in this self-limited disease. Codeine sulfate may be useful in the amelioration of headache and myalgia and is effective in the management of cough. Analgesics and antipyretics many be useful. Fluids should be encouraged. Bright light is not an ocular hazard, but photophobia may require darkening of the patient's room.

Antimicrobial Prophylaxis. The course of uncomplicated measles is not influenced by antimicrobial drugs, and their use during the acute illness has resulted in no decrease of secondary bacterial complications (otitis, sinusitis, pneumonia). Instead, the same rates of complications (about 10 to 15 per cent) have been observed, but with organisms resistant to the antibiotics used during the viral illness. If careful observation of the patient is possible, rational therapy is based on the prompt recognition and etiologic definition of complications, followed by initiation of the appropriate antimicrobial drug in proper dosage.

PREVENTION. *Vaccination.* A highly effective vaccine available for the prevention of measles is derived from the Edmonston strain of virus isolated originally in the laboratory of Dr. John Enders. This live virus vaccine produces immunity by infection. A second dose now is recommended routinely. In children over 1 year of age, seroconversion after vaccination in recent years is about 98 to 99 per cent. Measles vaccine usually is given as a single preparation as measles, mumps, and rubella (MMR) vaccine. Failure of measles immunization was much more common prior to 1980. The reasons for this are unclear. It may be due to poor recall or faulty documentation of immunization, age of immunization, use of immune globulin with the vaccine, receipt of killed rather than live vaccine, or the type of live vaccine.

Vaccine recommendations vary depending upon the measles experience in the community. The first dose is usually given at 15 months of age as MMR. In hyperendemic areas it is given at 12 months of age. During epidemics it may be given as monovalent measles vaccine to infants as young as 6 months of age. In the latter case, it should be repeated in combination with mumps and rubella (MMR) after the first birthday. The second routine dose of MMR is given between 5 and 12 years of age. All entering college students and beginning health care workers born after 1956 should show evidence of measles immunity, e.g., positive serologic test, physician-documented measles, or receipt of two doses of measles vaccine or preferably MMR. The immune status of those contemplating foreign travel should be reviewed. A large number of military personnel have been reimmunized without significant side effects.

Contraindications to live virus vaccine include pregnancy, immunodeficiency, leukemia, and other systemic malignant diseases, active tuberculosis, and administration of resistance-depressing drugs such as corticosteroids and antimetabolites.

Annunziato D, Kaplan MH, Hall WW, et al.: Atypical measles syndrome: Pathologic and serologic findings. Pediatrics 70:203, 1982. *Excellent clinical description and explanation of a syndrome now seen in young adults.*

Centers for Disease Control: Measles prevention: Recommendations of the Immunization Practices Advisory Committee (ACIP). MMWR 38:1–18, 1989. *Everything you want to know about the use of measles vaccine.*

Gilad M.: Measles in adults: A prospective study of 291 consecutive cases. Br Med J 295:1313, 1987. *A brief summary of findings in a large number of adults.*

Gremillioin DH, Crawford GE: Measles pneumonia in young adults. Am J Med 71:539–542, 1981. *A large series of cases of measles pneumonia in young adults and other features of measles in this group.*

Gustafson TL, Brunell PA, Lievens AW, et al.: Measles outbreak in a "fully-immunized" secondary school population. N Engl J Med 316:771–774, 1987. *School outbreaks are described in a presumably well-immunized population.*

Katz SL, Krugman S, Quinn TC (eds.): International symposium on measles immunization. Rev Infect Dis 5:389, 1983. *An all-inclusive presentation of measles and its prevention throughout the world.*

Panum PL: Observations Made During the Epidemic of Measles on the Faroe Islands. Delta Omega Society, 1940. *A classic clinical epidemiologic description of measles introduced into an isolated population with disease among all susceptibles born since the previous epidemic 65 years earlier.*

368 Rubella (German Measles)

Philip A. Brunell

DEFINITION. Rubella is an acute, usually benign infectious disease characterized by a 3-day rash, generalized lymphadenopathy, and minimal or no prodromal symptoms. Since 1941 it has been known to cause congenital malformations when infection occurs during the early months of pregnancy.

ETIOLOGY. Rubella is a small, spherical, enveloped virus containing single-stranded RNA of positive polarity. The structural proteins consist of membrane glycoproteins and a nucleocapsid protein. The virus is classified as a togavirus, genus rubivirus. It multiplies in a variety of primary cell culture systems and in some continuous cell lines in most systems without detectable cytopathic effects. Hemagglutination of avian erythrocytes provides a convenient method for virus assay, and by inhibition of this hemagglutination the presence and titer of antibody are readily measured.

EPIDEMIOLOGY. Prior to the availability of rubella vaccines, the disease was worldwide in distribution, produced major epidemics at 6- to 9-year intervals, and was recognized mainly in school-age children; it also produced outbreaks in settings such as military recruit bases and college campuses where large numbers of susceptible young adults gathered in relatively crowded conditions. Since licensure in 1969 in the United States there has been strikingly altered epidemiology. There has been no major epidemic since 1964–1965. In other nations, where rubella vaccine has not been widely utilized, the epidemiology has remained unchanged. Because the disease may be quite nonspecific clinically, with nearly one third of adults undergoing infection without rash, epidemiologic reporting tends to underestimate its prevalence. Since 1966, congenital rubella has been a reportable disease. It is probable that rubella is spread by the respiratory route and by close and sustained personal contact. The incubation period in experimentally infected individuals was found to be 12 to 19 days, with most cases occurring 14 to 15 days following exposure. Although virus was isolated as early as 7 days prior to and as late as 21 days following onset of rash, infectivity probably is greatest throughout the period of prodromal symptoms and for as long as 7 days after the appearance of rash. Infants with congenitally acquired infection may excrete virus in respiratory secretions and in urine for months after birth and are contagious during this time. In hospital environments, especially in nurseries, the congenital rubella baby has been a source of nosocomial infection of personnel involved in his care.

Immunity is lifelong in duration after initial infection. Authenticated second attacks are exceedingly rare and require serologic documentation because of the nonspecific nature of the clinical syndrome. Subclinical reinfection demonstrated by increase in IgG serum antibody has been documented. Such reinfections are not associated with viremia and thus pose little threat to pregnant women. IgM response has been used to distinguish primary infection from reinfection. Immunity that follows artificial immunization with live virus vaccine is apparently of equal duration even though the antibody titers induced may be somewhat lower.

PATHOLOGY. Death from postnatal rubella is usually due to encephalitis. Thus, most autopsies describe only the brain findings. Since 1962 it has been possible to investigate the pathogenesis and to correlate clinical findings with virologic events. After initial invasion of the upper respiratory tract, virus spreads to local lymphoid tissue, where it multiplies and initiates a viremia of approximately 7 days' duration. Respiratory tract shedding of virus and the viremia rise to peak levels until the onset of rash, at which time the latter becomes undetectable, whereas respiratory secretions contain diminishing quantities of virus over the succeeding 5 to 15 days. Specific serum antibodies can be demonstrated with the onset of rash, and circulating immune complexes are detectable soon thereafter.

Congenital Rubella. Necropsies of fetal and neonatal victims of intrauterine infection have shown a variety of embryonal defects related to developmental arrest involving all three germ layers.

The virus establishes chronic persistent infection of many tissues, with resultant intrauterine growth retardation. Delayed and disordered organogenesis produces embryopathic structural defects of the eye, brain, heart, and large arteries; continued viral infection during the fetal and postnatal period causes organ and tissue damage, e.g., hepatitis, nephritis, myocarditis, pneumonia, osteitis, meningitis, cochlear degeneration, and pancreatitis.

CLINICAL MANIFESTATIONS. _Postnatally Acquired Rubella._ Twelve to 19 days after exposure, the onset of rubella is manifested by the appearance of a rash with mild accompanying constitutional symptoms of malaise and occasionally sore throat. Enlargement of the postauricular and suboccipital nodes generally appears about a week prior to rash. Moderate fever, coryza, and faint conjunctivitis may accompany or precede the rash. Generalized peripheral lymphadenopathy and, more rarely, splenomegaly may occur.

The exanthem of rubella is usually apparent within 24 hours of the first symptoms as a faint macular erythema that first involves the face and neck. Characterized by its brevity and evanescence, it spreads rapidly to the trunk and extremities, sometimes leaving one site even as it appears at the next. The pink macules that constitute the rash blanch with pressure and rarely stain the skin. Rubella virus has been isolated from the skin lesions as well as from uninvolved sites. The truncal rash may coalesce, but the lesions on the extremities remain discrete. The eruption usually vanishes by the third day. Rubella may occur without rash. In the absence of an epidemic and of serologic or virologic confirmation, the clinical diagnosis of rubella is not reliable.

COMPLICATIONS. Recovery is almost always prompt and uneventful. In contrast to measles, secondary bacterial infections are not encountered in rubella. Transient polyarthralgia and polyarthritis are more common among adolescents and adults with rubella, particularly females. They appear 3 or more days after onset of rash and may last 5 to 10 days. The knees and joints of the hands and wrist are most often involved. Surveys during urban epidemics have revealed rates of 5 to 15 per cent in males and 10 to 35 per cent in females.

Thrombocytopenia, when sought by serial platelet counts, is common but rarely of clinical consequence. A meningoencephalitis of short duration may occur 1 to 6 days after the appearance of rash. Its incidence is estimated at 1 in 5000 cases, and it is fatal in approximately 20 per cent of those afflicted. Rubella encephalopathy is not associated with demyelinization, in contrast to other postviral encephalitides. Survivors may have electroencephalographic abnormalities, but intellectual function seems to be preserved. A progressive panencephalitis following congenital or postnatal rubella has been described. Its onset generally is during the second decade.

Congenital Rubella. Congenital transplacental infection of the fetus occurs as a consequence of maternal infection, usually in the first 4 months of pregnancy. Virus is demonstrable in placental and fetal tissues obtained by therapeutic abortion at that time. If pregnancy is not interrupted, fetal infection persists, and upon delivery of the infant, virus is recoverable from the throat, urine, conjunctivae, bone marrow, and cerebrospinal fluid of the living infant and from most organs at autopsy. From 20 to 80 per cent of infants born to mothers infected in the first trimester of pregnancy have stigmata of infection readily recognizable in the first year of life. These include cardiac lesions and eye defects, e.g., cataracts, glaucoma, retinitis, microphthalmia. Many infants in whom virus is detectable do not have evidence of disease at birth or may simply have intrauterine growth retardation. In others, more severe disease occurs. Most prominent of these manifestations is thrombocytopenic purpura, which disappears soon after birth. Hepatosplenomegaly with active hepatitis may persist for months. Other involvement includes interstitial pneumonia, meningoencephalitis, hearing loss of varying extent, and lesions of the long bones. Recently, a progressive panencephalitis simulating subacute sclerosing panencephalitis has been observed in the second decade following congenital infection. The long-term sequelae for infants with congenital rubella include psychomotor retardation, hearing loss, retinopathy, and diabetes.

A striking finding has been the persistence of virus in the pharynx, urine, and cerebrospinal fluid for as long as 1 year after birth in 7 per cent of infants. Infective virus was found in a congenital cataract after 3 years and in the urine of a victim of congenital rubella 29 years after her birth. This evidence of continuing viral synthesis occurs coincidentally with circulating antibody. The character of the antibody changes during the first months from maternal IgG to IgM, indicating a primary response of the infant to the persisting viral antigen. Studies of older infants and children with stigmata of congenital rubella show them to be free of demonstrable virus and to possess the IgG immunoglobulins that characteristically persist after other viral infections.

DIAGNOSIS. Rubella may be diagnosed clinically with assurance only during an epidemic. Distinction from measles may be made on the basis of fainter, nonstaining rash, the milder course, and the minimal or absent respiratory complaints. Sore throat is a more prominent complaint in scarlet fever; the course of infectious mononucleosis is often more protracted, and splenomegaly is more frequent than in rubella. Specific diagnosis of rubella is made by isolation of the virus in any of several cell culture systems or by demonstration of a rise in hemagglutination-inhibiting (HI), ELISA, or complement-fixing antibody during infection.

PROGNOSIS. Complete recovery from postnatally acquired rubella is almost invariable. The rare deaths attributable to rubella follow the infrequent complication of meningoencephalitis. Infection in pregnancy constitutes a grave hazard to the fetus but not to the mother.

TREATMENT. There is no specific antiviral therapy. Few patients suffer discomfort severe enough to warrant symptomatic medication. Headache and myalgia or arthritis may be controlled by analgesics.

PREVENTION. _Passive Immunization._ Administration of gamma globulin to the pregnant woman may only mask her symptoms of infection and not protect the fetus from viral invasions. Thus, its use may only obscure the picture and confound decision about the need to terminate the pregnancy if this is an option.

Active Immunization. Rubella may be prevented in children and adults by the parenteral administration of attenuated live virus vaccines produced in cell cultures. Seroconversion rates after immunization are at least 98 per cent with the current RA 27/3 vaccine. Joint symptoms are less common than with the older HPV 7-DE strain, occurring in about 2.5 per cent of adults. Arthritis occurs 13 to 19 days following immunization and lasts 2 to 11 days. The fingers are most often affected, with the wrists and knees less commonly involved. Arthralgias generally begin 10 to 25 days following vaccination and last 1 to 9 days. Joint symptoms are less common in men than in women. In children, vaccination is attended by little or no reaction.

It was initially recommended in the United States that immunization be carried out principally in childhood. There now is a more aggressive attempt to immunize those remaining susceptible women and adolescent girls. Current policy recommends vaccination of all such persons who have no history of previous rubella immunizations. Postpartum immunization of those found to be seronegative during pregnancy is encouraged. Although there occasionally has been transmission of vaccine virus to the newborn by breast milk, this has proven to be of little consequence. Only nonpregnant individuals should be immunized, and contraception, when appropriate, should be carried out for at least 3 months after vaccination. The inadvertent administration of vaccine to pregnant women has occasionally resulted in attenuated vaccine virus infection of the fetus. In more than 500 such cases studied, no infant has been observed with congenital malformations as a result. The frequency of fetal infection with the RA 27/3 vaccine currently used is less than with the previous rubella vaccine. The use of vaccine in the United States prevented a large epidemic of rubella expected in the early 1970's and has reduced the reported annual occurrence from more than 50,000 cases annually, with epidemic peaks of 200,000 to 500,000, to an all-time low in 1988 of 221 cases.

Burke JP, Hinman AR, Krugman S (eds.): International symposium on prevention of congenital rubella infection. Rev Infect Dis 7(Suppl):1, 1985. _Fifteen years of vaccine use summarized by investigators from the developed nations._
Centers for Disease Control: Rubella and congenital rubella syndrome—United States. MMWR 38:173, 1989. _A summary report of progress in rubella "eradication" in the United States._

Gregg NM: Congenital cataract following German measles in the mother. Trans Ophthal Soc Aust 3:35, 1941. *The original "classic" report associating rubella in pregnancy with congenital malformations.*

Proceedings of the International Conference on Rubella Immunization. Am J Dis Child 118, July 1969. *A compendium on rubella and congenital rubella.*

Sherman FE, Michaels RH, Kenny FM: Acute encephalopathy (encephalitis) complicating rubella. JAMA 192:675, 1965. *A clinical, pathologic, and epidemiologic study of rubella encephalitis.*

Townsend JJ, Stroop WG, Baringer JR, et al.: Neuropathology of progressive rubella panencephalitis after childhood rubella. Neurology 32:185, 1982. *A review of the clinical and neuropathologic findings.*

Weibel RE, Vilarejos VM, Klein EB, et al.: Clinical and laboratory studies of live attenuated RA 27/3 and HPV 77-DE rubella virus vaccines (40931). Proc Soc Exper Biol Med 165:44, 1980. *A description of the clinical and serologic response to rubella vaccine.*

369 Foot-and-Mouth Disease

John W. Gnann, Jr.

Foot-and-mouth disease virus (FMDV) is an extremely important pathogen of cloven-hoofed animals (e.g., cattle, swine, sheep, and goats) and a rare cause of disease in humans. Foot-and-mouth disease (FMD) should not be confused with hand-foot-and-mouth disease caused by coxsackieviruses. FMD is endemic in parts of Europe, Asia, Africa, and South America but is not currently present in North America or Australia. Strict regulations are in place to prevent importation of FMDV or FMDV-infected animals into the United States.

Because of the huge economic impact of FMD on the livestock industry, FMDV has been intensively studied and consequently is one of the best-characterized animal viruses. The three-dimensional ultrastructure of FMDV has been determined by x-ray diffraction studies. A highly immunogenic synthetic peptide based on a FMDV coat protein (VP1) sequence may prove to be the basis for an enhanced FMD vaccine. FMD is currently controlled among livestock herds either by test-and-slaughter procedures or by use of an inactivated virus vaccine.

FMDV is a member of the family Picornaviridae and the genus *Aphthovirus*. FMDV is a nonenveloped icosahedral virus with a diameter of about 25 to 30 nm. The genome consists of one linear molecule of positive-sense single-stranded RNA. Seven major serotypes have been identified; most well-documented human infections have been caused by type O.

FMD is extremely contagious and spreads rapidly among susceptible animals. Infected animals develop papular and vesicular eruptions of the mouth and other mucous membranes and of the skin around the hooves. FMDV can be isolated from the skin lesions, saliva, urine, and milk of infected animals. Although not usually fatal, infection renders the animal economically worthless.

Humans are not very susceptible to infection by FMDV, as evidenced by the rarity of infection among veterinarians, abattoir workers, and laboratory personnel who study the virus. Older literature contains many case reports of human infection with FMDV, but these were not confirmed serologically or virologically. However, there have been several cases of human FMD which have been documented by viral isolation. FMDV can apparently be transmitted to humans by direct skin contact with infected animal materials, by ingestion of virus (e.g., in contaminated milk), or possibly by inhalation. Following an incubation period of 3 to 8 days, human infection is characterized by fever, malaise, increased salivation, and vesicles in the mouth, on the perioral area, and sometimes on the hands and feet. The vesicles ulcerate, then slowly heal over a period of 10 days to 2 weeks. Virtually all infected individuals recover without sequelae. Human-to-human transmission of FMDV has not been documented. The diagnosis can be established either by isolation of the virus from vesicle fluid or by serologic testing. No specific therapy is available.

Armstrong R, David J, Hedger RS: Foot-and-mouth disease in man. Br Med J 4:529, 1967. *Report of a culture-proven case of human FMD.*

Bittle JL, Houghten RA, Alexander H, et al.: Protection against foot-and-mouth disease by immunization with a chemically synthesized peptide predicted from

the viral nucleotide sequence. Nature 298:30, 1982. *Immunization of animals with synthetic VP1 peptides induces serotype-specific virus-neutralizing antibody.*

370 Mumps

John W. Gnann, Jr.

Mumps is an acute systemic viral infection that is usually self-limited, occurs most commonly in school-age children, and is clinically characterized by nonsuppurative parotitis.

VIROLOGY. Mumps virus is classified as a member of the family Paramyxoviridae in the genus *Paramyxovirus*. Mumps virions are pleomorphic, roughly spherical, enveloped particles with an average diameter of 200 nm. Glycoprotein spikes project from the surface of the envelope, which encloses a helical nucleocapsid composed of RNA and nucleoproteins. The mumps virus genome is contained in a linear molecule of nonsegmented, single-stranded, negative-sense RNA. The virus is composed of five major proteins: Nucleocapsid protein (NP) is the major structural protein; polymerase protein (P) appears to have RNA-dependent RNA-polymerase activity; matrix (M) protein is important in the assembly of virions; and two surface glycoproteins mediate hemagglutinin-neuraminidase (HN) and fusion (F) activity. An additional large (L) nucleocapsid-associated protein has been observed by some investigators. There is only one serologic strain of mumps virus.

Humans are the only known natural hosts for mumps virus, although infection can be experimentally induced in a wide variety of mammalian species. In vitro, mumps virus can be cultured in many mammalian cell lines, including monkey kidney, BSC-1, Vero, and HeLa cells, as well as in embryonated hens' eggs.

EPIDEMIOLOGY. In unvaccinated urban populations, mumps is a disease of school-age children. Mumps infrequently occurs in infants less than 1 year of age, presumably because of transplacentally acquired antibody. The largest number of mumps cases occurs in children between 4 and 7 years of age. By age 15, 92 per cent of children have mumps antibodies. Prior to the release of the live attenuated mumps vaccine in the United States in 1967, mumps was an endemic disease with a seasonal peak of activity between January and May. Mumps epidemics occurred at 2- to 5-year intervals. The largest number of cases reported in the United States was in 1941, when the incidence of mumps was 250 cases per 100,000 population. In 1968, when the live attenuated vaccine was first entering clinical usage, the incidence of mumps was 76 cases per 100,000 population. In 1985, a total of only 2982 cases of mumps was reported, an incidence of 1.1 per 100,000 population, representing a 98 per cent decline from the number of cases reported in 1967.

Between 1985 and 1987, the incidence of mumps in the United States increased fivefold to 5.2 cases per 100,000 population. More than one third of the cases reported between 1985 and 1987 occurred in adolescents and young adults, reflecting the slow acceptance of universal mumps vaccination during the 1970's when this cohort of children grew up. This is an important trend, since mumps generally causes a more severe disease in adults than in children. The increased incidence of mumps in susceptible young adults was most prominent in those states without comprehensive school immunization laws.

PATHOGENESIS. Mumps can be experimentally transmitted by inoculation of virus onto the nasal or buccal mucosa, suggesting that most natural infections result from droplet spread of upper respiratory secretions from infected individuals. The average incubation period for mumps is 18 days. During this interval, primary viral replication is thought to take place in epithelial cells of the upper respiratory tract, followed by spread of virus to regional lymph nodes and subsequent viremia and systemic dissemination. Virus can be isolated from saliva for 5 to 6 days before and up to 5 days after the onset of clinical symptoms, meaning that an infected individual is potentially able to transmit mumps for a period of about 10 days.

Mumps is highly contagious, although some studies have suggested that it is less contagious than varicella or measles. This clinical observation may be skewed by the fact that up to 30 per cent of all mumps infections are subclinical and asymptomatic. Over 90 per cent of adults who give negative histories for mumps are seropositive when tested for mumps antibody, indicating prior subclinical infection.

CLINICAL MANIFESTATIONS. *Parotitis.* Mumps is a systemic infection, and the virus has been demonstrated to replicate in epithelial cells of multiple visceral organs. Mumps usually begins with a short prodromal phase characterized by low-grade fever, malaise, headache, and anorexia. Young children may initially complain of ear pain. The patient then develops the typical salivary gland enlargement and tenderness. The parotid glands are most commonly involved, although other salivary glands may occasionally be enlarged. Parotitis may initially be unilateral, with swelling of the contralateral parotid gland occurring 2 to 3 days later; bilateral parotitis eventually develops in most patients with symptomatic salivary gland involvement. Painful parotid gland enlargement progresses over about 3 days, lifting the ear lobe outward and obscuring the angle of the mandible. The orifice of Stensen's duct is often edematous. Parotid gland swelling and tenderness peak on about the third day of the illness, followed by defervescence and resolution of parotid pain and swelling within about 7 days. Long-term sequelae of parotitis are uncommon.

Meningitis. Symptomatic meningitis occurs in 15 per cent of cases and is the second most common manifestation of mumps. Studies with animal models indicate that mumps virus is clearly neurotropic and replicates well in the ependymal cells of the choroid plexus. Studies have shown that half of patients with mumps parotitis without signs or symptoms of meningitis have cerebrospinal fluid (CSF) pleocytosis. Mumps virus can be recovered from CSF.

Symptoms of meningeal irritation (headache, neck stiffness, vomiting, and lethargy) usually develop 4 to 5 days after the onset of parotitis, although the meningitis may occasionally precede the parotitis. Indeed, 40 to 50 per cent of all cases of documented mumps meningitis occur in patients who never develop clinical parotitis. Symptomatic central nervous system involvement with mumps is 2 to 3 times more common in males than in females. Examination of the CSF usually reveals a normal opening pressure and a mononuclear cell pleocytosis with an average cell count of 250 per cubic millimeter, although cell counts as high as 1000 to 2000 per cubic millimeter are not uncommon. A polymorphonuclear leukocyte predominance may be seen in some patients early during the course of mumps meningitis. The CSF protein is usually normal or mildly elevated (<100 mg per 100 ml). Hypoglycorrhachia, which is not usually seen in viral meningitis, may be present in 10 to 30 per cent of patients with meningitis due to mumps virus. Although the symptoms of mumps meningitis usually resolve within a week, the CSF abnormalities may persist for up to 5 weeks. The meningitis is usually benign, and significant neurologic complications are rare.

Encephalitis. The spectrum of mumps-induced central nervous system disease ranges from mild "aseptic" meningitis (which is common) to severe encephalitis (which is relatively rare). The pathogenesis of mumps encephalitis is not precisely understood. Some cases of encephalitis develop concurrently with the parotitis and are thought to result from direct extension of viral infection from the choroid plexus ependyma into parenchymal neurons. Other cases of mumps encephalitis occur 1 to 2 weeks after the onset of parotitis and may represent an autoimmune parainfectious encephalitis. Clinical findings in mumps encephalitis include obtundation (and less commonly delirium), generalized seizures, and high fever. Other neurologic findings, including focal seizures, aphasia, paresis, and involuntary movements, have been reported. Recovery from mumps encephalitis is usually complete, although complications such as aqueductal stenosis with hydrocephalus, seizure disorders, and psychomotor retardation have been noted. The overall mortality from mumps encephalitis is 0.5 to 2.3 per cent.

Orchitis. Epididymo-orchitis is rare in boys with mumps but occurs in 25 to 30 per cent of postpubertal men with mumps infection. Orchitis results from replication of mumps virus in seminiferous tubules with resulting lymphocytic infiltration and edema. Orchitis is most often unilateral, but bilateral involvement occurs in 17 to 38 per cent of cases. Orchitis typically develops within 1 week after the onset of parotitis, although orchitis (like mumps meningitis) can develop prior to or even in the absence of parotitis. Mumps orchitis is characterized by marked testicular swelling and severe pain, accompanied by fever, nausea, and headache. The pain and swelling resolve within 5 to 7 days, although residual testicular tenderness can persist for weeks. Testicular atrophy may follow orchitis in about 35 to 50 per cent of cases, but sterility is an uncommon complication even among patients with bilateral orchitis.

Other Manifestations. Mumps can cause inflammation of other glandular tissues, including pancreas and thyroid. Oophoritis and mastitis have been reported in postpubertal women with mumps. Renal function abnormalities are common in mumps, and virus can be readily isolated from urine, but significant renal damage is rare. Other infrequent manifestations of mumps include sensorineural deafness (either transient or permanent), arthritis, myocarditis, and thrombocytopenia.

Mumps During Pregnancy. Maternal mumps infection during the first trimester of pregnancy results in an increased frequency of spontaneous abortions. However, no clear association between congenital malformations and maternal mumps has been demonstrated.

IMMUNE RESPONSE. Transient IgM antibody responses are detected early in the course of mumps infection, followed by the appearance of IgG antibody and cytotoxic T lymphocytes (CTL). The relative contributions of humoral and cell-mediated immunity to viral clearance have not been precisely determined. Life-long immunity follows natural infection. Patients who report more than one episode of mumps probably had parotitis due to infection with a different virus.

A variety of serologic tests have been designed to determine susceptibility to mumps. The neutralizing antibody (NA) assay has been considered the "gold standard" test but is technically demanding. The hemagglutination inhibition (HAI) assay is simple to perform but less specific owing to cross-reactivity with other paramyxoviruses. Detection of complement fixing (CF) antibodies against V antigen (hemagglutinin-neuraminidase) has previously been the routine method for determining immune status but is being replaced by a sensitive and specific enzyme-linked immunosorbent assay (ELISA). The mumps skin test is not a reliable indicator of immune status.

DIAGNOSIS. The diagnosis of mumps is most often made on clinical grounds in a patient who presents with parotitis, particularly if the individual is known to be susceptible and has been exposed to mumps during the preceding 2 to 3 weeks. However, an atypical clinical presentation (e.g., meningitis or orchitis without parotitis) may require laboratory confirmation. Culturing for mumps virus is definitive but frequently not available. Testing of paired acute and convalescent sera should demonstrate a diagnostic fourfold rise in mumps antibody titer. Alternatively, demonstration of mumps IgM antibody provides good evidence of recent infection. In the past, a CF test for detecting antibodies against S (nucleocapsid) and V antigens has been the most commonly used diagnostic test, but ELISA is now becoming the standard assay.

Parotitis can be caused by other viruses such as influenza A, parainfluenza virus, coxsackievirus, lymphocytic choriomeningitis virus, and bacteria such as *Staphylococcus aureus*. Parotid gland enlargement can also be associated with Sjögren's syndrome, sarcoidosis, thiazide ingestion, iodine sensitivity, tumor, or salivary duct obstruction. A careful examination should distinguish parotitis from lymphadenopathy.

THERAPY. Management of the patient with mumps consists of conservative measures to provide symptomatic relief and to ensure adequate hydration and nutrition. Therapy of orchitis includes bed rest, scrotal support, analgesics, and ice packs. Patients with significant central nervous system involvement require hospitalization for observation and supportive care. There is currently no established role for antiviral drugs, steroids, or passive immunotherapy.

PREVENTION. Children with mumps are usually isolated for about 1 week after the appearance of parotitis, although this practice is of dubious benefit to classmates, since the virus is known to be excreted for several days prior to the onset of clinical symptoms. The cornerstone of mumps prevention is active immunization using the live attenuated mumps vaccine. This vaccine is administered in the United States to infants during the second year of life and produces protective antibody levels in more than 97 per cent of recipients. The vaccine is given subcutaneously in combination with the live measles and rubella vaccines and has virtually no side effects. Booster immunizations are not required.

Administration of the live mumps vaccine is relatively contraindicated in pregnant women, in persons with a history of anaphylactic reaction to eggs or neomycin (the vaccine is produced in chick-embryo cell culture), in persons who have received immunoglobulin therapy within the preceding 3 months (which might interfere with the immune response to the vaccine), or in persons with severe systemic immunosuppression. Mumps immunization is recommended for asymptomatic HIV-infected children.

Questions regarding prevention often arise when an individual with no history of mumps (typically an adult male) is exposed to a patient with active mumps. The immune status of the exposed individual can be determined by serologic testing, although this may involve some delay. Mumps vaccine can be safely administered to an individual of unknown immune status, although vaccine given to a susceptible individual after exposure to mumps may not provide protection. Mumps immune globulin is not of proven value and is no longer commercially available. The vast majority of adults born in the United States before 1957 have been naturally infected and are therefore immune.

ACIP: Mumps prevention. MMWR 38:388, 1989. *Current vaccination recommendations from the Immunization Practices Advisory Committee.*

Shehab ZM, Brunnell PA, Cobb E: Epidemiologic standardization of a test for susceptibility to mumps. J Infect Dis 149:810, 1984. *Development of an ELISA for detection of mumps antibody.*

371 Herpes Simplex Virus Infections

Mark Middlebrooks and Richard J. Whitley

Herpes simplex virus (HSV), a member of the family Herpesviridae, has been implicated in human infections since descriptions of cutaneous spreading lesions in ancient Greek times.

Scholars of Greek civilization define the word *herpes* to mean "to creep or crawl," in reference to the spreading nature of the observed skin lesions. More recent scholars have further described the spectrum of illnesses caused by HSV and have made significant discoveries in the molecular biology of HSV infection. A major advance was the detection of differences between herpes simplex virus types. Although suggested by clinical and laboratory observation for many years, it was not until 1968 that well-defined antigenic and biologic differences were demonstrated between herpes simplex virus type 1 (HSV-1) and herpes simplex virus type 2 (HSV-2). Nahmias and Dowdle demonstrated that HSV-1 was more frequently associated with nongenital infection and HSV-2 with genital disease. Further study has revealed that, of all the herpesviruses, HSV-1 and HSV-2 are the most closely related, with approximately 60 per cent genomic homology. These two viruses can be distinguished most reliably by DNA restriction enzyme analyses; however, differences in antigen expression and biologic properties also serve as methods for differentiation.

STRUCTURE. Membership in the family Herpesviridae is based on the structure of the virion (Fig. 371–1). Herpes simplex virus contains double-stranded DNA at the central core, has a molecular weight of approximately 100 million, and encodes at least 70 polypeptides. The DNA core is surrounded by a capsid that consists of 162 capsomers, arranged in icosapentahedral symmetry. The capsid is approximately 100 to 110 nanometers in diameter. Tightly adherent to the capsid is the tegument, which appears to consist of amorphous material. Loosely surrounding the capsid and tegument is a lipid bilayer envelope derived from host cell membranes. The envelope consists of polyamines, lipids, and glycoproteins. These glycoproteins confer distinctive properties to the virus and provide unique antigens to which the host is capable of responding. Notably, glycoprotein G (gG) provides antigenic specificity to HSV and therefore results in an antibody response that allows for the distinction between HSV-1 (gG-1) and HSV-2 (gG-2).

A fascinating feature of HSV DNA is its genomic sequence arrangement. The genome consists of two components, L (long) and S (short), each of which contains unique sequences that can invert upon themselves, leading to four isomers. The ability to exist as one of four isomers is a unique property of HSV. Viral DNA extracted from virions of infected cells consists of four equimolar populations, differing only with respect to the relative orientation of the two unique components. The biologic relevance of this phenomenon is unknown.

REPLICATION. Replication of HSV is a multistep process (Fig. 371–2). Following the onset of infection, DNA is uncoated and transported to the nucleus of the host cell. This is followed

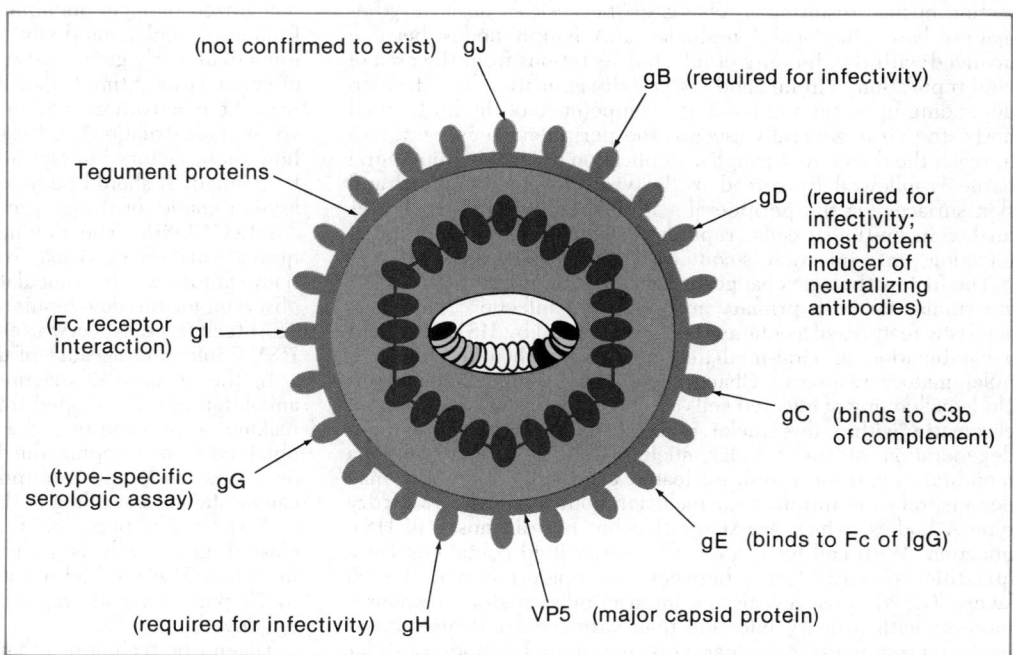

FIGURE 371–1. Schematic diagram of the HSV virion.

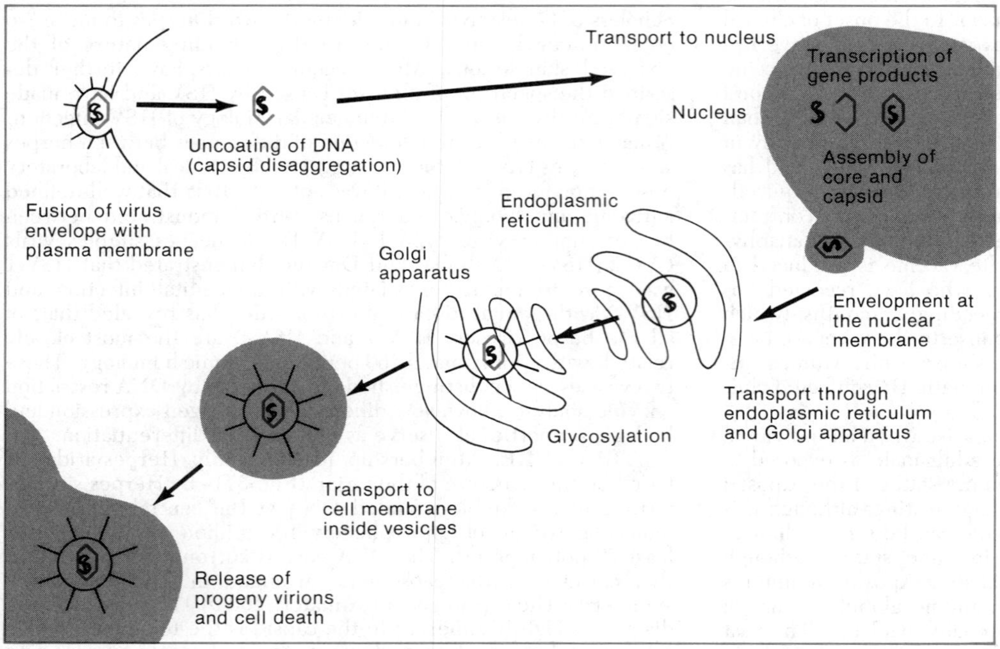

FIGURE 371–2. Schematic diagram of HSV replication.

by transcription of immediate-early genes, which encode for the regulatory proteins. Expression of immediate-early gene products is followed by the expression of proteins encoded by early and then late genes. These proteins include enzymes necessary for viral replication and structural proteins.

Assembly of the viral core and capsid takes place within the nucleus. This is followed by envelopment at the nuclear membrane and transport out of the nucleus through the endoplasmic reticulum and the Golgi apparatus. Glycosylation of the viral membrane occurs in the Golgi apparatus. Mature virions are transported to the outer membrane of the host cell inside vesicles. Release of progeny virus is accompanied by cell death. Replication for all herpesviruses is considered inefficient, with a high ratio of noninfectious to infectious viral particles.

PATHOGENESIS AND LATENCY. A critical factor for transmission of HSV, regardless of virus type, is intimate contact between a person who is shedding virus and a susceptible host. With inoculation onto the skin or mucous membrane, HSV replicates in epithelial cells; the incubation period is 4 to 6 days (Fig. 371–3). As replication continues, cell lysis and local inflammation ensue, resulting in characteristic vesicles on an erythematous base. Regional lymphatics and lymph nodes become involved with the draining of infected secretions from the area of viral replication. Viremia and visceral dissemination may develop depending upon the immunologic competence of the host. In all hosts, the virus generally ascends the peripheral sensory nerves to reach the dorsal root ganglia. Replication of HSV within neural tissue is followed by spread of the virus to other mucosal and skin surfaces via the peripheral sensory nerves. Virus replicates further in epithelial cells, reproducing the lesions of the initial infection, until infection is contained through host immunity.

The histopathologic changes induced by the replication of HSV are similar for both primary and recurrent infection. The characteristic features of a cutaneous lesion induced by HSV represent a combination of viral-mediated cellular death and associated inflammatory response. Changes induced by viral infection include ballooning of infected cells and the appearance of condensed chromatin within the nuclei of cells, followed by subsequent degeneration of the cellular nuclei. Cells lose intact plasma membranes and form multinucleated giant cells. They also may demonstrate the intranuclear inclusion bodies known as Cowdry type A bodies, which are suggestive but not diagnostic of HSV infection. With cell lysis, a clear vesicular fluid containing large quantities of virus forms between the epidermis and dermal layer. The dermis reveals an intense inflammatory response, more so with primary infection than with recurrent disease. As healing progresses, the clear vesicular fluid becomes pustular

with the recruitment of inflammatory cells. The pustule then forms a scab, with scarring being uncommon.

The vascular changes in the area of infection include perivascular cuffing and hemorrhagic necrosis. These changes are particularly prominent when organs other than skin are involved, as is the case with herpes simplex encephalitis or disseminated neonatal HSV infection. Local lymphatics can show evidence of infection with intrusion of inflammatory cells due to the draining of infected secretions from the area of viral replication. As host defenses are mounted, an influx of mononuclear cells can be detected in infected tissue.

A unique characteristic of the herpesviruses is their ability to establish latent infection, persist in an apparently inactive state for varying amounts of time, and then be reactivated (Fig. 371–4). The latent viral genome may be either extrachromosomal or integrated into host-cell DNA.

Latency is established when HSV reaches the dorsal root ganglia after retrograde transmission via sensory nerve pathways. Latent virus may be reactivated and enter a replicative cycle at any point in time. The reactivation of latent virus is a well-recognized biologic phenomenon but not one that is understood from a molecular standpoint. An antisense message to one of the immediate-early genes (α-O) may be involved in the maintenance of latent virus. Stimuli that have been observed to be associated with the reactivation of latent herpes simplex virus have included stress, menstruation, and exposure to ultraviolet light. Precisely how these factors interact at the level of the ganglia remains to be defined. It should be noted that reactivation may be clinically asymptomatic, or it may produce life-threatening disease.

DIAGNOSIS. The definitive diagnosis of HSV infection requires isolation of virus. Swabs of clinical specimens or other body fluids can be inoculated into susceptible cell lines and observed for the development of characteristic cytopathic effects. This technique is very useful for the diagnosis of HSV-1 and HSV-2 infection because of the short replicative cycles.

In the absence of diagnostic virology facilities, cytologic examination of cells scraped from a clinical lesion may be useful in making a presumptive diagnosis of HSV infection. Material obtained from scraping the base of a lesion should be smeared on a glass slide and promptly fixed in cold enthanol. The slide can be stained according to the methods of Papanicolaou, Giemsa, or Wright. The presence of intranuclear inclusions and multinucleated giant cells is indicative, but not diagnostic, of HSV infection. This method has a sensitivity of only approximately 60 to 70 per cent and should not be the sole diagnostic method employed.

Diagnostic techniques that are still being evaluated for clinical

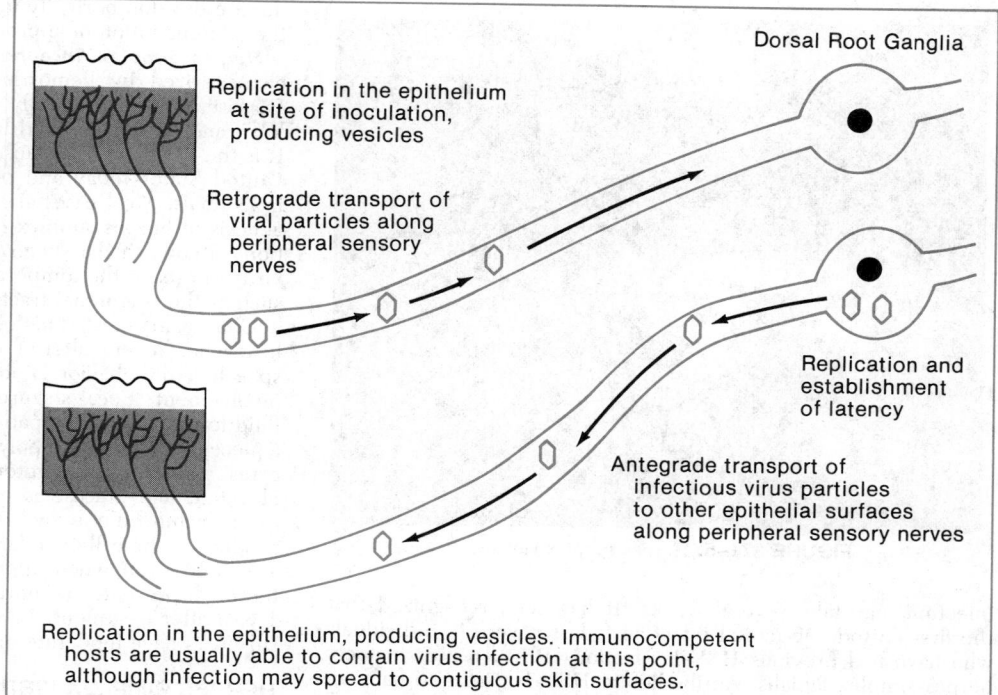

FIGURE 371–3. Schematic diagram of primary HSV infection.

Replication in the epithelium at site of inoculation, producing vesicles

Retrograde transport of viral particles along peripheral sensory nerves

Dorsal Root Ganglia

Replication and establishment of latency

Antegrade transport of infectious virus particles to other epithelial surfaces along peripheral sensory nerves

Replication in the epithelium, producing vesicles. Immunocompetent hosts are usually able to contain virus infection at this point, although infection may spread to contiguous skin surfaces.

utility include in situ and dot-blot hybridization, as well as DNA amplification by polymerase chain reaction. The potential for DNA amplification is significant, owing to its ability to detect small amounts of specific genomic material. However, its applicability to diagnostic assays is not well defined at the present time. A concern of many investigators is the specificity of these reactions owing to the possible amplification of contaminant DNA, which leads to false-positive results.

In addition to new tests for virus gene products and viral DNA, improved serologic assays are also becoming available. However, these tests are useful only for making a diagnosis in retrospect.

CLINICAL MANIFESTATIONS. *Mucocutaneous Infections.*
Gingivostomatitis. Gingivostomatitis, which is usually caused by HSV-1, occurs most frequently in children less than 5 years of age. This illness is characterized by fever, sore throat, pharyngeal edema, and erythema, followed by the development of vesicular

or ulcerative lesions on the oral and pharyngeal mucosa. Recurrent HSV-1 infections of the oropharynx are most frequently manifest as herpes simplex labialis (cold sores) and usually appear on the vermillion border of the lip (Fig. 371–5). Intraoral lesions as a manifestation of recurrent disease are uncommon.

Genital Herpes. Genital herpes is most frequently caused by HSV-2. Primary infection in women usually involves the vulva, vagina, and cervix. In men, initial infection is most often associated with lesions on the glans penis, prepuce, or penile shaft. In individuals of either sex, primary disease is associated with fever, malaise, anorexia, and bilateral inguinal adenopathy. Women frequently have dysuria and urinary retention due to urethral involvement. As many as 10 per cent of individuals develop an aseptic meningitis with primary infection. Sacral radiculomyelitis may occur in both men and women, resulting in neuralgias, urinary retention, or obstipation. The complete healing of primary

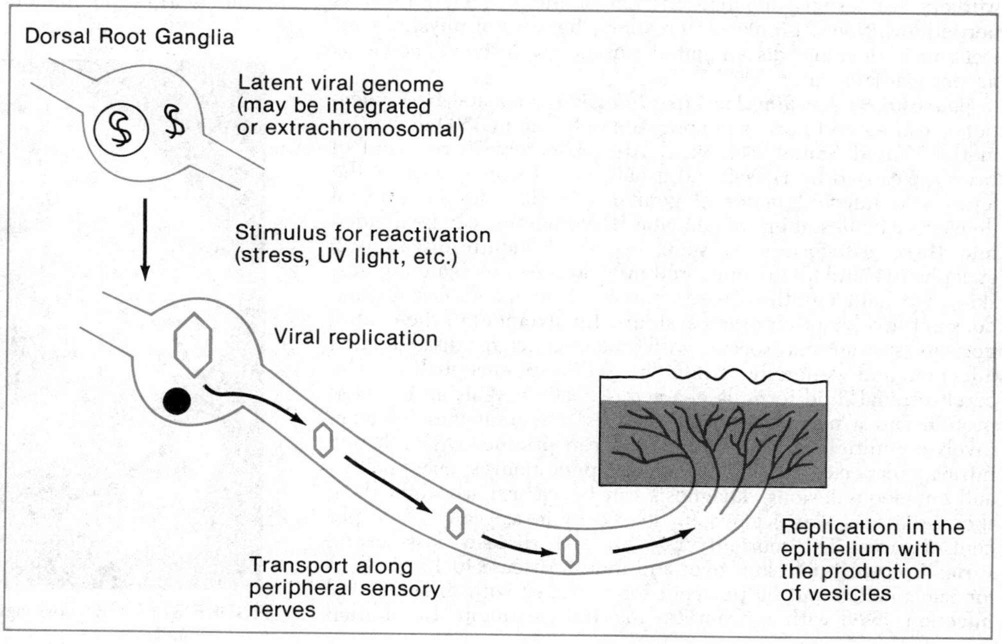

Dorsal Root Ganglia

Latent viral genome (may be integrated or extrachromosomal)

Stimulus for reactivation (stress, UV light, etc.)

FIGURE 371–4. Schematic diagram of HSV latency and reactivation.

Viral replication

Transport along peripheral sensory nerves

Replication in the epithelium with the production of vesicles

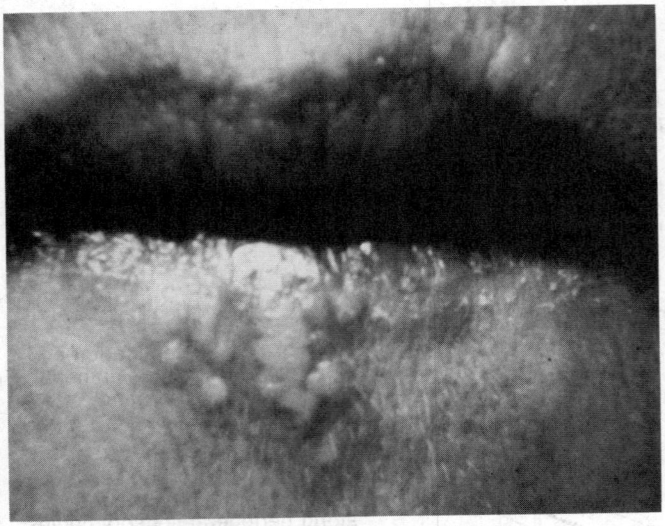

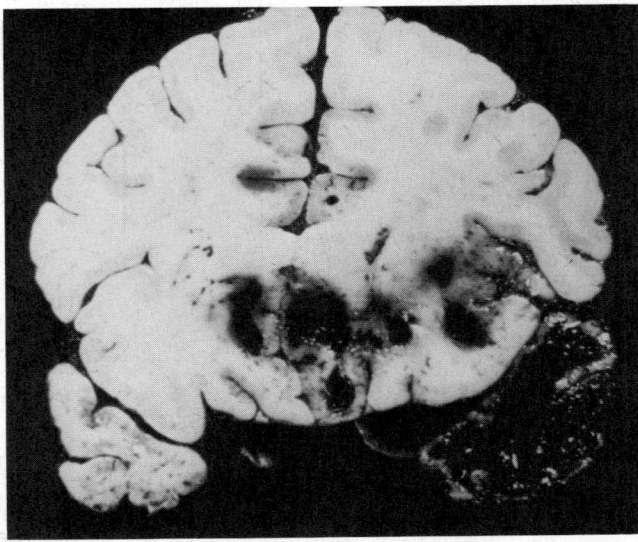

FIGURE 371–5. Herpes simplex labialis.

infection may take several weeks. It has been recognized that the first episode of genital infection is less severe in individuals who have had previous HSV-1 infections at other sites, namely herpes simplex labialis. Antibodies to HSV-1 appear to have an ameliorative effect on the expression of HSV-2 clinical disease.

Recurrent genital infections in either men or women can be particularly distressing. The frequency of recurrence varies significantly from one individual to another. It has been estimated that one third of individuals with genital herpes have virtually no recurrences, one third have approximately three recurrences per year, and another third have more than three per year. Seroepidemiologic studies have found that between 25 and 65 per cent of individuals in the United States in 1978 had antibodies to HSV-2 and that seroprevalence is correlated with the number of sexual partners.

Herpetic Keratitis. Herpes simplex keratitis is usually caused by HSV-1 and is accompanied by conjunctivitis in many cases. It is considered the most common infectious cause of blindness in the United States. The characteristic lesions of herpes simplex keratoconjunctivitis are dendritic ulcers best detected by fluorescein staining. Deep stromal involvement has also been reported and may result in visual impairment.

Other Cutaneous Manifestations. Herpes simplex virus infections can manifest at any skin site. Common among health care workers are lesions on abraded skin of the fingers, known as herpetic whitlows. Similarly, wrestlers, because of physical contact, may develop disseminated cutaneous lesions known as herpes gladiatorum.

Neonatal Herpes Simplex Virus Infection. Neonatal HSV infection is estimated to occur in approximately one in 3500 deliveries in the United States each year. Approximately 70 per cent of cases are caused by HSV-2 and usually result from contact of the fetus with infected maternal genital secretions at the time of delivery. Manifestations of neonatal HSV infection can be divided into three categories: (1) skin, eye, and mouth disease, (2) encephalitis, and (3) disseminated infection. As the name implies, skin, eye, and mouth disease consists of cutaneous lesions and does not involve other organ systems. Involvement of the central nervous system may occur with encephalitis or disseminated infection and generally results in a diffuse encephalitis. The cerebrospinal fluid formula characteristically reveals an elevated protein and a mononuclear pleocytosis. Disseminated infection involves multiple organ systems and can produce disseminated intravascular coagulation, hemorrhagic pneumonitis, encephalitis, and cutaneous lesions. Diagnosis can be particularly difficult in the absence of skin lesions, which occur in as many as 36 per cent of cases. The mortality rate for each disease classification varies from zero for skin, eye, and mouth disease to 15 per cent for encephalitis and 60 per cent for neonates with disseminated infection, even with appropriate antiviral treatment. In addition

to the high mortality associated with these infections, morbidity is significant in that children with encephalitis or disseminated disease develop normally in only 40 per cent of cases, even with the administration of appropriate antiviral therapy.

Herpes Simplex Encephalitis. Herpes simplex encephalitis is characterized by hemorrhagic necrosis of the temporal lobe. Disease begins unilaterally, spreads to the contralateral temporal lobe, and is characterized by hemorrhagic necrosis (Fig. 371–6). It is the most common cause of focal, sporadic encephalitis in the United States today and occurs in approximately 1 in 150,000 individuals. Most cases are caused by HSV-1. The actual pathogenesis of herpes simplex encephalitis requires further clarification, although it has been speculated that primary or recurrent virus can reach the temporal lobe by ascending neural pathways, such as the trigeminal tracts or the olfactory nerves.

Clinical manifestations of herpes simplex encephalitis include headache, fever, altered consciousness, and abnormalities of speech and behavior, findings characteristic of temporal lobe involvement. Focal seizures may also occur. The cerebrospinal fluid formula for these patients is variable but usually consists of a pleocytosis with both polymorphonuclear leukocytes and monocytes present. The protein concentration is characteristically elevated, and glucose is usually normal. A definitive diagnosis can be achieved only by brain biopsy, since other pathogens may produce a clinically similar illness. The mortality and morbidity are high, even when appropriate antiviral therapy is administered. At present, the mortality rate is approximately 30 per cent 1 year after treatment. In addition, approximately 50 per cent of survivors have moderate or severe neurologic impairment.

HERPES SIMPLEX VIRUS INFECTIONS IN THE IMMUNOCOMPROMISED HOST

Herpes simplex virus infections in the immunocompromised host are usually due to reactivation of latent infection and are clinically more severe, may be progressive, and require a longer time to heal. Manifestations of HSV infections in this patient population include pneumonitis, esophagitis, hepatitis, colitis, and disseminated cutaneous disease. Individuals suffering from human immunodeficiency virus infection may have extensive perineal or orofacial ulcerations. Herpes simplex virus infections are also noted to be of increased severity in individuals with extensive burns.

EPIDEMIOLOGY. Herpes simplex viruses are distributed worldwide and have been reported in both developed and underdeveloped countries. Animal vectors for human HSV infections have not been described, and there is no seasonal variation in the incidence of HSV infections. The virus is transmitted from infected to susceptible individuals during close personal contact, and virus must come in contact with mucosal surfaces or abraded skin for infection to be initiated. Since approximately one third of the world's population has recurrent HSV infections, and

FIGURE 371–6. Hemorrhagic necrosis in herpes simplex encephalitis.

because infection is rarely fatal, a large reservoir of HSV exists in the community.

Although HSV-1 and HSV-2 are usually transmitted by different routes and involve different areas of the body, there is a great deal of overlap between the epidemiology and clinical manifestations of infections caused by these viruses. The mouth and lips are clearly the most common sites of HSV-1 infection. Primary HSV-1 infection in the young child is usually asymptomatic but may be manifest as gingivostomatitis. Primary infection in young adults has been associated with pharyngitis and sometimes a mononucleosis-like syndrome. Seroprevalence studies have demonstrated that acquisition of HSV-1 infection is related to socioeconomic factors. Antibodies, which indicate past infection, are found early in life among individuals of lower socioeconomic groups. This presumably is a consequence of crowded living conditions that provide a greater opportunity for direct contact with infected individuals. As many as 75 to 90 per cent of individuals from lower socioeconomic populations develop antibodies by the end of the first decade of life. In contrast, only 30 to 40 per cent of persons in middle and upper socioeconomic groups are seropositive by the middle of the second decade of life.

Because infections with HSV-2 are usually acquired through sexual contact, antibodies to this virus are rarely found until the onset of sexual activity. There is a progressive increase in infection rates with HSV-2 in all populations beginning in adolescence. As with HSV-1 infections, the rate of acquisition of HSV-2 infection appears related to socioeconomic factors. The number of sexual contacts is also an important risk factor for the acquisition of HSV-2. Importantly, genital herpes infection has recently been found to be a risk factor for another sexually transmitted virus, the human immunodeficiency virus (HIV).

Localized, recurrent HSV-2 infection is the most common form of HSV infection during gestation. Transmission of infection to the fetus is most frequently related to the shedding of virus at the time of delivery. Since HSV infection of the fetus is usually the consequence of contact with infected maternal genital secretions at the time of delivery, the determination of viral excretion at this time is of utmost importance. The incidence of cervical shedding in pregnant women with asymptomatic HSV infection is approximately 1 per cent. Interestingly, most infants who develop neonatal disease are born to women who are completely asymptomatic for genital HSV infections at the time of delivery and who have neither a past history of genital herpes nor a sexual partner reporting a genital vesicular rash. These women account for 60 to 80 per cent of all women whose children develop neonatal HSV infection.

PREVENTION. At present, there are no licensed vaccines directed against HSV. However, experimental vaccines for HSV-1 and HSV-2 entered phase 1 and phase 2 trials in mid-1990. Acyclovir is currently being given to recipients of solid organ and bone marrow transplants in the immediate post-transplant period in an effort to prevent reactivation of latent disease.

TREATMENT. Infections caused by HSV-1 and HSV-2 are amenable to therapy with antiviral drugs (see Ch. 359). Both vidarabine and acyclovir have proved useful for the management of specific infections caused by these viruses. At present, acyclovir is the treatment of choice for mucocutaneous HSV infections in the immunocompromised host, herpes simplex encephalitis, and neonatal herpes simplex virus infections. Intravenous administration is preferred for therapy of life-threatening disease. Intravenous acyclovir is also recommended for treatment of clinically severe initial genital herpes in the immunocompetent host. This includes patients with complications such as urinary retention or aseptic meningitis, and they should receive 5 mg per kilogram every 8 hours for 5 to 7 days. Caution must be exercised when acyclovir is used intravenously, because it may crystallize in the renal tubules when given too rapidly or to dehydrated patients.

Immunocompromised individuals with mucocutaneous HSV infections that are not life-threatening may be given oral acyclovir. Oral acyclovir is also useful in the treatment of initial genital herpes. Recurrent episodes, however, are not as responsive to acyclovir. For individuals who experience severe or frequent recurrences of genital herpes, a "suppressive" regimen of acyclovir in doses of 600 to 800 mg per day may be useful. The efficacy of acyclovir for the treatment of primary or recurrent oropharyngeal HSV in the immunocompetent host has not been well established.

Corey L, Spear P: Infections with herpes simplex viruses. N Engl J Med 314:686–691, 749–757, 1986. *This two-article series is a concise review of herpes simplex virus infections.*

Goldsmith SM, Whitley RJ: Herpes simplex encephalitis. In Lambert HP (ed.): Infections of the Central Nervous System. Philadelphia, B. C. Decker, 1991, pp 283–299. *This chapter describes the clinical presentations, diagnostic evaluation, and treatment of herpes simplex virus encephalitis.*

Nahmias AJ, Lee FK, Bechman-Nahmias S: Sero-epidemiological and sociological patterns of herpes simplex virus infection in the world. Scand J Inf Dis 69:19–36, 1990. *A comprehensive analysis of herpes simplex virus seroepidemiology, utilizing new techniques for HSV-2–specific antibody.*

Roizman B: Herpesviridae: A brief introduction. In Fields BN, Knipe DM, Chanock E, et al. (eds.): Virology, 2nd ed. New York, Raven Press, 1990, p 1787. *This chapter provides an overview of the herpes family of viruses.*

Straus SE: Clinical and biological differences between recurrent herpes simplex virus and varicella-zoster virus infections. JAMA 262:3455–3458, 1989. *A concise article that emphasizes the distinctions between recurrent herpes simplex virus infections and recurrent varicella-zoster infections.*

Whitley RJ: Herpes simplex viruses. In Fields BN, Knipe DM, Chanock E, et al. (eds.): Virology, 2nd ed. New York, Raven Press, 1990. *A comprehensive text that includes a detailed analysis of the molecular biology and clinical manifestations of herpes simplex virus.*

372 Cytomegalovirus Infection

David J. Lang

DEFINITION. Infections caused by cytomegalovirus (CMV) may be asymptomatic or may cause disseminated and even fatal multisystem disease, depending upon the mode and timing of virus acquisition and the immunocompetence of the host. CMV infections occur commonly, although with variable severity, in the fetus, the neonate, and immunocompromised individuals.

ETIOLOGY. CMV is a species-specific member of the herpesvirus group. Like other herpesviruses, CMV has the capacity to replicate persistently in the face of normal host immunity and to establish latent infections subject to reactivation. Replication of the virus in vitro yields characteristic focal cytopathology and is largely limited to cell cultures of species-specific fibroblasts. In vivo, however, CMV replicates in epithelial as well as fibroblastic elements. Subtypes of CMV can be distinguished, although the variants do not seem to be associated with a unique clinical presentation.

EPIDEMIOLOGY. CMV is worldwide in distribution, and infection shows no seasonal preference. Persistence, latency, and reactivation of CMV make it difficult to interpret the etiologic significance of the recovery of the virus.

The age of acquisition of CMV is variable. In less developed parts of the world, CMV infection is acquired universally in infancy, probably at or shortly after parturition. Where interpersonal contact is reduced and sanitation is more advanced, acquisition of CMV infection is delayed and occurs gradually through infancy, childhood, and adulthood. Transmission of CMV is associated with close interpersonal (including sexual) contact or with direct introduction of cells or body fluids. CMV has been recovered from virtually all organs and tissues and can be found in urine, saliva, blood, semen, milk, secretions of the uterine cervix, and stool. CMV is opportunistic; it reactivates in, is transmitted to, and spreads from hosts whose defenses are compromised. Since these patients are often found in hospital settings, this virus poses a theoretic risk for nosocomial spread. However, no substantial evidence has been found for patient-to-patient or patient-to-staff transmission.

Transmission of CMV occurs with blood (estimated 5 per cent of whole-blood units) and with a proportion of organ transplants. Horizontal interpersonal transmission of CMV occurs, but not in epidemics. Young children, infected as neonates from blood or as toddlers by contact in day care centers, can serve as a source of family infection. Thus in a reversal of the usual pattern, the child attending day care may prove a risk factor for the pregnant, previously seronegative mother. Day care workers experience the acquisition of CMV infections more frequently than do matched controls. Young women working in a day care setting should be appropriately counseled about the risks of CMV infection and means to reduce that risk.

Prenatal CMV infection is the most common known congenital infection of humans. It occurs in about 1 per cent of infants born in the United States (0.5 to 8 per cent depending upon the population studied). Most of these infections reflect prenatal transmission of CMV reactivated during pregnancy in otherwise healthy immune women. As many as 30 per cent of pregnant women may shed CMV at some time and from some site during pregnancy.

PATHOGENESIS AND PATHOLOGY. CMV replicates slowly in vitro. Infected cells swell and develop characteristic intranuclear and paranuclear inclusions. CMV infections in vitro are accompanied by some changes associated with morphologic transformation. It has been possible to transform cells permanently by infecting with irradiated virus and in this way interfering selectively with the full cycle of virus replication and cytopathology. These CMV-transformed cells have malignant potential in certain animals. Whether CMV plays a role in the pathogenesis of malignancy in humans is unresolved.

CMV can and frequently does reactivate in immune hosts. When immune function is immature or compromised, reactivated virus can spread, causing significant injury and functional impairment. The pathogenesis of transplacental spread in the presence of intact maternal immunity remains unclear.

That CMV is carried in circulating cells of healthy individuals appears certain on the basis of epidemiologic observations. Nevertheless, it has been difficult to recover this virus from the circulating cells of healthy individuals. The use of CMV antibody–negative blood units has been recommended for transfusion in high-risk groups such as selected newborns (especially premature infants) and patients with compromised cell-mediated immunity (including those on chemotherapy and allograft recipients). There is evidence that certain blood filters can substantially reduce the risk of CMV transmission with transfusions.

CLINICAL MANIFESTATIONS. *Postnatal CMV Infection in Normal Hosts.* In healthy individuals CMV infection is usually asymptomatic or unrecognized. Occasionally primary CMV infection is accompanied by a self-limited, mononucleosis-like syndrome characterized by fever, splenomegaly, mild hepatocellular dysfunction, lymphoid hyperplasia (including the presence of atypical lymphocytes), occasional thrombocytopenia, hemolysis, and inconsistent skin rash. Pharyngitis may occur. The fever may range from 39°C to over 40°C and in some instances is accompanied by night sweats and chills. Between febrile episodes the patient, although tired, does not feel very ill.

Some cases of mild to moderate hepatitis have been associated with CMV infection, and infrequently a normal host experiences an interstitial pneumonitis caused by this virus. There have been reports associating prior CMV infection with the Guillain-Barré syndrome. CMV infections have also been associated with isolated thrombocytopenia, hemolytic anemia, and ulcerative gastrointestinal disease.

Postnatal CMV Infection in Abnormal Hosts. Individuals undergoing open heart surgery requiring perfusion and others receiving multiple units of blood may experience a mononucleosis-like illness about 3 to 6 weeks later. The illness can be mistaken for bacterial sepsis or endocarditis, a particularly important distinction in recipients of cardiac prostheses.

CMV infections have been a major problem for allograft recipients. Latent virus may be reactivated in connection with the response to the allograft (either host-versus-graft or graft-versus-host). Immunosuppression limits the ability of the host to restrict virus spread. CMV infections may enhance graft rejection, although the mechanism mediating this process remains uncertain. CMV infections have been prominently associated with bone marrow transplantation (BMT), and CMV interstitial pneumonitis has been an important cause of mortality following BMT. Viremia has been shown to be predictive of clinical disease in BMT recipients. CMV infections occur frequently among recipients of all forms of allograft, and infection can be associated with interstitial pneumonitis, hepatitis, encephalitis, retinitis, and diffuse cytomegalic inclusion disease. Both newly acquired (from transplant, blood cell components, or both) and endogenous (reactivated in host) CMV infections occur. The progress and

effect of these infections may be mediated by direct cytopathology or by immunopathologic mechanisms.

CMV infections are very common among male homosexuals and have been found prominently in the acquired immunodeficiency syndrome (AIDS), which occurs in response to infection with human immunodeficiency virus (HIV). Evidence indicates that reciprocal interactions may exist between CMV and HIV infections such that CMV may transactivate HIV and HIV infections may be associated with reactivation of CMV. Overall, CMV infections associated with AIDS are likely to be opportunistic, although since CMV infections are often associated with some depression of the helper-suppressor T-cell ratio, as well as suppression of natural killer (NK) cell activity and depression of T-cell proliferation, the precise distinction between cause and effect, opportunism and pathogenesis, remains to be elucidated. Much of the morbidity and some mortality associated with AIDS has been ascribed to CMV infections of the liver, brain (associated with glial nodules), gastrointestinal tract (ulcerative lesions), lungs (diffuse interstitial pneumonitis often coexisting with *Pneumocystis carinii* infection), and eyes (retinitis).

It has been proposed that CMV may play a role in atherogenesis, and supportive epidemiologic data have been presented. CMV infections can be shown to infect and injure endothelial cells of arterial walls, and it has been hypothesized that this may be followed by local cellular proliferation, injury, and cholesterol deposition.

Prenatal and Perinatal CMV Infection. Prenatal CMV infections were first appreciated through retrospective pathologic studies, and it was initially concluded that these infections were rare and always fatal. The severe, disseminated infection was termed *cytomegalic inclusion disease* (CID). Subsequently, cytologic and virologic techniques identified CMV infection in living infants, and it became apparent that infants congenitally infected with CMV could survive. In some cases these infected infants exhibited intracerebral calcifications, hepatosplenomegaly, chorioretinitis, thrombocytopenia with purpura, macular rash, hemolytic anemia, and a variety of structural and functional organ impairments.

Prospective studies determined that congenital infections with CMV were not rare. Overall, about 1 per cent of babies were found to be prenatally infected with CMV. Women who are immune prior to conception may give birth to CMV-infected infants. The birth to a woman of more than one CMV-infected infant with identical viral strains has been documented. Most prenatal CMV infections are acquired from latent maternal virus reactivated during gestation, and most CMV-infected infants appear normal at birth. Nonetheless, as many as 10 to 20 per cent of these apparently healthy babies ultimately display learning disabilities, hearing impairment, or evidence of cognitive dysfunction. In contrast, primary maternal infection during pregnancy, a much less common event, is associated in some cases with devastating CID.

Perinatal acquisition of CMV infection (from infected cervix, breast milk, or saliva) is usually asymptomatic. However, an infant born to a CMV-seronegative woman may develop significant postnatal pneumonia or hepatitis if infected with CMV via transfusion. This is a particularly important risk among markedly premature infants who may acquire no maternal immunoglobulins.

DIAGNOSIS. The laboratory isolation of CMV is accomplished in tissue culture and requires the prompt transportation of refrigerated specimens to a prepared virus laboratory. Weeks can be required for recovery and identification of virus. However, although the evolution of cytopathology may be slow, some viral antigens appear rapidly (hours) in inoculated cells. Furthermore, CMV replication in cell culture can be enhanced by centrifugation of specimens on monolayers in shell vials. The use of monoclonal antibodies to early CMV antigens, coupled with labeled antiglobulin preparations applied to inoculated centrifuged shell vials, can provide rapid and specific virus detection. The recovery of cloned subgenomic fragments of CMV DNA has permitted detection of CMV directly and specifically by hybridization procedures. Currently the polymerase chain reaction (PCR) is being explored as a means for rapid and specific CMV isolation and identification.

Regardless of the technique used, occasional prolonged shedding of virus and the intermittent reactivation of latent CMV can confuse the interpretation of virus recovery. The isolation of

CMV at certain times (from urine taken during the first days of life) or from unusual sites (blood, spinal fluid, or tissues specifically involved in the disease process) makes the etiologic association of virus and clinical condition more likely. Demonstration of simultaneous seroconversion or significant (fourfold or greater) serologic change further strengthens the association. CMV serology may be assessed by complement fixation, immunofluorescence, and enzyme-linked immunosorbent assay (ELISA) procedures. The detection of CMV-specific IgM serology is useful to identify recent infections.

DIFFERENTIAL DIAGNOSIS. Postnatally acquired CMV infections in normal hosts may be difficult to distinguish from those caused by Epstein-Barr virus (EBV). However, EBV mononucleosis is often associated with a positive heterophil-agglutination reaction, whereas CMV mononucleosis is always heterophil-negative. CMV mononucleosis tends to occur in older individuals and is associated with more prominent fever and night sweats and less adenopathy than EBV mononucleosis. Hepatitis associated with CMV infection is generally milder than that associated with hepatitis A, B, or C or other hepatitis viruses. The ultimate distinction between these conditions depends upon the results of virus-specific tests.

CMV interstitial pneumonitis, similar to that caused by *Pneumocystis carinii*, cannot be identified on clinical grounds alone but requires the use of virologic studies applied to clinical samples, especially those from lung biopsies, needle aspirations, bronchoscopy, and bronchoalveolar lavage. Accurate and rapid identification of CMV infections may be made in these specimens by application of histologic and cytologic techniques as well as by procedures employing monoclonal antibodies, immunofluorescence, DNA hybridization, and PCR.

Congenital infections caused by toxoplasmosis, rubella, syphilis, and herpes simplex virus (HSV) may be difficult to distinguish from those caused by CMV. All may be associated with intrauterine growth retardation, hepatic and splenic enlargement, purpura, thrombocytopenia, and hemolysis. Congenital toxoplasmosis can be associated as well with chorioretinitis and intracerebral calcifications.

Congenital rubella is associated with glaucoma, microphthalmia, cataracts, and cardiac malformations more frequently than is congenital CMV infection. The retinitis of congenital rubella, unlike that of CMV, is often marked by punctate retinal pigmentation.

HSV can be transmitted transplacentally, although usually neonatal HSV infection reflects perinatal acquisition. HSV infections are often associated with vesicular skin lesions, although systemic visceral and central nervous system infection may occur without rash.

In all of these instances the distinctions are made ultimately by laboratory studies. Specific IgM determinations are available for CMV, toxoplasmosis, rubella, and HSV. The presence of a positive test for specific IgM to only one of these agents is usually diagnostic. The recovery of the specific agent in the case of CMV, rubella, or HSV is also a rigorous means of identification. Differentiation of all of these conditions is important, since specific treatment is available for HSV and toxoplasmosis, and specific anti-CMV therapy is becoming available and is already applicable in some clinical settings. The distinction between congenital syphilis and bacterial sepsis, other potentially confusing entities in the neonate, is also important to facilitate specific therapy.

PROGNOSIS. Among individuals with acquired CMV infections, the prognosis depends upon the immune status of the host. In otherwise healthy persons, acquired CMV infections are self-limited and generally not associated with late complications. Among immunocompromised individuals, including patients with AIDS, those with disseminated neoplasms, and transplant recipients, the outlook may vary from those who recover, maintain (allograft) function, and are without sequelae, to those who die with progressive interstitial pneumonitis. Disseminated CMV may also predispose to significant life-threatening bacterial infections.

The outlook for normal development is variable in infants who are infected prenatally with CMV. Even among those with apparently symptomless congenital CMV infections, by school age as many as 20 per cent may manifest significant sensorineural dysfunction.

TREATMENT. Until recently, a variety of nucleoside analogues, other antiviral drugs, transfer factor, antiserum, and steroids have been administered in an effort to treat CMV infections without any conclusive success. The most that was achieved was the transient depression of virus titer without alteration of the clinical condition or ultimate course of the virus infection. The intensive use of interferon in renal transplant recipients has reduced the shedding of virus and apparently improved the associated clinical conditions. Withdrawal of immunosuppression has been used as a means to control CMV infections in allograft recipients. Recent preliminary studies have shown improvement in some immunodeficient patients with severe CMV infections when treated with 9-(1,3 dihydroxy-2-propoxymethyl) guanine (DHPG). Those who received DHPG for retinitis or gastrointestinal disease fared better than did patients with CMV pneumonitis. Foscarnet, a pyrophosphate analogue, is an investigational antiviral agent that inhibits CMV DNA polymerase and is being explored as a therapeutic alternative to DHPG in CMV retinitis. Concomitant treatment with DHPG and azidothymidine (AZT) is also under study in CMV-infected AIDS patients.

PREVENTION. CMV infections have been prevented in seronegative at-risk patients (newborns, allograft recipients) by the use of CMV-seronegative blood products and allografts. The administration to BMT patients of acyclovir (given to prevent HSV and varicella-zoster virus infections) has been shown to reduce the risk of CMV-associated disease and to improve survival. The use of CMV-specific intravenous immunoglobulin with and without DHPG has been associated in some studies with the reduction of CMV-associated symptoms in BMT recipients. Attenuated CMV vaccine strains have been produced in England, the United States, and France. These candidate vaccine strains have been administered to volunteers, including health care workers, and to some individuals prior to allograft. The vaccines are immunogenic and have not been associated with detectable virus shedding or reactivation. Inoculated individuals who later received transplants and were immunosuppressed did nevertheless experience CMV reinfection and associated virus shedding but seemed to have fewer sequelae of the infections.

Since evidence indicates that immunity does ameliorate, if not prevent, prenatal and postnatal CMV infections, and since some questions and concerns are associated with the production and use of attenuated CMV strains, attention is also being directed to the development of subunit and peptide immunogens.

Emanuel D: Treatment of cytomegalovirus disease. Semin Hematol 27(2)(Suppl 1):22–27; discussion 28–29, 1990. *Review of the treatment of CMV infections especially as they impact bone marrow transplantation.*

Ho M: Cytomegalovirus: Biology and Infection. New York, Plenum Publishing Corporation, 1982. *Treatise covering all aspects of CMV infection in humans. Small but thorough section pertinent to murine CMV. Very comprehensive bibliography.*

Jacobson MA, Mills J: Serious cytomegalovirus disease in the acquired immunodeficiency syndrome (AIDS). Clinical findings, diagnosis, and treatment. Ann Intern Med 108(4):585–594, 1988. *Experience with CMV-associated disease in patients with AIDS. Attention is given to therapeutic modalities, current and anticipated.*

Melnick JL, Adam E, DeBakey ME: Possible role of cytomegalovirus in atherogenesis. JAMA 263:2204–2207, 1990. *Hypothesis and review of evidence for the role of CMV in atherogenesis.*

Meyers JD, Reed EC, Shepp DH, et al: Acyclovir for prevention of cytomegalovirus infection and disease after allogeneic marrow transplantation. N Engl J Med 318:70–75, 1988. *Demonstration that prophylaxis with intravenous acyclovir significantly reduces the risk of CMV infection and disease and improves survival.*

Meyers JD: Management of cytomegalovirus infection. Am J Med 85(2A):102–106, 1988. *Management of CMV infections among immunocompromised patients from a center with extensive experience.*

Meyers JD, Ljungman P, Fisher LD: Cytomegalovirus excretion as a predictor of cytomegalovirus disease after marrow transplantation: Importance of cytomegalovirus viremia. J Infect Dis 162:373–380, 1990. *This study demonstrates that viremia in bone marrow transplant recipients is predictive of clinical disease.*

Pass RF: Daycare centers and transmission of cytomegalovirus: New insight into an old problem. Semin Pediatr Infect Dis 1:245–251, 1990. *A current review with complete discussion of background, mechanisms, means for control, and a complete reference list.*

Rubin RH (ed.): Cytomegalovirus infections: Epidemiology, diagnosis, and treatment strategies. Rev Infect Dis 12(Suppl 7):S691–S860, 1990. *An up-to-date series of reviews.*

373 Infectious Mononucleosis (Epstein-Barr Virus Infection)

Elliott D. Kieff

DEFINITION. Infectious mononucleosis is a clinical syndrome characterized by malaise, fever, pharyngitis, pharyngeal lymphatic hyperplasia, lymphadenopathy, atypical lymphocytosis, and heterophil antibody. The syndrome occurs most commonly in adolescents and young adults.

ETIOLOGY. Primary Epstein-Barr virus (EBV) infection is the cause of almost all typical infectious mononucleosis syndromes. EBV is a herpesvirus. In vitro, it infects only human B lymphocytes. Virus infection results in B lymphocyte proliferation and immunoglobulin secretion. EBV usually remains latent in the infected B lymphocyte.

EPIDEMIOLOGY. The usual mode of EBV infection is oropharyngeal inoculation. Virus in saliva from infected persons is infectious in nonimmune persons. Infection in infancy commonly results from eating food premasticated by an infected mother, whereas infection in adolescents or adults is usually from salivary transfer during kissing. Virus survival in expectorated saliva is probably brief, since infection does not spread to susceptible roommates. Spread among young children sharing toys has not been studied.

Following salivary inoculation, the virus replicates in oropharyngeal epithelial cells, including salivary gland epithelium. Although the amount of virus in saliva is highest in the months following primary infection, virus replication in the oropharynx persists indefinitely. EBV has also been found in cervical secretions, suggesting hematogenous dissemination to other epithelial surfaces. In the course of primary oropharyngeal infection, EBV infects tonsillar and peripheral blood B lymphocytes. Virus persists indefinitely in a small fraction of the peripheral blood B lymphocytes. Transfusion of whole blood, bone marrow, blood fractions, or tissue containing viable B lymphocytes to susceptible (nonimmune) persons may result in symptomatic primary infection. Following bone marrow transplantation, the donor's virus may predominate in the recipient, indicating that a bone marrow or blood cell is a site of persistent or latent infection. Previously infected normal persons are immune to the development of infectious mononucleosis. In less industrialized societies or among lower socioeconomic groups in industrialized societies, most children experience primary infection in the first decade of life. Among middle and higher socioeconomic groups, primary infection usually occurs as a consequence of adolescent or postadolescent kissing. More than 90 per cent of adults in all human populations have serologic evidence of EBV infections and are carriers. Although EBV infection is limited to humans, each Old World primate species is endemically infected with a related virus characteristic of that species. New World primates are free of EBV-related viruses and can be experimentally infected. Experimental infection of some species with a sufficient EBV inoculum results in acutely fatal lymphoproliferation.

CLINICAL MANIFESTATIONS. The syndrome of infectious mononucleosis was a distinctive clinical entity for at least 40 years before the discovery of its etiologic agent. After a 2- to 5-week incubation period, most infected nonimmune adolescents and young adults develop malaise, fever, pharyngitis, and lymphadenopathy lasting from one to several weeks. Temperatures may reach 40°C. Tonsillar or cervical lymph nodes may be quite enlarged, painful, and tender. Laboratory findings include a relative or absolute lymphocytosis and a high titer of heterophil antibody to horse or ox red blood cells. A substantial fraction of the peripheral lymphocytes is an atypical large cell with unusually abundant cytoplasm, large pale nucleus, and variable nuclear shape. Other common manifestations include splenomegaly (50 per cent), mild hepatitis or hepatomegaly (20 per cent), headache (20 per cent), vomiting (20 per cent), jaundice (5 per cent), palatal petechiae, skin rash (4 per cent), and albuminuria (10 per cent). Less frequent (0.5 to 1 per cent) manifestations include cough,

pneumonitis, neck stiffness, aseptic meningitis, cerebritis, cerebellar dysfunction, mono- or polyneuritis, transverse myelitis, Guillain-Barré syndrome, uveitis, subcapsular splenic hemorrhage or rupture, myocarditis, pericarditis, cardiac conduction abnormalities, diarrhea, hemolytic anemia with anti-I antibody, thrombocytopenia, agranulocytosis, pancytopenia, or a hemophagocytic syndrome. Malaise or weakness may recur over several months. Rashes are significantly more common in patients with primary EBV infection receiving penicillin or ampicillin treatment than in untreated patients or patients with other diseases who are treated with penicillin. Persistence of illness beyond several months is unusual. Almost all normal people completely recover from acute infectious mononucleosis. Persistent hematalogic, neurologic, or cardiac abnormalities are rare.

Outside of the adolescent and young adult populations, primary EBV infection frequently does not result in the full infectious mononucleosis syndrome. In younger children, fever and pharyngitis from primary EBV infection may be clinically indistinguishable from upper respiratory tract infections caused by other viruses, mycoplasma, or streptococci. At any age cerebritis, neuritis, pneumonitis, hepatitis, carditis, or autoimmune hemolytic anemia or thrombocytopenia may be the predominant clinical manifestation. Atypical lymphocytosis or heterophil antibody may be less prominent or absent.

Severe, progressive, and sometimes fatal primary EBV infections occur in children with X-linked lymphoproliferative disease (Duncan's syndrome). Non–X-linked, sporadic cases also occur. Although these children have no obvious pre-existing immune deficiency, primary EBV infection leads to massive lymphoproliferation, fever, anemia, hepatitis, or fulminant hepatic necrosis. The proliferating B lymphocytes are EBV-infected cells that express EBV latent infection associated proteins. The early proliferation is polyclonal. Fulminant hepatic failure is a frequent cause of death. Recovery may be accompanied by persistent anemia, hypogammaglobulinemia, or pancytopenia. Some patients present with agammaglobulinemia, anemia, or pancytopenia. Oligoclonal or uniclonal EBV-infected B lymphomas may occur during primary infection or after recovery. Similar illnesses occur in other immunosuppressed patients with primary EBV infection. The administration of high-dose cyclosporine as part of immunosuppressive regimens for organ or bone marrow transplantation has also been associated with severe EBV infection. Moreover, children with human immunodeficiency virus (HIV) infection are also at risk for severe EBV infection and lymphoproliferative disease (see Ch. 419). Lymphocytic interstitial pneumonitis may be prominent in such patients. In AIDS patients, replicating EBV has also been found in hairy leukoplakia of the tongue, a proliferative epithelial lesion.

Rare cases of chronic progressive primary EBV infection in young adults have been well documented. These patients have severe acute mononucleosis which persists, with clinical manifestations that include lymphadenopathy or visceral organ involvement and abnormally high antibody titers to EBV replicative cycle antigens. Some patients have lacked antibody to EBV nuclear antigens. Most patients eventually recover without specific treatment. In one patient, acycloguanosine treatment produced a clinical remission. Persistent active EBV infection was initially proposed to be the cause of a more common chronic mononucleosis or chronic fatigue syndrome. This syndrome is characterized by recurrent episodes of malaise and weakness, sometimes accompanied by myalgias, arthralgias, pharyngitis, lymphadenitis, or mild fever. Careful documentation of the lack of significant objective clinical or laboratory abnormalities distinguishes most patients with this poorly defined syndrome from those with known infectious, autoimmune, oncologic, metabolic, or neurologic diseases. EBV-specific antibody titers in most patients with the chronic fatigue syndrome do not differ significantly from those of normal infected adults (see below). Thus, there is little to support the initial hypothesis that EBV is a frequent cause of this syndrome.

Longstanding EBV infection is associated with B lymphomas in immunosuppressed patients, with Burkitt-type lymphoma in African children, and with anaplastic nasopharyngeal carcinoma. A substantial fraction of B lymphomas occurring in immunocompromised patients have EBV DNA in the tumor cells. In B lymphomas in which the virus is latent in all of the tumor cells, the virus probably provided an initial stimulus for cell proliferation. Malignant conversion in these late postinfection lymphomas requires at least one additional factor, since these cells also have a chromosome translocation that enhances c-*myc* oncogene expression. In a prospective study of African children, a correlation was noted between the EBV antibody response in the years between infection and tumor onset and the Burkitt tumor incidence, suggesting that the extent of EBV replication is an important parameter in tumor induction. In retrospective and prospective clinical studies, high levels of IgA antibody to EBV antigens have been closely associated with anaplastic nasopharyngeal carcinoma. EBV has also been uniformly found in each of the tumor cells of anaplastic nasopharyngeal carcinomas. The uniclonality of the virus genomes in these tumor cells indicates that the tumors arise in a single virus-infected cell. The virus is, therefore, likely to be necessary for this oncogenic conversion. Chinese and some native North American populations have a high incidence of nasopharyngeal carcinoma. Other factors in the pathogenesis of nasopharyngeal carcinoma have not been defined.

PATHOLOGY AND PATHOGENESIS. EBV first infects pharyngeal epithelial cells and then spreads to subepithelial circulating B lymphocytes. Infection may be confined to epithelial and B lymphocyte tissues, since only these cells have EBV receptors. The EBV receptor is also the receptor for the C3d fragment of complement. Tonsils and regional and systemic lymph nodes enlarge because of follicular hyperplasia, due in part to virus-infected B lymphocytes, and, because of infiltration of sinuses and paracortex with reactive, atypical T lymphocytes. Loss of normal architecture and the presence of Reed-Sternberg–like cells may make EBV infection difficult to distinguish from Hodgkin's disease. Similar changes occur in the spleen. In patients with significant hepatitis, hepatic lobules or portal areas may be infiltrated with mononuclear cells. The bone marrow is usually unaffected. Early in the illness, up to 1 or 2 per cent of the circulating leukocytes may be EBV-infected B lymphocytes. The predominant atypical lymphocyte in the peripheral blood, however, is a reactive T cell. EBV-infected B lymphocytes can be detected by their expression of EBV nuclear proteins (EBNA's) or by their ability to proliferate continuously in vitro or in SCID mice, a property that normal B lymphocytes lack. EBV infection of B lymphocytes stimulates both B-cell proliferation and Ig secretion, particularly IgM.

Lymphoproliferation following EBV infection of normal B lymphocytes in vitro is associated with the expression of six EBNA proteins, two membrane proteins (LMP's), and two small RNA's. The same repertoire of genes appears to be expressed in EBV-associated lymphoproliferative diseases. In vivo, primary infection results in transient hypergammaglobulinemia. The hypergammaglobulinemia results from direct and indirect effects of virus infection on B lymphocytes. The induction of antibodies that react with a heterologous erythrocyte glycoprotein antigen is the basis for the heterophil test. The pre-existence of B lymphocytes with heterophil antibody specificity remains an enigma, perhaps explainable by cross-reactivity of some of these antibodies with bacterial polysaccharides. The acute, non–B lymphocyte response to EBV infection is multifunctional. Some T lymphocytes suppress both B lymphocyte proliferation and Ig secretion. Other peripheral blood T lymphocytes and natural killer cells from patients with infectious mononucleosis are cytotoxic to autologous EBV-infected B cells. The cytotoxic T lymphocytes are largely CD8+ and recognize EBNA or LMP epitopes in the context of class I histocompatibility molecules. Other T lymphocytes may augment the T and B lymphocyte immune responses. Two EBV types are endemic in humans. These two types differ in their EBNA proteins and in their ability to transform B lymphocytes in vitro. Some cytotoxic T lymphocyte clones are specific for EBNA proteins. Some of these EBNA-specific cytotoxic T lymphocytes recognize only the EBNA protein of one virus type.

After recovery from acute infectious mononucleosis, the proportion of circulating B lymphocytes infected with EBV is one in 10^5 to 10^6. Latently infected B lymphocytes or B-lymphocyte precursors are likely to be the site of virus persistence, since long-term suppression of virus replication with antiviral chemotherapy does not decrease the number of circulating EBV-infected B lymphocytes; and following bone marrow transplantation, the donor's rather than the recipient's virus may persist. T lymphocytes also circulate which can suppress or kill HLA-related EBV-infected cells that express EBNA's or LMP's. EBV-infected B lymphocytes and reactive T cells circulate in the peripheral blood indefinitely after primary infection. Cyclosporine indirectly inhibits the EBV-specific T lymphocyte immune response, thereby enabling EBV-infected B lymphocytes to overgrow in transplantation recipients receiving high doses of cyclosporine and other immunosuppressive drugs. In this patient group EBV-associated lymphoproliferative diseases have been a significant, albeit unusual, problem.

DIAGNOSIS. In normal adolescents, the diagnosis of acute infectious mononucleosis can usually be made on clinical grounds and confirmed by the laboratory findings of atypical lymphocytosis and heterophil antibody to ox or horse erythrocytes. Bacterial throat culture should be done in patients with significant pharyngitis to exclude concomitant β-hemolytic streptococcal infection. The rapid heterophil tests are more than 95 per cent sensitive and more than 95 per cent specific in an adolescent or young adult population. Titers are substantially diminished by 3 months after primary infection and not detectable by 6 months. In patients with equivocal or absent heterophil antibodies, EBV-specific serologic testing should be done. The differential diagnosis may include streptococcal (pharyngeal) or gonococcal infection, cytomegalovirus, hepatitis virus A or B, HIV, HHV6, adenovirus, or toxoplasma infection, leukemia, and lymphoma. Most heterophil-negative infectious mononucleosis with pharyngitis is also caused by EBV. In the absence of pharyngitis, however, cytomegalovirus, toxoplasmosis, hepatitis virus, or HIV infections are likely causes of heterophil-negative or low-titer heterophil-positive infectious mononucleosis. In some patient populations, acute HIV infection is a significant cause of typical or atypical infectious mononucleosis syndromes. HIV antigen or nucleotide sequence–specific detection may be necessary to diagnose HIV infection early in the illness. Later, seroconversion may establish the diagnosis.

Specific serologic testing for EBV infection involves determining antibody titers to latently infected (anti-EBNA), early replication cycle (anti-EA), or late replication cycle (anti-VCA) viral proteins. This is usually done by indirect immunofluorescence microscopy or by enzyme-linked immunoassay. With acute primary infection, EA and IgM VCA titers are high and IgG VCA and EBNA titers are low. Patients recovering from primary infection have lower EA or IgM VCA titers, higher IgG VCA titer, and low EBNA titer. After several months, EA and IgM VCA titers are low or negative, whereas IgG VCA and EBNA titers are high. The high IgG VCA and EBNA titers frequently persist for many years. Those rare patients with chronically progressive EBV infection tend to have abnormally high titers of antibodies to some or many EBV antigens. On the other hand, serologic diagnosis may be misleading in immunosuppressed patients, including children with X-linked immunodeficiency. These infected children may have high or low antibody titers. EBV serologies are helpful in following patients with anaplastic nasopharyngeal carcinoma or in screening for early detection of this malignancy in high-risk populations. Patients at risk for primary anaplastic nasopharyngeal carcinoma or for recurrences have high IgG or IgA EA antibody titers.

TREATMENT. No treatment is necessary for most EBV infections. Rest during the period of acute symptoms and slow return to normal activity are commonly advised, although the therapeutic efficacy of this regimen has not been firmly established. Patients with splenomegaly should restrict their involvement in sports to avoid traumatic rupture. Acetaminophen or aspirin may be used to reduce temperature and pharyngeal pain. Very brief courses of glucocorticoid treatment (e.g., 60 mg prednisone per day for 4 days followed by rapidly decreasing doses) have been effective in shrinking obstructing tonsils, probably by ameliorating an overactive T-cell response. Autoimmune hemolytic anemia, granulocytopenia, and thrombocytopenia usually respond to longer courses of glucocorticoid therapy. The use of glucocorticoids for other manifestations of EBV infection is less certain to be beneficial. Glucocorticoids have no antiviral activity and are contraindicated in most herpesvirus infections. A few patients with severe hemorrhagic thrombocytopenia refractory to glucocorticoids have responded to intravenous immunoglobulin. Early plasmapheresis is indicated in patients with Guillain-Barré syndrome. Acycloguanosine and its derivatives have activity against EBV in vitro but are not approved for use against EBV. These drugs should not be used in normal patients with EBV infections but can be considered for AIDS patients with oral hairy leukoplakia or for patients with well-documented chronically progressive EBV infection. Acycloguanosine has not affected the outcome of EBV-associated lymphoproliferative syndromes in immunosuppressed patients. No effect on EBV DNA in latently infected cells has been seen. Partial restoration of immune function by lowering immune suppression has been beneficial. In one patient with X-linked lymphoproliferative disease, recombinant interferon-γ produced a rapid clinical remission.

Duncombe AS, Amos RJ, Metcalfe P, Pearson TC: Intravenous immunoglobulin therapy in thrombocytopenic infectious mononucleosis. Clin Lab Haematol 11(1):11–15, 1989. *Effect of Ig in two cases of refractory hemorrhagic thrombocytopenia.*

Ernber I, Andersson J: Acyclovir efficiently inhibits oropharyngeal excretion of Epstein-Barr virus in patients with acute infectious mononucleosis. J Gen Virol 67:2267–2272, 1986. *Effect of acycloguanosine on EBV infection.*

Kieff E, Liebowitz D: Epstein-Barr virus and its replication. *In* Fields B, Knipe D (eds.): Virology, 2nd ed. New York, Raven Press, 1990, pp 1889–1920. *Review of the biochemistry of Epstein-Barr virus and its effect on lymphocytes.*

Miller G: Epstein-Barr virus: Biology, pathogenesis and medical aspects. *In* Fields B, Knipe D (eds.): Virology, 2nd ed. New York, Raven Press, 1990, pp 1921–1958. *Review of EBV-associated diseases.*

Schooley RT, Carey RW, Miller G, et al.: Chronic Epstein-Barr virus infection associated with fever and interstitial pneumonitis. Clinical and serologic features and response to antiviral chemotherapy. Ann Intern Med 104:636–643, 1986. *Illustrative case of chronic EBV.*

374 Varicella

Philip A. Brunell

DEFINITION. Varicella, or chickenpox, is an acute communicable disease characterized by a generalized vesicular rash. Because it is highly contagious, most individuals contract it in childhood. Herpes zoster, due to reactivation of varicella-zoster virus (VZV), is a dermatomal cutaneous eruption (see Ch. 476.3).

ETIOLOGY. Varicella is caused by VZV, a member of the α-herpesvirinae subfamily. This enveloped herpesvirus contains at least five glycoproteins, some of which bear some homology to those of other members of the human herpesvirus group. The double-stranded DNA has a molecular weight of approximately 80 million. There is some diversity in the restriction enzyme patterns among wild isolates; there is only a single serotype. Although the human is the only known natural host, a closely related virus has been identified in a simian species.

EPIDEMIOLOGY. Varicella is a highly contagious disease. After continuing household exposure, as would occur in a family, almost all susceptibles are infected. The subclinical attack rate is believed to be no more than 4 per cent. The results of nonhousehold exposure are less certain. Although chickenpox is believed to be contagious prior to the onset of rash, this has been difficult to prove. Virus has not been isolated from respiratory secretions prior to onset of rash and is difficult to isolate following rash. Chickenpox is contagious for as long as 5 days after the appearance of the first lesion. Patients are customarily isolated for 5 days. The incubation period is usually about 14 days. Ninety-nine per cent of the cases occur 10 to 20 days following exposure. The disease is known to be spread by direct contact. Airborne spread also has been demonstrated, most notably in hospitals.

Nosocomial spread of varicella has been well documented. This has occurred room to room by airborne spread as well as by patient-to-patient or staff-to-patient contact. Adults with herpes zoster who are hospitalized are less likely to cause secondary cases of chickenpox among adult contacts than among children. The reason is that hospitalized children are more likely to be susceptible to chickenpox than hospitalized adults. Strict isolation is recommended for hospitalized patients with varicella and for children or immunocompromised adults with herpes zoster.

Adults with localized herpes zoster require less stringent isolation procedures.

Most cases of chickenpox occur in childhood. Most children contract chickenpox either in day care situations or shortly after they enter school. Fewer than 2 per cent of the cases occur following the second decade. Approximately 2.5 per cent of entering professional students were found to be seronegative. Approximately 10 per cent of hospital workers with a negative history are seronegative. Almost all individuals with a positive history are seropositive. A single attack of chickenpox usually confers lifetime immunity.

There appears to be more efficient transmission of disease in temperate than in tropical climates. The reason for this is uncertain but may be due to temperature rather than urbanization. Varicella occurs most commonly during the late winter and spring months, the peak being about in March. Sporadic cases occur into the early summer and start in late fall.

Varicella is more common than other childhood diseases during the early months of life. In this situation the disease is generally mild. Maternal antibody transferred across the placenta may not be as effective in protecting infants against this disease as are antibodies against other viruses. However, nursery outbreaks have been rare. Children who develop varicella during the early months of life, or are exposed in utero, have a greater risk of developing herpes zoster in childhood.

PATHOGENESIS. VZV produces a disseminated rash, which indicates that bloodstream distribution must have occurred. Virus has been isolated from white blood cells just prior to and during the first 1 or 2 days following the appearance of rash. After clinical recovery, the virus infection continues in the absence of clinical symptoms in a latent phase. During this time, virus deoxyribonucleic acid (DNA) or messenger ribonucleic acid (RNA) can be demonstrated in non-neuronal cells in dorsal root ganglia. The segmental distribution of herpes zoster (see Ch. 476.3), which usually occurs decades after the initial VZV infection, is consistent with a dorsal root ganglion site for the latent virus. In uncomplicated chickenpox, rises in serum transaminase levels have been demonstrated. This suggests that there is visceral involvement in the normal course of this disease.

The vesicular lesions of varicella contain a predominance of polymorphonuclear leukocytes even during the early phase of vesicle formation. Multinuclear giant cells are occasionally found in the base of the lesions, often containing eosinophilic intranuclear inclusions. Large amounts of virus can be demonstrated in vesicular fluid by electron microscopy.

Postmortem descriptions of patients with varicella have usually involved immunocompromised subjects. In these cases inflammatory changes are usually found in multiple organs, including the lung, liver, spleen, and skin, together with anoxic changes in the brain. Similar involvement is found in the newborn. Focal areas of necrosis and intranuclear eosinophilic inclusions in mononuclear cells are common. Changes in otherwise normal individuals usually include myocardial and pulmonary lesions. On microscopic examination, the brain has demonstrated edema with some lymphocyte cuffing around the cerebral vessels.

CLINICAL MANIFESTATIONS. Varicella is characterized by a generalized eruption that is centripetal in distribution; erythematous macules, papules, vesicles, and scabbed lesions may be present at the same time. The vesicles are superficial, with varying amounts of erythema at their bases. Adults tend to have considerably more erythema than children. During the early phase of the eruption, lesions are found on the face, scalp, and trunk. By running the fingers through the hair, one often detects lesions that were not visible. Later, new lesions appear on the extremities. By this time, the earlier lesions have dried and crusted. Excoriations are common, attesting to the pruritic nature of the lesions. Mucous membranes of the conjunctiva, oropharynx, and vagina are more frequently involved in adults than in children. New lesions continue to appear over a 3- or 4-day period, after which the rate of their appearance decelerates markedly.

There is a striking variation in the extent of systemic symptoms associated with varicella. Most children have a mild illness with few systemic complaints and an average maximal temperature of about 38.3°C. It is more common for adults to have considerable malaise, muscle ache, arthralgia, and headache. These may precede the first skin lesions by 24 to 48 hours.

In the immunocompromised subject, the disease often is very severe. Approximately 30 per cent of children with leukemia or lymphoma who get varicella develop "progressive varicella." Vesicles continue to erupt into the second week of illness, accompanied by high fever. Lesions tend to be deep seated rather than superficial. Toward the end of the first week and the beginning of the second week, the lesions are more common on the extremities than on the trunk. Indeed, the distribution and lesions may resemble those with smallpox. Visceral involvement occurs in about 30 per cent of these patients. The lung, liver, pancreas, and brain may be involved. Death occurs in about 9 per cent of immunocompromised patients who develop varicella. The death usually is due to pulmonary involvement.

Varicella in pregnant women is believed to be more serious than in nongravid females; fatalities have been reported. The rate of fetal wastage is not increased. Seven to 9 per cent of infants born to mothers who have had varicella early in pregnancy, however, have been found at birth to have "varicella embryopathy." These infants are born with cerebral damage and a variety of ocular findings and characteristically have a scarred, atrophic limb. They are generally small for gestational age and may have other abnormalities as well. When mothers develop chickenpox within a few days of delivery, "varicella of the newborn" may occur. If the onset of varicella is between 5 and 10 days after birth, it is associated with a higher risk of serious disease and even death.

Bacterial infections of the skin are the most common complication of chickenpox in childhood. The rate of complications is much higher in adults than in children. Although fewer than 2 per cent of the reported cases occur after the second decade, almost a quarter of the deaths occur in this group. A disproportionate rate of hospitalization also is found in adults. The major complications of varicella in adults are encephalitis and pneumonia.

Approximately 1 in 400 adults with chickenpox are hospitalized for pneumonia. In a prospective study, however, it was found that only 6 per cent of young adults with chickenpox had respiratory symptoms, whereas 16 per cent had roentgenographic evidence of pulmonary involvement.

Infection produces a diffuse interstitial type of pneumonia with hypoxia resulting from poor diffusion of gases. Diffuse calcification of the lung parenchyma may be found years after recovery.

Encephalitis in childhood is most commonly manifested by a cerebellitis, which usually occurs at the end of the first week or during the second week following onset of rash. This complication is almost always self-limited. In contrast, an acute form of encephalitis usually occurring soon after the onset of rash often has a fulminating course; it is characterized by severe brain swelling. It has been estimated that as many as 20 per cent of cases of Reye's syndrome may be preceded by chickenpox. A variety of other neurologic complications, including optic neuritis, transverse myelitis, and Guillain-Barré syndrome, may be associated with chickenpox. Hemorrhagic complications of chickenpox include thrombocytopenic purpura and purpura fulminans. Nephritis, myocarditis, and arthritis also have been described.

DIAGNOSIS. There is usually little difficulty in recognizing typical forms of chickenpox, particularly if there has been a history of exposure. The disease is seen more commonly by pediatricians than internists. The latter may not consider the diagnosis or may be less familiar with its clinical characteristics. The diagnosis may be more difficult in immunocompromised hosts, as they may have features of progressive varicella with visceral involvement. Modified cases of chickenpox may occur following passive or active immunization. These cases may require laboratory confirmation. The most common sources of confusion are insect bites; generalized herpes in the immunocompromised host; rickettsialpox; or "hand, foot, and mouth disease" caused by an enterovirus. The differentiation of disseminated herpes zoster from chickenpox may be difficult. The former usually has dermatomal involvement initially. Generalization usually does not occur until 3 to 5 days after onset of the zosteriform rash. In severely immunocompromised patients, e.g., bone marrow recipients, generalization may occur earlier and the clinical differentiation may be difficult.

The Tzanck smear is a frequently used laboratory aid for diagnosis. Multinucleated giant cells identify the lesions as being caused by one of the herpesviruses, but this is not specific for varicella. A properly stained smear also contains eosinophilic intranuclear inclusions. Virus can usually be isolated during the first 3 or 4 days after the onset of lesions. The virus is quite labile; it must be stored at $-70°C$ if cultures cannot be inoculated immediately. Our preference is to collect vesicular fluid in unheparinized capillary tubes and put the specimen directly into human embryonic lung fibroblasts at the bedside. A high isolation rate is found during the first 3 days of rash. Specimens from throat, urine, or stool are of little value for isolation of virus. PCR has been used to identify virus in vesicular fluid and respiratory secretions.

Serologic confirmation of diagnosis can be made using a variety of techniques. The enzyme-linked immunosorbent assay (ELISA) and complement fixation are the most generally available. The laboratory director should be consulted regarding appropriate time of collection of specimens as well as interpretation of data. Because complement-fixing antibody generally does not persist, a single high titer often is confirmatory evidence of recent infection.

Determining the immune status of contacts can be done with the ELISA or fluorescent antibody against membrane antigen (FAMA). The ELISA is a much simpler and technically less demanding test. Because complement-fixing antibody is lost rapidly after infection, it cannot be used for determining susceptibility. Fluorescence antibody tests using fixed cells sometimes yield false-positive results. A number of laboratories have developed tests for VZV immunoglobulin M (IgM). It was hoped that these might differentiate varicella from herpes zoster in cases in which this was unclear. Unfortunately, these tests have not been very useful, as VZV IgM is present in the sera of many patients with acute herpes zoster.

TREATMENT. Major therapeutic objectives are the prevention of superinfection and relief of pruritus. The latter can be accomplished frequently by application of calamine lotion. Occasionally this does not suffice, and a systemic antipruritic agent such as trimeprazine may be necessary. It is advisable to trim and file nails to reduce the damage from scratching. Bacterial superinfection can best be prevented by encouraging daily bathing with soap or hexachlorophene. Following this with a colloidal starch bath may also be useful in relief of pruritus.

Relief of systemic symptoms may require additional medication such as acetaminophen. Salicylates are contraindicated, as there is an association between their use and development of Reye's syndrome in children. Special care should be taken to be certain that over-the-counter medications containing salicylates are avoided.

Some patients, particularly those who are immunocompromised, may require antiviral therapy. Acyclovir has been shown to be effective in immunocompromised children with varicella. A dose of 500 mg per square meter repeated every 8 hours has been used. VZV is generally less sensitive to acyclovir than herpes simplex. For this reason, larger doses are probably required. Doses of 10 to 20 mg per kilogram have been shown to shorten the course of varicella by about 1 day if used early. The rate of complications was not affected. Patients who are sick enough to require antiviral therapy probably should be treated with parenteral rather than oral medication. In comparative studies, acyclovir appears to be somewhat safer and probably more effective than vidarabine.

Patients on high doses of steroids or other immunosuppressive drugs who have been exposed to chickenpox are at high risk of developing progressive varicella. Steroids appear to be most deleterious when given during the incubation period. They have been used without any obvious deleterious effects in the treatment of pneumonia after the eruption has occurred.

PREVENTION. Immune serum globulin does not prevent varicella. Massive doses are required to produce measurable modification. If prevention or modification is indicated, varicella zoster immune globulin (VZIG) should be given. Candidates are those who (1) are susceptible, (2) are at high risk of developing complicated varicella, and (3) have had an adequate exposure to the disease. Any individuals fulfilling the first two criteria who have had a household exposure should receive prophylaxis. It is often difficult to judge the degree of intimacy in other types of exposure. Reference to guidelines published by the Academy of Pediatrics or Centers for Disease Control (CDC) may be helpful.

Patients considered at high risk are (1) those who are immunocompromised by virtue of either disease or immunosuppressive therapy, (2) infants born to mothers who have had varicella less than 5 days prior to or 2 days following delivery, (3) premature infants of mothers with no history of varicella, (4) bone marrow transplantation recipients regardless of susceptibility, and (5) certain adults.

A history of varicella is usually reliable in both adults and children. Children who have a negative history are usually susceptible. Serologic testing of adults who have a negative history is useful if it does not delay administration of VZIG. VZIG should be given as soon as possible following exposure and should not be delayed more than 96 hours.

Nosocomial infection following herpes zoster or varicella has been well documented. These outbreaks may result in significant morbidity and cause disruption of hospital routine. These situations are best managed by serologic screening of personnel and by permitting only those who are seropositive to care for patients with varicella or herpes zoster. Patients who are hospitalized with varicella should be isolated for 7 days. Susceptible persons who are exposed to active cases should be isolated from the tenth to the twenty-first day after the last exposure if they cannot be discharged. Whenever possible, patients with chickenpox should be isolated in a room with negative pressure in order to prevent dissemination of infectious virus to other patients. Airborne spread in hospitals has been documented.

An attenuated live vaccine has been licensed for use abroad and is being considered for licensure in the United States. Susceptible adults who receive the vaccine have some local reactions and occasionally develop a varicelliform rash. Protection against infection is less complete than in children. In normal children, the vaccine is virtually benign and appears to offer very good protection. Initial data suggest that herpes zoster would be no more frequent and perhaps less common following immunization than following natural infection. Live varicella vaccine also has been used to protect children with acute lymphocytic leukemia. Protection is less complete than in normal children. Some of these vaccinated children develop a varicelliform illness from the vaccine.

Advisory Committee on Immunization Practice: Varicella-zoster immune globulin for the prevention of chickenpox. MMWR 33:84, 95, 1984. *Guidelines for passive immunization against chickenpox.*

Brunell PA: Fetal and neonatal varicella-zoster infections. Semin Perinatol 7:47, 1983. *A critical review of fetal, neonatal, and maternal varicella.*

Brunell PA: Varicella vaccine—where are we? Pediatrics 78:721, 1986. *A symposium on the epidemiology, cost burden, and complications of varicella and on varicella vaccine.*

Shehab ZM, Brunell PA: Varicella-zoster virus. *In* Rose NR, Friedman H, Fahey JL (eds.): Manual of Clinical Laboratory Immunity, 3rd ed. Washington, DC, American Society for Microbiology, 1986, pp 502–503. *A review of serologic tests for varicella-zoster antibody.*

Takahashi M: Chickenpox virus. Adv Virus Res 28:285, 1983. *A comprehensive review of both basic science and information on the vaccine.*

Varicella-zoster infections. Report of the Committee on Infectious Diseases, 21st ed. Evanston, IL, American Academy of Pediatrics, 1988, pp 456–462. *A useful guide to management of patients exposed to varicella, including control of nosocomial infection.*

Weller TH: Varicella and herpes zoster. N Engl J Med 309:1362, 1983. *A review of immunology, immunization, and therapy.*

375 Variola and Vaccinia

Donald A. Henderson

The Thirty-third World Health Assembly "declares solemnly that the world and all its peoples have won freedom from smallpox . . . an unprecedented achievement in the history of public health. . . ." (Resolution 33.3, May 8, 1980, Geneva, Switzerland).

This announcement was made some 30 months after the last known endemic case, in Somalia, on October 26, 1977. In 1978, two additional cases of smallpox occurred in Birmingham, Eng-

land, as a result of a laboratory infection, but except for these cases no others have been found.

To confirm that eradication had been achieved, each country where smallpox had been endemic since 1967 and those at risk of importations conducted a search for cases for at least 2 years after the last known case. At the end of this period, World Health Organization (WHO)–appointed International Commissions reviewed the records of work and conducted extensive field visits to confirm the results. Between 1973 and 1979, 21 different commissions visited and certified eradication in 49 countries.

Finally, a Global Commission for the Certification of Smallpox Eradication reviewed the findings and made special field visits. After satisfying itself that eradication had been achieved, the commission reported its findings to the World Health Assembly. The assembly members concurred and recommended that "smallpox vaccination be discontinued in every country except for investigators at special risk," and advised that "an international certificate of vaccination against smallpox should no longer be required of any traveller."

Thus concluded the first successful global program to eradicate a disease—one that had proved to be one of the most devastating known to man.

HISTORY. Because of the need for variola virus to spread continually from person to person to survive, historians speculate that it emerged after the first agricultural settlements, about 10,000 B.C. A distinctive smallpox rash has been identified on the mummy of Pharaoh Ramses V (1160 B.C.). In ancient times, only a few populated areas, probably in India, could have sustained its transmission. In the early Christian era descriptions suggestive of smallpox appear in historical accounts of western Asia, and by the eighth century it had established itself in Europe. Central and southern Africa were probably infected sometime later. In 1520, Spanish conquistadors brought the disease to the Americas.

Case-fatality rates of 20 per cent and greater were characteristic, and where population densities permitted the disease to become endemic virtually all persons eventually contracted smallpox. At the end of the eighteenth century, it was killing an estimated 400,000 Europeans each year and was responsible for one third of all cases of blindness.

VACCINATION. Edward Jenner discovered in 1796 that smallpox could be prevented by "vaccination" with material from a cowpox lesion. Before his discovery, the only defense against smallpox was deliberately to inoculate (variolate) scabs or pustular material from smallpox patients into the skin of susceptible persons. The resulting infection was usually less severe than infection acquired naturally by inhalation. Although case-fatality rates among those with induced infection were sometimes as low as 1 per cent, they readily transmitted infection to others.

Within 3 years after Jenner first published his findings, more than 100,000 had been vaccinated in England. By 1803, the new vaccine had been transported to the Americas, Asia, and Africa. During the nineteenth century, vaccination was increasingly widely practiced in temperate-climate countries, but the difficulties of sustaining the virus through arm-to-arm inoculation resulted in an uncertain supply. The discovery, late in the nineteenth century, that vaccinia virus could be propagated on the flank of a calf was an important advance. However, such vaccine remained viable for only a few days at ambient temperature. Finally, in the 1950's a commercially feasible technique was developed for producing a dried, heat-resistant vaccine.

In the industrialized countries, smallpox incidence declined steadily, and Europe and North America succeeded in interrupting smallpox transmission after World War II. In these areas, the impetus for vaccination had diminished early in the century when a less virulent strain, variola minor, with a case-fatality rate of about 1 per cent, replaced variola major. In most of Africa, however, 5 to 15 per cent died of smallpox, and in Asia the virulent variola major prevailed. Neither in Africa nor in Asia was vaccination widely practiced.

ERADICATION OF SMALLPOX. Smallpox was a problem to all countries. Even those without disease feared importations and conducted vaccination programs. Although the global control of smallpox was in everyone's best interests, progress was slow. Finally, in 1959, the World Health Assembly decided that a global eradication program should be undertaken. During the succeeding 7 years, a number of countries undertook campaigns, but few succeeded in interrupting smallpox transmission.

In 1966, the assembly decided that one further effort should be made. A 10-year goal was proposed. The program commenced on January 1, 1967 (Fenner and colleagues). In 1967, smallpox was endemic in 31 countries, and 13 additional countries reported importations. Although 131,768 cases were officially reported, the true number was about 10 to 15 million. Four geographic reservoirs of smallpox were identified: (1) Africa south of the Sahara; (2) a group of Southeast Asian countries, extending from Bangladesh through India, Nepal, Pakistan, and Afghanistan; (3) Indonesia; and (4) Brazil. The estimated population of these countries was more than 1 billion persons.

WHO's strategy called for each country to undertake a program of vaccination with the objective of reaching at least 80 per cent of the population during a 2- to 3-year period. During this time, a reliable reporting system was to be developed to identify foci of smallpox that would be eliminated by isolation of patients and vaccination of contacts. Extensive vaccination was believed necessary to increase population immunity and so reduce the number of cases to permit disease surveillance and containment activities to be effective.

Experience soon showed that the surveillance-containment strategy was more effective than had been thought, and this proved to be a key to success. In part, this was due to the unique characteristics of smallpox. An infected patient was able to transmit infection only from the time of first appearance of rash until the last scabs had separated. There were no chronic carriers or individuals with latent, transmissible infection and no animal reservoir. The rash was sufficiently characteristic to be diagnosed with a high degree of accuracy. The presence or absence of smallpox in an area could thus be reliably determined without laboratory studies. Moreover, approximately two thirds of recovered patients had characteristic residual facial scars. Thus, it was possible to determine both the present status of smallpox and its past history in an area.

To persist, smallpox virus had to be transmitted from patient to susceptible contact. By isolation of the patient and by vaccination of contacts, a barrier to transmission was created. In small villages and in scattered populations, chains of transmission often terminated without intervention. Because smallpox did not spread rapidly, and then only to those in close contact, secondary cases usually were found among neighbors and relatives. A patient rarely infected more than two to three others. Because of these factors, early detection of outbreaks and their containment proved effective in stopping transmission.

Smallpox vaccine that conferred excellent and durable immunity was an important factor in the program's success. Studies revealed vaccine efficacy ratios of more than 90 per cent after 20 years. Because the lyophilized vaccine retained its potency after incubation at 37°C for at least 1 month, the logistics of vaccine storage and distribution were comparatively simple. Vaccination was greatly facilitated by the inexpensive, newly developed bifurcated needle. Vaccine was held between the tines by capillarity. Fifteen rapid punctures were made with the needle held perpendicular to the skin. The technique was learned quickly and produced a high proportion of successful vaccinations.

PROGRESS IN THE PROGRAM. By 1969, eradication programs were in progress in all of the infected and immediately adjacent countries except for Ethiopia, whose program began in 1971. By 1970, the number of endemic countries had decreased from 31 to 18. Brazil registered its last case in 1971 and Indonesia and Afghanistan in 1972. By 1973, all of Africa had become smallpox free except for Ethiopia and Botswana. In Asia, there remained only four smallpox-endemic countries: India, Pakistan, Nepal, and Bangladesh. However, the population of these four was over 700 million, and the techniques of surveillance and containment that had been applied in other areas proved to be less successful.

A new strategy in India began in the autumn of 1973 (Basu and colleagues). Far more rapid case detection and more effective containment of outbreaks were required. Accordingly, for 1 week each month more than 100,000 health workers were mobilized to search house by house to detect cases. Hundreds of special teams contained the outbreaks that were found. Between searches, the teams asked questions at markets and in schools to uncover rumors of cases. By the summer of 1974, new cases began to decline, and a cash reward was offered to anyone who reported a case. In May 1975 the last case was detected in India, and on October 16, 1975, the last case in Asia.

The only remaining endemic country was Ethiopia. With the end of smallpox in Asia, resources were shifted to Ethiopia. In August 1976, the last case was isolated. Unfortunately, Somalian guerrilla forces had meanwhile introduced the disease into neighboring Somalia, and yet another year was to elapse before finally, on October 26, 1977, the last case occurred.

POSSIBLE SOURCES FOR A RETURN OF SMALLPOX. As of 1990, variola virus was known to exist in only two laboratories, where it was kept under high-security conditions.

Extensive studies had been conducted since 1967 to discover a possible animal or other natural reservoir of the virus. None was found. However, some 400 cases of a newly recognized disease that is clinically indistinguishable from smallpox but caused by the related monkeypox virus occurred in seven central and west African countries between 1970 and 1990. Genome maps of this and other animal poxviruses reveal many differences between them and variola, suggesting that mutation to variola would be highly unlikely.

The recurrence of smallpox resulting from a deliberate release of variola virus cannot be ruled out. However, the potential damage of such an act should not be exaggerated. Smallpox does not spread rapidly, and an outbreak caused in this manner should be able to be contained within 3 to 4 weeks.

As insurance against unforeseen events, WHO has established vaccine storage reserves of some 200 million doses of vaccine. Additional stocks are being retained by a number of governments.

Barring improbable circumstances, a human case of smallpox will never again be seen. However, the problem of mistaken diagnosis is a real one. For this reason, WHO medical officers with expertise in diagnosis remain on call to investigate rumors, and an expertise in laboratory diagnosis is maintained by WHO Diagnostic Reference Laboratories (Centers for Disease Control, Atlanta, and the Institute for Virus Preparations, Moscow).

VARIOLA (Smallpox)

ETIOLOGY. Variola virus is one of a group of orthopoxviruses that includes vaccinia, monkeypox, rabbitpox, cowpox, camelpox, buffalopox, and ectromelia. The poxviruses are the largest viruses so recognized. The virions are brick-shaped structures with a diameter of about 200 mμ. The genome consists of a single molecule of a double-stranded DNA.

INCIDENCE AND PREVALENCE. The disease was declared to be eradicated on May 8, 1980.

PATHOLOGY AND PATHOGENESIS. The site of entry of the smallpox virus was probably the respiratory tract. In the 12-day incubation period the virus multiplied in the regional lymphoid tissues. Viremia occurred at the onset of fever and continued during the first 2 or 3 days of the pre-eruptive phase. During this time, the virus localized in mucous membranes, skin, and internal tissues. Virus multiplication in the epithelial cells of the skin and mucous membranes caused pustulation. Antibodies appeared as early as the fourth day of disease.

CLINICAL MANIFESTATIONS. The incubation period of smallpox was about 12 days with a range of 7 to 17 days. The illness began with severe malaise, prostration, head- and backache, and high fever lasting 2 to 5 days (Rao). Following the initial febrile period, a macular rash developed, which quickly became papular, and within 2 days the papules developed into vesicles and then pustules. On the eighth or ninth day of rash, crusting began. The scabs separated over the succeeding 2 to 3 weeks, leaving pigment-free skin. Subsequently, scarring or pitting developed. The eruption was characteristically more severe on the face and the distal parts of the arms and legs, and less severe over the trunk and abdomen. Lesions were often found on the palms of the hands and the soles of the feet.

VARIOLA MINOR AND INTERMEDIATE FORMS. In the early twentieth century, a milder clinical form of smallpox (variola minor, or alastrim) became prevalent in the Americas, Europe, and parts of southern and eastern Africa. Case-fatality rates were 1 per cent or less. Variola major and minor were distinct although at times coexisting. Each of the two types gave rise to illnesses with a wide spectrum of severity. There was cross-protection between each of these forms and vaccinia.

DIFFERENTIAL DIAGNOSIS. Most cases of smallpox could

readily be identified by the typical deep-seated rash, the centrifugal distribution of lesions, and the fact that in any area on the body all lesions were at the same stage of development. The infrequent severe hemorrhagic cases were frequently mistakenly diagnosed as meningococcemia, acute leukemia, or drug toxicity. Mild cases with few lesions were confused with varicella. Most problematic were severe cases of chickenpox in adults. Of help in diagnosis, however, was the fact that in any outbreak 80 per cent or more of the cases were clinically typical.

LABORATORY TESTS. Diagnosis of a poxvirus infection can be rapidly established by electron microscopic identification of virus particles in vesicular or pustular fluid or scabs. Differentiation among poxviruses requires that the virus be isolated on chick chorioallantoic membrane and its properties characterized by specific biologic tests. WHO Reference Laboratories are prepared to undertake necessary diagnostic studies. For patients who have recovered, neutralizing antibody in serum specimens serves to identify which poxvirus was responsible for the illness.

TREATMENT. No specific treatment is available.

IDENTIFICATION OF A SUSPECT CASE OF SMALLPOX. Because smallpox has been eradicated, the occurrence of a single case has profound international implications. Should a suspect case be identified, *immediate notification of local, state, and national health officials is essential.* Most suspected cases in recent years have been cases of varicella in adults. Should a case prove to be smallpox, the source of virus must be assumed to be inadvertent or deliberate release from a laboratory. A suspect patient should be placed under strict isolation. Additional measures will be dictated by epidemiologic circumstances.

VACCINIA (Vaccination)

No countries now require international certificates of vaccination, and none conducts civilian vaccination programs. Several countries, including the United States, continue to vaccinate military personnel. Vaccination is recommended only for investigators who are working with poxviruses in the laboratory.

THE VACCINE. Vaccinia virus is grown in tissue culture or on the scarified flank of a calf. After purification and the addition of stabilizing agents, the suspension is freeze dried. Inoculated intradermally, vaccinia virus induces a mild infection and confers protection against all orthopoxviruses known to infect man—monkeypox, variola, and cowpox.

VACCINE PROTECTION. Following successful vaccination, protection against variola is virtually complete for 5 years, but effectiveness wanes over time. In poxvirus laboratories, vaccination at least every 3 years has been customary.

RISKS OF VACCINATION. Those who are candidates for vaccination are adults, a diminishing proportion of whom have received primary vaccinations as children. Although the risk of complications following revaccination is very low, primary vaccination of adults has been thought to be associated with a higher incidence of serious complications. However, a special study of vaccination complications among military recruits failed to document any cases of the most important, postvaccinal encephalitis, among an estimated 2 million primary vaccinees.

FIRST VACCINATION (PRIMARY TAKE). Three days after vaccination a papule appears at the vaccination site; the papule changes to a vesicle and by the seventh day is a fully developed pustule. It is whitish, umbilicated, and multilocular and contains clear lymph. An erythematous areola expands to reach a maximal diameter about 9 days after vaccination. A crust forms and falls off about 3 weeks after vaccination, leaving a scar.

REVACCINATION. When persons are vaccinated a second time, a gradation of cutaneous responses is observed. Individuals who have not been vaccinated for several decades may develop what appears to be a primary take. In persons with an intermediate level of immunity, development of the lesion is more rapid, and the maximal diameter of erythema is reached in 3 to 7 days. In the highly immune person, virus multiplication may not occur. In such persons, a hypersensitivity response to vaccinial protein may occur. A papule and sometimes a vesicle with erythema may develop, reaching its peak in 48 hours.

To distinguish the hypersensitivity type of reaction, which may be caused by heat-inactivated vaccine, from one in which virus multiplication has taken place, the site of inoculation is examined between the sixth and eighth days. If there is evidence of induration or congestion, virus multiplication may be assumed.

CONTRAINDICATIONS. Four groups of persons are at special risk of complications: (1) persons with eczema or other forms of chronic dermatitis; (2) pregnant women; (3) patients with leukemia, lymphoma, other reticuloendothelial malignancies and the acquired immunodeficiency syndrome (AIDS); and (4) those receiving immunosuppressive drugs, especially glucocorticosteroids. Vaccinees in close contact with persons with eczema may infect them, sometimes with serious consequences. If vaccination is required for persons at special risk, vaccinia immune globulin (0.3 ml per kilogram intramuscularly) should be administered simultaneously.

COMPLICATIONS. *Postvaccinal Encephalitis.* Encephalitis following vaccination is a rare event and occurs between the eighth and fifteenth days. Paralysis, when it occurs, is generally spastic in type. Residual paralysis and other central nervous system symptoms may persist. There is no treatment. Studies conducted in the United States in 1963 and 1968 (Neff and colleagues, Lane and associates) revealed 28 cases, 9 fatal, among 11.3 million primary vaccinees. No cases occurred among 16.3 million revaccinees.

Progressive Vaccinia (Vaccinia Gangrenosa). Progressive vaccinia is an exceedingly rare but often fatal complication among vaccinated persons who have deficient immune responses. The initial vaccinial lesion fails to heal and progresses to involve adjacent skin with necrosis of tissue. Dissemination may result in metastatic vaccinial lesions in other parts of the skin, bones, or viscera. Treatment with vaccinia immune globulin is beneficial.

Eczema Vaccinatum. Eczema vaccinatum is sometimes a serious complication, which may occur in vaccinated persons with active or healed eczema, or in subjects in contact with recent vaccinees. The disease tends to localize at sites where eczematous lesions are or have been present. Vaccinia immune globulin is of help in therapy.

Generalized Vaccinia. Generalized vaccinia represents a secondary eruption resulting from bloodborne dissemination of vaccinia virus. Almost all cases occur after primary vaccination. The lesions become evident between 6 and 9 days after vaccination. The number of lesions may range from a few to a generalized involvement of the skin. It is a self-limited illness, and complete recovery occurs without specific therapy.

Fetal Vaccinia. Fetal vaccinia results from a bloodborne dissemination of vaccinia virus in the pregnant woman given primary vaccination. It may occur during any trimester of pregnancy and frequently results in death of the fetus.

Miscellaneous Complications. A great variety of rashes have been reported to be caused by vaccination. Most common are erythema multiforme and variously distributed urticarial, maculopapular, blotchy erythematous eruptions.

Basu RN, Jerek Z, Ward NA: The Eradication of Smallpox from India. New Delhi, India, World Health Organization, 1979. *A well-written, detailed, profusely illustrated book describing the epidemiologic and operational aspects of the program in India.*

Fenner F, Henderson DA, Jerek Z, et al.: Smallpox and its Eradication. Geneva, Switzerland, World Health Organization, 1988. *This 1400-page, extensively illustrated and referenced book is the definitive text, providing an historical account of smallpox control and eradication as well as a summary of current knowledge regarding the epidemiology, virology, and pathogenesis of the disease.*

Hopkins DR: Princes and Peasants: Smallpox in History. Chicago, University of Chicago Press, 1983. *The only comprehensive history of smallpox prepared in this century, this interesting and readable book complements the book by Fenner and associates.*

Lane JM, Ruben FL, Neff JM, et al.: Complications of smallpox vaccination, 1968. N Engl J Med 281:138, 1969. *With the paper by Neff and co-workers, one of the few detailed studies of the frequency of complications following smallpox vaccination.*

Neff J, Lane JM, Pert JH, et al.: Complications of smallpox vaccination. N Engl J Med 276:1, 1967. *With the paper by Lane and associates, one of the few detailed studies of the frequency of complications following smallpox vaccination.*

Rao AR: Smallpox. Bombay, India, Kothari Book Depot, 1972. *Written by a clinician who treated more than 3000 cases, this book is an excellent reference on the clinical aspects of variola major.*

376 Retroviruses That Cause Human Disease*

William A. Blattner

The decade of the 1980's ushered in a new age of medical virology with the discovery and characterization of human oncornaviruses and lenti-retroviruses. These discoveries began with the search for human cancer viruses in the early decades of this century and were propelled by the studies of cancer-causing retroviruses in mammals from the 1950's to 1970's. During the 1960's and 1970's molecular retrovirology established the replication cycle and the nature and function of viral genes and proteins, along with basic technology to assay reverse transcriptase and grow key target cells using newly discovered growth factors such as interleukin 2 (IL2). Within a few years of the first detection of a human retrovirus, HTLV-I in 1978, systems for their study in vitro were developed; their modes of transmission and geographic prevalence were determined; their genomes were analyzed and some novel genes were found; the mechanism of their effects on cells was partly unraveled; and, most importantly, some were causally linked to fatal human diseases, including diverse malignancies and the pandemic of acquired immunodeficiency syndrome (AIDS). In this chapter, some of the general properties of this remarkable virus class are considered.

DEFINITION, GENERAL FEATURES, AND CLASSIFICATION. Retroviruses are ribonucleic acid (RNA) viruses consisting of an outer envelope and an inner core that contains two molecules of a single-stranded RNA. The genome is relatively small (8.0 to 9.5 Kb) and simple (three to eight genes). Envelope and core structural proteins of the virus are produced from spliced viral RNA coded message and as the virus assembles at the cell membrane, the envelope incorporates the cell's lipid

---

*This chapter is based in part on a chapter written by Dr. Robert C. Gallo and his colleague Dr. Howard Z. Streicher in the 18th edition of the *Cecil Textbook of Medicine*. They have given permission to update portions of that chapter and have assisted, in conjunction with Drs. Dani Bolognasi and Thomas Palker of Duke University, in the preparation of this chapter.

bilayer during the budding process, producing an infectious virion of about 100 nm. The life cycle of a human retrovirus is schematically portrayed in Figure 376–1.

The hallmark of a retrovirus is the replication of viral RNA through a deoxyribonucleic acid (DNA) intermediate called a provirus. The initial step in virus infection is attachment of the virus envelope glycoproteins to a cell surface receptor. For HIV-1 the receptor is the CD4 molecule, but other components including major histocompatibility molecules may also play a role in this high-affinity binding step. In addition to T lymphocytes, monocyte/macrophages that express CD4 may also be infected. The other human retroviruses, HTLV-I and -II, which preferentially infect and transform CD4+ cells, use another as yet unknown receptor. Following uptake and uncoating, viral RNA is transcribed by reverse transcriptase into double-stranded DNA. This unique mechanism is catalyzed by viral *reverse transcriptase*, an RNA-dependent DNA polymerase that is complexed to the RNA in the core of the virus particle. This double-stranded viral DNA is integrated by the virally encoded integrase into the host cell nucleus, resulting in cell infection that may be lifelong. Essential to integration are the viral long terminal repeat (LTR) elements. Depending on the specific retrovirus, the LTR's are sequences of 300 to 900 nucleotides that flank both ends of the viral genome. They form the sites of covalent attachment of the provirus to cellular DNA and are the site of important viral regulatory elements. The virus may remain "hidden" (unexpressed, nonreplicative) in cells for very long periods, and this may contribute to the long interval (sometimes many years to decades) between the time of infection and disease. Factors that control viral replication (viral regulatory genes, cell stimulation, and possibly coinfections) may also be cofactors in disease progression. When the DNA provirus is expressed (transcribed by a cellular RNA polymerase), viral genomic and messenger RNA and subsequently viral proteins are made by the cell. These assemble at the cell membrane to be packaged and released, thereby completing the replication cycle.

Retroviruses are found in many different vertebrates. Their principal target cells in most animals are those of the hematopoietic, immune, and central nervous systems. Consequently, they induce a wide range of diseases, including malignancies, which chiefly consist of leukemias and lymphomas. Yet retrovirus

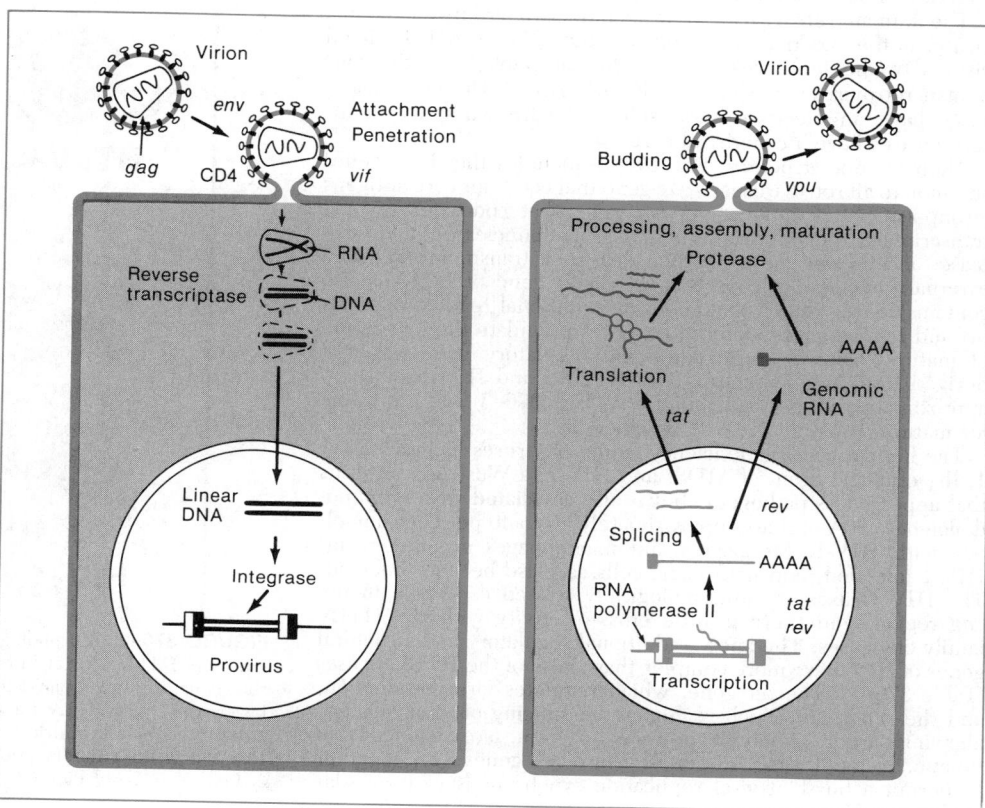

FIGURE 376–1. Life cycle of HIV. *Left,* Attachment of the virus involves binding to the CD4 receptor of the cell. The virus uncoats in an endosome transcribed to double-stranded viral DNA. Linear viral DNA is transported to the nucleus and integrated into host genome by virally encoded integrator. The proviral DNA can remain latent in the cell or serve as a template for production of new virions (*right*). Under the influence of viral regulatory proteins *tat* and *rev*, viral message is expressed either as structural proteins involving translation or as genomic RNA. New virions are produced with the viral protease modulating processing, assembly, and maturation. Particles bud through the cell membrane and incorporate into the cell lipid bilayer in which are embedded the viral transmembrane and external proteins. (Reprinted with permission from Gallo RC: Mechanism of disease induction by HIV. J AIDS 3:380–389, 1990.)

infection can produce quite the opposite effect. Sometimes they interfere with cell growth, leading to aplasias of various cell types (e.g., aplastic anemia of feline leukemia virus). Some infections are cytopathic, killing the infected cells (AIDS), and some may alter cell function. The kind of disease induced by a retrovirus depends in part upon its major target cell, (which is determined by viral envelope binding to cell receptor) and sometimes upon interaction of proviral LTR regulatory elements with cellular genes (e.g., *cis* activation of a cellular oncogene).

Retroviruses are named and classified according to their species, their mode of transmission (endogenous, exogenous), the type of disease produced (e.g., leukemia viruses, sarcoma viruses), their morphology and mode of maturation (types C,D,B, foamy, and lenti), the organization of their genome, and the genetic relatedness of one to another. Many of these terms and descriptions are no longer useful and are not considered here. For example, the ubiquitous endogenous retroviruses, sometimes known as spuma or foamy virus of the chimpanzee, are transmitted in the germ line as genetic elements and have no known role in the origin of disease except in a few highly inbred strains of laboratory mice. By contrast, exogenous viruses are transmitted by infection of a somatic cell like any other virus and frequently cause disease.

There are three general groups of retroviruses. The first are those with the three genes necessary for virus replication (*gag* gene for core proteins, *pol* gene for reverse transcriptase, and *env* gene for envelope). The majority of known animal retroviruses are of the first type. The mechanisms by which they induce disease often involve extensive replication of the virus and random integration of transcribed DNA into target-cell DNA with occasional chance integration in a region in which the viral LTR may promote altered expression of one or more nearby cellular genes important to cell growth or differentiation. This process is sometimes called *cis*-activation and may result in leukemia. The second group are those carrying a cellular *onc* gene that codes for a protein that transforms each infected cell; viruses belonging to this second type are rare and usually defective and have never been found in humans. The third group contains the three requisite genes for viral replication plus one or more additional genes (e.g., *tax* of HTLV-I) that regulate virus expression and also may directly or indirectly alter cell function. This third type includes all of the known human retroviruses.

The human retroviruses now include two groups, leukemia viruses of the oncornavirus family and the AIDS or AIDS-related viruses of the lentivirus family. The morphology of the four human retroviruses is shown in Figure 376–2. The oncoronaviruses have an electron-dense spherical core while the lentiretroviruses have a cylindrical core.

Their genetic structure (Fig. 376–3) includes the three genes common to all retroviruses: a *gag* gene that codes for core antigens (group-associated antigens); a *pol* gene that codes for reverse transcriptase (polymerase), integrase (endonuclease), and protease; and an *env* gene which codes for a transmembrane and external envelope glycoprotein. The *env* gene of HTLV-I also contains a "pX" region that codes for additional regulatory genes *tax* and *rex*, which function in concert to regulate the expression of mature virions. These additional regulatory genes are not derived from cellular genes. The HTLV-I and II viruses share approximately 60 per cent homology (Fig. 376–3) and are tropic for mature, usually CD4+ T lymphocytes.

The human immunodeficiency family of viruses includes HIV-1, the etiologic agent of AIDS, and HIV-2, a West African virus that appears less pathogenic but is also associated with immunodeficiency. HIV-2 shares approximately 30 to 40 per cent homology with HIV-1. Monocytes and macrophages are targets for HIV-1 infection, and neurologic cells can also become infected. The HIV viruses are immunologically related especially in the *gag* region, and there is little cross-reactivity with the HTLV family of viruses. The known additional regulatory and structural genes of HIV-1 are more complex than those of the HTLV viruses (Table 376–1). The *tat* gene, which regulates virus production, and the *rev* gene, which regulates the splicing of viral message allowing larger structural proteins to form, are analogous in function to the *tax* and *rex* genes. These two genes work together to permit a burst of viral replication synchronous with cellular

replication. They are essential for viral expression and may provide targets for future therapy. The function of other expressed small viral genes has been deduced primarily from deletion mutations and are essential in some cases for mature virion expression.

EPIDEMIOLOGY AND MODES OF TRANSMISSION OF HUMAN RETROVIRUSES. *Origin of Human Retroviruses.* The origin of human retroviruses is unclear. Retroviruses related to HTLV-I/II and HIV-1/2 have been isolated from several primate species, especially from Africa, suggesting the possibility of enzootic transmission to man. An African origin of HTLV-I is also supported by the fact that HTLV-I clusters among persons of African descent in the Caribbean but not in other populations. However, clusters of HTLV-I in southern Japan and northeastern Iran as well as elsewhere make the origin of this class of virus more difficult to discern. Although HTLV-I often appears in endemic clusters in a population, the pattern for HIV-1 is that of an epidemic contagion that is spreading worldwide. HIV-1 may be derived from a older virus, since its replicated mechanisms of cell infection and pathogenic function are highly evolved and adapted to complex human T-cell structures such as the CD4 molecule. Yet surveys of many populations have identified no evidence for widespread HIV-1 infection prior to the mid-1970's, when the epidemic of positivity first became evident in high-risk U.S. populations. There are only sporadic examples of putative infection in some rare individuals as early as the 1960's in Africa, a single putative positive in the United States with a possible history of male homosexual contact in the late 1960's, and a polymerase chain reaction–proven case of a British seaman from 1959.

Features of HTLV. The epidemiology of retroviruses has been largely defined through the use of antibody testing. Since virus-positive antibody-negative individuals could be missed by antibody tests, the true prevalence of virus may be underestimated. However, small-scale surveys employing polymerase chain reaction have not detected large numbers of virus-positive, antibody-

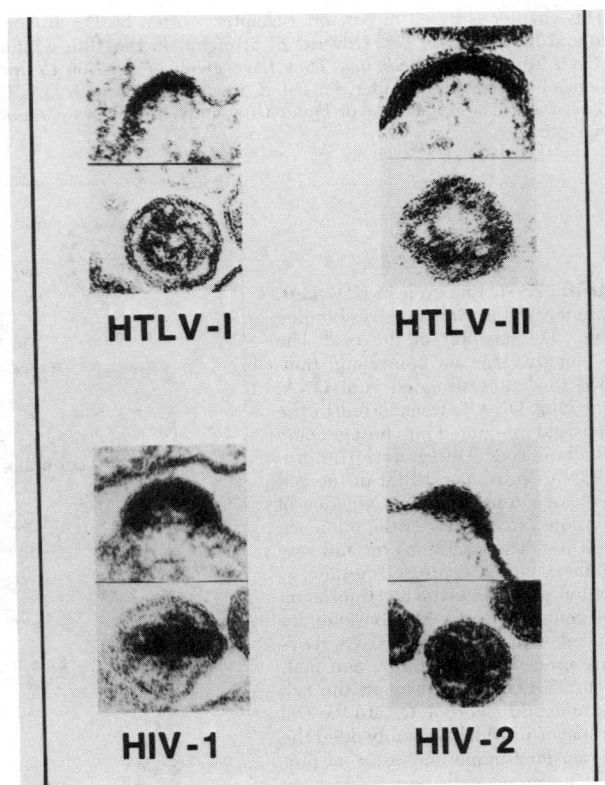

FIGURE 376–2. Morphology of human retroviruses. Electron micrographs of HTLV and HIV human retroviruses. The budding particles are shown in the upper panel for each virus and the mature virion in the lower panel. The HTLV-I and -II viruses have a spherical core and HIV-1 and -2 have a cylindrical core. (From Blattner WA: Retroviruses. *In* Evans A (ed.): Viral Infections of Humans, Epidemiology and Control, 3rd ed. New York, Plenum Publishing, 1989, pp 545–592.)

FIGURE 376-3. Genomic structure of human retroviruses. LTR = Long terminal repeat, which is organized into three regions: U5, R, and U3, which house the polyadenylation site; and the *rev*—responsive element—and the transactivating response (TAR) element, which are involved in controlling virus expression. *gag* = Gene for core protein. *pol* = Gene for reverse transcriptase, integrase, and protease. *env* = Envelope gene. *tax/tat* = Transactivating genes of HTLV and HIV. *rex/rev* = Viral regulatory genes involved in promoting genomic RNA production. *vif, vpr, vpu, vpx,* and *nef* = Additional regulatory genes whose functions are summarized in Table 376-1. (Reprinted by permission from *Nature*, Vol. 333, p. 504. Copyright © 1988 Macmillan Magazines Limited.)

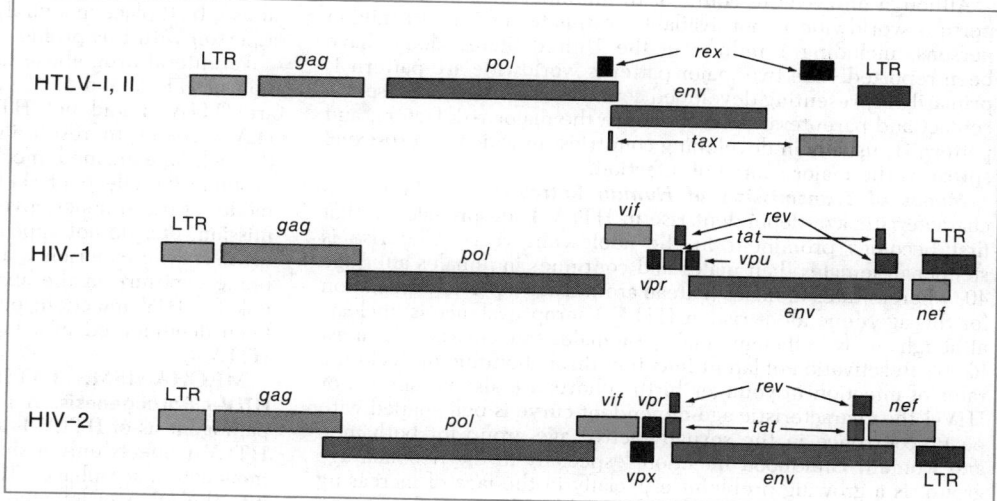

negative individuals, although some instances have been reported. Epidemiologic studies of HTLV-I are complicated by the inability of current serologic assays to distinguish HTLV-I from the closely related HTLV-II virus.

The distribution of antibody positivity in populations varies by region and risk group. Geographic clustering of HTLV-I is exemplified by endemic foci of HTLV-I in southern Japan (Kyushu, Shikoku, and the islands of the Ryukyu chain, including Okinawa) but not in Honshu and other areas of Japan. Extensive surveys of China, Korea, Taiwan, and Vietnam are also largely negative; high rates are reported from Papau New Guinea, but serologic and epidemiologic data raise the possibility that this reactivity is associated with a new variant of HTLV-I. A major focus of HTLV-I infection occurs in the Caribbean region. In Trinidad and Tobago, seropositivity is restricted almost exclusively to persons of African descent, even though individuals of Indo-Asian ethnic background have shared a common environment for over 100 years. In Jamaica highest rates of positivity are observed in the lowland, high-rainfall areas. In Colombia, HTLV-I clusters along the Pacific Coast in an area with an unusually high rate of the associated neurologic syndrome. Other areas of South America with documented foci of HTLV-I include Brazil, Venezuela, Surinam, and Guyana. In Panama, a cluster of HTLV-II was recently reported in an isolated Indian population, representing the first known endemic focus for this orphan virus.

Recent surveys of the African continent (Nigeria, Zaire, Kenya, Tanzania) document that rates of HTLV-I seropositivity are similar to those in the Caribbean region, with documented examples of a microgeographic clustering in Zaire. Recently a focus of HTLV-I was found among Iranian Jews from northeastern Iran residing in Israel and New York.

Migrant populations often acquire infection early in life and carry their virus infection to nonendemic areas where disease may appear years later. Migrant populations from Okinawa to Hawaii and from the Caribbean to the United States and the

United Kingdom are risk groups for HTLV positivity, as are Americans who experience exposure through sexual contact or transfusion in viral endemic areas.

Appearance and Nature of AIDS (see Ch. 412). Acquired immunodeficiency syndrome was recognized as a new disease among United States homosexual males in 1981. The disease was associated with a loss of T4 cells, progressive immunodeficiency manifesting with opportunistic infections, frequent development of certain tumors (particularly the peculiar multifocal proliferation known as Kaposi's sarcoma), and frequent impairment of the central nervous system. It was soon learned that the causal agent could also be transmitted by blood, plasma, and Factor VIII concentrate, and additional risk groups were identified (hemophiliacs, recipients of blood, and intravenous drug abusers and their sexual partners). The same disease was reported in central Africa and in Haiti, largely affecting sexually active heterosexual populations. By 1983 there were many theories on the cause of AIDS. One of these, the hypothesis that AIDS was caused by a new human T4 lymphotropic retrovirus, was proposed in 1982 and turned out to be correct. This idea was based on information derived from experiences with HTLV-I (and II) and from the feline leukemia virus. The latter virus causes a T-cell leukemia of cats, but a minor variant (of the envelope gene) causes an AIDS-like disease in cats. With the use of the same basic technology that had been employed for the isolation of HTLV-I, a new retrovirus termed LAV was identified in a patient with lymphadenopathy in 1983. In early 1984, numerous isolates of a new human retrovirus (termed HTLV-III) were described, and the virus was characterized, produced in permanent cell lines, used for development of a successful test to screen blood prior to transfusion, and unambiguously shown to be the cause of AIDS. In addition, reagents specific for this virus were developed and the virus was shown to be the same as the isolate obtained in 1983. The virus could now properly be called the AIDS virus or the human immunodeficiency virus (HIV-1).

TABLE 376-1. ROLE OF THE HIV ACCESSORY GENES FOR VIRUS REPLICATION

	Immunogenicity	Size	Cellular Localization	Function	Replication Competence of (−) Mutants
Viral infectivity factor (*vif*)	+	p23	Cytoplasm/inner membrane	Infectivity	±
Transactivating protein gene (*tat*)	+	p14	Nucleus/nucleolus	Transcriptional and post-transcriptional activation	−
Regulation of expression of virion gene (*rev*)	+	p19	Nucleus/nucleolus	Expression of structural proteins; modulation of transcription	−
Negative regulator factor gene (*nef*)	+ +	p27	Cytoplasm	Negative regulator	+ +
Viral protein R gene (*vpr*)	+	p18	Nucleus	Rapid viral growth (?)	+ +
Viral protein U gene (*vpu*) (HIV-1)	+	p15	Cytoplasm/membrane	Assembly and release (?)	+
Viral protein R gene (*vpx*)	+	p15	Cytoplasm	?	+ +

Although an accurate count of the number of HIV-1 infected persons worldwide is not available, estimates of 5 to 10 million persons, including 1 million in the United States alone, have been reported. The two major patterns worldwide are pattern I, primarily representing developed countries, in which homosexual contact and parenteral drug abuse are the major risk factors, and pattern II, usually in developing countries, in which heterosexual spread is the major source of infection.

Modes of Transmission of Human Retroviruses. There is a characteristic age-dependent rise in HTLV-I seroprevalence that first becomes prominent in the adolescent years. The rise is steeper in females than males and continues in females after age 40, whereas rates in males plateau around age 40. The explanation for this age-dependent rise in HTLV-I seroprevalence is unclear, although more efficient male-to-female transmission is most likely. Reactivation of latent infection throughout life or declining rates of infection in younger birth cohorts are also possible. For HIV-1 the characteristic age-dependent curve is bell-shaped with peak occurrence in the sexually active age group for both men and women. Childhood infection, especially in the neonatal age group, is a growing problem, especially in the face of increasing heterosexual spread. Summarized in Table 376–2 are the routes, cofactors, and viral characteristics associated with transmission of human retroviruses. The basic modes of transmission of HTLV-I are quite analogous to those of HIV-1.

Sexual transmission of HTLV-I from male to female and female to male as well as from male to male has been documented. HIV-1, which can be transmitted cell free (whereas HTLV-I is cell-associated) appears to be at least an order of magnitude more infectious than HTLV-I. Another cofactor for sexual transmission of HTLV and HIV is the coincidence of other sexually transmitted diseases, particularly ulcerative genital lesions such as occur in syphilis. Higher HIV-1 virus load, as measured by free p24 virus antigen and by quantitative PCR, is associated with heightened efficiency of transmission. For HTLV-I, elevated antibody titer, which also may correlate with virus load, is linked to heightened transmission.

The second major route of transmission is from mother to child. For HTLV-I, breast feeding, as documented from Japanese studies, is more efficient than perinatal transmission. For example, whereas 20 per cent of breast-fed infants seroconvert to HTLV-I, only 1 to 2 per cent of bottle-fed infants of HTLV-I–positive mothers become infected. In this regard HTLV-I differs from HIV-1 because perinatal transmission of HIV-1 appears to be associated with up to 30 per cent of neonatal (transplacental and/or perinatal) infections. The rate of breast milk–associated HIV-1 transmission is unknown because most HIV-1–positive mothers in the United States are discouraged from breast feeding.

A third major route of transmission is parenteral, via either transfusion or intravenous drug abuse. In the case of transfusion transmission, cellular components are associated with transmission of HTLV-I, whereas HIV-1 can be transmitted by cells, plasma, or plasma products. Approximately one half of recipients of HTLV-positive blood seroconvert, while for HIV-1 the percentage is over 95 per cent. Whereas AIDS results from HIV-1 transfusion transmission in a large percentage of cases, the only documented illness linked to HTLV-I transfusion transmission is the HTLV-associated demyelinating neurologic syndrome de-

TABLE 376–2. MODES OF HUMAN RETROVIRUS TRANSMISSION

Route
  Sexual: Male-to-female, female-to-male, and male-to-male
  Parenteral: Transfusion or IV drug abuse
  Mother-to-child transplacental, perinatal, and breast feeding
Cofactors
  Sexual
    Large number of sexual partners
    Traumatic sexual practice
    Coincident sexually transmitted diseases
  Needle sharing
Infectivity
  Virus replication
  Immune status—activated T-cell targets

scribed below. Among blood donors in the United States who are confirmed HTLV positive (approximately half are HTLV-I and the other half HTLV-II), the major risk factors are drug abuse, birthplace in a viral endemic area, and sexual contact with a person with this profile.

Parenteral drug abuse has also been associated with transmission of HTLV and HIV virus. The majority of HTLV positives are HTLV-II and not HTLV-I. Coinfection with HTLV-I and HIV-1 seems to result in a more rapid progression to AIDS through unexplained mechanisms possibly related to the cell-proliferative effects of HTLV-I on HIV-1 infected T cells. Other modes of transmission involving "casual contact," mosquito transmission, etc. do not appear to occur. Health care and laboratory workers who experience a needle stick or skin or mucous membrane exposure in the absence of protective barriers are at low risk for HIV infection; only a single case of such infection has been documented in a Japanese health care worker exposed to HTLV-I.

MECHANISM, PATHOGENESIS, AND PATHOLOGY.
HTLV-I Pathogenesis. A great deal has been learned about the pathogenesis of HTLV-I–associated leukemia. Early in infection, HTLV-I infects only a small number of T cells and perhaps the monocyte/macrophage. The DNA provirus randomly integrates into the DNA of infected cells. Whereas HTLV-I may exist as a latent virus, the genes of the virus promote cell proliferation by direct and indirect mechanisms including various lymphokine pathways. For example when lymphocytes from HTLV-I–infected normal persons are placed in tissue culture, they undergo spontaneous (in the absence of exogenous antigens or mitogens) lymphocyte proliferation. At some point, a clone of transformed, but not malignant, cells emerges, probably from a polyclonally transformed population. Such polyclonal, oligoclonal, and monoclonal expansions have been noted to appear and sometimes disappear spontaneously. After a long latent period (years to several decades), a monoclonal malignancy may develop, presumably involving additional oncogenic mutations. The reasons why only a small percentage of infected individuals develop malignancy (1 to 3 per cent lifetime risk), the disease takes so long to develop, and T4 cells are selectively involved (although T8 cells can also be infected) remain unknown. When malignancy develops, the HTLV-I provirus is found integrated in the DNA of the leukemic cells in a clonal fashion. The tumor contains one copy (or occasionally two copies) of the provirus integrated in the same chromosomal location in each cell. This means that the tumor was derived from a single transformed cell and that the virus infection occurred before transformation and clonal expansion, rather than later as a passenger virus. Tumors from different patients, however, have the provirus in different locations. This means that the mechanism cannot be a *cis*-activation of a nearby cellular gene by the LTR of the virus, as occurs with some animal leukemia viruses. It is postulated that transformation may involve at some stage the viral up-regulatory *tat* protein encoded by the px gene of HTLV-I. The *tat* protein induces expression of cellular genes critical for T-cell proliferation, including IL2 and its receptor (IL2R). The cells apparently both produce and respond to these growth factors (autocrine or autostimulation). This is probably the first step in leukemogenesis, and it leads to polyclonal T-cell proliferation. For the development of malignancy, one or more additional genetic changes are probably required because these cells become independent of IL2 requirements for growth. The continued expression of these growth factor receptors is likely to be a major abnormality in this leukemia. The nature and cause of the additional genetic changes are unknown, but these changes do not appear to require unique environmental factors, since the incidence of ATL is similar, for example, in the Caribbean region and Japan.

The pathogenesis of the HTLV-associated demyelinating neurologic syndrome, tropical spastic paraparesis/HTLV-associated myelopathy (TSP/HAM), is uncertain but appears to occur with a much shorter latency (sometimes acutely following transfusion-associated infection) than does ATL. Some researchers postulate a direct mechanism involving infection of nervous system cells, whereas others suggest an indirect mechanism involving immune- and autoimmune-mediated responses due to HTLV-I infection of regulatory T-cell populations.

Pathogenesis and Mechanisms of HIV-1. HIV-1 may be transmitted either as free extracellular virus or by virus-infected cells.

When transmitted by an infected cell, this "donor" cell may contact a target cell, the viral genes may then become activated, and virus is transmitted directly to the recipient cell. This route could avoid immune detection or exposure of the virus to antibodies. This mechanism may explain documented cases of virus-positive antibody-negative individuals as detected by virus culture and PCR. The duration of this latency is controversial and may vary from weeks to months. However, in general several weeks to months after exposure, a humoral immune response usually develops. High titers of antibodies are often made against every viral protein. This includes antibodies to the envelope of the virus, but the critical neutralizing antibodies (against one or more epitopes of the envelope) made after infection do not appear to prevent disease, presumably because the titers are too low or the response is too late, or both. Furthermore, it is now well documented that certain epitopes of the viral external envelope are hypervariable so that a series of quasispecies of viruses emerge which are resistant to immune inactivation. Cellular immunity (T-cell cytotoxicity against infected cells) has been well documented and appears to involve, among other sites, the same hypervariable neutralizing epitope that is shared by antibodies. The major target cells of HIV are the T4 cell and the monocyte/macrophage. Cells of the reticuloendothelial system, such as the Langerhans cells of the skin and follicular dendritic cells of the lymph node germinal centers and neuroglial cells of the brain, may also be infected. It appears that most target cells have CD4 on the cell surface. The mechanism by which HIV brings about destruction of the immune system is complex. In contrast to the immunostimulating effects of HTLV, HIV is immunoablative through both direct and probably indirect mechanisms.

For example, when the CD4 cell containing integrated HIV-1 DNA is immunostimulated, the HIV-1 provirus is activated, virus particles are formed, the CD4+ cell dies, and the virus spreads to reinitiate the process, which in time leads to a progressive depletion of the T4 cells. Other indirect mechanisms involving subversion of T-cell regulatory pathways, autoimmune phenomena, and immune paralysis have also been invoked to explain the discrepancy between the relatively small number of infected cells and the severity of the immune defect associated with HIV-1 infection. Infected macrophages may bring the virus to the brain, or free virus may cross the blood-brain barrier and infect microglial and possibly other non-neuronal cells. These cells may release factors that cause the major pathologic changes in the brain.

For HIV, the incubation period between infection and disease is estimated to range from 2 to 15 years or more, with a median of 8 to 10 years. In contrast to HTLV, which has a relatively low attack rate (3 to 5 per cent lifetime risk), HIV is projected to cause serious morbidity in over 60 to 80 per cent or more of infected persons. Prospective cohort studies document that 90 per cent of infected people progress from their presenting stage to a more advanced disease stage within 1.5 to 3 years. The major cofactor influencing progression is age. Newborns tend to progress more rapidly than adults, and older children and adolescents progress more slowly than adults or infants. The adolescent–young adult group tends to progress more slowly to immune depletion (e.g., CD4 count less than 200) than do adults, and once impaired they tend to take much longer to manifest clinical disease. A role for other cofactors has been postulated, including the occurrence of other viral infections, variation in HIV strain, difference in dose of inoculum, and nutritional status. Interestingly HTLV-I, perhaps owing to its shared regulatory structure or its immunostimulating effects, appears to accelerate progression to AIDS in HIV/HTLV-coinfected individuals. Some herpesviruses, including cytomegalovirus and human virus type 6 (HHV-6), may also accelerate progression, but the findings are controversial. Ultimately the fact that progression to AIDS shows a similar curve (controlling for age) in all risk groups suggests that most cofactor effects are less important than HIV-1 infection itself.

CLINICAL MANIFESTATIONS AND DIAGNOSIS. The list of HTLV-I–associated diseases has grown since adult T-cell leukemia/lymphoma (ATL) was first etiologically linked to HTLV-I (Table 376–3). The most common malignancy caused by HTLV-I is adult T-cell leukemia/lymphoma (ATL). The worldwide prevalence of these HTLV-I–associated leukemias is unknown; the incidence in any population depends on the prevalence of viral infection. In endemic areas such as southern Japan and the

TABLE 376–3. HTLV-ASSOCIATED DISEASE

Diagnosis	Nature of Syndrome	Strength of Association
Adult T-cell leukemia/lymphoma	Aggressive lymphoproliferative malignancy of mature T lymphocytes	Strong
B-cell chronic lymphocytic leukemia	Tumor-associated immunoglobin reacts to HTLV antigen	2 cases reported
Tropical spastic paraparesis (TSP)/HTLV-associated myelopathy (HAM)	Chronic progressive demyelinating syndrome of long motor tracks of spinal cord	Strong
Polymyositis	Degenerative inflammatory syndrome of skeletal muscles	Probable
Infective dermatitis	Chronic generalized eczema of skin; potential for preleukemia and immunodeficiency	Probable
Immune deficiency	Anecdotal reports of AIDS-like illness in HTLV-I positives; subclinical (e.g., decreased PPD response) or clinical (e.g., poor response to therapy for symptomatic strongyloidiasis)	Possible
Miscellaneous clinical conditions	Case reports or case series of polyarthropathy, interstitial pneumonitis, small cell lung cancer with monoclonal HTLV-I integration, and invasive cervical cancer in Japan	Uncertain

Caribbean islands, the annual incidence of virus-associated leukemia is approximately 3 per 100,000 per year and may account for one half of adult lymphoid malignancies in HTLV-I–endemic areas. The chance of an infected individual's developing malignancy over a lifetime is 1 to 5 per cent, with early-life exposure associated with the greatest risk for subsequent disease.

As further experience with ATL has been gained in viral endemic areas, the breadth of clinical variants has become more evident. The acute form of ATL as first described in Japan is characterized by an aggressive mature T-cell lymphoma whose clinical course is often associated with high white count, hypercalcemia, and cutaneous involvement. Other cases resemble T-cell chronic lymphocytic leukemia and are termed chronic ATL. Smoldering ATL may clinically resemble mycosis fungoides/Sezary syndrome with cutaneous involvement presenting as erythema or as infiltrative plaques or tumors. Sometimes a long prodrome of symptoms is noted before transformation to an acute, rapidly fatal form of disease occurs. Sometimes ATL presents as a T-cell non-Hodgkin's lymphoma with no clinical features of ATL except monoclonal integration of HTLV-I in proviral DNA in the tumor cells. Most patients with acute ATL die within 6 months of diagnosis. The cause of death is usually an explosive growth of tumor cells, hypercalcemia, and various opportunistic infections including *Pneumocystis carinii* pneumonia and other infections observed in AIDS patients. The age group ranges from adolescence to a peak in middle-aged adults. The diagnosis should be considered in adults with mature T-cell lymphoma and hypercalcemia and/or cutaneous involvement, particularly if the individual is from a known risk group or known endemic region. The diagnosis is established by testing serum for HTLV-I antibodies and finding leukemic T cells with the provirus in the blood or in biopsy specimens.

Other HTLV-I–Associated Diseases. An association between HTLV-I and some cases of B-cell chronic lymphotropic leukemia is now recognized. In this case, the role of the virus appears to be indirect. No viral sequences are found in the tumor, but the immunoglobulins of the tumor cell react to HTLV-I–specific antigens. It may be that chronic stimulation of B-cell proliferation by viral antigens, coupled with virus-induced impairment of T4-cell function, leads to an increase in the probability of malignant transformation in B cells.

HTLV-I has been linked to a neurologic syndrome called TSP/HAM. This disease is characterized by the usually chronic, slowly progressive development of spastic paraparesis resulting from the demyelination of the long motor neurons of the spinal cord. Symptoms often begin with a stiff gait progressing (usually slowly) to increasing spasticity and weakness, with incontinence and impotence developing later during the course of the illness. Sometimes ataxia develops. On nuclear magnetic resonance scan isolated lesions of the central nervous system are detected in some cases. The syndrome differs from classic multiple sclerosis because of the generally slow, progressive course and absence of waxing and waning of symptomatology. However, some cases are acutely progressive and such cases are sometimes associated with the transfusion of HTLV-I–positive blood. The incidence of disease is thought to be approximately twice that of ATL, and an indirect mechanism of pathogenesis, possibly immune-mediated, has been postulated, although direct viral infection of nervous system tissue has not been ruled out. The diagnosis is suspected in unexplained central nervous system disease with loss of pyramidal tract functions and is confirmed by testing sera for HTLV-I antibodies. There is no known treatment. Recently HTLV-I has also been linked to some cases of polymyositis of skeletal muscle in viral endemic areas. There are no features of these cases which distinguish this syndrome from polymyositis seen in HTLV-I–nonendemic areas. Possible links of HTLV-I to immunosuppression come from clinical and laboratory observations. Cases from Japan of patients with AIDS-like illnesses associated with HTLV-I (in the absence of underlying malignancy) have been reported. The association of HTLV-I with parasitic infestations (e.g., strongyloides) refractory to treatment have also been interpreted to suggest that HTLV-I may have immunosuppressive effects. Decreased skin test response to recall antigens has also been reported among HTLV-I–infected, especially older, individuals. The infective dermatitis syndrome in Jamaica may represent the first childhood HTLV-I syndrome, and immunosuppression and preleukemia are possible features. Other clinical syndromes mentioned as possible HTLV-associated diseases include large joint polyarthropathy and interstitial pneumonitis. A case of small cell lung cancer with monoclonal HTLV integration is of interest as well as the finding in Japan that invasive cervical cancer may also be HTLV-I–associated.

HTLV-II and Leukemia. This virus has been found in several cases of T-cell hairy cell leukemia and frequently among parenteral drug abusers. Recently a focus of HTLV-II was reported in an isolated tribe of Central American Indians in Panama. While molecular biologic studies of the leukemia cells from the HTLV-II–positive leukemia cases strongly suggest that HTLV-II is causally involved, surveys of hairy cell leukemia including some with T-cell phenotype have failed to document an association. HTLV-II, like HLTV-I, induces spontaneous lymphocyte proliferation in vitro but at a lower level than HTLV-I. HTLV-II remains a true orphan virus without clear disease association. The recognition of a naturally occurring endemic focus of HTLV-II in Panama and the development of new techniques for distinguishing HTLV-I from HTLV-II should make it feasible in coming years to characterize the epidemiology and clinical outcomes of infection.

CLINICAL MANIFESTATIONS OF HIV INFECTIONS.
The spectrum of clinical outcomes, particularly opportunistic infection linked to HIV infection, is quite broad as detailed in Part XXI. While contributing to a relatively smaller percentage of AIDS-associated morbidity and mortality, certain malignancies such as Kaposi's sarcoma, B-cell lymphomas, and some carcinomas are more common in HIV-infected persons in association with varying levels of immune impairment. These malignancies are not directly due to HIV as a transforming virus, since viral genes are not present in the DNA of the cells of any of these tumors. Kaposi's sarcoma associated with HIV is composed of endothelial cells, fibroblasts, and other infiltrating cells, and recently indirect HIV-mediated growth factors have been defined which contribute to pathogenesis. Since Kaposi's sarcoma is very common in HIV-1–infected homosexuals but much less so in other HIV-infected individuals, another still unknown etiologic factor may be involved. The B-cell lymphomas are of several types, including some with rearranged c-*myc* genes in association

with Epstein-Barr virus analogous to the pattern reported in Burkitt's lymphoma. Recently, a new virus called human herpesvirus type 6 (HHV6) was isolated from some cases, but its pathogenic role is unclear. The study of HIV-associated lymphomas provides a unique opportunity to gain fundamental etiologic insights, especially since the number of lymphoma cases may be increasing in association with prolonged survival in HIV-infected persons on antiretroviral therapy.

TREATMENT AND PREVENTION. *HTLV-I.* There is no proven effective therapy for ATL; however, some cases do respond, occasionally with prolonged remission, to multidrug regimens for advanced-stage aggressive lymphoma. Exciting experimental approaches that employ monoclonal antibodies to the IL2 receptor which can be linked with cell toxins, selectively targeted to the leukemic cells, are one example. Other approaches involving antiretroviral therapy and various lymphokines are under consideration. Treatment of the complicating hypercalcemia often responds to standard methods but may be refractory, and opportunistic infections are frequent. Prevention is achieved by avoiding infection: testing blood prior to transfusion, care in sexual practices, and avoidance of mother-infant transmission by discouraging breast feeding.

Vaccines containing recombinant HTLV-I envelope produced in *Escherichia coli* and vaccinia virus–based expression vectors have been used successfully to prevent HTLV-I infection in monkeys and rabbits. Various sites that represent important biologic and immunologic epitopes of HTLV-I envelope have been mapped. The envelope gene of HTLV-I encodes a 63- to 67-kilodalton (kd) glycoprotein precursor that is proteolytically processed to give rise to a mature gp46 external envelope glycoprotein and a 21-kd transmembrane protein designated as p21E. Using rabbit antisera to the N- and C-terminal portions of HTLV-I gp63 envelope precursor, Japanese investigations have neutralized both American and Japanese HTLV-I isolates in vitro. Results indicate the presence of at least two neutralizing sites on HTLV-I envelope, one associated with the external gp46 envelope glycoprotein and a second associated with the p21E transmembrane glycoprotein. A vaccine consisting of an envelope subunit of HTLV generated protective immunity in cynomolgus monkeys against primary infection by HTLV-I. Of interest is that this study employed HTLV-I–infected cells as the challenge vehicle, which is a step closer to natural transmission than free virus itself. Protection correlated with the presence of neutralizing antibodies, indicating that humoral immunity can be an effective barrier against infection. More intensive studies are currently being carried out in a rabbit model of HTLV-I infection. This approach enables the optimization of candidate HTLV vaccines in terms of immunogenicity and efficacy. Since human or animal antisera to Japanese and American HTLV-I envelope cross-neutralize, it is likely that the envelope antigens of HTLV-I represent a single serotype worldwide. Thus, unlike the isolate-specific neutralizing epitopes of HIV, a synthetic vaccine against one HTLV-I isolate should protect against other HTLV-I isolates.

HIV. As detailed in Ch. 411, an understanding of the fundamental biology of HIV has also led to therapeutic breakthroughs. Nucleotide analogues, which can be used as antimetabolites against the error-prone virus reverse transcriptase, have already resulted in substantial benefit to patients with AIDS and ARC and with depressed T cells. Examples of this class of drugs with proven efficacy include azidothymidine (AZT) and dideoxyinosine (DDI). Combinations of these and other drugs may also show the type of benefit first noted in combination chemotherapy for cancer. Other promising approaches, such as hybrid molecules that block CD4 binding of the virus, are the subject of ongoing therapeutic research. The major preventive strategies for HIV, in the absence of an effective vaccine, are to promote public health programs that decrease the likelihood of transmission. This includes educational campaigns which emphasize that HIV is a sexually transmitted agent. For parenteral drug abusers, elimination of needle sharing or, better yet, elimination of needle use through drug abuse treatment, as well as safe sex has also been promoted. A successful prevention strategy has been the implementation of screening of the blood supply for HIV, which has virtually eliminated this source of infection for hemophiliacs and blood recipients. HIV-1–positive women, whose children have a risk of infection from perinatal transmission of approximately 30 per cent, are encouraged not to breast feed their babies if they do conceive.

The goal of vaccine development is to generate an immune response that will be broadly reactive against all variants of the AIDS virus. A variety of approaches, including whole virus and subunit vaccines based on viral envelope proteins and *gag* antigen, are being tried (see Ch. 413). Type-specific neutralizing antibodies can be induced in many species, including primates, using native envelope glycoprotein, but no broadly reactive immunity has yet been achieved in animal studies. There are some early indications that some vaccine approaches are working in primate models. However, results are not yet reproducible, and the variation in virus strains, particularly at critical neutralizing sites, presents formidable barriers that need to be overcome.

SUMMARY

The story of human retrovirology is in its infancy, but it is already one of the most fascinating and important chapters in contemporary medicine. These viruses seem destined to open many doors to our knowledge of disease causation and provide conceptual advances in our understanding of disease pathogenesis. The human retroviruses—or viruses with similar properties of long latency, minimal replication, lymphotropism, and neurotropism—may be at the heart of some of our important unexplained autoimmune, immunodeficiency, and neurologic diseases. Some may be involved in other human malignancies.

Blattner WA (ed.): Human Retrovirology: HTLV. New York, Raven Press, 1990. *Comprehensive update of human T-cell leukemia virus, including chapters on virology, immunology, epidemiology, clinical features, and management.*

Bolognasi D: Immunobiology of the HIV envelope and its relativity to vaccine strategies. Mol Biol Med 7:1–15, 1990. *An updated review of HIV vaccine prospects and pitfalls.*

Ensoli B, Salahuddin SZ, Gallo RC: AIDS-associated Kaposi's sarcoma: A molecular model for its pathogenesis. Cancer Cells 1:93–96, 1989. *In this paper are reviewed new concepts of growth factor–mediated Kaposi's sarcoma carcinogenesis.*

Gallo RC, Montagnier L: AIDS in 1988. Sci Am 259:41–48, 1988. *The entire October, 1988 issue of Scientific American provides a readable and well-illustrated review of AIDS and HIV-related issues.*

Gallo RC, Wong-Staal F (eds.): Retrovirus Biology and Human Disease. New York, Marcel Dekker, Inc., 1990. *This scholarly book includes comprehensive reviews of the biology and molecular biology of human retroviruses.*

Goedert JJ, Kessler CM, Aledort LM, et al.: A prospective study of human immunodeficiency virus type 1 infection and the development of AIDS in subjects with hemophilia. N Engl J Med 321:1141–1148, 1989. *The natural history of HIV infection, particularly the role of age in progression to AIDS, is analyzed in this paper.*

Mitsuya H, Yarchoan R, Broder S: Molecular targets for AIDS therapy. Science 249:1533–1544, 1990. *A comprehensive review of current and future approaches to anti-HIV therapy which evaluates the basic molecular biology of the virus and the potential targets for therapeutic benefit.*

377 Enteroviral Diseases

Michael N. Oxman

Enteroviruses, so named because they generally infect the alimentary tract and are shed in the feces, cause a wide variety of diseases in humans and lower animals. They comprise one of the four major genera of the *Picornavirus* (pico, small; *rna,* ribonucleic acid) *Family.* The other picornavirus genera, distinguished from each other primarily by difference in sensitivity to acid and in buoyant density in cesium chloride, are *rhinoviruses,* which inhabit the upper respiratory tract and include the principal recognized etiologic agents of the common cold (see Ch. 360); *cardioviruses,* recovered chiefly from rodents and only very rarely implicated in human disease; and *aphthoviruses,* named for the vesicular lesions that they produce in cloven-footed animals. Only the enterovirus and rhinovirus genera contain important human pathogens.

Enteroviruses are differentiated from rhinoviruses primarily by their resistance to acid; they are fully infectious at pH 3 or even lower. Consequently, enteroviruses that have undergone limited replication in the oropharynx survive passage through the stomach and implant in the lower intestinal tract, where they undergo more extensive multiplication. In contrast, rhinoviruses are acid labile; they begin to lose infectivity at pH 6 and are completely inactivated at pH 3. They are further distinguished from enteroviruses by their lower optimal temperature of replication (33°C versus 37°C for enteroviruses) and higher buoyant density in cesium chloride. Since rhinoviruses inhabit the nasopharynx, they have no obvious need for acid stability, and their preferential replication at lower than body temperature probably reflects their adaptation to the cooler nasal passages.

Species of enteroviruses are distinguished immunologically by the ability of specific antisera to neutralize only the homotypic virus. There are now 68 recognized human enterovirus species (*serotypes* or *immunotypes*), as well as numerous enteroviruses of lower animals. Humans appear to be the only natural host for the human enteroviruses, and, in general, the enteroviruses of lower animals are not natural pathogens for humans.

Historically, human enteroviruses have been subclassified into *polioviruses,* group A and group B *coxsackieviruses,* and *echoviruses* on the basis of antigenic relationships, differences in host range, and type of disease produced (Table 377–1). By 1969, 67 species (serotypes) of human enteroviruses had been identified and classified according to these criteria, although reclassification and redundancy have reduced this number to 63. The distinguishing characteristics of these enterovirus subgroups are outlined below.

Polioviruses. The first human enteroviruses to be recognized, polioviruses produce characteristic lesions when inoculated into the central nervous system of primates. Clinical isolates replicate only in primates and in primate cell cultures (see Ch. 475). There are three poliovirus serotypes.

Coxsackieviruses. In contrast to polioviruses, coxsackieviruses produce paralysis and death when inoculated into suckling mice. This property was responsible for their detection and differentiation from polioviruses when they were first recovered in 1948 from the feces of two children in the village of Coxsackie, New York, who were suffering from a poliomyelitis-like paralytic illness. With the isolation of additional serotypes, it was recognized that when inoculated into suckling mice, some coxsackieviruses, designated *group A coxsackieviruses,* produced generalized myositis of skeletal muscles that resulted in flaccid

TABLE 377–1. CLASSIFICATION OF HUMAN ENTEROVIRUSES[a]

Enterovirus Group	Number of Serotypes	Numerical Designation	Growth in Primate Cell Culture	Pathogenicity for Suckling Mice	Pathogenicity for Monkeys
Poliovirus	3	1–3	+	–	+
Coxsackievirus, group A	23	A1–22, A24[b]	+/–[c]	+	–[d]
Coxsackievirus, group B	6	B1–6	+	+	–
Echovirus	31	1–9, 11–27, 29–34[e]	+	–	–
Enterovirus	5	68–72[f]	+[g]	Variable[h]	Variable[i]

[a]Many enterovirus strains have been isolated that do not conform to these criteria.
[b]Coxsackievirus A23 has been reclassified as echovirus 9.
[c]Except for a few serotypes (e.g., A7, A9, A16), primary isolates of group A coxsackieviruses grow poorly or not at all in cell culture; virus isolation requires inoculation of suckling mice.
[d]Coxsackievirus A7 is neurovirulent in monkeys.
[e]Echovirus 10 has been reclassified as reovirus type 1. Echovirus 28 has been reclassified as rhinovirus 1A.
[f]Hepatitis A virus has been classified as human enterovirus 72.
[g]Enterovirus 72 (hepatitis A virus) replicates in monkey kidney cell cultures without producing cytopathic effects.
[h]Enteroviruses 70 and 71 are pathogenic for suckling mice.
[i]Enteroviruses 70 and 71 are neurovirulent in monkeys.

paralysis, whereas others, designated *group B coxsackieviruses*, produced only focal myositis but caused an encephalitis that resulted in spastic paralysis and a generalized infection that involved the myocardium, brown fat, pancreas, and other organs. Moreover, group B coxsackieviruses could be readily propagated in primate cell cultures, whereas group A coxsackieviruses grew poorly or not at all. Twenty-three group A and six group B coxsackievirus serotypes have been identified.

Echoviruses. The use of the cell culture techniques developed by Enders and his associates led to the recovery from the feces of healthy children of additional enteroviruses that produced cytopathic effects in primate cell cultures but failed to produce disease in suckling mice or in the central nervous system of primates. There agents, initially considered "orphan" viruses because they were unrelated to any disease, were called *echoviruses* (enteric *c*ytopathic *h*uman *o*rphan). Echoviruses have now been associated with a variety of diseases, and 31 serotypes have been identified. Most echoviruses are readily propagated in primate cell cultures.

The detailed comparison of enterovirus genomes supports the validity of this classification scheme. Different serotypes within the same human enterovirus subgroup, e.g., group B coxsackieviruses, generally have 30 to 50 per cent of their nucleotide sequences in common, whereas serotypes from different subgroups generally share fewer than 20 per cent of their nucleotide sequences. About 5 per cent of the nucleotide sequences are conserved among all human enteroviruses.

Over the years, however, an increasing number of enterovirus isolates were identified that could not be subclassified unambiguously by these criteria (e.g., viruses serologically related to known echoviruses but with a host range characteristic of coxsackieviruses). Consequently, it was agreed in 1970 that newly recognized human enteroviruses would be simply designated "enterovirus" and numbered sequentially, beginning with enterovirus 68. To avoid confusion with the older literature, the original classification (poliovirus, group A and group B coxsackievirus, and echovirus) has been retained for the first 63 serotypes. Since adoption of this simplified taxonomic scheme, five new human enteroviruses, enteroviruses 68 to 72, have been recognized.

Enteroviruses 68 to 72. Enterovirus 68 was initially isolated from the throat of an infant with bronchiolitis and pneumonia. Few isolates have since been reported, and the agent is little studied. Enterovirus 69 was recovered from the feces of an asymptomatic child, and this serotype has not yet been associated with disease. Enterovirus 70 is the principal cause of acute hemorrhagic conjunctivitis, a disease that was first recognized in 1969 and has subsequently affected tens of millions of persons throughout the world. Enterovirus 70 has an unusually broad host range; it causes meningoencephalitis in humans and experimentally infected monkeys and infects both primate and nonprimate cell cultures. Genome analysis and serologic surveys raise the possibility that it may be a zoonotic enterovirus that has recently extended its host range to include humans. Enterovirus 70 is discussed in Ch. 381. Enterovirus 71, first recognized as the cause of an outbreak of aseptic meningitis and encephalitis in California between 1969 and 1972, is neurovirulent in monkeys and produces a myositis in suckling mice typical of that produced by group A coxsackieviruses. Enterovirus 71 has been recovered throughout the world in association with a variety of clinical manifestations and many fatal infections. These have included respiratory infections, aseptic meningitis, hand-foot-and-mouth disease, maculopapular exanthems, encephalitis, and poliomyelitis-like paralytic disease. Hepatitis A virus has been classified as enterovirus 72 on the basis of its physical, biochemical, and biologic characteristics. However, differences between the nucleotide sequence of its genome and the genomes of other enteroviruses suggest that it may belong in a separate genus. Hepatitis A virus (enterovirus 72) is discussed in Ch. 117.

The enteroviruses have many features in common, and thus they are discussed as a group before considering the special features of individual members. Since polioviruses are the subject of Ch. 475, this discussion is limited to the nonpolio viruses.

CHARACTERISTICS OF NONPOLIO ENTEROVIRUSES

PHYSICAL AND BIOCHEMICAL CHARACTERISTICS. The enteroviruses share with all picornaviruses certain important physical and biochemical characteristics: They are small, spherical, nonenveloped viruses approximately 30 nm in diameter. Their genome consists of a linear, single-stranded, unsegmented molecule of RNA with a molecular weight of about 2.6×10^6 daltons (approximately 7500 nucleotides) which has the same polarity as messenger RNA; i.e., it is plus (+) stranded and is thus infectious and can also be translated in vitro. The viral genome is tightly packed within an icosahedral protein shell or *capsid* composed of 60 identical subunits or *protomers*, each of which has a molecular mass of 90,000 to 100,000 daltons and is itself composed of four nonidentical virus-encoded polypeptides (VP1, VP2, VP3, and VP4). VP1, VP2, and VP3 are exposed on the virion surface, whereas VP4 lies buried in association with the RNA core. Like all picornaviruses, enteroviruses exhibit a unique pattern of replication in which the viral genome is translated into a single giant *polyprotein*, which is then cleaved by endogenous viral proteinases into the individual viral structural and nonstructural proteins.

Enteroviruses are stable over a wide range of pH (pH 3 to 10) and retain infectivity for days at room temperature, weeks at refrigerator temperature, and indefinitely when frozen at $-20°C$ or lower. They are readily inactivated at temperatures above 50°C, but this inactivation is inhibited by molar magnesium chloride, which greatly enhances the stability of enteroviruses at all environmental temperatures. Thus, magnesium chloride is widely employed as a stabilizer for oral poliovirus vaccines.

Enteroviruses are resistant to proteolytic enzymes and to inactivation by organic solvents (e.g., ether, alcohol, chloroform), disinfectants (e.g., Lysol, quaternary ammonium compounds), deoxycholate, and various detergents that destroy lipid-containing enveloped viruses such as herpesviruses, orthomyxoviruses, and paramyxoviruses. Enteroviruses are inactivated by formaldehyde, chlorination, and ultraviolet light but are protected from inactivation by dissolved organic matter, the formation of virus aggregates, and adsorption to particulate matter. Consequently, enteroviruses survive secondary sewage treatment and chlorination as generally practiced and are abundant in raw sewage and treated waste water. The agricultural use of treated sewage and recycled waste water may thus contaminate food and water supplies. Since sewage treatment that destroys fecal coliform bacteria does not eliminate enteroviruses, the use of fecal coliform counts to assess the sanitary quality of water is inadequate with respect to its potential for transmission of enteroviral diseases. Enteroviruses are often detectable in samples of recreational water judged acceptable on the basis of fecal coliform counts. Although person-to-person (fecal-oral) spread is the dominant mode of transmission, and waterborne outbreaks of enterovirus infection have rarely been documented, the hazard associated with the discharge of virus-laden sewage into coastal waters is demonstrated by the occurrence of shellfish-associated outbreaks of hepatitis A (caused by enterovirus 72). Clams, mussels, and oysters are filter-feeders that concentrate virus and function as passive virus carriers. Most of the enteroviruses in sewage are associated with suspended solids, and virus adsorbed to sediment remains infectious for long periods in the marine environment. The reintroduction of specific enteroviruses into coastal populations when marine sediments are disturbed by storms or dredging might explain the sudden occurrence of epidemics and the reappearance of certain enterovirus serotypes after years of absence from the human population.

EPIDEMIOLOGY. Human enteroviruses are worldwide in distribution, and humans are their only known reservoir. The prevalence of enterovirus infection varies markedly with season and climate and with the age and socioeconomic status of the population studied. In tropical and semitropical regions, enterovirus infections are frequent throughout the year. In temperate climates, the incidence of infection is markedly increased in the summer and early fall; 80 to 90 per cent of enterovirus isolates are recovered during the period from June through October, with peak recovery in August. Even within the United States, climatic and socioeconomic factors can be seen to affect the prevalence of enterovirus infections. Enterovirus isolation rates from young children are two- to threefold higher in southern than in northern cities and three- to sixfold higher in lower than in middle and upper socioeconomic districts. In developed countries, usually only one to three enterovirus serotypes are highly prevalent in a given community each year, with different serotypes prevalent in different years, and isolation rates in young children rarely exceed 10 per cent. In developing countries with poor sanitation, a greater number of enterovirus serotypes circulate simultaneously, and isolation rates in children regularly exceed 75 per cent, with many fecal specimens yielding three or more enterovirus serotypes.

Some enteroviruses appear to be endemic, being isolated at low frequency in the same locality each year, whereas others produce local or regional epidemics and then disappear, only to return again years later. Occasionally, an enterovirus spreads worldwide, infecting tens of millions of persons and producing pandemic disease. This pattern was observed with echovirus 9 in the late 1950's and with enterovirus 70, which caused a pandemic of acute hemorrhagic conjunctivitis beginning in 1969 (see Ch. 381).

Enteroviruses exhibit a high rate of mutation during replication in the human gastrointestinal tract, and this can lead to the appearance of antigenic variants, as well as virus strains with altered tissue tropism, host range, and virulence. Such mutations are readily detected within days after the administration of attenuated poliovirus vaccines to normal children. They have also been observed in a number of nonpolio enteroviruses. Recently isolated strains of several coxsackieviruses, echoviruses, and enterovirus 70 have been found to differ in many epitopes from the corresponding *prototype* strains isolated more than a decade earlier, a pattern of "antigenic drift" not unlike that seen with influenza viruses. In addition, recombination between the genomes of different enterovirus serotypes is a frequent occurrence in multiply infected individuals, e.g., in young children in developing countries, and in recipients of trivalent oral poliovirus vaccines. Antigenic changes and alterations in cell tropism produced by mutation and recombination may help to account for the ability of individual enterovirus serotypes to persist in nature and to cause a variety of clinical syndromes.

Transmission of human enteroviruses is chiefly by the fecal-oral route directly from person to person or via fomites; spread by respiratory secretions plays a lesser role. After infection by most serotypes, virus can be recovered from the oropharynx and intestine of both symptomatic and asymptomatic individuals, but virus is shed in greater amounts and for a longer period (a month or more) in the feces.

Young children have the highest rates of infection, and enteroviruses are most efficiently disseminated by infected children less than 2 years of age. Spread is from child to child and then within family groups, and it is facilitated by crowding and poor hygiene. Introduction of virus into the household by one family member results in a high rate of infection among others lacking type-specific neutralizing antibodies; family surveillance studies have demonstrated secondary attack rates of approximately 90 per cent for polioviruses, 75 per cent for coxsackieviruses, and 50 per cent for echoviruses. Middle-class parents with children in day care centers are at particular risk. Reared in circumstances that minimized their childhood exposure, they are likely to be susceptible to infection by many of the enteroviruses brought home from day care centers by their asymptomatically infected toddlers. This is well illustrated by day care center–based outbreaks of hepatitis A (see Ch. 117).

Although the epidemiology of most enteroviruses is similar, patterns of infection with some serotypes are distinctive. Enterovirus 70 and coxsackievirus A24, etiologic agents of acute hemorrhagic conjunctivitis (see Ch. 381), are transmitted by direct inoculation of the conjunctivae by fingers and fomites contaminated with infected tears. Replication of these viruses in the alimentary tract, if it occurs at all, is limited. Coxsackievirus A21 is also shed primarily from the upper respiratory tract, where it produces a rhinovirus-like illness.

The incubation period for illnesses caused by enteroviruses may vary from less than 1 day to more than 4 weeks, but it is generally 2 to 10 days. It is shortest when symptoms are the direct result of virus replication at the portal of entry (e.g., acute hemorrhagic conjunctivitis caused by enterovirus 70) and longest when they reflect tissue injury that involves immunopathology in target organs infected following viremia (e.g., hepatitis A and some forms of coxsackievirus myocarditis).

PATHOGENESIS. The pathogenesis of enterovirus infections is best understood for polioviruses, which have been extensively studied in experimentally infected primates and in humans infected with attenuated vaccine strains. The pathogenesis of most nonpolio enterovirus infections appears to be similar, except for the principal target organs affected.

Following ingestion of fecally contaminated material by individuals lacking type-specific neutralizing antibodies, virus implants and replicates in susceptible tissues of the pharynx and distal small intestine. These probably include mucosal epithelial cells and lymphoid tissues in the lamina propria, tonsils, and Peyer's patches. Within a day or two virus spreads to regional lymph nodes, and on about the third day small quantities escape into the blood stream (the "minor viremia") and are disseminated throughout the reticuloendothelial system (liver, spleen, bone marrow, lymph nodes) and to other receptor-bearing target tissues. None of the replicative events up to this point produce symptoms and, in most cases, infection is contained by host defense mechanisms without further progression, resulting in asymptomatic infection. In a minority of infected persons, replication continues in reticuloendothelial tissues, producing, by about the fifth day, a heavy sustained viremia (the "major viremia") that coincides with the "minor illness" of poliovirus infection (see Ch. 475) and with the "nonspecific febrile illness" caused by other human enteroviruses. The major viremia also disseminates large amounts of virus to target organs, such as the spinal cord, brain, meninges, heart, and skin, where further virus replication results in inflammatory lesions and cell necrosis. In most such patients, host defense mechanisms quickly terminate the major viremia and halt virus replication in target organs; only rarely is virus replication in target organs extensive enough to be clinically manifest. Although other host defense mechanisms (e.g., macrophages, interferon production) are doubtless involved, neutralizing antibodies play a major role in terminating viremia and limiting enterovirus multiplication in target tissues. Serotype-specific neutralizing antibodies may be detected in the serum within 4 or 5 days of the infection, and they generally persist for life. Evidence for the critical role of antibodies in terminating infection is provided by the occurrence of chronic persistent enterovirus infections in agammaglobulinemic children. Host defenses do not, however, terminate virus replication in the intestine, and fecal shedding continues for weeks after both symptomatic and asymptomatic enterovirus infections. Reinfection (i.e., virus excretion by a person with pre-existing homotypic antibodies) is relatively uncommon. When it occurs, infection is confined to the alimentary tract and is not associated with illness, and the duration of virus shedding is markedly reduced.

The clinical syndrome(s) caused by a given enterovirus reflects the particular target organs and tissues that it infects, i.e., its *cell tropism*. All of the determinants of cell tropism have not been elucidated, but a major factor is the presence on the cell surface of specific *receptor* molecules to which the virus attaches. Different groups of enteroviruses utilize different receptors, most or all of which are encoded by genes on human chromosome 19. Distinct receptors have already been identified for the polioviruses, a subset of group A coxsackieviruses, group B coxsackieviruses, and echoviruses, as well as for two subsets of human rhinoviruses.

The presence and density of various receptor molecules on the surface of cells are profoundly influenced by such factors as species, cell type, physiologic state, degree of differentiation, innervation, and exposure to extracellular signals such as hormones, lymphokines, and growth factors. Thus, for example, the susceptibility of primates and the resistance of mice to poliovirus infection are correlated with the presence of poliovirus receptors only on primate cells; and the ability of group A coxsackieviruses to produce myositis only in suckling mice is correlated with the presence of specific receptors on differentiating myoblasts, but not on the fully differentiated myocytes of older animals.

Several of the enterovirus receptors that have been characterized are members of the immunoglobulin superfamily; for example, intracellular adhesion molecule-1 (ICAM-1), which binds to an integrin (LFA-1) on lymphocytes and promotes their adherence to a variety of nonlymphoid cells, serves as the receptor for several of the group A coxsackieviruses as well as for the majority of human rhinoviruses. These receptor molecules appear to extend from the cell surface and mediate virus attachment by binding to a specific site located on the floor of canyon-like depressions on the surface of the virus capsid. Because these canyons are too narrow to admit antibody molecules, neutralizing antibodies are not directed at the receptor attachment site itself but at epitopes on or near the canyon rim. Antibody molecules bound to these epitopes prevent virus attachment indirectly by preventing the receptor molecule from reaching its attachment site within the canyon. Since these "neutralizing" epitopes are unique in each enterovirus serotype, neutralizing antibodies are serotype-specific (e.g., antibody to coxsackievirus B2 does not neutralize coxsackievirus B5) despite the fact that a number of enterovirus serotypes (e.g., all group B coxsackieviruses) share the same cellular receptor. In contrast to virus-specific neutralizing antibodies, monoclonal antibody to a cellular receptor can prevent infection by all of the enterovirus serotypes that utilize

it. Similarly, soluble preparations of receptor molecules can neutralize the infectivity of all enterovirus serotypes that utilize that particular receptor. These observations suggest new approaches to the prevention and treatment of enteroviral diseases.

CLINICAL MANIFESTATIONS. The majority of nonpolio enterovirus infections (50 to 80 per cent) are asymptomatic. Most symptomatic infections consist of "undifferentiated febrile illnesses" ("summer grippe"), often accompanied by upper respiratory symptoms. These are generally mild and last only a few days. This syndrome is totally nonspecific; it can be caused by virtually any enterovirus serotype, as well as by members of several other virus families (e.g., adenoviruses, paramyxoviruses, orthomyxoviruses). The so-called characteristic enterovirus syndromes, such as aseptic meningitis, hand-foot-and-mouth disease, and pleurodynia, are in fact unusual manifestations of enterovirus infection. They represent the "very small tip of a very large iceberg."

Some clinical syndromes are highly associated with certain enterovirus serotypes or subgroups (e.g., hand-foot-and-mouth disease with coxsackievirus A16, myopericarditis with group B

TABLE 377–2. CLINICAL MANIFESTATIONS OF NONPOLIO ENTEROVIRUS INFECTIONS[a]

Clinical Syndrome	Group A Coxsackieviruses[b]	Group B Coxsackieviruses	Echoviruses	Enteroviruses
Asymptomatic infection	All serotypes	All serotypes	All serotypes	All serotypes
Undifferentiated febrile illness ("summer grippe") with or without respiratory symptoms	All serotypes	All serotypes	All serotypes	68, 70, 71
Aseptic meningitis	1, 2, 3, 4, 5, 6, 7, 8, 9, 10, 11, 14, 16, 17, 18, 22, 24	1, 2, 3, 4, 5, 6	1, 2, 3, 4, 5, 6, 7, 8, 9, 10, 11, 12, 14, 16, 17, 18, 19, 20, 21, 22, 23, 25, 30, 31, 33	70, 71
Encephalitis	2, 4, 5, 6, 7, 9, 10, 16	1, 2, 3, 4, 5	2, 3, 4, 6, 7, 9, 11, 14, 17, 18, 19, 22, 25, 30, 33	70, 71
Paralytic disease (poliomyelitis-like)	4, 5, 6, 7, 9, 10, 11, 14, 16, 21	1, 2, 3, 4, 5, 6	1, 2, 4, 6, 7, 9, 11, 14, 16, 17, 18, 19, 30	70, 71
Myopericarditis	1, 2, 4, 5, 7, 8, 9, 14, 16	1, 2, 3, 4, 5, 6	1, 2, 3, 4, 6, 7, 8, 9, 11, 14, 16, 17, 19, 22, 25, 30	
Pleurodynia	1, 2, 4, 6, 9, 10, 16	1, 2, 3, 4, 5, 6	1, 2, 3, 6, 7, 8, 9, 11, 12, 14, 16, 19, 23, 24, 25, 30	
Herpangina	1, 2, 3, 4, 5, 6, 7, 8, 9, 10, 16, 22	1, 2, 3, 4, 5	6, 9, 11, 16, 17, 22, 25	
Hand-foot-and-mouth disease	4, 5, 7, 9, 10, 16	2, 5		71
Exanthems	2, 4, 5, 6, 7, 9, 10, 16	1, 2, 3, 4, 5	2, 4, 5, 6, 9, 11, 16, 18, 25	71
Common cold	2, 10, 21, 24	1, 2, 3, 4, 5	2, 4, 9, 11, 20, 25	
Lower respiratory tract infections (broncheolitis, pneumonia)	7, 9, 16	1, 2, 3, 4, 5	4, 8, 9, 11, 12, 14, 19, 20, 21, 25, 30	68, 71
Acute hemorrhagic conjunctivitis[c]	24			70
Generalized disease of the newborn	3, 9, 16	1, 2, 3, 4, 5	3, 4, 6, 7, 9, 11, 12, 14, 17, 18, 19, 20, 21, 22, 30	

[a]A great many enterovirus serotypes have been implicated in most of these syndromes, at least in sporadic cases. The serotypes listed are those that have been clearly and/or frequently implicated. Serotypes with the strongest association are underlined.
[b]Because isolation of many of the group A coxsackieviruses requires suckling mouse inoculation, they are likely to be underreported as causes of illness.
[c]Conjunctivitis without hemorrhage is frequently seen in association with other manifestations in patients infected with many group A and group B coxsackieviruses and echoviruses, especially coxsackieviruses A9, A16, and B1 to 5; and echoviruses 2, 7, 9, 11, 16, and 30.

coxsackieviruses), but these associations are not specific. The same syndrome may be caused by a number of enterovirus serotypes. Conversely, a single enterovirus serotype may cause several different syndromes, even within the same outbreak (Table 377–2). The more important syndromes are discussed below.

Aseptic meningitis is the most common significant illness caused by nonpolio enteroviruses, and these viruses are responsible for more than 80 per cent of the cases of aseptic meningitis in which an etiologic agent is identified. Almost every enterovirus serotype has been implicated, but those most frequently associated include coxsackieviruses A2, A4, A7, A9, A10, and B1 to 5; echoviruses 3, 4, 6, 9, 11, 14, 16 to 19, 25, 30, and 33; and enteroviruses 70 and 71, all of which have been responsible for outbreaks as well as sporadic cases. Attack rates are generally highest in children, but cases also occur in adults, especially during larger outbreaks. Initial symptoms, which are typical of *undifferentiated febrile illness* (e.g., fever, headache, malaise, myalgias, and sore throat) are followed, usually within a day, by signs and symptoms of meningitis, including a more severe headache that is often retrobulbar, photophobia, meningismus, stiffness of the neck and back, and nausea and vomiting, especially in children. The illness is sometimes biphasic like poliomyelitis. In some cases, especially those caused by echoviruses and enterovirus 71, meningitis may be accompanied by a rash which, if petechial, may raise the specter of meningococcemia. The cerebrospinal fluid is clear and under slightly increased pressure. The total cell count, which can vary from less than 10 per cubic millimeter to more than 3000 per cubic millimeter, averages 50 to 500 per cubic millimeter. Initially, neutrophils may predominate (although they rarely exceed 90 per cent), but they are quickly replaced by mononuclear cells. The glucose concentration is usually normal, and the protein concentration is normal or slightly elevated (<100 mg per deciliter). Fever and signs of meningeal inflammation subside in 3 to 7 days, although cerebrospinal fluid pleocytosis may persist for an additional week or more. The great majority of children and adults recover fully without sequelae. However, enteroviral meningitis during the first year of life may, in up to 10 per cent of affected infants, result in permanent neurologic damage as evidenced by reduced head circumference, spasticity, and impaired intellectual function.

Paralytic disease may occur in the course of many nonpolio enterovirus infections, but it is generally less severe than that caused by polioviruses. Muscle weakness is far more common than frank paralysis and recovery is nearly always complete, although occasional patients suffer cranial nerve palsies or severe, sometimes fatal, bulbar involvement. Frequently implicated serotypes include coxsackieviruses A7, A9, and B2 to 5; echoviruses 2, 4, 6, 9, 11, and 30; and enteroviruses 70 and 71. In contrast to paralytic poliomyelitis, which in the prevaccine era occurred in epidemics, cases of paralysis associated with nonpolio enteroviruses are generally sporadic. However, several nonpolio enteroviruses produce paralytic disease with sufficient frequency to cause local outbreaks and epidemics. A variant of coxsackievirus A7 has caused outbreaks, as well as numerous sporadic cases of paralytic disease. In fact, it was once thought to be a fourth serotype of poliovirus. Paralytic disease resembling poliomyelitis, with a significant incidence of residual paralysis and muscle atrophy, has been observed in patients with acute hemorrhagic conjunctivitis caused by enterovirus 70 (see Ch. 381). Enterovirus 71 has caused outbreaks and epidemics of cutaneous and central nervous system disease in temperate regions around the world since its initial isolation in California in 1969. These have included epidemics of poliomyelitis-like paralytic disease with residual flaccid paralysis and of encephalitis, with significant mortality.

Encephalitis is a well-recognized but uncommon manifestation of enterovirus infection. Thus, despite their prevalence, enteroviruses account for only 10 to 20 per cent of the cases of encephalitis of proven viral etiology in the United States. The most frequently implicated serotypes include coxsackieviruses A9, B2, and B5; echoviruses 4, 6, 9, 11, and 30; and enterovirus 71. In most cases, encephalitis complicates the course of aseptic meningitis; parenchymal involvement is indicated by the onset of confusion, coma, abnormalities of motor function, hemiparesis, vasomotor instability, cranial nerve palsies, cerebellar ataxia, and focal or generalized seizures, singly or in various combinations. Cerebral involvement is usually generalized, but focal encepha-

litis does occur and may occasionally be clinically indistinguishable from herpes simplex encephalitis. Recovery is usually complete, although neurologic sequelae and deaths occur, especially in young infants and during enterovirus 71 epidemics.

Other neurologic complications, including Guillain-Barré syndrome, transverse myelitis, and Reye syndrome, have been reported in patients with enterovirus infections. However, no clear epidemiologic or etiologic linkage to enteroviruses has been established and, given the high prevalence of enterovirus infections, the associations may be only coincidental.

Enterovirus infections tend to be more severe in the newborn infant than in older children and adults. Asymptomatic infections and undifferentiated febrile illnesses are still common, but many infections, especially those caused by group B coxsackieviruses and echovirus 11, result in a fulminant, frequently fatal, generalized disease. This *generalized disease of the newborn* is often clinically indistinguishable from bacterial sepsis or neonatal herpes simplex virus infection. Manifestations include myocarditis, meningoencephalitis, hepatitis, pancreatitis, adrenal involvement, and disseminated intravascular coagulation with hemorrhage and circulatory collapse. Virus is frequently acquired transplacentally when the mother is infected just prior to birth, but it may also be acquired by contact during delivery or nosocomially in the newborn nursery. Once an enterovirus is introduced into a newborn nursery, usually by a transplacentally infected infant, it is often spread to other infants on the hands of nursery personnel.

Enteroviruses, primarily echoviruses, have been responsible for a syndrome of chronic meningoencephalitis in patients with inherited or acquired defects in B-lymphocyte function, most often children with X-linked agammaglobulinemia. The majority of these patients have a dermatomyositis-like syndrome and many also have chronic hepatitis. Surprisingly, despite the presence in their cerebrospinal fluid of abundant virus, a lymphocytic pleocytosis and an elevated protein concentration, these patients generally exhibit few if any clinical signs of meningitis. The pathogenesis of this often fatal disease remains to be elucidated.

Several important syndromes caused by nonpolio enteroviruses are discussed in subsequent chapters and thus are not considered here. These include epidemic pleurodynia (Ch. 378), myopericarditis (Ch. 379), a variety of exanthems and enanthems (Ch. 380), and acute hemorrhagic conjunctivitis (Ch. 381).

A number of enteroviruses have been associated with mild upper respiratory tract illness in children and adults, especially coxsackieviruses A21, A24, and B1 to 5; and echoviruses 2, 4, 9, 11, 20, and 25. Enteroviruses have also been associated with lower respiratory tract illnesses in infants and children, although rarely in adults. These include tracheitis, bronchitis, croup, bronchiolitis, and pneumonia. Frequently implicated serotypes include coxsackieviruses A9, A16, and B1 to 5; echoviruses 4, 8, 9, 11, 12, 14, 19 to 21, 25, and 30; and enterovirus 68. In addition, respiratory tract symptoms frequently accompany the undifferentiated febrile illnesses ("summer grippe") caused by most enteroviruses. The respiratory illnesses caused by enteroviruses are clinically indistinguishable from similar illnesses caused by viruses more commonly considered to be respiratory tract pathogens, such as rhinoviruses, influenza viruses, parainfluenza viruses, respiratory syncytial virus, and adenoviruses. However, infections with these viruses occur most frequently during the winter, whereas enterovirus infections occur primarily in the summer and early fall.

DIAGNOSIS. The enteroviral etiology of a disease may be suspected on clinical and epidemiologic grounds, but the multiplicity of agents capable of causing most clinical syndromes makes it impossible to establish a specific etiologic diagnosis on the basis of such information alone. Virus isolation and/or serologic evidence is required. Most enteroviruses can be isolated from the pharyngeal secretions and feces of infected patients. However, the high prevalence of asymptomatic enterovirus infections and the prolonged period (up to 3 months) of virus shedding following both symptomatic and asymptomatic infections make it difficult to assess the etiologic significance of an enterovirus isolated concurrently with an episode of disease; it may merely reflect an etiologically unrelated antecedent or intercurrent infection. The development of serotype-specific antibodies, demonstrated by assay of acute and convalescent sera, indicates that the enterovirus infection occurred concurrently with the episode of disease, but even this does not prove that the enterovirus was causal. The following criteria are generally used to establish the etiologic association of an enterovirus with a given disease: (1) There is a much higher rate of isolation of the virus from patients with the disease than from healthy controls matched for age, socioeconomic status, area of residence, and time; (2) antibodies against the virus develop during the course of the disease; (3) virologic and serologic evidence of concurrent infection by other agents known to cause a similar clinical syndrome is negative; (4) the virus is isolated from pathologically involved tissues or body fluids that are not normally sites from which asymptomatic virus shedding occurs (e.g., from cerebrospinal fluid in patients with aseptic meningitis; from the myocardium in patients with myopericarditis). Only the isolation of virus from pathologically involved tissues constitutes proof of causation. An alternative to the isolation of virus from pathologically involved sites is the identification in these sites of viral proteins or viral RNA. It is now possible to detect enteroviral RNA in tissues directly by nucleic acid hybridization or following amplification by the polymerase chain reaction (PCR) using probes and primers from regions of the genome that are common to all human enteroviruses.

In the individual patient, the diagnosis of enterovirus infection is most readily established by virus isolation. Rising titers of serotype-specific neutralizing antibodies in paired acute and convalescent sera are confirmatory, but serologic diagnosis cannot generally substitute for virus isolation. This is because group-reactive antigens are lacking, and it is impractical to perform serotype-specific tests (e.g., neutralization tests) for each of the 68 recognized human enteroviruses. Of necessity, serologic assays are generally limited to neutralization tests against the patient's virus isolate (if one has been obtained), against one or two serotypes then prevalent in the community, or against a very limited number of enterovirus serotypes suspected on the basis of the nature of the clinical illness, e.g., the three poliovirus serotypes in a patient with paralytic disease, coxsackievirus A24 and enterovirus 70 in a patient with acute hemorrhagic conjunctivitis, or coxsackieviruses B1 to 6 in a patient with myopericarditis. Because of the importance of demonstrating seroconversion, or at least a marked rise in antibody titer, it is imperative that specimens of acute serum be obtained as early in the course of disease as possible; convalescent serum is obtained 2 to 4 weeks later. Serotype-specific IgM assays, already developed for enteroviruses 70 and 72 (hepatitis A virus), and the use of new techniques for the detection of enterovirus RNA, can be expected to improve the speed and accuracy of enteroviral diagnosis.

TREATMENT AND PREVENTION. Specific antiviral chemotherapy and chemoprophylaxis are not yet available for enterovirus infections. Treatment is symptomatic and, in severe disease, supportive. Corticosteroids, which have a deleterious effect on coxsackievirus-infected mice, should not be administered during acute enterovirus infections. Strenuous exercise and intramuscular injections, both of which appear capable of precipitating paralysis of the involved muscles during poliovirus and enterovirus 70 infections, should probably also be avoided during the acute, presumably viremic, phase of symptomatic enterovirus infections. Administration of immune serum globulin, which contains high titers of neutralizing antibodies to many enteroviruses, appears to have been useful in some agammaglobulinemic patients with chronic enteroviral meningoencephalitis. Immune serum globulin may also have a role in the treatment of enteroviral infections in other patients with severely compromised B-lymphocyte function. Infants with generalized neonatal enterovirus infections are unlikely to have received antibodies to the causative virus from their mothers. Consequently, it seems reasonable to administer immune serum globulin to such infants in an attempt to terminate their viremia and limit virus replication in infected tissues.

Live attenuated and inactivated poliovirus vaccines have been remarkably successful in preventing paralytic poliomyelitis (see Ch. 16), and live, inactivated, and synthetic vaccines produced by recombinant DNA technology are being developed for hepatitis A (caused by enterovirus 72). However, the large number of nonpolio enterovirus serotypes and the benign nature of most nonpolio enterovirus infections have precluded the development of vaccines for these agents. Pre-exposure administration of immune serum globulin reduces the risk of paralytic poliomyelitis. Since immune serum globulin also contains neutralizing antibodies to many nonpolio enteroviruses, it would probably prevent many nonpolio enteroviral diseases as well. This approach has proven effective for pre- and postexposure prophylaxis of hepatitis A and probably reduces the frequency of severe enteroviral infections in agammaglobulinemic patients receiving replacement therapy. However, the benign nature of most enterovirus infections, the fact that exposures are rarely recognized (most result from contact with an asymptomatically infected person), and the relatively short half-life of exogenous immune serum globulin make this approach to prevention impractical in most situations. Nursery outbreaks of severe enteroviral disease provide an exception; the administration of immune serum globulin to all infants in the nursery offers protection to those infants without transplacentally acquired neutralizing antibody who have not yet been infected.

In general, control of enterovirus infections is best effected by hygienic measures, such as handwashing, and improvements in sanitation. Isolation of patients with enteroviral illnesses is generally not helpful because of the simultaneous existence of a large reservoir of unidentified asymptomatically infected patients who are excreting virus.

Cherry JD: Enteroviruses: Polioviruses (poliomyelitis), coxsackieviruses, echoviruses, and enteroviruses. In Feigin RD, Cherry JD (eds.): Textbook of Pediatric Infectious Diseases. Philadelphia, W.B. Saunders, 1987, pp 729–790. *A thorough review of enteroviral diseases with an emphasis on infections of children and newborn infants and a comprehensive bibliography.*

McKinney RE, Katz SL, Wilfert CM: Chronic enteroviral meningoencephalitis in agammaglobulinemic patients. Rev Infect Dis 9:334–356, 1987. *An excellent review of this interesting syndrome with thoughtful discussion of pathogenesis and management.*

Melnick JL: Enteroviruses. In Fields BN, et al. (eds.): Virology, 2nd ed. New York, Raven Press, 1990, pp 549–605. *An authoritative review with an extensive bibliography and an emphasis on epidemiology.*

Modlin JF: Coxsackieviruses, echoviruses, and newer enteroviruses. In Mandel GL, Douglas RG Jr, Bennett JE (eds.): Principles and Practice of Infectious Diseases. New York, Churchill Livingstone, 1990, pp 1367–1383. *An extensive review of the epidemiology and clinical manifestations of nonpolio enterovirus infections, with an excellent bibliography.*

Rotbart HA: Nucleic acid detection systems for enteroviruses. Clin Microbiol Rev 4:156–168, 1991. *A practical and authoritative review of the newest and most promising approaches to the diagnosis of enteroviral diseases.*

Rueckert RR: Picornaviridae and their replication. In Fields BN, et al. (eds.): Virology, 2nd ed. New York, Raven Press, 1990, pp 507–548. *A detailed summary of our current knowledge of picornavirus structure, replication, and virus-cell interactions.*

378 Epidemic Pleurodynia (Bornholm Disease)

Michael N. Oxman

DEFINITION. Epidemic pleurodynia is an acute febrile viral illness characterized by the sudden onset of intense paroxysmal lower thoracic or abdominal pain. Synonyms include Bornholm disease, devil's grip, epidemic myalgia, epidemic benign dry pleurisy, and Sylvest's disease. The name *pleurodynia* (*pleura*, side; *odyne*, pain) reflects the characteristic intercostal location of the pain and does not connote disease of the pleura. Pleurodynia is usually an epidemic disease, but sporadic cases do occur.

ETIOLOGY. The enteroviral etiology of epidemic pleurodynia was established in 1949. Group B coxsackieviruses, especially B3 and B5, are the principal cause. Other viruses associated with epidemic disease include echoviruses 1 and 6. Sporadic cases have also been associated with these viruses, as well as with many other enteroviruses, including coxsackieviruses A1, A2, A4, A6, A9, A10, and A16 and echoviruses 2, 3, 7 to 9, 11, 12, 14, 16, 19, 23, 24, 25, and 30.

EPIDEMIOLOGY. Epidemics of pleurodynia have been recognized in Scandinavian countries for more than two centuries, but the disease was little known elsewhere until 1933, when a

Danish physician, Ejnar Sylvest, published a classic monograph describing an epidemic on Bornholm, a Danish island in the Baltic Sea. Since then, epidemics and sporadic cases have been recognized in many parts of the world. As with other enteroviral infections, the majority of illnesses occur in summer and early fall. However, in contrast to the annual outbreaks of enteroviral aseptic meningitis, epidemics of pleurodynia are much less frequent, generally occurring at intervals of 10 to 20 years.

Transmission is primarily from person to person, and multiple family members may be attacked almost simultaneously or in rapid succession at intervals of 2 to 5 days. In epidemics, disease is observed in children and adults of both sexes. The peak age of incidence is somewhat older than with other enterovirus syndromes, but the majority of cases occur in persons under 30 years of age. The incubation period is generally 2 to 5 days.

PATHOGENESIS. Pleurodynia is a disease of skeletal muscle, not of the pleura or peritoneum. As in most enteroviral diseases, infection is initiated in the alimentary tract. Skeletal muscle is probably most often infected during the primary ("minor") viremia, although it may be infected later, during the "major" viremia in the minority of patients in whom pleurodynia is preceded by a prodromal illness. Host immune responses terminate viremia and halt virus replication in the tissues, but they also contribute to the severity of local inflammation. Muscle tenderness and occasionally swelling can be detected at the site of pain, and characteristic paroxysms of pain can often be elicited by pressure on the affected muscles. In contrast, pleural friction rubs have been infrequently noted, and peritonitis has generally not been observed in patients who have come to laparotomy. Histopathologic data in humans is lacking because of the benign nature of the disease, but studies in murine models of coxsackievirus infection suggest that the myositis results from a combination of direct virus-induced cytolysis and immunopathology mediated by sensitized T lymphocytes.

CLINICAL MANIFESTATIONS. Pleurodynia is characterized by the abrupt onset of fever and sharp, paroxysmal pain over the lower ribs or upper abdomen. In about 25 per cent of patients, this is preceded by a 1- or 2-day prodrome of headache, malaise, anorexia, sore throat, and diffuse myalgia. The pain varies in intensity but is often severe. It is accentuated, sometimes elicited, by deep breathing, coughing, and movement. The pain of pleurodynia has been described as "catching" (a "stitch" in the side), "stabbing," "knife-like," "lancinating," "crushing," or "vice-like." In adults, the pain is primarily in muscles of the thorax, especially the intercostals. In children, abdominal muscles are more often involved. Occasionally, it may involve muscles in the neck or limbs. The pain is often unilateral and is generally experienced in only one or two locations.

During paroxysms of severe pain, the patient lies still in bed, sweating profusely and appearing acutely ill and apprehensive. Respiration, limited by pain, is shallow, rapid, and grunting, suggesting pneumonia or pleural inflammation. Fever of 38 to 40°C is present at the onset of pain, reaches its peak during the episode, and resolves between paroxysms. Multiple paroxysms of pain occur, each lasting from a few minutes to several hours. The initial paroxysm is usually the most severe, and patients frequently appear relatively well between paroxysms.

The acute illness generally lasts for 2 to 6 days, with a range of 12 hours to 3 weeks. The disease is often biphasic; the initial pain and fever resolve and the patient is asymptomatic for a day or more, and then the pain and fever recur, frequently at the same site. Rarely, patients have several recurrences over a period of several weeks or have a late recurrence after being symptom-free for a month or more.

LABORATORY DIAGNOSIS. A specific diagnosis can be established by isolating virus (usually a group B coxsackievirus) from the throat or feces during the acute illness and demonstrating the concurrent development of serotype-specific neutralizing antibodies by testing acute and convalescent sera. Virus is most readily isolated from samples taken early in the illness. The level of creatine phosphokinase in the serum may be elevated, reflecting injury to striated muscle. Other laboratory values are usually normal, although there may be a mild leukopenia in some patients.

DIFFERENTIAL DIAGNOSIS. The most useful distinguishing feature of pleurodynia is the intermittent paroxysmal character of the pain. Epidemiologic information, such as the occurrence of similar illnesses in family members or in the community, may also suggest the diagnosis. Nevertheless, depending upon the location of the pain, pleurodynia may be confused with any of a number of more serious diseases. When the pain is thoracic, these include pneumonia, pulmonary infarction, rib fracture, costochondritis, and myocardial infarction. The absence of physical and roentgenographic evidence of fracture, costochondritis, or pulmonary parenchymal disease; lack of sputum production; absence of leukocytosis; and normal electrocardiogram help to exclude these diagnoses. When the pain is abdominal, it can be difficult to differentiate pleurodynia from serious causes of acute abdominal pain, such as peritonitis, cholecystitis, appendicitis, perforated peptic ulcer, and acute intestinal obstruction. Thus, during epidemics of pleurodynia, it is common to have as many children with the disease admitted to surgical wards as to medical wards, and in one epidemic 9 of 49 of these children underwent laparotomy with negative findings before the nature of their disease was recognized. The absence of signs of peritonitis and the normal white blood cell count are helpful in excluding these diagnoses, as are normal ultrasound and roentgenographic studies. Pleurodynia may also be confused with the pain of pre-eruptive herpes zoster, herniated intervertebral disc, and renal colic. However, the pain of pre-eruptive herpes zoster is usually more constant, and the localization of pain and tenderness to the affected muscle, normal roentgenographic and neurologic examinations (except, perhaps, for a local area of hyperesthesia over the affected muscle), and the absence of hematuria help to exclude the other two diagnoses.

TREATMENT AND PREVENTION. Treatment of pleurodynia is symptomatic. Episodes of pain can usually be controlled with salicylates or other mild analgesics, but opiate analgesics are recommended for severe pain once serious intra-abdominal processes have been excluded. Application of heat to affected muscles may also be useful. Despite the tendency of the disease to relapse, patients with epidemic pleurodynia eventually recover completely. Occasionally, convalescence may be prolonged, with malaise or asthenia persisting for several months. Complications, which reflect dissemination of virus to other tissues, are relatively uncommon. When they do occur, they generally become apparent within several days after the onset of the disease. Aseptic meningitis is observed in approximately 5 per cent of cases and orchitis in a similar proportion of postpubertal males. Pericarditis and myocarditis are rare complications of epidemic pleurodynia.

Bain HW, McLean DM, Walker SJ: Epidemic pleurodynia (Bornholm disease) due to coxsackie B5 virus. The interrelationship of pleurodynia, benign pericarditis and aseptic meningitis. Pediatrics 27:889–903, 1961. *A good discussion of epidemic pleurodynia and its complications.*

Fin JJ Jr, Weller TH, Morgan HR: Epidemic pleurodynia: Clinical and etiologic studies based on one hundred and fourteen cases. Arch Intern Med 83:305, 1949. *An excellent clinical review of epidemic pleurodynia.*

Huebner RJ, Risser JA, Bell JA, et al.: Epidemic pleurodynia in Texas: A study of 22 cases. N Engl J Med 248:267–274, 1953. *Demonstration of the viral etiology of a local epidemic of pleurodynia.*

Pickles NW: Sylvest's disease (Bornholm disease). N Engl J Med 250:1033, 1954. *A vivid account of the clinical presentation of epidemic pleurodynia.*

Sylvest E: Epidemic Myalgia: Bornholm Disease. Transl. by H. Andersen. London, Oxford University Press, 1934, pp 1–155. *The classic monograph and still the best clinical description of the disease.*

Warin JF, Davies JBM, Sanders FK, et al.: Oxford epidemic of Bornholm disease, 1951. Br Med J 1:1345–1351, 1953. *An excellent description of an epidemic of pleurodynia, including its complications.*

Weller TH, Enders JF, Buckingham M, et al.: The etiology of epidemic pleurodynia: A study of two viruses isolated from a tropical outbreak. J Immunol 65:337–346, 1950. *The original study establishing the viral etiology of epidemic pleurodynia.*

---

379 Myocarditis and Pericarditis Caused by Enteroviruses

Michael N. Oxman

Myocarditis and pericarditis have long been known to occur in association with epidemic viral diseases, including measles, mumps, rubella, varicella, influenza, poliomyelitis, and pleurodynia. As many of these diseases have been controlled by the use of vaccines, enteroviruses have emerged as the major recognized infectious cause of myocarditis and pericarditis in North America and Western Europe. The pathogenesis, clinical manifestations, and outcome of enteroviral infections of the heart vary markedly depending upon properties of the virus and characteristics of the host, especially age. Neonatal infections frequently result in severe myocarditis, widespread involvement of other organs, and high mortality, whereas in older children and adults, pericarditis often predominates, and the disease is generally benign and self-limited. In fact, it appears that the clinical manifestations are generally so subtle that cardiac involvement during enteroviral infections is often unrecognized. However, there is increasing evidence that idiopathic dilated cardiomyopathy may, in many cases, be a late sequela of both recognized and unrecognized enteroviral myocarditis.

ETIOLOGY. The evidence linking specific enteroviruses with myocarditis or pericarditis varies markedly. Proof of causation requires the isolation of virus from, or the demonstration of viral proteins or nucleic acids in, the myocardium, pericardium, or pericardial fluid. Except in neonatal myopericarditis, virus is rarely isolated from cardiac tissue or pericardial fluid, and detection of viral proteins has been difficult, primarily because lack of specificity has led to false-positive results. However, the increasing use of endomyocardial biopsy and the application of new techniques for the detection and amplification of enteroviral nucleic acid should significantly improve our ability to establish the etiology in cases of myocarditis and pericarditis. In most instances, the association of a particular enterovirus with myocarditis or pericarditis is based upon the isolation of virus from noncardiac sources (e.g., feces) and/or serologic evidence of recent or concurrent enterovirus infection. Because of the high prevalence of enteroviral infections and the prolonged period of fecal virus shedding, these associations may often be coincidental rather than causal. On the other hand, because routine serologic testing is available for group B but not for group A coxsackieviruses or echoviruses, and because many group A coxsackieviruses are not readily isolated by routine cell culture techniques, the true contribution of group A coxsackieviruses and echoviruses is probably underestimated.

Coxsackieviruses B1 to 6, A4, and A16, and echoviruses 9, 11, and 22 have been proven to cause myopericarditis in children and adults. Coxsackieviruses A1, A2, A5, A7 to A9, and A14, and echoviruses 1 to 4, 6 to 8, 14, 16, 17, 19, 25, and 30 have also been implicated. The group B coxsackieviruses are the most common etiologic agents of myocarditis and pericarditis. They appear to account for approximately 50 per cent of sporadic cases of acute myocarditis and for virtually all cases that have occurred in epidemics. Group B coxsackieviruses also appear to account for 30 per cent or more of sporadic cases of acute nonbacterial pericarditis.

The newborn is particularly susceptible to severe, frequently fatal, enteroviral infections (*generalized disease of the newborn*), and myocarditis is invariably a major component. These overwhelming systemic enterovirus infections occur in nursery epidemics and as sporadic cases. They are most frequently caused by coxsackieviruses B2 to 5 and echovirus 11, but other echoviruses have also been implicated, including echoviruses 4, 6, 7, 9, 12, 14, 17 to 22, and 31. Coxsackieviruses A3, A9, and A16 have occasionally been associated with sporadic cases.

EPIDEMIOLOGY. Enteroviral myocarditis and pericarditis occur most frequently in the summer and early fall. Idiopathic myopericarditis also peaks during this period of maximum enterovirus prevalence, an observation that is consistent with the notion that most cases of idiopathic myopericarditis are caused by enteroviruses. The incidence of myocarditis and pericarditis has been observed to increase during periods of group B coxsackievirus prevalence, and epidemics of myopericarditis were observed during coxsackievirus B5 epidemics in a number of countries in 1965. However, except in the newborn, epidemic myopericarditis is unusual; most reported cases of enteroviral myopericarditis beyond the neonatal period have been sporadic.

The incidence of myopericarditis during enteroviral infections depends upon the virus and characteristics of the host, especially age. Myopericarditis has been the predominant manifestation of

infection in only about 3 per cent of group B coxsackievirus infections reported to the World Health Organization. However, 5 to 10 per cent of infected adults and children over 9 years of age who sought medical care during coxsackievirus B5 epidemics were found to have evidence of acute myopericarditis. The incidence of myocarditis and disseminated disease during group B coxsackievirus infection is very high during the neonatal period. It drops to a minimum (e.g., 1 per cent or less of symptomatic coxsackievirus B5 infections) in children 1 to 9 years of age and then increases again in older children and adults. Thus, despite the higher frequency of enterovirus infections in younger children, enteroviral myopericarditis is primarily a disease of adolescents and young adults. At least two thirds of the cases occur in males, but the risk of cardiac involvement also appears to be increased during pregnancy and immediately following delivery. An unknown but probably significant proportion of enteroviral myopericarditis appears to be asymptomatic or unrecognized. Postmortem examinations have revealed evidence of previously unsuspected myopericarditis in 2 to 10 per cent of unselected cases, with a higher incidence in young persons who have died suddenly. However, questions have been raised about the pathologic criteria employed, and thus the significance of these observations is unclear. The application of new techniques for detection and amplification of enteroviral nucleic acid may help clarify the situation.

Transmission of enteroviruses associated with myocarditis and pericarditis is the same as that of enteroviruses in general (see Ch. 377). In children and adults, it is primarily fecal-oral. The majority of neonatal enteroviral infections are acquired perinatally from an infected mother. Virus is frequently acquired transplacentally when the mother is infected shortly before birth, but it may also be acquired by contact during or after delivery. During nursery epidemics, virus is transmitted nosocomially on the hands of nursery personnel.

PATHOGENESIS. Enteroviruses reach the heart during the viremia that follows infection and replication in the alimentary tract. When enteroviral infections involve the heart they almost always cause an inflammatory response in both the myocardium (*myocarditis*) and the pericardium (*pericarditis*). Although one or the other usually predominates, the term *myopericarditis* best describes the pathologic process. The hallmark of enteroviral myopericarditis is injury to myocytes with an adjacent inflammatory infiltrate. The pathologic changes may be acute or chronic, and they vary in extent depending upon the severity of the disease and the point in its course at which tissue is obtained. Early in infection there are often hypereosinophilic myocytes, widespread edema, and only a few inflammatory cells, many of which are polymorphonuclear leukocytes. Later there is loss of striation, nuclear degeneration, and fragmentation of myocytes. The degenerating and partially necrotic myocytes are surrounded by lymphocytes, plasma cells, and macrophages. The acute process may resolve completely or progress. Healing and progression are reflected by the development of interstitial fibrosis and loss of myocytes. Enteroviral pericarditis is almost always accompanied by focal subepicardial myocarditis, which has these same pathologic characteristics.

The inflammatory process may affect myocytes, vascular elements, the conducting system, autonomic nerves, and/or the interstitium. One or more of at least four mechanisms appear to be involved: (1) cytolytic enteroviral infection; (2) cytotoxicity caused by infection-induced immune responses; (3) indirect nonspecific damage to myocytes caused by adjacent interstitial inflammation; and (4) indirect damage to myocytes caused by infection and inflammation of small blood vessels. Cardiac myocytes, which bear receptors that are shared by all six group B coxsackievirus serotypes, are infected and lysed by these viruses. Interestingly, this same receptor is utilized by several adenoviruses, which have also been implicated in some cases of myocarditis. It appears that other cell types are also infected, e.g., vascular endothelial cells.

Mouse models of myocarditis induced by coxsackievirus B3 have revealed several possible pathogenic mechanisms. Susceptibility to coxsackievirus B3–induced myocarditis is age dependent and genetically determined. Mechanisms of injury vary in different mouse strains. In susceptible animals, acute myocarditis results from direct infection and cytolysis of myocytes. In surviving animals, neutralizing antibody, perhaps in conjunction with interferon, macrophages, and natural killer (NK) cells, appears to terminate virus replication within 7 to 9 days after infection. Exercise and corticosteroids markedly enhance mortality during the early stages of infection, and nonsteroidal anti-inflammatory agents may also have deleterious effects. Mice surviving the acute replicative phase of infection may recover completely or go on to develop severe myocarditis in the absence of recoverable virus. This second phase of virus-induced myocardial destruction depends upon the presence of cytolytic T lymphocytes, which appear as virus replication ceases. Some of these cytolytic T lymphocytes recognize and lyse both infected and uninfected myocytes, and their presence correlates with myocardial damage. The severity of myocardial damage caused by this immune mechanism is greatest in male and pregnant female mice and is reduced in castrated males. In some strains of mice less prone to myocarditis, suppressor T lymphocytes appear to inhibit this cytolytic T-lymphocyte response. Variants of coxsackievirus B3 that do not elicit cytotoxic T lymphocytes directed at both infected and uninfected myocytes fail to cause myocarditis, even though they are indistinguishable from myocarditic strains in their ability to replicate in the myocardium and stimulate the production of interferon and neutralizing antibodies. Mice infected with coxsackievirus B3 also develop antibodies that react with cardiac tissue but do not cross-react with the virus, and these antibodies may contribute to myocyte destruction in some mouse strains. Certain strains of mice infected with coxsackievirus B3 go on to develop chronic dilated cardiomyopathy, primarily as a result of ongoing immunopathology that occurs in the absence of detectable virus. Enterovirus-associated myopericarditis in humans appears to involve a comparable spectrum of pathogenic mechanisms and outcomes.

In neonatal enteroviral myopericarditis, the relatively short incubation period, the widely disseminated infection, and the presence of high titers of virus in the heart and other organs indicate that the primary pathogenic mechanism is direct cytolytic virus infection of the tissues involved. In myopericarditis in older children and adults, the longer incubation period, the presence of virus-specific antibodies and T lymphocytes at clinical presentation, the low frequency of virus isolation from the heart and pericardial fluid, and the later occurrence of relapses suggest that immunopathologic mechanisms are involved. Idiopathic dilated cardiomyopathy may represent the end stage of an immunologically mediated chronic progressive enteroviral myocarditis. This notion is supported by observations in the mouse model of coxsackievirus B3 myocarditis, by the development of chronic cardiomyopathy in approximately 10 per cent of patients followed long term after group B coxsackievirus myocarditis, by the demonstration of progressive fibrosis in such patients by serial endomyocardial biopsies, and by the failure to isolate enterovirus from these biopsy specimens. The association of idiopathic dilated cardiomyopathy with group B coxsackievirus myocarditis has been further strengthened by the recent demonstration of group B coxsackievirus RNA in some myocardial biopsies obtained from patients with the disease. These observations need to be confirmed and extended.

CLINICAL MANIFESTATIONS. Although the term *myopericarditis* best describes the pathologic process observed in enteroviral infections of the heart, *myocarditis* or *pericarditis* usually predominates, and the two syndromes are sufficiently distinct in clinical presentation and pathophysiology to warrant separate consideration. They are discussed in detail in Ch. 50 and 51.

Neonatal Myocarditis. Most severe neonatal enterovirus infections begin during the first week of life; the infant's mother has frequently been infected shortly before delivery and has transmitted the virus transplacentally or by contact during or soon after delivery. However, the disease can be present at birth or, when acquired later, may present at any time during the first 3 months of life following a 2- to 8-day incubation period. The disease usually begins with the abrupt onset of fever, listlessness, and anorexia. This is often followed within a day or two by respiratory distress, rapid tachycardia, cardiomegaly, systolic murmur, and electrocardiographic evidence of myocarditis, which may rapidly progress to circulatory collapse and congestive heart failure manifested by cyanosis, hepatomegaly, pulmonary hemorrhage, and edema. Symptomatic meningoencephalitis usually accompanies myocarditis in fatal cases, and there is virus dissem-

ination to other organs, including the liver, lungs, pancreas, and adrenal glands. The disease is biphasic in about one third of patients; the initial symptoms are followed by 1 to 7 days of relative well-being, after which the signs and symptoms of myocarditis develop. The syndrome of neonatal myocarditis is simply a common manifestation of generalized enteroviral disease of the newborn, which is usually caused by group B coxsackieviruses, but it is also seen with echovirus 11 infection and is occasionally associated with other enteroviruses. The mortality in recognized infections appears to be nearly 50 per cent. Death usually occurs within a week of onset, but it can occur within hours in fulminant cases. In survivors, improvement is rapid following defervescence. A second syndrome, characterized by increasing jaundice, hypotension, profuse hemorrhage, and hepatic necrosis, with mortality exceeding 80 per cent, has been described in newborns with disseminated echovirus infections (usually echovirus 11). Severe myocarditis is present at postmortem examination, together with involvement of many other organs. These life-threatening neonatal enterovirus infections are more common in males and in premature infants.

Myocarditis and Pericarditis in Older Children and Adults. In contrast to the neonate, enteroviral infections of the heart in older children and adults often present clinically as pericarditis rather than myocarditis, although the myocardium is almost always involved to some degree. Approximately 60 per cent of older children and adults with symptomatic group B coxsackievirus–associated heart disease present with a clinical diagnosis of pericarditis; approximately 40 per cent present with a clinical diagnosis of myocarditis. More than two thirds of the patients are male. The clinical features of myocarditis and pericarditis are discussed in Ch. 50 and 51.

In 60 to 70 per cent of patients, a mild influenza-like illness with fever, malaise, myalgia, arthragias, and often upper respiratory tract symptoms precedes the manifestations of heart disease by 7 to 10 days. Presenting signs and symptoms may be those of pericarditis, progressive heart failure, or coronary artery occlusion. Some patients present with a nonspecific febrile illness and no signs or symptoms of heart disease; they are diagnosed only when typical electrocardiographic abnormalities are detected. The most common symptoms are chest pain, dyspnea, malaise, fever, and tachycardia, each of which occurs in the majority of patients. Chest pain is present in most patients who present with pericarditis. It is typically retrosternal and radiates to the left trapezius ridge, shoulder, and neck. It is usually exacerbated by breathing, swallowing, and lying supine, and relieved by sitting up and leaning forward. The classic physical finding is the three-component pericardial friction rub that reflects cardiac motion during atrial systole, ventricular systole, and rapid diastolic ventricular filling. The three-component rub is heard in 50 per cent of patients presenting with acute enteroviral pericarditis, and one or more component can be heard in more than 90 per cent. The rub is often intermittent, position-dependent, and brought out by maximum inspiration or expiration, and it may disappear as pericardial effusion accumulates. Patients presenting with acute myocarditis may also have chest pain. This is often dull and oppressive, but it may also resemble the pain of angina or have the character of pericardial pain when there is coexistent pericarditis. Many patients with enteroviral myocarditis present only with signs and symptoms of heart failure or with arrhythmias. Supraventricular tachycardia and ventricular extrasystoles are common, and varying degrees of heart block signal involvement of the conducting system and are responsible for the occurrence of sudden death in patients with enteroviral myopericarditis. Cardiomegaly is present in about 50 per cent of patients with enteroviral myopericarditis, reflecting either pericardial effusion or cardiac dilatation. Pleural effusions, generally left-sided, are present in about one third of patients. Other clinical manifestations of systemic enteroviral infection sometimes accompany myopericarditis, including aseptic meningitis, rash, pleurodynia, and orchitis. Death may occur as a consequence of arrhythmia or congestive heart failure, but this is uncommon in acute enteroviral myopericarditis.

LABORATORY DIAGNOSIS. The enteroviral etiology of myopericarditis is established by isolating virus from, or detecting viral proteins or nucleic acid in, the myocardium, pericardium, or pericardial fluid. Isolation of virus from the throat or feces, together with serologic evidence of recent or concurrent infection with the same enterovirus serotype, provides circumstantial evidence associating enterovirus infection with the cardiac disease.

Diagnosis of neonatal enteroviral infection is most rapidly accomplished by isolating virus, which is present in high titer and widely disseminated. Virus is readily recovered from the throat, feces, and urine. It can also be recovered from the blood, cerebrospinal fluid, ascitic fluid, and multiple tissues obtained by biopsy or at postmortem examination. Characteristic cytopathic effects can often be seen in cell culture within 2 or 3 days of inoculation. Serologic diagnosis is readily accomplished in surviving infants if a viral isolate has been obtained or if a particular enterovirus serotype is suspected.

In older children and adults, etiologic diagnosis of enteroviral myopericarditis is difficult. Virus is rarely isolated from the heart or pericardial fluid, and patients present late in the course of enterovirus infection when virus shedding has ceased and high stable levels of antiviral antibody are already present. The increasing use of endomyocardial biopsy combined with the application of new methods for the detection and amplification of enteroviral nucleic acid, as well as the increasing use of serotype-specific IgM antibody assays, should improve significantly our ability to establish the etiology of viral myopericarditis.

Electrocardiographic (ECG) abnormalities are present in virtually every patient with enteroviral myopericarditis. In pericarditis there is a characteristic progression of abnormalities. Initially, ST-segment elevation is observed in multiple leads without change in QRS morphology, reflecting diffuse subepicardial inflammation. There may also be depression of the PR segment. After a few days, the ST segment returns to baseline and there is T-wave flattening or inversion, which may persist for months. Large pericardial effusions may be associated with reduced QRS voltage and electrical alternans. The presence of nonspecific ST-segment and T-wave abnormalities is frequently used as the basis for the diagnosis of myocarditis. However, these same changes are often seen, in the absence of myocarditis, with fever, hypoxia, tachycardia, and electrolyte disturbances. Thus acceptance of ECG abnormalities alone as sufficient evidence of myocarditis may result in overdiagnosis. In severe myocarditis, Q waves, tachyarrhythmias, ventricular extrasystoles, and conduction disturbances are seen. Serum levels of myocardial enzymes are usually elevated in patients with severe myocarditis. Echocardiography is extremely useful for detecting and quantitating impaired ventricular function, identifying and quantitating pericardial effusion, and demonstrating early hemodynamic compromise.

The widespread use of endomyocardial biopsy was expected to compensate for the difficulty in clinically diagnosing myocarditis, but the introduction of this technique may have created as many problems as it has solved. In addition to the problem of sampling error, the question of whether small foci of lymphocytic infiltration, which have been observed on postmortem examination in 4 to 10 per cent of healthy young accident victims, are a manifestation of viral myocarditis or a normal finding is crucial but as yet unanswered. On the one hand, scattered small collections of inflammatory cells with focal necrosis of myocytes may occur in response to stress or the administration of vasopressors, and their presence in patients with heart failure may not be indicative of viral myocarditis. On the other hand, a single small focus of myocarditis in the conducting system may be responsible for a fatal arrhythmia in someone with little or no evidence of myocarditis elsewhere in the myocardium.

DIFFERENTIAL DIAGNOSIS. Neonatal myocarditis is sometimes mistaken for congenital heart disease, but fever, electrocardiographic evidence of myocarditis, and the involvement of other organ systems help to differentiate the two. Neonatal myocarditis and the generalized enteroviral infection that usually accompanies it are often indistinguishable from bacterial sepsis. Antimicrobial chemotherapy should be initiated and continued until bacterial sepsis is ruled out by appropriate cultures. Neonatal myocarditis is also difficult to distinguish from neonatal herpes simplex virus infection with visceral dissemination if cutaneous lesions are absent. In this situation, therapy with acyclovir should be initiated until herpes simplex virus

infection can be ruled out by virus isolation and antigen detection assays.

PROGNOSIS. With aggressive supportive therapy, the mortality of neonatal myocarditis appears to be less than 50 per cent. Long-term follow-up of survivors is lacking, but the frequent involvement of other organ systems, including the central nervous system, suggests that sequelae are likely to occur.

The majority of children and adults with enteroviral myopericarditis recover without obvious sequelae. Acute mortality is low (0 to 5 per cent), and deaths occur as a result of arrhythmias or congestive heart failure in patients with myocarditis; cardiac tamponade is rare in enteroviral pericarditis.

Approximately 20 per cent of patients experience one or more episodes of recurrent myopericarditis within 1 year of their initial illness, and persistent electrocardiographic abnormalities are observed in 10 to 20 per cent of patients. Cardiomegaly persists in 5 to 10 per cent of patients, and long-term follow-up suggests that 10 per cent or more may develop chronic cardiomyopathy. Constrictive pericarditis rarely occurs following enteroviral pericarditis.

TREATMENT AND PREVENTION. Specific antiviral chemotherapy is not yet available for enterovirus infections. Infants with neonatal myocarditis are unlikely to have received antibodies to the causative virus from their mothers. Thus it seems reasonable to administer human immune serum globulin, which contains high titers of neutralizing antibodies to a number of enterovirus serotypes, in an attempt to terminate viremia and limit further virus replication in infected tissues.

Treatment of enteroviral myopericarditis in older children and adults is primarily supportive. It should include control of pain with analgesics; careful monitoring for arrhythmias, heart failure, and hemodynamic compromise; and prompt treatment of these complications if they arise. Bed rest is an important component of therapy because of clear evidence in mice with coxsackievirus B3 myocarditis that exercise markedly increases the extent of myocardial necrosis and mortality during the acute phase of the disease. Adequate oxygenation should be assured and fluid overload avoided and promptly treated if it develops. In severe cases cardiac-assist devices may be lifesaving.

Corticosteroids should not be administered to patients with suspected enteroviral myocarditis or pericarditis. Their use during the acute phase of viral myocarditis has been associated with rapid clinical deterioration, and their deleterious effects have been clearly demonstrated during the acute phase of coxsackievirus B3 myocarditis in mice.

In uncontrolled trials, some patients with myocarditis who have been treated with immunosuppressive agents have shown improvement, but others have not, and early immunosuppressive therapy has increased myocardial damage in murine coxsackievirus myocarditis. Thus, because of the potential for harm, the use of immunosuppressive therapy for enteroviral myopericarditis should await the results of controlled trials now in progress.

Older children and adults with enteroviral myopericarditis do not require isolation. In neonatal myocarditis, the infected infant should be isolated and careful attention given to routine nursery infection control procedures, especially handwashing before and after handling each infant, in order to prevent nosocomial transmission. In nursery outbreaks, human immune serum globulin should be administered to all infants in an attempt to prevent disease.

Billingham M: Acute myocarditis: A diagnostic dilemma. Br Heart J 58:6–8, 1987. *A clear and concise discussion of the problems inherent in the use of endomyocardial biopsies for the diagnosis of myocarditis.*

Kaplan MH, Klein SW, McPhee J, Harper RG: Group B coxsackievirus infections in infants younger than three months of age: A serious childhood illness. Rev Infect Dis 5:1019–1032, 1983. *A thorough account of the clinical presentation, course, and outcome of neonatal myocarditis caused by group B coxsackieviruses.*

Koontz CH, Ray CG: The role of coxsackie group B virus infections in sporadic myopericarditis. Am Heart J 82:750–758, 1971. *A clinical and serologic study of 63 consecutive patients with suspected myopericarditis*

Savoia MC, Oxman MN: Myocarditis, pericarditis and mediastinitis. In Mandel GL, Douglas RG Jr, Bennett JE (eds.): Principles and Practice of Infectious Diseases. New York, Churchill Livingstone, 1990, pp 721–732. *A well-referenced review of the etiology, pathogenesis, clinical manifestations, and diagnosis of myocarditis and pericarditis.*

Woodruff JF: Viral myocarditis: A review. Am J Pathol 101:427–478, 1980. *A comprehensive review of all aspects of viral myocarditis.*

380 Mucocutaneous Syndromes Caused by Enteroviruses

Michael N. Oxman

Enteroviruses are the leading cause of exanthematous disease in the United States and most other developed countries. Almost all enteroviruses can cause maculopapular eruptions, and most serotypes are occasionally responsible for petechial or papulovesicular exanthems and enanthems as well. Moreover, a given enterovirus may cause more than one pattern of mucocutaneous disease, even within a single infected household. Consequently, except for hand-foot-and-mouth disease, which is usually caused by coxsackievirus A16 or enterovirus 71, there are no clinical or epidemiologic characteristics of any given enteroviral rash that point to a specific enterovirus as its cause.

EPIDEMIOLOGY. The epidemiology of enteroviral exanthems and enanthems is the epidemiology of enteroviral infections in general (see Ch. 377). The vast majority occur during the summer and early fall. The incidence of enanthems and exanthems in infected persons varies among different enteroviruses and even among different strains of the same enterovirus. For example, enanthems and exanthems are often seen in more than 50 per cent of infected children during outbreaks of infection caused by echovirus 9 or coxsackievirus A16 but are rare during outbreaks caused by echovirus 6 or coxsackievirus A7. Host factors, especially age, are also important; infants and young children are more likely to develop mucocutaneous lesions, whereas other manifestations of enterovirus infection, such as aseptic meningitis, are more likely to develop in older children and adults. Thus, during outbreaks of echovirus 9 infection, rash is often seen in the majority of infected children under 5 years of age but in less than 5 per cent of infected adults, and it is not uncommon when evaluating an adult with aseptic meningitis and no rash to find that a child in the same household is convalescing from an illness characterized by a maculopapular rash. Enteroviral exanthems and enanthems occur in outbreaks and as sporadic cases. Asymptomatic infections are common and are often the source of virus for symptomatic infections. Attack rates are highest in young children, who frequently introduce the virus into households where several members may become infected simultaneously or sequentially, with an incubation period of 3 to 10 days.

PATHOGENESIS. Enteroviral lesions in the oropharyngeal mucosa and skin are manifestations of a systemic virus infection. They result from the secondary infection of endothelial cells of small vessels in the underlying lamina propria and dermis, which occurs during the viremia that regularly follows enteroviral infection and replication in the alimentary tract. Their pathogenesis thus resembles that of the mucocutaneous lesions of measles, rubella, and varicella and contrasts with the pathogenesis of the lesions of acute herpetic gingivostomatitis, human papillomavirus infections (warts), and acute hemorrhagic conjunctivitis, which are the direct result of exogenous virus infection and replication in epithelial cells at the portal of entry. The nature of the enteroviral lesions reflects the nature and extent of local inflammatory changes in and around these small vessels. Vascular dilatation alone produces an erythematous macular eruption. Vascular dilatation plus edema and cellular infiltration results in erythematous papules. Endothelial damage with extravasation of red blood cells produces a petechial eruption. Infection and necrosis of cells in the surrounding dermis or overlying epidermis, together with the influx of fluid and inflammatory cells, produces vesicular lesions. When a vesicle forms in the mucosa of the oropharynx, the overlying layer of epithelial cells is rapidly macerated, producing a shallow ulcer that is usually surrounded by a zone of erythema. Although cytolytic virus replication is the predominant factor in the pathogenesis of enteroviral enanthems and exanthems, damage may be accentuated, at least in some cases, by host immune responses to enterovirus antigens in the infected tissues.

The obligatory occurrence of alimentary tract replication and viremia prior to the development of mucocutaneous lesions explains the 3- to 10-day incubation period and the frequent occurrence of prodromal signs and symptoms. Moreover, the simultaneous dissemination of virus to a number of target organs explains the concurrent appearance of other manifestations of enterovirus infection, such as aseptic meningitis and pericarditis.

CLINICAL MANIFESTATIONS. *Enanthems.* The oropharyngeal mucosa is involved to some degree during most symptomatic enteroviral infections. This is usually manifest by mild pharyngitis and mucosal erythema, but it may also result in a variety of enanthems. These may consist of macules, papules, vesicles, petechiae, or ulcers, and they may occur alone or in association with exanthems and other manifestations of systemic enteroviral infection. They are often transient and frequently unrecognized, but they occasionally lead to diagnostic confusion, for example, when they resemble Koplik's spots and accompany a morbilliform exanthem in a child infected by echovirus 9. Two enanthems are sufficiently unique to warrant separate description:

Herpangina (*herpes*, vesicular eruption; *angina*, inflammation of the throat) is a syndrome characterized by the sudden onset of fever, sore throat, pain on swallowing, and a vesicular enanthem of the posterior pharynx. It is seen primarily in children between 3 and 10 years of age. The disease begins abruptly, after a 3- to 10-day incubation period, with fever ranging from 38 to 41°C, sore throat, and pain on swallowing. Fever tends to be higher in younger children, who may suffer febrile convulsions; older children and adults frequently complain of headache and myalgia. On examination, there is pharyngeal erythema but little or no tonsillar exudate. The characteristic lesions are discrete 1- to 2-mm vesicles and ulcers surrounded by 1- to 5-mm zones of erythema. Lesions are few in number, averaging four or five per patient, with a range of 1 or 2 to 20. They occur most frequently on the anterior tonsillar pillars, the posterior edge of the soft palate and the uvula, and less frequently on the tonsils, the posterior pharyngeal wall, and the posterior buccal mucosa. They begin as small papules, progress to vesicles, and ulcerate within 24 hours. The shallow ulcers, which are moderately painful, may enlarge over the next day or two to a diameter of 3 to 4 mm. Symptoms generally disappear in 3 or 4 days, but the ulcers may persist for up to a week. Most cases are mild and resolve without complications, but herpangina is occasionally associated with exanthems, aseptic meningitis, or other serious manifestations of enterovirus infection. Outbreaks of herpangina are common during the summer, and sporadic cases are also observed. Group A coxsackieviruses (A1 to 6, A8, A10, and A22) account for the majority of outbreaks, but outbreaks have also been caused by other enteroviruses, including coxsackievirus B1 and echoviruses 16 and 25. In addition, these viruses, as well as coxsackieviruses A7, A9, A16, and B2 to 5, and echoviruses 6, 9, 11, 17, and 22, have been isolated from sporadic cases. A variant of herpangina has been described in children infected with coxsackievirus A10. The lesions have the same distribution as in typical cases of herpangina, but instead of evolving into vesicles and ulcers they remain papular and are infiltrated with lymphocytes to form 2- to 3-mm gray-white nodules surrounded by narrow zones of erythema. The disease, which has been called *acute lymphonodular pharyngitis*, is otherwise indistinguishable from herpangina.

Hand-foot-and-mouth disease (vesicular stomatitis with exanthem) is a mild enteroviral disease characterized by a vesicular eruption in the mouth and over the extremities. It occurs most frequently in children less than 5 years of age. After an incubation period of 3 to 6 days, the disease begins with mild fever ranging from 38 to 39°C, anorexia, malaise, and often a sore mouth. Within a day or two, vesicular lesions appear in the oral cavity, most frequently on the anterior buccal mucosa and the tongue but also on the labial mucosa, gingivae, and hard palate. The oral lesions begin as erythematous macules and quickly evolve into 2- to 4-mm vesicles surrounded by zones of erythema. Some vesicles ulcerate, forming 4- to 6-mm shallow painful ulcers surrounded by erythema; others coalesce to form bullae; and still others are absorbed without ulcerating. In the majority of preschool children, but in only about 10 per cent of infected adults, the oral lesions are accompanied by vesicular skin lesions, most often on the dorsal or lateral surfaces of the hands and feet and on the fingers and toes, but not infrequently on the palms and soles. Less often, lesions occur on the buttocks or more proximally on the extremities, and rarely on the genitalia. They are generally 3 to 7 mm in diameter and surrounded by a narrow zone of erythema. They range in number from two or three to 30 or more and consist of subepidermal vesicles containing a mixed inflammatory infiltrate of lymphocytes, monocytes, and neutrophils and accompanied by acantholysis and cellular degeneration in the overlying epidermis. The cutaneous lesions are generally not pruritic or painful, and they resolve without ulcerating, crusting, or scarring within about a week. Hand-foot-and-mouth disease is caused most frequently by coxsackievirus A16, less frequently by enterovirus 71 and coxsackieviruses A5, A9, and A10, and occasionally by coxsackieviruses A4, A7, B2, and B5. Outbreaks and sporadic cases occur primarily in the summer and early fall. Attack rates are highest in young children, and during epidemics more than half of the children in affected households may develop disease. Hand-foot-and-mouth disease itself is benign, but it may occasionally be associated with one of the more severe manifestations of systemic enterovirus infection, such as aseptic meningitis, encephalitis, or myocarditis. This has been especially true during epidemics of enterovirus 71 infection, in which a number of patients with hand-foot-and-mouth disease also developed serious central nervous system disease.

Exanthems. Enterovirus exanthems themselves are benign, but they are clinically important for at least three reasons: (1) They constitute direct evidence of enterovirus dissemination and thus provide a clue to the presence and the etiology of coexistent disease referable to other potentially infected target organs, such as the heart and the central nervous system; (2) they represent the "tip of an iceberg" of enterovirus infection in the community; and (3) they are often confused with other infectious exanthems, some of which have more serious consequences, require specific control measures, or are amenable to specific anti-infective therapy. Since enteroviral rashes are not sufficiently distinctive to permit an etiologic diagnosis to be made on clinical grounds, identification of the responsible agent requires laboratory diagnosis. However, the problem of confusing enteroviral rashes with other infectious exanthems can be approached by comparing the enterovirus rashes to the nonenterovirus rashes that they resemble.

The most common cutaneous manifestation of enterovirus infection is an erythematous maculopapular rash that appears together with fever and other manifestations of systemic infection. This is also a common manifestation of infection by a variety of other organisms, but it is more often caused by enteroviruses than by any other infectious agent. Only certain enteroviruses (e.g., echovirus 9) cause this syndrome with high frequency, but almost all can produce it, at least occasionally. The rash begins on the face and quickly spreads to the neck, trunk, and extremities. It consists of 1- to 3-mm erythematous macules and papules that may be discrete (*rubelliform*, resembling rubella) or confluent (*morbilliform*, resembling measles). It usually lasts for 2 to 5 days and does not itch or desquamate. Enteroviral exanthems are generally not accompanied by significant posterior cervical, suboccipital, or postauricular lymphadenopathy, but there are many exceptions. For example, posterior cervical and suboccipital lymphadenopathy similar to that seen in rubella has been observed in many children with exanthems caused by coxsackievirus A9.

When the enteroviral rash consists of discrete erythematous macules and papules (i.e., when it is rubelliform), it is most likely to be confused with rubella. When the lesions are confluent (i.e., when the rash is morbilliform), it is more likely to be confused with measles. Confusion with measles is accentuated when the rash is accompanied by an enanthem that resembles Koplik's spots, something that has often been seen in children infected with echovirus 9 and is occasionally seen in children infected with a number of other enteroviruses.

Enteroviral rashes are sometimes petechial and occasionally purpuric. Although this pattern is seen most frequently in echovirus 9 and coxsackievirus A9 infections, it is observed occasionally with many other enterovirus serotypes. When an enteroviral infection is accompanied by a petechial or purpuric rash, it is easily confused with meningococcemia, and when it is also associated with aseptic meningitis, as it often is in echovirus 9 and coxsackievirus A9 infections, it is clinically indistinguishable

from meningococcal meningitis. In this situation it is usually prudent to initiate antimicrobial chemotherapy pending the results of laboratory investigations.

Vesicular exanthems are most often seen as a component of hand-foot-and-mouth disease (see above), but several enteroviruses, including echovirus 11 and coxsackievirus A9, cause vesicular exanthems without an associated enanthem. The lesions resemble those caused by varicella-zoster and herpes simplex viruses. In contrast to varicella, however, vesicular rashes caused by enteroviruses are usually peripheral in distribution and consist of relatively few lesions that heal without crusting. When they are not associated with hand-foot-and-mouth disease, vesicular lesions caused by enteroviruses are often confused with insect bites or poison ivy. Echovirus 11 and several coxsackievirus serotypes have been associated with skin lesions resembling papular urticaria, lesions that usually result from insect bites.

Enteroviral rashes are generally accompanied by fever; they develop at or within a day or two of its onset. In some cases, however, the rash does not develop until the fever subsides, a pattern resembling that of *roseola infantum* (exanthem subitum), a benign sporadic disease of infants 6 to 24 months of age now known to be caused by human herpesvirus 6. These roseola-like enterovirus infections are typified by the "Boston exanthem," caused by echovirus 16 and first described during an epidemic in Boston in 1951. It is characterized by fever (to 38 to 39°C) lasting 2 to 4 days, followed by defervescence and then by the appearance of a salmon-pink maculopapular rash on the face and upper chest. The rash resolves in 1 to 5 days without sequelae. Frequently, multiple cases occur sequentially in households; the illness is mild in children and more severe in adults, who often develop high fever and aseptic meningitis without rash. In addition to echovirus 16, a number of other enterovirus serotypes have occasionally been associated with roseola-like illnesses.

DIFFERENTIAL DIAGNOSIS. Herpangina is most often confused with bacterial pharyngitis or tonsillitis or with pharyngitis caused by other viruses. Other considerations include hand-foot-and-mouth disease, herpes simplex virus infections, and herpes zoster involving the palate. In bacterial pharyngitis and tonsillitis there is usually a more extensive tonsillar exudate, more prominent cervical lymphadenopathy, and more signs of systemic illness. Bacterial pharyngitis and pharyngitis caused by most viruses other than enteroviruses are not ordinarily associated with vesicular lesions. However, in individual cases, bacterial pharyngitis may be difficult to distinguish from enteroviral pharyngitis on clinical grounds, and the two may even coexist. Thus, throat cultures and assays for group A β-hemolytic streptococcal antigens are often warranted. Herpangina is a disease of the posterior oropharynx, whereas hand-foot-and-mouth disease and primary herpes simplex gingivostomatitis involve the anterior oropharynx. The former is also generally accompanied by cutaneous lesions, and herpetic gingivostomatitis is characterized by more extensive and painful lesions, prominent gingivitis, cervical lymphadenopathy, and more severe systemic signs and symptoms. Recurrent herpes simplex (herpes labialis) generally involves the vermilion border of the lip or the adjacent skin rather than the palate, and it is often preceded by tingling or burning neuralgia. There is also usually a history of recurrent episodes. Palatal herpes zoster may sometimes mimic herpangina, but it generally occurs in older individuals, is preceded and accompanied by pain and sensory abnormalities, and is unilateral. Vesicular lesions caused by herpes simplex and varicella-zoster viruses contain multinucleated giant cells, which are not present in enteroviral lesions.

The vesicular lesions of hand-foot-and-mouth disease resemble those caused by herpes simplex and varicella-zoster viruses. Patients with primary herpetic gingivostomatitis are usually more toxic and have cervical lymphadenopathy and more prominent gingivitis. Their cutaneous lesions are usually perioral but may occasionally involve a finger that has been in the mouth. Lesions of herpes labialis usually involve the vermilion border of the lip or the adjacent skin, are rarely accompanied by lesions on the hands or feet, often have a neuralgic prodome, and frequently have a history of recurrent episodes. The cutaneous lesions of varicella are generally more extensive and are centrally distributed, sparing the palms and soles. Oral lesions are far less prominent in varicella, and its prevalence in winter and spring further distinguishes it from hand-foot-and-mouth disease.

Aphthous stomatitis is distinguished from hand-foot-and-mouth disease by the absence of fever and other signs of systemic illness, the absence of cutaneous lesions, and often a history of recurrence.

Maculopapular exanthems caused by enteroviruses are distinguished from measles and rubella by their summertime occurrence, the usual absence of posterior cervical, suboccipital, and postauricular lymphadenopathy, and their relatively short incubation period. The absence of significant coryza and conjunctivitis further distinguishes the typical enteroviral exanthems from measles. In addition, the probability of measles and rubella is markedly reduced in persons with a well-documented history of adequate immunization.

When enteroviral rashes are maculopapular they may be confused with drug reactions; when they are petechial they may be confused with bacterial or rickettsial rashes. In addition to obvious differences in epidemiologic and exposure histories, the maculopapular and petechial (but not vesicular) rashes caused by enteroviruses are distinguished by their tendency to spare the palms and soles, which are usually involved in drug reactions and bacterial and rickettsial rashes.

When enteroviral rashes are petechial, it is impossible to rule out meningococcemia on clinical grounds alone. Laboratory investigation is required, even during proven outbreaks of enteroviral disease, because concurrent enteroviral and meningococcal infections can occur.

Vesicular rashes caused by enteroviruses can be confused with varicella, herpes simplex virus infections, insect bites, and poison ivy. They can be distinguished from varicella by their occurrence during the summer and early fall, their relatively short incubation period, their peripheral distribution, and their tendency to heal without crusting. The various forms of herpes simplex virus infection have unique characteristics that distinguish them from enteroviral infections. Cutaneous dissemination occurs occasionally in patients with primary genital herpes or acute herpetic gingivostomatitis, but the clinical picture is dominated by genital or oral signs and symptoms. Primary cutaneous herpes simplex infections are uncommon, and the lesions are localized at the site of inoculation. Recurrent cutaneous herpes simplex (e.g., herpetic whitlow) is generally localized within a single dermatome and accompanied by neuralgia but not by fever or other signs of systemic infection. The vesicles of recurrent herpes simplex are grouped, whereas those of enteroviral exanthems are scattered, and there is often a history of previous episodes at the same site. The presence of fever and other signs of systemic infection distinguishes enteroviral exanthems from insect bites and poison ivy, whether the enteroviral rash is vesicular or urticarial.

Roseola-like enteroviral infections can be distinguished from roseola infantum by their occurrence in outbreaks and epidemics during the summer and early fall and by the involvement of older children and adults.

LABORATORY DIAGNOSIS. As with other enterovirus infections, the etiology of mucocutaneous syndromes caused by enteroviruses is established by virus isolation and demonstration of the concurrent development of serotype-specific neutralizing antibodies (see Ch. 377). Virus can be isolated from the throat, feces, blood, and vesicular lesions early in the disease, and it can also be isolated from the cerebrospinal fluid of many patients with aseptic meningitis. Vesicular lesions can be differentiated from those caused by herpes simplex and varicella-zoster viruses by the absence of multinucleated giant cells on Tzanck smears, as well as by immunofluorescent or immunoperoxidase staining for viral antigens. It is often essential to exclude other potential pathogens, such as *Neisseria meningitides* and the group A β-hemolytic streptococcus, by using appropriate cultures and antigen detection tests.

TREATMENT AND PREVENTION. Enteroviral enanthems and exanthems are benign, self-limited illnesses that require only symptomatic therapy for headache and sore throat. More serious manifestations of disseminated infection, such as aseptic meningitis or encephalitis, may require supportive treatment. When illness mimics meningococcemia or meningococcal meningitis, antimicrobial chemotherapy should be initiated until bacterial infection is ruled out by appropriate cultures and antigen detection assays.

Control of enterovirus infections is best accomplished by hygienic measures such as handwashing and improved sanitation.

Isolation of patients with enteroviral enanthems or exanthems is generally not helpful because of the simultaneous existence of a large reservoir of asymptomatically infected persons who are excreting virus. The generally benign nature of these infections and the large number of enterovirus serotypes that cause them preclude the development of vaccines.

Adler JL, Mostow SR, Mellin H, et al.: Epidemiologic investigation of hand-foot-and-mouth disease. Infection caused by coxsackievirus A16 in Baltimore, June through September, 1968. Am J Dis Child 120:309–313, 1970. *A detailed investigation of an outbreak of hand-foot-and-mouth disease caused by coxsackievirus A16.*

Cherry JD: Skin infections: Cutaneous manifestations of systemic infections. *In* Feigen RD, Cherry JD (eds.): Textbook of Pediatric Infectious Diseases. Philadelphia, W. B. Saunders, 1987, pp 786–817. *An excellent review of the etiology and differential diagnosis of the mucocutaneous manifestations of systemic infections.*

Cherry JD, Jahn CL: Herpangina: The etiologic spectrum. Pediatrics 36:632–634, 1965. *A review of herpangina and its various enteroviral causes.*

Hall CB, Cherry JD, Hatch MH, et al.: The return of Boston exanthem: Echovirus 16 infections in 1974. Am J Dis Child 131:323–326, 1977. *An excellent description of the roseola infantum–like disease produced by echovirus 16.*

Huebner RJ, Cole RM, Beeman EA, et al.: Herpangina. Etiologic studies of a specific infectious disease. JAMA 145:628–633, 1951. *The initial association of herpangina with group A coxsackievirus infections.*

Neva FA, Feemster RF, Gorbach IJ: Clinical and epidemiological features of an unusual epidemic exanthem. JAMA 155:544–548, 1954. *The original description of the Boston exanthem.*

Robinson CR, Doane FW, Rhodes AJ: Report of an outbreak of febrile illness with pharyngeal lesions and exanthem, Toronto, summer 1957-isolation of a group A Coxsackie virus. Can Med Assoc J 79:615–621, 1958. *An early description of hand-foot-and-mouth disease and its association with coxsackievirus A16.*

Sabin AB, Krumbiegel ER, Wigand R: ECHO type 9 virus disease. Virologically controlled clinical and epidemiologic observations during a 1957 epidemic in Milwaukee with notes on concurrent similar diseases associated with coxsackie and other ECHO viruses. Prog Pediatr 96:197–219, 1958. *A detailed review of the spectrum of disease associated with echovirus 9 infections and a comparison with diseases caused by other enteroviruses.*

381 Acute Hemorrhagic Conjunctivitis
Michael N. Oxman

DEFINITION. Acute hemorrhagic conjunctivitis (AHC) is an acute, highly contagious, self-limited disease of the eye characterized by the sudden onset of pain, photophobia, conjunctivitis, swelling of the eyelids, and prominent subconjunctival hemorrhages. Since its first appearance in 1969, AHC has occurred in explosive epidemics throughout the world. The disease was initially nicknamed "Apollo 11 disease" because its appearance in Ghana coincided with the Apollo 11 moon landing.

ETIOLOGY. Enterovirus 70, a new enterovirus isolated from patients during the initial pandemic of AHC that began in Ghana in 1969, has been responsible for tens of millions of cases that have occurred in widespread epidemics during the past 20 years. A variant of coxsackievirus A24, which first appeared at about the same time as enterovirus 70, has been responsible for hundreds of thousands of cases of the disease that have occurred in a number of more circumscribed epidemics during the same period. Both viruses have been involved concurrently in some epidemics. To date, coxsackievirus A24 has been responsible for fewer cases of epidemic conjunctivitis than enterovirus 70, and it does not cause subconjunctival hemorrhages in as high a proportion of patients. Nucleic acid hybridization and serologic studies have shown that the two viruses are genetically and antigenically unrelated.

EPIDEMIOLOGY. Although mild conjunctivitis may occur as a minor manifestation of infection by many enteroviruses, especially in children, its occurrence as the major clinical manifestation of enterovirus infection was not observed until 1969, when explosive epidemics of AHC occurred in Ghana and almost simultaneously in Indonesia. The responsible agent proved to be a new enterovirus, designated enterovirus 70. Over the next 2 years the disease assumed pandemic proportions, with large epidemics occurring in many areas of Africa, Southeast Asia, the Far East, India, and Japan and involving tens of millions of people. A number of smaller outbreaks also occurred in Europe. Scattered epidemics of AHC continued to occur in these same areas during the remainder of the decade, and the recurrence of epidemics in the same geographic areas suggests that immunity to AHC may be short-lived. In 1981 a new pandemic began, with epidemics again occurring in Africa and Asia, but this time it extended to Australia and the South Pacific, and to the Americas, including the United States, where its arrival was marked by an explosive outbreak of AHC in Miami, Florida. Some outbreaks in Europe and the United States have been initiated by infected travelers and then spread nosocomially within eye clinics.

Another enterovirus, subsequently identified as a variant of coxsackievirus A24, was responsible for a large epidemic of AHC in Singapore in 1970. This virus has subsequently been responsible for a number of epidemics in many of the same regions invaded by enterovirus 70, including Africa, Southeast Asia, India, the Far East, and the Americas. Both viruses have been involved together in several epidemics.

AHC is a highly contagious disease. In contrast to most enteroviral infections, it is transmitted by direct inoculation of the conjunctivae with virus-contaminated fingers or fomites (i.e., transmission is eye-finger or fomite-eye). Enterovirus 70 and the coxsackievirus A24 variant are both naturally occurring, temperature-sensitive viruses that replicate optimally at 33 to 35°C, the temperature of the conjunctivae. There appears to be little or no virus replication in the alimentary tract. Virus is abundant in the conjunctivae and in the ocular exudate, from which it can be readily isolated early in infection. Virus is less readily isolated from pharyngeal secretions and only very rarely recovered from feces. In contrast to most other enteroviruses, there does not appear to be a prolonged period of virus excretion following acute infection. Transmission is favored by crowding and unhygienic living conditions and also by warm, humid coastal climates. During epidemics all age groups are affected; attack rates of clinical illness are highest in young adults, but infection rates are highest in children under 10 years of age, many of whom experience mild or inapparent infections. Infection rates are also substantially higher among the poor than in middle and upper socioeconomic groups. School-age children are most likely to introduce infection into households, where secondary attack rates often exceed 50 per cent. During the 1969–1971 pandemic, postepidemic serologic surveys revealed enterovirus 70 neutralizing antibody prevalence rates to be nearly 50 per cent in affected populations in Ghana, Indonesia, and other developing countries, but only about 5 per cent in affected populations in Japan and other developed countries. These results were consistent with the more limited spread of AHC observed when the disease was introduced into developed countries, and they also confirmed the widespread occurrence of subclinical infections.

Enterovirus 70 is a most unusual enterovirus. In addition to being a naturally occurring temperature-sensitive virus that causes disease at its portal of entry and is not transmitted by the fecal-oral route, it has an exceptionally broad host range. It replicates in a wide variety of nonprimate as well as primate cells and causes paralytic disease in monkeys. Moreover, neutralizing antibodies to enterovirus 70 have been detected in a number of animal species, including cattle, sheep, goats, swine, chickens, dogs, and wild monkeys. Oligonucleotide mapping of a series of epidemic strains suggests that they all evolved from a hypothetical ancestor strain that was not in existence before 1967. Serologic studies have reinforced the notion that enterovirus 70 has only recently emerged as a human pathogen; neutralizing antibodies to enterovirus 70 have generally not been found in human sera collected prior to 1969, even sera from elderly persons. Detailed analysis of the enterovirus 70 genome, which has recently been cloned and sequenced, shows that except for its 5′ noncoding region, which is very similar to that of poliovirus type 3, the enterovirus 70 genome is more closely related to the genomes of bovine enteroviruses and swine vesicular disease virus than to the genomes of other human enteroviruses. Finally, neutralizing antibodies to enterovirus 70 have been detected in animal sera from Japan and West Africa collected prior to 1969, indicating

that enterovirus 70 or a very similar virus was circulating in animals before the first appearance of AHC in humans. Taken together, these observations suggest that enterovirus 70 may represent a zoonotic picornavirus that extended its host range to humans, perhaps as a consequence of recombination with poliovirus type 3.

PATHOGENESIS. In contrast to other enteroviral infections (see Ch. 377), AHC is transmitted by direct inoculation of the conjunctivae with virus on contaminated fingers or fomites (e.g., ophthalmologic instruments, shared towels). Disease results from local virus replication at the portal of entry; prior replication in the alimentary tract and viremia are not required to disseminate virus to ocular tissues. This explains the unusually short incubation period, which is generally 24 hours or less (range, 12 to 72 hours). There is, in fact, little evidence of alimentary tract infection or fecal virus shedding in AHC, and constitutional symptoms are observed in only a small minority of cases. This behavior is consistent with the preferential growth of enterovirus 70 (and coxsackievirus A24) at 33 to 35°C, which would be expected to limit its capacity to replicate and spread systemically. Conjunctival infection terminates spontaneously within 4 to 7 days of onset.

The major complication of AHC is a poliomyelitis-like flaccid paralysis, which occurs rarely in patients with AHC caused by enterovirus 70, but apparently not at all in patients with AHC caused by coxsackievirus A24. The pathogenesis of this AHC-associated paralytic disease is not clear. While enterovirus 70 has not been isolated from the cerebrospinal fluid, all of the affected patients have aseptic meningitis and evidence of local production of antibodies to enterovirus 70 within their central nervous system, findings not observed in patients with uncomplicated AHC. This suggests that AHC-associated paralytic disease probably reflects enterovirus 70 infection and destruction of motor neurons. The relatively high frequency of bulbar involvement (see below) further suggests that the route of infection of the central nervous system may be axonal rather than viremic.

CLINICAL MANIFESTATIONS. AHC begins with the sudden onset of eye pain and foreign body sensation, lacrimation, photophobia, blurred vision, and bulbar conjunctivitis. Signs and symptoms rapidly increase in severity with the development of palpebral conjunctivitis, conjunctival edema, swelling of the eyelids, subconjunctival hemorrhages in the bulbar conjunctivae, and a serous or seromucoid ocular discharge containing large numbers of polymorphonuclear leukocytes. The subconjunctival hemorrhages, which are the hallmark of the disease, range from discrete petechiae to confluent hemorrhages that occupy virtually the entire bulbar conjunctiva. They are present, usually within 24 hours of onset, in 70 to 90 per cent of patients with AHC caused by enterovirus 70, but are much less frequent in AHC caused by coxsackievirus A24. AHC often begins unilaterally, but it rapidly spreads to the other eye. Signs and symptoms peak within 24 to 36 hours of onset, by which time most patients have also developed hypertrophy of palpebral follicles and papillae, preauricular lymphadenopathy, and punctate epithelial keratitis with tiny corneal erosions that are often seen only by slit lamp examination after fluorescein staining. Clinical improvement usually begins by the second or third day, and recovery is generally complete without sequelae within 7 to 10 days. Constitutional symptoms, including headache, low-grade fever, and malaise, occur in a minority of patients.

A poliomyelitis-like motor paralysis occurs as a rare complication of AHC caused by enterovirus 70, but not in AHC caused by coxsackievirus A24. It occurs predominantly in adult males. The neurologic disease generally does not begin until 2 to 5 weeks after AHC (range, 5 to 60 days or more), and thus its relationship to the conjunctivitis is often overlooked by physicians, as well as by patients themselves. Radicular pain and paresthesia, usually accompanied by headache, fever, and malaise, are followed in 1 to 3 days by acute asymmetric areflexic paresis or paralysis of one or more limbs. Proximal muscles are usually affected more than distal muscles and lower limbs more than upper limbs. Bulbar involvement, as evidenced by paralysis of one or more cranial nerves, is observed in one third or more of affected patients. The cerebrospinal fluid is characterized by a mononuclear pleocytosis and elevated protein concentration. Permanent paralysis and muscular atrophy occur in approximately 25 per cent of affected patients. More than 200 cases have been reported to date, and the long interval between AHC and paralysis almost certainly accentuates underreporting. Nevertheless, in view of the many tens of millions of cases of AHC that have occurred since 1969, the incidence of this neurologic complication is probably less than 1 in 10,000 cases of AHC.

DIFFERENTIAL DIAGNOSIS. During major epidemics, AHC is unlikely to be confused with other eye infections. However, small outbreaks and sporadic cases may be mistaken for adenovirus infections, either acute follicular conjunctivitis or the more severe epidemic keratoconjunctivitis (EKC). This is especially likely when subconjunctival hemorrhages are not a prominant feature, as is often the case when AHC is caused by coxsackievirus A24. In addition, some outbreaks involve more than one agent (e.g., enterovirus 70 and adenovirus 11). Acute follicular conjunctivitis may occur as a separate entity or as one component of pharyngoconjunctival fever (PCF), in which case fever, malaise, pharyngitis, and cervical lymphadenopathy are prominent features. The adenovirus infections are more gradual in onset; in AHC, conjunctivitis generally reaches its peak within a day of onset and resolves in less than a week, whereas in adenovirus infections conjunctivitis slowly increases in intensity over several days and lasts for 2 weeks or more. Preauricular lymphadenopathy and conjunctival follicular hypertrophy are usually more prominent in adenovirus infections than in AHC, and in EKC epithelial keratitis is much more extensive than it is in AHC and is associated with subepithelial corneal opacities that persist for weeks to months after the epithelial lesions have resolved. Subconjunctival hemorrhages and eyelid ecchymosis may develop in EKC, producing an appearance suggesting previous eye trauma, but these manifestations do not appear until at least 4 or 5 days after onset, by which time AHC is always well on its way to resolution. EKC, which is often transmitted nosocomially during ophthalmic procedures such as tonometry or slit-lamp examination, is frequently unilateral, whereas AHC is almost always bilateral. Adenovirus is readily cultured from conjunctival scrapings or swabs in both EKC and acute follicular conjunctivitis.

Conjunctivitis caused by herpes simplex virus is most often associated with primary infection. Herpetic vesicles and ulcers often appear on the eyelids, and acute herpetic gingivostomatitis is typically present before the onset of the eye infection. Extensive subconjunctival hemorrhages are not a characteristic feature of herpes simplex virus infections of the eye. Recurrent ocular herpes usually produces characteristic dendritic corneal ulcers and little or no conjunctivitis. Tzanck smears of corneal scrapings reveal multinucleated giant cells, which are not observed in AHC, and herpes simplex virus is readily cultured from conjunctival swabs.

Bacterial and chlamydial infections are quite different from AHC in their epidemiology, presentation, and clinical course. A variety of noninfectious conditions can produce the signs and symptoms of conjunctivitis. These include chemical and radiation exposure (e.g., ultraviolet light from sunlamps or welders arcs), overwearing of contact lenses, and foreign bodies. Although none of these produces the extensive subconjunctival hemorrhages typically seen in AHC, their symptoms are sufficiently like the initial symptoms of AHC to cause confusion. The presence of a foreign body should be ruled out by careful examination, including eversion of the upper lid and fluorescein staining to highlight areas of epithelial disruption.

LABORATORY DIAGNOSIS. Enterovirus 70 and coxsackie-virus A24 can be isolated from conjunctival swabs and scrapings in a high proportion of patients with AHC if these specimens are obtained during the first 2 or 3 days of illness. In contrast to other enteroviral infections, virus is only occasionally isolated from the throat and almost never from the feces. The diagnosis is supported by the development of serotype-specific neutralizing antibodies, demonstrated by assay of acute and convalescent sera.

In AHC-associated paralytic disease, virus cannot be isolated from the cerebrospinal fluid or from the eye, throat, or feces. Serum antibodies to enterovirus 70 have generally already reached their maximum level before the onset of neurologic symptoms. The enterovirus 70 etiology of the paralytic disease can be supported by demonstrating serotype-specific antibodies in the cerebrospinal fluid at levels indicative of local central nervous system production and by documenting the absence of serologic evidence of poliovirus infection.

Appropriate cultures, conjunctival smears, and serologic assays can be used to exclude other infectious agents.

TREATMENT AND PREVENTION. AHC almost always resolves spontaneously without sequelae, and treatment is symptomatic. Topical application of antihistamine/decongestant eye drops and cold compresses may be used to reduce discomfort. Antimicrobial agents are not indicated unless there is bacterial superinfection (which should be documented by Gram's stain and culture). Corticosteroids, a component of many topical ophthalmic preparations, are contraindicated.

Transmission of AHC can be prevented by careful handwashing, avoidance of contaminated washcloths and towels, and sterilization of all ophthalmologic instruments. These practices should be routine in eye clinics.

Specific antiviral chemotherapeutic agents are not currently available, nor are vaccines for either enterovirus 70 or coxsackievirus A24.

Christopher S, Theogaraj S, Godbole S, et al.: An epidemic of acute hemorrhagic conjunctivitis due to coxsackievirus A24. J Infect Dis 146:16–19, 1982. *Clinical description and virologic studies of AHC caused by coxsackievirus A24*

Hierholzer JC, Hilliard KA, Esposito JJ: Serosurvey for "acute hemorrhagic conjunctivitis" virus (enterovirus 70) antibodies in the southeastern United States, with review of the literature and some epidemiologic implications. Am J Epidemiol 102:533–544, 1975. *A detailed review of the seroepidemiology and spread of enterovirus 70 infection*

Kono R: Apollo 11 disease or acute hemorrhagic conjunctivitis: A pandemic of a new enterovirus infection of the eyes. Am J Epidemiol 101:383–390, 1975. *An excellent description of the first pandemic of AHC.*

Kono R, Miyamura K, Tajiri E, et al.: Virologic and serologic studies of neurological complications of acute hemorrhagic conjunctivitis in Thailand. J Infect Dis 135:706–713, 1977. *Description of the poliomyelitis–like paralytic disease associated with AHC caused by enterovirus 70.*

Patriarca PA, Onorato I, Sklar VEF, et al.: Acute hemorrhagic conjunctivitis. Investigation of a large-scale community outbreak in Dade County, Florida. JAMA 249:1283–1289, 1983. *Excellent description of an epidemic of AHC in Miami, Florida.*

Ryan MD, Jenkins O, Hughes PJ, et al.: The complete nucleotide sequence of enterovirus type 70: Relationships with other members of the Picornaviridae. J Gen Virol 71:2291–2299, 1990. *A detailed comparison of the genome of enterovirus 70 to the genomes of other human and animal enteroviruses, with evidence for its unique nature and origin.*

Wadia NH, Katrak SM, Misra VP, et al.: Polio-like motor paralysis associated with acute hemorrhagic conjunctivitis in an outbreak in 1981 in Bombay, India: Clinical and serologic studies. J Infect Dis 147:660–668, 1983. *Description of the poliomyelitis-like paralytic disease associated with AHC and evidence linking it to enterovirus 70.*

Arthropod-Borne Viral Diseases

382 Introduction

Robert E. Shope

Arthropod-borne viruses (arboviruses) are transmitted biologically by an arthropod to a vertebrate host, either a human or a lower animal. The viruses replicate during an extrinsic incubation period in the arthropod, which may be a mosquito, tick, phlebotomine sandfly, or culicoid midge. The viruses are then transmitted by bite to the vertebrate, which becomes viremic and is in turn capable of infecting another biting arthropod. Some arboviruses also are transmitted vertically through the egg of the arthropod and may be maintained this way between seasons.

There are nearly 500 arthropod-borne viruses and at least 100 of these infect humans. These viruses contain RNA and all except the Reoviridae have lipid-containing envelopes. They are classified by biologic, physical, and chemical properties. Most fit into five families—Togaviridae, Flaviviridae, Bunyaviridae, Rhabdoviridae, and Reoviridae. Within each family are one or more genera, the genus usually corresponding to an antigenic group. These groups are important, because the clinician must rely heavily on the laboratory for a serologic diagnosis or identification of an isolate.

Table 382–1 lists some of the arboviruses that cause disease in humans. The viruses described in this section were selected as a few of the more important of approximately 100 that are known to infect people.

Most infections are inapparent. The remainder are associated with one or more of four major syndromes: (1) undifferentiated fever, (2) fever with rash and/or arthritis, (3) encephalitis, and (4) hemorrhagic fever (see Ch. 390).

The diseases described in this section are nearly all zoonoses (i.e., diseases caused by viruses transmitted from animals to man). The diseases are more prevalent in the tropics and subtropics and are usually focal because of ecologic restrictions on their transmission (Table 382–1). Diagnosis depends on a careful

TABLE 382–1. SOME PROPERTIES OF RNA VIRUSES CAUSING FEVER, ARTHRITIS, ENCEPHALITIS, OR HEMORRHAGIC FEVER

Family (*Genus*) Virus	Human Disease	Distribution	Vector
Togaviridae (*Alphavirus*)			
Mayaro	Fever, arthritis, rash	South America	Mosquito
Ross River	Arthritis, rash, sometimes fever	Australia, S. Pacific	Mosquito
Chikungunya	Fever, arthritis, hemorrhagic fever	Africa, Asia, Philippines	Mosquito
Eastern encephalitis	Fever, encephalitis	Americas	Mosquito
Western encephalitis	Fever, encephalitis	Americas	Mosquito
Venezuelan encephalitis	Fever, sometimes encephalitis	Americas	Mosquito
Flaviviridae (*Flavivirus*)			
Dengue (4 types)	Fever, rash, hemorrhagic fever	Worldwide (tropics)	Mosquito
Yellow fever	Fever, hemorrhagic fever	Tropical Americas, Africa	Mosquito
St. Louis encephalitis	Encephalitis, hepatitis (rare)	Americas	Mosquito
Japanese encephalitis	Encephalitis	Asia, Pacific	Mosquito
West Nile	Fever, rash, hepatitis, encephalitis	Asia, Europe, Africa	Mosquito
Kyasanur Forest	Hemorrhagic fever, meningoencephalitis	India	Tick
Omsk hemorrhagic fever	Hemorrhagic fever	U.S.S.R.	Tick
Tick-borne encephalitis	Encephalitis	Europe, Asia	Tick
Bunyaviridae (*Bunyavirus*)			
LaCrosse encephalitis	Encephalitis	North America	Mosquito
Oropouche	Fever	Brazil, Panama	Midge
Bunyaviridae (*Phlebovirus*)			
Sandfly fever viruses	Fever	Asia, Africa, tropical Americas	Sand fly, mosquito
Rift Valley fever	Fever, hemorrhagic fever, encephalitis, retinitis	Africa	Mosquito
Bunyaviridae (*Nairovirus*)			
Crimean-Congo hemorrhagic fever	Hemorrhagic fever	Asia, Europe, Africa	Tick
Bunyaviridae (*Hantavirus*)			
Hantaan	Hemorrhagic fever, renal syndrome	Asia	Rodent-borne
Puumala	Hemorrhagic fever, renal syndrome	Europe	Rodent-borne
Arenaviridae (*Arenavirus*)			
Junin	Hemorrhagic fever	Argentina	Rodent-borne
Machupo	Hemorrhagic fever	Bolivia	Rodent-borne
Lassa	Hemorrhagic fever	West Africa	Rodent-borne
Reoviridae (*Orbivirus*)			
Colorado tick fever	Fever	Western U.S.A.	Tick
Filoviridae (*Filovirus*)			
Marburg	Hemorrhagic fever	Africa	Unknown
Ebola	Hemorrhagic fever	Africa	Unknown

history encompassing exposure to vertebrate animals and arthropod vectors, age, season, and travel, including geographic site of exposure. The physician must have a high index of suspicion. Fevers may often be diagnosed erroneously as malaria; indeed, in malaria-endemic regions the patient frequently has malaria concomitantly with an arboviral infection.

Laboratory confirmation of infection is essential. Classically the virus was isolated from acute phase serum or whole blood in laboratory animals such as the mouse or in tissue culture. The neutralization, complement fixation, and hemagglutination-inhibition tests of acute and 3-week convalescent sera also led to the correct diagnosis. Now the fluorescent antibody and enzyme-linked immunosorbent assays (ELISA) are supplanting the classic techniques. Antigen detection and IgM capture ELISA permit diagnosis on the initial visit to the physician in many cases, and at least within a week of onset of the illness in most cases.

Control can be achieved by interrupting the cycle, including vaccination of reservoir animals, vector control, and education on methods to avoid the vector. Vaccines are available or under development for some of the agents such as Rift Valley fever, Venezuelan encephalitis, yellow fever, Japanese encephalitis, and dengue.

Beaty BJ, Calisher CH, Shope RE: Arboviruses. *In* Schmidt NJ, Emmons RW (eds.): Diagnostic Procedures for Viral, Rickettsial and Chlamydial Infections, 6th ed. Washington, D.C., American Public Health Association, 1989, pp 797–855. *Detailed description of diagnostic technology with clearly defined explanation of indications and limitations of procedures.*

Karabatsos N (ed.): International Catalogue of Arboviruses Including Certain Other Viruses of Vertebrates, 3rd ed. San Antonio, TX, American Society of Tropical Medicine and Hygiene, 1985. *Encyclopedic listing of 504 arboviruses and rodent-borne viruses with detailed description of epidemiologic, serologic, biochemical, and physical properties.*

383 Dengue

Jay P. Sanford

DEFINITION. Dengue is an acute arbovirus infection that presents chiefly with fever, malaise, lymphadenopathy, and rash. The first epidemic of a disease resembling dengue, which occurred in Philadelphia in 1780, was described by Benjamin Rush. Epidemics which now occur worldwide over large areas of the tropics and subtropics, including the Pacific basin, Southeast Asia, and Africa, were also common in North America in the nineteenth and early twentieth centuries, although many of these outbreaks more likely were Chikungunya virus disease. Outbreaks recurred in the Caribbean, including Puerto Rico and the U.S. Virgin Islands, in 1969. Indigenous infections were recognized in the continental United States for the first time in 35 years in 1980. Transmission by the mosquito *Aedes aegypti* was initially described by Bancroft (1906). *A. aegypti* has reappeared along the U.S. Gulf Coast; hence, the threat of reappearance of dengue in the United States again is real.

ETIOLOGY. Dengue viruses, members of the family Flaviviridae, are single-stranded, nonsegmented RNA viruses. There are four distinct serogroups of dengue viruses, types 1 through 4, each of which has now been documented in the western hemisphere.

EPIDEMIOLOGY. The cycle of dengue virus transmission involves primarily humans and mosquitoes. *A. aegypti* is the most important vector, but other species of *Aedes* are involved in Asia and the Pacific. *A. aegypti* is peridomestic, biting humans readily or even preferentially. Feeding is frequently interrupted, with the female taking multiple blood meals and thus enabling multiple infections by a single mosquito. Breeding occurs in small collections of water such as backyard litter, especially tires. Surveys in Texas have revealed containers with water in which *A. aegypti* were breeding in up to 25 per cent of premises. Zoonotic cycles of dengue virus transmission involving monkeys and forest *Aedes* species occur in Malaysia and West Africa. The mechanism for maintenance of the virus between epidemics has not been defined, but vertical transmission in *Aedes* has been experimentally documented. Nonimmune individuals are uniformly susceptible, and susceptibility is not influenced by age, sex, or race. During outbreaks attack rates in nonimmune individuals may be high; in Puerto Rico and the U.S. Virgin Islands, the overall rate of clinical disease was 20 per cent, with infection rates as determined by serologic surveys as high as 79 per cent. Immunity against homotypic reinfection is complete and probably lifelong, but cross-protection between different serotypes lasts less than 3 months.

PATHOLOGY. Dengue viruses multiply in the midgut epithelium and salivary glands of mosquitoes without producing pathologic changes. Mosquitoes remain infectious for life. The virus replicates in the female mosquito genital tract and may enter the ovum, enabling vertical transmission. In humans, in whom the classic disease is self-limited, biopsy of skin lesions shows swelling of endothelial cells and perivascular mononuclear cell infiltrates.

CLINICAL FEATURES. Dengue virus infection is often inapparent. When disease occurs, three overlapping clinical forms are recognized: classic dengue, a mild atypical form; dengue hemorrhagic fever (DHF), a severe form; and the dengue shock syndrome (DSS). Classic dengue (breakbone fever) occurs primarily in nonimmune individuals who are often nonindigenous children and adults. Disease begins abruptly after a 2- to 7-day incubation. Initial symptoms include a severe splitting headache, retro-orbital pain, backache especially in the lumbar area, leg pain, and arthralgia. At least three fourths of patients complain of pain on moving their eyes. True rigors are common during the illness but usually do not herald the onset. Other common symptoms include insomnia, nausea, anorexia with taste aberrations, cutaneous hyperesthesia, and generalized weakness. Mild rhinopharyngitis occurs in one fourth of patients. Findings on examination include a relative bradycardia, scleral injection (30 to 90 per cent), tenderness on pressure on the ocular globes, and pharyngeal injection. A transient macular rash may occur on the first or second day. Within 2 to 3 days after onset, the temperature may decrease to nearly normal and other symptoms subside. The remission typically lasts 2 days. Fever then recurs, giving the "saddle-back" or biphasic course. During the second phase, symptoms may return, although they are generally less severe. On the third to fifth day (with the second phase) a more definite maculopapular rash usually appears on the trunk and then spreads to the arms and legs while sparing the palms and soles. The rash is often characterized by 2- to 5-mm "islands of white in a sea of red." The rash is accompanied in some cases by complaints of burning in the palms of the hands and soles of the feet. On resolution, the rash may desquamate. Concurrently, generalized nontender lymphadenopathy, typically including posterior cervical, epitrochlear, and inguinal chains, develops. The biphasic febrile course is considered characteristic but often is not encountered. The entire illness lasts 5 to 7 days and terminates abruptly. Complaints of fatigue and depression for an additional several weeks are common.

In addition to the classic syndrome, an atypical mild illness characterized by fever, anorexia, headache, myalgia, and evanescent rashes occurs. The atypical syndrome is usually not associated with lymphadenopathy.

At the onset in both classic and mild dengue, leukocyte counts may be normal or low; however, by the third to fifth day leukocyte counts are decreased (less than 5000 per cubic millimeter with granulocytopenia). Thrombocytopenia (less than 100,000 per cubic millimeter) also may be a feature. Urinalysis may show moderate albuminuria.

DIAGNOSIS. A history of travel to dengue-endemic areas and occurrence of other cases in a community are important reminders to include dengue in the differential diagnosis. Specific diagnosis depends upon virus isolation or serologic tests. Viremia can be detected for the initial 3 to 5 days with dengue types 1, 2, and 3 by inoculation of mosquito tissue cell cultures. Viral titers in patients with dengue 4 are considerably lower than in patients with types 1, 2, and 3, making viral isolation less common. Of serologic tests, plaque-reduction neutralization is most specific. IgM antibodies indicate recent dengue infection but do not provide a type-specific diagnosis and cross-react with other flavivirus antibodies, including those following immunization with yellow fever vaccine.

TREATMENT. Treatment is entirely symptomatic—bed rest, antipyretics, and analgesics.

PROGNOSIS. In the absence of dengue hemorrhagic fever or the dengue shock syndrome, mortality is nil.

PREVENTION. Live attenuated vaccines against types 1, 2, and 4 are in various stages of development, but all are still investigational. Prevention of epidemics relies principally on reduction or eradication of *A. aegypti* by breeding site elimination and use of larvacides. Ultra low volume aerial spraying of organophosphate insecticides (malathion) to reduce the population of adult female mosquitoes has been used successfully for emergency control of epidemics.

Carey DE: Chikungunya and dengue: A case of mistaken identity. J Hist Med 26:243–262, 1971. *An in-depth review emphasizing clinical features. Not only interesting but provides useful clinical information.*

Ehrenkranz NJ, Ventura AK, Cuadrado RR, et al.: Pandemic dengue in Caribbean countries and the Southern United States—past, present and potential problems. N Engl J Med 285:1460–1469, 1971. *Summarizes the recent Caribbean pandemic and potential for reintroduction into the United States.*

Halstead SB: Pathogenesis of dengue: Challenges to molecular biology. Science 239:476–481, 1988. *The pathobiology of DHF and DSS versus that of classic dengue has remained unproved. Dr. Halstead reviews alternative hypotheses.*

Sabin AB: Research on dengue during World War II. Am J Trop Med Hyg 1:30–50, 1952. *This old paper still provides the best available summary of clinical features.*

384 West Nile Fever

Jay P. Sanford

DEFINITION. West Nile fever, like dengue, is a mosquito-transmitted, acute, self-limited illness that presents chiefly with fever, malaise, lymphadenopathy, and rash.

ETIOLOGY. West Nile fever virus is a member of the flaviviruses—single-stranded, nonsegmented RNA viruses. Viral strains from Africa, Europe, the USSR, and the Middle East are antigenically distinct from strains isolated in India and the Far East.

EPIDEMIOLOGY. The cycle of West Nile fever virus transmission involves mosquitoes and wild birds, with mammals, including man, as incidental end-stage hosts. The mosquito vector species vary between areas: *Culex univittatus, C. pipiens,* and *C. molestus* in the Middle East and Africa, *Mansonia metallicus* in Uganda, and *C. tritaeniorhynchus* in Asia. In many areas, human infections are extremely common, with over 60 per cent of young adults having antibodies. This indicates that in endemic areas there is a high prevalence of inapparent or undifferentiated febrile illness in children. There is no sex predominance.

CLINICAL FEATURES. Following an incubation period of 1 to 6 days, the onset is usually abrupt without prodromal symptoms. The temperature rises quickly to 38.3 to 40°C, with rigors in one third of patients. Symptoms include drowsiness, severe frontal headache, ocular pain, myalgia, and pain in the abdomen and back. A small number of patients have dryness of the throat, anorexia, and nausea. Cough is uncommon. Examination shows facial flushing, conjunctival injection, and coating of the tongue. The prominent finding is generalized lymphadenopathy. Nodes are of moderate size and nontender and usually include the occipital, axillary, and inguinal chains. The spleen and liver are occasionally slightly enlarged. The temperature curve may be biphasic. In one half of patients a pale roseolar maculopapular rash, predominantly truncal and on the upper arms, appears from the second to fifth day. The rash may be evanescent (several hours) or persist until defervescence. It clears without desquamation. Rarely vesicular lesions may occur. The illness is self-limited and lasts 3 to 5 days in 80 per cent of patients. Generally the illness in children is milder than in adults.

Infection may also result in aseptic meningitis or meningoencephalitis, especially in the elderly. Spinal fluid examinations may reveal a lymphocytic pleocytosis with some increase in protein concentration. Other rare complications include myocarditis, pancreatitis, and hepatitis. Convalescence is often prolonged, lasting several weeks with prominent symptoms of fa-

tigue. Lymph node enlargement requires several months to regress. Laboratory findings include leukopenia (less than 4000 per cubic millimeter in one third of patients).

DIAGNOSIS. Clinically West Nile fever resembles dengue. West Nile virus can be isolated from blood of three fourths of patients on the first day, with viremia persisting but decreasing over 5 days. Serologic diagnosis is possible using a number of tests; however, cross-reactions with other flaviviruses complicate interpretation.

TREATMENT AND PROGNOSIS. Treatment is symptomatic. Ribavirin has activity against West Nile fever virus, but since the disease is self-limited and almost never fatal its use does not seem indicated.

PREVENTION. There is no vaccine.

Flatau E, Kohn D, Daher O, et al.: West Nile fever encephalitis. Isr J Med Sci 17:1057–1059, 1981. *A brief but adequate description of encephalitis in older patients.*

Marberg K, Goldblum N, Sterk VV, et al.: The natural history of West Nile fever. 1. Clinical observations during an epidemic in Israel. Am J Hyg 64:259–269, 1956. *A good description of the clinical illness.*

Southam CM, Moore AE: Induced virus infections in man by the Egypt isolates of West Nile virus. Am J Trop Med Hyg 3:19–50, 1954. *A detailed paper that includes clinical and laboratory features of West Nile fever.*

385 Phlebotomus Fever

Jay P. Sanford

DEFINITION. Phlebotomus (sandfly, pappataci, or 3-day fever) is an acute, relatively mild, self-limited infection transmitted by *Phlebotomus* flies. It is characterized by fever, malaise, headache, and myalgia and caused by at least five immunologically distinct phleboviruses (Naples, Sicilian, Punto Toro, Chagres, and Candiru).

ETIOLOGY. The sandfly fever group of viruses, within the *Phlebovirus* genus, are enveloped, single-stranded, trisegmented RNA viruses.

EPIDEMIOLOGY. Phlebotomus fever viruses are transmitted by phlebotomine flies. In the Mediterranean, Middle East, and northwest India, *Phlebotomus papatasii*, which breeds in dry sandy areas and feeds in early evening, is the principal vector. In Central America, *Lutzomyia*, a forest-dwelling species, is the principal vector. In interepidemic intervals sandfly fever viruses are presumably maintained in a vector-host wildlife cycle, but this has not been defined. During epidemics man may act as the major host. Transovarial transmission probably serves as an alternative mechanism for virus perpetuation. Sandflies are small (2 to 3 mm), which enables them to penetrate screens and mosquito netting. There is no pain or itching after the bite; hence only about 1 per cent of patients remember being bitten. Epidemics occurred among allied troops in Italy in 1942–1944.

CLINICAL FEATURES. The best descriptions of clinical illness come from the study of experimentally infected human volunteers (Sabin). After an incubation period of 2 to 6 days, symptoms develop abruptly in over 90 per cent. Temperatures rise to 37.8 to 40.1°C. Headache is nearly always present and often is accompanied by pain on ocular movement and retro-orbital pain. Myalgia is common and may be localized, for example to the abdomen; if to the chest it resembles pleurodynia. Other symptoms include vomiting, photophobia, alteration or loss of taste, and arthralgia. Conjunctival injection is seen in one third of patients. With severe illness, mild papilledema has been seen. Small vesicles occur on the palate. Macular or urticarial rashes may occur. The spleen is rarely palpable and lymphadenopathy is absent. The pulse is proportional to the temperature on the first day; subsequently there is a relative bradycardia. Fever persists for 2 to 4 days in most patients, with gradual defervescence. Weakness and feelings of depression are common during convalescence. Second attacks occur 2 to 12 weeks after the first in 15 per cent of cases. Aseptic meningitis may occur. In one series, 12 per cent of patients had lumbar punctures; findings included pleocytosis (average cell counts of 90 per cubic millimeter with either mononuclear or neutrophilic leukocytes).

Laboratory findings include leukopenia (less than 5000 per cubic millimeter) in 90 per cent of patients. The leukopenia may not occur until the third day. Early there is lymphopenia with an increase in band neutrophils. Subsequently a relative lymphocytosis (40 to 65 per cent) occurs. Urinalyses are usually normal.

DIAGNOSIS. Diagnosis is made on clinical and epidemiologic findings. Sandfly fever viruses replicate and produce plaques in Vero cell cultures. Serologic tests are not available.

TREATMENT AND PROGNOSIS. Treatment is symptomatic. No fatalities have been reported.

PREVENTION. During World War II phlebotomus fever was controlled in the Mediterranean theater by the use of DDT, to which sandflies are sensitive.

Sabin AB, Philip CB, Paul JR: Phlebotomus (pappataci or sandfly) fever: A disease of military importance. JAMA 125:603–606, 693–699, 1944.

Oldfield EC, Wallace MR, Hyams KC, et al.: Endemic infectious diseases of the Middle East. Rev Infect Dis 13(Suppl 3):S199–S217, 1991. *The most recent review, which includes investigational use of oral ribavirin in experimentally infected volunteers.*

386 Rift Valley Fever

Jay P. Sanford

Rift Valley fever (RVF) is an acute disease principally of livestock—sheep, goats, cattle, and camels—caused by the Rift Valley fever virus, an RNA virus that is transmitted by mosquitoes. It belongs to the genus *Phlebovirus*, which contains more than 30 viruses. The other medically important phleboviruses are the sandfly fever (phlebotomus fever) group of viruses. RVF was originally recognized as a cause of epizootic hepatitis in sheep in 1912. In cattle and sheep, most pregnant ewes and cows abort, and mortality in newborn lambs is over 90 per cent. It was first described in humans in 1930 during an extensive epizootic of hepatitis in sheep in Kenya. During an epizootic in South Africa in 1950–1951, an estimated 20,000 humans were infected. Fatal human disease, four cases of hemorrhagic disease and hepatitis, was first reported during an epizootic in South Africa in 1975. In 1977–1978 Rift Valley fever virus appeared for the first time in Egypt with a major outbreak involving cattle, sheep, goats, and buffalo. Two hundred thousand cases of human disease were estimated, with 598 deaths reported in 1977. RVF appears to have disappeared from Egypt after 1981.

ETIOLOGY. Rift Valley fever virus is an enveloped, single-stranded, trisegmented RNA virus. The virus multiplies readily in most common cell cultures, is cytopathic, and forms plaques.

EPIDEMIOLOGY. Rift Valley fever virus can be transmitted by a number of mosquito species; in Egypt *Culex pipiens*, in South Africa *C. theileri*, and in East Africa *Aedes* species are the major vectors. Epizootics in large domestic animals have been associated with particularly wet rainy seasons and high mosquito density. A wildlife-mosquito cycle during interepizootic periods has been postulated but not confirmed. Transovarial vertical transmission is an alternative. During an epizootic, disease occurs first in animals and then in humans. Direct transmission to man by contact with blood or tissues of infected animals may be more important than mosquito transmission. Laboratory-acquired infections presumably due to aerosols are common. In addition to eastern and southern Africa, Rift Valley fever virus has been isolated in West Africa. Zinga virus, a cause of sporadic human disease in central Africa, has been shown to be a strain of Rift Valley fever virus.

CLINICAL FEATURES. The incubation period is usually 3 to 6 days. It is an influenza-like illness with an abrupt onset, malaise, occasionally rigors, headache, myalgia, and backache. The temperature rises rapidly to 38.3 to 40°C. Later complaints include anorexia, loss of taste, photophobia, and epigastric pain. On examination findings may include flushing of the face and conjunctival injection. The course of fever is often saddle-back, with the initial elevation lasting 2 to 3 days, followed by remission and then a second febrile period. The total duration of fever is usually about 1 week. Convalescence is usually rapid. Prior to

the outbreak in Egypt, RVF was considered to be a benign illness with almost no fatalities. In Egypt, approximately 1 per cent of patients developed severe complications—meningoencephalitis, retinopathy, or hepatic or hemorrhagic manifestations. Encephalitis with intense headache, confusion, and stupor appeared as the acute infection subsided. The cerebrospinal fluid showed a lymphocytic pleocytosis with normal CSF glucose values. Some survivors had severe residuals. Ocular complications were characterized by visual loss occurring 2 to 7 days after the onset. Findings on ophthalmoscopic examination included macular edema, cotton-wool exudates on the macula, hemorrhages, retinitis, and vascular occlusion. One half of such patients had some permanent loss of visual acuity. Hepatic and hemorrhagic manifestations also occurred during the acute illness. Deaths from massive hepatic necrosis occurred 7 to 10 days after onset. Hemorrhagic manifestations include epistaxis, hematemesis, melena, and intracranial hemorrhage. The fatality ratio in severely ill patients exceeded 50 per cent. Laboratory features include initial normal to increased total leukocyte counts followed by leukopenia with granulocytopenia but an increase in band forms. Thrombocytopenia and clotting defects occur.

DIAGNOSIS. The diagnosis is confirmed by isolating virus from blood by inoculation of mice. Three fourths of patients are viremic (up to 10^8 mouse intraperitoneal lethal doses per milliliter of blood) at onset of illness. Neutralizing antibodies appear as early as 4 days.

TREATMENT. Treatment has been symptomatic. In patients with hemorrhagic manifestations, transfusion of platelets and fresh frozen plasma may be beneficial. In experimentally infected animals, ribavirin has been partially protective. Given the experience including minimal toxicity with intravenous ribavirin in patients with Lassa fever and Korean hemorrhagic fever (Hantaan), one might consider administration of ribavirin in similar dosage (2.0-gram loading dose IV, then 1.0 gram IV every 6 hours for 4 days, then 0.5 gram IV every 8 hours for 6 days) to patients with severe disease.

PREVENTION. Because the virus can be spread by contact with blood and tissues, and humans show high levels of viremia, blood and needle precautions are essential. An inactivated Rift Valley fever vaccine, although not yet licensed for man, has been produced and is protective in animals.

Kark JD, Aynor Y, Peters CJ: A Rift Valley fever vaccine trial. I. Side effects and serologic response over a six-month follow-up. Am J Epidemiol 116:808–820, 1982.

Kende M, Alving CR, Rill WL, et al.: Enhanced efficacy of liposome-encapsulated ribavirin against Rift Valley fever virus infection in mice. Antimicrob Agents Chemother 27:903–907, 1985.

Laughlin LW, Meegan JM, Strausbaugh LH, et al.: Epidemic Rift Valley fever in Egypt: Observations of the spectrum of human illness. Trans Roy Soc Trop Med Hyg 73:630–633, 1979. *If you are going to read one paper on RVF, this one provides the best overall recent experience.*

Siam AL, Meegan JM, Gharbawi KF: Rift Valley fever ocular manifestations: Observations during 1977 epidemic in Egypt. Br J Ophthalmol 64:366–374, 1980.

387 Alphaviruses Associated with Polyarthritis

Jay P. Sanford

DEFINITION. The alphaviruses (previously designated group A arboviruses) are a genus within the Togaviridae family. They are single-stranded RNA viruses with common antigenic determinants. At least nine alphaviruses, including six which cause acute arthropathy, have been associated with epidemics. The cycle for all is mosquito-vertebrate-mosquito. Those alphaviruses associated with systemic febrile illness (Venezuelan equine encephalitis) and primarily encephalitis (eastern equine encephalitis and western equine encephalitis) are discussed in Ch. 389.

This section reviews the epidemiology and clinical features of the alphaviruses associated with acute arthropathy.

CHIKUNGUNYA VIRUS

DEFINITION. The name chikungunya is a local tribal word, "that which bends up," which was used to describe an epidemic of acute arthropathy in Tanzania in 1952–1953.

EPIDEMIOLOGY. Today Chikungunya (CK) virus is of major importance in Africa and Asia. It was probably responsible for disease in the southern United States in the early nineteenth century. In Africa CK virus is transmitted by *Aedes* mosquitoes. In the forests of tropical Africa the mosquitoes belong to the subgenera *Stegomyia* and *Diceromyia*. The vertebrate hosts are nonhuman primates—monkeys or baboons. Transmission occurs primarily in the rainy season. Human involvement is largely secondary. In villages and urban areas, *Aedes aegypti* also serves as a vector. In these circumstances humans may serve as the vertebrate host. In sub-Saharan Africa, except in the dry areas and below 18° latitude, antibody prevalence surveys range from 20 to greater than 90 per cent. In Asia, transmission is primarily human to human by *A. aegypti*. CK virus is present in India, Southeast Asia, and the Philippines. Seroprevalence rates in Bangkok of 31 per cent were observed. The potential for CK virus transmission outside of the current distribution, i.e., Central and South America as well as the southern United States, exists.

CLINICAL FEATURES. The incubation period is usually 2 to 3 days but may be as long as 12 days. The onset is usually abrupt, with temperatures rising to 38.3 to 40°C, often accompanied by rigors and incapacitating arthralgia. The arthralgias are polyarticular and migratory, involving predominantly the small joints of the hands, wrists, ankles, and toes. Pain is increased with motion and worse in the morning. Joint swelling is common, but effusions are uncommon. The arthralgia is associated with generalized myalgia. Other symptoms include headache, photophobia, sore throat, anorexia, and vomiting, but these do not dominate the clinical picture. Cutaneous manifestations are typical. At onset there is flushing of the face and neck. Other signs include conjunctival injection and lymphadenopathy. A maculopapular rash usually involving the trunk and limbs typically occurs on the second to fifth day. The rash lasts 1 to 5 days and may just fade or may desquamate. On the second or third day, the fever may remit for 1 to 2 days, then recur, giving a biphasic "saddle-back" course. However, the biphasic course is not as striking as that seen with dengue. Laboratory findings include occasional leukopenia with relative lymphocytosis, although most leukocyte counts are normal. Mild thrombocytopenia may occur. The joint symptoms may persist for long periods, only one third of individuals being asymptomatic within a few weeks. About 5 per cent of patients have persistent joint pain, stiffness, and recurrent effusions. Persistence may be more common in HLA B27 positive patients. In African children disease is milder, with arthralgia less prominent. In Asia CK virus is responsible for a hemorrhagic fever syndrome closely resembling dengue hemorrhagic fever or the dengue shock syndrome. About 8 per cent of patients with the hemorrhagic fever syndrome had CK virus. Other features may include encephalitis and myocarditis.

DIAGNOSIS. CK virus disease should be suspected clinically given the appropriate epidemiologic history and the triad of fever, acute arthralgia/arthritis, and rash. Viremia is present in most patients during the first 48 hours. Hemagglutination inhibition (HI) antibodies appear by day 5 to 7.

TREATMENT. Treatment is symptomatic.

PREVENTION. A promising live attenuated vaccine is under clinical investigation.

Deller JJ Jr, Russell PK: Chikungunya disease. Am J Trop Med Hyg 17:1007–1111, 1968.

Fourie ED, Morrison JGL: Rheumatoid arthritis syndrome after chikungunya fever. S Afr Med J 56:130–132, 1979.

Halstead SB, Udomsakdi S, Singharaj P, et al.: Dengue and chikungunya virus infection in man and virologic observations on disease in non-indigenous white persons. Am J Trop Med Hyg 18:984–996, 1969.

Robinson MC: An epidemic of virus disease in Southern Province Tanganyika Territory in 1952–53. I. Clinical features. Trans R Soc Trop Med Hyg 49:28–32, 1955.

O'NYONG-NYONG VIRUS

DEFINITION. O'nyong-nyong (ON) virus first appeared in February 1959 as an epidemic of polyarthritis in Uganda. The name o'nyong-nyong means "weakening of the joints." The epidemic spread to involve at least 2 million people, with clinical attack rates of 9 to 78 per cent in different villages. The epidemic ceased in the mid-1960's, although the virus was again isolated from mosquitoes in Kenya in 1978.

EPIDEMIOLOGY. The vectors of ON virus are mosquitoes, *Anopheles funnestus* and *A. anogambiae*. The nonhuman vertebrate reservoir, if there is one, is unknown.

CLINICAL FEATURES. The clinical features are similar to those of chikungunya virus disease. The incubation period may be somewhat longer, at least 8 days. Fever is less prominent, exceeding 38.3°C in only one third of patients. Rash occurred in 60 to 70 per cent. In contrast to CK virus disease, generalized lymphadenopathy was a common feature. There appears to be less residual arthropathy with ON than CK disease.

DIAGNOSIS. Diagnosis is based on virus isolation. Patients seroconvert by hemagglutination inhibition assays, but cross-reactions with CK virus make interpretation difficult.

Shore H: O'nyong-nyong fever: An epidemic virus disease in East Africa. III. Some clinical and epidemiological observations in the northern province of Uganda. Trans R Soc Trop Med Hyg 55:361–373, 1961.

MAYARO VIRUS

DEFINITION. Mayaro (MY) virus has been associated with epidemics of acute polyarthritis in Brazil and Bolivia.

EPIDEMIOLOGY. MY virus has been recognized in the forested areas of Central and South America with annual infection rates of 10 to 60 per cent. There is usually a 2:1 male predominance. The vectors for MY virus are *Haemagogus* mosquitoes. The virus causes high-level viremia in marmosets and other primates. Whether or not marmosets are the major vertebrate host has not been confirmed.

CLINICAL FEATURES. The incubation period is about 1 week. Ages of patients have ranged from 2 to 62 years with both sexes involved. Illness begins abruptly with fever, chills, severe frontal headache, myalgia, and dizziness. Arthralgia occurs uniformly and is very prominent and occasionally incapacitating and in some patients precedes the fever. Small joints, wrists, fingers, ankles, and toes predominate. Temperatures usually exceed 40°C. Other initial symptoms (less than one third of patients) include nausea, vomiting, and diarrhea. Initial clinical features include occasional conjunctival suffusion, inguinal lymphadenopathy (one half of patients), and joint swelling (one quarter of patients). About the fifth day maculopapular rash develops over the chest, back, arms, and legs. Rash appeared in 90 per cent of children and one half of adults and lasted about 3 days. The clinical course is usually 3 to 5 days except for the arthralgia, which may persist for several months. Laboratory findings include leukopenia (as low as 2500 per cubic millimeter). Urinalyses revealed albuminuria (2+) in one fourth of patients. Some patients showed increases in SGOT levels. In Brazil no relapses were observed and no deaths have been recognized. In Bolivia, several fatalities have been reported.

DIAGNOSIS. Diagnosis is confirmed by virus isolation, preferably in Vero cells. MY-specific IgM responses have been observed.

Pinheiro FP, Freitas RB, Travassos da Rosa JF, et al.: An outbreak of Mayaro virus disease in Belterra, Brazil. I. Clinical and virological findings. Am J Trop Med Hyg 30:674–681, 1981.

ROSS RIVER VIRUS

DEFINITION. Epidemics of fever, polyarthritis, and rash were noted in rural Australia in 1928.

ETIOLOGY. Ross River (RR) virus is a typical alphavirus.

EPIDEMIOLOGY. Outbreaks occur almost entirely between December and June. RR virus infection was limited to Australia, New Guinea, and the Solomon Islands until 1979, when a major outbreak occurred in Fiji and then spread to the Samoan, Cook, and some Melanesian Islands. The natural vector-reservoir relationships have not been well established. *Culex annulirostris* is probably the major vector, although other species of mosquitoes may be involved. Several mammalian species, especially the New Holland mouse and wallabys, are important hosts in Australia. In the Pacific outbreak *Aedes vigilax* may also have been an important vector. In the Pacific, man-mosquito-man transmission was likely. In the Fiji outbreak, infection rates were equal at all ages and in both sexes, but clinical disease rates were 4 per cent in patients under 20 years of age and 42 per cent in those over 20 years of age. The clinical attack rate of males to females was 1:1.7.

CLINICAL FEATURES. In Australia, the incubation is estimated to be 7 to 9 days, while in the Pacific the incubation period was shorter. The illness at onset is characterized by headache, myalgia, nausea and vomiting, and occasionally tenderness of the palms of the hands and soles of the feet. Initially fever may be absent or minimal (highest 38°C). In about one half of patients arthritis involving mainly the small joints, wrists, and ankles occurs. Knee involvement also is common. The joint swelling and paresthesias may precede a rash by 1 to 15 days. In the other half of patients the rash precedes the arthralgia. The rash, which is usually maculopapular, appears on the cheeks and forehead, occasionally spreads to the trunk, or may be restricted to extremities. The rash may be pruritic. Vesicles occur rarely. Tender lymphadenopathy occurs in one fifth of patients. Most patients are unable to work. Recovery is slow, only one half being able to return to work by 1 month and 10 per cent still having joint symptoms at 3 months. Laboratory findings are not striking; leukocyte counts are normal or minimally decreased. The erythrocyte sedimentation rate is increased acutely but normalizes over several weeks even with continued joint symptoms. Antinuclear antibodies and rheumatoid factor tests are negative. Synovial fluid changes are not striking—cell counts of 1,000 to 60,000, predominantly mononuclear, normal viscosity. Urinalyses are normal, although recently RR virus has been associated with segmental sclerosing glomerulonephritis.

DIAGNOSIS. The diagnosis is usually based on clinical features. In Australia patients seldom have viremia on presentation, while in the Pacific outbreak viremia was readily detected. Hemagglutination inhibition antibodies appear early.

TREATMENT. Treatment is symptomatic.

Aaskov JG, Mataika JU, Lawrence GW, et al.: An epidemic of Ross River virus infection in Fiji, 1979. Am J Trop Med Hyg 30:1053–1059, 1981.

Clarke JA, Marshall ID, Gard G: Annually recurrent epidemic polyarthritis and Ross River virus activity in the coastal area of New South Wales. I. Occurrence of the disease. Am J Trop Med Hyg 22:543–550, 1973.

Davies DJ, Moran JE, Niall JF, et al.: Segmental necrotising glomerulonephritis with antineutrophil antibody: Possible arbovirus etiology. Br Med J 285:606, 1982.

Fraser JRE: Epidemic polyarthritis and Ross River virus disease. Clin Rheum Dis 12:369–388, 1986. *If one is reading only one paper on RR virus, this is the most inclusive.*

SINDBIS VIRUS (Okelbo Disease, Pogosta Disease, Karelian Fever)

DEFINITION. Sindbis virus, a prototype alphavirus, was isolated from *Culex* mosquitoes collected in the Egyptian village of Sindbis in 1952. Initially it was thought only rarely to produce clinical disease. It has now been recognized elsewhere in Africa, in Europe, and in Australia. In the U.S.S.R. it is known as Karelian fever, in Sweden as Okelbo disease, and in Finland as Pogosta disease.

EPIDEMIOLOGY. The vector-host relationships have been best defined in Africa and the Middle East. *Culex univittatus* is the principal vector. The major hosts are birds. Human infection is common where birds and *Culex* mosquitoes are in close proximity. Human antibody rates are commonly 20 to 30 per cent in the Nile Valley of Egypt. Since Sindbis and West Nile fever virus share the same transmission cycles, Sindbis transmission often parallels West Nile fever virus. In northern Europe symptomatic disease is recognized between 60° and 65° north latitude. The virus has been isolated from *Culiseta*, *Aedes*, and *Culex* mosquitoes. In Europe it occurs in late summer in adults with forest occupations. The host has not been defined.

CLINICAL FEATURES. The incubation period has not been defined. Disease more closely resembles Ross River virus disease than chikungunya or o'nyong-nyong disease. Clinically fever is low grade and accompanied by malaise, myalgia, rash, and arthralgia. Joint involvement is multiple, involving wrists, ankles, knees, and elbows. Periarticular involvement and tendinitis are common. The rash begins on the trunk as scattered macules and spreads to the extremities, palms, and soles. The rash may precede or follow the joint symptoms by 1 to 2 days. Unlike that caused by other alphaviruses, the rash frequently becomes vesic-

ular, especially on the feet and hands. The rash fades within a week. In Europe, persistence of joint complaints is a common feature. In Sweden more than 20 per cent had joint symptoms longer than 1 month after onset.

DIAGNOSIS. Antibodies can be detected by hemagglutination inhibition tests within 7 to 10 days of onset.

TREATMENT. Treatment is symptomatic.

Espmark A, Niklasson B: Okelbo disease in Sweden: Epidemiological, clinical and virological data from the 1982 outbreak. Am J Trop Med Hyg 33:1203–1211, 1984.

Lvov DK, Skvortsova TM, Berezina LK, et al.: Isolation of Karelian fever agent from *Aedes communis* mosquitoes. Lancet 2:399–400, 1984.

Malherbe H, Strickland-Cholmley M: Sindbis virus infection in man. S Afr Med J 37:547–552, 1963.

IGBO-ORA VIRUS

DEFINITION. Igbo-ora virus is a closely related alphavirus isolated from a child in Nigeria. The virus was also isolated from a Peace Corps volunteer with a clinical illness resembling chikungunya disease.

Moore DL, Causey OR, Carey DS, et al.: Arthropod-borne viral infections of man in Nigeria, 1964–1970. Ann Trop Med Parasitol 69:49–64, 1975.

388 Colorado Tick Fever

Theodore C. Eickhoff

DEFINITION. Colorado tick fever (CTF) is an acute, benign, tick-transmitted viral infection that occurs throughout the Rocky Mountain area and is characterized by headache, myalgia, a biphasic febrile course lasting about 1 week, and leukopenia.

ETIOLOGY. CTF virus is an RNA virus in the orbivirus genus of the reoviruses; it is unrelated to other major arbovirus groups. The virus is transmitted to humans by the bite of the hard-shelled wood tick, *Dermacentor andersoni*. Human cases appear to be limited to the combined geographic distribution of the tick vector and the major mammalian rodent reservoirs, ground squirrels and chipmunks. Some antigenic variation of CTF virus has been documented.

EPIDEMIOLOGY. The disease occurs during the spring and summer months, when tick exposure in the mountains is common. Disease activity appears to follow springtime in the mountains, for cases occur at lower altitudes during April and May, and at higher altitudes during June and July, presumably reflecting the slower emergence of ticks at higher altitudes. Most patients give a history of having found attached ticks, but others are not aware of the tick attachment and bite, even though they may have seen ticks on their body or clothing. Cases may occasionally be encountered in other areas of the country as a result of travel outside the endemic area during the incubation period or accidental transportation of infected adult ticks in clothing or bedding.

CTF virus has been recovered from as many as 14 per cent of *Dermacentor andersoni* collected in endemic areas. The virus overwinters in hibernating nymphal and adult ticks and in infected hibernating rodent hosts. Infected nymphal ticks feed on ground squirrels and chipmunks in the spring, and since the resulting viremia in the rodent reservoirs lasts for weeks or months, the virus is amplified in a cycle involving larval and nymphal ticks and the chipmunk and ground squirrel hosts. Humans are accidental hosts, resulting from the bite of an adult tick.

INCIDENCE AND PREVALENCE. The disease has been reported from most states in the Rocky Mountain area and from western Canadian provinces. Several hundred cases are diagnosed annually in the endemic area, but it is likely that this represents only a fraction of the total. Mild or wholly subclinical infections probably do occur, but their frequency has not been systematically evaluated.

The virus has been isolated from other species of ticks and

from numerous species of small mammals, suggesting that the disease may occur over a wider geographic area than is currently appreciated.

PATHOGENESIS. There is no unusual local reaction at the site of the tick bite inoculation, and the site of initial localization of the virus is unknown. The virus replicates in hematopoietic stem cells. Symptoms begin 3 to 6 days after tick exposure. Viremia can be demonstrated at the time of onset of fever, not only persisting during the febrile illness itself, but remarkably persisting in red blood cells long after the virus has disappeared from serum and neutralizing antibody has appeared. The virus can be demonstrated within erythrocytes by fluorescent antibody staining for up to 120 days and has been grown from washed erythrocytes 100 days after the original infection. Transfusion-transmitted CTF has been documented.

Few pathologic data in humans are available, since fatal cases are rare. In experimental animals, the heart, lungs, spleen, bone marrow, and lymph nodes are important sites of viral replication. Occasional patients have clinical evidence of central nervous system or meningeal involvement, and CTF virus has been recovered from cerebrospinal fluid.

CLINICAL MANIFESTATIONS. The disease begins abruptly, with chilly sensations, fever of 38 to 40°C, myalgias most prominent in the back and legs, headache, retro-orbital pain, and photophobia. Malaise and nausea may occur, but vomiting is uncommon. Physical findings during the first 2 to 3 days of illness are nonspecific. The patient may be flushed, with conjunctival and pharyngeal erythema. Lymphadenopathy is not prominent, although mild splenomegaly is sometimes present. Rashes have been reported in up to 12 per cent of patients, commonly macular or maculopapular and distributed over the entire body, sometimes petechial and involving primarily the extremities. Tachycardia is in proportion to the temperature elevation.

In approximately one half of cases, a distinctly biphasic illness occurs, the so-called "saddleback" fever. Symptoms abate after 2 to 3 days, temperature becomes normal or nearly so, and the patient feels relatively well for 1 or 2 days, following which there is an abrupt return of fever, headache, and back pain, often more intense than in the first phase. The second phase lasts 2 to 4 days and then subsides, leaving the patient with weakness and lassitude that disappear during the succeeding week or two. Convalescence may be prolonged in patients over 30 years of age to 3 weeks or more. Some patients do not exhibit the typical biphasic course and experience only one bout of fever or have a typical illness but with a third phase of fever or have a single prolonged febrile illness lasting 5 to 8 days.

Central nervous system involvement has occurred in some patients, usually children. The presenting findings have been those of aseptic meningitis with nuchal rigidity and mononuclear pleocytosis or of encephalitis with a depressed sensorium or stupor. Hemorrhagic manifestations have been described in a few children with encephalitis.

Laboratory findings very early in the illness are generally not helpful, but leukopenia is usually present by the third day of illness and becomes even more pronounced during the second phase, reaching levels as low as 1000 per cubic millimeter. The most striking decrease is in the granulocyte series, with a relative lymphocytosis, and there is frequently an accompanying thrombocytopenia. Atypical, vacuolated lymphocytes are frequently observed. Bone marrow examination reveals a maturation arrest in the granulocyte series. The white blood count returns to normal during convalescence.

DIAGNOSIS. The diagnosis should be suspected in any person with a history of tick exposure in the endemic area 3 to 7 days prior to the onset of a febrile illness. Findings during the first phase, however, cannot be differentiated from many other acute febrile illnesses. A brief symptom-free interval followed by a second febrile illness should strongly suggest CTF. Profound leukopenia is usually present by that time and lends support to the diagnosis.

The diagnosis is confirmed by isolation of the virus from red blood cells, via inoculation of suckling mice, or in tissue culture. More rapid diagnosis is possible by direct immunofluorescent staining of virus in the patient's erythrocytes. A diagnostic rise in antibody titers can be detected by indirect immunofluorescence or by neutralization test; an enzyme-linked immunoassay is available also.

The differential diagnosis can be troublesome, inasmuch as Rocky Mountain spotted fever is transmitted in the tick fever endemic area by the same vector, *Dermacentor andersoni*. Paradoxically, Rocky Mountain spotted fever has become an unusual disease in the state of Colorado and is outnumbered by CTF in Colorado by at least 20-fold. Nevertheless, differential diagnosis may be impossible early in the course of disease, before the characteristic rash of Rocky Mountain spotted fever appears. A relatively symptom-free interval after 2 or 3 days would be most unusual in Rocky Mountain spotted fever and strongly favors the diagnosis of CTF.

TREATMENT. Therapy is entirely supportive, there being no specific therapy. Salicylates or acetaminophen may be necessary to minimize headache and myalgias but are neither required nor advisable in most patients.

PROGNOSIS. The disease is almost invariably benign, and the prognosis is excellent. Severe illness, complicated by central nervous system involvement, is seen infrequently and only in children.

PREVENTION. Both inactivated and live attenuated vaccines have been studied, but the modest number of cases and the benign nature of the disease suggest little need for active immunization.

The most effective means of preventing the disease is the use of protective clothing or repellents by people outdoors in endemic areas during the spring and summer months, together with frequent body inspection and prompt removal of ticks. Transfusion-associated disease can be prevented by exclusion of convalescent donors for a minimum of 6 months.

Anderson RD, Entringer MA, Robinson WA: Virus-induced leukopenia: Colorado tick fever as a human model. J Infect Dis 151:449, 1985. *An interesting exploration of the pathogenesis of the profound leukopenia observed in CTF.*

Emmons RW: Ecology of Colorado tick fever. Annu Rev Microbiol 42:49–64, 1988. *A comprehensive recent review.*

Goodpasture HC, Poland JD, Francy DB, et al.: Colorado tick fever: Clinical, epidemiologic and laboratory aspects of 228 cases in Colorado in 1973–1974. Ann Intern Med 88:303, 1978. *The most recent descriptive clinical study.*

Oshiro LS, Dondero DV, Emmons RW, et al.: The development of Colorado tick fever virus within cells of the haematopoietic system. J Gen Virol 39:73, 1978. *Recommended for those interested in the unusual host-parasite relationship in CTF.*

389 Arthropod-Borne Viral Encephalitides

R. Gordon Douglas, Jr.

Arboviral encephalitis is a significant health problem in Europe, the Soviet Union, parts of Asia, and Central and South America but not Africa. The disease is of particular concern in the Americas, not only because of its multiple etiologic agents and widespread occurrence, but also because of its concurrent affliction of domestic animals and humans and its potential for epidemic spread.

Only a few of the more than 500 arboviruses belonging to the Togaviridae, Bunyaviridae, and Reoviridae families are responsible for epidemic or endemic encephalitis (Table 389–1). These viruses, which circulate in the blood of vertebrate hosts, are transmitted between wild or domestic animals by mosquitoes or ticks. Once replication of the virus has taken place in the salivary glands of the arthropod vector (a week or more after ingestion of infectious blood), transmission by bite can occur. Humans are not essential hosts. Only a small fraction of persons experience severe central nervous system manifestations, and human infection is most often subclinical (Table 389–2). The ratio of inapparent to clinically overt infections is a distinctive, age-dependent quality of each disease. The neurologic disease usually begins after a variable period of nonspecific systemic symptoms and may take the form of aseptic meningitis, meningoencephalitis, or encephalitis. These syndromes are not distinguishable on clinical grounds alone from similar syndromes caused by other infectious agents.

PATHOLOGY AND PATHOGENESIS. Two pathologic processes are common to the arboviral encephalitides: (1) neuronal and glial damage mediated by intracellular viral infection, and (2) migration of immunologically active cells into the perivascular space and brain parenchyma. Endothelial cell swelling and proliferation, destruction of myelin sheaths in deep white matter areas, and vasculitis are present in some arboviral encephalitides.

After a bite by an infected arthropod, viral replication occurs in local tissues and in regional lymph nodes. Viremia, which seeds extraneural tissues, occurs and persists depending on the extent of replication in extraneural sites, the rate of viral clearance by the reticuloendothelial system, and the appearance of humoral antibodies. Sites of extraneural infection vary from virus to virus. Many alpha- and flaviviruses involve striated muscle and vascular endothelium, whereas Venezuelan encephalitis virus is associated with myeloid and lymphoid tissue invasion. During this viremia, the neural parenchyma may be invaded, but the mode of penetration of virus across the blood-brain barrier is not completely understood. Possible mechanisms include passive movement of virus across vascular membranes and virus replication in cerebral capillary endothelial cells. Factors that increase vascular permeability promote neuroinvasion. In experimental animals infected

TABLE 389–1. ARTHROPOD-BORNE VIRUSES THAT CAUSE ACUTE CENTRAL NERVOUS SYSTEM INFECTION AND ENCEPHALITIS

Virus by Group	Mode of Transmission	Geographic Distribution	Disease in Domestic Livestock
Viruses principally associated with the encephalitis syndrome; epidemic and endemic			
Togaviridae, alphavirus			
Eastern equine encephalitis	Mosquito	Eastern North America, Caribbean, South America	Equines, penned pheasants
Western equine encephalitis	Mosquito	Western North America, South America	Equines
Venezuelan equine encephalitis	Mosquito, possibly other modes (see text)	Florida, Central and South America	Equines
Flaviviridae, flavivirus			
St. Louis encephalitis	Mosquito	North America, Caribbean, Central and South America	None
Japanese encephalitis	Mosquito	East and Southeast Asia, India	Equines, swine
Rocio encephalitis	Mosquito	Brazil	None
Murray Valley encephalitis	Mosquito	Australia	(Equines)*
Tick-borne encephalitides: Russian spring-summer and Central European encephalitis	Tick, ingestion of milk	Europe, U.S.S.R.	None
Louping ill	Tick	British Isles	Sheep, equines, cows
Powassan	Tick	North America	None
Bunyaviridae, California subgroup			
California encephalitis, LaCrosse, Jamestown Canyon, snowshoe hare	Mosquito	North America, China, U.S.S.R.	None
Viruses principally associated with other syndromes, but occasionally causing encephalitis; epidemic and endemic			
Togaviridae, alphavirus			
Sindbis (febrile illness with rash)	Mosquito	Africa, Europe	None
Semliki Forest (febrile illness)	Mosquito	Africa, Southeast Asia	(Equines)*
Flaviviridae, flavivirus			
West Nile (febrile illness with rash)	Mosquito	Africa, Middle East	(Equines)*
Kyasanur Forest disease†	Tick	India	None
Omsk hemorrhagic fever†	Tick	Central Asia	None
Bunyaviridae, phlebovirus			
Rift Valley fever (febrile illness, hemorrhagic fever, retinitis)	Mosquito, direct contact	Africa	Sheep, cows, goats
Crimean hemorrhagic fever†—Congo	Tick	Eastern Europe, U.S.S.R., Africa	None
Reoviridae, orbivirus			
Colorado tick fever (febrile illness)	Tick	Western North America	None
Rare and sporadic infections associated with encephalitis			
Flaviviridae, flavivirus			
Ilheus‡	Mosquito	South America	None
Negishi	Tick	Japan, China	None
Langat†	Tick	Asia	None
Orthomyxovirus			
Thogoto	Tick	Africa	None

*Disease rare or suspected but not well documented.
†Tick-borne hemorrhagic fevers.
‡Encephalitis recorded in laboratory infections or experimental infections of cancer patients only; significance in naturally acquired infections unknown.

with some flaviviruses, virus enters the central nervous system by way of the olfactory neuroepithelium.

The immature brain is more susceptible to damage by Western equine, Venezuelan equine, and California encephalitis viruses (Table 389–2). St. Louis encephalitis principally affects the elderly, whereas Japanese encephalitis and eastern equine encephalitis have a bimodal incidence, striking both children and elderly persons. In endemic areas, immunity accumulated with increasing age may reduce the incidence of disease in older persons for some viruses; however, the reasons for increased severity of illness with other viruses are unknown.

DIFFERENTIAL DIAGNOSIS. The most important consideration in diagnosis is to differentiate arthropod-borne viral encephalitis from acute central nervous system infection due to treatable organisms. The early prodromata resemble those of influenza, dengue, or other influenza-like illness. Bacterial meningitis (especially early or partially treated), infective bacterial endocarditis, brain abscess, subdural empyema, and cerebral thrombophlebitis may mimic viral encephalitis, and cerebrospinal fluid changes are sometimes similar. Other infections that occasionally cause meningoencephalitis resembling arthropod-borne viral encephalitis include tuberculosis, cryptococcosis, histoplasmosis, coccidioidomycosis, Rocky Mountain spotted fever, leptospirosis, falciparum malaria, trichinosis, *Naegleria* meningitis, typhoid fever, Lyme disease, and *Mycoplasma* pneumonia.

Acute meningoencephalitis may result from infections with other viruses, including herpesviruses, human immunodeficiency virus, mumps virus, enteroviruses, lymphocytic choriomeningitis virus, rabies, influenza, and the exanthematous viral infections of childhood. Exposure history, presence of an outbreak of similar disease in the community, and summer-fall occurrence are principal clues to an arboviral etiology. Enteroviruses also cause summer-fall outbreaks, but the predominant syndrome is aseptic meningitis, and the occurrence of rash or pleurodynia is a helpful clue. Herpes simplex encephalitis presents an important diagnostic challenge, since chemotherapy is available. The presence of localizing neurologic signs, localizing findings on computed tomography or magnetic resonance imaging scans, or brain biopsy may help distinguish herpes simplex encephalitis from that due to arthropod-borne viral encephalitides.

Noninfectious diseases of the central nervous system such as *cerebrovascular accident* may be confused with viral encephalitis. For example, St. Louis encephalitis, a disease of the elderly, has been misdiagnosed as a stroke. Subarachnoid hemorrhage produces meningismus, fever, headache, and neurologic signs that mimic an infectious etiology. *Metabolic encephalopathies* may present features suggesting infectious encephalitis. *Neoplastic* or *granulomatous diseases* involving the central nervous system and a variety of diseases of uncertain etiology (cat scratch disease, Behçet disease, Reye syndrome, acute multiple sclerosis, and systemic lupus erythematosus) must be considered in the differential diagnosis as well.

WESTERN EQUINE ENCEPHALITIS (WEE)

ETIOLOGIC AGENT. WEE virus is a member of the alphavirus genus of the Togaviridae family.

EPIDEMIOLOGY. Incidence and Prevalence. Since 1955, the number of cases of WEE reported annually in the United States has varied from 0 to 200. Most affected in recent years has been the area from the Mississippi River west to the Rocky Mountains. Mixed outbreaks of WEE and St. Louis encephalitis are common. Epidemics occur in early or midsummer and may follow heavy snow melt or flooding, conditions favorable for breeding of mosquitoes. Cases of encephalitis in equines often precede the appearance of human disease. The disease principally affects residents of rural communities, and the incidence is higher in males than in females. WEE is most severe in infants and young children. The case-fatality rate is between 3 and 5 per cent. The ratio of inapparent to apparent infection is also age-dependent, ranging from about 1:1 in infants under 1 year, to 58:1 in children 1 to 4 years old, to over 1000:1 in persons over 14 years of age.

WEE virus also occurs in South America. Equine epizootics in Argentina have been associated with human cases.

Transmission. WEE virus circulates between wild birds and *Culex tarsalis* mosquitoes. *C. tarsalis* is responsible for infection of humans and equines, which develop low or undetectable viremias and do not perpetuate the chain of transmission. In temperate areas, transmission ceases during the winter months.

CLINICAL FEATURES AND PATHOLOGY. The disease usually begins with an influenza-like illness consisting of fever, headache, malaise, and myalgias lasting 1 to 4 days. Somnolence, lethargy, photophobia, vomiting, and neck stiffness may follow; neurologic involvement may rapidly progress to stupor, coma, and convulsions. Paresis, cranial nerve deficits, tremors, and abnormal reflexes may be present. In fatal cases, patients die 1 to 2 days after development of coma. Survivors generally experience a sudden and rapid recovery. However, about one third of surviving infants suffer retardation, cerebellar damage, choreoathetosis, and spastic paralysis. Children with protracted illnesses who develop convulsions during the acute stage are more likely to suffer long-term neurologic impairment. Adults may have a prolonged convalescent syndrome, but objective residua are rare. Congenital infections are documented and result in severe and progressive neurologic deterioration.

Leukocytosis and shift to the left are common. The cerebrospinal fluid contains less than 500 white cells (at first polymorphonuclear, then mononuclear) per cubic millimeter and elevated protein concentration (usually 90 to 110 mg per deciliter).

Pathologic examination of the brains of infants reveals massive neuroparenchymal destruction; children dying months or years after the acute insult often have large cystic lesions in many areas of the brain. In older children and adults, acute WEE is characterized by focal necrosis and perivascular cuffing, predominantly in the basal ganglia and thalamic nuclei but also in deep cerebral white matter.

DIAGNOSIS. Viral isolation from blood or cerebrospinal fluid is almost never successful. Diagnosis is achieved by demonstration of a rise in hemagglutination inhibition (HI), fluorescent, complement-fixing (CF), enzyme-linked immunosorbent assay (ELISA), or neutralizing antibody titers in appropriately timed (10 to 14 days apart) paired sera. Demonstration of immunoglobulin M (IgM) antibodies in serum or cerebrospinal fluid by ELISA provides a presumptive diagnosis.

TABLE 389–2. DIFFERING FEATURES OF ARTHROPOD-BORNE ENCEPHALITIDES IMPORTANT IN THE UNITED STATES

	Western Equine Encephalitis	Eastern Equine Encephalitis	Venezuelan Equine Encephalitis	St. Louis Encephalitis	California Encephalitis
Incidence	0–200/year, mostly infants and children	15/year	Rare in U.S.; mostly children	0–2000/year, mostly adults	50–100/year, mostly children
Time of year	Early or midsummer	Late summer, early fall	Summer	Mid- to late summer	July–September
Case-fatality	3–5% in children	50–70%, highest in children <15 years and adults >55 years	35% in children <10% in older persons	9% overall; 0% <20 years, 30% >65 years	<1%
Residual damage	33% in infants	30–50%, especially in children	Frequent in children	Frequent in elderly	Probably rare
Cerebrospinal fluid	<500 cells	500–2,000 cells PMNs*	<500 cells	<500 cells	<500 cells

*Polymorphonuclear leukocytes.

TREATMENT. As with most types of arboviral encephalitis, there is no specific therapy for WEE. Supportive care is essential and may reduce mortality. Control of high fever, convulsions, fluid and electrolyte imbalances, and airways is critical. Prevention and treatment of secondary bacterial infections, good pulmonary toilet, and care of urinary catheters also are essential. If clinical signs suggest cerebral edema or if the cerebrospinal fluid pressure is very high (>400 mm H_2O), measures to reduce brain swelling are indicated.

PREVENTION AND CONTROL. An experimental formalin-inactivated vaccine grown in chick embryo cell cultures has been used for protection of laboratory workers but is not indicated for others. In threatened or ongoing epidemics, residents should be advised to use protective clothing, insect repellents, and window screens and to restrict outdoor activity in the early morning, late afternoon, and evening (times of greatest mosquito activity). Public health measures include spray applications of insecticides aimed at the adult *C. tarsalis* vector.

EASTERN EQUINE ENCEPHALITIS (EEE)

ETIOLOGIC AGENT. EEE virus is a member of the Togaviridae family, alphavirus genus.

EPIDEMIOLOGY. *Incidence and Prevalence.* The disease in humans is relatively rare, with fewer than 15 cases occurring each year in the Gulf Coast and Atlantic states, usually associated with a predominantly equine epizootic involving 100 to 300 animals. Outbreaks usually occur during the late summer and early fall. The occurrence of equine cases or outbreaks of fatal encephalitis in penned exotic birds (pheasants, chukar partridges) precedes the appearance of human cases by several weeks or more. Epizootics of EEE have been reported in the Caribbean (Hispaniola) and South America.

Despite the small size of EEE epidemics, the severity is high. The case-fatality rate is 50 to 70 per cent. Incidence and mortality are highest in children under 15 and in persons over 55 years, with no sex predilection.

Transmission. In temperate areas, EEE virus circulates between wild birds and *Culiseta melanura* mosquitoes in freshwater swamp habitat. Equine epizootics and associated human cases result from extension of the transmission cycle to involve *Aedes* and *Coquillettidia* mosquitoes, which feed on horses and humans.

CLINICAL FEATURES AND PATHOLOGY. The disease is more acute and rapidly progressive than the other arboviral encephalitides. Onset is abrupt, with high fever, vomiting, and somnolence. Stupor, coma, myoclonus, and generalized convulsions appear within 24 to 48 hours. Autonomic disturbances (sialorrhea) may be prominent, and respiratory difficulty and cyanosis are frequent. In children, facial, periorbital, or generalized edema may be present. Death usually occurs during the first week; in surviving patients, recovery begins during the second week and may progress rapidly. Good functional recovery is associated with a long prodromal course and absence of coma. Residual damage, found in 30 to 50 per cent of the patients, is often severe, especially in children, and is characterized by retardation, spastic paralysis, and atrophy of brain substance.

A striking peripheral leukocytosis and shift to the left are frequent findings in patients with EEE. Examination of the cerebrospinal fluid reveals 500 to 2000 white cells (predominantly polymorphonuclear) per cubic millimeter. As the total cell count falls, polymorphonuclear cells persist as a significant fraction. Red blood cells may be present, the protein is elevated, and glucose is normal.

In contrast to St. Louis encephalitis and WEE, the brain is grossly edematous and congested, and the inflammatory response is predominantly polymorphonuclear. The areas most affected are basal ganglia, thalamus, hippocampus, and frontal and occipital cortex. Focal vasculitis, endothelial cell swelling, intravenous and arteriolar thrombus formation, demyelination, necrosis, neuronolysis, and neuronophagia are prominent.

SPECIFIC DIAGNOSIS. Isolation of virus from blood and spinal fluid is rarely successful. Serologic diagnosis by demonstration of a rise in antibody titer using appropriately timed paired sera is the most practical and available test. Because of the rapid course of the clinical disease, sera should be obtained at 2- to 3-day intervals during the acute phase of illness.

TREATMENT. Treatment is supportive (see previous discussion of WEE).

PREVENTION AND CONTROL. An experimental formalin-inactivated chick embryo cell culture vaccine is used to protect laboratory and field workers. Reduction of mosquito populations by appropriate use of insecticides may be effective in threatened or established outbreaks.

VENEZUELAN EQUINE ENCEPHALITIS (VEE)

ETIOLOGY. The causative agent of VEE is a member of the Togaviridae family, alphavirus genus. Six antigenic subtypes (I to VI) and multiple antigenic variants of subtypes I and III are recognized by serologic tests. Subtypes IAB and IC are responsible for epidemics involving humans and equines. In Florida, subtype II is enzootic and produces sporadic human disease.

EPIDEMIOLOGY. *Incidence and Prevalence.* Prior to 1973, large equine epizootics occurred at 5- to 10-year intervals in Venezuela, Columbia, Ecuador, and Peru, involving many thousands of animals and incurring mortality rates as high as 40 per cent. Associated human morbidity also was great (up to 32,000 clinical cases). No outbreaks of equine or human disease have been recognized in over 12 years.

The predominant syndrome is a self-limited influenza-like illness; only about 4 per cent of infected persons, principally children under 15 years, develop encephalitis. Subclinical infections are rare. The case-fatality rate in children up to 5 years old with encephalitis is approximately 35 per cent, but in older persons it is less than 10 per cent. Laboratory infections are common in unvaccinated persons working with the virus or infected animals.

Transmission. A large variety of mosquito vectors, including species of the genera *Aedes*, *Psorophora*, and *Mansonia*, transmit subtypes IAB and IC during epizootic epidemics. Equines are the principal viremic hosts. Virus may be present in pharyngeal excretions of human patients; contact or aerosol person-to-person spread, although possible, is not epidemiologically important.

The other members of the VEE viral complex, including subtype II in Florida, have enzootic transmission cycles involving *Culex (Melanoconion)* species mosquitoes and small forest rodents and marsupials. Equines are not involved in transmission. Human disease is sporadic and relatively uncommon.

CLINICAL FEATURES AND PATHOLOGY. After an incubation period of 2 to 5 days, there is sudden onset of fever, chills, malaise, and headache, followed by myalgias, nausea, vomiting, and occasionally diarrhea. Physical examination reveals fever, tachycardia, conjunctival injection, and, in some cases, nonexudative pharyngitis. The acute illness generally subsides in 4 to 6 days, and convalescent symptoms may last up to 3 weeks. A biphasic course has sometimes been noted; acute symptoms reappear after a brief remission, within a week after the initial onset.

Some patients exhibit evidence of mild central nervous system involvement (photophobia, somnolence, confusion) during the typical influenza-like illness. When it occurs, severe encephalitis is characterized by meningeal signs, convulsions, tremor, stupor, coma, spastic paralysis, abnormal reflexes, cranial nerve palsies, and central respiratory failure. Residual neurologic damage occurs in severe cases. Infections of pregnant women acquired during the first and second trimesters may result in fetal encephalitis and death.

The peripheral leukocyte count is often low, with decrease in both lymphocytes and neutrophils, or normal, with a relative lymphopenia. In patients with central nervous system signs, the cerebrospinal fluid contains up to 500 cells, predominantly lymphocytes, per cubic millimeter. The serum lactic dehydrogenase and glutamic-oxaloacetic transaminase levels may be elevated.

Pathologic changes in the central nervous system include edema, congestion, meningeal and perivascular inflammation, intracerebral hemorrhages, neuronal degeneration, and vasculitis. In addition, hepatocellular degeneration and necrosis, widespread lymphoid depletion and follicular necrosis, and interstitial pneumonitis are frequent findings. In the congenitally infected fetus, there are massive and widespread necrosis of brain tissue, hemorrhages, and resorption of brain material, resulting in hydranencephaly.

DIAGNOSIS. In contrast to the other arthropod-borne encephalitides, VEE virus can be isolated from the blood or from throat swabs or washings during the first 3 or 4 days of illness. Serodiagnosis is usually more practical and is achieved by testing appropriately timed paired sera by HI, CF, ELISA, neutralization, or IgM immunoassay.

TREATMENT. No specific therapy is available, and treatment of encephalitis cases is supportive (see WEE discussion).

PREVENTION AND CONTROL. An experimental live attenuated vaccine made from subtype IAB is used for adult laboratory personnel. It provides solid immunity to subtype IAB and its closest relative (IC) but incomplete protection against infection with other heterologous VEE viruses. Epidemics and epizootics can be prevented by effective vaccination of equines. Spraying insecticides to reduce adult (infective) mosquito populations is the only means of immediate control in the face of an ongoing epidemic. Individual protection against mosquitoes also is advised (see WEE discussion).

ST. LOUIS ENCEPHALITIS (SLE)

ETIOLOGY. St. Louis encephalitis virus, a member of the family Flaviviridae, shares close antigenic relationships with Japanese encephalitis, Murray Valley encephalitis, and West Nile viruses and is related to yellow fever and dengue viruses. Strains associated with *Culex pipiens*–borne epidemics in the eastern United States are distinct from endemic strains transmitted by *C. tarsalis* in the western states.

EPIDEMIOLOGY. *Incidence and Prevalence.* The virus is present in all parts of the western hemisphere, but epidemics occur only in North America and some Caribbean islands. During epidemic years, the virus has been responsible for up to 80 per cent of all reported cases of encephalitis of known etiology in the United States. In recent years, epidemics of up to 2000 cases have taken place, mainly in urban-suburban localities of the Ohio-Mississippi River basin, in eastern and central Texas, and in Florida. Small outbreaks also have occurred in the western United States. Epidemics usually occur between July and September but may arise later in the year in warm areas such as Florida. Prior exposure and immunity to dengue may provide a degree of cross-protection against clinical SLE.

The overall case-fatality rate is approximately 9 per cent. Mortality is negligible in persons under 20 years but rises steeply after age 55 to approximately 30 per cent in patients over 65 years of age. The ratio of inapparent to apparent infection is 800:1 in children up to 9 years, 400:1 in persons 10 to 49 years, and 85:1 in persons over 60 years.

Transmission. In most of the eastern United States, SLE virus circulates between wild birds and *C. pipiens* mosquitoes, which breed in polluted water. In Florida and in parts of the Caribbean, *C. nigripalpus* is the principal vector. The cycle in the western United States also involves wild birds, but the vector is *C. tarsalis*, the vector of WEE. Because of the similar ecology of SLE and WEE viruses in the west, mixed outbreaks occur, mostly in rural, agricultural areas.

Above-average summer temperatures and conditions such as deficient rainfall, which create stagnant pools suitable for *C. pipiens* breeding, are associated with epidemics in the eastern United States. SLE in the western states is favored by warm spring temperatures, heavy snow melt, and flooding (see WEE).

CLINICAL FEATURES AND PATHOLOGY. Three clinical syndromes are recognized: febrile headache, aseptic meningitis, and encephalitis. After an incubation period of 4 to 21 days, a variable period of nonspecific symptoms occurs, including fever (38 to 41°C), headache, malaise, drowsiness, myalgias, and sore throat. This may be followed by the acute or subacute onset of meningeal or encephalitic signs or both. Nausea, vomiting, and photophobia are common. Neurologic abnormalities occur in up to 25 per cent of patients. Extrapyramidal abnormalities (tremor of tongue, face, and limbs) and an altered state of consciousness are the most significant findings. Others include altered sensorium, meningismus, cranial nerve deficits (particularly of cranial nerve VII), abnormal reflexes, tremors, myoclonic twitching, nystagmus, and ataxia. Motor abnormalities are infrequent and sensory changes extremely uncommon. Convulsions occur in 10 per cent of patients and are a poor prognostic sign, as is a

persistent high temperature of 40 to 41°C. Signs of markedly increased intracranial pressure are very unusual. Guillain-Barré syndrome has occasionally been associated with SLE, both as an acute presentation and during the convalescent period. Approximately half of the patients with fatal outcome succumb during the first week and 80 per cent within 2 weeks after onset.

In uncomplicated cases of SLE, there is a moderate peripheral neutrophilic leukocytosis and shift to the left. Cerebrospinal fluid pressure is elevated, protein mildly elevated, and sugar normal. Pleocytosis up to 500 cells per cubic millimeter is present. Polymorphonuclear cells predominate early, the change to lymphocytes occurring within several days. Serum creatinine phosphokinase, glutamic-oxaloacetic transaminase, and serum aldolase are frequently elevated. The electroencephalogram typically shows amorphous δ-wave activity and diffuse generalized slowing most prominently in the frontal and temporal regions, but brain scans are normal. Inappropriate secretion of antidiuretic hormone is present in one third of patients.

Genitourinary tract symptoms (urgency, frequency, incontinence, and retention), microscopic hematuria, pyuria, and proteinuria, and elevated blood urea nitrogen are frequent. SLE viral antigen in cells of the urinary sediment has been detected by fluorescent techniques and virus-like particles in urine by immunoelectronmicroscopy.

A convalescent syndrome, characterized by weakness, fatigue, nervousness, tremulousness, sleeplessness, irritability, depression, difficulty in concentrating, and headaches, occurs in 30 to 50 per cent of older persons and clears in 80 per cent of these within 3 years.

Pathologic changes in fatal cases are limited to microscopic findings. Leptomeningitis is characterized by lymphocytic inflammation. Parenchymal changes consist of lymphocytic perivascular cuffing, cellular nodule formation, and neuronal degeneration. Changes are most pronounced in substantia nigra, thalamus and hypothalamus, cerebellar cortex, cerebral cortex, and basal ganglia.

DIAGNOSIS. SLE virus is rarely isolated from blood or spinal fluid obtained during the acute phase of illness. Serologic diagnosis is achieved by demonstration of changing antibody titers; the HI, fluorescent, ELISA, and neutralizing tests demonstrate antibody within the first week after onset, and titers rise during the ensuing 2 weeks. CF antibodies appear 10 to 20 days after onset. Rapid, early diagnosis is possible by detection of IgM antibodies by ELISA in serum and cerebrospinal fluid. Serologic cross-reactions may occur in persons with prior exposures to dengue and other related flaviviruses.

TREATMENT. Treatment is supportive (see WEE).

PREVENTION AND CONTROL. No vaccine is available for SLE. Surveillance of viral activity in vectors and avian hosts is used to define the risk of human infection and initiate vector control efforts. In an established outbreak, avoidance of mosquito bites and spraying to reduce infected adult mosquitoes are the only effective means of control (see WEE discussion).

CALIFORNIA ENCEPHALITIS

ETIOLOGY. At least four members of the California serogroup of the Bunyaviridae family (*Bunyavirus* genus)—LaCrosse, California encephalitis, Jamestown Canyon, and snowshoe hare virus—cause encephalitis. California encephalitis virus occurs in the western United States (California, New Mexico, Utah, Texas) and has been implicated in only three human cases. In contrast, LaCrosse virus, distributed more widely in the eastern half of the United States and southern Canada, is a major human pathogen. Recently, Jamestown Canyon and snowshoe hare viruses have been implicated in sporadic human encephalitis cases in the northern central United States and Canada. California serogroup viruses have been implicated in human disease in the People's Republic of China and the U.S.S.R.

EPIDEMIOLOGY. *Incidence and Prevalence.* California encephalitis occurs as an endemic rather than an epidemic disease, with individual or small clusters of cases scattered across the affected areas. An average of 80 cases are reported each year, generally occurring between July and September with peak incidence in August. The virus primarily affects persons less than 15 years of age living in rural and suburban areas characterized by deciduous hardwood forests. It is most prevalent in the northern central states, where it is responsible for as many as 20 per cent of cases of acute central nervous system infection in children. Focal "hot spots" (communities, even backyards) of recurrent summertime viral activity are recognized. The case-fatality rate is less than 1 per cent. The ratio of inapparent to apparent infection has been estimated variably at between 26:1 and 157:1.

Transmission. The vector of LaCrosse virus is *Aedes triseriatus,* which breeds both in forest tree-holes and in peridomestic artificial containers. The vector also serves as a reservoir of LaCrosse virus. Wild rodents (squirrels, chipmunks) contribute to a cycle of transmission as viremic hosts. Humans acquire the disease through the bite of an infected mosquito.

Aedes communis, A. stimulans, A. triseriatus, and possibly anopheline mosquitoes are involved in transmission of Jamestown Canyon virus, and deer are the principal vertebrate hosts.

CLINICAL FEATURES. The clinical spectrum of California virus infection includes nonspecific febrile illness, aseptic meningitis, and meningoencephalitis. The disease begins with fever, headache, sore throat, and gastrointestinal symptoms, with appearance of the neurologic disorder within 1 to 3 days. In mild cases, central nervous system signs appear on the third day after onset and subside within 7 to 8 days. In the more severe form, neurologic signs appear within 24 to 48 hours of onset, usually in the form of generalized seizures and altered consciousness, and are more prolonged. Papilledema or abnormal optic disc margins have been noted. Encephalitis may be quite severe in the acute stage, but the disease is almost always self-limited and death is extremely uncommon. The question of permanent sequelae is unsettled. Many researchers believe LaCrosse virus infection is responsible for residual psychologic problems, emotional lability, hyperkinesis, infantilism, compulsive behavior, and auditory and visual perceptual problems. There are case reports of hemiparesis and persistent seizure disorders.

The peripheral white cell count is elevated, with a predominance of polymorphonuclear cells and a shift to the left. The cerebrospinal fluid contains up to 500 lymphocytes per cubic millimeter, normal or mildly elevated protein, and normal glucose concentrations. The electroencephalogram reveals generalized slowing in the δ and θ range, indicating diffuse cortical dysfunction. Focal δ-wave activity related to cortical destruction or focal seizures is also a common finding.

Histopathologic features in the central nervous system are qualitatively similar to those of other viral encephalitides; however, absence of inflammatory lesions in cerebellum, medulla, and spinal cord has been postulated to be a distinguishing feature of LaCrosse infection.

DIAGNOSIS. The virus cannot be recovered from blood or spinal fluid obtained during the acute phase. Diagnosis is best achieved by tests for antibody in paired acute and convalescent sera using counterimmunoelectrophoresis, HI, CF, fluorescent, ELISA, and neutralization tests. The most practical, sensitive, and reliable methods are the HI test using the LaCrosse viral antigen and IgM antibody-capture ELISA.

TREATMENT. Treatment is supportive (see WEE).

PREVENTION AND CONTROL. There is no vaccine for California encephalitis. Vector-control methods are of uncertain usefulness in this disease. In defined "hot spots" of recurrent viral activity, efforts to eliminate breeding sites for *A. triseriatus* should be made. Parents should protect children by limiting exposure and using mosquito repellents (see WEE).

JAPANESE ENCEPHALITIS (JE)

ETIOLOGY AND EPIDEMIOLOGY. Incidence and Prevalence. Japanese encephalitis virus is a member of the Flaviviridae family. It causes epizootics of clinical encephalitis in equines. The disease occurs throughout Asia, including Japan, the Korean peninsula, Taiwan, People's Republic of China, Okinawa, Vietnam, the Philippines, Burma, Malaysia, Bangladesh, east and south India, Sri Lanka, Thailand, and Indonesia. Over 30,000 cases occur annually. JE is a summertime disease in temperate areas but occurs sporadically year-round in the tropics. Epidemics have been most frequent at the northern fringe of the tropical zone. JE is predominantly a rural disease, and the incidence in males is often higher than in females. In hyperendemic areas, over 70 per cent of adult populations surveyed have antibodies,

and children under 15 years old principally are affected by the disease. In areas without a high prevalence of background immunity (e.g., northern India), however, all age groups are affected. In Japan, where school children have been protected by vaccination campaigns targeted at this age group, occurrence of encephalitis in the elderly has become prominent. The ratio of inapparent to apparent infection is over 500:1 in children and decreases with age; in Korea, the ratio among American servicemen was estimated at 25:1. The case-fatality rate probably is about 25 per cent, but rates of 50 per cent or more have been reported, which may reflect underrecognition of nonfatal cases.

Transmission. The natural cycle involves *Culex* mosquito vectors and wild birds and swine. Humans and equines are incidental hosts.

CLINICAL FEATURES AND PATHOLOGY. Manifestations of JE include febrile headache, aseptic meningitis, and meningoencephalitis. Onset is abrupt, with fever, headache, and gastrointestinal symptoms. Meningeal irritation develops within 24 hours and is followed on the second or third day by the appearance of irritability, impaired consciousness, convulsions (especially in children), muscular rigidity, masklike facies, ataxia, coarse tremor, involuntary movements, cranial nerve deficits, paresis, hyperactive deep tendon reflexes, and pathologic reflexes. Weight loss and dehydration are often striking findings. In mild cases, fever subsides after the first week and neurologic signs resolve by the end of the second week after onset. In severe cases, hyperpyrexia, progressive neurologic dysfunction, and coma result in death, usually between the seventh and tenth days. About 25 per cent of patients undergo a prolonged recovery, often leaving permanent sequelae. Cardiorespiratory complications are frequent during the acute stage in these patients. A poor prognosis is associated with protracted high fever, frequent or prolonged seizures, high protein content in the cerebrospinal fluid, Babinski signs, and early appearance of respiratory depression. Fetal death and abortion due to transplacental JE infection have been reported.

The occurrence of sequelae correlates with severity of the acute stage of illness. Young children are most susceptible, and sequelae such as mental impairment, emotional lability, choreoathetosis, tremor, parkinsonism, autonomic disturbances, motor paralysis, and pathopsychologic syndromes (including schizophrenia) have been reported in up to 75 per cent of patients.

A moderate peripheral leukocytosis and neutrophilia occur early in the disease. Cerebrospinal fluid pleocytosis, protein elevation, and normal glucose are usual findings.

Neuropathologic changes and distribution of lesions are similar to those described for St. Louis encephalitis (see earlier discussion of SLE).

DIAGNOSIS. Isolation of JE virus from blood is uncommon; virus may be recovered from cerebrospinal fluid of about one third of patients who progress to a fatal outcome, but rarely from patients who live. HI and neutralizing antibodies appear during the first and CF antibodies during the second week after onset. Cross-reactions with other flaviviruses make serodiagnosis difficult. Specific IgM antibodies in serum or cerebrospinal fluid are detectable by immunoassays in over three fourths of patients at the time of hospital admission.

TREATMENT. Treatment is supportive (see WEE). Uncontrolled trials of intrathecal interferon suggest a beneficial effect but require confirmation.

PREVENTION AND CONTROL. Inactivated, partially purified mouse brain vaccines produced in Japan are safe and effective in preschool- and school-age children. Although not yet licensed for use in the United States, a vaccine produced in Japan is available on a limited scale to United States citizens traveling to high-risk areas. Information should be sought from state health departments or the Centers for Disease Control. Since three doses of the inactivated vaccine are used, and approximately 1 month is required to confer protection, vaccination is not a practical measure in the face of an ongoing epidemic. Live attenuated vaccines are under study in China. Reduction of vector mosquito populations by application of insecticides may help to abort outbreaks (see WEE). Immunization of swine is an ancillary control strategy.

MURRAY VALLEY ENCEPHALITIS AND ROCIO ENCEPHALITIS

Murray Valley encephalitis and Rocio encephalitis are similar to Japanese encephalitis in pathogenesis and clinical features and are caused by closely related flaviviruses. Murray Valley encephalitis has occurred in small epidemics in the Murray and Darling River valleys of Victoria and New South Wales, Australia. The virus is endemic in northern Australia and New Guinea, where it is maintained in a bird-mosquito cycle. Rocio encephalitis has caused epidemics of 1000 cases in São Paulo State, Brazil.

TICK-BORNE ENCEPHALITIS (TBE)

ETIOLOGIC AGENTS. A complex of six antigenically related tick-borne flaviviruses cause encephalitis: Powassan, tick-borne encephalitis, louping ill, Kyasanur Forest disease (KFD), Omsk hemorrhagic fever (OHF), and Langat viruses. The predominant syndrome in KFD and OHF is hemorrhagic fever (see Ch. 393), but meningoencephalitis may be a component of the disease spectrum. Two subtypes of TBE virus (Central European encephalitis and Russian spring-summer encephalitis) are distinguished by special serologic tests, are ecologically distinct, and differ in virulence for humans. Powassan and louping ill viruses are rare causes of encephalitis in North America and the British Isles, respectively. These viruses are serologically easily distinguished from mosquito-borne flaviviruses but induce cross-reactions within the complex.

Tick-borne Encephalitis (TBE). TBE occurs in Europe (including European Russia), southern Scandinavia, and the far eastern U.S.S.R. during summer months, corresponding to peak tick vector populations. Several hundred to 2000 cases are reported annually, with morbidity rates of up to 20 per 100,000 inhabitants. Inapparent infections are common. Adults over 20 years are mainly affected, and persons frequenting wooded areas that are heavily tick infested are at highest risk. In Europe, the disease is relatively mild (case-fatality rate 1 to 2 per cent), but in the Far East, it is severe (20 to 25 per cent).

In Europe, the vector of TBE is *Ixodes ricinus*, and in the Far East, *I. persulcatus*. The tick vector also serves as a reservoir of the virus. Larval ticks parasitize small rodents, which serve as amplifying viremic hosts during the spring and summer. Large vertebrates (goats, sheep, cattle) are hosts for nymphal and adult ticks. Outbreaks have occurred in families or groups of individuals ingesting unpasteurized milk or cheese from goats or sheep.

TBE in Europe typically (but not invariably) has a diphasic course, beginning 7 to 14 days after exposure with an influenza-like illness lasting 1 week, followed by a period of clinical remission for several days, and then abrupt onset of aseptic meningitis or meningoencephalitis. The latter is usually benign, although severe paralytic illness, myelitis, myeloradiculitis, and bulbar forms may occur. Convalescence is often prolonged, and residual paralysis may follow in severe cases. In the Far East, TBE begins suddenly with fever, headache, and gastrointestinal symptoms, followed rapidly by appearance of depressed sensorium, coma, convulsions, and paralysis. Bulbar paralysis and cervical myelitis are frequent findings. In fatal cases, death occurs in the first week after onset. Survivors have a high incidence of residual paralyses, especially lower motor neuron paralysis of upper extremities or shoulder girdle. Aseptic meningitis and milder forms of encephalitis also occur. Chronic forms of TBE have been described, with active clinical and pathologic abnormalities a year or more after onset.

In TBE, virus isolation from blood is also possible during the early phase of illness. Serologic diagnosis is achieved by the HI, CF, N, or ELISA techniques.

Treatment is supportive (see WEE).

In eastern Europe and the U.S.S.R., TBE vaccines are used in high-risk groups (forestry and agricultural workers, military personnel). In Austria, immunization of the general population has resulted in a marked decline in incidence. Avoidance of tick exposure by use of protective clothing and repellents may be recommended in areas of high TBE activity.

Louping ill Encephalitis. Louping ill causes encephalitis in sheep (rarely in cattle, horses, and swine) in Scotland and in northern England and Ireland. Sporadic human cases have been recognized. Louping ill virus is maintained in nature by *I. ricinus* ticks and a variety of hosts, including small mammals, ground-dwelling birds (grouse), and probably sheep. The clinical features of louping ill resemble the European form of TBE.

Powassan Virus Encephalitis. Powassan virus encephalitis has been documented in a total of 15 cases in the northeastern United States and eastern Canada, with a case-fatality rate of 50 per cent. The virus is not associated with animal disease. The transmission cycle of Powassan virus involves *I. cookei*, *I. marxi* (and possibly other tick species), and mammals, particularly rodents and carnivores. Powassan encephalitis is characterized by fever and nonspecific symptoms, followed by encephalitic signs, which are frequently severe. Residual paralysis may occur. Peripheral blood and cerebrospinal fluid changes are similar to those described in other forms of flaviviral encephalitis.

Calisher CH, Thompson WH (eds.): California Serogroup Viruses. New York, Alan R. Liss, Inc., 1983. *Symposium covering all aspects of this virus group.*

Day JF, Curtis GA, Edman JD: Rainfall-directed oviposition behavior of *Culex nigripalpus* (Diptera: Culicindae) and its influence on St. Louis encephalitis virus transmission in Indian River County, Florida. J Med Entomol 27(1):43–50, 1990. *Correlation between rainfall patterns and transmission of SLE virus by infected mosquitoes in the field.*

Hardy JL, Winkelstein W Jr, Milby MM (eds.): Symposium: The epidemiology of mosquito-borne virus encephalitis in the United States, 1943–1987. Am J Trop Med Hyg 37:1S–100S, 1987. *A thorough discussion of mosquito-borne viral encephalitis.*

Hoke CH, Nisalak A, Sangawhipa N, et al.: Protection against Japanese encephalitis by inactivated vaccines. N Engl J Med 319(10):608–614, 1988. *Report of protective efficacy of Japanese encephalitis vaccines. This study and the accompanying editorial (see Monath) raise the question of the advisability of widespread vaccination in Asia as well as vaccination of travelers to Asia.*

Holmgren EB, Forsgren M: Epidemiology of tick-borne encephalitis in Sweden 1956–1989: A study of 1116 cases. Scand J Infect Dis 22(3):287–295, 1990. *A recent description of epidemiologic and clinical factors of tick-borne encephalitis.*

Matthews CG, Chun RWM, Grabow JD, et al.: Psychological sequelae in children following California arbovirus encephalitis. Neurology 18:1023, 1968. *Useful to the physician facing questions from patients about sequelae in children recovering from this infection.*

Monath TP: Japanese encephalitis—a plague of the Orient (editorial). N Engl J Med 319(10):641–643, 1988. *See comment under Hoke.*

Monath TP (ed.): The Arboviruses: Epidemiology and Ecology. Boca Raton, CRC Press, 1988. *An up-to-date source of critical information.*

Monath TP (ed.): Saint Louis Encephalitis. Washington, D.C., American Public Health Association, 1980. *Encyclopedic coverage of all aspects of St. Louis encephalitis, including clinical features and differential and definitive laboratory diagnosis. Contains references to all previously published studies.*

Przelomski MM, O'Rourke E, Grady GF, et al.: Eastern equine encephalitis in Massachusetts. Neurology 38:736–739, 1988. *Review of 16 cases of EEE in Massachusetts showing increased frequency in older persons.*

Rosato RR, Mancaseet FF, Jahrling PB: Enzyme-linked immunosorbent assay detection of immunoglobulins G and M to Venezuelan equine encephalomyelitis virus in vaccinated and naturally infected humans. J Clin Microbiol 26(3):421–425, 1988. *Use of ELISA to detect antibody to VEE induced by injection or vaccination.*

Schlesinger S, Schlesinger MJ (eds.): The Togaviridae and Flaviviridae. New York, Plenum Publishing, 1986. *An authoritative source of epidemiologic and virologic information.*

Viral Hemorrhagic Fevers

Robert E. Shope

390 Introduction

The viral hemorrhagic fevers encompass syndromes that vary from febrile hemorrhagic disease with capillary fragility to acute severe shock leading rapidly to death. The causative agents include arthropod-borne and rodent-borne viruses. The rodent-borne viruses do not require an arthropod vector but are transmitted directly to vertebrates by aerosol spread or contact with infected excreta or body secretions of the rodent. The reservoir and natural mode of transmission for the African hemorrhagic fever viruses, Marburg and Ebola, are not known.

There are at least 15 viruses that cause human hemorrhagic fevers (see Table 382–1). They are in the families Flaviviridae, Bunyaviridae, Arenaviridae, and Filoviridae. All contain RNA, and all are zoonoses.

The hemorrhagic fevers form a special group of diseases characterized by viral replication in lymphoid cells, followed by fever and myalgia and leading to hemorrhagic manifestations and hypovolemic shock. The basic physiologic defect in most is capillary leakage. In some, such as yellow fever, hepatocellular damage is prominent. In others, such as hemorrhagic fever with renal syndrome, renal lesions are striking. The mortality rates may be high, and the pathogenesis is poorly understood. Disseminated intravascular coagulopathy (DIC) is a feature in some cases, but probably not all. Antigen-antibody complexes may lead to release of mediators of shock in some cases, and direct effects of viral replication on capillary permeability in some have not been ruled out. It is important to understand the pathogenetic mechanism in order to manage the patient, but our knowledge is sparse at present.

Control can be achieved by interrupting the cycle, including peridomestic rodent control (Bolivian hemorrhagic fever), and, in those that are arboviruses, by vaccination of reservoir animals (Rift Valley fever), vector control, and education on methods to avoid the vector (dengue). Vaccines are available or under development for some of the agents such as Rift Valley fever, yellow fever, dengue, and Junin viruses. For others such as Lassa virus, we now have an antiviral drug, and for still another (Junin) preexposure and postexposure protection is afforded by human immune plasma.

391 Yellow Fever

DEFINITION. Yellow fever is an acute viral disease caused by infection with yellow fever virus. The disease is exemplary of the viral hemorrhagic fevers described in the following sections (Table 391–1). The infection is often subclinical but may lead to disease whose severity varies from mild and self-limited to a fulminant fatal outcome. Classic yellow fever is characterized by sudden onset, moderately high fever, nausea, bradycardia, prostration, vomiting of altered blood, jaundice, oliguria, and albuminuria. Natural cycles of the infection occur periodically in mosquitoes and primates of tropical South America as far north as Panama and in tropical west, central, and east Africa.

ETIOLOGY. Yellow fever virus is in the genus *Flavivirus* of the family Flaviviridae. Members of the family are single-stranded, negative-sense RNA viruses, spherical and approximately 40 nm in diameter. Particles form in the cytoplasm in close association with endoplasmic reticulum. They contain a lipid envelope and replicate in both arthropod and vertebrate cells. Other members of the Flaviviridae, including dengue, West Nile, and St. Louis encephalitis, cross-react with yellow fever virus in serologic tests and may confound the diagnosis. Minor antigenic differences exist between strains of yellow fever virus from Africa and South America, and among strains from different regions of Africa; however, the 17D yellow fever vaccine protects against all strains. The virus can be isolated in mosquitoes, arthropod and vertebrate tissue cultures, baby mice, and several monkey species. Rhesus monkeys regularly succumb following experimental inoculation and mimic severe human disease.

EPIDEMIOLOGY. Two epidemiologic types of yellow fever are distinguished: the urban and the sylvan (jungle) forms. Urban yellow fever is transmitted by *Aedes aegypti* mosquitoes from person to person, whereas sylvan yellow fever is maintained in a forest cycle of monkeys and forest-canopy mosquitoes; humans are infected when they enter the forest. The two types do not differ clinically.

A. aegypti is a peridomestic mosquito that breeds in abandoned tires, jars, cans, water storage containers, roof catchments, and drains in and around houses. Urban yellow fever was a major killer until the early 1900's, when mosquito control in Havana, Rio de Janeiro, Guayaquil, and the other large urban centers eliminated the disease. The last recorded urban case in the Americas was in Trinidad in 1954. *A. aegypti* continues to be prevalent in African cities, and *A. aegypti*–transmitted outbreaks still occur there. Major epidemics were recorded in Ethiopia, 1960–1962; Nigeria, 1969; Senegal, 1965 and 1979; Gambia, 1978; and Ghana and Burkina Faso, 1983. In 1986, an epidemic involving at least 3000 persons occurred in Nigeria, in Benue and Cross River States, and extended into Oyo and Niger States in 1987. An estimated 39,000 cases, with 8400 deaths, were recorded.

Yellow fever virus in Africa is transmitted by *A. aegypti* not only in the cities but also in semirural areas. In addition, some African epidemics are maintained by other *Aedes* species, such as *simpsoni* and the tree hole–breeding *africanus, leuteocephalus,* and *furcifer-taylori*, which transmit the virus in savannah and the transition forest-savannah zones of west Africa.

Sylvan yellow fever was recognized initially in Brazil in 1932. After urban yellow fever had been controlled in the Americas, sporadic cases continued to occur in persons exposed to mosquitoes in the jungles of South America and Africa. This sylvan form is maintained in tropical America by *Haemagogus* mosquitoes and forest primates, and sometimes by other sylvan animals. Evidence favors the hypothesis that the virus moves through the forest, cycling in one place until the monkeys are immune, then dying out and moving to areas where there are susceptible monkeys. People entering the forest are at risk. Sylvan yellow fever extends periodically outside the enzootic zone into forests such as those in Panama and Central America. The virus can be maintained over dry periods by transovarial transmission in mosquitoes, although it remains to be shown whether maintenance in mosquito eggs is more than a temporary mechanism.

The sylvan cycle in Africa is more complicated than in the Americas; in tropical Africa the virus cycles between *A. africanus* and monkeys. Another African mosquito, *A. simpsoni*, which feeds on both humans and monkeys, serves in some areas as a link between primates in the deep forest and people in the African villages.

A. aegypti was once carried on sailing ships between tropical ports and into temperate-zone cities. Modern ocean-going ships no longer harbor mosquito breeding sites, but the mosquito continues to travel by small boats, airplanes, cars, and especially in the form of dried eggs transported by used tires. Cities such as Rio de Janeiro, which were once freed of the mosquito, are now reinfested. Dengue fever reappeared there in 1986. To control the mosquito again in this area will be difficult because of insecticide resistance and the high price of labor and materials. Jungle yellow fever continues to cycle, reappearing in the same locale every 5 to 40 years. The scene is thus set again for emergence of the virus from the jungle to reinitiate the urban cycle in the Americas.

A. aegypti is easily identified. It has white thoracic scales in the shape of a lyre and black legs with white bands. Mosquitoes that have fed on a viremic vertebrate become infective after an extrinsic incubation period of 9 to 30 days, the shorter periods correlating with higher ambient temperatures. This extrinsic incubation period in the mosquito accounts for the delay from the first human infection in an urban outbreak to subsequent clusters of infection.

Yellow fever is not found in Asia, although large areas harbor *A. aegypti* that are capable of transmitting the virus, should it be introduced. India and other Asian nations require vaccination of travelers from yellow fever–endemic regions.

All age groups and races are susceptible. However, sylvan yellow fever is found almost always in young males because they are the individuals who venture into the forest. Immunity following vaccination or infection is long-lasting. During an epidemic, the population at risk, therefore, may be limited to age groups not covered by prior immunization or those born since a prior outbreak. There is also some evidence that persons may be protected by antibody to heterologous flaviviruses.

During the 24-year period from 1965 to 1988, there were 3324 cases of yellow fever reported in the Americas, and 7701 in Africa. The numbers of cases are greatly underestimated, probably by a factor of at least 10. Case-fatality rates are usually about 20 per cent but are higher in some epidemics. Ratios of apparent to inapparent infection, estimated at 1:10, may vary greatly.

PATHOLOGY AND PATHOGENESIS. The lesions of yellow fever involve primarily the liver, heart, kidneys, and lymphoid tissues. Grossly, the skin is icteric, and there may be multiple hemorrhages or petechiae of the skin, mucous membranes, and multiple organs. The liver is normal in size, icteric, and fatty. The heart is soft and flabby, and the kidneys are swollen and a pink-gray color. Small peritoneal and pleural effusions are sometimes observed.

Histology is often characteristic in patients who die before the ninth day of illness, but the lesions are not always pathognomonic. The most striking lesion is the eosinophilic degeneration and coagulation of hepatocytes (Councilman's bodies). Hepatocyte destruction is most marked in the midzone of the lobule, with relative sparing of the central vein and portal areas. Intranuclear eosinophilic granular inclusions or enlarged nucleoli (Torre's bodies) are also described. Both microvacuolar- and multivacuolar fatty changes are prominent, especially after the first week of illness. Inflammation is uncommon, and the reticulum framework is unaffected, probably accounting for the absence of postnecrotic fibrosis in convalescence and the regeneration of hepatocytes in recovered cases. The kidneys show cloudy swelling of tubular epithelium leading to acute tubular necrosis. The glomeruli are not obviously affected, but special stains indicate Schiff-positive

alterations in the basal membranes, and proteinaceous material accumulates in the capsular spaces and lumina of the proximal tubules. The myocardium is characterized by granular or fatty infiltration of muscle fibers and of the atrioventricular (AV) conduction system and cloudy swelling and degeneration of myocytes without inflammation. Large monocytes replace lymphocytic cells in the splenic follicles and lymph nodes. Encephalitis is rare, although petechial hemorrhage in the brain stem and cerebral edema are observed.

Knowledge of the pathogenesis of yellow fever is sparse. Yellow fever cases occur in remote areas, and pathophysiologic studies of yellow fever patients are usually done with only rudimentary laboratory facilities. The virus replicates in the hepatocytes and myocytes, and it is presumed that lesions in these target cells are a direct effect of the virus. Jaundice and prolonged prothrombin time can be explained by hepatocellular damage; bradycardia and arrhythmias, by myocyte and AV node perturbation. The etiology of renal tubular necrosis is not clear, but it may be secondary to hepatic changes. Some, but not all, fatal cases are associated with thrombocytopenia; increased prothrombin, partial thromboplastin, and thrombin times; diminished factor VIII and fibrinogen; and the presence of fibrin split products. The bleeding in these cases may be secondary to disseminated intravascular coagulopathy, but this is not generally accepted by all investigators. Hypoglycemia, metabolic acidosis, and hyperkalemia characterize the terminal stage and are probably the result of multiple organ system failure.

CLINICAL MANIFESTATIONS. Severe yellow fever is a fulminant febrile illness with 50 per cent or greater mortality. There is a great deal of variation, however; most cases are mild with a better prognosis, and only about 10 to 20 per cent are in the severe category. The intrinsic incubation period is 3 to 6 days, exceptionally as long as 10 days.

The clinical syndrome is classified as very mild, mild, moderately severe, or malignant. Patients with very mild cases have fever and headache, and the patient recovers in 48 hours or less. Those with mild cases have sudden fever and headache with nausea, sometimes bleeding of the gums or epistaxis, bradycardia, or albuminuria. The patient recovers in 2 or 3 days. Those with moderately severe cases have more marked manifestations of bleeding, definite bradycardia in relation to the fever, nausea and vomiting, jaundice, and striking albuminuria. The illness may be aborted after 3 to 4 days or may develop serious hemorrhagic manifestations, such as black vomit, melena, and metrorrhagia. Moderately severe yellow fever may last 1 week or even longer.

Classic yellow fever is characterized as malignant and is divided into three periods. The period of infection involves sudden onset of fever and headache, with initial rapid pulse, but by day 2, the pulse slows in spite of continued fever (Faget's sign). Headache, back, and muscle pain may be severe, blood oozes from the gums, and other signs of bleeding become prominent. The face is flushed, the tongue is reddened (strawberry tongue), and the conjunctivae are injected; the patient is irritable, unable to sleep, and frequently constipated. The temperature is often 40°C or higher. On the third day of illness, there is nausea, vomiting of coffee-ground material, and notable albuminuria. The bleeding

TABLE 391-1. CLINICAL PARAMETERS OF VIRAL HEMORRHAGIC FEVERS

Disease	Viral Agent	Incubation Period (Days)	Clinical Syndromes				Case-Fatality Rate (%)
			Hemorrhage	*Hepatitis*	*Encephalitis*	*Nephropathy*	
Yellow fever	Yellow fever	3–6	major	major	absent	moderate	2–20
Dengue hemorrhagic fever	Dengue 1–4	5–8	moderate	moderate	absent	absent	2–5
Rift Valley fever	Rift Valley fever	3–6	major	major	moderate	absent	30–50
Crimean-Congo hemorrhagic fever	Crimean-Congo hemorrhagic fever	2–9	major	major	minor	absent	30–50
Kyasanur Forest disease	Kyasanur Forest disease	3–8	minor	minor	moderate	absent	5–10
Omsk hemorrhagic fever	Omsk hemorrhagic fever	3–8	minor	minor	moderate	absent	0.4–2.5
Hemorrhagic fever with renal syndrome	Hantaan	2–42	moderate	rare	minor	major	2–5
Argentine hemorrhagic fever	Junin	10–14	minor	rare	moderate	minor	1–15
Bolivian hemorrhagic fever	Machupo	7–14	moderate	rare	moderate	minor	15–30
Lassa fever	Lassa	3–16	minor	major	minor	minor	10–25
African hemorrhagic fever	Marburg	3–9	major	major	minor	absent	20–30
	Ebola	3–18	major	major	minor	absent	60–90

is usually gastric, not lower intestinal. In the period of remission, often on day 4, the patient feels better, the fever drops, and headache and nausea subside. Remission lasts a few hours to 2 days. It is followed by the period of intoxication in which the classic signs of fever, epigastric tenderness with vomiting of altered blood, nosebleeds, and albuminuria leading to oliguria or anuria occur. Dehydration may predispose to suppurative parotitis; the lungs are usually normal, but bacterial pneumonia may complicate the disease. Intoxication lasts from 3 days up to 2 weeks and may be accompanied by heart failure with drop in blood pressure, hiccough, coma, and death. Sometimes the patient is lucid until the end.

The clinical syndrome may be predominantly one of hepatic, renal, or cardiac failure. Meningoencephalitis has also been recorded. Death usually occurs between the seventh and the tenth day of illness. Patients who survive generally recover completely, although the convalescence may be prolonged, and late death from cardiac failure or arrhythmias is a rare complication.

CLINICAL LABORATORY FINDINGS. Early in the course there may be leukopenia with relative neutropenia (but sometimes with normal or elevated leukocyte count), decreased prothrombin time, and elevation of the serum bilirubin level. After the third day of illness, full-blown yellow fever is associated with abnormalities referable to the liver, kidneys, and heart. The total and conjugated bilirubin concentration values are elevated and rise together. The mean bilirubin value is 9 to 10 mg per deciliter but averages 15 to 20 mg per deciliter in severe cases and may be much higher. There are increased prothrombin and partial thromboplastin times and decreased platelets, blood glucose, and clotting factors II, V, VII, IX, and X. Alkaline phosphatase levels are normal. Aminotransferase levels are of prognostic value; serum aspartate aminotransferase and alanine aminotransferase levels are consistently elevated in jaundiced patients.

Albuminuria usually appears on the fourth day, reaching levels of 3 to 5 mg per liter (in severe cases much higher). Blood urea averages 109 mg per deciliter, and creatinine averages 5.9 mg per deciliter in fatal cases; the averages are 59 and 2.6 mg per deciliter, respectively, in nonfatal yellow fever. The urine may contain bile and casts. Electrocardiogram abnormalities are sometimes present, including abnormal ST-T waves and prolonged PR and QT intervals. The cerebrospinal fluid is under increased pressure and may contain increased protein with normal cell counts.

DIAGNOSIS. Diagnosis can be made by histopathologic examination of the liver, by isolation of yellow fever virus from blood during life and from liver and other tissues post mortem, by demonstration of specific nucleic acid, or by serologic tests. Yellow fever should be suspected in any febrile patient from endemic zones of Africa and the Americas and in areas of high A. aegypti prevalence where yellow fever may be introduced. Diagnosis post mortem by examination of liver taken by a viscerotome was successfully used in South America routinely for many years. Liver biopsy should not be attempted because of the danger of uncontrolled bleeding.

Yellow fever virus can be isolated from serum and blood during the first 4 days of fever by inoculation intracerebrally into baby mice or onto mammalian or mosquito cell cultures. Mice are observed for death; the virus causes cytopathic effect in Vero cells and is detected by immunofluorescence tests in mosquito cells 3 to 6 days after inoculation. The most rapid method of diagnosis is detection of antigen in acute phase blood by the antigen-capture enzyme-linked immunosorbent assay (ELISA). The test can be completed in a few hours, although detection of antigen by ELISA is less sensitive than virus isolation.

Serologic diagnosis is made by demonstrating immunoglobulin M (IgM) by the antibody-capture ELISA. Since IgM is relatively specific and is detectable for only a short time after infection, this technique is reliable using a single convalescent serum specimen. Alternatively, tests of sera collected during the acute and convalescent phases are diagnostic if they show a fourfold or greater rise (or fall) of yellow fever antibody. The neutralization test is highly specific, but the complement fixation, hemagglutination-inhibition, and ELISA methods are usually used because they are quicker and lend themselves to field laboratory use. The laboratory must also rule out cross-reacting antibody by related viruses such as dengue. A radiolabeled RNA probe detected

yellow fever RNA in fixed human liver stored for more than 20 years.

DIFFERENTIAL DIAGNOSIS. The mild form of yellow fever is not clinically distinguishable from other tropical fevers. Severe yellow fever simulates viral hepatitis, including delta hepatitis; other hemorrhagic fevers; leptospirosis; rickettsial fevers; malignant malaria; and drug- and toxin-related conditions.

PROGNOSIS. Two to 20 per cent of patients with clinically evident yellow fever die, although as many as 50 per cent of severely ill patients succumb. It is not clear whether these patients would survive if they received the most modern supportive treatment, because most cases are treated in primitive clinics in Africa and South America. Patients who enter the period of intoxication have a guarded prognosis, especially if they develop anuria, high levels of albuminuria and bilirubinemia, a prothrombin time prolonged beyond 25 per cent of normal, a rapid, weak pulse, uncontrolled bleeding, persistent hiccough, delirium, hypotension, or coma.

TREATMENT. The treatment consists of complete bed rest, fluid and blood replacement, and supportive care, including monitoring of vital signs. Analgesics and antiemetics may be useful, but aspirin is contraindicated because it may exacerbate bleeding. Patients are placed under bed nets to prevent possible mosquito transmission to other patients and to hospital personnel. Malaria and bacterial complications should be treated if diagnosed. Electrolyte imbalance should be corrected. Dialysis has not been used in cases of renal tubular damage but on theoretical grounds may benefit patients in renal failure. If disseminated intravascular coagulopathy is evident by laboratory tests, heparin may be used cautiously, although there is insufficient experience to date to predict its efficacy. Interferon and other antiviral substances have not been tried in patients with yellow fever.

PREVENTION AND CONTROL. Yellow fever can be prevented by inoculation of 17D attenuated vaccine. This vaccine is safe and in over 90 per cent of vaccinees induces antibody that persists at least 10 years, and usually for life. The vaccine is produced in eggs and should not be given to persons with egg allergies. Travelers should be vaccinated at least 10 days before arrival in yellow fever–endemic areas. Since the presence of yellow fever often goes undetected and unreported in tropical Africa and South America, the vaccine should be given to travelers whether or not there is known active transmission. Human immunodeficiency virus (HIV) infection is not a contraindication to vaccination. Unless the risk of exposure to yellow fever is great, vaccine is not recommended during pregnancy; however, it is not known to have caused fetal damage. In an epidemic, mosquito control measures and use of bed nets and repellents are recommended until vaccine can be obtained.

392 Hemorrhagic Fever Caused by Dengue Viruses

DEFINITION. Dengue hemorrhagic fever (DHF) is an acute febrile illness characterized by decreased platelet counts and hemoconcentration in patients infected with any one of the four serotypes of dengue virus. The disease affects children mainly and, sometimes, adults. Capillary permeability and coagulation defects lead to hemorrhagic manifestations and, in the more severe cases, to hypovolemic shock (dengue shock syndrome), with death in 40 to 50 per cent of untreated shock syndrome patients. The disease has been endoepidemic in Southeast Asia since 1953 and is increasing in prevalence. It was restricted to Asia and the Pacific until 1981, when epidemic DHF appeared in Cuba; it reappeared in Venezuela in 1990.

ETIOLOGY. DHF is caused by infection with dengue viruses, but it is not yet established why one patient develops hemorrhagic fever and another develops classic dengue fever. Initially, it was hypothesized that strains of dengue virus that caused DHF were more virulent than others; another current theory holds that infection is enhanced and the disease is more severe when the host has been sensitized by a prior dengue infection of different serotype.

EPIDEMIOLOGY. The epidemiology of DHF is that described for dengue fever with some added features. Epidemics of DHF are limited to Southeast Asia, the Pacific Islands, and, since 1981, the Caribbean and northern South America. It is estimated that fewer than 5 per cent of individuals with dengue develop DHF. The attack rate in Thailand is highest in children, with a minor peak in infants, when maternal antibody is waning, and a major peak at 4 to 12 years of age, when second dengue infections are most common; adults as well as children develop DHF in some outbreaks, such as that in Cuba in 1981. Well-nourished children in Southeast Asia appeared to be at higher risk than the undernourished, and blacks in the Cuban epidemic had milder illness than whites; well-controlled studies are needed to substantiate these observations.

PATHOLOGY. Post mortem there are focal hemorrhages, vascular congestion, and edema in multiple organs. The spleen and lymphoid tissues show marked lymphocytolysis and phagocytosis of lymphocytes, primarily in the T cell–dependent zones. There is also proliferation of lymphoblasts and young plasma cells. Monocytic and lymphocytic nonnecrotizing perivascular infiltration is found in skin lesions, resembling an antibody-dependent Arthus reaction.

PATHOGENESIS. Dengue virus infects the macrophages, lymphocytes, and endothelial cells. On rare occasions, DHF occurs in primary dengue, indicating that direct infection of these cells with the virus can lead to the syndrome; however, the vast majority of cases are secondary infections. In these cases there is a rapid anamnestic antibody response, with formation of antigen-antibody complexes. Experimentally, formation of complexes enhances infectivity of the virus for monocytes through attachment of complexes at the Fc receptor site and entry of virus into the cell. Between 0.05 and 0.1 per cent of monocytes in the peripheral blood can be visualized carrying dengue antigen. The replication of dengue virus in the monocyte is postulated to be the effector pathway leading to vascular permeability. Monocyte infection is presumably responsible for the observed complement activation and consumption via the classic and perhaps the alternate pathway. This process may result in formation of C3a and C5a, which are anaphylatoxins, or some other as yet unknown mediator of vascular permeability may be activated. Another effector pathway leads to coagulation defects, including thrombocytopenia and abnormal clotting. The entire process is rapid. It may evolve in a few hours to shock and death or, if managed effectively, to complete recovery. Although the pathogenesis is not understood, the pathophysiologic events are known and can be treated rationally.

CLINICAL MANIFESTATIONS. DHF usually starts with sudden onset of high fever and the signs and symptoms of dengue fever, which include facial flush, anorexia, headache, nausea, and pains in the muscles and joints. Hepatic tenderness, epigastric or generalized abdominal pain, and sore throat are frequent. The liver is usually palpable, and the spleen is characteristically prominent on radiographs. The temperature continues high for 2 days to a week. A positive tourniquet test result, easy bruising, and fine petechiae on the face, soft palate, and extremities indicate a hemorrhagic disorder. Sometimes gum bleeding and epistaxis are noted. The majority of cases are moderately severe or mild, and the patients recover after lysis of fever. The lysis may be associated with sweating, coolness of extremities, and transient lowering of blood pressure.

More severe cases are associated with shock. The fall in blood pressure occurs suddenly on the third to the seventh day of illness and is accompanied by cool, blotchy skin, circumoral cyanosis, and tachycardia. The patient becomes restless and may complain of acute abdominal pain. The pulse pressure drops to 20 mm Hg or less, and in severe cases the blood pressure and pulse may not be detectable. Uncorrected shock may lead to metabolic acidosis and severe bleeding from the gastrointestinal tract and other sites. Death or recovery usually occurs in 12 to 24 hours. Surviving patients do not usually have sequelae. The white blood cell count is normal or slightly elevated, with lymphocytosis and atypical lymphocytes commonly seen. There is hemoconcentration and elevated serum aspartate aminotransferase and blood urea nitrogen levels.

DIAGNOSIS. The laboratory diagnosis is that of dengue fever, which is usually made retrospectively. DHF with shock syndrome is a medical emergency, and therefore early clinical diagnosis is essential. DHF presents with (1) acute onset of fever, which is high, continuous, and lasts 2 days or more; (2) positive tourniquet test result, with spontaneous petechiae or ecchymoses; bleeding from gums or nose; hematemesis or melena; (3) hepatomegaly, observed in more than 90 per cent of Asian patients; (4) hypotension with cold, clammy skin, restlessness, and pulse pressure less than 20 mm Hg; (5) thrombocytopenia; (6) hematocrit increased 20 per cent over the convalescent value; and (7) radiographic evidence of pleural effusion. Fever, hemorrhagic phenomena, thrombocytopenia, and hemoconcentration are the hallmarks of DHF, and, with hypotension or narrow pulse pressure, of dengue shock syndrome (DSS). Hepatoencephalopathy sometimes develops as a late manifestation. Bacterial endotoxic shock and meningococcemia can mimic DHF/DSS.

TREATMENT. There is no specific treatment. The object of therapy is to maintain hydration, to combat acidosis, and to correct coagulation abnormalities. Salicylates may contribute to bleeding and acidosis and are contraindicated. Paracetamol may be used. Steroids should not be used. Hematocrit should be determined frequently, at least daily, to measure the degree of plasma loss and the need for intravenous fluid. Fluid should be started at 20 ml per kilogram of body weight. One third to one half of fluid should be physiologic saline and the remainder, 5 per cent glucose in water. If acidosis is present, one quarter of fluid should be 0.167 mol per liter of sodium bicarbonate. In shock cases, one should use Ringer's lactate, 5 per cent glucose in physiologic saline, 5 per cent glucose in one-half physiologic saline, 5 per cent glucose in one-half Ringer's lactate, or 5 per cent glucose in one-third physiologic saline (depending on degree of dehydration and age). One should monitor for signs of cardiac failure during rapid fluid administration.

In case of shock, one should administer fluid rapidly and under pressure if necessary. One should give plasma or another volume expander if shock persists and should follow the vital signs and hematocrit. The hematocrit should decline with fluid therapy, which is continued until the hematocrit is under 40 per cent, urine output is adequate, and the appetite returns. If electrolytes and blood gases indicate acidosis, sodium bicarbonate should be administered. Heparin for intravascular coagulopathy (prolonged prothrombin and partial thromboplastin times) is usually not needed but may be used cautiously in refractory cases. Chloral hydrate for sedation, oxygen for shock, and blood should be administered as needed.

PROGNOSIS. Case fatality from DHF is 2 to 10 per cent; deaths occur in shock cases. Most patients survive when treated early by experienced health care workers. Recovery is rapid and without sequelae.

PREVENTION. Prevention is as described for dengue fever.

393 Tick-Borne Flavivirus Diseases: Kyasanur Forest Disease and Omsk Hemorrhagic Fever

DEFINITION. Kyasanur Forest disease (KFD) of India and Omsk hemorrhagic fever (OHF) of western Siberia are tick-transmitted flavivirus fevers characterized by hemorrhage or encephalitis. Some patients manifest both syndromes.

ETIOLOGY. KFD and OHF viruses belong to the tick-borne complex of flaviviruses, which also encompasses the closely related viruses of central European tick-borne encephalitis, Russian spring-summer encephalitis, and Powassan encephalitis of North America and Asia.

EPIDEMIOLOGY. KFD was originally limited to the forests of Shimoga District of Karnataka State, India, but since its discovery in 1957 it has spread in an unpredictable fashion to three other neighboring forested districts. The largest and most recent outbreak occurred during 1982–83 in a new focus in Nidle Forest. Many tick species are involved in transmission, especially nymphal *Haemaphysalis spinigera*. Small terrestrial mammals as well as birds and bats are infected in nature. When the forest is felled for plantations, the ecology is upset. Cattle brought in to graze at the forest fringe are not infected but serve as hosts that greatly increase the numbers of ticks. Infected ticks feed on black-faced langur monkeys and South Indian bonnet macaques, which become viremic, serve as amplifiers of infection, and often die. At the same time, epidemics occur in persons involved in forest occupations. People are infected incidentally and do not form part of the transmission cycle.

OHF occurs in the forest-steppe areas of the lake region of western Siberia. Epidemics of as many as 600 cases were recorded in the 1940's, but in recent years the disease has virtually disappeared. Numbers of cases peak in May and again in August and September. The virus is transmitted by *Dermacentor pictus* ticks and is maintained in small-mammal populations. Muskrats, which were introduced for hunting in the 1920's, are susceptible and apparently transmit OHF virus to other muskrats and to hunters by direct contact. Lake water contaminated by dead muskrats is said to be responsible for water-borne disease. Both KFD and OHF are transmitted transovarially and trans-stadially in ticks.

CLINICAL MANIFESTATIONS AND PATHOLOGY. The incubation period is 3 to 8 days. Onset is sudden, with fever up to 40°C, headache, papulovesicular lesions of the soft palate, myalgia, and prostration lasting 1 to 2 weeks. In more severe cases, there may be nasal, enteric, uterine, or pulmonary hemorrhage. Leukopenia, thrombocytopenia, and albuminuria are found. Some patients have a diphasic course, with a more severe illness and meningoencephalitis after a 1- or 2-week afebrile period. The second phase is characterized by fever, severe headache, meningismus, mental disturbances, and tremors. Hemorrhagic manifestations or pneumonia may also be prominent in the second phase. The case fatality rate of KFD is 5 to 10 per cent; that of OHF is 0.4 to 2.5 per cent. There are no sequelae. Infections in laboratory workers are common but are usually mild. Histopathology is minor in comparison to the gravity of the clinical disease. Findings include extravasation of red blood cells, edema, and thrombi in the small vessels.

DIAGNOSIS AND TREATMENT. Diagnosis is by isolation of virus from the blood during the first 10 days of illness and by demonstration of antibody rise or presence of specific immunoglobulin M (IgM) during convalescence. There is no specific treatment, but fluid and electrolyte balance should be maintained and blood transfused if needed. Analgesics other than aspirin may be indicated.

PREVENTION. Tick repellents, protective clothing, and spraying of forest tracts with acaricides are the only measures available for prevention.

394 Crimean-Congo Hemorrhagic Fever

DEFINITION. Crimean-Congo hemorrhagic fever (CCHF) is an acute febrile hemorrhagic tick-borne disease of Asia, Europe, and Africa. Mortality is high and hospital-based outbreaks are common.

ETIOLOGY. The disease is caused by CCHF virus of the *Nairovirus* genus, family Bunyaviridae. The virus kills baby mice and replicates in CER cells and several other cell culture systems.

EPIDEMIOLOGY. CCHF virus is transmitted in nature principally by hard ticks of the genus *Hyalomma*, but also by ticks in the genera *Rhipicephalus*, *Boophilus*, and *Amblyomma*. Virus is maintained by transovarial and trans-stadial passage in the tick

and is amplified by hares and possibly hedgehogs, sheep, and cattle. Giraffe, rhinoceros, eland, buffalo, kudu, zebra, and dogs in southern Africa have antibody to CCHF virus.

The virus or its antibody is found in the distribution of *Hyalomma* ticks. Foci occur in the Soviet Union, the Balkan nations, Iraq, Iran, Pakistan, Afghanistan, western China, the Middle East, and most of sub-Saharan Africa, including South Africa. Outbreaks occur among military personnel, campers, and persons tending sheep and cattle. Medical workers are at high risk because of frequent spread in hospitals from infected human blood and tissues.

CLINICAL MANIFESTATIONS. The incubation period is usually between 2 and 9 days. Onset is sudden, with severe headache, fever, chills, myalgia, especially in the back and legs, sore throat, abdominal pain, nausea, vomiting, diarrhea, photophobia, and conjunctival injection. The fever is constant but may be remitting. The patient is often confused or aggressive with a marked mood change. Leukopenia and thrombocytopenia are usually observed. On days 3 to 6, hemorrhagic manifestations and a petechial rash on the trunk, limbs, and oral cavity appear. Epistaxis, hematemesis, melena, and uterine bleeding may be severe and require transfusion. The liver is sometimes enlarged and tender. In severe cases, hepatorenal failure or multiple organ system failure leads to death, usually on days 6 to 14 of illness. Death may also result from blood loss, cerebral hemorrhage, dehydration after diarrhea, or pulmonary edema. Patients recover gradually starting on day 10 when the rash fades. Asthenia may last for a month or more. Recovery is usually complete, although neuritis may persist for months. Liver function tests are abnormal, especially the aspartate aminotransferase, and serum bilirubin levels are often elevated late in the illness. Abnormal prothrombin, activated partial thromboplastin, and thrombin times, as well as increased fibrin degradation products, are indicative of disseminated intravascular coagulation (DIC).

DIAGNOSIS. Virus is easily isolated during the first 8 days of illness. Antibodies are detectable by the immunofluorescence and enzyme-linked immunosorbent assays in surviving patients. Specific immunoglobulin M (IgM) and immunoglobulin G (IgG) are present by days seven to nine of illness.

TREATMENT AND PROGNOSIS. Patients suspected of having CCHF should be housed in an isolation facility with needle and blood precautions. Health care personnel should use respirators and protective clothing. Treatment is supportive, including monitoring and correction of fluid and electrolyte imbalance and treatment of DIC. The vital signs and hematocrit should be tested frequently, and blood should be replaced by transfusion. Case-fatality rates range from 30 to 50 per cent.

PREVENTION. Protection from tick bites and care in handling blood and tissues of sick sheep and cattle are the only preventive measures available in the case of exposure in natural foci.

395 Hemorrhagic Diseases Caused by Arenaviruses (*Argentine and Bolivian Hemorrhagic Fevers and Lassa Fever*)

DEFINITION. Argentine and Bolivian hemorrhagic fevers and Lassa fever are acute febrile diseases characterized by hemorrhagic diatheses, marked myalgia, and, in severe cases, shock. Case-fatality rates are between 5 and 30 per cent.

ETIOLOGY. The diseases are caused by the viruses Junin (Argentina), Machupo (Bolivia), and Lassa (West Africa) of the family Arenaviridae.

EPIDEMIOLOGY. The reservoirs are rodents that excrete virus in urine and possibly other body fluids. The rodents involved are Junin virus, *Calomys musculinus*, *Calomys laucha*, and *Akodon arenicola*; Machupo virus, *Calomys callosus*; and Lassa virus, *Mastomys natalensis*. People are believed to be infected by inhaling or eating contaminated excreta or by passage of virus through abraded skin or mucous membranes. In Argentina, exposure to Junin virus is primarily in workers harvesting corn in Cordoba and Buenos Aires provinces in the north. In Bolivia, domestic and peridomestic exposure to Machupo virus occurs in Beni province. Lassa virus is endemic in west and central Africa, especially in Liberia, Sierra Leone, and parts of Nigeria, where it is transmitted in and around homes that have an abundance of domestic rats.

Argentine hemorrhagic fever epidemics involving hundreds to thousands of farm workers are recorded annually. Bolivian hemorrhagic fever epidemics were common in the 1960's, but after institution of rodent control measures, the disease has not been reported since 1974. Lassa fever was recognized first in 1969 in a nosocomial outbreak in Nigeria. Several other nosocomial outbreaks were subsequently diagnosed, but studies in Sierra Leone established the basic endemic nature of the disease. In the eastern province, 8 to 52 per cent of the population have antibody, and the annual seroconversion rate in susceptible subjects ranges between 5 and 22 per cent. It is estimated that 5 to 14 per cent of the fevers are Lassa virus infections and that Lassa fever accounts for 10 to 16 per cent of the adult hospital admissions.

PATHOGENESIS AND PATHOLOGY. The diseases are characterized by multiple organ impairment, yet specific lesions are absent. The prominent findings are focal diapedesis and capillary hemorrhage, but inflammation is minimal. Focal areas of liver necrosis in Lassa fever are not sufficient to account for the profound shock and death. It is postulated that the virus infects cells of the reticuloendothelial system, including the B and T cells. It causes temporary inhibition of immune cell function leading to prolonged and high-titered viremia. It is not known whether subsequent capillary damage and parenchymal edema are direct or indirect effects of the virus.

CLINICAL MANIFESTATIONS. The three diseases have many similarities. The incubation period of Lassa fever is 3 to 16 days; of Argentine hemorrhagic fever, 10 to 14 days; and of Bolivian hemorrhagic fever, 7 to 14 days. Onset is insidious, initially with fever, chills, malaise, asthenia, headache, retroocular pain, anorexia, nausea, vomiting, and muscle pain, (especially at the costovertebral angle in the South American forms and the legs in Lassa fever). Fever is nonremitting between 39° and 40.5°C. Sore throat is not prominent in the Argentine and Bolivian diseases, but purulent pharyngitis and aphthous ulcers are common in Lassa fever.

Signs include conjunctivitis, facial edema, enanthem with pharyngeal vesicles, exanthem of the face, neck, and upper thorax, tenderness of thighs, laterocervical and other polyadenopathy, and petechiae, especially in the axillae. There is no jaundice or hepatosplenomegaly. Leukopenia, thrombocytopenia, and albuminuria with casts are characteristic.

Late in the first week of illness, the signs and symptoms become more pronounced. Signs of dehydration, decreased blood pressure, and relative bradycardia are prominent. Hemorrhage from the gums, nose, stomach, intestines, uterus, and urinary tract indicates a severe hemorrhagic diathesis. Bleeding was observed commonly in the South American forms, but in only 17 per cent of Lassa fever cases. Blood loss is not massive enough to account for the shock. The acute phase usually lasts 7 to 15 days. Death is the result of uremia or hypovolemic shock, usually in the second week of illness. Recovery is heralded by lysis of fever; there is usually a prolonged convalescence marked by periods of sweating, flush, and postural hypotension, but patients suffer no permanent nonneurologic sequelae.

Neurologic signs are prominent in Bolivian hemorrhagic fever; nearly 50 per cent of patients have an intention tremor of the tongue and hands at about the fifth day of illness, and 25 per cent of these progress to more serious encephalopathy with delirium and convulsions. The cerebrospinal fluid is normal in these patients. A similar syndrome is occasionally seen in Lassa fever, and about 5 per cent of patients develop unilateral or bilateral eighth cranial nerve damage, which may be permanent. Other transient complications are loss of hair and Beau's lines of the nails.

Most patients have leukopenia with depression of both lymphocytes and neutrophils; however, some Lassa fever patients have markedly elevated white counts. Thrombocytopenia is present during the first week of illness.

DIAGNOSIS. The diagnosis can be made definitively only with laboratory tests. Fever, muscle pain, and diminished white cell count in the endemic areas should alert the physician to the diagnosis. Virus can be isolated in Vero cells from blood, cerebrospinal fluid, and throat washings during life and from most tissues at necropsy. Virus is recoverable even in the presence of antibody. Isolation of virus from Bolivian hemorrhagic fever cases is more difficult than from the Argentine or West African form. Virus isolation should be attempted only in laboratories with high biosecurity containment equipment because of the risk of infection of laboratory workers. Serologic diagnosis is made by the immunofluorescence test. Immunoglobulin G is present in 53 per cent of Lassa fever patients on admission to hospital and immunoglobulin M (IgM), in 67 per cent. The IgM test is useful for early and rapid diagnosis.

TREATMENT. Supportive therapy, including attention to electrolyte and fluid balance, is essential. Hematocrit and urine protein measurements aid in detection of hypovolemic shock. Plasma expanders are effective if used early but may precipitate pulmonary edema late in the clinical course.

Specific Junin virus–immune human plasma given during the first 8 days of Argentine hemorrhagic fever reduced the case-fatality rate from 16 to 1 per cent. A neurologic illness was observed about 3 weeks after the acute attack in some patients receiving this therapy. Most of these persons recovered completely.

Ribavirin given to Lassa fever patients early in the illness significantly reduced mortality. The drug was administered intravenously, 60 mg per kilogram per day for the first 4 days, and then orally, 30 mg per kilogram per day for 6 days more. Immune plasma was not effective in Lassa fever patients in controlled trials.

PROGNOSIS. In Lassa fever, bleeding manifestations, high levels of circulating virus in the blood, and elevated aspartate aminotransferase levels in serum are predictive of death. There are no such predictors for the South American arenavirus hemorrhagic fevers. Shock or abnormal neurologic findings indicate a poor prognosis.

PREVENTION AND CONTROL. Environmental sanitation, including rodent-proofing of homes, and proper storage of grains and other foods to diminish rodent populations are the only community control measures now available. An experimental vaccine for Junin virus has proved efficacious in Argentina. Barrier nursing with use of gloves and gowns should be instituted in suspected cases of arenaviral hemorrhagic fevers. Blood and other tissues are infective and should be decontaminated.

396 African Hemorrhagic Fever (Marburg-Ebola Disease)

DEFINITION. African hemorrhagic fever is an acute, often fatal, hemorrhagic disease. Fever, rash, hemorrhage, hepatic and pancreatic inflammation, and prostration are hallmarks of the illness.

ETIOLOGY. The disease is caused by Marburg and Ebola viruses of the family Filoviridae. The two viruses are distinct antigenically but of very similar morphology.

EPIDEMIOLOGY. Marburg disease was described in 1967 in Germany and Yugoslavia, where workers in vaccine manufacturing facilities sickened and died after they were exposed to infected tissues of African green monkeys from Uganda. Where the monkeys became infected is not known, although Marburg virus is indigenous to Africa. (Additional isolated cases in South Africa and Kenya are recorded.) Ebola virus epidemics in Sudan and Zaire in 1976 were traced to contact with infected patients and, in Zaire, to spread by needle. The disease recurred in Sudan in

1979, and there was an isolated case in Kenya in 1980. The source of the outbreaks is unknown, and the natural history remains a mystery. A third filovirus, most closely related to Ebola virus, was isolated in 1989 from sick cynomolgus monkeys recently imported to the United States from the Philippines. Animal handlers in the United States seroconverted to the virus without associated illness.

PATHOLOGY. African hemorrhagic fever is a systemic disease with multiple organ involvement, most prominently the lymphatic system, testes, ovaries, and liver. Liver cell necrosis with eosinophilic inclusions, unlike that in yellow fever, is random and focal. Fibrin deposits are found in the renal glomeruli, consistent with disseminated intravascular coagulopathy. There is edema and diffuse inflammation in the brain.

CLINICAL MANIFESTATIONS. The incubation period is 3 to 9 days for Marburg virus infection and 3 to 18 days for Ebola. Onset is abrupt, with severe headache, backache, muscle pains, and sometimes abdominal pain. At this stage, the disease is not readily differentiated from malaria, typhoid fever, and other bacterial, rickettsial, or viral illnesses. On about the third day, nausea, vomiting, and profuse watery diarrhea with mucus and blood commence. Diarrhea may continue for several days. A maculopapular rash appears on the trunk and spreads to the rest of the body. On day 4 or 5, the patient's status becomes critical, with high, unremitting fever and an altered mental state, including confusion, aggression, or lethargy. There is spontaneous bleeding from injection sites, hematemesis, melena, hemoptysis, and, in pregnant patients, abortion, often with massive blood loss. Renal failure may be a terminal event. Death occurs from day 8 to 17, often on day 8 or 9. Recovery is marked by fatigue, anorexia, weight loss, hair loss, and, sometimes, psychological problems.

The pathophysiology is characterized by leukopenia, thrombocytopenia, increased prothrombin time, and other abnormalities in the liver function tests, increased serum amylase, proteinuria, and electrocardiographic changes indicative of myocardial disease. Disseminated intravascular coagulopathy has been documented in some cases.

DIAGNOSIS. Virus is isolated from acute phase blood, liver, and other organs by inoculation into guinea pigs or cell culture. The immunofluorescence assay becomes positive during the second week of illness.

TREATMENT AND PROGNOSIS. There is no specific treatment. Supportive therapy consists of maintenance of fluid and electrolyte balance and administration of blood, platelets, or fresh frozen plasma to control bleeding. Peritoneal dialysis for renal failure and heparin for disseminated intravascular coagulopathy have been recommended, but their value in African hemorrhagic fever is not established. The presence of bleeding indicates a poor prognosis. The case-fatality rate under relatively sophisticated hospital conditions in Marburg, Germany, was 22 per cent in 1967, and under Third World rural conditions in Zaire during 1976, it was 90 per cent.

PREVENTION. Control activities are not carried out because the natural reservoir is unknown. Nosocomial spread can be minimized by barrier nursing and handling of blood and tissues in isolator laboratory units with proper decontamination.

397 Hemorrhagic Fever with Renal Syndrome

DEFINITION. Hemorrhagic fever with renal syndrome (HFRS) is a disease of Europe and Asia characterized by fevers, capillary dilatation, leakage of blood leading to hemorrhagic manifestations, and, in severe cases, shock and renal tubular disease.

ETIOLOGY. HFRS is caused by any one of several closely related viruses of the genus *Hantavirus*, family Bunyaviridae. The prototype is Hantaan virus, originally isolated from *Apodemus agrarius* field mice in the endemic region of Korea.

EPIDEMIOLOGY. The virus is transmitted from rodents. *Apodemus agrarius* in Korea and other parts of Asia, *Clethrionomys glareolus* in Finland and west of the Ural Mountains, and *Rattus rattus* and *R. norvegicus* in cities of Japan, Korea, and Belgium serve as reservoirs. The rodent excretes virus in urine, saliva, and feces for weeks, and sometimes for months, after infection. Transmission is presumably by respiratory spread or direct contact with fomites contaminated by rodent excretions. Persons at risk include soldiers in field operations, campers, farmers, woodsmen, and, especially in the winter, family groups in houses harboring field rodents that seek shelter from the cold. Outbreaks have also occurred in laboratories housing field rodents or housing laboratory rats that carry the virus as an inapparent infection. Nosocomial infections are not reported. Viruses of the genus *Hantavirus* have been isolated from rodents in the Americas, but HFRS is absent.

PATHOLOGY. Patients who die of shock in the early stages demonstrate retroperitoneal gelatinous edema. There are macroscopic hemorrhages in the pituitary and right auricle. The renal medulla is congested and hyperemic, and patients who die later in the course of the disease have marked renal tubular necrosis. Petechial hemorrhages found in the skin and in multiple organs indicate widespread capillary fragility.

CLINICAL MANIFESTATIONS AND PATHOLOGIC PHYSIOLOGY. The incubation period ranges from 2 to 42 days but is usually about 2 weeks. Eighty per cent of cases are mild (demonstrating only fever, facial flush, backache, and muscle aches) or moderate (fever plus proteinuria, and petechial hemorrhages). The remaining 20 per cent are severe. They progress through five characteristic phases: febrile, hypotensive, oliguric, diuretic, and convalescent. The febrile phase lasts about 5 days, during which fever, facial flush, conjunctival injection, and backache precede the appearance of petechial hemorrhages and albuminuria. In the hypotensive phase, the temperature returns to baseline, and the patient manifests nausea, vomiting, abdominal pain, and about 3 days of capillary leakage with a rising hematocrit, heavy proteinuria, leukocytosis, thrombocytopenia, and decreased renal clearance. This is followed for about 4 days by the oliguric phase, when extravascular fluid is resorbed, leading to relative hypervolemia, hypertension, metabolic acidosis, and sometimes pulmonary edema and/or acute renal failure. The diuretic phase is accompanied by return of renal clearance to normal, but with marked electrolyte and fluid imbalance, which may lead to death if not adequately managed. The convalescent phase may last 1 to 3 months, with slowly recovering renal function. The clinical diagnosis may be reliable during an outbreak with classic severe cases but not with mild infections; serologic confirmation is obtained by the immunofluorescence and neutralization tests, which become positive at the end of the first week of illness. Antibody titers peak at 2 weeks and last for many years.

TREATMENT AND PROGNOSIS. Management includes careful monitoring of electrolytes and fluid intake and output with correction, especially during the oliguric and diuretic phases. Plasma expanders can be used for shock, and hemodialysis in cases of renal failure with hyperkalemia. Ribavirin improves survival if given within 5 days of onset. The case fatality in Korea is about 5 per cent with hospital management; the disease in northern Europe is milder with a more favorable prognosis.

PREVENTION. Rodent control should be practiced where feasible, especially in urban settings.

Halstead SB: In vivo enhancement of dengue virus infection in rhesus monkeys by passively transferred antibody. J Infect Dis 140:527, 1979. *The definitive experimental evidence conferring credibility to the secondary infection hypothesis of dengue hemorrhagic fever.*

Hoogstraal H: The epidemiology of tick-borne Crimean-Congo hemorrhagic fever in Asia, Europe, and Africa. J Med Entomol 15:307, 1979. *Extensive description and bibliography of natural history of CCHF.*

Maiztegui JI, Fernandez NJ, deDamilano AJ: Efficacy of immune plasma in treatment of Argentine hemorrhagic fever and association between treatment and a late neurological syndrome. Lancet 2:1216, 1979. *Definitive study showing that immune plasma is efficacious for treatment of Argentine hemorrhagic fever.*

Monath TP: Lassa fever—new issues raised by field studies in West Africa. J Infect Dis 155:433, 1987. *An up-to-date perspective on Lassa fever surveillance, treatment, and research.*

Monath TP: Yellow fever: A medically neglected disease. Report on a seminar. Rev Infect Dis 90:165, 1987. *Excellent summary of state-of-the-art yellow fever case management and diagnosis.*

Pattyn SR (ed.): Ebola Virus Haemorrhagic Fever. New York, Elsevier/North-Holland, 1978. *Descriptions of the outbreaks of African hemorrhagic fever in 1976 in Zaire and Sudan.*

Reviews of Infectious Diseases, Vol. II, Suppl 4, May–June 1989, pp 5669–5896. *A comprehensive compilation of reviews of the viral hemorrhagic fevers, including DHF, Crimean-Congo hemorrhagic fever, arenaviral hemorrhagic fevers, African hemorrhagic fevers, and HFRS.*

Strode GK (ed.): Yellow Fever. New York, McGraw-Hill Book Company, 1951. *Classic description of history, epidemiology, and clinical details of yellow fever cases.*

Swanepoel R, Shepherd AJ, Leman PA, et al.: Epidemiologic and clinical features of Crimean Congo hemorrhagic fever in Southern Africa. Am J Trop Med Hyg 36:120, 1987. *Current clinical description and review of recent CCHF literature.*

Symposium on epidemic hemorrhagic fever. Am J Med 16:617, 1954. *Detailed information on the pathophysiology of HFRS.*

WHO Expert Committee Report: Viral Haemorrhagic Fevers. WHO Tech Rep Ser No 721, 1985. *Excellent review of hemorrhagic fevers by an international group of experts with detailed guide to management of patients, investigation of outbreaks, and vector control.*

WHO Scientific Group Report: Arthropod-borne and rodent-borne viral diseases. WHO Tech Rep Ser No. 719, 1985. *Authoritative discussion of epidemiologic principles, laboratory safety, vector control, and epidemic preparedness.*

WHO Technical Advisory Group Report: Dengue haemorrhagic fever: Diagnosis, treatment and control. Geneva, World Health Organization, 1986. *A most comprehensive manual for the physician faced with management of DHF patients.*

SECTION FOUR / THE MYCOSES

398 Introduction

William E. Dismukes

Fungi are classified as eukaryotic microorganisms, in contrast to bacteria, which are considered prokaryotic. Eukaryotes, such as fungi, possess a discrete nuclear membrane and a nucleus that contains several chromosomes, whereas prokaryotes have no nucleus or nuclear membrane and possess only a single chromosome. Fungi also differ from bacteria in the ability of the former to reproduce sexually or asexually. Most fungi reproduce by asexual spore formation. When sexual mating of two closely related species, e.g., *Cryptococcus neoformans*, serotypes A and D, takes place, the "perfect state" (*Filobasidiella neoformans* var. *neoformans*) is produced. Fungi for which a perfect state has not been identified are referred to as Fungi Imperfecti (e.g., *Candida albicans* and *Coccidioides immitis*). The cell walls of fungi are rigid, usually containing chitin and polysaccharides, another feature that distinguishes fungi from bacteria. In addition, the inner cytoplasmic membrane of fungi contains sterols, which are the site of action of the polyene antifungal agents amphotericin B and nystatin.

The terms "fungal diseases" and "mycoses" are used interchangeably. Fungal infections that involve only the skin and its appendages are referred to as cutaneous or superficial mycoses (e.g., ringworm of the scalp or groin and tinea versicolor). By contrast, fungal infections that are acquired primarily by inhalation and spread via lymphohematogenous dissemination to involve one or more organs, such as the lungs, skin, liver, spleen, and central nervous system, are referred to as systemic mycoses (e.g., blastomycosis, coccidioidomycosis, cryptococcosis, and histoplasmosis). Candidiasis is a mycosis that may cause superficial disease (e.g., intertrigo, oral thrush, and vaginitis) or systemic disease (e.g., candidemia and hepatosplenic candidiasis).

Fungi causing systemic disease may also be classified by the morphologic or structural form of the organism. For example, *Aspergillus* species and zygomycetes (*Mucor* and *Rhizopus* species) are molds that grow as a hyphal structural form both in the laboratory (and nature) and in humans. By contrast, other fungi are dimorphic, i.e., they have the ability to transform morphologically into either a mold or a yeast form, depending on the environmental conditions. *Blastomyces dermatitidis*, *C. immitis*, *Histoplasma capsulatum*, *Paracoccidioides brasiliensis*, and *Sporothrix schenckii* exist as hyphal or filamentous forms in nature, but as yeasts (*B. dermatitidis*, *H. capsulatum*, *S. sporothrix*) or endosporulating spherules (*C. immitis* and *P. brasiliensis*) in humans. *Cryptococcus neoformans* is a true yeast, growing as the same spherical form in both nature and humans.

The route (or routes) of transmission and the geographic distribution of the major systemic mycoses are shown in Table 398–1. Detailed discussions of these epidemiologic features of each mycosis are provided in the individual chapters that follow. As a rule, mycoses are not transmissible from human to human. The natural habitat of several fungal pathogens is limited to specific geographic areas. Consequently, persons living in these areas are at highest risk of acquiring infection. The diseases caused by such organisms are referred to as endemic mycoses. As shown in Table 398–1, the endemic systemic mycoses are blastomycosis, coccidioidomycosis, histoplasmosis, and paracoccidioidomycosis. These diseases, which are acquired by inhalation of spores, typically are associated with asymptomatic or mild pulmonary infection that heals spontaneously. Progressive pulmonary infection or spread to extrapulmonary sites occurs less frequently.

TABLE 398–1. EPIDEMIOLOGIC FEATURES OF COMMON SYSTEMIC MYCOSES

Disease	Geographic Distribution	Route of Transmission
Candidiasis	Worldwide (part of normal flora of skin, oropharynx, gastrointestinal tract, vagina)	Endogenous Contact (less commonly)
Cryptococcosis	Worldwide (avian habitats)	Respiratory
Aspergillosis	Worldwide (ubiquitous in nature)	Respiratory Cutaneous (rarely)
Zygomycosis (Mucormycosis)	Worldwide (ubiquitous in nature)	Respiratory Cutaneous (rarely)
Blastomycosis	South and North Central United States Mexico, Central and South America, Africa (occasionally)	Respiratory Cutaneous (rarely)
Coccidioidomycosis	Southwestern United States, Mexico, Central and South America	Respiratory
Histoplasmosis	Worldwide (along river basins, especially Mississippi, Tennessee, Ohio, and St. Lawrence—bird and bat habitats)	Respiratory
Paracoccidioidomycosis	Mexico, Central and South America	Respiratory
Sporotrichosis	Worldwide (soil and vegetation)	Cutaneous Respiratory (rarely)

TABLE 398–2. ALTERED HOST DEFENSE AND OPPORTUNISTIC FUNGAL DISEASE

Alteration in Host Defense	Opportunistic Fungal Disease
Interruption of mechanical barriers or indwelling foreign bodies	Candidiasis
Granulocyte dysfunction (quantitative or qualitative)	Aspergillosis Candidiasis Zycomycosis
Depressed cell-mediated immunity	Candidiasis (mucosal) Coccidioidomycosis Cryptococcosis Histoplasmosis

Some fungal organisms are considered opportunistic pathogens and are especially prone to cause disease in the setting of altered host defense (Table 398–2). Common predisposing conditions or factors include interruptions in anatomic barriers (burns and endotracheal tubes) or indwelling foreign bodies (arterial or central venous catheters, urinary catheters, and prosthetic heart valves or joints); granulocyte dysfunction secondary to hematologic malignancies (leukemia) or cytotoxic chemotherapy; and depressed cell-mediated immunity associated with organ transplantation, acquired immunodeficiency syndrome (AIDS), or immunosuppressive therapy, such as corticosteroids and azathioprine. Other conditions that may predispose to systemic mycoses include diabetic ketoacidosis (rhinocerebral mucormycosis) and intravenous drug abuse (*Candida* endocarditis and basal ganglia mucormycosis).

Culture for fungus and histopathologic studies using special stains of infected body fluids (sputum, blood, urine, and cerebrospinal fluid [CSF]) and tissues (skin, lung, liver, bone marrow, and lymph nodes) are the mainstays of diagnosis of the mycoses. If fungal disease is suspected, the microbiology laboratory should be alerted to use appropriate culture media. Skin testing with fungal antigens has no place in the diagnosis of individual infections, although skin tests are useful as indicators of prior infection in epidemiologic studies of prevalence. Although most serologic tests for mycoses have limited value in diagnosis because of either low sensitivity and specificity or poor standardization of assay reagents and methods, there are two exceptions. A positive latex agglutination test for cryptococcal antigen in CSF or blood

is a highly reliable indicator of cryptococcal disease; similarly, a positive titer for complement-fixing antibody in serum or CSF is a reliable marker of coccidioidal disease. Widely available serologic tests that are both sensitive and specific would be very useful in the diagnosis of invasive aspergillosis and candidiasis.

Table 398–3 provides an overview of the currently recommended treatment regimens for the common systemic mycoses. Although amphotericin B remains the "gold standard" of therapy for most fungal diseases, much progress in antifungal therapy has been made over the past two decades, especially with regard to antifungal azoles. Miconazole, the first of this class of drugs and a parenteral formulation, is associated with considerable toxicity, which has limited its usefulness. The approval in 1981 of ketoconazole represented a major breakthrough. Ketoconazole is an oral formulation with broad-spectrum activity and less toxicity than either miconazole or amphotericin B. Fluconazole, approved in 1990, possesses several advantages over ketoconazole, including availability as either an oral or a parenteral preparation, significant urinary excretion of active drug, good to excellent penetration into CSF (60 to 80 per cent of serum concentrations), and minimal toxicity, with no documented suppression of endogenous steroid synthesis. Promising investigational azole compounds include itraconazole and saperconazole.

The only other antifungal drug currently approved for the treatment of systemic mycoses is flucytosine, an oral preparation, which is often used in combination with amphotericin B to provide a synergistic effect against *C. neoformans* and *Candida* species and sometimes used alone as therapy for chromomycosis. Unfortunately, flucytosine is potentially toxic to the bone marrow and liver; in addition, its use, especially as a single agent, may be associated with rapid emergence of resistant organisms. Research efforts are currently ongoing to standardize and commercially prepare new formulations of amphotericin B, either encapsulated in liposomes or complexed with lipids. Preliminary evidence indicates that these investigational lipid preparations will offer several advantages over currently available amphotericin B (Fungizone), including less toxicity, increased tropism for reticuloendothelial organs, and possibly increased dosing of active drug.

Gallis HA, Drew RH, Pickard WW: Amphotericin B: 30 years of clinical experience. Rev Infect Dis 12:308, 1990. *A practical up-to-date review of the pharmacology, clinical uses, and adverse effects of amphotericin B, the most important systemic antifungal agent (190 references).*

Rippon JW: Medical Mycology. 3rd ed. Philadelphia, W.B. Saunders Company, 1988. *A comprehensive text that considers most fungal pathogens and their diseases, including the superficial mycoses.*

TABLE 398–3. THERAPY FOR THE COMMON SYSTEMIC MYCOSES

Disease	First Choice	Alternative(s)
Aspergillosis	Amphotericin B ± rifampin or flucytosine	Itraconazole*
Zygomycosis (Mucormycosis)	Amphotericin B	None
Candidiasis		
Candidemia, invasive, disseminated	Amphotericin B ± flucytosine	? Ketoconazole ? Fluconazole
Urinary tract	Fluconazole	Amphotericin B Flucytosine
Cryptoccocosis	Amphotericin B ± flucytosine	Fluconazole Itraconazole*
Coccidioidomycosis	Amphotericin B or ketoconazole	Fluconazole Itraconazole* Miconazole
Blastomycosis	Amphotericin B or ketoconazole	Itraconazole* ? Fluconazole
Histoplasmosis	Amphotericin B or ketoconazole	Itraconazole* ? Fluconazole
Paracoccidioidomycosis	Amphotericin B or ketoconazole	A sulfonamide Miconazole Itraconazole*
Sporotrichosis		
Cutaneous	Potassium iodide	Itraconazole* ? Fluconazole
Extracutaneous	Amphotericin B	Itraconazole*

*Investigational.
Adapted with permission from The Medical Letter 32:58–60, 1990.

399 Histoplasmosis

William E. Dismukes

DEFINITION. Histoplasmosis, the most common endemic systemic mycosis in the United States, is associated with a variety of clinical syndromes, the most frequent of which is an asymptomatic or self-limited influenza-like respiratory infection. Less frequently, histoplasmosis manifests as chronic cavitary pulmonary disease, progressive disseminated disease involving multiple organs, or immune-mediated disease of the mediastinum or eye.

ETIOLOGY. *Histoplasma capsulatum* is the imperfect state of a dimorphic fungus that grows as a mycelial form at temperatures below 35°C in the laboratory and in soil, its natural habitat, and as a yeast form at 37°C and in infected hosts. The perfect state is *Emmonsiella capsulata*. The mycelial form bears two types of infectious spores, macroconidia and microconidia, both of which are readily airborne, but the smaller microconidia (2 to 6 μm versus 8 to 14 μm) more easily reach alveoli or small bronchioles upon inhalation. The oval yeast cells (2 to 3 × 3 to 4 μm) reproduce by single narrow-based buds, are unencapsulated, and are usually found within macrophages in viable tissue. A variant strain, *H. capsulatum* var. *duboisii*, which is found solely in

Central Africa, is characterized by a larger yeast form (7 to 15 μm).

EPIDEMIOLOGY. Results of skin test surveys using histoplasmin antigen indicate that histoplasmosis is worldwide in distribution, with greatest prevalence in tropical and temperate zones. The disease is endemic in the South Central and North Central United States, especially along the Mississippi, Tennessee, Missouri, Ohio, and St. Lawrence River basins. A high prevalence has also been noted in selected areas of the eastern United States. In these endemic areas, over 80 per cent of persons are infected by 20 years of age. *Histoplasma capsulatum* can be readily recovered from soil, especially that enriched by bird and bat guano. Because of high body temperatures, birds are not infected, whereas bats are. Soil contaminated by chicken, pigeon, blackbird, or starling droppings and areas frequented by bats, such as caves, hollow trees, old buildings, and attics, are frequently identified sources of outbreaks. The disturbance of soil or sites by wind, bulldozing, demolition, or other construction-related activities may greatly increase the number of airborne spores and result in exposure of both nearby and distantly located persons. Although *H. capsulatum* is more prevalent in bird- or bat-related microenvironments, aerosolized microconidia are commonly present as "air pollutants" in endemic areas and may account for the majority of sporadic infections.

Pulmonary infection does not convey protective immunity; consequently, reinfection may occur. However, reactivation of quiescent or dormant disease appears to be more likely than reinfection as an explanation for second-episode disease or disease that develops after a person has left an endemic area. Person-to-person transmission of histoplasmosis is not known to occur. Although age, sex, and race do not significantly affect susceptibility to infection, middle-aged white men with pre-existing chronic obstructive pulmonary disease appear to be at highest risk of developing chronic pulmonary histoplasmosis. Over recent years, *H. capsulatum* has emerged as an opportunistic fungal pathogen, especially in hosts with altered cellular immunity secondary to organ transplantation, corticosteroid or cytotoxic drugs, or infection with human immunodeficiency virus (HIV). In some endemic areas, disseminated histoplasmosis is the most common acquired immunodeficiency syndrome (AIDS)–defining opportunistic infection.

PATHOGENESIS AND PATHOLOGY. Aerosolized microconidia of *H. capsulatum*, after inhalation into the lungs, undergo transformation into yeast forms at body temperature and are promptly phagocytized by macrophages. In nonimmune persons, macrophages are initially unable to kill the yeasts, which multiply intracellularly. These infected macrophages migrate to the mediastinal lymph nodes and to other organs of the mononuclear phagocyte system (reticuloendothelial system), such as the spleen. Recent evidence indicates that L3T4$^+$ cells are a critical determinant of an effective host response to *H. capsulatum*. In normal hosts, once antigen-specific cellular immunity becomes established, infection is usually contained by a sequence of events including a vasculitic response, granuloma formation with caseation necrosis, enlargement of regional lymph nodes followed by fibrosis, and, ultimately, calcification. By contrast, in persons with impaired cell-mediated immunity, the mononuclear phagocyte system is unable to contain the infection, and viable *H. capsulatum* organisms disseminate widely to macrophage-rich tissues, including liver, spleen, visceral lymph nodes, and bone marrow. In these individuals, because the normal reaction of host tissue to parasitized macrophages is either minimal or absent, infection goes unchecked, and progressive disseminated disease ensues. The pathogenesis of mediastinal fibrosis and ocular histoplasmosis, two uncommon but clinically significant complications of infection with *H. capsulatum*, is presumed to be immune mediated, at least in part. Mediastinal fibrosis appears to develop in hypersensitive persons with a large antigen load in caseous mediastinal nodes. Exuberant fibrous encapsulation of nodes and adjacent tissues may lead to bronchial or vascular occlusion or erosion.

In histopathologic specimens stained with periodic acid–Schiff (PAS), Giemsa, or Gomori methenamine silver (GMS), the characteristic ovoid yeast forms of *H. capsulatum*, surrounded by a clear space resembling a capsule but actually due to fixation artifact, are generally found in macrophages. Organisms are more difficult to visualize in tissue stained with hematoxylin-eosin. The likelihood of identifying organisms in tissue sections is directly related to the effectiveness of cellular immunity in a given host. In immune individuals with an intact host defense, fungi are rare, granuloma formation is well developed, and extent of disease is limited. By contrast, in compromised hosts with impaired cellular immunity, macrophages, including those in peripheral blood, are filled with intracellular yeasts; granulomas are poorly developed or absent; and disease is extensive.

CLINICAL MANIFESTATIONS. Pulmonary disease in histoplasmosis is conveniently classified into acute and chronic forms. Acute disease, which results from primary infection, most often resolves spontaneously but may be associated with early and late complications.

Acute Pulmonary Infection. The vast majority of primary infections with *H. capsulatum* are either asymptomatic or associated with a flulike illness, manifested by fever, chills, headache, nonproductive cough, pleuritic or substernal chest pain, malaise, and myalgias. The incubation period and severity of illness are directly related to the inoculum of inhaled spores and the prior immune status of the individual. In nonimmune persons with a heavy exposure, respiratory symptoms tend to be more severe and progressive and include severe dyspnea. Radiologic findings also vary, depending on the inoculum size and the pre-exposure immunity of the host. A normal chest x-ray film is most common, but abnormalities range from one or two patchy infiltrates, with or without mediastinal and hilar adenopathy, to diffuse miliary opacities, which frequently heal in a pattern of "buckshot" calcifications. Pleural effusion and cavitation are uncommon. Extrapulmonary symptoms and signs, including arthralgias, erythema nodosum, and erythema multiforme, may be present, especially in young women. Early and late complications of acute or primary pulmonary infection may result from vigorous host reactions causing enlarged mediastinal or hilar nodes and exuberant encapsulating fibrosis, which in turn lead to compression or erosion of adjacent mediastinal structures. These rare complications include acute pericarditis; tracheal, bronchial, or esophageal obstruction; esophageal diverticuli; bronchoesophageal fistula; broncholithiasis (secondary to erosion of a calcification into a bronchus); mediastinal granuloma; mediastinal fibrosis or fibrosing mediastinitis; and enlarging histoplasmoma (usually located in the peripheral lung parenchyma and recognized by concentric laminations of calcium). Mediastinal granuloma, which tends to develop more often in the right paratracheal area, is more circumscribed, smaller in size, and associated with fewer sequelae than is mediastinal fibrosis. Both entities are recognized causes of superior vena cava syndrome.

Chronic Pulmonary Infection. Chronic pulmonary histoplasmosis often occurs in men with underlying chronic obstructive pulmonary disease and resembles pulmonary tuberculosis in symptomatology and radiographic manifestations, although the course of this type of histoplasmosis tends to be milder and more indolent than that of tuberculosis. The pathogenesis and course of chronic pulmonary histoplasmosis are highly complex; pathologic studies indicate two basic lesions. An interstitial pneumonitis featuring mononuclear infiltration, periarteriolar inflammation, areas of infarct-like necrosis, and few organisms is characteristic of the early lesion. The inflammatory process often surrounds apical emphysematous blebs and bullae. In contrast, the chronic lesion is manifested by organization of diseased tissue, with prominence of giant cells and progressive cavitation. Cavities are surrounded by an area of vascular granulation tissue, and their inner linings are often necrotic. Organisms are typically found in the necrotic lining or in surface exudate. In the thicker walled cavities, infection is persistent, with continuing necrosis, leading to progressive cavity enlargement (marching cavity) at the expense of the surrounding lung parenchyma. In general, the symptoms and roentgenographic findings reflect the two types or stages of disease, namely, pneumonitis and progressive cavitation. Although symptoms overlap, they tend to be more abrupt in onset, with more severe constitutional symptoms, such as fever, night sweats, and malaise, in the pneumonitis stage; hemoptysis and progressive dyspnea are more typical of the cavitation stage. In 80 per cent of cases, the pneumonitis stage tends to resolve spontaneously over 2 to 3 months, with a small fibrotic residuum, whereas the cavitation stage, especially that associated with thick-walled cavities, tends to be relentlessly progressive, leading to destruction and diminution of lung parenchyma, fibrosis, and, eventually, respiratory insufficiency.

Disseminated Histoplasmosis. This less common form of histoplasmosis develops primarily in persons with defective host immunity, including infants with immature immune systems; compromised hosts, such as corticosteroid-treated organ recipients and HIV-infected persons; and individuals with either no measurable defect or a highly selective defect, such as the failure of host lymphocytes to undergo in vitro blast transformation upon exposure to *H. capsulatum* antigen. The severity of the symptoms and signs of disseminated disease and the attendant histopathologic findings in a given patient mirror the level of immunocompetence of the individual. For example, in patients with the mildest and most chronic forms of disseminated disease, well-developed tuberculoid granulomas, typical of the response in normal hosts, can be found in reticuloendothelial tissues. In contrast, in patients with overwhelming multiorgan histoplasmosis superimposed on a severely immunocompromising condition, such as AIDS, the host response is suboptimal, with the pathologic findings consisting of large numbers of diffusely scattered macrophages filled with yeast forms and minimal or no granuloma formation.

Fever, chills, and other nonspecific constitutional symptoms, including malaise and weight loss, predominate. On initial presentation, many patients satisfy criteria for fever of unknown origin. Enlargement of the liver and spleen is common; less frequently, peripheral lymphadenopathy is present. Mucous membrane ulceration, especially of the oropharynx, occurs in about 25 to 75 per cent of patients with subacute disease and should alert the physician to the possibility of histoplasmosis. Laboratory clues may include anemia, leukopenia and thrombocytopenia as evidence of impaired bone marrow function or replacement of the marrow, elevated alkaline phosphatase levels, elevated erythrocyte sedimentation rate, and electrolyte abnormalities suggestive of adrenal insufficiency. In some patients, adrenal hypofunction may not be clinically manifest until years later. Chest x-ray films may be normal or show findings suggestive of earlier primary infection or an interstitial pneumonitis consistent with hematogenous spread of infection. Unusual syndromes, including cardiac involvement with culture-negative endocarditis associated with large emboli, gastrointestinal involvement with bleeding secondary to mucosal ulceration, or central nervous system involvement with chronic lymphocytic meningitis, occasionally dominate the clinical course. Cutaneous lesions, manifested by diffusely scattered papulonodules on an erythematous base, and central nervous system disease are more likely in HIV-positive persons. In some AIDS patients, disseminated histoplasmosis represents reactivation of dormant foci, as evidenced by the development of symptoms and signs during a period of residence in a nonendemic area, years after having lived in an endemic region.

Ocular Histoplasmosis. Vision loss associated with the triad of punched-out choroidal lesions or "spots," macular neovascular membranes, and peripapillary atrophy or scarring, in the absence of inflammatory changes in the vitreous or anterior chamber, has been labeled presumed ocular histoplasmosis syndrome (POHS). Although no direct relationship to active ongoing infection with *H. capsulatum* has been established, POHS is believed to represent a localized hypersensitivity response to *Histoplasma* antigen. In almost all instances, the syndrome occurs in young adults with no evidence of pulmonary or disseminated histoplasmosis. Antifungal therapy, either systemic or intraocular, is not indicated. Laser photocoagulation appears to be the most beneficial therapeutic modality to prevent or reduce vision impairment.

DIAGNOSIS. The diagnostic approach varies in part with the clinical syndrome under consideration. Histoplasmosis in many ways resembles tuberculosis and is as clinically diverse in its myriad manifestations. Special features or presentations that should raise suspicion of histoplasmosis include atypical pneumonia syndrome that occurs in a resident of an endemic area, right paratracheal adenopathy, superior vena cava syndrome secondary to adenopathy or a mediastinal mass, an oral ulcer resembling carcinoma, chronic progressive upper lobe cavitation associated with negative sputum smears and cultures for tuberculosis, adrenal insufficiency, "buckshot" calcifications in the lungs or spleen, and persistent unexplained fever in an HIV-infected person. In most instances, diagnosis should be based on demonstration of *H. capsulatum* by culture or by histopathologic study of involved organs. The histoplasmin skin test, while important in epidemiologic studies, is not recommended for diagnostic purposes, owing to the high positivity rate among persons residing in endemic areas. In addition, the skin test may falsely elevate titers of serum antibodies.

Among the three serologic tests to detect serum antibody to *H. capsulatum*, complement fixation is the most widely used. Although a titer of 1:32 or more or a fourfold rise in titer provides presumptive evidence of active infection, a negative or lower titer does not exclude histoplasmosis. Similarly, titers do not parallel disease activity, correlate with response to therapy, or predict outcome. Testing of serum by immunodiffusion to detect precipitin bands to M and H antigens appears to be a more specific but less sensitive serologic method than complement fixation. The presence of both bands, while infrequent, is highly specific, provided the patient has not been previously skin tested with histoplasmin. A positive M band alone is more frequent than a positive H band and is moderately specific. The M band may persist for several years, while the H band usually clears within 6 months; thus, a positive H band signifies active infection. Radioimmunoassay is the most sensitive of the three methods for detection of antibody but is also the least specific. All three methods are associated with frequent false-positive reactions to *Histoplasma* antigens among patients with tuberculosis and other fungal diseases, especially blastomycosis and coccidioidomycosis. Because these cross-reactions are most commonly observed by testing with radioimmunoassay, this methodology for detecting antibody cannot be recommended over complement fixation and immunodiffusion. On the other hand, use of radioimmunoassay to detect *H. capsulatum* polysaccharide antigen in body fluids such as serum and urine appears to provide a relatively sensitive and specific marker of disseminated histoplasmosis. Antigen levels fall with treatment; consequently, this test is useful for both diagnosis and evaluation of response to therapy. At present, the availability of the antigen test is limited because of technical difficulties.

The diagnosis of primary pulmonary histoplasmosis should be suspected on the basis of clinical, radiographic, and epidemiologic clues, e.g., an acute febrile respiratory illness accompanied by scattered patchy infiltrates and hilar adenopathy in an individual with high risk of exposure to *Histoplasma* spores. An elevated complement fixation titer and/or precipitin bands in serum provide presumptive evidence. Whereas sputum cultures are rarely positive (only 10 to 20 per cent) in primary pulmonary disease, the likelihood of positive sputum cultures is significantly higher in chronic pulmonary histoplasmosis. Among patients with chronic disease, about 60 per cent with marching thick-walled cavities have positive cultures, and a significant percentage of these also have positive smears of stained sputum. Although serologic tests for antibody are only moderately helpful (positive results in only 50 per cent of cases), an elevated complement fixation titer in a patient with characteristic radiographic findings provides strong supportive evidence. Definitive diagnosis of chronic pulmonary histoplasmosis must be based on a positive sputum culture or smear or on histopathologic studies and special stains of lung tissue obtained by bronchoscopy.

The diagnosis of disseminated histoplasmosis depends on either demonstration of intracellular yeast forms by histopathologic study or a positive culture of blood, bone marrow, lymph node, skin or mucous membrane, liver, lung, or other involved site. A Wright-stained smear of peripheral blood is positive in more than 50 per cent of acute or subacute cases. If possible, serum and urine should be examined for *H. capsulatum* antigen by radioimmunoassay. The cerebrospinal fluid of patients with chronic unexplained culture-negative lymphocytic meningitis should be tested by complement fixation for antibodies to *H. capsulatum*.

TREATMENT. For most patients with primary pulmonary histoplasmosis, no antifungal therapy is necessary. For those with severe or progressive primary infection, short-course intravenous amphotericin B (a total dose of around 1000 mg) or oral ketoconazole, 400 mg daily for 3 to 6 months, is recommended, although neither therapeutic regimen has been prospectively evaluated in this setting. The treatment of chronic pulmonary histoplasmosis is less standardized, in large part owing to the relative difficulty in clinically and radiologically distinguishing the pneumonitic and cavitary stages of disease. While the early pneumonitic form of chronic pulmonary disease has been reported to resolve spontaneously in 80 per cent of cases, rest and inactivity clearly promote healing. Traditionally, antifungal therapy has been advocated only for patients with progressive or marching cavitary disease, manifested by persistent or enlarging thick-walled cavities larger than 2 mm. Both amphotericin B (total dose, 2.0 to 2.5 grams) and ketoconazole (400 mg daily for at least 6 months) are effective therapy. There may be merit in liberalizing criteria for treatment in patients with chronic pulmonary disease. Rather than reserving therapy only for patients with advanced cavitary disease, some authorities suggest that oral ketoconazole or a newer, better tolerated oral triazole may be indicated for all patients with chronic pulmonary disease, regardless of the stage.

In contrast to the somewhat controversial guidelines regarding therapy for pulmonary histoplasmosis, there is no question that all patients with disseminated histoplasmosis should be treated. For patients with severe, life-threatening disease, immunocompromised hosts, such as organ transplant recipients or corticosteroid-treated patients, and the rare patients with central nervous system or cardiac histoplasmosis, amphotericin B (total dose, 2.0 to 2.5 grams) is the drug of choice. Ketoconazole, 400 mg daily for 6 to 12 months, is an effective alternative in immunocompetent patients with mild to moderate subacute disease. Experience over the past decade with histoplasmosis in AIDS patients indicates that a more aggressive approach to treatment is necessary to prevent relapse. Intensive "induction" therapy with intravenous amphotericin B (total dose, 1.0 to 2.0 grams) is used to gain control of disease and reduce the organism load and is followed by lifelong maintenance or suppressive therapy with either weekly amphotericin B (1 mg per kilogram) or an oral antifungal azole, given daily. Among the azole drugs, itraconazole, an investigational triazole, appears to be the most promising therapy for AIDS patients. Ketoconazole is an inadequate primary or maintenance therapy in patients with AIDS. The approach of initiating therapy with intravenous amphotericin B and completing it with an oral agent may prove applicable to selected other patients with either chronic pulmonary or disseminated histoplasmosis.

The management of mediastinal fibrosis presumed secondary to *H. capsulatum* infection is largely unsatisfactory, as evidenced by progressive morbidity in many patients and a mortality rate of at least 30 per cent. Antifungal chemotherapy is generally not recommended. In selected cases, surgical extirpation may be beneficial in alleviating entrapment or obstructive syndromes.

PROGNOSIS. Although primary pulmonary histoplasmosis may be associated with acute or chronic intrathoracic complications, this form of disease is usually self-limited. In contrast, chronic cavitary pulmonary histoplasmosis is usually progressive, resulting in respiratory insufficiency and death. Disseminated histoplasmosis is variable in its severity and course, depending on the immune status of the host. Although a single course of therapy may be curative in some patients, long-term maintenance therapy to prevent relapse is required in others, especially HIV-positive individuals.

Dismukes WE, Cloud G, Bowles C, et al., National Institute of Allergy and Infectious Diseases Mycoses Study Group: Treatment of blastomycosis and histoplasmosis with ketoconazole: Results of a prospective randomized clinical trial. Ann Intern Med 103:861, 1985. *This study showed that ketoconazole is effective therapy for immunocompetent patients with non–life-threatening, nonmeningeal forms of histoplasmosis.*

Goodwin RA, Owens FT, Snell JD, et al.: Chronic pulmonary histoplasmosis. Medicine (Baltimore) 55:413, 1976. *This monograph, which describes the clinical, radiographic, and pathologic findings in 228 cases, remains the definitive commentary on this complex form of histoplasmosis.*

Loyd JE, Tillman BF, Atkinson JB, et al.: Mediastinal fibrosis complicating histoplasmosis. Medicine (Baltimore) 67:295, 1988. *An excellent review, with emphasis on clinical and radiographic manifestations plus management of this immune-mediated syndrome.*

McKinsey DS, Gupta MR, Riddler SA, et al.: Long-term amphotericin B therapy for disseminated histoplasmosis in patients with the acquired immunodeficiency syndrome (AIDS). Ann Intern Med 111:655, 1989. *A report of the results of amphotericin B treatment in 22 patients, indicating efficacy of long-term maintenance therapy in the prevention of relapse.*

Wheat LJ: Diagnosis and management of histoplasmosis. Eur J Clin Microbiol

Infect Dis 8:480, 1989. *A comprehensive, up-to-date review that includes an excellent perspective on the currently available serologic tests used to detect either antibody or antigen; includes 78 references.*

Wheat LJ, Connolly-Stringfield PA, Baker RL, et al.: Disseminated histoplasmosis in the acquired immunodeficiency syndrome: Clinical findings, diagnosis, treatment, and review of the literature. Medicine (Baltimore) 69:361, 1990. *A thorough, thoughtful, and current review that is especially valuable to physicians caring for AIDS patients at risk for histoplasmosis.*

400 Coccidioidomycosis

John N. Galgiani

DEFINITION. Coccidioidomycosis is a systemic infection due to *Coccidioides immitis*, a fungus that is endemic to certain desert regions of the Western Hemisphere.

ETIOLOGY. *C. immitis* is dimorphic, both forms of which grow asexually. Outside humans or other mammalian hosts, mycelia with true septations mature to produce arthroconidia, single-cell structures approximately 2 to 5 μm in length. After infection, an arthroconidium sheds its outer wall and enlarges as spherules, sometimes to as much as 75 μm in diameter, and undergo septation internally to produce scores of endospores. When spherules rupture, packets of endospores are released, and these produce more spherules in infected tissue or revert to mycelia if removed from the body.

EPIDEMIOLOGY. *C. immitis* can be recovered from the soil of the low deserts of Arizona; the Central Valley of California; parts of other states, including New Mexico and Texas; and parts of Central and South America. Endemic regions follow the climatologic Sonoran life zone, which is characterized by modest rainfall, mild winters, and low humidity. In such regions, *C. immitis* grows in a soil layer a few centimeters below the surface, and disruption of the dirt by windstorms or construction equipment increases the release of fungal particles into the air. The risk of sporadic exposure is seasonally more likely in dry periods. Primary infection outside the endemic regions has rarely occurred from exposure to contaminated soil carried on bales of cotton or other fomites. Person-to-person transmission of coccidioidomycosis has not been reported, and isolation precautions for patients are unnecessary.

INCIDENCE AND PREVALENCE. Dermal hypersensitivity to coccidioidal antigens is an indicator of prior infection. The frequency of skin test conversion is approximately 3 per cent per year within strongly endemic areas. This represents a lower estimate than that of 40 years ago, and the change is presumed to be the result of urbanization and the concurrent reduction of exposure to dust. However, in situations where exposure is unusually intense, such as at archeology sites or during military maneuvers within endemic regions, infections can develop in the majority of persons exposed for only a matter of days. The prevalence of reactive coccidioidal skin tests ranges as high as 60 per cent in certain populations, depending upon factors such as age, occupational exposure, and years of residence within the endemic area.

PATHOGENESIS AND PATHOLOGY. Virtually all coccidioidal infections are the result of inhalation of arthroconidia into the lung, and only rarely does direct cutaneous inoculation of the skin occur. Within the small airways, proliferation engenders both acute inflammation, including eosinophils, associated with spherule rupture, and granulomatous inflammation, associated with mature, nonproliferating spherules. Tissue damage results from the consequences of inflammation rather than the elaboration of specific fungal toxins. Focal pneumonia is often associated with ipsilateral hilar adenopathy, and less frequently, infection produces enlargement of peritracheal, supraclavicular, and cervical nodes. Lesions occurring elsewhere are the result of hematogenous dissemination from a pulmonary source and usually develop within months of the initial infection. Although extrapulmonary lesions occur in well below 1 per cent of all those infected, subclinical spread of the fungus beyond the chest may not be rare, since as many as 8 per cent of persons with self-limited infection are left with chorioretinal scars. In most persons, immunity develops within weeks after infection, arresting fungal proliferation and allowing inflammation to resolve. Despite apparent control of the infection, immunity may not sterilize lesions, and *C. immitis* may persist for long periods in a dormant state. The precise mechanisms responsible for these events are not understood but require competent T lymphocytes. Reactivation of dormant infection or second infections are infrequent, except in patients whose cell-mediated immunity becomes deficient.

CLINICAL MANIFESTATIONS. Two of every three infections are subclinical and are detectable by finding dermal hypersensitivity to coccidioidal antigens. Those who become ill usually experience a self-limited pulmonary syndrome. However, a minority of patients develop complications or progressive forms of infection that display a broad variety of manifestations and pose difficult problems for the clinician.

Primary Pulmonary Infections. Five to 21 days after exposure, symptoms develop; these may include fever, weight loss, fatigue, a dry cough, or pleuritic chest pain, and they are difficult to differentiate from those caused by other respiratory pathogens. Arthralgias without associated joint effusions are also frequent. Skin manifestations may also occur as a short-lived nonpruritic maculopapular rash, erythema multiforme, or erythema nodosum. The arthritic and dermatologic manifestations are thought to be mediated by circulating immune complexes or other immunologic phenomena and are referred to as "desert rheumatism." Roentgenographs of the chest may show no abnormalities or may demonstrate pulmonary infiltrates, either segmental or lobar. Hilar adenopathy is often a distinctive finding. Peripneumonic pleural effusions may occur and usually resolve without intervention, even though *C. immitis* is usually recoverable from the pleura. Eosinophilia is frequently a prominent finding in differential leukocyte counts of peripheral blood, and the erythrocyte sedimentation rate is usually elevated. Symptoms may persist for several weeks before improvement is clearly under way, and the illness, especially lassitude, may persist for months.

The primary pulmonary process produces a variety of sequelae. The most frequent is the development of a pulmonary nodule (Fig. 400–1A and B), typically measuring 1 to 4 cm and lying

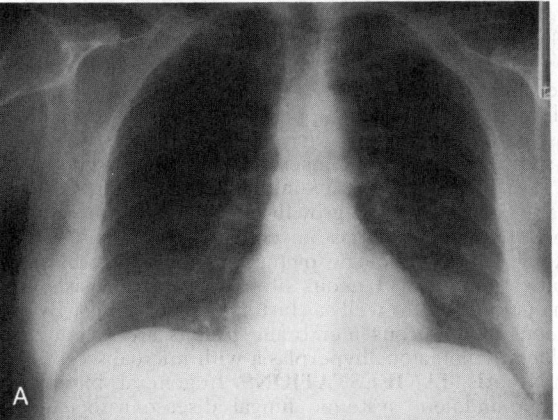

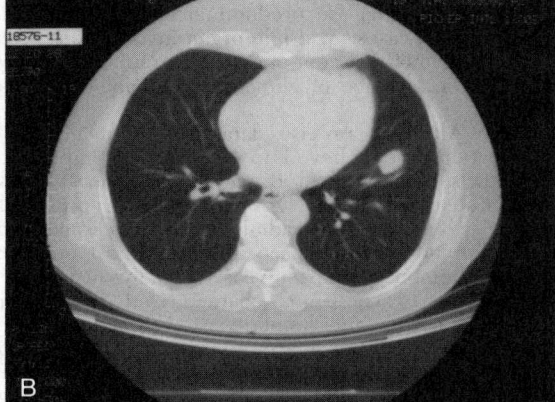

FIGURE 400–1. *A*, Benign nodule due to coccidioidomycosis. *B*, Computed tomographic (CT) image of the nodule shown in *A*.

within 5 cm of the hilus. Despite their harmless nature, coccidioidal nodules may engender concern because of their similarity to a malignant mass. For this reason, management usually requires percutaneous needle aspiration or resection. Another consequence of pulmonary coccidioidomycosis is cavitation of the infiltrate, which occurs in approximately 5 per cent of pneumonias. Cavities are usually single, thin walled, in an upper lobe, and close to the pleura; they may cause pain, produce hemoptysis, or develop associated infiltrates. Infrequently, a cavity ruptures, forming a pyopneumothorax. This usually is the first symptom of coccidioidal infection and commonly occurs in otherwise healthy young males. An air-fluid level, detectable by roentgenography in the pleural space, often helps differentiate this problem from a spontaneous pneumothorax. Surgical resection of the cavity with closure of the bronchopleural fistula is the preferred treatment for this complication. The least common pulmonary complication is persistent fibrocavitary infection that progresses from one lobe to another, involving both lungs.

Extrapulmonary Dissemination. Coccidioidomycosis usually results in dissemination beyond the lungs in immunosuppressed patients, such as organ recipients or those with acquired immunodeficiency syndrome (AIDS) or lymphoma. However, some patients have no underlying disease and do not manifest heightened susceptibility to other infections. The most common locations for disseminated lesions are skin (cutaneous papules or subcutaneous nodules); joints (especially the knee); bones, including vertebrae; and the basilar meninges. Such infections may produce one or many lesions and frequently are subacute or chronic in their presentation. When infections are more fulminant, they are usually in broadly immunosuppressed patients and produce fungemia detectable with blood cultures and diffuse reticulonodular embolic pulmonary infiltrates. Although the kidneys and the urinary bladder are rarely involved, *C. immitis* may be recovered from concentrated specimens of urine, because of either transient fungemia or focal dissemination to the prostate. In contrast to histoplasmosis, the gastrointestinal tract is rarely involved in coccidioidomycosis.

DIAGNOSIS. The diagnosis is firmly established by recovering *C. immitis* from clinical specimens. Growth of the fungus is supported by most routinely available microbiology media and may be evident by the first week of incubation. Spherules can be seen as large structures with doubly refractile walls and internal organization in KOH preparations or cytologic stains of respiratory secretions and also on hematoxylin-eosin, silver, or periodic acid–Schiff stains of histologic preparations. The Gram stain does not detect spherules. Except in the case of coccidioidal meningitis, in which positive cerebrospinal fluid (CSF) cultures are usually negative, isolation of the fungus is nearly always possible in patients with infections sufficiently severe to warrant therapy. In contrast, recovery of *C. immitis* may be difficult in patients who have only scant respiratory secretions associated with the initial pneumonia.

The presumptive diagnosis of coccidioidal infection is often based on detecting specific antibodies in serum. Within the first weeks of initial infection and occasionally with recurrent infections, a precipitin-type antibody is detected, usually by immunodiffusion techniques. Later in the course of infection, complement fixing (CF)–type antibodies are often detected. When reported quantitatively, CF antibodies generally are found to be highest in the most extensive infections and decrease in concentration in patients whose infections are controlled. An important means of diagnosing coccidioidal meningitis is by detection of CF antibodies in the CSF, along with other abnormalities, such as leukocytosis, elevated protein concentration, or low glucose concentration.

TREATMENT. Treatment has been limited to those with more serious forms of coccidioidal infection, since the primary pneumonia is usually self-limited, and until recently, amphotericin B was the only antifungal drug available. Amphotericin B has been used successfully in cumulative doses of 1.0 to 3.0 grams for treating all types of coccidioidomycosis. However, it has not been uniformly effective and frequently has produced treatment-limiting morbidity and toxicity. Treatment of coccidioidal meningitis has necessitated intrathecal administration, which imposes additional toxicity and risks. Binding amphotericin

B in liposomes or lipid complexes has been explored as a means of improving the therapeutic to toxic profile. However, to date, such efforts have been hindered by difficulties in producing stable, uniform material for clinical trials and hence remain investigative.

During the past 15 years, azole antifungals have been extensively studied as alternative therapy for coccidioidomycosis. Miconazole was found to be effective, but its use has necessitated multiple daily parenteral administrations, and frequent relapses were found upon cessation of therapy. Ketoconazole has also been found to be effective and is administered orally. However, absorption is variable; gastrointestinal intolerance is frequent; dose-dependent hormonal suppression and gynecomastia occur in some patients, especially at dosages above 400 mg per day; and as with miconazole, relapses after stopping therapy remain a significant limitation. Currently, triazoles such as itraconazole and fluconazole are under investigation and show promise. Although these agents appear nearly identical in terms of their mechanism of action, they differ significantly in their metabolism and disposition. Fluconazole achieves CSF concentrations approximately 80 per cent of that in serum during chronic therapy, and this finding has prompted hopes that triazole antifungals may be useful therapy for coccidioidal meningitis. It is not known if the use of ketoconazole or any other oral agent shortens the course of the primary coccidioidal pneumonia or changes the likelihood of later complications.

PROGNOSIS. After resolution of the initial untreated infection, most patients maintain lifelong immunity, and second infections are very infrequent. Similarly, late recurrence is unlikely in the absence of intercurrent profound immunosuppression. The disease in those who are unable to resolve the initial infection frequently follows a protracted course. Although infection is more debilitating than fatal, fulminant respiratory failure can occur, and if untreated, coccidioidal meningitis is nearly always fatal within 2 years.

Ampel NM, Wieden MA, Galgiani JN: Coccidioidomycosis: Clinical update. Rev Infect Dis 11:897, 1989. *Major review of recent literature of coccidioidomycosis. A previous comprehensive review was Drutz DJ, Catanzaro A: Coccidioidomycosis. State of the art. Am Rev Respir Dis 117:559, 727, 1978.*

Fish DG, Ampel NM, Galgiani JN, et al.: Coccidioidomycosis during human immunodeficiency virus (HIV) infection: A retrospective review of 77 patients. Medicine (Baltimore) 69:384, 1990. *In Arizona, coccidioidomycosis is the third most common opportunistic infection in patients with AIDS. Manifestations are usually severe in patients with CD4 counts less than 0.250×10^6 cells per liter.*

Graybill JR, Stevens DA, Galgiani JN, et al.: Itraconazole treatment of coccidioidomycosis. Am J Med 89:282, 1990. *Itraconazole is the first of several triazole antifungals likely to prove effective for the treatment of coccidioidomycosis.*

Labadie EK, Hamilton RH: Survival improvement in coccidioidal meningitis by high-dose intrathecal amphotericin B. Arch Intern Med 146:2013, 1986. *Cure of coccidioidal meningitis with intrathecally administered amphotericin B appears to be more likely if higher doses are given. This report antedates more recent experience using suppressive therapy with oral triazole antifungal agents such as fluconazole.*

Pappagianis D, Zimmer BL: Serology of coccidioidomycosis. Clin Microb Rev 3:247, 1990. *Authoritative review of serologic testing in relation to the clinical manifestations of coccidioidomycosis.*

401 Blastomycosis

William E. Dismukes

DEFINITION. Blastomycosis (North American blastomycosis, Gilchrist's disease) is an endemic systemic mycosis that occurs primarily in noncompromised hosts. As with the other important endemic mycoses, such as coccidioidomycosis and histoplasmosis, infection follows inhalation of the aerosolized spore form of the fungus. Clinical disease most commonly involves the lungs, skin, skeletal system, and male genitourinary tract.

ETIOLOGY. *Blastomyces dermatitidis*, the imperfect or asexual stage of *Ajellomyces dermatitidis*, is a dimorphic fungus, growing as a mycelial form in the environment and in the laboratory at room temperature and as a yeast form in mammalian tissue and in the laboratory at 37°C. The yeast cells, which are identical in vitro and in vivo in tissue and fluid specimens, vary from 8 to 15 μm in diameter, have a thick, highly refractile cell wall, and reproduce by single broad-based buds. In the laboratory, growth of *B. dermatitidis* is somewhat slow; mold colonies may not appear for 1 to 3 weeks.

EPIDEMIOLOGY. Because no sensitive and specific skin test exists, the epidemiology of blastomycosis is less well understood than that of coccidioidomycosis and histoplasmosis. The incidence of clinical disease as a manifestation of blastomycosis appears to be lower than the incidence of clinical disease associated with the two other endemic mycoses. The prevalence of subclinical blastomycosis is largely unknown. Isolated cases of blastomycosis have been reported worldwide, including Africa and Central and South America; however, the disease is concentrated or endemic in the South and North Central United States, especially in areas bordering the Mississippi and Ohio River basins, and the Great Lakes. In these endemic areas, small point-source outbreaks of blastomycosis have been associated with recreational or occupational activities occurring in wooded areas along waterways. Current evidence indicates that *B. dermatitidis* exists in warm, moist soil enriched by organic debris, including decaying vegetation or wood. It is not surprising, therefore, that persons with occupational or avocational exposure to soil and the outdoors appear to be at highest risk of acquiring infection. Data from point-source outbreaks indicate that the median incubation period from exposure to infection is about 43 days. Animals, especially dogs and horses, are also susceptible to infection, which may progress to clinical disease. Among humans, clinical illness is most common among middle-aged men. *Blastomyces dermatitidis*, in contrast to the other dimorphic fungi, rarely is an opportunistic pathogen in immunosuppressed hosts, e.g., human immunodeficiency virus (HIV)–infected individuals. This observation and other limited data suggest that reactivation blastomycosis is uncommon.

PATHOGENESIS AND PATHOLOGY. Humans and animals, for the most part, acquire infection by inhalation of aerosolized conidia that convert to the yeast form in the lungs at body temperature. Percutaneous inoculation of *B. dermatitidis* has been documented rarely, as a result of either a laboratory accident or a dog bite. The clinical manifestations of disease at body sites other than lung (and rarely skin) result from the hematogenous spread of organisms.

Cell-mediated immunity appears to be the most important arm of host defense against *B. dermatitidis*. Recent in vivo and in vitro studies indicate that macrophages, stimulated by lymphokines, are more effective in inhibiting or killing the organism than are granulocytes. A growth-inhibiting or protective role of humoral immunity in blastomycosis has not been established. The typical histopathologic picture of pulmonary blastomycosis and other nonmucocutaneous sites of disease consists of noncaseating granulomas as well as clusters of neutrophils. By contrast, cutaneous and mucous membrane lesions are characterized by pseudoepitheliomatous hyperplasia with microabscesses.

CLINICAL MANIFESTATIONS. In general, blastomycosis is a chronic indolent systemic fungal disease associated with a variety of pulmonary and extrapulmonary manifestations. Among the latter, cutaneous disease predominates, occurring in about 40 to 80 per cent of cases. Multiple organ involvement occurs in approximately 50 to 60 per cent of cases. Extrapulmonary disease may occur in the absence of clinical or radiologic evidence of lung disease.

Pulmonary. Although precise data are not available, most primary infections are believed to be either asymptomatic or unrecognized as being due to *B. dermatitidis* on the basis of nonspecific flulike symptoms. In patients with proven acute pulmonary blastomycosis, the radiologic findings usually consist of infiltrative or nodular air space opacities, most often in the lower lobes. Pulmonary blastomycosis usually manifests as a chronic pneumonia syndrome, characterized by productive cough, pleuritic chest pain, hemoptysis, weight loss, and low-grade fever. Although there are no distinguishing radiologic characteristics, one or more fibronodular infiltrates or mass lesions with or without cavitation are common, often mimicking the findings in other granulomatous diseases or bronchogenic carcinoma. Although hilar adenopathy and pleural effusions occur, they are uncommon. Rarely, patients with fulminant hematogenous dissemination may develop a miliary pattern on the chest radiograph and clinical evidence of acute respiratory distress syndrome.

Skin. The cutaneous lesions, which often prompt the patient with blastomycosis to seek medical evaluation initially, are of two general types, verrucous and ulcerative; both types tend to occur more commonly on exposed parts. The verrucous lesions, which begin as papulopustules, are more characteristic; these progress slowly over weeks to months to become crusted, heaped-up, and warty in appearance, often with a reddish-black or violaceous hue, an area of central healing and scarring, and a well-circumscribed outer border. Microabscesses, manifested by black dots on the surface, are typically located at the periphery of verrucous lesions; removal of the crusted eschar often reveals purulent material in which the yeast form of the organism can be demonstrated by wet preparation. Ulcerative lesions overlying a bed of friable red granulation tissue are less common. Occasionally, mucosal ulcerations may be found in the mouth, nose, or larynx, mimicking the mucocutaneous lesions of histoplasmosis. Lymphadenopathy in the region corresponding to the skin lesion or lesions is distinctly uncommon in patients whose cutaneous disease is secondary to hematogenous spread of organisms from a primary pulmonary focus.

Other. After lung and skin disease, bone and joint involvement is next most common and is seen in 10 to 50 per cent of cases. Osteolytic lesions, with or without sclerotic margins, are typically located in long bones and vertebrae. Often, patients with bone disease present as a result of overlying chronic draining sinuses or contiguous soft tissue lesions rather than bone pain. Septic arthritis, which is much less common than osteomyelitis, is frequently secondary to contiguous extension. Up to one third of men with blastomycosis have genitourinary tract disease, manifested most commonly by prostatic enlargement with obstructive symptoms and less frequently by epididymitis. Central nervous system disease in the form of either granulomatous meningitis or a mass lesion (intracerebral blastomycoma) occurs in fewer than 5 per cent of cases. Clinically apparent blastomycotic involvement of other organs, e.g., gastrointestinal tract, liver, spleen, adrenals, and kidneys, is unusual, except in patients with fulminant disseminated disease.

DIAGNOSIS. As is true for all systemic mycotic diseases, the definitive diagnosis of blastomycosis requires a positive fungal culture from clinical specimens. A presumptive diagnosis may be based on the finding of characteristic yeast forms in a wet preparation of sputum, pus, or other body fluid or in a histopathologic section of tissue, e.g., skin, lung, bone, or prostate. *Blastomyces dermatitidis* in wet preparations of fluid specimens mixed with 10 per cent KOH appears as a broad-based single budding yeast and in fixed-tissue specimens stained with hematoxylineosin or periodic acid–Schiff (PAS) reagents as single or budding yeast cells with a doubly refractile cell wall. Because a presumptive clinical diagnosis based on "characteristic" skin lesions or radiologic findings is associated with an unacceptably high error rate, obtaining fluids or tissue from involved sites for culture and histopathologic study is mandatory in the evaluation of all patients with suspected blastomycosis. Moreover, documented cutaneous and/or pulmonary disease should signal the possibility of bone or genitourinary disease and lead to appropriate diagnostic studies, such as bone scan and prostate examination and massage. As a diagnostic test, the blastomycin skin test lacks sensitivity and specificity and should not be used. Similarly, the complement fixation assay for serum antibody is highly cross-reactive and of no diagnostic value. Recent studies suggest that immunodiffusion or enzyme immunoassay tests for the A antigen of *B. dermatitidis* have potential as serologic markers of disease.

TREATMENT. At present, two drugs, amphotericin B and ketoconazole, are approved for the treatment of blastomycosis. Although intravenous amphotericin B has been traditionally considered the drug of choice for all forms of disease, studies and experience gained over the past decade indicate that oral ketoconazole is highly effective, especially in patients with chronic indolent disease and noninvolvement of the central nervous system. Oral ketoconazole should be initiated at a dosage of 400 mg per day, advanced by 200-mg increments at monthly intervals, up to a maximum of 800 mg per day in patients with progressive disease, and continued for a minimum of 6 months. Amphotericin B, a total dose of 1.5 to 2.5 grams, should be reserved for patients with overwhelming life-threatening or central nervous system disease, those rare patients who are immunocompromised, and those in whom ketoconazole has failed. In selected situations, some investigators advocate an induction course of amphotericin B (total dose of approximately 500 mg) for a rapid fungicidal effect to gain control of disease, followed by maintenance or "consolidation" therapy with ketoconazole for 3 to 6 months. Newer oral antifungal azoles, such as itraconazole and fluconazole, show promise and appear to be less toxic than ketoconazole. Although controversy exists about whether or not to treat patients with acute pulmonary blastomycosis who are identified as part of point-source outbreaks, available data suggest that most such patients do not require therapy. However, careful long-term follow-up of untreated patients is important to monitor for evidence of disease activity.

PROGNOSIS. In contrast to the past, now most patients with blastomycosis are identified and treated before the development of overwhelming or fatal disease. Both amphotericin B and ketoconazole are associated with cure rates of 80 per cent or better and relapse rates of less than 10 per cent. Relapse in a few ketoconazole-treated patients has been manifested by either central nervous system or genitourinary disease, not surprising in view of the poor penetration of ketoconazole into cerebrospinal fluid and the low level of active drug in urine.

Bradsher RW: Blastomycosis. Infect Dis Clin North Am 2:877, 1988. *A comprehensive, up-to-date review, with a nice perspective on treatment and 116 references.*

Dismukes WE, Cloud G, Bowles C, et al., National Institute of Allergy and Infectious Disease Mycoses Study Group: Treatment of blastomycosis and histoplasmosis with ketoconazole: Results of a prospective randomized clinical trial. Ann Intern Med 103:861, 1985. *Results of this study of 80 patients with blastomycosis indicate that ketoconazole is effective therapy for immunocompetent patients with non–life-threatening, nonmeningeal disease.*

Klein BS, Vergeront JM, Davis JP: Epidemiologic aspects of blastomycosis, the enigmatic systemic mycosis. Semin Respir Infect 1:29, 1986. *A valuable review that focuses on seven point-source epidemics and the ecologic niche of the organism.*

Sarosi GA, Davies SF, Phillips JR: Self-limited blastomycosis: A report of 39 cases. Semin Respir Infect 1:40, 1986. *This study provides evidence that acute pulmonary blastomycosis in most patients resolves spontaneously without therapy and with no sequelae.*

402 Paracoccidioidomycosis

William E. Dismukes

DEFINITION. Paracoccidioidomycosis is a chronic granulomatous disease typically involving the lungs, skin, mucous membranes, and lymph nodes and limited to an endemic area extending from Mexico south to Argentina.

ETIOLOGY. The causative agent, *Paracoccidioides brasiliensis*, is a dimorphic fungus that grows as a mycelial form in nature and as an oval or round yeast form in tissues or at 37°C. Identification of characteristic multiple budding or "pilot wheel," thick-walled yeast cells, 10 to 40 μm in diameter, in tissue provides presumptive evidence of disease. Because the organism grows slowly on primary isolation, fungal cultures should be held for at least 4 weeks before discarding.

EPIDEMIOLOGY. Most cases occur in persons living in or with a history of prior exposure to southern Mexico, Central America, or South America; in these areas, paracoccidioidomycosis is the most common systemic mycosis. Owing to the long period of latency, overt disease may develop in persons many years after they have left the endemic region. Infection is acquired via inhalation of spores. Neither human-to-human transmission nor common-source outbreaks have been documented. The majority of cases occur in adult males, especially those who labor in the outdoors. The preponderance of cases in men may also be related to the observation that estrogens inhibit the mycelium-to-yeast transformation of the organism. Although cases have been reported in compromised hosts, in general, paracoccidioidomycosis is not considered an opportunistic fungal disease.

PATHOGENESIS AND PATHOLOGY. After inhalation of

spores, infection may remain confined to the lungs or may spread by lymphohematogenous dissemination to multiple organs. The host pathologic response caused by *P. brasiliensis* is similar to that caused by tissue invasion with *Blastomyces dermatitidis* and *Coccidioides immitis*, i.e., both granulomas and suppuration may develop. The type of tissue pathology and the spectrum of clinical disease are in large part dictated by the integrity of the cell-mediated defenses of the host.

CLINICAL MANIFESTATIONS. Pulmonary paracoccidioidomycosis may be asymptomatic or result in symptomatic acute or chronic disease. Whereas the acute form of pulmonary paracoccidioidomycosis is usually nonspecific and indistinguishable from other influenza-like illnesses, the clinical and radiographic features of the chronic form often resemble those of chronic pulmonary coccidioidomycosis. Any or all lobes may be infected, but the upper lobes tend to be less frequently involved. In addition, cavities, if present, are usually small (so-called microcavities). Extrapulmonary disease, especially in persons less than 30 years old, may be acute in onset, is often manifested by lymphadenopathy and hepatosplenomegaly, and carries a poor prognosis. More typically, extrapulmonary disease in older adults is an indolent illness, manifested by oropharyngeal and laryngeal mucous membrane ulcers; verrucous, ulcerative, or nodular skin lesions, often on the face or mucocutaneous borders; and enlarged or necrotic, draining lymph nodes, especially in the cervical region. Other sites of less frequent involvement are the gastrointestinal tract, adrenal glands, testes, epididymis, and skeletal system. Central nervous system and eye disease secondary to *P. brasiliensis* are rare. A few cases of paracoccidioidomycosis have been observed in human immunodeficiency virus (HIV)–infected persons.

DIAGNOSIS. Demonstration of the characteristic "pilot wheel," multiple-budding *P. brasiliensis* yeast cells by wet mounts or KOH preparations of sputum, pus, or other body fluids or by special fungal stains of biopsy or cell-block specimens provides presumptive evidence of paracoccidioidomycosis. A positive culture of body fluid or tissue specimens is diagnostic. Two different serologic tests (agar gel immunodiffusion and complement fixation) are available through the Centers for Disease Control in Atlanta. Precipitin bands appear early in the course of active infection and may persist for years, even after successful therapy. Complement-fixing antibodies appear later and are more useful in evaluating response to treatment. Both tests have high specificity. Alternative serologic tests, including enzyme-linked immunosorbent assay (ELISA) and counterimmunoelectrophoresis (CIE) as well as newer ones for detection of a 43-kD glycoprotein antigen and for antibodies to this antigen, are under investigation. Skin tests have no role in diagnosis.

TREATMENT. In the past, oral sulfonamides were the mainstay of therapy; however, these have two major drawbacks, namely, a high rate of relapse even after prolonged suppression therapy and a high frequency of adverse reactions, especially skin rashes. Intravenous amphotericin B is effective therapy and is usually employed for more severe forms of paracoccidioidomycosis, such as pulmonary or disseminated multiorgan disease, and for more refractory cases. Follow-up chronic suppression therapy with sulfonamides is recommended. Oral antifungal azole drugs represent a significant advance in the treatment of this disease. Ketoconazole, an imidazole, is highly effective in both in vivo animal models and humans. Cure is usually achieved with dosages of 200 to 400 mg per day, given for at least 1 year. Recent trials indicate that itraconazole, a triazole, given in a dosage of 50 to 100 mg daily for 6 to 12 months, is as effective as ketoconazole and better tolerated. Because of the tropism of *P. brasiliensis* for the adrenal glands and the possibility of adrenal insufficiency during active disease or even after discontinuation of therapy, periodic tests of adrenal function are recommended.

PROGNOSIS. Untreated disseminated paracoccidioidomycosis is generally fatal. In general, the more common indolent forms of adult disease, usually associated with reactivation, are amenable to prolonged therapy, given over months to years.

Franco M: Host-parasite relationships in paracoccidioidomycosis. J Med Vet Mycol 25:5, 1987. *A thorough discussion of virulence factors, mechanisms of host defense, and granuloma morphogenesis, with 71 references.*

Naranjo MS, Trujillo M, Munera MI, et al.: Treatment of paracoccidioidomycosis with itraconazole. J Med Vet Mycol 28:67, 1990. *Forty-five of 47 patients had the chronic form of disease. Itraconazole, 100 mg per day, given for a mean duration of 6 months, was highly effective, as measured by radiographic and cultural responses, falling serologic titers, and improvement in clinical severity scores.*

Negroni R, Palmieri O, Koren F, et al.: Oral treatment of paracoccidioidomycosis and histoplasmosis with itraconazole in humans. Rev Infect Dis 9 (Suppl 1):S47, 1987. *Another study demonstrating the efficacy of itraconazole in 25 patients with paracoccidioidomycosis.*

Restreppo A, Robledo M, Giraldo R, et al.: The gamut of paracoccidioidomycosis. Am J Med 61:33, 1976. *An older review with emphasis on pulmonary and extrapulmonary manifestations.*

Sugar AM: Paracoccidioidomycosis. Infect Dis Clin North Am 2:913, 1988. *A recent comprehensive review.*

403 Cryptococcosis

William E. Dismukes

DEFINITION. Cryptococcosis is a systemic mycosis that most often involves the lungs and central nervous system and, less frequently, the skin, skeletal system, and prostate gland. *Cryptococcus neoformans*, the causative organism, is the most common etiologic agent of fungal meningitis, and since the onset of the acquired immunodeficiency syndrome (AIDS) epidemic in the early 1980's, it has been increasingly recognized as an opportunistic fungal pathogen.

ETIOLOGY. *Cryptococcus neoformans* is a yeastlike round or oval fungus, 4 to 6 μm in diameter, which is surrounded by a polysaccharide capsule and reproduces by budding. There are four different serotypes—A, B, C and D—based on the antigenic specificity of the capsule; biochemical differences also exist in serotypes. Nomenclature of the perfect or sexual states is based on mating properties. For example, serotypes A and D, which include the majority of clinical isolates, can be mated to produce the perfect state (*Filobasidiella neoformans* var. *neoformans*). In the laboratory on solid media, *C. neoformans* grows at 37°C as smooth yellow or tan colonies, usually within a week after inoculation. By contrast, nonpathogenic *Cryptococcus* species do not grow at 37°C. Other characteristics used to distinguish *C. neoformans* from nonpathogenic species include no pseudomycelial growth on cornmeal or rice-Tween agar, glucose assimilation but not fermentation, use of creatinine as a nitrogen source, and production of melanin and urease.

EPIDEMIOLOGY. Cryptococcosis is worldwide in distribution. Serotypes A and D are found in soil and other environmental areas, especially those contaminated by pigeon droppings; pigeons themselves are not infected. Less is known about the ecologic niche of serotypes B and C. Although humans and animals acquire infection after inhalation of aerosolized spores, clusters of cases or mini-outbreaks of cryptococcosis rarely occur, as they do in aerosol-transmitted mycoses such as blastomycosis and histoplasmosis. Animal-to-human and human-to-human transmission of cryptococcosis has not been documented, with one exception; active cryptococcosis in a corneal transplant donor is believed to have resulted in cryptococcal endophthalmitis in the recipient. There is no obvious age, sex, or occupational predilection. Conditions or factors that predispose to cryptococcosis include corticosteroid therapy, lymphoreticular malignancies (especially Hodgkin's disease), sarcoidosis (even in the absence of corticosteroid therapy), human immunodeficiency virus (HIV) infection, and perhaps diabetes mellitus (data are conflicting). The association of cryptococcosis and organ transplantation probably relates in large part to immunosuppression with corticosteroids. Cyclosporine, at least in a murine model, inhibits growth of *C. neoformans*. Among HIV-positive individuals, the incidence of cryptococcosis varies from 5 to 10 per cent, and *C. neoformans* ranks in frequency behind only *Pneumocystis carinii*, cytomegalovirus, and mycobacteria as an opportunistic systemic pathogen in this high-risk population group. Although cryptococcosis frequently occurs in immunosuppressed hosts, approximately one third of patients with the disease have no apparent underlying condition or predisposing factor.

PATHOGENESIS AND PATHOLOGY. After inhalation of aerosolized spores, most infections begin with an asymptomatic pulmonary focus. Subsequently, hematogenous spread to extrapulmonary organs occurs. Initially, neutrophils and, later, monocytes clear cryptococci from inflammatory sites. Phagocytosis by neutrophils and macrophages is mediated in part by complement, interferon, and other T cell–derived lymphokines. Cryptococcal polysaccharide capsule is a major virulence factor and may be immunosuppressive, induce T-suppressor cells, suppress both specific and nonspecific antibody response, inhibit phagocytosis, and impair migration of leukocytes. Paradoxically, cryptococcal polysaccharide has also been shown to activate the alternative complement pathway. In general, immunity depends on functioning, sensitized T cells and an intact cell-mediated arm of host defense. Consequently, patients with defective or altered T cell immunity, such as those with HIV infection, are highly susceptible to infection with *C. neoformans* and progressive disease. The preferential involvement of *C. neoformans* for the central nervous system is explained partially by the absence of complement and soluble anticryptococcal factors (present in normal serum) in normal cerebrospinal fluid (CSF), as well as a decreased to absent inflammatory response to cryptococci in brain tissue. As a result, well-formed granulomas are generally absent in histopathologic sections of infected tissue. The characteristic lesion in cryptococcal meningoencephalitis consists of cystic clusters of fungi; the basal ganglia and the cortical gray matter are the sites of heaviest involvement. In other organs such as the lung, the inflammatory response varies in intensity from minimal to heavy and consists of an array of cells, including organism-containing macrophages, giant cells, plasma cells, and lymphocytes. No necrosis is present, and tissue is usually displaced by multiplying organisms. Yeastlike cryptococci with characteristic narrow-based buds stain poorly with hematoxylin-eosin but are easily visualized with Gomori methenamine silver (GMS) or periodic acid–Schiff (PAS) stains. Mucicarmine stain further aids in identification by giving a rose color to the polysaccharide capsule.

CLINICAL MANIFESTATIONS

Pulmonary Cryptococcosis. The pattern of pulmonary cryptococcal infection is highly variable, ranging from the extremes of saprophytic airway colonization without clinical or radiographic evidence of disease to full-blown acute respiratory distress syndrome in compromised hosts, such as AIDS patients. More typically, radiographic findings include either patchy pneumonitis or solitary or multiple small nodules in asymptomatic persons or those with mild to moderate symptoms, e.g., fever, malaise, cough, scant sputum, pleuritic pain, or rarely hemoptysis. Although tumor-like masses mimicking carcinoma are not uncommon, cavitation and pleural effusions are less likely. The course of pulmonary cryptococcosis is also variable. In patients with normal host defenses, spontaneous regression of both clinical and radiographic manifestations is the rule, although chronic stable infection is known to occur. In contrast, pulmonary cryptococcosis in immunocompromised patients is more likely to progress and therefore requires antifungal therapy. Pulmonary disease may occur in the absence of extrapulmonary cryptococcosis, and, conversely, extrapulmonary disease, such as meningitis, may develop in the absence of apparent lung involvement.

Central Nervous System Cryptococcosis. Meningitis, usually subacute or chronic in nature, is the most common manifestation of central nervous system (CNS) cryptococcosis. Complications include hydrocephalus, encephalitis, involvement of the optic pathways, brain stem vasculitis, and mass lesions (cryptococcomas) of the brain parenchyma or spinal cord. The clinical presentation and course of cryptococcal meningitis vary greatly, related in part to the underlying condition and immune status of the host. In "normal" hosts, the onset is usually insidious, whereas in compromised hosts, such as HIV-infected or corticosteroid-treated patients, the onset tends to be more acute and the course more rapidly progressive. The most common symptoms are headache and alteration in mental status, e.g., confusion, lethargy, obtundation or coma, and personality change. Nausea and vomiting are frequent; fever and stiff neck are less common. Ocular symptoms, such as blurred vision, photophobia, vision loss, and diplopia, secondary to perineuritic adhesive arachnoiditis, papilledema, optic nerve neuritis, chorioretinitis, or retino-

vitreal abscess, are present in 30 to 50 per cent of patients. Other findings include hearing deficits, seizures, ataxia, aphasia, and choreoathetoid movements. Dementia is important to recognize as a potential sequela, since it may be curable. Because cryptococcomas reportedly accompany cryptococcal meningitis in as many as 20 per cent of cases, an imaging study (computed tomography [CT] or magnetic resonance imaging [MRI]) should be considered in the evaluation of all patients. Rarely, CNS cryptococcomas can be seen in the absence of meningeal disease. The mortality rate varies from 20 to 30 per cent; most deaths occur in the first 6 weeks of illness in patients with fulminant deterioration.

Miscellaneous. After the lungs and CNS, the next most commonly involved organs in patients with disseminated cryptococcosis are the skin and skeletal system. Cutaneous manifestations occur in 10 to 15 per cent of cases and usually take the form of papules, pustules, nodules, ulcers, or draining sinuses. Typically, cellulitis with prominent erythema and induration is seen in corticosteroid-treated transplant recipients, and umbilicated papules resembling molluscum contagiosum are observed in AIDS patients. Oral mucosal chancres have been reported rarely. Osteomyelitis is more common than septic arthritis. Less commonly involved sites of cryptococcal disease include pericardium, myocardium, muscle, liver, peritoneum, adrenal glands, kidneys, and prostate gland. Infections of these organs are being increasingly identified in AIDS patients. For example, the prostate has been reported to be a nidus of residual infection in this population group.

DIAGNOSIS. As with other systemic mycoses, the definitive diagnosis of cryptococcosis depends on demonstration of the characteristic yeastlike organism with its surrounding capsule in tissue or fluid obtained from involved sites, together with cultural confirmation. In addition, in patients with suspected cryptococcosis, the latex agglutination test for detection of cryptococcal polysaccharide antigen in serum and CSF is an extremely important adjunct to diagnosis, unlike the situation for most other fungal diseases, in which serologic tests lack specificity and sensitivity. Cryptococcal antigen is found in CSF in more than 90 per cent and in serum in about 75 per cent of patients with meningitis, especially if serial specimens are examined over time. Titers are particularly high in patients with AIDS. In patients with extraneural cryptococcal disease, antigen is detected in only 25 to 50 per cent of cases. Proper controls are necessary to eliminate rheumatoid factor, which may give rise to a false-positive result. Serum of patients with disseminated infection caused by *Trichosporon beigelii* may also test positive for cryptococcal antigen. False-negative tests for cryptococcal antigen may be due to low numbers of cryptococcal organisms invading tissue or in CSF, unencapsulated or poorly encapsulated strains, or a prozone phenomenon. Tests for cryptococcal antibody are not useful for diagnosis.

Pulmonary cryptococcosis is difficult to diagnose in most cases without obtaining lung tissue via bronchoscopy or open lung biopsy. Wet preparations of sputum are only occasionally helpful, and sputum cultures are positive for *C. neoformans* in only 20 per cent of cases. In patients with pleural effusions, test of the fluid for cryptococcal antigen may be positive, thereby obviating a more invasive procedure. In every patient with established pulmonary cryptococcosis, a lumbar puncture should be performed, whether or not CNS disease is apparent. Blood cultures and tissue for culture and histopathologic study of any other suspected sites of involvement, e.g., skin or bone, should also be obtained.

The diagnosis of cryptococcal meningitis is easier to establish than the diagnosis of cryptococcal pulmonary disease. Once the diagnosis of meningitis is considered, a lumbar puncture should be performed. Most patients, except for those with AIDS, have significant CSF abnormalities, including elevated opening pressure, depressed glucose levels (hypoglycorrhachia) in half the cases, elevated protein levels, and a low-grade lymphocytic pleocytosis. The India ink preparation of centrifuged CSF to detect budding yeast cells and surrounding capsule is positive in 50 to 75 per cent of cases; because the incidence of false-positive smears is high, confirmation of findings by culture is imperative. Culturing of centrifuged sediment of large volumes (5 to 10 ml) of CSF obtained by repeated lumbar punctures is associated with a positive culture rate of 90 to 95 per cent. In AIDS patients, the CSF formula is often normal or only minimally abnormal, owing to a diminished or absent inflammatory response. Yet in most cases, cultures are positive, cryptococcal antigen titers are high, and India ink preparations reveal organisms. The chest roentgenogram may or may not be abnormal. Blood should be cultured and tested for antigen in all patients. In addition, CT or MRI of the head is indicated in most patients, especially those with coma, suspected hydrocephalus, focal neurologic findings, seizures, or clinical deterioration after initial improvement. Cisternal puncture for CSF analysis, culture, and cryptococcal antigen testing may be rewarding in patients with chronic lymphocytic meningitis in whom an etiology has not been established over a period of weeks to months, despite serial testing of lumbar CSF.

TREATMENT. Approaches to therapy for cryptococcosis vary according to the site (or sites) of involvement and the underlying host status. Whereas all patients with CNS cryptococcosis or other forms of extrapulmonary disease require treatment, the majority of cases of pulmonary cryptococcosis alone, especially in the "normal" host, resolve without antifungal therapy. Every patient with pulmonary disease deserves thorough evaluation for the possibility of disseminated infection. In addition, malignancy such as bronchogenic carcinoma or metastases must be excluded. In the absence of extrapulmonary cryptococcal disease in the normal host, therapy may be safely withheld, provided careful follow-up evaluation can be done. By contrast, other patients with pulmonary cryptococcosis, including immunocompromised patients, those with accompanying extrapulmonary disease, and those with progressive disease, require antifungal therapy. Although specific guidelines are poorly defined, amphotericin B (total dose, 1.0 to 1.5 grams) is generally recommended. Fluconazole, recently approved by the Food and Drug Administration for treatment of cryptococcal meningitis (see below), appears to be more effective against C. neoformans than does ketoconazole, the other orally available antifungal azole. Fluconazole (200 to 400 mg per day for 3 to 6 months) is a promising alternative to amphotericin B, especially in patients with mild to moderate forms of pulmonary disease; however, data about its efficacy in this form of cryptococcosis are limited. Controversy also exists over the management of patients who have undergone thoracotomy with resection of a nodule or mass lesion that is subsequently proved to be caused by C. neoformans. In the past, if evidence of extrapulmonary infection was lacking, no antifungal therapy was advocated. Now, with the availability of a well-tolerated and potentially effective oral agent such as fluconazole, this approach deserves reconsideration; a 2- to 6-month course of fluconazole may be merited.

In terms of chemotherapy, cryptococcal meningitis has been more extensively studied than any other systemic fungal disease. Data indicate that (1) all patients require treatment; (2) a combination of amphotericin B and flucytosine for 4 to 6 weeks is the regimen of choice; and (3) combination therapy is more effective than therapy with amphotericin alone. Although recommendations are based on studies using a 0.3 mg per kilogram per day dosage of amphotericin B and a 150 mg per kilogram per day dosage of flucytosine, dosing regimens should be individualized, balancing the risk of toxicities associated with higher doses versus the potential benefits of enhanced efficacy. For example, some authorities recommend higher dose amphotericin B (0.5 to 0.7 mg per kilogram per day) and lower dose flucytosine (100 mg per kilogram per day). Regardless of regimen, both renal function and serum flucytosine levels should be closely monitored, and flucytosine doses should be regulated to maintain serum concentrations in the range of 50 to 100 µg per milliliter. Potential toxic effects of flucytosine include bone marrow suppression, hepatitis, diarrhea, and rash. Intrathecal therapy with amphotericin B is usually reserved for patients who relapse or whose disease is refractory to prolonged courses of high-dose intravenous amphotericin B.

Because cryptococcal meningitis in AIDS patients may be highly refractory and associated with a relapse rate of 50 to 60 per cent if therapy is stopped, more aggressive primary or initial therapy, as well as long-term maintenance therapy, is required.

For primary therapy, higher dose amphotericin B (0.5 to 1.0 mg per kilogram per day), preferably with flucytosine (approximately 100 mg per kilogram per day), should be administered until there is clinical and mycologic response. Some AIDS patients may not tolerate flucytosine because of a high incidence of drug-induced cytopenias, often superimposed upon pre-existing bone marrow suppression secondary to zidovudine, cytotoxic chemotherapy, and opportunistic infectious diseases. In addition, flucytosine should not be used unless serum levels can be monitored. Recent studies indicate that fluconazole (200 to 400 mg per day) may be an effective alternative to amphotericin B as primary therapy. Although limited clinical data also suggest a potential role for itraconazole, another triazole, fluconazole, is favored in cryptococcal meningitis because of its pharmacologic properties, including water solubility, minimal protein binding, and good to excellent penetration into CSF (60 to 80 per cent of serum concentration). In addition, an intravenous formulation of fluconazole is available. A major disadvantage of fluconazole is less rapid sterilization of CSF when compared with amphotericin B. As a result, amphotericin B should be preferentially used as primary therapy in more seriously ill patients, such as those who are obtunded or comatose or those who have widespread disseminated cryptococcosis.

Ventricular shunting of CSF should be performed in obtunded or comatose patients with hydrocephalus demonstrated by imaging studies. Since not all patients with abnormal mental status, blindness, hearing loss, or other neurologic complications have documented hydrocephalus, serial lumbar punctures or temporary ventricular drainage with monitoring of intracranial pressure plus observation of clinical response is often indicated in this setting.

Once primary therapy has sterilized the CSF, i.e., converted the fungal culture from positive to negative, some form of maintenance therapy should be initiated. Recent evaluation of maintenance therapy in AIDS patients with cryptococcal meningitis indicates that fluconazole (200 mg daily) is more effective in preventing relapse than is amphotericin (1 mg per kilogram per week) and is much better tolerated, resulting in better patient compliance. Regardless of which drug is used, chronic suppressive therapy must be continued for life.

PROGNOSIS. The outcome of cryptococcosis is significantly worse in AIDS patients than in the non-AIDS population. The mortality rate of treated cryptococcal meningitis approaches 30 per cent and is even higher among AIDS patients. Among non-AIDS patients treated with amphotericin B, the relapse rate is 20 per cent. Because the relapse rate of cryptococcal disease in persons with AIDS is 50 per cent or more, all such individuals must receive lifetime maintenance therapy. Prognostic factors, in addition to HIV infection, that adversely affect outcome include corticosteroid therapy or lymphoreticular cancer; absence of headache as a presenting symptom; pretreatment altered mental status, as evidenced by obtundation, stupor, or coma; a pretreatment CSF white cell count that is 20 per cubic millimeter or less; pretreatment cryptococcal serum antigen titer that is 1:32 or higher and end-of-therapy CSF and serum antigen titers that are 1:8 or higher; and positive India ink preparation at end of therapy. Some, but not all, studies indicate that high pretreatment CSF antigen titers also predict a poor outcome. Abnormalities of CSF, such as hypoglycorrhachia and elevated protein levels, may persist for months after therapy has been discontinued and do not appear to correlate with relapse.

PREVENTION. Because an environmental source of infection cannot be determined in the vast majority of patients who develop cryptococcal disease, attempts at elimination of C. neoformans from soil or other habitats are not feasible or practical. With the availability of effective, safe, orally administered antifungal agents, future consideration may be given to their use as prophylactic agents in groups at high risk of developing cryptococcosis, such as HIV-positive persons.

Bozette SA, Larsen RA, Chin J, et al.: A placebo-controlled trial of maintenance therapy with fluconazole after treatment of cryptococcal meningitis in the acquired immunodeficiency syndrome. N Engl J Med 324:580, 1991.

Chuck SL, Sande MA: Infections with Cryptococcus neoformans in the acquired immunodeficiency syndrome. N Engl J Med 321:794, 1989. A retrospective review of 106 cases of cryptococcosis in AIDS patients, with emphasis on management.

Dismukes WE, Cloud G, Gallis HA: Treatment of cryptococcal meningitis with combination amphotericin B and flucytosine for four as compared to six weeks. N Engl J Med 317:334, 1987. *The largest prospective clinical trial (194 patients) reported to date that deals with therapy for a systemic fungal disease. Focuses primarily on non-AIDS patients.* Stamm AS, Diasio RB, Dismukes WE, et al.: Toxicity of amphotericin B plus flucytosine in 194 patients with cryptococcal meningitis. Am J Med 83:236, 1987. *The companion paper, which addresses toxicity of the two mainstay drugs, amphotericin B and flucytosine.*

Miller GP: The immunology of cryptococcal disease. Semin Respir Infect 1:45, 1986. *A concise overview of the complex interaction between C. neoformans and host.*

Perfect JR: Cryptococcosis. Infect Dis Clin North Am 3:77, 1989. *A comprehensive, up-to-date review with 244 references.*

404 Sporotrichosis

William E. Dismukes

DEFINITION. Sporotrichosis is a chronic mycotic disease that typically involves skin, subcutaneous tissue, and regional lymphatics as a result of cutaneous inoculation of *Sporothrix schenckii*. Extracutaneous disease secondary to either lymphohematogenous dissemination or inhalation of organisms is rare.

ETIOLOGY. *Sporothrix schenckii* is a dimorphic fungus that grows in nature and in the laboratory on Sabouraud's agar as a white mold, which, with time, becomes brownish black. In tissue and at 37°C, the organism exists as yeastlike cells, which appear as round, spherical, or cigar-shaped budding forms, 2 to 6 μm in size.

EPIDEMIOLOGY. Sporotrichosis is worldwide in distribution. *Sporothrix schenckii* appears to be ubiquitous in soil and in both living and decaying vegetation. Although the organism does not appear to infect plants, it may infect animals, especially cats and dogs, as well as humans, especially those who frequently handle or come in contact with mulch, sphagnum moss, hay, timber, and thorny bushes. Consequently, sporotrichosis is considered an occupational disease of certain groups, including farmers, nursery or forestry workers, gardeners, florists, landscapers, and carpenters. Transmission almost always results from the percutaneous introduction of organisms. In the majority of patients with extracutaneous disease, the route of acquisition is unclear. Rarely, pulmonary sporotrichosis may result from inhalation of aerosolized conidia. Although person-to-person transmission is not known to occur, transmission from animals, especially cats, to humans has been documented. The number of cases of cutaneous disease in males and females is similar; gender and age appear to play less of a role than does environmental exposure. By contrast, extracutaneous sporotrichosis is more common in males. *Sporothrix schenckii* is not considered an opportunistic fungal pathogen, although sporotrichosis in compromised hosts is being increasingly recognized. For example, cases have been observed in human immunodeficiency virus (HIV)–infected persons.

PATHOGENESIS AND PATHOLOGY. Cutaneous inoculation may follow either inapparent or obvious penetrating trauma. In the majority of patients, clinical disease does not extend beyond the site of inoculation or the draining lymphatics. Localized disease may persist for years, and cell-mediated immunity appears to be responsible for preventing or limiting the spread to extracutaneous sites. Conversely, multiorgan disease involving skin and distant sites, such as lungs, bones, and joints, is more common in immunosuppressed hosts.

The basic histopathologic pattern in cutaneous sporotrichosis is a combination of suppuration and granulomas, often accompanied by pseudoepitheliomatous hyperplasia. This pattern is not diagnostic, as it may also be seen in malignancy as well as other fungal diseases, such as blastomycosis, coccidioidomycosis, and chromomycosis. Since the yeastlike cells, typical of *S. schenckii*, are uncommonly identified in tissue sections, cultural confirmation is usually necessary for diagnosis. The finding of large asteroid bodies (radiate eosinophilic material surrounding fungal yeast cells) provides presumptive evidence of sporotrichosis.

CLINICAL MANIFESTATIONS. Sporotrichosis is manifested by two distinctive clinical forms of cutaneous and extracutaneous disease, which differ in management and prognosis.

Cutaneous. This form of sporotrichosis can be further divided into two types: plaque (or fixed) and lymphocutaneous. Plaque sporotrichosis, which is less common, consists of a single ulcerative or nodular lesion at the site of primary inoculation, usually on an exposed extremity or the face. The lesion begins as a small, painless, red papule, which gradually enlarges and finally ulcerates (sporotrichotic chancre). A violaceous hue and intermittent serosanguineous drainage are characteristic. Lymphocutaneous sporotrichosis, which is the more typical type and is found in about 75 per cent of cases, represents an extension of the primary lesion. Subcutaneous nontender nodular lesions appear proximally along thickened lymphatics over days to weeks and occasionally ulcerate. Lymph nodes are rarely enlarged. Similarly, constitutional symptoms, such as fever and chills, are usually absent. This type of sporotrichosis, which usually remains confined to the primary site and its regional lymphatics, may wax and wane over years if untreated. Lymphohematogenous spread to distant organs is uncommon.

Extracutaneous. The pathogenesis of the majority of cases of extracutaneous sporotrichosis is uncertain, since most cases are not accompanied by clinically apparent cutaneous disease. The skeletal system is the most commonly involved extracutaneous organ. Although indolent monarticular arthritis of the knees, ankles, wrists, and elbows is most frequent, osteomyelitis (especially of the tibia), tenosynovitis, and carpal tunnel syndrome have been reported. Multiarticular arthritis is more likely in compromised hosts with widespread hematogenous spread to multiple organs. Pulmonary sporotrichosis is far less common than osteoarticular disease. Fewer than 100 cases of pulmonary disease have been reported. This form of insidious infection occurs primarily in older male alcoholics and mimics reactivation tuberculosis. Thin-walled cavitary lesions in a single upper lobe are characteristic; bilateral fibrocavitary disease may be seen occasionally. Extrapulmonary spread of disease is uncommon. Ocular sporotrichosis results from traumatic inoculation of the conjunctiva or cornea; endophthalmitis is unusual. Chronic lymphocytic meningitis may be a complication of sporotrichosis, even in the absence of obvious extraneural disease. Testing of cerebrospinal fluid (CSF) for antibody to *S. schenckii* should be performed in any patient with chronic meningitis of unknown etiology.

DIAGNOSIS. As a rule, the diagnosis of sporotrichosis must be based on cultural demonstration of the organism in tissue or fluid obtained from involved sites, e.g., skin, subcutaneous nodule, joint, or lung. Histopathologic findings are usually nonspecific, and the characteristic yeastlike cells are often not identified by special stains such as Gomori methenamine silver (GMS) or periodic acid–Schiff (PAS). Direct immunofluorescence, if available, may be helpful. Although testing of serum of CSF by latex agglutination or enzyme immunoassay for antibody to *S. schenckii* may be useful, especially in patients suspected of having extracutaneous disease, positive low-level antibody titers may be observed in normal persons. No skin test is commercially available.

TREATMENT. Conventional therapy for cutaneous sporotrichosis is saturated solution of potassium iodide, which is begun at a dosage of 5 drops three times a day and increased in a dropwise fashion (3 to 5 drops per day) up to a maximum of 120 drops per day or until the development of iodine toxicity (manifested by rash, lacrimation, parotid swelling, or nonspecific gastrointestinal symptoms). Iodide therapy should be continued for at least 1 month after clinical resolution of the disease. Itraconazole, an investigational oral triazole, in a dosage of 100 to 200 mg per day, is more effective than ketoconazole, an imidazole; is better tolerated than potassium iodide; and offers promise as the drug of choice for cutaneous sporotrichosis. Amphotericin B should be given to patients with cutaneous disease in whom iodide or azole therapy fails and to all patients with extracutaneous disease (total dose, 2.0 to 3.0 grams). Cure rates may be improved in selected patients with bone and joint disease or single-cavity pulmonary disease by surgical resection of synovial tissue, bone, or lung, as an adjunct to amphotericin B. Intra-articular amphotericin B may also be useful. The role of itraconazole in the treatment of extracutaneous disease has not been established.

PROGNOSIS. Although untreated cutaneous sporotrichosis may remit and relapse for years, and rarely disseminate, the likelihood of cure with iodide or itraconazole therapy is high. In contrast, extracutaneous disease is more refractory, even to therapy including amphotericin B and surgery; significant morbidity and mortality are frequent sequelae.

Dunstan RW, Langham RF, Reimann KA, et al.: Feline sporotrichosis: A report of five cases with transmission to humans. J Am Acad Dermatol 15:37, 1986. *Seven humans exposed to five cats developed disease, illustrating the potential importance of animal-to-human transmission.*

Pluss JL, Opal SM: Pulmonary sporotrichosis: Review of treatment and outcome. Medicine (Baltimore) 65:143, 1986. *A comprehensive review of 58 cases, with emphasis on management.*

Restreppo A, Robledo J, Gomez I, et al.: Itraconazole therapy in lymphangitic and cutaneous sporotrichosis. Arch Dermatol 122:413, 1986. *Total resolution without relapse was achieved in 82 per cent of patients treated for 3 to 5 months with 100 mg per day.*

Scott EN, Kaufman L, Brown A, et al.: Serologic studies in the diagnosis and management of meningitis due to *Sporothrix schenckii*. N Engl J Med 317:935, 1987. *A description of seven cases, all of whom had antibody to S. schenckii in CSF and serum.*

Winn RE: Sporotrichosis. Infect Dis Clin North Am 2:899, 1988. *An up-to-date literature review, emphasizing the varied clinical manifestations of sporotrichosis. Includes 74 references.*

405 Candidiasis

William E. Dismukes

DEFINITION. *Candida* species can cause a variety of clinical syndromes that are generically termed candidiasis and are usually categorized by site of involvement. Broadly speaking, the two most common syndromes are mucocutaneous candidiasis (e.g., stomatitis or thrush, esophagitis, and vaginitis) and invasive or deep organ candidiasis (e.g., fungemia, endocarditis, and endophthalmitis). In most patients, candidiasis is an opportunistic disease.

ETIOLOGY. Among more than 150 recognized species of *Candida*, *C. albicans* is the most commonly identified pathogen in humans. Other clinically important species include *C. tropicalis, C. parapsilosis, C. krusei, C. pseudotropicalis,* and *C. guilliermondi. Candida* organisms share two morphologic features: small, spherical yeast forms (4 to 6 μm), which reproduce by budding; and pseudohyphae (pseudomycelia), which are chains of elongated yeasts separated by constrictions. In body fluids or tissue, both budding cells and fragments of pseudohyphae may be visualized. Identification and speciation in the microbiology laboratory are based on both morphologic characteristics and results of metabolic tests. The ability of *C. albicans* to produce germ tubes in serum allows presumptive identification. The yeast form of *Torulopsis glabrata* resembles the yeast forms of other *Candida* species; because it does not produce a pseudomycelial form, *T. glabrata* is generally not considered a member of the genus *Candida*.

EPIDEMIOLOGY. Candidiasis occurs worldwide. *Candida albicans* is part of the normal human flora of the mouth, gastrointestinal tract, and vagina; normally lives in balance with other microorganisms in the body; and, in most individuals, exists as a saprophytic colonizer or commensal. When various drugs or conditions, such as broad-spectrum antibiotics, corticosteroids, diabetes mellitus, or human immunodeficiency virus (HIV) infection, upset this balance, *C. albicans*, arising from an endogenous source, may assume the role of pathogen and cause either mucocutaneous or deep disease. *Candida albicans* may also be recovered from soil, hospital environments, food, and other substrates. In contrast to *C. albicans*, the other *Candida* species that are pathogenic for humans may colonize skin but usually not the gastrointestinal tract or vagina of normal individuals. These species more often reside in the environment and on inanimate objects and thus reach the body from exogenous sources; consequently, they are generally regarded as opportunistic fungal pathogens. Unlike other fungi, *Candida* species may be transmitted from person to person, e.g., between sexual partners, by hands of medical personnel, and during birth from colonized vagina to neonatal oropharynx.

Candidiasis, both mucocutaneous and deep forms, has emerged as the most common opportunistic fungal disease over recent decades, owing to the progressively increasing use of antibiotics (both prophylactic and therapeutic); immunosuppressive and cytotoxic drugs; indwelling foreign bodies, including prosthetic heart valves, prosthetic joints, and intravascular monitoring devices; venous, arterial, urinary, and peritoneal catheters; and organ transplantation. In addition, the ongoing acquired immunodeficiency syndrome (AIDS) epidemic has been highly contributory.

PATHOGENESIS AND PATHOLOGY. Several components of the host defense system are important in protecting against infection with *Candida* species. An intact integumentary barrier, including skin and mucous membranes, prevents invasion of normally colonizing organisms, which possess adherence properties as yet not fully understood. *Candida albicans* and *C. tropicalis* appear to be more adherent than other species, accounting in part for the frequency of these organisms as pathogens. Disruption or loss of normal barriers as a consequence of percutaneous catheters, endotracheal tubes, severe burns, or abdominal surgery is a common predisposing factor, especially to deep invasive or disseminated disease. Polymorphonuclear leukocytes and monocytes are the major cellular defenses against *Candida* species; intracellular killing is largely dependent upon the myeloperoxidase, hydrogen peroxide, and superoxide anion systems. While the role of tissue macrophages is unclear, lymphocytes and cell-mediated immunity appear to play a role. Abnormalities of host defense include T cell dysfunction, which predisposes to mucocutaneous disease (oropharyngeal or esophageal candidiasis in HIV-infected persons as well as chronic mucocutaneous candidiasis), and granulocytopenia secondary to underlying disease or therapy, which predisposes to deep disease (candidemia or invasive candidiasis). In cutaneous candidiasis, histopathologic evidence of chronic dermatitis with yeasts confined to the stratum corneum is characteristic. By contrast, microabscesses interspersed in normal tissue are the characteristic pathologic finding in visceral candidiasis. Neutrophils appear initially, followed by histiocytes and giant cells and, in some cases, a readily apparent granulomatous response. In severely immunocompromised patients, the inflammatory response may be minimal or absent. Both yeasts and pseudohyphae can usually be visualized by special stains, such as periodic acid–Schiff (PAS) or Gomori methenamine silver (GMS).

CLINICAL MANIFESTATIONS

Mucocutaneous Infections. Thrush or oropharyngeal candidiasis is manifested by creamy white curdlike exudative patches on the tongue, buccal mucosa, palate, or other oral mucosal surfaces. These patches are actually pseudomembranes, which, upon removal, may leave a raw, bleeding, painful surface. Poorly fitting dentures may be a predisposing factor. Cheilosis, an inflammatory reaction at the corners of the mouth, and atrophic changes, either acute or chronic, are less common presentations of oropharyngeal disease. Esophagitis, which may occur as an extension of thrush or may occur in the absence of thrush in up to one third of patients, is manifested typically by odynophagia, dysphagia, or substernal chest pain and uncommonly by bleeding. Thrush or esophagitis, occurring in the absence of any known predisposing condition, should raise the suspicion of HIV infection. Gastrointestinal candidiasis involving the mucosa of the stomach and small and large bowel is most common in patients with cancer and is an important source of disseminated infection.

Intertrigo, a cutaneous *Candida* infection involving warm, moist surfaces, such as the axillae, gluteal and inframammary folds, and groin, may be variable in appearance but is usually manifested as well-marginated, erythematous, exudative patches surrounded by satellite vesicles or pustules. Paronychia, a painful, tense, reddened swelling at the base of the nail or along the sides, is commonly caused by *Candida* species, especially in diabetics and persons whose hands are chronically immersed in water. Although *Candida* species may cause onychomycosis, this chronic deforming infection of the nails is most frequently due to one of the genera of superficial dermatophytes, such as *Trichophyton* or *Epidermophyton*. Vulvovaginitis, probably the most common *Candida* mucocutaneous infection in women, especially in association with pregnancy, antibiotic therapy, and diabetes, is characterized by thick, creamy vaginal discharge, erythematous labia, and intense pruritus. Balanitis in males, often acquired through sexual intercourse, is manifested by superficial vesicles and exudative patches, usually on the glans penis. *Candida* cystitis, which at cystoscopy resembles oral thrush, is most often a complication of an indwelling bladder catheter. Chronic mucocutaneous candidiasis, a rare condition manifested by a heterogeneous group of persistent, often disfiguring *Candida* infections involving skin, mucous membranes, hair, and nails, occurs primarily in persons with altered T cell function or an endocrinopathy such as hypoparathyroidism or hypoadrenalism.

Deep Organ Candidiasis. Numerous diagnostic categories or labels for serious or deep *Candida* infection exist, including candidemia, disseminated candidiasis, systemic candidiasis, invasive candidiasis, visceral candidiasis, and terms indicating involvement of specific organs, such as hepatosplenic candidiasis and ocular candidiasis. Here, discussion focuses on two major categories: candidemia, which may or may not be associated with visceral organ involvement; and disseminated candidiasis, which implies systemic multiorgan disease and encompasses other subgroups, such as visceral, invasive, and hepatosplenic disease.

Candidemia. Candidemia, which is usually defined as more than one positive blood culture for *Candida* species, may occur in the presence or absence of clinical manifestations, e.g., fever or skin lesions. The incidence of candidemia has risen dramatically over recent years in association with the increased number of compromised hosts (e.g., those with AIDS, cancer, or burns, those in the postsurgical intensive care unit, and organ transplant recipients) managed by aggressive interventions, including empiric antibiotics, cytotoxic chemotherapy, hemodialysis, intravenous and intra-arterial catheters, other intravascular devices, and parenteral alimentation. In many hospitals, *Candida* has become one of the three to five most common microorganisms isolated from blood cultures. Previously, "transient candidemia" was used to imply short duration (<24 hours) of fungemia and indicate either clearing of the candidemia upon removal of an infected intravascular catheter or a benign condition that did not require antifungal therapy. Recent data argue against this concept and suggest that catheter removal alone is insufficient, even in the noncompromised patient, to prevent metastatic hematogenous dissemination to visceral organs. Accordingly, most investigators now believe that all patients with candidemia, regardless of duration or circumstances, deserve some form of antifungal treatment. Controversy at present centers on which drug, at what dose, and for how long (see Treatment below).

Candida albicans is the most common species identified in blood. Studies from multiple medical centers indicate that *C. tropicalis* is the most likely species in the leukemic population, while *C. parapsilosis* fungemia occurs most frequently in patients with solid tumor or nononcologic diseases, especially in association with cannula-related sepsis and hyperalimentation. *Torulopsis glabrata* resembles *C. parapsilosis* in its predilection for patients with solid tumors or nononcologic disorders.

Cannulas of various types are the most important portals of entry, accounting for more than one half of the episodes of candidemia. In almost all cases, removal of cannulas, either peripheral or central, is necessary for eradication of candidemia. Other common sources of infection are the gastrointestinal tract, especially in granulocytopenic patients, and surgical wounds. The urinary and respiratory tracts, while frequently colonized by *Candida* species, are less common sources of bloodstream infection. The mortality rate of candidemia caused by all species is high, ranging from 40 to 80 per cent; *T. glabrata* is associated with the highest mortality. The mortality rate in cannula-associated candidemia is lower than in candidemia related to other sources.

The frequency with which candidemia results in localized single-organ disease (e.g., ocular candidiasis) or widespread disseminated multiorgan disease is unknown. Premortem diagnosis of invasive or disseminated candidiasis must be based on histopathologic demonstration of *Candida* organisms invading tissue. Since blood cultures are negative in at least 50 per cent of patients with disseminated candidiasis and there are no other reliable markers, such as serologic tests, systemic *Candida* disease

may not be suspected and appropriate invasive diagnostic procedures may not be performed. Autopsy series indicate that disseminated disease involving kidneys, liver, spleen, brain, myocardium, and eyes is most likely in patients with some rapidly fatal underlying disease, such as leukemia complicated by neutropenia, and is least likely in patients with candidemia in the setting of nononcologic disease, especially cannula-related sepsis. In addition, patients whose candidemia is treated are less likely to develop disseminated disease.

Cutaneous Lesions of Disseminated Candidiasis. Papulopustules or macronodules on an erythematous base, usually widely distributed over the trunk and extremities, are the hallmark lesions associated with persistent candidemia. Hemorrhagic bullae have also been reported.

Ocular Candidiasis. This form of localized candidiasis may result from either hematogenous spread or direct inoculation, e.g., after cataract extraction or implantation of an intraocular lens. Any eye structure may be infected; endophthalmitis is the most fulminant manifestation and may result in blindness. Single or multiple fluffy white cotton ball–like chorioretinal lesions, often extending into the vitreous, are characteristic. These lesions can be easily recognized on fundoscopic examination and should be serially looked for in all patients with known candidemia.

Renal Candidiasis. Infection of the kidneys may be secondary to ascending extension from the bladder (*Candida* cystitis), resulting in papillary necrosis, caliceal invasion, or formation of a fungus ball in the ureter or renal pelvis. More commonly, renal candidiasis is secondary to hematogenous spread, in patients with either documented or undocumented candidemia, resulting in pyelonephritis with diffuse cortical and medullary abscesses. The triad of candidemia, candiduria, and *Candida* organisms within casts in urinary sediment provides presumptive evidence of upper urinary tract involvement.

Hepatosplenic Candidiasis. This visceral form of deep infection occurs most commonly in patients with hematologic malignancies, especially leukemia, who are in remission after prolonged chemotherapy-induced neutropenia. Gastrointestinal candidiasis complicated by portal fungemia is the source in most patients; documented candidemia or evidence of disease in other organs is usually absent. Persistent unexplained fever, right upper quadrant tenderness and pain, elevated alkaline phosphatase levels and multiple, scattered "bull's eye" lesions in the liver and spleen, demonstrated by abdominal ultrasonographic examination or computed tomography (CT), are features. Diagnosis is established by characteristic histopathology on liver biopsy.

Pulmonary Candidiasis. Whereas colonization by yeasts of the tracheobronchial tree is common in seriously ill, debilitated intensive care unit patients on ventilators, bona fide pneumonia caused by *Candida* species is rare. Diagnosis should be based on histopathologic evidence of yeast invasion.

Cardiac Candidiasis. Disseminated candidiasis is complicated frequently by *Candida* myocarditis (more than 50 per cent of cases) and occasionally by *Candida* pericarditis. *Candida* is the most common cause of fungal endocarditis and should be suspected in the setting of indwelling cardiac prostheses, intravenous drug abuse, and prolonged use of central intravenous catheters for chemotherapy, hyperalimentation, or hemodynamic monitoring. Because fungal valvular vegetations are large and friable, major embolic events involving the central nervous system, coronary arteries, and large peripheral arteries are common.

Central Nervous System Candidiasis. Meningitis and intracerebral microabscesses as well as macroabscesses frequently complicate disseminated candidiasis. Cerebrospinal fluid pleocytosis, most often lymphocytic, hypoglycorrhachia, and elevated protein levels are typical; yeast organisms can be identified by wet preparation, Gram stain, or culture, in fewer than one half of cases. *Candida* meningitis may be a complication of ventricular shunt infection.

Musculoskeletal Candidiasis. Manifestations include myositis (abscess) in neutropenic patients and costochondritis, arthritis, and osteomyelitis (special predilection for vertebrae and intervertebral discs) in intravenous drug users. All of these complications may develop in any patient with disseminated candidiasis, whatever the setting or source.

DIAGNOSIS. Mucocutaneous lesions are diagnosed on the

basis of clinical appearance and by examination of potassium hydroxide wet mounts or Gram-stained smears of lesion material obtained by scraping or swabbing. Masses of spherical budding yeast forms and pseudohyphae are characteristic. Patients suspected of having *Candida* esophagitis should undergo not only endoscopy and brushing but also biopsy in an attempt to demonstrate, histopathologically, mucosal invasion of *Candida* organisms. Esophagitis caused by either herpes simplex virus or cytomegalovirus may mimic the symptoms and appearance of *Candida* esophagitis; infection in a single patient caused by more than one microorganism is not unusual. Fungal blood cultures in patients with suspected candidemia or disseminated candidiasis should be performed using the highly sensitive lysis centrifugation method; this technique also allows more rapid detection of growth. Multiple serial cultures should be obtained. A patient with a single positive blood culture for *Candida* species poses a difficult clinical dilemma. Such a patient should be carefully evaluated for evidence of disseminated disease; foreign bodies, especially intravascular catheters, should be removed and additional blood cultures obtained. Two or more positive blood cultures should be assumed to represent clinically significant disease, which warrants antifungal therapy. The finding of heavy growth of *Candida* species in cultures of sputum, tracheal aspirate, wounds, or urine may increase the likelihood of bloodstream invasion but does not prove that dissemination has occurred. Since blood cultures may be negative in as many as 50 per cent of patients with disseminated candidiasis, diagnosis must often depend on the results of histopathologic study and fungal cultures of tissue obtained by biopsy. Diagnostic procedures that should be considered include CT of the head, thorax, and abdomen; echocardiography; thoracentesis; arthrocentesis; lumbar puncture; and biopsy of skin, liver, kidney, myocardium, bone, muscle, or lung. Although quantitative or semiquantitative cultures of selected tissue specimens have been advocated as useful predictors of disseminated disease, no correlative data support this concept. Skin testing with *Candida* antigen may be useful in assessing for anergy but has no role in diagnosing candidiasis. Although much effort has been devoted to the development of reliable, simple, sensitive, and specific serologic assays for detection of serum antibodies to *Candida* or circulating *Candida* antigen, controversy persists about the value of these serodiagnostic procedures. Because false-positive and false-negative results are common, the decision to initiate treatment cannot be based on results of serologic tests alone.

TREATMENT. In most patients with mucocutaneous infections, any one of several topical preparations, including nystatin, clotrimazole, miconazole, econazole, butoconazole, and ketoconazole, provides effective therapy. Nystatin suspension and clotrimazole troches appear to be equal in efficacy as therapy for oral thrush, but clotrimazole is better tolerated. Although the clinical manifestations of *Candida* vulvovaginitis are usually eliminated by local topical therapy with nystatin, clotrimazole, butoconazole, or miconazole administered for 3 to 7 days, the disease tends to recur frequently in some patients. Newer approaches to the management of acute vulvovaginitis utilize single-dose therapy, e.g., clotrimazole, 500-mg vaginal pessary; miconazole, 1200-mg ovule; or fluconazole, 150-mg oral tablet. In refractory cases, prolonged therapy with a topical agent or an orally absorbed azole, such as ketoconazole or fluconazole, provided that pregnancy has been excluded, may be beneficial. Oral ketoconazole, 200 to 400 mg daily, is the treatment of choice for chronic mucocutaneous candidiasis and must be continued indefinitely to avoid relapse. HIV-infected patients with mucocutaneous forms of candidiasis respond less rapidly than other patient groups and often with incomplete clearance of exudative patches. Nystatin suspension appears to be less effective than either clotrimazole troches or an oral drug, e.g., ketoconazole or fluconazole, in AIDS patients with oropharyngeal or esophageal candidiasis. Fluconazole appears to be more effective than ketoconazole. In refractory cases with severe disease, low-dose intravenous amphotericin B can be employed.

Therapy for serious *Candida* disease, such as candidemia or disseminated candidiasis, remains highly controversial. Although most authorities consider amphotericin B to be the mainstay of treatment, there have been no large prospective clinical trials to delineate optimal daily dose, total dose, or duration of amphotericin B therapy. Consequently, present guidelines are largely empiric. In most patients with catheter-related candidemia, the catheter, if still present, should be removed. In patients with suppurative peripheral thrombophlebitis, surgical segmental venous resection may be necessary. Because of the high risk of metastatic complications of candidemia, such as endophthalmitis, osteomyelitis, arthritis, and endocarditis, there is increasing evidence to support the approach that all patients with candidemia, even nonneutropenic hosts, should have a course of antifungal chemotherapy. Both low-dose amphotericin B regimens, 0.3 to 0.4 mg per kilogram per day or a 200- to 400-mg total dose, and high-dose regimens, 0.5 to 0.8 mg per kilogram per day or a 500- to 800-mg total dose, have been advocated. Until clearer guidelines are forthcoming from ongoing prospective studies, the decision regarding which regimen to employ must be based on the host defense status of the patient, underlying conditions, predisposing factors, and results of serial blood cultures and physical examinations to search for complications of candidemia.

Patients with documented disseminated disease, manifested either as localized deep disease (hepatosplenic candidiasis, central nervous system candidiasis, renal candidiasis, or *Candida* endocarditis) or as multiorgan disease, should be treated with amphotericin B (total dose, 2.0 to 3.0 grams) plus flucytosine (100 to 150 mg per kilogram per day). Because flucytosine may be associated with significant toxicity, including bone marrow suppression, hepatitis, diarrhea, and rash, serum flucytosine levels should be regularly monitored and the dosage adjusted to maintain levels in the range of 50 to 100 μg per milliliter. Valve replacement is a necessary adjunct to chemotherapy in patients with *Candida* endocarditis.

Current data do not justify the treatment of candidemia or disseminated candidiasis with newer oral antifungal azoles such as fluconazole. Prospective studies are ongoing to address this issue. Similarly, the role of immunomodulators, e.g., human granulocyte colony-stimulating factor, in the therapy of serious *Candida* disease has not yet been defined.

Candida cystitis, in contrast to renal candidiasis, can be cured by removal of the bladder catheter in the majority of cases. Therapeutic options available for the management of candiduria that is persistent after catheter removal or in diabetic patients include oral flucytosine, 75 to 100 mg per kilogram per day for 7 to 10 days, or oral fluconazole, 100 to 200 mg per day for 7 to 10 days. Although both of these antifungal agents are excreted by the kidneys, fluconazole is preferred because it is less toxic. Eradication of candiduria in patients whose condition justifies a persistent indwelling catheter can be attempted with amphotericin B (50 μg per milliliter) or miconazole (50 μg per milliliter) bladder rinses.

Therapy for *Candida* peritonitis, which most often is a complication of peritoneal dialysis, is less straightforward. Ideally, the peritoneal catheter should be discontinued, and either intravenous amphotericin B or oral fluconazole should be administered until clinical symptoms and signs resolve and cultures become negative. For patients in whom the catheter must be maintained, instillation of amphotericin B, 2 to 4 μg per milliliter in the dialysate fluid, has been successfully employed.

The management of ocular candidiasis requires close cooperation with an ophthalmologist experienced in eye infections. Although reports indicate that hematogenously acquired *Candida* eye disease not involving the vitreous may heal spontaneously, for most cases, systemic amphotericin B, with or without flucytosine, plus vitrectomy to remove vitreous abscesses is required. Findings at vitrectomy may also be used to confirm the diagnosis. Oral ketoconazole is reportedly effective, especially in endophthalmitis secondary to intravenous heroin use, but ketoconazole cannot be recommended over amphotericin B.

PREVENTION. Given the increasing incidence of nosocomial candidemia, with its high mortality rate, excess length of hospital stay, and potential for multiorgan complications, focus on awareness of the problem and development of measures aimed at prevention assume increasing importance. In selected clinical situations as discussed above, suspicion of candidemia or deep organ candidiasis should be high, and appropriate diagnostic studies pursued. Once the diagnosis is established, intensive antifungal therapy must be given. In addition, factors that predispose to *Candida* disease should be controlled or avoided, whenever possible. For example, the frequency and duration of use of intravascular catheters and monitoring devices should be reduced, and central catheters should be changed at least weekly. Special care should be paid to long-term access devices for chemotherapy, such as Hickman or Broviac catheters. Similarly, the frequency, breadth, and duration of courses of antibiotics should be reduced. Prophylactic regimens of oral nystatin, clotrimazole, ketoconazole, or fluconazole are widely employed in granulocytopenic patients to prevent *Candida* infection. Two problems, however, are associated with their use. First, their efficacy has not been unequivocally established. Second, azole-containing regimens may be associated with development of resistance of *Candida* species to amphotericin B.

Crislip MA, Edwards JE Jr: Candidiasis. Infect Dis Clin North Am 3:103, 1989. *A comprehensive, up-to-date review, with a nice perspective on clinical syndromes and treatment and 182 references.*

Jones JM: Laboratory diagnosis of invasive candidiasis. Clin Microbiol Rev 3:32, 1990. *A thorough, thoughtful perspective on the role of the microbiology laboratory, with a good analysis of the current status of serologic tests for candidiasis. Includes 131 references.*

Komshian SV, Uwaydah AK, Sobel JD, et al.: Fungemia caused by *Candida* species and *Torulopsis glabrata* in the hospitalized patient: Frequency, characteristics, and evaluation of factors influencing outcome. Rev Infect Dis 11:379, 1989. *Detailed univariate and multivariate analyses of the risk factors for development of candidemia and predictors of outcome among 135 cases occurring between 1983 and 1986. The findings lead the authors to argue against the concept of cannula-related candidemia as a benign disease.*

Thaler M, Behram P, Shawker T, et al.: Hepatic candidiasis in cancer patients: The evolving picture of the syndrome. Ann Intern Med 108:88, 1988. *A review of 68 cases with emphasis on diagnosis and therapy.*

Wey SB, Mori M, Pfaller MA, et al.: Hospital-acquired candidemia: The attributable mortality and excess length of stay. Arch Intern Med 148:2642, 1988. Wey SB, Mori M, Pfaller MA, et al.: Risk factors for hospital-acquired candidemia: A matched case-control study. Arch Intern Med 149:2349, 1989. *Two comparison papers that further our understanding of this increasingly recognized nosocomial infection.*

406 Aspergillosis

David A. Stevens

DEFINITION. Aspergillosis refers to infection with any of the species of the genus *Aspergillus*. These are in mold form in the environment, on artificial media, and when invading tissues.

ETIOLOGY AND EPIDEMIOLOGY. Aspergilli are ubiquitous in the environment and have been isolated with ease from fertile soil and air, and even swimming pools and saunas. They are associated with decaying matter and may grow well in any self-heating organic composting process; these processes attain temperatures of 40 to 50°C. The ease with which they are isolated from sewage sludge composting, from silos, and from the cooling canals of nuclear power plants has been an environmental and industrial concern. They are easily isolated from the human habitat, e.g., in houses, particularly from basements, crawl spaces, bedding, and house dust; and in surveys they have been found in, for example, 94 per cent of pasta samples and 92 per cent of marijuana samples. This pervasiveness should not make it surprising that they are found in 16 per cent of normal expectorated sputa. They are important pathogens of insects (of economic importance to beekeepers) and of birds, both domesticated and wild, in which the air sacs and lungs are targets. They are also important because of the production of toxins, particularly aflatoxin, one of the most potent carcinogens known, which are products of their growth and which contaminate the food chain, posing a risk to animals and humans. Their threat to hospitalized patients has been revealed in outbreaks of infection, particularly pulmonary infection in compromised hosts, associated with renovation and new construction. The suspected vector has been unfiltered air, as from inlets contaminated with bird excreta and fireproofing materials.

The most common species infecting humans are *A. fumigatus, A. flavus, A. niger,* and *A. terreus.* Some are speciated by the clinical laboratory only with difficulty, and they may be reported to the clinician only as "*Aspergillus* species." In tissues they may be seen as septate hyphae, dichotomously branched (resembling the divergence of fingers from one another), and they may produce their characteristic conidia in tissues or artificial media, which is one means of their differentiation. If the septation can be seen, they can be differentiated from the zygomycetes; they may be confused with *Pseudallescheria boydii,* however, unless the characteristic terminal spores of the latter are seen.

Aspergillosis generally results from airborne conidia and is not contagious.

SYNDROMES. The main forms of clinical aspergillosis are shown in Table 406–1.

The *invasive* form of the disease is generally a problem of immunocompromised hosts (Ch. 287), and more aggressive immunosuppression and anticancer therapy are the most important factors contributing to the rise of *Aspergillus* infections. Series have reported an incidence as high as 41 per cent in those with acute leukemia at autopsy, and in 89 per cent of these cases it played a significant role in the death of the patient. In 97 per cent, pulmonary involvement was present, and in 25 per cent, the infection was disseminated widely to various organs. Similarly, in a group of heart transplant patients, the incidence of infection was 28 per cent. This is also a problem in diabetics and patients with the neutrophil defect of chronic granulomatous disease. Diagnosis is difficult because aspergilli are frequently contaminants in sputum and even in other cultures when handled in the laboratory. In patients with leukemia, there is particularly an association with relapses of the malignancy, and usually three or four of the following factors are present: leukopenia, steroid therapy, cytotoxic chemotherapy, and broad-spectrum antibacterials. In addition, hypogammaglobulinemia is common. The classic picture is that of fever and pulmonary infiltrates or nodules, especially progressing to a cavity (usually when granulocytopenia is reversed), or wedge-shaped densities resembling infarcts. The pulmonary pathology in all these entities is that of hemorrhagic infarction and pneumonia. Pulmonary emboli are common because of the organism's tendency to invade blood vessel walls. These processes often combine to produce a "target lesion" pathologically, consisting of a necrotic center surrounded by a ring of hemorrhage. The sputum culture is positive in only 8 to 34 per cent of cases, and obtaining tissue is necessary to make the diagnosis. Prospective culturing of the nose of granulocytopenic patients has been of some value, because a positive nasal culture (and particularly the presence of nasal *Aspergillus* lesions) has led to the early diagnosis of concurrent pulmonary disease. However, negative nasal cultures are common in pulmonary aspergillosis.

Targets of *disseminated disease* include the central nervous system, where abscesses are characteristic. The cerebrospinal fluid (CSF) glucose level is normal, and cultures of the CSF are negative. Mycelia invading blood vessels may produce a microangiopathic hemolytic anemia. Dissemination can result in Budd-Chiari syndrome, myocardial infarction, gastrointestinal disease, or skin lesions. Esophageal ulcers may produce gastrointestinal bleeding. Abscesses are common in the kidney, liver, and myocardium.

Seventy-two per cent of *endocarditis* cases have occurred after cardiac surgery, and 69 per cent of these were associated with prostheses. Intravenous drug addicts are also susceptible. Eighty-three per cent of affected individuals have major arterial emboli, and neurologic presentations are common. Only 8 per cent have positive blood cultures, and this positivity is usually delayed 14 to 20 days, contributing to the poor record of diagnosis ante mortem (23 per cent), which is usually made on histologic examination of an embolus. Overall survival is about 5 per cent, or 22 per cent of those diagnosed ante mortem, and these individuals have had valve replacement. The disease should be suspected in any post–cardiac surgery patient who presents with endocarditis or emboli and negative blood cultures.

TABLE 406–1. ASPERGILLOSIS SYNDROMES

Invasive disease	Allergic bronchopulmonary disease
Aspergilloma (mycetoma)	Pleural disease
Superficial bronchial disease	Local disease
Extrinsic allergic alveolitis	Endocarditis
Mixed disease	

The typical picture of a *mycetoma* (aspergilloma) is a fungus ball (matted hyphae and debris) in a cavity in an upper lobe (Fig. 406–1). The mycetoma has been reported as a complication in as many as 11 per cent of old tuberculous cavities. The patients present with cough (87 per cent), hemoptysis (81 per cent), dyspnea (61 per cent), weight loss (61 per cent), fatigue (61 per cent), chest pain (31 per cent), or fever (25 per cent). The sputum culture is positive in most. Total immunoglobulin G (IgG) and immunoglobulin A (IgA) levels are elevated. Invasion of the parenchyma is rare.

Pleural disease is associated with tuberculosis and bronchopleural fistulas. It may occur after surgery or spontaneously.

Allergic bronchopulmonary aspergillosis is usually seen superimposed on a background of chronic asthma (see Ch. 57) or cystic fibrosis. It is characterized by episodic airway obstruction, fever, eosinophilia, mucous plugs, positive sputum cultures, and the presence of grossly visible brown flecks in the sputum (hyphae), transient infiltrates and parallel "tram-line" or ring markings on chest radiographs, proximal bronchiectasis, upper lobe contraction, and elevated levels of total IgA and immunoglobulin E (IgE) (especially when the patient is symptomatic). It is more common in agricultural areas and in the winter, presumably representing an association with stored agricultural products (especially moldy hay) and spore production. The eosinophilia is present in blood, sputum, and the lung on biopsy. The mucous plugs contain mycelia, and the plugs may be the cause of the infiltrates, with collapse and inflammation occurring peripherally, or inflammatory edema may be responsible. The parallel or ring markings are caused by thickened ectatic bronchi, and the upper lobe changes are a result of progressive apical fibrosis. The infiltrates may be nonsegmental and transient, with a clinical presentation of "eosinophilic pneumonia" and asthma, with eosinophils in blood and sputum; alternatively, they may be segmental, associated with the blocking of bronchi by plugs, and asthma and eosinophilia may be absent. A biphasic skin test response may assist in the diagnosis. A scratch test with *Aspergillus* antigens produces an immediate type I wheal and flare reaction, mediated by IgE and blocked by antihistamines, but not by corticosteroids. An intracutaneous test with the antigens produces a later (6 to 8 hours) Arthus-type reaction, mediated by IgG antibody and complement and blocked by steroids. Similarly, bronchial challenge with the antigens can produce a biphasic response. Immediate, short-lived wheezing may result, reproducing the asthmatic symptoms and associated with increased airways resistance; this can be blocked by isoproterenol, antihistamines, and cromolyn, but not by steroids. There may be a later (2 to 6 hours) reaction, of two types. One is increased airways resistance, as described. The other is a restrictive defect occurring peripherally, which may be associated with influenza-like symptoms, fever, leukocytosis, and infiltrates. These reactions are associated with IgG precipitins and are believed to account for some transient infiltrates.

Extrinsic allergic alveolitis is an unusual form of *Aspergillus* lung disease and has been most associated with *A. clavatus* in malt workers. The patients develop dyspnea and fever 4 hours after exposure, and the clinical picture resembles that of the better known bird-fancier's lung or farmer's lung (due to other allergens). Diffuse micronodular infiltrates may be present at the time of symptoms. The patients have IgG precipitins and cell-mediated immune reactions against *Aspergillus* antigens, and granulomas are present on biopsy. Eosinophilia is not a feature. The scratch test is negative, although an intradermal test produces a reaction in 4 hours, with immunoglobulins and complement present on biopsy. Bronchial challenge produces a reaction in 4 hours, with systemic symptoms and a restrictive defect but without airways resistance. The entity can progress to irreversible fibrosis. The same pathophysiology may be involved in episodes following massive inhalation of spores, usually in farm environments. Symptoms are present within 24 hours, and granulomas are found on biopsy.

Superficial bronchial disease, with features similar to those of acute or chronic bronchitis due to bacterial pathogens, may occur. Brown-flecked sputum and positive sputum cultures are associated. The allergic bronchopulmonary, alveolitis, and superficial forms rarely progress to invasive disease. *Chronic necrotizing pulmonary aspergillosis* is a poorly defined entity that usually occurs in patients with underlying lung disease, often with features of invasive disease and mycetoma.

Examples of *locally invasive disease* abound and are usually severe. These include invasion of burn wounds, keratitis or external otitis (particularly in the tropics), sinusitis (particularly in immunosuppressed and/or granulocytopenic hosts), and osteomyelitis or endophthalmitis (after fungemia, trauma, or surgery). Cutaneous ulcers have been associated with the use of adhesive tape. Bloodborne disease in addicts can produce foci of dissemination that are similar to those associated with the invasive pulmonary form of the disease. A noninvasive form of sinus disease with a predominantly allergic component and eosinophilia, responsive to drainage and corticosteroids, has also been described.

DIAGNOSIS. Some of the modalities of diagnosis have been mentioned in connection with specific syndromes. Common to several of the syndromes mentioned is the use of serodiagnosis. Antibody assays have been reported most commonly using radioimmunoassay, complement fixation, and immunodiffusion, but techniques such as immunofluorescence, counterimmunoelectrophoresis, passive hemagglutination, and enzyme-linked immunosorbent assay (ELISA) also show promise. A variety of methods for preparing antigen have been used. Data from the more commonly reported techniques suggest a high degree of sensitivity in allergic disease or aspergillomas, but generally a low sensitivity in invasive disease. As the frequency of false-positive reactions, even in the presence of other mycoses, is low (although a majority of marijuana smokers in one study had precipitins), a positive test in invasive disease may be useful. IgE antibody specific to *Aspergillus* antigens is another serodiagnostic adjunct in allergic disease. Detection of antigenemia, most commonly studied by radioimmunoassay, and detection of antigen in bronchoalveolar lavage fluid are also promising in the diagnosis of invasive disease. The problem at present with all serodiagnostic modalities is the lack of a generally available, standardized technique. The physician should know the background data for the laboratory to which the specimens may be sent, i.e., the sensitivity and specificity of the assay in the various syndromes. Serial antibody testing in groups of patients predisposed to aspergillomas (i.e., those with lung cavities), to endocarditis (cardiac surgery patients), or to invasive disease may increase the utility of otherwise problematic serodiagnostic methods.

In invasive disease, an aggressive, invasive approach, as well as making a tissue diagnosis early in the illness, appears to be a key to survival. In the appropriate clinical setting, a positive bronchial lavage or other endobronchial culture, or a repeated isolation of the same species in culture, correlates with invasive disease and may have to be the stimulus for therapy if invasive procedures cannot be done. Negative cultures (other than tissue) do not rule out invasive disease.

THERAPY. In invasive disease, prompt, aggressive chemotherapy has produced superior survival statistics at some institutions, although recovery from neutropenia is a necessary accompaniment of recovery in almost every success. The role of granulocyte transfusions is unclear. In endocarditis, in addition to prompt, aggressive chemotherapy, valve replacement appears necessary. Locally invasive disease in other sites also requires

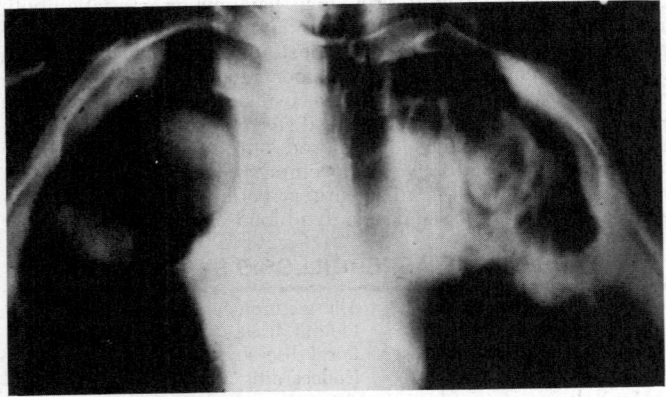

FIGURE 406–1. Tomogram of pulmonary aspergillosis mycetomas.

systemic or local chemotherapy, particularly intravitreal therapy or nephrostomy irrigation in renal disease. Surgical excision has an important role in the invasion of bone, burn wounds, epidural abscesses, vitreal disease, sinus disease of noncompromised hosts, and removal of catheters for peritonitis and of silk sutures in bronchial stump (postpneumonectomy) aspergillosis. It may have a function in invasive pulmonary disease for which chemotherapy has failed.

In cases involving mycetoma, there is evidence that patients with fever, cough, weight loss, malaise, and hemoptysis have an element of allergy, which can be demonstrated by bronchial challenge or the presence of cytophilic IgG and IgE. These patients symptomatically improve if given steroids. Intravenous amphotericin B therapy of patients with mycetoma produces results no better than those with routine pulmonary toilet. Intracavitary amphotericin, instilled through a catheter, is a heroic form of therapy that has been attempted in some patients. The role of surgery in this entity is controversial. Seven to 10 per cent of mycetomas undergo spontaneous lysis. The overall operative mortality aggregated from several series is 7 per cent but may be as high as 14 per cent in some large series. The frequency of various operative complications is 22 per cent, aggregated from several series, with a range of 7 to 60 per cent. Furthermore, new aspergillomas have later developed after surgical successes. On the other hand, in various series, 18 to 26 per cent of patients with adequate follow-up treated without surgery died of disease complications, usually hemoptysis, whereas 50 per cent have shown significant improvement symptomatically and radiographically. If any consensus exists, it is that surgical resection has a role in recurrent, significant hemoptysis. An alternative therapy, particularly for the nonsurgical patient, is selective bronchial arterial embolization to the bleeding vessel.

In pleural disease, local instillation of nystatin, amphotericin, or miconazole has resulted in successes. In allergic disease, measures that have *not* worked include hyposensitization, avoidance of sites in the environment, and aerosolized corticosteroids. Cromolyn is inadequate in most patients. Aerosolized antifungals have produced remissions but do not prevent recurrences. Treatment of the clinical disease is more complicated than the effects of drug blockade demonstrable in challenge tests. The continuous use of systemic corticosteroids can prevent the infiltrates and some accompanying symptoms. Intermittent use of steroids, or raising the dose in patients on chronic therapy, can produce rapid resolution of marked symptomatic episodes. The long-term beneficial effects of steroids are less clear; they are not so useful in arresting dyspnea or wheezing in the long term, and they do not prevent the development of the accompanying bronchiectasis. The proper approach to extrinsic alveolitis is avoidance of the stimulus.

For those entities in which systemic chemotherapy is indicated, almost all clinical experience has been with amphotericin B. Its track record is generally poor in invasive or disseminated disease in compromised hosts (especially so in those with cerebral or hepatic disease or in bone marrow transplant patients). In the compromised host, it should be used aggressively, with prompt progression to a full therapeutic dose, which should be about 1 mg per kilogram per day, if tolerated. Prophylactic therapy may have a role in patients who have survived invasive disease and will become neutropenic again. Rifampin almost always, and flucytosine sometimes, potentiates the activity of amphotericin in vitro against aspergilli. Moreover, animal models have shown an enhanced effect of combinations of these drugs over that with amphotericin alone. Clinical data to support combination therapy are limited, but given the poor record of amphotericin alone in invasive disease, combination therapy appears a logical avenue to explore, particularly if synergy can be demonstrated. A few cures have been reported in invasive disease with flucytosine (which may have a role in cerebral or renal disease) or miconazole alone. Of the new azole drugs, itraconazole is clearly the most promising and as sole therapy has produced responses in invasive disease. Other azoles, lipid-complexed amphotericin B, and other classes of drugs have demonstrated anti-*Aspergillus* activity in vitro, in models, and in a few patients and may represent future avenues of exploration. Comparative clinical trials are needed to assess all alternative forms of systemic therapy.

Denning DW, Stevens DA: The treatment of invasive aspergillosis. Rev Infect Dis 12:1147, 1990. *Reviews and tabulates data from more than 2000 published cases in 497 articles to give a current picture of therapeutic results.*

Gerson SL, Talbot GH, Hurwitz S, et al.: Discriminant scorecard for diagnosis of invasive pulmonary aspergillosis in patients with acute leukemia. Am J Med 79:57, 1985. *The Pennsylvania group published several studies defining the presentation of disease in the granulocytopenic patient. This paper ties many of their observations together in a useful form, presenting an approach to diagnosis when invasive procedures are not possible.*

Patterson R, Greenberger PA, Halwig JM, et al.: Allergic bronchopulmonary aspergillosis: Natural history and classification of early disease by serologic and roentgenographic studies. Arch Intern Med 146:916, 1986. *A recent review of diagnosis and treatment.*

Young RC, Bennett JE, Vogel CL, et al.: Aspergillosis: The spectrum of the disease in 98 patients. Medicine (Baltimore) 49:147, 1970. Meyer RD, Young LS, Armstrong D, et al.: Aspergillosis complicating neoplastic disease. Am J Med 54:6, 1973. *These classic reviews focus on the invasive form of the disease.*

407 Zygomycosis *(Mucormycosis)*

Sandy F. S. Chun and David A. Stevens

DEFINITION. Zygomycosis is generally an acute and rapidly developing fungal infection caused by fungi of the class Zygomycetes. In healthy hosts, these organisms seldom cause infection. However, in debilitated or immunosuppressed hosts, they produce a fulminant opportunistic infection resulting in marked tissue destruction. Several predisposing conditions have been identified. The infection is most commonly associated with the acidotic patient, especially those in diabetic ketoacidosis. Prolonged treatment with antibiotics, corticosteroids, and cytotoxic drugs and, most recently, the use of deferoxamine in the dialysis patient have also been associated, as have severe malnutrition, hematologic malignancies, and extensive burns.

THE PATHOGENS. The pathogenic zygomycetes are largely in the order Mucorales, which is related to the older (and more familiar) term for this infection, mucormycosis. Phycomycosis is another older term in the literature describing the same infections. The zygomycetes are morphologically distinct. Their hyphae are nonseptated, broad, and variable in size and shape. Furthermore, the branching of the hyphae is usually irregular and at right angles. Species of the genera *Rhizopus* and *Mucor* are the common pathogens of this group. Other genera, including *Absidia, Cunninghamella, Rhizomucor, Mortierella, Saksenaea, Syncephalastrum, Entomophthera,* and *Apophysomyces,* have also been reported to cause disease. These fungi cannot be differentiated histopathologically. Further speciation requires culturing of the pathogen and characterization of the isolates by their morphologic and physiologic features.

EPIDEMIOLOGY. The zygomycetes are ubiquitous saprophytic fungi and are abundant in nature. They have been recovered from bread, fruits, vegetables, soil, and manure. These fungi have been isolated from the nose, stool, and sputum of healthy individuals. Despite their widespread distribution, they cause disease infrequently. Fortunately, even in the severely immunocompromised hosts, zygomycosis remains a rare opportunistic infection. The disease is not contagious.

PATHOGENESIS AND PATHOLOGY. Currently, there is no unifying concept of the pathogenesis of zygomycosis. In diseases of the airways (sinus, lung), the infection is presumed to originate from inhaled spores, although the lung may also be involved secondary to bloodstream invasion. Diabetic patients appear to be more frequently colonized. While normal human serum can inhibit their growth, serum obtained from patients with diabetic ketoacidosis is not inhibitory and may even promote fungal growth. Undefined defects of macrophages and neutrophils contribute to the loss of immunity against this infection in the susceptible host. Corticosteroids weaken normal inhibitors of spore germination in tissue. Unlike most pathogenic fungi, these can grow in the absence of oxygen.

Invasion, thrombosis, and necrosis are the characteristic findings in this disease. Once the fungal spores have germinated at the site of infection, the hyphal elements are very aggressive and tend to invade blood vessels, nerves, lymphatics, and tissues. The infarction leads to further tissue hypoxia and acidosis, resulting in a vicious cycle enhancing rapid growth and infection. The paucity of a granulomatous reaction is quite characteristic. The fungal hyphae sometimes have little or no inflammation around them. In contrast to most fungi, these organisms are readily seen in hematoxylin and eosin–stained tissue. The Gomori methenamine silver stain is usually adequate, but some special fungus stains, such as periodic acid–Schiff, do not demonstrate the organism well.

CLINICAL MANIFESTATIONS. Zygomycosis can be manifested as at least six distinct clinical entities, dependent upon the types of predisposing factors of the patient and the portal of entry of the organism (Table 407–1).

Rhinocerebral zygomycosis is the most frequent form of presentation, accounting for more than 75 per cent of the cases in the literature. It commonly affects the poorly controlled diabetic patient who is also in ketoacidosis. It has also been reported in patients with hematologic malignancies who have been neutropenic for an extended period and who have received broad-spectrum antibacterial drugs or immunosuppressive therapy, in other acidotic patients, and in those with azotemia. This is one of the most rapidly fatal fungal diseases if left undiagnosed. Hyphae invade the paranasal sinuses and palate from the oronasal cavity. From the sinuses, especially the ethmoid sinus, the infection spreads to involve the retro-orbital region or the central nervous system. Epistaxis, severe unilateral headache, alteration in mental status, and eye symptoms such as lacrimation, irritation, or periorbital anesthesia are common symptoms. Examination of the nose may reveal the classic black necrotic turbinates (too often mistaken for dried blood) or even nasal septum perforation. However, at the early stage of infection, the nasal mucosa may appear only inflamed and friable. Facial cellulitis and palatal necrosis may be seen. The early eye findings include mild proptosis, periorbital edema, decreased visual acuity, or lid swelling. In more advanced orbital involvement, exophthalmos, complete ophthalmoplegia, conjunctival hemorrhage, blindness, fixed and dilated pupil, and corneal anesthesia may be found. These conditions result from fungal invasion of the roof of the orbit, affecting the nerves (third, fourth, and sixth cranial nerves and the ophthalmic branch of the fifth cranial nerve), muscles, and orbital vessels, a condition also known as the orbital apex syndrome. The infection can spread through the superior orbital fissure or the cribriform plate to involve the brain. Cavernous sinus thrombosis is a frequent complication usually resulting from hematogenous spread from the ophthalmic veins.

This hematogenous spread leads to additional cranial nerve involvement outside the orbital apex, specifically the trigeminal nerve ganglion and the root of the facial nerve, leading to ipsilateral paresthesia of the face or peripheral facial palsy. Internal carotid artery thrombosis, from retrograde spread from the ophthalmic artery or invasion from the cavernous sinus, is another late complication, leading to cerebral infarction. The middle ear may be involved via the blood, cerebrospinal fluid, or eustachian tube.

The radiographic manifestations are nonspecific. Plain roentgenograms of the sinuses and orbits may reveal nodular thickening of the mucosa of multiple sinuses, usually without air-fluid levels, or spotty destruction of the bone through the walls of the sinuses or into the orbit. Computed tomography is useful in better defining the bone destruction and soft tissue involvement, which could be important in guiding subsequent surgical intervention. The cerebrospinal fluid findings are usually nonspecific and often normal even in the presence of central nervous system involvement. The common findings are pleocytosis, with about 50 per cent polymorphonuclear cells and slight protein elevation; hypoglycorrhachia is rare. Smear and culture of cerebrospinal fluid are usually negative for fungus even in cases with documented meningeal involvement. Several infectious diseases can present

TABLE 407–1. CLINICAL MANIFESTATIONS OF ZYGOMYCOSIS

Rhinocerebral	Gastrointestinal
Pulmonary	Widely disseminated
Cutaneous	Central nervous system

a similar picture. Black necrotic lesions may also be seen with invasive aspergillosis and with infections by *Pseudomonas aeruginosa* or *Pseudallescheria boydii*. The only definitive method of differentiating between these possibilities is by examination of tissue. Cavernous sinus thrombosis due to *Staphylococcus aureus*, as well as rhinoscleroma, aggressive orbital tumor, midline granuloma, and other fungal infections, can mimic the disease as well.

Pulmonary zygomycosis occurs most frequently in patients with hematologic malignancies being treated with antibacterial drugs or immunosuppressive therapy. The presentation is usually acute, and the patients are often profoundly ill, with variable complaints of cough, fever, and sputum production. There is no specific lobar predilection. Pulmonary vascular thrombosis and infarction are universal findings. No pathognomonic clinical or radiographic findings exist. Sputum culture is usually negative. In fact, antemortem diagnosis is seldom made because of the acuteness of the illness, the lack of consideration of the diagnosis, and the need for tissue to establish the diagnosis.

Invasive pulmonary candidiasis, aspergillosis, or nocardiosis, other bacterial infections, such as *Pseudomonas* infection, malignant invasion, hemorrhage, or pulmonary embolism and infarction may mimic the presentation of pulmonary mucormycosis.

Cutaneous zygomycosis is rare and is primarily a nosocomial infection in burn victims. Local infection has also resulted from the use of contaminated elastic bandages. The involved area is erythematous and painful, with varying degrees of central necrosis. This form of infection can also occur as a result of dissemination from another site of involvement. Skin and subcutaneous infection in diabetics can occur.

Gastrointestinal zygomycosis is the rarest form of infection. It is seen primarily in patients suffering from intrinsic abnormalities of the gastrointestinal tract or severe malnutrition. The infection is thought to arise from fungi entering the body with food. Any part of the gastrointestinal tract is susceptible to infection, with the stomach, terminal ileum and colon being the most common sites. Wall invasion, ischemic infarction, and ulceration are characteristic. The diagnosis is frequently made at autopsy.

Disseminated zygomycosis is defined as infection occurring in two or more noncontiguous organ systems. The distant sites are infected by bloodstream invasion from a local site. Although any organ can be affected, the lungs and central nervous system are the two common sites. The outcome of this infection is almost invariably fatal.

Isolated central nervous system zygomycosis results from hematogenous spread and is seen primarily in intravenous drug addicts.

DIAGNOSIS. The diagnosis of any form of zygomycosis is dependent on direct and histologic examinations of scrapings and biopsies of necrotic material. Fixed tissue can be stained with hematoxylin and eosin, and fungal hyphae can be seen with this routine histologic stain. However, a more rapid but preliminary diagnosis can sometimes be made by demonstrating hyphal elements after potassium hydroxide digestion of fresh tissue scraping. The alkali digests some of the tissue debris, but not the fungus, and makes the identification of the fungi easier. Swabs of discharge or abnormal tissue are not adequate and can give erroneous information. Fungal cultures are occasionally positive, but a negative culture result does not exclude the diagnosis nor make it less likely. The media used for culturing these fungi should not contain cycloheximide. At present, no skin tests or serologic methods are adequate for diagnosing zygomycosis. Blood cultures are not helpful.

THERAPY. The hallmarks of successful outcome in this aggressive infection rely on early diagnosis by invasive procedures, immediate correction of the underlying predisposing condition, aggressive surgical debridement, and early rapid systemic amphotericin therapy. Amphotericin B is the only drug with proven clinical efficacy, and a high therapeutic dosage (such as 1.0 to 1.5 mg per kilogram per day, if tolerated) should be achieved as soon as possible. This may be reduced to alternate-day dosing once the patient is stabilized. Typically, a cumulative dose of 2 to 5 grams may be needed to achieve cure. Although local irrigation of infected sites with amphotericin is an unproven adjunct, given the difficulties in perfusion of infected areas because of the tendency to thrombosis, this measure seems logical. Similarly, potentiation of amphotericin with other drugs (such as rifampin, flucytosine) is of unproven benefit, but given the poor results with conventional therapy, this should be considered if susceptibility testing can be done in vitro with the patient's isolate to show synergy and exclude antagonism. The newer orally administered azole derivates have no proven activity against these fungi. Improvement of survival may necessitate repeated major surgical debridement of necrotic tissue, resulting in significant disfiguring. If the patient survives, major reconstructive surgery may be needed.

PROGNOSIS. Since its first description by Paltauf in Germany in 1885, zygomycosis remains a disease with guarded prognosis. It is difficult to ascertain accurately the effectiveness of any therapeutic approach because the disease is relatively rare and there is a general bias toward reporting cases only if therapy is effective. With the introduction of amphotericin B in 1961, it is generally accepted that the survival rate significantly improved. Rhinocerebral zygomycosis is the most common form of infection and is thought to have an overall mortality rate of about 50 per cent. Patients who develop hemiplegia, facial necrosis, or nasal deformity have a higher mortality. Pulmonary or disseminated zygomycosis frequently escapes antemortem diagnosis, and only a handful of patients have been reported to recover from these infections.

At this time, the most aggressive approach we can take toward this lethal disease is rapid diagnosis and immediate institution of surgical debridement plus systemic and local chemotherapy.

Bigby TD, Serota ML, Tierney LM, et al.: Clinical spectrum of pulmonary mucormycosis. Chest 89:435, 1986. *This review emphasizes the pulmonary form and includes discussion of the microbiology, pathology, predisposing factors, clinical presentation, diagnosis, and treatment.*

Ferry AP, Abedi S: Diagnosis and management of rhino-orbitocerebral mucormycosis. Ophthalmology 90:1096, 1983. *This article reports the personal experience of the senior author with 16 patients. All the patients had one or more predisposing factors, with diabetes mellitus being the most common.*

Ingram CN, Sennesh J, Cooper JN, et al.: Disseminated zygomycosis: Report of four cases and review. Rev Infect Dis 11:741, 1989. *A presentation of four cases of disseminated disease and a comprehensive review of 181 cases reported in the English language literature. Hematologic malignancy is the major predisposing factor for dissemination. More than 90 per cent of disseminated infections were diagnosed at autopsy.*

408 Mycetoma

Michael S. Saag

DEFINITION. Mycetoma is a chronic, localized, subcutaneous infection characterized by draining sinus tracts that frequently discharge purulent material containing granules. The disease most often affects the lower extremities, with the majority of cases involving the foot. Originally described in the mid-1800's, the disease was initially referred to as "Madura foot," named after the region in India where it was first identified. Although still referred to as maduromycosis, the preferred name and the term used most often to describe the disorder is mycetoma.

ETIOLOGY. More than 20 species of fungi and bacteria have been implicated as etiologic agents of mycetoma. Approximately 40 per cent of cases are due to true fungi (eumycetoma), and 60 per cent are caused by aerobic actinomycetes (actinomycetoma). The organisms are distributed throughout the world, and the predominant organisms responsible for disease are subject to regional variation. Etiologic agents of eumycetoma and actinomycetoma may be presumptively identified based on the characteristic pigment of their granules. A listing of the predominant causative organisms is given in Table 408–1.

EPIDEMIOLOGY. Mycetomas have been reported from all over the world but are endemic in tropical regions of Africa, India, Central and South America, and the Far East. The geographic distribution of the disease is more related to rainfall than any other climatic factor. Most of the etiologic agents have been cultured from the soil in endemic areas, and occasionally organisms have been identified on plant thorns, which may be responsible for intradermal inoculation. *Pseudallescheria boydii* is the most common cause of mycetoma in the United States and is readily isolated from the soil in the United States and Canada.

TABLE 408–1. CAUSATIVE ORGANISMS OF MYCETOMA AND THE CHARACTERISTIC PIGMENT OF THEIR ASSOCIATED GRANULES

Eumycetoma	Actinomycetoma
White to yellow grains	
Pseudallescheria boydii	*Nocardia brasiliensis*
Acremonium species	*Nocardia asteroides*
Trichophyton species	*Nocardia cavae* (tiny grains)
Microsporum species	*Actinomadura madurae* (large grains)
Fusarium species	
Aspergillus nidulans	
Yellow to brown grains	
Neotestudina (Zophia) rosatii	*Streptomyces somaliensis*
Black grains	
Madurella mycetomatis	*Streptomyces paraguayensis*
Madurella grisea	
Exophiala jeanselmei	
Leptosphaeria senegalensis	
Leptosphaeria thompkinsii	
Red to pink grains	
	Actinomadura pelletieri

Nocardia brasiliensis and *Actinomadura madurae* are the most frequently isolated organisms in Central America, South America, and the Caribbean.

The majority of cases occur in males, many of whom are field laborers or herdsmen who encounter repeated trauma to their feet while in wet or swampy soil. Although the disease afflicts people of all ages, most cases are reported in young adults. Person-to-person transmission is not believed to occur, and the disease is unrelated to animal contact.

PATHOGENESIS AND PATHOLOGY. In contrast to systemic mycoses, which are usually established via the respiratory route, mycetomas are initiated through direct inoculation of the organism into the skin or mucosal surface, frequently as a consequence of trauma. Although the foot is the most common site of infection, direct inoculation of organisms into the hand, back, neck, and back of the head can occur in individuals who carry loads contaminated with soil.

The precise mechanism of pathogenesis remains unknown. Once inoculated, the organism induces a subacute to chronic suppurative inflammatory response that is primarily neutrophilic in nature but that may be associated with a granulomatous reaction. Over time, localized necrosis, fibrosis, abscess formation, and, frequently, bone and joint disease ensue. Deep sinuses with fistulas commonly develop and present as draining sinus tracts on the skin surface. The purulent drainage from those tracts often contains grains or granules, which consist of the causative organism embedded in a host-derived, proteinaceous matrix. The size, character, and color of the granules suggest the underlying etiologic agent (Table 408–1).

The inflammatory process usually extends along fascial planes and may result in substantial regional destruction of deep tissues and bone. Distal spread of disease via the lymphatics or the bloodstream may occur but is distinctly uncommon.

CLINICAL MANIFESTATIONS. Most cases of mycetoma present late in the course of a longstanding, chronic inflammatory disease. The initial lesion appears as a small, painless nodule several weeks to months after primary inoculation. The patient generally cannot recall a precipitating event or specific traumatic incident. The lesions slowly extend into deep tissues, and the resultant lymphatic obstruction, fibrosis, and tissue thickening give the foot a shortened, raised appearance. Skin nodules may break down, yielding granulomatous tissue with serosanguineous to purulent discharge. Later in the course of disease, sinus tracts begin to appear through which the characteristic fungal granules are expelled onto the skin surface. The sinus tracts spontaneously heal, only to be replaced by new tracts at nearby sites. Eumycetomas tend to be more circumscribed, remain localized, and progress more slowly than actinomycetomas, which have less well defined margins, merge with surrounding tissue, and progress more rapidly. The lesions tend to remain painless until deep bone involvement occurs, although many patients may complain of a deep itching sensation during active disease progression. Systemic involvement is rare, and patients feel remarkably well even in the presence of advanced localized disease.

DIAGNOSIS. The definitive diagnosis of mycetoma depends on culture of the causative organism from tissue specimens. The disease is suspected in the appropriate clinical setting, especially when grains are identified in the purulent discharge. Examination of the grains can establish a differential diagnosis of eumycetoma or actinomycetoma based on the presence of characteristic broad (fungal) or narrow (actinomycete) filaments. The characteristics of the granules, when combined with geographic and epidemiologic information, can yield a presumptive identification of the specific organism. However, cultural data are required for confirmation. Serologic tests are not routinely available.

TREATMENT. The response to therapy is dependent on the underlying etiologic agent. Eumycetomas are unresponsive to antimicrobial therapy, although partial responses to amphotericin B, miconazole, ketoconazole, and thiabendazole have been reported. Fortunately, eumycetomas tend to be well circumscribed, yielding ready access to surgical approaches. If the lesion is not removed in its entirety and residual disease is present, relapse is inevitable.

Actinomycetomas are more responsive to antimicrobial therapy. Regimens consisting of high-dose penicillin (10 to 12 million units per day), sulfadiazine (3 to 10 grams per day), or minocycline (150 mg twice daily) have been reported to have some effect. The most successful regimens consist of trimethoprim-sulfamethoxazole (160 mg of trimethoprim and 800 mg of sulfamethoxazole given twice daily), combined with either streptomycin (1 to 3 grams per day for 3 weeks) or rifampin (600 mg per day for 3 to 4 months); or dapsone (100 mg twice daily) combined with streptomycin (1 gram per day for 1 month, given intramuscularly). The dapsone regimen is often preferred owing to its low cost. The duration of therapy with either the trimethoprim-sulfamethoxazole or the dapsone regimen is usually 9 months, depending on response.

PROGNOSIS. If the disease is diagnosed early, the prognosis for mycetoma is good. Unfortunately, many cases are not identified until late in the course of disease, when response to therapy is limited, and amputation may be required. When disease is located on the back, neck, trunk, or abdomen, very little therapeutic intervention can be offered. The prognosis for survival is quite good; however, the quality of life may be dramatically lessened.

Magana M: Mycetoma. Int J Dermatol 23:221, 1984. *A thorough review of clinical aspects of mycetoma and therapeutic approaches.*
Mahgoub ES: Medical management of mycetoma. Bull WHO 54:303, 1976. *Summarizes general principles of diagnosis and management.*
Smego RA Jr, Gallis HA: The clinical spectrum of *Nocardia brasiliensis* infection in the United States. Rev Infect Dis 6:164, 1984. *An important review of the pathogenesis, diagnosis, and therapy of the most common cause of mycetoma worldwide.*
Tight RR, Bartlett MS: Actinomycetoma in the United States. Rev Infect Dis 3:1139, 1981. *A comprehensive review that focuses on diagnosis, antibiotic susceptibility, and protracted therapy in disease management.*

409 Dematiaceous Fungal Infections

Michael S. Saag

DEFINITION. The term "dematiaceous" is applied to fungi that produce an intrinsic characteristic pigment. Diseases caused by dematiaceous fungi are divided into two groups: chromomycosis (chromoblastomycosis) and phaeohyphomycosis.

ETIOLOGY. Chromomycosis is caused by several species of related fungi, most notably *Fonsecaea, Phialophora, Cladosporium,* and *Acrotheca* species. These agents are brown-pigmented saprophytes commonly found in soil and wood. The clinical appearance, which is virtually identical for all of the causative agents, consists of thick-walled, dark brown bodies ("sclerotic cells" or "copper pennies"), which may be single or clustered. Sclerotic cells represent an intermediate form between yeasts and hyphae and multiply by horizontal and vertical separation, not by budding.

Phaeohyphomycosis may be caused by several organisms, frequently referred to as "black" fungi. They differ from the agents of chromomycosis in their clinical appearance and the absence of sclerotic cells. The black fungi usually exist in tissues as yeastlike cells (solitary or in small chains), as septated hyphae (branched or unbranched), or as a combination of yeast and hyphae. The hyphal forms are frequently confused with *Aspergillus* species but may be distinguished by using the Fontana-Masson staining procedure (a melanin-specific stain) or via in vitro culture. The most common agents of phaeohyphomycosis identified in humans include *Curvularia* species, *Bipolaris* species, *Exserohilum* species, *Alternaria* species, *Mycocentrospora* species, *Pyrenochaeta* species, *Trichomaris* species, *Wangiella* species, *Xylohypha* species, and *Exophiala* species.

EPIDEMIOLOGY AND PATHOGENESIS. The organisms causing chromomycosis and phaeohyphomycosis are worldwide in distribution. Chromomycosis occurs predominantly in young males and is usually inoculated into the skin via thorns, splinters, and other penetrating wounds. The disease is more prevalent in rural populations, especially among those with suboptimal nutritional status and personal hygiene. Chromomycosis appears to be endemic in certain areas, such as Madagascar and Costa Rica.

Phaeohyphomycosis is becoming an important disease among immunocompromised hosts. Despite the ubiquity of black fungi in the environment, disease due to these organisms had, in the past, been sporadic. More recently, however, clusters of cases have been reported from major medical centers as opportunistic infections in transplant recipients, especially bone marrow transplant patients.

CLINICAL MANIFESTATIONS. Chromomycosis initially manifests as a wart-like papule that slowly enlarges into a verruciform plaque. The lesions may progress to ulceration with or without an exudate. Over time, the lesions become dry and crusted with a raised border, which may be serpiginous. Large plaques frequently develop central scarring. Occasionally, the lesions become pedunculated and acquire a cauliflower-like appearance. Systemic spread to distal sites is distinctly uncommon, although spread through autoinoculation or via lymphatic drainage may occur. Rarely, widespread disseminated disease to the pancreas, liver, bowel, lymph nodes, meninges, and brain is noted.

Phaeohyphomycosis may occur as a wide spectrum of clinical disease. Superficial phaeohyphomycosis is the most benign and is found in the stratum corneum or around the hair shaft. Tinea nigra and black piedra are examples of this disorder. More invasive skin disease involving nonliving layers of keratinized epithelium include the dermatomycoses and onychomycoses. Mycotic keratitis may result in extensive corneal damage and subsequent blindness. Subcutaneous disease usually results from direct inoculation of fungi through intact skin. Cystic lesions with well-defined walls and central abscess formation, occasionally surrounding a foreign body such as a splinter, are characteristic.

Invasive phaeohyphomycosis is a potentially life-threatening disease that occurs predominantly in immunocompromised hosts. Localized invasive disease frequently occurs in the paranasal sinuses, lower respiratory tract, and bone. Disease due to *Cladosporium, Curvularia, Bipolaris, Xylohypha,* and *Exserohilum* species is especially prone to invade the central nervous system.

DIAGNOSIS. The diagnosis of chromomycosis and phaeohyphomycosis is made by histopathologic examination of tissue biopsy specimens or KOH (10 per cent) preparations. The brown sclerotic cells of chromomycosis are readily identified, and special stains are not usually required. Phaeohyphomycosis is best diagnosed using the Fontana-Masson technique, which distinguishes organisms producing phaeohyphomycoses from *Aspergillus* species. Cultures are required to identify the specific genera causing chromomycosis and phaeohyphomycosis. All cultures should be held for at least 8 weeks, since some of the organisms grow slowly. No serologic or skin tests are available.

TREATMENT. Surgical excision, when feasible, is the most effective mode of therapy for subcutaneous or deeply invasive disease. Unfortunately, unless lesions are diagnosed and treated early, the rate of relapse is high. Systemic antifungal therapy with amphotericin B is often used; however, the results are generally disappointing. Flucytosine (5-FC; 150 mg per kilogram per day) has been used on an investigational basis in patients with chromomycosis, with some success (16 of 23 patients cured); however, resistance developed in several treated patients. The response to therapy of phaeohyphomycosis is highly dependent on the causative organism. Many black fungi are resistant to 5-FC, and amphotericin B therapy yields variable results. Newer triazole antifungal agents show some promise as effective agents.

Adam RD, Paquin ML, Petersen EA, et al.: Phaeohyphomycosis caused by the fungal genera *Bipolaris* and *Exserohilum*. Medicine 65:203, 1986. *These fungi have been previously misclassified as* Helminthosporium *or* Drechslera *species, but the latter fungi appear not to produce human disease. This paper serves as an excellent review.*

Anaissie EJ, Bodey GP, Rinaldi MG: Emerging fungal pathogens. Eur J Microbiol Infect Dis 8:323, 1989. *An up-to-date overview of phaeohyphomycoses prevention in immunocompromised patients.*

Bennett JE, Bonner H, Jennings AE, et al.: Chronic meningitis caused by *Cladosporium trichoides*. Am J Clin Pathol 59:398, 1973. *Comprehensive review of cerebral infection with dematiaceous fungi.*

McGinnis MR: Chromoblastomycosis and phaeohyphomycosis: New concepts, diagnosis and mycology. J Am Acad Dermatol 8:1, 1983. *Clear-cut exposition of clinical and mycologic criteria for these diagnoses. A very important review.*

PART XXI

HIV AND ASSOCIATED DISORDERS

Introduction

Michael S. Saag

In June 1981 the sentinel cases of the acquired immune deficiency syndrome (AIDS) were reported. Throughout the remainder of that year, additional cases were identified in the major metropolitan centers of the United States. By 1982, the syndrome was beginning to be identified with certain "high-risk" groups, including homosexual men, heroin users, hemophiliacs, and Haitians (the four H's). As details from carefully performed epidemiologic studies became available, it was clear that the epidemic was most likely due to an infectious agent that was transmissible through intimate sexual contact or blood contact. In 1983, the human immunodeficiency virus (HIV-1; previously referred to as LAV, HTLV-III, and ARV) was identified, and by 1985 a blood test was established that could identify HIV-infected individuals prior to the development of AIDS. As a result, the term *AIDS* became important primarily as a useful epidemiologic description, but most clinicians began to think of the disorder as HIV disease, a spectrum of illness that ranges from asymptomatic seropositivity to full-blown AIDS.

The latest epidemiologic evidence strongly indicates continuing spread of the disease into rural areas of the United States and continued spread of infection through all types of sexual contact, both homosexual and heterosexual. As the number of cases continues to grow, it is inevitable that every primary care physician will encounter an HIV-infected patient in his or her practice. The approach to diagnosis and treatment in HIV-infected patients is no different than for uninfected patients: a careful history and physical examination, appropriate use of laboratory tests, development of a differential diagnosis, and initial approach to therapy are all still required. Although some of the opportunistic pathogens that are so common in HIV infection may be unfamiliar to the practicing primary care physician, information regarding current approaches to diagnosis and therapy of these pathogens is contained within this part. Still, the care of HIV-infected patients does present some unique challenges. The vast array of journal articles related to the care of AIDS patients can overwhelm a busy clinician in practice. Office staff and perhaps physicians themselves may be apprehensive in providing care for HIV-infected patients owing to fear of becoming infected. Most notably, however, providing care for HIV-infected patients is complicated by social problems that are unique to that group. Many patients encounter discrimination in the workplace, at schools, in housing, and in obtaining access to care. There are many psychological hurdles patients must overcome to truly focus on *living* with their infection in a positive way.

In the latter part of the 1980's, information regarding the natural history of the disease, approaches to the common manifestations of HIV-related disorders, and clinical experience in caring for HIV-infected patients began to grow in proportion to the exponential growth of the epidemic itself. New therapeutic modalities, earlier interventions of therapy, and application of preventive therapy led to a substantial increase in overall survival and improved quality of life for HIV-infected patients. The dramatic accumulation of knowledge, however, created problems for clinicians who were providing care. Publications, books, audio and video cassettes, and monographs regarding AIDS have flooded into physicians' offices at unprecedented rates. It is difficult, if not impossible, for even the "AIDS specialist" to keep up with state-of-the-art therapies for HIV infection. Owing to the rapid rate of development of new knowledge, sources of information regarding care of AIDS patients become rapidly outdated, sometimes even before the pages hit the press. In short, it is difficult to find a single best source for updated HIV information.

The goal of this part is to provide state-of-the-art information regarding the care of HIV-infected patients—"a single best source" of information on HIV infection for the practicing clinician. The chapters provide information on the basic biology of the virus, the epidemiology of its transmission and spread, approaches to antiretroviral therapy, common clinical manifestations of HIV-related disorders, approaches to therapy by organ systems, and approaches to prevention and counseling. HIV disease is indeed a spectrum of illness that challenges the physician to develop both breadth and depth of knowledge in science and medicine as well as psychosocial and political issues—a dynamic blend of the science and art of medicine.

410 Immunology Related to AIDS

Bruce D. Walker

Since the first cases of the acquired immune deficiency syndrome (AIDS) were reported in 1981, infection with the human immunodeficiency virus 1 (HIV-1) has become a global medical crisis. An estimated 5 to 10 million persons worldwide have become infected with HIV-1 and related retroviruses through sexual, parenteral, or perinatal exposure. The vast majority of infected individuals, if not all, can be expected eventually to develop symptomatic disease, characterized by progressive and ultimately profound immunosuppression. The clinical consequences of infection are due to the ability of this virus to disarm the host immune system, a process that occurs by virtue of the fact that the primary target for the virus is the helper-inducer subset of lymphocytes. This lymphocyte subset, defined by its surface expression of the CD4 molecule, acts as the pivotal orchestrator of myriad immune functions (see Ch. 242). HIV infection can therefore be considered a disease of the immune system, characterized by the progressive loss of CD4+ lymphocytes, with ultimately fatal consequences for the infected host.

Despite this immunosuppression induced by HIV, a number of specific immunologic defenses against the virus are generated in infected individuals and may contribute to the long asymptomatic phase following infection by keeping the virus at least partially contained. The potential significance of such responses is also underscored by the recent demonstration in animal AIDS models that a state of vaccine-induced protective immunity can be achieved against retroviruses related to HIV. An understanding of the immunology related to HIV provides insight not only into the clinical sequelae of infection but also into the prospects for development of an effective vaccine against HIV.

THE VIRUS LIFE CYCLE (see also Ch. 376, 411, and 421)

The basic molecular structure of HIV is similar to that of other retroviruses, with three major genes termed *gag* (group-specific antigen), *pol* (polymerase), and *env* (envelope), in addition to a number of regulatory genes (*nef, rev, tat*) and others (*vif, vpu, vpr*) with as yet undetermined function. The ability of HIV to infect cells is mediated through the viral envelope protein. The envelope gene encodes a precursor protein gp160, which is subsequently proteolytically cleaved to two smaller proteins, gp41 and gp120, which associate at the infected cell surface. Gp41 is a transmembrane protein that serves as a membrane anchor for gp120, the mature exterior envelope glycoprotein. The first step in virus infectivity is the binding of gp120 to the CD4 (also called T4) cell surface protein, which is the specific cellular receptor for the virus. The CD4 protein is found predominantly on the helper-inducer subset of lymphocytes but also to a lesser degree on monocytes/macrophages and some other nucleated cells (Fig. 410–1). Following binding to CD4, the viral membrane fuses with the host cell membrane and the virus is uncoated and enters the cell cytoplasm. The viral enzyme reverse transcriptase then transcribes the viral RNA into DNA. This double-stranded DNA can remain unintegrated in the cellular cytoplasm or can become integrated into the host chromosomal DNA, in which case it is termed proviral DNA. Through processes of transcription and translation, new viral RNA and proteins are produced, which are subsequently assembled into new virions. As the newly synthesized envelope precursor gp160 is glycosylated and cleaved, mature envelope glycoprotein knobs (gp41/gp120) are embedded in the cellular membrane. As mature capsid proteins containing viral RNA bud at the cell surface, the envelope coating is completed and mature infectious virions are released.

The majority of cell-associated virus in blood is contained within CD4+ lymphocytes. Despite a numerical decline in the absolute number of these cells with disease progression, the actual proportion of cells infected with HIV increases. In patients with AIDS, as many as 1 per 100 CD4+ lymphocytes have been demonstrated to harbor the provirus. Viral replication occurs continuously in HIV-infected persons, and there appears to be no truly latent phase when replication ceases altogether. A number of factors may, however, act to increase viral production in vitro by infected cells. Among these are other viruses (cytomegalovirus [CMV], Epstein-Barr virus [EBV], HTLV-I, and human herpesvirus VI [HHV-6]), mitogens, and lymphokines (GM-CSF, TNF-α, and interleukin 6), suggesting that these may serve as cofactors in disease induction.

HIV-INDUCED IMMUNOSUPPRESSION

The hallmark of HIV infection is progressive depletion of the CD4 helper-inducer subset of lymphocytes. Owing to the central role of these cells in immunologic functioning, the clinical disease manifestations of immunosuppression and susceptibility to opportunistic infections and neoplasms are not surprising. The immunologic deficits associated with HIV infection are wide-spread and involve numerous interdependent effector arms of the immune system, involving both cellular and humoral elements.

DIRECT IMMUNOSUPPRESSIVE PROPERTIES OF VIRAL PRODUCTS. Protein products of a number of retroviruses have been shown to have direct immunosuppressive properties independent of viral infection. A synthetic peptide corresponding to a highly conserved region in the HIV-1 gp41 transmembrane protein has been demonstrated to inhibit lymphocyte proliferative responses to mitogenic or antigenic stimuli in vitro. This region is analogous to a highly conserved immunosuppressive protein of HTLV-I, and similar inhibitory transmembrane proteins have been identified in other animal retroviral infections such as feline leukemia virus (FeLV). Whether such a phenomenon contributes to the global immunosuppression seen in HIV-infected individuals has not been determined, but the possibility that HIV proteins may be immunosuppressive has raised concerns about inclusion of such sequences in potential HIV vaccine candidates.

T-LYMPHOCYTE ABNORMALITIES. Lymphocyte abnormalities associated with HIV infection can be classified as both quantitative and qualitative. Qualitative deficiencies become apparent soon after infection and before CD4 depletion is evident and are largely related to intrinsic functional defects in the helper-inducer subset of lymphocytes. Studies using purified subpopulations of lymphocytes from AIDS patients have demonstrated a selective defect in soluble antigen (e.g., tetanus toxoid) recognition, although these cells are still able to undergo a normal degree of blast transformation and lymphokine production after exposure to mitogen (e.g., phytohemagglutinin). In other words, the weapon is loaded, but only mitogens and not antigens cause the trigger to be pulled. These studies also indicate that the central defect is the lack of helper cell function rather than an overabundance of suppressor cell activity. Other lymphocyte abnormalities observed with HIV infection include decreased lymphokine production, decreased expression of interleukin 2 (IL2) receptors, decreased alloreactivity, and decreased ability to provide help to B cells. The functional T-lymphocyte abnormalities also likely contribute to the loss of delayed-type hypersensitivity reactions, which become more prevalent as disease progresses.

The quantitative abnormality of T lymphocytes is the result of a progressive depletion of the CD4+ helper T-lymphocyte population, which begins soon after primary infection (Table 410–1). This downhill trend continues until the normal levels of 800 to 1200 CD4 cells per cubic millimeter drop below 50 and sometimes below 10 cells per cubic millimeter in the later stages of disease. CD4 cell depletion cannot be attributed solely to direct cytotoxic effects of virus infection, as only a minority of

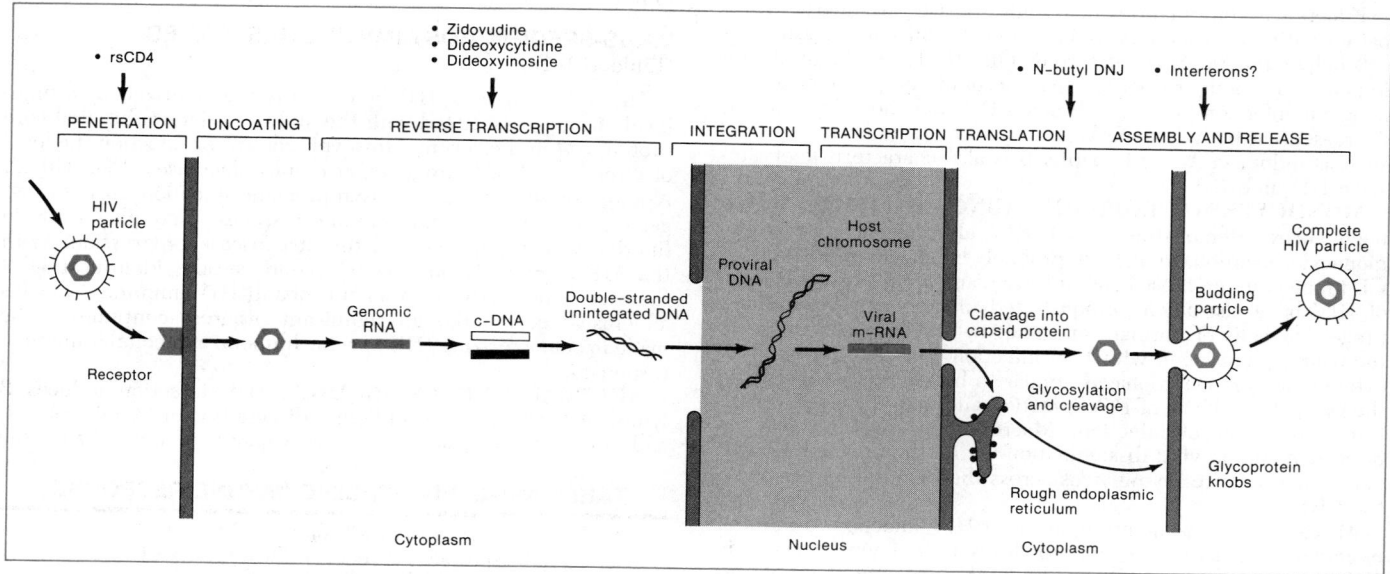

FIGURE 410–1. The life cycle of HIV. The target sites for antiretroviral agents are listed. (Reprinted from Johnson VA, Hirsch MS: *In* Volberding P, Jacobson M (eds.): AIDS Clinical Review 1990. New York, Marcel Dekker, 1990, p 238. By courtesy of Marcel Dekker, Inc.)

TABLE 410–1. POTENTIAL CAUSES OF CD4 CELL DEPLETION

1. Direct toxic consequences of infection
2. Syncytia formation
3. Innocent bystander destruction of cells with adsorbed gp120
4. HIV infection of stem cells
5. Autoimmune destruction

helper cells are actually infected, even in later stages of illness. Other factors potentially contributing to CD4 depletion include (a) syncytia formation, in which a single infected cell fuses via its surface gp120 with the CD4 molecule on uninfected cells, forming multinucleated giant cells, (b) "innocent bystander" destruction of uninfected CD4 cells that have bound free gp120 to the CD4 molecule, rendering them susceptible to immune attack, (c) HIV infection of stem cells, resulting in decreased helper cell production, and (d) autoimmune mechanisms, whereby cross-reactive antibodies or cellular immune responses to the virus result in killing of uninfected CD4 cells. Whatever the mechanisms of the CD4 cell depletion, the resultant consequence to immune function is so profound that total CD4 number is currently the best measure of disease progression. The risk of certain opportunistic infections increases significantly when the total CD4 cell number is less than 200 per cubic millimeter, which is why routine prophylaxis against *Pneumocystis carinii* pneumonia is instituted at this stage. At levels below 100 per cubic millimeter the risk for other complications, such as disseminated *Mycobacterium avium* or CMV infection, increases dramatically.

B-LYMPHOCYTE ABNORMALITIES. As with T-lymphocyte abnormalities in HIV infection, the B-lymphocyte abnormalities are both quantitative and qualitative. Most characteristic, particularly in the early stages of infection, is an intense polyclonal activation of B cells, evidenced clinically by elevated levels of immunoglobulins G and A, the presence of circulating immune complexes, and an increased number of peripheral blood B lymphocytes that secrete immunoglobulin spontaneously. These B-cell abnormalities are unlikely to be a direct consequence of HIV infection of B cells. Whereas B cells can express low levels of CD4 and have been infected in vitro, there are no conclusive data indicating that these cells became infected in vivo. Rather, the virus itself or viral proteins appear to interact directly with and stimulate uninfected cells. Other potential contributors to this polyclonal activation include concurrent viral infections. For example, CMV and EBV infections occur with greatly increased frequency in HIV-infected individuals and can lead to B-cell hyperactivity.

Functional abnormalities of B cells consist particularly of impaired antibody responses to antigenic stimuli, and impaired T-cell helper function may also contribute to this problem. These impaired antibody responses may account for the increase in pyogenic infections seen in advanced HIV infection. In addition, decreased antibody responsiveness to vaccination against viruses such as influenza A and hepatitis B is also characteristic of late-stage HIV infection.

MONOCYTE/MACROPHAGE ABNORMALITIES. It has been clearly demonstrated that HIV also infects cells of the monocyte/macrophage lineage, probably by attachment to surface CD4 molecules on these cells. Infection and high-level replication of HIV have also been demonstrated in monocyte/macrophage progenitor cells of normal bone marrow and may contribute to the pancytopenia seen with HIV infection. Unlike CD4 lymphocytes, however, macrophages appear to be relatively resistant to the cytopathic effects of HIV infection and may therefore constitute a reservoir of infection. Macrophages may also play an important role in viral dissemination within the infected individual, in particular carrying virus across the blood-brain barrier to the CNS.

At least in part as a consequence of HIV infection, a number of monocyte/macrophage abnormalities have been detected in HIV-seropositive persons. The ability of monocytes/macrophages to act as antigen-presenting cells is impaired, particularly in later stages of illness. Some defects in these cells in AIDS patients may be a consequence of chronic in vivo activation, such as

increased IL2 receptor expression, IL1 secretion, and increased chemotactic ligand receptor expression. The reasons for this chronic activation are likely multifactorial and may relate to exposure to viral proteins or lymphokines or to direct effects of HIV infection. These abnormalities may have immunopathogenic consequences, since defects in the ability to present antigens could ultimately impair the ability to sustain an immune response against HIV or other pathogens.

In the brain, cells of the macrophage lineage appear to be the major cell type infected with HIV and directly or indirectly may contribute to the CNS dysfunction observed in this disease. In the lung, infected alveolar macrophages may stimulate HIV-specific immune responses, the by-products of which have been postulated to contribute to the observed alveolitis. Deficient T4 helper cell function may also indirectly contribute to the observed defects in monocytes/macrophages, since a minority of monocytes/macrophages appear to be actually productively infected in vivo.

NATURAL KILLER CELL ABNORMALITIES. Natural killer (NK) cells are thought to be an important component of immunosurveillance against virus-infected cells, allogeneic cells, and tumor cells. NK cells are typically large granular lymphocytes that recognize foreign antigens on cells, resulting in activation of lytic machinery. NK cells are phenotypically and numerically normal in AIDS patients, but they are functionally defective. This may relate in part to an observed defect in the trigger mechanism necessary to deliver the lethal blow to a target cell. In addition, defective lymphokine production in HIV-infected persons may also contribute to NK cell dysfunction. However, addition of IL2 to these cells in vitro only partially restores NK function.

AUTOIMMUNE ABNORMALITIES. Autoimmune phenomena are also part of the immunologic derangement in HIV infection and may also contribute to the disease manifestations seen clinically. When sensitive assays are used, circulating immune complexes can be detected in the majority of HIV-infected individuals. These may help to explain the occurrence of HIV-related arthralgias, myalgias, renal disease, and vasculitis. Anti-HIV antibody complexes attached to platelets of persons with HIV-related thrombocytopenia may be the cause of this defect, although specific antiplatelet membrane antibodies have also been proposed as the cause of this thrombocytopenia.

Autoimmune mechanisms may also directly contribute to the immune suppression seen in AIDS. Sequence similarities exist between the HIV envelope transmembrane protein and HLA Class II proteins, and antibodies that cross-react with these two proteins have been detected in HIV-infected persons. Such autoantibodies could impair functioning of cells bearing Class II antigens, either by directly eliminating these cells through antibody-dependent cellular cytotoxicity or by inhibiting their ability to interact with other cells.

VIRUS-SPECIFIC HOST IMMUNE RESPONSES
(Table 410–2)

The initial phase of HIV infection is characterized by a high-level viremia, associated with the ability to detect the viral core protein p24 in the serum. However, soon after infection the level of viremia and p24 antigenemia rapidly decreases (Fig. 410–2). A long period of relatively asymptomatic infection ensues, suggesting that virus-specific immune responses may play a role in limiting viral replication and thereby disease progression. With the AIDS epidemic now in its second decade, identification of the precise protective components of anti-HIV immunity remains an elusive goal, although significant progress continues to be made in characterizing HIV-specific humoral and cellular immune responses.

NEUTRALIZING ANTIBODIES. HIV infection induces B lymphocytes to produce antibodies directed against viral proteins, and some of these antibodies are capable of neutralizing the

TABLE 410–2. HIV-SPECIFIC IMMUNE RESPONSES

1. Neutralizing antibodies
2. Antibody-dependent cellular cytotoxicity
3. Natural killer cells
4. Cytotoxic T cells
5. Cellular proliferative responses

virus. Antibody responses are typically observed 1 to 3 months following infection, although longer periods before the development of antibody responses have been documented in rare instances. Neutralizing antibodies directly neutralize free virus at a stage before the virus has entered the cell and become uncoated. In a number of viral infections, neutralizing antibody induced by immunization correlates with protection from subsequent viral infection. HIV-1 infection results in the production of HIV-specific antibodies directed at a number of viral proteins, and some of these antibodies demonstrate neutralizing activity. The primary target of neutralizing antibodies is the envelope glycoprotein, in particular a loop structure within a relatively hypervariable region of the gp120 glycoprotein termed the principal neutralizing domain.

Neutralizing antibodies have been demonstrated to be present at all stages of HIV infection, and although titers are generally lower in later stages of illness, attempts to correlate neutralizing antibody titers with disease progression have yielded conflicting results. In one study, chimpanzees given high-titered neutralizing antibody intravenously were not protected from subsequent challenge with HIV-1, although a possible explanation for this lack of protection is that the high virus inoculum used to challenge these animals may have overwhelmed the amount of neutralizing antibody present. In addition, titers of antibodies directed at the principal neutralizing domain were low in the immunoglobulin preparation used in this experiment.

The ability of HIV-specific neutralizing antibodies to confer protection may be impaired in part by the high degree of antigenic variation exhibited by HIV. This antigenic variation is particularly pronounced in the envelope region of the virus, and virus variants may emerge within an infected individual which are neutralization resistant. This antigenic variation also has significant implications for vaccine design, since neutralizing antibodies generated in response to a single immunizing strain of virus are likely to neutralize only very closely related viruses, a phenomenon known as type specificity.

Antibodies also constitute the first line of defense at mucosal surfaces, in the form of secretory IgA. Such secretory antibodies have been found in blood, saliva, and other body fluids of persons infected with HIV, but their potential role as a protective immune response in HIV infection remains undetermined.

In sharp contrast to proposed protective attributes, HIV-specific antibodies have also been shown to promote HIV infection under certain experimental conditions. Antibody binds to virions, and this complex appears to be taken up by some cells by binding of antibody through the cellular Fc receptor. This in vitro evidence for antibody-dependent enhancement is orders of magnitude less than what is observed, for example, in dengue virus infection, and the clinical significance of this phenomenon is not known.

ANTIBODY-DEPENDENT CELLULAR CYTOTOXICITY (ADCC). Another mechanism whereby the immune system can act to limit the spread of infection is ADCC, which involves both cellular and humoral components. ADCC is a process in which virus-specific antibodies bind directly to viral proteins expressed on the surface of infected cells, thereby sensitizing these cells for lysis by cells that bind to the exposed Fc portion of the antibody. The cells mediating this response are typically NK cells, which express the CD16 Fc receptor for IgG. Antibodies capable of mediating ADCC have been identified in the majority of HIV-infected individuals; these are present soon after seroconversion and are maintained throughout the disease course. The major ADCC target antigens are the envelope glycoproteins gp120 and gp41; *gag* proteins may also be involved. It has been postulated that ADCC may limit cell-to-cell spread of virus by providing an early cytotoxic host defense. ADCC may correlate with better clinical stage in children born to infected mothers, and ADCC titers have been shown to be higher in early stages of infection in some studies. However, the contribution of this immune response to protection from disease remains unclear.

NATURAL KILLER CELLS. In vitro evidence suggests that NK-type cells are not only important in ADCC, but also may bind free HIV-specific antibodies through their Fc receptors, arming them for attack against HIV-infected cells.

CYTOTOXIC T LYMPHOCYTES (CTL). Cytotoxic T lymphocytes have been demonstrated to be one of the protective host defenses generated in response to a number of viral infections. CTL's are able to kill virus-infected cells by recognizing viral protein fragments on the infected cell surface, where these proteins form a binary complex with a surface human leukocyte antigen (HLA) molecule (see Ch. 250). CTL recognition of this complex leads to lysis and elimination of the infected cell.

Although the hallmark of HIV infection is the development of profound immunosuppression, extremely vigorous HIV-specific CTL responses have been detected in the peripheral blood of infected individuals. These responses are directed not only against the major viral structural proteins, but also against the reverse transcriptase protein and regulatory proteins such as *vif* and *nef*. These responses appear to be mediated predominantly by CD8+ lymphocytes, which recognize processed HIV proteins on the surface of infected cells in conjunction with HLA Class I (A, B, C) molecules. In addition to this so-called HLA-restricted CTL population, other cells capable of recognizing HIV envelope protein on infected cells in an HLA-unrestricted fashion also appear to exist. These cells may be T cells or cells of the NK phenotype. Some studies have also suggested the existence of HIV-specific, CD4+ CTL restricted by HLA Class II molecules.

Although a protective role for CTL has been demonstrated in numerous experimental models of viral infection, the question remains unresolved as to the possible protective role of CTL in HIV infection. There is at least indirect evidence to suggest that the CTL response might indeed retard disease progression. For example, CD8+ lymphocytes from HIV-infected individuals are able to inhibit HIV replication in autologous CD4 lymphocytes in vitro. Similar inhibitory CD8 cells have also been identified in the simian immunodeficiency virus (SIV)–infected macaque monkeys, and since cell contact is necessary for this inhibition to occur, it suggests that the cell mediating this response may be a classic CTL. Other indirect evidence that CTL may be important in retarding disease progression stems from studies quantifying

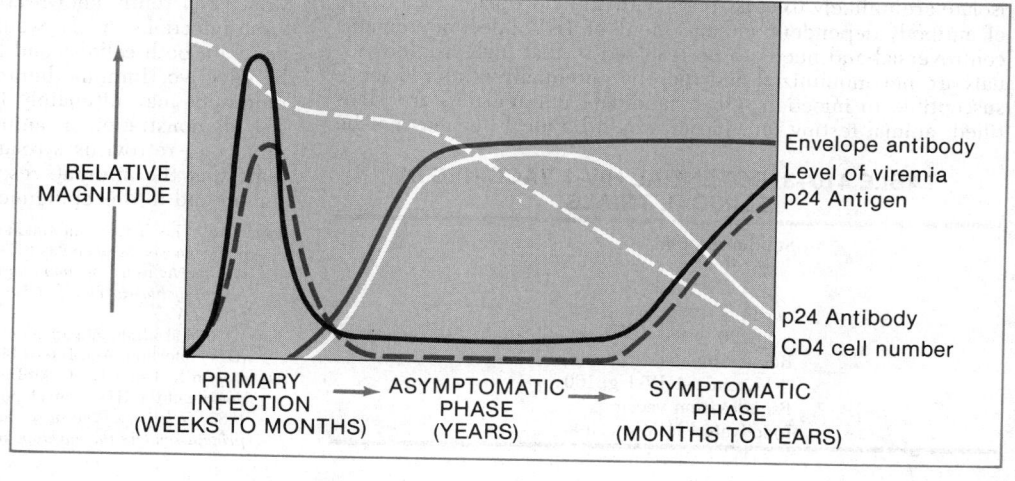

FIGURE 410–2. Schematic representation of immunologic parameters during the course of HIV infection. Note that the asymptomatic phase of infection typically lasts for years.

RELATIVE MAGNITUDE

Envelope antibody
Level of viremia
p24 Antigen

p24 Antibody
CD4 cell number

PRIMARY INFECTION (WEEKS TO MONTHS) → ASYMPTOMATIC PHASE (YEARS) → SYMPTOMATIC PHASE (MONTHS TO YEARS)

HIV-specific CTL in infected persons. As clinical disease progresses, CTL numbers decline, which could help to explain the increase in viremia observed in later stages of illness.

Conversely, HIV-specific CTL's have also been postulated by others to be deleterious to the host. These cells have been recovered from the lungs of subjects with lymphocytic alveolitis, suggesting that they may be inducing the alveolitis by attacking HIV-infected alveolar macrophages. In addition, CTL's have been detected in the CSF of HIV-infected individuals with neurologic disorders, prompting the hypothesis that CTL-mediated inflammatory reactions may contribute to the observed neurologic dysfunction. CTL's could also contribute to the progressive decline in CD4 cells by eliminating those cells that become HIV infected.

CELLULAR PROLIFERATIVE RESPONSES. T-cell immunity to viral pathogens consists not only of cytotoxic T lymphocytes, but also helper T-cell proliferation and cytokine production in specific response to viral antigens. This CD4+ proliferative response is generally triggered by recognition of viral antigen in association with Class II (HLA-D) molecules on the surface of antigen-presenting cells or B cells to be helped. Although HIV-specific proliferative responses are characteristically depressed in HIV-infected individuals, a number of epitopes eliciting these responses have been identified, particularly in the envelope glycoprotein gp120. Unfortunately, as with other HIV-specific immune responses, the precise contribution as a protective mechanism remains unclear.

PROSPECTS FOR VACCINE DEVELOPMENT
(Table 410–3)

Ultimate global control of the HIV epidemic likely will require a vaccine capable of eliciting protective immunity. Although efforts to define the components of protective immunity in infected persons have been unsuccessful thus far, recent data from animal models of retrovirus infection indicate that a state of protective immunity may be an attainable goal. When immunized with formalin-inactivated whole SIV, eight of nine rhesus monkeys were protected from infection when subsequently challenged with live SIV. The one animal that became infected developed a clinically attenuated form of disease, indicating a protective effect of the vaccine even when it is unable to prevent infection.

Despite these promising results in the SIV model of HIV infection, a number of potential obstacles exist to the development of an effective AIDS vaccine (Table 410–4). Foremost among these is the diversity of the viral genome. Most of this diversity occurs in the envelope gene, with as much as 20 per cent divergence in nucleotide sequence among field isolates. Even within a single individual, multiple divergent strains of virus have been identified, reflecting an extremely high intrinsic mutation rate for the virus. The implications of such diversity for vaccine development are profound, since the virus acts as a moving target for any immune response that is generated. Another obstacle to be overcome is the type specificity of immune responses generated to candidate vaccines, since immune responses generated by an immunogen representing a single field isolate are unlikely to cross-react with all field isolates. The issue of antibody-dependent enhancement of HIV infection remains controversial and needs to be resolved so that high-risk individuals are not immunized and thereby potentially rendered more susceptible to infection. Once candidate immunogens are identified, animal testing for efficacy would be ideal but may not be

TABLE 410–3. POTENTIAL HIV-1 VACCINES IN CLINICAL TRIALS

Soluble proteins
    gp160
    p24
    p17
    gp120
Recombinant live vaccines
    Vaccinia–HIV-1 gp160
Pseudovirion vaccines
Inactivated HIV vaccine

TABLE 410–4. POTENTIAL OBSTACLES TO HIV VACCINE DEVELOPMENT

Diversity of the viral genome
Type specificity of immune responses
Potential generation of enhancing antibodies
Lack of animal models of HIV infection and
    AIDS
Field trials to demonstrate efficacy
Indemnification of vaccinees from discrimination

possible for a number of reasons. Unfortunately there is no good animal model of HIV infection. Although chimpanzees become infected with HIV, they do not develop disease. Rhesus macaques develop an immunodeficiency disease similar to AIDS when infected with SIV but cannot be infected with HIV, are expensive to maintain, and are in limited supply. The potential utility of immunodeficient mice reconstituted with human fetal tissues, providing them with a "human" immune system, remains to be demonstrated. Perhaps the biggest obstacle will be demonstration of efficacy, which will require large field trials in populations demonstrating a high enough incidence of new infection that statistically significant data can be generated in a reasonable period of time. Demonstration of efficacy in one population may not translate to other populations. For example, protection of persons infected by sexual exposure will not necessarily imply that such a vaccine would protect intravenous drug abusers as well, who may be exposed to a higher initial inoculum of virus. As with HIV-infected persons, the potential for discrimination against vaccinees due to a positive serology will have to be addressed.

Although these obstacles exist, a number of preliminary clinical trials are already under way with a variety of vaccine candidates. These include soluble *gag* or envelope proteins, recombinant vaccina virus containing the HIV-1 envelope gene, pseudovirion vaccines that resemble whole HIV particles but are modified to exclude the viral genome or render it harmless, and whole killed virus vaccines. The latter approach is currently being investigated as an immunotherapy in HIV-infected persons. Combinations of some of these approaches are also under investigation. In subjects immunized with vaccinia–HIV-1 gp160, dramatic increases in HIV-1 envelope antibodies were observed when vaccines were boosted with recombinant gp160 protein. Other approaches in various stages of preclinical development include the use of recombinant BCG-HIV vectors and the use of attenuated salmonella-HIV recombinants.

SUMMARY

Since the identification of HIV as the cause of AIDS, it has been firmly established that the virus is able to induce disease because of its ability to disarm the host immune response. Despite this profound degree of immunosuppression, both humoral and cellular immune responses have been shown to be triggered by this infection, and these defenses may contribute to the prolonged asymptomatic period characteristic of this infection by keeping the virus at least partially contained. The precise components of protective immunity against HIV infection are yet to be determined, and an effective immunogen is yet to be identified. Given what is currently known about host responses to this and other viral infections, most would agree that vaccines designed to generate both cellular and humoral responses are most likely to be effective. Immunotherapies designed to bolster HIV-specific immunity may ultimately help those persons already infected. The demonstration in animal models that vaccine-induced immunity to retroviruses related to AIDS can be protective offers hope that the immune response can ultimately be harnessed to put an end to this epidemic.

Fauci AS: The human immunodeficiency virus: Infectivity and mechanisms of pathogenesis. Science 239:617–622, 1989. *An excellent review of viral infectivity, mechanisms of immunosuppression, cellular tropism, pathogenesis of neuropsychiatric manifestations of disease, and the interaction of cytokines with HIV.*

Fauci AS, et al.: Immunopathogenic mechanisms in human immunodeficiency virus (HIV) infection. Ann Intern Med 114:617, 1991.

Javerherian K, Langlois AL, McDanal C, et al.: Mapping the principal neutralizing domain of the HIV-1 envelope protein. Proc Natl Acad Sci USA 86:6768–6772, 1989. *Deletion of the principal neutralizing determinant of the HIV envelope protein renders the envelope unable to elicit neutralizing antibodies.*

Koff WC, Schultz AM: AIDS vaccines 1990: A brief update. AIDS 4(Suppl 1):S179–S184, 1990. *A review of vaccine trials in progress or planned.*

Levy JA: Changing concepts in HIV infection: Challenges for the 1990's. AIDS 4:1051–1058, 1990. *A review of recent advances in understanding of the immunopathogenesis of HIV infection and AIDS.*

Murphy-Corb M, Wyand MS, Kodama T, et al.: A formalin-inactivated whole SIV vaccine confers protection in macaques. Science 246:1293–1297, 1989. *Evidence of vaccine protection against a retrovirus related to HIV.*

Schnittman SM, Psallidopoulous MC, Lane HC, et al.: The reservoir for HIV-1 in human peripheral blood is a T cell that maintains expression of CD4. Science 245:305–308, 1989. *The major cell infected with HIV is the CD4-expressing helper T lymphocyte, and evidence indicates that these cells are present in higher numbers in later stages of illness.*

Shioda T, Levy JA, Cheng-Mayer C: Macrophage and T cell line tropism of HIV-1 are determined by specific regions of the envelope gp 120 gene. Nature 345:167–169, 1991.

Walker BD, Plata F: Cytotoxic T lymphocytes against HIV-1. AIDS 4:177–184, 1990. *A review of cell-mediated immune function in HIV infection, with discussion of the potential protective versus pathogenic role of such cells.*

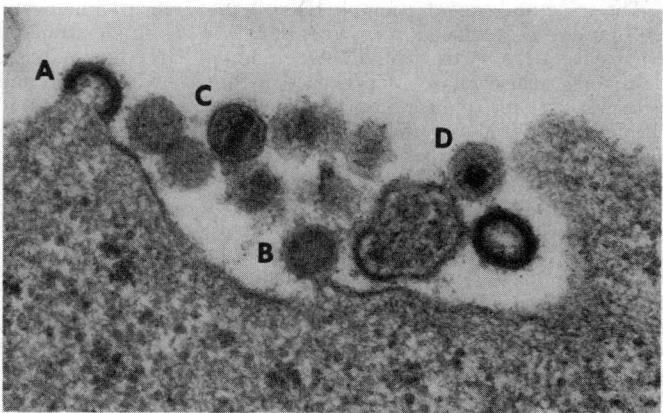

FIGURE 411–1. Transmission electron micrograph of HIV-1. Virions are shown at all stages of morphogenesis: early (A) and late (B) budding forms and cell-free mature virions (C and D) with condensed central cores. The diameter of virions is approximately 110 nm.

411 Biology of Human Immunodeficiency Viruses

George M. Shaw

DISCOVERY OF HUMAN IMMUNODEFICIENCY VIRUSES

The identification of HIV-1 as the causative agent of AIDS just 3 years after the initial description of the clinical syndrome represents a remarkable scientific achievement that had its roots in earlier discoveries of animal and human retroviruses. In the early 1900's, Ellerman, Bang, and Rous first showed that cell-free filtrates from tissues of leukemic chickens could induce leukemias and sarcomas in normal animals. Forty years later, Gross isolated the first mammalian retrovirus (murine leukemia virus) from inbred mice, and Jarrett observed that household cats were infected by a retrovirus, feline leukemia virus, that caused both leukemia and an AIDS-like immunosuppressive disease. However, it was not until 1970 when Temin and Baltimore independently reported the discovery of the retroviral enzyme reverse transcriptase that the unique replicative life cycle of these viruses was elucidated (RNA→DNA→RNA) and the molecular tools were made available to search for human retroviruses.

The first human retrovirus, human T-cell leukemia virus type I (HTLV-I), was discovered by Gallo in 1979 and has since been shown to be the causative agent of adult T-cell leukemia and a myelopathy termed tropical spastic paraparesis. In 1982, Gallo and co-workers reported the discovery of a second human retrovirus, HTLV-II, which is genetically related to HTLV-I but whose clinical significance is currently unknown. This conceptual framework of a family of phylogenetically related human retroviruses and the experimental approaches developed for their isolation in T-lymphocyte cultures were instrumental in the subsequent discovery of HIV-1 as the causative agent of AIDS.

Early suggestions that AIDS might be caused by an infectious agent were supported by epidemiologic evidences: (1) The AIDS epidemic was new in 1981; (2) the disease first appeared in a limited geographic region and subsequently spread to other areas; (3) the disease occurred in socially, economically, and geographically disparate groups that shared a propensity for communicable diseases; (4) clusters of disease were identified in individuals linked by common sexual contacts and by receipt of blood products; (5) children of affected individuals developed AIDS despite having no other risk factors for infection; (6) filtered Factor VIII coagulant transfused to hemophiliacs resulted in disease transmission. That AIDS might be caused by a retrovirus was suggested by the selective loss of CD4+ helper T lymphocytes in patients with the disease, implicating an agent with T-lymphocyte cell tropism reminiscent of infection with HTLV-I and HTLV-II. AIDS originated in Africa, where other human and simian retroviruses were known to be endemic. And a retrovirus in cats, feline leukemia virus, was known to cause an AIDS-like illness as well as leukemia. Based on this circumstantial evidence, investigative teams led by Montagnier at the Pasteur Institute in Paris and by Gallo at the National Institutes of Health undertook studies to isolate and identify retroviruses from patients with AIDS and pre-AIDS conditions. In 1983-84, the two groups reported the isolation and serologic detection of a novel retrovirus, at that time designated HTLV-III or LAV but now denoted HIV-1, in patients with AIDS and pre-AIDS conditions. As expected for an etiologic agent, HIV-1 was shown to be uniformly present in subjects with AIDS and to reproduce the hallmark of disease, destruction of T lymphocytes, in tissue culture.

GENERAL BIOLOGIC PROPERTIES OF HIV-1

Soon after its discovery, HIV-1 was shown to be biologically, structurally, and genetically distinct from HTLV-I and HTLV-II. Unlike the leukemia viruses, which lead to immortalization of lymphocytes in vitro and in vivo, HIV-1 exhibits pronounced cytopathic properties for lymphocytes, causing syncytia formation and cell death. Morphologically, HIV-1 differs from HTLV-I and other type C oncogenic retroviruses and more closely resembles the lentivirus subfamily of retroviruses, which exhibit a characteristic dense, cylindrical core surrounded by a lipid envelope (Fig. 411–1).

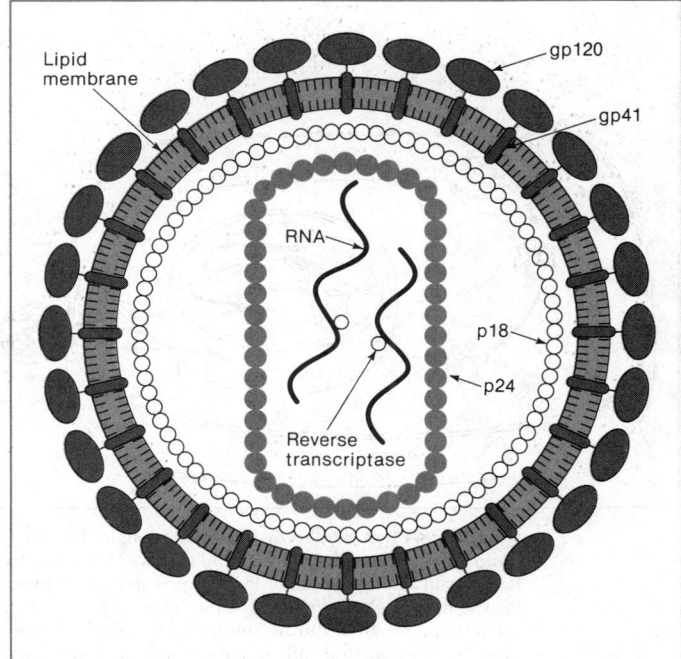

FIGURE 411–2. Structure of HIV-1. (Adapted from R.C. Gallo. Copyright © 1987 by Scientific American, Inc., and George V. Kelvin. All rights reserved.)

The structural organization of HIV-1 is shown diagrammatically in Figure 411–2. Like all retroviruses, HIV-1 is a single-stranded plus-sense RNA virus. The RNA-dependent DNA polymerase, or reverse transcriptase, is packaged within the virion core and is responsible for replication of the single-stranded RNA genome through a double-stranded DNA intermediate, which in turn serves as the precursor molecule for proviral integration within the host cell genome. The major structural core proteins of HIV-1 are the p24 capsid protein and the p18 matrix protein, as shown. Surrounding the viral core protein structures is a bilayered lipid envelope that is derived from the outer limiting membrane of the host cell as the virus buds from the cell surface during replication. Studding this outer viral membrane are the envelope glycoproteins, gp120 and gp41, which are encoded by viral-specific genes and are responsible for cell attachment and entry.

The life cycle of HIV-1 is shown diagrammatically in Figure 411–3. Features of this life cycle distinguish retroviruses from all other viruses. The cell-free virion first attaches to the target cell through a specific interaction between the viral envelope and the host cell membrane. The specificity of this interaction between virus and cell has been shown to be due to a high-affinity specific interaction between the viral gp120 envelope glycoprotein and the target cell–associated CD4 molecule. Following virus adsorption, fusion of the viral and cellular membranes occurs, resulting

in internalization of the nucleoprotein viral complex. Reverse transcription catalyzed by the viral reverse transcriptase generates a linear double-stranded DNA copy of the viral RNA within the nucleoprotein complex, and this migrates to the nucleus where covalent integration of viral DNA into the host chromosomes leads to formation of the provirus. Subsequent expression of viral DNA is controlled by a combination of viral and host cellular proteins that interact with viral DNA and RNA regulatory elements. Transcribed viral mRNA is translated into viral proteins, and new virions are assembled at the cell surface where genomic-length viral RNA, reverse transcriptase, structural and regulatory proteins, and envelope glycoproteins are assembled. Because the HIV-1 provirus is covalently integrated within the host cell chromosome, it represents a stable component of the host genome and is replicated and transmitted to daughter cells in synchrony with cellular DNA. Relevant to subsequent discussions of viral pathogenesis, the integrated provirus is thus permanently incorporated into the host cell genome and may remain transcriptionally latent or may exhibit high levels of gene expression with explosive production of progeny virus.

MOLECULAR STRUCTURE AND FUNCTION OF HIV-1

The genomic organization of HIV-1 is shown diagrammatically in Figure 411–4. The HIV-1 genome, like other retroviral genomes, is diploid, consisting of two identical viral RNA molecules assembled in a hydrogen-bonded 70S complex. These genomic subunits are plus strands of viral RNA in that they have the same

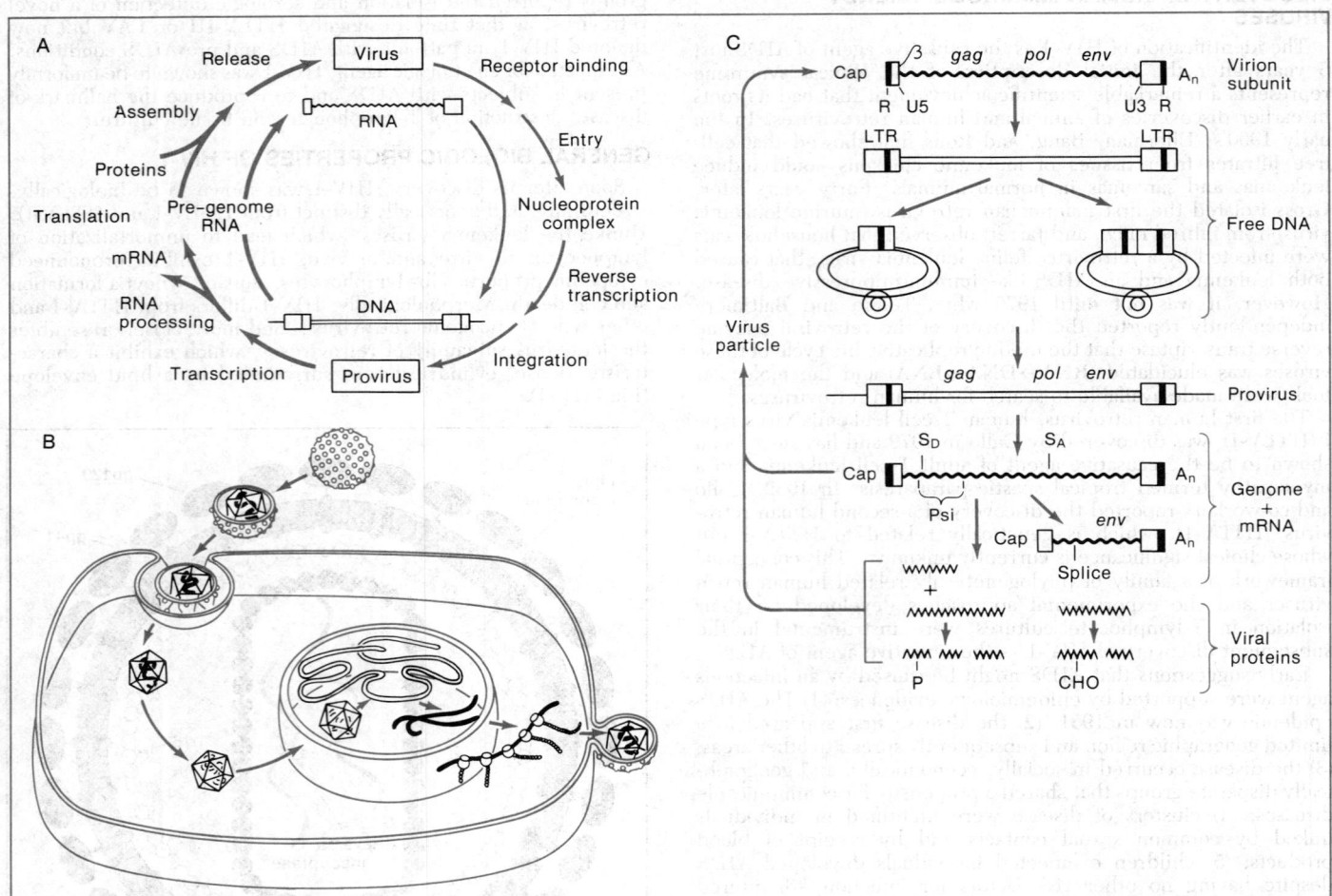

FIGURE 411–3. Different representations of the HIV-1 life cycle. *A,* An outline of the virus life cycle is shown, with thick arrows denoting amplification of viral products that may occur in the latter half of the replication cycle as a result of stimulation of virus expression. *B,* A pictorial overview of the virus life cycle outlined in *A,* beginning at the upper left and ending at the lower right. *C,* A detailed illustration of the major transformations of retroviral genetic information during the life cycle of HIV-1. Cap denotes the 5′ methyl-G-nucleotide, A_n the poly (A) tract, and S_D and S_A the splice donor and acceptor sites. Psi denotes the viral packaging signal sequence, P a phosphorylation site, and CHO a glycosylation site. (See text for discussion.) (Reprinted with permission from Varmus H, Brown P: Retroviruses. *In* Berg DE, Howe MM [eds.]: Mobile DNA. Washington, D.C., American Society for Microbiology, 1989, pp 53–108.)

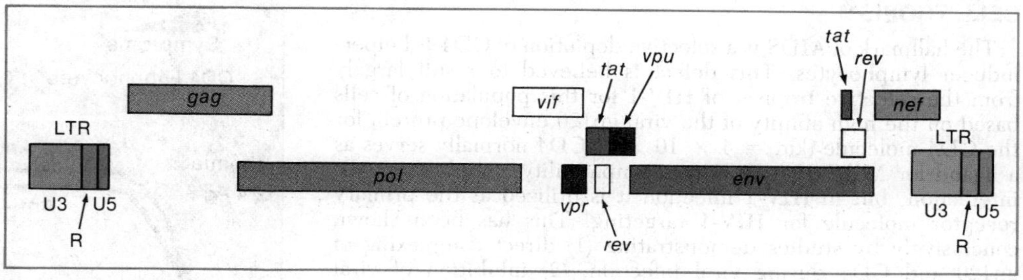

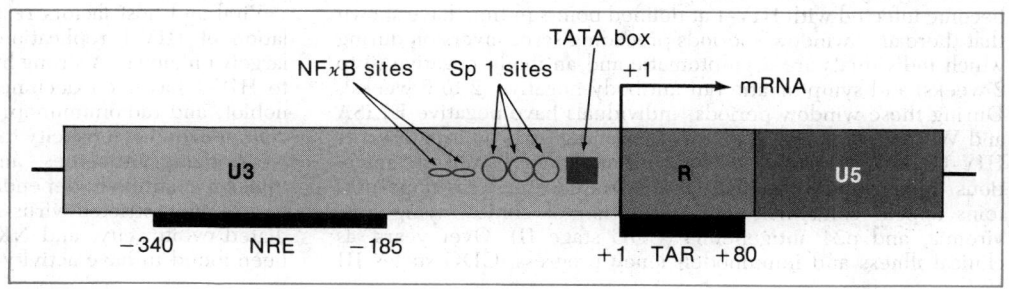

FIGURE 411–4. Genomic organization of HIV-1.

chemical polarity as the mRNA from which viral products are translated. Like eukaryotic mRNA's, the genomic viral RNA contains a 5' methylated-G nucleotide, a poly(A) tract of 100 to 200 nucleotides at its 3' end, and a number of methylated(A) residues. Host cell–derived tRNA incorporated within the virion is base paired over a stretch of 18 nucleotides to the primer binding site of the genomic viral RNA near its 5' terminus and serves to prime the synthesis of minus-strand DNA during the initial stages of viral replication following infection.

The HIV-1 genome is bounded by long terminal repeat (LTR) elements and contains genes encoding structural and enzymatic proteins (gag, pol, and env) found in all other replication-competent retroviruses. In addition to these, however, HIV-1 contains genes (tat, rev, vif, vpu, and nef) encoding other viral functions unique to this family of viruses that are responsible for their biologic behavior.

The LTR sequences of HIV-1 direct and regulate expression of the viral genome (Fig. 411–5). Deletion mutant studies of the LTR have identified at least five regions important for gene expression, including the TATA box and promotor where RNA polymerase binds and transcription is initiated (+1); a negative regulatory element (NRE) located between nucleotides −340 and −185, deletion of which increases the level of gene expression directed by the viral LTR; enhancer elements (NFκB and Sp1) located between nucleotides −137 and −17; and a trans-acting responsive region (TAR) located between nucleotides +1 and +80 which represents the putative binding region for regulatory factors responsible for tat-mediated transcriptional activation.

The gag gene encodes a precursor protein of 53 kDa (pr 53) which is cleaved into four smaller products with the linear order NH₂-p18-p24-p7-p9-COOH. These proteins constitute the core protein structure of the virus and also subserve nucleic acid and lipid membrane binding functions. The gag proteins of HIV-1, like those of other retroviruses, are synthesized as a polyprotein precursor that is subsequently cleaved during the viral maturation process. This facilitates the assembly of the different components of the virus core structure into a three-dimensional configuration that, when cleaved by a specific virus-derived protease, acquires the specialized functions characteristic of the mature virion. The polymerase gene products are translated from the same genomic RNA message as the gag proteins but in a different, overlapping reading frame as a result of ribosomal frame shifting. The pol gene encodes three proteins that are cleaved from a larger precursor polypeptide. These genes include NH₂–protease(p13)–reverse transcriptase (p66/p51)–integrase(p31)–COOH. The HIV-1 protease plays a critical role in virus biology, acting specifically to cleave gag and pol precursor polypeptides into functionally active proteins. The reverse transcriptase of HIV-1 is a magne-

sium-requiring RNA-dependent DNA polymerase responsible for replicating the RNA viral genome. The integrase protein is required for proviral integration into the host cell genome. The envelope gene (env) encodes a glycosylated polypeptide precursor (gp160) that is processed to form the exterior envelope glycoprotein (gp120) and the transmembrane glycoprotein (gp41), which anchors the envelope complex to the virus surface. It is the viral envelope that is responsible for CD4 binding, fusion, and virus entry.

Within the HIV-1 genome, there are additional genes that serve important viral functions and which distinguish HIV-1 and its related viruses from other retroviruses. These include the vif, vpr, and vpu genes located between pol and env; the nef gene located 3' to the env and extending into the U3 region of the viral LTR; and the tat and rev genes, both of which exist as bipartite coding exons in the central and 3' end of the virus. The tat gene encodes a 14-kDa protein that is essential for HIV-1 replication, upregulating HIV-1 expression at both transcriptional and post-transcriptional levels. The target sequence for tat-mediated upregulation of HIV-1 expression is the TAR region of the LTR, which apparently interacts with cellular factors induced by tat, since the tat protein itself has not been shown to bind TAR directly. The rev gene is also absolutely required for HIV-1 replication, facilitating transport of unspliced viral mRNA species from the nucleus to cytoplasm. In the absence of rev, gag and env mRNA transcripts are multiply-spliced such that gag and env proteins are not made. Recent studies have also shown that rev may possess an additional function of downregulating viral mRNA transcription when it is expressed at high levels. The vif gene encodes a protein product of 23 kDa, which, although not part of the virion itself, is required for the production of virions that are fully infectious. The vpr gene encodes a protein of 15 kDa which exhibits transactivating properties on viral and heterologous promoter sequences. The vpu gene encodes a 16-kDa protein that is involved in virus assembly and release. The nef gene encodes a 27-kDa protein that interacts with the NRE region of the LTR to downregulate viral transcription in vitro but whose function in vivo is uncertain. Interestingly, the nef protein shares structural homology with the ATP-binding site of protein kinases, is phosphorylated by protein kinase C, displays GTPase, autophosphorylation, and GTP binding activities, and has been reported to downregulate CD4 expression.

In summary, HIV-1 encodes the usual structural and enzymatic proteins typical of other replication-competent retroviruses, including gag, pol, and env, but in addition it encodes a group of at least six additional regulatory proteins (vif, vpr, vpu, tat, rev, and nef) whose activities are critically important in regulating the life cycle and pathogenesis of the virus.

FIGURE 411–5. Regulatory regions in the long terminal repeat (LTR) of HIV-1.

CELL TROPISM

The hallmark of AIDS is a selective depletion of CD4+ helper-inducer lymphocytes. This defect is believed to result largely from the selective tropism of HIV-1 for this population of cells based on the high affinity of the viral gp120 envelope protein for the CD4 molecule (km = 4×10^{-9}M). CD4 normally serves as a ligand for MHC II (major histocompatibility complex type II) interaction, but in HIV-1 infection it is utilized as the primary receptor molecule for HIV-1 targeting. This has been shown conclusively by studies demonstrating (1) direct complexing of gp120 and CD4 during viral infection; (2) inhibition of viral attachment and infection by anti-CD4 monoclonal antibodies that prevent gp120 binding; (3) the ability of recombinant CD4 to confer susceptibility to HIV-1 infection to transfected human cells that normally do not express CD4 (e.g., HeLa cells).

A variety of cell types other than helper-inducer lymphocytes are known to express CD4 on their surface and are capable of replicating HIV-1. These include blood monocytes, tissue macrophages, follicular dendritic cells in lymph nodes, Langerhans cells in skin, and microglial and multinucleated giant cells in the central nervous system. These cells generally express smaller amounts of CD4 on their cell surface but nonetheless have been shown to represent important reservoirs for HIV-1 in vivo. Infection of such cells, in fact, may play an important role in the pathogenesis of AIDS by sequestration of the virus as described for other lentiviruses such as visna. Other cell types, including neurons, glial cells, B lymphocytes, colorectal epithelial cells, and myeloid precursors, which may or may not express small amounts of CD4 or CD4-related mRNA, have occasionally been shown to support HIV-1 replication, but the pathophysiologic significance of such findings in regard to viral pathogenesis in vivo is uncertain. However, such studies have raised the possibility of the existence of cellular receptor molecules for HIV-1 in addition to CD4.

VIRAL PATHOGENESIS

Retroviral diseases are typically characterized by restricted viral gene expression, latency, and lifelong persistence of virus in the face of substantial host immune responses. These features are characteristic of natural infections with visna virus in sheep, equine infectious anemia virus in horses, caprine arthritis-encephalitis virus in goats, and HTLV-I and HTLV-II infection in humans. From cohort studies of individuals infected with HIV-1 at known points in time, it is estimated that between 26 and 36 per cent of infected individuals develop AIDS within 7 years of infection and that an additional 40 per cent develop lesser signs of immune dysfunction. This protracted clinical course suggests that expression of the HIV-1 genome in vivo is downregulated as compared to in vitro infection by lymphocytes by HIV-1, which is characterized by explosive lytic viral infection.

Figure 411–6 depicts the natural history of HIV-1 infection of humans in relationship to clinical symptoms, immune function, and viral replication. Initial infection with HIV-1 frequently causes an acute viral syndrome (CDC stage I) with protean manifestations most frequently characterized by fever, lymphadenopathy, pharyngitis, and rash. Other symptoms and signs that may occur with acute HIV-1 infection include myalgias and arthralgias, leukopenia, thrombocytopenia, nausea, diarrhea, headache, and encephalopathy. During this primary phase of infection, symptoms are accompanied by high-level HIV-1 plasma viremia, with peak virus titers reaching 10^3 to 10^4 infectious units per milliliter. Viremia is also accompanied by high levels of circulating HIV-1 p24 antigen. Studies of individuals who have become infected with HIV-1 at defined points in time have shown that there are "window" periods preceding seroconversion during which individuals are asymptomatic and antibody negative (0 to 2 weeks) and symptomatic but antibody negative (2 to 6 weeks). During these window periods, individuals have negative ELISA and Western blot antibody tests (screening and confirmatory) for HIV-1, yet they are virally infected and their tissues are infectious. Subsequently, antibodies to viral core and envelope proteins appear coincident with resolution of clinical symptoms, viremia, and p24 antigenemia (CDC stage II). Over years, as clinical illness and immunodeficiency progress (CDC stages III

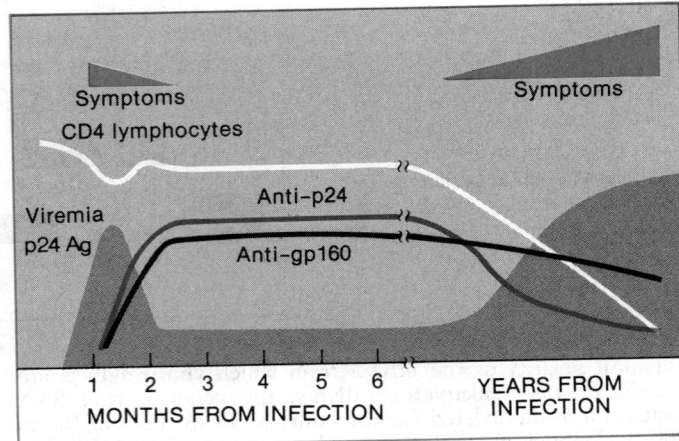

FIGURE 411–6. Natural history model for HIV-1 infection. Viremia denotes cell-free infectious virus in plasma, p24 Ag denotes circulating viral p24 antigen in plasma, and anti-p24 and anti-gp 160 correspond to antibodies to viral core and envelope proteins.

and IV), plasma viremia, p24 antigenemia, and intracellular virus burden increase.

The protracted clinical course of HIV-1 infection raises clinically relevant questions regarding viral pathogenesis: What are the molecular mechanisms responsible for CD4+ cell loss in vivo? What are the viral and host mechanisms underlying the chronicity of HIV-1 infection? The precise biologic mechanisms responsible for the cytopathic effects of HIV-1 in vivo are not known. Molecularly cloned HIV-1 proviral DNA, transfected into human cells, has been shown in cell culture experiments to contain all necessary information to generate infectious and cytopathic virus. Thus, there is no question that HIV-1 alone has the potential for direct cytopathic activity against CD4+ lymphocytes in vitro and in vivo. Expression of only the HIV-1 envelope on lymphocytes is sufficient for inducing fusion of cells with normal uninfected CD4+ bystander cells, suggesting that syncytium formation mediated by gp120–CD4 interaction may also contribute to cell loss in vivo. However, the relatively low proportion of virally infected cells in vivo at any one time has suggested that other mechanisms of CD4 cell loss may also be operative. Cell-free HIV-1 gp120 envelope protein has been shown to adsorb to CD4+ cells and serve as an effective antigen for mediating antibody-dependent cell-mediated cytotoxicity, and when processed by antigen-presenting cells, to constitute a target for direct T-cell cytotoxicity. The possibility has also been raised that since both HIV-1 gp120 and the cellular MHC class II molecule bind to the same ligand, CD4, the two molecules could share certain antigenic determinants. If so, then antibodies directed to gp120 could cross-react with MHC class II molecules, resulting in autoimmunity. Such autoantibodies reactive both with the HIV-1 gp120 and gp41 glycoproteins and with MHC II have been described. The relative importance of these processes to CD4 cell loss in vivo remains to be determined. Viral pathogenesis within the central nervous system of infected individuals, wherein the predominant cell types infected with HIV-1 are cells of the monocyte/macrophage lineage, is likely to involve additional mechanisms. Possibilities include the elaboration of cytotoxic factors from infected cells, interference with neurotropic factors, direct viral infection of neurons or oligodendrocytes, and stimulation of other viral infections. Although a great deal has been learned about the molecular structure and biology of HIV-1, the actual mechanisms of disease pathogenesis are still unclear.

Viral and host factors responsible for the apparent downregulation of HIV-1 replication following initial infection are also largely unknown. A strong humoral and cellular immune response to HIV-1 has been documented on the basis of ELISA, immunoblot, and radioimmunoprecipitation assays of patient sera and cell-mediated cytotoxicity to target cells displaying viral antigens. Neutralizing antibodies, antibody-dependent cell-mediated cytotoxicity, antibody-dependent complement-mediated cytotoxicity, MHC-restricted virus-specific cytotoxic T-lymphocyte–mediated cytotoxicity, and NK cell–mediated cytotoxicity have all been found to have activity against HIV-1 in vitro and may play an important role in the initial downmodulation of viral replication. However, the relative efficacy of the various immune effector arms and the changes that occur with time which eventually allow uncontrolled viral replication are unknown. Another factor believed to influence viral replication of HIV-1 in vivo, aside from the immune response, is the level of cell activation and the interaction of the normal immune cytokine network with viral transcriptional elements in infected cells. The importance of cell activation in the expression and propagation of HIV-1 has been demonstrated by treatment of lymphocytes and lymphoid cell lines with mitogens, antigens, and anti-CD3 monoclonal antibodies. Activation of HIV expression by mitogens is believed to follow a pattern similar to that of eukaryotic gene regulation with cellular transcription factors interacting with specific regions of gene promotors and enhancers, resulting in increased mRNA synthesis. Activation of T lymphocytes involves the induction of cellular factors that bind to specific enhancer elements, termed NFκB, present in both interleukin 2 and interleukin 2 receptor genes as well as in the LTR region of HIV-1 (see Fig. 411–5). Thus, mitogen and antigen activation of T cells resulting in the induction of NFκB binding proteins also stimulates HIV-1 enhancer elements to initiate transcription of viral mRNA. The induction of HIV-1 expression by T-cell activating mitogens and antigens also raises the possibility that specific cytokines may be directly involved in the activation of HIV-1. TNF-α and TNF-β (tumor necrosis factor) along with IL6 and GM-CSF have been shown to induce HIV-1 expression. TNF-α, in particular, is suspected to play an instrumental role in HIV-1 activation in vivo, since it is produced by monocytes/macrophages in response to naturally occurring infections and has been shown to act in both an autocrine and a paracrine fashion to activate macrophages and to further stimulate mitogen- and antigen-induced proliferation of T cells. Elevated levels of TNF-α are produced by monocytes from HIV-1–infected individuals, and such patients have elevated levels of TNF-α in their blood. Infection by other viruses such as herpes simplex virus, cytomegalovirus, Epstein-Barr virus, and HTLV-I and HTLV-II frequently coincides with HIV-1 infection and, by stimulating TNF-α and other cytokines, may enhance HIV-1 replication. In addition, coinfection of cells by HIV-1 and these other viruses may increase HIV-1 replication directly by heterologous enhancement of viral transcription.

One of the most striking properties of HIV-1 is the extent of genetic variability evident in independent isolates of the virus. The variability of the HIV-1 genome is characteristic of retroviruses in general, since reverse transcription of viral RNA into proviral DNA and transcription of proviral DNA into genomic viral RNA are not subject to cellular proofreading mechanisms, and the rate of nucleotide misincorporation by the viral reverse

transcriptase is of the order of 10^{-4} per nucleotide per replication cycle. Since the HIV-1 genome is 10^4 nucleotides in length, this high rate of nucleotide misincorporation means that virtually no two viruses are identical and that HIV-1 isolates must, by definition, be described in terms of a "quasispecies" composed of populations of highly related but distinct viral genomes. Direct nucleotide sequence analysis of uncultured, virally infected human tissues using polymerase chain reaction amplification has confirmed these findings. Different genomic regions of HIV-1 typically vary among independent isolates by 5 to 20 per cent in amino acid sequence, with gene products that correspond to structural or enzymatic proteins being more highly conserved than others such as envelope. During natural infection, different viral genomes evolve in parallel and result in the emergence of multiple distinct genotypic forms. Such variation of HIV-1 is comparable to that found for another lentivirus, equine infectious anemia virus, for which it is clear that such genotypic changes are responsible for biologically important alterations in viral antigenicity, allowing the virus to elude host immune defenses. For HIV-1, the full significance of HIV-1 variation has not yet been determined. However, virus strains have been isolated from patients before and after treatment with zidovudine, demonstrating the emergence of drug-resistant variants. Thus, it is believed that genotypic variability of HIV-1 may serve as an important source of antigenic and biologic variation relevant to immunologic control and to vaccine and antiviral drug development.

HUMAN IMMUNODEFICIENCY VIRUS TYPE II

Following the discovery of HIV-1 as the cause of epidemic AIDS in the United States, Europe, and central Africa, patients in West Africa with AIDS-like symptoms were identified whose sera reacted more strongly with an immunodeficiency virus (SIV$_{MAC}$) isolated from captive rhesus macaques in United States primate centers than with HIV-1. The identification of patients with serologic reactivity for SIV$_{MAC}$ raised the possibility that certain African human and simian populations could be infected with immunodeficiency viruses distinct from HIV-1. An extensive survey of African primate species for such viruses led to the identification of distinct SIV species present in African green monkeys (SIV$_{AGM}$), mandrills (SIV$_{MND}$), sooty mangabeys (SIV$_{SM}$), and chimpanzees (SIV$_{CPZ}$) (Fig. 411–7). West African patients with AIDS-like symptoms and healthy individuals at risk for AIDS were identified who were infected with a virus closely related to SIV$_{SM}$. This virus was isolated, molecularly cloned and characterized, and shown to represent a second major class of human immunodeficiency viruses termed HIV-2. Although originally limited geographically to West Africa, HIV-2 has now been

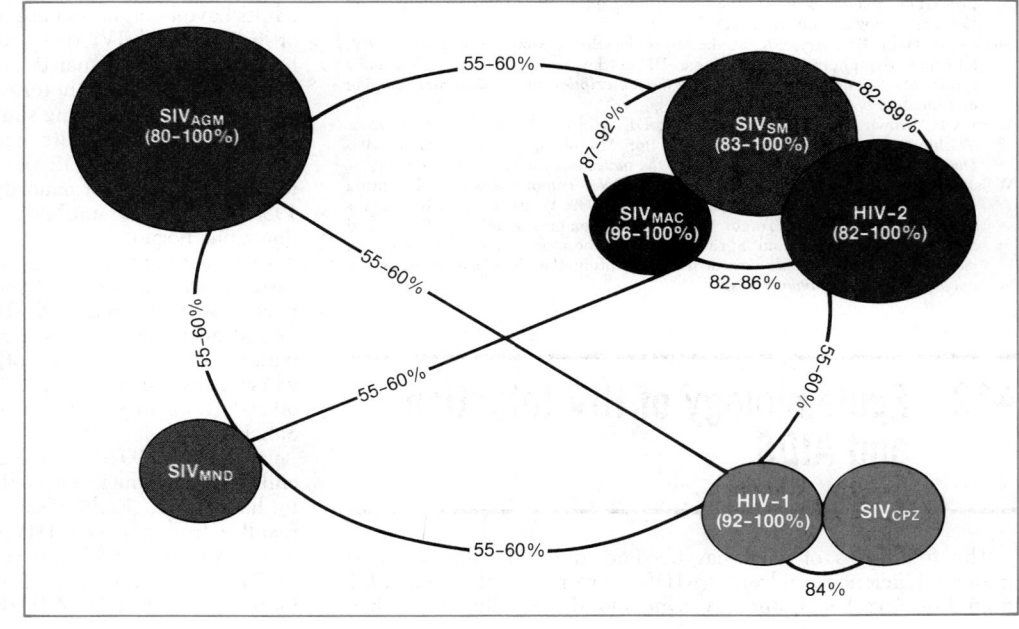

FIGURE 411–7. Primate lentivirus taxonomy. Percentages in lines represent amino acid identities in the *pol* gene product of the respective virus groups, whereas those in parentheses correspond to identities in this gene product among different virus isolates within each group. (Reprinted by permission from *Nature*, Vol. 345, pp. 288. Copyright © 1990 Macmillan Magazines Limited.)

identified infrequently in AIDS patients in Europe, the United States, and South America. HIV-2 is approximately 40 to 50 per cent similar to HIV-1 in overall nucleotide sequence homology. There are two major differences in the genomic organization of HIV-1 and HIV-2. The *vpu* gene of HIV-1 is not present in HIV-2, and HIV-2 contains an additional gene, *vpx*, in its central region that is not present in HIV-1. Although the function of *vpx* is not entirely clear, HIV-2 strains deficient in *vpx* replicate as well in primary lymphocyte cultures. Antigenically, HIV-2 and HIV-1 are distinct, with greatest cross-reactivity in structural proteins and least in envelope proteins. Like HIV-1, HIV-2 selectively infects CD4+ cells. Of clinical relevance, although HIV-2 can cause profound immunodeficiency and an AIDS syndrome indistinguishable from that caused by HIV-1, there is evidence to suggest that HIV-2 may in general be less virulent than HIV-1 and cause disease over a more prolonged period of time. Also, because of the antigenic differences between HIV-1 and HIV-2, currently licensed serologic tests for identification of HIV-1 detect only about half of individuals infected with HIV-2. It is anticipated that in the future diagnostic tests will be developed and licensed that will detect both HIV-1 and HIV-2 infections and distinguish them from each other.

The identification of SIV's in African primates that are genetically closely related to HIV-1 (SIV$_{CPZ}$) and HIV-2 (SIV$_{SM}$) (Fig. 411–7) suggests the possibility of a simian origin for these viruses followed by cross-species transmission. At the present time, genetic sequence information of virus strains from wild-caught African monkey species is insufficient to prove conclusively the pattern or timing of cross-species transmission of these viruses. However, such issues are fundamentally important to the elucidation of the origin of the current AIDS epidemic, the molecular basis for the pathogenicity of HIV's and SIV's in natural and unnatural host species, and an explanation for the relatively recent appearance of AIDS as an epidemic.

Barre-Sinoussi F, Chermann JC, Rey F, et al.: Isolation of a T-lymphotropic retrovirus from a patient at risk for acquired immune deficiency syndrome (AIDS). Science 220:868, 1983. *First description of HIV-1.*

Clark SJ, Saag MS, Decker WD, et al.: High titers of cytopathic virus in plasma of patients with symptomatic primary HIV-1 infection. N Engl J Med 324:954, 1991. *First study describing virologic determinants of HIV-1 natural history and the clinical findings associated with acute HIV-1 infection.*

Fauci AS: The human immunodeficiency virus: Infectivity and mechanisms of pathogenesis. Science 239:617, 1988. *Excellent review of immunopathogenic mechanisms of HIV-1 infection.*

Gallo RC, Salahuddin SZ, Popovic M, et al.: Frequent detection and isolation of cytopathic retroviruses (HTLV-III) from patients with AIDS and at risk for AIDS. Science 224:500, 1984. *Initial report conclusively identifying HIV-1 as the etiologic agent responsible for AIDS.*

Greene WC: The molecular biology of human immunodeficiency virus type 1 infection. N Engl J Med 324:308, 1991. *Excellent review of HIV-1 molecular biology and pathogenesis.*

Popovic M, Sarngadharan MG, Read E, et al.: Detection, isolation, and continuous production of cytopathic retroviruses (HTLV-III) from patients with AIDS and pre-AIDS. Science 224:497, 1984. *First description of the large-scale production and biologic analysis of HIV-1.*

Shaw GM, Hahn BH, Arya SK, et al.: Molecular characterization of human T-cell leukemia (lymphotropic) virus type III in the acquired immunodeficiency syndrome. Science 226:1165, 1984. *First description of the molecular cloning and analysis of the HIV-1 provirus.*

Varmus H, Brown P: Retroviruses. In Berg DE, Howe MM (eds.): Mobile DNA. Washington, D.C., American Society for Microbiology, 1989, pp 53–108. *Detailed and comprehensive review of the molecular biology of retroviruses.*

Weiss R, Teich N, Varmus H, Coffin J (eds.): RNA Tumor Viruses. Cold Spring Harbor, NY, Cold Spring Harbor Laboratory, 1982. Weiss R, Teich N, Varmus H, Coffin J (eds.): RNA Tumor Viruses 2/Supplements and Appendixes. Cold Spring Harbor, NY, Cold Spring Harbor Laboratory, 1985. *Textbooks on current knowledge of all retroviruses, including the three major groups of onco-, lenti- and spumaviruses.*

412 Epidemiology of HIV Infection and AIDS

James W. Curran

The first cases of what has become known as the acquired immunodeficiency syndrome (AIDS) were reported in mid-1981 from Los Angeles, California. One month following these five reports of *Pneumocystis carinii* pneumonia (PCP) in young homosexual men, 26 cases of Kaposi's sarcoma (KS) in homosexual men in New York and California and additional cases of PCP and other opportunistic infections were reported. Reports of cases in the United States continued to rise, and soon the occurrence of PCP, KS, or other serious opportunistic infections in a person with unexplained immune dysfunction became known as AIDS. In retrospect, sporadic cases may have occurred in the United States, Europe, or Africa as much as three decades earlier, but the worldwide epidemic was not apparent until much later. Extensive retrospective surveillance in the United States revealed several cases diagnosed in 1978 or 1979 with a clear increase in 1980–1981. For all practical purposes, AIDS was a new disease in the United States and throughout the world.

The initial occurrence of AIDS in homosexual men and intravenous drug users suggested by 1982 that a transmissible agent was the likely cause. In the absence of proof, other hypotheses abounded. The transmissible agent hypothesis gained credence by early 1983 with the documented occurrence of AIDS in persons with hemophilia and in recipients of blood transfusions. Within a year, the retrovirus, now termed human immunodeficiency virus (HIV), was isolated and shown to be the cause of AIDS.

HIV INFECTION AND AIDS IN THE UNITED STATES

Since 1981, more than 300,000 cases of AIDS have been reported from 156 countries. Slightly over half of these were reported from the United States, reflecting the relatively high incidence of the syndrome here and a well-established national active surveillance system. All 50 states require reporting of AIDS to state health departments, and subsequently without names to the Centers for Disease Control (CDC). The surveillance case definition for AIDS was initially developed before the etiology of AIDS was known but was revised following the development of diagnostic tests for HIV infection. The current definition provides a consistent method to accurately monitor trends of serious HIV-associated morbidity and mortality (Table 412–1). Patients infected with HIV exhibit a spectrum of manifestations ranging from no symptoms to AIDS. Systems have been developed to classify these manifestations in children and adults (Table 412–2). In states that require reporting of all HIV infections, use of a standardized classification system is encouraged.

INCIDENCE AND TRENDS OF AIDS IN THE UNITED STATES

By March 1991, 167,803 cases of AIDS in adults and children had been reported to the CDC; 106,361 (62 per cent) were reported to have died, including over 80 per cent of those diagnosed before 1987. Nearly sixty per cent of reported cases in adults have been in homosexual or bisexual men without a history of intravenous (IV) drug use, and 7 per cent have been in homosexual or bisexual IV drug users. More than 63 per cent of the reported cases in heterosexual men and women had a history of IV drug use, including slightly over half of the cases in women. One per cent of adults with AIDS had hemophilia or other coagulation disorders; 2 per cent of cases were associated with transfusions, the vast majority of which had been received before 1985, when HIV antibody screening of all blood and plasma donations began.

Five per cent of the total cases of AIDS and 34 per cent of cases in women were attributed to heterosexual contact with a person with documented HIV infection or in one of the other main transmission categories. Also included in this category are patients reported with no other risk who were born in countries where heterosexual contact has been shown to be the major route of HIV transmission (such as Haiti and most countries in sub-Saharan Africa).

By March 1991, 2903 cases of AIDS had been reported in children less than 13 years of age, with over 51 per cent reported to have died. Eighty-four per cent of pediatric AIDS cases resulted from perinatal HIV infection, 9 per cent were attributed to transfusions, and 5 per cent occurred in children with hemophilia. In 50 per cent of the perinatally acquired cases, the mother had a history of IV drug use, and in an additional 21 per

TABLE 412–1. SURVEILLANCE DEFINITION FOR AIDS, CENTERS FOR DISEASE CONTROL (REVISED SEPTEMBER 1987)*

A. Indicator diseases diagnosed definitively in the absence of other causes of immunodeficiency and laboratory tests for HIV

   Candidiasis of the esophagus, trachea, bronchi, or lungs
   Cryptococcus, extrapulmonary
   Cryptosporidiosis with diarrhea >1 month
   Cytomegalovirus disease exclusive of liver, spleen, or lymph nodes in patients >1 month of age
   Herpes simplex virus infection causing a mucocutaneous ulcer >1 month or bronchitis, pneumonitis, or esophagitis in patients >1 month of age
   Kaposi's sarcoma in patients <60 years of age
   Lymphoma of the brain (primary) in patients <60 years of age
   Lymphoid interstitial pneumonia and/or pulmonary lymphoid hyperplasia in patients <13 years of age
   Mycobacterium avium complex or *M. kansasii* disease, disseminated *Pneumocystis carinii* pneumonia
   Progressive multifocal leukoencephalopathy
   Toxoplasmosis of the brain in patients >1 month of age

B. Indicator diseases diagnosed definitively regardless of other causes of immunodeficiency and laboratory evidence of HIV present

   All indicator diseases listed in Section A
   Specified bacterial infections, recurrent or multiple, in patients <13 years of age that are caused by *Haemophilus, Streptococcus,* or other pyogenic bacteria
   Coccidioidomycosis, disseminated
   HIV encephalopathy
   Histoplasmosis, disseminated
   Isosporiasis with diarrhea >1 month
   Kaposi's sarcoma at any age
   Primary lymphoma of the brain at any age
   Non-Hodgkin's lymphoma of B cell or unknown immunologic phenotype, including small noncleaved lymphoma or immunoblastic sarcoma
   Mycobacterial disease exclusive of *M. tuberculosis*, disseminated
   M. tuberculosis, extrapulmonary
   Salmonella septicemia, recurrent
   HIV wasting syndrome

C. Indicator diseases diagnosed presumptively with laboratory evidence of HIV infection

   Candidiasis, esophageal
   Cytomegalovirus retinitis with loss of vision
   Kaposi's sarcoma
   Lymphoid interstitial pneumonia and/or pulmonary lymphoid hyperplasia in patients <13 years of age
   Mycobacterial disease, disseminated
   Pneumocystis carinii pneumonia
   Toxoplasmosis, brain, in patients >1 month of age

D. Indicator diseases diagnosed definitively in the absence of other causes of immunodeficiency and negative laboratory test results for HIV

   Pneumocystis carinii pneumonia
   Other indicator diseases listed in Section A and T helper-inducer (CD4) lymphocyte count <400 cubic millimeter

*From MMWR 36(Suppl 1):1–15, 1987.

---

cent, the mother was reported to be the sexual partner of an IV drug user.

AIDS has disproportionately affected black and Hispanic minority populations in the United States. Twenty-seven per cent of adult and 52 per cent of pediatric cases were blacks and 15 per cent of adult and 26 per cent of pediatric cases were Hispanic. In contrast, blacks and Hispanics are estimated to account for 11.6 per cent and 6.5 per cent of the United States population, respectively. This disproportionate AIDS rate for black and Hispanic Americans to a large extent reflects the much higher rates of reported AIDS cases in black and Hispanic IV drug users, their heterosexual partners, and infants (Table 412–3). The relatively higher rates of AIDS in blacks were greatest in the northeast and southeast regions of the country and in Hispanics among Puerto Rican Americans from the same regions. This reflects the high prevalence of HIV infection in IV drug–using populations in these areas.

Three quarters of cases of AIDS are reported among young adults in the 25- to 44-year-old age group, leading to substantial decreases in life expectancy. In 1988, AIDS accounted for 11 per

TABLE 412–2. CLASSIFICATION SYSTEM FOR HUMAN IMMUNODEFICIENCY VIRUS INFECTIONS IN ADULTS AND ADOLESCENTS (CENTERS FOR DISEASE CONTROL, 1986)*

Group I.   Acute infection
Group II.   Asymptomatic infection
Group III.   Persistent generalized lymphadenopathy
Group IV.   Other diseases
   Subgroup A.   Constitutional disease including HIV wasting syndrome in the CDC surveillance definition for AIDS
   Subgroup B.   Neurologic disease including HIV encephalopathy in the CDC surveillance definition for AIDS
   Subgroup C.   Secondary infectious diseases
     Category C-1.   Specified secondary infectious diseases in the CDC surveillance definition for AIDS
     Category C-2.   Other specified secondary infectious diseases
   Subgroup D.   Secondary cancers in the CDC surveillance definition for AIDS
   Subgroup E.   Other conditions

*From MMWR 35:334–339, 1986.

---

cent of deaths in men and 3 per cent of deaths in women in these age groups. In 1987, HIV infection and AIDS ranked seventh among contributors to premature mortality nationally, behind unintentional injuries, cancer, heart disease, suicide/homicide, congenital anomalies, and premature birth.

TRENDS IN AIDS AND PROJECTIONS FOR THE FUTURE

Reported cases of AIDS continued to increase in the United States throughout the 1980's. Cases diagnosed and reported in 1989 exceeded those in the previous year by 14 per cent. Although reported cases increased in all groups, proportional increases were greater for blacks and Hispanics than whites and substantially greater for women than men. Cases associated with heterosexual contact and pediatric cases resulting from perinatal transmission had the largest increases in the late 1980's.

Long-term trends in AIDS cases are depicted in Figure 412–1. Beginning in mid-1987, trends in reported AIDS cases in the United States shifted, primarily reflecting a slowdown in the increase in reported cases in homosexual/bisexual men (Fig. 412–1A). This slowing of the upward trend in AIDS cases that occurred in 1987, particularly in homosexual/bisexual men, is thought to be due to a combination of factors, including (1) a decline in the incidence of new HIV infections in homosexual/bisexual men in the early 1980's, leading to a subsequent decline in AIDS incidence; (2) use of antiretroviral and other therapies by mid-1987, leading to a lengthening of the incubation period from

TABLE 412–3. ANNUAL INCIDENCE (PER MILLION POPULATION) OF AIDS AND RELATIVE RISK BY RACIAL AND ETHNIC GROUPS, AGE, AND TRANSMISSION CATEGORY, 1989*

Category	White	Black	Hispanic	Other
Adult/adolescent men	243.9 (1.0)	788.1 (3.2)†	586.8 (2.4)†	121.8 (0.5)†
Adult/adolescent women	12.5 (1.0)	163.8 (13.1)†	80.1 (6.4)	14.1 (1.1)
Adult/adolescent total‡	124.4 (1.0)	454.8 (3.7)	331.4 (2.7)	66.3 (0.5)†
Homosexual men	177.9 (1.0)	289.0 (1.6)†	256.6 (1.4)†	64.7 (0.4)†
Bisexual men	30.2 (1.0)	106.5 (3.5)†	71.9 (2.4)†	23.0 (0.8)†
Heterosexual IV drug abusers	11.4 (1.0)	181.7 (15.9)†	117.0 (10.2)†	8.0 (0.7)†
Hemophilia	1.6 (1.0)	0.8 (0.5)†	1.3 (0.9)	0.9 (0.6)
Transfusion	3.6 (1.0)	5.5 (1.5)†	4.6 (1.3)†	2.2 (0.6)
Pediatric, total‡	3.5 (1.0)	47.9 (13.6)†	27.4 (7.8)†	4.2 (1.2)
Mother, IV drugs	1.3 (1.0)	19.9 (15.4)†	11.2 (8.7)†	0.5 (0.4)
Mother's partner, IV drugs	0.5 (1.0)	7.3 (14.9)†	7.0 (14.3)†	0.5 (1.0)
Transfusion-associated	0.7 (1.0)	1.1 (1.6)	1.1 (1.6)	0.5 (0.7)
Hemophilia	0.5 (1.0)	0.7 (1.4)	0.6 (1.2)	1.1 (2.2)

*Relative risk, shown in parentheses, is the ratio of the incidence in each race or ethnic group to the incidence in whites.
†Relative risk significantly different from 1.0 (P < 0.05).
‡For all men, homosexual men, and bisexual men, the denominator consisted of all men ≥13 years; for all women, the denominator was all women ≥13 years. For pediatric categories, the denominator consisted of all children <13 years.

infection to AIDS; and (3) possible decreases in the completeness or timeliness of reporting. Cases in adult transmission recipients and persons with hemophilia had likely reached their peak by 1989, reflecting the dramatic decline in new HIV infections from blood transfusions after 1985 (Fig. 412–1B). By 1989, a dramatic decline had been noted in pediatric cases of AIDS associated with blood transfusions. In contrast, cases associated with IV drug use (Fig. 412–1A), heterosexual transmission (Fig. 412–1C), and perinatal transmission (Fig. 412–1D) continued to increase.

Cases of AIDS are projected to continue to increase through 1993 in each of the principal transmission categories (Fig. 412–2). Including adjustments for underreporting, it was estimated that 390,000 to 480,000 persons will be diagnosed with AIDS by the end of 1993, including 61,000 to 98,000 cases in that year alone (Table 412–4). A minimum of 250,000 deaths are projected to have resulted from AIDS in the United States by 1993, just 12 years after the syndrome was first reported.

PREVALENCE AND INCIDENCE OF HIV INFECTION IN THE UNITED STATES

Trends in reported AIDS cases do not provide a complete picture of the prevalence of the public health problem HIV infection poses for a population group, community, or nation, since HIV infection per se precedes the clinical diagnosis of AIDS by many years. In some groups, reported AIDS continues to increase after HIV infection has declined. For example, despite very dramatic declines in HIV incidence associated with blood and plasma transfusions after 1985, when antibody screening of blood donations was instituted in the United States, reported cases of AIDS associated with transfusions and in persons with hemophilia continued to increase until 1989. Conversely, reported AIDS case rates may grossly underestimate the future impact of HIV infection, especially in communities or populations more recently affected by the epidemic. Most notable are the emerging epidemics of HIV infection in Thailand, India, and other areas of Asia where few cases of AIDS have reached the clinical horizon. For this reason, AIDS surveillance must be accompanied by carefully conducted HIV serosurveys to accurately monitor the public health problem.

The U.S. Public Health Service estimated that approximately 1 million persons were infected with HIV in the United States by the end of 1989, up from approximately 750,000 in 1986. These estimates were based both on available HIV seroprevalence data and on statistical models utilizing AIDS surveillance data and information on the natural history of infection.

National data on HIV prevalence are directly measured from HIV testing of first-time blood donors, military recruit applicants, job corps applicants, and surveys of antibody status of newborn infants. The prevalence of HIV infection in both military recruit applicants and blood donors grossly underestimates true HIV prevalence rates, since homosexual men, IV drug users, and persons with hemophilia are discouraged from applying for military service and actively deferred from donating blood.

Extensive analyses of HIV prevalence rates in military recruit applicants have been published. The crude HIV seroprevalence rates were similar to reported AIDS rates for 1989, with a remarkable similarity in geographic distribution (Fig. 412–3). After age adjustment, HIV prevalence rates in applicants are higher than AIDS rates but still greatly underrepresent the magnitude of the HIV problem. HIV prevalence rates were two to three times higher in male than female applicants and three to ten times higher in black and Hispanic than in white applicants. In limited studies of risk factors in military recruit applicants and blood donors, more than 85 per cent of those interviewed had recognized risk factors for HIV.

The highest HIV prevalence rates detected have been among homosexual or bisexual men, IV drug users, and persons with hemophilia. Prevalence rates in these groups ranged widely in studies—homosexual/bisexual men (10 to 70 per cent), IV drug users (0 to 70 per cent), and persons with hemophilia (15 to 90 per cent). Since most surveys in homosexual men and IV drug users were conducted among persons seeking medical care for sexually transmitted diseases (STD's) or treatment for drug abuse, the data may not be completely representative of these popula-

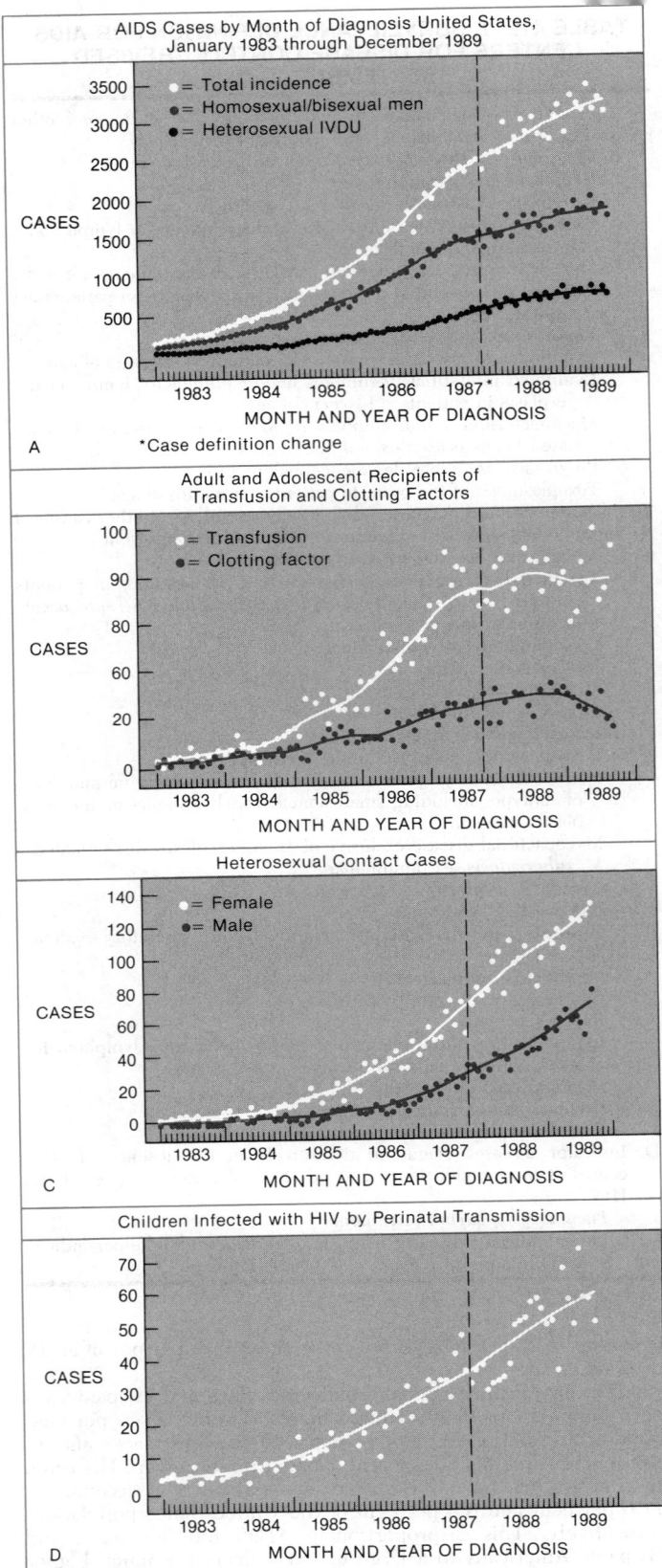

FIGURE 412–1. AIDS cases by month of diagnosis, United States, January 1983 through December 1989. Figures have been adjusted for reporting delays, by mode of transmission. Points represent monthly incidence; lines represent smoothed incidence. The vertical lines depict the date of change in the AIDS case definition. A, All cases, homosexual/bisexual men, and heterosexual intravenous drug users (IVDU). B, Adult and adolescent recipients of transfusions and clotting factors. C, Men and women infected with HIV through heterosexual contact (excludes persons born in countries where heterosexual transmission predominates). D, Children infected with HIV by perinatal transmission.

FIGURE 412–2. Cases of AIDS in the United States with projections through 1993. The projections, made for a U.S. Public Health Service meeting in late October 1989, are based on cases diagnosed through June 1989 and reported through September 1989. Projections were made as a range; for comparison with reported cases (*shaded bars*), the midpoint of the range is also shown (*open bars*). The range shown is the range of predictions obtained from two analyses using extrapolation and five analyses using back-calculation. Reported cases have been adjusted for estimated delays in reporting. Reported cases and projections include an adjustment for incomplete reporting of diagnosed cases, based on an assumption that 85 per cent of diagnosed cases are eventually reported.

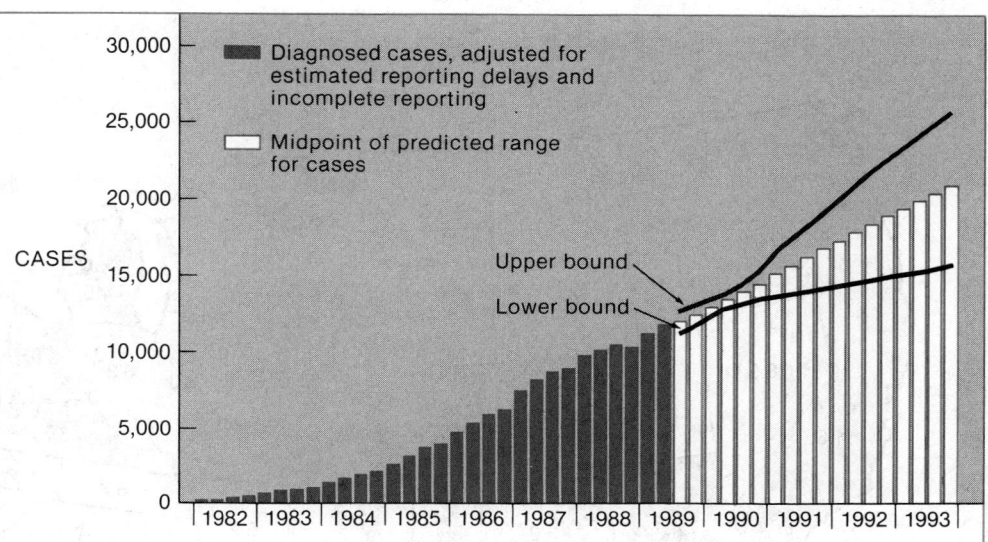

tions. HIV prevalence rates in persons with hemophilia A and B were directly related to the amount of clotting factor received prior to 1985 and were, hence, highest in those with severe hemophilia. HIV seroprevalence rates among female prostitutes varied widely from 0 to over 50 per cent, with the differences largely attributed to the extent of IV drug use in the population surveyed and the HIV prevalence among IV drug users in the community at that time. HIV prevalence rates in male prostitutes parallel rates in homosexual and bisexual men seen in STD clinics in the same communities.

HIV seroprevalence rates in childbearing women have been measured by blinded testing of blood samples collected on filter paper from newborns to measure maternal antibody. Seroprevalence rates varied widely among states, from less than one per thousand to greater than 1 to 3 per cent in northeastern urban areas. The survey results in New York State (HIV prevalence of 0.67 per cent statewide and greater than 1.4 per cent in New York City in childbearing women in 1989) resulted in a state policy that encourages HIV counseling of all women of childbearing age and offers counseling and HIV testing to women contemplating pregnancy or already pregnant.

Because incident HIV infections seldom cause persons to seek medical care, direct measurement of HIV incidence is very difficult in most populations. Using a combination of approaches, the U.S. Public Health Service estimated that between 40,000 and 80,000 new HIV infections occurred in adults and adolescents in 1989 and 1500 to 2000 HIV-infected infants were born that same year. HIV incidence estimates must be refined to measure

TABLE 412–4. PROJECTED NUMBERS OF AIDS CASES, DEATHS ATTRIBUTABLE TO AIDS, AND LIVING PERSONS WITH AIDS, UNITED STATES, 1989–1993*

Year	AIDS Cases		Deaths
	New Cases†	*Alive*‡	
1989	44,000–50,000	92,000–98,000	31,000–34,000
1990	52,000–57,000	101,000–122,000	37,000–42,000
1991	56,000–71,000	127,000–153,000	43,000–52,000
1992	58,000–85,000	139,000–188,000	49,000–64,000
1993	61,000–98,000	151,000–225,000	53,000–76,000
Through 1993§	390,000–480,000		285,000–340,000

*Projections are adjusted for unreported diagnoses of AIDS by adding 18 per cent to projections obtained from reported cases (corresponding to 85 per cent of all diagnosed cases being reported: 1/0.85 = 1.18) and rounded to the nearest 1000.
†Number of cases diagnosed during the year.
‡Persons with AIDS alive during the year.
§Rounded to the nearest 5000. Includes an estimated 120,000 AIDS cases diagnosed through 1988, 48,000 persons alive with AIDS at the end of 1988, and 72,000 deaths in diagnosed patients through 1988.
Adapted from MMWR 39:110–112; 117–119, 1990. CDC: Estimates of HIV prevalence and projected AIDS cases: Summary of a workshop.

the growth of the epidemic as well as the effectiveness of prevention efforts.

MODES OF TRANSMISSION OF HIV

HIV is transmitted primarily through sexual contact, parenteral exposure to blood or blood products, and perinatally from infected mothers to their infants.

Sexual Transmission

The predominant mode of HIV transmission throughout the world is sexual contact. The risk of acquiring HIV infection during a single sexual contact depends upon several factors. Most important, of course, is the likelihood that the contact is with an HIV-infected partner. Since the prevalence of HIV varies widely among populations within countries as well as among countries, the rates of sexual transmission also vary. Other factors affecting the efficiency of sexual transmission include the type of sexual practice, the infectivity of the source partner, coexisting genital infections, particularly those causing genital ulceration, and possibly others. HIV transmission has been attributed to vaginal, anal, and, less frequently, oral intercourse.

In epidemiologic studies among homosexual men, the risk of HIV acquisition increases with the number of sexual partners and the frequency of receptive anal intercourse, and practices associated with rectal trauma such as receptive "fisting" and anal douching. No sexual activity potentially involving the exchange of semen or blood, however, should be considered without risk. The relative efficiency of HIV transmission through various sexual practices was difficult to estimate precisely, since most HIV-infected homosexual men in epidemiologic studies had engaged in multiple practices. Although the frequency of female-to-female transmission would seem to be quite low, such HIV infections associated with traumatic sexual practices have been reported.

Most heterosexual transmission of HIV occurs during vaginal intercourse, although some studies suggest that receptive anal intercourse increases the risk of HIV transmission from an infected man to a woman. Some infected persons may be more efficient transmitters than others, perhaps owing to differences in viral strains or other factors. Transmission efficiency is probably inversely related to the immunologic status of the infected partner. In studies conducted among spouses and other steady sexual partners of HIV-infected persons with hemophilia, male-to-female sexual transmission of HIV increased as the index partner's T-helper lymphocyte numbers declined. These findings are not surprising, since the quantity of HIV in blood (and probably semen) increases as the disease progresses and the immune system weakens. Several studies have documented that infections such as *Haemophilus ducreyi, Treponema pallidum,* herpes simplex virus, and other pathogens causing genital or anal ulcers facilitate acquisition or transmission of HIV through sexual

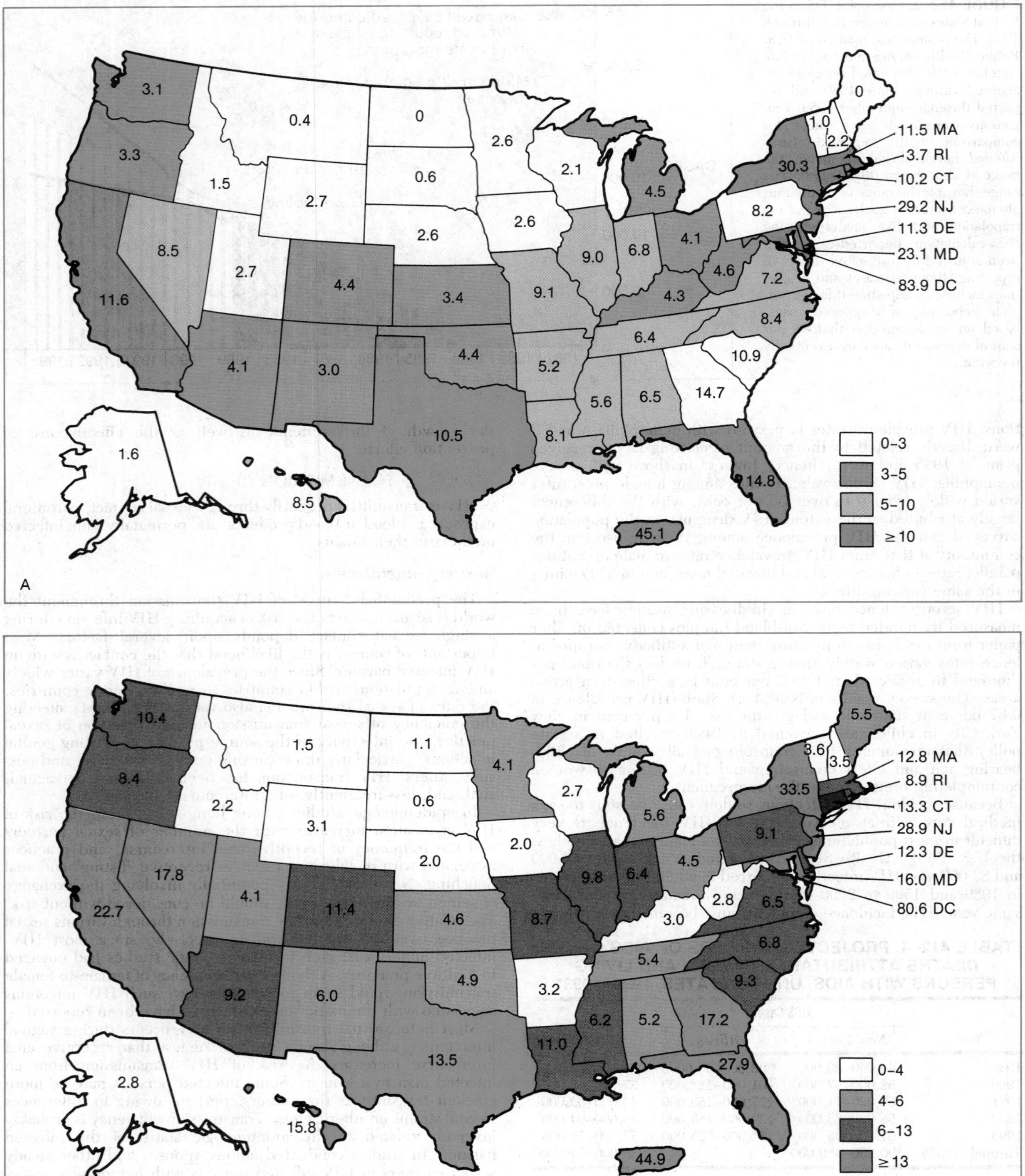

FIGURE 412–3. *A,* HIV seroprevalence in U.S. military recruit applicants, by state, 1989. *B,* Reported annual incidence of AIDS, by state, 1989. Rates shown are per 100,000 population (AIDS) or per 100,000 population tested (HIV); recruit applicants data are sex-adjusted.

contact, most likely by disrupting the genital or anal skin and mucous membranes. Undoubtedly, the higher rates of untreated genital ulcer disease contribute to the high rates of sexual transmission of HIV observed in some areas of the developing world. Not yet confirmed are preliminary observations associating increased risks of HIV acquisition for women with cervical infections with *Neisseria gonorrhoeae* or *Chlamydia trachomatis* and with cervical ectopy. To the extent that coexisting sexually transmitted infections increase the rate of HIV transmission, populations throughout the world with higher rates of these infections will be at higher risk of HIV infection. Conversely, prevention and treatment of other sexually transmitted infections should have a beneficial effect on preventing HIV transmission.

Transmission Through Parenteral Exposure to Blood or Blood Products

HIV is transmitted to IV drug users by parenteral exposure to contaminated injection equipment, including needles. Risk factors for infection include frequency of needle sharing, duration of IV drug use, use of drugs in "shooting galleries," and living in a community with a high prevalence of HIV infection in IV drug users. HIV has been transmitted by whole blood, plasma, cellular components, and clotting factors but not by other products produced in the United States from blood. No HIV transmission has been linked to receipt of immune serum globulin, hepatitis B immune globulin, Rh_o (O) immune globulin, or hepatitis B vaccine. The latter products have been produced by fractionation and other processes that remove and inactivate HIV. On the other hand, receipt of whole blood, packed cells, or plasma from an HIV-infected donor has been shown to transmit HIV virtually 100 per cent of the time. It has been estimated that over 12,000 living persons in the United States were infected with HIV through blood transfusions and that several thousand additional persons with hemophilia were infected from clotting factor concentrates between 1978 and 1985. In the United States and most industrialized countries, screening of all donated blood and plasma for HIV donor deferral procedures and heat treatment of clotting factor concentrates have minimized the risk of HIV transmission through transfusions. The exceptions occur largely in donors very recently infected who have yet to develop detectable antibody. The rate of HIV transmission from HIV-seronegative donors is estimated to range from 1 in 40,000 to 1 in 250,000 units transfused. Since HIV transmission has been reported in recipients of organs, tissue, and semen from HIV-infected donors, the U.S. Public Health Service recommends that potential donors be screened for HIV antibody and that organs, tissue, and semen not be used for transplantation or insemination.

Health Care and Laboratory Workers

Exposure to HIV-infected blood poses a definite occupational risk of HIV infection for health care, laboratory, and theoretically other workers. Large prospective collaborative studies have found the risk of seroconversion following needle stick or other parenteral exposures to the blood of HIV-infected persons to be approximately 0.3 per cent. In addition, there are a few well-documented and published reports of infections in health care workers following mucous membrane or extensive skin exposures. Such transmission can occur, but since transmission has not been observed following mucous membrane or skin exposures to HIV-infected blood in thousands of exposures in prospective studies, the risk is much lower than that following parenteral exposures. Finally, three cases of transmission of HIV from a single dentist to patients during an invasive procedure have been published. The epidemiologic and laboratory investigations, which involved comparison of the viral DNA sequences from the patients and the dentist, indicated that transmission during the invasive dental procedure was the most likely source of the patients' infections.

The risk of transmission of HIV, hepatitis B and C viruses, and other bloodborne pathogens to and from health care workers and patients can be minimized by close adherence to recommendations, which include universal precautions when caring for all patients.

Perinatal Transmission

HIV is transmitted from an infected woman to her fetus or newborn during pregnancy or delivery or through breast feeding.

Detection of HIV in fetal tissues and the isolation of HIV in cord blood provide suggestive evidence that most transmission occurs in utero, but definitive evidence is lacking. There are several reports of mothers who were infected through postpartum transfusions and subsequently transmitted HIV to their infants through breast feeding. For that reason, the U.S. Public Health Service strongly recommends that HIV-positive mothers avoid breast feeding in the United States where nutritionally adequate and safe substitutes are available. In prospective studies, perinatal transmission rates have varied from 15 to 40 per cent. In one study, the risk of perinatal transmission increased with the progression of HIV clinical illness and immunosuppression in the mothers. Obtaining precise estimates of perinatal transmission rates has been hampered by the lack of a reliable test to diagnose HIV infection in the newborn infant. The polymerase chain reaction (PCR) and specific serologic techniques are being applied in attempts to predict perinatal outcome during pregnancy as well as to rapidly diagnose HIV infection in the newborn.

Other Modes of Transmission

Throughout the world, the above routes of transmission have accounted for the overwhelming majority of HIV infections, but there has been considerable concern about other theoretical modes of transmission, especially through "casual" contact with HIV-infected persons, exposure to saliva or aerosols, or insect vectors. More than 700 nonsexual household contacts of adults or children with HIV infection have been evaluated in prospective studies. In thousands of person-years of close contact, including sharing bathroom and kitchen facilities, and frequent personal interactions including kissing and hugging, no transmission other than sexual or perinatal occurred. HIV has been isolated from saliva but less frequently than in blood. There have been no documented transmissions of HIV from exposure to saliva alone, either through kissing or through occupational exposures in dental, medical, or laboratory settings. Although a single case report of HIV transmission between siblings suggested a bite as the possible route of transmission, the precise mode of transmission in this case was unclear, since seroconversion was not documented and the bite did not break the skin or result in bleeding. Other small studies have failed to document HIV transmission following bites. Available evidence suggests that the risk of HIV transmission through normal exposures to saliva is extremely low, if it occurs at all. However, since saliva can contain other pathogenic organisms, appropriate precautions for health care and dental workers remain important, including universal precautions if gross contamination with blood is present. Aerosols have never been reported to transmit bloodborne pathogens such as HIV or hepatitis B in the health care or other settings. Extensive laboratory and epidemiologic studies of hepatitis B have failed to detect HBsAg in respirable particles in air samples in dental operatories or dialysis units during procedures on infected patients when aerosols were generated. Since the concentration of HBsAg in body fluids is much higher than that of HIV, it is unlikely that HIV would be detected. Extensive laboratory studies have failed to demonstrate replication of HIV in insects who were fed high concentrations of HIV or injected with HIV-contaminated blood. Epidemiologic studies in the United States, Haiti, and central Africa show no evidence of insect-borne HIV transmission.

The possibility of previously unrecognized modes of HIV transmission cannot be entirely excluded, but they are likely to be rare, if found.

NATURAL HISTORY OF HIV INFECTION

The time period between HIV infection and the development of severe immunosuppression and AIDS is long and variable. In a cohort study of homosexual men conducted at the San Francisco City Clinic, approximately 50 per cent of men were diagnosed with AIDS after 10 years of follow-up. An additional 30 per cent of infected homosexual men had less severe signs or symptoms and only 20 per cent were asymptomatic after 10 years. In contrast to studies in homosexual men, 49 per cent of patients infected with HIV through blood transfusions and followed in a national collaborative study developed AIDS after only 7 years

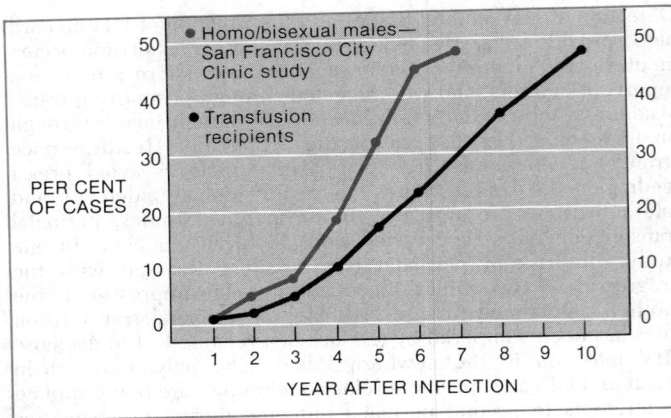

FIGURE 412–4. Estimate of the risk for development of AIDS, by year, after HIV infection in infected adult transfusion recipients and homosexual/bisexual men.

(Fig. 412–4). The authors of the latter study also found that transfusion recipients developed clinical illness more quickly if they had received transfusions from HIV-infected donors who themselves developed AIDS shortly after the donation. They hypothesized that these recipients received a larger inoculum of HIV and that the size of the inoculum affects disease progression, or, alternatively, that they had been inoculated with a more pathogenic strain of HIV. The more rapid rates of progression to AIDS in transfusion recipients may reflect the inoculum size, the older age, the immunologic status of the infected recipient, or all of these factors. Progression rates to AIDS are similar for persons with hemophilia over age 21 years to those observed in homosexual men. In contrast, children and adolescents with hemophilia and HIV infection progressed at a slower rate. Prospective studies of HIV infection in intravenous drug users and persons living in central Africa suggest progression rates at least as rapid as those in homosexual men, but the data are insufficient to make accurate comparisons.

Infants infected with HIV perinatally progress faster than adults. Whereas relatively few infected adults develop AIDS during the first 3 years after infection, the highest incidence of perinatally acquired AIDS occurs during the first year of life, with the median period of progression to AIDS thought to be 3 to 5 years. This difference is thought to reflect the immaturity of the fetal or neonatal immune system at the time of HIV infection. The incidence of AIDS in the first year of life is higher among children born to infected mothers than among children transfused as neonates, perhaps providing indirect evidence for in utero transmission, although other nutritional and socioeconomic factors may play a role.

Several clinical and/or laboratory findings have been shown to predict more rapid progression to AIDS among adults with HIV infection. Persons with oral or severe vaginal candidiasis, hairy leukoplakia, or severe disseminated herpes zoster developed AIDS more rapidly than infected persons without these findings. The single best laboratory predictor of disease progression is the T4 lymphocyte count. Persons with low T4 lymphocytes (e.g., T4 < 200 cells/cubic millimeter) progress much more rapidly to AIDS than those with normal (e.g., > 500 cells/cubic millimeter) counts, while persons with intermediate T4 counts progress at an intermediate rate. Other laboratory markers directly associated with disease progression include persistent HIV antigen in the blood, reductions in antibody to p24 (core protein), and elevated serum β_2-microglobulin, plus others. Other than age, and perhaps route of transmission, there are very few data to support specific cofactors relating to disease progression. Factors studied include coinfection with other organisms, behavioral factors, and genetic factors.

Population-based epidemiologic studies of HIV-infected homosexual men or active duty military personnel with HIV infection showed that the majority of infected adults already showed evidence of immunosuppression secondary to HIV infection. By 1989, approximately 58 to 64 per cent of persons with HIV infection had T4 lymphocyte counts below 500 per cubic millimeter.

In the future, the progression rates to AIDS as well as survival rates for those already diagnosed with AIDS will likely be favorably affected by antiviral therapy and the prophylactic treatment of opportunistic infections in those groups with access to these interventions.

AIDS AND HIV INFECTION OUTSIDE THE UNITED STATES

Within 3 years after recognition of the syndrome in the United States, cases of AIDS were reported from every continent. By July 1990, over 270,000 cases had been reported from 157 countries to the World Health Organization (WHO) (Table 412–5). AIDS case reports from North America, Europe, and Oceania fulfill the CDC/WHO surveillance definition of AIDS (see Table 412–1). The less sensitive and specific WHO clinical definition is often used in developing countries where facilities or resources are less adequate to consistently diagnose opportunistic infections, cancers, or HIV infection. AIDS case reporting from developing countries is often delayed and much less complete than in industrialized countries. Extensive HIV serosurveys in Africa and South and Central America provide evidence that AIDS case reports greatly underestimate the magnitude of the HIV problem in many countries in these regions. Serosurveys in drug users and prostitutes have recently revealed extensive epidemics of HIV infection in Thailand and India, foretelling major public health problems related to AIDS in the future in these regions of Asia.

Modes of transmission of HIV are similar throughout the world, but the relative frequency varies considerably between countries and regions. In North America, Europe, Australia, New Zealand, and some areas of South America, the majority of HIV infections have occurred in homosexual men and IV drug users; heterosexual and perinatal transmission has resulted mostly from transmission from IV drug users and their partners. In most countries in Africa and some in the Caribbean and South America, most HIV infections have occurred through heterosexual transmission. HIV seroprevalence rates are highest in urban prostitutes and sexually active young adults. High rates of infection in young women translate into a substantial perinatal transmission. In some areas of Africa, pediatric HIV infection has significantly increased already high infant mortality rates. In many developing countries, transfusion of HIV-infected blood remains a substantial problem owing to inadequate blood banking and serologic testing capacity. Reuse of nonsterile needles and syringes and other medical practices have caused major HIV outbreaks in the Soviet Union and Romania. Such transmission accounts for an undetermined but probably small proportion of HIV infection in developing countries. In Asian countries such as Thailand and India, emergence of HIV infection as a major public health problem began in IV drug users and prostitutes, respectively. In yet other countries, primarily in Eastern Europe, the Middle East, Asia, and the Pacific region, HIV has not yet been recognized as an important public health problem. The future course of HIV in these countries may depend upon their ability to anticipate and respond to the problem; it can be approximately predicted by the extent and pattern of sexually transmitted and transfusion-associated infections and the extent of IV drug use which currently exists in each country.

A second human immunodeficiency virus, HIV type 2 (HIV-2), was first described in asymptomatic West Africans with AIDS

TABLE 412–5. ACQUIRED IMMUNODEFICIENCY SYNDROME (AIDS) REPORTED TO THE WORLD HEALTH ORGANIZATION THROUGH JULY 1990

Continent	Number of Countries or Territories Reporting		Total Number of Cases Reported
	Zero Cases	*One or More Cases*	
Africa	2	51	66,978
Americas	0	44	167,014
Asia	12	25	665
Europe	1	29	36,635
Oceania	8	8	2,133
TOTALS	23	157	273,425

in 1986. HIV-2 infection remains most prevalent in West Africa, although well-documented cases have been reported from Western Europe, Canada, Brazil, the United States, and central Africa. HIV-1 and HIV-2 are closely related; tests for antibody for one virus often cross-react with the other. For example, licensed enzyme immunoassays for detecting HIV-1 detect HIV-2 antibody in 60 to 90 per cent of infected patients. As of 1990, HIV-2 infection remained rare in the United States, with nearly all cases detected in persons from West Africa.

SUMMARY

HIV infection and AIDS are already major causes of morbidity and mortality throughout the world. Owing to the large number of persons already infected and continuing high transmission rates, worldwide mortality will continue to increase for the foreseeable future. In both developed and developing countries, long-term commitments are needed to prevent further sexual contact, IV drug use, and perinatal transmission.

AIDS and human immunodeficiency virus infection in the United States: 1988 Update. MMWR 38(S-4):1–38, 1989. HIV infection in the United States: A review of current knowledge. MMWR 36(S-6):1–48, 1987. Gwinn M, Pappaionou M, George JR, et al.: Prevalence of antibody to the human immunodeficiency virus in women delivering infants in the United States. JAMA, in press. The sentinel HIV seroprevalence surveys—special section. Pub Health Rep 105:113–172, 1990. *These articles summarize recent methods and data on HIV seroprevalence throughout the United States.*

Castro KG, Berkelman RL, Jaffe HW, et al.: Revised classification system for human immunodeficiency virus infection in adolescents and adults. MMWR, in press. Redfield RR, Wright DC, Tramont EA: The Walter Reed staging classification for HTLV-III/LAV infection. N Engl J Med 314:131–132, 1986. *These are the most widely used classification systems in the United States. The systems are subject to revision.*

Estimates of HIV prevalence and projected AIDS cases: Summary of a workshop. MMWR 39:110–119, 1990. Karon JM, Devine OJ, Morgan WM: Predicting AIDS incidence by extrapolating from recent trends. In Castillo-Chavez C (ed.): Mathematical and Statistical Approaches to AIDS Epidemiology. Lecture Notes in Biomathematics 83:58–88, 1989. Gail MH, Rosenberg PS, Goedert JJ: Therapy may explain recent deficits in AIDS. J AIDS 3:296–306, 1990. Update: AIDS—United States, 1989. MMWR 39:81–86, 1990. *These papers detail recent trends and future projections of AIDS in the United States.*

Goedert JJ, Eyster EE, Biggar RJ, et al.: Heterosexual transmission of HIV: Association with severe depletion of T-helper lymphocytes in men with hemophilia. AIDS Res Hum Retroviruses 3:355–361, 1988. Holmberg SD, Horsburgh CR, Ward JW, et al.: Biologic factors in the sexual transmission of human immunodeficiency virus. J Infect Dis 160:116–125, 1989. *These papers summarize available information on factors related to the heterosexual transmission of HIV.*

Lifson AR, Rutherford GW, Jaffe HW: The natural history of HIV infection. J Infect Dis 158:1360–1367, 1988. Eyster ME, Gail MH, Ballard JO, et al.: Natural history of HIV infection in hemophiliacs: Effects of T-cell subsets, platelet counts, and age. Ann Intern Med 107:106, 1987. Ward JW, Bush TJ, Perkins HA, et al.: The natural history of transfusion-associated infection with HIV. N Engl J Med 321:947–952, 1989. *These manuscripts summarize data and factors associated with progression to AIDS in HIV-infected persons.*

Update: Universal precautions for prevention of transmission of HIV, hepatitis B virus, and other bloodborne pathogens in health care setting. MMWR 37:337–388, 1988. Public Health Service statement on management of occupational exposure to HIV including considerations regarding zidovudine postexposure use. MMWR 39(RR-1):1–14, 1990. Possible transmission of HIV to a patient during an invasive dental procedure. MMWR 39:489–493, 1990. Update: Transmission of HIV infection during an invasive dental procedure—Florida. MMWR 40:21–33, 1991. *These documents summarize data on transmission of HIV in the health care setting and list recommended precautions.*

413 Prevention of HIV Infection

Michael S. Saag

Prevention of HIV infection requires a thorough understanding of the modes of viral transmission, the populations at risk, and the established guidelines to avoid high-risk exposures. HIV has been identified in virtually every body fluid and tissue, including blood, semen, vaginal secretions, saliva, tears, breast milk, cerebrospinal fluid, amniotic fluid, urine, and fluid obtained from bronchoalveolar lavage. In most instances, the virus resides in lymphocytes present within body fluids; therefore, any fluid that contains lymphocytes could be implicated theoretically in the spread of the virus. Nonetheless, no cases of HIV transmission

have been documented through any body fluids except blood and fluids grossly contaminated with blood, semen, vaginal secretions, and, rarely, breast milk. HIV has been transmitted through transplanted organs, including kidney, liver, heart, pancreas, and bone.

MODES OF HIV TRANSMISSION AND PREVENTION

SEXUAL TRANSMISSION. HIV infection is a sexually transmitted disease (STD). Like other STD's, HIV spreads bidirectionally and appears to be transmitted from male to female and female to male with approximately equal efficiency. Although the majority of sexually transmitted cases reported in the United States occur via male homosexual activity, heterosexual transmission is one of the fastest growing modes of transmission reported in the United States and is the primary mode of disease acquisition in many African countries, where male-to-female prevalence ratios are approximately 1.1:1.

Certain cofactors are associated with an increased risk of acquiring HIV infection. Among homosexual men, receptive anal intercourse and contact with a large number of different sexual partners are the most important risk factors. Activities that may lead to damage of the rectal mucosa, such as rectal douching, manual penetration of the rectum ("fisting"), and concomitant ulcerative STD's, increase the likelihood of disease acquisition. Insertive rectal intercourse, fellatio, and ingestion of semen are associated with HIV transmission to a lesser degree. The likelihood of heterosexual acquired disease increases with a higher number of sexual partners, contact with intravenous drug users (IVDU's), prostitution, sexual practices that damage vaginal or rectal mucosa, and a previous history of other STD's. Female-to-female transmission has been reported via orogenital contact.

Prevention. Abstinence is the only absolute way of preventing sexual acquisition of HIV infection. Persons who have been engaged in a mutually monogamous relationship since the mid-1970's are at extremely low risk of acquiring disease; however, the assurance that both partners have remained "faithful" is sometimes difficult to confirm. For the majority of sexually active individuals it should be assumed that their partner is seropositive until demonstrated otherwise. Verbal claims of seronegativity should be viewed with skepticism. When a couple, heterosexual or homosexual, is establishing a long-term relationship, it may be recommended that they undergo serologic testing to determine their HIV status. However, the decision to be tested should be of mutual consent and viewed in the context that exposures outside the relationship may lead to seropositivity in the future.

In situations in which a decision to engage in sexual activity has been made and the HIV status of the partner is unknown or in doubt, safe sexual practices ("safe sex") should be implemented (Table 413–1). Mutual masturbation is considered "safe," assuming it is nontraumatic and not followed by ingestion of body fluids such as semen or vaginal secretions. Transmission of HIV has never been documented to occur through saliva; however, no group of patients has ever been studied who engage in deep "French" kissing as their sole means of sexual activity. Since HIV exists in saliva, albeit in very low titers, deep French kissing cannot be considered absolutely safe even though the likelihood of HIV transmission is extremely low. Condom use is the most

TABLE 413–1. SAFE AND UNSAFE SEXUAL PRACTICES IN ORDER OF "SURENESS" OF SAFETY

Safe
Abstinence
Monogamous relationship with confirmed seronegative partner
Manual sex (mutual masturbation)
Kissing
Intercourse with latex condom (used in combination with nonoxynol-9)

Unsafe
Intercourse with "natural skin" condom
Intercourse with latex condom lubricated with petroleum-based lubricants
Unprotected orogenital sex
Unprotected vaginal intercourse
Unprotected anal intercourse

effective means of preventing HIV infection among individuals who engage in vaginal or anal intercourse. To be effective, however, the condom should be made of latex and must be used properly. Natural skin condoms have been shown to leak in laboratory studies, whereas latex condoms maintain their integrity and are more durable. Nonoxynol-9, a spermicide with some antiviral activity, enhances the protective effects of condoms and should be used in conjunction with condoms either as a spermicidal jelly or impregnated into the latex condom itself. Petroleum-based lubricants enhance the likelihood of latex condom rupture and should be avoided. If needed, water-based lubricants such as K-Y Jelly should be used.

Both partners should be knowledgeable about the correct use of condoms. Discussions regarding condom use should occur before the need arises, and ideally, condom placement should be practiced in advance. A new condom should be used for each act of intercourse and each condom should be used only one time. Even under the best of circumstances, a 5 to 15 per cent failure rate has been noted among couples using condoms as their sole means of contraception, and HIV transmission has been reported in discordant couples using condoms. Condom ineffectiveness is most often due to improper placement, falling off during intercourse, and rupture. Therefore, while condom use during intercourse is considered "safer" sex, it is not absolutely safe.

HIV TRANSMISSION IN INTRAVENOUS DRUG USERS. The primary mode of HIV transmission in IVDU's is sharing of contaminated needles and syringes. Sharing of injection paraphernalia ("works") is commonplace among IVDU's and is reinforced by the cultural, economic, and legal environment in the IVDU community. Users often purchase and inject drugs in socalled shooting galleries, underground locations where addicts feel insulated from police surveillance. "Works" are rented or shared among several individuals and, in certain instances, sharing equipment represents an important social bond between users. The risk of HIV transmission is highest among IVDU's who share needles and use drugs that are injected more often, such as cocaine. HIV is frequently transmitted from IVDU's to their sexual partners through both heterosexual and homosexual activity, and ultimately, the virus may be transmitted to their children via perinatal exposure. Many cases of heterosexual transmission, including transmission from prostitutes, are associated with intravenous drug use.

Prevention. The primary mode of preventing HIV transmission in IVDU's is to prevent the use of intravenous drugs in the first place. Education programs that are culturally sensitive and geared to young audiences have the best chance of preventing drug use. Access to treatment centers is the best approach for those individuals already using IV drugs. Unfortunately, there is a critical shortage of such centers throughout the United States, and those that do exist are frequently understaffed, underfunded, and overworked. For those IVDU's who do not wish to seek treatment or who are unable to gain access to treatment, the most effective way to prevent HIV infection is to avoid sharing needles and works. Where works are in short supply, needles and syringes should be cleaned after each use, preferably with readily accessible virucidal cleansers such as chlorine bleach (diluted 1:100). Some communities have adopted programs that provide free needles and syringes for IVDU's. Voluntary HIV testing and outreach programs that rigorously maintain confidentiality can be effective in reducing transmission to sexual partners of IVDU's. In order to be effective, antibody testing should be combined with intensive pretest and post-test counseling.

The efficacy of many community programs is limited, however, by cultural barriers, including lack of trust, fear of prosecution, misconceptions regarding the prevalence of HIV infection within the local drug-using population, and the use of ineffective language in delivering anti-HIV messages by program staff. When combined with the relative paucity of IV drug treatment resources, HIV education among IVDU's which ultimately results in behavioral changes represents the most challenging HIV prevention goal.

TRANSMISSION OF HIV THROUGH BLOOD PRODUCTS. HIV has been transmitted via transfusion of single-donor blood and blood products, including whole blood, fresh frozen plasma, packed red blood cells, cryoprecipitate, clotting factors,

and platelets. Prior to May, 1985, when the Red Cross began testing the blood supply for evidence of HIV antibodies, an estimated 10,000 to 12,000 individuals received blood products from HIV-infected donors. Most recipients develop infection after transfusion with HIV-tainted blood products, and recent data suggest that the time to development of advanced disease is shorter among transfusion recipients than among those who acquired their disease via sexual contact.

Since 1985, the rate of HIV transmission through transfusion has dropped precipitously. The current estimated rate of transmission is 1 in 40,000 to 1 in 200,000 units of blood, depending on the prevalence of HIV infection in the community where the blood was collected. Pooled plasma components often require 2000 to 30,000 donors per lot and represent a higher potential risk of transmission than single-donor blood products if the pooled product is not treated to eliminate infectious virus.

Prevention. Aggressive efforts by the American Red Cross have greatly reduced the risk of HIV transmission via transfusion in the United States. Voluntary self-deferral of donors at risk for HIV acquisition in the community was initiated in 1983. The effectiveness of self-deferral is limited, however, by social pressures. Some high-risk individuals view blood donation as a means of being tested for HIV and provide erroneous screening information in order to receive free, confidential evaluation of their HIV status. Other at-risk individuals may be coerced to participate in blood donation drives at work. Potentially infected donors may feel uncomfortable excusing themselves from donation and provide false information on screening in order to avoid possible disclosure of a high-risk lifestyle to their co-workers. Self-deferral programs are most effective when free, voluntary testing centers are readily available elsewhere in the community and when blood drives encourage potential donors to come to donation centers by themselves and not in groups.

The institution of HIV antibody testing of donated blood and blood products in 1985 has had the most dramatic effect on lowering the incidence of transfusion-related transmission. When used in combination with voluntary self-deferral, the blood supply has become relatively free of HIV. The use of heat inactivation processes for cryoprecipitate and clotting factor concentrates has virtually eliminated transmission of HIV through use of these products. Other products, such as immune globulin preparations and hepatitis B vaccines, are produced via methods that inactivate HIV and have never been associated with transmission of HIV.

TRANSMISSION OF HIV TO HEALTH CARE WORKERS. Transmission of HIV in the health care delivery setting has been the subject of intense investigation throughout the course of the epidemic. Retrospective analysis of over 53,000 AIDS cases with known employment histories revealed that 5.3 per cent of the reported cases occurred in individuals who worked in a health care or laboratory setting; by comparison, health care workers made up 5.7 per cent of the work force during the same time period. Other epidemiologic studies provide additional evidence of the low likelihood of HIV transmission in the health care setting. The percentage of health care workers with AIDS who have "no identified risk" for HIV infection has remained low (<10 per cent) and has not increased over time, despite the dramatic increase in the number of AIDS cases and concomitant exposure of health care workers to patients with HIV disease. More importantly, detailed studies examining the risk of specific exposures, such as needle stick injuries and mucous membrane exposures, have demonstrated very low risk of disease acquisition in the workplace. Over 1300 health care workers have been examined prospectively in carefully designed surveillance studies at 10 high-incidence medical centers. The overall risk of seroconversion after a percutaneous needle stick from a known HIV-positive source is 0.30 per cent per exposure (95 per cent confidence interval 0.13 to 0.70 per cent). Although mucous membrane exposures to HIV-positive blood have resulted in seroconversion in at least three health care workers, prospective studies of over 900 splash exposures have failed to identify any seroconverters, implying that the risk of infection is even less after mucous membrane exposure than through percutaneous needle stick. To date, no transmission has occurred after exposure to body fluids other than blood or fluids heavily contaminated with blood. When combined with studies of household contacts demonstrating no transmission of HIV to family members living with an infected patient through usual activities of daily living, available evidence strongly argues against "casual contact" as a mode of HIV transmission. Therefore, while the potential for HIV transmission to health care providers clearly exists, the risk of infection is inherently low and can be further minimized by following routine precautions to prevent transmission.

Prevention. In August 1987, the Centers for Disease Control (CDC) published guidelines designed to minimize health care worker exposure to blood and body fluids which may be infected with blood-borne pathogens, such as HIV. These so-called universal precautions are based on the premise that any patient may be infected with blood-borne infectious agents and it may be difficult, if not impossible, to differentiate those with infection from their uninfected counterparts. Thus, all specimens containing blood or blood-tinged fluids obtained from *any* patient should be considered hazardous and handled as such (Table 413–2).

Handwashing is the cornerstone of universal precautions, as it is with all infection control practices. Gloves should be worn when spillage of blood or body fluids is likely. Gloves should *never* be washed and should be changed after soiling or after gross contamination, with handwashing immediately after the gloves are removed. Gowns, protective eyewear, and masks are usually not needed except in circumstances in which splattering or splashing of blood-containing fluids is likely to occur. Masks should always be worn in situations in which eyewear is required. Reusable equipment should be cleansed of visible organic material, placed in an impervious bag, and returned to central supply for decontamination. Although heat is the single best decontamination method, chemical agents that possess mycobactericidal activity are effective against both hepatitis B and HIV and are acceptable alternatives when heat inactivation is impractical. Blood spills should be cleaned with appropriate caution. After placement of gloves and other appropriate barrier precautions, excess blood should be removed with absorbent materials (e.g., paper towels), the area then cleaned with soap and water, and the area disinfected with a 1:10 solution of sodium hypochlorite (household bleach) and water. Health care workers with denuded skin, open lesions, or active dermatitis should avoid direct patient contact and should not process contaminated equipment or materials. Private rooms are generally not required for patients known to be HIV infected unless a concomitant opportunistic disease is present which requires respiratory, enteric, or contact isolation. Food service should be provided as usual on reusable dishware.

Since *all* blood and body fluids should be handled as potentially hazardous and *all* patients presumed to be infected, it makes little sense to identify infected patients or their specimens with

TABLE 413–2. SUMMARY OF UNIVERSAL PRECAUTIONS

Specimens, including blood, blood products, and body fluids, obtained from *all* patients should be considered hazardous and potentially infected with transmissible agents.

Handwashing should be performed before and after patient contact; after removing gloves; and immediately if hands are grossly contaminated with blood.

Gloves should be worn when hands are *likely* to come in contact with blood or body fluids.

Gowns, protective eyewear, and masks should be worn when splashing, splattering, or aerosolization of blood or body fluids is *likely* to occur.

Sharp objects ("sharps") should be handled with great care and disposed of in impervious receptacles.

Needles should never be manipulated, bent, broken, or recapped.

Blood spills should be handled via initial absorption of spill with disposable towels, cleaning area with soap and water, followed by disinfecting area with 1:10 solution of household bleach.

Contaminated reusable equipment should be decontaminated using heat sterilization, or when heat is impractical, using a mycobactericidal cleanser.

Pocket masks or mechanical ventilation devices should be available in areas where cardiopulmonary resuscitation procedures are likely.

Health care workers with open lesions or weeping dermatitis should avoid direct patient contact and should not handle contaminated equipment.

Private rooms are not required for routine care; select circumstances, however, such as the presence of concomitant transmissible opportunistic diseases, may warrant respiratory, enteric, or contact isolation.

"blood and body fluid" labels. The use of such labels on *known* infected patients implies that unlabeled specimens or specimens from patients of unknown status are less hazardous and may be handled with less care. Indeed, studies have shown that over half of the specimens containing antibodies to either HbsAg or HIV went to the laboratory unlabeled. The handling of sharp instruments ("sharps") represents the greatest risk of HIV transmission to health care workers. Although sharp injuries cannot be entirely eliminated, the number of exposures can be reduced substantially by adhering to guidelines put forth in universal precautions. Before a sharp instrument is used, thought should be given regarding where the instrument will be disposed after use. Impervious containers should be readily available in all patient care areas and identified by the health care worker *prior to* "sharp" utilization. The containers should be checked frequently and should not be allowed to overfill. Used needles should never be manipulated, bent, broken, or recapped. Recapping of needles is the single most common activity that results in needle stick injuries.

Despite their logical basis and relative ease of implementation, universal precautions have not been accepted by many medical centers and health care providers. Recent studies have shown that over 50 per cent of health care workers engage in inadequate infection control practices, even in high-impact AIDS centers, and up to 40 per cent of the needle stick exposures were judged to be preventable. Although lack of adequate education may partly explain these findings, implementation of infection control practices has been generally poor historically. Between 200 and 400 health care workers die each year as a result of hepatitis B infection acquired on the job. The use of universal precautions helps minimize the transmission of many transmissible diseases in addition to HIV.

Even in the best of circumstances, accidental mucous membrane and percutaneous exposures to blood from HIV-infected patients do occur. Each institution and health care facility should adopt procedures for management of these exposures based on guidelines published by the CDC. The essential elements of management following needle stick or mucous membrane exposure include definition of the type of exposure, appropriate evaluation of the donor (patient) and recipient (health care worker) at the time of exposure, and follow-up of the health care worker for at least 1 year after exposure.

Proposed definitions of the types of exposure are summarized in Table 413–3. Health care workers with any kind of parenteral exposure should be counseled and evaluated for possible acquisition of HIV and receive routine prophylaxis against hepatitis B. The source patient (donor) should be evaluated for HIV infection; if the donor's HIV status is unknown, the donor should be informed abut the incident and encouraged to allow voluntary, confidential screening of his blood for HIV and hepatitis B antibody. If the patient refuses or cannot give consent, he should be considered to be infected. In cases where exposure to HIV is documented or presumed to have occurred, the health care worker should be evaluated serologically for the presence of HIV as soon as possible after the exposure (baseline) and again at 6 weeks, 12 weeks, 24 weeks, and 1 year after the exposure to determine whether HIV transmission has occurred. The health care worker should report any acute illnesses that occur during the follow-up period, especially during the first 6 to 12 weeks after exposure. Exposed workers should follow the recommended guidelines for preventing HIV transmission, including use of safe sexual practices, refraining from blood, semen, and organ donation, and avoidance of breast feeding. If the source patient is seronegative for HIV and has no clinical manifestations of HIV disease, no further follow-up of the exposed health care worker is necessary, although some workers prefer follow-up for their own peace of mind. Serologic testing should be made available to all health care workers who are concerned about potential on-the-job exposure.

The use of zidovudine (AZT) prophylaxis following parenteral exposure to HIV remains controversial. Many clinicians favor use of prophylactic AZT after massive or definite exposures based on the proven antiviral effect of AZT, the relatively infrequent and apparently reversible nature of serious adverse drug effects, and the demonstration in some animal models of retroviral infection

TABLE 413–3. DEFINITIONS OF EXPOSURES TO BLOOD AND BODY FLUIDS FROM HIV-INFECTED PATIENTS*

Massive parenteral exposure
  Transfusion of blood
  High-inoculum injection of blood (>1 ml) or laboratory materials containing high viral titers

Definite parenteral exposure
  Deep intramuscular injury with a needle contaminated with blood or a body fluid
  Small volume injection of blood or body fluid (<1 ml)
  Laceration caused by instrument contaminated with blood or body fluids
  Laceration inoculated with blood, body fluids, or virus samples (research materials)

Possible parenteral exposure
  Subcutaneous or superficial injury with an instrument or needle contaminated with blood or body fluids
  Injury with a contaminated instrument or needle which does not cause visible bleeding
  Previous wound or skin lesion contaminated with blood or body fluids
  Mucous membrane exposure to blood or body fluids

Doubtful parenteral exposure
  Subcutaneous injury by instrument or needle contaminated with noninfectious fluids†
  Contamination of a wound, previous skin lesion, or mucous membrane with noninfectious fluids
  Intact skin visibly contaminated with blood

*Modified from Gerberding JC, Conte JE: Counseling and Testing Service, Center for Municipal Occupational Safety and Health, San Francisco General Hospital, University of California San Francisco, and the California Consortium for Health Care Workers. In Gerberding JL: AIDS and Health Care Workers. Chicago, American Medical Association, 1989, pp 35–46; with permission.
†Body fluids considered to be potentially infectious include blood, blood products, cerebrospinal fluid, amniotic fluid, menstrual discharge, inflammatory exudates, pleural fluid, peritoneal fluid, pericardial fluid, and any fluid visibly contaminated with blood. All other fluids are considered noninfectious.

that AZT, when given early after inoculation, modifies the course of disease. Others believe that AZT should not be administered based on the absence of postexposure prophylaxis data, the lack of information regarding toxicity in uninfected individuals, and the unknown long-term carcinogenic potential of AZT use. Unfortunately, it is unlikely that any clinical trials will be able to resolve the issue owing to the large number of participants required (based on low rates of seroconversion) and the difficulty of enrolling exposed health care workers into placebo-controlled studies. Although zidovudine prophylaxis cannot be considered an established standard of practice at this time, the option of zidovudine prophylaxis should be offered to all health care workers with massive or definite exposures and discussed with those encountering possible parenteral exposures. Health care workers with doubtful parenteral or nonparenteral exposures generally should not take zidovudine prophylaxis. Those workers with massive or definite exposures who elect to take zidovudine prophylaxis should sign an informed consent that outlines the risks and benefits of AZT prophylaxis prior to initiation of therapy. The optimal timing and dosage of AZT prophylaxis are unknown; however, animal studies suggest that higher doses given as soon as possible after exposure have the best chance of being effective. Therefore, most centers that offer zidovudine prophylaxis to their employees have established mechanisms whereby the health care worker can be evaluated and the drug administered within 2 to 4 hours after the exposure. Dosing regimens vary from center to center but usually consist of 100 mg to 200 mg of AZT every 4 hours, with or without a 4 A.M. dose, for 4 to 6 weeks.

VACCINE DEVELOPMENT

Education is the only means of HIV prevention currently available. Over the past few years significant efforts have been directed toward the development of an effective vaccine against HIV. Although substantial progress has been achieved, several obstacles still remain. Despite enormous advances in understanding the immunopathogenesis of HIV infection, the precise mechanism of protective immunity remains unknown. Without such knowledge, it is difficult to develop vaccines that are assured of targeting the appropriate arm of the immune system that confers long-term protective immunity. Another obstacle is that no animal

models currently exist to test the effectiveness of candidate vaccines. Therefore, even if an effective vaccine were available it would take years of human testing to demonstrate its effectiveness. Moreover, once a candidate vaccine is in human trials, the relatively low rate of HIV transmission, and in some cases, the difficulty in determining whether HIV infection has actually occurred will complicate the evaluation process. Nonetheless, several candidate vaccines have been developed and are now entering Phase I trials. Recombinant gp160 vaccines expressed in a baculovirus vector and a vaccinia virus vector have been developed. A whole killed HIV vaccine is being evaluated in HIV-infected patients.

In view of the enormous progress made in vaccine development over the last few years, the establishment of an effective vaccine is a viable possibility; unfortunately, it will take several more years before efficacy can be established. Until such time, education remains the primary mode of HIV prevention. Never before has so much been known about an epidemic during the time it was occurring. The challenge is to disseminate the knowledge to populations at risk in language they can understand and, ultimately, to modify activities so that the risk of transmission is minimized.

Brickner PW, Torres RA, Barnes M, et al.: Recommendations for control and prevention of human immunodeficiency virus infection in intravenous drug users. Ann Intern Med 110:883–887, 1989. *Thoughtful discussion of unique problems associated with prevention of HIV transmission in IVDU's.*
Centers for Disease Control: Recommendations for prevention of HIV transmission in health care settings. MMWR 36(2S), 1987. *Original description of universal precautions. Critical reading for all health care workers.*
Centers for Disease Control: Public health service statement on management of occupational exposure to human immunodeficiency virus, including considerations regarding zidovudine post-exposure use. MMWR 39 (RR-1), 1990. *State-of-the-art review of issues regarding use of prophylactic zidovudine after needle stick exposure to HIV.*
Fauci AS, Gallo RC, Koenig S, et al.: Development and evaluation of a vaccine for human immunodeficiency virus infection. Ann Intern Med 110:373–385, 1989. *Overview of HIV vaccine development: progress, obstacles, and future directions.*
Henderson DK, Fahey BJ, Willy M, et al.: Risk for occupational transmission of human immunodeficiency virus type-I associated with clinical exposures. Ann Intern Med 113:740–746, 1990. *Prospective study of health care workers at risk for HIV infection. Establishes risk of transmission to be 0.3 per cent per needle stick exposure.*
Sacks HS, Rose DN: Zidovudine prophylaxis for needle stick exposure to human immunodeficiency virus: A decision analysis. J Gen Intern Med 5:132–137, 1990. *A helpful discussion of how to approach risk analysis of zidovudine use after needle sticks.*
Wofsy CB: Prevention of HIV transmission. In Sande MA, Volberding PA (eds.): The Medical Management of AIDS. Philadelphia, W.B. Saunders, 1988, pp 29–43. *A practical review of HIV prevention in different risk groups with specific recommendations for counseling those at risk.*

414 Neurologic Complications of HIV-1 Infection

Richard W. Price

The neurologic complications of HIV-1 infection are both common and varied. Indeed, only rarely do the central and peripheral nervous systems of HIV-infected patients remain unaffected through the course of their disease. Because each of the individual neurologic disorders is discussed in more detail elsewhere in this volume, the major purpose of this chapter is to provide an overview and a general guide to differential diagnosis. It is important to emphasize that differential diagnosis in these patients is far from an "academic exercise," since many of these conditions can be reversed, stabilized, or even cured with specific therapy.

Although the major susceptibility to neurologic complications occurs in the late phase of HIV-1 infection, at the time when immunosuppression leads to a marked increase in vulnerability to a host of conditions, patients may also manifest certain neurologic afflictions early in infection. Because the neurologic complications of early and late HIV-1 infection differ, they are considered separately. Indeed, because of these stage-related differences in susceptibility, when approaching diagnosis in HIV-infected patients it is important to characterize their "background" systemic HIV-1 infection, either clinically with respect to the presence or absence of previous opportunistic infections indicating compromised immunity or by assessment of surrogate markers, particularly the blood CD4+ lymphocyte count.

EARLY HIV-1 INFECTION

Although less common than in the late stages of HIV-1 infection, the nervous system may also be afflicted earlier, indeed as early as the stage of primary infection and seroconversion. Thus, individual reports have described examples of focal or diffuse encephalopathy, ataxia, myelopathy, and meningitis presenting either within the context of the mononucleosis-like HIV-1 seroconversion reaction or with minimal associated systemic symptoms. These conditions appear to evolve acutely or subacutely, to pursue a monophasic course, and to be followed by good, although not always complete, recovery. Peripheral nervous system disorders, including mononeuropathy involving cranial or segmental nerves, brachial plexopathy, and polyneuropathy, have also been reported during this phase. At times these peripheral and central nervous system (CNS) disorders occur together.

Subsequently, during the "asymptomatic seropositive" phase of infection, several neurologic conditions have been reported. Among these is the Guillain-Barré syndrome and its more protracted counterpart, chronic idiopathic demyelinating polyneuropathy (CIDP), both of which are clinically indistinguishable from demyelinating polyneuropathies affecting non–HIV-1–infected individuals, except for higher cerebrospinal fluid (CSF) cell counts and perhaps a poorer prognosis. Response to treatment with corticosteroids and plasma exchange has been noted, supporting presumption of an autoimmune pathogenesis. Because of the potential hazards of corticosteroids, plasma exchange is the preferred therapy.

An additional important aspect of HIV-1 infection, with both diagnostic and pathogenetic implications, is the early development of CSF abnormalities, which presumably relate to early asymptomatic HIV-1 infection of the CNS soon after initial systemic infection. Several prospective studies have reported that the majority of asymptomatic HIV-1–infected individuals exhibit mild CSF changes, including elevations in the cell count and protein and immunoglobulin levels as well as evidence of local "intra–blood-brain barrier" synthesis of anti–HIV-1 antibody. Additionally, in a substantial number of asymptomatic patients HIV-1 can be isolated from the CSF using culture techniques. These findings have not been shown to have an adverse prognostic significance for the subject; indeed, it is clear that patients with such abnormalities can continue to function without symptoms or signs of neurologic impairment. These "background" abnormalities may confound CSF analysis.

LATE HIV-1 INFECTION

The evolving, and eventually severe, impairment of immune defenses caused by HIV-1 renders the nervous system highly vulnerable to a broad spectrum of disorders. The following overview emphasizes general principles of pathogenesis and approach to diagnosis.

Pathophysiology

A number of pathophysiologic processes may lead to neurologic dysfunction in the late phase of HIV-1 infection (Table 414–1). These include conditions that distinguish the AIDS patient from other groups, such as *opportunistic infections, opportunistic neoplasms,* and several conditions that appear to relate to more *direct effects of HIV-1* itself. AIDS patients are also susceptible to the neurologic conditions that affect other acute and chronically ill populations, including metabolic brain disease resulting from systemic organ dysfunction, stroke related to nonbacterial thrombotic endocarditis or coagulopathies, toxic effects of medications, and primary psychiatric disturbances. Here we focus on the first group of disorders, those that particularly distinguish AIDS patients.

OPPORTUNISTIC NERVOUS SYSTEM INFECTIONS. As with other organ systems, the spectrum of opportunistic infections of the nervous system results from the intrinsic vulnerabilities of the tissue (fertile soil) and the pattern of immunosuppression, in

TABLE 414–1. PATHOPHYSIOLOGIC CLASSIFICATION OF THE NEUROLOGIC COMPLICATIONS OF LATE HIV-1 INFECTION

Underlying Process	Examples
Opportunistic infections	Cerebral toxoplasmosis
	Cryptococcal meningitis
	Progressive multifocal leukoencephalopathy
	Cytomegalovirus encephalitis, polyradiculitis
Opportunistic neoplasms	Primary central nervous system lymphoma
	Metastatic lymphoma
Conditions possibly related to HIV-1 itself	AIDS dementia complex
	Aseptic meningitis
	Predominantly sensory polyneuropathy
Metabolic and vascular complications of systemic disease	Hypoxic, sepsis-related encephalopathies
	Stroke (nonbacterial thrombotic endocarditis, coagulopathies)
Toxic reactions	Dideoxyinosine, dideoxycytidine neuropathies
	Zidovudine myopathy
Functional (psychiatric) disorders	Anxiety disorders
	Psychotic depression

this case impaired T-cell/macrophage defenses. The patient's long-term history of exposure to particular organisms is also important because most of the opportunistic infections result from reactivation of latent infections rather than from new encounters with pathogens. An important implication of the preeminence of reactivated infection relates to serologic testing. Serology is most useful for assessing prior exposure to an organism and hence susceptibility to clinically important reactivation, but not for defining active infection. For example, patients with cerebral toxoplasmosis virtually always exhibit antecedent positive *Toxoplasma gondii* blood serology, and therefore a negative serum IgG antibody titer mitigates against this diagnosis; on the other hand, these serum antibody titers most often do not rise before or during the course of disease and therefore a fourfold increase cannot be relied upon to establish disease activity. Moreover, as long as immunosuppression persists and therapy remains incapable of eliminating latent infection, suppressive antibiotic therapy must be maintained for the remainder of the patient's life.

The reason for the intrinsic vulnerability of the nervous system to certain infections (e.g., *T. gondii*) and not others (e.g., *Pneumocystis carinii*) in many cases remains uncertain. However, in some instances susceptibility relates to the capacity of local cells to support intracellular replication. Thus, the virus causing progressive multifocal leukoencephalopathy (PML), JC virus, causes a productive and lytic infection of oligodendrocytes and hence leads to spreading infection and demyelination as the processes of these myelin-producing cells disappear. In the case of HIV-1, productive infection appears to involve monocyte-derived macrophages and perhaps local microglial cells.

The circumscribed nature of the immunologic defect in AIDS determines the range of opportunistic infections, which therefore differs somewhat from that of other immunosuppressed states. For example, AIDS patients are particularly susceptible to cerebral toxoplasmosis but, unlike patients with certain organ transplants, are very unlikely to develop cerebral *Candida* or *Aspergillus* infections. For this reason, AIDS patients present a unique set of disease probabilities.

OPPORTUNISTIC NEOPLASMS. The major consideration in this category is primary brain lymphoma. These B-cell lymphomas arise in the CNS, usually are multicentric (at least microscopically), and only rarely metastasize systemically. Characteristically, they develop late in HIV-1 infection when blood CD4+ lymphocytes are low, i.e., in the same setting as major opportunistic infections. Radiation therapy usually results in tumor regression, but overall prognosis is poor, principally because of the development of other complications; the role of chemotherapy is uncertain, but aggressive treatment is often not possible because of reduced bone marrow reserves. Systemic lymphoma can also spread to the CNS, although usually to the leptomeninges rather than brain parenchyma. Although Kaposi's sarcoma has been reported to metastasize to brain, this is exceedingly rare.

EFFECTS OF HIV-1 ON THE NERVOUS SYSTEM. Several disorders have been suggested to relate in a more direct or fundamental way to HIV-1 infection. These include the AIDS dementia complex, aseptic meningitis, and perhaps predominantly sensory neuropathy. While there is still considerable uncertainty regarding their etiology and pathogenesis, the seeming uniqueness of these conditions in HIV-1–infected compared with other immunosuppressed patients, as well as more direct evidence of virus infection in some patients with the AIDS dementia complex, lends support to this contention.

Diagnosis: Neuroanatomic Approach

As with other neurologic disease, diagnosis in AIDS patients begins with localization of symptoms and signs and hence involves neuroanatomic classification (Table 414–2).

MENINGITIS AND HEADACHE. Several disorders may involve the leptomeninges in patients with advanced HIV-1 disease. The most important of these is infection by *Cryptococcus neoformans* (see Ch. 403). This condition usually presents sub-

TABLE 414–2. NEUROANATOMIC CLASSIFICATION OF THE LATE COMPLICATIONS OF HIV-1 INFECTION

Meningitis and headache
  Cryptococcal meningitis
  Aseptic meningitis (HIV-1)
  Idiopathic, "HIV-1–related" headache
  Tuberculous meningitis (*Mycobacterium tuberculosis*)
  Syphilitic meningitis
  Lymphomatous meningitis (metastatic)
Diffuse brain diseases
  With preservation of consciousness
    AIDS dementia complex
  With concomitant depression of arousal
    Metabolic encephalopathies (alone or as an exacerbating influence)
    Toxoplasmosis ("encephalitic" form)
    Cytomegalovirus encephalitis
    Herpes encephalitis
Focal brain diseases
  Subacute
    Cerebral toxoplasmosis
    Primary CNS lymphoma
    Progressive multifocal leukoencephalopathy
    Tuberculous brain abscess (*M. tuberculosis*)
    Cryptococcoma
    Varicella-zoster virus encephalitis
    Herpes encephalitis
  Acute
    Vascular disorders
Myelopathies
  Subacute/chronic, progressive
    Vacuolar myelopathy
    HTLV-I–associated myelopathy
  Acute/subacute
    Transverse myelitis
      Varicella-zoster virus (herpes zoster)
      Spinal epidural or intradural lymphoma
    With polyradiculopathy
      Cytomegalovirus
Peripheral neuropathies
  Predominantly sensory polyneuropathy
  Toxic neuropathies (dideoxycytidine, dideoxyinosine)
  Autonomic neuropathy
  Cytomegalovirus polyradiculopathy
  Mononeuritis multiplex
  Herpes zoster
  Mononeuropathies associated with aseptic meningitis
  Mononeuropathies secondary to lymphomatous meningitis
Myopathies
  Polymyositis
  Noninflammatory myopathy
  Zidovudine myopathy

acutely with headache, nausea, vomiting, and confusion, just as in non-AIDS patients. However, importantly, in some patients initial symptoms can be remarkably benign, with only mild headache or fever. Likewise, the CSF findings may be bland, with few or no cells and little or no perturbation in either glucose or protein levels. For this reason the clinician should have a low threshold for lumbar puncture and should routinely examine CSF for *Cryptococcus* (India ink stain, cryptococcal antigen determination, culture). Initial treatment is usually gratifying, although sterilizing the CSF is difficult and continued chronic therapy is required.

The syndrome of aseptic meningitis, presumably relating to direct HIV-1 infection of the leptomeninges, may complicate advanced HIV-1 infection but most often develops in the period of transition from AIDS-related complex (ARC) to AIDS. Both acute and chronic forms are accompanied by headache and meningeal symptoms, whereas signs of meningeal irritation are more characteristic of the acute group. Cranial nerve palsies affecting the seventh and, less often, the fifth and eighth nerves may complicate the course. The CSF shows a modest mononuclear pleocytosis, usually with normal glucose and mildly elevated protein. The presumption that this condition is due to direct HIV-1 infection of the meninges derives from the fact that the virus can be readily isolated from the CSF and no other cause has been identified. The syndrome itself is characteristically benign but may imply a poor prognosis in relation to impending progression to AIDS. The efficacy of antiretroviral or other therapies in this disorder has not been studied.

Other, less common meningeal disorders (including meningeal lymphoma, tuberculous meningitis, meningovascular syphilis) resemble their counterparts in the non-AIDS patient. A number of other conditions may present with symptoms resembling meningitis; for example, parenchymal brain diseases such as toxoplasmosis and primary CNS lymphoma may initially manifest with headache as an important symptom. More common, however, is the development of headache of uncertain cause. Although not well studied, headache is a common symptom in late HIV-1 infection and at times can be a severe, debilitating problem. While acute headache in some patients may relate to the onset of systemic infection such as *P. carinii* pneumonia, in others the explanation is elusive.

PREDOMINANTLY FOCAL BRAIN DISORDERS. In approaching diagnosis of parenchymal brain disease, it is useful to separate the conditions that cause predominantly focal symptoms and signs from those producing more generalized brain dysfunction. Patients in the former group present with hemiparesis, aphasia, apraxia, hemisensory abnormalities, visual field loss, and the like, as a result of focal macroscopic lesions in cortical or subcortical brain regions. The most important of these are cerebral toxoplasmosis, which complicates the course of AIDS in 7 to 15 per cent of patients, primary cerebral lymphoma developing in up to 5 per cent, and PML, which occurs in perhaps 3 per cent. Less common are a miscellany of other infections and cerebrovascular disorders.

Although the three major focal disorders all characteristically have a subacute onset and may be clinically indistinguishable, they tend to have somewhat different temporal profiles (Table 414–3). Thus, cerebral toxoplasmosis typically progresses most rapidly (over a few days) and progressive multifocal leukoencephalopathy (PML) evolves most slowly (over a few weeks), with primary CNS lymphoma somewhere in between. Each may cause similar neurologic deficits, but there are often differences in the associated findings. Thus, toxoplasmosis commonly presents with a combination of focal deficit and generalized encephalopathy with confusion or clouding of consciousness; fever and headache may also be present. This contrasts with PML, at least at onset, in which focal neurologic deficits are unaccompanied by either diffuse brain dysfunction or evidence of a systemic toxic state. CNS lymphoma, when accompanied by significant mass effect or when deep in the frontal or periventricular region, may cause more global mental dysfunction, but, again, these patients are usually afebrile without constitutional symptoms or signs.

Once the focal nature of patient's symptoms and signs is recognized, use of neuroimaging techniques, including computed tomography (CT) and more recently magnetic resonance imaging (MRI), is critical both to confirm the presence of macroscopic focal disease and to determine the nature of the abnormalities

TABLE 414-3. COMPARATIVE CLINICAL AND RADIOLOGIC FEATURES OF CEREBRAL TOXOPLASMOSIS, PRIMARY CNS LYMPHOMA, AND PROGRESSIVE MULTIFOCAL LEUKOENCEPHALOPATHY

	Clinical Onset			Neuroradiologic Features		
	Temporal Profile	*Level of Alertness*	*Fever*	*Number of Lesions*	*Type of Lesions*	*Location of Lesions*
Cerebral toxoplasmosis	Days	Reduced	Common	Multiple	Spherical, ring-enhancing	Basal ganglia, cortex
Primary CNS lymphoma	Days to weeks	Variable	Absent	One or few	Irregular, weakly enhancing	Periventricular
Progressive multifocal leuko-encephalopathy	Weeks	Preserved	Absent	Multiple	Nonenhancing	White matter

(Table 414-3). Multiple lesions involving the cortex or deep brain nuclei (thalamus, basal ganglia) surrounded by edema strongly favor cerebral toxoplasmosis. In most cases *Toxoplasma* abscesses exhibit ringlike contrast enhancement on CT scan. Double-dose contrast CT studies, or preferably MRI, may help in more clearly defining these lesions and detecting additional characteristic spherical lesions. Cerebral lymphoma may produce a similar CT appearance, although the lesions of lymphoma are usually less numerous (one or two definable lesions), commonly exhibit more diffuse or less clear-cut contrast enhancement, and are more often located in the white matter adjacent to the ventricles. PML characteristically involves the white matter, most often adjacent to the cortex, and is without mass effect or contrast enhancement on CT.

After neuroimaging, the next step in diagnosis of focal mass lesions often involves a trial of anti-*Toxoplasma* therapy. Pyrimethamine and sulfa therapy characteristically results in clinical improvement within a few days and distinct reduction of lesions on neuroimaging by 1 or 2 weeks. This rapid and consistent improvement allows treatment response to serve as a basis for diagnosis and thereby obviates the need for brain biopsy in virtually all patients with toxoplasmosis. Biopsy is then reserved for cases with atypical clinical or laboratory features (including atypical neuroimaging appearance or negative *Toxoplasma* blood serology) along with those who fail to improve with treatment. It is important in the context of such therapeutic trial that, if possible, corticosteroids be avoided. Since the signs and symptoms, and even the CT or MRI abnormalities, of cerebral lymphoma may improve with corticosteroids, such treatment can confuse interpretation of the anti-*Toxoplasma* therapeutic trial. However, if cerebral edema threatens brain herniation, judicious short-term corticosteroids may be instituted along with appropriate specific therapy and subsequently tapered rapidly once the patient improves.

PREDOMINANTLY NONFOCAL BRAIN DISORDERS. The disorders presenting with more general or diffuse brain dysfunction and without focal features can be further divided into those in which consciousness remains fully preserved and those accompanied by a concomitant decrease in alertness. Most important among the former is the *AIDS dementia complex*, a clinical syndrome characterized by cognitive, motor, and, at times, behavioral dysfunction. A number of terms have been used to encompass this clinical syndrome, including the recent designation by the World Health Organization (WHO) as the HIV-1–associated cognitive/motor complex, with three subtypes: HIV-1–associated dementia, HIV-1–associated myelopathy, and HIV-1–associated minor cognitive/motor disorder.

Both the incidence and severity of the AIDS dementia complex increase with advancing immunosuppression. The clinical syndrome is somewhat variable, and its pathologic substrate is heterogeneous. At least in part, it appears to relate to effects of HIV-1 infection on the CNS rather than involving secondary opportunistic infection. Its early, mild form is usually characterized by impaired concentration and attention along with reduced mental agility, resulting in complaints of forgetfulness and slowness in performing complex mental tasks. In those who progress to more severe involvement, cognitive dysfunction worsens and involves other domains, and motor dysfunction becomes clinically manifest with gait unsteadiness and difficulty with rapid, fine movements of the hands. Personality change with apathy, lack of

initiative, or, at times, hyperactivity and agitation may be part of the syndrome. In its most severe form, global dementia, paraplegia, and virtual mutism may evolve with resultant incapacity. Although it is in part a diagnosis of exclusion, the symptoms and signs of the AIDS dementia complex are sufficiently distinct to allow bedside diagnosis in most patients on the basis of their stereotypy. Neuroimaging using CT or MRI characteristically reveals cerebral atrophy, and MRI may additionally demonstrate increased signal in white matter or basal ganglia. Several studies now suggest that zidovudine can partially reverse the symptoms and signs of the AIDS dementia complex. Whether newer antiretroviral drugs will demonstrate a similar therapeutic effect remains to be evaluated.

In the AIDS dementia complex there is relative preservation of alertness in relation to cognitive loss. This contrasts with most metabolic encephalopathies developing as sequelae of the systemic diseases suffered by AIDS patients; for example, hypoxia and sepsis are characteristically accompanied by a degree of lethargy and confusion which parallels the decline in cognition. Likewise, CNS-active drugs often cloud mentation and alertness together. While such metabolic and toxic disorders may present alone, they also commonly have an exacerbating or unmasking influence on the AIDS dementia complex, resulting in a mixture of the two conditions. HIV-1–infected patients may also be more sensitive to neuroleptics and thereby manifest parkinsonian or other movement disorders as side effects at seemingly low doses.

Brain infections may also produce diffuse brain dysfunction. Although CNS toxoplasmosis characteristically causes focal neurologic symptoms and signs, in some patients generalized encephalopathy predominates. Similarly, CNS lymphoma may infiltrate deep structures and impair cognition and motor function without prominent focal symptoms or signs. The clinical importance of CNS cytomegalovirus (CMV) infection in this regard remains imprecisely defined. Scattered CMV infection of the brain is common at autopsy, but the clinical correlate of this finding is not clear, and likely it is often silent or mild. On the other hand, in a small number of patients CMV encephalitis may be severe with subacute clouding of consciousness and, at times, seizures. Herpes simplex virus types 1 and 2 may also cause subacute nonfocal encephalitis.

MYELOPATHIES. The most common spinal cord affliction in AIDS patients is the pathologically defined vacuolar myelopathy, which has been included within the broader clinical designation of the AIDS dementia complex because it is usually accompanied by evidence of concomitant brain dysfunction. The disorder is generally of subacute or slow onset and progression with painless gait disturbance characterized by ataxia and spasticity. Bladder and bowel difficulty usually follow deterioration of gait, and sensory symptoms and signs are less prominent than gait dysfunction unless there is concomitant neuropathy. Patients do not manifest a distinct sensory or motor "level" as in transverse myelopathies but rather distal loss of large-fiber modalities accompanied by increased deep tendon reflexes (again, in the absence of neuropathy) and Babinski signs. The efficacy of zidovudine or other antiretrovirals in this subgroup of AIDS dementia complex patients is uncertain.

An additional, emerging cause of clinically similar myelopathy in HIV-1–infected patients relates to coinfection with a second retrovirus, human T-lymphotropic virus I (HTLV-I). Double infection results from the convergent epidemiologies of these infections related to intravenous drug abuse. Although pathologically distinct, clinical differentiation of vacuolar myelopathy and HTLV-I–associated myelopathy (HAM) may be very difficult. Diagnosis begins with suspicion based on risk and is supported by serologic documentation of HTLV-I infection, but the relative clinical contributions of the two viruses is problematic antemortem. In AIDS patients with myelopathy, laboratory diagnostic studies are principally directed at ruling out spinal cord disease other than vacuolar myelopathy. Neither myelography nor spinal MRI has allowed clear imaging of vacuolar myelopathy or HAM. However, these procedures are often needed to document focal intraspinal processes, including epidural masses.

PERIPHERAL NEUROPATHIES. The most common neuropathy in the late stages of HIV-1 infection is a distal, predominantly sensory, axonal neuropathy. Characteristically, sensory symptoms exceed both sensory and motor dysfunction. Although its prevalence has not been well defined, likely a mild form of this type of neuropathy is very common. In some patients these sensory symptoms become severe, and painful paresthesias and "burning feet" are disabling. Although suspected to relate to direct HIV-1 infection of nerve or dorsal root ganglia, this has not been directly confirmed, and the pathogenesis of this neuropathy is uncertain. Anecdotal experience suggests that it does not generally respond to zidovudine, and treatment therefore relies on symptom management with tricyclics and analgesics. Autonomic neuropathy has also been reported in AIDS patients, with presentation ranging from postural hypotension to cardiovascular collapse in the setting of surgery.

Likely to be of increasing importance in the next several years are the toxic neuropathies caused by some of the newer antiretroviral nucleoside drugs, including dideoxyinosine and dideoxycytidine. These drugs cause dose-dependent axonal neuropathies with clinical features very similar to the AIDS-related sensory polyneuropathy discussed above, often heralded by distal extremity pain.

CMV causes an uncommon but therapeutically important infection of nerve roots. This polyradiculopathy is usually of subacute but fulminant onset, with pain and sacral sensory loss followed by ascending progression to flaccid paralysis. The CSF reveals a characteristic pleocytosis with polymorphonuclear cell predominance. Early diagnosis and prompt institution of ganciclovir treatment can lead to arrest and clinical improvement.

Less common than these polyneuropathies is mononeuritis multiplex, with onset most commonly in the setting of ARC rather than far-advanced AIDS. Favorable response to plasma exchange has been reported.

MYOPATHIES. Several types of myopathy may complicate HIV-1 infection. Although classification and characterization of these conditions remain imprecise, both inflammatory and noninflammatory myopathies have been described, ranging in severity from asymptomatic creatine kinase elevation to severe proximal weakness. Improvement of patients with inflammatory, polymyositis-like illness has been reported following steroid therapy.

Zidovudine can also cause proximal weakness and loss of muscle mass. This toxic myopathy appears to develop only after prolonged use of the antiretroviral and perhaps relates to the drug's effect on mitochondria; muscle biopsy may reveal excessive or abnormal mitochondria. Drug discontinuation usually results in clinical improvement.

Baumbartner JE, Rachlin JR, Beckstead JH, et al.: Primary central nervous system lymphomas: Natural history and response to radiation therapy in 55 patients with acquired immunodeficiency syndrome. J Neurosurg 73:206–211, 1990. *Describes an extensive experience with primary CNS lymphoma in AIDS.*

Berger JR, Kaszovitz B, Post JD, et al.: Progressive multifocal leukoencephalopathy associated with human immunodeficiency virus infection. Ann Intern Med 107:78, 1987. *A review of experience with PML in AIDS.*

Dalakas MC, Illa I, Pezeshkpour GH, et al.: Mitochondrial myopathy caused by long-term zidovudine therapy. N Engl J Med 322:1098–1105, 1990. *Describes zidovudine myopathy and considers other myopathies in AIDS patients.*

Hollander H, Stringari S: Human immunodeficiency virus–associated meningitis: Clinical course and correlations. Am J Med 83:813, 1987. *Describes the aseptic meningitis complicating HIV-1 infection.*

Miller RG, Storey JR, Greco CM: Ganciclovir in the treatment of progressive AIDS-related polyradiculopathy. Neurology 40:569–574, 1990. *Reports experience in CMV-related polyradiculopathy and also discusses other neuropathies in HIV-1–infected patients; full bibliography.*

Navia BA, Cho ES, Petito CK, et al.: Cerebral toxoplasmosis complicating the acquired immune deficiency syndrome: Clinical and neuropathological findings in 27 patients. Ann Neurol 19:224, 1986. *Describes clinical features of cerebral toxoplasmosis in AIDS.*

Navia BA, Jordon BD, Price RW: The AIDS dementia complex. I. Clinical features. Ann Neurol 19517, 1986. *Report characterizing the clinical features of the AIDS dementia complex.*

Petito CK, Navia BA, Cho ES, et al.: Vacuolar myelopathy pathologically resembling subacute combined degeneration in patients with acquired immunodeficiency syndrome (AIDS). N Engl J Med 312:874, 1985. *Describes clinical and pathologic findings associated with vacuolar myelopathy.*

Price RW, Brew B: Management of the neurologic complications of HIV-1 infection and AIDS. In Sande MA, Volberding PA (eds.): The Medical Management of AIDS. Philadelphia, W.B. Saunders Company, 1990, pp 161–181. *An expanded general review with full bibliography.*

Zuger A, Louie E, Holzman RS, et al.: Cryptococcal disease in patients with the acquired immunodeficiency syndrome: Diagnostic features and outcome of treatment. Ann Intern Med 104:234–240, 1986. *Describes the clinical features of cryptococcal meningitis in AIDS.*

415 Pulmonary Manifestations of AIDS: Special Emphasis on Pneumocystosis

Fred R. Sattler

Protozoan, viral, fungal, and bacterial infections and tumors such as Kaposi's sarcoma cause most of the deaths in patients with AIDS. All of these complications may involve the lung and often require initial treatment in the hospital. Chest tightness, breathlessness, hacking cough, pleuritic pain, high fevers, drenching sweats, drug-induced rashes, and secondary bacterial infections result in considerable discomfort and anxiety for patients, their partners, and their families. Pneumothoraces, which may occur spontaneously or after bronchoscopy, often prolong hospitalization and contribute further morbidity.

Patients with AIDS are hospitalized two or three times per year for management of these complications. The cost for each hospitalization ranges from $10,000 to $20,000; in many large urban-metropolitan areas where AIDS is highly endemic, medical personnel and hospital services are being consumed and rapidly depleted. Prompt diagnosis and early treatment of these complications facilitates early discharge from the hospital by hastening clinical response and reducing the risks and severity of toxic drug effects. Of equal import, as prophylactic therapies for various infections are established to be effective for HIV-positive patients, the incidence of these pulmonary complications will be reduced. It is imperative, therefore, that medical providers implement a global strategy of prevention and early therapy of these life-threatening complications if the human suffering and progressive depletion of health care resources caused by AIDS are to be alleviated.

PATHOGENESIS AND RISK FOR INFECTION

The risk for HIV-positive persons developing opportunistic pulmonary complications is related to deficiencies in their T-helper (CD4 surface phenotype) lymphocytes, since these cells control or regulate virtually all components of immunity (see Ch. 242 and 410). Thus, host defenses become progressively compromised as the CD4 cells are destroyed during the course of HIV infection. Figure 415–1 shows that the CD4 lymphocyte count is generally below 100 cells per cubic millimeter (or less than 10 per cent of the total T lymphocytes, latter data not shown) for pneumonia due to *Pneumocystis carinii*, Kaposi's sarcoma, *Mycobacterium avium* complex, cytomegalovirus, and *Cryptococcus neoformans*. By contrast, nonspecific interstitial pneumonitis occurs at various levels of CD4 immunity, and pulmonary infection due to *Mycobacterium tuberculosis* most often occurs in HIV-positive persons when their CD4 count is in the range of 200 to 400 cells per cubic millimeter. Thus, the absolute or relative concentration of CD4 lymphocytes is related to the pathogenesis of many of the pulmonary complications and is

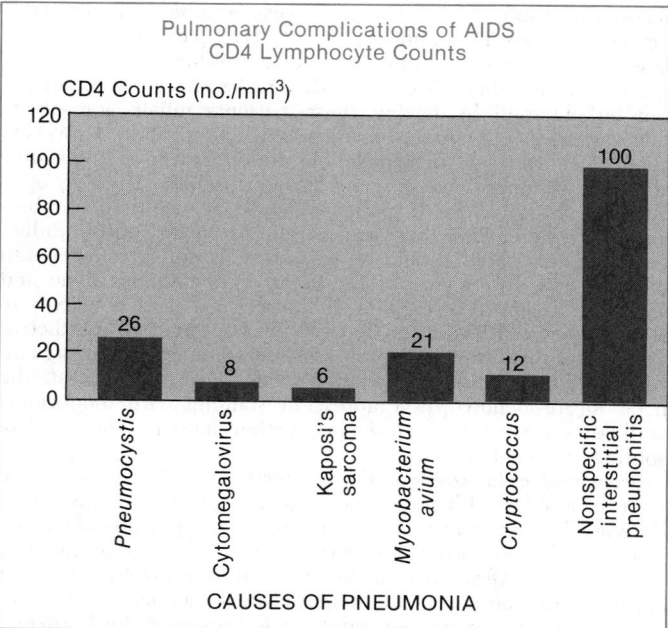

Figure 415–1. Median number of CD4 lymphocytes for various opportunistic pulmonary complications occurring in patients with AIDS. (Adapted from Masur H, Ognibene FP, Yarchoan R, et al.: CD4 counts as predictors of opportunistic pneumonias in human immunodeficiency virus (HIV) infection. Ann Intern Med 111:223–231, 1989.)

useful in assessing the relative risk of the various pulmonary disorders in HIV-positive patients.

Pneumocystis carinii Pneumonia (PCP)

Pneumonia due to *P. carinii* is the most common pulmonary complication in patients infected with HIV. Since the beginning of the epidemic in the United States, PCP has occurred in 50 to 60 per cent of patients as the initial opportunistic complication resulting in the Centers for Disease Control case definition of AIDS. Ultimately 70 to 80 per cent of AIDS patients experience one or more episodes of PCP, and without prophylaxis approximately 60,000 AIDS-related cases will occur in the year 1991 alone. Moreover, 10 to 50 per cent of episodes are fatal, depending on the severity of illness at presentation. In fact, PCP accounts for nearly half of the deaths due to opportunistic complications in patients with AIDS. Thus, considerable emphasis is given here to the diagnosis, treatment, and prevention of this devastating infection.

ETIOLOGY. *P. carinii* was long believed to be a protozoan organism because of its morphologic features and response to drugs used to treat other protozoan infections. However, the genetic composition of the ribosomal RNA of this organism suggests that it is similar to a fungus and phylogenetically may belong to the Ascomycetes yeasts. The immediate importance of this observation is unclear, since PCP does not respond to available antifungal drugs. Better understanding of the molecular composition of *P. carinii* will, however, ultimately provide valuable insights into pathogenic mechanisms and development of better therapies for infections caused by this organism.

CLINICAL SYNDROME. The onset of PCP in AIDS patients is usually insidious. The cardinal manifestation is chronic cough, which often has been present for weeks and sometimes months. The cough is usually nonproductive but occasionally is associated with mucoid sputum. Retrosternal chest tightness, which is intensified with inspiration and coughing, is a second nearly global symptom. Fever occurs in 80 to 90 per cent of patients but may have been present for a shorter duration than the cough and chest tightness. Dyspnea on exertion and breathlessness at rest occur late in the infection when oxygenation is moderately to severely impaired.

Abnormalities on physical examination are usually limited and nonspecific. Elevated temperature and respiratory rate may be present. With mild episodes there may be no tachypnea, but patients with severe episodes are often in respiratory distress and

are using their accessory chest wall muscles. The lungs are frequently clear to auscultation, as rales are detected in only 30 to 40 per cent of cases and are usually a late finding in severe episodes. Indeed, absence of adventitial breath sounds should not be used to exclude the possibility of PCP in persons who are at risk for AIDS.

Physical findings outside the lung are even less specific, but their presence or absence may assist the clinical assessment. For example, in patients with a forme fruste presentation who have not been treated with topical or oral antifungal drugs, a thick coating of thrush on the dorsal aspect of the tongue is a nearly universal finding. Seborrheic dermatitis involving the face between the brows, forehead, and upper cheeks is also common with PCP and unusual with other pulmonary complications of AIDS. By contrast, generalized adenopathy with lymph nodes greater than 1 cm in diameter is rare, since patients with PCP usually have severe immune deficiency and their lymph nodes are hypoplastic. Thus, the presence of large lymph nodes should suggest the occurrence of other opportunistic complications, although concurrent infection with *P. carinii* may occur.

EXTRAPULMONARY PNEUMOCYSTOSIS. *P. carinii* infection outside the lung may occur without prior or concurrent PCP, although most cases have occurred during prophylaxis with aerosolized pentamidine and the lung is frequently involved. It is unlikely that pentamidine is directly related to the pathogenesis of extrapulmonary pneumocystosis. Rather, it is probably an epiphenomenon associated with the lack of protection provided by aerosolized pentamidine for sites of infection outside the lung. Clinical presentations have included external auditory polyps, mastoiditis, choroiditis, digital necrosis secondary to vasculitis, obstruction of the small intestine, ascites with gross nodules in the stomach and duodenum, hepatitis, splenitis, hilar or mediastinal lymphadenopathy, and involvement of the bone marrow. Disseminated infection may also occur in virtually every organ including brain, heart, kidneys, and adrenal glands. Histologic examination of affected organs shows a striking resemblance to the pathology usually found in the lung. There are typical foci of eosinophilic frothy exudates which upon special staining reveal the presence of *P. carinii* cysts. Unlike the lung, these lesions are often calcified and there may be vasculitis with invasion of vessel walls by *P. carinii* organisms.

Signs and symptoms of extrapulmonary pneumocystosis are nonspecific, and the diagnosis usually requires histologic confirmation. *P. carinii* choroiditis is, however, associated with unique features. Lesions consist of slightly elevated, yellow-white plaques, generally limited to the choroid without evidence of intraocular inflammation. Identification of these typical lesions may provide the first clue to the diagnosis of *P. carinii* infection and mandates that therapy include systemic drugs active against *P. carinii*.

LABORATORY ABNORMALITIES. Most patients with PCP are anemic because of the advanced stage of their HIV infection, other concurrent diseases, or treatment with myelosuppressive drugs such as zidovudine. For similar reasons the white blood cell count (WBC) is usually depressed or in the low normal range. An elevated WBC or marked increase in the percentage of band forms should suggest a bacterial pneumonia or other pyogenic process. The serum albumin is often depressed by 0.5 to 1.0 gram per deciliter below normal and is probably a reflection of the poor overall nutritional status of these patients. Serum lactate dehydrogenase (LDH) is a sensitive but not specific marker of PCP and is elevated in more than 90 per cent of patients with PCP, whereas LDH values are usually only minimally elevated or normal in individuals with other pulmonary complications of AIDS.

The absolute or relative number of CD4 lymphocytes is the single most useful test in evaluating patients at risk for PCP. As shown in Figure 415–1 and confirmed by several other studies, more than 90 per cent of individuals when first diagnosed with PCP have less than 200 CD4 lymphocytes per cubic millimeter. However, in one large natural history investigation of ambulatory subjects at risk for AIDS, 26 per cent of individuals had CD4 counts above 200 (all but one had counts between 201 and 350) within 6 months prior to the diagnosis of PCP. The diagnosis is very unlikely in an individual with a normal or nearly normal (generally > 500) number of CD4 cells.

PULMONARY FUNCTION TESTS. Hypoxemia with PaO_2 less than 80 torr occurs in more than 80 per cent and an alveolar-arterial oxygen difference [$(A\text{-}a)DO_2$] of greater than 15 torr occurs in more than 90 per cent of patients with PCP. In patients with PCP in whom these tests are normal or nearly normal, oxygen desaturation can be documented with pulse oximetry during exercise and the $(A\text{-}a)DO_2$ generally widens. The carbon monoxide diffusing capacity (DL_{CO}) is less than 80 per cent of predicted in nearly all patients with PCP, since the transmembrane diffusion of carbon monoxide is impaired (alveolar capillary block) by the intra-alveolar exudate associated with this infection. The test is not specific, since it may be abnormal in other pulmonary disorders and in patients who use intravenous drugs. However, in patients with respiratory symptoms whose arterial blood gases and chest radiographs are not helpful, a normal DL_{CO} makes PCP unlikely at that time. The test is also helpful in AIDS patients with asthma, since results should be normal in subjects whose hypoxemia is due to bronchospasm.

RADIOGRAPHIC ABNORMALITIES. Typically in PCP, infiltrates on chest radiographs are interstitial and begin in the perihilar areas and spread to the lower and upper lung fields, although the apices are usually spared. As the disease progresses, an alveolar pattern with air bronchograms may be superimposed on the interstitial process, although alveolar patterns may be the initial presentation in up to 10 per cent of cases. In 10 to 30 per cent of cases the radiographic presentation is atypical, with asymmetric or predominantly upper lobe infiltration, lobar or segmental consolidation, cystic lesions (with a honeycombed appearance), overt cavitation, and rarely solitary parenchymal nodules or postobstructive infiltration secondary to endobronchial nodules of *P. carinii*. Pleural effusions and hilar adenopathy have only rarely been documented to be due to *P. carinii*, although both have reportedly disappeared during therapy for PCP, whereas Kaposi's sarcoma frequently involves the pleural space and hilar nodes may be enlarged with mycobacterial infection and cryptococcosis.

Lung cavitation is not uncommon in AIDS patients with PCP. Lesions are generally thin walled without air-fluid levels and may be solitary or more generalized, resulting in regional areas of honeycombed lung. These lesions may occur in nonsmokers, at initial presentation of the first episode of PCP, prior to bronchoscopy, prior to aerosol therapy, and prior to intubation. Thus, in most cases cavitation is not due to underlying lung disease, specific diagnostic or therapeutic interventions, or barotrauma. It may be due to activated pulmonary macrophages and release of elastase as a consequence of chronic infection with *P. carinii* per se. Regardless of the mechanism, cavitation and cystic lesions, which occurred in just over 10 per cent of patients in one large series, may be complicated by spontaneous pneumothoraces and bronchopleural fistulas that are refractory to closure. Moreover, cavitation is unusual in HIV-positive patients with pulmonary tuberculosis. Thus, radiographic appearance of cavitation or cystic disease should not be a deterrent to pursuing a diagnosis of PCP.

Ten to 20 per cent of patients with documented PCP have had normal chest radiographs at presentation. These patients generally have early, mild episodes and respond well to appropriate and prompt therapy. Thus, every effort should be made to diagnose PCP early when there is minimal or no infiltration present on the chest radiograph.

Gallium-67 accumulates in areas of lung inflammation, but pulmonary uptake is not specific for PCP. Specificity is reportedly improved if scans are designated positive only when gallium uptake in the lungs equals or exceeds that in the liver. However, patients with mild PCP may have minimal or no lung uptake, and other pulmonary complications may produce positive scans. In addition, the test is expensive and images are not produced until 48 to 72 hours after patients have been injected with gallium. However, gallium imaging is useful for patients with chronic lung disease who have worsening respiratory symptoms, since blood gases and radiographs are often not useful in these patients, and for detecting relapses when other tests are not diagnostic.

DIAGNOSIS. Sputum Induction. Unlike PCP in other immunocompromised patients in whom organisms are often difficult to find in lung tissue and are rarely present in tracheobronchial secretions, there are commonly excess numbers of organisms present in secretions obtained from AIDS patients with PCP. Unfortunately, most patients with PCP produce minimal or no sputum despite their chronic cough. Tracheobronchial secretions can be obtained by having these patients inhale aerosols of hypertonic saline generated by ultrasonic nebulization. However, even concentrates of such specimens are difficult to examine after adequate staining because of background debris. Thus, to optimize the diagnostic yield, patients should cleanse their oropharynx by brushing their teeth and gargling prior to sputum induction, and specimens should be treated with mucolytic agents to dissolve oral debris prior to staining. When this is done and slides are reviewed by experts, the procedure has a sensitivity of 50 to 80 per cent but only a 39 to 63 per cent negative predictive value. The procedure is laborious for respiratory therapists and laboratory technicians, but positive specimens usually obviate the need for bronchoscopy. Fluorescent staining with monoclonal antibodies against *P. carinii* may further increase the yield of sputum examination.

Bronchoalveolar Lavage. The cornerstone of diagnosis of PCP is bronchoscopy with bronchoalveolar lavage (BAL). This procedure involves wedging the bronchoscope into a peripheral airway. Aliquots of nonbacteriostatic saline of 20 to 30 cubic millimeters are instilled. After each instillation, fluid is aspirated. After approximately 50 cubic millimeters of fluid has been recovered, the specimen is centrifuged and the pellet is stained for *P. carinii*. In 86 to 97 per cent of cases *P. carinii* organisms are detected by this procedure.

Transbronchial Biopsy. When transbronchial biopsies are obtained and specimens are without crush artifact and contain at least 25 alveoli, this procedure results in a diagnostic yield similar to that achieved with BAL. If both BAL and transbronchial biopsies are obtained, the diagnostic sensitivity is additive and approaches 100 per cent. However, pneumothoraces or bleeding may occur in up to 10 per cent of subjects undergoing transbronchial biopsy. Thus, many pulmonologists prefer to perform only BAL with the initial bronchoscopy. If the first procedure fails to provide a diagnosis, BAL is repeated and transbronchial biopsies are obtained. If specimens from both procedures are adequate and fail to show *P. carinii* organisms with standard histologic and cytologic stains, the diagnosis is confidently excluded.

Open Lung Biopsy. Open lung biopsy is rarely needed in AIDS patients to diagnose PCP because of the high yield of sputum induction and bronchoscopy. It is usually reserved for patients in whom bronchoscopy has been nondiagnostic because of technical problems with the procedure or transbronchial biopsies are contraindicated because of bleeding disorders or concurrent management with mechanical ventilation. Open lung biopsy is safer than bronchoscopy for patients with abnormal coagulation, since hemostasis is more reliably achieved intraoperatively than at bronchoscopy.

TREATMENT. Initial Therapy. The key to successful treatment of PCP is early therapy, since mild episodes are more likely to respond favorably. In particular, patients with minimal infiltration on their chest radiographs, minimal elevation of serum LDH, and normal or nearly normal $(A\text{-}a)DO_2$ generally have greater than 90 per cent chance of responding to treatment. By contrast, patients with extensive infiltration, LDH in excess of 500, and $(A\text{-}a)DO_2$ greater than 35 torr have a risk for death during treatment that is greater than 40 per cent. If the $(A\text{-}a)DO_2$ exceeds 55 to 60 torr, the risk for a fatal outcome is in the range of 60 to 80 per cent.

Since sputum induction and bronchoscopies are generally not done at night or on weekends or holidays and results of cytologic stains are often not available for 24 hours or more after specimens have been collected, most patients with typical clinical features of PCP should be treated empirically, especially if there is moderate to severe impairment in gas exchange as measured by the PaO_2 or $(A\text{-}a)DO_2$. This does not impair the ability to make a histologic or cytologic diagnosis, as large numbers of *P. carinii* cysts and trophozoites remain in lung tissues and pulmonary secretions for weeks to months after the onset of therapy. There are several reasons why every effort should be made to confirm the diagnosis even if the patient appears to be responding promptly to treatment. Bacterial bronchopneumonia may respond to the antibiotic properties of the sulfonamide and sulfone drugs used to treat PCP, and nonspecific interstitial pneumonitis may

TABLE 415–1. TREATMENTS FOR PNEUMOCYSTIS CARINII PNEUMONIA

	Dosages*
Standard drug therapies	
Trimethoprim-sulfamethoxazole (IV or oral)	5 mg/kg q6h or q8h of trimethoprim
Pentamidine (IV or IM)	4 mg/kg/day
Trimethoprim-dapsone (both oral)	5 mg/kg q8h of TMP 100 mg/day of dapsone
Adjunctive corticosteroids (prednisone)†	60–80 mg/day for 5–7 days with tapering doses over 2–3 weeks
Experimental therapies	
Aerosolized pentamidine	600 mg/day via Respirgard II jet nebulizer
Trimetrexate-leucovorin (IV or IV/oral)	45 mg/M²/day of trimetrexate 20 mg/M²/q6h of leucovorin
Eflornithine (DFMO) (IV and oral)	100 mg/kg/q6h intravenously 75 mg/kg/q6h orally
Primaquine-clindamycin (oral-parenteral/oral)	15–30 mg/day primaquine base 0.6–0.9 gram IV or 450–600 mg orally of clindamycin q6–8h

*Dosages are once daily unless designated otherwise.

†To be administered concurrently with specific anti-*Pneumocystis* therapy for patients who present with (A-a)DO₂ > 35 mm Hg or PaO₂ < 70 mm Hg.

improve spontaneously. Both situations give the false impression that the patient has responded to anti-*Pneumocystis* therapy. Moreover, bacterial pneumonia can often be treated with a brief course of oral antibiotic therapy, and nonspecific interstitial pneumonitis should not be treated with antimicrobial agents.

Mycobacteriosis, cytomegalovirus pneumonia, and Kaposi's sarcoma may also closely resemble PCP. However, each of these pulmonary complications requires a different therapy. In addition, by the time patients fail to respond to empiric therapy for PCP, they may be too ill for bronchoscopy or open lung biopsy, thus denying them the opportunity to receive specific therapy.

For psychological reasons it is important for patients and their loved ones to know for certain whether they have AIDS. Results of empiric therapy may provide presumptive evidence for the diagnosis, although the uncertainties may be emotionally devastating for individuals who have not met the rigorous U.S. Public Health Service case definition for AIDS. Moreover, access to many community services and financial benefits requires a definitive diagnosis of AIDS, which can usually be established by documenting the presence of a pulmonary opportunistic complication (other than tuberculosis).

Finally, standard therapies for PCP are associated with a high rate of adverse and often serious drug reactions, which may prolong hospitalization. It is difficult to justify these toxic reactions and additional hospitalization for patients who do not have PCP. Thus, there are compelling reasons to establish a definitive diagnosis whenever possible.

Initial therapy should be given parenterally for patients with severe impairment in oxygen exchange as arbitrarily defined by an (A-a)DO₂ of greater than 30 torr. In non-AIDS patients with PCP, trimethoprim (TMP) and sulfamethoxazole (SMX), which have nearly complete bioavailability when administered orally, were erratically absorbed from the gut in subjects with severe hypoxemia. Patients who failed treatment often had serum TMP concentrations less than 5 μg per milliliter. The problem is further complicated by the fact that AIDS patients may have nonspecific malabsorption in the absence of overt diarrhea. The principle of beginning initial treatment with parenteral drugs for moderate to severe episodes should also apply to other anti-*Pneumocystis* therapies. Table 415–1 shows the drugs and dosages generally prescribed to treat PCP.

Trimethoprim-sulfamethoxazole. The antifolate combination of TMP-SMX was the first therapy licensed by the U.S. Food and Drug Administration for the therapy of PCP. In the largest prospective controlled study involving AIDS patients with moderate to severe PCP, subjects were prospectively randomized to receive a full 3-week course of either TMP-SMX or pentamidine without being crossed over to the opposite therapy for apparent treatment failure or adverse drug reactions. This allowed the relative efficacy and inherent toxicities of these two therapies to be fully assessed. In this investigation, 86 per cent of individuals

treated with TMP-SMX survived, compared to 61 per cent treated with pentamidine; this difference was statistically significant. An average of 2.4 adverse reactions were ascribed to study therapy in 89 per cent of individuals treated with TMP-SMX. Severe hematologic toxicities were prevented through pharmacokinetic monitoring. By reducing the initial dose of 15 to 20 mg per kilogram per day of the TMP component to maintain serum TMP concentrations in the 5 to 8 μg per milliliter range, dosage-terminating neutropenia or thrombocytopenia did not occur. With this approach the final average dosage was 12 mg per kilogram per day, yet efficacy was not compromised. In addition, therapy was continued despite hypersensitivity reactions of drug-induced fever or morbilliform rash. This was accomplished by concurrent therapy with acetaminophen for fever and antihistamines for rashes. In each case fever ultimately subsided and rashes coalesced and faded, although this occasionally took several weeks. There were no severe complications such as Stevens-Johnson syndrome or exfoliative dermatitis, and other adverse effects associated with TMP-SMX were tolerable. The spectrum and frequency of these toxic drug reactions are shown in Table 415–2. The approach of dosage reduction based on pharmacokinetic monitoring and continuing treatment despite manageable hypersensitivity reactions allowed patients to be switched to oral TMP-SMX once their respiratory status was improved and to complete therapy on an outpatient basis.

Pentamidine. Parenteral pentamidine is the other licensed therapy for PCP. In the aforementioned study involving individuals with moderate to severe PCP, survival was inferior with pentamidine compared to TMP-SMX. However, the dosage of pentamidine was reduced when nephrotoxicity occurred such that the final average dosage was approximately 3 mg per kilogram per day. It is possible that dosage reduction compromised outcome. In one study involving individuals with less severe PCP, 3 mg per kilogram per day resulted in a good outcome. However, until rigorous controlled studies are done to compare this lower dosage with the standard dosage, the initial dosage of pentamidine should be 4 mg per kilogram per day, especially for more severe episodes.

Toxic reactions are also frequent with parenteral pentamidine (Table 415–2). In the study mentioned earlier, an average of 2.9 adverse drug effects occurred in 97 per cent of the individuals treated with pentamidine. Nephrotoxicity (64 per cent), hypotension (27 per cent), and hypoglycemia (21 per cent) were the most frequent serious adverse effects. Impaired renal function, which

TABLE 415–2. TOXIC SIDE EFFECTS ASSOCIATED WITH TREATMENTS FOR PNEUMOCYSTIS CARINII PNEUMONIA*

Adverse Effect†	Trimethoprim-Sulfamethoxazole (%)	Pentamidine (parenteral) (%)
Fever (>37.7°C)	78	82
Leukopenia (<4 × 10⁹/L)	72	47
Rash—generalized	44	15
Anemia (↓ >3 g/dl)	39	24
Nausea/vomiting	25	24
Elevated ALT (↑ >5X)	22	15
Azotemia‡	14	64
Thrombocytopenia (<100 × 10⁹/L)	3	18
Hypotension (sys. <80 mm Hg)	0	27
Hypoglycemia (<70 mg/dl)	0	21
Hypocalcemia (<7 mg/dl)	0	3
Total percentage of subjects with adverse reactions	89	97
Average number of reactions per subject (range)	2.4 (0–5)	2.9 (0–7)

*Adapted from Sattler FR, Cowan R, Nielsen DM, Ruskin J: Trimethoprim-sulfamethoxazole compared with pentamidine for treatment of *Pneumocystis carinii* pneumonia in the acquired immunodeficiency syndrome: A prospective noncrossover study. Ann Intern Med 109:280–287, 1988. Thirty-six patients were treated with TMP-SMX and 33 with pentamidine.

†Adverse effects occurring during treatment (e.g., fever = increase in temperature >37.7°C after patient had been afebrile more than 24 hours).

‡Azotemia = increase in serum creatinine greater than 0.5 mg/dl if less than 2.0 at baseline or increase by greater than 1.5 if baseline value was greater than 2.0 mg/dl.

does not usually occur until the second week of therapy and may occasionally progress to renal failure, generally resolves after therapy is discontinued. Hypotension usually occurs in association with intravenous infusions and lasts up to several hours, although modestly low blood pressures may persist for several months after the last dose. The acute drop in blood pressure is corrected by placing the patient in the supine position and providing hydration therapy.

Hypoglycemia, which occurs in 10 to 30 per cent of AIDS patients treated with pentamidine, is a consequence of sudden increases in serum insulin concentrations due to lysis of pancreatic β cells. This is potentially the most serious complication of therapy for *P. carinii* pneumonia. The risk of hypoglycemia is directly related to the cumulative dose of drug administered, since the drug is bound avidly to tissues and is released intact slowly over weeks to months. Therefore, the risk increases with the duration of therapy and the number of courses of treatment. Symptoms are frequently absent until serum glucose concentrations decline to less than 20 mg per deciliter. Moreover, this toxic effect may occur precipitously up to 2 weeks after the last dose has been administered. When any degree of hypoglycemia is detected in patients receiving pentamidine, treatment with the drug should be discontinued and the patient should be monitored closely for several weeks with capillary glucose measurements taken several times daily. These patients must also be instructed to ingest extra glucose whenever symptoms of hypoglycemia occur or glucose measurements are low. Occasionally, patients must remain in the hospital to receive concentrated infusions of glucose for up to several weeks to keep their serum glucose concentrations above 40 mg per deciliter. Depletion of pancreatic insulin may also result in the ultimate need for treatment with oral hypoglycemic agents. Ketoacidosis and hyperosmolar coma have also occurred in some patients after treatment with pentamidine.

When the drug is administered intramuscularly, painful sterile abscesses occur frequently and often limit the usefulness of this mode of therapy for outpatient treatment. Other toxic effects occur less frequently and have included myositis and myoglobinuria, gross hematuria, fatal pancreatitis, ventricular tachycardia, and torsades de pointes.

EXPERIMENTAL THERAPIES. Severe Episodes.
For severe episodes of PCP (defined as $[A-a]DO_2$ greater than 30 torr) which are associated with high case fatality rates, more potent therapies are needed. Trimetrexate, eflornithine, and adjunctive therapy with corticosteroids are undergoing evaluation for such episodes. Trimetrexate (an antifolate, anticancer drug similar to methotrexate) binds the dihydrofolate reductase of *P. carinii* approximately 1500 times more avidly than TMP and because of its high lipid solubility is concentrated in protozoan cells. In an open study, 69 per cent of patients treated initially with 30 mg per square meter of intravenous trimetrexate once daily and 80 mg per square meter per day of leucovorin had a favorable response. In a dosage range investigation, 45 mg per square meter per day of trimetrexate and 80 mg per square meter per day of leucovorin proved to be the best regimen for initial therapy, resulting in a 92 per cent survival rate for episodes of various severity. In addition, all patients were able to receive a full 21-dose course of treatment; hypersensitivity reactions and hematologic toxicity were tolerable. Multicenter studies are underway to prospectively compare trimetrexate with TMP-SMX.

Eflornithine (also known as DFMO) is an irreversible decarboxylase inhibitor with efficacy against murine PCP. When this drug was administered to 345 patients who had failed or were intolerant to standard therapies, 66 per cent of nonventilated patients survived. However, only 10 per cent of respirator-dependent patients survived. The most serious toxicities have been thrombocytopenia, which may occur in up to 50 per cent of recipients, and a clinically relevant hearing loss in approximately 10 per cent. Eflornithine has not been adequately tested as initial therapy for PCP and should not be used for that purpose.

Use of corticosteroids as adjunctive therapy appears to benefit patients when instituted early in the course of therapy. In one unblinded study involving 326 patients who were treated with standard therapies, subjects were randomized within 36 hours of beginning therapy for PCP to receive 40 mg of prednisone twice daily for 5 days with tapering doses over the next 2 to 3 weeks or no treatment with corticosteroids. Patients treated with prednisone were significantly less likely to develop oxygenation failure or require intubation, and their chance for survival was increased from 80 per cent to 90 per cent after 31 days and 12 weeks. In a smaller study of similar design that was conducted in Canada, acute clinical respiratory failure defined by a decrease in oxygen saturation of more than 10 per cent occurred significantly less often in patients who received 60 mg of prednisone each day for 7 days followed by tapering doses over the next 14 days than in individuals who did not receive steroid therapy. In both studies there was no difference in the rate of secondary opportunistic complications, nosocomial infections, or adverse drug effects in the treatment groups.

By contrast, there is currently no evidence that corticosteroids are beneficial for "salvage" therapy. A double-blind comparison of adjunctive therapy with 60 mg of intravenous methylprednisolone every 6 hours versus placebo initiated anytime in the course of therapy (generally more than 3 days after beginning specific anti-*Pneumocystis* treatment) when the PaO_2 declined to less than 50 torr resulted in a different outcome. The trial was discontinued after 41 patients had been enrolled. There was no difference in survival between the two groups, but more secondary opportunistic infections occurred in patients receiving methylprednisolone. However, the power to determine clinically relevant differences in survival was severely limited by the small sample size.

Mild Episodes.
For mild episodes (defined by an $[A-a]DO_2$ less than 30 torr), new treatments should be relatively nontoxic and suited for home therapy, since these patients have at least a 90 per cent response rate to standard therapy with TMP-SMX or pentamidine. Aerosolized pentamidine is one such therapy. Drug is delivered directly to the alveolar airspaces, which are the primary sites of infection, and very little drug is absorbed systemically. Thus, systemic toxicities occur infrequently. In a multicenter investigation, 364 patients were randomized to receive either 600 mg of aerosolized pentamidine once daily via the Respirgard II jet nebulizer or TMP-SMX at 15 mg per kilogram per day (TMP). There was no difference in survival between the two groups after 21 days of treatment, but there were more deaths in the group receiving TMP-SMX by day 35. In addition, drug-related toxicities occurred significantly more often in patients treated with TMP-SMX. By contrast, PaO_2 improved significantly faster in patients treated with TMP-SMX. Aerosolized pentamidine alone is not well suited for patients who develop appreciable tachypnea, since alveolar deposition is related to minute ventilation and decreases significantly in individuals with rapid shallow breathing. Moreover, deposition is likely to be impaired in areas of densely consolidated lung. In fact, in two smaller studies, parenteral pentamidine was more effective than aerosol therapy in more severe episodes. In light of these data, aerosolized pentamidine should be prescribed as primary therapy only for patients who are not severely tachypneic and have mild PCP.

Dapsone (a sulfone drug used to treat leprosy and dermatitis herpetiformis) has potent activity against murine PCP. In uncontrolled studies, dapsone alone at 100 mg per day was not as effective as historical use of TMP-SMX, and 200 mg per day has been associated with a high rate of severe methemoglobinemia and respiratory distress. Thus, dapsone should not be used alone to treat PCP. However, at a dosage of 100 mg per day dapsone has been highly effective and well tolerated when combined with 20 mg per kilogram per day of TMP. In one comparative trial, this combination was as effective as TMP-SMX, which caused severe neutropenia and liver test abnormalities significantly more often. In addition, concentrations of dapsone were 40 per cent higher and TMP levels were 48 per cent higher when the drugs were used in combination than when patients were treated with either agent alone. This suggests that there is a bidirectional interference with clearance of both agents and that lower dosages may be effective and may reduce the risk for toxic reactions with the combination. Studies are under way to determine whether this combination is as effective as TMP-SMX and associated with less toxicity.

Clindamycin plus the antimalarial compound primaquine is another promising combination. In tissue cultures and the rat model of PCP, neither agent is effective alone but the combination has excellent activity. In the first clinical investigation of this combination, 23 of 25 patients treated with 600 mg of clindamycin intravenously every 6 hours and 15 mg of primaquine once daily were cured. However, 17 of the subjects had been treated with conventional therapies and the contribution of these other therapies to the ultimate outcome could not be ascertained. In a study of 22 patients with $(A-a)DO_2$ less than 30 torr, 900 mg of clindamycin intravenously every 8 hours and 30 mg of primaquine base orally once daily improved 20 patients by day 7 of treatment. These patients received no other anti-*Pneumocystis* therapies. Generalized rash was the most common toxicity and occurred in 15 cases but required cessation of therapy in only 3 patients. Whether this toxicity will limit the usefulness of this promising treatment is unknown.

OUTCOME AND PROGNOSIS. Several clinical parameters have been associated with an increased risk for a fatal outcome. These include at presentation an elevated serum LDH generally in excess of 500 IU per deciliter, a baseline $(A-a)DO_2$ greater than 35 torr on room air, and BAL neutrophils in excess of 10 per cent at presentation. Lack of clinical improvement and progressive increase in serum LDH during therapy have also been associated with ultimate fatality. During therapy it is often difficult to know when a given patient is failing a specific treatment and is destined for a fatal outcome. Persistence of fever is a poor indicator of treatment failure, since fever may be due to other opportunistic infections, nosocomial bacterial complications, HIV infection per se, drug allergy even in the absence of rash or eosinophilia, and catheter-associated phlebitis as well as PCP. Lack of improvement on chest radiographs is common, and persistence or progression of infiltrates frequently occurs even in patients who ultimately are cured. Repeat bronchoscopy in a patient failing to improve often is not helpful unless a second infection is detected, since *P. carinii* organisms may be present for weeks to months even after successful therapy. Patients are often switched from their initial therapy on a purely empiric basis. It may be that alveolar damage, as with the adult respiratory distress syndrome, which has a similar histologic pattern, is the most important determinant of outcome, and failure to improve promptly is not the result of antibiotic failure per se. Indeed, patients with more severe episodes often continue to deteriorate for 7 to 10 days before they stabilize and begin to show improvement, whether the initial therapy is continued or changed. The fact that nearly 90 per cent survived in one study of moderate to severe episodes despite continuation of TMP-SMX in the face of apparent early failure in many patients supports this contention. Switching therapy may serve only to expose patients to additional drug toxicities. Admittedly, except for patients who rapidly develop respiratory failure, it is often difficult to know when to change therapy.

For patients who survive their episodes, approximately 5 per cent per month, or 60 per cent after 1 year, have a recurrent bout of PCP despite therapy with zidovudine. Thus, effective prophylaxis is needed for such patients.

PROPHYLAXIS. The most desirable approach to therapy is to prevent PCP. Two controlled studies have suggested that the attack rate can be reduced by 5- to 10-fold in HIV-infected patients who are at highest risk, namely those individuals with less than 200 CD4 lymphocytes and those who have already experienced an episode of PCP.

The most compelling study involved 408 high-risk subjects at 14 community treatment centers in San Francisco who were randomly assigned to one of three dosage regimens of aerosolized pentamidine given by the Respirgard II jet nebulizer. A subset of these subjects had already experienced an episode of PCP. Three hundred milligrams once monthly was significantly more protective than the other two dosages in patients with prior episodes. Of equal import, toxicity was limited to transient dysgeusia and cough which generally lasted no more than 1 to 2 hours after treatment. More prolonged coughing and even bronchospasm may occur occasionally, but these toxicities are generally limited to smokers and patients with asthma and are usually prevented by pretreatment with an aerosol bronchodilator. Although very little pentamidine is absorbed into the systemic circulation during aerosol therapy, pancreatitis and hypoglycemia have occurred. Contact dermatitis on the face, conjunctiva, and upper torso may also occur. However, these other toxicities are exceedingly uncommon with aerosol pentamidine. The disadvan-

tages of aerosolized pentamidine include the cost of the drug, need for supervised therapy and a compressed air source for the jet nebulizers, lack of systemic prophylaxis against extrapulmonary *P. carinii* infection, and incomplete protection provided for patients who have already experienced PCP (20 per cent of patients treated with 300 mg once monthly in the San Francisco study relapsed within 12 months).

The need for supervised therapy and compressed air is obviated with the use of portable ultrasonic nebulizers. In a double-blind, placebo-controlled study conducted in Canada using the Fisons ultrasonic nebulizer, a dosage of 60 mg twice monthly was superior to placebo. Whether use of different, more efficient nebulizers or different dosage regimens will improve the efficacy of aerosolized pentamidine for secondary prophylaxis remains to be determined.

By contrast, TMP-SMX is inexpensive, is well suited for self-administration at home, and has been established to provide complete protection against PCP in pediatric cancer patients. The combination has been studied less well for prophylaxis in AIDS. In one study involving patients with Kaposi's sarcoma who were receiving chemotherapy, there were no episodes of PCP in subjects receiving one double-strength tablet twice daily, compared with 16 episodes in 30 subjects who received no prophylaxis. Of concern, gastric intolerance or rash occurred in 50 per cent of subjects treated with TMP-SMX, but these "toxicities" also occurred to a lesser extent in patients who were not given preventive therapy. Unfortunately, the protective efficacy and tolerability of TMP-SMX, especially in combination with zidovudine, which like the antifolate drugs is also myelosuppressive, is currently under examination in controlled studies of other HIV-infected populations. Whether treatment with 5 or 10 mg of oral folinic acid each day can prevent the neutropenia commonly associated with TMP-SMX is unknown.

Other antifolate drugs, dapsone and pyrimethamine-sulfadoxine (Fansidar, used for malaria prophylaxis), have also appeared highly protective in uncontrolled studies involving patients at high risk for PCP. The most serious potential toxicities associated with dapsone are hemolytic anemia and methemoglobinemia, although the exact frequency of these adverse effects in patients infected with HIV is unknown. In contrast to dapsone and TMP-SMX, hematologic toxicities have been relatively infrequent with pyrimethamine-sulfadoxine. However, fatalities have resulted from Stevens-Johnson syndrome during prophylaxis for malaria (although this has occurred in only one patient infected with HIV), which has dampened enthusiasm for prophylaxis with this combination.

The relative efficacy of aerosolized pentamidine and the antifolate drugs for prophylaxis of PCP will be determined in two large multicenter studies sponsored by the National Institutes of Health. The results of these trials should be available in 1991 or 1992. Until then physicians should follow guidelines outlined by the U.S. Public Health Service which currently endorse either aerosolized pentamidine or oral TMP-SMX for patients at high risk for PCP. The selection of either therapy depends in part on the patient's tolerance of these agents, health insurance and patient resources, and individual preferences of physicians and patients.

For patients with 200 to 500 CD4 lymphocytes per cubic millimeter, specific prophylaxis for PCP does not appear necessary if patients are taking 500 to 600 mg of zidovudine daily. Two large placebo-controlled trials established that zidovudine significantly reduced the risk for asymptomatic patients or those with early ARC who had 200 to 500 CD4 cells per cubic millimeter from progressing to advanced ARC or AIDS. Protection against PCP was excellent, thereby obviating the need for specific prophylaxis until CD4 counts decline to less than 200 per cubic millimeter or the percentage of CD4 cells decreases to less than 20 per cent.

KAPOSI'S SARCOMA

Kaposi's sarcoma (see Ch. 163) is the second most common opportunistic complication resulting in a case definition of AIDS in persons infected with HIV and occurs in 20 to 25 per cent of patients with AIDS. The lung is clinically involved in approximately 20 per cent of these patients, commonly when there are extensive cutaneous lesions, although pulmonary involvement has been documented in up to 50 per cent of cases at autopsy. Pulmonary Kaposi's sarcoma occasionally occurs when there is no mucocutaneous involvement.

CLINICAL SYNDROME. The majority of patients with pulmonary Kaposi's sarcoma have nonproductive cough, dyspnea, and fever, although any of these findings have been absent in up to 40 per cent of cases. Large endobronchial lesions may cause localized wheezing, and laryngeal involvement may result in stridor. Owing to the propensity of these lesions to bleed, some patients may present with hemoptysis. Moderate to severe hypoxemia, widened $(A-a)DO_2$, and impaired DL_{CO} (less than 80 per cent of normal) are associated with Kaposi's sarcoma in most patients, although lung volumes are usually normal.

RADIOGRAPHIC ABNORMALITIES. Interstitial infiltrates are the most common abnormalities detectable on chest radiographs and are present in approximately 80 per cent of patients with Kaposi's sarcoma. Pulmonary nodules with or without interstitial infiltrates are present in 20 to 60 per cent, pleural effusions in 20 to 90 per cent, and hilar or paratracheal adenopathy in 50 to 90 per cent of cases. Gallium imaging of the lung has little utility. However, nodules, effusions, and adenopathy not present on plain radiographs may be demonstrable by computed tomography.

DIAGNOSIS. In patients with pleural effusions due to Kaposi's sarcoma, thoracentesis usually produces an exudative fluid but rarely yields a diagnosis, since there is not a particular cell type associated with the tumor. Diagnosis requires the presence of a characteristic histologic architecture. However, pleural biopsies are rarely positive, perhaps owing to the patchy involvement of the pleural surfaces as detected at autopsy.

Bronchoscopy is the single most useful test in confirming the suspicion of pulmonary Kaposi's sarcoma. In most cases one or more typical violaceous or cherry red, plaquelike lesions are distributed throughout the tracheobronchial tree. Despite their raised appearance these lesions are generally submucosal, and, thus, superficial bronchial biopsies frequently are not diagnostic. Transbronchial biopsy of parenchymal disease is also unfruitful, with yields as low as 10 per cent, probably owing to the fact that lung infiltration is patchy with lesions generally less than 1 cm in diameter. In addition, endobronchial lesions may bleed profusely if biopsied. Thus, if typical endobronchial lesions are seen during bronchoscopy and there is histologic confirmation of Kaposi's sarcoma elsewhere, this is sufficient evidence of pulmonary involvement and biopsy is not indicated. In cases in which there are no endobronchial lesions, open lung biopsy may be necessary to establish the diagnosis.

TREATMENT. Most patients with pulmonary Kaposi's sarcoma survive only several months after the diagnosis is established, whereas patients who present with limited cutaneous disease generally have higher CD4 counts and often survive for several years until serious complications of AIDS occur. In one investigation, chemotherapy with bleomycin and vincristine with or without doxorubicin increased survival from 6 to 10 months in responders versus nonresponders. Survival was shortened in patients with pleural effusions and CD4 counts less than 100 per cubic millimeter. Total lung irradiation improved symptoms and pulmonary function tests in one series. Thus, palliative therapy is available for some patients with pulmonary Kaposi's sarcoma and supports a reasonably aggressive approach to establish the diagnosis.

MYCOBACTERIUM AVIUM COMPLEX

EPIDEMIOLOGY. *Mycobacterium avium* complex (*M. avium–M. intracellulare*) (see Ch. 333) appears to be the most frequent cause of systemic bacterial infection in patients with AIDS. This organism is ubiquitous in soil and water. The portal of entry probably involves either the gastrointestinal tract (macrophages laden with acid-fast bacilli are frequently identified in the lamina propria of the small bowel) or the respiratory tract (since the organism was isolated from respiratory secretions in 17 of 23 patients in one study).

Infection is generally widespread at the time of clinical diag-

nosis. Although disseminated disease is AIDS defining or results in the initial case definition of AIDS in only 4 per cent of patients with AIDS, this infection is ultimately documented ante mortem in 18 to 29 per cent and is detected in 53 to 79 per cent of AIDS patients at autopsy. Moreover, the organism was recovered from the lung in 11 (34 per cent) of 32 patients with systemic infection documented at autopsy.

CLINICAL SYNDROME. *M. avium* complex generally causes disease late in the course of AIDS when patients are severely immunocompromised. Thus, patients are often coinfected with other opportunistic pathogens, making it difficult to ascertain whether various symptoms, clinical signs, or radiographic abnormalities are specifically related to *M. avium* complex. However, a systemic illness with fever, sweats, and weight loss and a gastrointestinal disorder with diarrhea and abdominal pain appear to be the most commonly associated clinical syndromes. However, cough was reported to have been present in 36 (70 per cent) of 51 patients and dyspnea in 27 (57 per cent) of 47 patients in one retrospective study.

RADIOGRAPHIC ABNORMALITIES. Chest radiographs may show interstitial, alveolar, or nodular infiltrates. Hilar or mediastinal adenopathy may occur together with or isolated from parenchymal abnormalities. Cavitation and pleural effusions are rare. It is difficult to know precisely how frequently these abnormalities are due specifically to *M. avium* complex because of other concurrent opportunistic complications.

DIAGNOSIS. Recovery of *M. avium* complex from standard automated blood cultures is the sine qua non of disseminated infection, with isolation rates of 90 to 100 per cent. Similarly, the organism is readily recovered from sputum. In one study 23 (92 per cent) of 25 patients with evidence of pulmonary disease had positive sputum cultures, although smears for acid-fast bacilli were positive in only 4 (16 per cent) of the patients. It is possible that some patients with negative blood but positive sputum cultures have infection limited to the lung. However, a positive culture from respiratory secretions may only indicate colonization if there is no clinical or radiographic evidence of disease. It is unknown whether such patients are more likely to develop a pneumonic illness or disseminated disease than those not colonized.

TREATMENT. Treatment of patients with positive blood cultures has provided conflicting results. Initial studies showed that treatment had minimal effect on the clinical illness or numbers of organisms in the blood of these patients. More recently, uncontrolled studies of four- and five-drug regimens indicate that treatment may be beneficial in terminating fever and sweats and decreasing the number of organisms in blood by several logarithms. Whether such therapies will increase survival in AIDS patients infected with *M. avium* complex must be determined in controlled studies.

For patients with pulmonary infiltrates and *M. avium* complex identified in respiratory secretions or specimens of lung in the absence of other identifiable opportunistic pathogens, consideration may be given for treatment. In vitro and in the immunodeficient beige mouse, ethambutol, ansamycin, clofazamine, quinolones (ciprofloxacin and sparfloxacin), macrolides (clarithromycin and azithromycin), and amikacin have activity against the majority of isolates at concentrations achievable in humans. Isoniazid and pyrazinamide have little to no activity as single agents or in combination, although rifampin (structurally similar to ansamycin) does improve the inhibitory effect of other drugs. Based on such laboratory data and several pilot studies showing efficacy, two regimens that are being tested clinically include ethambutol (15 mg per kilogram per day), rifampin (600 mg per day), clofazimine (100 or 200 mg per day), and ciprofloxacin (500 mg twice daily) with or without amikacin (10 mg per kilogram per day 5 days per week for 20 doses). Before the physician prescribes one of these or a similar regimen, patients should be advised that such therapy is unproven, may increase their risk for drug toxicity, but could improve their quality of life.

OTHER ATYPICAL MYCOBACTERIA

M. kansasii, M. haemophilum, M. scrofulaceum, M. fortuitum, M. flavescens, M. xenopi, and *M. gordonae* have caused disseminated disease in AIDS patients. Clinical manifestations are similar to those associated with *M. avium* complex, with involvement of the lung, liver, and bone marrow being especially common. Effective treatment regimens have not been established for these infections. However, the Centers for Disease Control and American Thoracic Society have recommended that disease caused by *M. kansasii* should be treated with isoniazid, rifampin, and ethambutol for a minimum of 18 months, or 15 months after culture conversion.

MYCOBACTERIUM TUBERCULOSIS (see Ch. 332)

EPIDEMIOLOGY. During the latter half of the 1980's, the annual incidence of tuberculosis increased compared to declining rates in the first half of the decade. The excess cases were focused largely in geographic areas where AIDS is highly endemic. Overall, nearly 4 per cent of AIDS patients have had tuberculosis, which represents an attack rate that is several hundred–fold greater than the average annual incidence in HIV-negative persons during the same period. The risk of tuberculosis has been greatest in AIDS patients who are black, Hispanic, Haitian, or intravenous drug users. The proportion of AIDS patients with tuberculosis composed of racial or ethnic minorities has ranged from 35 to 100 per cent in various areas of the United States; 7 to 69 per cent have been intravenous drug users.

PATHOGENESIS. Since latent tuberculous infection is contained by an intact cell-mediated immune system, it is not surprising that tuberculosis is common in AIDS patients. The fact that 14 per cent of HIV-positive intravenous drug users who were PPD positive developed tuberculosis over 2 years compared to no cases in HIV-positive persons with negative skin tests suggests that this opportunistic complication most often occurs as a reactivation process, although person-to-person spread also occurs.

Unlike *M. avium* complex, *M. tuberculosis* generally causes disease when cell-mediated immunity is normal or only modestly depressed. The median CD4 lymphocyte count was 354 cells per cubic millimeter in one study and the mean count in another investigation was 170 cells per cubic millimeter. In fact, tuberculosis occurred before the first nonmycobacterial AIDS-defining event in 48 (87 per cent) of 55 patients with AIDS and concurrently with an AIDS-defining event in the other 7 (13 per cent) patients in one study. This implies that *M. tuberculosis* is more virulent than *P. carinii* or *M. avium* complex, which generally do not cause disease in HIV-positive patients until CD4 counts are severely depressed.

CLINICAL SYNDROME. Pulmonary tuberculosis is the most common manifestation of tuberculous disease in HIV-positive patients. When tuberculosis precedes the diagnosis of AIDS, disease is usually confined to the lung, whereas, when tuberculosis is diagnosed after the onset of AIDS, the majority of patients also have extrapulmonary tuberculosis, most commonly involving the bone marrow or lymph nodes, or have disease confined to sites outside the lung. Fever, night sweats, wasting, cough, and dyspnea occur in the majority of patients but may be due to infection with HIV per se or other opportunistic infections. Lymphadenopathy, especially in patients with severe immune deficiency (namely, CD4 lymphocyte counts less than 200 per cubic millimeter), is likely to be due to tuberculosis or another opportunistic complication, since lymph nodes are generally hypoplastic at this stage of HIV infection. Other physical findings are rarely helpful.

RADIOGRAPHIC ABNORMALITIES. Although pulmonary tuberculosis in HIV-positive persons is usually a reactivation process, the radiographic abnormalities are more characteristic of primary infection and include hilar or mediastinal adenopathy with or without focal consolidation, which is frequently in the mid to lower lung fields. Upper lobe infiltrates, cavitation, and pleural effusions, which are typical of reactivation disease in HIV-negative persons, generally occur in less than 10 to 15 per cent of cases. In patients with more advanced immune deficiency, when extrapulmonary and disseminated infection are common, the chest radiograph may show a miliary pattern or diffuse interstitial infiltrates indistinguishable from PCP.

DIAGNOSIS. Although most patients with AIDS are anergic, 40 to 80 per cent of HIV-positive patients with tuberculosis have greater than 5 mm cutaneous induration in response to 5 tuberculin units. The "relatively" high rate of cutaneous reactivity likely reflects the fact that HIV-positive patients with tuberculosis

are often only modestly immunocompromised. Examination of respiratory secretions shows acid-fast bacilli in 50 to 80 per cent of patients with pulmonary tuberculosis. With disseminated disease, aspirates from 90 per cent of lymph nodes have shown acid-fast bacilli, and cultures of blood and diarrheal stools have each grown *M. tuberculosis* in approximately 40 per cent of patients.

TREATMENT. The U.S. Public Health Service and the American Thoracic Society recommend that HIV-positive patients with tuberculosis be treated with 10 to 15 mg per kilogram per day of isoniazid, 10 to 15 mg per kilogram per day of rifampin, and for the first 2 months of therapy, pyrazinamide (25 mg per kilogram per day) and/or ethambutal (25 mg per kilogram per day). Therapy with isoniazid should be continued for at least 9 months and at least 6 months after the last positive culture. Patients with extrapulmonary disease should be treated for at least 12 to 18 months.

Since *M. tuberculosis* and *M. avium* complex are indistinguishable morphologically, patients with body fluids containing acid-fast bacilli should be treated presumptively for tuberculosis. Some experts prescribe a regimen of isoniazid and rifampin along with several agents known to be active against *M. avium* complex and then modify the regimen when identification of the mycobacteria and drug susceptibilities have been established.

PREVENTION. In HIV-negative persons with latent infection due to *M. tuberculosis*, the risk of developing tuberculosis is approximately 10 per cent over the remainder of their lifetime and greatest in the first year after infection. The risk is likely to be greater in HIV-positive persons. Thus, the Centers for Disease Control and the American Thoracic Society have recommended that all HIV-positive patients be screened with the Mantoux skin test. Persons who have not been serotested for HIV but who are in risk groups for AIDS, especially intravenous drug users, should also be tested for tuberculous infection. Those with greater than 5 mm of cutaneous induration should have a chest radiograph and sputum induction for acid-fast bacilli and mycobacterial cultures. If there is no evidence of active disease, patients with positive skin tests should receive preventive therapy with 300 mg of isoniazid daily for 6 to 12 months.

PERSON-TO-PERSON TRANSMISSION. The potential for person-to-person transmission is great among AIDS patients. Since individuals receiving inhaled pentamidine frequently cough vigorously during and after treatment, patients with unsuspected tuberculosis are at risk of spreading this infection to other patients and medical personnel, especially in poorly ventilated areas. Thus, patients should be screened by skin testing (if not done previously) and chest radiographs prior to receiving aerosolized pentamidine.

FUNGAL INFECTIONS (see Ch. 398)

Generally fungi cause primary infection in the lung relatively infrequently in AIDS patients, unlike *P. carinii* or *M. tuberculosis*. However, they do cause pulmonary disease as part of disseminated fungal infection in these patients.

Histoplasma capsulatum

EPIDEMIOLOGY AND PATHOGENESIS. Progressive disseminated histoplasmosis occurs as a complication of impaired cell-mediated immunity in HIV-positive persons. As with tuberculosis, this infection occurs early in the course of HIV disease. In fact, disseminated histoplasmosis was the first manifestation of AIDS in 50 to 61 per cent of two groups totalling 125 patients. This suggests that *H. capsulatum*, like *M. tuberculosis*, is more virulent than other opportunistic pathogens, which generally cause infection only when CD4 immunity is more compromised.

Most cases are believed to result from reactivation of prior infection. Many cases have occurred outside the major endemic areas of the Mississippi and Ohio River valleys. However, these patients frequently have a history of travel or residence in other endemic areas such as Puerto Rico, the Dominican Republic, or South America. By contrast, histoplasmosis occurred with high frequency in AIDS patients during an outbreak in the midwestern United States, indicating that disseminated disease may also occur as a consequence of primary infection.

CLINICAL SYNDROME. Patients with disseminated histoplasmosis have usually been ill for 4 to 8 weeks with fever and weight loss. In one series involving 125 patients, respiratory symptoms were limited to cough in 28 per cent and dyspnea in 16 per cent, although both occurred in 60 per cent of the 72 patients with abnormal chest radiographs. Other patients present acutely with septic shock and disseminated intravascular coagulopathy. Important physical findings have included splenomegaly in 32 per cent, hepatomegaly in 26 per cent, and skin lesions in 7 per cent. Anemia, leukopenia, or thrombocytopenia has occurred in 30 per cent. The average PaO$_2$ is in the range of 84 torr, despite extensive involvement of the lung.

RADIOGRAPHIC ABNORMALITIES. Of the 72 patients described with reports of chest radiographs, 56 per cent have had either diffuse interstitial or diffuse small nodular infiltrates. Of note, 23 (31 per cent) of patients with these radiographic abnormalities had no respiratory symptoms. In addition, unlike disseminated histoplasmosis in HIV-negative persons, there are rarely pulmonary or splenic calcifications.

DIAGNOSIS. *H. capsulatum* has been recovered from the bone marrow in 54 to 70 per cent, blood in 37 to 55 per cent, lung or pulmonary secretions in 36 to 69 per cent, and other organs or body fluids less often. Isolation from blood is increased when lysis centrifugation is used to release *H. capsulatum* from circulating mononuclear cells. It is noteworthy that the organism is infrequently detected microscopically in smears of bronchoalveolar lavage fluid. Since *H. capsulatum* often takes 2 to 3 weeks to be identified in culture, transbronchial biopsy is also advocated by some investigators when histoplasmosis is suspected, since the yeast can be identified in up to 69 per cent of lung tissue sections. The polysaccharide antigen of *H. capsulatum* was detected in the urine of 98 per cent and serum of 75 per cent of 40 patients with histoplasmosis in one study. If the test becomes commercially available, it should facilitate diagnosis.

TREATMENT. Amphotericin B is the treatment of choice for disseminated histoplasmosis. Treatment with a cumulative dose of 2 grams or more results in a significantly greater survival than lower doses. Although ketoconazole alone has been ineffective, another oral triazole, itraconazole, has shown promise in a small number of patients. Studies are needed to determine if the new, inherently less toxic oral azoles are as effective as amphotericin B.

Relapse is common after completion of treatment with amphotericin B, suggesting that chronic suppressive therapy may be necessary. Weekly infusions of 50 to 100 mg of amphotericin B prevented relapse in 13 of 14 patients treated in this manner for a median of 9.5 months in one study. The role of newer oral agents for suppressive therapy is currently under study.

Cryptococcus neoformans

Cryptococcosis occurs in approximately 10 per cent of AIDS patients. Lung involvement has been documented in 4 to 39 per cent of these patients. More than 90 per cent of patients with pulmonary cryptococcosis also have meningitis or disseminated infection. Less than 10 per cent have primary lung infection. The most common symptoms are fever, headache, weight loss, cough, and dyspnea occurring in 42 to 66 per cent. These symptoms may have been present for a few days to a few months. Lymphadenopathy, which is unusual in AIDS patients, was present in 7 of 12 patients in one series and 3 also had splenomegaly without other cause. Patients are usually not severely tachypneic, as their average PaO$_2$ on room air is in the 70 torr range. Their chest radiographs show either diffuse or focal interstitial infiltrates in more than 90 per cent, with or without hilar or mediastinal adenopathy. Focal areas of consolidation, lung abscess, pleural effusion, and isolated adenopathy may also be detected on radiographs.

Diagnosis is usually not difficult. Cryptococcal antigen has been detected in serum, often in high titers, in virtually all patients with pulmonary cryptococcosis, and BAL specimens have been positive in each case. Moreover, the organism can be recovered from blood cultures in more than 90 per cent of cases. As with histoplasmosis, amphotericin B is the treatment of choice; 5-fluorocytosine may be added for patients who also have meningeal involvement. In a large multicenter comparison of ampho-

tericin B versus fluconazole, an oral triazole, for treatment of cryptococcal meningitis in AIDS patients, fluconazole resulted in a high failure rate during the first 2 weeks, although late failure rates were similar in the two groups. However, in a different study fluconazole prevented relapse in 14 of 15 patients following therapy with amphotericin B, which is comparable to weekly infusions of amphotericin B for suppressive therapy.

Coccidioides immitis

Coccidioidomycosis does not appear to occur as commonly as histoplasmosis or cryptococcosis in patients with AIDS, but it may involve the lung as part of disseminated infection in these patients. The clinical syndrome is, therefore, similar to that associated with histoplasmosis or cryptococcosis. However, cough and dyspnea have been reported in the majority of patients. Radiographs usually reveal diffuse nodular or interstitial infiltrates. Occasionally, isolated nodular lesions, cavities, or pulmonary adenopathy may be the only radiographic abnormalities detected. Complement or tube precipitin antibodies are detectable in most cases, and the fungus can usually be recovered from bronchoscopy specimens.

Other Fungi

Aspergillus, Candida, and other fungi are relatively infrequent causes of pulmonary complications in AIDS patients. Care must be taken not to ascribe pulmonary disease to *Aspergillus* or *Candida* when these fungi are cultured from bronchoscopy specimens, since *Aspergillus* is an ubiquitous environmental saprophyte and specimens may be contaminated with *Candida* from the oropharynx. A diagnosis of invasive fungal infection should not be made unless these fungi are demonstrated histologically within pulmonary tissues.

PYOGENIC BACTERIA

PATHOGENESIS AND EPIDEMIOLOGY. Pyogenic bacteria are responsible for 2 to 10 per cent of pulmonary complications in AIDS patients. HIV-associated defects in T cell–mediated immunity result in impaired activation and chemotaxis of macrophages and neutrophils. In addition, B cell–mediated antibody production necessary for opsonization and killing of certain bacteria is impaired in patients with AIDS. It is not surprising, therefore, that patients with AIDS have an increased incidence of pneumonias caused by encapsulated bacteria, in particular *Streptococcus pneumoniae* and *Haemophilus influenzae*. In fact, the attack rate of pneumococcal pneumonia is approximately sixfold greater and the incidence of pneumococcal bacteremia is increased nearly 100-fold in HIV-positive persons. The risk may be even greater in intravenous drug users, as 10 per cent of 144 HIV-seropositive patients had bacterial pneumonias, compared to only 2 per cent of 289 seronegative patients who also used intravenous drugs. Hospital-acquired pneumonias due to staphylococci and gram-negative bacilli are common in patients infected with HIV, but it is uncertain whether these nosocomial infections are more frequent than in HIV-negative patients.

CLINICAL SYNDROME. Fever and cough are nearly universal symptoms in HIV-positive patients with pyogenic pneumonia. Purulent sputum occurs in the majority and distinguishes these patients from those with other causes of pneumonia, albeit opportunistic complications such as PCP can occur together with pyogenic infection of the upper or lower respiratory tract. Unlike other pulmonary infections in AIDS patients, more than half of patients with bacterial pneumonia have lung signs of consolidation.

Most patients have white blood cell (WBC) counts of 6,000 to 12,000 per cubic millimeter with predominantly band forms. By contrast, in most other pulmonary complications of AIDS (other than tuberculosis) the WBC count is usually less than 5000 without a left shift. The serum LDH is minimally elevated in up to one third of patients, and oxygenation is modestly impaired, with room air PaO$_2$ averaging 60 to 80 torr.

RADIOGRAPHIC ABNORMALITIES. Focal infiltrates with lobar or segmental consolidation occur in 60 to 80 per cent. Infiltrates may be bilateral and there may be pleural effusions, but the frequency of these latter complications has not been established in HIV-positive patients. By contrast, diffuse infiltrates typical of other opportunistic processes are relatively common if the pneumonia is caused by *H. influenzae.*

DIAGNOSIS. The presence of polymorphonuclear neutrophils in sputum is useful in distinguishing bacterial pneumonia from other pulmonary complications. A predominance of either gram-positive or gram-negative bacteria in the presence of PMN's is helpful in selecting initial therapy. The yield of sputum cultures for bacterial pathogens has not been established in AIDS and ARC patients, but 50 to 80 per cent of patients reported to have pneumococcal pneumonia and 5 to 25 per cent with *H. influenzae* pneumonia have had positive blood cultures.

Other bacteria frequently isolated from sputum and occasionally blood of HIV patients with community-acquired infections include *S. pyogenes,* other streptococcal species, *Moraxella catarrhalis,* nonencapsulated *Haemophilus* species, and in intravenous drug users, *Staphylococcus aureus* (see Ch. 302). In hospitalized patients infected with HIV, the most common organisms associated with nosocomial pneumonias have been staphylococci and gram-negative bacteria, as with other patient populations.

TREATMENT. Initial treatment should be directed by the Gram's stain and whether the pneumonia was acquired in the community or the hospital. Ambulatory patients who are stable may be treated with oral antibiotics, since mortality with the most potentially lethal community-acquired bacterial pneumonia, bacteremic pneumococcal pneumonia, has been less than 10 per cent. With appropriate therapy most patients become afebrile with improvement in respiratory symptoms within 5 to 7 days. Patients with severe tachypnea and hypoxemia or evidence of sepsis should be hospitalized for intravenous therapy.

PREVENTION. Bacterial pneumonia may recur in HIV-infected patients, as with other populations who have defective humoral immunity. Thus, the Advisory Committee on Immunization Practices has recommended that all HIV-positive patients receive pneumococcal vaccine, although type-specific protective antibodies are infrequently produced in patients with less than 400 CD4 lymphocytes per cubic millimeter.

ATYPICAL BACTERIAL INFECTIONS

Legionella, Chlamydia, and other atypical bacteria have been associated with pneumonic illnesses in patients with AIDS, although these infections have been infrequent in this population (see Ch. 296 and 345).

CYTOMEGALOVIRUS AND OTHER VIRUSES

Cytomegalovirus, herpes simplex virus, varicella-zoster virus, and respiratory syncytial virus have all been documented to cause pneumonia in patients with AIDS (see Ch. 362, 371, 372, and 374). Although each of these viruses appears to cause opportunistic pulmonary disease only infrequently in HIV-infected patients, their identification as sole pulmonary pathogens is important, since effective therapies are available for these viruses. Influenza and other respiratory viruses such as the adenoviruses may also cause community-acquired pneumonia in AIDS patients, but whether these infections occur more frequently or are more severe in this population than in immunocompetent persons is unknown. HIV per se (and possibly Epstein-Barr virus) has been associated with lymphoid interstitial pneumonitis in children but probably has a limited role in the direct pathogenesis of pulmonary complications in adults.

Cytomegalovirus Pneumonia

Distinguishing actual disease caused by cytomegalovirus from clinically insignificant infection is often difficult in HIV-positive patients. The virus is nearly universal in AIDS patients. Cytomegalovirus viremia was documented in 56 per cent of these patients in one study. Moreover, the virus is commonly cultured from pulmonary secretions (especially bronchoalveolar lavage fluid) and lung tissue in the absence of histologic evidence of cytomegalovirus pneumonia and is often recovered in the presence of other pathogens such as *P. carinii.* Presumably many specimens are contaminated by virus shed in salivary secretions.

Even cytopathologic evidence of infection does not establish with certainty that cytomegalovirus is causally related to pulmonary illness in AIDS patients. In one multicenter study the virus was identified by culture or presence of characteristic cytologic abnormalities in 74 (17 per cent) of 441 bronchoscopy specimens.

Yet, cytomegalovirus was the sole pathogen identified in only 4 per cent of specimens. Similarly, cytomegalovirus infection has been detected at postmortem examination in 50 to 90 per cent of AIDS patients, and there was evidence of lung involvement in 58 per cent of 81 patients with cytomegalovirus infection in one autopsy series. However, another opportunistic infection or neoplasm was found in every patient and in no case was cytomegalovirus infection ascertained to be the direct cause of death. Thus, it is often difficult to know what role cytomegalovirus has in causing pulmonary disease in AIDS patients. Moreover, results of studies differ as to whether cytomegalovirus infection in the lung increases the morbidity or mortality of concurrent opportunistic complications such as PCP.

Strict criteria should, therefore, be defined to establish the diagnosis of cytomegalovirus pneumonia before instituting treatment for this infection with potentially toxic drugs. In particular, patients with hypoxemia (or widened $[\text{A-a}]\text{DO}_2$) and interstitial pulmonary infiltrates should have cytologic (namely, presence of typical intranuclear and intracytoplasmic inclusion bodies) or histochemical evidence of cytomegalovirus infection and histologic documentation of interstitial pneumonitis in the absence of other opportunistic pulmonary pathogens. All of these elements should be present, since some patients with typical cytomegalovirus inclusion bodies in lung tissue improve during specific treatment for other opportunistic pulmonary complications. With this strict definition, very few patients actually have disease caused by cytomegalovirus alone.

It is clear that antiviral therapy is effective for cytomegalovirus-related disease in other organs of AIDS patients, which also provides indirect evidence of the pathogenic potential of this virus in these patients. In fact, induction therapy with ganciclovir or foscarnet results in improvement of 70 to 90 per cent of patients with cytomegalovirus retinitis or colitis. For lung infection 30 (64 per cent) of 47 patients were reported to respond to treatment with ganciclovir. To what degree these patients would meet a rigorous case definition for cytomegalovirus pneumonia is uncertain. Until controlled studies are conducted to establish the effectiveness of specific antiviral therapy for this pulmonary complication of AIDS, most experts advise treating patients with ganciclovir or foscarnet when there is unequivocal cytomegalovirus pneumonia.

Other Viruses

The epidemiology, pathogenesis, clinical syndrome, severity and mortality, and response to therapy of other viral pulmonary infections have not been well defined in HIV-positive persons. Varicella-zoster, herpes simplex, influenza, respiratory syncytial, and adenoviruses have all been associated with nonproductive cough, dyspnea, hypoxemia, and diffuse interstitial radiographic infiltrates (occasionally mimicking *P. carinii* pneumonia) in other patient populations, including severely immunocompromised persons without HIV infection. By inference, these pathogens are likely to cause similar illnesses in patients with AIDS.

Pulmonary infection with varicella-zoster should be suspected in HIV-positive patients who present with lower respiratory symptoms and either primary varicella or disseminated zoster infection. Unlike findings in PCP, the radiographic infiltrate may be more reticulonodular. Herpes simplex infection must be considered in a patient with a *Pneumocystis*-like illness and hemoptysis, especially if tracheobronchial ulcerations are found at bronchoscopy. Community-acquired infections such as influenza, respiratory syncytial virus, and adenovirus are often associated with "flu"-like illnesses occurring in the winter months. Infection with these viruses should be sought, since specific therapy is available for all except adenovirus and the pulmonary complications caused by these viruses are likely to be more severe in AIDS patients, again emphasizing the need for early intervention. With influenza it is unlikely that amantadine will have much benefit if instituted more than several days after the onset. Thus, preventive therapy through vaccination is the most desirable approach, despite the fact that immunodeficient patients infected with HIV have defective antibody response to various immunogens.

INTERSTITIAL PNEUMONITIS

At least two forms of noninfectious interstitial pneumonitis occur in patients with AIDS and may mimic PCP and other opportunistic infections that cause diffuse infiltrates in these patients.

Nonspecific Interstitial Pneumonitis

In one study 32 per cent of 152 episodes of pneumonitis were associated with this entity. Typically, patients have nonproductive cough, dyspnea, fever, and mild to moderate widening of the (A-a)DO$_2$. The chest radiographs most commonly show interstitial infiltrates that are usually diffuse but may be focal. Infiltrates may also be reticulonodular or even alveolar. Approximately 50 per cent have no abnormalities on their chest radiographs. Lung biopsies generally reveal mild alveolar damage with interstitial edema, mononuclear cell infiltration, and type II alveolar cell proliferation. The clinical course is characterized by ultimate stabilization or resolution without specific therapy. The etiology is not clear, as opportunistic pathogens are not detectable in most cases and there is no evidence of local HIV infection by in situ hybridization, although approximately half of the cases have been associated with concurrent pulmonary Kaposi's sarcoma and other cases have occurred in patients who have used intravenous drugs or received experimental therapies, suggesting a role for antigenic stimulation.

Lymphoid Interstitial Pneumonitis

Lymphoid interstitial pneumonitis occurs in 10 to 40 per cent of children with AIDS and is case-defining in persons under 13 years of age but occurs in only 1 to 2 per cent of adult patients with AIDS and pulmonary complications. The clinical syndrome and radiographic abnormalities are indistinguishable from those associated with nonspecific interstitial pneumonitis. However, the histopathology of the lymphoid form differs and includes extensive infiltration of the alveolar septae with nonmalignant lymphocytes and plasma cells. In addition, HIV RNA has been detected in the lung of one patient and EBV DNA was present in the pulmonary tissue of 8 of 10 children with lymphoid interstitial pneumonitis, suggesting a possible etiologic role for these two viruses.

SUMMARY

Many of the opportunistic pulmonary complications described in this chapter cannot be distinguished on clinical grounds alone. Most cases require bronchoscopy for a definitive or expeditious diagnosis so that specific treatments can be administered and unnecessary toxic therapies avoided.

Conte JE Jr, Chernoff D, Feigal DW, et al.: Intravenous or inhaled pentamidine for treating *Pneumocystis carinii* pneumonia in AIDS. A randomized trial. Ann Intern Med 113:203, 1990. *One of two controlled studies suggesting that aerosolized pentamidine may be inferior for primary therapy of PCP compared with parenteral therapy.*

DeLorenzo LJ, Huang CT, Maguire GP: Roentgenographic patterns of *Pneumocystis carinii* pneumonia in 104 patients with AIDS. Chest 91:323, 1987. *Comprehensive description of the radiographic manifestations of PCP.*

Gill PS, Akil BA, Colletti P, et al.: Pulmonary Kaposi's sarcoma: Clinical findings and results of therapy. Am J Med 87:57, 1989. *Best overview of the clinical presentation, treatment, and survival of patients with pulmonary Kaposi's sarcoma.*

Hopewell PC: *Pneumocystis carinii* pneumonia: Diagnosis. J Infect Dis 157:1115, 1988. *Concise review of issues relating to the diagnosis of PCP.*

Johnson PC, Hamill RJ, Sarosi GA: Clinical review: Progressive disseminated histoplasmosis in the AIDS patient. Semin Respir Infect 4:139, 1989. *Most complete overview of histoplasmosis in AIDS patients.*

Masur H, Lane HC, Kovacs JA, et al.: Pneumocystis pneumonia: From bench to clinic. Ann Intern Med 111:813, 1989. *Discusses the immunologic, epidemiologic, taxonomic, diagnostic, and therapeutic aspects of PCP.*

Masur H, Meier P, McCutchan A, et al.: Consensus statement on the use of corticosteroids as adjunctive therapy for pneumocystis pneumonia in the acquired immunodeficiency syndrome. N Engl J Med 323:1500, 1990. *Reviews five controlled studies of adjunctive corticosteroid therapy for Pneumocystis pneumonia and summarizes the United States Public Health Service recommendations for this therapy.*

Medina I, Mills J, Leoung G, et al.: Oral therapy for *Pneumocystis carinii* pneumonia in the acquired immunodeficiency syndrome. A controlled trial of trimethoprim-sulfamethoxazole versus trimethoprim-dapsone. N Engl J Med 323:776, 1990. *Describes the relative efficacy and safety of two all-oral therapies for treatment of Pneumocystis pneumonia in AIDS patients.*

Modilevsky T, Sattler FR, Barnes PF: Mycobacterial disease in patients with human immunodeficiency virus infection. Arch Intern Med 149:2201, 1989. *Compares the clinical, laboratory, and radiographic features of tuberculosis and M. avium infection in patients with HIV.*

Murray JF, Felton CP, Garay SM, et al.: Pulmonary complications of the acquired immunodeficiency syndrome: Report of a National Heart, Lung, and Blood Institute workshop. N Engl J Med 310:1682, 1984. *Excellent description of types and frequency of pulmonary disorders in 441 patients with AIDS and the yield of diagnostic tests.*

Phair J, Munoz A, Detels R, et al.: The risk of *Pneumocystis carinii* pneumonia among men infected with human immunodeficiency virus type I. N Engl J Med 322:161, 1990. *Describes the relationship of CD4 counts over time and the occurrence of fever and oral thrush to the risk of PCP.*

Pitchenik AE, Fertel D, Bloch AB: *Mycobacterial* disease: Epidemiology, diagnosis, treatment, and prevention. Clin Chest Med 9:425, 1988. *Best overview of the epidemiology and treatment of tuberculosis and M. avium infections in patients with HIV.*

Sattler FR, Allegra CJ, Verdegem TD, et al.: Trimetrexate-leucovorin dosage evaluation study for treatment of *Pneumocystis carinii* pneumonia. J Infect Dis 161:91, 1990. *Establishes the dosage of trimetrexate and leucovorin resulting in the least dosage-modifying toxicity and excellent efficacy for PCP.*

Sattler FR, Cowan R, Nielsen DM, Ruskin J: Trimethoprim-sulfamethoxazole compared with pentamidine for treatment of *Pneumocystis carinii* pneumonia in the acquired immunodeficiency syndrome: A prospective noncrossover study. Ann Intern Med 109:280, 1988. *Only study comparing efficacy and toxicities of TMP-SMX to pentamidine when patients are not crossed over for failure or drug toxicity.*

Suffredini AF, Ognibene FP, Lack EE, et al.: Nonspecific interstitial pneumonitis: A common cause of pulmonary disease in the acquired immunodeficiency syndrome. Ann Intern Med 107:7, 1987. *Describes incidence, clinical features, and histologic findings of nonspecific interstitial pneumonitis in AIDS patients with pneumonia.*

United States Public Health Service: Guidelines for prophylaxis against *Pneumocystis carinii* pneumonia for persons infected with human immunodeficiency virus. MMWR 38 (S-5):1, 1989. *Summarizes risk factors and effective therapies for prevention of PCP in HIV-positive patients.*

Wallace JM: Pulmonary infection in human immunodeficiency disease: Viral pulmonary infections. Sem Respir Infect 4(2):147, 1989. *Excellent overview of viral lung infections in AIDS.*

416 Gastrointestinal Manifestations of AIDS

John G. Bartlett

The gastrointestinal tract is an especially common site for clinical expression of HIV infection and represents an important factor in morbidity, including malnutrition. Large-scale studies indicate that most patients with AIDS have oral candidiasis, many have severe periodontal infections, up to one third have perirectal lesions due to herpes simplex, 30 to 60 per cent complain of chronic or intermittent diarrhea, and the average weight loss following an AIDS-defining diagnosis is 12 to 15 kg. Most of these complications represent opportunistic infections that occur only with advanced stages of immunosuppression when the T4 lymphocyte count is less than 300 per cubic millimeter.

ORAL LESIONS. Oral candidiasis ("thrush") is encountered at some time in 80 to 90 per cent of all patients with advanced stages of HIV infection. The usual finding is white patches that show yeast forms and pseudohyphae on KOH preparation. The diagnosis is usually made by visual appearance. Thrush is the most common form of AIDS-related complex (ARC), and when found in an otherwise asymptomatic person with HIV infection heralds the probability of an AIDS-defining diagnosis within 2 to 3 years. The lesions usually respond to nystatin, clotrimazole troches, ketoconazole, or fluconazole, but relapse rates are high so that continuous therapy is often necessary. Oral hairy leukoplakia (OHL) is a newly recognized condition found almost exclusively in persons with HIV infection. The cause is unknown, but in situ hybridization implicates Epstein-Barr virus. Typical lesions are patches of white fibrillar projections that are usually located on the tongue and often confused with thrush. OHL is usually asymptomatic, but occasional patients complain of pain or voice changes and respond to treatment with acyclovir. Herpes simplex virus often causes painful oral lesions that have the typical appearance of vesicles on an erythematous base and break down to form ulcers. Herpetic lesions tend to be more severe and prolonged in patients with HIV infection. The usual treatment is acyclovir given orally or parenterally. The major source of confusion is aphthous ulcers of unknown etiology that seem to respond best to topical or systemic administration of corticosteroids. Patients with Kaposi's sarcoma often have involvement of the oral cavity, most frequently with typical erythematous purplish raised lesions on the palate, although any site in the oral cavity may be involved. Most are asymptomatic; symptomatic lesions generally respond to radiation or laser treatments. Periodontal disease is relatively common with either gingivitis or periodontitis. Treatment consists of topical chlorhexidine (Peridex) or systemically administered metronidazole.

ESOPHAGITIS. Dysphagia or odynophagia generally indicates an esophageal lesion. The most common cause is candidiasis, and most patients also have thrush. Alternative causes include herpes simplex, cytomegalovirus, or aphthous ulcers. The diagnosis is optimally made with endoscopy showing grayish white plaques, and smears or biopsy to demonstrate the etiologic agent. A presumptive diagnosis of *Candida* esophagitis is made in patients with thrush combined with dysphagia. Preferred drugs for *C. albicans* esophagitis are ketoconazole or fluconazole by mouth, or a brief course of amphotericin B by vein. Herpes simplex may be treated with acyclovir, cytomegalovirus often responds to ganciclovir, and aphthous ulcers are optimally treated with systemic corticosteroids.

GASTRIC LESIONS. Patients with AIDS often have gastric achlorhydria; less common gastric lesions are Kaposi's sarcoma and opportunistic infections.

SMALL BOWEL AND COLON LESIONS. Acute and/or chronic diarrhea is a frequent complication, usually in the relatively late stages of HIV infection. In many instances, diarrhea is accompanied by severe weight loss, a combination referred to as "diarrhea-wasting syndrome" that is now included as an AIDS-defining diagnosis according to WHO and CDC definitions. The frequency of chronic diarrhea is usually reported at 30 to 60 per cent for patients with AIDS, many have intermittent symptoms, and the small bowel is the most common site of pathologic changes. The most common opportunistic pathogens responsible for chronic diarrhea are *Cryptosporidium*, Microsporida, *Mycobacterium avium*, and cytomegalovirus (CMV).

Cryptosporidia tend to cause intermittent diarrhea that persists for months and may be responsible for severe fluid losses, dehydration, and electrolyte abnormalities. Small bowel biopsies show villous atrophy, crypt hyperplasia, and intraepithelial lymphocytes with typical schizonts that appear adherent to the brush border. Functional tests show D-xylose malabsorption and stools show no fecal leukocytes. The usual diagnostic test is a stool examination for oocysts that appear like yeast but are easily detected using modified acid-fast stains. Complications include papillary stenosis and obstruction of the common bile duct. No therapy has proven effective.

Microsporidia are a group of extremely small unicellular parasites, with the most frequent species in AIDS patients being *Enterocytozoon bieneusi*. The organism cannot be easily detected in stool, so small intestinal biopsy with electron microscopy is often required. Histopathologic changes are similar to those noted with cryptosporidiosis except for the unique morphologic features and location of the organism within the cytoplasm of the enterocyte. No treatment has established merit.

M. avium may cause pathologic changes in the small bowel which appear identical to those of Whipple's disease, with foamy macrophages distended by vesicles containing periodic acid–Schiff (PAS)–positive material in the lamina propria. However, unlike Whipple's disease, the putative agents in the macrophage are acid fast and do not cross-react with antibacterial typing sera. *M. avium* is resistant to most antimicrobial agents, and the utility of aggressive treatment using multiple drugs in combination is controversial.

CMV commonly causes disseminated infection in the late stages of HIV infection at any level of the gastrointestinal tract including the mouth, esophagus, stomach, small bowel, colon, and perirectal region. The most common is a diffuse colitis with superficial ulcerations. Symptoms ascribed to this infection include diarrhea, abdominal pain, or bloody stools. Less common are a solitary ulcer, toxic megacolon, or intestinal perforation. The diagnosis is generally established by demonstrating typical viral inclusions in intestinal biopsies, but the role of this organism as a cause of symptomatic disease is often controversial even when seen. A large number of inclusion bodies per square millimeter of tissue and the presence of high-grade inflammation or typical CMV

vasculitis are possible important correlates in interpretation. Ganciclovir is sometimes effective, although many patients do not respond.

Another enteric pathogen that is found with increased frequency among patients with advanced stages of HIV infection is *Isospora belli*, a protozoan parasite that may cause symptoms similar to those described for cryptosporidiosis. The diagnosis is established by recognition of large acid-fast oocysts (20 to 30 × 10 to 20 μm) in stool. This organism responds well to treatment with trimethoprim-sulfamethoxazole, although the relapse rate is high, so that long-term maintenance treatment is often necessary. With regard to other protozoa, *Entamoeba histolytica* and *Giardia lamblia* are occasionally encountered in this population and both represent treatable pathogens. *Blastocystis hominis* is found in stools of 10 to 15 per cent of healthy heterosexual persons and 35 to 50 per cent of asymptomatic homosexual men; its role as an enteric pathogen is unclear. Nonpathogenic ameba (*E. hartmani, E. coli, E. nana*, and *Iodamoeba butchii*) play no established role in diarrhea in persons with or without HIV infection.

Among bacterial pathogens, *Salmonella*, especially *S. typhimurium*, is found at least 20-fold more frequently in patients with AIDS than in the general population. Unusual features include the lack of an identifiable source of infection in most, a high rate of bacteremia (enteric fever), and the propensity of the infection to recur when treatment is discontinued. The favored drugs include ampicillin or amoxicillin, trimethoprim-sulfamethoxazole, third-generation cephalosporins, and quinolones. Antibiotic-associated diarrhea or colitis is also relatively common in patients with HIV infection owing to their high rate of antibiotic consumption. Additional bacterial agents to consider in this patient population include *Shigella, Campylobacter jejuni*, and other *Campylobacter* species including *C. fetus, C. laridis, C. cinaedi*, and *C. fennelliae*.

Tumors of the gastrointestinal tract associated with HIV infection include Kaposi's sarcoma, non-Hodgkin's lymphoma, cloacogenic carcinoma of the rectum, and squamous cell carcinoma of the rectum and anus. The most common of these is Kaposi's sarcoma, which has been found in gut tissue at autopsy in 40 to 50 per cent of persons with typical cutaneous lesions. Endoscopy typically shows raised red nodules, but histologic confirmation is difficult owing to the depth of pathologic changes. The great majority are asymptomatic; less common presentations include diarrhea, subacute intestinal obstruction, protein-losing enteropathy, and rectal ulcer. The lymphomas associated with HIV infection are usually high-grade B-cell lymphomas that are extranodal in origin. The gastrointestinal tract is affected in up to 20 per cent, and there may be involvement of any site from the oral cavity to the rectum.

AIDS ENTEROPATHY. Endoscopy in patients with advanced AIDS often shows morphologic changes in the small bowel in the absence of evidence for a superimposed opportunistic infection. Characteristic features are villous blunting, a reduced villus:crypt ratio, and an inappropriately low number of mitotic figures. In the absence of an enteric pathogen the findings are sometimes referred to as "AIDS enteropathy." Studies of gastrointestinal function in the presence of AIDS enteropathy usually show malabsorption with abnormal D-xylose and ^{14}C-glycerol-tripalmitin absorption tests. The cause of these changes is not known, but the major considerations include direct invasion by HIV, an opportunistic infection that has not been detected, or a consequence of immune suppression.

MANAGEMENT GUIDELINES FOR PATIENTS WITH DIARRHEA. Recommended tests should be tailored to the specific clinical findings and likely etiologic agents. For most patients with HIV infection and diarrhea that is severe or prolonged, the initial evaluation should include cultures for bacterial pathogens (*Salmonella, Shigella* and *Campylobacter jejuni*), direct examination for ova and parasites, and a *Clostridium difficile* toxin assay. Previous studies indicate that a likely etiologic agent will be detected in 30 to 50 per cent of patients, the most common in chronic diarrhea being *Cryptosporidium*. Those with persistent and unexplained diarrhea or disabling abdominal pain may undergo additional testing, including radiography with contrast, abdominal computerized tomography, and/or endoscopy. Extensive use of upper or lower endoscopy in this setting is controversial, since the conditions most often found cannot be readily treated, giving a poor cost-benefit ratio. These conditions include AIDS enteropathy and infections with cytomegalovirus, *M. avium,* and Microsporida. The treatment of diarrhea in the patient with advanced infection should include appropriate antimicrobial agents directed against identified pathogens (Table 416–1). Nonspecific agents such as imodium or loperamide, indomethacin, somatostatin, or bismuth salts are sometimes useful. Nutritional consequences of chronic diarrhea need to be addressed as described below.

NUTRITIONAL SUPPORT. The average patient with AIDS loses 15 to 20 per cent of his or her baseline weight during the course of the infection. Protein-calorie malnutrition is a common and important sequela to late disease that may accelerate progressive immunosuppression. Contributing factors to malnutrition include a hypermetabolic state associated with chronic infection (especially with fever), oral lesions causing pain, esophageal lesions resulting in dysphagia, reduced taste sensation, depression, HIV-associated subcortical dementia, gastrointestinal side effects of medications, and enteropathy. Therapeutic approaches are optimally based on the cause. Patients with chronic diarrhea should receive small, frequent meals that are low in fiber, residue, lactose, fat, and caffeine. These patients often require additional nutritional support. Enteral feedings are preferred using the oral route, transnasal feeding tubes, or percutaneous endoscopic jejunostomy. Supplementary enteral nutritional feedings may include polymeric formulas or, for patients with severe enteropathy, elemental formulas.

"GAY BOWEL SYNDROME." This term is used in reference to the enteric and perirectal infections that are commonly encountered in homosexual men. Relevant in the context of HIV infection is the fact that the homosexual lifestyle is a risk category for both. However, the pathogens observed with gastrointestinal lesions in immunocompetent homosexual men and immunosuppressed patients with HIV infection are very different (Table 416–2). The former includes a number of sexually transmitted diseases combined with several conventional enteric pathogens. By contrast, the listing for patients with HIV infection is largely restricted to opportunistic infections and opportunistic tumors, reflecting immunosuppression. The single pathogen encountered in both lists is herpes simplex virus, although this infection is distinctive in the two groups; herpes simplex virus infections in patients with AIDS are usually more extensive, more severe, and more prolonged.

HEPATOBILIARY DISEASE. The prevalence of markers for hepatitis B (HBsAg, anti-HBs, or anti-HBc) is 35 to 80 per cent in AIDS patients, reflecting their prevalence among homosexual

TABLE 416–1. TREATMENT OF ENTERIC PATHOGENS IN AIDS

Pathogen	Treatment
Candida albicans	
Thrush	Nystatin, clotrimazole, or ketoconazole
Esophagitis	Ketoconazole, fluconazole, or amphotericin B
Herpes simplex	Acyclovir
Cytomegalovirus	
Esophagitis	Ganciclovir
Enteritis/colitis	Ganciclovir (?)
Oral hairy leukoplakia	Acyclovir (symptomatic only)
Mycobacterium avium	Clofazimine, ethambutol, rifampin, ciprofloxacin ± amikacin (?)
Salmonella species	Ampicillin/amoxicillin, quinolone, trimethoprim-sulfamethoxazole, or third-generation cephalosporin
Clostridium difficile	Metronidazole or vancomycin
Campylobacter species	Erythromycin or quinolone
Entamoeba histolytica	Metronidazole + diloxanide
Giardia lamblia	Quinacrine or metronidazole
Isospora	Trimethoprim-sulfamethoxazole
Cryptosporidium	None

TABLE 416–2. GASTROINTESTINAL LESIONS IN HOMOSEXUAL MEN AND PATIENTS WITH HIV INFECTION

Site	Immunocompetent Homosexual Men	Immune Deficiency with HIV Infection
Oral cavity	*Neisseria gonorrhoeae* Herpes simplex	*Candida albicans* Oral hairy leukoplakia Herpes simplex Aphthous ulcers Necrotizing gingivitis Kaposi's sarcoma
Esophagitis		*Candida albicans* Cytomegalovirus Herpes simplex Aphthous ulcers
Small bowel	*Giardia*	*Cryptosporidium* *Isospora* Microsporida *Mycobacterium avium* Cytomegalovirus *Salmonella typhimurium* "AIDS enteropathy" Lymphoma, B cell
Colon	*Chlamydia trachomatis* LGV serovars *Campylobacter* species *Shigella* *Entamoeba histolytica*	Cytomegalovirus
Anus, rectum	*Neisseria gonorrhoeae* *Treponema pallidum* Condyloma acuminatum Herpes simplex	Herpes simplex Cytomegalovirus

men, intravenous drug abusers, and hemophiliacs. Hepatitis surface antigen (HBsAg) is found in 5 to 10 per cent. Nevertheless, chronic active hepatitis and cirrhosis are relatively unusual, possibly reflecting the role of cell-mediated immunity in hepatitis B–associated hepatocellular damage. Other viral causes of hepatitis include herpes simplex virus and CMV. Granulomatous hepatitis is most often due to *M. avium;* less common are histoplasmosis and cryptococcosis. Hepatotoxic drugs commonly taken by HIV-infected patients include sulfonamides, ketoconazole, isoniazid, and rifampin. Cholestasis due to papillary stenosis and sclerosing cholangitis are most often due to *Cryptosporidium* or cytomegalovirus.

ABDOMINAL SURGERY. The most common clinical syndromes in persons with HIV infection that require abdominal surgery are peritonitis associated with perforation due to CMV infection; lymphoma of the gut (most frequently with involvement of the terminal ileum with obstruction or bleeding); Kaposi's sarcoma; and *M. avium* infection involving retroperitoneal lymph nodes or spleen. Patients with cholangiopathy due to CMV or cryptosporidiosis often respond to endoscopic retrograde cholangiopancreatography. The experience to date indicates that patients with HIV infection tolerate surgical procedures well and do not have an unusually high incidence of postoperative complications.

Greenson JK, Belitsos PC, Yardley JH, et al.: AIDS enteropathy: Occult infections and duodenal mucosal alterations in chronic diarrhea. Ann Intern Med 114:366, 1991. *The authors review histopathologic changes in AIDS patients with chronic diarrhea.*

Johanson JF, Sonnenberg A: Efficient management of diarrhea in the acquired immunodeficiency syndrome (AIDS). Ann Intern Med 112:942–948, 1990. *Review of efficacy and cost-effectiveness of various strategies for evaluating diarrhea in AIDS patients suggests that endoscopy and other costly tests are infrequently warranted.*

Kotler DP, Clayton F, Scholes JV, Orenstein JM: Small intestinal injury and parasitic diseases in AIDS. Ann Intern Med 113:444–449, 1990. *The authors review histopathologic findings including electron microscopy in AIDS patients with cryptosporidiosis and microsporidiosis.*

Laughon BE, Druckman DA, Vernon A, et al.: Prevalence of enteric pathogens in homosexual men with and without acquired immunodeficiency syndrome. Gastroenterology 94:984–993, 1988. *This is an exhaustive study of stool to detect bacterial, viral, fungal, and parasitic pathogens in homosexual men without AIDS, with AIDS, and with proctitis or diarrhea.*

Soave R, Johnson WD Jr: Cryptosporidium and Isospora belli infections. J Infect Dis 157:225–229, 1988. *The authors review* Cryptosporidium *and* Isospora *with particular attention to their causing infections in AIDS patients.*

417 Cutaneous Signs of AIDS

Neal S. Penneys

Cutaneous signs and symptoms associated with AIDS are primarily those found with more advanced disease. However, initial infection by human immunodeficiency virus (HIV) may produce a transient macular roseola-like eruption. Infectious processes and neoplastic disease are most commonly seen as the infection progresses. Occasionally, patients have symptoms such as pruritus without visible skin lesions.

Cutaneous infections are a common feature of AIDS. Common superficial infectious processes may be extensive and may have altered appearances because of the immunosuppression associated with HIV infection. Disseminated scabetic infestations may resemble Norwegian scabies. Cutaneous dermatophyte infections have a range of clinical appearances and need not be annular or have an associated scale. These infections may not be clinically recognizable (tinea incognito) or may occur in unusual areas such as the face. Superficial fungal infections may coexist with other pathogens such as herpesvirus or cytomegalovirus (CMV) to produce unusual complex cutaneous infections. These lesions are analogous to oral hairy leukoplakia in that there is more than one infectious agent present in the lesion.

Cutaneous viral infections may also have bizarre presentations. Molluscum contagiosum occurs commonly and is persistent. Lesions may become quite large. A variety of papillomavirus-induced lesions occurs. Persistent common warts occur. Plantar warts may be quite large, painful, and difficult to treat. Anal/genital warts may be a marker of HIV infection. Huge condylomata have been described (see Color Plate 12A). Verrucae may be widespread and have the clinical and histologic morphology of epidermodysplasia verruciformis. Molluscum contagiosum and papillomavirus lesions frequently occur in cosmetically sensitive areas. Locally destructive treatment methods such as curettage and cryotherapy are effective, but lesions almost always recur or new lesions develop.

Herpesvirus infections produce the most significant cutaneous findings in HIV-seropositive patients (see Color Plate 12B). Coinfection by herpesvirus may activate HIV and alter its expression in an infected cell. The development of herpes zoster may be a reliable sign of progression of HIV infection in an otherwise asymptomatic person. With the diminution of the immune response, herpetic infections may become chronic and fail to heal. Chronic herpetic lesions may not exhibit the characteristic morphology of acute lesions in immunocompetent individuals. Both herpes simplex and herpes zoster viruses may produce disseminated skin lesions in HIV-infected individuals. The diagnosis of herpetic infections can be made by morphology of the clinical lesion, Tzanck preparation, skin biopsy, and/or viral culture. For localized persistent herpetic infection, topical acyclovir has some benefit. For symptomatic or severe herpetic infections, systemic acyclovir therapy is helpful. Lastly, viral processes that normally do not affect the skin can occur in the skin of patients with AIDS. Examples include CMV and disseminated vaccinia infections involving the skin.

Unusual primary and disseminated infections occur in the skin. Mucosal and cutaneous lesions of histoplasmosis and cryptococcosis can be signs of disseminated infection in AIDS patients. Mycobacterial infections produced by *M. tuberculosis, M. avium-intracellulare, M. haemophilum,* and others affect the skin in patients with AIDS. Unusual or unique infections such as disseminated amebiasis, sporotrichosis, *Strongyloides* infection, alternariosis, and superficial phaeohyphomycosis have also occurred. Reiter's syndrome is found with increased frequency in patients with AIDS. These patients have all of the characteristics normally associated with Reiter's syndrome, including keratoderma blennorrhagicum (see Color Plate 12C). The treatment approach to Reiter's syndrome in these patients must be cautious. Patients have developed Kaposi's sarcoma and fulminant AIDS after receiving methotrexate as therapy for Reiter's syndrome. It is safe to predict that unusual presentations of disseminated infectious diseases will continue to be described in the skin of AIDS patients.

Mucous membranes are commonly affected by infectious processes in patients with HIV infection. Oral candidiasis may be present and is one harbinger of the progression of HIV infection. White plaques of yeast can be confluent on the palate. Papillomavirus and herpesvirus can produce lesions in the oral cavity. Oral hairy leukoplakia, a mixed infectious process, produces a characteristic "hairy" appearance to the sides of the tongue. This infection contains several pathogens, including Epstein-Barr virus, herpesvirus, and others. Lastly, disseminated infectious disease can affect the mucous membranes.

Neoplastic processes have been associated with AIDS. The most common is Kaposi's sarcoma, and the skin is the most common location for initial recognition of this neoplasm (see Color Plate 12D). In patients with AIDS, however, lesions may be solitary or disseminated, variable in color from light tan to deep purple; variable in appearance from macules to tumor nodules; arranged in a follicular, zosteriform, or linear pattern; and are generally atypical when compared to the lesions of Kaposi's sarcoma occurring in non-AIDS individuals. Kaposi's sarcoma found in AIDS patients frequently affects the mucosae. The risk of development of Kaposi's sarcoma in patients with AIDS does not appear to be uniformly distributed, being highest in homosexual men and lowest in blacks. Other malignant tumors have an increased incidence in these patients, including squamous cell carcinoma and a variety of lymphomas, and these may have cutaneous involvement.

A number of poorly classified eruptions occur in AIDS patients. The best known is seborrheic dermatitis, which occurs in the usual locations but can be persistent and difficult to treat. Patients with AIDS may also have persistent pruritic eruptions that resemble papular urticaria, annular eruptions that resemble granuloma annulare, folliculitis, yellow nail syndrome, vasculitis, alopecia areata, vitiligo, prophyria cutanea tarda, eosinophilic pustular folliculitis, and hypertrichosis of the eyelashes. Certain well-characterized dermatoses such as psoriasis and atopic dermatitis appear to be worsened by the presence of HIV infection. Lastly, many AIDS patients receive a panoply of therapeutic agents that in turn produce a spectrum of cutaneous reactions ranging from macular eruptions to toxic epidermal necrolysis. The etiologic agents that produce certain reactions, such as discolored nails from azidothymidine and interferon (see Color Plate 12E) therapy and palmoplantar thickening from glucan administration, are readily identifiable.

Greenspan J, Greenspan D, Lennette E, et al.: Replication of Epstein-Barr virus within the epithelial cells of oral "hairy" leucoplakia, an AIDS-associated lesion. N Engl J Med 313:1564–1571, 1985.

Klein RS, Harris CA, Butkus-Small C, et al.: Oral candidiasis in high-risk patients as the initial manifestation of the acquired immunodeficiency syndrome. N Engl J Med 311:354–358, 1984.

Lindskov R, Lindhardt BO, Weissmann K, et al.: Acute HTLV-III infection with roseolalike rash. Lancet 1:447, 1986.

Melbye M, Grossman RJ, Goedert JJ, et al.: Risk of AIDS after herpes zoster. Lancet 1:728–730, 1987.

Penneys NS: Skin Manifestations of AIDS. London, Martin Dunitz, 1990.

Redfield RR, Wright C, James WD, et al.: Disseminated vaccinia in a military recruit with human immunodeficiency virus (HIV) disease. N Engl J Med 316:673–676, 1987.

418 Ophthalmologic Manifestations of AIDS

Mark A. Jacobson

Infectious or noninfectious ocular disorders, some of which may lead to severe visual impairment, have been reported in 40 to 90 per cent of patients with AIDS referred for formal ophthalmoscopy. The true incidence of ophthalmic complications of AIDS is difficult to assess because of selection bias in most reported series. For example, in a population of 200 AIDS patients referred to ophthalmologists at Johns Hopkins University, 28 per cent had cytomegalovirus retinitis diagnosed. Smaller referral series have reported even higher percentages. However, the prevalence of this disease in 1986 was only 5.7 per cent in a population-based study of 760 patients with AIDS at San Francisco General Hospital.

The differential diagnosis of HIV-associated ocular disease is best considered by its anatomic location.

DISEASES OF THE CHOROID, RETINA, AND VITREOUS

RETINAL MICROVASCULAR DISEASE (Table 418–1). The most common ophthalmologic complication observed in patients with HIV infection is retinal microvascular disease, which usually manifests as asymptomatic cotton-wool spots or small retinal hemorrhages. Cotton-wool spots have been reported in at least half of patients with AIDS and in up to 40 per cent of patients with ARC. Histopathologically, these lesions represent areas of retinal ischemia. Both immune complex deposition and direct HIV retinal infection have been implicated in the pathogenesis of cotton-wool lesions. On funduscopic examination, they typically appear as white spots with feathered edges on the surface of the retina. A common location is near major posterior retinal vessels, and these lesions can have small associated retinal hemorrhages. It may be difficult to differentiate between cotton-wool spots and early lesions of cytomegalovirus retinitis, which can have a very similar appearance. Sometimes the distinction can be made only by serial ophthalmoscopic examination. Cotton-wool spots remain stationary or resolve, whereas the lesion of cytomegalovirus retinitis increases in size over time. Since cotton-wool spots virtually never cause symptomatic loss of vision and often spontaneously resolve, no treatment is indicated.

Small retinal hemorrhages and other microvascular abnormalities have been reported in up to 40 per cent of patients with AIDS. These lesions also are asymptomatic, except in the rare case where perifoveal involvement may result in visual blurring.

CYTOMEGALOVIRUS (CMV) RETINITIS. CMV retinitis is the most common sight-threatening ocular opportunistic infection in patients with AIDS. It usually occurs in patients with advanced AIDS; and among patients with CMV retinitis at San Francisco General Hospital, it was the index AIDS diagnosis in only 9 per cent. The typical appearance is a white, cottage cheese–like retinal exudate often associated with hemorrhage and frequently located adjacent to major retinal vessels. In tissue sections, full-thickness retinal necrosis and swollen retinal cells containing intranuclear and intracytoplasmic inclusions are observed.

Patients with CMV retinitis typically present with complaints of painless visual impairment—either blurred vision, decreased visual acuity, or visual field defects—almost always affecting one eye more than the other. Several studies of untreated CMV retinitis have demonstrated a natural history of progressive retinal destruction caused by new retinal lesions or increasing size of previous lesions, which is usually evident within 1 month of initial diagnosis.

CMV retinitis is diagnosed primarily by its typical clinical appearance. The differential diagnosis includes cotton-wool spots, retinal hemorrhages, choroidal granulomas, acute retinal necrosis syndrome, and toxoplasmic and syphilitic retinitis. Because differentiating between these entities may be difficult and the therapy of CMV retinitis is expensive, time-consuming, and toxic, the diagnosis of CMV retinitis must be confirmed by an experienced ophthalmologist. In a majority of patients with advanced AIDS, cytomegalovirus can be isolated from urine or blood; hence, viral cultures are of value only in monitoring the efficacy of specific anti-CMV therapy.

The current standard therapy for CMV retinitis is ganciclovir, a nucleoside analogue prodrug that is preferentially phosphorylated within CMV-infected cells to an active drug, ganciclovir triphosphate, which inhibits CMV replication. Although intravenous ganciclovir therapy is effective in halting retinitis progression in 80 to 90 per cent of cases, most AIDS patients progress within 1 month after discontinuing therapy. Hence, therapy must be given indefinitely to minimize further visual impairment. Recently, ganciclovir-resistant strains of CMV have emerged and have been associated with therapeutic failure. Foscarnet, a pyrophosphate analogue that does not require phosphorylation for activity, may be effective in controlling retinitis in such cases and in patients who cannot tolerate ganciclovir therapy because of drug toxicity (Table 418–2).

Since atrophy occurs in areas of active CMV retinitis, patients are susceptible to rhegmatogenous retinal detachment (resulting from a scar in a thinned portion of the retina). This complication often occurs during the healing stage, even in patients whose active retinitis has been controlled with antiviral therapy.

TOXOPLASMIC CHORIORETINITIS. Toxoplasmic chorioretinitis is rare compared with cytomegalovirus retinitis but may complicate up to 20 per cent of cases of AIDS-associated toxoplasmic encephalitis. Unlike toxoplasmic retinitis in immunocompetent individuals, which typically results from reactivation of congenitally acquired cysts latent in the retina, AIDS-associated toxoplasmic chorioretinitis does not appear to originate in pre-existing retinochoroidal scars but from dissemination of organisms from nonocular sites of disease. Necrotizing retinal lesions are often bilateral and multifocal, and (as in cytomegalovirus retinitis) may result in rhegmatogenous retinal detachment. Vitreous inflammation and anterior uveitis are more common and associated hemorrhage less common than in cytomegalovirus retinitis. Since nearly all cases of toxoplasmic chorioretinitis are associated with toxoplasmic encephalitis, a computed tomographic or magnetic resonance scan of the brain should be done whenever this diagnosis is considered. Specific antiparasitic therapy (pyramethamine and sulfadiazine, or pyramethamine and clindamycin, in the same doses used to treat toxoplasmic encephalitis) is usually effective in preventing further retinal necrosis, but chronic maintenance therapy must be continued indefinitely to prevent relapse.

ACUTE RETINAL NECROSIS SYNDROME. Widespread, often bilateral, necrotizing retinitis caused by herpes simplex or varicella-zoster virus is now a well-characterized, although rare, AIDS-associated condition. Unlike cytomegalovirus retinitis, this disease is often associated with ocular pain and concomitant keratitis or iritis. Many individuals have had recent or concurrent trigeminal zoster or orolabial herpes simplex infection, and evidence of concurrent viral meningoencephalitis may be present. On funduscopic examination, widespread, pale or gray, peripheral retinal lesions are noted. Although intravenous acyclovir is effec-

TABLE 418–1. DIAGNOSTIC FEATURES OF IMPORTANT CAUSES OF HIV-ASSOCIATED RETINITIS*

Feature	Cytomegalovirus	Acute Retinal Necrosis (VZV, HSV)	Toxoplasmosis	Syphilis
Ocular symptoms	Floaters, visual field defect, or decreased visual acuity. Painless.	Floaters, visual field defect, or decreased visual acuity. Pain common.	Floaters, visual field defect, or decreased acuity. ± Photophobia.	Floaters, visual field defect, or decreased acuity. ± Photophobia.
Associated clinical findings	AIDS	Orolabial herpes, trigeminal herpes zoster	AIDS, encephalitis	Rash, hearing loss
Typical retinal lesion	Cottage-cheese exudate with hemorrhage	Confluent, gray or pale retina	White or yellow exudate	Variable
Typical retinal location	Adjacent to major vessel	Peripheral	Multifocal	Focal or posterior retina
Risk of retinal detachment	+ + +	+ + + +	+ +	+
Serology, culture	Not helpful	Viral culture of skin lesion	*Toxoplasma gondii* IgG titer	VDRL, FTA-ABS

*Modified with permission from Int Ophthalmol Clin 29:108–118, 1989.

TABLE 418–2. GANCICLOVIR THERAPY FOR CYTOMEGALOVIRUS (CMV) RETINITIS

I. Standard ganciclovir dosing regimen for CMV retinitis
   A. Induction therapy: 5 mg/kg IV q12h × 14 days
   B. Chronic maintenance therapy: 5–6 mg/kg every day or 5 days per week
II. Common adverse effect of ganciclovir
   A. Granulocytopenia (absolute neutrophil count < 500 cells/μl occurs in 16% of patients)
   B. Thrombocytopenia (platelet count < 20,000 cells/μL occurs in 5% of patients)
   C. Azoospermia
III. Clinical considerations for initiating ganciclovir therapy
   A. Proximity of retinal lesions to critical anatomic areas (fovea, optic nerve head)
   B. Patient's baseline absolute neutrophil count and marrow reserve
   C. Necessity for concurrent therapy with other myelosuppressive drugs
   D. Practicality of caring for a chronic indwelling venous catheter

tive in preventing further retinal necrosis, subsequent retinal detachment is a frequent, sight-threatening complication.

OTHER CAUSES OF CHORIORETINITIS AND VITRITIS. Cases of syphilitic retinitis have been reported in individuals with AIDS, ARC, and asymptomatic HIV infection. There is no characteristic ophthalmologic appearance, but nearly all reported cases have had markedly positive serologic tests for active syphilis and dermatologic or central nervous system manifestations of secondary syphilis. Generally, response to intravenous penicillin therapy has been good. Disseminated pneumocystosis and *Mycobacterium avium* complex infections with choroidal infiltrates have been described, but these lesions generally have not been sight-threatening. Recently, several cases of indolently progressive retinitis have been attributed to endogenous bacterial infection on the basis of retinal histopathology and response to broad-spectrum antibiotics. Also, vitritis (i.e., endophthalmitis) due to disseminated candidiasis may occur in parenteral drug users who are HIV infected or AIDS patients with indwelling central venous catheters.

OPTIC NEUROPATHY

Opportunistic infectious diseases affecting the optic nerve of patients with ARC or AIDS may result in visual impairment or blindness. The most common cause of optic neuropathy is CMV infection. When CMV retinitis involves the optic disc, swelling of the optic nerve head (papillitis) leads to decreased visual acuity. This may occur in the presence or absence of other areas of retinitis and alternatively may affect the intraorbital optic nerve (optic neuritis) or retrobulbar nerve (retrobulbar neuritis). The acute retinal necrosis syndrome caused by herpes simplex or varicella-zoster virus infection may cause papillitis, and syphilis may cause papillitis, optic neuritis, or retrobulbar neuritis in patients at any stage of HIV disease. The most serious ocular complication of cryptococcal meningitis is an arachnoiditis compressing the retrobulbar optic nerve and occasionally causing blindness. The cause of optic neuropathy can usually be established by seeking the other characteristic features of the specific infection. However, specific antimicrobial therapy for the cause of optic neuropathy often fails to improve vision once significant visual loss has occurred.

ANTERIOR UVEITIS

Severe anterior uveitis is uncommon in patients with HIV disease, but when such cases occur, syphilis or varicella-zoster virus infection is the most common cause. Mild, asymptomatic anterior uveitis commonly is observed in patients with CMV retinitis, but inflammation severe enough to cause symptoms is extremely rare. Occasional cases of toxoplasmic anterior uveitis have also been reported.

KERATITIS

Inflammatory disease of the cornea (keratitis) is most frequently caused by varicella-zoster or herpes simplex virus, and the clinical features usually make diagnosis relatively simple. Patients with advanced HIV disease who develop this complication may require intravenous acyclovir therapy in addition to topical trifluridine.

DISEASES OF THE CONJUNCTIVA AND ADNEXA

Kaposi's sarcoma has a predilection to involve ocular structures. Twenty of 100 patients with Kaposi's sarcoma examined at UCLA had ophthalmic lesions, 16 involving the eyelid and 7 the conjunctiva. In four of these patients, the ophthalmic lesion was the first and only clinically identified manifestation of Kaposi's sarcoma. Conjunctival Kaposi's lesions appear as bright red subepithelial nodules, and small lesions may be mistaken for subconjunctival hemorrhages. Periorbital edema may be caused by lymphangitic Kaposi's sarcoma, even in the absence of apparent ocular or cutaneous lesions. Most ocular lesions respond to local irradiation.

Nonspecific, nonpurulent conjunctivitis that often is self-limited has been reported in up to 10 per cent of AIDS patients. Topical steroid and sulfa therapy may be beneficial for this condition. Other rare causes of conjunctivitis include syphilis and molluscum contagiosum infection. Orbital Kaposi's sarcoma or Burkitt's lymphoma may present with ptosis and diplopia.

Bloom JN, Palestine AG: The diagnosis of cytomegalovirus retinitis. Ann Intern Med 109:963–969, 1988. *Reviews the clinical presentation and natural history of CMV retinitis.*

Jabs DA, Green WR, Fox R, et al.: Ocular manifestations of acquired immune deficiency syndrome. Ophthalmology 96:1092–1099, 1989. *A series of 200 AIDS patients evaluated for ophthalmologic disease.*

Jacobson MA: Ganciclovir therapy for opportunistic cytomegalovirus disease in AIDS. *In* Volberding PA, Jacobson MA (eds.): AIDS Clinical Review 1990. New York, Marcel Dekker, 1990, pp 149–163. *Reviews clinical pharmacology and rational therapeutic use of ganciclovir.*

Krieger AE, Holland GN: Ocular involvement in AIDS. Eye 2:496–505, 1988. *A practical clinical review that organizes ophthalmic complications of AIDS by pathogenic mechanisms (microvascular disease, opportunistic infections, neoplasms, and neuro-ophthalmic abnormalities).*

Winward KE, Hamed LM, Glaser JS: The spectrum of optic nerve disease in human immunodeficiency virus infection. Am J Ophthalmol 107:373–380, 1989. *A series of four patients with HIV-associated optic neuropathies (syphilitic, CMV, varicella-zoster virus, and cryptococcal).*

419 Hematology/Oncology in AIDS

Jerome E. Groopman and David T. Scadden

HEMATOLOGIC ASPECTS OF HIV INFECTION

Hematologic abnormalities are frequent in HIV infection, and their pathogenesis is a subject of intense study. Cytopenias are often the limiting factors in delivery of anti-infective and antineoplastic therapy for patients with AIDS and ARC. Several newly available recombinant hematopoietic growth factors have been employed to ameliorate anemia and neutropenia and are likely to be important components of therapeutic regimens for such patients.

CYTOPENIA. HIV infection is associated most prominently with a decline in the number of CD4 lymphocytes over time. However, other cytopenias are also frequent, with anemia reported in 60 per cent, thrombocytopenia in 40 per cent, and neutropenia in 50 per cent of patients with AIDS. These cytopenias occur in conjunction with progressive deterioration of immune function and are less common in the earlier stages of HIV infection. Thrombocytopenia is the exception to this generalization and may constitute a manifestation of HIV infection during the asymptomatic phases. Multiple etiologies are frequently operative in causing the cytopenia in advanced HIV infection. Direct and indirect effects of HIV, opportunistic infections, neoplasms, and toxic antiretroviral, antimicrobial, or antitumor chemotherapy are the major factors to be considered. The differential diagnosis of cytopenia in HIV infection should primarily consider these etiologies. Evaluation of patients with low blood counts should focus on infectious processes and attendant myelotoxic effects of therapy. In addition to the usual laboratory approaches to diagnosis of cytopenia based on impaired production, excess consumption, and/or sequestration, blood and marrow cultures and stains for fungi and mycobacteria, and buffy coat cultures for cytomegalovirus (CMV) should be performed. *Mycobacterium avium-intracellulare* (MAI), *Mycobacterium tuberculosis*, *Cryptococcus neoformans*, and *Histoplasma capsulatum* may be found within the marrow and lead to hematologic abnormalities. CMV does not generally cause specific histopathologic changes of the bone marrow but may suppress hematopoiesis and is best cultured from the circulating buffy coat. Neoplastic involvement of the marrow by B-cell lymphoma is frequent in AIDS patients with this malignancy, whereas Kaposi's sarcoma has only rarely been found in the bone marrow.

Bone marrow aspirate and biopsy in HIV-infected patients with low blood counts is recommended, particularly in cases of fever of otherwise unknown cause and in staging of patients with non-Hodgkin's lymphoma.

Morphologic abnormalities of myeloid and erythroid lineages are often present in the bone marrow of patients with AIDS and ARC in the absence of infection or neoplasm. These changes are nonspecific and include hypercellularity, dysplasia with frequent megaloblastosis, lymphoid aggregates, and increased eosinophils, plasma cells, and reticulin. The pathogenetic mechanisms for these morphologic abnormalities and the associated impaired hematopoiesis are not well defined. Laboratory studies of hematopoiesis in HIV infection have yielded variable and differing results. Bone marrow cell progenitor number has been quantitated using in vitro colony growth assays. Normal or decreased numbers of progenitors have been reported in such assays using marrow cells from HIV-infected patients. Although differences in experimental methods may account for these contradictory findings, a significant decrease in progenitor cell number due to HIV does not appear to occur. Similarly, the susceptibility to direct HIV infection of bone marrow progenitors bearing the CD34 surface antigen was reported, but subsequent studies indicated that such infection occurs rarely if at all.

The stage of myeloid maturation during which cells may be infected with HIV is not yet rigorously defined. Similarly, the issue as to HIV infection of bone marrow progenitors with resultant direct impairment of blood cell development is unresolved.

The dysregulation of expression of trophic and/or suppressive factors important in control of hematopoiesis has been postulated to occur in HIV infection. T cells and macrophages are important cellular components of the bone marrow which produce such regulatory factors (cytokines) and are major in vivo targets of HIV (see Ch. 242). In vitro, another source of hematopoietic growth regulatory cytokines, the bone marrow fibroblast, may also be infected with HIV. Again, there are conflicting studies on alteration of cytokine production by these cells due to HIV infection. Growth-suppressive factors that impair hematopoiesis have been reported, including an inhibitor within the immunoglobulin fraction of AIDS patients' serum in one study and an 84-kDa glycoprotein derived from AIDS patients' mononuclear cells in another study. T-cell depletion of AIDS patients' bone marrow prior to in vitro culture has been reported to increase colony growth, suggesting that T cells may elaborate inhibitory factors. Further investigation is needed to delineate the pathogenesis of impaired hematopoiesis due to HIV given the lack of consensus from these initial studies.

THROMBOCYTOPENIA (see Ch. 154). Thrombocytopenia may be a presenting laboratory finding in an otherwise asymptomatic HIV-infected person. Consideration should be given to HIV infection in the differential diagnosis of thrombocytopenia, and the medical history should include questions regarding risk factors for this retrovirus. Clinically asymptomatic but thrombocytopenic HIV-infected patients have a similar rate of progression to ARC and AIDS as asymptomatic HIV-seropositive persons without thrombocytopenia. Thrombocytopenia is not a criterion for more advanced HIV disease according to the staging system developed by the Centers for Disease Control. Multiple etiologies need to be considered in evaluating thrombocytopenia in HIV infection. Immune-mediated destruction and ineffective hematopoiesis may both be operative. In addition, cases of AIDS with apparent hemolytic-uremic syndrome or thrombotic thrombocytopenic purpura have been described but are rare. Isolated thrombocytopenia is most often clinically similar to classic autoimmune thrombocytopenic purpura. Bone marrow examination

reveals an increased number of megakaryocytes, and there are elevated levels of bound immunoglobulin on the platelet surface. Both platelet-bound immune complexes and a specific antibody against a 25-kDa platelet-associated antigen have been described. The immune complexes may contain anti-HIV antibodies and antibodies directed against them. Several platelet-associated autoantibodies appear to be anti-idiotypic antibodies. The detection of such immune complexes or antiplatelet antibodies does not correlate with low platelet numbers in HIV-infected patients. One possible explanation for normal platelet numbers despite coating of platelets with immune complexes or autoantibodies is dysfunction of the reticuloendothelial system in HIV infection. Impaired Fc receptor–mediated clearance of coated platelets could allow sufficient compensatory production in some patients to sustain a normal platelet count.

The thrombocytopenia in HIV-infected patients has similar sequelae to classic immune thrombocytopenia, yet special attention to the issue of thrombocytopenia should be given in HIV-infected hemophiliacs. The pathogenesis of thrombocytopenia in HIV-infected hemophiliacs appears similar to that in other groups of HIV-infected patients, and the diagnostic study of bone marrow aspiration and biopsy should be performed following administration of factor component, as for other invasive procedures. Complications from thrombocytopenia may be more severe in the setting of hemophilia, so that therapy may need to be initiated at a higher platelet count than in HIV-infected patients without other coagulation defects.

An important observation has been the improvement in platelet count due to treatment with zidovudine (AZT) in HIV-infected patients with significant thrombocytopenia, regardless of risk group. Nearly half of such patients may respond to antiretroviral therapy and increase their platelet counts (mean of threefold increase) within 12 weeks of initiating treatment. If there is no response to zidovudine, then several treatment modalities may be considered, including splenectomy, corticosteroids, danazol, intravenous gamma globulin, anti-RhD preparations, or vincristine. Many of these have been successful in classic immune thrombocytopenia, particularly corticosteroids. There is a theoretical risk of steroid use in an HIV-infected individual, including exacerbation of fungal infection, Kaposi's sarcoma, and activity of HIV itself. Nonetheless, most patients have tolerated corticosteroids for short treatment intervals in studies reported to date. Their long-term use in HIV-associated thrombocytopenia is problematic and cannot be recommended.

ANEMIA. Anemia increases in incidence in HIV-infected patients as their degree of immune dysfunction worsens. The anemia is usually characterized as normochromic and normocytic, and iron studies are either normal or indicative of chronic disease. Occasionally the vitamin B_{12} level is decreased. The anemia rarely is due to vitamin B_{12} deficiency; rather, transcobalamin transport may be altered and therapy with the vitamin does not lead to improved erythropoiesis. Should a low vitamin B_{12} level be found, then a true deficiency needs to be ruled out by a Schilling test and other studies (see Ch. 128).

The Coombs' test (antiglobulin) may be positive in the majority of patients with AIDS or ARC and in about a third of asymptomatic HIV-infected individuals. Although anti-i or other specific antibodies may occur, nonspecific binding of antiphospholipid antibodies or immune complexes to erythrocytes is more common. True hemolysis is unusual in HIV-infected patients as a cause of anemia.

Impaired erythropoiesis accounts for anemia in most HIV-infected individuals. Serum erythropoietin levels are often disproportionately low for the degree of anemia in the patient without renal abnormalities and is of unclear etiology. Parvovirus infection has been reported in HIV-infected patients and may result in red cell aplasia. Gamma globulin therapy has been reported to reverse this unusual cause of severe anemia.

The impairment in erythropoiesis due to HIV infection per se may be due to release of inhibitors and/or impaired production of trophic cytokines, as discussed above. Drug-induced anemia is frequent in HIV-infected patients. Zidovudine is associated with both dose-related and idiosyncratic suppression of erythropoiesis. In the AZT Collaborative Working Group Study, anemia occurred in one third of AIDS patients following 6 weeks of treatment. This occurred at relatively high doses of zidovudine, and patients with severe immunosuppression were least tolerant of the drug. In other studies of zidovudine at doses of 300 to 600 mg per day, the decline in hemoglobin levels was less severe and the need for transfusion less frequent. The reductions in the recommended dosing of zidovudine have reduced the frequency and severity of anemia, but the toxicity profile for prolonged (longer than 2 years) usage at lower doses is not yet defined.

Macrocytic changes occur in the erythrocytes with zidovudine therapy. The mechanism of impaired erythropoiesis due to the drug appears to be impairment of DNA synthesis in developing progenitors. Recombinant erythropoietin therapy may decrease the transfusion requirement and increase the hemoglobin in anemic AIDS patients on zidovudine therapy. The response to recombinant erythropoietin treatment is most clearly seen in patients with pretreatment serum erythropoietin levels below 500 mµ per ml. Some anemic AIDS patients receiving zidovudine have developed red cell aplasia that does not improve with recombinant erythropoietin therapy.

NEUTROPENIA. Neutropenia occurs in the HIV-infected patient in concert with decreases in other cell counts with progressive deterioration of the immune system. As with the other cytopenias, neutropenia may be caused by impaired production and/or increased destruction of leukocytes. Antibody bound to granulocyte membrane structures has been observed in nearly one third of HIV-infected individuals. The presence of neutrophil-associated antibodies has not predicted the development of neutropenia. Impaired hematopoiesis is presumed to be the major etiology of neutropenia due to HIV. In addition to neutropenia, neutrophil destruction has been reported in AIDS and ARC. The extent to which neutrophil defects, particularly in microbial killing, contribute to host immune impairment is unknown, but infections associated with other clinical states of neutrophil dysfunction are unusual in AIDS patients, suggesting that dysfunction is rarely of clinical significance.

Neutropenia is most commonly caused by myelosuppressive therapy in AIDS patients. Zidovudine treatment is at times limited by neutropenia. Other important therapies including trimethoprim-sulfamethoxazole for *Pneumocystis carinii* pneumonia, pyrimethamine-sulfadiazine for CNS toxoplasmosis, ganciclovir (DHPG) for CMV retinitis, and acyclovir for disseminated herpes simplex or herpes zoster may be myelotoxic and result in neutropenia.

HEMATOPOIETIC GROWTH FACTORS. Suppression of leukocyte, as well as erythrocyte, production is a major issue in treatment of both HIV infection and its complicating infectious or neoplastic diseases. This problem may become less limiting as new antiretroviral therapies are developed and hematopoietic growth factors are employed to override myelotoxicity. Several studies have been conducted on the activity and safety of hematopoietic growth factors used to increase blood cell number in cytopenic HIV-infected individuals. The results of these studies have been quite encouraging with respect to the erythroid growth factor, erythropoietin, and the myeloid growth factors, granulocyte colony stimulating factor (G-CSF) and granulocyte macrophage colony stimulating factor (GM-CSF). It is clear that in most patients with anemia due to HIV infection and/or concomitant zidovudine therapy, with baseline serum erythropoietin concentrations that are inappropriately low compared with the degree of anemia, recombinant erythropoietin increases the hemoglobin and reduces the transfusion requirement. In many patients, this allows for treatment with zidovudine that would otherwise be difficult to sustain. The use of the myeloid growth factors, G-CSF or GM-CSF, to ameliorate leukopenia due to HIV infection and/or therapy with zidovudine, interferon-α, or ganciclovir has also been relatively successful. The myelotoxicity of these agents can be overcome using relatively low doses of G-CSF or GM-CSF. It is clear that with the myeloid growth factors as well as with erythropoietin, there is no sustained increase in blood cell production, so that therapy with the growth factor must be continued so long as the myelotoxic agent is administered.

The side effects of growth factor therapy seen in patients with AIDS or ARC have been similar to those in other patients treated with these recombinant proteins. The major issue in the safety profile of the myeloid growth factors relates to their potential effects on replication of HIV. The preponderance of data indicate the stimulation of HIV replication in vitro by GM-CSF but not G-CSF. This is most clearly seen when isolates of HIV that are tropic for monocytes are studied. One clinical report has provided data suggesting increased serum HIV antigen levels during GM-CSF therapy. On the other hand, there is also laboratory evidence that the antiretroviral effects of zidovudine in monocytes can be significantly augmented by the presence of GM-CSF. It appears that the growth factor increases the uptake and phosphorylation of zidovudine, resulting in higher intracellular concentrations of active drug. It is believed that GM-CSF should be considered for therapy only in combination with zidovudine based on these in vitro studies. G-CSF and erythropoietin do not appear to alter HIV expression and have been successfully combined with zidovudine, as stated above. Further clinical trials are required to demonstrate that addition of the erythroid or myeloid growth factor not only will allow for concomitant therapy with myelotoxic agents but will significantly alter the natural history of patients with AIDS or ARC.

Karpatkin S, Nardi M, Lennette ET, et al.: Anti-human immunodeficiency virus type 1 antibody complexes on platelets of seropositive homosexuals and narcotic addicts. Proc Natl Acad Sci USA 85:9763, 1988. *Detailed study of immune complexes in HIV-associated thrombocytopenia.*

Koyanagi Y, O'Brian WA, Zhao JQ, et al.: Cytokines alter production of HIV-1 from primary mononuclear phagocytes. Science 241:1673, 1988. *Important laboratory study of cytokine effects on HIV in monocytes.*

Ratner L: Human immunodeficiency virus–associated autoimmune thrombocytopenic purpura: A review. Am J Med 86:194, 1989. *Excellent review of mechanisms and management.*

Richman DD, Fischi MA, Grieco MH, et al.: (AZT Collaborative Working Group): The toxicity of azidothymidine (AZT) in the treatment of patients with AIDS and AIDS-related complex: A double-blind, placebo-controlled trial. N Engl J Med 317:192, 1987. *A major study detailing the hematologic side effects of zidovudine therapy.*

Scadden DT, Zon LI, Groopman JE: Pathophysiology and management of HIV-associated hematologic disorders. Blood 74:1455, 1989. *A comprehensive review with emphasis on pathophysiology; extensive bibliography.*

Stricker RB, Abrams DI, Corash L, Shuman MA: Target platelet antigen in homosexual men with immune thrombocytopenia. N Engl J Med 313:1375, 1985. *Report of antiplatelet antibody in HIV infection.*

Volberding PA, Lagakos ST, Koch MA, et al.: Zidovudine in asymptomatic human immunodeficiency virus infection: A controlled trial in persons with fewer than 500 CD4-positive cells per cubic millimeter. N Engl J Med 322:941, 1990. *An important trial of zidovudine demonstrating improved hematologic tolerance at lower but effective doses.*

Walker RE, Parker RI, Kovacs JA, et al.: Anemia and erythropoiesis in patients with the acquired immunodeficiency syndrome (AIDS) and Kaposi's sarcoma, treated with zidovudine. Ann Intern Med 108:372, 1988. *Detailed clinical and pathologic study focusing on anemia.*

ONCOLOGIC MANIFESTATIONS OF AIDS

Neoplasms, particularly Kaposi's sarcoma and B-cell lymphoma, are frequent in HIV-infected persons. Their development demonstrates the relationship of immune function to suppression of certain oncogenic events and provides a model to study the pathogenesis of these tumors. Clinical management of AIDS-associated neoplasia is complex, since therapy should optimally address HIV and concurrent opportunistic infections as well as the tumors.

KAPOSI'S SARCOMA (see Ch. 109, 154, 417, and 525). Kaposi's sarcoma is the most frequent neoplastic manifestation of HIV infection. Indeed, it forms one of the Centers for Disease Control criteria that define an HIV-infected individual as having AIDS. Kaposi's sarcoma has been recognized in a number of other clinical and epidemiologic settings. The "classic" form of the neoplasm was described over a century ago in predominantly elderly men of Mediterranean and Jewish extraction. It generally involves lower extremities and is an indolent neoplasm. This form of Kaposi's sarcoma was also recognized in association with other malignancies, particularly lymphoma. This latter observation led to the hypothesis that immune surveillance was important in restricting the development of Kaposi's sarcoma. Another form of Kaposi's sarcoma was recognized in certain geographic locations of Central Africa and has been termed the "endemic" form of the neoplasm. This occurrence in Africa was not related to infection with HIV. Again, the neoplasm was more frequently seen in men than in women but was generally more aggressive and involved lymph nodes and viscera.

Patients receiving immunosuppressive therapy, particularly for renal and hepatic transplants, were recognized to have a markedly increased incidence of Kaposi's sarcoma. This further supported the hypothesis that immunocompetence is important with respect to pathogenesis of this neoplasm. Of particular note has been well-documented resolution of Kaposi's sarcoma upon discontinuation of immunosuppressive therapy in these patients. Other disorders of the immune system, including systemic lupus erythematosus and pemphigus vulgaris, have also been associated with Kaposi's sarcoma.

Epidemiologic studies in classic Kaposi's sarcoma, endemic African Kaposi's sarcoma, and among transplant patients all suggest that there are likely to be genetic and environmental factors involved in tumorigenesis in addition to the level of immune competence per se. The clearest genetic association has been with the HLA DR-5 phenotype in classic Kaposi's sarcoma.

The incidence of Kaposi's sarcoma has been estimated to be 20,000 times greater among HIV-infected individuals than in the general population. Although the neoplasm was originally diagnosed in 40 per cent of AIDS patients when first reported in 1981, the incidence may be declining and is believed to constitute 15 per cent of all AIDS patients in the United States diagnosed in 1989. It is not believed that this reduced incidence of the neoplasm is simply due to incorrect diagnosis or altered reporting patterns. AIDS-associated Kaposi's sarcoma is more frequently seen among homosexual or bisexual men with HIV than in other risk groups with the virus. This suggests that HIV infection itself is not sufficient to account for the increased incidence of the disease, but there may be other factors important in the pathogenesis of the neoplasm. Early in the AIDS epidemic, it was suggested that cytomegalovirus infection or the use of volatile nitrites could potentiate the development of Kaposi's sarcoma. However, careful studies have not verified the importance of such candidate cofactors in the development of the neoplasm. A current hypothesis is that other cofactors of an infectious nature may be transmitted in tandem with HIV during intercourse and possibly during use of intravenous drugs. Molecular studies have failed to demonstrate HIV or cytomegalovirus genome in Kaposi's sarcoma lesions. A model of a neoplasm that distantly resembles Kaposi's sarcoma has been established in transgenic mice using the *tat* gene of HIV, but the significance of this to clinical Kaposi's sarcoma in AIDS is still unclear. It has been speculated that certain cytokines, such as interleukin 6, may be elaborated by the Kaposi's sarcoma cells and lead to autocrine proliferation. The recent reports of the development of Kaposi's sarcoma in homosexual men who are not infected with HIV has provided further support to the hypothesis of an independent sexually transmitted infectious agent as an important cofactor in this neoplasm.

Histopathologically, these lesions are a mixture of different cell types. Endothelial cells are quite prominent within the Kaposi's sarcoma lesions, and there is usually a prominent spindle cell proliferation surrounded by extravasated erythrocytes and macrophages. The cell of origin of the neoplasm is still debated, but permanent cell lines derived from the lesions suggest that the spindle cell is the primary neoplastic cell and is of mesenchymal origin. Others have suggested that the primary neoplastic cell is an endothelial cell originating from lymphatic endothelium.

Kaposi's sarcoma usually presents as a cutaneous nonblanching red macule. As lesions increase in size, they often have surrounding ecchymoses and become more of a violet hue than red. At times, the lesions may become nodular, pedunculated, or even necrotic. In advanced disease, the lesions may become confluent with large plaques developing, particularly on the legs. There is no orderly pattern of tumor progression, and presentation may be with lesions at multiple sites. There is no effect on the subsequent appearance of lesions if the primary lesion is excised. The rate of growth of the primary lesions, as well as the appearance of new lesions, can be quite variable from patient to patient. The control of the growth of lesions and of the distribution of lesions is not understood. The lesions may occur on any cutaneous site. Lymphatic involvement is not unusual, and Kaposi's sarcoma may present as lymphadenopathy. Visceral involvement, particularly of trachea, lungs, and gastrointestinal tract, may occur. Clinical symptoms associated with pulmonary involvement include dyspnea and fever and with gastrointestinal involvement, nonspecific abdominal complaints and low-grade blood loss. The most striking morbidity associated with Kaposi's

sarcoma is that of lymph node involvement and consequent lymphedema involving the lower extremities, groin, and head and neck.

The diagnosis of Kaposi's sarcoma is relatively straightforward in HIV-infected individuals presenting with an erythematous or violaceous cutaneous or mucosal lesion. On the other hand, the lesions may initially appear unimpressive and often are misdiagnosed as an insect bite, bruise, or inflammatory reaction. Biopsy is indicated to confirm the clinical diagnosis. Histopathology is generally diagnostic, although there are no specific stains that differentiate the neoplastic spindle cell in Kaposi's sarcoma from that of other proliferative lesions. Following diagnosis, an assessment should be made of the rate of growth and distribution of the lesions. The presence of visceral disease does not necessarily correlate with poor response of lesions to therapy, so that an extensive evaluation for gastrointestinal or lymphadenopathic Kaposi's sarcoma is not indicated unless there are specific symptoms referable to such involvement. It should be pointed out that AIDS patients in general do not die of Kaposi's sarcoma, except for pulmonary Kaposi's sarcoma, but usually succumb to infectious complications of immunosuppression. Thus, staging systems of the neoplasm have emphasized immunologic status and systemic symptoms in addition to the extent of the neoplasm. Recently, a classification system has been adopted by the AIDS Cooperative Trial Group (ACTG) and appears particularly useful in evaluation of such patients. This system proposes a tumor (T), immunologic status (I), and systemic symptoms (S) staging (Table 419–1).

The clinician should pursue therapy of Kaposi's sarcoma in patients with symptomatic visceral disease or rapidly evolving lesions associated with edema. Such patients usually require chemotherapy. The most active chemotherapeutic drugs appear to be doxorubicin, etoposide, vinblastine, bleomycin, and vincristine. Combinations of these agents, particularly doxorubicin, bleomycin, and vincristine, have been associated with a response rate of 50 per cent or greater. The combination of bleomycin and vincristine has been recommended for patients with borderline marrow function, since the drugs are minimally myelotoxic and may be given in conjunction with zidovudine. Response to chemotherapy usually occurs within the first few weeks of treatment. Unfortunately, the lesions regrow when the chemotherapy is stopped so that treatment needs to be chronic.

Patients with Kaposi's sarcoma who do not have rapidly progressive disease and therefore do not require immediate intervention may be treated with several other approaches. These include observation, single-agent interferon-α, local radiation, intralesional chemotherapy, or combinations of these. Zidovudine alone is not effective as an antineoplastic therapy for Kaposi's sarcoma. Selection of the optimal therapeutic approach involves

TABLE 419–1. KAPOSI'S SARCOMA (KS): RECOMMENDED STAGING CLASSIFICATION

	Good Risk (0) (All of the Following)	Poor Risk (1) (Any of the Following)
Tumor (T)	Confined to skin and/or lymph nodes and/or minimal oral disease*	Tumor-associated edema or ulceration Extensive oral KS Gastrointestinal KS KS in other non-nodal viscera
Immune system (I)	CD4 cells ≥ 200/μl	CD4 cells < 200/μl
Systemic illness (S)	No history of OI† or thrush No "B" symptoms‡ Performance status ≥ 70 (Karnofsky)	History of OI and/or thrush "B" symptoms present Performance status < 70 Other HIV-related illness (e.g., neurologic disease, lymphoma)

*Minimal oral disease is non-nodular KS confined to the palate.
†OI = Opportunistic infection.
‡"B" symptoms are unexplained fever, night sweats, >10% involuntary weight loss, or diarrhea persisting more than 2 weeks.
Modified from Krown SE, Metroka C, Wernz J: Kaposi's sarcoma in the acquired immune deficiency syndrome: A proposal for uniform evaluation, response, and staging criteria. J Clin Oncol 7:1201–1207, 1989.

determining the clinical status of the patient, particularly utilizing the ACTG staging classification, as well as lifestyle issues. Patients who are categorized as "good risk" by the TIS staging system are also excellent candidates for response to interferon-α. Interferon-α has been shown to have not only antineoplastic but also anti-HIV effects. Therapy of Kaposi's sarcoma with single-agent interferon-α requires relatively high doses of the agent (18 to 36 million units daily). Recently, it has been recognized that similar benefit may be obtained utilizing lower doses of interferon-α in combination with zidovudine, although hematologic toxicity may be dose limiting. Such hematologic side effects may be overcome by use of myeloid and erythroid growth factors. Interferon-α is associated with flulike side effects, and many patients were not able to tolerate prolonged therapy. It is unclear whether the antiviral as well as the antitumor properties of interferon-α make it a superior agent in the therapy of AIDS-associated Kaposi's sarcoma compared with chemotherapy alone or zidovudine in combination with chemotherapy (Table 419–2).

"Poor risk" patients by TIS staging should be given antiretroviral therapy, since their major life-threatening complication of AIDS is related to immune suppression and opportunistic infection. Local treatment of disfiguring Kaposi's sarcoma lesions may be achieved using radiation therapy (either photon or electron beam) or chemotherapy in these patients. Radiotherapy should be used in low-dose fractions, since the skin of many AIDS patients is unusually sensitive. Radiotherapy is often avoided for oral Kaposi's sarcoma lesions, since severe mucositis may result.

NON-HODGKIN'S LYMPHOMA. B-cell lymphoma frequently occurs in immunosuppressed individuals. Genetic disorders of the immune system such as Wiskott-Aldrich syndrome, as well as immunosuppressive therapy used in organ transplantation, are associated with malignant transformation of B cells and an oligoclonal or monoclonal lymphoma. Non-Hodgkin's B-cell lymphoma is emerging as a frequent manifestation of HIV infection as individuals with the retrovirus live longer as a result of AZT and anti-infective prophylaxis. The initial relative risk of lymphoma in HIV-infected individuals compared with matched uninfected controls was 850 times; it is likely that this is an underestimate of the current risk. Thus, we expect to see an increasing incidence of B-cell lymphoma in this population.

Etiologic factors operative in the development of lymphoma in AIDS are likely to be multiple (see Ch. 147). The Epstein-Barr virus has been suggested as an important agent that induces B-cell proliferation, leading initially to polyclonal expansion of the

TABLE 419–2. TREATMENT OF KAPOSI'S SARCOMA

Interferon-α		
Single agent	Alpha-2a (Roche)	18–36 mU SC daily for 8 weeks, then three times weekly
	Alpha-2b (Schering)	30 mU SC three times weekly
Combined therapy	Zidovudine	Zidovudine 100 mg PO every 4 hours while awake, interferon-α 5–10 mU SC three times weekly
Chemotherapy		
Single agent	Doxorubicin	20–40 mg/m² IV every 3 weeks
	VP-16	100 mg/m² IV every 3 weeks
	Vinblastine	4–8 mg IV weekly
Combined therapy	Vincristine/vinblastine	2 mg IV vincristine every 2 weeks
		4–8 mg IV vinblastine on alternate weeks
	Doxorubicin/bleomycin/ vincristine	Doxorubicin 10–20 mg/m² IV every 3 weeks
		Bleomycin 15 mg/m² IV every 3 weeks
		Vincristine 2 mg IV every 3 weeks
	Bleomycin/vincristine	Bleomycin 15 mg/m² IV every 2–3 weeks
		Vincristine 2 mg IV every 2–3 weeks

B-cell population (see Ch. 373). This expanded population may provide targets for genetic abnormalities that lead to malignant transformation and emergence of several dominant clones. The oligoclonal populations of malignant B cells seen in some HIV-infected individuals with lymphoma support such a model. Ultimately, a single malignant clone may emerge, leading to a monoclonal neoplasm. The chromosomal abnormalities frequently seen in B-cell lymphoma involve chromosome 8 and chromosomes 14 and 22, with translocation of loci encoding the immunoglobulin genes. There is often overexpression of the c-myc oncogene. Genomic evidence of Epstein-Barr virus is found in about one third to one half of B-cell lymphomas in AIDS patients. Cytogenetic abnormalities are found in the majority of such individuals. There is likely to be a number of interacting factors that are important in the pathogenesis of lymphoma in individuals with HIV infection.

Clinically, B-cell lymphoma in AIDS patients tends to be of high-grade histologic pattern and follows an aggressive clinical course. Small, noncleaved or immunoblastic histologies are most frequent and account for nearly three fourths of all lymphomas in this setting. The remaining are usually a diffuse, large-cell type of more intermediate grade. The lower-grade lymphomas reported among HIV-infected individuals may represent background rather than neoplasm directly associated with immunosuppression. Rarely, B-cell acute lymphoblastic leukemia has been reported.

The majority of patients have extranodular disease involving the gastrointestinal tract, central nervous system, liver, soft tissues, and bone marrow. In one large series, nearly two thirds of all patients diagnosed with B-cell lymphoma in AIDS had nonnodular involvement. Lymphoma strictly confined to lymph nodes is uncommon. Gastrointestinal lymphoma may occur anywhere from the esophagus to the anus. Primary central nervous system lymphoma is usually immunoblastic in histologic type (see Ch. 414). Such patients generally present with solitary mass lesions in the parenchyma of the brain, whereas central nervous system involvement in conjunction with systemic lymphoma is more often meningeal in location. All AIDS patients diagnosed with systemic non-Hodgkin's lymphoma should undergo careful assessment of the central nervous system.

The majority of AIDS patients with B-cell lymphoma are classified as having stage III (involving both sides of the diaphragm without visceral involvement) or stage IV (visceral involvement). Systemic "B" symptoms are frequent, but fever should not be immediately ascribed to lymphoma in AIDS patients and secondary infectious etiologies need to be ruled out. Staging of patients should follow the approach used in other settings of non-Hodgkin's lymphoma, with particular attention to the gastrointestinal tract, bone marrow, and central nervous system. It is not clear in the setting of AIDS that prognosis of lymphoma is better among stage III than among stage IV patients.

The major differential diagnosis to be considered with primary central nervous system lymphoma is Toxoplasma gondii infection or progressive multifocal leukoencephalopathy (PML) (see Ch. 414). PML can usually be distinguished from central nervous system lymphoma by its lack of enhancement with gadolinium on MRI. Central nervous system lesions due to lymphoma may be isodense or hypodense and contrast-enhancing on CT scan, and enhance on MRI, thereby resembling toxoplasmosis. Nonetheless, toxoplasmosis usually presents with multiple lesions throughout the neuraxis, whereas primary CNS lymphoma tends to be a single lesion located in a paraventricular site. Accessible lesions should be biopsied to distinguish between lymphoma and toxoplasmosis; lesions that are difficult to approach surgically may be empirically treated with antitoxoplasmal therapy for a limited period of time, generally 1 to 2 weeks. If no response is seen, then lymphoma becomes more likely.

The treatment of AIDS-related B-cell lymphoma is controversial owing to the poor prognosis of the neoplasm and the limited tolerance of aggressive chemotherapy in this patient population. Both opportunistic infection and bone marrow suppression often limit the delivery of adequate dosage of chemotherapy on schedule. Patients with prior AIDS-defining illness, particularly a history of opportunistic infection, have a poor prognosis compared with patients who present with lymphoma as their initial manifestation of AIDS. Similarly, more severely immunocompromised patients with low CD4 cell numbers have a poor outcome and are less tolerant of chemotherapy than are those patients with more intact immune function.

Among "good prognosis" patients with relatively intact immune function and/or those presenting with lymphoma as their AIDS manifestation, aggressive therapy with combination regimens is indicated. For those patients who do not have central nervous system involvement at the time of presentation, it is not clear that prophylactic therapy to the central nervous system offers any long-term benefit. The response rate in these good-prognosis patients is similar to that of non-Hodgkin's lymphoma patients of stage IIIB or IVB without HIV (see Ch. 421), but the long-term survival rate is still poor. Nonetheless, some patients have survived 12 months or longer disease free following complete remission.

Patients with poor prognosis based on severe immune suppression and/or complicating opportunistic infections pose a particularly complex treatment dilemma. Some patients have opted for palliative therapy with corticosteroids, since intensive chemotherapy may lead to further immune compromise and infection. Yet lymphoma is generally rapidly growing and fatal in patients who are not aggressively treated. Thus, the clinician needs to pursue therapy in such patients only with an informed discussion of the risks and benefits of treatment, honestly emphasizing the poor prognosis with or without chemotherapy.

Addition of zidovudine to chemotherapeutic regimens has been difficult owing to myelosuppression. Nonetheless, this approach has appeal in that it provides one way to potentially limit HIV spread and stabilize immune function. As less myelotoxic antiretroviral drugs are developed, or as results of current experimental programs incorporating erythroid or myeloid growth factors into lymphoma therapy are available, this particular approach is likely to become feasible.

The outlook is generally poor for patients with lymphoma, and the majority die within 6 months. No chemotherapeutic regimen has been identified as superior to others for AIDS patients with this neoplasm. The survival is even poorer for those with primary central nervous system lymphoma, on the order of 2 to 4 months. Therapy for central nervous system lymphoma may lead to complete response but does not necessarily alter survival outcome.

OTHER MALIGNANCIES. There is currently active clinical surveillance to determine whether neoplasms other than Kaposi's sarcoma and B-cell lymphoma may ultimately arise at an increased incidence in immunocompromised patients with HIV infection. The incidence of Hodgkin's disease is not clearly increased among HIV-infected individuals. Nonetheless, there may be important differences in the course of Hodgkin's lymphoma in such patients, including a higher incidence of advanced disease, mixed cellularity histology, and extranodular disease. Furthermore, HIV-infected individuals with Hodgkin's disease appear to tolerate chemotherapy less well and have a higher incidence of tumor relapse than do those without HIV infection. This is likely due to their impaired hematopoiesis and the potential for opportunistic infections in such patients. In general, patients have a survival of less than 12 months when presenting with HIV infection and Hodgkin's disease. Further work is needed to better understand the altered pattern of Hodgkin's disease in the setting of HIV infection.

Therapy of Hodgkin's disease among HIV-infected patients is similar to that of uninfected individuals (see Ch. 148). The major difference is to incorporate prophylaxis against opportunistic infections, particularly *Pneumocystis carinii* pneumonia, and to be particularly alert to infectious complications during therapy.

There has been speculation that anal cancer and cervical cancer, neoplasms associated with papillomavirus infection, may increase in incidence in HIV-infected patients. This is due to the high prevalence of papillomavirus infection in groups at risk for HIV (see Ch. 335). A careful cervical examination including colposcopy is indicated in HIV-infected women to detect early malignant change. Ongoing surveillance programs of HIV-infected individuals using Pap smears on cells from the transitional zone of the anus and cervix should provide important data as to the increased incidence, if any, of this cancer in this population.

Although anecdotal reports abound of other malignancies in HIV-infected individuals, it is unclear whether these occur above that of the background prevalence in the general population. Nonetheless, consideration should be given to the significance of the HIV infection in clinical management. These patients have a propensity to develop opportunistic infections upon initiation of chemotherapy or radiotherapy and, in general, have fared poorly because of these infectious complications.

Ensoli B, Nakamura S, Salahuddin SZ, et al.: AIDS-Kaposi's sarcoma–derived cells express cytokines with autocrine and paracrine growth effects. Science 243:223, 1989. *Characterization of Kaposi's sarcoma cells; interesting basic science study.*

Gill PS, Levine AM, Krailo M, et al.: AIDS-related malignant lymphoma: Results of prospective treatment trials. J Clin Oncol 5:1322, 1987. *Detailed analysis of therapeutic trials in AIDS lymphoma.*

Groopman JE, Scadden DT: Interferon therapy for Kaposi's sarcoma associated with the acquired immunodeficiency syndrome (AIDS). Ann Intern Med 110:335, 1989. *Balanced discussion of treatment options in Kaposi's sarcoma.*

Krown SE, Metroka C, Wernz J: Kaposi's sarcoma in the acquired immune deficiency syndrome: A proposal for uniform evaluation, response, and staging criteria. J Clin Oncol 7:1201, 1989. *Kaposi's sarcoma staging system presented and explained.*

Levine AM: Lymphoma in acquired immunodeficiency syndrome. Semin Oncol 17:104, 1990. *Review of lymphoma in AIDS; excellent bibliography.*

Ziegler JL, Beckstead JA, Volberding PA, et al.: Non-Hodgkin's lymphoma in 90 homosexual men: Relationship to generalized lymphadenopathy and acquired immunodeficiency syndrome (AIDS). N Engl J Med 311:565, 1984. *Large clinical study describing lymphoma in AIDS.*

420 Renal, Cardiac, Endocrine, and Rheumatologic Manifestations of HIV Infection

Michael S. Saag

Infection with the human immunodeficiency virus type 1 (HIV) is a multisystem disease that affects every organ system. Manifestations of pulmonary, gastrointestinal, neurologic, hematologic, and oncologic disease are well described in the literature, owing in large part to their high prevalence and often dramatic modes of presentation. In contrast, HIV-related renal, cardiac, endocrine, and rheumatologic diseases are more insidious in presentation. As overall survival of HIV-infected individuals continues to improve and therapeutic regimens become more sophisticated, clinicians will undoubtedly encounter disorders of the latter organ systems with increasing frequency.

RENAL DISEASE

Renal disease associated with HIV infection may present as fluid-electrolyte and acid-base abnormalities, acute renal failure, coincidental renal disorders, or a glomerulopathy directly related to underlying HIV infection, the so-called HIV-associated nephropathy (HIVAN). Originally observed in patients with AIDS and referred to as AIDS-associated nephropathy, recent studies have described the characteristic renal changes of HIVAN in both asymptomatic HIV-infected individuals and those with AIDS-related complex (ARC), thereby broadening the definition to include all HIV-infected patients.

FLUID, ELECTROLYTE, AND ACID-BASE DISORDERS. Fluid-electrolyte disorders are common in patients with advanced HIV infection. Hyponatremia is noted in up to 40 per cent of hospitalized AIDS patients and occurs in the setting of both hypovolemia and euvolemia. Hypovolemia, most often due to gastrointestinal fluid losses, is the most common cause of hyponatremia among this group of patients. The syndrome of inappropriate antidiuretic hormone release (SIADH) is responsible for the majority of cases of euvolemic hyponatremia and is most often due to underlying *Pneumocystis carinii* infection, malignancy, or central nervous system disease. The presence of hyponatremia is associated with increased morbidity and mortality, especially in conjunction with certain opportunistic infections, such as cryptococcosis.

Adrenal insufficiency is a less frequent cause of hyponatremia. Although abnormalities of the adrenal glands are frequently reported at autopsy, overt adrenal insufficiency occurs in less than 5 per cent of patients. The typical findings of hyponatremia, hyperkalemia, non–anion gap metabolic acidosis, hypovolemia, renal salt wasting, and mild renal insufficiency are usually present in some combination.

Drugs are an important cause of fluid and electrolyte disorders in HIV-infected patients and can mimic the abnormalities associated with adrenal dysfunction. Hyperkalemia and non–anion gap metabolic acidosis have been noted in patients receiving parenteral pentamidine. Amphotericin B is associated with hypokalemia, hypomagnesemia, renal tubular acidosis, and renal insufficiency. Chemotherapeutic agents used to treat AIDS-associated malignancies may lead to fluid and electrolyte disturbances through direct nephrotoxicity or gastrointestinal losses associated with prolonged vomiting or diarrhea.

ACUTE RENAL FAILURE. As with most chronic illnesses, acute renal dysfunction may develop as a complication in the management of HIV-infected patients. Prerenal azotemia often results from hypovolemia secondary to poor fluid intake, increased gastrointestinal losses, or both. Acute tubular necrosis can be ischemic in origin, usually secondary to hypotension or sepsis, or due to nephrotoxic agents. Acute interstitial nephritis is another complication associated with drugs used to treat HIV-related diseases. A listing of agents with nephrotoxic potential commonly used in HIV-infected patients is presented in Table 420–1.

Opportunistic infections, invasion of renal parenchyma with lymphoma or Kaposi's sarcoma, and amyloidosis, which occurs as a complication of subcutaneous narcotic abuse, all may result in interstitial nephritis. Other renal lesions, such as hepatitis B–induced membranous glomerulonephritis, acute glomerulonephritis secondary to bacterial infection, direct infection of the renal parenchyma with cytomegalovirus, fungi, or mycobacteria, and the hemolytic-uremic syndrome, have all been associated with renal dysfunction in HIV-infected individuals. The diagnosis and management of acute renal failure are no different in HIV-infected patients than in their uninfected counterparts.

HIV-ASSOCIATED NEPHROPATHY. *Definition.* HIV-associated nephropathy (HIVAN) was first established as a unique clinical entity in 1984. Because it was originally called AIDS-associated nephropathy (AAN), many investigators questioned whether AAN was indeed a unique manifestation of AIDS or simply represented heroin-associated nephropathy (HAN) occurring in intravenous drug users who also happened to be infected with HIV. Although the lesions and clinical manifestations of HAN are similar to those of AAN, further studies have established clear distinctions between the two entities. Of note, AAN occurs in individuals, including children, who have never used intravenous drugs. More recently, the manifestations of AAN have been reported in a significant number of HIV-infected patients who are otherwise asymptomatic. Therefore, HIV-associated nephropathy (HIVAN) has replaced AIDS-associated nephropathy (AAN) as the most appropriate name for this entity.

Epidemiology. The first cases of HIVAN were described in major urban centers, such as New York and Miami, which also had a large proportion of intravenous drug users among their HIV patient population. In contrast, centers whose HIV population consisted primarily of homosexual and bisexual men, such

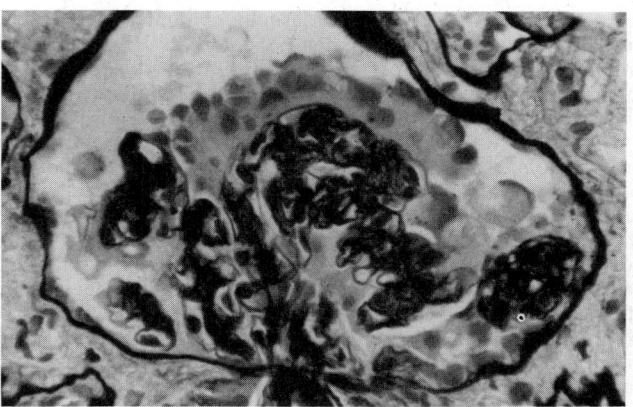

FIGURE 420–1. Glomerulus from a patient with HIV-associated nephropathy demonstrating global collapse of the glomerular capillaries, increased mesangial sclerosis, and a proliferative "cap" of visceral epithelial cells. (Silver methenamine; magnification × 400. Courtesy of Dr. William L. Clapp.)

as San Francisco and the National Institutes of Health, were not observing the renal changes of HIVAN in their patients, thereby implying that HIVAN was a manifestation of HAN. More recent epidemiologic data indicate that 60 per cent of patients with HIVAN are IV drug users, with the remaining cases occurring in homosexual and bisexual men, immigrants from Haiti, women who have acquired HIV from heterosexual contacts, and children born to infected mothers, many of whom did not use intravenous drugs.

Over 90 per cent of patients with HIVAN are black. No explanation regarding the high prevalence of cases among blacks has been established, although many investigators have speculated that cofactors such as superimposed infection(s) or specific immune response genes may be responsible.

Pathology and Pathogenesis. Focal and segmental glomerulosclerosis (FSGS) is the characteristic renal lesion identified in patients with HIVAN, occurring in 80 to 90 per cent of patients. On gross inspection, the kidneys are usually enlarged and the cortical surface is smooth, even in advanced uremia. Microscopic examination of early lesions reveals diffuse mesangial hyperplasia with minimal glomerular sclerosis over time. A variable number of glomeruli develop segmental sclerosis characterized by hyperplastic visceral epithelial cells with coarse cytoplasmic vacuoles, collapsed capillary walls or capillaries obliterated by protein deposits (hyalinosis), and foam cells (lipid-filled monocytes) in the lumina (Fig. 420–1). Bowman spaces are usually dilated and tubular damage is universal. Microcystic dilation of tubules is a unique feature of HIVAN not reported in the FSGS of HAN (Fig. 420–2). Interstitial changes consisting of mild edema with

TABLE 420–1. DRUGS WITH NEPHROTOXIC POTENTIAL COMMONLY USED IN THE TREATMENT OF HIV-RELATED DISEASE

Acyclovir	Nonsteroidal anti-inflammatory
Aminoglycosides	agents
Amphotericin B	Penicillins
Aspirin	Pentamidine
Cephalosporins	Phenytoin
Cimetidine	Rifampin
Cis-platinum	Spiramycin
Dapsone	Sulfonamides
Ethambutol	Tetracyclines
Foscarnet*	Thiazides
Ganciclovir	Trimethoprim

*Investigational

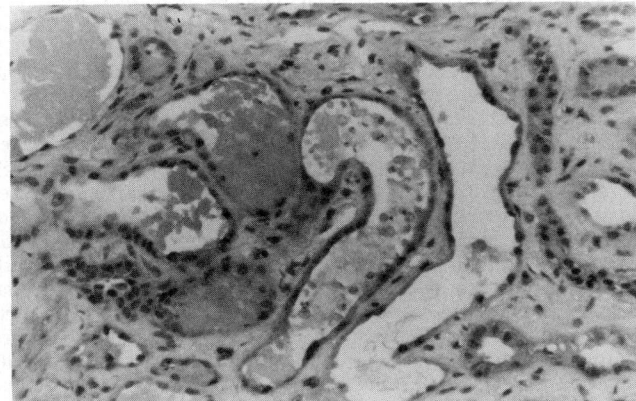

FIGURE 420–2. Dilated degenerated tubules demonstrating flattened epithelium and loss of nuclei and containing proteinaceous casts from a patient with HIV-associated nephropathy. (Hematoxylin-eosin; magnification × 200. Courtesy of Dr. William L. Clapp.)

scattered mononuclear cells are usually evident in HIVAN kidneys but not nearly to the degree noted in HAN. Similarly, although interstitial fibrosis may be present in advanced HIVAN disease, it is not nearly as prominent as the marked interstitial fibrosis noted in HAN disease.

The etiology of HIVAN remains unknown; however, many investigators suspect that an infectious agent is responsible. Ultrastructural studies have demonstrated tubuloreticular structures in vascular endothelium as well as in circulating and tissue lymphocytes. Other findings, such as a large number of nuclear bodies existing as budding forms in renal and lymphoid tissues, have been interpreted by some investigators to suggest a viral etiology. In situ hybridization studies have demonstrated proviral HIV DNA in renal tubular and glomerular epithelial cells, implicating HIV as the causative agent. However, the predominance of HIVAN in blacks and the relative paucity of cases among Caucasian homosexual men suggest that other factors not yet identified must play a role in the pathogenesis of HIVAN.

Clinical Manifestations. HIVAN is characterized by the development of proteinuria, nephrotic syndrome, and rapidly progressive irreversible azotemia. The proteinuria is typically heavy and presents as an early manifestation. The time to the development of end-stage renal disease (ESRD) from the initial diagnosis of proteinuria is 4 to 16 weeks in patients with HIVAN, compared to 20 to 40 months among patients with HAN. Another clinical distinction between HIVAN and HAN is the relative absence of significant hypertension among patients with HIVAN. Accelerated hypertension is a hallmark of HAN. Peripheral edema and anasarca are conspicuously absent in a large number of HIVAN patients with high-grade proteinuria and hypoalbuminemia.

Nephropathy has been documented in patients months to years before the onset of clinical symptoms of ARC or AIDS. In some studies up to 50 per cent of the patients with HIVAN were either asymptomatic or in early stages of ARC. HIVAN is being reported with increasing frequency among HIV-infected children and appears to be independent of the risk factors for HIV infection in their mothers. It is anticipated that the incidence of HIVAN will continue to grow and should be considered as a diagnostic possibility in any HIV-infected patient who presents with unexplained proteinuria regardless of the stage of disease.

Diagnosis. Quantitative measurement of the amount of protein excreted in the urine along with estimation of the creatinine clearance via a 24-hour urine collection should be performed early in the course of evaluation. Other reversible causes of renal insufficiency such as bacterial infection, crystalluria, and obstructive uropathy should be ruled out using urine culture, urinalysis, and ultrasonography. The kidneys are enlarged early in HIVAN and remain enlarged throughout the course of disease. The decision to perform renal biopsy should be made on a case-by-case basis depending on the clinical presentation, the likelihood of other diagnoses, and the therapeutic options available. Since a variety of other renal lesions, such as membranous nephropathy related to hepatitis B, membranoproliferative disease, and immune complex–related glomerular damage, may also present as nephrotic syndrome in HIV-infected patients, renal biopsy should be encouraged. The presence of the typical features of FSGS with tubular involvement as described above establishes the diagnosis of HIVAN when renal tissue is obtained.

Treatment. The lesions of HIVAN respond poorly if at all to currently available treatment regimens. Corticosteroids and other immunosuppressive agents usually have no effect on FSGS. Therefore the treatment of HIVAN is largely supportive in nature. Nutritional support along with appropriate dosage adjustments of nephrotoxic drugs is critical in daily management. Hemodialysis is of marginal benefit in prolonging survival of patients with advanced HIV disease once they have reached end-stage renal disease. Among patients with AIDS, hemodialysis provides short-term prolongation of life for 3 to 11 months. Patients who are asymptomatic or have ARC survive longer, with some patients living over 2 years on chronic hemodialysis. The use of peritoneal dialysis should be considered in patients who are suitable candidates. Chronic ambulatory peritoneal dialysis (CAPD) may offer several advantages over hemodialysis, including avoidance of leukopenia caused by the hemodialysis membranes, fewer problems with anemia, and theoretical advantages of less stimulation of HIV-infected T lymphocytes via membrane-induced cytokine release. A potential disadvantage of CAPD is the higher incidence of peritonitis. Renal transplantation is not considered a viable option in HIV-infected patients owing to the intensive immunosuppressive regimens required to prevent rejection. In some patients with advanced HIV infection or AIDS who develop HIVAN it may be appropriate to withhold dialysis support based on the generally poor prognosis. As always, such decisions should be individualized, taking into account the wishes of the patient, the family, and significant others.

CARDIAC DISEASE

A wide variety of cardiac abnormalities have been reported in HIV-infected patients, including ventricular dysfunction, myocarditis, pericarditis, endocarditis, and arrhythmias. Most often, cardiac involvement is clinically silent and is noted as an incidental finding at autopsy. When clinical symptoms are present, however, disease manifestations can be debilitating, and, in many cases, life threatening. Unlike HIV-associated renal disease, no specific cardiac syndrome or disease state has been described.

Epidemiology. Cardiac abnormalities have been observed in 25 to 75 per cent of HIV-infected patients studied at autopsy. Myocardial disease is noted most frequently, occurring in over 90 per cent of subjects with cardiac findings. Pericardial disease, often with adjacent myocardial involvement, is observed in over 20 per cent of cases with cardiac abnormalities. Endocarditis is evident histologically in 3 to 5 per cent of cases reported in autopsy series. No characteristic epidemiologic factor, such as age, sex, race, or means of acquiring HIV infection, has been identified which predisposes patients to develop cardiac disease. Although cardiac abnormalities are observed more frequently in AIDS patients, up to 30 per cent of patients with ARC are noted to have abnormal findings on echocardiograms and electrocardiograms.

Pathology and Pathogenesis. HIV-related heart disease may result from metastatic extension of a concomitant opportunistic infection or malignancy but most often is seen as lymphocytic infiltration of the myocardium or as an unspecified myocarditis. The mechanism responsible for the myocarditis remains unknown, although many investigators believe that HIV itself may be directly responsible. Preliminary reports have demonstrated immunologic evidence of HIV antigens (p17, p24, and gp120) in cardiac tissue, molecular evidence of HIV in heart tissue using Southern blot techniques, and virologic evidence of myocardial involvement through culturing HIV-1 from an endocardial biopsy obtained from an AIDS patient with end-stage cardiomyopathy. None of these studies clearly establishes HIV-1 as an etiologic agent of cardiomyopathy, however, since the virus is known to exist in the lymphocytes that invade the myocardium. Other viruses, such as cytomegalovirus, may be responsible for the development of myocarditis, although the typical "owl's eye" inclusion bodies are rarely seen in patients with HIV-associated cardiomyopathy. Additional mechanisms, such as postviral myocarditis or catecholamine-induced myocarditis, have been postulated, but little evidence exists to support their role.

A broad range of opportunistic infections and malignant diseases has been described in cardiac tissue examined at autopsy. Among the infectious disorders, fungal and viral pathogens are identified most often, followed by bacterial and protozoal infections (Table 420–2). Although the invading pathogen is frequently diagnosed at another primary site ante mortem, cardiac involvement is rarely (<2 per cent) identified prior to autopsy. This is due in large part to the clinically silent nature of cardiac disease in HIV infection and a low index of suspicion by clinicians. Kaposi's sarcoma and metastatic lymphoma are the most common neoplastic diseases reported which invade the heart. Primary cardiac lymphoma has been reported rarely.

Pericardial disease is almost invariably associated with adjacent myocardial involvement. Pericarditis is usually nonspecific in origin, but when an etiologic process is identified, Kaposi's sarcoma or a pathogen such as *Mycobacterium tuberculosis* or *Cryptococcus neoformans* is responsible most often. Drugs used to treat HIV-associated disorders, such as doxorubicin for Kaposi's sarcoma, may cause myocardial damage. Other toxins, vitamin deficiencies, or metabolic abnormalities (e.g., hypothyroidism) may also result in myocardial dysfunction or pericardial disease.

TABLE 420–2. INFECTIOUS CAUSES OF CARDIAC DISEASE IN HIV-INFECTED PATIENTS

Bacteria
  Bacteria (endocarditis)
  Mycobacterium tuberculosis
  Mycobacterium avium-intracellulare
  Nocardia asteroides
  Actinomyces
Fungi
  Cryptococcus neoformans
  Histoplasma capsulatum
  Coccidioides immitis
  Candida species
  Aspergillus species
Viruses
  Cytomegalovirus
  Herpes simplex virus
  Human immunodeficiency virus
Protozoa
  Toxoplasma gondii
  Pneumocystis carinii

Endocardial disease has been described in up to 3 per cent of cases studied at autopsy and usually presents as either nonbacterial thrombotic (marantic) endocarditis or healed bacterial endocarditis. The precise etiology of marantic endocarditis is unknown, but it has been reported in other long-term wasting illnesses and malignant diseases. Vegetations are usually located on the mitral valve, although lesions on the tricuspid valve have been noted in up to 29 per cent of AIDS patients with this disorder. Significant embolization to the spleen and brain was noted in over 50 per cent of patients with marantic endocarditis studied at autopsy. Bacterial endocarditis is reported rarely in AIDS patients. Healed lesions from previous bouts of bacterial endocarditis have been reported in autopsy series but are of little clinical significance.

Clinical Findings. Most cardiac disease in HIV-infected patients is clinically silent. When symptoms are present they usually consist of the ordinary findings noted in non–HIV-infected patients with myocarditis or pericarditis, such as fever, dyspnea, chest pain, fatigue, cough, and orthopnea. Hepatomegaly and jugular venous distention are the most common signs noted on physical examination, followed by rales, systolic murmurs, and the presence of an S3 gallop. Signs of advanced pericardial disease with impending tamponade are among the most common clinical manifestations observed in patients who present with clinical symptoms of cardiac disease.

Diagnosis. The demonstration of cardiomegaly on a chest roentgenogram is an important marker of underlying cardiac disease in HIV-infected patients. Right ventricular enlargement is usually the result of pulmonary artery hypertension, which in AIDS patients is often due to severe or recurrent opportunistic pneumonia. Left ventricular or biventricular enlargement is a characteristic finding of congestive cardiomyopathy due to any cause. Echocardiography is a more sensitive and specific noninvasive test that is used to assess the degree of ventricular dysfunction and to characterize the extent of pericardial effusion, if present. Several series have demonstrated echocardiographic abnormalities in up to 50 per cent of HIV-infected patients who had no cardiac symptoms at the time of study. Ventricular enlargement, pericardial effusion, and ventricular hypokinesis were the abnormalities noted most frequently. In view of the overall silent nature of cardiac disease, the high likelihood that infiltrative processes will be evident and diagnosed at another site, and the often limited therapeutic options available for treating cardiac disease in HIV-infected patients, routine echocardiography should be discouraged in patients without cardiac symptoms. The experience with endomyocardial biopsies in HIV-infected patients is quite limited; however, in those individuals who show signs of cardiac disease and have not had a specific diagnosis established, endomyocardial biopsy is a viable option that may lead to a definitive diagnosis.

Treatment. Supportive treatment consisting of diuretic therapy, preload and afterload reduction when appropriate, and correction of cardiac arrhythmias is the obvious initial approach to the treatment of myocardial disease. Pericardial disease requires careful volume management with avoidance of aggressive diuresis or preload reduction. In the case of pericardial tamponade, surgical intervention is warranted. When the underlying etiology of the cardiac disease is known, appropriate targeted therapy directed at the specific infectious agent or malignancy is indicated.

ENDOCRINE DISORDERS

Endocrine dysfunction has not been a prominent clinical manifestation of HIV infection. Nonetheless, all glands of the endocrine system may be infiltrated with opportunistic infections or malignancies or may be affected by drugs used to treat HIV-related disorders. The subtle presentations of endocrine diseases create difficult diagnostic challenges.

ADRENAL GLAND DYSFUNCTION. The adrenal gland is the endocrine gland most commonly affected in patients with AIDS examined at autopsy, although clinical evidence of adrenal insufficiency is observed in less than 8 per cent of AIDS patients. Widespread lipid depletion and varying degrees of adrenal necrosis are the most prevalent pathologic findings in postmortem examinations. Adrenal invasion by cytomegalovirus is noted in up to 50 per cent of patients with adrenal pathology. *Mycobacterium avium* complex, Kaposi's sarcoma, *C. neoformans*, and *Histoplasma capsulatum* involve the adrenal glands in 5 to 12 per cent of cases. Drug therapy with agents such as ketoconazole or rifampin may also result in adrenal dysfunction. Fatigue, anorexia, nausea, vomiting, orthostatic hypotension, and hyponatremia are symptoms frequently noted in many HIV-infected patients; however, only a few patients with these symptoms are actually adrenal insufficient when evaluated using standard laboratory criteria.

Basal 8 A.M. plasma cortisol levels are usually higher in patients with advanced HIV disease than in ARC patients and uninfected healthy controls. However, other ACTH-dependent steroids, such as desoxycorticosterone (DOC), compound B, and 18-hydroxy-DOC, are not elevated and show a blunted response to ACTH stimulation, implying subnormal adrenal reserves. Patients who fail to achieve plasma cortisol levels greater than 20 μg per deciliter 60 minutes after corticotropin (ACTH) stimulation should be considered to have, or be at high risk of developing, adrenal insufficiency. Plasma corticotropin levels are frequently normal or subnormal even when plasma cortisol levels are depressed, suggesting that adrenal insufficiency in some HIV-infected patients is due to a primary pituitary or central nervous system disorder. Treatment of adrenal insufficiency in HIV-infected patients is no different than in other individuals with abnormal adrenal function.

HYPOGONADISM. The most common abnormality of endocrine function noted clinically is hypogonadism. Decreased libido occurs in over one half of male patients with AIDS, and impotence, usually associated with low serum testosterone levels, is reported in up to 30 per cent of AIDS patients. Serum gonadotropin levels may be below normal or inappropriately within normal limits in hypogonadal men with AIDS. When pituitary responsiveness to gonadotropin-releasing hormone is assessed in these hypogonadotropic males, normal release of luteinizing hormone (LH) and follicle-stimulating hormone (FSH) has been observed, suggesting a hypothalamic basis for the central hypogonadotropism. Other studies have demonstrated appropriately elevated levels of LH and FSH in hypogonadal men, implying primary testicular dysfunction. Studies of gonadal function in women are limited, although menstrual irregularities are common in women with advanced HIV disease.

THYROID DISEASE. Thyroid function remains remarkably normal throughout the course of HIV disease. Low levels of thyroxine (T_4), triiodothyronine (T_3), and free-thyroxine index (FTI) in the setting of low concentrations of thyrotropin (TSH), the so-called euthyroid sick syndrome, are remarkably uncommon among ambulatory HIV-infected patients. Decreased levels of T_3 resin uptake and elevated levels of T_4-binding globulin are frequently noted in ambulatory patients with advanced disease; however, concentrations of T_3 and T_4 are most often within normal limits. Invasive disease due to cytomegalovirus, *P. carinii*, *C. neoformans*, Kaposi's sarcoma, and lymphoma has been described in the thyroid. Remarkably, even patients with infiltrating opportunistic diseases of the thyroid gland usually remain euthyroid throughout the course of their disease. Nonetheless, despite the relative infrequency of clinical disease, hypothyroidism represents a potentially reversible cause of fatigue, malaise, altered mental status, and "failure to thrive" in HIV-infected individuals and should be routinely evaluated.

Less common causes of hypothyroidism in HIV-infected patients include adverse effects of medications. Ketoconazole has been associated with primary hypothyroidism on rare occasions. In addition, drugs that are strong inducers of hepatic microsomal enzymes, such as rifampin, may lead to increased clearance of T_4.

METABOLIC ABNORMALITIES. Hyponatremia is the most common electrolyte disturbance noted in HIV-infected individuals (see discussion in renal section). Disorders of carbohydrate metabolism have been reported in association with direct pancreatic invasion by opportunistic processes and with drug therapy. Pancreatic lesions caused by cytomegalovirus, toxoplasmosis, Kaposi's sarcoma, and lymphoma are noted in up to 35 per cent of cases at autopsy. Yet the development of type I diabetes mellitus has been reported in only a few instances. Hypoglycemia is the most common alteration in glucose metabolism. Direct toxic effects of drugs may induce premature release of insulin by β cells, resulting in hypoglycemic episodes that may be severe and prolonged. Pentamidine isothionate is the most common cause of hypoglycemia, occurring in 4 to 33 per cent of treated patients. Renal insufficiency is a predisposing factor in the development of pentamidine-induced hypoglycemia. Although most hypoglycemic episodes result from parenteral administration of pentamidine, several cases have been reported in patients receiving aerosolized drug.

Disorders of calcium metabolism are relatively uncommon but do occur. Hypercalcemia is associated with HIV-related leukemia and lymphoma. Hypocalcemia usually is the result of drug therapy with agents, such as amphotericin B and aminoglycosides, which induce magnesium wasting. Cytomegalovirus has been observed in parathyroid tissue; however, CMV-induced hypoparathyroidism is extremely rare.

RHEUMATOLOGIC DISEASE

Rheumatologic manifestations of HIV disease are being recognized with increased frequency. Musculoskeletal complaints are reported in 33 to 75 per cent of HIV-infected patients and may present as a wide variety of rheumatologic disorders (Table 420–3). The severity of disease ranges from intermittent arthralgias to debilitating arthritis and vasculitis. An array of autoimmune antibodies, including antinuclear, antiplatelet, antilymphocyte, antigranulocyte, and antiphospholipid (anticardiolipin and lupus anticoagulant) antibodies, are associated with HIV infection along with circulating immune complexes, rheumatoid factor, and cryoglobulins. Despite the presence of these antibodies in some patients, the precise mechanisms by which the rheumatologic abnormalities develop have not been elucidated and most likely are different for each particular disorder.

ARTHRALGIAS. Arthralgia is a common manifestation of acute HIV seroconversion, in addition to fever, myalgia, headache, sore throat, abdominal cramps, and lymphadenopathy. Generalized arthralgias are reported in up to one third of HIV-infected patients with minimally symptomatic disease. Some patients develop arthralgias and myalgias upon initiation of zidovudine therapy; however, these symptoms are usually self-limited and abate within 4 to 6 weeks after starting treatment. The "painful articular syndrome" is characterized by severe articular pain of 2 to 24 hours' duration. Although uncommon, this disorder is quite incapacitating and usually unresponsive to oral nonsteroidal anti-inflammatory agents or narcotic analgesics. The etiology of this disorder remains unknown. With the exception of the painful articular syndrome, most of the arthralgias associated with HIV disease are treated with nonsteroidal agents.

MYOPATHIES. Polymyositis-like illnesses, characterized by myalgias, proximal muscle weakness, and wasting, have been reported in several HIV-infected patients and have been the initial HIV-defining presentation in a few. The findings of creatinine phosphokinase (CPK) elevation (greater than five times

TABLE 420–3. RHEUMATOLOGIC DISEASES ASSOCIATED WITH HIV INFECTION

Autoimmune phenomena
  Anticardiolipin antibodies
  Antigranulocyte antibodies
  Antilymphocyte antibodies
  Antinuclear antibodies
  Antiplatelet antibodies
  Circulating immune complexes
  Cryoglobulins
  Rheumatoid factor
Dermatologic disorders
  Dermatomyositis
  Malar flush
  Psoriasis
Joint disease
  Arthralgias
  Arthritis
  Enthesopathies
  HIV-associated arthritis
  "Painful articular syndrome"
  Psoriatic arthritis
  Reactive arthropathy
  Reiter's disease
  Septic arthritis
  Systemic lupus erythematosus (lupus-like syndrome)
Myopathies
  Infectious (septic) myositis
  Myalgias
    Idiopathic
    Zidovudine-associated
  Necrotizing, noninflammatory myopathy
  Nemaline rod polymyositis
  Polymyositis
Sjögren's syndrome
  Sicca complex
Vasculitis
  Central nervous system angiitis
  Eosinophilic vasculitis
  Leukocytoclastic vasculitis
  Polyarteritis nodosa

normal) and abnormal electromyography are indistinguishable from those of idiopathic polymyositis. Muscle biopsies reveal necrosis, fibrosis, and inflammation, but usually to a lesser extent than is noted in non–HIV-infected individuals. The presence of nemaline rods, often noted in muscle biopsies of older adults with myositis, suggests the likelihood of underlying HIV infection when noted in biopsy specimens obtained from younger adults, especially in the absence of inflammation.

Although virus-like particles have been demonstrated on rare occasions in synovial tissue and HIV p24 antigen has been noted in the cytoplasm of degenerating muscle cells, no specific viral etiology has been determined. All attempts to culture HIV-1 from muscle tissue of patients with myositis have been unsuccessful.

Patients receiving long-term zidovudine therapy may develop myositis characterized by muscle weakness, elevated CPK levels, myalgias, and evidence of myopathy with a paucity of inflammatory cells on biopsy. Zidovudine-associated myositis usually responds to drug discontinuation and may recur on rechallenge. No definitive therapy exists for HIV-associated polymyositis, although corticosteroid therapy has been successful in reversing symptoms in some patients. If corticosteroid therapy is contemplated, the potential risks of superimposing immunosuppressive therapy on an immunocompromised host must be considered.

REITER'S SYNDROME. Reiter's syndrome is noted in up to 10 per cent of HIV-infected patients who develop arthritis, and an additional 10 to 20 per cent of patients are classified as having "reactive arthritis" because they lack the nonarticular features of Reiter's. Severe, persistent oligoarticular arthritis associated with urethritis, conjunctivitis, painless oral ulcerations, keratoderma blennorrhagicum, or circinate balanitis is the hallmark of Reiter's disease in both HIV-infected and noninfected individuals. Clinical manifestations of Reiter's syndrome may precede or occur at the time of the initial diagnosis of HIV infection but most often follow the onset of immunodeficiency. HLA-B27 positivity is noted in

65 to 75 per cent of HIV-infected patients with Reiter's syndrome. However, studies of African HIV patients with Reiter's disease or reactive arthritis revealed no increased incidence of HLA-B27, suggesting involvement of other gene markers in this group (see Ch. 259). *Shigella, Campylobacter, Ureaplasma,* and other bacterial species associated with the development of reactive arthropathies are rarely described in HIV patients with Reiter's syndrome. However, underlying concomitant sexually transmitted disease(s) may prove to be an important etiologic factor.

Treatment options for HIV patients with Reiter's disease are quite limited. Responses to nonsteroidal anti-inflammatory agents are minimal, and more potent immunosuppressive agents, such as methotrexate and azathioprine, frequently lead to the development of opportunistic diseases and Kaposi's sarcoma shortly after initiation of therapy.

SJÖGREN'S SYNDROME. Xerophthalmia and xerostomia, the characteristic symptoms of Sjögren's syndrome (SS), have been reported with increasing frequency in AIDS patients. Features that closely resemble idiopathic SS, including sicca symptoms, a positive Schirmer test, abnormal salivary gland emptying, and abnormal salivary gland biopsies, have been reported in HIV-infected patients. As a result, it has been suggested that AIDS be an exclusionary disease for the diagnosis of idiopathic SS. The predominance of male patients, the absence of anti-Ro/SS-A and anti-La/SS-B antibodies, the absence of a well-defined connective tissue disease, the presence of HLA-DR52 and DR5 alleles instead of the characteristic A1, B8, DR3, DR2, and DQ1/DQ2 antigens, and a predominance of CD8+ lymphocytes instead of CD4+ cells infiltrating salivary tissue are the characteristic features of AIDS-associated SS, which differs from classic idiopathic SS. Treatment is primarily symptomatic.

SEPTIC ARTHRITIS. Joint space infection is remarkably uncommon in HIV-infected patients. Sporadic case reports have been published of septic arthritis due to fungal pathogens, such as *C. neoformans, H. capsulatum,* and *S. schenkii,* mycobacteria, and routine pyogenic organisms. The approach to diagnosis and treatment of septic arthritis is no different for HIV-infected patients than non–HIV-infected individuals.

HIV-ASSOCIATED ARTHROPATHY. A relatively uncommon arthritis has been described in patients with moderately advanced HIV disease who demonstrate no other signs of any recognizable rheumatologic disease. The so-called HIV-associated arthropathy (HIVAA) presents as a mono- or pauciarticular arthritis. The arthritis is usually severe, affects primarily the knees and ankles, and lasts from 1 week to 6 months. No extra-articular manifestations have been noted. The synovial fluid is noninflammatory in nature, although a mild synovitis consisting of a chronic mononuclear cell infiltrate is noted on biopsy. Rheumatoid factor, antinuclear antibodies, anti-DNA antibodies, and antibodies against RNP, Sm, Ro/SS-A, and La/SS-B are negative. No predominant HLA pattern has been described. Nonsteroidal anti-inflammatory agents are of some benefit, but some patients require intra-articular steroid injections.

VASCULITIS. Several varieties of vasculitis have been reported in association with HIV infection. Necrotizing vasculitis of the polyarteritis nodosa type is reported most commonly and presents as a peripheral sensory or sensorimotor neuropathy. The vasculitis involves the medium-sized vessels of the nerves, skin, and muscle. None of the reported patients with HIV-related PAN were hepatitis B surface antigen positive. Primary angiitis of the central nervous system has been noted in two patients, one of whom had persistent varicella-zoster virus infection. Lymphomatoid granulomatosis has also been reported in HIV-infected patients.

It is unclear whether HIV-associated vasculitis is the result of direct HIV invasion of the vessels, an immunologic reaction to an underlying viral infection, or a response to an opportunistic viral pathogen that invades vascular tissue. As with other serious rheumatologic manifestations of HIV disease, treatment options are limited by the underlying immunodeficiency of the host.

Acierno LJ: Cardiac complications in acquired immunodeficiency syndrome (AIDS): A review. J Am Coll Cardiol 13:1144–1154, 1989. *An in-depth review of potential pathogenic mechanisms responsible for HIV-associated cardiac disease.*

Aron DC: Endocrine complications of the acquired immunodeficiency syndrome. Arch Intern Med 149:330–333, 1989. *An overview of common endocrine disorders in HIV-infected patients.*

Calabrese LH: The rheumatic manifestations of infection with the human immunodeficiency virus. Semin Arthritis Rheum 18:225–239, 1989. *Comprehensive review of rheumatologic disease in HIV-infected patients with special emphasis on autoantibodies and disease pathogenesis.*

Dobs AS, Dempsey MA, Ladenson PW, et al.: Endocrine disorders in men infected with human immunodeficiency virus. Am J Med 84:611–616, 1988. *A review of AIDS-related endocrine abnormalities with special emphasis on hypogonadism and pituitary function.*

Glassock RJ, Cohen AH, Danovitch G, et al.: Human immunodeficiency virus (HIV) infection and the kidney. Ann Intern Med 112:35–49, 1990. *A comprehensive overview of renal disorders associated with HIV infection.*

Kaye BR: Rheumatologic manifestations of infection with human immunodeficiency virus (HIV). Ann Intern Med 111:158–167, 1989. *Clinically relevant review of rheumatologic diseases in AIDS patients.*

Nyamathi A: AIDS-related heart disease: A review of the literature. J Cardiovasc Nurs 3(4):65–76, 1989. *A thorough review of the cardiac manifestations of HIV infection.*

Sreepada Rao TK, Friedman EA: AIDS (HIV)-associated nephropathy; does it exist? Am J Nephrol 9:441–453, 1989. *A nice discussion comparing HIVAN to HAN; it establishes a strong argument for HIVAN as a distinct entity.*

---

421 Treatment of AIDS and Related Disorders

Robert Yarchoan and Samuel Broder

The last several years have seen a dramatic change in the approach to the treatment of AIDS and related disorders. In 1984, therapy was either entirely supportive or directed at a bewildering array of infectious and oncologic complications. Since that time, the identification of human immunodeficiency virus (HIV) as the causative agent of AIDS and the elucidation of the life cycle of this virus has enabled the development of specific antiretroviral therapy. Such therapy is now recognized as central to the treatment of these diseases. In addition, there is now an intense effort to evaluate new agents and combinations of agents, and the majority of AIDS patients at least consider experimental treatment at some time in the course of their illness. In this chapter, we review the current recommendations for AIDS therapy. In addition, we discuss certain experimental approaches that are now under active clinical development. In AIDS as perhaps in no other disease, the line between approved and experimental therapy is difficult to draw.

The immunodeficiency in AIDS results, either directly or indirectly, from the progressive destruction of the immune system by HIV. In addition, HIV infection affects other organ systems (such as the central nervous system). T lymphocytes bearing CD4 antigen on their surface (CD4 cells or T4 cells), monocytes, macrophages, and monocyte-derived cells such as microglial cells are now recognized as the principal cellular targets for HIV. Although other cells are also susceptible to infection, the clinical significance of this phenomenon is unclear. In infected individuals, the development and progression of disease require at least some level of ongoing infection of new cells by HIV. Thus, one could reason that interference with HIV replication in vivo could halt or even reverse the progression of disease to AIDS. Indeed, the successful development of antiretroviral therapy has shown this to be the case.

AZIDOTHYMIDINE (ZIDOVUDINE) AND OTHER DIDEOXYNUCLEOSIDES

The first antiretroviral drug to be developed and approved for the therapy of HIV infection was 3′-azido—2′,3′-dideoxythymidine, also called azidothymidine, zidovudine, or AZT (Fig. 421–1). This drug was initially synthesized by Jerome Horwitz as an anticancer drug in 1964. At the National Cancer Institute in 1985 it was found to inhibit HIV replication in human T cells in vitro and was later found to have anti-HIV activity in monocytes and macrophages. AZT is a member of a family of compounds called dideoxynucleosides, in which the 3′-hydroxy (-OH) group is replaced by another group that does not form phosphodiester linkages. In the case of AZT, the 3′-hydroxy group of thymidine

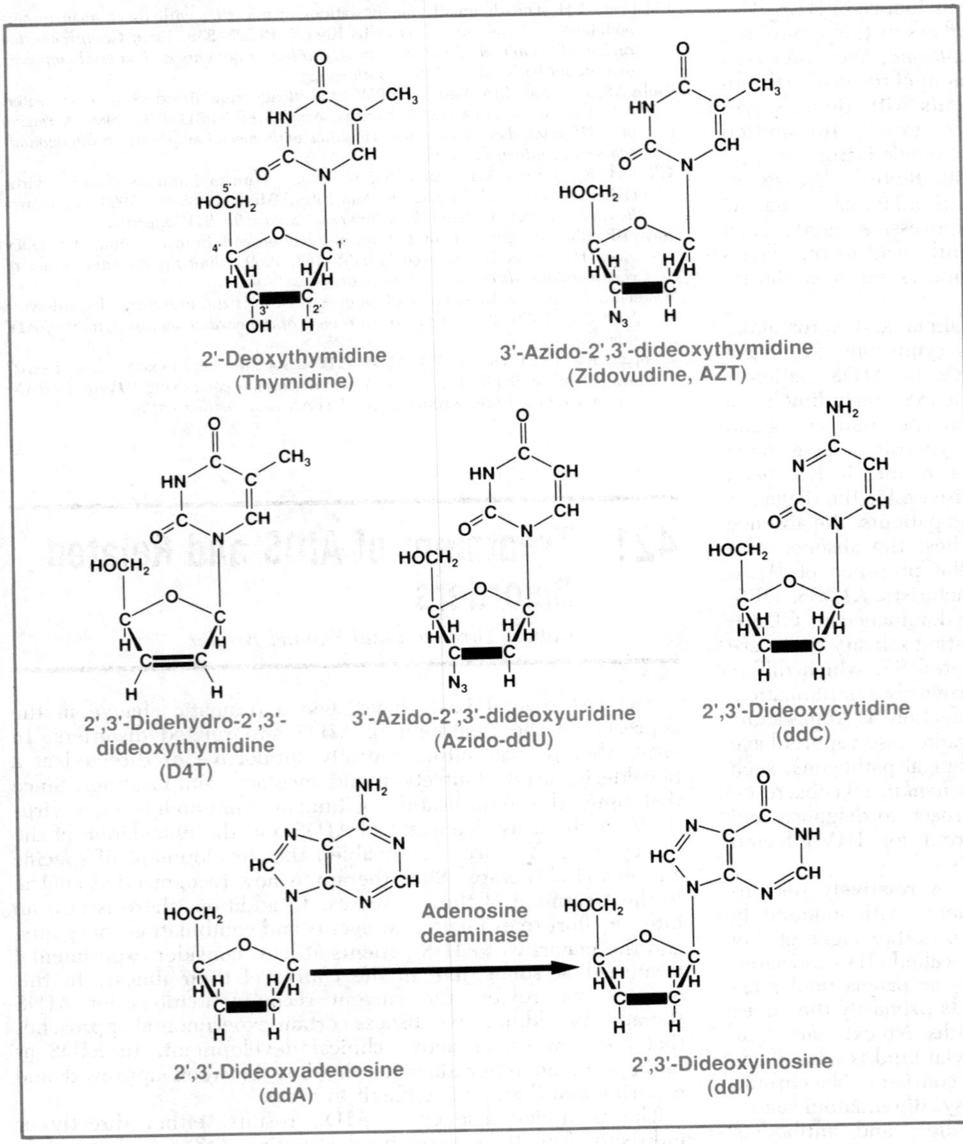

FIGURE 421–1. *Top,* Structures of thymidine (*left*) and AZT (*right*). The 3'hydroxy (-OH) group of thymidine is replaced by an azido (-N₃) group to form AZT. *Middle,* Three other dideoxypyrimidines undergoing clinical testing as anti-AIDS drugs. *Bottom,* Two dideoxypurines undergoing clinical testing as anti-AIDS drugs. Dideoxyadenosine (ddA) is rapidly converted to dideoxyinosine (ddI) by the ubiquitous enzyme adenosine deaminase, and these can be considered alternate forms of the same drug for many purposes. (Modified from Yarchoan R, Mitsuya H, Myers CE, Broder S: Clinical pharmacology of 3'-azido-2',3'-dideoxythymidine (zidovudine) and related dideoxynucleosides. N Engl J Med 321:726–738, 1989. Reprinted by permission of the New England Journal of Medicine.)

is replaced by an azido (-N₃) group. A number of members of this family have been found to be potent inhibitors of HIV replication in vitro, and several, including AZT, have been shown to have clinical activity in patients with HIV infection.

Upon entering human cells, AZT and other dideoxynucleosides are activated (phosphorylated) to form a 5'-triphosphate moiety. This activation process, called anabolic phosphorylation, utilizes a series of enzymes (kinases) which usually serve to phosphorylate deoxynucleosides (Fig. 421–2). There are substantial differences in the rates at which human cells phosphorylate these compounds and in their enzymatic pathways, and these differences may be important in their antiretroviral activity and differing toxicity profiles. AZT, for example, is much more potent than 2',3'-dideoxythymidine (ddT) in human cells because of differences in the rate of phosphorylation. Also, the rates of phosphorylation vary markedly between species, and one cannot draw conclusions about the activity of dideoxynucleosides in human cells on the basis of animal models.

As triphosphates, dideoxynucleosides act as inhibitors at the level of HIV DNA polymerase (reverse transcriptase). This unique viral enzyme catalyzes the conversion of HIV genetic information from RNA to DNA and subsequently catalyzes the formation of a second viral DNA strand, i.e., a copy complementary to the first. The activity of reverse transcriptase is essential for HIV replication to occur. As 5-triphosphates, dideoxynucleosides are believed to inhibit reverse transcriptase in two ways. First, they can act as DNA chain terminators: Once added to the end of a growing chain of viral DNA, the chain is elongated by exactly one residue and no further nucleotides can be added because of the 3'-modification. Also, as triphosphates they act as competitive inhibitors for the binding of the physiologic nucleoside-5'-triphosphates to relevant sites within reverse transcriptase. Reverse transcriptase, but not mammalian DNA polymerase α, preferentially utilizes dideoxynucleoside-5'-triphosphates in place of the respective physiologic 5'-triphosphates, and this is most likely the basis for their selective antiretroviral activity. However, human mitochondrial DNA polymerase (γ) is relatively sensitive to inhibition by certain of these drugs, and this may be a basis for certain toxicities. As with virtually any explanation for the mechanism of action for a new drug, the physician should always bear in mind that new knowledge could modify or supplant any working theory.

Clinical Activity of AZT (Zidovudine)

Phase I and II clinical trials of AZT conducted during the years 1985 and 1986 convincingly showed that the drug could be administered to patients and was effective at reducing morbidity and mortality in patients with severe HIV infection (Fig. 421–3). Patients with AIDS or severe ARC had an increase in the number of T4 cells, improved immunologic function, and a decrease in the viral load (as assessed by HIV p24 antigenemia) upon receiving AZT. In addition, patients had increased appetite, gained

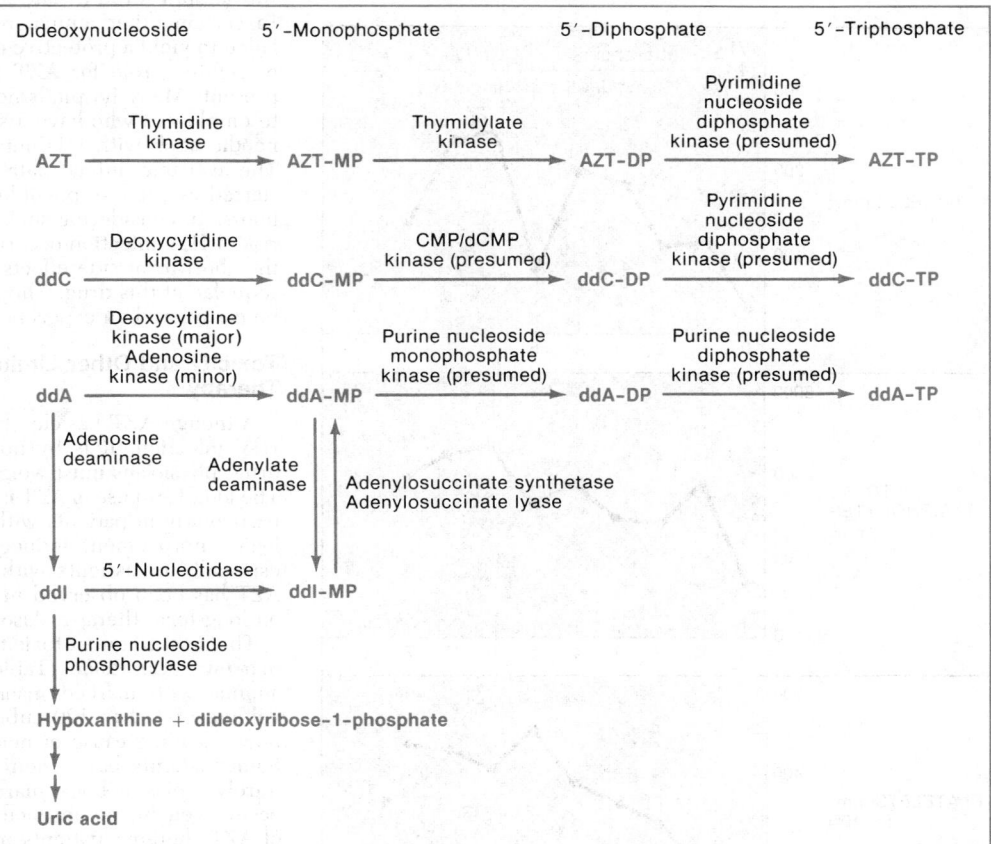

FIGURE 421–2. Activation pathways for AZT, ddC, ddA, and ddI to the active triphosphate moieties in human cells. MP = 5'-monophosphate; DP = 5'-diphosphate; TP = 5'-triphosphate.

weight, and often reported feeling better at least temporarily. In a multicenter randomized trial in which AZT was compared with placebo, patients who had severe ARC or who had had *Pneumocystis carinii* pneumonia (PCP) were found to have a markedly reduced mortality and incidence of opportunistic infections upon receiving AZT as compared with patients on the placebo arm. Some (but not all) of this reduced mortality could be attributed to the T4 increases induced by AZT. Based on these studies, AZT was initially approved for patients with severe HIV infection at a recommended dosage of 200 mg every 4 hours (1200 mg per day) around the clock. Since that time, it has been found that a maintenance regimen of 100 mg every 4 hours (600 mg per day), initiated after a month's therapy with 200 mg every 4 hours, is as effective as the initially recommended regimen and is associated with less toxicity. This is the currently recommended dosage schedule. Many physicians are now suggesting that their patients omit waking up to take their nighttime dose; however, while this 500-mg daily regimen has been found to be effective in asymptomatic patients with fewer than 500 T4 cells per cubic millimeter (see below), it has not formally been proven in patients with AIDS. Studies are now underway to examine the effectiveness of even lower dosages of AZT, and physicians should be keenly alert for possible future modifications of the recommended dosage of this drug.

The pharmacokinetic profile of AZT is one of the factors that guides its usage. AZT is well absorbed by mouth; the average oral bioavailability is 63 per cent. The circulating half-life is approximately 1.1 hours. It is because of this relatively short half-life that a dosing schedule of every 4 hours was initially recommended. However, other dosing regimens are now being examined. Fifteen to 20 per cent of an administered dose of AZT is excreted unchanged in the urine, while approximately 75 per cent undergoes glucuronidation to an inactive form in the liver. AZT glucuronidation can be inhibited by certain other drugs, such as probenecid, which share this pathway, and these drugs can prolong the half-life of AZT. However, certain other drugs that undergo hepatic glucuronidation (e.g., acetaminophen) have no such effect. Studies are underway to evaluate the interactions

of other drugs with AZT. Finally, AZT penetrates effectively into the cerebrospinal fluid.

Two large randomized studies recently conducted by the AIDS Clinical Trials Group of the National Institutes of Allergy and Infectious Diseases showed that AZT could reduce the short-term progression to AIDS or severe ARC in patients with 200 to 500 T4 cells per cubic millimeter. One of these trials involved asymptomatic patients, and the other involved patients with minimal symptoms. As a result of these studies, AZT (100 mg every 4 hours) is now recommended for HIV-infected patients with less than 500 T4 cells per cubic millimeter. Physicians should be aware, however, that patients in those studies were followed only for 3 months to 2 years and that no improvement in overall survival was formally proven. As noted above, a formal survival benefit had been shown in advanced AIDS or ARC. Long-term AZT therapy may be associated with cumulative toxicity and the development of viral resistance, and it is not proven at this point whether early intervention with AZT improves long-term survival. We will return to these points below.

AZT was made widely available in the United States in the fall of 1986 for patients who had had PCP, and it was approved as a prescription drug in the spring of 1987. There are epidemiologic data that the widespread use of AZT since that time has played a role in substantially lengthening the survival of patients with AIDS. In New York State, the 18-month survival of homosexual men with AIDS increased from 34.8 per cent in patients diagnosed in 1985 to 62.9 per cent in patients diagnosed in 1987. It is likely that other advances in the diagnosis, prevention, and treatment of complications of AIDS (particularly chemoprophylaxis for PCP) have contributed to this effect. However, where this specific factor has been looked at, the effect of AZT on survival has been observed over and above any contribution from *Pneumocystis* prophylaxis. Also, although AZT has only recently been approved specifically for patients with 200 to 500 T4 cells per cubic millimeter, it has been widely used in such patients during the past several years by physicians practicing in the community. There is now epidemiologic evidence that by delaying the development of fulminant AIDS in HIV-infected individ-

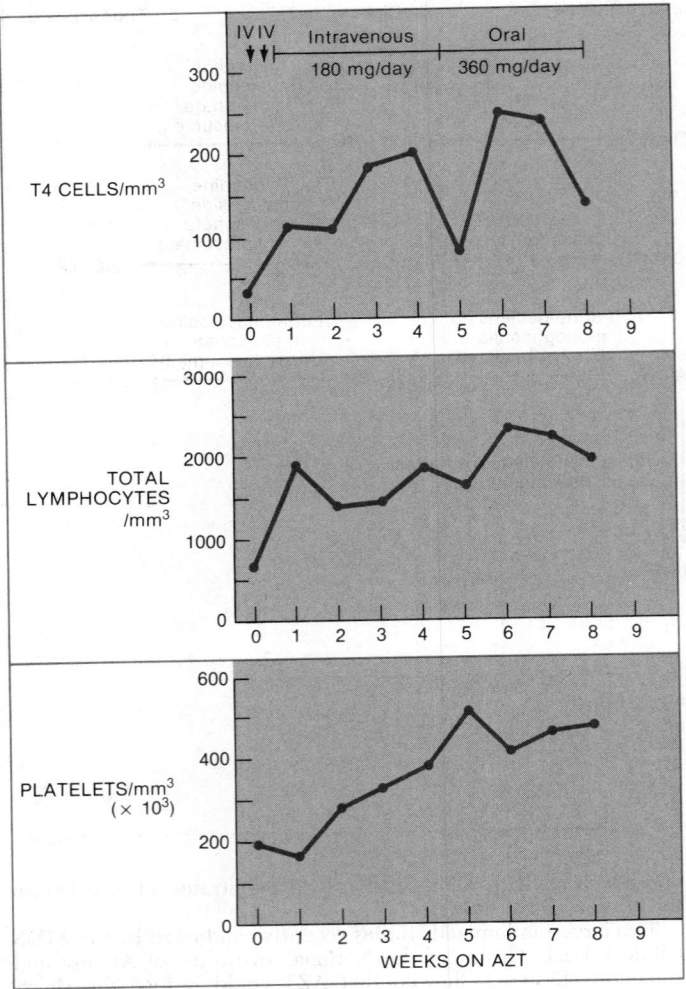

FIGURE 421–3. Course of the first patient ever to receive AZT. This patient, who had recently recovered from *Pneumocystis carinii* pneumonia, was treated on the National Cancer Institute service of the National Institutes of Health Clinical Center with 180 mg per day of AZT intravenously for 4 weeks, followed by 360 mg per day orally for 4 weeks.

uals, this early use of AZT may have led to an unexpected decline in the incidence of new AIDS cases (Fig. 421–4).

As mentioned above, AZT can penetrate into the cerebrospinal fluid. Several studies have shown that AZT can reverse HIV-induced cognitive dysfunction or even frank dementia. Patients have been observed to have improvement on psychometric testing, and, in several cases studied by positron emission tomography, there has been a normalization of the pattern of glucose metabolism in the brain (see Color Plate 12F). The reversal of HIV dementia has been particularly striking in HIV-infected children. In this population, neurologic dysfunction is a particularly prominent feature of HIV infection. It is possible that the ability of AZT to reverse HIV-induced dementia results in part from its ability to protect monocyte-derived cells in the brain (such as microglial cells) from HIV infection. However, much more needs to be learned about the pathogenesis of HIV dementia and the mechanism of AZT's effect on this disorder.

An unresolved question at present is whether AZT given at the time of exposure can protect against HIV infection. In several animal retroviral systems, a short course of AZT given at the time of inoculation was found to prevent infection from occurring. More recently, this issue has been examined by McCune and colleagues in mice with genetically determined severe combined immunodeficiency disease reconstituted with a human immune system (SCID-hu mouse). When a 2-week course of AZT was administered to such mice within 2 hours of an intravenous inoculum of HIV, no evidence of viral infection was detected. In

certain instances, protection was conferred even when the drug was administered as late as 36 hours after the viral inoculation. In certain other animal retroviral systems, however, AZT has failed to yield a protective effect, and there are no data to confirm or refute a role for AZT as a prophylactic drug in humans at present. Many hospitals now offer a 4- to 6-week course of AZT to employees who have a substantial exposure to HIV, such as a needle stick with HIV-infected blood or a laboratory accident. The available animal data suggest that if used, AZT should be started as soon as possible after the exposure, ideally within 2 hours. In considering such therapy, physicians should weigh the risk of HIV infection occurring (about 1 in 200 for a needle stick), the short-term side effects of AZT, and the unknown long-term sequelae of this drug. They should also be aware that this should be considered an experimental use of AZT.

Toxicity and Other Limitations of AZT (Zidovudine) Therapy

Although AZT has clearly been shown to benefit patients with HIV infection, it is by no means a perfect drug. As with any drug, physicians must weigh the risks versus benefits of therapy. The long-term use of AZT is associated with a number of toxicities, particularly in patients with advanced AIDS. Also, the immunologic improvement induced by AZT may be only temporary, especially in patients with AIDS, and a reduced sensitivity to AZT has been observed in strains of HIV isolated from patients on long-term therapy. Also, AZT does not cure AIDS.

The most frequent toxicity associated with AZT therapy is bone marrow suppression (Table 421–1). The earliest sign is often anemia with marked macrocytic changes; a mean corpuscular volume of 110 to 120 cubic microns is not uncommon. AZT is now a leading cause of macrocytosis in several medical centers. Some patients have been observed to develop hypocellular or (rarely) aplastic bone marrows while receiving AZT. This can occur even in the absence of macrocytosis. Later in the course of AZT therapy, patients may become neutropenic or thrombocytopenic. In some patients, the platelet count remains stable or paradoxically increases for some time, perhaps reflecting an effect against underlying HIV-induced thrombocytopenia. AZT-induced bone marrow suppression is most common in patients with advanced AIDS, low T4 counts, pretherapy anemia, and pretherapy neutropenia. It is less problematic with the recently recommended dosage of 600 mg per day; however, even with this dosing schedule, it can occur in 30 per cent or so of patients with advanced disease during the first year of therapy. It is unclear at the present time whether it is preferable to continue the same dose of AZT once patients become anemic and to provide transfusion therapy or to reduce the dose of AZT. It is possible that monitoring of HIV p24 antigenemia will be found to be useful in guiding individual therapy in such situations. HIV-infected patients often have vitamin deficiencies, particularly of vitamin B_{12}, and megaloblastic anemia from folic acid or vitamin B_{12} deficiency bears a certain similarity to AZT toxicity. It may thus be prudent to measure serum levels of folic acid and vitamin B_{12} and give replacement therapy if they are low; however, this intervention has not been shown to prevent or reverse AZT toxicity. It has been shown that administration of genetically engineered erythropoietin (epoetin alfa) can partially ameliorate AZT-induced anemia, particularly in patients who do not have markedly elevated erythropoietin levels. For such patients (with erythropoietin levels of <500 mU per millimeter) epoetin alfa should be considered at starting doses of 100 U per kilogram administered intravenously or subcutaneously three times per week. Other hematopoietic cytokines are now being investigated for AZT-induced marrow suppression.

Myalgias are also common in patients receiving AZT. In addition, after long-term therapy (e.g., a year or more), a subset of patients may develop frank myopathy with muscle wasting and sometimes (but not always) elevations of creatine kinase. In rare cases, this side effect can lead to a catastrophic failure of systemic muscles. AZT-induced myositis can usually be distinguished from myositis caused by HIV by the presence of "ragged red" fibers on biopsy, indicative of abnormal mitochondria (see Color Plate 12G). Paracrystalline inclusions in the mitochondria can be seen on electron microscopy. It is believed that this toxicity results from the inhibitory effect of AZT-5′-triphosphate on mammalian

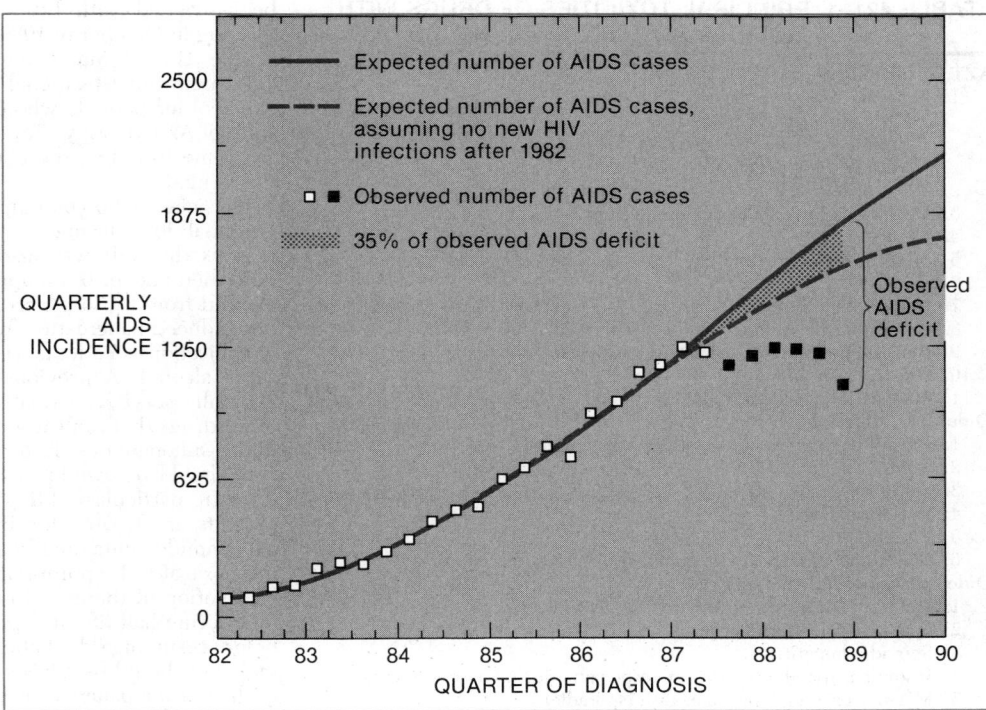

FIGURE 421–4. Decrease in the observed number of cases of AIDS in homosexual men in San Francisco, Los Angeles, and New York since the middle of 1987. The solid line depicts the number of AIDS cases expected. The dashed line depicts the number of AIDS cases that would be expected if one makes the extreme assumption that, as a result of safe sex practices and other public health measures, no patients became infected with HIV after 1982. It was about this time that sexual practices began to change in response to the awareness that AIDS was a sexually transmitted disease. As can be seen, the deficit in AIDS cases since the middle of 1987 is largely attributed to changes in the therapy of HIV-infected individuals before they develop AIDS, including the administration of AZT. Only 35 per cent of the AIDS deficit could be explained by an absence of new infections with HIV after 1982. AZT became a prescription drug in March, 1987. (Reproduced with permission from Gail MH, et al: J AIDS 3:296–306, 1990.)

γ DNA polymerase, an enzyme found in the mitochondrial matrix. Some patients with this toxicity respond to a nonsteroidal anti-inflammatory drug, with or without a reduction in the dose of AZT. In other cases, it may be necessary to discontinue the AZT. Certain patients who do not respond to the above interventions have been reported to respond to therapy with prednisone (40 to 60 mg daily). However, this potentially dangerous immunosuppressive drug should be used only as a last resort in severe cases.

Patients receiving AZT frequently complain of malaise, fatigue, nausea, or headaches. These often become less severe after several weeks on the drug. However, in a subset of patients, these symptoms are intolerable. Some patients, particularly blacks, develop bluish fingernail coloration as a result of AZT therapy (see Color Plate 12E). Finally, clinicians should be aware that AZT has been found in animal studies to be mutagenic and to cause an increased incidence of vaginal tumors in rodents administered life-long high-dose drug. At the present time, the implications of such findings to the treatment of HIV infection are still unclear; however, they do suggest that AZT should not be casually administered to patients without specific indications or outside of an approved clinical trial. AZT should be used in pregnant HIV patients with great caution and preferably only in the context of a clinical trial.

Improved survival from antiretroviral therapy may permit AIDS patients to live long enough to develop certain HIV-related complications. In particular, an unexpectedly high incidence of non-Hodgkin's lymphoma, in some instances approaching 10 per cent of patients per year, has been observed in AIDS patients who have been followed for several years on AZT-containing regimens. These are almost certainly not caused by AZT, but instead appear to represent the development of opportunistic tumors in immunosuppressed patients. The situation is analogous to that of certain genetic immunodeficiency diseases in which the cumulative incidence of tumors was observed to increase when survival is enhanced by improved anti-infective therapy.

Even in patients who tolerate AZT, there are limitations to its long-term use. Although a majority of patients have increases in the number of T4 cells during the first several weeks of therapy, the increases are often transient, particularly in patients with advanced AIDS. In the original Phase II trial of AZT, there was no final difference in the number of T4 cells between the AZT-treated group and the placebo-treated group after 6 months of

therapy. It is conceivable that lower-dose regimens (perhaps by reducing cumulative toxicity in lymphocytes) could yield better performance in this regard.

Some patients who initially have a decrease in their p24 antigenemia upon starting AZT may have late increases while continuing on therapy. Isolates of HIV from patients who have received AZT for over 1 year frequently have reduced sensitivity to AZT. There is suggestive evidence that this may occur as a result of a defined set of mutations in the reverse transcriptase. Interestingly, strains of HIV which have become resistant to AZT have been found to preserve their sensitivity to most other dideoxynucleosides. The clinical significance of these changes in in vitro sensitivity is not clear at this time.

Clinicians frequently ask whether AZT should be continued in patients on long-term therapy who had initial T4 rises but subsequent falls to or below baseline on long-term treatment. There are at present no controlled trials to address this issue. However, one could argue that as long as the drug is reasonably tolerated, suppression of HIV replication to some degree is probably beneficial and AZT therapy should be continued. Such patients will of course be likely beneficiaries of any new effective anti-HIV therapies that may become available.

Other Dideoxynucleosides

As noted above, AZT is one member of the family of compounds called dideoxynucleosides (see Fig. 421–1). More than a score of other dideoxynucleosides have been found to be active against HIV in the laboratory. Of these, 2′,3′-dideoxycytidine (ddC), 2′,3′-dideoxyadenosine (ddA), 2′,3′-dideoxyinosine (ddI), 2′,3′-didehydro-2′,3′-dideoxythymidine (D4T), and 3′-azido-2′,3′-dideoxyuridine (azido-ddU) have entered clinical testing, and trials of others are planned. Several halogenated congeners of these drugs are quite interesting. As noted above, these compounds are believed to inhibit HIV by the same general mechanism as AZT. However, because of differences in their intracellular or extracellular metabolism and effects on normal nucleotides, various dideoxynucleosides may have fundamentally different activity and toxicity profiles. Each must be considered a different drug.

ddC, the first of these other dideoxynucleosides to be tested in vivo, was found to reduce the viral load and improve virologic parameters in patients with AIDS or ARC. The drug has excellent bioavailability. Patients receiving ddC generally did not develop bone marrow suppression. However, a reversible painful periph-

TABLE 421–1. PRINCIPAL TOXICITIES OF DRUGS WITH ANTIRETROVIRAL ACTIVITY USED IN AIDS

AZT (Zidovudine)
1. Bone marrow suppression
   Red cells usually affected more than white cells or platelets
   Prominent increase in red cell mean corpuscular volume
   Marrow may become hypocellular
2. Malaise, fever, fatigue (especially during first few weeks)
3. Headaches (especially during first few weeks)
4. Myalgias
5. Myositis (in approximately 10% of patients after long-term use)
6. Seizures (can be fatal)
7. Nausea, vomiting
8. Confusion, tremulousness (especially with high doses)
9. Bluish pigmentation of nails (especially in blacks)
10. Hepatic transaminase elevations
11. Stevens-Johnson syndrome (very rare)

Dideoxycytidine (ddC)
1. Painful peripheral neuropathy (involving feet)
2. Aphthous stomatitis
3. Skin rash (transient)
4. Fevers, malaise
5. Diarrhea
6. Thrombocytopenia, neutropenia (at high doses)

Dideoxyinosine (ddI, didanosine)
1. Painful peripheral neuropathy (involving feet)
2. Sporadic pancreatitis (can be fatal)
3. Sporadic hepatitis
4. Insomnia, irritability, anxiety (especially during first few weeks)
5. Macular erythematous skin rash (sporadic)
6. Increases in uric acid (from ddI metabolism)
7. Hyperamylasemia, hypertriglyceridemia
8. Diarrhea, hypokalemia (from citrate/phosphate/sucrose vehicle)
9. Neutropenia, thrombocytopenia (rare, relationship to drug unclear)
10. Seizures (relationship to drug unclear)
11. Dry mouth
12. Confusion (especially when administered with triazolam)

Interferon-α
1. Flulike symptoms very common (fatigue, fever, chills, myalgias)
2. Headaches (common)
3. Nausea, vomiting, anorexia, weight loss (common)
4. Diarrhea (common)
5. Bone marrow suppression
6. Hepatitis, hepatic transaminase and alkaline phosphatase elevations
7. Rash, dry skin, pruritus
8. Congestive cardiopathy (sporadic)
9. Decreased mental status, depression, visual disturbances
10. Hypotension
11. Inflammation at injection sites

eral neuropathy was found to be the dose-limiting toxicity. Additional studies have shown that the development of this neuropathy can be delayed or prevented by administration of a carefully selected regimen of low-dose ddC or through intermittent dosing. Some patients receiving ddC also developed aphthous stomatitis or skin rashes; these generally subsided even with continued ddC administration. ddC is now being studied further, both as a single agent and in combination with AZT. In addition, it is being made available, under the mechanism of an open label protocol, to certain patients with advanced disease who have failed or cannot tolerate AZT.

Another dideoxynucleoside, ddI, was also found in initial clinical testing to be well absorbed by the oral route when given with appropriate buffers (oral bioavailability 40 per cent) and to have antiviral activity in patients with AIDS or ARC. In addition, patients not heavily pretreated with AZT had increases in T4 cells upon receiving ddI. At high doses, ddI was found to cause painful peripheral neuropathy. The drug can also cause acute pancreatitis. ddI can be catabolized to hypoxanthine and subsequently to uric acid, and asymptomatic hyperuricemia has been observed in some patients receiving very high doses of ddI. Other adverse reactions were generally not severe enough to warrant discontinuation of therapy (Table 421–1). In contrast to AZT, bone marrow toxicity was not prominent, even in patients

receiving high doses. Also, intermediate doses of ddI (e.g., 500 to 750 mg per day) were found to have anti-HIV activity but to be associated with little long-term toxicity in most patients. Starting in October of 1989, ddI was made available to physicians in the United States under the regulatory mechanisms of a Treatment Investigational New Drug Program or Open Label Protocol for patients who cannot tolerate AZT or were failing in spite of AZT therapy. Several large studies of ddI were begun at that time to define the efficacy and long-term toxicity profile of this drug.

Physicians who contemplate using ddI should be aware of its potential for causing acute pancreatitis. During the initial 6 months that ddI was made available under the two programs described above, 6 of approximately 7000 patients receiving ddI expired from acute pancreatitis. It can be difficult to distinguish ddI-induced pancreatitis from that caused by HIV infection or its complications. Patients receiving ddI should be counseled to avoid alcohol. A previous history of pancreatic disease should generally serve as a relative contraindication for ddI use. Also, other drugs that can cause pancreatitis, such as systemic pentamidine, sulfonamides, furosemide, and thiazide diuretics (see Ch. 106) should be avoided whenever possible in patients receiving ddI. In particular, ddI should be temporarily stopped when patients are treated for PCP with intravenous pentamidine or sulfonamide-containing regimens (including trimethoprim-sulfamethoxazole). If appropriate, ddI can then be restarted after the completion of therapy. In the case of pentamidine, which has a long serum half-life, it is probably prudent to wait at least 1 week before resuming ddI. Patients receiving ddI who develop abdominal pain should be advised to stop the drug immediately and be evaluated for pancreatitis. Physicians should probably avoid administering cimetidine or ranitidine along with ddI, as those drugs have the potential of increasing the absorption of ddI and can cause pancreatitis in their own right. Although ddI has a serum half-life of only 40 minutes, it remains a long time in lymphocytes after being metabolized to a triphosphate. For these reasons, it is currently being administered every 12 hours. The recommended oral doses of ddI for adults are now 334 to 750 mg per day, depending on the patient's weight. However, it is likely that the recommendations for ddI therapy will be modified as we learn more about this drug.

OTHER ANTI-HIV THERAPIES

The development of anti-HIV therapy is currently an area of intense laboratory and clinical research activity, and developments are occurring at a rapid rate. There are now many ongoing clinical trials of anti-AIDS drugs, and physicians who treat AIDS patients may be called upon to counsel their patients about the advisability of entering a particular experimental protocol. A basic knowledge of the strategies being considered to inhibit HIV replication at various steps in its life cycle may therefore be of use (Table 421–2).

As described in Ch. 411, the first step in the infection of a cell by HIV is its binding to a cellular receptor. The principal receptor for HIV binding is the first domain of CD4 glycoprotein. CD4 is an important molecule found on helper T cells and certain other cells. There is some experimental evidence that under certain circumstances, CD4-independent entry mechanisms may exist, although the clinical significance of this finding is unknown. Several groups have shown that genetically engineered soluble recombinant CD4 (containing the extracellular domains) can prevent the binding and infection of cells by laboratory strains of HIV in vitro. These preparations were generally safe to administer to patients. However, recombinant soluble CD4 was found to have a short serum half-life, and it has proved difficult to maintain levels associated with anti-HIV activity in vivo. More recently, hybrid proteins combining the pertinent domain(s) of CD4 with the constant portion of immunoglobulin heavy chain have been created. Such molecules, which are often referred to as immunoadhesins, likewise had anti-HIV activity in the laboratory. In addition, they were found to have substantially longer serum half-lives than unmodified soluble CD4. Initial clinical trials, however, have not shown clear evidence of anti-HIV activity in vivo. It has been found that fresh isolates of HIV are relatively resistant to these agents, and this may in part explain their lack of clinical activity. As another approach, CD4 has been linked

TABLE 421–2. SELECTED DRUGS (EXPERIMENTAL AND APPROVED) FOR THE THERAPY OF AIDS

Site of Effect	Name	Status (Spring 1991)	Comments
Viral binding	Soluble CD4	Experimental	Genetically engineered HIV receptor
	CD4-IgG chimera (immunoadhesin)	Experimental	Longer half-life than CD4
	CD4-toxin hybrids	Preclinical	May selectively kill HIV-producing cells
	Dextran sulfate	Experimental	Poor oral absorption; prototype for polyanionic polysaccharides with anti-HIV activity
	Anti-HIV antibodies	Experimental	May block HIV fusion and entry
Reverse transcriptase	AZT (zidovudine)	Approved	Optimal use still under study
	ddA and ddI	Treatment IND	Available for patients who cannot tolerate or have failed AZT therapy; can cause pancreatitis or peripheral neuropathy at high doses
	ddC	Open label protocol	Peripheral neuropathy is dose-limiting toxicity
	D4T	Experimental	Can cause peripheral neuropathy
	Azido-ddU	Experimental	Cross-reactive resistance with AZT
	Phosphonoformate (Foscarnet)	Experimental	Also has activity against cytomegalovirus
	TIBO derivatives	Experimental	Benzodiazepine derivatives
Replicative efficiency	Tat inhibitors	Experimental	Inhibitors of Tat, a virally encoded protein required for efficient replication
Protein modification	Protease inhibitors	Experimental	An intense effort is now under way to identify selective inhibitors of HIV protease
	Castanospermine and other trimming glucosidase inhibitors	Experimental	Affects sugar moiety of HIV envelope, reducing its ability to infect new cells
Viral budding	Interferon-α	Approved for Kaposi's sarcoma	Antitumor activity against Kaposi's sarcoma; may also have anti-HIV activity

with certain toxins (such as ricin or *Pseudomonas* endotoxin) with the idea of selectively killing cells that are producing HIV. Other approaches being considered to inhibit HIV binding or fusion include polyanionic polysaccharides (such as dextran sulfate or pentosan) or anti-HIV antibodies. In regard to the latter, however, it should be remembered that patients can progress to AIDS in spite of having neutralizing antibodies against HIV.

As discussed above, much of the effort in developing anti-AIDS drugs has focused on reverse transcription. All of the dideoxynucleosides (as triphosphates) are thought to act at this step. In addition, phosphonoformate (Foscarnet), a drug originally developed for the treatment of cytomegalovirus, inhibits HIV replication at the level of reverse transcription. Finally, several benzodiazepine derivatives (TIBO derivatives) have been found to have potent anti-HIV activity and are believed to act at this step.

There is now a substantial research effort directed at inhibiting certain late steps in HIV replication. The proteins of HIV are first produced as large polyproteins and later undergo a variety of modifications to form active proteins or glycoproteins. One of these steps is cleavage by an HIV protease. In the absence of effective protease activity, infectious virions cannot be produced. The structure of this enzyme has recently been determined by x-ray crystallography, and several selective inhibitors have been identified. Clinical trials of these agents are now under way.

HIV replication is regulated by certain genetic elements (long terminal repeats) on either end of the viral genome and by several small proteins encoded by the viral genome. Efficient viral replication requires the proper function of these regulatory elements, and as such they may also be targets for therapy. An inhibitor of the transactivating protein (Tat) has been identified and is expected to enter clinical trials in the near future. Another approach to this step has been the construction of "antisense" segments of modified DNA (e.g., phosphorothioate oligodeoxynucleotides). These are strands of DNA, modified to prevent degradation by cellular nucleases, with sequences complementary to those of HIV RNA. They are believed in part to prevent the movement of ribosomes along the RNA and thus prevent viral proteins from being formed. Phosphorothioate oligodeoxynucleosides can also inhibit HIV replication in a sequence-nonspecific manner.

The last step in the replication of HIV is viral budding. There is evidence that interferon-α can prevent HIV replication in vitro, in part by acting on this final step. Interferons may have other sites of activity as well. Interferon-α has been found to have antitumor activity against Kaposi's sarcoma, particularly in patients with over 100 T4 cells per cubic millimeter who have

disease limited to the skin, and it has recently been approved for HIV-associated Kaposi's sarcoma. It has been found to have synergistic anti-HIV activity with AZT in vitro, and this combination is now being explored in patients with HIV infection.

A final word should be said about strategies to boost the immune system of individuals with HIV infection. The progression of HIV infection to fulminant AIDS represents an interplay between the infective potential of the virus and the ability of the immune system to interfere with this process. In most if not all patients, the virus eventually prevails in the absence of specific therapy and fulminant AIDS develops. Even so, the immune response against HIV certainly slows down this process, and a boosting of the immune system (or of the specific response to HIV) might prove to be advantageous to HIV-infected patients. However, there are also some theoretical considerations to suggest that T-cell activation could trigger viral replication and thereby harm the patient. A variety of experimental approaches to this have been explored, including administration of cytokines (such as interleukin 2) and immunostimulatory drugs. Trials of some of these approaches are still ongoing, but none has so far been definitively shown to offer clinical benefit. Recently, progress has been made in understanding the specific aspects of the immune response which control HIV infection and in eliciting such responses, and it is possible that such an approach will be found to be beneficial in combination with antiretroviral therapy.

Combinations of drugs may potentially offer several advantages over a given single agent. Indeed, it is likely that as individual drugs are developed, combination regimens will become the mainstay of therapy for HIV infection. The use of several agents may help delay the development of HIV resistance. Also, certain combinations, particularly those that act at different steps in the viral replicative cycle, may have synergistic anti-HIV activity. Moreover, combinations of drugs with different toxicity profiles, for example AZT and ddC, may permit a sustained anti-HIV effect with reduced toxicity from either drug. The various agents could be administered either sequentially (e.g., alternating weekly) or simultaneously, and clinical studies will be needed to sort out the relative merits of these approaches. For example, an alternating regimen of AZT and ddC may provide rest periods from each drug, while there is some evidence that they may be synergistic if used simultaneously. Certain drugs may be useful in suppressing certain opportunistic infections and thus have a secondary effect on HIV infection. For example, acyclovir can suppress herpesviruses and might thus indirectly reduce HIV infection (a nuclear regulatory protein of herpesviruses can activate HIV replication). The combination of AZT and acyclovir is usually tolerated and is now used by a number of physicians, particularly for patients who are troubled by recurrent herpes infection. However, it remains to be seen whether this regimen offers any advantages over AZT as a single drug. Combination therapy of AIDS will be an important area for clinical investigation in the near future. However, physicians should be cautioned against ad hoc experimentation in this area, as unexpected drug interactions may occur.

CLINICAL TRIALS OF AIDS DRUGS

Since AIDS-related therapeutics is a rapidly evolving field, it may be worthwhile to provide a brief summary of some principles for developing new drugs and biologics. The clinical evaluation of new drugs generally involves three phases of clinical trials. The first, called Phase I, typically involves toxicity testing. Groups of three to six patients are each administered increasing doses of the drug until a toxic dose is reached; the dose immediately below that level is considered the "maximal tolerated dose." Phase II studies conventionally involve determinations of activity in small groups of patients using doses selected from the Phase I experience. Phase III studies involve definitive testing of efficacy in large groups of patients and generally involve comparison with placebo or with accepted treatment. Such trials also provide useful information on the long-term toxicity profile of the drug in large numbers of patients.

Because of the urgent need to develop effective drugs for AIDS, this process has been compressed somewhat. Phase I studies of new AIDS drugs are now often examined for evidence of a possible anti-HIV effect (activity) in addition to toxicity data. Changes in the number of T4 lymphocytes or other measures of immune function are monitored. HIV p24 antigenemia or related measures of viremia have been useful in detecting effects of HIV replication. Other tests, such as quantitative polymerase chain reaction analyses for HIV genome or plasma culture of HIV, are now being studied for their ability to detect an anti-HIV effect. Laboratory tests per se, however, as "surrogate markers" for a clinical effect, have generally not yet been accepted by regulatory agencies for demonstrating the efficacy of AIDS drugs. Clinical endpoints, such as an effect on survival, disease progression, or the development of opportunistic infections, have so far been required. However, this issue is now being actively studied. There are recent data, for example, to indicate that patients receiving AZT-based therapy in a research setting rarely die until their T4 count falls below 50 cells per cubic millimeter.

Along with the extraction of activity data from Phase I trials, there is a trend toward combining Phase II and Phase III trials for anti-AIDS drugs so that potentially the agents can be approved after two rounds of testing. In the case of AZT, for example, Phase I testing provided strong evidence that the drug had anti-HIV activity. A 282-patient randomized placebo-controlled trial subsequently showed clear evidence that patients taking AZT had a survival advantage over those taking placebo, and the drug was approved at that point. There are a number of risks to patients and society at large from such an accelerated drug development, and clinical researchers are at present trying to grapple with the best balance between speed, safety, and accuracy in developing AIDS drugs, as well as the imperative to provide compassionate therapy for dying patients.

Before the development of AZT, there was no effective antiretroviral therapy for AIDS, and the Phase II AZT trial was designed to show a difference between patients taking AZT and those taking placebo with respect to survival and the development of opportunistic infections. Trials of new therapies may now be designed to show that the therapy is superior to AZT (or other standard therapy) or alternately may be designed to show that the new treatment is equivalent to the standard treatment but may possess fewer side effects or offer other benefits. In efficacy studies, it is important that each patient be followed for a sufficiently long period of time for potential differences to appear. For example, there are data to suggest that AZT requires 6 weeks or so to bring about immunologic improvements, and only after this period can a difference in the development of opportunistic infections be observed.

In determining the optimal sample size for such efficacy studies, it is important to consider two potential types of error which may occur. The first, called a type I error, happens when investigators conclude that two treatments have different effects when in fact the effects are equivalent. In general, studies are designed and carried out so that the probability of a type I error (called α) is 5 per cent or less. This is usually denoted as $P < 0.05$. The second type of error, called type II, occurs when an investigator concludes that two treatments have the same effect when in fact they are different. The probability that this will occur (called β), depends on the specified difference in outcome required in order for the results to be considered different and on the number of subjects entered into the study. A trial may be designed, for example, to permit a 20 per cent type II error in detecting a 10 per cent survival difference at 1 year. This means there is one chance in five of not observing a difference, even though there is a "real difference" between the drugs under study. In such a case the "power" of the study to detect this 10 per cent difference in 1-year survival is $1-\beta$, or 80 per cent. Studies with a power of less than 80 per cent run the serious risk of missing real differences between treatments. Careful study design, including appropriate numbers of patients, can ensure an adequate power in a clinical trial.

Once one has estimated the likelihood of events occurring in the control population in a given period of time, chosen the differences in event rates required to conclude that the treatments are different, and chosen rates of type I and type II errors which one will accept, it is possible to estimate the sample size required. It is important to remember, however, that even in large studies, there is always some possibility of an incorrect conclusion being reached, and clinicians should be aware of these limitations. Such considerations are particularly important in the testing of AIDS drugs, in which there has been an attempt to compress the development process.

GENERAL RECOMMENDATIONS

At the present time, AZT is the only specific antiretroviral therapy formally approved for HIV infection. It is recommended for patients with HIV infection with less than 500 T4 cells per cubic millimeter. For adults with symptomatic HIV infection, including AIDS, the recommended dose is 200 mg every 4 hours for 1 month and then 100 mg every 4 hours. For patients with asymptomatic HIV infection and less than 500 T4 cells per cubic millimeter, a dose of 100 mg administered every 4 hours while awake (500 mg per day) is recommended. There is clear-cut evidence that AZT can increase survival when administered to symptomatic HIV-infected patients with less than 200 T4 cells per cubic millimeter. There is also evidence that short-term progression to AIDS or severe ARC can be decreased by administration of AZT to patients with 200 to 500 T4 cells per cubic millimeter. For patients who develop toxicity on AZT, dose reductions may be necessary. Epoetin alfa can be considered for those patients who develop anemia and have circulating erythropoietin levels of less than 500 mU per milliliter.

In addition to AZT, interferon-α (which may have anti-HIV activity) is approved for its anti-Kaposi's activity, and ddC and ddI are now available under restricted conditions for patients who cannot tolerate or who have failed AZT. AIDS patients may develop many complications that require therapy in their own right, and physicians should be vigilant to monitor unexpected drug interactions.

Yearly vaccinations with killed influenza virus are advisable; however, vaccinations with attenuated viruses should generally be avoided in this population. Because of the high incidence of cervical carcinoma in sexually active HIV-infected women, yearly pelvic examinations and Pap tests are advised in this population. Chemoprophylaxis for PCP, generally with aerosolized pentamidine or trimethoprim-sulfamethoxazole, is now recommended for patients with less than 200 T4 cells per cubic millimeter. Finally, some physicians have found megestrol acetate to be useful in stimulating the appetite of patients with progressive wasting. Perhaps most importantly, physicians should be attuned to diagnose and treat the myriad complications that can develop in this immunosuppressed population (see Ch. 422 as well as other relevant chapters for specific complications).

Through the combination of antiretroviral therapy and improvements in the prevention, diagnosis, and treatment of the complications of HIV infection, much progress has been made in the last several years. Given the agents now in laboratory and clinical development, physicians will likely have an expanding armamentarium of anti-AIDS drugs in the near future. The pace of research in this area is rapid, and physicians treating patients with AIDS should remain alert to ongoing developments that may dramatically alter accepted medical practice with very little advance notice.

Review Articles

Hirsch MS, Kaplan JC: Treatment of human immunodeficiency virus infections. Antimicrob Agents Chemother 31:839–843, 1987. *Overview of approaches to AIDS therapies.*

Mitsuya H, Yarchoan R, Broder S: Molecular targets for AIDS therapy. Science 249:1533–1544, 1990. *Detailed review article discussing the variety of approaches that can be taken to inhibit HIV infection.*

Yarchoan R, Mitsuya H, Myers CE, Broder S: Clinical pharmacology of 3'-azido-2',3'-dideoxythymidine (zidovudine) and related dideoxynucleosides. N Engl J Med 321:726–738, 1989. *Review article stressing the metabolism and clinical pharmacology of dideoxynucleosides. Extensive bibliography.*

In Vitro Studies of Dideoxynucleosides

Furman PA, Fyfe JA, St. Clair M, et al.: Phosphorylation of 3'-azido-3'-deoxythymidine and selective interaction of the 5'-triphosphate with human immunodeficiency virus reverse transcriptase. Proc Natl Acad Sci USA 83:8333–8337, 1986. *Describes the anabolic phosphorylation of AZT and its effects on cellular kinases.*

Hartshorn KL, Vogt MW, Chou T-C, et al.: Synergistic inhibition of human immunodeficiency virus in vitro by azidothymidine and recombinant alpha A interferon. Antimicrob Agents Chemother 31:168–172, 1987. *Discussion of synergy in anti-HIV therapy.*

Mitsuya H, Broder S: Inhibition of the in vitro infectivity and cytopathic effect of human T-lymphotropic virus type III/lymphadenopathy virus-associated virus (HTLV-III/LAV) by 2',3'-dideoxynucleosides. Proc Natl Acad Sci USA 83:1911–1915, 1986. *Description of potent anti-HIV activity of a variety of dideoxynucleosides.*

Mitsuya H, Weinhold KJ, Furman PA, et al.: 3'-Azido-3'-deoxythymidine (BW A509U): An antiviral agent that inhibits the infectivity and cytopathic effect of human T-lymphotropic virus type III/lymphadenopathy-associated virus *in vitro.* Proc Natl Acad Sci USA 82:7096–7100, 1985. *Description of in vitro anti-HIV activity of AZT.*

Clinical Studies of AZT (Zidovudine)

Dalakos MC, Illa I, Pezeshkpour GH, et al.: Mitochondrial myopathy caused by long-term zidovudine therapy. N Engl J Med 322:1098–1105, 1990. *Description of the clinical and pathologic features of AZT-induced myopathy.*

Dournon E, Matheron S, Rozenbaum W, et al.: Effects of zidovudine in 365 consecutive patients with AIDS or AIDS-related complex. Lancet 2:1297–1302, 1988. *Discussion of the activity and toxicity profile of AZT therapy in a general AIDS population.*

Fischl MA, Richman DD, Grieco MH, et al.: The efficacy of azidothymidine (AZT) in the treatment of patients with AIDS and AIDS-related complex: A double-blind, placebo-controlled trial. N Engl J Med 317:185–191, 1987. *Efficacy data from the Phase II trial of AZT that demonstrated an effect on the survival of patients with AIDS.*

Fischl M, Parker C, Pettinelli C, et al.: A randomized controlled trial of a reduced daily dose of zidovudine in patients with acquired immunodeficiency syndrome. N Engl J Med 323:1009–1014, 1990. *Article providing the basis for the current dose recommendation of AZT in AIDS.*

Fischl M, Richman DD, Hansen N, et al.: The safety and efficacy of zidovudine (AZT) in the treatment of subjects with mildly symptomatic human immunodeficiency virus type I (HIV) infection. A double-blind, placebo controlled trial. Ann Intern Med 112:727–737, 1990. *Data that AZT reduces the short-term progression to AIDS in mildly symptomatic patients with 200 to 500 T4 cells per cubic millimeter.*

Larder BA, Darby G, Richman DD: HIV with reduced sensitivity to zidovudine (AZT) isolated during prolonged therapy. Science 243:1731–1734, 1989. *Presents evidence that HIV isolated from patients on long-term AZT therapy often has reduced sensitivity to AZT.*

Pizzo PA, Eddy J, Falloon J, et al.: Effect of continuous intravenous infusion zidovudine (AZT) in children with symptomatic HIV infection. N Engl J Med 319:889–896, 1988. *Effect of AZT on HIV infection and in particular HIV-induced neurologic dysfunction in children with HIV infection.*

Richman DD, Fischl MA, Grieco MH, et al.: The toxicity of azidothymidine (AZT) in the treatment of patients with AIDS and AIDS-related complex: A double-blind, placebo-controlled trial. N Engl J Med 317:192–197, 1987. *Data on AZT toxicity from the Phase II trial.*

Volberding PA, Lagakos SW, Koch MA, et al.: Zidovudine in asymptomatic human immunodeficiency virus infection. A controlled trial in persons with fewer than 500 CD4-positive cells per cubic millimeter. N Engl J Med 322:941–949, 1990. *Describes the efficacy of AZT in preventing progression to AIDS when administered to asymptomatic HIV-infected patients.*

Yarchoan R, Berg G, Brouwers P, et al.: Response of human-immunodeficiency-virus-associated neurological disease to 3'-azido-3'-deoxythymidine. Lancet 1:132–135, 1987. *Describes the activity of AZT on AIDS dementia and its ability to reverse HIV-induced abnormalities of cerebral glucose metabolism.*

Yarchoan R, Klecker RW, Weinhold KJ, et al.: Administration of 3'-azido-3'-deoxythymidine, an inhibitor of HTLV-III/LAV replication, to patients with AIDS or AIDS-related complex. Lancet 1:575–580, 1986. *First description of the clinical activity of AZT.*

Clinical Studies of Other Dideoxynucleosides

Butler KM, Husson RN, Balis FM, et al.: Dideoxyinosine (ddI) in symptomatic HIV-infected children: A phase I–II study. N Engl J Med 324:137–144, 1991. *Data showing effect of ddI on HIV infection and in particular on HIV-induced neurologic dysfunction in children.*

Cooley TP, Kunches LM, Saunders CA, et al.: Once-daily administration of 2',3'-dideoxyinosine (ddI) in patients with the acquired immunodeficiency syndrome or AIDS-related complex. N Engl J Med 322:1340–1345, 1990. *Study showing the short-term activity and toxicity of ddI given once daily.*

Lambert JS, Seidlin M, Reichman RC, et al.: 2',3'-Dideoxyinosine (ddI) in patients with the acquired immunodeficiency syndrome or the AIDS-related complex. A Phase I trial. N Engl J Med 322:1333–1340, 1990. *A study showing the short-term activity and toxicity profile of ddI given twice daily.*

Merigan TC, Skowron G, Bozzette SA, et al.: Circulating p24 antigen levels and responses to dideoxycytidine in human immunodeficiency virus (HIV) infections. Ann Intern Med 110:189–194, 1989. *More detailed profile of the effect of ddC on HIV p24 antigenemia in patients with severe HIV infection.*

Yarchoan R, Pluda JM, Thomas RV, et al.: Long-term toxicity/activity profile of 2',3'-dideoxyinosine in AIDS or AIDS-related complex. Lancet 2:526–529, 1990. *Data showing the long-term toxicity profile of ddI and its ability to induce sustained T4 elevations.*

Yarchoan R, Perno CF, Thomas RV, et al.: Phase I studies of 2',3'-dideoxycytidine in severe human immunodeficiency virus infection as a single agent and alternating with zidovudine (AZT). Lancet 1:76–81, 1988. *Data from Phase I trial of ddC.*

Other Agents

Capon DJ, Chamow SM, Mordenti J, et al.: Designing CD4 immunoadhesions for AIDS therapy. Nature 337:525–531, 1989. *Discussion of rCD4-IgG immunoadhesions and the general approach of engineered CD4 as a therapy for AIDS.*

Lane HC, Kovacs JA, Feinberg J, et al.: Anti-retroviral effects of interferon-alpha in AIDS-associated Kaposi's sarcoma. Lancet 2:1218–1222, 1988. *Article showing evidence of an anti-HIV effect of interferon in certain patients with Kaposi's sarcoma.*

Meek TD, Lambert DM, Dreyer GB, et al.: Inhibition of HIV-1 protease in infected T-lymphocytes by synthetic peptide analogues. Nature 343:90–92, 1990. *Discussion of the approach of inhibiting HIV protease.*

Effects of Therapy on the Epidemiology of HIV Infection

Gail MH, Rosenberg P, Goedert J: Therapy may explain recent deficits in AIDS incidence. J AIDS 3:296–306, 1990. *Describes a decline in the incidence of AIDS in homosexual men since 1987 and provides evidence that this is an effect of improvements in therapy, particularly the introduction of AZT.*

Lemp GF, Payne SF, Neal D, et al.: Survival trends for patients with AIDS. JAMA 263:402–406, 1990. *Shows improvement in survival in patients with AIDS since 1986 and a correlation of this effect with AZT therapy.*

Clinical Trial Methodology

Freiman JA, Chalmers TC, Smith H Jr, Kuebler RR: The importance of beta, the type II error and sample size in the design and interpretation of the randomized clinical trial. Survey of 71 "negative" trials. N Engl J Med 299:690–694, 1978. *Good discussion of type I and type II errors and the power of the statistical test of significance in clinical trials.*

422 Chronic Management and Counseling for Persons with HIV Infection

John A. Bartlett

HISTORICAL PERSPECTIVE

The clinical syndrome of Kaposi's sarcoma and *Pneumocystis carinii* pneumonia (PCP) occurring in previously healthy young homosexual men was originally described in 1981. For the next 3 years efforts focused upon the epidemiology of this immunodeficiency state and identification of the responsible infectious agent. The clinical care for these patients was extremely limited and consisted of the delayed treatment of complications with little ability to provide early intervention, preventive treatment, or treatment aimed at the underlying retroviral infection. The past 10 years have witnessed an unprecedented growth of knowledge about AIDS and its causative agent, human immunodeficiency virus (HIV). Early treatment aimed at HIV or the complications of the immunodeficiency state can now delay the onset of full-blown AIDS. For persons with severe AIDS-related complex (ARC) or AIDS, zidovudine can prolong survival, with the preservation of meaningful and productive time. For example, the median survival for a patient with PCP prior to the advent of zidovudine or PCP prophylaxis was 10.5 months; the same patient now has an almost 90 per cent chance of survival at 1 year. AIDS has truly become an illness to be "managed" medically on a chronic basis.

INTRODUCTION

Providing health care to persons with HIV infection represents a tremendous challenge to the involved medical personnel. This challenge is very broad and contains facets involving significant medical, psychological, and social issues. The optimal care for persons with HIV infection must include a comprehensive approach to all of these issues, and therein lies the essential principle for their successful clinical management.

Between 1 and 1.5 million Americans are infected with HIV, and to date only 10 per cent of those infected have been diagnosed with AIDS. As HIV infection progresses within this population and as new HIV infections occur, the burden of their health care needs will increase tremendously. It is doubtful that any health care provider will not have the opportunity to care for HIV-infected persons in the coming 10 years.

NATURAL HISTORY

Understanding the natural history of HIV infection is essential prior to beginning a discussion of medical management. HIV infection is a chronic viral illness characterized by progressive immunologic impairment. The immunologic damage can be directly measured through the determination of lymphocyte subsets, specifically in the absolute number and percentage of CD4 (or T-helper) lymphocytes. The CD4 lymphocyte is the primary target of HIV infection, and declines in the number and percentage of CD4 lymphocytes correlate most closely with clinical progression of HIV infection. It must be emphasized that HIV infection is a chronic illness with a median delay of approximately 10 years between acute infection and progression to AIDS (Fig. 422–1). Full-blown AIDS is a clinical syndrome defined by the occurrence of complicating opportunistic infections and neoplasms and severe HIV-related symptoms. It is simply a clinical manifestation of the underlying immunologic deficit and repre-

sents the end-stage of many years of progressive immunologic damage. Once an individual has been diagnosed with AIDS, there is an anticipated series of complications which can occur. Grossly these can be categorized into relatively early and late complications (Fig. 422–2). Although significant advances have occurred in the treatment of AIDS and its complications, it remains a fatal illness.

MEDICAL MANAGEMENT

Based upon the understanding of the natural history of HIV infection, the medical management of HIV infection focuses upon two major goals: delay in the progression of HIV infection to AIDS and improvement in the quantity and quality of life for persons who have progressed to AIDS. Four aspects of medical management are discussed: the initial evaluation, assessing the need for antiretroviral therapy, assessing the need for preventive therapy, and evaluating the febrile patient with HIV infection.

Initial Evaluation

Each person with HIV infection should undergo an initial comprehensive evaluation of his or her HIV infection to serve as a foundation for subsequent decisions (Table 422–1). Obviously this evaluation begins with a careful history. Specific points to be addressed include the duration of HIV infection, previous evaluations, HIV-related symptoms, HIV-related complications, history of sexually transmitted diseases, previous tuberculin testing or tuberculosis exposure, previous residential and travel history, and medication allergies. Because HIV infection and its complications involve all organ systems, a thorough physical examination is essential. The areas of greatest concern include the skin, eyes, oropharynx, lymphatics, genital and perirectal areas, and neurologic system.

The initial laboratory examination should include a complete blood count with differential, electrolytes, liver and kidney chemistries, lymphocyte subset analysis, and VDRL. Persons with a past history of a negative PPD more than 1 year previously should have a 5TU PPD placed. Persons with a current or past positive PPD should receive 1 year of isoniazid owing to their high risk of tuberculosis reactivation. Persons with HIV infection are at an increased risk for pneumococcal disease and complications of influenza. Currently both vaccinations are recommended, although the serologic response of this population has not been well documented. Based upon this initial evaluation of HIV infection, careful staging can be performed and the relevant therapeutic issues addressed.

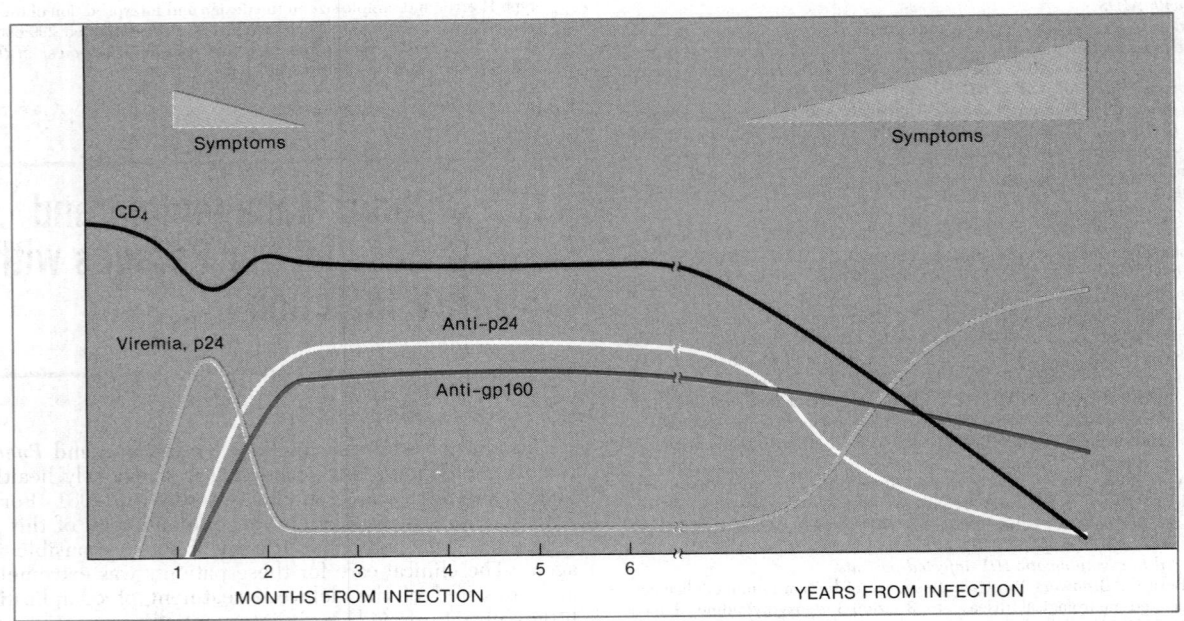

FIGURE 422–1. Model of the time course of HIV-1 infection. (Modified from Clark SJ, et al.: High titer of cytopathic virus in plasma of patients with symptomatic primary HIV-1 infection. N Engl J Med 324:954–960, 1991. By permission of the New England Journal of Medicine.)

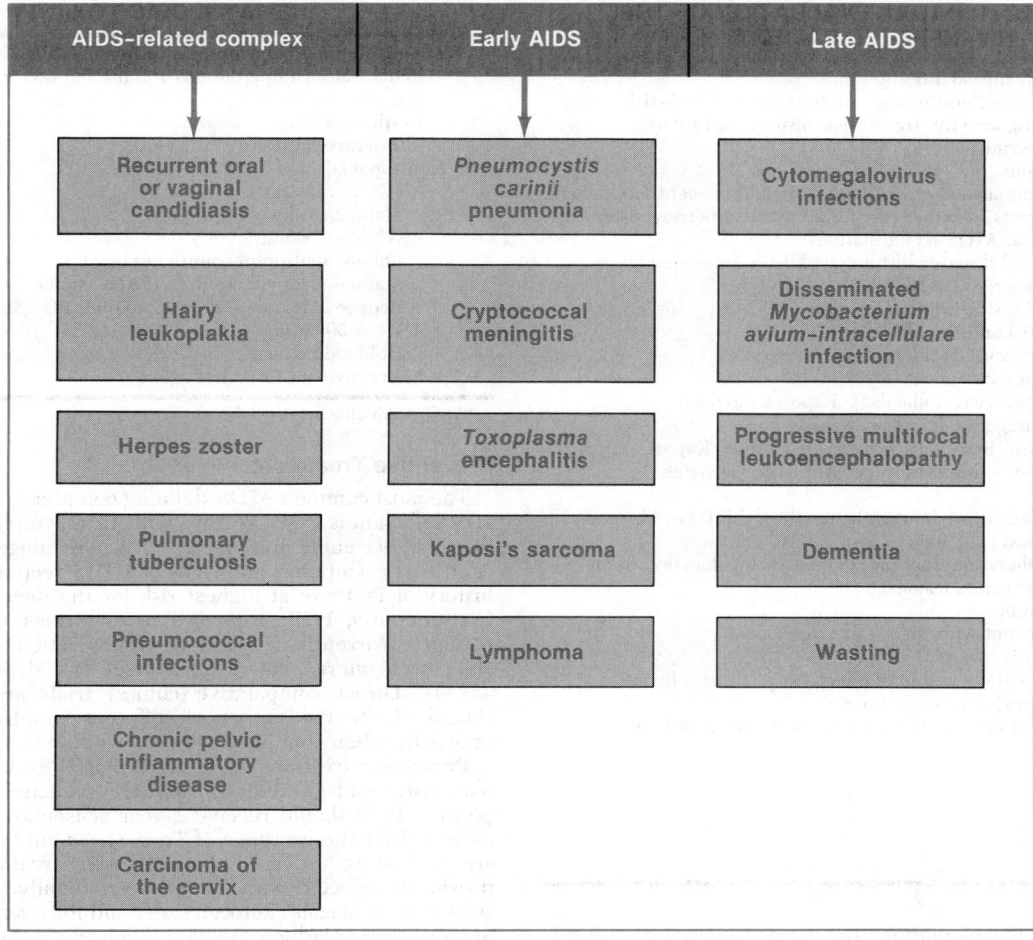

AIDS-related complex	Early AIDS	Late AIDS
Recurrent oral or vaginal candidiasis	*Pneumocystis carinii* pneumonia	Cytomegalovirus infections
Hairy leukoplakia	Cryptococcal meningitis	Disseminated *Mycobacterium avium-intracellulare* infection
Herpes zoster	*Toxoplasma* encephalitis	Progressive multifocal leukoencephalopathy
Pulmonary tuberculosis	Kaposi's sarcoma	Dementia
Pneumococcal infections	Lymphoma	Wasting
Chronic pelvic inflammatory disease		
Carcinoma of the cervix		

FIGURE 422–2. Time line of AIDS-related complications.

Antiretroviral Therapy (see Ch. 421)

Antiretroviral therapy is currently in its infancy. Only one approved treatment is available—zidovudine (previously known as azidothymidine or AZT). Fortunately, zidovudine has shown significant antiretroviral and clinical activity across a spectrum of persons with HIV infection.

Zidovudine has also demonstrated clinical efficacy in the treatment of patients with severe ARC and AIDS. This efficacy is defined as both a prolongation in survival and an improvement in quality of life as assessed by increased Karnofsky performance status, weight gain, neurocognitive functioning, and fewer opportunistic infections. Zidovudine may also increase platelet counts in HIV-associated idiopathic thrombocytopenic purpura and improve the dermatologic and rheumatologic manifestations associated with HIV.

The optimal dosing schedule for zidovudine remains to be defined (see Ch. 421). A dose of 100 mg orally five times per day is currently recommended, but the best schedule and lowest effective dosage are uncertain. Persons with HIV-associated neurologic disease may benefit from a higher dose of 200 mg orally five times daily.

Zidovudine may cause significant toxicity in persons with HIV infection, predominantly involving suppression of erythropoiesis and myelopoiesis. The occurrence of toxicity is clearly related to the stage of HIV infection, pretreatment hemoglobin and neutrophil counts, and zidovudine dosage. Nonhematologic toxicities may include nausea, headaches, alterations in mental status, myositis, fevers, rash, hepatitis, and seizures.

All persons with HIV infection and a CD4 lymphocyte count of less than 500 per cubic millimeter should receive zidovudine (Table 422–2). If an individual's CD4 lymphocyte count is greater than 500 per cubic millimeter, his or her CD4 lymphocyte count should be repeated at intervals of 6 months to closely monitor the need for zidovudine. It is also likely that the therapeutic efficacy of zidovudine may be demonstrated in HIV-infected persons with greater than 500 CD4 lymphocytes per cubic millimeter in the future, and consequently the threshold value of CD4 lymphocytes may be altered. Once zidovudine is begun, complete blood counts and chemistries should be followed every other week for 2 months, then monthly thereafter provided that these parameters remain stable. The management of zidovudine-related toxicity can be very challenging (Table 422–3). Anemia may be managed through dosage reduction, transfusions, or the administration of erythropoietin. Zidovudine-associated neutropenia is generally well tolerated down to absolute neutrophil counts of 500 per cubic millimeter and may respond to dosage reduction or the administration of granulocyte colony stimulating factors when necessary. As a general therapeutic principle, most clinicians attempt to maintain patients on zidovudine whenever possible without interruptions. Concern about frequent discontinuations of therapy originates in the observations of increases in p24 antigen levels and virus culture positivity in patients who have recently discontinued zidovudine. CD4 lymphocyte counts in persons with pretreatment counts greater than 200 per cubic millimeter receiving zidovudine are followed at least every 6 months owing to the need for initiation of PCP prophylaxis when counts fall below 200 per cubic millimeter. In persons with pretreatment counts of less than 200 per cubic millimeter on zidovudine and PCP prophylaxis, the follow-up of CD4 lymphocyte counts adds little to therapeutic decisions, given the lack of currently available therapeutic alternatives.

Zidovudine-resistant HIV isolates were recently identified from persons with ARC or AIDS who had received prolonged zidovudine treatment. However, there were no clinical or laboratory correlations with the isolation of resistant virus. The clinical significance of zidovudine-resistant isolates, the effect of disease stage on the frequency of resistant isolates, and the ramifications

TABLE 422–1. INITIAL EVALUATION OF THE HIV-INFECTED PATIENT

Medical history with special attention to:
  Duration of HIV infection (timing and geography of high-risk sexual or needle-sharing activity, transfusion history, history of mononucleosis syndrome)
  Previous evaluations
  HIV-related symptoms and complications (fatigue, weight loss, fevers, chills, night sweats, diarrhea, dementia, thrush, herpes zoster, hairy leukoplakia, AIDS manifestations)
  Sexually transmitted diseases history (syphilis, herpes simplex, hepatitis B, gonorrhea, chlamydia)
  Previous tuberculosis testing or exposure
  Previous residential and travel history
  Medication history and allergies
Physical examination with special attention to:
  Skin (seborrhea, psoriasis, folliculitis, Kaposi's sarcoma)
  Lymphatics (extrainguinal lymphadenopathy)
  Oropharynx (thrush, hairy leukoplakia, ulcerations, Kaposi's sarcoma)
  Genitalia (ulcerations, Kaposi's sarcoma, penile discharge, epididymitis)
  Rectum (ulcerations, condylomata, hemorrhoids, fistulas, abscesses, prostatitis, Kaposi's sarcoma)
  Neurologic (peripheral neuropathy, dementia, myelopathy, focal central nervous system lesions)
Laboratory examination
  Complete blood count with differential (leukopenia, thrombocytopenia, anemia)
  Electrolytes with kidney and liver chemistries (chronic hepatitis, renal insufficiency, Addison's disease)
  Lymphocyte subset analysis (number and percentage of CD4 lymphocytes)
  VDRL
  PPD
Vaccinations
  Pneumovax
  Influenza

for the initiation of zidovudine treatment remain to be determined. Many other drugs to treat HIV infection are in the process of laboratory or clinical development (see Ch. 421).

Access and entry into HIV treatment trials are important issues for patients and health care providers. Participation is increasingly available through both academic and private medical centers. Many persons with HIV infection are well informed regarding their illness and potential treatments, and access to new agents is an extremely important issue in their health care. The efficient entry of interested patients into well-designed clinical trials serves to advance the development of improved treatment most rapidly.

Persons with HIV infection not enrolled in clinical trials may choose to pursue complementary or alternative treatments to zidovudine. Such treatments, it is hoped, are not to the exclusion of zidovudine. Given the recognition that many of these treatments are of unproven benefit but also of little potential harm to patients, most AIDS clinicians accept their patients' desires to pursue complementary treatments.

TREATMENT OF HIV-RELATED COMPLICATIONS

All patients with progressive HIV infection can be anticipated to have a series of complications due to their immune compromise. These complications can be broadly categorized as early or late (Fig. 422–2). Treatment may be preventive in patients identified as high risk for a given complication, or it may begin after the complication has occurred.

TABLE 422–2. THERAPEUTIC DECISIONS IN HIV INFECTION

CD4 Count (per mm³)	Recommendation
>500	Follow CD4 count every 3–6 months
≤500, >200	Begin zidovudine, follow CD4 count every 3–6 months
≤200	Begin zidovudine and PCP prophylaxis

TABLE 422–3. SUGGESTED SCHEME FOR THE MANAGEMENT OF ZIDOVUDINE-ASSOCIATED HEMATOLOGIC TOXICITY

Anemia defined by symptoms or hemoglobin ≤ 8 grams/dl
  Reduce zidovudine dose to 100 mg PO q8h
  Transfuse as needed
  Erythropoietin
  Alternative antiretroviral agent
Neutropenia
  ANC* > 750/mm³
    Maintain zidovudine dosage
  ANC 500–750/mm³
    Follow neutrophil count closely
    Maintain zidovudine dose if ANC stable
    Reduce zidovudine dose to 100 mg PO q8h if ANC falling
  ANC < 500/mm³
    Hold zidovudine
    Alternative antiretroviral agent

*ANC = Absolute neutrophil count.

Preventive Treatment

The most common AIDS-defining complication in persons with HIV infection is PCP. Persons with CD4 lymphocyte counts less than 200 per cubic millimeter, CD4 percentage less than 20 per cent, early symptoms and signs of HIV infection, and a previous history of PCP are at highest risk for the development of PCP. Consequently, PCP prophylaxis is now recommended for these patients. Currently a variety of prophylactic regimens are available; each offers relative advantages and disadvantages (Table 422–4). Direct comparative clinical trials are underway and should clarify the merits of different prophylactic regimens, especially when combined with zidovudine.

Preventive treatment is being explored for tuberculosis, toxoplasmosis, and candidiasis. All HIV-infected persons with a positive PPD should receive 1 year of isoniazid. They may also be tested for the presence of *Toxoplasma* antibody; clinical trials are evaluating the role of suppressive treatment for persons previously infected with *Toxoplasma*. Finally, antifungal agents such as clotrimazole, ketoconazole, and fluconazole may be given in a preventive fashion to avoid oropharyngeal candidiasis.

Acute and Chronic Treatment

Many of the complications of HIV infection are infectious illnesses caused by opportunistic pathogens. Three principles are important in prescribing treatment for complicating infections: The infections are frequently widely disseminated at the time of diagnosis, the host immune response is minimal, and without chronic suppressive therapy many infections relapse. Chronic therapy is important for many bacterial, protozoal, fungal, and viral infections. As the number of infectious complications increases, the complexity of an individual's chronic suppressive treatment increases. With the improved recognition of infectious complications, the improved treatment options for these complications, and the use of survival-prolonging antiretroviral drugs such as zidovudine, many persons with AIDS are now developing multiple chronic infections necessitating lifelong suppression.

Neoplasms are also common complications of progressive HIV infection. Although the incidence of Kaposi's sarcoma has de-

TABLE 422–4. PROPHYLACTIC REGIMENS FOR PNEUMOCYSTIS CARINII PNEUMONIA

	Advantages	Disadvantages
Sulfamethoxazole-trimethoprim	Low cost Systemic	Hematologic toxicity Fever Cutaneous reactions
Dapsone	Systemic	Hematologic toxicity Hepatic toxicity Fever Cutaneous reactions
Aerosolized pentamidine	Topical	High cost Bronchospasm Upper lobe or extra-pulmonary *Pneumocystis*

TABLE 422–5. EVALUATION OF THE FEBRILE PATIENT WITH HIV INFECTION

A. History
  1. Duration, severity, and pattern of fever
  2. Localizing symptoms (headache, visual changes, central nervous system abnormalities, pharyngitis, odynophagia, cough, chest pain, abdominal pain, changes in bowel habits or stools, urinary tract symptoms, skin abnormalities, or changes in lymph nodes)
  3. Previous febrile episodes and associated causes
  4. CD4 lymphocyte counts
B. Physical examination
  1. Vital signs
  2. Special emphasis
    a. Eye—retinitis, papilledema
    b. Oropharynx—thrush, ulcerations, Kaposi's sarcoma
    c. Lungs—physical findings of pneumonia
    d. Abdomen—hepatobiliary disease, gastroenteritis, colitis
    e. Genitalia—prostatitis, sexually transmitted diseases
    f. Rectum—ulcerations, abscesses
    g. Skin—ulcerations, abscesses
    h. Central nervous system—nuchal rigidity, focal abnormalities
C. Laboratory studies
  1. General
    a. Complete blood count with differential
    b. Blood cultures
      Routine bacterial
      Lysis/centrifugation tubes—fungi, mycobacteria
    c. Serum cryptococcal titer
    d. Urinalysis
  2. Respiratory symptoms
    a. Chest radiograph
    b. Arterial blood gas
    c. Sputum induction with special stains
    d. Bronchoscopy
  3. Central nervous system abnormalities
    a. Head computed tomography or magnetic resonance scanning
    b. Lumbar puncture

creased, it remains a frequent complication of AIDS. Isolated lesions are usually not treated, and locally symptomatic disease may respond to radiation therapy. When disseminated cutaneous or visceral disease is present, interferon-α or combination chemotherapy may be useful. Non-Hodgkin's lymphomas may occur in persons with AIDS and may be treated with traditional chemotherapy and/or radiation therapy. Unfortunately, the use of chemotherapy may prohibit the concomitant prescription of zidovudine owing to combined myelosuppression.

The neurologic complications of HIV infection are also relatively common. Among the most problematic are HIV-associated peripheral neuropathy and dementia. The neurocognitive and behavioral abnormalities may respond to antiretroviral therapy with zidovudine, especially in high doses. The treatment of HIV-associated peripheral neuropathy is more difficult and may respond only to symptomatic treatment such as amitriptyline.

As the longevity of persons with AIDS increases, the number of complications also increases. Given the need for chronic suppressive treatment, one person with AIDS may be receiving many oral, intravenous, and aerosolized medications. This plethora of drugs forces the clinician to be keenly aware of drug interactions and also raises difficult issues of patient compliance and pharmaceutical costs.

Evaluation of the Febrile Patient

The most common reason for an unscheduled clinic visit of a person with HIV infection is the development of fever. The clinician must begin the evaluation with a careful history (Table 422–5). Important elements of fever include its severity (low grade versus hectic), duration, and pattern. The discovery of localizing symptoms (headache, visual changes, central nervous system abnormalities, pharyngitis, odynophagia, cough, chest pain, abdominal pain, changes in bowel habits or stools, urinary tract symptoms, skin abnormalities, or changes in lymph nodes) is very useful in identifying a fever source. The history of previous febrile episodes and associated causes is essential. Patients may frequently offer insightful hypotheses about the etiology of their fever. Finally, recent CD4 counts may be helpful in grossly assessing the likelihood of an opportunistic infection. For exam-

ple, a person with a recent CD4 lymphocyte count of less than 250 per cubic millimeter is clearly at risk for an opportunistic infection. Conversely, a person with a recent CD4 lymphocyte count greater than 250 per cubic millimeter is less likely to have an opportunistic infection.

A careful physical examination begins with vital signs. Obviously the temperature is important in a febrile patient, but pulse, blood pressure, and especially respirations need close attention. In patients complaining of dyspnea, it is frequently useful to stress the patient by walking or climbing stairs and observe the respiratory response. On physical examination, special emphasis should be placed upon the eye, oropharynx, lungs, abdomen, genitalia, rectum, skin, and central nervous system.

Laboratory studies should be tailored to the significant historical and physical findings. In general, blood counts, blood cultures including the use of lysis/centrifugation tubes for the isolation of fungi and mycobacteria, and serum cryptococcal antigen titers are useful tests when no specific etiology for the fever is apparent. For the patient with respiratory symptoms, a chest radiograph and arterial blood gas measurement are important. Remember that the most common radiographic appearance of PCP is a normal chest radiograph, although other radiographic appearances of PCP (upper lobe disease, unilateral or nodular infiltrates) may be found. Sputum induction with the use of rapid special stains for microorganisms can be performed immediately in the clinic. In some centers, the use of sputum induction with stains employing monoclonal antibodies against P. carinii can detect greater than 90 per cent of cases of proven PCP. Bronchoscopy can be performed if necessary in patients with a nondiagnostic sputum examination. In patients with headaches or central nervous system abnormalities, imaging of the brain with computed tomography or magnetic resonance scanning and lumbar puncture is essential.

The evaluation and treatment of febrile patients may frequently be accomplished on an outpatient basis. Many opportunistic infections including PCP, cryptococcal meningitis, Toxoplasma encephalitis, and cytomegalovirus retinitis can be treated on an outpatient basis. However, important elements of outpatient care must include a medically stable, compliant, and well-informed patient with easy access to the health care provider, the availability of personal care providers within the home, and home health care agencies to provide nursing, pharmaceutical, and technical care when necessary. Potentially home-based care can be beneficial to both patients and the health care system. Patients may be more comfortable and have an increased sense of control at home. Tremendous cost savings may also be realized through home-based care, and limited resources such as hospital beds may be reserved for the most acutely ill patients.

COUNSELING AND PSYCHOSOCIAL ISSUES

The proper recognition of the complex psychosocial issues in the care of persons with HIV infection offers the clinician an opportunity to truly excel in providing patient care. As a biologic process, HIV infection is simply a chronic viral infection resulting in progressive immunologic impairment. However, the person with HIV infection faces daily problems owing to the powerful psychological and social responses that accompany the diagnosis. Frequently persons with HIV infection may have been rejected by other health care providers, and the clinician must begin with an attitude of compassion, tolerance, and patience. The successful clinician caring for persons with HIV infection must adopt a comprehensive approach to patient care.

Counseling

Counseling for persons with HIV infection begins with a description of the biologic processes relevant to transmission and natural history. As a general principle, the clinician should not assume that patients are already familiar with these issues and should begin with a basic discussion. Modes of HIV transmission should be frankly discussed, with ample opportunity for patient-initiated questions. Prevention must be encouraged through safer sex measures, the avoidance of needle sharing, needle cleansing, and certain methods of birth control (Table 422–6). Frequently discussions of prevention are most productive when the patient

TABLE 422–6. MEASURES TO PREVENT HIV TRANSMISSION

Means of Transmission	Preventive Measures
Sexual contact	Use of condoms; use of spermicidal foams containing nonoxynol-9; limiting the number of sexual partners; informing sexual partners; no exchange of body fluids
Shared needles	No sharing of needles; cleaning needles with bleach; needle exchanges; education of health care workers about avoiding needle sticks
Blood or blood products	Screening of all donated blood and blood products for the presence of HIV antibody; heat treatment of clotting factors
Perinatal transmission	Certain means of birth control
Breast milk	Bottle feeding

is accompanied by his or her sexual partner, friends, or family. Prevention can be a successful means of interrupting HIV transmission. The homosexual community has engaged in an active program of self-education regarding prevention of HIV infection, and both indirect and direct evidence strongly suggest a decreased incidence of new HIV infections. Reaching intravenous drug users with educational campaigns presents a much greater challenge, but modest effects in decreasing the incidence of new HIV infections have been realized in areas where intense efforts are concentrated. Counseling about prevention is the most important intervention that can be offered until a vaccine or truly effective treatment becomes available.

The natural history of HIV infection should be reviewed with all HIV-infected persons. Explanation of the need for regular medical follow-up and the potential symptoms of HIV infection and its complications serve to improve their care. Persons with HIV infection may be well educated with regard to their medical illness, treatment, and prognosis. These patients frequently request an increased level of self-participation in their medical care. Although this desire for increased self-control may be perceived as threatening to the clinician, significant benefits can be gained by allowing this participation. Persons with HIV infection must be viewed within the context of young persons diagnosed with a chronic and perhaps ultimately fatal viral illness for which the therapeutic options are of limited benefit. In many respects, they have very little control over their illness. However, to the extent that any sense of control can be encouraged, a patient's anxiety level will be reduced. The successful sharing of control with patients requires a mature and understanding clinician who is not threatened by his or her patient's independence.

Psychological Issues

A proper consideration of the psychological issues of HIV infection begins with the understanding of risk behaviors. The issues of sexuality, intravenous drug use, transfusions, and parenthood must be acknowledged and accepted. Frequently these issues have resulted in important personality traits that antedate the development of HIV infection and continue to resurface during its course. They may lead to feelings of guilt, low self-esteem, isolation, mistrust, and discrimination which need to be addressed. Each risk category and each individual has a different

mix of these feelings. In addition, the clinician must not allow his or her own reaction to risk behaviors to interfere with the provision of patient care.

Certainly an awareness of one's own HIV infection and its prognosis can lead to anxiety. Anxiety is a very common finding among persons with HIV infection across risk group categories and disease stages. Additional anxiety can result from concerns about sexuality; sharing the knowledge of one's infection with others and the potential for negative reactions; the loss of one's job, appearance, material possessions, and significant others; fear of the unknown; and loss of control in the waning stages of one's illness. Anxiety may lead to the difficulties with substance abuse commonly seen in persons with HIV infection. Alleviating anxiety may be accomplished by involving the patient actively in his or her own care, through frequent clinic visits, and through participation in peer support groups.

Once an individual is diagnosed with AIDS and the attendant recognition of AIDS as a terminal illness follows, a curious psychological paradox may occur for both the person with AIDS and his or her health care provider. Naturally persons with AIDS become bereaved as they recognize the finite period of their lives. They must develop personal priorities that incorporate the prognosis of AIDS. Preparing for death involves the difficult issues of the aggressiveness of health care interventions including cardiopulmonary resuscitation, writing a will, assigning durable power of attorney, identifying primary home care providers, and decisions about burial or cremation. However, persons with AIDS need a hopeful approach to the immediate demands of their health care whenever possible. Hope can be maintained by focusing on short-term health care goals and helping persons with AIDS to focus on short-term personal goals. In addition, currently available treatments for AIDS on both a practicing and research basis provide some opportunity of hope for a more prolonged survival with an improved quality of life. The navigation of this paradox may be very difficult for both persons with AIDS and health care providers, and the balance may tip in excessively depressed or hopeful directions. The use of community-based support groups may be helpful in maintaining this balance, and occasionally psychiatric consultation is necessary. Health care providers should also recognize that they may face their own fears about mortality as they aid their patients.

Clinicians must also investigate the social supports available to their patients. Significant issues include interpersonal support (lovers, spouses, family, and friends), insurance information (availability of coverage, limits of coverage, the ability to extend health insurance coverage beyond the period of employment, home care benefits, disability and life insurance), employment, and housing. Each of these issues may impact tremendously on the life of a person with HIV infection or AIDS. The contributions of a social worker may be invaluable in these areas.

SUMMARY

For the clinician caring for HIV-infected persons, both HIV infection and AIDS have become chronic illnesses to be managed over a period of years. The potential therapeutic interventions are rapidly increasing and have thus far contributed significantly to the improved quantity and quality of life for persons with HIV infection and AIDS. The clinician also has the opportunity to become involved with the complex social and psychological responses to HIV infection. In the future, all must hope for continued improvements in the treatment of HIV infection and for a more educated and enlightened response from society.

PART XXII

DISEASES CAUSED BY PROTOZOA AND METAZOA

423 Introduction to Protozoan and Helminthic Diseases

Adel A. F. Mahmoud

Human infections with parasitic protozoa and helminths account for a major proportion of the diseases caused by infectious agents. The magnitude of these infections is staggering; malaria infects 600 million, and ascariasis and trichuriasis 1 billion each, and 600 million are estimated to be infected with either schistosomiasis or filariasis. In spite of some worldwide efforts to control the spread and consequences of these infections, the associated morbidity and mortality have not been appreciably reduced. Furthermore, in the developed countries, infection with protozoa and helminths is being seen with increasing frequency in immigrants and is also among the more important causes of disease in the growing number of patients with depressed immune responses. Exciting developments have recently been reported concerning our understanding of the host-parasite relationship and the introduction of new and safe wide-spectrum chemotherapeutic agents.

BIOLOGY OF PARASITIC PROTOZOA AND HELMINTHS

This group of infectious agents belongs to the animal kingdom, unlike bacteria, viruses, or fungi. Such distinction led to restricting the term "parasite" to include only protozoa and helminths, whereas it should include all infectious agents because of their specialized dependent mode of life. The host-parasite relationship in protozoan and helminthic infections is complex because of the distinctive biologic features of the organisms. Although protozoa are unicellular pathogens and are mainly microscopic in size, they are far larger than viruses and bacteria. Protozoa multiply within mammalian hosts, as do viruses, bacteria, and fungi. Infection, therefore, can be initiated by a relatively small inoculum of organisms, which then multiply within the host and reach the numbers that cause disease.

By contrast, helminths are multicellular organisms with well-developed organ structures. They vary in size from 1 cm to approximately 10 meters. Unlike other infectious agents, helminths do not multiply within mammalian hosts. Re-exposure is, therefore, necessary to increase the number of helminths in a host. This distinguishing feature has important clinical significance, as disease in most helminthiasis is closely related to intensity of infection. For example, anemia results from hookworm infection only if the individual is harboring a significant worm load or there are other reasons for nutritional deficiencies. In rare circumstances, such as strongyloidiasis in the immunosuppressed, the worm can increase its population through an autoinfection cycle. This leads to life-threatening infection that necessitates aggressive medical attention.

Eosinophilia, when present, is a useful clinical manifestation of worm infections that migrate in host tissues. Worms that reside exclusively in body cavities, such as adult cestodes in the lumen of small intestines, are not associated with eosinophilia. Increased eosinophil counts may be observed in peripheral blood or affected tissues of infected individuals. Specific chemotherapy is usually followed by an increase in cell count before it subsides to normal levels. Eosinophilia in helminthic infections may be related to their ability to kill multicellular organisms. Because of the large size of most invading worms, killing of these targets by eosinophils occurs extracellularly and is mediated by a combination of oxidative and nonoxidative mechanisms.

Parasitic protozoa and helminths have developed elaborate mechanisms for evasion of host-protective responses. One of the best studied is antigenic variation noted in African trypanosomiasis. Parasitemia in infected individuals declines with the development of a protective antibody response but is followed by the emergence of a new parasite variable antigen; the organisms are therefore capable of avoiding the host response and increasing their numbers. The trypanosomes are capable of expressing at least 100 different variable antigens, allowing a long chronic course of infection. The organisms contain individual genes for all the different variable glycoproteins, but only one is expressed at a time. The multiplicity of trypanosome variable glycoprotein genes and of mechanisms for introducing mutations in them illustrates the complexity and sophistication of these pathogens.

The constantly changing nature of infectious disease is best illustrated in parasitic protozoan and helminthic infections. For example, new human pathogens such as *Isospora* and *Cryptosporidium* species have been appreciated only recently as causes of diarrheal illness, particularly in the immunosuppressed. These new developments add to difficulties in the treatment and control of parasitic protozoa and helminths. Recently, new chemotherapeutic agents have been developed, such as praziquantel and ivermectin, which are safe and effective broad-spectrum antihelminthics. However, the ever-spreading resistance of the parasites causing malaria and their mosquito vectors to most available compounds is imposing a considerable challenge to clinicians and public health specialists.

APPROACH TO THE PATIENT WITH PROTOZOAN OR HELMINTHIC INFECTION

Since most of the clinical manifestations of protozoan and helminthic diseases are not specific or pathognomonic, a high degree of suspicion is essential. The simple question "Where have you been?" and knowledge of the general geographic distribution of parasitic protozoa and helminths often save exhaustive and costly diagnostic workups and may spare human lives. Furthermore, inquiry into the immune status of individual patients, other drug therapies, or other diseases may be helpful in establishing the diagnosis of an opportunistic protozoan or helminthic infection.

The next phase in attempting to reach correct diagnosis involves interpretation of the presenting symptoms and signs. Peripheral blood eosinophilia remains an important and early indication of infections with tissue-invading worms. Definitive diagnosis in most cases requires isolation and identification of the specific pathogen. Since the number of cases seen by any single laboratory in North America is limited, expertise is required for correct identification that may not be available to many practicing physicians. Serologic testing for evidence of exposure to specific protozoa or helminths is currently available in many clinical or state laboratories or by consultation with the Centers for Disease Control. Although positive serologic results do not usually differentiate between past or present exposure, they are particularly helpful to physicians practicing outside areas endemic to these infectious diseases.

Centers for Disease Control: HHS Publication No. (CDC) 90–8280. Health Information for International Travel, Atlanta, Georgia, 1990, 164 pp. *A review of the geographic distribution of worldwide infections, updated yearly. It also contains the most recent recommendations for prophylaxis.*

Drugs for parasitic infections. Med Lett Drugs Ther 32:23, 1990. *A review of antiparasitic drugs published and updated annually. It includes dose, availability, and alternative choices.*

Mahmoud AAF: Parasitic protozoa and helminths: Biological and immunological challenges. Science 246:1015, 1989. *A selected review of some of the unique biologic, immunologic, and molecular aspects of malaria and schistosomes that accounts for the ability of these organisms to invade and establish themselves as parasites in humans.*

Warren KS, Mahmoud AAF (eds.): Tropical and Geographical Medicine, 2nd ed. New York, McGraw-Hill, 1990. *Detailed description of the biology and molecular understanding of protozoa and helminths and the diseases they cause in individuals and in populations.*

424 Malaria

Donald J. Krogstad

DEFINITION. Malaria is a disease characterized by recurrent fever and chills associated with the synchronous lysis of parasitized red blood cells. Its name is derived from the belief of the ancient Romans that malaria was caused by the bad air of the marshes surrounding Rome.

ETIOLOGY. Malaria is produced by intraerythrocytic parasites of the genus *Plasmodium.* Four plasmodia produce malaria in humans: *Plasmodium falciparum, Plasmodium vivax, Plasmodium ovale,* and *Plasmodium malariae.* The severity and characteristic manifestations of the disease are governed by the infecting species, the magnitude of the parasitemia, and the cytokines released as a result of the infection.

INCIDENCE, PREVALENCE, AND RESURGENCE. Incidence. Although precise data are difficult to obtain, malaria is unquestionably one of the most common infectious diseases. At least 200 to 300 million cases of malaria occur each year, with 2 to 3 million deaths. Most deaths are due to *P. falciparum* infection and occur among children less than 5 years old in sub-Saharan Africa. One of the major unanswered questions about malaria is how plasmodia produce repetitive infections without stimulating an effective (protective) immune response.

Prevalence. The prevalence of malaria varies widely; it may reach 10 per cent or more in hyperendemic areas. Thus its impact on the health of the developing world is enormous.

Resurgence. The major factors responsible for the resurgence of malaria are drug resistances: (1) the widespread resistance of the anopheline vector to economical insecticides such as chlorophenothane (DDT) and (2) the increasing prevalence of chloroquine resistance in *P. falciparum,* which is now endemic in South America, Southeast Asia, and Africa.

LIFE CYCLE AND EPIDEMIOLOGY. Life Cycle. The life cycle can be viewed as beginning with synchronous asexual replication of the erythrocytic stage of the parasite (Fig. 424–1; see Color Plate 11*A* to *D*). During the asexual erythrocytic cycle, the parasites mature from rings to trophozoites to schizonts, which ultimately rupture the red cell and release merozoites that enter uninfected red cells via receptors such as Duffy factor in *P. vivax;* the cycle is then repeated. By contrast, some erythrocytic parasites mature to sexual forms (gametocytes) that are ingested by the female anopheline mosquito. Within the mosquito intermediate host, male and female gametocytes mature to gametes, fuse to form an ookinete that matures to a zygote and ultimately produces the sporozoites that are infectious for humans. When an infected mosquito bites a human, sporozoites travel via the bloodstream to the liver, where they enter hepatocytes and mature to tissue schizonts, which release merozoites that are infectious for red cells and produce the asexual erythrocytic cycle. Two of the four species that infect humans (*P. vivax* and *P. ovale*) produce dormant (hypnozoite) forms in the liver,

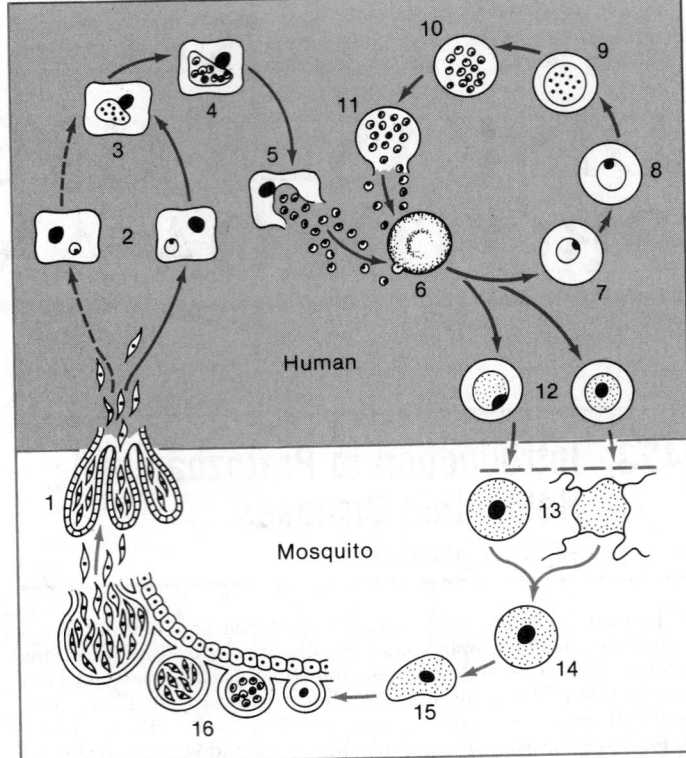

FIGURE 424–1. Life cycle of the malaria parasite. The lower and upper halves of the diagram indicate the anopheline mosquito and human parts of the cycle, respectively. Sporozoites from the salivary gland of a female *Anopheles* mosquito are injected under the skin (1). They then travel through the bloodstream to the liver (2) and mature within hepatocytes to tissue *schizonts* (4). Up to 30,000 parasites are then released into the bloodstream as *merozoites* (5) and produce symptomatic infection as they invade and destroy red blood cells. However, some parasites remain dormant in the liver as *hypnozoites* (2, *dashed lines from 1 to 3*). These are the parasites that cause relapsing malaria (in *P. vivax* or *P. ovale* infection). Once within the bloodstream, merozoites (5) invade red cells (6) and mature to the *ring* (7,8), *trophozoite* (9), and *schizont* (10) asexual stages. Schizonts lyse their host red cells as they mature and release the next generation of merozoites (11), which invade previously uninfected red cells. Within the red cell some parasites differentiate to sexual forms (male and female *gametocytes*) (12). When taken up by a female *Anopheles* mosquito, the gametocytes mature to *male* and *female gametes*, which produce *zygotes* (14). The zygote invades the gut of the mosquito (15) and develops into an *oocyst* (16). Mature oocysts produce *sporozoites*, which migrate to the salivary gland of the mosquito (1) and repeat the cycle. The dashed line between 12 and 13 indicates that absence of the mosquito vector prevents natural transmission via this cycle. Infection by the injection of contaminated blood bypasses this constraint and permits transmission among intravenous drug addicts or to recipients of blood transfusions. (Reproduced with permission from Krogstad DJ: Blood and tissue protozoa. *In* Schaecter M, Medoff G, Schlessinger D [eds.]: Mechanisms of Microbial Diseases. © 1989, the Williams & Wilkins Company, Baltimore.)

which mature 6 to 11 months or more after the initial infection and thus produce relapsing malaria.

Two characteristics of the life cycle are essential for the long-term survival of the parasite: multiplicity of replication and antigenic variability. *Multiplicity of replication* is apparent at each stage of the life cycle. The mature asexual erythrocytic schizont releases 8 to 32 merozoites when it ruptures its host red cell; up to 10,000 sporozoites result from one zygote; and 10,000 to 30,000 merozoites are released from one tissue (exoerythrocytic) schizont in the liver. This multiplicity of replication provides a redundancy that protects the parasite against losses from both immune and nonimmune host factors. *Antigenic variability* is associated with the morphologic changes that occur during the parasite's life cycle and similarly protects the parasite against the host immune response. For example, antibodies against sporozoites are ineffective against the asexual erythrocytic stages of the infection. Similarly, immune responses directed against asexual erythrocytic stages have no effect against the sexual (gametocyte) stages of the parasite. In addition, antigenic variation exists among strains of the same species. These observations are critically relevant to the development of a malaria vaccine (see below).

Epidemiology. The epidemiology of malaria is determined by the distributions of the anopheline mosquito vectors required for natural transmission and of the infected human reservoir. Both factors are present in endemic areas throughout the tropics. Important determinants of transmission include the vector population (vectors such as the *Anopheles gambiae* complex in Africa are more efficient), temperature (elevated temperatures shorten the life of the vector and hasten the maturation of the parasite within the vector), and control programs (which reduce both the vector population and the prevalence of human infection).

Competent mosquito vectors are present in the United States (*A. albimanus* in the east and *A. freeborni* in the west). Transmission in the United States is limited by the absence of infected humans, but natural mosquito-borne transmission can and does occur with the importation of infected humans (e.g., the return of soldiers after their exposure in endemic areas). Mosquito-borne transmission (*introduced malaria*) occurred in the United States after World War II, the Korean War, the Vietnam War, and, most recently, the arrival of refugees from Southeast Asia.

PATHOGENESIS. Species-Dependent Factors. Malaria is a multifactorial disease that can be explained in part, but not completely, by the magnitude of the parasitemia. *Plasmodium falciparum* is the most lethal parasite because it can invade red cells of any age and can thus produce unrestricted parasitemias involving 10^6 or more parasitized red cells per cubic millimeter of blood (≥ 20 per cent of circulating red cells). Conversely, *P. vivax* and *P. ovale*, which invade only young red cells, are limited to parasitemias of 25,000 or less per cubic millimeter, and *P. malariae*, which invades only older red cells, is limited to parasitemias of 10,000 or less per cubic millimeter.

The Host Immune Response. Because millions of people experience repetitive episodes of malaria throughout their lives in the tropics, the immune response to natural infection is inadequate by definition. Thus the term *semi-immune*, rather than immune, is used for residents of malaria-endemic areas. The reasons for the inadequate host immune response are only partially clear and are likely to be central to the development of a successful vaccine. For example, most exposed persons make antibodies directed against the repetitive epitope or epitopes on the surface of the sporozoite, and antibodies to asexual stages have been shown to reduce the magnitude of the parasitemia in children. However, cell-mediated immune responses are less frequent and may be essential for effective immunity. At least two factors have been identified that may be relevant to the poor cell-mediated response to sporozoite antigen: (1) The sites that determine the cell-mediated response are in the hypervariable region of the molecule, and (2) the ability to produce a cell-mediated response may be restricted by the individual's human leukocyte antigen (HLA) haplotype (immune restriction).

Peripheral Sequestration of Parasitized Red Cells. With maturation, red cells containing *P. falciparum* parasites develop knobs that contain histidine-rich proteins. In vivo, these knobs adhere to endothelial cells in the peripheral microvasculature via proteins such as thrombospondin, ICAM-1, or CD36. This phenomenon has at least two consequences: (1) It enhances the microvascular obstruction and pathology produced by the parasite, and (2) it removes mature *P. falciparum* parasites from the circulation, so that only early asexual erythrocytic stages, such as rings, are seen on peripheral blood smears.

Cytokines in the Pathogenesis of Malaria. Recent studies suggest that the release of cytokines in malaria is a central factor in the pathogenesis of the disease. Cytokines that have been shown to be important include tumor necrosis factor–α (TNF–α). Serum levels of TNF–α are elevated in severe *P. falciparum* infection and correlate with complications such as cerebral malaria and death, although a direct cause-and-effect relationship has not been established. Interferon-γ (IFN-γ) has antiparasitic activity against the exoerythrocytic stages of the parasite in the liver. However, neither TNF-α nor IFN-γ has been shown to inhibit the replication of asexual erythrocytic stages of the parasite in vitro.

PATHOLOGY. The pathology of severe malaria is that of a microvascular disease involving the brain, lung, and kidney.

Postmortem examination in fatal *P. falciparum* infection demonstrates parasitized red cells in the capillaries of the brain and other affected organs. In severe cases, acute tubular necrosis may be present, and the liver, spleen, and other sites in the reticuloendothelial system may be filled with dark malarial pigment from the phagocytosis of parasitized red cells. This predominantly microvascular pathology is consistent with the importance of sequestration and cytokine release in the pathogenesis of severe *P. falciparum* malaria (see above). By contrast, the other malarias that infect humans produce lower parasitemias, do not sequester, and are rarely fatal.

CLINICAL MANIFESTATIONS. Fever and Chills. Most patients with malaria present with recurrent fever and chills (at 48-hour intervals for *P. vivax* and *P. ovale* and at 72-hour intervals for *P. malariae*). By contrast, patients with *P. falciparum* infection typically have irregular fever and chills and rarely present with a regular 48-hour cycle of symptoms despite the 48-hour cycle of the parasite.

Coma. Coma (cerebral malaria) is the most feared complication of *P. falciparum* infection and has a substantial fatality rate. Although it has been attributed to the blockage of capillaries with parasitized red cells, both hypoglycemia and the effects of cytokines such as TNF-α are important factors. Hypoglycemia in *P. falciparum* malaria may have at least three causes: (1) the release of insulin from the pancreatic β cell by quinine or quinidine during treatment, (2) glucose consumption by the massive numbers of parasites present in the patient, and (3) depletion of liver glycogen stores in persons who have not eaten for several days before seeking medical care because they were ill with malaria. Hypoglycemia is particularly important to consider because it is treatable. Although the effects of TNF-α undoubtedly contribute to cerebral malaria, it is difficult to separate them from the magnitude of the parasitemia because the concentration of TNF-α and the magnitude of the parasitemia correlate with each other.

Renal Failure. Patients with massive parasitemias may have dark urine from the free hemoglobin produced by hemolysis (blackwater fever) and may later develop renal failure. Although hemolysis alone should not produce renal failure, some degree of renal impairment is typical in such patients. In most instances, the patients recover uneventfully; however, acute renal failure may occur with a time course similar to that of other causes of acute tubular necrosis.

Pulmonary Edema. This complication also occurs in patients with high *P. falciparum* parasitemias (≥ 5 per cent of circulating red cells). Hemodynamic measurements indicate that this is a noncardiogenic form of pulmonary edema with normal pulmonary arterial and capillary pressures. These findings and the association with high TNF-α levels suggest that the pathogenesis of this pulmonary edema may be similar to that of bacterial septicemia.

Gastrointestinal Manifestations. Diarrhea is common among children with *P. falciparum* infection. Although the pathogenesis of this complication is unclear, postmortem studies of children with diarrhea demonstrate parasitized red cells in the microvasculature of the intestine.

DIAGNOSIS. Giemsa-Stained Thick and Thin Smears. The most direct way to diagnose malaria is to prepare and examine Giemsa-stained thick or thin smears using oil immersion magnification ($\times 1000$). Giemsa's stain is preferable to Wright's stain, especially for persons with *P. vivax* or *P. ovale* infection, because the Schüffner's dots characteristic of those infections are often not visible with Wright's stain. Thick smears are more sensitive than thin smears because the red cells have been lysed. As a result, approximately 10 times as much blood can be examined per field and thus per unit of time. However, because the red cells have been lysed, it is not possible to determine the effect of the parasite on red cell size or the position of the parasite within the red cell on a thick smear (Table 424–1). Therefore, persons without previous experience in reading thick smears should consider using thin smears to identify the infecting parasite or parasites. A common mistake is to require characteristic gametocytes for a diagnosis of *P. falciparum* infection. Because gametocytes require longer to develop than asexual parasites (7 to 10 versus 2 days), they are usually not present in the peripheral blood when nonimmune tourists or expatriates first become symptomatic. Conversely, gametocytes are frequently present in

TABLE 424–1. MALARIA PARASITES THAT INFECT HUMANS

	Parasitemia (per μl blood)	Complications
P. falciparum	≥10⁶	Coma (cerebral malaria) Hypoglycemia Pulmonary edema, renal failure Anemia
P. vivax	25,000	Late (2–3 mo) splenic rupture
P. ovale	25,000	—
P. malariae	10,000	Immune complex nephrotic syndrome

	Morphology		
	Red Blood Cell Size	Schüffner's Dots	Stages
P. falciparum	No RBC enlargement	Absent	Rings, occasionally gametocytes
P. vivax	Enlarged host RBC	Present	All forms
P. ovale	Enlarged host RBC	Absent	All forms
P. malariae	No RBC enlargement	Present	All forms

	Relapse from Hypnozoites	Antimalarial Resistance
P. falciparum	No	Chloroquine and pyrimethamine-sulfadoxine
P. vivax	Yes	Possibly chloroquine
P. ovale	Yes	None known
P. malariae	No	None known

RBC = red blood cell

the blood of semi-immune residents of endemic areas with few or no symptoms or asexual parasites. A second common mistake is to assume that the patient can have only one kind of parasite: Approximately 5 per cent of persons with malaria have more than one type of parasite.

Fluorescent Staining with Acridine Orange. Fluorescence microscopy is one of two new techniques for detecting malaria parasites in peripheral blood specimens. This technique takes advantage of the fact that parasitized red cells are less dense than unparasitized red cells. A finger stick specimen is taken into a capillary tube prepared with acridine orange (to stain the nucleic acid in the parasite) and an anticoagulant. After centrifugation, parasitized red cells are found at the top of the red cell layer just below the buffy coat. Experienced investigators can examine a blood specimen in 30 to 40 seconds (less time than necessary to examine a thick or thin smear).

DNA Probes. Several investigators have developed *Plasmodium* and species-specific (e.g., *P. falciparum*–specific) DNA probes that can detect 40 to 100 parasites per microliter of blood (similar to the 1 to 10 parasites per microliter threshold of the thick smear). Problems that remain to be solved in the application of this technology include the development of signal systems as effective as ³²P that are not radioactive and the role, if any, of the polymerase chain reaction in enhancing the sensitivity of the assay under field conditions.

Serology (Antibody Testing). Testing for antibodies to plasmodia is of limited value. In endemic areas, most persons have antibody titers from previous infections whether or not they were infected recently. In addition, 3 to 4 weeks may be required to develop a diagnostic rise in antibody titer, whereas the decision to treat must be made in the first few hours of evaluation. However, serology may be of value retrospectively in nonimmune persons (expatriate tourists) who have been treated empirically for malaria without a microscopic diagnosis. For example, a high titer of antibodies against *P. vivax* suggests that the patient has had a recent *P. vivax* infection and should receive primaquine if it has not been given previously (see the section on treatment, below).

PREVENTION. The acquisition of malaria by exposed nonimmune persons may be prevented by taking antimalarials prospectively (chemoprophylaxis); by using insect repellents and otherwise reducing contact with the anopheline vector; and possibly, in the future, by a malaria vaccine (immunoprophylaxis).

Chemoprophylaxis. Drugs used for chemoprophylaxis should be safe because they are given to healthy persons for long periods. They should also have long serum half-lives so that they can be given infrequently. On the basis of these criteria, chloroquine is an excellent drug for chemoprophylaxis in areas without chloroquine-resistant *P. falciparum* (Table 424–2). It is the only chemoprophylactic agent safe for pregnant women and does not produce retinal toxicity at the doses used for antimalarial chemoprophylaxis. Unfortunately, chloroquine-resistant strains of *P. falciparum* are now established in Southeast Asia, South America, and Africa. For areas with chloroquine-resistant *P. falciparum*, mefloquine is now the recommended chemoprophylactic agent, although resistance to mefloquine is developing in Southeast Asia. Doxycycline is an alternative, with the advantage that it also reduces the frequency of traveler's diarrhea. The disadvantages of doxycycline include the need to take it daily, photosensitivity reactions, and vaginitis. Because of hypersensitivity reactions to pyrimethamine-sulfadoxine (Fansidar) and both agranulocytosis and hepatitis with amodiaquine, neither of these agents is recommended for chemoprophylaxis.

Vector Control. Because of widespread drug resistance in *P. falciparum*, increasing emphasis is placed on reducing exposure to the anopheline vector, especially in hyperendemic areas such as Africa. Strategies that are successful and should be considered include DEET *(N,N'-diethyl toluamide)–containing insect repellents and insecticide (pyrethrin)–impregnated bed nets. DDT is no longer effective in most regions of the world because of widespread resistance.

Immunoprophylaxis—Development of a Malaria Vaccine. Although a malaria vaccine is not available, it is hoped that this goal will ultimately be achievable. Because the three major parasite stages in humans are antigenically distinct, a successful vaccine will likely need to contain at least three parasite antigens (sporozoite, merozoite, and gametocyte). A vaccine need not be 100 per cent effective to be valuable. For example, a vaccine that requires boosting could be quite effective because of the repetitive exposure to natural infection in endemic areas. In addition, a vaccine that limits the magnitude of the parasitemia could have a marked effect on survival even if it had no effect on the incidence of infection, because severe morbidity and death are associated with high parasitemias.

TREATMENT. Successful treatment of patients with malaria depends primarily on effective antimalarial drugs. However, it is also dependent on ancillary measures as diverse as the infusion of glucose and exchange transfusion. Monitoring of the blood glucose level is important because hypoglycemia is a common cause of coma and because both quinine and quinidine stimulate the release of insulin directly from the pancreatic β cell. Steroids are contraindicated in cerebral malaria because they prolong the duration of coma.

The treatment of chloroquine-susceptible malaria (*P. vivax*, *P. ovale*, or *P. malariae* malaria, and chloroquine-susceptible *P. falciparum* malaria) is satisfactory (Table 424–3) because chloroquine is a safe and effective antimalarial. However, the treatment of chloroquine-resistant *P. falciparum* malaria is unsatisfactory. Potential choices include quinidine, quinine, and mefloquine. For comatose patients, intravenous quinidine may be the safest treatment. With the measurement of serum quinidine levels (2.0 to 5.0 μg per milliliter is usually adequate; ≥6 μg per milliliter is potentially toxic) and cardiac monitoring (for a QT interval greater than 0.6 second or QRS widening beyond 25 per cent of baseline) during intravenous infusion, the risk of quinidine cardiovascular toxicity is low. Although pyrimethamine-sulfadoxine

TABLE 424–2. CHEMOPROPHYLAXIS OF MALARIA*

For Areas without Chloroquine-Resistant *Plasmodium falciparum*:

Chloroquine phosphate (Aralen)	500 mg/wk (300 mg chloroquine base) during exposure and for 4 wk after leaving the endemic area

For Areas with Chloroquine-Resistant *Plasmodium falciparum*:

Mefloquine (Lariam)	250 mg/wk during exposure and for 4 wk after leaving the endemic area
Doxycycline	100 mg/d during exposure and for 4 wk after leaving the endemic area

*Updated recommendations on malaria chemoprophylaxis may be obtained 24 hours a day, 7 days a week, through the Centers for Disease Control (CDC) Hot Line at (404) 639-1610.

TABLE 424–3. TREATMENT OF MALARIA

P. vivax, P. ovale, P. malariae, and Chloroquine-Susceptible P. falciparum:

For patients unable to take oral medications:

IM chloroquine: 2.5 mg/kg IM q 4 hr or 3.5 mg/kg q 6 hr (total dose not to exceed 25 mg/kg base)

IV chloroquine: 10 mg/kg base over 4 hr, followed by 5 mg/kg base q 12 hr (given in a 2-hr infusion; total dose not to exceed 25 mg/kg base)

For patients able to take oral medications:

PO chloroquine: 10 mg/kg = 600-mg base, followed by an additional 300-mg base after 6 hr and 300-mg base again on days 2 and 3

Chloroquine-Resistant *P. falciparum*:

For patients unable to take oral medications:

IV quinidine: 6.25 mg/kg quinidine base (10 mg/kg quinidine gluconate) IV over 1 to 2 hr, followed by a constant infusion of 0.0125 mg/kg quinidine base (0.02 mg/kg quinidine gluconate) IV per minute until the parasitemia is < 1% or oral treatment is tolerated

For patients able to take oral medications:

PO quinine*: 650 mg quinine sulfate (540 mg quinine base) q 8 hr until significant improvement, or for 10 d

PO mefloquine: 750 mg as a single oral dose

PO pyrimethamine + sulfadoxine: 3 tablets (75 mg pyrimethamine plus 1500 mg sulfadoxine) as a single dose

To Prevent Relapse in *P. vivax* or *P. ovale* Infection:

PO primaquine†: 15 mg primaquine base (26.3 mg primaquine phosphate) daily × 14 d

---

*A number of investigators recommend tetracycline (250 mg PO q 6 hr for 7 to 10 days), pyrimethamine plus sulfadiazine or sulfisoxazole (25 mg twice daily plus 500 mg q 6 hr PO for 5 days), or 3 tablets of pyrimethamine-sulfadoxine (total of 75 plus 1500 mg PO once) in addition to oral quinine. These regimens have not been shown to be more effective than quinine alone.

†To prevent potentially severe hemolysis, patients should be tested for glucose-6-phosphate dehydrogenase deficiency prior to treatment with primaquine.

IM = Intramuscular; IV = intravenous.

(Fansidar) has been used for treatment, it is now controversial because of the increasing prevalence of resistance in areas of chloroquine resistance.

Patients with *P. vivax* or *P. ovale* infection should be tested for glucose-6-phosphate dehydrogenase deficiency before treatment with primaquine, which is used to eradicate persistent hypnozoites in the liver so that relapse may be prevented.

PROGNOSIS. Virtually all patients with *P. vivax, P. ovale,* or *P. malariae* infection respond well to chloroquine and make an uneventful recovery. Although chloroquine-resistant strains of *P. vivax* have been reported from Indonesia, these reports have not yet been confirmed. For patients with *P. falciparum* infection, the quantitative parasite count is the best predictor of the outcome. Patients with 5 per cent or greater parasitemia (≥250,000 parasites per microliter of blood) are at increased risk of severe and complicated malaria, including death. In addition to standard antimalarial treatment (outlined above), such patients should be considered for more heroic measures, such as exchange transfusion, if they do not improve within the first 12 to 24 hours of treatment.

Canfield CJ, Chongsuphajaisiddhi T, Danis M, et al.: Severe and complicated malaria. Trans R Soc Trop Med Hyg 89 (Suppl 2):1, 1990. *A comprehensive review of the pathogenesis and treatment of severe falciparum malaria.*

Good MF, Pombo D, Quakyi IA, et al.: Human T-cell recognition of the circumsporozoite protein of *Plasmodium falciparum:* Immunodominant T-cell domains map to the polymorphic regions of the molecule. Proc Natl Acad Sci USA 85:1199, 1988. *Evidence that the determinants of T cell reactivity are in hypervariable regions of the circumsporozoite protein.*

Grau GE, Taylor TE, Molyneux ME, et al.: Tumor necrosis factor and disease severity in children with falciparum malaria. N Engl J Med 320:1586, 1989. *Serum levels of TNF are increased in children with severe falciparum malaria.*

Krogstad DJ, Gluzman IY, Klye DE, et al.: Efflux of chloroquine from *Plasmodium falciparum:* Mechanism of chloroquine resistance. Science 238:1283, 1987. *The basis of chloroquine resistance is rapid efflux of the drug from the resistant parasite.*

Miller KD, Greenberg AE, Campbell CC: Treatment of severe malaria in the United States with a continuous infusion of quinidine gluconate and exchange transfusion. N Engl J Med 321:65, 1989. *Efficacy and safety of the continuous intravenous infusion of quinidine.*

Miller LH, Howard RJ, Carter R, et al.: Research toward malaria vaccines. Science 234:1249, 1986. *A review of the rationale for a vaccine and of the problems that will need to be addressed in producing a vaccine.*

Udeinya IJ, Schmidt JA, Aikawa M, et al.: Falciparum malaria–infected erythrocytes specifically bind to cultured human endothelial cells. Science 213:555, 1981. *Knobs on falciparum-infected cells bind to endothelial cells and thus explain the sequestration of red cells with mature falciparum parasites.*

White NJ, Warrell DA, Chanthavanich P, et al.: Severe hypoglycemia and hyperinsulinemia in falciparum malaria. N Engl J Med 309:61, 1983. *Hypoglycemia may result from quinine or quinidine treatment, which releases insulin from the pancreatic β cell.*

425 African Trypanosomiasis (Sleeping Sickness)

Thomas C. Quinn

DEFINITION. Known widely as sleeping sickness, African trypanosomiasis is an acute and chronic disease caused by *Trypanosoma brucei*. The parasites are transmitted to humans through the bite of tsetse flies located in regions of Africa between 15 degrees north and 15 degrees south latitude. In humans, there are two distinct forms of the disease, East African trypanosomiasis caused by *T. brucei rhodesiense* and West African trypanosomiasis caused by *T. brucei gambiense*. Although there is some clinical overlap, East African trypanosomiasis primarily causes an acute febrile illness with myocarditis and meningoencephalitis that is rapidly fatal if not treated, while West African trypanosomiasis is characterized as a chronic debilitating disease with mental deterioration and physical wasting (Table 425–1). A closely related variant, *T. brucei brucei*, is noninfectious for humans, but causes a chronic wasting illness in cattle, called nagana, which has a considerable indirect effect on human nutrition in sub-Saharan Africa.

ETIOLOGY AND LIFE CYCLE. Trypanosomes are motile hemoflagellates with a single undulating membrane that passes along the length of the parasite, terminating in an anterior flagellum (Color Plate 11*E*). Located anteriorly is a kinetoplast, an organelle containing topologically interlocked circular DNA molecules and mitochondria. In the peripheral blood of humans, trypanosomes vary in length from 10 to 40 μm. Both short stumpy and long slender forms can be present in a patient at the same time. The different variants of *T. brucei* cannot be distinguished morphologically but can be identified by differences in pathogenicity for certain animals, as well as in biochemical

TABLE 425–1. A COMPARISON OF GAMBIAN AND RHODESIAN SLEEPING SICKNESS

	Gambian (West African)	Rhodesian (East African)
Etiologic agent	*Trypanosoma brucei gambiense*	*Trypanosoma brucei rhodesiense*
Vector	*Glossina palpalis* or *tachinoides* (riverine tsetse)	*Glossina morsitans* (savanna tsetse)
Distribution	West and Central Africa	East Africa
Reservoir	Humans (domestic animals)	Wild game
Course of infection	Slow (months–years)	Rapid (<1 yr)
Clinical features		
Lymphadenopathy	+ + (Winterbottom's sign)	±
Myocarditis, heart failure	−	+ +
Neurologic symptoms	+ +	+
Disseminated intravascular coagulation	−	+
Parasitemia	Low	High

requirements, electrophoretic pattern of component enzymes, and DNA hybridization.

T. brucei is transmitted by the tsetse fly *Glossina*, within which it undergoes several developmental changes. During the bite of an infected host, trypanosomes are ingested and within the insect midgut rapidly differentiate into procyclic forms with loss of their dense surface coat, composed of variant surface glycoprotein. After 2 to 3 weeks of multiplication within the midgut the procyclic trypanosomes migrate to the insect's salivary glands, where they change morphologically into epimastigotes. These forms further undergo multiplication and ultimately differentiate into metacyclic trypanosomes that are coated with characteristic variant surface glycoprotein and are infectious to mammalian hosts. When a new host is bitten by the tsetse fly, the trypanosomes present in the salivary glands are injected into the connective tissue and blood. Within the human host they divide by binary fission and undergo antigen variation, a process by which they continually change their surface glycoproteins and evade the immune system of the host. With the bite of another tsetse fly, ingestion of the parasite occurs, and the life cycle of the organism is completed (Fig. 425–1). Mechanical transmission can theoretically also occur via blood transfusion or by interrupted biting of a tsetse fly feeding on an infectious person and directly thereafter biting an uninfected individual.

EPIDEMIOLOGY. It is estimated that African trypanosomiasis infects more than 20,000 Africans annually and that approximately 50 million people live at risk of acquiring trypanosomiasis because of the presence of the disease and its vector. Approximately 4 million square miles in Africa remain unpopulated because of the presence of *T. brucei brucei* infection, which results in the loss of domestic and wild animals, including cattle, waterbuck, bushbuck, and buffalo.

T. b. gambiense occurs primarily in the west and central regions of sub-Saharan Africa. Although it primarily infects humans, there may be animal reservoirs, such as pigs, dogs, and sheep. Gambian sleeping sickness is spread mainly by three species of tsetse fly, *Glossina palpalis*, *G. tachinoides*, and *G. fuscipes*. Distribution of these flies includes shaded areas along rivers and streams, where the conditions of temperature, darkness, and moisture are optimum.

T. b. rhodesiense differs from *T. b. gambiense* in that it is primarily a parasite of wild game, with humans serving only as occasional hosts. The geographic distribution of *T. b. rhodesiense*

is primarily East Africa from Ethiopia and eastern Uganda south to Zambia and Botswana. Rhodesian sleeping sickness is spread by tsetse flies of the *G. morsitans* group, including *G. pallidipes* and *G. swynnertoni*. These flies can survive in the open savanna, and Rhodesian sleeping sickness usually occurs among individuals visiting or traveling through an endemic area. Consequently, hunters, fishermen, and tourists are at risk, exposing themselves to vectors that usually feed on wild animals.

Imported African trypanosomiasis is a rare disease, with only 15 cases diagnosed in Americans since 1967. Most of these cases were among Americans who had been on safari in East Africa for a very brief period. Nearly all of these cases were initially misdiagnosed because of the unfamiliarity of American physicians with this disease. With an increase in international travel, 20,000 Americans are now estimated to visit endemic areas yearly, and approximately 10,000 aliens enter the United States each year from countries in Africa where the infection is endemic.

PATHOGENESIS AND PATHOLOGY. Following the bite of the tsetse fly, trypanosomes accumulate in the connective tissue, where they multiply to produce a local chancre (trypanoma). The organisms subsequently spread through the lymphatics, resulting in enlargement of lymph nodes secondary to reactive plasma cell and macrophage infiltration. The trypanosomes eventually disseminate to the circulatory system, where the parasitemia usually remains at low intensity and the organisms multiply by binary fission.

The host immune response plays an integral role in the pathogenesis of African sleeping sickness, although the exact nature of the immunopathogenic reactions has not been clearly defined. Trypanosomes survive by periodically altering their surface antigenic coat, avoiding successful eradication by the host. One organism can produce multiple antigenic variants (100 or more), each genetically determined and selected by the host antibody response. Consequently trypanosomes occur in the peripheral blood of infected individuals in waves, with each parasite wave consisting of a serologically distinct organism.

Tissue damage is induced by either toxin production or immune complex reaction with release of proteolytic enzymes. Immune complexes consisting of variant antigens of the organism and complement-fixing antibodies have been demonstrated in both the circulation and the target organs of infected patients. The production of autoantibodies is a prominent feature, and they are frequently directed against antigen components of red cells, brain, and heart. Anemia secondary to autoimmune hemolysis can be severe, resulting in anoxia and further tissue destruction. Thus the host-parasite interaction can result in generalized febrile episodes, lymphadenopathy, and myocardial and pericardial inflammation, along with anemia, thrombocytopenia, disseminated intravascular coagulation, and renal disease primarily during the acute stage of the disease.

During this period of circulatory dissemination, trypanosomes localize in the small vessels of the central nervous system (CNS). Pathologic changes in the CNS are most prominent in chronic cases of Gambian sleeping sickness. The meninges are thickened and infiltrated with lymphocytes, plasma cells, and morular cells. Morular cells are modified plasma cells (up to 20 mm in diameter) with large granular inclusions that have been shown to consist of immunoglobulin. These cells may play an important role in the local production of immunoglobulin M (IgM) in the cerebrospinal fluid. Edema, hemorrhages, and granulomatous lesions are frequently present, along with thrombosis as a result of endoarteritis and with neuronal degeneration.

African trypanosomes appear to induce a state of B cell polyclonal activation caused either by interference with host T cell control of antibody production or by a B cell mitogen released by the parasite. Polyclonal hypergammaglobulinemia, with very high levels of IgM, is commonly seen. High levels of nonspecific heterophile antibody, rheumatoid factor, and autoantibodies are also produced.

CLINICAL FEATURES. The signs and symptoms of sleeping sickness differ according to the infecting organism (Table 425–1). Rhodesian sleeping sickness, due to *T. b. rhodesiense*, causes a rapid progressive disease often resulting in cardiac failure and acute neurologic manifestations. Gambian sleeping sickness, caused by *T. b. gambiense*, is typically a more chronic illness with primarily neurologic features. However, this difference is not absolute; in some cases Gambian sleeping sickness can

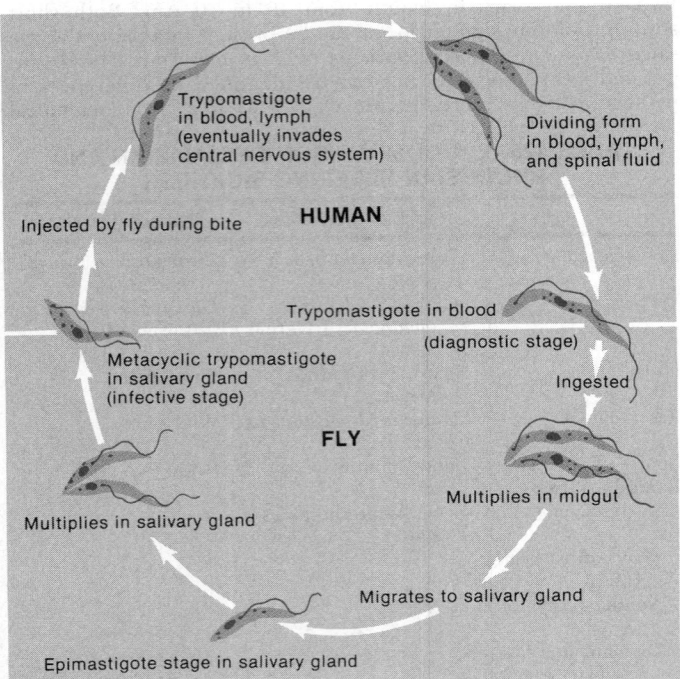

FIGURE 425–1. Life cycle of *Trypanosoma (Trypanozoon) brucei*, *T. (T.) B. gambiense*, and *T. (T.) b. rhodesiense*.

Trypomastigote in blood, lymph (eventually invades central nervous system)

Dividing form in blood, lymph, and spinal fluid

Injected by fly during bite

HUMAN

Trypomastigote in blood

(diagnostic stage)

Metacyclic trypomastigote in salivary gland (infective stage)

Ingested

FLY

Multiplies in salivary gland

Multiplies in midgut

Migrates to salivary gland

Epimastigote stage in salivary gland

progress rapidly, and occasionally Rhodesian sleeping sickness may follow a more chronic course.

Gambian Sleeping Sickness. Within several days following the bite by an infected tsetse fly, a trypanosomal nodule or chancre develops, typically on the exposed parts of the body. Within a week the lesion becomes a hard, painful nodule surrounded by erythema and swelling, which persists for 1 to 2 weeks. After this incubation period, clinical features develop after systemic, lymphatic, and circulatory invasion of the trypanosomes. Fever, headache, dizziness, and weakness occur in the majority of these patients. Febrile episodes may last 1 to 6 days, alternating with afebrile periods. Lymphadenopathy with prominent supraclavicular and posterior cervical enlargement is seen in more than 80 per cent of infected individuals. Known as Winterbottom's sign, these enlarged lymph nodes are usually discrete, rubbery, and painless. Moderate splenomegaly may occur, and urticaria and erythematous rashes have also been observed. Electrocardiograms are often abnormal, but clinical signs of heart disease are unusual.

Six months to several years after the first appearance of symptoms, the clinical features of this early hemolymphatic stage progress to a late meningoencephalitic stage. Behavioral and personality changes are often the first signs of CNS involvement. Later, more florid psychological changes may occur, with hallucinations and delusions. Reversion of sleep rhythm is characteristic, with drowsiness during the day, a feature from which the disease derives its name. Other nervous symptoms include tremor, most characteristically of the face and lips, and hyperesthesia, causing some patients to avoid common practices such as closing (Kerandel's sign) or locking doors (key sign). Without treatment, the patient's level of consciousness progressively deteriorates until he or she finally lapses into stupor. Alterations in thermoregulation may lead to hypothermia or hyperthermia, and progressive neurologic alterations lead to convulsions, chorea, and athetosis. The cerebrospinal fluid shows an increase in cells and protein, much of which is IgM. Free immunoglobulin light chains may be present. Most of the cells are lymphocytes, but a few are plasma cells and morula cells. Trypanosomes may also be evident within the cerebrospinal fluid.

Rhodesian Sleeping Sickness. This disease is more acute than Gambian sleeping sickness, and symptoms usually occur a few days after the victim has been bitten by the tsetse fly. Alternating periods of high fever, malaise, and headache, followed by several days of well-being, are often misinterpreted as acute malaria infection. Lymphadenopathy is not prominent in this variety of the disease, and Winterbottom's sign is usually absent. Tachycardia with arrhythmias and extrasystoles is common. Anemia, thrombocytopenia, and disseminated intravascular coagulation are usually evident within the first several weeks of infection. Liver enzyme values are often elevated, and electrocardiograms are abnormal, usually reflecting underlying myocarditis. Neurologic features are similar to those described for Gambian sleeping sickness, but they occur much earlier and with more rapid deterioration. Without treatment the disease may result in death within a matter of weeks to months, without clear distinction into an early and late phase, as described for Gambian trypanosomiasis.

DIAGNOSIS. Although a presumptive diagnosis of trypanosomiasis is based on clinical suspicion, history of travel to areas where this disease is endemic, and tsetse fly exposure, confirmation of the diagnosis is based solely on the demonstration of trypanosomes. These organisms may be found in the blood (Color Plate 11*E*), bone marrow, centrifuged cerebrospinal fluid, lymph node aspirates, and scrapings from the chancre. Giemsa's or Wright's stain of the buffy coat of centrifuged heparinized blood make identification easier, since the trypanosomes are often concentrated in the buffy coat. In patients with Gambian sleeping sickness, in which trypanosomes are found less frequently in the blood, concentration methods such as ion exchange chromatography, diethylaminoethyl (DEAE) filtration, culture, or animal inoculation should be used.

All patients should have a lumbar puncture prior to and following therapy to determine whether CNS involvement is present. Documentation of CNS involvement is imperative, since suramin, a drug effective against the hemolymphatic stage of *T. brucei*, does not penetrate the spinal fluid. CNS disease is manifested by pleocytosis and elevation of spinal fluid total protein and IgM levels. Trypanosomes can be found in most patients, provided that the cerebrospinal fluid is examined immediately after collection and that clean glassware is used. For those patients in whom trypanosomes cannot be found, measurement of the cerebrospinal fluid IgM is often of great diagnostic help. A high cerebrospinal fluid IgM value and a modest increase in total protein are almost pathognomonic of sleeping sickness.

Several immunodiagnostic tests have been developed for African trypanosomiasis, including an indirect hemagglutination test, indirect fluorescent antibody test, and enzyme-linked immunosorbent assay (ELISA), that are useful for epidemiologic surveys. A simple direct agglutination test for stained trypanosomes performed on cards (CATT) has been developed and is commercially available. However, at present, no serologic test provides sufficient definitive information for treatment of a patient without demonstration of the organism.

TREATMENT. Suramin* is the drug of choice for the early hemolymphatic stage of both *T. b. gambiense* and *T. b. rhodesiense* infections before CNS invasion has occurred. Suramin does not cross the blood-brain barrier in increased amounts, and it will not cure the disease once CNS invasion has occurred. The dose is 20 mg per kilogram of body weight given intravenously up to a maximum single dose of 1 gram. Suramin is freshly prepared as a 10 per cent aqueous solution. Intramuscular injection is not advised because of local irritation and pain. Suramin binds to plasma proteins and may persist in the circulation at low concentrations for as long as 3 months. A test dose of 200 mg is given initially; if no adverse side effects are noted, then full doses of the drug may be given on days 1, 3, 7, 14, and 21. A single course for an adult is usually 5 grams; it should not exceed 7 grams.

Suramin is a toxic drug that may result in idiosyncratic reactions in some individuals (1 in 20,000). The drug is excreted entirely by the kidneys; renal damage may result because of deposition of the drug in the renal tubules. The urine should be examined prior to administration of each dose of suramin, and if proteinuria or casts are present, treatment should be stopped. Other side effects include a papular eruption, photophobia, arthralgias, peripheral neuritis, fever, and agranulocytosis.

Pentamidine isethionate* is an alternative drug for the treatment of early hemolymphatic African trypanosomiasis, but it is much less active against *T. rhodesiense* than is suramin. The dose is 4 mg per kilogram of body weight; it is given every other day by intramuscular injection for a total of 10 injections. Pentamidine is also ineffective in the treatment of CNS trypanosomiasis.

The arsenical melarsoprol* (Mel B) is the treatment of choice for both Gambian and Rhodesian sleeping sickness once involvement of the CNS has occurred. The drug is given in three courses of 3 days each. The recommended dosage is 2.0 to 3.6 mg per kilogram per day given intravenously in three divided doses for 3 days, followed 1 week later by 3.6 mg per kilogram per day in three divided doses for 3 days. This latter course is then repeated 10 to 21 days later. Melarsoprol is a highly toxic drug and should be administered with great care. If signs of arsenical toxicity occur, the drug should be discontinued.

The most important side effects involve the CNS. A reactive encephalopathy, probably due to release of trypanosomal antigens, may occur early in the course of treatment, and its incidence has been reported to be as high as 18 per cent. It may develop very rapidly or insidiously, and its mortality is about 50 per cent. Clinical indications of reactive encephalopathy include high fever, headache, tremor, seizures, and finally coma. It has been suggested that corticosteroids protect patients from melarsoprol encephalopathy, but this assertion has not been clearly documented. Alternative drugs for CNS involvement include tryparsamide, melarsonyl potassium (Mel W), and nitrofurazone. These drugs appear either to be more toxic than Mel B or less effective in the treatment of CNS disease. Difluoromethylornithine (eflornithine, DFMO), a specific, irreversible inhibitor of polyamine biosynthesis, has been shown to be curative in animal models inoculated with *Trypanosoma* species. In a preliminary open field trial, 20 patients, 18 of whom had CNS infection with *T. b.*

*Available from the Centers for Disease Control, Atlanta, GA.

gambiense, had a clinical response with parasitic clearance of the CSF. The recommended dosage is 400 mg per kilogram per day given intravenously in four divided doses for 2 weeks, followed by 300 mg per kilogram per day given orally in four doses for 30 days. Frequent side effects include diarrhea and anemia. Further studies are under way to define optimal treatment regimens, and its efficacy in *T. b. rhodesiense* has not been determined. Regular follow-up with clinical examination and lumbar puncture is necessary for all patients for at least 1 year after treatment.

PROGNOSIS. Untreated African sleeping sickness is almost invariably fatal. Many patients with early Gambian sleeping sickness may remain relatively well for months to years without treatment, but once CNS involvement has occurred, death is inevitable unless treatment is given. Death frequently results from pneumonia in Gambian sleeping sickness and from heart failure in Rhodesian sleeping sickness. Treatment with suramin in the early phase of sleeping sickness results in a cure rate of over 90 per cent. A few patients may subsequently develop CNS involvement and require further treatment. Mel B achieves a parasitologic cure in at least 90 per cent of cases of advanced disease, and many patients may recover completely. Unfortunately, some patients are left with irreversible neurologic damage. Approximately 5 per cent of patients may die during the course of Mel B therapy.

CONTROL AND PROPHYLAXIS. Measures to prevent and control African trypanosomiasis can be instituted at three different levels: surveillance and treatment, chemoprophylaxis, and vector control. Surveillance with treatment is necessary to reduce the human reservoir of infection, particularly in areas where epidemics have occurred in the past. Pentamidine has been successfully used as a chemoprophylactic in Gambian sleeping sickness when given as a single intramuscular injection of 4 mg per kilogram every 3 to 6 months. However, the drug is generally not recommended for mass use, and it appears to be ineffective against Rhodesian trypanosomiasis.

Vector control requires destruction of tsetse fly habitats by selective clearing of vegetation and spraying with insecticides, which are effective only temporarily. Because of the wide range of the tsetse fly, these vector control measures are not economically feasible except when it is necessary to break transmission in epidemics. For individual protection, avoidance of contact with infected tsetse flies is best achieved by the use of repellents and protective clothing.

A vaccine is not currently available because of the occurrence of antigenic variation. However, the potential for development of a vaccine has increased with the progress in cultivation of *T. brucei* in vitro and analysis of the chemical structure of its variant antigens.

Donelson JE, Rice-Ficht AC: Molecular biology of trypanosome antigenic variation. Microbiol Rev 49:107, 1985. *A review of the genetic control of host-parasite interaction in trypanosomiasis.*

Jennings FW: Future prospects for the chemotherapy of human trypanosomiasis. Combination chemotherapy and African trypanosomiasis. Trans R Soc Trop Med Hyg 84:618, 1990. *A review of the different drug regimens for treatment of trypanosomiasis and discussion of their advantages and toxicities.*

Kirchhoff LV: Agents of African trypanosomiasis (sleeping sickness). *In* Mandel GL, Douglas RJ, Bennett JE (eds.): Principles and Practice of Infectious Disease, 3rd ed. New York, John Wiley & Sons, 1990, pp 2085–2090. *An excellent chapter on the biology and clinical features of African trypanosomiasis.*

Molyneux DH: Selective primary health care: Strategies for control of disease in the developing world: VIII. African trypanosomiasis. Rev Infect Dis 5:945, 1983. *A review of the various chemotherapeutic, vector, and environmental control measures for sleeping sickness.*

Pepin J, Milord F, Guer C, Schechter PJ: Difluoromethylornithine for arseno-resistant *Trypanosoma brucei gambiense* sleeping sickness. Lancet 2:1431, 1987. *Successful use of this less toxic drug (DFMO) in the treatment of* T. gambiense.

Poltera AA: Pathology of human African trypanosomiasis with reference to experimental African trypanosomiasis and infections of the central nervous system. Br Med Bull 41:169, 1985. *A review of the clinical and pathologic findings of CNS disease in both human and animal models infected with African trypanosomiasis.*

Van Nieuwenhove S, Schechter PJ, DeClercq J, et al.: Treatment of gambiense sleeping sickness in the Sudan with oral DFMO, an inhibitor of ornithine decarboxylase; first field trial. Trans R Soc Trop Med Hyg 79:692, 1985. *A successful clinical treatment trial of 20 patients with chronic Gambian trypanosomiasis with DFMO, a new nontoxic trypanosomicidal drug.*

World Health Organization: Epidemiology and control of African trypanosomiasis. Report of a WHO Expert Committee. WHO Tech Rep Ser 739:36, 1986. *An excellent review on the topic of African trypanosomiasis.*

426 American Trypanosomiasis (Chagas' Disease)

Franklin A. Neva

DEFINITION. Chagas' disease, resulting from infection with the protozoan parasite *Trypanosoma cruzi*, is named after the Brazilian physician Carlos Chagas, who discovered the parasite. Distinction should be made between infection caused by the parasite, as manifested by positive serologic findings, and clinical disease. Chronic disease manifestations develop years after initial infection in the form of chronic cardiomyopathy with conduction defects or with dysfunction of the esophagus or colon (mega syndromes).

LIFE CYCLE OF THE ETIOLOGIC AGENT. The causative agent, *T. cruzi*, is usually transmitted as a zoonosis. Various species of blood-sucking reduviids become infected when they take a blood meal from animals or humans who have circulating parasites, trypomastigotes, in the blood. The ingested parasites transform into epimastogotes and multiply in the midgut of the insect vector, where they later transform once again into metacyclic trypomastigotes in the hindgut of the bug. When the infected bug takes a subsequent blood meal, it frequently defecates during or after feeding, so that the infective metacyclic forms are deposited on the skin. Transmission to a second vertebrate host occurs when the feeding puncture site or a mucous membrane is inadvertently contaminated with infective bug feces. The parasites can penetrate a variety of host cell types, within which they transform into intracellular amastigote forms. In contrast to certain other intracellular organisms, amastigotes of *T. cruzi* are not enclosed in phagolysosomes. They multiply in the cytoplasm, elongate, transform into motile trypomastigotes, and rupture out of the cells. Liberated organisms penetrate new cells or are carried into the bloodstream to initiate further cycles of multiplication, preferentially in muscle cells, or are ingested by new vectors to maintain the cycle (Fig. 426–1).

Asymptomatic infected individuals with low-level parasitemia can transmit *T. cruzi* via blood transfusion. Another route of transmission of the parasite is congenital infection.

EPIDEMIOLOGY. *T. cruzi* and its arthropod vectors are widely distributed from the southern United States through Mexico and Central America into South America down to central Argentina and Chile. The parasite is restricted to the Western Hemisphere. In most countries where it occurs, the parasite cycle is sylvatic; i.e., it takes place in wild animals and vector bugs that associate with them. Human contact with sylvatic vectors is sporadic and accidental. A peridomestic cycle occurs under conditions in which infected animals, such as opposums and rats, live close to human habitations, and vector bugs may invade houses to seek a blood meal. Certain species of triatomine bugs, such as *Triatoma infestans*, *Rhodnius prolixus*, and *Panstrongylus megistus*, have a great propensity to invade, live, and breed in houses if suitable microenvironments are present. Cracks and holes in adobe mud huts or in crude wooden walls, thatched roofs, and household rubble provide ideal hiding and breeding places for the bugs, which venture out at night to feed upon sleeping inhabitants. Under these conditions *T. cruzi* is transmitted from person to person—a domiciliary cycle—and Chagas' disease becomes a public health problem. Thus, human trypanosomiasis in Latin America is primarily an infection of poor people living in substandard housing in rural areas.

The prevalence of antibodies to the parasite in human populations varies widely in different countries, as well as within regions of a country. A recent nationwide survey in Brazil found about 10 per cent of the rural population to be infected. It is not unusual for up to half of all inhabitants in selected villages to be antibody positive. Countries with the highest incidence of both infection and disease due to *T. cruzi* include Brazil, Argentina, Chile, Bolivia, and Venezuela. It is estimated that in all of the Americas a total of 15 million people are infected. In many Latin American countries, positive serologic findings for *T. cruzi* constitute a social stigma; a lower socioeconomic background is implied, and employers are reluctant to hire someone who may later develop chronic Chagas' disease.

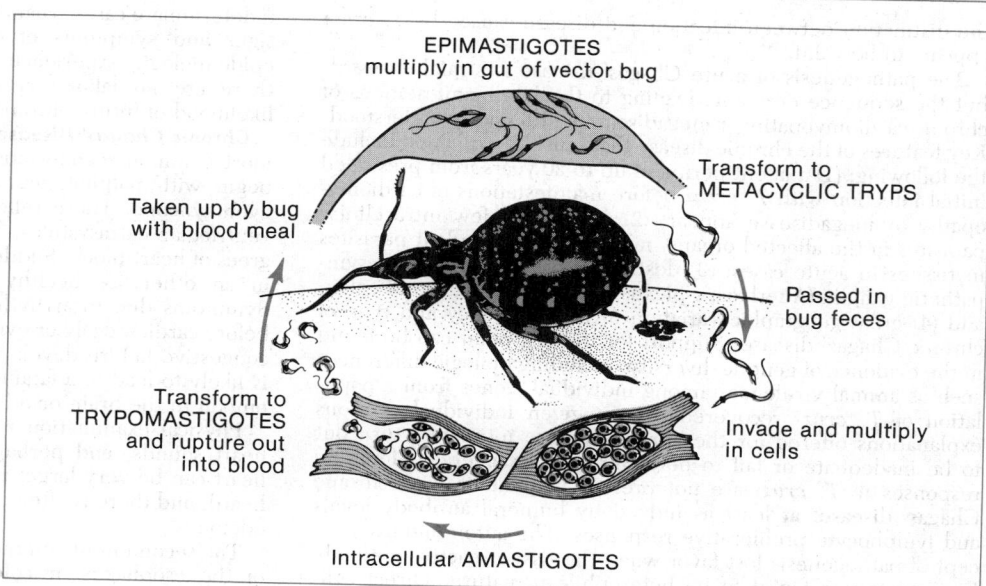

FIGURE 426–1. Life cycle of *Trypanosoma cruzi.*

EPIMASTIGOTES
multiply in gut of vector bug

Taken up by bug
with blood meal

Transform to
METACYCLIC TRYPS

Passed in
bug feces

Transform to
TRYPOMASTIGOTES
and rupture out
into blood

Invade and multiply
in cells

Intracellular AMASTIGOTES

Considerable geographic variation exists in both the prevalence and the type of chronic disease manifestations. In Brazil, for example, cardiomyopathy and megadisease are common, and often a patient has both types of involvement. However, chagasic megaesophagus and megacolon are virtually unknown in Venezuela, Colombia, and Panama, whereas cardiomyopathy is relatively high, moderate, and low in prevalence, respectively. In general, the frequency of cardiac disease in Central America and Mexico in seropositive persons is low, even though rates of seropositivity may be substantial. Also in these countries heart disease tends to develop later in life than in Brazil.

The situation regarding Chagas' disease in the United States is interesting because only four autochthonous acute cases have been recognized despite the presence of *T. cruzi* in vector bugs as well as in animal reservoirs. The lack of transmission of *T. cruzi* to humans in this country is probably due to preference of the vectors for sylvatic habitats and their tendency to defecate late after feeding. Yet in some areas of the West, bites from aggressive and abundant reduviid bugs can be a source of annoyance to, and allergic reactions in, suburbanites and outdoorspeople. Because of increased Hispanic immigration in recent years, sporadic cases of chronic Chagas' disease will probably be encountered in the United States.

PATHOLOGY AND PATHOGENESIS. In *acute Chagas' disease,* a local inflammatory lesion called a chagoma may develop at the site of entry of the parasite. Histologically, the chagoma shows mononuclear cell infiltration, interstitial edema, and intracellular aggregates of amastigotes in cells of the subcutaneous tissue and muscle. Other pathologic changes in the acute disease are known only for the severe cases that come to autopsy, since the great majority of cases are subclinical and self-limiting. Biopsy specimens from enlarged lymph nodes show hyperplasia, and amastigotes may be present in reticular cells. Skeletal muscle tissue from muscle biopsies have shown organisms and focal inflammation. In acute cases that have a fatal outcome there is invariably myocarditis with an enlarged heart. Microscopically, there is degeneration of cardiac muscle fibers and prominent but patchy areas of inflammation with nests of amastigotes in the muscles. The brain and meninges may also be parasitized in acute Chagas' disease. Virtually all organs and cell types can be invaded by *T. cruzi.*

The organs primarily affected in *chronic Chagas' disease* are the heart and certain hollow viscera, such as the esophagus and colon. Surprisingly, the intracellular *T. cruzi* usually cannot be found in the affected organs, or a few may be demonstrable after protracted search of many tissue sections. The heart in those patients with chronic disease who die suddenly, presumably of ventricular arrhythmias or heart block, may be normal in size or only moderately enlarged. Other patients with chronic chagasic

cardiomyopathy develop cardiomegaly and die of intractable failure. The hearts are both hypertrophied and dilated, with thinning, especially at the apex to form a characteristic apical aneurysm. Mural thrombi, with subsequent embolization of the lungs and peripheral organs, are frequently seen. The coronary arteries are generally normal.

Microscopic findings in the heart are not specific, consisting of focal mononuclear cell infiltrates, hypertrophy of cardiac fibers with patchy areas of necrosis, variable fibrosis, and edema. The components of the conduction system of the heart most often involved by inflammatory changes are the sinoatrial and atrioventricular nodes, as well as the right branch and left anterior branches of the bundle of His. Andrade's detailed studies of these pathologic changes indicated that they correlated well with electrocardiographic (ECG) changes during life but were diffusely scattered without specific localization to the conducting system.

When either the esophagus or the colon is affected in chronic Chagas' disease, the gross appearance is of dilatation and hypertrophy of the affected organ. The microscopic pathologic changes are disappointingly similar to those in the heart, again with no or very few organisms. However, myenteric ganglion cells are strikingly reduced in number. This type of parasympathetic denervation may also be found in other hollow viscera, such as duodenum, ureters, or biliary tree.

The significant pathology of *congenital Chagas' disease* is chronic placentitis, with inflammatory changes and focal necrosis in the chorionic villi. Amastigotes of *T. cruzi* are present in the lesions. The presence of lesions and organisms in the placenta may be associated with abortion, stillbirth, or acute disease in the fetus. However, pregnancy may result in a normal fetus, even though placental lesions are present.

The extent and clinical significance of pathologic changes in those individuals with antibodies to *T. cruzi* but without evidence of disease, i.e., the *indeterminate form,* are not yet clear. Such indeterminate cases may have significantly reduced numbers of esophageal or colonic ganglion cells. It has been claimed that endocardial biopsy specimens from indeterminate cases have recognizable pathologic changes. In addition, in some indeterminate cases there is a chronic low level of parasitemia. Therefore, one point of view is that everyone with positive serologic findings has a continuing subclinical disease process that will become manifested with time. On the other hand, even in those areas where chronic Chagas' disease is common, one half or more of those with a positive serology will die of causes other than Chagas' disease. In most Latin American countries, where endemicity is much lower, a positive serologic finding constitutes a relatively small risk factor for later chronic disease. Until better information on this issue becomes available and, more important, until the pathogenesis of chronic Chagas' disease is unraveled, the distinction between infection and disease caused by *T. cruzi* appears to be valid.

The pathogenesis of acute Chagas' disease is straightforward, but the sequence of events leading to the late manifestations of chronic cardiomyopathy or megadisease is still poorly understood. Key features of the chronic disease that must be explained include the following: (1) a latent period of up to 20 years from presumed initial infection with *T. cruzi* before manifestations of cardiomyopathy or megadisease appear; (2) no or very few intracellular parasites in the affected organs, in contrast to abundant parasites in tissues in acute cases; (3) destruction of autonomic parasympathetic ganglia (Auerbach's plexus) of the esophagus and colon; and (4) great geographic variation in the frequency and type of chronic Chagas' disease. Support for the last point can be found in the evidence of genetic diversity, including biologic differences such as animal virulence, among individual clones from a population of *T. cruzi* recovered from a given individual. Various explanations offered for the chronic disease ultimately turn out to be inadequate or fail to be confirmed. Exaggerated immune responses to *T. cruzi* are not present in patients with chronic Chagas' disease, at least as judged by humoral antibody levels and lymphocyte proliferative responses. The autoimmunity concept of pathogenesis lost favor when the tissue reactive antibody in patients was found to be heterophile in nature. Direct cell-mediated cytotoxicity to heart muscle has also been proposed as a mechanism for the chronic disease. An even more complicated type of autoimmune response involving anti-idiotypic antibodies as T cell antigens, as well as differential responses in antigen presentation, has also been proposed to explain chronic Chagas' disease. But a unifying concept of pathogenesis for chronic Chagas' disease is still lacking.

Some insight into the host-parasite balance that exists in individuals chronically infected with *T. cruzi* is provided by observations on the influence of intercurrent infections or interventions affecting the immune status. One such experience concerns the development of acute disease observed in a number of recipients of heart transplants for chagasic cardiomyopathy, presumably because of the heavy immunosuppression required. On the other hand, although the experience is still early, there are no reports that human immunodeficiency virus (HIV) infection precipitates either acute or chronic manifestations of Chagas' disease.

CLINICAL PRESENTATION. In endemic areas, first exposure to *T. cruzi* generally is subclinical and goes unnoticed. When those initially exposed do develop clinical manifestations, the disease is an acute systemic infection. Chronic Chagas' disease, in contrast, evolves as a later sequel with specific organ involvement and no systemic features.

Acute Chagas' Disease. Although acute Chagas' disease is most commonly seen in children, it can occur at any age, depending upon the nature of exposure to the causative organism. The incubation period under natural conditions cannot be established accurately but is probably at least a week. A local area of erythema and induration (chagoma) may develop in the skin at the site of parasite entry. When infection takes place via the conjunctival route, as it frequently does, the local periorbital swelling is referred to as Romaña's sign. The chagoma is often accompanied by regional adenopathy and persists for several weeks. Other signs of acute Chagas' disease include fever, generalized lymphadenopathy, hepatosplenomegaly, and transient skin rashes.

Myocarditis, accompanied by tachycardia and nonspecific ECG changes, can occur in the acute stage. Meningoencephalitis is another serious complication, particularly in very young patients. Fatal outcome in acute Chagas' disease is rare, but when it does occur, it is due to myocarditis and congestive failure or to meningoencephalitis.

Signs and symptoms of acute disease gradually subside within a few weeks to several months even without treatment. Trypanosomes, which have been demonstrable by direct microscopy in the peripheral blood during the acute phase, become more difficult to find and then disappear. The patient then enters the *indeterminate phase*, which is characterized by the presence of antibodies to *T. cruzi* and often also by the presence of low-level parasitemia in the blood demonstrable only by special sensitive methods. This state of apparent complete recovery with positive serologic findings may continue indefinitely without further evidence of disease or sequelae. However, a variable proportion of indeterminate cases, years to a decade or more later, will develop signs and symptoms of chronic Chagas' disease. Except for epidemiologic experience from a particular geographic region, there are no laboratory or clinical indicators to predict the likelihood of future chronic disease.

Chronic Chagas' Disease. Cardiac signs and symptoms are the most common manifestations of chronic disease and are apt to begin with palpitations, dizziness, precordial discomfort, and even syncope. These reflect a variety of arrhythmias, including ventricular extrasystoles, bouts of tachycardia, and various degrees of heart block. Sudden death due to ventricular tachycardia in an otherwise healthy young adult is not at all unusual. Symptoms due to arrhythmias may be present for a long time before cardiomegaly or evidence of cardiac failure appears. When congestive failure develops, it is predominantly right sided and is likely to lead to a fatal outcome within a few years. Peripheral emboli to the brain or other organs are frequent.

Physical examination reveals only an irregular pulse, distant heart sounds, and perhaps a gallop rhythm. With failure, the heart can be very large, functional regurgitant murmurs may be heard, and there is often congestive hepatomegaly and peripheral edema.

The second most common chronic manifestation is megadisease of the esophagus or colon, most frequently the former. The symptoms are indistinguishable from those of idiopathic achalasia and include dysphagia, feeling of fullness after eating or drinking only small amounts, chest pain, and regurgitation. Aspiration with secondary pneumonia is a common complication in advanced cases, as are weight loss and cachexia. Salivary gland hypertrophy secondary to hypersalivation is sometimes seen. Esophageal cancer is reported to be more frequent in patients with chagasic megaesophagus, as with idiopathic achalasia.

Patients with chagasic megacolon suffer from chronic constipation and abdominal pain. Volvulus, obstruction, and perforation of the bowel may occur. An astonishing history of going several weeks between bowel movements can be obtained from some patients with severe megacolon. Megaesophagus and megacolon may both be present in the same patient, and cardiomyopathy can occur with either form of megadisease.

DIAGNOSIS. For both acute and chronic Chagas' disease, a history of possible exposure to *T. cruzi* should be sought. Usual tourist travel to endemic areas is not likely to provide sufficient exposure to infected vectors. Blood transfusion from a chronically infected donor can be a source of infection.

For *acute Chagas' disease* direct microscopic examination of anticoagulated blood or a buffy coat preparation for motile trypanosomes is the most important procedure. Organisms are more difficult to find on stained thin or thick blood films, but the morphology of organisms seen on direct microscopy should be confirmed in a stained preparation. Red cells may be lysed, using 0.083 per cent NH₄Cl to concentrate parasites by centrifugation. If parasites cannot be found in the peripheral blood and acute disease is still suspected, blood can be cultured on NNN (Novy, MacNeal, and Nicolle's medium) or other suitable media. Inoculation of mice with patient's blood may sometimes result in recovery of the parasite. Biopsy of an enlarged lymph node or of skeletal muscle for culture and/or histologic examination is another possibility.

The most sensitive technique for recovery of trypanosomes from the blood is a procedure referred to as xenodiagnosis. It is basically a form of blood culture using the insect vector, by allowing up to 40 normal, laboratory-reared reduviid bugs to feed directly upon the patient or on the patient's blood through a membrane. Circulating parasites ingested by the bugs multiply in the gut and can be detected when the intestinal contents are examined 30 days later. Under experimental conditions, polymerase chain reaction techniques to demonstrate low levels of parasitemia appear promising, but no simple and specific methods are yet available for routine use.

Serologic testing is generally not needed for the diagnosis of acute disease. Parasite-specific immunoglobulin M (IgM) antibodies detected by immunofluorescence or direct agglutination do not become positive until 20 to 40 days after the onset of symptoms. In certain situations this delayed antibody response permits the demonstration of seroconversion. Other laboratory tests often show nonspecific changes, such as a lymphocytic leukocytosis, elevated sedimentation rate, or transient electrocardiographic abnormalities. Reversible cardiomegaly and even pericardial effusion may occur.

The diagnosis of *chronic Chagas' disease* requires demonstration of antibodies to *T. cruzi* in the presence of the characteristic cardiac abnormalities and/or megadisease. Thus, except for the positive serologic findings, the diagnosis relies heavily upon clinical judgment in excluding other causes of heart disease or gastrointestinal dysfunction. A positive xenodiagnosis is strongly suggestive, but not in itself diagnostic, of chronic disease, since patients in the indeterminate phase may have low-level parasitemia. A variety of assays for specific antibody are available, and generally the results of different tests are comparable. However, there are cross-reactions in some tests with sera from patients with leishmaniasis or syphilis, for example. Therefore, in individual cases it may be very helpful to confirm the presence of antibody to specific antigens of *T. cruzi* with more sophisticated tests, such as immunoblots.

Symptomatic heart involvement in the chronic disease is manifested by characteristic ECG abnormalities, often without cardiomegaly. The most common of these is complete right bundle branch block. Other frequent ECG findings are left anterior hemiblock, ventricular extrasystoles, and even complete heart block. If heart failure is present, radiographs and echocardiograms will show generalized cardiomegaly with a reduced ejection fraction (Fig. 426–2).

Chagasic megaesophagus in the early stages shows only delayed emptying and minimal dilatation on studies after a barium swallow. With more advanced disease, retention of swallowed material and eosophageal dilatation are progressively increased. Manometric studies show spasm of the esophageal sphincter and uncoordinated peristaltic movements. Endoscopy should be performed to rule out malignant disease. However, all of these findings are indistinguishable from idiopathic achalasia. Barium enema with air contrast shows the dilated colon with impaired peristalsis, but other causes of colonic obstruction must be ruled out.

DIFFERENTIAL DIAGNOSIS. When acute Chagas' disease is symptomatic and severe, it can resemble a variety of acute systemic infections. Romaña's sign must be distinguished from other causes of unilateral orbital edema, such as the reaction to an insect bite, trauma, or orbital cellulitis.

Congenital infections are virtually indistinguishable from congenital toxoplasmosis, cytomegalic inclusion disease, and syphilis.

Various cardiomyopathies, such as postpartum, alcoholic, and endomyocardial fibrosis, can resemble chronic Chagas' heart disease. Endocardial biopsy is of dubious diagnostic value because of the nonspecific pathologic changes in chagasic cardiomyopathy; it might, however, identify other causes of heart disease. The characteristic heart murmurs of rheumatic valvular disease are helpful in differentiating this entity from chagasic cardiomyopa-

thy. The value of positive serologic findings for *T. cruzi* in the differential diagnosis of both heart and megadisease will depend upon the background prevalence of antibodies in the general population.

TREATMENT. Two drugs with reasonable antitrypanosomal activity are currently in use for the treatment of Chagas' disease. One of these is a nitrofuran derivative, nifurtimox (Lampit, Bayer 2502), which has been extensively evaluated. Nifurtimox* is the only drug available in the United States for treatment of Chagas' disease; it is used in a dose of 8 to 12 mg per kilogram per day. The second drug, benznidazole (Radinil, Roche 7-1051), is a nitroimidazole derivative that appears to be equal to nifurtimox in efficacy, although there is less experience with its use. The exact mechanism of antitrypanosomal action of both of these drugs is not known.

There is now considerable evidence that if patients with acute Chagas' disease are treated with either nifurtimox or benznidazole, the likelihood of future chronic disease is reduced. Many patients treated in the acute phase never develop antibodies to *T. cruzi*, or do so only transiently. From this observation, plus the fact that xenodiagnosis in such treated patients often does not indicate parasites, it is assumed that parasites can be eliminated and the patient cured if treated in the acute stage. However, nifurtimox is not uniformly effective in producing these results, and parasite strains from certain geographic areas (Brazil) appear to be less responsive to treatment than do strains from other countries (Argentina and Chile).

The frequency of side effects from both nifurtimox and benznidazole is high, and since they are administered for 60 to 90 days, drug toxicity is a serious problem. The most common adverse effect with nifurtimox is gastrointestinal intolerance, with anorexia, nausea, vomiting, and abdominal pain. Neurologic symptoms include restlessness, insomnia, disorientation, paresthesias, polyneuritis, and even seizures. Skin rashes can also occur. Peripheral neuropathy and bone marrow suppression have been reported with benznidazole. These side effects subside when the dosage of the drugs is reduced or treatment is stopped.

Since these drugs have shown effectiveness in treatment of acute Chagas' disease, some Latin American physicians are also treating chronic and indeterminate cases. There is no evidence that the established pathologic changes of chronic Chagas' disease can be reversed by nifurtimox or benznidazole therapy. The question of whether drug treatment in the indeterminate case, i.e., the asymptomatic patient with positive serologic findings, would prevent development of later chronic disease is controversial. Although it would not be easy, the issue ideally could be settled by a controlled, long-term prospective study. Some data

*An investigational drug that must be obtained from the Centers for Disease Control Drug Service (404-639-3356).

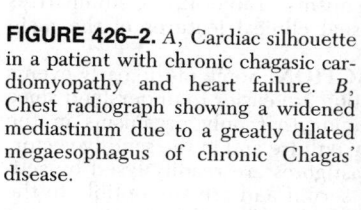

FIGURE 426–2. *A*, Cardiac silhouette in a patient with chronic chagasic cardiomyopathy and heart failure. *B*, Chest radiograph showing a widened mediastinum due to a greatly dilated megaesophagus of chronic Chagas' disease.

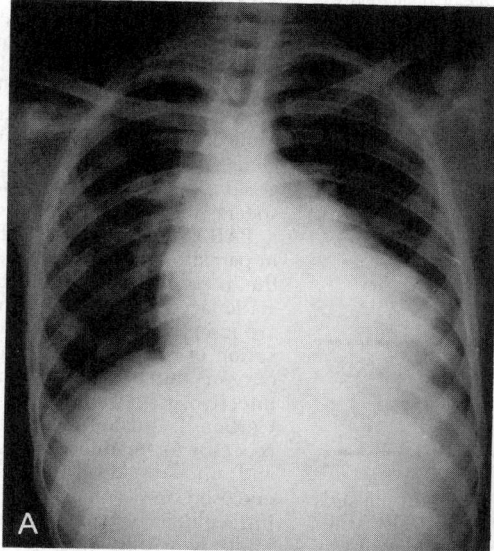
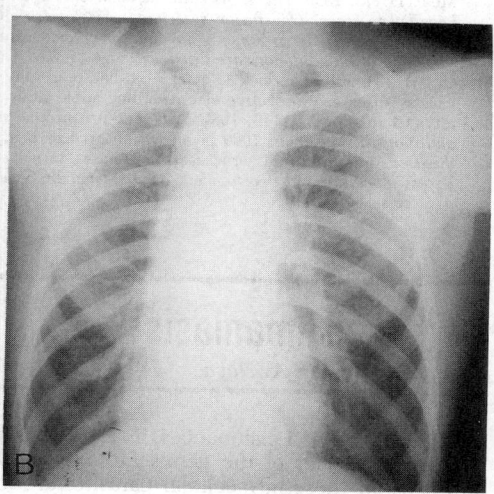

suggest that low-level parasitemia, as assessed by xenodiagnosis, can be reduced or eliminated after treatment with antitrypanosomal drugs, including allopurinol. But such studies require critical confirmation to establish their ultimate influence on the development of chronic disease, as well as risk versus benefit evaluation.

The treatment of patients with established chronic heart disease is supportive. Patients with frequent ventricular premature beats can benefit from antiarrhythmic drugs such as amiodarone. Cardiac pacemakers may prolong survival of those with complete heart block. The congestive failure of chagasic cardiomyopathy is disappointingly refractory to the usual cardiotropic drugs.

More options are open for the management and treatment of megadisease. In the early stages of megaesophagus, pneumatic dilatation of the sphincter is probably more effective than bougienage. For more advanced cases, various surgical procedures involving myotomy of the sphincter or partial resection are necessary. Early stages of megacolon can be managed by manipulation of diet and use of laxatives and occasional enemas. Sometimes resection of an aperistaltic section of the colon can be done in more severe cases.

PREVENTION. Chagas' disease could be eliminated as a serious health problem for the rural poor of Latin America by adequate housing and education. But stark socioeconomic realities dictate another approach to control. This consists mainly of the use of residual insecticides directed at domiciliary vectors. The use of benzene hexachloride (BHC), sprayed once or twice a year, has been very effective when used systematically.

Serologic testing in blood banks to avoid the use of seropositive donors is carried out in endemic areas. Another precaution is to add 1:4000 gentian violet to blood 24 hours before use to kill trypanosomes that may be present. With the recent occurrence of several transfusion-associated cases of acute Chagas' disease in North America, the question of serologic screening of blood donors has been raised for areas of the country with large Latin American populations. The development of vaccines is still in the research stage.

American Trypanosomiasis Research. PAHO Scientific Publication 318, 1975. *Proceedings of an international symposium with useful reviews on all aspects of the subject, including the vector bugs and control of the disease.*

Amorin DS, Manco JC, Gallo L Jr, et al.: Chagas' disease as an experimental model for studies of cardiac autonomic function in man. Mayo Clinic Proc (Suppl) 57:48, 1982. *A careful evaluation of cardiac autonomic function (changes in heart rate after vagal blockade with atropine and after Valsalva maneuver and hand grip exercise) that indicates that some individuals infected with T. cruzi, but without overt signs of heart disease, show evidence of cardiac autonomic denervation. There are many references to previous similar studies by the first author.*

Dias JCP: The indeterminate form of human chronic Chagas' disease. A clinical epidemiological review. Rev Soc Bras Med Trop 22:147, 1989. *A well-balanced review in English by a Brazilian expert. It documents the important point that infection with T. cruzi does not invariably progress to chronic disease.*

Dvorak J, Gibson C, Maekelt A: A bibliography on Chagas' disease (1968–1984). Washington, D.C., National Institutes of Health, Pan American Health Organization and World Health Organization, 1985. *This Medlars-based computer-processed bibliography is a complete listing of references on an annual basis, by author and subject for the period indicated. For real students of the subject!*

Kirchhoff LV: Is *Trypanosoma cruzi* a new threat to our blood supply? Ann Intern Med 111:773, 1989. *This short editorial comments upon the circumstances that have led to recent transfusion-associated cases of acute Chagas' disease in the United States. The arguments for and problems associated with serologic screening of blood donors are discussed.*

Maguire JH, Hoff R, Sherlock I, et al.: Cardiac morbidity and mortality due to Chagas' disease: Prospective electrocardiographic study of a Brazilian community. Circulation 75:1140, 1987. *A 6-year prospective study of ECG changes and mortality in about 1000 people in an area of Brazil endemic to Chagas' disease. Antibodies to T. cruzi were present in 42 per cent of the population. Excess mortality and development of abnormal ECGs were clearly related to positive serology.*

427 Leishmaniasis

Franklin A. Neva

DEFINITION. Leishmaniasis is a protozoan infection caused by various species of the genus *Leishmania*. Paradoxically, the host cells for these intracellular parasites are mononuclear phagocytes, cells that normally destroy microorganisms. In nature the infection is usually a zoonosis, with transmission of the parasite by sandflies to wild or domestic animals, especially rodents and canines, with humans as incidental hosts.

Human leishmanial infections can result in three main forms of disease, sometimes with dual manifestations in the same patient. The *visceral* form (kala-azar) is a systemic disease with parasites in the reticuloendothelial system, characterized by hepatosplenomegaly, fever, weight loss, leukopenia, and ultimately death if the disease is untreated. The *cutaneous* disease is generally manifested by one or more indolent ulcers, but a wide spectrum of skin involvement can occur. When parasites from skin lesions sometimes metastasize to produce later destructive lesions of the oronasopharynx, the result is *mucocutaneous* leishmaniasis. Although parasite species are the main determinant for the form of disease, clinical manifestations and outcome are also dependent upon the immune response of the host.

ETIOLOGY. *Leishmania* exist in two morphologic forms, a motile flagellate, or *promastigote*, and a smaller, nonmotile intracellular form, the *amastigote*. Promastigotes are found in the sandfly vector as well as in cultures, both habitats requiring temperatures of about 22 to 26°C. Also called *Leishman-Donovan* or *LD bodies* after their describers, amastigotes are the form of parasite found in humans or other vertebrate hosts. In addition to a nucleus, these 2 by 5 μm round or oval bodies contain a characteristic rodlike structure of extranuclear DNA, the *kinetoplast*, a useful structure in morphologic identification and differentiation from other intracellular organisms.

In the infected animal, leishmania are found only in monocytes and macrophages, where they multiply by binary fission. An appropriate sandfly vector becomes infected by ingesting organisms during a blood meal from tissue juice or cells in the skin or blood. In the gut of the sandfly, the parasites transform to promastigotes and multiply as spindle-shaped flagellates 15 to 26 μm long and 2 to 3 μm wide. In vectors ultimately capable of transmitting the parasite, promastigotes tend to migrate into the pharynx and buccal cavity. At least 7 days are needed before the sandfly becomes infective. The actual mechanism by which infective promastigotes are transferred to a new vertebrate host is not clear—possibly by regurgitation into the bite wound during a blood meal or perhaps even by being rubbed into abrasions after a successful swat. Once inoculated, the promastigotes are taken up by macrophages; they transform into amastigotes and begin to multiply. A vasoactive factor in sandfly salivary glands that enhances parasite infectivity has been described. Amastigotes that rupture from infected macrophages are taken up by adjacent cells; some infected cells may be transported to distant sites via the blood or lymphatics.

Classification of *Leishmania* is based primarily upon patterns of parasite isoenzymes separated by electrophoresis and immunologic reactions of surface and parasite-soluble (EF or excretion factor) antigens with monoclonal and polyclonal antisera. Additional taxonomic criteria include hybridization of kinetoplast DNA after treatment with restriction endonucleases and the type of disease produced in experimental animals. For example, *L. donovani* produces a progressive disease in hamsters similar to human visceral disease, and strains of *L. major* produce cutaneous ulcers in BALB/c mice with later visceralization and death. The most meaningful classification of *Leishmania* will probably come from correlating biochemical and immunologic results with biologic characteristics of the organisms. Table 427–1 summarizes geographic distribution and usual clinical features of the main species of *Leishmania*.

PARASITE-HOST INTERACTION. Some of the early events in parasite-macrophage interaction are easier to understand since the recent finding with *L. major* that only organisms in the stationary growth phase, both in culture and in the sandfly vector, are infective. Log-phase promastigotes are readily lysed by activation of complement in fresh serum and are susceptible to the oxygen burst of macrophages when ingested. Stationary, or infective, stages are more resistant to both of these host defenses. Certain ligands on macrophage membranes, such as CR3 and the receptor for mannose-fucose, are involved in parasite attachment and uptake. After ingestion by macrophages, leishmania are enclosed in a phagocytic vacuole. In contrast to some other intracellular organisms, leishmania not only survive but also multiply within phagolysosomes into which lysosomal enzymes

TABLE 427–1. GEOGRAPHIC DISTRIBUTION AND CLINICAL DISEASE CAUSED BY DIFFERENT SPECIES OF *LEISHMANIA*

Species	Geographic Distribution	Clinical Manifestations
L. mexicana complex (L. m. mexicana, L. m. amazonensis, L. m. venezuelensis, ? others)	New World—from southern U.S. through Central America, northern and central South America, Dominican Republic	Cutaneous ulcers; small proportion of patients may develop diffuse cutaneous (DCL) or mucocutaneous (MCL) leishmaniasis
L. braziliensis complex (L. b. braziliensis, L. b. panamensis, L. b. guyanesis, L. b. peruviana)	New World—from Central America through various parts of South America, including Brazil, Venezuela, Bolivia, Peru to northern Argentina	Cutaneous ulcers; some cases may later develop MCL (probably more likely if cutaneous lesion not treated adequately)
L. major	Northern Africa, Middle East, Central Africa, and southern Asia	Cutaneous ulcers
L. tropica	Middle East and southern Asia	Cutaneous ulcers and chronic relapsing cutaneous disease (recidivans form); rarely kala-azar
L. aethiopica	Ethiopia	Cutaneous ulcers, rarely DCL
L. donovani	Old World—East Africa and south of Sahara, southern Asia, including India and Iran	Visceral leishmaniasis; small proportion may develop post–kala-azar dermal leishmaniasis
L. infantum (? separate species)	Old World—North Africa and southern Europe	Visceral leishmaniasis; rarely cutaneous
L. chagasi (? separate species)	New World—foci in several areas of Brazil, Venezuela, Honduras, and Colombia, and isolated cases elsewhere in Central and South America	Visceral leishmaniasis; also nonulcerative cutaneous

*DCL = Diffuse cutaneous leishmaniasis; MCL = mucocutaneous leishmaniasis.

are discharged. The parasite is probably protected from this enzyme assault by the presence of abundant membrane-bound acid phosphatase. Leishmanial parasites within macrophages in vitro can be destroyed by activating cells or exposure to certain lymphokines, such as interferon-γ.

The variation in temperature sensitivity of various species of leishmania is a critical factor that determines clinical expression of the disease. For example, *L. donovani* can survive and multiply in macrophages at higher temperatures than can cutaneous strains. Among isolates causing cutaneous disease in the Americas, most members of the *L. mexicana* complex are inhibited to a greater extent at 37°C than are strains of the *L. braziliensis* complex. These differences in temperature tolerance probably explain why some varieties of cutaneous leishmaniasis can be treated successfully by local heat.

IMMUNOLOGY. The pattern of humoral and cell-mediated immune responses that normally develops during or after leishmanial infection varies with the clinical form of disease. Serum antibody can be demonstrated by a variety of tests, usually indirect immunofluorescence assay (IFA) or enzyme-linked immunosorbent assay (ELISA), in patients with established visceral or cutaneous leishmaniasis. Cell-mediated immunity in leishmaniasis can be evaluated by a delayed hypersensitivity skin test (leishmanin or Montenegro test) or by lymphocyte proliferation to leishmanial antigen. Positive skin test results and lymphocyte proliferation are normally present in patients with cutaneous disease, but only after recovery or effective treatment in patients with visceral disease. Cell-mediated immunity is absent or suppressed during active visceral infections.

Resistance to leishmaniasis is best correlated with the presence of cell-mediated immunity. Its absence in visceral disease has already been noted, and it is dramatically demonstrated in a rare form of disease called *diffuse cutaneous leishmaniasis* (DCL). In patients with DCL, not only is there specific anergy to the skin test but also parasites are very abundant in lesions, lymphocytes are scanty, lesions do not ulcerate, and response to chemotherapy is poor. Antigen-specific suppressor cells have been demonstrated in DCL. In contrast, a normal immune response in cutaneous leishmaniasis is generally associated with lesions that ulcerate and show relatively few parasites but abundant lymphocytes and even giant cells, plus a positive skin test. This relationship of immune response to clinical forms of disease in leishmaniasis is similar to that in leprosy (see Ch. 334).

VISCERAL LEISHMANIASIS (Kala-Azar)

EPIDEMIOLOGY. The visceral form of leishmaniasis, caused by *L. donovani* and related organisms, has worldwide distribution. Certain regions continue to be endemic areas of this disease. These include the following: northeastern India, especially Assam

and Bihar states; Kenya, Sudan, and Ethiopia in eastern Africa; northeastern China; the shores of the Caspian Sea and Iran in southern Asia; the countries of Europe, North Africa, and the Middle East surrounding the Mediterranean; and northeastern Brazil. In addition to these macrofoci, smaller foci occur outside these areas. In the Western Hemisphere, for example, visceral leishmaniasis is sporadically seen in southern Brazil, Paraguay, and northern Argentina, as well as in the vicinity of Belém at the mouth of the Amazon. In addition, there are foci of transmission in Venezuela, Colombia, and Honduras. Isolated cases occur in other Central American countries and Mexico.

With such a wide geographic distribution of the disease, it is not surprising that different species of phlebotomine flies are involved in the various regions. What is surprising is that the causative organisms from these widely separated regions are relatively uniform in their properties. The organisms causing visceral leishmaniasis in the Mediterranean region (*L. infantum*) and those in the Americas (*L. chagasi*) are very similar to one another, but sufficiently different from *L. donovani* to be considered separate species. *L. chagasi* was probably introduced to the New World by explorers or their dogs.

FACTORS AFFECTING TRANSMISSION. A common transmission cycle for *L. donovani* that takes place close to people involves dogs as reservoir hosts and sandfly vectors that will also feed on humans. The domestic dog, as well as wild canines such as the fox, develop a chronic systemic disease very similar to that of humans when infected with *L. donovani*. But an additional unique feature of leishmanial infection in canines is the frequent presence of organisms in the skin, including the nose and ears, which are favorite feeding sites of sandflies. An epidemiologic cycle of the parasite involving wild foxes, domestic dogs, and humans via the vector *Lutzomyia longipalpis* has been documented in northeastern Brazil. The domestic dog has also been incriminated as an important reservoir host for visceral leishmaniasis of the Mediterranean region and in certain areas of China.

Rodents are the likely reservoir in the Sudan, and the activity of the vector, *Phlebotomus orientalis,* is high in clumps of acacia woodland near villages. In Kenya, transmission of disease is associated with termite hills, which serve as resting places for the vector, *P. martini,* and around which village men gather in the evening. However, the animal reservoir in Kenya has not been identified. In some regions such as northeastern India, humans appear to be their own reservoir, and several factors serve to facilitate person-to-person transmission. The vector, *P. argentipes,* has a preference for human blood. The parasite is found in circulating monocytes in Indian cases of kala-azar more frequently than usual. Dermal lesions that develop after the initial disease in Indian patients may be an additional source of parasites for the vector.

The past few decades have seen a resurgence of visceral leishmaniasis in regions where it had disappeared after the widespread use of chlorophenothane (DDT) for malaria control. Phlebotomine populations were greatly reduced around houses, but zoonotic transmission was not affected. When the use of residual insecticides was discontinued, transmission to people was re-established. This has occurred in the countries around the Mediterranean, with an epidemic reported in western Italy.

Outbreaks of visceral leishmaniasis have often followed famine, wars, and civil or political disturbances resulting in malnutrition and mass migration of people. It is not known whether this is due to greater exposure to infected vectors, defective immune response, reactivation of latent infection, or a combination of these and other factors.

PATHOLOGY. The organs mainly affected are the liver, spleen, bone marrow, and elements of the reticuloendothelial system in diverse sites. These organs and tissues hypertrophy, with the increased cells made up of parasitized macrophages and histiocytes, but with little or no lymphocytic response. Generalized enlargement of lymph nodes is not a consistent finding (see below), but hyperplasia of lymphoid tissue in the nasopharynx and in the Peyer's patches of the gut is common. Endothelial proliferation occurs in certain organs as within septa of pulmonary alveoli and in renal glomeruli.

The spleen is enlarged, sometimes to tremendous size, but is firm and has a thick capsule. Although the splenic pulp is friable and there may be infarcts, the nature and chronic course of the enlargement make the spleen relatively resistant to tears from an aspirating needle. Enlargement of the liver is due to hyperplasia of the Kupffer cells, which are packed with amastigotes. Only rarely are parenchymal cells of the liver parasitized. There may be focal granulomas and some fibrosis in the liver in chronic untreated cases.

The bone marrow is infiltrated with parasitized macrophages, a process that may later impair red and white cell production. The enlarged spleen undoubtedly also contributes to the anemia and leukopenia. There is a striking polyclonal B cell activation that results in high immunoglobulin G (IgG) and total serum protein values. Some organs, most notably the kidneys, may show pathologic changes secondary to deposition of immune complexes.

CLINICAL FEATURES. The incubation period is long, generally 1 to 3 months, but it may be as short as 10 to 14 days. There are well-documented instances of activation of latent infection several years after exposure to the parasite, under conditions of immunosuppression. The onset is usually insidious and difficult to date, especially among people who regard intermittent fevers and lassitude as normal. Fever, accompanied by sweating, weakness, and weight loss, gradually becomes noticeable. These symptoms, perhaps including nonproductive cough and abdominal discomfort produced by an enlarging liver and spleen, may continue for months with the patient still up and about. In some patients the course of disease is more rapid, with high temperature and chills, simulating typhoid fever or acute brucellosis. The most prominent physical findings are fever, splenomegaly, and cachexia, which is especially evident in the thorax and shoulder girdle (Fig. 427–1). Although the fever pattern can be variable, ultimately it often exhibits characteristic twice-daily elevations to 38 to 40°C for some time. Generalized adenopathy is common in patients from some geographic areas, but it is seldom striking. In light-skinned patients, hyperpigmentation of the skin may be noted; the term *kala-azar* is Hindi for black sickness. Splenic enlargement can be extreme in this disease, often reaching the iliac fossa, and the organ is firm and nontender. Some otherwise typical cases may involve only modest hepatosplenomegaly.

COURSE AND COMPLICATIONS. There is increasing evidence from skin test and serologic surveys, as well as prospective epidemiologic studies, that asymptomatic and subclinical infections with spontaneous recovery are more common than is overt disease. Poor nutritional state is a critical predisposing factor. When infection becomes clinically apparent, manifestations of systemic disease include fever, weight loss, fatigue, and anemia. Subcutaneous edema, ascites, and other evidence of hypoalbuminemia may develop. Bleeding from the nose or gums can

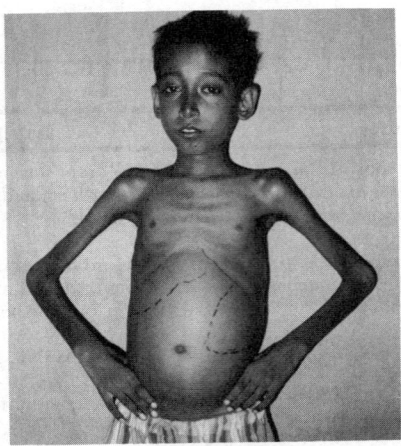

FIGURE 427–1. Indian patient with kala-azar. Note wasting of thorax and shoulder girdle and hepatosplenomegaly as outlined.

occur. Finally, after an illness that may be as short as a few months or as long as a year, the patient becomes emaciated and exhausted. In the great majority of instances, death is due to intercurrent infections such as pneumonia, tuberculosis, dysentery, and gangrenous stomatitis. Advanced cases are particularly susceptible because of leukopenia and undoubted impairment of cell-mediated immunologic function, although specific mechanisms have not been defined. Another cause of death is massive gastrointestinal bleeding.

SKIN LESIONS ASSOCIATED WITH KALA-AZAR. In the early stages of visceral leishmaniasis, small nodules in the skin containing parasites have been described at or near the inoculation site. There are scattered reports of the demonstration of parasites even in apparently normal skin. A somewhat more common type of cutaneous lesion, although variable by geographic location, is post–kala-azar dermal leishmaniasis (PKDL). This is the development in some patients, weeks or months after recovery from disease, of papular or nodular lesions containing many parasites. Depigmentation of the skin resembling vitiligo may occur as a sequel to PKDL. The presence of chronic, nonulcerative, papular lesions, often located on the face of children and young adults, has been described from endemic areas for kala-azar in Honduras. Although these patients had no history of kala-azar, *L. chagasi* was cultured from the lesions. No systemic evidence of disease or consistent immunologic abnormalities are demonstrable in cases of PKDL or the atypical cutaneous disease.

SPECIFIC LABORATORY DIAGNOSIS. Since other clinical states may mimic certain features of visceral leishmaniasis, demonstration of the parasite, preferably by culture, is essential before treatment is undertaken. In addition, presence or absence of the parasite can be used to monitor response to treatment. Organisms are most readily recovered by aspiration from bone marrow, spleen (see Color Plate 11F), liver, lymph nodes, or blood. Material obtained is:

1. Used to make smears and slides stained with Giemsa or other Romanovsky stains for examination under oil immersion for amastigotes. Although bone marrow aspiration is usually the method of choice, splenic aspiration can be done if the spleen is readily palpable, if prothrombin and bleeding times are normal, and if proper technique is used (see Chulay and Bryceson for details).

2. Inoculated into appropriate culture media.

3. Inoculated into hamsters, but 3 to 4 months may be required before organisms are found in their liver or spleen, so this method is not very practical.

Immunologic Tests. By the time patients with visceral leishmaniasis come to clinical attention, they invariably have readily demonstrable antileishmanial serum antibodies. For this, the ELISA test using promastigotes as antigen is probably the most practical; it can be read visually if necessary and is applicable for testing large numbers of sera, including specimens eluted from filter paper. The IFA test employing either amastigotes or promastigotes as antigen has been used, as has direct agglutination of fixed promastigotes. In certain areas of Latin America, there may be cross-reactions with sera from people infected with *Trypanosoma cruzi*. The leishmanin skin test for delayed hypersensitivity is negative in cases of active visceral leishmaniasis but becomes positive after recovery.

Laboratory Findings. Most of the laboratory abnormalities involve the hematopoietic system. Leukopenia, with absolute reductions in neutrophils and eosinophils and a relative increase in lymphocytes and monocytes, is characteristic. In one series the total white cell count was below 4000 in 90 per cent of cases by 1 month after onset of symptoms, and it frequently may be around 2000. Thrombocytopenia is also present, and the erythrocyte sedimentation rate is increased. A moderately severe normocytic and normochromic anemia, unless complicated by blood loss or deficiency states, is very common, caused by increased red cell destruction. In late stages of the disease prothrombin, bleeding, and clotting times are prolonged.

Total serum proteins are increased to levels of 9 to 10 grams per deciliter, virtually all IgG, because of polyclonal B cell activation. Serum albumin levels, especially in advanced cases, are normal or low. The striking hyperglobulinemia is the basis for the old recommended diagnostic tests, such as the formol-gel test and Chopra reaction, before specific serodiagnosis was available. Evidence for circulating immune complexes, based upon C1q binding in the serum, is readily demonstrable. Liver function tests show only mild abnormalities, if any.

DIFFERENTIAL DIAGNOSIS. Chronic malaria in endemic regions may present some problems in differential diagnosis. In malaria-immune individuals, the presence of malaria parasites in the blood does not rule out the additional diagnosis of leishmaniasis. Conversely, an enlarged spleen is hardly enough on which to base the diagnosis. Tropical splenomegaly syndrome (an exaggerated immune response to malaria) could easily be confused with the clinical picture of visceral leishmaniasis. Several different forms of schistosomiasis may also mimic visceral leishmaniasis: the acute disease with fever and hepatosplenomegaly, the severe chronic variety with Symmers' fibrosis and portal hypertension, and chronic relapsing enteric fever that can be a complication of schistosomiasis. Other diseases that may resemble kala-azar include lymphoma, cirrhosis of the liver with hypersplenism, miliary tuberculosis, brucellosis, typhoid fever, and subacute bacterial endocarditis.

TREATMENT. The drug of choice for treatment has been and remains pentavalent antimony (Sb), even with novel approaches to possible use of other drugs. The Sb preparation available in the United States* and some European countries is sodium stibogluconate (Pentostam), a preparation containing 100 mg of Sb per milliliter. The dose is 20 mg per kilogram of body weight, given daily by intramuscular or intravenous injection, not exceeding 1000 mg of Sb per day. Another pentavalent Sb preparation used in Latin America, meglumine antimonate (Glucantime), is virtually identical but contains a slightly lower concentration of Sb per milliliter. The total dose required for cure varies in different parts of the world; Mediterranean kala-azar generally responds to 10 or 15 doses, whereas the disease in Kenya requires 30 injections, and up to 30 per cent of cases may still relapse within 6 months. Pentavalent Sb is relatively nontoxic in comparison to trivalent Sb, except for local pain at the injection site when given intramuscularly. Other side effects are cumulative with dose and include arthralgias, weakness, nausea, vomiting, slight elevation of liver enzyme values, and nonspecific T wave changes if electrocardiograms are obtained.

Response to treatment is not dramatic and may not be apparent for several weeks. Useful indicators to follow are temperature, spleen size, hemoglobin, and white blood cell count. Weekly splenic aspirates were used by one group, with "cure" defined as two successively negative aspirates a week apart. Since relapse may occur up to a year after apparent cure, monthly follow-up for 6 months and then follow-up after a year are recommended.

Primary unresponsiveness to Sb, that is, little or no improvement during or after the first course, occurs in up to 10 per cent of cases. Actual resistance of the parasite to Sb has been difficult to document in humans; therefore, lack of response may reflect

ineffective immune mechanisms of the host. Allopurinol combined with Sb is reported to be of benefit in some unresponsive patients. Pentamidine is a second-line drug. The dosage of pentamidine† is 4 mg per kilogram given intramuscularly three times weekly for 10 doses, but severe pain at the injection site is common, and sterile abscess formation can occur. Additional systemic side effects of anorexia, nausea, abdominal pain, hypotension, and development of diabetes in 10 per cent of patients make the decision to use pentamidine a difficult one. Another second-line drug, amphotericin B, must be given intravenously on alternate days at 1 mg per kilogram each time over many weeks to achieve the recommended total dose of 1.5 to 2.0 grams. This drug regularly produces chills, fever, and nausea with each dose and a cumulative reduction of hemoglobin and renal function. New approaches to treatment include incorporation of drugs in liposomes for more efficient uptake by macrophages and use of interferon-γ combined with Sb.

Supportive treatment can be very important, especially in the malnourished and debilitated. These patients are prone to develop complicating bacterial infections for which proper treatment must be instituted. Fluid and electrolyte imbalance must be corrected, and hemorrhagic complications may require blood transfusion. Good nursing care, attention to oral hygiene, adequate diet, and correction of nutritional deficiencies are, of course, desirable.

PREVENTION. Since the epidemiology of kala-azar varies among different geographic areas, the local conditions responsible for transmission must be understood to implement preventive measures. Where sandflies are in or around houses, vector control with insecticides is appropriate. If an animal reservoir such as the domestic dog is involved, destruction of infected dogs, especially strays, can be instituted. If focal sites of infected flies are known, they can be destroyed or avoided. Personal protection by wearing protective clothing in the evenings, using insect repellents, and sleeping under fine mesh netting is applicable under some circumstances.

CUTANEOUS LEISHMANIASIS OF THE OLD WORLD (Oriental Sore) AND NEW WORLD (Including Mucocutaneous or Espundia)

EPIDEMIOLOGY. Although basically the same disease, there are differences in epidemiology and clinical course in cutaneous leishmaniasis of the Old and New Worlds. In the Mediterranean basin, Middle East, and southern Asia, the disease tends to be clinically more benign and occurs in semiarid and desert climates; transmission can become established in villages and cities. Cutaneous leishmaniasis in the Americas is acquired by workers in the jungle or by farmers and their families living at its edges. The New World disease sometimes produces later metastatic and destructive lesions of the mucous membranes.

The epidemiology of cutaneous leishmaniasis is best understood in southern Russia, Iran, and Middle Eastern countries where infected desert rodents (*Rhombomys opimus* and *Psammomys obesus*) live in burrows with phlebotomine vectors (often *Phlebotomus papatasii*). People are infected with *L. major* when they invade this environment to establish settlements or excavate archaeologic ruins. If settlements are established, the parasite may adapt to a new transmission cycle with dogs and humans as reservoirs and an urban sandfly such as *P. sergenti* as vector. Parasite species from such locations are often identified as *L. tropica*. The commonness of typical face scars in adults in Iran, Afghanistan, Syria, and Iraq indicates the high frequency of cutaneous leishmaniasis in these countries.

The epidemiology of cutaneous leishmaniasis in West Africa and the sub-Sahara belt is less clear. Human cases are sporadic, with a rural transmission cycle, and the parasite species is often *L. major*. In Ethiopia and Kenya, however, the animal reservoir is often the hyrax (*Procavia*), the vector is *Phlebotomus longipes*, and the parasite species is *L. aethiopica*.

In the Americas, cutaneous leishmaniasis occurs from Texas to northern Argentina (see Color Plate 10C), with only Chile free of the disease. Except for some areas of Peru, where the domestic dog is a reservoir, New World cutaneous leishmaniasis is a forest or jungle zoonosis, with forest rodents or sloths serving as animal reservoirs. Western Hemisphere sandfly vectors are now classified as members of the genus *Lutzomyia*.

The organism in Texas (10 human cases), Mexico, and northern Central America is mainly *Leishmania m. mexicana*. Members of the *L. braziliensis* complex are predominant in the remainder of Central America, Panama, and northern South America. This species complex also extends into Brazil, Bolivia, and tropical regions of Peru, with complex ecologic combinations of jungle animal reservoirs and sandfly vectors. Yet within the major distribution of a group, there may be isolated pockets of a second species complex, such as *L. b. braziliensis* in Belize, where *L. mexicana* predominates, or *L. mexicana* on the Atlantic coast of Panama, and *L. m. amazonensis* in many sites of central Brazil. Additional members of the two major complexes, or even new species, are likely to be described as newer methods of taxonomy are applied.

PATHOLOGY. The earliest changes at the site of inoculation have not been described. Established lesions show a large accumulation of macrophages containing amastigotes, with variable numbers of lymphocytes and plasma cells. There may be focal accumulations of polymorphonuclear cells, especially in areas of necrosis, but the exact mechanism for ulceration of the epithelium is not clear. With time, numbers of parasites diminish and the lesion heals. In other instances the lesion persists and a granulomatous histologic reaction is seen, including multinucleated giant cells. This is the type of pathology seen in *chronic relapsing cutaneous leishmaniasis*, also known as the *lupoid* or *recidivans* form. Delayed skin test reactivity to leishmanial antigen is present in normally healing and recidivans leishmaniasis.

The unusual complication known as diffuse cutaneous leishmaniasis (DCL), associated with anergy to leishmanial antigen, has a different histologic picture. DCL lesions show a heavy infiltrate of foamy or vacuolated macrophages containing large numbers of amastigotes with only scant numbers of lymphocytes. Moreover, the overlying epithelium is not ulcerated.

The lesions of mucocutaneous leishmaniasis (espundia) represent the metastatic spread of organisms via the bloodstream to mucous membranes of the nose, mouth, and upper pharyngeal tissues. The histology is a confusing mixture of granulomatous inflammatory cell reaction with necrosis, fibrosis, and often response to secondary bacterial infection. Organisms are usually scanty. Tissue destruction can involve cartilage with perforation of the nasal septum, loss of much of the nose and palate, and even involvement of the larynx.

CLINICAL MANIFESTATIONS. The lesion begins as a small erythematous papule on exposed areas, often the face or extremities, within 2 to 8 weeks after infection. The papule develops a tiny vesicle that opens and oozes some serous fluid and enlarges to form an ulcer with firm, raised, and reddened edges. The ulcer can remain relatively dry with a central crust (dry form) or may ooze (wet form). Lesions can be single or multiple; small satellite papules may occur at the edge of a larger lesion. Subcutaneous nodules in a centripetal alignment from an ulcer may develop (sporotrichoid form). Cutaneous leishmanial lesions generally heal spontaneously, but the process can take a few months to a year or more. The result is a depressed, depigmented scar. *Recidivans* or *lupoid leishmaniasis* may sometimes develop months or years after healing of a primary lesion and may persist for years. This lesion exhibits central healing with nonulcerative papules developing in the periphery or center of the scar. Regional adenopathy may or may not occur with cutaneous leishmaniasis; this finding is not helpful in differential diagnosis.

COMPLICATIONS. Metastatic spread of parasites and development of destructive naso-oropharyngeal lesions is a serious later sequel to cutaneous disease. This mucous membrane involvement occurs almost exclusively in the Western Hemisphere and is said to be associated primarily with *L. braziliensis* infections. Mucocutaneous disease due to *L. mexicana amazonensis* does occur, so until more data correlating parasite type with clinical disease are available, this complication can also be related to geographic region as well as to parasite species. Thus, mucocutaneous leishmaniasis is most common in central Brazil and adjacent portions of Bolivia, Peru, and Ecuador, and is relatively uncommon in Panama and Central America. Mucosal involvement generally does not become manifest until the initial skin lesion has healed, even many years later, and presumably is more likely to occur if there has been no or inadequate treatment of the original ulcer.

Earliest signs and symptoms of mucosal disease commonly involve the nose, with epistaxis and obstruction. Perforation of the nasal septum is common, or the upper lip may be involved. The process can destroy cartilaginous structures of the nose and palate and extend to the larynx. Death may result from aspiration pneumonia or suffocation. Distinction should be made between the mucuous membrane involvement that occurs as direct extension from a facial lesion, as in Ethiopia, and the late metastatic form seen in South America.

DCL is a rare complication that offers insight into immunity to leishmaniasis because it features antigen-specific anergy and cell-mediated immunosuppression. DCL seems to occur more commonly in certain countries (Dominican Republic, Venezuela, Mexico, and Ethiopia) and in the Americas is caused by organisms belonging to the *L. mexicana* complex. The disease begins with one or only a few nodular lesions that do not ulcerate but go on to metastasize to other cutaneous sites, primarily the face and extensor surfaces of the limbs. The subcutaneous nonulcerative nodular lesions are not associated with fever or other systemic symptoms and do not involve visceral organs. The appearance, distribution, and chronic nature of DCL have often led to the erroneous diagnosis of lepromatous leprosy (Fig. 427–2). No mortality is associated with DCL, but disfigurement and ulceration secondary to trauma at pressure points lead to chronic morbidity, since this disease is notoriously unresponsive to the usual antileishmanial drugs.

DIAGNOSIS. Leishmaniasis can be suspected in anyone who develops one or more chronic ulcers on exposed areas of skin after recently visiting or working at archaeologic sites in the Middle East, at Mayan ruins, or in jungle or rural areas of Latin America. Ideally, diagnosis should be confirmed by culture of the organism in NNN (Novy, MacNeal, and Nicolle's medium) or other appropriate media from a biopsy or aspirated specimen obtained from the edge of the lesion. Culture is the most sensitive method for detection of organisms. Excisional or punch biopsy offers an additional advantage of providing a portion of the specimen for histopathologic examination and routine bacteriologic, fungal, and acid-fast cultures in cases in which a wider differential diagnosis is required. Appropriate impression smears can also be made and stained from biopsy material, whether culture is possible or not. If biopsy is not possible because of circumstances or location of the lesion, scrapings from a slit made in involved skin or from the debrided base of an ulcer can be cultured or stained for organisms. The characteristic amastigotes

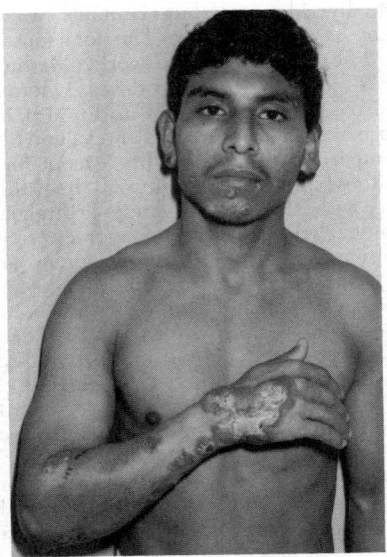

FIGURE 427–2. Patient with diffuse cutaneous leishmaniasis of 5 years' duration. Note nonulcerative lesions of chin, ear lobes, right arm, and hand.

in lesions appear larger and are more easily recognized in smears than in tissue sections. A recent technique that may permit direct and rapid diagnosis, as well as species differentiation of leishmania, is blotting with radiolabeled DNA probes. The numbers of parasites present and ease of culture vary with the strain, but the concentration of parasites in lesions tends to diminish with time as healing occurs, and they are also reduced if the ulcer is secondarily infected with bacteria. It is usually more difficult to culture or demonstrate organisms in lesions of mucocutaneous disease.

A positive leishmanin skin test and serum antibody can usually be demonstrated in patients by the time a cutaneous lesion has ulcerated. These tests remain positive in mucocutaneous disease. Serologic tests are not very useful in diagnosis because antibody levels are low. It must also be remembered that positive skin and serologic tests can reflect a previous rather than a current leishmanial infection.

Cutaneous leishmaniasis must be differentiated from the following conditions, with decreasing likelihood of occurrence: nonspecific tropical or traumatic ulcers due to bacterial infection or stasis; fungal infections, especially sporotrichosis and blastomycosis; mycobacterial infections such as *Mycobacterium marinum* and *tuberculosis;* syphilis and other treponematoses of the skin; sarcoidosis; and neoplastic ulcers. Mucocutaneous leishmaniasis is especially likely to mimic infection with *Paracoccidiodes brasiliensis*, histoplasmosis, Wegener's disease, midline granuloma, or rhinoscleroma.

TREATMENT. As described earlier for visceral leishmaniasis, the standard and recommended treatment for cutaneous leishmaniasis is pentavalent Sb, available in the United States as Pentostam.* The dose is 15 to 20 mg of Sb per kilogram by intramuscular or intravenous injection, not exceeding 1000 mg per dose. The drug is given daily for 15 to 20 days. Modest elevation of liver enzymes and/or mild, nonspecific ST or T wave electrocardiographic changes may occur during therapy, especially after six or eight doses. These changes are generally not associated with symptoms, but it may be prudent to monitor them.

Old World cutaneous leishmaniasis, especially in patients from the Middle East, often heals spontaneously within 6 months. Since leishmaniasis in this region does not metastasize to mucosal tissues, treatment may justifiably be withheld if the lesion is not extensive and appears to be healing.

In contrast, if the infection is known or suspected to originate from an endemic area of mucocutaneous disease, some authorities recommend longer (20 to 30 days) or multiple-course therapy. However, healing of the lesion is the ultimate clinical criterion for successful treatment.

Regardless of the infecting species of parasite, it is not unusual for cutaneous leishmanial lesions to require a second course of Sb treatment. Two weeks of rest and clinical observation are generally allowed between courses of treatment. Although different strains of leishmania can vary in their susceptibility to Sb, there is no evidence of drug resistance. Yet the circumstances required to eliminate the organisms from a lesion are not fully understood, and probably a normal immunologic response on the part of the host is required.

Amphotericin B is indicated in cases in which antimonials have failed to control the disease. Side effects are common and can be severe. The effective total dose is lower than for many systemic mycoses, with a total dose of 1.5 to 2.0 grams for a 60-kg adult often being sufficient.

A number of other drugs with varying degrees of antileishmanial activity may be useful in treatment under certain circumstances. Ketoconazole,† in a daily dose of 400 or 600‡ mg, may be effective against certain species of parasites but must be given for 4 weeks. Other orally administered drugs, such as rifampin or metronidazole, have been touted on the basis of limited or uncontrolled trials, but they are clearly inferior to Sb. Innovative approaches to therapy are under way with liposome-encapsulated compounds and even topically applied drugs containing paromomycin; their ultimate usefulness remains to be established.

---

*Available from Centers for Disease Control, Atlanta, GA.
†This use is not listed in the manufacturer's directive.
‡Exceeds the dose recommended by the manufacturer.

The application of local heat (40° to 41°C) for 25 hours or more over a period of 4 or 5 days may be effective for lesions caused by the *L. mexicana* complex organisms.

PREVENTION. Transmission of leishmaniasis in cities can be prevented by control of sandfly populations with insecticides or destruction of breeding sites. Where reservoirs and vectors are sylvatic, other measures must be employed, such as insect repellents and use of protective clothing over exposed parts of the body. Vaccines should theoretically be effective, since immunity to second episodes of cutaneous disease does exist. However, the effectiveness of immunization with either viable or killed organisms has been difficult to evaluate.

Badero R, Jones TC, Carvalho EM, et al.: New perspectives on a subclinical form of visceral leishmaniasis. J Infect Dis 154:1003, 1986. *A prospective epidemiologic study in Brazil that documents a feature of kala-azar long suspected—namely, that subclinical infection is common and some infected individuals recover spontaneously.*

Chulay JD, Bryceson ADM: Quantitation of amastigotes of *L. donovani* in smears of splenic aspirates from patients with visceral leishmaniasis. Am J Trop Med Hyg 32:475, 1983. *This reference outlines a way to follow patients for response to treatment, including details of their technique for splenic aspiration.*

Marsden PD: Mucosal leishmaniasis ("espundia" Escomel, 1911). Trans R Soc Trop Med Hyg 80:859, 1986. *An excellent review of the clinical aspects of the subject by a real student of the disease. The paper is thoroughly referenced.*

Ponce C, Ponce E, Morrison A, et al.: *Leishmania donovani chagasi*: New clinical variant of cutaneous leishmaniasis in Honduras. Lancet 337:67, 1991. *A description of a benign skin disease in endemic areas for kala-azar, caused by the same organism that produces visceral disease.*

Sacks DL: Metacyclogenesis in leishmania promastigotes (minireview). Exp Parasitol 69:100, 1989. *A short review of the immunologic and biochemical events that occur and confer infectivity to leishmanial parasites as they grow in culture and in the gut of the sandfly vector.*

Sacks DL, Lal SL, Shrivastova SN, et al.: An analysis of T cell responsiveness in Indian kala-azar. J Immunol 138:908, 1987. *Documentation of the antigen-specific T cell unresponsiveness in Indian kala-azar patients during active disease.*

Velasco D, Savarino SJ, Walton BC, et al.: Diffuse cutaneous leishmaniasis in Mexico. Am J Trop Med Hyg 41:280, 1989. *Although this paper concerns an unusual complication of cutaneous leishmaniasis, it stimulates thinking about the factors involved in pathogenesis of this disorder.*

428 Toxoplasmosis

Henry Masur

Toxoplasmosis is a common disease of birds and mammals caused by the protozoan *Toxoplasma gondii*. The name *T. gondii* is derived from the Greek word *toxon*, meaning arc, and from the North African rodent *gondi*, in which the organism was first recognized. *T. gondii* currently infects over 500 million humans around the world. This obligate intracellar protozoan can proliferate readily and cause clinically important disease in individuals with normal or abnormal immune function. A clear distinction must be kept in mind between *T. gondii* infection, which is defined by the presence of viable organisms in a patient, and toxoplasmosis, a relatively uncommon occurrence that indicates an active disease process.

THE PROTOZOA. Three forms exist in the life cycle of *T. gondii*: the *cyst*, the *trophozoite (tachyzoite)*, and the *oocyst*. The trophozoite has an arc or oval form and is about 3 to 7 μm in size. It is an obligate intracellular form that proliferates in acute infection. Trophozoites can enter cytoplasmic vacuoles in any nucleated mammalian cell. They divide by endodyogeny, an asexual process whereby two daughter cells are formed within one parent cell. Division continues until the cell ruptures, releasing trophozoites to infect adjacent cells. As the host develops immunity, trophozoite proliferation slows.

Toxoplasma cysts are 10 to 200 μm forms that contain several thousand very slowly dividing organisms; these appear to develop within host cells. Cysts can be seen in any tissue, but they are most common in brain, skeletal muscle, and cardiac muscle. Cysts are more resistant to environmental conditions than are trophozoites and remain viable after exposure to digestive enzymes.

Oocysts are 10 to 12 μm oval forms that exist uniquely in the intestinal mucosa of cats. Toxoplasma released from cysts or oocysts in the cat intestine enter epithelial cells, where they proliferate and then mature by gametogony into microgametocytes or macrogametocytes. A zygote is formed by the union of the gametocytes; this zygote matures in 1 to 4 days into an oocyst. Large quantities of oocytes (up to 10 million per day) are excreted by the cat for 1 to 3 weeks, beginning 3 to 5 days after ingestion of the Toxoplasma cysts or oocysts. Cats also get a concurrent systemic infection. Oocysts are not infectious until they undergo sporogony outside the body, a process that requires 1 to 21 days, depending on environmental conditions. Oocysts are quite hardy: They can exist outside the body for at least a year in warm, moist soil.

EPIDEMIOLOGY. Toxoplasma infection is a worldwide zoonosis. Natural infection occurs by ingestion of cysts or oocysts and by transplacental transmission. In nature the cycle of infection is probably maintained by cats, birds, and small mammals. Primary human infection usually occurs by accidental ingestion of infected cat feces or by consumption of inadequately cooked meat. The relative importance of these primary routes probably depends on the amount of rare meat consumed, hygienic practices, climate, and the proximity of a feline population. When cats consume infected animals or inadequately cooked meat scraps, they become infected and excrete oocysts. Children are particularly likely to come into contact with contaminated cat feces when playing in sand or to inhale aerosolized dried feces under dusty conditions. Cockroaches and flies have also been shown to transfer oocysts to uncovered food.

In North America and Western Europe, where many cats are confined to the home and eat only processed foods, and where food is usually covered and refrigerated, the consumption of rare meat is probably of greater epidemiologic importance than contact with cats or insects. Pork and lamb are more likely to contain cysts than is beef. If meat is not cooked to 60°C, or frozen to −20°C (a temperature not reliably reached by most commercial freezers), the cysts may be infective.

Toxoplasma has been transmitted rarely by needle stick accidents involving laboratory workers, by accidental inoculation during autopsy procedures, by transfusion of infected blood products, and by transplantation of an infected heart or kidney. A few immunodeficient patients (particularly some with acquired immunodeficiency syndrome [AIDS]) have parasitemia, and persistent parasitemia for a year has been described in an apparently healthy individual.

Secondary Toxoplasma infection can occur by transplacental transmission. Such transmission occurs only if an immunocompetent mother acquires Toxoplasma infection during the pregnancy or perhaps during the few months prior to conception. Some women with human immunodeficiency virus (HIV) infection can probably have persistent parasitemias that reflect reactivation of latent infection and that can be persistent over many months or several years. It is only this unique group of women who could have more than one pregnancy complicated by congenital toxoplasmosis. The frequency of congenital toxoplasmosis is thus dependent on the frequency with which women of childbearing age acquire Toxoplasma infection. In the United States and Europe, 0.5 to 1 per cent of women show high or rising antitoxoplasma titers during pregnancy. The likelihood of transmission increases progressively during successive trimesters of pregnancy, from 17 to 65 per cent.

The frequency of Toxoplasma infection in any population depends on a variety of sociologic, economic, and environmental factors. Among both men and women, there is increasing prevalence of positive serologic results with increasing age. In the United States fewer than 1 per cent of infants have congenital Toxoplasma infection; the incidence rises abruptly during the teenage years; and from age 15 to 50 years, there is an increase of approximately 1 per cent per year. Thus, about 20 to 70 per cent of adults in this country have positive serologic tests for Toxoplasma infection, the precise number depending on the specific population studied. Individuals in cold, arid, or mountainous regions tend to have a lower frequency than do those in tropical areas. There are isolated communities that have little or no Toxoplasma infection. The regional variations cannot all be explained on the basis of meat-eating habits, the presence of felines, or climatic extremes.

PATHOGENESIS AND PATHOLOGY. Toxoplasma organisms are liberated from cysts or oocysts in the gastrointestinal tract, where they multiply in the mucosal cells. Trophozoites then disseminate via the bloodstream or lymphatics to infect any nucleated host cell. Multiplication of the trophozoites within host cell vacuoles does not appear to disturb host cell function until the dividing organisms cause the cell to rupture. As adjacent cells are infected and they are themselves ruptured, progressive tissue necrosis occurs and an inflammatory response is elicited. The inflammatory response typically consists of mononuclear cells, a few polymorphonuclear cells, and edema. How extensive the tissue necrosis and dissemination become depends on the effectiveness of both humoral and cellular immune mechanisms. Although any organ can be involved, small foci of infection are most often established in lymph nodes, skeletal muscle, myocardium, and brain. Even after effective immunologic response, the organisms are not eradicated; a few cysts form in these organs as early as the first week of infection and remain dormant for the lifetime of the host unless host immunity is diminished, in which case active proliferation of the organisms can again cause substantial local disease and dissemination. In some patients, primary infection can be associated with widely disseminated disease, since most of these patients have defects in cell-mediated immune mechanisms.

The histopathologic changes in lymph nodes are so characteristic that they are virtually diagnostic even in the absence of a visualized or cultivated organism. The lymph node shows reactive follicular hyperplasia with irregular clusters of epithelioid histiocytes. Trophozoites or cysts are rarely seen in lymph nodes, although promptly performed cultures grow the organism in many cases.

When other organs are involved, the pathologic findings can vary from a few isolated cysts to a marked inflammatory response associated with extensive necrosis. In skeletal muscle or brain, an isolated cyst can be found unassociated with any inflammatory response or with any clinical manifestations of organ dysfunction; this response is most often seen in chronic latent infection without active disease. In patients with disseminated disease, however, the heart, brain, liver, spleen, kidney, pancreas, or other organs can manifest an intense inflammatory response surrounding areas of necrosis that can vary greatly in size. The inflammatory response consists of lymphocytes, plasma cells, and monocytes in association with edema. Perivascular mononuclear inflammatory changes are often seen contiguous to the necrotic areas. Intracellular and extracellular trophozoites are usually found in the periphery of the lesion rather than in the necrotic center; these trophozoites can be very difficult to distinguish from inflammatory debris.

The central nervous system may contain single or multiple necrotic lesions with margins of mononuclear cells. Periaqueductal and periventricular necrosis in congenital infection may lead to obstruction of the aqueduct of Sylvius or the foramen of Monro, resulting in obstructive hydrocephalus. The necrotic areas may ultimately calcify. In the eye, single or multiple necrotic lesions in the retina are the first manifestations of Toxoplasma infection. Mononuclear cell infiltrates are seen in association with cysts or trophozoites. Granulomatous inflammation occurs secondary to the necrotizing retinitis. The disease involves the posterior chamber almost exclusively and may be complicated by iridocyclitis, glaucoma, or cataracts.

In immunocompetent patients, primary Toxoplasma infection is associated with both a humoral and a cellular immune response. Antibodies (both IgG and IgM) against various Toxoplasma antigens can be detected in the blood. These specific antibodies have roles in producing extracellular killing of organisms (in conjunction with alternate complement pathway) and in promoting intracellular killing when opsonized organisms are ingested by mononuclear phagocytes. Subsequently, lymphocytes become responsive to Toxoplasma antigens and produce lymphokines. These lymphokines, especially interferon-γ and interleukin 2, which are secreted by antigen-sensitized CD4-positive (helper) T cells, enable mononuclear phagocytes to inhibit Toxoplasma replication and to kill the intracellular organisms. Even immunocompetent individuals are not able to eliminate all Toxoplasma organisms from the body; cysts characteristically form in brain and muscle and remain viable for the lifetime of the host. With the exception of those in the retina, these cysts do not cause disease unless host immune function is altered.

CLINICAL MANIFESTATIONS.

Acquired Toxoplasmosis in the Immunocompetent Individual. The vast majority of individuals who are infected with *T. gondii* after birth have no apparent clinical symptoms. In the small number of individuals with a symptomatic illness, lymphadenopathy (90 per cent), fever (40 per cent), and malaise (40 per cent) are the common manifestations. The lymphadenopathy is classically symmetric in the posterior auricular, anterior cervical, or posterior cervical chains. Generalized lymphadenopathy or localized unilateral enlargement or enlargement of a solitary node can also be seen. The nodes are characteristically rubbery and nontender. Splenomegaly occurs in about 30 per cent of patients. Fever is usually low grade, but on occasion can be high, rapidly fluctuating, and prolonged. Fatigue can be a prominent feature. A minority of patients have a sore throat, maculopapular rash, myalgias, arthralgias, urticaria, or headache. The sore throat presents as hyperemia rather than as an exudative pharyngitis. For most patients with clinically apparent disease, toxoplasmosis is self-limiting over a period of several weeks. Toxoplasmosis can, however, be a prolonged, severely debilitating disorder that may prevent the patient from working for many weeks or months. The lymph nodes may fluctuate in size during the recovery period.

In immunocompetent adults, specific organ involvement can lead to clinically significant disease involving the lungs, myocardium, pericardium, liver, skin, and skeletal muscle. These manifestations may dominate the clinical picture. Glomerulonephritis has been reported. Death due to toxoplasmosis in immunocompetent individuals is extremely rare.

Laboratory evaluation reveals a normal leukocyte count with a slight lymphocytosis or monocytosis. When atypical lymphocytes are present, they are found only in small numbers. The hemoglobin is usually normal, although a Coombs-negative hemolytic anemia has occasionally been reported. Serum transaminase levels are rarely elevated to more than twice normal. The chest radiograph is usually normal; hilar adenopathy is unusual. On the electrocardiogram ST and T wave abnormalities may be seen if myocarditis is present.

Ocular Involvement in the Immunocompetent Individual. *Toxoplasma* has been estimated to cause 20 to 35 per cent of cases of retinochoroiditis in children and adults. This ocular disease is almost always a consequence of congenital infection; there are very few well-documented cases of eye disease caused by infection acquired after birth.

Symptoms of retinochoroiditis are usually noted initially during the second or third decade of life. Symptoms and the degree of vision loss depend on the location and the extent of retinal involvement. Patients may complain of blurred vision, scotomas, pain, or epiphora. Strabismus may be an early sign in children. The lesions appear acutely as white or yellow cotton-like patches that have indistinct, elevated margins. Inflammatory exudate in the vitreous may obscure visualization of the fundus. As the lesions age, they become atrophic with whitish-gray plaques, more distinct borders, and black spots of choroidal pigment. Lesions may be peripheral, but characteristically they occur near the posterior pole of the retina. They are usually multiple and vary in age, but single lesions do occur. Panuveitis and papillitis with optic atrophy can occur. Exclusively anterior uveitis has never been proved to be caused by *Toxoplasma*.

Patients with *Toxoplasma* retinochoroiditis have an unpredictable clinical course. Episodes of active disease may occur once or many times but usually stop after the age of 40. Recurrent episodes are often associated with progressive loss of vision.

Toxoplasmosis in the Immunodeficient Patient. Toxoplasmosis can occur as a disseminated disease in patients with immunodeficiencies. In most cases, it probably represents reactivation of latent infection rather than primary infection. The disease occurs with particular frequency in patients with AIDS but is also seen occasionally in patients with hematologic malignant conditions (particularly Hodgkin's disease) and organ transplants. The clinical manifestations are variable. Fever, hepatosplenomegaly, pneumonitis, maculopapular rash, myositis, myocarditis, meningoencephalitis, and central nervous system mass lesions may be seen. The lymphadenopathy characteristic of acquired disease in the

immunocompetent patient is often absent. This syndrome is usually fulminant and rapidly fatal. It is very difficult to distinguish from numerous other infectious and noninfectious processes that can present in a similar fashion. The most common manifestation, particularly in patients with AIDS, is central nervous system involvement with fever, headache, confusion progressing to coma, focal neurologic signs, and seizures. The cerebrospinal fluid shows nonspecific changes that usually include pleocytosis and moderately increased protein and normal glucose content. Computed tomography usually shows one or more lesions that are contrast enhancing in a ring or nodular pattern.

Toxoplasmosis has been serologically associated with progressive polymyositis. It is unclear whether the association reflects the etiology of the muscular disorder or whether the disorder activates *Toxoplasma* infection. A few patients with polymyositis and high antitoxoplasma antibody titers have responded symptomatically to antitoxoplasma therapy.

Congenital Disease. Congenital toxoplasmosis is the result of acute infection acquired by the mother just before or during gestation. These *Toxoplasma* infections in the mother are usually asymptomatic, as is *Toxoplasma* infection acquired by other immunocompetent hosts, and thus there is nothing to warn the mother or her physician unless serologic testing is routinely performed. The likelihood that the fetus will become infected and the severity of the congenital infection are largely dependent on when during the gestation the infection is acquired. When the infection occurs late during gestation or involves very few organisms, the infant will probably have no immediate clinical manifestations but will have positive humoral and cellular immune responses to *Toxoplasma*. Cysts of *Toxoplasma* organisms persist in the retina, brain, myocardium, and/or skeletal muscle for the infant's lifetime. If the infant remains immunocompetent during its lifetime, the subsequent clinical manifestations that might occur are retinochoroiditis, which usually flares during the second or third decade of life; seizures; and mild retardation. In infants who are infected early during gestation or with large inocula, the clinical sequelae can be severe. Spontaneous abortion, stillbirth, and prematurity may result. The infant may be born with microphthalmia, microcephaly, seizures, cerebral calcifications, bilateral retinochoroiditis, rash, lymphadenopathy, pneumonitis, fever, or hepatosplenomegaly, which can result in severe incapacity. If the cerebral inflammatory response involves the aqueduct of Sylvius, hydrocephalus may result. Clinical manifestations of these complications may be apparent at birth or may become obvious several months later when the infant fails to reach normal milestones.

DIAGNOSIS.

The diagnosis of toxoplasmosis can be based on serologic tests, lymph node histology, the demonstration of trophozoites in body tissues or fluids, or isolation of *T. gondii* from certain sites. Which diagnostic test is most appropriate depends on the clinical situation.

Serology. Measurement of antitoxoplasma antibody titers is the most commonly employed mechanism for diagnosing toxoplasmosis. The *Sabin-Feldman dye test*, which uses live *T. gondii*, is the most sensitive and specific serologic test but is only available at a few centers. The Sabin-Feldman dye test and the indirect fluorescent antibody (IFA-IgG) test give comparable titers that measure IgG antibodies. Titers begin to rise 1 to 2 weeks after infection and reach a peak after 2 to 8 weeks that is almost always 1:1000 or higher. Titers drift down slowly over several years and persist at low levels (1:16 to 1:64) for the patient's lifetime. The height of the initial peak does not correlate with severity of clinical disease. IFA-IgG titers are positive at stable low levels in adults with reactivated ocular disease and in most immunoincompetent patients with disseminated toxoplasmosis. Titers in infants may be elevated because of passively transferred maternal antibodies. Sequential studies over 4 to 6 months must be performed to determine whether the infant's titers are rising, suggesting that the infected infant is producing antibody, or whether they are falling (usually by 50 per cent per month) and attributable to passively transferred maternal antibodies.

Tests for IgM antibody (IgM fluorescent antibody or double-sandwich enzyme-linked immunosorbent assay [ELISA] techniques) are particularly useful for establishing recent *Toxoplasma* infection because titers appear early (as early as 5 days after infection) and disappear within several months. IgM tests have not been carefully standardized; the significance of specific titers needs to be evaluated by the laboratory performing the test. IgM titer elevations are recognized in 80 per cent of immunocompetent individuals with acute disease and in infants with congenital disease, but they are not elevated in adults with reactivated ocular disease or in most immunoincompetent individuals with disseminated toxoplasmosis.

The indirect hemagglutination (IHA) test as performed in most laboratories measures antibodies that increase very late in the course of infection (and persist for years). Thus the test is a poor screening device for identification of pregnant women who have acquired Toxoplasma infection early during gestation and who might otherwise have elected abortion. The IHA tests that are available in commercial kits are often poorly standardized and difficult to interpret.

False-positive results are not known to occur with the Sabin-Feldman dye test. The IFA-IgG and IgM-IFA tests may produce false-positive results if antinuclear antibody is present. Rheumatoid factor can also cause false-positive IgM-IFA titers.

In general, acute acquired toxoplasmosis is suggested serologically by the Sabin-Feldman dye test or IFA-IgG titers of 1:1000 or higher and proved convincingly by the documentation of elevated IgM-IFA or IgM-ELISA titers or by the documentation of a two-tube (or greater) titer rise in the Sabin-Feldman dye test, IFA-IgG test, and perhaps the IHA test. Thus, a pregnant woman with stable IFA-IgG titers below 1:1024 is presumed to have chronic, latent infection acquired prior to conception. A stable IFA-IgG titer of 1:1024 or higher may represent recent infection, acquired during pregnancy, and the woman should thus be assessed by other techniques such as the IFA-IgM. Serial IFA-IgG titers that rise by two tubes or more would confirm very recent acquisition of Toxoplasma infection. Congenital toxoplasmosis in infants is documented by demonstrating elevated complement fixation or IgM-IFA titers or by showing that the Sabin-Feldman dye test or IFA titers are stable or rising over 4 to 6 months. Ocular toxoplasmosis or toxoplasmosis in the immunoincompetent host cannot be diagnosed with certainty by antibody testing. A negative Sabin-Feldman dye test result or IFA-IgG test titer (<1:4) excludes Toxoplasma as a cause of the ocular disease in the immunocompetent patient. In immunosuppressed patients, serology is not highly useful. Since most cases of toxoplasmosis in this population appear to represent reactivation of latent infection, seropositive individuals are much more likely to develop Toxoplasma disease than are seronegative individuals. A typical serologic pattern for a patient with Hodgkin's disease or AIDS and active cerebral toxoplasmosis would be a stable IFA-IgG titer of 1:16 to 1:256 and a negative IgM-IFA. Cerebral toxoplasmosis has probably occurred in a few seronegative AIDS patients, however. The host may not produce specific antibody in some such cases either because of inadequate humoral response to primary infection or because of deficiencies in antibody production despite chronic, latent infection.

Isolation of the Organism. T. gondii can be isolated from leukocytes, body fluids, or tissue by direct inoculation of the specimens subcutaneously or intraperitoneally into mice. The mice are then examined periodically for the presence of antibody to Toxoplasma, for the presence of trophozoites in the peritoneum, or for the presence of cysts in the brain. Isolation can also be performed by tissue culture. The isolation of the Toxoplasma organisms from leukocytes or body fluids is convincing evidence of acute infection, although parasitemia persisting for a year has been described, especially in immunodeficient patients. The isolation of Toxoplasma organisms from tissue does not provide convincing evidence of acute infection because a tissue cyst may have been present for many years and may be irrelevant to the active disease process. Isolation of Toxoplasma organisms requires several weeks to carry out.

Histologic Diagnosis. The histologic findings in the lymph nodes of patients with acute toxoplasmosis, described earlier, are so characteristic as to be diagnostic. The inflammatory reaction in other tissues is much less specific. In nonlymphoid tissue, free or intracellular tachyzoites must be demonstrated for the diagnosis of toxoplasmosis to be established. The demonstration of Toxoplasma cysts proves that the patient was infected by T.

gondii at some time in the past but does not document that the current clinical disease is related. Histologic diagnosis is the preferred technique for patients with urgent clinical syndromes, especially immunoincompetent patients with cerebral mass lesions. The diagnosis of cerebral toxoplasmosis can be established by assessing empiric response to a 2-week course of pyrimethamine (Daraprim) and sulfadiazine, especially in patients with HIV infection and circulating CD4+ lymphocyte counts below 200 per cubic millimeter. A guided needle biopsy (if such a procedure is technically feasible) is preferable when there is considerable diagnostic uncertainty, i.e., in most patients without HIV infection.

DIFFERENTIAL DIAGNOSIS. The differential diagnosis of a patient with lymphadenopathy includes lymphoma, Hodgkin's disease, AIDS, sarcoidosis, mycobacterial disease, cytomegalovirus disease, mononucleosis, brucellosis, tularemia, cat scratch disease, and many other infectious processes. Toxoplasmosis can be distinguished from mononucleosis by the absence of atypical lymphocytosis, exudative pharyngitis, increased serum transaminase levels, and heterophile antibodies. Appropriate serologic tests, cultures, and lymph node biopsies are necessary to distinguish the other processes. Toxoplasmosis in immunosuppressed patients may mimic other disseminated infections. The central nervous system mass lesions need to be distinguished by biopsy from neoplastic or other infectious processes in non-AIDS patients; an empiric trial of therapy is probably sufficient diagnostically if response is prompt in patients with HIV infection and low CD4+ lymphocyte counts.

Toxoplasma retinochoroiditis needs to be distinguished on the basis of lesion morphology, serology, and appropriate cultures from cytomegalovirus, herpes, tuberculosis, histoplasmosis, syphilis, and sarcoidosis. Congenital toxoplasmosis must be distinguished from cytomegalovirus disease, syphilis, herpes simplex infection, rubella, erythroblastosis fetalis, and bacterial sepsis.

THERAPY. The need and duration of therapy depend on the clinical setting. Most immunocompetent adults with lymphadenopathic disease do not need specific antitoxoplasma therapy. Patients with severe or prolonged constitutional symptoms, patients with specific organ dysfunction, immunoincompetent patients, and probably patients infected by direct inoculation (laboratory workers and transfusion recipients) merit treatment. Treatment for patients with retinochoroiditis or for pregnant patients is more controversial.

A combination of pyrimethamine and sulfadiazine is effective in inhibiting the replication of trophozoites. There are no drugs that will kill trophozoites or eradicate the cyst form. Pyrimethamine can only be given orally. In adults an initial dose of 75 mg is given, followed by 25 mg daily. Infants should be given 1 mg per kilogram for 3 days, followed by 0.5 mg per kilogram per day. Sulfadiazine, 1.0 to 1.5 grams orally every 6 hours, is the adult dose. Infants should receive 100 mg per kilogram per day. Triple sulfonamides (sulfamerazine, sulfamethazine, and sulfadiazine) can be substituted for sulfadiazine, but sulfisoxazole (Gantrisin) is ineffective. Good urine flow should be maintained by adequate fluid intake to prevent crystalluria. Since sulfa drugs and pyrimethamine inhibit folate synthesis, folinic acid (leucovorin), 5 to 10 mg, should be administered two to three times weekly to reduce bone marrow toxicity. Platelet counts and white blood cell counts should be monitored at least twice weekly during therapy. Pyrimethamine is a potential teratogen and is not desirable to use in pregnant women.

Evaluation of the effectiveness of sulfadiazine and pyrimethamine therapy in immunocompetent patients has been limited by the marked variability in clinical course and the frequency of spontaneous improvement. There is considerable anecdotal experience, however, that specific therapy can shorten the symptomatic period of fever and fatigue (although not the lymphadenopathy) in immunocompetent patients with acquired disease and is probably effective in hastening the resolution of serious organ dysfunction. Often a 4- to 6-week course of therapy is given and then the clinical situation re-evaluated. In Toxoplasma retinochoroiditis, primary therapy should be directed at controlling the hypersensitivity response with anti-inflammatory drugs such as corticosteroids if the lesions are extensive or central. Pyrimethamine and sulfadiazine should be used to prevent local proliferation of the organisms and potential dissemination during periods when corticosteroids are given.

Sulfadiazine and pyrimethamine have been effective in immunosuppressed patients with disseminated disease in controlling systemic symptoms and specific organ dysfunction. For AIDS patients, some authorities advocate the use of higher daily doses of pyrimethamine (50 to 100 mg) in conjunction with sulfadiazine, but the benefits of these higher doses have not been established. Long-term therapy should be strongly considered for the duration of immunosuppression; for AIDS patients, therapy should probably be continued for life. Some authorities recommend reduced dosages for long-term suppression in AIDS patients after the initial lesion resolves radiologically, but whether such reduced doses are equally effective as full doses is uncertain. Bone marrow toxicity and skin rash are major management problems in many of these patients, particularly those with AIDS or those treated with antineoplastic chemotherapy.

In pregnant women who plan to complete their pregnancy despite the acquisition of *Toxoplasma* infection during gestation, pyrimethamine has been used despite its teratogenic potential. There is some evidence that sulfadiazine alone may be effective therapy. In Europe spiramycin* has been used, but its efficacy has not been clearly established. Congenital toxoplasmosis should be treated aggressively, whether or not the infant is symptomatic, because organism proliferation can continue after birth. Antitoxoplasma therapy does not reverse damage that has already occurred.

For patients who cannot tolerate sulfadiazine and pyrimethamine, there are several promising alternatives. For AIDS patients, the combination of intravenous clindamycin (2.4 grams per day) plus pyrimethamine appears to be quite efficacious but associated with considerable toxicity. Other promising regimens being assessed include oral clindamycin plus pyrimethamine; newer macrolides, such as azithromycin or clarithromycin or roxithromycin, either alone or in combination with pyrimethamine; and the new hydroxynaphthoquinone 566C80.

PREVENTION. Effective prevention should be directed against minimizing consumption of undercooked meat or exposure to oocyst-infected cat feces. Pet cats should be kept in the house and should not be fed raw meat or have access to wild rodents or birds. Susceptible individuals or pregnant women who are seronegative should avoid sandboxes or moist soil where outdoor cats may defecate.

Congenital toxoplasmosis can be largely avoided if pregnant women follow the aforementioned precautions carefully. Serologic testing at the time of the mother's first prenatal examination and again at 16 to 18 weeks of gestation permits recognition of mothers who have acquired toxoplasmosis early in pregnancy and allows consideration of therapeutic abortion.

Brooks RG, McCabe RE, Remington JS: Role of serology in the diagnosis of toxoplasmic lymphadenopathy. Rev Infect Dis 9:1055, 1987. *Serologic results in 92 cases of toxoplasma lymphadenopathy diagnosed by lymph node biopsy.*

Daffos F, Forestier F, Capella-Pavlovsky M, et al.: Prenatal management of 746 pregnancies at risk for congenital toxoplasmosis. N Engl J Med 318:271, 1988. *Prenatal diagnosis, maternal therapy, and postnatal follow-up for a large series of women are reviewed.*

Leport C, Raffi F, Matheron S, et al.: Treatment of central nervous system toxoplasmosis with pyrimethamine/sulfadiazine combination in 35 patients with the acquired immunodeficiency syndrome. Efficacy of long term continuous therapy. Am J Med 84:94, 1988. *Detailed information about the efficacy and toxicities of treatment with sulfadiazine-pyrimethamine.*

McCabe RE, Brooks RG, Dorgman RF, et al.: Clinical spectrum in 107 cases of toxoplasmic lymphadenopathy. Rev Infect Dis 9:754, 1987. *Extensive compilation of clinical data from lymph node biopsy–proven cases with 14 illustrative case reports.*

Schlaegel TF: Ocular Toxoplasmosis and Pars Planitis. New York, Grune and Stratton, 1978. *A comprehensive survey of the history, epidemiology, clinical features, and laboratory aspects of ocular toxoplasmosis.*

*Spiramycin is available from the National Center for Orphan Drugs and Rare Diseases (703–522–2590) in Virginia and (1–800–336–4797) in Washington, D.C.

429 Cryptosporidiosis
Rosemary Soave

Cryptosporidiosis is a gastrointestinal infection characterized by watery diarrhea, abdominal cramps, malabsorption, and weight loss. It is usually a severe, unrelenting illness in immu-

nocompromised patients, particularly those with the acquired immunodeficiency syndrome (AIDS), and a self-limited disease in the immunologically normal host. It is caused by the coccidian protozoan *Cryptosporidium,* long associated with disease in animals. In 1981–82, identification of *Cryptosporidium* in 47 AIDS patients with severe enteritis brought the protozoan to the attention of the medical community. As more physicians have looked for this parasite, the number of reported cases of cryptosporidiosis has continued to rise, and it has come to be recognized as an important public health problem worldwide. There is currently no known effective therapy.

THE PROTOZOAN. *Cryptosporidium* (which means "hidden spore") belongs to the class Sporozoa and the suborder Eimeriorina, or true coccidia. Other pathogens of humans in this group include *Toxoplasma gondii, Isospora belli,* and *Sarcocystis* species. Although many species within the genus *Cryptosporidium* have been described, recent cross-transmission experiments suggest that little or no host specificity exists. Because the number of cryptosporidial species is not known, the organism is commonly referred to as *Cryptosporidium* sp.

The 4- to 5-μm, spherical, acid-fast *Cryptosporidium* oocyst is the environmentally resistant form of the parasite that is identified in fecal specimens (Fig. 429–1). Sporulated (mature) oocysts contain four elliptical (2 to 4 × 6 to 8 μm), flat, aflagellar but motile sporozoites that are released (excystation) in the host intestinal tract upon dissolution of the oocyst's outer wall. Sporozoites implant on the host mucosal epithelium and undergo asexual and sexual development within a parasitophorous vacuole. The parasite-host cell relationship is unique in that the parasite is intracellular, i.e., enveloped by a host cell membrane, but extracytoplasmic. Sporozoites develop into trophozoites and subsequently undergo asexual multiplication (merogony), formation of macrogametes and microgametes (gametogony), fertilization, and oocyst formation. Newly formed oocysts that are expelled in the feces are immediately infective. The ability of *Cryptosporidium* to develop completely within one host (monoxenous life cycle) imparts a tremendous potential for reinfection and may contribute to the refractory nature of the illness that is seen in *Cryptosporidium*-infected AIDS patients.

EPIDEMIOLOGY. Although more than 40 reports of cryptosporidial infection have emanated from at least 35 countries spanning 6 continents, the true prevalence of cryptosporidiosis in either immunocompetent or immunocompromised hosts is unknown. These surveys of selected populations have revealed infection rates ranging from 0.6 to 20 per cent in the developed world and 4 to 32 per cent in the developing world. Available reports indicate that *Cryptosporidium* is ubiquitous and a major cause of diarrhea worldwide. They also suggest that higher infection rates are associated with young age (<2 years); warm, wet weather; and overcrowding. In addition, several studies have revealed higher than expected rates of seropositivity, suggesting that active or recent cryptosporidial infection may be common in the general population. As of 1986, the Centers for Disease Control estimated that 3 to 4 per cent of AIDS patients had cryptosporidiosis. In recent studies conducted at the National Institutes of Health and The Johns Hopkins Hospital, approximately 16 per cent of AIDS patients with diarrhea were found to be infected. By contrast, more than 50 per cent of AIDS patients

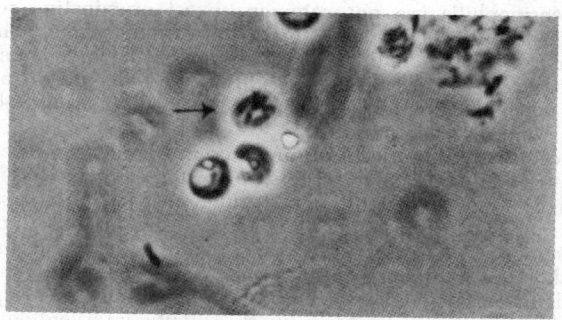

FIGURE 429–1. Wet mount of human stool showing three cryptosporidial oocysts and sporozoites (*arrow*) (×630).

in Haiti and parts of Africa have cryptosporidiosis. Asymptomatic carriage of the parasite has been documented in immunocompetent and immunocompromised subjects, but the frequency with which it occurs and its significance have yet to be determined.

Transmission of *Cryptosporidium* between humans and domestic animals has been well documented, and it is likely that both serve as reservoirs of the disease. For humans, however, spread from person to person and via contaminated water may be more common than zoonotic transmission. Spread of the parasite via sexual contact or aerosolization has been suggested but not confirmed. Person-to-person transmission has been implicated in day care center outbreaks, clusters of infection among contacts of index cases, and nosocomial spread of infection among patients and health care workers. Contaminated water appears to be responsible for infection in travelers and swimmers, and in at least four major community outbreaks in the United States and two in the United Kingdom. *Cryptosporidium* oocysts have been found in surface and drinking waters, as well as in sewage effluent samples from different geographic regions of the United States. Like *Giardia lamblia*, the environmentally resistant *Cryptosporidium* oocyst is not affected by the chlorine concentrations used to decontaminate drinking water. Infectivity of *Cryptosporidium* appears to be destroyed by freeze-drying; a 30-minute exposure to temperatures above 60°C or under −20°C; or treatment with 50 per cent ammonia, full-strength bleach, or 10 per cent formalin for 30 minutes.

PATHOLOGY AND PATHOGENESIS. *Cryptosporidium* has been found in the pharynx, esophagus, stomach, duodenum, jejunum, ileum, appendix, colon, rectum, gallbladder, pancreas, bile, and pancreatic ducts, as well as within colonic submucosal vessels of infected immunocompromised (primarily AIDS) patients. The parasite has also been detected in sputum, tracheal aspirates, bronchoalveolar lavage, and lung tissue of a small number of immunocompromised patients with gastrointestinal cryptosporidiosis. Light microscopic evaluation of Giemsa-stained or hematoxylin-eosin–stained *Cryptosporidium*-infected tissue reveals small, spherical, basophilic structures along the epithelial cell brush border. Ultrastructural studies reveal the entire spectrum of endogenous stages of the organism adherent to the enterocyte surface and enveloped by a membrane, believed to be derived from the host cell. Histologic changes are nonspecific and minimal, resembling those described for giardiasis, i.e., villous atrophy, crypt elongation, and minimal subjacent inflammatory infiltrates of the lamina propria. By contrast, marked histologic changes ranging from acute inflammation to gangrenous necrosis of the gallbladder and biliary duct epithelium have been described for patients with cryptosporidial cholangitis or cholecystitis.

The pathogenic mechanisms by which *Cryptosporidium* causes enteritis are unknown. The secretory nature of the diarrhea and the presence of malabsorption suggest that an enterotoxin-mediated mechanism and/or physical destruction of the brush border may be operative.

CLINICAL MANIFESTATIONS. The spectrum of cryptosporidial infection ranges from asymptomatic infection to fulminant diarrhea. Cryptosporidiosis is characterized by watery diarrhea, cramping abdominal pain (often exacerbated by food ingestion), weight loss, and flatulence. Nausea, vomiting, anorexia, myalgias, and malaise may also be present. Fever, leukocytosis, and eosinophilia are not common. Fecal examination reveals cryptosporidial oocysts and mucus, but no leukocytes or blood. Vitamin B$_{12}$, xylose, and fat malabsorption has been documented. Radiographic abnormalities are nonspecific and include prominent mucosal folds, intestinal wall thickening, small bowel dilatation, and disordered motility.

The incubation period for human cryptosporidiosis appears to be between 2 and 14 days. The severity and course of the illness are determined by host immunocompetence. In the immunologically normal host, infection is often explosive in onset and lasts an average of 10 to 14 days. Clearance of the parasite from stool lags behind clinical resolution by 2 to 3 weeks, thus creating problems for infection control. Although self-limited, symptoms are often severe enough to justify therapeutic intervention, were it available. Infection in AIDS patients often begins insidiously and escalates in severity as the underlying immune defect be-

comes more profound. Frequent (6 to 25), voluminous (1 to 25 liters) daily bowel movements, profound weight loss, and stool oocyst shedding often persist for months.

Biliary cryptosporidiosis has been documented only in immunocompromised patients. Because invasive procedures that may not be justified in the absence of treatment options are a prerequisite for definitive diagnosis, the incidence of this complication is not known. Most patients with biliary cryptosporidiosis have classic signs of cholangitis, including severe right upper quadrant pain, nausea, and vomiting. Serum levels of alkaline phosphatase and γ-glutamyl transpeptidase are elevated, but serum bilirubin and transaminase levels are normal. Radiographic evaluation may reveal a dilated gallbladder, thickened gallbladder wall, and dilated bile ducts with luminal irregularities. Patients undergoing endoscopic retrograde cholangiopancreatography (ERCP) are often found to have cryptosporidia studding the surface epithelium and in the bile. In certain instances, cholecystectomy or endoscopic papillotomy has resulted in transient improvement of both symptoms and laboratory abnormalities.

DIAGNOSIS. The diagnosis of cryptosporidial enteritis is based on identification of the oocyst form of the parasite in fecal specimens. Since 1981, various staining techniques for detecting oocysts have been popularized, including several modifications of the acid-fast stain (Kinyoun, Ziehl-Neelsen), the fluorescent auramine-rhodamine stain, and the periodic acid–Schiff (PAS) and carbol fuchsin–negative stains. With the acid-fast stain, acid-fast (red) oocysts may be easily distinguished from yeast that are similar in size and shape but are not acid fast (they stain green). The sensitivity, specificity, and relative merits of the various staining methods have not been determined. Most recently, a method for detecting cryptosporidial oocysts that uses a fluorescein-labeled immunoglobulin (IgG) monoclonal antibody was made available commercially (Meridien Diagnostics, Cincinnati, OH). This method appears to be more sensitive and specific than other currently available techniques, and its role in the clinical laboratory is currently being investigated. Since the pattern of fecal oocyst shedding in human cryptosporidiosis has not been determined, and the sensitivity of the various methodologies is also not known, the optimal number of negative stool specimens required to confirm the absence of cryptosporidia has yet to be defined. Stool concentration techniques do not appear to be necessary for routine diagnosis but are most useful in detecting oocysts in follow-up specimens, asymptomatic contacts, or environmental samples.

Although the sensitivity and specificity of stool examination compared with small intestinal biopsy have not been determined, stool examination appears to be more sensitive. In addition to being invasive and costly, intestinal biopsies may be falsely negative owing to autolysis during processing and sampling difficulties related to the parasite's patchy distribution and the paucity of inflammatory changes to guide the endoscopist.

Anticryptosporidial IgG and IgM have been detected in both immunocompetent persons and patients with AIDS by immunofluorescent assay (IFA) and enzyme-linked immunosorbent (ELISA) assay. Antibody titers rise within 6 to 8 weeks after the onset of infection and decline within 1 year. Immunocompetent hosts generally have higher titers. The IgM response is often absent or minimal in patients with AIDS. Serologic studies are not useful in the diagnosis of acute cryptosporidiosis but do have a role in defining the epidemiology of the disease.

TREATMENT. In contrast to all the other opportunistic infections of AIDS patients, there is currently no known effective therapy for cryptosporidiosis. Identification of potentially active agents has been severely hampered by the absence of an asymptomatic, small-animal model of the chronic disease and by an inability to cultivate the organism in vitro. Investigational therapy has not been given to the immunocompetent host with cryptosporidial enteritis because illness in these patients is usually self-limited. Persons receiving corticosteroids or cytotoxic agents may be successfully managed by discontinuation of the immunosuppressive drugs.

Because of the severe nature of the illness in AIDS patients with cryptosporidiosis, a vast array of antidiarrheal, antimicrobial, and immunomodulating agents have been administered in an unprecedented manner with few preclinical data to support their use. Early anecdotal reports of success using the antitoxoplasma macrolide spiramycin led to two controlled studies with this agent. A placebo-controlled clinical trial of oral spiramycin in 54 AIDS patients with cryptosporidiosis failed to show any difference between placebo and drug. Subsequent pharmacokinetic studies suggested that this may have been due to suboptimal drug absorption. As a result, the intravenous form of spiramycin is being evaluated in a single-blind placebo-controlled trial. In a recently concluded study, the benzeneacetonitrile derivative diclazuril, known for its activity against the animal pathogen *Eimeria*, was found to have some promise as an anticryptosporidial agent. Since lack of absorption appeared to be a significant problem, future trials employing a more absorbable congener of diclazuril are being planned. Anecdotal reports of amelioration of cryptosporidial infection with paromomycin are also being verified. α-Difluoromethylornithine, an irreversible ornithine decarboxylase inhibitor that is active against a number of protozoa, has been found to be moderately efficacious against *Cryptosporidium*, but toxicity (bone marrow suppression and gastrointestinal irritation) has limited its use.

The mechanisms by which the immunocompetent host successfully deals with cryptosporidial infection are poorly understood but appear to include both intact T cell– and B cell–mediated immunity. Novel attempts at modulating immune function in *Cryptosporidium*-infected patients centered on the use of immune bovine colostrum, bovine milk globulins, and bovine transfer factor have provided interesting and promising results that require further investigation.

In the absence of any proven effective therapy for cryptosporidiosis, careful management of fluid and electrolyte balance is of paramount importance. All classes of nonspecific antidiarrheal agents, including the long-acting, parenterally administered somatostatin analogue octreotide acetate, may be useful, when used in trial-and-error fashion, for individual patients. However, their safety in *Cryptosporidium*-infected patients is not known. Total parenteral nutrition often provides major benefits, but its use is controversial owing to the need for an invasive procedure and its high cost.

Crawford FG, Vermund SH: Human cryptosporidiosis. CRC Crit Rev Microbiol 16:113, 1988. *This exhaustive review covers all aspects of cryptosporidiosis in humans.*

Fayer R, Ungar BLP: *Cryptosporidium* spp. and cryptosporidiosis. Microbiol Rev 50:458, 1986. *This thoroughly referenced review emphasizes the biologic and veterinary aspects of Cryptosporidium.*

Jokipii L, Jokipii AM: Timing of symptoms and oocyst excretion in human cryptosporidiosis excretion in human cryptosporidiosis. N Engl J Med 315:1643, 1986. *A clinical and parasitologic study of 68 immunocompetent patients with cryptosporidiosis in Finland.*

Soave R: Treatment strategies for cryptosporidiosis. Ann NY Acad Sci 616:442, 1990. *A thoroughly referenced up-to-date review of the approaches to treating cryptosporidiosis.*

430 Giardiasis

David P. Stevens

DEFINITION. Giardiasis is an infection of the small intestine caused by the flagellated protozoan *Giardia lamblia*. When symptomatic, it results in diarrhea, malabsorption, and weight loss.

ETIOLOGY. The organism exists in two forms: the motile, flagellated, pear-shaped trophozoite, 12 to 15 μm in length, or the smaller, tough-walled oval cyst. Trophozoites either attach to the microvilli of the intestinal epithelium or move about in the unstirred layer of mucus just above the epithelial surface. The trophozoites, carried caudally by peristalsis, eventually encyst and pass into the environment. The cyst is resistant to many environmental stresses, including concentrations of chlorine normally found in treated municipal water supplies. It is ingested eventually by a subsequent host. Excystation occurs in the acid environment of the stomach, and infection is again established in the small intestine.

EPIDEMIOLOGY. Giardiasis is present in all climates. It spreads by two routes: water-borne infection, particularly in contaminated community water supplies, and direct person-to-person transmission. Dozens of epidemics have been described in the United States consequent to breakdown of community water filtration systems. Epidemics in day care centers for children and among promiscuous male homosexuals indicate that direct person-to-person spread can occur. Household contacts must be tested for infection, even if they are asymptomatic.

A role for animal reservoirs of infection has been suggested by the demonstration of *Giardia*-infected beaver upstream from communities where outbreaks of human infection have occurred. It is likely that both beaver and dogs carry *Giardia* species infectious for humans. Campers must be particularly mindful of the risk of drinking untreated water, no matter how pristine the water source. The American Rockies are areas of particularly high risk.

Giardia is a frequent source of diarrhea in travelers returning from endemic areas. Twenty-three per cent of North American travelers returning from Leningrad have been shown to have giardiasis. The incubation period is 7 to 21 days. Typically, the infected traveler develops symptoms several weeks after returning home, and on this basis the infection may be distinguished from that caused by toxigenic *Escherichia coli* and other forms of infectious traveler's diarrhea with shorter incubation periods.

PATHOGENICITY. Jejunal mucosal biopsies from infected persons range in appearance from normal to marked subtotal mucosal atrophy with submucosal inflammatory cell infiltration, reduced villus height, and elongated crypts. Electron microscopic observation of epithelial cells beneath overlying adherent trophozoites shows deformation and blunting of the individual microvilli.

CLINICAL MANIFESTATIONS. *Giardia* infection is frequently asymptomatic. In those persons who are ill, disease ranges from mild diarrhea to severe, debilitating malabsorption and weight loss. Reversible lactase deficiency as well as malabsorption of fat and vitamin B_{12} has been documented. The majority of symptoms result from malabsorption and include abdominal distention, cramps, nausea, flatulence, borborygmi, and frequent loose, bulky, foul, and urgent stools. Fever and chills may be present. Blood or mucus in the stool is *not* typical of giardiasis. Upper gastrointestinal symptoms such as nausea and epigastric pain may distinguish giardiasis from infectious disorders of the colon. Although the infection is frequently self-limited, many persons have a prolonged, indolent illness with waxing and waning symptoms and progressive weight loss.

DIAGNOSIS. The diagnosis is established by demonstration of cysts or trophozoites in stools or of trophozoites in small bowel contents. Because excretion of the organism in stool is episodic and its demonstration elusive, at least three stool specimens should be examined before a negative conclusion is drawn. If no organisms are seen, the small bowel contents may be sampled. This can be achieved by aspiration or passage of a string that will absorb sufficient jejunal fluid for examination. Microscopic examination of a wet preparation of jejunal contents usually reveals motile organisms in the infected person. Small bowel biopsy may be reserved for situations in which these measures are unsuccessful. The small bowel roentgenogram usually shows an edematous mucosa, but this finding is nonspecific. Hematologic values are normal. Eosinophilia should not be expected, since this is a finding associated with infections by worms, not protozoa.

TREATMENT. All infected persons should be treated. There is occasional justification for a trial of therapy in the patient with typical signs and symptoms of giardiasis but in whom efforts to demonstrate the organism fail. Therapy is achieved with quinacrine hydrochloride, 100 mg three times per day for 10 days. When this drug is contraindicated, metronidazole,* 250 mg three times per day for 7 days, is an alternative. Treatment with either drug may be unsuccessful in 5 to 20 per cent of patients, requiring a second course of therapy.

Stevens DP: Selective primary health care: Strategies for control of disease in the developing world: XIX. Giardiasis. Rev Infect Dis 7:530, 1985. *A review of epidemiologic, clinical, and therapeutic aspects of giardiasis.*

Stevens DP: Giardiasis: Host-pathogen biology. Rev Infect Dis 4:851, 1982. *A detailed review of the sparse knowledge available on the pathogenesis of this infection.*

---

*This use is not listed in the manufacturer's directive but is recommended by the Centers for Disease Control.

431 Amebiasis

Jonathan I. Ravdin

Human amebiasis is due to infection with the enteric protozoan *Entamoeba histolytica*. This parasite infects 10 per cent of the world's population, with the disease burden highest in poor, developing areas. To manage patients with amebiasis appropriately, physicians must have knowledge of the biology of the organism, risk factors for infection, mechanisms of disease, pathogenesis and host immunity, the presenting manifestations of the invasive syndromes, the correct diagnostic approach, alternative therapeutic drug regimens, and strategies for prevention of infection.

BIOLOGY OF *E. HISTOLYTICA* AND EPIDEMIOLOGY. Infection results from ingestion of the fecally excreted acid-resistant cyst form. Excystation occurs in the small bowel, leading to colonization of the colon with *E. histolytica* trophozoites. Transmission of infection results from fecal contamination of water or food or direct fecal-oral contact because of poor hygiene or anal-oral sexual practices. Epidemiologic and molecular biology studies indicate that there are distinct pathogenic and nonpathogenic strains. Infection with the latter does not result in systemic invasive disease or antigenic exposure. Approximately 10 per cent of those with pathogenic infection present clinically with invasive amebiasis, although all manifest a serum antibody response. The relative frequency of pathogenic and nonpathogenic infection varies, depending on geographic area. Regions of the world with a high incidence of invasive amebiasis include Mexico, parts of South America, Western and South Africa, the Indian subcontinent, the Middle East, and Southeast Asia. High-risk groups in the United States include sexually promiscuous male homosexuals, the institutionalized mentally retarded population, and travelers or emigrants from areas of high prevalence (especially Mexican-Americans). Groups that, when infected, can experience an increased severity of invasive amebiasis are the very young (under age 2 years), pregnant women, malnourished individuals, and patients on corticosteroids.

PATHOGENESIS AND HOST IMMUNITY. *E. histolytica* trophozoites cause disease by sequentially adhering to colonic mucus, disrupting mucosal barriers with proteolytic enzymes, and producing contact-dependent lysis of host cells, including responding inflammatory cells. Trophozoite adherence to colonic mucins is mediated by a galactose-binding surface protein; attachment by this protein is the first step in the amebic lysis of human cells. Tissue destruction is enhanced following parasite lysis of responding polymorphonuclear leukocytes, owing to release of toxic neutrophil components. Intestinal infection with nonpathogenic *E. histolytica* usually clears within 8 to 12 months without evidence of a specific immune response. Cure of invasive amebiasis is associated with resistance to recurrent disease, but not necessarily immunity to asymptomatic intestinal infection. Protective immunity is apparently mediated by development of an amebicidal cell-mediated immune response with lymphokine-activated macrophages and a CD8 subset of cytotoxic lymphocytes serving as effector cells. It is unclear whether the serum or secretory antiamebic antibody response that develops after pathogenic infection has any protective role. Acute amebiasis is associated with the occurrence of antigen-specific suppression of cell-mediated responses to *E. histolytica*, facilitating parasite survival in tissues.

CLINICAL DISEASE SYNDROMES. The disease syndromes caused by *E. histolytica* are summarized in Table 431–1. It is unknown whether health is impaired by asymptomatic infection with nonpathogenic *E. histolytica*; unfortunately, there is as yet no clinically applicable means to differentiate between pathogenic and nonpathogenic infection. Occasionally, infected patients present with nonspecific gastrointestinal complaints, such as bloating and cramps, without evidence of invasive colitis. Amebic rectocolitis is characterized by the subacute onset of bloody diarrhea over days, abdominal tenderness, weight loss, and fever in only one third of cases. Fulminant colitis with perforation is uncom-

TABLE 431–1. CLINICAL SYNDROMES ASSOCIATED WITH *E. HISTOLYTICA* INFECTION

Intestinal Disease
Asymptomatic infection
Symptomatic noninvasive infection
Acute rectocolitis (dysentery)
Fulminant colitis with perforation
Toxic megacolon
Chronic nondysenteric colitis
Ameboma

Extraintestinal Disease
Liver abscess
Liver abscess complicated by:
    Peritonitis
    Empyema
    Pericarditis
Lung abscess
Brain abscess
Genitourinary disease

Modified with permission from Mandell GL, Douglas RG Jr, Bennett JE (eds.): Principles and Practices of Infectious Diseases. 3rd ed. New York, Churchill Livingstone, 1989.

mon; patients are in a toxic state, are acutely ill, and have a rigid, tender abdomen. Toxic megacolon is an unusual complication that is associated with the inappropriate use of corticosteroids when amebic colitis is mistaken for idiopathic inflammatory bowel disease. Chronic nondysenteric amebic colitis can manifest with years of intermittent bloody diarrhea, a syndrome symptomatically indistinguishable from ulcerative colitis. Ameboma is a rare segmental form of chronic amebic colitis that is more common in the cecum and ascending colon and presents as a tender abdominal mass that can be confused with colonic carcinoma.

Extraintestinal disease consists mainly of amebic liver abscess, which can occur up to 5 months after intestinal infection. Two types of presentation have been observed. One is an acute presentation of fewer than 10 days' duration that consists of high fever and marked right upper quadrant tenderness. Alternatively, with more than 10 days of symptoms, pain and weight loss predominate, with fever being less frequent. Fewer than a third of patients have concurrent diarrhea. Extension of an amebic liver abscess into the peritoneum or pericardium is more likely with a left lobe abscess and results in a very acute clinical presentation. Disease can extend to the pleura, causing empyema, and, less likely, can disseminate hematogenously to the lung and brain.

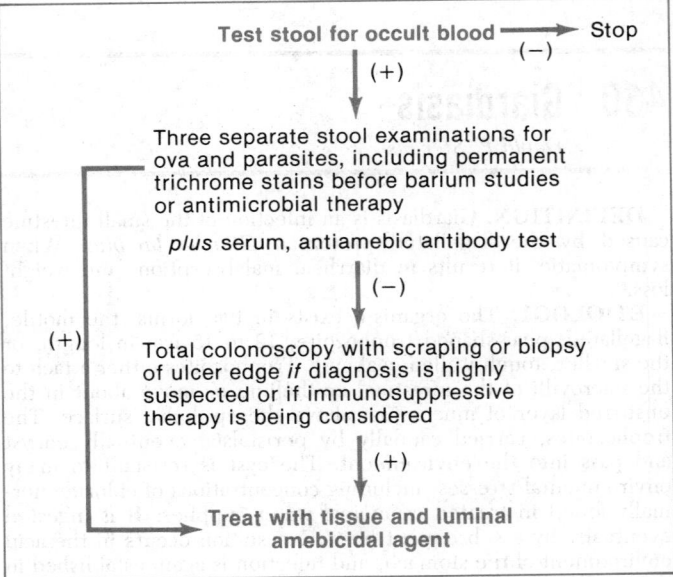

FIGURE 431–1. Diagnostic evaluation for acute amebic rectocolitis in a patient with suggestive epidemiology and clinical manifestations. (Reproduced with permission from Kass EH, Platt R [eds.]: Current Therapy in Infectious Disease—3. Philadelphia, B. C. Decker, 1990.)

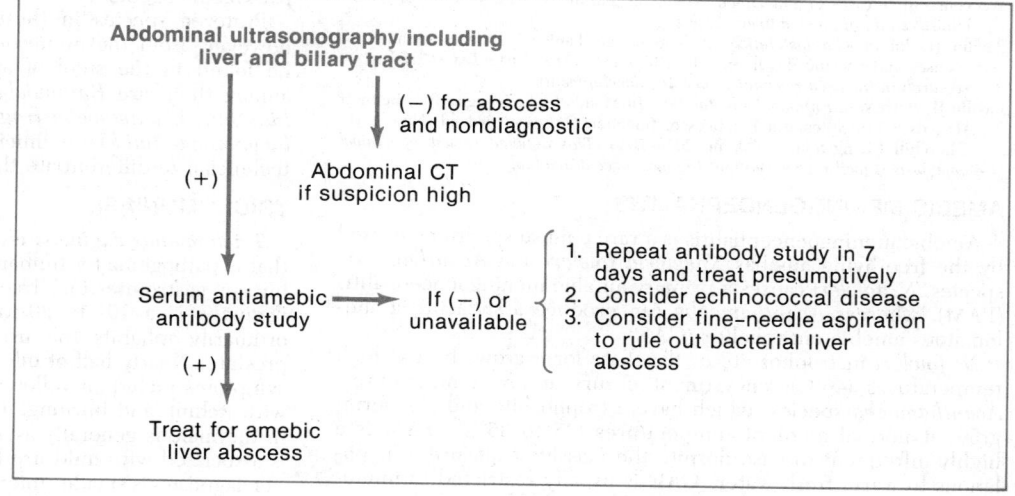

FIGURE 431–2. Diagnostic evaluation for amebic liver abscess in a patient with suggestive epidemiology and clinical manifestations. (Reproduced with permission from Kass EH, Platt R [eds.]: Current Therapy in Infectious Disease—3. Philadelphia, B. C. Decker, 1990.)

DIFFERENTIAL DIAGNOSIS AND WORKUP. Algorithms for the diagnosis of amebic colitis and liver abscess are provided in Figures 431–1 and 431–2, respectively. The differential diagnosis of acute amebic colitis includes infection due to *Shigella*, *Campylobacter*, *Salmonella*, *Yersinia*, and invasive *E. coli* species or to *Clostridium difficile* toxin-mediated disease. Amebiasis is one cause of inflammatory colitis in which fecal leukocytes may be absent, owing to the ability of trophozoites to lyse human neutrophils. Unfortunately, the diagnosis of intestinal amebiasis still rests upon the morphologic identification of trophozoites in fecal specimens (see Color Plate 11*H*). At least three stool samples are necessary to reach a 90 per cent yield; samples should be refrigerated or placed in fixative if they cannot be processed immediately. Laboratories in the United States frequently falsely identify fecal leukocytes as trophozoites; careful study with skilled microscopy is necessary. Serology for antiamebic antibodies is positive in more than 85 per cent of patients with amebic colitis and is very helpful. Interpretation of results can be difficult in highly endemic areas, where up to 25 per cent of the population is seropositive owing to the persistence of serum antibodies for years after pathogenic *E. histolytica* infection. Endoscopy with biopsies of the ulcer edge is diagnostic in 90 per cent of cases; this is helpful if a rapid diagnosis is needed, if serology results are nondiagnostic, or to differentiate amebiasis from idiopathic inflammatory bowel disease.

The key study in the diagnosis of amebic liver abscess is abdominal ultrasonography, a rapid, noninvasive procedure that should differentiate between biliary tract disease and a cavity in the liver. The differential diagnosis can then be narrowed to amebic liver abscess, pyogenic bacterial abscess, echinococcal cyst, and hepatoma. Attention to epidemiologic risk factors and detection of serum antiamebic antibodies are usually sufficient to establish the diagnosis, with the caveat that serology may be negative in patients with fewer than 7 days of symptoms. However, if concern exists regarding a bacterial abscess and a serologic study is not immediately available, then a "skinny-needle" aspiration, guided by ultrasonography, or computed tomography, can be performed. This procedure is diagnostic of bacterial abscess; aspiration of an amebic abscess normally yields a yellow proteinaceous fluid without white blood cells or amebas. The trophozoites are found in tissue at the periphery of the liver lesion.

THERAPY. Regimens for the treatment of amebiasis are summarized in Table 431–2. Therapy usually requires a tissue-active agent followed by a drug effective in the bowel lumen. In pregnant women, the use of nonabsorbable agents (paromomycin) or the judicious use of metronidazole is advisable. It is controversial whether therapy is necessary for asymptomatic *E. histolytica* intestinal infection without evidence of tissue invasion; however, this may be advisable in areas where pathogenic infection is likely or reinfection is not expected. Careful follow-up of stool examination is necessary, as all available agents are incompletely effective in eradicating intestinal infection. Patients with amebic liver abscess respond gradually with decreased pain and fever after 3 to 5 days of therapy. A small minority do not respond at all within 3 days or have a very large abscess that appears close to rupture; needle aspiration is indicated in such patients. After aspiration, continued therapy with metronidazole alone should be adequate. There is no evidence that the addition of other therapeutic agents is necessary. Although fewer than 20 per cent of patients with liver abscess have trophozoites found in their stool, follow-up with a luminally active agent is advisable.

PREVENTION. *E. histolytica* infection can be prevented by the availability of clean water, adequate sanitation, and avoidance of sexual practices or living conditions that facilitate direct fecal-oral contamination. Boiling is the only reliable way of killing cysts; halide solutions are not reliable. In endemic areas, uncooked foods such as salads and vegetables should be avoided. No vaccine or acceptable form of chemoprophylaxis is available; however, current research on the pathogenesis of amebiasis and the host immune response has led to the identification of multiple *E. histolytica* antigens that are candidates for vaccine development.

Healy GR: Diagnostic techniques for stool samples. *In* Ravdin JI, (ed.): Amebiasis: Human Infection by *Entamoeba histolytica*. New York, Churchill Livingstone, 1988, pp 106–119. *A recent authoritative review of the diagnosis of amebiasis using fecal specimens; the text contains more than 50 chapters on all aspects of* E. histolytica *infection.*

Katzenstein D, Rickerson V, Braude A: New concepts of amebic liver abscess derived from hepatic imaging, serodiagnosis, and hepatic enzymes in 67

TABLE 431–2. THERAPEUTIC REGIMENS FOR TREATMENT OF AMEBIASIS*

Cyst Passers
Diloxanide furoate, 500 mg tid × 10 days, or
Paromomycin, 30 mg/kg/day in 3 divided doses × 5–10 days, or
Tetracycline, 250 mg qid × 10 days, then diiodohydroxyquin, 650 mg tid × 20 days

Invasive Rectocolitis
Metronidazole, 750 mg tid × 5–10 days
  or 2.4 grams qd × 2–3 days
  or 50 mg/kg × 1 dose
  plus diloxanide furoate or paromomycin or
Dehydroemetine, 1–1.5 mg/kg/day × 5 days plus diloxanide furoate or paromomycin

Liver Abscess
Metronidazole, 750 tid × 5–10 days or 2.4 mg qd × 1–2 days plus diloxanide fuorate or paromomycin or
Dehydroemetine, 1–1.5 mg/kg/day × 5 days plus diloxanide furoate or paromomycin or
Chloroquine (base), 600 mg qd × 2 days, 300 mg base qd × 2–3 weeks (can be added to other regimens)

*All dosages are for oral administrtion except dehydroemetine, which is given intramuscularly; metronidazole can be used intravenously.

Adapted with permission from Mandell GL, Douglas RG Jr, Bennett JE (eds.): Principles and Practices of Infectious Diseases. 3rd ed. New York, Churchill Livingstone, 1989.

consecutive cases in San Diego. Medicine (Baltimore) 61:237, 1982. *Excellent clinical study of amebic liver abscess.*

Ravdin JI: *Entamoeba histolytica:* Pathogenic mechanisms, human immune response, and vaccine development. Clin Res 38:215, 1990. *Latest update on research in the area relevant to vaccine development.*

Ravdin JI, Petri WA: *Entamoeba histolytica. In* Mandell GL, Douglas RG, Bennett JE (eds.): Principles and Practices of Infectious Disease. 3rd ed. New York, Churchill Livingstone, 1990, pp 2036–2048. *This detailed review of clinical amebiasis is well referenced and the most recent available.*

AMEBIC MENINGOENCEPHALITIS

Amebic meningoencephalitis is a rare clinical syndrome caused by the free-living amebas *Naegleria fowleri* and *Acanthamoeba* species. *N. fowleri* causes a primary amebic meningoencephalitis (PAM), whereas *Acanthamoeba* can produce a subacute granulomatous amebic encephalitis (GAE).

N. fowleri in trophozoite or flagellate form grows best at high temperatures (46°C); encystment occurs at low temperatures. *Acanthamoeba* species, which have a trophozoite and cyst form, grow at normal ambient temperatures (25 to 35°C). PAM is a highly infrequent disease despite the massive exposure of populations to warm fresh water. GAE is usually restricted to immunosuppressed populations, such as those with acquired immunodeficiency syndrome (AIDS) or those with organ transplants. *N. fowleri* enters the central nervous system by penetrating the nasal mucosa and cribriform plate and is highly cytolytic. GAE probably results from hematogenous dissemination and can be distinguished from PAM by the presence of cysts in tissue.

PAM is characterized by the abrupt onset of headache, fever, and meningismus, with rapid development of focal neurologic findings, including olfactory loss. A neutrophilic cerebrospinal fluid (CSF) pleocytosis is frequently associated with increased CSF protein and hypoglycorrhachia. A negative CSF Gram stain result, India ink preparation, culture for bacteria, and cryptococcal antigen study in a patient with acute meningitis who has a history of exposure to fresh water suggests the need to examine the CSF for motile trophozoites (10 to 30 μm), a finding that is diagnostic. In contrast, GAE manifests subacutely over weeks with focal central nervous system signs, headache, fever, and depressed mental status and is often complicated by seizures. The presence of *Acanthamoeba* organisms in a nodular or ulcerative skin lesion is helpful; study of the CSF usually reveals a nonspecific lymphocytosis with abnormally elevated protein levels. A brain biopsy is necessary to differentiate GAE from toxoplasmosis, pyogenic brain abscess, and other causes of focal central nervous system disease.

There is no treatment known to be efficacious for PAM or GAE. Treatment with systemic and intrathecal amphotericin B was associated with survival in two patients with PAM. *Acanthamoeba* organisms are usually susceptible in vitro to ketoconazole, miconazole, 5-flucytosine, and pentamidine. After determination of susceptibility of the patient's isolate in vitro, the above agents and amphotericin B can be considered. These are rare disorders, and the risk of PAM from diving or waterskiing in warm fresh water cannot be quantified. Opportunistic infections other than those caused by *Acanthamoeba* are much more frequent in immunosuppressed patients.

Petri WA, Ravdin JI: Free Living Amebas. *In* Mandell GL, Douglas RG, Bennett ED (eds.): Principles and Practices of Infectious Diseases. 3rd ed. New York, Churchill Livingstone, 1990, pp 2049–2055. *This is an up-to-date, well-referenced review of disease caused by free-living amebas.*

432 Other Protozoan Diseases

David P. Stevens

The human host provides an ever changing environment for protozoan infections. With the increasing prevalence of immunodeficiency, caused by either immunosuppressant drugs or the acquired immunodeficiency syndrome (AIDS), protozoan infections that were previously considered rare or exotic are now observed more frequently. With this changing epidemiologic setting, additional protozoa will play the opportunist's role as pathogenic agents.

Protozoa species in these settings should be distinguished, however, from the numerous nonpathogenic protozoa that may be found in the stool of apparently healthy persons. Notable among them are *Entamoeba coli, Endolimax nana, Iodamoeba bütschlii, Dientamoeba fragilis, Trichomonas hominis,* and *Chilomastix mesnili.* The clinician must rely on a skilled laboratory technician to differentiate these agents from pathogenic species.

TRICHOMONIASIS

Trichomonas vaginalis is the only species of the trichomonads that is pathogenic for humans. *T. tenax* and *T. hominis* infect the human gastrointestinal tract but are harmless commensals. *T. vaginalis* is a 10- to 20-μm motile, flagellated organism that ordinarily inhabits the urethra, urinary bladder, vagina, and prostate. Nearly half of infections are asymptomatic. Recognized symptoms include a yellow, creamy vaginal discharge associated with itching and burning. Dysuria may be prominent. Infection in the male is generally asymptomatic. Occasionally, however, it is associated with mild urethral burning of brief duration.

Diagnosis is made microscopically by identification of the organism in a wet preparation of the exudate. Long-term complications are unrecognized in otherwise healthy persons. Treatment of both partners is advised for this sexually transmitted disease. Treatment with a single 2-gram dose of metronidazole is as effective as metronidazole, 250 mg three times daily for 7 days. It is frequently associated with side effects of nausea, a metallic taste, or alcohol intolerance.

Lossick JG: Sexually transmitted vaginitis. Urol Clin North Am 11:141, 1984. *An authoritative clinical report for further detailed study.*

BALANTIDIASIS

Balantidium coli is a large, motile, oval ciliate, some 5 to 10 times the size of an erythrocyte. The trophozoite form resides as a facultative anaerobe in the colon. The great majority of infections in humans are noninvasive, asymptomatic, and self-limited. Infrequently a cause of disease, this protozoan can penetrate the colonic mucosa with formation of deep ulcers. Illness consists of dysentery, usually bloody, often with resulting dehydration and prostration. Complications include colonic perforation at the site of the ulcers. Infection may extend to mesenteric lymph nodes and, less commonly, the appendix and terminal ileum. Isolated reports of infection of the vagina, liver, lung, and pleura have documented that extraintestinal migration of the organism is rare.

Balantidia infect numerous nonhuman reservoirs, particularly swine. It is said that 80 per cent of pigs in England carry this organism. The relevance of various other animal reservoirs, such as rats, to human infection is debated. The importance of porcine infections to human disease is borne out, however, by the documented high incidence of balantidiasis in communities where swine and humans live together closely, e.g., in New Guinea, Micronesia, Peru, and southern Russia. Poor nutrition and debilitating illness seem to predispose to symptomatic balantidiasis. Person-to-person spread probably occurs in settings where crowding and poor hygiene exist.

Ingestion of *Balantidium* cysts—resistant to drying and other environmental stresses—leads to infection in the susceptible host. Excystation occurs at an unknown location in the gastrointestinal tract, and multiplication occurs in the colon. Encystation occurs in the distal colon or after expulsion into the environment.

The diagnosis is confirmed by microscopic demonstration of trophozoites in fresh wet preparations of liquid stool or scrapings of colonic ulcers. Cysts are less frequently observed in stool, and concentration techniques are usually required. Differentiation from amebiasis and idiopathic ulcerative colitis must always be considered.

Therapy is reserved for the patient with symptomatic infection and consists of tetracycline, 500 mg four times daily for 10 days. Metronidazole, 250 mg four times daily for 7 days, is probably effective and may serve as alternative therapy when tetracycline is not tolerated.

Knight R: Giardiasis, isosporiasis, and balantidiasis. Clin Gastroenterol 7:31, 1978. *There are few useful clinical reviews on balantidiasis; this is the best of the lot.*

Babesiosis is an uncommon febrile illness spread by the northern deer tick, *Ixodes dammini*. Babesiosis and Lyme disease are both spread by this same vector and are found most frequently in Massachusetts—including the off-shore islands—portions of New Jersey, New York, Maryland, Minnesota, and Wisconsin. The illness typically includes fever, malaise, headache, chills, weakness, arthralgias, and nausea. Splenomegaly is uncommon. There is no rash. Parasitemia is demonstrated by observation of typical intraerythrocytic forms. Confirmation of elevated convalescent antibody titers to the infectious organism, *Babesia microti*, may be obtained through the Centers for Disease Control. Contaminated blood transfusions have been implicated as the cause of a few rare cases. Infection is usually self-limited but may be severe in splenectomized patients. Therapy with quinine sulfate, 650 mg every 6 hours, combined with clindamycin, 300 mg every 6 hours, given intravenously, has been successful in severely ill patients.

Ruebush TK, Cassady PB, Marsh HJ, et al.: Human babesiosis on Nantucket Island. Ann Intern Med 86:6, 1977. *This report summarizes well the clinical aspects of this infection.*

SARCOSPORIDIOSIS

Infections with *Sarcocystis hominis* (previously designated *Isospora hominis*) may be associated with abdominal pain, diarrhea, and nausea. The human is the definitive host, with sexual reproduction taking place in the small intestine; cattle are the intermediate host, where the sarcocyst resides in skeletal or cardiac muscle with little or no reaction. While infection in humans is relatively common in areas of the world where undercooked beef is ingested, the definition of the precise role of this agent in human disease remains clouded by its frequent coincidence with other pathogenic agents.

Beaver PC, Gadgil RK, Morera P: Sarcocysts in man: A review and report of five cases. Am J Trop Med Hyg 28:810, 1979. *This reference provides a good starting point into the available clinical literature.*

433 Cestode Infections
Charles H. King

Humans are infected by a number of different cestodes of the phylum Platyhelminthes (flatworms). The species most commonly causing human infection are summarized in Table 433–1.

One key to understanding the broad spectrum of cestode-associated disease is to recall that tapeworm parasites divide their life cycle between two or more different animal hosts. The first, or *intermediate*, host is typically an insect or herbivorous vertebrate that ingests parasite eggs in fecally contaminated food or water. The tapeworm eggs hatch into invasive oncospheres in this primary host's intestinal tract and then migrate into the host viscera or muscles to develop into immature cystic forms, called cysticerci or cysticercoids (for Cyclophyllidea cestodes such as *Taenia* and *Hymenolepis*), or procercoid larvae (for Pseudophyllidea cestodes such as *Diphyllobothrium*). For the latter parasite group, the procercoid forms become infectious for humans if they are consumed by a second intermediate host (usually a fish or reptile) and become plerocercoid cysts.

The *definitive* host for a tapeworm species is a carnivorous or omnivorous mammal that acquires infection by consuming larval cysts in the uncooked tissues of an intermediate host. Upon exposure to stomach acid and bile salts in the digestive tract, larvae excyst and develop into mature tapeworms within the intestinal lumen. Adult tapeworms contain two sections: a *scolex* (or head), used to adhere to the wall of the intestine, and a *strobila*, or tapelike chain of developing segments called proglottides. The hermaphroditic segments produce large numbers of fertile, infectious parasite eggs that reach the environment either free or enclosed within segments in the host's feces.

In general, humans serve as *either* definitive *or* intermediate hosts for a given cestode species. For example, we are strictly definitive hosts for the tapeworms *Diphyllobothrium latum* (the "fish" tapeworm) and *Taenia saginata* (the "beef" tapeworm). These adult tapeworms do not enter the tissues of the human body and cause only minimal clinical symptoms. In contrast, we are solely intermediate hosts for *Echinococcus granulosus* (hydatid cyst disease), *E. multilocularis* (alveolar cyst disease), *T. multiceps* (coenurosis), and *Spirometra* species. In the human body, these parasites develop as larval cysts and cause significant, symptomatic tissue damage.

There are two exceptions to this rule. First, patients with *T. solium* infection may be infected with larval cysts (cysticercosis), adult tapeworms ("pork" tapeworm), or both. Second, in the case of the dwarf tapeworm, *Hymenolepis nana*, complete egg-to-tapeworm development can take place within a single human host. *H. nana* can thus be transmitted directly from person to person, and internal autoinfection may substantially increase the tapeworm burden of an infected individual. For all other cestode infections, increases in parasite burden occur only by means of continued exposure to egg-contaminated or larvae-infested foods and water.

INTESTINAL CESTODE (TAPEWORM) INFECTIONS
Diphyllobothrium latum

D. latum tapeworms are the largest parasites that infect humans, ranging up to 10 meters in length. Infection is acquired by ingestion of parasite cysts in the tissues of smoked or uncooked freshwater fish (e.g., as sushi, sashimi, or ceviche). Tapeworms develop to maturity within 3 to 6 weeks after exposure and may survive for up to 20 years. Infection is prevalent (up to 2 per cent of local residents) in many parts of the world; endemic foci are found in lake or delta regions of Scandinavia, the C.I.S., Japan, Europe, Chile, and North America. Contamination of freshwater bodies by raw sewage increases the risk for *D. latum* infection, but stable transmission may also occur owing to local infection of alternate definitive hosts, such as foxes, wolves, minks, and bears.

TABLE 433–1. COMMON HUMAN CESTODE INFECTIONS

Species	Infective Stage for Humans	Common Name	Pathology	Therapy
Diphyllobothrium latum	Adult	Fish tapeworm	Pernicious anemia	Niclosamide or Praziquantel
Hymenolepis nana	Adult	Dwarf tapeworm	Rarely symptomatic	
Taenia saginata	Adult	Beef tapeworm	Rarely symptomatic	
Taenia solium	Adult	Pork tapeworm	Rarely symptomatic	
	Larva	Cysticercosis	Brain and tissue cysts	Albendazole* Praziquantel Surgery
Echinococcus granulosus	Larva	Hydatid cyst disease	Solitary tissue cysts	Surgery Albendazole*
Echinococcus multilocularis	Larva	Alveolar cyst disease	Multilocular cysts	Surgery Albendazole*
Taenia multiceps	Larva	Bladderworm, coenurosis	Brain and eye cysts	Surgery
Spirometra mansonoides	Larva	Sparganosis	Subcutaneous larvae	Surgery

*This drug has not been approved by the Food and Drug Adminstration at the time of publication.

CLINICAL MANIFESTATIONS. For most patients, *D. latum* infection produces few, if any, symptoms. These are typically limited to nonspecific complaints of weakness, dizziness, craving for salt, diarrhea, and intermittent abdominal discomfort. Occasional patients may experience vomiting, severe abdominal pain, and weight loss. In cases of multiple infection, biliary or intestinal obstruction may occur. One to 2 per cent of patients with *D. latum* infection develop significant vitamin B_{12} deficiency, resulting in megaloblastic anemia and/or neurologic disease. Folate deficiency may also occur. Vitamin B_{12} deficiency is a product of extensive vitamin uptake by the worm as well as worm-induced interference with gastrointestinal uptake by the host (despite normal gastric acidity and intrinsic factor production). Vitamin B_{12} deficiency is most common among older patients and is more likely to occur in patients with low dietary intake of vitamins, multiple tapeworms, or a tapeworm in the proximal jejunum. In the debilitated host, nervous system complications can be quite extensive and can range from peripheral neuropathy to the syndrome of severe combined degeneration (see Ch. 456).

DIAGNOSIS. The diagnosis of *D. latum* infection is made by stool examination for characteristic operculated eggs that are 65 by 45 μm. Recovery of proglottides is infrequent owing to segment degeneration during intestinal transit.

TREATMENT. Treatment is with niclosamide or praziquantel, as summarized in Table 433–2. Severe vitamin B_{12} deficiency can be rapidly treated by parenteral vitamin injections.

PREVENTION. Fish tapeworm infection is prevented by avoiding consumption of raw, smoked, or salted fish from endemic areas. Parasite cysts may be killed by cooking (above 56°C for 5 minutes) or by freezing (−20°C for 24 hours). Control of human sewage and frequent screening of high-risk populations help to eliminate the human reservoir (but not the zoonotic reservoirs) of infection.

Hymenolepis nana

H. nana, or dwarf tapeworm, is found frequently in warm, dry climates and is prevalent in Southern and Eastern Europe, Asia, Africa, Central and South America, and Australia. It is the only human tapeworm that does not require an intermediate host. In the small intestine, hatching eggs release oncospheres that penetrate the villi of the mucosa. Four to 5 days later, the developed cysticercoid ruptures out of the villus and a parasite scolex attaches to the lining of the ileum, maturing in 10 to 12 days. Mature worms are small, measuring 25 to 40 mm long by 1 mm wide. Autoinfection can occur internally, i.e., within the small bowel, or externally, via the fecal-oral route, resulting in heavy infection. With time, however, a regulatory immunity to infection may develop, so that *H. nana* infection can be spontaneously cleared. Intensive infection is more common in institutionalized, malnourished, or immunodeficient individuals.

CLINICAL MANIFESTATIONS. The clinical manifestations of *H. nana* vary with intensity and may include diarrhea, anorexia, abdominal pain, and pallor. A statistical association with phlyctenular keratoconjunctivitis has been observed and has been tentatively ascribed to the immune response to infection.

DIAGNOSIS. The diagnosis of *H. nana* infection is made by stool examination for eggs of 30 to 47 μm that have a characteristic double membrane. Proglottides are usually not seen in the stool.

TREATMENT. Treatment is with niclosamide or praziquantel, as outlined in Table 433–2. In comparison to the treatment of other tapeworm infections, longer courses of niclosamide and higher doses of praziquantel are recommended for the therapy of *H. nana* infection because of the relative resistance of larval cysticercoids to drug therapy. Because of the potential for late emergence of worms from viable cysticercoids remaining in the ileum, heavily infected individuals should be retested for infection and retreated 10 to 14 days after initial therapy.

PREVENTION. Because *H. nana* is easily transmitted from person to person, sanitation and hand washing are essential to control this parasite. Mass chemotherapy may also be used to suppress endemic transmission, particularly within closed institutions.

Taenia saginata

T. saginata, or beef tapeworm infection, is widespread in cattle-breeding areas of the world. Endemic foci (defined as prevalence greater than 10 per cent) are found in the southern C.I.S., in the Near East, and in central and eastern Africa. Infection is less common in other parts of the world but is found at prevalence rates of 0.1 to 5 per cent in Europe, Southeast Asia, and South America. Infection is acquired by the consumption of cysticerci in the muscle tissue of infected cattle. The consumption of dishes such as steak tartare, "bleu" or rare steak, and undercooked shish kebabs is associated with infection in North American travelers to endemic areas.

CLINICAL MANIFESTATIONS. *T. saginata* infection may cause nonspecific complaints of weakness and mild abdominal discomfort in a minority (one third) of patients. Because *T. saginata* proglottides are motile, they may cause acute abdominal symptoms by migrating into and obstructing the appendix or the pancreatic and biliary ducts. A psychologically distressing feature of infection (and often the first symptom reported by the patient) occurs when motile proglottides migrate out of the anus onto skin or clothing or when they are observed moving in the feces.

DIAGNOSIS. The diagnosis of taeniasis is most readily established by stool examination and perianal inspection for parasite proglottides and eggs. It is not possible, however, to distinguish *T. saginata* eggs from those of *T. solium* morphologically, and the definitive diagnosis of *T. saginata* infection requires pathologic examination of proglottid features or DNA hybridization studies. In practice, because patients with *T. solium* are at risk for self-infection with cysticercosis (see below), and because medical therapy for taeniasis is both safe and highly effective, treatment of an undetermined *Taenia* species infection should not be delayed pending speciation of the infecting tapeworm.

TREATMENT. Treatment of beef tapeworm infection is with praziquantel or niclosamide, as outlined in Table 433–2. Both medications are highly effective in eliminating infection, and no special preparation or purgation is required. After therapy, the parasite scolex is digested within the gastrointestinal tract before it is passed in the feces. Although with the highly effective medications currently in use one no longer needs to collect the scolex to be assured that the parasite head has been expelled, digestive destruction of the head limits our ability to establish a species-specific clinical diagnosis for individual *Taenia* infections.

TABLE 433–2. THERAPY FOR INTESTINAL CESTODE (TAPEWORM) INFECTION

	Niclosamide	Praziquantel

Dosage
  Adults
  Children > 34 kg
  Children 11–34 kg
	2 grams (4 tablets)
	1.5 grams (3 tablets)
	1 gram (2 tablets)
		10–20 mg/kg for all age groups
		(25 mg/kg for *H. nana*)

Administration	For most tapeworm species, taken as a single dose; tablets must be thoroughly chewed before swallowing to obtain complete therapeutic effect; a 7-day course of drugs is used for *H. nana*, with reduced pediatric doses on days 2–7	Taken as a single dose for all species; may repeat after 7 days for heavy *H. nana* infections
Side effects	Nausea, vomiting, abdominal pain, diarrhea, drowsiness, dizziness, headache, pruritus	Mild but frequent, including dizziness, myalgias, nausea, vomiting, diarrhea, abdominal pain
Pregnancy	No known mutagenic effects; considered safe if indicated; because of risk of cysticercosis by autoinfection in *T. solium* tapeworm infection, therapy should not be delayed	

PREVENTION. *T. saginata* infection is prevented by avoidance of foods containing undercooked or raw beef. As for the fish tapeworm, cooking to 56°C for 5 minutes or freezing at −20°C for 7 to 10 days destroys the infective larvae. Because humans are the sole reservoir for infection, effective sanitation and periodic treatment of those in contact with cattle can have a significant impact on transmission.

Taenia solium

T. solium, also known as pork tapeworm, causes human infection in two different forms. Individuals who consume undercooked pork containing intermediate parasite cysts will develop intestinal *T. solium* tapeworms. Individuals who consume parasite eggs may develop intermediate parasite cysts within the tissues of the body. (This condition, called *cysticercosis*, is described in more detail in the section on tissue cestode infections.) Autoinfection, most likely via the fecal-oral route, is possible, and a single patient may harbor both adult tapeworm and tissue cysticerci. *T. solium* infection is prevalent in Mexico, Central and South America, Africa, Southern Europe, Southeast Asia, and the Philippines. Most infections seen in the United States and Canada are found in immigrants from these endemic foci.

CLINICAL MANIFESTATIONS. *T. solium* tapeworms are relatively short (3 meters) but may survive for several decades once established in the human jejunum. Generally, tapeworm infections with *T. solium* produce minimal or no symptoms, being limited to mild, nonspecific abdominal complaints. Unlike *T. saginata* proglottides, the segments of *T. solium* are nonmotile and are unlikely to cause obstruction.

DIAGNOSIS. The diagnosis of intestinal infection with *T. solium* tapeworm is made by examination of the stool for eggs and proglottides. Since the eggs are morphologically indistinguishable from those of *T. saginata*, study of the proglottid or head of the tapeworms is required for species identification. Stool samples and proglottides should be handled with care because of the risk of acquiring cysticercosis by accidental ingestion of *T. solium* eggs.

TREATMENT. *T. solium* tapeworm infection is treated with either niclosamide or praziquantel, as outlined in Table 433–2. Once diagnosis is established, therapy should be instituted as soon as possible because of the risk of autoinfection with cysticercosis. Therapy for cysticercosis is substantially longer and more intensive than that for intestinal infection and is described in detail in the section on tissue cestode infections.

PREVENTION. Individuals may avoid *T. solium* tapeworm infection by avoiding foods containing raw or undercooked pork. Meat inspection and improvements in pork-raising practices have successfully reduced transmission in some areas. In endemic areas, periodic chemotherapy of human populations may reduce the reservoir of egg production and reduce pork infestation.

Other Intestinal Cestodes

Other tapeworms that occasionally infect humans include the dog tapeworm *Dipylidium caninum* and the rodent tapeworm *Hymenolepis diminuta*. These are most common in children and are acquired by inadvertently ingesting the intermediate larval forms of these parasites in the bodies of fleas or other insects. Usually, *D. caninum* and *H. diminuta* infections produce minimal symptoms. Diagnosis is established by stool examination, and infections are readily treated with standard doses of niclosamide or praziquantel.

TISSUE CESTODE (CYST) INFECTION
Echinococcosis

Human echinococcosis causes significant morbidity and mortality in livestock-raising regions in all parts of the world. The causative agents of "hydatid" and "alveolar" cyst disease in humans are the intermediate larval forms of the tapeworms *Echinococcus granulosus* and *E. multilocularis*, respectively.

Like other cestodes, *Echinococcus* tapeworms have both intermediate and definitive hosts. For *Echinococcus* species, dogs and other canines are the definitive hosts. Tapeworm-infected animals pass eggs in their feces, which contaminate the local environment. Contamination of grazing areas and foodstuffs results in egg ingestion by intermediate hosts, e.g., humans, sheep, goats, camels, and horses for *E. granulosus* and mice or other small rodents for *E. multilocularis*. Life cycle transmission is completed when the definitive carnivore host consumes meat or offal of the intermediate host that contains hydatid or alveolar cysts. Protoscolices within the cysts mature in the lumen of the canine gut to become adult, egg-bearing tapeworms. Because the cysts of *Echinococcus* contain a germinal layer that can produce multiple internal "daughter" cysts by asexual budding, an individual dog may develop infection with dozens of tapeworms after consumption of a single large cyst. Once the tapeworms mature, a heavily infected dog may contaminate 10 or more hectares of ground with infectious eggs in the space of a week.

In most areas of the world, burial practices make humans a "dead-end" host for *Echinococcus*, i.e., human infection does not perpetuate transmission in the local ecosystem. Nevertheless, the "inadvertent" hydatid cyst disease caused by *E. granulosus* and the more aggressive alveolar cyst disease caused by *E. multilocularis* are severe or even fatal illnesses for a significant minority of infected individuals.

EPIDEMIOLOGY. *E. granulosus* is common in livestock-raising areas of both developed and developing countries. Sheep- and goat-herding populations that keep dogs as pets or work animals are at highest risk for hydatid cyst disease. Until recently, hydatid disease was common in Australia, New Zealand, Argentina, Chile, Ireland, Scotland, the Basque country, the Mediterranean basin, and throughout middle Europe. Currently, the area with the highest prevalence in the world is the Turkana and Samburu regions of northwestern Kenya, where domestic and feral transmission of *E. granulosus* is perpetuated among nomadic farmers by poor hygienic practices. Occasional hydatid disease transmission is also found in central Asia, Mexico, the United States, and South America.

Alveolar cyst disease due to *E. multilocularis* is usually transmitted by wild animals, e.g., foxes and bush dogs, and is found in the arctic regions of the United States, Canada and the C.I.S.

CLINICAL MANIFESTATIONS. Human disease caused by *Echinococcus* species results from bloodborne invasion of the liver (50 to 70 per cent of patients), lungs (20 to 30 per cent), or other organs by developing parasite oncospheres. As these mature, they grow within tissues by concentric enlargement (*E. granulosus*) or by extension through adjacent host tissues (*E. multilocularis*). At any given time, most infected individuals are asymptomatic, and it may take 5 to 20 years for a cyst to grow to sufficient size (3 to 15 cm) to cause symptoms. When present, symptoms and findings refer to the anatomic site of involvement and derive from local inflammation, secondary bacterial infection, obstruction, or local mass effect. In hydatid cyst disease, the growing cyst becomes surrounded by a fibrous capsule formed by host immune reaction. Within this primary unilocular cyst, multiple daughter cysts, each containing an infective protoscolex, develop by asexual budding of the germinal layer. In alveolar cyst disease, the parasite cyst is not well separated from surrounding tissues, and lateral budding and malignancy-like growth (including distal metastasis of daughter cysts) may occur.

Patients with symptomatic hydatid liver cysts may complain of abdominal discomfort or mass in the right upper quadrant. Cyst leakage into the peritoneal cavity or pleural space may be associated with fever, urticaria, or a severe anaphylactoid reaction. Invasion of the biliary system often leads to the passage of daughter cysts into the common bile duct, with clinical and chemical evidence of intermittent obstruction resembling choledocholithiasis. Individuals with symptomatic hydatid involvement of the lungs present with cough, hemoptysis, and pleurisy. Spontaneous rupture of the cyst may lead to intrathoracic spread or to evacuation of daughter cysts via the bronchus. At either lung or liver sites, bacterial superinfection may cause an acute presentation with symptoms of sepsis. Hydatid involvement of the brain is marked by slow-onset mass effect, hydrocephalus, and often seizures. Cysts of the bone frequently fail to form a discrete capsule but rather cause local erosion of the cortex, resulting in pathologic fracture.

Symptomatic alveolar cyst disease most frequently refers to liver involvement and manifests as vague, mild upper quadrant and epigastric pain. Signs of hepatomegaly or obstructive jaundice may be present. Occasionally, metastatic lesions in the lung or brain are the first to cause symptoms by local inflammation or mass effect.

DIAGNOSIS. Laboratory evaluation may show marked eosinophilia, but this finding is inconstant (30 per cent prevalence). In hydatid cyst disease, radiographic and ultrasonographic studies typically show characteristic large, avascular cysts containing internal structures consistent with daughter cysts. Detection of mural calcification strongly favors the diagnosis of hydatid cyst. The differential diagnosis includes hemangioma, metastatic carcinoma, and remote bacterial or amebic liver abscess. Confirmatory evidence of infection may be obtained by serology (sensitivity of 60 to 90 per cent, depending on the test used). Serologic testing is available commercially or from the Centers for Disease Control, Atlanta, GA (through local state health departments). Until recently, it has not been recommended to perform closed aspiration on the cyst for diagnosis, as cyst leakage has the potential to initiate a severe allergic reaction and may result in the metastatic spread of daughter cysts. However, a recent clinical series has reported successful computed tomography (CT)–guided thin-needle aspiration of hydatid cysts for diagnosis. This procedure, when followed by immediate instillation of ethanol to kill viable protoscoleces, was associated with minimal side effects and was followed by apparent regression of cysts on CT scans. Further trials of this simplified approach to diagnosis and therapy appear warranted.

With alveolar cyst disease due to *E. multilocularis,* the organism's appearance on radiographic and sonographic imaging often mimics that of hepatic carcinoma. A definitive diagnosis may require either angiography or open biopsy at surgery. Precautions must be taken to prevent metastatic dissemination of daughter cysts at the time of surgery.

TREATMENT. Stable, asymptomatic, calcified cysts do not require specific therapy but should be monitored by serial imaging over several years to ensure a benign resolution. When technically feasible, expanding, symptomatic, or infected cysts are best removed in toto at surgery, with care taken to isolate and kill the cyst with hypertonic saline (25 to 30 gm per deciliter) or other cidal agents (such as iodophor, ethanol, or 10 per cent formalin) prior to excision, to avoid secondary spread or parasite cysts. Surgical resection should include careful closure of biliary and enteric fistulas and extensive postoperative drainage of the cyst bed to prevent fluid accumulation and secondary bacterial infection. Alveolar cyst disease may require wide resection, i.e., total lobectomy of liver or lung, to remove all cyst material.

In many cases, symptomatic echinococcal cysts are not amenable to resection. In such cases, oral drug therapy with the anthelminthics, either long-term mebendazole (40 mg per kilogram of body weight per day in three divided doses for 6 to 12 months) or albendazole* (400 mg twice a day for one to eight periods of 28 days each, separated by drug-free rest intervals of 14 to 28 days), has been recommended for cure or palliation. Cure rates, particularly for difficult cases with recurrent or extrahepatic/extrapulmonary cysts, have been low (less than 33 per cent), although a majority of patients show some improvement. Because the efficacy of drug therapy is limited, a combined medical-surgical approach should be individualized for each patient.

PREVENTION. The transmission of echinococcal disease has been prevented by regular praziquantel treatment of tapeworm-infected dogs in endemic areas. This approach, used in New Zealand and other endemic areas, has markedly reduced the prevalence of hydatid cyst disease in these areas over the past three decades. Related emphasis has been put on isolated butchering of livestock hosts to reduce transmission to working and feral dogs. Currently, human transmission is most common in the least-developed areas of the world, where veterinary practices are limited or nonexistent and butchering is done in the home environment. Research is focusing on means to identify infected populations rapidly and on finding the most effective ways to treat feral vectors.

---

*This drug has not been approved by the Food and Drug Administration at the time of publication. In the United States, compassionate use may be available through Smith Kline & French Laboratories, Philadelphia, PA.

Cysticercosis

Cysticercosis represents human tissue infection with the intermediate cyst forms of the pork tapeworm *T. solium*. Cysticercosis is acquired by ingestion of *T. solium* eggs in contaminated foods. Infection prevalence is approximately 1 to 10 per cent in endemic areas of Latin America, India, Asia, Indonesia, and parts of Africa. Because of its potentially life-threatening complications, cysticercosis has greater clinical significance than does intestinal *T. solium* tapeworm infection, particularly if cyst disease involves the central nervous system, the eyes, the heart, or other vital organs.

CLINICAL MANIFESTATIONS. The clinical manifestations of cysticercosis depend on the location and number of infecting cysts. Cysticerci are bladder-like, fluid-filled cysts containing an invaginated protoscolex. They are often surrounded by a dense fibrous capsule of host origin. In infected humans, cysticerci are usually multiple, 0.5 to 2 cm in size, and distributed widely throughout the body. Many patients have minimal, if any, symptoms of infection. However, symptomatic *neurocysticercosis* (i.e., cerebral cysticercosis, eye or spinal cord involvement) requires medical attention. This syndrome has an estimated mortality of up to 50 per cent, and any neurologic, cognitive, or personality disorder in an individual from an endemic area should be considered a possible manifestation of undiagnosed neurocysticercosis. In the past decade, diagnosis of this condition has been facilitated by the advent of CT scanning and magnetic resonance imaging (MRI), both of which are highly sensitive in detecting central nervous system cysticerci. Patients with central nervous system involvement have an average of 10 cysts distributed throughout the brain and spinal cord. These cysts may be in different stages of development, with symptoms commonly arising when older cysts begin to die, lose osmoregulation, and release antigenic material to provoke significant host inflammatory response.

In practice, neurocysticercosis may be divided into six discrete syndromes for management. In the *acute invasive* stage of cysticercosis, immediately after infection, the patient may experience fevers, headache, and myalgias associated with significant peripheral eosinophilia. Heavy infection at this stage may result in a clinical picture of "cysticercal encephalitis" associated with coma and rapid deterioration. This presentation should be treated aggressively with antiparasitic agents and anti-inflammatory drugs. After cysticerci become established, *parenchymal central nervous system cysticercosis* (50 per cent of cases) is associated with seizures, intellectual impairment, and personality changes. Compression due to swelling or inflammation around the cysts may result in focal deficits, signs of cerebral edema, and/or hydrocephalus. Seizures may be focal (jacksonian), referring to the specific cortical locus of involvement, or may be generalized. *Subarachnoid cysticercosis* (30 per cent of cases) is frequently associated with obstruction of cerebrospinal fluid (CSF) flow. Intracranial hypertension may manifest as vomiting, headache, and visual disturbances. Sensorial changes may include apathy, amnesia, dementia, hallucination, and emotional disturbance. Like other forms of basilar meningitis, pericysticercal inflammation at the base of the brain may cause obstruction or vasculitis of the cerebral arteries, leading to intermittent ischemia or stroke. *Intraventricular cysticercosis* (15 per cent of cases) is, because of its location, the most difficult to diagnose and treat. Symptomatic cysts are most frequent in the fourth ventricle, where they cause outflow obstruction and increased intracranial pressure without localizing signs. An aggressive variant of ventricular neurocysticercosis, called racemose cysticercosis, frequently involves the basal cisterns. This form of cysticercosis has been noted most often in young women and involves multiple, rapidly spreading cysts in the cerebrum and around the base of the brain. Whereas symptoms due to isolated cysts may remit, racemose cysticercosis usually has a progressive, deteriorating course if therapy is not given. Those with *spinal cysticercosis* may present with cord compression, radiculopathy, transverse myelitis, or signs of meningitis, depending on the location of involvement. *Ocular cysticercosis* is a distinct syndrome that manifests as eye pain, scotomata, and decreasing vision due to iridocyclitis, clouding of the vitreous, and retinal inflammation or detachment.

DIAGNOSIS. A definitive diagnosis of cysticercosis requires examination of biopsy material obtained from a tissue cyst. However, a presumptive diagnosis may be made on the basis of a history of residence in an endemic area, the presence of characteristic radiographic findings on plain films (calcified cysts in soft tissues) or scans (multiple, low-density, enhanced, and unenhanced lesions on CT or MRI), and suggestive laboratory findings. Infection with *T. solium* tapeworm is present in about 25 per cent of neurocysticercosis cases. In neurocysticercosis, examination of the cerebrospinal fluid may show hypoglycorrhachia, elevated total protein levels, and lymphocytic and eosinophilic pleocytosis (5 to 500 cells per microliter). Serum and CSF enzyme-linked immunosorbent assay (ELISA) and Western blot testing for specific immunoglobulin M (IgM) and immunoglobulin G (IgG) anticysticercal antibodies have a sensitivity of 75 to 100 per cent. These tests are available through commercial laboratories or from the Centers for Disease Control, Atlanta, GA (samples should be sent through state health departments). It should be noted, however, that antiparasite antibodies may persist long after infection, and a positive IgG serology merely indicates prior *Taenia* exposure, not necessarily active disease. The differential diagnosis of neurocysticercosis includes tumor, hydatid cyst disease, vasculitis, and chronic fungal and mycobacterial infection.

TREATMENT. Given the high prevalence of cysticercosis in some areas of the world, it is evident that most cysticerci do not cause significant symptoms. For *symptomatic* cysts outside the central nervous system, the optimal therapy is surgical removal, as this ensures complete elimination of the cyst. In the case of symptomatic neurocysticercosis, which carries an associated mortality of up to 50 per cent, therapy is definitely indicated, but surgery may be risky or technically unfeasible. An alternative approach to the control of some forms of neurocysticercosis has been demonstrated in recent clinical studies: Drug therapy with either praziquantel (50 mg per kilogram per day in three divided doses for 14 to 30 days) or albendazole* (15 mg per kilogram per day for 30 days) has been associated with alleviation of symptoms and regression of cyst size and number in patients with viable (nonenhancing) cysts in the cerebral parenchyma. However, drug therapy has provided only limited improvement in patients with arachnoiditis and no improvement in patients with intraventricular cysts. For these latter presentations, the treatment of choice remains surgery and/or palliation with shunting, anticonvulsants, and anti-inflammatory agents. It should be noted that in about 20 per cent of treated cases, the initiation of drug therapy is associated with a severely symptomatic, increased inflammatory response at the site of the cyst. This inflammation may be controlled with corticosteroids, but corticosteroids are not recommended for routine use in all patients, as they may significantly alter the pharmacokinetics of the anthelminthics used to treat infection. Follow-up tomographic scanning should be repeated 3 months after the cessation of therapy to ensure adequate response. If necessary, a repeat course of drug therapy with the alternate agent may be given to improve response. Because parasite-induced ocular inflammation does not respond well to systemic anti-inflammatory agents, patients with cysticercosis of the eye (20 per cent of cases of neurocysticercosis) should not receive drug therapy until the eye disease has been controlled surgically.

PREVENTION. As discussed earlier, the prevention of *T. solium* transmission requires control of human tapeworm infections, careful personal hygiene, and a high level of community sanitation.

Coenurosis

A different, but more rare, form of tissue cysticercosis may be caused by larval stages of the dog tapeworms *T. multiceps* and *T. serialis*. Lesions tend to be solitary and are distinguished pathologically from *T. solium* cysticerci on biopsy. Ocular involvement is common, and surgical resection is currently the only effective mode of therapy.

Sparganosis

Sparganosis is a tissue cestode infection caused by the plerocercoid larval stages of *Spirometra* species tapeworms of cats and other carnivores. Humans may become infected by ingestion of

---

*This drug has not been approved by the Food and Drug Administration at the time of publication.

infected water fleas (*Cyclops*), by ingestion of uncooked meat from infected animals (reptiles, birds, or mammals), or by cutaneous exposure (e.g., via traditional skin or eye poultices) to uncooked, infected meat. Usually, the larva encysts within the intestinal submucosa or skin. In some cases, however, parasites may invade the eye or central nervous system and cause significant inflammatory pathology at the site of encystment. Occasionally, proliferation into surrounding tissues occurs by lateral budding of the parasite (termed *sparganum proliferum*). The treatment of choice for sparganosis is ethanol injection and/or surgical removal, as limited experience with medical anthelminthic therapy has shown no beneficial effect.

Bia FJ, Barry M: Parasitic infections of the central nervous system. Neurol Clin 4:171, 1986. *Explores the range of parasite infections of the brain and their differential diagnosis.*

Davis A, Dixon H, Pawlowski Z: Multicentre clinical trials of benzimidazole carbamates in human cystic echinococcosis (phase 2). Bull WHO 68 67:503, 1989. *Up-to-date review of experience in multicenter trials of medical therapy for hydatid and alveolar cyst disease.*

Del Brutto OH, Sotelo J: Neurocysticercosis: An update. Rev Infect Dis 10:1075, 1988. *Extensive review of the diagnosis and treatment of this varied and complex disease. Contains a useful flow diagram on therapy for neurocysticercosis.*

Filice C, Di Perri G, Strosselli M, et al.: Parasitologic findings in percutaneous drainage of human hydatid liver cysts. J Infect Dis 161:1290, 1990. *Description of a small series of patients undergoing CT-guided diagnosis and treatment of hydatid cyst disease.*

Flisser A, Reid A, Garcia-Zepeda E, et al.: Specific detection of *Taenia saginata* eggs by DNA hybridization. Lancet 2:1429, 1988. *Description of a promising technique for species-specific diagnosis of* Taenia *infections from stool samples.*

King CH, Mahmoud AAF: Drugs five years later: Praziquantel. Ann Intern Med 110:290, 1989. *A summary of new data on the anthelminthic agent praziquantel since its release in the United States. Includes a listing of doses recommended for cestode therapy; with references.*

Pau A, Perria C, Turtas S, et al.: Long-term follow-up of the surgical treatment of intracranial coenurosis. Br J Neurosurg 4:39, 1990. *Recent review of treatment of this rare cestode infection.*

Pawlowski ZS: Cestodiases: Taeniasis, cysticercosis, diphyllobothriasis, hymenolepiasis and others. *In* Warren KS, Mahmoud AAF (eds.): Tropical and Geographical Medicine. 2nd ed. New York, McGraw-Hill, 1990, pp 490–504. *A detailed and current review of cestode infections (excluding* Echinococcus *species).*

Schantz PM, Okelo GBA: Echinococcosis (hydatidosis). *In* Warren KS, Mahmoud AAF (eds.): Tropical and Geographical Medicine. 2nd ed. New York, McGraw-Hill, 1990, pp 505–518. *Up-to-date review of human infection with Echinococcus species. Useful for hydatid disease as well as less common E. multilocularis and E. vogeli infections.*

Sotelo J, Escobedo F, Penagos P: Albendazole vs praziquantel for therapy for neurocysticercosis. A controlled trial. Arch Neurol 45:532, 1988. *A small head-to-head comparison of these two agents. Overall results were comparable (76 versus 73 per cent) for the two drugs in terms of cyst regression. A later study by the same group favors albendazole therapy, but flaws in study design make its analysis and conclusions unconvincing.*

Teitelbaum GP, Otto RJ, Lin M, et al.: MR imaging of neurocysticercosis. AJR 153:857, 1990. *Important description of a noninvasive modality for diagnosing parenchymal and ventricular neurocysticercosis.*

---

434 Schistosomiasis *(Bilharziasis)*

Adel A. F. Mahmoud

DEFINITION. Schistosomiasis, a chronic worm infection, affects more than 200 million people in the world; several hundred million more live in endemic areas and are at risk of exposure to the parasites. In view of its prevalence and the morbidity it causes, schistosomiasis ranks among the most important public health problems of tropical and subtropical areas. The schistosomes are blood flukes that parasitize the venous channels of the definitive human host; infection is transmitted via freshwater snails. Humans may be infected by one of five species: *Schistosoma haematobium, S. mansoni, S. japonicum, S. intercalatum,* or *S. mekongi.* Each species is endemic in specific geographic areas of the world; infection in humans may result in defined clinical syndromes. Other species that occasionally infect humans include *S. bovis, S. matthei,* and some avian schistosomes. In many parts of the world, enhanced agricultural productivity involving water conservation schemes is an economic necessity.

Inadvertently, these projects create ideal breeding places for the snail intermediate host, thus increasing prevalence of schistosomiasis in the population and possibly causing its spread to new areas. Currently, schistosomiasis is endemic in various areas of Africa, Asia, South America, and the Caribbean islands. In the United States, there are approximately 400,000 infected individuals; these include Puerto Ricans, and immigrants or travelers who have been exposed while in endemic areas. Because of the absence of susceptible snails, the life cycle of the schistosomes cannot be established in this country.

ETIOLOGY. The schistosomes differ from other trematodes that infect humans in having separate sexes. The species of schistosomes that infect humans share some common features, although they are morphologically distinctive. Each worm has two suckers (anterior and ventral), and the bifurcate intestinal ceca unite posteriorly. The larger male (0.6 to 2.2 cm × 2 to 4 mm) has a ventral gynecophoric canal in which the female is held during copulation. The slender female worm (1.2 to 2.6 cm × 1 to 2 mm) has a rounded body with pointed ends.

Adult schistosome worms parasitize defined sites of the venous vasculature of humans. *Schistosoma haematobium* worms inhabit the venous plexus around the lower end of the ureters and the urinary bladder, whereas *S. mansoni*, *S. japonicum*, *S. intercalatum*, and *S. mekongi* are located in the mesenteric veins. Sexual maturity of female worms requires the presence of living mature males; when ready to deposit eggs, the worms move against the bloodstream toward the small venous radicles. The female schistosomes deposit ova singly or in bunches, depending on the species of the parasite, and retreat in the direction of blood flow. Egg deposition has been estimated at 300 per day for female *S. haematobium* and *S. mansoni* worms and 3000 per day for *S. japonicum*. The ova of each species have characteristic morphologic features, which are of diagnostic importance. Once deposited in the host, eggs attempt to penetrate the venous capillaries and escape to the bladder or intestinal lumen; enzymatic secretions are thought to aid egg migration. The proportion of ova escaping from infected individuals varies in each species and also may depend on the extent of pathology and state of resistance in the host. Eggs that fail to reach the lumen of urinary tract or gut are trapped in these organs or may be carried by portal blood to the liver; these ova result in inflammatory and immunopathologic changes that are a major cause of disease in schistosomiasis.

The schistosome eggs, upon deposition by female worms, contain immature miracidia; they take approximately 10 to 12 days to develop while migrating through the host tissues. Once mature, miracidia have a mean lifespan of 11 to 12 days. Promiscuous urination and defecation by infected individuals result in dissemination of the parasite eggs in the environment. In fresh water the schistosome ova hatch within a few hours. Miracidia escape head first and swim, usually near the surface of water; they remain infective to the snail intermediate host for approximately 8 hours. On encountering the specific snail, the miracidia penetrate its tissues and undergo tremendous asexual multiplication and transformation into hundreds of cercariae. Schistosome infection of snails causes varying degrees of pathology in their liver and sexual organs and reduces their lifespan. Development of schistosomes inside the snail takes approximately 4 to 6 weeks, but it varies with the species of the parasite and mollusc and with changes in environmental conditions. Cercariae, the infective forms to humans, emerge from the snails under specific conditions of light and temperature; they are elongate with a pear-shaped body and a long forked tail and measure approximately 400 to 600 μm in length. They can survive in fresh water for almost 72 hours but lose their infectivity considerably within the first 24 hours. Cercariae attach to skin of mammalian hosts by their oral or ventral suckers. Burrowing of the skin is helped by vertical vibratory movements of their bodies and secretions of the cephalic penetration glands; the process is usually completed within a few minutes. During penetration, the cercariae shake off their tails and change into the next stage of the life cycle, the schistosomula, which lie in tunnels in the stratum corneum parallel to the skin surface. Schistosomula are covered by a heptalaminar membrane (instead of the trilaminar cercarial membrane) and can no longer survive in fresh water. They are thought to remain in the skin for 1 to 3 days before migrating to the lungs, finally reaching the liver in 2 to 4 weeks. In the intrahepatic portal system, the worms complete the major digestive and sexual stages of their development. Adult worms start their migration to their final habitat in 2 weeks and mate; viable eggs can be seen in the excreta 5 to 9 weeks after cercarial penetration.

The mean lifespan of adult schistosome worms inside the human host is not exactly known. Several individual case reports indicate that worms may live 20 to 30 years. This, however, represents extreme cases, as examination of infected individuals who migrate to nonendemic areas indicates that the mean lifespan of the worms is in the range of 3 to 10 years.

EPIDEMIOLOGY. The endemicity of schistosomiasis in any specific area is dependent upon the unsanitary disposal of urine and feces, the presence of suitable snail hosts, and human exposure to cercaria-infected bodies of water. Furthermore, the epidemiology of schistosomiasis is complex because of the existence of several stages of the life cycle of the parasite and the multitude of factors affecting each. Since adult schistosomes, like many parasitic worms, do not multiply in the human body, a close correlation obtains between worm load and fecal or urinary egg counts; estimates of intensity of infection can therefore be obtained by ova-enumerating procedures. Quantifying worm loads is important epidemiologically as well as for the individual patient, as it determines the potential of participation in transmission of schistosomiasis and predicts, to a large extent, the risk of morbidity and pathologic outcome.

In endemic areas, schistosomiasis prevalence and intensity show characteristic association with age. Schistosomiasis is acquired early in childhood; prevalence and intensity gradually increase to a peak in the second decade of life. In older individuals, a modest reduction of prevalence may be seen along with a sharp fall in intensity of infection. The marked drop in intensity in adults may be due to a decrease in their water-related activities. Development of immunity may also explain the age-related decrease in intensity. Intensity of infection in endemic communities shows another characteristic feature: Most infected individuals harbor low worm loads, and only a small proportion acquire heavy infection. The underlying mechanism of this clustering of heavy infection in schistosomiasis is not known but may be due to varying degrees of susceptibility and/or response of humans to the parasites.

Observations in endemic areas suggest that the schistosomiasis transmission rate is slow. Several ecologic as well as host factors help maintain this slow rate. For example, the prevalence of schistosomal infection in the snail intermediate host is usually low, ranging between 0.6 and 2 per cent. Cercarial dispersion in water bodies is considerable; cercariae appear in significant numbers only during certain hours of the day and lose their infectivity shortly thereafter. Once within the human host, no more than 40 per cent of cercariae mature into adult worms. In addition, attempts to measure incidence rates in endemic areas have confirmed the relatively slow rate of transmission, ranging from 2 to 4 per cent per year.

In some areas, the endemicity of schistosomiasis may be maintained by animal reservoirs; this is especially the case with *S. japonicum*, which infects dogs and cows. Although both *S. haematobium* and *S. mansoni* can infect primates and rodents, the role of these animals as reservoirs does not seem to be epidemiologically important.

PATHOGENESIS. Schistosomiasis is initiated by cercarial penetration of skin; inside the host three maturational forms of the parasite evolve: schistosomula, adults, and eggs. These stages are associated with morphologic, biochemical, and antigenic changes of the worm, which add to the complexity of the host-parasite relationship. Disease caused by schistosomiasis occurs mainly in those with high egg counts. This relationship, however, is not exact, as the roles of other factors such as genetic background and immunologic modulatory mechanisms are now being elucidated.

Three distinct disease syndromes caused by schistosomiasis have been described; each corresponds roughly to a stage in the parasite development in the host. Cercarial dermatitis, or swimmer's itch, may be seen in infections with human schistosomes but is more common when avian or other nonhuman cercariae penetrate the skin. Swimmer's itch caused by nonhuman schistosomes is commonly seen in the North Central United States, where some lakes are infected. The condition has also been reported in subjects exposed to *S. mansoni* or *S. haematobium* but rarely after exposure to *S. japonicum*. Primary exposure to these larvae results in either no reaction or immediate pruritic macular rash. On repeated exposures, sensitization occurs, and a more pronounced papular eruption develops with erythema, edema, and pruritus. Histopathologically, edema, round cell infiltrate, and eosinophilia can be seen in the dermis and epidermis. Although the mechanism of this reaction is not known, it is probably due to the host response to dying larvae and the subsequent development of humoral and cellular immunity.

Acute schistosomiasis, or Katayama fever, is a serum sickness–like syndrome that occurs 3 to 9 weeks after infection. This period coincides with the onset of egg production and its associated increase in antigenic challenge to the host. Clinically significant acute schistosomiasis occurs more often with *S. japonicum* infections but has also been reported with the other species. It is seen in previously unexposed individuals; the severity of symptoms and signs correlates with intensity of infection. Very little is known of the mechanism of this syndrome; it manifests itself as fever, abdominal pain, and headache with hepatosplenomegaly and eosinophilia. Elevations of serum immunoglobulin (Ig)G, IgM, IgE, and specific antischistosomal antibodies have also been observed, leading to the suggestion that the syndrome is a form of immune complex disease.

The basic pathologic lesion in chronic schistosomiasis is the egg granuloma. Although the schistosomes do not multiply in the definitive host, they continually produce eggs; some of these are trapped in the tissues. Enzymes and antigens are subsequently released from the eggs to facilitate their migration out of the body. These parasite products sensitize the host lymphocytes, which migrate to areas of egg deposition and recruit other cells through the secretion of lymphokines, and a compact cellular infiltrate "granuloma" is formed. Several cell types are prominent in the schistosome egg granuloma: lymphocytes, macrophages, eosinophils, and fibroblasts. The size of these granulomas and the resulting fibrosis lead to most of the chronic fibro-obstructive lesions in schistosomiasis. In *S. haematobium* infection, granulomas at the lower end of the ureters impede urine flow and cause hydroureter and hydronephrosis. In infections with other schistosome species, granulomas in the intestinal wall are associated with the abdominal manifestations of the disease, and those in the liver result in presinusoidal obstruction of portal blood flow, portal hypertension, splenomegaly, and esophageal varices. Less commonly, eggs may be carried to almost any organ or tissue in the body, eliciting granuloma formation and its pathologic sequelae. The size of the granulomatous response represents a delicate balance between sensitizing and modulating mechanisms. In chronic schistosomiasis, granulomas spontaneously modulate—i.e., their size decreases significantly—which may result in slowing the progression of disease manifestations. Modulation has been shown to be mediated by several arms of the host's immune system, including serum antibodies, anti-idiotypic antibodies, immune complexes, suppressor lymphocytes, and macrophages. Functionally, granulomas serve to destroy the parasite eggs. Among the cells constituting the granulomatous response, eosinophils play a key role in egg destruction.

The immune response of individuals with schistosomiasis includes humoral as well as cellular components. The degree and extent of these responses provide the balance between asymptomatic infection and disease manifestations. Furthermore, mechanisms that control the host immune response, such as genetic background, have been demonstrated to influence the extent of granuloma formation and consequently disease. The host immune response to schistosome antigens also is inversely related to intensity of infection; impaired responses are seen only in those with heavy worm loads. Whether the defect in immunity is a cause or consequence of infection is not yet clear. Another aspect of the host's immune response in schistosomiasis relates to the development of peripheral blood as well as tissue eosinophilia. Schistosomiasis, similar to other worm infections with tissue phases, results in a significant increase of peripheral blood eosinophils, especially during the acute phase of infection. Later, in the chronic stage, the eosinophil count may not be significantly elevated. Eosinophils are seen in subcutaneous tissues around the entry points of cercariae, and they constitute approximately 50 per cent of the cells in egg granulomas. Eosinophils have been shown to play a central role in host defenses against the invading

stage of the parasite (schistosomula) and the phase (ova) retained in the tissues.

Acquired immunity to schistosomiasis may explain the drop in intensity of infection observed in older individuals in endemic areas. This phenomenon may be explained equally by the differences in patterns of contact with infected waters and by changes in the rate of egg production by adult worms. Studies in vitro have demonstrated that several human cells—eosinophils, neutrophils, basophils, monocytes, cytotoxic T lymphocytes and platelets—may alone or in combination with complement components or antischistosomal antibodies damage the larvae of the parasite. The biologic relevance of these observations in humans is not yet clear.

MANAGEMENT. Diagnosis of schistosomiasis must be based on the clinical presentation, positive geographic history, and finding the parasite eggs in the excreta or biopsy material. Quantification of infection and assessment of viability of the eggs are important procedures not only for planning therapy but also for prognostic evaluation. For physicians practicing in nonendemic areas, e.g., North America, most infected individuals present with the early acute and nonspecific features of the infection. Eosinophilia and serologic evidence of exposure to schistosome infection are two particularly helpful laboratory findings. Safe chemotherapeutic antischistosomal agents are now available and provide high cure rates (e.g., praziquantel). Appropriate management of individuals with schistosomiasis must take into consideration the extent of disease and intensity of infection. Antischistosomal therapy, if given early during the course of disease, may lead to reversal of pathologic lesions. In late cases, chemotherapeutic measures may be useful only in preventing further damage from the presence of the parasite.

CONTROL. The intimate relationship between humans and bodies of fresh water in their environment leads to schistosomiasis endemicity. In addition, the lack of precise knowledge of the epidemiology of infection and disease has hampered efforts for its control. Several developments, such as single-dose oral chemotherapeutic agents and better appreciation of transmission dynamics, have led to a clearer definition of strategies for control of schistosomiasis. Ideally, eradication of infection should be the target, but this is impossible to achieve with the currently available tools and the economic and social structure of the endemic areas. Research toward antischistosome vaccine is progressing, but not to the extent of contemplating human trials soon. A more realistic approach is based on control of disease and reduction of transmission. The most cost-effective measure currently advocated is targeted chemotherapy, combined with focal mollusciciding if needed. Because of the specific features of infection dynamics, treated individuals persist with low egg counts for a few years. In addition, health education, attempts at raising socioeconomic standards, providing privies, and abandoning obsolete agricultural practices offer means for achieving progress in containing this infection.

Those traveling to endemic areas should be given proper advice. There are virtually no safe freshwater bodies in most of the areas endemic for schistosomiasis. Avoiding contact with these water sources is strongly recommended.

Capron A, Dessaint JP, Capron M, et al.: Immunity to schistosomes. Progress toward vaccine. Science 238:1065, 1987. *A detailed description of evidence in vitro and components of protective effector mechanisms against schistosomiasis.*

Chapman PJ, Wilkinson PR, Davidson RN: Acute schistosomiasis (Katayama fever) among British air crew. Br Med J 297:1101, 1988. *A description of the acute clinical, parasitologic, and laboratory findings in 10 British subjects who swam in fresh water in Ghana. The article emphasizes the nonspecific nature of the clinical presentation. Peripheral blood eosinophilia and enzyme-linked immunosorbent assay (ELISA) were most helpful in establishing the diagnosis.*

King CH, Mahmoud AAF: Drugs five years later: Praziquantel. Ann Intern Med 110:290, 1989. *A review of the clinical applications of praziquantel as a safe, oral, broad-spectrum antihelminth.*

Mahmoud AAF (ed.): Clinical Tropical Medicine and Communicable Diseases. Vol. 2: Schistosomiasis. London, Bailliere's Tindall, 1987. *A concise review of the biology, immunology, and clinical features of human schistosomiasis written by physicians and scientists.*

Mahmoud AAF: Strategies for vaccine development: Schistosomiasis. Ann NY Acad Sci 589:136, 1989. *A summary of the available protective monoclonal antibodies and purified schistosome antigens with promise as vaccines.*

Mahmoud AAF, Arap Siongok TK, Ouma J, et al.: Effect of targeted mass treatment on intensity of infection and morbidity in schistosomiasis mansoni. Lancet

1:849, 1983. *Evaluation of the clinical and parasitologic effects of targeting chemotherapy to those with hepatosplenomegaly and heavy infection.*

Mahmoud AAF, Warren KS, Peters PA: A role for the eosinophil in acquired resistance to *Schistosoma mansoni* infection as determined by antieosinophil serum. J Exp Med 142:805, 1975. *Demonstration of the in vivo protective function of eosinophils in animals with schistosomiasis.*

World Health Organization: Atlas of the Global Distribution of Schistosomiasis. Geneva, World Health Organization, Parasitic Diseases Programme, 1987. *Detailed information on the geographic distribution of the different schistosome infections in humans.*

World Health Organization: The Control of Schistosomiasis. Technical Report Series 728, pp 1–113, World Health Organization, Geneva, Switzerland, 1985. *An up-to-date examination of the epidemiology, morbidity, and methods of control of schistosomiasis. The report also includes a summary of control programs in endemic areas and an outline for a strategy of morbidity control.*

SCHISTOSOMIASIS HAEMATOBIA (Urinary Bilharziasis)

S. haematobium infection is endemic in Africa and some parts of the Middle East; it is highly prevalent in the Nile Valley and extends along the Mediterranean coast of the continent. In West Africa it is more widely disseminated than *S. mansoni*; its distribution in East and South Africa is patchy. In Southwest Asia the endemic area includes most countries of the Middle East and Arabian peninsula. Clinically, infection with *S. haematobium* is the most significant of the human schistosome infections because symptoms such as hematuria and dysuria occur early and affect approximately two thirds of infected individuals. In endemic areas, extensive hydroureter and hydronephrosis can be demonstrated in a considerable proportion of infected children; the natural history of these lesions and the course of disease in adults have not been clearly defined.

Adult male *S. haematobium* worms are distinguished by their finely tuberculate surface and by the presence of four to five large testes. The ovaries are found in the posterior half of the female body and contain 20 to 30 eggs. Mature *S. haematobium* eggs measure approximately 143×50 μm and are spindle shaped with a rounded anterior end and a conical posterior end that tapers to a terminal delicate spine. Eggs are mainly found in urine of infected individuals but may occasionally be seen in stools or rectal biopsy material. The main intermediate hosts of *S. haematobium* in North Africa and the Middle East are freshwater snails of the genus *Bulinus*; in Africa south of the Sahara they belong to the subgenus *Physopsis*.

PATHOLOGY AND CLINICAL MANIFESTATIONS. In the urinary bladder, the formation of egg granulomas leads to hyperemia, tubercles, ulcers, and polyps; as healing proceeds, sandy patches and scarring may be seen. Obstructive uropathy is the main functional disturbance caused by schistosomiasis haematobia. Other urinary tract disorders, such as bacteriuria, calculi, and bladder cancer, have been epidemiologically associated with *S. haematobium* infection, but no causal relationship has yet been confirmed. Ova of *S. haematobium* have occasionally been found in the lungs with subsequent focal pulmonary arteritis and diffuse hypertensive arteriolar changes; chronic cor pulmonale may occur in these patients.

Swimmer's itch and acute schistosomiasis have rarely been described in *S. haematobium* infection. By contrast, symptoms related to the urinary tract, including dysuria, hematuria, or frequency, occur in a large proportion of infected individuals. Hematuria is characteristically terminal, but with extensive ulceration the whole stream of urine may be bloody, along with passage of clots. In late cases, symptoms related to secondary infection of the urinary tract, severe obstructive uropathy, or neoplasia may appear. Urine examination reveals proteinuria and hematuria; both signs are closely related to intensity of infection. An association between *S. haematobium* infection and bacteremia, mainly caused by *Salmonella* organisms, has been reported. Renal function may be compromised in patients with obstructive uropathy. Cytoscopic examination shows some degree of pathology in almost all infected individuals, the most common being hyperemia near the ureteral openings and the bladder trigone. Sandy patches, tubercles, ulcers, and polyps are less frequently seen. Radiographically, bladder calcification is a characteristic feature of urinary schistosomiasis; it is found in approximately 50 to 80 per cent of infected individuals. Other pathologic lesions are also frequently seen in 40 to 60 per cent of patients, including obstructive uropathy, hydroureter, hydronephrosis, and filling defects in the bladder and ureters. Ultrasonographic examination of the urinary tract confirms the bladder lesions and their obstructive sequelae.

DIAGNOSIS. Urine examination for *S. haematobium* eggs can be performed by direct or concentration methods. Excretion of the parasite eggs is maximal around mid-day, when samples should optimally be obtained. Diagnosis and quantification of infection can be achieved by filtering 10 ml of urine through a Nuclepore membrane. Examination of more than one urine sample may be necessary to establish the diagnosis; rectal biopsy may be done in suspected cases with negative urine results. Serology may be needed to diagnose early or light infection. Once *S. haematobium* infection is diagnosed, assessment of urinary tract pathology by ultrasonography is recommended. In addition, care must be taken in some endemic areas for early detection of bladder cancer by appropriate cytologic and histologic examinations.

TREATMENT. See Management of Schistosomiasis, below.

King CH, Lombardi G, Lombardi C, et al.: Chemotherapy based control of schistosomiasis haematobia. II. Metrifonate vs. praziquantelin control of infection associated morbidity. Am J Trop Med Hyg 42:587, 1990. *The article presents data on long-term effects of metrifonate and praziquantel on the clinical as well as ultrasonographic manifestations of* S. haematobium *infection in school-aged children.*

Mott KE, Dixon H, Osei-Tutu E, et al.: Relation between intensity of *Schistosoma haematobium* infection and clinical hematuria and proteinuria. Lancet 1:1005, 1983. *Correlation of proteinuria and hematuria with counts of* S. haematobium *eggs in urine.*

Warren KS, Mahmoud AAF, Muruka JF, et al.: Schistosomiasis haematobia in Coast Province, Kenya. Am J Trop Med Hyg 28:864, 1979. *Correlation of morbidity, with egg counts in schistosomiasis haematobia; even in lightly infected children disease manifestations are significant.*

Wilkins A, Gilles H: Schistosomiasis haematobia. *In* Mahmoud AAF (ed.): Clinical Tropical Medicine and Communicable Diseases. Vol. 2: Schistosomiasis. London, Bailliere's Tindall, 1987, pp 333–348. *A comprehensive review of the epidemiology, pathology, and clinical features of schistosomiasis haematobia based on wide experience in Africa.*

SCHISTOSOMIASIS MANSONI (Intestinal or Hepatosplenic Bilharziasis)

Infection with *S. mansoni* is endemic in Africa, the Middle East, South America, and some Caribbean islands. The distribution of schistosomiasis mansoni in Africa overlaps with that of schistosomiasis haematobia. In Southwest Asia, it occurs in Yemen and Saudi Arabia. *S. mansoni* is sporadically distributed all over the northern part of South America and is endemic in several Caribbean countries and islands and in many parts of Puerto Rico.

Adult male *S. mansoni* worms have a grossly tuberculate surface and usually contain seven small testes. In the female, the ovary occupies the anterior half of its body, with a short uterus containing one to four ova. Mature eggs measure 155×66 μm and are oval with a lateral, long spine. The intermediate snail hosts of *S. mansoni* are species of the genus *Biomphalaria* in Africa and *Australorbis tropicorbis* in the Americas.

PATHOLOGY AND CLINICAL MANIFESTATIONS. Acute schistosomiasis mansoni is the most common early presentation encountered by physicians in North America. Symptoms appear between 3 and 7 weeks after exposure and include fever, anorexia, abdominal pain, and headache. Less often, diarrhea, nausea, and vomiting may occur. Hepatosplenomegaly, eosinophilia, and increased serum immunoglobulins are the main clinical signs. Most of these manifestations correlate significantly with intensity of infection as evaluated by stool egg counts.

Schistosoma mansoni eggs are primarily deposited in the small veins around the large intestine; some of the eggs may be trapped in the gut wall or break loose into the portal circulation to be carried to the small intrahepatic portal venules. On examination, the intestinal mucosa appears red and granular with pinpoint elevations surrounded by hyperemic zones. There may be minute hemorrhages and ulcerations. Sessile and pedunculated polyps, mainly in the rectosigmoid area, have been reported in Egyptians infected with *S. mansoni*, but not in persons from other endemic areas. Pathologic examination of the liver in lightly infected individuals shows schistosome eggs with and without granulomas and mild portal inflammation. In advanced cases, the typical picture of Symmers' fibrosis is seen; the eggs are concentrated in and around large portal tracts with marked fibrosis and obstructive portal venous lesions. The lobular arrangement of liver parenchyma and its function are usually maintained. However, these structural changes lead to marked alteration of hepatic hemodynamics, such as obstruction of portal blood flow through the liver and increase in number and size of intrahepatic arterial branches, thus shifting the blood flow through the liver from mainly portal to arterial sources. Portal hypertension leads to congestive splenomegaly and formation of portosystemic venous shunts at the lower end of the esophagus and other sites. In these patients, schistosome eggs may find their way to the pulmonary circulation, bypassing the obstructed portal blood flow. In the lungs, granulomas form around the trapped eggs, leading to arteriolar fibrosis and pulmonary hypertension.

Nervous system involvement in schistosomiasis mansoni is rare; the main clinical presentation, as in schistosomiasis haematobia, is transverse myelitis. The preferential involvement of the spinal cord may be due to the anatomic location of adult worms. The underlying pathologic lesions are usually granulomas forming around eggs in the spinal cord.

Infection with *S. mansoni* does not have characteristic or specific symptomatology. Early symptoms of acute schistosomiasis, as described earlier, are all nonspecific in nature. This is particularly the case in travelers who are accidentally exposed to infection in endemic areas. In chronic schistosomiasis mansoni, infected individuals have a slightly higher incidence of crampy abdominal pain (21 to 48 per cent) and bloody diarrhea (4 to 28 per cent) than do matched uninfected controls from the same endemic area. Other frequently mentioned nonspecific symptoms and signs, such as weakness, inability to work, or diarrhea, have not been convincingly demonstrated in any controlled studies. Significant enlargement of the liver is seen in 4 to 11 per cent of infected subjects, and splenomegaly occurs in 3 to 7 per cent. Patients with schistosomal hepatosplenomegaly present with a unique form of liver disease. The pathophysiologic changes are based on alteration of hemodynamics, fibrosis of large portal tracts, and very little derangement of liver function. Enlargement of the liver usually occurs in the left lobe, but later, in the course of infection and particularly in adults, uniform hepatomegaly may be seen. Ultrasonographic examination of the liver shows evidence of specific patterns of fibrosis, which distinguishes this syndrome from other causes of hepatomegaly. Simultaneously, gross enlargement of the spleen may occur; the organ is characteristically rubbery hard. Laboratory examination may show indications of anemia and a low degree of eosinophilia but no changes in liver function test results until late in the course of disease. Total serum proteins are usually normal, but gamma globulin increases are common. An association between schistosomal hepatosplenomegaly and hepatitis B antigen and antibody presence has been described, but its pathophysiologic significance is not clear. Although hepatosplenomegaly usually occurs in heavily infected individuals, other underlying mechanisms may be involved. An association between human leukocyte antigen (HLA) haplotypes and schistosomal hepatosplenomegaly has been demonstrated. In patients with pure schistosomal fibrosis uncomplicated by cirrhosis or viral hepatitis, liver function is preserved for a long time. These individuals often present clinically with an episode of hematemesis caused by rupture of esophageal varices without prior complaints. Bleeding may recur several times while the liver parenchyma maintains its normal functions. Finally, however, symptoms and signs of liver cell failure ensue, along with the development of stigmata of chronic liver disease and ascites.

Several less defined clinical syndromes have been associated with schistosomiasis mansoni. Formation of antigen-antibody complexes and their deposition in the kidney glomeruli have been demonstrated in infected laboratory animals as well as in individuals with chronic schistosomiasis mansoni. However, the prevalence of this syndrome and the rate at which it occurs in schistosomiasis are unknown, since proteinuria and nephrotic syndrome are not particularly prevalent in schistosomiasis-endemic areas. Cor pulmonale in schistosomiasis is a better defined disease entity, although its incidence is not known. It usually occurs in patients with advanced hepatosplenic schistosomiasis mansoni or japonica because of the development of collateral circulation. In *S. haematobium*–infected individuals, the anatomic location of adult worms may help eggs reach the systemic circulation directly and become trapped in the pulmonary arterioles. Patients with schistosomal pulmonary hypertension present clinically with symptoms and signs similar to those in cor pulmonale of other causes. Aneurysmal dilation of the pulmonary artery and its branches, along with right ventricular hypertrophy, may occur.

DIAGNOSIS. Stool examination for the characteristic *S. mansoni* eggs is the definitive diagnostic procedure. Because assessing intensity of infection is essential, quantitative techniques are recommended. The Kato thick smear method involves examination of sieved 50-mg stool samples placed on glass slides and spead under a cellophane cover slip presoaked in 50 per cent glycerol. The slides should be left at least 24 hours to allow for clearing of fecal material; the embryo within the ovum also clears, but the characteristic shape of the eggshell is retained. Rectal biopsy or serologic testing may be used for diagnosis of stool-negative cases, particularly in lightly infected individuals.

TREATMENT. See Management of Schistosomiasis, below.

Abdel-Salam E, Abdel Khalik A, Abdel-Meguid A, et al.: Association of HLA class I antigens (A1, B5, B8, and CW2) with disease manifestations and infection in human schistosomiasis mansoni in Egypt. Tissue Antigens 27:142, 1986. *A large-scale, population-based study of association between certain HLA haplotypes and hepatosplenomegaly due to schistosomiasis mansoni.*

Mahmoud AAF, Abdel Wahab MF: Schistosomiasis. *In* Warren KS, Mahmoud AAF (eds.): Tropical and Geographical Medicine. 2nd ed. New York, McGraw-Hill, 1990, pp 458–473. *Detailed description of the clinical manifestations of S. mansoni infection and its characteristic features in ultrasonographic examination of the liver.*

Prata A: Schistosomiasis mansoni in Brazil. *In* Mahmoud AAF (ed.): Clinical Tropical Medicine and Communicable Diseases. Vol. 2: Schistosomiasis. London, Bailliere's Tindall, 1987, pp 349–369. *A review of the clinical features as seen in an endemic area, with emphasis on diagnostic methods.*

SCHISTOSOMIASIS JAPONICA

On the main Asian continent, schistosomiasis japonica is prevalent in some parts of China, Thailand, Laos, Cambodia, and Malaysia. It is also endemic in Taiwan, Japan, the Philippines, and Celebes. This schistosome species characteristically infects humans and domestic animals such as cats, dogs, and cattle, thus providing reservoir hosts that may contribute to its endemicity in certain areas of the Far East.

Adult *S. japonicum* male worms have a nontuberculate surface and seven medium-sized testes. The ovary occupies the middle part of the body of female worms and contains 50 to 100 ova. *S. japonicum* eggs are found in stools of infected individuals; they measure 89×67 μm and are oval or rounded with a lateral short, sometimes curved spine. The intermediate hosts for *S. japonicum* are snails of the genus *Oncomelania*.

PATHOLOGY AND CLINICAL MANIFESTATIONS. Cercarial dermatitis is not a prominent feature of schistosomiasis japonica. Katayama fever, or acute schistosomiasis, was named after the district in Japan endemic for *S. japonicum* infections. Symptoms usually begin 5 to 7 weeks after infection and are similar to those associated with schistosomiasis mansoni. The clinical features usually subside in a few days but may last for several months, and fatalities have been reported. The chronic manifestations of schistosomiasis japonica are related to ova deposited in the intestines and liver; adult worms produce 10 times more eggs than those of *S. mansoni*. These ova are laid in aggregates and remain so in the intestinal wall or when carried to the liver by the portal blood flow. In addition, *S. japonicum* eggs differ from those of *S. mansoni* in their tendency to calcify in tissues. Schistosomiasis japonica granulomas vary in size tremendously and tend to show signs of necrosis.

Individuals with chronic schistosomiasis japonica may present with no symptoms or several nonspecific complaints. Controlled surveys in endemic areas have shown no particular increase in complaints of weakness, abdominal pain, or diarrhea in infected individuals. Clinical signs of hepatosplenomegaly are more frequently seen in infected than in uninfected individuals, but they are not uniformly correlated with intensity of infection. Severe hepatosplenic disease caused by schistosomiasis japonica may be seen in endemic areas, but its prevalence and relationship to intensity of infection and other complicating factors are unknown.

Cerebral schistosomiasis japonica is a unique syndrome reportedly occurring in 2 to 4 per cent of infected individuals in the endemic countries. *S. japonicum* infection of the central nervous system preferentially affects the brain. The lesions consist of large aggregates of eggs in the cerebral venous system, but adult worms have never been found in the brain. Cerebral schistosomiasis japonica presents clinically early in the course of the infection; the most frequent manifestation is focal jacksonian epilepsy; less commonly, generalized encephalitis may be the presenting feature.

DIAGNOSIS. Stool examination for *S. japonicum* eggs is the only reliable diagnostic procedure. The Kato thick smear technique provides both diagnosis and quantitative assessment of infection. Rectal biopsy or serologic testing may be used in individuals with light infections, particularly when a less common manifestation, such as cerebral schistosomiasis, is encountered.

TREATMENT. See Management of Schistosomiasis, below.

Olveda RM, Domingo EO: Schistosomiasis japonica. In Mahmoud AAF (ed.): Clinical Tropical Medicine and Communicable Diseases. Vol. 2: Schistosomiasis. London, Bailliere's Tindall, 1987, pp 397–417. *Description of epidemiology, clinical features, and diagnostic methods. The article is based on wide experience with schistosomiasis japonica in the Philippines.*

Warren KS, Su DL, Xu CY, et al.: Morbidity in schistosomiasis japonica in relation to intensity of infection; study of 2 royal brigades in Anhui Province, China. N Engl J Med, 309:1533, 1983.

OTHER HUMAN SCHISTOSOMES

Endemic foci for *S. intercalatum* are found in Central and West Africa. Adult worms inhabit the mesenteric blood vessels, and terminal spine eggs are seen in stools of infected individuals. Symptoms usually ascribed to this species of schistosome include abdominal pain, diarrhea, and blood in stools. Diagnosis is based on positive geographic history and finding parasite ova upon fecal examination.

S. mekongi is the most recent schistosome species to be described as a cause of infection and disease in humans. The parasite is endemic in some parts of the mainland of Southeast Asia. Adult worm and eggs are similar to those of *S. japonicum*; ova of *S. mekongi* are, however, smaller. In symptomatic patients, a syndrome not unlike that due to *S. japonicum* has been observed. It includes abdominal pain, diarrhea, and heptosplenomegaly. Diagnosis is established by fecal examination for parasite ova.

Hofstetter M, Nash TE, Cheever AW, et al.: Infection with Schistosoma mekongi in Southeast Asian refugees. J Infect Dis 144:420, 1981. *Description of clinical and parasitologic features of schistosomiasis mekongi.*

MANAGEMENT OF SCHISTOSOMIASIS

Chemotherapy is the major antischistosome strategy for eradication of parasites in infected individuals and for reducing incidence, intensity, and morbidity in populations of endemic areas. The current drug of choice is praziquantel, a pyrazinoisoquinoline derivative that is effective against all species of schistosomes that infect humans. Praziquantel has several advantages as the chemotherapeutic agent of choice, including oral administration, low incidence of toxicity and side effects, and marked antiparasitic activity. The recommended dose of praziquantel for treatment of infections with *S. haematobium*, *S. intercalatum*, or *S. mansoni* is 40 mg per kilogram of body weight administered once. For *S. japonicum* infection, it is recommended to administer 30 mg per kilogram twice in 1 day, and for *S. mekongi*, 20 mg per kilogram three times in one day. These dosages have been shown to result in parasitologic cure in approximately 80 per cent of treated individuals and in a highly significant reduction of intensity of infection. Side effects of praziquantel are rare, usually mild, and self-limiting. These include abdominal pain, headache, dizziness, and skin rashes.

The effect of antischistosome chemotherapeutic agents on disease manifestations is variable. It is dependent on the duration of infection and extent of disease. Treatment is expected to result in reversal of pathology, e.g., hematuria and hepatosplenomegaly, in infected children. By contrast, adults with established fibroobstructive disease in the liver and urinary tract may not show significant clinical improvement following chemotherapy. Other therapeutic or surgical methods may therefore be necessary to correct the anatomic lesions. Furthermore, medical management of the chronic sequelae of schistosomiasis, such as liver fibrosis, portal hypertension, and esophageal varices, should be conducted according to established practices and taking into consideration

the unique pathophysiologic characteristics of disease due to schistosomiasis.

Mahmoud AAF: Praziquantel for the treatment of helminthic infections. Adv Intern Med 32:193, 1987. *A summary of the known anthelminthic effects of praziquantel in experimental animals and humans.*

435 Hermaphroditic Flukes
S. K. K. Seah

The hermaphroditic flukes are unlike the *Schistosoma* flukes in that they have male and female organs in the same worm and self-fertilize. The ones that are of medical importance are (1) flukes that parasitize the biliary tract, i.e., *Clonorchis sinensis*, *Opisthorchis viverrini*, *Opisthorchis felineus*, *Fasciola hepatica*, *Dicrocoelium dendriticum*, and *Metorchis conjunctus;* (2) flukes that parasitize the intestinal lumen, i.e., *Fasciolopsis buski*, *Heterophyes heterophyes*, *Echinostoma ilocanum*, *Gastrodiscoides hominis*, and *Metagonimus yokogawai;* (3) flukes that parasitize the lung, i.e., *Paragonimus westermani* and other species; and (4) the mesocercarial stage of *Alaria americana*, which causes generalized systemic infection.

The more important of these flukes, such as *Clonorchis* and *Opisthorchis*, affect many millions of people in Asia and Eastern Europe. All of these flukes parasitize other mammals, and some of them, such as *Fasciola hepatica*, are of major importance in veterinary medicine. Although most of these flukes have limited geographic distribution, with the migration of people around the world, human infections are often seen in nonendemic areas.

The hermaphroditic flukes are leaflike, nonsegmented, and bilaterally symmetric, ranging in size from a few millimeters to several centimeters. On one end is the anterior or oral sucker, and just behind it is the ventral sucker or acetabulum. The acetabulum acts as a holdfast to the epithelial tissue of the final host.

Eggs appear in bile and stool or, in the case of the lung fluke, in sputum and stool. The eggs are operculated. Some are fully embryonated when passed; others may require time for embryonation. The embryonated egg contains the first-stage larva, or miracidium. After hatching in fresh water, the miracidium penetrates, or is ingested by, a suitable first intermediate host, a snail. In the snail, the miracidium develops into thousands of cercariae, which are released into the water. The cercariae attach themselves to or penetrate the second intermediate hosts, which, depending on the flukes, may be freshwater fish, crustaceans, frogs, or aquatic plants. The final definitive hosts (humans or animals) acquire the infection by ingesting encysted metacercariae.

Infection by digenetic or hermaphroditic trematodes is treated by the broad-spectrum anthelminthic praziquantel. Personal prevention of infection includes eating only well-cooked fish or crustaceans and avoiding raw watercress in endemic areas. Community prevention consists of cleaning up the environment and preventing infection of the intermediate hosts.

Seah SKK: Digenetic trematodes. Clin Gastroenterol 7:98, 1978. *A good review of all the hermaphroditic flukes.*

HEPATIC HERMAPHRODITIC FLUKES
Clonorchiasis (*Clonorchis sinensis*)

This infection is very common in the Far East, especially southern China, Taiwan, Hong Kong, Japan, and Korea, where raw or undercooked fish has long been considered a delicacy. *Opisthorchis* is almost identical to *Clonorchis* in its morphology, epidemiology, and clinical manifestations. Opisthorchiasis is very common in Thailand, Laos, the Philippines, and Eastern Europe. In some areas, virtually the whole population is infected. Even infants are infected, as they are fed chopped raw fish as a dietary supplement. More than 40 species of freshwater fish, mainly the carp and salmon group, harbor metacercariae.

Clonorchis sinensis has a very long lifespan (probably up to 50 years), and this parasitic infection will likely remain important in endemic areas for many years. Clonorchiasis occurs in all parts of the world where there are Asian immigrants. Many hundreds of thousands of Southeast Asian refugees and other Asian immigrants have come to North America in recent years, and surveys show that a large percentage of these have asymptomatic liver fluke infection.

After the contaminated fish is ingested, the metacercariae excyst in the duodenum. Most of the larval flukes ascend the biliary tree directly, but some may pass via the portal circulation to the liver. During maturation of the fluke, marked desquamation of the biliary epithelium takes place. The fluke matures in 2 to 3 weeks and begins to lay eggs. Flukes prefer to reside in the second-order bile ducts, but in heavy infection they are found throughout the biliary system, including the gallbladder, and sometimes in the pancreatic duct. Adult flukes are grayish-brown and 15 mm by 3 mm. They feed on secretions of the bile duct mucosa. They cause low-grade inflammatory changes in the biliary tree, proliferation of the biliary epithelium, and progressive portal fibrosis. As a rule, there is no parenchymal damage, and cirrhosis does not result from uncomplicated clonorchiasis.

CLINICAL MANIFESTATIONS. Acute clonorchiasis occurs 1 to 3 weeks after the ingestion of encysted metacercariae. The condition is only rarely diagnosed and is a flulike illness. Fever, chills, abdominal pain, diarrhea, tender hepatomegaly, and mild jaundice may be present. The white cell count is elevated, and there is marked eosinophilia. The serum alkaline phosphatase, aspartate aminotransferase (AST) (SGOT), alanine aminotransferase (ALT) (SGPT), and bilirubin levels are elevated. The clinical presentation is often confused with acute viral hepatitis, which is even more common in these tropical endemic areas. Acute clonorchiasis is therefore rarely recognized. The ova of *C. sinensis* appear in the stool or bile 3 or 4 weeks after ingestion of the metacercariae. The history of eating raw fish in the endemic area and the eosinophilia should suggest the diagnosis.

The majority of people with the ova of *C. sinensis* in their stool have no symptoms even when heavily infected. It is impossible to predict who will develop the complications of chronic clonorchiasis. A small percentage of infected individuals will develop the symptoms of chronic clonorchiasis, which include inflammation, infection, stones, obstruction, and neoplastic changes in the biliary tree. Acute suppurative cholangitis is a serious febrile illness often associated with hypoglycemia and *Escherichia coli* bacteremia. The biliary system is blocked by numerous flukes and becomes secondarily infected. The condition carries a high mortality rate. Recurrent pyogenic cholangitis is a recurrent febrile illness associated with clonorchiasis and intrahepatic bile duct calculi. During surgical operation or autopsy, *Clonorchis* flukes are not consistently found, as in the case of acute suppurative cholangitis. With recurrent pyogenic cholangitis, cirrhosis may eventually develop. The flukes occasionally block the pancreatic ducts and induce pancreatitis. Cholangiocarcinoma is a late complication of chronic clonorchiasis. Clonorchiasis has no causal relation to hepatocellular cancer.

DIAGNOSIS. The diagnosis is made by finding the characteristic light bulb–shaped, operculated eggs in the stool or duodenal aspirate. The eggs average 29 μm by 16 μm. Unfortunately, the *C. sinensis* egg is almost identical to those of *Opisthorcis*, *Heterophyes*, and *Metagonimus*. To be absolutely certain of the diagnosis, one must examine the adult fluke. However, geographic distribution may help in separating *Clonorchis* from *Opisthorcis*. In a patient with abdominal or other symptoms and *C. sinensis* eggs in the stool, it is often difficult to decide if the complaint is due to clonorchiasis. It is often necessary to eliminate other current illnesses before attributing the symptoms to clonorchiasis. As a rule, in uncomplicated established clonorchiasis, there is no eosinophilia, elevation of sedimentation rate, anemia, or abnormal liver function test results, and radioisotope scan and ultrasonography (B scan) of the liver are normal.

In acute clonorchiasis, leukocytosis, marked eosinophilia, and abnormal liver function test results are present. This condition must be distinguished from hepatic amebiasis and visceral larva migrans. In the former, eosinophilia is absent and serology for amebiasis is positive. In the latter, the serology for toxocariasis is positive. The presence of the flukes provokes irregular antibody response, and a large variety of serologic and skin tests are available in some centers. However, these are not sufficiently specific and sensitive for clinical use.

TREATMENT. Praziquantel has revolutionized the treatment of this condition. The recommended dose is 75 mg per kilogram of body weight, divided in three doses on the same day (this dose of praziquantel exceeds the manufacturer's recommendation). This drug is very well tolerated, and no long-term toxicity has been shown. At the dose recommended, some gastrointestinal disturbance and transient headaches may occur. Because this drug is safe, it is recommended that all cases of clonorchiasis, symptomatic or not, be treated. The cure rate of a single-day treatment is almost 100 per cent. Stool should be checked for ova of the fluke 1 month, 6 months, and 1 year after treatment. Retreatment may be necessary. In parts of the endemic areas, mass treatment is showing encouraging results by reducing the prevalence of this infection.

The treatment of complications such as calculi, suppurative cholangitis, recurrent pyogenic cholangitis, and pancreatitis is both medical and surgical. Conservative treatment consists of broad-spectrum antibiotics and intravenous fluids. If this is not effective, a permanent and adequate drainage procedure, such as choledochoduodenostomy, is required. A course of praziquantel should be given when the patient is able to swallow the tablets.

PREVENTION. In endemic areas, freshwater fish should be well cooked before being eaten. In hyperendemic areas, where a large proportion of the population is infected, mass chemotherapy with a single dose of praziquantel (40 to 50 mg per kilogram of body weight at bed time) is recommended. The local people should be educated regarding how this infection is acquired and should change the habit of eating raw fish.

Opisthorchiasis (*Opisthorchis viverrini* and *felineus*)

Opisthorchis felineus is common in Eastern and Central Europe, India, Japan, and the Philippines. *O. viverrini* is common in Thailand, Laos, and Kampuchea. In parts of Thailand and the U.S.S.R., the infection rate is as high as 90 per cent of the population. Many animals, especially cats, are natural reservoirs. The life cycle, mode of transmission, pathology, clinical manifestations, treatment, and prevention are similar to those of *Clonorchis sinensis*. Cholangiocarcinoma can also result from chronic opisthorchiasis.

Dicroceliasis

Dicrocoelium dendriticum is a lancet-shaped fluke, measuring 10 mm by 2 mm, that normally lives in the biliary tree of sheep, cattle, and other herbivores. The operculated eggs are passed in the feces and are ingested by land snails. Cercariae are released in slime balls shed by the snails, which act as the first intermediate host. The slime is ingested by ants, the second intermediate host. Herbivores become infected by eating the ants. Very rarely, true human infection occurs when such ants are ingested. Less rarely, spurious infection in humans occurs when raw infected liver is eaten. This infection is seen in Europe, the Mediterranean basin, and Asia. The maturing flukes move from the biliary vasculature into the biliary tree and gallbladder and may give rise to symptoms of abdominal pain and vomiting. The diagnosis is made by finding the characteristic ova in the stool. Praziquantel, given in a dose similar to that for clonorchiasis, is the treatment of choice.

Fascioliasis (*Fasciola hepatica*)

Fasciola hepatica is a common parasite in the biliary tract of sheep and cattle, but it may also infect all types of mammals, including humans. It has worldwide distribution in sheep and is prevalent in low, wet pastures, where suitable species of snails are present. The cercariae, discharged from the snails, attach themselves to water plants and encyst as metacercariae. Humans are infected mainly as a result of eating watercress and other aquatic plants gathered in these pastures. In the duodenum, the immature fluke penetrates the mucosa, enters the abdominal cavity, and through some unexplained hepatotropism penetrates Glisson's capsule. The immature flukes migrate throughout the liver for some weeks until they reach the biliary tract, where they mature in about 2 months. The fluke is 3.0 cm by 1.3 cm, and the eggs are large, ovoid, and operculated, measuring 140 μm by 75 μm.

CLINICAL MANIFESTATIONS. *Acute Fascioliasis.* Invasion and maturation occur during the first 3 months after ingestion of the metacercariae. The immature flukes produce small necrotic foci along the migration paths. There may be no significant symptoms, or there may be abdominal pain, hepatomegaly, fever, vomiting, and jaundice. Leukocytosis and marked eosinophilia are present, but *F. hepatica* eggs are not found in the stool at this stage.

Established Infection. The mature flukes now produce metabolites that irritate the biliary passages, resulting in hyperplasia. Obstruction and dilation of the biliary passage and cholecystitis may occur. There may be abdominal pain, hepatomegaly, recurrent urticaria, jaundice, irregular fever, diarrhea, and weight loss. Anemia from blood loss can be severe. The obstruction and irritation may produce thickening of the biliary tree, atrophy of the hepatic cells, and biliary cirrhosis. Cholelithiasis is common. A relationship between fascioliasis and biliary cancer is not proved.

Extrabiliary Fascioliasis. Ingestion of raw sheep and goat liver containing young flukes causes the condition called halzoun (suffocation). This pharyngeal fascioliasis is due to the lodgment of flukes in the upper respiratory and digestive tracts. Inflammation and edema may lead to dysphagia, dyspnea, and even asphyxiation. Cutaneous fascioliasis, usually in the upper abdomen, manifests as migratory nodules that are 2 to 5 cm. Rarely, the flukes may be found in the lung, peritoneum, muscles, eye, and brain.

DIAGNOSIS. In acute infection, the diagnosis is made in an endemic area by a high index of suspicion and the clinical triad of fever, hepatomegaly, and marked eosinophilia. A history of ingestion of wild watercress supports the diagnosis. At this stage, the stool does not contain eggs. Serologic tests, such as complement fixation, are helpful. In chronic infection, the stool contains the characteristic large, operculated eggs (140 μm × 75 μm). Duodenal and biliary aspirate provides a higher yield than does fecal examination. Liver function test results reflect the degree of hepatic cellular damage and biliary obstruction. Intravenous or percutaneous cholangiography, B scan, and magnetic resonance imaging (MRI) scan may show filling defects. The diagnosis is often made during surgical operation for biliary disease. The diagnosis of halzoun in an endemic area is made by the history of ingestion of raw liver and the finding of a pharyngeal mass.

TREATMENT. Praziquantel is effective, and the dosage is 75 mg per kilogram of body weight divided into three doses per day for 2 days. Ectopic flukes are removed surgically. Prevention consists of not eating raw watercress and raw sheep and goat liver in the endemic areas.

Fasciola gigantica

This large fluke is a liver parasite of herbivorous animals and occasionally of humans in Asia and Africa. The life cycle, mode of infection, clinical manifestations, and treatment are similar to those of *F. hepatica*.

Bunnag D, Harinasuta T: Trematode infections excluding schistosomiasis. *In* Gilles HM (ed.): Recent Advances in Tropical Medicine. No. 1. Edinburgh, Churchill Livingstone, 1984, pp 223–227. *A good review especially of opisthorchiasis.*

Gibson JB, Sun T: Clonorchiasis. *In* Marcial-Rojas RA (ed.): Pathology of Protozoal and Helminthic Diseases. Baltimore, The Williams & Wilkins Company, 1977, pp 546–566. *Profusely illustrated; very good on all aspects, especially on epidemiology and pathology as seen in Hong Kong.*

Schwartz DA: Cholangiocarcinoma associated with liver fluke infections: A preventable source of morbidity in Asian immigrants. Am J Gastroenterol 81:76, 1986. *Emphasizes the importance of early diagnosis and treatment of all liver fluke infections in the prevention of bile duct cancer in the high-risk group.*

LUNG HERMAPHRODITIC FLUKES (Paragonimiasis)

Paragonimiasis is due to infection with the adult *Paragonimus westermani* and other species. As a rule, the infection is in the lung, where the flukes are encapsulated in the parenchyma. The disease is also called pulmonary diastomiasis, endemic hemoptysis, and Oriental lung fluke disease. Human paragonimiasis occurs most commonly in the Far East, especially central China, Japan, Korea, Vietnam, Thailand, and the Philippines. It also occurs in the Indian subcontinent, Central and South America, and West Africa. In addition to *P. westermani*, more than 30 species may affect humans. Most of these flukes are parasites of mammals, especially of the cat family, foxes, dogs, cattle, and pigs.

The adult flukes live singly or in pairs encapsulated in the cystic spaces in the lung. They are ovoid, plump, and leaflike and measure about 1.0 cm by 0.5 cm by 0.4 cm. Oval, yellowish-brown, operculated ova (90 μm × 55 μm) are coughed up and expelled in the sputum or are swallowed and passed in the feces. The flukes have a lifespan of 5 to 6 years. In fresh water, the miracidia escape from the ova and penetrate the first intermediate host, a suitable snail. After several weeks, the cercariae emerge and penetrate the second intermediate host, the crayfish or crab. Humans or animals acquire the infection by eating raw meat or viscera of the freshwater crustacean. In Korea and West Africa, fresh crab juice is used as a home remedy in the treatment of measles. In the duodenum the metacercariae excyst, enter the abdominal cavity, migrate through the diaphragm into the pleural space, and end up in the lung parenchyma, where they mature and begin to lay eggs about 2 months after ingestion of the crayfish. This circuitous route of migration explains the extrapulmonary cysts of *Paragonimus*.

PATHOLOGY. The migratory larval flukes tunnel into the lung at the periphery. This condition is accompanied by an inflammatory reaction with many eosinophils. They finally encyst with a fibrous tissue wall. The cyst may communicate with a bronchus and may often be secondarily infected with abscess formation. The death of the fluke is followed by calcification. Flukes in the abdominal cavity may cause abscess and adhesion and intestinal ulceration, resulting in bloody diarrhea with mucus and ova. In the brain, the temporal and occipital lobes are the favored sites of eosinophilic granulomas containing flukes or ova. Lodgment of the flukes in the spinal cord causes transverse myelitis. Adult flukes have been found in other organs.

CLINICAL MANIFESTATIONS. In the rare case of acute paragonimiasis, there may be fever, chills, and chest pain. The symptoms and physical signs are indistinguishable from those of bronchopneumonia. As a rule, the onset is insidious, and the symptoms are those of chronic bronchitis and bronchiectasis. Cough, especially in the morning, that is productive of thick, gelatinous, blood-tinged sputum, is the most prominent symptom. Exertional dyspnea and night sweats are common. Frank hemoptysis often occurs after a paroxysm of coughing. Chest pain and pleural effusion may be present, and clubbing of the fingers may occur. The most characteristic finding is persistent moist, coarse rales over the area of involvement. Chest radiographs early in the disease show patchy, cloudy infiltrations, but later dense, nodular opacities or ring shadows indicate the site of the cysts. Pleural thickening and calcification may be seen late in the disease.

Abdominal paragonimiasis occurs when the flukes localize in the abdomen. The symptoms are nonspecific dull ache, tenderness, and diarrhea, which may be bloody and accompanied by mucus. An abdominal mass with lung disease in a patient from an endemic area should raise suspicion of this disorder. On rare occasions, the fluke localizes in the brain, resulting in a seizure disorder similar to cysticercosis. There may be pareses of varying degrees and optic atrophy with papilledema. The cerebrospinal fluid shows a raised protein concentration, and eosinophils are present. Children with cerebral paragonimiasis are usually mentally retarded. Subcutaneous localization of the fluke results in abscess formation.

DIAGNOSIS. The diagnosis rests mainly on finding ova in the sputum and stool. The differential diagnoses based on the chest radiographs are bronchopneumonia, bronchiectasis, tuberculosis, tumor, and the rarer fungal infections. In practice, the most important differential diagnosis is tuberculosis. Active tuberculosis and paragonimiasis often are present in the same individual from the endemic area.

Abdominal paragonimiasis must be differentiated from intestinal parasitic and nonparasitic infections and other intra-abdominal disorders. The finding of ova in the stool does not necessarily indicate abdominal paragonimiasis. The cerebral presentation must be differentiated from other causes of seizure disorder, space-occupying leisons, cysticercosis, hydatid disease, and meningoencephalitides.

Moderate eosinophilia is usual in early cases, but in established cases there may be no abnormal hematologic findings. As with other helminthic infections, serologic testing is not useful.

TREATMENT. Praziquantel is the treatment of choice. The dosage is 75 mg per kilogram of body weight divided into three doses daily for 2 days. Paragonimiasis of the central nervous system requires surgery. Praziquantel should be given before surgery. Subcutaneous flukes should also be surgically removed.

PREVENTION. In theory, prevention is simple. Freshwater crustaceans must be well cooked before eating, and hands and utensils should be thoroughly washed after contact with raw crabs and crayfish. However, in endemic areas it is difficult to persuade people to relinquish long-established cooking and eating habits and the use of raw crab juice for medicinal purposes.

Chung CH: Human paragonimiasis. *In* Marcial-Rojas RA (ed.): Pathology of Protozoal and Helminthic Diseases. Baltimore, The Williams & Wilkins Company, 1971, pp 504–535. *Profusely illustrated and very detailed description of the pathologic changes in this condition.*

Higashi K, Aoki H, Tatebayashi K, et al.: Cerebral paragonimiasis. J Neurosurg 33:515, 1971.

Monson MH, Koenig JW, Sach R: Successful treatment with praziquantel of six patients infected with the African lung fluke *Paragonimus uterobilateralis.* Am J Trop Med Hyg 32:371, 1983. *Describes the use of this drug in the West African species of Paragonimus.*

INTESTINAL HERMAPHRODITIC FLUKES

Fasciolopsiasis (*Fasciolopsis buski*)

Fasciolopsis buski is the largest intestinal fluke and is normally a parasite of pigs. Human infection is widespread in southern China, Southeast Asia, and the Indian subcontinent. The eggs are passed in the feces, and the miracidia are released and penetrate a snail. The cercariae encyst as metacercariae on edible water plants. Often the edible plants are peeled to remove the "skin," and the metacercariae are swallowed in the process. The larvae attach themselves to the upper small intestine, where they mature in about 4 weeks. The adult fluke measures about 3.0 cm by 1.2 cm.

CLINICAL MANIFESTATIONS. Many light infections are asymptomatic, but heavy loads of flukes produce symptoms, especially in children. The worm load may be up to several thousand. The flukes attach themselves to the duodenal and jejunal mucosa and produce symptoms by trauma, obstruction, and toxin production. Abdominal pain, gastrointestinal hemorrhage, diarrhea, and intestinal obstruction may occur. In severe cases, edema of the face, trunk, and legs, as well as ascites, may be present.

DIAGNOSIS. This rests on finding the large ova (135 μm × 80 μm) or on recovering the characteristic adult flukes in the stool. Difficulty may be encountered in distinguishing the ova of *F. hepatica* and *F. buski.* Eosinophilia is common and may exceed 50 per cent of the white cell count. In some centers, serologic and skin tests are available, but these are not sensitive and specific. Facial edema may require differentiation of fasciolopsiasis from trichinosis or the nephrotic syndrome.

TREATMENT. Praziquantel is the treatment of choice. The dosage is 75 mg per kilogram of body weight divided into three doses per day for 2 days. Personal prevention consists of avoidance of eating raw aquatic plants in endemic areas. Community prevention consists of eradicating the snails with molluscacides, public education, and prevention of fecal contamination of ponds.

Other Intestinal Hermaphroditic Flukes

Heterophyes heterophyes and *Metagonimus yokogawai* are small flukes that are acquired by eating raw or undercooked fish that contain the metacercariae. The former is found in Egypt, Tunisia, southern China, India, and the Philippines, and the latter in the Far East and Indonesia. The adult fluke is 2 to 3 mm long and attaches itself to the intestinal mucosa. Usually, the infection is light, and there are few symptoms. Very rarely, the eggs gain access to the circulation and may be found in the organs. As a rule, the eggs are passed in the stool; they closely resemble *Clonorchis* eggs. Infection by both flukes can be treated with praziquantel. Differentiation of the two species requires examination of the adult flukes by experts. Many species of the genus *Echinostoma* infect humans in the Far East, but they rarely produce symptoms. *Gastrodiscoides hominis* occurs in India and Malaysia and may cause diarrhea. In western Canada,

the eggs of *Metorchis conjunctus,* which are somewhat similar to those of *Clonorchis,* are occasionally found in the stools of humans who eat raw fish. If treatment is required, praziquantel (75 mg per kilogram of body weight in three divided doses for 1 day) is the treatment of choice.

Alaria americana is an intestinal trematode of carnivores, such as the fox, wolf, lynx, or skunk. Two cases of human infection by the mesocercariae of this fluke have been reported in Ontario. The mesocercaria is a stage of development between the cercaria and the metacercaria. The cercariae emerging from the snail penetrate tadpoles. As the tadpole grows into a frog, the mesocercariae tend to concentrate in the hind legs. When the frog is eaten by a carnivore, the mesocercariae develop into metacercariae and adult flukes in the lung and the gut, respectively. When humans, who are not the normal host, eat the frog, the mesocercariae migrate all over the body. In the first reported case, the mesocercaria was surgically removed from the retina of the eye. The second case was a fatal systemic infection manifested by severe respiratory distress, coma, coagulation abnormality, and vasculitis. At autopsy, mesocercariae were found in all organs. The diagnosis is made by biopsy of affected organs. No effective treatment is known, although praziquantel may be useful.

Faust EC, Beaver PC, Jung RC: Intestinal flukes. *In* Faust EC, Beaver PC, Jung RC: Animal Agents and Vectors of Human Disease. 4th ed. Philadelphia, Lea & Febiger, 1975, pp 134–141. *A good reference for the less important parasites. Emphasis is on the parasitology, life cycles, and morphology.*

Fernandes BJ, Cooper JD, Cullen JB, et al.: Systemic infection with *Alaria americana* (Trematoda). Can Med Assoc J 115:1111, 1976. *The first report of generalized infection with mesocercariae of this fluke. Good description of the clinical course and autopsy findings.*

436 Nematode Infections

James W. Kazura

Nematodes (phylum Nematoda), or roundworms, include a vast number of species of free-living and parasitic helminths of plants and animals. These multicellular organisms differ markedly from unicellular bacteria and protozoa in that they have well-differentiated organ systems with specialized nervous, muscular, gastrointestinal, and reproductive functions. Parasitic nematodes are nonsegmented worms varying in length from several millimeters to approximately 2 meters. Nematodes have four larval stages and adult worms of both sexes. With the exception of *Strongyloides* and a few other helminths of medical importance, larval forms are produced after mating of sexually mature adult parasites, which by themselves are incapable of multiplying in the mammalian host. The inability of adult worms to replicate has important implications for the propensity of this class of organism to establish an infection and cause disease. Unlike the situation pertaining to bacterial, viral, or protozoan infections, casual or a low degree of exposure to infective stages of helminthic parasites generally does not result in patent infection or pathologic manifestations. Repeated or intense exposure to a large number of infective larvae is required for establishment of infection and development of disease.

Nematode infections are endemic in both temperate and tropical climates. They are transmitted either by the fecal-oral route or by inoculation of infective larvae into the skin, primarily by blood-feeding intermediate insect vectors. The prevalence of infection is greatest in circumstances conducive to the development and transmission of infective forms of the parasites, i.e., overcrowded, perennially warm geographic areas with poor sanitation, such as in many less developed countries of Africa, Asia, and Latin America and economically poor areas of North America and Europe.

The epidemiology of human nematode (as well as trematode and cestode) infections has several unique features. The infection in an endemic area has a negative binomial distribution, i.e., the majority of individuals in an endemic area have low parasite burdens and a small number harbor relatively high burdens.

Persons in the latter group have the greatest significance from an epidemiologic perspective in that they contribute most substantially to transmission and are most likely to develop pathologic manifestations. This characteristic implies that transmission in an endemic area may be decreased or interrupted by reduction of the parasite burden in a small proportion of the population. In addition, because total worm load correlates directly with the propensity to develop disease, treatment of lightly infected persons may not be indicated or may be unnecessary, especially if the available chemotherapy has major side effects.

Nematode infections of medical importance may be broadly classified into those in which the route of infection, larval migration, and disease manifestations are primarily gastrointestinal and those that affect other tissues. The former group includes hookworms (*Ancylostoma duodenale, Necator americanus*), the roundworm *Ascaris lumbricoides*, the pinworm *Enterobius vermicularis*, and the whipworm *Trichuris trichiuria*. Animal intestinal nematodes such as *Trichostrongylus* and *Anisakis* species also occasionally infect and cause disease in humans. *Trichinella spiralis, Strongyloides stercoralis*, and *Angiostrongylus cantonensis* infect humans by the oral route, but disease manifestations are due primarily to migration in other tissues. Tissue-invasive nematodes include lymphatic filariae (*Wuchereria bancrofti, Brugia malayi*, and *B. timori*), skin-dwelling *Onchocerca volvulus* and *Loa loa*, and the guinea worm, *Dracunculus medinensis*.

Anderson RM, May RM: Helminthic infections of humans: Mathematical models, population dynamics, and control. Adv Parasitol 24:1, 1985. *An excellent discussion of the relationship of the biology of parasitic helminthic infections to their epidemiology and control strategies.*

INTESTINAL NEMATODES

These infections include hookworm disease, ascariasis, enterobiasis, trichuriasis, and rarely animal nematodiases. They are prevalent in temperate and tropical areas of the world, especially those that are overcrowded and have poor sanitation. Intestinal nematode infections have little morbidity in most cases and are easily treated with mebendazole.

Hookworm Disease

ETIOLOGY AND EPIDEMIOLOGY. The major hookworms that infect humans are *Ancylostoma duodenale* and *Necator americanus*. *A. ceylonicum* infection is less common and occurs primarily in the South Pacific. Animal hookworms such as *A. braziliense* and *Uncinaria stenocephala* do not undergo full development in incidentally exposed humans. Infection occurs when exposed skin maintains contact for several minutes with soil contaminated with parasite eggs containing viable larvae. Larvae penetrate the skin and subsequently migrate to and mature in the lungs. The parasites then break into the air spaces, ascend the trachea, and are swallowed. Adult worms mature in the upper small intestine and attach to the mucosa by their buccal capsules. Female worms release more than 10,000 eggs per day, which are passed in the stools and deposited in the soil. The prepatent period (duration of time between infection and passing of eggs in the feces) is 40 to 105 days. Adult hookworms have a lifespan of 2 to 5 years.

Hookworms infect over 1 billion persons worldwide. The highest prevalences of infection (80 to 100 per cent) occur in tropical and less developed countries, where environmental and socioeconomic conditions are especially favorable to transmission. These include warm, moist soil; lack of public sewage disposal systems; and the habit of walking barefoot. The higher prevalence of hookworm infection in children than adults results from more frequent exposure of skin to larvae in soil among children. As is the case in other intestinal nematode infections, acquired resistance is minimal or does not develop at all as a consequence of previous infection.

PATHOGENESIS AND CLINICAL MANIFESTATIONS. Hookworm disease is due primarily to gastrointestinal blood loss and attendant iron deficiency anemia. The latter correlates directly with the total worm burden. Adult worms attached to the mucosa of the upper small intestine digest ingested blood as well as cause focal bleeding mediated by helminth-derived proteases. *A. duodenale* is estimated to cause a blood loss of 0.3 ml per day

per worm; *N. americanus* induces loss of approximately 0.03 ml per day. Nutritional deficiencies secondary to coexisting conditions that result in low iron stores (e.g., malabsorption, insufficient dietary intake in children, and multiparous women) contribute significantly to morbidity. Hypoproteinemia has been reported in children with hookworm disease in less developed countries. This complication is most likely due to coexisting malnutrition rather than gastrointestinal disease caused by hookworm infestation per se. Abdominal signs or symptoms are not caused by hookworm infection.

Pruritus at the site of larval skin penetration ("ground itch") occurs occasionally. In the case of primary exposure, local itching and erythematous papules lasting 1 week develop. More intense pruritus, vesiculation, and edema of 2 to 3 weeks' duration may occur after repeated exposure to infective larvae. Migration of hookworm larvae through the lungs rarely causes pulmonary symptoms.

DIAGNOSIS. Hookworm infection is diagnosed by identification of the characteristic round eggs containing convoluted larvae. Direct smears of freshly passed stool using the Kato or other techniques are satisfactory for the diagnosis of moderately to heavily infected cases (more than 400 eggs per gram).

TREATMENT AND PREVENTION. Mebendazole, administered orally at a dosage of 100 mg twice daily for 3 days, is the treatment of choice. Iron supplementation should be included if the degree of anemia and complicating illnesses warrant it. Administration of mebendazole to pregnant women should be delayed until after delivery. Light infections (feces with fewer than 400 eggs per gram) do not cause blood loss sufficient to induce iron deficiency. Therefore, in the absence of the complicating factors discussed above, individuals with such infections do not require anthelminthic chemotherapy. The ideal method for preventing hookworm infection is improvement of hygienic conditions. Use of footwear, especially by children, is currently the only practical means of avoiding infection.

Ascariasis

ETIOLOGY AND EPIDEMIOLOGY. *Ascaris lumbricoides* are roundworms 2 to 3 cm in length that reside in the lumen of the jejunum and in the mid-ileum. Infection occurs by the oral route when soil containing embryonated eggs is ingested. Larvae are released from eggs in the small intestine, penetrate the gut, and migrate to the liver and then lungs via the blood or lymphatic circulation. Following maturation in the lungs over a 4-week period, the parasites ascend the respiratory tract and are swallowed. Adult worms reach sexual maturity (i.e., female worms release eggs that are detectable in feces) approximately 60 days after infection.

Ascariasis affects approximately one quarter of the world's population and is likely the most prevalent helminthiasis of humans. Infection is common in Africa, Asia, and Latin America, especially in areas of high population density and unhygienic conditions. The use of human feces as fertilizer, defecation in soil, and hand-to-mouth contact with contaminated soil are major factors that contribute to the spread of *Ascaris*. The ability of *Ascaris* eggs to remain viable in harsh environmental conditions (embryonated eggs remain infectious after exposure to freezing temperatures and desiccation for several weeks) also facilitates transmission.

PATHOGENESIS AND CLINICAL MANIFESTATIONS. Disease caused by *A. lumbricoides* is infrequent and generally correlates with the intensity of infection. The majority of infected individuals are asymptomatic.

Symptomatic cases can be divided into two broad categories based on the phase of infection and site of pathology, i.e., pulmonary or gastrointestinal tract. Pulmonary disease is caused by the migration of larvae in the small vessels of the lung and their subsequent rupture into alveoli. Tissue damage is thought to be due to the host immune response, which includes production of immunoglobulin E (IgE) and eosinophilia. Transient pulmonary infiltrates, fever, cough, dyspnea, and eosinophilia lasting 1 to several weeks are the major clinical manifestations. This complex of symptoms and signs is frequently seasonal and coincidental with environmental changes that favor development of infective-stage larvae in eggs (e.g., spring rains that follow cold and dry periods). Intestinal signs and symptoms are due either to obstruction caused by the presence of an exceptionally large number of parasites in the small intestine or to migration of adult worms to unusual sites, such as the biliary tree or pancreatic duct. Intestinal obstruction almost always occurs in children less than 6 years old. The onset is sudden and characterized by colicky abdominal pain and vomiting. Heavily infected children are also prone to biliary disease or pancreatitis secondary to lodging of *Ascaris* in the ducts draining these organs. A malabsorption syndrome characterized by steatorrhea and low vitamin A levels has been reported in Latin American children with ascariasis.

DIAGNOSIS. Intestinal infection is diagnosed by the presence of the typical oval, thick-shelled *Ascaris* eggs in thick smears of fecal specimens. The existence of adult worms in pancreatic or biliary ducts should be suspected in children who have high egg outputs in conjunction with jaundice or pancreatitis. Pulmonary ascariasis cannot be diagnosed on the basis of identification of ova in feces because adult worms have not yet matured and reached the intestinal tract. Biopsy of the lung is unlikely to demonstrate larvae and is not recommended.

TREATMENT AND PREVENTION. Uncomplicated intestinal ascariasis is treated with mebendazole (100 mg orally twice per day for 3 days). Children with heavy infections or those with biliary tract obstruction should be given piperazine (50 to 75 mg per kilogram of body weight per day for 2 days), which causes neuromuscular paralysis of the worms and expulsion of intact helminths. No specific treatment is recommended for pulmonary ascariasis because the condition is self-limited.

The major means of preventing *Ascaris* infection is improvement of hygienic and socioeconomic conditions. Mass chemotherapy has been successful in reducing worm loads, but frequent retreatments are required.

Enterobiasis

Enterobius vermicularis or pinworm infection is cosmopolitan in its distribution. It is especially common in overcrowded settings and spreads rapidly in conditions in which person-to-person contact is frequent, such as in institutions for children.

Infection occurs by the fecal-oral route. Embryonated eggs carried on the fingernails, bed clothing, or bedding are ingested and hatch in the upper small intestine. Larvae subsequently pass distally and develop in the large bowel into adult parasites measuring 2 to 5 mm in length. Female worms migrate nightly out of the rectum and deposit large numbers of ova (11,000 per worm) in the perianal and perineal areas. Larvae in the deposited eggs become infective within several hours of exposure to ambient oxygen. Infectivity is usually maintained for 1 to 2 days.

The vast majority of pinworm infections are asymptomatic or associated with perianal pruritus and consequent sleep deprivation. *E. vermicularis* is a rare cause of appendicitis and, when the adult worms follow an aberrant path of migration, vulvovaginitis, urethritis, or peritonitis.

The diagnosis of pinworm infection is easily made by identification of ova on a piece of cellophane tape applied to the perirectal area in the morning. *E. vermicularis* eggs are oval and slightly flattened on one side. It is unusual to find eggs in feces or adult worms in the perianal area. Repeated examinations may be necessary.

Treatment is by administration of a single dose of mebendazole (100 mg one time) to affected individuals as well as close associates, such as family members. Several treatments may be required (every 3 to 4 months) if exposure continues, such as in institutional settings. Although personal cleanliness is recommended as a means of limiting transmission of enterobiasis, there is no clear-cut demonstration that it prevents infection.

Trichuriasis

Trichuris trichiura or whipworm infection is similar to pinworm infection in that it is limited to the gastrointestinal tract and does not have a tissue migratory phase. Eggs containing infective larvae mature in warm, moist soil over a 2-week period. Ingested eggs hatch in the small bowel and subsequently develop in epithelial cells of the cecum and ascending colon into adult worms that are 40 mm in length. The body of the parasite protrudes into the colonic lumen. Its anterior portion has a whiplike shape.

As is the case with most intestinal nematode infections, trichuriasis is most common in overcrowded areas with poor sanitation. The estimated prevalence worldwide is 800 million, with approximately 2 million cases in the southern United States. Children are more frequently infected than adults and also more likely to have higher worm burdens.

Adults with trichuriasis are usually asymptomatic. In children with heavy infections (more than 10,000 eggs per gram of feces), a syndrome of dysentery, growth retardation, and rectal prolapse has been described. The pathologic manifestations include infiltrates of eosinophils and neutrophils accompanied by epithelial denudation. Complicating diseases such as shigellosis and amebiasis may contribute to this condition in children.

Whipworm infection is diagnosed by identification of football-shaped eggs in direct smears of fecal specimens. Mebendazole at the same dosage indicated for ascariasis is satisfactory treatment.

Other Animal Nematodiases

Humans may serve as paratenic hosts for several nematodes that ordinarily parasitize the intestine of other mammals. Able to complete their life cycle in their natural hosts, these helminths are incapable of doing so in humans and display aberrant immigration patterns in both intestinal and nonintestinal tissues.

Several species of the genus *Trichostrongylus* infect both humans and domestic ruminants. The infection is found widely in the Middle and Far East and Australia. Ova are passed in the stool of ruminants and hatch in the soil. Humans are incidentally infected when larvae are ingested with leafy vegetables. The adult worms live in the intestines and suck small amounts of blood; heavy infections result in anemia. Diagnosis is made by identifying ova, which resemble those of hookworm, in the stool. Treatment is with thiabendazole, 25 mg per kilogram of body weight twice a day for 2 days.

Anisakis is an intestinal nematode of marine mammals. Several species of saltwater fish are intermediate hosts. Human infection occurs when raw fish is eaten. The larvae of both *Anisakis* and *Phocanemia decipiens* have been implicated. Most cases have been reported in Japan or Western Europe, particularly Scandinavia. The larvae invade the wall of the small intestine or stomach, causing pain and, rarely, intestinal obstruction or perforation. Gastric anisakiasis can be diagnosed endoscopically and treated by removal of the worms. Intestinal anisakiasis often resembles an acute abdomen, leading to laparotomy. Thiabendazole, 25 mg per kilogram twice a day for 3 days, may be given if surgical intervention is not required. Infection is prevented by cooking or freezing fish prior to eating.

Capillaria philippinensis infection has been reported from the Philippines and Thailand. This nematode is thought to parasitize birds, with fish and crustaceans serving as intermediate hosts. Humans are infected by eating the raw intermediate hosts. The ingested larvae mature and live in the crypts of the small intestine, where they reproduce. The result is often a heavy infection; up to 40,000 adult worms have been recovered at one autopsy. The clinical syndrome includes severe malabsorption and protein-losing enteropathy. The diagnosis is made by finding eggs or larvae in the stool; an intradermal test is also available. The treatment of choice is mebendazole, 200 mg twice a day for 20 days; an alternative is thiabendazole, 25 mg per kilogram daily for 30 days. Supportive care, such as fluid and electrolyte replacement and a high-protein diet, is also important.

Gnathostoma spinigerum is an intestinal nematode of dogs and cats; fish are intermediate hosts. The infection is endemic in rodents in the Far East and Thailand. Human infection has also been reported in South America. Infective larvae are ingested by humans in raw or undercooked fish. The larvae do not complete their life cycle in humans but migrate through the body. The most frequent site is subcutaneous tissues, where larvae are found in eosinophilic granulomas. A few weeks after infection, pruritic or painful subcutaneous nodules and swellings appear. These may be migratory and develop into abscesses. In central nervous system gnathostomiasis, hemorrhagic tracts may be found in the brain. Fever, vomiting, and abdominal pain occur a few days after ingestion of larvae. Paralysis of the extremities, encephalitis, and subarachnoid hemorrhage have been reported. Eye involvement with uveitis and orbital cellulitis represents a third variety.

Peripheral eosinophilia is usual in cutaneous gnathostomiasis; the diagnosis may be established by biopsy. In central nervous system infection, blood eosinophilia is an inconstant feature, but eosinophils are present in the cerebrospinal fluid, as in the case of angiostrongyliasis. Treatment of subcutaneous lesions consists of surgical removal. For central nervous system infection, mebendazole, 200 mg every 3 hours for 6 days, may be given. The infection may be prevented by cooking fish thoroughly before eating.

Several nematodes that ordinarily parasitize the intestine of monkeys occasionally infect humans. *Oesophagostomum* has been reported from Africa, Asia, and Brazil; it is responsible for the formation of granulomas in the intestinal wall. *Ternidens diminutus* is sometimes found in the human colon in Africa and Asia; a heavy infection may cause anemia. *Physaloptera mordens,* also reported from Africa, may attach itself to the esophagus, stomach, or small intestine of humans. The definitive host of *Lagochilascaris minor* is unknown. About 30 human cases have been reported from Central and South America, usually with worms invading the soft tissues of the neck and throat and sinuses.

Khuroo MS, Zargar SA, Mahajan R: Sonographic appearances in biliary ascariasis. Gastroenterology 93:267, 1987. *A discussion of the ultrasound appearance of this unusual but clinically important aspect of ascariasis.*
Pawlowski ZS: Ascariasis: Host-pathogen biology. Rev Infect Dis 4:806, 1982. *Reviews the basic biology and host interactions of Ascaris.*
Schad GH, Banwell JG: Hookworms. *In* Warren KS, Mahmoud AAF (eds.): Tropical and Geographical Medicine. New York, McGraw-Hill, 1990. *A general review of biology, clinical aspects, and epidemiology of hookworm infection. Synthesizes a large amount of confusing literature.*
Schultz MG: Ascariasis: Nutritional implications. Rev Infect Dis 4:815, 1982. *Reviews the basic biology and host interactions of Ascaris.*
Smith JW, Wootten R: Anisakis and anisakiasis. Adv Parasitol 16:93, 1978. *An exceptionally complete review.*

TOXOCARIASIS

DEFINITION. Visceral larva migrans (VLM) and ocular larva migrans (OLM) are caused by ingestion and subsequent development and migration of embryonated eggs of the canine roundworm *Toxocara canis.* Roundworms of cats (*T. cati*) and raccoons (*Baylisascaris procyonis*) also rarely cause VLM.

ETIOLOGY. In its normal canine host, *T. canis,* ingested embryonated eggs follow a route of migration similar to that described for *Ascaris,* i.e., larvae penetrate the small intestinal mucosa, migrate to the lungs, are reswallowed, and develop into adult worms in the small intestine; the adult worms lodge there and release eggs that are passed in the feces. When embryonated *T. canis* eggs are ingested by humans, larvae also migrate throughout the body (lung, liver, brain, muscles, and occasionally eyes) but fail to complete development to the adult stage. Tissue necrosis secondary to penetrating larvae and associated host inflammatory reactions, such as eosinophil-rich granulomas, are the underlying cause of disease.

EPIDEMIOLOGY. Toxocariasis is endemic in both temperate and tropical areas of the world. The vast majority of symptomatic cases occur in young children. This age group is most likely to be infected by virtue of frequent and intimate handling of dogs (especially newborn puppies that may be hyperinfected), playing in areas where dogs and cats defecate (e.g., public sandboxes), and the habit of geophagia. The potential of exposure to embryonated eggs is high in that *T. canis* infection is common in dogs (a 20 per cent infection rate in dogs in the United States).

CLINICAL MANIFESTATIONS. The vast majority of children who ingest *T. canis* eggs are asymptomatic. VLM is the most common clinically defined entity attributable to *T. canis.* It is most frequent in children less than 5 years old (there are no published series of adults with VLM) and is characterized by fever less than 39°C; pulmonary symptoms, including wheezing and cough; and, less frequently, pain in the right upper quadrant. These symptoms have a gradual onset and resolve over 4 to 8 weeks. Physical signs include wheezing and hepatomegaly in about one quarter of cases. Larvae less commonly migrate to the brain and heart and cause focal neurologic defects and heart failure.

OLM has an incidence approximately one-tenth that of VLM and affects children older than 8 to 10 years. Visual disturbances due to VLM are not distinguishable from other causes of focal intraretinal granulomas or space-occupying lesions, such as tuberculosis and retinoblastoma. *T. canis* larvae may migrate intraretinally and produce transient and recurrent impairment of vision.

DIAGNOSIS AND TREATMENT. VLM is diagnosed on the basis of suspicion of ingestion of *T. canis* eggs in a child with the symptoms described above. Eosinophilia, elevated erythrocyte sedimentation rate, and generalized hypergammaglobulinemia are also consistent with the diagnosis. Biopsy to document the presence of larvae is insensitive and not recommended. An enzyme-linked immunosorbent assay (ELISA) for measurement of anti-*Toxocara* antibodies is helpful if elevated immunoglobulin M (IgM) antibodies and a rise in titer between acute and convalescent phases are documented. Most cases of VLM are not life threatening and are self-limited. Treatment is therefore not required. In persons with severe pulmonary, cardiac, or neurologic involvement and high-grade eosinophilia (more than 10,000 per cubic millimeter of blood), albendazole (200 mg twice daily for 10 to 20 days) and corticosteroids may be used with the aim of reducing symptoms and shortening the course of the illness. No controlled studies, however, demonstrate the efficacy of this approach.

OLM represents a diagnostic dilemma in that it must be distinguished from intraretinal neoplasms and infections. Expert ophthalmologic consultation is necessary. Computerized tomography and fluorescein angiography are helpful in diagnosis. Elevated anti-*Toxocara* antibody titers in aqueous fluid relative to serum values are consistent with OLM. It is unclear if administration of anthelminthics is useful for the treatment of OLM.

VLM and OLM may be prevented by periodic deworming of dogs, especially puppies, and limiting their defecation in public places.

Glickman LT, Schantz PM, Cypess RH: Epidemiologic characteristics and clinical findings in patients with serologically proven toxocariasis. Trans R Soc Trop Med Hyg 73:254, 1979. *An excellent description of the major clinical manifestations of toxocariasis.*

CUTANEOUS LARVA MIGRANS

Animal hookworms, most frequently the dog parasite *Ancylostoma braziliense* and less commonly *Uncinaria stenocephala* and *Bunostomum phlebotomum,* are the major etiologic agents of cutaneous larva migrans, or creeping eruption. *Ancylostoma duodenale, Necator americanus,* and *Strongyloides stercoralis* may produce a similar syndrome during the phase of infection that involves penetration of the skin.

The disease occurs when skin comes into direct and prolonged contact with hookworm larvae contained in the feces of dogs, cats, or humans. Moist areas visited by animals, such as vegetation near beaches and exposed soil covered by porches, are common sites in which humans may be infected. Cutaneous larva migrans in the United States is most prevalent in southern coastal regions.

Clinical manifestations result from penetration and migration of larvae in the epidermal-dermal junction of the skin. Within several hours of contact with exposed skin, the patient notes pruritus and development of raised erythematous serpiginous lesions. The lesions migrate approximately 1 cm per day and evolve into bullae. Multiple lesions may appear if large areas of the body have been exposed, as in sunbathing. The extremities are the most common area of the body affected.

Creeping eruption may be treated by topical application of thiabendazole oral suspension. This may be prepared by trituration of a 500-mg tablet in 5 grams of petroleum jelly. If untreated, cutaneous larva migrans is self-limited, with resolution of signs and symptoms in several weeks to 2 months.

ANGIOSTRONGYLIASIS

Angiostrongylus cantonensis is a cause of eosinophilic meningitis in Asia and the South Pacific. Small numbers of cases have also been reported in Cuba and Africa. *Angiostrongylus costaricensis* is a rare cause of gastrointestinal bleeding. The nematode is limited in its distribution to Central and South America. Humans are infected with these rodent (primarily rat) nematodes following ingestion of poorly cooked or raw intermediate mollusc hosts, such as snails, slugs, and prawns. Fresh vegetables may also be contaminated with infective larvae and serve as a vehicle of infection.

In the case of *A. cantonensis* infection, ingested infective larvae penetrate the gut wall and migrate to small vessels of the meninges and, less commonly, the spinal cord and eye. An intense local inflammatory reaction ensues within 1 week. Fever, meningismus, and headache develop in association with eosinophilic pleocytosis of the cerebrospinal fluid. Strabismus, paresthesias, and vomiting have been observed in a minority of cases. Diagnosis is based on a history of ingesting potentially contaminated foodstuffs and the presence of eosinophils in cerebrospinal fluid. Larvae are usually not found in cerebrospinal fluid. Other less common causes of eosinophilic meningitis of infectious etiology include *Trichinella spiralis*, *Taenia solium*, *Toxocara canis*, *Gnathostoma spinigerum*, and *Paragonimus westermani*. Symptomatic *A. cantonensis* infection resolves over a 2-week period. The value of administering specific anthelminthic therapy or corticosteroids has not been established.

A. costaricensis larvae penetrate the mucosa of the terminal ileum, appendix, and ascending colon. The larvae subsequently develop into adult worms in the local lymphatics and mesenteric arterioles. Eggs released by the female worms elicit multiple eosinophil-rich granulomatous reactions that cause edematous, thickened bowel and necrosis (secondary to mesenteric blood vessel obstruction). Clinical presentations typically include right-sided abdominal pain, vomiting, and fever. Abnormal laboratory findings include leukocytosis with eosinophilia (at least 10 per cent, with a white cell count greater than 10,000 per cubic millimeter). Parasite larvae and eggs are not present in stools. A palpable mass secondary to granulomatous lesions may be present and cause intestinal obstruction. Less frequently, gastrointestinal bleeding is the principal manifestation. Treatment is surgical. There is no demonstrated benefit of specific anthelminthic chemotherapy.

Koo J, Pien F, Kliks MM: *Angiostrongylus (Parastrongylus) eosinophilic meningitis.* Rev Infect Dis 10:1155, 1988. *An excellent discussion of the biology of the helminth and the clinical manifestations of human infection.*

Silvera CT, Ghali VS, Heimann J, et al.: Angiostrongyliasis: A rare cause of gastrointestinal hemorrhage. Am J Gastroenteral 84:329, 1988. *A case report of* A. costaricensis *infection and excellent discussion of clinical manifestations of this uncommon infection.*

TRICHINOSIS

DEFINITION. Infection of humans by *Trichinella spiralis* occurs when viable infective larvae are eaten in undercooked pork or other meats. The majority of infected individuals are asymptomatic. Clinical manifestations in heavily infected persons include diarrhea, myalgias, fever, and, less commonly, myocarditis and neurologic disease. Trichinosis occurs in all areas of the world, including the Arctic and temperate regions. The incidence of trichinosis in the United States has decreased markedly over the past several decades.

ETIOLOGY. Infection is initiated by ingestion of infective larvae encysted in striated muscle. Excystment occurs in the acid-pepsin environment of the stomach, and parasites develop into sexually mature adult worms in the upper to middle small intestine of the human host. Completion of the enteric phase of the parasite life cycle takes about 1 week, with adult worms remaining viable and productive of larval offspring for an additional 3 to 5 weeks. The systemic phase commences 1 week after infection, when larvae released by female worms migrate through blood vessels and lymphatics and invade multiple organ systems. Mature third-stage larvae develop in host-derived nurse cells in striated skeletal and cardiac muscle, where they become encysted and remain viable for years. As is the case with most helminthiases, the severity of symptoms is related to the total parasite load. Because adult worms are incapable of reproducing themselves, the number of infective larvae ingested is the most important determinant of worm load (i.e., number of larvae that invade muscle and other tissues).

EPIDEMIOLOGY. *T. spiralis* infection is enzootic in omnivorous and carnivorous animal populations, including rats, bears, and aquatic mammals of the Arctic. The nematode is introduced into domestic animals such as pigs and horses by feeding them garbage containing carcasses of these animals, most commonly rats. Human infection usually occurs in two settings: first, when undercooked or smoked pork products or beef contaminated with nematodes are eaten, and second, when flesh of poorly cooked wild game, such as bear or boar meat, is ingested. An important

source of infection in Alaskan and Canadian Arctic native populations is uncooked walrus meat.

The annual incidence of human trichinosis in the United States has decreased from more than 450 in 1947–1949 to fewer than 56 between 1982 and 1986. This decline is primarily due to fewer cases related to ingestion of commercial pork products. Recent cases in the United States occur in point-source outbreaks associated with ingestion of game or noncommercial pork products.

PATHOGENESIS AND CLINICAL MANIFESTATIONS. Tissue-invasive *T. spiralis* larvae elicit an eosinophilic granulomatous reaction that may result in significant end-organ tissue damage and dysfunction. Skeletal muscle is the most frequent site involved. Myocardial damage, pulmonary infiltration, and focal neurologic damage secondary to invasion by larvae are seen in only the most heavily infected persons. The systemic phase of infection usually occurs 2 to 3 weeks after ingestion of infective larvae and may last for 2 months. Clinical manifestations typically include myalgias (especially of the gastrocnemius and masseter), periorbital edema, and fever. Myocardial damage may manifest as heart failure or dysrhythmias.

The enteric phase of infection may also cause gastrointestinal signs and symptoms, such as diarrhea and abdominal cramps. These typically occur within 1 week of eating contaminated meat and last less than 2 weeks. Reports from the Canadian Arctic suggest that the *T. spiralis* larvae that infect walrus meat may cause diarrhea of 1 to 3 months' duration in the absence of myalgias or other signs of larval invasion of deeper tissues.

DIAGNOSIS. A diagnosis of trichinosis should be considered in individuals with generalized myalgias and eosinophilia (more than 600 eosinophils per cubic millimeter). Serologic testing for *T. spiralis* antibodies is available at the Centers for Disease Control. Elevation of IgM antibodies or a more than fourfold rise in titer between acute and convalescent phases of infection is helpful in diagnosis. The levels of creatine phosphate kinase and of serum immunoglobulins and the erythrocyte sedimentation rate are also increased for several weeks after infection. Muscle biopsy (e.g., of the gastrocnemius) may demonstrate larvae, although their absence does not exclude the diagnosis. Most important to consider in the differential diagnosis of trichinosis are the eosinophilia-myalgia syndrome associated with L-tryptophan and idiopathic hypereosinophilic syndrome.

TREATMENT AND PREVENTION. If patients present at a time when adult parasites are in the intestine (i.e., during the initial 1 to 2 weeks after infection, when gastrointestinal symptoms are prominent), thiabendazole is recommended at a dosage of 25 mg per kilogram of body weight twice a day for 1 week. Larvae in muscle are not killed by this drug, and treatment is primarily symptomatic with antipyretics and analgesics. Although there are too few recent cases to establish clearly a possible beneficial effect of corticosteroids, they may be useful to diminish the severity of inflammation when signs of myocarditis, neurologic disease (e.g., seizures, focal weakness), or pulmonary insufficiency develop. *T. spiralis* infection is prevented by killing larvae in meat products. This is achieved by heating to 80.5°C. Freezing, smoking, or exposure to microwave does not reliably kill the helminth.

Bailey TM, Schantz PM: Trends in the incidence and transmission patterns of trichinosis in humans in the United States. Comparisons of the periods 1975–1981 and 1982–1986. Rev Infect Dis 12:5, 1990. *A comprehensive review of the epidemiology of trichinosis.*

MacLean JD, Viallet J, Law C, et al.: Trichinosis in the Canadian Arctic: Report of five outbreaks and a new clinical syndrome. J Infect Dis 160:513, 1989. *Excellent description of severe gastrointestinal manifestations of* T. spiralis *in a population in which the prevalence of trichinosis is among the highest in the world.*

STRONGYLOIDIASIS

DEFINITION. *Strongyloides stercoralis* infection is endemic in warm climates worldwide, including the southern United States. In immunologically normal individuals, infection is usually asymptomatic or causes gastrointestinal dysfunction, manifest as abdominal pain, bloating, or bleeding. Persons who have deficient cell-mediated immunity are permissive for development of an autoinfective and hyperinfective life cycle of the nematode that markedly increases the total worm load. Life-threatening acute pulmonary disease and organ dysfunction due to dissemination of larvae to aberrant sites such as the brain, pancreas, and kidneys may result in immunocompromised hosts.

ETIOLOGY. *S. stercoralis* infection occurs when skin contacts free-living filariform larvae in the soil. After penetrating the skin, the parasite embolizes to the small vessels of the lungs via the venous circulation. Rhabditiform larvae then break into the alveolar spaces, ascend the respiratory tree, and are swallowed. Further development to adult worms occurs in the duodenum and upper jejunum, where egg-laying parasites live in the mucosa and submucosa. Rhabditiform larvae are released from eggs and are passed from the body in stools. Infective filariform larvae develop in the soil by two alternative means, either by direct transformation from rhabditiform larvae or indirectly from free-living intermediate forms.

Several unusual features of the life cycle of *S. stercoralis* are critical to understanding how this parasitic nematode causes life-threatening disease. First, unlike the vast majority of human helminthic parasites, adult worms are only of the female sex and reproduce parthogenetically in the gastrointestinal tract. The total worm burden in the host may therefore be greatly expanded in the absence of repeated exposure to infective larvae in the environment. Second, rhabditiform larvae may develop into infective filariform larvae in the gastrointestinal tract as well as after passage in feces, as described above. Occurrence of the former process in immunocompromised hosts allows autoinfection, whereby larvae pass directly through the bowel (internal autoinfection) or perianal skin (external autoinfection) to reinitiate migration and development in the lungs. When this event is frequent, a hyperinfection syndrome ensues. Disseminated strongyloidiasis refers to a situation of hyperinfection in which the organisms also migrate to and cause pathology in organs not usually traversed by larvae, such as those of the central nervous system.

EPIDEMIOLOGY. *S. stercoralis* infection is endemic in Africa, Asia, Latin America, and areas of Eastern and Southern Europe. Prevalence rates based on examinations of stools for rhabditiform larvae vary from more than 40 per cent in areas of sub-Saharan Africa to 1 to 7 per cent in rural Eastern Europe. In the United States, the infection is endemic in rural Appalachia and other parts of the South. Prevalences range from 0.4 to 3 per cent in the United States. Refugees from Asia have a higher prevalence of infection than do indigenous Americans. Surveys of homosexual men conducted before 1980 indicate a frequency of infection of 3.9 per cent. It is likely that most studies of prevalence underestimate infection because they are based on examination of a single stool specimen, which is less sensitive than multiple examinations performed over days or weeks.

Strongyloidiasis is especially common in overcrowded situations in which sanitation and personal hygiene are poor, such as in institutions for retarded children and camps for prisoners of war. An unusually high frequency of *S. stercoralis* infection has also been reported in persons with asymptomatic human T cell lymphotropic virus (HTLV)–I infection.

PATHOGENESIS. Adult worms and larvae penetrating the upper small bowel cause an enteritis characterized histopathologically by eosinophil and mononuclear cell infiltration of the lamina propria. Edema and mucosal atrophy are present on gross examination. Ulcerative lesions with hemorrhages are present in the most severe cases. Filariform larvae in the lungs elicit an inflammatory response in the alveoli consisting of mononuclear cells and eosinophils. In hyperinfection syndrome, these may coalesce and result in alveolar hemorrhage.

Autoinfection leading to exceptionally high worm loads (hyperinfection) and disseminated strongyloidiasis occur in persons with deficient cell-mediated immunity. Groups at risk include persons who are chronically taking corticosteroids, renal transplant recipients, patients with Hodgkin's disease and other lymphomas, and leukemic patients. Because *S. stercoralis* may persist and remain asymptomatic for decades after exposure (e.g., in military veterans who were imprisoned in the South Pacific during World War II), it is important to keep in mind that a change in immune status may convert a previously asymptomatic infection to hyperinfection. Surprisingly, there is no clear-cut evidence that persons with acquired immunodeficiency syndrome (AIDS) have a propensity to develop disseminated strongyloidiasis, despite a higher frequency of infection in homosexual men.

CLINICAL MANIFESTATIONS. More than 50 per cent of immunocompetent infected persons are asymptomatic. The frequency of clinical manifestations among infected immunocompromised subjects is not known.

Signs and symptoms of *S. stercoralis* infection are attributable to the presence of adult worms in the upper gastrointestinal tract and larval invasion and attendant host pathologic responses in the lung, skin, and aberrant sites of migration, such as the brain, eyes, pancreas, and kidney. Immunocompetent individuals rarely develop signs or symptoms attributable to larval migration outside the gut.

Gastrointestinal disease usually manifests as abdominal bloating, vague epigastric pain, and diarrhea with nausea. Symptoms are exacerbated by eating. Hematochezia and melena occur in fewer than 20 per cent of subjects with intestinal strongyloidiasis. Major causes of morbidity related to *S. stercoralis* infection of the intestine are paralytic ileus, small bowel obstruction, and a malabsorption syndrome.

Pulmonary signs and symptoms in immunocompromised persons with hyperinfection syndrome are similar to those seen in the adult respiratory distress syndrome, i.e., acute onset of dyspnea, productive cough, and hemoptysis. These are accompanied by fever, tachypnea, hypoxemia, and respiratory alkalosis. *Strongyloides* larvae may also invade the central nervous system, pancreas, eye, and so on and cause signs and symptoms attributable to tissue destruction in these sites.

Dermatologic manifestations include self-limited creeping eruption and, more commonly, larva currens. The latter is due to migration of filariform larvae produced by a process of external autoinfection as described above. The larvae elicit serpiginous erythematous papules and occasionally urticaria around the buttocks, upper thigh, and lower abdomen. The lesions migrate approximately 10 cm per hour. Larva currens has been noted among former prisoners of war in the South Pacific.

DIAGNOSIS. The unequivocal diagnosis of *S. stercoralis* infection is dependent on identification of larvae in host tissues or gastrointestinal and pulmonary secretions. The existence of filariform larvae in stools implies an active autoinfection.

Intestinal strongyloidiasis is most easily diagnosed by identification of parasites in direct smears of freshly passed stools. Rhabditiform larvae are 225 to 380 μm in length. Repeated examinations and concentration of stools increase the sensitivity of this method from approximately 25 to 80 per cent. Examination of fluid obtained by duodenal aspiration or passage of a swallowed string into the upper small bowel may also be used if stool examinations are negative. Serologic tests are sensitive but not generally available. The differential diagnosis of intestinal *S. stercoralis* infection includes sprue, peptic ulcer, regional enteritis, and ulcerative colitis.

Hyperinfection syndrome and disseminated strongyloidiasis are diagnosed by identification of filariform larvae (500 to 600 μm in length) in gastrointestinal secretions, as described above, or in pulmonary tissues, secretions, or washings, such as those obtained by bronchoalveolar lavage or in sputum. Larvae have also been recovered from cerebrospinal fluid, peritoneal washings, kidneys, urine, skin, and brains of immunocompromised persons.

Accompanying laboratory abnormalities frequently include eosinophilia. However, eosinophilia may not develop in immunocompromised hosts. Lack of eosinophilia is therefore not helpful in excluding strongyloidiasis in the differential diagnosis. The differential diagnosis of hyperinfection and disseminated strongyloidiasis includes overwhelming bacterial or fungal sepsis.

COMPLICATIONS. Disseminated strongyloidiasis is frequently accompanied by fungal or bacterial sepsis. Gram-negative enterococcal and polymicrobial septicemia has been observed. These infections likely result from translocation of gut organisms by migrating larvae.

TREATMENT. Uncomplicated intestinal strongyloidiasis should be treated with thiabendazole (25 mg per kilogram of body weight twice daily for 2 days with a maximum of 3 grams per day). Parasitologic cure rates are greater than 90 per cent. Thiabendazole at the same daily dosage should be given to immunocompromised patients with hyperinfection syndrome (i.e., pulmonary disease) or disseminated disease. The drug should be continued for a minimum of 5 to 7 days, although 1 to 2 weeks may be required if organ dysfunction and larval recovery persist. Symptomatic improvement and failure to detect larvae in gastrointestinal secretions or other sites are indicative of cure. Corticosteroids and other immunosuppressive agents should be discontinued when possible.

PREVENTION. Infection is preventable by avoiding skin contact with contaminated soil. Immunocompromised patients in endemic areas should be advised to avoid walking barefoot. Persons residing in endemic areas who are to become immunosuppressed (e.g., for renal transplantation) should have their stools examined three times for the presence of larvae, and they should be treated if the examination is positive. Because infected individuals may be incorrectly categorized as uninfected by this test, it is suggested by some authorities that prophylactic thiabendazole (25 mg per kilogram of body weight daily for 2 days) be given in the month preceding iatrogenic immunosuppression. Positive serology for *S. stercoralis* is also an indication for thiabendazole administration prior to immunosuppression.

Cook GC: *Strongyloides stercoralis* hyperinfection syndrome: How often is it missed? Q J Med 64:625, 1987. *Discusses in detail the differential diagnosis and pitfalls in diagnosis of strongyloidiasis in the immunocompromised host.*

Neva FA: Biology and immunology of human strongyloidiasis. J Infect Dis 153:397, 1987. *An overview of the biology of* Strongyloides stercoralis *and utility of serodiagnostic tests.*

DeVault GA Jr, King JW, Rohr MS, et al.: Opportunistic infection with *Strongyloides stercoralis* in renal transplantation. Rev Infect Dis 12:653, 1990. *Excellent discussion of clinical presentation and management of hyperinfection in immunocompromised hosts.*

Genta RM: Global prevalence of strongyloidiasis: Critical review with epidemiologic insights into the prevention of disseminated disease. Rev Infect Dis 11:755, 1989. *Well-balanced synthesis of the validity of multiple epidemiologic surveys of strongyloidiasis in the United States and other areas of the world.*

437 Filariasis

437.1 INTRODUCTION

Eric A. Ottesen

Eight filarial parasites commonly infect humans (Table 437–1), but three are responsible for most of the pathology associated with these infections. These are the lymphatic dwelling filariae *Wuchereria bancrofti* and *Brugia malayi* and the subcutaneous filarid *Onchocerca volvulus.*

All eight species are transmitted by biting arthropods (Table 437–1) and go through complex life cycles that include a slow maturation phase of 3 to 18 months from the time infective larvae are introduced by the vector until the adult worms mature and reside in the lymph nodes, subcutaneous tissue, or body cavities. The offspring of these adults (microfilariae) are 200 to 300 μm long and 5 to 7 μm wide. They either circulate in the blood or migrate through the skin, awaiting ingestion by the appropriate arthropod in which they develop over 1 to 2 weeks to infective forms capable of initiating this life cycle again. Adult worms are long lived (probably up to 15 years), while microfilariae probably live about 6 months. Patent infection is generally not established unless exposure to infective larvae is intense and prolonged, and manifestations of disease usually develop slowly.

Diagnosis can be extremely difficult because in endemic populations it relies almost exclusively on parasitologic techniques to demonstrate microfilariae in the blood or tissue, and at present, there are no completely satisfactory methods for making a definitive diagnosis in states of "amicrofilaremic filariasis" (before or after the microfilaremic state). When microfilariae circulate in the blood, they do so with or without a distinct periodicity (Table 437–1). Some are garbed in sheaths while others are sheathless. These two features, as well as other more subtle morphologic distinctions, are helpful diagnostically. Microfilariae can be identified either by direct observation of Giemsa-stained blood smears or, more sensitively, by concentration techniques using Knott's method (examination of centrifuged sediment after mixing 1 ml of blood with 9 ml of 2 per cent formalin) or membrane filtration of 1 ml or more of blood through a 3-μm or 5-μm pore Nuclepore membrane filter. Skin microfilariae are best sought by performing skin snips either as described in Ch. 437.4 or using a corneal-scleral biopsy punch. Antibody detection, although helpful in certain situations, is generally nondiagnostic because it cannot differentiate current from past infection or exposure and because of antigenic cross-reactivity between the filariae and other helminth parasites.

Diethylcarbamazine (DEC)* has been the single mainstay of treatment for all filarial infections since the late 1940's; however, it shows variable effectiveness for the different conditions. The new drug ivermectin,† because of greater efficacy and fewer side effects, has replaced DEC as the drug of choice for onchocerciasis; it is currently under evaluation for use in lymphatic and other filariases. Suramin,† although extremely toxic, is also used for onchocerciasis.

Filariasis. Ciba Found Symp: 127:305, 1987. *A multiauthored compendium of the current forefronts of understanding in most aspects of the filarial diseases.*

Greene BM: Onchocerciasis. *In* Warren KS, Mahmoud AA (eds.): Tropical and Geographic Medicine. 2nd ed. New York, McGraw-Hill, 1990, pp 429–439. *Detailed clinical, parasitologic, and epidemiologic discussion of onchocercal infection and the new developments in its treatment and control.*

Ottesen EA: The filariases and tropical eosinophilia. *In* Warren KS, Mahmoud AA (eds.): Tropical and Geographical Medicine. 2nd ed. New York, McGraw-Hill, 1990, pp 407–429. *Detailed clinical, parasitologic, and epidemiologic discussion of filarial disease.*

*Not commercially available in the United States but may be obtained in special circumstances from Lederle Laboratories, Pearl River, NY.

†Available from the Centers for Disease Control, Parasitic Disease Drug Service, Atlanta, GA.

437.2 LYMPHATIC FILARIASIS

Eric A. Ottesen

ETIOLOGY. There are three lymphatic-dwelling filarial parasites of humans, *Wuchereria bancrofti*, *Brugia malayi*, and *Brugia timori*. Adult worms are threadlike in form (2 to 10 cm

TABLE 437–1. THE COMMON FILARIAL PARASITES OF HUMANS

Species	Distribution	Vector	Primary Pathology	Microfilariae Primary Location	Microfilariae Periodicity	Microfilariae Presence of Sheath
Wuchereria bancrofti	Tropics worldwide	Mosquitoes	Lymphatic, pulmonary	Blood, hydrocele fluid	Nocturnal, subperiodic	+
Brugia malayi	Southeast Asia	Mosquitoes	Lymphatic, pulmonary	Blood	Nocturnal, subperiodic	+
Brugia timori	Indonesia	Mosquitoes	Lymphatic	Blood	Nocturnal	+
Onchocerca volvulus	Africa; Central and South America	Black fly	Skin, eye, lymphatic	Skin, eye	None or minimal	−
Loa loa	Africa	Horse fly	Allergic	Blood	Diurnal	+
Mansonella perstans	Africa; South America	Midge	? Allergic	Blood	None	−
Mansonella streptocerca	Africa	Midge	Skin	Skin	None	−
Mansonella ozzardi	Central and South America	Midge	Vague	Blood	None	−

long by less than 0.4 cm wide) and usually reside in the lymph nodes or afferent lymphatic channels. The female worms produce large numbers of microfilariae (200 to 300 μm long), which circulate in the peripheral blood awaiting ingestion by mosquito intermediate hosts, which are necessary to continue the parasite's life cycle. After about 2 weeks in these mosquitoes, the microfilariae develop into infective third-stage larvae (L_3's). When infected mosquitoes feed, these L_3's leave the mosquito mouth parts and come to rest on the surface of the host's skin. Only if they manage to penetrate the skin through the puncture at the site of the bite can transmission be successful; after a further developmental period lasting as long as 4 to 12 months, adult worms can again be found in the lymphatic tissues, where they mate and produce another generation of microfilariae. The adult parasites may remain viable in the human host for decades.

EPIDEMIOLOGY. For *W. bancrofti,* humans are the only definitive host and thus the natural reservoir for infection. Indeed, considerable experimental effort to establish the parasite in a wide variety of mammalian hosts has met with minimal success. *W. bancrofti* is found throughout the tropics and subtropics, including areas of South America and the Caribbean, Africa, Asia, and the Pacific. Two forms of the parasite are distinguished by the periodicity of their circulating microfilariae. Nocturnally periodic forms have microfilariae detectable in peripheral blood primarily at night, whereas in the subperiodic forms the microfilariae are usually present in the blood at all hours but with maximal levels often in the late afternoon. Generally, subperiodic bancroftian filariasis is found only in the Pacific islands east of 160 degrees E longitude (including New Caledonia, Fiji, Samoa, Ellis and Cook Islands, Society Islands, and the Marquesas); elsewhere *W. bancrofti* is nocturnally periodic. The natural vectors are *Culex fatigans* in urban settings and usually anopheline or aedean mosquitoes in rural areas.

The distribution of brugian filariasis is much more restricted, being limited primarily to parts of Malaysia, Indonesia, India, China, Korea, the Philippines, and Japan. Again, there are both nocturnally periodic and subperiodic forms of the parasite. The former is more common and is transmitted in coastal rice fields primarily by mansonian and anopheline mosquitoes; mansonian mosquitoes, found in swamp forests, are the major vectors of the subperiodic form. Unlike *W. bancrofti, B. malayi* can be a natural infection of cats and can be established in a number of laboratory animals. *B. timori* has been described from only two Indonesian islands.

PATHOLOGY. Most of the pathology of bancroftian and brugian filariasis is initiated in the lymphatics. Although details of the pathogenesis are lacking, the progression of pathologic changes is clear. Damaged lymphatics lead first to reversible lymphedema and then to chronic obstructive changes (elephantiasis) in the limbs, breasts, or genitalia, or to chyluria. The location of lymphatic damage determines the site and type of pathology expressed.

Adult worms, residing in the afferent approaches or cortical sinuses of the lymph nodes, induce local reactions by undefined mechanisms that result in dilatation of the lymphatics and hypertrophy of the vessel walls. Endothelial and connective tissue proliferation leads to polypoid growths that protrude into the lymphatic lumen, but even while the vessels remain patent, normal lymphatic function is not ensured. Indeed, lymphangiographic studies have clearly documented the development of a characteristic tortuosity of the lymph vessels with loss of valvular function and backflow of lymph leading to lymph stasis and lymphedema even during this "preobliterative phase."

Because of a still undefined interplay between the host immune system and the parasite, local inflammatory and granulomatous reactions subsequently develop around the adult worms, with infiltration of plasma cells, eosinophils, and giant cells. Fibrosis occurs, and the fragmented parasites are either completely resorbed or partially calcified. Lymphatic obstruction develops, and associated endophlebitis may further complicate the lymphatic obstruction. Although there is subsequent formation of collateral lymphatics and some recanalization of obstructed vessels, lymphatic function remains compromised. Repeated infection with increasing host response to the parasite leads to the chronic changes of advanced elephantiasis.

CLINICAL MANIFESTATIONS. Though previously not well recognized, a major distinction exists between the clinical presentation of lymphatic filariasis in individuals native to the endemic regions (whose exposures have been lifelong) and that of those entering such areas and meeting the infection for the first time. In these latter (e.g., long-term visitors, military personnel, settlers) the most common presentations are localized inflammatory reactions, especially adenolymphangitis, and evidence of immediate hypersensitivity responses to the parasites (i.e., urticaria, eosinophilia, and immunoglobulin E [IgE] elevations). Only rarely do such individuals present with the contrasting set of findings characteristic of the infection in those native to the endemic areas, i.e., asymptomatic microfilaremia, "filarial fevers," lymphatic obstruction, and, less commonly, the tropical pulmonary eosinophilia syndrome (Ch. 437.3).

Patients manifesting asymptomatic microfilaremia rarely come to the physician's attention except through an incidental finding of microfilariae in the peripheral blood smear during mass surveys in endemic regions, or when blood eosinophilia leads to a diagnostic evaluation for filariasis. Such asymptomatic persons appear to be clinically unaffected by the parasites. Though unproven, it is likely that in some of these individuals the infections clear spontaneously, whereas the infections of others subsequently progress and become symptomatic, but what determines such clinical changes is unclear.

"Filarial fevers" are acute febrile episodes characterized by high temperature (often with shaking chills), lymphatic inflammation (i.e., lymphadenitis and lymphangitis), and transient local edema. They occur as often as 6 to 10 times per year in affected persons and usually last 3 to 7 days before subsiding spontaneously. The factors that initiate these episodes are unknown, but they are definitely parasite related. The lymphangitis characteristically develops in a retrograde fashion, extending peripherally *from* the draining node where the adult parasites reside. Regional nodes are enlarged and painful, and the entire lymphatic tract often becomes indurated and inflamed. Concomitant local thrombophlebitis is common. In brugian filariasis especially, a single local abscess may form along the inflamed lymphatic and subsequently rupture to the surface, leaving a characteristic scar. Neither the lymphatic inflammation nor the characteristic abscesses appear to be bacterially induced. Such lymphadenitis and lymphangitis occur in the upper and lower extremities with both bancroftian and brugian filariasis, but involvement of the genital lymphatics is almost exclusively a feature of *W. bancrofti* infection. Thus, acute *bancrofti* episodes may also involve funiculitis, epididymitis, scrotal pain, and tenderness. Patients with filarial fevers may be microfilaremic but more often are not.

As lymphatic damage progresses, the edema and anatomic distortion that were initially transient develop into the permanent changes of elephantiasis. Pitting edema yields to brawny edema, and both thickening of subcutaneous tissue and hyperkeratosis develop. Fissuring of the skin develops along with nodular and papillomatous hyperplastic changes. Superinfection (especially with the dermatophytes) becomes a problem. In addition, in bancroftian filariasis, obstructed genital lymphatics may lead to scrotal lymphedema or hydrocele, whereas obstruction of the retroperitoneal lymphatics can increase hydrostatic pressure in the renal lymphatics, causing their rupture into the renal pelvis or tubules and leading to chyluria. Characteristically, chyluria is intermittent, sometimes lasting for days or weeks before abating spontaneously and then recurring; often it is most prominent in the morning, after the patient first arises.

DIAGNOSIS. Definitive diagnosis of filariasis can be made only by the demonstration of parasites, either adult worms associated with the lymphatics (rarely observed) or microfilariae in the blood, hydrocele fluid, or chylous urine. These fluids can be examined directly (20 cu mm on a slide with or without red blood cell lysis), after concentration of the parasites by centrifugation in 2 per cent formalin (Knott's technique), or after filtration through a membrane (3- to 5-μm Nuclepore) filter. The time of blood collection should take into account the parasite's possible nocturnal periodicity.

Because many persons with filariasis (especially those with chronic pathology) are not microfilaremic, diagnosis must often be made clinically. The differential diagnosis is broad but in the acute episodes primarily includes thrombophlebitis, infection, and trauma. The edema and other lymphatic obstructive changes associated with chronic filariasis must be distinguished from the manifestations of congestive heart failure, malignant disease, trauma, postsurgical scarring, and a number of less common congenital and idiopathic abnormalities of the lymphatic system. The many disorders associated with serum immunoglobulin E (IgE) and blood eosinophil elevations must be considered in evaluating asymptomatic filarial infections. Several specific points may help in this differential diagnosis: (1) Exposure to filariae must be prolonged or intense (for at least several months) before persons become infected; (2) the physical finding or history of *retrograde* lymphangitis can often aid in distinguishing filarial from bacterial lymphangitis; (3) although lymphadenopathy is characteristic of filariasis, alone it is never diagnostic; (4) lymphangiographic patterns of elephantiasis and chyluria are well defined, so that even though not always diagnostic, lymphangiography is sometimes useful in distinguishing filarial from congenital or neoplastic lymphatic abnormalities; (5) although total serum IgE and blood eosinophil levels are often elevated in filarial infections, they cannot distinguish filarial from other helminth infections except in the case of the tropical eosinophilia syndrome (see Ch. 437.3); and (6) because most residents of endemic regions have been immunologically "sensitized" to filarial antigens through years of bites by infected mosquitoes and because filarial antigens cross-react extensively with those of other nematode parasites, positive results in the numerous serologic and skin tests that have been developed are of little diagnostic value *except* in those individuals who are not native to endemic areas.

TREATMENT. Available chemotherapy for lymphatic filariasis is both limited and inadequate. Diethylcarbamazine* (DEC, 6 mg per kilogram per day given in single or divided doses for 2 to 3 weeks) rapidly kills microfilariae in vivo, but its effect on adult parasites is less dramatic. Thus, following treatment with DEC, although the blood is temporarily free of microfilariae, the infection itself has often not been terminated, and several courses of DEC or long-term intermittent treatment with low doses of DEC are often required to kill the adult parasites. Early trials with ivermectin† in bancroftian and brugian filariasis indicate excellent effectiveness in clearing microfilaremia after a single oral dose, but its effects on adult parasites and its optimal dosing schedules are still under study.

Side effects of DEC treatment, although not so frequent or severe as those seen in onchocerciasis, can be troublesome, especially in brugian filariasis. These include fever, chills, headache, dizziness, nausea, vomiting, and arthralgias, all usually occurring in the first 24 to 36 hours. Both the likelihood of developing such reactions and the degree of their severity are directly related to the number of circulating microfilariae. Thus, the side effects of DEC administration at these dosage levels are due not to direct drug toxicity but to allergic or immunologic responses of the host to dying parasites. To avoid these reactions in highly parasitemic persons, one can initiate treatment with very small doses of DEC or premedicate the patients with steroids, as suggested for onchocerciasis (see Ch. 437.4). A very few patients may also develop filarial fever episodes with lymphangitis and lymphadenitis in the first days after DEC treatment. All of these side effects occur early in treatment and generally subside even with continued administration of the drug.

Severe chronic lymphatic damage has recently been shown to have a surprising degree of reversibility. All such affected patients should receive long-term low-dose DEC (to eradicate persistent or new filarial infections) and diligent attention to local care of the lymphedematous extremity through limb elevation, use of special massage techniques and elastic stockings, and prevention of superficial bacterial and fungal infection. More severely affected patients may benefit remarkably from surgical decompression of the lymphatic system through "nodovenous shunt" surgery followed by excision of redundant tissue. Hydroceles can be repeatedly drained or managed surgically. Chyluria also can sometimes be corrected surgically, but, interestingly, many cases have been reported in which diagnostic lymphangiography itself

appears to have terminated the leak of chyle into the urine, probably as a result of its sclerosing effects.

PREVENTION. DEC kills developing preadult forms of many filarial species, and its value as a prophylactic agent in humans (10 mg per kilogram on 2 consecutive days each month) has recently been established. In addition, for public health programs DEC has been used successfully as a protective measure to reduce infection rates in selected populations. Because of its microfilaricidal effects, small doses administered intermittently (or even as an additive to common table salt) to all residents of an endemic region‡ (e.g., 3 mg per kilogram monthly) reduce the number of bloodborne microfilariae in the community to levels so low that successful transmission of the infection by mosquitoes cannot occur. Other approaches to filariasis control designed to eradicate the mosquito vectors have also proved effective for the short term but have been difficult to sustain.

Filariasis. Ciba Found Symp 127:305 1987. *A multiauthored compendium of the current forefronts of understanding in most aspects of the filarial diseases.*

Ottesen EA: Efficacy of diethylcarbamazine in eradicating infection with lymphatic-dwelling filariae in humans. Rev Infect Dis 7:341, 1985. *A thorough review of observations from the literature, finally concluding that the more DEC administered (preferably over an extended period), the greater the likelihood that lymphatic filarial infections will be eradicated.*

Ottesen EA: Filariasis now. Am J Trop Med Hyg 41(Suppl):9, 1989. *A review of recent advances in our understanding of the immunopathogenesis, diagnosis, and treatment of lymphatic filarial infections.*

World Health Organization: Lymphatic pathology and immunopathology in filariasis: Report of the twelfth meeting of the scientific working group on filariasis. TDR/FIL-SWG(12)/85.3, 1986, p 33. *A report available through WHO that summarizes the most recent advances in understanding the pathogenesis and optimal management of the consequences of filaria-induced lymphatic obstruction.*

---

‡This use is not listed in the manufacturer's directive.

437.3 TROPICAL EOSINOPHILIA

Eric A. Ottesen

Tropical eosinophilia is a syndrome of acute and chronic lung disease first defined in the 1940's but not generally recognized as being of filarial etiology until the 1960's. Its main clinical features are a history of residence in a filaria-endemic region; paroxysmal cough and wheezing, which generally occur at night; scanty sputum production; occasional weight loss, low-grade fever, and adenopathy; and extreme blood eosinophilia (>3000 per microliter). It is more common in men than in women. Chest roentgenograms can be normal but generally show increased bronchovascular markings, diffuse interstitial lesions, or mottled opacities primarily involving the mid and lower lung fields. Tests of pulmonary function almost always indicate restrictive abnormalities and usually obstructive defects as well. The association of the syndrome with filarial infection was first recognized by finding very high levels of antifilarial antibody in these patients and by noting the favorable response to treatment with antifilarial drugs (now diethylcarbamazine* [DEC], 6 to 10 mg per kilogram per day for 3 to 4 weeks). Later, several reports described microfilariae or their degenerating remnants in lung biopsy specimens. Most recently, extremely high levels of total serum IgE (usually 10,000 to 100,000 ng per milliliter) have been found in these patients, and an appreciable fraction of this IgE has been shown to be directed against filarial antigens.

Because of these and other findings, tropical eosinophilia is now considered a form of "occult filariasis" in which host immunologic hyperresponsiveness to the parasite results in such rapid clearance of microfilariae from the blood that this stage of the parasite is essentially never detectable. Generally, this microfilarial clearance takes place in the lungs, and the clinical symptoms appear to result largely from the allergic and inflammatory reactions elicited by the cleared parasites. In some subjects, however, trapping of the microfilariae occurs predominantly in

---

*Not commercially available in the United States but may be obtained in special circumstances from Lederle Laboratories, Pearl River, NY.

†Available in the United States from the Centers for Disease Control, Atlanta, GA.

---

*Not commercially available in the United States but may be obtained in special circumstances from Lederle Laboratories, Pearl River, NY.

other organs of the reticuloendothelial system (liver, spleen, lymph nodes), and in these persons the major clinical manifestations are those resulting from hepatomegaly, splenomegaly, or lymphadenopathy. It has been postulated that infection with nonhuman filarial parasites is the major cause of tropical eosinophilia. Almost certainly, however, the syndrome is caused not by an "abnormal parasite" but rather by an abnormal host response to those same parasites (*Wuchereria bancrofti* and *Brugia malayi*) that commonly cause lymphatic filariasis (see Ch. 437.2). In this respect, tropical eosinophilia may be similar to another pulmonary eosinophilic disorder, allergic bronchopulmonary aspergillosis, both in its clinical expression and in its pathogenesis (see Ch. 406).

Diagnosis depends primarily on distinguishing tropical eosinophilia from the other important eosinophilic syndromes with pulmonary involvement, namely, Löffler's syndrome, chronic eosinophilic pneumonia, allergic aspergillosis, certain vasculitic syndromes, the idiopathic hypereosinophilia syndrome, drug allergies, and some helminth infections. Although there is no one clinical or laboratory criterion that will distinguish tropical eosinophilia from these other conditions, a history of residence in the tropics, high levels of specific filarial antibodies, and a response to DEC therapy are the most helpful differential points. Within 3 to 7 days after initiation of DEC, there is almost always marked improvement or disappearance of symptoms. Resolution may not be complete, however, and relapse may occur months to years later and require retreatment. DEC will not, of course, reverse permanent pulmonary damage (primarily an interstitial fibrosis), which frequently develops prior to successful diagnosis and treatment of the disorder.

Pinkston P, Vijayan VK, Nutman TB, et al.: Tropical pulmonary eosinophilia: Characterization of the lower respiratory tract inflammation and its response to therapy. J Clin Invest 80:216,1987. *Clinical and bronchoalveolar lavage studies probing the pathologic and immunopathologic mechanisms of the pulmonary pathology in this disorder.*

Rom WN, Vijayan VK, Cornelius MJ, et al.: Persistent lower respiratory tract inflammation associated with interstitial lung disease in patients with tropical pulmonary eosinophilia following conventional treatment with diethylcarbamazine. Am Rev Respir Dis 142:1088, 1990. *Bronchoalveolar lavage evidence that despite 3 weeks of DEC treatment (6 mg per kilogram per day), there was a persistent low-grade eosinophilic alveolitis in most patients 6 to 36 months after treatment; the recommendation for alternative treatment regimens is made.*

437.4 ONCHOCERCIASIS (River Blindness)

Bruce M. Greene

Onchocerciasis is a disease, most commonly manifest by skin and ocular damage, resulting from chronic infection with the filarial parasite *Onchocerca volvulus*.

ETIOLOGY. Onchocerciasis is a vector-borne disease, transmitted from person to person by the bite of the black fly, *Simulium* species. The female black fly ingests microfilariae from the skin of an infected person while taking a blood meal. Within the vector, microfilariae develop into infective larvae over a period of 6 to 8 days, and these larvae are transmitted to another person when the fly bites again. Over a period of several months, the larvae undergo a series of transformations leading to the development of adult worms that coil up into spherical bundles located in the subcutaneous tissues and deeper fascial planes. After a prepatent period of 9 to 18 months, the adult male and female worms reproduce sexually to yield millions of microfilariae that migrate through the skin and ocular tissues.

Microfilariae are highly motile, are unsheathed, and measure 210 to 320 μm in length and 6 to 9 μm in width. Infective larvae measure approximately 600 μm in length and in the human host undergo a molt to stage 4 larvae after a period of several days. Adult female worms are 23 to 70 cm in length, while the males are 3 to 6 cm long and weigh only 1 per cent as much as the female.

The lifespan of the adult worm in humans is known not to exceed 18 years, and the average survival is probably 8 to 10 years.

PREVALENCE AND EPIDEMIOLOGY. *Onchocerca volvulus* infects an estimated 20 to 40 million persons, principally in equatorial Africa in a broad belt extending from the Atlantic coast on the west to the Red Sea and Indian Ocean on the east. In the Western Hemisphere, the major focus is in Guatemala, on the Pacific slope of the Sierra Madre. Additional foci exist in Yemen, southwestern Saudi Arabia, southern Mexico, Venezuela, and northwestern Brazil, Colombia, and Ecuador.

Endemicity of *O. volvulus* in human populations is dependent upon habitation of fly-infested areas by sufficient, but not excessive, numbers of people who are exposed to human-biting flies during daily activities such as farming, fishing, bathing and washing, and water collection. Black flies deposit eggs on vegetation, rocks, sticks, and debris in freely flowing streams and rivers, and these develop into larvae and pupae that attach to vegetation and continuously filter the water to obtain oxygen and nutrients. Because of the dependency of the fly on waterways for reproduction, flies concentrate around streams and rivers. As a result, infection in human populations and disease tend to be similarly distributed; hence the term *river blindness*. The vector usually flies only a few kilometers from waterways but may fly as many as 20.

Approximately 1 to 4 per cent of infected persons become blind, and onchocerciasis ranks as the fourth leading cause of blindness in humans. In hyperendemic areas, more than one half of adults become blind. A much higher percentage of persons develop skin disease and/or some ocular involvement. Because blindness or serious ocular involvement, or severe debility resulting from skin disease, typically occurs during the third and fourth decades of life, the impact of the disease on the community is particularly devastating, frequently incapacitating the heads of households.

PATHOLOGY AND PATHOGENESIS. The disease affects primarily the skin, lymph nodes, and ocular tissues. In the skin, histopathology reflects a low-grade chronic inflammatory process. The end stage shows loss of elastic fibers, atrophy, and fibrosis. The onchocercomata, which are fibrous subcutaneous nodules containing adult worms, show a rim of chronic inflammation with fibrosis and extensive capillary infiltration surrounding the worms themselves. Lymph nodes show chronic inflammatory changes and, in some cases, fibrosis and atrophy. In the eye, neovascularization and scarring of the cornea lead to loss of transparency and blindness. The remainder of the eye is frequently involved by a chronic nongranulomatous inflammatory process that leads to anterior uveitis and associated chronic complications, chorioretinitis with damage to the retinal pigment epithelium, and optic atrophy.

The basis for the pathologic changes of onchocerciasis is believed to be the host reaction to chronic infestation with microfilariae. A multiplicity of factors appears to contribute to the pathologic changes; these include toxic or tissue-altering products of host granulocytes and lymphoid cells, which are reacting to the parasite, and perhaps products of the microfilariae themselves.

CLINICAL MANIFESTATIONS. The earliest signs of infection include pruritus and intermittent papular rash with some thickening of the skin, which may be localized to one area of the body, and conjunctivitis. In nonresidents of endemic areas, who are usually lightly infected, these are frequently the only manifestations. Onchocercomata are firm, 0.5- to 3-cm subcutaneous nodules that are nontender and freely movable if not attached to periosteum. These frequently occur in clusters that can be disfiguring. Common locations include the skin overlying bony prominences, including the superior iliac crests, the coccyx, the greater trochanter of the femur, the bony thorax, and the scalp and head region. With chronic infection, permanent skin changes occur, including loss of elasticity, a chronic, scaling hyperkeratotic maculopapular pruritic rash with mottled hypopigmentation or hyperpigmentation, and, finally, atrophy, leading in some cases to areas of breakdown with the risk of superinfection. Chronic skin manifestations are unpredictably punctuated by transient episodes of localized rash, erythema, and edema. In Central America the dermal manifestations are most prominent around the head and neck, while in Africa they more commonly involve the trunk, buttocks, and lower extremities. Lymph node involvement is usually manifested by enlargement, particularly in the inguinal and femoral regions, and in some cases by secondary obstructive changes in the groin region or in an extremity. Early ocular manifestations include punctate keratitis and anterior uveitis. Chronic changes include sclerosing keratitis, chorioretinitis (which leads to progressive constriction of visual fields), optic atrophy, and complications due to persistent anterior uveitis, including meiosis, pupillary distortion, and glaucoma. In general, the severity of disease correlates with intensity and duration of infection.

DIAGNOSIS. The diagnosis can be made clinically by the presence of onchocercomata, typical skin changes, or eye findings of onchocerciasis, including microfilariae in the cornea or anterior chamber in otherwise normal-appearing eyes. The diagnosis is confirmed by finding microfilariae of *O. volvulus* in the skin of the patient. This is done by biopsy, using a corneoscleral biopsy instrument or a razor blade, to yield approximately 1 to 2 mg of skin, including superficial dermis. The skin is weighed and incubated in tissue culture medium or saline, and the microfilariae that emerge are counted after a 3-hour or overnight incubation. These must be distinguished from the smaller *Mansonella streptocerca* microfilariae. The skin-snipping technique has the inherent advantage of providing a measure of intensity of infection, with fewer than 10 microfilariae per milligram of skin constituting a light infection and greater than 100, a heavy infection. For greatest reliability, four to six biopsies are done in different areas, including the hips, calves, and shoulders. Although elevated titers of antifilarial antibodies may support the diagnosis of onchocerciasis, a definitive immunodiagnostic technique has not yet been developed.

TREATMENT. Ivermectin,* a newly developed semisynthetic macrocyclic lactone, is now the drug of choice to treat onchocerciasis. The dosage is 150 µg per kilogram, given in a single dose on an empty stomach, once every year or every 6 months. The retreatment interval depends upon parasite burden, disease severity, and rapidity of recurrence of symptoms. Nonresidents of endemic countries often require more than once-a-year treatment because of rapid recurrence of pruritus in these hyperreactive individuals. Ivermectin should not be given to pregnant women, individuals with a serious central nervous system disorder or an acute illness, children less than 5 years of age or 15 kg in weight, and mothers who are nursing children within a week of delivery. Ivermectin causes killing of microfilariae but does not kill adult worms effectively. Therefore, retreatment is necessary over a period of years.

Diethylcarbamazine citrate† (DEC) was previously the standard drug used to treat onchocerciasis. Although well tolerated in uninfected persons, DEC frequently causes complications and side effects when given to individuals infected with *O. volvulus;* these complications appear to result in part from the massive killing of microfilariae that occurs over a few days after initiation of DEC therapy. This results in fever, intense pruritus, lymph node pain and swelling, prostration, hypotension, and arthralgias. In the eye, a worsening of ocular inflammation occurs transiently, and permanent sight-threatening lesions may occur in the posterior segment of the eye. In an effort to minimize these complications, patients should be given corticosteroids (e.g., prednisone 40 to 60 mg per day) starting the day before initiation of DEC therapy and continuing for 4 to 7 days as needed. DEC therapy should be started with a test dose of 25 to 50 mg and then increased to 4 mg per kilogram per day to complete a 10-day course. Because of the superior safety and tolerability of ivermectin, DEC should be reserved for persons who cannot be treated with ivermectin. Suramin, although it does kill adult worms, should *not* be used except in rare circumstances, as it is toxic and impractical.

Removal of nodules containing adult worms in the head region is indicated because of the increased risk of ocular involvement. Other palpable nodules should also be removed if feasible.

PROGNOSIS. With treatment, the early ocular and cutaneous changes are reversible, but for persons living in an endemic area, therapy must be given repeatedly, since neither DEC nor ivermectin is curative of the infection, and reinfection usually

occurs continuously. The atrophic skin changes, sclerosing keratitis, and disease in the posterior segment of the eye are not helped by therapy.

PREVENTION. There is no proven chemoprophylaxis. Vector control is difficult and expensive but has achieved remarkable success in some areas of Africa. Protective clothing, insect repellents, and avoidance of areas harboring the vector are useful measures for visitors to endemic areas.

Anderson J, Fuglsang H, Hamilton PJS, et al.: Studies on onchocerciasis in the United Cameroon Republic: II. Comparison of onchocerciasis in rain-forest and sudan-savanna. Trans R Soc Trop Med Hyg 68:209, 1974. *Detailed analysis of clinical manifestations with comparison of forest and savanna types of disease.*

Greene BM, Dukuly ZD, Muñoz B, et al.: A comparison of 6, 12, and 24 monthly dosing with ivermectin for treatment of onchocerciasis. J Infect Dis 163:376, 1991. *Retreatment at 6-month, as opposed to yearly, intervals may provide an advantage in the first 1 to 2 years, but very little thereafter.*

Greene BM, Taylor HR, Cupp EW, et al.: Comparison of ivermectin and diethylcarbamazine in the treatment of onchocerciasis. N Engl J Med 313:133, 1985. *Shows that ivermectin is better tolerated, more effective, and safer than diethylcarbamazine.*

WHO Expert Committee on Onchocerciasis: Third Report. Technical Report Series No. 752. Geneva, World Health Organization, 1987. *Comprehensive summary of the disease and its distribution and impact.*

437.5 LOIASIS

Eric A. Ottesen

Loa loa is indigenous only to the rain forest belt of western and central Africa. Mature female parasites, about twice the size of the males, are 50 to 70 mm long and 0.5 mm wide. They live wandering through the subcutaneous tissue in humans, usually attracting attention only when they cross the eye subconjunctivally. The sheathed microfilariae produced by these females circulate with a diurnal periodicity that peaks at about noon.

Clinical loiasis presents in two primary forms, one more common among individuals native to endemic regions and the other more common in visitors to these areas who acquire infection. Among the natives, loiasis is often entirely asymptomatic until an adult worm appears moving across the eye or blood examination reveals microfilaremia. Such individuals may also have occasional episodes of Calabar swellings. These are characteristic localized areas of erythema and angioedema (up to 5 to 10 cm in diameter) that occur primarily on the extremities and last 1 to 3 days before regressing spontaneously. These swellings appear to be a hypersensitivity reaction to the adult worm, whose presence can also be detected in some patients by either a subcutaneous crawling sensation or the appearance of a fine vermiform hive in the skin. When the inflammation extends to nearby joints or peripheral nerves, corresponding symptoms may develop. Rarely, nephropathy (probably immune complex mediated) and encephalopathy have been reported.

The major difference between this presentation and that seen in outsiders who acquire infection is the greater predominance of allergic or hyperreactive symptoms in the latter. Episodes of angioedema are likely to be more frequent and debilitating, and patients are much less likely to have microfilariae in the blood. In addition, they often present with extensive blood eosinophilia (30 to 60 per cent of an elevated total leukocyte count), much like patients with tropical eosinophilia (Ch. 437.3). Diagnosis in these patients often cannot be made parasitologically and must be based on the characteristic history, clinical presentation, blood eosinophilia, and elevated filarial antibody titers. If untreated, a small (but undefined) percentage of such patients develops severe cardiomyopathy, presumably secondary to the hypereosinophilia elicited by the infection.

Treatment is with diethylcarbamazine* ([DEC], 6 to 10 mg per kilogram per day for 2 to 3 weeks). The drug is extremely effective against microfilariae but less so against adult worms, so that multiple courses of treatment are often necessary before there is complete resolution of signs and symptoms. In cases of

---

*Available in the United States from the Centers for Disease Control, Atlanta, GA.

†Available in the United States from Lederle Laboratories, Pearl River, NY.

---

*Available in the United States from Lederle Laboratories, Pearl River, NY.

heavy microfilaremia (greater than several hundred microfilariae per milliliter of blood), allergic and other inflammatory side effects of treatment may be so severe that a regimen of 0.5 to 1.0 mg per kilogram DEC per dose (with or without simultaneous steroids) is safer for initiating treatment. DEC is effective in preventing loiasis when taken in prophylactic doses of 300 mg weekly.

Klion AD, Massougbodji A, Sadeler BC, et al.: Loiasis in endemic and non-endemic populations: Immunologically-mediated differences in clinical presentation. J Infect Dis, in press. *A clinical and immunological study contrasting the presentations of Loa loa infection in patients who have lived their entire lives in the endemic areas and patients who acquired their infections while visiting these areas.*

Nutman TB, Miller KD, Mulligan M, et al.: Diethylcarbamazine prophylaxis for human loiasis: Results of a double-blind study. N Engl J Med 319:752, 1988. *A placebo-controlled study in Peace Corps volunteers showing clearly that clinical loiasis can be prevented by weekly DEC in long-term visitors to endemic countries.*

437.6 DRACUNCULIASIS

Donald R. Hopkins

Dracunculiasis, or guinea worm disease, is caused by infection with the parasite *Dracunculus medinensis*. It occurs in the Indian subcontinent and Africa, where up to 5 million persons living in rural areas are thought to be affected annually and more than 100 million persons are at risk of infection.

Diagnosis of patent infections is easy. The thin adult female worms, each up to 1 meter long, emerge directly through the skin, usually of the lower leg, ankle, or foot. The worms emerge 10 to 14 months after victims have drunk water containing infected *Cyclops*, a barely visible crustacean that serves as the parasite's intermediate host. When persons harboring such emerging worms enter a stagnant source of drinking water, such as a step well or pond, larvae are released into the water, where some are ingested by *Cyclops*. When humans drink water containing *Cyclops* with infective larvae, the larvae penetrate the intestinal or stomach wall, mature, and mate, after which the male worms die.

The adult worms emerge slowly, over a period of weeks or months. Emergence may be preceded by generalized allergic symptoms and is usually accompanied by a blister that ruptures to form an ulcer at the site of emergence. Some worms present first as a serpentine cord just beneath the skin or at the center of an abscess. No immunity develops, so persons in endemic areas are infected year after year.

The great social and economic significance of dracunculiasis, which rarely is fatal, derives from the fact that emergence of the worm is very painful and is often associated with swelling, local arthritis, and secondary infection. Thus, victims are often unable to farm or sometimes even walk for weeks or months. Over half of the adults in a village may be crippled at the same time, and the seasonal infection tends to occur precisely when villagers need to harvest or plant their crops. School attendance is also affected.

Treatment is difficult because anthelminthics such as thiabendazole or metronidazole only marginally reduce the duration of emergence and associated pain. Aspirin can help relieve the pain. Emerging worms are best rolled around a small stick as their predecessors have been for centuries, care being taken not to break the worm (which would exacerbate the inflammation). Some worms can be removed surgically. Victims should be immunized against tetanus, which is sometimes caused by secondary infection of the ulcer around the emerging worm. Persons at risk should be taught to boil their drinking water or filter it through a cloth and to avoid entering sources of drinking water when the infection is patent.

Since the most effective intervention against this infection is to provide safe drinking water, efforts began during the International Drinking Water Supply and Sanitation Decade (1981–1990) to provide safe water to dracunculiasis-endemic areas as a priority and thereby eliminate the disease. By the end of 1990, India had reduced its reported dracunculiasis cases by 90 per cent, Pakistan had almost eliminated the disease altogether, and most of the remaining major endemic countries had begun programs to eradicate the disease by 1995.

Hopkins DR, Ruiz-Tiben E: Dracunculiasis Eradication: Target 1995. Am J Trop Med Hyg 43:296–300, 1990. *A recent review of all aspects pertaining to control and eradication of dracunculiasis.*

Muller R: *Dracunculus* and dracunculiasis. *In* Dawes B (ed.): Advances in Parasitology. Vol 9. New York, Academic Press, 1971, pp 73–151. *A thorough consideration of the parasite's biology, life cycle, and the disease it produces.*

437.7 OTHER FILARIAL INFECTIONS

Eric A. Ottesen

PERSTANS FILARIASIS

Mansonella perstans (formerly *Dipetalonema perstans, Acanthocheilonema perstans*) is distributed in a broad belt across the center of Africa and in northeast South America. Adult worms, up to 70 to 80 mm long, reside in the body cavities (pleural, peritoneal, and pericardial) and in the mesentery, perirenal, and retroperitoneal tissues. Microfilariae are liberated *unsheathed* from the females and circulate in the blood without regular periodicity.

M. perstans infection was long thought to be asymptomatic, because up to 90 per cent of individuals with the parasite appeared to have no difficulty with it. Subsequent studies, however, indicate clearly that *M. perstans* is capable of inducing a variety of symptoms, including angioedematous swellings much like the Calabar swellings of loiasis; fever; headache; pain in bursae and/or joint synovia, in serous cavities, or over the liver; neurologic or psychological symptoms; and extreme exhaustion. There is some evidence that symptoms are more prominent in outsiders coming to endemic regions, but in all series at least a quarter of the patients were asymptomatic despite persistent microfilaremia.

Treatment with diethylcarbamazine* ([DEC], 5 to 6 mg per kilogram per day for 2 to 3 weeks) is often ineffective, with multiple courses usually necessary to achieve cure. When the parasites are eliminated, however, patients characteristically lose their symptoms (no matter how vague), lose their eosinophilia, and regain a sense of well-being.

Adolph PE, Kagan IG, McQuay RM: Diagnosis and treatment of *Acanthocheilonema perstans* filariasis. Am J Trop Med Hyg 11:76, 1962. *Results from a series of patients observed in the United States after returning from missionary work in Africa.*

Clarke V deV, Harwin RM, MacDonald DF, et al.: Filariasis: *Dipetalonema perstans* infections in Rhodesia. Cent Afr J Med 17:1, 1971. *Discussion of the clinical expression of* M. perstans *filariasis in Africans and Europeans living in East Africa.*

STREPTOCERCIASIS

Mansonella streptocerca is transmitted by midges, especially *Culicoides grahami*. It occurs in the tropical forest belt of Africa from Ghana to Zaire. The adult worms are subcutaneous, especially over the torso; and the microfilariae, which have characteristic shepherd's-crook tails, are found in the skin (see Ch. 437.4 for skin-snipping technique).

Infection is usually symptomless, but the adult worms may produce hypopigmented macules (to be distinguished from leprosy), and the microfilariae occasionally cause itching papular rashes similar to those of onchocerciasis. Both adult worms and microfilariae are killed by diethylcarbamazine* (e.g., 7 to 10 days of treatment at 6 mg per kilogram per day).

Meyers WM, Connor DH, et al.: Human streptocerciasis: A clinicopathologic study of 40 Africans (Zairians) including identification of the adult filaria. Am J Trop Med Hyg 21:528, 1972. *Covers the clinical aspects and gives references to other aspects.*

MANSONELLA OZZARDI INFECTION

M. ozzardi is restricted in distribution to Central and South America and certain islands of the Caribbean. Adult worms have

---

*Not commercially available in the United States but may be obtained in special circumstances from Lederle Laboratories, Pearl River, NY.

been recovered in humans only twice, both times from the peritoneal cavity. *Unsheathed* microfilariae circulate in the blood with little or no periodicity.

Many investigators consider these parasites to be nonpathogenic, but in one of the fullest clinical studies of an affected population it was asserted that the major clinical presentation is severe articular pain or dysfunction, especially in the arms and shoulders. Headache, fever, pulmonary symptoms, adenopathy, hepatomegaly, and pruritic skin eruptions also occurred in a small number of patients with a frequency greater than that in nonparasitized individuals in the same population. Diethylcarbamazine* has little or no effect on this infection, but a single case report suggests that ivermectin† is effective therapy.

Marinkelle CJ, German E: Mansonelliasis in the comisaria del Vaupes of Colombia. Trop Geogr Med 22:101, 1970. *A very complete and interesting account of clinical manifestations ascribed to* M. ozzardi *infections in South American Indians.*

Nutman TB, Nash TE, Ottesen EA: Ivermectin in the successful treatment of a patient with *Mansonella ozzardi* infection. J Infect Dis 156:662, 1987. *A single case report presenting clinical and immunologic evidence for the effectiveness of ivermectin (140 μg per kilogram given once) in an* M. ozzardi *infection.*

HUMAN DIROFILARIASIS

Dirofilaria species are filarial parasites mostly of dogs, cats, and raccoons that sometimes infect humans but almost never fully develop to complete their life cycles in this abnormal host. The distribution of cases is worldwide and reflects the distribution of the parasites in animals.

Two general types of clinical presentation predominate. Pulmonary dirofilariasis, caused by the dog heartworm *D. immitis,* usually presents as an asymptomatic solitary pulmonary nodule but occasionally with chest pain, cough, or hemoptysis. Microscopically there is local eosinophilia and granuloma formation accompanied by infarction and thrombosis around an impacted, immature worm. The second common clinical presentation is that of a subcutaneous nodule found anywhere on the body (or within the eye) that results usually from infection with the subcutaneous dwelling filarids of dogs (*D. repens*) or raccoons (*D. tenuis*) but occasionally from infection with *D. immitis.* Local lesions again are granulomatous and eosinophilic and are sometimes accompanied by bacterial superinfection.

Definitive diagnosis and treatment most often result from the same surgical (excisional) procedure. Blood eosinophilia is not a regular finding in these patients nor are detectable antifilarial antibodies. Furthermore, since the worms are usually incompletely developed, microfilaremia occurs only in the rarest of circumstances. These "abnormal" parasite infections do not respond to DEC, and their treatment is primarily surgical.

Dissanaike AS: Zoonotic aspects of filarial infections in man. Bull WHO 57:349, 1979. *A scholarly, readable discussion of the human's interaction with zoonotic filarial infections.*

---

*Not commercially available in the United States but may be obtained in special circumstances from Lederle Laboratories, Pearl River, NY.

†Available in the United States from the Centers for Disease Control, Atlanta, GA.

---

438 Arthropods and Leeches

William L. Krinsky

ARTHROPODS AS AGENTS OF DISEASE

Disease associated directly with arthropods results from toxins, or allergic responses to the organisms or their products when humans are exposed by bites or stings, simple contact, or invasion through the skin or natural orifices. Arthropods most often involved in these types of exposure are listed in Table 438–1.

Physicians usually become aware of insects and their relatives (spiders, mites, ticks, scorpions, millipedes, and centipedes) when patients present with skin lesions caused by arthropods, when infestations of the creatures themselves are seen, when

TABLE 438–1. ARTHROPODS CAUSING HUMAN PATHOLOGY

Human Exposure	Arthropod	Antigens or Toxins
Bites	Insects (lice, bedbugs, and other true bugs; fleas; flies including mosquitoes, black flies, biting midges, sandflies, horse and deer flies, stable flies, tsetse flies, keds; ants)	Salivary secretions, venoms
	Arachnids (chigger and other rodent and bird mites; ticks; spiders)	
	Centipedes	
Stings	Insects (some ants, wasps, and bees)	Venoms
	Arachnids (scorpions)	
Invasion	Insects (fly larvae, *Tunga* fleas)	Salivary secretions, excretions
	Arachnids (scabies mites)	
Simple contact	Insects (caterpillars, pupae, or adults of moths and butterflies; blister and some rove beetles)	Setae, spines, secretions (venoms) and excretions
	Arachnids (stored product mites)	
	Millipedes	

foreign bodies extracted from skin or sense organs are identified as arthropods, or when respiratory symptoms develop in response to arthropods or their products. Dermatoses associated with arthropods and human infestations with arthropods (e.g., lice, mites, fly larvae) are discussed in detail in this chapter. Arthropods as vectors are mentioned here; detailed discussions of arthropod-borne pathogens may be found elsewhere in this book.

Alexander JO: Arthropods and Human Skin. Berlin, Springer-Verlag, 1984. *This is the first comprehensive text devoted to dermatologic problems associated with arthropods.*

Harwood RF, James MT: Entomology in Human and Animal Health. 7th ed. New York, The Macmillan Company, 1979. *This is a comprehensive textbook that provides detailed references to the diverse arthropod-associated problems discussed here.*

Biting Arthropods

Louse Infestations (Pediculosis)

Pediculosis is infestation of the body with lice. The observation of louse eggs (nits) cemented to hairs of the scalp or lice themselves confirms the diagnosis of head louse (*Pediculus capitis*) infestation. Nits (or lice) attached to the seams of clothing (often in undergarments) indicate the presence of body lice (*P. humanus*), and nits or lice attached to pubic hairs indicate a pubic (crab) louse (*Phthirus pubis*) infestation.

The eggs are pearly yellow-white and opaque, elongate-oval, about 0.8 mm long and 0.3 mm wide, and are attached singly to each hair or clothing fiber. After hatching, the nits appear translucent and opalescent. Although nits may be numerous, usually not more than 10 to 20 lice are associated with infested persons. The head louse egg is cemented on a hair about 1 mm above the scalp surface.

Head and body lice are very similar in appearance. Adult head lice are 2.5 to 3.5 mm long, and adult body lice are 3.0 to 4.5 mm long. Each immature and adult head and body louse has three pairs of about equal-sized legs bearing claws for gripping hairs or fibers. Adult pubic lice, somewhat crablike in appearance, are 1 to 2 mm long, about as broad, grayish-white or yellowish-brown, and they have forelegs narrower than the other pairs. All immature lice (three stages in each species) resemble their respective adults except in size, and all immature lice and adults are obligate bloodsucking ectoparasites. The body louse is the only known natural vector of the pathogens of louse-borne typhus, trench fever, and louse-borne relapsing fever.

Head lice and their nits are found most frequently in the hair over the postauricular and occipital regions. Body lice are usually seen in clothing, with nits in the seams and creases in areas that contact the body. Crab lice and nits are found on hairs in the pubic and perianal regions, sometimes on hairs on the thighs and abdomen, less commonly on axillary hairs, beard, mustache, eyebrows, and eyelashes, and rarely on the scalp. Pubic infestations are found only in postpubertal individuals.

The skin lesions produced by the bites of lice are erythematous papules that may be accompanied by urticaria or lymphadenopathy. Extensive erythema and pruritus result from hypersensitivity to louse saliva. Crab lice typically induce nonpruritic small gray-blue macules (0.3 to 1.0 cm in diameter) with irregular borders (maculae ceruleae) that may persist for months. The lesions produced by any of the species may be covered with hair matted with eggs, dried serous secretions, and dark louse excrement. The latter, seen on the body or in underclothing, should trigger a search for lice. Excoriations from scratching disguise bite lesions and may lead to impetigo or to furuncular or eczematous lesions. The possibility of louse infestation should be considered when pyoderma is seen. The combination of lichenification and pigmentation in chronically infested individuals is called vagabond's disease (morbus vagabondus). A nondescript macular or papular erythematous rash on the trunk may be the presenting sign for an undiscovered head louse infestation. Postauricular and posterior cervical lymphadenopathy in the absence of other node enlargement should suggest head lice. Body louse infestation may be differentiated from scabies by the absence of lesions on the hands and feet and the common occurrence of lesions in the intrascapular region. The differential diagnosis of louse-induced dermatitis from various mite-induced lesions or non–arthropod-associated dermatoses is made by finding nits or lice.

Treatment for lice includes shampoos, creams, and lotions containing insecticides. The most often used preparations contain lindane (γ benzene hexachloride) or pyrethrins with piperonyl butoxide. Malathion and permethrin, a synthetic pyrethrin, are being used more frequently because of their apparent ovicidal effect. One effective treatment for head lice or pubic lice is a 4-minute shampoo of the affected areas with about 25 ml of 1 per cent lindane shampoo. This may not be ovicidal; therefore, the treatment may be repeated 7 to 10 days later if lice or new nits are seen. Patients infested with body lice may apply lindane (1 per cent) lotion or cream to affected areas. This should be thoroughly washed off 6 to 8 hours later. Lindane should be used with caution on infants, children, and pregnant women. Infested clothing and linen should be washed in hot water (60°C) for 20 minutes or dry cleaned.

After being treated, lice and nits can be removed with a metal comb with teeth 0.1 mm apart. Moisture or oil rinses may make removal easier. Mechanical removal is recommended for facial pubic louse infestations.

Prevention of recurrence involves treatment of infested human contacts and materials (fomites). Pillow cases, hats, scarves, and other items should be washed or cleaned. Infested combs and brushes should be cleaned and boiled or soaked for 1 hour in lindane shampoo or Lysol (2 per cent). Head and body lice survive only about 3 days (10 days maximum) away from the body. Sexual partners of persons with pubic lice should be treated, and bedding, towels, and clothing should be washed or dry cleaned. Pubic lice do not survive longer than 24 hours away from a body. Transmission via toilet seats is unlikely. Fumigation after any louse infestation is unnecessary, but vacuuming is helpful to remove stray lice and shed hairs with affixed nits.

Arnold HL, Odom RB, James WD: Andrews' Diseases of the Skin. 8th ed. Philadelphia, W. B. Saunders Company, 1990, pp 512–515. This text has excellent photographs of nits, lice, and skin lesions seen in pediculosis.
Raber IM: Pediculosis cilaris. In Parish LC, Nutting WB, Schwartzman RM (eds.): Cutaneous Infestations of Man and Animal. New York, Praeger, 1983, pp 138–143. This is a lucid description of the clinical aspects and treatment of pubic louse infestation of the eyelashes.
Witkowski JA, Parish LC: Pediculosis. In Parish LC, Nutting WB, Schwartzman

RM (eds.): Cutaneous Infestations of Man and Animal. New York, Praeger, 1983, pp 125–137. A concise, well-documented discussion of clinical louse infestations.

Flea Bites

Most fleas, unlike lice, do not infest the body. The common flea species that suck blood from humans visit the body for a few minutes to hours, during which time feeding occurs. As in louse infestations, flea bites generally cause pruritus. Each bite lesion is an erythematous papule with a hemorrhagic punctum. Sensitization of an individual to flea saliva may result in papular urticaria (common in affected children), bullous eruptions, or erythema multiforme–type lesions. Bites are usually multiple and irregularly grouped. Bites in adults appear as widespread papules that become lichenified or as grouped papules overlying erythema or edema. Persons entering a previously infested room that has been vacant for weeks or months often suffer from multiple bites on the ankles and legs as hungry fleas emerge from pupal cocoons in floor crevices, debris, or carpeting. As with louse bites, excoriated lesions may become infected and furuncular.

Flea eggs are usually laid off the host, and larvae live off the host, feeding on organic debris. Adults reach their hosts by jumping. Flea species that most often bite humans are the cat flea (Ctenocephalides felis), the dog flea (C. canis), and somewhat less commonly the so-called human flea (Pulex irritans). Occasionally, household infestations with fleas may arise from abandoned wild animal nests built near houses.

Treatment of flea bites is symptomatic and involves the use of antipruritic and anti-inflammatory creams or lotions or oral antihistamines. Secondary infections may require antibiotic therapy. Infested pets should be treated with specific insecticides. Floors, carpets, upholstered furnishings, and pets' sleeping quarters should be sprayed or dusted with insecticides to kill larval, pupal, and adult fleas. A thorough cleaning, including vacuuming, of infested premises should eliminate the insects. Because fleas at all stages can live for weeks or months, a repeat insecticide application may be necessary.

Persons may protect themselves from fleas with repellents containing diethyl metatoluamide. Wild animal (especially rodent) fleas that feed on humans may transmit the bacilli of plague or tularemia, as well as the less virulent rickettsia of murine (flea-borne) typhus. Less common pathogens transmitted by accidental ingestion of fleas (mostly by children) are the dwarf tapeworm Hymenolepis diminuta and the dog tapeworm Dipylidium caninum.

Bagnall B, Rook A: Arthropods and the skin. In Rook A (ed.): Recent Advances in Dermatology. No. 4. Edinburgh, Churchill Livingstone, 1977. This review includes information about the ecology of fleas and pathogenesis and clinical features of infestations.
Smit FGAM: Siphonaptera (fleas). In Smith KGV (ed.): Insects and Other Arthropods of Medical Importance. London, British Museum (Natural History), 1973. This is a careful overview of the medical importance of fleas.

Bedbugs and Kissing Bugs

Bedbugs (Cimicidae) are flat, mahogany-brown, wingless insects (5 to 7 mm long). Most species are bloodsucking ectoparasites of birds and bats. Two species (Cimex lectularius and C. hemipterus) feed almost exclusively on humans; the former is cosmopolitan; the latter has a tropical distribution. Both species cause irritating, pruritic bite lesions in sensitized individuals. The bugs become engorged with blood in 3 to 15 minutes and feed only at night or in subdued light. They hide in crevices of bedding, beds, floors, and furnishings and in wood and paper trash accumulations during the day. The bites are often seen in short linear groups and vary from small urticarial lesions to large erythematous papules or bullae. The lesions are often excoriated, and eczematous reactions and pyoderma may be seen. Hypersensitivity reactions may include asthma, generalized urticaria, and arthralgia. While some affected persons complain of being awakened at night, most are troubled by the lesions on arising in the morning. Treatment is symptomatic. Prevention includes removal of debris that harbors the bugs, use of insecticides in crevices and cleaning of infested furnishings.

Triatomine kissing bugs (Reduviidae) that suck blood from a diversity of hosts are found in the New World subtropics and tropics and in Asia. Most of these cone-nosed bugs (8 to 38 mm long) are tan, brown, or black, with yellow or red spots around the dorsal edge of the abdomen. The bugs feed rapidly at night. Sensitive individuals may develop papular lesions, small vesicles, or, in the extreme, large urticarial or hemorrhagic nodular to bullous lesions. Generalized anaphylactoid reactions, including shock and angioneurotic and laryngeal edema, have occurred. Kissing bugs may feed anywhere on the body. Domesticated species in the tropics are found most often in thatched houses or those with mud floors. In the southwestern United States, a species (*Triatoma protracta*) living in wood rat nests in desert areas occasionally invades homes. Treatment of bites or allergic reactions is symptomatic. In Central and South America, these insects are vectors of Chagas' disease trypanosomes.

Crissey JT: Bedbugs—an old problem with a new dimension. Int J Dermatol 20:411, 1981. *This review article discusses bedbug biology and the possible role of these bugs in human disease.*

Ryckman RE: Host reactions to bug bites (Hemiptera, Homoptera): A literature review and annotated bibliography. Parts I, II. Calif Vector Views 26, Nos. 1–2, 1979. *This is an excellent source of specific references about all bugs that prey on humans.*

Mosquitoes and Other Bloodsucking Flies

Mosquitoes (Culicidae) are found worldwide, breeding wherever there is stagnant water. While biting, a female mosquito (3 to 6 mm long) induces a pruritic wheal that becomes an erythematous papule. In sensitive persons, bullous lesions, cellulitis, or hemorrhagic necrotic reactions may follow the bites. Systemic anaphylactic reactions are rare. The most serious medical problems associated with mosquitoes relate to their transmission of the agents of yellow fever, dengue, arboviral encephalitides, malaria, and filariasis.

Biting midges (Ceratopogonidae), also called "punkies" or "no-see-ums" because of their minute size (most are 0.6 to 2 mm long), give a painful bite. The resulting erythematous punctiform lesions may become papular and pruritic. Vesicles may develop that ooze fluid for days. These midges, especially *Culicoides* species, bite mostly on exposed parts of the body and may be pestiferous in sandy seashore or marshy areas where they breed. Biting occurs mostly at dawn or dusk.

Black flies (Simuliidae), also called buffalo gnats, are small (1 to 5 mm long), humpbacked, tan to black insects that breed only in running water. They are troublesome bloodsuckers in northern temperate regions. The bites may become hemorrhagic papules that ooze blood for hours. These lesions may be painful and cause recurrent pruritus. Lymphadenopathy is common in sensitive individuals, who may develop localized edema. Cephalalgia, fever, and nausea may occur following large numbers of bites. Black fly species found at high elevations in Central and South America and along rivers in Africa transmit *Onchocerca volvulus*, the etiologic agent of river blindness.

Phlebotomine sandflies (Psychodidae) are delicate, small (2 to 3 mm long), hairy flies found mainly in subtropical and tropical areas. Various species are abundant in rain forests in the New World and in arid areas in the Mediterranean region and Asia. Biting occurs at night or in subdued light. The bites may be painful, occur usually on the extremities, and cause pruritus and elevated pale urticarial lesions that become papular. Vesicular or bullous lesions may occur. Phlebotomine flies are vectors of sandfly (pappataci) fever, bartonellosis, and leishmaniasis.

Other flies that may attack humans and cause painful bites are horse and deer flies (Tabanidae), stable flies, and tsetse flies. Tsetse flies, found only in Africa, transmit the trypanosomes of African sleeping sickness.

Treatment of any of these fly bites is symptomatic and includes the use of topical corticosteroids and oral antihistamines to reduce itching. Personal protection from biting flies involves the use of screen enclosures, headnets, and insect repellents. Protective clothing and open mesh jackets impregnated with repellents are effective.

Allen JR: Mosquitoes and other biting flies. *In* Parish LC, Nutting WB, Schwartzman RM (eds.): Cutaneous Infestations of Man and Animal. New York, Praeger, 1983, pp 344–355. *This is a concise, clearly presented review of the pathogenesis and clinical aspects of fly bites.*

Chiggers and Other Biting Mites

Chiggers are the larvae (six-legged stage) of trombiculid (itch or harvest) mites. These larvae (0.15 to 0.40 mm long) are white to yellow or orange-red and are found on many vertebrates.

Human infestation occurs following contact with grassy or shrubby vegetation inhabited by the mites. First exposure may not produce dermatitis or may produce only slightly irritating, transient erythematous macules or papules (1 to 2 mm). The more commonly seen skin reactions to chigger feeding are extremely pruritic, papular, papulovesicular or papulourticarial lesions (4 to 20 mm) that persist with burning and itching for days to weeks. The lesions may fade and flatten or become hemorrhagic, purpuric, or vesicular. Diagnosis is dependent upon morphology and distribution of lesions, exposure history, and observation of the mites. Engorging chiggers may be apparent as minute reddish blebs embedded in hair follicles. The mites most often attach to skin covered by clothing, especially near belts, straps, or elastic bindings. Scrub itch mites of Asia and South Pacific Islands usually do not cause dermatitis, but they are vectors of scrub typhus rickettsiae.

Other mites that bite humans, but that are rarely recovered from the lesions they cause, are pyemotid (straw, hay, or grain itch) mites, cheyletoid (cat or dog fur and predatory) mites, and dermanyssid (chicken, red, house mouse, tropical rat, fowl, and rodent) mites. All of these mites are extremely small (about 0.4 to 1 mm long), and depending on the species, the six-legged larvae or eight-legged nymphs and adults may attack humans. The resulting skin lesions may be extremely variable.

The differential diagnosis of mite-induced dermatitis depends on associating the patient with a source of mites. Sources include wild and domestic animals, agricultural commodities, dried floral arrangements, infested furniture, and, in chigger-associated cases, particular outdoor habitats.

Treatment of dermatitis associated with biting mites is symptomatic. Antipruritic lotions and creams or oral antihistamines are useful. Secondary infections may require antibiotic therapy. Rare allergic reactions, including edema and asthma, require emergency treatment.

Prevention of recurrences is dependent on destruction or fumigation of the mite source. Personal repellents (containing sulfur or diethyltoluamide) are helpful in preventing chigger infestation, although avoidance of infested areas is the best prevention. *Rickettsia tsutsugamushi* is the only pathogen of major medical importance specifically associated with mite transmission. *R. akari*, the etiologic agent of rickettsialpox, is transmitted by the house mouse mite.

Krinsky WL: Dermatoses associated with the bites of mites and ticks (Arthropoda: Acari). Int J Dermatol 22:75, 1983. *This review includes a list of mites causing human dermatitis and discusses clinical findings.*

Parkhurst HJ: Trombidiosis (infestation with chiggers). Arch Dermatol Syphilol 35:1011, 1937. *This is an extensive review of the biology and clinical importance of chiggers.*

Tick Bites and Tick Paralysis

Ticks, like mites, are arachnids that have six-legged larvae and eight-legged nymphs and adults. Ticks, found worldwide, are grouped in two major families, soft ticks (Argasidae) and hard ticks (Ixodidae). The former, which have rugose integuments, are associated with restricted habitats, such as rodent burrows and bird nests, and rarely feed on humans. When they do, most attach for only a matter of minutes and produce maculate, erythematous lesions (6 to 30 mm in diameter). Some species in Africa cause extensive ecchymosis; pain, pruritus, edema, ulceration, and necrotic lesions have also been observed. The pajaroello (talaja) tick (*Ornithodoros coriaceus*), found in Mexico, California, and Oregon, is known to produce hemorrhagic, painful lesions. Soft ticks are of primary medical importance as vectors of the borreliae of relapsing fevers.

Hard ticks have smooth, hard, shiny integuments and are found on a diversity of animals and in grass and forests. Ticks carried on dogs, cats, or other animals sometimes drop off and attach to humans. Hard ticks remain embedded in the skin for days while becoming engorged with blood and usually do not cause pain or discomfort. Engorging ticks, mistakenly identified as pedunculated moles or warts, are usually noticed only by chance observation. Typical tick bite lesions are small indurations with peripheral erythema. Unusual manifestations of hard tick bites include various forms of nonspecific dermatitis, acrodermatitis chronica atrophicans, necrotic ulcers, and alopecia. Most hard ticks attach, feed, drop off, and are never noticed. Nodular lesions that may persist for years at the sites of bites must be differentiated from malignant conditions, such as lymphomas. Hard ticks are vectors of the etiologic agents of various arboviral hemorrhagic fevers and encephalitides, several kinds of tick-borne typhus (including Rocky Mountain spotted fever), tularemia, babesiosis, ehrlichiosis, and Lyme disease. An engorging tick itself may induce tick paralysis (discussed below).

Attached soft ticks may be easily removed by gentle traction with a forceps. Hard ticks require strong constant traction. Use of heat, flames, or caustic substances is ill advised and may cause unnecessary damage to the patient. Hard ticks, embedded in sensitive sites, such as the ear canal or genitals, may be covered with petrolatum. The ticks then detach within about 2 hours and can be gently removed. Complete extraction of the mouthparts lessens the chance of secondary infection. Persistent nodules that cause discomfort should be surgically excised.

Tick paralysis is an unusual form of ascending flaccid paralysis that occurs while a tick is attached to the body. Mostly children (especially girls) are affected. Tick paralysis in humans has been associated with only a small number of hard tick species in North America, Europe, South Africa, and Australia. Most cases have been caused by female wood ticks, the Rocky Mountain wood tick (*Dermacentor andersoni*) in western North America and the common dog tick (*D. variabilis*) in eastern North America. Although nonspecific numbness or irritability may occur before the onset of paralysis, the initial consistent sign is *weakness in the legs*. Leg tendon reflexes are reduced or absent, and Romberg's sign is often present. Sensory changes are rarely noted. Blood counts and lumbar puncture usually give no indication of the disease. Complete paralysis of the extremities may occur within a few days after a tick attaches. If the cause is unrecognized, paralysis usually progresses, causing speech dysfunction, dysphagia, and ultimately death from aspiration or respiratory paralysis. If a tick is found, removal usually results in reversal of paralysis with a return to normal function in hours to weeks, depending on the severity of the neurologic deficit. The patient should be examined for other ticks, with special attention to concealed areas, such as the scalp, ear canals, axillae, popliteal fossae, anus, and genitals. Even after all ticks are removed, death may occur in patients who exhibit bulbar or respiratory paralysis.

The clinical presentation of tick paralysis may suggest poliomyelitis, Guillain-Barré syndrome, diphtheritic polyneuropathy, transverse myelitis, botulism, or other acutely developing neuropathies. The specific etiologic agent of *Dermacentor* tick paralysis is unknown.

Prevention of tick bites and tick paralysis includes avoidance of tick-infested habitats. Individuals and their pets who enter such habitats should be thoroughly examined for ticks. Personal measures that may prevent ticks from reaching the skin include wearing long-sleeved shirts and long pants, tucking pants legs into socks, and using chemical repellents.

Gothe R, Kunze K, Hoogstraal H: The mechanisms of pathogenicity in the tick paralyses. J Med Entomol 16:357, 1979. *This review lists the tick species that have been associated with paralysis, general clinical aspects, and experimental observations.*
Krinsky WL: Dermatoses associated with the bites of mites and ticks (Arthropoda: Acari). Int J Dermatol 22:75, 1983. *This is a review of skin lesions caused by acarines and epidemiologic and clinical factors helpful in diagnosis.*

Spider Bites

All spiders are eight-legged arachnids that use venom to immobilize their prey. Relatively few species have mouthparts (chelicerae) large and strong enough to inject venom into human skin. Among the better known spiders that cause moderate to severe reactions in humans are the widows (*Latrodectus* species) of the Old and New World, brown spiders (*Loxosceles* species) of the Americas and southern Africa, wandering spiders (*Phoneutria* species) in South America, species of *Chiracanthium* in both hemispheres, and funnel web spiders (*Atrax* species) in Australia.

The black widow (shoe button) spider (*Latrodectus mactans*) female may bite if it or its web is disturbed. Its abdomen is 6 mm wide and 9 to 13 mm long and is shiny black with a reddish hourglass marking or less well defined markings on the underside. The spider lives in sheltered, dark, dry places, such as in garages

and in old stone walls and outhouses. The bite, which may not be felt, may become slightly swollen and appear as two erythematous puncture marks. Within a few hours, a bitten person develops intense muscle pains and commonly a tightening feeling in the chest. Abdominal (boardlike) rigidity and waves of excruciating cramping pain are characteristic. Respiratory distress, nausea, vomiting, profuse perspiration, headache, vertigo, paresthesias of the extremities, and hyperactive reflexes are common. Speech difficulty and visual dysfunction may occur. In untreated adults, the pathologic effects of the venom usually disappear within 2 to 3 days. Death from cardiac or respiratory arrest occurs mostly in very young children and elderly or hypertensive persons.

The differential diagnosis requires consideration of various abdominal and vascular crises, such as perforated ulcer, acute appendicitis or pancreatitis, cholelithiasis, nephrolithiasis, splenic, renal, or mesenteric embolism, volvulus, porphyria, tetanus, and strychnine and lead poisoning. The generalized muscle pain, the lack of abdominal tenderness, and the peripheral sensory changes help to differentiate the widow spider bite.

Treatment with muscle relaxants temporarily relieves muscle pains. A specific antivenin available from Merck Sharp and Dohme is effective against all *Latrodectus* venom and neutralizes the effects of the venom. Because the antivenin is derived from horses, horse serum sensitivity testing is required before the antivenin is administered.

The brown (violin or fiddleback) spiders, including *Loxosceles reclusa* (brown recluse) and *L. laeta* of the western hemisphere, are also secretive, living in secluded places in houses and nesting in clothing, and they may bite when disturbed. They are 10 to 15 mm long and have a dark violin-shaped mark on the brown to gray cephalothorax. Their bites are most often recognized when a serious condition, *necrotic arachnidism*, is the result. The sometimes painful lesion that develops 2 to 6 hours after a bite is a bulla or pustule surrounded by concentric rings of ischemia and erythema. Within 24 to 48 hours, the lesion becomes cyanotic, and a central necrotic area begins to form. This area may slowly expand (up to 20 cm) over days to weeks. The resulting ulcer may not heal for weeks or months. Systemic reactions to the bite include fever, chills, edema, nausea, vomiting, dizziness, myalgias, and arthralgias; morbilliform and petechial eruptions may occur within 48 hours of the bite. A fatal complication, most often seen in children, is *intravascular hemolysis*, followed by hemoglobinuria and acute renal failure.

Treatment of necrotizing lesions is mainly symptomatic and may include antibiotic therapy for secondary infection. Dapsone is effective in promoting healing.

Lucas S: Spiders in Brazil. Toxicon 26:759, 1988. *This review describes the most venomous species in Brazil and their habitats and behavior, as well as clinical aspects of envenomation, epidemiology, and prevention.*
Southcott RV: Arachnidism and allied syndromes in the Australian region. Rec Adelaide Child Hosp 1:99, 1976. *This detailed review treats basic biology and clinical aspects of arachnid bites and infestations and is relevant to much of the world's fauna.*
Wong RC, Hughes SE, Voorhees JJ: Spider bites. Arch Dermatol 123:98, 1987. *This detailed review gives accounts of the most venomous North American spiders and discusses recent approaches to diagnosis and treatment.*

Centipede Bites

Centipedes are multilegged, elongated (up to 30 cm) arthropods with one pair of legs on each body segment. The first pair of legs is modified as poison claws that are used to inject venom into prey. Centipedes, which shun the light and are found under rocks and forest litter, rarely bite. The characteristic bite lesion has two punctate hemorrhages in the center of an erythematous swelling. Centipede bites may cause severe (fiery) local pain that may be followed by inflammation, edema, and superficial necrosis. Systemic reactions may include headache, dizziness, and vomiting. The transient effects of a bite may be accompanied by irregular pulse, muscle spasm, or lymphadenopathy. In general, centipede bites cause no long-term pathologic effects.

Southcott RV: Arachnidism and allied syndromes in the Australian region. Rec Adelaide Child Hosp 1:99, 1976. *This includes a careful review (pp 174–177) of clinical aspects of centipede bites and some case histories.*

Stinging Arthropods

Bee, Wasp, and Ant Stings

Bees, wasps, and ants (order Hymenoptera) are insects that include solitary and social species. Females have an egg-laying tube (ovipositor) that has been modified as a sting that secretes venom from abdominal glands. Social bees include honeybees and bumblebees, which all have two pairs of membranous wings and are stocky, hairy, and often yellow and black or brown. The honeybee (*Apis mellifera*) and its close relatives are found worldwide and often are responsible for human sting reactions. The honeybee has a barbed sting that becomes embedded in skin, and as the bee tries to escape, it leaves its venom apparatus and other abdominal organs and soon perishes. Vespid wasps (yellow jackets, hornets, paper wasps) are smooth insects, sleeker than bees and often yellow and black or with combinations of yellow, red, brown, or black. These wasps make the paper nests found in trees, under eaves of houses, or underground. Honeybees and bumblebees may sting when disturbed while seeking nectar or pollen at flowers. Vespid wasps may become pestiferous around food, being especially attracted to sweet or fermented liquids, fruit, fish, and meats. Mutillid wasps (velvet ants, cow killers), which are hairy and wingless, sometimes sting persons in sandy, arid environments.

Human reactions to stings usually include intense local pain, followed by the appearance of a red punctum surrounded by a blanched area and erythema. A wheal forms and the swelling and erythema, accompanied by pruritus, may last for a few hours. Multiple stings, especially on the face, may cause extensive edema, multiple vesicles, bullae, or purpura. Treatment includes gentle removal of the sting by scraping with a sharp blade (in cases of honeybee envenomation), application of ice, and topical hydrocortisone or oral antihistamines. Severe and sometimes fatal allergic reactions to stings of bees and wasps that occur in sensitized individuals are discussed in Ch. 248.

Ants (Formicidae) of some species can sting, causing severe pain. Two groups of New World stinging ants are the fire ants (*Solenopsis* species) and harvester ants (*Pogonomyrmex* species). These ants build ground nests that protrude as large mounds. An ant may grip the skin with its mandibles and then insert its sting. The ant may pivot and sting many times. This behavior, compounded by the common occurrence of mass attacks, leads to a clustering of lesions. The usual reaction to the sting is fiery, sharp pain, followed by a wheal and flare response. A clear vesicle appears that becomes pustular after about 24 hours. This sterile pustule may persist for 3 to 10 days and dry as a crust that sloughs, leaving a macule, scar, or fibrous nodule. Systemic reactions such as dizziness, nausea, vomiting, profuse perspiration, cyanosis, and asthma occur in allergic individuals but may also be seen in cases of multiple stings. Symptomatic treatment of local reactions is similar to that for bee and wasp stings.

Harwood RF, James MT: Venoms, defense secretions, and allergens of arthropods. *In* Entomology in Human and Animal Health. 7th ed. New York, The Macmillan Company, 1979. *This is a review of the biology and clinical importance of stinging Hymenoptera.*
Paull BR: Imported fire ant allergy. Perspectives on diagnosis and treatment. Postgrad Med 76:155, 1984. *A well-illustrated review of the distribution and clinical aspects of fire ant stings.*

Scorpion Stings

Scorpions are mostly subtropical and tropical arachnids that have a pair of lobster-like claws (pedipalps) anteriorly and a curved spine posteriorly that is an outlet for the proteinaceous venom produced by a pair of venom glands. Scorpions are nocturnal predators that sting quickly and repeatedly when disturbed in their hiding places under rocks, lumber, and vegetation or in shoes, bedding, or clothing left on the ground. In the United States, one scorpion species, *Centruroides sculpturatus*, of about 40 native species causes severe pathologic effects in humans. This small (about 6 cm long), straw-colored species is found only in Arizona. The arid regions that extend from North Africa to India are inhabited by the most abundant and dangerous scorpions.

The nature and severity of human reactions to scorpion stings are not consistent with the size, appearance, or aggressiveness of different species. Intense and immediate pain at the site of a sting is common to all cases. When a mildly toxic scorpion such as *C. vittatus*, a common southern United States species, is involved, the pain may be followed by local swelling and perhaps skin discoloration, regional lymphadenopathy, pruritus, or paresthesias, and less commonly by nausea and vomiting. These reactions are transient, lasting for minutes to as long as 24 hours.

The more toxic species cause local pain but little or no skin response, and systemic effects are usually noted within a few minutes to 24 hours after the sting. Symptoms may include anxiety, drowsiness, syncope, increased salivation, lacrimation, perspiration, diminished vision, photophobia, numbness and sluggishness of the tongue, vomiting, diarrhea or involuntary defecation and micturition, priapism, muscular fibrillations or spasms, and convulsions. Clinical signs may include hypotension or hypertension, irregular pulse, tachycardia and arrhythmias, irregular respiration, rapid shifts in body temperature, oliguria or polyuria, and hemiplegia. Laboratory tests may reveal hyperglycemia, glycosuria, serum glutamic-oxaloacetic transaminase (SGOT) increase, hematuria, and melena. Pathologic changes that may lead to death include myocarditis, pulmonary edema, and shock. Respiratory paralysis is the usual immediate cause of death. In the most toxic cases, death may occur within minutes of the sting or not for over 40 hours later, but most deaths occur in 2 to 20 hours after the sting. The mortality is highest in children. Close monitoring of affected patients is important because sudden relapses, often involving acute respiratory distress, may occur after a patient's condition seems to have stabilized.

The most important treatment for moderate to very toxic stings is administration of an antivenin. Antivenin to *C. sculpturatus* is available in Arizona from the Antivenom Production Laboratory, Arizona State University, Tempe, Arizona 85281 (602-965-6443 or 602-965-1457) and Poison Control in Phoenix (602-253-3334). Antivenins against other species are available from laboratories in Mexico, Brazil, Europe, Africa, and Asia. In India, where antivenin is not available, acute pulmonary edema and hypertension have been successfully treated with vasodilators, such as prazosin hydrochloride.

Early treatment of stings may include cooling of the sting site for up to 2 hours and use of a local anesthetic. Oxygen administration or artificial respiration, sodium phenobarbital injection, and parenteral solutions, including blood plasma, may be needed to treat respiratory distress, convulsions, and shock, respectively. Calcium gluconate (10 ml of 10 per cent solution) given as a slow intravenous injection reduces muscle spasms. In the United States, morphine and meperidine are contraindicated because they enhance the toxic effects of *C. sculpturatus* venom. Morphine and barbiturates are not recommended for treatment of any scorpion stings because these drugs inhibit the bulbar respiratory centers.

Personal protection includes wearing heavy gloves and boots when reaching into hidden areas in which scorpions may hide. Shaking out shoes and other materials left on the ground before using them is essential. Removal of litter from around houses, sealing cracks in foundations, and selective use of pesticides are helpful means of preventing scorpions from inhabiting houses and gardens.

Chippaux JP, Goyffon M: Producers of antivenomous sera. Toxicon 21:739, 1983. *Addresses of antivenom suppliers are listed in this article by type of venomous animal and continent.*
Keegan HL: Scorpions of Medical Importance. Jackson, University of Mississippi Press, 1980. *This book reviews scorpion morphology, taxonomy, biology, and geographic distribution, as well as clinical aspects and prevention of scorpion envenomation.*

Invasive Arthropods

Scabies

The scabies mite (*Sarcoptes scabiei*), unlike the other mites discussed, burrows into the skin and, because it reproduces on humans, can maintain a continuous infestation. Fertile female mites burrow into the skin and lay their eggs as they tunnel. Immature stages (larvae and nymphs) move out to the surface and enter hair follicles. Further development and mating take place near the skin surface. The mite burrows are slightly raised, curved, or tortuous gray lines, 5 to 15 mm long, and at the end of each is a female, a minute pearly bleb. The burrows are restricted to the horny layer of the skin and occur most often in the sides of the fingers, the interdigital webs, flexor surfaces of the wrists, elbows, skin around the nipples, and penis. Other lesions, including erythematous papules, lichenified patches, and pustules, which occur in sites other than the burrows, may be seen on the abdomen, thighs, and buttocks. In infants and young children, burrows may occur in the palms and soles, and papular lesions may be seen on the scalp, face, and neck.

Intense pruritus begins from 2 to 6 weeks after first exposure to the mite. Definitive diagnosis of the lesions is often difficult because of excoriations. In very clean individuals, few lesions may be present, and burrows may not be clearly visible. Generalized urticarial papules may result from previous treatment with fluorinated corticosteroids. Some patients have pruritic inflammatory nodules (≤12 mm in diameter) that occur on covered skin, especially the axillae, abdomen, scrotum, and penis. A severe form of scabies most often seen in immunologically compromised persons is called *crusted scabies* (originally called Norwegian scabies). As the name implies, warty plaques occur frequently on the hands and feet, and extensive scaling covers the scalp to the trunk or below. Horny debris collects under the fingernails, which are usually distorted and thickened. Pruritus, erythema, and lymphadenopathy may occur.

Diagnosis of any scabies infestation depends on observation of a mite in skin scrapings of a burrow or in situ, by gently raising the top of a burrow with a sterile needle and looking with a magnifier. In most scabies cases, only 10 to 15 mites are present on the body. In crusted scabies, large numbers of mites are present. To obtain a scraping of a burrow, an area suspected of infestation is scraped with a scalpel blade. The scraped material is examined at 50 to 100 times magnification. The movements of a living mite may be observed if the material is placed on a slide without any mounting media. Otherwise, the scraping may be cleared in potassium hydroxide (20 per cent) or suspended in mineral oil under a coverslip on the slide. The adult female mite is about 300 to 400 μm long, oval, with the dorsum convex and venter flattened. It has four pairs of legs, two pairs directed anteriorly and two posteriorly. Each anterior leg ends in an unjointed stalk with a distensible thin-walled sac at its tip; each posterior leg ends in a long, thick bristle. The size of the mite egg is about 100 × 150 μm.

Scabies lesions initially may be diagnosed as those of other skin conditions, e.g., neurodermatitis, dermatitis herpetiformis, lichen planus, and various other kinds of mite-associated dermatitis, such as that caused by *Cheyletiella* fur mites. The distribution of lesions and observation of the mite rule out these other diagnoses. Secondary infections appearing as pyoderma are common, and nephrogenic strains of streptococci infecting the lesions may cause acute glomerulonephritis.

Treatment of uncomplicated scabies involves application of one of various acaricides. Permethrin (5 per cent in dermal cream) in a single-dose regimen has recently been used with success. Lindane (1 per cent) cream or lotion is often used in a manner similar to that suggested for pediculosis, namely, an 8- to 12-hour treatment for adults, followed by thorough washing. Use of lindane on infants and pregnant women is discouraged. Pruritus and dermatitis may persist for days after adequate treatment. Antipruritic medications are often prescribed.

Transmission occurs during contact with infested persons or with clothing recently worn by such persons. Transmission between bed partners is common and does not require body contact. All household and intimate contacts should be treated to prevent recurrence or continued transmission. The female mite survives for only 2 to 3 days away from a host; therefore, as with louse infestations, fumigation of premises is unnecessary. Clothing, especially undergarments, bedding, and towels should be laundered in hot water.

Scabies mites infesting domestic animals, including dogs and cats, occasionally cause dermatitis in humans, but the lesions are usually limited to the areas that contact the animals. These mites are usually not recovered from humans.

Green MS: Epidemiology of scabies. Epidemiol Rev 11:126, 1989. *This article reviews clinical and epidemiologic aspects of scabies.*
Mellanby K: Scabies. Middlesex, England, E. W. Classey (1943), 1972. *This classic work, available in this reprinted form, is a comprehensive review of the basic biology, clinical evolution, and treatment of scabies.*

Myiasis and Tungiasis

Myiasis is the infestation of living vertebrate tissue by fly larvae. Many flies (order Diptera) that normally deposit eggs or larvae on carrion, manure, or decaying organic matter sometimes deposit their immature stages in open wounds or infected human tissues. These include blow flies, also called greenbottle or bluebottle flies (Calliphoridae), flesh flies (Sarcophagidae), and house flies (Muscidae). The larvae of some of these flies are attracted to draining infections or to clothing stained with urine or feces. The larvae crawl into lesions or natural orifices when an infected person sleeps on the ground or is otherwise exposed to flies. Individuals immobilized because of physical illness or old age who have such open lesions or infections, and especially those who are living in poor sanitary conditions, are particularly susceptible. Urogenital myiasis may cause dysuria, hematuria, and pyuria.

Some fly larvae invade intact skin of domestic animals or humans; species in this group include the human bot fly (*Dermatobia hominis*) found in Central and South America, the African tumbu fly *Cordylobia anthropophaga*, and some species of *Wohlfahrtia* that have a predilection for the tender skin of infants.

Fly larvae that live in food, e.g., vinegar flies (Drosophilidae) and cheese skippers (Piophilidae), are sometimes accidentally ingested and may cause gastrointestinal discomfort.

Wound or dermal myiasis often results in furuncular lesions, and an infested individual notices a swelling and feels pain or movement under the skin where the larvae are feeding on tissue fluids. Careful observation of the top of a lesion enables one to see two dark respiratory openings (spiracles) through which the larva breathes. Treatment consists of gentle compression of the swelling and removal of the larva with a forceps. A local anesthetic may be helpful because recurved spines may hold the larva tightly under the skin. Topical antibiotics are used to control or prevent secondary infections. Removal of larvae that crawl into sensory openings or urogenital and anal orifices may require irrigation or surgical intervention. Intestinal myiasis is usually self-limited, ceasing when the larvae are passed in the stool. Dermal myiasis of most kinds, if untreated, progresses until the mature larvae back out of the skin and drop to the ground to pupate. The physical and emotional distress caused by the presence of living larvae can be prevented if a physician considers the possibility of such an infestation and removes the larvae early in the infestation. Warble fly larvae, which normally migrate from the legs of cattle through the body to the back, in human infestations also migrate dorsally and, unless they reach a cutaneous exit site, may cause extensive tissue damage that leads to chronic illness or death.

Prevention of myiasis requires frequent changing of dressings on wounds and use of screening.

Tungiasis is the infestation of vertebrate, including human, skin by the female flea *Tunga penetrans* (chigoe, jigger, or sand flea). This flea occurs in sandy soil in subtropical and tropical regions of the Americas, the West Indies, and Africa. It usually feeds between the toes, under a toenail, or in the sole of the foot and becomes embedded as it gorges on blood. The flea, which remains embedded permanently, may cause irritation, pain, or pruritus, and the resulting swelling is often pustular. Secondary skin infections and tetanus are complications of infestations, and autoamputation of digits in Africans is apparently caused by inflammatory reactions to the flea.

Treatment of tungiasis includes removal of the flea with a sterile needle or blade, tetanus vaccination, and application of topical antibiotics. Personal protection against *T. penetrans* includes wearing footwear and using insect repellent. Sleeping above the ground surface usually prevents the flea from reaching the body.

Brothers W, Heckmann R: Tungiasis (*Tunga penetrans*) in Utah. J Parasitol 65:782, 1979. *This note succinctly describes the clinical problem and gives references to cases.*
Harwood RB, James MT: Myiasis. *In* Entomology in Human and Animal Health. New York, The Macmillan Company, 1979. *This is a thorough review of different clinical forms of myiasis.*

Arthropods and Contact Dermatitis

Various species of nonbiting mites found in stored products may cause dermatitis when they contact human skin. These microscopic foodstuff mites (Acaridae, Glycyphagidae) are found in commodities, including grains, cereals, seeds, bulbs, dried herbs, copra, dried vegetables, cured meats, mushrooms, humus, cheese, and animal and plant material used for stuffing furniture, pillows, and mattresses. Dried fruit mites (Carpoglyphidae) are found not only in dried fruits but also in jams, jellies, spoiled fruit, wine, caramel, flour, and dried milk products. The skin reactions to these mites vary, but pruritic diffuse erythema with urticarial wheals or erythematous papular eruptions are common. Laborers in granaries, food-processing plants, and commercial kitchens and dockworkers are most susceptible.

Another form of pruritic dermatitis is caused by contact with various caterpillars, pupae, adults, and some egg masses of moths and butterflies (order Lepidoptera). Urticating setae and spines on these life forms may cause mechanical irritation of the skin or may have toxic effects. Contact with setae, spines, or hairs may cause intense stinging or fiery pain, followed by the formation of wheals, local edema, erythema, and pruritus. Less common reactions include lymphadenopathy, cephalalgia, shocklike symptoms, or convulsions.

Treatment of dermatitis caused by foodstuff and dried fruit mites or lepidopteran spines or setae is symptomatic. Antipruritic substances, including antihistamines, corticosteroids, and anesthetics, have been used. Commodities containing mites must be fumigated or destroyed. Spines or setae of lepidopterans may be removed from the skin with fine forceps. Use of protective clothing and thorough washing of exposed materials help prevent continuation of these forms of dermatitis.

A third form of contact dermatitis results from vesicants produced by blister beetles (Meloidae) and some rove beetles (Staphylinidae). Cantharidin, first isolated from the meloid called the Spanish fly, is found in all species of blister beetles. Contact with this substance causes mild to severe vesicular dermatitis.

Similar lesions, which usually follow a burning sensation and tanning of the skin, result from contact with millipedes. Some species of these herbivorous myriapods exude a fluid from pores along the length of the body. Secretions from the aforementioned beetles or millipedes cause burning pain and conjunctivitis if they are rubbed into the eyes.

Treatment of toxic dermatitis associated with beetles or millipedes includes rapid washing of the skin or eyes, if affected, and use of local anesthetics. The dermal reactions caused by contact with mites, lepidopterans, beetles, and millipedes are usually transitory and do not have long-lasting effects.

Harwood RB, James MT: Vesicating Coleoptera. In Entomology in Human and Animal Health. New York, The Macmillan Company, 1979, pp 441–443. This section discusses the nature of vesicant chemicals from beetles and reviews clinical cases.
Radford AJ: Millipede burns in man. Trop Geogr Med 27:279, 1975. Geographic distribution, toxicology, pathogenesis, clinical features, and treatment of millipede envenomation are carefully reviewed.
Southcott RV: Lepidoptera and skin infestation. In Parish LC, Nutting WB, Schwartzman RM (eds.): Cutaneous Infestations of Man and Animal. New York, Praeger, 1983, pp 304–343. This chapter gives a comprehensive review of worldwide lepidopterism, including pathogenesis and clinical presentations.

PENTASTOMIASIS (Linguatuliasis)

Pentastomiasis is infestation with pentastomids, little-known invertebrates called tongue worms, which have been variously classified as arthropods or helminths. These bloodsucking endoparasites are found as adults in the lungs of reptiles and birds or in the nasal cavity of carnivores, especially cats and dogs. Herbivores are normal intermediate hosts, but humans and other mammals can be dead-end aberrant hosts for the larvae. Ingested eggs hatch, and the larvae burrow through the intestine and migrate to diverse tissues, where they molt several times and become encysted as third-stage larvae.

Human infestations have occurred in Europe, Africa, and North, Central, and South America. Two species account for most cases, Armillifer armillatus, found in pythons and other vipers in tropical Africa, and Linguatula serrata, found in canids in Europe and the Near and Middle East.

Infection occurs by accidental ingestion of tongue worm eggs contaminating food or drink, by ingestion of eggs picked up on fingers from handling infected snakes or lizards, or by ingestion of improperly cooked or raw reptiles. The third-stage larvae (20 to 25 mm long) encysted in fibrous capsules occur most often in the liver and are rarely noted except incidentally at autopsy or as calcified cysts (3 to 6 mm in diameter) on radiographic examination. Rarely, a mass of cysts in the intestinal wall may cause obstruction. Cysts compressing vital structures such as bile ducts or bronchi may lead to infections or obstructions.

Linguatuliasis, the direct infection of humans with third-stage larvae of Linguatula species, occurs most often in Lebanese people who eat raw or inadequately cooked liver or lymph nodes of goats and sheep. The ingested larvae migrate to the nasopharynx from the stomach. These larvae (5 to 10 mm long) cause Halzoun's syndrome, characterized by paroxysmal coughing, sneezing, and nasal and lacrimal discharge, accompanied by pain and itching in the throat. Other symptoms may include hoarseness, dyspnea, dysphagia, and vomiting. Submaxillary and cervical lymph nodes may be enlarged. Recovery in most cases is spontaneous in 7 to 10 days; however, death from asphyxiation due to tonsillar edema has been reported. A similar syndrome seen in Sudan, Turkey, and Greece is called Marrara's syndrome.

Prevention of pentastomiasis includes proper cooking of exotic foods such as herbivore organs and reptiles, improved hygiene of persons handling reptiles, and ingestion only of clean water and thoroughly washed raw vegetables.

Drabick JJ: Pentastomiasis. Rev Infect Dis 9:1087, 1987. This review discusses biology, parasitology, clinical manifestations, pathology, diagnosis, treatment, and epidemiology.
Herzog U, Marty P, Zak F: Pentastomiasis: Case report of an acute abdominal emergency. Acta Trop 42:261, 1985. This report reviews clinical and epidemiologic information.

LEECHES AS AGENTS OF DISEASE (Hirudiniasis)

Leeches of medical importance are bloodsucking annelid worms. Each has a ventral anterior or posterior sucker. The former encloses teeth that cut through the skin after the leech attaches. Feeding occurs within a half-hour or more.

The leeches most often feeding on humans are aquatic (freshwater) species of Hirudo, the cosmopolitan medicinal leeches; Limnatis, the nasal leeches found from the Canary Islands east through Europe, Africa, and Asia; Dinobdella, found in Asia; and terrestrial species of Haemadipsa, found in Asia, Indonesia, Australia, Pacific Islands, and Central and South America. Humans are subject to attack by large leeches in tropical rain forests or to infestation with aquatic species while wading or swimming.

Wounds produced by leeches often go unnoticed, except for the oozing blood or prolonged bleeding caused by an anticoagulant, hirudin. Pruritus is common at bite sites, and although leeches are not known to transmit any human pathogens, secondary infections may occur. Immature aquatic leeches may be ingested with water and infest the upper respiratory and digestive tracts or may invade the mouth, nose, eyes, vagina, urethra, or anus of swimmers.

Attachment of leeches to the nasal passages may cause epistaxis. Attachment to the larynx may cause hoarseness, dyspnea, and hemoptysis, and attachment to the pharynx or esophagus may cause dysphagia and hematemesis. Hemorrhaging from leech infestations may be so severe, especially in children, that anemia occurs, leading to death.

Techniques used for removing leeches from the respiratory and digestive tracts include a steady pull on the specimen with a forceps or hemostat or narcotizing the leech with a spray of 5 per cent cocaine hydrochloride before removal. In genitourinary infestations, irrigation with a strong salt solution may cause the leeches to detach. A leech attached to skin or respiratory or digestive tract surfaces may be induced to release its grip by holding it in a hemostat and touching the exposed part of the worm with a small flame or other cauterant.

Prevention of attack by aquatic and land leeches includes use of protective clothing and of insect repellents. Repellents applied to boots, trouser legs, and exposed skin are quite effective, but, because they are water soluble, must be reapplied every few hours in wet tropical regions where leeches are commonly found.

Keegan HL, Radke MG, Murphy DA: Nasal leech infestation in man. Am J Trop Med Hyg 19:1029, 1970. This paper discusses two cases and reviews other clinical reports and treatment.

439 Snake Bites

Jay P. Sanford

EPIDEMIOLOGY. Of the nearly 3500 species of snakes, fewer than one tenth are venomous. The poisonous varieties belong to five families (Table 439–1). Throughout the world, snake bites are estimated to account for 30,000 to 40,000 deaths annually. The largest number occur in Burma (Russell's viper) and Brazil (*Bothrops jararaca*). In the United States, the number of snake bites is estimated at 8000 per year. Twenty to 60 per cent of the bites by venomous snakes in the United States result in little or no envenomation (poisoning). Most bites occur in the states bordering on the Gulf of Mexico. Despite the large number of bites with envenomation, fewer than 15 deaths occur, and almost all of these are due to rattlesnake bites. This low case fatality ratio reflects the virtual absence of members of the families Elapidae and Hydrophidae in the United States.

Coral snakes, eastern and western varieties, are found in southern and western states (North Carolina, South Carolina, Georgia, Florida, Alabama, Mississippi, Louisiana, Arkansas, Texas, New Mexico, and Arizona). Their fangs are short and permanently erect. They envenomate through chewing movements. Since they are nocturnal and shy, they rarely bite humans.

The pit vipers (Crotalidae) are identified by a small depression between the eyes and nostrils. Their fangs are long and hinged, folding back when the mouth is closed and erect when open. Upon contact, venom is expressed by muscular contraction. The pit vipers are generally aggressive. The eastern (*Crotalus adamanteus*) and western (*C. atrox*) diamondback rattlesnakes are the largest and most dangerous in the United States. Their distribution includes the aforementioned states plus California, Nevada, and Oklahoma. Cottonmouths (*Agkistrodon piscivorus*), or water moccasins, are found along streams in the southern and southeastern states. They may inflict facial bites when disturbed while resting on tree branches. Contrary to lore, they can bite under water. Copperheads (*A. contortrix*), or highland moccasins, have a geographic distribution similar to that of the cottonmouths. Their bite is painful but rarely fatal.

PATHOGENESIS. Snake venoms are probably the most complex of all poisons. Because of the heterogeneous composition and multiplicity of effects, snake venoms cannot be classified simply as neurotoxic, cardiotoxic, myotoxic, or hematotoxic on the basis of the snake family (Table 439–2).

Venoms from Elapidae and Hydrophidae snakes contain basic polypeptides that produce presynaptic and/or postsynaptic neuromuscular block with resultant flaccid paralysis, including respiratory paralysis. Cobra cardiotoxin, an additional basic polypeptide, depolarizes cell membranes of skeletal, cardiac, and smooth muscles, thus contributing to paralysis. Venom of the South American rattlesnake (*Crotalus durissus*) contains an acidic protein with nondepolarizing curare-like neuromuscular blocking effects. Viperatoxin isolated from the Palestine viper causes a

TABLE 439–1. VENOMOUS SNAKES OF THE WORLD

Family	Common Varieties	Geographic Distribution
Crotalidae	Pit vipers (rattlesnakes, water moccasins, copperheads), fer-de-lance, bushmaster	Americas, Asia
Elapidae	Cobras, kraits, mambas, coral snakes, death adder	Worldwide except Europe
Columbridae	Boomslangs, bird snakes	Africa
Hydrophidae	Sea snakes	Indo-Pacific waters
Viperidae	True vipers (Russell's viper), puff adder	Worldwide except Americas

TABLE 439–2. BIOCHEMISTRY OF SNAKE VENOMS

Toxins	Family	Mechanism of Injury/Death
Neurotoxin (basic polypeptide)	Elapidae, Hydrophidae, South American rattlesnake (*Crotalus durissus terrificus*), Palestine viper (*Vipera palestinae*)	Respiratory paralysis
Cardiotoxin	Elapidae	Cardiovascular depression

Enzymes
  Phospholipase A
  5-Nucleotidase
  Phosphodiesterase
  Deoxyribonuclease II
  Ribonuclease
  Adenosine-triphosphatase
  Nucleotide pyrophosphatase
  Exopeptidase
  Hyaluronidase
  L-Amino acid oxidase
	Elapidae, Hydrophidae, Crotalidae, Viperidae
	
	(Absent in spitting cobra)
		Hemolysis

Proteases	Crotalidae, Viperidae	Hypotension due to release
Acetylcholinesterase	Elapidae (absent in spitting cobra, mamba, coral snake)	
Alkaline phosphatase		
Acid phosphatase		

peripheral nerve conduction block. A variety of enzymes, mostly hydrolases and phospholipase A, are present in most venoms. Bradykinin is released from bradykininogen by most crotalid and viperid venoms but not by Elapidae except the king cobra (*Ophiophagus hannah*). The venom of a single snake seldom contains all of the toxins. The composition and potency of venom are highly variable and differ not only among species but even among individual snakes.

SYMPTOMS AND SIGNS. *Pit Viper Envenomation.* In the United States, most victims reach a physician within 15 minutes to 3 hours. At that time, it is essential to determine whether or not envenomation has occurred and, if it has occurred, to determine the severity; this has important therapeutic implications. The clinical effects are summarized in Table 439–3. The most important early findings of envenomation are swelling at the bite, usually occurring within 10 minutes, and pain, although pain may be absent. Mild envenomation is characterized by local edema (1 to 5 inches in diameter) and pain without systemic symptoms or signs. With moderate envenomation, local findings are more extensive—edema of 6 to 12 inches in diameter. Systemic findings occur: weakness, sweating, nausea, faintness, dizziness, ecchymoses, and tender regional lymph nodes. With severe envenomation, systemic involvement includes tachycardia; tachypnea; hypothermia; hypotension; ecchymoses; paresthesias of the scalp and finger and toe tips; and muscle fasciculations. With very severe envenomation, gingival bleeding, hematemesis, hematuria, melena, oliguria, and coma occur.

Over the first 12 hours, the skin develops a tense, discolored appearance and bullae, which may be either serous or hemorrhagic.

Coral Snake Envenomation. The bite wound usually resembles scratch marks and is somewhat painful, but there is little or no edema. The onset of systemic manifestations is usually delayed 1 to 6 hours. Paresthesias around the bite may occur within several hours. Systemic symptoms may include weakness, apprehension, giddiness, nausea, vomiting, excess salivation, and even a sense of euphoria. Bulbar and cranial nerve paralysis may develop with ptosis, diplopia, papillary dilation, excess salivation, dysphagia, dysphonia, and respiratory failure. Paralysis may last 6 to 14 days, and muscular strength may not be fully regained for 6 to 8 weeks.

LABORATORY FINDINGS. Proteolytic enzymes in venoms not only produce tissue damage but also have a marked effect on coagulation, thrombin-like activity being most prominent. Within the first few hours, there is a drop in platelets owing to local consumption (occasionally to fewer than 10,000 per milliliter), a decrease in fibrinogen, and an increase in fibrin degradation products. Striking increases in prothrombin time and partial thromboplastin time occur with severe envenomation. Erythrocytes show a peculiar "burring," indicating membrane damage, and drops in hematocrit and hemoglobin concentration occur.

With pit viper envenomation, baseline laboratory tests should include complete blood count, platelet count, prothrombin time, partial thromboplastin time, bleeding time, urinalysis, and serum electrolytes. Blood should be obtained for typing and crossmatching. In patients with envenomation of moderate or greater severity, arterial blood gas determinations and an electrocardiogram are indicated. Hematologic studies should be repeated every 4 to 6 hours for the first day or until the coagulopathy has stabilized. With coral snake envenomation, repetitive coagulation studies are not indicated.

TREATMENT. *First Aid.* The initial goal of first aid is to minimize systemic absorption of the toxin. This is accomplished by restraining the patient to minimize muscular activity, application of compressive dressings, and transport to the hospital with as little effort exerted by the patient as circumstances permit. With neurotoxic venoms, absorption may result in respiratory arrest, for which resuscitation is essential. Respiratory paralysis may develop within 15 minutes following cobra bites. The snake should be killed if this can be done quickly and safely and taken along with the patient to allow accurate identification; this may obviate unnecessary therapy. The dead snake must be handled with care, since the head of an apparently dead snake can deliver a venomous bite for up to an hour after being severed. The potential value of incision and suction is less than the risks, which include delay in antivenin (antivenom) administration. The site of the bite should be wiped but not incised. Incisions can aggravate bleeding; damage nerves and tendons; introduce infection, especially with mouth suction; and delay healing. An absorption-delaying compressive bandage, preferably crepe (not a tourniquet) should immediately be applied firmly, as for a sprain, over the bite site and up the entire limb. The affected part should be immobilized (splinted) promptly. If available, an inflatable splint provides both compression and immobilization. The patient should be promptly transported to the nearest medical treatment facility. The compressive bandage should not be released during transit. The affected area should not be placed in ice. Cryotherapy results in greater tissue damage with the potential for necessitating amputation.

Hospital Care. On admission it is important to determine, if possible, if the bite was inflicted by a pit viper—specifically, rattlesnake, moccasin, or copperhead—or a coral snake and whether envenomation has occurred. The mainstay of therapy is physiologic monitoring in an intensive care unit and, for rattlesnake bites with envenomation, antivenin, which is a horse serum product; hence it has a high potential of causing serum sickness later. There are two antivenins: one polyvalent for North American pit vipers and another for eastern coral snakes. Water moccasin and copperhead bites can be managed without antivenin, avoiding immediate anaphylactic reactions and later serum sickness. With rattlesnake bites, for minor envenomation, antivenin is not indicated. For more serious rattlesnake envenomation, antivenin should be administered. For mild envenomation, three to five ampules of antivenin should be diluted (10 ml each) and then added to 500 ml of intravenous fluid. Skin or conjunctival sensitivity tests are unreliable in predicting early reactions to antivenin. Treatment should not be delayed 20 to 30 minutes to await results. All patients given antivenin should be regarded as likely to have a reaction; the incidence ranges from 3 to 54 per cent. Epinephrine should be available in a syringe before the infusion is started. At the first sign of anaphylactoid reaction, bronchospasm, hypotension, or angioedema, the infusion should be stopped and 0.5 ml of 1:1000 epinephrine injected intramuscularly. This is almost always effective, and the antivenin infusion can be restarted. A history of allergy to horse serum contraindicates antivenin unless the risk of death from envenomation is high and the patient is pretreated with epinephrine. The 500 ml should be given intravenously over 60 minutes. If the amount is adequate, the swelling will not progress and paresthesias will decrease. If progression occurs, the dose should be repeated. For moderate envenomation 5 to 10 vials, for severe envenomation 10 to 20 vials, and for very severe envenomation up to 40 vials (400 ml) may be required. In one series, the average dose required for adults with severe bites was 16 vials. Larger doses are required for bites in children and for those involving the fingers. Antivenin neutralizes both the local and the systemic effects of the venom.

In coral snake bites, if any symptoms or signs develop within the first several hours, 3 to 5 vials of antivenin (*Micrurus fulvius*) should be given intravenously. Even in the absence of symptoms, patients should be observed in the hospital for approximately 48 hours because onset of symptoms may be delayed and insidious. If neurotoxic signs appear (Table 439–3) an edrophonium test should be done: atropine sulfate (0.6 mg) given by slow intravenous infusion, followed by edrophonium chloride (10 mg) given intravenously over 2 minutes. If improvement occurs, neostigmine methylsulfate should be administered (beginning with 25 µg per kilogram of body weight per hour) by continuous infusion.

Antibiotics are usually recommended. Bacteriologic cultures of rattlesnake venom and fangs show growth from over 90 per cent. Aerobic gram-negative bacilli (*Enterobacter* sp., *Pseudomonas* sp., and *Citrobacter* sp.) and histotoxic clostridia (*Clostridum perfringens*) are the predominant isolates. On the basis of the microbiologic results, administration of one of the newer beta-lactam antibiotics—piperacillin, ceftazidime, or carbenicillin clavulanate—is most appropriate. A tetanus toxoid booster is recommended.

In the severely envenomated patient, concurrent supportive measures include the management of shock and of respiratory and renal failure. Glucocorticoids have been recommended, but a controlled trial of prednisone therapy helped neither local nor systemic effects of viperine poisoning. Despite the hypofibrinogenemia and increase in fibrin degradation products, heparin is not of benefit.

Decompressive fasciotomy is indicated only if edema within closed muscular compartments is inadequately controlled, compartmental pressures are 30 mm Hg or higher, and arterial blood supply is compromised. From the end of the first to the third week, the majority of patients will develop serum sickness, the prevalence approximating 1 per cent per milliliter of horse serum administered. Steroids are useful for treatment of serum sickness reactions.

TABLE 439–3. PIT VIPER ENVENOMATION: SYMPTOMS AND SIGNS (PERCENTAGE)

Local		Systemic						
		Generalized		*Hematologic*		*Neuromuscular*	
Fang marks	100	Weakness	70	Thrombocytopenia	42	Paresthesia of scalp, fingertips	63
Edema	74	Tachycardia	60	Increased clotting time	37	Faintness, dizziness	57
Pain	65	Hypotension	54	Decreased hemoglobin	37	Paresthesias of affected part	57
Vesicles	40	Sweating	43	Burring of RBC	18	Fasciculations	41
Necrosis	27	Nausea/vomiting	42	Thrombocytosis	16		
		Hypothermia	42	Bleeding	15		
		Tachypnea	40				
		Regional adenopathy	40				

Adapted, with permission, from the Annual Review of Medicine, Vol. 31, © 1980 by Annual Reviews, Inc.

PROGNOSIS. If adequate antivenin has been administered intravenously, mortality is virtually nil. If cryotherapy has been avoided, amputation or serious resultant deformities are uncommon.

BITES CAUSED BY SNAKES NOT FOUND IN THE UNITED STATES

VIPER (VIPERIDAE) BITES. Bites by Russell's viper are the leading cause of fatal snake bite in Pakistan, India, Bangladesh, Sri Lanka, Burma, and Thailand. They are an occupational hazard of rice farmers. Up to 70 per cent of the protein content of the venom is phospholipase A2, which can induce hemolysis, rhabdomyolysis, presynaptic neurotoxicity, and shock. Geographic variation in clinical manifestations is striking. The most common systemic signs are those of neurotoxicity; external ophthalmoplegia, ptosis, difficulty in opening the mouth ("pseudotrismus"), and inability to protrude the tongue are observed. Symptoms include drowsiness, headache, vomiting, and abdominal pain. Incoagulable blood commonly leads to spontaneous hemorrhage, often massive. Generalized muscle tenderness, myoglobinuria, and oliguria also are common. In some countries, viper bite envenomation is the most common cause of acute renal failure. Management requires intensive supportive therapy and specific antivenin. Antivenin is most effective when administered within 4 hours, 400 to 500 ml often being required. Adequate doses restore blood coagulability but do not reverse shock, nephrotoxicity, or myotoxic signs. Causes of death include shock; pituitary, intracranial, and gastrointestinal hemorrhage; and tubular or renal cortical necrosis. Individuals who recover often show clinical or laboratory evidence of hypopituitarism.

COBRA (ELAPIDAE) BITES. Bites are almost invariably painful. Local necrosis is often preceded by bullae, which may not develop for 2 to 4 days after the bite. Neurotoxic symptoms may appear as early as 3 minutes after a bite, with onset rare after 6 hours. Respiratory paralysis may occur within 15 minutes. Responses to intravenous edrophonium chloride (administered as above) usually occur. The effectiveness of cobra antivenin is inconsistent. Maintenance of adequate ventilation is essential. In survivors, neurotoxic manifestations usually resolve within a week.

Burch JM, Agarwal R, Mattox KL, et al.: The treatment of crotalid envenomation without antivenin. J Trauma 28:35, 1988. *A report of 81 patients managed by close physiologic monitoring in an intensive care unit without antivenin or surgical therapy. Excellent results were obtained.*

Curry SC, Kraner JC, Kunkel DB, et al.: Noninvasive vascular studies in management of rattlesnake envenomations to extremities. Ann Emerg Med 14:1081, 1985. *Provides details for monitoring, using noninvasive arterial studies. All but 1 of 25 patients received antivenin, and none underwent early surgical decompression.*

Malasit P, Warrell DA, Chanthavanich P, et al.: Prediction, prevention and mechanism of early (anaphylactic) antivenom reactions in victims of snake bites. Br Med J 292:17, 1986. *A study demonstrating the futility of intradermal and conjunctival tests for hypersensitivity.*

Minton SA: Neurotoxic snake envenoming. Semin Neurol 10:52, 1990. *An excellent brief summary of clinical manifestations.*

Russell FE: Snake venom poisoning in the United States. Annu Rev Med 31:247, 1980. *An excellent general review by one of the foremost authorities on the subject in the United States. An excellent source of clinical features.*

Stewart RM, Page CP, Schwesinger WH, et al.: Antivenin and fasciotomy debridement in the treatment of the severe rattlesnake bite. Am J Surg 158:543, 1989. *An experimental study in rabbits showing superior survival and preservation of muscle function in animals treated with antivenin alone.*

Tun-Pe, Phillips RE, Warrell DA, et al.: Acute and chronic pituitary failure resembling Sheehan's syndrome following bites by Russell's viper in Burma. Lancet 2:763, 1987. *A study of 33 patients; of 24 survivors, 46 per cent had evidence of pituitary insufficiency.*

Warrell DA: Snake venoms in science and clinical medicine. 1. Russell's viper: Biology, venom and treatment of bites. Trans R Soc Trop Med Hyg 83:732, 1989. *If you are going to read only one paper, select this one. A thorough, succinct review with good bibliography.*

Warrell DA, Looareesuwan S, Theakston RGD, et al: Randomized comparative trial of three monospecific antivenoms for bites by the Malayan pit viper (Calloselasma rhodostoma) in southern Thailand: Clinical and laboratory correlations. Am J Trop Med Hyg 35:1235, 1986. *The authors' clinical observations are very helpful in understanding management and complications.*

Watt G, Meade BD, Theakston RDG, et al.: Comparison of tensilon and antivenom for the treatment of cobra-bite paralysis. Trans R Soc Trop Med Hyg 83:570, 1989. *Results of a double-blind study of edrophonium versus placebo and a study of antivenin.*

440 Venomous and Poisonous* Marine Animals

John Williamson

The story of the effects of venomous and poisonous marine creatures on humankind dates from antiquity, but their scientific study remains relatively neglected. The animals are found in greatest variety and profusion in warmer tropical and subtropical waters—the very seas that attract human activities. Communities dependent on the seas as a food source or as a tourist attraction are typically foremost in studying the subject. Current research is being conducted in Australia, French Polynesia, Japan, China, Southeast Asia, Greece, India, Russia, and the United States (including Hawaii). Although the subject has emerged from the realm of folklore, lack of objectivity still exists. *Human injury by venomous marine creatures results from accidental or intentional human interference with the animal or its territory.*

TAXONOMIC CLASSIFICATION

Taxonomic classification has been customary but is of limited practical value to those responsible for treatment and prevention of marine envenomation. The animals listed in Table 440–1 have accounted for the majority of human deaths and a significant number of the poisonings and injuries that are documented to date.

ANIMALS CAUSING HUMAN FATALITIES

Table 440–1 lists marine invertebrates and vertebrates that have caused fatalities by envenomation and animals responsible for fatal poisonings in humans.

Box Jellyfish

The northern Australian box jellyfish (*Chironex fleckeri*) and the Phillipines' closely related *Chiropsolmus quadrigatus* have been responsible for 80 documented human deaths since 1884; many more fatalities remain unconfirmed. Found only in tropical West Indo-Pacific waters, they are true jellyfish, carrying up to 60 extendable tentacles. These tentacles bear a vast number of nematocysts (stinging capsules, including microbasic mastigophores) that discharge massively when a person blunders into them and becomes entangled. The animals are difficult to see under natural conditions. This massive envenomation produces rapid systemic venom delivery that is enhanced by struggling, and collapse occurs within minutes in serious cases. Seventy per cent of fatalities occur in women and children (small body mass and hairless skin). The venom of *Chironex fleckeri* at least is a high

---

*The currently held view is that the administration of venoms requires mechanical penetration, whereas the term *poison* implies oral ingestion. The term *toxins* (here marine zootoxins) refers to both venoms and poisons.

TABLE 440–1. MARINE ANIMALS CAUSING HUMAN FATALITIES

I. From Envenomation
A. Invertebrates
  1. Box jellyfish (*Chironex fleckeri, Chiropsolmus quadrigatus*)
  2. Blue-ringed octopuses (Family Octopodidae)
  3. Portuguese man-of-war (Bluebottle) (*Physalia* ssp.—Atlantic Ocean only)
  4. Venomous cone shells (Family Conidae)
B. Vertebrates
  1. Venomous sea snakes (Family Hydrophidae)
  2. Scorpionfishes, including stonefishes (Family Scorpaenidae)
  3. Stingrays (Order Rajiformes)
  4. Catfish (Suborder Siluroidei)

II. From Poisoning
A. Ciguatoxic fishes
B. Tetrodotoxic fishes
C. Shellfish
D. Sea turtles
E. Viscera of whales, porpoises, polar bears, walruses, seals

molecular weight protein mixture containing "lethal" and dermatonecrotic factors. Death in massive envenomations is by myocardial systolic standstill. Respiratory depression also can occur. Intravenous verapamil (dose titrated) may revert the myocardial effects.

The densely adherent tentacles produce whip wheals with a diagnostic ladder pattern on the envenomated skin. Treatment is immediate resuscitation on the beach, vinegar dousing, compressive bandaging, and injection of the specific antivenom, intravenously if possible, in a dosage large enough to be effective. The antivenom is sheep antiserum; therefore, appropriate precautions are necessary.

Blue-Ringed Octopus

At least two species (*Hapalochlaena maculosa* and *H. lunulata*) have produced morbidity and mortality. The venom is located in the salivary glands and is injected by a bite that may be painless. The salivary toxin contains tetrodotoxin (M.W. 319), a unique biologic material also found in the flesh of puffer fish (see below). It inhibits action potentials (Fig. 440–1) by specific blockade of sodium ion transport. Clinically, the danger is respiratory failure and hypoxia. Airway protection and expired air resuscitation are lifesaving. There is no antivenom. First aid is as for snakebite (see Ch. 439) and must include early compression-immobilization bandaging.

Portuguese Man-of-War (Bluebottle)

This is the world's best known jellyfish and probably the most common source of human stings. Thousands of stings occur annually the world over, usually during the summer months. *Physalia* exists in at least two different forms, an Atlantic (large, two long tentacles) and a Pacific (smaller, single long tentacle) form. The Atlantic form has caused human death (at least five in the United States the past 3 years). No fatalities from the Pacific form are yet known. Sting pain is immediate and severe. The sting pattern is a linear white beaded wheal. Allergic reactions to the protein-mix venom are possible. Mechanisms of death are unknown. The uncommon death usually occurs within minutes. Vinegar dousing for *Physalia* stings remains controversial. Ice packs are recommended for analgesia. Compression-immobilization bandaging is not recommended. There is no antivenom. Regional lymphadenopathy and vomiting may occur. *Physalia* occurs in numbers, or "navies"; hence stings among swimmers and divers are usually multiple.

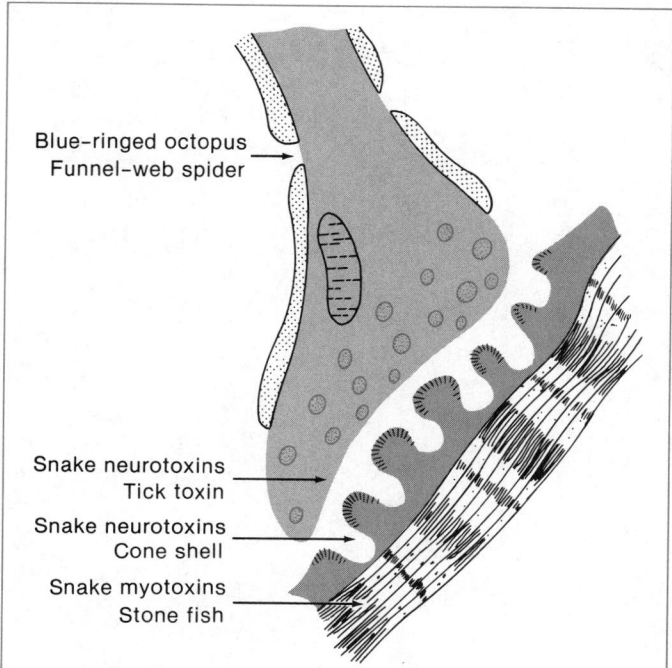

FIGURE 440–1. Scheme of a somatic neuromuscular junction, showing sites of action of a number of animal toxins. (Courtesy of Dr. V. Callanan, Townsville, North Queensland, Australia.)

Venomous Cone Shells

There are 37 cases of cone shell envenomation in the literature, 8 of them fatalities. Seven species of cone shells are considered dangerous. The injected venom produces postsynaptic neuromuscular blockade (Fig. 440–1) and thus death from hypoxia (respiratory failure). On-the-spot airway protection and expired air resuscitation are lifesaving. No antivenom exists. First aid is as for snakebite and must include compression-immobilization bandaging.

Venomous Sea Snakes

Apart from the predominance of these snakes in warmer waters, the proven lethality of several species, and the availability of an antivenom that is effective against all sea snake venoms (*Enhydrina schistosa* antivenom—Melbourne and Bombay), the subject of sea snakebite can be considered as for land snakebite. Early application of compression-immobilization bandages to the bite site is crucial first aid treatment for sea (and most terrestrial) snakebites.

Scorpionfishes and Stonefishes

Deaths from zebrafish stings have been documented. No firm record of a fatality from stonefish (*Synanceja*) stings has been located in Australia, where these stings are not uncommon. In this group of animals dorsal spines inject the venom. The ensuing pain is devastating, with intense local tissue swelling and discoloration. Immersion of the envenomated part in hot water offers partial pain relief. Medical management is for pain relief (conduction anesthesia), prevention of wound infection, tetanus immunization and, in the case of stonefish stings, specific antivenom injection, with appropriate precautions. Tourniquets or compressive bandages should not be used.

Catfish and Stingrays

Despite their ubiquity, catfish rarely cause human death. Stingrays certainly do! Documented deaths are all associated with barb penetration of the chest or abdomen. The deposited venom is powerfully tissue necrosing. No antivenom is available. All such wounds should be referred to early and sophisticated medical assessment. Pieces of the brittle stingray spines may break off in wounds, necessitating radiography and perhaps careful exploration with the patient under anesthesia, prior to local wound debridement.

Ciguatera (Poisoning by Fish in the Tropics)

This poisoning occurs in all tropical and subtropical seas and is a major public health and economic problem in the Pacific. About 1500 cases of ciguatera poisoning occur annually in the South Pacific alone. Deaths have occurred. The search for a simple chemical test of fish flesh to reveal the presence of ciguatoxin is proceeding. Symptoms are gastrointestinal (nausea, abdominal pain, vomiting, and diarrhea) and peripheral neurologic (paresthesias, especially circumoral and intraoral, dental discomfort, and a classic confusion of peripheral temperature sense; that is, hot and cold are confused). A generalized skin itch that is potentiated by alcohol consumption occurs.

Ciguatoxin is believed to be passed along in the food chain. One source may be a dinoflagellate, *Gambierdiscus toxicus*. Treatment is symptomatic. Symptoms may persist for months. Following a serendipitous clinical observation, recent use of intravenous mannitol for acute ciguatoxin poisoning (1 gm per kilogram of body weight administered over 30 minutes) is encouraging; the mechanism of mannitol's action in this setting is unclear (molecular scavenger?). The precise chemical structure of ciguatoxin remains uncertain.

Tetrodotoxic Fishes

These include toad fish and puffer fish. Ingestion of the toxin in the fish flesh produces symptoms and signs characteristic of tetrodotoxin's action potential blockade (Fig. 440–1), viz.: numbness, motor weakness, ataxia, and respiratory failure. Tetrodotoxin is one of the most toxic of known poisons and is the active component in blue-ringed octopus envenomation (see above).

There is no specific antidote, so management of a patient is symptomatic.

Shellfish Poisoning

Paralytic shellfish poisoning is due to the ingestion of saxitoxin and is associated with a fatality rate of about 8.5 per cent. This condition should be distinguished from the gastrointestinal and the allergic types of shellfish poisoning. Like ciguatoxin (see above), saxitoxin is thought to originate in dinoflagellate organisms, at the beginning of the marine food chain. Treatment is symptomatic. No specific antidote is known.

Whales, Porpoises, Polar Bears, Walruses, and Seals

Poisoning results from the ingestion of the viscera of these animals, notably liver or kidneys. The intoxication from such organs of polar bears, walruses, and seals is believed to be due to hypervitaminosis A.

SOME NONFATAL ENVENOMATIONS (Table 440–1)

Numerous, sometimes serious, nonfatal envenomations continue to occur from true jellyfish (Class Scyphozoa), including *Carybdeid medusae* (notably *Carukia barnesi*—"*Irukandji*"), and the "hydroids" (Class Hydrozoa), including the Pacific *Physalia* species (bluebottle, or Portuguese man-of-war; see above), sea nettle (*Chrysaora quinquecirrha*), mauve stinger (*Pelagia noctiluca*), moon jellyfish (*Aurelia aurita*), and *Gonionemus*. Others have included corals and anemones (Class Anthozoa) and toxic sponges (Class Demospongiae).

A vast array of marine animals continue to be involved in less serious human envenomations, accompanied by symptoms ranging from mild local pain and itching to serious allergic manifestations. Certain management principles are becoming established.

1. Household vinegar inactivates undischarged nematocysts of several medically significant species of jellyfish (*Irukandji, Carybdia tamoya, C. rastoni*, and *Chironex*). Vinegar does nothing for the pre-existing pain of these stings.

2. In general, ethyl alcohol should not be applied to serious marine stings.

3. Nematocyst inhibition appears to be a "species-specific" phenomenon.

4. Allergic phenomena can play a significant role in some marine envenomations, such as jellyfish stings and toxic sponge contacts. Susceptible patients are those with a history of atopy.

5. Immediate pain relief continues as a major research goal. Local cooling (ice) helps in some jellyfish stings.

6. Serum-specific immunoglobulins (especially immunoglobulin G [IgG]) are detectable in stung patients, assist in sting identification, and may persist for years.

Burnett JW, Calton GJ: Jellyfish envenomation syndromes updated. Ann Emerg Med 16:1000, 1987.

Burnett JW, Calton GJ, Fenner PJ, et al.: Serological diagnosis of jellyfish envenomations. J Comp Biochem Physiol 91C:79, 1988. *Authoritative and to the point.*

Burnett JW, Othman IB, Endean R, et al.: Verapamil potentiation of *Chironex* (box-jellyfish) antivenom. Toxicon 28:242, 1990. *The advancing front in therapy.*

Fenner PJ, Williamson JA, Skinner RA: Fatal and non-fatal stingray envenomation. Med J Aust 151:621, 1989. *The situation at present.*

King GK: Acute analgesic and cosmetic benefits of box-jellyfish antivenom. Med J Aust 154:365, 1991. *Illustrates the short- and long-term value of appropriate Chironex antivenom administration.*

Martin CJ, Audley I: Cardiac failure following *Irukandji* envenomation. Med J Aust 153:164, 1990. *A serious new syndrome in the Indo-Pacific; with references.*

Sutherland SK: Australian Animal Toxins. 2nd ed. Melbourne, Australia, Oxford University Press, 1990. *This detailed and profusely illustrated work is a hallmark in the subject of animal envenomation and poisoning, both marine and terrestrial. The definitive work on snake and spider bite management.*

Williamson J: Ciguatera and mannitol: A successful treatment. Med J Aust 153:306, 1990. *The use of mannitol in acute ciguatoxin poisoning.*

Williamson J, Fenner P, Burnett J: The Marine Stinger Book. 4th ed. Brisbane, Surf Life Saving Association of Australia, Queensland State Centre, 1991. *A concise illustrated account of the subject.*

PART XXIII

NEUROLOGY

SECTION ONE / PRINCIPLES OF CLINICAL NEUROLOGIC DIAGNOSIS

441 Clinical Study of the Patient

441.1 APPROACH TO THE PATIENT
Fred Plum and Jerome B. Posner

The great, continuing triumphs of genetic, cellular, and molecular biology that have marked the past 20 years have added greatly to our understanding of neurologic-neuromuscular function and the etiology and mechanisms of neurologic diseases. At last count, more than 95 distinct genetic disorders of the nervous system have been assigned to specific chromosomal or mitochondrial loci. In 39 of these, the particular enzymatic abnormality has been delineated, and hardly a month passes without new discoveries in this realm. Efforts to transfer missing genes to deficient hosts have been started, and functionally effective nerve cell transplants have been placed successfully in the human brain in efforts to correct parkinsonism. These triumphs presage entirely new and potentially remarkable approaches to future neurologic therapy.

Despite these advances, the fundamental challenge in successfully diagnosing and treating patients with neurologic symptoms or disease remains in (1) understanding the genesis of their complaints, (2) parsimoniously but effectively utilizing laboratory aids to rule in or out the presence of structural-chemical disease, and (3) managing them with full recognition that the individual physician still represents the most important component in improving the health and spirits of another, suffering human being. This section particularly addresses the third principle.

The evaluation of patients whose complaints potentially implicate the nervous system challenges the physician on several levels. At the outset, patients often arrive frightened at the prospect of neurologic disease. They are afraid of pain, often disturbed by the threat of visible crippling, and terrified of chronic disorders such as Alzheimer's and other degenerative diseases. Often they use misleading or incorrect terminology to describe their symptoms, and some repress critical information because they fear its implications. Another issue is the ambiguity of many neurologic complaints. Ultimately, all symptoms of whatever origin are neurologic, since they necessarily require abnormal stimulation of either peripheral or central nervous pathways to make themselves felt. Separating primary neurologic symptoms from those reflecting trouble in other bodily organs represents only a first small step down the diagnostic trail. Even seemingly direct neurologic complaints such as headache, nausea, dizziness, tinnitus, fatigue, and generalized weakness are as likely to signal the presence of an emotional disorder as a somatic neurologic abnormality, and the distinction often evades laboratory investigation. To assign the basis of such complaints accurately requires that the physician know why *this* symptom occurred in *this* patient at *this* particular time. To reach such answers often takes time and repeated questioning, but until the physician fully understands these matters he or she can neither treat present disability nor anticipate future developments.

Even more important than separating emotional from somatic

neurologic complaints is recognizing the urgency for prompt diagnosis and treatment of serious neurologic disorders. If nerve cells die they cannot regenerate or be repaired. Furthermore, the older the patient, the less likely the brain is able to substitute a new, learned function for one damaged or destroyed by disease. The guiding principle in treating neurologic illness is that the more rapidly the doctor can reach an accurate diagnosis, the more likely he or she is to prevent progression and reduce future disability. The mandate is clear: In seriously and acutely ill patients with neurologic abnormalities, life- or brain-threatening complications must be treated immediately even while proceeding with diagnostic procedures that may take much longer to complete. By contrast, patients whose diseases lack quick and specific remedies (e.g., most psychosomatic disorders, degenerative diseases, or residua of severe trauma) usually need far more from the doctor than the local pharmacy can supply.

Several important maxims apply to all treatment situations: Protect the brain first, no matter what successive steps must follow; relieve pain even while proceeding with diagnosis; and give reassurance, hope, and explanation at every step along the way. In order to plan long-term management effectively and economically, try to construct an accurate prognosis as early as possible. In acute, self-limited illnesses, such as meningococcal meningitis or most cases of acute inflammatory polyneuritis, for example, one usually can predict the probable outcome within a few days of onset. One even knows for most such patients the difference in convalescent time required before they return to their former occupations. With diseases with intermediate outcomes, such as multiple sclerosis, full recovery is less certain and the risk of relapse or chronic disability requires the physician to appraise all aspects of the patient's life in order to give proper guidance. At the worst extreme are patients who become severely aphasic and hemiplegic from stroke or demented from Alzheimer's disease. They may never recover independence, and their proper early management often requires that one guide families through major social and financial readjustments in planning for the future. How the doctor manages such complexities determines his or her effectiveness as a physician.

441.2 CLINICAL DIAGNOSIS
Fred Plum and Jerome B. Posner

A logical approach to neurologic problems yields high clinical dividends in accuracy of diagnosis and selection of appropriate therapy. The following imperatives outline a widely used strategy.

Focus strongly on the relevant history, weighing the biologic implications of the patient's symptoms in order to link such descriptions to known neuroanatomic and physiologic perturbations. Vague symptoms can sometimes reflect educational problems or mental decline in the patient. Alternatively, they may hint at a distressed psyche more than a diseased soma. By contrast, perturbations of specific sensory, motor, or language pathways often produce symptoms that almost immediately hint at the general nature of "where and what" the neurologic abnormality may be.

Pay attention to chronology. The identification of remote, temporary sensorimotor or visual symptoms in a 35 year old who now, several years later, develops an "acute" paraparesis suggests an exacerbating and remitting disorder such as multiple sclerosis rather than a new spinal neoplasm. Conversely, a several-year history of sharply episodic, brief experiences of depersonalization accompanied by automatic behavioral activity in a patient with a recently developing unilateral headache suggests temporal lobe seizures heralding the recent expansion of an intracranial mass lesion rather than the onset of a migraine syndrome late in life.

Try to place the origin of symptoms and signs on at least a crude neuroanatomic map. Taken together, do the findings fit a common-sense interpretation? Do they suggest disease in a single anatomic locus or do they reflect dysfunction affecting several different anatomic areas? Do they suggest a system disorder (e.g., motor neuron disease or neuromuscular disease) rather than a focal structural lesion, e.g., a single spinal neoplasm producing focal lower motor neuron changes at one level accompanied by upper motor neuron abnormalities below that level?

Are the symptoms and signs consistent with known physical disorders? For example, chronic weakness and fatigue lasting more than 6 months unaccompanied by physical or laboratory abnormalities suggest chronic anxiety-depression rather than structural disease or systemic metabolic dysfunction. Beware, however; some diseases affecting the nervous system move so slowly that their early symptoms and signs may not be readily localizable. A corollary to not overdiagnosing somatic disorders is that it is equally important not to jump to conclusions regarding psychiatric diagnoses unless other findings by history or physical or projective tests support such conclusions. For example, low-grade astrocytomas of the frontal lobe may produce new-onset behavioral abnormalities long before they cause focal abnormalities on the neurologic examination or unequivocal alterations in magnetic resonance images.

Form etiologic hypotheses logically, apply common sense, and consider the common before the rare. Age, previous symptoms, epidemiologic frequency, gender in X-linked diseases (e.g., muscular dystrophy or adult-onset optic atrophy) as well as personal changes in the home and workplace all can contribute important elements that must be weighed in the evaluation.

Reach ultimate diagnoses deliberately, basing conclusions on their capacity to satisfy known principles of anatomy, perturbed neurologic function, and disease mechanisms. Avoid undue efforts to fit collections of signs and symptoms into inexact syndromes. Physicians who too rapidly attempt to match selected symptoms and signs into an iteratively constructed diagnosis often find it difficult to surrender prematurely made conclusions. A more open mind, aware that early working diagnoses are necessarily probablistic, is in a better position to modify preliminary hypotheses in order to meet unexpected changes as they evolve in the clinical course or the laboratory findings. Lastly and importantly, order tests sparingly, armed with knowledge of what each procedure can or cannot provide and how it specifically may help to diagnose or confirm the particular patient's problem.

441.3 THE NEUROLOGIC HISTORY

Jerome B. Posner

The neurologic history usually supplies a greater proportion of the diagnostically relevant information than does either a medical history or the neurologic examination. Many neurologic diseases (e.g., migraine and, often, epilepsy) are not accompanied by abnormal physical or laboratory findings, and in these instances the physician must depend solely on the history to reach an appropriate diagnosis. Even when the patient suffers from a neurologic disease marked by physical signs and/or laboratory abnormalities, the history usually supplies about 80 per cent of the total diagnostic information. Furthermore, because neurologic abnormalities affect such important functions as thinking, moving, and feeling, it is unusual to have significant abnormal signs that have not been reflected in symptoms. (Exceptions occur in

demented patients and those with lesions of the nondominant parietal lobe, characterized by denial of disability. In these instances, abnormal behavior may be recognized by family and friends.) Thus, findings on examination not recognized by the patient or family are likely to be irrelevant or even misleading. By contrast, symptoms complained of by the patient, such as mild weakness or alterations of sensation, are probably significant even if too subtle to be detected by the examination. Because patients so keenly appreciate neurologic symptoms, a meticulous history often allows a physician to localize the disease anatomically and to understand its pathophysiology even before he begins the physical examination.

Taking the neurologic history usually occupies the majority of time spent in an initial visit with a patient suffering a neurologic disorder. At the completion of the history, the physician should be able either to make a definite diagnosis or to formulate three or four hypotheses which can be tested by the physical and laboratory examinations. To reach this goal, the experienced physician gradually develops a targeted approach, similar to that which follows.

BE INTERESTED AND SUPPORTIVE. Try not only to gain diagnostic information but also to learn enough about the patient's psychologic and social background to establish a satisfactory doctor-patient relationship. Diagnostic information is often lost when the patient does not volunteer symptoms that he believes would not interest the physician or that are too intimate to tell to an "unsympathetic stranger." Such information is more readily forthcoming if the physician demonstrates interest, reassurance, and support.

BE ALERT TO NONVERBAL CUES. What the patient does is often as important as what he or she says. The patient's overall appearance and demeanor, tone of voice, or tendency to sigh or shed a tear in discussing what appear to be relatively trivial symptoms may be important clues to an underlying depression or severe anxiety over those symptoms.

REQUIRE PRECISION. Do not accept jargon or names of diseases from the patient. Jargon terms such as "dizziness" or diagnostic appellations such as "sinus headache" require an exact definition.

MAINTAIN A BALANCE BETWEEN LISTENING AND ASKING. Elicit the history in the patient's own words and, whenever possible, allow the patient to tell the story without interruption. Excessive interruptions imply impatience or disinterest and may lead to the exclusion of vital information. However, the physician must ask direct questions to encourage relevance, achieve precision, and place each symptom in its correct context. If the information is not volunteered, the physician must ask about the intensity and frequency of the complained symptoms, their duration, events and factors that precipitate or relieve them, and any other symptoms associated in time with the patient's major complaint.

FORM HYPOTHESES. Do not be a passive recipient of the patient's story. While taking the history, one must sift and distill the information in order to retain the relevant and discard the irrelevant. Concurrently, one must form hypotheses about the nature of symptoms as they are presented and test those hypotheses by asking pertinent questions. Hypotheses are tested and refined during the course of taking the history, so that by the end the physician has three or four potential diagnoses to guide the physical and laboratory examinations. The best hypotheses are broad explanations of the patient's symptoms in anatomic and/or pathophysiologic terms, which are gradually refined into etiologic terms as the history develops. Hypotheses should give preference to illnesses that are probable (i.e., common diseases are more likely than rare diseases), serious (e.g., brain tumors should be considered before tension headache), treatable (e.g., spinal cord meningioma and vitamin B_{12} deficiency should be ruled out before making a diagnosis of multiple sclerosis), and novel (some patients have rare diseases, and these should not be forgotten).

ALWAYS TAKE A COMPLETE HISTORY. Even if the diagnosis seems clear from the chief complaint and the present illness, elicit other aspects of the patient's history in order to rule in or out other physical or psychologic disabilities that could contribute to the patient's discomfort. In particular, inquire about the patient's mood (e.g., is he depressed or suicidal?), his usual daily activities (and whether the illness interferes with them), his sexual activities, the nature of psychologic and physical support at home, and his or her view of the illness and its effects.

END BY SUMMARIZING. At the end of the history, summarize the history as you understand it, asking the patient if the summary is correct and if anything has been overlooked.

OBTAIN FURTHER HISTORY FROM THE PATIENT'S FAMILY AND FRIENDS. If the history appears incomplete, and particularly if part of the illness involves changes in mental state or episodic unconsciousness, ask family, friends, and colleagues to supply missing elements, giving their views on how the signs and symptoms affect the patient's daily life.

441.4 THE NEUROLOGIC EXAMINATION
Fred Plum

Several texts contain detailed techniques of bedside neurologic examinations. In most clinical circumstances, however, an understanding of a few fundamental principles about the nervous system plus the mastering of a brief but systematically thorough approach to the examination can give reliable and effective answers. The secret is to learn well an approach that covers the main elements of nervous system function and to be familiar with ways to seek out more exhaustive evaluations if and when the history or examination suggests special abnormalities. Under all circumstances, however, the details of how one examines the patient should be geared to evaluating clinical hypotheses derived from the history.

An effective neurologic examination proceeds from general to specific in its principles and rostral to caudal in its anatomy. The examination checks on the integrity of major functions but avoids details that do not relate to the complaints of most patients. In awake and talking patients, begin to evaluate mental status and language as they give their histories. Apply at least a brief mental examination on everyone, but be gentle and understanding: "How has your memory been? Can I just check a couple of points with you?" Check orientation. Examine memory for recent events, for public figures, and for three unrelated words after a 5-minute interval. Review the capacity to handle abstractions (boy—dwarf, small tree—bush, proverbs). Provide a problem in simple arithmetic (the number of nickels in $1.35). Check serial sevens. Have the patient repeat five numbers or the spelling of "world" backwards. Be patient and remember that anxiety can compromise the performance of even a normally good mind, but if in doubt, perform a minimental status evaluation (see Table 450–3). Have the patient stand and walk; bear in mind that the nervous system is the organ of communication and behavior, and that one learns most about human beings by watching them attempt natural tasks. To detect apraxia (see Ch. 449) watch the patient at least partially dress and undress; remark on alertness-dullness; hyperactivity-apathy; adventitious movement–akinesia; visible deformities, asymmetries, or weaknesses in functional tasks; hypertrophies-atrophies; cutaneous abnormalities (pox, birthmarks, café au lait spots, pigmented or hair spots over spinal defects); a straight, flat, or crooked spine. Learn to observe constantly and closely, comparing what you see with what you already have encountered in thousands of people living everyday lives. Wise physicians gain experience not only from their patients but from the everyday world in which they live.

Examine cranial functions. Palpate the skull and test the neck gently for suppleness and length. Then examine the following in every patient: vision, the optic fundi, pupillary activity, ocular movements, corneal reflexes, jaw movement, facial movement, hearing, swallowing, speaking, and breathing. One can omit examinations of smell, taste, facial sensation, labyrinthine-vestibular activity, sternocleidomastoid function, or detailed tongue movements unless symptoms suggest the involvement of these areas. Examine in everyone the extremities and trunk for hypertrophy or atrophy, size, gross strength, muscle tone, adventitious movements (e.g., tremors, fasciculations, tics), coordination (rhythmic movements and point-to-point tests), and reflexes. If the patient has no sensory symptoms, he or she is unlikely to have abnormal sensory signs. Nevertheless, check the distal extremities briefly for the threshold perception of vibration and

pin prick. Examine the plantar responses. Evaluate autonomic and sphincter functions as part of the general medical examination. Get in the habit of examining the neck over the carotid arteries for bruits that may herald partial stenoses. Above all, be systematic and consistent in the approach and *do not jump at diagnosis until all the evidence is in.* Doctors tend to make diagnoses quickly and surrender wrong ones reluctantly. By contrast, they view even partial unknowns as challenging problems. Try to choose the latter approach until matters become certain.

USE OF LABORATORY TESTS. Advances in laboratory methods during recent years have remarkably increased the accuracy of diagnosis and physiologic evaluations. At the same time, excessive technology raises the costs of medical care unnecessarily. More than anything else, the physician's ordering practices influence this aspect of health care costs. The doctor must recognize the precise advantages for both positive and negative knowledge that derive from each test, then gear his or her ordering to hypotheses gained from the history and whatever additional clues come from the neurologic examination. For example, when managing an adult with recent onset of headache, the results of a computed tomographic scan, whether normal or abnormal, commonly help management and provide the patient with great reassurance. However, to repeat scans unnecessarily or to order irrelevant tests just for the sake of "a complete workup" wastes the time and resources of all concerned.

De Jong RN: The Neurologic Examination. New York, Harper and Row, 1979. *The standard, detailed text describing the bedside evaluation of patients.*
Landau WM: Strategy, tactics and accuracy in neurological evaluation. Ann Neurol 27:86, 1990. *A master clinician expounds his approach.*

441.5 NEUROLOGIC DIAGNOSTIC PROCEDURES
Jonathan D. Victor

LUMBAR PUNCTURE

Sampling the cerebrospinal fluid (CSF) is indispensable in diagnosing infections of the central nervous system and needs to be performed on an emergency basis when bacterial meningitis is suspected. Table 441–1 lists other indications for lumbar puncture, as well as major contraindications.

ELECTRODIAGNOSTIC STUDIES

Examinations performed in the clinical neurophysiology laboratory are best viewed as extensions of the bedside neurologic examination. The neurologic examination, fundamentally, is a series of observations of the patient's response to a traditional set of standard stimuli. The techniques of clinical neurophysiology allow one to detail the responses with a greater temporal reso-

TABLE 441–1. COMMON INDICATIONS AND CONTRAINDICATIONS FOR LUMBAR PUNCTURE

Diagnostic indications
 Known or suspected meningitis and encephalitis
  Acute: bacterial, viral
  Subacute: tuberculous, syphilitic, fungal, neoplastic
  Chronic: syphilitic, granulomatous, neoplastic
 Intracranial or intraspinal hemorrhage, if CT or MRI is not available
 Multiple sclerosis
 Acute polyneuropathy
 Suspected benign intracranial hypertension (pseudotumor), if CT or MRI is negative
Therapeutic indications
 Intrathecal administration of antimicrobial or chemotherapeutic agents
 CSF drainage in benign intracranial hypertension or communicating hydrocephalus
Contraindications
 Intracranial hypertension due to mass lesion or obstructive hydrocephalus
 Bleeding diathesis
 Local skin or epidural infections

lution, to demonstrate the activity of single cells and cell populations that underlie the responses, and to quantify the observations.

It is important to remember that neurophysiologic tests are not etiologic tests. They do not replace the basic neurologic paradigm of reasoning from localization to possible etiologies but rather add to the precision and sensitivity with which functional pathology can be defined.

Electroencephalography

The electroencephalogram (EEG) is a record of the spontaneous electrical activity of the brain as recorded on the scalp. The clinical EEG is typically recorded from 8 to 16 pairs of electrodes (called "derivations"). The "international 10-20" system of electrode placement provides coverage of the scalp at standard locations denoted by the letters F (frontal), C (central), P (parietal), T (temporal), and O (occipital) with subscripts (odd for left-sided placements, even for right-sided placements, and "z" for midline placements).

Recorded in this fashion, electrical potentials due to normal brain activity have a typical amplitude of 30 to 100 μV and an irregular wavelike variation in time (Fig. 441-1A). The main generators of the EEG are thought to be postsynaptic potentials, with the largest contribution arising from pyramidal cells in cortical layer III. The minute amplitude of the EEG compared with the ECG is a consequence of two facts: The normal ECG is generated by cells that are synchronously activated and geometrically aligned, whereas the normal EEG is generated by cells that are asynchronously activated and, in general, not geometrically aligned. Thus, the EEG is a composite record of fluctuating correlations between the activities of many populations of cells.

Ongoing EEG activity, called the *background*, is described in terms of frequency ranges: less than 3.5 Hz (delta), 4 to 7.5 Hz (theta), 8 to 13 Hz (alpha), and greater than 13.5 Hz (beta). In awake but relaxed normal adults, the background consists primarily of alpha activity in occipital and parietal areas and beta activity in central and frontal areas. Variations in this pattern occur as a function of age (particularly in the first years of life)

and behavioral state (e.g., vigilant versus relaxed versus drowsy versus asleep; eyes open versus eyes closed).

EEG ABNORMALITIES. EEG abnormalities can be divided into two categories: alterations in the background activity and paroxysmal activity. Global abnormalities in the EEG background are seen in diffuse brain dysfunction associated with developmental delay, metabolic disturbances, infections, and degenerative diseases. EEG background abnormalities are never specific enough to establish a diagnosis. For example, the "burst-suppression" pattern illustrated in Figure 441-1B may be seen in severe anoxic brain injury as well as in coma due to barbiturates. Several encephalopathies, however, have characteristic EEG features that suggest a diagnosis. For example, an excess of beta activity suggests intoxication with barbiturates, benzodiazepines, and related drugs. Triphasic slow waves (Fig. 441-1C) are typical of metabolic encephalopathies, particularly those due to hepatic and renal dysfunction. Creutzfeldt-Jakob disease and subacute sclerosing panencephalitis have characteristic EEG signatures, consisting of background alterations along with periodic paroxysmal discharges (see below).

Psychiatric illness is not associated with prominent changes in the EEG. Thus, a normal EEG helps to distinguish pseudodementia from dementia and psychogenic unresponsiveness from neurologic disease.

Thalamocortical connections play a major role in establishing the normal EEG background. Thus, although brain stem and diencephalic activity is not directly registered in the EEG, structural lesions of the brain stem may cause diffuse changes in background activity via their effect on thalamocortical relays.

The EEG is an adjunctive test in the determination of brain death. An active EEG readily distinguishes de-efferented or locked-in states (such as severe Guillain-Barré syndrome and basal pontine infarction) from cortical inactivity (see Ch. 445). Electrocerebral silence, however, does not necessarily imply brain death, since it may be produced by reversible conditions such as barbiturate intoxication and hypothermia.

Focal or lateralized abnormalities in the EEG background imply similarly localized disturbances in brain function and thus suggest the presence of underlying structural lesions. CT and MRI imaging have largely supplanted the EEG as a localizing technique. An important exception is herpes simplex encephalitis,

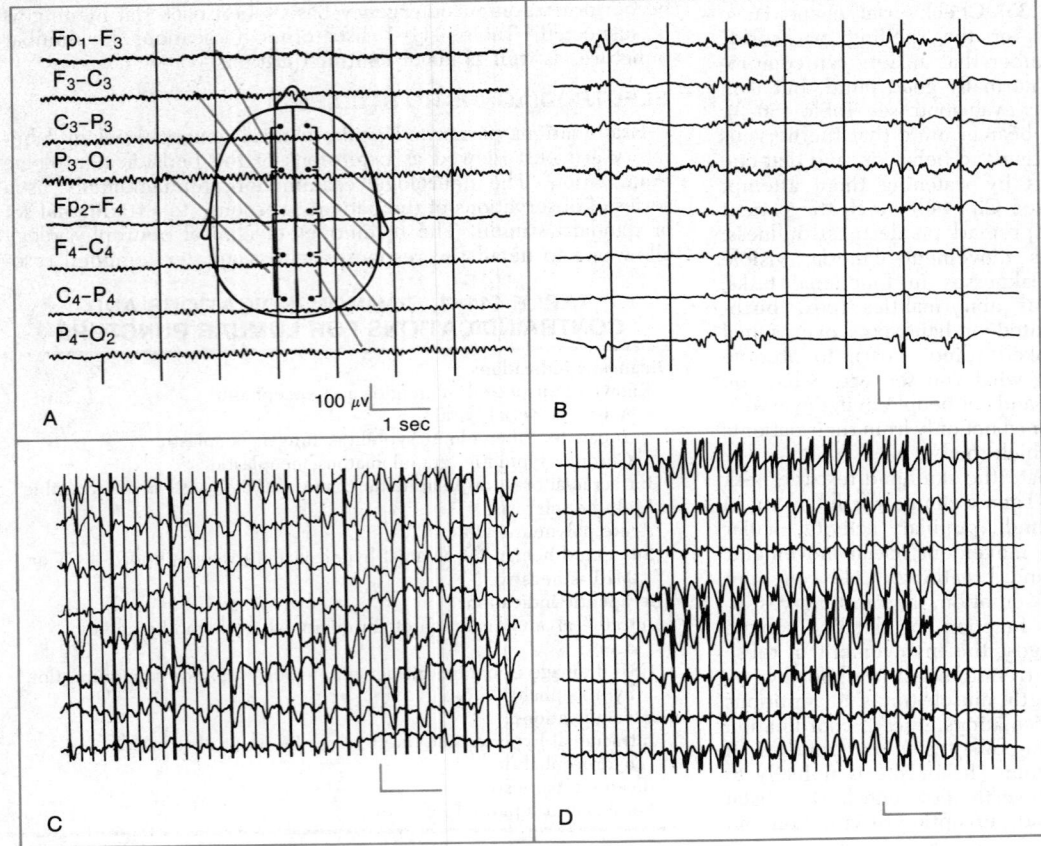

FIGURE 441-1. Normal and abnormal EEG's. *A,* The EEG of a normal alert adult. *B,* Burst-suppression, a pattern seen in severe cerebral dysfunction. *C,* Triphasic slow waves, seen in metabolic encephalopathies. *D,* A brief spike-and-wave seizure. In each record, the top four tracings are from parasagittal left-sided bipolar electrode placements (Fp_1-F_3, F_3-C_3, C_3-P_3, P_3-O_1); the lower four tracings are from the corresponding right-sided placements (Fp_2-F_4, F_4-C_4, C_4-P_4, P_4-O_2). The scale represents 1 sec and 100 μV. Note the reduced vertical scale in *D.*

which may produce focal abnormalities in temporal leads before imaging techniques demonstrate structural changes.

Paroxysmal EEG activity ("spikes" and "sharp waves") reflects pathologic synchronization of neurons. As such, this finding implies a brain region with epileptogenic potential. Spikes and sharp waves commonly appear in the EEG records of epilepsy patients during the interictal period. Along with routine clinical information, the location and character of EEG paroxysms and their relationship to the background help to classify the epileptic disorder, guide rational anticonvulsant therapy, and assist prognosis. Some patients with epilepsy may not show paroxysmal activity on a routine EEG, either because the focus is infrequently active or because it is too small or too deep to be evident in scalp recordings. The diagnostic yield of the EEG can be increased by *activation procedures*, such as hyperventilation and photic stimulation, by prolonged ambulatory monitoring, or through the use of special recording sites, including nasopharyngeal leads, anterior temporal leads, and surgically placed subdural and depth electrodes.

During a seizure, paroxysmal EEG activity becomes continuous and rhythmic and replaces normal background activity (see Ch. 483). In partial seizures with secondary generalization, paroxysmal activity begins in one brain region and spreads to uninvolved regions. The EEG identifies a focal onset of seizures more accurately than clinical observation alone. In primary generalized seizures, paroxysmal EEG activity is bilateral at onset. An example is shown in Figure 441–1D.

Whether focal or generalized, seizures with motor manifestations are unlikely to be subtle clinical events. However, sensory seizures, psychomotor seizures, and other forms of seizures without major motor manifestations may require an EEG for identification and diagnosis.

Evoked Potentials

External stimuli evoke changes in the ongoing electrical activity of the brain that may be extracted from scalp recordings by signal-averaging techniques. The three modality-specific evoked potentials discussed below form the bulk of clinical practice.

VISUAL EVOKED POTENTIALS (VEP). The VEP is commonly elicited by stimulating the retina with repetitive reversals of black-and-white checkerboard patterns. The most robust component is an occiput-positive wave several microvolts in amplitude, occurring approximately 100 msec after pattern reversal. Termed the P-100, its cellular origins include a mixture of excitatory and inhibitory synaptic signals. The VEP is recorded separately for each eye. Interocular differences in P-100 latency imply prechiasmal conduction abnormalities, and bilateral delay in the P-100 latency implies bilateral conduction defects in the visual system. Since VEP's measure central response time rather than visual resolution, they may be abnormal in patients with normal visual acuity and visual fields. VEP's are particularly useful in identifying unsuspected optic nerve or cerebral abnormalities in patients whose clinical signs point to disease affecting the brain stem or spinal cord. Demonstration of such multifocal lesions in the appropriate setting fortifies the clinical diagnosis of multiple sclerosis. Delayed optic nerve conduction may also be due to compressive lesions (e.g., pituitary tumor), metabolic disorders (e.g., vitamin B_{12} deficiency), and other neurodegenerative diseases (e.g., olivopontocerebellar atrophy). In infants and patients who cannot cooperate with behavioral tests, VEP's elicited by a graded series of stimuli provide a measure of visual resolution and contrast sensitivity.

BRAIN STEM AUDITORY EVOKED POTENTIALS (BAEP). The BAEP is commonly elicited by brief clicks presented to one ear while random noise is presented to the other ear. The normal response, recorded by an electrode at the ear referenced to the vertex, consists of a series of submicrovolt waves at approximately 1-msec intervals. Wave I is generated at the distal end of the eighth nerve, wave III is generated along auditory pathways at the level of the superior olive, and wave V is generated at the level of the inferior colliculus. BAEP abnormalities commonly accompany mass lesions in the cerebellopontine angle and intraparenchymal brain stem lesions affecting the auditory pathways. Since the BAEP shows a stereotyped maturational pattern in the first 2 years of life, it is a valuable means of assessing the developmentally delayed or at-risk neonate.

BAEP's elicited by a sequence of increasingly intense click stimuli provide a measure of auditory threshold in infants and patients who cannot cooperate with behavioral tests. In the appropriate clinical setting, absence of BAEP potentials rostral to wave II accompanied by still-remaining peripherally generated potentials supports the diagnosis of brain death.

SOMATOSENSORY EVOKED POTENTIALS (SEP). An SEP may be elicited by brief electrical stimulation delivered to any of several sensory nerves and dermatomes, but median, peroneal, and posterior tibial nerves are most commonly used. Scalp electrodes placed over somatosensory areas record submicrovolt potentials, and the spinal cord volley and peripheral nerve action potential often can be recorded by appropriately placed electrodes. With median nerve stimulation, potentials generated at medullary and midbrain-thalamic levels can be identified. Compressive, demyelinating, or metabolic disturbances affecting central sensory pathways delay centrally generated potentials but not potentials generated prior to entry to the spinal cord. Upper- and lower-extremity SEP's, in conjunction with nerve conduction studies and EMG, can help to identify radiculopathies and plexopathies.

OTHER PHYSIOLOGIC MEASURES OF BRAIN ACTIVITY. The limitations of the EEG have motivated many approaches to provide functional images of the brain with better spatial resolution. Two of these techniques deserve mention here.

Positron emission tomography (PET) is an isotopic, computed tomographic method for imaging regional cerebral blood flow and metabolism. It provides a spatial resolution of somewhat better than 1 cm. In normal subjects, PET has identified local brain regions activated by specific sensory, motor, and cognitive tasks. In vegetative and demented patients, PET demonstrates characteristic global patterns of metabolic derangements. In patients with epilepsy, PET may demonstrate focal metabolic abnormalities even when structural changes are not apparent. At present, the main limitations of PET are the high doses of radioisotope required, its relatively poor temporal resolution, and its high cost.

Magnetoencephalography (MEG), the recording of magnetic fields generated by intracranial current loops, achieves a higher spatial resolution than the EEG because magnetic fields are virtually unaffected by the volume-conduction effects that distort the brain's electrostatic fields. Since MEG retains excellent temporal resolution, it adds to the ability of electrical recordings to localize the generators of evoked potentials and epileptic spikes. Unfortunately, the minute size of the brain's magnetic fields and the costly and cumbersome nature of present-day detectors limit MEG to investigational use.

Nerve Conduction Studies and Electromyography

NERVE CONDUCTION STUDIES. Many motor and sensory peripheral nerves can be stimulated percutaneously at one or more points along their length. The induced electrical activity of muscles can be recorded with surface electrodes or with appropriately inserted needle electrodes. The *conduction velocity* of motor nerves can be calculated from the difference in latency of the motor response evoked by stimulation at two or more points along their length. Conduction velocity in sensory nerves can be determined by recording sensory nerve action potentials elicited by electrical stimulation at proximal or distal sites.

The function of nerve roots and segments of peripheral nerves that lie too close to the spinal cord to be studied directly may be assayed by the F-response and H-reflex. The *F-response* describes a muscle action potential that results from antidromic conduction of a volley along a motor nerve to the anterior horn cell body and back again to muscle. The *H-reflex*, a muscle response that represents the electrical equivalent of the monosynaptic stretch reflex, is elicited by stimulating sensory fibers in the corresponding peripheral afferent nerve. Under normal circumstances, it is readily recorded only in the soleus after stimulation of the tibial nerve. It thus serves to test the S1 root only.

Compound nerve action potentials are elicited by electrical stimulation of a peripheral nerve and are recorded by electrodes placed at a second site along the nerve. The response is dominated by the larger and more rapidly conducting myelinated nerve fibers. Accordingly, demyelinating neuropathies characteristically slow the conduction velocities. By contrast, axonal neuropathies, in which individual cell bodies or axons fail, decrease the amplitude of evoked motor and sensory responses but preserve normal conduction velocities until all of the largest myelinated fibers are affected.

Routine clinical tests cannot readily assess the function of unmyelinated fibers. Percutaneous microneurographic recording from single nerve fibers in the intact peripheral nerve represents an investigational approach to study unmyelinated and small myelinated fibers.

Electromyography (EMG) is performed by inserting a needle electrode into the muscle. At rest, a normal muscle with normal innervation remains electrically silent. With denervation, spontaneous activity occurs, consisting predominantly of fibrillation potentials and positive sharp waves. Fasciculation potentials, representing synchronous firing of entire motor units, occur mainly in anterior horn cell disorders and mechanical disturbances affecting motor nerve roots and may result in fasciculations that visibly dimple the overlying skin. Fibrillation potentials, representing electrical activity of single muscle fibers, and positive sharp waves occur predominantly in neurogenic lesions but can also be seen in dystrophies and inflammatory myopathies.

After the muscle's resting activity is observed, the patient is asked to gradually contract the muscle. This permits observation of individual motor units and their pattern of *recruitment*. In myopathies, degeneration of muscle fibers leads to a decrease in the size of motor units: Voluntary contraction recruits a normal number of units but with small amplitude and short duration. In denervated muscle, voluntary activity recruits a decreased number of units. With chronic denervation, collateral sprouting by remaining motoneurons leads to residual motor units of abnormally large amplitude and duration. Myotonic discharges, abnormal repetitive discharges that vary in amplitude and frequency, are seen in a variety of specific myopathies.

Table 441–2 summarizes how nerve conduction studies and EMG distinguish myopathies from neuropathies and indicate whether a neuropathy is demyelinating or axonal. Note that radiculopathies are distinguished from polyneuropathies on the basis of the distribution of the affected nerves and muscles rather than the findings in the affected areas. Detailed analysis of EMG activity may also help define central disturbances of motor control.

TABLE 441–2. TYPICAL ELECTROPHYSIOLOGIC FEATURES OF NEUROPATHIES AND MYOPATHIES

	Nerve Conduction Velocity	F-response	H-reflex	Electromyography
Inflammatory myopathy or dystrophy	Normal	Normal	Normal	Fibrillations; positive sharp waves; small motor units
Metabolic myopathy	Normal	Normal	Normal	Small motor units
Axonal neuropathy	Normal	Normal	Normal	Fibrillations; positive sharp waves; fasciculations; large motor units with distal predominance
Demyelinating neuropathy	Slowed diffusely	Delayed or absent diffusely	Delayed or absent	Normal motor units
Radiculopathy	Normal	Delayed or absent in damaged root	Delayed or absent if S1 is involved	Fibrillations; positive sharp waves; fasciculations; large motor units if chronic
Motoneuron disease	Normal	Normal	Normal	Fibrillations; positive sharp waves; fasciculations; large motor units diffusely

NEUROMUSCULAR TRANSMISSION STUDIES. Diseases of the neuromuscular junction are identified by the presence of abnormal neuromuscular transmission in the setting of otherwise normal nerve conduction studies. At the normal neuromuscular junction, the amount of acetylcholine released exceeds severalfold the requirements for activating the muscle. Repetitive action potentials cause a mild decrement in acetylcholine release, but the safety factor prevents a decrement in the postsynaptic response. In myasthenia gravis, immunologic blockade reduces the safety factor of the postsynaptic receptors. As a result, repetitive stimulation of a motor nerve elicits a rapid diminution of the evoked muscle action potential, paralleling the decreasing amounts of acetylcholine released. In botulism and Eaton-Lambert syndrome, repetitive stimulation overcomes a presynaptic blockade and produces a gradual increase in the size of the evoked muscle action potential.

Pathologic reductions in the safety factor magnify the normal variability of the time interval between nerve action potential and depolarization of the postsynaptic fiber. This increased variability, or "jitter," can be assayed by simultaneously recording two muscle fibers in the same motor unit with single-fiber EMG electrodes. The jitter study is a more sensitive test of defective neuromuscular transmission than repetitive stimulation.

Aminoff MJ (ed.): Electrodiagnosis in Clinical Neurology, 2nd ed. New York, Churchill Livingstone, 1986. *Comprehensive introduction to EEG, EP, EMG, and other modalities.*

Chiappa KH: Evoked Potentials in Clinical Medicine. New York, Raven Press, 1983. *Emphasis on practical matters and interpretation.*

Kimura J: Electrodiagnosis in Diseases of Nerve and Muscle: Principles and Practice, 2nd ed. Philadelphia, F. A. Davis, 1989. *A standard reference.*

Niedermeyer E, Lopes da Silva F: Electroencephalography: Basic Principles, Clinical Applications, and Related Fields, 2nd ed. Baltimore, Urban and Schwartzenberg, 1987. *Encyclopedic, authoritative.*

Regan D: Human Brain Electrophysiology. New York, Elsevier, 1989. *Encyclopedic, emphasis on fundamentals and evoked potentials.*

Spehlmann R: EEG Primer. New York, Elsevier, 1981. *Clear and concise.*

Spehlmann R: Evoked Potential Primer. New York, Elsevier, 1985. *Clear and concise.*

441.6 RADIOLOGIC IMAGING TECHNIQUES

Michael Deck

Neurologic patient care has improved dramatically in the last 20 years because of a revolution in imaging techniques such as computed tomography (CT) introduced in 1972, magnetic resonance imaging (MRI) in the late 1970's, and positron emission tomography (PET) and single-proton emission computed tomography (SPECT), which have been the subject of increasing interest over the last 10 years. Improvements in ultrasound equipment with digital processing of the image and superimposed Doppler imaging have facilitated the diagnosis of intracranial cerebrovascular disease in adults as well as brain damage in neonates. Magnetic resonance spectroscopy (MRS), currently being evaluated, measures various aspects of regional brain metabolism that may complement the findings of PET and SPECT.

Interventional radiology of the brain also has developed to the point that it is now possible to place microcatheters directly into the feeding arteries of arteriovenous malformations or arteriovenous fistulas, so as to treat the lesion with rapidly polymerizing glues such as *N*-butyl-cyanoacrylate, with platinum microcoils, or with detachable liquid-filled microballoons. Similarly, balloon dilatation techniques can now be used to treat intracranial arterial stenosis due to atheroma and intracranial vasospasm resulting from subarachnoid hemorrhage.

THE SKULL AND BRAIN

PLAIN RADIOGRAPHY. Plain radiographs of the skull are routinely taken in frontal, lateral, and half-axial projections. Such films are useful principally in the initial evaluation of head trauma, in which demonstration of fractures of the vault and base may influence subsequent management. Depressed bone fragments may require elevation, and involvement of the paranasal sinuses or mastoid air cells may result in meningitis, requiring prophylactic antibiotics. Most skull radiographs are taken for medicolegal reasons. Their diagnostic and prognostic value is limited because of poor correlation with injury of the underlying brain, a condition that is much better demonstrated by CT or MRI.

CT and MRI have supplanted plain radiographs in the evaluation of intracranial mass lesions such as tumors, hematomas, and infarcts, as well as in the detection of optic foramen enlargement due to tumors and bony sclerosis due to meningiomas. Tumors and inflammatory lesions of the paranasal sinuses and abnormalities of the craniovertebral junction also are demonstrated better by CT or MRI than plain radiography.

COMPUTED TOMOGRAPHY (COMPUTED AXIAL TOMOGRAPHY, CAT). CT employs an x-ray source with a tightly collimated beam passing through the anatomic area under study. An array of x-ray detectors numbering from 520 to 4800 measure the radiation absorbed by the organs targeted by the x-ray beam during a 360-degree rotation lasting 1 to 6 seconds. The analogue output from each detector is digitized and then computed to calculate a coefficient of absorption for each "pixel" in the field, using a mathematical process called filtered backprojection. The resulting computed image is displayed on a cathode-ray tube monitor that may be viewed directly or photographed onto transparent film. CT images from current equipment demonstrate anatomic structures in the skull and brain with high spatial resolution. Fresh hemorrhages within either the brain or the subarachnoid, subdural, or epidural spaces can be identified because of the greater x-ray attenuation of clotted blood. Areas of calcification may have similar appearances but are usually more irregular and have a higher attenuation value. Many CT examinations employ contrast enhancement with intravenous iodinated material to demonstrate normal vascular structures as well as the abnormal endothelial permeability that accompanies certain types of tumors and inflammatory processes.

Although contrast enhancement can add critical information in many CT examinations of the brain, the material also carries a small risk of adverse anaphylactic reactions. The general population has about a 1 in 10,000 chance of serious anaphylactic reaction and a 1 in 40,000 chance of death. These dangers increase fourfold in patients with previous allergic history to iodinated contrast material, iodine, or shellfish. The risk may be reduced by administering an antihistamine drug immediately before or 50 mg of prednisone orally 24, 12, and 6 hours before the injection. Special techniques can be used to improve the resolution of CT and generate physiologic data. These include the following:

1. Coronal projections to image the floor of the skull, the sella turcica, and the petrous bones.
2. Image reformatting to generate coronal or sagittal images from multiple axial images. The technique, which depends on absolute immobilization of the patient, produces good resolution but results in greater amounts of radiation to the brain and potentially the eye. Three-dimensional reformatting may be useful for displaying surfaces and contours and is increasingly utilized by craniofacial surgeons to evaluate facial trauma and congenital anomalies.
3. Ultrathin sections of 1.5 mm or less to examine areas requiring high detail, such as the sella turcica, orbits, and petrous bones.
4. Bone targeting, which employs a special reconstruction algorithm to define fine anatomy such as the ossicles and osseous labyrinth of the petrous bone.
5. Dynamic scanning achieved by performing rapid sequence scans after rapidly injecting a bolus of contrast agent. The subsequent contrast enhancement and washout can help to differentiate an aneurysm or arteriovenous malformation from a vascular tumor.
6. CT cisternography and myelography performed by injecting water-soluble nonionic contrast material (iohexol or iopamidol) into the subarachnoid space and running the contrast material to scan the area of suspected abnormality. This technique may help to delineate tumors of the sella region, the foramen magnum, and the spinal canal. It may also be used to investigate CSF rhinorrhea and CSF dynamics in hydrocephalic patients.

MAGNETIC RESONANCE IMAGING (MRI, NUCLEAR MAGNETIC RESONANCE IMAGING). MRI, a rapidly developing technology, has replaced CT as the examination of choice for most neurologic conditions. Nuclear magnetic resonance occurs when hydrogen atoms or certain other elements with an odd number of nuclear particles, such as sodium or phosphorus, are placed in an intense magnetic field varying between 3,000 and 15,000 gauss (0.3 to 1.5 tesla). The nuclei behave like small magnets and align themselves in the field. When stimulated by a pulse of radioenergy of a specific frequency (the Larmor frequency), determined by the intensity of the main magnetic field, the nuclei flip off axis. While in this energized state, the nuclei spin in phase as they subsequently relax into their original alignment with the main magnetic field, thereby emitting a small radiofrequency signal. The image is generated by a number of such magnetic resonance signals, transformed by a computer using techniques similar to those employed in CT. The resulting images demonstrate a high contrast between various tissues due largely to differences in the rate at which magnetized nuclei in tissues of different chemical composition resume their original state (T1 and T2).

The intensity of the MR image may be measured on the viewing console using a movable cursor similar to that on a CT scanner. Using standard "spin-echo" imaging sequences, a short T1 relaxation time (e.g., fat) results in high intensity (bright) while a long T1 relaxation time (e.g., cerebrospinal fluid) results in low signal intensity. Conversely, a short T2 relaxation time (fat) results in a low signal intensity and a long T2 relaxation time (CSF) results in a high signal intensity.

Thus the appearance of fat, brain, and CSF on a T1-weighted spin echo (TE 30, TR 500) reverses on a T2-weighted spin echo (TE 80, TR 2000). The concentration of protons also affects intensity, as it is the signal from the proton that is being measured. Other factors affecting the signal intensity include flow, magnetic susceptibility, paramagnetic effects, and the static field strength of the device.

MR images may be obtained in axial, coronal, sagittal, or oblique planes simply by changing the switching of the instrument's several magnetizing coils. Paramagnetic contrast agents developed for use with magnetic resonance imaging contain unique elements such as gadolinium that, because of the large number of unpaired electrons in their outer shells, have a marked effect on the T1, or spin-lattice relaxation time, of protons. Gadolinium chelated to DTPA is used in a manner similar to iodinated contrast media in CT to define areas of increased vascularity and/or capillary permeability. Recently, methods have been developed to quantify pulsatile and nonpulsatile flow of blood within the arteries and veins. The resulting images have a resolution similar to those of intravenous digital subtraction angiography techniques. Other methods permit quantitation of the flow of CSF through the aqueduct and posterior fossa in various disease entities such as aqueduct stenosis, communicating hydrocephalus, and transtentorial brain herniation.

MRI is contraindicated for patients who harbor cardiac pacemakers or ferrous foreign bodies such as shrapnel. Intracranial aneurysm clips provide a relative contraindication unless made from nonmagnetic titanium or stainless steel.

The presence of metal prostheses, spinal rods, certain metallic dental implants, and metallic cranioplastic prostheses may produce interfering artifacts but carry no risk of injury to the patient.

CEREBRAL ANGIOGRAPHY. Most cerebral angiograms are performed with an intra-arterial catheter inserted over a guide wire into the femoral artery and passed upward to the aortic arch or into the carotid or vertebral arteries. Although cerebral angiography is a relatively safe procedure in experienced hands, complications, such as arterial damage, emboli to the brain, and contrast neurotoxicity, occur in 1 to 2 per cent of procedures. New, less toxic non-ionic contrast agents are now replacing traditional ionic contrast materials, and the use of smaller catheters facilitates performing the examination on outpatients.

Arterial digital subtraction angiography (DSA) uses computerized imaging enhancement to improve the contrast of the injected contrast agent and lower the dose required.

Intravenous DSA is performed using similar equipment and rapid injections of contrast material into a peripheral vein or the right atrium. The procedure may be performed as an outpatient procedure for demonstrating the aortic arch and great vessels in the neck, as well as the intracranial cerebral arteries and veins. Intravenous DSA is not satisfactory for demonstrating small

TABLE 441–3. IMAGING MODALITY OF CHOICE IN DISEASES OF THE CNS

	CT	CT + C	MRI	MRI + Gd
Brain				
Gliomas	+	+ +	+ + +	+ + + +
Metastases	+	+ + +	+ + +	+ + + +
Meningiomas	+	+ + +	+ +	+ + + +
Lymphoma	+	+ +	+ + +	+ + + +
Postoperative tumor recurrence and radiation necrosis	+	+ +	+ +	+ + + +
Hematomas	+ + +	–	+ + + +	–
Subarachnoid hemorrhage	+ + +	–	+	–
Aneurysm and arteriovenous malformation	+	+ +	+ + +	–
Head trauma	+ + +	–	+ + +	–
Infarcts	+ +	+	+ + +	+ +
Abscess	+	+ +	+ + +	+ + + +
AIDS	+	+ + +	+ + +	+ + + +
Multiple sclerosis	–	+	+ + + +	+ + + +
Hydrocephalus/atrophy	+ +	+ +	+ + + +	–
Congenital anomalies	+	+	+ + + +	–
Sellar tumors	+	+ +	+ + + +	+ + +
Posterior fossa				
Acoustic neurinomas	+	+ +	+ + + +	+ + +
Meningiomas	+	+ + +	+ + +	+ + + +
Epidermoid tumors	+	+	+ + + +	–
Cholesterol granuloma	+	+	+ + + +	–
Basilar artery aneurysm	+	+ +	+ + + +	–
Arachnoid cysts				
Craniovertebral junction		+	+ + + +	
Intra-axial gliomas	+	+ +	+ + + +	+ + +
Cerebellar tumors	+	+ + +	+ + +	+ + + +
Spine				
Trauma	+ + +	–	+ + +	–
Degenerative disc disease	+ + +	–	+ + + +	–
Postoperative disc disease	+ +	+ + +	+ + +	+ + + +
Metastatic bone disease	+ +	–	+ + + +	+ + +
Arteriovenous malformation of the cord	–	+	+ + +	+ + +

CT = Computed tomography; C = contrast enhancement; MRI = magnetic resonance imaging; Gd = gadolinium enhancement; – = no additional value.

aneurysms of the circle of Willis or intracranial arterial abnormalities such as occlusions from emboli or vasculitis. Its rate of complications is about the same as that of arterial angiography.

THE SPINE

RADIOGRAPHY (PLAIN FILMS). *Conventional radiography of the spine* demonstrates bony abnormalities such as degenerative disc disease, primary and metastatic tumors, and fractures of the vertebral bodies. Plain radiographs are the best method for demonstrating osteophytes in the neural foramina in the cervical, thoracic, and lumbar spine. Plain films should be obtained prior to myelography, CT, or MRI to identify segmentation anomalies at the thoracolumbar and lumbosacral junctions.

COMPUTED TOMOGRAPHY. CT of the spine demonstrates abnormalities of the spinal cord, meninges, vertebral bodies, and intervertebral articulations as well as those affecting paravertebral and prevertebral soft tissues. CT supplemented with intravenous contrast enhancement may be used to demonstrate vascular tumors of the spinal cord and meninges and can be valuable in distinguishing recurrent herniation of lumbar intervertebral discs from postsurgical scarring.

Postmyelogram CT or CT with intrathecal contrast improves delineation of subtle nerve root displacement due to posterolateral herniation of the intervertebral discs and associated osteophytes. It is also useful in demonstrating cysts and hydromyelia of the spinal cord, conditions in which CT may detect entry of contrast agent into the cavity 12 to 24 hours after intrathecal injection.

MAGNETIC RESONANCE IMAGING. MRI of the spine has replaced CT as the examination of choice because it gives better resolution of the spinal cord, subarachnoid space, and vertebral anatomy and clearly depicts the intervertebral discs, showing the state of hydration of the nucleus pulposus and the condition of the annulus with usually clear and unequivocal demonstration of any rupture of the annulus.

MRI of the spine with enhancement by Gd-DTPA defines spinal cord tumors and inflammatory processes of the meninges and differentiates recurrent disc herniation from postoperative scar tissue.

MYELOGRAPHY. Myelography is the most sensitive examination for demonstrating intradural mass lesions and can be helpful when an MRI is equivocal or shows multilevel disc disease without a predominant level of pathology. Iodinated water-soluble non-ionic contrast agent (iohexol, iopamidol) is introduced by lumbar puncture or if indicated by lateral cervical puncture (C1–C2). The contrast is hyperbaric and flows by gravity. By tilting the patient on a radiographic table, the contrast may be manipulated under fluoroscopic control from the lumbosacral region to the base of the skull.

Complications of myelography are rare, and the study is often performed as an outpatient procedure. Nevertheless, neurotoxic and other complications rarely can occur. They include injury to nerve roots by the lumbar puncture needle; subarachnoid, subdural, or epidural bleeding; infection; and aggravation of spinal cord compression by mass lesions due to changes of pressure in the subarachnoid space.

IMAGING TECHNIQUES IN SPECIFIC DISEASE CATEGORIES (Table 441–3)

Tumors of the Cerebral Hemispheres

GLIOMAS (Fig. 441–2). Gliomas are demonstrated better with MRI than with CT because the superior sensitivity of MRI to slight changes in water content produces a focal area of hyperintensity on T2-weighted images. Tumors adjacent to the skull are seen better on MRI because of the absence of bone artifact. Differentiation of tumor from peritumoral edema may be obvious or difficult depending on the tumor margin but is improved with Gd-DTPA enhancement, which may demonstrate the areas of blood-brain barrier disruption or hypervascularity. Pre-gadolinium T1-weighted images may demonstrate hyperintensity due to hemorrhage into the tumor.

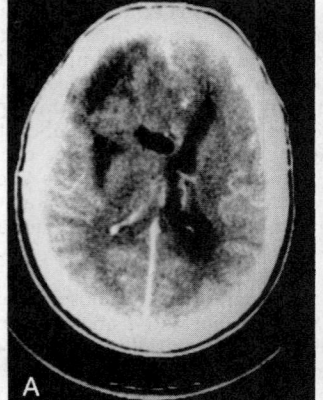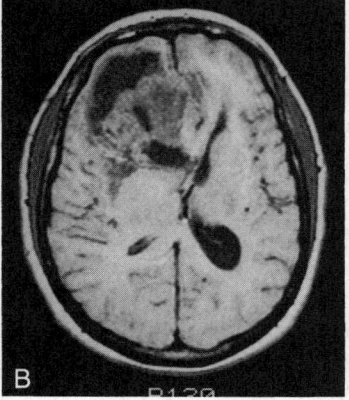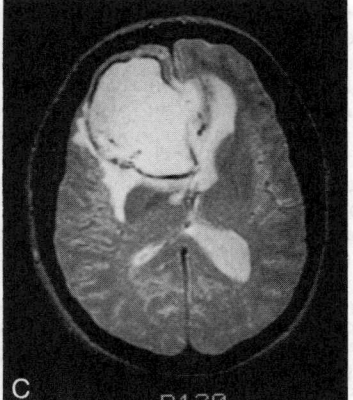

FIGURE 441–2. Right frontal glioblastoma multiforme. *A,* CT axial section with iodinated contrast enhancement. *B,* MRI axial section, 500/30 SE (T1-weighted). *C,* MRI axial section, 2000/80 SE (T2-weighted).

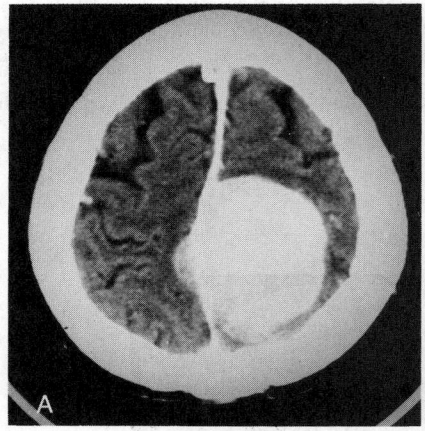 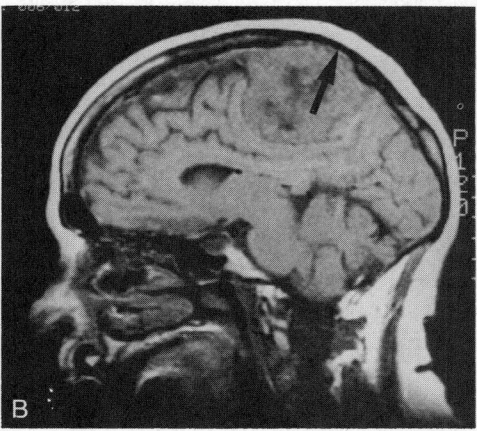 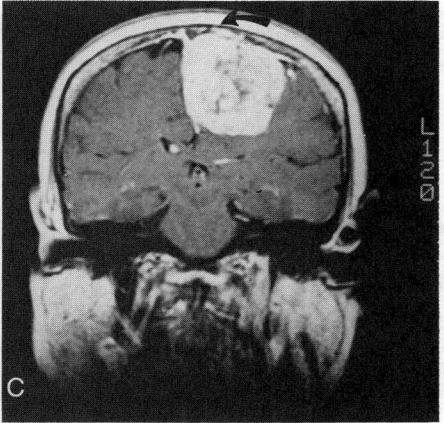

FIGURE 441–3. Left parietal parasagittal meningioma. *A,* CT axial section with iodinated contrast enhancement. *B,* MRI sagittal 500/30 SE section demonstrates invasion of the superior sagittal sinus *(arrow). C,* MRI coronal 500/30 SE section after intravenous administration of gadopentetate dimeglumine demonstrates intense enhancement of the tumor, dural extension, and invasion of the superior sagittal sinus *(arrow).*

METASTASES. Metastases usually show better by MRI than by contrast-enhanced CT. Occasionally metastases may be missed on a regular MRI or contrast-enhanced CT but image clearly on a postcontrast MRI. Since gadolinium-enhanced MRI is the superior examination, it should be performed when metastases are suspected or when evaluating "extent of disease."

Multiple metastases may resemble other disease processes such as *Toxoplasma* abscesses or even the active stage of multiple sclerosis. An accurate history is always required and sometimes even a biopsy.

MENINGIOMAS (Fig. 441–3). Meningiomas are usually well demonstrated on contrast-enhanced CT but if small they may be difficult to identify on MRI without contrast. Almost all meningiomas, however, exhibit intense homogeneous gadolinium enhancement; visualization, particularly of the components adjacent to the inner table of the skull, may be superior. MRI scans in multiple planes increase the examiner's confidence of the extracerebral location of these tumors.

Postoperatively, enhanced MRI is superior to enhanced CT for demonstrating residual tumor, invasion of the venous sinuses, and surgical scar formation.

LYMPHOMAS. Primary and secondary lymphoma of brain is shown better by MRI than CT, although the changes may sometimes resemble meningiomas or gliomas, thus requiring a biopsy for ultimate diagnosis. Patients with AIDS may simultaneously harbor lymphoma and *Toxoplasma* granulomas that cannot be differentiated by MRI except as part of evaluating the response to anti-*Toxoplasma* therapy.

TUMOR STATUS. Postoperative evaluation of tumor recurrence and radiation necrosis may be difficult with either CT or MRI if only a single examination is available. Contrast enhancement on CT and MRI may persist for several months after surgery, and radiation therapy may open the blood-brain barrier to contrast agent in such a way as to result in a deteriorating appearance of associated images. Chronic postradiation changes with demyelination of white matter are detected better on MRI than on CT. True radiation necrosis may be indistinguishable from recurrent tumor by either enhanced MRI or CT, but positron emission tomography (PET) utilizing fluorodeoxyglucose as a measure of regional cerebral metabolic rate typically demonstrates hypoactivity in areas of radionecrosis and hyperactivity in recurrent tumor. Some gliomas, however, may have low metabolic activity due to cystic components or a low grade of malignancy so that differentiation is not absolutely certain.

Other Brain Lesions

HEMATOMAS AND HEMORRHAGE. CT plays an important role in the diagnosis of intracranial hemorrhage (Fig. 441–4) and is routinely performed as an emergency procedure following recent severe head injury or stroke. Acute hemorrhages appear as areas of increased density depending on the anatomic location

(spherical or irregular if intracerebral, lentiform if chronic subdural, and concavo-convex if acute subdural or epidural). The CT-recorded increased density of clot fades so that by 10 to 14 days after bleeding occurs the area may be isodense relative to brain but has a thin rim of contrast enhancement. Subacute subdural hematomas (Fig. 441–5) are frequently visualized better after contrast because of enhancement of the adjacent brain surface. Subsequently the aging clot, although unchanged in size, becomes hypodense, approaching the density of the CSF.

Intracranial hemorrhages cause complex changes with resultingly rapid dramatic changes of MRI signal intensity during the first 4 days. Accordingly the appearance of such bleeding depends upon time of onset, source (arterial or venous), location (subarachnoid, subdural, intraparenchymal), and whether or not rehemorrhage occurs. Other factors affecting MRI reliability include the pulse sequences used and the field strength of the magnet.

An acute hemorrhage in any location is isointense or slightly hyperintense on T1-weighted spin-echo images but is hyperintense or heterogeneous on T2-weighted spin-echo techniques. At this stage such hemorrhage resembles an acute infarct, tumor, or abscess/granuloma, but the presence of blood may be inferred by a gradient-echo scan that accentuates the magnetic susceptibility effect of the iron in hemoglobin.

During the first 24 hours after clot formation oxyhemoglobin in the intact red cells changes to deoxyhemoglobin and methemoglobin, resulting in a decreased signal intensity on the T2-weighted spin-echo images.

Between 3 and 6 days after clot formation there is lysis of red cells with accumulation of extracellular deoxyhemoglobin and methemoglobin that results in a shortening of the T1 relaxation time, leading to increased signal intensity on T1-weighted spin-echo images.

After about 5 days, when red cell lysis is complete, there is complete conversion of deoxyhemoglobin to methemoglobin, resulting in a marked decrease in T1 relaxation time and an increase in the T2 relaxation time. This produces high signal intensity on T1- and T2-weighted spin-echo images, the unmistakable hallmark of hemorrhage. This appearance remains for 30 to 40 days, after which the T1 hyperintensity gradually decreases. Finally, the aging hemorrhage approaches the signal intensity of CSF, but the margin may remain hypointense (dark) owing to the paramagnetic effect of hemosiderin in the surrounding macrophages, resulting in a "tattoo" at the site of hemorrhage.

Because of these complex changes, CT is often easier to interpret during the first 48 hours after a hemorrhage. If gradient-echo techniques are used, however, it appears that MRI may be more sensitive than CT during this time, although fresh hemorrhage may be indistinguishable from old hemorrhage or areas of abnormal brain mineralization.

ANEURYSMS AND ARTERIOVENOUS MALFORMATIONS. Aneurysms and arteriovenous malformations may be

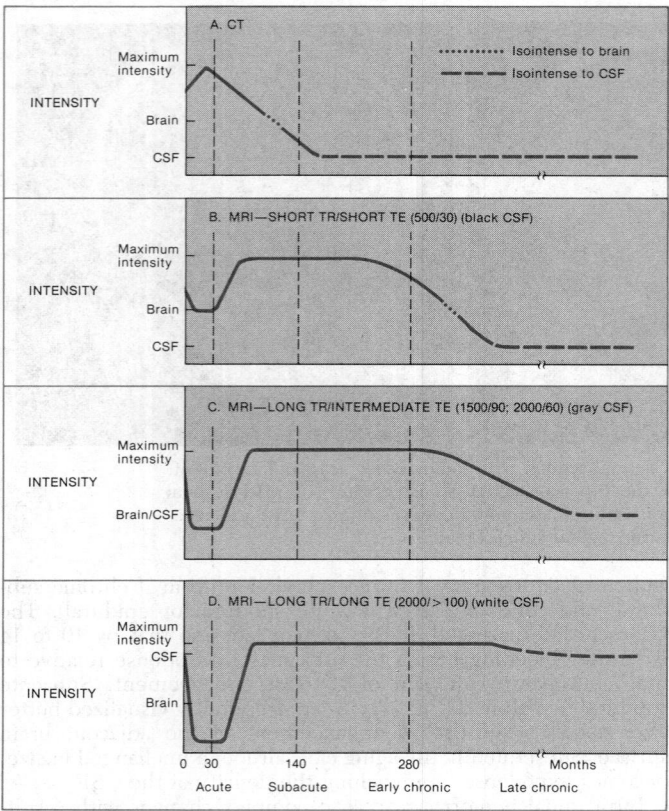

FIGURE 441–4. Appearance of hemorrhage on computed tomography (CT) and magnetic resonance imaging (MRI) with different techniques over time.

HEAD TRAUMA. Following significant head trauma, conventional radiographs of the skull are obtained to detect fractures of the skull vault and associated fractures of the facial bones and cervical spine. Particular attention to the upper cervical spine is required in the elderly patient because of the possibility of a fractured odontoid process or a "bamboo" fracture of a spine affected by ankylosing spondylitis.

CT is the best examination for demonstrating acute brain

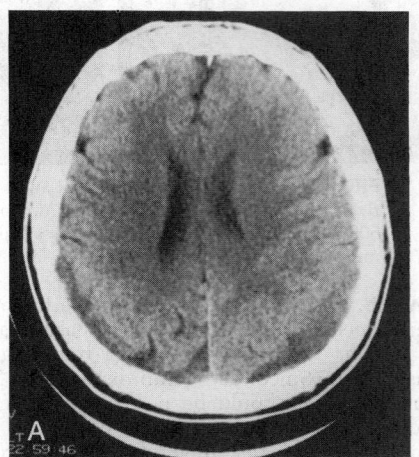

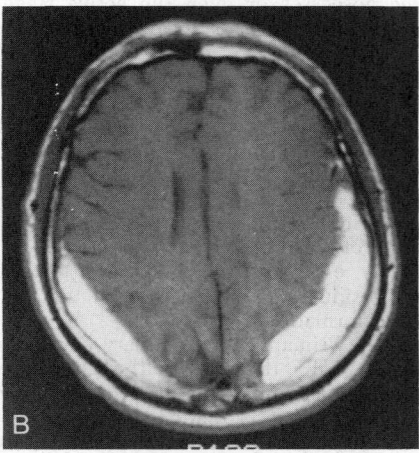

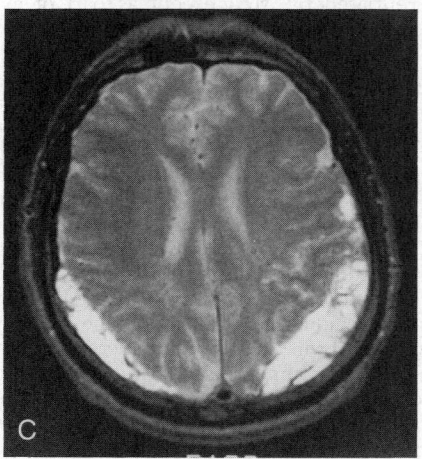

FIGURE 441–5. Bilateral subacute subdural hematomas. *A*, CT axial section shows low-attenuation biparietal extracerebral collections. *B*, MRI axial 500/30 SE section reveals biparietal hyperintense collections. *C*, MRI axial 2000/40 SE section demonstrates hyperintense collections with heterogeneous centers due to fibrous bands in the clot.

diagnosed by CT because of curvilinear calcifications, contrast enhancement of the lumen, and mass effect. MRI is superior to CT, however, because the rapidly flowing blood in the lumen of the aneurysm or the nidus of a malformation results in a "signal void." Aneurysms as small as 3 mm may be detected, and surrounding hemorrhage in the brain is readily identified. Giant aneurysms greater than 1 cm in diameter may have turbulent flow, leading to heterogeneous signal intensity with an appearance similar to that of mural thrombosis.

Subarachnoid hemorrhage, usually due to rupture of an aneurysm, is better shown on CT than on MRI because of the effects of CSF on clot formation, deoxyhemoglobin accumulation, and resolution of the hemorrhage (Fig. 441–6). *In suspicious cases, however, subarachnoid hemorrhage should never be excluded unless a lumbar puncture is normal.*

Cerebral arteriography remains essential to demonstrate the precise anatomy of the aneurysm neck, to exclude multiple aneurysms, and to demonstrate flow patterns and anatomic anomalies of the circle of Willis prior to surgical or endovascular intervention.

Most arteriovenous and venous malformations can be differentiated on MRI, but cerebral arteriography is required to differentiate a venous malformation from a small "high-flow" arteriovenous malformation and also to demonstrate the dural component of an arteriovenous malformation.

Cavernous hemangiomas, small benign tumors that can arise in the cerebral hemispheres, cerebellum, or brain stem, cause gradual neurologic deterioration owing to small recurrent hemorrhages. On CT they appear as hyperdense masses with variable contrast enhancement. On MRI they produce a pathognomonic appearance with heterogeneous hyperintensity on T1-weighted spin-echo and a dark rim on T2-weighted images. A cerebral arteriogram may be normal except for a faint homogeneous stain without a mass effect.

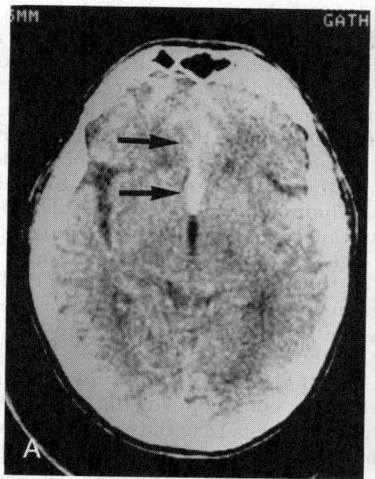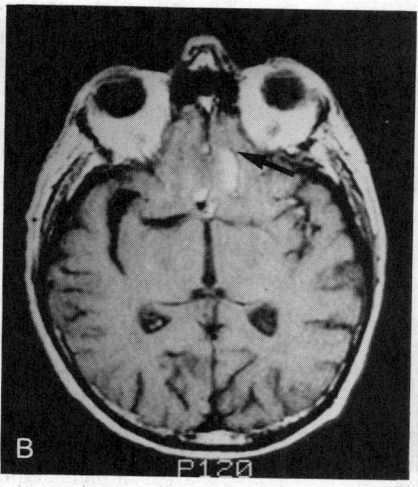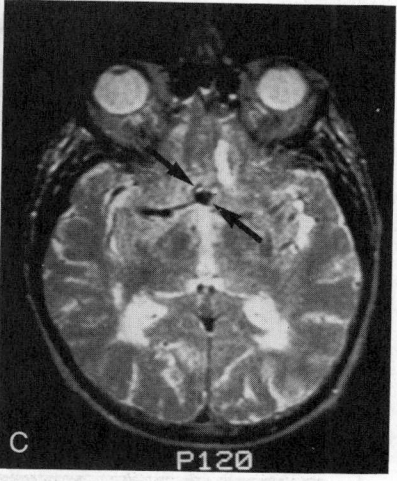

FIGURE 441–6. Subarachnoid hemorrhage due to rupture of anterior communicating artery aneurysm. *A,* CT axial section demonstrates hyperdense blood in the interhemispheric fissure *(arrows)*. *B,* MRI axial 500/30 SE section demonstrates hyperintense blood along the olfactory groove *(arrow)*. *C,* MRI axial 2000/80 SE section (T2-weighted) scan demonstrates the aneurysm of the anterior communicating artery *(arrows)*.

contusions or intracranial hemorrhages during the first 48 hours. Later MRI is superior for imaging small hemorrhagic collections revealing cerebral contusions, and axonal shearing injuries.

CEREBRAL INFARCTS (Fig. 441–7). CT is currently the imaging modality of choice in acute stroke. Any degree of significant hemorrhage can be detected, permitting an early decision for use of anticoagulants.

MRI, however, demonstrates changes in the brain parenchyma earlier and also is superior for detecting thrombosis of the carotid artery or intracerebral arteries. Venous sinus occlusion leading to infarction also is demonstrated better with MRI.

An acute infarct appears as an area of hyperintensity on T2-weighted spin-echo images within 4 hours after onset of stroke; CT images may remain normal for the first 12 to 24 hours. After 4 days, areas of contrast enhancement may be detected with CT or even better with MRI owing to the development of pial and subpial collateral arteries and capillaries. Old infarcts with areas of focal brain atrophy or "encephalomalacia" are seen better with MRI than CT, and areas of old hemorrhage are also demonstrated.

In elderly patients with hypertension or arteriosclerosis and in patients with vasculitis such as lupus erythematosus, foci of hyperintensity on T2-weighted images often appear in the hemispheres or cerebellum, even though the CT remains normal.

INFLAMMATORY BRAIN LESIONS. CT and MRI demonstrate inflammatory changes due to herpes simplex encephalitis, progressive multifocal leukoencephalopathy, and cytomegalovirus infection because of brain edema, mass effect, and occasionally

contrast enhancement. MRI is superior to CT for demonstrating multiple granulomas such as those that affect AIDS victims (Fig. 441–8); the use of gadolinium enhancement increases their detectability. Unfortunately, it is not always possible by either CT or MRI to differentiate concurrent inflammatory lesions such as *Toxoplasma* granulomas from tuberculomas or from neoplasms such as primary lymphomas.

MRI with gadolinium enhancement is superior to CT for demonstrating acute and chronic meningitis as well as subdural and epidural empyemas. Intracerebral abscesses are demonstrated equally well with contrast-enhanced MRI and contrast-enhanced CT, but abscesses adjacent to the ethmoid sinuses and petrous temporal bones may be demonstrated best on coronal MRI images with contrast enhancement.

MULTIPLE SCLEROSIS AND WHITE MATTER DISEASE. MRI is much better than CT for detecting hyperintense areas of demyelination due to multiple sclerosis (Fig. 441–9). Contrast enhancement after Gd-DTPA differentiates acute plaques from old healed lesions. Lesions are identified by MRI in about 80 per cent of patients with multiple sclerosis, whereas CT demonstrates lesions in only 25 per cent of such patients.

Focal hyperintensities similar to those of multiple sclerosis are seen frequently in elderly patients and are usually due to ischemic demyelination or to multiple small infarcts. Similar lesions also can follow radiation therapy, Lyme disease, and, occasionally, severe recurrent migraine headaches. Small disseminated metastases may have a similar appearance.

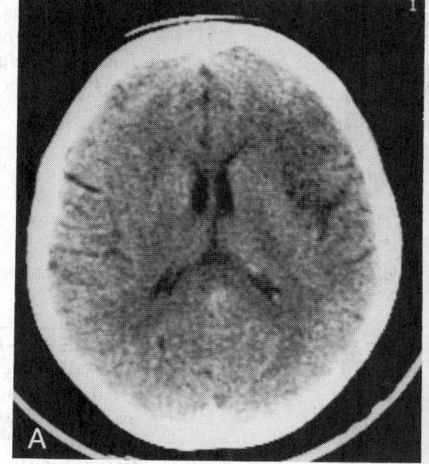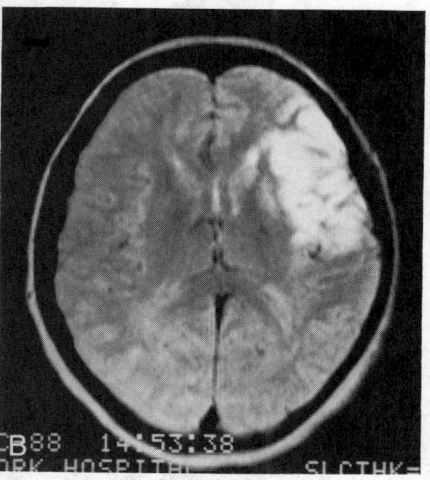

FIGURE 441–7. Acute left frontal infarct. *A,* CT axial section at 24 hours demonstrates a vague area of decreased attenuation of the left frontal lobe. *B,* MRI axial 2000/30 SE section reveals a very hyperintense area of the left frontal lobe with involvement of the cerebral cortex and adjacent basal ganglia due to a partial occlusion of the middle cerebral artery.

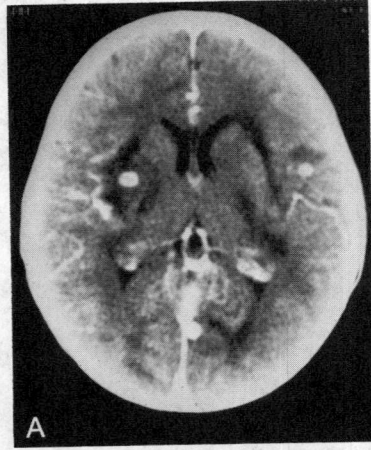

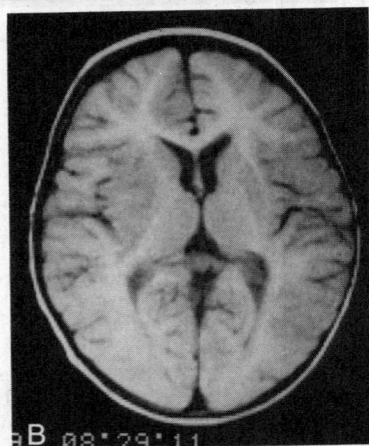

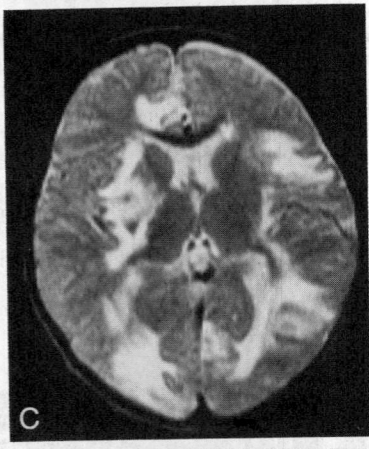

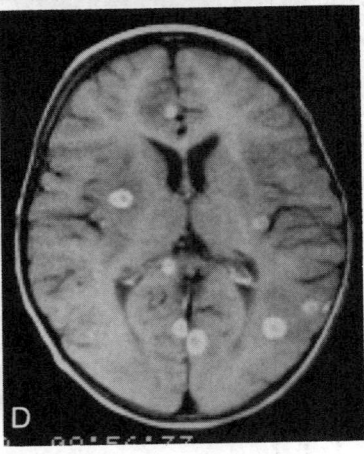

HYDROCEPHALUS AND ATROPHY. Both hydrocephalus and atrophy are associated with loss of brain volume and increased volume of CSF. Hydrocephalus results from obstruction to the flow of CSF from the site of production (the choroid plexus of the lateral third and fourth ventricles) to the site of absorption at the cranial and spinal arachnoid granulations. Rarely, overproduction of CSF has been claimed to be due to a papilloma of the choroid plexus. MRI is the examination of choice for differentiating hydrocephalus from atrophy and for determining whether the site of obstruction is at the foramen of Monro or the aqueduct of Sylvius. MRI with gadolinium enhancement should be performed to detect small infiltrating tumors or chronic meningitis.

In the presence of large cerebral tumors, chronic aqueduct stenosis, or colloid cysts obstructing the third ventricle, caudal herniation of the brain stem through the tentorium may be demonstrated on sagittal MRI images and may precede the usual clinical signs of that condition.

CONGENITAL ANOMALIES. MRI is superior for demonstrating and understanding certain developmental anomalies of the brain. The multiplanar coronal sagittal and axial images make structural changes more apparent, and MRI better distinguishes areas of damaged or injured brain following perinatal anoxia.

SELLAR TUMORS. MRI is superior to CT in delineating tumors of the pituitary glands (Fig. 441–10), the suprasellar region, and the optic chiasm. Contrast enhancement is essential in CT studies of this region and is increasingly used with MRI examination.

MR images in the sagittal and coronal planes demonstrate the normal pituitary gland, including the hyperintense posterior pituitary. Microadenomas are detected reliably using thin-section T1-weighted spin-echo sequences in the coronal plane. They show up as hypointense nodules with mass effect, resulting in displacement of the pituitary stalk, upward bulging of the diaphragma sellae, and erosion of the adjacent sellar floor. Large adenomas extending into the suprasellar cisterns may displace the optic nerves and chiasm superiorly and the cavernous internal carotid arteries laterally. Cerebral arteriograms no longer are required to exclude an aneurysm.

Analysis of the signal intensity (on T2-weighted images) separates solid fibrous adenomas from soft or cystic ones. Craniopharyngiomas and meningiomas may be differentiated from each other by their suprasellar location, tissue characteristics, and enhancement pattern after administration of gadolinium. The precise location of adjacent cranial nerves and cerebral arteries may be identified, aiding the preoperative planning and surgical removal of the tumor.

POSTERIOR FOSSA LESIONS. MRI is superior to CT for all posterior fossa studies because of its multiplanar capabilities, absence of bone artifacts, and superior contrast detection between gray and white matter and CSF. Tumors arising outside the cerebellum and brain stem provide a clearly differentiated image from primary intra-axial tumors. Tumors arising in the skull base and clivus are detected because of the normal high signal intensity of fat-containing bone marrow. The MRI examination should be modified for the posterior fossa to include high-resolution coronal and axial images with T1-weighted spin echo. Gadolinium enhancement is increasingly employed to demonstrate the total extent of meningiomas and to rule out additional tumors.

Acoustic Neurinomas. These benign tumors usually originate from the superior vestibular division of the eighth cranial nerve

FIGURE 441–8. Multiple tuberculous granulomas in a child with AIDS. *A,* Axial CT section with iodinated contrast enhancement reveals scattered small, dense nodules. *B,* MRI axial 500/30 SE section is normal. *C,* MRI axial 2000/80 section demonstrates multiple areas of "brain edema." *D,* MRI axial 500/30 SE section after gadopentetate dimeglumine administration reveals multiple small "ring-enhancing" lesions. The appearance is similar to that of *Toxoplasma* abscesses and metastases.

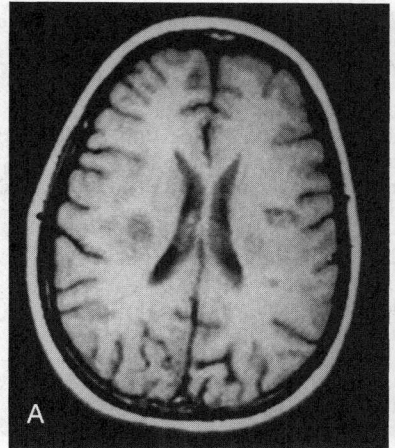
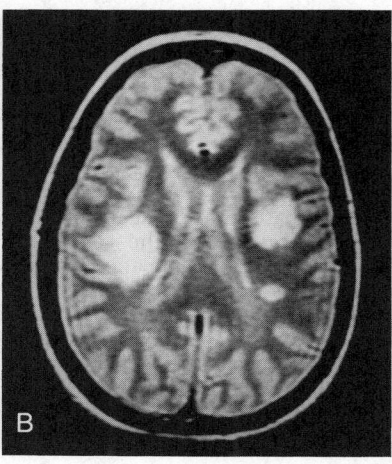

FIGURE 441–9. Multiple sclerosis. *A*, MRI axial 500/30 SE section reveals several areas of low signal intensity due to plaques of demyelination. *B*, MRI axial 2000/40 SE (proton-density) section demonstrates that the areas of demyelination are more numerous and larger.

in the internal auditory canal of the petrous temporal bone. They cause sensorineural hearing loss and vertigo, symptoms that can be caused by tumors as small in diameter as 5 mm or less or as large as 4 cm, a size at which they can distort and compress the brain stem and produce secondary hydrocephalus.

MRI demonstrates acoustic neurinomas as slightly hypointense or isointense masses in the internal auditory canal with extension into the adjacent cerebellopontine angle cistern. On T2-weighted images the tumor becomes hyperintense but may be obscured by the hyperintensity of the surrounding CSF. The separate divisions of the seventh and eighth cranial nerves are visible on the contralateral side. Such tumors show marked enhancement after gadolinium administration. Acoustic neurinomas can be bilateral in 5 per cent of patients, most of whom suffer from neurofibromatosis type 2.

Meningiomas of the Posterior Fossa. Meningiomas can grow anywhere in the posterior fossa. Those in the cerebellopontine angle appear similar to acoustic neurinomas but rarely extend into the internal auditory canal. Meningiomas frequently have a "beaklike" extension along the dura that is never seen with acoustic neurinomas. Gadolinium enhancement is necessary to visualize the dural beak. Meningiomas may infiltrate and obstruct the adjacent venous sinuses, resulting in a loss of signal void. Such sinus-contained tumors show up well on postcontrast images.

Epidermoid Tumors. These interesting tumors consist of glittering white folds of epidermal tissue surrounded by CSF. The tumors produce a mass effect and insinuate themselves into the basal cisterns, wrapping around blood vessels and cranial nerves. On CT the lesions appear as fluid densities, sometimes resembling an arachnoid cyst. Epidermoid tumors show no contrast enhancement.

MRI demonstrates the full extent of the tumor, and subtle

changes in signal intensity on T2-weighted spin-echo images usually clearly differentiate the growth from surrounding CSF. Considerable deformity of the brain stem can occur before abnormal neurologic signs develop.

Cholesterol Granulomas of the Petrous Apex. These unusual lesions are of uncertain etiology but often contain brown fluid with cholesterol crystals, thought to be the result of an inflammatory response to hemorrhage into infected petrous apical air cells. The clinical effects are usually due to compression of adjacent cranial nerves V, VI, VII, or VIII.

Basilar Artery Aneurysms. Both saccular and fusiform aneurysms may be difficult to diagnose using CT in the axial plane. Diagnosis is straightforward on MRI because of the characteristic signal void of the lumen and the clear anatomic localization. The lumen, however, may be heterogeneous owing to turbulent slow flow resembling extensive thrombosis.

Arachnoid Cysts. Primary arachnoid cysts of the posterior fossa occur in the prepontine cistern, cerebellopontine angle, and cisterna magna. On MRI they demonstrate a signal intensity identical to that of CSF. The associated mass effect of the cyst usually differentiates it from an enlarged cisterna magna.

Craniovertebral Junction. MRI is superior to CT for demonstrating basilar impression, whether due to congenital anomalies at the craniovertebral junction or to soft bone collapse such as occurs in Paget's disease or osteogenesis imperfecta. Brain stem compression caused by atlantoaxial subluxation due to rheumatoid arthritis or trauma is also well shown. Abnormal cerebellar tonsils due to Chiari I malformation or the Arnold-Chiari malformation are easily detected.

Intra-axial Posterior Fossa Tumors. Intracranial tumors of the brain stem such as gliomas, ependymomas, cavernous hemangiomas, and metastases often present with progressive unilateral or bilateral cranial nerve palsies similar to those caused by

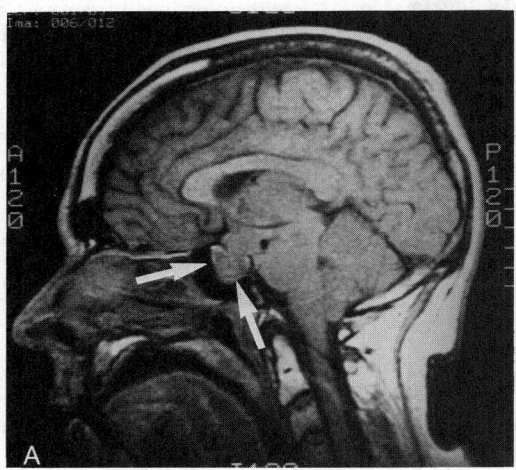
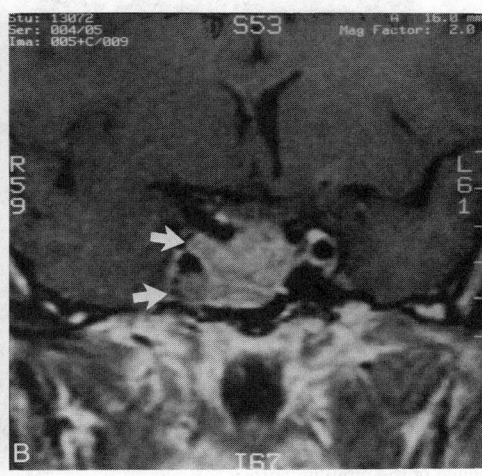

FIGURE 441–10. Pituitary adenoma. *A*, MRI 500/30 SE sagittal section demonstrates enlargement of the sella (*arrows*), with an isodense mass extending from the sella to occupy the interpeduncular cistern and the anterior half of the third ventricle. *B*, MRI 500/30 SE coronal section after gadopentetate dimeglumine administration. The tumor is enhanced and extends into the right cavernous sinus (*arrows*) as well as to the suprasellar cistern.

extracranial tumors. Imaging techniques are crucial in the diagnosis and usually determine treatment such as radiation or chemotherapy, as surgical biopsy may have a high complication rate.

MRI examination with multiple planes, multiple sequences, and contrast enhancement demonstrates the intra-axial location and extent of the mass with a high degree of confidence. Differentiation between a glioma and ependymoma may be possible based on the sharply defined edge of an ependymoma and its location near the ventricular surface. Metastases of the brain stem vary in appearance depending upon the site of origin and may be mistaken for granulomas or lymphoma.

CEREBELLAR TUMORS. Medulloblastomas as well as solid and cystic astrocytomas are usually well demonstrated with CT or MRI with contrast enhancement. Hemangioblastomas, often cystic, are better shown on MRI with contrast enhancement. The upper spinal cord should be included in the study, since the area may contain additional hemangioblastomas.

The Spine

TRAUMA. Conventional radiographs are performed initially to demonstrate fracture and dislocation. Following a neck injury radiographs of the cervical spine are usually taken in flexion and extension to detect instability due to ligamentous injury after midposition views with a collar have revealed normal alignment and an intact odontoid process. CT is helpful in demonstrating fractures of the neural arch and articular facets as well as transverse fractures of the vertebral body and post-traumatic disc herniations that may result in cord nerve root compression. If spinal cord injury is evident clinically, MRI examination may be used to elucidate the cause, such as hematomyelia or epidural hematoma, and may assist in the decision for conservative or surgical management.

DEGENERATIVE DISC DISEASE. Plain radiographs should be taken to demonstrate the vertebrae and disc spaces. Views in flexion and extension are often helpful in showing instability at the intervertebral articulation.

MRI is the study of choice for demonstrating degeneration or prolapse of the discs (Fig. 441–11). Images are obtained in the sagittal plane and in the oblique axial planes through the intervertebral discs using various T1- or T2-weighted spin-echo sequences or gradient-echo techniques. Disc prolapse is identified and the annular deficit is usually clearly seen. Spinal stenosis, if present, is easily identified, and spinal cord or cauda equina compression may be detected.

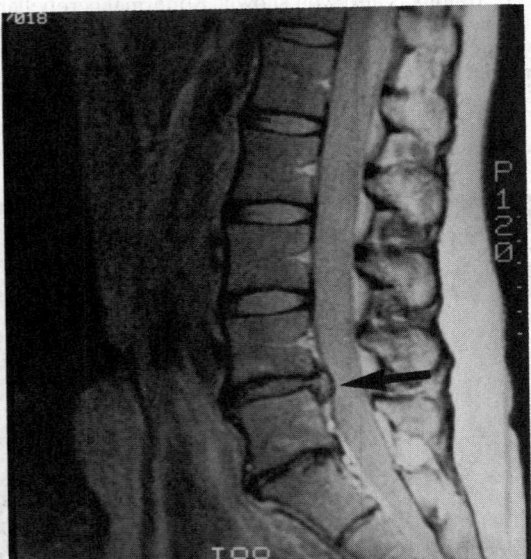

FIGURE 441–11. Herniation of a lumbar intervertebral disc. MRI 1500/30 SE sagittal section reveals a midline posterior prolapse of the nucleus pulposus of the L4/5 intervertebral disc (arrow) with an obvious dehiscence of the annulus fibrosis.

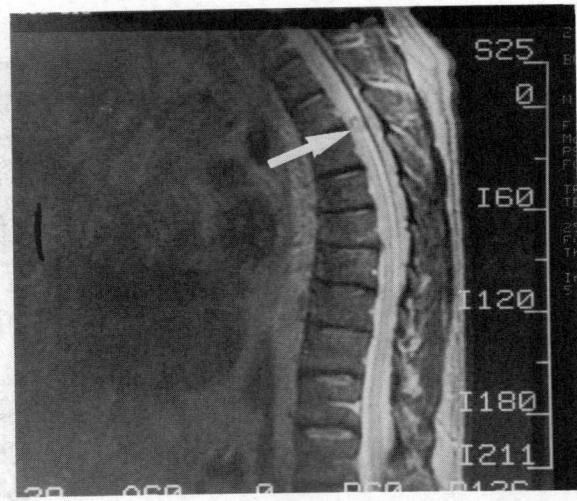

FIGURE 441–12. Thoracic neurofibroma. MRI 2000/80 SE sagittal section demonstrates an ovoid tumor (arrow) overlying the thoracic spinal cord.

In the cervical region, spinal stenosis with instability of the intervertebral joints may lead to cystic changes in the spinal cord that are easily seen on MRI.

In the postoperative patient with recurrent symptoms, MRI with gadolinium enhancement is necessary to differentiate recurrent disc prolapse from postoperative scarring in the epidural space.

If MR images are degraded by implanted metallic clips or patient motion, a CT examination of the area may be used in the postoperative patient. Intravenous iodinated contrast is used to differentiate enhancing epidural scars from recurrent disc disease.

PRIMARY TUMORS, HYDROMYELIA, AND DEMYELINATING DISORDERS OF THE SPINAL CORD. MRI is the study of choice (Fig. 441–12). Gadolinium enhancement is required to demonstrate areas of increased vascularity in the spinal cord due to inflammatory and neoplastic processes. In cases of an apparent hydromyelia, small intramedullary tumors with extensive associated cysts may be overlooked on nonenhanced studies. Meningeal metastases either from systemic cancer or from central nervous system tumors show enhancement after gadolinium on MRI.

METASTATIC BONE DISEASE. MRI is the most accurate technique for detecting osseous metastases and epidural masses that may result in cord or cauda equina compression. The approach is replacing emergency myelography and is usually sufficient to direct radiotherapy to the appropriate areas. MRI or CT may be used to direct needle biopsies of suspected metastases of the vertebrae.

ARTERIOVENOUS MALFORMATIONS OF THE SPINAL CORD. Although large arteriovenous malformations may be identified on MRI or MR angiography, myelography is necessary to identify small malformations. Selective spinal arteriography with injections of contrast into multiple intercostal and lumbar arteries is required to identify the precise feeding artery and nidus of the malformation.

Brant-Zawadski M, Norman D (eds.): Magnetic Resonance Imaging of the Central Nervous System. New York, Raven Press, 1987. *An up-to-date atlas of MRI demonstrating the classic appearances of a variety of brain lesions.*

Huk WJ, Gademann G, Friedmann G: Magnetic Resonance Imaging of Central Nervous System Diseases. Berlin, Springer-Verlag, 1990.

Newton TH, Potts DG (eds.): Advanced Imaging Techniques: Modern Neuroradiology. Vol. 2. San Anselmo, Calif., Clavedel Press, 1983. *Contains, among other useful information, an excellent description of the physics and techniques of various imaging modalities written for nonphysicians.*

Stark DD, Bradley WG (eds.): Magnetic Resonance Imaging. St. Louis, CV Mosby, 1988. *A comprehensive text containing detailed technical and clinical descriptions of MRI.*

442 Neurologic Problems Associated with Aging

Fred Plum

Persons older than 60 years are predisposed to several specific neurologic diseases discussed elsewhere in this section (Table 442–1). In addition, aging-related changes in the peripheral and central nervous systems produce worrisome symptoms in a far larger number. The process of aging importantly affects neurologic structures governing mood, intellectual processing, skilled movement, and the perceptions mediated by the special senses (Table 442–2). Symptoms of mild autonomic insufficiency, including constipation, nocturia, relative insomnia, sexual inadequacy, mild orthostatic hypotension, and increased susceptibility to hypothermia, affect many, if not most, persons more than 70 years of age. Almost half of those who survive beyond age 85 develop signs and symptoms of clinically diagnosable Alzheimer's disease, stroke, or both. Not surprisingly, many of the remainder become apprehensive about developing these conditions. Furthermore, many drugs employed to ameliorate symptoms in various body systems also can cause brain dysfunction in the elderly. These considerations can make difficult the problem of distinguishing benign neurologic symptoms from those related to disease (Table 442–3).

Many, perhaps most, persons living beyond age 70 have at least some recent memory loss, many have lost their life-long regular occupations, and few have developed active social, recreational, or athletic diversions to fill their time. Despite even television's lulling immanence, many become anxious and some depressed. Severe depression affects more than 15 per cent of those older than 65 years, striking men more than women. Antidepressant medication often is effective but may be tolerated only at doses substantially lower than those indicated for younger persons. Chapter 451 discusses this problem at greater length.

No effective treatment for organic memory loss has appeared, but due to anxiety or inattention may be helped by counseling or referral to appropriately concerned lay or religious associations. The merely anxious do best with reassurance; benzodiazepines or other tranquilizers seldom provide enduring benefit and sometimes make matters worse. Physiologic sleep in the elderly becomes less satisfying; deep, stage 4 sleep disappears and the remainder becomes more fitful and less lengthy. Furthermore, natural circadian rhythms intensify their effects, increasing the urge to postprandial drowsiness. A postlunch siesta can minimize or prevent the latter, heading off embarrassment and the appearance of senility that surround those who uncontrollably doze off at meetings or social gatherings. Otherwise, reassurance is all that is needed to alleviate concern about reduced ability to sleep. Sedative use for sleep problems in the elderly is almost never helpful and sometimes harmful. For the already addicted, it may be impossible to discontinue such drugs. Otherwise their use should be confined briefly to emergencies or travel that extends beyond more than four to six time zones. In such instances, one can use one-half the smallest available (0.125 mg) triazolam tablet, i.e., a dose of approximately 0.060 mg, which usually brings at least brief sleep with no or minimal toxic side effects.

Postural and musculoskeletal problems abound in the elderly.

TABLE 442–1. NEUROLOGIC DISORDERS ESPECIALLY RELATED TO AGING

Alzheimer's disease and related dementias
Cerebrovascular disease
"Idiopathic" degenerative disorders
   Parkinson's disease
   Senile tremor and allied movement disorders
   Motor neuron diseases
   Late-life ataxias
Spinal arthropathies with nerve root or spinal cord entrapment
Cranial arteritis
Herpes zoster
"Idiopathic" peripheral neuropathy
Drop attacks and falls

TABLE 442–2. AGING CHANGES IN THE NERVOUS SYSTEM (65 TO 80 YEARS)

Brain shrinks and neuron counts decrease
   Frontal lobe (30%)
   Temporal lobe (45%)
   Basal ganglia (30%)
Cerebral blood flow and metabolism eventually decline
Speed of central and peripheral neural processing slows
Autonomic and muscle stretch reflexes lose sensitivity
Central and peripheral cholinergic systems decay
Olfactory, visual, and auditory-vestibular systems deteriorate
Susceptibility increases to degenerative, vascular, and immune-mediated disorders

Joint and muscle-tendon pain sometimes can be difficult to separate from nerve root pain. Except for hip and knee replacements, however, few patients benefit from surgical treatment. Most of the symptoms derive from longstanding wear and tear on joints and tendons, but changes in basal ganglia, postural reflexes, and perceptual functions contribute. Even in the absence of true parkinsonism, standing and walking become more stooped; the restless, normal, spontaneous muscular activity that characterizes more youthful life disappears; and physiologic tremor intensifies. Inadvertent falls become an increasing risk. The skeletal muscles lose their tone, reflex speeds slow down, and strength declines. All these changes reduce the sense of well-being but can be ameliorated somewhat by postural education and exercise. Even walking with briskly swinging arms can reduce discomfort and improve the sense of vigor. More extensive muscular activity must be appropriately individualized.

Chronic feelings of dizziness, "spaciness," or giddiness plague the elderly. True vertigo is uncommon (see Ch. 453), but slowed or reduced baroceptor reflexes frequently induce brief orthostatic dysequilibrium. Similarly, contradictions among visual, labyrinthine-vestibular, and proprioceptive perceptions develop and often generate a sense of giddiness or unsteadiness during standing or walking. Extending the head and looking skyward while walking or standing accentuates the contradictions between visual and proprioceptive signals, making matters worse. Among the very old, extremes of head extension (e.g., women leaning backward to the hairdresser's sink, men painting the ceiling) can induce true vertigo, which may derive from vertebral artery compression. All but the last of the above symptoms can be minimized by careful explanation, since anxiety plays a role in every case. No drugs help the symptoms and many worsen them. Maneuvers that induce true vertigo should be specifically advised against.

Population surveys indicate that symptom-producing high-pitched, ringing tinnitus affects about 25 per cent of all persons aged over 60, probably reflecting gradual high-tone hearing loss. Only rarely is this distressing, and there is no effective treatment. The finding of progressive nerve deafness deserves referral to an otologist or neurologist. Most serious visual impairment in the elderly stems from cataracts, glaucoma, or macular degeneration (see Ch. 511 to 513). Once these conditions are excluded or treated by ophthalmologic evaluation, the physician can deal with nonspecific symptoms of visual fatigue or intermittent impairment of acuity by reassurance and common sense.

A variety of medications cause unwanted neurotoxic side effects in the elderly, including depression of mood, delirium, dyssomnia, and incoordination. Many produce side effects even at

TABLE 442–3. COMMON NONSPECIFIC SYMPTOMS OF NEUROLOGIC AGING

1. Recent memory loss
2. Depression or hopelessness
3. Insomnia-fatigue
4. Postural unsteadiness, giddiness, "spaciness," vertigo
5. Hearing difficulty—tinnitus, high-tone deafness, nerve deafness
6. Dimmed vision—cataracts, glaucoma, macular degeneration, presbyopia
7. Nocturia and/or incontinence
8. Vulnerability to drugs

TABLE 442–4. POTENTIAL NEUROTOXIC DRUG REACTIONS IN THE ELDERLY, MOSTLY DOSE-RELATED

Analgesics	
Aspirin (large doses)	Tinnitus, confusion
Nonsteroidal anti-inflammatory drugs	Confusion, aseptic meningitis
Opiates	Increased vulnerability to known effects
Anticholinergics	
Includes many agents employed for gastric difficulties (e.g., metoclopramide, atropine), urinary frequency, or parkinsonism; also tricyclic antidepressants and several tranquilizers	Confusion, hallucinations, glaucoma, urinary retention, constipation, hypothermia
Antihypertensives	Postural hypotension, erect giddiness, falls
Anticonvulsants	
Carbamazepine; phenytoin	Lethargic confusion; ataxia, mild confusion
Benzodiazepines	Depression, amnesia, confusion, drowsiness, falls
Cimetidine and other H_2 blockers	Confusion
Corticosteroids	Delirium
Digitalis	Confusion, hallucinations
Dopaminergic agents	
Levodopa	Dyskinesias, postural hypotension, confusion
Bromocriptine	

dosages and measured drug levels that lie within the "therapeutic ranges." Table 442–4 lists major pharmacal offenders, which should be prescribed cautiously.

The neurologic examination in healthy elderly patients reflects the inevitable decay that sooner or later affects nearly all neurologic systems. In addition, three fourths of those who live beyond 70 years have a major disorder of at least one other bodily system which reduces their sense of well-being. Nearly all have at least some difficulty with recent memory compared with their younger years. Nevertheless, "normal" old persons retain sufficient cognitive and verbal activity to perform bedside mental status examinations at a normal level. Old-age changes in station, gait, mood, and neuromuscular functions have been mentioned above. As many as half of the very old have difficulty converging the eyes, and a substantial fraction show functionally unimportant limitations of conjugate upgaze. Pupillary miosis is common. As the skeletal muscles weaken, interosseous atrophy gradually, unavoidably affects the hands and feet. The capacity to perform rapid skilled movements slows, and many persons develop a mild, non-parkinsonian tremor of the head or hands. Deep-tendon reflexes decline in amplitude and Achilles tendon jerks often disappear. Extensor plantar responses are *not* a normal finding. In asymptomatic patients, however, they sometimes can reflect benign osteoarthritic spinal cord encroachment rather than serious brain or spinal cord dysfunction. Perception of pain, touch, and proprioceptive sensation remain essentially intact in normal elderly persons, but most have reduced vibratory perception in the distal lower extremities. A few develop peripheral neuropathy demonstrable more in the lower than the upper extremities and characterized chiefly by annoying paresthesias and a degree of proprioceptive impairment. Such patients should be evaluated for metabolic disorders or possible nerve root compression, but for most the cause remains unknown and the treatment is symptomatic.

Creasey H, Rapoport SI: The aging human brain. Arch Neurol 17:2–10, 1985. *Succinctly summarizes morphologic and chemical changes in the aging brain. Despite these, brain blood flow, metabolic rate, and "crystallized" intelligence frequently remain within normal limits because of the plasticity of the organ.*

Hale WE, Perkins LL, May FE, et al.: Symptom prevalence in the elderly. An evaluation of age, sex, disease and medication use. J Am Geriatr Soc 34:333–340, 1986. *Among 1927 women and 1140 men over age 65 years, nocturia affected 80 per cent, over 20 per cent had tinnitus, more than 15 per cent had dizziness or "spaciness," and 7 per cent (men) to 14 per cent (women) had frequent headaches.*

Hazzard WR, Andres R, Bierman EL, Blass JP (eds.): Principles of Geriatric Medicine and Gerontology, 2nd ed. New York, McGraw-Hill, 1990. *Part 3, Section 1 provides a good background to the neurobiology of the aging brain and the specific diseases that affect the central and peripheral nervous systems.*

Katzman R, Terry R: The Neurology of Aging. Philadelphia, F. A. Davis, 1983. *An excellent small monograph concentrating especially on principles of age-related symptoms, with less attention to specific disorders.*

SECTION TWO / DISORDERS OF CEREBRAL FUNCTION

443 Disturbances of Consciousness and Arousal

Fred Plum

DEFINITIONS AND MECHANISMS OF ALTERED CONSCIOUSNESS

Consciousness is a brain-generated psychological state expressed in two dimensions: wakefulness and the self-aware cognition of past events and future anticipations which accompanies the normal wakeful state. Disease or dysfunction that impairs this combination usually causes readily identifiable conditions as defined in Table 443–1. Occasionally, however, either certain forms of neurologic damage or the presence of a severe psychiatric disorder can mimic an unconscious state. A later section discusses these potentially deceptive conditions.

Impaired consciousness can be *sustained*, i.e., prolonged for periods lasting for hours or more, or *brief*, with the lapse enduring for no more than a few seconds to an hour or so. The longer the duration of an abnormal state of consciousness, the more likely it is to reflect structural damage to the brain rather than a transient alteration in its function. Sustained alterations of consciousness are discussed in Ch. 444. Brief loss of consciousness is considered in Ch. 446.

The normal capacity to awaken and direct attention depends upon ontogenetically primitive arousal mechanisms lodged within or in close association with the ascending reticular activating system (ARAS). The ARAS consists of a loosely organized, fairly dense column of neurons which extends forward along the brain's central core from approximately the upper third of the pons to the deep reaches of the hypothalamus and the thalamus. The system includes cholinergic, adrenergic, and serotonergic fibers as well as others employing still undefined neurotransmitters. The self-aware, cognitive aspects of consciousness depend largely on the interconnected neural networks of the cerebral hemispheres, including their cortical mantles and their extensive interconnections with the thalamus, basal ganglia, and cerebellum. Normal conscious behavior depends on the continuous,

TABLE 443–1. STATES OF ALTERED CONSCIOUSNESS OR UNRESPONSIVENESS

Coma: A state of unarousable unresponsiveness; even strong exteroceptive stimuli fail to elicit recognizable psychological responses.

Stupor: Spontaneous unarousability interruptable only by vigorous, direct external stimulation.

Hypersomnia, pathologic drowsiness, obtundation: Terms applied to an increase above the patient's normal sleep/wake ratio, often accompanied during wakefulness by reduced attention and interest in the environment.

Delirium: An acute or subacute reduction in awareness, attention, orientation, and perception ("clouding of consciousness"), usually fluctuating and accompanied by abnormal sleep/wake patterns and often psychomotor disturbances.

Syncope: Brief loss of consciousness due to global failure of cerebrovascular perfusion.

Dementia: A sustained or permanent multidimensional or global decline in cognitive functions.

Vegetative state: A sustained, complete loss of cognition, with wake/sleep cycles and other autonomic functions remaining relatively intact. The condition can either follow acute, severe bilateral cerebral damage or develop gradually as the end stage of a progressive dementia.

Locked-in state: Preservation of intellectual activity accompanied by severe or total incapacity to express voluntary responses due to damage to or dysfunction of descending motor pathways in the brain or peripheral motor nerves. Most, but not all, such patients can use vertical eye movements to signal by code.

---

effective interaction between these cerebral systems and the subcortical activating mechanisms.

Impaired consciousness can be partial or complete, acute or chronic. By definition, acute disturbances of consciousness always include at least some change of the normal wake-sleep cycle toward a reduction in alertness and attention. These reductions often are accompanied by diffuse impairments of normal cognitive activity, reflecting a close interdependence between cortical and cognitive mechanisms and the ascending activating systems. Accordingly, acute lesions that affect either the ascending system or diffusely impair large amounts of the cortex reduce the level of consciousness. Since its anatomic subcortical cross-sectional area is small, yet the system projects diffusely to the cortex and subcortical structures, acute damage to or depression of the ARAS carries a high risk of blocking cortical arousal. By contrast, any given region of cortex feeds back to only a limited subcortical area so that disease or dysfunction at the cerebral level usually must impair extensive areas of cerebral activity bilaterally to cause stupor or coma. The tempo of the damage also is important. With disease that gradually affects either the cortex or the ascending activating mechanisms alone, arousal mechanisms tend to adapt so rapidly that wakefulness never is altogether lost. Accordingly, slowly advancing, diffuse cerebral disease causes a multifaceted dementia rather than the clouded consciousness with fluctuating or reduced arousal that results from acute disturbances. Among subcortical reticular structures, the posterior hypothalamus is essentially the only locus where a chronic lesion produces a permanent loss or severe reduction of the capacity to reawaken.

---

444 Sustained Impairments of Consciousness

Fred Plum

Three classes of neurologic disorders may produce sustained impairment of consciousness. These include (1) supratentorial mass or destructive lesions that either secondarily compress or directly destroy deep midline thalamic-hypothalamic activating structures, (2) posterior fossa mass or destructive lesions that compress or destroy the brain stem's upper pontine–mesence-

phalic reticular formation, and (3) metabolic-diffuse abnormalities that acutely or subacutely impair the functions of the two cerebral hemispheres, the brain stem, or both. Metabolic abnormalities especially tend to affect both cerebral and ascending arousal mechanisms concurrently. Table 444–1 enumerates the more common specific causes of stupor and coma according to these mechanisms.

PATHOPHYSIOLOGY AND CATEGORICAL DIAGNOSIS OF DELIRIUM, STUPOR, AND COMA

INTRACRANIAL MASS LESIONS. Intracranial mass and destructive lesions that immediately or eventually impair consciousness can arise either above or below the tentorium, the fibrous structure that divides the diencephalon and forebrain from the brain stem. Whether such lesions are supra- or subtentorial in location, their effects and outcome depend on (1) the geographic anatomy of the abnormality, (2) its size and rate of enlargement, and (3) any reactive changes it causes in surrounding brain. These reactive changes include tissue edema and vasodilatation as well as proliferative inflammatory and glial responses. Their volume and effect can be as dangerous as the primary lesion itself, since they can triple the size of the primary lesion. Such severe reactions are especially prominent in and around malignant neoplasms, acute infarctions, hemorrhages, or abscesses. Since the skull is inexpansible, all enlarging masses eventually cause intracranial shifts and compressions that endanger the vitality of adjacent and remote brain areas.

As mass lesions form and enlarge within the cranial cavity, local intracranial compliance declines, cerebrospinal fluid flow and absorption are impeded, and the intracranial pressure rises, first within tissues adjacent to the abnormality and then more generally. If the process is not interrupted, intracranial distortion and pressure eventually increase sufficiently to impede the blood supply in areas of compressed tissue. When this occurs, arteriolar resistance intermittently fails, leading to temporary increases in intracranial blood volume which produce brief but potentially dangerous episodes of greatly increased intracranial pressure, called *pressure waves*.

As could be expected, functional neurologic abnormalities accompanying the above pathophysiologic changes occur earliest in regions in and adjacent to the primary lesion, then gradually affect more remote brain areas made vulnerable by being compressed against unyielding edges of bone or dura. Particularly at risk of this complication are structures that become squeezed against the falx cerebri or herniate into the restricted apertures of the tentorial notch or foramen magnum, thereby impacting areas critical to consciousness and even survival (Fig. 444–1).

TABLE 444–1. THE COMMON CAUSES OF STUPOR AND COMA

Supratentorial lesions (causing secondary upper brain stem dysfunction)
  Cerebral hemorrhage
  Large cerebral infarction
  Subdural hematoma
  Epidural hematoma
  Brain tumor
  Brain abscess (rare)
Subtentorial lesions (compressing or destroying the rostral reticular formation)
  Pontine or cerebellar hemorrhage
  Brain stem infarction
  Brain stem or cerebellar tumor
  Cerebellar abscess
Metabolic and diffuse lesions (see also Table 444–5)
  Exogenous poison
  Infections
    Meningitis
    Encephalitis
  Concussion and postictal states
  Anoxia or ischemia
  Hypoglycemia
  Ionic and electrolyte disorders
  Endogenous toxin due to organ failure or deficiency
  Nutritional deficiency
Psychogenic unresponsiveness

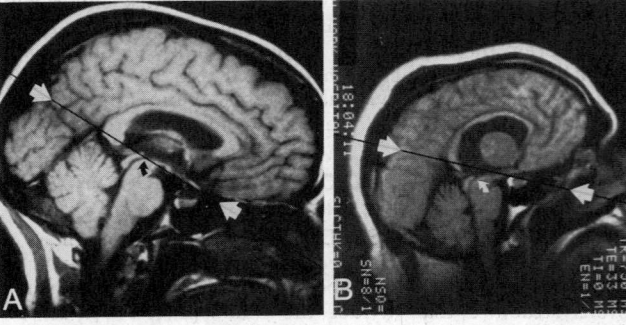
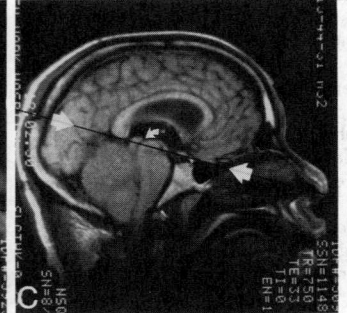
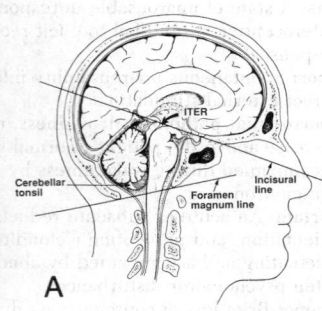
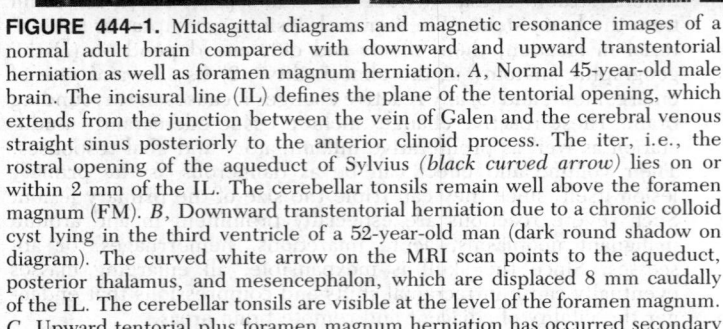
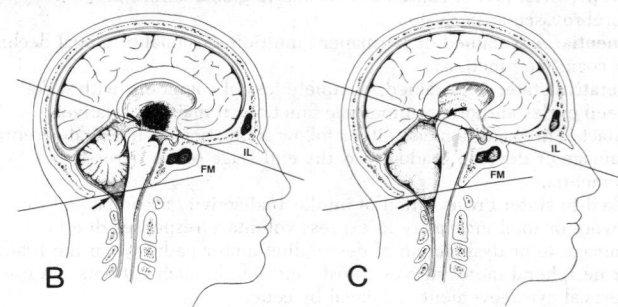

FIGURE 444–1. Midsagittal diagrams and magnetic resonance images of a normal adult brain compared with downward and upward transtentorial herniation as well as foramen magnum herniation. *A,* Normal 45-year-old male brain. The incisural line (IL) defines the plane of the tentorial opening, which extends from the junction between the vein of Galen and the cerebral venous straight sinus posteriorly to the anterior clinoid process. The iter, i.e., the rostral opening of the aqueduct of Sylvius *(black curved arrow)* lies on or within 2 mm of the IL. The cerebellar tonsils remain well above the foramen magnum (FM). *B,* Downward transtentorial herniation due to a chronic colloid cyst lying in the third ventricle of a 52-year-old man (dark round shadow on diagram). The curved white arrow on the MRI scan points to the aqueduct, posterior thalamus, and mesencephalon, which are displaced 8 mm caudally of the IL. The cerebellar tonsils are visible at the level of the foramen magnum. *C,* Upward tentorial plus foramen magnum herniation has occurred secondary to a cerebellar lymphoma in a 32-year-old man with HIV-I infection. The cerebellum is enlarged. The iter *(black curved arrow)* and the rostral mesencephalon have herniated 6 mm above the IL, and the brain stem is flattened against the base of the skull. The cerebellar tonsils have herniated into the foramen magnum.

SUPRATENTORIAL MASS LESIONS CAUSING COMA.

Enlarging supratentorial lesions that affect the cerebral hemispheres or diencephalon most often produce stupor or coma by shifting brain tissue either horizontally across the midline or caudally toward the tentorium. Either way, the process compresses and displaces the diencephalon, producing distinctive clinical features (Table 444–2). Localizing symptoms such as frontal headache, focal seizures, or other changes consistent with unilateral hemispheric disease almost always appear first, followed, as the lesion enlarges, by the development of altered consciousness. In keeping with this sequence, most patients demonstrate a combination of *focal* hemispheric signs, e.g., sensorimotor abnormalities, aphasia, or visual field defects, followed by signs of *diffuse* supratentorial dysfunction, consisting of nonfocal headache, reduced attention, confusion, and somnolence. If untreated, the process eventually produces stupor and evidence of bilateral corticospinal tract dysfunction reflecting secondary distortion and compression of the opposite hemisphere and the deep-lying diencephalon. Decerebrate responses to noxious stimuli emerge in these circumstances as late and dangerous events.

Some supratentorial masses can arise and enlarge in neurologically silent areas such as the frontal lobes or the subdural space. In such instances, signs and symptoms of diffuse cerebral dysfunction and increased intracranial pressure can predominate, consisting of papilledema, confusion, apathy, or hypersomnolence (see Ch. 447). In either event, computed tomography (CT) or magnetic resonance (MR) images of coma-causing supratentorial masses disclose a large, space-occupying lesion, characteristically associated with evidence of displacement of adjacent tissues caudally, across the midline, or both. An important negative finding is that, unless the brain already has begun to herniate into the tentorial notch, no clinical evidence of brain stem dysfunction can be found; pupillary and oculovestibular reflexes remain intact, and decerebrate motor responses develop only as a late sign.

Stupor or coma with supratentorial lesions implies that the deeply located diencephalon is already compressed or distorted, threatening the advent of potentially irreversible midbrain compression. Such impaction-herniation begins either with downward displacement of the diencephalon (central herniation) or with the uncus of the temporal lobe squeezing against the midbrain in the tentorial notch (uncal herniation). Either way, characteristic syndromes evolve (Table 444–3). With impending *central* herniation, stupor becomes gradually deeper, and patients sigh, yawn, or develop periodic breathing. The pupils shrink to 1 to 2 mm

TABLE 444–2. CHARACTERISTICS OF SUPRATENTORIAL LESIONS LEADING TO COMA

Initiating symptoms usually cerebral-focal: aphasia; focal seizures; contralateral hemiparesis, sensory change, or neglect; frontal lobe behavioral changes; headache.

Dysfunction moves rostral to caudal: e.g., focal motor → bilateral motor → altered level of arousal.

Abnormal signs usually confined to a single or adjacent anatomic level (not diffuse).

Brain stem functions spared unless herniation develops.

TABLE 444–3. SIGNS OF INCIPIENT DOWNWARD HERNIATION

	Central	Uncal
Arousal	Impaired early, before other signs	Impaired late, usually with other signs
Breathing	Sighs, yawns, sometimes Cheyne-Stokes respirations	No early change
Pupils	First small reactive (hypothalamus), then one or both approach midposition	Ipsilateral pupil dilates, followed by somatic third nerve paralysis
Oculocephalic responses	Initially sluggish, later tonic conjugate	Unilateral third nerve paralysis
Motor signs	Early hemiparesis opposite to hemispheric lesion followed late by ipsilateral motor paresis and extensor plantar response	Motor signs late, sometimes ipsilateral to lesion

in diameter, reflecting hypothalamic dysfunction, but retain their light reflexes. Later, one or both pupils may ominously dilate. Loss of forebrain inhibition on the brain stem results in the development of brisk oculomotor reflexes (see Ch. 453). Until mesencephalic insufficiency develops, oculovestibular reflex responses (cold caloric test) are marked by tonic deviation of the eyes toward the stimulated side. Bilateral dysfunction develops in corticospinal motor pathways, causing hyperactive deep tendon reflexes, spasticity, extensor plantar responses, and, eventually, decerebrate or decorticate reflex posturing, worse on the body side contralateral to the brain mass.

With *uncal* herniation, signs generally resemble the above except that as the uncus slides over the tentorial edge, it may compress the third nerve ahead of it before the diencephalon is squeezed (Table 444–3). Shortly afterward, somatic oculomotor functions of the third nerve usually deteriorate, and the involved eye turns outward. If the herniating process continues, the opposite third nerve becomes involved, and other mesencephalic functions begin to fail. Effective treatment of impending diencephalic-midbrain compression-herniation must be initiated before these late signs of deterioration appear.

SUBTENTORIAL MASS OR DESTRUCTIVE LESIONS CAUSING COMA. Subtentorial mass or destructive lesions cause stupor or coma if they directly damage or compress the ascending activating systems that arise from the paramedian rostral pontine tegmentum and mesencephalon. Since such coma-causing abnormalities almost always affect adjacent neuro-ophthalmologic centers, they often produce tell-tale neurologic signs that pinpoint the anatomy of damage (Table 444–4).

Subtentorial lesions that cause coma by directly injuring the upper brain stem (e.g., infarcts or hemorrhages) usually produce coma from the outset. The pupils are always abnormal, owing to dysfunction or destruction of pontine sympathetic pathways, third nerve nuclei, or their fibers. Dysconjugate eye movements are common, as are nystagmus, bizarrely or independently moving eyes, ocular bobbing, or rotating ocular deviation. Unilateral facial anesthesia involving both the brow and lower face, absent caloric responses to either side, and conjugate eye deviation toward the paralyzed arm and leg all suggest a subtentorial lesion. The combination of flaccidity in the arms and flexor responses in the legs signifies pontine-midbrain damage. CT scans in such cases reveal cerebellar or pontine hemorrhage as well as expanding cerebellar hematomas, neoplasms, or, sometimes, infarctions. MR produces even better images of the cerebellum and brain stem, readily identifying even small areas of infarction or other damage.

Compressive lesions of the posterior fossa, such as hemorrhages, abscesses, or tumors of the cerebellum or fourth ventricle, rarely cause coma until late in their course, at which time they may cause the mesencephalon to herniate upward through the tentorial notch or force the cerebellar tonsils to impact downward into the foramen magnum. These developments produce deepening stupor, failure of upward gaze, unequal or fixed pupils, and irregularly irregular breathing patterns. In such instances, occipital headache, nystagmus, diplopia, nausea, vomiting, cranial nerve signs, and ataxia usually precede unconsciousness. The circumstances call for immediate treatment consisting of shrinking the brain and, in most instances, surgical decompression of the lateral cerebral ventricles.

METABOLIC AND DIFFUSE BRAIN DISTURBANCES CAUSING STUPOR AND COMA. Definition. The term *metabolic* or *diffuse encephalopathy* describes the behavioral state produced by a group of brain-affecting disorders that impair predominantly the organ's higher functions and usually pursue a

TABLE 444–4. TELLTALE SIGNS OF PRIMARY SUBTENTORIAL LESIONS CAUSING COMA

Onset of coma often sudden
Symptoms of brain stem dysfunction may precede coma
Localizing brain stem signs always present
  Caloric responses disconjugate or absent
  Pupil(s) abnormal: pinpoint (pons), fixed (midbrain), irregular and/or unequal (midbrain-pontine)
  Often "bizarre" signs: ocular bobbing, ataxic breathing, etc.
  Often signs of cerebellar or bilateral motor dysfunction

temporary, reversible course. They all produce clouding of consciousness, characterized by impaired attention, difficulty in concentration, reduced intellectual capacity, and altered sleep-wake patterns (Table 444–5). Metabolic encephalopathy is a major comorbidity factor in a variety of serious medical and surgical illnesses, and its effects complicate patient management both in and out of hospital. Especially susceptible to metabolic encephalopathy are patients who are critically ill from systemic disease or major surgery as well as the aged. If one includes examples of the toxic effects of abused and therapeutic drugs, the metabolic encephalopathies make up the largest category of illnesses causing confusion, stupor, or coma.

Disorders or drugs affecting several neurochemical and neuropharmacologic systems can cause a metabolic encephalopathy. Prominent examples are those with anticholinergic and sedative effects. Other common causes include a number of inflammatory or infectious illnesses, physiologic disturbances such as epilepsy or complicated migraine, diffuse brain trauma, and disseminated structural lesions such as certain forms of cancer or cerebral thromboembolism. Diffuse, acute or subacute, bilateral, multi-level cerebral and subcerebral dysfunction that almost always spares pupillary reactivity is the hallmark of metabolic encephalopathy and is a combination only rarely produced by structural brain disease.

Terminology. Classic neurologic thinking has employed the term *delirium* or *acute toxic psychosis* for the more blatantly agitated and severely disoriented, hallucinatory-delusional forms of metabolic encephalopathy. Quieter, less severe disturbances have been termed *acute* or *subacute confusional states*. This chapter often employs these terms as being more descriptively informative than the usage adopted by the American Psychiatric Association's Diagnostic Manual, which applies the term *delirium* to all examples of acquired confusion, agitation, disorientation, or hallucinations occurring in the setting of structural or known neurochemical brain disease.

Clinical Features. The clinical evaluation of confused or delirious states attempts first to determine whether observed changes in consciousness are due to metabolic rather than structural brain disease or psychiatric dysfunction. One then proceeds to define the particular metabolic or structural defects and treat them. Evaluations of the history, the pattern of impaired consciousness, motor activity, and autonomic activity help answer the first question, whereas the general physical examination, evaluation of pulmonary ventilation, and laboratory tests assist with the second (Table 444–6). The history is especially important and should inquire into previous systemic medical illnesses, psychiatric history, access to potentially intoxicating drugs or alcohol, and recent changes in behavior.

State of Consciousness and Mental Content. Disorders of attention are the earliest sign and the hallmark of metabolic brain disease. Some patients act quietly perplexed, preoccupied, and unable to concentrate sufficiently to deal with significant stimuli in the environment. Others appear hypervigilant and distractible, picking at the bedclothes and attending briefly to each new environmental stimulus no matter how trivial or irrelevant. Still others lose contact with the environment, becoming completely preoccupied and often frightened by vivid fragmentary hallucinations or delusions. Early attentional deficits may be subtle and easily mistaken for normal, slightly odd behavior. Soon, however, other symptoms emerge, including emotional lability, insomnia or drowsiness, and often vivid nightmares. As delirium worsens, some patients express the fear of "going crazy." Others lie quietly or sleep when left alone. None reads for substance or attends with any interest to the surrounding world. With more severe metabolic disturbances, patients become drowsy and finally stuporous or comatose. The prevailing affect depends partly on the nature of the illness and partly on how rapidly it develops. Remarkably, previous personality often has surprisingly little influence on delirious behavior. Rapidly developing metabolic abnormalities are more likely to produce agitation or stupor than are those that evolve more slowly.

Disturbances in cognition consistently accompany altered alertness and awareness, causing difficulties with immediate recall and the ability to abstract. Normal subjects readily recall and repeat six or seven digits forward and five or six backward and

TABLE 444–5. COMMON CAUSES OF METABOLIC OR DIFFUSE BRAIN DYSFUNCTION CAUSING DELIRIUM OR COMA

I. Exogenous poisons
  A. Alcohol–sedative drug abuse, acute or chronic, immediate or withdrawal
  B. Acid poisons or poisons with acidic breakdown products:
    Paraldehyde
    Methyl alcohol
    Ethylene glycol
  C. Psychotropic drugs, acute or chronic:
    Opiates and their congeners
    Cocaine
    Amphetamines
    Tricyclic antidepressants and anticholinergic drugs
    Lithium
    Phenothiazines
    LSD-mescaline
    Monoamine oxidase inhibitors
  D. Other drugs:
    Anticonvulsants
    Steroids
    Cardiac glycosides
    Cimetidine
    Salicylates
II. Mixed metabolic encephalopathy
  Age + drugs + intensive care unit + postoperative state + fracture, etc.
III. Deprivation of oxygen, substrate, or metabolic cofactors
  A. Hypoxia (interference with oxygen supply to the entire brain; cerebral blood flow normal)
    1. Decreased oxygen tension (usually $PaO_2 < 35$ mm Hg) and content of blood: pulmonary disease, alveolar hypoventilation, decreased atmospheric oxygen tension (e.g., high altitude)
    2. Decreased oxygen content of blood—normal tension:
      Anemia (Hb < 40% normal)
      Carbon monoxide poisoning
      Methemoglobinemia
  B. Ischemia (diffuse or widespread multifocal interference with blood supply to brain)
    1. Decreased cerebral blood flow resulting from decreased cardiac output:
      Hemorrhagic or septic shock
      Stokes-Adams syndrome, cardiac arrest, cardiac arrhythmias
      Myocardial infarction
      Aortic stenosis
      Pulmonary embolism
    2. Decreased cerebral blood flow resulting from decreased systemic peripheral resistance:
      Syncope: orthostatic, vasovagal
      Carotid sinus hypersensitivity
      Hypovolemia
    3. Decreased cerebral blood flow due to generalized or multifocal increase in cerebrovascular resistance:
      Hyperventilation syndrome
      Increased blood viscosity (polycythemia, cryo- and macroglobulinemia, sickle cell anemia)
      Bacterial meningitis and encephalitis
      Subarachnoid hemorrhage

    4. Decreased local cerebral blood flow due to widespread small vessel occlusion or tissue necrosis:
      Disseminated intravascular coagulation
      Systemic lupus erythematosus
      Subacute bacterial endocarditis
      Cardiopulmonary bypass
      Small emboli (fat, fibrin, platelets)
      Acute viral encephalitis
    5. Alterations of blood flow due to failure of autoregulation:
      Hypertensive encephalopathy
  C. Hypoglycemia:
    Hyperinsulinism: exogenous; endogenous
  D. Cofactor deficiency:
    Thiamine (Wernicke's encephalopathy)
    Pyridoxine
    Vitamin B_{12}
IV. Diseases of organs other than brain
  A. Nonendocrine organs:
    Liver (hepatic coma)
    Kidney (uremic coma)
    Lung (CO_2 narcosis)
  B. Hyper- and/or hypofunction of endocrine organs:
    Panhypopituitarism
    Thyroid (myxedema-thyrotoxicosis)
    Parathyroid (hyper- and hypocalcemia)
    Adrenal (Addison's disease, Cushing's disease)
  C. Other systemic diseases:
    Diabetes
    Cancer and its treatments
    Porphyria
    Sepsis
V. Abnormalities of fluid, ionic, or acid-base environment of CNS
  A. Water and sodium (hyper- and hyponatremia; hypo- and hyperosmolality)
  B. Acidosis (metabolic and respiratory)
  C. Calcium (hyper- and hypocalcemia)
VI. Disordered temperature regulation
  A. Hypothermia
  B. Heat stroke, fever, malignant neuroleptic syndrome
VII. Infections or inflammation of CNS
  A. Leptomeningitis
  B. Encephalitis
  C. Acute "toxic" encephalopathy
  D. Parainfectious encephalomyelitis
  E. Cerebral vasculitis
  F. Subarachnoid hemorrhage
VIII. Miscellaneous diseases of uncertain pathophysiology
  A. Seizures and postictal states
  B. Concussion

---

can identify the common denominator between such pairs as an apple and an orange or a fly and a tree; confused patients cannot. But the examiner must be cautious; innate intelligence and education also determine cognitive abilities. Unless the physician already knows the patient, it may be difficult to attribute mild mental changes to a metabolic defect. Loss of memory for recent

TABLE 444–6. CHARACTERISTICS OF METABOLIC ENCEPHALOPATHY

Confusion, lethargy, delirium often precede or replace coma
Motor signs, if present, usually symmetric
Bilateral asterixis, myoclonus appear
Pupillary reactions usually preserved; tonic calorics often present
Sensory abnormalities usually absent
Hypothermia common
Abnormal signs reflect incomplete brain dysfunction at multiple anatomical levels

events and disorientation for time are hallmarks of organic brain disease. Orientation to place and time should be specifically tested by asking the date and year, the day of the week, and the present location.

Perceptual errors, e.g., mistaking the physician for someone else, as well as illusions and hallucinations, are more serious symptoms. Hallucinations are common and usually animate. They frighten and agitate some patients, but others tolerate them quietly and must be asked about their presence. Delirious hallucinations or delusions may be visual, auditory, or tactile, alone or in combination; rarely are they systematic. By contrast, schizophrenic delusions or hallucinations are usually systematic in pattern and consist almost exclusively of endogenous auditory perceptions.

Characteristically, the mental status examination fluctuates in metabolic encephalopathy, with patients out of contact one moment and lucid the next. Such intervals appear unpredictably and last for minutes or hours. Delirious patients typically become more disoriented at night and in unfamiliar surroundings. The presence of restraints, intermittent background noise, and unfamiliar activity accentuates their confusion.

Motor Activity. Bilateral tremor, asterixis, and multifocal myoclonus are hallmarks of metabolic brain disease. The *tremor* ranges from fine to coarse, is irregular at a rate of about eight to ten per second, and involves the distal more than proximal parts of the extremities. Fine tremor usually disappears at complete rest and is best brought out in the fingers of the outstretched hands. Coarse tremor such as accompanies certain drug withdrawals or intoxications may be so heavy that it shakes the bed.

Asterixis describes an abnormal, irregular, distal involuntary jerking movement, best elicited with arms outstretched, hands pronated, and fingers extended. Severe examples border on myoclonus. Asterixis is encountered rarely, and then unilaterally, in patients with structural brain disease.

Multifocal myoclonus consists of sudden nonrhythmic, nonpatterned coarse jerks affecting resting groups of muscles. The movements most often affect the face and shoulders but can occur anywhere in the body. They are accentuated by voluntary or passive movement. Multifocal myoclonus occurs most frequently in uremia, in hypercarbic-anoxic encephalopathy, with penicillin or lithium overdose, and in association with the progressive dementia of Creutzfeldt-Jakob disease (see Ch. 478).

Psychomotor activity in delirium can range from extremes of picking at the bedcovers, sustained restlessness, and thrashing about to total immobility. Increased psychomotor activity is typical of acute deliria such as delirium tremens and other drug withdrawal states. More commonly, toxic confusional states are marked by lethargy, drowsiness, and general bradykinesia. Some acutely delirious patients alternate over a few hours between psychomotor overactivity and quiet apathy. Others may be unwilling or unable to stay in bed. They pace the halls, move constantly, and often shout vulgarities or aggressive threats. Unless restrained, many confused patients fall in trying to walk or during efforts to climb out of bed.

Speech is often abnormal. Patients with increased psychomotor behavior often speak rapidly, muttering or slurring speech into an incomprehensible jumble. Bradykinetic patients may speak slowly, monotonously, and so softly as to be barely heard.

Seizures, hyperactive stretch reflexes, and *signs of mild focal brain dysfunction* frequently accompany severe metabolic brain disease, especially after alcohol-sedative withdrawal. The seizures are usually generalized and the motor abnormalities usually symmetric. Nevertheless, focal paresis and focal seizures occasionally occur, especially with hypoglycemia, hepatic encephalopathy, or postanoxic encephalopathy.

Autonomic Activity. *Pupillary light reactions are preserved in metabolic coma with rare exceptions, and their absence requires a specific search for a pre-existing or acute structural lesion.* Nevertheless, a few exceptions exist; the ingestion of drugs possessing an anticholinergic action can paralyze the pupils transiently in either mid-position or dilation. Also, exposure to severe anoxia or asphyxia can produce fixed mid-position or dilated pupils. If sustained, these imply irreversible brain stem damage. In general, the pupils usually remain symmetric in metabolic brain disease, but are often asymmetric and sometimes fixed in patients comatose from structural brain disease.

Hypothermia is common in sedative intoxication as well as with hypoglycemia and myxedema. *Hyperthermia* with profuse perspiration and tachycardia accompanies most agitated deliria and is especially common with delirium tremens. Hyperthermia without perspiration suggests anticholinergic drug ingestion, infection, heat stroke, or the malignant neuroleptic syndrome that sometimes develops with neuroleptics or anesthetic drugs. Less severe, unexplained hyperthermia can reflect idiosyncrasy to a variety of widely used drugs, including salicylates.

Laboratory Tests. The causes of metabolic coma are legion. In many instances the history (e.g., of drug abuse, systemic disease, exposure to toxins) immediately suggests the cause. When this is uncertain, tests listed in Table 444–7 should be performed immediately to establish the presence of life-threatening metabolic defects. Unless strong evidence indicates a specific metabolic or infectious process causing the delirium, diagnostic CT or MR brain imaging is desirable. Imaging shows no immediately pertinent abnormalities in metabolic encephalopathy, although

TABLE 444–7. LABORATORY EVALUATION OF METABOLIC BRAIN DISEASE

Test	Reason for Test
Immediate	
Glucose	Hypoglycemia, hyperosmolar coma
Na^+	Osmolar abnormalities
Ca^{++}	Hyper- or hypocalcemia
BUN	Uremia
Arterial blood pH, P_{CO_2}, P_{O_2}	Acidosis, alkalosis, hypoxia
Lumbar puncture	Infection, hemorrhage, meningeal carcinomatosis
Later	
Liver function tests	Hepatic coma
Sedative drug levels	Overdose
Blood and CSF culture	Sepsis, encephalitis, meningitis
Full electrolytes, including Mg^{++}	Electrolyte imbalance
Coagulation profile	Intravascular coagulation
EEG	Seizure disorder

one can detect pre-existing abnormalities such as chronic subdural hematoma or previous brain damage, the effects of which can mimic or accentuate metabolic delirium.

PSYCHIATRIC DISORDERS. Psychiatric disorders capable of producing the behavioral appearance of impaired consciousness include delirious stages of acute schizophrenic or manic attacks, the nearly total withdrawal of severe depression or certain forms of catatonia, and the pseudocoma of hysteria and malingering (Table 444–8). Especially in the early stages of such disorders, distinction from physiologic alterations of consciousness sometimes can be difficult. Psychiatric amnesia is the most common pseudo-organic symptom and the most readily diagnosed. One should suspect psychiatric amnesia especially when the experience covers sharply delineated periods of time, has an abrupt onset and offset with total amnesia in the middle, is nonprogressive in nature, and relates either to experiences that provoked severe anxiety or to potentially punishable behavior. Catatonic withdrawal states or psychotic deliria in psychiatric illness sometimes can be difficult to differentiate from those of metabolic origin, but applying the guidelines given in Table 444–9 usually provides the answers. As a general rule, however, if the patient's cooperation can be elicited to obtain satisfactory answers, recent memory and cognitive functions usually turn out to be preserved in the functional psychoses. Hallucinations are auditory rather than visual or tactile, and neither asterixis nor multifocal myoclonus occurs. Patients with extreme anxiety may hyperventilate, producing respiratory alkalosis, a diffusely slow electroencephalogram, and sometimes tetany. Otherwise, physical and laboratory evaluations in psychogenically altered consciousness remain normal.

TABLE 444–8. PSYCHIATRIC STATES RESEMBLING ACUTE IMPAIRMENT OF CONSCIOUSNESS

1. **Catatonic states.** Uncommon conditions occurring in either schizophrenic or severe depressive illness which may resemble organic stupor. Mutism, bilateral motor resistance, hypokinesia, and even rigidity are common. Absent are pathologic reflexes, as well as abnormal brain images, EEG's, and laboratory chemical tests.
2. **Acute psychotic deliria.** Uncommon. Involves adult patients of any age, more frequently those older than 50 years. The state can arise with either affective or schizophrenic disorders. Agitation, fear, and hypermobility are prominent. Auditory or visual hallucinations occur, not necessarily paranoid but usually systematized. Fast, coarse tremor can be present and tends to last longer than drug-alcohol withdrawal tremors. Verbal responses, when elicitable, usually reflect orientation for time and place, but distractibility or muteness often limits more detailed mental testing. Pathologic reflexes are lacking. EEG and laboratory chemical tests remain normal in the absence of medical complications. The condition can be difficult to diagnose, but an agitated delirium that lasts longer than 2 weeks almost always reflects psychiatric disease.
3. **Hysteria-malingering.** Unarousable unresponsiveness, usually of brief duration, unaccompanied by physiologic abnormalities and often associated with obviously factitious responses to stimulation.

TABLE 444–9. ORGANIC AND FUNCTIONAL PSYCHOSES COMPARED

Variable	Organic	Functional
Onset	Usually > 30 years	Usually < 40 years
Family history	Usually negative	Often abnormal psychiatrically
Immediate history	Drugs, alcohol, acute medical or neurologic illness	No established medical or neurologic features
Psychology of history	Psychologically coherent	Psychologically incoherent
	Agitation, tremor, noisiness, inattention	Same
Major (psychotic) symptoms		
Orientation and memory	Abnormal	Normal if answers obtained
Delusions or hallucinations	Visual, sometimes olfactory or auditory; nonsystematic (chaotic)	Mainly auditory; systematic: tell a story
Mood	Fearful or apathetic; delusions often regarded as unwanted	Consistent with psychotic symptoms
Coma or akinetic (catatonic) state	Systemic and/or neurologic signs present; EEG abnormal	Neurologic signs absent; EEG normal
Fever, leukocytosis	Signs of medical illness often present	Absent (except malignant hyperthermia or catatonia)
Alcohol-drug intoxication or withdrawal	Often present	Absent
Clinical or EEG seizures	Often present	Absent

Patients with hysterical pseudocoma have normal somatic neurologic examinations. Breathing is eupneic or voluntarily hyperpneik. Most such patients lie supine and quietly unresponsive, with limbs remaining either flaccid or resisting movement in unpredictable patterns. Eyelids usually are closed, actively resist opening, and may spontaneously flutter. Furthermore, the eyelids are incapable of the slow closure that follows passive raising of the lids of patients with physiologic coma. The pupils in psychiatric unresponsiveness are briskly responsive or, if cycloplegics have been self-instilled, widely dilated. Oculocephalic responses are unpredictable, but if the diagnosis is doubtful, irrigating the tympanum with 50 ml of cold water produces physiologic nystagmus rather than the tonic eye deviation or absent responses shown by comatose patients with structural or metabolic disease. Sometimes, the eyes may deviate toward the bed when the patient is turned to one side.

Occasionally, psychiatric pseudodelirium or unresponsiveness can be superimposed on underlying physical illness. An example is the patient hospitalized with a severe medical or neurologic illness who becomes so anxious that he or she is unable to cope and withdraws psychologically to the point of unresponsiveness. In such doubtful instances, slow infusions of small amounts of sodium amobarbital (Amytal interview) may allow the physician to establish contact and rapport with the patient. Since the drug may similarly awaken patients rendered unconscious by continuous focal seizures, close clinical observation and, if possible, an EEG are best done before the test.

ACUTE CENTRAL NERVOUS SYSTEM POISONING. Table 444–10 lists the most frequent acute neurotoxic poisonings in the United States, gives their principal signs of toxicity, and outlines their treatment. To find descriptions of poisons not included in this section, especially chronic neurotoxic agents, the reader should consult the textbooks listed in the references. Almost all drugs in overdose amounts are likely to be mixed with intoxicating amounts of alcohol, thereby making their clinical signs more difficult to appraise. Nevertheless, clinical appraisal must be used to diagnose the specific agent causing several of these reaction patterns, since chemical tests are in many instances either unavailable or impractically slow. When any doubt exists, one should keep admission serum samples for possible later analysis. With most of the drugs, tolerance develops to chronic ingestion and individuals may react differently to similar doses. Accordingly, blood levels and size of the dose are unreliable guides to the potential depth of coma or other complications. The mixing of agents adds to the unreliability. Only the opiates and some of the sedatives create an immediate risk of death; concurrent alcohol ingestion enhances both these risks. Opiate poisoning is discussed in greater detail in Ch. 15.

Pathogenesis. All sedative drugs depress the central nervous system, although not equally on a gram-molecular weight basis, and not to the same degree so far as different central structures are concerned. The duration of action varies widely and depends largely on how the particular drug is detoxified or eliminated. The benzodiazepines, short-acting barbiturates, pentobarbital, secobarbital, and amobarbital are detoxified by the liver, as is methaqualone. They exert their maximal effects promptly after being absorbed and, even in huge doses, seldom cause neurologic depression lasting longer than 3 to 5 days. Barbital and phenobarbital are partially detoxified by the liver and partially excreted in the urine. Severe poisoning with the latter agent can cause coma lasting 10 to 14 days. Glutethimide, nowadays seldom used, has a short duration of action comparable to that of secobarbital, but it is poorly absorbed from the gut and may degenerate into more long-lasting neurotoxic metabolites. Meprobamate has an intermediate duration of effect lasting for days. Bromide rarely causes full coma, but, once it reaches high levels, it replaces chloride in the blood and tissues and persists for weeks to cause symptoms without further ingestion.

Although the sedatives have few important effects outside the nervous system, barbiturates, glutethimide, and meprobamate in toxic doses tend to produce hypotension. Glutethimide possesses anticholinergic properties and is the only sedative that predictably produces light-fixed pupils in only moderately heavy anesthetic doses.

A withdrawal syndrome consisting of tremulousness, agitation, and sometimes delirium and convulsions can develop after prompt withdrawal from chronic exposure to any of the hypnotic sedatives. Convulsions are a particular problem after withdrawal from barbiturates, meprobamate, and methaqualone.

Clinical Manifestations. Stupor or coma caused by depressant drug poisoning usually presents the characteristic picture of acute general anesthesia. The depression of the central nervous system tends to be bilateral and symmetric and the drug affects simultaneously many levels, including the spinal cord. Respiratory and circulatory controlling mechanisms in the lower brain stem are affected only with very high doses or not at all, and, except with glutethimide or extremely large doses of barbiturates, the pupillary light reflexes are preserved. Early in the course of acute poisoning, patients can demonstrate muscular hypertonus or even spasticity as the result of uneven depression of different neurologic levels. Within a short time, usually an hour or less, flaccidity supervenes, and the stretch reflexes tend to disappear. Even moderate degrees of drug depression can depress or block the oculovestibular reflexes.

As mentioned, blood levels are a poor index to the depth of coma. Generally speaking, however, blood levels of short-acting barbiturates of more than 2.5 mg per deciliter and phenobarbital blood levels of more than 12 mg per deciliter are associated with very deep coma to the level at which apnea and hypotension become management problems. Apnea rarely supervenes with the benzodiazepines, even at very high doses.

Diagnosis. The combination of acutely occurring unresponsiveness, with preserved or sluggish pupillary reactions, absent oculovestibular reactions, motor areflexia, hypothermia, and relative depression of respiration and circulation is clinically diagnostic of sedative-anesthetic drug poisoning. Only infarction or hemorrhage of the pons resembles this clinical state, and with lesions of the pons the pupils are usually small or pinpoint, the stretch reflexes are generally preserved or hyperactive, and the plantar responses are extensor. Specific chemical tests detect barbiturates, glutethimide, meprobamate, methaqualone, and bromides in blood or urine, and can be done as emergency measures.

TABLE 444-10. COMMON DRUG POISONINGS, SIGNS OF TOXICITY, AND TREATMENT

| Drug | Signs and Symptoms | | Diagnostic Test | Treatment |
	Mild	Severe		
Opiates Heroin Morphine Meperidine Methadone Hydromorphone Oxycodone Levorphanol	"Nodding" drowsiness, small pupils, urinary retention, slow and shallow breathing; skin scars and subcutaneous abscesses; duration 4–6 hours; with methadone, duration to 24 hours	Coma; pinpoint pupils, slow irregular respiration or apnea, hypotension, hypothermia, pulmonary edema	Response to naloxone Urine	Naloxone, 0.4 mg intravenously or intramuscularly; repeat at 15-minute intervals if patient responds and gradually increase intervals; repeat in 3 hours if necessary; if no response by second dose, suspect another cause; treat shock; find and detect infection
Depressants Alcohol Barbiturates Chloral hydrate Glutethimide (Doriden) Meprobamate (Equanil)	Confusion, rousable drowsiness, delirium, ataxia, nystagmus, dysarthria, analgesia to stimuli	Stupor to coma; pupils reactive, usually constricted; oculovestibular response absent; motor tonus initially briefly hyperactive, then flaccid; respiration and blood pressure depressed; hypothermia; with glutethimide, pupils moderately dilated, can be fixed; with meprobamate, withdrawal seizures common; with methaqualone, coma, occasional convulsions, tachycardia, cardiac failure, bleeding tendency	Blood, urine, breath Blood Blood Blood	Intubate, ventilate, lavage; drainage position; antimicrobials; keep mean blood pressure >90 mm Hg and urine output >300 ml per hour; avoid analeptics; hemodialyze severe phenobarbital poisoning
Methaqualone (Quaalude, Sopor, Mandrax)	Hallucinations, agitation, motor hyperactivity, myoclonus, tonic spasms		Blood	As above; diuresis of little help
Benzodiazepines (Librium, Valium, Tranxene, Ativan, Dalmane, etc.) Ethchlorvynol (Placidyl)	Usually taken with another sedative if poisoning is attempted	Coma seldom severe if drug taken alone	Blood	As above; diuresis of little help
Stimulants Amphetamines Methylphenidate	Hyperactive, aggressive, sometimes paranoid, repetitive behavior, dilated pupils, tremor, hyperactive reflexes; hyperthermia, tachycardia, arrhythmia Acute torsion dystonia	Agitated, assaultive and paranoid excitement; occasionally convulsions; hypothermia; circulatory collapse	Blood	Chlorpromazine
Cocaine	Similar but less prominent than above; less paranoid, often euphoric	Twitching; irregular breathing, tachycardia, arrhythmia, occasionally convulsions	Blood, urine	Diazepam plus specific symptomatic
Psychedelics (LSD), mescaline, psilocybin, phencyclidine (PCP, angel dust)	Confused, disoriented, perceptual distortions, distractable, withdrawn or eruptive, leading to accidents or violence; wide-eyed, dilated pupils; restless, hyperreflexic; less often, hypertension or tachycardia	Panic		Reassure; diazepam satisfactory; avoid phenothiazines
Scopolamine-atropine (knockout drops, Transderm delirium)	Agitated or confused, visual hallucinations, dilated pupils, flushed and dry skin	Florid toxic disoriented delirium, visual hallucinations; later, amnesia, fever, dilated fixed pupils, hot flushed dry skin, urinary retention		Reassure; sedate lightly, (1) avoid phenothiazines; (2) do not leave alone

Table continued on following page

TABLE 444–10. COMMON DRUG POISONINGS, SIGNS OF TOXICITY, AND TREATMENT *Continued*

Drug	Signs and Symptoms		Diagnostic Test	Treatment
	Mild	*Severe*		
Antidepressants				
Tricyclics (Tofranil, Elavil, Desipramine, etc.)	Restlessness, drowsiness, tachycardia, ataxia, sweating	Agitation, vomiting, hyper-pyrexia, sweating, muscle dystonia, convul-sions, tachycardia or arrhythmia	Blood	Symptomatic; gastric lavage Intensive care, anticonvul-sants, and antiarrhythmics for severe cases
MAO inhibitors (Parnate, Nardil, Eutonyl, etc.)	Hypertensive crises, agitation, drowsiness, ataxia	Hypotension; headache; chest pain; agitation; coma, seizures and shock	Clinical	Symptomatic; gastric lavage
Neuroleptics (phenothia-zines, butyrophen-ones, etc.)	Acute dystonia, somno-lence, hypotension	Coma; convulsions (rare); arrhythmias; hypotension	Blood	Anticholinergics; diphenhydra-mine; symptomatic; gastric lavage
Lithium	Mild lethargy	Sustention-intention tremor, lethargy; mute-ness with appearance of distraction; coma; multi-focal seizures; slow or fluctuating course	Blood	Hydrate if mild; hemodialyze for delirium, coma, or con-vulsions
Acid-forming intoxicants				
Methanol (formic); ethylene glycol (oxalic and hippuric); other organic alcohols	Inebriation with hyperpnea	All produce progressive hyperventilation, drunkenness, stupor, eventually convulsions and death. Early blind-ness with methanol	Blood shows increas-ingly severe anion-gap acidosis	Inhibit hepatic alcohol dehy-drogenase by giving alcohol until acidosis controlled; treat acidosis vigorously
Salicylate				
Aspirin	Tinnitus, dyspnea	Older persons: confusional state or toxic delirium leading to stupor, convulsions, coma	Blood salicylate > 60 mg/dl	Alkaline diuresis

CLINICAL EVALUATION OF DELIRIUM, STUPOR, OR COMA

The immediate step consists of assuring vital cardiorespiratory systems and protecting against further damage to the central nervous system. Once these measures are taken, the keys to diagnosis, specific treatment, and prognosis lie in carefully ex-amining the patient, systematically seeking the answers to a few central questions:

Is the process neurogenic or psychogenic in origin?

If neurogenic, is (are) the lesion(s) supratentorial, subtento-rial, focal, or multifocal-diffuse?

Once the immediate cause of loss of consciousness is under control, is the appropriate treatment medical or surgical?

If the illness is nonstructural, is it exogenously toxic or endogenously metabolic, already maximal (e.g., postanoxic, post-intoxicant), or progressive; is it worsening or improving?

Which immediate treatment best halts the pathologic process and sustains the patient?

DIFFERENTIAL HISTORY. If sudden unconsciousness is not an expected consequence of an already known illness, wit-nesses to the onset provide the most helpful immediate infor-mation. Was the onset gradual or abrupt? Was it preceded by headache and, if so, of what location and duration? Was paralysis or seizure activity observed? Were antecedent or prodromal symptoms noted? Did the onset occur in a circumstance or geographic area in which drugs, trauma, or foul play could be suspected? What medications might the patient have taken? Beyond these immediacies, what has been the patient's physical and mental health for the past few days, weeks, or months?

PHYSICAL AND NEUROLOGIC EXAMINATION. In cases of deep unresponsiveness, one first carries out steps 1 to 5 described below under Emergency Management, then proceeds with the physical examination. Under urgent circumstances, the physician should be able to conduct a highly focused, pertinent physical and neurologic examination on patients in coma in less than 5 minutes. This includes appraising cardiopulmonary status

as indicated above and systematically carrying out the main features of the examination outlined in Table 444–11. In the course of the above, trauma or seizures make themselves evident. In patients with coma of unknown cause, clues should be sought to drug exposure, as well as to past serious medical or psychiatric problems. Companions should be asked about recent neurologic function and dysfunction.

For patients presenting with less severe impairments, i.e., acute-subacute confusion, delirium, or hypersomnolence, the examiner can take a more deliberate approach. Usually, a detailed history can precede the exigencies of stabilizing vital functions and a thorough organ-by-organ physical examination can be conducted. Either way, by the end of the initial examination, the findings should begin to indicate which of the four major causes of coma, as listed in Table 444–1, is responsible for the patient's acute problem. At that juncture, one can move toward obtaining supplementary or reinforcing laboratory tests as indicated below.

LABORATORY STUDIES. Unless the acutely obtained clin-ical findings make the diagnosis and appropriate treatment immediately obvious, blood should be drawn for laboratory tests listed in Table 444–7. Lumbar puncture is best deferred until after a contrast-enhanced brain CT or an MRI is obtained, so long as the images can be obtained promptly as an emergency procedure. If imaging is not available and the findings suggest acute, treatable meningitis or encephalitis, the physician has no choice but to proceed cautiously with lumbar puncture, using a No. 20 or 22 needle. The EEG (see Ch. 441) is diagnostically indispensable for detecting delirious states caused by continu-ously recurring partial complex seizures. A normal EEG rules out organic causes of acute unresponsiveness.

EMERGENCY MANAGEMENT OF COMA. Faced with acute coma of uncertain origin, one must treat the patient first, even as the history and initial diagnostic tests are being applied. Certain measures apply to the care of all patients:

1. *Assure an adequate airway and oxygenation.* Immediately check and clean out the upper airway. If the patient is deeply

TABLE 444–11. THE NEUROLOGIC EXAMINATION IN COMA

1. Guarantee vital functions as indicated in text.
2. Feel the scalp for hematomas (overlying fracture lines); be sure the neck is not fractured; test *gently* for stiff neck.
3. Test language. Test arousability by words, loud sounds, noxious stimuli. If vocalizations occur, check quickly for appropriate phrases, actual words, and presence or absence of aphasia.
4. Do a neuro-ophthalmologic examination.
   Funduscopy (if difficult can be deferred until patient is stabilized)
   Papilledema? (increased intracranial or venous sinus pressure)
   Hemorrhages (subarachnoid hemorrhage; hypertensive encephalopathy; diabetes; hypoxic-hypercarbic encephalopathy)
   Pupils
   Light reaction. Use bright flashlight and, if necessary, magnifying glass to be certain. Absence means potentially fatally deep sedative poisoning or acute or chronic structural brain stem damage (e.g., tabetic pupils).
   Equality. 15% of normals have mild anisocoria but new or >2 mm dilation means parasympathetic (third nerve) palsy.
   Extraocular movements. Absence acutely means deep drug poisoning, severe brain stem damage, Wernicke's encephalopathy, polyneuropathy, or botulism.
   Dysconjugate at rest means an acute third, fourth, or sixth nerve palsy or internuclear ophthalmoplegia. Tonic conjugate deviation toward a paralytic arm and leg means forebrain seizures or a contralateral pontine destructive lesion; away from the paralytic arm and leg means forebrain gaze paralysis.
   Spontaneous eye movements. In coma patients, nystagmus, bobbing, independently moving eyes all mean brain stem damage.
   Oculocephalic (away from direction of head turning) or oculovestibular (toward cold caloric irrigation) responses. Absence of responses means drugs or severe brain stem disease; dysconjugate responses with equal pupils mean internuclear ophthalmoplegia, with unequal pupils mean third nerve disease.
5. Examine the motor systems.
   Strength
   Unilateral weakness or motionlessness of arm and leg means contralateral supraspinal upper motor neuron lesion, most often cerebral; if of arm, leg, and face, contralateral cerebral lesion. Occasionally arm and leg weakness can reflect contralateral brain stem lesion.
   All four extremities weak or motionless implies metabolic disease; less likely is brain stem disease (tone and reflexes increased) or peripheral disease (tone and reflexes decreased).
   Attempt to elicit reflex posturing
   Arm flexed, leg extended—contralateral deep cerebral-thalamic lesion
   Arm and leg extended—thalamic or mesencephalic lesion
   Arms extended and legs flexed or flaccid—pontine lesion
   Legs flexed, arms flaccid—pontomedullary or spinal lesion
   Compare side-to-side reflexes and examine plantar responses.
6. Seek seizure activity or abnormal movements. (1) Generalized? (2) Focal? (3) Multifocal? (4) Myoclonic?
   Control 1 immediately, 2 and 3 deliberately; if 4, treat underlying disease.
   Acute tremor, asterixis, multifocal myoclonus—seek metabolic cause.
7. Inspect breathing.
   Regular hyperpnea: metabolic acidosis; pulmonary infarction; congestive failure or alveolar infiltration; sepsis; salicylism; hepatic coma
   Cyclically irregular (Cheyne-Stokes): low cardiac output plus bilateral cerebral or upper brain stem dysfunction
   Irregularly irregular gasping, slow or weak: lower brain stem dysfunction (including hypoglycemia, drug effects), less often peripheral ventilatory paralysis
8. Proceed with laboratory tests and emergency management as described in text.

unresponsive, insert an endotracheal airway, but first give 1 mg of atropine intravenously to guard against hypoxigenic vagal-induced asystole. Be sure that no neck fracture exists before extending the head for intubation. Auscultate both lung bases to assure that the lower airway is open. Ventilate if necessary and keep arterial PaO_2 greater than 80 mm Hg and $PaCO_2$ 30 to 35 mm Hg. To empty the stomach in comatose patients suspected of acute orally ingested drug poisoning, initiate lavage only after the cuffed airway tube is in place.

2. *Maintain circulation.* Insert venous line(s) and start Ringer's lactate solution. Determine and maintain a satisfactory cardiac rate and rhythm. Avoid overhydration but keep mean blood pressure at 80 to 90 mm Hg, using dopamine if necessary. In poisoning cases maintain urine flow at 300 ml or more per hour. In any patient during the early stages of coma, check electrolytes acutely and at 12-hour intervals thereafter.

3. *Draw blood for emergency laboratory analysis.* Give IV Narcan to protect against opiate intoxication and 50 mg thiamine to prevent accentuation of Wernicke's encephalopathy.

4. *Give glucose.* If hypoglycemia is a possible diagnosis, give 50 ml of 50 per cent glucose. Draw blood first in order not to lose evidence for the diagnosis. The glucose does not appreciably intensify serum hyperosmolality.

5. *Stop generalized motor seizures.* Repetitive convulsions can result from either cerebral structural lesions, pre-existing epileptic disorders, or acquired metabolic-diffuse encephalopathies. In either event, status epilepticus can cause coma and within a short period of time produces irreversible brain damage as well. Start treatment with intravenous diazepam. Give 5 to 10 mg or more, if necessary, at a rate of 1 to 2 mg per minute, keeping a ventilator available to treat depressed breathing. As soon as convulsions stop, give between 500 and 1000 mg of phenytoin intravenously at a rate of less than 50 mg per minute. If seizures continue, give more diazepam or resort to barbiturate general anesthesia. Repetitive focal seizures and myoclonus are less damaging to brain than are generalized convulsions, and their continuation does not require the use of general anesthesia.

6. *Restore blood acid-base and osmolar balance.* Extremes of either acidosis or alkalosis usually reflect profound metabolic problems, severe circulatory insufficiency, the postictal state (muscular lactic acidosis), or hyperadrenocorticism. Since severe metabolic acidosis can precipitate cardiovascular irregularity and alkalosis depresses breathing, they should be corrected. Extreme hypo- and hyperosmolality are equally dangerous to brain and should be corrected, the first by withholding fluids (except water by mouth) and stopping diuretics and the second by administering fluids (and insulin for hyperglycemia). Beware of too rapid reversal. Osmotic delays across the blood-brain barrier during treatment can lead to large fluid shifts in or out of the brain. Also, too rapid correction of hyponatremia can produce central pontine myelinolysis (Ch. 456). A reasonable goal in treating osmolal shifts is to correct blood by about 0.5 mOsm per hour.

7. *Treat infection.* Several kinds of infection can cause or intensify delirium and coma. Obtain nose, throat, blood, and wound cultures, and perform lumbar puncture if indicated. With any sign of infection, begin antimicrobial treatment after obtaining the cultures cited above, based on either the results of smears or the most probable clinically suggested organism.

8. *Treat extreme body temperatures.* Hyperthermia above 40°C or hypothermia below 34°C should be brought to within 3°C of normal.

9. *Consider specific antidotes.* Many, if not most, patients admitted to emergency rooms in coma have taken an overdose of drugs, often in combination. For narcotic overdose, give 0.4 mg of naloxone intravenously every 5 minutes until the subject awakens. If the subject may be an addict, dilute the dose in 10 ml of saline and give slowly, trying to minimize withdrawal phenomena. Remember that naloxone's duration of action of 2 to 3 hours is shorter than that of several narcotics, and the dose may require repeating. Analeptics of any kind are contraindicated.

Recently, flumazenil, a benzodiazepine antagonist, has been found useful in treating patients with benzodiazepine overdose, with or without concurrent ingestion of other depressant drugs. Length of unresponsiveness was shortened, and complications were reduced. The agent has not yet been released for use in the United States.

10. *Control agitation,* avoiding barbiturates but employing diazepam or haloperidol as necessary.

11. *Prevent complications.* If possible, keep unconscious patients semiprone in the drainage position and change their position from side to side, but never place them fully supine. In most instances, treat potential pulmonary infection with a broad-spectrum antibiotic. Poisoned patients and many with head injuries are unconscious for only a few days, and the risk of

emergence of drug-resistant bacterial infections is less of a concern than is pneumonia caused by already aspirated material. It is wise to protect the corneas against abrasions, using ophthalmic ointment and, if necessary, taping the lids shut.

RECOVERY AND PROGNOSIS. Patients recovering from coma require close medical supervision. Severe pneumonitis can develop as late as 3 to 4 days after recovery. If antimicrobial drugs were started during coma, they are best continued for at least 48 hours after it ends. Permanent physical sequelae are rare. Among 356 of our own cases of sedative drug overdose, residual brain injury was observed only once (in a patient who suffered an acute cardiac arrest). Peripheral nerve injuries from pressure developed in 6 subjects, and 14 subjects had pressure skin lesions leaving scars. There were no other physical residua.

Convalescent management varies according to the patient's underlying psychiatric disorder and attitudes. Suicide attempts are never accidents, and reports of near-fatal ingestion caused by misunderstanding the dose or forgetting previous doses carry little validity. The expert opinion of a psychiatrist should be sought before deciding whether to release or to institutionalize a patient. The immediate prognosis is good, but there is a high incidence of recurrent attempts over the years.

PROGNOSIS IN SEVERE BRAIN DAMAGE

An important part of the physician's responsibility includes forecasting the outcome of illness. Modern medical advances currently save many lives that only a few years ago would have been lost to severe disease or trauma. Unfortunately, however, when severe brain dysfunction accompanies acute illness, these advances create the risk that if the cerebrum fails to recover, vigorous treatment may be followed by an unwanted outcome. According to Harris polls, most persons in the United States prefer death to a life of severe, permanent neurologic disability and often express this view in the form of a living will. Several empirically based guidelines can help the physician's decisions in such instances by predicting with a high degree of certainty between good and very poor neurologic outcomes following illnesses causing severe brain damage or coma.

Nontraumatic Coma

The outcome from medical coma depends upon (a) its cause, and (b), excepting only depressant drug poisoning, the initial

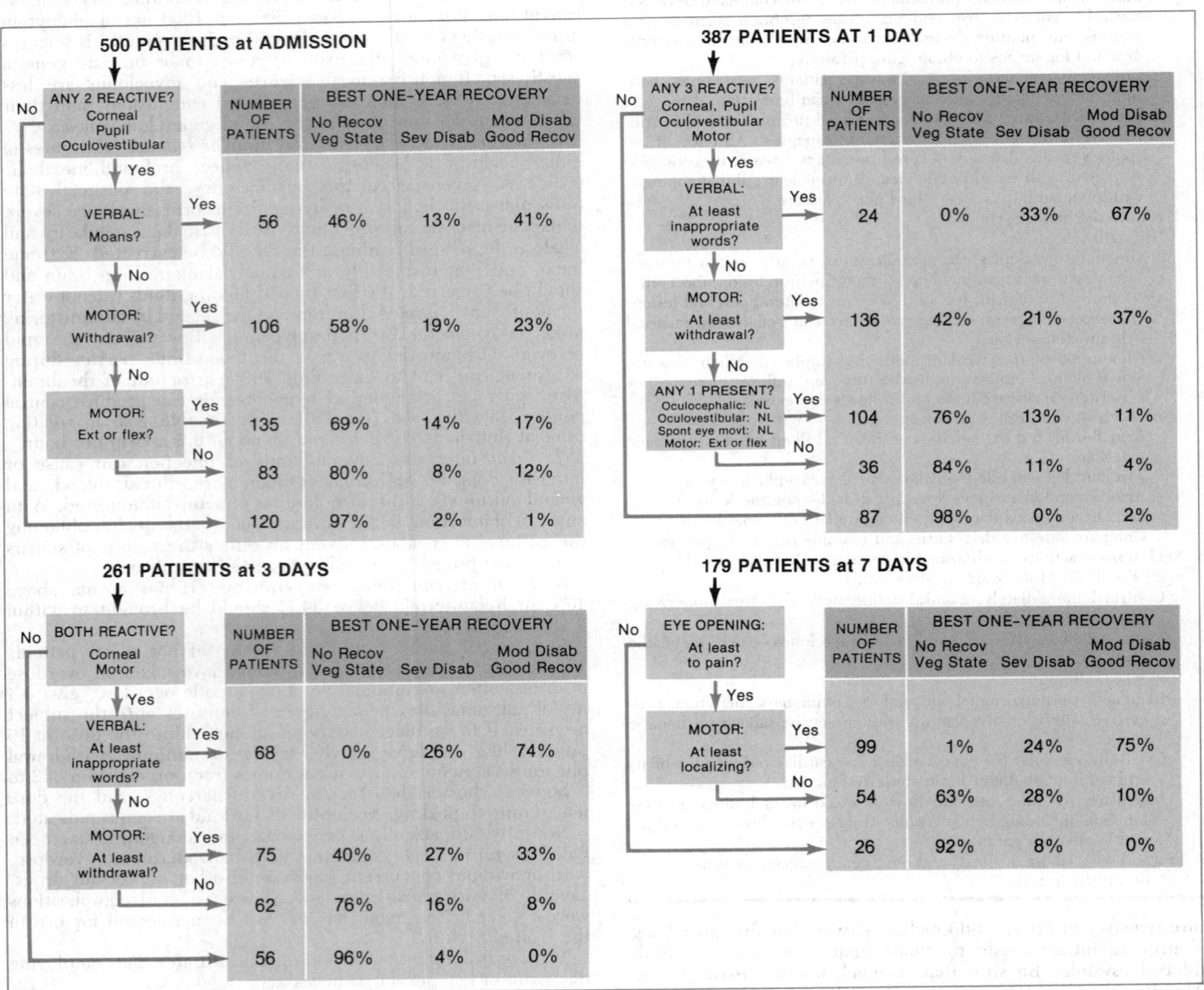

FIGURE 444–2. The best 1-year outcome for 500 optimally treated patients in coma from nontraumatic causes. For each time period following onset, the diagram correlates the degree of recovery with clinical signs observed at that point. Although the diagrams describe actual events in a specific population, the numbers in most instances are sufficiently large to provide a basis for estimating prognosis among similarly affected patients in the future. (From Levy DE, Bates D, Caronna JJ, et al.: Prognosis in nontraumatic coma. Ann Intern Med 94:293, 1981, with permission.)

severity and extent of neurologic damage as revealed by clinical neurologic signs obtained within the first few days of illness.

Depressant drug poisoning, no matter how deep the coma, reflects a state of general anesthesia. Barring severe complications, almost all patients with drug intoxication who reach medical attention recover completely. This favorable prognosis applies even when coma is so profound that normal brain stem reflexes and the EEG temporarily disappear. Since most comas of unknown origin leading to emergency house calls or emergency room visits are due to drug ingestion, such initially undiagnosed patients should receive maximal treatment unless direct evidence points to severe structural brain damage and the use of drugs by ingestion or for therapy has been ruled out.

Aside from drug poisoning, the acute or subacute development in the course of medical illness of loss of consciousness lasting more than a few hours carries a poor prognosis, with only about 15 per cent of patients making a good recovery. The major problem in making early treatment decisions lies in discriminating between patients who have a chance of reaching a good outcome and those whose chances of neurologic recovery are extremely small. In making such early decisions, clinical signs of abnormal forebrain and/or upper brain stem function have been found to be the most powerful available discriminating indicators. The nature of the underlying illness and age have secondary influences but do not modify importantly the accuracy of early signs in distinguishing between probably good and poor outcomes. No laboratory determinants have been found to predict outcome accurately.

The clinical tests most valuable for estimating the capacity for recovery after medical coma are identical to those used in making the initial diagnosis and in following the later course of the patient in coma. In most instances, early functional changes evolve so rapidly that one cannot reliably estimate the outcome of coma within the first minutes to hours, a time when improvement often occurs. After about 6 hours, however, so long as the patient has not received heavy doses of sedative drugs or alcohol, certain neurologic findings begin to correlate increasingly with the potential for neurologic recovery or otherwise. By the end of the first day, clinical signs accurately predict about two thirds of the patients who actually will do well. With each successive day, the signs develop greater predictive power. When considered appropriate to the patient's expressed wishes, treatment can be adjusted accordingly.

Figure 444–2 provides a series of algorithms that describe the actual outcome of 500 patients in coma from medical illness (mostly cardiac arrest) related to their neurologic findings at 6 hours and on days 1, 3, and 7 following onset. The charts disclose that signs of brain stem dysfunction (absent pupillary or corneal responses, imperfect or absent oculocephalic responses, or abnormal motor responses to stimulation) worsened the prognosis and, in combination, indicated a nearly hopeless outlook when they persisted beyond the third day.

Following an acute diffuse brain injury such as follows cardiac arrest, a few patients become immediately vegetative following the ictus and remain so as the days pass into weeks. Most who fail to speak until after the end of the second week are left with prominent intellectual defects, especially in recent and anterograde memory, even if sensorimotor activities return to normal. Persistence of coma or the vegetative state in an adult for more than 4 weeks almost never is associated with later complete recovery and the longer the mindless state lasts, the greater the chance of permanent disability. Care must be taken in such instances to rule out a locked-in state (see Table 443–1).

Traumatic Coma

Coma following head injury has a statistically better outcome than that associated with medical illness. About 50 per cent of patients in coma from head injury die, many instantly. Acute treatment may somewhat improve the outcome of those who reach hospital. Recovery in traumatic cases is closely linked to age: the younger the better. As with medical coma, severely abnormal neuro-ophthalmologic signs reflecting brain stem dysfunction imply a poor prognosis, with approximately 90 per cent of such patients either dying or remaining in near-vegetative states.

Dreisbach RH, Robinson WO: Handbook of Poisoning, 11th ed. Norwalk, CT, Appleton and Lange, 1987. *Succinct and handy, an excellent quick source to consult in emergencies, especially for poisoning in children.*

Feldmann E, Gandy SE, Becker R, et al.: MRI demonstrates descending transtentorial herniation. Neurology 38:697, 1988. *Sagittal images of brain demonstrate the physical basis of the herniation syndromes described in this text.*
Gilman AG, Rall TW, Nies AS, Taylor P (eds.): Goodman and Gilman's The Pharmacological Basis of Therapeutics, 8th ed. New York, Pergamon, 1990. *The "bible" of pharmacology and associated toxicology addresses major drug poisonings in authoritative chapters.*
Goetz CG: Neurotoxins in Clinical Practice. New York, SP Medical and Scientific, 1985. *A useful guide, classified by agent and syndrome, to all forms of exogenous toxins affecting the nervous system.*
Plum F: Coma and related global disturbances of the human conscious state. *In* Jones EG, Peters A (eds.): Cerebral Cortex. Vol. 9, Altered Cortical States. New York, Plenum Press, 1991. *A recent chapter describing current advances in pathophysiology.*
Plum F, Posner JB: Diagnosis of Stupor and Coma, 3rd ed., rev. Philadelphia, F. A. Davis, 1982. *Provides more discussion of the material described in this chapter.*

445 Brain Death
Fred Plum

Modern resuscitative devices can maintain the functions of the heart, lungs, and visceral organs for hours or days after the life-maintaining centers of the brain stem tissue have stopped functioning. The economic waste of this hopeless condition, as well as the increasing success of organ transplant programs, has led countries worldwide to adopt the principle that death of the person occurs when either the brain or the heart irreversibly fails in its functions. In the United States the time of brain death has been accepted as the time of the person's death in legal terms. Many states accept the brain death concept by statute, and in no state has the principle failed to meet legal challenge. The Presidential Commission set as the criterion for brain death the "irreversible cessation of all functions of the entire brain, including the brain stem." Guidelines for the practical application of these principles are listed in Table 445–1. One of the supplementary criteria often is particularly desirable when making decisions at 6 hours to facilitate organ transplant.

Certain points in the diagnosis of brain death must be emphasized. *Recoverable drug depressant poisoning can in all ways resemble brain death and must be explicitly ruled out.* In any doubtful case, any evidence of EEG activity or of reflex activity of the brain stem means that the brain is not dead and contravenes immediate discontinuation of life support. However, purely spinal reflex activity can persist after brain death, including reflexes of the limbs and even some remarkably complex movements, including flexion of the trunk and raising of outstretched arms.

TABLE 445–1. CRITERIA FOR DIAGNOSIS OF BRAIN DEATH

1. **Nature and duration of coma must be known**
   a. Known structural disease or irreversible systemic metabolic cause
   b. No chance of drug intoxication or hypothermia; no paralyzing or potentially anesthetizing drugs recently given for treatment
   c. Body temperature must be above 34°C
   d. Six-hour observation of no brain function is sufficient in cases of known structural cause when no drug or alcohol is involved in causation or treatment; otherwise, 12 hours plus negative drug screen required
2. **Absence of cerebral and brain stem function**
   a. No behavioral or reflex response to noxious stimuli above foramen magnum level
   b. Fixed pupils
   c. No oculovestibular response to 50 ml ice water calorics
   d. Apneic off ventilator with oxygenation for 10 minutes
   e. Systemic circulation may be intact
   f. Purely spinal reflexes may be retained
3. **Supplementary (optional) criteria**
   a. EEG isoelectric for 30 minutes at maximal gain
   b. Brain stem–evoked responses reflect absent function in vital brain stem structures
   c. No cerebral circulation present on angiographic examination

It is recommended that physicians faced with applying and acting upon the diagnosis of brain death familiarize themselves with the additional pertinent material listed in the references and whenever possible obtain confirmation with an experienced consultant.

Abrams MB, et al.: Deciding to Forego Life-Sustaining Treatment. A Report on the Ethical, Medical, and Legal Issues in Treatment Decisions. President's Commission for the Study of Ethical Problems in Medicine and Biomedical and Behavioral Research. Washington, D.C., United States Government Printing Office, March, 1983. *A long and thoughtful report on the problems associated with the terminally ill and the neurologically hopelessly damaged patient.*

Barber J, et al.: Guidelines for the determination of death: Report of the medical consultants on the diagnosis of death to the President's Commission for the Study of Ethical Problems in Medicine and Biomedical and Behavioral Research. Neurology 32:395, 1982. *The detailed report describing that cardiac death and brain death are equivalent and giving criteria for each.*

Council on Scientific Affairs and Council on Ethical and Judicial Affairs: Persistent vegetative state and the decision to withdraw or withhold life support. JAMA 263:426, 1990. *The article provides criteria for the diagnosis of permanent unconsciousness and summarizes the data that support their reliability.*

Levy DE, Caronna JJ, Singer BH, et al.: Predicting outcome from hypoxic-ischemic coma. JAMA 253:1420, 1985. *Prospective correlations were obtained between early neurologic signs and eventual course in 210 patients, mostly with cardiac arrest. By 72 hours, signs accurately selected between good or poor eventual outcome in over 75 per cent of patients.*

446 Brief Loss of Consciousness

Fred Plum

Brief loss of consciousness (BLOC), defined as loss of self-awareness lasting from a few minutes to as much as an hour, is a relatively common symptom. If one excludes conditions readily diagnosed by circumstances or history such as acute traumatic concussion, a known recurrent minor seizure disorder, or accidental insulin-induced hypoglycemia, most such cases are due to causes listed in Table 446–1. As the table indicates, *syncope*, defined as brief unconsciousness due to a temporary, critical reduction of cerebral blood flow, is by far the most common cause of BLOC. With any of the conditions, however, reliable observations of the attack itself often are unavailable. Under such circumstances, a careful history and physical examination, including any possible information gained from witnesses, generally give more diagnostic information than any other approach.

Certain immediate guidelines aid in differential diagnosis. Patients under age 50 years with no previous history of cardiac disease, seizures, antihypoglycemic medication, or drug-alcohol abuse almost all turn out to have either benign syncope or a disorder undiagnosable from available evidence. Such patients rarely require an evaluation more elaborate than a careful history and physical examination plus standard blood counts and blood chemistry determinations. For those over age 40, an electrocar-

TABLE 446-1. PRINCIPAL CAUSES AND APPROXIMATE FREQUENCIES OF BRIEF LOSS OF CONSCIOUSNESS OF UNKNOWN ORIGIN

Syncope	
Primarily neurogenic-vasodepressor	55%
Primarily cardiogenic	10%
Central Nervous System	<10%
First seizure	
Cerebral vascular insufficiency	
Subarachnoid hemorrhage	
Intracranial pressure waves	
Drugs-Metabolic	<10%
Alcohol-sedative blackouts	
Narcotic overdose	
Hypoglycemia—exogenous or endogenous	
Antihypertensive drugs	
Diagnosis Unknown	15–20%

diogram (ECG) should be obtained. Computed tomography and electroencephalographic examinations are not cost-effective in the absence of abnormal neurologic symptoms or signs.

446.1 SYNCOPE

ETIOLOGY AND INITIAL CONSIDERATIONS. A brief dysfunction of vasodepressor cardiovascular reflexes causes most syncope. Less frequent causes include primary cardiovascular disease or the drugs employed to treat it, primary or secondary orthostatic hypotension, and, rarely, cerebral arterial vascular disease. Seizure disorders or psychiatric episodes represent possibly confusing conditions when only a retrospective history can be obtained. Acute, severe vertiginous attacks sometimes can induce secondary, reflex syncope. Hysterical unresponsiveness, although not uncommon, cannot be diagnosed reliably in retrospect. Diagnostic signs of such attacks are given in Table 446–2.

Among patients over age 50 with no historical or physical features suggesting cardiac, neurologic, or systemic illness, benign syncope remains the most common cause of unexplained BLOC. Nevertheless, most authorities recommend at least 24 hours of prolonged ECG monitoring in such instances. In Kapoor's study of 433 mostly older patients (mean age, 56 years) with presumed syncope, prolonged ECG recording independently provided important diagnostic information in approximately 20 per cent.

MECHANISMS OF SYNCOPE. Unconsciousness results when generalized cerebral blood flow declines to approximately 40 per cent of normal. Such a drop usually reflects a fall in cardiac output by half or more, and a fall in mean erect arterial blood pressure to below 40 to 50 mm Hg. Given this principle, it comes as no surprise that posture contributes importantly to the event. Syncope of any cause is far more common in the sitting or standing position than during recumbency. Indeed, recumbent syncope must be regarded as reflecting either serious cardiovascular disease or neurologic disease until proved otherwise.

Pathophysiologic changes in several bodily systems, acting alone or together, can cause the changes in global cerebral blood flow necessary to induce syncope. These include (1) temporarily or permanently abnormal neural reflexes acting on an otherwise normal cardiovascular system; this category includes the most common causes of fainting in persons who have no history of serious cardiovascular disease; (2) abnormal intrinsic cardiovascular function, including especially disease of the conduction system predisposing to malignant arrhythmias; (3) impaired right heart filling secondary to functionally increased resistance to venous return; (4) acute or subacute loss of blood volume; (5) increased resistance of cervical or intracranial arterial vascular beds; (6) subacute or chronic autonomic insufficiency producing severe orthostatic hypotension. Table 446–3 lists subcategories of these disorders which are discussed more fully in the following paragraphs.

Neurogenic Mechanisms in Normal and Abnormal Cardiovascular Control. Sympathetic and parasympathetic influences on the cardiovascular system normally act in a finely tuned and balanced manner to slow the heart (vagal) and regulate the degree of constriction of the large venous capacitance vessels of the trunk and extremities (sympathetic outflow). Imbalance, be it a reflection of paralysis or excessive activity in either system, can perturb heart rhythm and rate, slacken venomotor tone, and lead to either reduced left ventricle output, reduced right heart filling, or the two combined. Depending on the degree of blood pressure

TABLE 446-2. SIGNS OF PSYCHOGENIC PSEUDOSYNCOPE

Lids close actively, may flutter, and often resist examiner's attempt to open them.
Breathing: eupnea or acute hyperventilation.
Pupils responsive or dilated (self-administered cycloplegic).
Oculocephalic responses unpredictable; calorics produce quick nystagmus.
Motor responses unpredictable, often bizarre and self-protecting.
No pathologic reflexes. EEG normal in awake patient.

I. Mainly impaired right heart filling
  A. Reflex abnormalities
    1. Vasodepressor ("vasovagal"): capacitance veins dilated, cardiac rate normal or slow
      a. Psychophysiologic (limbic) stimuli, including hyperventilation
      b. Visceral reflex (micturition, pain, gastrointestinal dilatation, acute labyrinthine vertigo)
      c. Carotid baroreceptor sensitivity
    2. Primary or secondary autonomic insufficiency (Ch. 452)
  B. Hypovolemia: hemorrhage, acute salt-water loss, protein loss, enteropathy, burns
  C. Mechanically impaired right heart return: Valsalva maneuver, tussive excess, abrupt chest compression; term pregnancy; pulmonary embolism; pericardial tamponade
II. Globally impaired cardiac output
  A. Reflex abnormalities
    1. Vagal sinus arrest
      a. Psychophysiologic (rare)
      b. Visceral stimulation: glossopharyngeal neuralgia, swallow syncope, direct tracheal stimulation, dilatation of hollow viscus
      c. Carotid baroreceptor sensitivity
  B. Intrinsic cardiac disease (with or without reflex enhancement) (Table 446-4).
III. Primary cerebral ischemia (uncommon)
  A. Multivessel cervical arterial obstructive disease
  B. Transient acute increase in intracranial pressure (plateau waves)
  C. Basilar migraine (rare in adults)
  D. Vertebral-basilar TIA's (rare)

fall and the patient's age and posture, hypoperfusion sufficient to produce vagal reflex syncope can require as much as 30 seconds or more to evolve or can be so abrupt as to produce immediate unconsciousness. To produce primary cardiac syncope, sinus bradycardia in most healthy persons must fall below about 30 to 35 beats per minute in order to cause functionally important cerebral blood flow changes; asystole for longer than 3 to 5 seconds usually causes fainting in the erect position at any age. Higher rate and shorter duration thresholds apply to older patients and those with diseased hearts. Atrioventricular arrest, however, is extremely uncommon in persons with healthy hearts, possible exceptions being overtrained athletes and rare "hypervagal" subjects undergoing severe psychophysiologic threats.

PHYSIOLOGIC REFLEX (VASOVAGAL) SYNCOPE. Most functionally benign syncope stems from reduced right heart filling resulting from venomotor failure and dilatation of the capacitance veins of the splanchnic-innervated abdominal cavity and the lower extremities. Relaxation of arterial resistance vessels plays a lesser role. Since gravitational factors contribute importantly to the impaired venous return, fainting caused by impaired right heart filling always occurs in the erect or, occasionally, sitting position.

Acute vasodepressor syncope is the most common cause of fainting and typically is marked by a diphasic course. During an initial brief period of apprehension and anxiety, heart rate, blood pressure, total systemic resistance, and cardiac output all may increase. This initial sequence, however, often is lacking. The vasodepressor phase follows, during which heart rate slows and blood pressure falls, cardiac output declines, and the cerebral blood flow eventually drops. Both sympathetic and parasympathetic abnormalities are involved, since atropine prevents the bradycardia but not the depressor response. Symptoms of palpitation, salivation, and anxiety characteristically mark the first phase, whereas progressive sensations of lightheadedness, giddiness, abdominal sinking sensations, nausea, urinary urgency, and finally "gray-out" or faintness accompany the vasodepressor component. Occasionally the reflex suppression of sympathetic tone comes so rapidly that the affected subject topples like a log. Rarely, with a severe attack of vasodepressor syncope, as with other forms of profound reduction of cardiac output and cerebral ischemia, brief tonic convulsive movements result (convulsive syncope).

During vasodepressor syncope, subjects appear pale (but not dead-white or cyanotic), and the accompanying parasympathetic hyperactivity characteristically induces piloerection and sweating. Since cardiac action continues, awareness and normal cardiovas-

cular reflexes usually return promptly once the subject becomes supine. Vomiting or explosive diarrhea may follow. Occasionally, emotionally generated dysautonomic influences on the heart can be so profound as to induce arrhythmia. Engel and others have speculated that this mechanism can cause sudden death associated with sudden grief or fright.

Fainting is more likely in circumstances of emotional perturbation, in hungry subjects, after a heavy, alcohol-supplemented meal, in a warm, moist environment, and after prolonged standing. A few individuals give a history of lifelong susceptibility to fainting attacks. Rarely, one gets a history suggesting predisposition to vasodepressor syncope based on an autosomal dominant trait, with family members in several generations having been susceptible to recurrent vasodepressor attacks.

Visceral reflex syncope acts via the same medullospinal pathways as the examples cited above. A sense of faintness or even complete syncope can follow immediately after any of the following: emptying a full bladder from the standing position (*micturition syncope*), acute visceral pain (as occurs with a suddenly distended gut or an abrupt joint or ligament injury), an attack of severe vertigo (as occurs with Ménière's disease), or a migraine attack.

Carotid sinus syncope type 2 describes a severe vasodepressor response to carotid sinus massage. The condition is seldom a practical consideration except with neoplasms of the neck that directly irritate afferent glossopharyngeal fibers.

The diagnosis of vasodepressor syncope is made largely by history; rarely are the events medically witnessed. Among young persons who lack histories or physical findings of neurologic or cardiovascular disease, treatment is symptomatic. When impending sensations of faintness threaten, persons should be promptly placed in the supine position. Placing the head far forward in a sitting position is usually ineffective because it fails to empty the enlarged pool of blood located in the muscles and veins of the lower extremities. Subjects who have fainted should be mobilized slowly, because the reflex abnormality occasionally can persist for as long as 2 hours. Prophylactic treatment has little value except when fainting occurs in response to a disease or injury that requires attention. Occasionally, overtrained athletes with chronically slow hearts and a history of syncope during exertion are helped by a regimen of reduced training combined with oral anticholinergic agents.

SYNCOPE DUE PRIMARILY TO CARDIAC CAUSES. Pathologic reflex (vagovagal attacks) result primarily from failure of left heart output associated with reflexly induced changes in the cardiac rhythm, including nodal or sinus arrest, atrioventricular asystole, atrioventricular block, sinoatrial block, and ventricular arrhythmias. Usually these are accompanied by relatively minor vasodepressor changes in the peripheral vasculature, implying a lesser sympathetic abnormality. Most patients with vagovagal attacks belong to the older population and have associated heart disease, resulting in abnormally intense cardiac responses to a relatively normal degree of increased parasympathetic stimulation or sympathetic inhibition. Vagal bradycardia or arrest occasionally is induced by sudden emotional stimuli, but more commonly follows acute noxious or abnormal visceral stimulation. Severe bradycardia or arrest especially accompanies glossopharyngeal neuralgia, swallowing in patients with mechanical esophageal lesions, sudden painful dilatations of a hollow viscus, prostatic manipulation, tracheal stimulation, or visceral wounds. *Carotid sinus syncope type 1* is a rare phenomenon in which massage or pressure of the sinus induces transient asystole.

Cardiac syncope almost always reflects serious heart disease. As already noted, to cause syncope, cardiac output must fall by at least half. In the absence of severe heart disease, this rarely occurs from primary alterations in cardiac rhythm or myocardial strength. Given a normal heart, neither bradycardia above 30 beats per minute nor tachycardia up to 200 beats per minute causes syncope in the supine or seated position so long as functioning vasomotor reflexes remain. Analyses of large series of patients show serious associated cardiac risk factors, including those listed in Table 446-4. In the case of patients over 40 years of age or those showing such risk factors, prolonged (Holter) monitoring of cardiac activity is indicated. In the absence of specific predisposing abnormalities discovered by history, physi-

TABLE 446–4. CARDIOVASCULAR ABNORMALITIES FREQUENTLY ASSOCIATED WITH SYNCOPAL ATTACKS

Myocardial infarction	Ventricular tachycardia
Aortic stenosis	Sick sinus syndrome
Severe cardiomyopathy	Complete heart block
Severe hypertension	Asystole ($> \pm 3$ sec erect, ± 8 sec supine)
Pulmonary embolism	
Pulmonary hypertension	Bradycardia <44/min
Dissecting aortic aneurysm	Tachycardia >160–180/min
Pacemaker malfunction	

cal examination, and such ECG monitoring, additional studies such as direct electrophysiologic studies of the heart, cardiac catheterization, coronary or cerebral angiography, brain CT scanning, and electroencephalography seldom add helpful information. Management of cardiac syncope depends upon the nature of the underlying heart disease, although affected persons should be considered for pacemaker insertion.

OTHER CAUSES OF FAINTING. *Orthostatic Hypotension.* Acute orthostatic hypotension occasionally can occur in normal persons after acute blood loss, e.g., cryptic gastrointestinal hemorrhage, or following prolonged standing as with soldiers at parade rest in a hot sun; affected subjects undergo a sudden collapse of sympathetic reflex tone. Recurrent symptoms of syncope or faintness accompanying the erect position usually can be traced to the presence of the chronic use of diuretics and vasodepressor drugs or to neurologic disorders involving the peripheral or central nervous system. Chronic hypovolemia, such as occurs in the elderly cardiac or systemically ill patient, also predisposes to syncope, especially following periods of bed rest or prolonged sitting. Increased age as well as many drugs accentuate tendencies to orthostatic hypotension. The latter include most antihypertensive agents and many of the antidepressants, phenothiazines, and sedatives. Neurogenic causes of autonomic insufficiency are discussed in Ch. 452.

Orthostatic hypotension sufficient to cause cerebral symptoms can occur either rapidly upon standing or develop insidiously over seconds or minutes. Although symptoms of faintness and giddiness predominate, some patients lack such prodromal warnings, presumably because of the absence of strong efferent parasympathetic activity. Sometimes when chronically ill patients sit for long periods or stand, they become confused or tremulous without the usual sensations of faintness or collapse. Diagnosis comes from observing an acute or progressive decline in the mean blood pressure of more than 10 to 15 mm Hg in the erect position. Autonomic insufficiency can be inferred by observing an unchanging pulse rate despite the hypotension, and confirmed by tilt-table tests or by identifying other autonomic impairment. The simplest way to evaluate sympathetic tone at the bedside is to take the pulse while the supine patient performs a vigorous Valsalva maneuver for a matter of 30 seconds or so. The normal response consists of a palpable post-Valsalva slowing of pulse and a 10 to 30 mm Hg rise in mean blood pressure.

Treatment of orthostatic hypotension depends upon the cause. Symptomatic treatment requires eliminating drugs that cause hypotension, searching for and correcting causes of blood volume depletion, and applying elastic stockings to the lower extremities. When other measures fail, an increased salt intake and, subsequently, administering the salt-retaining steroid fludrocortisone, 0.3 to 0.8 mg per day in divided doses, can be cautiously initiated. The chronic use of vasopressor agents seldom helps. Just as vasomotor reflexes can be deconditioned by excess bed rest, they can be at least partially reconditioned by erect activity. Every effort should be made to keep susceptible patients up and walking.

Mechanically Impaired Right Heart Filling. In patients with congestive heart disease or cardiopulmonary failure, a strong *Valsalva maneuver* or sustained coughing (*tussive syncope*) raises intrathoracic pressure sufficiently to impede venous return and induce syncope. *Term pregnancy* causing compression of abdominal veins can occasionally induce a similar, posturally related effect. *Pulmonary embolism* and *acute cardiac tamponade*, due most often to subpericardial aortic dissection, act similarly to reduce the right heart filling and critically reduce cardiac output.

Recurrent symptoms of chronic hypovolemia are common in the chronically ill, especially in cardiac patients, the elderly, and those kept at bed rest for sustained periods (in whom baroceptor reflexes also become blunted). Syncope is a risk in all these groups, especially with prolonged motionless sitting.

Cerebral Vascular Disease. Intrinsic cerebral vascular diseases only rarely cause episodes of brief loss of consciousness. Although syncopal episodes might be expected on anatomic grounds as part of the symptom complex associated with vertebral-basilar insufficiency, such is rarely the case. Several reports describing symptoms in large numbers of patients with vertebral-basilar insufficiency do not mention a single example, nor have we encountered such in the extensive New York Hospital experience. By contrast, brief periods of confusion or even unconsciousness do occasionally mark the course of patients with severe stenosis or occlusion of one or both internal carotid arteries; they may or may not show concurrent narrowing of the vertebrobasilar system. In a few such patients, pulse and blood pressure have been monitored through the attacks, which are marked by brief unresponsiveness associated with transient amnesia but no seizures or EEG changes. Surgical removal of carotid stenoses have helped some, but not all, affected patients. Presumably the spells reflect transient, global blood flow reductions to the cerebral hemispheres associated with hemodynamic insufficiency in cervical arterial circulations.

446.2 NONSYNCOPAL CAUSES OF BRIEF ALTERATIONS OF CONSCIOUSNESS

HYPERVENTILATION. The disorder is mechanistically closely related to syncope in that a globally reduced cerebral blood flow gives rise to sensations of giddiness, faintness, and other distress. Full unconsciousness rarely occurs without some additional abnormal maneuver. The abnormal state is most often part of an anxiety response and often is accompanied by sensations of suffocation, pressure on the chest, and a sense of being unable to obtain the satisfaction of a lung-filling deep breath. Extreme or prolonged hyperventilation can produce feelings of unreality with anxiety bordering on panic.

In healthy subjects, only a modest increase in respiratory rate and depth is required to drop $PaCO_2$ levels promptly to 25 mm Hg or less; once a new steady state develops, little more than the normal level of breathing is sufficient to match bodily CO_2 production and maintain hypocapnia. Casual inspection may show no more than a respiratory rate of 16 to 18 per minute, interrupted perhaps by occasional sighs. Hypocapnia induces cerebral vasoconstriction. This reduces the amount of oxygen delivered to the brain and is the presumed basis of the accompanying sensations.

Symptoms and signs include feelings of unreality, difficulty in concentrating, and several hard-to-explain sensory complaints, such as unilateral or bilateral chest pain or paresthesias involving the body and extremities. Symptoms of facial twitching, carpal spasm, and perioral paresthesias are more easily understood as part of alkalotic tetany.

Diagnosis is easy when otherwise structurally healthy patients complain of the aforementioned symptoms in settings of anxiety or dyspnea but necessarily is conjectural when made in retrospect. Some patients can reproduce their symptoms by voluntarily overbreathing and the maneuver can be helpful in guiding treatment. Most often the symptoms are observed as part of a larger pattern of anxiety and must be treated accordingly.

Hyperventilation occasionally precipitates syncope under special circumstances. Children sometimes voluntarily hyperventilate, then perform a vigorous Valsalva maneuver to induce syncope (fainting lark). Athletes may repeat a similar sequence in contests such as weight lifting or squat jumps. More dangerous is a pattern wherein underwater swimmers hyperventilate before diving, then exhaust their oxygen reserves before producing sufficient carbon dioxide to produce dyspnea. The ensuing cerebral hypoxia can induce fatal submersion syncope.

SEIZURE DISORDERS. Seizure disorders, discussed fully in Ch. 483, produce a diagnostic problem under four principal circumstances:

1. *Rapid, profound syncope* may induce a single brief tonic seizure or series of clonic twitches as a result of abrupt cerebral ischemia (*convulsive syncope*). The response is more likely when the subject has made maximal efforts to stand or sit despite premonitory symptoms. Differential diagnosis rests on identifying the following as more consistent with syncope than epilepsy: the attendant psychologic circumstances and physical appearance, the associated medical conditions and body position, the brief quality of the seizure, rapid recovery, and the presence of a normal neurologic examination and interictal EEG.

2. *Akinetic seizures* consist of attacks of suddenly falling or pitching to the ground, starting in early childhood. Similar episodes occur in the supine position and are marked by unresponsiveness accompanied by generalized muscular hypotonia or brief body spasm. Diagnosis rests on the typical history, the age of onset, and the presence of an abnormal EEG. *Absence (petit mal) seizures* rarely provide a diagnostic problem, since children with petit mal, although out of contact, neither fall nor turn pale and usually have no memory of the episode. The EEG is abnormal and frequently diagnostic.

3. *Partial complex (psychomotor) seizures* sometimes include brief behavioral automatisms in which the subject recalls only being out of contact and may retrospectively consider himself to have suffered a state of unconsciousness. Usually the presence of a characteristic, self-recognized aura or set of incipient symptoms indicates the diagnosis. Falling to the ground rarely occurs unless a generalized seizure develops. Witnessed attacks and the abnormal EEG usually are typical.

4. *Postictal unresponsiveness* from grand mal attacks produces unconsciousness lasting minutes, the duration usually depending on the severity of the preceding convulsion. Diagnosis is a problem only if the seizure was unwitnessed, in which case the state may look like concussion or profound fainting. Even so, the postictal state is marked initially by flushing (cyanosis), giving way to pallor, hyperpnea, and deep unresponsiveness, none of which occurs in syncope.

HYPOGLYCEMIA (see Ch. 219). Hypoglycemia, usually caused by excess exogenous insulin, less often by insulin secreted from endogenous tissues, can produce a variety of relatively brief episodes of neurologic dysfunction. These can consist, variably, of brief confusional episodes, seizures of a variety of types, narcolepsy-like syndromes, and focal or tetraparetic weakness with or without coma but not resembling syncope. Diagnosis depends on suspicion plus the detection of blood sugars of less than 30 to 40 mg per deciliter during an attack.

DRUG OR ALCOHOL BLACKOUTS. Drug or alcohol blackouts consist of episodes of such severe intoxication that they anesthetize memory for the event, leaving the subject with an episode of focal amnesia. Many are accompanied by "passing out," consisting of deep, barely arousable sleep.

CONCUSSION-POSTCONCUSSION AMNESIA. Variable periods of memory loss for immediate subsequent events can follow brief periods of concussive unconsciousness. The usual question is whether an intrinsic malady caused the fall or whether the fall represented the whole illness. Only diagnostic diligence can solve the issue.

ACUTE INTRACRANIAL HYPERTENSION. Plateau waves, associated with this condition, can produce brief episodes of loss of consciousness that resemble syncope, as described above. Occasionally, such brief unconsciousness may accompany the onset of acute subarachnoid hemorrhage. The unconscious episode, which is syncopal in its abruptness and often accompanied by either a tonic extensor spasm or brief clonic jerks, is most often due to an acute cardiac arrhythmia or asystole accompanying the onset of bleeding. Cerebral hemorrhage with intraventricular rupture can produce similar events.

DROP SPELLS. As discussed in Chapter 454, these are poorly understood attacks affecting older persons. The legs suddenly and unexplainedly give way, and the women fall, often injuring themselves but experiencing no observed interruption of consciousness. The cause is unknown.

CONVERSION REACTIONS OR MALINGERING (PSEUDOSYNCOPE). Hysterical or other forms of psychogenic unresponsiveness are almost impossible to diagnose in retrospect. If such a condition occurs during the physical examination, the diagnosis can be reached by the absence of physiologic abnor-

mality and the presence of additional, often bizarre features (see Table 446–2). Most subjects awaken with gentle but firm confrontation. A few do so only when advised that psychiatric admission lies in store. Mutilating stimuli are neither justified nor often successful in proving the diagnosis.

Aminoff MJ, Scheinman MM, Griffin JC, Herre JM: Electrocerebral accompaniments of syncope associated with malignant ventricular arrhythmias. Ann Intern Med 108:791, 1988. *Ten of 17 episodes of syncope caused by electrically induced ventricular tachycardia or arrhythmia had accompanying tonic seizures or irregular muscular twitching. The results illustrate the high incidence of convulsive syncope.*

Engel GL: Psychological stress, vasodepressor (vasovagal) syncope and sudden death. Ann Intern Med 89:403, 1978. *Must reading for the internist by one of the pioneers in understanding of both the physiology and emotion of cardiovascular responses.*

Evans DW, Lum LC: Hyperventilation: An important cause of pseudoangina. Lancet 1:155, 1977. *A clinical article, emphasizing the often misleading symptoms of the disorder.*

Kapoor WN: Evaluation and outcome of patients with syncope. Medicine 69:160, 1990. *Among 433 medically studied patients with a median age of 61, one quarter had a cardiac cause. In another 40 per cent exact cause was uncertain but their findings resembled those of the remaining one third who were concluded to have noncardiac causes.*

Mandis AS, Linzer M, Salem D, Estes NA: Syncope. Current diagnostic evaluation and management. Ann Intern Med 112:850, 1990. *A comprehensive review of the problem identifying rare as well as common causes and emphasizing laboratory evaluations, especially of cardiovascular mechanisms.*

Savage DD, Corwin L, McGee DL, et al.: Epidemiologic features of isolated syncope: The Framingham Study. Stroke 16:626, 1985. *In a population of 5209 men and women aged 30 to 62 years and then followed for a mean of 26 years, 3.3 per cent developed syncope without evidence for concurrent cardiovascular or neurologic disease. Such isolated syncope was not associated with any subsequent increased incidence of stroke, cardiovascular disease, or early mortality compared with the remainder of the cohort.*

Yanagihara T, Klass DW, Piepgras DG, Houser OW: Brief loss of consciousness in bilateral carotid occlusive vascular disease. Arch Neurol 46:858, 1989. *Briefly describes three cases and reviews this uncommon disorder.*

447 Sleep and Its Disorders

Anthony Kales

Humans spend at least one third of their lives asleep, yet physiologists little understand the specific biologic events that explain why we need sleep and what mechanisms underlie sleep's sense of joyous reward. Certain empiric features, however, provide useful guides to the evaluation and management of most of the sleep complaints that arise in standard clinical practice.

PHYSIOLOGY OF SLEEP. Natural sleep-wake rhythms cycle at about 25 hours rather than coinciding with the solar 24-hour schedule. As a result, many persons depend on external cues to keep their diurnal cycle "on time." The normal diurnal clock resists natural changes in its pattern by more than about 1 hour per day, which explains the sleep irregularities that often accompany adaptation to new time zones or switches in work shifts.

Individuals differ considerably in their natural sleep patterns. Normal adults can average as little as 4 to as much as 11 hours of sleep per day. Most adults in nontropical areas are comfortable with 6.5 to 8 hours daily, taken in a single period. Children and adolescents sleep more than adults, and young adults more than older ones. Normal sleep consists of a series of behaviorally and electroencephalographically (EEG) defined cycles, including neurophysiologically active periods accompanied by rapid eye movements, called REM sleep, interspersed with four progressively deeper, quieter sleep stages graded 1 to 4 on the basis of increasingly slow EEG patterns. Stages 3 and 4 (deep) sleep gradually lessens with age and usually disappears after age 55.

SLEEP DISORDERS. Both functional and organic disorders can perturb sleep. Insomnia, the most common of the sleep disorders, most often reflects psychological disturbances; hypersomnia can have similar origins but often reflects organic dysfunction of the brain. The parasomnias, including sleep walking, night terrors, and nightmares, similarly most often have a func-

TABLE 447–1. GUIDELINES FOR TAKING A SLEEP HISTORY

Define the specific sleep problem.
Assess the clinical course of the condition.
Distinguish among sleep disorders.
Reassess previous diagnoses.
Evaluate 24-hour sleep/wakefulness patterns.
Question the bed partner.
Determine the presence of other sleep disorders.
Obtain a family history of sleep disorders.
Evaluate the impact of the sleep disorder.

tional basis. They usually have benign associations in childhood but often reflect psychopathology in adolescents and adults. By contrast, narcolepsy and sleep apnea are exclusively of organic origin, the first being a chronic genetically related disorder and, the second occurring predominantly in middle-aged men and associated with obesity and cardiovascular problems. Accordingly, the first step in evaluating a sleep complaint is to obtain a thorough history (Table 447–1).

Sleep complaints are common at all ages and range widely in their nature and biologic importance, a natural variation that sometimes makes it difficult for the physician to distinguish trivial from serious problems and to appraise their medical importance.

INSOMNIA

Insomnia is by far the most common sleep complaint, affecting as many as one fifth of all patients who consult general physicians. Short-term insomnia often results from stressful life events or the recent onset of medical disorders. Chronic, severe insomnia, by contrast, often becomes a central complaint and the focus of distress and is perceived by the patient as a distinct disorder itself.

CLINICAL FEATURES. Most patients with chronic insomnia report difficulty in falling asleep, either alone or in combination with difficulty in staying asleep or early final awakening. Compared with normal sleepers, insomniacs feel worse in the morning than late at night and arise feeling sleepy, groggy, physically and mentally tired, depressed, worried, tense, anxious, and irritable. Characteristically, these symptoms persist during the day and contribute to feelings of depression, hopelessness, and fears of losing self-control. As bed time approaches, they become even more tense, anxious, and ruminative about health, death, work, and personal problems. Many such persons show autonomic hyperactivity evidenced by increased heart rate, muscle tension, increased body temperature, and peripheral vasoconstriction.

ETIOLOGY. Acute or short-term insomnia can be associated with a variety of situational (work-related, interpersonal, or financial difficulties) or medical problems including ascent to high altitudes, pain, cardiopulmonary disorders, thyrotoxicosis, or the febrile prodromes to influenza. Drugs of a variety of kinds, including caffeine, cigarettes, alcohol, steroids, amphetamines and other stimulants, energizing antidepressants, central adrenergic blockers, and bronchodilators, can impair both falling asleep and staying asleep.

Notwithstanding the above possible causes, psychological distress is the most common cause of chronic insomnia. Patients with longstanding sleep difficulties show less than adequate coping mechanisms to stressful life events. Many display specific personality patterns characterized by chronic anxiety, rumination, neurotic depression, inhibition of emotions, and an inability to discharge anger outwardly. They generally handle external stress and conflicts by internalizing their emotions, generating a combination of emotional arousal and autonomic activation. This state of hyperarousal leads to difficulty in initiating sleep, whether at the beginning of the sleep period or when returning to sleep following nocturnal or other awakenings. Fear of sleeplessness further intensifies the emotional arousal, thus insidiously conditioning and perpetuating insomnia.

DIAGNOSIS. Evaluation of transient or situational insomnia focuses on identifying the stressful factors and providing reassurance about those that interfere with restful sleep. When addressing chronic insomnia, the evaluation should include a complete

history that assesses various sleep, drug, medical, and emotional factors (Table 447–1). It is important to assess sleep/wakefulness patterns on a 24-hour basis, particularly in the elderly. Widespread insomnia affecting this age group results in their ingesting a high proportion of all the sedatives prescribed in this country.

In taking the general medical and drug history, conditions and medications that are known to be associated with disturbed sleep should be identified. Although *sleep apnea* and *nocturnal myoclonus* only rarely serve as causes for the primary complaint of insomnia, symptoms of these disorders should stimulate a detailed inquiry, including obtaining information from the bed partner. Most importantly, underlying emotional factors contributing to chronic sleep difficulty must be identified.

MANAGEMENT. The successful and effective treatment of chronic insomnia usually requires attention to several factors, including general measures for improving sleep hygiene and lifestyle; supportive, insight-oriented, or behavioral psychotherapeutic techniques; adjunctive use of hypnotic medication; or use of antidepressant medication.

Measures for improving sleep hygiene and lifestyle include regularizing the patient's schedule; emphasizing that the bedroom should be the handmaiden of rest and sleep rather than of conflict and worry; and improving the sleep environment by minimizing noise and disruptions. Providing a gradually increasing daily activity and exercise program has been shown to increase early night slow-wave sleep.

Allowing for modest variation, times to retire and awaken should be regularized. In counseling the insomniac, it is helpful to explain how anxiety participates in the vicious circle that exacerbates and maintains the condition. Patients can be taught to reduce stress and anxiety by managing emotions more effectively through pertinent stress management techniques (Table 447–2). Most patients with severe, chronic insomnia require psychotherapy.

Benzodiazepine hypnotics have largely replaced other drugs in the adjunctive pharmacologic treatment of insomnia, primarily owing to their greater margin of safety and degree of effectiveness. Five benzodiazepines are marketed currently as hypnotics: flurazepam, temazepam, triazolam, quazepam, and estazolam; the last has been recently introduced, and significant data are lacking regarding its safety, particularly in terms of long-term use, drug dependence, and withdrawal issues. In adults, for the long-term adjunctive drug treatment of chronic insomnia, intermittent use of flurazepam, 15 mg, and quazepam, 15 mg, is recommended. These agents maintain their efficacy very well with continued use and produce few adverse reactions, and their intermittent use minimizes the occurrence of daytime sedation. In the elderly, or when a mild, short-term hypnotic effect is desired, temazepam, 15 mg, may be used. Triazolam is not recommended because of frequent and severe adverse reactions, including the following:

TABLE 447–2. GENERAL MEASURES IN TREATING INSOMNIA (STRESS- AND DRUG-INDUCED DISTURBANCES)

Recommendation	Implementation
Manage stress properly	Recognize association between stressful events and sleeplessness.
	Ventilate conflicts and anger to avoid internalization.
	Be tolerant of occasional sleeplessness.
	Avoid rumination over sleep difficulty.
	Relaxation exercise may be helpful.
Avoid drug-induced sleep disturbances	Minimize use of caffeine, cigarettes, stimulants, and other medications.
	Recognize that alcohol may cause fragmentation of sleep.
	Be aware of hyperexcitability states (early morning insomnia and daytime anxiety) caused by hypnotics with a short half-life.
	Recognize sleep disturbances following drug withdrawal.

hyperexcitability states (early morning insomnia and daytime anxiety) and cognitive impairment (memory impairment/amnesia, confusion, delusions, hallucinations, and delirium), both occurring during drug administration; and withdrawal difficulties (rebound insomnia) following drug termination. These serious safety concerns and the lack of efficacy of the recommended starting dose (0.25 mg) result in a very narrow benefit-to-risk ratio for triazolam.

When depression contributes a major factor to insomnia, antidepressants with sedative side effects, such as tricyclics, are generally indicated. Neuroleptics with sedative effects are preferred for psychotic patients who have insomnia.

PARASOMNIAS: SLEEPWALKING, NIGHT TERRORS, AND NIGHTMARES

These conditions are common. About 15 per cent of children, for example, have had at least one sleepwalking episode, and 1 to 3 per cent report night terrors. Nightmares are a current problem for approximately 5 per cent of the general population and a past problem for another 5 per cent.

CLINICAL FEATURES. Sleepwalking (somnambulism) occurs in episodes lasting for several minutes. During this period, patients generally have blank expressions, behave as if they are indifferent to the environment, and exhibit low levels of awareness and reactivity, manifested by clumsiness and purposeless activity. They rarely recall the events upon awakening. Night terror episodes have the additional and often dramatic characteristics of extreme vocalization and movement, excessive autonomic discharges, and panic. Sleepwalking and night terrors appear to fall along a pathophysiologic continuum and share many clinical and physiologic similarities (Table 447–3).

Nightmares are most often associated with fears of attack, falling, or death, and in many patients the nightly themes recur. Nightmares occur during REM sleep and may take place at any time during the night but are more likely during the late night when REM sleep periods increase in length. Patients typically report considerable sleep disruption and have vivid recall of the dream content, characteristics that easily differentiate nightmares from the more dramatic but forgotten night terrors.

ETIOLOGY. Genetic, developmental, organic, and psychological factors have been proposed as causing parasomnias. Maturational components are implicit in their frequent onset in childhood and termination by late adolescence. Febrile episodes and brain tumors occasionally have been implicated but are rare causes. Somnambulism-like episodes also have been pharmacologically induced by lithium, high doses of neuroleptic drugs, and triazolam. Furthermore, withdrawal of certain drug treatments, resulting in an increase in REM sleep (REM rebound), may be associated with a temporary increase in the intensity of dreaming and the possible occurrence of nightmares.

Psychological abnormalities seldom accompany early childhood parasomnias. When the disorders begin in late childhood or adolescence, however, they often persist into adulthood, usually associated with significant psychopathology.

DIAGNOSIS. Sleepwalking or night terror–like activity that begins in middle or old age should prompt the physician to rule out brain tumor or other cerebral disorders, including sedative intoxication. Night terrors should be differentiated from temporal lobe epilepsy, which, however, rarely expresses itself during sleep. Most "sleepwalking" in elderly persons reflects episodes of confusion and nocturnal wandering rather than a parasomnia. A careful drug history is important in the evaluation of persons who have nightmares. This is because administration or withdrawal of certain drugs, including alcohol, induces marked

TABLE 447–3. CLINICAL CHARACTERISTICS OF SLEEPWALKING AND NIGHT TERRORS

Episodes early in the night when stages 3 and 4 of sleep predominate
Confusion on awakening and minimal recall of event
High risk of injury
Often a family history of sleepwalking or night terrors
Onset usually in childhood or early adolescence
Usually outgrown by late adolescence
Psychopathology suspected with adult onset
Some elderly patients have central nervous system pathology

TABLE 447–4. INDICATIONS FOR SLEEP LABORATORY RECORDING

Always
    Sleep apnea

Sometimes
    Narcolepsy

Infrequent
    Insomnia
    Nocturnal myoclonus
    Parasomnias

changes in the frequency, intensity, and disturbing content of dreaming. Many patients are unaware of such connections.

Adult patients with chronic parasomnias commonly show serious psychopathology deserving psychiatric consultation. It is important to differentiate night terrors, and particularly sleepwalking, from hysterical dissociative phenomena such as amnesia, fugue states, and multiple personalities. Most patients experiencing the latter conditions demonstrate complex and purposeful behaviors and describe longer episodes that may last as long as several hours compared with the minutes-long duration of parasomniac sleepwalking.

Sleep laboratory recordings are seldom useful in evaluating parasomnias (Table 447–4), an exception being when nocturnal epilepsy is strongly suspected.

MANAGEMENT. The most important consideration in managing episodic sleepwalking or night terrors is protection from injury. Attempts to interrupt the episodes should be avoided, since intervention often confuses and frightens the patient even more. Minimizing children's exposure to potentially traumatic experiences, such as terrifying movies and television programs or frightening bedtime stories, can help to reduce the frequency of nightmares. Parents should be counseled and reassured that affected children usually outgrow the conditions by late adolescence, if not sooner. Drugs such as diazepam and flurazepam that suppress stages 3 and 4 sleep may be prescribed as adjuncts to psychotherapy for adults who experience night terrors or sleepwalking. Psychotropic medication is not recommended in children. Depression, especially in men with nightmares, deserves special attention because these persons may be at higher risk for suicide. Overtly psychotic behavior associated with nightmares is best treated with neuroleptic drugs.

NARCOLEPSY

Narcolepsy is a serious clinical problem that usually begins before age 25 years and persists throughout life. The estimated incidence is about one person per thousand population, with men and women equally affected.

CLINICAL FEATURES. Narcolepsy is characterized by excessive daytime sleepiness and irresistible sleep attacks that usually occur in conjunction with one or more of three auxiliary symptoms: cataplexy, sleep paralysis, and hypnagogic hallucinations. The sleep attacks may last from a few seconds to half an hour and may be precipitated by sedentary, monotonous activity of any kind, including driving, sitting in lectures, or even eating meals. Excessive daytime sleepiness and sleep attacks usually usher in the disease, with the auxiliary symptoms appearing several years later.

About three fourths of narcolepsy patients have *cataplexy*, a brief and sudden loss of muscle control without loss of consciousness. The severity of cataplectic attacks ranges from light knee buckling or drooping of the jaw to complete collapse. Episodes are precipitated by strong emotions such as fear, surprise, laughter, or anger.

Sleep paralysis and *hypnagogic hallucinations* describe short (a minute or less) episodes that occur during the transition between wakefulness and sleep. Sleep paralysis consists of a transient experience of being unable to move any muscle (breathing persists). Hypnagogic hallucinations are vivid hallucinatory perceptions (usually visual or auditory) that appear particularly while drifting into sleep. About half of narcoleptic patients complain of disturbed nocturnal sleep, which may be a direct

TABLE 447–5. DIFFERENTIAL DIAGNOSIS OF SLEEP APNEA AND NARCOLEPSY

	Sleep Apnea	Narcolepsy
Age of onset	Middle age	Adolescence
Sex distribution	Predominantly male	Equal sex distribution
Daytime sleepiness	+ +	+ +
Sleep attacks	+ +	+ + +
Auxiliary symptoms	– –	+ + +
Snoring/snorting	+ + +	– –
Nocturnal breath cessation	+ + +	– –
Disturbed nocturnal sleep	+ + +	+ +
Associated medical conditions (hypertension, obesity, etc.)	+ +	– –
Family history	+	+ + +
Adverse psychosocial consequences	+ + +	+ + +

effect of the disorder or due to the use of stimulant medication to control daytime sleep, or both.

ETIOLOGY. Family studies showing a 10 to 50 per cent incidence of affected first-degree relatives and a high incidence of HLA concordance imply a strong genetic predisposition. The pattern must be multifactorial, however, since monozygotic twins have a high rate of discordance. The sleep attacks and other manifestations of the auxiliary symptoms of narcolepsy appear to be closely related to aberrations in the neurophysiologic mechanisms of REM sleep, since REM sleep ushers in a large proportion of narcoleptic sleep patterns, in contrast to those of normals, in whom the first REM period occurs after about 70 to 90 minutes of nonrapid eye movement (NREM) sleep.

Many narcoleptics show a high level of psychopathology that is a secondary reaction to the disorder, resulting in considerable psychosocial disturbances that need to be addressed.

DIAGNOSIS. Usually, the history is typical. Passing consideration should be given to hysteria (rarely expressed as brief, episodic hypersomnia), seizures (characterized by automatisms but not brief sleep states), or true neuropathologic hypersomnia (sleep episodes last longer). Narcolepsy must be differentiated from sleep apnea (Table 447–5). A history of cataplexy and the other auxiliary symptoms make the diagnosis certain. In questionable instances, especially in the absence of cataplexy, multiple daytime nap recordings may detect sleep-onset REM periods and/or extremely short sleep latencies in narcoleptics. A sleep latency of less than 5 minutes on at least two of five 20-minute opportunities to sleep between 10:00 A.M. and 6:00 P.M. strengthens the diagnosis.

MANAGEMENT. Therapy begins nonpharmacologically by prescribing therapeutic naps to enhance alertness for daytime tasks. Patients should be warned about the potential dangers of driving or other activities requiring full alertness and muscle control. Physicians should check with their local department of motor vehicles regarding the legal responsibility for reporting narcolepsy. One must advise and educate patients gently but honestly that this is a frequently misunderstood chronic disorder. All concerned must learn that narcolepsy is a physical illness and not under voluntary control.

Pharmacotherapy involves separate treatments for the sleep attacks and cataplexy. Methylphenidate is the preferred drug for treating sleep attacks because of its prompt onset of action and relatively few side effects. Other potential agents include amphetamines, modafinil, mazindol, and selegiline.

Imipramine and other nonsedating antidepressants can be helpful in preventing cataplexy; the drugs also alleviate sleep paralysis but have little effect on the sleep attacks. Imipramine acts rapidly and requires a lower dose than when treating depression. Stimulants and antidepressants can be combined for patients who require treatment for both sleep attacks and auxiliary symptoms. Because this combination may produce serious side effects such as hypertension, careful titration and monitoring are necessary.

SLEEP APNEA

This disorder affects men more than women and is often associated with obesity and hypertension. The clinical diagnosis of sleep apnea syndrome includes quantification of the number of apneic events, the degree of associated oxygen desaturation, and the patient's total clinical picture. Apneas are characterized as central (i.e., neurogenic), obstructive (peripheral), or mixed. In central apnea, an uncommon condition related to central nervous system disorders, breathing efforts cease or become minimal, whereas in obstructive apnea, the most common form of sleep apnea, respiratory efforts persist and even become unusually prominent but are rendered ineffective by upper airway blockage. Sleep apnea also can occur as a late manifestation of chronic peripheral neuromuscular diseases, including myotonic muscular dystrophy and motor neuron disorders.

CLINICAL FEATURES. Patients with obstructive sleep apnea characteristically provide a history of excessive daytime sleepiness, sleep attacks, and repetitive nocturnal breath cessations followed by brief arousals (probably related to choking or hypercapnia); breathing resumes accompanied by loud snorting and gasping sounds. The disorder usually has its onset before the age of 40.

In most patients, the bed partner or roommate observes episodes of breath cessation followed by snorting and gasping. Some patients become self-aware of nighttime choking experiences. Excessive body movements during sleep, diaphoresis, secondary enuresis, early morning headaches, and sexual impotence may occur.

Most patients with symptomatic obstructive sleep apnea have at least moderate systemic hypertension and obesity. The hypoxia and carbon dioxide retention associated with the nocturnal apneic events eventually can induce polycythemia, pulmonary hypertension, cardiomegaly, right-sided heart failure, and persistent cardiac dysrhythmias as well as cognitive impairment, psychological distress, and psychosocial disruption.

ETIOLOGY. Multiple factors in addition to obesity can contribute to the etiology of sleep apnea, including inherent predisposition, hypothyroidism, and a menopausal lessening of the respiratory stimulating effects of progestational hormones. Clinical inspection usually detects no anatomic abnormalities of the upper airway. Nevertheless, smaller pharyngeal areas have been demonstrated in some cases. Chronic vasomotor and nasal obstruction may increase the frequency of apneic episodes in others. Alcohol ingestion, smoking bronchitis, and sleep deprivation can increase the number and severity of sleep apneic events.

DIAGNOSIS. Thorough assessment of suspected sleep apnea begins with a complete sleep history (see Table 447–1). When a patient reports excessive daytime sleepiness, sleep attacks, or unusual snorting or gasping sounds during sleep, families or roommates should be questioned about severe snoring or interrupted breathing. A complete medical history and a physical examination with otorhinolaryngologic evaluation should follow, as well as measurements of hematocrit, chest radiography, electrocardiography, and 24-hour ECG monitoring. A family history

TABLE 447–6. TREATMENT OF SLEEP APNEA

Method	Response	Disadvantages
Mild apnea		
Weight loss	Delayed and limited	None
Pharmacologic (protriptyline, medroxyprogesterone)	Limited and inconsistent	Side effects
Moderate/severe apnea		
Continuous positive air pressure	Effective initially Long-term efficacy uncertain	Compliance (?) Mechanical problems Discomfort
Dental appliance	60%–80% effective Long-term efficacy not determined	Discomfort and compliance (?) Cannot use with full dentures
Uvulopalatopharyngoplasty	50% effective Delayed relapse	Possible operative morbidity Irreversible
Tracheostomy	100% effective	Operative and postoperative morbidity

of loud snoring or excessive daytime sleepiness provides an important clinical clue. The patient's psychosocial and vocational functioning should be assessed. Ultimately, the clinician depends on the result of a sleep laboratory evaluation with recording of respiration and ear oximetry (Table 447–4) to confirm the diagnosis and its severity.

MANAGEMENT. Treatment options depend upon severity, specific type of apneic events, and level of daytime functioning (Table 447–6). Steps should be taken to improve underlying medical illnesses or complications such as congestive heart failure, chronic reversible respiratory disorders, and metabolic abnormalities that could impair upper airway functioning. Drugs that depress the central ventilatory drive, such as sedative/hypnotics, barbiturates, narcotics, sedating analgesics, and alcohol, should be avoided.

Severe cases of sleep apnea syndrome can interfere with many aspects of normal life. While initiating treatment, physicians should counsel the patient, his family, and, if appropriate, his employer that the excessive daytime sleepiness and associated symptoms are beyond volitional control and are likely to improve. Patients who fail to improve with dietary and conservative drug efforts should receive the advice of an experienced consultant before embarking on surgical therapy.

Kales A, Kales JD: Evaluation and Treatment of Insomnia. New York, Oxford University Press, 1984. *An excellent, comprehensive monograph on the subject.*

Kales A, Soldatos CR, Kales JD: Sleep disorders: Insomnia, sleepwalking, night terrors, nightmares and enuresis. Ann Intern Med 106:582–592, 1987. *A very useful and clear clinical description of the various sleep disorders.*

Kales A, Vela-Bueno A, Kales JD: Sleep disorders: Sleep apnea and narcolepsy. Ann Intern Med 106:434–443, 1987. *A very useful clinical description of these sleep disorders.*

Parkes JD: Sleep and Its Disorders. Philadelphia, W. B. Saunders Company, 1985. *An excellent, detailed textbook on the subject.*

Roth B: Narcolepsy and Hypersomnia. Revised and edited by R. Broughton. Basel, S. Karger, 1980. *A comprehensive monograph on this important disorder.*

448 Diagnosis of Regional Cerebral Dysfunction

Antonio R. Damasio

Localizing the site of neurologic dysfunction based on clinical signs and symptoms is a crucial step in the assessment of neurologic diseases. Although advanced and noninvasive neuroimaging techniques localize many brain lesions, the abnormalities associated with some diseases often elude all but research-level imaging procedures. For instance, in most degenerative diseases, the regional anatomic defect can be defined only on the basis of clinical signs. The diagnosis of most epileptogenic foci, a key element in the therapeutic management of epileptic patients, is another example.

Figure 448–1 diagrams the regional neuroanatomy of the adult human brain. The accuracy of regional clinical diagnosis depends on numerous factors. First, elementary motor and sensory disorders, which are related to dysfunction in motor and sensory pathways and in primary motor and sensory cortices, can be detected earlier than disorders of language or thinking, which result from dysfunction in association cortices. The localization of the underlying lesions is generally more precise in the former than in the latter. This difference reflects the fine anatomic and functional modularity of the primary sensory and motor systems and the fact that cognitive processes depend on far more complex and distributed anatomic systems. Furthermore, the neural substrate for integrative processes is prone to vary individually, different individuals having different endowments for specific abilities. For instance, language or visuospatial skills are linked to a variety of genetic and epigenetic factors and are influenced by age, educational background, and even gender. Second, the pathologic type of lesion and its rate of development influence the rate of appearance and the extent of symptoms. Most infarcts cause their damage rapidly and lead to an abrupt onset of signs followed by at least some improvement. By contrast, most

intracranial tumors generate symptoms gradually and the brain adapts to the tumor enlargement. Some slow-growing meningiomas can reach the size of a plum before they cause detectable dysfunction, while small brain metastases from a carcinoma elsewhere in the body may cause major symptoms rapidly. Thirdly, the mass effect and the edema that accompany large infarcts and some tumors may cause a shift of brain structures and thereby compress remote and otherwise intact areas of the brain against the rigid frame of the skull and dural meninges. Compression can generate false localizing signs and lead to impairment in attention, motivation, and wakefulness which can, in turn, mask or aggravate other symptoms (see Ch. 446).

OCCIPITAL LOBES

The occipital cortices are solely dedicated to visual processing. Information from both lateral geniculate nuclei arrives in each primary visual cortex (Brodmann's area 17); these cortices occupy the superior and inferior banks of the calcarine fissure (see also Ch. 454.2). This region contains a retinotopic projection of visual information. The inferior visual field maps onto the superior calcarine cortex and vice versa; the right visual field maps into the left calcarine region and conversely for the left visual field; the central part of the retina projects onto the caudal part of the calcarine region, at the occipital pole, while progressively more peripheral sectors of the retina project to more anterior sectors of the calcarine region. Beyond area 17, visual information is widely distributed by a large number of functionally distinct regions, located within the association cortices of Brodmann's areas 18 and 19. The main goals of these parallel processing units are (1) to generate representations of the form, volumetric shape, texture, movement, color, and spatial location of stimuli in the external world, and (2) to serve as the distributed storage sites for the records of visual perception that become committed to memory and are later used in the processes of visual recall, recognition, imagetic thinking, and dreaming.

Damage to the calcarine cortices (Table 448–1) or to the optic radiations as they approach the calcarine region, causes varied field defects for form vision (hemianopias or quadrantanopias) depending on the region affected (e.g., damage to the left superior calcarine region causes a right inferior quadrantanopia; damage to an entire calcarine region leads to a hemianopia). When damage is confined to inferior occipital cortices but spares the calcarine regions, patients may develop achromatopsia, a disturbance of color perception without compromise of form vision (damage to the left side causes right hemiachromatopsia and vice versa). Damage to left occipital cortices and underlying periventricular white matter combined with destruction of the interhemispheric visual pathways, often causes a disorder of reading without concomitant impairment of writing (alexia without agraphia). This may be accompanied by an impairment of color naming without impairment of color perception (color anomia). Bilateral damage to inferior visual association cortices causes agnosia, a selective impairment of visual recognition (see Ch. 449). However, lesions that extensively involve the right occipital cortices (inferior *and* superior) can cause agnosia for unique faces and places, and lesions that involve left occipital cortices (inferior *and* superior) can cause agnosia for manipulable objects. Bilateral damage to superior visual association cortices leads to disturbances of visual attention (visual disorientation or simultanagnosia) and stereo vision (astereopsis). Visual disorientation can also result from bilateral superior parietal lesions, as a component of Balint syndrome (see Parietal Lobe, below). Lesions that involve the lateral occipital cortices about their middle tier can cause defects of motion perception. Infarctions in the territory of one or both posterior cerebral arteries are the most common cause of pathology in the occipital lobes.

TEMPORAL LOBE

The temporal lobes contain structures necessary for visual and auditory perception, language, memory, and affect. The most characteristic signs of temporal lobe damage are impairments of memory, which can be caused by lesions of either side, and impairments of language, usually related to dominant hemisphere lesions (see Ch. 449). The cortical structures related to vision are located in the inferior and lateral aspects of the lobe (part of area 37, areas 20 and 21). They are higher-order association cortices that receive information from the occipital association cortices. The inferior component of the geniculocalcarine pathway (Meyer's loop) courses in the depth of the temporal lobe (see Ch. 453).

The primary auditory cortices (areas 41 and 42) are located in the first temporal gyrus at the end of the most complex chain of subcortical processing stations of any sensory portal of the brain. Their purpose is the representation of acoustic frequencies and intensities for a large range of pitched and unpitched sounds (speech, music, environmental noises) so as to permit their recognition and spatial localization. The record of those representations is contained in the auditory association cortices which surround the primary cortices bilaterally, in the superior temporal gyrus (largely area 22). Although the auditory input from the contralateral ear prevails functionally over the ipsilateral input, each cortex receives information from both ears, so unilateral temporal lesions never cause deafness.

The medial temporal lobes contain cortical and subcortical structures of the limbic system, e.g., the entorhinal cortex (area 28) located in the anterior part of the parahippocampal gyrus; the hippocampal formation; and the amygdala. These highly inter-connected structures are privy to information emanating from all sensory cortices as well as the diencephalon, and they project back to both. They correlate perceptual inputs, ongoing verbal and nonverbal thought operations, and the status of the internal milieu. This correlation is indispensable for memory, affective experience, and emotional expression. Lesions of this region severely compromise those functions.

The temporal lobes can be compromised by numerous pathologic processes (Table 448–2). Epileptogenic scars and intracranial tumors are common; head injury often damages anterior temporal structures, and herpes simplex encephalitis has a predilection for the region; the highest and earliest concentration of cytoskeletal pathology in Alzheimer's disease is in entorhinal cortex and hippocampus; the hippocampus is selectively vulnerable to anoxia. Patients with temporal epileptogenic lesions experience a variety of affective, sensory, and visceral disturbances and exhibit emotional and motor disturbances that can appear before or during a seizure. In some patients, more subtle but longer-lasting behavioral changes develop between seizures. Tables 448–3 and 448–4 list the major ictal and interictal symptoms. Although violent behavior is often blamed on temporal lobe dysfunction, the evidence indicates that temporal lobe epilepsy should not be regarded as a medical explanation for criminal aggression. Bilateral removal of this region in animals causes the Klüver-Bucy

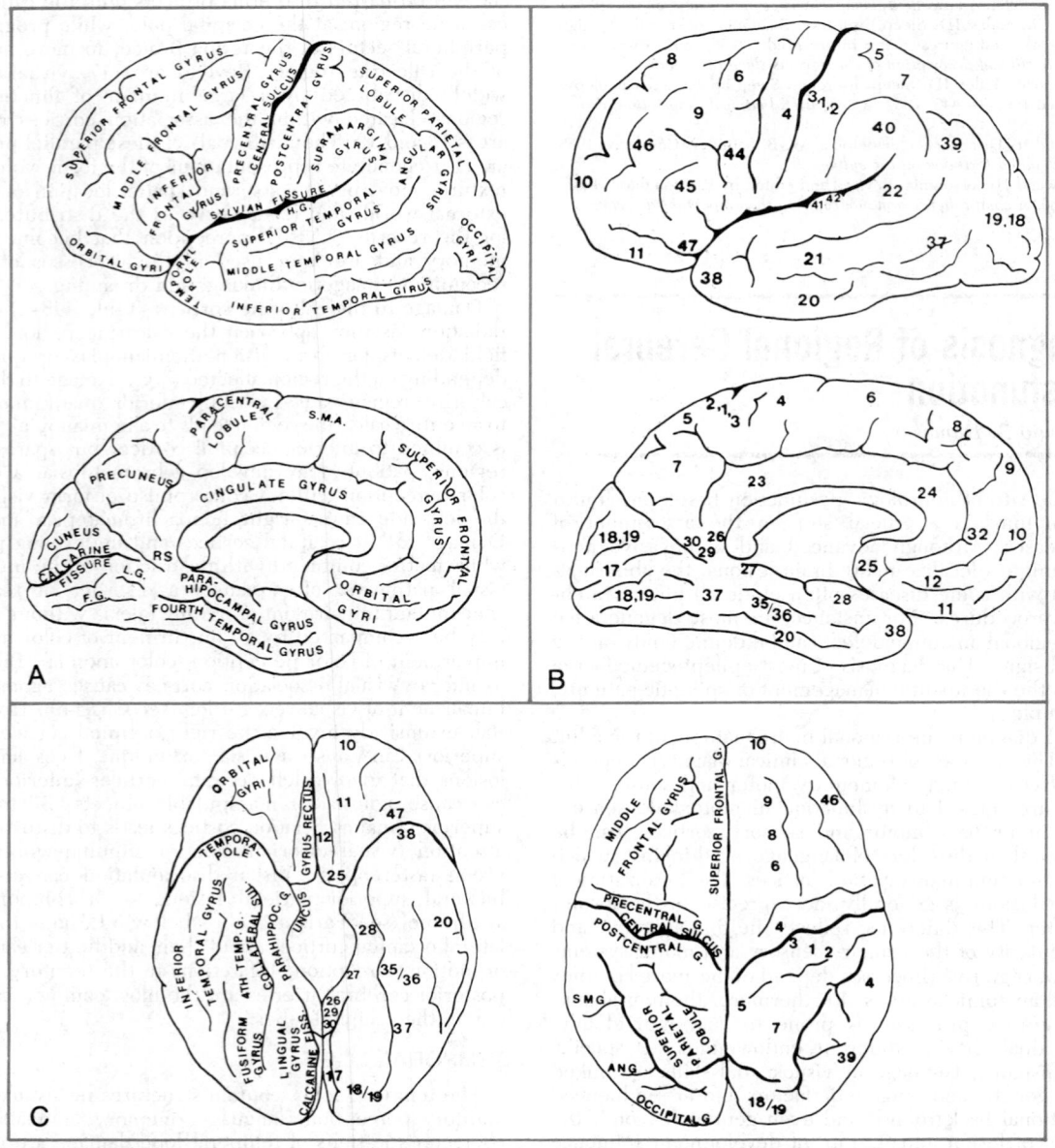

FIGURE 448–1. The principal gyri, sulci, and Brodmann's cytoarchitectonic areas of the human brain. *A*, Gyri and sulci in lateral (*top*) and mesial (*bottom*) view. *B*, Brodmann's areas in lateral (*top*) and mesial (*bottom*) view. *C*, Gyri, sulci, and Brodmann's areas in orbital (*left*) and superior (*right*) view.

TABLE 448–1. CHARACTERISTIC MANIFESTATIONS OF OCCIPITAL LOBE DAMAGE

Sign	Qualification	Lesion
Hemiachromatopsia	Right or left field (whole hemifield affected)	Left or right inferior mesial cortex and white matter
Pure alexia	Noted anywhere in intact field	Left inferior cortex and white matter (including outflow of callosum)
Color anomia	Seen only in left visual field in combination with right hemianopia	Left inferior and mesial
Visual agnosia	Noted anywhere in intact field	Usually bilateral inferior (but right occipital may involve faces and places and left occipital may involve manipulable objects)
Visual disorientation	Noted anywhere in intact field	Bilateral superior
Astereopsis	Noted anywhere in intact field	Bilateral superior
Impaired movement detection	Noted anywhere in intact field	Bilateral superior

syndrome, a disorder characterized by indiscriminate sexual behavior, excessive orality, and placidity. The full syndrome rarely develops in humans, but some components are often noted in patients with extensive bilateral temporal damage caused by herpes simplex encephalitis and the dementias of degenerative or post-traumatic etiologies.

PARIETAL LOBE

The anterior aspect of the parietal lobe contains the postcentral gyrus where Brodmann's areas 3, 1, and 2 receive somatosensory information obtained from nerve terminals in the contralateral half of the body (the projections are somatotopically organized with the largest share given to the phonatory apparatus and hand). These cortices are interlocked with the primary motor cortex in the precentral gyrus (area 4), and project to the superior parietal lobules (area 5 and 7), and inferior parietal lobules (areas 39 and 40, respectively, the angular and supramarginal gyri). A second source of somatic sensation is area S2, located in the upper bank of Sylvian fissure, which receives bilateral information and distributes it to ipsilateral parietal cortices. These cortices generate representations of the perceiver's body and of three-dimensional stimuli as apprehended by somatosensory processing and interweave such representations with appropriate motor programs as well as pertinent visual and auditory information.

Damage to the hand projection sector of the postcentral somatosensory cortex in either hemisphere impairs the ability to recognize form (astereognosia), scale, texture, and weight of objects in the contralateral hand. (The thresholds for touch, pain, vibration, and temperature are generally not disturbed.)

TABLE 448–2. MANIFESTATIONS OF TEMPORAL LOBE DAMAGE

	Unilateral	Bilateral
Posterolateral	Aphasia* Pure-word deafness* Amusia†	Global auditory agnosia (includes aphasia, amusia, and agnosia for environmental sounds)
Medial	Verbal* or nonverbal memory impairment Complex seizures	Amnesia
Anterolateral and inferior	Anomia* Nonverbal memory impairment Visual agnosia Complex seizures	Amnesia

*Usually left hemisphere
†Right hemisphere only

TABLE 448–3. ICTAL MANIFESTATIONS OF TEMPORAL LOBE EPILEPTIC FOCI

Medial Basal Structures	Lateral Structures
Olfactory hallucinations Memory disturbances (dejà vu or jamais vu); forced thinking, dreamy state	Language impairment; hissing, roaring or clicking hallucinations; vertigo

Epigastric distress
Blank staring
Repetitive somatic automatisms

Damage to the dominant or nondominant inferior parietal lobule causes diverse manifestations. The dominant somatosensory cortex develops dynamic representations of (a) the body and of its movements (especially those of the hand and phonatory apparatus) and (b) the shapes of objects located within arm's reach (in so-called intrapersonal space). Dysfunction in the area of the dominant angular gyrus disrupts reading and writing, planning and execution of representational hand movements in specific contexts (apraxia), arithmetic skills (acalculia), finger recognition (finger agnosia), right-left orientation and the ability to copy drawings, diagrams, and execute three dimensional constructions (constructional apraxia). Dysfunction in the dominant supramarginal gyrus is mainly associated with aphasia (Table 448–5).

The nondominant parietal cortices hold a dynamic representation of extrapersonal space (the space beyond arm's reach) based on somatosensory, visual, and auditory cues. *Both* hemispaces are represented in this region. The attentional survey of external sensory events and projected movements in both hemispaces also depend on this nondominant region, damage to which leads to complex defects in spatial processing. The defects are especially pronounced in the hemispace opposite the lesion and cause the commonly encountered neglect syndrome. Not only is the left hemispace inappropriately attended but the left side of the body itself may be neglected and left hemiplegia or hemisensory loss may be ignored or actively denied (anosognosia). The ability to negotiate a route without hitting obstacles placed to the left side of the body, the skill to follow a previously known and automated route (in a house or town), and the capacity to learn a new route are all compromised by nondominant inferior parietal lesions. So is constructional ability, which is far more disturbed than with equivalent lesions on the dominant side. Unlike their counterparts with left-sided lesions, patients with such nondominant injuries show little concern for their condition and often offer an indifferent affect. An adequate rehabilitation program must take into account this reduced motivation. When these structures are affected on the right side together with the right nearby auditory cortices (as a result of extensive cerebrovascular damage affecting the nondominant middle cerebral artery territory), patients may become acutely confused.

Bilateral damage confined to superior parietal lobules causes ocular apraxia (the inability to direct gaze voluntarily toward new visual stimuli appearing in the periphery of the visual field), bilateral optic ataxia (the inability to generate precise contralateral hand movements toward an outbound target under visual guidance), and an impairment of visual attention, a breakdown in the ability to apprehend the visual panorama in a coherent, seamless manner (this is known as visual disorientation or simultanagnosia). The combination of ocular apraxia, optic ataxia, and visual disorientation constitutes the Balint syndrome. Common causes are bilateral infarctions in the border zone between the posterior and

TABLE 448–4. INTERICTAL TRAITS OF PATIENTS WITH TEMPORAL LOBE EPILEPTIC FOCI

Lack of humor
Sadness
Obsessiveness
Metaphysical preoccupation
Hyposexuality
Dependence

TABLE 448–5. MANIFESTATIONS OF PARIETAL LOBE DAMAGE

Superior parietal lobule		Bilateral damage causes Balint syndrome. Unilateral damage causes mainly optic ataxia and transient abnormalities of pursuit eye movements.
Inferior parietal lobule	left	Aphasia; alexia; agraphia; acalculia; constructional apraxia; right/left disorientation; finger agnosia
	right	Neglect; anosognosia; inappropriate affect
Post-Rolandic cortices		Subjective alterations in somatic sensation. Astereognosia

middle cerebral artery territories and bilateral metastases. Unilateral damage to the superior parietal lobule causes optic ataxia and defective pursuit eye movements.

FRONTAL LOBES

The human frontal cortices encompass nearly half of the entire cortical mantle and include a large number of diverse anatomic fields. Their operations assist with movement control; general problem solving; decision making; planning; generation of willful responses; regulation of social behaviors, emotion, affect, and autonomic function; and regulation of language and thought processes. Understanding of the correspondence between structure and function is less advanced for frontal cortices than for other cerebral regions. Furthermore, impairments of the functions outlined above are less easy to detect in clinical and laboratory settings than in real life.

The motor sector of the frontal lobe (the precentral and premotor cortices) is located mainly in the lateral frontal surface but spills into the mesial surface as well. The precentral cortex (area 4 or M1) contains a somatotopic representation of contralateral body movements in which the phonatory apparatus and hand are accorded the largest share. It is the principal target of re-entrant projections from cerebellum and motor thalamus. The premotor region (area 6) is part of a network for motor programming, and it receives re-entrant projections from basal ganglia as well as projections from the posterior sensory cortices. It integrates incoming movement-related information for final transmission to the corticospinal tract. Part of the nearby area 8, known as the frontal eye field, controls voluntary eye movements (seizures originating in this area cause the eyes to *deviate away from the lesion;* damage by an infarction makes the eyes deviate *toward the lesion*). The mesial aspect of area 6 contains the supplementary motor area (SMA or M2). The SMA is anatomically contiguous with the rest of the premotor cortex but constitutes a functionally separate region. (It contains a whole body map in its relatively small cortical surface.) Damage to area 4 causes varied degrees of focal paralysis in the contralateral side of the body or face (involvement of corticospinal projections in corona radiata or internal capsule causes less focal paralysis). Damage to the lateral aspect of area 6 causes impairments of motor learning and execution as well as transient forms of neglect, while involvement of the SMA leads to mutism and contralateral akinesia. Infarctions and parasagittal tumors in this region often compromise part of both SMA and the nearby cingulate gyrus (area 24) located immediately beneath the cingulate sulcus. The cingulate is a limbic cortex and its acute damage also causes akinesia, mutism, transient neglect, and an impairment of motivation (abulia). Tumors impinging in this region may cause speech arrest and seizures characterized by vocalization and may trigger involuntary movement synergies involving contralateral limbs and trunk. Motor symptoms of frontal lobe lesions are presented in Table 448–6.

The frontal lobes also contain limbic cortices in the posterior orbital surface. Involvement of this region is associated with disturbances of social behavior. These include inability to recognize the social value of real-life situations and an inability to plan future social actions appropriately. On occasion, especially with large lesions, patients may exhibit inappropriate demeanor (facetiousness). During the acute phase of frontal limbic damage patients are generally akinetic and inattentive and may exhibit inappropriate behavior regarding their sphincters. They may urinate or defecate in public although sphincter function per se is preserved.

Areas 44 and 45 on the dominant side are known as Broca's area. Their damage causes aphasia (see Ch. 449). Damage to the nondominant side of this area alters the prosodic qualities of speech. The most anterior regions of the frontal lobe accommodate the prefrontal cortices (areas 46, 9, 10, 11, 12), damage to which impairs decision making and planning, reduces creativity, and alters the regulation of affect and emotion. With permanent damage, the magnitude of the deficit relates directly to the bilaterality or unilaterality of the lesion, the size of the lesion, and the previous intellectual caliber and occupation of the patient. Relatively small unilateral lesions produce minor impairments that are difficult to detect and tend to recover. Large bilateral prefrontal lesions, however, although they leave motor, perceptual, and language functions intact, are incompatible with maintaining a socially adapted, fully self-conscious and creative personality. The defects are most noticeable in patients who undergo bilateral prefrontal ablations for the treatment of large midline brain tumors. Even then, however, the impairments can be better sensed by appraising social and occupational behavior than by neuropsychologic tests, most of which may be passed flawlessly.

The frontal lobes are especially vulnerable to closed head injury resulting in many of the signs described above as well as in the formation of cortical scar tissue and the appearance of seizures. The lateral sectors are frequently compromised by infarctions and meningiomas. The mesial sector is often struck by infarctions or hemorrhages, mostly as a consequence of ruptured anterior communicating or anterior cerebral artery aneurysms. Meningiomas arising in the falx are another common cause of damage. The posterior orbital sector is often involved by herpes simplex encephalitis, by hemorrhages from ruptured anterior circulation aneurysms, and by meningiomas arising in the sphenoid and ethmoid regions. The brunt of the effects of normal-pressure hydrocephalus reflect damage to the frontal white matter. Finally, all prefrontal cortices are markedly involved in Pick's disease, and both prefrontal and frontal limbic cortices are involved to some extent in Alzheimer's disease. When involvement of frontal lobe structures is caused by large tumors, especially by malignant gliomas which often arise in the white matter of one hemisphere but traverse the corpus callosum to involve the other, patients exhibit the florid disturbances outlined above and also impairments of attention and balance (see Ch. 454), along with primitive reflexes (grasp reflex, Gegenhalten or paratonia, echopraxia).

TABLE 448–6. MOTOR SYMPTOMS OF FRONTAL LOBE DISEASE*

	Structural Damage	Seizure
Precentral gyrus	Focal distal weakness, maximal in lower face, hand, less often foot; increased reflexes, mild spasticity, Babinski sign	Jacksonian: focal onset on face, thumb, foot. "March" toward proximal limb and trunk.
Corona radiata or internal capsule	Hemiplegia; increased spasticity	
Premotor (lateral)	Ocular ipsiversion; paratonic resistance to passive motion; grasping; hypokinesia; optic ataxia, aphasia	Adversive: ocular contraversion.
Premotor (mesial)	Mutism	Involuntary synergies (elevated arm and leg, body turning); speech arrest and/or vocalization

*All arise contralateral to the brain lesion.

Bear DM, Fedio P: Quantitative analysis of interictal behavior in temporal lobe epilepsy. Arch Neurol 34:454, 1977. *An effort to quantify the personality traits of epileptics.*

Damasio H, Damasio AR: Lesion Analysis in Neuropsychology. New York, Oxford University Press, 1989. *A method to study the anatomic location of cerebral lesions, and a review of advances in neuropsychology.*

Eslinger PJ, Damasio AR: Severe disturbance of higher cognition after bilateral frontal lobe ablation. Neurology 35:1731, 1985. *An example of the extreme dissociation of behavior caused by frontal lobe damage. The lesions prompted a variety of socially unacceptable behaviors but did not interfere with language or memory. The intelligence quotient remained superior.*

Gazzaniga M, Le Doux J: The Integrated Mind. New York, Plenum Press, 1978. *A brief and lucid survey of the integration of higher functions and of the role the cerebral commissures play in it.*

Heilman K, Valenstein E (eds.): Clinical Neuropsychology. Oxford, Oxford University Press, 1985. *A multiauthored collection of essays on major aspects of neuropsychology.*

Hier DB, Mondlock J, Caplan LR: Behavioral abnormalities after right hemisphere stroke. Neurology 33:337, 1983. *An analysis of a large series of patients with damage to the right parietal lobe.*

Mesulam M-M: (ed.): Principles of Behavioral Neurology. Philadelphia: F. A. Davis Co., 1985, pp. 125–168. *Another collection of comprehensive reviews on neuropsychology.*

Penfield W, Jasper W: Epilepsy and the Functional Anatomy of the Human Brain. Boston, Little, Brown, and Company, 1954. *The classic monograph on what epilepsy and the electrical stimulation of the cerebral cortex tell us about the neural substrates of higher brain function.*

449 Disturbances of Memory and Language

Antonio R. Damasio

The concerted operation of multiple but relatively specific cortical systems is the basis for the most complex human abilities: the acquisition and categorization of knowledge (learning and memory), the translation of knowledge in a verbal code (language), the manipulation of nonverbal and verbal knowledge in thought processes, the ability to select responses and solve problems (decision-making, planning, creativity), and the reflection upon ongoing cognitive activities in the perspective of one's autobiography (self-consciousness). These functions presume the normal operations of attention (the ability to concentrate willfully on a specific mental content to the exclusion of others) as well as motivation (the affective impetus to sustain a given mental activity or action).

MEMORY AND ITS IMPAIRMENTS

Memory is the ability to make a record of perceptions of the external world, usually combined with perceptions of the perceiver's body and movements. Memory also encompasses the ability to store concepts derived from the categorization of those records and to manipulate the records internally for recall and recognition. The terms "learning" and "memory" are used almost interchangeably, although learning should be used only to denote "memory acquisition."

Unless the process of consolidation takes over, the memory of objects or events that we perceive is retained only briefly (less than 60 seconds). The material held during that period is said to be in *short-term memory* or *immediate memory* (Table 449–1). (Immediate memory is preserved in most amnesias.) If those materials are to be recorded into permanent or *long-term memory*, an active physiologic process must start promptly. The process of consolidation takes time, and recently acquired memories are more vulnerable to decay than those that have been

TABLE 449–1. TYPES OF MEMORY

Factual (declarative)
Skill (procedural)

Short-term (immediate)—less than 60 seconds
Long-term—more than 60 seconds

Recent
Remote

held long and internally rehearsed. Newer memories are known as *recent* memories, and older memories as *remote*.

Memory for unique faces, objects, or events is often termed *episodic* (e.g., the memory of a personal friend or a favorite landscape), whereas memory for classes of objects or events is usually known as *generic* or *semantic* (e.g., the knowledge that allows us to categorize a car as a transport vehicle, a dog as an animal, or a given locale as urban or rural). Episodic and semantic memories pertain to factual knowledge and are known as *declarative*. Declarative memory contrasts with *procedural* memory, which is based on skills rather than facts and refers to actions rather than to the knowledge necessary to acquire those actions. Dancing, the playing of instruments, typing, and swimming are examples of *procedural* memory. Procedural memory is spared in most amnesias.

MEMORY MECHANISMS. The thesaurus of facts and rules acquired in a lifetime is stored in the association cortices of every lobe of both hemispheres. Memories are dynamically and flexibly distributed in overlapping neuron ensembles linked by patterned, highly specific, and hierarchically organized corticocortical and commissural connections. Access to single-modality memories depends on association cortices near the primary sensory cortex that conveyed the information in the first place (the impaired access or partial destruction of those cortices causes an *agnosia*—Table 449–2). Access to memories of polymodal events depends on cortices farther away from sensory sources. Finally, access to unique and complex polymodal episodes depends on inferior and anterolateral temporal cortices (impaired access or partial damage to such cortices causes *amnesia*).

The ability to lock sensory events into neural structures to form a permanent record depends on the normal operation of the hippocampal system, the basal forebrain, and the diencephalon, as well as several brain stem nuclei. The elucidation of the respective roles of these components is imperfect, but it appears that the hippocampus, which is informed about relationships between components of an event via connections from the higher-order association cortices, binds and stabilizes information according to its appropriate temporal and spatial links. The stabilization appears to involve molecular and cellular changes during long-term potentiation. Through the interconnected amygdala the hippocampus also influences basal forebrain, diencephalon, and brain stem nuclei. The basal forebrain and brain stem, in turn, provide the cerebral cortex with neurochemical inputs that probably also contribute to stabilize records at the cellular level (acetylcholine from the nucleus basalis of Meynert in the basal forebrain, noradrenaline from the locus coeruleus in the brain stem, and other, still ill-defined mediators and modulators). The hippocampal interconnections with the diencephalon sample the status of the internal milieu at the time of a given sensory experience, informing on the value of a particular stimulus or event in the context of instinctual goals. Finally, the ascending brain stem reticular formation contributes importantly because

TABLE 449–2. DISTINGUISHING AMNESIA FROM OTHER IMPAIRMENTS

Agnosia	Impaired recognition of stimuli presented in one sensory channel (e.g., object, face, voice, melody) that cannot be explained by defective perception.
Anomia	Impaired retrieval of the name for a stimulus (e.g., object or face) that is otherwise properly perceived and properly recognized.
Amnesia	A pervasive impairment of the ability to recall and recognize unique events and unique stimuli. The defect is independent of the sensory channel used to probe memory (e.g., given a unique person, *neither* the face *nor* the voice is recognizable).
Aphasia	A pervasive impairment of linguistic processing; (e.g., structure of sentences; assembly of phonemes in a word; retrieval of words from the lexicon).
Dysarthria	Defective articulation of speech sounds without compromise of linguistic processing. When the articulation breakdown is complete, the term *anarthria* applies.

most learning presumes attention and arousal. The neural structures and systems involving the acquisition of procedural memories are different: After bilateral destruction to hippocampus and basal forebrain, most motor skills remain intact and new motor skills can be learned. The motor and sensory cortices generate those memories and so do the cerebellum, the neostriatum, and the motor nuclei of the thalamus. A discussion of the molecular and cellular changes related to memory is outside the scope of this chapter.

MEMORY DISORDERS. Table 449–3 lists several terms that are helpful in describing and classifying the amnesias. The terms *anterograde* and *retrograde* are especially important. Anterograde designates the time compartment *since* the amnesia began. Retrograde refers to the time compartment *prior* to the onset of amnesia and to information previously acquired that may not be retrievable in recall or recognition. Retrograde amnesia can be as short as hours or days, as is often the case in post-traumatic situations, or may extend back years or even decades, as in Korsakoff's amnesia or the amnesias that follow herpes simplex encephalitis.

Some middle-aged and elderly persons have an increasing but isolated difficulty in recalling proper names and recent events of limited importance. This "benign forgetfulness" is not a predictor of the progressive dementias and is best treated with prompt and vigorous reassurance. The most frequent causes of incapacitating memory loss are the degenerative dementias, head injury, cerebrovascular disease, encephalitis, brain anoxia and ischemia, and nutritional impairment (Table 449–4).

A major part of our knowledge about the critical contribution to memory of the hippocampal formation and its input and output stations came from a single, well-studied patient who underwent *bilateral medial temporal lobe resection* to treat epilepsy. He became severely amnesic postoperatively and has remained unable to learn factual memories to this day. His severe anterograde amnesia contrasts with a largely spared retrograde memory and with preserved generic memories and procedural learning. The amnesias caused by *postanoxic encephalopathy*, in which anterograde memory is heavily involved, also are caused by hippocampal damage in which the CA1 sector is selectively damaged. Together with the evidence that specific areas of the entorhinal cortex and subiculum are damaged in amnesic patients with *Alzheimer's disease*, these findings underscore the importance of hippocampus in memory (see Ch. 450). *Herpes simplex encephalitis* commonly damages the hippocampal region bilaterally, but it involves other anterolateral and inferior regions of the temporal cortices. Such patients suffer not only an anterograde memory defect but also a severe retrograde amnesia that can span virtually their entire lives, especially when the right hippocampal area is heavily involved. Bilateral damage to hippocampus can also be caused by infarctions in the territory of the posterior cerebral arteries. Infarctions in the area of the basal forebrain (septal nuclei, nucleus accumbens, nucleus basalis of Meynert) due to ruptured aneurysms in the anterior circulation are also associated with amnesia. Both anterograde and retrograde memory are involved, but unlike temporal lobe amnesia, the defect is mild, tends to improve, and appropriate cueing helps recall. *Head injury* is another major cause of amnesia. Even modest head trauma results in transient dysfunction of the hippocampus and diencephalon. *Korsakoff's*

TABLE 449–3. TYPES OF AMNESIA

Retrograde	Amnesia for information learned before the onset of illness
Anterograde	Amnesia for information that presented itself after onset of illness
Global	Information cannot be retrieved through *any* sensory channel
Modality-specific	Same as associative agnosia; information cannot be retrieved through the affected channel, e.g., vision
Permanent	
Stable	Example: postencephalitic
Progressive	Example: Alzheimer's disease
Transient	Examples: transient global amnesia, post-traumatic amnesia

TABLE 449–4. ETIOLOGIES OF AMNESIA

Alzheimer's disease and other degenerative dementias
Head injury
Herpes simplex encephalitis
Ruptured anterior circulation aneurysms with infarction in basal forebrain
Infarctions in other memory-related systems, e.g., medial thalamic nuclei; temporal cortices
Anoxic/ischemic encephalopathy
Wernicke-Korsakoff encephalopathy
Psychogenic amnesia

syndrome is a severe amnesia that compromises both anterograde and retrograde memories and is accompanied by confabulation and lack of insight. It is caused by attacks of severe thiamine deficiency, generally in the setting of alcoholism, and often accompanies or follows acute Wernicke encephalopathy (see Ch. 456), or delirium tremens (see Ch. 14), although it can occur whenever thiamine-free calories are the mainstay of nutrition. Thiamine deficiency results in bilateral damage to diencephalic structures, including the dorsal medial nucleus of the thalamus and the hypothalamic mamillary bodies. The consistent presence of these lesions in Korsakoff's amnesia established the diencephalon as a crucial component of the memory-related network.

Transient global amnesia (TGA) is a self-limited memory impairment during which the patient can identify himself but is unable to recall events preceding the episode and generally cannot recognize places. Patients with TGA remain attentive, have normal language and reasoning, and are generally distressed by their disorientation. They tend to ask repeatedly where they are, what they have been up to, and what is going on. Most TGA episodes last about 4 or 5 hours (but may be shorter or longer), and the disorientation gradually clears. The attacks leave no residual impairment and are generally nonrecurrent. Status epilepticus with complex partial or petit mal seizures may mimic TGA but can be distinguished because patients with seizures are generally noninquisitive and inattentive. Most TGA attacks occur in middle-aged or older persons and presumably reflect transient vascular insufficiency affecting memory-related areas in the temporal lobe or thalamus.

Psychogenic amnesia is generally greatest for emotionally important events and may erase circumscribed epochs of the past while leaving intact epochs immediately preceding or following the amnesic period. It may include disorientation to self. Questions such as "Who am I?" or "What is my name?", unless uttered during delirium or a seizure, raise the possibility of a psychogenic process. Psychogenic amnesia must be distinguished from emotional upheaval (which often impairs attention and produces inconsistent performance in psychological testing), from depression (which may reduce communication to monosyllables), and from organic amnesias (in which emotionally reinforced material tends to be recalled better than neutral events, and disorientation is worst for time, less for place and persons, and never for self).

Treatment. Patients with acute post-traumatic amnesia tend to recover spontaneously. The same is true of amnesia caused by overmedication or delirium. Memory loss caused by depression (pseudodementia) has a good prognosis when psychological and psychiatric treatment is effective. A less fortunate prognosis accompanies amnesia following prolonged post-traumatic coma. When coma lasts more than 2 or 3 weeks, most patients over 25 years old tend not to recover from the memory loss. Patients with amnesia due to herpes encephalitis recover only when the lesions are mostly or solely unilateral and even those persons retain substantial impairments. In most amnesias the recovery is inversely proportional to the initial severity and is constrained by the extent and placement of lesions. The bulk of improvement usually takes place within the first year after onset, especially within the first 6 months. Neuroactive peptides, neurotransmitter precursors, neurotransmitters, and special dietary agents have no proven usefulness in chronic organic amnesia.

AGNOSIA. Agnosia is the inability to recognize a previously familiar sensory stimulus despite the integrity of elementary perception of the stimulus and the absence of defects of intelligence, motivation, or attention. It is "a percept stripped of its meaning." The disorder is a form of monomodal amnesia, a disability that prevents a perceived stimulus from triggering pertinent, previously acquired information whose evocation would reveal its identity. Agnosia results from dysfunction of association cortices of the affected sensory modality, which contain records of purely modal processing. *Visual agnosia* is the most frequent example. It consists of the failure to recognize familiar faces (prosopagnosia) or objects (visual object agnosia), despite the ability to describe their physical structures, copy them, or recognize the stimulus by sound (prosopagnosics can recognize the possessor of a face by voice). The phenomenon is generally associated with bilateral occipitotemporal lesions, although visual object agnosia can be caused by *left* unilateral lesions of the occipital lobe, and *right* unilateral lesions reduce the efficiency of face recognition.

LANGUAGE AND ITS DISORDERS

Verbal languages are arbitrary symbolic codes in which words stand for properties of external stimuli, actions, and relationships, as well as for the intellectual and emotional reactions that such stimuli evoke in the perceiver. The normal brain acquires and stores a dictionary of such words in at least one language, a lexicon, and develops a highly automated process of two-way translation between the mechanism to reconstruct word representations and the mechanism to reconstruct nonverbal representations of objects, actions, or concepts. The process of language comprehension is the translation of sentences (structured sequences of words) into sequences of approximate nonverbal counterparts whose ongoing manipulation is known as thought. Nouns, verbs, or adjectives have fairly direct referential nonverbal equivalents. On the contrary, functor words (conjunctions, prepositions and adverbs, verb endings) refer to abstract relationships. Functors, together with word order, are the key to the grammatical organization of sentences (syntax) and their nonverbal counterparts in thought. The formulation of speech or writing is the rendering of a nonverbal thought process in a syntactic frame filled with appropriate lexical elements. The lexical and syntactic operations of language depend on phonemic and graphemic devices, which can enact correspondences between sounds, their visual representations, and the articulatory patterns that permit their sensorimotor implementation in phonetic utterances or writing. Oral verbal expression also depends on word stress and the intonational contour of sentences, i.e., the fundamental frequency of the sounds in an utterance as well as the durational elements of speech. The term *prosody* subsumes the latter qualities of verbal expression.

NEURAL SUBSTRATES OF LANGUAGE. Verbal language is characteristically human, and its experimental study is restricted to human beings. Considerable knowledge has been gathered about the neural substrates of language from the cognitive and neuroanatomic study of patients with acquired impairments caused by focal brain lesions (aphasias). Most such studies have relied largely on postmortem, computed tomography, and magnetic resonance imaging analysis, although more recent evaluations have been conducted using positron emission tomography (PET). Electrical stimulation of different regions of the cerebrum during surgery for seizures or motor disorders also has provided information on the neural representation of language. The preoperative precaution of pharmacologically inactivating part of the hemispheres with the intracarotid injection of a barbiturate (Amytal) has also contributed important clues. A salient finding, first noted more than a century ago and thoroughly confirmed since, is that the left hemisphere of more than 95 per cent of individuals is especially adroit at language processing. In left language–dominant persons all aspects of language depend largely on left-hemisphere processing, with the partial exception of some aspects of prosody. Handedness is an imperfect but clinically useful indicator of language dominance. In almost all right-handed persons the left hemisphere is dominant for language, and its damage in key areas leads to severe aphasia. Most left-handed and ambidextrous persons (about 70 per cent) are also left language–dominant, although they may have additional language representation in the right hemisphere. About one third of left-handers have either bilateral language representation or right-hemisphere language representation. Such persons are at a disadvantage in that lesions of either side can cause aphasia, although the disability tends to be less severe and to improve. Even extreme right-handed individuals with full language domi-

nance in the left hemisphere possess some language representation in the opposite hemisphere (especially for nouns and verbs; adjectives are poorly represented and functor words probably not at all). The right hemisphere of such a person has little access to speech output and little syntactic capability. It has been suggested that gender is an important variable in language representation, but the available data do not permit conclusive statements. Certainly both men and women can develop aphasia with similar signs and following similar lesions. Language representation is definitely different in children, however. Most children who suffer severe brain lesions up to age 5 or 6 years can recover from aphasia and continue to develop language to nearly normal levels. Left-hemisphere lesions sustained later, especially after puberty, have the same consequences as for adults.

Some asymmetric abilities of the cerebral hemispheres have been related to neuroanatomic asymmetries. The left planum temporale, the area of association cortex located immediately behind the transverse gyrus (the primary auditory cortex), is far larger than the right in about 70 per cent of individuals. The sizable difference is visible on gross inspection and in the microscopic cytoarchitectonic structure of the area. In the same individuals, the left sylvian fissure is longer on the left than on the right so as to accompany the larger extent of the posterior temporal region, and more horizontally placed so as to accommodate a more voluminous left lower parietal lobule (supramarginal gyrus and angular gyrus). Fetuses show these anatomic symmetries as early as the sixteenth week of gestation, and the changes can be identified by MRI as well as in the vascular patterns of cerebral angiographies.

Language depends on a wide network of cortical and subcortical processing units, and its knowledge and operations are distributed within key cortical regions (see Fig. 448–1). The principal set of language areas is located around the left sylvian fissure (the perisylvian language region). In its posterior aspect lies Wernicke's area (the posterior auditory association cortex, or Brodmann's area 22; it includes the planum temporale and the posterior portion of the first temporal gyrus). Immediately below and behind lies area 37, the lateral aspect of which, in the posterior sector of the second and third temporal gyri, is committed to language. Above and behind the sylvian fissure lie the supramarginal gyrus (area 40) and the angular gyrus (area 39). In the anterior aspect of the perisylvian region in the inferior and posterior aspect of the frontal operculum lie areas 44 and 45, also known as Broca's area. Between sit the motor and sensory regions associated with sensory motor phonatory representations. Also contributing to the language network are components of the basal ganglia (especially in the head of the caudate nucleus and parts of the putamen), some thalamic nuclei, the supplementary motor areas (especially the one on the left), and the anterior cingulate gyri.

THE APHASIAS. Aphasia (or dysphasia) is a disturbance of the comprehension or formulation of verbal messages caused by newly acquired brain disease. Although developments in cognitive science have led to a linguistic-based approach to aphasia, Geschwind's diagnosis of aphasic disorders in terms of the comprehension of language, the fluency of output, and the ability to repeat sentences remains clinically useful because of the strong relationship between these traits and the anatomic sites of the underlying lesions. Table 449–5 summarizes the important clinical clues.

Damage to the posterior sector of the left superior temporal gyrus and its surround causes *Wernicke aphasia*. Patients speak fluently, with normal melodic contour, and even a normal syntactic frame. However, they select wrong words (semantic paraphasias), so the intelligibility of their otherwise well-formed verbal messages may be low (jargon aphasia). Likewise, their comprehension of verbal message is poor because of their inability to translate words into nonverbal meanings. Wernicke aphasics with severe comprehension defects may develop paranoid reactions and become homicidal or suicidal. Wernicke aphasia must be distinguished from *auditory agnosia*, the inability to recognize objects or actions by the characteristic sounds they made (due to bilateral lesions in auditory cortex), and *pure word deafness*, an agnosia restricted to words which allows patients to recognize nonspeech sounds and to produce normal speech (owing to

TABLE 449-5. DIAGNOSTIC POINTERS TO THE MOST FREQUENT APHASIA TYPES

	Speech	Comprehension	Repetition	Other Signs	Localization
Broca	Nonfluent; effortful	+	−	Right hemiparesis worse in arm; aware of defect; frustrated	Lower posterior frontal
Wernicke	Abundant; fluent; well articulated	−	−	Often none; may be euphoric and/or paranoid	Posterior and superior temporal
Conduction	Fluent with some articulatory defects	+	−	Often none; cortical sensory loss in right arm	Usually supramarginal gyrus; may extend to insula and primary auditory cortex
Global	Scant; nonfluent	−	−	Right hemiparesis worse in arm; may present *without* hemiparesis	With hemiparesis: massive perisylvian lesion; without hemiparesis: separate Broca and Wernicke area damage
Transcortical motor	Nonfluent; explosive	+	+		Anterior or superior to Broca area
Transcortical sensory	Scant; fluent	−	+		Surrounding Wernicke area, posteriorly or inferiorly
Atypical ("basal ganglia")	Fluent dysarthric	−	−/+	Right hemiparesis worse in arm	Head of caudate; anterior limb of capsule
Atypical ("thalamus")	Fluent	−	+	Attentional and memory defects in acute phase	Anterolateral thalamus

+ = Intact or largely preserved
− = Impaired

dominant lesions undercutting the auditory cortex). It is also different from the logorrhea of manic states, the logical thought derailment of schizophrenia, and the rare verbal salads of chronic schizophrenics.

Posterior lesions outside the Wernicke area produce more restricted disturbances. Lesions of the supramarginal gyrus give rise to *conduction aphasia*, a disorder in which the patient speaks fluently, has relatively preserved comprehension, but makes sound substitution errors (phonemic paraphasias). The major impairment of repetition stands out among these comparatively milder defects. Other strategically placed lesions of the posterior dominant hemisphere selectively compromise reading or writing. Alexia (inability to comprehend written language while retaining relatively normal vision) without concomitant writing impairment results when a lesion destroys the left visual cortex and, in addition, involves the outflow of the splenium of the corpus callosum. This placement cuts off projections that otherwise connect the unaffected right visual cortex to language areas of the left. Despite their inability to comprehend the written word, patients with "pure" alexia can speak and write normally, in contrast to those with a combination of *alexia with agraphia* (impairment of writing despite normal motor function of the hand), in whom both reading and writing are compromised. In its pure form the abnormality is rare and follows lesions of the left angular gyrus. More frequently alexia and agraphia are accompaniments of Wernicke aphasia.

Broca aphasia is characterized by nonfluent, effortful, melodically flat speech, often shorn of functor words and marred by poor word order. The syntactic defect far outweighs the lexical impairment. Comprehension is well preserved in conversation. Broca aphasia must be distinguished from dysarthria, a disorder of speech articulation that does not impair the linguistic structure of communication. Many Broca aphasics are mute in the first hours or days after the onset of the disorder and only gradually develop the characteristic verbal signs. The intent to communicate, however poorly, is rarely in question. The lesion compromises Broca's area and adjacent cortical and subcortical territories. Because of patterns of vascular supply, many such patients also suffer a contralateral hemiparesis. Apraxia is added when the lesion involves the adjacent premotor cortex. Aphasia caused by lesions confined to Broca's area has a comparatively good prognosis.

Global aphasia consists of a severe loss of all aspects of language operation. Acutely, patients are often mute and have a right hemiplegia. The paucity of speech may become chronic, the patient being able neither to comprehend nor to produce language (except in the form of expletives or brief phrases). Despite rehabilitation efforts, the prognosis is poor, and patients often become depressed and listless, more so than Wernicke aphasics.

As indicated in Table 449–5, two possible localizations can be associated with global aphasia.

With all the aphasias described above, patients are unable to repeat long sentences after the examiner. With some language defects, however, repetition is preserved. The dissociation between intact repetition and disturbed comprehension or speech output implies that Wernicke and Broca regions, as well as their interconnections, must be intact and that the causative lesions may lie near but outside those areas. There are two frequently encountered aphasias of this type: *transcortical motor* and *transcortical sensory* (Table 449–5).

Mutism accompanies a variety of conditions. It may describe the initial state of patients who evolve into Broca or global aphasia but produce no speech at all acutely. It may describe patients with bilateral premotor lesions who often remain chronically mute. Mutism has been applied to the paroxysmal speech arrest caused by seizures arising out of the supplementary motor or Broca areas, generally as an irritative response to an overlying tumor, and to the absence of speech in acute psychoses. Prominent mutism affects patients with lesions of the dominant-sided supplementary motor area and/or nearby cingulate, who not only do not speak but show no inclination to communicate through facial expression or gestures. Those patients also are generally motionless and when they recover do not exhibit aphasic symptoms. Mutism is not *anarthria*, a severe impairment of articulation that prevents speech but allows both the vivid expression of the intent to communicate and the frustration of not being able to do so (anarthria is caused by bulbar or pseudobulbar defects and can be confirmed by the presence of other signs of nuclear and supranuclear paralysis of lingual–vocal cord functions). Nor is mutism the same as *aphonia*, in which the phonatory apparatus is locally inoperative for mechanical or psychogenic reasons.

Some aphasias can be caused by infarcts in the dominant basal ganglia, especially when they involve the head of the caudate and the anterior limb of the internal capsule, and by infarcts in anterolateral nuclei of the dominant thalamus. Their appearance indicates that subcortical structures contribute to language processing, probably by assisting cortical units. The basal ganglia aphasias most often show a combination of fluent, dysarthric speech accompanied by impaired auditory comprehension and a right hemiparesis. The thalamic aphasias resemble transcortical sensory aphasia.

Although seizures or transient vascular insufficiency can cause brief language disturbances, the development of a selective disturbance in language that lasts more than a few hours always reflects a structural and focal lesion. The most common causes are infarction and hemorrhage in the distribution of a major cortical artery branch. Less frequent causes are head trauma and space-occupying lesions.

Damasio H: Neuroimaging contributions to the understanding of aphasia. In Boller F, Grafman J (eds.): Handbook of Neuropsychology, Vol. 2. Amsterdam, Elsevier, 1989, pp. 3–46. *A description of different aphasia types and their localization.*

Damasio AR: Time-locked multiregional retroactivation: A systems level proposal for the neural substrates of recall and recognition. Cognition 33:25–62, 1989. *A testable and nontraditional model of neural systems underlying memory in humans.*

Damasio AR, Tranel D, Damasio H: Amnesia caused by herpes simplex encephalitis, infarctions in basal forebrain, Alzheimer's disease, and anoxia. In Squire L (ed.): Handbook of Neuropsychology, Vol. 3. Amsterdam, Elsevier, 1989, pp. 149–166. *A review of the profiles and anatomic correlates of the amnesias.*

Damasio AR, Tranel D, Damasio H: Face agnosia and the neural substrates of memory. Annu Rev Neurosci 13:89–109, 1990. *A discussion of the cognitive and neuropsychological aspects of this intriguing phenomenon, with information applicable to the understanding of memory.*

Dudai Y: The neurobiology of memory: Concepts, findings, trends. Oxford, Oxford University Press, 1989. *A comprehensive review of the neuroscience of memory.*

Geschwind N: Disconnection syndromes in animals and man. Brain 88:237, 585, 1965. *A seminal discussion on the anatomic basis of memory.*

Ojemann GA, Creutzfeldt OD: Language in humans and animals: Contribution of brain stimulation and recording. In Plum F, Mountcastle VB, et al. (eds.): Handbook of Physiology, Section 1: The nervous system. Vol. V, Higher functions of the brain, Part 2. Bethesda, MD, American Physiological Society, 1987, pp. 675–699. *Electrical stimulation and recording from the cerebral cortex provide clues to the neural basis of language.*

Raichle ME: Exploring the mind with dynamic imaging. Semin Neurosci 2:307–315, 1990. *A review of recent findings on language based on PET research.*

Scoville WB, Milner B: Loss of recent memory after bilateral hippocampal lesions. J Neurol Neurosurg Psychiatry 20:11, 1957. *Removal of the uncus and underlying amygdaloid complex resulted in little behavioral change. When the hippocampus was removed bilaterally, memory loss ensued.*

Victor M, Adams RD, Collins GH: The Wernicke-Korsakoff Syndrome and Related Neurologic Disorders Due to Alcoholism and Malnutrition, 2nd ed. Philadelphia, F. A. Davis Company, 1989. *The classic monograph on the subject provides evidence for the role of the diencephalon in memory.*

450 Alzheimer's Disease and Related Dementias

Antonio R. Damasio

Introduction

The term *dementia* describes a pervasive decline in a number of crucial functions resulting in the loss of personal and social independence in a previously competent individual. Although a defect in memory is often the core impairment in dementia, the term applies only to patients who have additional impairments in intellect as reflected by defective problem-solving, decision-making, and judgment. Those impairments are usually accompanied by disturbances in language and spatial orientation. Isolated defects in memory (amnesia) or in language (aphasia) do not qualify for the diagnosis of dementia even when their severity curtails normal behavior. The term *dementia* also does not apply to mentally retarded individuals who have never become intellectually competent (the term *amentia* may be used instead) and should not be applied to disturbances of attention, regardless of how profound they may be, for which the terms *confusional state* or *delirium* should be reserved.

From a physiopathologic standpoint, dementia occurs when several of the cerebral systems that support learning, memory, decision-making, and language are rendered dysfunctional by *any* neurologic disease process. Dementia can be a stable state when the disease is self-limited (such as may follow brain damage from cardiac arrest or result from multiple cerebral lesions following head trauma). In most instances, however, the dementia develops insidiously, as a result of diseases such as Alzheimer's or communicating hydrocephalus. Although the term *dementia* is equally appropriate for either stable or evolving mental decline, in practice dementia generally denotes a progressive condition of gradual and often slow course.

Table 450–1 lists the most frequent causes of progressive dementia. Dementia has never been a rare occurrence but of late its frequency has been rising steeply. In part, this may reflect public and physician awareness of the condition, but far more important is the remarkable rise of longevity in the indus-

TABLE 450–1. THE MOST FREQUENT CAUSES OF PROGRESSIVE DEMENTIA

Alzheimer's disease
Other degenerative diseases, e.g., Pick's, Parkinson's, Huntington's; progressive supranuclear palsy
Multiple cerebral infarcts
Chronic drug use
Depression
Intracranial mass lesions
Communicating hydrocephalus
Endocrine and metabolic disorders
CNS infections, e.g., HIV opportunistic, syphilis, Creutzfeldt-Jakob disease

trialized world. Progress in medicine and the environment over the past four decades has extended life expectancy by about 15 years, dramatically increasing the incidence of late-life neurologic diseases, with degenerative diseases and especially Alzheimer's disease topping the list. Some recent studies have claimed that as many as 50 per cent of individuals over the age of 80 develop Alzheimer's disease. Even assuming some exaggeration in those predictions, the impact of this disease in medicine and society cannot be overemphasized. Furthermore, all dementia is not Alzheimer's dementia: Many patients so affected have conditions that are partially or completely reversible (Table 450–2). The diagnosis of dementia must be rigorously made, followed by an attempt to uncover its probable etiology.

Diagnosing Dementia

The imperative first step lies in establishing that there is indeed a decline in cognitive and behavioral capacities indicative of underlying neurologic disease. Many normal older individuals inappropriately sense that their mental abilities are diminishing. It is equally important to reassure such persons about the benign nature of their complaints as to make a diagnosis of dementia in those who suffer it. Forgetfulness, especially of proper names, is common at any age and is accentuated by anxiety, fatigue, and depression in late life. Benign forgetting, however, is accompanied neither by amnesia for recent social and personal events nor by impaired judgment and decision-making (although depression may severely impair decision-making and planning). A probing history and interview, together with a normal neurologic examination, can rapidly exclude the possibility of dementia. In addition, brief tests such as the Minimental Status Examination or the Iowa Battery for the Detection of Mental Decline offer simple measures of psychological ability that can be used to reassure the concerned patient (Table 450–3 and references).

If the brief examinations and detection tests suggest that dementia exists, the next step is to establish a premorbid baseline, something that the patient may be unable to provide and may depend on testimony from a reliable relative or escort. What is the patient's education and cultural background? What have been his or her professional and social achievements? Whenever possible, specific information should be sought about years of education, degrees achieved, professional positions, and the judgment of colleagues, friends, and relatives.

The examination should evaluate the following: (1) orientation, (2) attention, (3) social appropriateness, (4) affect, (5) memory, and (6) language. Most of these emerge almost automatically as the evaluation proceeds. What is the patient's attitude toward the examiner? Is he or she cooperative? Socially appropriate? Attentive and able to communicate verbally? Oriented to time and place? Can the patient relate recent public and personal

TABLE 450–2. TREATABLE CAUSES OF DEMENTIA

Inappropriate or excessive use of medications or alcohol
Resectable intracranial tumors
Subdural hematomas
Depression
Communicating hydrocephalus
Endocrine and metabolic disorders, e.g., hypothyroidism, vitamin B$_{12}$ deficiency
CNS infections

TABLE 450–3. OUTLINE OF MINIMENTAL STATUS EXAMINATION*

Test	Score
What is the year, season, date, day, month?	5
Where are you: state, county, town, place, floor?	5
Name three objects: State slowly and have patient repeat (repeat until patient learns all three)	3
Do reverse serial 7's (five steps) or spell "WORLD" backwards	5
Ask for the three unrelated objects above	3
Name from inspection a pencil, a watch	2
Have patient repeat "No if's, and's, or but's"	1
Follow a three-stage command (1 pt each) ("Take a paper in your hand, fold it, and put it on the floor.")	3
Read and obey, "Close your eyes."	1
Write a simple sentence	1
Copy intersecting pentagons	1

*Reprinted by permission from Folstein MF, Folstein SE, McHugh PR: Minimental state. A practical method for grading the cognitive state for the clinician. J Psychiatr Res 12:189, 1975. The authors found that out of a possible total score of 30, mean score for dementia was 9.7, depression with cognitive impairment was 19.0, and uncomplicated affective depression was 27.6.

events (the accuracy of the latter corroborated by an escort)? Patients with early Alzheimer's disease tend to be cooperative, socially appropriate, and attentive, but their recent memory clearly shows a decline. Patients with dementia due to brain tumors, CNS infections, or hydrocephalus are more often distractible, less appropriate, and careless of appearances.

Some traditional mental status tests such as the recall of three unrelated words at 5 minutes, the reverse spelling of WORLD, or the backwards subtraction of serial 7's, can give helpful hints but are not reliable. Many nondemented patients with aphasia, amnesia, parietal lobe dysfunction, or mere emotional distraction can fail such tests; conversely some patients with early dementia can pass them. The popular Minimental Status Examination fares better (Table 450–3).

A formal neuropsychological evaluation conducted by a trained neuropsychologist offers the most reliable means to diagnose the presence and severity of dementia. Such evaluations quantify intellectual and problem-solving ability, memory, speech and language, perception, attention and concentration, and personality. Many of the standardized tests, such as the Wechsler Adult Intelligence Scale—Revised, the Wechsler Memory Scale—Revised, and the Benton Visual Retention Test, permit a level of diagnostic precision that cannot be approximated by bedside evaluations or screening batteries. Formal neuropsychological examination is especially useful in distinguishing dementia from depression.

Differential Diagnosis

There are more than 50 possible causes of dementia, but many are rare and the most frequent, Alzheimer's disease, has a fairly distinctive profile. Nonetheless, only histologic analysis of brain tissue at autopsy offers an absolute confirmation of Alzheimer's disease, so that clinical diagnosis remains one of exclusion. Because some of the less frequent causes of dementia can be treated and occasionally may mimic Alzheimer's disease, it is important to rule them in or out. The distinction depends largely on the results of a small group of critical tests (Table 450–4).

ALZHEIMER'S DISEASE

PATHOGENESIS AND MANIFESTATIONS. Alzheimer's disease is caused by a progressive and selective degeneration of neuron populations in the entorhinal cortex, the hippocampus, the high-order association cortices of the temporal, frontal, and parietal regions, and some subcortical nuclei in the basal forebrain (septal nuclei and nucleus basalis) and brain stem (locus coeruleus). The neuronal damage and the attending loss of synaptic density disable several neuronal networks essential to learning and retrieval of memories. By itself, the cortical component of the damage would explain the prominent memory defects of Alzheimer patients. In addition, however, damage to cholinergic neurons in the basal forebrain results in a loss of delivery of acetylcholine to the cerebral cortex, whereas damage to the brain

stem's locus coeruleus precludes the delivery of norepinephrine to the cerebral cortex. Those neurochemical defects are likely to worsen, if not independently explain, many of the behavioral changes seen in Alzheimer patients. At autopsy, the brains of Alzheimer patients are atrophied, especially in the regions where most neurons die. Characteristically, the motor and primary sensory cortices remain unaffected, as do the basal ganglia and cerebellum. Histologically, the diseased neurons show up as containing cytoplasmic neurofibrillary tangles composed of paired helical filaments visible with stains such as Congo red and thioflavin S. The most prominent anatomic change, however, consists of prominent amyloid plaques containing degenerated neuronal fragments, all surrounding a small, dense core of amyloid material. The neuropathologic diagnosis of Alzheimer's disease, however, depends not only on the presence of neurofibrillary tangles and neuritic plaques but also on their anatomic distribution and quantity. Neurofibrillary tangles are present in other diseases, including the dementia that follows repeated boxing injuries. Indeed, neuritic plaques are present in the brains of normal aged persons, only the number of abnormalities being different from the Alzheimer brain. Such findings lead some investigators to believe that Alzheimer's dementia may represent an accelerated form of brain aging rather than a conventional disease.

In about 25 per cent of cases of Alzheimer's disease, the history reveals a relative affected by the disease, and in some rare families the disease can start early (fifth or sixth decade) and affect the offspring in an autosomal dominant pattern. Also, patients with trisomy 21 (Down syndrome) invariably develop the neuropathologic changes of Alzheimer's disease in their third or fourth decades. These findings have stimulated a major effort to identify a chromosomal defect responsible for the condition, but to date no such linkage has been found. The search for toxins, infectious agents, and nutritional or environmental factors has been equally disappointing.

Clinically, Alzheimer's disease is characterized by a relentless impairment of memory and decision-making that generally begins insidiously and can progress for a decade or longer. Most Alzheimer's disease starts after age 60 and the incidence increases with each decade thereafter. Analyses show a greater incidence in women, some of which may reflect their increased longevity compared to men. In most patients the gradual impairment of memory dominates the early clinical picture. They fail to learn new recent events, both public and personal. A defect in recognition of previously known familiar places or situations is often an inaugural sign. As time passes, the impairments worsen. Despite preserving their speech, their motor performances, and their social graces, patients are not able to retain employment and sooner or later become unable to cope with the activities of daily living. A loss of affective resonance is common, which relatives may describe as shallowness or lack of interest. Unwise decisions regarding property or investments are often made during these early stages of the disease, especially if a protective family member is not available to intervene. Signs of poor judgment and a deterioration of social relationships commonly ensue.

Sometimes Alzheimer's disease takes other forms of onset (Table 450–5). Some patients become suspicious of friends, employers, or spouse, developing paranoid ideas, especially during the evening and night hours. They may awaken in the middle of the night disoriented to place and time and behaving in acute psychotic fashion. In another variant, language may be especially compromised. In those instances memory for words

TABLE 450–4. USEFUL TESTS IN THE EVALUATION OF DEMENTIA

Brain computed tomography or magnetic resonance imaging
Neuropsychological evaluation
Complete blood count and erythrocyte sedimentation rate, serologic test for syphilis
Metabolic screen (SMA 12–16)
Serum thyroxine, vitamin B_{12} level
Chest radiograph
Cerebrospinal fluid analysis: cells, protein
Electroencephalography

TABLE 450–5. VARIETIES OF ALZHEIMER'S DISEASE ONSET

Amnesic form	Gradual decline for episodic learning and deficient episodic recall.
Psychiatric form	Delusional ideation, especially severe during the night, dominates the presentation.
Aphasic form	A severe anomia of gradual onset precedes other aspects of mental decline by at least 2 years.

suffers the most, with patients displaying a remarkable anomia that precludes naming of specific objects and people. Finally, the disease occasionally begins by compromising visual attention. Patients report an inability to perceive simultaneously more than one object in the visual field and become unable to orient themselves along previously familiar routes. Whatever the variants, however, a pervasive impairment of memory eventually sets in. In striking contrast to the intellectual decay, motor performance (strength, coordination) remains preserved in most cases during the first years of the disease. Some patients with Alzheimer's disease can even learn *new* motor skills despite their otherwise ravaged ability to retain new factual information. (Nevertheless, rare exceptions exist. A patient has recently been described with left hemiplegia and dementia whose autopsy revealed neuropathologic changes entirely characteristic of Alzheimer's disease.)

Despite the fact that Alzheimer's disease is the most common cause of dementia and that rich neurochemical and neuropathologic characterizations are now available for the disease, no reliable antemortem marker exists for the diagnosis. Accordingly, diagnosis must be formulated in terms of probability, based on the identification of a typical profile and the exclusion of other potentially similar conditions.

A detailed diagnostic codification for Alzheimer's disease is listed in the references. In order to diagnose probable Alzheimer's disease, one must (1) document the dementia by neuropsychological tests revealing scores significantly below the range commensurate with the patient's age and educational level; (2) verify that impairment of memory is a critical component; and (3) verify that the onset of dementia was not sudden or rapidly progressive. A diagnosis of Alzheimer's disease should not be entertained if early in the presentation (1) there are motor signs such as hemiparesis or gait disorder (but see exception above); (2) there is loss of somatic sensation; (3) there is a visual field defect; and (4) seizures have occurred. The EEG should be normal early in the course of the disease, although as the disease progresses it may reveal a nonspecific pattern of slowing. The cerebrospinal fluid should also be normal, containing no cells and either a normal or mildly elevated protein level. CT or MR may be normal early in the course or reveal enlargement of sulci. The enlargement can become quite pronounced in late stages of the disease but is generally more symmetric and severe than in Pick's disease (see below). Positron emission tomography has revealed a consistent pattern of diminished metabolic activity in the temporoparietal regions.

MANAGEMENT. There is no cure for Alzheimer's disease, and no drug tried so far can alter the progress of the disease.

Tacrine (tetrahydroaminoacridine) exerts a modest central cholinesterase inhibition effect and has been found to produce limited improvement in selective mental status tests in patients with Alzheimer's disease. Thus far, at least, beneficial effects have been demonstrated for activities of daily living. Liver toxicity is a risk and must be guarded against.

There are numerous nonpharmacologic ways in which caregivers can ameliorate the manifestations or consequences of Alzheimer's disease and reduce the heavy burdens of caretaking that fall on families. During early stages of the disease, when patients can remain at home, strategically placed cue cards around the house can help patients orient themselves and carry on tasks relating to their self-care. Variations of such a strategy also can help patients cope with nondemanding social activities. An emphasis on tasks that require motor skills (music playing, dancing, card playing, typing, drawing) can help to make the days more pleasurable to the patient and less frustrating to caretakers.

Appropriate drugs help to cope with bouts of anxiety, depression, or paranoid ideation that some patients show. Drugs also can be used to regulate the sleep cycle and avoid nighttime waking and "sundowning." Reduction of environmental stresses and random sensory stimuli can yield surprisingly good results in this regard. Eventually a decision may be needed regarding nursing home placement and the securing of appropriate medical care in such a setting. The Alzheimer's Disease and Related Disorders Association has chapters in every state which can guide physicians and patients to services dedicated to these patients. The references also contain a valuable guide to management. A comprehensive discussion of the diagnosis and prognosis of the disease, as well as of the limited knowledge currently available about it, probably constitutes the greatest help a physician can render to relatives.

DISTINGUISHING ALZHEIMER'S DISEASE FROM OTHER DEMENTIAS

Treatable Dementias

INAPPROPRIATE OR EXCESSIVE USE OF MEDICATIONS. This is perhaps the most frequent and most amenable to correction. Naturally, it can coexist with Alzheimer's disease, but it is important to determine that it is not the cause of dementia when the diagnosis of Alzheimer's disease is entertained in a patient who is taking target drugs. Cough suppressants, barbiturates, benzodiazepines, tricyclic antidepressants, monoamine oxidase inhibitors, anticholinergics, and digitalis are the common offenders. The combination of some of these drugs with alcohol in an elderly and frail individual can easily mimic Alzheimer's disease.

DEPRESSION. This should always be considered in the differential diagnosis because it can present as mental decline, in which case it is known as masked depression or pseudodementia. As noted, expert psychological testing is the key to the diagnosis. A number of neuropsychological tests are capable of discriminating depression from Alzheimer's disease with high specificity. The Benton Visual Retention Test, for example, is passed by nearly all patients who are eventually diagnosed as having pseudodementia, whereas patients who are eventually confirmed to have Alzheimer-type dementia fail or perform at the borderline level. Antidepressant medication, psychotherapy, and, if needed, electroconvulsive therapy can effectively solve the problem.

BRAIN TUMORS AND SUBDURAL HEMATOMAS. Tumors that involve structures of the limbic system, e.g., meningiomas that compress frontal lobe structures or gliomas that infiltrate the white matter of frontal and temporal cortices, often present as dementia. Distractibility, bradykinesia, and apathy dominate the clinical picture and a CT or MR scan easily confirms the suspicion. In most instances, meningiomas can be resected with success. The elderly are prone to develop subdural hematomas after relatively minor, and thus easily forgettable, head injuries. Such hematomas, especially when bilateral, can lead to dementia, often with little in the way of a telltale history. CT or MRI is diagnostic.

COMMUNICATING HYDROCEPHALUS. Communicating hydrocephalus of the so-called normal-pressure variety is another late-life condition easily detected by brain imaging. The lateral ventricles and the third ventricle are enlarged, the sulci may be effaced, and the sampling of cerebrospinal fluid pressure in a routine lumbar puncture may fail to reveal an elevation because the pressure waves that pound the ventricular walls are intermittent. Not uncommonly the past history reveals a significant neurologic antecedent such as bacterial meningitis, subarachnoid hemorrhage, or severe head injury. The dementia is probably due to pervasive dysfunction in white matter pathways surrounding the ventricles. The clinical picture is dominated by impaired attention and flatness of emotional expression and always includes a gait disorder and urinary incontinence, neither of which affects early Alzheimer's patients. The gait disorder consists of a loss of the automatic motor patterns that are normally engaged in walking (apraxia) combined with a broad-based ataxia. An intraventricular shunt may reverse the symptoms in selected patients.

OTHER CAUSES. Endocrine and metabolic disorders, especially hypothyroidism and vitamin B_{12} deficiency, also cause dementia. They are easily detectable and largely correctable. Syphilis and fungal infections can cause reversible dementias. In the appropriate setting syphilis is an especially important diagnostic consideration. Many other dementias exist that can be reversed upon correcting the conditions to which they are secondary. Chronic liver disease, chronic lung disease, and uremia are obvious examples.

Nontreatable Forms of Dementia

PICK'S DISEASE. In spite of its low frequency, the number of Pick's disease cases appears to be rising. This is a degenerative condition characterized by a markedly asymmetric loss of neurons in the frontal and anterior temporal regions. In some cases, the involvement is virtually unilateral and may be largely confined to either the temporal or frontal lobe (hence the term *lobar atrophy*). An intriguing preponderance for involvement of the left hemisphere has been noted. Histologic analysis reveals loss of cortical neurons in the atrophied areas. Two signs that assist with the microscopic diagnosis are the presence of Pick's neurons (pale, swollen neurons that fail to take conventional stains and are thus achromatic) and Pick's bodies (a silver-staining cytoplasmic inclusion easily distinguishable from a neurofibrillary tangle). Pick's neurons are more commonly found in the frontal region, whereas Pick's bodies are virtually found only in the temporal region. Neurofibrillary tangles and neuritic plaques are not a histologic feature of the disease.

Pick's disease has two prevalent profiles. Both usually begin in the sixth or seventh decade and affect women more frequently than men. In one profile, the patient has a gradual mental decline not unlike that seen in Alzheimer's disease but in which impairments of judgment, decision-making, and affect predominate over the recent memory defect. Social appropriateness deteriorates more rapidly than learning and memory. Not uncommonly, these patients make unwise business decisions and if they live alone they may care little about their appearance. Eventually, memory impairment sets in. This profile correlates with preponderant involvement of the frontal lobe. In the other prevalent profile, patients begin by complaining of a problem with name finding. Few specific names for objects or people can be produced, although speech articulation, syntactic processing, memory, and judgment may be intact. In most instances, within 2 to 5 years, memory and judgment begin to decline. The anatomic correlate is involvement of the *left* temporal lobe. Incidentally, Pick's original description was of the latter profile, although the former has become the textbook standard.

The left temporal form of Pick's brings into the discussion an elusive entity known as *progressive aphasia without dementia*. The pattern observed in some of the patients resembles Pick's disease, but the language disorder has remained the most prominent or sole symptom. It is possible that these cases are examples of Pick's disease in which involvement beyond the left temporal cortices is minimal or delayed. Other evidence suggests that the condition reflects either a variant of Alzheimer's disease or a nonspecific spongiform degeneration. The diagnosis of Pick's disease in the early stages is hazardous, although after about 2 years of evolution the clinical profile becomes suggestive. By then, state-of-the-art CT or MR should provide evidence of asymmetric lobar atrophy.

PARKINSON'S DISEASE. Dementia complicates a mounting number of cases of idiopathic parkinsonism. From a clinical standpoint it is important to ensure that the mental decline is not due to the effects of anticholinergic medication or to the multifarious cognitive changes induced by levodopa. Histologic study of brain tissue of demented patients with Parkinson's disease has shown in many but not all instances abundant neurofibrillary tangles and neuritic plaques identical to those encountered in Alzheimer's disease.

HUNTINGTON'S DISEASE. Patients with Huntington's disease are prone to a host of cognitive and behavioral changes (see Ch. 461). Depression and psychotic states are part of the clinical picture. They may precede chorea and dystonia and persist into the later stages, producing a high suicide rate. Measurable mental decline is often found as the disease progresses. Distractibility and slowness of cognitive processing hallmark the presentation.

The dementia is best explained by extensive cortical dysfunction secondary to neuron loss in the basal ganglia, especially in the caudate.

MULTIPLE VASCULAR LESIONS. A variety of conditions resulting in multiple strokes, large and small, can cause dementia. The following should be considered:

1. Multiple small infarcts (multiple infarct dementia), occurring at different points in the history and involving cortical or subcortical gray matter, especially in the territories of middle cerebral and anterior cerebral arteries. The history and physical examination of such patients invariably reveal systemic hypertension, diabetes, signs of widespread vascular disease, or a combination of the above. The age range is similar to that during which degenerative diseases strike, but a careful history and neurologic examination disclose distinctive clues. For instance, the development of the dementia is stepwise, punctuated by datable events. The patient, family, or relatives can describe specific events during which disturbances of speech, orientation, or motor impairment developed, often followed by some recovery. In short, the mental decline is cumulative but not really gradual. Naturally, if the information source does not have proper insight, or if the events occurred a long time before, there is the risk of smoothing out the history profile and misleading the examiner. Helpful clues under such circumstances are the finding of focal motor defects, especially weakness, ataxia, or urinary incontinence. Alzheimer's disease shows none of these abnormalities during its early clinical course.

2. Multiple demyelinating lesions occurring in the surround of a blood vessel are revealed by MRI in the subcortical white matter. This puzzling condition, sometimes called Binswanger's disease or subcortical arteriosclerotic encephalopathy, can have a dementia profile indistinguishable from that of Alzheimer's disease. Most affected patients are hypertensive, however, although the condition has been described in normotensive individuals. Both CT and MRI reveal enlargement of the lateral ventricles disproportionate to the enlargement of the cortical sulci. MRI also reveals an abundance of periventricular lucencies, which show up as white on T2-weighted images. It should be noted that similar lucencies can be seen in normal older individuals but generally without ventricular enlargement of the same magnitude.

3. Multiple infarcts caused by vasculitis such as congophilic angiopathy, isolated angiitis of the central nervous system, and systemic lupus erythematosus. These are all rare conditions that present in a far more severe and dramatic way than degenerative diseases, multiple infarct dementia, or Binswanger's disease. Such patients usually become acutely ill and are more likely to be admitted to an inpatient service than to remain ambulatory patients. The severity of the condition usually is paralleled by a relatively rapid course compared to the longer time scale of most of the other dementias discussed above. Other clues help the diagnosis. For instance, congophilic angiopathy causes medium to large *hemorrhagic* infarctions. Congophilic angiopathy often coexists with Alzheimer's disease for reasons that are not clear. Lupus is rare in the elderly, and the signs of systemic involvement are diagnostic. Isolated angiitis is more elusive, but the severity and rapidity of the course help the diagnosis.

CENTRAL NERVOUS SYSTEM INFECTIONS. Until recently, the most frequent form of nontreatable infectious dementia has been the transmissible form of Creutzfeldt-Jakob disease, a spongiform encephalopathy (see Ch. 478.6). This rapidly evolving dementia is hallmarked by defects in attention, visual perception, and motor coordination. Once the disease is established, myoclonus is a consistent sign and can be easily evoked by a sudden unexpected noise (startle myoclonus). Myoclonus occurs, albeit infrequently, in advanced stages of Alzheimer's disease but is otherwise uncommon. Triphasic waves in the EEG support the diagnosis. The cerebrospinal fluid is normal. Over the past decade, immune suppression in the setting of HIV infection has become the most common infectious cause of dementia. In some cases the dementia is due to direct HIV involvement of the cerebral parenchyma; in others it is caused by opportunistic infections.

Cummings JL, Benson DF: Dementia: A Clinical Approach. Boston, Butterworths, 1983. *A monograph that discusses the differential diagnosis of the dementias.*

Eagger SA, Levy R, Sahakian BJ: Tacrine in Alzheimer's disease. Lancet 337:989–992, 1991.

Eslinger P, Damasio AR, Benton A, Van Allen M: Neuropsychological detection of abnormal mental decline in older persons. JAMA 253:670–674, 1985. *A brief neuropsychological test for the screening of early dementia.*

Folstein MF, Folstein SE, McHugh PR: Minimental state. A practical method for grading the cognitive state for the clinician. J Psychiatr Res 12:189, 1975. *The authors found that out of a possible total score of 30, mean score for dementia was 9.7, depression with cognitive impairment was 19.0, and uncomplicated affective depression was 27.6.*

Katzman R, Terry R: The Neurology of Aging. Philadelphia, F. A. Davis, 1983. *A discussion on aspects of the many needs of the aging patient, including conditions that must be differentiated from dementia.*

Mace NL, Rabin PV: The 36-hour Day. A Family Guide to Caring for Persons with Alzheimer's Disease, Related Dementing Illnesses, and Memory Loss in Later Life. Baltimore, Johns Hopkins University Press, 1981. *An invaluable book for families and friends of the affected.*

McKhann G, Drachman D, Folstein M, et al.: Clinical diagnosis of Alzheimer's disease. Report of the NINCDS-ADRDA Work Group under the auspices of Department of Health and Human Services Task Force on Alzheimer's disease. Neurology 34:939–944, 1984. *A codification of criteria for the diagnosis of Alzheimer's disease.*

Van Hoesen GW, Damasio AR: Neural correlates of cognitive impairment in Alzheimer's disease. *In* Plum F (ed.): Handbook of Physiology: Higher Functions of the Nervous System. Bethesda, MD, American Physiological Society, 1987, pp. 871–898. *A review of the neuropsychological and neurobiologic characteristics of the disease.*

451 Psychiatric Disorders in Medical Practice

Gary J. Tucker

Perhaps of most concern to the nonpsychiatric physician is the process of psychiatric diagnosis. When does the wide range of human behavior become a pathologic process needing intervention and when is it a variation of normal response to life events? Lacking clear laboratory tests, precise anatomic dysfunctions, or specific pathologic findings, the diagnostic process in psychiatry has followed traditional medical practice for such conditions, i.e., to delineate syndromes and to categorize patterns of symptomatology. However, these syndromes and categories until recently have been broad, often regional, and idiosyncratic. A massive revision of diagnostic practice in psychiatry occurred in 1980 with the publication by the American Psychiatric Association of the third edition of the *Diagnostic and Statistical Manual of Mental Disorders (DSM III)*, now revised. The key components of this nomenclature represent diagnostic criteria that are descriptive and data based, and they require that the clinician view psychiatric disorders from a number of different aspects or axes. The specific symptoms not only include those that must be present but also identify explicit symptoms that must be excluded before a diagnosis can be made. For example, to make the diagnosis of "schizophrenia," one must exclude depressive illness. The clinician must also stipulate the role of biologic, characterologic, and sociologic factors that affect the illness in terms of five axes. Axis I is the specific syndrome, such as schizophrenia, affective disorder, etc. Axis II includes specific personality disorders such as antisocial, dependent, and specific developmental disorders, language disorders, reading disorders, etc. Axis III consists of contributing physical disorders and medical conditions. Axis IV consists of psychosocial stressors. Axis V designates the highest level of adaptive functioning the patient manifested in the past year. All of these axes add to the diagnostic description of the patient and are important in understanding and treating the specific condition. For example, a 50-year-old lawyer with a major depression may be described as follows: Axis I—major depression; Axis II—obsessive personality; Axis III—diabetes, hypertension; Axis IV—marital discord; Axis V—good social and work functioning.

At various times most people experience anxiety, depression, sleep disturbance, and/or somatic preoccupation. In most cases such symptoms are transient, and the precipitants to such symptoms are often evident—an upcoming examination, a new job, marriage, divorce, work or family problems. In these instances the physician has no difficulty in reassuring the patient that the symptoms are transient and situational. However, when these symptoms persist and/or when they occur in situations that have no clear precipitants, they should become of concern to the physician. In order to classify someone as having a psychiatric illness, one must consider the following factors: (1) Do the signs and symptoms fit a psychiatric diagnosis? For example, when patients say they are sad or depressed, do they meet the diagnostic criteria for a diagnosis of depression or dysthymic disorder (see Tables 451–7 and 451–9)? (2) Is there a family history of similar symptoms? Many psychiatric illnesses tend to have a genetic or familial basis. (3) Is the longitudinal pattern of the symptoms consistent with the natural history of a psychiatric disorder? Emotional symptoms associated with specific situations are usually classified as reactions to the situation (see grief reactions); they do not usually become psychiatric disorders. (4) Are the symptoms incapacitating? All persons have enduring patterns of relating, perceiving, and reacting to others. These constitute various components of a person's personality and may take the form of such patterns as obsessive, passive, or antisocial personality traits. When such characteristics interfere with the individual's ability to function, however, the condition is regarded as a personality disorder, named for the predominant personality characteristic. (5) Do delusions and hallucinations exist? Delusions and hallucinations in the absence of other medical causes always indicate major psychiatric illness. Although illusory phenomena can often occur at times of tiredness, intoxication, fever, etc., their occurrence in clear states of consciousness should alert one to the presence of major psychiatric illness.

The proper delineation of psychiatric disorders from normal emotional reactions rests on a careful history, a mental status evaluation, and a knowledge of psychiatric syndromes. If the findings of the history and mental status evaluation do not fit into any of the known psychiatric syndromes, the physician should reserve judgment and follow the patient. In many cases, the symptoms neither persist nor return and all can be reassured. If the symptoms continue, one may recognize a clear psychiatric syndrome. With all persistent emotional and behavioral symptoms, however, the physician must first rule out systemic medical disorders.

DIFFERENTIATING PSYCHIATRIC DISORDERS FROM MEDICAL DISORDERS

While it has always been evident that the central nervous system mediates behavior, there has been a reluctance to look at major psychiatric illnesses as disorders of the central nervous system. However, as biologic studies of psychiatric patients progress and specific psychopharmacologic agents are found to affect behavior, it becomes increasingly evident that psychiatric disorders are disorders of central nervous system functioning. This awareness includes recognition that the central nervous system has a limited number of ways of responding to stress. For example, hallucinations can arise from psychological causes, from toxins in the blood, from head trauma, from seizure disorders, and from fever. With such potentially diverse etiologies, it is imperative that the physician seek clues to differentiate the causes of the behavior change (Table 451–1).

Many clues in the history can suggest something other than an intrinsic psychiatric illness as a cause of abnormal behavior. Most patients with psychiatric illnesses have had psychiatric symptoms or reveal seeds of the current disturbance in their histories. When a patient presents with a good premorbid social history, a good work history, a warm and supportive family, and well-preserved personality, one should seek nonpsychiatric factors to

TABLE 451–1. CLUES TO NONPSYCHIATRIC DISORDERS AFFECTING BEHAVIOR

1. The signs and symptoms do not fit into an established psychiatric diagnostic category.
2. There is no prior psychiatric history or symptoms.
3. The patient demonstrates an abrupt change in behavior or personality.
4. Signs and symptoms fluctuate rapidly.
5. The condition does not respond to treatment.

explain the behavior change. Many physicians tend erroneously to view behavior changes only in a psychological framework. Abrupt changes in behavior, personality, mood, or ability to function should be evaluated for possible organic causes. As indicated, most decompensating patients with psychiatric illness describe similar, albeit less severe, symptoms in the past. To give an example: A 60-year-old man who has been formal and proper his entire life but abruptly becomes bawdy and flirtatious is probably not experiencing the onset of a major psychiatric illness but rather is showing personality changes associated with a new disturbance of the central nervous system, such as brain tumor, vascular disease, endocrine abnormality, or drug reaction. Rapid fluctuations in mental status also suggest a new disturbance rather than a psychiatric disorder. Patients with psychiatric disease occasionally are delusional and hallucinating in the morning but free of these symptoms the same evening (or vice versa). By contrast, the resolution of the delusions and hallucinations associated with schizophrenia typically requires days to weeks. Similarly, motor behavior does not change rapidly in psychiatric illness. Patients with encephalopathies, by contrast, often have a "motor drivenness" with episodic desires to move about, to get up and walk. This restlessness is particularly prominent in delirious states. Lastly, and perhaps most subtly, when a patient does not respond to the usual interventions one should suspect the possibility of an incorrect diagnosis. For example, when a patient with hallucinations and delusions has been treated unsuccessfully with adequate doses of neuroleptic medications for an appropriate period of time with no change in the symptoms, one should consider the possibility of a disorder other than schizophrenia. These simple guidelines often alert the clinician to multiple diagnostic possibilities.

Goodwin D, Guze S: Psychiatric Diagnosis, 4th ed. New York, Oxford University Press, 1989. *An excellent overall text on descriptive psychiatry and the basis for diagnostic groupings.*
Lishsman W: Organic Psychiatry, 2nd ed. Oxford, Blackwell, 1987. *A comprehensive description of neurologic and medical complications of behavioral disorders.*
Pincus J, Tucker G: Behavioral Neurology, 3rd ed. New York, Oxford University Press, 1985. *This monograph discusses differential diagnosis and behavioral aspects of neurologic disease as well as neurologic aspects of psychiatric disorders.*
Schiffer RB, Klein RF, Sider RC: The Medical Evaluation of Psychiatric Patients, New York, Plenum Press, 1989. *A detailed explication of the comorbidity of medical illnesses and behavioral symptoms.*
Spitzer RL (ed.): Diagnostic and Statistical Manual of Mental Disorders, 3rd ed., rev. Washington, D.C., American Psychiatric Association, 1987. *A useful, widely accepted outline of diagnostic features of the gamut of psychiatric disorders.*

SCHIZOPHRENIC DISORDERS

Schizophrenia and some forms of affective disorders comprise the major psychotic illnesses. (Psychosis is defined as the presence of hallucinations and/or delusions.) Kraepelin, a noted German psychiatrist, observed that among hospitalized psychotic patients there were two longitudinal patterns. The first seemed to be characterized by exacerbations and remissions in mood and cognitive functioning which he labeled "manic-depressive illness," and the second was characterized by a chronic psychotic course with its onset in youth and deteriorating social function, which he labeled "dementia praecox" (a dementing illness of young people). In 1911 Eugene Bleuler, a Swiss psychiatrist, changed the name of dementia praecox to "schizophrenia." He described the central features of schizophrenia as a psychotic process manifested by disturbed thinking, changes in the emotional responsiveness of the patient, and a preoccupation with their own inner life, or autism. By schizophrenia he did not mean a "split personality" but more a splitting of psychological functions. While some functions, such as the ability to communicate, were often impaired, others, such as memory and mathematical abilities, were sustained. In essence, this early concept remains a good definition of the schizophrenic process.

Schizophrenia most often has its onset in late adolescence. The course of the illness is usually marked by a decline in psychosocial functioning, with a tendency for the patient to become downwardly mobile in social class. The introduction of neuroleptics in 1954 brought about some improvement in the treatment of these patients, but the observations of Kraepelin of an ultimate dete-

riorating course still hold true. Current treatment aims toward shorter hospitalizations for schizophrenics with more vigorous attempts to retain the patient in a community setting. Physicians encounter two principal groups of schizophrenic patients, one with an acute florid psychotic illness and the other suffering chronic illness with less florid symptoms. The care of these two groups differs in that the acute management is simple, whereas the care and rehabilitation of the chronic patient can be extremely difficult. The nationally pursued process of "deinstitutionalization" has thrust this latter patient population into our everyday world.

DIAGNOSTIC CRITERIA AND CLINICAL SIGNS AND SYMPTOMS. Table 451–2 lists the clinical symptoms of schizophrenia. Note the emphasis on hallucinations and delusions. The ones cited are typical of schizophrenia, although similar hallucinations and delusions can occur in affective disorders and organic conditions; however, the course of these later illnesses is different. A study by Cloninger et al. (1985) demonstrates the importance of the presence of delusions and hallucinations in the diagnosis of schizophrenia. They found that the greater the number of delusions and hallucinations present, particularly persecutory delusions, delusions of control, firmly fixed mood incongruent delusions, and auditory hallucinations, the more likely was the person to progress to a chronic psychotic condition. Other prominent symptoms of schizophrenia are the presence of incoherence and the inability of the patient to communicate with others in a logical and goal-directed fashion. As an example of the speech of a schizophrenic, the patient may respond as follows when asked why he was brought to the hospital: "You are a Nazi; God sent me to save the world; I have a lovely apartment; your eyes are blue."

The stipulation that these criteria must last for a 6-month period (demonstrating a deterioration from a previous level of functioning) defines a more chronic population (Table 451–3). When the duration of symptoms is shorter than 6 months, it is inadvisable to use the diagnosis of schizophrenia. This allows the clinician to withhold judgment and encourages a search for other disorders. This is particularly important with the first episode of psychotic illness, in that it is difficult to differentiate an acute manic episode from an acute schizophrenic episode. Psychotic episodes due to toxic drug reactions, sleep deprivation, and medical causes invariably last less than 6 months (Table 451–4).

In the past many subtypes of schizophrenia have been described, but their predictive validity has been poor except for catatonia and paranoia. Catatonic symptoms include either markedly retarded motor behavior (often to the point of no voluntary movement, the patient retaining any posture into which he is passively placed) or markedly agitated motor behavior. The importance of a catatonic diagnosis, in either the retarded or the agitated form, has retained some validity in conferring a better

TABLE 451–2. SCHIZOPHRENIA*

A. Characterized by psychotic symptoms during the active phase of illness. One of the major symptom categories below must be present for at least 1 week (or less if symptoms respond to treatment):
　1. Two of the following:
　　a. Delusions
　　b. Prominent hallucinations (throughout the day for several days or several times a week for several weeks; each hallucinatory experience is not limited to a few brief moments)
　　c. Incoherence of speech or marked loosening of verbal associations
　　d. Catatonic behavior
　　e. Flat or grossly inappropriate affect
　2. Bizarre delusions (i.e., involving a phenomenon that the individual's subculture would regard as totally implausible, e.g., thoughts being broadcast out loud, being controlled by a dead person)
　3. Prominent hallucinations of a voice keeping up a running commentary on the individual's behavior or thoughts, or two or more voices conversing with each other
B. During the course of the disturbance, a decrease in functioning in such areas as work, social relations, and self-care.
C. Major depressive or manic syndrome and medical conditions ruled out.
D. Continuous psychiatric symptoms for at least 6 months.

*Modified from American Psychiatric Association: Diagnostic and Statistical Manual of Mental Disorders, 3rd ed., rev. Washington, DC, APA, 1987. Used with permission.

TABLE 451–3. PRODROMAL OR RESIDUAL SYMPTOMS IN SCHIZOPHRENIA*

1. Marked social isolation or withdrawal
2. Marked impairment in role functioning as wage-earner, student, or homemaker
3. Markedly peculiar behavior (e.g., collecting garbage, talking to self in public, hoarding food)
4. Marked impairment in personal hygiene and grooming
5. Blunted, flat, or inappropriate affect
6. Digressive, vague, overelaborate, or circumstantial speech; poverty of speech; or poverty of content of speech
7. Odd beliefs or magical thinking, e.g., superstitiousness, belief in clairvoyance, telepathy, "sixth sense," "others can feel my feelings," overvalued ideas, ideas of reference
8. Unusual perceptual experiences, e.g., recurrent illusions, sensing the presence of a force or person not actually present
9. Marked lack of initiative, interests, or energy

*Modified from American Psychiatric Association: Diagnostic and Statistical Manual of Mental Disorders, 3rd ed., rev. Washington, DC, APA, 1987. Used with permission.

prognosis, but there is also evidence that catatonia may be more related to affective disorders than to schizophrenia. The paranoid forms of schizophrenia also show some unique features in that the paranoid delusions are often the only major symptoms and they tend to remain stable over time.

EPIDEMIOLOGY. The prevalence of schizophrenia in the general population is about 1 per cent for lifetime risk, or about an 0.5 in 1000 incidence of recorded or treated cases per year in the United States. The schizophrenic syndrome has a similar worldwide incidence, the only cultural difference being that prognosis for recovery seems better in rural environments than in urban settings. The prevalence rate is eight times higher in the lower than in the higher socioeconomic classes. Since the parents of schizophrenics have a social class distribution similar to that of the general population, the lower position of the patients appears to be a result of the illness rather than the cause of it.

Since the highest incidence of schizophrenia is in younger people, whose illness often becomes chronic, the number of cases is constantly increasing. Seventy per cent of schizophrenics become ill between ages 15 and 35, and the illness affects males slightly more than females. Peak onset in males lies between 15 and 24 years and in females between 25 and 34 years. There are slight ethnic differences, with a higher incidence in Scandinavian countries and in nonwhites. The chronicity of the illness presents an enormous cost. A recent study notes that although schizophrenia affects only one-twelfth as many persons as does myocardial infarction, the cost is six times as great.

PATHOPHYSIOLOGY. The pathophysiology of schizophrenia is unknown, nor has an anatomic origin of the symptoms been determined. Nevertheless, a number of conditions (including trauma, seizure disorders, and Huntington's disease) can produce schizophrenia-like hallucinations and delusions. Many authors have reported a higher than normal incidence of nonlocalizing neurologic abnormalities in schizophrenia, changes that are not present in other psychiatric conditions. These include defects in stereognosis, graphesthesia, and various skilled motor activities. Minor vestibular system defects, usually consisting of a reduction in the nystagmus response unrelated to medication use, have been noted in schizophrenic patients. Deficits in smooth-pursuit

TABLE 451–4. USUAL SYMPTOMATIC PATTERNS OF PSYCHOTIC DISORDERS

	Acute Schizophrenia	Mania	Major Depression	Delirium
Delusions	+ + + +	+ + + +	+ + +	+ +
Hallucinations	+ + + +	+ +	+ +	+ + +
Disorientation/ confusion	0	0	0	+ + + +
Incoherent speech	+ + + +	+ + +	0	+ + + +
Depressed mood	+	0	+ + + +	+
Grandiosity	+ +	+ + + +	0	0

eye movements during pendulum tracking have been reported in schizophrenia as well as in other psychoses. Other evidence of organic damage, including EEG abnormalities, is tantalizingly frequent.

Twenty-five per cent of hospitalized schizophrenic patients show abnormally slow EEG tracings using standard recording techniques; with more complex instrumentation the incidence rises as high as 80 per cent. Since the development of pneumo-encephalography, reports of gross anatomic cerebral changes in subgroups of schizophrenic patients have been frequent. With the rapid developments of computed tomography (CT), magnetic resonance imaging (MRI), and more dynamic measures such as single photon emission (SPECT) and positron emission tomography (PET), these reports have been more consistent and refined. CT and MRI studies have both shown lateral ventricle and third ventricle enlargement, widened cortical sulci, cerebellar atrophy, cerebral asymmetry, and decreased brain density consistently in many, but not all, studies in subgroups of schizophrenic patients. Not all of these changes occur in the same subgroups. Although it is not yet clear what the implications of these findings are, there have been correlative studies of these abnormalities with increased cognitive disturbance, poorer premorbid adjustment, and longer duration of illness. However, as with most new techniques, there is great variation of the instruments and methodologies used in these studies as well as the definitions of the populations. As more standardization of the techniques and diagnostic criteria occur, there should be greater consistency of findings. Using the more dynamic measures, changes have been reported in the cerebral blood flow in the anterior frontal regions, the temporal cortex, and the globus pallidus, as well as decreased D2 receptor sites in schizophrenics. Neuropsychological testing shows a great deal of overlap between the findings in patients with clear-cut organic disease and those with schizophrenia to the point where the tests often fail to distinguish between the two conditions.

Most of the above-described dysfunctions imply an abnormality in the functional integration of sensory and cognitive information in schizophrenia.

Strong evidence implicates a genetic factor in schizophrenia to a degree that 10 to 15 per cent of the offspring of a schizophrenic parent are at risk for the disease. Furthermore, the coincidence of schizophrenia in monozygotic twins is roughly 60 per cent. Additional evidence for a genetic factor comes from studies of children of schizophrenic parents, who are raised by either their natural or adoptive, nonschizophrenic parents: The chance of developing the disease is identical, regardless of the developmental environment. While genetic factors are evident in the transmission of schizophrenia, the family has been implicated in other ways in its development. Previous theories relate to the "schizophrenogenic mother," but little scientific documentation has been provided. A more likely hypothesis of family interaction was developed by Leff and others, who noted that certain family environments had a great deal of "expressed emotion." In these families with much highly charged emotional interaction, schizophrenic patients seemed to do very poorly. Those environments that were less stimulating emotionally allowed the schizophrenic to function better. Hogarty et al. discuss these familial factors more extensively.

Additional indirect evidence for biologic mechanisms in schizophrenia derives from pharmacologic studies: (1) Most of the neuroleptic drugs effective in controlling schizophrenic symptoms act as dopamine blockers in the central nervous system. (2) Many psychoactive drugs such as mescaline and amphetamines are dopaminergic and also have the potential for creating psychotic reactions. Further suggestions of altered dopamine metabolism in schizophrenic patients come from the inconsistent findings of both elevated and reduced levels of homovanillic acid, its major metabolite in the CSF and urine. As yet, most of these biologic findings, as well as the results of parallel animal studies, are too inconsistent or incomplete to permit unifying hypotheses.

PROGNOSIS AND TREATMENT. Prognosis in schizophrenia is poor and specific therapy lacking. Over a 25- to 30-year period, approximately one third of cases show some recovery or remission, and the remainder either have major residual symptoms or are still hospitalized. The major treatment is neuroleptic medication.

Table 451–5 lists the drugs most commonly used in the treatment of schizophrenia. The goal of treatment is to decrease as many of the symptoms as possible. As long as hallucinations, delusions, and disorganized thinking persist, the accepted practice is to increase the dose of medication until reaching a maximum decrease in symptoms. The response is usually achieved in a period of 2 to 3 weeks, with decreases in hallucination and thought disorder and a variable response of delusions. The most frequent limiting factor is the appearance of extrapyramidal side effects, the most common of which are dystonia, akathisia (restlessness), and parkinsonism. These occur most commonly in the first 2 to 4 months of drug use.

There is little difference in efficacy in the neuroleptics (Table 451–5), and lack of efficacy usually reflects too low a dose. If, however, no response occurs to a phenothiazine-type drug (e.g., chlorpromazine), one usually changes to another class of neuroleptics, such as a butyrophenone (haloperidol) or a thioxanthene. The physician should become familiar with one drug from each of these classes of neuroleptics for acute and maintenance use. The major long-term hazard in the use of these medications is tardive dyskinesia.

Tardive dyskinesia is a syndrome of involuntary movements, usually choreoathetoid, that may affect the mouth, lips, tongue, extremities, or trunk. Although usually associated with use of neuroleptics for 6 months or more, tardive dyskinesia can occur with shorter administration. Patients on neuroleptics should be periodically evaluated for these abnormal movements. A frequent early sign consists of vermicular movements of the tongue. Anticholinergic drugs do not help this condition. The symptoms may decrease with an increase of the medication, but such improvement usually is only temporary and may lead to a vicious circle of worsening chorea and increased drug dosages. The cause of tardive dyskinesia is not known, but it is believed to represent the development of dopaminergic hypersensitivity. Although no effective treatment has been found, in many instances gradually decreasing the dose of neuroleptics induces a slow remission of the symptoms (see also Ch. 462).

Despite the above conditions, the use of neuroleptics is effective, and the drugs should be used to help the patient function with as few symptoms as possible despite the potential side effects. Removing schizophrenic patients from medication greatly increases the chances of hospitalization within the following 6 months. This lag represents a major problem in that most patients immediately feel and do better without the medications. As a result, families and patients often fail to associate the cessation of medication with the subsequent relapse.

In spite of the fact that typical neuroleptics are the treatment of choice for schizophrenia, they are not a panacea and there are alternative or adjunctive agents that the clinician may consider. At this stage these agents should be regarded as novel. They include medications such as anticonvulsants, benzodiazepines, calcium channel blockers, and monoamine agonists and antagonists. Additionally, the recent FDA approval of clozapine (Clozaril), an atypical antipsychotic with potent serotonergic, adrenergic, and histaminergic blocking activity and relatively weak

TABLE 451–5. DRUGS COMMONLY USED FOR TREATMENT OF SCHIZOPHRENIA*

	Daily Dosage Range (mg)
Phenothiazines	
Chlorpromazine (Thorazine)	300–1500
Thioridazine (Mellaril)	150–800
Perphenazine (Trilafon)	8–64
Trifluoperazine (Stelazine)	4–60
Fluphenazine (Prolixin)†	2–20
Butyrophenones	
Haloperidol (Haldol)†	2–40
Thioxanthenes	
Thiothixene (Navane)	6–60

*Owing to untoward extrapyramidal reactions, one often needs to administer these drugs along with such drugs as benztropine mesylate (Cogentin), trihexyphenidyl HCl (Artane), diphenhydramine HCl (Benadryl).

†Comes in two injectable slow-release forms that can be given every 10 days to 3 weeks.

TABLE 451–6. DRUGS USED IN ACUTELY AGITATED STATES

Drug	Dose*	24-hr Maximum
Haloperidol (Haldol)	5–10 mg every 1–2 hr I.M. or P.O.	50 mg
Thiothixene (Navane)	5–10 mg every 2–4 hr I.M. or P.O.	40 mg
Lorazepam (Ativan)	0.5–1.0 mg every 1–2 hr I.M. or P.O.	10 mg

*Doses should be 50 to 75 per cent reduced in the elderly or medically ill.

and equivalent D_1 and D_2 dopamine-blocking activity, represents a significant advance in the treatment of schizophrenia. It should be reserved for those patients with treatment-resistant illness, those who are unable to tolerate good trials of neuroleptics due to side effects, or those with tardive dyskinesia. The fact that there is a cumulative incidence of agranulocytosis of 2 per cent after a year of treatment with clozapine necessitates weekly CBC monitoring of patients treated with this medication. It has minimal risk for producing extrapyramidal symptoms (EPS), probably does not cause tardive dyskinesia, and is reported to be efficacious in 30 per cent of treatment-resistant schizophrenics.

Most criteria for judging prognosis in schizophrenia are related to short-term outcome and can be summarized by saying that the more acute and florid the early symptoms or, as some have phrased it, the more the patient has "positive" symptoms (delusions, hallucinations, agitation, and depressive symptoms), the more likely he is to recover from the acute episode. The more insidious the onset and the more lacking in emotional display (negative symptoms), the worse the short- and long-term prognoses. The natural history of the illness (even in treated patients) seems to be of two major types: (1) an episodic, relapsing course with each episode resulting in a lower level of psychosocial functioning; and (2) a gradual, slow decline in functional ability. Both courses eventually result in a progressive loss of psychosocial capacities (see Table 451–3). Recent treatment efforts in schizophrenia have taken a rehabilitative, or psychoeducational, approach in which the family is educated about the problems of schizophrenia and issues of living are openly dealt with.

ACUTE USE OF NEUROLEPTIC MEDICATION. Neuroleptic drugs are also useful for patients who are markedly agitated with or without delusions and hallucinations (Table 451–6). They also help to control agitated states associated with organic delirium and dementia. In elderly patients and in those with delirium and/or dementia, the doses should be much lower until the patient's reaction is ascertained. Since acutely agitated psychotic patients respond to lorazepam as well as to neuroleptics, the initial use of benzodiazepines is probably safer in cases in which the source of the agitation is not known and in manic states for which long-term neuroleptic medication is not planned.

Andreasen N (ed.): Brain Imaging: Applications in Psychiatry. Washington, D.C., American Psychiatric Press, 1989. *A comprehensive review of CT, MRI, SPECT, PET, and EEG investigations of behavioral disorders.*

Cloninger C, Martin R, Guze S, et al.: Diagnosis and prognosis in schizophrenia. Arch Gen Psychiatry 42:15–25, 1985. *An excellent study of the implications of symptoms for prognosis in schizophrenia.*

Hogarty G, Anderson C, Reiss A, et al.: Family psychoeducation, social skills training, and maintained chemotherapy in the aftercare treatment of schizophrenia. Arch Gen Psychiatry 43:633–642, 1986. *A convincing review and study of the role of psychosocial factors in the treatment of schizophrenia.*

Kaplan H, Saddock B: Comprehensive Textbook of Psychiatry, 5th ed. Baltimore, Williams & Wilkins, 1989. *An excellent and detailed overview of all aspects of schizophrenia.*

Schulz C, Tamminga C: Schizophrenia: A Scientific Focus. New York, Oxford Press, 1989. *A comprehensive review of current knowledge about schizophrenia.*

Strauss J, Carpenter W: Schizophrenia. New York, Plenum Press, 1981. *A comprehensive presentation of major aspects of schizophrenic disorders.*

AFFECTIVE DISORDERS

A difficulty in clinical psychiatric diagnosis is that similar terms are used to describe feeling states that differ greatly in degree and sometimes in kind. Such is the case with the term *depression.* In common use the meaning may extend from a description of a brief pang of regret to profound feelings of futility and suicidal despair. At what point along this spectrum does one label the condition "illness"? When does normal grief become pathologic? This section discusses these questions.

Many have attempted to classify depressive illnesses based on *symptomatology*, e.g., psychotic versus neurotic; *supposed etiology*, e.g., endogenous versus reactive; or *age*, e.g., childhood, involutional. None of these distinctions has resisted careful investigation. The most recent characterization of depressive illness has been simplified into *bipolar disorders*, identifying wide swings of mood; *major depressive illness*, marked by severe depressive symptoms but without manic swings; and two milder forms, *cyclothymic disorder* and *dysthymic disorder* (formerly called depressive neurosis). These latter two terms describe milder forms of bipolar disorders and depression that fall short of the specific diagnostic criteria for the more serious disorders.

Symptoms of depression also are classified by the company they keep. The psychiatric condition alone would be classified as a primary affective disorder, but when symptoms of affective disorders accompany medical conditions, they are termed secondary affective disorders. Marked depressive symptoms have been noted with various endocrine disorders, tumors, seizure disorders, vitamin deficiencies, and particular neurologic disorders such as multiple sclerosis, Parkinson's disease, and stroke. Depressive symptoms also can be associated with drugs used to treat medical conditions. In at least some instances, the consistency of the symptoms may reflect the fact that similar neurotransmitter systems are altered in both the primary and secondary affective disturbances.

Major Depression

The symptomatology and diagnostic criteria for major depression are listed in Table 451–7. Although many patients have single episodes of major depressive illness, the condition also can be repetitive, and this recurrent condition is frequently called unipolar depressive illness. Fifty per cent of patients with a single episode of major depression eventually have another depressive episode.

The key features of major depression are a markedly gloomy mood in which there is a loss of interest in life, a lack of pleasure in almost all activities, and a general feeling of hopelessness and worthlessness. The illness takes the form of a cognitive change in which the patient seemingly looks at the world with "black glasses," and everything thought about or accomplished is minimized or negated: The wealthy and successful career person talks about his or her impending financial doom and general lack of accomplishment in life; the gifted artist dismisses his creations as trivial. When vegetative functions (sleep, appetite, psychomotor activity) are markedly impaired and a complete loss of pleasure accompanies almost all activities with no reactions to pleasurable stimuli, we often add the term *melancholia*.

Depressive symptoms range in severity from mild mood swings to severe delusions about self-worth, accomplishments, and the future. The "blackness" of the presentation in the depressed

TABLE 451–7. MAJOR DEPRESSIVE EPISODE*

A. At least five of the following symptoms have been present during the same 2-week period; at least one of the symptoms was either 1 or 2 below and not related to a physical condition. These symptoms can be subjective reports or reported by others and must occur nearly every day.
  1. Depressed mood most of the day (e.g., the patient feels "down" or "low")
  2. Loss of interest or pleasure in all or almost all activities
  3. Significant weight loss or weight gain when not dieting or binge-eating (e.g., more than 5 per cent of body weight in a month), or decrease or increase in appetite
  4. Insomnia or hypersomnia
  5. Psychomotor agitation or retardation
  6. Fatigue or loss of energy
  7. Feelings of worthlessness or excessive or inappropriate guilt (which may be delusional)
  8. Diminished ability to think or concentrate, or indecisiveness
  9. Thoughts that he or she would be better off dead, or suicidal ideation, nearly every day; a suicide attempt
B. 1. An organic etiology has been ruled out
  2. Not a normal reaction to the loss of a loved one
C. Not superimposed on schizophrenia

*Modified from American Psychiatric Association: Diagnostic and Statistical Manual of Mental Disorders, 3rd ed., rev. Washington, DC, APA, 1987. Used with permission.

patient is most often accompanied by severe motor retardation with profound sleep and appetite disturbance and suicidal ideation. Nevertheless, some severe depressions can present in a highly anxious, agitated state. The history of previous episodes (either manic or depressive) aids in the diagnosis.

Affective Disorders in the Elderly

The increasing precision of psychiatric diagnosis has made it evident that at the two ends of life, i.e., childhood and aging, the psychopathology of affective disorders is less distinct than during the years between. Elderly patients may have many dysphoric symptoms but not meet the precise diagnostic criteria for major affective disorder. Diagnosis in the elderly is also complicated by two factors: (1) the behavioral and cognitive changes caused by the aging of the central nervous system (although, other than minor memory impairments, the presence of cognitive impairments should make one consider a more comprehensive workup for dementia), and (2) the presence of other medical illnesses and their attendant medications.

The most common psychiatric symptoms in community populations of older adults are those of depression (15 per cent), hypochondriasis (14 per cent), suspiciousness (17 per cent), and persecutory ideation (4 per cent). As many as one third complain of difficulty in falling asleep, awakening during the night, or being sleepy during the day. All these symptom rates increase for the institutionalized elderly. By contrast, cases fulfilling the specific diagnoses of major depression, dysthymia, and schizophrenia occur at a much lower rate than in younger populations.

Although the aged patient may not meet full diagnostic criteria for affective disturbance, persistent symptomatology nevertheless deserves a trial of cautious pharmacologic intervention. This is particularly true when one looks at elderly patients who have cognitive impairments. Community samples of aged populations show about a 4 to 5 per cent prevalence of severe cognitive impairment. The figure may not entirely reflect degenerative brain disease, however, since the biologic changes that occur with affective illness also can cause cognitive impairments detected by both neuropsychological testing and clinical neurologic examination. This is true in younger populations as well. The abnormalities can include not only problems with memory and orientation, but signs of minor neurologic impairment as well; all may clear after a trial of antidepressive medication. The term "pseudodementia" has been used for these potentially treatable cognitive changes in elderly affectively disordered patients.

DIAGNOSIS. The diagnosis is made on clinical grounds as discussed above. Many tests to aid the diagnosis of depression have been introduced, including the dexamethasone suppression test (DST), the thyroid-stimulating hormone (TSH) response (see below), and many measures of disturbed sleep function such as rapid eye movement (REM) latency. Unfortunately, none has proved to be diagnostically reliable or specific for affective disorder. In diagnosing depression, the interview is central.

EPIDEMIOLOGY. The sex distribution of major depression is almost two-to-one female to male. The peak incidence for women is 35 to 45 years, whereas the age pattern is less clear for men. There may also be an increased incidence in women in their early 50's. The prevalence is about 3.2 per 100 males and about 4.5 to 9.3 per 100 females. Incidence is 82 to 201 new cases per 100,000 for men and 247 to 598 new cases per 100,000 for women. The mean duration of first attack of an untreated depressive illness is about 13 months. The episodes, if they recur, are likely to be similar in nature and respond to treatment in a similar fashion. As with bipolar illness, alcoholism is a frequent complication of depressive illness, particularly when it has a recurring course.

Patients in primary care clinics (5 to 10 per cent) and on medical inpatient services (15 per cent) show an increased prevalence of depression.

PATHOPHYSIOLOGY. Pathophysiologic theories of affective disorders have developed along three major lines: (1) endocrine studies; (2) neurotransmitters; and (3) electrophysiologic studies. Depressed patients frequently have elevated levels of cortical steroids in the blood and urine and at least half fail to suppress cortisol secretion after dexamethasone administration. Thyroid-stimulating hormone (TSH) response to thyrotropin-releasing hormone also has been found to be aberrant in many depressed patients, even though their blood T_3 and T_4 levels are normal. Growth hormone, prolactin, gonadal hormones, CRF, and melatonin have all been shown to have diminished responses in subgroups of affective disorders. Although none of these findings is specific for any type of depressive illness or consistent in all depressive illnesses, they nevertheless suggest the presence of pituitary-hypothalamic dysfunction in affective disorders.

Studies of neurotransmitters in depression have been stimulated largely by the success of pharmacologic agents used to treat affective disorders. Many of the tricyclic compounds and the MAO inhibitors effective in the treatment of depression increase the availability of catecholamines and indolamines in the central nervous system. L-Dopa, used to treat Parkinson's disease, is a major catecholamine (dopamine) precursor and may in itself induce mania. These and other observations have given rise to the catecholamine-indolamine hypothesis of depression. The theory postulates that a certain level of amines and/or receptor sensitivity to catecholamines functions to generate a normal mood. Receptor insensitivity, a depletion of amines, or a decrease in their synthesis or storage leads to depression. Conversely, if the amines are in excess or the receptors are hypersensitive, mania may develop. Recently, the acetylcholine system has also been implicated in affective disorders, a "balance" between adrenergic and cholinergic function being postulated as necessary for the stabilization of mood. Neither theory, however, is entirely satisfactory, since it has been found that the tricyclic drugs affect many receptor systems and that their main action may be one of changing or regulating the sensitivity of the receptor rather than acting directly as neurotransmitters. Furthermore, newer drugs that have antidepressant effects do not affect these transmitter systems. One study, for example, has found that the anticonvulsant carbamazepine favorably affects the course of certain patients with bipolar illness.

Electrophysiologic studies on affective illness have concentrated on changes in sleep functions, especially the presence of changes in the REM sleep pattern during episodes of active illness. A subgroup of patients with affective disorder shows a shortened REM latency. Furthermore, analyses of circadian rhythms provide increasing evidence for autumn and winter precipitation of some bipolar disorders, with depressive illnesses apparently related to diminished ambient light in winter climates. The change has been correlated with alterations of melatonin metabolism.

TREATMENT. In most cases the physician is presented with someone who seems mildly sad and self-deprecating, with perhaps slight sleep and appetite disturbances. In such patients an attempt at counseling about the events in their lives and helping delineate appropriate priorities and activities, along with prescriptions for adequate exercise, diet, rest, and general health measures, may suffice. When symptoms become more marked, particularly when they disturb sleep and appetite, and the person becomes unable to perform work, school, or household tasks, one should consider adding antidepressant medication to the above regimen (Table 451–8). If the mild symptoms have been present for a number of years, a trial of medication may be in order. With prominent depressive symptomatology hospitalization may be necessary, the major indication being to prevent suicide (15 per cent of patients with major affective disorders commit suicide). As discussed in a later section, it is a wise step in medicine to ask all patients with depression of mood, apathetic fatigue, or ill-defined somatic symptoms if they have ever considered the situation sufficiently unbearable that suicide becomes an option.

The approach and response to drug therapy in depression vary considerably among both physicians and patients. Perhaps the best prediction of a favorable response is if a blood relative has responded well to a similar agent. In patients who present primarily with insomnia and marked vegetative disturbances as well as some agitation, amitriptyline (or nortriptyline) is somewhat more sedating, particularly if given at bedtime. Imipramine (or desipramine) is less sedating and often avoids the drowsiness that amitriptyline causes. After initial CBC, liver profiles, and in older patients an ECG, it is best to start these medications in single

TABLE 451–8. ANTIDEPRESSANT DRUGS

Dose	Daily Dosage Range (mg)*	Anticholinergic Effects
Tricyclics		
Imipramine (Tofranil)	50–150	+ +
Amitriptyline (Elavil)	50–150	+ + +
Nortriptyline (Aventyl)	50–150	+ +
Desipramine (Norpramin, Pertofrane)	50–150	+
Doxepin (Sinequan)	150	+ +
Tetracyclic		
Maprotiline (Ludiomil)	50–225	+
Other		
Fluoxetine (Prozac)	20–80	0
Buproprion (Wellbutrin)	300–450	0
Trazodone (Desyrel)	150–600	0
MAOI's†		
Phenelzine (Nardil)	15–90	+ +
Tranylcypromine (Parnate)	20–30	+ +

*In most cases the dose should be reduced 30 to 50 per cent in the elderly and medically ill.
†Monoamine oxidase inhibitors.

doses at bedtime. An initial starting dose of 50 mg may be rapidly increased every several days until a total dosage of 150 mg per night is reached. As stated earlier, with elderly patients all psychotropic drugs should be used cautiously, and doses of antidepressants should be decreased by 30 to 50 per cent from the above. For example, one would start an elderly patient on 10 or 25 mg of an antidepressant such as amitriptyline (nortriptyline) at bedtime or even every other night. For prolonged treatment the elderly may often respond to smaller doses (10 to 75 mg). However, if after 6 weeks the elderly patient has not responded to doses as high as 75 mg and there are no marked side effects, doses can be slowly increased. In the normal adult without medical illness, if there is no response to 150 mg per day within 6 weeks, then the dosage can often be increased to as much as 200 to 300 mg (this is beyond manufacturers' guidelines). It is wise, however, to obtain the counsel of a specialist prior to using these doses. If there is still no response one could switch to another tricyclic or immediately to an MAOI. Blood level measurements are available for most of the tricyclic antidepressants, although their main usefulness is to indicate that the person is taking and absorbing the drug. Only nortriptyline has had an effective therapeutic window (50 to 140 ng per milliliter) established.

It is useful to caution patients that the antidepressants do not produce an immediate response, although if given at bedtime they may improve sleeping immediately. Also, the prominent anticholinergic side effects and hypotension are often a bother, and patients should be forewarned. Some of the supposed side effects of the medication are also accompaniments of the depressive illness, and patients, if questioned, may reveal that they have had many of the symptoms prior to taking the medication. Several of the new antidepressants, fluoxetine and buproprion, have entirely different actions and have succeeded when traditional medications have failed. One must recognize that the tricyclics have a quinidine-like effect and have been used to treat some cardiac arrhythmias.

For patients who fail to respond to tricyclic antidepressants, psychiatric consultation is critical. However, some have found it useful to add 0.25 µg per day of triiodothyronine (T_3) to the tricyclic dosage, particularly in female patients. Also, the addition of lithium to tricyclic regimens has been found to have a marked augmenting effect on the response to antidepressant tricyclics (neither of the above is in FDA-approved use).

The monoamine oxidase inhibitors (MAOI's) have enjoyed a return to usage recently with the introduction of fluoxetine and buproprion. They had been underutilized in the United States owing to their tendency to cause hypertensive crises following the ingestion of foods containing tyramine. However, for patients not responding to tricyclic medications or those with atypical depressions marked predominantly by anxiety symptoms, they are quite effective. Patients can be started on MAOI drugs immediately following tricyclic cessation. The reverse, however, does not hold, and patients stopping an MAOI drug must wait 7 to 14 days before starting a tricyclic antidepressant. If dietary restrictions are followed and sympathetic amine medications are avoided, MAOI's are usually safe, their major side effects being hypotension and insomnia. They have milder anticholinergic effects and often are easier to tolerate than the tricyclic antidepressants, but the specific side effects and indications for use are still being delineated.

In older patients, in those who fail to respond to pharmacotherapeutic interventions, and in those with complicated medical conditions which the drugs might adversely affect, electroconvulsive therapy (ECT) is probably the safest treatment. Whereas 60 per cent of most affective disturbances respond to pharmacotherapy, close to 80 per cent improve after ECT. There are few contraindications: When ECT is administered in association with modern anesthetic techniques, the morbidity is reduced to that of the anesthesia alone. With careful monitoring, even patients with recent cerebral or myocardial insults can be treated with ECT.

PROGNOSIS. Antidepressant drugs should be continued for 6 to 20 weeks after patients become free of symptoms. More prolonged treatment is desirable for those who have had recurrent episodes. Many patients have been maintained for years on tricyclic antidepressants and MAOI's without major impairment. Nevertheless, in spite of the best treatment, between 15 and 20 per cent of depressives go on to a chronic course. Most patients with a single episode continue to function well and, in fact, often tend to use the depressive episode as a chance to reorient and reorganize their lives and proceed to function better than they had previously.

Dysthymic Disorder (Depressive Neurosis)

DEFINITION. The symptoms consist of a depressed mood of longstanding duration with a severity less intense than in a major depressive disorder. These patients often seem to have situational reasons for their illness. Many present primarily with physical complaints to physicians. Substance and drug abuse, as well as personality profiles that involve dependency and obsessional symptomatology, are often part of the clinical picture. The diagnostic criteria are outlined in Table 451–9.

EPIDEMIOLOGY. As this condition is treated in many settings, the epidemiologic distribution is difficult to determine. One estimate of prevalence is 60 per 1000. Women predominate and familial patterns have not been established.

PATHOPHYSIOLOGY. There is evidence that various personality conflicts and situational precipitants are related to these conditions more than to the other affective disorders.

TREATMENT. Many types of short-term psychotherapy have been effective in treating these conditions. Patients who respond poorly to psychotherapy often benefit from antidepressant medication.

GRIEF REACTIONS

Physicians often find it emotionally difficult to deal with the relatives of patients who have died or been seriously injured, yet

---

TABLE 451–9. DYSTHYMIA*

A. At least 2 years (1 year for children and adolescents) during which there has been depressed mood most of the day, more days than not (either by subjective account, e.g., feels "down" or "low," or is observed by others to look sad or depressed) and at least two of the following:
1. Poor appetite or overeating
2. Insomnia or hypersomnia
3. Low energy or fatigue
4. Low self-esteem
5. Poor concentration or difficulty making decisions
6. Pessimism
B. During that 2-year period the patient is never without the above symptoms for more than 2 months at a time.
C. No clear evidence of a major depressive episode during the first 2 years of the disturbance.
D. Has never had a manic episode.
E. No psychotic symptoms and symptoms not the residual phase of schizophrenia.
F. Not sustained by a specific organic factor or substance, e.g., prolonged administration of an antihypertensive medication.

*Modified from American Psychiatric Association: Diagnostic and Statistical Manual of Mental Disorders, 3rd ed., rev. Washington, DC, APA, 1987. Used with permission.

---

such contacts provide important preventive medicine. Grief should be looked upon as a biologic process with psychological roots. Issues of loss and attachment are extremely prominent in bereavement. In normal bereavement 50 per cent of persons experience depressed mood, sleep disturbances, and crying lasting anywhere from 2 to 6 months. Furthermore, many grief reactions resolve only slowly over a number of years. This is particularly true in older persons who have lost spouses of many years' duration.

During bereaved states general health deteriorates, and there is often an increase in serious illness. A decrease in lymphocyte responses in husbands during mourning has been described. Some persons lose contact with reality and blame themselves, constantly asking, "Why did this happen?" Others even have difficulty in accepting that the person is dead. Anger and withdrawal can prevail. Some survivors, particularly when the death was violent, experience stress responses similar to those of combat veterans, who in addition to the symptoms related above may have frequent and often violent intrusive mental images.

These normal reactions can blur into a more serious state with intense and prolonged symptoms lasting 6 months or more. Some survivors undergo a delayed response, functioning well immediately after the event but experiencing later symptoms of bereavement, often precipitated by the death of another person or the anniversary of the death of the loved one. Others can develop hypochondriacal symptoms resembling those of the deceased. Panic attacks and depressive illness may develop also in prolonged grief reactions.

The prevention and treatment of grief reactions can often be undertaken by the physician in his normal contact with the bereaved survivor. Lindeman has outlined several valid principles: (1) Allow the patient to share his feelings about the death of the relative. The physician can be extremely helpful in discussing the normal process of grief and the reactions that people experience. (2) Review the relationships of the deceased with the important people in their lives. (3) Help grieving persons to accept their feelings and fears about things such as their ability to cope, their fears about "going crazy," anger, etc. (4) Discuss with the bereaved how they are adapting to the stress and what modes they are using to cope. (5) Attempt to formulate the future relationships between the bereaved and others in their lives. (6) Find new persons with whom the bereaved can develop relationships.

While the above matters can only be touched on in the acute situation, they often can be dealt with over time. Even the gathering of information about these areas is often seen as useful by the patient. If the condition progresses to an abnormal degree, the use of medications for the appropriate conditions, e.g., affective disturbance or panic disorder, is indicated. The use of mild sedation and hypnotics at the acute stage is also useful. Support groups have been organized to deal with both the normal and excessive processes of grieving and appear to be useful.

SUICIDAL BEHAVIOR

About 75 per cent of patients who actually commit suicide will have seen a physician within the previous 6 months. Most practicing physicians encounter half a dozen potentially suicidal patients per year, among whom 10 to 12 actually do away with themselves over the ensuing years. The figures illustrate how important it is for the physician to detect various clues. Suicide is higher in patients with psychiatric problems, with the highest incidence occurring in those with affective disorders or alcoholism or those who are in the early post-hospital phase of schizophrenic disorders. Suicidal behavior is not specific to any one major psychiatric disturbance. For example, about the same percentage of schizophrenic patients commit suicide as do patients with major depression. Suicidal behavior occurs across a spectrum of mental illness, and a good argument can be made that it should be treated as a distinct problem separate from the major psychiatric disorders. Effective pharmacologic treatments for depression and schizophrenia have been available since the 1950's, yet there is no evidence that these treatments have reduced the suicidality of either population. Therapy that may be pertinent in reducing suicidality includes techniques to enhance one's social supports, development of problem-solving and other coping skills, and treatments designed to reduce alcohol use, especially during periods of stress. Pharmacologic interventions aimed specifically at suicidal behavior, interventions that, for the most part, involve manipulation of the serotonergic system, are now being investigated.

The typical patient who makes a suicide attempt is a white female, 20 to 40 years of age, who ingests pills, usually after an interpersonal conflict. By contrast, the typical successful suicide victim is a white male, 45 years of age or older, often separated, widowed, or divorced, who lives alone and may be unemployed or retired. Patients who commit suicide suffer a high incidence of poor physical health, medical care within the past 6 months, and evidence of some psychiatric disturbance. Many have a previous history of suicide attempts or threats.

Doctors often feel more awkward than their patients in discussing suicidal thoughts or intent. It must be done understandingly, but almost all seriously ill adults should be asked gently if they have had thoughts about death or suicide. Comments patients make about feeling they would be "better off dead" or "people would be better off without me" should be taken seriously. Preoccupations with funerals, cemetery lots, and the buying of weapons should make one suspicious. Any patient who presents with vague complaints should be asked about his or her emotional state. If any indication of suicidal intent is forthcoming, one must immediately evaluate its seriousness, inquiring about the following: (1) Has the person considered actual suicide? If so, what plans have been made and how specifically? The more specific, the more worrisome. (2) What other psychopathology exists? Is the patient agitated, seriously depressed, etc.? (3) What precipitating stresses exist? (4) Are there people in the environment whom the person trusts and who could help? (5) Will the person agree to work with you and contact you if his suicidal feelings intensify? (6) If no reassurance comes from the patient or relatives that the situation can be managed at home, hospitalization may be necessary.

An even more difficult evaluation is how to treat those who have made a recent unsuccessful suicide attempt. After a suicide attempt there often is a brief period of days to weeks of lightening of the depressive mood, after which strong self-destructive feelings reappear. The more lethal the risk (i.e., the higher was the potential risk of death in the initial suicide attempt), the more determined should be the effort to provide psychiatric treatment, preferably in a hospital. If patients express an explicit intent to die, often stated with determination and conviction, there is no question about the necessity for hospitalization.

Most patients after suicide attempts should have a psychiatric consultation, but sometimes this may not be possible and the nonpsychiatric physician must assess the suicidal potential. Part of the evaluation of the patient can also serve as the initial formation of a doctor-patient relationship. If they have a supportive environment and will keep contact, some of these patients can be managed as outpatients. Physicians should be aware of writing potentially lethal prescriptions for patients who may have suicidal tendencies. For example, for a routine dosage schedule of tricyclic antidepressants (150 mg per day), even a week's supply provides a potentially lethal overdose.

SUICIDE IN ADOLESCENTS. Nine to 18 per cent of children and adolescents have made suicide attempts. This astoundingly high figure correlates with turmoil in the family as well as disturbed parent/child interactions. There are also significant correlations with substance abuse, depressive illness, and conduct disorders in children and adolescents as well as histories of physical and sexual abuse. Many of these children and adolescents had threatened suicide previously. Many have done poorly in school and have records of chronically aggressive behavior. One of the most difficult questions which faces the psychiatrist is whether to hospitalize an adolescent at risk for suicide. The answer relates primarily to the severity of the suicidal behavior and the patient's intent to "be dead." Interestingly, in adolescents, it also relates to the presence of assaultive behavior in that the hostility toward self can also be directed against others. The enviromental supports available to see someone through a depressive episode also mitigate the need for hospitalization. It is extremely important in treating the adolescent to provide some

form of individual counseling, usually centered around coping skills and cognitive therapy as well to work with the environmental support system or the patient's family. Pharmacologic treatment is quite effective for affective illness in adolescents.

SUICIDE AND AGING. Age groups over age 70 years have a higher suicide rate, with single males at the peak. Some of the risk factors are unemployment, isolation, poor health, pain, feelings of being rejected, history of mental illness, and previous suicide attempts. A history of alcoholism is a high comorbid factor within suicidal behavior. Many elderly pursue indirect suicide by stopping eating or necessary medications. Electroconvulsive therapy is often the most effective form of treatment for suicidal behavior in geriatrics.

Bipolar Disorders

Bipolar disorders (previously called manic-depressive disorders) are probably the most homogeneous diagnostic grouping in psychiatry, as they consist of a marked change in mood that varies from major depressive episodes (as discussed) (see Table 451–7) to significant manic episodes as defined below. There is usually a return to normal behavior between episodes. There is little difficulty in recognizing the illness if one looks at the longitudinal course. However, if patients are examined only briefly, at a particular moment in time, manic excitement can be confused with schizophrenic psychosis. The depressive phase of bipolar illness can also be misconstrued as a catatonic state.

DIAGNOSTIC CRITERIA AND CLINICAL SIGNS AND SYMPTOMS. The manic phase of the illness is characterized by an expansive euphoric mood in which grandiose plans and ideas predominate. It is important to be aware that despite this expansiveness and grandiosity, patients who are frustrated or disagreed with can often become quite irritable and at times aggressive. The major diagnostic criteria are listed in Table 451–10. The patient can be psychotic in the manic phase, with delusions and hallucinations that are consistent with the grandiosity; however, persecutory delusions, feelings of being controlled, etc., can also be present. At times it is difficult to distinguish an excited schizophrenic patient from a manic one. As already stated, one must examine the longitudinal course of the illness, either until the occurrence of a depressive episode or a deteriorating course after remission of the acute symptom, in order to diagnose a schizophrenic process. In all instances, it is crucial to rule out organic factors.

The average age of onset of bipolar disorder is about 30 years, but about 20 per cent of patients have an onset below the age of 20. In females, the onset of the condition seems to have a bimodal distribution, with one peak falling between 20 and 30 years and the other between 40 and 50 years. The peak age of onset of schizophrenia is much younger, but the age of onset of bipolar

TABLE 451–10. MANIC EPISODE*

A. A distinct period (lasting at least 1 week) when mood was abnormally and persistently elevated, expansive, or irritable.

B. During the period of mood disturbance, at least three of the following symptoms have been present to a significant degree:
1. Inflated self-esteem (grandiosity, which may be delusional)
2. Decreased need for sleep, e.g., feels rested after only 3 hours of sleep
3. More talkative than usual or pressure to keep talking
4. Flight of ideas or subjective experience that thoughts are racing
5. Distractibility, i.e., attention too easily drawn to unimportant or irrelevant external stimuli
6. Increase in activity (either socially, at work, or sexually) or physical restlessness
7. Excessive involvement in activities that have a high potential for painful consequences which is not recognized, e.g., buying sprees, sexual indiscretions, foolish business investments, reckless driving

C. The episode of mood disturbance was sufficiently severe to cause marked impairment in occupational functioning, usual social activities, or relationships with others.

D. At no time during the disturbance have there been delusions or hallucinations for as long as 2 weeks in the absence of prominent mood symptoms (i.e., before the mood symptoms developed or after they have remitted), which would be more indicative of schizophrenia.

*Modified from American Psychiatric Association: Diagnostic and Statistical Manual of Mental Disorders, 3rd ed., rev. Washington, DC, APA, 1987. Used with permission.

illness overlaps enough so that the differential diagnosis of a psychotic illness in a young person is difficult and may change as the clinical picture evolves over time. Almost half the patients with bipolar disorders have at least two to three episodes of illness, and as many as one third experience seven or more episodes of illness once the pattern has started. Each episode of illness, whether it is a manic or a depressive phase, can last from 4 to 13 months; some of these go on to chronicity and some are over much sooner. The course of the illness, however, has been modified significantly with the advent of lithium therapy, especially with respect to diminishing both the severity and the frequency of the episodes. The shorter durations are usually related to the effectiveness of the treatment. Although some patients rapidly alternate between extremes over 2 to 4 days, most episodes have a longer duration and, frequently, after a manic phase there can be a subsequent depressive phase. Chronicity, again as opposed to schizophrenia, is not a major problem with manic-depressive illness, being cited as low as 1 per cent in some studies. Mortality with bipolar illness averages between two and two and one-half times the expected rate for that age; suicide occurs in about 8 to 10 per cent.

EPIDEMIOLOGY. The lifetime risk for developing bipolar illness ranges from 0.6 to 0.9 per cent of the population. The incidence per hundred thousand per year in men is from 9 to 15 new cases and for women from 7.4 to 32 new cases. The risk increases with a family history of bipolar illness. The exact mechanism of the genetic transmission in bipolar illness is uncertain but suggests autosomal dominance with incomplete penetration. There is a 72 per cent concordance in monozygotic twins and a 19 per cent concordance in same-sex dizygotic twins. Both the course of illness and the response to treatment are similar among blood relatives. In one well-studied Amish family, the abnormal gene has been identified on chromosome 11. Other families with equally strong genetic patterns, however, have not possessed this particular chromosomal alteration.

PATHOPHYSIOLOGY. Most of what is known about the pathophysiology of bipolar illness is similar to what is known about the biology of the major depressive disorders.

DIAGNOSIS AND TREATMENT. The treatment of bipolar disorders has three distinct aspects: the manic episode, the major depressive episode, and long-term maintenance therapy. Prior to any specific therapy, an adequate medical workup is necessary in order to be certain that the patient suffers from a primary affective illness. The patient in an acute manic state is delusional, grandiose, and hyperactive and in this condition looks similar to any patient with psychosis. If this is the first episode, one cannot differentiate this state phenomenologically from the first episode of schizophrenia or a psychosis due to physical illness. The major differential diagnosis of the first episode rests on a careful history, family history, and physical and laboratory examination (see Table 451–3). The past history and the nature of onset of the illness are important, as noted previously. Furthermore, most psychiatric disorders have a familial pattern. A psychiatrist should be involved in the evaluation of patients who present with their first psychotic episode.

The treatment of the acute manic phase is usually undertaken in the hospital, as it is imperative to protect the patient from his own misdeeds, e.g., spending inordinate amounts of money, making embarrassing speeches, etc. If the family is supportive, however, and feels it can control the situation, treatment can be started outside of the hospital. Lithium is not useful for the acute management of mania and if the patient is severely agitated, sedation is necessary. Neuroleptics are not used in the long-term treatment of bipolar illness, but the use of benzodiazepines, particularly lorazepam, effectively controls most acute manic states (see Table 451–6). If the agitation is marked and not controlled with medication, one should obtain psychiatric consultation to consider using ECT to control the manic excitement. Manic excitement creates a medical emergency in which patients can die from exhaustion.

Although most general physicians treat acute mania rarely, the use of lithium is something they may encounter more often. Lithium effectively prevents relapses in over 60 per cent of bipolar illnesses. The drug is slightly more effective in preventing manic relapses than the depressive episodes, and its most specific use seems to be in preventing manic recurrences. Nevertheless, its use should be considered with any repetitive affective disturbance.

Prior to the beginning of lithium therapy, a CBC, urinalysis, electrolytes, creatinine, BUN, thyroid studies, and a baseline ECG and EEG should be obtained. Chronic medical illnesses, especially renal insufficiency, can contraindicate use of the agent. Lithium has a half-life of 24 to 36 hours, and it takes at least 4 days to achieve a steady state. The specific therapeutic effectiveness is not evident until at least 4 to 10 days after institution of therapy. Consequently, lithium is not a good medication for the acutely agitated or manic patient but should be started early in anticipation of maintenance use. It is necessary to monitor the serum level of lithium, adequate levels for acute illness being in the range of 0.8 to 1.4 mEq per liter. For maintenance therapy, satisfactory responses accompany blood levels of 0.4 mEq per liter. Dose and blood level, however, should be titrated against clinical effectiveness for each patient. Once maintenance levels are reached patients usually can be maintained for long periods with minimal contact. Doses usually are given twice daily, as absorption from the gastrointestinal tract is rapid and the drug peaks in the serum within 1 to 2 hours. Serum lithium levels of more than 2 mEq per liter are highly dangerous and represent a medical emergency requiring immediate hospitalization and, sometimes, hemodialysis. Of most concern with regard to side effects in the long-term use of lithium is the development of mild leukocytosis, hypothyroidism, diabetes insipidus, and, occasionally, renal tubular damage. While these long-term side effects are not trivial, they are uncommon and must be weighed against the propensity of untreated patients to be chronically hospitalized. For patients who do not respond to lithium therapy or cannot tolerate it, increasingly encouraging reports describe the effective use of carbamazepine and other anticonvulsants in treating bipolar conditions.

The depressive phase of bipolar illness is treated the same as any major depressive disorder, as outlined previously.

Patients with bipolar disorders are often reluctant to continue with their medications, particularly lithium, as they feel it inhibits them, decreases their energy, or even affects their creativity. Consequently, a good deal of discussion about these issues is pertinent for the patient and especially for the family. The enlistment and assistance of the family of the patient with bipolar disorder are important. During either acute mania or severe depressive reactions, verbal interventions are often difficult, and it is useful simply to repeat some major reassuring statements—that they are a patient, that they are going to get better, and that this is not their normal state. While the role of precipitants is not clear in the onset of bipolar illness, it is important for patients to remain in treatment, and this can often be accomplished by helping them understand what situations seem to be stressful in their lives. Family and marital counseling often is useful.

PROGNOSIS. The more episodes a patient has had, the more likely he is to have another. Nevertheless, if one takes as indices of outcome successful marital and occupational adjustment, approximately two thirds of patients do well. About 15 per cent have some improvement, and the remainder do poorly. While manic or depressive episodes may cause much acute social disruption, including job loss and marital strife, the wide spacing of episodes often spares long-term social decay. Patients with bipolar disease usually function normally between episodes. Accordingly, a major goal of treatment is to protect the patient during episodes so as to minimize social disruption. Nevertheless, while the prognosis is not as devastating as in schizophrenia, it is still fraught with a significant amount of periodic and, sometimes, long-term functional disability.

Busse E, Blazer D: Geriatric Psychiatry. Washington, D.C., American Psychiatric Press, 1989. *An excellent and comprehensive review of geriatric psychiatry.*

Conte H, Plutchik R, Wild K, et al.: Combined psychotherapy and pharmacotherapy for depression. Arch Gen Psychiatry 43:471–480, 1986. *A good review of treatment of unipolar depression.*

Hodgkinson S, Sherrington R, Gurling H, et al.: Molecular genetic evidence for heterogeneity in manic depression. Nature 325:805, 1987. *Study of three large Icelandic kindreds indicates that although a single autosomal dominant allele predisposes to bipolar illness, linkage analysis does not incriminate the abnormal gene locus on chromosome 11. Genetic heterogeneity appears to underlie the expression of the manic-depressive phenotype.*

Katon W, Roy-Burne P: Antidepressants in the medically ill. Clin Chem 34:829–836, 1980. *A useful and necessary article for treating depressed medical patients.*

Michels R (ed.): Psychiatry. Philadelphia, J.B. Lippincott Company, 1985. *Excellent and detailed overview of affective disorders, especially with respect to treatment.*

Parkes CM, Weise RS: Recovery from Bereavement. New York, Basic Books, 1983. *Excellent summary of treatment of grief.*

Pfeffer CR: Clinical perspectives on treatment of suicidal behavior among children and adolescents. Psychiatr Ann 20:143–153, 1990. *An excellent general article on the management of suicidal behavior in children, adolescents, applicable to adults as well.*

Post RM, Ballenger J: Neurobiology of Mood Disorders. Baltimore, Williams & Wilkins, 1984. *A comprehensive overview of biologic and pharmacologic aspects of affective disorders.*

Shucter S, Zisook S.: Treatment of spousal bereavement. Psychiatr Ann 16:295–308, 1986. *An excellent discussion of treatment of bereavement.*

Simons A, Murphy G, Levine J, et al.: Cognitive therapy and pharmacotherapy for depression. Arch Gen Psychiatry 43:43–50, 1986. *A study of the use of cognitive therapy in depression.*

ANXIETY DISORDERS

Anxiety is the most ubiquitous psychiatric symptom. It occurs as part of most major psychiatric syndromes, particularly depressive ones, and represents several semidistinct entities. Anxiety also accompanies at least some aspects of most normal lives, and it can be an effective stimulus to improved performance. The performance curve follows an inverted U: A little anxiety can improve performance, performance then plateaus as the anxiety increases, and eventually too much anxiety causes a decrease in the ability to function. Currently, anxiety disorders are divided into two major categories: (1) panic disorders, which are episodic, "attack-like" symptoms; and (2) generalized anxiety disorder, which is a persistent state of anxiety.

Most patients with anxiety symptoms, including those with panic disorder, consult a general physician first. Such patients, who are extremely high users of medical services, usually complain vaguely that "something is wrong." A retrospective study of 55 patients with panic disorder referred for psychiatric consultation from primary care physicians revealed that 89 per cent initially presented with one or two somatic complaints and, in most, somatic misdiagnoses continued for months or years. The most frequent symptom patterns were (1) cardiac (chest pains, tachycardia, irregular heartbeat); (2) gastrointestinal (epigastric distress); and (3) neurologic (headache, dizziness/vertigo, syncope, or paresthesias). In a random survey of 195 patients in a primary care practice screened with structured interviews, 13 per cent met DSM-III criteria for panic disorder.

DIAGNOSTIC CRITERIA AND CLINICAL SIGNS AND SYMPTOMS. A panic attack produces a distinct symptomatic event. There is a precipitous sensation of feelings of fear, impending doom, or imminent death, accompanied by a potential host of physical symptoms (Table 451–11). Affected patients often complain of the physical symptoms in an agitated state. These circumstances differ markedly from chronic anxiety states, in which symptoms are more gradual and do not create life-threatening fears. Generalized anxiety disorder is a pervasive feeling of anxiety or "nervousness" that lacks the attack-like characteristics of panic disorder. The symptoms of generalized anxiety disorders are mainly muscle tension, autonomic hyperactivity, and apprehensive hypervigilant behavior.

A strong association links agoraphobia and panic attacks. Agoraphobia is defined as a morbid fear and avoidance of being alone or being in public places, resulting in a marked restriction of travel, often to the point of becoming housebound. In many cases the agoraphobia is secondary to panic attacks: The patient restricts activities for fear of having a panic attack and thereby develops an agoraphobic profile. Consequently, one looks for the presence of panic attacks or panic attack–like symptoms in patients with agoraphobia, as they often respond to the same treatment given for panic attacks. Simple phobias, e.g., fear of flying, heights, snakes, respond better to behavioral management than to drug treatment and are usually associated with generalized anxiety rather than panic-like episodes.

EPIDEMIOLOGY. Recent epidemiologic studies of panic disorder have noted a prevalence rate of 0.4 to 1.2 per 100. The rates are highest in persons aged 25 to 44 years and in the separated and divorced. The rates are lowest in persons over the age of 64 and bear no relationship to race or education. For agoraphobia the prevalence rates are between 2.5 and 5.8 per 100. There is a marked prevalence for women (two to four times that of men), with an age range of 18 to 64 years. The rates for generalized anxiety disorder range from 2.5 to 6.4 per 100, again slightly more common in young women. Genetic studies have shown that monozygotic twins have higher concordance for anxiety disorders than do dizygotic twins when the proband has panic disorder but not when he has a generalized anxiety disorder.

PATHOPHYSIOLOGY. Panic attacks can be precipitated in susceptible patients by sodium lactate infusions, caffeine (P.O.), CO_2 inhalation, yohimbine (P.O.), isoproterenol (I.V.), and benzodiazepine receptor antagonists. All of these agents interact with the noradrenergic system and particularly the locus coeruleus system, which contains most of the brain's noradrenergic cell bodies. Recent studies of cerebral blood flow and metabolism in patients with panic disorder show asymmetric changes in the parahippocampal region.

TREATMENT. There are two major treatments available for panic attacks, one pharmacologic, the other psychological. The key to treatment is the establishment of a supportive relationship with the patient. Affected patients are often frightened, concerned about "going crazy" and/or dying, and somewhat ashamed of the symptoms. It is useful for the physician immediately to reassure the patient by clarifying that what he experiences is part of a well-known illness that causes these feelings. It is often useful to educate patients with appropriate reading material.

Well-controlled studies have demonstrated the effective treatment of panic attacks with tricyclic antidepressants (particularly imipramine), MAOI's (particularly phenelzine), and the benzodiazepines (particularly alprazolam). The doses and treatment pattern of the tricyclics and the MAOI's are similar to those used for affective disorders, and the dose of alprazolam is usually between 4 and 6 mg per day.* At times the β-blocking agents offer relief, but they are not as dramatic and effective as the antidepressants and alprazolam. The doses of the antidepressants may need to be somewhat higher for these conditions than for affective disorders (tricyclics are usually used in the range of 150 to 300 mg; the MAOI's in the range of 60 mg or more per day—both higher than manufacturers' guidelines). Pharmacologic treatment should last for 6 months to 1 year after response, with the drugs then gradually tapered. β-Blocking agents can be useful for treating the tachycardia and palpitations associated with panic attacks. β Blockers can also be used to decrease the cardiac symptoms associated with tricyclic use, which is often reassuring to the patient.

The treatment of generalized anxiety disorders has less clear guidelines. Although benzodiazepines and psychological interventions are commonly emphasized, their benefit is more difficult to evaluate. A patient on benzodiazepines for 6 to 12 months may experience withdrawal symptoms on cessation of medication.

TABLE 451–11. PANIC DISORDER*

A. At some time during the disturbance, one or more panic attacks (discrete periods of intense discomfort or fear).

B. Either four attacks within a 4-week period, or one or more attacks were followed by a period of persistent fear of having another attack.

C. At least four of the following symptoms during the attacks:
1. Shortness of breath (dyspnea) or smothering sensations
2. Choking sensation
3. Palpitations or accelerated heart rate (tachycardia)
4. Chest pain or discomfort
5. Sweating
6. Dizziness, unsteady feelings, or faintness
7. Nausea or abdominal distress
8. Depersonalization or derealization
9. Numbness or tingling sensations (paresthesias)
10. Flushes (hot flashes) or chills
11. Trembling or shaking
12. Fear of dying
13. Fear of going crazy or of doing something uncontrolled

D. An organic etiology (e.g., amphetamine or caffeine intoxication, hyperthyroidism) has been ruled out.

*Modified from American Psychiatric Association: Diagnostic and Statistical Manual of Mental Disorders, 3rd ed., rev. Washington, DC, APA, 1987. Used with permission.

*Exceeds manufacturer's recommended dosage.

Furthermore, one must be concerned and cautious about the addicting potential of the benzodiazepines and to some extent the tricyclics. Consequently, the treatment of generalized anxiety disorders should rely heavily on counseling, relaxation techniques, behavioral modification, exercise, etc., rather than on prolonged pharmacologic interventions.

Certain medical conditions can simulate panic attacks and must be excluded. These include arrhythmias, angina, respiratory illnesses, asthma, obstructive pulmonary disease, various endocrine disturbances (hyperthyroidism, pheochromocytoma), seizure disorders, vertiginous conditions, and pharmacologic stimulants and caffeine. Withdrawal syndromes can simulate panic-like states, particularly withdrawal from central nervous system depressants (e.g., barbiturates and, occasionally, benzodiazepines). Medical conditions that are often noted in patients with severe panic attacks include episodic hypertensive episodes, peptic ulcer disorder, and mitral valve prolapse.

Sequelae of the Vietnam conflict caused considerable interest on *post-traumatic stress disorders*. The basic differentiation of post-traumatic stress disorder from generalized anxiety disorder is the presence of a clear antecedent that is recognizable as potentially causing symptoms of distress in almost anyone. Another major characteristic of post-traumatic stress disorder is the feeling of re-experiencing the trauma, through either recurring or intrusive recollections, dreams, or sudden feelings that the event is about to recur. Patients often exhibit a lack of emotional responsiveness or involvement with the world after the trauma. Other symptoms may include hyperalertness, "startle responses," sleep disturbance, guilt, and memory and concentration difficulties. Affected persons may avoid activities that could evoke recollections of the traumatic event. While medications are sometimes useful for acute symptoms (especially if accompanied by panic attacks or depressive symptoms), the major treatment of post-traumatic stress is psychotherapeutic, particularly group sessions. At times narcosynthesis has been used successfully.

PROGNOSIS IN ANXIETY DISORDERS. The ubiquity of anxiety symptoms and the blurring of panic disorder into generalized anxiety or chronic anxiety and phobic states, as well as a strong association with depressive illness, make a prognosis difficult to establish. In general, panic disorder may run a limited course with episodic patterns; long periods of remission can intervene with no symptomatology at all. Only about one quarter of patients with panic disorder are treated, implying a high incidence of spontaneous remission in cases that do not come to medical attention. Nevertheless, many patients become housebound for a significant part of their lives. Follow-up studies of 5 to 20 years' duration show that about 50 to 60 per cent of the patients recovered or were much improved. Drug abuse and alcoholism are potentially serious complications.

Katon W, et al.: Chest pain: Relationships of psychiatric illness to coronary arteriographic results. Am J Med 84:1–9, 1988. *An excellent overview of the relation between anxiety and somatic symptoms.*

Klerman G (ed.): Update on anxiety and panic disorders. J Clinic Psychiatry, Supplement to Vol. 47, 1986. *This whole issue is an up-to-date review of all aspects of anxiety disorders, diagnosis, treatment, and research.*

Roy-Burne P, Katon W: An update of treatment of anxiety disorders. Hosp Commun Psychiatry 38:835–843, 1987. *A complete update of treatment.*

Sonnenberg S, Blank A, Talbott J: The Trauma of War. Washington DC, American Psychiatric Press, 1985. *A good review of current knowledge on post-traumatic stress disorder.*

SOMATIZATION DISORDERS

Somatization disorders consist of psychologically engendered symptoms suggesting organ dysfunction for which associated physical or laboratory dysfunction is either absent or trivial in relation to the degree of complaint. If physicians can find no clear biologic mechanism for a set of symptoms because they are too vague, diffuse, or disparate (or even anatomically impossible) and the symptoms could fulfill some purpose in the patient's life (e.g., would help to avoid some area of responsibility, deny failure, evoke increased attention by the family or others, etc.), they should have a high index of suspicion of a purely psychological disorder. However, these patients should not be treated lightly. Many vague symptoms arise early in organic disease, and patients must be examined carefully, supported, and followed. For example, among one group of 85 patients diagnosed as hysterical, 42 were given a diagnosis 10 years later of an organic

TABLE 451–12. COMMON FEATURES IN THE HISTORIES OF PATIENTS WITH SOMATIZATION SYMPTOMS

1. Developmental histories of gross neglect, child abuse, and/or sexual abuse
2. Unstable adult relationships characterized by multiple divorces and often physical violence
3. Past family histories of alcoholism
4. A past history of alcohol abuse prior to the start of somatization
5. Past history of substance abuse
6. A positive review of systems on medical history
7. A polysurgery history
8. A history of litigious relationships with authority figures
9. Past history of psychiatric illness
10. Modeling of pain behavior in their families as ways of solving problems and coping with intimate relationships

disease that could have explained their initial symptoms. In a similar manner patients with unfounded symptoms should also be evaluated for major depression and panic disorder, as those conditions can present primarily with somatic complaints. Patients who tend to present with somatization often have histories that are characterized by disturbed interpersonal relations and emotional disruptions (Table 451–12).

Diverse disorders can present with medically unfounded somatic symptoms, including such disparate conditions as somatization disorder (Briquet's syndrome), hypochondriasis, conversion disorder (hysteria), psychogenic pain disorders, factitious disorders, and malingering. What ties these conditions together are the following characteristics: (1) symptoms that suggest a physical disorder; (2) no demonstrable clinical signs or clear physiologic mechanism evident; (3) some evidence that the symptoms may be associated with psychological factors; (4) symptoms that do not seem to be under voluntary control (except in malingering and factitious disorder).

Somatization disorder, or Briquet's syndrome, has been studied in most detail and is a condition manifested by frequent and recurrent multiple somatic complaints, usually beginning before the age of 30.

DIAGNOSTIC CRITERIA AND CLINICAL SIGNS AND SYMPTOMS. If one looks at the diagnostic criteria for somatization disorder, the number and variety of somatic symptoms are impressive (Table 451–13). It is also evident from the range of these symptoms that patients meeting these criteria have all types of somatic symptoms, from conversion reactions to pain syndromes; it is the number of symptoms over time and their persistence that are important diagnostically. While the minor symptoms may seem common to everyone, they are reported

TABLE 451–13. SOMATIZATION DISORDER*

A. Many physical complaints or a belief that he or she has been sickly, for several years beginning before the age of 30.
B. At least 13 symptoms from the following list:
   1. *Gastrointestinal symptoms*, e.g., vomiting (other than during pregnancy), abdominal pain (other than when menstruating), nausea (other than motion sickness), bloating (gassy), diarrhea, intolerance of (gets sick on) several different foods
   2. *Pain symptoms* such as pain in extremities, back pain, joint pain, pain during urination, other pain (other than headaches)
   3. *Cardiopulmonary symptoms*, e.g., shortness of breath when not exerting oneself, palpitations, chest pain, dizziness
   4. *Conversion symptoms*, e.g., amnesia, difficulty swallowing, loss of voice, deafness, double vision, blurred vision, blindness, fainting or loss of consciousness, seizure or convulsion, trouble walking, paralysis or muscle weakness, urinary retention or difficulty urinating
   5. *Psychosexual symptoms*, e.g., burning sensation in sexual organs or rectum (other than during intercourse), sexual indifference, pain during intercourse, impotence
   6. *Female reproductive symptoms*, e.g., painful menstruation, irregular menstrual periods, excessive menstrual bleeding, vomiting throughout pregnancy

*Modified from American Psychiatric Association: Diagnostic and Statistical Manual of Mental Disorders, 3rd ed., rev. Washington, DC, APA, 1987. Used with permission.

with such vigor and intensity that the physician almost feels obligated to investigate them. This constellation of symptoms was described in 1859 by Briquet and has been confirmed over and over again, most convincingly in a series of studies by Guze in the early 1960's.

EPIDEMIOLOGY. The syndrome occurs mostly in females. About 1 per cent of the population is estimated to suffer from somatization disorder. The condition runs in families, but in males it correlates significantly with the occurrence of sociopathy and alcoholism rather than somatic symptoms.

PATHOPHYSIOLOGY. The condition is marked by an empiric collection of symptoms, the exact etiology and pathophysiology of which are not understood. Most patients come from a low education level and lack sophistication; however, there are many exceptions to this characterization. Most explanations have been sociologic and psychological and center on the somatization as a signal of personal distress. Consequently the behavior is often interpreted as a way to obtain help from caregivers or as a mechanism of obtaining social supports and, perhaps, manipulating relationships. It has also been postulated to represent a cognitive style whereby somatic symptoms are used in place of emotional expression.

TREATMENT. These patients are difficult to treat. Perhaps the most important factor should be the attempt to rule out depressive and panic disorders, as there is a high correlation of depressive symptomatology with many of these conditions. Patients with somatization disorders can make the physician feel that there is an urgent need to intervene; however, this temptation should be resisted. Careful evaluation of the history is extremely important for, as is evident, most of them do not respond to treatment. It is not that these patients enjoy their pain but that they are seeking other things, e.g., attention, relief from other problems. Perhaps the most important thing the physician can convey to patients is that they will neither seriously worsen nor die, and although the physician may not know the cause of the complaint he is willing to see them through the illness episode. In fact, it is almost paradoxic that by scheduling these patients for frequent regular visits the physician often not only saves time but may decrease the patient's need to develop symptoms in order to be seen. After one becomes certain of the diagnosis and of the absence of a pathologic process, the diagnostic workup should be kept to a minimum, as the more the physician investigates the more the patient becomes convinced that something is wrong. There is a tendency to dispense medications to these patients, and one of the complications is not only addiction but such a confusion and plethora of drugs that they become a cause of untoward symptoms. The major goal of treatment should be to keep to a minimum the medical and surgical interventions. A general attempt should be made to substitute inquiry into the patient's life as opposed to procedures. A helpful attitude on the part of the physician is that he is more interested in maintaining the relationship than in curing the symptoms and that a successful outcome is the reduction in the number of physicians the patient sees and medications prescribed.

In summary, treatment of these difficult patients should include (1) recognizing the disorder; (2) listening to the patient to determine what has been helpful or harmful in the past; (3) defining a clear contract for continued supervision with no assurances for dramatic cure (or attempts at dramatic intervention beyond what the symptoms warrant). The scheduling of visits can be based on the frequency of visits over the past 2- to 3-month period; (4) empathizing with patients about their suffering, avoiding statements such as "It's all in your head" or "There is nothing wrong with you"; (5) openly discussing the risks of too much medical intervention and avoiding opiates and benzodiazepines owing to their potential for abuse. Tests should be ordered on the basis of objective symptoms, not just complaints; and (6) expecting a long-term relationship with slow improvement.

PROGNOSIS. Somatization disorders are more a way of life than a discrete episodic illness. The patient maintains a propensity for expression of emotional need or distress with somatic symptoms. While the episodes may wax and wane, it is clear that these patients are wedded to the medical establishment.

Other Conditions Associated with Somatic Symptoms

Somatization disorder has been extensively studied, but there are other conditions that are similar to somatization disorder that can be confusing to the physician. Although the term *hysteria* has been dropped from official use and such conditions are now termed *conversion reactions*, such patients present commonly to physicians and make up about 1 per cent of a neurologist's practice. The predominant disturbance in conversion disorder is a loss or alteration in physical functioning suggesting a physical disorder. Often the loss or distortion of neurologic function is not fully explained by any known disease process as determined by physical and laboratory examination. Much of what has been covered with regard to somatization disorder is true of hysterical conditions. These patients do not necessarily have histrionic personalities (overly dramatic, attention seeking, shallow manipulative relationships, etc.). They do have physical complaints, but when examined closely their symptoms conform more to a psychological than a physiologic reaction.

Hypochondriasis is often simple to recognize in that the patient presents with a belief that a disease is present for which diagnosis and treatment are necessary. The complaints are more circumscribed, with often minute examination and description of bodily functions to the physician. As the physician talks to the patient he becomes increasingly aware that the patient is more concerned about the belief of illness than the discomfort from symptoms. In fact, the symptoms are not especially distressing or painful. This is in marked contrast to the patient with chronic pain whose pain is often out of proportion to the physical findings.

In patients with chronic pain, the continuation of the pain often allows the avoidance of activities in the patient's life or the obtaining of emotional or financial support from others. Affected patients frequently have histories of addiction, seeing many physicians, and undergoing multiple surgical procedures.

The genesis of many of the above conditions lies at an involuntary level in that the symptoms and the motivation for them are not in the control of the patient. Two conditions, factitious disorder and malingering, are voluntarily controlled by the patient. These patients, often described as having *Munchausen's syndrome*, induce illnesses in themselves, e.g., fevers (by injection), dermatitis, blood disease (anemia), or seizures. Affected patients are often associated with the health professions, and one can discern no clear goal or gain from their behavior. They frequently are peripatetic, traveling from hospital to hospital. When a factitious disorder is diagnosed, these patients should be confronted openly as to their behavior and what treatment (as some may be necessary) will be provided and not provided. In true malingering, the goal of the illness behavior is often evident (or evident after extensive inquiry), and the condition is usually less a chronic than a factitious disorder. In most cases we see partial malingering, in which an individual exaggerates symptoms of a real disease or attributes a voluntarily induced disability to an accident or injury. In both these conditions there is a tendency to be angry with the patient, but it is best to confront him about the situation in a nonjudgmental rather than an angry manner. Particularly when compensation issues surround the case, treatment is pointless until any legal questions or damage awards are settled.

Katon W, Egan K, Miller D: Chronic pain: Lifetime psychiatric diagnosis and family history. Am J Psychiatry 142:1156–1160, 1985. *An interesting study of the relationship between pain syndromes and psychiatric problems.*

Lipsitt P: Medical and psychologic characteristics of "crocks." Psychiatry Med 1:15–25, 1970. *Still one of the best discussions of the management of patients with many somatic complaints.*

Marsden CD: Hysteria—A neurologist's view. Psychol Med 16:277–288, 1986. *An excellent review of hysteria.*

Quill T: Somatization disorder. JAMA 254:3075–3079, 1985. *A good discussion of the physician's role in the treatment of patients with somatic disorder.*

Ries R, Balcon J, Katon W: The medical abuser: Differential diagnosis and management. J Fam Pract 3:257–265, 1981. *Good differential diagnosis of somatic complaints.*

Slater E, Glithero E: A followup of patients diagnosed as suffering from "hysteria." J Psychosomatic Res 9:9–13, 1965. *A classic article discussing the potential hazards in the diagnosis of hysteria.*

Smith R, Mouson RA, Ray DC: Psychiatric consultation in somatization disorders. N Engl J Med 314:1407–1413, 1986. *Emphasizes the importance of diagnosis of somatization.*

452 Autonomic Disorders and Their Management

Clifford B. Saper

The autonomic nervous system consists of collections of nerve cell bodies (ganglia) associated with the cranial and spinal nerves that innervate all of the internal organs and contribute to the regulation of their function. Disorders of the autonomic nervous system are of great importance to internal medicine, as they can present as disorders of virtually any organ system in the body. Furthermore, the central regulation of autonomic response is closely tied to neuroendocrine control, and both are often involved by central disorders. Aspects of neuroendocrine disease are discussed in Ch. 209, 211 to 215, and 229. This chapter focuses on disorders of the autonomic nervous system (Table 452–1) and discusses them in the overall context of diseases affecting basic integrative functions of the nervous system.

DISORDERS OF PERIPHERAL AUTONOMIC FUNCTION

Organization of Peripheral Autonomic Regulation

The peripheral autonomic nervous system consists of three main divisions. The *parasympathetic* division includes the outflow from the cranial nerves and the low lumbar and sacral spinal cord. The cholinergic preganglionic fibers synapse upon cholinergic ganglion cells that are located in or near the tissues that are innervated. The *sympathetic* division comprises the autonomic outflow from the thoracic and high lumbar segments of the spinal cord. Cholinergic preganglionic fibers end in paravertebral or prevertebral ganglia upon noradrenergic or in some cases cholinergic ganglion cells and also innervate the adrenal medulla. Postganglionic fibers may travel a considerable distance with various peripheral nerves to innervate their target tissues. The *enteric* nervous system includes neurons, many cholinergic, that are intrinsic to the wall of the gut. These neurons form an independent network that is loosely under the control of the other two divisions of the autonomic nervous system. Neurons in all three divisions of the autonomic nervous system commonly employ a wide variety of peptide neuromodulators. Under specific physiologic conditions, these peptides may enhance or suppress the activity induced by the primary neurotransmitter. In some cases, different functions in a peripheral tissue may be subserved by different transmitters released by the same set of neurons (e.g., in the salivary gland, parasympathetically mediated secretion is caused by acetylcholine, but the concomitant vasodilatation is due to vasoactive intestinal peptide).

Knowledge about the different neurotransmitter and receptor types associated with the peripheral autonomic nervous system has resulted in the availability of a wide range of drugs to modify autonomic responses. Some key autonomic drugs and their clinical uses are listed in Table 452–2. These are covered in detail in clinical pharmacology texts.

Pandysautonomias

ACUTE PANDYSAUTONOMIA. Widespread failure of the autonomic nervous system may evolve acutely or subacutely as part of a parainfectious inflammatory polyneuropathy (of the Guillain-Barré type). In rare cases, the autonomic neuropathy predominates. In most patients, however, the autonomic changes are easily overlooked, as the clinical course is dominated by motor paralysis. In severe cases, once the patient is intubated and artificially ventilated, the autonomic neuropathy becomes the chief life-threatening complication. Wide swings in blood

TABLE 452–1. DISORDERS OF THE AUTONOMIC NERVOUS SYSTEM

Peripheral Autonomic Disorders	Genitourinary disorders
Pandysautonomias	Incontinence
Acute pandysautonomia	Urinary retention
Tetanus	Spastic bladder
Chronic autonomic neuropathy	Impotence
Familial dysautonomia	**Disorders of Central Autonomic Integration**
Idiopathic autonomic insufficiency (Shy-Drager syndrome)	Emotional disorders
	Panic disorder
Regional dysautonomia	Psychosomatic illness
Horner's syndrome	Cardiac arrhythmias
Paraspinal tumors	Thermoregulatory disorders
Somatosympathetic dysreflexia	Poikilothermia
Reflex sympathetic dystrophy (causalgia)	Paroxysmal hypothermia
Disorders of specific autonomic functions	Hyperthermia and fever
Pupillary disorders	Malignant hyperthermia
Horner's syndrome	Feeding disorders
Oculomotor paresis	Hyperphagia and obesity
Cardiovascular disorders	Hypophagia and inanition
Glossopharyngeal neuralgia	Disorders of fluid and electrolyte regulation
Carotid sinus hypersensitivity	Hypernatremia, hyperosmolality, and absence of thirst
Sweating disorders	Hyperdipsia, hyponatremia, and water intoxication
Hyperhidrosis	Paroxysmal hyponatremia
Anhidrosis	Central reproductive disorders
Gastrointestinal disorders	Arousal disorders
Disorders of motility	Hypersomnolence
Vomiting	Insomnia

TABLE 452–2. SYSTEMIC EFFECTS OF SOME COMMONLY USED AUTONOMIC DRUGS

Receptor Type	Drug Type (Example)	Tissue	Effect
Muscarinic cholinergic	Antagonist (atropine)	Pupil	Mydriasis
		Salivary gland	Dry mouth
		Bronchi	Dilation
		Heart	Tachycardia
		Gut	Decreased motility and secretion
α-Adrenergic	Antagonist (phenoxybenzamine)	Blood vessels	Vasodilation
α₁-Adrenergic	Agonist (phenylephrine)	Blood vessels	Vasoconstriction
	Antagonist (prazocin)	Blood vessels	Vasodilation
α₂-Adrenergic	Agonist (clonidine)	Blood vessels	Vasoconstriction
β-Adrenergic	Agonist (isoproterenol)	Heart	Increased rate and contractility
β₁-Adrenergic	Antagonist (metoprolol)	Heart	Decreased rate and contractility
β₂-Adrenergic	Agonist (terbutaline)	Bronchi	Dilation

pressure and heart rate occur but usually reverse themselves in a few minutes. Generally, putting the patient into the Trendelenberg position is sufficient to maintain cerebral perfusion during hypotensive periods. Cardiac arrhythmias of all types may occur, presumably as a result of the instability of autonomic innervation of the cardiac conducting system. These must be treated gingerly, as the underlying conduction abnormality may change very rapidly.

TETANUS. A similar subacute pandysautonomia is also seen in severe cases of tetanus. Tetanus toxin, elaborated by *Clostridium tetani* organisms in an infected wound, is transported by autonomic as well as motor axons back to the spinal cord, where it is taken up by and inactivates the terminals of inhibitory interneurons. Treatment of the motor manifestations of tetanus by paralyzing and sedating the patient does little to abate the autonomic storm. Up to 40 per cent of patients with tetanus in an intensive care environment may suffer cardiac arrest as a result of arrhythmias. They are generally easily resuscitated with standard measures.

CHRONIC AUTONOMIC NEUROPATHY. The axons of the peripheral autonomic nervous system generally are of small caliber and poorly myelinated or unmyelinated. Certain polyneuropathies that have a predilection for small-diameter axons can result in autonomic changes. *Amyloid neuropathy*, for example, often includes a major autonomic component that may present as a gastrointestinal motility disorder or orthostatic hypotension. Similarly, *diabetic neuropathy*, although it is often dominated by sensory or motor complaints, may cause widespread autonomic failure. The neuropathy of *acute intermittent porphyria* and certain toxic agents, such as *Vacar* (a rat poison), may have a prominent autonomic component. Acute poisoning with *organophosphate insecticides* that block acetylcholinesterase results in a hypercholinergic state, including miosis and cardiac slowing, that lasts for several days. The neuropathy that follows several weeks later usually does not have a strong autonomic component. Other peripheral neuropathies that may have an autonomic component are listed in Table 452–3.

CHRONIC DYSAUTONOMIA. Recessively inherited *familial dysautonomia* of the Riley-Day type is most commonly seen in

TABLE 452–3. PERIPHERAL NEUROPATHIES THAT MAY HAVE AN AUTONOMIC COMPONENT

Autonomic symptoms often prominent
  Guillain-Barré syndrome
  Amyloid neuropathy
  Diabetic neuropathy
  Acute intermittent porphyria
  Vacar (rat poison)
Autonomic symptoms may occur
  Renal failure
  Toxic neuropathies
    Vinca alkaloids
    Perhexiline maleate
    Thallium

Arsenic
Mercury
Organic solvents
Acrylamide
Vasculitis
Systemic lupus erythematosus
Rheumatoid arthritis
Mixed connective tissue disease
Thiamine deficiency
Leprosy
Charcot-Marie-Tooth disease
Fabry's disease

Ashkenazi Jewish children. Symptoms referable to the autonomic nervous system and relative indifference to pain are present from birth.

Idiopathic autonomic insufficiency of the *Shy-Drager* type may develop as a chronic degenerative condition in middle age or late adult life. The presenting complaint is often orthostatic hypotension, but signs or symptoms of pupillary, gastrointestinal, genitourinary, sweating, or other autonomic abnormalities are elicited on history and physical examination. A summary of tests of the autonomic nervous system is presented in Table 452–4. Idiopathic autonomic insufficiency is part of a spectrum of disorders, ranging from isolated orthostatic hypotension, with or without parkinsonian features, to *multisystem atrophy* with evidence of cerebellar and extrapyramidal involvement. At autopsy, degenerative changes may be seen in the autonomic ganglia as well as in the preganglionic cell groups in the medulla and the spinal cord. Additional cell loss is seen in other affected areas in multisystem atrophy.

Idiopathic autonomic insufficiency is distinguished from nonneurologic causes of orthostatic hypotension by the lack of compensatory tachycardia, indicating impairment of either the peripheral or central components of the baroreceptor reflex. Severe autonomic neuropathy affecting the glossopharyngeal or vagus nerves may also impair the baroreceptor response but is typically associated with other evidence of sensory or motor neuropathy. Other cardiovascular signs include loss of sinus arrhythmia and absence of normal overshoot in the diastolic blood pressure during phase IV of the Valsalva maneuver. An abnormally accentuated blood pressure response to intravenous infusion of norepinephrine is consistent with widespread denervation supersensitivity.

Pupils are often small and poorly responsive to light. Pharmacologic testing (Table 452–4) can determine whether the deficit is central or peripheral. Sweating impairment also may be either of central or peripheral origin. Absence of axon reflex sweating indicates a peripheral lesion. Gastrointestinal impairment may include diarrhea, constipation, incontinence, or abdominal pains. There may also be urinary hesitancy, urgency, or incontinence or impotence in men.

Orthostatic hypotension is generally the most disabling aspect of autonomic degeneration. Indomethacin may be effective in selected patients. Other patients require elastic stockings or even entire lower body suits to reduce blood pooling in the lower extremities during standing. Treatment with mineralocorticoids, such as fludrocortisone, can expand intravascular blood volume and cause elevation of blood pressure in all positions. In such patients, the head of the bed should be elevated in recumbency to minimize hypertensive effects on the brain. Occasionally, oral sympathomimetic agents, such as ephedrine, or monoamine oxidase inhibitors are employed. The latter must be used with caution, as the ingestion of vasoactive amines present in many common foods, including certain wines, cheeses, pickled foods, and smoked meats, can cause severe hypertension.

When idiopathic autonomic insufficiency is associated with a multisystem neurologic degenerative disease, it may be accompanied by ataxia, rigidity, bradykinesia, tremors, weakness, or other neurologic disturbances.

The segmental organization of the sympathetic nervous system can result in regional disturbances of function. The most common of these is caused by injury to the cranial sympathetic innervation arising from the superior cervical ganglion, or *Horner's syndrome.* Miosis, ptosis, and anhydrosis may occur if the ascending sympathetic fibers are injured below the level at which they enter the skull with the internal carotid artery. Damage to sympathetic fibers along the course of the intracranial carotid artery produces only oculosympathetic paresis (Raeder's syndrome). Unfortunately, this difference is only of marginal value clinically, as the Horner's syndrome produced by extracranial lesions is often incomplete. Lesions of the central descending sympathoexcitatory pathway, running through the lateral portions of the brain stem from the hypothalamus to the spinal cord, may produce a central Horner's syndrome, in which there is miosis and ptosis as well as loss of sweating over the entire ipsilateral body. Postganglionic Horner's syndrome can be differentiated from preganglionic or central lesions by pharmacologic testing (Table 452–4). The most common cause of Horner's syndrome is atherosclerotic disease affecting the vasa nervorum originating in the carotid artery. However, Horner's syndrome may also be seen when an intrathoracic or cervical tumor involves the sympathetic chain. Hence, evaluation of Horner's syndrome should include radiographic or magnetic resonance examination of the pulmonary apices and paracervical area.

Paraspinal tumors at lower levels along the sympathetic chain may cause loss of sweating over the involved dermatomes. This deficit can be appreciated by running the handle of a tuning fork down the skin in the paraspinal region. The smooth movement is interrupted by the dry skin at the level of the lesion. Occasionally, compression of a midthoracic spinal root, which carries visceral sensory fibers, by a disc or tumor may present as abdominal pain.

Stimulation of pain fibers at any level results in both local (spino-spinal) and generalized (spino-bulbo-spinal) *somatosympathetic reflex responses,* including sweating, vasoconstriction, and pupillodilatation. In patients with a pre-existing spinal cord transection, a noxious stimulus below the level of the transection may produce only local sympathetic reflex responses. Hence it is important in the paraplegic patient to investigate asymmetric sympathetic responses for a local lesion that might cause pain in an intact individual.

Following injury to peripheral nerves, aberrant regeneration

may result in *reflex sympathetic dystrophy.* It is believed that the sympathetic efferent fibers form excitatory synapses along the course of damaged peripheral sensory nerves. Normally innocuous sensory stimulation, such as covering the affected limb with a sheet or with clothing, may cause excruciating burning pain, associated with variable autonomic changes. Atrophic changes in the skin and bone may reflect abnormal sympathetic innervation or disuse. Relief can sometimes be obtained with guanethidine or phenoxybenzamine. If regional sympathetic block alleviates pain, removal of the affected ganglion can produce permanent relief.

Disorders of Specific Autonomic Functions

PUPILS. Anisocoria, asymmetry of pupillary size, may reflect a deficit of sympathetic innervation of the smaller pupil (causing miosis) or parasympathetic innervation of the larger one (causing mydriasis). As both the oculosympathetic and oculomotor (parasympathetic) innervations participate in lid elevation, ptosis if present generally indicates the abnormal eye. Anisocoria may be longstanding and of little clinical significance, but pupillary asymmetry of recent onset should be evaluated by a neurologist. Impairment of sympathetic innervation of the iris (pupillodilator) muscle is not always accompanied by ptosis or a sweating deficit (Horner's syndrome). The pupilloconstrictor fibers travel in the dorsomedial part of the oculomotor nerve, where they may be selectively affected by temporal lobe herniation or by an aneurysm of the posterior communicating artery. Pharmacologic testing may aid in the identification of the pupillary abnormality (Table 452–4). The most common cause of a large pupil is instillation of atropinic eye drops or application of a scopolamine patch near the face (to prevent motion sickness); the pharmacologically dilated pupil does not respond even to strong solutions of pilocarpine. Another common cause of a large, poorly reactive pupil is *Adie's syndrome,* an idiopathic condition involving degeneration of the ciliary ganglion. The pupil usually shows sector paralysis and constriction with accommodation, and it dilates and responds to light after a period in complete darkness. The abnormal pupil responds briskly to 0.1 per cent pilocarpine (Table 452–4), and there is concomitant loss of tendon reflexes in most cases.

CARDIOVASCULAR. The baroreceptor reflex is an important protective response, causing bradycardia and peripheral vasodilatation to counteract an acute increase in blood pressure, or the

TABLE 452–4. TESTS OF AUTONOMIC FUNCTION*

Test	Interpretation
Pupillary responses	
4% cocaine	
1% hydroxyamphetamine	Pupillodilatation indicates release of normal catecholamine stores.
1% phenylephrine	
0.1% epinephrine	Pupillodilatation indicates denervation supersensitivity.
0.1% pilocarpine	
2.5% methacholine	Pupilloconstriction indicates denervation supersensitivity.
Sweating responses	
Thermal sweating	Regional absence of sweating indicates sympathetic cholinergic denervation.
Galvanic skin response	Increased conductivity under mild stress indicates normal adrenergic innervation.
1:1000 pilocarpine	
1:10,000 acetylcholine	Intradermal injection causes axon reflex sweating.
Axon reflex	
1:1000 histamine	Intradermal injection normally causes wheal and flare.
Cardiovascular responses	
Orthostatic challenge	Pulse normally increases and diastolic blood pressure falls <15 mm Hg.
Carotid sinus massage	Normally causes fall in blood pressure and heart rate.
R-R interval	Normally increases during inspiration (sinus arrhythmia).
Valsalva maneuver	Longest to shortest R-R interval ratio normally is ≥1.4.
Cold pressor test	Immersing hand in ice water normally increases blood pressure and heart rate.
Plasma catecholamines	Normally increase response to standing or stress.
Norepinephrine infusion 0.05 µg/kg/min	Diastolic blood pressure increase ≥20 mm Hg indicates supersensitivity.
Genitourinary, rectal responses	
Cremasteric reflex	Stroking skin of thigh normally causes testicular retraction.
Anal wink reflex	Scratching perianal skin normally causes anal sphincter contraction.
Bulbocavernosus reflex	Squeezing glans penis or clitoris normally causes anal contraction.

*For details see McLeod and Tuck, 1987.

reverse response during hypotension. The afferent fibers for the response run in the glossopharyngeal (carotid sinus) and vagus (aortic depressor) nerves, while the efferent response includes both parasympathetic and sympathetic components. Injury to the glossopharyngeal or carotid sinus nerves in the neck (often by a tumor) can cause episodic attacks of hypotension and bradycardia, which often present as syncope. In most cases, there is an associated pain or paresthesia in the cutaneous distribution of the glossopharyngeal nerve (in the external auditory meatus or the pharynx), known as *glossopharyngeal neuralgia*. The situation is analogous to tic doloreaux, in which there are intermittent volleys of firing in the affected nerve. Atropine or a transvenous pacemaker may prevent the bradycardia associated with the attacks, but loss of vasoconstrictor tone sometimes results in symptomatic hypotension despite these maneuvers. Anticonvulsants, particularly phenytoin and carbamazepine, may prevent the attacks.

Carotid sinus syncope (see Ch. 446) is a condition seen most commonly in elderly individuals with carotid atherosclerosis. Even mild pressure over the carotid bulb, such as a tight shirt collar, can produce a full-blown carotid sinus response, resulting in syncope. The diagnosis is made by gently compressing the carotid artery below the angle of the jaw while the electrocardiogram (ECG) is monitored. Facilities for cardiac resuscitation must be immediately available, as the compression may result in sinus arrest. Vigorous massage should be avoided, as it may dislodge an embolus, resulting in a transient or even permanent neurologic deficit. Treatment of carotid sinus hypersensitivity is the same as that for glossopharyngeal neuralgia.

SWEATING. Human sweat glands are innervated by both noradrenergic sympathetic fibers (mediating emotional responses) and cholinergic sympathetic fibers (thermal sweating). Certain somatosympathetic reflexes can produce generalized or regional sweating, in response to innocuous or noxious somatosensory stimuli. *Paroxysmal localized hyperhidrosis* is a rare condition that probably represents an exaggeration of normal somatosympathetic reflexes. Generalized hyperhidrosis, particularly involving the hands and the soles of the feet, is most likely a normal variant. Drugs directed at interrupting α-adrenergic transmission (phenoxybenzamine, clonidine) have been useful in some cases of localized hyperhidrosis. In extreme cases, regional sympathectomy has been performed.

Idiopathic anhydrosis may be segmental or generalized. This rare condition is sometimes associated with Adie's syndrome (Ross syndrome), but in other cases there are no other signs of autonomic impairment. In some cases the impairment is preganglionic and in others postganglionic, as judged by the axon reflex sweating response (Table 452-4). In most recorded patients, the deficits have been stable and did not go on to involve other autonomic functions.

GASTROINTESTINAL. Disorders of intestinal motility, which may be due to damage to the parasympathetic innervation of the gut or to dysfunction of the enteric nervous system itself, are discussed in Chapter 100. Specific abnormalities of esophageal contraction and colonic tone have been noted in patients suffering from depression and may predict response to antidepressant medication.

Vomiting is a neurally mediated gastrointestinal reflex that is coordinated by neurons in the medullary reticular formation. Chemical emetic agents such as certain narcotics or dopaminergic agonists act at the area postrema, a chemosensory zone on the fourth ventricular surface of the medulla, to elicit the vomiting reflex. Local dopaminergic connections are thought to mediate the response, and antidopaminergic drugs such as prochlorperazine may act at the level of the area postrema to suppress vomiting. Intractable vomiting without any gastrointestinal abnormalities has been reported in certain patients with tumors involving the medullary cell groups controlling vomiting or their connections. Treatment of the tumor with steroids and radiation therapy generally results in improvement.

GENITOURINARY. The urinary bladder is composed of interlacing smooth muscle fibers of the detrusor covered by an internal mucous membrane and an outer serosa. The detrusor is innervated by parasympathetic neurons whose preganglionic cell bodies are located in the intermediolateral column at the second through fourth sacral segments. Parasympathetic fibers travel through the pelvic plexus and nerve. Additional motor neurons located in the ventral horn at the same levels constitute Onuf's nucleus. Their axons run through the pelvic nerve to innervate striated accessory muscles of micturition (including the external urethral sphincter) in the pelvic floor. Neurons of Onuf's nucleus are strikingly preserved in motor neuron disease but are lost along with autonomic preganglionic cells in idiopathic autonomic insufficiency. The internal sphincter at the bladder neck is innervated via the hypogastric nerve by sympathetic prevertebral pelvic ganglia whose preganglionic innervation arises from the intermediolateral column at the T12–L1 level.

During bladder filling the intravesical pressure remains relatively constant as a result of sympathetically mediated relaxation of the detrusor muscle and inhibition of parasympathetic tone in response to bladder stretch sensation. Bladder relaxation during filling and subsequent coordination of micturition are under the control of Barrington's nucleus, located in the floor of the fourth ventricle at the pontine level. Brain stem control of micturition is, in turn, under voluntary regulation by areas within the cerebral sensory and motor cortex lying along the medial wall of the cerebral hemisphere. When bladder fullness is sensed and the environmental conditions are appropriate, micturition is initiated by Barrington's nucleus, under forebrain control. There is a fall in external sphincter pressure, resulting in reflex relaxation of the internal sphincter and contraction of the bladder.

Forebrain impairment results in loss of voluntary control of micturition but does not otherwise affect the complex sensory and motor program that results in normal voiding. Incontinence in such patients can be managed by using adult diapers or external urinary collection devices without risk of frequent urinary tract infections or damage to the upper urinary tract. Injury to the bulbospinal pathway from Barrington's nucleus to the sacral intermediolateral column, however, causes major disruption of coordinated bladder function. Acutely following spinal cord injury there is a period of spinal shock, during which the bladder does not undergo reflex contraction as it fills. The bladder may overfill, overstretching the muscular wall, and elevation of bladder pressure above 40 mm H_2O can result in hydronephrosis. Such patients require urinary catheterization to prevent vesical and renal damage.

One to 2 weeks following injury, spinal reflex control of the bladder returns. Some patients can induce reflex bladder emptying by somatosensory stimulation, such as stroking the skin over the thigh. The spastic bladder reflexively contracts at a lower volume and, because detrusor action is not coordinated with sphincter opening, rarely empties completely. Postvoid residual urine in excess of 25 to 50 ml is an important sign of impairment of supraspinal pathways controlling the bladder. Injury to sensory nerves supplying the bladder also may cause overfilling and incomplete emptying, indicating the importance of sensory feedback in bladder control. Patients with significant postvoid residual urine are at increased risk for urinary tract infections, but bladder overfilling with elevated pressures may ultimately be a greater problem. It is important to monitor bladder pressure in such patients with cystometrography. Elevations in pressure above 40 mm H_2O may require continuous or intermittent catheterization to prevent damage to the upper urinary tract.

Pharmacologic intervention, aimed at augmenting or suppressing autonomic motor responses of the bladder or internal sphincter, cannot reconstitute the coordinated control of the different components of the lower urinary tract. Bethanacol, a cholinergic agonist, is used to augment bladder contraction to improve emptying. It is most effective in combination with an α-adrenergic blocker, such as phenoxybenzamine or prazocin, that simultaneously reduces pressure of the internal sphincter. Baclofen may be used to decrease spastic contraction of the external sphincter. Drugs that have atropinic properties, including a surprising variety of antiarrhythmic, antihistamine, neuroleptic, and antidepressant medications, may inhibit bladder contraction, resulting in overfilling and urinary retention (Table 452–5).

Erectile function in males is under parasympathetic control by the same sacral levels as the urinary system. Sensory afferent fibers travel via the pudendal nerve, while parasympathetic motor fibers run in the pelvic nerve. Sympathetic innervation via the

TABLE 452–5. SOME COMMONLY PRESCRIBED DRUGS THAT MAY IMPAIR URINARY FUNCTION

Antiarrhythmics	Chlorpromazine	Dopa/carbidopa
Atropine	Antidepressants	Bromocriptine
Diisopyramide	Amitriptyline	Benztropine
Antihistamines	Imipramine	Trihexiphenidyl
Diphenhydramine	Antiparkinsonian agents	Antispasmodics
Neuroleptics	Amantadine	Baclofen
Haloperidol		

hypogastric nerve contracts the seminal vesicles during ejaculation and closes the bladder neck to prevent retrograde emission. Although supraspinal influences are of great importance, reflex erection and ejaculation can occur in patients after spinal injury. Neurogenic impotence can result either from damage to descending pathways relaying forebrain influence from the hypothalamus to the sacral preganglionic neurons or from injury to the sensory or parasympathetic motor innervation of the penis. A variety of drugs that block either parasympathetic or sympathetic function can interfere with erectile function (Table 452–6). As erections normally occur several times nightly during periods of rapid eye movement sleep, it is possible to document organic disorders of erection by measuring penile tumescence overnight. Disorders of male sexual dysfunction are considered in Ch. 222.

DISORDERS OF INTEGRATIVE CONTROL OF THE AUTONOMIC NERVOUS SYSTEM

ORGANIZATION OF CENTRAL AUTONOMIC AND ENDOCRINE REGULATION. The autonomic nervous system is under three levels of central control. The *preganglionic* neurons located in the medulla and the spinal cord provide the final common pathway for central autonomic control. Each of these neurons integrates the inputs from many sources, including afferents from higher levels of the nervous system and local reflex responses. A series of *brain stem and spinal* cell groups coordinates *reflex control* of the autonomic nervous system. These nuclei receive cranial (parasympathetic) and spinal (sympathetic) afferent information and control a variety of important reflexes (e.g., swallowing, maintaining blood pressure, initiation of voiding). Both the preganglionic neurons and the brain stem reflex neurons are under the control of *forebrain integrative* cell groups that coordinate autonomic function with behavior and with endocrine control.

The hypothalamus is the most important area for integration of behavior with autonomic responses and with neuroendocrine control of the anterior and posterior pituitary glands (Fig. 452–1). Because the hypothalamus consists of tightly packed, interwoven pathways and cell groups, it is unusual for an injury to involve selectively a single functional system. Nevertheless, considerable progress has been made in determining the anatomic substrates for specific integrative functions, and disorders of these systems are occasionally encountered (Table 452–7). In addition, autonomic dysfunction is a frequent concomitant of emotional disorders.

Emotional Disorders

Portions of the insular and cingulate areas of the cerebral cortex and the amygdala are believed to regulate autonomic responses to emotional stress. In healthy individuals, stress can induce sympathetic responses, such as pupillodilatation, dry mouth, and increases in blood pressure. In patients with *panic disorder* (see Ch. 451), such autonomic responses can become overwhelming and convince the patient that there is a serious organic problem.

TABLE 452–6. SOME COMMONLY PRESCRIBED DRUGS THAT MAY IMPAIR ERECTILE FUNCTION

Drugs causing impotence	Propranolol	Drugs causing priapism
Parasympatholytics	Prazocin	
Atropine	Vasodilators	Chlorpromazine
Amitriptyline	Hydralazine	Thioridazine
Sympatholytics	Diuretics	Trazadone
Methyldopa	Hydrochlorothiazide	Prazocin
Guanethidine	Antihistaminergic	Dopa/carbidopa
Clonidine	Cimetidine	

PET studies show increased metabolism in the structures of the medial temporal lobe and the insular cortex during panic attacks. After eliminating the possibility of pheochromocytoma (see Ch. 229), anxiolytic or antidepressant drugs are usually found helpful.

In some individuals under chronic emotional stress, a variety of syndromes are seen implicating autonomic control of the internal organs. While *psychosomatic illness* is often thought to be nonorganic and may respond to psychotherapeutic drugs, there is considerable evidence that some organic disorders that are seen in anxious patients also may be caused by autonomic dysregulation. For example, swallowing disorders often represent abnormal control of peristalsis. Erosive gastritis and even frank ulceration may occur as a result of autonomic dysfunction. Perhaps the most serious problems are encountered in patients with pre-existing cardiac abnormalities, who may have cardiac arrhythmias under stressful conditions. Retrospective studies of victims of sudden death due to lethal ventricular arrhythmias indicate a much higher incidence of behavioral stress in the period preceding the attack. The protective effect of β-adrenergic blockers against sudden death in the post–myocardial infarction patient may be due in part to the reduction in such arrhythmias.

Thermoregulatory Disorders

Thermoresponsive neurons in the medial preoptic area monitor brain temperature and activate autonomic, endocrine, and somatomotor responses to match body temperature to a set-point, which is normally 37°C in humans. Control of body temperature requires shifting blood flow between deep and superficial vascular beds and regulating conservation of body fluids (increased urination in the cold, increased sweating in the heat). Hence, thermoregulation is tightly linked to control of blood pressure, volume, and electrolyte composition, which are also regulated by neurons around the anteroventral tip of the third ventricle (see below).

Poikilothermia, defined as a fluctuation in body temperature of more than 2°C with changes in ambient temperature, is the most common disorder of heat regulation in humans. Lesions in the posterior hypothalamus or midbrain result in severe damage to the hypothalamic pathways for autonomic as well as behavioral thermoregulation. Relative poikilothermia can also result from metabolic disorders such as sedative drug ingestion, hypoglycemia, or hypothyroidism, and in a mild form is often seen in old age. Such patients are dangerously susceptible to lowered environmental temperature. Conversely, patients with relative poikilothermia or those taking anticholinergic drugs that prevent thermal sweating may experience dangerously elevated body temperatures during periods of hot weather. *Heat stroke*, in which body temperature may exceed 42°C, is often fatal and requires prompt treatment by cooling the patient in an ice bath and expanding body fluids. Death is often a result of ventricular arrhythmia (see also Ch. 532).

PAROXYSMAL HYPOTHERMIA. Occasional patients are encountered who suffer episodic attacks during which they thermoregulate in a nearly normal fashion but around a lowered set-point. During an attack, a body temperature of 32°C or lower is maintained for a period of several days to 2 weeks. Attacks occur up to several times per year and may be accompanied by fatigue, malaise, somnolence, hypoventilation, hypotension, cardiac arrhythmias, lacrimation, ataxia, and asterixis. During the attacks, the patient may behaviorally thermoregulate to maintain the lowered set-point. In some patients, the serum sodium may decrease in tandem with the body temperature, to levels of 110 mEq per liter or even lower. Attacks subside spontaneously and are followed by heat conservation measures to bring body temperature up to the normal set-point. Nearly all such patients have evidence of injury to the preoptic area of the hypothalamus. Paroxysmal hypothermia is sometimes seen in patients with agenesis of the corpus callosum, most likely because the corpus callosum and the preoptic area are both embryologic derivatives of the lamina terminalis, which fails to form normally. Anticonvulsants have been prescribed to alleviate attacks but have rarely been effective.

HYPERTHERMIA AND FEVER. During an immune re-

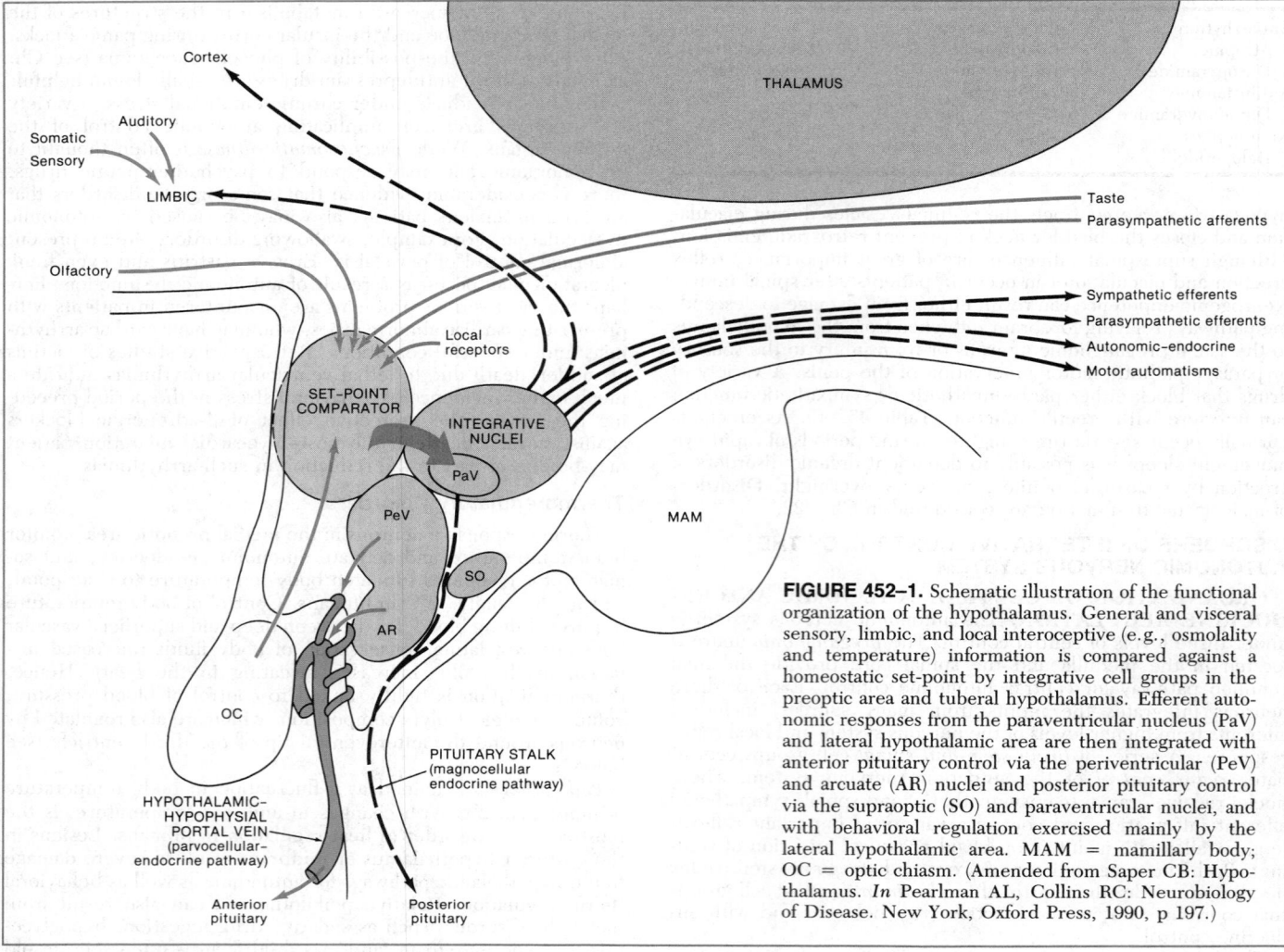

FIGURE 452–1. Schematic illustration of the functional organization of the hypothalamus. General and visceral sensory, limbic, and local interoceptive (e.g., osmolality and temperature) information is compared against a homeostatic set-point by integrative cell groups in the preoptic area and tuberal hypothalamus. Efferent autonomic responses from the paraventricular nucleus (PaV) and lateral hypothalamic area are then integrated with anterior pituitary control via the periventricular (PeV) and arcuate (AR) nuclei and posterior pituitary control via the supraoptic (SO) and paraventricular nuclei, and with behavioral regulation exercised mainly by the lateral hypothalamic area. MAM = mamillary body; OC = optic chiasm. (Amended from Saper CB: Hypothalamus. *In* Pearlman AL, Collins RC: Neurobiology of Disease. New York, Oxford Press, 1990, p 197.)

sponse, macrophages release cytokines, such as interleukin-1 and tumor necrosis factor, that act on neurons or glial cells at the organum vasculosum of the lamina terminalis, a vascular structure outside the blood-brain barrier that sits in the anteroventral tip of the third ventricle, to cause a febrile response. Prostaglandins are a critical mediator for producing fever and some of the endocrine and metabolic changes that accompany it. Fever, an upward resetting of the thermoregulatory set-point, is achieved by normal heat conservation mechanisms, including shivering and behavioral thermoregulation. Drugs that inhibit the generation of prostaglandins are the mainstay of treatment of fever, but there is considerable debate on the wisdom of treating low-grade fever (<38.5°C) during an infectious illness. An elevated body temperature may improve the function of certain immune cells while impairing the defenses of invading microorganisms.

Any physical injury to the brain that allows the entry of macrophages or activates microglial cells to produce cytokines induces a febrile response as well. Hence, fever may be seen after head trauma, intracranial surgery, or cerebral hemorrhage or infarction. Central neurogenic fever is often proposed as a mechanism for fever of unknown origin, but careful investigation generally demonstrates that most if not all of these cases are normal cerebral responses to cytokine generation by immune cells or tumors.

Malignant hyperthermia can occur in patients who have been exposed to certain drugs. During induction of anesthesia, partic-

TABLE 452–7. REGIONAL HYPOTHALAMIC SYNDROMES

Region	Normally Regulates	Disorders
Preoptic	Blood volume, pressure, and electrolytes	Paroxysmal hyponatremia
		Essential hypernatremia
	Thermoregulation	Paroxysmal hypothermia
Tuberal	Gastrointestinal tract and feeding	Hyperphagia (ventromedial lesions)
		Hypophagia (lateral lesions)
	Reproduction	Hypogonadism
	Emotions	Rage responses
Posterior	Arousal	Hypersomnolence
	Descending autonomic and motor pathways	Poikilothermia

ularly with halothane and succinylcholine, certain patients sustain sudden massive muscle contractions accompanied by a rapid rise in body temperature to 42°C or greater. The response is believed to be due to the anesthetic's causing the release of calcium stores from the sarcoplasmic reticulum. Circulatory and respiratory collapse and death can ensue unless immediate treatment with intravenous dantrolene and supportive measures are instituted. A similar picture of muscular rigidity and elevated body temperature can occasionally be seen following treatment with neuroleptic drugs. The pathogenesis of the *neuroleptic malignant syndrome* is not understood, but such patients can sometimes be improved by administering dopaminergic agonists such as bromocriptine.

Feeding Disorders

To provide a constant supply of substrate for energy metabolism, it is necessary to balance bodily requirements against the daily intake of nutrients and body stores of glycogen, fat, and protein. To accomplish this task, the hypothalamus monitors blood glucose, fatty acids, and perhaps other nutrients and attempts to match blood glucose to a set-point. Body weight, which is regulated within a rather narrow range in most people, is also thought to be matched to a set-point, but this is clearly secondary to the immediate need for metabolic substrate. The neural mechanisms regulating energy metabolism and feeding are mainly coordinated in the region of the ventromedial nucleus of the hypothalamus and the nearby paraventricular nucleus. The control of feeding is closely related to autonomic control of the gastrointestinal system.

HYPERPHAGIA AND OBESITY. Lesions in the region of the ventromedial nucleus of the hypothalamus can result in massive overeating and obesity. Experimental studies indicate that overeating is largely in response to parasympathetically mediated hyperinsulinemia, causing a chronically lowered blood glucose. Transection of the vagus nerve below the diaphragm corrects insulin secretion and overeating. Hence, hypothalamic hyperphagia is mainly a disorder of autonomic control of the pancreas, with a resultant attempt to defend the blood glucose set-point.

The *Klein-Levin syndrome* is a poorly understood disorder in which patients, typically adolescent boys, have episodic attacks of somnolence, often sleeping up to 20 hours per day. When awake, they appear dull and often confused and consume enormous quantities of food. Attacks may last up to 2 weeks and can recur several times per year. Pathologic verification of the site of the lesion in typical cases is lacking, but a similar syndrome may be seen acutely in encephalitis involving the hypothalamus.

The *Prader-Willi syndrome* is a congenital disorder due to a deletion in chromosome 15, which includes mental retardation, hypogonadism, and hyperphagia, often with massive obesity. The cause of the overeating is not known.

HYPOPHAGIA AND INANITION. Large lesions in the region of the lateral hypothalamic area, at the level of the ventromedial nucleus, result in aphagia, which may recover to hypophagia and regulation around a new, lower body weight set-point. Such lesions, which must be bilateral, are usually devastating, and selective impairment of eating on this basis has rarely been reported in adults. More often, patients with hypothalamic damage and inanition are somnolent and show a variety of endocrine abnormalities. There is no evidence for injury to the hypothalamus in anorexia nervosa.

Children may demonstrate a quite different response to congenital hypothalamic tumors or malformations. In the diencephalic syndrome of infancy, there is profound emaciation, despite good feeding and linear growth. The affected children are often exceptionally good-natured. The difference from adults with similarly placed tumors probably reflects the capacity for plasticity and formation of new neuronal connections during development.

Central Disorders of Fluid and Electrolyte Regulation

The medial preoptic area, around the anteroventral tip of the third ventricle, plays a critical role in regulating blood pressure, volume, and electrolyte composition. Endocrine control (mineralocorticoids and especially vasopressin), autonomic regulation (control of blood flow in different vascular beds, innervation of sweat glands and kidney, especially the juxtaglomerular apparatus controlling renin release), and behavioral response (drinking) all play important roles in this process. Disorders of the release of vasopressin, by neurons whose cell bodies are located in the supraoptic and paraventricular nuclei, are discussed in Ch. 75 and 214. Coordinated central disorders of fluid regulation are rare.

HYPERNATREMIA, HYPEROSMOLALITY, ABSENCE OF THIRST. Neurogenic hypernatremia is a rare disorder marked by impairment of the normal responses to osmolar stimuli. Hence, there is a deficit in vasopressin response to increased sodium and osmolality and an absence or relative deficiency of thirst. Vasopressin response to hypovolemia may be maintained, and there is preservation of habitual drinking of water (often related to meals) which may be sufficient to maintain serum osmolality under normal conditions. During hot weather, when there is increased loss of water through evaporation of sweat, patients often fail to increase their water consumption adequately and may suffer attacks of fatigue, fever, muscle cramps and tenderness, and even myoglobinuria (associated with hypokalemia). With serum sodium in excess of 180 mEq per liter, patients may experience confusion or even become stuporous, and some may die.

The hypothalamic injury giving rise to essential hypernatremia has been accurately localized in only a few cases but in all of these seems to involve the preoptic area in the region of the anteroventral third ventricle. Treatment consists of training the patient to drink adequate amounts of fluids, particularly during hot weather. Spironolactone, chlorpropamide, and thiazide diuretics have been used to reduce serum sodium and increase potassium. During an attack of severe hypernatremia, when it becomes necessary to provide intravenous fluid and potassium supplementation, it is important not to reduce serum sodium by more than 20 mEq per liter per day. More rapid correction has been associated with central pontine myelinolysis, which may leave the patient quadriplegic.

HYPERDIPSIA, HYPONATREMIA, AND WATER INTOXICATION. Excessive water drinking in the absence of either hypovolemia or serum hyperosmolality is termed primary hyperdipsia and must be distinguished from the compensatory hyperdipsias of diabetes insipidus, diabetes mellitus, and polyuric renal failure. In the absence of inappropriate vasopressin secretion, symptoms of water intoxication, such as stupor, delirium, or convulsions, are infrequent. Most severe hyperdipsia occurs in persons who have psychiatric disturbances. We have seen only one case of primary hyperdipsia, in a patient who had suffered an attack of encephalitis involving the hypothalamus during childhood.

PAROXYSMAL HYPONATREMIA. Many of the patients with paroxysmal hypothermia (see above) suffer simultaneous hyponatremia, which may be sufficiently severe (serum sodium <110 mEq per liter) to cause symptoms of confusion or even convulsions. The serum sodium is regulated around the reduced set-point but may respond to fluid restriction.

Central Reproductive Disorders

Reproductive hormonal control, behavior, and the associated autonomic responses are controlled by poorly defined mechanisms in the medial basal hypothalamus overlying the pituitary stalk. To the extent that it relies upon control of blood flow in specific vascular beds, the autonomic regulation of sexual function must be coordinated with control of body temperature and fluid balance. The change in body temperature that accompanies ovulation and the fluid shifts seen in the perimenstrual period in women are examples of this integration.

Reproductive endocrine disorders are covered in Ch. 213 and 224. Male erectile function, which is dependent upon sacral parasympathetic innervation of the penis, may be affected by diseases of the peripheral autonomic nervous system (see above) as well as psychogenic factors acting at the level of the forebrain. Diagnosis and treatment of male sexual dysfunction are discussed in Ch. 222.

Arousal Disorders

The function of the autonomic nervous system is to augment the activity of various organ systems to deal with perturbations of internal homeostasis. Of all the body's organs, the single most important one to activate during an external threat is the brain. The ascending activating system, running from the brain stem reticular formation to the diencephalon, increases the responsiveness of the forebrain to external stimuli and may be considered a cerebral component of the autonomic system. Ch. 443, 444, and 446 describe the details of altered states of consciousness. We discuss here briefly disorders associated with lesions of the ascending arousal system. Sleep disorders are discussed in Ch. 447.

HYPERSOMNOLENCE. Following lesions of the ascending activating system at the level of the rostral brain stem, there is typically impairment of level of consciousness acutely. After a few weeks, the forebrain recovers spontaneous wake-sleep cycles. Prolonged sleeplike stupor lasting longer than a few weeks is seen only when lesions involve the posterior diencephalon. It is not clear whether this continued somnolence results from injury to the thalamus, to the hypothalamus, or to the connections of these structures. Methylphenidate, amphetamine, and bromocriptine have been used in these patients, with some anecdotal reports of success.

INSOMNIA. Sleep is an active process, requiring the participation of hypnogenic influences arising from the lower brain stem and serotoninergic neurons in the midbrain raphe. We have seen one patient in whom destruction of the medulla, below the level of the ascending activating system, resulted in a chronically wakeful state. Lesions of the preoptic area may also cause a decrease in sleep, but this may be secondary to the deficit in thermoregulation.

Peripheral Autonomic Disorders

Krane RJ, Goldstein I, Saenz de Tejada I: Impotence. N Engl J Med 321:1648–1659, 1989. *A thorough review of the physiology and pathophysiology of erectile function.*

McGuire EJ: The innervation and function of the lower urinary tract. J Neurosurg 65:278, 1986. *A thoughtful review of the physiology and pathophysiology of micturition.*

McLeod JG, Tuck RR: Disorders of the autonomic nervous system: Part 1. Pathophysiology and clinical features. Ann Neurol 21:419, 1987. *A recent review of autonomic physiology and pathophysiology.*

McLeod JG, Tuck RR: Disorders of the autonomic nervous system: Part 2. Investigation and treatment. Ann Neurol 21:519, 1987. *A guide to pharmacologic testing and treatment of autonomic dysfunction.*

Schwartzmann RJ, McLellan TL: Reflex sympathetic dystrophy. A review. Arch Neurol 44:555, 1987. *A review of the pathophysiology and clinical aspects of reflex sympathetic dystrophy.*

Central Autonomic Disorders

Greenberg HS, Rocher LL, Clavin DB, et al.: Episodic hyperhidrosis, hypothermia, and agenesis of the corpus callosum. Neurology 33:1122, 1983. *A review of paroxysmal hypothermia.*

Loewy AD, Spyer KM: Central Regulation of Autonomic Functions. New York, Oxford Press, 1990. *A comprehensive series of reviews on the central components of the autonomic nervous system.*

Plum F, Posner JB: The Diagnosis of Stupor and Coma, 3rd ed., rev. Philadelphia, F. A. Davis, 1982. *A comprehensive review of mechanisms of arousal and evaluation of neurologic impairments in comatose patients.*

Plum F, van Uitert R: Non-endocrine diseases and disorders of the hypothalamus. Res Publ Assoc Res Nerv Ment Dis 56:415, 1977. *A comprehensive review of the integrative disorders of autonomic function.*

Saper CB: Hypothalamus. *In* Pearlman AL, Collins RC: Neurobiology of Disease. New York, Oxford Press, 1990, p 197. *A review of hypothalamic regulation of integrated functions and their disorders.*

Talman WT: Cardiovascular regulation and lesions of the central nervous system. Ann Neurol 18:1, 1985. *A review of central control of the circulation and the effects of nervous system lesions on cardiac arrhythmias and blood pressure control.*

453 The Special Senses

Robert W. Baloh

453.1 SMELL AND TASTE

Approximately 2 million American adults suffer from disorders of taste and smell, yet there is relatively little information available on how to evaluate or treat these patients. These disorders have been neglected because they are seldom fatal and, unlike abnormalites of vision and hearing, are not considered serious handicaps. Chemosensory disorders, however, often reduce the enjoyment and quality of life and are important to patients who suffer from them. Disorders of taste interfere with digestion because taste stimulants alter salivary and pancreatic flow, gastric contractions, and intestinal motility. Smell also contributes to the anticipation and ingestion of food, since much of what we taste derives from olfactory stimulation during ingestion and chewing. The inability to detect noxious tastes and odors can result in food or gas poisoning, particularly in elderly subjects. In the extreme, chemosensory disorders can lead to overwhelming stress, anorexia, and depression.

DEFINITIONS. Disorders of taste and smell are defined as follows: *Ageusia*, absence of taste; *hypogeusia*, diminished sensitivity of taste; *dysgeusia*, distortion of normal taste; *anosmia*, absence of smell; *hyposmia*, diminished sensitivity of smell; and *dysosmia*, distortion of normal smell. *Hypergeusia* and *hyperosmia* (increased sensitivity of taste and smell) also occur, but little is known about their cause or significance.

ANATOMY. The sensory receptor for taste, the taste bud, is made up of approximately 50 cells arranged to form a pearshaped organ. The life span of these cells is about 10 days, and they are constantly being renewed from dividing epithelial cells surrounding the bud. Taste buds are located on the tongue, soft palate, pharynx, larynx, epiglottis, uvula, and the upper one third of the esophagus. The taste buds located on the anterior two thirds of the tongue and on the palate are innervated by the seventh cranial nerve. The ninth cranial nerve innervates the posterior one third of the tongue and the folds or clefts on the lateral border of the tongue. The ninth and tenth nerves innervate taste buds in the pharynx. Afferent signals from the taste buds project to the nucleus of the solitary tract in the medulla and then via a series of relays to the thalamus and postcentral somatosensory cerebral cortex. Free nerve endings of the fifth cranial nerve are found on the tongue and in the oral cavity, and lesions involving these pathways also can alter taste perception.

Olfactory receptors lie in a roughly dime-sized area of specialized pigmented epithelium that arches along the superior aspect of each side of the nasal mucosa. Specialized bipolar sensory cells in this region thrust short receptor hairs into the overlying mucosa to detect aromatic molecules as they dissolve. As with taste buds, the specialized receptor portion of the bipolar neuron undergoes continuous renewal, turning over approximately every 30 days. Thin axons of the bipolar neurons course through small holes in the cribriform plate of the ethmoid bone to form connections in the overlying olfactory bulb on the ventral surface of the frontal lobe. From here second- and third-order neurons project directly and indirectly to the prepiriform cortex and parts of the amygdaloid complex of both sides of the brain, representing the primary olfactory cortex.

PATHOPHYSIOLOGY OF CHEMOSENSORY DISORDERS. Disorders of taste and smell can be divided into local, systemic, and neurologic (Table 453–1). The taste buds and the specialized receptor portion of the bipolar olfactory cells are constantly being renewed, and the process of renewal can be affected by nutritional, metabolic, and hormonal states, therapeutic radiation, drugs, and age. For example, with interruption of mitosis by antiproliferative agents, a return of normal taste

TABLE 453–1. COMMON CAUSES OF LOSS OF TASTE AND SMELL

	Taste	Smell
Local	Radiation therapy	Allergic rhinitis, sinusitis, nasal polyposis, bronchial asthma
Systemic	Cancer, renal failure, hepatic failure, nutritional deficiency (B_{12}, zinc), Cushing syndrome, hypothyroidism, diabetes mellitus, infection (influenza), drugs (antirheumatic and antiproliferative)	Renal failure, hepatic failure, nutritional deficiency (B_{12}), Cushing syndrome, hypothyroidism, diabetes mellitus, infection (viral hepatitis, influenza), drugs (nasal sprays, antibiotics)
Neurologic	Bell's palsy, familial dysautonomia, multiple sclerosis	Head trauma, multiple sclerosis, Parkinson's disease, frontal tumor

function takes a minimum of 10 days, while a return to normal olfactory function takes more than 30 days. Numerous local conditions such as colds and allergies, chronic sinusitis, and nasal polyposis can influence the sense of smell by restricting airway patency. Accidental blows to the head can shear the fine axons of the bipolar olfactory neurons, resulting in loss of smell. Lesions of the fifth, seventh (*chorda tympani*), and ninth cranial nerves can lead to disordered taste sensation. Olfactory and gustatory disturbances can serve as important diagnostic signs for focal neurologic lesions (e.g., frontal lobe tumors). Hallucinations of smell and taste occur with epileptogenic lesions affecting the mesial temporal lobe and insular region, respectively. Finally, olfactory disturbances and hallucinations occur with a number of psychiatric illnesses (particularly depressive illness and schizophrenia).

EXAMINATION OF TASTE AND SMELL. Olfaction can be tested grossly at the bedside with a few easily recognized odors such as coffee, chocolate, and the roselike aroma of the compound phenylethyl alcohol. (Avoid nasal irritants.) Each nostril is tested separately to determine whether the problem is unilateral or bilateral. More detailed testing can be obtained in specialized clinics in which a variety of qualitatively distinct substances that span a number of established odor classes are presented with a forced-choice paradigm. Gustatory sensation is typically tested with weak solutions of sugar, salt, and acetic acid, or vinegar. The patient must keep his tongue protruded and respond to questions either by nodding the head or pointing to names of the tastes written on cards. The protruding tongue is dried and a drop of test solution is applied to the lateral border of each side. The anterior two thirds and posterior one third of the tongue should be tested separately.

COMMON CAUSES OF LOSS OF SMELL AND TASTE. The most frequently encountered causes of loss of smell are local obstructive disease, viral infections, head injuries that sever the neurons crossing through the cribriform plate, and normal aging. Patients can lose their sense of smell not only from chronic allergies and sinusitis but also from the nasal sprays and drops that they use to treat these conditions. The most common cause of loss of the sense of taste is drug ingestion, particularly antirheumatic and antiproliferative drugs and drugs containing sulfhydryl groups in their molecular structure, such as penicillamine and captopril. Patients with poor dental hygiene commonly complain of distortions of taste. Many of the systemic disorders listed in Table 453-1 probably have their effect by decreasing the rate of turnover of sensory receptors on the tongue and olfactory epithelia. Disturbances of smell and taste in malnourished patients have been attributed to specific deficiencies in vitamins and minerals, such as zinc. However, it is possible that the loss of protein and calorie intake impairs the functioning of taste buds and olfactory cells in the same manner that it impairs the regeneration of intestinal epithelia. Viral illnesses such as influenza and viral hepatitis produce disorders of both taste and smell. The loss of olfactory sensation after viral illnesses may be due to scarring of the subepithelial tissue and the replacement of olfactory epithelium with respiratory epithelium. Multifocal neurologic disorders such as multiple sclerosis can affect the central olfactory and gustatory pathways at multiple levels, and therefore abnormalities of taste and smell are common in such patients. Treatment, other than avoiding drugs known to affect taste or smell, is unsatisfactory.

Estrem SA, Renner G: Disorders of smell and taste. Otolaryngol Clin North Am 20:133, 1987. *Concise clinical review.*
Schiffman SS: Taste and smell in disease. N Engl J Med 308:1275, 1337, 1983. *A well-referenced two-part short review.*
Taste and smell disorders: parts 1 and 2. Ear Nose Throat J 68:286, 291, 297, 316, 331, 352, 354, 362, 373, 386, 393, 398, 1989. *Two issues devoted to diagnosis and management.*

453.2 NEURO-OPHTHALMOLOGY

The mechanistic understanding of vision impairment along with disturbances of pupillary and oculomotor control lies close to the heart of diagnosing neurologic disorders. Diseases of the eye itself are further considered in Part XXIV.

VISION

One of the most difficult diagnostic problems is vision loss that cannot be explained by obvious abnormalities of the eye. In order to properly evaluate such a patient the examining physician must be familiar with the anatomy and physiology of the afferent visual system. The afferent visual pathways cross at right angles to the major ascending sensory and descending motor systems of the cerebral hemispheres and in their anterior portion are intimately related to the vascular and bony structures at the base of the brain. Not surprisingly, localization of lesions within the afferent visual pathways has great localizing value in neurologic diagnosis.

DEFINITIONS. *Amblyopia* refers to dimness or partial loss of vision, *amaurosis* to blindness. *Scotomas* are areas of relative or complete vision loss isolated within a comparatively better total field of vision for the particular eye. Involvement of the macular area or its projections produces *central scotomas*. Scotomas that lie near the macular visual area are sometimes called *paracentral*, whereas those that extend into macular vision from the more peripheral field may be termed *cecocentral*.

Visual field defects impairing half or nearly half of a field are termed *hemianopic*. Those affecting less than this extent are called *partial field defects*, often with the additional designation of *quadrantic* or *altitudinal* (superior or inferior), depending on the abnormality. A vision defect that affects similar points of the right or left half-field in both eyes is called *homonymous*; identical areas of involvement from the two eyes are termed *congruent*.

ANATOMY OF THE VISUAL PATHWAYS. Light entering the eye falls on the retinal rods and cones, which transduce the stimulus into neural impulses to be transmitted to the brain. The distribution of visual function across the retina takes a pattern of concentric zones increasing in sensitivity toward the center, the fovea. The fovea consists of a "rod-free" central grouping of approximately 100,000 slender cones. The ganglion cells subserving these cones send their axons directly to the temporal aspect of the optic disk, forming the papillomacular bundle. Axons originating from ganglion cells in the temporal retina must curve above and below the papillomacular bundle, forming dense arcuate bands.

The arteries supplying the optic nerve and retina both derive from branches of the ophthalmic artery. The central retinal artery approaches the eye along each optic nerve and pierces the inferior aspect of the dural sheath about 1 cm behind the globe to enter the center of the nerve. The artery emerges in the fundus at the center of the nerve head, from which it nourishes most of the retina by superior, medial, inferior, and lateral branches. Anastomotic branches derived from the choroidal and posterior ciliary arteries supply the nerve head itself and the macular region. Venous drainage from the retina and nerve head flows primarily via the central retinal vein, whose course of exit from the eye parallels that of the entry of the artery. The venous anatomy explains why inflammatory lesions of or adjacent to the optic nerve head cause venous distention and ipsilateral papilledema (optic neuritis), whereas inflammation lying posterior to the point where the vein leaves the nerve produces only visual loss without swelling of the nerve head (retrobulbar neuritis).

What each eye "sees" is termed its visual field (Fig. 453-1). The nasal side of the left eye and the temporal side of the right eye see the left side of the world, and the upper half of each retina sees the lower half of the world. Behind the eye, the optic nerve passes through the optic foramen and sphenoid bone to reach the optic chiasm. In the chiasm, nerves from the nasal half of each retina decussate and join the fibers from the temporal half of the contralateral retina. From the chiasm, the optic tracts pass around the cerebral peduncles to reach the lateral geniculate ganglia of either side. At the level of the geniculus, fibers serving corresponding points in each retinal half visual field lie adjacent to each other, and this proximity is maintained in the subsequent relay to the calcarine cortex. The geniculocalcarine radiation initially fans out into superolateral and inferolateral projections, the latter passing around the lateral ventricle and for a short distance into the temporal lobe (Meyer's loop) before turning posteriorly to head for the striate cortex of the occipital lobe. At the occipital pole, the striate cortex (Area 17) lies along the superior and inferior bands of the calcarine fissure, with macular

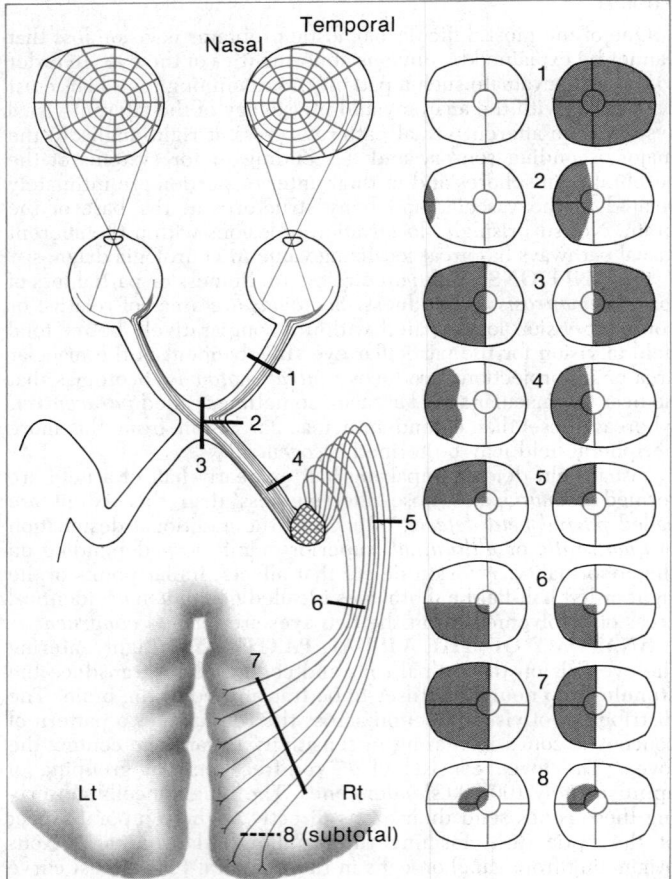

FIGURE 453–1. Visual fields that accompany damage to the visual pathways. 1. Optic nerve: Unilateral amaurosis. 2. Lateral optic chiasm: Grossly incongruous, incomplete (contralateral) homonymous hemianopia. 3. Central optic chiasm: Bitemporal hemianopia. 4. Optic tract: Incongruous, incomplete homonymous hemianopia. 5. Temporal (Meyer's) loop of optic radiation: Congruous partial or complete (contralateral) homonymous superior quadrantanopia. 6. Parietal (superior) projection of the optic radiation: Congruous partial or complete homonymous inferior quadrantanopia. 7. Complete parieto-occipital interruption of optic radiation. Complete congruous homonymous hemianopia with psychophysical shift of foveal point often sparing central vision, giving "macular sparing." 8. Incomplete damage to visual cortex: Congruous homonymous scotomas, usually encroaching at least acutely on central vision.

fibers projecting most posteriorly to the occipital pole and more peripheral retinal projections lying more anteriorly. Each occipital pole "sees" the opposite half of the world. Fibers serving the superior retinal quadrants project to the superior bank of the calcarine fissure, and those from the inferior quadrants project to the inferior bank. The macular field is represented strictly unilaterally.

LOCALIZATION OF LESIONS WITHIN THE VISUAL PATHWAYS. Monocular vision loss is due to a lesion of one eye or its retina or optic nerve. Binocular visual loss, on the other hand, can result from disease located anywhere in the visual pathways from the retinae to the occipital poles. Lesions involving or compressing the optic chiasm produce nonhomonymous visual abnormalities that affect the unilateral visual fields incongruously (e.g., the bitemporal hemianopia illustrated by Lesion 3 in Fig. 453–1). Optic tract abnormalities are comparatively rare but produce characteristic visual changes. The fibers serving identical points in the homonymous half fields do not fully commingle in the anterior optic tract, so lesions encroaching on this structure produce incongruous and usually incomplete homonymous hemianopias. Lesions of the geniculate ganglia, visual radiations, or visual cortex produce congruent hemianopic field defects that may go unrecognized unless the hemianopia intrudes on macular vision. Bilateral damage to the visual radiations or optic cortex

produces cortical blindness. Postgeniculate amaurosis can be differentiated from pregeniculate amaurosis by (1) a normal funduscopic appearance, (2) intact direct and consensual pupillary light reactions, and (3) the presence of anatomically appropriate lesions by brain imaging.

EXAMINATION OF THE AFFERENT VISUAL SYSTEM. Visual function for neurologic purposes consists of "best corrected visual activity." If the visual acuity is not normal, then it must be determined whether acuity can be improved with lenses or at least with the use of a pinhole. Patients with uncorrected myopia or presbyopia correct vision to nearly normal by gazing at the test chart through a pinhole in a card held immediately over the eye. The tiny aperture overcomes any aberration created by failure of the lens to accommodate. The normal reference is a recognition of letters at an idealized 20 feet, and acuity charts are designed with even larger letters that normally are recognized at proportionally greater distances. Thus, if one reads at 20 feet letters no better than those normally perceived at 40 feet, vision is recorded as 20/40. Small visual charts that are easily carried in the physician's case permit quick and fairly accurate bedside appraisals of acuity. Finger counting is a reasonable approximation of an acuity of 20/200, and the greatest distance at which this can be accomplished should be recorded.

Visual fields can be tested at the bedside by confrontation, and rough estimates of their integrity can be made even in patients with reduced alertness. The fields should be tested individually for each eye, since the pattern of visual field defects can provide important localizing information. A quick screen of the visual fields can be made by having the patient fixate on the examiner's nose and identify the number of fingers flashed in each of the four visual field quadrants. With practice and a cooperative subject, accurate confrontation fields can be obtained that outline even scotomas. The examiner should place the test object (e.g., a red match head) midway between his eye and the patient's eye and test the patient's unilateral visual field against his own. Ophthalmoscopic examination permits direct visualization of the cornea, lens, vitreous, retina, and optic disk. Ophthalmologists routinely dilate the pupil to examine the optic fundus, but this step should be avoided in acutely ill patients or those suspected of neurologic diseases until one is certain that an intrinsic pupillary abnormality will not be important in reaching a diagnosis or in following the patient's course. Corneal, lenticular, or vitreous opacities large enough to produce visual symptoms almost always can be detected with the ophthalmoscope.

COMMON CAUSES OF VISUAL LOSS. (See also Ch. 510 and 513.) *Eye.* The cause of monocular vision loss due to ocular and retinal lesions often can be detected with ophthalmoscopic examination or with measurement of intraocular pressure. *Glaucoma* caused by impaired absorption of the aqueous humor results in a high intraocular pressure that usually produces gradual visual loss, "halos" seen around illuminated lamps, and, often, pain and redness in the affected eye. Infrequently, rapid vision loss can occur with few premonitory symptoms. Diagnosis comes from the tonometric measurement of a high intraocular pressure and may be suspected by palpating an abnormally firm globe and observing a deep, pale optic cup and attenuated blood vessels. *Retinal tears and detachments* give rise to unilateral distortions of the visual image seen as sudden angulations or curves of objects containing straight lines (metamorphopsia). *Hemorrhages* into the vitreous humor or unilateral *infections* or *inflammatory lesions* of the retina can produce scotomas that in all ways resemble those resulting from primary disease of the central visual pathway.

Binocular vision loss due to retinal disease in younger subjects is usually due to *heredodegenerative conditions.* Vascular diseases, diabetes, idiopathic (senile) macular degeneration, and bilateral retinal detachments are causes in older age groups. In the *pigmentary retinal degenerations* visual loss begins peripherally and proceeds centrally, and often very slowly, before acuity (central vision) is impaired. By contrast, *macular degenerations* impair central vision early in their course. Most of the retinal degenerations produce characteristic and recognizable ophthalmoscopic appearances. With pigmentary degenerations the visual fields shrink progressively in size. With macular degenerations, on the other hand, the fields show noncongruent central scotomas.

Optic Nerve. Acute or subacute monocular vision loss due to optic nerve disease is most commonly produced by demyelinating disorders, vascular obstruction, or neoplasm. Demyelinating disease of the nerve head (*optic neuritis* or *papillitis*) produces papilledema along with loss of central vision in the affected eye only; subjectively unrecognized scotomas sometimes may be found in the other eye. Demyelination in the optic nerve behind where the retinal vein emerges (*retrobulbar neuritis*) initially leaves a normal-looking disk but a central or paracentral scotoma. With chronic demyelinating disorders the optic disk becomes pale and atrophic. More than 50 per cent of patients who initially present with optic neuritis or retrobulbar neuritis go on to develop typical symptoms and signs of multiple sclerosis. Vascular lesions produce either total amaurosis or a sector field defect consistent with an intraocular arterial occlusion (*ischemic optic neuropathy*). The common causes of transient monocular vision loss and their differential features are listed in Table 453–2. *Tumors* invading the optic nerve or space-occupying lesions compressing it anywhere between the orbit and the chiasm cause gradually decreasing central vision (intrinsic or far advanced lesions) or a sector defect of the peripheral visual field. With such chronic lesions the affected optic nerve becomes visibly atrophic.

Acute binocular vision loss due to bilateral optic nerve disease is most often caused by demyelinating disease and less frequently by optic nerve or retinal vascular disease or by toxic or nutritional optic neuropathies. In younger persons and those lacking a clear history of toxic exposures demyelinating lesions overwhelmingly predominate (optic neuritis). Symptoms are of abrupt or subacute onset with visual blurring or loss of acuity, which may progress rapidly to blindness within hours or days. There may be pain about the eyes, particularly on eye movement.

Papilledema resulting from increased intracranial pressure occasionally causes vision loss under one of three circumstances: (1) Acute transient episodes of amaurosis lasting a few seconds and attributable to acute increases in intracranial pressure (plateau waves) that interfere with retinal venous drainage into the cavernous sinus or with vascular irrigation of the occipital lobe; (2) acute bilateral sustained amaurosis following abrupt surgical relief of longstanding, severely increased, intracranial pressure (a rare cause); (3) progressive loss of peripheral vision with longstanding, severe papilledema, presumably owing to pressure atrophy of the most peripherally lying fibers in the tightly sheathed optic nerve. Table 453–3 gives the main differential points between papilledema and optic neuritis. Subacute or chronic binocular vision loss due to optic nerve disease results mainly from *toxic nutritional* causes and the *inherited optic atrophies*. The latter sometimes accompany spinocerebellar degeneration or selectively affect the optic nerves in both juveniles and adults (Leber's forms). With either cause visual loss is moderate or severe and primarily or initially affects central vision; ophthalmoscopy shows mild to moderate primary optic atrophy.

TABLE 453–2. COMMON CAUSES OF TRANSIENT MONOCULAR VISION LOSS

Category (Typical Duration)	Causes	Differential Features
Thromboembolism (1–5 min)	Atherosclerosis	Other atherosclerotic vascular disease, associated crossed hemiparesis, angiography (carotid atheromata)
	Cardiac	Valvular disease, mural thrombi, atrial fibrillation, recent MI
	Blood dyscrasia	Blood tests + for sickle cell anemia, macroglobulinemia, multiple myeloma, polycythemia, etc.
Vasospasm (5–30 min)	Migraine	Ipsilateral headache, other classic aura, and family history
Vascular compression (few sec)	Papilledema	Precipitated by position change, Valsalva maneuver, or pressure waves
	Tumor	Associated slowly progressive monocular visual loss
Vasculitis (1–5 min)	Temporal arteritis	Associated headache, polymyalgia rheumatica, palpable temporal artery, elevated sedimentation rate

TABLE 453–3. DIFFERENTIATION OF OPTIC NEURITIS FROM PAPILLEDEMA

	Optic Neuritis	Papilledema
Central-cecocentral vision loss	Present	Absent
Distribution	Usually unilateral	Usually bilateral
Ocular pain on movement	Present	Absent
Direct light reflex	± Reduced	Intact
CT or MRI scan of head	Normal	Often abnormal
Visual evoked responses	Abnormal	Normal
Lumbar puncture pressure	Normal	Elevated

Chiasm and Optic Tract. Patients with lesions of the optic chiasm and optic tract are often unaware of visual impairment until the deficit encroaches on central vision in one or both eyes. Intrinsic or extrinsic neoplasms and parachiasmal arterial aneurysms are the most common lesions in this location. *Gliomas* that arise in the chiasm are rare in adulthood but, when they occur, impair central vision early. Extrinsic space-occupying lesions compressing the chiasm can arise from the superior, lateral, or inferior aspect and include *dysgerminomas*, *craniopharyngiomas*, *pituitary adenomas*, *meningiomas* arising from the sphenoid bones, and large *aneurysms* of the carotid artery. The diagnosis rests on finding the characteristic visual field abnormalities (bitemporal hemianopsia for chiasm and incongruous homonymous hemianopsia for optic tract lesions) and identifying the specific lesion with computed tomography (CT) or magnetic resonance imaging (MRI). Pituitary apoplexy (due to acute hemorrhage into the gland, occurring most frequently in patients with unrecognized pituitary adenomas) can result in sudden vision loss. Prompt neurosurgical intervention under steroid coverage is required for most patients.

Visual Radiations and Occipital Cortex. Lesions involving the postgeniculate visual pathways most often result from *vascular damage, traumatic injuries, neoplasms* or, rarely, *inflammatory* or *degenerative disorders* involving the cerebral white matter. Their localization can be deduced by the resulting visual field defects (see Fig. 453–1). Vascular disease of the occipital lobes is the most common cause of homonymous visual field defects in the middle-aged and elderly population. Typically, the onset of such field defects is associated with other signs and symptoms of transient ischemic episodes in the vertebrobasilar distribution. Bilateral damage to the visual radiations or occipital cortex produces *cortical blindness*. Most often, there are other signs of vascular disease including focal neurologic findings. *Anton's syndrome* refers to cortical blindness with denial of visual defect. Affected patients not only deny the fact that they are blind but confabulate details of their visual environment from memory. Autopsy studies reveal lesions of the medial, temporal, and parietal lobes as well as the calcarine cortex. *Tumors* are rarely confined to the limits of the occipital lobes; therefore neurologic deficits with occipital tumors are rarely only visual.

PUPILLARY CONTROL

The neuromechanisms that control pupil size and reactivity are complex, yet they can be evaluated by simple clinical procedures. The diameter of the pupil is determined by the antagonistic actions of the iris sphincter and dilator muscles with the latter playing a minor role. If the sphincter muscle is severed or ruptured it does not retract toward one quadrant but rather continues to function except in the altered segment. Therefore, the pupillary response can be evaluated even in the presence of significant damage to the iris.

DEFINITIONS. A difference in the size of the pupils is called *anisocoria*. *Mydriasis* refers to a dilated pupil while *miosis* refers to a constricted pupil. *Hippus* refers to a pupil that is constantly changing in size (a physiologic phenomenon that has no pathologic significance). *Light-near dissociation* refers to a pupil that responds to accommodation but not to light. An *afferent pupil* is a pupil that responds poorly, or not at all, to direct light but has a normal consensual response when a light is shined in the opposite eye.

ANATOMY AND LOCALIZATION OF LESIONS WITHIN PUPILLARY PATHWAYS. The size of the pupil is governed by tonic balance between sympathetic and parasympathetic innervation of the muscles of the iris. Sympathetic stimulation dilates the pupil, and parasympathetic stimulation constricts it. In the normal resting state, light entering the eye provides the major stimulus governing the size of the pupil (Fig. 453–2). Light activates the retinal rods and cones with maximal sensitivity in the macular area. The optic nerve fibers follow the crossed and uncrossed visual pathways to the pregeniculate portion of the optic tracts, where the receptor fibers for light diverge to the pretectal nucleus located at the midbrain diencephalic junction. Interneurons project from this nucleus to the Edinger-Westphal nuclei atop the midbrain third nerve complex of either side. From that point paired parasympathetic efferents leave the midbrain with the third nerves to travel in the interpeduncular space across the petroclinoid ligament and edge of the tentorium, where, after traversing the cavernous sinus, they enter the superior orbital fissure. In the orbit the parasympathetic efferents synapse in the ciliary ganglion from which short ciliary nerves enter the eye to reach the pupillary muscles.

Lesions of the retina or optic nerve result in an ipsilateral afferent pupillary defect. Pretectal lesions commonly produce light-near dissociation; i.e., the pupils respond to accommodation but not to light. Damage to a third nerve or its parasympathetic postganglionic fibers results in a dilated pupil that does not respond to direct or consensual stimulation.

The principal sympathetic control of the pupil originates in the ventral lateral hypothalamus (first-order neuron) from which fibers descend ipsilaterally to the lower brain stem tegmentum and thence to the cervical cord, where they lie superficially and synapse with the preganglionic neurons in the intermedial lateral column of the upper three thoracic segments. Preganglionic fibers (second-order neurons) emerge with the ventral roots of C8, T1, and T2 and ascend in the neck to synapse in the superior cervical ganglion adjacent to the base of the skull. Postganglionic (third-order neurons) pupillary fibers accompany the internal carotid artery through the skull, leaving it to follow the ophthalmic branch of the trigeminal nerve to reach the pupillodilator muscle of the eye.

Sympathetic paralysis of the eye with ptosis and miosis (Horner's syndrome) can result from lesions anywhere along the course of the pathway described above. Topical diagnosis is made best by identifying associated signs in the brain stem or neck or along the carotid artery.

EXAMINATION OF THE PUPIL. The pupillary response to light should be examined in a dimly lighted room, in which case the pupils are in a semidilated state. First, the size and symmetry of the pupils are assessed by shining a dim light onto the face from below so that both pupils are seen simultaneously in the indirect illumination. To test light reactivity, gaze is directed at a distant object and first one and then the other pupil is illuminated with a very bright light source. If a pupil reacts poorly to direct light, it is observed as the opposite eye is illuminated (consensual response). Pupils that react poorly to light should be tested for activity to the near reflex. This is done by first having the patient gaze at a distant object and then quickly fixate on his fingertip just in front of his nose.

COMMON CAUSES OF PUPILLARY ABNORMALITIES. The differential features for distinguishing between several common causes of a dilated pupil are illustrated in the logic tree shown in Figure 453–3. With so-called benign pupillary dilatation or *physiologic anisocoria* there is a lifelong difference in the size of the two pupils with normal reflex reactions; the disparity remains constant during constriction and dilatation. Lesions compressing or damaging the tectal region interrupt the afferent light reflex bilaterally to produce dilated (>5 mm) and light-fixed pupils (e.g., Lesion 2, Fig. 453–2). Pupillary constriction on accommodation is preserved until late stages. Tumors of the pineal gland (e.g., dysgerminomas) and *localized infarctions* are the most common lesions in this location. *Adie's tonic pupil* is a medium-to-large (3 to 6 mm) pupil that constricts little or not at all to light and slowly to accommodation but constricts with the instillation of dilute pilocarpine (0.125 per cent). The abnormal pupil is associated with diminished or absent deep tendon reflexes in the extremities. The condition usually affects one eye (occasionally both), is more common in women 25 to 45 years of age, and carries no serious implications. Its cause is unknown. Unexplained unilateral or bilateral dilated pupil as an isolated finding can result from the *accidental or intentional instillation of mydriatics.* The recent widespread use of transdermal scopolamine has increased the problem. Failure of the pupil to constrict promptly with pilocarpine (1 per cent) gives the diagnosis if the history is unclear. Interruption of the emerging third nerve in the ventral midbrain or along the proximal part of its course produces a mid-dilated pupil 6 to 7 mm in diameter. Important causes of compression of the third nerve in this region are *aneurysms, neoplasia,* and *brain herniation* due to increased intracranial pressure. In nearly all cases the pupillary involvement is associated with other signs of third nerve involvement, as

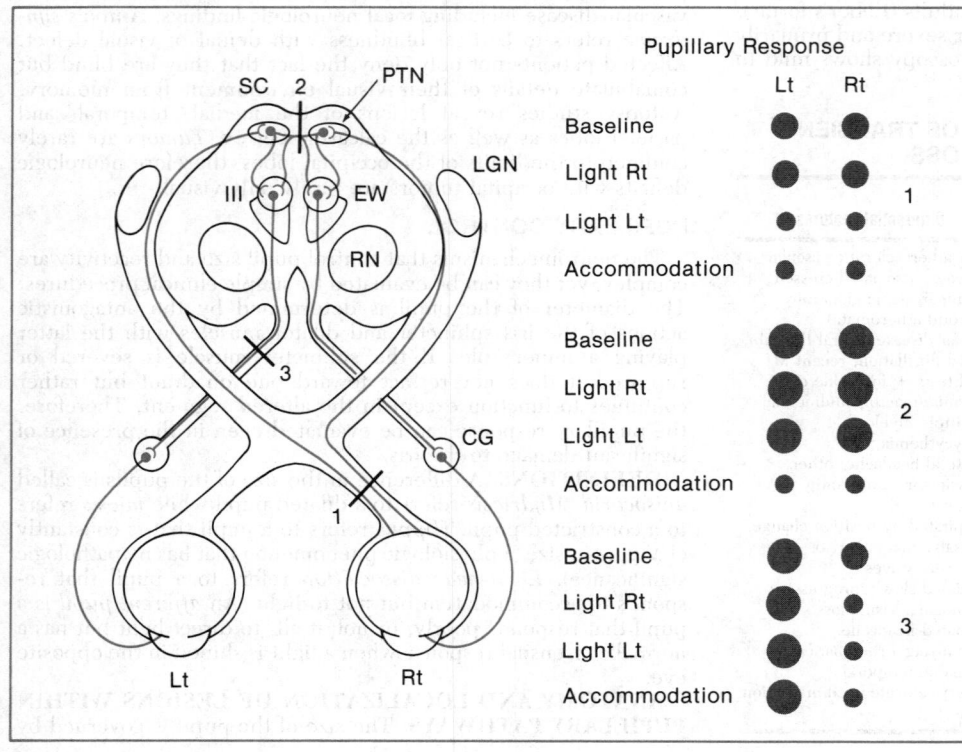

Pupillary Response

FIGURE 453–2. Pupillary responses associated with lesions of the (1) optic nerve, (2) pretectum, and (3) oculomotor nerve. SC = Superior colliculus; PTN = pretectal nucleus; EW = Edinger-Westphal nucleus; LGN = lateral geniculate nucleus; RN = red nucleus; CG = ciliary ganglion.

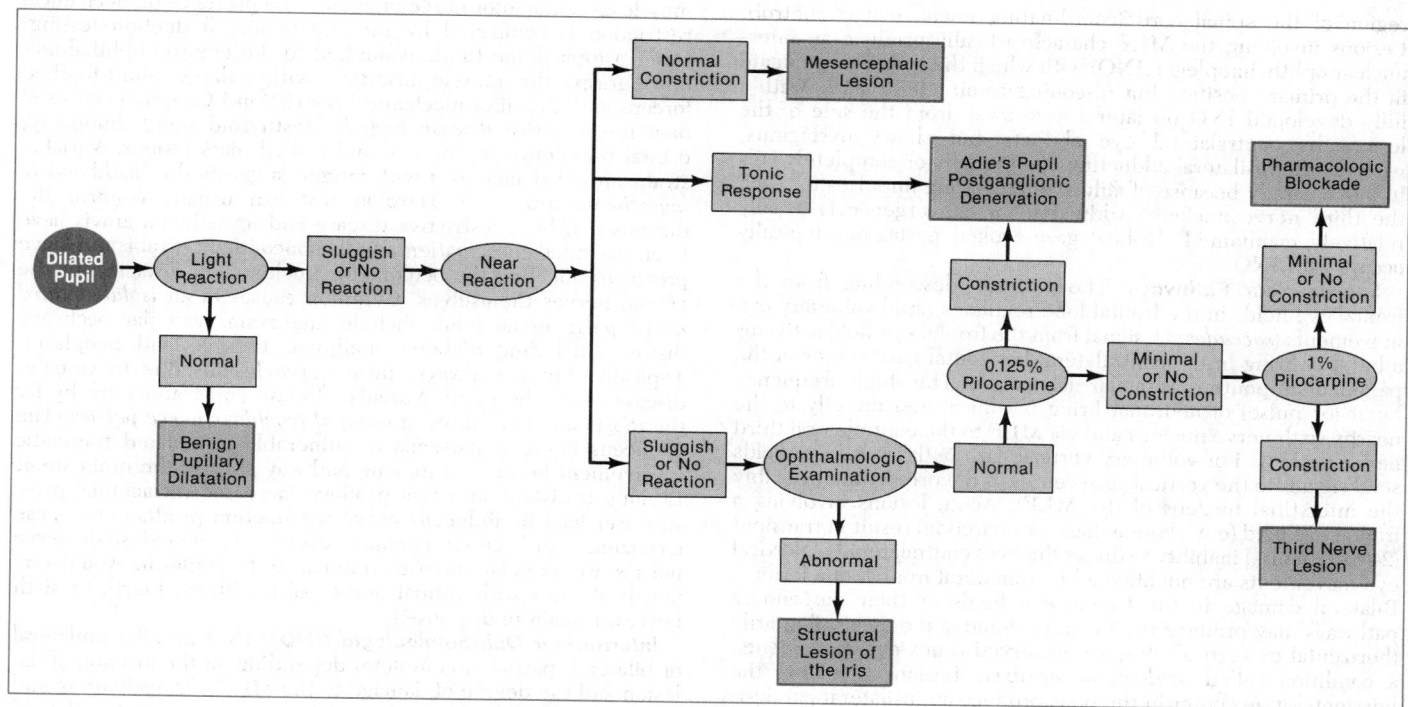

FIGURE 453–3. Evaluation of a dilated pupil.

described in the section below dealing with localization of lesions in oculomotor pathways. Rarely, compressive lesions such as a posterior communicating artery aneurysm can present with an isolated dilated pupil.

As noted above, the causes of *Horner's syndrome* are numerous because of the long course of sympathetic innervation to the eye. It is unlikely that a patient with a central nervous system lesion will present with an isolated Horner syndrome. The most common lesions producing Horner syndrome involve the ascending second-order neuron in the neck or the extracranial postganglionic neuron; *malignant tumors in the apex of the lung* are by far the most common. *Argyll Robertson pupils* are small (1 to 2 mm), unequal, irregular, and fixed to light; they constrict to accommodation. Their principal cause is tertiary neurosyphilis, although partial Argyll Robertson changes occur with diabetes and certain of the autonomic neuropathies.

OCULOMOTOR CONTROL

Abnormal eye movements can result from disturbances at several levels. Disconjugate eye movements result from lesions of the individual ocular muscles, the myoneural junctions, the oculomotor nerves and their three paired nuclei in the brain stem, and the internuclear medial longitudinal fasciculus (MLF) that yokes the eyes in parallel movements. Supranuclear lesions typically produce disorders of conjugate gaze (gaze palsies).

DEFINITIONS. The term *strabismus* describes an involuntary deviation of the eye from its normal physiologic position. *Nonparalytic strabismus* is due to an intrinsic imbalance of ocular muscle tone and is usually congenital. *Paralytic strabismus* results from defects in ocular muscle innervation. Strabismus is called *comitant* when the relationship between the two ocular axes remains constant in all directions of gaze, *noncomitant* when they change, and *latent* when the imbalance is brought out only by covering one eye to prevent fixation. Latent strabismus can become *manifest* during great fatigue or in association with high fever in systemic illness. Congenital comitant strabismus present at birth or soon thereafter carries with it the strong risk that if uncorrected the subject will suppress vision in the nondominant eye during the developmental period when it usually forms its connections with the visual cortex. The result is unilateral, permanent reduction of vision in the nondominant eye (*amblyopia ex anopia*). Strabismus beginning after binocular fusion has developed does not lead to permanent visual loss. *Nystagmus* is an involuntary rhythmic oscillation of the eyes that usually has clearly defined fast and slow components. By convention, the direction of the fast component defines the direction of nystagmus. Physiologic nystagmus refers to nystagmus that occurs in normal subjects, while pathologic nystagmus implies an underlying abnormality. *Physiologic nystagmus* may be vestibular induced (rotational or caloric), visual induced (optokinetic), or end point (occurring on extreme lateral gaze). *Pathologic nystagmus* may be spontaneous (present in the primary position with the patient seated), positional (induced by change in head position), or gaze evoked (induced by change in eye position).

ANATOMY AND LOCALIZATION OF LESIONS WITHIN THE OCULOMOTOR PATHWAYS. *Nuclear and Internuclear Pathways.* The abducens nerve supplies the lateral rectus muscle. Selective involvement of the abducens nerve anywhere along its pathway leads to isolated weakness of abduction of the affected eye. Destruction of the abducens nucleus in the brain stem leads to a conjugate gaze paralysis (ipsilateral) because, in addition to oculomotor neurons, the nucleus contains interneurons destined for the contralateral medial rectus nucleus. The trochlear nucleus supplies the contralateral superior oblique muscle which intorts the eye and moves it down. Patients with superior oblique weakness note an increase in diplopia with head tilt toward the side of weakness and often tilt the head in the opposite direction. At rest there is slight upward deviation of the involved eye and downward movement is impaired when the affected eye is turned in. The third cranial nerve supplies the remaining ocular muscles. Involvement of the third nerve nucleus in the midbrain always produces at least some bilateral oculomotor weakness; the superior rectus division of the nucleus supplies the contralateral superior rectus muscle (all other divisions supply ipsilateral muscles). Peripheral third nerve paralysis can result from lesions damaging the structure anywhere from its origin from the ventral midbrain to where it enters the orbit via the superior orbital fissure. Depending on its completeness, a third nerve palsy produces a widely dilated pupil, severe ptosis, and an externally deviated eye held in position by the unopposed contraction of the lateral rectus muscle. In such conditions, the continued trochlear action reveals itself by intorsion of the eye when the subject attempts to look down and in.

The MLF interconnects the abducens nucleus in the pons with the contralateral oculomotor nuclear complex in the midbrain. It terminates cephalad in the interstitial nucleus in the rostral midbrain and can be traced as far caudad as the thoracocervical region of the spinal cord (coordinating nuchal-ocular control). Lesions involving the MLF characteristically produce an internuclear ophthalmoplegia (INO) with which the eyes are conjugate in the primary position but disconjugate on lateral gaze. With a fully developed INO on lateral gaze away from the side of the lesion the contralateral eye abducts and shows nystagmus, whereas the ipsilateral adducting eye partially or completely fails to move nasally because of failure of ascending impulses to reach the third nerve nucleus. Adduction for convergence is usually relatively maintained. Upbeat gaze-evoked nystagmus typically occurs with INO.

Supranuclear Pathways. The pathway descending from the frontal eye fields in the frontal lobe regulates rapid voluntary eye movements (*saccades*). A signal from the frontal eye field activates a burst of firing in the contralateral horizontal gaze center in the paramedian pontine reticular formation. This high frequency burst (or pulse) of neuronal firing is transmitted directly to the nearby sixth nerve nucleus and via MLF to the contralateral third nerve nucleus. For voluntary vertical gaze both frontal eye fields send signals to the vertical gaze center in the pretectum (probably the interstitial nucleus of the MLF). Acute lesions involving a frontal eye field (e.g., hemorrhage or infarction) result in transient (24 to 72 hours) inability to direct the eyes contralaterally. Vertical eye movements are not affected by unilateral frontal lobe lesions. Bilateral damage to the frontal eye fields or their descending pathways may produce the inability to move the eyes voluntarily (horizontal or vertical) despite preserved reflex eye movements, a condition called *oculomotor apraxia*. Lesions involving the horizontal-gaze center in the pons produce an ipsilateral paralysis of conjugate gaze and tonic deviation of the eyes to the contralateral hemiorbit. Lesions of the pretectum selectively impair vertical gaze with the vertical up-gaze center being slightly rostral and dorsal to the vertical down-gaze center.

Pathways descending from the parieto-occipital region of the two hemispheres subserve slow visual tracking or *smooth pursuit movements*. The exact location of these descending pursuit pathways is not completely known, but there are strong projections to the ipsilateral superior colliculus and ipsilateral pons. The cerebellar flocculus is also a critical relay station for smooth pursuit pathways. Lesions of the parieto-occipital region, pons, and cerebellum impair smooth pursuit and optokinetic slow phases when the target moves ipsilateral to the lesion. The *convergence* center is located in the rostral-dorsal midbrain near the vertical-gaze center. Lesions in this region typically impair convergence and voluntary vertical gaze (particularly up-gaze). Pathways for cortical control of convergence have not been identified. The fourth supranuclear oculomotor control system, the *vestibulo-ocular reflex*, and its examination are discussed below.

EXAMINATION OF EYE MOVEMENTS. Fixation and gaze holding are tested by having the patient look center, right, left, up, and down. Each position should be held steady and unwavering with the observer documenting carefully abnormal movements or ocular disconjugacies. Each supranuclear oculomotor control system is examined separately. *Saccades* are tested by having the patient fixate alternately on two targets such as the examiner's finger and nose; the speed and accuracy are noted. *Smooth pursuit* is tested by slowly moving a target back and forth and up and down and observing the patient's ability to produce smooth tracking movements. If the target velocity is low (less than 30 degrees per second) normal subjects should be able to pursue without requiring catch-up saccades. *Convergence* is tested by having the patient follow a target moving from far to near. The degree of normal convergence varies considerably and depends on the cooperation of the patient. A clear sign that the patient is attempting to converge is simultaneous pupillary constriction.

COMMON CAUSES OF ABNORMAL OCULOMOTOR CONTROL. *Strabismus.* The flow chart in Figure 453–4 outlines the logic for determining the common causes of strabismus. A comitant strabismus present since childhood is usually a benign *congenital disorder*. As noted earlier, latent congenital strabismus can become manifest in adulthood in association with a systemic illness. An acquired skew deviation (vertical displacement of the ocular axes) can result from any number of lesions involving the

brain stem and has little localizing value. Noncomitant strabismus can result from restrictive disease of the orbit or from abnormal muscle or oculomotor nerve function. The presence of mechanical restriction is confirmed by the use of forced duction testing. (After a topical anesthetic is applied to the eye the ophthalmologist grasps the muscle insertion with a large blunt-toothed forceps and identifies mechanical restriction.) Common causes of *orbital restrictive disease* include dysthyroid ophthalmopathy, orbital pseudotumor, trauma, and orbital mass lesions. Variable strabismus that increases with fatigue suggests the likelihood of *myasthenia gravis*. A Tensilon test can usually confirm the diagnosis. If both restrictive disease and myasthenia gravis have been excluded most patients with noncomitant strabismus have processes affecting the oculomotor nuclei, their fascicles, or the cranial nerves themselves. Common causes of an *isolated third nerve palsy* in an adult include aneurysm, vascular occlusive disease (including diabetes mellitus), trauma, and neoplasm. Typically, but not always, third nerve lesions due to vascular disease spare the pupil. Vascular disease and trauma are by far the most common causes of *isolated trochlear nerve palsies*. The abducens nerve is particularly vulnerable to isolated traumatic involvement because of its long pathway outside the brain stem. Lesions at distant sites that produce increased intracranial pressure can lead to abducens nerve dysfunction producing a "false localizing sign." Other common causes of *isolated sixth nerve palsies* are vascular disease, trauma, and neoplasm. About one fourth of cases with cranial nerve palsies (third, fourth or sixth nerves) remain undiagnosed.

Internuclear Ophthalmoplegia (INO). INO may be unilateral or bilateral, partial or complete, depending on the location of the lesion and the degree of damage to the MLF. *Demyelinating* and small *vascular lesions* are the most common cause of unilateral INO unaccompanied by other ocular palsies or brain-stem signs. Larger brain-stem lesions that damage one or more oculomotor nuclei plus the MLF often produce bizarre combinations of disconjugate eye movements coupled with nuclear oculomotor palsies. Myasthenia gravis can produce an ophthalmoparesis resembling INO owing to the greater involvement of the medial rectus compared to the lateral rectus. Demyelinating diseases are by far the most common causes of bilateral INO involvement.

Disorders of Conjugate Gaze. As noted earlier, infarction of the frontal cortex results in transient contralateral gaze paresis. Tumors and infarction of the paramedian pontine reticular formation produce ipsilateral horizontal gaze paralysis. With the so-called locked-in syndrome (secondary to basilar artery thrombosis) voluntary horizontal eye movements are absent; the patient's only remaining motor functions are vertical eye and lid movements. Lesions of the pretectum typically affect only vertical eye movements, although the descending pathways from the frontal eye fields to the horizontal gaze centers in the pons can also be affected. With the *dorsal midbrain syndrome* (Parinaud syndrome) patients present with a conjugate up-gaze paresis. When they attempt to make upward saccades they develop convergence retraction nystagmus. As noted earlier, impaired convergence and light-near dissociation of the pupillary reflexes are also part of the syndrome. The most common causes of the dorsal midbrain syndrome include tumors of the pineal gland (dysgerminomas), aqueductal stenosis, and localized infarction.

Nystagmus. *Spontaneous nystagmus* can be congenital or acquired. *Congenital nystagmus* typically has a high frequency and variable wave form (occasionally pendular) and is highly fixation-dependent. It is usually not associated with a structural brain lesion. The lifelong history confirms the diagnosis. Spontaneous nystagmus due to a *peripheral vestibular* lesion (i.e., in the labyrinth or vestibular nerve) usually has combined horizontal and torsional components and is strongly inhibited with fixation (Table 453–4). Acquired persistent spontaneous nystagmus that is not inhibited by fixation indicates a lesion in the brain stem and/or cerebellum (*central vestibular*). The latter is often purely vertical or horizontal, since the vertical and horizontal vestibulo-ocular pathways separate beginning at the vestibular nuclei. Spontaneous *downbeat nystagmus* is commonly seen with lesions of the medulla or cervicomedullary junction (e.g., Arnold-Chiari malformation).

Gaze-evoked nystagmus is always in the direction of gaze and is usually present with and without fixation. It is most commonly

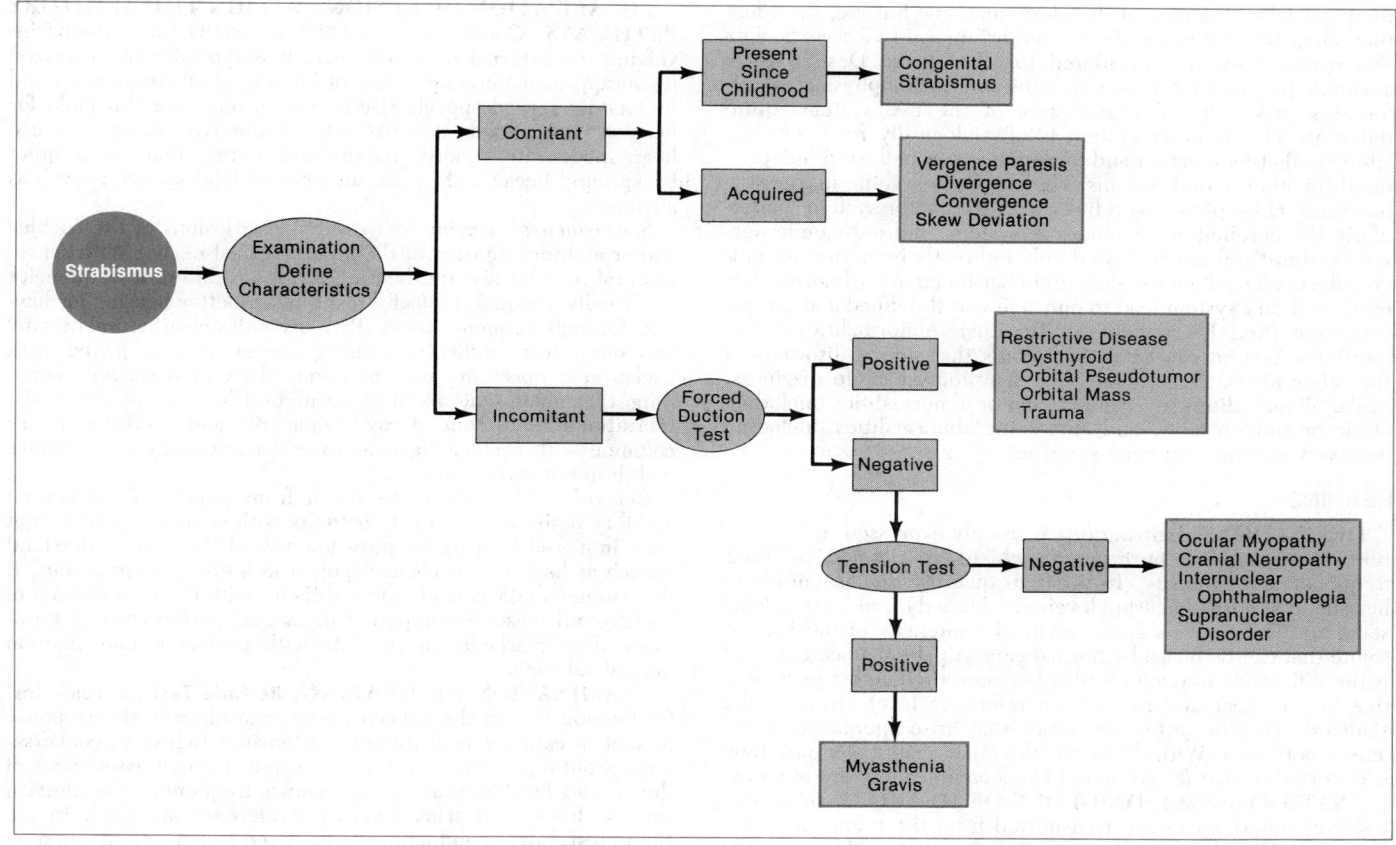

FIGURE 453–4. Diagnostic approach to strabismus.

produced by ingestion of *drugs* such as phenobarbital, phenytoin, alcohol, and diazepam. It can also occur in patients with such varied conditions as myasthenia gravis, multiple sclerosis, and cerebellar atrophy. Asymmetric horizontal gaze-evoked nystagmus indicates a structural brain-stem or cerebellar lesion (particularly at the cerebellopontine angle) with the lesion usually being on the side of the larger amplitude nystagmus. *Rebound nystagmus* is a type of gaze-evoked nystagmus that either disappears or reverses direction as the eccentric gaze position is held. When the eyes are returned to the primary position nystagmus occurs in the direction of the return saccade. Rebound nystagmus occurs in patients with cerebellar atrophy and focal structural lesions of the cerebellum; it is the only variety of nystagmus thought to be specific for cerebellar involvement. *Disconjugate gaze-evoked nystagmus* most commonly results from lesions of the MLF (see above), but it can also occur with other lesions of the brain stem involving the oculomotor nuclei. Positional nystagmus is discussed on page 2110.

TABLE 453–4. KEY DISTINGUISHING FEATURES OF PERIPHERAL AND CENTRAL TYPES OF SPONTANEOUS AND POSITIONAL NYSTAGMUS

Type of Nystagmus	Peripheral (End Organ and Nerve)	Central (Brain Stem and Cerebellum)
Spontaneous	Unidirectional, fast phase away from lesion, combined horizontal torsional, inhibited with fixation	Bidirectional or unidirectional; often pure horizontal, vertical, or torsional; *not* inhibited with fixation
Static positional	Direction-fixed or direction-changing, inhibited with fixation	Direction fixed or direction-changing, *not* inhibited with fixation
Paroxysmal positional	Vertical-torsional, occasionally horizontal-torsional, vertigo prominent, fatigability, latency	Often pure vertical, vertigo less prominent, no latency, nonfatigable

Other Ocular Oscillations. *Ocular bobbing* consists of a fast conjugate downward eye movement followed by a slow return to the primary position. The phenomenon accompanies severe displacement or destruction of the pons or, much less often, metabolic CNS depression. *Ocular myoclonus* consists of continuous rhythmic pendular oscillations, most often vertical, with a rate of 2 to 5 beats per second. Often it accompanies palatal myoclonus and has a similar pathogenesis. *Square wave jerks* and *ocular flutter* consist of brief, intermittent, horizontal oscillations (saccades) arising from the primary gaze position. These types of ocular oscillation are most commonly seen with cerebellar disease but can also accompany more diffuse central nervous system disorders. *Opsoclonus* consists of rapid, chaotic, conjugate, repetitive, saccadic eye movements (dancing eyes). One type of opsoclonus accompanies cerebellar dysfunction, but the most chaotic varieties are associated with brain-stem encephalitis or the remote effects of systemic neoplasm, especially neuroblastoma in children. *Ocular dysmetria* refers to over- and undershooting of saccadic eye movements often followed by multiple attempts at refixation. It reflects cerebellar dysfunction.

Burde RM, Savino PJ, Trobe JD: Clinical Decisions in Neuro-ophthalmology. St. Louis, The C. V. Mosby Company, 1985. *Liberal use of flow charts to help the clinician answer the question, "Given the symptom and signs, what is the disease?"*

Glaser JS: Neuro-ophthalmology, 2nd ed. Hagerstown, MD, Harper & Row, 1990. *An excellent one-volume didactic introductory text.*

Leigh RJ, Zee DS: The Neurology of Eye Movement, 2nd ed. Philadelphia, F. A. Davis Company, 1991. *An up-to-date monograph that gives the clinical and physiologic details of modern investigations on ocular control.*

453.3 HEARING AND EQUILIBRIUM

The neural pathways subserving hearing and those most important for equilibrium and spatial orientation are anatomically proximate in much of their course from their end organs in the inner ear to their termination in the superior portion of the temporal lobe. Because of the close anatomic linkage, disorders that affect hearing often affect equilibrium, and vice versa. For this reason they are considered together here. Despite their anatomic propinquity, however, substantial pathophysiologic differences make clinical examination of the two systems quite different. The auditory system is physiologically relatively isolated, so that its function and dysfunction can be tested independently of other neural systems. The vestibular system, in contrast, has many close physiologic links with the motor system (particularly the cerebellum, oculomotor system, and autonomic nervous system) and can be tested only indirectly by noting secondary effects on oculomotor and cerebellar functions. Abnormalities of the auditory system lead to only a few well-defined and unique symptoms (i.e., hearing loss or tinnitus). Abnormalities of the vestibular system can cause symptoms that mimic disorders of the other neural structures. Such symptoms include dizziness, ocular abnormalities (nystagmus), motor abnormalities (including ataxia or sudden falls), and autonomic abnormalities (including nausea, vomiting, and even syncope).

HEARING

DEFINITIONS. *Hearing loss* is usually expressed in terms of the ability to hear *pure tones*, which are defined by their frequency and intensity. In order to quantify the magnitude of hearing loss, normal hearing levels are defined by an international standard. These levels approximate the intensity of the faintest sound that can be heard by normal ears. A patient's hearing level is the difference in decibels (dB) between the faintest pure tone that he can hear and the normal reference level given by the standard. *Tinnitus* refers to noises that arise spontaneously in one or both ears. With *diplacusis* the tonal quality of a pure tone is distorted so that it may sound like a complex mixture of tones.

ANATOMY AND PHYSIOLOGY OF HEARING. In normal hearing, sound waves are transmitted from the tympanic membrane via the three ossicles of the air-filled middle ear (air conduction) to the oval window and the basilar membrane of the fluid-sealed cochlea. The ossicles serve to increase the gain from the tympanum to oval window about 18-fold, compensating for the loss that sound waves moving from air to fluid would otherwise suffer. In the absence of this system, sound may reach the cochlea by vibration of the temporal bone (bone conduction) but with much less efficiency (approximately 60 dB loss). Hair cells lying along the cochlear basilar membrane detect the vibratory movement of that membrane and transduce vibration into nerve impulses. The nerve impulses are relayed via nerve cells that synapse at the base of hair cells and have their bodies in the spiral ganglion to the cochlear nucleus of the ipsilateral pontine tegmentum. The spiral cochlea mechanically analyzes the frequency content of sound. For high-frequency tones, only sensory cells in the basilar region are activated, whereas for low-frequency tones all or nearly all sensory cells are activated. Therefore, with lesions of the cochlea and its afferent nerve the hearing levels for different frequencies are usually unequal, typically resulting in better hearing sensitivity for low-frequency than for high-frequency tones. Within the brain stem, auditory signals ascend from the ventral and dorsal cochlear nuclei to reach the superior olivary nuclei of both sides. Thus nervous system lesions central to the cochlear nucleus do not cause monaural hearing loss, and, conversely, unilateral central lesions do not cause deafness. From these structures the pathway projects by way of the lateral lemnisci to the inferior colliculi. Each inferior colliculus transmits to the other and to its ipsilateral medial geniculate body, which in turn sends the final projection to the transverse auditory gyrus lying in the superior portion of the ipsilateral temporal lobe.

The normal ear can detect sound frequencies ranging between 20 and 20,000 hertz (Hz); the upper range drops off fairly rapidly with advancing age. The ear is most sensitive between 500 and 4000 Hz, which roughly corresponds to the frequency range most important for understanding speech. The hearing level in this range has several practical implications in terms of the degree of handicap and the potential for useful correction with amplification. A 30 to 40 dB hearing level in the speech range would impair normal conversation, whereas an 80 dB hearing level

would make everyday auditory communication almost impossible (the social definition of deafness).

LOCALIZATION OF LESIONS WITHIN THE AUDITORY PATHWAYS. *Conductive hearing loss* results from lesions involving the external or middle ear. It is typically characterized by an approximately equal loss of hearing at all frequencies and by well-preserved speech discrimination once the threshold for hearing is exceeded. Patients with conductive hearing loss can hear speech in a noisy background better than in a quiet background because they can understand loud speech as well as anyone.

Sensorineural hearing loss results from lesions of the cochlea and/or auditory division of the eighth cranial nerve. With sensorineural hearing loss the hearing levels for different frequencies are usually unequal, typically resulting in better hearing for low-than for high-frequency tones. Patients with sensorineural hearing loss often have difficulty hearing speech that is mixed with background noise and may be annoyed by loud speech. Three important manifestations of sensorineural lesions are diplacusis, recruitment, and tone decay. Diplacusis and recruitment are common with cochlear lesions; tone decay usually accompanies eighth nerve involvement.

Central hearing disorders result from lesions of the central auditory pathways. As a rule patients with central lesions do not have impaired hearing for pure tones, and they can understand speech as long as it is clearly spoken in a quiet environment. If the listener's task is made more difficult with the introduction of background noise or competing messages, performance deteriorates more markedly in patients with central lesions than in normal subjects.

EXAMINATION OF HEARING. Bedside Test. A quick test for hearing loss in the speech range is to observe the response to spoken commands at different intensities (whisper, conversation, shouting). Tuning fork tests permit a rough assessment of the hearing level for pure tones of known frequency. The clinician can use his own hearing level as a reference standard. In the Rinne test, nerve conduction is compared to bone conduction by holding a tuning fork (preferably 512 Hz) against the mastoid process until the sound can no longer be heard. It is then placed 1 inch from the ear and in normal subjects can be heard about twice as long by air as by bone. If bone conduction is better than air conduction, the hearing loss is conductive, but care must be taken to assure that the bone conduction is not heard in the normal ear. In the Weber test, the tuning fork is placed on the patient's forehead or upper teeth. Normally this sound is referred to the center of the head. If it is referred to the side of unilateral hearing loss, the hearing loss is conductive; if it is referred away from the side of unilateral hearing loss, the loss is sensorineural. The Weber test is often unreliable in conductive hearing loss because the patient cannot accept the fact that he hears better in what he knows to be the diseased ear.

Audiometry. *Pure tone testing* is the nucleus of most auditory examinations. Pure tones at selected frequencies are presented via either earphones (air conduction) or a vibrator pressed against the mastoid portion of the temporal bone (bone conduction), and the minimal level that the subject can hear is determined for each frequency. Two speech tests are routinely used. The *speech reception threshold* (SRT) is the intensity at which the patient can correctly repeat 50 per cent of the words presented. The SRT is a test of hearing sensitivity for speech and should reflect the hearing level for pure tones in the speech range. The *speech discrimination test* is a measure of the patient's ability to understand speech when it is presented at a level that is easily heard. In patients with eighth nerve lesions speech discriminations can be severely reduced, even when pure tone thresholds are normal or nearly normal, whereas in patients with cochlear lesions discrimination tends to be proportional to the magnitude of hearing loss.

Recruitment is usually measured by the alternating binaural loudness balance (ABLB) test (if the hearing loss is unilateral). This test compares the loudness for tones of varied intensities as perceived by the pathologic ear and the normal ear. Recruitment is present if smaller increases in stimulus intensity are required in the poorer ear than in the better ear to maintain equal loudness. Otologists employ a variety of special tests to evaluate hearing loss, including tone decay, distorted speech testing and dichotic stimulation, acoustic impedance, tympanometry, and stapedius muscle contraction. The text by DeWeese and Saunders gives details.

Brain stem auditory evoked responses (BAER) can be recorded from scalp electrodes at 0 to 10 msec (early), 10 to 50 msec (middle), and 50 to 500 msec (late) following a click stimulus. The early potentials reflect electrical activity at the cochlea, eighth cranial nerve, and brain stem; the later potentials reflect cortical activity. Computer averaging of the responses to 1000 to 2000 clicks separates the evoked potential from background noise. Early evoked responses may be used to estimate the magnitude of hearing loss and to differentiate among cochlea, eighth nerve, and brain-stem lesions.

CAUSES OF HEARING LOSS. Conductive Hearing Loss. The logic for identifying common causes of hearing loss is shown in Figure 453–5. The history, examination, and audiometry usually provide the key differential features. The most common cause of conductive hearing loss is *impacted cerumen* in the external canal. This benign condition is usually first noticed after bathing or swimming when a droplet of water closes the remaining tiny passageway. The most common serious cause of conductive hearing loss is inflammation of the middle ear, *otitis media*, either infected (suppurative) or noninfective (serous). Fluid accumulates in the middle ear, impairing the conduction of airborne sound. Since the air cavity of the middle ear is in direct connection with the mastoid air cells, infection can spread through the mastoid bone and, occasionally, into the intracranial cavity. Chronic otitis media with perforation of the tympanic membrane can result in an invasion of the middle ear and other pneumatized areas of the temporal bone by keratonizing squamous epithelium (*cholesteatoma*). Cholesteatomas can produce erosion of the ossicles and bony labyrinth, resulting in a mixed conductive-sensorineural hearing loss. *Otosclerosis* commonly produces progressive conductive hearing loss by immobilizing the stapes with new bone growth in front of and below the oval window. The hearing loss is typically conductive, although in some persons the cochlea may be invaded by foci of otosclerotic bone, producing an additional sensorineural hearing loss. Otosclerosis usually stabilizes when the hearing level reaches 50 to 60 dB and rarely progresses to deafness. Other common causes of conductive hearing loss include trauma, congenital malformations of the external and middle ear, and glomus body tumors.

Sensorineural Hearing Loss. Genetically determined deafness, usually from hair cell aplasia or deterioration, may be present at birth or may develop in adulthood. The diagnosis of *hereditary deafness* rests on the finding of a positive family history. In many instances the inheritance is through a recessive gene or a dominant gene with low penetrance, making it difficult to determine the genetic nature of the disorder. *Intrauterine factors* resulting in congenital hearing loss include infection (especially rubella);

toxic, metabolic, and endocrine disorders; and anoxia associated with Rh incompatibility and difficult deliveries.

Acute unilateral deafness usually has a cochlear basis. *Bacterial or viral infections* of the labyrinth, *head trauma* with fracture or hemorrhage into the cochlea, or *vascular occlusion* of a terminal branch of the anterior inferior cerebellar artery all can damage extensively the cochlea and its hair cells. An acute idiopathic, often reversible, unilateral hearing loss strikes young adults and is presumed to reflect an isolated viral infection of the cochlea and auditory nerve terminals. Sudden unilateral hearing loss often associated with vertigo and tinnitus can result from a *perilymphatic fistula*. Such fistulae may be congenital or may follow stapes surgery or head trauma. *Drugs* cause acute and subacute bilateral hearing impairment. Salicylates, furosemide, and ethacrynic acid have the potential to produce transient deafness when taken in high doses. More toxic to the cochlea are aminoglycoside antibiotics (gentamicin, tobramycin, amikacin, kanamycin, streptomycin, and neomycin). These agents can destroy cochlear hair cells in direct relation to their serum concentrations. Some antineoplastic chemotherapeutic agents, particularly cisplatin, cause severe ototoxicity.

Subacute relapsing cochlear deafness occurs with *Meniere syndrome*, a condition associated with fluctuating hearing loss and tinnitus, recurrent episodes of abrupt and often severe vertigo, and a sensation of fullness or pressure in the ear. Recurrent endolymphatic hypertension (hydrops) is believed to cause the episodes. Pathologically, the endolymphatic sac is dilated, and the hair cells become atrophic. The resulting deafness is subtle and reversible in the early stages but subsequently becomes permanent and is characterized by diplacusis and loudness recruitment. The disorder is usually unilateral, but in about 20 to 40 per cent of patients bilateral involvement occurs.

The gradual, progressive, bilateral hearing loss commonly associated with advancing age is called *presbycusis*. Presbycusis is not a distinct disease entity but rather represents multiple effects of aging on the auditory system. It may include conductive and central dysfunction, although the most consistent effect of aging is on the sensory cells and neurons of the cochlea. The typical audiogram of presbycusis is a symmetric high-frequency hearing loss gradually sloping downward with increasing frequency. The most consistent pathology associated with presbycusis is degeneration of sensory cells and nerve fibers at the base of the cochlea. The recurrent trauma of *noise-induced hearing loss* affects approximately the same cochlear region and is almost as common, particularly among those with exposure to loud explosive or industrial noises. Loud, blaring, modern music has become a recent offender. The loss almost always begins at 4000 Hz and does not affect speech discrimination until late in the

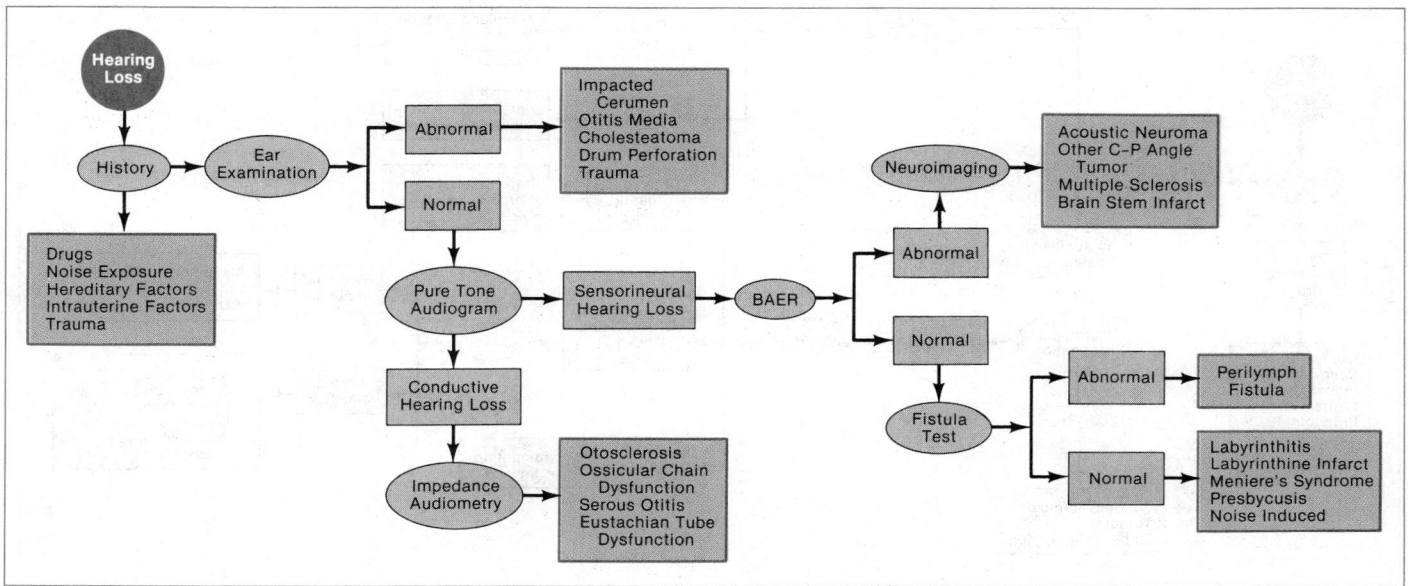

FIGURE 453–5. Evaluation of hearing loss.

disease process. With only brief exposure to loud noise (hours to days) there may be only a temporary threshold shift, but with continued exposure permanent injury begins. The duration and intensity of exposure determine the degree of permanent injury.

Hearing loss from direct damage to the acoustic nerve in the petrous canal occasionally results from infection within or trauma to the surrounding bone; severe deafness of abrupt onset marks the event and is usually associated with acute vertigo due to concurrent vestibular nerve injury. Progressive unilateral hearing loss that arises insidiously and worsens by almost imperceptible degrees is characteristic of benign neoplasms of the cerebellopontine angle, such as *acoustic neuromas.* In about 10 per cent of cases the hearing loss can be acute, apparently owing to either hemorrhage into the tumor or compression of the labyrinthine vasculature.

Central Hearing Loss. Central hearing loss is unilateral only if it results from damage to the pontine cochlear nuclei on one side of the brain stem. Such can occur with *ischemic infarction* of the lateral brain stem (e.g., occlusion of the anterior inferior cerebellar artery), a plaque of *multiple sclerosis,* or, rarely, invasion or compression of the lateral pons by a *neoplasm* or *hematoma.* Bilateral *degeneration* of the cochlear nuclei accompanies some of the rare recessive inherited disorders of childhood. As noted, clinically important unilateral hearing loss never results from neurologic disease arising rostrad to the cochlear nucleus. Although bilateral hearing loss could, in theory, result from bilateral destruction of central hearing pathways, in practice this is rare since involvement of neighboring structures in brain stem or hemisphere would usually produce overwhelming neurologic disability.

TREATMENT OF HEARING LOSS. If an underlying disorder has not yet destroyed the auditory system and can be ameliorated medically or surgically, hearing may be improved or preserved. Most patients with otosclerosis respond to stapedectomy. Closure of a perilymph fistula may improve hearing. Antibiotic and decongestive treatment of otitis media should prevent permanent hearing loss. A low-salt diet and diuretics are effective in selective cases of Meniere syndrome, particularly if episodes are precipitated by premenstrual water retention. The surgical treatment of Meniere syndrome is still controversial. Hearing aids amplify sound, usually with the goal of making speech intelligible. Patients with conductive hearing loss require simple amplification, but those with sensorineural hearing loss often need frequency-selective amplification in order to make hearing aids useful. Recent advances in acoustic technology have markedly improved the outlook for the latter. Monitoring audiograms in patients with exposure to noise or ototoxic drugs is critical for prevention of permanent hearing loss.

TINNITUS. The flow chart in Figure 453–6 outlines the logic for determining the common causes of tinnitus. A careful history should be taken to identify common offending drugs (Table 453–5). With *objective tinnitus* the patient hears a sound arising external to the auditory system, a sound that can usually be heard by the examiner with a stethoscope. Objective tinnitus usually has benign causes such as noise from temporomandibular joints, opening of eustachian tubes, or repetitive muscle contractions. Sometimes, in a quiet room, the patient can hear the pulsatile flow in the carotid artery or a continuous hum of normal venous outflow through the jugular vein. The latter can be obliterated by compression of the jugular vein or extreme lateral rotation of the neck. Pathologic objective tinnitus occurs when patients hear turbulent flow in vascular anomalies or tumors (e.g., glomus jugulare tumor). Objective tinnitus may also be an early sign of increased intracranial pressure. Such tinnitus, which is usually overshadowed by other neurologic abnormalities, can be obliterated by pressure over the jugular vein. It probably arises from turbulent flow through compressed venous structures at the base of the brain.

Subjective tinnitus can arise from sites anywhere in the auditory system. The sounds most frequently complained of are metallic ringing, buzzing, blowing, roaring, or, less often, bizarre clanging, popping, or nonrhythmic beating. Tinnitus heard as a faint, moderately high-pitched, metallic ring can be observed by almost anyone who concentrates attention on auditory events in a quiet room. Sustained louder tinnitus accompanied by audiometric evidence of deafness occurs in association with both conductive and sensorineural hearing loss. Tinnitus observed with otosclerosis tends to have a roaring or hissing quality, while that associated with Meniere syndrome often produces sounds that vary widely in intensity with time and quality, sometimes including roaring or clanging. Tinnitus with other cochlear or auditory nerve lesions tends to be higher pitched and ringing in quality. Audiometric and brain stem–evoked response testing can help distinguish between lesions involving the conducting apparatus, the cochlea, and the auditory nerve.

Tinnitus without observable deafness appears sporadically and

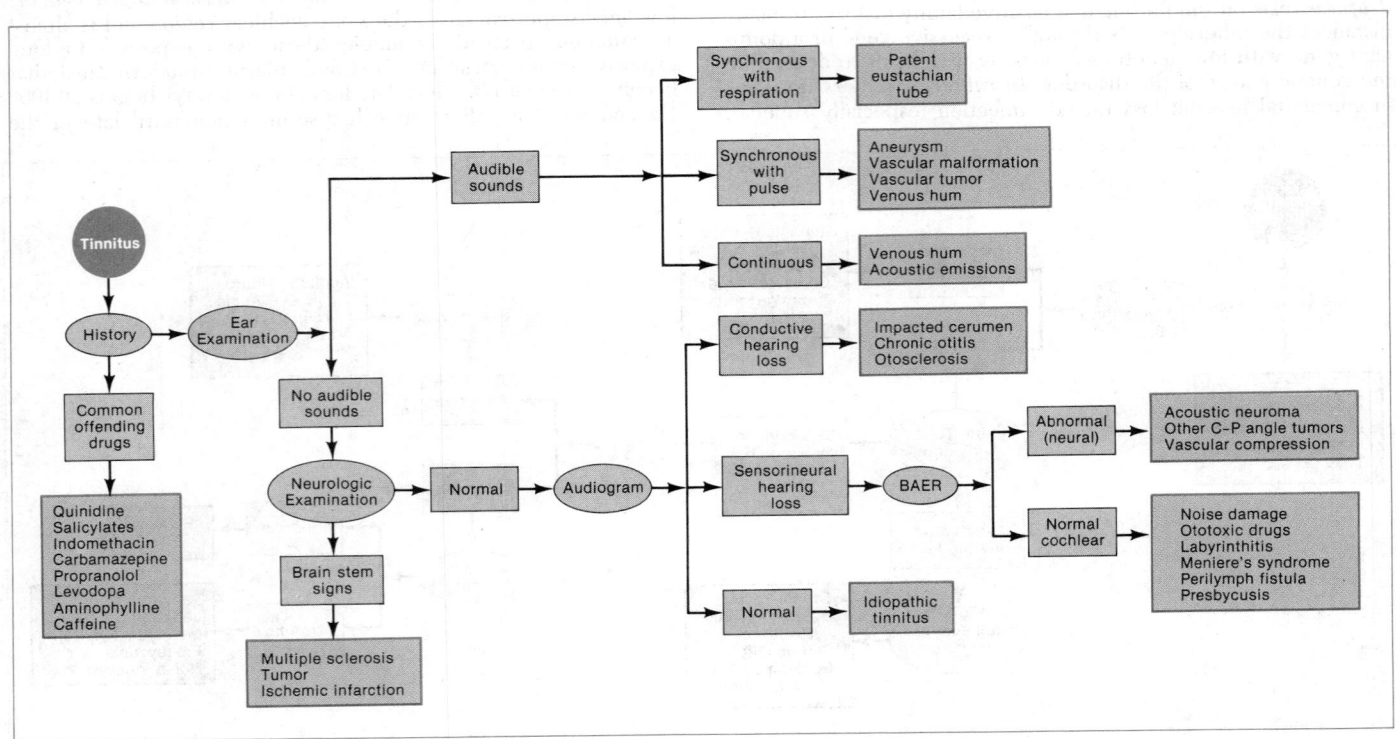

FIGURE 453–6. Evaluation of tinnitus.

TABLE 453–5. DRUGS COMMONLY ASSOCIATED WITH TINNITUS

Quinidine	Propranolol
Salicylates	Levodopa
Indomethacin	Aminophylline
Carbamazepine	Caffeine

for variable lengths of time in many persons without other evidence of an ongoing pathologic process. In many instances one suspects that the auditory experience is no more than an anxious preoccupation with normal auditory physiology.

TREATMENT OF TINNITUS. Most patients with tinnitus can be helped by detailed interview together with the relevant examination and laboratory investigations followed by reassurance where this can be given. Often exacerbating factors such as chronic anxiety and depression can be identified. In patients with hearing loss and tinnitus a hearing aid may improve communication in two ways, as amplification of ambient sound may effectively mask the tinnitus. This mechanism probably explains the frequent observation that removal of cerumen from the external auditory canal to improve ambient hearing also improves tinnitus. Also, when cerumen is attached to the tympanic membrane, tinnitus may result from local mechanical effects on the conductive system. For patients who find their tinnitus most obtrusive when trying to sleep, a bedside FM clock radio tuned between stations can provide an effective masking sound that will switch itself off after the patient falls asleep. A careful drug history should be taken, and a drug-free trial period should be considered when possible. Some patients who notice that caffeine, alcohol, or nicotine exacerbates their tinnitus experience significant relief when these drugs are discontinued.

Surgical treatment of tinnitus has been disappointing. Even when a lesion can be localized to the inner ear or cochlear nerve, removing these structures often has little effect on the tinnitus. A single exception to the generally dismal record of surgical treatment of tinnitus is complete cure of objective tinnitus after surgical correction of a vascular malformation or tumor in the mastoid.

EQUILIBRIUM—VESTIBULAR SYSTEM

DEFINITIONS. *Vertigo* is a subtype of dizziness in which there is an illusion of movement, most commonly rotation. *Physiologic vertigo* occurs in normal subjects when there is a mismatch among the vestibular, visual, and somatosensory systems induced by some external stimulus. The most common example is coming to a sudden stop after several whirling turns. The vestibular signals arising from the semicircular canals are in conflict with the visual signals that indicate a stable surround. *Pathologic vertigo* occurs when there is an imbalance in the vestibular system caused by a lesion within the vestibular pathways anywhere from the inner ear to the cerebral cortex. *Oscillopsia* refers to an illusion of oscillation of the environment.

ANATOMY AND PHYSIOLOGY OF THE VESTIBULAR SYSTEM. The paired vestibular end organs lie within the temporal bones next to the cochlea. Each organ consists of three semicircular canals that detect angular acceleration and two otolith structures, the utricle and saccule, that detect linear acceleration (including gravitational). Like the cochlea, these organs possess hair cells that act as force transducers, converting the forces associated with head acceleration into afferent nerve impulses. The hair cells of the three semicircular canals, each of which is oriented at right angles to the others, are concentrated in the crista, where they are embedded in a gelatinous mass called the cupula. Movement of the head causes the endolymph to flow either toward or away from the cupula, bending the hair cells and, depending on the direction of endolymphatic movements, either exciting or inhibiting the afferent nerve firing. Since the afferent nerves arising from the semicircular canals are tonically active, the baseline activity can be increased or decreased depending on the direction of hair cell bending. Furthermore, the two sets of semicircular canals are approximately mirror images of each other, so that rotational movement of the head that excites one canal inhibits the analogous canal on the opposite side. The hair cells of the utricle and saccule are concentrated in an area called the macule. The macule of the

utricle lies approximately in the plane of the horizontal canal and the macule of the saccule is approximately in the plane of the anterior canal. The hair cells are embedded in a membrane that contains calcium carbonate crystals or otoliths; the density of otoliths is considerably greater than that of the endolymph. Linear accelerations of the head combine with the linear acceleration of gravity to distort the otolith membrane, thereby bending the underlying hair cells and modulating the activity of the afferent nerve terminals at the base of the hair cells.

The afferent vestibular nerves have their cell bodies in Scarpa's ganglion. The nerve fibers travel in the vestibular portion of the eighth cranial nerve contiguous to the acoustic portion. Fibers from different receptor organs terminate in different vestibular nuclei at the pontomedullary junction. There are also direct connections with many portions of the cerebellum, the greatest representation being in the flocculonocular lobe, the so-called vestibular cerebellum. Efferent fibers from the brain stem travel through the vestibular nucleus to reach hair cells of the semicircular canals and macules. Efferent fibers are inhibitory in nature and, like the efferent fibers of the cochlea, may function to enhance inputs to which the brain attends. From the vestibular nuclei second-order neurons make important connections to the vestibular nuclei of the other side, to the cerebellum, to motor neurons of the spinal cord, to autonomic nuclei in the brain stem, and, most importantly for the examining clinician, to the nuclei of the oculomotor system. Fibers from the vestibular nuclei also ascend through the brain stem and thalamus to reach the cerebral cortex bilaterally. The exact site of cortical representation is unclear. Clinical evidence points to both superior temporal and inferior parietal lobes as likely sites.

LOCALIZATION OF LESIONS WITHIN THE VESTIBULAR PATHWAYS. Vertigo can be caused by either the peripheral or central vestibular apparatus. In general, peripheral vertigo is more severe, is more likely to be associated with hearing loss and tinnitus, and often leads to nausea and vomiting. Nystagmus associated with peripheral vertigo is usually inhibited by visual fixation. Central vertigo is generally less severe than peripheral vertigo and is often associated with other signs of central nervous system disease. The nystagmus of central vertigo is not inhibited by visual fixation and frequently is prominent when vertigo is mild or absent.

EXAMINATION OF THE VESTIBULAR SYSTEM. Most vestibular problems presenting to the physician are episodic, and often there are neither symptoms nor signs when the physician examines the patient. The history, therefore, can become paramount for identifying vestibular dysfunction. The history should attempt to distinguish vertigo (the illusion of movement in space) from light-headedness (presyncope), ataxia (disequilibrium of the body without true movement in space), and psychogenic symptoms (the feeling of dissociation or, sometimes, dysequilibrium). If the history is not clear, bedside provocative tests to mimic the symptom may assist in making a pathophysiologic diagnosis. Hyperventilation, which lowers the Pa_{CO_2} and decreases cerebral blood flow, causes a light-headed sensation associated with syncope. Ask the patient to hyperventilate maximally for 1 to 3 minutes to cause light-headedness. If the episode mimics the patient's symptoms it suggests that anxiety and hyperventilation may be playing an important role. In addition, during the course of hyperventilation the patient may suffer dry mouth, chest tightness, and paresthesias, which he may recognize as part of his spontaneous attacks, thus helping in diagnosis.

Bedside tests of vestibulospinal function are often insensitive because most patients can use vision and proprioceptive signals to compensate for any vestibular loss. Patients with acute unilateral peripheral vestibular lesions may past point or fall toward the side of the lesion, but within a few days balance returns to normal. Patients with bilateral peripheral vestibular loss have more difficulty compensating and usually show some imbalance on the Romberg and tandem walking tests, particularly with eyes closed.

The vestibulo-ocular reflex can be tested at the bedside by inducing physiologic nystagmus and searching for pathologic nystagmus. In an alert human, rotating the head back and forth in the horizontal plane induces compensatory horizontal eye movements that are dependent on both the smooth pursuit and vestibular systems. Because of the combined visual and vestibular input, a patient with complete loss of vestibular function and normal pursuit may still have normal compensatory eye movements on this test. The doll's-eye test is a useful bedside test of vestibular function in a comatose patient, however, since such patients cannot generate pursuit or corrective fast components. In this setting slow conjugate compensatory eye movements indicate normally functioning vestibulo-ocular pathways. Since the vestibulo-ocular reflex has a much higher frequency range than the smooth pursuit system, a qualitative bedside test of vestibular function can be made by having the patient shake his head back and forth at frequencies above 1 Hz while reading a standard visual acuity chart. A decrease in visual acuity of more than one line compared to testing with the head still indicates an abnormal vestibulo-ocular reflex.

The caloric test uses a nonphysiologic stimulus to induce endolymphatic flow in the horizontal semicircular canal and horizontal nystagmus by creating a temperature gradient from one side of the canal to the other. With a cold caloric stimulus the column of endolymph nearest the middle ear falls because of its increased density. This causes the cupula to deviate away from the utricle (ampullofugal flow) and produces horizontal nystagmus with the fast phase directed away from the stimulated ear. A warm stimulus produces the opposite effect causing ampullopedal endolymph flow and nystagmus directed toward the stimulated ear (mnemonic: COWS—cold opposite, warm same). Because of its ready availability ice water (approximately 0° C) is usually used for bedside caloric testing. To bring the horizontal canal into the vertical plane the patient lies in the supine position with head tilted 30 degrees forward. Infusion of 10 ml of ice water induces a burst of nystagmus usually lasting from 1 to 3 minutes. A comatose patient shows only a slow tonic deviation toward the side of stimulation. Greater than a 20 per cent asymmetry in nystagmus duration suggests a lesion on the side of the decreased response. This should always be confirmed, however, with standard bithermal caloric testing and electronystagmography (see below).

Examination for pathologic vestibular nystagmus should include a search for spontaneous and positional nystagmus (see Table 453–4). Since vestibular nystagmus secondary to peripheral vestibular lesions is inhibited with fixation, the yield is increased by impairing fixation (such as with +30 lenses, Frenzel glasses). Two general types of positional nystagmus can be identified on the basis of nystagmus regularity: static and paroxysmal. One induces static positional nystagmus by slowly placing the patient into the supine, then right lateral, and then left lateral position. This type of positional nystagmus persists as long as the position is held. Since direction-changing and direction-fixed static positional nystagmus occur with both peripheral and central vestibular lesions, their presence indicates only a dysfunction somewhere in the vestibular system. As with spontaneous nystagmus, however, lack of suppression with fixation and signs of associated brain-stem dysfunction suggest a central lesion.

Paroxysmal positional nystagmus is induced, after a brief delay, by a rapid change from erect sitting to supine head-hanging left, center, or right position (the so-called Hallpike maneuver). It is initially high in frequency but dissipates rapidly (within 30 seconds to 1 minute). The most common variety of paroxysmal positional nystagmus, benign positional nystagmus, usually has a 3 to 10 second latency before onset and rarely lasts longer than 30 seconds. The nystagmus is always torsional with fast phase directed upward (i.e., toward the forehead). It is usually prominent in only one head-hanging position, and a burst of nystagmus

in the reverse direction occurs when the patient reassumes the sitting position. Another key feature is that the severe vertigo and nystagmus that the patient experiences with the initial positioning rapidly disappear with repeated positioning (fatigability). Benign positional nystagmus is a sign of vestibular end-organ disease (probably damage to the posterior semicircular canal, see p. 2111).

Electronystagmography (ENG) is a technique for recording eye movements that allows precise quantification of both physiologic and pathologic nystagmus. A standard ENG test battery includes (1) tests of visual ocular control (saccades, smooth pursuit, and optokinetic nystagmus); (2) a careful search for pathologic nystagmus with fixation and with eyes open in darkness; and (3) measurement of induced physiologic nystagmus (caloric and rotational). ENG can be helpful in identifying a vestibular lesion and localizing it within the peripheral and central pathways.

EVALUATING THE "DIZZY" PATIENT. The history is key, since it determines the type of dizziness (vertigo, light-headedness, feeling of dissociation, disequilibrium), associated symptoms (neurologic, audiologic, cardiac, psychiatric), precipitating factors (position change, trauma, stress, drug ingestion), and predisposing illness (systemic viral infection, cardiac disease, cerebrovascular disease). Features that distinguish between vestibular and nonvestibular types of dizziness are summarized in Table 453–6. The examination should include complete neurologic, head and neck, and cardiac assessments. When focal neurologic signs are found, neuroimaging usually leads to a specific diagnosis. When vertigo is present without focal neurologic symptoms or signs, audiometry and electronystagmography aid in localizing the lesion to the labyrinth or eighth nerve. Patients with hyperventilation syndrome and/or acute anxiety should be identified after the history and examination so that needless tests are not obtained. A detailed cardiac evaluation (including Holter monitoring) often identifies the cause of episodic presyncopal light-headedness.

COMMON CAUSES OF VERTIGO. The logic for identifying common causes of vertigo is shown in Figure 453–7.

Physiologic Vertigo. Physiologic vertigo includes common disorders such as *motion sickness*, *space sickness*, and *height vertigo*. In these conditions vertigo (defined as an illusion of movement) is minimal or absent while autonomic symptoms predominate. With height vertigo, patients often experience acute anxiety and panic reaction. Subjects with motion sickness and space sickness typically develop perspiration, nausea, vomiting, increased salivation, yawning, and generalized malaise. Gastric motility is reduced and digestion impaired. Even the sight or smell of food is distressing. Hyperventilation is a common sign, and the resulting hypocapnia leads to changes in blood volume, with pooling in the lower parts of the body predisposing to postural hypotension and syncope. An unusual variant of motion sickness continues when the subject returns to stationary conditions after prolonged exposure to motion. Typically, affected patients report that they feel the persistent rocking sensation of a boat long after returning to solid ground. Rarely, the syndrome can last for months to years after exposure to motion and can even be incapacitating. The cause is unknown.

Physiologic vertigo can often be suppressed by supplying sensory cues that help to match the signals originating from different sensory systems. Thus, motion sickness, which is exacerbated by sitting in a closed space or reading (giving the visual system the miscue that the environment is stationary), may be improved by looking out at the environment and watching it move. Height vertigo, caused by a mismatch between sensation of normal body sway and lack of its visual detection, can often be relieved either by sitting or by visually fixating a nearby stationary object.

TABLE 453–6. DISTINGUISHING BETWEEN VESTIBULAR AND NONVESTIBULAR TYPES OF DIZZINESS

	Vestibular	Nonvestibular
Common descriptive terms	Spinning (environment moves), merry-go-round, drunkenness, tilting, motion sickness, off-balance	Light-headed, floating, dissociated from body, swimming, giddy, spinning inside (environment stationary)
Course	Episodic	Constant
Common precipitating factors	Head movements, position change	Stress, hyperventilation, cardiac arrhythmia, situations
Common associated symptoms	Nausea, vomiting, unsteadiness, tinnitus, hearing loss, impaired vision, oscillopsia	Perspiration, pallor, paresthesias, palpitations, syncope, difficulty concentrating, tension headache

Reprinted with permission from Baloh RW, Honrubia V: Clinical Neurophysiology of the Vestibular System, 2nd ed. Philadelphia, F. A. Davis Company, 1990.

Benign Positional Vertigo (BPV). BPV is by far the most common cause of pathologic vertigo. Patients with this condition develop brief episodes of vertigo (less than 1 min) with position change, typically when turning over in bed, getting in and out of bed, bending over and straightening up, or extending the neck to look up. BPV can result from *head injury, viral labyrinthitis,* and *vascular occlusion,* or it may occur as an isolated symptom of unknown cause (in about 50 per cent of cases). The latter is particularly common in the elderly. This syndrome is important to recognize, since, in the vast majority of patients, the symptoms spontaneously remit within 6 months of onset. It does commonly recur, however. The diagnosis rests on finding characteristic fatigable paroxysmal positional nystagmus after a rapid change from the sitting to head-hanging position (described on p. 2110). The pathophysiology of BPV is not established, but some investigators have postulated that debris from the utricular macule may become attached to the cupula of the posterior semicircular canal and artificially stimulate that canal when it is in the dependent position. Consistent with this theory, the burst of paroxysmal positional nystagmus is in the plane of the posterior canal of the "down ear," and the positional nystagmus disappears after the ampullary nerve has been surgically resected from the posterior canal on the diseased side. If the history and physical findings are typical, no further evaluation is necessary. If the history or findings are atypical, the condition must be distinguished from other causes of positional vertigo that may occur with tumors or infarcts of the posterior fossa. Typical BPV is not associated with such conditions. The treatment for most patients is simple reassurance. Since the vertigo can be extinguished by fatigue, many patients find that exercises involving repetitive position changes that initially produced the vertigo provide prolonged relief.

Acute Peripheral Vestibulopathy ("Acute Labyrinthitis"). One of the most common clinical neurologic syndromes at any age is the acute onset of vertigo, nausea, and vomiting lasting for several days and not associated with auditory or neurologic symptoms. Most affected patients gradually improve over 1 to 2 weeks, but some develop recurrent episodes. A large percentage report an upper respiratory tract illness 1 to 2 weeks prior to the onset of vertigo. This syndrome occasionally occurs in epidemics (epidemic vertigo), may affect several members of the same family, and more often erupts in the spring and early summer. All of these factors suggest a viral origin, but attempts to isolate an agent have been unsuccessful, except for occasional findings of a herpes zoster infection. Pathologic studies showing atrophy of one or more vestibular nerve trunks, with or without atrophy of their associated sense organs, are evidence of a vestibular nerve site and, probably, viral etiology for many patients with this syndrome (*viral neurolabyrinthitis*). In some patients attacks of acute vestibulopathy (usually less severe) recur over many months or years. There is no way of predicting whether a person who suffers a first attack will have repetitive attacks.

Meniere Syndrome. The typical clinical features of Meniere

syndrome are described on page 2107. This disorder accounts for about 10 per cent of all patients with vertigo. The diagnosis is based on documenting episodic severe attacks accompanied by tinnitus, ear fullness, and fluctuating hearing levels on audiometric testing.

Post-traumatic Vertigo. Vertigo, hearing loss, and tinnitus often follow a blow to the head that does not result in temporal bone fracture, the so-called *labyrinthine concussion.* Although they are protected by a bony capsule, the delicate labyrinthine membranes are susceptible to blunt trauma. Blows to the occipital or mastoid region are particularly likely to produce labyrinthine damage. *Transverse fractures* of the temporal bone typically pass through the vestibule of the inner ear, tearing the membranous labyrinth and lacerating the vestibular and cochlear nerves. Complete loss of vestibular and cochlear function is the usual sequela, and the facial nerve is interrupted in approximately 50 per cent of cases. Examination of the ear often reveals hemotympanum, but bleeding from the ear seldom occurs, since the tympanic membrane usually remains intact. As noted above, *benign positional vertigo* is also a common sequela of head trauma. *Fistulae* of the oval and round windows can result from impact noise, deep-water diving, severe physical exertion, or blunt head injury without skull fracture. The mechanism of the rupture is a sudden negative or positive pressure change in the middle ear or a sudden increase in cerebrospinal fluid pressure transmitted to the inner ear via the cochlear aqueduct and internal auditory canal. Clinically, the rupture leads to the sudden onset of vertigo or hearing loss, or both. Surgical exploration of the middle ear is warranted when there is a clear relationship between the onset of vertigo or hearing loss, or both, and the onset of severe exertion, barometric change, head injury or impact noise.

Postconcussion Syndrome. The so-called postconcussion syndrome refers to a vague dizziness (rarely vertigo) associated with anxiety, difficulty in concentrating, headache, and photophobia induced by a head injury resulting in concussion. Occasionally, similar, less pronounced symptoms are associated with mild head injury judged to be trivial at the time. The cause is unknown, but animal studies indicate that small multifocal brain lesions (petechiae) commonly occur after concussive brain injury.

Other Peripheral Causes of Vertigo. Vertigo can be associated with *chronic bacterial otomastoiditis,* either from direct invasion of the inner ear by the bacteria or by erosion of the labyrinth by a cholesteatoma. Radiographic studies of the temporal bone readily identify these disorders. Just as *otosclerosis* can result in sensorineural hearing loss it can also produce vertigo by involving the bony labyrinth. The typical audiometric findings of a combined conductive and sensorineural hearing loss should suggest this diagnosis. Several *drugs* that damage the auditory system (see p. 2107), such as the aminoglycosides, may also damage the vestibular labyrinth. The patient may suffer acute vertigo, either along with or independent of hearing loss and tinnitus, if the

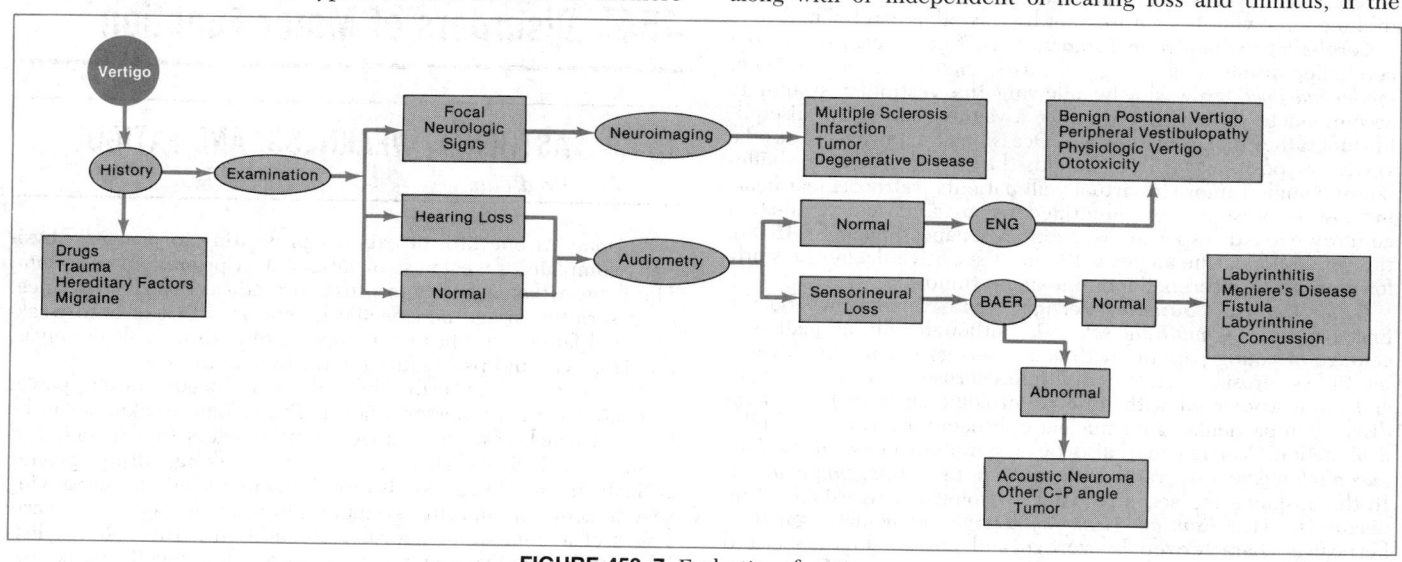

FIGURE 453–7. Evaluation of vertigo.

toxic effect is asymmetric. More often there is a progressive symmetric loss of vestibular function leading to imbalance but not vertigo. Unfortunately, many patients being treated with ototoxic drugs are initially bedridden and unaware of the vestibular impairment until they recover from their acute illness and try to walk. Then they discover that they are unsteady on their feet and that the environment tends to jiggle in front of their eyes (oscillopsia). Younger patients adapt after weeks to the labyrinthine failure; older ones may be left permanently disabled. Usually there is no nystagmus (because of the symmetric involvement), but the patient is ataxic. Caloric and rotational tests during electronystagmography can document impairment or absence of vestibular function. The best treatment is prevention. If the drug is discontinued early during the course of symptoms the disorder may stabilize or improve.

Vascular Insufficiency. Vertebrobasilar insufficiency is a common cause of vertigo in the elderly (see also Ch. 469). Whether the vertigo originates from ischemia of the labyrinth, brain stem, or both structures is not always clear, since the blood supply to the labyrinth, eighth cranial nerve, and vestibular nuclei originate from the same source, the basilar vertebral circulation. Vertigo with *vertebrobasilar insufficiency* is abrupt in onset, usually lasting several minutes, and is frequently associated with nausea and vomiting. Associated symptoms resulting from ischemia in the remaining territory supplied by the posterior circulation include visual illusions and hallucinations, drop attack and weakness, visceral sensations, visual field defects, diplopia, and headache. These symptoms occur in episodes either in combination with the vertigo or alone. Vertigo may be an isolated initial symptom of vertebrobasilar ischemia, but repeated episodes of vertigo without other symptoms should suggest another diagnosis. Vertebrobasilar insufficiency usually is caused by atherosclerosis of the subclavian, vertebral, and basilar arteries. Occasionally, episodes of vertebrobasilar insufficiency are precipitated by postural hypotension, Stokes-Adams attacks, or mechanical compression from cervical spondylosis. Diagnostic studies including CT scans are usually normal, since the vascular insufficiency is transient and function returns to normal between episodes. Angiography can be helpful in confirming the diagnosis but carries a risk and rarely leads to definitive therapy.

Vertigo is a common symptom associated with *infarction of the lateral brain stem or cerebellum,* or both. The diagnosis usually is clear, based on the characteristic acute history and pattern of associated symptoms and neurologic findings. Occasionally cerebellar infarction or hemorrhage presents with severe vertigo, vomiting, and ataxia without associated brain-stem symptoms and signs that might suggest the erroneous diagnosis of acute peripheral vestibular disorder. The key differential point is the finding of clear cerebellar signs (extremity and gait ataxia) and gaze-evoked nystagmus. Such patients must be watched carefully for several days, since they may develop progressive brain-stem dysfunction owing to compression by a swollen cerebellum.

Cerebellopontine-Angle Tumors. Most tumors growing in the cerebellopontine angle (e.g., *acoustic neuroma, meningioma, epidermal cyst*) grow slowly, allowing the vestibular system to accommodate so that they produce a vague sensation of disequilibrium rather than acute vertigo. Occasionally, however, episodic vertigo or positional vertigo heralds the presence of a cerebellopontine-angle tumor. In virtually all patients, retrocochlear hearing loss is present, best identified by an abnormal brain-stem auditory evoked response. Magnetic resonance imaging (MRI) of the cerebellopontine angles is the most sensitive diagnostic study for identifying a cerebellopontine-angle tumor.

Other Central Causes of Vertigo. Acute vertigo may be the first symptom of *multiple sclerosis,* although only a small percentage of young patients with acute vertigo eventually develop multiple sclerosis. Vertigo in multiple sclerosis is usually transient and often associated with other neurologic signs of brain stem disease, in particular, internuclear ophthalmoplegia or cerebellar dysfunction. Vertigo may also be a symptom of *paroxysmal encephalomyelitis* or, rarely, *parainfectious cranial polyneuritis.* In this instance the accompanying neurologic signs establish the diagnosis. The *Ramsay Hunt syndrome* (geniculate ganglion herpes) is characterized by vertigo and hearing loss associated with facial paralysis and, sometimes, pain in the ear. The typical

lesions of herpes zoster, which may follow the appearance of neurologic signs, are found in the external auditory canal and, sometimes, over the palate. Rarely is herpes zoster responsible for vertigo in the absence of the full-blown syndrome. *Granulomatous meningitis* or *leptomeningeal metastasis* and cerebral or systemic *vasculitis* may involve the eighth nerve, producing vertigo as an early symptom. In these disorders cerebrospinal fluid analysis usually suggests the diagnosis. Patients suffering from *temporal lobe epilepsy* occasionally experience vertigo as the aura. Vertigo in the absence of other neurologic signs or symptoms is never caused by epilepsy or other diseases of the cerebral hemispheres.

TREATMENT OF VERTIGO. Treatment of vertigo can be divided into two general categories: specific and symptomatic. Specific therapies include antibiotics for bacterial or syphilitic labyrinthitis, anticoagulants for vertebrobasilar insufficiency, and surgery for acoustic neuroma. When possible, treatment should be directed at the underlying disorder. In most cases, however, symptomatic treatment is either combined with specific therapy or is the only one available (e.g., with acute peripheral vestibulopathy). Many different classes of drugs have been found to have antivertiginous properties, and in most instances the exact mechanism of action is uncertain. All of these agents produce potentially unpleasant side effects, and the decision on which drug or combination to use is based on their known complications and on the severity and duration of the vertigo. An episode of prolonged, severe vertigo is one of the most distressing symptoms that one can experience. Affected patients prefer to lie still with eyes closed in a quiet, dark room. Antivertiginous drugs with sedation such as phenergan (25 mg four times daily [q.i.d.]) or diazepam (5 mg q.i.d.) may be helpful. Prochlorperazine suppositories (25 mg) may stop vomiting. In more chronic vertiginous disorders, when the patient is trying to carry on normal activity, less sedating antivertiginous medications such as meclizine (25 mg q.i.d.) or transdermal scopolamine (0.5 mg every 3 days) may provide relief. Transdermal scopolamine has also been shown to prevent motion sickness. To be most effective, the patch must be in place several hours before exposure to motion. Scopolamine should be used cautiously in elderly subjects because it tends to produce confusion, memory loss, and even hallucinations.

Baloh RW: Dizziness, Hearing Loss and Tinnitus: The Essentials of Neurotology. Philadelphia, F. A. Davis Company, 1984. *More details in a similar format.*
Baloh RW, Honrubia V: Clinical Neurophysiology of the Vestibular System, 2nd ed. Philadelphia, F. A. Davis Company, 1990. *Monograph reviewing basic and clinical aspects of vestibular function.*
DeWeese DD, Saunders WH: Textbook of Otolaryngology, 6th ed. St. Louis, The C. V. Mosby Company, 1982. *A good text with chapters on hearing loss, tinnitus, dizziness, and vertigo.*
Hazell JWP: Tinnitus I, II and III. J Otolaryngol 19:1, 6, 11, 1990. *Up-to-date clinical review.*

454 Disorders of Motor Function

454.1 ASTHENIA, WEAKNESS, AND FATIGUE
Fred Plum

As many as one fifth of patients presenting to primary physicians complain of weakness or fatigue as a prominent symptom. The term *asthenia* finds more use in medical than lay parlance. Its descriptive usage nonspecifically overlaps that of both weakness and fatigue and has been applied to both neurologic (myasthenia gravis) and psychiatric (neurasthenia) disorders.

Weakness is arbitrarily defined as reduced muscle power compared with the person's norm. Physiologic weakness can be focal, in which case the individual often refers to a specific loss of strength during particular acts, e.g., walking, lifting, playing an instrument. Weakness also can be generalized, accompanying several acute or subacute systemic disorders as well as the early stages of a number of neurologic conditions. Table 454–1 lists levels of disease that may result in more or less specific weakness.

TABLE 454–1. CAUSES OF ACUTE OR SUBACUTE WEAKNESS

Condition	Examples or Mechanisms
Joint or muscle injury-inflammation	Movement of the part induces pain.
Primary muscle disease	Genetically transmitted muscle or mitochondrial disorders; inflammatory or granulomatous myopathies; corticosteroid administration
Neuromuscular junction	Myasthenia gravis; Lambert-Eaton myasthenic syndrome
Peripheral motor or sensorimotor pathways (lower motor neuron)	Damage to peripheral motor nerves, spinal motor roots, anterior horn cells *N.B.:* Dysfunction of proprioceptive sensory pathways can produce the illusion of weakness secondary to impaired position sense.
Corticospinal pathways (upper motor neuron)	Disease or injury to the system anywhere from above the anterior horn cell to frontal lobe motor areas
Basal ganglia	Hypokinesia, slow starting, and weakness in parkinsonism
Cerebellum	Sense of incomplete strength with neocerebellar damage
Hysterical or pretended weakness	Signs inconsistent with specific physiologic failure

Table 454–2 defines several particular acute or subacute disorders that may cause generalized weakness. Beyond these classes of specifically identifiable disorders, however, most chronic weakness unaccompanied by diagnosable neurologic or appropriate medical conditions is more likely to have a psychiatric than a neurologic genesis.

Fatigue, as employed in medical terms, describes a reduction in performance due to an experienced deterioration in capacity. Fatigue can be local or general, acute or chronic, and, depending on circumstance, the sense of exhaustion may follow, accompany, or precede attempts at either motor or intellectual effort. Most short-term fatigue lasting for minutes to as much as a few weeks in duration can be traced to recognized antecedents, such as acute systemic illness, severe emotional perturbation, or intense effort of either a physical or intellectual nature. Recurrent, rapidly developing fatigue involving local or generalized striated muscle is typical of myasthenia gravis or, less often, the metabolic myopathies (see Ch. 498). Multiple sclerosis and Parkinson's disease characteristically are accompanied by chronic feelings of fatigue, usually worse at the end than at the beginning of the day. Still-cryptic processes such as tuberculosis, systemic cancer, subacute endocarditis, collagen vascular disease, and certain endocrinopathies represent less frequent causes. Subacute, disabling fatigue also can accompany early HIV involvement of the brain, but that condition also causes recognizable abnormalities in cognitive capacities.

As a group, subacutely or chronically fatigued patients compared with nonexhausted controls have not shown higher long-term antibody titers against Epstein-Barr virus, Lyme borreliosis,

TABLE 454–2. MEDICAL-NEUROLOGIC ILLNESSES COMMONLY ASSOCIATED WITH ACUTE-SUBACUTE GENERALIZED WEAKNESS OR FATIGUE

Systemic	Neurologic
Acute bacterial-viral infections	Myasthenia gravis
Thyrotoxicosis	Early polyneuropathy
Post–myocardial infarction	Multiple sclerosis
Addison's disease	Parkinsonism
Disseminated malignancy	Postconcussion syndrome
Anticancer chemotherapy	Sustained drug use
Acute hepatitis; acute Epstein-Barr virus or Lyme disease	
Severe anemia	

or other organisms. A condition defining "chronic fatigue of recent onset" with a duration of greater than 6 months but less than 1 year and accompanied by objectively verified signs of low-grade fever, painful lymph nodes, and nonexudative pharyngitis recently has been set aside as a distinct syndrome deserving of complex medical evaluation. Such studies as exist to date, however, find few relevant physical or laboratory abnormalities in most chronically fatigued patients. Furthermore, little evidence has been advanced that the physical signs cited above identify any specific somatic illness that might respond to medicinal measures.

All well-analyzed studies of patients with chronic debilitating fatigue emphasize the frequency of the symptoms (up to 25 per cent or more of primary care patients), the lack of identifiable medical abnormalities, and a high incidence of psychiatric disorder. Symptoms of chronic anxiety, personality disorders, or depression have been identified in as many as 80 per cent of such cohorts. The condition frequently includes somatoform complaints unaccompanied by physical or laboratory abnormalities as well as expressions of autonomic dysfunction including breathlessness, palpitations, tachycardia, constipation-diarrhea, sexual impairment, inappropriate sweating, and unsatisfactory sleep patterns. Prospective and retrospective studies in these patients consistently have identified significantly more manifestations of depression, somatic anxiety, and emotional maladjustment than were expressed by nonfatigued controls chosen from patients with neuromuscular disease or recovering from known viral illnesses. No satisfactorily evaluated treatment program has been forthcoming for persons with chronic fatigue. Most patients with somatoform disorders of this kind have sustained better outcomes when "floated" by physicians providing repeated reassurances at short intervals than by psychiatrists attempting intense psychotherapy. Advisory psychiatric consultation, as well as modest doses of tricyclic antidepressants for some, have at times been found to reduce an otherwise high rate of incapacitating somatoform complaints.

Holmes GP, Kaplan JE, Gantz NM, et al.: Chronic fatigue syndrome: A working case definition. Ann Intern Med 108:387, 1988. *Definition of a syndrome in search of a medical cause.*

Kroenke K, Wood DR, Mangelsdorff AD, et al.: Chronic fatigue in primary care. Prevalence, patient characteristics and outcome. JAMA 260:929–934, 1988. *Among 1159 consecutive outpatients in primary care clinics, 24 per cent described chronic fatigue as a major problem. Screening psychometric instruments identified depression, somatic anxiety, or both among 80 per cent of fatigued patients versus 12 per cent of controls.*

Rowland LP: Weakness: The syndromes caused by weak muscles. *In* Rowland LP (ed.): Merritt's Textbook of Neurology, 8th ed. Philadelphia, Lea and Febiger, 1989, pp 50–54. *A systematic explanation of patterns of weakness accompanying disease entities ranging from muscle to brain.*

Smith GR, Monson RA, Ray DC: Psychiatric consultation in somatization disorder. A randomized controlled study. N Engl J Med 314:1407–1413, 1986. *Psychiatric consultation offering suggestions on management to primary physicians reduced quarterly health care charges in the treatment groups by 49 to 53 per cent.*

454.2 ATAXIA AND RELATED GAIT DISORDERS
Fred Plum

Any neurologic illness that affects sensorimotor functions in the lower extremities can interfere with the coordinated act of walking. Accordingly, an introductory analysis of the differential features of certain gait abnormalities may prove helpful in diagnosis. Other chapters provide descriptions of the specific abnormalities that characterize parkinsonism, chorea, athetosis, spastic paraparesis, and various forms of poly- and mononeuritic motor weakness.

ATAXIA. Ataxia is a failure of muscular coordination expressed as irregularity or awkwardness of movement. Common usage has applied the term most often to an unsteadiness of walking, but the same principles apply to disturbances in coordinated movements affecting the upper extremities, the speech mechanisms, or even the eye movements. In the literal sense, ataxia can result from any abnormality in motor function, whether induced by faulty peripheral sensory mechanisms or by disturbances of descending corticospinal, basal ganglion, or cerebellar control.

Most often the analysis of ataxia as a diagnostic problem lies in distinguishing disturbances in proprioceptive control from those caused by weakness, cerebellar-vestibular abnormalities, or the influence of toxic drugs.

PROPRIOCEPTIVE (SENSORY) ATAXIA. Proprioceptive ataxia can result from abnormalities anywhere along the afferent pathway from peripheral nerve, dorsal root, dorsal spinal funiculus, or, less often, the brain stem lemniscal system or the sensory projection from the thalamus to the parietal lobe cortex. The functional defect results from an impaired perception of the location of the body part combined with relatively preserved strength in the member. Afferent peripheral nerve, dorsal root, and spinal lesions are most often caused by inflammatory-demyelinating neuropathy, diabetic neuropathy, syphilitic tabes dorsalis, or meningomyelopathy, as well as any of several inherited forms of spinocerebellar degeneration (see Ch. 463). Cobalamin (B_{12}) deficiency involves both the peripheral nerve and the dorsal column of the cord, whereas multiple sclerosis and compressive cord diseases affect the cord alone.

Nerve or root lesions cause a bilateral defect that characteristically (1) affects the lower more than the upper extremities; (2) involves position sense as much as or more than vibratory sensation; (3) shows absent or greatly reduced deep tendon reflexes; and (4) produces a broad-based, weaving gait that with severe sensory loss becomes lurching, sometimes leg flinging, or pounding, and is worse in the dark (rombergism). Spinal dorsal column lesions produce similar symptoms except that position loss may be more profound, the signs may be less equally symmetric, the tendon reflexes can be preserved, and pathologic reflexes may be present if the abnormality also involves the descending corticospinal tract. By contrast, spinal cord compression tends to impair vibration sensation more than position. Brain stem lemniscal involvement resembles spinal impairment but is seldom bilateral; position sense loss may outstrip vibratory impairment. Patients with peripheral or spinal sensory ataxia are subjectively well aware of their deficits. They are also aware that their lack of coordination is not due to "dizziness," which distinguishes them from patients with vestibular disorders. Parietal or thalamoparietal proprioceptive impairment produces an ataxia that is usually unilateral and (1) affects the contralateral upper extremity as severely as the lower, (2) impairs position sense disproportionately more than vibration, and (3) may go partially unrecognized or be denied by the patient (anosognosia).

CEREBELLAR ATAXIA. The motor abnormality associated with cerebellar lesions depends on the localization of the abnormality in the cerebellum and whether or not adjacent or related neural structures are involved. Thus midline, lateral-hemispheric, and cerebellar outflow lesions tend to produce somewhat distinct syndromes. These differences become blurred when cerebellar tumors compress the adjacent brain stem to produce additional dysfunction or when diseases such as disseminated sclerosis or spinocerebellar degeneration affect neurologic structures that lie remote from the cerebellum.

Spinocerebellar disorders produce a predominantly sensory ataxia superimposed on which is a variable degree of cerebellar dyssynergia, depending on the extent of specific cerebellar inflow and outflow pathway involvement.

Midline cerebellar dysfunction results principally from degenerative (nutritional-alcoholic) or neoplastic (e.g., medulloblastoma, hemangioblastoma, metastasis) disease. The gait is characteristic with legs thrust widely apart and extended, the arms extended in compensatory balance, and walking accomplished by short steps. Affected patients usually look at the ground for additional sensory stabilization and turn en bloc. With extension into the anterior midline cerebellum, stretch reflexes become hyperactive. In the early stages of the illness, the upper extremities and cranial nerves can be affected little or not at all, even in the presence of substantial lower extremity ataxia. As the disorder advances, rhythmic truncal titubation appears, as can difficulty in rhythmic movements of the upper extremities and, eventually, even nystagmus. Posterior midline space-occupying lesions may add retropulsion (see below) to this symptom complex.

Lateral cerebellar hemispheric abnormalities produce ipsilateral hypotonia and incoordination of the limbs, an irregular

swaying gait and a tendency to drift toward the side of the lesion. The feet are spread apart, although not so broadly as with midline lesions, and patients characteristically cannot manage close-footed tandem walking. Rombergism is absent, but, as with all ataxias, distorted vision or closing the eyes accentuates the patient's unsteadiness. Rhythmic movements and point-to-point tests are impaired in both the upper and lower extremities. If classic intention tremor appears, it implies that the abnormality includes the outflow from the dentate nucleus or its projection through the superior cerebellar peduncle to the red nucleus of the midbrain.

DRUNKENNESS. Drunkenness, whether due to alcohol or depressant drug intoxication, results mainly from bilateral labyrinthine-vestibular dysfunction and is accompanied by sensations of both vertigo and dizziness. Few patients with cerebellar disease suffer as much incapacity as the reeling, lurching, twisting, and falling inebriate. Lesser degrees of intoxication produce unsteadiness, a tottering, cautious gait with the feet placed moderately widely apart, clumsiness, dysarthria, and nystagmus in all directions.

VESTIBULAR ATAXIA. Chronic unilateral impairment of the vestibulosensory system can occur with lesions anywhere along the peripheral eighth nerve pathway from labyrinth to brain stem. Patients with such abnormalities tend to drift toward the side of impairment and then quickly correct the deviation in the opposite direction. Turning accentuates their unsteadiness and induces missteps. Bilateral damage or degeneration of the vestibular nuclei in the brain stem results in a narrow-based ataxia with poor compensating movements in the limbs. Patients may drift or fall to either side, and some show a tendency to retropulsion and falling backward. Patients with vestibular dysfunction depend heavily on visual proprioception, so closing the eyes accentuates the gait disorder.

SPASTIC ATAXIA. Combined abnormalities of the spinal dorsal columns and cortical spinal tracts produce a characteristic broad-based tottering and sometimes pounding gait with the knees held high but the legs moving stiffly. The condition occurs with demyelinating diseases and other intrinsic spinal disorders such as vascular malformations, cobalamin deficiency, arachnoiditis, and, occasionally, neoplasms.

FRONTAL LOBE GAIT DISORDERS. Patients with frontal lobe disease can suffer any of several gait disorders, depending upon the anatomic distribution of the lesions. Unilateral injury to the foot-leg area of the somatosensory cortex produces a focal monoparesis, whereas bilateral motor-premotor damage results in a relatively narrow-based, stiff-legged impairment, sometimes with scissoring of the legs. More anteriorly placed premotor and prefrontal abnormalities arise in association with deep bilateral tumors, multiple cerebral infarctions, or communicating, "low pressure" hydrocephalus. The ensuing ataxia consists of a severe difficulty in initiating walking or otherwise using the lower extremities so long as the patient is in the erect position. The feet appear glued to the floor (magnet reaction), and attempts to walk often consist of short shuffles or even hops, before the legs get moving. Walking, once (or if) it begins, proceeds as a halting and broad-based movement made easier by guidance or support. Advanced cases tend to retropulse or fall backward, even from a sitting position. At least some dementia almost always accompanies the gait disorder.

Patients with frontal ataxia of this type show a considerably greater ability to move their legs when lying supine than when standing. Examination of the lower extremities discloses an increased paratonic resistance to passive movements coupled with bilateral plantar grasp responses, extensor thrust responses, and usually accentuated tendon reflexes. These reflex abnormalities and physiologic dysfunctions best explain the difficulty in movement.

HEMIPARESIS. Both pyramidal-corticospinal and extrapyramidal motor disorders may have a hemiparetic pattern, potentially confusing their early differentiation. Severe spastic hemiplegia from damage to the corticospinal tract or the full-blown stooped, festinating, semishuffling gait of parkinsonism is so well known and readily recognized as to require no discussion. In their initial stages, both pyramidal and extrapyramidal disorders produce mild or inconstant weakness, a susceptibility to easy fatigue in the affected member, and a sense of stiffness. Both corticospinal hemiparesis and parkinsonian hemiparesis incipiently produce a gait disorder marked by a slack arm and a reduction of automatic accessory movements on the affected side, a tendency to scuff the toe, and a measure of bodily akinesia. Both may result in an increase in muscular resistance to passive stretch on the involved side. The following points help in differential diagnosis. Patients with early pyramidal tract dysfunction tend to have unilaterally increased reflexes on the affected side. When walking, they flex the wrist and fingers, circumduct the lower extremity, and hold the foot in an equinovarus position. Patients with early hemiparetic parkinsonism, on the other hand, tend to have greater facial and bodily hypokinesia, to stoop, to have difficulty in performing two independent motor acts simultaneously, and to show at least some mild cogwheel resistance on rotary movements of the elbow or wrist. They extend the affected wrist and step the weak foot forward rather than circumducting it. The foot itself is held in simple varus position. The deep tendon reflexes may or may not be slightly asymmetric.

GAIT DISTURBANCES IN THE ELDERLY. Any of several specific visual, somatosensory, or motor diseases may impair walking in elderly persons. Less easily classified but fairly typical walking difficulties include a tendency to walk with slow, short, mincing, and unsteady steps (marche à petits pas). Fairly common is a stooped position coupled with a moderately broad-based, unsteady gait, sometimes associated with computed tomographic evidence of a chronic communicating hydrocephalus (see Ch. 486).

RETROPULSION. A tendency to step backward from the standing position or to fall backward while sitting can be a symptom of several serious, acquired midline abnormalities of the brain. The physiology is poorly understood. The abnormality accompanies midline tumors of the posterior cerebellum as well as degenerative disorders affecting the central vestibular mechanisms bilaterally, and has been reported in association with bilateral lesions affecting the sides of the third ventricle, the basal ganglia, and the frontal lobes. Occasionally the abnormality is associated with large, unilateral frontal lobe neoplasms that produce an increase in intracranial pressure and intracranial shift. Retropulsion of posterior fossa origin is especially dangerous, as it often comes on suddenly and is accompanied by a loss of the normal postural protective mechanisms that guard against injury during falling.

HYSTERICAL GAIT. Hysteria can mimic a variety of hemiparetic, steppage, or ataxic gait disorders. With a hemiparetic type, the pattern usually reveals its genesis by an atypical dragging behind of the affected leg during a series of hops or supported steps. The most obviously factitious hysterical disorder is a lurching, irregularly based, sometimes bent-forward walk in which the patient grasps any object in reach for support and reels from side to side inconsistently. Such patients may sink to the floor, but almost never endure an unsupported, self-injuring fall. Other than the examination of gait, the neurologic examination is normal in these patients. Signs of altered muscular tonus or abnormal reflexes are absent, and the bizarre movements not only differ from the expected pattern of sensory or cerebellar dysfunction but often change from examination to examination.

Garcin R: Coordination of voluntary movement and the ataxias. *In* Vinken PJ, Bruyn GW, Garcin R (eds.): Handbook of Clinical Neurology, Vol 1, Disturbances of Nervous Function. Amsterdam, North Holland, 1969, pp 293, 309. *A detailed and thoughtful exposition of clinical and physiologic principles.*

Keane JR: Hysterical gait disorders: 60 cases. Neurology 39:586, 1989. *A lively and perceptive evaluation of the problem finds that dystonia and chorea are most likely to be overlooked, and that prompt diagnosis leads to the best outcomes.*

454.3 EPISODIC LOSS OF MOTOR FUNCTION

Jerome B. Posner

Sometimes patients, especially in their older years, report episodic loss of motor function affecting one or more extremities unilaterally or bilaterally. The motor loss is brief in duration and is followed quickly by a return to normal. When the legs are affected bilaterally, the patient, if erect, falls (drop attacks). Episodic loss of motor function can be caused by several pathophysiologic abnormalities. Because the symptoms are episodic,

TABLE 454–3. CAUSES OF FALLING IN THE ELDERLY

Drop Attacks	Other Causes
Cryptogenic (see text)	Generalized weakness
Cardiac arrhythmias	Orthostatic hypotension
Transient cerebral ischemia	Sedative drugs
Cataplexy (Ch. 447)	Visual loss
Plateau waves (Ch. 486)	Gait disorders (Ch. 454.2)
Vestibular failure	
Seizures	
Psychogenic	

most such persons are normal by the time the physician sees them, so preliminary diagnosis depends on obtaining an accurate description of the event. The paragraphs below describe some causes of episodic loss of motor function.

DROP ATTACKS AND FALLS

The most perplexing diagnostic problem associated with episodic loss of motor function is the so-called drop attack (Table 454–3). A drop attack is a falling spell that occurs without warning and is not accompanied by changes in sensorium or by other neurologic symptomatology. In a classic drop attack, the patient, usually elderly, does not lose consciousness, has not tripped or otherwise lost his balance, and is able to resume normal activity immediately or shortly following the fall. Affected persons suffer no accompanying neurologic signs but sometimes fall with sufficient suddenness and force to cause injury. The attacks are more common in women and can occur episodically for months or years without the development of other nervous system disease. Although the falls sometimes produce injury, most drop attacks have a benign prognosis, either responding to treatment when a cause can be identified or resolving spontaneously when no cause is identified. The stroke rate and overall survival of elderly patients with drop attack are no different from those of age-matched controls. The pathophysiology of drop attacks is poorly understood. Abnormal tonic, long-loop, posture-controlling reflexes to extensor muscles have been postulated, but the mechanism lacks proof. In most elderly patients, a specific cause is never identified (cryptogenic drop attacks). When a cause is identified, cardiac arrhythmia or cerebral ischemia is usually the offender.

Transient cerebral ischemia produces bilateral leg weakness when motor pathways are involved bilaterally but only rarely causes sudden collapse. Bilateral weakness is likely only when the ischemia occurs in the distribution of either the anterior spinal or the vertebrobasilar arterial system. Episodic spinal cord ischemia is usually accompanied by sensory as well as motor symptoms, and with vertebrobasilar ischemia, most patients suffer other signs of brain stem ischemia as well (see Ch. 469).

Cataplexy, the sudden loss of motor tone without paralysis or change in consciousness, is an occasional cause of drop attacks. The fall to the ground is usually slower than with the classic drop attacks, and the patient rarely hurts himself (Ch. 447). Cataplexy can occur in young adults as part of the narcoleptic-cataplectic disorder (Ch. 447). Otherwise, cataplexy occasionally occurs as an isolated symptom of the sudden rises of intracranial pressure (*plateau waves*) that sometimes accompany brain tumors or hydrocephalus (Ch. 486). Because there are important connections between the vestibular system and pathways controlling muscle tone, sudden *labyrinthine-vestibular failure* such as occurs in Meniere's disease can cause drop attacks. Such episodes are almost always accompanied by vertigo and usually by nausea and vomiting as well. *Akinetic or myoclonic seizures* causing drop attacks are common in childhood but rare in adults. However, drop attacks occasionally have been reported in adults which appear to be epileptic in origin and respond to anticonvulsant drugs.

Falls in the elderly are extremely common, annually affecting one third of elderly persons living at home and as many as half of the residents in nursing homes. Ten to 20 per cent of these falls result in body-damaging injury. A minority of falls in the elderly are due to drop attacks (Table 454–3). Careful evaluation often detects previously unrecognized medical problems, the

TABLE 454–4. CAUSES OF TRANSIENT FOCAL MOTOR PARALYSIS

Transient carotid or basilar ischemia
Nonconvulsive seizures
Complicated migraine
Plateau waves (rare)

identification of which, although not always preventing future falls, substantially decreases future emergency hospitalizations.

DIAGNOSIS. The first task is to determine whether the patient was truly unconscious at any time during the episode. If so, the first diagnosis should be syncope, and the diagnostic evaluation is directed toward that disorder (see Ch. 446.1). If the patient was conscious throughout the episode and the disorder cannot be attributed to tripping or loss of balance, the physician should probe carefully for accompanying symptoms or signs that may help to localize the cause. Back pain, lower extremity paresthesias or sensory loss, or sudden changes in bladder or bowel function accompanying the drop attacks suggest spinal cord dysfunction. Headache, diplopia, and dysarthria accompanying the attack suggest brain stem dysfunction, probably caused by vertebrobasilar arterial insufficiency. Tinnitus or vertigo suggests a vestibular disorder. Severe headache, particularly if accompanied by nausea and vomiting, suggests plateau waves from increased intracranial pressure.

Magnetic resonance imaging (MRI) can rule out brain tumor or hydrocephalus (plateau waves). In the absence of demonstrated syncope or a cause of increased intracranial pressure, the most serious potential diagnoses are cardiac arrhythmias and vertebrobasilar transient ischemic attacks. These diagnoses require appropriate laboratory evaluation.

OTHER TRANSIENT PARALYSES

Episodic loss of motor function in one or more extremities can be a perplexing problem (Table 454–4). Affected patients may complain of sudden or rapid loss of motor function involving an arm or a leg or both, with or without associated sensory symptoms, but without abnormal motor movements of either the arm or the leg. The most common cause is transient cerebral ischemia in the distribution of the internal carotid artery (see Ch. 469). All patients suffering episodic loss of motor function on one side of the body should be considered to be suffering from transient ischemic attacks until proven otherwise. In transient ischemic attacks and the much less frequent plateau waves of increased intracranial pressure, there is usually sudden loss of motor function lasting 5 to 15 minutes and, in the instance of plateau waves, often an accompanying headache and sometimes some clouding of consciousness. With atonic seizures and migraine, the onset of motor dysfunction is usually, but not always, slower, but it, too, persists for 5 to 20 minutes. The motor weakness in late-life migraine may or may not be accompanied by a contralateral headache that appears as the paralysis disappears.

MRI can identify intracranial abnormalities while noninvasive ultrasonography or angiography can detect carotid vascular lesions. Electroencephalography may assist in the diagnosis of a seizure disorder, but the EEG is often normal between episodes. A past or family history of migraine assists in the diagnosis of late-life migraine. Therapeutic trials directed successively at treatment of the several causes of these episodic attacks sometimes help in reaching a definitive diagnosis.

Fisher CM: Late-life migraine accompaniments as a cause of unexplained transient ischemic attacks. Can J Neurol Sci 7:9, 1980. *A classic paper describing neurologic abnormalities, including episodic paralyses in patients with late-life migraine.*

Meissner I, Wiebers DO, Swanson JW, et al.: The natural history of drop attacks. Neurology 36:1029, 1986. *A comprehensive analysis of 108 mostly elderly patients with drop attacks, defining the diagnostic approach, treatment, and prognosis.*

Rubenstein LZ, Robbins AS, Josephson KR, et al.: The value of assessing falls in an elderly population. A randomized clinical trial. Ann Intern Med 113:308–316, 1990. *A randomized clinical trial of the prophylactic value of assessing nursing home patients who fall.*

455 Disorders of Sensation

Jerome B. Posner

455.1 MAJOR SENSORY SYMPTOMS

An organism perceives its environment through its sensory systems. When a sensory system is disordered, sensation may be diminished, increased, or distorted. Table 455–1 lists definitions for major sensory abnormalities.

Anatomy and Physiology of Sensory Pathways

Two major sensory pathways subserve exteroception (cutaneous sensation) and conscious proprioception. The first pathway subserves the sensations of pain, temperature, and crude touch. The receptors are naked nerve endings (nociceptors and thermoreceptors) connected either to small (5 μ), thinly myelinated, "A delta" fibers, which conduct at about 35 meters per second, or to unmyelinated "C" fibers (1 to 2 μ), which conduct at about 0.5 meter per second. (This dual set of fibers explains the phenomenon of "double pain." A noxious stimulus elicits first a sharp, pricking, well-localized pain mediated by the more rapidly conducting fibers, and the C fibers mediate a burning, poorly localized, exceedingly unpleasant "second pain.") Those sensory fibers, all of which have their cell borders in the dorsal root ganglia, enter the spinal cord and synapse in the dorsal horn. The ascending (second order) pain pathways cross the spinal cord and divide into two groups: the neospinothalamic tract, which is believed to subserve the perception of intensity and localization of pain, temperature, and crude touch, and the phylogenetically older paleospinothalamic tract, which is believed to subserve the arousal and emotional components of pain. The axons of the neospinothalamic tract arise from the dorsal horn, cross the anterior commissure, and ascend in the anterolateral quadrant of the spinal cord. The axons terminate in the ventral basal complex of the thalamus, principally within the ventral posterolateral nucleus (VPL) ipsilateral to the side of their ascent. The thalamic terminations of these fibers coincide to a large extent with those of the dorsal column. Third-order neurons from the thalamus project to somatosensory area 1 (sensorimotor cortex), with the same somatotopic localization as other sensory modalities. Lesions at the brain stem or thalamic level often lead to chronic so-called "thalamic pain." The paleospinothalamic tract, whose cells of origin in the dorsal horn receive C-fiber input, also crosses in the anterior commissure and ascends in the spinal cord closely applied to but more ventral than the neospinothalamic tract. Many of the fibers of the paleospinothalamic tract send collaterals to the reticular formation of the brain stem.

The second system subserving the functions of light touch, position sense, and tactile localization begins as encapsulated terminals (mechanoreceptors) connected to larger myelinated fibers. These large fibers enter the spinal cord via the dorsal root ganglion, lying in a position medial to the smaller fibers that subserve pain and temperature. Most of the large fibers ascend without synapsing in the posterior and to a lesser extent lateral columns of the spinal cord to reach the gracile and cuneate nuclei in the low brain stem. Second-order neuron fibers then decussate and ascend in the medial lemniscus to reach the contralateral ventral posterolateral thalamus. Third-order neurons projected

TABLE 455–1. MAJOR SENSORY SYMPTOMS DEFINED

Hypesthesia, anesthesia: reduction or loss of cutaneous touch sensation
Hypalgesia, analgesia: reduction or loss of cutaneous pain sensation
Hyperesthesia: lowered sensory threshold to cutaneous touch
Hyperalgesia: lowered cutaneous threshold to noxious stimuli
Hyperpathia: elevated threshold to noxious stimuli with accentuated discomfort above the threshold
Paresthesias: spontaneously arising exteroceptive sensation (e.g., pins and needles sensations, burning sensations)
Dysesthesias: unpleasant distortion of innocuous afferent stimuli
Allodynia: the perception of an ordinarily nonpainful stimulus as painful or excruciating

from the thalamus terminate in the cerebral cortex, predominantly in the sensorimotor strip surrounding the Rolandic fissure. Lesions of this system lead to loss of sense of position of the limbs and body in space, inability to localize tactile stimuli or to distinguish between one and two closely placed stimuli (two-point discrimination), and inability to describe accurately the size, shape, and texture of objects (stereoanesthesia). Subcortical lesions of the system also cause loss of the ability to recognize vibratory sensation (pallesthesia).

The two major exteroceptive systems are anatomically separated through much of their course, particularly in the spinal cord, and they differ physiologically as a result of fiber size. Thus, lesions at different sites in the nervous system and lesions of different physiologic natures cause unique sensory syndromes that assist in localizing the site and nature of the disorder. A discussion of the principles of pain management can be found in Ch. 26.

Localization of Sensory Disorders

PERIPHERAL NERVES. Sensory perception begins when a physical or chemical stimulus alters the activity of a *sensory receptor* in such a way that the stimulus is transduced into an electrical potential (receptor potential). Many diseases of peripheral nerves affect both large and small fibers, leading to a diminution of all sensory modalities to approximately equal degree. In some disorders of peripheral nerves, however, small or large fibers can be involved preferentially, leading to a "dissociated sensory loss." When small fibers are predominantly affected, pain and temperature sensation are involved out of proportion to light touch, vibration, and position sense. Spontaneous pain and burning dysesthetic sensations are common and often provide the presenting complaints. Because autonomic fibers are also small, trophic changes in skin and joints may accompany such a small-fiber peripheral neuropathy, but because motor fibers and the afferent portion of the stretch reflex are subserved by large fibers, these functions may be relatively preserved despite sometimes profound loss of pain and temperature sensation. Such selective small fiber damage is sometimes encountered in diabetes and is common in some of the hereditary neuropathies as well as in toxic-nutritional neuropathies (Ch. 499 and 500).

Large fiber damage, more common in demyelinating neuropathies, is characterized by profound loss of localizing touch and proprioception, with relative preservation of crude touch, pain, and temperature sensation. Paresthesias are common. The deep tendon reflexes are lost because of damage to large afferent fibers from muscle, and there is usually weakness as well.

The diagnosis of a peripheral neuropathy (see Ch. 495 to 502) involving sensory fibers is established by the distribution of the sensory loss, which may be in the distribution of a single nerve, multiple individual nerves, or a symmetric distal stocking-and-glove distribution. Polyneuropathies are distributed distally because longer axons are more vulnerable to disease than shorter ones. In general, mononeuropathies are caused by local disease (e.g., compression entrapment), mononeuritis multiplex by vascular disorders (e.g., polyarteritis), and polyneuropathies by immunologic or metabolic disorders (e.g., demyelinating-inflammatory neuropathy, diabetes, uremia, nutritional neuropathy).

SPINAL CORD. True dissociation of sensory loss is more common in spinal cord disorders than in those originating in peripheral nerves or roots. Lesions of the posterolateral columns produce profound loss of position and vibration sense with normal crude touch, pain, and temperature sensation. Usually corticospinal tracts are involved as well as sensory pathways, and thus many such patients often have hyperactive reflexes and extensor plantar responses. Lesions of the spinothalamic tract or of crossing fibers from the posterior horn to the spinothalamic tract cause loss of pain and temperature sense with preservation of vibration, position, and localizing touch. Such dissociated sensory loss is common in syringomyelia and may occur with infarction of the anterior portion of the spinal cord from occlusion of the anterior spinal artery. In both of these disorders, motor function may be relatively well preserved. When only one side of the spinal cord is involved, one finds loss of proprioceptive sensation on the ipsilateral side and loss of pain and temperature sensation on the contralateral side, both below the level of the lesion. There is

usually a small band of decreased sensation to all modalities resulting from damage to the posterior horn at the level of the lesion. This so-called Brown-Séquard syndrome is sometimes seen with tumors either compressing or invading the spinal cord and is a common presenting syndrome in radiation myelopathy. Lesions of the spinal cord are rarely confused with those of peripheral nerves, even when the latter show dissociated sensory loss, because the sensory loss in spinal cord lesions is usually proximal as well as distal and restricted to those segments below the spinal cord level damaged. Thus, by the time a polyneuropathy causes substantial sensory loss above the knees, nerve fibers supplying the fingertip are usually involved as well, whereas with a thoracic spinal cord lesion the arms are always spared. Furthermore, motor signs of upper motor neuron disease, particularly extensor plantar responses, usually correctly identify the central nature of a spinal cord disorder rather than pointing to a peripheral disturbance.

BRAIN STEM. In the lower brain stem, spinothalamic and proprioceptive pathways remain separated, lateral lesions of the medulla causing loss of pain and temperature sensation on the ipsilateral side of the face (a result of damage to the descending root of the trigeminal nerve) and the contralateral side of the body. This sensory abnormality is usually accompanied by other signs of lateral medullary damage (Wallenberg's syndrome) and spares proprioceptive pathways. Higher in the brain stem, as the two pathways converge in their route toward the thalamus, damage causes contralateral sensory loss to all modalities, usually accompanied by cranial nerve palsies, ataxia (from the cerebellar outflow), and motor weakness.

CEREBRUM. In the thalamus, damage to the ventral posterolateral nucleus causes decreased sensation of all modalities on the contralateral side of the body and face. Sensory loss is often accompanied by dysesthesias. A *thalamic syndrome* often appears 4 to 6 weeks after acute thalamic damage and has been attributed to denervation hypersensitivity of sensory neurons in the midbrain reticular formation. The patient develops spontaneous pain in the distribution of the sensory loss, usually associated with a dysesthetic response to touch and a hyperresponsiveness to pinprick once threshold is exceeded. The thalamic syndrome is rare but causes a particularly unpleasant pain intractable to most therapeutic endeavors. Conversely, surgical lesions of the intralaminar nuclei, which receive fibers from the paleospinothalamic tract, often decrease pain without affecting sensory thresholds.

Lindblom U, Ochoa JL: Somatosensory function and dysunction. *In* Asbury AK, McKhann GM, McDonald WI (eds.): Diseases of the Nervous System, 2nd ed. Philadelphia, WB Saunders, 1991, in press.

455.2 HEADACHE AND OTHER HEAD PAIN

Headache ranks ninth among the causes of visits to physicians and is a major source both of time lost from work and of medical diagnostic procedures. The frequency of disabling headache is explained in part by the rich nerve supply to the head (including afferent nerve fibers from trigeminal, glossopharyngeal, vagus, and upper three cervical nerves) and in part by the psychological significance of head pain, causing anxiety about even modest discomfort, whereas a pain of equal severity elsewhere in the body might be ignored. Head pain can result from distortion, stretching, inflammation, or destruction of pain-sensitive nerve endings as a result of intra- or extracranial disease in the distribution of any of the aforementioned nerves. However, most head pain arises from extracerebral structures and carries a benign prognosis. The physician's twofold task is first to distinguish the very much more common, benign head pain from rarer but more serious causes and then to administer appropriate treatment. The diagnosis can usually be established by history and physical findings alone; skull radiographs, computed tomographic (CT) and magnetic resonance (MR) images, and other diagnostic tests are seldom required. Table 455–2 is a simplified classification of the pathogenesis of head pain; the overwhelming majority of

TABLE 455–2. PATHOPHYSIOLOGIC CLASSIFICATION OF HEADACHE

Vascular Headache	**Tension Headache**
Migraine headache	Common tension headache
Classic migraine	Depressive equivalent
Common migraine	Conversion reaction
Complicated migraine	Temporomandibular joint
Variant migraine	dysfunction
Cluster headache	Atypical facial pain
Episodic cluster	
"Chronic" cluster	**Traction-Inflammation Headache**
Chronic paroxysmal hemicrania	Cranial arteritis
Miscellaneous vascular headaches	Increased or decreased
Carotidynia	intracranial pressure
Hypertension	Extracranial structural lesions
Orgasmic, exertional, and	Pituitary tumors
cough headache	
Hangover	**Extracranial Structural Lesions**
Toxins and drugs	Paranasal sinusitis and tumors
Occlusive vascular disease	Dental infections
	Otitis
Cranial Neuralgias	Ocular lesions
	Pituitary tumors
	Cervical osteoarthritis

headaches are either migraine or so-called tension headaches, with both abnormalities frequently playing a role in a given individual. Other forms of headache are much less common.

Migraine and Other Vascular Headaches

The term *vascular headache* applies to a group of clinical syndromes of unknown etiology in which the final step in pathogenesis of the pain appears to be dilatation of one or more branches of the carotid artery, leading to stimulation of nerve endings supplying that artery. There may be a release of noxious substances by either the arterial wall or nerve endings, causing a substantially lowered pain threshold. Such substances as serotonin, substance P, bradykinin, histamine, and prostaglandins alone or in combination have all been implicated in the pathogenesis of vascular headache. Most vascular headaches are unilateral, often but not always throbbing, and recurrent over months or years. Individual headaches are precipitated in some by identifiable environmental, dietary, or psychological factors. During the course of a vascular headache, the involved arteries may be tender to the touch, and pain may be relieved temporarily by compression of the carotid artery, only to return with increased intensity when compression is released. Most vascular headaches can be relieved by prompt administration of ergotamine; recurrent headaches can often be prevented by one of several prophylactic drugs (see below). So-called common migraine may affect as many as 25 per cent of the population. Other vascular headache syndromes are less common, but each has distinctive clinical findings.

CLASSIC MIGRAINE

Classic migraine is distinguished by well-defined symptoms of neurologic dysfunction that precede or, less often, accompany the headache. Neurologic symptoms are usually visual, consisting of bright flashing lights (scintillation or fortification scotomata) beginning in the center of a homonymous visual half-field and radiating over 10 to 30 minutes outward toward the periphery. Less commonly, the visual abnormalities are monocular (retinal) or consist of hemianoptic loss of vision in place of or following the scintillating scotomata. Other neurologic disturbances that can occur in classic migraine include unilateral paresthesias, usually involving the hand and perioral area, aphasia, hemiparesis, and hemisensory defects. An uncommon variant named *basilar artery migraine* occurs predominantly in children and adolescents and is characterized by vertigo, ataxia, and diplopia, along with hemiparesis or hemisensory changes. Rarely, confusion, stupor, or even coma may develop. Neurologic symptoms of classic migraine usually last no longer than 30 minutes and generally clear before the headache phase begins. However, in some instances neurologic signs may persist for hours or, rarely, for days, throughout and even beyond the headache phase of the illness.

The pathogenesis of the neurologic dysfunction is not fully understood. Measurements of regional cerebral blood flow during episodes of classic migraine have shown a wave of focal hyperemia followed by abnormally low flow spreading from posterior to anterior over the cerebral cortex. The flow reduction may be sufficient to cause the neurologic symptoms and, rarely, cerebral infarction. In most cases, however, the reduced cerebral blood flow is insufficient to account for the neurologic symptoms. One explanation is that there may be a wave of physiologic "spreading" depression that spreads across the cortex, accounting for both the neurologic symptoms and the changes in blood flow. Changes in brain blood flow do not accompany common migraine, even though the headache phase of the illness is similar. Thus, it is likely that if "spreading depression" is the cause of the neurologic symptoms of migraine, it is only one of several precipitating factors that may produce the headache.

The syndrome of classic migraine has four parts: (1) The *prodromal phase* occurs in a minority of patients and consists of an alteration of mood, often occurring for 24 or more hours before the headache. Patients may complain of increased hunger or thirst, drowsiness, euphoria, or depression. In some patients, known precipitants such as red wine commonly induce an attack. (2) The second phase consists of the *neurologic symptoms* described above. The neurologic symptoms may occur without subsequent headache (termed migraine equivalent), particularly in older people. (3) The third phase usually begins as the neurologic symptoms clear and characteristically consists of a unilateral throbbing frontotemporal *headache* on the side opposite the neurologic symptoms. The headache is frequently accompanied by nausea, photophobia, vomiting, diarrhea, phonophobia (noise intolerance), and a general feeling of being unwell. The headache commonly lasts 4 to 6 hours but may persist for 1 or more days. If the headache is prolonged, it may change into a dull, aching, bilateral pain extending back into the neck and shoulders. The headache phase is often terminated either by vomiting or by a period of sleep. (4) The *postheadache* phase is characterized by a feeling of exhaustion, tenderness of the scalp at the site of the headache, and recurrence of headache on sudden head movement.

The diagnosis of classic migraine is made by history; physical findings are absent, and laboratory evaluation is not helpful. When the attacks are atypical, particularly when neurologic disability is severe or prolonged, CT or MR imaging may be required to rule out structural lesions of the brain. However, such instances are rare. The treatment of classic migraine is similar to that of common migraine (see below), except that classic migraine attacks usually occur no more than four or five times a year and rarely more than once a month.

COMMON MIGRAINE

Common migraine is similar to classic migraine except that neurologic symptoms are absent. Many patients with classic migraine also have episodes of common migraine. Common migraine is characterized by recurrent headaches, often severe, frequently beginning unilaterally, and usually associated with malaise, nausea and/or vomiting, and photophobia. The disorder often begins in childhood, affects women more often than men, and runs in families (70 per cent of patients give a family history). Identifiable factors that often precipitate individual headaches are holidays and weekends, menstrual periods, foods (especially red wine, chocolate, nuts, and aged cheese), environmental stimuli (such as bright sunlight, too much sleep, and undue emotional stress or resentment). Medical conditions and their treatment may also precipitate attacks. Vasodilators such as nitroglycerin and antihypertensives and serotonin releasers such as reserpine, as well as estrogens and oral contraceptives, have been reported to cause migraine attacks in susceptible individuals. The diagnosis of common migraine is usually made by the history. Important historical points that help distinguish migraine from the equally common tension headaches (see below) include their unilaterality, their association with nausea or vomiting, the tendency of migraine to awaken one from sleep, a positive family history, and a positive response to ergot preparations. When the diagnosis is in doubt, treatment of the patient for common migraine often clarifies the issue.

TREATMENT. The best treatment for migraine is prevention.

The patient should avoid known precipitating factors. Medications known to cause migraine should be withdrawn if others can be substituted. Foods commonly implicated may also be withdrawn and, if withdrawal is effective, replaced one at a time to determine the specific precipitant. The patient should attempt to avoid undue stress or fatigue and not to sleep excessively on weekends. If these methods fail and severe headaches occur frequently (once a week or more), pharmacologic prophylaxis is indicated. Several agents have been reported effective in the prophylaxis of migraine, but not every patient responds to each agent. Perhaps the safest and most effective class of drugs are the β-adrenergic blockers, particularly propranolol. The drug is begun at a dose of 80 mg a day in divided doses and increased as tolerated until headaches are controlled. Recent reports suggest that calcium channel blockers such as verapamil* (80 mg three to four times daily) sometimes are effective. Amitriptyline* in gradually increasing doses from 25 to 125 mg daily may be useful if the above drugs fail. Methysergide, a serotonin antagonist, is effective at a dose of 2 mg three to four times daily. Methysergide must be employed cautiously because it can cause serious side effects, including vascular insufficiency, retroperitoneal or pleural fibrosis, and fibrotic thickening of heart valves. The side effects can be minimized by gradually withdrawing the drug for 1 month after every 4 to 6 months of treatment.

Acute attacks, if mild, often respond to analgesic agents and bedrest. More severe attacks are best treated by ergot preparations such as ergotamine tartrate. The drug, given parenterally, is sufficiently effective (85 to 90 per cent) to be useful as a diagnostic test. Oral ergot 1 to 2 mg given at the onset of a headache is effective in about 50 per cent of patients. However, during the headache, absorption of the oral form of the drug is often poor, and better results can be achieved with sublingual or rectal preparations. The best nonparenteral results are generally achieved by the insertion of half of a 2-mg ergotamine rectal suppository. The side effects of *ergotism* (muscle pain, vasoconstriction, mottled skin, peripheral gangrene, multifocal encephalopathy) make it unwise to treat frequent migraine headaches in this way, and one should switch to prophylaxis if the headaches occur more than once a week. For patients who present to emergency rooms with very severe headaches, intravenous phenothiazines (e.g., prochlorperazine 10 mg IV or chlorpromazine) have proved to be superior to narcotics, as has droperidol, 0.5 cc IM.

MIGRAINE VARIANTS

Several migraine syndromes differ sufficiently from classic and common migraine to earn separate names. *Ophthalmoplegic migraine* is the name given when an ocular motor palsy develops during the course of a severe migraine attack. Ophthalmoplegic migraine usually begins in childhood and is characterized by unilateral pupillary dilatation, ptosis, and paralysis of ocular muscles occurring 12 to 24 hours *after* the beginning of an attack of severe migraine. The ophthalmoplegia usually clears within hours to days but frequently recurs. Angiography may be required to rule out a carotid aneurysm. *Hemiplegic migraine* is a familial syndrome in which aphasia, confusion, and hemiparesis or hemiplegia precede or more often accompany the migraine attack. Repetitive episodes alternating from side to side may occur over many years. *Complicated migraine* is a term applied to attacks of migraine prodromes in which the focal neurologic defects may last for the entire headache attack and may even leave permanent residua. The few available anatomic studies of such patients have shown ischemic brain infarction involving the functionally impaired region.

CLUSTER HEADACHE

Cluster headaches are short-lived attacks of severe, acute, and intense unilateral head pain that occur in clusters lasting several weeks, only to disappear for months or years. The disorder affects men much more than women and usually begins between the third and sixth decades. Clusters characteristically occur in the spring and fall and last 3 to 8 weeks. The individual headaches occur one to several times a day, particularly at night, awakening the victim from sleep. They frequently have a clock-setting

predictability. Each attack, which lasts 30 minutes to 2 hours, is characterized by rapid onset of a knife-like pain in the nostril or behind the eye which spreads to involve the forehead. During the attack, the ipsilateral nostril may water and the eye tear. In about 20 per cent of instances, homolateral Horner's syndrome develops. During the course of the headache, the patient is usually unable to lie still (the opposite of the situation with migraine) and restlessly paces the floor. The pain may be so severe that the patient bangs his head against the wall or threatens suicide. The headache disappears as abruptly as it arises, usually leaving no residua. Unlike the patient with migraine, the patient with cluster headaches does not feel systemically ill, and there is no nausea, vomiting, or sense of exhaustion when the headache ceases. During the time when clusters are occurring (but not between) alcohol invariably induces an attack. When the headaches occur frequently, Horner's syndrome may outlast the head pain.

The pathogenesis of cluster headache is unknown, although it is believed to be a vascular headache related to migraine. The diagnosis is established by the characteristic history. Treatment of an acute attack is usually not worthwhile, since by the time the patient absorbs the analgesic agents the attack is over. In some patients the headache rapidly responds to oxygen inhalation. Several drugs prevent attacks of cluster headache. Ergotamine tartrate given prophylactically in a dose of 1 mg four times a day, or 2 mg at bedtime if the attacks are all nocturnal, is often effective. The drug should be withdrawn every seventh day to prevent the symptoms of ergotism and to see if the cluster has ceased. Methysergide 2 mg three to four times daily is also often effective; since the cluster rarely lasts more than 8 weeks, the drug can be discontinued and therefore is safe. Prednisone 40 mg daily in divided doses may also work and can be added to methysergide if the former is only partially effective. Lithium carbonate in daily doses of 0.9 to 1.5 grams sometimes works.

CLUSTER VARIANTS

Several variants of cluster headache should be recognized by the physician, since their treatment may be different. The most striking is *chronic paroxysmal hemicrania*, a rare disorder consisting of painful episodes similar to cluster headaches that appear many times a day and recur unremittingly for years. There may be as many as 10 to 20 headaches daily, each lasting 10 to 30 minutes. Indomethacin* orally in doses of 75 to 150 mg daily has relieved all subjects. A cluster variant characterized by daily cluster headache without remission, multiple brief jabs of pain in the head, and a background of continuous unilateral headache of variable severity exacerbated by exertion has recently been described and is said to respond to indomethacin in most instances. Patients who did not respond to indomethacin did so to tricyclic antidepressants.

OTHER VASCULAR HEADACHES

Several vascular headache variants deserve mention so that the physician may recognize them as benign and treat them appropriately. Included are *orgasmic headaches*, several short-lived bilateral throbbing headaches occurring in either sex and appearing abruptly at orgasm. The attack can be differentiated from subarachnoid hemorrhage because the headache usually disappears within minutes to an hour or more and may recur repetitively. Usually the illness is self-limited, but if not it may respond to 1 mg of ergot given an hour before sexual activity. *Exertional headache* occurs, as the name implies, during active exercise. Like orgasmic headaches, these are usually bilateral and throbbing, and may last several hours. They respond well to indomethacin. Vascular headaches have been reported to follow minor *trauma* to the carotid artery in the neck and to *carotid endarterectomy*. These headaches are unilateral, recurrent, and severe and usually respond to prophylaxis with propranolol. *Carotidynia* is the name given to spontaneous vascular headaches associated with unilateral anterior neck pain and/or carotid tenderness. They usually respond to the same treatment as vascular headaches. When attacks of carotid pain and/or headache recur, the diagnosis

*This use is not listed in the manufacturer's directive.

*This use is not listed in the manufacturer's directive.

is not difficult, but the first attack must be distinguished from a spontaneous dissection of the carotid artery and may require intravenous angiography for diagnosis.

Hangover headache is part of a larger syndrome, usually including premature awakening from an evening of overindulging and often accompanied by a fine tremor of the extremities and mild gastric distress or nausea, mental dulling, and mild incoordination. The pathogenesis is related to alcohol withdrawal, dehydration, and the toxic effect of various congeners found with different intoxicants. *Nitrites* can induce pulsating headache and, occasionally, facial flushing, most often after the ingestion of processed foods ("hot dog" headache). *Monosodium glutamate* has been blamed for the "Chinese restaurant syndrome," characterized by postprandial headache, tight sensations about the face and head, and, less often, giddiness and diarrhea.

Cough headache is, as the name implies, sudden and often severe headache related to cough. The headache may last only seconds or may persist minutes to hours after a single cough or a coughing paroxysm. In some patients, cough headache is a symptom of an intracranial mass lesion. Most patients, however, do not have underlying structural disease; in these patients the disorder is probably similar to exertional and orgasmic headaches and has a vascular origin. *"Ice pick"* headaches are brief (1 to 2 seconds), sharp focal head pains occurring at unpredictable intervals and at different areas of the head. They do not indicate intracranial disease. *Thunderclap* headaches are sudden, severe, "exploding" pains that involve the entire head and resolve slowly over hours. Although these headaches may indicate an unruptured cerebral aneurysm, most are without pathologic significance. A severe thunderclap headache probably deserves evaluation with CT or MR to look for a cerebral aneurysm. In some patients angiography may be indicated.

Hypertensive headaches occur only in patients with very severe or episodic hypertension. They are characterized by early-morning, usually throbbing, occipital headache that responds to the treatment of the hypertension.

Tension Headaches

Tension headaches are characterized by a steady, nonpulsatile, unilateral, or bilateral aching pain, beginning in the occipital, frontal, or temporal regions. The headaches are also called "muscle contraction headaches" because they are frequently accompanied by tight and tender muscles at the site of most severe pain. They are probably the most common cause of headache in the adult. Tension headaches are recurrent, often present every day, and usually begin in early afternoon or evening, with a dull occipital or frontal pain that may spread to grip the entire head "in a vise." Unique among headaches, the pain may be constantly present for days, weeks, or months and is often associated with tenderness in the posterior cervical, temporalis, or masseter muscles. The pain may be quite severe, but patients rarely complain of nausea, vomiting, or malaise, although modest dizziness, blurring of vision, and sometimes tinnitus may occur. These headaches are more frequent in women, in individuals who are tense and anxious, and in those whose work or posture requires sustained contraction of posterior cervical, frontal, or temporal muscles. The symptoms of common migraine and tension headaches overlap, and many patients suffer from both. The distinguishing features favoring tension headaches include pressure or tightness, which is worst at the back of the neck, increased severity of pain as the day progresses, and pain that is preceded by or associated with anxiety-producing situations. Tension headaches are less commonly unilateral than migraine and less commonly associated with nausea and vomiting. They seldom awaken the patient from sleep and do not respond to ergot preparations.

The pathogenesis of tension headaches is unknown. Electromyographic investigation shows no sustained muscle contraction in the tender muscles, nor are there changes in blood flow to the muscles to suggest the presence of ischemia. In many respects muscle pain and tenderness in tension headaches resemble the fibromyalgia syndrome. Some have suggested that the pathogenesis of both is the accumulation of substances in the muscles which sensitize nociceptive nerve endings. Because decreased pain perception thresholds have been identified in patients with chronic tension headaches, others have suggested that the process is a central one.

TREATMENT. The first step in treatment is to identify causal factors. If these include abnormalities of posture leading to sustained muscle contraction, they should be corrected. Many patients with tension headache, particularly chronic ones, are depressed and respond to treatment with antidepressant agents such as amitriptyline. Others are tense and anxious and respond to anti-anxiety agents such as diazepam. This drug, in a dose of 15 to 20 mg a day for 2 to 3 weeks, is often effective as a diagnostic test. The relief of chronic headache establishes the diagnosis for the physician and helps to convince the patient that tension and anxiety are playing a major role in the headache. In addition, these drugs frequently break up a cycle of anxiety–muscle tension–anxiety, so that a short course may give prolonged relief. Addiction, however, is a potential complication of chronic use.

An individual headache may be treated with aspirin. This drug is probably more useful for tension headaches than acetaminophen because of its anti-prostaglandin properties. Vasoactive agents used for the treatment of migraine have no role in this disorder unless vascular headaches are concomitantly present. Some clinics report that biofeedback treatments effectively relieve muscle contraction and thus the headache. For sharply localized, painful areas present at the site of headache, injection with local anesthetics may transiently relieve the headaches. Sometimes massage has a similar effect.

TENSION HEADACHE VARIANT

Several rather characteristic headache syndromes of unknown cause may have muscle contraction and psychological tension as part of their pathogenesis. The syndrome most clearly related to muscle contraction headache is the so-called temporomandibular joint syndrome. Patients complain of unilateral or bilateral head pain, usually in the temporal region and in the jaw, often radiating into the ear. The pain is often associated with tenderness of the masseter and temporalis muscles and may be exacerbated by chewing. Accompanying symptoms often include limitation of full movement at the temporomandibular joint when opening the jaw, bruxism, and malocclusion. The disorder sometimes responds to dental manipulation, particularly use of a mouth guard during sleep that prevents bruxism. However, for most patients analgesics and anxiolytic agents effectively treat muscle-contraction head pain. *Post-traumatic headaches* are dull, generalized, aching head pains that follow head injury. The injury is often mild. The patient suffering the "post-traumatic syndrome" complains of headache often coupled with unsteadiness, giddiness, difficulty concentrating, insomnia, and fatigue. Contrary to popular belief, the syndrome is not more common in patients seeking compensation for the injury. It often persists for months or years. Treatment, like that of muscle contraction headaches, consists of psychological support and reassurance and the use of mild analgesics and sometimes anxiolytic agents. Patients should be encouraged to return to work as soon as possible and to try to live a normal life despite the symptoms. The disorder can blend into *depressive headache*, a chronic generalized headache, usually vaguely described, sometimes associated with giddiness and unsteadiness, that occurs as a frequent and sometimes predominant manifestation of depression. The headache may have muscle contraction and tension as its pathogenesis or may be a *somatic delusion* in a severely depressed patient. In either event, the treatment of choice is an antidepressant drug.

ATYPICAL FACIAL PAIN

Atypical facial pain or atypical facial neuralgia is a term used to describe a syndrome characterized by steady aching facial pain, usually unilateral, localized to the lower part of the orbit, maxillary area, and sometimes the jaw. The pain begins without a known precipitating episode and may last for hours to days. It may spread to involve the head or neck, and muscles of the jaw and neck are often tender. Sometimes autonomic symptoms including sweating, flushing, rhinorrhea, and pallor are present. The disorder usually affects women, often in early middle age. Patients affected with the disorder are tense, anxious, and often chronically depressed. The pathogenesis of the illness is unknown. The autonomic changes have led some to suggest that the syndrome is a migraine variant, and the muscle tenderness and depression have led others to suggest that it be classified with musculoskeletal tension pain. Patients suffering from atypical facial pain should be examined carefully for local pathology of the eyes, nose, teeth, sinuses, and pharynx, but such is rarely found. Careful psychological evaluation often reveals a masked depression. Treatment is usually unsatisfactory. Analgesic agents are usually not helpful, and patients respond poorly to psychotherapy. In some patients, ergot preparations or propranolol is effective, suggesting a vascular pathogenesis for the face pain. Others respond to physical methods such as massage and biofeedback. Antidepressants sometimes help. It is important to recognize that the syndrome is not caused by structural disease and that patients require no invasive diagnostic or therapeutic procedures. Dental extraction does more harm than good. This disorder should not be confused with trigeminal neuralgia, discussed below; carbamazepine is ineffective.

Head Pain Due to Traction or Inflammation

CRANIAL ARTERITIS

This condition receives detailed consideration in Ch. 267 but deserves mention here as an important cause of headache in the elderly. The illness almost always appears after age 60 and usually later. It usually begins with unilateral or bilateral temporal, occipital, or fronto-occipital head pain of variable intensity, often coupled with tenderness of the painful areas. Many patients have pain in the jaw muscles, making chewing uncomfortable. Nodules occasionally are palpable on affected vessels. The great risk is occlusion of retinal arteries secondary to untreated inflammation. Diagnosis depends on suspicion and usually on the presence of an elevated erythrocyte sedimentation rate. Diagnosis should be confirmed by arterial biopsy because definitive steroid treatment, once started, often must be maintained for many months. Since migraine, vascular headaches, and depressive headaches also can have their onset in the elderly, a confirmed diagnosis is essential.

MENINGITIS AND SUBARACHNOID HEMORRHAGE

Acute and subacute meningitis cause headache by inflammation of the pain-sensitive meninges surrounding the brain. The headache is usually generalized, throbbing, and very severe. It may be rapid or gradual in onset, and by the time it is fully developed is associated with nuchal rigidity. The diagnosis is established by lumbar puncture. In patients suspected of harboring an intracranial mass lesion, MR scan of the brain should be performed first and lumbar puncture deferred, unless the physician suspects that the patient is suffering from acute bacterial meningitis, in which case lumbar puncture must be done immediately. In *subarachnoid hemorrhage*, the initial sudden headache is caused by alteration of intracranial pressure. This headache is succeeded by a chronic persistent headache, often accompanied by nuchal rigidity that results from inflammation of the meninges caused by the blood. In a patient suspected of having suffered a subarachnoid hemorrhage, a CT scan should be performed first. The presence of extravascular blood establishes the diagnosis and obviates the need for lumbar puncture, which may exacerbate the bleeding by altering intracranial dynamics. The absence of identifiable hemorrhage on CT scan, however, does not rule out a small subarachnoid hemorrhage, and lumbar puncture then must be performed to establish or rule out the diagnosis definitively.

ALTERATIONS OF INTRACRANIAL PRESSURE

Headache from altered intracranial pressure is caused by compression or traction of pain-sensitive vascular and neural structures over the apex and base of the brain. In the instance of *intracranial hypotension,* the loss of spinal fluid decreases the buoyancy of the brain so that the organ descends when the upright position is assumed, exerting traction on structures at its apex and compression on structures at its base. (In rare instances, the small bridging veins that enter the sagittal sinus may rupture and cause subdural hematomas.) In *intracranial hypertension,* the source of pain is probably compression of vascular and neural structures at the base of the brain by tumor or edematous brain.

INTRACRANIAL HYPERTENSION. Increased intracranial pressure per se does not lead to headache unless pain-sensitive

structures are distorted. Many patients with high intracranial pressure from brain tumors, jugular venous obstruction, hydrocephalus, or pseudotumor cerebri do not suffer headache. If headache is present, it may be mild or severe, throbbing or steady, localized or generalized. When localized, it usually overlies the site of the lesion, but posterior fossa lesions may cause bifrontal headache. The headache is characteristically at its worst early in the morning, although, unlike cluster headache, it usually does not awaken the patient from sleep. It is exacerbated by stooping, coughing, moving the head suddenly, or straining at stool. Many patients prefer to sleep in the sitting position. The headache is rarely continuously intense. Transient rises of intracranial pressure called plateau waves (see Ch. 486) sometimes cause 5 to 20 minutes of severe headache accompanied by nausea, vomiting, or other neurologic signs. These episodes are commonly precipitated by assuming the upright posture but can also be precipitated by coughing, sneezing, or straining.

The treatment of headache related to increased intracranial pressure is the treatment of the underlying disease. Mild analgesics produce temporary relief; narcotic analgesics should not be used because of their tendency to produce respiratory depression and further raise the pressure in neurologically compromised individuals.

INTRACRANIAL HYPOTENSION (see Ch. 486) **AND LUMBAR PUNCTURE HEADACHE.** Intracranial hypotension usually follows a lumbar puncture and is due to continued leakage of cerebrospinal fluid through a rent in the dural sheath. The syndrome develops 12 hours to several days after the lumbar puncture and is characterized by headache on assuming the upright position. There is no evidence that a period of recumbency after a lumbar puncture prevents subsequent development of the headache. The headache usually begins as a dull ache in the posterior cervical area, radiating laterally toward the shoulders and cephalad toward the frontal area. It persists, often growing more severe, as long as the patient remains upright, and when most severe it may be associated with perspiration, nausea, and vomiting. Persistent headache of intracranial hypotension can lead to diplopia, probably a result of traction on the abducens nerves. The diagnosis of post–lumbar puncture headache is made by history; spontaneous intracranial hypotension is suspected by the history of positional headache and confirmed by low (<30 mm H_2O) or even negative CSF pressure on attempted lumbar puncture. The fluid is usually normal, but there may be an elevated protein concentration if the needle has entered a subdural or epidural fluid collection. Analgesics relieve the mildest headaches; the most severe ones can be controlled only by assuming the recumbent position. The headaches usually clear within a few days to a few weeks; in rare instances, surgical repair of the torn dura is necessary.

Extracranial Structural Causes of Headache

NASAL AND SINUS HEADACHE

Although acute or chronic inflammation and neoplasms of the paranasal sinuses can cause headache, most patients who have been physician- or self-diagnosed as having sinus headaches are in fact suffering from either vascular or tension headache. Most true paranasal sinus headaches result from acute inflammation causing pain localized over the involved sinus and associated with stigmata of acute infection, including fever, swelling, and tenderness over the sinus and engorgement of the turbinates, ostia, nasofrontal ducts, and superior nasal spaces. Most of the discomfort comes from the ostia, which are many times more sensitive than the poorly innervated walls of the sinuses. Typically, "sinus" headache commences in the morning (frontal) or early afternoon (maxillary) and subsides in the early or late evening. The pain is dull and aching, is made worse by changing head position, and is seldom associated with nausea and vomiting. Sinus headache is best treated with decongestants and analgesics. Persistent purulent discharges should be cultured and appropriate antimicrobial drugs employed. Chronic suppurative disease in the frontal, ethmoid, and sphenoid sinuses, or in the mastoid air cells, may result in osteomyelitis and inflammation of adjacent cranial tissues. Headache persisting after surgical drainage of the diseased sinus is evidence for extradural and possibly subdural infection. More chronic inflammation and neoplasms, particularly when they occur in the sphenoid sinus, may not be accompanied by the usual physical signs of sinusitis. In such instances, sinus radiographs or MR scan may be required to establish the diagnosis.

DENTAL PAIN

Noxious stimuli in a tooth usually evoke local toothache, but severe dental pain can be extremely difficult to localize. Afferent fibers from the teeth are contained in the second and third divisions of the trigeminal nerve, and tooth pain can be referred to areas of the head supplied by these nerves. More commonly, in association with toothache, tooth extraction, or a tender, diseased tooth, distant tissues exhibit surface hyperalgesia, tenderness, and vasomotor reactions, such as tender eyeballs, reddening of the conjunctivae, and tenderness of the auricular and temporal tissues. Because of secondary muscle contraction, other sites of tenderness and pain may be noted behind the ears, behind the lower border of the mastoid process, and in the muscles of the occiput, neck, and shoulders. The upper teeth frequently hurt in association with disease of the nasal and paranasal structures. Occasionally, in coronary insufficiency, pain is experienced in the lower jaw. One should beware of ascribing bizarre pains in and around the jaws to a dental origin unless unequivocal acute inflammatory dental lesions are present. Dental extraction rarely ameliorates neuralgias or atypical facial pain. However, hysterical or delusional face pain is often attributed by the patient to prior dental work. Headache should not be attributed to a diseased tooth unless the injection of procaine into the tissues about the suspected tooth greatly reduces the intensity of, or eliminates, such headache.

AURAL PAIN

Severe pain in the vicinity of the ear can be caused by disease of the teeth, acute tonsillitis, inflammatory and neoplastic disease of the larynx and nasopharynx, temporomandibular joint disorders, tumors, inflammation in the posterior fossa, and disease of the cervical spine and its soft tissues. Pain in the ear is also associated with vascular headaches, atypical facial pain, and herpes zoster of the fifth and seventh cranial nerves and, rarely, the glossopharyngeal nerve. True glossopharyngeal neuralgia causes severe pain radiating from the tonsil into the ear. It has the usual timing feature of "tic" (see Cranial Neuralgias, below).

Primary ear disease is an infrequent but important source of headache, because it almost always indicates inflammation or destructive disease. Acute otitis media (purulent or nonpurulent), furunculosis of the ear canal, traumatic rupture of the tympanum, and fracture of the anterior wall of the bony canal all cause pain in the ear associated with tenderness of adjacent skeletal muscles. Osteomyelitis of the mastoid bone may be associated with inflammation of the nearby periosteum as well as of dura and adjacent tissues (epidural abscess)—both sources of pain in or behind the ear. Pain in this region also accompanies tumors of the acoustic nerve and inflammation and thrombosis of the lateral sinus.

EYE PAIN AND HEADACHE

Errors of *refraction* (hypermetropia, astigmatism, anomalies of accommodation), disturbances of ocular muscle equilibrium, and glaucoma are universally described as causing headache, but most such headaches are probably tension headaches rather than truly related to "eye strain." Refractive errors are also said to give origin to such other symptoms as aching of the eyes, "sandy" feeling in the eyes, pulling sensations in and about the orbit, and conjunctival congestion. Headache is mild in degree and usually starts around and over the eyes and subsequently radiates to the occiput and back of the head.

The pain of *glaucoma* at first remains localized in the eyeball, then extends along the rim of the orbit and, finally, throughout most of the area supplied by the ophthalmic division of the trigeminal nerve. Nausea and vomiting sometimes accompany such headaches, which can become prostratingly severe if not treated promptly.

With inflammation of the iris and ciliary body, light may cause intense pain in the eye and adjacent areas because of movement of the inflamed iris. When the iris is immobilized, pain is allayed.

PITUITARY PAIN

Headache caused by pituitary tumors is the result of compression and distortion of pain-sensitive structures at the base of the skull, particularly the diaphragma sella. Pain is generally referred to the frontal or temporal regions bilaterally and may on occasion be referred to the vertex or occipital regions. Because the pain is not related to intracranial pressure, it does not have the same temporal characteristics of most brain tumor headaches and instead can occur at any time and is frequently chronic and unremitting. The diagnosis can be established by endocrine examination and by an MRI of the pituitary fossa employing 1-mm cuts. Acute headache occurring with known pituitary lesions *(pituitary apoplexy)* usually results from infarction or hemorrhage into the tumor. Sudden expansion of the tumor may compromise the overlying optic chiasm, leading to visual loss, or invade the laterally lying cavernous sinus, producing ocular palsies. Pituitary apoplexy should be treated surgically by emergency drainage of the hemorrhagic or infarcted material.

NECK PAIN

Osteoarthritis of the zygapophyseal joints of the upper cervical spine is an occasional cause of perplexing headache. The pain is generally constant, aching, and perceived in the upper cervical and occipital areas. It may radiate to the vertex of the head or even the orbit. At times, vertex or orbital pain is more severe than occipital and neck pain, leading to confusion in diagnosis. The pain probably results from entrapment of the C3 root by overgrowth of the C2 zygapophyseal joint. A syndrome of unilateral upper nuchal and occipital pain accompanied by ipsilateral numbness of the tongue occurring on sudden turning of the head is probably explained by compression of the second cervical root in the atlanto-occipital space. Such acute pain can be prevented by restricting neck movement with a cervical collar. Upper cervical nerve blocks relieve more chronic pain and are useful diagnostically as well as therapeutically. A few reports suggest that severe headache and neck pain affecting young male weight lifters (weight-lifter's headache) may result from pull or tear of cervical ligaments during the strain of exertion.

Cranial Neuralgias

The term cranial neuralgias refers to several distinctive head pains that appear to result from sudden and excessive discharge from the involved nerve. The best-known cranial neuralgia is trigeminal neuralgia. The concept of cranial neuralgias has been expanded to include the chronic burning pain that frequently follows herpes zoster infection of the nerve. Some also include atypical facial pain and temporomandibular joint syndrome under the cranial neuralgias, but these probably have tension or vascular disturbances as their pathogenesis and in this chapter are included under those headings.

TRIGEMINAL NEURALGIA. Trigeminal neuralgia (tic douloureux) is characterized by sudden, lightning-like paroxysms of pain in the distribution of one or more divisions of the trigeminal nerve. Most trigeminal neuralgia is caused by compression of the trigeminal nerve by arteries or veins of the posterior fossa. In some patients there is no identifiable structural disease. Occasionally trigeminal neuralgia may be a symptom of a gasserian ganglion tumor, multiple sclerosis, or a brain-stem infarct involving the descending root of the trigeminal nerve.

The history is diagnostic. The pain occurs as brief, lightning-like stabs, frequently precipitated by touching a trigger zone around the lips or the buccal cavity. At times, talking, eating, or brushing the teeth serves as a trigger. The pains rarely last longer than seconds, and each burst is followed by a refractory period of several seconds to a minute in which no further pain can be precipitated. The pains, however, often occur in clusters so that the patient may report somewhat erroneously that each pain lasts for hours. The pain is limited to one or more divisions of the trigeminal nerve, usually the second, or third, or both. Spontaneous remissions and exacerbations are common, the exacerbations tending to occur in spring and fall. Between paroxysms of pain, the patient is asymptomatic. Tic pain rarely occurs at night. In idiopathic trigeminal neuralgia, the neurologic examination is entirely normal. In symptomatic trigeminal neuralgia, there may be sensory changes in the distribution of the trigeminal nerve, and such a finding should prompt a careful search for structural disease of the nervous system.

Carbamazepine is the drug of choice for the treatment of trigeminal neuralgia. The anticonvulsant drug is given in doses varying from 400 to 800 mg a day, but because of its sedative properties the initial dose is 100 mg twice daily, gradually increased to the required maintenance dose. No more than 1200 mg should be taken daily. The drug is not an analgesic and is only effective for specific kinds of pain such as trigeminal neuralgia, glossopharyngeal neuralgia, and the lightning pains of tabes dorsalis. Side effects include dizziness, sedation and, rarely, aplastic anemia. Phenytoin* in doses of 400 mg a day is also effective in trigeminal neuralgia but less so than carbamazepine. Occasionally the two drugs appear to be synergistic. Baclofen* 60 to 80 mg daily has also been found to be a useful agent. If medical treatment fails, surgical intervention is necessary.

The most popular operations consist of lesioning of the gasserian ganglion (either by radiofrequency or glycerol injections) and posterior fossa craniotomy to relieve the compression of the trigeminal nerve by vascular structures. Gasserian ganglion lesions can be made under local anesthesia, are generally effective initially, but have a high relapse rate. Posterior fossa craniotomy is as effective as gasserian ganglion lesions and appears to have a lower relapse rate. The purpose of both operations is to relieve pain with little or no loss of sensation, thus preventing the dreaded complications of anesthesia dolorosa. Either of these operations is preferable to section of the nerve root proximal to the ganglion. However, that operation affords permanent relief. If surgery on the ganglion is contemplated, a prior test of local anesthesia of the ganglion or the peripheral branches of the nerve is desirable because some patients find the sensory loss less tolerable than the pain itself.

GLOSSOPHARYNGEAL NEURALGIA. Glossopharyngeal neuralgia is characterized by pain similar to that of trigeminal neuralgia but in the distribution of the glossopharyngeal and vagus nerves. The trigger zone is usually in the tonsil or posterior pharynx, and the pain spreads toward the angle of the jaw and the ear. Occasional patients suffer cardiac slowing or arrest during these attacks as a result of the intense afferent discharge over the glossopharyngeal nerve. Carbamazepine is often effective, but if it fails, glossopharyngeal nerve roots are sectioned in the posterior fossa. Symptomatic glossopharyngeal neuralgia is occasionally the presenting complaint of a tonsillar tumor, and careful examination of the pharynx and tonsillar fossa must be carried out.

OTHER NEURALGIAS. Similar but much rarer disorders than trigeminal or glossopharyngeal neuralgia have been reported to involve the greater occipital nerve and the nervus intermedius portion of the facial nerve. The clinical features and treatment of these rare disorders are similar to those for trigeminal neuralgia.

Diagnostic Evaluation

Headache is an extremely common disorder, and the excessive application of expensive and highly technical laboratory procedures to the diagnosis and management of benign head pain has been a substantial cause of unnecessary medical costs. Set against this truism is the fact that in some instances a timely MRI or lumbar puncture can give life-saving information about an otherwise undiagnosable problem. Given these antitheses, the following principles may help in the management of the individual patient:

1. Patients with chronic classic or common migraine or with chronic tension headache rarely require more than a careful history and examination. Even when the unilateral prodromes and headache of longstanding, classic migraine consistently affect the same side, the incidence of associated intracranial lesions remains so low that scans are unnecessary and arteriography unjustified.

2. Headaches that are of recent origin or progression deserve investigation. This principle especially applies to headaches that have a consistently focal distribution, follow trauma, or begin after the age of 30 years. MRI is more sensitive than CT.

3. The EEG is almost never useful in the diagnosis of diseases causing headache and can be omitted. Skull radiographs are useful in diagnosing headache only (a) when searching for abnormalities involving the base of the brain such as sellar and suprasellar lesions or (b) immediately following head trauma. CT scans have discriminating capacities superior to those of plain films and, when available, make radiographs unnecessary.

4. Diagnostic lumbar puncture should be performed with any acute headache that (a) is accompanied by fever or (b) is explosive or the most severe headache ever suffered (a history typical of acute subarachnoid hemorrhage—but see thunderclap headache, p. 2120). Lumbar puncture should, if possible, be deferred until after CT scanning with other forms of acute headache, especially if stiff neck but no fever is present. (This combination may indicate partial herniation of cerebellar tonsils into the foramen magnum secondary to an intracranial mass lesion.)

5. Now that CT and MRI are widely available, radioisotopic brain scanning rarely if ever adds useful information and is expensively superfluous.

Bonica JJ: The Management of Pain, 2nd ed. Philadelphia, Lea and Febiger, 1990. *A two-volume multiauthored encyclopedia of the causes of pain and its management. Individual chapters describe anatomy, physiology, pathology, and pain disorders affecting head, neck, back, and the remainder of the body. Everything you wanted to know about pain and more.*

Cady RK, Wendt JK, Kirchner JR, et al.: Treatment of acute migraine with subcutaneous sumatriptan. JAMA 265:2831, 1991. *A first North American report on a potentially favorable drug for migraine.*

Diamond S (ed.): Headache. Med Clin North Am 75:521, 1991. *The latest monograph on all aspects of the problem.*

Mathew NT (ed.): Headache. Philadelphia, W.B. Saunders Company, 1990, Vol. 8, No. 4. *A multiauthored monograph describing pathophysiology, diagnosis, and management of headaches and other head pain.*

455.3 SOME SPECIFIC PAIN SYNDROMES

Some chronic painful disorders are associated with a specific constellation of signs and symptoms which establishes them as identifiable pain syndromes. Those most commonly encountered in clinical practice include the *neuropathic pain* disorders of diabetic polyneuropathy (see Ch. 498), sympathetically maintained pain, postherpetic neuralgia, phantom limb pain, and the *non-neuropathic pain* syndromes, fibromyalgia and myofascial pain. Taken together, these syndromes cause chronic, usually unremitting pain that is often disabling and difficult and frustrating to treat.

SYMPATHETICALLY MAINTAINED PAIN. This term applies to severe pain, usually burning in quality and associated with autonomic changes including swelling, vasomotor instability, and abnormalities of sweating. The pain syndrome usually follows an injury, often minor, to an extremity. If the injury has involved a peripheral nerve, particularly the sciatic or median nerve, the syndrome is called *causalgia*. If the injury does not involve a peripheral nerve, if there has been no trauma, or if the syndrome follows a visceral illness (e.g., myocardial infarction), the term applied is *reflex sympathetic dystrophy*. (Older and outmoded terms include post-traumatic painful osteoporosis, Sudek's atrophy, post-traumatic spreading neuralgia, minor causalgia, and shoulder-hand syndrome.) The exact pathophysiology of the disorder is unknown, but, as the name implies, abnormal activity of the sympathetic nervous system plays an important role in both the pain and the autonomic symptoms.

The disorder is characterized by severe and continuous pain exacerbated by emotional stress and is usually associated with severe hyperpathia so that moving or touching the limb is often intolerable. At first the pain is localized to the site of injury or the distribution of the nerve injured, but with time it spreads to involve the entire extremity. Spread to other areas of the body sometimes occurs. Along with the pain go vasomotor changes including vasodilatation (warm and dry skin) or vasoconstriction (cyanosis, cool skin). Other autonomic changes may include edema and either hypo- or hyperhidrosis; trophic changes of the skin, subcutaneous tissues, muscles, and bone (osteoporosis) also occur. The entire symptom complex rarely affects any one patient,

---

*This use is not listed in the manufacturer's directive.

and one sign or symptom usually predominates. Untreated, the disorder can lead to muscle atrophy, fixation of joints, and a useless extremity. The diagnosis is largely a clinical one but can be supported by laboratory tests that document autonomic instability or trophic changes including increased uptake in involved bones on radionuclide bone scan, bone atrophy or plain radiographs, and temperature abnormalities on thermography.

The earlier the treatment, the more effective it is likely to be. Treatment is directed at blocking sympathetic outflow to the involved site while stimulating and mobilizing the painful site. To that end, a combination of repetitive sympathetic ganglionic blocks with lidocaine and vigorous physical therapy is used. In addition, sympatholytic agents (e.g., phenoxybenzamine up to 120 mg a day in divided doses) and short courses of corticosteroids have been reported to be effective. How often these techniques afford permanent relief is unknown, and many patients fail to respond. In refractory patients pharmacologic agents directed at neuropathic pain, including tricyclic antidepressants (e.g., amitriptyline, 50 to 150 mg at bedtime), anticonvulsants (e.g., carbamazepine, 600 to 800 mg a day in divided doses), and oral local anesthetics (e.g., mexiletine 300 mg three times a day) can be tried. The disorder is often difficult and frustrating to treat, and in such cases the physician is advised to consider referral to a multidisciplinary pain clinic.

POSTHERPETIC NEURALGIA. Postherpetic neuralgia refers to severe and prolonged burning pain with occasional lightning-like stabs in the involved dermatome after an attack of herpes zoster. Severe postherpetic neuralgia is usually a disease of elderly patients and, like most chronic pain, is exacerbated by emotional upset and relieved to some degree by distraction. Touching the involved area sometimes exacerbates the pain. Treatment of postherpetic neuralgia is not entirely satisfactory. The initial treatment should be directed toward stimulating the painful area. In some patients brisk rubbing applied repeatedly with a terrycloth towel or stimulation of the dermatome with a cutaneous electrical stimulator often brings relief which long outlasts the stimulus and is occasionally permanent.

Most patients, however, require multimodality therapy, which includes not only stimulation of the area but physical therapy, psychological support, and pharmacologic treatment. The application of topical pharmacologic agents, such as lidocaine, sometimes gives temporary relief, and anecdotal evidence claims that topical application of capsaicin is useful. Lancinating pains, which are usually a minor component, usually respond to anticonvulsants (e.g., carbamazepine, 400 to 600 mg a day in divided doses), but anticonvulsants do not affect the continuous pain. The latter may be treated by tricyclic antidepressants or mexiletine (see above); neuroleptics (e.g., fluphenazine 1 to 3 mg daily) may also be helpful. When these conservative approaches fail, one should consider either anesthetic approaches with subcutaneous local injection or sympathetic blockade. The only surgical approach that has proved at all useful is the dorsal root entry zone lesion. Adrenocorticosteroids and acyclovir, both of which may diminish pain in the acute stage, have little or no effect on the development of postherpetic neuralgia. In many patients, the disease runs its course and, after a year or two, disappears spontaneously.

The pharmacologic approach is the same as that described for the neuropathic pains above and includes tricyclic antidepressants, anticonvulsants, neuroleptics, and sometimes sympathetic blockade. Referral to a multidisciplinary pain center may be helpful.

PHANTOM LIMB PAIN. Phantom limb pain is a chronic and severe pain appearing to be localized in an amputated or totally denervated limb. All patients suffer phantom sensations after amputation and as many as 60 to 70 per cent suffer significant pain, especially if there has been severe preamputation pain. The pain is frequently similar to that suffered before amputation, or at times it may resemble muscle pain with the phantom seeming to be in a cramped or uncomfortable position. In most instances, the pain lessens and disappears with time, but sometimes it becomes a chronic and severe problem. Therapy is difficult. A search should be made for painful neuromas, but these are an uncommon cause, and even if small neuromas are found and removed, the pain is not usually relieved. Surgical procedures directed at the central nervous system are often not helpful. The pain may be triggered by touching the amputation stump, and eventually even touching healthy areas may trigger pain. Phantom pain is sometimes permanently abolished by cutaneous stimulation, either rubbing or electrical stimulation, or by repeated anesthetic blocks of peripheral nerves proximal to the stump. The pharmacologic approach is the same as that described for the neuropathic pains above and includes tricyclic antidepressants, anticonvulsants, neuroleptics, and sometimes sympathetic blockade. Referral to a multidisciplinary pain center may be helpful.

FIBROMYALGIA AND MYOFASCIAL PAIN. Fibromyalgia (also called fibrositis) is characterized by widespread or generalized musculoskeletal pain associated with morning stiffness, disturbed sleep and fatigue (nonrestorative sleep) and at times by vague complaints of a feeling of swelling or paresthesias. On examination, *tender points* can be found at multiple sites over muscles and ligaments, particularly at the upper borders of the trapezius, supraspinatus, and upper gluteal area and below the lateral epicondyle of the elbow and the medial epicondyle of the femur. The disorder usually occurs in middle-aged women and is often associated with anxiety and depression. Tension headaches and irritable bowel syndrome are common in these patients and may have a similar pathogenesis.

The myofascial pain syndrome refers to chronic pain in a regional distribution associated with trigger point(s). *Trigger points* are tender, sometimes hardened areas in a muscle which, when palpated, reproduce the distribution of the spontaneous pain. When injected with a local anesthetic, both the local and referred pain are relieved.

The pathophysiology of these syndromes is poorly understood. Some observers have reported microscopic changes at trigger points (so-called fibrous nodules), suggesting that a tonic contraction of muscle has led to structural changes. Others have suggested that release of noxious substances, such as lactic acid, potassium, or kinins from chronically contracted muscles, may be responsible for the pain and tenderness associated with the syndromes.

Treatment is often difficult and frustrating. In some patients, mild analgesic drugs, heat, and massage yield temporary or long-term relief. In patients with trigger points (myofascial pain), massage or even injection of trigger points with local anesthetics may give relief. Biofeedback, with the patient trying consciously to relax contracted muscle recorded by surface EMG, has been reported to be useful. Antidepressants are modestly effective and produce at least a short-term remission in about 20 per cent of patients. For most patients, a combination of the above physical methods with investigation and treatment of associated psychological disorders is necessary if long-term relief is to be achieved.

Bonica JJ: The Management of Pain, 2nd ed. Philadelphia, Lea and Febiger, 1990. *A two-volume multiauthored encyclopedia of the causes of pain and its management. Individual chapters describe each of the pain syndromes mentioned in this section.*

Fricton JR, Awad EA (eds.): Myofascial Pain and Fibromyalgia. Advances in Pain Research and Therapy. Volume 17. New York, Raven Press, 1990. *A comprehensive analysis of the pathophysiology, diagnosis, and treatment of fibromyalgia and myofascial pain.*

Payne R: Neuropathic pain syndromes, with special reference to causalgia and reflex sympathetic dystrophy. Clin Pain 2:59, 1986. *A thorough review of the pathogenesis and management of a perplexing pain problem.*

Thompson JM: Tension myalgia as a diagnosis at the Mayo Clinic and its relationship to fibrositis, fibromyalgia, and myofascial pain syndrome. Mayo Clin Proc 65:1237–1248, 1990. *Outlines specific criteria for various forms of this disorder and appropriate approaches to treatment.*

456 Nutritional Disorders of the Nervous System

Ivan Diamond

The neurologic effects of either general or specific nutritional deprivations are common worldwide (Table 456–1). In the developed countries of Western Europe and North America, many of these disorders are observed most frequently in association with chronic alcohol abuse. Other major causes include food faddism; chronic starvation such as can occur with cancer, infantile malnutrition, or psychiatric illness; intestinal malabsorption; and the complicated postoperative state. The conditions are relatively common, especially in large public hospitals that serve the underprivileged. More important, they often go undiagnosed. One recent study, for example, determined that only 20 per cent of patients found at autopsy to have Wernicke's encephalopathy had their condition correctly diagnosed and treated during life.

Although conditions such as Wernicke's encephalopathy can develop in as little as a few weeks after an acute illness such as hyperemesis gravidarum, most nutritional syndromes among alcoholics develop only following prolonged severe abuse with years of proportional semistarvation. Binge drinkers who eat well between bouts of intoxication seldom suffer neurologic complications. Genetic predisposition also may contribute to neurologic vulnerability. Ch. 201 and 204 more extensively discuss nutritional requirements and the systemic effects of their deprivation.

THE WERNICKE-KORSAKOFF SYNDROME

Wernicke's Encephalopathy

This acute disorder occurs most commonly in chronic alcoholics but also can accompany the other conditions listed in Table 456–2. This is the only alcohol-related neurologic disorder that can be corrected by a specific vitamin—thiamine.

CLINICAL MANIFESTATIONS. A clinical triad of ophthal-moplegia, ataxia, and global confusion is characteristic, although the condition should be suspected and treated in any chronically malnourished subject suffering from a confusional state of recent onset. Affected patients may complain of double vision or difficulty with balance. There is almost always horizontal nystagmus on lateral gaze. Vertical nystagmus, usually on upward gaze, occurs in about 50 per cent of cases. Bilateral, often asymmetric, lateral rectus palsies are characteristic and may develop rapidly. Defects in conjugate gaze are common. Bilateral ptosis and total external or an apparent internuclear ophthalmoplegia occur rarely. Light-fixed pupils should suggest an alternate or additional diagnosis.

Virtually all patients have an ataxic gait due to cerebellar involvement. This can vary widely in severity. Peripheral neuropathy and vestibular dysfunction frequently complicate Wernicke's encephalopathy. Intention tremor is less common, and speech disturbances are rare.

Most patients have an acute confusional state characterized by inattention, disorientation, and sleepiness. Stupor or coma occurs but is rare. Sometimes patients may be hyperactive and agitated (alcohol withdrawal, see Ch. 14), but most are apathetic, indifferent, and amnesic.

Associated physical abnormalities related to chronic alcoholism or poor nutrition are often present (see Ch. 118). Tachycardia and orthostatic hypotension are common. Hypothermia occurs less frequently; any fever should prompt a search for concomitant infection. Patients with Wernicke's encephalopathy do not develop beriberi heart disease (see Ch. 204).

PATHOLOGY. The major lesions occur in the periventricular regions of the diencephalon, mid-brain, and brain stem and in the superior vermis of the cerebellum; they may consist of areas of demyelination and glial proliferation. Microglia are prominent in acute lesions and fibrous astrocytes in older ones. Acute lesions show capillary dilation with occasional petechial hemorrhages. In experimental animals, defects in serotonergic transmission can be demonstrated in affected areas.

TREATMENT. Thiamine is specific. Because intestinal absorption is impaired in malnourished alcoholics, thiamine (50 or 100 mg) is given parenterally before starting infusions. Glucose administered prior to giving thiamine can precipitate or worsen the encephalopathy. Recovery begins promptly. Ophthalmoplegia and gaze palsies often begin to resolve during the first day. Nystagmus, gait ataxia, and confusion may improve within days to weeks, although many patients are left with residual nystagmus or gait ataxia. Nearly all patients with Wernicke's encephalopathy recover from the global confusional state, but many are left with a residual disorder of memory—Korsakoff's amnestic syndrome.

TABLE 456–1. MAJOR ACQUIRED NUTRITIONAL SYNDROMES AFFECTING THE NERVOUS SYSTEM

Vitamin A (carotene)	Night blindness, possibly pseudotumor in children
Vitamin B	
B₁ (thiamine)	Peripheral neuropathy, Wernicke-Korsakoff syndrome
	Possibly amblyopia, cerebellar degeneration, cerebral atrophy
B₂ group	
Panthothenic acid	Possibly burning feet syndrome
Nicotinic acid	Pellagra, polyneuropathy, spastic ataxia, amblyopia, psychosis-dementia
Riboflavin	Possibly burning feet syndrome, amblyopia
B₆ (pyridoxine)	Convulsions in B₆-deprived babies and older children, possibly peripheral neuropathy
B₁₂ (cyanocobalamin)	Combined systems disease, peripheral neuropathy, dementia
Folic acid	Impaired peripheral nerve function, possibly neuropathy and encephalopathy
Vitamin C (ascorbic acid)	Retinal and occasionally cerebral hemorrhages
Vitamin E (α-tocopherol)	Peripheral neuropathy and cerebellar degeneration
Starvation	Possibly developmental neurologic defects in infants

TABLE 456–2. CONDITIONS PREDISPOSING TO WERNICKE'S ENCEPHALOPATHY

Chronic alcoholism
Starvation
Persistent vomiting
    Hyperemesis gravidarum
    Gastric malignancy
    Gastritis
    Intestinal obstruction
    Digitalis intoxication
Systemic diseases
    Malignancy
    Hepatic failure
    Disseminated tuberculosis
    Uremia
Iatrogenic
    Inadequate parenteral nutrition
    Chronic hemodialysis

Korsakoff's Syndrome

CLINICAL MANIFESTATIONS (see also Ch. 452). There is a characteristic defect in forming new memories (anterograde amnesia) and in summoning previously established memories (retrograde amnesia). Patients are usually disoriented for place and time. Immediate recall is intact, but patients are unable to remember the same items several minutes later. Unhesitating confabulation often occurs early in the course. Other aspects of cognitive function, including arousal, language, praxis, and judgment, are spared.

PATHOLOGY. The findings are of active or remote Wernicke's encephalopathy. Damage to the dorsal medial nucleus of the thalamus probably accounts for the memory deficits.

TREATMENT. Patients with Korsakoff's syndrome should be given thiamine to treat coexistent Wernicke's encephalopathy and to prevent progression of the amnesia. About 20 per cent of patients recover completely, but more than half show little or no change. Improvement may take 1 to 3 months to be recognizable.

METABOLIC CONSIDERATIONS. Thiamine (vitamin B_1) in human tissues is derived entirely from dietary sources, is absorbed in the small intestine (see Ch. 204), and is transported into the brain by a saturable, energy-dependent transport system. Alcohol inhibits thiamine absorption. A series of reactions produces phosphorylated thiamine derivatives, and thiamine pyrophosphate (TPP) is a required co-enzyme for pyruvate dehydrogenase, α-ketoglutarate dehydrogenase, branched-chain α-keto acid dehydrogenase, and transketolase. The affinity of transketolase for TPP appears reduced in Wernicke's encephalopathy. Individuals with this enzyme abnormality are at greater risk to develop functional thiamine deficiency when dietary levels are compromised, as in alcoholism.

The confusional state and oculomotor disturbances seen in Wernicke's encephalopathy respond to thiamine treatment, and it is said that recovery may proceed during thiamine therapy whether or not alcohol consumption continues. However, calorie-containing ethanol appears to be an important contributing factor to the neurologic deficits. Calorie-deprived prisoners of war who developed Wernicke's encephalopathy rarely exhibited the irreversible amnestic syndrome. Moreover, nystagmus, ataxia, and the memory deficits often fail to improve after thiamine therapy, indicating that some areas of the brain have become irreversibly damaged. Serotonin deficiency may play a role in the memory disorder, but the molecular metabolic defect that precedes tissue damage in Wernicke's encephalopathy and Korsakoff's amnestic syndrome is not known.

ALCOHOLIC CEREBRAL ATROPHY

Many chronic alcoholics develop cerebral atrophy that increases with age and that can be visualized on computed tomographic (CT) scans of the brain. There is usually symmetric enlargement of the lateral ventricles and an increase in the size of cerebral sulci and the width of interhemispheric and sylvian fissures. The abnormalities may lessen if drinking is discontinued. Many chronic alcoholics also show deficiencies on psychometric examination. The CT scan abnormalities, however, correlate poorly with such specific cognitive defects. The specific mechanisms of these cerebral abnormalities are not known.

ALCOHOLIC-NUTRITIONAL NEUROPATHY

CLINICAL MANIFESTATIONS. Polyneuropathy is common among alcoholic patients. The most typical complaints are weakness, pain, and paresthesias in the hands and especially the feet. Symptoms usually begin insidiously in the legs and progress proximally and symmetrically. Abnormal motor and sensory signs develop concomitantly. Patients may complain of burning pain and heat sensations on the plantar surfaces of the feet and aching pain in the calves. Dysesthesias can become so severe that light touch and deep pressure are intensely unpleasant. Burning pain made worse by contact can interfere with walking despite adequate strength.

On examination, muscle weakness and wasting are usually more prominent distally, affecting legs more than arms and never the latter exclusively. The muscles may feel tender to pressure. Weakness can be so severe that contractures develop at the ankles and knees. Sensory abnormalities usually involve all modalities, but especially the pain and temperature modalities early in the course, and are more prominent distally. The deep tendon reflexes are usually absent to diminished in a distal to proximal distribution. Even asymptomatic patients often show mild sensory loss in the feet and absent Achilles tendon reflexes.

Involvement of the vagus nerve and thoracoabdominal sympathetic chain occurs rarely and can produce hoarseness, dysphagia, vocal cord paralysis, and hypotension. Cerebrospinal fluid protein levels are usually normal.

PATHOPHYSIOLOGY AND TREATMENT. The classic pathologic findings in alcoholic neuropathy are axonal degeneration and demyelination. Alcoholic-nutritional neuropathy, since it first affects smaller sensory fibers, is characterized by axonal degeneration, with electromyographic signs of denervation and normal nerve conduction velocities often present at an early stage. Later, additional nutritional change may result in slow nerve-conduction velocities.

A specific vitamin deficiency has not been identified in alcoholic neuropathy. Treatment consists of a balanced diet with supplemental B vitamins. Recovery is slow and often incomplete. Several weeks may be needed for motor improvement to begin, and it may take a year before patients with marked weakness begin to walk.

ACUTE AND CHRONIC ALCOHOLIC MYOPATHY

ACUTE MYOPATHY. This is a dramatic and life-threatening condition that develops in chronic alcoholics during prolonged heavy drinking. Symptoms begin abruptly with pain, cramps, tenderness, weakness, and swelling of the legs. Muscle involvement may be generalized or confined to one limb. Creatine phosphokinase activity in blood is elevated, and muscle biopsy shows acute rhabdomyolysis. Myoglobinuria often occurs and may lead to acute renal failure, hyperkalemia, and death. Electromyography usually shows evidence of a primary myopathy (see Ch. 441.5). Recovery usually follows days to weeks of abstinence, occasionally leaving residual proximal muscle weakness in its wake.

CHRONIC MYOPATHY. This is a chronic, painless disorder of proximal muscle weakness and atrophy that occurs rarely in alcoholics and develops only after excessive drinking. It can be mild or severe. Muscles of the pelvic girdle and thighs are involved most frequently; weakness of shoulder girdle muscles is less common. Alcoholic myopathy and cardiomyopathy (Ch. 50) often develop concurrently. Improvement usually occurs within 2 to 3 months after ethanol withdrawal. A coexistent peripheral neuropathy may contribute to the weakness.

ALCOHOLIC CEREBELLAR DEGENERATION

Cerebellar cortical degeneration occurs frequently in chronic alcoholics and in several presumably nutritional disorders in underdeveloped countries. About half the patients have an associated peripheral neuropathy. Men are affected more often than women. Most patients give a history of episodic binge drinking superimposed on heavy consumption extending over many years. Some complain of progressive unsteadiness and difficulty in walking, but these more insidiously developing symptoms often reflect a superimposed peripheral neuropathy that may clear with treatment. Abnormalities of gait and station are the most common findings. Initially, unsteadiness occurs during rapid turns, and tandem walking is difficult or impossible. Gradually, the feet become more widely based, walking becomes hesitant, and truncal ataxia is added. Ataxia of the legs may be demonstrable on heel to shin tests, but nystagmus, dysarthria, and tremor are rare. Often the syndrome develops abruptly or rapidly over several weeks and then remains stable. Sometimes the disorder evolves more slowly, with exacerbation following a binge or during an intercurrent illness. The most prominent pathologic abnormality is degeneration of the neurons of the anterior and superior cerebellar vermis with loss of Purkinje cells. CT or magnetic resonance (MR) images confirm cerebellar vermis atrophy. Abstinence, dietary treatment, and supplemental B vitamins may produce moderate improvement in the gait ataxia as peripheral neuropathy resolves.

NUTRITIONAL AMBLYOPIA

The condition involves retrobulbar neuritis affecting maculopapillary fibers, caused by a nutritional deficiency and encountered primarily in alcoholics. Patients complain of dim or blurred vision that evolves gradually over weeks to months. Decreased visual acuity occurs in one or both eyes, accompanied by bilateral symmetric central or centrocecal scotomas. Peripheral visual fields are usually unaffected, and funduscopic examination is normal. Treatment consists of abstinence, diet, and supplemental B vitamins. The extent of recovery varies inversely with the severity of impairment before therapy.

CENTRAL PONTINE MYELINOLYSIS

Central pontine myelinolysis (CPM) is a rare disorder that affects alcoholics primarily but also occurs in children and adults with severe electrolyte disorders, liver disease, malnutrition, anorexia, burns, cancer, Addison's disease, sepsis, and Wilson's disease.

PATHOPHYSIOLOGY, SIGNS, AND SYMPTOMS. The signs and symptoms relate closely to the pathologic change, which consists of a varying extent of symmetric focal myelin destruction involving the basal central pons, with similar lesions occasionally affecting extrapontine areas (Fig. 456–1). There is no associated inflammation or nerve cell destruction, and the lesions appear to be reversible with time and proper nutritional and fluid balance.

Typically, CPM evolves within days or weeks in severely ill patients. Almost always, the condition follows by 1 to 3 days a period of profound hyponatremia followed by rapid osmolal correction of greater than 20 mEq per liter. Mental symptoms often are prominent and consist of clouded consciousness or exacerbation of pre-existing delirium. Reflecting interruption of corticospinal pathways in the pons, a flaccid or spastic quadriparesis ensues, accompanied in many instances by bulbar difficulties of speaking and swallowing. Some patients develop a supranuclear ophthalmoplegia, and the mortality is high. Reflecting the sparing of the pontine tegmentum, sensory abnormalities usually fail to develop. The characteristic story has recently led to the diagnosis of many cases during life, confirmed by abnormalities on CT or MRI scan. Some patients recover; others remain tetraplegic. Treatment consists of meticulous maintenance of electrolytes, especially sodium balance and adequate nutrition.

MARCHIAFAVA-BIGNAMI DISEASE

This is a rare disorder consisting of symmetric demyelination of the corpus callosum and adjacent white matter. The lesions can be imaged by CT scan. The disorder affects mainly middle-aged men, severely addicted to various kinds of alcoholic beverages. Patients may have a progressive dementia accompanied by agitation or apathy, hallucinations, and emotional disorders until seizures, stupor, and coma supervene. Clinical findings such as rooting and sucking responses, grasp reflexes, paratonic rigidity, incontinence, and a slow hesitant gait suggest bilateral frontal

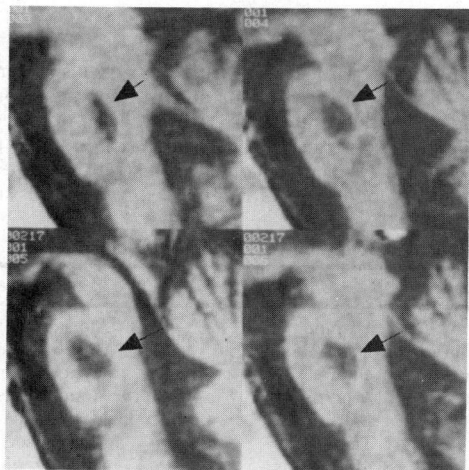

FIGURE 456–1. Central pontine myelinolysis. Magnetic resonance images were obtained in the sagittal plane using a "T₁-weighted" pulse sequence. An area of decreased signal is seen in the pons (*arrows*). (Photographs courtesy of Drs. Michael E. Charness and Robert L. DeLaPaz.)

lobe involvement. Recovery is rare, and the specific etiology is unknown.

VITAMIN E DEFICIENCY

Vitamin E deficiency is a complication of intestinal malabsorption in patients with chronic steatorrhea often due to cholestatic liver disease or cystic fibrosis (see Ch. 64). Patients with vitamin E deficiency develop a slowly progressive, distinctive neurologic syndrome with areflexia, cerebellar ataxia, ophthalmoplegia, pigmentary retinopathy, loss of vibratory sensation, and muscle weakness. Neurologic signs usually begin in childhood or adolescence with a loss of deep tendon reflexes followed by mild reduction in vibratory sensation; position sense is less affected, and pain and temperature sensation may be normal. Babinski signs are variable. A progressive external ophthalmoplegia is commonly associated with limitation of upward gaze. There may be impaired visual acuity and night vision because of pigmentary retinopathy. Muscle weakness and atrophy are often late complications, affecting muscles diffusely, distally, or in a proximal myopathic distribution. Untreated patients can become severely disabled. Vitamin E deficiency probably is responsible for the similar neurologic syndrome that develops in abetalipoproteinemia (see Ch. 463).

Vitamin E is an antioxidant that appears to protect unsaturated fatty acids of membrane phospholipids from oxidative degradation. The major pathologic findings in vitamin E deficiency are axonal degeneration of peripheral nerves and dorsal columns, reduced numbers of large myelinated fibers in peripheral nerves, and breakdown of the outer rod segments of the retina. Deposition of lipopigment, perhaps due to polymerization of peroxidized fatty acids, occurs in selected neurons and nonneural tissue. Similar neurologic abnormalities have been produced in animals with experimental vitamin E deficiency.

Serum vitamin E levels are low, particularly when related to serum lipids or cholesterol. Neurophysiologic studies usually show evidence of an axonal neuropathy with abnormal sensory nerve conduction velocities or amplitudes, and abnormal H-reflexes. Motor nerve conduction is altered less often or less severely, but evidence of denervation may be found in the tongue and somatic muscles. Central somatosensory conduction is often delayed, consistent with posterior column axonal degeneration. Electroretinograms and visual evoked potentials are abnormal according to the severity of the neurologic findings.

Treatment with vitamin E often improves the neurologic condition, but high oral doses or parenteral administration may be necessary. Early treatment of unaffected children with cholestasis probably prevents the neurologic complications of vitamin E deficiency (Ch. 204).

COBALAMIN (VITAMIN B₁₂) DEFICIENCY

Cobalamin (vitamin B₁₂) deficiency causes subacute degeneration of white matter in the dorsal and lateral columns of the spinal cord, peripheral nerves, optic discs, and cerebral hemispheres. The neurologic findings usually accompany a macrocytic (pernicious) anemia, but anemia need not be present. Hematologic and pathophysiologic considerations of cobalamin deficiency and details of treatment are discussed in Ch. 204.

CLINICAL MANIFESTATIONS. Neurologic symptoms develop in most patients with long untreated pernicious anemia, especially those in whom anemia has been masked by folate ingestion. Occasional examples can occur with cobalamin deficiency due to intestinal malabsorption, gastrectomy, or inadequate diet. Patients first complain of paresthesias in the hands or legs, such as tingling, numbness, and "pins and needles" sensations. Stiffness and weakness of the legs with unsteadiness in walking may be bothersome, particularly in the dark. Neurologic symptoms progress relentlessly if untreated; ataxia and stiffness eventually are followed by paraplegia and dysfunction of bowel and bladder. Psychological symptoms are frequent and include apathy and depression, irritability and paranoid tendencies, nocturnal confusion, and dementia. Intellectual deterioration does not usually develop in the absence of other neurologic signs. Failing vision with central scotomas occurs rarely.

Initially, one may find few objective changes despite complaints of paresthesias. Later, symmetric distal impairment of vibratory sensation occurs, usually first in the legs but eventually reaching the trunk and arms. Position sense is affected less prominently, although Romberg's test may be positive. The earliest changes are those of a peripheral neuropathy. The patellar and Achilles tendon reflexes are diminished or absent, and there may be decreased perception of touch, pain, and temperature in the feet and ankles. In the intermediate advanced case, one finds symmetric weakness in the legs associated with spasticity, clonus at the knees and ankles, increased or decreased deep tendon reflexes, and extensor plantar responses. Tingling distal paresthesias may follow flexion of the neck (Lhermitte's sign). Recent studies attributing a wide variety of vague neuropsychiatric difficulties to cobalamin deficiency in the absence of either reduced serum B$_{12}$ levels or abnormal Schilling tests remain to be verified by independent, controlled studies.

PATHOLOGY. The most prominent findings are in the peripheral nerves and dorsal and lateral columns of the spinal cord. Fragmentation and spongy degeneration of myelin usually begin in the lower cervical and upper thoracic regions; in untreated patients the disease progresses up and down the spinal cord and reaches into the ventral columns. Myelin sheaths and axons are destroyed, and wallerian degeneration is found in the spinal cord funiculi. Cerebral white matter is affected late. Peripheral nerves may show distal degeneration.

DIAGNOSIS AND PATHOPHYSIOLOGY. Serum vitamin B$_{12}$ levels are low and appear to correlate with the severity of the neurologic findings. The cerebrospinal fluid (CSF) protein concentration may be increased slightly. Neurologic disorders that can be confused with cobalamin deficiency include multiple sclerosis, cervical spondylosis, spinal cord tumors, and syphilitic meningomyelitis. A virtually identical syndrome has been reported after chronic abuse of nitrous oxide.

PATHOGENESIS. The molecular pathogenesis of the neurologic lesion in cobalamin deficiency is unknown. Cobalamin exists in different forms, some of which are required for at least two enzymes: N-5-methyltetrahydrofolate homocysteine methyltransferase, which catalyzes the synthesis of methionine and regeneration of tetrahydrofolate, and methylmalonyl-CoA mutase, which generates succinyl-CoA. Cobalamin deficiency produces elevated serum levels of homocysteine and methylmalonic acid. Prolonged exposure to nitrous oxide, which produces a neurologic disorder resembling combined system disease, also inhibits methionine synthesis.

TREATMENT. Intramuscular administration of cobalamin is the only treatment for cobalamin deficiency due to pernicious anemia or other malabsorptive states. Therapy should be started immediately and continued throughout the patient's lifetime. Early neurologic changes can be rapidly and completely reversed if treatment with cobalamin is begun promptly within the first few weeks or months of symptoms. If the neurologic manifestations have reached the stage of spinal cord dysfunction, therapy will halt progression, but improvement cannot be guaranteed.

Blass JP: Vitamin and nutritional deficiencies. In Siegel GJ, Agranoff BW, Albers RW, Molinoff PB (eds.): Basic Neurochemistry. 4th ed. New York, Raven Press, 1989. A clear discussion of the basic neurochemistry of the vitamins.

Charness ME, Simon RP, Greenberg D: Ethanol and the nervous system. N Engl J Med 321:442, 1989. A scholarly review with many references.

Diamond I: Alcohol neurotoxicity. In Asbury AK, McKhann GM, McDonald WI (eds.): Diseases of the Nervous System. 2nd ed. Philadelphia, W. B. Saunders Company, 1992. A comprehensive discussion of recent advances and the pathophysiology of alcohol-related neurologic disorders. A helpful bibliography.

Harper CG, Giles M, Finlay-Jones R: Clinical signs in the Wernicke-Korsakoff complex: A retrospective analysis of 131 cases diagnosed at necropsy. J Neurol Neurosurg Psychiatry 49:341, 1986. In this large series from Australia, correct antemortem diagnosis was reached in only 20 per cent of cases; most of the missed cases lacked ophthalmoplegia.

Lindenbaum J, Mealton EB, Savage DG, et al.: Neuropsychiatric disorders caused by cobalamin deficiency in the absence of anemia or macrocytosis. N Engl J Med 318:1720, 1989. A recent report of 141 patients suggesting that neurologic symptoms occur commonly without anemia and that measurement of serum methylmalonic acid and total homocysteine is useful in the diagnosis.

Satya-Murti S, Howard L, Krohel G, et al.: The spectrum of neurologic disorders from vitamin E deficiency. Neurology 36:917, 1986. A recent study of nine patients with more variable features. A helpful bibliography.

Sterns RH, Riggs JE, Schochet SS: Osmotic demyelination syndrome following correction of hyponatremia. N Engl J Med 314:1535, 1986. A recent report of eight patients and a review of the literature suggests that to avoid myelinolysis serum sodium should be raised by less than 12 mmol per liter per day.

SECTION FIVE / THE EXTRAPYRAMIDAL DISORDERS

Joseph Jankovic

457 Introduction

The term extrapyramidal refers to the anatomic and functional characteristics that distinguish the basal ganglia–regulated motor system from the pyramidal (corticospinal) and cerebellar systems. Extrapyramidal movement disorders are divided descriptively into hypokinesias, characterized by poverty and slowness of movement; hyperkinesias, manifested by abnormal involuntary movements; and miscellaneous motor disturbances (Table 457–1). Before discussing the clinical, pathophysiologic, and therapeutic aspects of the different movement disorders, it is important to review the anatomic and functional organization of the basal ganglia.

FUNCTIONAL AND NEUROCHEMICAL ANATOMY OF THE BASAL GANGLIA

The six paired nuclei that constitute the basal ganglia include the caudate nucleus, putamen, globus pallidus (or pallidum),

nucleus accumbens, subthalamic nucleus, and substantia nigra (Fig. 457–1). The caudate nucleus and putamen, although separated by the internal capsule, share cytoarchitechtonic, chemical, and physiologic properties; they are often referred to as the corpus striatum, neostriatum, or simply striatum. The striatum is a highly inhomogeneous structure composed of subregions

TABLE 457–1. MOVEMENT DISORDERS

Hypokinesias	Hyperkinesias	Miscellaneous
Parkinsonism	Tremor	Ataxia
Hypomimia	Dystonia	Gait disorders
Dysarthria	Chorea	Hyperekplexia
Sialorrhea	Athetosis	Hemifacial spasm
Micrographia	Ballism	Myokymia
Shuffling gait	Tics	Stiff-person syndrome
Other signs of	Myoclonus	Psychogenic
bradykinesia	Stereotypy	
and rigidity	Akathisia	
	Restless legs	
	Paroxysmal dyskinesias	

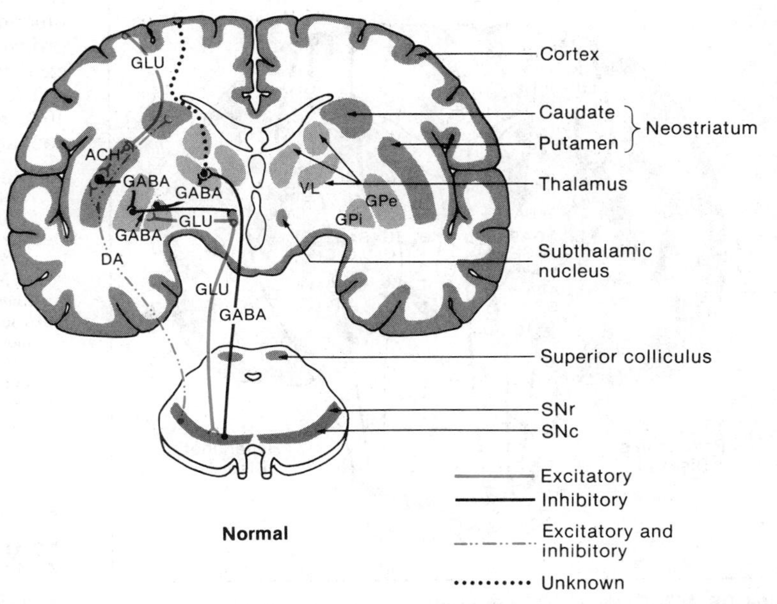

FIGURE 457-1. Anatomy of the basal ganglia and their connections. ACH = acetylcholine; GABA = γ-aminobutyric acid; GLU = glutamate; GP = globus pallidum (e = external, i = internal); DA = dopamine; SN = substantia nigra (c = compacta, r = reticulata); VL = ventrolateral.

termed striosomes and matrix. The limbic system provides major input to the striosomes, whereas neocortical areas primarily project to the matrix. Although the internal capsule separates the internal segment of the globus pallidus (GPi) and the pars reticulata of the substantia nigra (SNr), evidence suggests that these nuclei should be regarded as a single functional structure. The term *lenticular nucleus* refers to the putamen and globus pallidus combined because of their lenslike shape.

Recent anatomic and physiologic data suggest a complex organization of the basal ganglia and related structures (Fig. 457-1). According to this schema, the sensorimotor, association, and limbic cortical areas provide anatomically and functionally segregated inputs to the dorsal (the caudate and putamen) and ventral (nucleus accumbens, not shown) striatum. The somatosensory, motor, and premotor cortical areas project mainly to the putamen, while the posterior parietal and temporal and frontal association cortical areas project largely to the caudate and nucleus accumbens. The anatomy is consistent with the concept that the putamen is primarily concerned with motor function and the caudate is more involved with emotional and cognitive processes. The corticostriatal afferents are mediated by the excitatory neurotransmitter glutamic acid. The other major striatal afferents originate in the substantia nigra pars compacta (SNc), which provides major dopaminergic inhibitory input to the basal ganglia via the nigrostriatal pathway. Other inhibitory inputs to the striatum arise from the brain stem raphe nuclei (serotonergic) and from the locus ceruleus neurons (noradrenergic). The striatum is composed largely of cholinergic neurons, and some excitatory cholinergic projections to the striatum originate in the midline intralaminar thalamic nuclei.

The striatal nuclei project somatotopically to the external segment of the globus pallidus (GPe) and the GPi-SNr complex. The striatal efferents utilize the inhibitory neurotransmitter γ-aminobutyric acid (GABA). The subthalamic nucleus (STN) regulates the output of the basal ganglia to the thalamus by modulating the inhibitory GABAergic afferents from the GPe and the excitatory glutamatergic efferent projections to the GPi-SNr complex. The efferent inhibitory GABAergic projections from the GPi terminate in the thalamus. The thalamic nuclei in turn project to the supplementary motor area of the cortex and the primary motor cortex.

MOVEMENT DISORDERS

Single-cell recordings in behaving animals and other physiologic studies have demonstrated that one of the primary roles of the basal ganglia is to scale the movement amplitude and velocity rather than to initiate movements. Besides their critical role in

the execution of movement, the basal ganglia also seem to be involved in the preparation for movement.

In addition to impaired voluntary movements, dysfunction in the basal ganglia can also cause a variety of abnormal involuntary movements. Correlations between the various types of abnormal movements and sites of experimental and pathologic lesions have provided helpful insights into and better understanding of the function of the basal ganglia. The remainder of this section is organized according to the major categories of movement disorders into hypokinetic (parkinsonian), hyperkinetic, and miscellaneous movement disorders (Table 457-1).

HYPOKINESIAS (PARKINSONIAN DISORDERS)

Bradykinesia is manifested clinically by slowness of automatic and spontaneous movements and impaired ability to initiate voluntary movements (akinesia). This typical parkinsonian symptom presumably results from loss of the inhibitory dopamine input to the striatum and hypoactivity of the GPe neurons. This, in turn, causes functional disinhibition (excitation) of the STN, inducing an increase of neuronal activity in the GPi, thereby raising the tonic inhibitory output from the basal ganglia (GPi) to the thalamus and to the cortical projection areas (Fig. 457-2). The altered activity in the "motor" circuit is manifested by increased movement time, which becomes particularly prolonged when a parkinsonian subject performs sequential movements.

Rigidity, another cardinal sign of parkinsonism, is demonstrated clinically by increased resistance against passive movement of a body part, usually associated with the "cogwheel" phenomenon. A parkinsonian patient perceives rigidity as a feeling of joint stiffness and muscle tightness. The pathophysiologic mechanisms of rigidity have been attributed to pallidal disinhibition resulting in increased suprasegmental activation of normal spinal reflex mechanisms.

Postural instability due to loss of righting reflexes can cause propulsion (tendency to fall forward) and retropulsion (tendency to fall backward). It is one of the most disabling symptoms of Parkinson's disease. The mechanism of postural instability is unknown, but it has been attributed primarily to involvement of the pallidum. Other hypokinetic manifestations are listed in Table 457-1.

HYPERKINESIAS (ABNORMAL INVOLUNTARY MOVEMENTS)

Tremor is a rhythmic oscillatory movement produced by alternating or synchronous contractions of opposing muscle groups. Tremors are divided into rest or action tremors; the latter are further subdivided into postural or contraction tremors (e.g.,

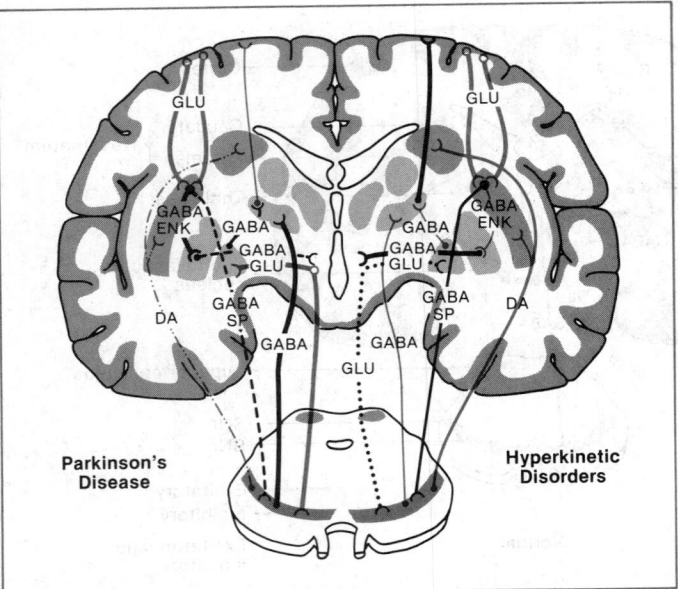

FIGURE 457–2. Functional organization of the basal ganglia in parkinsonian disorders and hyperkinetic movement disorders. ACH = acetylcholine; GABA = γ-aminobutyric acid; GLU = glutamate; DA = dopamine; ENK = enkephalin; SP = substance P.

arms outstretched in front of the body or in a "wing-beating" position) and kinetic or intention tremors (e.g., during target-directed movement, such as the finger-to-nose maneuver). *Rest tremor,* usually asymmetric at onset, is the typical tremor of Parkinson's disease. When it involves the hands, it causes a supinating-pronating oscillatory (pill-rolling) movement at approximately 4- to 6-Hz frequency. Parkinsonian tremor also often involves the legs, feet, lips, tongue, chin, and voice but almost never affects the head or neck. *Postural tremor,* with frequency ranging between 4 and 12 Hz, is most typically seen in patients with essential tremor. *Kinetic (intention) tremors* are slow and more irregular movements with a rate of 1.5 to 3 Hz. Kinetic tremors usually indicate an abnormality of the cerebellum or its outflow pathways (the dentate nucleus, the superior cerebellar peduncle, and contralateral red nucleus).

Dystonia is produced by involuntary, sustained (tonic) or spasmodic (rapid or clonic), patterned, and repetitive muscle contractions, frequently causing twisting (e.g., torticollis), flexing or extending (e.g., writer's cramp, retrocollis), and squeezing (e.g., blepharospasm, writer's cramp) movements or abnormal postures. Dystonia is usually constant but occurs in some cases only during particular activities. Examples of task-specific dystonias include writer's or typist's cramp and inversion of a foot while running. As dystonia progresses, the involuntary contractions also appear at rest. A characteristic feature of dystonia is that the spasms lessen in intensity with "sensory tricks," such as touching one side of the face to maintain a primary position, thus counteracting involuntary torticollis. Dystonia can fluctuate in intensity and is exacerbated by stress, fatigue, activity, or a change in posture. It subsides during sleep, relaxation, and hypnosis. These features and the bizarre nature of dystonic patterns sometimes are wrongly attributed to psychogenic causes. About half of patients with dystonia have a coexistent postural tremor, identical to essential tremor. The anatomic substrate for dystonia is unknown. Clinicopathologic studies of patients with secondary dystonias most often implicate the putamen and the rostral brain stem in its genesis.

Chorea consists of continuous, abrupt, rapid, brief, flowing, unsustained, irregular, and random jerklike movements. Choreic patients frequently mask the abnormal movements by voluntary semipurposeful activities. A characteristic feature of chorea is the inability to maintain voluntary sustained contraction. Examples include an inability to sustain manual grip or tongue protrusion and the dropping of objects. Muscle stretch reflexes are usually

"hung up" and "pendular." Affected patients typically have a peculiar, irregular, and dancelike gait. The pathogenesis of chorea is unknown. Some findings point to abnormalities in caudate function. A selective loss of the GABA-enkephalin striatal neurons projecting to the GPe, found in Huntington's disease, results in excessive inhibition of STN neurons.

The movement disorders of athetosis (Ch. 461), ballism (Ch. 461), myoclonus (Ch. 462), tics (Ch. 462), and stereotypies (Ch. 462) are discussed in later chapters of this section.

Albin RL, Young AB, Penney JB: The functional anatomy of basal ganglia disorders. TINS 12:366, 1989. *An excellent review of current understanding of the basal ganglia connections in the normal and diseased brain.*
DeLong MR: Primate models of movement disorders of basal ganglia origin. TINS 13:281, 1990. *A review of the MPTP model of parkinsonism used in the study of basal ganglia circuitry. Hyperactivity of the STN is associated with bradykinesia, and a chemical lesion in the STN reduces this cardinal sign.*
Jankovic J, Tolosa E (eds.): Parkinson's Disease and Movement Disorders. Baltimore-Munich, Urban and Schwarzenberg, 1988. *A comprehensive review of hypokinetic, hyperkinetic, and miscellaneous movement disorders.*
Marsden CD, Fahn S: Movement Disorders 3. London, Butterworths Scientific, 1991. *A comprehensive review of different movement disorders by recognized experts.*

458 Parkinsonism

Parkinsonism is a clinical syndrome dominated by four cardinal signs: tremor at rest, bradykinesia, rigidity, and postural instability. Less prominent manifestations concern the mood and intellect, oculomotor control, autonomic function, and the sensory system (Table 458–1). The average age at onset is 55 years, with about 1 per cent of persons 60 years of age or older having the disease. Men are affected more frequently than women by a ratio of 3:2. At least two major subtypes of Parkinson's disease (PD) have been identified: One subtype is characterized by tremor as the dominant parkinsonian feature, and the other is dominated by postural instability and gait difficulty (PIGD). The *tremor subtype* of PD is associated with relatively normal mental status, earlier age at onset, and slower progression of the disease than is the *PIGD subtype,* which shows more bradykinesia, dementia, and a more rapidly progressive course.

Resting tremor and bradykinesia are the most typical parkinsonian signs and are virtually synonymous with the diagnosis. Bradykinesia accounts for most of the associated parkinsonian symptoms and signs: general slowing down of movements and of activities of daily living; lack of facial expression (hypomimia or masked facies); staring expression due to decreased frequency of blinking; impaired swallowing, which causes drooling; hypokinetic and hypophonic dysarthria; monotonous speech; small handwriting (micrographia); difficulties with repetitive and simultaneous movements; difficulty in arising from chair and turning

TABLE 458–1. NONMOTOR DISTURBANCE IN PARKINSON'S DISEASE

Neurobehavioral Abnormalities in Parkinson's Disease
Personality changes (apathy, lack of confidence, fearfulness, anxiety, emotional lability and inflexibility, social withdrawal, dependency)
Dementia (tip-of-the-tongue phenomenon [partial anomia], spatial disorientation, paranoia, psychosis, hallucinations)
Bradyphrenia (slow thought processes, loss of concentration, difficulty with concept formation)
Depression
Sleep disturbance
Sexual dysfunction
Psychiatric side effects of therapy

Other Nonmotor Manifestations of Parkinson's Disease
Autonomic dysfunction (orthostatic hypotension, respiratory dysregulation, flushing, "drenching sweats," constipation, sphincter and sexual dysfunction)
Sensory symptoms (paresthesias, pains, akathisia; visual, olfactory, and vestibular dysfunction)
Seborrhea, pedal edema, fatigue, weight loss

over in bed; shuffling gait with short steps; decreased arm swing and other automatic movements; and start hesitation and freezing. Freezing, manifested by sudden and often unpredictable inability to move, is one of the most disabling of all parkinsonian symptoms.

Several disorders other than PD can cause at least part of the parkinsonian syndrome (Table 458–2). Non-PD parkinsonian disorders can be distinguished clinically from PD by the presence of atypical findings, absence or paucity of tremor, and poor response to levodopa. The last feature may be partly explained by the fact that postsynaptic dopamine receptors are preserved in PD, but they are decreased in the other parkinsonian syndromes.

PARKINSON'S DISEASE

Pathogenesis

The most typical pathologic hallmarks of PD are (1) neuronal loss with depigmentation of the substantia nigra (SN) and (2) Lewy bodies, which are eosinophilic cytoplasmic inclusions in neurons consisting of aggregates of normal filaments. These abnormalities are most prominent in the ventrolateral region of the SN that projects to the putamen. At least an 80 per cent loss of dopaminergic neurons in the substantia nigra and the same degree of dopamine depletion in the striatum must appear before clinical symptoms of PD become evident.

Motor symptoms of PD result chiefly from degeneration of the nigrostriatal pathway, causing a deficiency of dopamine in the putamen and, to a lesser degree, the caudate nucleus. The cognitive deficits and some neurobehavioral symptoms have been attributed to degeneration of the dopaminergic mesocortical and mesolimbic pathways, and the associated autonomic dysfunction may be partly caused by dopamine depletion in the hypothalamus. Besides dopamine deficiency, impairment of the other neurotransmitters may be responsible for some of the associated findings. For example, degeneration of the noradrenergic locus ceruleus may contribute to the "freezing" phenomenon and to depression. Degeneration of the cholinergic nucleus basalis probably relates to the dementia that eventually affects about a third of all PD patients.

Although several hypotheses are currently being investigated, the etiology of PD is still unknown. Genetic factors may increase its risk, but the contribution is more complex than simple mendelian inheritance. The "environmental" hypothesis of PD is primarily based on the observation that the meperidine analogue 1-methyl-4-phenyl-1,2,3,6-tetrahydropyridine (MPTP), originally used by heroin addicts, causes parkinsonism in humans and in animals. MPTP must be oxidized to a pyridine MPP+ to be neurotoxic, and antioxidants such as deprenyl (a selective monoamine oxidase [MAO]–B inhibitor) prevent MPTP-induced experimental parkinsonism. As a result, it has been postulated that some environmental MPTP-like toxin might be responsible for human PD. An alternative hypothesis is that an endogenous toxin, such as dopamine, damages susceptible neurons. During the process of oxidative deamination, dopamine generates hydroxyl radicals and hydrogen peroxide, which, in the presence of iron deposits in the brain, could lead to lipid peroxidation and neurotoxicity, possibly by interfering with mitochondrial oxidative metabolism. Observed abnormalities in mitochondrial complex I activity have stimulated renewed interest in the role of genetic susceptibility in PD.

Treatment

The finding that deprenyl prevents MPTP-induced parkinsonism has stimulated interest in antioxidative therapy as a means of retarding the progression of PD. Some studies have found that deprenyl slows the development of motor disability and the rate of disease progression when used in the early stages of PD. These findings, if confirmed, suggest the possibility of favorably altering the natural course of the disease.

In addition to its possible protective effect, deprenyl may provide moderate symptomatic relief. After starting deprenyl, many patients report improvement in their energy level and bradykinetic symptoms. The effect may be due to deprenyl's ability to increase striatal concentrations of dopamine by blocking its metabolism by MAO. The addition of one of the anticholinergic drugs, such as trihexyphenidyl, may provide additional symptomatic relief, particularly in younger patients and patients in whom tremor predominates. Associated depression, present in many parkinsonian patients, can be treated with tricyclic antidepressants, such as amitriptyline or nortriptyline. Because the anticholinergics, including the tricyclics, can produce undesirable psychological symptoms as well as side effects, such as dry mouth, blurring of vision, and urinary hesitancy, amantadine may offer a useful alternative, particularly in elderly patients. Amantadine, however, while helpful in controlling both tremor and bradykinesia, can also cause adverse effects, including livedo reticularis, ankle edema, exacerbation of congestive heart failure, and mild anticholinergic side effects.

Many neurologists favor employing combinations of deprenyl, the anticholinergics, and amantadine until they no longer provide a satisfactory control of parkinsonian symptoms. At that point, in socially or occupationally disabled patients, levodopa combined with carbidopa, a peripheral dopa decarboxylase inhibitor, is added to the antiparkinsonian regimen. The starting dosage of carbidopa/levodopa is 25 mg/100 mg twice daily, to be gradually increased over 3 weeks to three times per day. The dosage is then adjusted, depending on the severity of symptoms and occupational demands. Some patients require as much as 25/250 four or five times daily; others tolerate no more than 25/100 four times daily. Although levodopa can suppress tremor, it is most useful in controlling bradykinesia and rigidity. Postural instability may be ameliorated by levodopa in early stages, but dopaminergic therapy is usually ineffective later on. Levodopa is contraindicated in patients with diagnosed melanoma and should be used with caution in those with prominent psychosis or dementia, peptic ulcer disease, and cardiac arrhythmias.

About 15 per cent of parkinsonian patients fail to improve with levodopa. Most of these nonresponders probably suffer from a form of postsynaptic parkinsonism rather than PD. A failure to respond to levodopa should also suggest the possibility of a wrong diagnosis, a drug interaction (concomitant use of dopamine receptor blocking agents, such as antipsychotic and antiemetic drugs), and pharmacokinetic reasons, such as insufficient dosage, slow stomach emptying, and competition for absorption in the small intestine and at the blood-brain barrier by amino acids in protein meals. In any event, almost all patients who initially improve lose their response to levodopa sometime between 3 and 8 years after onset.

TABLE 458–2. CAUSES OF THE PARKINSON SYNDROME

I. Primary (Idiopathic) Parkinsonism
Parkinson's disease
Juvenile parkinsonism

II. Secondary (Acquired, Symptomatic) Parkinsonism
Infectious: postencephalitic, slow virus
Drugs: neuroleptics (antipsychotic, antiemetic drugs), reserpine, tetrabenazine, α-methyldopa, lithium, flunarizine, cinnarizine
Toxins: MPTP, CO, Mn, Hg, CS$_2$, methanol, ethanol
Vascular: multi-infarct, hypotensive shock
Trauma: pugilistic encephalopathy
Other: parathyroid abnormalities, hypothyroidism, hepatocerebral degeneration, brain tumor, normal-pressure hydrocephalus, syringomesencephalia

III. Heredodegenerative Parkinsonism
Autosomal dominant Lewy body disease
Huntington's disease
Wilson's disease
Hallervorden-Spatz disease
Olivopontocerebellar and spinocerebellar degenerations
Familial basal ganglia calcification
Familial parkinsonism with peripheral neuropathy
Neuroacanthocytosis

IV. Multiple-System Degenerations (Parkinsonism-Plus)
Progressive supranuclear palsy
Shy-Drager syndrome
Striatonigral degeneration
Parkinsonism-dementia-ALS complex
Corticobasal ganglionic degeneration
Alzheimer's disease
Hemiatrophy-parkinsonism

The two primary reasons why PD patients lose their response to levodopa are (1) natural progression of the disease and (2) development of complications as a result of chronic levodopa therapy. Although nonneuronal elements may participate in the conversion of levodopa to dopamine, the surviving striatal dopaminergic terminals are primarily responsible for this process. With progression of the disease and accompanying cellular degeneration, this capacity for conversion of levodopa to dopamine is lost, and the patient develops motor fluctuations and symptomatic deterioration.

The most challenging problem in the management of PD is the treatment of levodopa complications. Side effects caused by peripheral dopamine (and dopamine stimulation of the medullary vomiting center, which is not protected by the blood-brain barrier) include gastrointestinal symptoms, tachycardia, and orthostatic hypotension. The most common central side effects of levodopa therapy include psychiatric problems, dyskinesias (seen in about 80 per cent of patients after 3 years of therapy), and clinical fluctuations (seen in about 50 per cent of patients after 5 years of therapy). The most common form of clinical fluctuation is the wearing-off effect, characterized by end-of-dose deterioration and recurrence of parkinsonian symptoms as a result of shorter (sometimes only 1 to 2 hours) duration of benefit after a given dose of levodopa. Slow-release preparations of levodopa (e.g., Sinemet CR, Madopar CR) have been shown to prolong the plasma (and presumably brain) levels and may be useful in the treatment, and possibly prevention, of motor fluctuations. Deprenyl can also prolong the duration of benefit from each levodopa dose.

Because the onset of levodopa-induced complications seems to be related to the duration of levodopa therapy, some authorities delay initiating levodopa therapy until the patient's symptoms begin to interfere with normal activities. Once levodopa treatment is initiated, the dose should be maintained as low as possible (Fig. 458–1). Therefore, instead of increasing the dosage of levodopa, dopamine agonists such as bromocriptine or pergolide should be introduced early in the course of anti-PD therapy. These drugs directly activate the dopamine receptors. Initially, dopamine agonists were used primarily as adjunctive therapy in patients with levodopa-induced fluctuations. The role of dopamine agonists in the treatment of PD has broadened, however, and these agents are now recommended in the early phases of

therapy in an attempt to delay or reduce the risk of levodopa side effects. In experimental studies, pergolide has been shown to exert its dopaminergic effects on both D_1 and D_2 receptors without presynaptic dopamine, and it may improve parkinsonian symptoms even before levodopa is given. Some authorities, therefore, give pergolide as the first dopaminergic drug. However, as symptoms increase, dopamine agonists must be combined with levodopa. The starting dosage for bromocriptine is 1.25 mg twice a day and for pergolide, 0.05 mg twice a day. The dosage should be increased slowly to prevent gastrointestinal, psychiatric, autonomic, and other side effects. The side effects of dopamine agonists are similar to those of levodopa, although dopamine agonists may produce hallucinations, delusions, and other psychiatric symptoms more often than does levodopa. They also can cause erythromelalgia manifested by painful erythema of the legs, which is not usually seen with levodopa. Other motor and nonmotor symptoms of PD may require more specific therapy.

Surgical treatment of PD remains of unproven long-term value, although stereotaxic thalamotomy is occasionally employed in an attempt to ameliorate disabling tremor. Surgical transplantation of autologous adrenal medulla or fetal substantia nigra into the striatum remains under investigation.

As with all progressive, disabling diseases, psychological support of patients and family offers important help. Patients should be encouraged to learn about their disease (by reading educational material provided by the national and local support organizations) and to be physically and socially active.

SECONDARY PARKINSONISM

POSTENCEPHALITIC PARKINSONISM. Many individuals who survived the acute febrile illness and encephalopathy during the pandemics of encephalitis lethargica (von Economo's encephalitis) between 1919 and 1926 later developed a variety of movement disorders, including parkinsonism. The postencephalitic syndrome was also manifested by hemiparesis, involuntary ocular deviations (oculogyric crises), dystonia, chorea, tics, and behavioral problems. Postencephalitic parkinsonism has a slower progression and is more sensitive to levodopa therapy. Although the virus or viruses responsible for encephalitis lethargica were never isolated, infections caused by coxsackie, Japanese B, and western equine encephalitis viruses have since been identified as being complicated by parkinsonism.

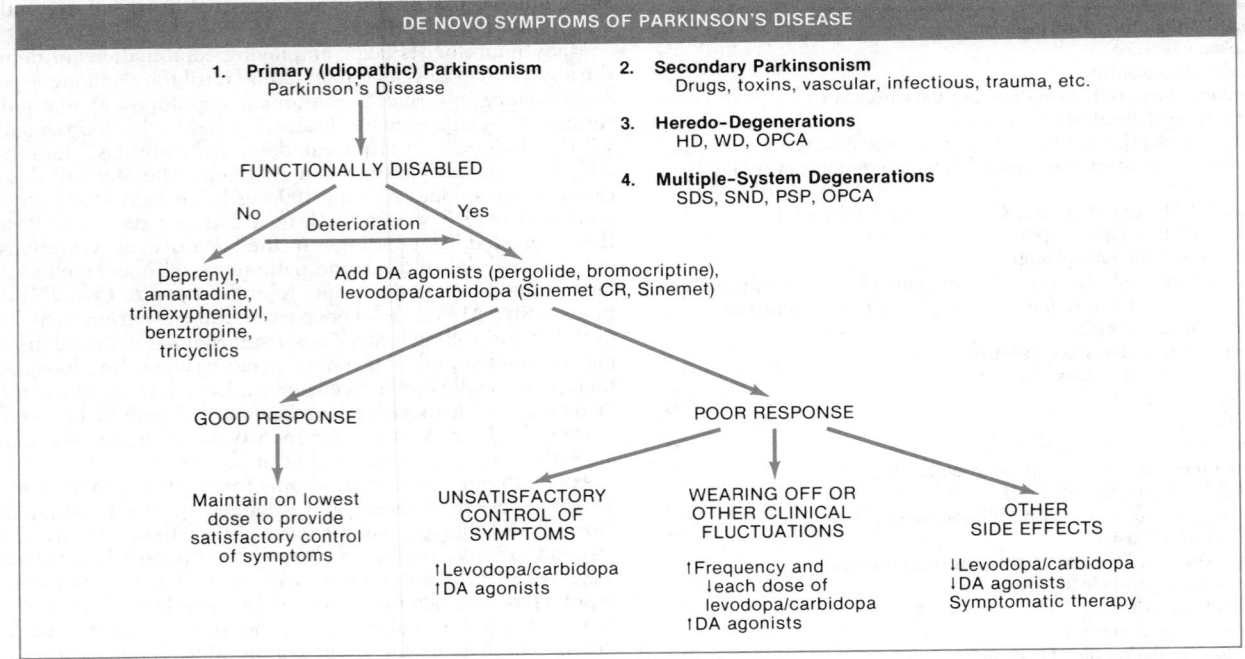

FIGURE 458–1. Diagrammatic representation of therapeutic approach to patients with parkinsonism. DA = dopamine; HD = Huntington's disease; OPCA = olivopontocerebellar atrophy; PSP = progressive supranuclear palsy; SDS = Shy = Drager syndrome; Sinement CR = controlled = release levodopa/carbidopa; SND = striatonigral degeneration; WD = Wilson's disease.

DRUG-INDUCED PARKINSONISM. After PD, drugs that deplete dopamine stores or block dopamine receptors are the most common causes of parkinsonian findings. Drugs that deplete the presynaptic stores of dopamine, such as reserpine and tetrabenazine (an investigational drug not available for general use in North America), and drugs that block the dopamine receptors, such as antipsychotic and antiemetic agents, can cause a parkinsonian syndrome clinically indistinguishable from idiopathic parkinsonism (PD). The same drugs can also cause a variety of other movement disorders, such as akathisia, dystonic reactions, and various tardive syndromes (e.g., tardive stereotypy, tardive dystonia, and tardive akathisia).

VASCULAR PARKINSONISM. Cerebrovascular disease accounts for only a small proportion of parkinsonism. Single strokes rarely cause parkinsonian findings, although multiple small infarctions involving the striatum can produce the syndrome. Brain imaging is helpful in the diagnosis. One form of vascular parkinsonism is the so-called "lower body parkinsonism," manifested chiefly by gait disturbance with short steps, "freezing," and difficulties with turning. (Chronic communicating, "low-pressure" hydrocephalus causes a similar clinical picture.) Patients with vascular parkinsonism may have dementia, hyperactive reflexes, and urinary incontinence, but tremor is rare. Levodopa therapy usually fails, probably because ischemia damages the striatal postsynaptic receptors. The diagnosis is suggested by these atypical findings in patients with a history of stroke risk factors.

HEREDODEGENERATIVE PARKINSONISM

Very few parkinsonian patients have a family history suggesting a specific pattern of inheritance. With such a history, the differential diagnosis should include one of the heredodegenerative disorders (Table 458–2).

HALLERVORDEN-SPATZ DISEASE. This rare condition is manifested by childhood or adult-onset progressive dementia, bradykinesia, rigidity, and spasticity, variously combined with dystonia, choreoathetosis, ataxia, seizures, amyotrophy, and retinitis pigmentosa. Most reported cases have suggested an autosomal recessive inheritance. Neuropathologically, iron accumulates in the globus pallidus (GP) and SN, accompanied by axonal swelling and neuronal degeneration in the basal ganglia, corticospinal tract, and cerebellum. Cysteine, found to be increased in the GP, possibly chelates iron, causing a generation of free radicals and subsequent neuronal degeneration.

FAMILIAL BASAL GANGLIA CALCIFICATIONS. Calcium may accumulate in the basal ganglia in association with hypoparathyroidism or as a result of a familial disorder, sometimes referred to as Fahr's disease. Affected patients exhibit parkinsonism, chorea, dementia, and palilalia. Brain imaging may detect basal ganglia calcification in clinically unaffected relatives.

OLIVOPONTOCEREBELLAR AND SPINOCEREBELLAR DEGENERATIONS. The combination of parkinsonism and cerebellar ataxia characterizes olivopontocerebellar degeneration or atrophy (OPCA), a heterogeneous group of neurodegenerative disorders most often inherited in an autosomal dominant pattern, but occasionally occurring sporadically. In addition to the parkinsonism-ataxia complex, patients with OPCA often exhibit marked dysarthria, neuro-ophthalmologic signs, and a variable degree of upper and lower motor neuron signs (see Ch. 465).

MULTIPLE-SYSTEM DEGENERATIONS (PARKINSONISM-PLUS)

Approximately 10 to 15 per cent of all patients with parkinsonian findings have a more widespread disorder classified clinically as "parkinsonism-plus syndrome" and pathologically as a "multiple-system degeneration." In addition to parkinsonism, such patients suffer from additional findings that may include supranuclear ophthalmoparesis (progressive supranuclear palsy), dysautonomia (Shy-Drager syndrome), ataxia (OPCA), laryngeal stridor (striatonigral degeneration), apraxia and alien hand (corticobasal degeneration), dementia (Alzheimer's disease with parkinsonism and diffuse Lewy body disease), and a combination of dementia and motor neuron disease (parkinsonism–dementia–amyotrophic lateral sclerosis [ALS] complex). The etiology for all forms of this syndrome is unknown.

PROGRESSIVE SUPRANUCLEAR PALSY. Progressive supranuclear palsy (PSP) is the most common of the parkinsonism-plus syndromes, accounting for about 8 per cent of all parkinsonian patients evaluated in a PD clinic. PSP has its onset in the seventh decade, about 10 years after the usual onset of PD. Initial symptoms consist of a gradual onset of postural instability, unsteady gait, and supranuclear vertical ophthalmoparesis, first expressed by impairment of downward gaze. Later, upward and then lateral conjugate gaze also become impaired, but until the advanced stage, the external ophthalmoparesis can be overcome by labyrinthine stimulation via the oculocephalic maneuver. Patients with PSP often exhibit axial rigidity, nuchal dystonia, and a rigid-dystonic facial expression with deep nasolabial folds (in contrast to the flattened facies seen in patients with PD). Mild to moderate dementia is a late sign; tremor almost never occurs. Neither the hypokinetic rigidity nor the other changes respond to antiparkinsonian drugs. The poor response to these drugs is partly explained by the loss of postsynaptic D_2 receptors.

Pathologically, PSP is characterized by selective neuronal loss and gliosis affecting the midbrain tegmentum and tectum, the internal segment of the globus pallidus (GPi), the subthalamic nucleus (STN), the vestibular and dentate nuclei, the basal nucleus of Meynert, and the pedunculopontine nucleus. Neurofibrillary tangles, somewhat different from those in Alzheimer's disease, and granulovacuolar degeneration involve nerve cells in these areas.

SHY-DRAGER SYNDROME. When patients with atypical parkinsonism (usually without tremor) complain of orthostatic light-headedness, incontinence, sexual impotence, and other autonomic symptoms, the diagnosis of Shy-Drager syndrome should be considered (see Ch. 452).

Cedarbaum JM: Pharmacokinetic and pharmacodynamic considerations in management of motor response fluctuations in Parkinson's disease. Neurol Clin 8:31, 1990. *A review of the pharmacology of levodopa, deprenyl, and dopamine agonists.*

Jankovic J: Parkinsonism plus syndromes. Movement Disord 4:S95, 1989. *A survey of most of the secondary forms of parkinsonism.*

Jankovic J: Clinical aspects of Parkinson's disease. In Marsden CD, Fahn S (eds.): New Trends in the Treatment of Parkinson's Disease. Carbforth, England, Parthenon Publishing, 1990, pp 51–73. *A review of the pathophysiologic mechanisms of parkinsonian signs and symptoms.*

Jankovic J, McDermott M, Carter J, et al.: Variable expression of Parkinson's disease: An analysis of the DATATOP database. Neurology 40:1529, 1990. *An analysis of clinical correlates in 800 patients in early stages of PD, not yet treated with dopaminergic drugs.*

Marsden CD: Parkinson's disease. Lancet 1:948, 1990. *A critical review of the current knowledge about the pathogenesis and therapeutics of PD.*

459 Tremors

ESSENTIAL TREMOR

Essential tremor is the most common type of symptomatic tremor, affecting about 0.5 per cent of the American population. The tremor is inherited in an autosomal dominant pattern with high penetrance. Affected patients lack the hypokinetic features and rigidity of Parkinson's disease (PD), discussed in the preceding chapter. Essential tremor typically produces flexion-extension oscillation of the hands at the wrists or adduction-abduction movements of the fingers when arms are outstretched in front of the body. Although frequently referred to as "benign essential tremor," it may be disabling, often causing spilling of liquids and interfering with handwriting. Essential tremor also frequently involves the head and voice, which helps to differentiate it from parkinsonian tremor. Another useful distinguishing feature is the occurrence of essential tremor during maintenance of posture; parkinsonian tremor is usually present when the affected body part is at relative rest. Parkinsonian patients, however, often exhibit postural tremor, and patients with essential tremor may have tremor at rest, suggesting an overlap between PD and essential tremor.

The frequency of essential tremor ranges from 4 to 12 Hz, and the oscillation may be produced by either alternating or synchronous contractions of antagonistic muscles. Some forms occur only during a specific activity, such as writing or holding an object in a particular position. Such *focal task-specific tremors* may be associated with task-specific dystonias ("occupational cramps") or with generalized essential tremor and dystonia. Nearly half of all patients with essential tremor show evidence of an associated dystonia. The nature of the link is unknown.

Essential tremor has many variants, including isolated head, voice, tongue, facial, and chin tremors and orthostatic tremor. Although considered a variant of essential tremor, orthostatic tremor usually does not respond to propranolol; clonazepam, however, provides satisfactory control in most patients. Focal tremor may be rarely induced by trauma to the affected body part. This peripherally induced tremor is often associated with focal dystonia and reflex sympathetic dystrophy.

β-Adrenergic blocking drugs (e.g., propranolol at 80 to 240 mg per day) are the most effective agents in the treatment of essential tremor. Modest doses of alcohol also reduce the tremor in most instances, but this is an impractical approach to treatment. Other occasionally useful drugs include primidone (starting dosage is 25 mg at bedtime; the daily dosage can be gradually increased to 750 mg per day), lorazepam, and alprazolam. Patients with a disabling essential tremor that does not respond satisfactorily to medications sometimes improve with local injections of botulinum toxin. Thalamotomy is used as a last resort.

Hubble JP, Busenbark KL, Koller WC: Essential tremor. Clin Neuropharmacol 12:453, 1989. *A comprehensive review of physiology, pharmacology, and clinical aspects of tremors.*

Lou J-S, Jankovic J: Essential tremor: Clinical correlates in 350 patients. Neurology 41:234, 1991. *A comprehensive analysis of clinical features of a large cohort of patients with essential tremor.*

Rosenbaum F, Jankovic J: Focal task-specific tremor and dystonia: Categorization of occupational movement disorders. Neurology 38:522, 1988. *A review of 28 patients with dystonia, tremor, or a combination present only during specific activities, such as writing or typing.*

Tasker RR: Tremor of parkinsonism and stereotactic thalamotomy. Mayo Clin Proc 62:736, 1987. *A review of current experience with surgical treatment of tremors.*

460 Dystonias

DEFINITION

Dystonia may be defined as a syndrome dominated by involuntary, sustained (tonic) or spasmodic (rapid or clonic), patterned, and repetitive muscle contractions, frequently causing twisting (e.g., torticollis), flexing or extending (e.g., writer's cramp, retrocollis), and squeezing (e.g., blepharospasm) movements or abnormal postures. Dystonia is frequently associated with other movement disorders, particularly tremor, myoclonus, and parkinsonism. About 1 of 3000 people is diagnosed as having dystonia, but the true prevalence is probably much higher.

CLASSIFICATION

Dystonia may vary in severity, and it may progress as follows: task-specific (occurring only during a specific activity, such as writing or typing) → action (present only during, not necessarily specific, activity) → overflow (involving adjacent muscles) → at rest (present even during rest) → fixed postures (joint contractures). Dystonia is exacerbated by stress, fatigue, activity, or a change in posture and is relieved by sleep, relaxation, hypnosis, and a variety of sensory tricks. While the vast majority of dystonias are continual, some occur paroxysmally and some have marked diurnal variations (Fig. 460–1). Partly because of fluctuations in severity, sometimes influenced by the emotional state of the patient, dystonia is often mistakenly attributed to psychogenic causes.

Dystonia can be classified according to its *distribution* as focal, segmental, multifocal, generalized, or unilateral (hemidystonia). Most childhood-onset dystonias begin focally, usually in one foot; other body parts become involved later, eventually resulting in generalized dystonia. In contrast, adult-onset dystonias tend to remain focal or segmental. Examples of focal dystonia include blepharospasm, oromandibular dystonia, torticollis, spasmodic dysphonia, and occupational (e.g., writer's, typist's, pianist's)

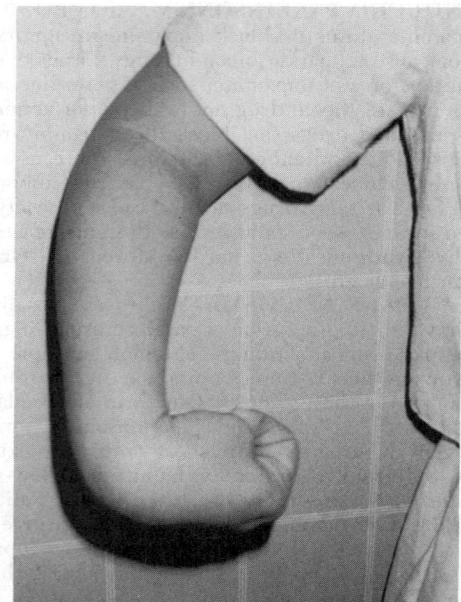

FIGURE 460–1. Focal dystonia of the distal right arm.

cramps (Fig. 460–1). Blepharospasm is categorized as a *focal dystonia* when it occurs alone (essential blepharospasm). However, blepharospasm is often associated with dystonic movements in the adjacent facial, oromandibular, laryngeal, and neck muscles. This *segmental dystonia* is sometimes referred to as Meige's syndrome, but the term "*cranial-cervical dystonia*" is more descriptive.

The most common form of dystonia is *cervical dystonia* (Table 460–1). According to the position of the head, cervical dystonia can be categorized as torticollis, laterocollis, anterocollis, retrocollis, or a combination of these abnormal postures. There is a 3:2 female preponderance, and the onset is usually in the fifth decade. Local pain is reported by about half the patients, and radiculopathy complicates cervical dystonia in about 20 per cent. Half of all patients with cervical dystonia have an associated head-neck tremor. The tremor can be dystonic, seen only when the patient attempts to keep the head straight; essential, in which case the tremor persists irrespective of the position of the head; or a combination of dystonic and essential. About half the patients report a movement disorder such as tremor or dystonia in family members. The etiology of most cervical dystonias is unknown. In 15 per cent of cases, however, cervical dystonia can be attributed to either local trauma or an exposure to neuroleptic drugs.

PATHOGENESIS

The pathoanatomy of dystonia is unknown, but studies suggest a predominant involvement of the basal ganglia, particularly the putamen, and the brain stem. Brain imaging and autopsy examinations usually yield normal findings. Electrophysiologic studies suggest increased excitatory drive from the basal ganglia to brain stem interneurons. Postmortem biochemical analyses have found evidence of enhanced noradrenergic transmission in the rostral brain stem. Some cases of dystonia appear to be caused or triggered by peripheral nerve or root injury.

TABLE 460–1. DISTRIBUTION OF DYSTONIA

Distribution	N*
Cervical	326
Blepharospasm and oromandibular dystonia	228
Generalized	169
Blepharospasm	109
Focal (distal)	79
Spasmodic dysphonia	67
Hemidystonia	51
Oromandibular dystonia	48

*N = 1000 at Baylor College of Medicine.

PRIMARY DYSTONIA

This category accounts for 85 per cent of cases. Primary dystonias with onset in childhood have been previously termed *dystonia musculorum deformans.* Childhood-onset dystonias are often inherited, usually in an autosomal dominant pattern; about half of adult-onset cases seem to have a genetic basis. Other members of the family may have only partial manifestations, such as club foot, scoliosis, torticollis, writer's cramp, bruxism, or essential tremor. Genetic dystonia seems to have a higher prevalence among Ashkenazi Jews, but both Jewish and non-Jewish dystonias have been linked to a marker in the q32–q34 region of chromosome 9. An X-linked dystonia has been recently described in Filipino families.

SECONDARY DYSTONIA

Occasionally, a specific, and potentially treatable, cause of dystonia can be identified (Fig. 460–1). One of the most important examples is *Wilson's disease.* Neurologic symptoms represent the first manifestations in about 50 per cent of patients with this autosomal recessive disorder, appearing during their second or third decade. Changes usually consist of a gradual onset of dysarthria; drooling; dementia; clumsiness, often affecting handwriting; postural tremors; gait disturbance; and various forms of dystonia affecting distal and proximal body parts. Dystonia of facial and bulbar muscles is responsible for the dysarthria and drooling as well as the typical fixed pseudo-smile (risus sardonicus), inspiratory noises, and dysphagia. Other motor abnormalities include parkinsonism, cerebellar findings, a wing-beating proximal tremor, and other movement disorders. All patients with neurologic findings have a Kayser-Fleischer ring, a greenish-brown copper infiltration of the cornea near the scleral junction. Further details are given in Ch. 192.

Tardive dystonia is a persistent form of dystonia caused by exposure to dopamine receptor blocking drugs, such as major tranquilizers (e.g., chlorpromazine, thioridazine, fluphenazine, thiothixene, haloperidol, loxapine, amoxapine) and certain antiemetics (e.g., prochlorperazine, metoclopramide) (Fig. 460–2). Curiously, levodopa can also cause intermittent dystonia (and focal dystonia may be the presenting symptom of Parkinson's

disease). In all drug-induced dystonias, the offending drug should be withdrawn or the dosage reduced whenever possible. In contrast to focal, segmental, or generalized dystonia, hemidystonia is associated with an identifiable etiology in a majority of cases. These etiologies include subcortical infarction, arteriovenous malformation, abscess, tumor, and other lesions, some of which can be treated surgically. There are many other causes of secondary dystonia, but only a few are amenable to therapy.

TREATMENT

The treatment of most dystonias consists of supportive therapy (e.g., relaxation techniques, prostheses), medications, botulinum toxin injections, and surgery. The anticholinergic drugs are sometimes beneficial. Trihexyphenidyl, the most frequently used anticholinergic, must be started in low doses and slowly increased to tolerance, perhaps up to 60 mg per day. Some children can tolerate such high doses, but anticholinergic side effects usually limit adult tolerance to 20 to 25 mg daily or less. In advanced cases, dopamine-depleting and dopamine receptor blocking drugs may be added. Muscle relaxants (e.g., diazepam or lorazepam), baclofen, and carbamazepine sometimes provide benefit. About 10 per cent of patients with childhood or adolescence dystonia improve with use of levodopa. Diurnal fluctuations with exacerbation of the movement disorder toward the end of each day are typical in this form of dystonia. In patients with refractory focal dystonia and, less often, segmental dystonia, injection of the paralysis-inducing botulinum A toxin (Botox) into the contracting muscles provides effective, albeit temporary, relief. Such approaches are best left to those with experience in this treatment.

Patients who are socially and occupationally disabled by dystonia despite optimal medical therapy, including botulinum toxin, sometimes can be helped surgically. Surgical procedures include orbicularis myectomy for blepharospasm, cervical rhizotomy for neck dystonia, and thalamotomy for hemidystonia or generalized (predominantly distal) dystonia. Such procedures are effective in a majority of patients but have both potentially serious complications and high rates of symptom recurrence, making them a last resort.

Fahn S, Marsden CD, Calne DB: Dystonia 2. Advances in Neurology, Vol. 50. New York, Raven Press, 1988. *A series of papers presented at a symposium on dystonia, summarizing current knowledge about all aspects of this disorder.*

Fletcher NA, Harding AE, Marsden CD: A genetic study of idiopathic torsion dystonia in the United Kingdom. Brain 113:379, 1990. *A review of inheritance in dystonic families in England suggests that 85 per cent are inherited in an autosomal dominant pattern with 40 per cent penetrance.*

Jankovic J, Brin M: Therapeutic applications of botulinum toxin. N Engl J Med, April 25, 1991. *A critical review of studies using botulinum toxin in different dystonic and other disorders.*

Jankovic J, Leder S, Warner D, Schwartz K: Cervical dystonia. Clinical findings and associated movement disorders. Neurology, in press. *Largest reported series of patients with cervical dystonia (torticollis).*

Nygaard TG, Marsden CD, Fahn S: Dopa-responsive dystonia: Long-term treatment response and prognosis. Neurology 41:174, 1991. *A comprehensive review of a potentially treatable dystonia that affects up to 10 per cent of children with dystonia.*

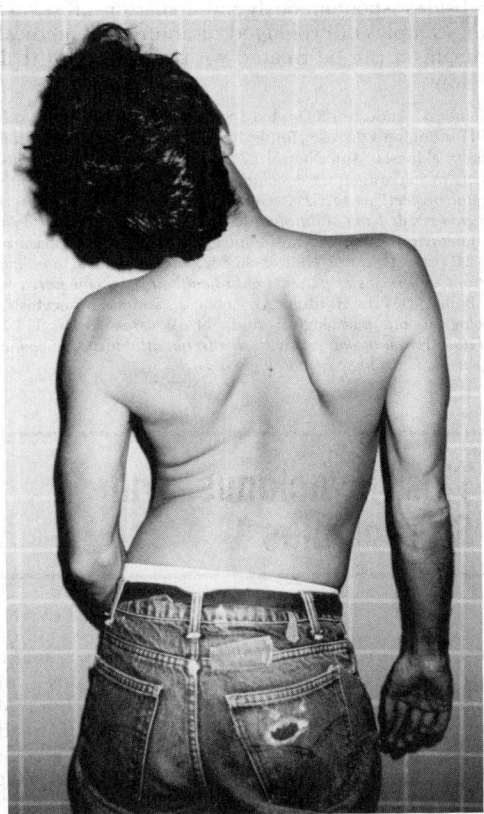

FIGURE 460–2. Truncal dystonia in a manic-depressive patient with tardive dystonia secondary to a variety of antipsychotic drugs.

461 Choreas, Athetosis, and Ballism

HUNTINGTON'S DISEASE

Huntington's disease (HD), an autosomal dominant disorder with complete penetrance, is the most common form of hereditary chorea. Besides chorea, the other two components of the HD triad are a decline in cognitive functioning leading to dementia and various emotional and psychiatric disturbances. A major milestone in HD research has been the identification of a gene marker on chromosome 4. Treatment, however, remains as ineffective as it was in 1872, when George Huntington first described the disease. The estimated prevalence of HD in the United States is 4 to 8 per 100,000 people. Although about 10 per cent of HD cases begin before age 20, the peak age at onset is in the fourth and fifth decades. Juvenile HD often first manifests with progressive parkinsonism, dementia, and seizures. In contrast, adult HD often starts with the insidious onset of clumsiness and adventitious, fidgety, random, brief movements. Initially, these purposeless movements may be incorporated into and masked by normal intentional acts, delaying the recognition of chorea. Chorea often begins distally, but as the disease progresses, it becomes generalized and can interrupt voluntary movements. Characteristically, patients with HD have difficulty in maintaining tongue protrusion or a steady grip, and their gait is often irregular, hesitant, unsteady, and dancelike. Other motor symptoms include dysarthria, dysphagia, and postural instability.

Neurobehavioral symptoms may precede motor changes and usually consist of personality changes, apathy, social withdrawal, agitation, impulsiveness, depression, mania, paranoia, delusions, hostility, hallucinations, or psychosis. Cognitive changes are manifested chiefly by loss of recent memory and impaired judgment. Progressive motor dysfunction, dementia, and incontinence eventually lead to institutionalization and death from aspiration, infection, and poor nutrition. The duration of illness from onset to death is about 15 years for adult HD and 8 to 10 years for the juvenile variant.

Postmortem changes in HD brains include neuronal loss and gliosis in the cortex and the striatum, particularly the caudate nucleus. Chorea seems to be primarily related to the loss of striatal neurons projecting to the lateral globus pallidus (GPe), whereas rigid-akinetic symptoms correlate with the additional loss of striatal neurons projecting to the medial globus pallidus (GPi). Loss of medium-sized spiny neurons, which normally constitute 80 per cent of all striatal neurons, is associated with a marked decrease in γ-aminobutyric acid (GABA) synthesis. There is also a decline in acetylcholine activity, presumably resulting from a degeneration of cholinergic striatal interneurons. The neuropeptides are markedly altered in HD: Levels of substance P, cholecystokinin, and metenkephalin are decreased, but somatostatin, thyrotropin-releasing hormone, neurotensin, and neuropeptide Y levels are increased. The number of dopamine, acetylcholine, and serotonin receptors is decreased in the striatum.

Reliable clinical diagnosis depends on the combination of chorea, emotional disturbances, progressive dementia, and a family history suggestive of autosomal dominant inheritance. Because spontaneous mutations are rare, lack of family history raises questions of paternity or misdiagnosis. The correct diagnosis of HD is supported by evidence of caudate atrophy on neuroimaging studies and hypometabolism in the basal ganglia by positron-emission scanning with fluoro-2-deoxyglucose. A specific marker for HD has been identified on the short arm of chromosome 4, making genetic diagnosis likely in the future.

Treatment is symptomatic only. The psychosis may improve with neuroleptics, such as haloperidol, pimozide, fluphenazine, and thioridazine, but these drugs can induce tardive dyskinesia and other adverse effects and should be used only if absolutely needed to control symptoms. Monoamine-depleting drugs, such as reserpine (0.25 mg to 8 mg per day) and tetrabenazine (an investigational drug not available for general use in North America), may relieve chorea, do not cause tardive dyskinesia, and may be as effective as the dopamine-blocking drugs. Unfortunately, these drugs can cause or exacerbate depression, sedation, akathisia, and parkinsonism. Anxiolytics and antidepressants may also be useful in some patients with psychiatric problems associated with HD. Genetic aspects of HD should be discussed openly with the patients to provide them and their relatives with nondirective counseling.

OTHER CHOREIC DISORDERS

Besides HD, other genetically transmitted choreas include *benign hereditary chorea*, a nonprogressive chorea with childhood onset, and *paroxysmal choreoathetoses*. *Senile chorea* is a rare symptom complex in which chorea begins after age 60 and is unaccompanied by the neurobehavioral symptoms or family history of HD. Some patients have been reported to have pathologic changes identical to those of HD; others have had predominant degeneration of the putamen rather than the caudate. *Neuroacanthocytosis*, also referred to as "chorea-acantho-

cytosis," usually presents in the third or fourth decade of life with a combination of self-mutilation manifested by lip and tongue biting, generalized chorea, lingual dystonia, and motor and phonic tics. Other features include seizures, amyotrophy, areflexia, and elevated levels of serum creatine phosphokinase. Wet blood or Wright-stained fast-dry smears reveal more than 15 per cent of red blood cells as acanthocytes. Neuroimaging usually demonstrates caudate atrophy. The condition may have a pattern of autosomal recessive inheritance but its genetics are still unclear. *Sydenham's chorea*, now an uncommon disorder, has an autoimmune basis, most often appearing as a consequence of infection with group A streptococcus. Unlike arthritis and carditis, which occur soon after such infection, chorea and various neurobehavioral symptoms may be delayed for 6 months or longer. Chorea appearing during pregnancy (chorea gravidarum), with use of birth control pills, or during the course of systemic lupus erythematosus probably has a similar pathogenesis.

ATHETOSIS

Athetosis is a slow form of chorea characterized by twisting, writhing movements. It most often accompanies static encephalopathy due to cerebral palsy, kernicterus, prematurity, glutaric aciduria, poststroke hemiplegia, and other causes of early life brain damage. In some cases, the movement disorder becomes progressive after decades of no apparent change. Athetosis usually does not respond to pharmacologic therapy.

BALLISM

Ballism is a form of forceful, flinging, high-amplitude, coarse chorea. Because the involuntary movement usually affects only one side of the body, the term hemiballism is used. The movement disorder is often preceded by hemiparesis associated with a hemorrhagic or ischemic stroke involving the contralateral subthalamic nucleus (STN) or adjacent structures. Less common causes of hemiballism include abscess, arteriovenous malformation, cerebral trauma, hyperosmotic hyperglycemia, tumor, and multiple sclerosis. Lesions produced by these pathologic processes usually involve the STN, but hemiballism has been described in patients with lesions outside the STN. Dopamine-blocking and -depleting drugs, used in the treatment of chorea, are beneficial in most patients with hemiballism, but the disorder usually subsides spontaneously in a matter of several weeks. Occasional examples of prolonged disabling and medically intractable hemiballism can be treated with contralateral thalamotomy or pallidectomy.

Albin RL, Reiner A, Anderson KD, et al.: Striatal and nigral neuron subpopulations in rigid Huntington's disease: Implications for the functional anatomy of chorea and rigidity-akinesia. Ann Neurol 27:357, 1990. *Using neuropeptide immunochemistry, the investigators conclude that chorea correlates with damage to the striatal projections to GPe, whereas parkinsonian signs observed in some HD patients result from additional damage in the projections to the GPi.*
Dewey RB, Jankovic J: Hemiballism-hemichorea: Clinical and pharmacologic findings in 21 patients. Arch Neurol 46:862, 1989. *Clinical and brain imaging correlations in a series of patients with hemiballism, hemichorea, or both.*
Hardie RJ, Pullon HWH, Harding AE, et al.: Neuroacanthocytosis. A clinical, haematological and pathological study of 19 cases. Brain 114:13, 1991. *A detailed description of patients with this frequently unrecognized and clinically heterogeneous neurologic-hematologic disorder.*

462 Tics, Myoclonus, and Stereotypies

TICS

Tics describe involuntary, abrupt, sudden, isolated, brief movements (*motor tics*); sounds produced by nose, mouth, or throat (*vocal/phonic tics*); or sensations (*sensory tics*). Motor tics may be simple (e.g., eye blinking, nose twitching, head jerking) or complex (e.g., repetitive touching, jumping, kicking, pelvic gyrations). Similarly, vocal/phonic tics may be simple (e.g., throat clearing, grunting, sniffing) or complex (e.g., echolalia, palilalia, coprolalia). Characteristics of tics include suppressibility, increase with stress and excitement, decrease with distraction and concentration, suggestibility, waxing and waning, and possible persistence during sleep.

The most common cause of tics is the *Gilles de la Tourette's syndrome*, an autosomal dominant disorder dominated by tics and a variety of behavioral manifestations. Transient tics of childhood and persistent simple tics probably represent fragmentary forms of Tourette's syndrome. The following criteria are required for diagnosis: (1) Both multiple motor and one or more phonic tics must be present at some time during the illness, although not necessarily concurrently; (2) the tics occur many times a day, nearly every day or intermittently through a period of more than a year; (3) the anatomic location, number, frequency, complexity, type, and severity of tics change over time; (4) onset is before age 21; and (5) involuntary movements and noises cannot be explained by other medical conditions. Because of the fluctuating, heterogeneous, and often bizarre manifestations of Tourette's syndrome, affected patients frequently have their illness misdiagnosed by physicians and are mistreated by schoolmates, teachers, co-workers, and strangers.

Epidemiologic studies suggest that Tourette's syndrome is mostly a genetic disorder, occurring commonly and with penetrance approaching 100 per cent, particularly in males. In addition, some cases are nongenetic and may be triggered or caused by neuroleptics, carbon monoxide poisoning, head trauma, viral encephalitis, cocaine abuse, or opiate withdrawal. Many patients with Tourette's syndrome suffer from obsessive-compulsive disorder and have problems with attention and learning. Sleep disorders are common and include parasomnias, bedwetting, and interruption of sleep by tics.

Therapy requires individual attention. Since most patients experience waxing and waning of symptoms and a generally favorable natural course, reassurance and behavioral therapy may be sufficient in mild cases. Drugs usually are indicated when tics cause physical discomfort or social embarrassment. Judicious use of dopamine receptor blocking drugs, such as fluphenazine, pimozide, and haloperidol, often reduces the frequency and severity of tics and may ameliorate impulsive and aggressive behavior. These drugs, however, cause sedation, depression, and weight gain. Furthermore, tardive dyskinesia is a potentially serious complication of chronic neuroleptic therapy. Clonazepam, clonidine, fluoxetine, and clomipramine seem to be particularly helpful in the treatment of obsessive-compulsive disorder and other behavioral problems frequently associated with Tourette's syndrome.

MYOCLONUS

Myoclonus describes a jerklike movement produced by a sudden, rapid, and brief contraction (positive myoclonus) or a muscle inhibition (negative myoclonus). Myoclonus may be focal, multifocal, segmental, or generalized. *Segmental myoclonus* usually involves either the branchial structures, innervated by the lower cranial nerves and upper cervical nerve roots, or other body parts innervated by the spinal roots and nerves; it consists of rhythmic (1 to 3 Hz) contractions caused by a lesion of the brain stem or spinal cord. *Palatal myoclonus* results from acute or chronic lesions involving the anatomic triangle linking dentate, red, and inferior olivary nuclei. *Generalized myoclonus* is believed to reflect discharges arising from the brain stem reticular formation and is categorized as physiologic, essential, epileptic, or symptomatic. Two forms of myoclonus are associated with sleep: physiologic sleep myoclonus, occurring normally during initial phases of sleep, and nocturnal myoclonus, now called *"periodic movements of sleep,"* often associated with *"restless legs syndrome"* as well as with abnormal involuntary movements while the person is awake.

Causes of myoclonus include acute and prolonged hypoxia and ischemia; various metabolic, infectious, and toxic factors; and exposure to neuroleptic drugs (tardive myoclonus). Myoclonus can be associated with familial chorea and dystonia and with many neurodegenerative disorders, including parkinsonism, progressive myoclonus epilepsy, and a variety of rare heredodegenerative disorders. Multifocal myoclonus often develops in the late stages of Creutzfeldt-Jakob disease and, less frequently, Alzheimer's disease.

The specific physiologic and pharmacologic pathogeneses of myoclonus are unknown; clinical studies suggest an abnormality in the brain stem reticular formation. Clonazepam, lorazepam,

TABLE 462–1. NEUROLEPTIC-INDUCED MOVEMENT DISORDERS

Acute-Transient	Chronic-Persistent
Dystonic reaction	Tardive stereotypy
Action tremor	Tardive chorea
Parkinsonism	Tardive dystonia
Akathisia	Tardive akathisia
Neuroleptic malignant syndrome	Tardive tics
	Tardive myoclonus
	Tardive tremor

valproate, carbamazepine, and 5-hydroxytryptophan have been reported to have antimyoclonic activity. Clonazepam, at a dosage of 1 to 9 mg per day, is the drug of first choice, but the development of adverse effects, such as drowsiness, ataxia, and sexual dysfunction, often limits its usefulness.

STEREOTYPIES

The term "stereotypy" describes a continuous or intermittent, involuntary, coordinated, patterned, repetitive, rhythmic, purposeless, but seemingly purposeful and ritualistic movement. Stereotypies may be simple (e.g., chewing movement, foot tapping, body rocking) or complex (e.g., complicated rituals, sitting down and arising from a chair). They can be volitionally suppressed. The stereotypic behavior displayed by some animals when placed in restraining environments has been used as an experimental model of hyperkinetic movement disorders. Stereotypies can accompany a variety of human behavioral disorders, such as anxiety, obsessive-compulsive disorders, Tourette's syndrome, schizophrenia, akathisia, autism, and mental retardation. Stereotypies and self-stimulatory or self-injurious behavior constitute the most recognizable symptoms in mentally retarded and autistic patients.

Tardive dyskinesia, a persistent movement disorder caused by exposure to dopamine receptor blocking drugs, is one of the most common causes of stereotypies. Many other tardive movement disorders can result from the use of dopamine receptor blocking drugs (neuroleptics) (Table 462–1). The term "akathisia" describes the combination of stereotypy and a sensory component, such as an inner feeling of restlessness. Akathisia, whether due to neuroleptics, Parkinson's disease, or other causes, is sometimes confused with the syndrome of *restless legs*. Both disorders are characterized by stereotypic movements and motor restlessness, but patients with restless legs complain more of paresthesias, particularly a creeping or crawling sensation in the legs associated with an irresistible urge to keep the limbs in motion. The restless legs syndrome is often worse at night, causing insomnia, and it may be associated with periodic movements of sleep. Elderly women appear to be at particularly high risk for tardive dyskinesia. The use of high doses and depot injections of neuroleptics carries an increased risk of tardive dyskinesia. The mechanism of the disorder is poorly understood but is believed to result from the development of supersensitive dopamine receptors caused by chronic neuroleptic blockade. Prevention is the best treatment for the drug-induced movement disorders. Whenever possible, drugs other than the neuroleptics should be used for psychiatric or gastrointestinal problems. When no alternative exists, the dosage and duration of exposure should be kept at a minimum. Spontaneous remissions of tardive dyskinesia occasionally follow withdrawal of the offending agent. Dopamine-depleting drugs, such as reserpine and tetrabenazine are the most effective drugs in the symptomatic treatment of tardive dyskinesia.

Jankovic J: Stereotypies. *In* Marsden CD, Fahn S (eds.): Movement Disorders 3. London, Butterworths, 1991. *A review of animal and clinical studies of stereotypic disorders.*

Kurlan R: Tourette's syndrome: Current concepts. Neurology 39:1625, 1989. *A critical review of current knowledge about the motor and behavioral aspects of Tourette's syndrome.*

Miller LG, Jankovic J: Drug-induced dyskinesias. *In* Appel SH (ed.): Current Neurology. Vol 10. Chicago, Year Book Medical Publishers, 1990, pp 321–355. *A comprehensive review of tardive dyskinesia and related disorders.*

Patel VM, Jankovic J: Myoclonus. *In* Appel SH (ed.): Current Neurology. Vol 8. Chicago, Year Book Medical Publishers, 1988, pp 109–156. *A comprehensive review of the classification, physiology, and pharmacology of myoclonus.*

SECTION SIX / DEGENERATIVE DISEASES OF THE NERVOUS SYSTEM

Robert B. Layzer

The term "degenerative diseases" refers to a varied assortment of central nervous system disorders characterized by gradual and progressive loss of neural tissue. This section deals with several degenerative diseases of unknown cause: the hereditary ataxias, paraplegias, and amyotrophies; the phakomatoses; syringomyelia; and amyotrophic lateral sclerosis. Several important diseases are discussed in other chapters concerned with dementia, extrapyramidal diseases, and autonomic disorders. Some degenerative diseases are difficult to classify because they involve multiple anatomic locations; these *multisystem atrophies* have arbitrarily been assigned to the chapters that deal with their principal symptom (see Table 463–1).

463 Hereditary Cerebellar Ataxias and Related Disorders

The symptoms of hereditary ataxia may be intermittent or progressive. *Intermittent or periodic ataxia* occurs in children with a variety of recessively inherited biochemical disorders, such as aminoacidurias and disorders of pyruvate metabolism. A rare, autosomal dominant disease known as hereditary periodic ataxia is characterized by attacks of vertigo, nystagmus, ataxia, and dysarthria, lasting several hours; it responds to prophylactic treatment with acetazolamide.

Progressive ataxia occurs in children with known biochemical disorders such as abetalipoproteinemia and some of the lipidoses, but most diseases in this category are of unknown etiology. Those that begin before age 20, including Friedreich's ataxia and ataxia-telangiectasia, are usually inherited in an autosomal recessive fashion, while most adult-onset types are autosomal dominant.

FRIEDREICH'S ATAXIA

This autosomal recessive disease, with a carrier frequency of nearly 1 in 100 and a prevalence of 2 in 100,000, is probably the most common type of hereditary ataxia. The biochemical mechanism is unknown, but the abnormal gene has been mapped to the short arm of chromosome 9.

PATHOLOGY. At autopsy the spinal cord is atrophic. There is loss of nerve cells in the dorsal root ganglia and Clarke's columns, and "dying-back" degeneration of nerve fibers in the dorsal columns, pyramidal tracts, spinocerebellar tracts, and peripheral nerves. Minor changes are present in the brain stem

and cerebellum. The heart shows chronic interstitial fibrosis and ventricular hypertrophy.

CLINICAL MANIFESTATIONS. Progressive ataxia of gait usually begins in childhood or adolescence and within a few years is accompanied by loss of deep reflexes, limb ataxia, Babinski signs, and cerebellar dysarthria. The ability to walk is lost about 15 years after onset. Most patients eventually exhibit scoliosis, pronounced impairment of vibration and position sense in the lower extremities, and pes cavus. Some develop wasting of distal limb muscles, a stocking-glove deficit of superficial sensation, nystagmus, deafness, or optic atrophy. Intellect remains normal. A hypertrophic cardiomyopathy is present in most patients and often leads to supraventricular arrhythmias; heart failure is probably the major cause of death. Insulin-dependent diabetes mellitus develops in 10 to 20 per cent of patients. The mean age at death is 37 years.

DIAGNOSIS. Sensory nerve action potentials are small or absent. Electromyography may show signs of denervation in distal limb muscles, but motor nerve conduction velocities are normal. The cerebrospinal fluid is normal except for mild elevation of the protein content in a few cases. Computed tomographic (CT) brain scans may show mild cerebellar atrophy late in the disease. Electrocardiography often shows inverted T waves, right- or left-axis deviation, and right or left ventricular hypertrophy; conduction disturbances are uncommon.

DIFFERENTIAL DIAGNOSIS. The constellation of progressive ataxia, areflexia, Babinski signs, and onset before age 25 is usually diagnostic. However, a similar picture can occur in vitamin B_{12} deficiency and in vitamin E deficiency (including abetalipoproteinemia). True Friedreich's ataxia is sometimes confused with a less common autosomal recessive type of early-onset progressive ataxia, in which the tendon reflexes are preserved; in the latter syndrome, optic atrophy, scoliosis, and electrocardiographic abnormalities are rare.

ATAXIA-TELANGIECTASIA

Ataxia-telangiectasia is an autosomal recessive, multisystem disease affecting the skin, nervous system, and immune system. Its prevalence has been estimated at 1 to 2 per 100,000. The gene mutation has been localized to the long arm of chromosome 11. Although the precise biochemical defect is not known, it appears to involve defective DNA repair, with an increased frequency of chromosomal breakage and translocations. The main neuropathologic abnormality is a severe loss of neurons in the cerebellar cortex, dentate nuclei, and inferior olives. The level of α-fetoprotein in the blood is elevated in nearly all cases.

Beginning at a few years of age, affected children show progressive cerebellar ataxia and incoordination, choreoathetosis, and a peculiar incoordination of head and eye movements known as oculomotor apraxia. Some develop opsoclonus. Later, fine venous telangiectases appear on the conjunctivae, ears, face, and

TABLE 463–1. THE MULTISYSTEM ATROPHIES

Disease	Heredity	Principal Feature	Associated Features	Chapter
Shy-Drager syndrome	Sporadic	Autonomic insufficiency	Parkinsonism, cerebellar ataxia, dysphagia, laryngeal stridor, amyotrophy	452
Progressive supranuclear palsy	Sporadic	Ophthalmoplegia, especially vertical	Gait ataxia, axial dystonia, parkinsonism, pseudobulbar palsy, dementia	460
Kearns-Sayre syndrome	Sporadic	Ptosis and ophthalmoplegia	Short stature, cerebellar ataxia, retinal degeneration, heart block, deafness, mitochondrial myopathy, mental deficiency, Babinski signs	504
Hereditary ataxias, adult type	Autosomal dominant	Cerebellar ataxia	Ophthalmoplegia, dementia, parkinsonism, dystonia, optic atrophy, retinal degeneration, dysphagia, amyotrophy	463

skin creases. The thymus gland and lymph nodes are underdeveloped, and serum immunoglobulin A (IgA) levels are usually low; the resulting impairment of immunity leads to repeated bacterial infections in the respiratory tract. An axonal polyneuropathy appears late in the disease. Lymphoreticular malignancies and other forms of cancer develop in 10 to 20 per cent of patients. Most patients die of infection or neoplasm in the second or third decade of life.

ADULT-ONSET CEREBELLAR ATAXIA

Hereditary ataxia starting in adult life is nearly always an autosomal dominant disorder with multiple neurologic manifestations, among which cerebellar signs are prominent. The classification of these diseases is difficult because the clinical features vary greatly even within the same family, and there is no agreement with regard to how many genetically distinct diseases exist in this category. In southern England, cases of this type are about one-tenth as numerous as cases of Friedreich's ataxia. Brain enzymes related to cholinergic synaptic transmission have been reported to be present in reduced amount.

PATHOLOGY. Many cases have the pathologic features of olivopontocerebellar atrophy, with loss of neurons in the inferior olives and pontine nuclei (which provide major afferent pathways to the cerebellum), as well as degeneration of the spinocerebellar tracts, corticospinal tracts, and posterior columns. Neuronal degeneration is sometimes found in the cerebellar cortex, dentate nucleus, basal ganglia, midbrain, cerebral cortex, and spinal cord, including the anterior horns. The pathology, however, is as variable as the clinical findings, even within a given family. In cases of Azorean origin (Machado-Joseph disease), the cerebellar cortex and olives are spared.

CLINICAL MANIFESTATIONS. The age of onset, though quite variable, is usually between 20 and 50. Cerebellar ataxia of gait, dysarthria, and incoordination of the limbs usually dominate the clinical picture, so that the ability to walk is lost within 15 years. The other manifestations are extremely variable. Babinski signs and increased reflexes are commonly present, and some patients have spastic weakness in the legs. Vibration and position sense are sometimes lost as the disease advances, and the reflexes may disappear as the primary sensory neurons degenerate. Extrapyramidal findings may include impassive facies, cogwheel rigidity, chorea, athetosis, dystonia, and facial dyskinesia. Many patients have supranuclear oculomotor disorders such as lid retraction, ptosis, nystagmus, slow eye movements, and gaze paresis, especially upgaze. Optic atrophy, with pale discs, is common. Personality change or dementia, muscle wasting and fasciculation in the tongue and distal extremities, and bulbar symptoms of dysphagia or hoarseness are other common manifestations. Death occurs approximately 20 years after onset, at an average age of 57.

Pigmentary degeneration of the retina, beginning in the macula, is an early and constant feature in some families, suggesting that these cases may be genetically distinct. A few families seem to have a "pure" cerebellar syndrome beginning in the seventh decade of life. There is much controversy about the status of Machado-Joseph disease, which affects mainly people of Portuguese and Azorean descent. Although the range of clinical manifestations in these patients is similar to that of patients who have typical olivopontocerebellar atrophy, the pathologic features are said to be distinct because the inferior olives are spared. However, only a few cases have come to autopsy.

DIAGNOSIS. CT or magnetic resonance (MR) images may show atrophy of the cerebellar folia and pons, with enlargement of the fourth ventricle and pontine cisterns. The cerebrospinal fluid is usually normal. Sensory nerve action potentials are small or absent in patients with absent reflexes; in patients with preserved reflexes, somatosensory evoked potentials may be abnormal.

DIFFERENTIAL DIAGNOSIS. Nonhereditary cases of late-onset cerebellar degeneration are at least as common as the hereditary kind. Some are associated with alcoholism or a visceral malignancy, but in many, no apparent cause can be established. These patients' cerebellar symptoms tend to begin between the ages of 40 and 60 and may be accompanied by dementia, extrapyramidal signs, or Babinski signs. Some cases of this kind have the pathologic features of olivopontocerebellar atrophy, but

whether there is any genetic link to the autosomal dominant ataxias is unclear. It should be noted that patients presenting with ataxia may later develop the typical signs of progressive supranuclear palsy or one of the other multisystem atrophies listed in Table 463–1.

Harding AE: The Hereditary Ataxias and Related Disorders. Edinburgh, Churchill Livingstone, 1984. *A detailed review of the hereditary cerebellar ataxias and spastic paraplegias, including the author's own study of several hundred patients and family members. A modern classic.*

464 Hereditary Spastic Paraplegias

This is a diverse group of uncommon diseases whose main symptom is an insidiously beginning, progressive spasticity of the lower extremities. Families with "pure" hereditary spastic paraplegia (Strümpell's disease) are the most numerous, but many rare variants have been reported in which spasticity is associated with other neurologic, ocular, or cutaneous manifestations, overlapping with the spinocerebellar degenerations. The prevalence of these diseases is not well established. Harding found 29 families with hereditary spastic paraplegia in southern England, compared with 11 families of autosomal dominant late-onset cerebellar ataxia. Rare examples of *primary lateral sclerosis*, although sporadic in incidence, may belong to this class.

PATHOLOGY. In the pure form, the spinal cord shows degeneration of the lateral corticospinal tracts and posterior columns, most severe in the thoracic region. Less often there is minor degeneration of the spinocerebellar tracts, anterior corticospinal tracts, anterior horn cells, and cortical Betz cells. The dorsal root ganglia, posterior roots, and peripheral nerves are normal, suggesting that the dorsal column degeneration is caused by "dying-back" of the central processes of the sensory neurons.

CLINICAL MANIFESTATIONS. Most patients with pure hereditary spastic paraplegia continue to walk for many years and have a normal lifespan. Many cases begin in infancy with delayed walking, but the onset can be as late as the seventh decade. Spasticity of the legs and a stiff, slow gait are the main symptoms. Affected persons walk on their toes, trip easily, and are unable to run. About one fourth have pes cavus. The legs are spastic with hyperactive reflexes, clonus, and Babinski signs, while the arms are usually normal. Later the legs may become weak, the arms may show increased reflexes, and distal muscle wasting may develop, especially in the hands. Vibration and position sense may become impaired in the legs, and many patients develop urinary frequency, urgency, and precipitancy, although sexual function remains normal. Most patients become unable to walk sometime in the sixth or seventh decade.

DIAGNOSIS. The cerebrospinal fluid is normal. Electromyography may show denervation in the distal limb muscles, but the sensory nerve action potentials are preserved, even in patients showing decreased vibration and position sense. Somatosensory evoked potentials, however, are consistently small or unobtainable, reflecting a degeneration of dorsal column fibers.

DIFFERENTIAL DIAGNOSIS. Hereditary spastic paraplegia must be distinguished from nonhereditary causes of slowly progressive myelopathy such as cervical spondylosis, intraspinal tumor, arteriovenous malformation of the spinal cord, multiple sclerosis, amyotrophic lateral sclerosis, and myelopathy associated with human T cell lymphotropic virus 1 (HTLV-1 tropical spastic paraparesis, Ch. 478.3). Magnetic resonance (MR) imaging has simplified the diagnosis of many of these conditions.

Harding AE: The Hereditary Ataxias and Related Disorders. Edinburgh, Churchill Livingstone, 1984. *A detailed review of the hereditary cerebellar ataxias and spastic paraplegias, including the author's own study of several hundred patients and family members. A modern classic.*

465 Hereditary and Acquired Intrinsic Motor Neuron Diseases

Degenerative diseases of several kinds can attack the large motor neurons of the spinal cord or the brain to produce selective impairment of muscle strength or motor skill. Those of childhood are largely hereditary, while the major adult disorder, amyotrophic lateral sclerosis, is nearly always sporadic, with few clues illuminating either its etiology or molecular pathogenesis. Table 465–1 lists the major disorders in this category, and the references provide greater detail on the many subtypes.

HEREDITARY AMYOTROPHIES

Hereditary spinal muscular atrophy is a syndrome of progressive muscular weakness and atrophy resulting from selective degeneration of the motor neurons of the spinal cord. A comparable disorder of the lower brain stem nuclei produces progressive bulbar palsy. Many different clinical syndromes have been delineated based on the age of onset, the pattern of muscular weakness, the rate of progression, and the mode of inheritance. Using this approach, at least 15 separate genetic disorders can be recognized. Pearn (1980) has estimated that 1 in 40 Caucasians carries a gene for spinal muscular atrophy. No consistent biochemical defect is known, although hexosaminidase deficiency has been identified in a few cases.

PATHOLOGY. At the time of postmortem examination in the spinal cases, the anterior horns show gliosis and loss of large neurons, and many of the remaining motor neurons are undergoing degeneration. The ventral roots are atrophic owing to loss of myelinated nerve fibers. Similar changes are observed in the motor nuclei of the brain stem in bulbar cases.

In the well-developed infantile and childhood types, microscopic examination of the skeletal muscles using histochemical techniques shows large groups of round, atrophic muscle fibers and large groups of hypertrophied fibers staining uniformly as either type 1 or type 2. These features reflect the continuing process of denervation and reinnervation. However, at an early stage of infantile spinal muscular atrophy the only finding may be uniform atrophy of all muscle fibers, with preservation of the normal "checkerboard" fiber-type pattern. In slowly progressive cases of juvenile or adult onset, atrophic muscle fibers are found mainly in small groups; most muscle fibers are of normal size but are arranged in groups of uniform fiber type. After many years some muscle fibers show secondary myopathic changes, such as internal nuclei, splitting, or degeneration.

ACUTE INFANTILE SPINAL MUSCULAR ATROPHY

Werdnig-Hoffmann disease is a fatal, early infantile form of spinal and bulbar muscular atrophy that appears to be a single genetic entity. Inherited as an autosomal recessive trait, it is one

TABLE 465–1. THE MAJOR INTRINSIC MOTOR NEURON DISEASES

Hereditary
Spinal muscular atrophy
  Type I. Acute, infantile (Werdnig-Hoffmann disease)
  Type II. Late infantile and childhood type
  Type III. Juvenile and adult types
Familial amyotrophic lateral sclerosis (ALS)
Acquired
Acute: anterior poliomyelitis
Chronic:
  ALS alone
  Anterior horn cell degeneration associated with spinocerebellar
    degeneration, Shy-Drager syndrome, parkinsonism, Creutzfeldt-
    Jakob disease
  Remote neoplasms, other
  Primary lateral sclerosis (rare)

of the most common fatal hereditary diseases of childhood, with an annual incidence of 1 in 20,000 live births and a carrier frequency in the general population of about 1 in 80. The abnormal gene is located on the long arm of chromosome 5.

In at least one third of the cases, there is a prenatal onset, with reduced fetal movements, weakness at birth, or congenital joint deformities. In the remainder of cases, the disease becomes apparent in the first 2 or 3 months of life. There is progressive, flaccid weakness of the trunk and limbs, with severe hypotonia, poor head control, and diminished movements of the limbs, more severe in the proximal muscles. Weakness of the intercostal muscles causes retraction of the chest during inspiration; the cry is weak, and coughing is ineffective. Bulbar weakness causes difficulty in sucking and swallowing. The tendon reflexes are usually absent. Death occurs before 3 years of age; 50 per cent of the patients die in the first 7 months of life and 95 per cent in the first 18 months.

The serum creatine kinase activity and the cerebrospinal fluid are normal. Electromyography shows reduced activation of motor unit potentials, many of which are of increased size, duration, and complexity. Fibrillations may be present, and in the majority of cases there is a spontaneous, regular discharge of motor unit potentials at a frequency of 5 to 15 Hz. It is important to distinguish this disease from treatable disorders such as infant botulism and chronic inflammatory polyneuropathy. The former is identified by repetitive nerve stimulation tests showing abnormal neuromuscular transmission and the latter, by abnormalities of nerve conduction and increased protein levels in the cerebrospinal fluid.

PROGRESSIVE MUSCULAR ATROPHY IN CHILDREN

Proximal Type. Clinically, this is a rather diverse disorder, but most cases are now thought to be caused by a single autosomal recessive gene, located on the long arm of chromosome 5, near or at the locus for Werdnig-Hoffmann disease. The incidence of this syndrome is 1 in 24,000 live births, and the carrier rate is approximately 1 in 90. A milder, autosomal dominant form is also known.

Weakness starts any time from birth to 8 years of age, usually before 1 year of age. The weakness affects the trunk and limbs and initially is more severe in proximal muscles. The limb muscles become atrophic, the tendon reflexes are lost, and joint contractures may develop. Fasciculations are not prominent but may be apparent in the fingers, producing a fine, irregular tremor. The face and jaws may be weak, and the tongue may be atrophic and show fasciculation.

Children with early onset may never be able to walk and often develop severe scoliosis, limb deformities, and respiratory insufficiency. Many eventually die of pulmonary infection, but some very weak patients survive into adult life, the progress of the disease apparently having arrested early in childhood. Children with a later onset of weakness tend to have a milder course, with slowly progressive proximal weakness, increased lumbar lordosis, and a waddling gait. Those with autosomal recessive inheritance rarely walk after age 20, while those with the rare autosomal dominant form may still be walking in middle age.

Serum creatine kinase activity may be mildly or moderately increased in patients with slowly progressive weakness, apparently because of secondary myopathic changes in muscle. The cerebrospinal fluid is normal. Electromyography shows the typical changes of chronic denervation and reinnervation as well as fibrillations and fasciculations, serving to distinguish these patients from similar patients with muscular dystrophy. Spontaneous, regular discharges of single motor unit potentials, like those found in infants with Werdnig-Hoffmann disease, are seen in children whose weakness began before age 2, but not in those with onset later in childhood.

Many of these children benefit from active and passive physical therapy and the judicious use of lightweight braces. Special attention should be given to spinal support to counteract scoliosis. Later in childhood, surgical immobilization of the spine may be indicated.

Distal Type. This category includes both dominant and recessive disorders and accounts for about 10 per cent of all cases of spinal muscular atrophy. Distal limb weakness and muscle wasting, more severe in the lower extremities, usually begins in early childhood and tends to be mild and slowly progressive. Three quarters of the patients have pes cavus, and, except for the absence of sensory deficits, the disorder is often clinically indistinguishable from Charcot-Marie-Tooth disease. However, patients with spinal muscular atrophy have normal conduction in motor and sensory nerves. A rare scapuloperoneal type, with autosomal recessive inheritance, is characterized by distal leg weakness and scapular winging, starting in infancy; there may also be bulbar symptoms such as laryngeal stridor.

Bulbar Type. The Fazio-Londe syndrome is a rare, fatal disorder of young children characterized by degeneration of the motor neurons of the brain stem resulting in progressive paralysis of the face, throat, larynx, and tongue and sometimes the ocular and jaw muscles. The cases have occurred sporadically or among siblings, suggesting autosomal recessive inheritance.

SPINAL MUSCULAR ATROPHY OF ADOLESCENT OR ADULT ONSET

Patients with late-onset spinal muscular atrophy have slowly progressive muscular weakness and usually continue to walk for two or three decades or more. Although much less common than the infantile and childhood types, the adult types include at least four clinical and eight genetic categories.

Proximal Type. These patients resemble patients with muscular dystrophy, and clinical examination may offer few clues to the neurogenic character of the proximal weakness. Fasciculations and muscle cramps are usually not prominent, and the serum creatine kinase activity may be substantially increased. To add to the confusion, males with onset of symptoms in their teens may have large calves. Some patients eventually develop mild bulbar symptoms, such as dysphagia. Electromyography serves to establish the neurogenic nature of the disorder, and muscle biopsy is rarely needed. Families with autosomal dominant and autosomal recessive inheritance have been described. A distinctive X-linked recessive variety, known as bulbospinal neuronopathy, is associated with gynecomastia and dysphagia.

Scapuloperoneal and Facioscapulohumeral Types. Both myopathic and neurogenic scapuloperoneal syndromes are known, and several varieties begin in the second or third decade of life. Autosomal dominant, autosomal recessive, and X-linked recessive forms have been described. The common feature of these disorders is progressive atrophy and weakness of the shoulder girdle and lower leg muscles, though weakness eventually may spread to the other limb muscles. Electromyography and muscle biopsy can distinguish the anterior horn cell diseases from the muscular dystrophies, but the prognosis is similar in both groups. A few families have an autosomal dominant form of spinal muscular atrophy resembling facioscapulohumeral muscular dystrophy.

Distal Type. This is usually a childhood disorder, but there are a few families with distal amyotrophy beginning in the third or fourth decade of life, inherited as an autosomal dominant trait. Some familial as well as adult cases exhibit onset in middle age and such a slow progression as never to be incapacitating, even in old age.

AMYOTROPHIC LATERAL SCLEROSIS

Amyotrophic lateral sclerosis (ALS) is a fatal degenerative disease of the central nervous system characterized by slowly progressive paralysis of the voluntary muscles. The French neurologist Charcot gave a detailed clinical and pathologic description in 1865. Little substantive knowledge about the cause and treatment of the disorder has been added since.

INCIDENCE. The annual incidence is about 1 case per 100,000 population, the prevalence being 4 to 6 cases per 100,000. Geographical pockets of much higher incidence in Guam, the Kii peninsula of Japan, and western New Guinea suggest possible, still unknown, exogenous causes. Ninety-five per cent of cases in the United States are sporadic, but a few families have several members with the typical clinical picture of sporadic ALS arising in an autosomal dominant pattern. Males are affected slightly more often than females. Although the disease can appear as early as the third decade of life, most cases begin after the age of 40, and the incidence increases with age into the eighth decade.

PATHOLOGY. Degeneration of the motor neurons of the spinal cord and lower brain stem is marked by extensive cell loss

and astrocytic gliosis. Swellings containing neurofilaments are often found on axons close to their cell bodies. As the Betz cells and large pyramidal neurons of the motor cortex disappear, the corticospinal tracts degenerate, leaving gliosis of the lateral columns of the spinal cord. The ventral spinal roots are depleted of large myelinated nerve fibers, but surviving axons develop distal sprouts that reinnervate some muscle fibers, so that skeletal muscle histopathology shows both muscle fiber atrophy and fiber-type grouping.

ETIOLOGY. Few clues exist to the cause of ALS. Some authors regard the disease as a manifestation of premature aging or a deficiency of a neurotrophic factor. Other speculations include toxic exposure to minerals such as lead or aluminum, deficiency of calcium or magnesium, infection by an unidentified virus, and autoimmunity. Benign paraproteinemia has been encountered in a small proportion of patients, and antiganglioside antibodies have been found in the serum in a majority of the cases, but the significance of these findings is unclear.

CLINICAL MANIFESTATIONS. The major symptom consists of slowly progressive muscle weakness involving the limbs, trunk, breathing muscles, throat, and tongue. Most patients have a mixture of lower and upper motor neuron symptoms, although either may predominate. The former include muscle weakness, wasting, fasciculations, and cramps; the latter include stiffness and slowness of movement, slow and clumsy speech, and explosive release of laughter and crying (pseudobulbar palsy). The ocular muscles are not affected except in patients who survive long times after bulbar paralysis has begun. No impairment affects bladder, bowel, or sexual function. The stretch reflexes are diminished in severely denervated muscles, but more often signs of lower motor neuron weakness are combined with brisk reflexes, a finding nearly specific to ALS. Babinski signs are often present. Sensation is normal except for an expected diminution of vibration sense in the feet in older patients, and mental function is nearly always normal.

The onset is insidious, and initial symptoms may be confined to a single limb (especially the distal muscles), both limbs on one side, or to lower cranial nerves. Gradually, however, the patchy and asymmetric weakness becomes widespread, and the patient becomes unable to walk, dress, or feed himself or herself. There is loss of weight because of muscle atrophy and impaired swallowing; the speech becomes unintelligible; choking interferes with eating and sleeping; and breathing becomes difficult even at rest. Death occurs from pulmonary infection and insufficiency. The average survival is 3 years after onset of symptoms, but a few patients live for 10 years or longer in a severely debilitated state.

DIAGNOSIS. Because there are no specific laboratory tests, the diagnosis is based principally on clinical criteria. The disease to be diagnosed as ALS should have a relentlessly progressive, gradual course; lower motor neuron signs should exist at widely separate levels of the nervous system, or upper motor neuron signs should be found well above the level of the lower motor neuron signs; and no conflicting findings such as sensory loss, incontinence, or ocular weakness should be present. The cerebrospinal fluid is normal except for a mild elevation of protein concentration in some cases. Computed tomography (CT) and magnetic resonance (MR) imaging of the brain and spinal cord are unrevealing. Electromyography shows active and chronic denervation in multiple muscles of the brain stem, upper and lower extremities, and trunk; motor nerve conduction velocity is normal or slightly reduced, and sensory nerve conduction is normal. Serum creatine kinase activity is normal or moderately increased.

DIFFERENTIAL DIAGNOSIS. Although ALS is nearly always fatal, a few patients stop deteriorating or even recover normal strength, but such cases are extremely rare. Other motor neuron disorders, treatable myelopathies and neuropathies, and even thyrotoxic myopathy must be distinguished from ALS (see Table 465–2).

TREATMENT. With a disease as grim as ALS, the physician must be careful to avoid premature misdiagnosis. Once the diagnosis is certain, however, some explanation must be given to the patient and the family. This requires considerable tact and gentleness; often it is best to convey the information gradually

TABLE 465–2. DIFFERENTIAL DIAGNOSIS OF AMYOTROPHIC LATERAL SCLEROSIS

Disease	Distinguishing Features
Benign fasciculations	No weakness, atrophy, or electromyographic (EMG) abnormality
Motor neuron diseases	
*Lead or mercury toxicity	Increased lead or mercury levels
Benign focal amyotrophy	Onset in youth, strictly focal, no upper motor neuron signs
Postpolio progressive muscular atrophy	Slow course, no upper motor neuron signs
Subacute motor neuronopathy in lymphoma	Plateau in few months, later improvement
*ALS in lung cancer or B cell dyscrasia	Improves on treatment of tumor
Hereditary spinal muscular atrophy	Symmetric, slow course, no upper motor neuron signs
*Thyrotoxic myopathy with fasciculations	Myopathic EMG
*Compressive myelopathy due to cervical spondylosis or extramedullary tumor	Sensory symptoms, no lower motor neuron signs in legs, cord compression on MRI or myelography
*Immune-mediated multifocal motor neuropathy	Multifocal nerve conduction block, very high antiganglioside antibody titers

*Treatable conditions

on successive visits, allowing the relentless progression of weakness to speak for itself.

No medication has been shown to be beneficial, and physical therapy does not delay the neuromuscular deterioration. Quack remedies surface periodically; for their own protection, patients who wish to try experimental forms of treatment should be referred to a reputable academic center.

Patients with impaired gait may benefit from using a cane or a walker, and patients who suffer from severe dysphagia without other disabling symptoms can be offered nasogastric tube feeding or a gastrostomy. The most difficult medical question, however, involves the therapeutic role of artificial ventilation. Most patients, understanding the hopeless prognosis, prefer not to be kept alive artificially in a state of total paralysis, unable to communicate except with eye movements. Nevertheless, some patients have survived for several years in this fashion, living at home with the help of a devoted and intelligent family. It is important to discuss these issues when patients are in the early stages of respiratory involvement, so that they can make decisions in advance about whether or not to accept emergency resuscitation during a respiratory crisis.

PRIMARY LATERAL SCLEROSIS

Primary lateral sclerosis (PLS) describes a relatively rare condition characterized by painless, insidiously beginning, and gradually progressing spastic weakness that involves first the lower limbs but that in some instances ascends the neuraxis to affect the upper extremities. Rarely, pseudobulbar palsy adds its limitations to the woes of quadriplegia. In most instances, the disease begins in middle or late life with a duration that occasionally lasts no more than a year but most often persists for well over a decade before complications or intercurrent illness causes death. Typically, neurologic examinations show a relatively symmetric spastic paraparesis or quadriparesis with heightened deep tendon reflexes and extensor plantar responses but no hint of sensory abnormality. Neither clinical nor electrical studies detect evidence of skeletal muscular denervation in PLS. Similarly, central nervous system imaging procedures disclose no relevant abnormalities involving either brain or spinal cord. The cerebrospinal fluid remains unremarkable, and appropriate tests fail to disclose HIV, HTLV, or other inflammatory processes. Autopsy examinations, performed in a number of cases, have revealed ascending bilateral demyelination of the thoracolumbar corticospinal tracts extending to levels anywhere from the lower cord up to and including the cerebral peduncles. Cerebral degeneration has not

been noted. The cause of PLS is not known, but sporadically arising familial spastic paraplegia cannot be excluded in cases selectively involving the lower extremities. No specific treatment exists, although baclofen may bring modest relief of stiffness.

Brzustowicz LM, Lehner T, Castilla LH, et al.: Genetic mapping of chronic childhood onset spinal muscular atrophy to chromosome 5q 11.2–13.3. Nature 344:540, 1990. *Evidence that the infantile and childhood types of spinal muscular atrophy are allelic disorders of a single gene.*
Dubowitz V: Muscle Disorders in Childhood. London, W.B. Saunders Company, 1978, pp 146–90. *A rich compendium of clinical observations on the spinal muscular atrophies, by a leading neuromuscular expert. Superb illustrations.*
Mitsumoto H, Hanson MR, Chad DA: Amyotrophic lateral sclerosis. Recent advances in pathogenesis and therapeutic trials. Arch Neurol 45:189, 1988. *An extensive review of putative variants and possible mechanisms or treatment for this devastating disorder; 336 references.*
Siddique T, Figlewicz DA, Pericak-Vance MA, et al.: Linkage of a gene causing familial amyotrophic lateral sclerosis to chromosome 21 and evidence of genetic-locus heterogeneity. N Engl J Med 324:1381, 1991. *Twenty-three kindreds with this rare condition were evaluated by polymorphic markers for possible specific chromosome markers. Positive linkage to chromosome 21 was found in about half, adding a crucial suggestion relating to cellular susceptibility in this devastating illness.*
Tandan R, Bradley WG: Amyotrophic lateral sclerosis: Part 1. Clinical features, pathology, and ethical issues in management. Part 2. Etiopathogenesis. Ann Neurol 18:271, 419, 1985. *A recent review of research and treatment, with an important discussion of the ethical issues involved in the use of respirators.*
Younger DS, Chou S, Hayes AP, et al.: Primary lateral sclerosis. A clinical diagnosis reemerges. Arch Neurol 45:1304, 1988.

466 Syringomyelia

Syringomyelia is a disorder of the spinal cord and, often, the lower brain stem, characterized by slowly progressive enlargement of a fluid-filled cyst (syrinx) within the cord or medulla. Most cases are congenital in origin, related to maldevelopment of the cervicomedullary junction; others are caused by arachnoiditis, intraspinal tumor, or trauma. A prevalence of 8.4 cases per 100,000 has been suggested.

PATHOLOGY. In congenital cases, the cyst is thought to represent an enormously dilated remnant of the fetal central canal, which usually does not communicate with the fourth ventricle. It is lined by glial tissue, and in places by remnants of ependyma, and contains clear fluid identical to cerebrospinal fluid. Extending from the high cervical level or medulla to the thoracic or lumbar cord, the cyst varies in shape and size at different levels and is variably associated with damage to the anterior horns, crossing spinothalamic fibers, and lateral columns. Most patients have a Chiari type of congenital cerebellar malformation, in which the flattened ectopic tonsils descend caudally and press against the dorsal aspect of the upper cervical cord so as to obstruct both the exit foramina of the fourth ventricle and the subarachnoid space at the foramen magnum.

Acquired syringomyelia may result from basal arachnoiditis, obstructing the cerebrospinal fluid pathways around the foramen magnum, or may develop in a segment of the cord rendered abnormal by an intramedullary tumor, spinal arachnoiditis, or severe traumatic injury. In nontumor cases the cavity is lined only by glia, whereas in tumor cases the cyst wall may contain both tumor and glial cells. The cyst fluid may have an increased protein concentration in post-traumatic and tumor cases.

PATHOGENESIS. The mechanism of cyst formation and expansion is poorly understood. In congenital syringomyelia the cavity probably originates before birth as a dilatation of the primitive central canal. Enlargement of the cyst is somehow related to obstruction of the subarachnoid space at the cervicomedullary junction by the ectopic cerebellar tonsils, causing a pressure gradient between the cyst and the subarachnoid space, especially during straining, coughing, or sneezing. The mechanism may be similar in cases of basal arachnoiditis. In patients with spinal arachnoiditis, the cyst may originate in an area of ischemic myelomalacia, and in cases associated with tumor or severe injury there is cystic degeneration of the spinal cord before the syrinx starts to expand. Why the cyst continues to enlarge in these noncommunicating cases is hard to understand, since there is no apparent pressure gradient between the cyst and the subarachnoid space. Obstruction of cerebrospinal fluid circulation due to spinal arachnoiditis may be an important factor.

CLINICAL MANIFESTATIONS. The classic clinical picture of congenital syringomyelia is of a slowly progressive, asymmetric, destructive process in the central portion of the cervical and thoracic spinal cord, damaging the anterior horn cells, the crossing spinothalamic tract fibers, and the lateral corticospinal tracts. This causes muscle weakness and wasting in the hands and arms; scoliosis owing to denervation of paraspinal muscles; loss of arm reflexes; spastic weakness of the lower extremities; and a *dissociated sensory loss* with impaired perception of pain and temperature in the neck, arms, and upper trunk and preserved light touch perception and proprioception. Some patients experience a deep, aching pain in the neck or arms. Symptoms usually begin between 25 and 40 years of age and advance relentlessly for decades, although one third of the patients have long periods of stability. The deficits may worsen suddenly after a fall or after coughing or sneezing. Ten per cent of patients develop a painless arthropathy (Charcot joint) of the shoulder, elbow, or hand. Extension into the medulla may cause nystagmus, dysphagia, or wasting of the tongue, and some patients have hydrocephalus or cerebellar signs related to an associated Chiari malformation.

The manifestations of acquired syringomyelia depend on the segment of the spinal cord affected. Posttraumatic syringomyelia, developing in paraplegic or quadriplegic patients months or years after the injury, is revealed by weakness and sensory impairment rising craniad from the transected level. The cases associated with arachnoiditis following previous purulent meningitis, subarachnoid hemorrhage, surgery, trauma, or spinal anesthesia tend to involve the thoracic and lower cervical segments. Syringes associated with intramedullary spinal cord tumor extend for variable distances rostrad or caudad to the tumor.

DIAGNOSIS. Myelography, once widely employed, has been rendered largely obsolete by magnetic resonance (MR) imaging, which is both safer and more informative. Such images outline the size and extent of the cavity as well as the presence of cerebellar ectopia, arachnoiditis, or an intraspinal tumor (Fig. 466–1). Electromyography reveals active and chronic denervation in wasted upper extremity muscles, but sensory nerve conduction is normal in the analgesic hand, since the lesion is located proximal to the dorsal root ganglia. The cerebrospinal fluid is normal except for a raised protein content in cases associated with tumor or arachnoiditis.

TREATMENT. Various surgical procedures have been devised in the hope of arresting the neurologic deterioration, but none has been reliably successful. For congenital syringomyelia associated with cerebellar ectopia, it is often sufficient to perform a posterior decompression of the foramen magnum, ensuring that

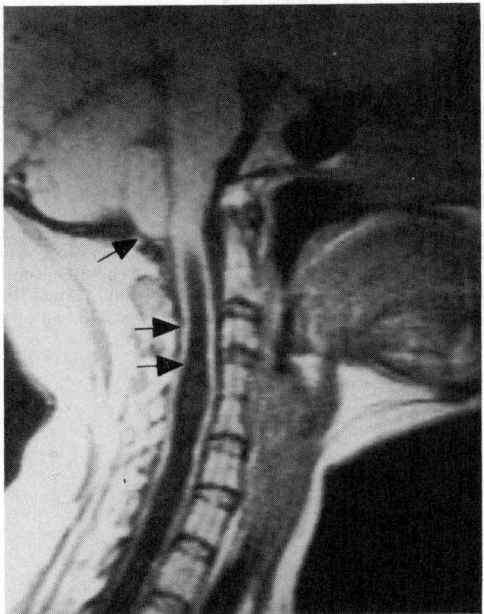

FIGURE 466–1. Magnetic resonance image of upper spine and foramen magnum in a patient with syringomyelia and a small Chiari I malformation (*single arrow*). The syrinx appears as a dark central area in the cervical and thoracic spinal cord (*double arrows*).

the fourth ventricle communicates with the subarachnoid space. Acquired syringomyelia is usually treated by decompressing the cyst via a syringoarachnoid, syringopleural, or syringoperitoneal shunt. It has not been satisfactorily established that the outcome of any of these procedures is superior to the natural history of the disease. Several neurosurgical reports, however, suggest that these operations often reduce chronic pain and arrest the progression of neurologic symptoms, especially if performed before severe neurologic disability develops.

Anderson NE, Willoughby EW, Wrightson P: The natural history and the influence of surgical treatment in syringomyelia. Acta Neurol Scand 71:472, 1985. *A thoughtful critique of the uncertain role of surgical treatment for syringomyelia.*

467 The Phakomatoses

The phakomatoses, or neurocutaneous syndromes, are congenital disorders characterized by disordered growth of ectodermal tissues, producing distinctive skin lesions and malformations or tumors of the nervous system. More than 20 syndromes have been described, the most important of which are neurofibromatosis 1 and 2, tuberous sclerosis, and Sturge-Weber disease.

NEUROFIBROMATOSIS 1 (von Recklinghausen's Disease)

Neurofibromatosis 1 is characterized by multiple café au lait spots on the skin, multiple peripheral nerve tumors, and a variety of other dysplastic abnormalities of the skin, nervous system, bones, endocrine organs, and blood vessels. It is one of the most common genetic diseases, occurring approximately once in every 3000 births and present in about 30 persons per 10,000 population. It is inherited as an autosomal dominant trait, but 40 to 60 per cent of cases are clinically sporadic. Even allowing for the difficulty of detecting the trait in mild cases, there seems to be a remarkably high mutation rate, on the order of 10^{-4} per locus per generation. The gene has been mapped to a large region (about 13 kilobases) of the long arm of chromosome 17.

PATHOLOGY. The peripheral nerve tumors are of two types, schwannomas and neurofibromas, the latter derived from both Schwann cells and perineural fibroblasts. Neurofibromas of sensory nerve twigs produce the distinctive subcutaneous nodules; in peripheral nerve trunks the tumor appears as a fusiform enlargement or plexiform neuroma. Schwannomas arise in cranial and spinal nerve roots and also in peripheral nerve trunks. Both types of tumor occasionally become malignant. The brain may show disordered architecture, hamartomas, gliomas, and meningiomas.

CLINICAL MANIFESTATIONS. Some manifestations are congenital, but most appear gradually during childhood and adult life. Café au lait spots become larger and more numerous with age; the majority of patients eventually have more than six spots greater than 1.5 cm in diameter. Other skin lesions include freckles (axillary freckles being specific to this disease); soft, pedunculated, cutaneous neurofibromas; and firm, subcutaneous neurofibromas.

Plexiform neurofibromas may grow to lemon or even melon size, leading to grotesque overgrowth of soft tissues and bone in a limb or around the orbit. Enlarging nerve trunk tumors may cause pain and impairment of motor and sensory function; intraspinal nerve root tumors do the same and also compress the spinal cord. Gliomas of the optic nerve and chiasm are the most frequent intracranial tumor; they usually behave in an indolent fashion as hamartomas do. A hamartoma of the hypothalamus may cause precocious puberty.

About 10 per cent of children are mentally deficient, and about 10 per cent develop seizures, half in association with an intracranial tumor. Kyphoscoliosis, dysplasia of the skull, bowed legs, and other bone abnormalities are common. Pheochromocytoma occurs in about 5 per cent of patients, usually in adult life, and hypertension may result from renal artery dysplasia.

DIAGNOSIS. The diagnosis of neurofibromatosis is usually evident on clinical grounds, but biopsy of a neurofibroma can be diagnostic in otherwise cryptic cases. Spinal nerve root tumors often have a dumbbell shape, with intraspinal and extraspinal components; these are most readily identified on magnetic resonance (MR) imaging. For diagnosis of intracranial tumors and hamartomas either computed tomographic (CT) or MR images are suitable.

TREATMENT. Most patients live a normal life with few or no symptoms. Small cutaneous or subcutaneous neurofibromas can be removed if they are painful or frequently irritated, but large plexiform neurofibromas should usually be left alone. A few become malignant with continued invasion and fatal outcome. Asymptomatic peripheral nerve trunk schwannomas can sometimes be removed safely by an experienced surgeon. Intraspinal and intracranial schwannomas are approached in the usual surgical fashion. Optic nerve gliomas are generally treated with radiation, but it is not clear whether this improves the outcome.

NEUROFIBROMATOSIS 2

Often called central neurofibromatosis, this rare disease is characterized by the occurrence of bilateral acoustic neuromas and often other intracranial tumors, such as meningiomas and ependymomas. A few café au lait spots are present in 42 per cent of cases. Inherited as an autosomal dominant trait, the disease has a prevalence of 0.1 per 100,000. The responsible gene has been assigned to the long arm of chromosome 22. Family members at risk for the disease should be screened regularly with hearing tests and brain stem auditory evoked responses.

TUBEROUS SCLEROSIS

The typical clinical triad of tuberous sclerosis consists of mental deficiency, epilepsy, and a characteristic facial eruption known as adenoma sebaceum. The disease is inherited as an autosomal dominant trait, but about 80 per cent of the cases are sporadic, owing to new mutations. The incidence is about 3 cases per 100,000 births, the prevalence is about 10 per 100,000 population, and the mutation rate is 10.5×10^{-6} per gene per generation. Recently, the gene has been mapped to the long arm of chromosome 11.

PATHOLOGY. The facial papules of adenoma sebaceum are angiofibromas. The cerebral hemispheres contain multiple hamartomas or tubers, which give the disease its name; these are characterized by disordered architecture, proliferating and abnormal astrocytes, and deposits of calcium. Occasionally a subependymal nodule forms a giant cell astrocytoma, obstructing the foramen of Monro. The common retinal hamartomas are also probably of glial origin. Visceral lesions include multiple rhabdomyomas of the heart, multiple angiomyolipomas of the kidneys, and cystic transformation of the lungs by proliferating fibrous, muscular, and vascular tissue.

CLINICAL MANIFESTATIONS. Mental deficiency may be mild or severe, but one third of affected individuals have normal or even superior intelligence. Seizures occur in 80 per cent of cases, usually starting before the age of 5, and are often difficult to control with medication. In infants the seizures often take the form of infantile spasms; these children tend to be more severely impaired mentally. Occasionally, diagnosis escapes attention until late adolescence or adult life, when investigation of a seizure disorder of new onset turns up subtle skin lesions or multiple retinal or intracranial hamartomas.

Nearly all patients have distinctive skin lesions. Hypopigmented spots are present from the time of birth in nearly 100 per cent of patients; they are more numerous on the trunk and are easier to see with a Wood lamp. The next most common is adenoma sebaceum, a papular, salmon-colored eruption on the center of the face, especially in the nasolabial folds. It usually appears around 4 years of age and becomes more prominent after puberty. Leathery "shagreen" patches over the lower back and fibromas of the nailbeds affect perhaps 40 per cent of patients.

Retinal hamartomas are present in about half the patients. About 30 per cent of patients have cardiac rhabdomyomas, which sometimes cause arrhythmia or congestive heart failure. Renal tumors occur in two thirds of patients and are usually asymptomatic, though pain and bleeding can occur. Cystic disease of the lungs, an uncommon complication, mainly affects women over the age of 20; the symptoms include pneumothorax, dyspnea, cyanosis, and cor pulmonale.

DIAGNOSIS. Calcified cerebral lesions and subependymal nodules are well seen on brain CT, but uncalcified cortical tubers may show up better with MRI. Adenoma sebaceum, ungual fibromas, and hypopigmented spots are diagnostically specific, but retinal hamartomas also occur in neurofibromatosis. In 85 per cent of patients the electroencephalogram (EEG) is abnormal, most often showing epileptiform activity.

Treatment is confined to symptomatic control of the epilepsy and to surgical therapy of the occasional hamartoma that undergoes gliomatous changes and enlarges to produce symptoms.

STURGE-WEBER SYNDROME

The Sturge-Weber syndrome is a nonhereditary, congenital disorder of facial and cerebral blood vessels characterized by a facial angioma (port-wine stain), seizures, and mental deficiency. The condition involves a defect of embryonic development, with persistence of a vascular plexus in the cephalic portion of the neural tube. The incidence is about 5 in 100,000 births.

The facial angioma is usually unilateral but may extend to the other side and conforms largely but not strictly to trigeminal nerve subdivisions. There may be cavernous angiomas of the tongue, gums, or mouth, and choroidal angiomas may cause congenital glaucoma. An angioma of the occipital and parietal leptomeninges accompanies the facial nevus on the same side, and the underlying cerebral hemisphere is atrophic, with degenerative changes and deposits of iron and calcium in the superficial layers of the cerebral cortex. The cortical calcifications and atrophy are easily seen on brain CT. Neurologic symptoms develop in infancy or early childhood, consisting of focal or generalized seizures. Half of the children become mentally impaired, and one third develop a hemiparesis. When seizures are difficult to control with medication, early surgical removal of the affected part of the brain may improve control and prevent intellectual deterioration.

Gomez MR (ed.): Tuberous Sclerosis. New York, Raven Press, 1979. *A compilation of the Mayo Clinic experience, with excellent illustrations of the skin and retinal lesions.*
Riccardi VM: Medical progress. Von Recklinghausen neurofibromatosis. N Engl J Med 305: 1617, 1981. *A good review of the multiform clinical manifestations.*
Wertelecki W, Rouleau GA, Superneau DW, et al.: Neurofibromatosis 2: Clinical and DNA linkage studies of a large kindred. N Engl J Med 319: 278, 1988. *Includes evidence assigning the gene to chromosome 22.*

468 Cerebrovascular Diseases— Principles

The family of cerebrovascular diseases can be classified according to whether they affect the brain's vascular supply either focally or diffusely (Fig. 468–1). The generic term *stroke* has come to signify the abrupt impairment of brain function caused by a variety of pathologic changes involving one (focal) or several (multifocal) intracranial or extracranial blood vessels. Approximately 80 per cent of all strokes are caused by too little blood flow (ischemic stroke), and the remaining 20 per cent are nearly equally divided between hemorrhage into brain tissue (parenchymatous hemorrhage) or the surrounding subarachnoid space (subarachnoid hemorrhage). In contrast, diseases that affect the heart or the systemic circulation cause generalized hypoperfusion and diffuse brain dysfunction or injury. Ischemic stroke and the hypoperfusion syndromes affecting the brain share much pathophysiology, and therefore both processes are considered together in Ch. 469; hemorrhagic stroke is addressed in Ch. 470.

Often cited as the third most frequent cause of death in the developed countries, stroke imposes an even greater impact on society in terms of the visible disability it causes. Many stroke victims survive for years with major impairments of speech, intellect, and motor or sensory function. Unlike survivors of myocardial infarction, who may be able to engage in most nonstrenuous activities, stroke victims often have difficulty with everyday acts like dressing, eating, walking, and communicating.

EPIDEMIOLOGY

The annual incidence and death rates for stroke have showed a steady decline in the United States throughout the twentieth century and for most European countries and Japan since approximately 1960. In the United States, a 1 per cent per year decrease in the annual mortality rate from stroke recorded since 1915 accelerated in the early 1970's to approximately 5 per cent per year. A recent analysis of a representative U.S. population indicates that the stroke incidence has stabilized at approximately 0.5 to 1.0 per 1000 population. Incidence rates in most European countries are only slightly higher (1.5 per 1000), but several Eastern European countries and Japan have rates of 3 per 1000, for unexplained reasons. At these current rates, stroke remains the third leading cause of medically related deaths and, after Alzheimer's disease, the most frequent cause of neurologic morbidity in developed countries.

Several other important facts about stroke incidence have emerged: a higher incidence and death rate for stroke among blacks than whites in the United States; approximately similar rates in men and women, in contrast to the male predominance for myocardial infarction; and importantly, a strikingly higher incidence (20 to 30 per 1000) for those over the age of 75. The last fact takes on particular significance in view of the aging population in North America, Europe, and parts of Asia.

CEREBROVASCULAR ANATOMY

Since most strokes are caused by abnormalities within the cerebral circulation, some understanding of cerebrovascular anatomy helps in arriving at the correct diagnosis and determining the underlying pathogenesis and prognosis. For example, symptoms that signal selective involvement of cortical blood vessels suggest cerebral emboli rather than atherothrombosis; clinical changes that cannot be attributed to a specific vascular territory may have causes other than a stroke; and transient ischemia of the vertebrobasilar system carries a better prognosis than does that of the carotid artery circulation.

The brain is supplied by four major arteries: the left and right internal carotid and vertebral arteries (Fig. 468–2). The left common carotid artery arises from the aortic arch, but the other vessels originate from branches of the aorta; the right common carotid artery stems from the innominate artery, and the left and right vertebral arteries take off from their respective subclavian arteries.

INTERNAL CAROTID ARTERIES. Each common carotid artery bifurcates in the majority of individuals just below the angle of the jaw and approximately at the level of the thyroid cartilage into an internal and external carotid artery (Fig. 468–2). The *internal carotid artery (ICA)* usually lies posterior and somewhat medial to the *external carotid artery* as the former ascends to the cranial vault. The ICA enters the cranium through the foramen lacerum and travels a short distance within the petrous portion of the temporal bone. It then enters the cavernous

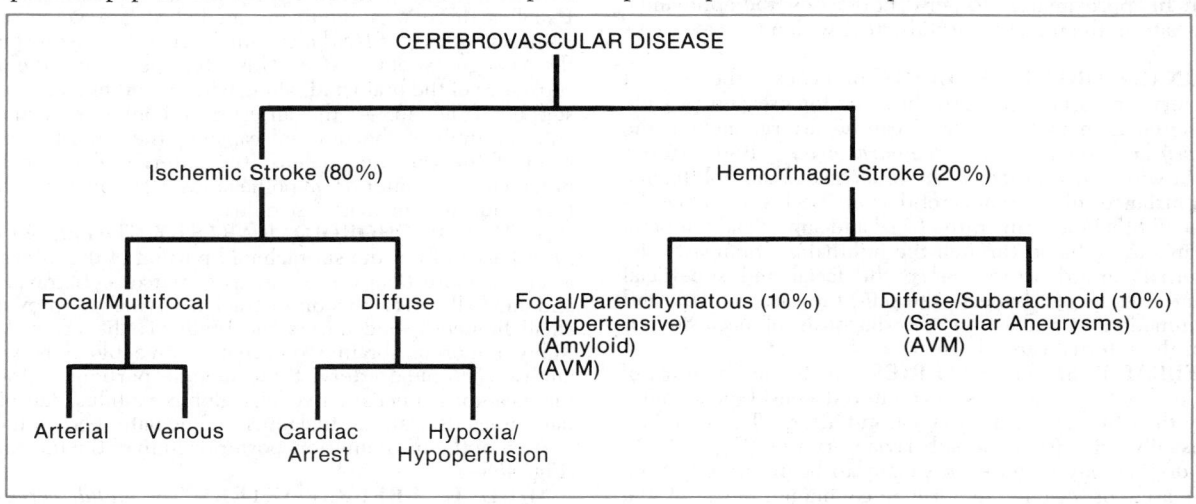

FIGURE 468–1. Classification of cerebrovascular disease.

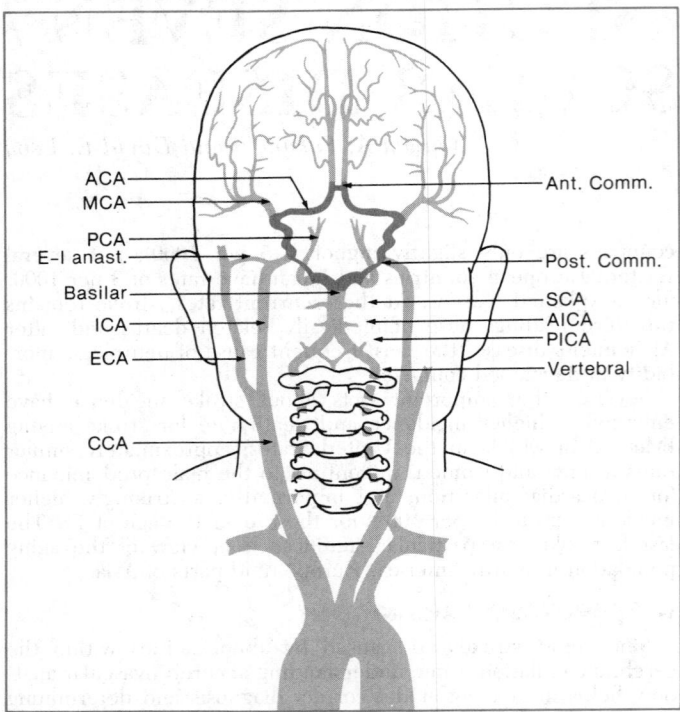

FIGURE 468–2. Extracranial and intracranial arterial supply to brain. Vessels forming the circle of Willis are highlighted in dark red. Abbreviations for intracranial and extracranial arteries are as follows: ACA = anterior cerebral artery; MCA = middle cerebral artery; PCA = posterior cerebral artery; E-I Anast = extracranial-intracranial anastomosis; ICA = internal carotid artery; ECA = external carotid artery; CCA = common carotid artery; Ant. Comm. = anterior communicating artery; Post. Comm. = posterior communicating artery; SCA = superior cerebellar artery; AICA = anterior inferior cerebellar artery; PICA = posterior inferior cerebellar artery. (Modified from Lord R: Surgery of Occlusive Cerebrovascular Disease. St. Louis, C.V. Mosby Company, 1986; with permission.)

sinus before penetrating the dura and ascends above the clinoid processes to divide into the *anterior* and *middle cerebral arteries.* The portion of the internal carotid artery that lies between the cavernous sinus and the supraclinoid process forms an **S** shape and is sometimes referred to as the carotid syphon by neuroradiologists. The internal carotid artery gives off no branches in the neck and a few nutritive branches within the petrous bone, and then at the supraclinoid level, the *ophthalmic, posterior communicating,* and *anterior choroidal arteries* usually arise in that order. In approximately 10 per cent of cases, the ophthalmic artery arises from the internal carotid artery within the cavernous sinus.

EXTERNAL CAROTID ARTERIES. Branches of the external carotid artery, important because they anastomose and provide collateral circulation to the internal carotid artery, include the *facial artery* and the *superficial temporal artery.* Both arteries anastomose with the *supratrochlear* branches of the ophthalmic artery. In instances of internal carotid artery occlusion below the level of the ophthalmic branch, the facial and superficial temporal arteries can supply blood through the ophthalmic branch to the distal internal carotid artery. Since the facial and superficial temporal arteries lie just beneath the skin, they are palpable and their examination can assist in the diagnosis of occlusion or stenosis of the internal carotid artery.

VERTEBRAL-BASILAR ARTERIES. Anatomic variation of the *vertebral artery* system is encountered considerably more frequently than that of the internal carotid artery. The vertebral arteries usually arise from the subclavian arteries (Fig. 468–2), but their origins may migrate proximally to begin directly from the aortic arch or distally to form a common branch of the thyrocervical trunk. The vertebral arteries enter the foramen of

the sixth cervical vertebra or, much less commonly, at the fourth, fifth, or seventh cervical vertebral level. The vertebral arteries ascend through the transverse foramina and exit at C1, where they turn 90 degrees posteriorly to pass behind the atlantoaxial joint before penetrating the dura and entering the cranial cavity through the foramen magnum. The portion of the vertebral artery that loops behind the atlantoaxial joint is prone to mechanical trauma, and rotation of the head to approximately 60 degrees may cause arterial narrowing and reduce blood flow to the ipsilateral vertebral artery.

Intracranially, the vertebral arteries lie lateral to the medulla oblongata and then course ventrally and medially, where they unite at the medullopontine junction to form the *basilar artery.* The basilar artery bifurcates at the pontomesencephalic junction into the *posterior cerebral arteries.*

In up to 20 per cent of persons, the right or left vertebral artery terminates before reaching the basilar artery, leaving the latter to be supplied inferiorly by a single vessel. Intracranial branches of the vertebral arteries include medial branches, which unite to form the *anterior spinal artery,* and lateral branches to the dorsolateral medulla and posterior cerebellum, called the *posterior inferior cerebellar arteries.*

CIRCLE OF WILLIS. The *circle of Willis* (Fig. 468–2) is formed by the union at the base of the brain of both anterior cerebral arteries via the *anterior communicating artery* and the middle cerebral arteries with the posterior cerebral arteries on each side via the *posterior communicating arteries* (Fig. 468–2). Anomalies of the circle of Willis occur frequently; in large autopsy series of normal individuals, more than half showed an incomplete circle of Willis. The most common sites for such abnormalities, which usually present as hypoplasia or atresia, are the posterior communicating arteries (22 per cent) and the anterior cerebral arteries (10 per cent).

ANTERIOR CEREBRAL ARTERY. The *anterior cerebral arteries* (ACA) pass medially above the optic chiasm and head rostrally toward the interhemispheric fissure, where they arc caudally to lie just dorsal to the corpus callosum (Fig. 468–3). In approximately 10 per cent of normal individuals, the A1 segment of the ACA (the portion between the middle cerebral and anterior communicating arteries) is atretic or absent, leaving its distal portion to be supplied by the opposite ACA via the anterior communicating artery. Branches of the ACA supply the frontal poles, the entire superior surfaces of the cerebral hemispheres where their distal branches anastomose with those of the middle cerebral artery, and all of the medial surfaces of both cerebral hemispheres with the exception of the calcarine cortex. Cortical areas served by the ACA include the motor and sensory cortex of the legs and feet, the supplementary motor cortex, and the presumed cortical micturition center lying in the paracentral lobule (Figs. 468–3 and 468–4).

The A1 and A2 segments (the portion between the anterior communicating artery and the genu of the corpus callosum) give off many small branches that penetrate the anterior perforated substance of the brain. These small penetrating branches include all of the *anterior* and some of the *medial lenticulostriate* arteries. Usually, there is a dominant medial striate vessel called the *recurrent artery of Heubner,* which arises in most instances from the A1 segment of the ACA. This artery penetrates the perforated substance of the brain and, along with the other small perforators, supplies (Fig. 468–4) the anterior and inferior portions of the anterior limb of the internal capsule, the anterior and inferior head of the caudate nucleus, the anterior globus pallidus and putamen, the anterior hypothalamus, the olfactory bulbs and tracts, and the uncinate fasciculus.

ANTERIOR CHOROIDAL ARTERY. The *anterior choroidal artery* arises from the supraclinoid portion of the internal carotid artery in more than three fourths of persons. It travels caudally and medially over the optic tract, to which it provides a few small branches, and enters the brain via the choroidal fissure. Many important brain structures receive blood flow from the anterior choroidal artery; these include portions of the anterior hippocampus, uncus, amygdala, globus pallidus, tail of the caudate nucleus, lateral thalamus, geniculate body, and a large portion of the most inferior, posterior limb of the internal capsule (Fig. 468–4).

MIDDLE CEREBRAL ARTERY. The *middle cerebral artery* (MCA) provides flow to most of the lateral surface of the cerebral

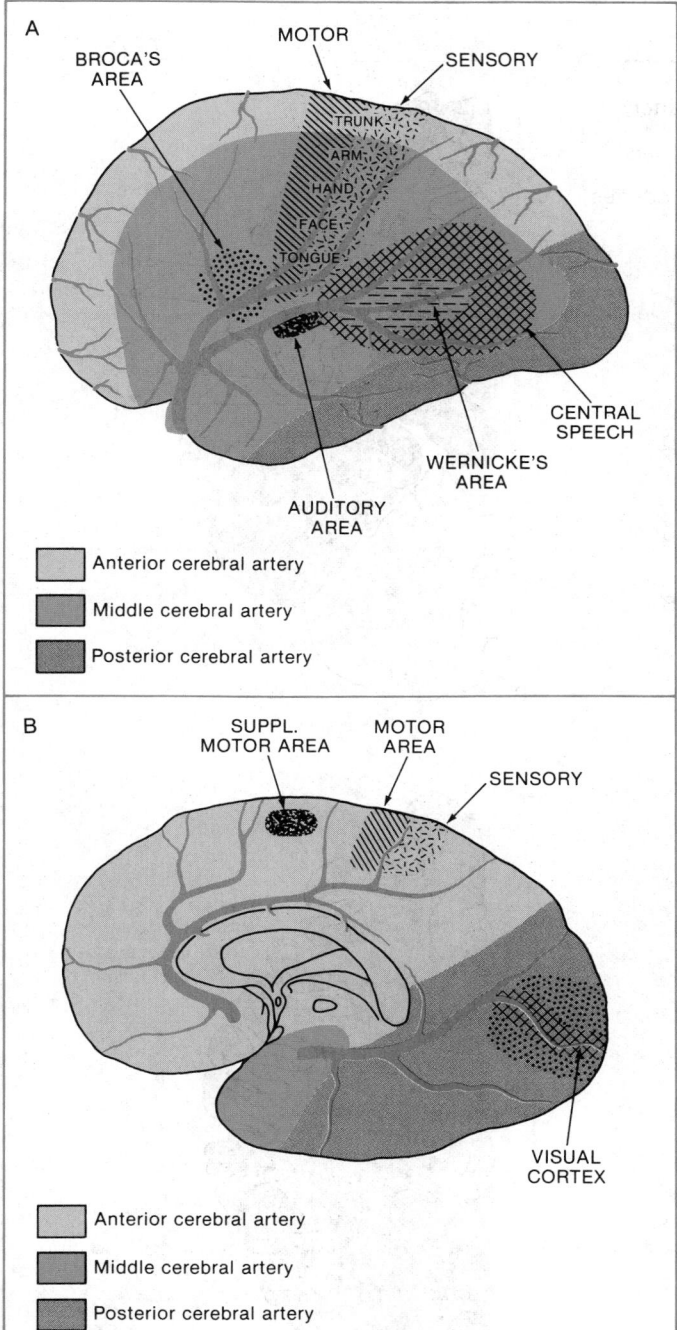

FIGURE 468–3. Lateral *(A)* and medial *(B)* views of the cerebral hemisphere showing the surface distributions of the anterior, middle, and posterior cerebral arteries.

hemispheres and is the vessel most frequently involved in ischemic stroke (Figs. 468–3 and 468–4). As the main MCA trunk passes laterally towards the sylvian fissure, it gives rise to some of the *medial* and all of the *lateral lenticulostriate* arteries. These arteries irrigate (Fig. 468–4) the putamen, the head and body of the caudate nucleus, the lateral globus pallidus, the full vertical extent of the anterior limb of the internal capsule, and a superior portion of the posterior limb of the internal capsule. The middle cerebral artery extends into the sylvian fissure, where it branches into several smaller arteries grouped into a superior division, which feeds the cortical surface above the fissure, and an inferior division, which supplies the cortical surface of the temporal lobe. The territory of the MCA includes the major motor and sensory areas of the cortex, the areas for contraversive eye and head movement, the optic radiations, auditory sensory cortex, and, in the dominant hemisphere, the motor and sensory areas for language.

POSTERIOR CEREBRAL ARTERY. Blood flow to both *posterior cerebral arteries* (PCA) is derived primarily from the basilar artery (70 per cent of the time) and from the internal carotid arteries (10 per cent of the time). In the remaining 20 per cent, one PCA is supplied by the internal carotid artery and the other by the basilar artery. The PCA pass dorsal to the third cranial nerves and across the cerebral peduncles and then ascend upward along the medial edge of the tentorium, where they branch into anterior and posterior divisions. The anterior division (Figs. 468–3 and 468–4) supplies the inferior surface of the temporal lobe, where its terminal branches anastomose with branches of the MCA. The posterior division supplies the occipital lobe, where its terminal branches anastomose with both the ACA and the MCA. In its most proximal course along the base of the brain, the PCA gives off several groups of penetrating arteries commonly referred to as the thalamogeniculate, the thalamoperforating, and the posterior choroidal arteries. The red nucleus, the substantia nigra, medial parts of the cerebral peduncles, the nuclei of the thalamus, the hippocampus, and the posterior hypothalamus all receive blood from these penetrating branches (Fig. 468–4).

BRAIN STEM BLOOD FLOW. At all rostrocaudal levels of the brain stem, the ventral medial portion is supplied by short paramedian vessels; the ventrolateral portion by short circumferential branches from the vertebral or basilar arteries; and the dorsolateral portion and cerebellum by long circumferential branches, which include the *posterior inferior cerebellar* arteries, which arise from the vertebral arteries, and the *anterior inferior* and *superior cerebellar* arteries, which arise from the basilar artery (Fig. 468–5A and B).

The pyramids, the inferior olives and medial lemnisci, the medial longitudinal fasciculi, and the emerging fibers of the hypoglossal nerve (Fig. 468–5A) derive blood from the vertebral arteries. Longer branches from the vertebral arteries and posterior inferior cerebellar arteries supply the spinothalamic tracts, the vestibular nuclei, the sensory nuclei of the fifth cranial nerve, the descending fibers of the sympathetic nervous system, the restiform body, and the emerging fibers of the vagus and glossopharyngeal nerves. The most cephalad and dorsal segment of the medulla includes the vestibular and cochlear nuclei, which, along with the posterior portion of the cerebellum, receive flow from the posterior inferior cerebellar artery.

The basilar artery gives rise to perforating branches as it spans the ventral midline pons and midbrain (Fig. 468–5B). These short perpendicular branches distribute blood to the paramedian structures, including the corticospinal tracts, the pontine reticular nuclei, the medial lemnisci, the medial longitudinal fasciculi, and the pontine reticular nuclei. The *anterior inferior cerebellar artery* feeds blood to the lateral pons, including the emerging seventh and eighth cranial nerves, the trigeminal nerve root, the vestibular and cochlear nuclei, and the spinothalamic tracts. It also branches to the most dorsal and lateral of these structures on its dorsal course toward the cerebellum.

At the midbrain level, the basilar artery lies in the midline in the peduncular fossa. Short branches pass laterally and dorsally to both sides to supply the cerebral peduncles, the emerging fibers of the third nerve, medial portions of the red nuclei, the medial longitudinal fasciculus, the oculomotor nuclei, and the midbrain reticulum. The superior cerebellar arteries contribute to the dorsal midbrain supply, including that of the colliculi and the superior portion of the cerebellum on each side.

VENOUS DRAINAGE. The veins in the brain, unlike those in many other parts of the body, do not accompany the arteries (Fig. 468–6). Cortical veins drain into the superior sagittal sinus, which runs posteriorly between the cerebral hemispheres. Deeper structures drain into the inferior sagittal sinus and great cerebral vein (of Galen), which join at the straight sinus. The straight sinus runs posteriorly along the attachment of the falx cerebri and tentorium and joins the superior sagittal sinus at the torcular Herophili, from which the two transverse sinuses arise. Each transverse sinus passes laterally toward the petrosal bone, to become the sigmoid sinus, which exits the skull into the internal jugular vein. Each cavernous sinus communicates with its contralateral twin and surrounds the ipsilateral carotid artery; both drain posteriorly into the petrosal sinuses, which in turn drain into the sigmoid sinus.

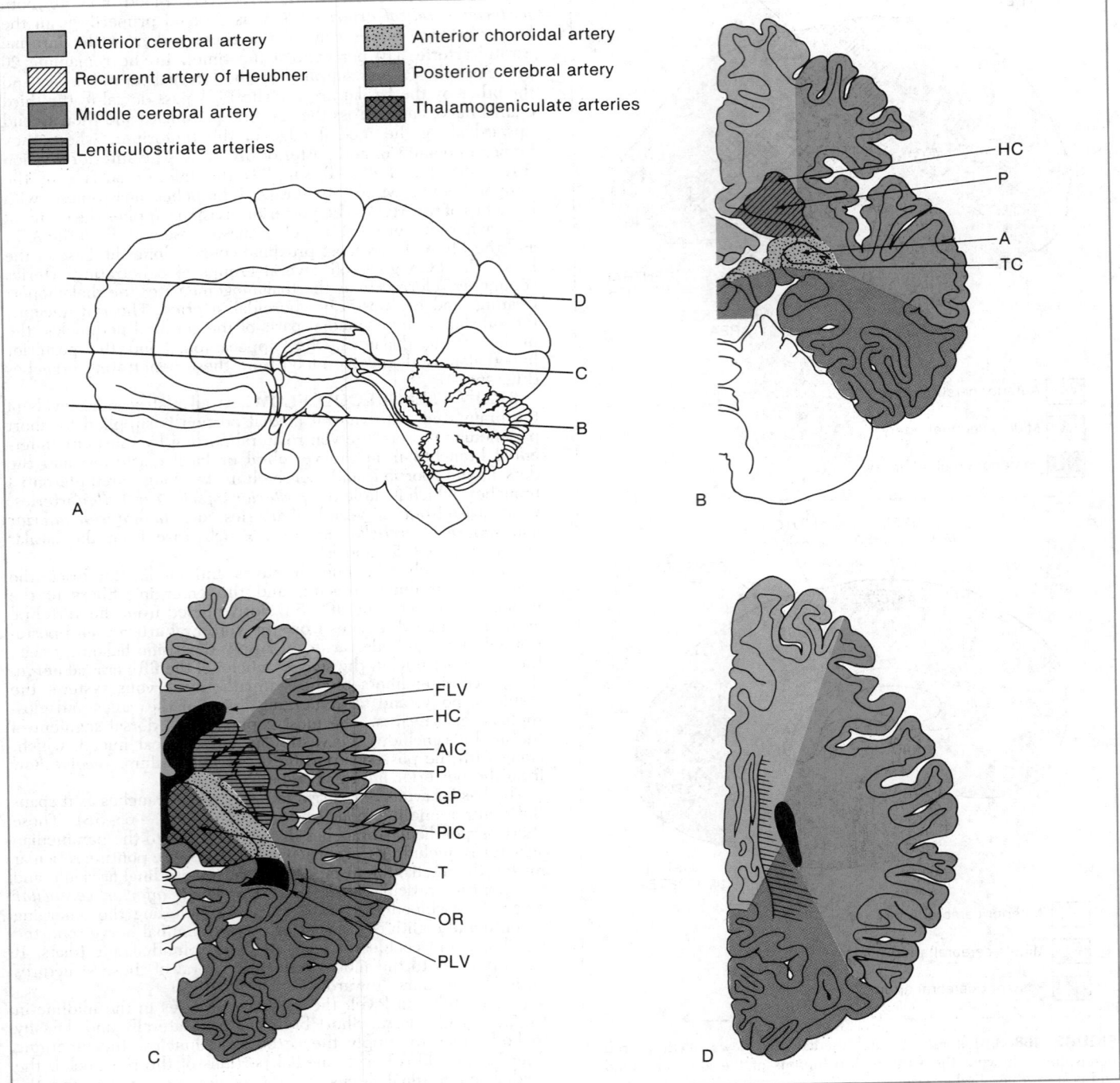

FIGURE 468–4. Arterial supply of deep brain structures. *A,* Sagittal view of the brain showing the computed tomographic (CT) planes through which views B,C, and D were taken. *B,* CT plane through the head of the caudate nucleus (HC), putamen (P), amygdala (A), tail of the caudate nucleus (TC), hypothalamus, temporal lobe, midbrain, and cerebellum. *C,* CT plane through the frontal horn of the lateral ventricle (FLV), head of the caudate nucleus (HC), anterior and posterior limbs of the internal capsule (AIC, PIC), putamen (P), globus pallidus (GP), thalamus (T), optic radiations (OR), and posterior horn of the lateral ventricle (PLV). *D,* CT plane through the centrum semiovale. (Modified from De Armond S, Fuso M, Dewey M: Structure of the Human Brain. New York, Oxford Press, 1989; with permission.)

NORMAL PHYSIOLOGY

CEREBRAL METABOLISM AND BLOOD FLOW. The brain performs no mechanical work; nevertheless, the energy demands to support normal electrophysiologic brain activity in conscious humans equal, on a per weight basis, those of metabolically active tissues like the heart and kidney. The energy demands necessary to drive membrane ion pumps, to synthesize, store, and release neurotransmitters, and to maintain tissue structure are met almost entirely by the aerobic metabolism of glucose to CO_2 and H_2O. The normal, conscious human consumes approximately 160 µmoles of O_2 and 30 µmoles of glucose per 100 grams of brain each minute (Table 468–1).

Approximately 10 per cent of available blood glucose is extracted and phosphorylated by the brain in a single pass, yet only 80 per cent of this glucose is used to generate energy. The 5:1 ratio of O_2 versus glucose consumption (Table 468–1) indicates

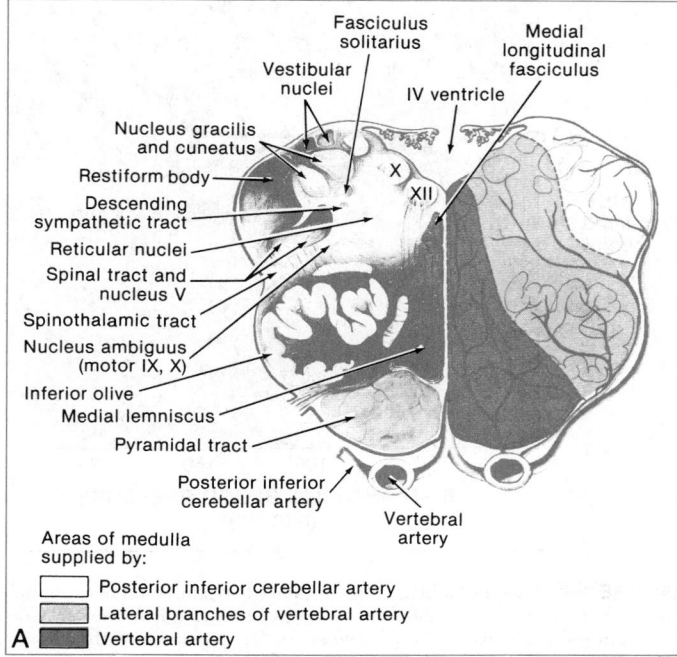

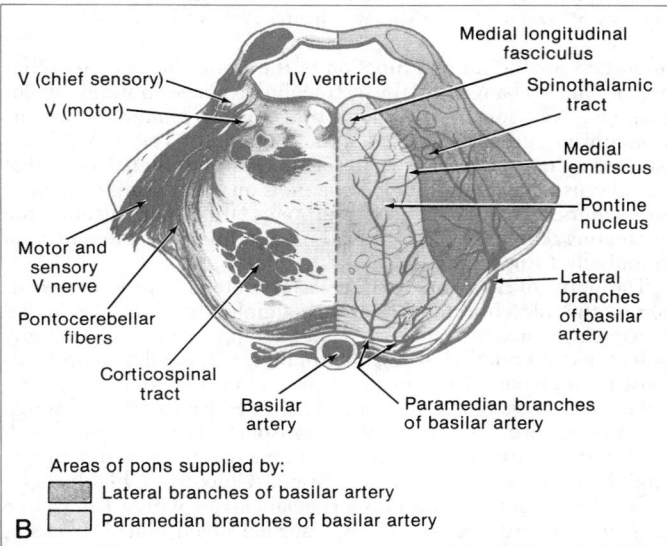

FIGURE 468-5. *A,* Cross-section of the medulla oblongata at the level of the hypoglossal nuclei (XII). Short branches of the vertebral and anterior spinal arteries supply the medial medulla. Longer circumferential branches, including the posterior inferior cerebellar artery, supply the lateral portions of the medulla. *B,* Cross-section of the mid-pons. The medial portion receives the blood supply from short, perforating basilar artery branches. More laterally, the blood supply comes from lateral basilar artery branches.

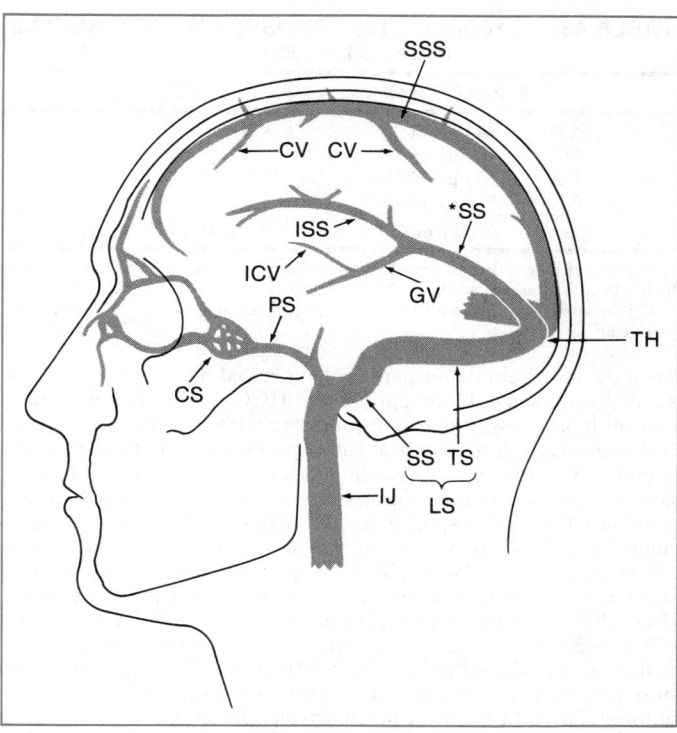

FIGURE 468-6. Venous drainage of intracranial structures. SSS = superior sagittal sinus; CV = cortical veins; ISS = inferior sagittal sinus; ICV = internal cerebral vein; GV = great vein of Galen; *SS = straight sinus; TH = torcular Herophili; PS = petrosal sinus; CS = cavernous sinus; TS = transverse sinus; SS = sigmoid sinus; LS = lateral sinus; IJ = internal jugular vein. (Amended with permission from Barnett JM: Venous disease: Cortical veins and sinuses. *In* Barnett H, Mohr JP, Stein BM, Yatsu FM [eds.]: Stroke: Pathophysiology, Diagnosis and Management. New York, Churchill Livingstone, 1986, p 731.)

that approximately 20 per cent of glucose carbons are not oxidized. Approximately 10 to 15 per cent of glucose is metabolized to lactate, which may be lost to the circulation; the remainder is used for the synthesis of neurotransmitters, fats, and, to a small degree, proteins. Each mole of glucose metabolized by the brain through glycolysis and the mitochondrial respiratory chain therefore yields approximately 30 moles of ATP instead of the expected 38.

Unlike muscle or other tissues, the brain stores few glucose, glycogen, or other high-energy phosphate (ATP, phosphocreatine) reserves (Table 468–2) but instead relies on a sizable and well-regulated blood flow to satisfy its immediate needs for energy. Cerebral blood flow (CBF) averages 60 ml per 100 grams of brain per minute in the normal, conscious human; in the absence of such flow, the brain has sufficient high-energy stores to support normal metabolic needs for only a few minutes. At normal arterial O_2 tensions and blood glucose concentrations, CBF delivers 350

μmoles of O_2 and 260 μmoles of glucose to 100 grams of brain each minute (see Table 468–1). These values exceed the brain's normal consumption rates of O_2 and glucose by factors of approximately 2 and 9, respectively, suggesting modest reserves of these molecules in the blood vascular compartment. In fact, the blood vascular reserves for both O_2 and glucose must be small, since changes of synaptic activity related to, for example, the normal acts of speaking or listening are tightly *coupled,* both temporally and spatially, to a proportional increase in CBF. As a consequence, the anatomic segregation of the brain's functional activities results in an ever-changing mosaic of regional metabolic/blood flow values that reflect moment-to-moment changes in electrophysiologic activity.

The coupling of CBF to regional synaptic activity and thereby to local metabolic activity represents only one of several important mechanisms regulating normal CBF. Changes in the respiratory rate or volume, which lead to even mild hypercapnia or hypocapnia, respectively dilate or constrict cerebral resistance vessels, so that CBF shows a linear relationship to Pa_{CO_2} (Fig. 468–7). This normal physiologic response to Pa_{CO_2} is exploited clinically to treat cerebral herniation syndromes. Mechanical hyperventilation to a Pa_{CO_2} of 20 to 25 mm Hg reduces CBF by approximately 40 to 45 per cent and normal adult cerebral blood volume from 50 ml to approximately 35 ml. While seemingly small, this 15 ml of additional intracranial volume is sufficient to retard the pro-

TABLE 468-1. METABOLIC ACTIVITY (NORMAL CONSCIOUS HUMAN)

	Consumed	Supplied
	(/100 gm brain/min)	
CBF	60 ml	—
O_2	156 μmol	350 μmol
Glucose	33 μmol	260 μmol

CBF = cerebral blood flow.

TABLE 468–2. HIGH-ENERGY PHOSPHATE METABOLISM (NORMAL HUMAN)

	~ P Stores (/100 gm)*	~P Use (/100 gm/min)
ATP	= 300 μmol	
PCr	= 400 μmol	
Glu	= 150 μmol (×2)	
Gly	= 500 μmol (×3)	
Total	= 2500 μmol	800 μmol

*Values are derived from anesthetized subjects and may therefore be slightly higher than in awake subjects.

ATP = adenosine triphosphate; PCr = phosphocreatine; Gluc = glucose; Gly = glycine.

gression of cerebral herniation. Unfortunately, the response is short lived, since brain and blood HCO_3^- and H^+ ions that control blood vessel tone re-equilibrate within 30 to 60 minutes.

A complex system of neural pathways involving both peripheral sympathetic and parasympathetic nerve fibers, plus intrinsic central nervous system fibers originating in the brain stem, regulates CBF in response to external stimuli. Some of these neural pathways may participate in *autoregulation,* a poorly understood process whereby CBF is maintained at a constant level despite wide fluctuations in cerebral perfusion pressure (Fig. 468–8). Cerebral perfusion pressure is defined as the difference between mean systemic arterial pressure and intracranial pressure; since the latter is relatively small (10 mm Hg) and normally nearly constant, it is common practice to describe autoregulation in terms of mean arterial pressure.

Autoregulation has both upper and lower limits (Fig. 468–8); at mean arterial pressures above 150 mm Hg, blood flow increases and capillary pressure rises, while at mean arterial pressures below 50 mm Hg, CBF falls. Increased capillary pressure in hypertensive patients may be a factor in intracerebral hemorrhage and hypertensive encephalopathy. In patients with chronic hypertension, the upper and lower autoregulatory limits are shifted toward higher systemic pressures (Fig. 468–8). Consequently, rapid therapeutic reduction of blood pressure to apparently normal levels carries with it the potential for further lowering of cerebral blood flow in hypertensive patients with ongoing cerebral ischemia. Chronic treatment with antihypertensive agents causes a readjustment of the autoregulatory curve toward more normal values.

BLOOD-BRAIN BARRIER. Regulation within narrow limits of the extracellular ionic and molecular composition is more

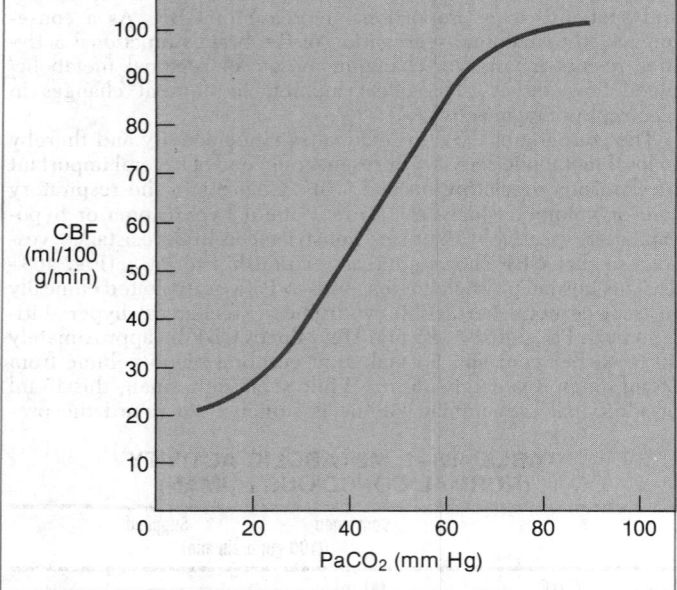

FIGURE 468–7. Cerebral blood flow response to changes in the arterial CO_2 tension. (From Lord R: Surgery of Occlusive Cerebrovascular Disease. St. Louis, C. V. Mosby Company, 1986; with permission.)

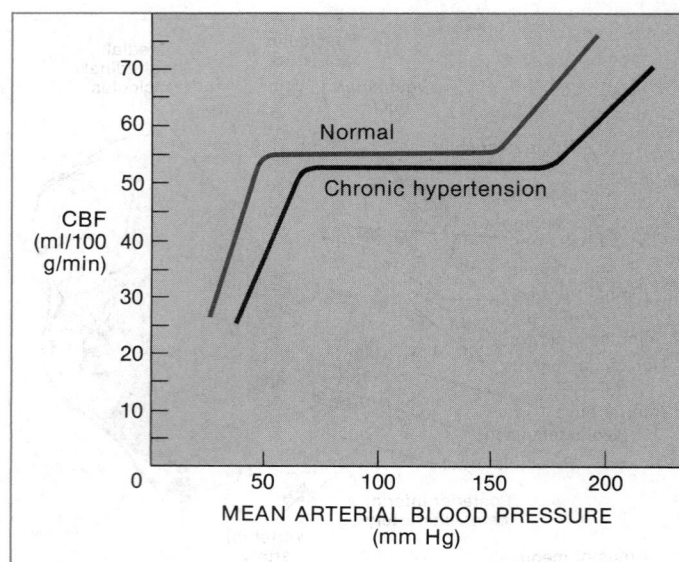

FIGURE 468–8. Cerebral blood flow response to changes in mean arterial pressure in normotensive and chronically hypertensive individuals. Note the shift of the curve toward higher mean pressures with chronic hypertension. (From Lord R: Surgery of Occlusive Cerebrovascular Disease. St. Louis, C. V. Mosby Company, 1986; with permission.)

important for the normal function of the brain than for any other organ. Small changes in the extracellular concentrations of, for example, Na^+ ions or the neurotransmitters glutamate or norepinephrine greatly alter neuronal function. The blood-brain barrier, composed anatomically of unique endothelial cells that lack the usual transendothelial channels and that seamlessly abut one another (tight junctions), protects the brain against the fluctuating composition of blood and minimizes the entry of potentially toxic compounds.

The entry of nutrients and egress of metabolic products occur across the blood-brain barrier via simple diffusion, facilitated transport, or active transport. Lipid-soluble compounds rapidly diffuse across endothelial cell membranes, while polar compounds must be transported on special carrier molecules that are driven either by concentration gradients (facilitated transport) or through the expenditure of energy (active transport). Gas molecules such as O_2 and CO_2 freely diffuse across plasma membranes and rapidly equilibrate between blood and brain. Glucose, a highly polar molecule, enters the brain on a special carrier with a Km (7 to 8 mM) just slightly higher than the normal blood glucose concentration. The rate of brain glucose transport is normally two to three times faster than the metabolism of glucose, but since glucose uptake depends so highly on its concentration, a reduction of blood sugar to one-third the normal amount, caused by either ischemia or hypoglycemia, may compromise normal metabolism (Table 468–3).

PATHOPHYSIOLOGY/PATHOLOGY OF CEREBRAL ISCHEMIA

The pathophysiologic consequences of failed O_2 and glucose delivery to the brain encompass a cascade of events that vary qualitatively and quantitatively with the severity of the ischemic insult. The severity of cerebral ischemia, defined as the degree and duration of blood flow loss, largely determines whether the brain suffers only temporary dysfunction, irreversible injury to a few highly vulnerable neurons (selective ischemic necrosis), or

TABLE 468–3. HUMAN HYPOXIC-ISCHEMIC THRESHOLD VALUES

	Pa$_{O_2}$ (mm Hg)	CBF (ml/100 gm/min)	Blood Glucose (mg/dl)
Normal	90	60	80
Stupor	30–40	20–30	25–30
Coma	20–30	15–20	20–25
Brain injury	<20	<15	<20

damage to extensive areas involving all cell types (cerebral infarction).

TYPES OF CEREBRAL HYPOXIA-ISCHEMIA.

Cerebral hypoxia-ischemia can be conveniently divided on the basis of clinical criteria into focal or multifocal ischemia from vascular occlusion, global ischemia from complete failure of cardiovascular pumping, and diffuse hypoperfusion-hypoxia caused by respiratory disease or reduced perfusion pressure. *Focal cerebral ischemia,* resulting most frequently from embolic or thrombotic occlusion of extracranial or intracranial blood vessels, variably reduces blood flow within the involved vascular territory. Blood flow to the central zone of the ischemic vascular bed usually is severely reduced but rarely reaches zero because of partial filling from collateral blood vessels. In the transition zones between normally perfused tissue and the severely ischemic central core, blood flow is moderately reduced. This rim of moderately ischemic tissue has been called the "ischemic penumbra," and although brain cells in this region remain viable longer than do those in the ischemic core, they too will die if left deprived of adequate blood flow.

Focal cerebral ischemia sufficient to cause clinical signs or symptoms and lasting only 15 to 30 minutes causes irreversible injury to specific, highly vulnerable neurons. If the ischemia lasts an hour or longer, infarction of part or all of the involved vascular territory is inevitable. Clinical evidence of permanent brain injury from such ischemia may or may not be detectable, depending upon the region and the amount of brain tissue involved (see Ch. 469).

Global cerebral ischemia, typically caused by cardiac asystole or ventricular fibrillation, reduces blood flow to zero throughout all of the brain. Global ischemia lasting more than 5 to 10 minutes is usually incompatible with recovery of consciousness in normothermic individuals. Brain damage from more transient global ischemia, uncomplicated by periods of prolonged hypotension or hyperglycemia, is limited to specific populations of highly vulnerable neurons. This "selective ischemic necrosis" of neurons involves, for example, the CA1 pyramidal neurons of hippocampus, the cerebellar Purkinje cells, and the pyramidal neurons in neocortical layers 3, 5, and 6 (Table 468–4). While selective ischemic necrosis of neurons is typical of transient global ischemia, such injury may also accompany prolonged hypoxemia, carbon monoxide poisoning, and focal cerebral ischemia of brief duration. Cardiac resuscitation complicated by prolonged hypotension or hyperglycemia may cause cerebral infarction, particularly in border zones that lie between the terminal branches of major arterial supplies.

Diffuse cerebral hypoxia, uncomplicated by cerebral ischemia, is limited to conditions of mild to moderate hypoxemia, since myocardial contractility and blood pressure fall with severe hypoxemia. As a consequence, pure cerebral hypoxia causes cerebral dysfunction but not irreversible brain injury. Individuals with pure cerebral hypoxia from altitude sickness, pulmonary disease, or severe anemia present with confusion, cognitive impairment, and lethargy; the onset of coma signals cardiovascular compromise and imminent brain damage. With relatively *acute* changes in arterial oxygen tension from normal to a Pa_{O_2} of 40 mm Hg (see Table 468–3) or with a fall in the hemoglobin concentration below 7 grams per deciliter, compensatory increases of cerebral blood flow become inadequate, and clinical signs and symptoms of cerebral hypoxia develop. Chronic exposure to such low oxygen or hemoglobin levels invokes other poorly defined compensatory mechanisms, which allow near-normal cerebral function. The climbers of Mount Everest, having slowly acclimatized to breathing ambient air, developed only minor impairments of short-term memory and motor function despite having arterial oxygen tensions of 28 mm Hg.

NEUROPATHOLOGY OF CEREBRAL ISCHEMIA.

Ischemic injury to the brain can be classified on the basis of cytopathologic criteria into four types. Cerebral *autolysis,* most frequently seen in brain-dead patients preserved on mechanical ventilators for several days, reflects complete and permanent loss of blood flow accompanied by enzymatic autodigestion of the tissue.

Cerebral *infarction,* usually caused by focal vascular occlusion, is characterized histopathologically by necrosis of neurons, glia, and, in some areas, endothelial cells. Microscopically, neurons within the infarct appear eosinophilic, are shrunken, and have pyknotic nuclei. The histologic appearance of cerebral infarction differs from that of autolysis. Such differences probably reflect the permanent and complete loss of blood flow and the early release of lysosomal proteolytic enzymes in the autolytic tissue. Cerebral infarcts are frequently described as pale (anemic) despite the fact that microscopically most of them harbor extravasated red blood cells. Ischemic infarcts that show gross petechial hemorrhages are termed "hemorrhagic infarctions." The hemorrhagic areas lie most often along border zones of partially perfused tissue and occur most frequently with transient embolic occlusion followed by reperfusion of the infarcted vascular bed. Presumably, exposure of the necrotic tissue to the full pressure head of arterial blood leads to hemorrhage.

Transient arrest of the cerebral circulation (global ischemia) for periods of a few minutes causes *selective ischemic necrosis of neurons* (see Table 468–4) that are highly vulnerable to ischemia for unexplained reasons. Microscopically, these neurons evolve through several stages of "eosinophilic or ischemic cell change" and eventually appear shrunken and eosinophilic, containing darkly staining, pyknotic nuclei. Although such injury may be limited to only a small percentage of the total neuronal population, profound neurologic deficits manifested as cognitive impairment and/or movement disorders can be associated.

The time required for histologic changes to reach their maximum in areas of cerebral infarction differs markedly from the time course of injury encountered in selective ischemic necrosis of neurons. Infarction usually requires only a few hours before histologic stains sharply outline the distinct margins between living and dying neurons and glia. By contrast, selective ischemic necrosis of neurons evolves more slowly and sometimes requires several days or more to mature fully. For example, pyramidal neurons in the CA1 zone of the hippocampus remain histologically normal for 24 hours following cardiac arrest and require 48 hours or more before all of the cells that are destined to die show signs of irreversible injury. This delayed onset and the slow progression of injury following transient cerebral ischemia have important implications for potential therapies that may be initiated even after the onset of the ischemic insult.

Another distinctive neuropathologic lesion due to ischemia is *demyelination* of the central hemispheric white matter. Such injury is usually the consequence of carbon monoxide poisoning or other prolonged periods of moderately severe hypoxemia or cerebral hypoperfusion. Within these lesions, nerve cell axons are demyelinated, and there is generalized loss of oligodendroglial cells.

MOLECULAR MECHANISMS.

In severely ischemic tissue—for example, the central ischemic vascular bed of an occluded MCA—energy-rich compounds remain sufficient to maintain normal function for only seconds, and glycogen, glucose, phosphocreatine, and ATP become depleted in a few minutes (see Table 468–2). Soon thereafter, the tissue begins to lose structural integrity. With the failure of energy-dependent membrane pumps, neuronal and glial cell membranes depolarize and allow the influx of Na^+ and Ca^{2+} ions and the efflux of K^+ ions. Elevated intracellular Ca^{2+} and other second messengers activate lipases and proteases, which in turn release membrane-bound free fatty acids and denature proteins. Depolarization of presynaptic terminals releases abnormally high concentrations of excitatory and inhibitory neurotransmitters, which may further exacerbate injury. If blood flow is restored in 15 to 30 minutes and no other complicating variables, such as hyperglycemia, are involved, most of these events are reversible, and only neurons selectively vulnerable to ischemia will die. If ischemia lasts hours

TABLE 468–4. ORDER OF DECREASING NEURONAL VULNERABILITY TO ANOXIA

Hippocampus
CA1, CA4 > CA3 > granule cells
Cerebellum
Purkinje > stellate and basket > granule > Golgi cells
Striatum
Small and medium-sized > large neurons
Neocortex
Layers 3,5,6 > layers 2,4

or more, cerebral infarction develops. What distinguishes ischemia-sensitive from ischemia-resistant neurons, why some of these neurons die rapidly, whereas others require days, and why glial cells are generally more resistant than neurons to ischemia remain challenging questions for basic research.

In contrast to the rapid cascade of events caused by severe ischemia, moderate ischemia triggers poorly defined mechanisms that sacrifice electrophysiologic activity to preserve brain structure, at least temporarily. Acute reduction of blood flow below one-half that of normal exceeds the capacity of compensatory mechanisms, such as increased O_2 and glucose extraction, to maintain normal synaptic function. The electroencephalogram (EEG) slows, and if ischemia is diffuse, the patient becomes confused, lethargic, or stuporous. The molecular mechanisms that suppress normal synaptic activity in the face of moderately compromised blood flow are unknown. Depletion of whole tissue energy reserves is not an explanation, since these remain normal, partly as a consequence of the decreased energy demand normally used to maintain membrane ion pumps and EEG activity. Some theorize that microregional reduction of the extracellular ATP concentration in the vicinity of the presynaptic terminals relieves the normal blockade of K^+ ion movement through ATP-sensitive K^+ channels and thereby hyperpolarizes the presynaptic membrane so as to inhibit synaptic transmission. With slightly greater ischemia, all synaptic activity ceases and the EEG becomes isoelectric. This too occurs with only partial depletion of high-energy stores, indicating that generalized energy failure cannot account for this early loss of synaptic activity. Prompt recovery of blood flow restores full function and structural integrity to the tissue. If moderate ischemia persists for several hours, however, irreversible injury will develop, probably as a consequence of compromised calcium homeostasis. Tissues with partial depletion of ATP and partial loss of calcium homeostasis may benefit from pharmacologic therapies that reduce calcium movement through voltage-dependent and neurotransmitter-dependent ion channels.

CEREBRAL EDEMA. Pathologic increases in the water content of the brain (edema) accompany all types of ischemic and hemorrhagic stroke. Brain swelling and raised intracranial pressure are proportionally related to the volume of the accumulated water; in many instances, they can cause neurologic deterioration and death by transtentorial herniation. Cerebral edema and herniation represent the immediate cause of death in one third of all ischemic and three quarters of all hemorrhagic strokes.

Brain edema is categorized on the basis of pathophysiologic and anatomic criteria as intracellular, interstitial, or periventricular. Intracellular edema, also called cytotoxic edema, represents an accumulation of intracellular osmoles and water causing cell swelling at the expense of the interstitial brain volume. Intracellular edema develops rapidly in ischemic brain tissue as energy-dependent membrane ion pumps fail and Na^+ ions and osmotically bound water derived from interstitial and the blood vascular compartment enter the cell. Cell swelling occurs predominantly in astrocytes, but neurons, oligodendroglial cells, and endothelial cells also are involved to a lesser degree. The osmolality of ischemic brain increases acutely from 310 mOsm to approximately 350 mOsm; 20 of these mOsm represent influx of ions, primarily Na^+. The identity of the remaining particles is unknown (idiogenic osmoles). The intracellular accumulation of water increases from a normal value of approximately 79 per cent to 81 per cent of brain weight. This 1 to 2 per cent increase in the volume of brain is insufficient in most instances to cause cerebral herniation. If cerebral circulation is re-established before permanent brain injury develops, intracellular brain edema resolves within a matter of hours without permanent sequelae.

Interstitial brain edema, also called vasogenic edema, is caused by the movement of large molecules and water from plasma into the interstitial spaces of the brain. Ischemia-induced damage to the endothelial cells making up the blood-brain barrier allows macromolecules such as plasma proteins to enter the interstitial space, carrying with them osmotically bound water. The bulk of this plasma filtrate accumulates preferentially in the interstitial spaces of the white matter. Interstitial brain edema that accompanies cerebral infarction progressively worsens for 3 to 4 days after a stroke. Fluid accumulation within the vicinity of damaged

endothelial cells and the zone of infarction can raise the local water content of brain by as much as 10 per cent. Such large volume increases can easily lead to transtentorial herniation and death.

Periventricular edema reflects the obstruction of cerebrospinal fluid (CSF) outflow pathways, the accumulation of CSF, and the transependymal movement of CSF into the white matter surrounding the periventricular regions. Such edema can be caused by intracerebral and subarachnoid hemorrhage if it interferes with CSF outflow pathways.

Barnett HJ, Stein BM, Mohr JP, et al. (eds.): Stroke: Pathophysiology, Diagnosis and Management. New York, Churchill Livingstone, 1986. *A comprehensive two-volume overview of all aspects of ischemic and hemorrhagic stroke.*

Caplan LR, Stein RW: Stroke: A Clinical Approach. Boston, Butterworths, 1986. *A pragmatic description of the diagnosis and treatment of stroke.*

Plum F, Pulsinelli WA: Cerebral metabolism in hypoxic-ischemic brain injury. *In* Asbury AK, McKann GM, McDonald IW (eds.): Diseases of the Nervous System. 2nd ed. Philadelphia, W.B. Saunders Company, 1992. *A contemporary review of the pathogenesis of ischemic injury to brain.*

Siesjo BK, Bengtsson F: Calcium fluxes, calcium antagonists, and calcium-related pathology in brain ischemia, hypoglycemia and spreading depression: A unifying hypothesis. J Cereb Blood Flow Metab 9:127, 1989. *A contemporary review of calcium homeostasis and the pathogenesis of calcium-related mechanisms in cerebral ischemia.*

West JB: Tolerance to severe hypoxia: Lessons from Mt. Everest. Acta Anaesth Scand 34(Suppl 94):18, 1990. *A description by the expedition leader of respiratory physiology and the effects of sustained hypoxemia during the ascent of Mt. Everest.*

469 Ischemic Cerebrovascular Disease

469.1 FOCAL ISCHEMIA

CLASSIFICATION

The clinical manifestations of focal ischemic stroke result from interference with blood circulation to the brain; the precise signs and symptoms depend on the region deprived of flow. For any brain region, however, focal ischemia can be classified into categories that have important pathologic and management implications.

STROKE VERSUS TRANSIENT ISCHEMIC ATTACK (TIA). *Stroke* is defined as a neurologic deficit lasting more than 24 hours caused by reduced blood flow in a particular artery supplying the brain. The usual pathologic outcome is infarction in the ischemic portion of the brain. A *transient ischemic attack,* or *TIA,* by contrast, is defined arbitrarily as a similar neurologic deficit lasting less than 24 hours. Originally, the time limit for transient neurologic deficits due to ischemia was less than 1 hour, but the definition was subsequently expanded to encompass events lasting up to 24 hours. Most TIA's resolve within an hour; thus once a deficit has lasted longer than an hour, it is likely to be classified as a presumptive stroke and is often associated with permanent brain injury. Computed tomographic (CT) brain scans frequently show cerebral infarction in areas affected by "TIA's" lasting longer than several hours. The relevant clinical distinction between a TIA and a stroke is whether the ischemia has caused brain damage (infarction or selective ischemic necrosis). Since no clear temporal threshold separates the two, decisions concerning the initiation of therapy and its type are unavoidably vague.

STABLE VERSUS UNSTABLE STROKES. Patients with *unstable strokes* are identifiable by either improvement or deterioration of their signs or symptoms. Deciding whether a stroke is unstable may be difficult, since in theory all strokes require some period to reach a stable maximum or minimum. The decision depends on an accurate history, on the interval between onset of symptoms and the first examination, and, later, on the frequency and duration of observation. Two thirds of patients with anterior circulation strokes and a higher number of those with vertebrobasilar strokes who are examined within a few hours of onset fluctuate in their signs and symptoms during the first week.

The identification of patients with worsening signs and symptoms, frequently referred to as *progressing stroke* or *stroke in evolution,* is particularly important, since if the cause can be identified, treatment to limit brain damage may be possible. The pathogenesis of progression may involve one or a combination of factors. Clot propagation has been suggested, but little direct evidence supports this conclusion. Other equally, if not more important, causes for progressing stroke include compromise of cardiac output due to myocardial ischemia, cardiac arrhythmias, and congestive heart failure. Systemic hypotension and increased blood viscosity can adversely affect the course of acute cerebral ischemia, as can associated pneumogenic hypoxemia or systemic electrolyte imbalance. Progression of cerebral edema, which usually maximizes by 3 to 4 days, contributes to neurologic deterioration with large strokes but not with smaller ones. Bleeding into the infarct affects as many as 40 per cent of patients but seldom causes new symptoms.

COMPLETE VERSUS INCOMPLETE STROKES. An important distinction is that made between a *complete* and an *incomplete stroke.* The terms refer to whether the affected vascular territory has been completely involved; if not, more brain remains at risk of additional focal ischemia, making treatment an urgent matter. The clinical distinction between complete and incomplete strokes can be difficult, especially soon after onset. As a practical matter, the distinction between a complete and incomplete stroke is often based on the severity of functional loss, for example, hemiplegia versus hemiparesis.

CLINICAL MANIFESTATIONS AND VASCULAR SYNDROMES
(Table 469–1)

INTERNAL CAROTID ARTERY. The carotid artery bifurcation and origin of the internal carotid artery provide the most frequent sites for atherothrombosis of cerebral blood vessels. Symptoms from such severe stenoses closely resemble those caused by middle cerebral artery disease (see below). Flow through the ophthalmic artery is often affected sufficiently to produce *transient monocular blindness* (also called amaurosis fugax). Severe bilateral internal carotid artery stenosis can sometimes cause cerebral hemispheric hypoperfusion and symptoms in *border zones* between the major vascular territories. Anterior circulation TIA's more frequently herald the presence of internal carotid artery disease than of intracranial atherosclerosis. Similarly, acute headache ipsilateral to an acutely ischemic hemisphere more frequently signals occlusion of the internal carotid artery than of the intracranial vessels.

ANTERIOR CEREBRAL ARTERY. Occlusion of one anterior cerebral artery (ACA) distal to the anterior communicating artery produces motor and cortical sensory symptoms in the contralateral leg and, less often, proximal arm. Other manifestations of ACA occlusion include gait ataxia and sometimes urinary incontinence from damage to the parasagittal frontal lobe. Language disturbances, manifested as decreased spontaneous speech, may accompany generalized depression of psychomotor activity. ACA occlusion does not typically cause paralysis of both legs, an acute syndrome more likely related to spinal cord disease or occlusion of the superior sagittal sinus, which drains the medial surfaces of both cerebral hemispheres.

ANTERIOR CHOROIDAL ARTERY. Brain image analyses suggest a clinical syndrome associated with occlusion of this vessel. Affected patients suffer a hemiparesis involving the face, arm, and leg; variable hemisensory loss; and in some instances hemianopsia from optic tract ischemia. The syndrome is difficult to distinguish from middle cerebral artery (MCA) ischemia.

MIDDLE CEREBRAL ARTERY. Most ischemic strokes involve part or all of the territory of the MCA, with emboli from the heart or extracranial carotid arteries accounting for most cases. Emboli may occlude the main stem of the MCA but more frequently produce distal occlusions of either the superior or the inferior branch. Occlusion of the superior branch causes weakness and sensory loss that are greatest in the face and arm; vision is spared, but an inferior quadrantanopsia may rarely coexist. Hemianopsias reported with MCA infarction more likely reflect hemineglect than true blindness, since deeply penetrating MCA branches supply only the dorsal, parietal half of the optic radiations. Voluntary gaze away from the side of the lesion may be impaired, but full-range oculocephalic or oculovestibular reflexes remain (Ch. 453.3). In the dominant hemisphere, the deficit includes an expressive (Broca's) aphasia with impaired fluency, naming, and writing, but relatively preserved comprehension. In the nondominant hemisphere, unilateral neglect, anosognosia (unawareness of the deficit), and spatial disorientation may be detected.

Occlusion of the inferior branches of the MCA infrequently produces sensory loss, most notably of integrated sensations, such as perception of shapes (stereognosis). In the dominant hemisphere, occlusion of the inferior division of the MCA causes receptive (Wernicke's) aphasia, with fluent speech characterized by jargon and paraphasias; comprehension, naming, reading, and writing are often abnormal.

The so-called deep MCA syndrome may occur from selective occlusion of the MCA main stem, causing ischemia in the territory of the lenticulostriate vessels but sparing the superior and inferior MCA branches. Collateral filling of the distal MCA cortical branches prevents cortical injury, but since the lenticulostriates are end-arteries, infarction of the deep MCA territory evolves. Alternatively, the lenticulostriates may be occluded by local atherosclerotic or hypertensive vascular disease. Patients with occlusion of the lenticulostriate arteries develop internal capsular infarction accompanied by hemiparesis or hemiplegia without visual, language, or sensory disturbances.

Proximal occlusions of the MCA may affect both superior and inferior branches as well as perforating branches to the internal capsule, optic radiations, and basal ganglia, thus resulting in contralateral hemiplegia, hemianesthesia, dense homonymous hemianopsia, and global aphasia with dominant or anosognosia with nondominant hemisphere involvement.

POSTERIOR CEREBRAL ARTERY. Occlusion of the posterior cerebral artery (PCA) distal to its penetrating branches most frequently causes complete contralateral loss of vision or a superior or inferior quadrantanopsia, depending upon whether the lower or the upper calcarine arteries are affected individually. Central (macular) vision may be spared owing to collateral supply from the MCA. If only the calcarine cortex is involved, the patient is usually aware of the vision loss, but denial of unilateral or bilateral blindness can ensue if one or both adjacent parietal cortices are affected (Ch. 449). Difficulty in reading (dyslexia) and performing calculations (dyscalculia) may follow ischemia of the dominant PCA territory.

TABLE 469–1. CLINICAL MANIFESTATIONS OF ISCHEMIC STROKE

Occluded Blood Vessel*	Clinical Manifestations
ICA	Ipsilateral blindness (variable)
	MCA syndrome (see below)
MCA	Contralateral hemiparesis, sensory loss (arm, face worst)
	Expressive aphasia (dominant) or anosognosia and spatial disorientation (nondominant)
	Contralateral inferior quadrantanopsia
ACA	Contralateral hemiparesis, sensory loss (leg worst)
PCA	Contralateral homonymous hemianopsia or superior quadrantanopsia
	Memory impairment
Basilar apex	Bilateral blindness
	Amnesia
Basilar artery	Contralateral hemiparesis, sensory loss
	Ipsilateral bulbar and/or cerebellar signs
Vertebral artery and/or PICA	Ipsilateral loss of facial sensation, ataxia
	Contralateral hemiparesis, sensory loss
Superior cerebellar artery	Gait ataxia, nausea, dizziness, headache progressing to ipsilateral hemiataxia, dysarthria, gaze paresis
	Contralateral hemiparesis, somnolence

*ICA = internal carotid artery; MCA = middle cerebral artery; ACA = anterior cerebral artery; PCA = posterior cerebral artery; PICA = posterior inferior cerebellar artery.

Proximal occlusion of the PCA causes ischemia of penetrating branches (thalamogeniculate, thalamoperforating, posterior choroidal) to thalamic and limbic structures. The results are hemisensory disturbances that may chronically change to intractable pain on the defective side (thalamic pain). Memory dysfunction may result, especially with bilateral occlusions. With involvement of the subthalamic nucleus, wild, uncontrolled, flailing limb movements called hemiballism may develop (Ch. 461).

VERTEBRAL AND BASILAR ARTERIES. Focal brain stem ischemia produces a group of so-called "crossed syndromes" in which contralateral (pyramidal, spinothalamic, dorsal column) long-tract abnormalities (e.g., hemiparesis or hemisensory deficit) are accompanied by signs of ipsilateral cerebellar or brain stem nuclear dysfunction (e.g., ataxia, lower motor neuron facial weakness, third cranial nerve paresis). Occlusion of a vertebral artery and interference with flow through the ipsilateral *posterior inferior cerebellar artery* cause the *lateral medullary syndrome*, consisting of severe vertigo, nausea, vomiting, nystagmus, ipsilateral ataxia, and ipsilateral Horner's syndrome. There is an ipsilateral loss of facial pain and temperature sense and a contralateral loss of the same sensory modalities in trunk and limb. Discrete lesions in the distribution of the *anterior inferior cerebellar artery* are less common.

The *superior cerebellar artery* supplies most of the cerebellar cortex. Occlusion of this vessel is the most common cause of *cerebellar infarction*, characterized initially by gait ataxia, headache, nausea, vomiting, dizziness, ipsilateral clumsiness, and dysarthria. Subsequent brain swelling may induce ipsilateral gaze paresis and/or nystagmus toward the side of the infarction; ipsilateral facial weakness is sometimes seen. With further progression, lethargy and stupor deepen, and contralateral hemiparesis sometimes develops. Cerebellar edema formation can obstruct the fourth ventricle, producing hydrocephalus, and can result in herniation of the cerebellum either upward across the tentorium or downward through the foramen magnum (see Fig. 444–7).

Vertebrobasilar ischemia often produces multifocal lesions, scattered on both sides and along a considerable longitudinal extent of the brain stem. Except for cerebellar infarction and the lateral medullary syndrome, the clinical syndromes of discrete lesions are thus seldom seen in pure form. *Vertebrobasilar ischemia (VBI)* manifests with various combinations of symptoms such as dizziness (usually vertigo), diplopia, facial weakness, ataxia, and long-tract signs. Distinguishing mild VBI from more banal causes of dizziness can be difficult; the solution lies in identifying other, more specific symptoms or signs of parenchymal brain stem disease. Rarely does the person with VBI present with "dizziness" in the absence of other brain stem signs or symptoms.

Basilar artery occlusion produces massive deficits. The *locked-in state* is one possible consequence; in this condition, paralysis of the limbs and most of the bulbar muscles means that the patient can communicate only by moving the eyes or eyelids to command. Normal intelligence can often be demonstrated through codes involving eye movements. *Occlusion of the basilar apex* (or *top-of-the basilar*) is usually caused by emboli that lodge at the junction between the basilar artery and the two PCA's. The condition produces an initial reduction in arousal followed by blindness and amnesia (from interruption of flow into the PCA's) and abnormalities of vertical gaze and pupillary reactivity (from tegmental damage).

DIAGNOSIS

HISTORY. The history should emphasize the precise onset of the clinical deficit and the course since onset (stable or unstable). Preceding TIA's are more likely to be associated with an ischemic than a hemorrhagic stroke. Headache more often occurs with hemorrhage and embolus than with atherothrombotic ischemic stroke. The possibility of other diagnoses (e.g., hypoglycemia or seizures) should be considered. A thorough search for vascular disease risk factors (see below) should be made in the initial evaluation, since their presence will strengthen the likelihood of an ischemic stroke and influence eventual management.

PHYSICAL EXAMINATION. The neurologic examination serves to localize the lesion site, but the general medical examination more frequently provides clues to pathogenesis. Specific attention should be given to the cardiovascular examination and to evidence of hematologic disease. The arterial blood pressure in both arms, cardiac rhythm, and other cardiac abnormalities, such as murmurs or opening snaps, should be carefully recorded. The vascular examination should include gentle palpation and auscultation (with a bell-type stethoscope) of the carotid arteries in the neck and sometimes also orbital auscultation. Ophthalmoscopy can detect retinal cholesterol or platelet-fibrin emboli as well as evidence of chronic hypertensive or diabetic disease. The presence of retinal hypertensive changes can indicate that hypertension has been chronic rather than transiently stroke associated. Except with posterior circulation insufficiency or previous strokes, loss of consciousness or confusion should prompt consideration of other diagnoses.

LABORATORY EXAMINATION. *Hematologic Tests.* These include a complete blood count and platelet count (to evaluate for polycythemia, thrombocytosis, bacterial endocarditis, and severe anemia); blood for glucose, prothrombin time, and partial thromboplastin time; and a lipid profile. In the elderly, determination of the erythrocyte sedimentation rate should be performed urgently to exclude giant cell arteritis; in the young, the presence of antiphospholipid antibodies helps to identify immune-related disease processes predisposing to stroke. Other blood tests (e.g., protein C, protein S, measurements of viscosity or platelet function, and tests for collagen vascular diseases) may be indicated in younger patients without other obvious causes for their strokes. The rising incidence of syphilis in urban areas makes a serum VDRL desirable. Tests of renal function and serum electrolyte measurements help to establish systemic illnesses as well as the milieu in which subsequent diagnostic tests (e.g., contrast injection) and treatments might be offered.

Cardiovascular Examination. All stroke patients require a standard 12-lead electrocardiogram (ECG) and rhythm strip at admission to exclude acute myocardial ischemia and arrhythmias. Authorities disagree over whether one should search with echocardiography for a cardiogenic source of emboli in acute focal stroke, since the yield is low in patients who have no history or physical evidence of cardiac disease. Our practice is to employ two-dimensional echocardiography or, less often, transesophageal echocardiography in patients with focal stroke who are (1) young; (2) have no detectable atherothrombosis of the appropriate extracranial vessel, regardless of age; and (3) have no detectable risk factors, including polycythemia or oral contraceptive use. In suitable patients, *stress testing* during convalescence may be recommended to evaluate possible ischemic cardiovascular disease.

Brain Imaging. Although routine blood, urine, and ECG analyses are obtained immediately upon hospital admission, brain imaging is the most important differential diagnostic test to identify other causes of focal neurologic dysfunction, such as neoplasms or subdural hematomas, and to distinguish ischemic from hemorrhagic stroke. CT scanning, the most commonly used imaging technique, has limitations that must be considered. CT cannot always detect cerebral infarction; the size, location, and age of the lesion affect the lesion's visibility. Infarcts less than 5 mm in diameter often escape detection, especially within the brain stem, where bone artifact may interfere with resolution. Further, only about 5 per cent are visible on CT scan within the first 12 hours; detection increases to approximately 50 per cent between 24 and 48 hours and approximately 90 per cent by the end of 1 week.

Infarcts appear as hypodense areas on non–contrast-enhanced CT scans with increasingly well demarcated margins as edema peaks between 3 and 5 days (Fig. 469–1). Contrast-enhancing agents carry a small risk of neurotoxicity, and they may normalize the CT density of an otherwise small hypodense infarct, making the infarct less visible. Accordingly, one should use contrast-enhancing agents during the acute phase of the ischemic stroke only to seek out a mass lesion and only after a noncontrast scan has been obtained.

CT scans immediately delineate primary cerebral hemorrhage, but hemorrhagic conversions of an ischemic infarct usually develop only after 1 to 2 days (Fig. 469–1), and a few continue to appear for up to 4 weeks.

Magnetic resonance imaging (MRI) is more sensitive than CT

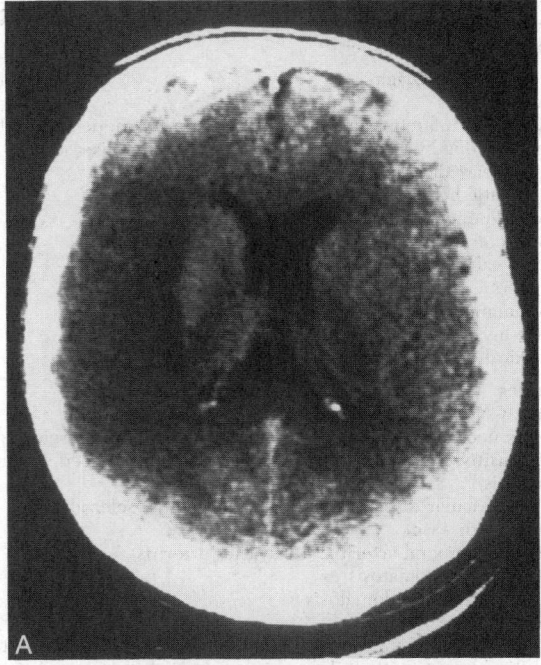

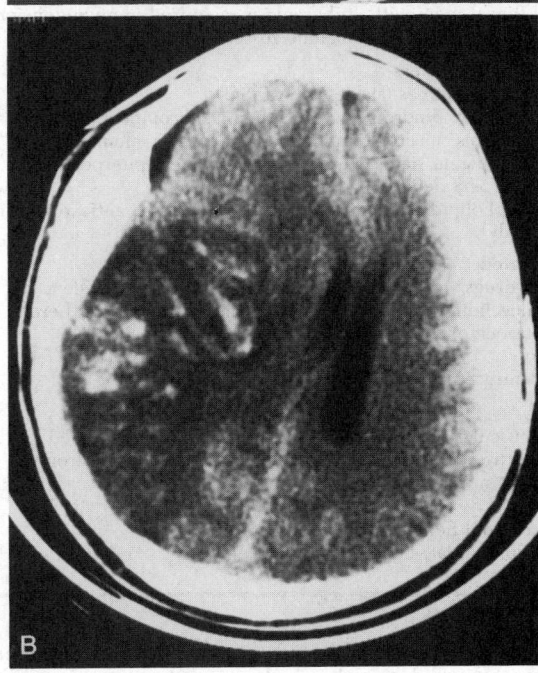

FIGURE 469–1. Right middle cerebral artery distribution infarctions shown on computed tomography (CT) at 24 hours. In *A*, hypodensity on the left side of the figure represents an ischemic infarction; in *B*, inhomogeneous areas of increased density interspersed with decreased density and mass effect on the left side of the figure represent a hemorrhagic infarction. This inhomogeneity distinguishes hemorrhagic infarction from primary brain hemorrhage (compare with Fig. 470–3).

to changes in tissue structure and may provide a more accurate and earlier measure of cerebral infarction. MRI, however, is more costly, and, with the present equipment, requires more time to perform than CT; in addition, the need to exclude ferromagnetic materials from the MRI suite, as well as the difficulty in monitoring patients in the scanner, makes MRI unsuitable for many acutely ill patients. If the diagnosis remains in doubt, MRI may be used after the acute phase to verify infarction.

Lumbar Puncture. Lumbar puncture (LP) is no longer widely used in routine stroke diagnosis because noninvasive CT or MRI detects cerebral hemorrhage and anticoagulation begun within 6

hours after a lumbar puncture risks causing a spinal epidural hematoma. An LP is important, however, in diagnosing neurosyphilis or meningitis, as, for example, in patients with acute stiff neck who show no blood on brain imaging. If an LP is to be done in those suspected of having had a stroke, it should be preceded by funduscopic examination and brain imaging if possible to rule out raised intracranial pressure.

Noninvasive Cerebrovascular Examination. Several noninvasive techniques help to evaluate the cerebrovascular supply. Indirect tests that examine blood flow in the periorbital or orbital circulation include *Doppler sonography* and *quantitative oculopneumoplethysmography* (OPG). Periorbital Doppler sonography measures the amplitude of pulsations and the direction of blood flow in the periorbital arteries. Normally, blood flows from the intracranial vault to the skin surface. In severe internal carotid artery disease, blood flow reversal can be detected by Doppler sonography. Quantitative OPG measures the systolic blood pressure and amplitude of pulsations in the ophthalmic artery. Internal carotid artery stenosis is detected by comparing the values between the eyes or the eye and the systemic systolic blood pressure. Both Doppler sonography and OPG do not easily distinguish between severe stenosis and occlusion of the internal carotid artery, and neither technique readily detects a less than 60 per cent stenosis of the artery.

Direct examination of the common, internal, and external carotid arteries is best achieved with *duplex ultrasonography.* Duplex ultrasonography consists of B-mode ultrasonography, which produces a real-time image of the carotid vessels and a range-gaited pulsed Doppler that is visually guided by the B-mode image to measure the frequency shift associated with increased blood velocity through a stenotic lumen. The combination of the precise location of the Doppler frequency signal and the B-mode image provides the most accurate noninvasive method for analyzing disease of the extracranial circulation. Limitations of the technique include (1) access to only the portion of the carotid circulation that lies between the clavicles and the mandible (in approximately 10 per cent of patients, the carotid bifurcation lies above the angle of the jaw, making ultrasonography difficult or impossible); (2) absorption of sound waves by calcium within a mural plaque, which may "shadow" and obscure a plaque on a distal vessel wall; and (3) echolucency of acute thrombi, which can be indistinguishable from flowing blood.

The direction and velocity of blood flow in the intracranial blood vessels originating from the circle of Willis may be examined with low-frequency *pulsed transcranial Doppler,* a technique still being evaluated for its usefulness as a diagnostic tool. The intracranial blood vessels can also be examined on reconstructed CT or MRI images. A still experimental technique involves the imaging of flowing blood using *magnetic resonance angiography.* The procedure produces images of the extracranial and intracranial blood vessels, as well as atherosclerotic abnormalities of the carotid bifurcation; some aneurysms can also be detected. Several different software programs are currently being evaluated, and the procedure remains investigational.

Cerebral Angiography. Intracranial and extracranial *cerebral angiography* of elderly patients prone to ischemic stroke carries a 2 to 4 per cent risk of producing a reversible neurologic deficit and a 0.5 to 1.0 per cent risk of permanent neurologic deficits or death. Accordingly, angiography should be reserved for specific indications in which it may reveal abnormalities amenable to therapy. Examples include a search for fibromuscular dysplasia, arterial dissection, or cranial arteritis or a preparation for cerebrovascular surgery. *Digital subtraction arteriography* permits use of smaller amounts of intravascular contrast material and may thus be of lower risk, especially in patients with marginal renal or cardiac function. *Digital subtraction venous angiography* is no longer widely used because of its unreliability in detecting plaque ulcerations and in differentiating carotid stenosis from complete occlusion.

Other Techniques. Methods for measuring CBF are still largely investigational; they include *positron emission tomographic (PET)* methods, usually using radiolabeled water or carbon dioxide; *single-photon emission computed tomography (SPECT)*; and radiolabeled and stable *xenon* inhalation techniques.

DIFFERENTIAL DIAGNOSIS OF ISCHEMIC STROKES AND TIA'S

The clinical diagnosis of ischemic or hemorrhagic stroke relies primarily on the clinician's understanding of brain function and pathology. Deficits that evolve over weeks are usually caused by a brain mass, either *primary or metastatic brain tumor* or *brain abscess*. *Subdural hematoma* should be distinguishable from stroke by the hematoma's more prolonged course and its combination of diffuse and focal dysfunction.

TIA's may be confused with classic or complicated *migraine*, the former being associated with scintillating scotomata and the latter with hemiparesis or other focal deficits; some of the underlying pathophysiology may be ischemic for both TIA's and migraine, but evidence is accumulating that nonischemic electrical disturbances (spreading depression) are involved in the pathophysiology of migraine.

Seizures can be confused with TIA's. Most such seizures produce motor activity or positive sensory phenomena, whereas most strokes and TIA's produce weakness and sensory loss, but seizures can sometimes produce these "negative" symptoms. The postictal state following (unobserved) seizures is even more likely to imitate an ischemic deficit. Serial observations usually permit the rapid differential diagnosis of stroke versus seizure, but prompt differentiation may be difficult and may interfere with early stroke treatment. As with migraine, stroke and seizure can coexist: A small proportion of strokes (about 10 per cent), especially embolic strokes, are associated at onset with seizures.

Hemorrhagic stroke often enters the differential diagnosis for ischemic stroke. Although the anatomic locations of the two may differ, with hemorrhage seldom involving a discrete vascular territory, clinical differentiation can be uncertain, making CT scan necessary. Other illnesses included in the differential diagnosis of vertebrobasilar ischemia include, as mentioned above, nonspecific dizziness, Ménière's disease, or peripheral vestibulopathy.

CAUSES AND PATHOGENESIS (Table 469–2)

ATHEROSCLEROSIS. Atherosclerosis of extracranial and intracranial arteries accounts for approximately two thirds of all ischemic strokes and an even greater proportion of those affecting patients over the age of 60. Atherosclerosis causes strokes either by *in situ stenosis* or *occlusion* or by *embolization* of plaque material to distal cerebral vessels. In either case, the clinical and pathologic effects depend on the adequacy of collateral circulation to the affected vascular territory. It is not uncommon for unilateral or, more rarely, bilateral occlusion of the internal carotid artery to develop without neurologic symptoms, especially if the stenosis or occlusion develops slowly. In instances of marked stenosis or occlusion of extracranial arteries that is combined with intracranial atherosclerosis, cerebral perfusion occasionally can relate closely to small changes in perfusion pressure. One effect can be a worsening stroke deficit associated with orthostatic blood pressure changes that would otherwise be considered normal.

The more common effect of atherosclerosis is that a platelet-fibrin embolus detaches from a plaque and floats distally, where it occludes a smaller branch. Such emboli are likely to produce symptoms, since the more distal the occlusion, the less likely can collateral filling prevent damage. In these cases of artery-to-artery embolization, the embolus usually emanates from a plaque at the bifurcation of the common carotid artery or at the point where the vertebral arteries originate from the subclavian arteries.

EMBOLI OF CARDIAC ORIGIN. Cerebral emboli of a cardiac source may account for up to one third of all ischemic strokes. Thrombus formation and the release of thromboemboli from the heart are promoted by arrhythmias and structural abnormalities of the heart valves and chambers.

Mural Thrombi. Mural thrombi typically form under areas of dyskinetic myocardium damaged by *myocardial infarction.* As many as 35 per cent of patients with recent anterior wall infarction harbor mural thrombi, and if not anticoagulated, nearly 40 per cent of these embolize systemically within 4 months after the myocardial infarction. *Cardiomyopathies* can also predispose to mural thrombi and embolization. They are defined as diseases of

TABLE 469–2. CAUSES OF ISCHEMIC STROKES

Atherosclerosis

Emboli of Cardiac Origin
Mural thrombus
  Myocardial infarction (anterior wall septum, akinetic segment)
  Cardiomyopathy (infectious, idiopathic, Chagas' disease)
Valvular heart disease
  Rheumatic heart disease
  Bacterial endocarditis
  Nonbacterial endocarditis (carcinoma, Libman-Sacks)
  Mitral valve prolapse
  Prosthetic valve
Arrhythmia (atrial fibrillation)
Cardiac myxoma
Paradoxical emboli

Vasculitides
Primary CNS vasculitis
Systemic necrotizing vasculitis (polyarteritis nodosa, allergic angiitis)
Hypersensitivity vasculitis (serum sickness, drug-induced, cutaneous vasculitis)
Collagen vascular diseases (rheumatoid arthritis, scleroderma, Sjögren's disease)
Giant cell (temporal arteritis, Takayasu's arteritis)
Wegener's granulomatosis
Lymphomatoid granulomatosis
Behçet's disease
Infectious vasculitis (neurovascular syphilis, Lyme disease, bacterial and fungal meningitis, tuberculosis, acquired immunodeficiency syndrome [AIDS], ophthalmic zoster, hepatitis B)

Hematologic Disorders
Hemoglobinopathies (sickle cell, HbSC)
Hyperviscosity syndromes (polycythemia, thrombocytosis, leukocytosis, macroglobulinemia, multiple myeloma)
Hypercoagulable states (carcinoma, pregnancy, puerperium)
Protein C or S deficiency
Antiphospholipid antibodies (lupus anticoagulant, anticardiolipin antibody)

Drug Related
"Street drugs" (cocaine, "crack," amphetamines, lysergic acid, phencyclidine, methylphenidate, sympathomimetics, heroin, pentazocine)
Alcohol
Oral contraceptives

Other
Fibromuscular dysplasia
Arterial dissection (trauma, spontaneous, Marfan's syndrome)
Homocystinuria
Migraine
Subarachnoid hemorrhage/vasospasm
Other emboli (fat, bone marrow, air emboli)
Moyamoya

the myocardium of variable, often unknown, cause and usually are characterized by cardiac enlargement, systemic embolism, and conduction abnormalities or arrhythmias. In one study, systemic emboli were found in approximately 15 per cent of patients with congestive or dilated cardiomyopathy, a subgroup of the condition that is usually caused by alcohol abuse or viral infections. Patients who also had atrial fibrillation had a higher incidence of embolism (33 per cent) than did those without (14 per cent). As a note of therapeutic importance, none of the cardiomyopathy patients on anticoagulation had systemic emboli.

Valvular Heart Disease. Although less common than previously, *rheumatic heart disease* often gives rise to systemic embolization. In one series, 20 to 25 per cent of patients with mitral stenosis developed systemic emboli, although most had coexisting atrial fibrillation.

Acute or subacute *infective endocarditis* produces vegetations on heart valves, debris that can embolize into the cerebral circulation. Many emboli are relatively small, but those associated with endocarditis caused by staphylococcus, fungi, or yeast often are large enough to occlude proximal intracranial arteries. In autopsy series, systemic emboli are found in as many as 30 per cent of patients with infective endocarditis. Prompt recognition of the heart lesion based on the presence of fever, a murmur, petechiae, and other characteristics, such as Osler's nodes and Roth spots, in patients with underlying valvular disease or intravenous drug use should prompt blood cultures and treatment with antibiotics to reduce the risk of embolism. Anticoagulation is not effective and may even increase the risk of parenchymal bleeding. Infective endocarditis is associated with other forms of cerebrovascular disease, including cerebral hemorrhage, subarachnoid hemorrhage, and mycotic aneurysm, as well as cerebral abscess.

Embolization from heart valves also occurs in *nonbacterial endocarditis (NBTE)*, in which predominantly platelet-fibrin vegetations form on the heart valves and then embolize into the systemic circulation. NBTE occurs commonly in association with cancer of the stomach, prostate, ovary, pancreas, and lung. In one autopsy series of patients with NBTE, cerebral emboli were found in one third. Clinically, diffuse encephalopathy as well as focal stroke is observed; associated disseminated intravascular coagulation accompanies about 20 per cent of cases.

Libman-Sacks (atypical verrucous) endocarditis is associated with systemic lupus erythematosus. In this condition, soft, friable vegetations form on the leaflets of any of the heart valves, not just the tricuspid valve, as believed earlier. Systemic (and cerebral) emboli are rare.

Mitral valve prolapse describes a billowing of the mitral leaflets into the left atrium during systole. Although usually asymptomatic, some patients experience palpitations or chest pain. The diagnosis is suggested by auscultatory and echocardiographic criteria, but normal standards are uncertain, making the true incidence of the condition unknown; it is estimated to be 6 to 10 per cent in healthy, young women. In part because of different diagnostic criteria, the role of mitral valve prolapse in cerebral embolism remains controversial: Several analyses of strokes in young adults suggest a disproportionately high representation of patients with mitral valve prolapse, but others indexed on patients with mitral valve prolapse suggest that systemic embolism is infrequent. In one of these latter studies, however, the risk of cerebral embolism was 5 to 10 per cent. Coexisting infective endocarditis or arrhythmia contributes to cerebral embolism.

Prosthetic heart valves carry a high risk of systemic (including cerebral) embolism, mechanical heart valves having a higher risk than biologic valves (e.g., porcine). The overall risk of embolism is roughly equivalent in anticoagulated patients with mechanical valves and in nonanticoagulated patients with biologic valves: 1 to 3 per cent per year for aortic prostheses, and 3 to 5 per cent per year for mitral substitutions.

Arrhythmias. *Atrial fibrillation*, with or without valvular disease, strongly increases the risk of embolic ischemic stroke, especially in patients over the age of 60. In one large series, the risk of ischemic stroke was 6 to 7 per cent per year. The risk is highest shortly after development of atrial fibrillation: Up to one third of emboli occur in the first month. Embolism can also accompany therapeutic cardioversion. About 35 per cent of patients with nonvalvular atrial fibrillation sooner or later will have an ischemic stroke. In some, embolism underlies the stroke; in others, the fault lies in coexisting intrinsic cerebrovascular disease associated with coronary artery disease. Even thyrotoxic, nonvalvular atrial fibrillation is associated with a 10 to 12 per cent risk of stroke. The one group without a strikingly increased risk is patients with lone atrial fibrillation, meaning those without other clinical evidence of cardiopulmonary disease.

Cardiac Myxoma. Cardiac tumors are uncommon, occurring in about 0.05 per cent of autopsies. *Myxomas* account for about 35 per cent of all intracardiac tumors but are the ones most likely to embolize, from either overlying thrombus or the tumor itself. In one series, about one quarter of patients with autopsy-proven cardiac myxomas had clinical evidence of strokes. Aneurysms and intracranial hemorrhage were also reported. The coexistence of hemolytic anemia due to red blood cell trauma and lysis sometimes suggests a cardiac tumor, but firm diagnosis requires echocardiography or angiography.

Paradoxical Emboli. Emboli of venous origin have long been known to cross a patent foramen ovale into the systemic circulation. Recent evidence employing bubble echocardiography found that 40 per cent of stroke patients under age 55 with a normal cardiac evaluation by history, examination, and ECG had a patent foramen ovale detected by bubble echocardiography.

VASCULITIDES. A group of disorders classified as vasculitides

cause focal or multifocal cerebral ischemia through inflammation and necrosis of extracranial and/or intracranial blood vessels. The pathogenesis of vascular inflammation differs among these disorders, but all involve, to some degree, deposition of humoral and cellular immune complexes and infiltration of polymorphonuclear and mononuclear cells in blood vessel walls. In most cases, the cause of the inflammatory response is unknown, but in others, infection, a postinfectious or neoplastic process, or a hypersensitivity immune reaction triggers the inflammation.

Segmental inflammation of cerebral blood vessels causes cerebral ischemia acutely at the site of involvement through platelet aggregation and/or clot formation or chronically through fibrinoid necrosis, which narrows the vessel lumen. Central nervous system (CNS) vasculitis, although a rare cause of stroke, is itself not uncommon and should enter the differential diagnosis whenever a young patient presents with a stroke or a patient of any age presents with a diffuse encephalopathy.

Symptoms of CNS vasculitis include cognitive disturbances, headache, and seizures (encephalopathy), which occur more frequently than with focal neurologic dysfunction. The differentiation from other causes of encephalopathy depends on the angiographic appearance of a "beadlike" segmental narrowing of cerebral blood vessels and/or the finding of characteristic inflammatory histopathology in leptomeningeal and cortical biopsy specimens. Cerebral angiograms may appear normal in 20 to 30 per cent of histologically positive cases of cerebral vasculitis. In addition, because of the segmental or "skip" nature of the inflammatory response, the histopathology may go undetected in the presence of a positive angiogram.

The diagnosis of CNS vasculitis is aided by the presence or absence of peripheral nervous system or systemic organ involvement and by identifying the underlying cause of the inflammation. Primary CNS vasculitis, Behçet's disease, Takayasu's arteritis, and temporal arteritis are notable for their infrequent involvement or noninvolvement of the peripheral nervous system. By contrast, the hypersensitivity and systemic necrotizing vasculitides frequently produce polyneuropathies.

Primary CNS arteritis, giant cell arteritis, and vasculitis associated with certain CNS infections deserve specific attention, since these may present initially or solely with neurologic signs and symptoms.

Primary CNS Arteritis. Primary arteritis of the CNS, also called granulomatous arteritis of the CNS, causes headache and other encephalopathic-like symptoms in young or middle-aged individuals. The course is usually insidiously progressive but may wax and wane for periods of several months. It is a diagnosis of exclusion.

Giant Cell Vasculitis. *Temporal arteritis* and *Takayasu's arteritis* are characterized by a granulomatous vasculitis of medium-sized and large arteries. Temporal arteritis affects predominantly patients over the age of 60, causing constitutional symptoms such as fever, malaise, weight loss, and headache. In half of the patients, symptoms consistent with polymyalgia rheumatica may coexist, including jaw, neck, and facial pain, as well as morning stiffness. Tenderness and pain over the temporal arteries and an elevated erythrocyte sedimentation rate are frequently, but not always, present. Biopsy of the superficial temporal artery provides the definitive diagnosis. Because of the segmental nature of the vasculitis, serial sections should be examined. Even then, typical features of fever, malaise, tender scalp vessels, and a grossly elevated sedimentation rate dictate the early initiation of corticosteroid therapy because of the high risk of acute ischemic blindness. A *dramatic* response to therapy is semidiagnostic.

Takayasu's arteritis affects primarily young women and involves mainly the aortic arch, the large brachiocephalic arteries derived from the arch, and the abdominal aorta. Mononuclear infiltrates and fibrous proliferation produce progressive narrowing of the lumen of these vessels, causing reduced flow into the upper extremities (hence the name "pulseless disease") and cerebral ischemia. Although initially diagnosed in Japanese women, in recent years its recognition in Western countries has led to more frequent diagnosis.

Infectious Vasculitis. Bacterial, fungal, and viral infections can induce CNS vasculitis and cerebral ischemia (Table 469–2). Neurosyphilis and its meningovascular complications have increased considerably in recent years (see Ch. 472) and should be considered in patients with atypical or unexplained cerebrovascular disease.

HEMATOLOGIC ABNORMALITIES. *Hemoglobinopathy.* Among the hemoglobinopathies, *sickle cell disease* is by far the most common cause of stroke. In sickle cell disease, a single substitution of the amino acid valine for glutamate at the sixth position of the β-globin molecule causes the mutant molecule HbSS to become highly insoluble and polymerize under deoxygenated conditions. The polymerization alters the erythrocyte's shape ("sickling") and decreases the cell's deformability, leading to increased blood viscosity, microvascular sludging, and microvascular infarction. Sickle cell disease also causes hyperplasia of fibrous tissue and muscle cells of the vascular intima, leading to stenosis and occlusion of some medium-sized to large cerebral arteries.

Ischemic stroke occurs in approximately 15 per cent of patients with HbSS and in a much smaller percentage of those with sickle cell trait (HbSA) or HbSC. At normal arterial oxygen saturations of 95 to 100 per cent in HbSS, some sickling is present, and at 65 per cent, i.e., just slightly lower than normal venous oxygen saturation, approximately 75 per cent of erythrocytes sickle. Ischemic stroke arises most frequently in children, whereas hemorrhagic stroke is more common in adults with HbSS; subarachnoid hemorrhage in patients with sickle cell disease is frequently the result of a ruptured saccular aneurysm.

Small changes in oxygen tension, dehydration, acidosis, or infection can precipitate sickle cell crisis and stroke. Cerebral angiography causes an increased risk for patients with sickle cell disease. In instances when such angiography is necessary to evaluate the source of intracerebral hemorrhage, the level of HbSS should be reduced to less than 20 per cent through transfusions.

Hyperviscosity Syndrome. Cerebral blood flow is inversely related to blood viscosity. The latter is directly proportional to the number of circulating red and white blood cells, the aggregation state, the number of platelets, and the plasma protein concentration. Blood flow is inversely proportional to the deformability of erythrocytes and blood velocity (shear rate). Patients with the hyperviscosity syndrome can present either with focal neurologic dysfunction or, more frequently, with diffuse or multifocal signs or symptoms, including headache, visual disturbances, cognitive impairment, and seizures.

Cellular hyperviscosity, associated with *polycythemia*, *thrombocytosis*, or *leukocytosis* of any cause, can reduce CBF below threshold levels for cerebral dysfunction and injury. Hematocrits above 50 per cent, white cell counts greater than 150,000 per microliter, and platelet counts in excess of 1 million per microliter increase the risk of stroke.

Elevated plasma protein concentrations caused by *macroglobulinemia* or *multiple myeloma* elevate plasma viscosity and increase stroke risk. Approximately 25 per cent of patients with macroglobulinemia experience some form of cerebral ischemia, and a lesser number of patients with multiple myeloma experience the hyperviscosity syndrome. Of the various forms of multiple myeloma, those with a predominance of immunoglobulin A (IgA) most frequently develop a hyperviscosity syndrome because this particular molecule is likely to form high molecular weight polymers.

Hypercoagulable States. Cancer, particularly the adenocarcinomas, pregnancy, and the puerperium have all been associated with a "hypercoagulable state" that predisposes to arterial and venous thrombosis. Despite the fact that any one of several abnormalities, including elevations of fibrinogen levels, alterations of partial thromboplastin or prothrombin times, and platelet aggregation, occurs in the hypercoagulable state, no tests have been devised to diagnose it specifically.

Protein C or S Deficiency. Proteins C and S are two naturally occurring anticoagulants synthesized in the liver via vitamin K–dependent mechanisms. Deficiencies of either are rare, dominantly inherited, and expressed phenotypically by incomplete penetrance. Homozygotes develop serious and frequently fatal clotting abnormalities at birth, while heterozygotes may show no signs of hypercoagulability. Proteins C and S act in concert to inactivate the activated coagulating Factors V and VIII; protein

C also triggers the endogenous fibrinolytic pathways. Deficiencies in either are associated with ischemic vascular disease. Because of incomplete penetrance, the occurrence of thrombosis and stroke in the adult is extremely rare.

Antiphospholipid Antibodies. A strong epidemiologic association links a group of antiphospholipid antibodies to cerebral ischemia manifested clinically as atypical migraine, TIA, recurrent strokes, or ischemic encephalopathy. These antibodies bind to membrane phospholipids and include anticardiolipin antibody, the lupus anticoagulant, and antibodies causing a false-positive VDRL. The pathogenetic relationship between the antibodies and enhanced cerebral thrombosis is unknown. The syndrome may manifest at any age but usually affects patients less than 50 years old. Antiphospholipid antibodies often accompany collagen vascular disease, especially systemic lupus erythematosus, as well as valvular heart disease. Circulating titers of phospholipid antibodies correlate poorly with either the incidence or the severity of cerebral ischemia.

DRUG-RELATED CAUSES OF STROKE. An extensive list of "street" drugs (Table 469–2) has been associated with stroke, reflecting as much the social patterns of drug abuse as the unique properties of the drugs themselves. The sharing of nonsterile needles to inject many of these drugs intravenously (e.g., heroin, cocaine) may precipitate infectious processes (bacterial endocarditis, hepatitis B, mycotic aneurysms) that lead to strokes. Several of the drugs are potent vasoconstrictors and may initiate cerebral vasospasm. Others have been associated with cerebral vasculitis caused either by immune responses to the primary drug or by hypersensitivity to contaminating adulterants. The intravenous injection of oral medications (pentazocine [Talwin], methylphenidate [Ritalin]) that have been crushed and suspended in water for intravenous injection can cause cerebral microemboli from particles of talc and cellulose used as ingredients in the pills. These particles are thought to be trapped by pulmonary arterioles, causing local arteritis and later arteriovenous shunts that allow the microemboli to reach the CNS.

Over-the-counter cold remedies and nasal decongestants containing sympathomimetics such as ephedrine, phenylpropanolamine, and phenoxazoline have been associated with ischemic stroke. Cases have been reported following the prolonged use of oral cold medications as well as in patients who chronically overuse nasal decongestants.

The risk of ischemic and hemorrhagic stroke is increased from 4- to 13-fold among users of high-dose estrogen contraceptives. The coexistence of hypertension, prolonged use of the pill, smoking, a previous history of migraine, and age exceeding 35 years seems to enhance the risk of contraceptive-related stroke. A clear association between stroke and the newer low-dose estrogen contraceptives has not been established.

OTHER CAUSES OF STROKE. *Fibromuscular dysplasia* (or hyperplasia) describes areas of segmental nonatherosclerotic arterial narrowing, usually caused by fibroplasia and smooth muscle proliferation, that alternate with rings of medial thinning. The condition affects the carotid and vertebral arteries, usually at the level of the second cervical vertebra rather than at the origin of the vessels; it also affects the renal arteries and is associated, therefore, with hypertension. Fibromuscular dysplasia predominates in women and occurs, on the average, in the sixth decade of life. The condition is uncommon: In one angiographic series, fibromuscular dysplasia was identified in fewer than 1 per cent of vessels studied. It produces ischemic stroke both by the hemodynamic effects of stenosis and by thromboembolism. The condition is also associated with aneurysm formation and with arterial dissection. Angiography usually enables one to make the diagnosis, although flow studies with MRI may prove increasingly useful. Because of its rarity, there is little information about treatment.

A *dissecting aortic aneurysm*, although uncommon, can occlude major branches of the aorta supplying the cranial circulation and produce ischemic strokes. Chest, back, or abdominal pain accompanying the stroke and differences in palpable pulses or in blood pressure in the limbs suggest the diagnosis. Emergency angiography is needed to confirm it.

Extracranial *dissections of the carotid artery* are increasingly recognized. Many follow relatively trivial trauma (e.g., pharyngeal injury with blunt objects in children and neck torsion, sometimes from chiropractic manipulation, in adults). Some are associated with fibromuscular dysplasia, others with a variety of childhood conditions, including Ehlers-Danlos and Marfan's syndromes as well as tuberous sclerosis. Pathologically, intraluminal blood enters the subintimal or medial vascular planes, and the lumen becomes progressively narrowed and thrombosed. Carotid artery dissections can sometimes be recognized clinically by intense ipsilateral pain. Angiography may be needed for diagnosis, but MRI is sometimes sufficient.

Homocystinuria is characterized by dislocated ocular lenses, bone deformities, a marfanoid appearance, mental retardation, accelerated atherosclerosis, and arterial or venous thromboses. Several different genetic defects can cause homocystinuria, but the most frequent is a deficiency of the enzyme cystathionine β-synthase. The pathogenesis of accelerated atherosclerosis and enhanced thrombosis associated with homocystinuria is unknown, but approximately one third of affected individuals have one or more strokes by the age of 15 years. In some studies, heterozygous homocystinuria has been reported in as many as one quarter of young persons who have suffered strokes. Treatment with pyridoxine or folic acid may limit disease progression.

Reactive vascular narrowing (*vasospasm*) causes ischemic strokes in two settings. One causes substantial disability in *subarachnoid hemorrhage* (Ch. 470.1). Vasospasm also presumably explains ischemic strokes seen in a small number of patients with *migraine* headaches. Migraineurs develop ischemic strokes, either in conjunction with migraine (in which case they appear to result from a prolonged migraine attack) or remote from the attack (in which case more traditional stroke mechanisms, such as atherosclerosis, are likely to be responsible).

Fat emboli typically occur several days after trauma and fracture of the long bones. Although focal ischemic strokes may occur, more typically the condition manifests with seizures and a diffuse encephalopathy consistent with disseminated embolization. Associated findings include petechiae and fat emboli visible on funduscopic examination. Fat globules may be identified in urine or CSF.

Air emboli can occur with open heart surgery, in patients with pneumothorax, or in divers who ascend too rapidly to the surface. Like fat emboli, air emboli cause altered mental status and seizures, but the changes are maximal immediately after the embolization. Segmental areas of pallor may be observed on the tongue, and there may be marbling of the skin and air emboli seen on funduscopic examination. When caused by sudden decompression, the condition is treated in a decompression chamber.

Moyamoya disease is a rare condition that is most common among the Japanese, in whom it has been reported to affect fewer than 0.1 per 100,000 of the general population. A "definite" diagnosis requires demonstration of bilateral terminal internal carotid artery occlusion that involves the origins of the MCA and ACA and an abnormal vascular network at the base of the brain that is believed to provide collateral circulation. The abnormal collateral channels appear on angiograms as a "smoky haze," hence the Japanese term "moyamoya." The cause of the vascular occlusion is unknown, but it occurs most commonly in children (peak incidence at age 6 years), in whom it may be associated with ischemic stroke; in adults, it more commonly causes hemorrhage. The diagnosis requires that no known predisposing cause exist, but a similar angiographic picture is seen occasionally with acute tonsillitis, atherosclerosis, meningitis, cancer, trauma, and radiotherapy.

A condition in which the walls of small arteries are thickened and disorganized, referred to by some as lipohyalinosis, was originally believed to underlie small, subcortical brain infarcts called *lacunes*. The condition was thought to be related to hypertension and to require management that differed from that for more conventional strokes. Lacunes were initially described as being associated with a restricted number of characteristic syndromes (e.g., pure motor stroke), but over the years, progressively more clinical syndromes have been attributed to lacunes. Moreover, traditional causes of stroke, including diabetes and hyperlipidemia, have appeared in these patients with almost the same frequency as in those with nonlacunar, ischemic stroke. Perhaps as a result, treatment recommendations, which initially differed for lacunar strokes, now parallel those for nonlacunar strokes.

PREVENTION AND TREATMENT OF STROKE

Currently, there are several promising but no proven therapies for acute ischemic stroke. Even when effective treatments become available, the physician's opportunity to deliver medical care and the utility of a particular pharmacotherapy will be hampered by time constraints; the evolution of irreversible brain damage occurs within 2 to 3 hours of focal vascular occlusion (see Ch. 468). Such considerations place a premium on preventing stroke.

The reduction of stroke risk factors, through therapy for hypertension, diabetes mellitus, smoking, atherosclerosis, and cardiac arrhythmias (Table 469–3) is largely responsible for the marked decline in the incidence of stroke over the past 30 to 40 years. Unfortunately, the effectiveness of stroke prevention is not well appreciated by either the medical or the lay community. Untreated or poorly treated hypertensives, diabetics, and smokers continue to enter the hospital with acute stroke.

Risk Factors and Primary Prevention Therapies

Stroke risk factors have been determined on the basis of mathematical abstractions of epidemiologic data that imply an association or a cause-effect relationship. This section categorizes such risk factors as *definite* or *presumed* and indicates whether they are related to *genetic* and *lifestyle* factors or to *disease processes*. Treatable risk factors are emphasized, and the expected outcome of such prophylactic therapy is presented.

DEFINITE GENETIC AND LIFESTYLE RISK FACTORS. *Hypertension.* This is the most powerful risk factor for stroke. Even within relatively "normal" ranges of blood pressure, the risk of stroke increases by approximately 50 per cent for every 5 mm Hg increase in diastolic pressure throughout the range of 70 to 110 mm Hg. All components of blood pressure (systolic, diastolic, mean) correlate with the incidence of stroke, and the elevation of the systolic pressure is probably a direct cause of stroke that is independent of the secondary complications of hypertension, such as atherosclerosis or arterial rigidity. The risk of stroke is approximately four times greater in patients with definite hypertension (160/95 mm Hg) than in normotensive individuals and is twofold higher in so-called borderline hypertensive individuals. Antihypertensive therapy that lowers the diastolic pressure by as little as 6 mm Hg reduces stroke risk by nearly one quarter in as little as 2 to 3 years. Data from the Framingham Study indicate that the control of hypertension is equally beneficial in reducing stroke risk in the eighth and ninth decades of life as at earlier ages.

Smoking. Smoking increases stroke risk twofold to fourfold. Those who stop smoking substantially reduce their risk of stroke over a period of 2 to 5 years, but their level of risk may not return completely to that of nonsmokers.

Age, Gender, and Race. Age, gender, and race are all unalterable risk factors for stroke, but they may signal treatable disease processes. The incidence of stroke approximately doubles with each decade between ages 45 and 85. Unlike cardiovascular ischemia, in which the incidence in men is approximately three times that in women, stroke occurs only 1.3 times more often in men than in women. The stroke risk in U.S. blacks is approximately 1.3 times that of whites. Some of the differences may be related to environmental or lifestyle factors, since southeastern blacks have a higher stroke rate than do northern ones. Similarly, the high incidence of stroke in the Japanese is not seen in their kindred living in Hawaii.

TABLE 469–3. PREVENTION OF STROKE

Treat hypertension and diabetes mellitus
Stop smoking
Limit alcohol intake
Control diet and obesity
Thoughtful use of oral contraceptives
Anticoagulants for atrial fibrillation and selected acute myocardial infarctions
Antiplatelet agents for carotid/vertebrobasilar atherosclerosis
Endarterectomy for symptomatic carotid artery atherosclerosis of 70–99%

POSSIBLE GENETIC AND LIFESTYLE RISK FACTORS.
Cholesterol, Lipids, Diet, and Obesity. Several dietary factors and obesity may play a role in stroke incidence, but the evidence is inconclusive. Diet and obesity may predispose toward diabetes mellitus and cardiovascular disease, and such patients have a higher chance of dying of stroke than do age-matched controls. Despite the incontrovertible relationship between elevated blood cholesterol and lipids and coronary artery disease, no conclusive evidence currently links lipid abnormalities to stroke. Nevertheless, most authorities strongly advise stroke-prone patients to lower elevated cholesterol and triglyceride levels. Because of the relationships that link obesity with diabetes mellitus, elevated blood pressure, and lipid abnormalities, weight control also is recommended for stroke-prone patients.

Alcohol. Moderate alcohol consumption relates inversely to the incidence of atherosclerosis and coronary artery disease, and a similar reduction of stroke risk with moderate alcohol consumption has also been suggested but not proved. By contrast, binge drinking may increase the incidence of both hemorrhagic and ischemic stroke, especially when combined with cigarette smoking. Much of the latter risk may be attributable to a combination of hemoconcentration and hypertension associated with heavy alcohol consumption.

Oral Contraceptives. Although formerly available high-dose estrogen oral contraceptives were related to stroke, the association is less clear for current preparations. Nevertheless, the combination of oral contraceptives with other risk factors, such as migraine, smoking, hypertension, and age greater than 35 years, may act in combination to raise stroke risk, and many recommend against oral contraceptives in such circumstances.

DEFINITE DISEASE-RELATED RISK FACTORS. Heart Disease. Rheumatic valvular disease plus atrial fibrillation increases the risk of stroke 17-fold. Chronic or paroxysmal atrial fibrillation without lesions of the heart valves is associated with a fivefold increase in the risk of stroke. Chronic anticoagulation with warfarin is recommended for most fibrillators, especially those with a history of prior embolism, the presence of a left atrial thrombus on two-dimensional echocardiography, or the coexistence of dilated or hypertrophic cardiomyopathy or of thyrotoxic heart disease, as well as prior to direct-current (DC) conversion. Asymptomatic individuals over the age of 60 may be considered for anticoagulation on an individual basis. Preliminary data from a U.S. study indicated that treatment of chronic atrial fibrillation with warfarin or aspirin reduced the risk of embolic stroke by approximately 80 per cent; other studies indicate that only warfarin confers such benefits. Furthermore, low-dose warfarin with a target prothrombin time ratio that is 1.2 to 1.5 times the control value conferred protection similar to that conferred by conventional warfarin therapy. Valvular disease related to bacterial or nonbacterial endocarditis, myxomatous degeneration of the mitral valve or other diseases causing mitral valve prolapse, mitroannular calcification, and prosthetic heart valve replacements all predispose toward cerebral emboli.

Myocardial infarction involving the anterior wall or septum is associated with a mural thrombus in up to one third of patients, and of these, approximately 15 per cent will suffer a cerebral embolus within a 2-year interval. Acute anticoagulation therapy with heparin, with later conversion to warfarin therapy, is recommended for patients with myocardial infarction involving the anterior or septal wall or in patients with an intramural thrombus detected by two-dimensional echocardiography. Anticoagulation should continue until the two-dimensional echocardiogram indicates resolution of the thrombus. Such therapy reduces the incidence of stroke by approximately one half.

Stroke and TIA. The occurrence of an initial stroke is a powerful predictor of recurrent stroke. Patients between the ages of 45 and 65 years have a 10- to 20-fold increased risk of having a recurrent versus an initial stroke. The comparative risk drops to eightfold for those over the age of 65. The apparent decrease in the incidence of recurrent stroke with age reflects the marked increase in the incidence of an initial stroke in patients over the age of 65. The annual stroke risk following a TIA is 5 per cent per year, which declines to 3 per cent after 3 years. After the occurrence of amaurosis fugax, the annual risk of stroke is 1 to 2 per cent.

Strong evidence derived from meta-analyses supports the use of prophylactic aspirin to protect against strokes in patients with prior strokes or TIA's. Similarly prophylactic antiplatelet therapy with ticlopidine has also been shown to protect against such secondary events. A decision to use antiplatelet or anticoagulant therapy in patients with prior strokes must take into account both the individual patient's risk of further functional loss and the risks of treatment.

Asymptomatic Carotid Stenosis. Individuals with asymptomatic carotid stenosis or carotid bruits have approximately a 1.5- to 2-fold increase in the risk of stroke compared with the general population. Cerebral infarction in this population, however, occurs as frequently in a vascular territory different from the stenotic artery as in the involved one. Asymptomatic carotid stenosis or bruit is a marker of cerebrovascular disease and signals an increased risk of stroke, but not necessarily one in the territory of the involved vessel. No large, randomized, placebo-controlled trial has determined the efficacy of prophylactic antiplatelet therapy in patients with asymptomatic carotid stenosis or bruits.

Other Diseases. Diabetes mellitus is a risk factor independent of hypertension and is associated with an approximate threefold increase in the risk of stroke. No present data indicate that normalization of the blood sugar level reduces the incidence of stroke. Polycythemia, sickle cell disease, migraine, CNS vasculitis, and several infectious diseases all somewhat increase the risk of stroke.

ASPIRIN TREATMENT FOR THE PREVENTION OF STROKE

Although prophylactic aspirin therapy in a healthy population of U.S. physicians reduced the incidence of myocardial infarction, no change occurred in the incidence of ischemic stroke, and a slight increase was detected in the incidence of hemorrhagic stroke. Antiplatelet agents cannot be recommended for stroke prophylaxis in healthy individuals.

SURGICAL TREATMENT FOR THE PREVENTION OF STROKE. The role of *prophylactic surgery* in the prevention of ischemic stroke is highly controversial. A multi-institutional, randomized trial of an external carotid artery–middle cerebral artery anastomosis showed no benefit, and the procedure has been largely abandoned. *Carotid endarterectomy*, designed to remove stenotic plaques from diseased carotid arteries, was developed in the mid 1960's, and from 1971 until about 1984 the number of such operations steadily increased, despite controversy concerning its efficacy. Several multicenter trials in North America are currently examining the indications and efficacy of carotid endarterectomy versus medical therapy in symptomatic and asymptomatic carotid stenosis. Preliminary results from one study indicate that endarterectomy significantly reduces ipsilateral stroke in patients with recent symptoms of ischemia and angiographically proven 70 to 99 per cent ipsilateral carotid artery stenosis. Only patients with a 50 per cent or greater 5-year life expectancy were entered in the study. The procedure is not appropriate for vertebrobasilar disease (Table 469–4). Although *angioplasty* is used widely for coronary artery disease, its utility for cerebrovascular atherosclerosis has not been established.

Surgery for *subclavian steal* is almost never indicated. This steal is a radiographic finding associated with occlusion or severe stenosis of a proximal subclavian artery, resulting in retrograde flow in the ipsilateral vertebral artery. The finding is only rarely associated with symptoms of vertebrobasilar ischemia when the ipsilateral arm is exercised; in most cases, it is merely a radiographic curiosity.

Management and Treatment of Acute Stroke

Patients clinically diagnosed as having an *acute ischemic stroke* should be admitted to the hospital unless the deficit has existed for several days and is stable. The initial history and physical

TABLE 469–4. GUIDELINES FOR CAROTID ENDARTERECTOMY

1. Recent ischemic symptoms (TIA, minor stroke)
2. Angiographically proven ipsilateral stenosis (70–99%)
3. Surgical risk ≤ 5%
4. Five-year cardiovascular life expectancy > 50%

examination emphasize the rapid diagnosis of ischemic cerebral ischemia (TIA or stroke) and the exclusion of seizures, hypoglycemia, tumor, and other alternative diagnoses. As already noted, a normal CT scan within the first several hours is consistent with an ischemic stroke. Admission is also advised for patients with *new-onset TIA's* or those in whom TIA's are occurring with markedly increasing frequency or severity (*crescendo TIA's*).

GENERAL MANAGEMENT. Once admitted, stroke patients should be maintained for at least 24 hours at bed rest to avoid postural hypotension. Since autoregulation (see Ch. 468) is usually ineffective in areas of ischemic brain, CBF will decline if systemic blood pressure falls because of postural changes or volume restriction. Hypertension, if present, should be treated, but with limited, stepwise reductions in blood pressure, for the same reason. If patients have bulbar dysfunction affecting chewing or swallowing, mouth feedings should be avoided to reduce the chance of aspiration. Virtually all patients should have intravenous catheters placed to facilitate urgent treatments. If oral feedings are restricted for prolonged periods, supplementation with intravenous thiamine becomes important to prevent Wernicke's disease; eventually, hyperalimentation or feeding by nasogastric or gastrostomy tube may be needed.

In the early days of an ischemic stroke, passive range-of-motion exercises to the affected limbs can help retain mobility and prevent contractures. Later, more intensive rehabilitation individualized to improve gait, speech, dexterity, and ability to manage activities of daily living is important. Patients often benefit from brief, intensive rehabilitation in specialized hospitals before being sent home. All patients at bed rest should be encouraged to flex and extend their ankles periodically to reduce the chances of deep venous thrombosis, and all should also take occasional deep breaths to combat atelectasis.

PHARMACOTHERAPY (Table 469–5). No pharmacologic therapy has been proved effective for acute ischemic stroke. Nonetheless, several agents are used, depending on the underlying pathophysiology. Intravenous *heparin* is frequently begun on an acute basis for progressing or incomplete stroke, but as already noted, results are difficult to determine. One recent, controlled study, for example, failed to demonstrate any effectiveness of modest heparinization when used in patients with stable, incomplete strokes. An important point is that none of the studies of heparin have examined the effect of beginning within the first hours after stroke onset, so that poor study design may have masked detection of any benefit. A current multicenter trial in North America of heparinoid therapy in acute stroke may provide better guidelines.

Despite underlying bleeding into the blood vessel wall, patients with vascular dissections are often treated with heparin in an effort to maintain patency of the vascular lumen and limit the likelihood of embolism; no proof of efficacy exists. Patients with lacunar strokes were previously considered not to benefit from heparin, but that view has been modified in recent years, possibly as the distinction from larger strokes has blurred.

Patients whose strokes are attributed to emboli of cardiac origin are sometimes treated acutely with heparin. As noted below, chronic oral anticoagulation is usually started concurrently, but debate surrounds the use of heparin until oral anticoagulation takes effect. Some advocate heparin because of concern about early re-embolization and the possibility that warfarin (Coumadin) sometimes enhances coagulability during the first 6 to 8 hours of therapy; others worry about the risks of hemorrhage into the initial stroke. It seems clear that the risk of bleeding is greater

TABLE 469–5. PHARMACOTHERAPY

Prophylactic
    Antiplatelet: aspirin, nonsteroidal anti-inflammatory drugs (NSAID's), ticlopidine
    Anticoagulant (for emboli of cardiac origin, some TIA's): Coumadin or other warfarin derivatives
Acute Treatment
    Anticoagulant (progressing stroke, some emboli): heparin
    Calcium channel blockers (vasospasm with subarachnoid hemorrhage): nimodipine
    Unproven agents or therapies: thrombolytics, antioxidants, glutamate/aspartate antagonists, possibly hypothermia
No Value: corticosteroids

for larger infarcts; a reasonable course is to withhold heparin from these patients and reserve it for those with smaller strokes. Heparin is generally not given to patients with bacterial endocarditis in whom embolization to the brain has occurred, since evidence suggests an increased risk of bleeding in such cases. Although not intended to reduce cerebral ischemia, low-dose heparin or heparinoids should be used in contraindication-free immobile patients to reduce the chance of peripheral thrombophlebitis.

As noted, *warfarin* anticoagulation is sometimes begun in patients with acute embolic strokes to prevent subsequent embolic strokes. The rationale is that therapeutic anticoagulation will not be achieved for several days after stroke onset, thereby reducing the risk of bleeding into the embolic infarct. This strategy is most useful in patients with large embolic infarctions, in whom the risk of secondary bleeding is greatest.

Patients with stable, complete strokes or those admitted with new-onset or crescendo TIA's are often placed on *aspirin* prophylactically at admission. It is advisable to observe these patients in the hospital for several days, however, until the situation has stabilized. When heparin might be initiated in response to subsequent deterioration, it may be wiser to use shorter-acting antiplatelet medications like nonsteroidal anti-inflammatory drugs (*NSAID's*, e.g., indomethacin or ibuprofen). Such agents share many of aspirin's antiplatelet actions, but unlike aspirin, which permanently inactivates platelet cyclo-oxygenase, NSAID's remain active only while in the bloodstream. Consequently, if necessary, heparin can be started and the NSAID held, thereby avoiding concomitant use of an anticoagulant and antiplatelet agent.

Because of their success in the treatment of myocardial infarction, *fibrinolytic agents*, such as tissue plasminogen activator (t-PA), are currently being tested in the management of acute stroke. Early evidence suggests that the rate of intracranial bleeding may be somewhat increased. Undoubtedly, some such hemorrhages simply reflect conversion of an ischemic to a hemorrhagic infarction without accompanying clinical worsening, an event known to occur in conventionally treated ischemic strokes. Symptomatic parenchymal hematomas develop in only 3 to 5 per cent of patients if fibrinolytic agents are given within 1 to 3 hours of stroke onset; this risk may be acceptable if benefit is established. Striking clinical improvement has been reported in some patients, but double-blind, randomized studies are only just beginning.

Several recent studies have shown that the calcium channel blocker *nimodipine*, 30 mg by mouth every 6 hours, favorably but modestly affects long-term neurologic outcome in ischemic stroke. The benefit has not been seen in all studies, however, and the drug's mechanisms remain unclear.

A trial of the opiate antagonist naloxone showed no benefit. Corticosteroid administration has no benefit in acute ischemic stroke and may be harmful. Experimental studies of acute stroke suggest that antioxidants and inhibitors of excitatory amino acid neurotransmitters may have promise, but neither class of agent has been tested clinically. Ultimately, stroke treatment may employ several of these modalities.

OUTCOME AND REHABILITATION

About 10 to 15 per cent of patients with ischemic stroke will die, some because of brain swelling or neurologic dysfunction directly related to the stroke (e.g., impaired respiration with medullary infarctions) but most because of systemic complications, such as myocardial infarction, pulmonary embolism, and pneumonia. Several studies show an association of stroke with subendocardial necrosis. Most large population studies report that about one fifth of patients surviving stroke require long-term institutionalization and one third to one half of the remaining are left with various disabilities. Most functional recovery takes place during the first 3 months, but some continued slow improvement is possible.

Probably because of overlapping risk factors, the leading cause of death in patients who survive the initial stroke is myocardial infarction, underscoring the importance of cardiac evaluation. Patients who have had one stroke are at increased risk of having additional ones, particularly those whose strokes are attributed to emboli of cardiac origin.

VENOUS STROKE

Although considerably less common than arterial cerebrovascular disease, venous occlusions can cause massive damage and death. As with ischemic strokes from arterial disease, the primary mechanism of brain damage is reduction in capillary blood flow, in this instance because of increased outflow resistance. Back-transmission of high pressure into the capillary bed usually results in early brain swelling from edema and superimposes a potentially severe degree of hemorrhagic infarction in subcortical white matter.

The most dangerous form of venous disease arises when the superior sagittal sinus is occluded, but obstruction of a transverse sinus or one of the major veins over the cerebral convexity (e.g., vein of Labbé) can also produce significant damage. Venous occlusions occur most commonly in association with coagulopathies, often in the puerperal period or in patients with disseminated cancer, and sometimes as a result of contiguous disease, such as infection or cancer. The transverse sinus can be occluded as a consequence of inner ear infections, producing a once common condition called otitic hydrocephalus.

With *superior sagittal sinus obstruction*, veins draining into the sinus from the superior and medial surfaces of both cerebral convexities are commonly obstructed, and thus in its early stages, the condition can result in bilateral weakness and sensory changes in the legs. This bilaterality should alert the clinician to the possibility of sinus thrombosis. Brain swelling and bilateral involvement can produce lethargy or stupor early in the course. Seizures occur more often with venous than with arterial occlusion, possibly because of the irritating effect of parenchymal blood on the cortex.

The differential diagnosis of venous obstruction can include traditional arterial strokes but more often extends to diffuse processes such as herpes simplex encephalitis and meningitis. Diagnosis of the disease depends on the recognition of impaired venous flow. Increasingly, this is detected by loss of flow artifact on MRI. On contrast CT scans, a nonenhanced triangular area surrounded by contrast in the posterior sinus (the empty "delta" sign) should suggest the diagnosis. Since MRI is not infallible, angiography is still the definitive way to make the diagnosis, but attention must be directed to films showing the venous phase.

The management of venous sinus thrombosis increasingly relies on the use of heparin anticoagulation, even in the presence of superimposed parenchymal hemorrhage. Venous occlusions are serious and often fatal, but acute anticoagulation started as soon as the diagnosis is recognized appears to lessen substantially the morbidity and mortality of the condition. Anticonvulsants should be used as needed to control seizures and limit concomitant increases in CBF that might otherwise aggravate brain swelling and bleeding. Without aggressive treatment, venous strokes can be very serious. Nonanticoagulated superior sagittal sinus occlusion that is not complicated by infection carries a mortality rate of 25 to 40 per cent. Uncontrolled series suggest that early heparin therapy can reduce the mortality and morbidity by more than half.

469.2 DIFFUSE ISCHEMIA

Brief diffuse cerebral ischemia causes syncope without any permanent sequelae (Ch. 443). Prolonged diffuse ischemia, by contrast, has devastating consequences. The most common cause is cardiac asystole or other forms of overwhelmingly severe cardiopulmonary failure. Aortic dissection and global hypoxia or carbon monoxide poisoning can cause a similar picture.

Diffuse hypoxia-ischemia typically kills neurons in the hippocampus, cerebellar Purkinje cells, the striatum, and cortical layers 3, 4, and 6. Clinically, it results in unconsciousness: coma followed in many instances by a chronic vegetative state. If patients do not regain consciousness within a few days, the prognosis for return of independent function becomes very poor. Early absence of pupillary light reflexes, corneal reflexes, and reflex eye movements also predicts a poor outcome. Patients lacking all of these responses even within the first day of hypoxic-ischemic coma have less than a 5 per cent chance of resuming independent activities within 1 year (see Ch. 443). Even if consciousness is regained, such patients often suffer long-term impairment of memory and sometimes a variety of sensorimotor syndromes consistent with lesions in a boundary zone distribution. One such abnormality produces weakness and sensory changes that are greatest in the proximal arm, the cortical representation of which lies between the territories of the ACA and MCA.

Other than prompt and aggressive efforts to restore cardiovascular circulation, no treatments have been found to help patients who are comatose after cardiac arrest. A randomized, multi-institutional trial of barbiturates was without benefit, and corticosteroids may even be harmful. In young patients hypoxic because of drowning, evidence suggests that hypothermia may prolong resistance to ischemic damage, but therapeutic hypothermia in adults can induce cardiac arrhythmias and has not yet been tested. Chronically unconscious patients have not been shown to benefit from either physical or electrical stimulation programs.

Antiplatelet Trialists' Collaboration: Secondary prevention of vascular disease by prolonged antiplatelet treatment. Br Med J 296:320, 1988. *A meta-analysis of 31 randomized trials concluding that aspirin reduces stroke risk by 22 per cent.*

Barnett HJ, Stein BM, Mohr JP, et al. (eds.): Stroke: Pathophysiology, Diagnosis and Management. New York, Churchill Livingstone. 1986. *A comprehensive review of the diagnosis and management of ischemic and hemorrhagic stroke.*

The Boston Area Anticoagulation Trial for Atrial Fibrillation: The effect of low-dose warfarin on the risk of stroke in patients with nonrheumatic atrial fibrillation. N Engl J Med 323:1505, 1990. *A multi-institutional study showing the striking effectiveness of low-dose warfarin in preventing stroke in patients with nonrheumatic atrial fibrillation.*

Classification of Cerebrovascular Diseases III. Special Report from the National Institute of Neurological Disorders and Stroke. Stroke 21:637, 1990. *A contemporary classification of stroke with brief descriptions of each category.*

Collins R, Peto R, MacMahon S, et al.: Blood pressure, stroke, and coronary heart disease, Part 2. Short-term reductions in blood pressure: Overview of randomised drug trials in their epidemiological context. Lancet 335:827, 1990. *A meta-analysis showing a strong association between even modest hypertension and stroke and striking benefits from blood pressure management.*

Del Zoppo GJ: Thrombolytic therapy in cerebrovascular disease. Stroke 19:1174, 1988. *A comprehensive review of animal and human studies of thrombolytics published up to 1988.*

Editorial: Left ventricular thrombosis and stroke following myocardial infarction. Lancet 335:759, 1990. *A brief summary of recommended anticoagulation therapy to reduce embolic stroke after myocardial infarction.*

Haas WK, Easton DJ, Adams HP Jr, et al.: A randomized trial comparing ticlopidine hydrochloride with aspirin for the prevention of stroke in high-risk patients. N Engl J Med 321:501, 1989. *A multicenter trial showing a significant but small advantage of ticlopidine over aspirin.*

Hachinski V, Norris JW: The Acute Stroke. Philadelphia, FA Davis, 1985. *A comprehensive review of the diagnosis and treatment of ischemic stroke.*

Pulsinelli WA, Jacewicz M, Buchan AM: Hypoxic-ischemic disorders in stroke. In Johnston MD, McDonald R, Young AB (eds.): Scientific Basis of Neurologic Drug Therapy. Philadelphia, FA Davis, 1992. *Contemporary review of the pharmacologic treatment of ischemic stroke.*

Recommendations on Stroke Prevention, Diagnosis, and Therapy: Special Report from the World Health Organization. Stroke 20:1407, 1989. *A contemporary review of stroke risk factors and their prevention.*

Sandercock P: Recent developments in the diagnosis and management of patients with transient ischemic attacks and minor ischemic strokes. Q J Med 78:101, 1991. *A review of current diagnosis and management of transient ischemic attacks and stroke.*

Stroke Prevention in Atrial Fibrillation Study: Preliminary report of the Stroke Prevention in Atrial Fibrillation Study. N Engl J Med 322:863, 1990. *Preliminary report of a multi-institutional study emphasizing the importance of warfarin or, at least in the nonelderly, aspirin to prevent stroke in atrial fibrillation.*

470 Hemorrhagic Cerebrovascular Disease

Approximately 20 per cent of all strokes consist of intracranial hemorrhages, half into the subarachnoid space and the remainder within the brain itself. The acute rise in intracranial pressure

1. Arterial aneurysms
   a. "Berry" aneurysm
   b. Fusiform aneurysm
   c. Mycotic aneurysm
   d. Aneurysm with vasculitis
2. Cerebrovascular malformations
3. Hypertensive-atherosclerotic hemorrhage
4. Hemorrhage into brain tumor
5. Systemic bleeding diatheses
6. Hemorrhage with vasculopathies
7. Hemorrhage with intracranial venous infarction

from arterial rupture causes loss of consciousness in approximately half the patients, and many of these die of cerebral herniation (see Ch. 443). However, since hemorrhage into the subarachnoid space or brain parenchyma causes less tissue injury than does ischemia, patients who survive often show a remarkable recovery.

Like ischemic stroke, hemorrhagic stroke can be thought of as diffuse (subarachnoid and/or intraventricular) or focal (intraparenchymal). Subarachnoid hemorrhage (SAH) is caused by rupture of surface arteries (aneurysms, vascular malformations, head trauma), with blood usually limited to the cerebrospinal fluid (CSF) space between the pial and arachnoid membranes (Table 470–1). Intracerebral hemorrhage is most frequently caused by the rupture of arteries lying deeply within the brain substance (hypertensive hemorrhage, vascular malformations, head trauma), but in some instances the force of blood from ruptured surface arteries may penetrate the brain parenchyma. Blood within the cerebral ventricles results either from reflux of subarachnoid blood through the fourth ventricular foramina or by extension from a site of intraparenchymal hemorrhage.

470.1 ANEURYSMAL SUBARACHNOID HEMORRHAGE

EPIDEMIOLOGY

Rupture of a saccular or "berry" aneurysm causes approximately 80 per cent of all SAH's, 5 per cent are caused by mycotic aneurysm rupture, and an even smaller percentage reflects bleeding from atherosclerotic, neoplastic, or dissecting cerebral aneurysms. The incidence of aneurysmal SAH is approximately 10 per 100,000 population, with 80 per cent of these occurring in persons 40 to 65 years old, 15 per cent in those 20 to 40 years old, and 5 per cent in those below 20 years of age. Women are slightly more likely than men (3:2) to suffer rupture of a cerebral aneurysm, especially during pregnancy.

ETIOLOGY AND PATHOGENESIS

SACCULAR ANEURYSMS. The pathogenesis of saccular aneurysms reflects a combination of congenital, acquired, and hereditary factors. Congenital defects in the muscle and elastic tissue of the arterial media, seen at autopsy in 80 per cent of normal vessels of the circle of Willis, gradually deteriorate as they are exposed over time to the hemodynamic stresses of pulsatile blood flow. These defects lead to microaneurysmal dilatations (<2 mm) of the circle of Willis arteries in 15 to 20 per cent of the population. Larger (>5 mm) aneurysms are found in 5 per cent of the population. These larger, potentially symptomatic saccular aneurysms are characteristically distributed at the arterial bifurcations, 80 per cent being located in the anterior, carotid artery–derived, arterial circulation and the rest lying along the bifurcation of the vertebrobasilar arteries (Fig. 470–1).

The remarkably high incidence of wall defects in the media of normal vessels, the high frequency of incidental microaneurysms, and the tendency for aneurysms to enlarge with time and rupture when they exceed 1 cm in diameter imply that both congenital and acquired factors influence the pathogenesis of rupture. On the other hand, the relative rarity of SAH suggests that other factors, possibly genetic, may predispose to aneurysm formation. A modest incidence of familial saccular aneurysms as well as their

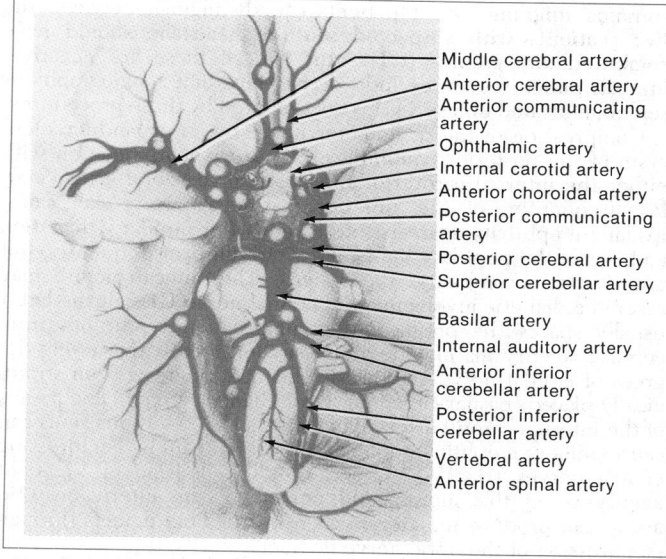

FIGURE 470–1. The common sites for berry aneurysms to develop at the bifurcation of arteries on the undersurface of the brain.

association with polycystic kidney disease, Ehlers-Danlos syndrome, and other connective tissue disorders implicates hereditary factors. Although hypertension per se is not a significant risk factor for aneurysmal SAH, aneurysms have been known to rupture under conditions associated with a sudden rise in blood pressure, including extremes of emotional excitement and physical exertion such as coitus and athletic events.

FUSIFORM ANEURYSMS. Fusiform or ectatic aneurysms acquire their name from the spindle-shaped dilatation and elongation that occur in large arteries at the site of arteriosclerotic narrowing. These aneurysms develop most frequently in the basilar artery but may also affect the internal, middle, and anterior cerebral arteries of individuals with widespread arteriosclerosis and hypertension. They rarely rupture and are difficult to treat when they do because their shape and stiff walls preclude easy surgical clipping. Progressive dilatation and the tortuous elongation of the vessel cause neurologic dysfunction most frequently by compressing surrounding structures. Typically, ectatic aneurysms of the basilar artery compress cranial nerves V, VII, and VIII, causing facial pain, hemifacial spasm, and hearing loss with vertigo, respectively. Fusiform aneurysms may imitate the features of cerebellopontine angle tumors, or they may mimic pituitary and suprasellar mass lesions. The underlying arteriosclerotic disease may cause ischemic stroke either through occlusion of the vessel or by producing cerebral embolism from a clot formed within the aneurysm. Rarely, ectasia of the basilar artery causes communicating hydrocephalus by interfering with normal CSF outflow at the level of the third ventricle.

MYCOTIC ANEURYSMS. Mycotic cerebral aneurysms are caused by septic degeneration of arterial wall muscle and elastic tissue. In contrast to saccular and fusiform aneurysms, which are located primarily in large arteries at the base of the brain, mycotic aneurysms form in more distal cerebral arteries at the point where small septic cardiogenic emboli lodge. They are frequently multiple and can be found in either the anterior or the posterior cerebral circulation.

CLINICAL PRESENTATION

Prodromal signs and symptoms caused by compression of surrounding brain structures, by warning or "sentinel" leaks, or by embolization of the aneurysmal clot to distal arteries frequently precede the catastrophic rupture of saccular aneurysms. Focal headaches may signal compression of pain-sensitive structures from an expanding aneurysm, in which case the headache is usually progressive, or by "sentinel" leaks that cause sudden, focal head pain. Such sentinel headaches are frequently severe and may be accompanied by nausea or vomiting or may cause meningeal irritation. Despite the similarity of these headaches to common migraine, most patients can distinguish between the two. Patients with suspected sentinel headache should have computed tomographic (CT) scans and, if these are negative, lumbar punctures to exclude active bleeding; angiography is seldom indicated unless SAH is documented by these procedures.

Compression of the oculomotor nerve by an expanding aneurysm of the posterior communicating artery at its junction with either the internal carotid or the posterior cerebral artery and, less frequently, of the superior cerebellar artery can cause ipsilateral ophthalmoparesis, ptosis, and later pupillary dilatation and loss of the pupillary light reflex. Orbital pain frequently, but not always, accompanies these signs. The clinical picture may resemble diabetic involvement of cranial nerve III, but the latter usually spares the pupil. Other compression syndromes from cerebral aneurysms include amnesia combined with varying degrees of cranial nerve III paresis and quadriparesis from strategically placed, basilar-tip aneurysms. Giant (>2.5 cm) aneurysms of the internal carotid artery lying within the cavernous sinus can cause unilateral ophthalmoplegia and orbital pain by compressing cranial nerves III, IV, VI, and the first division of V. Giant aneurysms of the supraclinoid portion of the internal carotid artery can produce unilateral vision loss or field defects through compression of the optic nerve or tracts.

Rupture of saccular aneurysms into the subarachnoid space seldom is associated with focal signs or symptoms. Nearly half of patients so affected lose consciousness, at least transiently, as intracranial pressure exceeds cerebral perfusion pressure. Approximately 10 per cent of patients remain in coma for several days, depending upon the location of the aneurysm and the amount of bleeding. Patients who remain conscious and those who awaken from coma commonly recall the sudden onset as producing the "most excruciating headache" of their life. Rupture of an intracranial aneurysm in the absence of headache is rare, and some reported cases probably reflect amnesia for the event.

In addition to the frequent change in the level of consciousness, acute SAH causes meningeal irritation, nuchal rigidity, and photophobia, symptoms that may require several hours to develop. Subhyaloid retinal hemorrhages occur in 20 to 30 per cent of patients as a result of increased intracranial pressure, raised retinal venous pressure, and dissection of blood along the optic nerve sheath. Blood pressure is frequently elevated, and body temperature usually rises, particularly during the early days after bleeding as blood products produce a chemical meningitis. Focal neurologic dysfunction is not a prominent feature of SAH unless there is associated compression by the aneurysm of surrounding brain structures, the jet of blood dissects directly into a clinically relevant brain region, or vasospasm occurs as a complication (see below).

LABORATORY EXAMINATION

Serum electrolytes should be measured at the time of admission to serve as a baseline for detecting later hyponatremia. A complete blood count, including platelets and clotting times, should be obtained to evaluate possible infection or hematologic or clotting abnormalities. The electrocardiogram (ECG) may show various abnormalities, including heightened T waves, shortened PR intervals, peaked or inverted T waves, and increased U waves. These ECG abnormalities and subsequent arrhythmias have been attributed to multifocal myocardial necrosis caused by elevated levels of circulating catecholamines.

CT scans reveal subarachnoid blood within the basal cisterns in about three quarters of patients within 48 hours of bleeding. Magnetic resonance (MR) images have a lower index of accuracy. Detection of intracranial blood on the CT scan, however, becomes more difficult with time as blood and its breakdown products become isodense. Blood localized to the basal cisterns, the sylvian fissure, or the intrahemispheric fissure more frequently indicates rupture of a saccular aneurysm, while blood lying over the convexities or within the superficial parenchyma of the brain is more consistent with either the rupture of an arteriovenous malformation or a mycotic aneurysm. The amount and location of blood within the subarachnoid space relate directly to an aneurysm's location and the likelihood of subsequent vasospasm. Importantly, an early CT scan also allows a baseline evaluation

of ventricular size to compare against later hydrocephalus caused by hemogenic obstruction of CSF outflow pathways. A contrast-enhanced CT scan may aid in the identification of an arteriovenous malformation and some large (>1.0 cm) aneurysms but should be obtained only after a noncontrast study has been completed, since contrast agents may obscure detection of subarachnoid blood.

If the CT scan fails to show blood, a lumbar puncture is diagnostic. To avoid puncture of the venous plexus lying on the anterior wall of the spinal canal, the spinal needle should be advanced slowly, with frequent removal of the trocar to detect first entry of the subarachnoid space. A traumatic lumbar puncture usually can be distinguished from SAH by the failure of the latter to show a decrease in the red blood cell (RBC) count between the first and last tubes of CSF (Table 470–2). In addition, in the presence of bloody fluid, one of the CSF samples should be centrifuged immediately and the supernate examined for the presence of xanthochromia by visual inspection and testing the fluid with a benzidene (Hemoccult) stick. Red blood cells in the spinal canal begin to lyse within 2 to 3 hours, and the centrifuged supernate will then appear pink. Later (10 hours) as the hemoglobin is converted to bilirubin, the fluid develops a yellow tinge (xanthochromia). The CSF pressure is usually elevated and may remain so for many days. Spinal fluid samples taken within the first 24 hours often show a white blood cell (WBC) count consistent with the normal circulating WBC-RBC ratio (ca. 1:1000); later samples contain increased polymorphonuclear and mononuclear cells secondary to chemical meningitis caused by breakdown products of subarachnoid blood. The CSF blood glucose level is usually normal early, but as chemical meningitis develops, the level may decrease, but rarely to less than 40 mg per deciliter. The protein content of the CSF is usually elevated, consistent with contamination by blood (1 mg per deciliter of protein for every 1000 RBC's).

Cerebral angiography remains the definitive study to detect the source of SAH. In instances in which the diagnosis of aneurysmal SAH is certain, the timing and need for a cerebral angiogram should be determined by surgical considerations (see below). When diagnostic doubt exists, the angiogram should be performed immediately. Since as many as one third of patients with aneurysmal SAH harbor multiple cerebral aneurysms, both carotid and both vertebral arteries should be examined. It is interesting that among patients with multiple cerebral aneurysms, almost half have identically placed aneurysms in the left and right circulation, so-called mirror aneurysms. Cerebral angiography fails to detect the source of bleeding in 10 to 20 per cent of cases. Such patients are thought to have a better prognosis, with only a 1 to 2 per cent chance of recurrent SAH. Failure to detect the source of bleeding may result from obliteration of an aneurysm through clotting; because bleeding was caused by rupture of a small, superficial venous angioma; or when hemorrhage has occurred from a spinal cord aneurysm or arteriovenous malformation (AVM). The presence of back pain or spinal cord symptoms at onset should prompt a search for a spinal source of hemorrhage. Repeat cerebral angiography is indicated 3 to 4 weeks later when the initial angiogram is negative and no other clues to the bleeding site can be found.

Cerebral angiography is recommended immediately in patients who have septic endocarditis and SAH to search for possible mycotic aneurysms. Since 25 per cent of patients with subacute bacterial endocarditis and evidence of systemic embolism harbor one or more cerebral mycotic aneurysms, they should also undergo cerebral angiography.

LATE MEDICAL AND NEUROLOGIC COMPLICATIONS

The medical complications of SAH include cardiac myonecrosis and arrhythmias attributed to abnormal levels of circulating

TABLE 470–2. "TRAUMATIC TAP" OR SUBARACHNOID HEMORRHAGE?

	"Traumatic Tap"	Spontaneous Subarachnoid Bleed
Xanthochromia	Absent	Onset: 4–6 hr Duration: approximately 6 wk
Red cell count (serial tubes)	Decreasing	Constant
Blood clot formation	Rapid	Slower

epinephrine. Symptomatic hyponatremia may also develop from the inappropriate secretion of antidiuretic hormone.

Late neurologic complications include *rebleeding* from the same aneurysm, cerebral *vasospasm* and its ischemic consequences, *hydrocephalus* caused by blockage of CSF outflow pathways, and occasionally *seizures*. Aneurysmal rerupture is suggested by new headache or neurologic worsening but can be diagnosed firmly only if a repeat CT scan or lumbar puncture shows the presence of new blood in the subarachnoid space. Approximately one third of patients with aneurysmal SAH rebleed during the first month, the incidence being highest during the first 2 weeks after the initial bleed. Patients with an unclipped aneurysm who survive their initial bleed for more than 1 month have a 2 to 3 per cent yearly risk of rebleeding.

Cerebral vasospasm as diagnosed by cerebral angiography is defined as an abnormal narrowing of cerebral arteries. Vasospasm has been reported in up to 75 per cent of patients with SAH, half of whom develop strokelike neurologic signs and symptoms. The peak onset for cerebral vasospasm is between days 3 and 14, but the complication can develop as late as 3 weeks after SAH. Arteries forming the circle of Willis and their major branches are the initial site of involvement, with more distal arteries becoming involved later. The amount and location of blood detected within the basal cisterns on CT scans correlate with the incidence and location of cerebral vasospasm.

The molecular mechanisms causing cerebral vasospasm are unknown but probably involve release of vasoactive amines and polypeptides, which pathologically influence vascular smooth muscle contraction. Vasospastic vessels show medial necrosis within the first few weeks, and later medial atrophy, subendothelial fibrosis, and intimal thickening.

Communicating hydrocephalus may develop as early as the first or second week after SAH. Patients with more extensive bleeding are more likely to develop the complication, but its incidence correlates with the amount of blood on CT images less clearly than does the development of vasospasm. Red blood cells and their breakdown products cause hydrocephalus by obstruction of CSF outflow pathways both at the level of the fourth ventricle and through the pacchionian granulations lining the venous sinuses. Seldom communicating hydrocephalus require surgical treatment early after SAH.

Seizures are infrequent but can complicate SAH. The presence of seizures usually signals cortical damage either from bleeding into the neocortex or from ischemic necrosis.

TREATMENT

SACCULAR ANEURYSMS. The definitive therapy for a ruptured saccular aneurysm consists of surgical clipping of the aneurysm to prevent rebleeding. Medical therapy aims to reduce the risk of rebleeding and cerebral vasospasm and to prevent other medical complications before and after surgical intervention. Patients should be kept quiet at bed rest, with the administration of appropriate analgesics for the treatment of headache and gentle sedation. Stool softeners minimize straining with subsequently increased intracranial pressure. Hypertension should be treated, but not aggressively, since some of the elevated pressure may represent normal compensatory mechanisms to maintain cerebral perfusion pressure in the face of increased intracranial pressure or cerebral arterial narrowing. Systolic pressures in the range of 160 to 170 mm Hg and diastolic pressures in the range of 90 to 100 mm Hg are acceptable. The voltage-regulated calcium channel antagonist nimodipine should be given orally in a dosage of 60 mg every 4 hours for 21 days. Although it does not reduce the frequency of vasospasm, nimodipine lowers by one third the incidence of cerebral infarction in patients suffering SAH and cerebral vasospasm.

The effects of cerebral vasospasm can also be partly overcome by raising cerebral perfusion pressure through plasma volume expansion and pressor agents, usually phenylephrine or dopamine. Such measures, however, may raise the risk of rebleeding and should be undertaken only in patients with surgically clipped saccular aneurysms.

Efforts to reduce the incidence of rebleeding with ε-aminocaproic acid, an inhibitor of fibrinolysis, have been successful. Such therapy is not recommended for routine use, since it increases the incidence of vasospasm, cerebral infarction, and subsequent hydrocephalus.

TABLE 470–3. HUNT CLASSIFICATION OF PATIENT'S CONDITION

Grade	Condition
0	Unruptured aneurysm
1	Asymptomatic or minimal headache and slight nuchal rigidity
1A	No acute meningeal or brain reaction but with fixed neurologic deficit
2	Moderate to severe headache, nuchal rigidity; no neurologic deficit other than cranial nerve palsy
3	Drowsiness, confusion, or mild focal deficit
4	Stupor, moderate to severe hemiparesis, possible early decerebrate rigidity and vegetative disturbances
5	Deep coma, decerebrate rigidity, and moribund appearance

The optimal time to clip a ruptured saccular aneurysm remains controversial. An increasingly accepted approach is to operate either within the first 3 days or after days 10 to 14. The logic relates to the timing of intrinsic rebleeding and the onset of cerebral vasospasm. Since the incidence of aneurysmal rebleeding is highest during the first 2 weeks after SAH and the mortality associated with each bleed approaches 40 to 50 percent, the aneurysm should be clipped as soon as possible. Nevertheless, undertaking aneurysmal surgery in the presence of active vasospasm has been associated consistently with poor neurologic outcomes. As a result, most surgeons avoid operating during days 3 to 10, when maximal cerebral vasospasm is likely. Patients in Hunt's grade 1 to 3 (Table 470–3) should, if possible, have their aneurysms clipped prior to 3 days if the cerebral angiogram shows little or no evidence of cerebral vasospasm. In patients whose aneurysm is clipped early, preliminary studies suggest that lysing blood clots in the basal cisterns with locally applied fibrinolytic drugs, followed by washing the blood out, may reduce subsequent vasospasm. Aneurysmal clipping should be delayed until 10 to 14 days after the last documented SAH in patients who present to hospital later than 3 days, who have active vasospasm on early cerebral angiograms, or who fall initially into a poor clinical grade (Hunt 4 and 5). In instances of delayed surgical intervention, most authorities recommend repeating the cerebral angiogram prior to surgery to rule out the continued presence of vasospasm. Some neurosurgeons also recommend postoperative angiograms to verify proper clip placement and obliteration of the aneurysm.

MYCOTIC ANEURYSMS. Unruptured mycotic aneurysms should be treated with antibiotics appropriate for the infecting organism and followed angiographically. Single aneurysms and those in surgically accessible areas should be considered for prompt surgical clipping.

PROGNOSIS

The mortality rate from aneurysmal SAH is 50 to 60 per cent after 1 year. Almost half such patients die before reaching the hospital, and most of the remaining die during the first month. An equally high mortality accompanies each episode of rebleeding. Approximately 25 per cent of survivors have persistent neurologic deficits.

Unruptured cerebral aneurysms detected incidentally during cerebral angiography bleed at a yearly rate of 1 to 3 per cent. Aneurysm size is strongly associated with the likelihood of rupture, so that saccular aneurysms less than 5 mm should be followed carefully, aneurysms between 5 and 10 mm may be considered for surgical clipping, and those greater than 10 mm should be clipped at the earliest convenience. The experience of the surgical team critically affects decisions and outcome concerning such treatment.

470.2 HEMORRHAGE FROM VASCULAR MALFORMATIONS

CLASSIFICATION AND EPIDEMIOLOGY

Congenital vascular malformations of the brain and spinal cord fall into five categories according to vessel size and type. *Venous angiomas*, the most common cerebrovascular malformations, are composed entirely of veins and usually lie close to the brain's surface. Hemorrhage from a venous angioma is uncommon and rarely fatal. Nevertheless, these lesions have gained considerable attention, since they are readily detected by CT scans. They seldom produce seizures and headaches. A cerebral *varix* is a single dilated vein and very rarely causes clinical symptoms.

Telangiectasias are uncommon vascular anomalies composed of tangles of small, capillary-like vessels. They are usually located deep in the brain (diencephalon, brain stem, cerebellum) and rarely produce symptoms. Because of their strategic location, hemorrhage from these small vessels can occasionally be fatal.

Cavernous angiomas are large sinusoidal channels served by large feeding arteries and veins. Many of the channels thrombose, and the remainder have very low blood flow, which makes their visualization on angiograms difficult. They are readily detected by CT scan and rarely bleed, but they may cause headaches and seizures.

The most common symptomatic vascular anomaly is the *arteriovenous malformation* (AVM). AVM's are composed of tangles of arteries connected directly to veins without intervening capillaries. The resulting vessels are thin walled owing to poorly developed elastic and muscle tissue within the media. The large arteries, which feed the AVM, usually show hypertrophy of the media and thickening of the endothelium. Brain tissue is usually absent from the AVM but when present is nonfunctional. AVM's can be located anywhere in the brain and can produce headaches, seizures, focal neurologic deficits, or intracranial hemorrhage. Intracranial hemorrhage from vascular malformations accounts for 1 per cent of all strokes and 10 per cent of all SAH's. The prevalence of AVM's among the general population is uncertain, but autopsy studies of unselected patients indicate that 4 to 5 per cent harbor some form of vascular malformation, of which only 10 to 15 per cent produce symptoms. Familial cases of AVM's are rare, indicating that the problem reflects sporadic abnormalities in embryologic development.

CLINICAL PRESENTATION

Most AVM's manifest with intracranial hemorrhage, a lower proportion causing seizures or progressive neurologic disability as first symptoms. The initial hemorrhage tends to occur during the second through fourth decades, with the risk of rebleeding averaging approximately 6 to 7 per cent the first year, 2 per cent after 5 years, and 1 to 2 per cent thereafter. The decline in the incidence of rebleeding with time may reflect the spontaneous thrombosis of arterial feeders. The initial and subsequent hemorrhages are associated with a 10 per cent chance of death. If the rebleed rate of 1 to 2 per cent is maintained for life, the young individual who presents with a hemorrhagic AVM faces a 50 to 60 per cent chance of an incapacitating or fatal repeat hemorrhage during a normal lifespan.

AVM's may bleed into the subarachnoid space, into the brain parenchyma, or into the ventricular system. Focal neurologic signs and symptoms depend upon the severity of the bleed and the extent to which brain parenchyma has been destroyed. Bleeding into the subarachnoid space is usually less severe than with saccular aneurysms, and blood tends to localize over the cerebral convexities rather than in the basal cisterns. The incidence of cerebral vasospasm with AVM hemorrhage appears less than for aneurysm SAH, perhaps because less blood accumulates around the large arteries at the base of the brain. No explanation has been provided for the observation that small AVM's (<2.5 cm) tend to bleed more frequently than do large AVM's (>5 cm).

Approximately one third of patients who harbor an AVM present with seizures, of which about half have a focal onset. Focal neurologic deficits independent of seizures also develop, resulting from vascular thrombosis and brain tissue hypoperfusion caused by either vascular compression or a "steal" syndrome. Shunting of blood through arteriovenous fistulas may draw blood away from normal brain tissue, causing hypoperfusion and dysfunction of the brain proximal to the AVM. With treatment of the AVM, either through surgical resection or by embolization of the feeding arteries, some of these focal neurologic signs may improve or disappear. Approximately 10 per cent of patients with AVM's have a history of headache, the location of which seldom

coincides with the site of the AVM. Some AVM-associated headaches closely resemble migraine, but unlike migraine, most AVM-associated headaches rarely alternate between the two sides of the head.

LABORATORY EXAMINATION

The laboratory evaluation for intracranial hemorrhage from an AVM is similar to that described for aneurysmal SAH. A CT scan with contrast is diagnostic in approximately 85 per cent of patients. MR images are equally, if not more, effective in diagnosis. Angiography remains the definitive test to identify the AVM and delineate its feeding arteries and draining veins. Since approximately 10 per cent of AVM's are associated with saccular aneurysms, four-vessel angiography is indicated even if the AVM is defined by unilateral carotid injection. In addition, extracranial or contralateral arteries occasionally supply intracranial AVM's and should be considered in the angiographic evaluation.

TREATMENT

Uncertainties concerning the natural history of unruptured AVM's, as well as the efficacy and complications associated with newer forms of interventional therapy, make it difficult to define a simple set of guiding therapeutic principles. Generally speaking, unruptured AVM's that manifest with either seizures or headache may be treated conservatively, especially in patients older than 55 to 60 years. In such patients, hypertension should be controlled, platelet antiaggregating agents and anticoagulants avoided, and anticonvulsants given to control the seizures.

Interventional therapeutic options include surgical resection of the AVM, embolization of the feeding arteries, or radiation-induced thrombosis. Various considerations, including age, the degree of neurologic dysfunction, and location of the AVM, must be considered when choosing treatment. The present custom is to treat younger patients (<55 years) more aggressively, resecting surgically accessible AVM's, since removal of the AVM and *all* its arterial feeders is curative. In older patients or if the AVM lies in language-vulnerable areas or deep in the brain, use of focused gamma x-rays or proton beam radiation is safer but only effective in lesions less than 3 cm in diameter. Embolization of the feeding arteries is rarely recommended as the sole interventional therapy, since such an approach totally obliterates the arterial feeders in only about 40 per cent of cases. Arterial embolization is frequently used in conjunction with either surgery or focused radiation therapy.

470.3 FOCAL CEREBRAL HEMORRHAGE

Focal hemorrhage occurs spontaneously in three common settings: hypertension, ruptured AVM's, and amyloid (or congophilic) angiopathy. Additional contributing causes are excessive anticoagulation, systemic bleeding diatheses, and trauma.

EPIDEMIOLOGY

In the United States, primary intracerebral hemorrhage occurs with an incidence of about 12 per 100,000 population, a rate similar to that for SAH but only 10 per cent that for ischemic stroke. Age-adjusted rates for men are about 50 per cent higher than for women, and rates for blacks are over twice those for whites. As with ischemic stroke, the incidence appears to be declining; excluding hemorrhage associated with anticoagulation, the rate in Rochester, Minnesota, fell from about 15 per 100,000 in 1945 to 5 per 100,000 in the early 1970's. Hypertension has declined in frequency during the same period, but no conclusive data link the two trends.

PATHOLOGY

The pathologic picture of primary intracerebral hemorrhage typically consists of a large confluent area of blood that clots and then weeks later begins slowly to be phagocytosed; after several months, the only residuum may be a small, collapsed cavity lined by hemosiderin-containing macrophages. Although hemorrhages may destroy brain tissue locally, histologic examination suggests that displacement of normal brain tissue and dissection along fiber tracts account for much of the pathology. Consequently, hemorrhage may be less destructive of brain tissue than is ischemic infarction.

In hypertensive persons at least, active bleeding probably occurs over a very short time; radiolabeled red cells injected intravenously in patients more than 2 hours after initial symptoms do not appear to leak into brain. This observation suggests that the source of bleeding is rapidly compressed, in part by extravascular blood, and that delayed clinical worsening in patients with primary hemorrhage is related to mechanisms such as brain swelling and not to continued bleeding.

PATHOGENESIS

Hypertension can produce hemorrhages throughout the brain, but usually they occur in four locations: external capsule-putamen, internal capsule-thalamus, central pons, and cerebellum (Fig. 470–2). A smaller number arise throughout the subcortical white matter. Bleeding in such instances is believed to result from rupture of microaneurysms in small, intracerebral arteries (50 to 150 μm in diameter). The pathology of the microaneurysms includes replacement of normal lining endothelium, media, and elastic tissue with fibrous tissue and fat. Similar changes can lead to necrotic vascular degeneration, which, along with microaneurysms, predisposes to hemorrhage. A strong relationship links microaneurysms to hypertension; in one autopsy series, microaneurysms were found in 46 of 100 hypertensive brains and in 85 per cent of hypertensive persons with hemorrhages, but in only 7 of 100 normotensive brains.

Amyloid (or congophilic) angiopathy is a pathologic diagnosis, increasingly encountered in the elderly. Unrelated to generalized amyloidosis and occasionally hereditary, the condition often appears in the brains of patients with Alzheimer's disease and has been associated with nonhypertensive hemorrhage. It is rare in patients under age 55. Amyloid deposits, chemically related to those in Alzheimer plaques, are seen in the media and adventitia of medium- and small-sized arteries. In contrast to hypertensive hemorrhages, bleeding in amyloid angiopathy most often occurs in the lobar subcortical white matter (Fig. 470–2). Multiple small hemorrhages may be associated with the condition.

Anticoagulation, fibrinolysis, and other hematologic abnormalities can be associated with intracerebral hemorrhages. Warfarin anticoagulation has been implicated in about 10 per cent of primary intracerebral hemorrhages. With the less aggressive programs of low-dose warfarin anticoagulation (target prothrombin time ratio of 1.2 to 1.5) now used for peripheral venous disease and to prevent arterial embolism, the rate of intracranial bleeding in one recent study had fallen to under 1 per cent with 2 years of treatment. Data from large-scale studies of fibrinolysis (e.g., tissue plasminogen activator, t-PA) in acute myocardial infarction indicate that at a total t-PA dose no greater than 100 mg, the rate of symptomatic intracerebral hemorrhage is only about 0.5 per cent (although in one small series, it was 5 per cent); at higher doses of 150 mg, the rate rises to about 1.5 per cent. Cerebral hemorrhages occur in *leukemia, polycythemia, hemophilia,* and other clotting abnormalities, and they also occur in patients using *amphetamines* and *cocaine*.

Although *trauma* causes intracerebral (as well as subarachnoid) hemorrhage, the diagnosis is usually aided by the history as well as by coexistent external signs of trauma, SAH, and, on CT scan, multifocal, inhomogeneous hemorrhages and areas of decreased density (see Ch. 487).

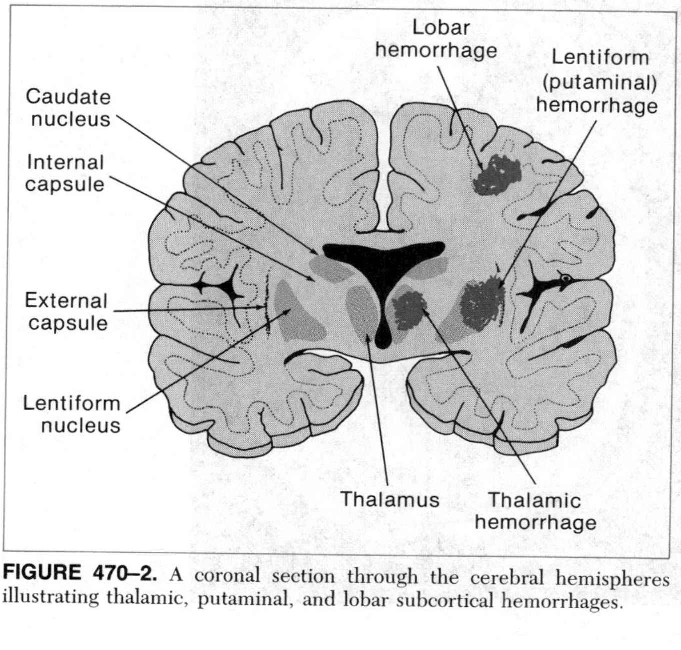

FIGURE 470–2. A coronal section through the cerebral hemispheres illustrating thalamic, putaminal, and lobar subcortical hemorrhages.

CLINICAL PRESENTATION

Large cerebral hemorrhages usually produce catastrophic, acute syndromes. The onset is often associated with physical (or emotional) activity; onset during sleep is rare. Common early features include alterations in consciousness, headache, nausea, and vomiting. Although uncommon, seizures occur, possibly reflecting cortical irritation by blood. With the increasing ability to recognize less dramatic hemorrhages by using CT and MRI, neurologists now realize that hemorrhages can also produce less severe dysfunction that may be indistinguishable clinically from ischemic stroke. Clinical evolution over hours is common and usually attributed to secondary brain swelling.

The clinician should be able to recognize common hemorrhagic syndromes (Table 470–4) to anticipate dangerous brain swelling and provide appropriate medical and supportive management. Hypertensive hemorrhages typically occur deep within the cerebral (or cerebellar) hemispheres, producing several well-described syndromes. In the following paragraphs, percentages indicate the approximate contribution of each specific syndrome to all primary intracerebral hemorrhages.

PUTAMINAL HEMORRHAGE (35 TO 50 PER CENT). Patients with massive putaminal hemorrhages (Fig. 470–3) become lethargic or comatose within minutes to hours of onset and concurrently develop contralateral weakness (including face) and a contralateral hemianopsia and gaze paresis (with eyes deviated toward the hemorrhage). For unknown reasons, some patients develop an ipsilateral gaze palsy (with the eyes deviated toward the paretic limbs). Brain stem reflexes remain intact, and the gaze paresis can be overcome with oculovestibular stimulation. A contralateral sensory deficit is often detectable. Pupillary size may be normal initially, but as the upper brain stem is compressed, pupils first constrict and then dilate, and limb posturing develops. Although some patients display their maximal deficit at onset, the majority progress over the first several hours.

THALAMIC HEMORRHAGE (10 TO 15 PER CENT). Some patients with thalamic hemorrhages lose consciousness early in the clinical course, but those who are awake often experience contralateral hemiparesis, sensory changes, and homonymous hemianopsia (the last often clearing quickly). A contralateral gaze palsy (as with putaminal hemorrhage) is occasionally present. Some patients develop fixed downward ocular deviation, presumably from compression of the adjacent midbrain tectum. Pupillary reactions to light are usually preserved, although pupils are often small, reflecting hypothalamic sympathetic disturbances.

PONTINE HEMORRHAGE (10 TO 15 PER CENT). Traditional teaching held that coma always accompanied the onset of pontine hemorrhage, but refined imaging shows that with smaller hemorrhages this is not always the case. In the comatose patient, small, reactive pupils are common, oculovestibular responses are lost early, and vomiting often occurs at onset. Patients usually have quadriplegia and bilateral extensor posturing. If facial weakness is present, it commonly has characteristics of a lower motor neuron weakness. Ocular bobbing is sometimes reported.

CEREBELLAR HEMORRHAGE (10 TO 30 PER CENT). Because cerebellar hemorrhage initially spares the brain stem, consciousness is usually preserved in the early stages. Occipital headache is usually the first symptom, followed by unsteady gait, clumsiness, nausea, and vomiting, which may be severe and repetitive. Motor weakness is seldom prominent at onset, but with progression and brain stem compression, contralateral hemiparesis and caloric-resistant ipsilateral gaze paresis help to localize the lesion to the posterior fossa. Pupillary reactions are usually

TABLE 470–4. CLINICAL FEATURES OF COMMON HYPERTENSIVE HEMORRHAGES

Clinical	Putaminal	Thalamic	Pontine	Cerebellar
		Site of Hemorrhage		
Unconsciousness	Later	Later	Early	Late
Hemiparesis	Yes	Yes	Quadriparesis	Late
Sensory change	Yes	Yes	Yes	Late
Hemianopic	Yes	Yes	No	No
Pupils:				
Size	Normal	Small	Small	Normal
Reaction	Yes	Yes or no	Yes or no	Yes
Gaze paresis:				
Side	Contralateral Sometimes ipsilateral	Contralateral	Ipsilateral	Ipsilateral
Response to calorics	Yes	Yes	No	Yes or no
Downward eye deviation	No	Yes	No	No
Ocular bobbing	No	No	Sometimes	Sometimes
Gait lost	No	No	Yes	Yes
Vomiting	Occasional	Occasional	Often	Severe

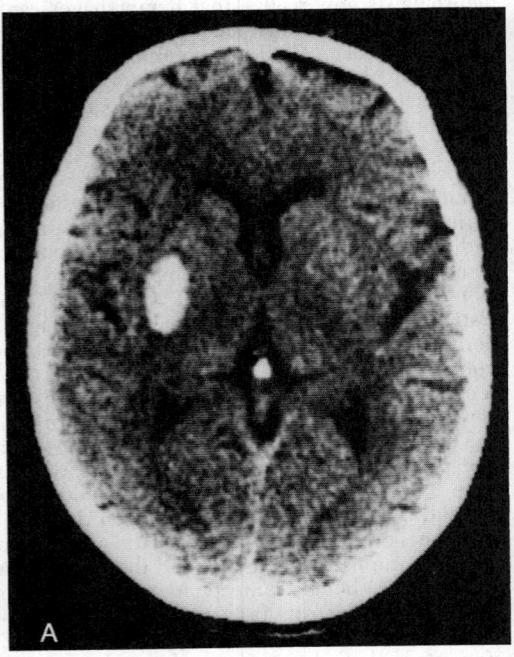

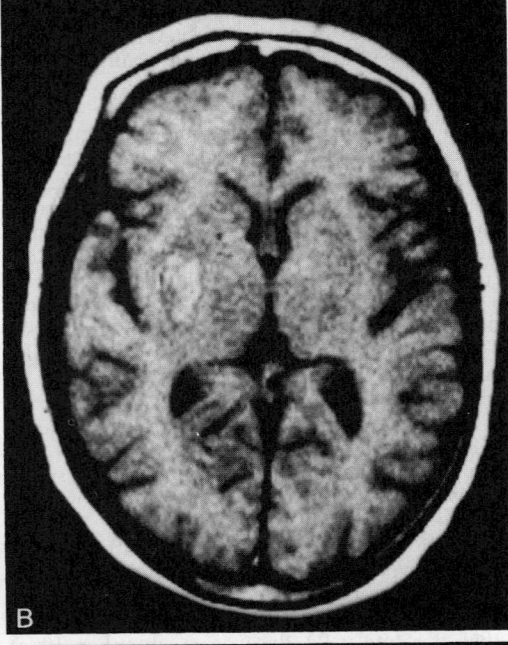

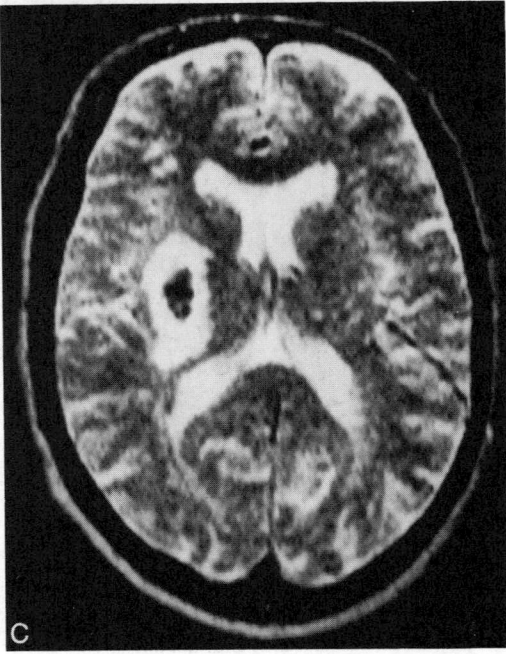

FIGURE 470–3. Hypertensive putaminal hemorrhage shown on CT at 24 hours (*A*), T₁-weighted magnetic resonance image (MRI) at 72 hours (*B*), and T₂-weighted MRI at 72 hours (*C*). Uniform hyperdensity on CT distinguishes primary hemorrhage from hemorrhagic and nonhemorrhagic infarction (compare with Fig. 469–1). The relative, though mild, hyperintensity on the T_1-weighted MRI image distinguishes hemorrhage from the hypointensity of nonhemorrhagic infarction; T_1-weighted MRI scans within 24 hours (not available for this patient) typically display more marked hyperintensity than at 72 hours. The core of the hematoma appears hypointense on the T_2-weighted MRI scan at 72 hours; T_2-weighted MRI scans within 12 hours (not available) typically show hyperintensity of greater degree than do concurrent T_1-weighted images. The rim of hyperintensity in *C* probably represents edema fluid. (Reproduced with permission from Zimmerman RD, Hier L, Snow R, et al.: Acute intracranial hemorrhage: Interval changes on sequential MR scans at 0.5 tesla. AJNR 9:47–57, 1988. © 1988, American Society of Neuroradiology.)

preserved. Further deterioration in arousal can result from several sources: extension into or compression of the brain stem, herniation of cerebellar tissue downward through the foramen magnum or upward across the tentorium, or hydrocephalus caused by obstruction of CSF flow into or out of the fourth ventricle. Prompt recognition and treatment of cerebellar hemorrhage before this stage can be life saving.

LOBAR CEREBRAL HEMORRHAGES. Lobar hemorrhages typically occur with amyloid angiopathy. The clinical presentation depends on the actual location of the hemorrhage, but there are some common features. Most patients are elderly; headache, nausea, and vomiting probably occur with about the same frequency but less intensity as in deep, hypertensive hemorrhages. Coma and seizures are less common, possibly because the bulk of the hemorrhage is in subcortical white matter.

LABORATORY EXAMINATION

Noncontrast CT scans demonstrate areas of hemorrhage as zones of increased density and rule out infarction (Fig. 470–3). Spontaneous hemorrhages typically display homogeneous areas of increased density and a mass effect, whereas hemorrhagic infarctions are characterized by areas of increased density (blood) interspersed with areas of decreased density (infarction). CT does not always distinguish reliably between a primary intraparenchymal hemorrhage and a hematoma resulting from a ruptured aneurysm. Similarly, some primary intracerebral hemorrhages dissect into the ventricular or subarachnoid system, inducing secondary intraventricular hemorrhage or SAH.

The MRI picture of hemorrhage depends on the precise sequence used and the age of the hemorrhage. At present, the advantages and disadvantages of MRI in this condition remain incompletely described, particularly in the early hours after onset. One known advantage of MRI is its ability to detect small hemorrhages, especially in the brain stem. Cerebral angiography is seldom used to evaluate acute hemorrhages, except those attributed to mycotic aneurysm being considered for surgical intervention.

TREATMENT

The management of acute parenchymal hemorrhage is supportive, but vigilance for transtentorial or foramen magnum herniation must be exercised, particularly with cerebellar hemorrhages. Herniation is initially treated with hyperventilation (which takes advantage of the vasoconstricting effect of hypocapnia; see Ch. 468) and osmotic agents (e.g., mannitol), but both of these interventions lose effectiveness with time. Corticosteroids have not been effective in treating brain edema from cerebral hemorrhage, and since they carry added risks (e.g., immunologic compromise, gastrointestinal hemorrhage), they are not advocated.

Direct surgical evacuation of acute spontaneous cerebral hemorrhage seldom is justified, occasional cerebellar hemorrhages providing a possible exception. What few comparative studies are available suggest that acute surgical evacuation of hematomas from the cerebral hemispheres does not substantially improve mortality and considerably increases the risk of severe residual neurologic disability if the patient survives. Cerebellar hemorrhages require surgical attention only if they are followed by signs indicating secondary brain stem compression. In such instances, lateral ventricular shunting appears to produce results as good as or better (fewer neurologic residua) than surgical removal of hematomas. Large lesions greater than 3 cm in diameter that continue to cause brain stem dysfunction after the shunt is placed occasionally benefit from clot evacuation.

As with ischemic strokes, blood pressure should not be lowered precipitously in patients with acute cerebral hemorrhage, since parenchymal blood and edema formation are likely to compress the tissue vascular bed and increase vascular resistance; an abrupt and steep reduction in systemic blood pressure could lower perfusion pressure below the critical threshold, thereby superimposing ischemic on hemorrhagic damage.

PROGNOSIS

The prognosis for patients with intraparenchymal hemorrhage is surprisingly good if they survive the acute illness, but mortality is higher (30 to 40 per cent) than in ischemic stroke (10 to 20 per cent). As with ischemic stroke, recent studies show that about one fifth of patients surviving hemorrhage require institutionalization; in contrast to ischemic stroke, however, most of the remaining survivors achieve a good status or complete recovery. Age and large hemorrhage size are associated with a worse prognosis, and prognosis after extensive brain stem hemorrhage is guarded. In contrast to SAH, the risk of recurrent hemorrhage is relatively low, the exception being that AVM's can rebleed at rates approaching 2 per cent per year within the first several years of the initial bleed.

PROPHYLAXIS

Epidemiologic data strongly suggest that control of hypertension reduces the risk of hypertensive intraparenchymal hemorrhage. Careful control of anticoagulation and avoidance of other agents known to be associated with hemorrhage (e.g., amphetamines) should reduce the risk of hemorrhage. At present, there is no way to control the risk of bleeding from amyloid angiopathy.

470.4 HYPERTENSIVE ENCEPHALOPATHY

Hypertensive encephalopathy is a syndrome that accompanies markedly elevated blood pressures. Clinically, the disorder is characterized by symptoms of increased intracranial pressure (headache, nausea, vomiting, visual blurring) and of focal neurologic dysfunction, along with seizures and progressive stupor and coma. Retinal changes characteristic of severe hypertension are common and often include hemorrhages or papilledema, but arteriolar narrowing may be the only abnormality.

The cause of neurologic dysfunction is not clearly established. One theory, largely discounted, was based on observed retinal vasospasm and hypothesized that similar intracerebral vasospasm caused focal ischemia and resultant neurologic dysfunction. More recent evidence rests on the observation that with severe hypertension the upper limit of cerebral arterial autoregulation is exceeded, and blood flow rises passively with further increases in systemic blood pressure. Coincident with this inability to maintain constant blood flow, progressively higher pressures are transmitted into the capillary system, causing movement of plasma and even some cellular elements from blood into surrounding brain tissue. Resulting local and diffuse edema is postulated to cause the focal and diffuse neurologic changes.

Uremia uncomplicated by hypertension can produce a similar clinical picture, but this is easily excluded by determining the blood urea nitrogen (BUN) or creatinine values. Other complications of hypertension to be considered in the differential diagnosis include hemorrhagic and ischemic stroke, but in these conditions, focal signs predominate, whereas in hypertensive encephalopathy they are accompanied by prominent signs of diffuse dysfunction. Increased intracranial pressure from obstructive hydrocephalus, brain tumor, or subdural hematoma, particularly if pressure is transmitted into the fourth ventricle, can elevate blood pressure and slow the pulse (Cushing's sign). Usually, the absence of retinal changes suggesting chronic hypertension and the presence of signs reflecting the underlying neurologic diagnosis differentiate such neurogenic hypertension from hypertensive encephalopathy.

Hypertensive encephalopathy is a medical emergency. Treatment should be directed to acute, deliberate lowering of blood pressure (e.g., with intravenous nitroprusside), avoiding hypotensive or even normal levels. In most patients with chronic hypertension, the upper and lower limits of autoregulation are shifted upward, and if systemic pressure is lowered below the lower limit of the patient's intrinsic autoregulation (which can rise as high as 120 mm Hg), cerebral ischemia can result. When associated with pregnancy (eclampsia), hypertensive encephalopathy usually responds well to prompt delivery of the fetus. Hypercapnia, by dilating cerebral blood vessels, can exacerbate the effects of hypertensive encephalopathy, and seizures also are associated with further increases in cerebral blood flow and capillary pressure. Both should be avoided by controlled ventilation, when required, and anticonvulsants such as intravenous diazepam, 10 to 20 mg given slowly in repeated doses as needed to control seizures, and followed by phenytoin or carbamazepine.

With prompt treatment, the prospect is excellent for full recovery from the immediate episode. Long-term management requires close supervision of and compliance with an effective antihypertension program.

Biller J, Godersky JC, Adams HP Jr: Management of aneurysmal subarachnoid hemorrhage. Stroke 19:1300, 1988. *A review of practice to 1988, at which time antifibrinolytics, now seldom used, were still advocated and calcium channel blockers were achieving acceptance.*

Brown RD Jr, Wiebers DO, Forbes G, et al.: The natural history of unruptured intracranial arteriovenous malformations. J Neurosurg 68:352, 1988. *A follow-up study of 168 patients to define the natural history of clinically unruptured intracranial AVM's.*

Dias MS, Sekhar LN: Intracranial hemorrhage from aneurysms and arteriovenous malformations during pregnancy and the puerperium. Neurosurgery 27:855, 1991. *A review article discussing the risks and medical and surgical management of intracerebral hemorrhage in pregnant women.*

Gilbert JJ, Vinters HV: Cerebral amyloid angiopathy: Incidence and complications in the aging brain. I. Cerebral hemorrhage. Stroke 14:915, 1983. *Eleven patients with fatal cerebral hemorrhage and amyloid angiopathy.*

Juvela S, Heiskanen O, Potanen A, et al.: The treatment of spontaneous intracerebral hemorrhage: A prospective randomized trial of surgical and conservative treatment. J Neurosurg 70:755, 1989. *A randomized trial of 52 patients with brain hemorrhage showing that while surgery saves lives, it does not improve function.*

Kassell NF, Torner JC, Haley EC, et al.: The International Cooperative Study on the timing of aneurysm surgery. Part I: Overall management results. J Neurosurg 73:18, 1990. *This manuscript summarizes the results of the International Cooperative Study on saccular aneurysms and documents the status of medical management in the 1980's.*

Kassell NF, Torner JC, Jane JA, et al.: The International Cooperative Study on the timing of aneurysm surgery. Part 2: Surgical results. J Neurosurg 73:37, 1990. *This manuscript describes 3521 patients with ruptured saccular aneurysms who came from 68 centers. It presents a contemporary discussion of the diagnosis of SAH, prevention of rebleeding, vasospasm, and early versus late surgical intervention.*

Mendelow AD: Spontaneous intracerebral hemorrhage. J Neurol Neurosurg Psychiatry 54:193, 1991. *An editorial reviewing current diagnosis and management of intracerebral hemorrhage.*

Vermeulen M, van Gijn J: The diagnosis of subarachnoid haemorrhage. J Neurol Neurosurg Psychiatry 53:365, 1990. *A review justifying the use of CT instead of lumbar puncture to diagnose SAH and the interpretation of CSF in patients with a negative CT.*

SECTION EIGHT / INFECTIONS AND INFLAMMATORY DISORDERS OF THE NERVOUS SYSTEM

Roger P. Simon

471 Parameningeal Infections

Parameningeal central nervous system infections include those that affect brain parenchyma directly (brain abscess), those that produce suppuration in potential spaces covering the brain and spinal cord (epidural abscess and subdural empyema), those that produce occlusion of the contiguous venous sinuses and cerebral veins (cerebral venous sinus thrombosis), and remote infectious processes (bacterial endocarditis and sepsis) that result in diffuse, multifactorial involvement of the central nervous system.

BRAIN ABSCESS

Brain abscess is an uncommon disorder, accounting for only 2 per cent of intracranial masses. Abscesses produce localized, circumscribed central nervous system infections that manifest clinically as an expanding mass lesion, with symptoms and findings similar to those of other space-occupying lesions, such as brain tumors. Brain abscesses, however, often progress more rapidly than tumors and more frequently produce meningeal involvement.

ETIOLOGY. Infections resulting in brain abscess originate or extend from extracerebral locations. Although the most frequent predisposing factors have changed over the past decades and vary with the given hospital's population and referral base, the most common (Table 471–1) are bloodborne metastases from unknown sources and from lung or heart, direct extension from parameningeal sites (otitis, cranial osteomyelitis, sinusitis), recent or remote head trauma or neurosurgical procedures, and infections associated with cyanotic congenital heart disease. Bloodborne infections seed the brain via hematogenous spread and produce abscesses in brain regions in proportion to the blood flow; accordingly, parietal lobe abscesses predominate. Extension of infection from otitis and mastoiditis involves contiguous brain regions of the temporal lobe and cerebellum, whereas abscesses resulting from sinusitis affect contiguous brain regions of the frontal and temporal lobes. Currently, the most common cause of brain abscess in many urban hospitals is toxoplasmosis occurring in immunodeficiency states due to co-infection with the human immunodeficiency virus (HIV).

PATHOLOGY. On the basis of findings of clinical and experimental research, most brain abscesses evolve over a number of stages, beginning with vascular seeding of brain parenchyma, producing early cerebritis during the first 1 to 3 days. Inflammatory infiltrates of polymorphonuclear cells, lymphocytes, and plasma cells follow within 24 hours. By 3 days, the surrounding area shows a marked increase in perivascular inflammation. The late cerebritis phase develops approximately 4 to 9 days after infection, during which time the center becomes necrotic, containing a mixture of debris and inflammatory cells. Neovascularity is maximal at this time. Early reactive astrocytes surround the zone of cerebritis and proceed to early capsule formation between approximately 10 and 13 days. At this time, the necrotic center shrinks slightly, and a well-developed fibroblast layer evolves. The late capsule stage continues to evolve between 14 days and 5 weeks, with continual shrinking of the necrotic center and a relative decrease in the inflammatory cells. The capsule thickens as reactive astrocytes proliferate.

BACTERIOLOGY. The pathogenic organisms vary considerably, depending on the clinical circumstances. *Staphylococcus aureus* is the most common isolate in trauma-related cases. In patients with HIV-associated disease, *Toxoplasma* is the most common offending organism and bacterial abscesses are rare. Among other abscesses, the most commonly isolated pathogens are anaerobic organisms, but aerobic and microaerobic streptococci, *Staphylococcus aureus*, *Bacteroides*, *Proteus*, and other gram-negative bacilli may also be found (Table 471–1). *Actinomyces*, *Nocardia*, and *Candida* are less frequent offenders. Infection is often polymicrobial. Culture-negative abscesses from surgical specimens occur in 30 per cent of antibiotic-treated patients and in 5 per cent of patients operated on before antibiotic administration.

CLINICAL PRESENTATION. Signs of infection may be

TABLE 471–1. SUMMARY OF UCSF CASES ACCORDING TO TIME PERIODS

	1970–1974	1975–1980	1981–1986	Total
Number of Cases	22(%)	33(%)	47(%)	102(%)
Etiology				
Local infection	2(9)	4(12)	13(28)	19(19)
Cardiac	6(27)	6(18)	5(11)	17(17)
Surgery	1(4)	7(2)	8(17)	16(16)
Trauma	2(9)	1(3)	6(13)	9(9)
Pulmonary	4(18)	4(12)	1(2)	9(9)
Immunocom- promise	2(9)	2(6)	2(4)	6(6)
Other	1(4)	4(12)	0(0)	5(5)
Unknown	4(18)	4(12)	13(28)	21(21)
Organisms				
Aerobic	16(73)	27(82)	34(72)	77(75)
Anaerobic	5(23)	8(24)	7(15)	20(20)
Multiple	5(23)	8(24)	7(15)	20(20)
None cultured	6(27)	6(18)	14(30)	26(25)
Deaths	9(41)	3(9)	2(4)	14(14)

Adapted with permission from Mampalam TJ, Rosenblum ML: Trends in the management of bacterial brain abscesses: A review of 102 cases over 17 years. Neurosurgery 23:451–457, 1988, © by Congress of Neurologic Surgeons.

minimal or absent. Almost half of affected patients maintain a normal body temperature, and fewer than a third show a peripheral white cell count above 11,000 per microliter. Neck stiffness is rare in the absence of increased intracranial pressure.

Otherwise, the presenting features resemble those of any expanding intracranial mass (Table 471–2). A headache of recent onset is the most common symptom, representing distortion or irritation of pain-sensitive structures within the cranial vault, especially those of the great venous sinuses and the dura about the base of the brain. If the process continues untreated, isolated headache will increase in severity and become accompanied by focal signs followed by obtundation and coma. Hemiparesis and aphasia represent involvement of motor and language brain regions. Lethargy progressing to stupor occurs especially with frontal abscesses or with mass effect compressing the contralateral hemisphere or rostral brain stem. Seizures may occur with abscesses involving the cortical gray matter. The period of evolution may be as brief as many hours or as long as many days to weeks with more indolent organisms.

CEREBROSPINAL FLUID EXAMINATION. Cerebrospinal fluid (CSF) examination is not useful in diagnosing brain abscess, since the findings range from normal to those of purulent meningitis, depending on the walling off of the brain abscess or its closeness to CSF compartments (Table 471–3). More important, since abscesses often expand rapidly, lumbar puncture may precipitate or aggravate impending transtentorial herniation. If possible, the procedure should be deferred until after brain images are obtained, which may eliminate the value of CSF analysis.

TABLE 471–2. BRAIN ABSCESS: PRESENTING FEATURES IN 43 CASES

Headache	72%
Lethargy	71%
Fever	60%
Nuchal rigidity	49%
Nausea, vomiting	35%
Seizures	35%
Ocular palsy	27%
Confusion	26%
Visual disturbance	21%
Weakness	21%
Dysarthria	12%
Stupor	12%
Papilledema	10%
Dysphasia	9%
Hemiparesis	9%
Dizziness	7%

Reproduced with permission from Chan CH, Johnson JD, Hofstetter M, et al.: Brain abscess, a study of 45 consecutive cases. Medicine 65:415–431, © by Williams & Wilkins, 1986.

NEUROIMAGING. Computed tomography (CT) and magnetic resonance imaging (MRI) are the laboratory studies of choice for diagnosing brain abscesses and monitoring their response to therapy. MRI may be especially useful for posterior fossa abscesses, as it provides an artifact-free view of the brain stem and cerebellum. In addition, MRI with intravenous gadolinium contrast is superior in demonstrating cerebritis, surrounding edema, and the extent of mass effect.

The evolution of the abscess can be estimated radiologically. In the early cerebritis stage, images reveal a low-density lesion with partial ring enhancement. In the late cerebritis and early capsule stage, well-formed ring-enhancing lesions are seen. The ring enhancement is typically thin walled and uniform, with subtle medial thinning adjacent to the ventricular system. Thick, nonuniform, or nodular enhancement should raise suspicion of an alternative etiology. Delayed scans show diffusion of contrast material into the lucent center, with gradual development of a homogeneous appearance. In the late capsule stage, well-formed ring enhancement may be seen with no delayed diffusion of contrast. Other ring-enhancing lesions that may mimic the image of brain abscess include primary and metastatic tumor, a resolving infarct or hematoma, and, rarely, demyelinating disease.

TREATMENT. Pyogenic brain abscess may be treated with antibiotic therapy alone or antibiotics combined with surgical aspiration or excision. Needle aspiration may be performed stereotactically with CT guidance while the patient is under local anesthesia; excision requires craniotomy. Aspiration offers the advantage of identifying the infecting organism. Initial surgical therapy may be preferred when significant mass effect is present, when the abscess adjoins the ventricular surface (raising the possibility of catastrophic rupture into the ventricular system), when abscesses arise in the posterior fossa (with the potential of brain stem compression), or when abscesses reach a large size (greater than 3 cm diameter) or become refractory to medical therapy. Medical therapy alone is indicated for surgically inaccessible, multiple abscesses (seen in 10 per cent of patients) or abscesses in the early cerebritis stage. With medical therapy alone, the causal organism is not identified, and antibiotic coverage directed toward the most likely organisms (streptococci and anaerobes) is needed. A suggested regimen includes penicillin G, 4 million units given intravenously (IV) every 4 hours, and metronidazole, 15 mg per kilogram IV over 1 hour, followed by 7.5 mg per kilogram given IV or orally every 6 hours. If staphylococcal infection is suspected (e.g., a history of trauma or intravenous drug abuse), oxacillin or nafcillin should be added at a dosage of 3 grams IV every 6 hours. Concomitant corticosteroid therapy may attenuate edema surrounding abscesses.

With medical therapy alone, the resolution of abscesses can be

TABLE 471–3. SUMMARY OF LUMBAR FLUID CHANGES ASSOCIATED WITH BRAIN ABSCESS*

	Number of Patients	Per Cent
Pressure		
<200 mm	38	38
200–300 mm	35	35
>300 mm	26	26
Total	99	
White cells per mm³		
<5	61	29
5–100	81	38
>100	71	33
Total	213	
Protein mg per dl		
<50	26	24
50–100	38	35
>100	44	41
Total	108	
Glucose mg per dl		
>40	89	79
<40	23	21
Total	112	

*Most of these data were obtained before brain imaging was widely available. Reproduced with permission from Fishman RA: Cerebrospinal Fluid in Diseases of the Nervous System. Philadelphia, W. B. Saunders Company, 1980, p 264.

followed by serial CT or MRI. Antibiotics must be continued until the abscess cavity resolves completely. A failure to demonstrate abscess shrinkage in 4 weeks constitutes an antibiotic failure; a surgical procedure should then be performed. Of note is that the ring enhancement may persist after clinical and CSF normalization. Treatment durations are approximately 4 weeks for surgically treated patients and 6 weeks for unoperated on patients.

Abscesses associated with HIV infection are assumed to be due to *Toxoplasma gondii*. The diagnosis is confirmed by response to empiric treatment with daily doses of sulfadiazine, 12 to 15 mg per kilogram, given orally, and pyrimethamine, 25 to 50 mg, given orally. An alternate regimen is pyrimethamine given orally and clindamycin, 900 to 1200 mg IV every 6 hours (or 600 mg orally every 6 hours) for patients allergic to sulfa drugs.

PROGNOSIS. The current mortality rate is 5 to 15 per cent, depending on locale and the nature of pre-existing illness. Outcome also correlates inversely with the abscess size and the degree of neurologic dysfunction at presentation. Age, cause, number of abscesses, or corticosteroid use does not affect outcome.

SPINAL EPIDURAL ABSCESS

Infection within the epidural space about the spinal cord is an uncommon but readily diagnosable and treatable cause of paralysis and death. Its incidence is 0.5 to 1.0 per 10,000 hospital admissions in the United States, but the frequency is substantially increased in the intravenous drug–using population.

CLINICAL PRESENTATION. Patients are usually systemically ill with fever (to 38° to 39°C) in virtually all acutely evolving cases and in the majority of those with a subacute evolution. The initial feature is acute or subacute back pain, with focal percussion tenderness being virtually universal; stiff neck and headache are common. As the infection progresses, over hours, days, or weeks, radicular pain occurs, the site varying with the location of the abscess. Accordingly, this radicular component can be mistaken for sciatica, a visceral abdominal process, chest wall pain, or cervical disc disease. If the condition is unrecognized at this stage, the symptoms rapidly evolve, over a few hours to a few days, to produce weakness and finally paralysis at the spinal level dictated by the site of the infection. This characteristic progression from focal pain and tenderness to pain with radicular signs or symptoms evolving to pain with signs of weakness or paralysis below the level of the lesion is highly typical of an expanding epidural process. In this clinical setting, spinal epidural abscess should be assumed, systemic antibiotics begun, and urgent neuroradiologic confirmatory diagnostic procedures pursued.

The differential diagnosis includes compressive and inflammatory processes involving the spinal cord (transverse myelitis, intervertebral disc herniation, metastatic tumor), which can usually be differentiated clinically by the absence of systemic infection. Transverse myelitis, however, may be associated with fever; the most useful differential feature is its rapid evolution to maximum deficit within 24 to 48 hours or less. Other infectious processes that may have back or neck pain or tenderness as a notable feature must be excluded as well (bacterial meningitis, perinephric abscess, disc space infection, bacterial endocarditis). *Spinal subdural empyema* produces a similar but rare syndrome that often cannot be differentiated clinically from epidural abscess.

ETIOLOGY. Although a specific source cannot always be identified, infections of the epidural space originate from contiguous spread or via hematogenous routes from a distant source. Cutaneous sites of infection are the most common remote sources, especially in intravenous drug users. Abdominal, respiratory tract, and urinary sources are also common. Osteomyelitis may be a cause by either direct extension or hematogenous spread, especially when associated with sepsis. Contiguous spread of infection occurs, most commonly from psoas abscesses, decubitus ulceration, perinephric and retropharyngeal abscesses, surgical sites, or epidurally placed catheters. Whether or not venous spread can occur from pelvic infections via Batson's plexus of spinal veins remains unsettled. Minor back trauma has been implicated in producing a cutaneous hematoma near the spine, which is subsequently seeded via hematogenous sources.

PATHOPHYSIOLOGY. The anatomy of the epidural space dictates the location of the abscess, the frequency of epidural infections being proportional to the volume of the epidural space. Because the size of the intravertebral canal remains relatively constant while the circumference of the spinal cord changes, this is maximal in the thoracic region, next largest in the lumbar region, and least at the cervical spine enlargement. Further, as the dura about the cord is adherent to the vertebral columns anteriorly, the potential epidural space lies posteriorly, as do most epidural abscesses. Anteriorly situated abscesses can occur from contiguous spread of osteomyelitis but represent less than a fifth of all epidural abscesses. Since no anatomic barriers separate spinal segments in the epidural space, such abscesses usually extend over three to five or more vertebral segments.

As the epidural space is not confined rostrocaudally, there is no clear abscess cavity or focal mass to provide a situation of simple compression for spinal cord compromise in epidural abscess. Clinical signs often are substantially greater than would have been predicted from the anatomic extent of pus or granulation tissue found at surgical exploration. Further, in many instances, no frank compression is found on postmortem examination. The spinal cord dysfunction then is likely to be multifactorial, involving toxic processes secondary to inflammation, as well as venous thrombosis, thrombophlebitis, ischemia, and edema. The lack of a clear compressive etiology has important implications for treatment.

BACTERIOLOGY. Causative organisms can be identified by culture or Gram stain from pus obtained at exploration (90 per cent of cases), blood cultures (60 to 70 per cent of cases), or CSF (20 per cent of cases). *Staphylococcus aureus* accounts for most infections, followed by streptococci and gram-negative anaerobes. Tuberculous abscesses remain common, representing as many as 25 per cent of cases in high-risk populations.

DIAGNOSIS. CSF examination is often performed because of associated fever and meningeal signs. The fluid usually is nonspecifically abnormal, containing normal glucose levels, a moderately elevated protein content (400 to 500 mg per milliliter), and a lymphocytic pleocytosis (22 to 150 per cubic millimeter). Spinal fluid cultures yield organisms in about 25 per cent of cases. Almost 90 per cent of patients show a peripheral blood leukocytosis.

Plain spine radiographs, with attention to the area of percussion tenderness, may show osteomyelitis/discitis, a compression fracture, or a paravertebral mass. MRI is considered the study of choice for the evaluation of a suspected epidural abscess because of its ability to demonstrate the craniocaudal extent of the extradural soft tissue mass, associated mass effect upon the cord or cauda equina, and potential signal abnormalities within the discs and vertebral body marrow. The additional advantage, if any, of an intravenous gadolinium contrast agent has not been defined. If MRI is unavailable or technically impossible, CT with myelography usually provides adequate information.

TREATMENT. The disease is fatal in the absence of antibiotic therapy. Unless culture and sensitivities dictate otherwise, penicillinase-resistant penicillin (nafcillin, 12 grams per day, or oxacillin, 12 grams per day) with an aminoglycoside (gentamicin, 5 mg per kilogram per day) should be started empirically as antistaphylococcal treatment for presumed bacterial infection. For confirmed *Staphlyococcus aureus* abscesses, penicillinase-resistant penicillin can be used alone, but many authorities add rifampin (300 mg every 12 hours) because of its ability to penetrate the abscess cavity. Therapy should be continued intravenously for 3 to 4 weeks in the absence of osteomyelitis and 6 to 8 weeks with associated osteomyelitis. Surgical decompression was once felt to be mandatory, but early diagnosis by CT or MRI, as well as the absence of clearly compressive lesions at surgery or postmortem examination, has revised the treatment approach. Many examples demonstrate that medical therapy alone can be curative, particularly in instances in which diagnosis can be established prior to neurologic abnormalities, associated medical complications exist that increase the surgical risk, and complete paraplegia (or quadriplegia) has been present for more than 48 hours. Needle aspiration of the abscess or laminectomy should be performed to determine the causative organism when blood cultures are negative. Medical management of cervical epidural abscesses requires close neurologic evaluation because of the small space available to the abscess and the potential for quadriparesis.

PROGNOSIS. The chances of partial or complete recovery relate inversely to the amount of neurologic dysfunction at the time of diagnosis. Patients with abnormalities limited to pain recover without deficit. Approximately half the patients with some weakness have complete resolution, and nearly half the patients with paralysis of less than 36 hours' duration show some recovery of motor function. In tuberculous epidural abscess, recovery of motor function has been reported even after paralysis lasting for weeks.

VENOUS SINUS THROMBOSIS SECONDARY TO INFECTION

Thrombosis of cerebral veins or sinuses may be of idiopathic origin (Ch. 469), may occur in the setting of hematologic disorders or coagulation abnormalities (Ch. 155), or may result from local or contiguous infectious processes. The last-named syndromes are dealt with here.

Venous drainage from the brain begins with venules and veins that drain into the great venous sinuses. The venous sinus system itself lacks valves, permitting retrograde propagation of clots or infections emanating from structures such as those located in the central portion of the face or the middle ear.

Septic Cavernous Sinus Thrombosis

The cavernous sinuses comprise the most caudal dural venous chambers at the skull base. The paired structures lie on either side of the pituitary fossa, immediately above the midline sphenoid sinus. The cavernous sinus encloses the "cavernous portion" of the internal carotid artery; the third, fourth, and sixth cranial nerves en route to the apex of the orbit; and the ophthalmic and maxillary branches of the trigeminal nerve, which supply sensation to the forehead, periocular regions, cornea, and malar area of the face. Septic cavernous sinus thrombosis most commonly results from extension of infections involving the neighboring sphenoid and ethmoid sinuses, the central portion of the face, or the pharynx or tonsils.

Presenting symptoms are headache and/or lateralized facial pain, followed in a few days to weeks by fever, and involvement of the orbit, producing proptosis and chemosis secondary to obstruction of the ophthalmic vein. Paralysis of oculomotor nerves follows rapidly. Sensory dysfunction in the first and second divisions of the trigeminal nerve and a decrease in the corneal reflex are less obvious. Further involvement of the contiguous orbital contents follows, with mild papilledema and decreased visual acuity, sometimes progressing to blindness. Extension to the opposite cavernous sinus or to other intracranial sinuses with cerebral infarction, or increased intracranial pressure secondary to impaired venous drainage can result in stupor, coma, and death.

The differential diagnosis includes carotid cavernous sinus fistula (diagnosed by ocular bruit and an afebrile state); idiopathic granulomatous involvement of the cavernous sinus (the Tolosa-Hunt syndrome) or orbit (orbital pseudotumor, diagnosed by relative sparing of the orbital contents); and orbital cellulitis (infection localized to the orbit but sparing the structures of the cavernous sinus). Some overlap often occurs between involvement of these contiguous structures of the orbit and involvement of the cavernous sinus.

The CSF is abnormal in almost all cases, sometimes with a profile resembling that of purulent meningitis or parameningeal infection.

The most common causative organism is *Staphyloccocus aureus*, with streptococci and pneumococci being less common; anaerobic infection has been reported. Radiologic evaluation includes sinus imaging, with attention to the sphenoid and ethmoid sinuses. MRI (with and without intravenous contrast) can often demonstrate venous thrombosis by illustrating the lack of the normal "flow void" within vascular structures. Cranial CT scans, employed with or without intravenous contrast material, are seldom helpful. Cerebral angiography is usually unnecessary but may demonstrate extrinsic narrowing of the intracavernous portion of the internal carotid artery.

Treatment relies on early diagnosis and consists of the prompt drainage of infected paranasal sinuses as well as specific antistaphylococcal agents, such as nafcillin or oxacillin, given intravenously. Heparin anticoagulation may reduce morbidity from associated brain ischemia, but this treatment remains controversial in cases involving infection.

Lateral Sinus Thrombosis

Septic thrombosis of the lateral sinus results from acute or chronic infections of the middle ear. The symptoms consist of ear pain followed by headache, nausea, vomiting, and vertigo, evolving over several weeks. On examination, most patients are febrile. An abnormality on otologic examination is nearly invariable; mastoid swelling may be seen. Sixth cranial nerve palsies can occur, but other focal neurologic signs are rare. Papilledema occurs in half the cases, and elevated CSF pressure is present in most, especially with occlusion of the right lateral sinus (which is the major venous conduit from the superior sagittal sinus). CSF contents are usually normal, although parameningeal inflammatory profile may be seen.

Treatment includes intravenous antibiotics to cover staphylococci and anerobes (nafcillin or oxacillin with penicillin or metronidazole). Surgical drainage (mastoidectomy) may be required. Increased intracranial pressure seldom needs direct treatment unless visual fields show progressive constriction. The outcome is usually favorable.

Septic Sagittal Sinus Thrombosis

This uncommon condition occurs as a consequence of purulent meningitis, infections of the ethmoid or maxillary sinuses spreading via venous channels, compound infected skull fractures, or, rarely, neurosurgical wound infections. Symptoms include manifestations of elevated intracranial pressure (headache, nausea, and vomiting) that evolve rapidly to stupor and coma. Seizures and hemiparesis may result from cortical infarction. The rate of progression, severity of symptoms, and prognosis are all related to the location of thrombosis involving the sinus. When only the anterior third of the sinus is obstructed, symptoms are less intense and evolve more slowly. If or when the thrombosis progresses to involve the middle and posterior thirds of the sinus, deterioration progresses more rapidly and outlook for recovery declines.

CSF abnormalities accompany well over half the cases. The opening pressure is increased in proportion to the extent of the sagittal sinus involvement, and a pleocytosis usually reflects the association of a meningeal or parameningeal process.

Radiologically, septic sagittal sinus thrombosis may be excluded by visualization of the normal sagittal sinus during the venous phase of cerebral angiography. Contrast-enhanced CT scanning may reveal a contrast void lying at the junction of the transverse and sagittal sinuses (the region of the torcula); this so-called "delta sign" represents an intraluminal clot surrounded by contrast material. An appropriately programmed MRI scan will demonstrate an abnormal increase in signal intensity (absent flow void) within the affected venous sinus.

Intravenous antibiotics should be directed at organisms recovered from the meningeal process or the parameningeal site. *Staphyloccocus aureus*, β-hemolytic streptococci, pneumococci, and *Klebsiella* are the most common organisms. Initial antibiotic treatment should include nafcillin and an aminoglycoside. Associated paranasal sinusitis should be drained surgically. Heparin use in septic venous thrombosis is controversial, as the mortality rate (resulting from cerebral infarction) still approaches 8 per cent. Experience with noninfected sinus thrombosis has shown that heparin therapy substantially reduces morbidity-mortality, even when CT scans show evidence of hemorrhagic infarction (Ch. 469).

NEUROLOGIC COMPLICATIONS OF INFECTIOUS ENDOCARDITIS

Neurologic complications occur in one third of patients with bacterial endocarditis and triple the general mortality rate of the disease. Most such complications derive from valvular vegetations. Cerebral (but not systemic) emboli are more common from mitral valve endocarditis, for reasons unknown. The time of embolization during the course of endocarditis depends upon the virulence of the organism and whether it produces acute or subacute disease. With acute endocarditis (predominantly staphylococci or enterococci), embolization occurs early, often during the first week, while in subacute disease (predominantly viridans group streptococci or enterococci) emboli occur over the full course of treatment and occasionally after treatment is completed. Emboli lodge in the peripheral branches of the middle cerebral artery, in most cases with resultant hemiparesis. Focal seizures may result.

Whether or not warfarin anticoagulation decreases the risk of embolization remains a controversial issue. This therapy was administered in an earlier period to decrease platelet fibrin vegetations that sequestered the bacteria away from the body's defenses. Current evidence suggests a high rate of hemorrhagic intracerebral complications from warfarin anticoagulation in native valve endocarditis, but not in prosthetic valve endocarditis. Mechanisms to explain the difference remain unknown. Nevertheless, most authorities believe that patients already receiving chronic anticoagulation at the time of diagnosis of endocarditis should be maintained on such therapy.

Mycotic aneurysms complicate endocarditis in 2 to 10 per cent of cases and are more common in acute than subacute disease. The middle cerebral artery is most commonly involved, with the aneurysms being located distally in the vessel, differentiating them from congenital berry aneurysms. The process by which the aneurysmal dilatation occurs remains in dispute, although embolization of infectious vegetations is accepted as the inciting event. Aneurysmal rupture results in 80 per cent mortality, and early diagnosis is therefore important. Whom to subject to angiography is uncertain. However, clinical or radiologic evidence of cerebral or other embolization defines the high-risk group. Other suggested indications for angiography include severe headache (presumably the result of aneurysmal leakage). When an unruptured aneurysm is identified by angiography, it may resolve with antibiotic therapy alone. Accordingly, following such patients with serial angiograms is indicated, as surgical therapy requires excision of the infected portion of the artery. Patients with proximal mycotic aneurysms have a greater risk of perioperative stroke than do those with distal involvement.

Small brain abscesses may complicate the course of endocarditis, but macroscopic abscesses are rare. Most occur in the setting of acute, rather than subacute, endocarditis. Multiple microabscesses, however, can result in a diffuse encephalopathy similar to that seen in sepsis. Such lesions may escape detection on CT scanning and are not amenable to surgical drainage. Antibiotic treatment of the primary disease is indicated.

A CSF pleocytosis occurs in 70 per cent of patients with neurologic complications, but in an unknown number of patients in whom the central nervous system is clinically spared. The CSF profile may be that of a purulent meningitis (polymorphonuclear predominance, elevated protein level, and low glucose level) or that of a parameningeal infection (lymphocytic predominance, modest protein elevation, and normal glucose level). A hemorrhagic component may be seen. Purulent CSF is associated with signs of meningeal irritation and infection with a virulent organism producing an acute endocarditis.

SUBDURAL EMPYEMA

Empyema refers to infection in a preformed space, in this case that separating the dura and arachnoid. Subdural empyema is responsible for one fifth of localized intracranial infections and results from direct extension from infected paranasal sinuses or, less frequently, untreated chronic otitis. Unilateral empyema is most common, as the falx prevents passage across the midline, but bilateral and/or multiple concurrent empyemas occur. Cortical venous thrombosis or brain abscess develops in approximately one fourth of cases; purulent meningitis is a less common accompaniment.

Symptoms initially reflect those of chronic otitis or sinusitis, upon which lateralized headache (a universal feature), fever, and obtundation become superimposed. Vomiting, meningeal signs, and focal neurologic abnormalities (hemiparesis or seizures) usually follow. If the disease remains untreated, obtundation progresses, and the septic mass and swollen underlying brain soon lead to venous thrombosis or death from herniation. The major differential diagnosis is that of meningitis. Nuchal rigidity and obtundation occur in both, but papilledema and lateralizing

deficits are more common in empyema. Lumbar puncture, if obtained because of the suspicion of meningitis, reveals an elevated intracranial pressure accompanied by an increased protein content and a polymorphonuclear pleocytosis with usually a normal glucose concentration in the CSF. Either CT or MRI can be diagnostic of empyema, showing an extra-axial, crescent-shaped mass with an enhancing rim lying just below the inner table of the skull over one or both hemispheres. MRI better detects underlying parenchymal edema.

Treatment requires both surgical drainage of the empyema cavity and high-dose intravenous antibiotics directed toward organisms found at the time of craniotomy. The bacteriology of subdural empyemas is similar to that of sinusitis and cerebral abscess, discussed above. Anticonvulsants should be administered prophylactically, as seizures are common.

If cortical infarction from venous thrombosis does not occur, the prognosis is surprisingly favorable, although chronic epilepsy results in one third of patients.

CRANIAL EPIDURAL ABSCESS

Infections of the epidural space coexist most often with subdural empyema and less frequently with chronic sinusitis or otitis alone. Symptoms and signs are headache and fever with focal neurologic abnormalities due to the coexistent subdural empyema or brain abscess. The diagnosis is made with MRI or contrast-enhanced CT scan (which demonstrate an enhancing lenticular lesion in the epidural space), and the abscess is treated by surgical drainage followed by systemic antibiotics. In uncomplicated cases, the prognosis is excellent.

MALIGNANT EXTERNAL OTITIS

This necrotizing osteitis occurs in elderly patients with diabetes. The associated organism, *Pseudomonas aeruginosa*, is a normal flora of the external ear. In this case, it produces an external otitis that fails to respect normal anatomic boundaries. The result consists of a rapidly evolving syndrome of ear pain, facial swelling, osteomyelitis, and purulent meningitis accompanied by multiple cranial nerve palsies. Urgent treatment with antipseudomonal penicillin (mezlocillin) or a third-generation cephalosporin (ceftazidime) and tobramycin, as well as surgical debridement and drainage, is essential. The mortality rate is high.

Brain Abscess

Haimes AB, Zimmerman RD, Morgello S, et al.: MR imaging of brain abscesses. AJR 152:1073, 1989. *Reviews MRI of brain abscesses and its differential diagnosis.*
Mampalam TJ, Rosenblum ML: Trends in the management of bacterial brain abscesses: A review of 102 cases over 17 years. Neurosurgery 23:451, 1988. *A recent review from a referral center with attention to the issue of corticosteroid therapy.*
Maniglia AJ, Goodwin WJ, Arnold JE, et al.: Intracranial abscesses secondary to nasal, sinus, and orbital infections in adults and children. Arch Otolaryngol Head Neck Surg 115:1424, 1989. *Association of sinus disease with brain abscesses is reviewed.*
Patel KS, Marks PV: Management of focal intracranial infections: Is medical treatment better than surgery? J Neurol Neurosurg Psychiatry 53:472, 1990. *Discussion of the issue of nonsurgical management.*

Spinal Epidural Abscess

Danner RL, Hartman BJ: Update on spinal epidural abscess: 35 cases and review of the literature. Rev Infect Dis 9:265, 1987. *An up-to-date review of all aspects.*
Del-Curling O Jr, Gower DJ, McWhorter JM: Changing concepts in spinal epidural abscess: A report of 29 cases. Neurosurgery 27:185, 1990. *A recent neurosurgical series.*
Lasker BR, Harter DH: Cervical epidural abscess. Neurology 37:1747, 1987. *Specific problems of cervical abscesses are reviewed and anatomic considerations are addressed.*
Leys D, Lesoin F, Viaud C, et al.: Decreased morbidity from acute bacterial spinal epidural abscesses using computed tomography and nonsurgical treatment in selected patients. Ann Neurol 17:350, 1985. *The issue of nonsurgical treatment is introduced.*

Venous Sinus Thrombosis Secondary to Infection

Southwick FS, Richardson EP, Swartz MN: Septic thrombosis of the dural venous sinuses. Medicine 65:82, 1986. *Complete review of all aspects.*

Neurologic Complications of Infectious Endocarditis

Davenport J, Hart RG: Prosthetic valve endocarditis 1976–1987. Antibiotics, anticoagulation, and stroke. Stroke 21:993, 1990. *Anticoagulation in prosthetic valve endocarditis is readdressed.*

Pruitt AA, Rubin RH, Karchmer AW, et al.: Neurologic complications of bacterial endocarditis. Medicine 57:329, 1978. *Major review of all aspects from a single referral center.*

Subdural Empyema

Kaufman DM, Miller MH, Steigbigel NH: Subdural empyema: Analysis of 17 recent cases and review of the literature. Medicine 54:485, 1975. *A complete discussion of clinical features from patients at a single center.*

Pathak A, Sharma BS, Mathuriya SN, et al.: Controversies in the management of subdural empyema. A study of 41 cases with review of literature. Acta Neurochir 102:25, 1990. *A recent large series and literature review.*

Weingarten K, Zimmerman RD, Becker RD, et al.: Subdural and epidural empyemas: MR imaging. AJR 152:615, 1989. *MRI is described.*

Cranial Epidural Abscess

Silverberg AL, DiNubile MJ: Subdural empyema and cranial epidural abscess. Med Clin North Am 69:361, 1985. *Reviews the topic.*

Malignant External Otitis

Johnson MP, Ramphal R: Malignant external otitis: Report on therapy with ceftazidime and review of therapy and prognosis. Rev Infect Dis 12:173, 1990. *A recent review of clinical and therapeutic aspects.*

472 Neurosyphilis

The resurgence of primary and secondary syphilis (now estimated to be 14.7 cases per 100,000) first occurred among promiscuous homosexual males but has more recently spread to heterosexual contacts via prostitutes. If untreated, approximately 7 per cent of patients with primary syphilis infection will develop some form of symptomatic neurosyphilis.

PATHOPHYSIOLOGY. Each of the neurologic manifestations of syphilis results from a chronic, insidious meningeal inflammatory process occurring as a reaction to treponemal invasion of the central nervous system (CNS). An inflammatory response in the cerebrospinal fluid (CSF) occurs in 34 per cent of asymptomatic persons with syphilis, with the CSF abnormalities peaking at 13 to 18 months after the primary infection. This CNS invasion dictates the risk of future symptomatic and asymptomatic neurosyphilis, which amounts to approximately 30 per cent following a primary infection but falls to 1 per cent or less if CSF examination is normal 5 years after the primary infection (Merritt, 1946).

CLINICAL SYNDROMES. The clinical manifestations of neurosyphilis are conventionally divided into acute syphilitic meningitis, cerebrovascular syphilis, syphilitic dementia (general paresis), and tabes dorsalis. These entities, however, form an overlapping spectrum. For instance, paresis and tabes may coexist (taboparesis). After primary infection, these clinical subtypes of neurosyphilis follow a predictable time course (Fig. 472-1) based on the evolution of the meningeal inflammatory process. Why this inflammatory process becomes symptomatic at a particular stage in a particular patient is unknown. Symptomatic syphilitic meningitis is the earliest manifestation of nervous system syphilis, often occurring coincident with a secondary rash. The meningeal inflammation later extends to involve the cerebral blood vessels and, when symptomatic, results in cerebrovascular neurosyphilis (usually seen within the first 5 years following primary infection). The so-called parenchymal forms of neurosyphilis (paresis and tabes) occur after a more protracted interval. Syphilitic meningitis and cerebrovascular syphilis, the earlier forms, are therefore the most frequently observed manifestations of neurosyphilis in the present epidemic.

Acute Syphilitic Meningitis. Symptomatic meningeal syphilis occurs during the first months to a year or two after the primary infection, with 10 per cent of cases occurring coincident with a secondary rash. The course is subacute. Headache is common, and asymmetric cranial nerve abnormalities are prominent (especially those involving auditory function, facial strength, eye movements, and vision, this last being secondary to unilateral or bilateral optic papillitis). Patients are afebrile; meningeal signs are often present, and some patients become confused. The CSF shows a lymphocytic pleocytosis. Accurate diagnosis is important, as relatively mild symptoms may resolve spontane-

ously without treatment, leaving the patient at risk for progression to the fixed deficits associated with the later forms of neurosyphilis.

Cerebrovascular Syphilis. As the meningeal inflammatory process progresses, a diffuse vasculitis evolves, compromising the cerebral arteries traversing the subarachnoid space and producing a subacute encephalopathy with ischemia-caused focal features. Associated symptoms include confusion, personality change, and intellectual decline, usually followed by the emergence of focal deficits resulting from occlusion of specific vessels. Arteries in the middle cerebral artery distribution are most often involved, but any cerebral or spinal vascular bed may be affected alone or in combination, the condition often evolving over a period of several hours or days. The resulting syndrome is distinct from thromboembolic stroke because of the associated encephalopathy, the multifocal pattern, and the subacute time course.

Diagnosis is confirmed by finding an inflammatory spinal fluid with a positive serology; angiography is unnecessary, but if performed demonstrates vasculitis of medium-sized arteries. Areas of ischemia observed on computed tomography (CT) or magnetic resonance imaging (MRI) in association with the characteristic CSF suggest the diagnosis. These ischemic areas most often arise in the deep cerebral white matter and follow the distribution of the lenticulostriate branches of the middle cerebral artery.

Syphilitic Dementia. Dementia paralytica, or general paresis of the insane, is the diffuse meningoencephalitic form of neurosyphilis. Affected patients usually present 10 to 20 (range, 3 to 30) years after the primary infection. General paresis affects men four to seven times more frequently than women, perhaps because the infectivity of *Treponema pallidum* declines during pregnancy.

Syphilitic dementia produces notoriously nonspecific symptoms, the pattern of which can be mimicked by almost any organic brain syndrome. The colorful descriptions of grandiose delusional states and psychosis are well known but were uncommon even in the prepenicillin era. Then, as now, a simple dementing illness predominated. Tremors of the hands, tongue, and lips, resulting in disordered handwriting and dysarthria, were classically described as characteristic; modern experience is insufficient to confirm the observations.

Several features help to differentiate paresis from other causes of dementia. Syphilitic dementia has a relatively early onset, most commonly beginning between ages 30 and 50, and it progresses rapidly if untreated, being fatal within months to a few years. An inflammatory CSF is always found, and the blood and CSF syphilis serologies are always positive.

Tabes Dorsalis. The term describes a myeloneuropathy that characteristically occurs 10 to 20 years after primary infection (range, 5 to 50 years). A sensory neuropathy results, with the primary lesions affecting either the proximal dorsal root entry zones or the dorsal root ganglia. As with paresis, a marked male predominance (7:1) was noted in the prepenicillin era.

The classic triad of symptoms includes lightning pains, sensory ataxia, and urinary disturbance. The triad of most common and earliest signs is that of pupillary abnormalities, lower extremity areflexia, and the Romberg sign. Lightning pains are transient, agonizing, shooting pains described as being "like the twanging of a single fiddle string," which are most common in the legs but which may affect any region of the body. Characteristic is an early loss of vibration and position sense attributed to secondary degeneration of the posterior columns of the spinal cord. The proprioceptive impairment engenders a wide-based, unsteady gait that is exacerbated by elimination of visual input (eye closure): the Romberg sign. Bladder hypotonia with overflow incontinence results from deafferentation of the lower sacral sensory nerve roots. Rectal incontinence is uncommon; genital sensory and autonomic impairment eventually results in impotence. Peripheral autonomic impairment often develops and, along with loss of peripheral nociceptive afferent fibers, is responsible for the development of trophic (Charcot) joint deformities and distal extremity ulcers. The sensory impairment is responsible for the loss of deep tendon reflexes.

Of the pupillary abnormalities, half have the classic Argyll Robertson pattern, being small, irregular, and bilaterally reacting

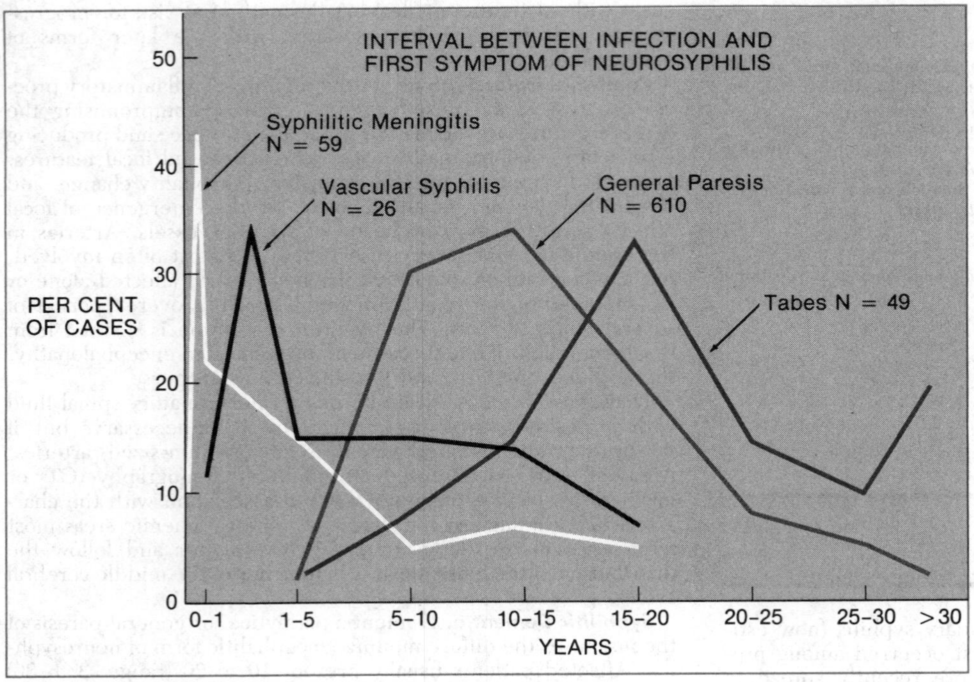

FIGURE 472–1. Interval between primary and symptomatic neurosyphilis by type (meningeal, vascular, paresis, tabes), abstracted from the literature and presented as per cent of total cases within type. (Reproduced with permission from Simon RP: Neurosyphilis. Arch Neurol 42:606–613, 1985. Copyright 1985, American Medical Association.)

poorly to light but constricting briskly to accommodation (the phenomenon of light-near dissociation). Other pupillary abnormalities in tabes include unilateral mydriatic pupils with loss of pupillary light reflex.

CEREBROSPINAL FLUID EXAMINATION. A chronic, insidious inflammatory response within the CSF (Table 472–1) accompanies each of the clinical syndromes of neurosyphilis and provides the ultimate diagnostic test establishing the presence of active neurosyphilis and/or its response to therapy. The absence of a CSF inflammatory response excludes a diagnosis of active neurosyphilis and therefore precludes a clinical response to antibiotic therapy. As with any chronic meningitis, the γ globulin portion of the protein content is commonly elevated, and oligoclonal bands may be present.

Active neurosyphilis causes an abnormal CSF. The possibility of a negative serology in neurosyphilis is difficult to ascertain from the classic literature because of the relatively insensitive Wasserman test and the unrecognized inclusion of nonsyphilitic syndromes of cerebrovascular disease and viral meningitis. When the clinical diagnosis was characteristic, however, only rare cases showed a negative CSF serology (even with the Wasserman reaction): In 100 paretic patients reported by Merritt (1946), the CSF Wasserman test was positive in every case. Wilson also reported universal CSF positivity in 77 cases of paresis. Theoretically, a negative CSF VDRL might occur in the presence of severe immunosuppression, as a prozone phenomenon, or, in an early case, as a manifestation of the CSF inflammatory response preceding seropositivity. This last situation may explain occasional recent reports of false-negative results or delayed conversions in early meningeal syndromes.

The role of the more sensitive treponemal test (fluorescent treponemal antibody [FTA]) in diagnosing CNS syphilis remains uncertain because of a high false-positive response and decreased sensitivity (75 per cent); without supporting clinical or laboratory data, the diagnostic value of a reactive CSF FTA is unknown. An additional confirmatory test is to inject CSF into rabbit testes; a reactive testicular swelling and recovery of spirochetes prove treponemal infectivity.

TREATMENT. Since neurosyphilis of all clinical types is associated with a CSF inflammatory response, the CSF cell count provides the ultimate monitor of the effectiveness of therapy. Normalization of the spinal fluid is the required endpoint of antibiotic therapy. Once the CSF remains normal for 2 years, relapses fail to occur.

Penicillin is the drug of choice. Various regimens from 12 to 24 mU per day have been suggested, but it is not clear that the higher doses alter the clinical outcome. Intramuscular benzathine penicillin usually results in undetectable levels in CSF and accordingly should not be used for treatment of neurosyphilis. Spirocheticidal levels (0.03 IU per milliliter, 0.018 µg per milliliter) in CSF are exceeded with 12 million units of IV penicillin daily in four divided doses. Some regimens include probenecid

TABLE 472–1. MODERN EXAMPLES OF CSF FINDINGS IN VARIOUS NEUROSYPHILITIC SYNDROMES

Syndrome	OP	WBC	Glu	Prot	Gamma Globulin*	VDRL Blood	VDRL CSF
Meningitis	170	154 (94% L)	29	95		1:64	1:4
Cerebrovascular	192	58 (87% L)	41	119	IgG index .93	1:512	1:16
Paresis		220	49	305	IgG index 1.99	1:128	1:8
Tabes (active)		62		140		1:16	1:28
Tabes (inactive)		2	76	43		1:16	1:2

*Normal IgG index = 0.23 to 0.64.

OP = Opening pressure; WBC = white blood cells; Glu = glucose; Prot = protein; VDRL = Venereal Disease Research Laboratory; CSF = cerebrospinal fluid; L = lymphocytes; IgG = immunoglobulin G.

TABLE 472–2. CSF RESPONSE TO PENICILLIN TREATMENT*

	Admission	Day 7	Day 21	6 Mo
Opening pressure, mm CSF	120	—	—	Normal
Cells/cu mm	207 (94% L)	100 (100% L)	24 (100% L)	0
Glucose, mg/dl	51	66	54	66
Protein, mg/dl	50 (14.4% gamma globulin)	38	48	34
Serology (VDRL)				
CSF	1:2	1:1	—	—
Blood	1:64	1:64	1:64	1:64

*Meningovascular syphilis treated with aqueous penicillin G, 24 million units daily for 21 days; data from Holmes MD, Brant-Zawadski MM, Simon RP: Clinical manifestations of meningovascular syphilis. Neurology 34:553–556, 1984.

to increase concentrations in CSF by decreasing reabsorption of penicillin through the choroid plexus. Probenecid, however, also decreases parenchymal penicillin concentrations by competing for uptake at membrane transport sites.

The optimal duration of penicillin treatment for neurosyphilis is uncertain. Complete normalization of CSF is uncommon during the usual 2- to 3-week course of intravenous treatment, but the spinal fluid continues to return to normal over the next weeks to months (Table 472–2). Proof of adequate treatment requires a normalized cell count and a falling protein content at 6 months.

HUMAN IMMUNODEFICIENCY VIRUS (HIV) INFECTION IN NEUROSYPHILIS. Neurosyphilis and HIV-associated disease may coexist, both being consequences of sexual promiscuity. It has been recently suggested that syphilis is an opportunistic infection in HIV disease, and that in such patients syphilis follows an atypical, penicillin-resistant, aggressive course. However, syphilitic syndromes described in these patients are not different in either time course or clinical presentation from those in the pre-AIDS era. Further, the apparent "penicillin resistance" may represent coexistent HIV-induced CSF pleocytosis that is not altered by penicillin therapy. In addition, the occasional recovery of treponemes following penicillin treatment for syphilis in HIV–co-infected patients was similarly observed in the pre-AIDS era. Antibody production to syphilis by plasma cells is impaired with progressive immunosuppression, however, which has resulted in a loss of FTA reactivity in 10 per cent of a San Francisco cohort. Accordingly, a decline in the immune capacity of patients with HIV infection does occur late in this disease, but its association with any continued activity nervous system syphilis in such patients remains speculative.

The principles of treating neurosyphilis in HIV–co-infected patients are similar to those used in patients without the retrovirus disease; intravenous penicillin should be used in spirocheticidal doses, and the spinal fluid should be monitored as an index of therapy. As noted, when the inflammatory response is due partly to syphilis and partly to HIV infection, only a portion of the pleocytosis will disappear, leaving a new plateau level of CSF cellularity. The Centers for Disease Control (CDC) recommends that patients co-infected with HIV and syphilis for more than 1 year should have an examination of their CSF, whether or not they have neurologic symptoms.

CDC: Recommendations for diagnosing and treating syphilis in HIV-infected patients. MMWR 37:600, 1988. *Current recommendations.*
Jordan KG: Modern neurosyphilis—a critical analysis. West J Med 149:47, 1988. *Review and critique of diagnostic, clinical, and laboratory criteria for neurosyphilis with and without HIV co-infection.*
Merritt HH, Adams RD, Solomon HC: Neurosyphilis. 2nd ed. New York, Oxford University Press, 1946. *The classic descriptive work of the prepenicillin era.*
Musher DM, Hamill RJ, Baughn RE: Syphilis in the presence of human immunodeficiency virus infection. Ann Intern Med 113:872–881, 1990. *A critique of the association between syphilis and HIV infection.*
Simon RP: Neurosyphilis. Arch Neurol 42:606, 1985. *A review of the clinical syndromes, CSF, and serologic diagnostic criteria.*
Wilson SAK: Neurology. Vol 1. London, E. Arnold Company, 1940, pp 455–459. *Extensive single-author experience with neurosyphilis in the prepenicillin era.*

SECTION NINE / VIRAL INFECTIONS OF THE NERVOUS SYSTEM

473 Introduction

Richard W. Price

Agents belonging to nearly all the major groups of animal viruses can infect the central nervous system. The spectrum ranges from the large, complex DNA herpesviruses to small, relatively simple viruses with DNA or RNA genomes, such as the papovaviruses and retroviruses. Also included are agents not yet fully characterized that cause the spongiform encephalopathies in which the nature of "transmissible material" remains uncertain. As a result, neurologic manifestations of viral infections can be almost equally diverse, extending from the typical acute febrile encephalitides to chronic progressive disorders that clinically resemble degenerative neurologic diseases.

In most cases, particularly in those infections presenting as acute encephalitis, nervous system involvement is an uncommon complication of a relatively common systemic infection. In adaptive terms, extension of infection to the central nervous system is "accidental" and may even preclude survival of the virus and its transmission to a new host. For example, the polioviruses cause enteric infections in which replication in the gut and fecal-oral transmission determine the essential survival and transmission of the organism; extension of infection to anterior horn cells of the spinal cord devastates the host but does not contribute to the "life cycle" of the virus. By contrast, the neurotropic herpesviruses, including herpes simplex virus type 1, are exquisitely adapted to cause latent and reactivated infection within the peripheral nervous system; in this case, the sensory neuron is the reservoir for latent virus, and reactivated virus exploits axoplasmic transport to reinfect the epithelium and consequently induce local shedding of virus. However, even in the case of the herpesviruses, central nervous system complications, such as acute herpes encephalitis, are "accidental" and not essential in the organism's adaptive strategy. Rabies illustrates an illness in which central nervous system infection plays a central role in the life cycle of the virus: Involvement of the brain produces "rabid," biting behavior that actually contributes to virus transmission.

Viruses can enter the nervous system along a number of avenues. Transport up peripheral nerves can allow direct passage from epithelium or viscera to the central nervous system, and once virus enters the brain, similar intraneural passage by axoplasmic transport can facilitate further spread. It has been demonstrated that a number of viruses are transported along nerve processes by both orthograde and retrograde axoplasmic transport systems. This mode of transport allows rapid passage over long distances and also provides an avenue that is protected from immunologic interference. Many, if not most, viruses, however, enter the brain via hematogenous dissemination, with passage across the vascular endothelium. As a general rule, agents that travel over neural routes tend to produce initially focal neurologic symptoms and signs, while those that disseminate hematogenously cause more diffuse clinical changes. Exceptions exist, however. One lies in the selective vulnerability of particular nervous system structures or cells to infection with particular agents. Focal or multifocal disease can also follow general hematogenous dissemination in a random seeding of brain regions. Many viruses preferably infect the meninges rather than the brain, gaining access via the choroid plexus.

While within the nervous system a number of viruses appear not to discriminate among neurons, glial, or endothelial cells, others choose selective targets. Such selectivity is probably determined to a great extent by cell-surface molecules, principally glycoproteins, that serve as receptors for viruses and determine the character of attachment and subsequent entry into cells. Different cell types may also vary in their capacity to support virus-directed metabolism and replication.

The character of virus-cell interactions can assume a number of courses: *abortive infection* results in little or no change in the cell and no virus replication; *acute productive/lytic infection* is characterized by a full replication cycle with production of progeny and subsequent cell death; *chronic productive infection* may allow prolonged release of progeny virus without cell death; in *latent infection*, the viral genome resides in the cell, either integrated into the host genome or as a separate genomic fragment with little or no gene transcription or translation but retention of the capacity to reactivate subsequently; *transforming infection* results in increased and characteristically abnormal cell proliferation, usually in the absence of virus replication; *defective infection* may result in nonproductive infection or production of incomplete particles, yet cause varying degrees of cell alteration and viral antigen expression.

Diagnostic approaches to viral diseases depend on the clinical setting and specific agents involved. Available methods of diagnosis include serologic assessment of host-antibody responses in serum or cerebrospinal fluid, direct identification of virus in brain or cerebrospinal fluid using viral isolation techniques or methods that identify viral antigens or nucleic acid, and histologic examination of infected tissue for pathognomonic reactions (e.g., formation of inclusion bodies or other specific cell changes).

In the past, limitations of treatment made specific virologic diagnosis either largely an academic exercise or important principally for epidemiologic purposes. Efforts to combat viral disease consisted exclusively of prevention through active, or at times passive, immunization. These time-honored methods still predominate, and the prevention of poliomyelitis remains a landmark of biomedical research. In the past two decades, however, antiviral chemotherapy has become a practical reality. Effective therapy is now available for neurotropic herpesviruses and for human immunodeficiency virus, and the promise exists not only for more effective treatments for infection by these groups of viruses but also for the development of chemotherapeutic agents that will act selectively against several other important viruses causing neurologic diseases.

Johnson RT: Viral Infections of the Nervous System. New York, Raven Press, 1982.
Although now outdated in certain details, this remains an excellent introduction to the general principles of viral infection of the nervous system.

474 Acute Viral Meningitis and Encephalitis

Richard W. Price

DEFINITIONS. The terms *viral meningitis* and *viral encephalitis* refer to infections of the leptomeninges and brain parenchyma, respectively. When the spinal cord is involved along with the brain, the term *viral encephalomyelitis* may be used. When both meninges and brain parenchyma appear to be involved, *viral meningoencephalitis* sometimes is employed, although viral encephalitis is almost always accompanied by meningeal inflammation. The nonspecific term *aseptic meningitis* refers to an inflammatory process of the meninges accompanied by a predominantly mononuclear cell pleocytosis and not caused by pyogenic bacterial infection. Although viral infections are the most common cause of aseptic meningitis, infections by other types of organisms, as well as chemical irritation of the meninges and reactions to certain medications, can cause a similar clinical picture and cerebrospinal fluid profile. Most viral meningitides are benign, self-limiting processes with a low acute morbidity and only rare long-term sequelae. While viral encephalitides are also often benign, they more often result in significant morbidity and mortality.

Acute central nervous system infections caused by a variety of viruses are appropriately considered together because their clinical aspects are largely indistinguishable. Viral infections causing more distinct neurologic symptoms and signs are considered separately in subsequent sections.

ETIOLOGIES. Many viruses can cause acute encephalitis or meningitis (Table 474–1). Table 474–2 indicates the most common virus groups and the syndromes they produce.

Enteroviruses are small, nonenveloped RNA viruses of the picornavirus family with numerous serotypes, over 50 of which have been associated with meningitis or encephalitis. This family includes members of the coxsackie A and B, echovirus, and newer enterovirus groups, as well as the three poliovirus subtypes (see Ch. 475).

The arboviruses include agents of several families that are transmitted by mosquitoes or ticks. More than 15 different arboviruses have been associated with encephalitis in varied geographic areas of the world. In the United States, the five most important are eastern and western equine encephalitis, St. Louis encephalitis, California encephalitis (with most cases involving the LaCross subtype), and Colorado tick fever. Less common within the continental states are Venezuelan equine encephalitis and Powassan encephalitis.

Herpes simplex virus type 1 causes severe encephalitis, but usually with characteristical focal features, while herpes simplex virus type 2 causes aseptic meningitis in association with primary or secondary genital herpes (see Ch. 476). Lymphocytic choriomeningitis (LCM) virus, an arenavirus, is a sporadic cause of meningitis and occasionally encephalitis. Aseptic meningitis has now been recognized as a complication of acute infection by the retrovirus causing the acquired immunodeficiency syndrome (AIDS; see Part XXI). Adenoviruses are respiratory viruses that only rarely cause meningitis or severe childhood encephalitis.

The acute neurologic disease associated with measles, vaccinia, and rubella infections in most cases represents postinfectious encephalomyelitis (see Ch. 479). This may also be true of the encephalitis that has occasionally been reported with influenza and parainfluenza virus infections.

EPIDEMIOLOGY. Viral meningitis and encephalitis are relatively common disorders. In one study in Rochester, Minnesota, for example, the incidence of aseptic meningitis was nearly 11 per 100,000 person-years, while that of viral encephalitis was more than 7 per 100,000 person-years. This finding was compared with a rate of 8.6 episodes of bacterial meningitis. A relatively low mortality rate in this study (3.8 per cent) may have reflected the inclusion of milder cases and the predominance of the LaCross type of viral encephalitis. In other epidemiologic settings, the mortality is considerably greater. In general, a specific etiologic diagnosis is identified in only about 10 to 15 per cent of cases of meningitis and encephalitis in the United States.

TABLE 474–1. VIRUSES ASSOCIATED WITH ACUTE CENTRAL NERVOUS SYSTEM INFECTIONS IN THE UNITED STATES

RNA Viruses
  Picornaviruses (enteroviruses)
    Polioviruses
    Coxsackieviruses, groups A and B
    Echoviruses
    Enteroviruses
  Togaviruses
    Eastern equine encephalitis*
    Western equine encephalitis*
    St. Louis encephalitis*
    Powassan*
    Tick-borne encephalitis
    Rubella
  Bunyavirus
    California encephalitis* (includes LaCross subtype)
  Orbivirus
    Colorado tick fever*
  Arenavirus
    Lymphocytic choriomeningitis
  Rhabdovirus
    Rabies
  Myxoviruses and paramyxoviruses
    Influenza
    Parainfluenza
    Mumps
    Measles
  Retroviruses
    Human immunodeficiency virus type 1

DNA Viruses
  Herpesviruses
    Herpes simplex, types 1 and 2
    Varicella zoster
    Epstein-Barr
    Cytomegalovirus
    Adenoviruses

*Arthropod-borne viruses (arboviruses).

Each of the viruses causing central nervous system infection has its own epidemiologic pattern. Because of the predominance of enteroviruses and arboviruses, the overall incidence of viral meningitis and encephalitis peaks in the late summer. Enterovirus epidemics in temperate climates characteristically take place in the summer, with transmission occurring by the fecal-hand-oral route, often involving young children, with rapid spread in family or social groups. The geographic and seasonal incidence of arbovirus infection relates to the life cycle of arthropod vectors and animal reservoirs (Ch. 389) and their contact with humans. Eastern equine encephalitis virus is limited largely to the Atlantic and Gulf coasts, while western equine encephalitis virus is confined to the western two thirds of the country, with the highest incidence in the middle states. The latter virus causes many more human infections than does the eastern virus, but only 1 in 100 of those infected develops encephalitis. St. Louis encephalitis virus causes disease in both rural and urban areas over a large part of the United States. In the rural areas, the virus has the same pattern as western encephalitis virus, but in urban areas more explosive outbreaks can occur. In recent years, the LaCross subtype of the California encephalitis virus has been related to encephalitis every year over a wide geographic area of

TABLE 474–2. RELATIVE FREQUENCY OF MENINGITIS AND ENCEPHALITIS OF KNOWN VIRAL ETIOLOGY

Viral Agent	Viral Meningitis (%)	Viral Encephalitis (%)
Enteroviruses	83	23
Arboviruses	2	30
Mumps	7	2
Herpes simplex	4	27
Varicella	1	8
Measles	1	<1

Modified with permission from Jubelt B: Enterovirus and mumps virus infections of the nervous system. Neurol Clin 2:187, 1984.

the eastern United States, particularly in the midwestern states, with disease confined largely to children. Colorado tick fever occurs in the Rocky Mountain area; about 18 per cent of infected patients develop meningitis, but encephalitis is rare. Venezuelan encephalitis has spread into Florida and the southwestern states and, in most of those infected, produces an influenza-like illness, but about 3 per cent develop acute meningitis or encephalitis. Powassan virus is a rare cause of encephalitis in Canada and along the northern border of the United States.

Lymphocytic choriomeningitis virus is the major zoonotic virus causing meningitis and encephalitis. Humans acquire the infection by contact with dust or food contaminated by excreta of the common house mouse. Human disease is more common in winter, when the natural host tends to move indoors. Lymphocytic choriomeningitis virus has also been found in hamsters, and human infections have been traced to laboratory and pet hamsters.

Mumps virus spreads by the respiratory route, with infection occurring throughout the year but increasing in incidence during the spring. Although mumps virus infects the two sexes equally, males develop meningitis three times more frequently than females.

PATHOGENESIS. Events leading up to the development of the acute viral encephalitides and meningitides can be divided into three stages. The first involves exposure of an external body surface to the virus, usually with local replication of the "inoculum." In the case of enteroviruses, the infecting virus is contained in body fluids or excreta from infected persons and transferred by direct contact or within contaminated environmental materials, while the arboviruses are introduced by an arthropod bite. The next stage involves systemic viremia and amplification of virus in visceral organs; a secondary viremia may then lead to invasion of and replication within the nervous system or meninges. With the exception of rabies virus, the neurotropic herpesviruses, and perhaps the polioviruses, agents that cause acute viral encephalitis or meningitis reach the nervous system hematogenously. This factor accounts for the widespread distribution of cerebral dysfunction associated with most of the encephalitides.

In viral encephalitis, infection of neurons, glial cells, and even vascular endothelium leads to cell dysfunction and sometimes cell death. Inflammatory responses follow, and lymphocytes and macrophages first line the blood vessels and then migrate into the parenchyma. Clinical symptoms and signs depend on the distribution of infection and on both the direct effect of the virus and the secondary inflammatory reactions in the tissue. The relative contribution of direct viral infection or secondary host reactions to the genesis of brain dysfunction varies, depending on the particular infecting virus. The remarkable degree of recovery in many patients suggests that secondary immune responses often play an important role in producing symptoms.

CLINICAL MANIFESTATIONS. The systemic accompaniments of most acute viral encephalitides and meningitides are similar but depend on the particular virus. Often central nervous system manifestations are preceded or accompanied by fever, malaise or myalgia, gastrointestinal disturbance, respiratory symptoms, or rash. These are followed in viral meningitis by the development of headache, photophobia, stiff neck, and other signs of meningeal irritation, usually with an intensity milder than that of bacterial meningitis.

When encephalitis is present, evidence of diffuse or, less commonly, focal brain dysfunction accompanies or overshadows the signs of meningeal irritation. Patients characteristically exhibit altered attention and consciousness, ranging from confusion to lethargy or coma. Motor function may also be abnormal, with weakness, altered tone, or incoordination, reflecting affliction of the cortex, basal ganglia, or cerebellum in varying degree. In severe cases, generalized or focal seizures may occur, and their control may be difficult. Some patients exhibit myoclonus or tremor. Hypothalamic involvement may lead to hyperthermia or hypothermia, autonomic dysfunction with vasomotor instability, or diabetes insipidus. Abnormalities of ocular motility, swallowing, or other cranial nerve functions are uncommon. Similarly, spinal cord infection is usually less conspicuous but can result in flaccid weakness, with acute loss of reflexes in the most severe cases. Focal symptoms other than seizures are usually minor and overshadowed by generalized brain dysfunction, but in some patients hemiparesis, visual disturbance, or sensory loss may be prominent. Such focal abnormalities are particularly characteristic of herpes encephalitis (see Ch. 476).

The time course of acute viral meningitis and encephalitis is variable. The onset may occur within a matter of hours or may evolve more slowly over a few days. Usually, maximum deficit appears within 1 to 4 days.

LABORATORY FINDINGS. Examination of the cerebrospinal fluid is essential. The presence of 10 to 1000 mononuclear cells per cubic millimeter is characteristic. On occasion, early examination may show acellular fluid or predominance of polymorphonuclear leukocytes, but the typical mononuclear pleocytosis soon evolves. The pressure may be elevated, while the glucose level is characteristically normal or only modestly reduced. The protein content is usually elevated (50 to 100 mg per deciliter) and may exhibit increased immunoglobulin concentration and the presence of oligoclonal bands. An increased protein content and number of cells may persist for weeks and perhaps months after convalescence, and the oligoclonal bands can be detected for an even longer period.

Systemic laboratory findings may vary, depending on the etiologic agent. Generally, the white blood cell count is not elevated, but either elevations or depressions can be seen, usually with a lymphocytic predominance. Involvement of salivary glands or pancreas in mumps may elevate the serum amylase level.

Neurodiagnostic tests usually reveal nonspecific abnormalities, with notable exception in the case of herpes simplex encephalitis (see Ch. 476). The electroencephalogram characteristically exhibits generalized slowing, but focal sharp-wave or spike activity can occur in association with seizures. Computed tomography (CT) and magnetic resonance imaging (MRI) are usually normal early in the course of the nonherpetic viral encephalitides, but focal edema and contrast enhancement may appear in the more severe cases. The greatest value of these neuroimaging procedures lies in excluding alternative diagnoses.

DIAGNOSIS. With a few exceptions, the neurologic and laboratory findings accompanying the acute viral meningoencephalitides are insufficiently distinct to allow an etiologic diagnosis, and it may even be difficult to distinguish these disorders from a number of nonviral diseases. The epidemiologic setting (e.g., time of year, exposure to insects, the local community) and accompanying systemic manifestations may be helpful in presumptive virologic diagnoses. Thus, involvement of the nervous system by mumps virus is usually suspected from associated clinical parotitis or pancreatitis, although the neurologic disease can be the sole or presenting clinical manifestation; conversely, a certain history of previous mumps eliminates this diagnostic possibility. Several enterovirus infections produce a rash, which usually accompanies the onset of fever and persists for 4 to 10 days. In infections by coxsackievirus A5, 9, and 16 and echovirus 4, 6, 9, 16, and 30, the rash is typically maculopapular and nonpruritic and may be confined to the face and trunk or may involve extremities, including the palms and soles. Echovirus 9 infections can cause a petechial rash resembling meningococcemia. Herpangina, characterized by grayish vesicular lesions on the tonsillar fossae, soft palate, and uvula, can accompany group A coxsackie infection. In coxsackievirus A16 and, rarely, other group A serotype infections, a vesicular rash may involve hands, feet, and oropharynx. As discussed below, the encephalitis related to Epstein-Barr virus occurs in the setting of acute mononucleosis, and the principally postinfectious encephalitides related to measles and varicella follow overt systemic diseases with characteristic rashes.

Because no specific treatment exists for acute viral meningitis and encephalitis (except herpes), and their signs and symptoms are often nonspecific, exclusion of other diagnoses becomes important. Potentially confusing are partially treated bacterial meningitis; rickettsial infections; Lyme disease; meningitis caused by a variety of nonpyogenic organisms, including *Mycobacterium tuberculosis* and *Cryptococcus neoformans* and other fungi; meningeal or parameningeal bacterial infections; brain abscess; subacute bacterial endocarditis; and the cerebral vasculitides. Among noninfectious causes, trimethoprim-sulfamethoxazole, nonsteroidal analgesics, OKT3 antibody given for immunosuppression,

intravenous immunoglobulin, and certain other drugs may occasionally cause a sterile meningeal reaction. Without a cerebrospinal fluid examination, the differential diagnosis becomes even broader, encompassing additional toxic and vascular diseases. Most alternative diagnoses can be suspected or eliminated by the cerebrospinal fluid profile or by appropriate brain imaging.

Despite the absence of effective treatment, specific virologic diagnosis is useful both for prognosis in the individual patient and for epidemiologic implications for the populations at risk. Diagnosis usually relies on serology, although direct detection of the organism in the cerebrospinal fluid, blood, or stool may also be achieved in some cases. Selection of tests and their interpretation depend upon the particular organism. Almost all acute viral syndromes occur in the setting of a first encounter with the agent, which then results in lasting immunity. In these cases, seroconversion documented by a fourfold or greater rise in antibody titers between acute and convalescent sera is a principal means of diagnosis. A notable exception is herpes simplex encephalitis, in which antibody titers must be more cautiously interpreted (Ch. 476). Attempts at direct viral isolation are of limited value in clinical management and must be tailored to the suspected agent. Arboviruses and enteroviruses can be isolated from the blood but are seldom recoverable at the time of clinically evident meningitis or encephalitis. During the acute disease, coxsackieviruses and echoviruses are most readily isolated from stool or cerebrospinal fluid and, in some cases, throat washings. Lymphocytic choriomeningitis virus can be isolated from blood or cerebrospinal fluid. Mumps virus may be isolated from saliva, throat washings, or cerebrospinal fluid. Type 2 herpes simplex virus may also be cultured from the cerebrospinal fluid or identified in genital lesions.

TREATMENT. Treatment of acute viral encephalitis and meningitis (except herpes) is directed at symptom relief, supportive care, and preventing and managing complications. Strict isolation is not essential, although when enteroviral infection is suspected, precautions in handling of stools and the practice of careful hand washing should be instituted. Those with measles, chickenpox, rubella, or mumps virus infections should observe the usual precautions of isolation from susceptible individuals. Arboviruses are not characteristically spread from person to person but require an intermediate insect vector.

The headache and fever of meningitis can usually be managed with judicious doses of acetaminophen. Severe hyperthermia (>40°C) may require vigorous therapy, but modest temperature elevations may serve as a natural defense mechanism and are best left untreated.

Patients with severe encephalitis often become comatose. Since, however, some may achieve remarkable recovery, vigorous support and avoidance of complications are essential. Meticulous care in an intensive care unit setting with respiratory and nutritional support is therefore usually justified.

Although seizures sometimes complicate encephalitis, prophylactic anticonvulsants are not routinely recommended. If seizures develop, they can usually be managed with phenytoin and phenobarbital. If status epilepticus ensues, appropriate vigorous therapy should be instituted to prevent secondary brain injury and attendant hypoxia (Ch. 483). Similarly, secondary bacterial infections should be sought and promptly treated.

Modest increases in intracranial pressure can be treated with mannitol or glycerol, but this is usually only of short-term benefit. Steroids should probably generally be avoided in the treatment of encephalitis because of their inhibitory effects on host immune responses, but they may be required for control of intracranial hypertension in some patients.

PROGNOSIS. Full recovery from viral meningitis usually occurs within 1 to 2 weeks of onset, although some patients describe fatigue, light-headedness, and asthenia persisting for months.

The prognosis of encephalitis is dependent on the etiologic agent. Arbovirus encephalitides have variable mortality rates; that with eastern equine encephalitis is approximately 50 per cent; with St. Louis, 10 per cent; with western equine, 10 per cent; with Venezuelan equine, 1 per cent; and with California, less than 0.5 per cent. The mortality rates for western equine encephalitis are greater in children under 1 year of age, and for St. Louis encephalitis they are greater in the elderly. Nonfatal encephalitis caused by eastern, western, and St. Louis viruses leaves a relatively high rate of neurologic sequelae. Encephalitis associated with mumps or LCM virus is very rarely associated with death, and sequelae are infrequent. Hydrocephalus has been reported as a late sequela of mumps meningitis and encephalitis in children.

Chonmaitree T, Baldwin CD, Lucia HL: Role of the virology laboratory in diagnosis and management of patients with central nervous system disease. Clin Microbiol Rev 2:1, 1989. *A review of laboratory procedures used in the diagnosis of acute viral diseases of the central nervous system.*

Evans AS: Viral Infections of Humans: Epidemiology and Control. 3rd ed. New York, Plenum Publishing Corporation, 1989. *A useful text dealing with the epidemiology of viral infections; contains individual chapters dealing with the major groups, including the arboviruses, enteroviruses, and herpesviruses.*

Johnson RT: Viral Infections of the Nervous System. New York, Raven Press, 1982. *A comprehensive monograph reviewing the pathogenesis, epidemiology, and clinical features of central nervous system viral infections.*

Jubelt B: Enterovirus and mumps virus infections of the nervous system. Neurol Clin 2:187, 1984. *A useful review of the pathogenetic and clinical aspects of enterovirus and mumps virus infections.*

Jubelt B, Miller JR: Viral infections. *In* Merritt's Textbook of Neurology. Philadelphia, Lea & Febiger, 1989. *An excellent general review with a useful bibliography of "classic" and recent articles on individual infections.*

Nicolosi A, Hauser WA, Beghi E, et al.: Epidemiology of central nervous system infections in Olmstead County, Minnesota, 1950–1981. J Infect Dis 154:399, 1986. *Provides incidence figures for viral meningitis and encephalitis.*

Rennels MB: Arthropod-borne virus infections of the central nervous system. Neurol Clin 2:241, 1984. *A review of the major epidemic arbovirus infections in the United States.*

Whitley RJ: Viral encephalitis. N Engl J Med 323:242, 1990. *A recent review that emphasizes herpes encephalitis management and differential diagnosis.*

475 Poliomyelitis

Richard W. Price

DEFINITIONS. Poliomyelitis (acute anterior poliomyelitis, infantile paralysis) is an acute illness caused by the three strains of poliovirus. The disease selectively destroys the motor neurons of the spinal cord and brain stem to cause flaccid asymmetric weakness. Until recently one of the most feared of all human infectious diseases, poliomyelitis is now almost entirely preventable by vaccination.

ETIOLOGY. The three antigenically different strains of poliovirus (types 1, 2, and 3) are classified in the genus *Enterovirus* within the family Picornaviridae. These are small (approximately 270 nm), roughly spherical particles with icosahedral symmetry containing a single-stranded RNA core and are surrounded by a protein capsid. Lacking a lipid envelope, the polioviruses are resistant to lipid solvents and stable at low pH.

INCIDENCE, PREVALENCE, AND EPIDEMIOLOGY. In the United States, the number of cases of paralytic poliomyelitis, which averaged 21,000 per year over the 5 years before the introduction of vaccines, has now fallen to just a few cases yearly. However, in less advanced regions of the world, polioviruses remain endemic, and paralytic polio continues to occur, with a seasonal incidence of infection in temperate zones but a more even distribution throughout the year in tropical areas. Poliovirus is acquired by the oral route and subsequently replicates in the oropharynx and lower gastrointestinal tract. It may be secreted for a week or two in saliva and for more prolonged periods in feces, which provides the major avenue of host-to-host transmission. Spread of polioviruses is greatly influenced by standards of hygiene, and greatest dissemination occurs within families or other crowded circumstances.

Paralysis is an unusual complication of poliovirus infection. During an epidemic, 95 per cent of infections are asymptomatic and only 1 to 2 per cent result in neurologic symptoms and signs; the remaining 4 to 8 per cent of affected individuals suffer nonspecific (minor) illness. Where poliovirus is endemic and among children during epidemics, the incidence of neurologic manifestations is even lower. A number of factors increase the incidence of paralytic disease, including advancing age, recent hard exercise, tonsillectomy, and pregnancy. Immunity to each of the three types of poliovirus is lifelong, but infection with one strain does not necessarily protect against subsequent infection

by another. In the United States, poliomyelitis due to live-attenuated strains is as common as disease related to wild-type virus.

PATHOGENESIS AND PATHOLOGY. Polioviruses selectively infect certain neuronal populations, inducing highly stereotyped pathology, and in this manner contrast with most of the viruses causing acute encephalitis or meningitis.

The poliovirus invades the nervous system only after prior systemic replication. An initial alimentary phase with local replication in the intestinal mucosa and spread to the local lymphatics is followed by a viremic phase, which results in seeding of the nervous system. Once within the central nervous system, poliovirus may disseminate along neural pathways, attacking principally motor neurons of the spinal cord and lower brain stem, the brain stem reticular formation, and, to a lesser extent, the precentral gyrus. Convalescent poliomyelitis is characterized by loss of motor neurons and denervation atrophy of their associated skeletal muscles.

CLINICAL MANIFESTATIONS. The incubation period from virus exposure to the neurologic phase characteristically lasts between 4 and 10 days but may be prolonged to 4 to 5 weeks. The major illness usually begins with fever and malaise and is followed within hours by generalized headache, vomiting, and within another day by the development of neck and back stiffness. Patients at this time often are drowsy but on arousal are irritable and apprehensive. Progression may stop at this point, making the illness indistinguishable from other enterovirus meningitides. When paralysis develops, it usually begins on the second to fifth day after the onset of headache. Weakness, however, may be among the initial symptoms or, rarely, especially in children, may be delayed for 7 to 10 days. Children generally exhibit less intense systemic symptoms than do adults, who characteristically appear acutely ill and are tremulous, flushed, and agitated. Their muscles are often sensitive and stiff.

Poliomyelitis preferentially damages the larger somatic motor neurons. In all but the most severe cases, the involvement tends to include the lumbar segments to a greater degree than the cervical, and the spinal cord more than the brain stem. The damage and consequent paralyses are usually asymmetric, weakness characteristically being more proximal than distal, and in mild cases affecting parts of muscles rather than the entire muscle or the distribution of a single motor root. The asymmetry may be such that one member is rendered useless yet the contralateral one is spared entirely. About 50 per cent develop acute urinary retention. The trunk musculature is least commonly affected. The affected muscles are flaccid, and the deep tendon reflexes may be absent. Atrophy develops rapidly, usually beginning within a week in paralyzed muscles and progressing over the ensuing weeks. Once it starts, progression of the motor deficit for more than 3 to 5 days is rare.

About 10 to 15 per cent of cases affect the lower brain stem motor nuclei. Involvement of the ninth and tenth cranial nerve nuclei leads to paralysis of pharyngeal and laryngeal musculature, with resultant difficulty in phonation and swallowing. Parts of the facial muscles can be involved, either unilaterally or bilaterally. Less often, the tongue and muscles of mastication are partially paralyzed. External oculomotor weakness occurs only rarely and never permanently. The pupils are spared. Direct involvement of the brain stem reticular formation can disrupt breathing and swallowing and can produce serious disturbances in cardiovascular control. Poliomyelitis seldom causes permanent functional paralysis of the bulbar muscles, probably because of the relatively small size of the motor units served by brain stem nuclei and because overwhelming disease in these critical segments usually kills the patient.

DIAGNOSIS AND DIFFERENTIAL DIAGNOSIS. Because of its rarity in the United States, poliomyelitis may present diagnostic difficulties. In its early phases, it may be difficult to differentiate from other acute meningitides, and when paralysis ensues, a major differential diagnosis is with the Guillain-Barré syndrome and other predominantly motor polyneuropathies. However, for practical purposes, no other acute disease produces headaches, stiff neck, fever, and asymmetric flaccid paralysis without sensory loss coupled with an increase in white blood cells in the cerebrospinal fluid (CSF). Diagnosis may be more difficult if these major findings are equivocal or lacking. The CSF rarely shows a persistence of significant pleocytosis in polyneuritis, and CSF protein levels above 100 mg per milliliter are frequent. Acute intermittent porphyria may cause an illness similar to that of postinfectious polyneuropathy. At times, acute transverse myelitis may be confused with poliomyelitis, but in the former a sensory and motor level at the appropriate spinal cord segment usually serves to separate an inflammatory cord transection from diffuse anterior horn cell involvement. Both epidemic neuromyasthenia (Iceland disease) and pleurodynia (Bornholm's disease) may be confused with mild attacks of poliomyelitis. The epidemiologic setting, the lack of CSF abnormalities, and the absence of clear motor paralysis serve to distinguish these entities. In rare cases, infection with other enteroviruses can produce a paralytic illness resembling mild paralytic poliomyelitis. Both coxsackievirus and echoviruses have been reported to cause encephalitides with prominent (but not extensive) motor neuron symptoms and signs. Diagnosis can be established by isolation of virus from blood or CSF or by serologic evidence of acute poliovirus infection. In cases related to vaccine strains, viral isolates can be distinguished in the laboratory.

TREATMENT. There is no specific treatment, but supportive care can be important in reducing suffering during the acute attack, in maintaining vital functions to ensure survival, and perhaps in modifying the overall outcome and disability. Important measures include preventing contractures, maintaining airway and cardiovascular stability, and preventing excessive calcium mobilization and bed sores.

PROGNOSIS. Death in poliomyelitis is usually the result of bulbar involvement and is attributable to respiratory and cardiovascular impairments. Death rates are higher in adolescents and adults than in children. Mortality also varies with individual epidemics and has been considerably reduced with modern management of respiratory insufficiency. Patients who survive an episode of acute paralytic poliomyelitis usually recover considerable motor function. Generally, motor improvement begins within the first weeks after onset, and 60 per cent of eventual recovery is achieved by 3 months and 80 per cent by 6 months. The degree of permanent paralysis cannot be assessed accurately until 2 to 3 months have passed.

The Postpolio Syndrome. A number of patients with previous poliomyelitis develop further functional deterioration later in life. In some this relates simply to musculoskeletal decompensation or other factors but does not involve new weakness. However, in others there is a true loss of strength; the condition in these patients has been referred to as postpoliomyelitis progressive muscular atrophy (PPMA). This disorder is characterized by progressive weakness beginning 30 or more years after an attack of poliomyelitis. Clinicians in the United States are now much more likely to see this late complication of poliomyelitis than the initial paralytic disease. Most commonly, it presents as a late-life progression of weakness in already affected muscles, or, less often, in muscles previously thought to be normal. This weakness is often accompanied by fasciculations, and there may be additional atrophy. Muscle biopsy shows type grouping consistent with active denervation-reinnervation. Overall, the prognosis is generally good, with only slow progression of further weakness, which may plateau and rarely leads to a severe increase in disability or to death. This development must be distinguished from motor neuron disease of a more malignant variety (Ch. 465), which has also been described many years after acute poliomyelitis but appears to be much less common than the more gradual and benign syndrome of PPMA.

PREVENTION. Poliomyelitis can be prevented by either live-attenuated or killed polio vaccines. These are now given routinely in Western cultures, although the practice of immunization has relaxed as the threat of developing paralytic poliomyelitis has become less conspicuous. If this trend is not reversed, a resurgence of the disease can be expected. An important consequence of accurate diagnosis of poliomyelitis is the prompt institution of local vaccination programs for communities at risk, including subcultures in which vaccination is avoided for religious or other reasons.

Dalakas MC, Elder G, Hallett M: A long-term follow-up of patients with postpoliomyelitis neuromuscular symptoms. N Engl J Med 314:959, 1986. *Describes the clinical and laboratory features of late-onset weakness in patients suffering poliomyelitis earlier in life.*

Price RW, Plum F: Poliomyelitis. In Vinken PJ, Bruyn GW (eds.): Handbook of Clinical Neurology. Vol. 32, Part I. Amsterdam, Elsevier North-Holland, 1978. *A general review of clinical and biologic aspects of poliomyelitis.*

Wyatt HV: Incubation of poliomyelitis as calculated from the time of entry into the central nervous system via the peripheral nerve pathways. J Infect Dis 12:547, 1990. *Discusses the pathogenesis of poliomyelitis, hypothesizing that axoplasmic transport of virus over motor nerves provides the major portal of entry into the central nervous system and explains the tropism for anterior horn cells.*

476 Herpesvirus Infections of the Nervous System

Richard W. Price

Three of the six human herpesviruses (see also Ch. 371 to 375) share an essential "neurotropism" in their adaptation for survival and transmission. Herpes simplex virus types 1 and 2 (HSV-1 and HSV-2) and varicella zoster virus all establish in sensory ganglion neurons a latent infection that can subsequently reactivate to release progeny virus into the territory of the ganglion's epithelial innervation. The major complications of these infections in adults include adult-type herpes simplex encephalitis caused by HSV-1; aseptic meningitis, radiculitis, and sacral autonomic insufficiency caused by HSV-2; and encephalitis, myelitis, radiculopathy, and vasculitis complicating herpes zoster. Prompt diagnosis of infections by these viruses is important, since they are now amenable to selective antiviral drug therapy. Two of the remaining human herpesviruses, Epstein-Barr virus and cytomegalovirus, although largely lymphotropic, can also cause neurologic disease in the setting of systemic illness.

476.1 HERPES SIMPLEX ENCEPHALITIS (HSE)

Adult-type HSE is a sporadic disease with a severe morbidity and high mortality. Both HSV-1 and HSV-2 are capable of causing encephalitis, but type 1 by far predominates. In contrast, HSV-2 accounts for the great majority of neonatal herpetic encephalitis, which is not considered here.

EPIDEMIOLOGY AND PATHOGENESIS. Although the most common identified cause of severe, sporadic viral encephalitis in the United States, HSE is nonetheless uncommon. The disease afflicts persons of all postneonatal ages, with peaks of incidence in late childhood and middle age. It occurs with approximately equal frequency throughout the year, and case-to-case transmission does not occur. Immunosuppression plays no apparent role.

HSV-1 is a ubiquitous organism; more than 90 per cent of adults exhibit serologic evidence of exposure, and most harbor latent ganglionic infection. Recurrent cold sores resulting from viral reactivation occur in perhaps one fourth of adults. Although HSE may occur as a primary infection, it likely more often results from reactivated virus or perhaps from reinfection by a new strain of virus.

The characteristic gross and microscopic pathology of herpetic infection, particularly its anatomic localization, distinguishes HSE from other encephalitides. Although often asymmetric, the disease is usually bilateral and afflicts the medial temporal and inferior frontal lobes and related "limbic" structures, including the hippocampus, amygdaloid nuclei, olfactory cortex, insula, and cingulate gyrus. Necrosis with petechial hemorrhage is so intense that the disease was once called *acute necrotizing encephalitis*. Microscopically, hemorrhagic necrosis with mononuclear inflammation characterizes involved areas, with neurons and glia often containing Cowdry type A intranuclear inclusions during the acute phase of infection. The gray matter is affected predominantly, but infection extends into the white matter as well.

CLINICAL MANIFESTATIONS. HSE most commonly presents as an abruptly beginning subacute illness causing local and diffuse cerebral dysfunction. Typically, patients are febrile, although in as many as 10 per cent fever may be absent, and thus herpes encephalitis warrants consideration even in afebrile patients who present with an acutely altered mental status. Severe headache, focal or generalized convulsions, and alterations in behavior and consciousness are the most prominent symptoms. Common symptoms including disorientation, delusions, agitation, personality changes, or dysphasia sometimes lead erroneously to psychiatric referral. Motor paralyses are present in fewer than half of affected individuals.

DIAGNOSIS. Evaluation of suspected HSE has been an area of controversy, principally related to the issue of diagnostic brain biopsy. Among the arguments for brain biopsy are that (1) it is the most sensitive and accurate diagnostic method, contrasting with the insensitivity and difficulty in early interpretation of serologic studies and neurodiagnostic procedures; and (2) this procedure results in identification of alternative diagnoses, some of which respond to specific treatment. Arguments against brain biopsy relate to its potential short- and long-term sequelae, the benignity of empiric therapy, and the improved sensitivity and accuracy of magnetic resonance imaging (MRI) compared with earlier diagnostic methods. Important issues regarding management also relate to the facilities, expertise, and experience available to the patient at the admitting hospital. This author feels that, all in all, in most instances patients are appropriately managed without biopsy and that the combination of clinical and laboratory features warrants an approach utilizing empiric therapy with persistent pursuit of alternative diagnoses.

The most important step in management involves prompt recognition of HSE as a diagnostic possibility and rapid institution of acyclovir therapy. Among the important neurodiagnostic evaluations in patients suspected of having HSE are MRI, cerebrospinal fluid (CSF) analysis, and electroencephalography. While computed tomographic (CT) scanning is surprisingly insensitive in detecting early HSE, with two fifths or more patients having normal scans, MRI, at least on the basis of anecdotal experience, more often detects characteristic abnormalities. The latter include virtually pathognomonic increased signal, particularly on T_2-weighted sequences, in the same regions showing pathology at autopsy: the medial temporal lobes, inferior frontal regions, insulae, and cingulate gyri, often bilateral (Fig. 476–1). The MRI also allows more sensitive detection of alternative diagnoses, such as brain abscess, vasculitis, or demyelination. Some patients are so ill or agitated that MRI may not be possible; in these patients, biopsy might be needed.

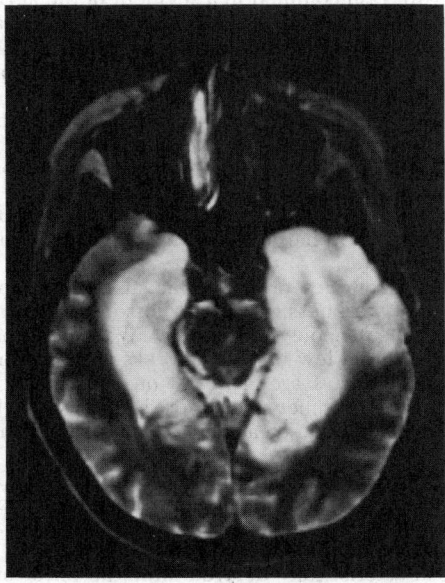

FIGURE 476–1. MRI scan of a 54-year-old woman with herpes simplex encephalitis who presented with fever, dysphasia, and confusion. The T_2-weighted image shows increased signal in both medial temporal lobes, with more extensive involvement on the left (right side of figure).

CSF examination is also important in detecting evidence of virus infection. Most patients exhibit a mononuclear pleocytosis with 50 or more leukocytes per cubic millimeter, although fewer or even a normal number of cells may be noted. The protein content is usually mildly elevated, and the glucose level is normal or only mildly reduced. Like MRI, cerebrospinal fluid analysis may also be useful in establishing alternative diagnoses, such as bacterial or fungal infection. In more than three fourths of patients, the electroencephalogram exhibits focal abnormalities, most often showing spike and slow-wave or sharp-wave patterns over the involved temporal lobes.

Attempts at isolating HSV-1 from CSF rarely succeed. Newer methods of diagnosis seeking detection of viral antigens (by enzyme-linked immunoassay) or nucleic acid (by polymerase chain reaction gene amplification) are under development. Isolation of the virus from the oropharynx is useless, since no relationship exists between symptomatic or asymptomatic viral shedding at such peripheral sites and brain infection. HSV-1 is often reactivated by other neurologic diseases eliciting fever, creating a source of false-positive serologic responses in patients suffering from nonherpetic encephalitis or meningitis.

In contrast to the epidemic encephalitides, in which documentation of seroconversion provides a major method of diagnosis, in HSE serologic testing is often inconclusive. This is particularly true at the onset, when prompt diagnostic decisions are critical. Even during convalescence, analyses of blood and CSF antibody titers can give false-negative or false-positive results.

TREATMENT. The introduction of antiviral therapy has greatly improved the outcome of HSE. This was first demonstrated with vidarabine, and even greater benefit has been shown with acyclovir, which has become the treatment of choice. HSE is treated by an intravenous infusion of 10 mg per kilogram given over a 1-hour period every 8 hours for 10 days. The therapeutic efficacy of acyclovir is restricted to the herpesviruses by virtue of the drug's selective interaction with two virus-coded enzymes, thymidine kinase and DNA polymerase; acyclovir is thus not a broad-spectrum antiviral. Because acyclovir is excreted principally by the kidney, caution must be exercised in patients with renal impairment. Side effects of acyclovir are generally few, although neurotoxicity rarely occurs, manifested as altered consciousness, tremors, hallucinations, and seizures. Other aspects of care also require meticulous attention. Optimally, patients with HSE should be managed in the intensive care setting of a tertiary referral center.

PROGNOSIS. Both age and initial neurologic status significantly influence the prognosis in HSE; even with antiviral therapy, patients who are comatose when first treated often fare poorly. Extensive infection and brain damage are present in most of these patients as a result of a more fulminant illness and, sometimes, a delay in beginning therapy. Many patients, however, particularly those younger than 30 years old who are neurologically intact when treatment begins, recover normal or nearly normal function. Patients with minor neurologic deficits may survive without severe long-term sequelae and return to normal function if diagnosis is made and specific treatment is instituted early in the course. In a few patients, and despite antiviral treatment, HSE can relapse within a few weeks after the acute disease, resulting in severe sequelae. The pathogenesis of such relapses is unknown.

476.2 NEUROLOGIC COMPLICATIONS OF GENITAL HERPES

Genital herpes, most often caused by HSV-2, may be complicated by local or radicular pain, aseptic meningitis, autonomic (bowel, bladder, and sexual) dysfunction, and rarely myelitis. These complications are more common in association with primary genital herpes but may occur with recurrent disease as well. Prodromal neuritic symptoms commonly precede recurrences and may involve the buttock, the groin, or, less commonly, the lower extremities.

Aseptic meningitis and autonomic dysfunction may occur either independently or together. Meningitic symptoms are associated with primary genital herpes in about one fourth of patients, but only a minority require hospitalization. Its course is benign, usually clearing in 4 to 10 days without residua. The CSF profile is typical of an aseptic meningitis, with a mononuclear pleocytosis, mild protein elevation, and normal, or occasionally reduced, glucose level. When the history clearly implicates an epidemiologic and temporal relationship with genital herpes and the CSF findings are those of a typical mononuclear profile, a clinical diagnosis can usually be made. Specific diagnosis can often be established by isolation of HSV-2 at lumbar puncture.

Urinary retention, constipation, and sexual impotence in association with genital herpes are less common than meningitis. Symptoms and signs of a sacral sensory radiculopathy sometimes accompany the autonomic changes. The pathophysiology of this disorder is uncertain, but direct herpetic infection of nervous system structures is likely. Fortunately, autonomic dysfunction is reversible, and patients can be assured that their symptoms will probably clear. Although unusual, these autonomic symptoms can recur. It is important to consider and pursue the diagnosis of HSV-2 infection in patients who present with isolated bladder, bowel, or sexual dysfunction. It is critical not to make an inappropriate diagnosis of spinal neoplasm or, especially, early multiple sclerosis. When there is a clear history of genital herpes, the cause of autonomic dysfunction is usually readily established clinically. Inspection and viral culture of genital lesions, plus accompanying antibody titers, which may appear and rise slowly only in primary HSV-2 infection, provide additional help.

In adults, HSV-2 only rarely produces adult-type herpes encephalitis indistinguishable from that caused by HSV-1. Transverse myelopathy due to HSV-2 is very rare.

Epithelial HSV-2 primary infections and recurrences can be treated with acyclovir, but the effect on the neurologic complications of genital herpes is uncertain. In the absence of adequate data, it appears appropriate to give acyclovir for neurologic complications of primary genital herpes.

In patients with frequent recurrent attacks of genital herpes, early, self-initiated treatment of recurrent lesions with oral acyclovir has been advocated, beginning therapy at the onset of prodromal symptoms. This approach is probably appropriate for the rare patient with recurrent herpetic meningitis.

476.3 NEUROLOGIC COMPLICATIONS OF VARICELLA ZOSTER VIRUS INFECTIONS

Herpes zoster (HZ) (shingles, zona) is a dermatomal cutaneous infection caused by reactivation of the varicella zoster virus that normally lies latent in sensory ganglia following an early attack of varicella. In addition to its cutaneous manifestations, zoster is accompanied by neuritic symptoms and may be complicated by an array of neurologic sequelae. The varicella zoster virus is distantly related to HSV, sharing only minor antigen cross-reactivity.

INCIDENCE AND EPIDEMIOLOGY. HZ is a common disorder, with an annual incidence estimated at 3.4 cases per 1000 persons. Unlike varicella, HZ occurs throughout the year, with neither significant clustering of cases nor seasonal or yearly preponderance. Case exposure in HZ is rarely identified. Two factors, age and immunosuppression, significantly influence its incidence. The disease is uncommon in childhood, relatively constant in those between 20 and 50 years of age (approximately 2.5 cases per 1000 annually), and thereafter doubles its incidence in those between the ages of 50 and 60 and redoubles it in those between age 80 and 90. Immunosuppression due to systemic disease (in particular, Hodgkin's disease and other lymphoreticular malignancies, cytotoxic drugs, corticosteroids, radiation therapy, or infection by human immunodeficiency virus (HIV) predisposes. In some cases, a history of neoplasm, radiation exposure, or physical injury in the proximity of the dorsal root ganglion or nerve is elicited.

Age is an important factor also in the development of postherpetic neuralgia, which develops almost exclusively in persons older than 50 years of age. The incidence of postherpetic pain varies, ranging between 15 and 75 per cent, depending on clinical definition of the syndrome and selection of patients. Immunosuppression predisposes to spread of virus beyond the ganglion-nerve-dermatome unit into the central nervous system or systemically.

PATHOGENESIS AND PATHOLOGY. Once the reactivation of latent varicella zoster virus occurs, it characteristically spreads within the sensory ganglion and travels centrifugally over the peripheral nerve processes of this ganglion, eventually seeding the skin with the resultant dermatomal vesicular rash.

Cell-mediated defenses rather than humoral immunity are critically involved in protecting the host during HZ. Pathologically, acutely infected dorsal root ganglia and nerve show the presence of a mononuclear inflammatory response, neuronal degeneration with intranuclear Cowdry type A inclusion bodies, and similar infection of surrounding satellite cells. The peripheral nerve may contain parallel changes. In more severe cases, dorsal root ganglia above and below the primarily affected ganglion also show active herpetic infection.

CLINICAL MANIFESTATIONS. Prodromal sensory symptoms include dermatomal pain, itching, or paresthesias, which often antecede by several days the eruption of the segmental rash. The early pain of zoster may be confused with other types of neuropathic or visceral pain. The most frequently involved dermatomes are those extending from the third thoracic to the second lumbar segments and the first (ophthalmic) division of the trigeminal nerve. The rash itself initially consists of erythematous macules that vesiculate over 12 to 24 hours. Normally the vesicular fluid pustulates within 72 hours; in a week the pustules begin to dry, and crusting takes place by 10 to 12 days. The crusts, in turn, fall off in 2 to 3 weeks. In the immunocompromised host, this time course may be protracted. In uncomplicated cases, the rash heals with a variable degree of superficial scarring, at times leaving areas of hyperpigmentation or depigmentation, which may be anesthetic. More severe cases may leave denervation of a large segment of the dermatome.

Zoster can affect any of several of the cranial nerves. The ophthalmic division of the trigeminal nerve is the most commonly affected, and the condition may be complicated by spread to orbital structures, resulting in acute and long-term ocular sequelae. Spread of cutaneous rash along the bridge of the nose to its tip should be taken as a signal of impending ocular infection, prompting early ophthalmologic consultation. Facial palsy, with or without accompanying loss of taste on the anterior two thirds of the tongue, may accompany either otic zoster (Ramsay Hunt syndrome), with rash confined to a segment of the auricle, or the second and third cervical dermatone (cervical collar zoster). Occasionally, infection of the ninth and tenth or fifth cranial nerve may antecede facial weakness. As with other motor syndromes (see below), weakness is often delayed for a variable period after the rash. Eighth nerve dysfunction with sensorineural hearing loss or vertigo occurs in the same setting as facial palsy but with less frequency. HZ may rarely cause facial palsy in the absence of rash (zoster sine herpete). Zoster of the ninth and tenth cranial nerves is unusual and may be overlooked without a careful search for the pharyngeal rash or ipsilateral laryngeal or pharyngeal palsy.

HZ of the extremities or trunk can also be complicated by segmental motor weakness, the motor loss usually corresponding to the involved cutaneous dermatome. Weakness characteristically develops from a few days to 2 weeks after the onset of the rash, and longer delays are rare. Its onset is characteristically abrupt, occurring over hours or 1 or 2 days, with little or no subsequent deterioration. Weakness abates or disappears in about 85 per cent of cases.

Myelitis of variable extent is a less common complication of HZ and results from direct viral invasion of the spinal cord, perhaps augmented by local inflammatory responses. It occurs most commonly in the immunosuppressed person and, like motor paresis, is characteristically delayed after the onset of the rash. The most common manifestation is bladder dysfunction. Other signs include mild or transient asymmetric reflexes, lower extremity weakness, and sensory disturbance. Severe myelopathy can produce a partial Brown-Séquard syndrome or total cord transection. Characteristically, involvement lies at the same spinal cord segment as the rash but may ascend to a higher level. Spinal MRI or myelography may be needed to rule out coexisting epidural tumor.

At least three types of brain involvement may complicate zoster: diffuse encephalitis, focal parenchymal infection, and vasculitis. Headache, stiff neck, and mild diffuse encephalitis often accompany acute HZ but are difficult to distinguish from the effects of fever, sepsis, narcotic analgesics, and other underlying medical problems. Most such patients recover. In more severe diffuse encephalitis, chances for recovery may also be good if other complications of the disease do not intervene. The clinical picture is that of an acute or subacute delirium accompanied by cerebrospinal fluid pleocytosis with few focal features.

Focal varicella zoster virus encephalitis is a rare complication in immunosuppressed patients that can resemble progressive multifocal leukoencephalopathy. The onset may be temporally remote from the cutaneous rash. The cerebral lesions involve principally the white matter. Brain biopsy is required for diagnosis, allowing identification of Cowdry type A inclusions or of varicella zoster virus antigens or nuclei acids.

Cerebral vasculitis is probably the most common serious post-zoster central nervous system complication. Affected patients usually develop delayed contralateral hemiplegic strokes following ophthalmic division zoster owing to inflammation or occlusion of the internal carotid artery and its major branches ipsilateral to the rash. The delay between the rash and the onset of cerebral dysfunction varies from none to as much as 6 months, with a mean interval of 7 weeks. A more widespread cerebral vasculitis following zoster in other locations has also been reported. The pathogenesis is still incompletely understood, but the characteristic involvement of local vessels innervated by the infected ganglion, in conjunction with reports suggesting the presence of viral nucleocapsids and viral antigens within vessels, suggests that the arteries are directly infected. Additional contributions may be made by secondary local inflammatory responses and thrombosis, leading to vascular occlusion or distal embolization. Arteriographic evidence of vasculitis or occlusions in the involved vessels and the clinical setting usually allow diagnosis.

DIAGNOSIS. The clinical diagnosis of HZ is seldom difficult. The dermatomal distribution and the evolution of the vesicular rash are characteristic, and only rarely does herpes simplex infection assume a similar pattern and confuse the diagnosis. Difficulty, however, may occur early in the disease, when pain or other sensory symptoms precede the rash. The rare case of zoster sine herpete may require additional methods of diagnosis, and, in cases with an occult rash, a careful search is necessary. When there is a question of the diagnosis, a Tzanck test examining lesion scrapings, a direct culture, or immunohistochemical identification of infected cells can provide specific identification of varicella zoster virus. Serology may also be helpful, although the commonly used complement fixation test can cross-react between HSV and varicella zoster virus.

THERAPY. The goals are to relieve the acute segmental infection, to curtail spread of infection either systemically or to other areas of the nervous system, and to prevent postherpetic neuralgia. The means available consist of using antiviral drugs to interrupt viral replication and perhaps corticosteroids to modify local inflammatory responses. Treatment of individual patients must take into account their background risk for particular complications.

Since involvement of the ophthalmic division of the trigeminal nerve risks spreading to orbital structures, such infections should receive early antiviral treatment. Systemic antiviral therapy should also be used for immunosuppressed patients, who are more susceptible to severe disseminated infection. In young patients with normal immune function, there is usually no requirement for specific therapy because zoster is usually mild with swift recovery and no residua. Older nonimmunosuppressed persons are susceptible to postherpetic neuralgia; two controlled studies of such individuals have suggested that a brief course of corticosteroids may reduce the subsequent incidence of pain without untoward complications. A reasonable course begins with a daily dose of 60 mg of prednisone (or the equivalent glucocorticoid) in four individual doses with rapid tapering so that patients are off medication within 7 to 10 days. Whether the addition of acyclovir to the corticosteroids is helpful has not been evaluated.

The antiviral treatment of choice for HZ is acyclovir. The nucleoside can abort the rash and prevent systemic spread when administered promptly by the intravenous route. The recommended intravenous dosages vary from 5 to 10* mg per kilogram infused every 8 hours for 5 days. More recently, the use of oral acyclovir has been suggested at a dosage of 800 mg* every 4 hours with omission of the nighttime dose, particularly in individuals who are not at marked risk of developing viral complications.

Intravenous acyclovir is indicated for patients in whom varicella zoster virus infection progresses to cause myelitis or encephalitis, although delay in institution reduces its overall effect. No satisfactory data indicate whether either acyclovir or steroids improve the outcome of HZ-associated motor weakness. Similarly, there is no proven effective treatment for zoster-associated cerebral vasculitis. Postherpetic neuralgia is discussed in Ch. 455.

476.4 NEUROLOGIC COMPLICATIONS OF CYTOMEGALOVIRUS AND EPSTEIN-BARR VIRUS INFECTIONS

Both human cytomegalovirus and Epstein-Barr virus infections can cause neurologic disease. While in children cytomegalovirus is an important and relatively common cause of congenital neurologic deficit, central and peripheral nervous system infections in adults occur almost exclusively in the setting of immunosuppression. Central nervous system complications of Epstein-Barr virus infections occur in the setting of acute mononucleosis. Both viruses have been implicated in triggering the Guillain-Barré syndrome.

Cytomegalovirus encephalitis and, less commonly, meningo-encephalitis or myelitis have been reported as opportunistic infections in adults suffering from impaired cell-mediated immunity. Earlier these complications were reported most commonly in patients undergoing organ transplantation, but more recently their occurrence has been noted principally in association with acquired immunodeficiency syndrome (AIDS). The clinical features of cytomegalovirus brain infection have been imprecisely characterized, but the major symptoms and signs appear to reflect diffuse brain dysfunction with concomitantly impaired levels of attention and cognition, paralleling the symptomatology of a metabolic encephalopathy. At times, focal deficits (e.g., hemiparesis) or seizures are superimposed. Pathologically, infection of the brain by this virus is marked by scattered microglial nodules, some of which contain typical cytomegalovirus intranuclear inclusions. As many as one fourth of autopsied AIDS patients have neuropathologic evidence of central nervous system cytomegalovirus infection, although in most the infection appears to be mild, and indeed its contribution to symptoms is uncertain. Some patients may exhibit ventricular subependymal abnormalities or small abscess-like lesions on MRI.

More recently, the role of cytomegalovirus in causing severe ascending polyradiculopathy has been delineated. This syndrome is usually characterized by the subacute evolution of severe, painful polyradiculopathy that begins with sacral or lumbar sensory, motor, and autonomic dysfunction and is accompanied by CSF pleocytosis with nearly diagnostic polymorphonuclear cell predominance.

The diagnosis of cytomegalovirus encephalitis is difficult. Most AIDS patients, particularly homosexual men, have circulating antibody to the virus, and in many it can be isolated from urine or blood, yet they do not suffer nervous system infection. For this reason, serologic evaluation and systemic virus isolation are not particularly helpful in diagnosis; rather, one must rely on clinical suspicion. Cytomegalovirus polyradiculopathy can be diagnosed by the CSF findings, including the prominence of neutrophils and the isolation of virus. Recently, the antiviral nucleoside ganciclovir been found effective in treating certain

*Exceeds manufacturer's recommended dosage.

manifestations of cytomegalovirus infection, including particularly the retinopathy that sometimes complicates AIDS. No information is yet available regarding the drug's efficacy in central nervous system infections caused by human cytomegalovirus, but individual case reports suggest that ganciclovir may be helpful in patients with cytomegalovirus polyradiculopathy.

The neurologic complications of Epstein-Barr virus infection range from symptoms of headache, photophobia, weakness, and fatigue, which occur relatively frequently in infectious mononucleosis, to more serious, but uncommon, complications that have been described principally in the context of individual case reports. These include encephalitis, meningoencephalitis, Guillain-Barré syndrome, Bell's palsy, acute cerebellar ataxia, and transverse myelitis. It is likely that most of these neurologic complications result from immune-mediated injury rather than direct viral infection.

Bale JF Jr: Human cytomegalovirus infection and disorders of the nervous system. Arch Neurol 41:310, 1984. *A general review of the nervous system complications of human cytomegalovirus, including both congenital and adult infections.*

Corey L, Spear PG: Infections with herpes simplex viruses. N Engl J Med 314:749, 1986. *A review of the clinical spectrum and treatment of HSV infections.*

Esiri MM: Herpes simplex encephalitis. An immunohistochemical study of the distribution of viral antigen within the brain. J Neurol Sci 54:209, 1982. *An excellent paper outlining the topography of HSV infection in brain, using immunohistochemistry.*

Hilt DC, Buchholz D, Krumholz A, et al.: Herpes zoster ophthalmicus and delayed contralateral hemiparesis caused by cerebral angiitis: Diagnosis and management approaches. Ann Neurol 14:543, 1983. *A report of four cases and review of the literature related to herpes zoster–associated cerebral angiitis.*

Horten B, Price RW, Jimenez D: Multifocal varicella-zoster virus leukoencephalitis temporally remote from herpes zoster. Ann Neurol 9:251, 1981. *A report of two immunosuppressed patients with multifocal varicella zoster virus encephalitis.*

Jemsek J, Greenberg SB, Taber L, et al.: Herpes zoster–associated encephalitis: Clinicopathologic report of 12 cases and review of the literature. Medicine 62:81, 1983. *A review of encephalitis complicating HZ.*

Miller RG, Storey JR, Greco CM: Ganciclovir in the treatment of progressive AIDS-related polyradiculopathy. Neurology 40:569, 1990. *Describes the clinical and therapeutic aspects of cytomegalovirus polyradiculopathy in AIDS patients.*

Price RW: Neurobiology of human herpesvirus infections. CRC Crit Rev Clin Neurobiol 2:61, 1986. *A general review of the pathophysiology of neurotropic herpesvirus infections and their neurologic complications.*

Whitley RJ: Viral encephalitis. N Engl J Med 323:242, 1990. *A review emphasizing HSE and favoring the role of brain biopsy.*

477 Rabies

Richard W. Price

DEFINITION. Rabies is a viral infection with nearly worldwide distribution that affects principally wild and domestic animals but also involves humans, resulting in a devastating, almost invariably fatal encephalitis.

ETIOLOGY, PATHOGENESIS, AND PATHOLOGY. Rabies virus is a bullet-shaped, enveloped, single-strand RNA virus classified in the rhabdovirus family and *Lyssavirus* genus. It has particular neurotropic properties, and unlike many of the other viruses causing acute encephalitis, it appears to require central nervous system infection as an essential part of its "life cycle."

Viral transmission to both animals and humans characteristically results from the bite of a rabid animal, although cases of transmission by aerosol in the laboratory or in a bat cave and by transplanted infected corneal tissue have also been recorded. Once the virus breaches the protective epithelium, it reaches the central nervous system via peripheral nerves, exploiting retrograde axoplasmic transport. The interval between the bite and the onset of disease is variable, ranging from days to a year or more, but in most cases lasting 1 to 2 months. This delay may relate to amplification of the virus in peripheral tissues, particularly skeletal muscle, before it gains access to the central nervous system over motor and sensory nerves. During this delay, the virus can be eliminated by host immune mechanisms; indeed, it is this delay that affords an opportunity for prophylactic postexposure immunization after the rabid bite. Evidence suggests a possible role for the nicotinic acetylcholine receptor and the neuromuscular junction in the concentration and access of rabies virus to the central nervous system. Once virus enters peripheral and central nervous system pathways, immune defenses are unlikely to be able to suppress further replication and spread of infection, which includes axoplasmic transport and perhaps transsynaptic transmission.

The central nervous system, in turn, is involved in the subsequent transmission of the virus by infected animals in two essential ways: (1) Infection of certain brain regions underlies the characteristic behavioral changes in the rabid animal, leading to increased biting activity; (2) antegrade transport of the virus to salivary glands leads to virus shedding. In concert, these two aspects of infection ensure transmission and survival of the virus in the wild. They also have practical diagnostic implications for the human disease. The characteristic altered behavior in humans often results in a distinct clinical picture distinguishing rabies from other viral encephalitides. Antegrade virus transport also affords a means of diagnosing rabies by isolation from saliva or immunohistochemical staining of infected cutaneous nerves innervating hair follicles.

Pathologic findings are variable and include both nonspecific and specific abnormalities. Perhaps most remarkable is the frequent apparent discrepancy between the degree of pathologic change, particularly neuronal loss, and the severe antemortem clinical state. Nonspecific changes include perivascular mononuclear infiltrates and microglial response, although inflammation may be scant in relation to the widespread distribution of infected cells detected immunohistochemically. Similarly, neuronal destruction is less prominent than the abundance of viral antigen, which is located principally in neurons but also in astrocytes. More specific changes include the presence of Negri bodies, eosinophilic neuronal intracytoplasmic inclusion composed of viral nucleoprotein. At autopsy, infection is usually widespread in the brain, but with prominent involvement of the brain stem and spinal cord and also involvement of the hippocampus, basal ganglia, cortex, and other structures. The relation of virus infection of neurons and the attendant inflammatory reaction to the clinical manifestations remains incompletely understood. Rabies virus infection of neurons may alter their membrane properties or synaptic transmission. Whatever the means by which infection perturbs neuronal function, patients eventually manifest widespread brain dysfunction that terminally impairs respiratory and autonomic control.

EPIDEMIOLOGY. The epidemiology of rabies varies in different parts of the world, falling into two patterns. In *sylvatic rabies*, infection is maintained in wildlife reservoirs. Thus, in the United States, rabies is endemic in the striped skunk in the central states, in the raccoon in the southeastern and mid-Atlantic states, and in the red fox in northern New York and adjacent regions of Canada; bat rabies has a wide geographic range. A similar pattern holds in other developed nations, where human rabies is rare and more often results from direct contact with wildlife than from secondary transmission to the domestic dog or cat and then to humans. This pattern contrasts with the one in much of Asia, Africa, and South America, where *urban rabies* is maintained as an epizootic infection in the domestic dog and human disease is far more common.

CLINICAL MANIFESTATIONS. After the silent incubation period, clinical rabies frequently begins with a prodromal phase, which may include nonspecific symptoms of malaise, fever, and headache but also more specific local symptoms related to the site of the original bite. These include itching, paresthesias, or other sensations beginning in the area of the healed wound and then spreading to a wider region and eventually involving the whole limb or side of the body.

Within a few days, the full-blown illness begins, taking one of two forms—encephalitic (*furious*) or paralytic (*dumb*) rabies—perhaps depending on the source and strain of the infecting virus. In its initial phase, encephalitic rabies is often distinguished from other viral infections by irritability of the patient and hyperactivity of a number of automatic reflexes. Periods of calm lucidity may alternate with confusion and seeming intense anxiety precipitated by internal or external stimuli. Hydrophobia, with reflexive intense contraction of the diaphragm and accessory respiratory and other muscles, is induced upon attempts to drink or even at the sight of water. Similarly, blowing or fanning air on the chest may induce intense laryngeal, pharyngeal, or other muscle spasms (aerophobia). High fever persists throughout the illness.

Paralytic rabies is less common and more readily misdiagnosed. Patients present with weakness, usually beginning in the bitten extremity and spreading to involve all four limbs and the facial muscles. Early in the course, both consciousness and sensory function are spared. Helpful signs include myoedema and pilo-erection, and fever is also present. As the disease progresses, it may converge with the encephalitic form, accompanied by some of the same irritative phenomena. Both forms evolve into lethargy and coma, with prominent alterations of respiratory and cardio-vascular function. Tachycardia may precede bradycardia with ectopic rhythms, and the breathing pattern becomes irregular with cluster or periodic respirations. Patients succumb to respi-ratory failure or cardiovascular collapse within a mean interval of 4 days from onset, although patients may survive as long as 3 weeks or more. Intensive supportive care may extend survival longer; in three clinically unusual cases, patients with partial vaccine-induced immunity have been reported to survive with intensive care. However, additional experience with vigorous support has not duplicated this overall effect on long-term sur-vival.

DIAGNOSIS. Rabies is usually suspected on the basis of a history of animal bite or other exposure, although in as many as one third of cases no such history is obtained. Definitive ante-mortem diagnosis is established by immunohistochemical iden-tification of rabies virus antigen in hair follicle nerve endings of biopsied skin, usually obtained from the nape of the neck. Isolation of virus from saliva or the presence of antirabies anti-bodies in blood in the absence of vaccination or in the cerebro-spinal fluid may also be used to establish diagnosis. Postmortem diagnosis is usually made by histologic or immunohistochemical examination of the brain.

The differential diagnosis depends on the clinical presentation and the epidemiologic setting. In the case of paralytic rabies, diagnosis is most often confused with the Guillain-Barré syn-drome, poliomyelitis, or other neuropathies or myelopathies, while the encephalitic form must be differentiated from other viral and infectious encephalitides, tetanus, and toxic encepha-lopathies. In regions where vaccine is prepared using neural tissue (still the practice in many regions of the world with the highest rates of rabies), allergic encephalomyelitis remains a principal differential diagnosis.

TREATMENT AND PREVENTION. Unfortunately, estab-lished central nervous system disease remains essentially untreat-able. Disease prevention relies on public health measures to reduce animal reservoirs and on postexposure immune prophy-laxis to abort viral penetration of the central nervous system after a rabid bite or other contact. Although clinical rabies is a rare disease in most developed countries such as the United States, the decision to administer active prophylaxis remains a relatively common clinical issue. The physician first determines the type of possible exposure; an open wound or disrupted mucous mem-brane exposed to saliva may warrant postexposure prophylaxis, whereas contact of saliva with intact skin may not. The first step in management is to administer prompt local wound care, thor-oughly washing with soap or iodine. The epidemiologic setting is important in determining the likelihood that the biting animal might be rabid and often requires consultation with local health authorities to ascertain which animals carry rabies in the geo-graphic setting. In the absence of previous vaccination, both passive (rabies immune globulin of human origin) and active (human diploid cell vaccine) immunizations are administered, whereas individuals with previous vaccination (e.g., laboratory workers) required only active vaccine. Fortunately, such tissue culture–derived vaccines are safe, with a very low incidence of major adverse reactions, in contrast to earlier nerve tissue–derived vaccines.

Baer GM, Bridbord K, Hui FW, et al. (eds.): Research towards rabies prevention. Rev Infect Dis (Suppl) 10:S5773, 1988. *A compendium of brief papers presented at a symposium dealing with various aspects of rabies, particularly strategies for prevention, but covering a broad range of related tissues.*

Centers for Disease Control: Rabies surveillance, United States, 1988. MMWR 38:1, 1989. *Reviews the animal and human epidemiology of rabies in the United States over the past four decades, providing a guide to risk after animal exposure.*

Fishbein DB, Baer GM: Animal rabies: Implications for diagnosis and human treatment. Ann Intern Med 109:935, 1988. *An editorial outlining current recommendations for prophylaxis and treatment as well as future prospects for control of animal and human infection.*

Hemachudha T: Rabies. *In* McKendall RR (ed.): Viral Disease. Elsevier Science Publishing Company, New York, 1989, pp 383–404. *A recent comprehensive review written from the perspective of a neurologist who has personal experi-ence with clinical rabies.*

Immunization Practices Advisory Committee: Rabies prevention—United States, 1984. MMWR 33:393, 407, 1984. *U.S. guidelines on prevention of rabies by vaccination.*

Kaplan C, Turner GS, Warrell DA: Rabies: The Facts. Oxford, England, Oxford University Press, 1986. *A brief, highly readable monograph.*

478 Slow Virus Infections of the Nervous System

478.1 INTRODUCTION

Richard W. Price

The term *slow infections* was first applied by Bjorn Sigurdsson to a group of transmissible diseases of sheep characterized by an incubation period and course measured in months or years rather than hours or days, as in typical acute viral or bacterial infections. Subsequently, several human diseases sharing these characteris-tics have been described. Although often considered together because of their chronic nature, these disorders are in fact heterogeneous with respect to their clinical manifestations, neu-ropathology, etiology, and pathogenesis. Although in some in-stances the infections are accompanied by inflammatory pathol-ogy, in several, symptoms and signs typical of the acute encephalitides are absent, and both clinically and pathologically they resemble degenerative or hereditary diseases of the nervous system. Two of the sheep diseases upon which Sigurdsson based his concept of slow infections, *visna* and *scrapie*, have subse-quently proved to have human counterparts. Visna is caused by a retrovirus and somewhat resembles the nervous system infec-tions caused by the human immunodeficiency virus type 1 (HIV-1) responsible for acquired immunodeficiency syndrome (AIDS) and tropical spastic paraparesis caused by human T cell lympho-tropic virus type I (HTLV-I), while scrapie closely parallels Creutzfeldt-Jakob disease and kuru.

The agents causing the slow infections are taxonomically diverse, as are the mechanisms by which they maintain chronic progressive infection and cause clinical symptomatology (Table 478–1). Thus, HIV is an RNA-containing retrovirus that codes for a DNA intermediary that can integrate into the host genome and persist for the life of the cell; progressive multifocal leuko-

TABLE 478–1. HUMAN SLOW VIRUS INFECTIONS OF THE CENTRAL NERVOUS SYSTEM

Disease	Etiologic Agent	
	Name	Classification
AIDS dementia com-plex	Human immunodefi-ciency virus type 1	Retrovirus (RNA)
Tropical spastic para-paresis	Human T cell lympho-tropic virus type 1	Retrovirus (RNA)
Progressive multifocal leukoencephalopathy	JC virus	Papovavirus (DNA)
Subacute sclerosing panencephalitis	Measles virus	Paramyxovirus (RNA)
Progressive rubella panencephalitis	Rubella virus	Togavirus (RNA)
Creutzfeldt-Jakob syn-drome, Gerstmann-Sträussler-Scheinker disease, kuru	—	Spongiform encepha-lopathy agents (cod-ing material uncer-tain), prions

encephalopathy is caused by a small, nonenveloped DNA-containing papovavirus; subacute sclerosing panencephalitis is due to the enveloped RNA measles virus; and Creutzfeldt-Jakob disease is caused by an agent that has not yet been definitively identified but may consist of a modified cell protein only (see Ch. 478.6). Contributions of host immune responses to the development and symptomatology of these diseases are similarly varied. In the case of progressive multifocal leukoencephalopathy, a conventional virus that circulates commonly in the human community and is ordinarily associated with little, if any, disease causes devastating central nervous system infection in the presence of depressed host cell–mediated immunity. HIV-1 causes profound systemic disease by virtue of its predilection for infecting the helper-inducer (T4) subset of lymphocytes, with the resultant systemic immunosuppression perhaps playing a role in the subsequent development of progressive brain disease by this same virus. The pathogenesis of myelopathy caused by HTLV-I most likely significantly involves immunopathologic mechanisms. Subacute sclerosing panencephalitis appears to result from defective replication in the brain of a once-common conventional virus and is accompanied by an exuberant but ineffective antibody response. In the case of Creutzfeldt-Jakob disease, immunosuppression plays no role in the development or progression of the disease, and indeed there is little evidence that the host recognizes the infectious agent as foreign.

The diversity of the agents causing these slow infections, along with their variable cell and tissue tropism, host susceptibility, and pathologic reactions, has led to speculation that viruses may play a role in several of the common neurodegenerative disorders, including multiple sclerosis, amyotrophic lateral sclerosis, parkinsonism, and Alzheimer's disease. To date, however, no direct evidence for such an infectious cause of any of these disorders has been identified.

Johnson RT: Viral Infections of the Nervous System. New York, Raven Press, 1982.
 Contains sections dealing with the general background as well as the specific slow virus infections of the nervous system.

478.2 HUMAN IMMUNODEFICIENCY VIRUS INFECTION AND THE AIDS DEMENTIA COMPLEX

Richard W. Price

DEFINITION. Among the common neurologic complications of human immunodeficiency virus type 1 (HIV-1) infection (see Ch. 414) is the *AIDS dementia complex*, which appears to relate pathogenetically in an elemental way to the AIDS virus itself rather than to secondary opportunistic infection. The nomenclature for this "subcortical" dementing syndrome is still in a state of flux, and several alternative terms have been used, including AIDS dementia, subacute encephalitis, HIV dementia, and HIV encephalopathy. Recently, the World Health Organization proposed new terminology, using the term *HIV-1–associated cognitive/motor complex* to encompass the full constellation of features and with subcategories referring to patients with predominantly cognitive (*HIV-1–associated dementia*) or myelopathic (*HIV-1–associated myelopathy*) presentations. The term *HIV-1–associated minor cognitive/motor disorder* was introduced to designate patients with mild symptoms and signs and only minimal functional impairment of work or activities of daily living. In this section, we continue to use the earlier AIDS dementia complex terminology.

Although this condition may relate to HIV-1 itself, and in some patients appears to be caused by productive HIV-1 infection within the CNS, it is important to distinguish the AIDS dementia complex, which refers to a clinical syndrome, from HIV-1 brain infection, a pathobiologic process. Although the syndrome and the infective process overlap, they are not equivalent.

CLINICAL MANIFESTATIONS. The AIDS dementia complex is characterized by a triad of cognitive, motor, and behavioral dysfunction. Patients' earliest symptoms usually consist of difficulties with concentration and memory. They complain of losing track of their train of thought or conversations and find that they need to keep lists to maintain their daily schedules. Many complain of "slowness" in thinking. Complex tasks at work or in the home, such as balancing the checkbook or reconciling other personal financial affairs, become increasingly difficult and take longer to complete.

Despite these complaints, early in the evolution of the illness, bedside screening or mental status testing may yield results within the normal range, although characteristically patients are slower and less facile than previously. With advancing disease, patients perform poorly on tasks requiring concentration and attention, such as word and digit reversals and serial subtraction. Eventually, a larger array of mental status tests are abnormal, and psychomotor slowing is more prominent.

Symptoms of motor dysfunction usually are less prominent than those of intellectual impairment. However, motor abnormalities, including, particularly, slowing of rapid successive and alternating movements of the extremities and eyes, are almost always noted on examination. Abnormal reflexes are common, with generalized hyperreflexia (in the absence of concomitant neuropathy) along with release signs such as snout or glabellar responses. With disease progression, symptomatic difficulty with balance or incoordination may be evident; patients may drop things more frequently or become slower and less precise with hand activities, including writing. Similarly, gait incoordination may result in more frequent tripping or falling or in a perceived need to exercise new care in walking. In more advanced disease, ataxia and, subsequently, leg weakness limit ambulation. Patients with early or predominating spastic-ataxic gait are usually shown to have vacuolar myelopathy pathologically (see below). Bladder and bowel incontinence is common in the late stages of the disease.

Psychological depression appears to be surprisingly infrequent in these patients, despite the prominence of psychomotor slowing. Patients appear uninterested and lack initiative but are not dysphoric. In a minority, a more agitated organic psychosis with manic features may be the presenting or predominant aspect of the illness.

In those with a severe progressive course, the end stage of the AIDS dementia complex is nearly vegetative; patients lie in bed with a vacant stare and with paraparesis or quadriparesis and incontinence. They may be mute or exhibit an extraordinary delay in making brief verbal responses. Unless intercurrent illness develops, the level of arousal is usually preserved.

DIAGNOSIS AND DIFFERENTIAL DIAGNOSIS. Diagnosis relies on identifying the characteristic clinical features of the AIDS dementia complex and excluding other conditions. No single laboratory test establishes the presence of the syndrome. In those with milder forms, perhaps the major difficulty is in distinguishing true cognitive impairment from the effects of fatigue and systemic illness or from psychiatric conditions, including anxiety and depression. The history is critical in establishing functional decline, and an observant friend or family member may be particularly helpful in judging change in performance. Neuropsychological testing can be helpful in providing objective evidence of characteristic impairment of attention and motor speed but must be interpreted, taking into account the patient's background, including age and education, as well as confounding conditions such as substance abuse, previous head trauma, and the effects of various medications. Formal neuropsychological studies are also useful for quantitatively following the patient's progression or response to treatment.

In those with more severe disease, the differential diagnosis most commonly centers on distinction from the other neurologic complications noted in HIV-1–infected patients (see Ch. 414) or, less commonly, from dementing or myelopathic neurologic disease observed in the normal population. Both neuroimaging procedures and cerebrospinal fluid (CSF) examination are essential aspects of evaluation, although principally to eliminate other conditions rather than to establish a diagnosis of the AIDS dementia complex. Computed tomography (CT) and magnetic resonance imaging (MRI) detect the nearly universal finding of cerebral atrophy with widened cortical sulci and enlarged ventricles. In some patients, MRI also shows patchy or diffuse signal changes in the hemispheric white matter and, less commonly, the basal ganglia or thalamus.

Routine CSF analysis is not specifically diagnostic, and findings may be indistinguishable from those in asymptomatic HIV-1–infected patients, with variable elevation of protein content or mononuclear cells. Elevations of CSF neopterin and β₂-microglobulin levels have been reported to correlate with the presence and severity of the AIDS dementia complex, but these markers of immune activation are also increased in central nervous system opportunistic infections and are therefore not specific. Unfortunately, HIV-1 isolation from the CSF is not diagnostically helpful, since the virus can also be cultured from asymptomatic seropositive subjects. The p24 core protein is seldom detected by immunoassay in the CSF of patients with milder clinical disease.

EPIDEMIOLOGY. The frequency of the AIDS dementia complex increases as the systemic effects of HIV-1 infection and resultant immunosuppression worsen. This complication is rare in patients who are otherwise entirely asymptomatic but begins to become more frequent in those manifesting constitutional symptoms (fever, weight loss, malaise). Its prevalence increases further as the helper (CD4+) blood lymphocyte counts fall and opportunistic infections develop, so that preterminally the majority of AIDS patients may manifest this neurologic syndrome. However, precise prevalence figures are not available, and, indeed, with the introduction of antiviral treatment, the epidemiologic pattern of this neurologic disease may be changing. In general, milder forms of the AIDS dementia complex, with a static or indolently progressive course, are more common in patients with preserved immune function (CF4+ lymphocyte counts above 200 per cubic millimeter), while the progressive and more severe forms characteristically develop in patients with advanced immunosuppression. In addition, although there is a general parallel between the onset and severity of this neurologic condition and the onset and severity of systemic complications, wide individual variability exists; at one extreme, the clinician encounters patients with little or no systemic disease but with severe AIDS dementia complex, while at the other end of the spectrum are patients with repeated episodes of opportunistic infection who remain neurologically preserved.

PATHOLOGY AND PATHOGENESIS. The neuropathologic findings in patients with the AIDS dementia complex include at least three "subsets" of major abnormalities: (1) central gliosis and white matter pallor, (2) multinucleated cell encephalitis, and (3) vacuolar myelopathy. In general, these findings correlate with the clinical severity. Central gliosis and white matter pallor are almost universal findings and, in isolation, are the major abnormality in patients with milder AIDS dementia complex. Rarely, they are the only abnormalities in patients with even more severe clinical symptoms and signs. Virologic studies to date have usually failed to detect evidence of productive HIV-1 brain infection in this subgroup of patients.

Multinucleated cell encephalitis is characterized by the presence of perivascular and, at times, parenchymal cell reactions that include macrophages and microglial cells along with multinucleated cells derived from fusion of these two cell types. These multinucleated cells are infected by HIV-1, and, indeed, the cell fusion likely results from interaction of the viral glycoproteins gp120 and gp41 with the CD4 cell receptor. Multinucleated cell encephalitis is thus properly referred to as *HIV-1 encephalitis* and is noted in patients with more severe and progressive AIDS dementia complex.

Vacuolar myelopathy, while defined pathologically, can also often be distinguished clinically on the basis of the predominant myelopathic symptoms and signs. Patients with this condition usually present with spastic-ataxic gait difficulty but with proportionally little sensory disturbance and usually no definable sensory "level." Histologically, the disorder closely resembles subacute combined spinal cord degeneration accompanying vitamin B₁₂ deficiency. Its pathogenesis is uncertain, and results conflict regarding the role of direct spinal cord HIV-1 infection, although clearly it is independent of the type of productive infection that produces multinucleated giant cells.

The pathogenesis of the neurologic injury underlying the AIDS dementia complex has been difficult to unravel from a number of aspects. Since the major "functional elements" of the brain, i.e., the neurons, oligodendrocytes, and astrocytes, do not appear to be infected, it remains uncertain how these cells are damaged. In both the gliosis-pallor and the vacuolar myelopathy subsets, overt HIV-1 brain infection is absent or undetectable, and even in multinucleated cell encephalitis the magnitude of neurologic dysfunction often appears to exceed the distribution and extent of productive infection. Speculation has centered on possible indirect mechanisms of injury involving toxic molecules of either viral (e.g., gp120) or cellular (e.g., cytokines elaborated by infected cells or by uninfected cells responding to infection) origin. It is also possible that nonproductive infection of glia or even neurons might lead to cell dysfunction without virus replication as a result of restricted viral genome transcription or translation. Whatever the mechanisms, however, HIV-1 infection, either of brain or of systemic organs, appears to be the *prime mover* in the pathogenesis of the AIDS dementia complex and thus the major target of therapy.

TREATMENT AND PROGNOSIS. Several reports now suggest that zidovudine (also azidothymidine, or AZT) relieves, at least partially, the symptoms and signs of the AIDS dementia complex. Therapeutic effect has been documented by improvement in neuropsychological test performance in two placebo-controlled trials (one in adults and the other in children with AIDS). Dose recommendations remain uncertain, but in the absence of precise information, conventional dosage (100 mg every 4 hours while the patient awake) is advised. Limitations of treatment most often relate to hematologic toxicity, but noninflammatory myopathy has also been reported (see Ch. 414). In patients whose neurologic condition deteriorates on these doses, the clinician may attempt to increase the dose, although toxicity is more likely. Additional antiretroviral drugs are currently being assessed with respect to their effect on this condition.

Symptomatic management is also important. In the subset of patients who present with mania, lithium or neuroleptics may be helpful. However, these patients may be unusually susceptible to the side effects of neuroleptics and other psychotropic drugs, and thus treatment should be cautious and begin with low doses.

Navia BA, Cho ES, Petito CK, et al.: The AIDS dementia complex: II. Neuropathology. Ann Neurol 19:525, 1986. Navia BA, Jordan BD, Price RW: The AIDS dementia complex: I. Clinical features. Ann Neurol 19:517, 1986. *Companion articles describing the clinical and pathologic features of the AIDS dementia complex.*

Price RW, Brew B, Sidtis J, et al.: The brain in AIDS: Central nervous system HIV-1 infection and the AIDS dementia complex. Science 239:586, 1988. *A review discussing the pathogenesis of the AIDS dementia complex.*

Sidtis JJ, Price RW: Early HIV-1 infection and the AIDS dementia complex. Neurology 40:323, 1990. *A review of the issue of the AIDS dementia complex in asymptomatic HIV-1 seropositive individuals.*

478.3 HUMAN T CELL LYMPHOTROPIC VIRUS TYPE I–ASSOCIATED MYELOPATHY AND TROPICAL SPASTIC PARAPARESIS

Richard W. Price

DEFINITION. Human T cell lymphotropic virus type I (HTLV-I) was the first human retrovirus to be identified in the laboratory and the second, after human immunodeficiency virus type 1 (HIV-1), to be etiologically implicated in neurologic disease. This connection was made when a survey in Martinique discovered that nearly 60 per cent of patients with tropical spastic paraparesis (TSP) were seropositive for HTLV-I. A similar serologic association was soon established in other tropical areas, and, concomitantly, Japanese workers implicated this virus in the etiology of a myelopathy occurring principally in the Kyushu district; because this is not a tropical region, they proposed the name HTLV-I–associated myelopathy (HAM). Although the two conditions were first considered to be clinically distinct, subsequent comparison of the clinical and laboratory features suggests that the tropical and Japanese conditions are, in fact, the same disease, and the combined term HAM/TSP has been advocated.

ETIOLOGY AND EPIDEMIOLOGY. HTLV-I is a genomically complex virus classified among the oncogenic retroviruses. Although infection is most often asymptomatic, the virus has been implicated in acute T cell lymphoma/leukemia (ATLL) as well as HAM/TSP. In Japan it is estimated that myelopathy develops in about 1 in every 2000 infected carriers and ATLL in perhaps 1 in 10,000 carriers, and the two conditions rarely coexist. Infection is widely prevalent in much of the Caribbean, in certain parts of South Africa, South India, Colombia, Peru, and the Seychelles Islands, as well as Japan. In the United States, endemic infection is found principally in certain parts of the Southeast, chiefly among blacks; however, the influx of Caribbean and other migrants, as well as perhaps transfusion-related transmission, has resulted in more widespread sporadic dispersion. Both HAM/TSP and ATLL follow this same geographic pattern. Infection is thought to be transmitted sexually from males to females, in breast milk, and by transfusion, the last factor having led to serologic blood donor screening. Although some preliminary observations suggested that multiple sclerosis might be associated with this retrovirus, numerous subsequent studies have failed to substantiate such a connection.

HAM/TSP usually afflicts individuals between 20 and 65 years old and most commonly begins between ages 35 and 45 years. For those infected early in life, this implies a very prolonged incubation period. In patients infected by transfused blood, however, the incubation period is as short as 5 or 6 months. Otherwise, most cases are sporadic, although there is an occasional familial incidence. The variability in disease expression among those infected has led to the suggestion that host factors, including histocompatibility immune response genes, might be cofactors in the development of HAM/TSP.

CLINICAL MANIFESTATIONS. The salient feature of HAM/TSP is spastic paraparesis or paraplegia. Typically, the onset is gradual, with steady disease progression over months to years and a tendency in many instances to stabilize later on. Occasionally, the disorder begins more abruptly and has a more irregular course. Patients almost universally exhibit spastic legs; bladder and bowel disturbance is present in more than three quarters, while only about half have position or vibratory sensory impairment. Low back stiffness and pain are common. The gait may at times appear ataxic, and probably fewer than one tenth of affected persons have symptoms of neurologic dysfunction outside the spinal cord. Optic atrophy, nerve deafness, peripheral neuropathy, a clinical picture of pseudo–amyotrophic lateral sclerosis with anterior horn cell disease, and polymyositis have all been noted. Patients may also have systemic findings involving the lung (lymphocytic alveolitis), skin, and eyes (cotton-wool spots).

Characteristic cerebrospinal fluid (CSF) findings include oligoclonal immunoglobulin bands and intrathecal synthesis of anti–HTLV-I antibodies. The CSF cell count may be normal or show a mild lymphocytic pleocytosis; lymphocytes with flower-like nuclear changes similar to those seen in ATLL may be present. About half of patients have abnormal signal in the cerebral white matter detected by magnetic resonance imaging (MRI), indicating subclinical involvement.

The diagnosis of TSP/HAM relies principally on the identification of the clinical manifestations and documentation of viral infection; CSF abnormalities, including the high level of antibodies to the virus, are also helpful. Because of the high rate of asymptomatic HTLV-I infection, other neurologic conditions are likely to develop in seropositive patients, and thus the diagnosis requires more than simply ascertaining the presence of antibodies in a patient with spinal cord or other neurologic abnormalities. In addition, current serologic screening methods may not discriminate between HTLV-I and the related retrovirus, human T cell lymphotropic virus type II (HTLV-II), which has not yet been clearly implicated in causing neurologic disease; additional testing with Western blot or direct characterization of viral isolates can be used to discriminate between the two viruses.

PATHOLOGY AND PATHOGENESIS. Neuropathologically, in the spinal cord the corticospinal tracts are most severely affected, although abnormalities are usually more widely distributed. Perivascular inflammation involving lymphocytes, macrophages, and plasma cells, along with fibrosis, is notable. Gliosis is prominent, with loss of myelin and, frequently, axons as well. While scattered perivascular inflammation is also present in the brain, parenchymal changes are usually minimal or absent. Immunologic studies show activation of major histocompatibility class I antigens in association with the inflammatory and gliotic responses.

Although HTLV-I antigens have been noted in at least one

case, most other attempts to identify infected cells have been negative, indicating that productive infection is minimal. This observation, along with the prominence of inflammation and the therapeutic response to corticosteroids and other immunosuppressive measures, suggests that immunopathologic processes are significantly involved in the genesis of spinal cord injury. HTLV-I infection is associated with a state of immune activation with circulating activated T cells. Whether the neurologic injury relates to immune reactions to HTLV-I antigens and consequent "innocent bystander" injury of adjacent neural tissue or to true autoimmunity with activation of immune responses against self-antigens is uncertain.

TREATMENT AND PROGNOSIS. Immunosuppression using corticosteroids, plasma exchange, or other measures has been reported, principally by the Japanese, to alleviate TSP/HAM, although remission may not be well sustained. Antiviral therapy (with zidovudine or newer antiretroviral drugs used for AIDS) has not yet been assessed in TSP/HAM. As noted above, the course and outcome are variable. Usually the disease becomes disabling, but not directly life limiting; thus supportive measures are of paramount important, as in other spinal cord diseases.

Jacobson S, Shida H, McFarlin DE, et al.: Circulating CD8 + cytotoxic T lymphocytes specific for HTLV-I pX in patients with HTLV-I associated neurological disease. Nature 348:245, 1990. *The cytotoxic lymphocytes were identified in HTLV-I–infected patients with neurologic manifestations of the disease but not in seropositive individuals who lacked neurologic involvement. HTLV-I–specific cytotoxic lymphocytes may contribute to the neurologic manifestations of the disease.*
Roman GC, Vernant J-C, Osame M (eds.): HTLV-I and the Nervous System. Proceedings of an international meeting organized by the Departments of Neurology of Texas Tech University and La Meynard Hospital, April 15–16, 1988, Fort-de-France, Martinique, French Antilles. New York, Alan R. Liss, 1989. *Contains reviews of the clinical, epidemiologic, and biologic aspects of TSP/HAM.*

478.4 SUBACUTE SCLEROSING PANENCEPHALITIS AND PROGRESSIVE RUBELLA PANENCEPHALITIS

Richard W. Price

Subacute sclerosing panencephalitis (SSPE), a "slow" infection caused by measles virus, usually affects children, but its onset can extend into young adulthood. Patients usually have a history of measles within the first 2 years of life, and it is speculated that such early host exposure allows emergence of persistent defective virus replication. Fortunately, its incidence has markedly decreased in recent years.

Clinically, SSPE usually begins with cognitive and behavioral changes; progresses to include motor dysfunction with prominent myoclonus, choreoathetosis, dystonia, and rigidity; and usually pursues a progressive course with steady deterioration over 1 to 3 years to eventual rigid quadriparesis and a vegetative state. The condition is more common in a rural setting and affects males more often than females. The electroencephalogram (EEG) reveals periodic complexes with synchronous bursts of two to three per second slow waves, recurring at 5- to 8-second intervals. The cerebrospinal fluid (CSF) is characterized by a high immunoglobulin concentration, oligoclonal bands, and abundant intrathecal synthesis of antibody to measles virus antigens. Serum measles antibody titers are also high. These findings are usually sufficiently characteristic for diagnosis, but brain biopsy may be needed for definitive diagnosis in some cases. The distinct pathology of SSPE includes gliosis, loss of myelin, and perivascular infiltrates of lymphocytes and plasma cells in white and gray matter. Intranuclear inclusions containing viral nucleocapsids are noted in both neurons and glia.

Measles virus may also cause a subacute encephalitis in the immunocompromised host. The prominence of cognitive and motor dysfunction in these patients resembles SSPE, but the clinical setting, its subacute onset and more rapid evolution, and the presence of seizures rather than myoclonus are distinctive. Brain pathology includes abundant intranuclear inclusions, but inflammation is minimal, and neither serum nor CSF antibody titers against measles virus are high. For this reason, brain biopsy is usually needed for diagnosis.

Progressive rubella panencephalitis is a rare disorder resembling SSPE but caused by rubella virus and developing as a complication of either the congenital rubella syndrome or, more typically, childhood rubella. A hiatus of years separates early infection from the onset of neurologic deterioration, which is characterized by behavioral changes, intellectual decline, ataxia, spasticity, and sometimes seizures. Myoclonus is not a prominent feature, as it is in SSPE. Serology or viral isolation from brain or peripheral blood lymphocytes confirms the etiology.

With the advent of widespread measles and rubella immunization, these disorders have been all but eliminated in the United States, although SSPE still occurs in less advanced parts of the world. There is no known treatment.

Graves M: Subacute sclerosing panencephalitis. Neurol Clin 2:267, 1984. *A thorough general review of SSPE.*

Wolinsky JS: Subacute sclerosing panencephalitis, progressive rubella panencephalitis, and multifocal leukoencephalopathy. *In* Waksman B (ed.): Immunologic Mechanisms in Neurologic and Psychiatric Disease. New York, Raven Press, 1990, pp 259–268. *A recent review of the pathogenesis of SSPE and subacute rubella encephalitis.*

478.5 PROGRESSIVE MULTIFOCAL LEUKOENCEPHALOPATHY

Richard W. Price

DEFINITION. Progressive multifocal leukoencephalopathy (PML) is an opportunistic viral infection of the central nervous system caused by a papovavirus, JC virus. Initially described in patients with a variety of underlying disorders accompanied by impaired T lymphocyte/macrophage–mediated immune defenses, it now most frequently occurs in patients with advanced human immunodeficiency virus type 1 (HIV-1) infection. It is one of the AIDS-defining opportunistic conditions. As the name implies, it is a disorder that affects principally the white matter of the brain, usually encompassing more than one lesion and pursuing an inexorably progressive course.

ETIOLOGY AND EPIDEMIOLOGY. Two factors are important in the development of PML: exposure to JC virus in the past and suppression of T cell–related immune defenses against the virus. With respect to the former, JC virus has a virtually worldwide distribution, and the majority of the population exhibits serologic evidence of exposure by the teenage years. Primary infection is benign, and, indeed, disease accompanying initial exposure has not been clearly defined. PML appears to result almost always from reactivation of latent JC virus infection rather than from recent exposure. The virus is thus innocent, except under circumstances in which the host's T lymphocyte–directed immunity is impaired and rendered unable to suppress JC virus reactivation and subsequent continued replication and spread. Recent studies indicate that JC virus infection in PML patients is not confined to the brain but also involves peripheral blood mononuclear cells, probably chiefly B lymphocytes.

While the incidence of PML has increased with the AIDS epidemic to complicate perhaps 2 to 5 per cent of cases, it may also complicate organ transplantation, lymphoreticular and hematologic malignancies (particularly in the context of cytoreductive chemotherapy), autoimmune disorders, and other immunosuppressed states associated with T lymphocyte dysfunction.

CLINICAL MANIFESTATIONS AND DIAGNOSIS. PML is characterized by the gradual onset and usually steady progression of focal neurologic dysfunction, usually involving the cerebral hemispheres. Thus, patients may present with homonymous visual field disturbance, hemiparesis, hemisensory disturbance, aphasia, apraxia, or other "cortical" dysfunction, depending on the location of the demyelinating focus. Posterior fossa abnormalities with cerebellar dysfunction or signs of brain stem involvement are less common. Most often the patient is otherwise well, without constitutional symptoms (e.g., fever, malaise), and consciousness is preserved. Headache or seizures are unusual, occurring in 10 per cent or fewer of patients.

Diagnosis is often suspected on the basis of the underlying condition (e.g., AIDS) and the clinical presentation of focal neurologic deficit. Neuroimaging is helpful in demonstrating loss of white matter rather than an expanding mass (as, for example, in toxoplasmosis or primary central nervous system lymphoma). Computed tomographic (CT) scanning is less sensitive than magnetic resonance imaging (MRI), both with respect to detecting multiple lesions and in distinguishing white matter localization, most commonly adjacent to the cerebral cortex. Characteristically, contrast enhancement is absent. Although MRI in the AIDS dementia complex may show multifocal abnormalities in the white matter that superficially resemble those of PML, patients with AIDS dementia complex usually do not have focal neurologic symptoms and signs.

Cerebrospinal fluid (CSF) is usually acellular, with normal or only mild elevation of protein content. Serologic studies usually document the presence of serum antibodies against JC virus, but this is of very limited diagnostic utility, since antibody titers are indistinguishable from those of the normal population and do not rise with the onset or progression of the disease. CSF JC virus antibodies are usually not detected. Culture of the virus from CSF or blood is very difficult, requiring specialized techniques, and thus is not useful for diagnosis. Identification of viral nucleic acid in the CSF, blood, or urine using in situ hybridization or the polymerase chain reaction is currently being explored, but the sensitivity and specificity of these methods have yet to be defined. For these reasons, brain biopsy is still necessary for definitive diagnosis. The distinct histologic abnormalities usually permit diagnosis on routinely processed and stained tissue, but immunohistochemical identification of JC antigens or in situ hybridization to identify viral nucleic acid may also be useful.

PATHOLOGY AND PATHOGENESIS. The pathology of PML provides an example of the selective effects of a virus on different cell populations within the brain. Thus, the major macroscopic finding of demyelination results from the progressive productive-lytic infection of oligodendrocytes. Infection of these cells is marked by enlargement of the nucleus by a nucleocapsid-filled inclusion. Lesions begin as microscopic centers of infection, which then spread concentrically outward; oligodendrocytes are lost in the center, and their nuclei are swollen, with inclusions at the periphery. Since myelin is composed of the elaborated cytoplasmic membranes of these cells, their lysis results in the characteristic demyelination; in mild lesions, axons are relatively spared, while in more severe, coalescent foci, frank cavitation may result. Macroscopic pathology consists of multiple foci of enlarging demyelinating "plaques." Astrocytes undergo marked alteration, with formation of bizarre nuclei resembling transformed cells, but without apparent real malignant potential. Neurons, on the other hand, are spared. Inflammation is usually minimal, but in perhaps 15 per cent of cases, perivascular mononuclear infiltrates may be more conspicuous.

TREATMENT AND PROGNOSIS. There is no established treatment for PML. Earlier anecdotes of response to cytosine arabinoside have not been confirmed by more recent observations. Spontaneous remissions have been reported, including two in patients with AIDS.

Berger JR, Kaszovitz B, Post MJD, et al.: Progressive multifocal leukoencephalopathy associated with human immunodeficiency virus infection: A review of the literature with a report of sixteen cases. Ann Intern Med 107:78, 1987. *A review of AIDS-associated PML.*

Houff SA, Major EO, Katz DA, et al.: Involvement of JC virus–infected mononuclear cells from the bone marrow and spleen in the pathogenesis of progressive multifocal leukoencephalopathy. N Engl J Med 318:301, 1988. *A report emphasizing the presence of systemic JC virus infection in PML.*

Walker DL: Progressive multifocal leukoencephalopathy: An opportunistic viral infection of the central nervous system. *In* Vinken PJ, Bruyn GW, Klawans HL (eds.): Handbook of Clinical Neurology. Vol. 34: Infections of the Nervous System, Part II. Amsterdam, Elsevier North-Holland, 1978. *A comprehensive review from the pre-AIDS era that emphasizes the virologic and clinical aspects of PML.*

478.6 CREUTZFELDT-JAKOB DISEASE

Paul E. Bendheim

DEFINITION. Creutzfeldt-Jakob disease (CJD) is a subacute central nervous system disorder characterized by a progressive dementia, myoclonus, and distinctive electroencephalographic and neuropathologic findings. Although uncommon, it is the most prevalent of the human subacute spongiform encephalopathies—fatal diseases caused by transmissible pathogens of uncertain type. Accumulating research data indicate that these disorders are probably unique in regard to their etiologic agents.

ETIOLOGY. CJD is closely related to kuru, scrapie, and a rare, inherited human disease termed the Gerstmann-Sträussler-Scheinker syndrome (GSS). *Scrapie* is a spongiform encephalopathy of sheep and goats experimentally transmissible to other animal species. The scrapie agent is not known to cause disease in humans. *Kuru* is a disease previously endemic among the Fore people inhabiting an area in the eastern highlands of Papua New Guinea. Cerebellar dysfunction, dementia, and progression to death within 2 years were typical. Women and children were affected much more frequently than men. Circumstantial evidence indicates that the kuru agent was transmitted through the ritual handling of affected tissues, especially brain, from deceased relatives. This cultural practice was discontinued, and the incidence of kuru has decreased dramatically since 1959. Brain tissues from patients dying of kuru were inoculated into the brains of chimpanzees, which, after a prolonged incubation period, developed a similar disease. Subsequently, the neuropathology of kuru and that of CJD as well as GSS were noted to be similar, and experimental transmission studies using CJD-affected or GSS-affected brain were undertaken successfully, eventually in a wide range of laboratory animals.

The CJD, GSS, kuru, and animal spongiform encephalopathy agents are unlike any known virus or other well-characterized transmissible pathogen. This has resulted in the terms *slow virus*, *virino*, and *prion* being used interchangeably with "agent" to refer to them. Prion proteins (PrP) in humans and animals are closely related, with the locus of the PrP genes in hereditary GSS lying on the short arm of chromosome 20. Current knowledge favors a direct role for abnormal PrP variants in the pathogenesis of both hereditary GSS and acquired CJD. The scrapie and CJD agents provoke no inflammatory response or specific antibody production. They are resistant to chemical and physical treatments that inactivate most viruses, including heat, formaldehyde, nuclease digestion, and ultraviolet and ionizing radiation. The agents can be inactivated by procedures that denature proteins. Unique fibrillar structures are observed in electron micrographs of samples prepared from brain tissue of individuals with CJD. They resemble the abnormal fibrils that accumulate in scrapie-affected animals and represent an aggregated form of the CJD protein.

INCIDENCE AND EPIDEMIOLOGY. On a worldwide basis, the incidence of CJD is one case per million population. This incidence peaks in the fifth through seventh decades, although cases have been documented as early as the second decade. The sexes are equally affected. Approximately 250 deaths occur in the United States each year. Higher rates have been noted in Israel among Libyan-born Jews and in circumscribed areas of Czechoslovakia and Chile.

CJD usually occurs sporadically in middle-aged adults without known exposure. A family history is evident in 8 per cent of patients and suggests common exposure or a genetic susceptibility. Several reports document iatrogenic human-to-human transmission by cornea transplants and via the reuse of stereotaxic electroencephalographic (EEG) electrodes that had unknowingly been previously implanted in a patient with CJD. Several cases have resulted from the use of dura mater allografts. Additional clusters of cases suggesting neurosurgical transmission have been reported. In the past 6 years, CJD has been diagnosed in 12 individuals in four countries who had received human pituitary gland growth hormone replacement therapy. It seems apparent that certain lots of the cadaveric hormone preparation were contaminated with the CJD agent. Incubation periods were between 4 and 21 years, emphasizing the astonishingly long incubation times of the spongiform encephalopathies. Additional cases may yet appear, since more than 10,000 patients worldwide received this form of human growth hormone prior to its discontinuation in 1985.

Worldwide, the incidence of CJD is the same in countries with endemic sheep scrapie as it is in those without scrapie, indicating that there is no apparent transmission to humans from this animal

reservoir. In the past 5 years, a major outbreak of a new veterinary disease, bovine spongiform encephalopathy (BSE), or *mad cow disease*, has appeared in Great Britain. BSE has not occurred in the United States. BSE appears to have had its origin in the use of food supplements contaminated with the sheep scrapie agent. Although unlikely, it is too early in the BSE epidemic in Great Britain to determine if the passage of the scrapie agent through cattle poses any increased risk to humans. Nevertheless, British authorities have taken measures to prevent human consumption of contaminated beef.

PATHOLOGY. The pathologic findings in CJD are limited to the central nervous system, although the transmissible agent can be detected in many organs. Cortical neuronal depletion, marked reactive astrocytosis, intracellular vacuolar or spongiform change, and the absence of inflammation are the major features. Amyloid fibrils and plaques occur in virtually all cases.

CLINICAL MANIFESTATIONS. Vague psychiatric or behavioral symptoms suggesting a personality change often herald the onset of CJD, but within a few weeks or months a relentlessly progressive dementia becomes evident. Myoclonus is usually present and often prominent at some time during the course. Deterioration is usually rapid, and 90 per cent of victims die within 1 year. CJD patients are afebrile and have normal blood and cerebrospinal fluid profiles. In the late stages, the EEG in at least 75 per cent of cases shows a diffusely slow background with superimposed complexes, which may or may not be associated with myoclonus.

The dementia can be accompanied by signs of involvement of any part of the central nervous system. Most patients develop signs of cerebellar and pyramidal tract dysfunction as the disease advances. Visual disturbances, extrapyramidal signs, and various dysphasias often occur. The terminal stage is marked by decorticate and decerebrate postures, stupor, and coma. Massive myoclonic responses to auditory or other sensory stimuli may create the false impression that the patient is alert and responsive.

Subtypes of CJD based on distinctive clinical presentations have been delineated. The optic type features visual disturbances, usually cortical blindness. The dyskinetic form has prominent extrapyramidal signs, while the ataxic variant resembles kuru with its marked cerebellar involvement. GSS is an autosomal dominant genetically transmitted form of CJD with slower progression and signs of spinocerebellar ataxia. A specific mutation in the gene that codes for the CJD precursor protein has been found in some patients with this familial form of CJD. This mutation results in a protein with leucine substituted for proline at PrP codon 102, a step that promotes its aggregation into the characteristic brain amyloid.

DIAGNOSIS. The diagnosis of CJD should be considered when a relatively rapidly progressive dementia develops in an adolescent or adult patient with normal spinal fluid. The presence of myoclonus or the characteristic EEG recording is strongly supportive, but often either or both are absent in early stages. All treatable diseases that can cause dementia need to be specifically tested for before a presumptive diagnosis of CJD or another untreatable dementia is made. Neither brain imaging nor laboratory evaluations are useful in diagnosis. Brain biopsy has been the usual method to establish definitive diagnosis. Research level, two-dimensional electrophoresis, however, has also provided accurate diagnosis in an increasing number of cases. In early cases, psychological depression, the AIDS dementia complex, and a number of rare dementias, including collagen vascular diseases and paraneoplastic limbic encephalitis, must be considered. Rarely, lithium toxicity can present with a clinical picture and EEG pattern resembling those of CJD. Discontinuation of the drug results in improvement within a few weeks.

Alzheimer's disease (see Ch. 450), the most common neurodegenerative dementia, usually has a more protracted course, without either the myoclonus or the typical EEG of CJD. Amyloid deposition in the brain is a pathologic hallmark of both Alzheimer's disease and CJD, but the amyloid proteins deposited in these two diseases are structurally unrelated. The development of specific antibodies for both these amyloid proteins allows rapid immunologic differentiation between CJD and Alzheimer's disease if a brain biopsy or postmortem examination is done.

TREATMENT AND PROGNOSIS. No effective treatment is available, and the disease appears to be uniformly fatal.

PREVENTION. Although CJD can be transmitted, the risk to health care workers and others having contact with patients is no higher than that to the general population. Isolation of patients is not indicated, but certain guidelines should be followed. Hospital workers should wear gloves when handling tissues, blood, and spinal fluid. Accidental skin contact with possibly contaminated fluids or materials should be followed by washing with 1N sodium hydroxide or a 1:10 dilution of 5 per cent household chlorine bleach (sodium hypochlorite). All laboratory samples should be clearly marked and needles disposed of properly. The agent can be inactivated on contaminated surfaces using a 1:10 dilution of bleach for 1 hour. Surgical and pathologic instruments should be steam autoclaved for 1 hour at 132°C. No organs, tissues, or tissue products from patients with CJD or with any ill-defined neurologic disease should be used for transplantation or replacement therapy.

Bock G, Marsh J (eds.): Novel infectious agents and the central nervous system. Ciba Foundation Symposium 135. Chichester, United Kingdom, Wiley-Interscience Publications, 1988. *A monograph from an international symposium with chapters on epidemiologic, pathologic, and research aspects of CJD and scrapie.*

Brown P, Cathala F, Castaigne P, et al.: Creutzfeldt-Jakob disease: Clinical analysis of a consecutive series of 230 neuropathologically verified cases. Ann Neurol 20:597, 1986. *Clinical features are detailed in this large series of documented cases.*

Harrington MG, Merril CR, Asher DM, Gajdusek DC: Abnormal proteins in the cerebrospinal fluid of patients with Creutzfeld-Jakob disease. N Engl J Med 315:279, 1986. *The original report showing that CJD, but not other dementias, is associated with specific abnormalities in CSF proteins.*

Prusiner SB: Molecular biology of prion disease. Science 252:1515, 1991. *A thorough summary of the epidemioloy in animals and humans of this still mysterious infectious disease plus a description of the molecular biology and genetics of sporadic and inherited forms of CJD.*

Rosenberg RN, White CL III, Brown P, et al.: Precautions in handling tissues, fluids, and other contaminated materials from patients with documented or suspected Creutzfeldt-Jakob disease. Ann Neurol 19:75, 1986. *Safety guidelines for health care workers and specific decontamination protocols for surgical and pathologic instruments.*

SECTION TEN / NEUROLOGIC DISORDERS ASSOCIATED WITH ALTERED IMMUNITY OR UNEXPLAINED HOST-PARASITE ALTERATIONS

Jerry S. Wolinsky

479 Central Nervous System Complications of Viral Infections and Vaccines

Central nervous system (CNS) symptoms and signs arising in the course of systemic infections usually reflect direct CNS invasion by the inciting organism. Less frequently, systemic infections, especially viral infections, or the administration of certain vaccines give rise to CNS abnormalities that do not appear to depend on direct invasion of the brain but rather reflect presumed autoimmune or toxic mechanisms. Several reasonably distinct patterns of involvement have been delineated. Two of these, *acute disseminated encephalomyelitis* and *acute hemorrhagic encephalomyelitis*, appear to be mediated by immune mechanisms and have a peripheral nervous system counterpart, *acute inflammatory polyneuropathy*, or the *Guillain-Barré syndrome*. The remainder, *Reye syndrome, acute toxic encephalopathy*, and *acute cerebellar ataxia of childhood*, are likely to be toxic in origin.

ACUTE DISSEMINATED ENCEPHALOMYELITIS (ADE)

DEFINITION. Acute disseminated encephalomyelitis (*parainfectious* or *postinfectious encephalomyelitis, acute demyelinating encephalitis, immune-mediated encephalomyelitis*) is an acute disease of the CNS that most commonly occurs in association with viral infections or as a complication of vaccination. Involvement of brain and spinal cord is usually widespread but may be limited clinically to discrete areas such as the optic nerves, as in optic neuritis or papillitis, or to a single spinal cord level, as in acute transverse myelitis.

ETIOLOGY AND PATHOGENESIS. Table 479–1 lists principal factors predisposing to ADE. The neurologic complications usually occur 6 to 10 days after the appearance of the exanthem or onset of other specific symptoms. However, ADE can occur prior to or concomitantly with systemic symptoms of infection. Characteristically, ADE begins 10 days to 3 weeks after initiation of the vaccination regimen. Perhaps the most easily understood form of ADE is that which followed vaccination against rabies with (now obsolete) inactivated inoculum of fixed rabies virus propagated in animal brain. These early vaccines were contaminated with CNS proteins, including the antigens associated with myelin. Both complement-fixing antibody and specific lymphocyte blast transformation responses to crude and purified CNS antigens have been measured in blood of patients receiving rabies vaccine, and the responses were highest in those whose vaccination was complicated by ADE; the incidence of neuroparalytic accidents was reported to be as high as 1:600 to 1:6000 persons. Current rabies vaccines derived from virus grown in human diploid cells appear to be essentially free of neural complications (Ch. 477).

A compelling analogy links rabies vaccine–related ADE to the animal experimental disorder *experimental allergic encephalo-*

TABLE 479–1. PRINCIPAL CONDITIONS PREDISPOSING TO ACUTE DISSEMINATED ENCEPHALOMYELITIS

Infections	
Measles	*Mycoplasma pneumoniae*
Varicella zoster	Respiratory agents
Influenza	Epstein-Barr
Rubella	

Vaccines: smallpox, measles, rabies (Semple vaccine)

myelitis (EAE). In EAE, brain homogenates, highly purified myelin components, or peptides containing the encephalogenic sequences of myelin basic protein (MBP) or proteolipid protein (PLP) can induce an acute CNS perivascular inflammatory and demyelinative reaction that is histologically identical to ADE. In affected animals, clinical disease begins 10 to 14 days after sensitization and is associated with both humoral and cellular immune responses directed against the inciting CNS antigen. Furthermore, EAE can be adoptively transferred to naive animals by T lymphocytes, suggesting that this cell type is of primary importance in the pathogenesis.

The occurrence of ADE following viral infections is more difficult to understand. Encephalitis is relatively frequent following measles (1:1000 cases), but there is little evidence to implicate invasion of the CNS by measles virus as an obligate prerequisite. Theoretical data support the possible importance of sequence similarities between measles virus and other viral antigens and CNS proteins such as MBP and PLP. Very early in the course of measles ADE, specific blast transformation responses to MBP are apparent in the lymphocytes of children, and measurable quantities of MBP are released into the cerebrospinal fluid (CSF). These findings support the hypothesis that acute measles transiently alters the immune system, which in some persons results in a breakdown of tolerance to CNS antigens. Despite the usual absence of CNS symptoms, this process appears to occur frequently, as reflected by a high incidence of abnormal-appearing electroencephalograms (EEG's). Both EEG abnormalities and clinical ADE can occur after vaccination with live-attenuated measles virus but at a markedly lower frequency, with ADE arising in about 1:1,000,000 vaccinated persons.

INCIDENCE. Valid incidence figures for ADE are difficult to derive. Encephalitis complicates about 1:1000 cases of measles. ADE following vaccination for smallpox is only of historical interest but occurred in the United States with a reported incidence of 2.9 per million primary vaccinations. ADE following other childhood viral illnesses or vaccinations is uncommon. Most adult cases of ADE have no identifiable antecedents.

PATHOLOGY. Neuropathologic change consists of perivenular infiltration by lymphocytic and mononuclear cells and variable amounts of primary demyelination extending in centripetal manner from involved vessels of the white matter. The axons are relatively spared. This primary lesion can occur throughout the neuraxis but tends to be most prominent in the centrum semiovale of the cerebrum and in the pontine white matter. The brain may appear somewhat swollen or grossly normal. Repair occurs through remyelination. In certain cases, large, confluent demyelination can take on a superficial resemblance to the plaques of multiple sclerosis, differing primarily in that all lesions reflect a similar time of onset.

CLINICAL MANIFESTATIONS. The clinical disorder can resemble almost any of the acute encephalitides. In adults, neurologic symptoms often first suggest the illness. With the childhood exanthemata, CNS symptoms usually begin about 5 days after the onset of the rash (range 0 to 24 days, with rare examples of ADE preceding the rash). The course of the preceding illness is in no way atypical for patients who subsequently develop ADE. Fever or recrudescence of fever is nearly universal. Headache, with or without meningismus, and lethargy occur in 20 to 80 per cent of cases. In about half of the cases, one or more generalized seizures occur. Usually the onset of altered consciousness is abrupt, occurring within a few hours, but CNS symptoms sometimes evolve over several days. Stupor, delirium, or coma develops in severe cases. Multifocal motor and sensory deficits of varied severity are common and often asymmetric.

The EEG is abnormal in appearance, with widespread slowing of background rhythms. The CSF in children almost invariably shows a modest mononuclear pleocytosis of 20 to 200 cells per cubic millimeter and occasionally higher. The fluid contains a slight elevation of protein content, a normal glucose level, and a raised myelin basic protein level. After several days, magnetic resonance imaging (MRI) characteristically defines scattered white matter lesions, at least some of which enhance with paramagnetic agents during the acute phases of the disease.

The duration of active CNS disease varies from days to weeks, often with a protracted convalescence. The overall mortality is about 20 per cent. About 90 per cent of survivors recover completely or nearly completely, although severe residual deficits can occur.

DIAGNOSIS. Diagnosis in ADE is by exclusion. First, encephalitis, meningitis, or meningoencephalitis must be excluded as a direct effect of a virus or other infectious agent. In the setting of a recent exanthematous illness or vaccination, ADE is more readily implied. However, in pathologic series of clinically diagnosed ADE occurring in the course of mass vaccination programs, postmortem examination proved the majority of patients to have had other illnesses, including potentially treatable CNS infections. Differentiation of an initial severe episode of multiple sclerosis can be challenging, even with MRI help, but subsequent recurrences eventually make the proper diagnosis clear.

TREATMENT. Treatment consists of supportive care, including the use of anticonvulsants and, when necessary, intensive care monitoring. Although sometimes employed clinically, neither corticosteroids nor other immunosuppressive drugs have proved beneficial.

ACUTE HEMORRHAGIC LEUKOENCEPHALITIS

Acute hemorrhagic leukoencephalitis is a fulminant and fatal syndrome believed to have an immunopathogenesis similar to that of ADE. Typically, the illness arises either spontaneously or following an uneventful upper respiratory illness. Sudden headache precedes the neurologic symptoms, which include seizures and rapid progression from lethargy to coma in a matter of a few hours to several days. Major focal neurologic abnormalities are common and may suggest lateralized cerebral involvement. Systemic signs and symptoms include fever and marked peripheral leukocytosis. The accompanying CSF pleocytosis usually shows a preponderance of polymorphonuclear cells and sometimes evidence of minor degrees of hemorrhage into the subarachnoid space. More than 80 per cent of all recognized cases of acute hemorrhagic leukoencephalitis are fatal, although these findings may be biased by selective reports of postmortem studies. The brain is usually swollen, and examination shows bilateral but asymmetric abnormalities, with petechial hemorrhages scattered throughout the white matter. Microscopic lesions consist of features reminiscent of hyperimmune forms of EAE. The clinical differential diagnosis includes ADE and acute viral encephalitis, especially herpes simplex encephalitis (see Ch. 476.1). Computed tomography (CT) or MRI may be diagnostically helpful in selected cases. Therapy is supportive.

Griffin DE: Monophasic autoimmune inflammatory diseases of the CNS and PNS. Res Publ Assoc Res Nerv Ment Dis 68:91, 1990. *A review of recent advances in unraveling parainfectious nervous system disease.*

Kesselring J, Miller DH, Robb SA, et al.: Acute disseminated encephalomyelitis— MRI findings and the distinction from multiple sclerosis. Brain 113:291, 1990.

480 Reye Syndrome

DEFINITION. Reye syndrome is a well-delineated biphasic disease in which one of several common viral illnesses is followed by an acute and sometimes fatal encephalopathy associated with fatty infiltration and dysfunction of the liver.

ETIOLOGY AND PATHOGENESIS. Reye syndrome most commonly occurs following influenza A, influenza B, herpes varicella zoster, and, to a lesser extent, several other common virus infections. Many other common viral illnesses have been implicated, each at a much lower frequency. Little evidence links the precipitating viral infection directly to either the CNS or hepatic involvement. A toxic origin is proposed for both types of involvement. The hepatic dysfunction appears to be the primary error and the direct result of a mitochondrial disturbance that causes secondary metabolic derangements, including hyperammonemia, lactic acidemia, and elevated levels of serum free fatty acids. These metabolic derangements have been implicated in the pathogenesis of the brain swelling and increased intracranial pressure that dominate the clinical course of severe cases. What causes the mitochondrial impairment remains to be clarified. Epidemiologic evidence suggests that aspirin plays a potentiating role in the pathogenesis of this syndrome.

INCIDENCE. Reye syndrome occurs most commonly among children between 1 and 15 years of age but has been reported in adolescents and is increasingly recognized in adults. Inner city black infants may be especially at risk for the disease. Prospectively derived incidence figures for the most susceptible age groups are as high as 6.2 per 100,000 children.

PATHOLOGY. The liver shows a noninflammatory, panlobular, hepatocellular accumulation of lipid droplets and both histochemical and ultrastructural evidence of inflammation. At postmortem examination, swelling of astrocytic foot processes and ultrastructural changes in mitochondria similar to those seen in hepatic mitochondria may be found in the greatly swollen brain.

CLINICAL MANIFESTATIONS AND COURSE. Reye syndrome is a biphasic disorder. As symptoms of the initial viral illness begin to wane or clear, the dramatic features begin, usually with intractable vomiting associated with lethargy or delirium. Early diagnosis is confirmed by the findings of nonicteric hepatic dysfunction, an elevated arterial blood ammonia level, and serum transaminase levels that exceed three times normal levels. Hepatic enlargement is present in about one half of the cases. Children under 1 year of age often show hypoglycemia. Signs of CNS deterioration include the development of generalized seizures, deepening obtundation, and transtentorial herniation. The CSF is under increased pressure but is acellular, with otherwise normal constituents.

DIAGNOSIS. Diagnosis rests on the clinical findings and appropriate biochemical abnormalities. Liver biopsy usually is not necessary. Central nervous system infection, inborn errors of metabolism, such as ornithine transcarbamylase deficiency and systemic carnitine deficiency, and the presence of known hepatotoxins, including valproate, salicylates, and paracetamol, among others, must be actively excluded. A childhood syndrome, distinguishable from Reye syndrome only by the absence of hepatic involvement and a high incidence of acute convulsions, can follow both banal viral infections and vaccination.

TREATMENT. Affected patients require intensive care monitoring until the course of the disease is well established. Hypoglycemia and electrolyte abnormalities must be corrected. Many authorities suggest hydration with solutions of high glucose content. Appropriate measures should be taken to monitor intracranial pressure continuously in the more severely affected cases, as judicious control of intracranial hypertension contributes to a favorable outcome. Mortality is about 10 per cent.

Ede RJ, Williams R: Reye's syndrome in adults. Br Med J 296:517, 1988. *Although uncommon, such cases do occur and need management different from that for children.*

Pranzatelli MR, DeVivo DC: Pharmacology of Reye syndrome. Clin Neuropharmacol 10:96, 1987. *A comprehensive review including detailed recommendations for medical management.*

481 Neurologic Complications in the Immunologically Compromised Host

Modern treatment of several previously fatal conditions in many instances leads to an immunocompromised state that is associated with opportunistic infections of the CNS. Such treatments include transplantation for organ failure, chemotherapy and radiotherapy of malignancies, and immunosuppressive treatment of autoimmune diseases. The epidemic emergence of the acquired immunodeficiency syndrome (AIDS) also has been associated with a marked increase in the number of unusual CNS infections likely to be encountered in routine practice.

CNS INFECTIONS IN TRANSPLANT RECIPIENTS. Renal transplantation is now commonplace, and bone marrow, cardiac, and other organ transplantations are performed with increasing effectiveness. Hospital-acquired bacterial species predominate in early infections in transplant recipients. Immunosuppression, especially lethal irradiation used in the preparation for marrow transplantation from nonidentical donors, almost predictably gives rise to reactivation of herpesviruses: first herpes simplex viruses types 1 and 2 (HSV), then herpes varicella zoster virus (HVZ), and finally cytomegalovirus (CMV). The systemic manifestations of each can be overwhelming, but symptomatic CNS dissemination has so far been remarkably infrequent. However, encephalitis or meningitis can complicate either HSV or HVZ infections. Also, while EEG, CT, or MRI findings evolve as anticipated in the intact host, the CSF pleocytosis is often absent, especially in patients with severe leukopenia. CNS involvement by CMV has been pathologically documented in transplant patients but has not been associated with a recognizable clinical syndrome and at present appears to be asymptomatic. The availability of effective antiviral chemotherapy now makes it imperative to attempt early diagnosis in cases of suspected HSV or HVZ meningoencephalitis (see Ch. 473).

Transplant patients are at greatest risk of infection by opportunistic agents after the second month of the transplant. They remain at risk while they are on most immunosuppressive regimens, if they are azotemic, and when there are ongoing graft-versus-host or chronic rejection reactions. *Listeria monocytogenes, Cryptococcus neoformans,* and *Aspergillus fumigatus* account for the overwhelming majority of infections. *Toxoplasma gondii, Candida* species, *Nocardia asteroides,* the rhinocerebral phycomycoses, and *Coccidioides immitis* are less frequently encountered.

The acute or subacute development of fever in the transplant patient should suggest *Listeria* meningitis even in the absence of meningeal signs. The CSF has the characteristics of a purulent meningitis, although occasionally patients with *Listeria* infection have misleading mononuclear pleocytosis (see Ch. 301). Otherwise unexplained headache of acute or chronic duration, even in the absence of a febrile response or confusion, should suggest the possibility of cryptococcal meningitis. A mononuclear pleocytosis with or without a low glucose content is the characteristic CSF finding (see Ch. 403). India ink preparations can provide immediate confirmation of diagnosis, and tests for cryptococcus antigen can be more helpful than direct culture of the organism from the CSF. Since both listerial and cryptococcal meningitis represent some of the most frequently encountered and more manageable infections that affect the immunocompromised host, careful attention must be given to symptoms that suggest infection of the CNS.

Aspergillus fumigatus infections of the CNS usually are manifested as acute fulminant disease with seizures, obtundation, and, frequently, apoplectic onset of focal neurologic deficits. The propensity of *Aspergillus* to invade and destroy blood vessels underlies the frequent strokelike appearance of infected patients. Low-density lesions with ill-defined, poorly contrast-enhancing borders may be seen on CT, but diagnosis depends on brain biopsy in the absence of systemic disease. Current diagnostic and therapeutic approaches to this CNS infection are inadequate (see Ch. 406).

CNS INFECTION IN PATIENTS WITH LYMPHOMA, LEUKEMIA, OR CHRONIC IMMUNOSUPPRESSIVE THERAPY. Splenectomy, often used in the staging of Hodgkin's disease, places patients at increased risk for conventional bacterial infections that may be complicated by meningitis. In community-acquired infections, *Haemophilus influenzae* and *Streptococcus pneumoniae* species predominate. Metastatic spread from various systemic sites by a wide spectrum of bacterial organisms is a continual threat for all immunosuppressed patients. The usual signs and symptoms of CNS infection can be obscured by the anti-inflammatory effect of therapy. The use of chronic immunosuppressive therapy for leukemia, lymphoma, or presumed autoimmune disorders can be complicated by *Listeria monocytogenes* in a manner similar to that described for transplant patients. The emergence of listerial meningitis often follows an increase in the intensity of the immunosuppressive regimen.

Cryptococcal meningitis and *Aspergillus* meningoencephalitis are significant sources of morbidity for this group of patients. Their clinical appearances parallel those seen in organ transplant patients. Segmental zoster, occasionally with dissemination, is a well-recognized problem among these patients, and CNS toxoplasmosis is occasionally encountered. Of special interest is *progressive multifocal leukoencephalopathy* (PML) (Ch. 478.5), which may account for up to 10 per cent of all CNS infections in this patient group. Progressive deterioration in mental status and the evolution of focal neurologic deficits in the absence of meningismus or CSF abnormalities characterize the clinical symptomatology of PML. Serial CT scans are usually diagnostic, but the recent observation that some patients with CNS infections by HVZ can have a clinical course similar to that of PML must be considered because HVZ is potentially responsive to antiviral chemotherapy.

Conti DJ, Rubin RH: Infection of the central nervous system in organ transplant recipients. Neurol Clin 6:241, 1988. *A comprehensive review of an extensive experience with opportunistic CNS infections.*

SECTION ELEVEN / THE DEMYELINATING DISEASES

482 The Demyelinating Diseases

Donald H. Silberberg

The demyelinating diseases affect myelin to a greater extent than other nervous system components. This section discusses disorders that primarily affect central nervous system (CNS) myelin; the demyelinating peripheral neuropathies are discussed in Ch. 497. A few disorders, such as the neurologic complications of vitamin B_{12} deficiency and some of the leukodystrophies, affect both central and peripheral myelin.

Since central myelin is an extension of the oligodendrocyte, which manufactures the myelin sheath, most demyelinating diseases include alterations in or disappearance of this glial cell. An oligodendrocyte process wraps around a segment of an axon in a concentric fashion to form myelin. One oligodendrocyte sends processes to as many as 20 or 30 axons within a surrounding area of several millimeters, myelinating axon segments of 1 mm or less on each fiber. The most active synthesis of myelin starts in utero and continues for the first 2 years of life; subsequently, slower synthesis continues until the adult CNS is achieved.

Each tightly compacted layer of mature myelin is a bimolecular lipid leaflet between parallel layers of hydrated protein, which is in close apposition to the polar groups of the lipid molecules. The lipids, which constitute about 75 per cent of the dry weight of myelin, include cerebroside, phospholipids, and cholesterol. Proteins include the distinctive molecule, myelin basic protein (the antigen capable of eliciting experimental allergic encephalomyelitis in experimental animals), myelin-associated glycoprotein, proteolipid proteins, and many others detectable by electrophoretic separation but not yet well characterized. Turnover of the components of mature myelin continues at a slower rate than the rate during development. Both developing and mature forms of myelin are readily susceptible to injury by many diseases.

CLASSIFICATION. Definitive classification awaits an understanding of the causes of these disorders. Failing that, a mixed temporal-etiologic-descriptive classification must serve as the scaffold. A useful distinction is to separate what seem to be acquired disorders from those that are errors in development (Table 482–1). Multiple sclerosis will be discussed first, since it is by far the most common of these problems.

MULTIPLE SCLEROSIS

DEFINITION. Multiple sclerosis (MS) is a disorder of unknown etiology, defined by its clinical characteristics and by typical scattered areas of brain, optic nerve, and spinal cord demyelination. Clinical diagnosis requires evidence on neurologic examination of two or more CNS white matter lesions, preferably with at least a month's interval between symptoms, in a patient of the appropriate age, in whom evidence is lacking of any other explanation for the signs and symptoms. MS usually produces its first clinical symptoms in those between ages 15 and 50 years. Occasional cases occur beyond these extremes, but the average age of onset is 33. Most patients recover clinically to some extent from individual bouts of demyelination, producing the classic remitting and exacerbating course of the early disease. Except for autopsy findings, currently available laboratory data may support the clinical diagnosis but cannot be used to define MS.

ETIOLOGY. The cause of MS remains unknown. The tissue response has features of an immunopathologic process, with perivenular mononuclear cell infiltration and absence of any overt histopathologic evidence of an infection. Two other lines of evidence point to either an immunologic cause or immunologic participation in the MS process: (1) the frequent elevation of cerebrospinal fluid (CSF) gamma globulin levels and the common oligoclonal pattern in the gamma globulin region on CSF electrophoresis, apparently synthesized by plasma cells in areas of demyelination, and (2) changes in the proportion of lymphocyte subclasses in the peripheral blood, CSF, and brain lesions. These changes are, however, nonspecific and may be the consequence of demyelination induced by some other disease mechanism, rather than the cause of the demyelination.

TABLE 482–1. DISORDERS SELECTIVELY AFFECTING MYELIN

I. **Demyelinating diseases (acquired destruction of preformed myelin)**
  A. Multiple sclerosis
    1. Uniphasic events presumably related to multiple sclerosis
      a. Optic neuritis
      b. Acute transverse myelopathy
  B. Parainfectious disorders
    1. Acute disseminated encephalomyelitis
    2. Acute hemorrhagic leukoencephalopathy
  C. Viral infections
    1. Progressive multifocal leukoencephalopathy
    2. Subacute sclerosing panencephalitis
  D. Nutritional disorders
    1. Combined systems disease (vitamin B_{12} deficiency)
    2. Demyelination of the corpus callosum (Marchiafava-Bignami disease)
    3. Central pontine myelinolysis
  E. Anoxic-ischemic sequelae
    1. Delayed postanoxic cerebral demyelination
    2. Progressive subcortical ischemic encephalopathy
II. **Dysmyelinating diseases (developmental failure to form or maintain myelin)**
  A. The leukocystrophies
    1. Metachromatic leukodystrophy
    2. Sudanophilic (Pelizaeus-Merzbacher disease)
    3. Globoid cell (Krabbe's disease)
    4. Adrenoleukodystrophy (Schilder's disease)
    5. Others (e.g., Alexander's, Canavan's, Seitelberger's disease)
  B. Aminoacidurias (e.g., phenylketonuria)
  C. Neonatal hypothyroidism

Epidemiologic studies suggest an infectious etiology. Perhaps the best evidence for this is the outbreak of MS that occurred in the Faroe Islands during the 20 years following the start of World War II. The Faroes were occupied by British troops during the war. No cases of MS had occurred prior to the occupation. The sudden appearance of MS starting several years after the arrival of the troops strongly suggests the presence of an infectious agent. The geographic areas where MS is prevalent are farther from the equator, suggesting the presence of an environmental factor, presumably an infectious agent. Efforts continue without confirmed success to recover a virus from MS tissues. MS is among the diseases with a strong linkage to certain human leukocytic antigen (HLA) haplotypes. The particular haplotype varies from one population group to another. In North America, haplotypes Dw2 and DR2, D locus markers, are found in about 65 per cent of MS patients, compared with 15 per cent of control subjects. Recent work suggests linkage to T cell receptor genes as well. Additional evidence for an immunogenetic component in the etiology of MS is the increase in frequency of MS among close relatives and the fact that MS is rare among Asians, even after emigration to the United States. A possible synthesis is that MS is an unusual consequence of infection by a common virus, or any of several viruses, with subsequent immunologic alterations in genetically susceptible individuals.

INCIDENCE AND PREVALENCE. The prevalence of MS in the northern United States and Canada and in northern Europe is at least 60 per 100,000 population, perhaps higher, based on recent data from Rochester, Minnesota. The risk is somewhat higher for women. MS is almost unknown among Asians and African blacks. There is little evidence for changing incidence or prevalence, except where population patterns are undergoing changes as the result of immigration.

EPIDEMIOLOGY. MS is more common farther from the equator in North America, in Europe, and in Australia and New Zealand. Regional population figures are punctuated by many reports of clusters of cases in a small area, such as particular cantons in Switzerland.

Many of the population studies were done before the availability of HLA typing, so that some of the observed regional differences may prove to have a genetic basis. MS occurs in both members of about 50 per cent of monozygous twin pairs when the disease has been identified in one. This finding supports the concept that genetic susceptibility may increase the chances of developing MS but is not sufficient to cause it and may not be required for its development.

PATHOLOGY. The lesions of MS consist of scattered areas of dissolution of CNS myelin, within which the axons remain intact. The border between histologically normal myelin and myelin dissolution is often sharp or may shade from normal to thinning before bare axons occur. Some areas show only partial myelin destruction. Lesions range in size from 1 mm to several centimeters in diameter and occur throughout the brain, optic nerves (which are central tracts of white matter), and spinal cord. Although plaques may occur anywhere within CNS myelin, predilections involve the optic nerves, periventricular regions within the cerebrum, and cervical spinal cord. Most plaques occur near blood vessels.

Oligodendrocytes disappear from within plaques initially. Subsequently, immature oligodendrocytes appear as attempts to remyelinate occur. However, remyelination is not nearly so complete as to explain the remissions of neurologic dysfunction that characterize MS. Astrocytes proliferate, forming the scar that lent the term "sclerosis" to multiple sclerosis. One always finds many more plaques at autopsy than could have been suspected on the basis of the clinical history and examination. Similarly, the sensitivity and resolution provided by magnetic resonance imaging (MRI) often reveal clinically unsuspected plaques. The acute lesion of MS may produce considerable edema, visible as cord swelling on myelography or as optic nerve enlargement on imaging studies. Occasionally, typical plaques of MS are found in previously asymptomatic individuals at autopsy.

B lymphocytes appear to synthesize much of the excess of gamma globulin that is found in and around plaques and in CSF. These plasma cells occur throughout affected tissue and persist in large numbers throughout a patient's lifetime, correlating with the observation that once CSF gamma globulin elevation appears, it persists. It is not known whether plasma cells and other

mononuclear cells precede, accompany, or follow myelin and oligodendrocyte destruction.

LABORATORY ABNORMALITIES. Cerebrospinal Fluid. Increased CSF gamma globulin synthesis occurs in 80 to 90 per cent of MS patients, more commonly after the first year following the onset of symptoms. Normal CSF gamma globulin is less than 13 per cent of total CSF protein by most testing methods. The gamma globulin is mostly immunoglobulin (Ig) G but often contains IgA and IgM as well. Separate discrete "oligoclonal" bands are seen in the gamma region on agarose or polyacrylamide gel electrophoresis in about 90 per cent of patients, including some with normal IgG quantitation. These abnormalities are helpful when other causes of the phenomenon are excluded; these include CNS syphilis, subacute sclerosing panencephalitis, chronic meningitis, and any disease associated with a peripheral blood paraproteinemia, such as human T cell lymphotropic virus I (HTLV-I) infection. Other CSF abnormalities in MS can include elevation in total protein, usually to no more than 100 mg per deciliter, and an increase in the number of mononuclear white cells, usually to 5 to 15 per cubic millimeter, rarely to more than 50 per cubic millimeter. Myelin destruction releases myelin basic protein (MBP) into the CSF, which can be detected by radioimmunoassay. The amount present correlates wtih disease activity and lesion size and location; none is detectable normally, or during quiescent periods in MS patients. MBP levels rise in association with acute attacks or rapid progression. This serves as an index of disease activity but is not specific to MS. Myelin destruction from any other cause, such as acute infarction, causes a similar elevation of MBP.

Alterations in the ratio of subclasses of peripheral blood and of CSF lymphocytes occur at the time of acute exacerbations. These changes, which may indicate abnormalities of immunoregulation, are currently of investigative interest only.

Neurophysiologic Function Studies. The presence of myelin enhances the propagation of the nerve impulse along the axon. Loss of myelin, from any cause, slows conduction velocity. This alteration in conduction velocity can be measured by timing the appearance of an evoked potential (visual, auditory, or somatosensory) after an appropriate stimulus. Measurement of the latency of the visual evoked response (VER) is used most widely (Ch. 441.5). The normal latency from stimulus to VER in most laboratories is less than 102 to 105 milliseconds. A prolonged latency indicates an abnormality in the visual system, most commonly within the optic nerve in patients with MS. An abnormality of the visual, auditory, or somatosensory evoked response is used to detect dysfunction (prolonged conduction velocity) either as an objective measurement of what has already been detected clinically or for detection of a presumed subclinical abnormality.

CT and MRI Scans. Hypodense areas seen with the computed tomographic (CT) scan reflect the presence of lesions in various stages, ranging from inflammation with edema to various degrees of demyelination. Edema, which may resemble a mass lesion, often occurs acutely. During this stage, leakage of intravenously injected iodinated contrast material into the lesion area reflects abnormal leakage of the blood-brain barrier. Atrophy is seen in instances of severe demyelination.

MRI provides a much more sensitive method for detecting abnormalities in MS, and often reveals many more areas of hyperintensity on T_2-weighted images than were suspected clinically. The use of intravenously injected paramagnetic agents, such as gadolinium, permits detection of alterations in the blood-brain barrier with MRI, which occur with new activity in a particular area. The abnormalities detected by CSF examination, by neurophysiologic testing, and by imaging are not specific for MS (see Role of Laboratory Aids, below).

CLINICAL MANIFESTATIONS. Onset. The random distribution of MS lesions leads to a variety of initial symptoms and signs, alone or in combination. Further, it must be kept in mind that lesions occur in clinically silent areas of CNS white matter so that the first lesion that announces itself clinically may not be the first that has occurred in an individual. Common initial problems include weakness of one or more extremities, unilateral vision loss (optic neuritis), incoordination, and paresthesias (Table 482–2). Urinary frequency, incontinence, hesitancy, or retention;

TABLE 482–2. FIRST SYMPTOMS OF MULTIPLE SCLEROSIS IN 937 PATIENTS*

Symptom	Per Cent†
Weakness	48
Paresthesias	31
Vision loss	25
Incoordination	15
Vertigo	6
Sphincter impairment	6

*Combined series of Carter et al.: Res Publ Assoc Nerv Ment Dis 28:471, 1950; Poser CM: Recent advances in multiple sclerosis. Med Clin North Am 56:1343, 1972; and McAlpine et al.: Multiple Sclerosis: A Reappraisal. 2nd ed. Edinburgh, Churchill Livingstone, 1972.

†Many patients experience more than one symptom at onset.

vertigo; hearing loss; facial, extremity, or truncal pain; dysarthria; and changes in intellectual function occur less commonly initially. Weakness most often affects the lower extremities and may produce a range of dysfunction from slight fatigability to paraparesis. The arm and hand may be involved alone or with the legs. Patients who develop paraparesis often develop urinary urgency and constipation. Incoordination as the result of cerebellar lesions, or loss of position sense, may occur independently of weakness and often leads to gait impairment or to tremor-like, clumsy movements of the arms and hands. Paresthesias range from the spontaneous perception of vague pins-and-needles discomfort, or girdle-like pressures, to the pain of classic trigeminal neuralgia. Loss of perception of vibration and position at the ankle and toes is common; loss of pain and touch perception is less frequent. Impairment of two-point discrimination over the palmar surface of the fingertips often accompanies cervical cord lesions.

Vision loss can vary in degree from slight blurring with a small central scotoma, slight decrease in acuity, and a slight impairment of color perception to no light perception. The patient often reports acute pain on eye movement. Other visual symptoms include blurring secondary to nystagmus on primary gaze, or explicit perception of nystagmus as spontaneous movement of objects (oscillopsia). Diplopia often occurs as the result of involvement of the pontine white matter. Horizontal nystagmus of the abducting eye on lateral gaze with paresis of the adducting eye, termed *internuclear ophthalmoplegia*, is common. It is often unilateral at first and is due to lesions involving the median longitudinal fasciculus in the pons. In rare instances, extensive midline lesions lead to alterations of consciousness.

The speed of onset of symptoms varies from minutes to days, and in patients with a chronic progressive course, symptoms may appear to increase gradually over many months. The timing of recovery (remission) varies enormously but usually occurs over the course of 2 to 8 weeks following an acute bout.

Clinical Course. At least 70 per cent of patients improve in the days to months following their initial bout, the degree ranging from slight to virtual disappearance of the neurologic dysfunction. Whether or not a particular patient will improve, and to what extent, is as unpredictable as whether or not more lesions will occur and when. Overall, about three fourths of patients experience exacerbations and remissions early in their course. In many, however, as time goes by, the recovery from individual bouts decreases, disability results from accumulated failures to improve, and the course becomes chronically progressive.

About 30 per cent of patients develop successive disabilities without remission, often with long periods of clinical stability between periods of deterioration. This chronic progressive course occurs more commonly in patients experiencing their first neurologic manifestations after age 45. Patients whose disease onset has occurred at an older age seem to compress the course of events and often develop the same degree of dysfunction within a few years that takes decades to occur in a patient whose onset has occurred at a younger age.

Most patients experience additional difficulties at some time after their initial symptoms; subsequent acute bouts or chronic progression may produce signs and symptoms in any combination. Several generalizations are of interest but help little when counseling the individual. Ten years after onset, about 50 per cent of patients are still able to carry out their household and/or employment responsibilities. Twenty years after onset about 25 per cent have these capacities. However, a fortunate few patients never develop significant disabilities, whereas others are bedridden within months after onset. One of the major psychological burdens borne by patients with MS is the uncertainty about their future. Most neurologists find it useful to emphasize the hopeful possibilities, allowing the patient's course to reveal its own manner of progression.

The average interval from clinical onset to death is 35 years; 75 per cent are living 25 years after diagnosis. Premature death is usually due to bacterial infection resulting from urinary retention, decubiti, or inability to handle pulmonary secretions. Rarely, primary respiratory failure from lower medullary lesions spells the terminal event.

Factors Possibly Affecting the Clinical Course. Elevation of body temperature by as little as 0.5°C noticeably reduces neurologic function transiently in some patients, particularly those with recent disease activity. Reduction in visual acuity, incoordination or weakness, and sensory or bladder dysfunction can be affected. This is the result of slowed axonal conduction induced by heating, and the alterations disappear within hours of regaining normal body temperature. This contributes to the fact that many patients' conditions worsen concomitantly with an intercurrent infection. However, it is likely that immunologic changes induced by infection are responsible, since the temperature effect is a transient one. Patients should be instructed to rest and respond to respiratory infections with more care than they might otherwise exercise and to use aspirin to reduce fever.

Pregnancy makes neither exacerbations nor progression of MS more likely. Decisions regarding childbearing should be made on the basis of the patient's overall situation, rather than on the basis of this concern alone.

DIAGNOSIS. Despite the availability of increasingly complex laboratory aids, MS remains fundamentally a clinical diagnosis (Table 482–3). Physical signs on examination providing solid evidence for two or more lesions of central white matter occurring at least a month apart in a patient between age 10 and the early 50's, in the absence of any other possible etiology, are required. If the evidence for a second lesion is history or a laboratory abnormality alone, the diagnosis should be considered possible or probable, rather than clinically definite MS. The differential diagnosis includes cervical cord compression resulting from tumor or cervical spondylosis; cerebral, cerebellar, brain stem, and pituitary tumors; familial spinocerebellar degenerations; acute systemic lupus erythematosus (SLE); sarcoidosis; brain stem atherosclerotic cerebrovascular disease; vitamin B_{12} deficiency; chronic barbiturate or other intoxications; and psychogenic disturbances (Table 482–4).

If all of the patient's signs can be attributed to a lesion in a single area of the nervous system, the working assumption must be that one is not dealing with MS. In patients with a persistent headache, seizures, persistent and progressive unifocal signs, or

TABLE 482–3. SCHUMACHER PANEL CRITERIA FOR DIAGNOSIS OF (CLINICALLY DEFINITE) MULTIPLE SCLEROSIS

1. Neurologic examination must reveal objective abnormalities that can be attributed to dysfunction of the central nervous system.
2. Examination or case history must supply evidence that two or more parts of the central nervous system are involved.
3. Evidence of central nervous system disease must reflect predominant involvement of white matter, that is, long-tract damage.
4. Involvement of the neuraxis must have followed one of two time patterns:
   a. Two or more episodes of worsening, each lasting at least 24 hours and each at least a month apart.
   b. Slow or stepwise progression of signs and symptoms over at least 6 months.
5. At onset the patient must be between 10 and 50 years old.
6. A physician competent in clinical neurology should decide that the patient's condition could not better be attributed to another disease.

Reprinted with permission from Schumacher G, Beebe G, Kibler R, et al.: Problems of experimental trials of therapy in multiple sclerosis: Report by the panel on the evaluation of experimental trials of therapy in multiple sclerosis. Ann NY Acad Sci 122:552–568, 1965.

TABLE 482–4. DIFFERENTIAL DIAGNOSIS OF MULTIPLE SCLEROSIS

Multifocal, CNS, relapsing and remitting course
Systemic lupus erythematosus, periarteritis nodosa
Primary CNS granulomatous angiitis
Sarcoidosis
Meningovascular syphilis
Atherosclerotic cerebrovascular disease, particularly vertebrobasilar distribution
Sjögren's syndrome
Drug intoxication
Lyme disease
Behçet's disease

Multifocal, CNS, progressive course
Familial or sporadic spinocerebellar degenerations
B_{12} deficiency myelopathy (subacute combined degeneration), optic neuropathy, cerebral dysfunction, and/or peripheral neuropathy
HTLV-I myelopathy

Single site, relapsing and remitting course
Brain tumors, particularly posterior fossa
Spinal cord tumor
Sarcoidosis
Arteriovenous malformation

Single site, progressive course
Brain, spinal cord tumors
Cervical spondylosis
Thoracic herniated intervertebral disc
Arnold-Chiari malformation
Paraspinous abscess
HTLV-I myelopathy
Human immunodeficiency virus (HIV) myelopathy
Idiopathic transverse myelopathy

papilledema (without a central scotoma), MRI is the most sensitive screening procedure. MRI examination of the spinal canal often obviates myelography to exclude cervical mass lesions.

Spinocerebellar degenerative diseases differ from MS by having associated abnormalities (such as the areflexia commonly seen with Friedreich's ataxia); by progressing slowly within a given neuroanatomic system, such as the cerebellum and its connections; and by exhibiting an abnormal family history. However, MS occurs more commonly in first-degree relatives of patients with MS, so that family history alone is not sufficient to make the distinction. Neurologic presentation of SLE in young women can be distinguished by appropriate immunologic testing. The neurologic manifestations of B_{12} deficiency may precede the peripheral red blood cell abnormalities by several years; the deficiency is detected by the serum B_{12} level, Schilling test, and methylmalonic acid levels. The correct diagnosis of brain stem arterial disease in patients in their 50's can sometimes be difficult; absence of CSF abnormalities associated with MS helps, as does the fact that all the abnormalities can be localized to a small anatomic area. The clinician's suspicion of chronic drug intoxication, often accompanied by nystagmus and ataxia, may be substantiated by appropriate blood levels or other evidence of disturbed behavior.

The total absence of objective neurologic signs at any time, together with apparent weakness or sensory loss or symptom patterns that fail to conform to known neuroanatomic systems, raises the suspicion of psychogenic illness. However, one must be wary, for many patients with urinary retention, urgency, or incontinence; ataxia; or vague sensory symptoms occurring in the early stages of MS have had their condition misdiagnosed as psychoneurotic. MRI, evoked response, or CSF abnormalities help exclude purely psychogenic disturbances but must not be overinterpreted.

Role of Laboratory Aids. The rational use of laboratory abnormalities requires an awareness of their limitations. Elevation of the CSF gamma globulin or the appearance of an oligoclonal pattern within the gamma region on electrophoresis is not specific for MS, although the non-MS causes can usually be readily excluded. However, these abnormalities fail to appear in 10 to 20 per cent of patients with clinically definite MS. Further, many patients who experience a single episode of neurologic abnormality, such as optic neuritis or transverse myelopathy, may

exhibit CSF gamma globulin abnormalities but do not develop a second clinically visible lesion after long follow-up. Thus it is not appropriate to make the diagnosis of MS with a first neurologic attack, even when one encounters CSF gamma globulin abnormalities.

Similarly, although evoked potential abnormalities serve to suggest the possibility of a lesion in that part of the CNS tested, the nonspecific nature of the electrophysiologic alterations makes it unwise to base a diagnosis on such data. A patient with paraparesis and prolonged latency of the VER may have MS but could possibly have two tumors, pernicious anemia, systemic vasculitis, or a spinal cord tumor plus an uncorrected refractive error. Similarly, multiple lesions detected via MRI may reflect many other multifocal disease processes. Despite these cautions, the discovery of CSF abnormalities commonly associated with MS, evoked potential evidence of a second lesion, and/or multiple lesions on MRI help greatly to focus on MS as a possible or probable diagnosis.

TREATMENT. Management of MS requires a combination of an understanding of the personal problems posed by an unpredictable disorder of unknown etiology; an awareness of the measures available to alleviate spasticity, urinary incontinence, and other dysfunctions; and a skeptical approach to "definitive" treatments that are proposed to alter the course of the illness. The fact that over 70 per cent of patients experience spontaneous improvement following an acute bout makes evaluation of proposed treatment difficult, time consuming, and expensive. Nevertheless, carefully conducted controlled trials are the only means for deciding whether or not an agent helps patients with MS. Testimonial-style reports should not be accepted as evidence until a controlled study has confirmed the findings. At present, no method for prevention of MS is known.

Dealing with patients affected by a chronic, sometimes disabling disease for which there is no specific treatment is frustrating to many physicians. Patients with MS often report that they must help alleviate their physician's depression by denying problems. Most patients respond well to an explanation of the disease, a discussion of those things that can be done, and assurance that vigorous research is under way to develop better treatment.

Acute bouts of neurologic dysfunction may be treated with short-term administration of corticosteroids. There is evidence that administration of adrenocorticotropic hormone (ACTH) for 10 to 14 days somewhat shortens exacerbations, although the ACTH (or other corticosteroid) does not alter the long-term course of MS. From 40 to 80 units of ACTH per day may be used; prednisone, 40 to 60 mg per day, or equivalent doses of other oral corticosteroids are often employed as alternatives. The period of treatment should not exceed 3 or 4 weeks, with appropriate precautions to avoid steroid complications. It must be emphasized that there is no evidence that corticosteroids (or any other agent) modify the MS pathogenic process. Beneficial effects are most probably due to anti-edema and anti-inflammatory effects. Many responsible clinicians choose not to treat patients in this manner, believing that minimal evidence favors steroid use.

Over 45 substances or other treatments are currently being evaluated in clinical trials, ranging from immunomodulators, such as interferons, to monoclonal antibodies directed at specific T lymphocyte subsets; none can be recommended at present.

Physical therapy plays an important role in several aspects of patient management, including developing alternative muscle strengths, preventing contractures, improving daily living, and providing supportive psychotherapy. Immersion in a cool bath or swimming pool improves neurologic function transiently by lowering body temperature and improving axonal conduction. Occupational therapy is often a key to the patient's adjustment to MS.

The chronic fatigue often associated with MS often responds to amantadine, 200 to 300 mg per day. Spasticity and flexor spasms can be alleviated with baclofen or with diazepam, which inhibits central synaptic transmission. Individual responses vary sufficiently that one must start with very low doses and increase slowly if needed. Many patients depend on spasticity for support while walking, so that removal of this aid or induction of weakness or drowsiness as temporary side effects limits treatment. Occasionally, leg contractures occur despite physical therapy and require orthopedic surgical relief for ease of handling the patient.

Bladder dysfunction is usually the result of incomplete emptying, accumulation of residual urine, and overflow frequency or incontinence and infection. Rational treatment requires careful urologic evaluation, often including urodynamic studies, to plan appropriate pharmacologic therapy. Uninhibited bladder contraction leading to urinary frequency or incontinence may be alleviated by controlling infection and restricting fluid intake prior to trips or several hours before sleep. Imipramine, oxybutynin chloride, or propantheline may help patients who cannot initiate urination or cannot fully empty their bladder. Attempts to void at fixed intervals and the Credé maneuver often help. If catheterization becomes necessary, many individuals can learn self-catheterization to avoid the complications of an indwelling catheter. Long-term urinary bacterial suppressant therapy is helpful in minimizing infection in patients carrying residual urine. The possibility of an ascending urinary tract infection must be sought and treated appropriately in any patient with recurrent cystitis.

Constipation usually responds to stool softeners and laxatives. Many patients must be reassured that no harm arises from the lack of a daily bowel movement.

Painful paresthesias and dysesthesias may occur and fortunately are usually transient. Carbamazepine, diazepam, or phenytoin usually provides relief. Prevention of decubiti in the paraplegic or desensitized patient requires constant vigilance.

Specific psychiatric support is often needed to aid patients and their families. The incidence of marital breakup, changes in roles within the family, and financial problems is exceeded only by the frequency of frustration over the unpredictability of MS. The physician often must call on a range of associates, including social workers, community agency workers, and psychiatrists, to help these patients cope.

Brown FR, Beebe GW, Kurtzke JF, et al.: The design of clinical studies to assess therapeutic efficacy in multiple sclerosis. Neurology 29:1, 1979. *A thorough review of the many factors that must be taken into consideration in designing a study to determine whether or not a proposed treatment benefits patients with MS.*

Gonzalez-Scarano F, Grossman RI, Galetta S, et al.: Multiple sclerosis disease activity correlates with gadolinium-enhanced MRI. Ann Neurol 21:300, 1987.

Kurtzke JF, Hyllested K: Multiple sclerosis in the Faroe Islands: I. Clinical and epidemiological features. Ann Neurol 5:6, 1979. *A lucid description of the remarkable, seemingly limited epidemic of MS in the Faroe Islands.*

McDonald WI, Silberberg DH (eds.): Multiple Sclerosis. London, Butterworths, 1986.

Poser C, Presthus J, Horstal O: Clinical characteristics of autopsy-proved multiple sclerosis. Neurology 16:791, 1966. *A valuable analysis of the presentation and signs and symptoms that developed among a large series of patients in whom MS was proved by autopsy.*

Poser S, Raun E, Wikstrom J, et al.: Pregnancy, oral contraceptives, and multiple sclerosis. Acta Neurol Scand 59:108, 1979. *The largest study of the possible effect of pregnancy or oral contraceptives on the course of MS; this study shows no relationship.*

Prineas J, Kwon E, Goldenberg P, et al.: Multiple sclerosis. Oligodendrocyte proliferation and differentiation in fresh lesions. Lab Invest 61:489, 1989. *One of a series of elegant descriptions of the tissue alterations produced by MS.*

MULTIPLE SCLEROSIS VARIANTS

Neuromyelitis Optica (Devic's Disease)

Neuromyelitis optica describes a syndrome characterized by the occurrence of partial or complete transverse myelopathy and optic neuritis. Loss of vision and paraplegia may occur in either disorder, and days or weeks may elapse between the onsets of the two symptom complexes. It is best considered a syndrome, in that it may occur as the result of MS, acute disseminated encephalomyelitis, SLE, or sarcoidosis. When this symptom complex occurs in the course of MS, its clinical and pathologic features are indistinguishable from those of MS.

Diffuse Sclerosis, Transitional Sclerosis

These terms describe a group of progressive neurologic disorders occurring primarily in young patients who manifest severe neurologic deficits of various types with progressive visual and mental deterioration. These are pathologists' terms, which were first used in the late nineteenth century. Schilder described three cases of what came to be known as Schilder's cerebral sclerosis,

or Schilder's disease. It is likely that three separate conditions have been included as Schilder's disease and that this eponymic designation should be discarded. Some cases represent the result of severe confluent extensions of large lesions of MS. Some represent white matter disease of known viral origin, such as subacute sclerosing panencephalitis and progressive multifocal leukoencephalitis (see Ch. 478). A third group includes the leukodystrophies (see later discussion). It is probable that adrenoleukodystrophy was the disorder identified by Schilder in one of his early cases.

Possibly Related Monophasic Disorders

ACUTE DISSEMINATED ENCEPHALOMYELITIS. This disorder is discussed in Ch. 481. It can be noted here that an episode of acute disseminated encephalomyelitis can closely resemble an attack of MS. Distinction may be impossible until sufficient time has elapsed to determine whether or not a second bout occurs. The distinction between acute disseminated encephalomyelitis and MS is blurred by the occurrence of typical exacerbations in the course of MS, concomitant with intercurrent viral infection.

OPTIC NEURITIS. Optic neuritis denotes partial or complete loss of vision in one or both eyes, attributable to one or more optic nerve lesions of unknown etiology. If a cause is known, it is more precise to describe, for example, syphilitic optic neuropathy or optic neuritis or neuropathy secondary to MS. Retrobulbar neuritis describes a lesion in the posterior two thirds of the optic nerve. The term papillitis indicates a lesion in the anterior portion of the optic nerve, leading to an ophthalmoscopic appearance indistinguishable from that of acute papilledema but differing from the papilledema of increased intracranial pressure by being associated with reduction of visual acuity early in its course. The vision loss usually, but not always, affects macular vision, with appearance of a central scotoma and a reduction in color perception. Pain on eye movement is frequent during the first few days of the event. Unless the patient has papillitis, ophthalmoscopic examination is normal for the first 2 to 3 weeks, after which disc pallor with loss of small vessels on the disc or more severe atrophy may develop.

Vision loss occurs over the course of hours to several days and almost always recovers to some degree within several weeks. Blindness as the result of the optic nerve demyelination of MS rarely occurs. Optic neuritis can occur as the presenting sign of MS (see Table 482–2) or at any time during the course of the disease. Practically all MS patients exhibit optic nerve demyelination at autopsy, which underlines the usefulness of the VER. Approximately 60 per cent of patients who develop idiopathic optic neuritis go on to develop the clinical manifestations of MS. The presence of CSF or MRI abnormalities associated with MS makes this course somewhat more likely but does not have firm predictive value; MS may develop in the absence of initial laboratory abnormalities, and conversely, no further clinical signs may occur despite CSF or MRI findings.

The illnesses that can mimic idiopathic optic neuritis include optic nerve compression on any basis, neurosyphilis, ischemic optic neuropathy (in older patients), pernicious anemia, Leber's optic atrophy (which is hereditary), tobacco-alcohol amblyopia, and chronic papilledema with optic atrophy and vision loss, associated with prolonged increased intracranial pressure.

LEUKODYSTROPHIES

The leukodystrophies are diseases of dysmyelination, rather than demyelination, in that the normal formation of myelin is interfered with by a genetically determined biochemical defect. The classification of leukodystrophies is based on their histopathology. A biochemical defect is known for several, but they remain relatively rare, incurable disorders, affecting individuals from the first months of life to the 20's.

Metachromatic Leukodystrophy

This, the most common of the leukodystrophies, describes diffuse dysmyelination, usually starting in the first 10 years of life. It produces personality changes leading to dementia, convulsions, cranial nerve abnormalities, and finally severe spasticity or rigidity. Death usually occurs in from 2 to 4 years, although longer survival is reported. Juvenile and adult-onset cases have been reported.

The appearance of metachromatic material (staining red with toluidine blue) in the urinary sediment and in peripheral nerves usually allows diagnosis during life. The metachromatic material also collects in the liver, gallbladder, kidneys, and spleen. The CSF protein is usually elevated above 100 mg per deciliter.

Metachromatic leukodystrophy is usually inherited as an autosomal recessive trait. The pathogenesis of the widespread loss of normal myelin is accumulation of sulfatides in glial cells, in Schwann cells, within myelin lamellae, and in the cytoplasm of some nerve cells. The underlying biochemical defect is abnormally low activity of arylsulfatase A, an enzyme in the system that normally reduces the concentration of cerebroside sulfate. An effort to prevent disease progression by bone marrow transplantation appears to have succeeded.

Sudanophilic Leukodystrophy

This subset includes a heterogeneous group of diseases that have in common only the fact that extensive CSF myelin destruction occurs, associated with products of myelin breakdown, cholesterol esters that stain bright red with the usual fat stains. This staining quality distinguishes these diseases from the metachromatic leukodystrophies. These pathologic characteristics are found in aminoacidurias, adrenoleukodystrophy, and Pelizaeus-Merzbacher disease.

ADRENOLEUKODYSTROPHY. This disorder causes diffuse and multifocal dysmyelination, and adrenocortical insufficiency. The X-linked form, occurring exclusively in males, is associated with a defective gene in the Xq28 region, leading to impairment of the degradation of very long chain fatty acids. The onset occurs most often in childhood but has been reported in adults, with a progression of symptoms similar to those of metachromatic leukodystrophy. CSF protein is elevated in most patients. Endocrine testing reveals primary adrenal failure. Instances of adrenal failure alone have been reported in relatives of patients with adrenoleukodystrophy, and paraparesis has been observed in female carriers.

Pathologic examination reveals widespread changes in CNS myelin and peripheral nerve demyelination, with numerous lipid lamellar inclusions throughout the tissue. An effort to prevent disease progression by bone marrow transplantation appears to have been successful.

PELIZAEUS-MERZBACHER DISEASE. This rare leukodystrophy affects males primarily, is inherited as an X-linked recessive trait, and starts in early infancy. It progresses slowly, producing extensive, diffuse, symmetric disturbances of myelin staining associated with gliosis within the cerebrum and cerebellum. The peripheral nervous system is not affected. The underlying biochemical defect is unknown. No treatment is available.

Globoid Cell Leukodystrophy (Krabbe's Disease)

This disease affects infants in the first 2 to 3 months of life, initially producing irritability and unexplained episodes of crying, sensitivity to light and noise, and failure to achieve developmental milestones. During the second year, these children become opisthotonic, developing myoclonic jerks, atypical seizures, and optic atrophy. Rare instances occur in late infancy or in adulthood.

Neuropathologic examination reveals marked loss of myelin throughout the brain with the presence of round or oval mononuclear cells the size of large glia or as large, irregular multinucleated cells. These globoid cells contain galactocerebroside (galactosyl ceramide), which accumulates in abnormal quantities. The disorder probably is transmitted as an autosomal recessive trait. No treatment is known.

Spongy Degeneration of White Matter

Many disorders can produce the pathologic changes leading to this label, including aminoacidurias and other metabolic disturbances. Instances affecting infants in whom no underlying metabolic defect is apparent are called Canavan's disease, with spastic paraplegia, severe mental retardation, optic atrophy, enlargement of the head, and death occurring by 18 months. Spongiform degeneration is also produced by exposure to large amounts of hexachlorophene in infancy and by Creutzfeldt-Jakob disease in adults (see Ch. 478.6).

Aubourg P, Blanche S, Jambaque I, et al.: Reversal of early neurologic and neuroradiologic manifestations of X-linked adrenoleukodystrophy by bone marrow transplantation. N Engl J Med 322:1860, 1990.
Krivit W, Shapiro E, Kennedy W, et al.: Treatment of late infantile metachromatic leukodystrophy by bone marrow transplantation. N Engl J Med 322:28, 1990.
Moser HW, Moser AB, Singh I, et al.: Adrenoleucodystrophy: Survey of 303 cases, biochemistry, diagnosis and therapy. Ann Neurol 16:628, 1984.
Seitelberger F: Pelizaeus-Merzbacher's disease. In Vinken P, Bruyn G (eds.): Handbook of Clinical Neurology. Vol 10. Amsterdam, North-Holland, 1970, p 150. An excellent review of this and related degenerative diseases of myelin.

THE SYNDROME OF ACUTE TRANSVERSE MYELITIS

CLINICAL DESCRIPTION. Acute transverse myelitis or myelopathy describes the rapid onset of paraparesis or paraplegia as the result of spinal cord dysfunction. The term transverse myelitis has a slightly more specific meaning, referring to acute transverse myelopathy of unknown etiology. The onset of weakness is often preceded by abrupt or rapidly developing, localized back pain or radicular pain, often in the thoracic region. This is followed by paresthesias of the toes and feet and rapidly ascending sensory loss and weakness. Urinary and fecal incontinence is common. The speed of progression varies from minutes, as with an infarction, to steady or stepwise progression over several days, as often occurs with compression due to a tumor or as a result of MS. It is often difficult to separate the patient who has developed an idiopathic transverse myelopathy from the one who has a detectable and often treatable underlying cause. Presentation of the syndrome of acute spinal cord dysfunction demands immediate and careful consideration of the differential diagnosis so as to undertake appropriate treatment if warranted.

DIFFERENTIAL DIAGNOSIS. Table 482–5 lists disorders that produce an acute or subacute transverse myelopathy with varying degrees of frequency.

Bacterial infections of the spinal cord and its surrounding spaces are considered in Ch. 471. HTLV-I myelopathy is considered in Ch. 478.3.

Viral infection of the spinal cord occurs with direct extension by the varicella (herpes) zoster or other viruses. Alternately, spinal cord inflammation and demyelination may follow a viral infection, such as measles or other common viruses, either as an isolated phenomenon or as part of the more widespread acute disseminated encephalomyelitis.

Spinal cord compression from metastatic tumor may present acutely, even though the tumor has been present for a longer time. Centrally *herniating intervertebral discs* may lead to acute cord compression with or without local pain. In each instance, myelography is usually required for diagnosis, although CT scans or MRI may be sufficient. Trauma often leads to an acute transverse myelopathy in what is usually an obvious setting.

Rapidly progressing myelopathy in a previously healthy person should always raise the question of *spontaneous epidural, subdural, or intraparenchymal bleeding*, as may occur from an arteriovenous malformation, or as a complication of anticoagulation or blood dyscrasia. CT or MR imaging visualizes the blood. Surgical decompression is often appropriate. Other vascular

TABLE 482–5. ACUTE OR SUBACUTE TRANSVERSE MYELOPATHY

Associated with infection
　Bacterial
　Spinal epidural abscess
　Intramedullary abscess
　Viral, e.g., herpes zoster
　Postviral, e.g., rubella with disseminated encephalomyelitis

Compression
　Tumor, especially metastatic
　Trauma
　Herniated intervertebral disc

Vascular
　Acute extradural, subdural, or parenchymal hemorrhage
　Dissecting aortic aneurysm
　Arteritis
　Lupus erythematosus

Idiopathic

causes of transverse myelopathy include interruption of spinal cord blood supply by dissecting aortic aneurysm or traumatic aortic rupture. Inflammatory disorders affecting blood vessels, such as disseminated lupus erythematosus or giant cell arteritis, may produce an acute myelopathy.

Subacute myelopathy is a common manifestation of MS, either as a first clinical manifestation or in a patient with previous clinical evidence of the disorder. Motor dysfunction is usually much more prominent than sensory loss, and complete cord transection syndrome only rarely occurs. When a patient with isolated transverse myelopathy has CSF oligoclonal bands, abnormal visual or brain stem auditory evoked response values, or MRI evidence of multiple lesions, one must suspect MS. However, the probability has not yet been established, and it is not appropriate to consider that combination with a single clinical event as having established the diagnosis of MS (see Table 482–2).

In many instances, no identifiable cause of acute transverse myelopathy is found even at autopsy, although some will prove to have an occult arteriovenous malformation or unsuspected MS. The degree of acute neurologic impairment among patients with the idiopathic syndrome ranges from partial to complete; the speed of onset ranges from hours to days. Patients who progress acutely to total paralysis are less likely to improve than those whose impairments develop over several days or longer. Idiopathic acute transverse myelopathy may leave a patient paraplegic regardless of treatment or may lead to complete or nearly complete recovery, probably depending on the degree of necrosis that occurs initially.

LABORATORY AIDS. An imaging procedure is essential in the evaluation of acute transverse myelopathy. Increasingly sensitive CT and MRI techniques are beginning to replace myelography. The CSF examination is usually obtained as part of or following the appropriate imaging procedure and is often essential.

PATHOLOGY. Idiopathic acute transverse myelopathy is associated with destruction of neurons, glia, and tracts at the level involved. A range of inflammatory cells have been seen acutely. Invasion by macrophages with subsequent cord atrophy and hypertrophy, and adhesion of the meninges to the spinal cord occur and sometimes lead to spinal block. The pathology of instances secondary to known causes depends on the disorder in question.

TREATMENT. Time is of the essence. Treatment may halt progression but may not restore function already lost. Diagnostic studies must be undertaken on an emergency basis, and when cord compression is present, surgical decompression and treatment with antibiotics or with corticosteroids are needed quickly. In idiopathic transverse myelopathy, MS, or cord compression, corticosteroids may reduce edema and lead to earlier restitution of function, although the effect on long-term outcome is problematic. Treatment of specific recognized etiologies is covered elsewhere. Urinary retention must be treated symptomatically with intermittent catheterization. Fecal impaction must be prevented. Patients with cervical lesions may require ventilatory assistance.

Berman M, Feldman S, Alter M, et al.: Acute transverse myelitis: Incidence and etiological considerations. Neurology 31:966, 1981. *A retrospective study of a well-defined population.*

Ropper AH, Poskanzer DC: The prognosis of acute and subacute transverse myelopathy based on early signs and symptoms. Ann Neurol 4:51, 1978. *Reviews the experience of a large general hospital with an excellent description of the clinical findings and follow-up.*

SECTION TWELVE / THE EPILEPSIES

483 The Epilepsies
Jerome Engel, Jr.

DEFINITION AND PREVALENCE. Epilepsy is the term applied to a group of disorders, sometimes called *the epilepsies*, that are characterized by the behavioral consequences of recurrent, spontaneous, transient paroxysms of abnormal brain activity. The epileptic attack or seizure, the common denominator of all of these conditions, may appear as impaired consciousness, involuntary movement, autonomic disturbance, or psychic or sensory experiences.

Epileptic disorders most commonly begin in early childhood but can appear at any time. Approximately 0.5 per cent of the United States population suffers from active seizures. It is estimated that 1 in 10 persons will experience at least one epileptic seizure during his or her lifetime. Prevalence is greater in areas of the world that have a higher incidence of brain injury due to high rates of infection, poor perinatal care, and frequent head trauma.

PATHOGENESIS. Most investigators believe that the fundamental abnormality in all epileptic conditions lies in the cerebral cortex, including the limbic cortex (hippocampus). In chronic epilepsy, the recurrent neuronal paroxysms that underlie ictal (seizure) events are transient expressions of a more permanently physiologically disordered cortex. Even though seizures themselves are intermittent, the physiologic abnormality persists throughout the interictal (between seizures) period.

An epileptogenic cortex in the interictal state is characterized by the appearance of brief, high-amplitude electrical discharges that usually can be recorded from the scalp by *electroencephalography (EEG)*. The typical interictal EEG discharge consists of a sharp negative transient followed by a slower wave, referred to as a *spike-and-wave complex*. Studies in animals indicate that the EEG spike-and-wave complex reflects the summation of highly synchronized abnormal neuronal membrane potentials: large paroxysmal depolarization shifts followed by prolonged after-hyperpolarizations. The depolarization shift results in enhanced neuronal excitation, while the after-hyperpolarization represents inhibition that may prevent ictal development. These abnormal membrane events reflect inherent pathologic properties of individual epileptic neurons as well as disturbances in interconnections of neuronal aggregates. However, the fundamental mechanisms that underlie spontaneous recurrent seizures in the various forms of chronic human epilepsy remain unknown.

Whatever the precise mechanism, ictal symptoms in human seizures reflect the functions of the cortex from which they arise, and the symptoms may gradually progress as the local discharge spreads to adjacent areas. Propagation to distant brain areas can proceed along fiber tracts to produce additional symptoms. With widespread or bilateral involvement, consciousness becomes impaired and generalized tonic-clonic convulsions can occur. *Partial seizures* are seizures initiated in only part of the cerebral cortex. They can, but do not always, spread to involve larger areas of the brain. *Generalized seizures* are seizures that begin bilaterally from the start, presumably as a result of synchronizing afferent influences from brain stem and diencephalon acting on diffusely epileptogenic cortex or on widespread, multiple cortical epileptogenic foci. This condition has been referred to as *corticoreticular epilepsy*.

Seizures stop not merely as a result of neuronal exhaustion but also because of self-activating inhibitory mechanisms. These events can depress neuronal function after a seizure, producing prominent postictal symptoms. Generalized convulsions and partial seizures with impaired consciousness are followed by diffuse EEG suppression and periods of confusion and fatigue that can last minutes to hours. Partial seizures may also be followed by transient, localized EEG suppression and focal neurologic deficits, known as *Todd's paralysis*, that reflect postictal dysfunction of cortical structures involved in the ictal event.

ETIOLOGY. Epileptic seizures can be a natural reaction to physiologic stress or transient systemic injury (*reactive seizures*), or they can indicate an epileptic disorder. This disorder can reflect intrinsic, nonprogressive, and presumably hereditary cerebral disturbances, with seizures as the only manifestation of abnormal brain function (*primary epilepsies*), or can be symptomatic of some known pathologic process affecting the brain (*secondary epilepsies*) (Table 483–1). Several factors often exist in the same patient, and commonly the combination of a cerebral insult and a genetic predisposition determines the appearance of epileptic seizures. Systemic illness or trauma may uncover a latent epileptic condition.

Genetic Factors. Genetic factors may contribute to the development of epilepsy in three ways: (1) An individual may inherit a low threshold for seizures; (2) genetic traits underlie certain specific primary epileptic conditions; and (3) many inherited diseases of the brain are associated with structural disturbances that produce seizures.

A number of poorly understood genetic factors determine the susceptibility of individual brains to the development of generalized convulsions. Under certain circumstances a single isolated generalized convulsion can occur as a reaction to insults such as sleep deprivation, alcohol or sedative drug withdrawal, use of convulsant drugs, fever, and acute head trauma. Recurrent generalized convulsions may also be induced by reversible infectious, toxic, or metabolic processes and are limited to the period of systemic illness. Occurrence of such reactive seizures generally indicates an inherited lowered threshold for seizures and not a chronic epileptic condition. The most commonly encountered reactive seizures are the *benign febrile convulsions* of infancy and early childhood. Persons with lowered convulsive thresholds are also more likely to develop chronic recurrent seizures of all types if irreversible brain injury occurs for other reasons.

Inherited primary epilepsies account for 30 per cent of chronic epileptic disorders. Autosomal dominant genetic traits have been identified as the basis of characteristic EEG patterns that underlie the generalized *petit mal epilepsy* and partial *sylvian epilepsy*, but not all individuals with these EEG traits have seizures. Primary epilepsies are relatively benign, and most remit spontaneously in adolescence or early adulthood.

Secondary epilepsies are most often due to acquired factors; however, inherited neurologic diseases can also produce brain lesions that give rise to chronic recurrent epileptic seizures. These include inborn errors of metabolism, such as phenylketonuria and the lipoidoses; other degenerative diseases, not only those that affect gray matter, such as the progressive myoclonus epilepsies, but also the leukodystrophies; and syndromes such as tuberous sclerosis and neurofibromatosis that are associated with the development of cerebral ectopic or alien tissue.

Acquired Factors. *Congenital lesions* due to prenatal and perinatal injuries are commonly encountered in epileptic patients.

Minor focal lesions that can give rise to partial seizures include microgyria, porencephalic cysts, areas of calcification, and atrophy. More severe trauma, anoxia, and infections such as toxoplasmosis, cytomegalic inclusion disease, rubella, herpes, and syphilis also can produce diffuse cerebral damage and secondary generalized seizure disorders.

Head trauma with cicatrix formation is an important cause of epileptic seizures. Chronic recurrent seizures occur in 30 per cent of patients with acute hematomas, 15 per cent of those with depressed skull fractures, and 5 per cent of those hospitalized for severe closed head trauma. Epilepsy is rare, however, after head trauma without loss of consciousness. Seizures occurring at the time of injury (contact seizures) or within the first week thereafter do not necessarily herald development of a recurrent epileptic disorder. Chronic posttraumatic seizures usually have a delayed onset, most often beginning 6 to 12 months following injury and occasionally starting even many years later.

Infectious processes involving the brain and its coverings can produce acute and chronic seizures. As with trauma, generalized seizures during active meningitis and encephalitis may not indicate a recurrent epileptic condition. Recurrent generalized and partial seizures occur with slow virus infections and are common late sequelae when adhesions or scars result from purulent meningitis, fungal infections, or destructive viral processes such as herpes simplex encephalitis. Partial seizures may be the first sign of focal bacterial encephalitis or abscess formation, lesions especially likely to produce chronic epilepsy. Tuberculomas and parasitic infestations, particularly cysticercosis and schistosomiasis, are common causes of partial seizures in some developing countries and because of increased international travel are sometimes found outside their endemic areas.

About half of all *brain tumors* located in the anterior and middle cranial fossae produce epileptic symptoms. Partial seizures are common with *Sturge-Weber syndrome* and often result from small cryptogenic hamartomas, ectopias, and angiomas.

Cerebrovascular diseases produce seizures in many ways. Partial seizures are rare during acute strokes and usually reflect embolic events with bleeding into the cortex rather than thrombosis. Completed strokes, however, often produce scar tissue that can become epileptogenic months or years later. Such a process is presumed to be the most common cause of unexplained recurrent partial seizures in the elderly. Partial and generalized seizures are early symptoms of cerebral venous thrombosis, cerebral arteritis, and hypertensive encephalopathy (now rare). Partial seizures often occur with arteriovenous malformations (AVM's), and small cortical hemorrhages of any cause can produce refractory partial seizures or focal myoclonic jerks.

Systemic toxic and metabolic disturbances, both exogenous and endogenous, as well as *ionic imbalance*, such as hyponatremia, can cause reactive generalized convulsions, which occasionally can lead to status epilepticus with subsequent brain damage or death. Toxic or metabolic disturbances may occasionally cause partial seizures when superimposed on unsuspected focal cerebral

TABLE 483–1. CAUSES OF EPILEPSY

Type of Disorder	Genetic Factors	Acquired Factors
Reactive seizures (transient reaction to stress or insult, not epilepsy)	Lowered threshold	Physiologic stress Sleep deprivation Alcohol or sedative drug withdrawal Convulsant drugs Fever Acute head trauma Toxic, metabolic, and infectious processes
Primary epilepsy (without structural lesions, usually benign)	Genetic trait	Little or none

Secondary epilepsy (with structural lesions and associated neurologic disturbances)	Lowered threshold
	Inherited diseases associated with epilepsy:
	  Inborn errors of metabolism
	  Degenerative diseases
	  Ectopic or alien tissue
		Congenital lesion
		Head trauma
		Infections
		Cerebrovascular diseases
		Brain tumors
		Systemic toxic and metabolic disorder
		Hippocampal sclerosis
		Miscellaneous disorders

lesions from old head injuries. These occur most commonly in alcohol and drug abusers who are undergoing withdrawal. Hyperosmolar conditions such as nonketotic hyperglycemia and uremia may also give rise to partial seizures, presumably because of brain shrinkage that tears bridging vessels and produces small areas of hemorrhage into the cortex.

Miscellaneous disorders that can cause seizures include systemic diseases that give rise to cerebral pathology, such as the collagen vascular diseases and blood dyscrasias; and cerebral gray matter degenerative diseases, such as allergic encephalopathies and, very rarely, the presenile and senile dementias. Demyelinating diseases occasionally produce lesions adjacent to cortex that cause epileptic attacks: seizures occur in 3 per cent of patients with multiple sclerosis.

Hippocampal sclerosis, consisting of largely unilateral neuronal loss often accompanied by astrocytic proliferation in the hippocampus and adjacent limbic structures, is found in over half the patients who have undergone temporal lobe resection for complex partial seizures. This may be the most common pathologic finding in epilepsy and, in some cases, could be both the cause and the result of seizures. Prolonged convulsive seizures are known to produce cell loss in the hippocampus, the neocortex, and the cerebellum. Some authorities believe that prolonged convulsions (lasting more than 30 minutes), such as those that occasionally accompany fever in infancy or childhood exanthems, can produce mesial temporal sclerosis and that this lesion becomes epileptogenic later in life. In any event, this form of epileptic brain damage suggests that in some situations epilepsy itself becomes a cause of progressive symptoms. For this reason, convulsive seizures should be controlled as promply as possible.

CLINICAL MANIFESTATIONS AND CLASSIFICATION. Classification of *epileptic seizures* is based on their clinical manifestations (Table 483–2). Partial seizures are more likely than generalized seizures to be associated with a localized cerebral lesion that could represent a curable cause of epilepsy. When a treatable underlying cause is not present, the choice of antiepileptic drugs is usually determined by the seizure type. Specific *epileptic syndromes* have also been defined on the basis of seizure manifestations and other clinical features (Table 483–3). Although the pathophysiologic mechanisms are unknown for most, diagnosis of an epileptic syndrome usually has important therapeutic and prognostic implications.

Partial Seizures. Although the expression of partial seizures depends on the areas of cerebral cortex that are involved, the precise anatomic origin of specific seizures cannot always be accurately inferred from ictal symptoms, since functional localization within the brain remains inexact. Moreover, epileptic

TABLE 483–2. CLASSIFICATION OF EPILEPTIC SEIZURES*

Partial seizures (focal, local)
  Simple partial seizures
    With motor signs
    With somatosensory or special sensory symptoms
    With autonomic symptoms or signs
    With psychic symptoms
  Complex partial seizures
    Simple partial onset followed by impairment of consciousness
    With impairment of consciousness at onset
  Partial seizures evolving to generalized tonic-clonic convulsions
    (secondarily generalized)

Generalized seizures (convulsive or nonconvulsive)
  Nonconvulsive seizures
    Absence seizures
    Atypical absence seizures
    Myoclonic seizures
    Atonic seizures
  Convulsive seizures
    Tonic-clonic seizures
    Tonic seizures
    Clonic seizures

Unclassified epileptic seizures

*Modified from Commission on Classification and Terminology of the International League Against Epilepsy: Epilepsia 22:489, 1981.

TABLE 483–3. SOME DISTINCTIVE EPILEPTIC SYNDROMES

Type of Disorder	Partial	Generalized
Reactive seizures		Febrile convulsions
Primary epilepsy	Sylvian epilepsy	Petit mal epilepsies
		Juvenile myoclonic epilepsy
Secondary epilepsy	Temporal lobe epilepsy	Lennox-Gastaut syndrome
	Epilepsia partialis continua	Progressive myoclonus epilepsies
		West's syndrome

manifestations may reflect dysfunction produced by propagation away from the primary focus as much as or more than from the area where the lesion lies.

Partial seizures are classified as simple when consciousness is preserved. *Simple partial seizures* reflect an ictal discharge that is localized within one hemisphere and can take many forms (Table 483–4).

Motor symptoms begin with clonic or tonic movements of a discrete body part. Areas of the body with large representation in the motor cortex, such as the face and hand, are involved most frequently. When spread occurs in an orderly fashion along the precentral gyrus, clonic motor symptoms can progress (e.g., from thumb or face), which is termed a *jacksonian march*. More commonly, however, ictal discharges in frontal cortex activate multiple muscle groups to produce complex versive movements, such as turning of the head, eyes, or body to one side and posturing with one or more extremities. Other simple motor manifestations include speech arrest or vocalizations when language areas are involved; eye or lid twitching, which is most often initiated from the frontal or occipital cortex; and inappropriate laughter unassociated with humor (*gelastic epilepsy*). Simple partial clonic or tonic motor seizures can be followed by a transient *Todd's paralysis* of involved muscles, which rarely persists longer than 48 hours.

Sensory symptoms occur with lesions in or connected to primary sensory cortex. Thus, localized paresthesias or numbness, unformed luminous visions, unpleasant olfactory and gustatory sensations, vertigo, and sounds can result from lesions of appropriate cortical areas. Postictal negative sensory phenomena, such as blindness and anesthesia, may occasionally occur.

Autonomic symptoms often are due to ictal involvement of limbic structures in the mesial temporal and frontal lobes that project to the hypothalamus and brain stem. They commonly consist of feelings of epigastric rising or distress, nausea, or vague light-headedness. In other autonomic seizures, ictal signs and symptoms such as pallor, flushing, sweating, piloerection, pupillary dilatation, cardiac arrhythmia, and incontinence may be apparent.

TABLE 483–4. SIGNS AND SYMPTOMS OF SIMPLE PARTIAL SEIZURES

Motor
  Focal without march
  Focal with march (jacksonian)
  Versive
  Postural
  Phonatory

Sensory
  Somatosensory
  Special sensory (visual, auditory, olfactory, gustatory, vertiginous)

Autonomic
  Any autonomic sign or symptom

Psychic
  Dysphasic
  Dysmnesic (e.g., déjà vu)
  Cognitive (e.g., dreamy state)
  Affective (e.g., fear, anger)
  Illusions
  Structured delusions

Psychic symptoms can accompany ictal discharges in limbic and association cortex and can mimic features of psychiatric disorders. These include dysmnesic symptoms, such as feelings of familiarity (déjà vu) and unfamiliarity (jamais vu) and forced thinking; cognitive disturbances, such as dreamy states, depersonalization, and time distortion; affective symptoms, such as fear and rage, which often are associated with appropriate autonomic changes, depression, and, on rare occasions, elation; illusions, such as multiple images (polyopia) or distortions of size (micropsia and macropsia); and hallucinations consisting of stereotyped mixed sensory experiences, such as visions of well-formed, recognizable faces or specific scenes accompanied by voices that can be understood, familiar smells, and emotional responses. Persistent psychic symptoms in epileptic patients may also be postictal.

Simple partial seizures are usually brief and do not interfere with daily living unless they occur frequently or evolve into other types of attacks. Simple partial seizures without obvious motor manifestations may be referred to as *auras* when the patient perceives them as a warning of impending, more noticeable epileptic symptoms. Patients who complain only of simple partial seizures may report having many seizures a week or many a day, with each lasting a few seconds.

Partial seizures are classified as complex when they impair consciousness. Approximately 40 per cent of patients with epilepsy experience *complex partial seizures* with impaired consciousness ranging from amnesia for the ictal event to behavioral unresponsiveness. Complex partial seizures usually reflect bilateral ictal involvement of limbic structures, particularly the hippocampus, amygdala, and their connections. The seizure may begin with impaired consciousness from the start or evolve from a simple partial event (aura). Because complex partial seizures most often originate in mesial temporal limbic areas, autonomic auras are common. Complex partial seizures preceded by olfactory auras are called *uncinate fits.* Such attacks may be more consistently associated with brain tumors than are other types of seizures.

The term complex partial seizure is not synonymous with *temporal lobe, psychomotor,* and *limbic seizures.* These latter designations have more specific anatomic implications and may involve ictal symptoms resulting from unilateral activation of mesial temporal limbic structures without impaired consciousness. Some atypical complex partial seizures, on the other hand, may not reflect primary activation of the limbic system. The typical complex partial seizure (temporal lobe or psychomotor attack) begins with a stare at the time consciousness is impaired and purposeless movements called *automatisms.* Oroalimentary automatisms, such as chewing, swallowing, sucking, and lip smacking, are most common and presumably reflect amygdala involvement. Other examples of automatisms include verbal utterances of sounds or words; gestural movements, such as fumbling, posturing, and picking at clothing; expressions of emotion; and ambulation. Ongoing activities such as washing dishes or even driving a car may continue automatically. Patients may undress, run, respond to commands, and demonstrate a variety of complicated automatisms that indicate a residual ability to relate to the environment despite the ictal state. In some types of complex partial seizures, patients can display irregular thrashing movements of the extremities, scream, fall, or exhibit bizarre behavior that can be difficult to differentiate from hysteria.

Complex partial seizures usually last from a few seconds to a few minutes and are followed by confusion as well as amnesia for the ictal event, although most patients remember an aura. Postictal anterograde amnesia and automatisms are common, and aphasia often occurs when seizures begin in the dominant hemisphere. In cases of unusually prolonged or recurrent complex partial seizures, postictal anterograde memory disturbance can persist for hours or days.

Complex partial seizures and postictal symptoms can severely disrupt daily life. While it is not uncommon for patients to have many complex partial seizures a week and several auras a day, even one or two seizures a year may prevent them from driving a car or destroy a chosen career.

Both simple and complex partial seizures can evolve into *secondarily generalized tonic-clonic convulsions.* Most patients with partial seizures experience at least some secondarily generalized seizures, but generalization usually occurs infrequently and is more easily controlled by drugs than are partial ictal

symptoms. Some patients, particularly those with lesions in the frontal lobes, have partial seizures that always generalize secondarily. When such secondarily generalized partial seizures begin in a silent area of the brain, their partial origin may be overlooked by both the patient and observers. When neither ictal symptoms nor signs provide a clue that a seizure is secondarily generalized, postictal focal or lateralizing signs and symptoms, such as reflex asymmetry, focal weakness, or aphasia, may indicate a partial seizure disorder. Differentiation from true generalized convulsions in these cases helps to identify potentially progressive or treatable focal lesions.

Partial Syndromes. *Sylvian* or *rolandic epilepsy* (benign partial epilepsy of childhood with centrotemporal spikes) is a familial disorder that can afflict as many as 20 per cent of children with seizures. It is characterized by nocturnal generalized convulsions and simple partial seizures that occur during the day. Typically, the partial seizures begin with perioral or lingual paresthesias, although other sensory or motor symptoms may occur, especially involving the face. The EEG demonstrates centrotemporal interictal spikes that may be unilateral or bilaterally independent. Associated neurologic deficits are lacking, and the seizures respond well to medication. The disorder almost always disappears during adolescence.

Temporal lobe (psychomotor, limbic) epilepsy is the most common chronic epileptic syndrome and may account for 40 per cent of adult epilepsies. The underlying lesion characteristically involves mesial temporal limbic structures and is most often hippocampal sclerosis. The syndrome can also be caused by lesions elsewhere that produce ictal discharges that preferentially propagate to mesial temporal structures. Patients experience auras and typical complex partial seizures, as described earlier. They may also have memory deficits and psychiatric symptoms and usually exhibit unilateral or independent bilateral anterior temporal EEG spikes. Seizures in this disorder can be difficult to control medically but may be abolished by surgical resection.

Continuous partial epilepsy (epilepsia partialis continua) also is often unresponsive to medication. This disorder occurs in adults after severe cerebral injury, such as anoxia or stroke, and occasionally with brain tumors. It can also begin in young children with a rare unilateral chronic cerebral inflammatory disorder of unknown cause (*Rasmussen's syndrome*). The continuous focal motor seizures usually reflect widespread or multiple rather than single lesions that usually are not amenable to localized surgical resection. Seizures can be abolished by large resections, such as hemispherectomy, and this procedure may be indicated in some children who already have hemiatrophy and hemiparesis.

Generalized Seizures. *Absences* are brief losses of consciousness that can be of two types. Both begin almost exclusively in childhood and take the form of a blank stare, which can also be associated with mild clonic movements of eyelids and face, more generalized jerks, alterations in motor tone, and simple automatisms. *Petit mal absences* affect about 10 per cent of epileptic children, last less than 10 seconds, and begin and end abruptly without preictal or postictal EEG or clinical disturbances. *Atypical absences* also occur in about 10 per cent of epileptic children, can last longer than 10 seconds, and produce some degree of postictal confusion. Petit mal and atypical absences must not be confused with each other or with complex partial seizures consisting only of brief lapses of consciousness, since cause, prognosis, and treatment differ for the three seizure types.

Absences can occur spontaneously hundreds of times a day. Petit mal absences respond well to appropriate medications, tend to disappear during adolescence, and are rarely disabling. Atypical absences may be refractory to therapy and can disrupt normal function. Children with atypical absences, however, are usually hampered more by other seizures and by neurologic and mental deficits.

Myoclonic seizures are single, rapidly recurrent, bilaterally synchronous shock-like jerks of the face, trunk, and extremities that are not associated with loss of consciousness. In most patients with myoclonic seizures, these events cluster shortly after waking or when falling asleep. A single myoclonic jerk that occurs while a person is falling asleep, however, is a normal physiologic event. A prolonged attack can terminate in a generalized tonic-clonic convulsion. Myoclonic seizures occur in certain rare benign genetic epileptic disorders of the primary generalized type, such as *juvenile myoclonic epilepsy (impulsive petit mal)*, and respond well to drug therapy.

In contrast to myoclonic seizures, there are many other types of myoclonic jerks that are not generalized and should not be considered epileptic. These include the following: asymmetric or sporadic jerks (involving first one area of the body and then another) that are spontaneous or induced by movement or sensory stimulation and that result from anoxic, toxic, and metabolic disturbances; similar events associated with the *progressive myoclonus epilepsies*, due to lesions of the diencephalon, brain stem, and cerebellar nuclei; regular rhythmic *palatal myoclonus* and *segmental myoclonus* that are caused, respectively, by medullary and spinal cord lesions; and *benign familial (essential) myoclonus* of unknown origin.

Tonic-clonic (grand mal) convulsions occur at least once in 80 per cent of epileptic patients and can be the expression of reactive seizures, partial seizures that secondarily generalize, or a generalized epileptic disorder. Convulsions that are not secondarily generalized from partial seizures never have auras, although patients may occasionally recognize nonspecific affective changes or experience a flurry of bilaterally synchronous myoclonic jerks some hours before a seizure occurs. The typical generalized convulsion begins with a sudden cry accompanied by loss of consciousness, falling, and bilateral tonic extensor rigidity of the trunk and extremities. After several seconds of rigidity, recurrent synchronous clonic muscular contractions ensue for 1 or 2 minutes, until the seizure ends, leaving the patient flaccid and unconscious. Cyanosis results from breath-holding during the tonic phase, and autonomic hyperactivity is prominent. The blood pressure increases abruptly, the body temperature rises, and patients salivate and may have urinary and fecal incontinence. Often they bite their tongue and the inside of their mouth. Occasionally, generalized convulsive attacks consist of either tonic or clonic activity alone.

Postictal depression can last many minutes, occasionally hours, and rarely a day or more. During this period, patients gradually regain consciousness but feel exhausted, frequently complain of headache, and wish to sleep. A few remain disoriented for some time. Focal or lateralized postictal symptoms do not occur following true generalized tonic-clonic convulsions.

Grand mal convulsions rarely occur more than a few times a year in primary generalized epileptic disorders but can occur daily in severe secondary generalized disorders. In both situations, however, the attacks tend to respond well to antiepileptic drugs.

Atonic seizures (drop attacks) begin almost exclusively in childhood and usually reflect diffuse lesions of the brain. The ictal episode consists of a sudden, extremely brief loss of tone. In its simplest form, the child's head drops for a second or less. More severe forms cause tone to disappear in the entire body, leading to collapse, sometimes with serious injuries, such as concussion, broken bones, and lost teeth. Atonic seizures occur many times a day and are refractory to drug therapy but do respond to corpus callosotomy; they can be the most debilitating ictal manifestation of secondary generalized epilepsies. Brief *tonic seizures* and myoclonic jerks also cause drop attacks in this patient population.

Generalized Syndromes. One or more *febrile convulsions* occur in 3 to 4 per cent of otherwise healthy children between the ages of 6 months and 5 years and consist of brief tonic-clonic reactive generalized seizures. Although febrile convulsions can be recurrent, the syndrome is benign. It is not considered an epileptic disorder, and treatment is usually not necessary. A genetic basis is certain but poorly defined. Affected children outgrow their vulnerability between 3 and 5 years of age, although 5 per cent develop seizures without fever later. Features that would discount the diagnosis of benign febrile convulsions are the following: seizures lasting longer than 10 minutes, focal abnormalities during or after the seizure, or an abnormal neurologic or mental status examination result. In such instances, an underlying neurologic disorder is likely and treatment is required.

The *petit mal epilepsies* are inherited conditions that account for 10 per cent of childhood epilepsies. Several varieties are recognized, depending on the age of onset, frequency of EEG spike-and-wave discharges, and occurrence of myoclonic seizures. Infrequent grand mal seizures can occur in all forms, or they may occur alone. They are characterized by frequent petit mal absences in an otherwise neurologically normal child. Response to appropriate medication is usually excellent, especially when onset is in early childhood. These disorders often remit in adolescence; juvenile-onset or myoclonic seizures tend to worsen the prognosis.

Juvenile myoclonic epilepsy is another common inherited epileptic condition. It begins in middle to late childhood with bilaterally synchronous myoclonic seizures. The paroxysms can be completely controlled with appropriate medication, and there are no other associated disturbances. The condition should not be confused with the myoclonic disorders characterized by sporadic, often stimulus-sensitive, myoclonic jerks, such as postanoxic myoclonus and the progressive myoclonus epilepsies. These last-mentioned sporadic myoclonic events are not epileptic, are extremely difficult to treat, and are usually associated with other evidence of diffuse cerebral injury.

The *Lennox-Gastaut syndrome* describes a nonspecific epileptic condition of children suffering from diffuse or multiple lesions of the brain. Although patients with the Lennox-Gastaut syndrome can have absences, convulsions, and myoclonic jerks identical to the primary generalized type, usually they also have or develop additional neurologic impairment, mental subnormality, and multiple seizure types, including drop attacks. Seizures associated with the Lennox-Gastaut syndrome and other secondary generalized epileptic disorders are difficult to control. The patients often are severely handicapped by the frequent attacks as well as other static or progressive interictal neurologic deficits.

The *progressive myoclonus epilepsies* constitute a group of familial cerebral degenerative disorders that affect both cortical and subcortical gray matter, leading to progressive neurologic deficits, dementia, sporadic multifocal myoclonic jerks, and secondary tonic-clonic convulsions. Whereas the epileptic seizures respond well to medication, patients are severely disabled by the nonepileptic sporadic myoclonus and other handicaps. The course may be rapid, with severe neurologic and mental impairment (*Lafora type*); intermediate (*Unverricht-Lundborg type*); or relatively slow, with little mental impairment or EEG disturbance (*Ramsay Hunt syndrome*, which is associated with cerebellar disturbances and may be considered a separate entity). A benign familial myoclonic syndrome (*essential myoclonus*) without epileptic seizures has an excellent prognosis and responds readily to treatment.

Unclassified Seizures. Certain *neonatal seizures* and *infantile spasms* (seen in *West's syndrome*) reflect severe diffuse disturbances of brain function from a variety of causes. These events are age dependent and have not been adequately classified as epilepsy, and some may be of subcortical origin. It is important to note here only that the underlying cerebral dysfunction often results in chronic secondary epileptic conditions later in life, usually the *Lennox-Gastaut syndrome*.

Patterns of Seizure Occurrence. Appreciation for precipitating factors and temporal patterns of certain epileptic seizures can influence approaches to management. In some of the primary generalized epileptic disorders, seizures may be induced by specific sensory stimuli, most commonly flashing light (*photosensitive epilepsy*). Reading, video games, music, and other specific complex stimuli may activate seizures in patients with rarer forms of primary and secondary *reflex epilepsy*. The seizures themselves range from brief absences through synchronous myoclonic jerking to partial seizures and occasional generalized convulsions. *Hyperventilation* is a potent activator of petit mal absence seizures and sometimes will precipitate other types of ictal events as well. Emotional stress, drowsiness, sleep deprivation, and withdrawal from alcohol and sedative drugs are well-established precipitants of partial and generalized convulsive seizures in patients with chronic epilepsy. Some patients have seizures that occur only at night or only during the day. Others exhibit regular cycles of seizures over days or months or patterns of seizure clusters followed by prolonged seizure-free periods. The term *catamenial epilepsy* is used when seizures regularly recur in women around the menstrual period. Women with all forms of epileptic disorders commonly experience more frequent seizures at this time of the month, and seizures may worsen or disappear during pregnancy. *Status epilepticus* refers to a condition of rapidly recurrent epileptic seizures or continuous ictal symptoms. The latter occur with continuous partial epilepsy and also in a form of *absence status (spike wave stupor)*, which is discussed further on. Of the rapidly recurrent forms, generalized convulsive status epilepticus is a life-threatening situation demanding immediate treatment, and complex partial status epilepticus requires prompt intervention.

Complex partial status epilepticus is a rare condition of rapidly recurring seizures characterized by a fluctuating level of consciousness, automatic behavior, and ictal EEG discharges recorded over the temporal lobe. The condition may be confused clinically with a psychosis or metabolic disturbance and must be included in the differential diagnosis of altered states of consciousness; failure to treat it promptly can be followed by prolonged memory deficits.

Absence status, or *spike wave stupor*, consists of a continuous state of dulled mentation, which is often of a subtle nature. Eye blinking and other associated movements can occur, and there is a characteristic EEG pattern of diffuse spike-and-wave discharges. The condition occurs fairly often in patients with atypical absences and is also seen with a juvenile form of primary generalized petit mal epilepsy. A rare type of absence status of unknown cause also affects older adults with no previous history of epilepsy. Absence status is not a medical emergency, since no secondary brain damage occurs. The benign and adult forms respond well to antiepileptic drugs, but atypical absence status associated with diffuse lesions of the brain may be extremely difficult to control.

Major motor status epilepticus exists when generalized tonic-clonic convulsions recur so frequently that consciousness is not regained between them. This condition can occur with the generalized disorders but is more commonly a result of partial seizures that secondarily generalize. In the latter instance, the partial onset often is not recognized because of the severity of the attacks. Toxic and metabolic disturbances, including drug and alcohol withdrawal, can precipitate major motor status epilepticus in epileptic patients as well as in nonepileptic individuals with genetically low seizure thresholds. Major motor status epilepticus can also be a presenting symptom of acute intracranial hemorrhage and infections, as well as brain tumors and other focal processes, especially in the frontal lobes. Major motor status epilepticus is a life-threatening situation demanding immediate treatment.

DIAGNOSIS. Diagnosis in epilepsy involves searching for treatable causes when possible and recognizing epileptic conditions that indicate a specific prognosis and therapy. When a treatable cause of epilepsy is not revealed, management of the seizures is determined by correct diagnosis of the type of epileptic disorder.

History. The history is overwhelmingly important. The patient's description of any auras should be recorded as well as the ictal behavioral changes observed by others. The occurrence of an aura or any focal signs at onset, during progression, or in the postictal period indicates a partial rather than a generalized seizure disorder. If more than one type of seizure occurs, each should be described separately. Often patients will report several seizure types, which after careful questioning are revealed to be variations of the same ictal phenomenon and not evidence of multiple lesions. For instance, when auras are not followed by further symptoms, they may be recognized as one event, while the same aura that spreads to become a complex partial seizure may be reported as another phenomenon. If on occasion there is evolution to a secondarily generalized seizure without postictal recall of the aura, a careful description of the initial ictal events by an observer will often verify that the generalized convulsion is a manifestation of the same epileptogenic lesion. When patients report only seizures that are generalized from the start, an attempt should be made to determine whether convulsive and nonconvulsive ictal manifestations resemble those of benign genetic disorders, generalized disorders caused by diffuse or multiple brain lesions, or secondarily generalized partial seizures caused by a focal lesion. Clues to differential diagnosis derive from the circumstances and age of the patient at onset of seizures and how they may have changed with time or treatment. If the patient has been treated previously, it is important to know what drugs have been used and the specifics of their therapeutic and toxic effects.

The history can provide crucial etiologic information. In children, patterns of early development may delineate the difference between a progressive degenerative disorder and a static lesion. There may be evidence of specific predisposing factors, such as perinatal injury, intracranial infections, or reactions to immunizations. A history of a prolonged childhood convulsion preceding the onset of complex partial seizures raises the possibility that hippocampal sclerosis is the cause of the subsequent chronic epileptic disorder. In older patients there may be hints of cerebrovascular disease or metastatic cancer. Prior head trauma is usually relevant only if it resulted in loss of consciousness. A specific injurious event, such as a fall, may be mistakenly interpreted as having generated traumatic epilepsy when it actually represented the first seizure.

The family history can reveal important genetic factors. The existence of relatives with similar seizures or other neurologic symptoms suggests a specific primary epileptic disorder. A family history of individuals with isolated seizures or varied epileptic conditions may indicate the inheritance of a lowered threshold for seizures.

The psychosocial history can give important clues to diagnosis and indicate the need for more specific evaluations. Patients with benign inherited epileptic disorders usually have normal school and work histories and no evidence of mental disturbance. A history of specific cognitive deficits suggests a focal lesion, while more generalized mental impairment suggests a diffuse abnormality. When the latter is progressive, more detailed laboratory, EEG, and psychometric examinations can determine whether the patient has an underlying degenerative disease, increasing dysfunction because of recurrent seizures, or toxic symptoms of overmedication.

Physical Examination. A careful physical examination can reveal evidence of systemic diseases responsible for seizures as well as stigmata of tuberous sclerosis, neurofibromatosis, hemangiomas, and other predisposing congenital disorders. Asymmetry (hemiatrophy) in the size of hands, feet, and face may indicate a longstanding abnormality in one cerebral hemisphere. Clumsiness, posturing, and hyperreflexia or a more marked diffuse impairment suggests a secondary rather than a primary generalized seizure disorder. Focal neurologic and mental status disturbances support a diagnosis of partial epilepsy. Poor attention span in patients on drug therapy may indicate side effects of medication rather than structural lesions. Increasing degrees of fixed neurologic and mental impairment confer a poor prognosis for both seizure control and psychosocial adaptation.

Many patients can be observed during a seizure. Status epilepticus usually lasts until hospitalization, absences can be provoked by hyperventilation, reflex seizures are easily induced (it is unwise to attempt to induce tonic-clonic convulsions), and spontaneous seizures may occur in the examining room. The initial manifestations and early development should be noted. Consciousness should be assessed by repeating a phrase to determine whether the patient can recall it after the seizure is over. Even if the seizure appears to be generalized at the start, postictal examination of neurologic and mental status may reveal focal deficits that indicate that a partial seizure has occurred.

Laboratory Studies. Epilepsy provides no diagnostic hematologic or chemical laboratory tracers, but such tests can help to diagnose underlying disease processes that give rise to seizures. One or more generalized epileptic attacks can mildly increase protein content and white cell count in the cerebrospinal fluid for 24 to 48 hours. Although up to 100 white cells per cubic millimeter have been reported after major motor status epilepticus, a lumbar puncture revealing more than 10 white cells per cubic millimeter should initiate a search for an intracranial inflammatory process. Complete blood count, liver function tests, blood urea nitrogen, and urinalysis are necessary in all patients about to begin antiepileptic drug therapy to establish a baseline for evaluating possible subsequent toxic side effects.

Structural Imaging. Magnetic resonance imaging (MRI) is preferred to x-ray computed tomography (XCT) unless a disorder associated with small calcified lesions is suspected. Structural imaging is necessary for adolescents and adults with the recent onset of seizures but may be avoided in younger children when history and other examinations indicate a primary generalized disorder or a nonprogressive lesion. Cerebral angiography should

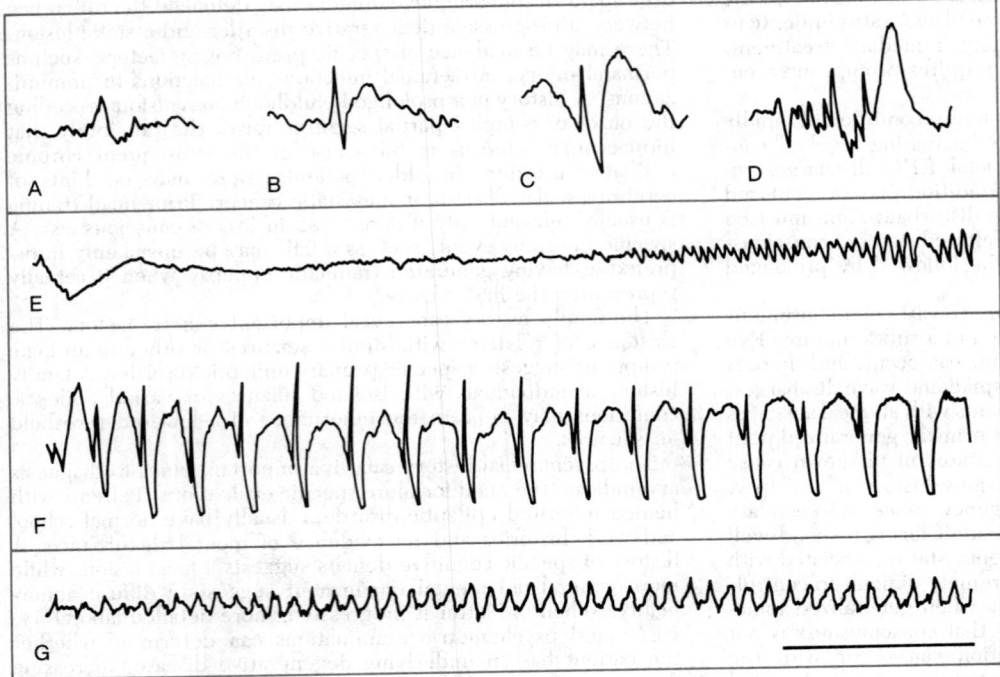

FIGURE 483–1. Examples illustrate waveforms of typical interictal electro-encephalographic (EEG) transients and ictal EEG discharges. *A*, Interictal sharp wave. *B*, *C*, Interictal spike-and-wave complexes. *D*, Interictal poly-spike-and-wave complex. *E*, Recruiting rhythm typical of generalized convulsion onsets. *F*, Repetitive spike-and-wave discharges typical of absence seizures. *G*, Rhythmic pattern seen with temporal lobe seizures. Line at the bottom right of the figure represents 1 second.

be confined to cases in which surgery is considered or a primary vascular disorder is suspected.

Psychometric Studies. Psychometric testing, including standard tests of attention, performance and verbal IQ, memory, language, and personality, can help verify the existence of a focal or diffuse brain disturbance. When there is concern that mental function is changing, serial testing can document the effects of disease or therapy. An astute psychometrician should also be able to offer advice for improving psychosocial adaptation.

Electroencephalography. The EEG is the most useful diagnostic laboratory test for epilepsy. However, overinterpretation of the EEG often generates an unwarranted diagnosis of epilepsy. A number of spike-like EEG events can be normal, and 2 per cent of the nonepileptic population may have abnormal, epileptiform spike-and-wave complexes on their EEG's but never develop seizures. Conversely, 20 per cent of patients with epilepsy do not demonstrate epileptic abnormalities on a routine interictal EEG. Whereas an EEG can help verify a clinical diagnosis of epilepsy, interictal epileptiform EEG abnormalities alone should be considered neither necessary nor sufficient information for arriving at this diagnosis. If a seizure occurs in the EEG laboratory, the association of an ictal EEG pattern with observed clinical behavior makes possible a definitive diagnosis.

The pattern of interictal EEG abnormalities may help determine the type of epileptic disorder (Figs. 483–1 and 483–2). Focal spike-and-wave discharges or slow waves indicate a partial

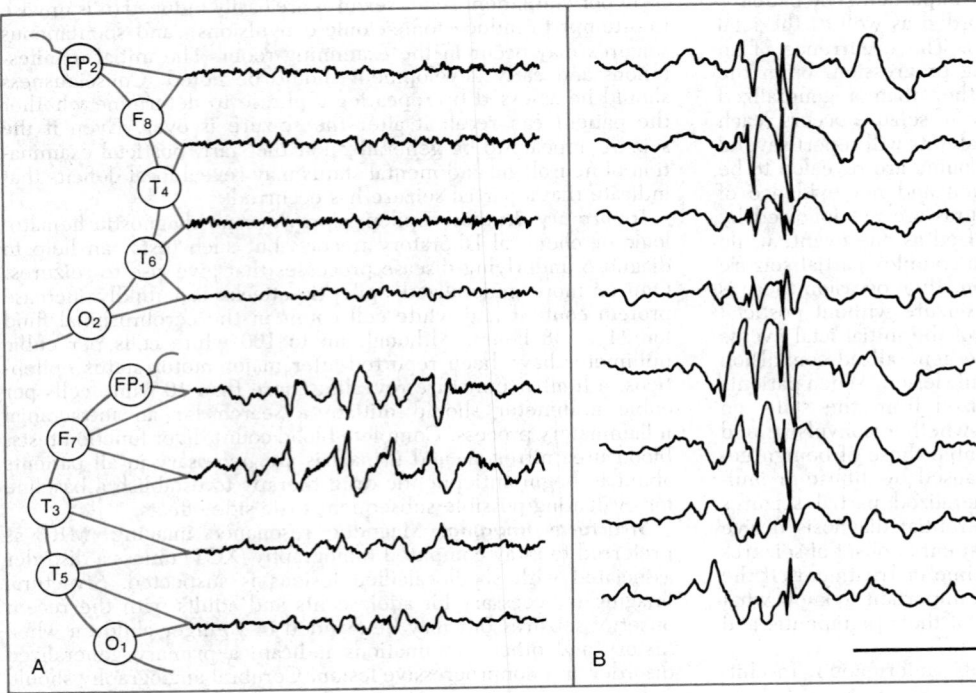

FIGURE 483–2. Examples illustrate the spatial distribution of typical focal (*A*) and generalized (*B*) epileptiform EEG discharges. *A*, Left anterior temporal spikes, sharp waves, and slowing. *B*, Generalized, frontally predominant, spike-and-wave burst. Line at the bottom right of the figure represents 1 second.

epileptic disorder. A diagnosis of benign sylvian epilepsy can be confirmed by the occurrence of characteristic centrotemporal spikes. While bilaterally synchronous EEG discharges can be seen with focal lesions (*secondary bilateral synchrony*), especially in the frontal lobes, such activity more often indicates a generalized epileptic disorder. Baseline nonepileptiform EEG abnormalities suggest a secondary epileptic disorder, although antiepileptic drugs can produce mild, diffuse EEG slowing.

Typical petit mal absences are associated with symmetric, synchronous, and regular *three-per-second* (or faster) *spike-and-wave* discharges that begin and end abruptly without postictal EEG changes. This EEG pattern is usually easily distinguished from the *slow and irregular spike-and-wave* discharges (2.5 per second or less) seen in the Lennox-Gastaut syndrome.

Activation procedures used in the EEG laboratory include hyperventilation for absences, photic stimulation for photosensitive epilepsy, and sleep. But there are major pitfalls: Hyperventilation in children and some normal adults can induce high-amplitude slowing resembling spike-and-wave discharges; photomyogenic responses of facial muscles to photic stimulation can occur in normal individuals and during drug and alcohol withdrawal and should not be considered evidence of epilepsy; a number of normal sharp transients that occur during sleep and on arousal often are misinterpreted as epileptic spikes.

Nonstandard techniques, available in some laboratories, may offer additional diagnostic advantages. Recordings from sphenoidal electrodes can clarify interictal EEG spike patterns originating in mesial temporal structures, but the same information often can be obtained more easily from ear lobe or lower temporal scalp electrodes. Special epilepsy centers throughout the country offer prolonged EEG telemetry and television monitoring to provide a precise electroclinical description of habitual seizures when diagnosis is in doubt. Ambulatory EEG monitoring is also useful, particularly to quantify ictal events that have already been characterized.

A repeat EEG may be indicated to determine whether behavioral deterioration is due to an increase in subclinical seizure activity, an increase in drug side effects, or a progressive underlying lesion. If necessary, long-term EEG recordings combined with frequent antiepileptic drug level determinations can improve medical management by allowing dose schedules to be tailored to individual patients' needs.

DIFFERENTIAL DIAGNOSIS. The diagnosis of epilepsy should be made only on firm clinical evidence. Such a diagnosis can have irreversible psychosocial effects resulting in the loss of a driver's license, a job, independence, and self-esteem. Consequently, a physician often does more harm by making an unjustified diagnosis than by reserving judgment until the nature of the disorder has declared itself adequately. When doubt exists, injury can be minimized by warning the patient to avoid the conditions that might have precipitated the event and to be aware of potentially dangerous situations, should another event occur. Systemic, neurologic, and behavioral disturbances can give rise to episodic events that might be mistaken for epileptic seizures (Table 483–5).

Systemic Disturbances. *Syncope* is the most common systemic disturbance confused with epilepsy (Ch. 443). Syncope can be associated with convulsive movements in susceptible individuals (*convulsive syncope*) but should still be treated as syncope, not as epilepsy. Because cardiogenic syncope can cause a convulsion, while seizures may be associated with cardiac arrhythmias, diagnostic monitoring in at-risk patients with blackout spells should ideally include both electrocardiographic (ECG) and EEG recordings.

Neurologic Disturbances. Transient ischemic attacks must be considered when intermittent neurologic symptoms occur in older patients. Prodromal migraine symptoms, particularly with basilar migraine, can resemble symptoms of epileptic seizures, and the distinction between migraine and epilepsy is not always completely clear. All-night polysomnography may be necessary to distinguish dyssomnias from nocturnal epileptic events. Although some forms of paroxysmal dyskinesia can be successfully treated with antiepileptic medication, they are not epileptic disorders.

Behavioral Disturbances. *Psychogenic seizures* (sometimes referred to as *pseudoseizures*) may be manifested in ways that have psychological significance. They may consist of pelvic thrusting and alternate thrashing of the limbs or may involve motor symptoms that do not fit with known anatomic spread patterns but they only rarely result in injury to the patient, despite risk. Nevertheless, it is usually impossible to make this diagnosis definitively from a description or even from observation of the seizure. Virtually any paroxysmal behavior, no matter how bizarre, could be an epileptic event. The diagnosis of psychogenic seizures can be made with some confidence, however, when ictal events are suggestive for the reasons just stated, EEG recordings are normal, antiepileptic medication is ineffective, and evidence of secondary gain is obtained during psychiatric interview. EEG telemetry and video monitoring of ictal events can help in this differential diagnosis. Clear EEG changes or an elevated postictal serum prolactin level can confirm the occurrence of an epileptic convulsion, but their absence does not necessarily rule out this possibility; simple partial ictal events usually have no EEG correlates that can be recorded from the scalp and only rarely elevate the serum prolactin level. Repeated bilaterally synchronous myoclonic jerks unassociated with loss of consciousness can be mistaken for psychogenic events. Even if a definite diagnosis of a psychogenic seizure disorder can be made, many such patients have epileptic seizures as well. When psychogenic seizures and epileptic seizures coexist, EEG and video monitoring can help to differentiate the two types and provide a basis for independently assessing the results of psychiatric and medical treatment.

Episodic dyscontrol is a poorly defined entity consisting of intermittent periods of inappropriately violent, occasionally destructive behavior. Confusion with epilepsy is compounded by the fact that some patients with this syndrome have epileptic seizures as well. If the episodic behavior lasts only several minutes, is uncharacteristic of the patient's interictal personality, and there is amnesia for the event with appropriate remorse afterward, this could conceivably reflect an epileptic disturbance. Although ictal EEG recordings have not supported this contention, an occasional patient with episodic dyscontrol may be helped by antiepileptic medication. Organized and directed violence is not seen during the epileptic seizures described earlier, and epilepsy is never the cause of premeditated criminal acts.

TABLE 483–5. NONEPILEPTIC EPISODIC DISORDERS

Systemic
Syncope
Breath-holding spells
Hyperventilation syndrome
Alcoholic blackouts
Intermittent porphyria
Hypoglycemia
Pheochromocytoma
Tetanus
Psychomimetic drugs

Neurologic
Trasient ischemic attacks
Vertebral basilar insufficiency
Transient global amnesia
Migraine
Narcolepsy
Hypersomnia (e.g., Kleine-Levin syndrome, sleep apnea)
Dyssomnias (e.g., sleep walking, bed wetting, night terrors)
Paroxysmal vertigo
Trigeminal neuralgia
Gilles de la Tourette's syndrome
Extrapyramidal disorders (e.g., hemiballism, chorea, athetosis)
Paroxysmal dyskinesias
Hemifacial spasms
Startle disease (hyperekplexia)
Myoclonic disorders

Behavioral
Psychogenic seizures
Attentional deficits
Episodic dyscontrol
Obsessive-compulsive behavior
Dissociative states (e.g., psychogenic fugue)
Panic attacks
Schizophrenia

TABLE 483–6. PHARMACOLOGIC DATA FOR THE COMMONLY USED ANTIEPILEPTIC DRUGS
(ORAL ADMINISTRATION)

Drug	Seizure Type	Adult Dose (mg/kg/d)	Therapeutic Range (µg/ml)	Half-life (hr)	Peak Time (hr)	Daily Doses
Carbamazepine (Tegretol)	P, GC	15–25	8–12	12	2–6	4
Phenytoin (Dilantin)	P, GC	3–8	10–30	24	3–12	2
Primidone (Mysoline)†	P, GC	10–20	5–15	12	2–4	4
Phenobarbital	P, GC	2–4	15–40	96	6–18	1
Clorazepate (Tranxene)	P, GC	0.7–1.0	1–2*	30*	1*	2
Ethosuximide (Zarontin)	A	10–30	40–100	40	2–3	2
Clonazepam (Klonopin)	A, M	0.03–0.3	0.01–0.05	30	1–2	2
Methsuximide (Celontin)	P, A	10–25	20–40*	40*	<3	2
Valproate (Depakene)	All	15–60	50–100	14	1–4	4
Divalproex sodium (Depakote)	All	15–60	50–100	14	3–5	4

*For derived metabolite.
†Substantial antiepileptic effect is also obtained from derived phenobarbital.
P = partial; GC = generalized convulsive; A = absence; M = myoclonus.
Modified with permission from Engel J Jr: Seizures and Epilepsy. Philadelphia, F.A. Davis, 1989.

Some epileptic symptoms can be confused with behavioral disturbances. Frequently occurring absences in children can be mistaken for attentional deficits, learning disabilities, and disciplinary problems, but the EEG should provide the correct diagnosis. Certain simple partial seizures with sensory or psychic symptoms may be interpreted as schizophrenic hallucinations. Epileptic hallucinations usually are more stereotyped and more likely to have visual components than are psychotic hallucinations. Rarely, dissociative states may represent continuous epileptic seizures or prolonged periods of postictal confusion.

TREATMENT. Treatable causes of epileptic seizures include intracerebral lesions that can be surgically removed and toxic, metabolic, infectious, and vascular diseases that require medical management. A treatable cause cannot be found in most patients with chronic recurrent seizures, however, and the objective of therapy is then to maximize useful function, ideally by complete eradication of seizures without introduction of unwanted side effects. Adequate control is usually possible with appropriate pharmacologic, surgical, and psychosocial management. However, only half of patients treated for chronic epilepsy can expect to become seizure free indefinitely.

Pharmacologic Therapy. Although many antiepileptic drugs are available, it is prudent to become familiar with and use the few that are most effective for each of the various seizure types (Table 483–6). Pharmacologic therapy is based on obtaining an accurate diagnosis of seizure type or epileptic syndrome, selecting the single most appropriate drug for that diagnosis (monotherapy), and correlating measurements of drug levels in the serum with patient reports to adjust dosages and dose schedules for the best control and fewest side effects. The best control does not necessarily mean the greatest reduction in seizure frequency. In certain patients, the disability caused by some continued seizures may be less than limitations induced by therapy. For example, the occurrence of a few absences a day for a child is preferable to an alternative of no seizures on a dose of medication that produces continuous sedation and impairs school performance. Similarly, aggressive therapy is not justified for a patient with refractory epilepsy when high drug levels exacerbate existing physical and mental handicaps without producing a worthwhile improvement in the seizure pattern.

Pharmocokinetic Principles. Dose planning for individual antiepileptic drugs depends on pharmacokinetic factors that determine the amount of available drug in the blood. The therapeutic ranges for individual antiepileptic drugs refer to the ranges of steady-state levels of each drug that by trial and error have been most effective in controlling seizures with minimal or no side effects. Average or approximate pharmacokinetic variables for the commonly used antiepileptic drugs appear in Table 483–6.

The proper dose schedule for a newly introduced drug depends on balancing the need for rapid control of seizures against the avoidance of side effects. If a patient has been warned about the possible occurrence of another seizure and takes appropriate precautions, it usually is not necessary to build a drug level rapidly at the risk of producing severe toxicity. It is more important that the patient accept the drug of first choice. Patients

can be encouraged to remain on medication by beginning a drug regimen slowly, taking the medication with meals when nausea is anticipated, using higher doses at bedtime when sedation is anticipated, and reducing doses transiently when untoward side effects occur. Most unpleasant dose-related side effects are temporary, and an appropriate regimen eventually can be instituted. A loading dose can be given practically for some drugs (phenytoin and phenobarbital) when the risk of repeated seizures requires therapeutic levels to be achieved rapidly despite side effects. A loading dose of 1.5 (rather than 2) times the calculated total daily dose may be an adequate compromise between obtaining rapid seizure control and producing minimal side effects if the planned maintenance schedule is begun less than one half-life after the loading dose.

Although a maintenance steady-state level of a drug can be achieved with an interdose interval of approximately one half-life time, in this situation drug levels will fall below the protective range if a single dose is missed. However, a dose schedule that requires a drug to be taken too frequently may be inconvenient and reduce compliance. An interdose interval of 0.5 half-life, which amounts to one to four times a day for the commonly used medications, is usually recommended. Failure to achieve a therapeutic drug level using recommended dose schedules most commonly reflects noncompliance by the patient but also may result from aberrant absorption and metabolism, and dose schedules must then be determined individually from measurements of serum drug levels.

The recommended therapeutic range for a given drug is based on average measures. One should use these values as a guide rather than a goal; therapeutic drug levels in individual patients may be well above or below the average. Once an effective maintenance schedule has been achieved, determinations of serum drug levels, always drawn at the same time after a given dose, provide a reliable long-term record of steady-state conditions. Such measurements are useful when recurrent seizures or side effects result from decreases or increases in available drug (Table 483–7).

Enzyme Induction and Inhibition. Enzyme induction by the

TABLE 483–7. INDICATIONS FOR SERUM ANTIEPILEPTIC DRUG LEVELS

To establish individual therapeutic range
  Initiation of treatment while seizures remain uncontrolled

To identify altered pharmacokinetics
  Loss of seizure control or appearance of toxic symptoms
  Addition of second antiepileptic drug or change in drug regimen
  Questionable change in drug efficacy during:
    Intercurrent illness
    Multiple drug therapy
    Altered physiologic state, such as pregnancy or puberty
  Unexplained behavioral or neurologic symptoms that might be evidence of toxicity

To document compliance

liver is a common reason for the late appearance of subtherapeutic serum drug levels after an effective maintenance schedule has been achieved. If seizures recur following a period of control, owing to enzyme induction, the dose of the initial anticonvulsant should be increased gradually to the desired blood level or to toxicity rather than immediately adding a new drug. The latter may merely enhance enzyme induction and further decrease serum drug levels. Addition of a second drug can also inhibit liver enzymes and cause toxic effects owing to increased levels of the first drug. If it is necessary to add a second anticonvulsant, serum levels of both agents require checking to ensure that adequate but not toxic levels of both have been attained. In general, if the first drug recommended for treatment has no effect on seizure control despite adequate serum levels or achieves control only at the expense of severe toxicity, it is best to replace it with a second drug. Gradual withdrawal of the first drug may induce a temporary exacerbation of seizure frequency, which does not necessarily indicate that the second drug is ineffective. Occasionally, the use of more than one drug becomes unavoidable, particularly when patients have more than one type of seizure.

Selection of Antiepileptic Drugs. Preferred Agents. While specific types of seizures respond to specific drugs (Table 483–8), many factors determine the choice of the best single drug for an individual patient. The trend today is to treat generalized convulsive and partial seizures first with either carbamazepine or phenytoin. While both drugs offer the same protection, phenytoin use is associated with a high incidence of disturbing cosmetic side effects.

Primidone and phenobarbital are also used for convulsive and partial seizures. They are less effective than carbamazepine and phenytoin, but phenobarbital is the least expensive of the available antiepileptic drugs and has the fewest dangerous side effects. Sedation is common but may not be a problem at lower doses and may subside over time even at higher doses. Furthermore, both carbamazepine and phenytoin can dull mentation at high doses. Phenobarbital commonly causes hyperkinetic activity and other undesirable behavioral disturbances in children. Most epileptologists now generally prefer carbamazepine for this age group. Phenobarbital should not be given to patients with depressive tendencies. It can exacerbate psychological depression and is the most common instrument of suicide in the epileptic population.

Valproate suppresses generalized seizures and is also occasionally effective against partial seizures as well. Consequently, the drug may be used to treat generalized convulsions even when they secondarily generalize from a partial seizure. Although valproate has few sedative and adverse cognitive side effects compared with other antiepileptic drugs and does not produce the cosmetic side effects associated with phenytoin, it has been associated with serious idiosyncratic hepatotoxicity. Most fatal hepatic dysfunction, however, has been encountered in small children on multiple drugs and is not a realistic concern in patients over the age of 10 who are on monotherapy. The enteric-coated form (divalproex sodium) is usually preferred to reduce the incidence of gastrointestinal side effects. Valproate increases serum levels of barbiturates, which can result in inadvertent sedation or even coma.

Ethosuximide and valproate are the drugs of choice for absence seizures. Since valproate is effective against generalized convul-

TABLE 483–8. THERAPEUTIC CLASSIFICATION OF EPILEPTIC SEIZURES

Seizure Type	Preferred Drugs
Partial seizures and generalized convulsions	Carbamazepine
	Phenytoin
	Phenobarbital
	Primidone
	Valproate
Absences	Ethosuximide
	Valproate
	Clonazepam
Myoclonus	Clonazepam
	Valproate

sions, it is used when absences and generalized convulsions coexist. It is also recommended by many in disorders such as petit mal epilepsy in which generalized convulsions might occur, even if they have not appeared by the time therapy is instituted. Valproate is the drug of choice for mixed seizure disorders and for juvenile myoclonic epilepsy because of its broad spectrum of action. It is also widely used for other types of generalized seizures.

The drugs of choice for nonepileptic forms of myoclonus are the benzodiazepine clonazepam, and valproate. Benzodiazepines tend to lose their effectiveness with time as tolerance develops. In progressive myoclonus epilepsy, in which myoclonic jerks and seizures are both present, valproate may be the best hope for control with monotherapy. If this is unsuccessful, clonazepam plus carbamazepine or phenytoin may be required. Clonazepam and valproate given together may interact to make seizures worse and produce unpleasant side effects.

If epileptic seizures do not respond to first-line antiepileptic medications, patients should be referred to specialized epilepsy centers for management. Additional medications that might be effective as primary epileptic drugs, or as adjunctive therapy, include clorazepate for partial and convulsive seizures, clonazepam for absences, and methsuximide for absence, atonic, and partial seizures. Acetazolamide can be a useful adjunctive medication when given from 10 days premenstrually through the end of menses to ameliorate catamenial accentuation of seizures.

Side Effects. Almost all antiepileptic drugs potentially produce undesirable side effects, and physicians should consult the *Physicians' Desk Reference* or a current textbook before first use. Common dose-related side effects of carbamazepine and the hydantoins include nausea, dizziness, diplopia, and ataxia. Sedation, impaired mentation, and hyperactivity occur most often with the barbiturates and benzodiazepines. These symptoms may abate with time. Drug-induced folic acid deficiencies may reach symptomatic levels in some patients and require vitamin supplements. Idiosyncratic side effects that usually affect skin, blood, liver, and kidneys are potentially more serious. When a new drug is introduced, complete blood counts and appropriate blood chemistry analyses should be obtained every 4 weeks for several months and then monitored every 3 to 12 months as long as therapy continues. Leukopenia with counts as low as 3000 per cubic millimeter with carbamazepine does not necessarily indicate impending agranulocytosis, but a neutrophil count of less than 1000 per cubic millimeter is cause for concern. Serum alkaline phosphatase levels are often elevated with antiepileptic drug use, but this finding alone does not indicate a hepatotoxic reaction. Mild pruritus may be treated medically. Evidence of blood dyscrasias, liver or kidney damage, or more serious skin rash requires prompt discontinuation of medication and referral to the proper specialist. Cosmetic side effects commonly associated with phenytoin include hirsutism, gingival hyperplasia, and coarsening of features; weight gain and alopecia are occasionally seen with valproate therapy. Carbamazepine can cause water retention and is not used for patients at risk for congestive heart failure. A paradoxical increase in seizure frequency may result from elevated drug levels, particularly with phenytoin, and can cause seizures to recur after a period of control.

Special Considerations. *Pregnancy* presents particular problems for women with epilepsy. Serum drug levels can fall as a result of noncompliance and increased elimination, so frequent drug level determinations are recommended. A decreased serum drug level need not be corrected, however, unless it is accompanied by an exacerbation of seizures. First-time convulsions in the third trimester usually indicate eclampsia. If required, short-term administration of appropriate antiepileptic agents poses little or no risk to the fetus at this point and should be used instead of the still common practice of therapy with magnesium sulfate. The risk of major and minor malformations in children born of mothers on antiepileptic medication is approximately twice that of untreated epileptic mothers, but this difference may be due to the severity of the disorder as well as to the teratogenic effects of these drugs. Valproate is believed to produce neural tube defects, and a teratogenic effect of trimethadione has also been well established; consequently, they are not recommended during the first trimester of pregnancy. Polypharmacy and unnecessarily high drug levels also increase the potential for problems during this period. Otherwise, there is no evidence that one antiepileptic medication is any worse than another during pregnancy. There is little to be gained from discontinuing effective medication once pregnancy has been determined, especially after the first trimester has been completed. The risk to mother and fetus from seizures may be greater than the risk from drugs. Hemorrhagic disease of the newborn occurs with the mother's use of phenobarbital and phenytoin and can be treated with vitamin K. Maternal drug levels can cause sedation and withdrawal in the newborn, but only rarely do they present a problem for breastfed infants.

Age is a factor that must be taken into account when planning pharmacotherapy. The rate of metabolism is slower, renal clearance is decreased, and protein binding is less in neonates and the elderly than in children and adults. Consequently, the half-life of drugs is longer and the percentage of free drug is greater for a given serum concentration at the extremes of age. In children, however, the metabolic rate is higher than in adults, and the half-life of drugs may be shorter, requiring more frequent doses to achieve a steady-state level. The risk of fatal hepatic dysfunction with valproate may be as high as 1 in 500 for children under the age of 2 who are on polytherapy. Elderly patients at risk for congestive heart failure should not be treated with carbamazepine, which can cause water retention. Barbiturates and, to a lesser extent, benzodiazepines, produce reversible hyperkinetic and aggressive behaviors in children as well as confusion, agitation, and depression in the elderly.

Surgical Therapy. *Resective surgery* has proved safe and beneficial and can cure a chronic epileptic condition when all else fails. At present, it is a greatly underutilized therapeutic modality. Most surgical facilities will consider epileptic patients potential candidates for resective surgical therapy if (1) a partial seizure disorder has been documented, (2) seizures continue at a frequency that seriously interferes with daily living despite adequate levels of appropriate antiepileptic medication, and (3) there is not substantial interictal mental retardation or psychosis. Patients with complex partial seizures of temporal lobe origin are ideal candidates for surgery. Worthwhile improvement occurs in over 85 per cent of such patients, and as many as two thirds may become seizure free after anterior temporal lobectomy. Local resection of an extratemporal focal epileptogenic lesion is also possible if the area of cortex can be identified precisely and removed safely. A history of generalized convulsions, a focus in the dominant hemisphere, or the presence of bilateral independent temporal spike foci on EEG does not contraindicate surgery.

Section of the corpus callosum has been particularly effective in controlling otherwise intractable drop attacks, and patients with other secondary generalized and partial seizure patterns have experienced improvement from this operation. While *hemispherectomy* is the most effective surgical procedure for epilepsy, it is justified only for children who have severely incapacitating unilateral seizures and hemiparesis with a useless hand.

Other Therapeutic Measures. Patients with some types of seizures may benefit from special management. Reflex seizures induced by specific stimuli can be treated by avoiding the stimuli. For example, epileptic photosensitivity can be abolished by patching one eye or wearing colored glasses, and desensitization is possible for many forms of reflex seizures. Spread of some simple partial seizures may be aborted by strong or painful sensory stimulation administered at onset. When seizures occur only at specific times of the day, medications can be adjusted to ensure maximum levels at those times, and daily schedules can be altered so that the patient is home or in a safe environment when at risk.

Patients with all types of seizures should remain active and maintain daily habits that ensure regular meals, adequate sleep, and a reduction in unnecessary stress. Alcohol or sedative drugs can be taken sparingly, but excessive use can provoke seizures during withdrawal. Patients who have seizures associated with an alteration in consciousness, particularly those that occur without warning, should be counseled to avoid hazardous situations: They should not swim alone, should shower rather than bathe, should not climb to unprotected heights, and should not operate potentially dangerous power-driven machines, including automobiles.

Emergency Treatment. First aid for a generalized tonic-clonic convulsion consists of protecting the patient from self-injury. Clothing should be loosened, sharp objects removed from the area, and the patient's head cushioned from impact. Hard objects or fingers must not be inserted into the patient's mouth—patients do not choke on their own tongues. When the seizure is over, turn the patient's head to drain oral secretions. Have someone stay with the patient during the postictal period until full consciousness has returned. It is not necessary to call an ambulance unless the patient has never had a seizure before, the seizure lasts longer than 10 minutes, another attack occurs before consciousness is regained, or there is evidence of injury, respiratory distress, or pregnancy. Patients should not be forcibly restrained during complex partial seizures but should be protected from surrounding hazards until ictal and postictal symptoms cease and they can care for themselves.

Status Epilepticus. The various forms of status epilepticus require specialized approaches to treatment. *Major motor status epilepticus* is a medical emergency requiring immediate intervention to prevent permanent brain damage or death. A recommended approach is given in Table 483–9. As soon as the airway is secured, a quick neurologic examination should be performed to appraise critical forebrain and brain stem functions. There may be evidence of an acute intracerebral lesion with herniation or other life-threatening conditions. Because the effects of diazepam are short lived, it should be administered simultaneously with a longer acting antiepileptic drug. Phenytoin usually is preferred, since it produces no sedative effects. This allows the patient to regain consciousness when seizures are terminated and facilitates neurologic evaluation. If seizures persist after the institution of appropriate therapy, high intravenous doses of phenobarbital or general anesthesia with short-acting barbiturates are recommended. When intubation and ventilation are necessary, the progress of treatment should be monitored closely with EEG

TABLE 483–9. MANAGEMENT OF CONVULSIVE STATUS EPILEPTICUS

Treatment Goal	Cumulative Time Since Arrival in Emergency Room
Restore homeostasis	0–15 min
Airway, blood pressure, nasal O_2; record ECG; intubate only if necessary	
Administer 50 ml 50% glucose and 100 mg thiamine IV	
Start isotonic saline slow drip IV	
Stop convulsive seizures	
Diazepam, 0.25 mg/kg IV up to 20 mg (<5 mg/min), followed immediately by phenytoin, 18 mg/kg IV (<50 mg/min); monitor blood pressure and ECG; repeat 7 mg/kg if necessary	
or	
Lorazepam, 0.1 mg/kg IV (<2 mg/min), with subsequent medication determined by serum drug levels or, if necessary, phenytoin IV as above	15–60 min
If seizures persist:	
Intubate; EEG should be used at this point Phenobarbital, 20 mg/kg IV (<100 mg/min)	60–120 min
If seizures persist:	
General anesthesia with short-acting barbiturates (e.g., pentobarbital, 5 mg/kg, then 1–3 mg/kg/hr); adjust dose to obtain burst suppression pattern on EEG without depressing blood pressure severely, and titrate to keep patient seizure-free	
Use additional anticonvulsants as necessary	After 2–3 hr
Obtain anticonvulsant blood levels	
Diagnostic evaluation (do concurrently with above)	
History, examination, urinalysis for toxic screen	

Modified with permission from Engel J Jr: Seizures and Epilepsy. Philadelphia, F.A. Davis, 1989.

recordings. Once status has been controlled, maintenance drug therapy is instituted. The most common cause of major motor status epilepticus is a sudden reduction or discontinuation of antiepileptic drugs in patients with known seizure disorders.

Absence status epilepticus can be aborted early by ethosuximide or valproate. Once under way, however, it is treated with intravenous diazepam followed by valproate, because parenteral preparations of antiabsence drugs are not available. An adult form of absence status, without previous history, and postictal absence-like status respond to the protocol outlined in Table 483–9. Complex partial status should be treated as aggressively as generalized convulsive status. Neither absence status nor complex partial status is life threatening, however, and general anesthesia may not be necessary. Both absence and complex partial status can be mistaken for psychiatric disturbances until EEG recordings demonstrate their typical ictal patterns. Simple partial status epilepticus (continuous partial epilepsy) may be effectively treated with intravenous diazepam or lorazepam followed by phenytoin, but this is not a medical emergency and usually does not warrant more aggressive measures.

Psychosocial Considerations. To some extent, psychosocial disturbances among epileptics are situational. Because most seizures occur spontaneously and unpredictably, many patients spend their lives anticipating inappropriate behavior, embarrassment, or serious injury. Epileptics are frequently unable to find work if they admit to a seizure disorder, so that their opportunities for rewarding social relationships are reduced. In most states, patients with seizures that impair consciousness are not allowed to drive. These factors contribute to a higher incidence of depression and suicide among epileptics than in the general population.

Although the evidence is controversial, aberrant personality traits, affective disorders, and psychoses, including late paranoid schizophrenia, have been reported to be more common among patients with epilepsy, particularly those with complex partial seizures of limbic origin. It is unclear to what extent these disturbances result from the underlying pathologic lesions or specific seizure activity, how much can be attributed to the effect of long-term antiepileptic drug therapy, and how much relates to limitations imposed on daily living and the stigma of being epileptic.

Only about one in four patients with uncontrolled epilepsy is handicapped by seizures alone. The others have physical, intellectual, and/or psychiatric disabilities that disrupt their daily lives. Epileptic seizures, perhaps more than any other neurologic symptom, are modified by internal and external influences that are under the control of the patient and other persons. For these reasons, treatment of the epileptic patient requires more than manipulation of anticonvulsant drugs, and outcome depends upon more than just seizure control. The physician must come to know the patient and the patient's family, their psychological interactions, and their social situation. Furthermore, improving psychosocial adaptation itself often leads to a reduction in seizure frequency. To provide the comprehensive care required by patients with seizure disorders, the physician must attend to the patient as well as to the neurologic disorder. The doctor must be friend as well as therapist.

Engel J Jr: Seizures and Epilepsy. Philadelphia, F. A. Davis, 1989. *A thorough overview of the field of epileptology and an introduction to the literature.*

Engel J Jr (ed.): Surgical Treatment of the Epilepsies. New York, Raven Press, 1987. *A comprehensive presentation of modern surgical therapy for epilepsy.*

Epilepsy Abstracts 1947–present. *Published now by Excerpta Medica, this monthly journal contains abstracts of all epilepsy-related papers and is an easy introduction to the literature on any subject.*

Levy RH, Dreifuss FE, Mattson RH, et al. (eds.): Antiepileptic Drugs. 3rd ed. New York, Raven Press, 1989. *A multiauthored compendium of recent concepts of pharmacologic therapy for epilepsy.*

Penfield W, Jasper H: Epilepsy and the Functional Anatomy of the Brain. Boston, Little, Brown and Company, 1954. *A classic by pioneers of modern epileptology; describes epileptic phenomena and applications of clinical data to the understanding of normal brain functions.*

Porter RJ: Epilepsy: 100 Elementary Principles. 2nd ed. Philadelphia, W. B. Saunders Company, 1989. *A small volume of clinical pearls.*

Roger J, Dravet C, Bureau M, et al.: Epileptic Syndromes in Infancy, Childhood and Adolescence. London, John Libbey Eurotext, Ltd., 1985. *Detailed descriptions of the currently recognized epileptic syndromes.*

SECTION THIRTEEN / INTRACRANIAL TUMORS AND STATES OF ALTERED INTRACRANIAL PRESSURE

484 Intracranial Tumors: General Considerations

Nicholas A. Vick

Approximately 14,000 new cases of primary brain tumors are treated each year in the United States. Metastases of the brain are even more frequent and contribute considerably to suffering and death from systemic cancer. The diversity of brain tumors makes it important to attend to what is characteristic about each histologic type, since attention to biologic specificity crucially guides present therapy and almost certainly will advance future understanding of these lesions and their treatment.

The classification of brain tumors is a subject often beset with confusing terminology, understood only by the knowledgeable. This text employs a simpler approach, classifying brain tumors into *metastatic, primary extra-axial,* and *primary intra-axial* (Table 484–1). These categories include all of the primary brain tumors listed in the World Health Organization classification (Table 484–2), adds pituitary and metastatic tumors, and is obviously simple. Moreover, it follows practical clinical thinking. This chapter deals with the general biology, clinical features, and treatment of brain tumors as an overall problem. The following

TABLE 484–1. THE COMMON BRAIN TUMORS IN ADULTS WITH PERCENTAGE INCIDENCE BY CATEGORY*

Metastatic	Primary Extra-axial	Primary Intra-axial
Lung (37)	Meningioma (80)	Glioblastoma (47)
Breast (19)	Acoustic neuroma (10)	Anaplastic astrocytoma (24)
Melanoma (16)	Pituitary adenoma (7)	Astrocytoma (15)
Colorectum (9)	Other (3)	Oligodendroglioma (5)
Kidney (8)		Lymphoma (2)
Other (11)		Other (7)

*These figures, given in parentheses, can be extremely variable from one center to another, depending on referral pattern. They are given here as general estimates based upon many published series.

TABLE 484–2. WORLD HEALTH ORGANIZATION CLASSIFICATION OF BRAIN TUMORS*

A. Astrocytic tumors
  1. Astrocytoma
    a. Fibrillary
    b. Protoplasmic
    c. Gemistocytic
  2. Pilocytic astrocytoma
  3. Subependymal giant cell astrocytoma (ventricular tumor or tuberous sclerosis)
  4. Astroblastoma
  5. Anaplastic (malignant) astrocytoma
B. Oligodendroglial tumors
  1. Oligodendroglioma
  2. Mixed oligoastrocytoma
  3. Anaplastic (malignant) oligodendroglioma
C. Ependymal and choroid plexus tumors
  1. Ependymoma
    Variants:
    a. Myxopapillary ependymoma
    b. Papillary ependymoma
    c. Subependymoma
  2. Anaplastic (malignant) ependymoma
  3. Choroid plexus papilloma
  4. Anaplastic (malignant) choroid plexus papilloma
D. Pineal cell tumor
  1. Pineocytoma (pinealocytoma)
  2. Pineoblastoma (pinealoblastoma)
E. Neuronal tumors
  1. Gangliocytoma
  2. Ganglioglioma
  3. Ganglioneuroblastoma
  4. Anaplastic (malignant) gangliocytoma and ganglioglioma
  5. Neuroblastoma
F. Poorly differentiated and embryonal tumours
  1. Glioblastoma
    Variants:
    a. Glioblastoma with sarcomatous component (mixed glioblastoma and sarcoma)
    b. Giant cell glioblastoma
  2. Medulloblastoma
    Variants:
    a. Desmoplastic medulloblastoma
    b. Medullomyoblastoma
  3. Medulloepithelioma
  4. Primitive polar spongioblastoma
  5. Gliomatosis cerebri

*This is one of several formal schemes that are based on neuropathologic criteria. Metastasis is not considered, and one can get no sense of a given tumor as a *clinical* problem, as suggested by the simple classification in Table 484–1.

chapter describes the particular behavior of the most important subtypes in accordance with the outline of Table 484–1.

"Is it benign or malignant?" is invariably the first question patients, families, and physicians ask when confronted with a diagnosis of brain tumor. About a third of primary brain tumors can be called benign. Meningiomas and acoustic neuromas are good examples, since they grow relatively slowly, often can be removed completely, and do not recur after such a removal.

Nevertheless, the concept of malignancy in the central nervous system has a different meaning from that which applies to systemic cancers. For one thing, the term "malignant" has nothing to do with metastasis out of the central nervous system, which is extraordinarily rare. It has, however, everything to do with anatomic location and the possibility of complete surgical removal. If a meningioma is so positioned that it cannot be completely removed, such as at the base of the brain, it is likely to kill the patient eventually, even though it may possess only indolent growth characteristics. Unless a tumor can be completely excised to the last cell, all intracranial neoplasms are potentially malignant in that they may recur, and often do.

INITIAL EVALUATION

SYMPTOMS AND SIGNS. Brain tumors present clinically in two patterns, not necessarily mutually exclusive. One pattern consists of nonfocal symptoms of *increased intracranial pressure*, such as headaches, nausea, vomiting, confusion, and lethargy. The other consists of symptoms or signs of *focal brain dysfunction*, such as hemianopia, hemiparesis, selected cranial nerve palsies, or focal motor seizures (Table 484–3). Such signs of focal brain dysfunction may have convincing localizing value even before an image of the brain is made by computed tomography (CT) or magnetic resonance imaging (MRI). Some tumors that arise in neurologically "silent" areas, such as the parietal or frontal association cortices, may produce only minor symptoms of headache, confusion, behavioral change, or, eventually, a seizure, despite growing to a considerable size. These symptoms may not indicate at all what part of the brain is affected or may lead to a localizing diagnosis only in the hands of a neurologically experienced consultant. Although the capacity to reach early diagnosis by CT or MRI has greatly reduced the numbers of patients in whom symptoms of increased intracranial pressure represent initial complaints, examples still remain, especially in association with fast-growing tumors and in children. The latter are particularly likely to have tumors in the posterior fossa that tend to obstruct spinal fluid pathways earlier than do supratentorial tumors. As implied, the tempo with which a brain tumor grows also influences the presenting symptoms. Despite the fixed space of the skull (once infantile sutures have closed), the human brain possesses a remarkable capacity to make room for a slowly growing tumor (Fig. 484–1). Because of this, and even allowing for the relative rapidity of growth of aggressive brain tumors such as glioblastomas, the rule is that the patient usually appears better clinically than might be expected from the degree of abnormality seen on CT or MRI scan.

DIFFERENTIAL DIAGNOSIS. Patients who present with symptoms and signs of increased intracranial pressure or a first convulsive seizure need to be hospitalized. Diagnosis and treatment measures must be started at once; it is a waste of time and may be unsafe to wait. On the other hand, those who present with focal neurologic impairment and who do not have symptoms of increased intracranial pressure may reasonably be evaluated in the outpatient setting for other conditions that are often considerations in the differential diagnosis of brain tumor (Table 484–4). The tempo of evolution of symptoms and signs of focal neurologic impairment, much more than their severity, governs urgency of evaluation. The tempo also strongly influences diagnostic considerations. Although an occasional brain tumor may manifest with such rapid onset of hemiparesis or aphasia that a stroke is mimicked, most do not. Further, most strokes do not evolve over several weeks, though some may do so. Associated aspects of the history, such as recent head trauma, previous episodes of reversible neurologic impairment, or recent infection and fever, should direct attention to diagnostic alternatives such as subdural hematoma, multiple sclerosis, or cerebral abscess. Simply stated, it is the careful history, not the neurologic examination, that usually points to the alternative diagnoses.

IMAGING AND OTHER DIAGNOSTIC PROCEDURES

Brain imaging by MRI or CT scans is an indispensable component of the modern diagnosis of brain tumors. Only seldom, however, are such images sufficient to offer tissue diagnoses, since one type of tumor can look like another or even resemble nonneoplastic mass lesions, such as brain abscesses, fungal infections, parasitic invasions, demyelinating diseases, and even strokes. For definitive diagnosis and adequate treatment planning, one must obtain a tissue diagnosis whenever possible. This can be made either by direct surgical biopsy or, in the case of some nonneoplastic conditions, by judging CT or MRI responses to particular therapies.

MRI is almost always superior to CT scanning in providing diagnostic information for all types of intracranial mass lesions. Several features account for this superiority. MRI resolution is slightly better, but, more important, discrimination between tissue components is greater. Furthermore, MRI outlines posterior fossa structures and tumors with a clarity that CT cannot achieve because of x-ray distortions due to the bony structure of that region. In several types of tumor, particularly the low-grade gliomas, MRI may show extensive brain infiltration in cases that fail to produce any image abnormality on CT or, at most, a vague low density. It should be noted that although either MRI or CT should be used with contrast enhancement in cases of suspected

TABLE 484–3. FOCAL CLINICAL MANIFESTATIONS OF BRAIN TUMORS

Frontal Lobe	**Corpus Callosum**	**Sella/Optic Nerve/Pituitary**
Generalized seizures	Dementia (anterior)	Endocrinopathy
Focal motor seizures (contralateral)	Behavioral changes (posterior)	Bitemporal hemianopia
Expressive aphasia (dominant side)	Asymptomatic (mid)	Monocular visual defects
Behavioral changes		
Dementia		
Gait disorders, incontinence		
Parietal Lobe	**Basal Ganglia**	**Pons/Medulla**
Receptive aphasia (dominant side)	Hemiparesis (contralateral)	Cranial nerve dysfunction
Spatial disorientation (nondominant side)	Movement disorders very rare	Ataxia, nystagmus
Cortical sensory dysfunction (contralateral)		Weakness, sensory loss
Hemianopia (contralateral)		Spasticity
Temporal Lobe	**Thalamus**	**Cerebellopontine Angle**
Complex partial (psychomotor) seizures	Sensory loss (contralateral)	Deafness (ipsilateral)
Generalized seizures	Behavioral changes	Loss of facial sensation (ipsilateral)
Behavioral changes	Language disorder (dominant side)	Facial weakness (ipsilateral)
Olfactory and complex visual auras		Ataxia
Occipital Lobe	**Midbrain/Pineal**	**Cerebellum**
Hemianopia (contralateral)	Paresis of vertical eye movements	Ataxia (ipsilateral)
Visual disturbances (unformed)	Pupillary abnormalities	Nystagmus
	Precocious puberty (boys)	

brain tumor, the passage of such contrast agents beyond the blood-brain barrier into the tissue does not necessarily imply the presence of a histologically malignant tumor. For example, although malignant gliomas almost always show contrast enhancement, so do meningiomas, which are entirely benign if they can be fully removed surgically.

It is now generally understood that a CT scan done without contrast enhancement is of little value in the diagnosis of brain tumors or other mass lesions. While it is true that hemorrhage, calcifications, hydrocephalus, and shift can be well seen on a noncontrast CT scan, the interpretation of even these conditions is tentative because each can have an underlying causative structural abnormality such as a brain tumor, which may fail to appear on a noncontrast CT study. Allergy to CT dye is rare and readily manageable. Currently available nonionic CT dyes have an extremely low incidence of side effects. There is little risk that currently used CT dyes will cause renal dysfunction in normally hydrated patients who are not known to have kidney disease.

MRI initially provided two types of images, designated T_1 and T_2. For brain tumors, the former generally showed a well-demarcated area of low density and the latter, bright whiteness that encompassed a more extensive region owing to the signal of the surrounding brain edema (Fig. 484–2). With the availability for general usage in 1988 of *gadolinium contrast for MRI*, a new set of criteria of usage and differential diagnostic considerations in brain imaging have quickly evolved (Table 484–5). T_1 gadolinium imaging is the most precise way to image a brain tumor, and often patients can be followed with that type of study alone. Such an approach is easier for patients because it reduces the length of time otherwise spent on T_2 scanning. Now and then, T_2 images are useful. For example, T_2 images, besides showing the extent of edema, also delineate the demyelinating effects of radiation upon white matter.

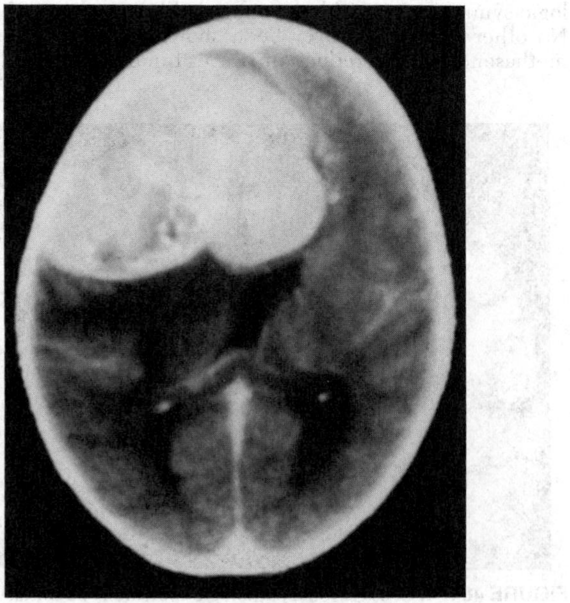

Cerebral angiography has become seldom used in the diagnosis of brain tumors. In a few circumstances, however, neurosurgeons, in preparation for surgery, require a more precise knowledge of the pattern and position of blood vessels that can be obtained only by angiography. The procedure is also used to embolize certain tumors, such as highly vascular meningiomas, or to study cerebral dominance by injection of sodium amytal into the carotid artery (the Wada test) in left-handed individuals who are to have surgery near language areas. Cerebral dominance in such persons is quite variable; preoperative determination of cerebral localization helps surgeons to plan the extent of surgery and avoid postoperative language deficits.

Examination of the *spinal fluid* has virtually been abandoned in the diagnosis of brain tumors. Several exceptions exist, however. One is that the patient may be thought to have an inflammatory disorder mimicking a brain tumor. Another is that a patient initially believed to have a brain tumor because of clinical symptoms and signs of increased intracranial pressure has negative MRI scans and needs the diagnosis of benign intracranial hypertension established (see Ch. 486). In addition, spinal fluid cytology may be useful for determining instances of malignant meningitis secondary to metastatic neoplasms, in association with spinal spread of medulloblastoma in some children and in identifying primary lymphomas of the brain in cases in which MRI changes are ambiguous.

FIGURE 484–1. CT scan with contrast of a meningioma in a patient who presented with mild cognitive deficits, illustrative of the size a slow-growing tumor can attain in the brain. The tumor was completely resected.

TABLE 484–4. THE MAIN DIFFERENTIAL DIAGNOSES OF BRAIN TUMORS

Hematomas, especially in tumors that have a tendency to bleed, such as melanoma
Abscesses, including fungal
Granulomas
Parasitic infections, such as cysticercosis
Vascular malformations, especially those without arteriovenous shunts
Solitary large plaques of multiple sclerosis
Seldom, progressive strokes

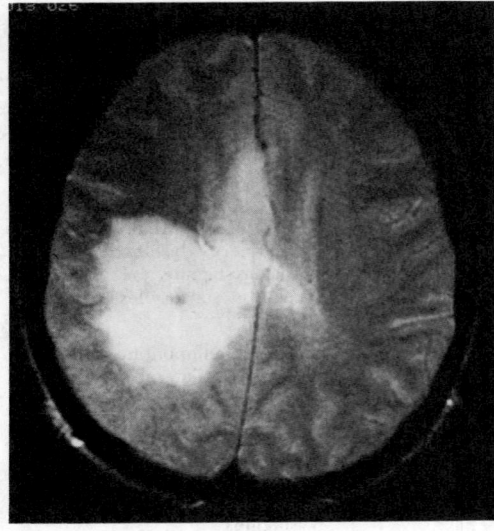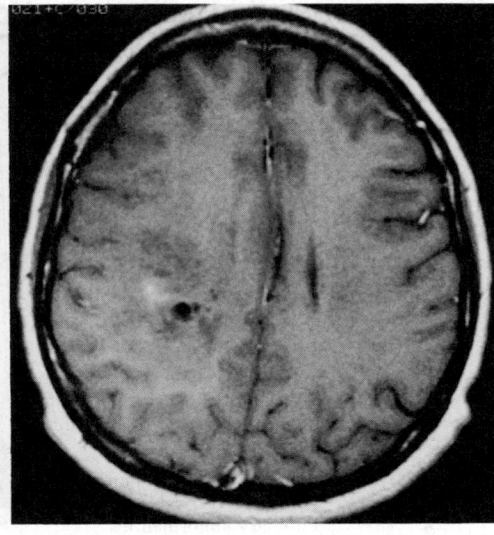

FIGURE 484–2. Low-grade astrocytoma as imaged by MRI. On the left, T_2-weighted image; on the right, T_1-weighted image, gadolinium contrast with minimal enhancement. The images are typical of this tumor, which is being detected with increasing frequency in seizure patients by MRI. Many are invisible on CT scans.

The electroencephalogram (EEG) has virtually no role in the diagnosis of brain tumors, although the procedure is sometimes useful in managing seizures in brain tumor patients. Furthermore, depth electrode studies as well as intraoperative monitoring can be of great importance in identifying and removing epileptogenic areas associated with certain tumors (see Ch. 483). The details of the EEG do not assist in the selection of anticonvulsant drugs in brain tumor patients.

Positron emission tomography (PET) is able to quantify biochemical functions, such as oxygen and glucose utilization, within tumors as well as normal brain tissue. PET scanning is a powerful research tool of limited availability for routine clinical purposes. Its actual spatial resolution is practically and theoretically inferior to that of both CT and MRI. It can differentiate radiation-induced brain injury and necrosis from recurrent tumor, which neither CT nor MRI can do. It is not an imaging tool for high-volume, regular clinical purposes.

TABLE 484–5. T_1 GADOLINIUM MRI CHARACTERISTICS OF BRAIN TUMORS

Metastases	These are remarkably variable (see Fig. 485–1). Some enhance brightly and solidly with gadolinium. Others are in ring configuration. Many are invisible with contrast CT.
Acoustic Neuromas	These are invariably intensely contrasted by gadolinium, even more reliably than by CT.
Meningiomas	Same as for acoustic neuromas.
Pituitary Adenomas	These always enhance less than the normal pituitary gland. MRI is superior in every way to CT, especially when thin slices and magnified views are ordered.
Glioblastoma	These are almost always in ring configuration (see Fig. 485–2).
Anaplastic Astrocytomas	These are sometimes solidly bright; they are often patchy, may be noncontrasting, and may look like low-grade astrocytoma.
Low-grade Astrocytomas	These do not enhance (see Fig. 485–2). They are often invisible by CT or are imaged only as vague low density.
Oligodendrogliomas	These generally do not enhance unless anaplastic and are often invisible on CT unless they are calcified.
Primary Brain Lymphomas	These usually exhibit homogeneous enhancement and are smoothly rounded. Periventricular location is common. They are multiple in about a fourth of cases. This lesion does not often look like glioblastoma but is easily mistaken for metastases if multiple.

TREATMENT

PREOPERATIVE CONSIDERATIONS AND MEDICAL MANAGEMENT. In almost every instance when a brain tumor is suspected on the basis of the combined results of history, physical findings, and imaging studies, the *first consideration is its surgical resectability*. There are exceptions, such as cases of multiple brain metastases in a patient with known systemic cancer. Patients with single brain metastases, defined by MRI, may be candidates for surgical resection of the metastasis, depending on their systemic medical status. It is unproductive to embark upon an extensive systemic evaluation in the search for an unknown primary cancer in patients with a single resectable presumed brain metastasis. If a primary tumor is not quickly revealed by a careful medical evaluation, with special attention to skin (for melanoma), breasts, and lungs, the pathologic diagnosis of the brain tumor will need to be disclosed by resection or, if unresectable owing to its position, by biopsy.

While small meningiomas or acoustic neuromas usually do not require treatment to reduce intracranial pressure, in the majority of brain tumor patients it is appropriate to start *dexamethasone* promptly. The purpose is to reduce intracranial pressure, which accompanies the majority of brain tumors, and to relieve neurologic symptoms caused by peritumoral brain edema (Fig. 484–3). No other steroid has ever been shown to be superior to dexamethasone for the reduction of peritumoral brain edema. The

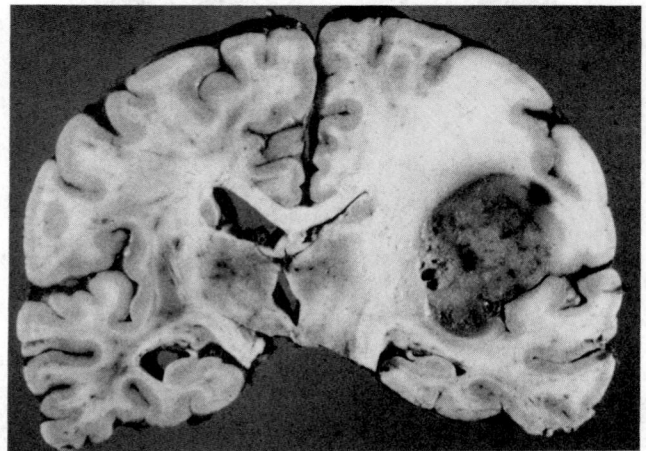

FIGURE 484–3. Gross coronal pathologic specimen of a solitary metastasis from a non–small cell lung carcinoma to the right cerebral hemisphere. The tumor is well circumscribed. It causes marked edema that greatly expands the cerebral white matter. Metastatic tumors such as this can often be surgically resected.

drug's long biologic half-life and steady action upon the brain have made it the steroid of choice for treating patients with brain tumors. It should be started with an immediate oral dose of 24 or 48 mg, followed with 8 or 12 mg twice daily. It is well absorbed by mouth, and its action by that route is almost as rapid as when given intravenously. Dexamethasone need not be given more than twice a day, since its biologic half-life is so long. Breakfast and dinner are convenient times; the presence of food in the stomach precludes the need for antacids. H_2 blockers should be given only if the patient has a prior history of peptic ulcer disease. If focal neurologic symptoms are due to peritumoral vasogenic edema, dexamethasone will induce improvement within 48 hours and usually sooner. If there is no benefit, the neurologic symptoms are likely to be due to damage of the brain tissue by the tumor and not to edema.

Edema associated with brain tumors is due chiefly to abnormally fenestrated endothelium in the tumor, which permits excess flow of fluid from capillaries into the growth. Normally, solutes are transported through capillaries into brain by dissolving in and diffusing through the cerebral endothelium, a phenomenon dependent on lipid solubility and molecular size. Endothelial cells also possess some facilitated or carrier-mediated processes that are stereospecific, saturable, and independent of lipid solubility and molecular size. In brain tumors, these selective properties of the blood-brain barrier are overwhelmed by increased bulk flow and hydraulic conductivity through the defective endothelium. The result is vasogenic edema, and it is this reaction that dexamethasone so greatly reduces.

In instances of extreme intracranial pressure, the speed and action of dexamethasone are not sufficient to reduce the brain swelling quickly enough to prevent complications. In such instances, hyperosmotic solutions of *mannitol* must be given. The usual dosage is 0.5 to 2.0 gm per kilogram given intravenously over 15 minutes, followed by additional boluses of 25 gm as needed. The osmotic action of mannitol occurs within minutes. Clinical improvement may be dramatic. It is unusual for preoperative brain tumor patients to decompensate so severely from increased intracranial pressure that intubation becomes necessary. Nevertheless, this does occur. In such cases the Pa_{CO_2} must be decreased by passive hyperventilation to approximately 25 mm Hg. The effect constricts the cerebral vasculature and promptly induces a major reduction of intracranial pressure, which can be life saving.

About 20 per cent of brain tumor patients develop *seizures* some time in their lives, even if they do not have seizures at the time of diagnosis. It is conventional and probably effective to treat all patients with supratentorial tumors with anticonvulsants before surgery. Most patients with acoustic neuromas or other posterior fossa tumors have a low probability of convulsive seizures and do not need such drugs. Phenytoin is the best initial drug because it can be administered either intravenously or orally, unlike either carbamazepine or valproic acid, which can be used only orally. An intravenous drug is especially useful for continuation during the perioperative period. If required, patients may be switched easily to alternative oral drugs later. Phenytoin should be started orally, giving 1000 mg over 12 hours, or intravenously, with 1000 mg given over 1 hour. Thereafter, the usual dosage is 300 to 400 mg daily, administered in one dose or split between breakfast and dinner, along with dexamethasone. Periodic blood levels need to be checked to adjust the dosage to ensure concentrations of 10 to 20 μg per milliliter.

SURGERY. Although complete excision of a brain tumor is the ultimate goal in every case, this is not always possible. Even potentially curable tumors, such as meningiomas or acoustic neuromas, may reside in positions that make complete resection technically impossible. Malignant gliomas lack microscopic boundaries, even though they may appear by imaging studies to have well-defined limits. How much surgical success can be achieved with these tumors depends on several factors, including the tumor's proximity to cognitively indispensable areas, the skill and experience of the neurosurgeon, and, to a degree, the general health of the patient and preoperative level of neurologic function. The combination of current standards of neurosurgical anesthesia, the capacity to control intracranial pressure, and the recent addition of lasers to other operative tools such as the operating microscope have greatly increased the surgeon's capacity for well-chosen radical resection. Correspondingly, the relative risks of surgery have become less age dependent than was previously the case. The greatest surgical risk is to neurologic function and the fear of unacceptable postoperative neurologic deficits. For this reason, radical operations upon tumors involving language areas, sensorimotor regions, the basal ganglia, corpus callosum, and brain stem are generally avoided. However, partial removal in these areas by specialized stereotaxic methods may be surprisingly effective. MRI facilitates such surgery by showing that the tumor has pushed aside functionally critical brain structures and that a macroscopic tumor edge can be delineated. As for the extent of surgery itself, it has been repeatedly shown that resection of the maximal possible amount of tumor consistent with functional preservation provides patients with better neurologic function and longer lives.

A number of patients have tumors that cannot be even partially resected because they invade language-related or other functionally indispensable areas of the brain. Most such lesions are intraaxial tumors, such as the gliomas. While current imaging techniques may produce a seemingly characteristic picture highly suggestive of a particular histologic diagnosis, effective treatment planning demands a tissue diagnosis. The only possible exception to this rule consists of certain brain stem tumors that are technically too dangerous on which to perform a biopsy. In some hands, even these may be approached by the method of MRI-guided stereotaxic biopsy, a technique that has considerably improved the opportunity to make unequivocal tissue diagnoses before treatment, regardless of the brain region. Most such stereotaxically guided biopsies are performed upon the cerebral hemispheres. The tissue specimens are small, but they are almost invariably adequate to establish a diagnosis. Morbidity, chiefly hemorrhage, occurs in about 2 per cent of cases. Patients usually need to remain in the hospital for less than 48 hours. Open biopsies of brain tumors are rarely justifiable. If the skull and dura are to be opened, the surgeon should be prepared to do a gross total resection or, at least, a major removal of as much tumor as is consonant with preservation of neurologic function.

The postoperative management of neurosurgical patients is now a relatively standard matter best left to specialized intensive care units. Deep leg vein thrombophlebitis leading to pulmonary embolism is a recurrent problem, only partially helped by prophylactic application of compression boots. Close observation and early passive exercises and mobilization are imperative. The staff must monitor and maintain anticonvulsant levels to prevent postoperative seizures. Dexamethasone should be administered at adequate levels for at least 5 days to minimize the further development of surgically induced brain edema. The drug can be tapered thereafter.

RADIOTHERAPY. All forms of external beam radiation, whether γ photons emitted from ^{60}Co sources or x-rays generated from linear accelerators, act similarly. They produce fast-moving electrons and free radicals in biologic tissue that interrupt chemical bonds between DNA base pairs. Affected cells either die or become so altered that their mitotic rate is greatly diminished. Radiotherapy is given in small daily fractions to build to a total dose. It appears safer and more effective to do this than to give larger fractions over shorter periods. Hyperfractionation, defined as two (or more) doses during a day, does not seem to be worthwhile. Therapeutic brain irradiation with particulate radiation such as neutrons has been attempted experimentally at facilities with cyclotrons. Such densely ionizing radiation, however, dissipates its energy in short path lengths, causes more damage in biologic media, and has shown no therapeutic advantage over γ photons or x-rays. Interstitial (implanted) radiotherapy (brachytherapy) is being tried and is of considerable interest. It is usually given in the form of $^{125}I_3$ or $^{192}Ir_4$ in "seeds" with placement by stereotaxic techniques. This method permits localized high-dosage radiation with sharp edges and sparing of the adjacent brain. Considerable controversy exists about the actual utility of such interstitial radiotherapy, but it can be effective in well-selected patients. The intense localized radiation of this technique, however, sometimes causes coagulative necrosis of the tumor being treated. This necrosis may create an additional mass, which can produce a dangerous degree of increased intracranial pressure, sometimes requiring further surgery for relief.

The *complications of radiotherapy* are usually said to be

infrequent, perhaps 2 to 5 per cent of cases. These figures, however, are unrealistically low if one includes effects on long-term survivors. They reflect the fact that most irradiated patients with brain tumor die before brain injury appears. Postradiation neurologic damage is unusual before a year after treatment and may not become apparent for several years. About 30 per cent of patients with glioblastomas who receive radiotherapy develop neurologic impairment with disturbed mobility and dementia if they live for twice the predicted survival time for their particular type of tumor. Another 30 per cent remain ambulatory but are unemployable owing to impairment of memory function. In these patients, while no evidence of tumor recurrence can be found by imaging studies, characteristic demyelinative changes of the white matter of the brain are evident. Dementia is a considerable problem in children who survive radiotherapy for medulloblastoma. This problem occurs because about 50 per cent survive treatment for 5 years. Such consequences emphasize the validity of waiting with radiotherapy for patients with low-grade astrocytomas and oligodendrogliomas until the progression of disease is unequivocal. Most of them will survive 5 to 10 years after the time of diagnosis, and there is little evidence to document that radiotherapy prolongs their survival.

Except in the few instances in which the process creates a surgically resectable necrotic mass, no useful treatment exists for postradiation neurologic damage. Clinical progression is the rule, though some patients stabilize with a restricted degree of impairment and do not become grossly impaired. Occasional individuals have episodic worsening that evolves in a strokelike pattern. Dexamethasone or anticoagulation or both have been found useful in some instances. The pathophysiology of these strokelike events is thought to be due to obliterative changes of small blood vessels induced by radiation, a process that may be independent of the demyelinating effects reflecting selective damage of oligodendrocytes. Neither CT nor MRI scanning definitively differentiates tumor recurrence from radiation necrosis of the brain. As noted earlier, PET can, since necrotic masses have very low glucose utilization compared with recurrent tumor.

Despite its limitations, external beam radiotherapy has proven value in controlling the growth of malignant gliomas and metastatic brain tumors. It doubles median survival time for both types of tumors. Radiation therapy, however, has little, if any, value for recurrent meningiomas and acoustic neuromas. These are almost invariably better handled by reoperation. Primary brain lymphomas are so responsive to radiotherapy that many neurologists and radiotherapists continue to use it alone despite the fact that chemotherapy may prove to provide superior initial treatment. It has already been mentioned that solitary brain metastases are best managed by surgical resection.

Radiotherapy is being studied to see whether, in fact, it actually adds to the survival of the latter group of patients. Strategies to limit the distribution of radiation to the tumor area and to increase dosage to the tumor itself are rational, as are efforts to enhance the radiation sensitivity of tumor compared with the surrounding brain. Neither approach has succeeded as yet.

CHEMOTHERAPY. Chemotherapy for brain tumors has had a disappointing record. The reasons are many, but inadequacy of drug delivery, tumor cell heterogeneity, and inherent resistance are among the important ones. Almost all efforts have been directed toward the primary brain tumors, especially the gliomas. Metastatic brain tumors regularly occur while systemic metastases are responding to chemotherapy. The alkylating agents have been the most useful drugs, although their bone marrow toxicity has been a limitation. BCNU (bischloroethylnitrosurea), the most frequently used drug, remains the most effective single agent available to treat the malignant astrocytomas. The combination of procarbazine, CCNU (cyclohexylchloroethylnitrosourea), and vincristine is the most effective multidrug regimen for the malignant astrocytomas, and it is probably superior to BCNU. It has an unusually beneficial effect against oligodendrogliomas. Overall, however, no more than 10 per cent of patients with malignant gliomas have meaningful and durable responses to chemotherapy, whether it is given immediately after radiotherapy (when its effect is especially hard to assess) or at the time of recurrence. Efforts to improve response to chemotherapy by delivering drugs through the carotid artery have not been successful. BCNU,

usually given intravenously, has intolerable toxicity when given by the intra-arterial route. Cisplatin is being studied for possible utility as an intra-arterial drug in highly selected patients.

The pharmacokinetics of drugs used in brain tumor chemotherapy are not well understood. Knowledge about their ability to gain adequate concentration within the tumors is minimal, and almost nothing is known about chemosensitivity. There have been efforts to explore these issues in animal models; the athymic (nude) mouse has been used extensively with human glioblastoma xenografts, but the observations in this model have proved to be overpredictive when tried clinically. Nonetheless, occasional remarkable responses to chemotherapy do occur in patients with glioblastomas or anaplastic astrocytomas, and as mentioned, oligodendrogliomas may be particularly responsive. The relative infrequency of ependymomas and other uncommon gliomas has left uncertain the efficacy of chemotherapy in their outcomes. Among other primary intra-axial brain tumors, primary brain lymphoma has a reasonably good response rate. The drugs used are those given regularly for systemic lymphoma. Patients with primary brain lymphoma do better with chemotherapy added than with radiotherapy alone. On average, 3- to 4-year survivals can now be expected.

Several additional forms of medical treatment for brain tumors have been attempted experimentally. These include slow release of BCNU from implanted biodegradable polymers and the administration of interferons, other biologic response modifiers, and radionuclides coupled with monoclonal antibodies. None have met with appreciable success to date. In all probability, much new biologic knowledge, such as the sequential genetic events that influence the malignant transformation and progression of brain tumors, will be required before new medical treatments become practical realities.

485 Specific Types of Brain Tumors and Their Management

Nicholas A. Vick

METASTATIC TUMORS

All systemic cancers are capable of metastasizing to the intracranial contents and skull, though some do so more readily than others. The most frequent are lung, breast, and melanoma. This is not surprising, since they are among the most common cancers. In many instances, brain metastases produce symptoms before the primary tumor is suspected. Furthermore, the primary cancer may not be found without considerable effort.

Patterns of metastasis to the nervous system have some variability, but none are truly characteristic. Non–small cell carcinoma of the lung and renal carcinoma tend to be associated with single metastases, whereas small cell carcinoma of the lung, breast carcinoma, and melanoma often generate multiple secondary deposits. The metastases may be miliary in melanoma. T_1 gadolinium magnetic resonance imaging (MRI) scans are critical in the imaging of brain metastases (Fig. 485–1). *Multiple metastases* may be revealed with this method, while T_2 MRI and contrast computed tomography (CT) may show only one or, in rare instances, none. For multiple metastases, whole-brain irradiation is the best form of treatment as long as the patient's systemic condition indicates a potential for high-quality survival. Patients with widespread systemic metastasis who are unlikely to survive more than a few months are best treated with dexamethasone alone.

The major benefit of aggressive surgery in patients with a *single brain metastasis* is for the quality of life that remains. Studies of evaluation of performance are compelling. Some of the best outcomes are in patients who present with non–small cell lung carcinoma and no other metastasis except for a single one in the brain ("solitary" brain metastasis) if both tumors are removed surgically. In patients with little, but potentially controllable, systemic tumor burden, the resection of a single metastasis is often worthwhile. However, no difference in mortality

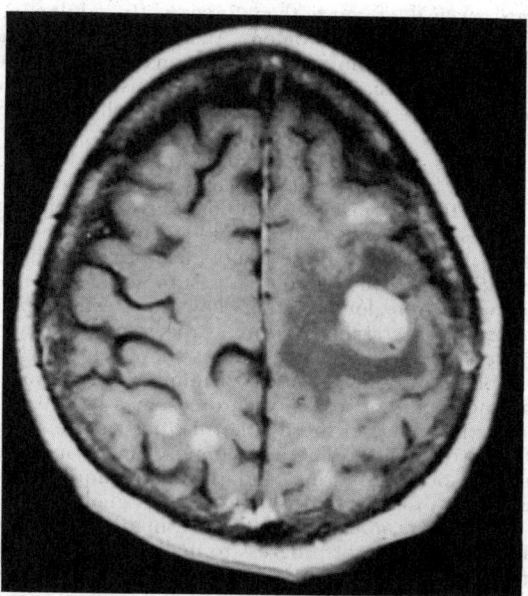

FIGURE 485–1. MRI scan, T₁ gadolinium, of multiple metastases from breast carcinoma. The tumors were not visible on CT, even after giving a contrast agent.

TABLE 485–1. METASTATIC BRAIN TUMORS

These tumors affect 10% of cancer patients (and still another 20% have dural meningeal involvement).

At least 50% are multiple.

If solitary (the only metastatic lesion in the body), surgery clearly provides best results in most cases. Surgery may be the best approach even if other metastases are present in patients in good condition.

Radiotherapy is useful palliation but not curative. Long-term survivors may have consequential side effects such as dementia.

at 2 years distinguishes patients who have been operated on from those who receive radiotherapy alone. This is because most patients with systemic metastases die of their systemic illness and not their brain metastasis.

Metastases to the dura and meninges are more common than generally recognized. Meningeal carcinomatosis manifests with headache, cranial nerve palsies, and stiff neck. These symptoms are due to the presence of tumor cells within the spinal fluid and to small deposits on the meninges around cranial nerves, at the base of the brain, and upon spinal roots. The diagnosis of meningeal carcinomatosis is made by cytologic examination of large-volume spinal fluid specimens. As many as three or more spinal taps may be needed to find the tell-tale cells in some cases. The spinal fluid protein level is generally elevated, and the glucose concentration may be low. The latter changes are sufficiently characteristic, in the absence of evidence of infection, to suggest the diagnosis. T₁ gadolinium MRI scanning may image the small deposits in the meninges. They are especially evident in the cauda equina even in the absence of clinical symptoms referable to lumbosacral nerve roots. The treatment of meningeal carcinomatosis includes irradiation of the brain and spinal cord, which usually provides benefit but rarely long remission. In patients with limited systemic metastases, intrathecal chemotherapy with methotrexate through an Ommaya reservoir is appropriate; occasional patients respond impressively. Most do not, however, and the effective treatment of meningeal carcinomatosis remains a difficult problem. In the future, the still experimental treatment of meningeal carcinomatosis with isotope-emitting radionuclides coupled to monoclonal antibodies may replace intrathecal chemotherapy.

Table 485–1 lists some key features of metastatic brain tumors.

PRIMARY EXTRA-AXIAL TUMORS

Meningiomas, acoustic neuromas, and pituitary adenomas are the most frequent in this group, which, by definition, are tumors that are not of the brain itself but of its coverings, the cranial nerves, and the adjacent structures. The primary extra-axial tumors differ from tumors of the brain in many ways. They are not of neuroectodermal origin, they are histologically unrelated, and most are truly benign, since they can be excised completely and cured. They exert effects upon the brain by pressure and only occasionally by actual invasion.

Meningiomas, which are growths of the fibroblast-like cells of the dura and arachnoid villi, account for about 15 per cent of all primary brain tumors. They occur more often in women. The biologic explanation is unknown, but the finding has stimulated interest in the presence of estrogen receptors in these tumors. Only a few causative factors are known. Meningiomas may occur

many years after radiation delivered to the head, in which setting they may be multiple. A relationship to head trauma has never been convincingly documented. Some examples follow a familial pattern. Such cases, as well as most apparently sporadic examples, are associated with a loss of a portion of chromosome 22.

Most meningiomas arise as solitary tumors in certain characteristic sites, such as over the cerebral convexities, attached to the sagittal sinus or at the base of the brain, attached to the dura of the sphenoid sinus, the olfactory grooves, or the region of the sella. In some of these areas, they may be difficult to remove completely without excessive risk and may recur slowly but repeatedly. Many meningiomas grow so slowly that serial CT or MRI images suggest no enlargement over many years. It is this slow growth that at times permits the brain to accommodate them with relatively modest symptoms even when the tumors are remarkably large (see Fig. 484–1). Many are detected incidentally. Small, asymptomatic meningiomas are often best watched by imaging studies at intervals; in the elderly, even large, asymptomatic ones may not require surgery.

Most *acoustic neuromas* consist of distinctive growths of Schwann cells (schwannoma) of the eighth cranial nerve. Almost all are unilateral and not apparently familial. Bilateral acoustic neuromas, which have a different tissue type, are rare, familial, and diagnostic of neurofibromatosis II. This autosomal dominant condition occurs with nearly 100 per cent penetrance in successive generations and derives from a gene deletion on chromosome 22.

Typically either form of acoustic neuroma grows on the nerve into a round mass just as the nerve emerges from the acoustic canal into the cerebellopontine angle. Some such tumors produce symptoms when they are extraordinarily small and confined within the canal. Others may go unsuspected until they grow to rather large size, filling the cerebellopontine angle and compressing the brain stem. Acoustic neuromas greatly surpass in frequency any other tumor of cranial nerves. Partial or complete nerve deafness is characteristic and is the usual presenting symptom. As acoustic neuromas gradually grow, they sequentially affect the fifth and then the seventh cranial nerves on the same side. When large, they cause cerebellar ataxia on the same side and, ultimately, symptoms of brain stem dysfunction. MRI scans accurately detect even very small acoustic neuromas. All patients who develop hearing loss in the middle years of life should be considered to have an acoustic neuroma until proved otherwise. Audiometry alone is suggestive but not diagnostic; caloric tests of labyrinthine function almost always show abnormalities, but the most efficient physiologic study is the auditory evoked response. Current microsurgical techniques yield remarkably good results, usually preserving the seventh nerve and, occasionally, preserving hearing as well.

Pituitary Adenomas

According to the hormones they produce, these tumors may cause endocrine symptoms, such as hypothyroidism, amenorrhea, galactorrhea, infertility, acromegaly, or Cushing's syndrome (Ch. 161). Null cell adenomas may manifest with the symptoms of hypopituitarism. With the exception of these hormonal impairments, early symptoms, if any, are usually limited to nonspecific headaches. As pituitary adenomas enlarge, they erode the sella turcica and extend above it to compress the optic nerves, eventually causing bitemporal visual field defects. Rare hemorrhages into large pituitary tumors can cause pituitary apoplexy, producing a characteristic syndrome that requires emergency decompression to preserve vision. Progressive headaches are usually the only warning of this catastrophic event.

Current endocrinologic and MRI techniques greatly facilitate the diagnosis of pituitary tumors, especially if 1-mm cuts and magnified views through the sella are obtained. Medical treatment with bromocriptine may be effective but is slow in yielding results. Its value can be determined by careful endocrinologic follow-up. The drug must be continued indefinitely. Only surgical removal can produce a cure. The safety and efficiency of transsphenoidal pituitary surgery warrant its consideration in all patients, including those with microadenomas that, in the past, could be approached only by a subfrontal craniotomy. Radiotherapy may be required in occasional patients who have large and incompletely removed macroadenomas.

Less common primary extra-axial tumors include *craniopharyngiomas*, related *suprasellar epidermoid cysts*, and *Rathke cleft cysts*. Although they reflect congenital abnormalities of the brain and most frequently become symptomatic in childhood, as many as one third can first appear in adult life, some as late as the sixth decade. In adults, craniopharyngiomas may compress the frontal lobes and are an infrequent cause of dementia. As a group, such tumors are almost always benign and surgically curable if they can be separated from adjacent parasellar structures, optic nerves, and hypothalamus. Pineal region tumors include *pineocytomas* and *pineoblastomas* derived from pineal parenchymal cells, as well as *teratomas* and *germinomas*. These two groups appear with about equal frequency, all having the capacity to be biologically aggressive, making them difficult to manage surgically. Characteristic symptoms and signs include increased intracranial pressure, paresis of upward gaze, pupillary dysfunction, convergence nystagmus, and hydrocephalus due to obstruction of cerebrospinal fluid outflow pathways. Precocious puberty occurs in young males, the result of destruction of the pineal by germinomas. The true pineal tumors may cause delayed puberty. Intracranial *chordomas*, tumors of residual notochordal tissue, are rare and usually arise within the skull at the base of the brain, on the clivus. They are regionally invasive and rarely can be controlled even with aggressive surgery and radiotherapy. *Lipomas* of the skull occur chiefly in midline structures, especially over the corpus callosum. *Arachnoid cysts* can arise anywhere on the surface of the brain; some grow to remarkable size. Most arachnoid cysts are incidental, cause no symptoms, and are best left alone. Their infrequency, as well as that of the other extra-axial tumors mentioned, stands in contrast to the frequency and clinical importance of meningiomas and acoustic neuromas (see Table 484–1).

PRIMARY INTRA-AXIAL TUMORS

This group comprises mainly tumors of the glioma family, including astrocytomas, oligodendrogliomas, ependymomas, medulloblastomas, less common neuroectodermal tumors, and primary brain lymphoma. They possess in common the quality of direct, invasive involvement of the substance of the brain, making them rarely curable by surgical excision owing to the difficulty or impossibility of defining their microscopic borders. Accordingly, gliomas are fundamentally malignant, although some may behave in an indolent manner.

Astrocytomas are the most common of the gliomas. Their cause is unknown, familial examples constituting only 1 per cent of cases. Astrocytomas have occurred as a late consequence of radiation to the head or skull. The most aggressive variant, *glioblastoma multiforme*, accounts for more than 50 per cent of all primary brain tumors. Glioblastoma (astrocytoma IV) is distinguished pathologically from the less aggressive *anaplastic astrocytoma* (astrocytoma II/III) on histopathologic grounds, and the two have important clinical differences. Glioblastoma is more common, is more characteristic of older age groups, and has a median survival time of less than 1 year even with aggressive treatment with surgery, radiotherapy, and chemotherapy. By contrast, patients with anaplastic astrocytoma have a median survival time of slightly more than 2 years. Age is an important variable for both of these tumors: The younger the patient, the better the prognosis. Glioblastoma in children, for example, has

a median survival of more than 2 years. In adults, men are affected more often than women. Anaplastic astrocytomas and glioblastoma occur in multicentric locations in about 5 per cent of cases. In these instances, they may be mistaken for multiple cerebral metastases or for primary brain lymphoma on imaging studies.

Glioblastomas and anaplastic astrocytomas produce a similar clinical picture, and CT or MRI images may be somewhat alike (Fig. 485–2). In most instances, the onset is relatively rapid and heralded by seizures, headaches, and focal neurologic deficits. A minority of patients with these tumors have relevant histories of seizures with onset years before; one assumes that such malignant growths evolve from long-existing, low-grade astrocytomas. Sequential genetic alterations occur in astrocytomas as they become more aggressive. Tissue culture studies show that a high proportion of glioblastomas have increased numbers of chromosome 7 and rearrangements or losses of chromosomes 9p, 10, 17p, and 22. A lower incidence of these abnormalities can be detected in anaplastic astrocytomas. These genomic changes may relate to the presence of an abnormal and possibly unique receptor to epidermal growth factor that is expressed on glioblastoma cells.

Low-grade astrocytomas can pursue a highly variable course, and many of them do not progress to malignancy. Indeed, some are extremely indolent in their growth, so that the median survival time of patients with low-grade astrocytomas is a full 7 years from the time of diagnosis. This prognosis means little in individual cases, however, because the course of these tumors is, as noted before, highly variable. In some patients, low-grade astrocytomas transform to glioblastoma within a few years, whereas other astrocytomas can remain indolent for 10 years or more. Many low-grade astrocytomas will have spread too extensively before diagnosis can be made to allow surgical resection (see Fig. 484–2). By contrast, smaller, favorably situated ones sometimes can be totally removed and the patient apparently cured. Paradoxically, astrocytomas associated with large cysts have a much better prognosis. This favorable circumstance occurs most often in the cerebellum in children and young adults but also in the cerebral hemispheres.

Low-grade astrocytomas, with or without cysts, are invariably solitary, though they may extend into several contiguous brain structures. Some may involve large adjacent areas of frontal and temporal lobe in one hemisphere. Others invade the brain stem, usually producing devastating symptoms and signs in children but sometimes pursuing a surprisingly indolent course in adults. Brain stem astrocytomas cannot be operated upon except in rare instances when they are exophytic. Most infiltrate the brain stem and enlarge it. In a similar way, optic nerve astrocytomas, an uncommon cause of vision loss that affects chiefly children, enlarge the optic nerves and may erode the optic foramina. They grow slowly, are sometimes associated with neurofibromatosis,

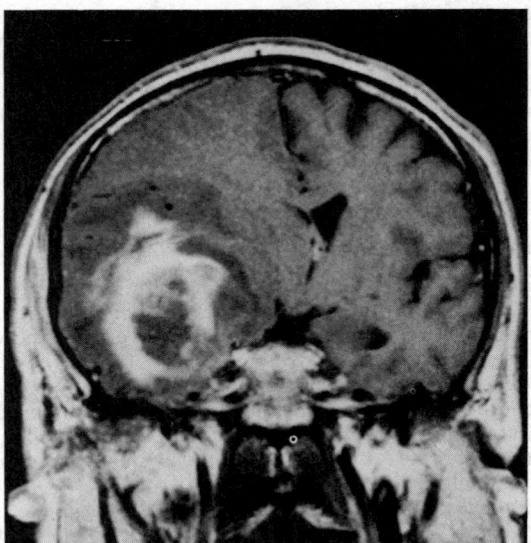

FIGURE 485–2. MRI scan, T_1 gadolinium enhanced, of a temporal lobe glioblastoma, showing typical ring configuration of contrast with central necrosis and marked mass effect.

and are often best left untreated until MRI scanning documents unequivocal tumor growth or vision declines. What to do at that point is controversial. Many authorities withhold radiation treatment for low-grade astrocytomas, at least until all other approaches fail and for as long as the quality of life can be maintained. Two important reasons support this position. One is that little well-controlled evidence indicates that radiation greatly shrinks these tumors, eradicates them, slows their growth, or prevents their conversion into malignant astrocytomas. The other, as already remarked upon, is that radiation damages the normal brain, producing selective neuronal injury, areas of radiation necrosis, or both.

Oligodendrogliomas are the most "benign" of the gliomas, although some develop anaplastic features. Their clinical manifestations usually are indistinguishable from those of low-grade astrocytomas. Seizures are an important early symptom. Oligodendrogliomas occur chiefly in the cerebral hemispheres and especially in the frontal lobes. Many contain flecks of calcium, demonstrable by brain imaging. Complete surgical resection is the therapeutic goal but often cannot be realized because of the size and location of the tumors. Despite their slow growth, most oligodendrogliomas respond well to chemotherapy. As many as 80 per cent improve with a regimen that combines procarbazine, CCNU, and vincristine. This response to chemotherapy seems to be superior to that observed with radiotherapy alone. Oligodendroglioma is the primary intra-axial tumor most likely to bleed spontaneously. In addition, anaplastic oligodendrogliomas tend to spread through the spinal fluid to the meninges. A few of these tumors eventually become so anaplastic that they histologically and clinically resemble glioblastomas.

Medulloblastomas occur chiefly in the region of the fourth ventricle and affect principally children and young adults. They cause characteristic symptoms of cerebellar and brain stem dysfunction. In children, aggressive surgery and radiotherapy yield a 5-year survival of 50 per cent, but many children treated in this manner suffer serious, permanent postradiation intellectual deficits. Several reports indicate that chemotherapy with cyclophosphamide and vincristine improves survival, and other drugs are being tried.

Medulloblastoma is characterized by an amplification of the *c-myc* oncogene and abnormalities of chromosome 17. Medulloblastomas arising in the cerebral hemispheres resemble, or may be the same as, *primitive neuroectodermal tumors* (PNET). These tumors are radiosensitive, like medulloblastomas of the fourth ventricle and cerebellum, and at times respond temporarily to aggressive chemotherapy.

Gangliogliomas are composed of neoplastic astrocytes and abundant dysmorphic neoplastic neurons. They occur chiefly in the temporal lobes of children and young adults, have an unusually slow growth rate, and may have a good prognosis even when untreated. Some are associated with tuberous sclerosis.

Primary brain lymphoma is increasing in frequency among both the acquired immunodeficiency syndrome (AIDS) and, for unknown reasons, the non-AIDS populations. These growths involve the brain diffusely, producing infiltrating and often multicentric tumors that tend to lie deep in the brain and adjacent to ventricular surfaces. Almost all of these tumors are B cell derived; the eye is the only other extranodal site that is regularly involved concomitantly. Only rare patients go on to develop systemic lymphoma, and that occurs late in the disease. Primary brain lymphoma is fundamentally unresectable. It responds temporarily to radiotherapy but is rarely cured. Steroids are an important component of treatment; dexamethasone is uniquely chemotherapeutic for this tumor. Median survivals of 3 years can now be expected with the addition of multidrug chemotherapy to radiotherapy.

Rare intra-axial brain tumors include *choroid plexus papillomas* and *carcinomas*, which are even less common than the benign but troublesome *colloid cysts* of the third ventricle. The last-mentioned lesion may cause hydrocephalus by blocking the outflow of cerebrospinal fluid from the lateral ventricle. *Capillary hemangioblastomas* arise in the cerebellum and elsewhere. They are sometimes associated with an autosomal dominant inherited disorder that includes retinal angiomatosis as well as cysts and tumors of the pancreas, kidneys, and adrenals (von Hippel syndrome). Some of these cerebellar capillary hemangioblastomas secrete erythropoietin and cause polycythemia.

Vascular malformations of the brain are more frequent and important than the above-named rare brain tumors and often can be mistaken for gliomas. They frequently manifest with nonhemorrhagic symptoms such as seizures. They sometimes resemble brain tumors in appearance on CT or MRI, and a distressing number, especially of the capillary variety (which lack large arteriovenous shunts), cannot be imaged by cerebral angiography. Many of these abnormalities lie in the brain stem and thalamus; because they are indistinguishable from brain tumors on even the best imaging studies, they may undergo biopsy as a diagnostic step, with devastating results. Vascular malformations of the brain involving large-caliber vessels are readily diagnosed by CT or MRI even without cerebral angiography.

Abscesses and *granulomas* of the brain cannot usually be distinguished from tumors by CT or MRI alone. If systemic evaluations fail to suggest a proper diagnosis, reliable management demands that biopsy be used. Even in the non-AIDS population, surprising alternatives to the clinical and radiologic diagnosis of a brain tumor are regularly revealed by biopsy. In many instances, potentially tragic errors of management can be avoided by taking a direct approach and studying the tissue of the intracranial lesion.

Fadul C, Wood J, Thaler H, et al.: Morbidity and mortality of craniotomy for excision of supratentorial gliomas. Neurology 38:1374, 1988. *A recent paper that documents convincingly the safety and efficacy of aggressive surgery for gliomas.*

Marks JE: Radiation treatment of brain tumors: Concepts and strategies. Crit Rev Neurobiol 5:93, 1989. *A short, clear, practical review.*

Patchell RA, Tibbs PA, Walsh JW, et al.: A randomized trial of surgery in the treatment of single metastasis to the brain. N Engl J Med 322:494, 1990. *An important paper, not only for its conclusion, which clearly supports surgery for a single metastasis, but also because it is an example of what careful clinical trials in neuro-oncology can achieve. Jerome Posner's editorial comments on this paper, and on metastasis in general, are in the same issue and are masterful.*

Russell DS, Rubinstein LJ: Pathology of Tumours of the Nervous System. 5th ed. Baltimore, The Williams & Wilkins Company, 1989. *The definitive text, indispensable, scholarly, complete, and beautifully redone by Professor Rubinstein just before his death in 1989.*

Shapiro WR: Brain tumors. Semin Oncol 13:1, 1986. *An issue devoted to the subject with wide-ranging and excellent review articles.*

Stewart DJ: The role of chemotherapy in the treatment of gliomas in adults. Cancer Treat Rev 16:129, 1989. *A comprehensive review with an exhaustive list of references.*

Vick NA, Bigner DD (eds.): Neuro-oncology. Neurol Clin 3:4, 1985. *A collection of excellent reviews of the important topics in the field, both clinical and in the basic sciences.*

486 Disorders of Intracranial Pressure

Nicholas A. Vick and David A. Rottenberg

INTRACRANIAL HYPERTENSION

GENERAL PRINCIPLES. Cerebrospinal fluid (CSF) pressure in excess of 250 mm CSF is usually a manifestation of serious underlying neurologic disease. Intracranial hypertension is most often associated with rapidly expanding mass lesions, CSF outflow obstruction, or cerebral venous congestion; however, a variety of systemic and central nervous system disorders may be accompanied by an increase in intracranial pressure (ICP) (Table 486–1). Lumbar CSF pressure may not accurately reflect ICP. In patients with intracranial mass lesions and brain herniation, lumbar CSF pressure may be normal or even low despite grossly elevated supratentorial CSF pressure. Kinking of the aqueduct of Sylvius by adjacent mass lesions, diencephalic–temporal lobe transtentorial herniation, or cerebellar compression of the fourth ventricle, with or without accompanying descent of the cerebellar tonsils into the foramen magnum, each can impede the free transmission of CSF into the lumbar subarachnoid space.

Headache is the principal symptom associated with intracranial hypertension. Headache is produced by traction on pain-sensitive

TABLE 486–1. PATHOGENESIS OF INCREASED INTRACRANIAL PRESSURE

Perturbation	Proximate Cause	Clinical Example
Increased dural sinus venous pressure	Sinus compression or occlusion	Sagittal sinus thrombosis Otitic hydrocephalus Brain tumors
	Increased sinus blood flow	CO_2 retention Arteriovenous malformation
	Increased peripheral venous pressure	Internal jugular vein occlusion Superior vena cava syndrome Congestive heart failure
Increased CSF outflow resistance	Ventricular outflow obstruction	Brain tumors Aqueductal stenosis
	Obliteration of the cisternal and/or convexity subarachnoid space	Meningitis Extradural or subdural masses Cerebral masses or edema
	Plugging of the arachnoid villi	Subarachnoid hemorrhage Infectious polyneuritis Spinal cord tumors
Increased rate of CSF formation	Increased choroidal CSF formation Increased extrachoroidal CSF formation	Choroid plexus papilloma Hypo-osmolality Cerebral edema
Unknown	Increased cerebral volume Increased sagittal sinus pressure Increased CSF outflow resistance	Benign intracranial hypertension

cerebral blood vessels or dura mater lying at the base or, less often, the vertex of the brain. Focal neurologic signs reflect the presence of impending herniation with intermittent vascular compression, midline shift, or axial distortion of the brain stem (see Ch. 443). In the absence of such shifts, increased ICP alone may be asymptomatic. *Papilledema* is the most reliable sign of ICP; but in many patients with increased ICP, it fails to develop. Moreover, in some patients with benign intracranial hypertension, papilledema develops and then subsides spontaneously, although CSF pressure remains pathologically elevated. Papilledema is not synonymous with increased ICP. Ocular hypotony, bilateral optic neuritis, orbital venous stasis, retrobulbar tumors, granulomatous inflammation, or cystic lesions of the optic nerve sheath may produce inflammatory changes in the optic disc indistinguishable from the papilledema caused by the absence of intracranial hypertension. Most papilledema caused by intracranial hypertension, however, is bilateral, whereas most of these other causes affect only one eye at a time. Retinal venous pulsations, when present, imply that CSF pressure is normal or not significantly elevated, but their absence is not helpful diagnostically. Patients with increased ICP, often complain of worsening symptoms, particularly headache, in the morning, perhaps because plateau waves (spontaneous elevations of ICP) occur more commonly during sleep.

The initial treatment of any patient with increased ICP whose neurologic status is deteriorating is aimed at reducing the volume of the intracranial contents in an attempt to prevent brain damage (Table 486–2). If ICP approaches the systolic blood pressure, the cerebral perfusion pressure decreases and irreversible ischemia may develop. Some believe that head elevation and fluid restriction are useful; furosemide, barbiturates, antihypertensives, and muscle relaxants are often used. Almost always, ICP is not the actual cause of the patient's distress; the definitive treatment of intracranial hypertension is ultimately determined by the nature of the underlying pathologic process.

TABLE 486–2. EMERGENCY TREATMENT OF IMPENDING HERNIATION IN ACUTELY DECOMPENSATING PATIENTS

Therapy	Dosage or Procedure	Onset (Duration) of Action
Hyperventilation	Lower Pa_{CO_2} to 25 to 30 mm Hg	Seconds (minutes)
Osmotherapy	Mannitol, 0.5 to 2.0 gm/kg intravenously over 15 minutes, followed by 25 gm as needed	Minutes (hours)
Corticosteroids	Dexamethasone, 50 mg intravenous push, followed by 50 mg daily in divided doses	Hours (days)

Benign Intracranial Hypertension

Benign intracranial hypertension is a syndrome of increased ICP unaccompanied by localizing neurologic signs, intracranial mass lesion, or CSF outflow obstruction in an alert, otherwise healthy-looking patient. These patients are almost always obese and considerably more often women. Benign intracranial hypertension (also called pseudotumor cerebri, serous meningitis, or otitic hydrocephalus) may be associated with a variety of systemic and iatrogenic disorders (Table 486–3). The cause is usually unknown. Chronically increased ICP may give rise to the "empty sella syndrome," which refers to a radiographically globular enlargement of the sella turcica, an incompetent diaphragma sellae, and a compressed but functioning pituitary.

The diagnosis of benign intracranial hypertension is one of exclusion. Intracranial masses (tumors, hematomas, infections) and CSF outflow obstruction must be excluded by computed tomography (CT) or magnetic resonance imaging (MRI). Cerebral angiography is occasionally necessary to rule out dural venous

TABLE 486–3. SYSTEMIC AND IATROGENIC DISORDERS ASSOCIATED WITH BENIGN INTRACRANIAL HYPERTENSION

Commonly Prescribed Drugs
Nalidixic acid
Nitrofurantoin
Phenytoin
Sulfonamides
Tetracycline
Vitamin A

Endocrine and Metabolic Disorders
Addison's disease
Cushing's syndrome
Hypoparathyroidism
Levothyroxine therapy
Menarche, pregnancy, oral contraceptives
Obesity and irregular menses
Steroid therapy/withdrawal

Hematologic Disorders
Cryoglobulinemia
Iron deficiency anemia

Miscellaneous Disorders
Dural venous sinus obstruction/thrombosis
Head trauma
Internal jugular vein ligation
Lupus erythematosus
Middle ear disease

sinus or cortical venous thrombosis. Lumbar puncture, which is usually deferred until CT or MRI has revealed a normal or small ventricular system, is required to confirm the diagnosis. Lumbar spinal fluid pressure is elevated, frequently above 300 mm CSF, but the composition of the fluid is normal; the protein content is usually in the low normal range, below 20 mg per deciliter.

PATHOPHYSIOLOGY. In most cases, the causal mechanism is unknown. Chronically elevated ICP necessarily implies an increase in dural sinus venous pressure, an increase in CSF outflow resistance, an increase in the rate of CSF formation (if it ever really occurs), or some combination of these factors. One or more of these mechanisms must elevate the CSF pressure. Pathogenetic hypotheses that postulate an increase in brain bulk consequent to an increase in cerebral blood volume or in brain water content (interstitial brain edema) do not provide an adequate explanation. The constancy of obesity, often extreme, has suggested the possibility of a disorder of the hypothalamus. But no data have emerged to support this idea. Despite decades of knowledge of the association with obesity, the link remains completely obscure. The strikingly greater incidence in women than in men (4:1) is also unexplained but surely important in some way.

CLINICAL MANIFESTATIONS. Most patients complain of headache. Other common early symptoms include nausea and vomiting, visual disturbances (blurring, obscuration of vision, scotomata), retro-ocular pain, diplopia, tinnitus, and vertigo. Bilateral papilledema, the cardinal feature, is almost invariably present and may be associated with peripapillary retinal hemorrhages, exudates, or both. Vision loss, the only serious complication of benign intracranial hypertension, may occur either early or late in the course of the disease but is seen less than feared. Transient obscurations of vision do not predict subsequent failure of vision. Characteristically, visual field testing reveals enlarged blind spots. Generalized constriction of the peripheral isopters and inferior nasal quadrantanopsia are less frequently observed, as are central and paracentral scotomata. Diplopia, caused by unilateral or bilateral abducens palsy, may develop as a false localizing sign. The remainder of the neurologic examination is always normal. It is important to distinguish pseudopapilledema—an anomalous elevation of the optic disc—from true papilledema, which is prima facie evidence of increased ICP. Anomalous elevation of the disc, which may be associated with identifiable hyaline bodies (drusen), should suggest the diagnosis of retinitis pigmentosa.

In some instances, benign intracranial hypertension is a self-limited disease in which CSF pressure returns to normal as clinical symptoms remit over several months. However, clinical improvement is not always accompanied by a reduction in CSF pressure, and there is a vexing subgroup of patients whose pressure remains persistently elevated after neurologic signs and symptoms have resolved. The course of such cases implies that clinical symptoms may be independent of the absolute magnitude of CSF pressure and that chronically raised ICP may be totally asymptomatic. In addition, despite persistently elevated CSF pressure, patients do not become hydrocephalic. The ventricular system remains small, or no larger than normal. This finding suggests that whatever mechanism "resets" CSF pressure above normal does not predispose to the development of communicating hydrocephalus and that the two conditions are biologically unrelated.

TREATMENT. Unfortunately, no convincing evidence exists that any of the frequently recommended treatment modalities are regularly efficacious. The high rate of spontaneous remission complicates the evaluation of various therapies. At present, four general approaches to symptomatic treatment are used: (1) repeated lumbar puncture, (2) pharmacologic treatment, (3) ventriculosystemic or lumboperitoneal shunting, and (4) incision of the optic nerve sheath.

Frequent (such as alternate day), large-volume lumbar punctures may provide relief of symptoms and document the occurrence of remission. Either it is beneficial or remission occurs independently during the period of treatment. Corticosteroids and diuretics have been the mainstay of medical treatment, and both are effective; or, again, the disease remits during the period of treatment. Dexamethasone, furosemide, and acetazolamide are often tried. CSF shunting procedures are not without risk, and their long-term efficacy remains to be established. Incision of the

optic nerve sheath for the relief of papilledema and vision loss is heroic and fortunately performed infrequently. Now and then, it is done because lumbar punctures, steroids, diuretics, and ventriculosystemic or lumboperitoneal shunting have failed in the rare patient with vision loss.

HYDROCEPHALUS

Hydrocephalus refers to the net accumulation of CSF within the cerebral ventricles and their consequent enlargement. Although acute obstructive hydrocephalus usually produces a sudden increase in intraventricular pressure, CSF pressure is frequently normal (or low) in patients with chronic hydrocephalus. It is customary to distinguish between "noncommunicating" and "communicating" hydrocephalus; the former is produced by lesions that obstruct the intracerebral CSF circulation at or proximal to the foramina of Luschka and Magendie, the latter by obstruction of the basal cisterns or convexity subarachnoid space in such a way that the ventricular system communicates with the spinal subarachnoid space but CSF cannot drain through the arachnoid villi into the superior sagittal sinus. Since both "noncommunicating" and "communicating" types of hydrocephalus are obstructive and both are treated by shunts, the distinction really has less meaning than that usually ascribed to it. Perhaps the important distinction should be between obstructive and nonobstructive hydrocephalus. Ventricular dilatation associated with severe cerebral atrophy, sometimes called "hydrocephalus ex vacuo," is the best example of nonobstructive hydrocephalus. It is so different from obstructive hydrocephalus that it is misleading to use the term hydrocephalus except in the setting of obstruction.

DIAGNOSIS. Hydrocephalus is easily diagnosed by CT or MRI. The diagnosis must take into account the increase in ventricular volume that accompanies normal aging and the presence or absence of cerebral atrophy. Enlargement of the temporal horns and an inability to visualize the sylvian and interhemispheric fissures or cerebral sulci, plus the presence of periventricular lucencies (CT) or periventricular hyperintensity (MRI), favor the diagnosis of hydrocephalus. A normal or small fourth ventricle in the presence of enlarged lateral and third ventricles suggests aqueductal stenosis.

ACUTE VERSUS CHRONIC HYDROCEPHALUS. Sudden, complete ventricular outflow obstruction leads to acute hydrocephalus, coma, and, if untreated, death; partial obstruction is more common and only moderately less dangerous (Table 486–4). Chronic hydrocephalus in the adult is most often caused by aqueductal stenosis or the complications of subarachnoid hemorrhage. Other reported causes and associations are listed in Table 486–4. In many instances, the cause of symptomatic chronic hydrocephalus ("normal-pressure hydrocephalus") cannot be determined. Unequivocally asymptomatic hydrocephalus may be found in approximately 4 per cent of patients over the age of 60 who consult a neurologist for assorted neurologic complaints and who undergo CT scanning.

CLINICAL MANIFESTATIONS. The patient with acute ob-

TABLE 486–4. CAUSES OF HYDROCEPHALUS

Acute
Cerebellar hemorrhage/infarction
Colloid cyst of the third ventricle
Exudative meningitis
Head trauma
Intracranial tumor/hematoma
Spontaneous subarachnoid hemorrhage
Viral encephalitis

Chronic
Aqueductal stenosis
Ectasia and elongation of the basilar artery (rare)
Granulomatous meningitis
Head trauma
Hindbrain malformations
Meningeal carcinomatosis
Brain and spinal cord tumors
Spontaneous subarachnoid hemorrhage
Syringomyelia

**TABLE 486–5. CAUSES OF ABNORMALLY LOW
(0–50 mm) CSF PRESSURE**

Dehydration-hypovolemia
Cranial-intraspinal CSF block
Post–CNS surgery
CSF fistula
Post–LP drainage
Spontaneous-idiopathic; dural nerve sheath tear

structive hydrocephalus may have severe headache, lethargy, signs of increased ICP, papilledema, abducens palsy, and signs of the causative lesion. Hyperactive reflex and bilateral extensor plantar responses are almost invariably present. Ventricular CSF pressure is markedly increased, but if CSF pathways are blocked, this increase may not be transmitted to the lumbar subarachnoid space. Patients with chronic communicating hydrocephalus, including normal-pressure hydrocephalus, have a progressive dementia characterized by forgetfulness and psychomotor retardation, an unsteady gait, and urinary incontinence. Bilateral pyramidal and extrapyramidal signs may be present. Some patients have an overtly parkinsonian disorder. The lumbar CSF pressure is usually normal or nearly normal in range, although overnight recording of ventricular CSF pressure may reveal intermittent waves of elevated pressure.

TREATMENT. Acute hydrocephalus responds dramatically to ventricular drainage and CSF diversion. Treatment of the primary lesion is the treatment of choice, although temporary ventricular decompression or ventriculosystemic shunt may be necessary in some cases. Ventricular shunting has also been used for patients with chronic communicating hydrocephalus. Unfortunately, not all patients respond, or response may be delayed for weeks or months; moreover, there are no reliable clinical or neuroradiologic predictors of shunt response. Recent onset and mild dementia remain better predictors than does isotope cisternography. Absence of cerebral atrophy and temporary improvement after lumbar puncture seem to correlate with benefit from a shunt operation.

INTRACRANIAL HYPOTENSION

CSF pressure measured at a lumbar puncture site, with the patient in the lateral decubitus position, normally ranges from 70 to 200 mm CSF (5 to 15 mm Hg). Low or zero lumbar CSF pressure can be recorded under several circumstances, as indicated in Table 486–5. Symptoms of the first two or three

circumstances on that list are likely to be dominated by the underlying illnesses. The remainder of the circumstances tend to cause a consistent syndrome characterized by severe, throbbing frontal and occipital headache, which usually appears within 30 seconds after the patient assumes an erect posture and which subsides completely upon the patient's lying flat. Associated complaints may include dizziness, nausea, stiff neck, photophobia, and, rarely, diplopia due to an associated abducens nerve palsy. The disorder often arises 3 to 21 days after lumbar puncture. The pathogenesis is similar to that of lumbar puncture headache (p. 2121).

Rare cases of CSF hypotension may occur spontaneously, producing, in previously healthy persons, symptoms similar to those already described. The onset can be acute or subacute and is occasionally precipitated by mild trauma, such as a fall on the buttocks or a casual bump to the head. The cause usually remains unknown, although spontaneous rupture of a dural nerve sheath has been postulated. Diagnosis can be difficult, since spontaneous pressure in the lumbar subarachnoid space can be zero, giving the false impression of missing the thecal sac. Treatment is symptomatic; spontaneous recovery usually requires days to a few weeks. When post–lumbar puncture symptoms are persistent, disabling, or both, an epidural "blood patch" may be indicated. The actual need for blood patches is far less than the frequency with which the procedure is done by worried physicians for impatient sufferers of post–lumbar puncture headache. This procedure involves the injection of 10 ml of the patient's own blood into the epidural space to seal a presumed dural leak. Rarely, in very long-lasting cases, surgical exploration has exposed the dural leak, which must be sutured.

Ahlskog JE, O'Neill BP: Pseudotumor cerebri. Ann Intern Med 97:249, 1982. *A critical review of the clinical syndrome. The section on patient management is excellent.*

Bell WE, Joynt RJ, Sahs AL: Low spinal fluid pressure syndromes. Neurology 10:512, 1960. *A detailed clinical account of the neurologic manifestations of intracranial hypotension. A classic.*

Corbett JJ, Savino PJ, Thompson HS, et al.: Visual loss in pseudotumor cerebri. Arch Neurol 39:461, 1982. *This paper provides a detailed and definitive discussion of the only serious complication, vision loss.*

Lyons HK, Meyer FB: Cerebrospinal fluid physiology and the management of increased intracranial pressure. Mayo Clin Proc 65:684, 1990. *A superb review with excellent references.*

Petersen RC, Bahram M, Laws ER Jr: Surgical treatment of idiopathic hydrocephalus in elderly patients. Neurology 35:307, 1985. *A clinically oriented review of the indications for, risks of, and benefits to be expected from the surgical treatment of normal-pressure hydrocephalus.*

Ropper AH, Kennedy SK: Neurological and Neurosurgical Intensive Care. 2nd ed. Rockville Md., Aspen Publishers Inc, 1988. *Chapter 3 is a brief but excellent resource, with 129 well-chosen references, on all aspects of the treatment of intracranial hypertension.*

SECTION FOURTEEN / INJURY TO THE HEAD AND SPINAL CORD

Lawrence F. Marshall

487 Head Injury

GENERAL CONSIDERATIONS

Head injury is a major public health problem. Not only is traumatic brain injury responsible for more than 50,000 deaths each year in the United States, but a veritable epidemic of less severe injuries results in long-term morbidity because of intellectual and behavioral changes. Although severe head injury is mainly a disease of the young, with its greatest frequency occurring between the ages of 15 and 30 years, it spares no age

or socioeconomic group. Missile injuries, particularly gunshot wounds that penetrate the skull and brain, are more frequent in urban regions of economic and social decay but are far from confined to such areas.

Head injury includes a spectrum of pathologic changes with varying degrees of severity. Underlying almost all nonpenetrating brain trauma is diffuse axonal injury, a condition in which axons are either sheared at the time of impact or degenerate soon after because of irreversible traumatic or ischemic damage to the fibers. Superimposed upon such white matter changes are contusions, which represent hemorrhage mixed into the tissue, and hematomas, more focal collections of blood. Hematomas can occur on the external surface of the dura (extradural hematoma), under the dura and over the underlying brain (subdural hematoma), or within the substance of the brain (intraparenchymal hematoma). In mild and moderate head injury the frequency of surgical hematomas is low. As the degree of neurologic injury increases, however, the severity of diffuse axonal injury rises in almost direct proportion, as does the frequency of intracranial hematomas. Most severe head injuries are characterized by a mixture of pathologic changes consisting of a combination of contusion, diffuse axonal injury, and, in approximately 40 per cent of the cases, hematomas of a size needing surgical attention.

MECHANISM OF BRAIN DAMAGE

Damage to the brain as a result of traumatic injury occurs through a variety of dynamic processes. The impact, in addition to causing immediately variable degrees of abnormality, sets into motion a series of events which, if left uninterrupted, may result in much more severe changes in the tissues and even death. The last 15 years have made it increasingly apparent that primary damage to the brain that at first seems moderate and compatible with a good recovery in many cases may give way to the later development of intracranial hematoma or ischemic brain damage as a result of shock and/or hypoxia.

PRIMARY DAMAGE

Primary traumatic damage to the brain can be separated into three basic processes: (1) diffuse axonal injury (DAI), (2) brain contusion, and (3) intracranial hematoma. DAI always occurs in severe head injury and has a predilection for the brain stem, corpus callosum, and deep white matter. Experimental studies suggest that minor degrees of DAI probably occur in patients who suffer only a *concussion*, i.e., a transient loss of consciousness usually associated with no or minimal residua. With more severe head trauma, the number of areas and the severity of DAI increase proportionally. Some patients with almost immediately fatal injury have shown white matter injuries that completely interrupted long sensorimotor pathways at the cervicomedullary junction.

Brain contusions as shown in Figure 487–1 are common. Traumatic contusions can occur throughout the brain but are more frequent on the cortical surface and in the superficial white matter. Contusions vary in size from less than 2 to 3 ml to much larger lesions. Such areas of tissue injury are important for several reasons. First, they represent areas of at least partially irreversible damage to the brain. Depending on the size and location of the contusions, the consequences can range from undetectable to a dense hemiplegia or aphasia. Second, contusions may act as mass

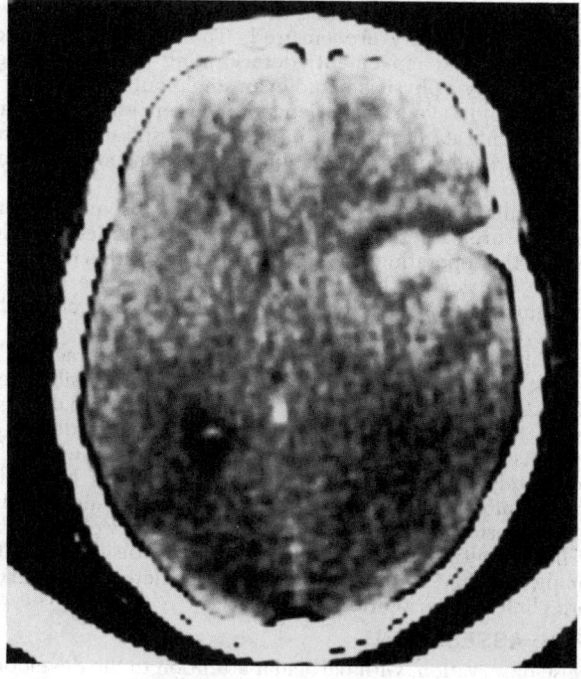

FIGURE 487–1. Brain contusion.

lesions because of the development of secondary edema in the surrounding tissues. Such mixtures of edema and hemorrhagic tissue may enlarge, progressively causing brain displacement and distortion.

The third type of primary injury to the brain, which can develop within hours or days following injury, is intracranial hemorrhage, resulting in epidural, subdural, or intraparenchymal hematomas.

Epidural hematomas usually result from moderate impact injuries. A baseball striking the head, an assault producing only a transient loss of consciousness, or a fall from a horse are typical precipitating events. Extradural hematomas characteristically follow fractures of the temporal bone associated with laceration of the middle meningeal artery. In some instances, the epidural hemorrhage may follow a fracture tearing one of the major draining venous sinuses of the brain. The clinical course of epidural hematoma is classically described as one of a transient loss of consciousness, followed by a period of lucidity and then a rather abrupt deterioration. Actually, this sequence occurs in only a minority of patients: Some lose consciousness immediately following impact, whereas others deteriorate abruptly without a history of initial loss of consciousness.

In the apparently minimally injured patient brought to an emergency room following an ostensibly minor head injury, skull radiographs considerably assist in triage. The absence of a skull fracture makes a hematoma sufficiently unlikely so that, with the exception of the elderly, it is usually safe to send the patient home. Elderly patients, who sometimes develop delayed, venous hematomas, or those with fractures should have computed tomography (CT) scans before being discharged. Such persons should be hospitalized for close observation if the neurologic examination is abnormal or if consciousness is altered in any way. The early detection of extradural hemorrhages is of utmost importance because most affected patients do not initially have irreversible brain damage.

Subdural hematomas are divided into three subgroups: acute, subacute, and chronic. An *acute subdural hematoma* almost always signifies severe brain injury and is associated with significant DAI and contusions in approximately 80 per cent of patients. Most patients with acute subdural hematomas are unconscious from impact, and half die. Nevertheless, approximately 20 per cent develop a more or less isolated subdural hematoma that can expand and cause abrupt deterioration. Recent studies have demonstrated that early surgery for acute subdural hematomas improves outcome, particularly in patients who show little other associated injury to the brain. The frequency of subdural hematomas increases with age, presumably because age-associated brain atrophy more readily allows the expansion of such venous bleedings. Most subdural hematomas are caused by laceration of the bridging veins that drain blood from the surface of the brain into the major sinuses or by laceration of cortical veins in the region of the sylvian fissure. Acute subdural hematomas are especially likely following assaults, falls (particularly in the elderly or in the alcoholic), and motor vehicle accidents when the head is decelerated suddenly on impact.

Subacute subdural hematomas consist of blood clots that underlie the dura on the surface of the brain, developing from 48 hours to 1 week following injury. Some must arise within a few hours of impact but do not reach a sufficient size to cause either depression of consciousness or a focal neurologic deficit. Patients with subacute subdural hematomas are usually older than age 50, occasionally have been taking anticoagulants, and usually have less serious head injuries than those with acute subdural hematomas. Only a small percentage are in coma when first seen and, if the hematoma is diagnosed promptly following its onset, most enjoy a good outcome.

Chronic subdural hematomas have distinct qualities. They usually occur between 1 and 6 weeks following injury, often bilaterally. Many follow trivial injuries, such as striking the head on a door, with no associated loss of consciousness. Indeed, affected patients often forget the inciting event. Patients with chronic subdural hematomas characteristically come from older age groups and many suffer from chronic illnesses, including alcoholism and dementia. Headache, worse in the morning, hypersomnolence or confusion, mild focal weakness, difficulty writing, and unsteadiness are common complaints. Chronic subdural hematomas, because of age-related shrinkage of the brain, may reach a substantial size in excess of 100 cc before the patient seeks medical attention. The mechanisms of this enlargement are poorly understood. Partly, they may be secondary to the development of an overlying capillary membrane which bleeds intermittently into the clot. In addition, tears in the arachnoid membrane may allow one-way entry of CSF from the subarachnoid space. The treatment is relatively straightforward. Some resolve spontaneously. For larger clots, a twist drill hole and puncture of the dura suffice for many patients. Many surgeons leave a drain in the subdural space to allow gravity drainage for 24 to 48 hours following evacuation of the clot. In some instances, particularly if CT scanning reveals an area of increased density, two burr holes are placed to allow irrigation of the subdural space. Craniotomy should be avoided if possible in elderly debilitated patients.

The third type of intracranial hematoma is the *intraparenchymal hemorrhage*, sometimes called intracerebral hemorrhage. These may vary in size from 1 to 100 ml, but they are usually considered for surgical drainage only when they exceed 15 to 20 ml. Intraparenchymal hemorrhages are usually caused by vascular disruption at the time of impact but may be exacerbated by arterial hypertension or coagulation disturbances, especially in alcoholic patients. Since hematomas generally enlarge by approximately 40 per cent during the first 24 hours after injury, those detected on a first CT scan but not operated on should be rescanned within 16 to 24 hours.

PREHOSPITAL CARE AND INITIAL RESUSCITATION

Head injuries often occur under circumstances that traumatize other organ systems as well. Fractures of the long bones and injuries to the chest and abdomen are common, particularly as a result of motor vehicle accidents or pedestrian-vehicle interactions. Until recently, concerns about secondary insults such as shock and hypoxia arose primarily among the more severely injured. Present evidence, however, indicates that even moderate levels of hypotension can convert a reversible brain injury to one with ischemic brain damage. Accordingly, immediate and adequate restitution of blood pressure and intravascular fluid volume and the institution of early steps to prevent or treat hypoxia represent essential preventive measures.

Utilization of the Glasgow Coma Scale (GCS) shown in Table 487–1 provides a simple and reproducible means for serially assessing the head-injured patient. This examination, which assesses the patient's ability to respond to pain, to speak, and to

TABLE 487–1. GLASGOW COMA SCALE

The Glasgow Coma Scale is a practical means of monitoring changes in level of consciousness, based upon eye opening and verbal and motor responses. The responsiveness of the patient can be expressed by summation of the figures. The lowest score is 3, the highest is 15.

Eyes open	Spontaneously (eyes open does not imply awareness)	4
	To speech (any speech, not necessarily a command)	3
	To pain (should not use supraorbital pressure for pain stimulus)	2
	Never	1
Best verbal response	Oriented (to time, person, place)	5
	Confused speech (disoriented)	4
	Inappropriate (swearing, yelling)	3
	Incomprehensible sounds (moaning, groaning)	2
	None	1
Best motor response	Obeys commands	6
	Localizes pain (deliberate or purposeful movement)	5
	Withdrawal (moves away from stimulus)	4
	Abnormal flexion (decortication)	3
	Extension (decerebration)	2
	None (flaccidity)	1
	Total Score	_____

open his or her eyes, when performed in concert with examination of the pupils, serves as an excellent field guide to the severity of injury. All four limbs must be tested for responsiveness either to verbal command or to pain in order not to overlook focal neurologic deficits, such as hemiparesis, paraparesis, or quadriparesis. Changes in pupillary responsiveness suggest brain stem compression, which must be detected early and dealt with promptly if treatment is to be successful.

Patients who cannot follow commands, do not open their eyes to noxious stimuli, and fail to utter words or comprehensible sounds are considered in coma (GCS score of 8 or less) and require early assurance of a secured airway. The frequency of shock and hypoxia increases in proportion to the severity of injury. Hypoxia occurs in approximately one third of all severe head injuries, and significant pulmonary shunting affects more than half. Because of these changes, early controlled intubation, often at the scene of the injury, is highly recommended for severe head injuries. Search for sources of hemorrhage is essential and should include the less obvious ones such as scalp lacerations and pelvic fractures. If such cannot be found, neurogenic hypotension should be suspected. Fluid resuscitation should begin at the scene, with recognition of the difficulties in administering large amounts of fluid under these conditions. Current evidence suggests that even with modern paramedic systems shock often receives inadequate treatment in the field and that newer strategies, utilizing hypertonic saline or pressor agents, may be required. Table 487–2 demonstrates the influence of shock on outcome in 699 head injury cases treated at four neurosurgical head injury centers. As noted, the presence of hypotension at outset almost doubled the mortality suffered by the entire cohort.

Once the airway has been secured and fluid resuscitation initiated, stabilization of the cervical spine and transport become the next priorities. In general, the neck should be placed in a neutral position. However, if the patient is awake and chooses to hold the neck in an unusual position, it should not be forced to the neutral position. Some patients with cervical spine fractures but no neurologic deficit have been made quadriplegic by ill-advised attempts to straighten the neck.

Upon arrival at the hospital the priorities of maintaining airway and circulation remain uppermost. Adequate oxygenation with a PaO_2 above 80 and moderate hyperventilation to $PaCO_2$ of 27 to 30 mm Hg to control brain swelling are initial objectives. A mean systolic blood pressure of at least 100 mm Hg is mandatory.

CT SCANNING

The availability of rapid-sequence CT scanning has revolutionized the care of the head injured. Patients with focal neurologic deficits and severe injuries, i.e., a GCS score of 8 or less, should receive immediate CT scanning as soon as a secured airway and hemodynamic stability are ensured. To minimize the risks of transportation and movement, deteriorating patients should be accompanied by a physician, and even stable but seriously injured patients should have an experienced emergency room or trauma nurse present at all times. Supervised respiratory assistance should assure adequate ventilation during transport and during the scan.

The results of CT scans heavily influence subsequent management. If a surgical lesion is demonstrated, the patient should be taken to the operating room immediately. Otherwise severe traumatic injuries are best treated in intensive care units, with lesser injuries being handled in units that provide close observation.

Several findings on the CT scan, other than intracranial hematomas, merit close attention and forewarn of possible deterioration. Compression or absence of the mesencephalic cistern augurs a high risk of intracranial hypertension and death, even in patients whose clinical examination at the time suggests only a moderately severe injury. Unilateral or bilateral hemispheric swelling almost always predicts the likelihood of dangerous intracranial hypertension. In patients showing such swelling or those who have multiple areas of hemorrhagic contusion, repeat CT scanning within 24 hours is essential to detect abnormalities before clinical deterioration takes place.

SERIAL ASSESSMENT

Close observation, with particular attention to the development of tachypnea and bradycardia, is important. Table 487–3 lists the

TABLE 487–2. OUTCOME RELATED TO SECONDARY INSULT AT TIME OF ARRIVAL AT HOSPITAL FOR MUTUALLY EXCLUSIVE INSULTS

Secondary Insults	Number of Patients	Per Cent of Total Patients	Outcome Percentages		
			Good–Moderate	*Severe–Vegetative*	*Dead*
Total cases	699	100.0	42.9	20.5	36.6
Neither	456	65.2	51.1	21.9	27.0
Hypoxia	78	11.2	44.9	21.8	33.3
Hypotension	113	16.2	23.7	14.2	60.1
Both	52	7.4	5.8	19.2	75.0

Hypoxia = PaO_2 <60 mm Hg; hypotension = SBP <90 mm Hg.

signs that portend potential intracranial catastrophe. An increase in systolic blood pressure of 15 mm Hg or more or a decline in heart rate of 15 beats per minute often gives the first hints of the development of an intracranial mass lesion.

Tachypnea holds particular importance. Respiratory rates over 20 per minute are abnormal in patients over 15 years of age and imply the development of pulmonary edema or infection. Similarly, increasing headache is often present but overlooked; it may reflect a rising intracranial pressure. The use of continuous flow sheets in an intermediate care setting or in a neurologic observation unit assists in monitoring the course and detecting subtle changes in vital signs.

THE INTENSIVE CARE MANAGEMENT OF THE SEVERELY HEAD INJURED

The overriding objective in the care of the severely head injured is to prevent further insults to the traumatized brain. The situation requires meticulous attention to detail and continuous vigilance to detect and counteract deterioration in hemodynamic, pulmonary, and neurologic function. The brain's vulnerability to secondary injury extends beyond shock and hypoxia. Fever increases the metabolic rate of the tissue by approximately 13 per cent for each degree Celsius, a demand that the already injured brain may not be able to meet. Seizures are a major threat—they increase tissue energy requirements and trigger a rise of up to 400 per cent in cerebral blood flow, accentuating any existing increase in the intracranial pressure.

The objectives in the critical care of head injury shown in Table 487–4 illustrate an approach that includes both the avoidance of systemic insults to the brain and the treatment of intracranial hypertension. Elevations of intracranial pressure above the normal of 15 mm Hg accompany most severe head injuries, and much evidence suggests that they contribute directly to further tissue damage if left untreated. Compression of the mesencephalic cistern, usually readily detected by CT scans and generally referred to as "diffuse swelling," is frequent in patients with even moderately severe injuries. Since mortality in such cases can be reduced from approximately 85 to 35 per cent with early and rapid intervention for intracranial hypertension, most academic neurosurgical centers record the intracranial pressure (ICP) continuously so as to treat intracranial hypertension whenever it develops. Several available techniques are discussed in the references to this chapter.

ICP monitoring should not be initiated in patients with coagulation disturbances. Patients in whom multiple contusions can be detected by a first CT scan can be assumed to have a trauma-related coagulopathy that will correct itself within a few hours, after which a ventricular cannula can be inserted.

The treatment of *traumatic intracranial hypertension* is central to the intensive care of the critically brain-injured patient. The cornerstone of management is to deliver moderate hyperventilation, maintaining a $PaCO_2$ in the 27 to 32 mm Hg range so as to obtain moderate intracerebral arterial vasoconstriction. Levels of more extreme hyperventilation may be counterproductive by producing excessive vasoconstriction. The head should be maintained in a neutral position because turning it to the right or left may introduce venous obstruction and a rise in ICP. Also, the head should be elevated to not more than 30 degrees. Intravascular volume must be maintained using balanced salt solutions. Dextrose and water should be avoided. Head trauma often induces salt retention initially so that half-normal saline may be

TABLE 487–3. SIGNS OF POTENTIAL INTRACRANIAL CATASTROPHE AND WHAT THEY MAY SIGNIFY

Signs	Changes	Implications
Respiration	Rate >20	Pulmonary edema or pneumonitis
Pulse	Change >10/min and/or heart rate <60	Each may indicate elevated ICP with transtentorial herniation
Blood pressure	Change in systolic >15 mm Hg and/or widening pulse pressure	
Headache*	Is it increasing?	Often indicates increased ICP
Pupils	Enlargement Asymmetry Irregular shape (oval) Decrease in reactivity Change from preresuscitation	Transtentorial herniation until proven otherwise
Motor	Decrease of 1 point on GCS New focal deficit	Increased mass effect New hemorrhage Recurrent hemorrhage
Level of consciousness	Abrupt decrease	Increased ICP Seizures Hypotension
	Transient	Seizures Hypoxia
	Progressive decrease	Rehemorrhage Brain stem involvement Septicemia Electrolyte imbalance Vasospasm Hydrocephalus

*All changes except headache may occur in both awake and unconscious patients. GCS = Glasgow coma scale; ICP = intracranial pressure.

TABLE 487–4. ICU MANAGEMENT OF SEVERE HEAD INJURY AND INTRACRANIAL HYPERTENSION

1. Head elevated 30 degrees and in neutral plane
2. Intubation with controlled ventilation to an arterial $PaCO_2$ of 27–30 mm Hg
3. Good pulmonary toilet
4. Maintain fluid balance with 0.5 normal saline
5. Maintain systolic arterial pressure between 100 and 160 mm Hg
6. Maintain cerebral perfusion pressure >70 mm Hg (CPP = MAP − ICP)
7. Adequate sedation
8. Muscle relaxants prn (must use sedation concurrently)
9. Maintain normothermia
10. Adequate anticonvulsant therapy
11. Ventricular drainage for intracranial hypertension
12. Mannitol, 0.25 mg/kg, if No. 11 fails or is not available
13. Hypnotic for elevated ICP in patients with diffuse or hemispheric swelling

most useful to meet fluid needs. Since hyperglycemia exacerbates ischemic brain injury in experimental animals and there is an important component of ischemia in many patients suffering head injury, it appears wise to avoid glucose infusions.

Muscle relaxants with vecuronium or other short-acting agents may be helpful in controlling ICP, but should not be used without adequate sedation. Morphine sulfate by continuous infusion of 2 to 8 mg per hour is the least complicated and most effective regimen. Details of ventricular drainage and other specialized techniques for controlling dangerous levels of intracranial pressure are discussed in the references to this chapter.

Anticonvulsants have a limited but important use in acute traumatic head injury. Temkin et al. found that phenytoin given for the first 7 days after injury reduced the incidence of post-traumatic epilepsy during that period, but no study has shown a protective effect when medication was continued beyond the first week.

THE LONG-TERM CONSEQUENCES OF SEVERE HEAD INJURY

Severe head injury causes serious long-term intellectual and behavioral impairment. Most such patients suffer from residual difficulties in recent memory, abstract thinking, and the rapidity of information processing. Depression, fatigue, and impetuosity accentuate these cognitive deficits. By contrast, long-term deficits of motor function are relatively uncommon and considerably less socioeconomically important. Many rehabilitation programs have been developed to assist the severely head injured in the management of these problems. Therapies tailored to individual needs often favorably influence the long-term outcome and can be cost-effective if appropriate objectives are defined early and the program is appropriately structured. Counseling of the family is essential. Divorce, suicide, and spouse abuse are common eventualities but can be reduced in frequency by early intervention.

MINOR HEAD INJURY

Minor head injury is defined as including a GCS score of 13 to 15 following emergency room or hospital admission combined with a return to a normal level of consciousness within 24 hours. Most but not all such patients have normal CT scans. Patients suffering minor head injuries characteristically experience early post-traumatic problems with recent memory, concentration, and abstract thinking. In most patients such problems subside within the first 1 to 3 months following minor injury, although approximately 15 per cent are left with cognitive deficits that, although improved, do not completely remit. Age is a specific risk factor, and many elderly persons develop chronic dizziness and disequilibrium after even minor trauma. Such symptoms are classified as a *post-traumatic or postconcussive syndrome*. Past medical opinion has regarded such symptoms as psychogenic or prompted by hopes for secondary gain. Recent evidence fails to support such associations and indicates that a small percentage of patients suffer modest but permanent residual cognitive impairment.

Many patients with minor head injuries suffer transiently from insomnia, depression, and headache. Early support and reassur-

ance from the physician often improve these symptoms. If headache persists for more than 60 to 90 days, propranolol, 30 to 60 mg in three divided doses, may bring relief.

MODERATE HEAD INJURY

Patients who have not been rendered comatose by their injuries but have a depressed level of consciousness for several hours or days following injury are classified as having suffered moderate head injuries. These patients have GCS scores of 9 to 12. Such patients almost always suffer measurable cognitive and behavioral difficulties over the long term. Nevertheless, many eventually return to gainful employment. Even so, the potential for social disruption is high, and traits of impetuousness and heightened irritability often create socioeconomic problems. Depression is frequent and may respond to tricylic antidepressants. Intervention, using a variety of psychological services including social workers and psychiatrists, has a more favorable impact if carried out early rather than after the problems have overwhelmed the patient and family.

Cooper P (ed.): Head Injury, 2nd ed. Baltimore, Williams & Wilkins, 1987. *A modern definitive discussion of head injury.*
Levin HS, Eisenberg HM, Benton AL: *In* Levin HS (ed.): Mild Head Injury. New York, Oxford University Press, 1989. *A comprehensive review of the sequelae of minor and moderate brain injury.*
Marshall SB, Marshall LF, Vos H, Chesnut R: Neuroscience Critical Care: Pathophysiology and Patient Management. Philadelphia, W. B. Saunders Co., 1990. *Particular emphasis on assessment of the neurologically impaired patient, modern neuroradiology, and intensive care.*
Stein SC, Ross SE: The value of computed tomographic scans in patients with low-risk head injuries. J Neurosurg 26:638, 1990. *Incidence of CT abnormalities in the patient with minor head injury.*

488 Spinal Cord Injury

The cervical spine sacrifices bony mass in order to allow tremendous flexibility and rotatory capacity. In contrast, the lumbar spine is ideally designed for its major function of weight bearing. Modern modes of transport and recreation have made the spine and its encased spinal cord particularly vulnerable to injury. Fortunately, most injuries to the spinal column do not result in spinal cord injury, but there are still approximately 35 spinal cord injuries per million Americans each year. In addition to the neurologic deficit that such injuries can produce, they often result in persistent and severe pain and, if not treated properly, bony deformity. The mortality rate of spinal cord injury has fallen to less than 5 per cent, so that long-term survival is now the rule. Associated with this, however, are tremendous costs stemming from medical treatment, lost occupations, and the need for life-long medical and emotional support systems for many paraplegics and nearly all quadriplegics.

NATURE OF THE INJURY

About half of all serious spinal injuries affect the cervical level, with nearly 50 per cent of such cases becoming quadriplegic. Next most frequent is high thoracic cord damage, with the remainder distributed variously at lower spinal levels. Three major abnormalities damage the tissue: destruction from either direct trauma, e.g., gunshot wounds, or secondary bone displacement; compression by displaced or broken bones; and ischemia due to compression or laceration of spinal arteries. Postinjury edema of both spinal soft tissues and the cord itself accentuates these changes. Reversal or prevention of such post-traumatic alterations may explain the beneficial effects of methylprednisolone mentioned below.

Spinal cord injuries can be categorized as complete or incomplete. Acute, complete injuries most often produce acute *spinal shock*, with loss of all sensorimotor functions including flaccidity and loss of reflexes at and below the level of injury. A few such cases may show sustained priapism. Less severe injuries can produce a *central cord syndrome* resulting from ischemia or hematomas of the cervical cord (Fig. 488–1), resulting in a syringomyelia-like clinical syndrome characterized by weakness in the distal upper extremities combined with impaired or lost pain and temperature sensations in the arms but sparing of touch and often of all functions below the cervical cord level. The upper extremity weakness generally improves in such cases. Other patterns of cord injury may produce an anterior spinal artery syndrome (see Ch. 493) or can result in partial hemisection, producing distal weakness and proprioceptive loss ipsilateral to the cord damage accompanied by contralateral pain and temperature impairment.

EMERGENCY MANAGEMENT

For the physician and internist, the most important elements in treating traumatic spinal cord injury arise at the scene of the accident or within the first few hours of arrival at the hospital. After that time, effective management increasingly depends on experienced neurosurgeons or orthopedists, supplemented if at all possible by the resources of a tertiary care center equipped to meet the needs of acute paraplegic or quadriplegic injuries.

At the site of injury three major concerns are paramount: maintenance of ventilation, protection against shock, and neck immobilization to prevent further spinal cord damage.

Damage to high thoracic or cervical spinal levels creates the immediate risk of ventilatory failure due to acute paralysis of intercostal-abdominal muscles, loss of diaphragmatic activity, or both. Untoward movement of the neck in such patients risks converting a partial injury to a complete one, making nasotracheal intubation preferable to standard orotracheal intubation. Tracheostomy or cricothyroidotomy should be avoided if possible because these procedures often put pressure on the vertebral column.

Severe hypotension often follows cervical injury because the lesion interrupts the descending sympathetic pathways; bradycardia characteristically accompanies the low blood pressure. Such neurogenic hypotension can be distinguished from hypovolemic shock by the tachycardia of the latter. In either case, the legs should be elevated gently to improve venous return and fluids delivered in amounts sufficient to counter both the traumatic and neurogenic aspects of the problem. It is not widely realized that severe hypotension during the early minutes or hours after injury is itself a potential cause of spinal cord damage.

The neck and spine should be immobilized as gently as possible at the injury site, using a carrying board, sandbags and adhesive tape, or a Philadelphia collar. Soft collars are ineffective. The head is best maintained in a neutral position but should not be forced into such an attitude lest the maneuver induce further spinal cord damage.

Recent controlled studies indicate that giving large doses of methylprednisolone within 8 hours of the onset of trauma appears to reduce the degree of eventual neurologic dysfunction in acute traumatic paraplegia. Dose levels used in the study trial included immediate intravenous administrations of 30 mg per kilogram of body weight of the steroid followed by continuous infusion of 5.4 mg per kilogram per hour for the next 23 hours. Treatment begun more than 8 hours after injury was not helpful.

HOSPITAL CARE

The medical care of spinal cord injuries is a specialty unto itself. Such patients often are critically ill owing to a combination of systemic injuries, blood and fluid loss, various fractures, and infections. Considerable expertise is required for the accurate interpretation of spinal radiographs. Patients with cervical fracture-dislocations usually are placed in strong traction prior to administering definitive surgical repair. Usually, the latter step is deferred until patients regain a stable medical course. Injuries to the thoracic or lumbar level provide an exception to this principle; since traction has little benefit, open surgery, when indicated, usually is carried out earlier.

Medical management of spinal injuries emphasizes the guiding principles of trauma care. Rotating beds reduce the risk of decubitus erosions, meticulous chest physiotherapy and pulmonary toilet can minimize lung complications, and cardiovascular as well as fluid-electrolyte stability requires continuous attention. Pneumatic antiembolism stockings, vigorous fluid replacement, and early mobilization have reduced the frequency of deep venous thromboses in such patients by one third. Anticoagulants should be considered for severely immobilized patients who do not require early surgery. Nearly all patients with traumatic cord injury require prolonged urinary bladder catheterization. Meticulous effort to prevent infection should be applied from the start and, whenever staff experience permits, indwelling catheters should be replaced by intermittent catheterization at 4- to 6-hour intervals. Acidification of the urine with vitamin C or cranberry juice helps to reduce the incidence of infection.

Trauma patients require heavy nutrition to feed the demands of wound healing and the efforts of rehabilitation. For those who cannot eat, enteral solutions sufficient to meet caloric need can be started within 3 to 4 days after injury. Every effort should be given to supplying appetizing food and vitamins subsequently.

Autonomic dysfunction complicates the convalescence of more than half of patients who suffer severe spinal cord injuries above the midthoracic level. Disconnected distal autonomic pathways can induce a variety of troublesome phenomena, including systemic hypertension, reflex sweating, skin flushing, headache, and painful flexor spasms of the lower extremities. Bladder distention and infection are frequent factors producing such reflex dysautonomia and require urgent treatment. Diazepam, in small doses initially, and baclofen given chronically may be useful for the treatment of reflex spasms. Some centers have successfully employed the continuous intrathecal administration of baclofen by an indwelling pump to prevent disabling reflex spasms of this type.

PHYSICAL AND OCCUPATIONAL THERAPY AND REHABILITATION

Almost all patients with spinal cord injury require prolonged postacute care. Those with complete transections have suffered a devastating injury with life-long functional and psychiatric con-

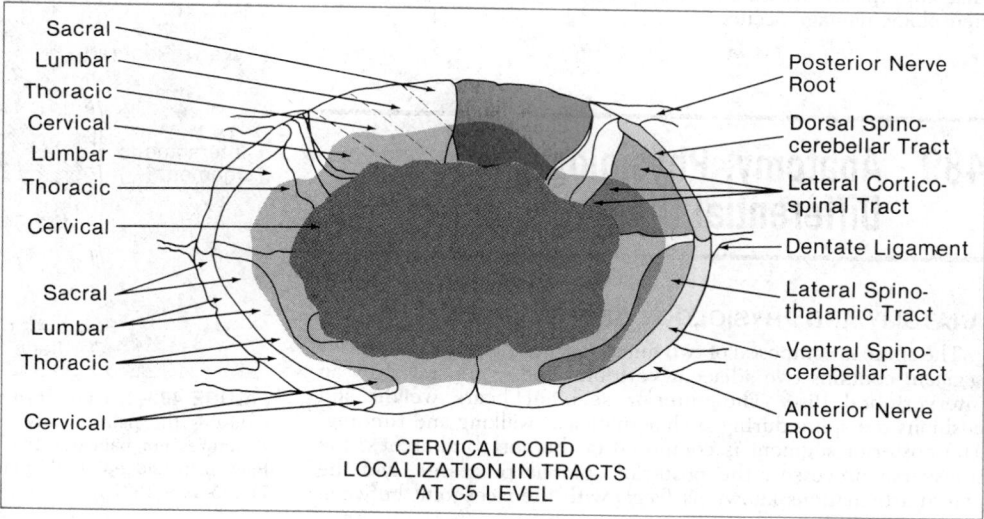

FIGURE 488–1. Diagrammatic description of the spinal pathways at the lower cervical level showing the usual distribution of the contusion-hemorrhage that causes a central cord syndrome.

Sacral
Lumbar
Thoracic
Cervical
Lumbar
Thoracic
Cervical
Sacral
Lumbar
Thoracic
Cervical

Posterior Nerve Root
Dorsal Spinocerebellar Tract
Lateral Corticospinal Tract
Dentate Ligament
Lateral Spinothalamic Tract
Ventral Spinocerebellar Tract
Anterior Nerve Root

CERVICAL CORD
LOCALIZATION IN TRACTS
AT C5 LEVEL

sequences. Early physical and emotional therapy is critical in minimizing these effects. Early range of motion prevents contractures, diminishes the risk of venous thrombosis, protects the skin, and boosts morale. A comprehensive and individualized management plan is essential. Patients and family members must be counseled in detail about probable changes in lifestyle. All of these features are best carried out in experienced rehabilitation centers that can provide assistance in home modification, driver retraining, and vocational rehabilitation. Depression following an initial period of denial occurs in almost all patients and may be masked by jocularity. If the rehabilitation team moves quickly to provide emotional as well as physical management, many patients with spinal cord injury can return to a competitive place in modern society. Most of the injured do best if a single physician

organizes the long-term aspects of urinary tract management, skin care, sexual problems, and emotional-vocational needs.

Bracken MB, Shepard MJ, Hellenbrand KG, et al.: A randomized, controlled trial of methylprednisolone or naloxone in the treatment of acute spinal cord injury. N Engl J Med 322:1405, 1990. *The first study to clearly demonstrate the efficacy of pharmacologic treatment for spinal cord injury.*

Cooper PR: Management of posttraumatic spinal instability. In Neurosurgical Topics. Park Ridge, IL, American Association of Neurological Surgeons, 1990. *Detailed, step-by-step management of spinal cord injury.*

Marshall LF, Knowlton S, Garfin SR, et al.: Deterioration following spinal cord injury. A multicenter study. J Neurosurg 66:400, 1987. *A demonstration that most patients have an identifiable cause of deterioration.*

Temkin NR, Dikmen SS, Wilensky AJ, et al.: A randomized, double-blind study of phenytoin for the prevention of post-traumatic seizures. N Engl J Med 323:497, 1990. *Four hundred and four patients with serious head trauma were randomly assigned to treatment with phenytoin or placebo within 24 hours of injury; significant reduction in seizure incidence (p < 0.001) occurred only between drug loading time and day 7.*

SECTION FIFTEEN / MECHANICAL LESIONS OF THE SPINE AND RELATED STRUCTURES

Jerome B. Posner

The vertebral column, its contents (spinal cord, exiting nerve roots) and surrounding structure (spinal ligaments, paraspinous muscles) are responsible for some of the most common afflictions of man. Neck and/or back pain originating from these structures affects almost every individual at some time of life. Each year 4 per cent of Americans suffer an episode of low back pain. The disorder ranks next to alcoholism as the leading cause of time lost from work. More than 200,000 spinal operations are performed in the United States annually.

Most back and neck pain is transient and neither life-threatening nor associated with obvious pathologic abnormalities. However, in the few patients who suffer from serious structural disease of the spine or spinal cord, severe neurologic abnormalities may develop which, unless correctly diagnosed and treated, may lead to paralysis, sensory loss, and incontinence. Because the pathophysiology of most neck and back pain is poorly understood, the physician often encounters patients in whom he can neither make a certain diagnosis nor prescribe rational therapy. From this vast group he must cull the small number of patients suffering potentially remediable structural disease of the spine so that appropriate treatment can be instituted before permanent neurologic damage occurs.

489 Anatomy, Physiology, and Differential Diagnosis

ANATOMY AND PHYSIOLOGY OF THE SPINE

The spine is composed of two functional segments. The *anterior segment* contains two adjacent vertebral bodies separated by an intervertebral disc. The anterior segment bears weight and cushions the spine during such activities as walking and running. The posterior segment is composed of the vertebral arches, the transverse processes, the posterior spinous processes, and the paired articulations known as *facets* with the facet joint between

them. The *posterior segment* is non–weight-bearing but protects the contained spinal cord and nerve roots and allows the spine to move in extension and rotation. The midcervical and lower lumbar levels are particularly mobile, making them susceptible to mechanical disorders such as osteoarthritis and herniated discs (see Ch. 490). Several ligaments offer the spine passive support and paravertebral muscles support the spine actively by voluntary and reflex contraction.

Only parts of the spine are pain-sensitive (Fig. 489–1). The *periosteum* of the vertebral body is pain-sensitive so that compression fractures are at least initially painful. The *intervertebral disc* is probably not pain-sensitive. However, if the disc bulges and compresses the outer layers of the annulus fibrosus or the posterior longitudinal ligament, pain may result even if the nerve root is not involved. Posteriorly, the synovium-lined *facet joints* are pain-sensitive and may be an important source of neck and back pain, although the intraspinal ligaments holding the poste-

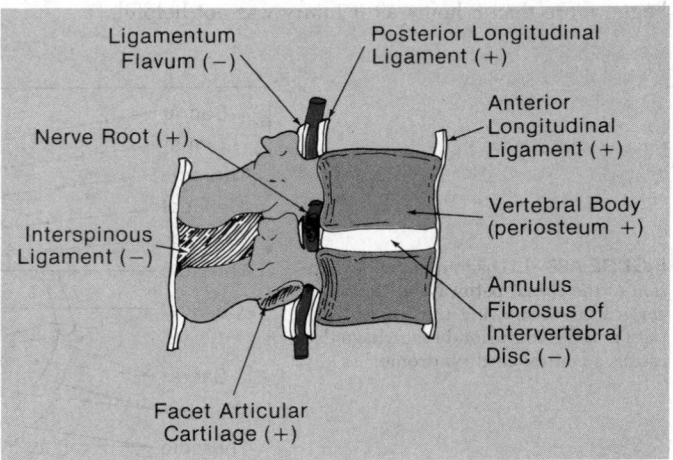

FIGURE 489–1. Pain-sensitive structures of the spine. This lateral view indicates the pain-sensitive structures with a plus sign (+) and those structures not pain-sensitive with a minus sign (−). (From Posner JB: Back pain and epidural spinal cord compression. Med Clin North Am 71:185–205, 1987.)

rior elements are not. Most of the pain-sensitive structures are innervated by the recurrent meningeal or sinuvertebral nerves, a branch of each spinal nerve that arises just distal to the dorsal root ganglion and re-enters the spinal canal through the intervertebral foramen. The sinuvertebral nerves also receive fibers from neighboring grey rami or directly from thoracic sympathetic ganglia. *Sympathetic nerves* contain sensory fibers and probably play a role in the transmission of pain. The *paravertebral muscles* surrounding and supporting the spine are also pain-sensitive, particularly when overstretched or in spasm. These muscles are probably the most common source of both acute and chronic neck and back pain (myofascial pain syndromes). The pain-sensitive *nerve root* usually occupies only a small portion of the intervertebral foramen through which it exits the spinal canal. When the spine is extended (i.e., hyperlordotic posture), the intervertebral foramen becomes smaller, potentially impinging on the nerve root and leading to overlap of the facet joints, giving potential irritation of pain-sensitive synovial membranes. Thus, pain in patients with intervertebral disc or facet joint disease may be exacerbated by extension and relieved somewhat by flexion of the spine. Additionally, hyperlordosis, a common postural abnormality, sometimes leads to chronic low back pain; most back exercises aim at developing a flat or slightly flexed, but not hyperlordotic, lumbar spine.

The spinal cord and its attached motor, sensory, and autonomic nerve roots are the primary occupants of the spinal canal. The spinal cord itself extends in the adult from the first cervical to the first lumbar vertebral body, and the spinal roots continue in the subarachnoid space to the second sacral vertebra. The caudal portion of the spinal cord is called the *conus medullaris*, and the bunched lumbar and sacral roots that exit below the cord are the *cauda equina*.

Within the canal several processes can compress or deform the spinal cord and its roots. The resulting signs and symptoms depend on the location of the abnormality, its speed of development, and whether it affects the nerve roots or the spinal cord alone. In the cervical spine, the spinal cord and vertebral segments lie at approximately the same level; thus, the C5 vertebral body marks the C5 spinal segment and emerging nerve roots are virtually horizontal. The more caudad spinal cord segments and vertebral segments move out of alignment so that thoracic spinal cord segments gradually become two to three levels higher than the corresponding vertebral segments (e.g., T8 vertebral body marks the T11 thoracic segment). Most of the lumbar and sacral cord is found between T10 and L1 lumbar segments. As a result, the nerve roots travel a descending pathway in the subarachnoid space before exiting via the vertebral foramen. In addition, because there is a C8 spinal segment and no C8 vertebral body, cervical spine nerve roots exit above the vertebral body with the same number (e.g., the C4 root exits between C3 and C4). Thus, a herniated C4–C5 disc may compress the C5 or C6 root but not the C4 root.

In the thoracic and lumbar spine, nerve roots leave the intervertebral foramen above the disc (e.g., the L4 root exits between L4 and L5 and the S1 root between L5 and S1) so that a herniated disc between L4–L5 vertebral bodies usually compresses the L5 nerve root; a herniated disc between L5 and S1 usually compresses the S1 root (Fig. 489–2). If the disc protrudes medially (less common than laterally protruding discs), an L4–L5 disc may compress sacral roots rather than the L5 lumbar root. Only if the disc completely extrudes into the vertebral canal does an L4–L5 disc compress the L4 root.

The size of the vertebral canal relative to the spinal cord varies from level to level and among persons. There is generally more space in the lumbar and cervical areas than in the thoracic area. Thus, herniated thoracic discs (uncommon) are more likely to cause myelopathy than cervical or lumbar herniations. In some individuals the spinal canal is congenitally small (spinal stenosis). Disc herniation or osteoarthritis is more likely to cause myelopathy in these individuals than in those with capacious canals.

TYPES OF PAIN

The cardinal symptom of lesions of the spine or its contents is pain. The type and location of pain often help substantially in diagnosis.

LOCAL PAIN. Local pain results from the irritation of nerve

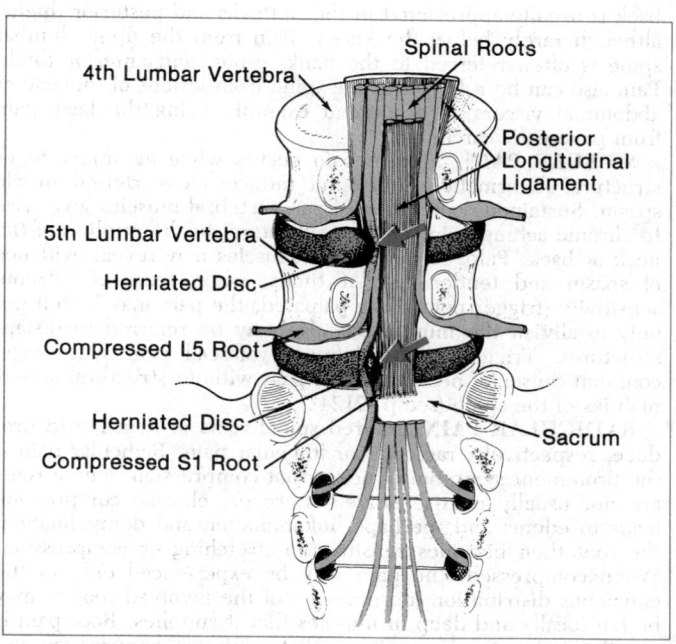

FIGURE 489–2. Nerve root compression by herniated disc. The figure illustrates that the posterior longitudinal ligament tapers as it reaches the lower lumbar area, leaving a weakened area laterally allowing disc herniation. An L4–L5 disc is shown lateral to the L5 root, displacing it medially; a herniated disc between L5 and S1 displaces the root laterally. (From Posner JB: Back pain and epidural spinal cord compression. Med Clin North Am 71:185–205, 1987.)

endings at the site of the pathologic process. Metastatic tumors and osteoporotic collapse of a vertebral body cause pain at the site of the lesion by irritation of nerve endings in the periosteum surrounding the vertebral body. Metastatic tumors involving the vertebral body that do not distort the periosteum are usually painless. Intervertebral discs cause local pain when they compress nerve endings in the anulus fibrosus or posterior longitudinal ligament. Local pain is usually steady and aching but may be intermittent, occurring particularly when the involved structure is moved. Local pain is usually associated with tenderness to palpation or percussion. The site of local pain is diagnostically helpful. Most spine pain from mechanical causes (e.g., herniated disc) occurs either in the neck or low back, since these structures are most mobile and more subject to injury. However, tumors often strike the thoracic area, and osteoporotic vertebral collapse often affects the structurally weaker thoracic vertebral bodies.

The *character* of the local pain is helpful diagnostically. Pain caused by lumbar muscle or ligamentous strain or by herniated disc usually disappears when the patient lies recumbent. Herniated lumbar disc pain is often exacerbated by sitting and relieved by standing or walking. The pain of spinal stenosis, on the contrary, is often absent when lying or sitting and occurs only when the patient walks. Vertebral metastases with or without epidural spinal cord compression cause pain that is often more prominent when lying and sometimes is relieved by sitting up; many patients with spinal cord compression elect to sleep in a sitting position. Even if pain is absent in the lying position, movement such as turning over in bed or arising may be particularly painful.

REFERRED PAIN. Referred pain arises from deep somatic or visceral structures and is perceived at a distant area within the same spinal segment but not necessarily in dermatomal distribution (radicular pain, see below). In many instances, the distribution is sclerotomal or myotomal. Referred pain, like local pain, has a deep aching quality and is often associated with tenderness of subcutaneous tissues and muscles at the site of referral. Maneuvers that affect local pain usually have the same effect on referred pain. Pain referred from pathologic abnormalities of the cervical spine often is either just medial to the scapula or over the lateral aspect of the arm; pain referred from the low back is usually appreciated in the buttocks and posterior thighs, although rarely below the knees. Pain from the upper lumbar spine is often referred to the flank, groin, and anterior thigh. Pain also can be referred to the spine from lesions of thoracic or abdominal viscera, a prominent example being the back pain from pancreatic carcinoma.

MUSCLE PAIN. Muscle pain occurs when an injury to or structural abnormality of the spine induces paravertebral muscle spasm. Sustained contraction of paravertebral muscles gives rise to chronic aching pain, usually felt lateral to the midline of the neck or back. Palpation of painful muscles may reveal evidence of spasm and tenderness. At times, when areas of extreme sensitivity (trigger points) are palpated, the pain may be felt not only locally in the muscle but also may be referred to distant structures. Trigger points define myofascial pain syndromes, common causes of neck and back pain without structural abnormalities of the spine (see p. 2124).

RADICULAR PAIN. Injured spinal roots or spinal cord produce, respectively, radicular or funicular pain. Radicular pain is the prominent symptom of nerve root compression. Nerve roots are not usually pain-sensitive. However, chronic compression leads to edema and, perhaps, inflammation and demyelination; the root then becomes sensitive to stretching or compression. When compressed, the pain may be experienced only in the cutaneous distribution (dermatome) of the involved root or may be felt locally and deep in muscles that it supplies. Root pain is usually least severe in positions that minimize compression and most severe in positions that compress or stretch the root. Root pain is usually exacerbated by increasing intraspinal pressure by coughing, sneezing, and straining.

FUNICULAR PAIN. Funicular pain is caused by compression of the long tracts of the spinal cord. Funicular pain is less sharp than radicular pain and is often described as a cold, unpleasant sensation in the extremity. Its distribution is more diffuse than that of radicular pain but like root pain is usually exacerbated by movements that stretch the cord (neck flexion, straight leg raising) or that increase intraspinal pressure.

In addition to pain, chronic compression of nerve roots can produce paresthesias, sensory loss, weakness, atrophy, and hyporeflexia in root-supplied areas, thus localizing the lesion. Knowing the myotomal and dermatomal distribution of spinal roots (Table 489-1) often allows one not only to localize the lesion but also to suggest its etiologic diagnosis: Involvement of a single root is more likely to occur with intervertebral disc herniation (Ch. 490), whereas multiple root dysfunction is likely to be caused by tumor or chronic inflammation. However, myotomal and dermatomal localization must be utilized cautiously. In the first place, not every body obeys the standard maps. Also, contiguous dermatomes overlap, and the apparent size of a dermatome can vary between examinations, depending on central nervous system excitability. Nevertheless, the localizing diagnosis of root lesions is usually accurate.

The clinical signs of spinal cord compression depend on the speed with which the compression develops, the transverse and longitudinal site of the lesion, and the vulnerability of the individual spinal fibers. The spinal cord accommodates considerably to gradually developing compression (e.g., from meningiomas); such disorders can cause the gradual onset of painless paraparesis or paraplegia. Because of this accommodation, subsequent decompression, even when patients are severely paraparetic, often leads to complete resolution of neurologic symptoms. On the other hand, rapidly developing lesions such as epidural hematomas, acute midline herniated discs, or epidural spinal cord compression from metastatic tumor are usually painful and cause rapidly developing neurologic signs that respond poorly to therapy once severe paraparesis has developed.

The site of compression in the transverse plane may determine clinical signs, particularly when the compression develops slowly. For example, laterally located lesions compressing one side of the spinal cord may cause the Brown-Séquard syndrome (ipsilateral hemiparesis, vibration and position sense loss, with contralateral pain and temperature loss); compression of the posterior portion of the cord may cause bilateral position and vibratory loss, with preservation of pain and temperature sensation and of

TABLE 489-1. DIAGNOSIS OF NERVE ROOT LESIONS

	C2-C3	C5	C6	C7	C8	Nerve T1
Pain	Back of head, lateral face, behind ear (occasionally vertex or orbit)	Medial scapula, lateral border of arm	Lateral forearm, thumb and index finger	Posterior arm, lateral hand, midforearm, and medial scapula	Medial forearm and hand	Deep aching in shoulder and axilla to olecranon
Sensory loss	Posterior scalp, pinna, lateral face	Lateral border of upper arm	Lateral forearm, including thumb	Mid-forearm and middle finger	Medial forearm and little finger	Axilla down to olecranon
Reflex loss	None	Biceps	Supinator	Triceps	Finger stretch	None
Motor deficit	None	Deltoid, supraspinatus, infraspinatus, rhomboids	Biceps, brachioradialis, brachialis (pronators and supinators of forearm)	Latissimus dorsi, pectoralis major, triceps, wrist extensors, wrist flexors	Finger flexors, finger extensors, flexor carpi ulnaris (thenar muscles in some patients)	*All* small hand muscles (in some thenar muscles via C8)
Some causative lesions	Tumor, injury	Brachial neuritis, cervical disc or spondylosis, upper plexus injury	Cervical disc or spondylosis	Cervical disc or spondylosis	Pancoast tumor, rare in disc lesions or spondylosis, metastatic tumor, thoracic outlet syndrome	Pancoast tumor, cervical rib, outlet syndromes, metastatic carcinoma in deep cervical nodes
Autonomic changes	Gustatory sweating					Horner's syndrome

motor power. However, most lesions twist the cord as they compress it and also interfere with the vascular supply to sites beyond the compression. Accordingly, one can depend only in a general way on the neurologic signs to evaluate the exact transverse site of compression. The longitudinal location of the lesion is more important. Cervical lesions cause quadriplegia, thoracic lesions, paraplegia; and upper lumbar lesions, normal motor function with bowel and bladder dysfunction and extensor plantar responses (conus medullaris syndrome). Lesions below the first lumbar vertebral body compress the cauda equina, causing loss of bowel and bladder function with lower motor neuron leg weakness and normal plantar reflexes.

Certain spinal tracts appear to be more vulnerable to compression than others. The corticospinal tracts and posterior columns are particularly vulnerable, the spinothalamic tracts and descending autonomic fibers less so. As a result, weakness, spasticity, and reflex hyperactivity tend to be the earliest signs of spinal cord compression, with paresthesias and vibratory and position sense loss occurring soon thereafter. Loss of pain and temperature sensation and of bladder and bowel function usually occurs late in the course of spinal cord compression. The spinocerebellar pathways are also sensitive to compression, and at times ataxia mimicking cerebellar disease may be the only sign of spinal cord compression.

APPROACH TO THE PATIENT

Most mechanical lesions of the spine and its contents begin with pain and only later produce other signs of neurologic dysfunction. There are many potential causes of neck or back pain. One survey listed over 100 causes (Table 489–2). The task for the physician is to separate those patients with potentially serious disease from those with more common, if unknown, causes of back pain who need only reassurance, sometimes coupled with bed rest, analgesics, and physical therapy.

HISTORY. The diagnostic evaluation begins with the history. Get a complete description of the pain. Most spine pain begins acutely or subacutely and often follows, by minutes to hours, some unaccustomed physical activity, particularly lifting or bending. Patients may awaken stiff and sore the morning after unusual exercise or may develop acute back pain on arising in the morning, without any obvious precipitating event. Most neck pain begins as a stiff neck, often on awakening, without a history of unusual activity. In many patients, neck or low back pain recurs episodically over many years. Most neck or back pain is dull and aching in quality, exacerbated by movement and relieved by rest. Pain that is present when the patient is immobile and cannot be relieved by positional manipulation should lead the physician to consider a more serious disorder (e.g., tumor or extruded disc). *Radicular pain*, particularly if accompanied by paresthesias or loss of sensation, indicates mechanical compression of the nerve root supplying that dermatome and implies identifiable structural disease (e.g., herniated disc). *Referred pain* does not imply compression of a root.

A history of serious systemic illness may suggest disease of vertebral bodies. Carcinoma of the breast or thyroid may cause back pain from bony metastases years after the primary tumor has been successfully treated. Previous systemic infection may lead to delayed onset of vertebral osteomyelitis or epidural abscess. A family history may also give clues to the etiology of back pain. Neurofibromas causing neck or back pain by compression of nerve root or the spinal cord may be associated with neurofibromatosis. Rheumatoid arthritis and ankylosing spondylitis are causes of familial back pain.

EXAMINATION. A careful general physical examination may reveal evidence of systemic disease such as cancer or infection. Urinary tract infections, pelvic disease, abdominal aneurysms, and other intra-abdominal or intrathoracic processes sometimes cause back pain by impinging on vertebral bodies or paravertebral structures. Special attention should be paid to mobility of the spine and paravertebral structures. Most patients who complain of a stiff neck have some limitation of movement of the cervical spine, but if gradual movement of the cervical spine causes intense pain, if pain on neck flexion is referred to the thoracic or lumbar area, or if neck flexion causes paresthesias radiating into the arms, legs, or back (Lhermitte's sign), spinal cord compression should be suspected. Most low back pain not caused by a herniated disc is exacerbated by flexion and relieved by lying down. The paravertebral muscles are often in spasm, are tender

TABLE 489–1. DIAGNOSIS OF NERVE ROOT LESIONS Continued

Roots							
T4	T10	L2	L3	L4	L5	S1	S2–S4
Anterior chest and/or upper back	Midback and/or anterior abdomen	Across thigh	Across thigh	Down to medial malleolus	Back of thigh, lateral calf, dorsum of foot	Back of thigh, back of calf, lateral foot	Buttocks, genitalia, back of thigh
Usually none (upper back and chest at nipple level)	Usually none (mid-back and abdomen at umbilicus level)	Often none	Often none	Medial leg	Dorsum of foot	Behind lateral malleolus	Buttocks, genitalia
None	Decreased abdominal reflex	None	Adductor reflex	Knee jerk	None	Ankle jerk	Bulbocavernosus
Not discernible	None	Hip flexion, adduction of thigh	Knee extension, adduction of thigh	Inversion of foot	Dorsiflexion of toes and foot (latter L4 also)	Plantar flexion and eversion of foot	Bladder and bowel
Intravertebral or paravertebral tumor, herpes zoster	Intravertebral and paravertebral tumor, herpes zoster	Neurofibroma, meningioma, neoplastic disease; disc lesions very rare except at L4 < 5 per cent			Disc lesions, metastatic malignancy, neurofibromas, meningioma		Tumor, midline disc
Chest wall, piloerection, hyperhidrosis, unilateral gynecomastia, galactorrhea	Chest wall, piloerection, hyperhidrosis, retrograde ejaculation	Alterations in temperature and color of all or parts of the leg or thigh					Incontinence, impotence, urinary retention

TABLE 489–2. SOME CAUSES OF BACK PAIN

Common Causes

Degenerative disorders
  Osteoarthritis, facet syndrome
  Herniated disc
  Spinal stenosis
  Nerve root entrapment
Muscle dysfunction
  Spasms, fatigue, fibromyalgia, and myofascial pain
Psychosomatic (e.g., stress, conversion reaction, tension states)
Trauma
  Lumbar strain (acute or chronic)

Less Common Causes

Congenital disorders
  Facet tropism (asymmetry)
  Transitional vertebra
  Spondylolysis and spondylolisthesis
Infections (e.g., disc space infection, tuberculosis, epidural and
  subdural abscess, herpes zoster, meningitis, sacroiliac joint
  infection)
Inflammatory diseases (e.g., ankylosing spondylitis, arachnoiditis,
  rheumatoid arthritis)
Metabolic disorders (e.g., osteoporosis, gout, diabetic neuropathy,
  Paget's disease)
Postoperative (e.g., sequelae of scar formation, arachnoiditis)
Scoliosis (e.g., idiopathic, postparalytic, aging)
Trauma
  Lumbosacral, sacroiliac strain
  Compression fracture (vertebral body or transverse process)
Dislocation or subluxation
Tumors
  Benign bone and neural tumors (e.g., neurinoma, ependymoma,
    meningioma, osteoid osteoma, hemangioma, osteoblastoma)
  Malignant bone and neural tumors
    Primary (e.g., multiple myeloma, osteosarcoma)
    Secondary (metastases)
Visceral disease (e.g., visceral inflammation, female pelvic pathology,
  retroperitoneal pathology, aortic aneurysm, prostatic disease)

to palpation, and straighten the normally lordotic lumbar spine. Almost any severe low back pain, particularly if it radiates into a lower extremity, can increase when the extended leg is raised from the bed (straight leg raising sign). However, pain referred to the contralateral back or leg when the non-painful leg is raised (crossed straight leg raising) implies root compression. Forced extension of the hip (reverse straight leg raising) can elicit pain from upper lumbar root disease (L4 and above). Point tenderness over a spinous process raises the suspicion of involvement of the vertebra by either tumor or infection.

The neurologic examination is important. Sensory loss, reflex diminution, and weakness all suggest neurologic disease that requires further evaluation. The distribution of abnormalities localizes the lesion. Remember, however, that patients in severe pain may be reluctant to move the painful part, making normal muscles appear weak. Likewise, guarding can affect deep tendon reflexes, either increasing or decreasing them with respect to the normal side. Repeating the neurologic examination after pain has been relieved by analgesics usually clarifies whether or not there is neurologic dysfunction. Clear and reproducible neurologic signs, particularly sensory loss in a dermatomal distribution or a diminished stretch reflex, imply root compression.

Careful examination can reveal inconsistencies (e.g., leg pain on straight leg raising that appears when the patient is recumbent but not when sitting) that suggest a psychological rather than a physiologic basis.

LABORATORY AIDS TO INVESTIGATION. For most patients with back or neck pain, laboratory tests are neither required nor helpful. Plain radiographs of the spine rarely reveal relevant, clinically unsuspected findings, and more sensitive tests (e.g., CT and MR) often identify abnormalities such as herniated discs in asymptomatic as well as in symptomatic patients. Radiographic examination of neck or back should be undertaken only when the history and examination suggest specific findings (e.g., fracture or dislocation). If the clinical examination points to other signifi-

cant disease of the neck or back (e.g., herniated disc) and if pain does not respond to conservative measures in a few weeks, the physician should proceed directly to MR imaging, which can identify all elements of the spinal column and its contents in multiple planes. Patients suspected of harboring tumors, infection, or vascular disease should be imaged without delay.

The only abnormalities not easily identified by MR are subluxations of vertebral bodies with movement. Flexion and extension plain radiographs of the neck or back settle that issue. Images of the neck and back must be interpreted with caution, since degenerative disc changes are frequently found in asymptomatic patients and increase with age. MR imaging, even though more expensive than CT and *radionuclide bone scan*, is so much more sensitive that it will probably replace these tests. Invasive tests, such as *myelograms, spinal angiography,* and *discography,* should be performed only in those special few instances when surgery is planned and MR does not give adequate information.

A committee of the American Academy of Neurology has determined that "based on the present medical literature, infrared *thermography* [does not] provide sufficiently reliable . . . [diagnostic] information . . . to accept it . . . for . . . neck or back pain and/or . . . radiculopathy. . . ."

Electromyography and nerve conduction studies, particularly using H and F responses, can help identify the presence and site of proximal sensory and motor root damage and anterior horn cell dysfunction. *Somatosensory evoked potentials* can be recorded along the spinal cord or in the brain after a peripheral nerve is stimulated and can sometimes identify the approximate site of a spinal cord lesion (see Ch. 441.2).

ANESTHETIC BLOCKS. Injections of local anesthesia into sites that are potential sources of neck or back pain sometimes aid diagnosis. Injection of facet joints may relieve both local and referred pain arising from osteoarthritis of those joints (see *facet syndrome,* p. 2236). Injection of trigger points may aid in the diagnosis of *myofascial back pain* (see p. 2124). Similarly, injections into and around the sacroiliac joint or intraspinal lesions may aid in diagnosis. Repetitive injections occasionally provide prolonged relief.

MANAGEMENT OF THE PATIENT WITH NECK AND BACK PAIN. If no clinical findings suggest serious structural disease of the spine, nerve roots, or spinal cord, patients should be treated as if they suffered from an acute neck or back strain, without further diagnostic evaluation. Because most patients recover within a few weeks without specific therapy, it is difficult to assess various therapeutic regimens. For severe pain, the best treatment probably consists of 2 to 3 days of bed rest on a firmly supported mattress in the position most comfortable. The best position for low back pain is usually semi-Fowler's position (head slightly elevated with pillows under the knees). For neck pain use a cervical pillow that maintains the normal lordotic curve rather than flexes the neck as regular pillows do. A soft cervical collar may be as effective in immobilizing the neck as bed rest. Bed rest may be combined with analgesic agents (usually aspirin or acetaminophen) and with local heat. Patients should be encouraged to stay recumbent, except to go to the toilet, until pain diminishes. As pain subsides, patients should gradually ambulate and start strengthening exercises for the paravertebral muscles of the neck and back, to prevent recurrence of pain. Other treatment modalities, including physical therapy, traction, procaine or saline injection into trigger points, transcutaneous stimulation, and spinal manipulation, are not more efficacious than the regimen described above. One recent study suggests that chiropractic manipulation of the back produces more rapid and prolonged relief of nonsciatic low back pain than does physical therapy with or without manipulation. Manipulation of the neck is potentially dangerous, however, because it can occlude the vertebral arteries as they enter the skull.

Using standard therapy, 70 to 80 per cent of patients become free of pain and able to return to full activity within a 4-week period. During the period of bed rest, repeated physical and neurologic examinations are unwise, since vigorous movement of the neck, back, and extremities can exacerbate pain and delay improvement. A small minority of patients continue to have chronic pain, and they, along with those whose initial examination has suggested more serious disease, need further evaluation.

The management of specific causes of nerve root and spinal cord compression, such as a herniated disc, is detailed in the chapters that follow.

Bonica JJ: Management of Pain, 2nd ed. Philadelphia, Lea and Febiger, 1990. *Excellent and detailed chapters on pain in the neck (Ch. 47) and in the low back (Ch. 71 and 72) which deal with management as well as diagnosis.*

Frymoyer JW: Back pain and sciatica. N Engl J Med 318:291–300, 1988. *A medical progress article reviewing acute and chronic low back pain.*

Reed TW, Dwyer S, Browne W, et al.: Low back pain and mechanical origin: Randomized comparison of chiropractic and hospital out-patient treatment. Br Med J 30:1431–1437, 1990. *A report sure to elicit continuing controversy on the medical management of low back pain.*

490 Intervertebral Disc Disease

HERNIATED DISC. Herniated intervertebral discs are the most common cause of neck or low back pain associated with a clearly defined structural abnormality. Lumbar and cervical strain and myofascial pain syndromes (see Ch. 489) are more common but not marked by clear pathologic abnormalities. Between each two vertebral bodies is a fibrocartilaginous intervertebral disc. The disc consists of a soft inner nucleus pulposus (a remnant of the notochord) surrounded by thicker fibrous tissue (the anulus fibrosus). The nucleus pulposus is gelatinous in structure and acts as a shock absorber between adjacent vertebral bodies. With advancing age, the nucleus loses fluid, volume, and resiliency, and the entire disc structure becomes more susceptible to trauma and compression. Tears develop in the anulus fibrosus as a result of repeated minor trauma, and eventually, if the tears become large enough, a portion of the soft nucleus pulposus herniates through the anulus. Asymptomatic herniation may occur into the center of the vertebral bodies bordering the disc (Schmorl's nodules). When, however, disc material herniates into the vertebral canal, it can compress nerve endings and nerve roots, causing pain and other symptoms. Generally, the disc herniates lateral to the posterior longitudinal ligament, thus compressing spinal roots as they enter the intervertebral foramen. Occasionally the disc herniates more centrally, compressing either the spinal cord in the cervical or thoracic area or the cauda equina in the lumbar area. The term *herniated disc* refers to a disc that maintains continuity with the nucleus pulposus; *extruded disc* refers to a fragment within the spinal canal that has lost continuity with the disc itself. The signs and symptoms of herniated discs are caused by compression of either nerve roots or the spinal cord. The specific signs and symptoms depend in part on whether the predominant compression is spinal cord or nerve root, and in part on the level at which the neural structures are compressed (see Ch. 489). The most common sites of disc herniation are in the lumbar area, between L4 and L5 and between L5 and S1, compressing the L5 and S1 roots, respectively. L3–L4 herniations are less common. In the cervical area, the common herniations occur between C5 and C6 (C6 root) and, especially, C6 and C7 (C7 root). Less commonly, herniations appear between C3 and C4, C4 and C5, and C7 and T1. Thoracic disc herniations are less common but can cause severe myelopathy because the thoracic area is the narrowest of the entire vertebral canal and the cord has a relatively poor vascular system, making it vulnerable to ischemic compression. Although clinical localization in diagnosis of disc disease is usually quite accurate, at times an extruded disc fragment may be large enough to affect several roots, or may migrate from the disc space in which it herniated, to cause signs at a distance.

The most common symptom of a herniated disc is pain. Local pain is felt as a dull aching in the neck or back, with an associated stiffness of those structures, frequently occurring episodically in response to minor trauma (or no discernible trauma at all) months or years prior to the development of radicular pain. The exact pathogenesis of the local pain in disc disease is not known, but some believe that it results from compression of the sinuvertebral nerve, a recurrent branch of the nerve root that supplies the dura mater. Radicular pain may occasionally be the first sign of disc disease but is far more likely to follow repeated bouts of local pain. Radicular pain is generally sudden in onset, often following minor trauma such as a twist, turn, or unusual bend. Radicular pain is perceived as sharp and well localized and may radiate from the back along the entire distribution of the involved root or affect only a portion of the root. Both local pain and radicular pain have the characteristics of being exacerbated by activity and relieved by rest.

With cervical disc herniation, most patients hold their necks stiffly and resist passive movement. Lateral bending either to or away from the side of the herniated disc frequently exacerbates both the local and radicular pain. The patient may be more comfortable with his neck slightly flexed but is usually comfortable only in the recumbent position. Patients with lumbar disc disease are most comfortable lying, most uncomfortable sitting, and a little less uncomfortable standing. The back is held stiffly, so that the normal lumbar lordotic curve is no longer apparent, and pain is usually exacerbated by extension of the back. Slow forward bending sometimes relieves the pain. Muscle spasm is prominent with both cervical and lumbar disc disease. Raising the intraspinal pressure, as by coughing, sneezing, or straining, increases the pain sharply. Stretching the compressed root also aggravates the pain. In the upper extremities, extending the arm and laterally flexing the neck away from the extended arm often reproduces radicular pain. In the lower extremities, raising the extended leg with the patient in the recumbent position frequently reproduces the pain of an L5 or S1 radiculopathy and, if the spontaneous pain is reproduced by raising the contralateral leg (crossed straight leg raising), the sign is very suggestive of herniated disc disease. Symptoms of L4 radiculopathy can often be reproduced by extending the hip (stretching the femoral nerve) when the patient is lying in the prone position. Often tenderness is present along the entire distribution of the nerve(s) supplied by the compressed root as well as in muscles supplied by the root. In patients with cervical disc disease, palpation or light percussion of the brachial plexus in the supraclavicular fossa or axilla often causes pain. In patients with lumbar disc disease, palpation over the femoral nerve (L4) in the groin or over the sciatic nerve (L5–S1) in the calf, thigh, or buttocks often causes severe pain. Occasionally tenderness in the calf (the posterior tibial nerve) is so striking as to suggest that the patient is suffering from thrombophlebitis rather than disc herniation. Other neurologic signs that commonly accompany disc disease include paresthesias and sensory loss in the distribution of the involved root and motor weakness in the myotome supplied by that root. The most important single sign is a diminished or absent reflex, giving objectively verifiable evidence of neurologic disease.

If an intervertebral disc herniates medially rather than laterally, it may spare the root and involve the spinal cord directly. When this occurs, there may be little or no pain or pain in a bilateral radicular distribution. Sometimes the pain is felt at a site far distant from the disc herniation as a result of compression of long sensory tracts in the spinal cord (funicular pain). The signs and symptoms of cord involvement are the same as those of compression of the spinal cord by other mass lesions. In contradistinction to diseases that arise within the spinal cord, compressive lesions tend to spare bladder and bowel function until late. (The exception is when the compression occurs either at the conus medullaris or in the cauda equina.)

The diagnosis of herniated disc is deduced from the characteristic clinical symptoms and findings. In many patients with radiculopathy, findings are minimal and the history must establish the diagnosis. When the patient complains of back pain, with or without a radicular component, but has no motor, sensory, or reflex changes to suggest the site of a radiculopathy, the differential diagnosis includes pain arising from pain-sensitive nerve endings in the muscles, ligaments, and joints of the vertebral bodies and the paravertebral structures. These structures must be examined carefully to determine which of them is responsible. MRI is helpful (see Ch. 489).

There is controversy about the management of herniated discs. Most physicians believe that the first step is bed rest. Some investigators have reported that adrenocorticosteroids, either taken orally or injected into the epidural space, may hasten resolution of pain and other symptoms. No controlled studies support this recommendation. Steroids injected into the epidural or subarachnoid space are contraindicated and may produce severe inflammatory reactions. Surgery is indicated when (1) bed rest fails, and the patient is incapacitated by severe, intractable pain; (2) a centrally placed lumbar disc compresses the cauda equina, producing urinary dysfunction; (3) motor weakness (e.g., foot drop) is severe and gets worse on bed rest; or (4) acute cervical or thoracic discs cause substantial myelopathy. Myelography may be performed before surgical extirpation to localize the site of disc herniation and to determine whether other disc lesions or tumors are present as well, but in many cases MRI suffices. The best operation removes the involved disc, leaving as much bone as possible intact. Fusion of the lumbar spine is rarely necessary. Lumbar disc operations are done posteriorly via a laminotomy. Cervical disc operations may be done either posteriorly to decompress the cord or anteriorly across the neck to remove the disc without disturbing posterior bony elements. The surgical approach for myelopathy should probably be anterior if the disc is in the cervical area and lateral if the disc is in the thoracic area.

Disc dissolution by the injection of the enzyme chymopapain directly into a lumbar disc space has received enthusiastic support from some centers and, in the best hands, appears as effective as surgery. Occasional, serious anaphylactic reactions can occur and the procedure's role remains uncertain. Percutaneous aspiration of disc material is usually safe and often effective in relieving root compression without a laminotomy.

SPONDYLOSIS. Spondylosis is a term applied to chronic degenerative disease of intervertebral discs associated with reactive changes in the adjacent vertebral bodies. Spondylotic changes in the neck and low back increase with age and are almost invariably present in the elderly. Spondylosis is usually asymptomatic except when the reactive tissue compresses a nerve root or the spinal cord. When this occurs, the signs and symptoms are similar to those of herniated disc disease, but the onset is less abrupt and the treatment often more difficult. In both the cervical and lumbar areas, spondylosis is more likely to produce spinal cord or cauda equina symptoms if the sagittal diameter of the spinal canal is congenitally narrow.

Cervical Spondylosis. Most patients suffer either radiculopathy or myelopathy, but not both. Pain is common but usually less acute and severe than with herniated discs. Even muscle spasm may be absent. However, the vertebral degenerative changes in the neck lead to limitation of movement in all directions. The classic picture of cervical spondylotic myelopathy is one of little or no pain but slowly developing weakness, atrophy, and fasciculations in the upper extremities, particularly the small muscles of the hand, accompanied by spastic paraparesis with decreased proprioception in the legs. At first the findings may suggest a diagnosis of amyotrophic lateral sclerosis. However, in cervical spondylosis there are sensory changes, particularly vibration loss in the lower extremities, and in amyotrophic lateral sclerosis fasciculations extend to innervated areas beyond the cervical level. The differential diagnosis also includes other compressive lesions of root and spinal cord as well as chronic multiple sclerosis.

The diagnosis of cervical spondylitic myelopathy is established with MRI, which accurately delineates the size of the cervical canal and the site of spinal cord and/or root compression.

The natural history of cervical myelopathy and radiculopathy is not well established. Many patients experience long periods of pain relief and remission or stabilization of neurologic symptoms, making it difficult to evaluate the effect of a particular treatment. Many physicians prefer, once having established the diagnosis, to begin with conservative treatment with a brief period of bed rest accompanied by cervical traction and stabilization of the neck with a soft collar. If collar and traction are successful, they should be continued. However, if the patient develops progressive neurologic signs in the face of conservative treatment, surgical therapy is indicated. Most neurosurgeons believe that if the spinal cord compression occurs at one or two segments, anterior removal of the disc material with spinal fusion is the preferred course. If more than a few segments are involved, laminectomy with foraminotomy is preferred.

In some patients with cervical spondylosis (or with congenital narrowing of the cervical spinal canal, or both), neurologic symptoms are exacerbated by exercise, with pain, numbness, and weakness appearing when a particular extremity is exercised. The pathogenesis is thought to be compression of the spinal cord so severe that the blood supply to the area cannot increase during its activity, leading to ischemia of cord and root structures (pseudoclaudication).

LUMBAR SPONDYLOSIS. Most of the considerations described above apply. The symptoms of lumbar spondylosis are similar to those of herniated disc, often occurring at multiple levels. One outstanding difference is the frequent presence of *pseudoclaudication* from cauda equina compression in patients with spinal stenosis due to either spondylosis or congenital narrowing. Typically, symptoms and signs are evoked or accentuated by walking and include pain, paresthesias, and weakness in the lower extremities. All of the symptoms may disappear when the patient ceases walking, even though he remains in the standing position. At times, however, the symptoms may be exacerbated by prolonged standing and relieved only by sitting or lying down. Pseudoclaudication of the cauda equina may be distinguished from intermittent vascular claudication in several ways. In vascular disease, the pulses in the lower extremities are usually absent or become absent as exercise begins. Also, the symptoms are usually reproducible and stereotypic, i.e., the patient can predict the exact distance he can walk at a given speed before symptoms develop. Symptoms of cauda equina pseudoclaudication are less stereotypic, so that on some days patients can walk much longer distances than on others. The reason for this variability is not known. In patients with pseudoclaudication, the narrowed lumbar canal is easily measured by MRI. With severe lumbar stenosis, conservative treatment usually fails, and decompressive laminectomy is the treatment of choice.

OTHER CAUSES OF BACK AND NECK PAIN. Several common pathophysiologically poorly understood disorders that produce pain in the back or neck can be confused with intravertebral disc disease or cervical or lumbar spondylosis. These include pain arising in lumbosacral, sacroiliac, or zygapophyseal joints that results from muscle spasm or muscle tension and the fibromyalgia and the myofascial pain syndromes (see p. 2124). These disorders usually cause chronic aching local pain that, when severe, may be referred to distant sites. Typical radicular pain never occurs. As a group, the diagnosis is usually suspected by finding tenderness at a specific muscle site or limitation of motion in a specific joint. The diagnosis is supported by a lidocaine block, which should completely relieve the pain if the presumptive diagnosis is correct.

The *facet syndrome* is believed to result from osteoarthritis or trauma of the zygapophyseal joints or their synovial membranes. In the low back it is characterized by pain in the back, buttocks, and thighs. It is often relieved by flexion and aggravated by extension of the spine and frequently accentuated by rest and relieved by movement. Characteristically the area is stiff and painful in the morning and improves somewhat as the day wears on. There is tenderness to palpation of the joint. Anesthetic blocks of the joint relieve both the local and referred pain. Similar chronic pain may have its origin in the lumbosacral or sacroiliac joints.

Musculoskeletal pain is also a common but poorly understood cause of low back and probably neck pain. In patients with painful muscle spasm the normal lordotic curve is usually straightened and tight, and tender muscles can be palpated by the examiner. Local anesthetic blocks, followed by gentle mobilization, usually relieve the spasm and the pain. Prolonged contraction of muscles, such as results from sustained posture or psychological stress, may produce similar pain and tenderness. Fibromyalgia and myofascial pain syndromes often affect the neck and back, as noted above and on p. 2124.

---

491 Neoplasms of the Spinal Canal

Neoplastic growths that cause nerve root or spinal cord compression can be paravertebral, extradural, intradural, or intramedullary (Fig. 491–1). Most of those causing spinal cord compression are extradural and metastatic. Most extradural neoplasms originate in the vertebral body surrounding the spinal cord and

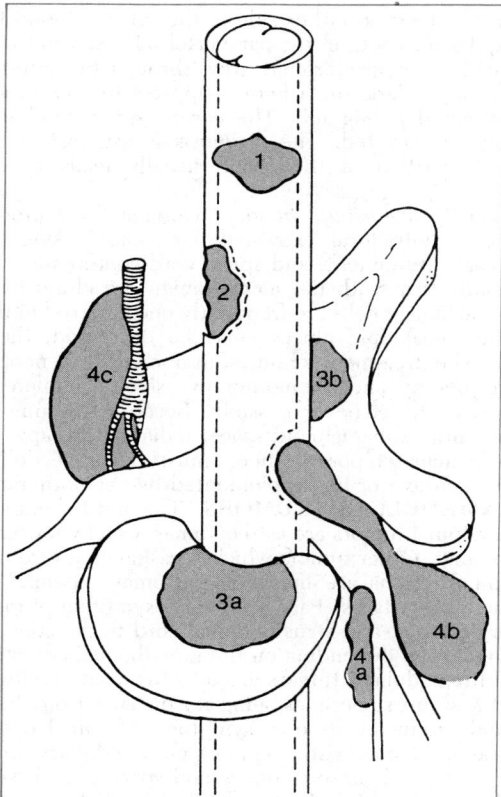

FIGURE 491–1. Pathophysiology of myelopathy caused by neoplasms. 1, The tumor may arise in or metastasize hematogenously to the substance of the spinal cord (intramedullary). 2, The tumor may be extraparenchymal but intradural. 3, The tumor may be extradural, extending either from the vertebral body (3a) or from a spinous process (3b), and cause symptoms by compressing the spinal cord. 4, The tumor may originate in or spread to the paravertebral space and produce its symptoms either by (4a) invading nerve roots, (4b) invading the epidural or subdural space through the intervertebral foramen, or (4c) compressing radicular arteries to cause spinal cord ischemia. (From Andreoli TE, Carpenter CCJ, Plum F, Smith LH Jr (eds.): Cecil Essentials of Medicine. Philadelphia, W. B. Saunders Company, 1986.)

compress spinal roots or cord without invading them. Most intradural neoplasms also cause symptoms by compressing spinal roots or cord without invading, but unlike extradural neoplasms the majority are benign and slow growing. Intramedullary neoplasms cause symptoms both by invading and by compressing spinal structures; the tumors may be either benign or malignant.

PARAVERTEBRAL TUMORS. Neoplastic lesions that begin in or metastasize to the paravertebral space often cause serious and perplexing neurologic problems. The tumor may extend longitudinally within the paravertebral space, progressively compressing or invading nerve roots. At times, such tumors grow through an intervertebral foramen and compress not only the nerve root but also the spinal cord. Rarely, spinal cord symptoms may be caused by paravertebral tumors compromising radicular arteries that supply the spinal cord. If the tumor is more lateral than the immediate paravertebral space, the brachial, lumbar, or sacral plexus may be compressed, causing symptoms similar to those of root compression but with a different pattern of sensory and motor loss. The symptoms of extravertebral tumor begin insidiously with severe, unremitting pain, often with a burning quality and usually localized just lateral to the spine, radiating in a bandlike pattern in the distribution of the involved dermatome(s). If the lesion involves abdominal or thoracic roots, motor and sensory changes are usually not appreciated by either the patient or the examiner. Autonomic changes may be a prominent or the only neurologic sign. Hyperhidrosis occurring in a band coinciding with the site of the pain strongly suggests the diagnosis. When the tumor involves cervical or lumbar roots, the pain may be soon followed by numbness in fingertips or toes, with accompanying weakness and reflex diminution, depending on the roots

involved. Autonomic changes, including anhidrosis or hyperhidrosis, may affect the arm or leg. Horner's syndrome or diaphragmatic paralysis often accompanies cervical or upper thoracic paravertebral tumors. The diagnosis is best established by MR scan of the level suggested by the clinical findings. The scans can also determine whether the lesion has grown through the intervertebral foramen or has eroded vertebral bodies.

The differential diagnosis of paravertebral tumor includes disorders that cause paravertebral pain with or without compression of nerve roots. *Myofascial pain syndromes* cause low back or neck paravertebral pain with referred pain into arms or legs. On examination there is often marked tenderness of muscles and, sometimes, trigger points identified by either their hardness to palpation or their ability to reproduce symptoms when compressed. Relief of pain in these instances can be produced by injecting the trigger point with saline solution or a local anesthetic. Temporary relief of pain after such injection does not imply that structural disease is absent; the trigger points may be a reaction to spinal or nerve root disease. In myofascial syndromes, autonomic, sensory, or motor changes are never present. Disease of kidneys and other viscera lying in the retroperitoneal space may cause pain similar to that of paravertebral tumors, but the pain usually does not radiate and is not associated with autonomic, motor, or sensory changes. Percussion of the involved viscera reproduces the pain that is described as a dull ache rather than a neurogenic burning pain. Spontaneous or induced *entrapment neuropathies* not caused by tumor occasionally mimic the symptoms of paravertebral tumor. Chronic pain after a thoracotomy (*post-thoracotomy pain*) probably results from entrapment of nerve roots at the time of surgery, perhaps with neuroma formation. The pain characteristically appears shortly after surgery and may be unremitting for many years. Motor, sensory, or autonomic changes are rare. The pain can sometimes be relieved by paravertebral anesthetic blocks.

The management of paravertebral masses depends on the diagnosis. In patients known to have cancer, particularly lymphomas or carcinomas of the breast or lung, the tumor can be assumed to be metastatic and should be treated with radiation therapy and, if available, chemotherapy. If the patient has no history of cancer, a biopsy is required and, depending on the site of the lesion, resection may be attempted both to establish a diagnosis and to decompress the nerve roots. Once the diagnosis is established by biopsy, further therapy such as radiation or chemotherapy may be indicated.

EXTRADURAL TUMORS. Extradural neoplasms compress spinal roots and cord in one of three ways. Either they arise in vertebrae surrounding the spinal cord and grow into the epidural space or they arise in the paravertebral space and grow through the intervertebral foramen to compress the cord laterally. Rarely, tumors may arise in the epidural space itself, without involving either vertebral or paravertebral structures. Most extradural neoplasms are metastatic (e.g., carcinomas of the breast, lung, prostate, or kidney). Some extradural neoplasms arise de novo in the vertebral bodies (e.g., chordoma, osteogenic sarcoma, myeloma, chondrosarcoma). A minority of extradural neoplasms are benign (e.g., osteoma, osteoid osteoma, angioma). Because extradural neoplasms usually destroy bone before producing spinal cord compression, local pain is the first symptom and may precede either radicular pain or other symptoms of spinal cord compression by weeks or months, depending on the rate of growth of the tumor. Rarely, extradural neoplasms may be painless and the first symptoms may be spinal cord dysfunction. As with other causes of spinal cord compression, extradural neoplasms cause symptoms first distally and later proximally. Thus, even thoracic and cervical neoplasms generally cause weakness and numbness in the legs before trunk and upper extremity muscles are involved. The diagnosis of extradural spinal cord compression must be suspected by the history of pain followed by signs and symptoms of spinal cord dysfunction and confirmed by radiographic study. In about 85 per cent of patients suffering from extradural spinal cord compression, there are bone lesions at the site of compression on plain radiographs. In those few patients with negative plain radiographs, radionuclide bone scan, CT, or MR scan may demonstrate a bone lesion. MRI usually also establishes the site and degree of spinal cord compression, often obviating the need for an invasive myelogram.

The differential diagnosis of extradural neoplasms includes inflammatory disease of bone and epidural abscess (e.g., vertebral tuberculosis, bacterial osteomyelitis), acute or subacute epidural hematomas, herniated intervertebral discs, spondylosis, and, very rarely, extramedullary hematopoiesis (in patients with severe and chronic anemias) or epidural lipomatosis (in patients on chronic steroid therapy). MRI often distinguishes those from tumor, but sometimes definitive diagnosis requires biopsy of the lesion either via decompressive laminectomy or by percutaneous needle biopsy.

The treatment of extradural neoplasms depends on the cause. Most neoplasms that cause extradural spinal cord compression are malignant and progress rapidly. Once spinal cord symptoms begin, paraplegia may develop in hours to days. Paraplegia is usually irreversible, whereas treatment often can correct mild to moderate spinal cord dysfunction. Thus, early diagnosis and effective emergency treatment of extradural spinal cord compression are mandatory. The treatment of patients known to be suffering from cancer who develop signs and symptoms of spinal cord compression from extradural metastases is radiation therapy. Therapy should begin with corticosteroids (dexamethasone, 16 to 100 mg daily) to decrease spinal cord edema, followed immediately by radiation therapy. If effective chemotherapeutic agents are available, they should be used in conjunction with steroids and radiation therapy for the treatment of metastatic or primary malignant tumors of the extradural space. In patients not known to be suffering from a primary cancer, metastatic disease is the most common cause of extradural spinal cord compression, but in these instances a definitive diagnosis must be made by biopsy. Such patients should begin corticosteroid therapy followed by surgery with removal of as much tumor as possible for both diagnostic and therapeutic purposes. If a malignant neoplasm is encountered at operation, radiation therapy should be begun as soon after the surgery as is practical. In a few patients in whom radiation therapy and chemotherapy are ineffective, resection of the vertebral body involved by tumor may delay the development of paraplegia. In some patients with extradural tumors and destruction of the vertebral body, subluxation may compress the cord and may be relieved by surgery. Benign extradural tumors require surgery.

INTRADURAL EXTRAMEDULLARY TUMORS. Most intradural tumors are benign. Meningiomas and neurofibromas are the two most common types. Teratomas, arachnoid cysts, and lipomas are less common. *Meningioma* occurs in middle-aged and elderly women, predominantly in the thoracic region of the spinal cord. Another common site is at the foramen magnum. Meningiomas are benign, slow growing, and usually located on the posterior aspect of the spinal cord. Pain is the first symptom in the majority of patients, but in about 25 per cent the meningioma is painless, the first symptoms being those of spinal cord compression. Because they are often located on the posterior aspect of the cord, paresthesias and sensory changes beginning distally in the lower extremities are a frequent early symptom and are often mistaken for peripheral neuropathy. As the disease progresses, however, corticospinal tract signs betray the spinal origin. Even when spinal cord signs and symptoms are obvious, the lack of pain may lead one to suspect a degenerative or demyelinating disease such as multiple sclerosis rather than a neoplasm. MRI usually settles the issue when contrast enhancement is used. Many meningiomas have a density similar to that of normal brain and spinal cord, making them difficult to identify on noncontrast MRI, but they all intensely contrast-enhance, making identification easy. The treatment of spinal cord compression from meningiomas is surgical removal. Because the tumor grows so slowly and the cord has an opportunity to adapt to compression, even patients with severe neurologic disability often make a full recovery after the lesion is removed.

The second common cause of intradural spinal cord compression is *neurofibroma*. Because these tumors usually arise from the dorsal root, radicular pain is often the first symptom, preceding signs of spinal cord compression by months or years. When spinal cord compression develops, it progresses slowly. Some patients with spinal neurofibroma suffer from neurofibromatosis. That diagnosis may be suspected either by a positive family history or by the cutaneous stigmata of the disease. A neurofi-

broma may extend on either side of the intervertebral foramen, involving the root both in the paravertebral space and within the spinal canal. As neurofibromas grow through the intervertebral foramen, they enlarge it, a finding appreciated by an appropriately positioned radiograph. The cerebrospinal fluid protein is almost always elevated. The diagnosis is established by MRI. Surgical extirpation of the lesion usually leads to complete recovery.

Occasionally, *metastatic tumors* involving the leptomeninges present with intradural extramedullary mass lesions. Pain is almost always prominent, and spinal cord compression develops more rapidly than with the more benign intradural tumors. In addition, malignant cells are frequently encountered in the spinal fluid. The spinal fluid glucose may be decreased, the protein elevated. The treatment of intradural malignant neoplasms is radiation therapy and chemotherapy, since complete surgical extirpation is almost never possible. Because the tumor usually seeds the entire subarachnoid space, radiation therapy, if it is to have more than temporary effect, must either be delivered to the entire neuraxis or be supplemented by chemotherapy.

INTRAMEDULLARY TUMORS. The most common intramedullary spinal tumors are astrocytomas (usually low grade) and ependymomas. Other tumors which occasionally cause intramedullary spinal lesions are hemangioblastomas, lipomas, and hematogenous metastases. Pain is an early symptom of most intramedullary tumors, and signs of spinal cord dysfunction progress rapidly or slowly, depending on the growth characteristics of the tumor. Intramedullary tumors are often associated with syringomyelia, the syrinx sometimes being at a distance from the primary tumor and producing its own symptoms of spinal dysfunction. The so-called characteristic signs of intramedullary spinal cord lesions (dissociated sensory loss, sacral sparing, and early onset of bladder and bowel dysfunction) are not reliable enough clinically to distinguish intramedullary from extramedullary lesions; that diagnosis is established by MRI. In some patients with longstanding benign intramedullary lesions, plain radiographs of the spine may show widening of the spinal canal and erosion of the pedicles. The differential diagnosis of intramedullary tumors includes intramedullary abscesses and syringomyelia without tumor. A definitive diagnosis is established by biopsy. Successful surgical removal of intramedullary tumors is possible, particularly with ependymomas and hemangioblastomas and sometimes with gliomas as well. Highly skilled and experienced surgeons are necessary for tumors to be removed without increasing neurologic symptoms. If the tumor cannot be totally excised, postoperative radiation therapy often delays recurrence.

Ependymomas have a predilection to involve the lower end of the spinal cord and the filum terminale. An unusual symptom sometimes produced by such tumors is hydrocephalus with headache, papilledema, and enlarged cerebral ventricles. The pathogenesis of the hydrocephalus is believed to be the plugging of pacchionian granulations by protein exuded from the tumor into the spinal fluid.

Byrne TN, Waxman SG (eds.): Spinal Cord Compression. Philadelphia, F.A. Davis, 1990. *Specific chapters cover non-neoplastic as well as neoplastic causes of spinal cord compression and noncompressive myelopathies simulating spinal cord compression.*

492 Inflammatory Diseases Compressing the Spinal Canal

Inflammatory diseases that compress nerve roots and spinal cord can be extradural, intradural, or intramedullary. Extradural inflammatory lesions include vertebral tuberculosis or bacterial osteomyelitis with extradural extension and primary extradural bacterial abscesses. These entities are discussed in Ch. 471. Intradural but extramedullary inflammatory diseases include bacterial, fungal, and parasitic meningitis, inflammatory disease of the leptomeninges of unknown cause such as sarcoidosis or Behçet's syndrome, and reactions to foreign substances such as myelographic contrast material, spinal anesthetics, or steroids. Occasionally, leptomeningeal infiltration with tumor or subarachnoid hemorrhage causes an inflammatory response of the leptomeninges that mimics subacute or chronic infection. All of these inflammatory intradural lesions can lead to spinal arachnoiditis. *Spinal arachnoiditis* is characterized by neck and back pain and by radicular pain in the distribution of the roots involved in the inflammatory process. Dysfunction of multiple roots, particularly in the lumbosacral area, is common; occasional patients go on to develop signs of spinal cord dysfunction (often caused by syrinx formation), which may progress to paraplegia. The diagnosis of spinal arachnoiditis is established by myelography. A myelogram reveals spotty and irregular collections of contrast material with impairment of the flow through the subarachnoid space. Sometimes there is a complete block to the passage of the myelographic contrast material. The spinal fluid may contain an increased cellular response and a decreased glucose concentration. The protein concentration is usually elevated. Sometimes a specific infectious organism can be identified either by microscopic examination or by culture. There is no therapy for spinal arachnoiditis unless a specific treatment-sensitive infective agent is identified.

Intramedullary infectious processes include bacterial and parasitic abscesses and acute transverse myelitis. These entities are discussed under the appropriate chapter headings.

Byrne TN, Waxman SG (eds): Spinal Cord Compression. Philadelphia, F.A. Davis Co., 1990. *Chapters discuss vascular and inflammatory causes of spinal cord compression and noncompressive myelopathies mimicking spinal cord compression.*

Caplan LR, Norohna AB, Amico LL: Syringomyelia and arachnoiditis. J Neurol Neurosurg Psychiatry 53:106–113, 1990. *A recent well-referenced discussion of chronic arachnoiditis and its sequelae.*

493 Vascular Disorders Compressing the Spinal Canal

Extradural, intradural, and intramedullary vascular disorders all can cause spinal cord compression. The most common and serious extradural vascular disease is *spinal epidural hematoma.* Hemorrhage into the spinal epidural space may occur spontaneously or be associated with trauma, a bleeding diathesis, or a vascular malformation. It is particularly common in patients being treated with anticoagulants. It may occasionally follow lumbar puncture, particularly in patients with bleeding abnormalities. Hemorrhage usually arises from the epidural venous plexus and tends to collect over the dorsum of the spinal cord covering several segments. The clinical picture is characterized by the sudden onset of severe localized back pain and the rapid development of spinal cord dysfunction, often leading to complete paraplegia in several hours. If the patient has a known bleeding disorder, the clinical diagnosis is easily established. In patients without known bleeding or clotting disorders, the differential diagnosis includes acute epidural abscess and acute transverse myelopathy. Although occasional patients recover from paraparesis related to epidural spinal cord compression spontaneously, the majority require emergency surgical evacuation if neurologic function is to be preserved. The more rapidly the paralysis develops and the longer the delay in decompression, the less likely is the patient to recover.

Intradural but extramedullary vascular lesions are usually caused by hemorrhage from *vascular malformations* on the surface of the spinal cord. *Spinal subarachnoid hemorrhage* is characterized by the sudden onset of back pain, often with a radicular component with or without the development of signs of spinal cord compression. Lumbar puncture reveals evidence of subarachnoid hemorrhage with red cells, xanthochromic spinal fluid, and usually an elevated protein concentration. In the absence of spinal cord signs, the differential diagnosis includes spontaneous intracerebral subarachnoid hemorrhage.

Vascular malformations also may lie within the substance of the spinal cord where they can give rise to intramedullary hemorrhage (hematomyelia) as well as subarachnoid hemorrhage. The sudden development of partial or complete transverse myelopathy is the most common onset. If blood leaks into the subarachnoid space, pain in the neck and back and other signs of meningeal irritation occur.

Arteriovenous malformations may also compress the spinal cord or give rise to hemodynamic changes that result in spinal ischemia. In such cases, distortion and compression of the cord by enlarged, abnormal vessels occur only gradually, producing slowly progressive symptoms of spinal cord dysfunction. Exacerbation of symptoms may accompany menstrual periods or pregnancy.

Complete or partial recovery of function can follow episodes of spinal cord ischemia or even small hemorrhages. The unchanging localization of the attacks and the prominence of pain help differentiate arteriovenous malformations from other recurrent neurologic disorders such as multiple sclerosis. Rarely, a bruit may be heard by auscultation over the site of the malformation. MRI identifies most hemorrhages and vascular malformations, but angiography with regional catheterization of radicular vessels is necessary to identify feeding vessels as a preliminary step to surgical treatment. Advances in microsurgery have increased the chances for satisfactory removal of these lesions. Embolization of the malformation or ligation of feeding arteries has been performed when the abnormality cannot be removed surgically.

Barnwell SL, Dowd CF, Davis RL, et al.: Cryptic vascular malformations of the spinal cord: Diagnosis by magnetic resonance imaging and outcome of surgery. J Neurosurg 72:403–407, 1990. *Description of a clinical entity usually not diagnosed before the advent of MRI.*

Gueguen B, Merland JJ, Riche MC, Rey A: Vascular malformations of the spinal cord. Neurology 37:969–979, 1987. *A good description of the anatomy and approach to treatment of these disorders.*

Mattle H, Sieb JP, Rohner M, Mumenthaler M: Nontraumatic spinal epidural and subdural hematomas. Neurology 37:1351–1356, 1987. *A recent paper with good references to the previous literature.*

494 Congenital Anomalies of the Craniovertebral Junction, Spine, and Spinal Cord

Congenital anomalies of the spine are common and are often encountered on radiographs of patients suffering from neck or low back pain. Some congenital anomalies such as *spina bifida occulta* can be considered variants of normal and are probably never responsible for low back pain. Others such as the *Klippel-Feil syndrome* (congenital fusion of two or more cervical vertebrae) are not responsible for neck pain or other neurologic symptoms except when associated with coexisting congenital anomalies of the central nervous system. Congenital abnormalities of the spine that are common and usually asymptomatic but that must be considered potential causes of neck or back pain include *facet tropism* (misalignment of the facets on the two sides of the corresponding vertebral body; several authorities believe that this increases rotational stress on the facet joints and may cause back pain); *transitional vertebrae,* such as in sacralization to a lumbar vertebra or lumbarization of a sacral vertebra (these alter spinal mechanics and result in instability and stress, sometimes producing back pain); and *spondylolisthesis* (forward slipping of one vertebral body onto another caused by a defect between the articular facets). A third group of congenital anomalies of the spine consists of those that are likely to cause not only neck or back pain but also neurologic disability. These include *basilar impression,* which is often associated with *Arnold-Chiari malformation* (see later discussion). Severe spinal *scoliosis* or *kyphosis,* congenital *stenosis* of the lumbar or cervical spinal canal, anterior and lateral spinal *meningoceles,* and *diastematomyelia* are other causes of back pain and neurologic disability. Diastematomyelia is a bony abnormality that divides the spinal canal, leading to duplication of the spinal cord. It is usually associated with evidence of spina bifida on plain radiographs, and sometimes the bony septum can be identified as well. Patients who become symptomatic in adulthood almost always have some cutaneous abnormality, especially hypertrichosis over the sacral area. The disorder may be associated with other congenital abnormalities of the central nervous system as well.

ARNOLD-CHIARI MALFORMATION

INFANTILE FORM. The Arnold-Chiari malformation is characterized by downward displacement of the cerebellum through the foramen magnum of the skull and by similar caudal elongation of the medulla. The infantile form is commonly associated with other midline defects such as spina bifida and meningocele, hydrocephalus caused by aqueductal or fourth ventricular obstruction, and other congenital malformations of the brain and cord. The infantile form of the Arnold-Chiari malformation usually occurs because of hydrocephalus in the early months of life, with evidence of spina bifida or frank paraparesis resulting from meningomyelocele. Therapy is directed toward surgical relief of the hydrocephalus with a ventricular shunting procedure and repair of the meningomyelocele. Prognosis is poor for patients with extensive defects.

ADULT FORM. The malformation may be asymptomatic until adult life, when the patient gradually develops symptoms and signs of dysfunction of the cerebellum, lower cranial nerves, pyramidal tracts, and posterior columns. Posterior cranial displacement may occur with coughing or straining. Downbeat nystagmus is characteristic. At times the initial signs may be those of hydrocephalus secondary to obstruction of the cerebrospinal fluid pathways or to coexisting syringomyelia of the cervical spinal cord and medulla (see Ch. 466). Commonly there is radiographic evidence of fusion of the cervical vertebrae, platybasia, or basilar impression, but MR scan establishes the diagnosis even when there are no coexisting bony abnormalities. The Arnold-Chiari malformation in adults may simulate syndromes produced by tumors near the foramen magnum or by multiple sclerosis. Surgical enlargement of the foramen magnum and decompression of the cervicomedullary junction benefit selected cases.

BASILAR IMPRESSION AND PLATYBASIA

Basilar impression refers to abnormal invagination of the cervical spine into the base of the posterior fossa of the skull. The diagnosis is made from sagittal MR reconstructions or lateral roentgenograms of the skull which show excessive protrusion of the tip of the odontoid process of the axis above Chamberlain's line, i.e., a line drawn from the back of the hard palate to the posterior margin of the foramen magnum. *Platybasia* refers to flattening of the base of the skull, wherein lateral roentgenograms of the skull reveal flattening of the angle between the orbital plates of the anterior fossa and the clivus, the sloping anterior floor of the posterior fossa. The abnormality by itself has no clinical significance.

These malformations are usually developmental in origin, and there may be hereditary transmission. Occasionally, basilar impression may result from metabolic bone diseases such as rickets, osteitis deformans, osteomalacia, osteogenesis imperfecta, or fibrous dysplasia. Minor degrees of deformity of the base of the skull give rise to no symptoms. The neck appears shortened, and its movements may be limited. With more severe invagination, there may be signs of impaired function of the cerebellum, lower cranial nerves, pyramidal tracts, and posterior columns. Syringomyelia and syringobulbia may be present. Increased intracranial pressure may develop owing to obstruction of the foramina of the fourth ventricle and the basal cisterns. The clinical manifestations must be differentiated from those caused by neoplasms in the region of the foramen magnum and multiple sclerosis. When neurologic signs are progressive, surgical decompression of the posterior fossa and upper cervical cord may be indicated.

Vinken PJ, Bruyn GW, Klawans HL, Myrianthopoulos NC (eds.): Handbook of Clinical Neurology. Volume 50, Malformations. New York, Elsevier Science Publishers, 1987. *A recent comprehensive review of congenital malformations of the brain and spine.*

SECTION SIXTEEN / DISEASES OF THE PERIPHERAL NERVOUS SYSTEM

Herbert H. Schaumburg

495 Introduction and Basic Terminology

The structure and function of the peripheral nervous system (PNS) appear deceptively simple when compared with the central nervous system (CNS). Actually, however, PNS diseases represent a potentially confusing jumble of conditions whose only common thread appears to be PNS dysfunction. Thus, while the anatomic diagnosis of peripheral neuropathy is readily established in nearly 100 per cent of cases by symptoms and signs, the correct cause is determined in less than one half of cases except in a few special centers. Recent clinical and experimental studies propose a simple, anatomic classification of most PNS disorders, suggesting that a working knowledge of the common peripheral neuropathies can be easily mastered. Since common diseases (diabetes or malignancy) produce more than one type of anatomic reaction in the PNS and most physicians are "etiology oriented,"

this chapter is organized according to individual diseases, stressing their common anatomic and pathophysiologic features whenever possible.

Certain terms associated with peripheral nerve disease have, by common usage, acquired set connotations. These include:

Radiculopathy. This term designates a selective abnormality of the dorsal (sensory) or ventral (motor) nerve root between the point where it joins the spinal cord or brain stem and the more distal point where the two roots fuse to form the peripheral nerve.

Neuropathy (peripheral neuropathy). This is the usual term for any disorder of peripheral nerves and replaces the term *peripheral neuritis.*

Polyneuropathy (symmetric polyneuropathy). This designates a generalized process resulting in widespread and symmetric effects on the peripheral nervous system.

Focal or multifocal neuropathy (mononeuropathy, mononeuropathy multiplex). These terms indicate local involvement of one or more individual peripheral nerves.

Dysesthesia. This term, like paresthesia, is poorly defined; it is commonly used to describe an unpleasant sensation produced by an ordinarily painless stimulus.

Paresthesia. This term indicates a spontaneous aberrant sensation such as pins and needles or tingling.

Hypoesthesia. This term refers to diminished sensation.

Hyperesthesia. This condition is an excessive response to sensory stimulus, even when the sensory threshold is elevated.

496 Anatomic Classification of Neuropathy

SYMMETRICAL GENERALIZED NEUROPATHY (Polyneuropathy)

DISTAL AXONOPATHY (DYING-BACK NEUROPATHY). This is the most common morphologic reaction of the peripheral nervous system (PNS) to toxins and underlies many metabolic and hereditary neuropathies.

The pathologic features include initial degeneration of the distal ends of large and long axons; the myelin sheath breaks down concomitantly with axonal disintegration. Axonal degeneration appears to advance slowly proximally toward the nerve cell body. Schwann cells and their connective tissue tubes remain in distal nerves, facilitating appropriate peripheral regeneration (Fig. 496–1).

Many prominent clinical phenomena closely correlate with the morphologic profile. Gradual onset reflects chronic metabolic disease or prolonged intoxication, stocking-glove sensorimotor loss reflects distal axonal degeneration in long nerves (sciatic, ulnar), normal cerebrospinal fluid (CSF) protein reflects the sparing of proximal sited nerve roots, and slow recovery corresponds to the indolent rate of axonal repair.

MYELINOPATHY. The term myelinopathy, when applied to the PNS, refers to conditions in which the lesion primarily affects myelin or the myelinating (Schwann) cell. Acute inflammatory demyelinating polyradiculoneuropathy (AIDP) is the only frequently encountered disease that primarily affects PNS myelin. It is likely that the demyelination of spinal roots and nerves in this disorder results from an immune system–mediated attack on PNS myelin.

The cardinal pathologic features, depicted in Figure 496–2, include primary destruction of the myelin sheath with the axon usually left intact. Demyelination initially affects multiple sites in nerves. The Schwann cell subsequently divides and rapidly remyelinates the axon to restore function.

TABLE 496–1. CLASSIFICATION OF PERIPHERAL NEUROPATHY

Symmetric generalized polyneuropathy

Distal axonopathy (associated with drugs, industrial chemicals, metabolic diseases, deficiency syndromes)

Myelinopathy (AIDP, CIDP associated with diphtheria, genetic leukodystrophies)

Neuronopathy (associated with motor neuron diseases, herpes zoster neuronitis, carcinomatous sensory neuronopathy)

Focal and multifocal neuropathies (mononeuropathy)

Ischemia (vasculopathy)

Trauma

Infiltration (granulomatous, malignancy)

Many prominent clinical findings correlate with the morphologic profile. Onset is rapid and recovery (once commenced) occurs steadily, reflecting the speed of demyelination and ease of remyelination. Initial changes may be distal or proximal or may affect cranial nerves. Generalized weakness and reflex loss are dominant features, reflecting the vulnerability of long myelinated fibers, and the CSF protein is usually elevated because inflammation in spinal roots results in leakage of protein into the surrounding subarachnoid space.

NEURONOPATHY. This term denotes conditions in which the initial morphologic changes occur in the neuron cell body. If the changes are intense, the affected neuron dies and permanent total motor or sensory dysfunction in the affected segment follows. The neuronopathies are a heterogeneous, poorly understood group of conditions and include many disorders of motor, sensory, and autonomic neurons. Infectious neuronopathies include familiar conditions such as poliomyelitis (motor neuronopathy) and herpes zoster ganglionitis (sensory neuronopathy). Some hereditary and toxic neuropathies probably are best conceptualized as neuronopathies. In general, a diffuse peripheral nerve disorder that is exclusively motor or sensory and that is characterized by little or no recovery should suggest the possibility of a primarily neuronal disorder.

An outline of the classification of peripheral neuropathy is provided in Table 496–1.

FOCAL AND MULTIFOCAL NEUROPATHIES (Mononeuropathy)

These conditions are characterized by dysfunction of an isolated peripheral nerve. Usually both motor and sensory symptoms are present. Trauma is the most common cause of monofocal neuropathy. Instances of nontraumatic focal neuropathies may pose

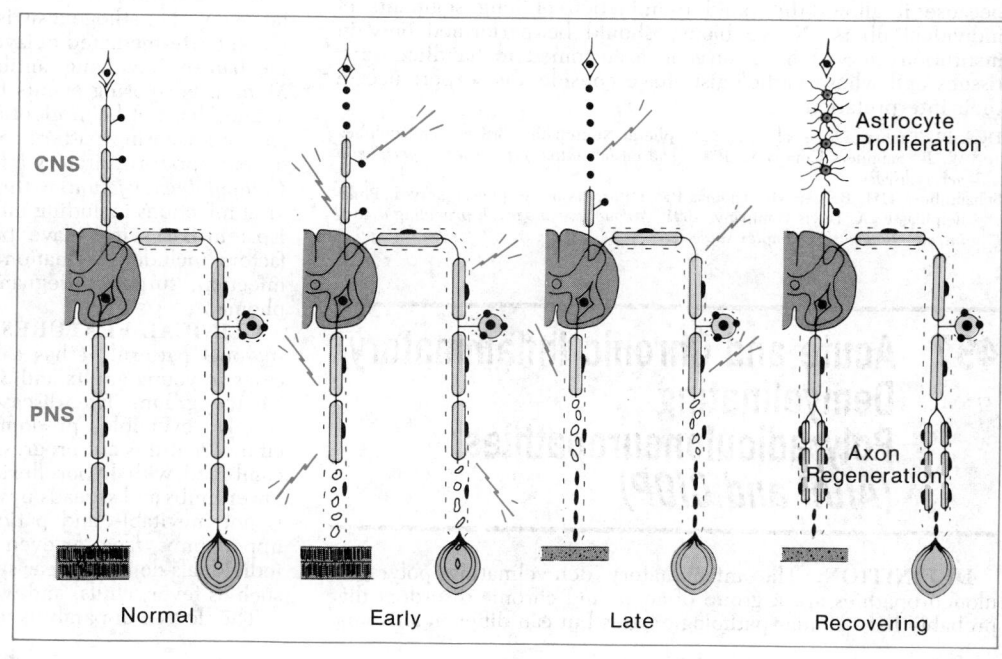

FIGURE 496–1. The cardinal features of a toxic distal axonopathy. The jagged lines (lightning bolts) indicate that the toxin is acting at multiple sites along motor and sensory axons in the PNS and CNS. Axon degeneration has moved proximally (dying-back) by the late stage. (From Schaumburg HH, Berger AB, Thomas PK: Disorders of Peripheral Nerves. Philadelphia, F. A. Davis Company, 1991; with permission.)

CNS

PNS

Astrocyte Proliferation

Axon Regeneration

Normal   Early   Late   Recovering

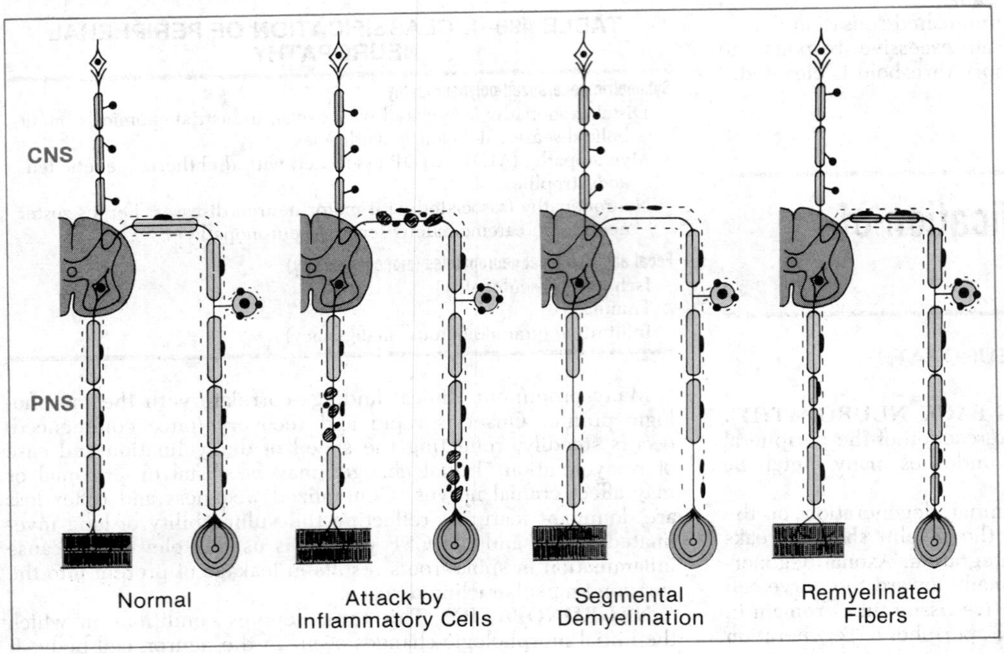

FIGURE 496–2. The cardinal pathologic features of an inflammatory myelinopathy. Axons are spared as is CNS myelin. After the attack, the remaining Schwann cells divide and remyelinate the denuded segments of axons. (From Schaumburg HH, Berger AB, Thomas PK: Disorders of Peripheral Nerves. Philadelphia, F. A. Davis Company, 1991; with permission.)

formidable diagnostic problems and usually require extensive evaluation for the underlying cause (ischemia, infiltration by tumor, amyloid, leprosy, among others).

DIAGNOSIS. Nerve conduction studies performed by an expert in neuromuscular disease are the initial diagnostic procedures (see Ch. 441). They are critical in determining the presence of neuropathy, whether suggested by clinical features or subclinical. Nerve conduction studies also establish the location of focal peripheral nerve lesions such as carpal tunnel or other entrapments. Also, they usually indicate whether a symmetric polyneuropathy is axonal or demyelinating, a crucial first step in diagnosis.

Nerve biopsy may be useful in identifying the cause of multiple mononeuropathy syndromes (amyloidosis, sarcoidosis, leprosy, and vasculitis). Conditions readily diagnosed on clinical grounds, such as diabetic neuropathy and AIDP, do not require biopsy. Biopsy is seldom helpful in distal axonopathies, since most display similar nonspecific findings.

Either the sural nerve at the ankle or the radial nerve at the wrist may be sampled under anesthesia. Tissue should be processed for routine histopathologic study, electron microscopy, and nerve fiber teasing. The latter technique is especially useful because it allows the rapid examination of long segments of individual fibers. Nerve biopsy should be performed only in institutions served by a surgeon accustomed to handling such tissues and whose pathologists have considerable experience in their interpretation.

Dyck PJ, Thomas PK, et al. (eds.): Peripheral Neuropathy, 3rd ed. Philadelphia, W. B. Saunders Company, 1991. *The authoritative reference on peripheral nerve disease.*

Schaumburg HH, Berger AB, Thomas PK: Disorders of Peripheral Nerves. Philadelphia, F. A. Davis Company, 1991. *A concise monograph providing a good introduction to this complex subject.*

497 Acute and Chronic Inflammatory Demyelinating Polyradiculoneuropathies (AIDP and CIDP)

DEFINITION. The inflammatory demyelinating polyradiculoneuropathies are a group of acute and chronic disorders that probably have similar pathologic bases but can differ in anatomic

sites and temporal profile. The most common is AIDP (Guillain-Barré syndrome), a rapidly evolving paralytic illness of unknown origin. Its salient morphologic feature is widespread inflammatory peripheral nervous system (PNS) demyelination, presumably secondary to a hypersensitivity reaction. The other, less common, form of inflammatory neuropathy is chronic inflammatory demyelinating polyneuropathy (CIDP). AIDP is the most common acute paralytic illness in young adults and almost the only form of inflammatory polyneuropathy encountered in general medical practice.

PATHOLOGY, PATHOGENESIS, AND PREDISPOSING FACTORS. Inflammatory cell infiltration (lymphocytes and plasma cells) followed by segmental demyelination is the hallmark of AIDP. Axons are relatively spared and blood vessels are normal. These reactions are most pronounced in spinal roots, limb girdle plexuses, and proximal nerve trunks; less intense changes are also present in distal nerves and autonomic ganglia. There is virtually no inflammatory change in the central nervous system (CNS). Within 2 to 3 weeks of the onset of acute demyelination, Schwann cell proliferation occurs as a prelude to remyelination and recovery.

It is generally held that AIDP is an autoimmune disorder; however, its pathogenesis is unclear. There is evidence for both lymphocyte-mediated delayed hypersensitivity and for a humoral mechanism involving antibodies to peripheral nerve myelin. Many predisposing events have been implicated, but a common antigen has not been identified, and HLA studies fail to disclose any predisposing pattern. Sixty per cent of cases have an antecedent upper respiratory infection or gastrointestinal illness (e.g., *Campylobacter jejuni*) within 1 month of onset. A host of common viral infections including infectious mononucleosis, hepatitis, and Epstein-Barr virus have been implicated. Other predisposing factors include vaccination against rabies and swine flu, HIV infection, surgery, pregnancy, and malignancy (especially lymphoma).

CLINICAL FEATURES. AIDP occurs worldwide in a nonseasonal pattern. It has a bimodal age distribution, with most cases in young adults and a lesser peak in incidence in the 45 to 64 age group. The disease consists of a rapidly progressive, largely reversible, predominantly motor neuropathy. Cardinal clinical features are progressive and usually symmetric weakness, combined with hyporeflexia. Weakness usually begins in distal lower limbs and spreads upward (ascending paralysis); this pattern is not inevitable and patients may have weakness of proximal upper limbs, face, or even extraocular muscles. Most weakened individuals do not appear systemically ill, and constitutional signs such as fever, chills, and weight loss are unusual.

The degree of paralysis varies from a mild footdrop to extreme weakness of all extremities and of the face. Severe involvement may lead to flaccid quadriplegia with inability to breathe, swallow, speak, or close the eyes. Limb weakness is generally symmetric and early muscle atrophy mild. Tendon reflexes usually disappear.

The presence of facial weakness helps to distinguish AIDP from most other neuropathies, apart from those related to sarcoidosis. Rarely, limb ataxia, paralysis of eye movements, and diffuse hyporeflexia may be the sole manifestations. Central nervous system involvement is not part of this illness. Increased intracranial pressure and papilledema rarely occur late.

Sensory symptoms, usually distal paresthesias, are present in most cases and rarely persist or progress (in contrast to weakness). Mild impairment of distal position and vibration sensation and slight loss of pinprick sensation over the toes are common.

Autonomic dysfunction accompanies most cases. Relative tachycardia is universal. Orthostatic hypotension and hypertension are frequent, difficult to treat, and can complicate the management of patients with respiratory compromise. Death can occur suddenly following unexplained fluctuations in blood pressure or cardiac dysrhythmias.

Cerebrospinal fluid (CSF) and electrodiagnostic studies are helpful. The CSF protein concentration is usually normal during the first 3 days of illness; it then steadily rises and may exceed 500 mg per deciliter. The CSF protein level may remain elevated even after recovery is under way. Mononuclear cells, usually less than 10 per cubic millimeter, are present in as many as half the cases.

At the commencement of illness, distal motor nerve conduction may be normal. Presumably, in such cases the disease process is confined to spinal roots and proximal nerves. If the demyelination affects distal nerves as well, slowing of motor conduction, characteristic of segmental demyelination, occurs. Analysis of the F response, a measurement of proximal motor conduction, can be useful in early diagnosis of patients who display normal distal motor conduction.

Differential diagnosis is not difficult, especially since the decline of poliomyelitis and diphtheria in North America. Hypokalemia, tick paralysis, botulism, acute myelitis, and cervical spine fracture should be ruled out rapidly.

COURSE AND PROGNOSIS. Rapid progression of weakness is characteristic of AIDP. Paralysis is maximal by 1 week in more than half, by 3 weeks in 80 per cent, and by 1 month in 90 per cent. In the other patients, weakness may progress for variable intervals up to 8 weeks.

Recovery usually begins 2 to 4 weeks after progression ceases. The pattern is variable, normally proceeding at a steady pace. Within 6 months 85 per cent of patients are ambulatory. Occasionally, individuals experience more rapid recovery and are able to return to work within 2 months following quadriparesis. Rare cases show little or no improvement.

Most patients eventually recover but one out of 20 dies and more than half suffer residual peripheral nervous system damage, with one sixth remaining handicapped by weakness. Some initial features help in predicting the eventual outcome. Older patients and those with electrodiagnostic evidence of axonal compromise do less well than individuals who experience only mild distal extremity weakness and subsequently improve within weeks of the first signs.

TREATMENT. Early and accurate diagnosis is crucial since plasmapheresis, the accepted therapy, when administered within the first 2 weeks shortens the clinical course and reduces morbidity. A continuous-flow regimen of 200 to 250 cc per kilogram is given within 2 weeks. Patients suspected of having AIDP must be admitted to the hospital even if involvement is minimal, since neuropathy may evolve rapidly and unpredictably. In general, they should be admitted to a unit where respiratory care is available, and remain until their condition stabilizes or improves. Tidal volume, oxygen saturation, vital capacity, blood pressure, and ability to cough and swallow should be closely monitored, since they can change without warning.

If a need for mechanical ventilation is anticipated (as determined by the degree of respiratory effort, the vital capacity, and the blood gases), it should be instituted early without waiting for decompensation.

Autonomic dysfunction may produce pupillary disturbances, neuroendocrine disturbance, peripheral pooling of blood, poor venous return, cardiac arrhythmias, and low cardiac output. Beat

to beat (R-R) variation of the heart rate during normal and deep breathing is a reliable index. Pharmacologic manipulation of blood pressure in AIDP patients is perilous and should be avoided unless absolutely necessary.

Some patients are unable to swallow or to gag. Feeding should be done through a small nasogastric tube. The patient should be sitting when food is given and for 30 to 60 minutes thereafter to minimize the risk of aspiration.

If patients with AIDP can be carried through the acute stage of progressive paralysis (usually 2 to 3 weeks), strength will gradually return. Since most patients achieve good recovery after months of weakness, the importance of fastidious supportive care in the acute stage cannot be overstressed. Glucocorticoids are contraindicated.

CHRONIC INFLAMMATORY DEMYELINATING POLYNEUROPATHY

DEFINITION, PATHOLOGY, AND PATHOGENESIS. Affected individuals initially have an illness similar to AIDP (although usually with a more gradual onset) but subsequently undergo either a chronic relapsing or progressive course. The salient histologic features of both chronic forms are similar to those of AIDP. Segmental demyelination, "onion bulb" formations areas of thickened nerves due to repeated demyelination-remyelination, and lymphocytic infiltration are prominent findings.

CLINICAL FEATURES. The progressive form is more common and, except for cases associated with HIV, there is rarely a clear temporal relationship to antecedent infections. The cardinal symptoms and signs reflect predominant motor involvement: weakness of the extremities, intercostal muscles, and lower cranial nerves. Sensory complaints are almost as common as weakness, and objective signs of sensory loss are more frequent in the chronic disorders than in AIDP. Hyporeflexia or areflexia occur in almost all cases.

The development and course of illness are the salient features that distinguish between the progressive and relapsing variants. Each has a protracted onset and an indolent progression.

The progressive form usually proceeds in stepwise fashion but may be gradual. If untreated, the condition may become disabling or fatal; the prognosis is uncertain. The course of the relapsing form may vary considerably in interval between episodes and rate and degree of recovery. With treatment, improvement is generally good between episodes. Life-threatening episodes with respiratory insufficiency are more common early in the illness.

The CSF protein level is elevated at some stage of the illness in almost every case. Slowed nerve conduction in both motor and sensory nerves is characteristic, although not always present. Nerve conduction studies can be extremely helpful in diagnosis, especially in the progressive form. The histologic picture is characteristic for these disorders. The differential diagnosis of the relapsing form is seldom a problem after several episodes have occurred. The differential diagnosis of the progressive disorder is sometimes extremely difficult. Unless nerve conduction studies display characteristic changes, it may be indistinguishable from a chronic axonopathy.

TREATMENT. Glucocorticoids are sometimes efficacious in treating chronic polyneuropathy, in contrast to the acute form. Human immune globulin therapy is gaining acceptance as a first-line treatment; it appears especially effective in HIV-associated cases. Plasma exchange may produce dramatic improvement in the relapsing form and is sometimes effective in the progressive disorder. It offers a useful alternative for individuals who cannot tolerate long-term corticosteroids or other immunosuppressive therapy.

McCombe PA, Pollard JD, McLeod JG: Chronic inflammatory demyelinating polyneuropathy. Brain 110:1617, 1987. *A detailed review of the clinical and therapeutic issues of the disorders.*
McKhann GM: Guillain-Barré syndrome: Clinical and therapeutic observations. Ann Neurol 27(Suppl 1):S13, 1990. *A timely review that thoughtfully analyzes the role of plasmapheresis and other therapies in AIDP.*
Ropper AH, Eelco FM, Wijdicks MD, Truax BT: Guillain-Barré Syndrome. Philadelphia, F. A. Davis Company, 1991. *A comprehensive monograph discussing the disorder.*

498 Diabetic and Other Endocrine Neuropathies

THE DIABETIC NEUROPATHIES

A variety of peripheral nerve disorders may occur in diabetes mellitus. Diabetic neuropathies may be classified as either mononeuropathies or symmetric polyneuropathies, but mixed syndromes often occur. For instance, an individual with symmetric sensory polyneuropathy may develop acute third-nerve palsy (a mononeuropathy). See Table 498–1.

Symmetric Polyneuropathy

PATHOLOGY. The experimental animal model of diabetic neuropathy exhibits only nerve conduction abnormalities without degeneration of nerve fibers; therefore, the early fundamental, pathologic diabetic changes in peripheral nerve are unclear. Previous human histopathologic studies were described in individuals with chronic neuropathy; nerves from biopsy or autopsy displayed a mixture of axonal loss and segmental demyelination. These observations suggested that axonal loss was primary and reflected an underlying metabolic disorder and that segmental demyelination was secondary to focal axonal change. Clearly fiber loss is the predominant change in chronic cases, restricting potential recovery. Postmortem histopathologic studies of long segments of nerves of diabetics indicate a multifocal pattern of fiber loss along nerves, suggesting that ischemia has a role in the symmetric neuropathies. Microangiopathic changes in the vasa nervorum are prominent in such nerve tissue. Sural nerve biopsies of diabetics contain abundant endoneurial capillary changes that include reduplicated basement lamina, closed lumens, and increased numbers of endothelial nuclei. These abnormalities appeared to correlate with degree of nerve fiber loss.

PATHOGENESIS. The clinical features of symmetric polyneuropathy, which often selectively involve particular fiber types, favor a metabolic basis. Elevated levels of neurotoxic ketones have been sought but not found. Distal axonopathy may be one of the mechanisms operating in individuals with the common progressive distal symmetric sensory neuropathy. No valid animal models are currently available to test this hypothesis.

Confounding a metabolic explanation is the inconsistent relationship of severity of neuropathy to control of blood glucose. There are many instances of "well-controlled" patients who develop severe sensorimotor neuropathy and others with "poor control" who have no evidence of neuropathy. The balance of recent evidence favors the notion that hyperglycemia is an important determinant of diabetic neuropathy and improved glycemic control is beneficial for nerve function.

Glycemic control does help two types of symmetric diabetic neuropathy. One affects the newly diagnosed, insulin-dependent diabetic whose nerve conduction velocity and distal sensation loss improve following institution of therapy. The other occurs in individuals with acute painful neuropathy associated with rapid weight loss (diabetic neuropathic cachexia) in whom institution of glycemic control is followed by weight gain and recovery from neuropathy.

Among the proposed biochemical mechanisms underlying diabetic neuropathy, accumulation of nerve sorbitol and depletion of nerve myoinositol have received most attention. Sorbitol accumulates in the lens of the eye, alters the state of hydration, and may, by this mechanism, lead to cataract formation. Sorbitol also accumulates in nerve, but not in sufficient quantities to lead to osmotic damage unless it is confined to a particular cell compartment. Controlled clinical trials of aldose reductase inhibitors (the enzyme responsible for sorbitol accumulation) have been inconclusive.

Myoinositol is a cyclic hexitol normally present in nerve and is a precursor of membrane polyphosphoinositides that may regulate the patencies of ion channels. Nerve myoinositol concentration is reduced in experimental diabetes but is normal in human nerve biospy specimens. Although the addition of small quantities of myoinositol to the diet of animals with experimental diabetes may prevent reduction in nerve conduction velocity, the administration of dietary inositol to humans with diabetic neuropathy has little beneficial effect.

It is suggested that prolonged hyperglycemia may induce nonenzymatic glycosylation of vessel membrane protein. These membrane changes possibly account for progressive alteration of both endoneurial capillary wall and the endoneurial matrix, producing ischemic change in multiple levels of nerve.

CLINICAL FEATURES. See Table 498–2. *Distal Sensory Polyneuropathy.* This is the most common type of diabetic peripheral nerve disorder, estimated to be present in about 40 per cent of individuals with diabetes of 25 years' duration. It is present in less than 10 per cent of patients at the time of diagnosis (which it may antedate) and is uncommon in children.

Neuropathy may be asymptomatic, with abnormal signs first detectable on routine examination, or there may be a variety of symptoms. There appear to be three consistent patterns:

1. A "large-fiber" pattern with paresthesias in legs, absent ankle jerks, and impaired senses of light touch, vibration, and position in the lower limbs. Slight distal weakness is common and the hands may become involved.

2. A "small-fiber" pattern with dull aching pain and impaired cutaneous pain, touch, and temperature sensations. Position and vibration sense, deep tendon reflexes, and strength are usually spared. Autonomic nervous system dysfunction may accompany this variant.

3. A rare "pseudotabetic" pattern associated with long-term diabetes. Severe reduction of cutaneous and deep senses permits ulceration of the feet and distal joint deformity. Romberg's sign is present, tendon reflexes are absent in the legs, and hypotension and Argyll Robertson pupils may be observed.

The course is variable in sensory neuropathy. Most often it fluctuates and then plateaus. The pseudotabetic variety of the illness has an especially bad prognosis. Electrodiagnostic tests usually reveal changes in sensory conduction and variable alteration in motor conduction. The cerebrospinal fluid protein is usually elevated, sometimes to a very high level.

There is no specific treatment. Simple analgesics rarely help the severe pain that accompanies sensory neuropathy. Trial treatment with phenytoin, carbamazepine, phenothiazine, and tricyclic antidepressants is advocated. Persons with pain and temperature insensitivity of hands and feet are vulnerable to injuries that potentially can cascade into ulceration, cellulitis, lymphangitis, osteomyelitis, and osteolysis. Similar abnormalities are seen in syphilitic tabes, leprosy, inherited amyloidosis, and other inherited and acquired neuropathies, with the aforementioned sensory loss. The goal in treatment is to prevent the onset of tissue damage or, when it has occurred, to promote healing and prevent further damage. Persons with loss of pain and temperature sensation should not engage in most forms of manual labor or perform potentially bruising tasks with the hands and feet. Repeated inspection of hands and feet is necessary. If any bruise or ulcer appears, weight bearing or rough use should be

TABLE 498–1. CLASSIFICATION OF DIABETIC NEUROPATHIES

Symmetric polyneuropathies
  Distal primary sensory neuropathy
  Autonomic neuropathy
  Rapidly reversible neuropathy

Mononeuropathy and multiple mononeuropathies
  Cranial neuropathies
  Focal nerve lesions (other than cranial)
  Proximal painful lower limb neuropathy (diabetic amyotrophy)

TABLE 498–2. SYMMETRIC DIABETIC POLYNEUROPATHY SYNDROMES

Distal sensory neuropathy
Autonomic neuropathy
Symmetric proximal lower limb neuropathy
Rapidly reversible neuropathy

stopped until healing occurs. Shoes should be wide and well constructed, with the insides inspected to remove retained objects or nails. Patients should soak the feet in lukewarm water for 15 minutes twice daily and cover them lightly with petrolatum lotion to retain moisture in the softened skin.

Autonomic Neuropathy. Diabetic autonomic neuropathy generally is associated with symmetric sensory neuropathy and occasionally predominates. Autonomic involvement can be asymptomatic or cause incapacitating disability. Three types of dysfunction are prominent: gastrointestinal, cardiovascular, and genitourinary. The common gastrointestinal disturbances are gastroparesis, episodic nocturnal diarrhea, and colonic dilatation. Gastroparesis is often asymptomatic; it is best identified by radiographic or nuclear scans that demonstrate delayed emptying. Cardiovascular manifestations include impaired vasomotor reflexes (postural hypotension), elevated heart rate, and loss of respiratory sinus arrhythmia. Genitourinary disturbances are especially distressing and include disordered micturition with large residual volume, retrograde ejaculation, and impotence. Impotence is sometimes the initial manifestation of autonomic neuropathy. It usually steadily worsens and rarely, if ever, is reversed by control of hyperglycemia, the use of testosterone, or penile implants.

Treatment of autonomic disturbances is difficult. Gastroparesis secondary to vagal denervation can be treated with either neostigmine or metoclopramide. Diabetic diarrhea may be helped by codeine phosphate or diphenoxylate, but not all cases respond favorably. A single 250-mg dose of tetracycline, if given at the outset, sometimes aborts the attack. Simple cases of postural hypotension may be helped by support stockings. More severe cases may require supplemental sodium in the diet plus sodium-retaining steroids.

Symmetric Proximal Lower Extremity Motor Neuropathy. This syndrome is most common in elderly diabetics but may appear at any age and occasionally heralds the onset of the metabolic disorder. Initial symptoms of low back and thigh pain are followed by slowly progressive weakness and atrophy of thigh and gluteal muscles. Loss of patellar reflexes is universal, but sensation is strikingly spared. Recovery is variable.

Rapidly Reversible Neuropathy. Newly diagnosed untreated diabetics may display asymptomatic slowing of nerve conduction velocity. This slowing is rapidly reversed by lowering blood sugar concentration to normal levels. It seems unlikely that this phenomenon is associated with structural breakdown in peripheral nerve fibers; it is not known whether such individuals are at greater risk of developing persistent symptomatic neuropathy.

MONONEUROPATHY AND MULTIPLE MONONEUROPATHY

PATHOLOGY AND PATHOGENESIS. It is believed that isolated peripheral nerve lesions in diabetics have a vascular basis. Several clinical facts support this notion: They have an abrupt onset, often recover spontaneously, and are most common in the elderly. Three careful autopsy studies, two of oculomotor palsy and one of femoral neuropathy, have demonstrated focal vascular lesions within the area of nerve damage.

CLINICAL FEATURES. See Table 498–3. *Cranial Nerve Lesions.* Isolated or multiple palsies of extraocular muscle nerves or lower cranial nerves may be the first indication of diabetes in asymptomatic older adults. The third nerve is most frequently affected. Onset is usually abrupt and associated with an intense, retro-orbital aching sensation. Sparing of the pupillomotor fibers in diabetic third-nerve palsy helps distinguish this condition from lesions that compress the nerve, such as aneurysm. Satisfactory recovery of nerve function usually occurs within several weeks.

Focal Limb Lesions. Almost every isolated peripheral nerve can be affected by diabetic mononeuropathy. Lesions of the ulnar, radial, sciatic, peroneal, tibial, and lateral cutaneous nerves of

TABLE 498–3. DIABETIC MONONEUROPATHY AND MULTIPLE MONONEUROPATHY

Cranial nerve lesions
Focal limb lesions
Truncal neuropathy
Asymmetric proximal lower extremity motor neuropathy

the thigh are especially common. Diabetic nerves are especially vulnerable to compression, and lesions frequently appear at such sites. Onset is abrupt and usually painful. Recovery is usually good in distally sited lesions and less satisfactory if the lesions are proximal. Treatment includes physical therapy and use of appropriate orthotic devices.

Truncal Neuropathy. The syndrome of acute unilateral pain in the distribution of one or more thoracic nerves occurs in older individuals and can appear in any diabetic state. Pain is often intense, poorly localized, and associated with hypersensitivity and loss of pain sense. Recovery over a 2-year period is usual.

Asymmetric Proximal Lower Extremity Motor Neuropathy. This syndrome usually appears after middle age, in the setting of substantial recent weight loss. Cardinal findings include rapidly progressive, painful, asymmetric weakness of thigh muscles, loss of knee jerks, and few sensory abnormalities. The spinal fluid protein level is usually elevated, and weakness is usually bilateral, differentiating the condition from acute nerve root disease. Recovery is gradual. There is considerable variation in the clinical features, and many patients display distal weakness as well. Treatment includes major analgesics for relief of the self-limited pain, and physical therapy.

OTHER ENDOCRINE NEUROPATHIES

Hypothyroidism is associated with both mononeuropathy and symmetric polyneuropathy. Clumsiness and limb ataxia of uncertain origin are common, probably due to cerebellar disease. Thyroid replacement therapy ameliorates the carpal and tarsal tunnel syndromes as well as the diffuse symmetric neuropathy.

Acromegaly produces entrapment neuropathies at wrist and elbow and a distal symmetric polyneuropathy. Proximal weakness occurs independently of the peripheral neuropathies and may make the clinical profile confusing. The carpal tunnel syndrome presumably results from compression by acral soft-tissue hyperplasia and osteoarthritis. Improvement follows removal of the pituitary tumor; surgery of the carpal ligament is seldom necessary. Symmetric polyneuropathy usually occurs late in the illness; it bears no relationship to plasma levels of growth hormone. No studies have been made on the effect of removal of the pituitary adenoma on neuropathy.

Aminoff MJ (ed.): Neurology and General Medicine. New York, Churchill Livingstone, 1989. *An excellent encyclopedic text covering the neurology of systemic diseases.*

Asbury AK: Understanding diabetic neuropathy. N Engl J Med 319:577, 1988. *A thoughtful summary of pathogenetic theories and treatment strategies for diabetic neuropathy.*

Dyck PJ, Thomas PK, Asbury AK, et al.: Diabetic Neuropathy. Philadelphia, W. B. Saunders Company, 1986. *A book that covers all aspects of diabetic neuropathy.*

499 Hereditary Neuropathies

Hereditary neuropathies represent a group of slowly progressive disorders characterized by the type of inheritance, their natural history, and the population of neurons involved. Predominant involvement of lower motor neurons (progressive muscular atrophy) is called *inherited motor neuropathy*; involvement of sensory neurons is *hereditary sensory neuropathy* (HSN); involvement of both motor and sensory neurons is *hereditary motor and sensory neuropathy* (HMSN); and involvement of autonomic neurons is *dysautonomia.*

Expression of clinical symptoms varies widely from patient to patient, and functional disability is frequently less than might be expected from the neurologic signs. Certain of these disorders (HMSN types I and II) are common and account for many cases of cryptogenic neuropathy. The number of correct diagnoses increases considerably when the patient's asymptomatic relatives are examined clinically and by nerve conduction studies.

TABLE 499–1. THE HEREDITARY MOTOR AND SENSORY NEUROPATHIES (HMSN)

Nomenclature	Heredity	Clinical Features	Pathology and Pathogenesis
HMSN type 1 (peroneal muscle atrophy; hypertrophic form of Charcot-Marie-Tooth disease)	Autosomal dominant	Common; many mild cases; childhood onset; slow progression; predominantly motor; deformed feet (pes cavus); extreme distal lower limb atrophy; very slow motor nerve conduction	Possibly a distal axonopathy but much segmental demyelination and remyelination ("onion bulbs"); nerves may be enlarged
HMSN type II (neuronal form of Charcot-Marie-Tooth disease or peroneal muscle atrophy)	Autosomal dominant	Less common than type I; onset in second decade; nerve conduction almost normal; otherwise, identical to type I	Possibly a motor and sensory neuronopathy syndrome; loss of fibers; little remyelination (no "onion bulbs")
HMSN type III (Déjérine-Sottas disease)	Autosomal recessive	Rare; infantile onset; short stature, scoliosis, pes cavus; steady progression to severe disability; very slow nerve conduction	Few studies; enlarged nerves; many "onion bulbs"; pathogenesis unclear

HEREDITARY MOTOR AND SENSORY NEUROPATHY

These disorders, previously described by various eponyms (Charcot-Marie-Tooth disease, Déjérine-Sottas disease) are now numerically subdivided into types I, II, and III. Table 499–1 outlines their salient features.

DISORDERS OF PERIPHERAL SENSORY NEURONS

Patients with disorders of peripheral sensory neurons characteristically suffer from pain, cutaneous injury from lack of sensation, unsteady movement from kinesthetic sensory loss, or combinations of these conditions. Frequently they also have autonomic dysfunction. The nature of these symptoms and the associated sensory loss correspond reasonably well with the populations of fibers affected. Thus patients with loss of pain and temperature sensation and with autonomic impairment have degeneration mostly of unmyelinated and small myelinated fibers, whereas patients with loss of touch-pressure sensation have degeneration of large myelinated fibers of cutaneous nerves. In advanced disease this selectivity of involvement by fiber size tends to be lost.

HEREDITARY SENSORY NEUROPATHY, TYPE I. Hereditary sensory neuropathy, type I, is a dominantly inherited sensory radicular neuropathy. It has been variously termed perforating ulcers of the feet, mutilating acropathy, acrodystrophic neuropathy, and hereditary sensory radicular neuropathy. The severity varies widely. Sensory loss is usually more severe over the feet and legs than in the hands and forearms, and some patients have lancinating pains. Pain and temperature sensation are affected more than touch-pressure sensation. Nerve conduction of motor fibers is usually normal, as is life expectancy in most cases. Late in the disorder, perforating ulcers of the foot may develop, especially in patients with poor foot care.

HEREDITARY SENSORY NEUROPATHY, TYPE II. This is a recessively inherited disorder, also called congenital sensory neuropathy, that usually manifests itself in infancy or childhood with a mutilating acropathy characterized by paronychia, whitlows, ulcers of the fingers and plantar surfaces of the feet, and, frequently, unrecognized fractures of the extremities. Sensory loss affects all types of cutaneous and sometimes kinesthetic sensation and is most marked distally in all four limbs. Tendon reflexes are usually absent.

HEREDITARY SENSORY NEUROPATHY, TYPE III (Dysautonomia of Riley-Day). Familial dysautonomia is a recessively inherited disorder of Jewish infants and children. It affects peripheral autonomic neurons, peripheral sensory neurons, peripheral motor neurons, and probably other central nervous system neurons. Characteristics are onset in infancy, poor feeding, repeated episodes of vomiting and pulmonary infections, autonomic disturbances, and premature death. Autonomic abnormalities include defective lacrimation, defective temperature control, skin blotching, excessive perspiration, hypertension, and postural hypotension. There is insensitivity to pain, areflexia,

corneal insensitivity, and absence of the fungiform papillae of the tongue. An abnormality of nerve growth factor is postulated.

Dyck PJ, Thomas PK (eds.): Peripheral Neuropathy, 3rd ed. Philadelphia, W. B. Saunders Company, 1991. *A large, multiauthored reference text.*
Schaumberg HH, Berger AB, Thomas PK: Disorders of Peripheral Nerves, 2nd ed. Philadelphia, F. A. Davis Company, 1991. *A succinct, clearly expressed, comprehensive monograph.*

500 Toxic Neuropathies

UREMIA

DEFINITION AND ETIOLOGY. Uremic polyneuropathy can be associated with chronic renal insufficiency of any type. The cause is unknown. It is believed that uremic neuropathy is related to dialyzable toxins or metabolites normally excreted by the kidneys. The responsible agent has a molecular weight exceeding that of urea or creatinine.

PATHOLOGY. Axonal degeneration is characteristic of this disorder, and the distribution suggests that it is a distal axonopathy. The nature of the axonal change is nonspecific.

CLINICAL FEATURES. Initially, sensory symptoms predominate, with especially frequent tingling paresthesias of the leg. Occasionally a "burning foot" or "restless leg" syndrome accompanies uremic polyneuropathy. Muscle cramps in the distal extremities are common. Diminished sensation in distal limbs is the most consistent feature, usually in combination with hyporeflexia and moderate weakness.

Uremic neuropathy has an insidious onset, and subclinical cases are common. Most cases progress over several months to reach a plateau despite worsening of the renal state. The prognosis of untreated uremic neuropathy is poor.

TREATMENT. Successful renal transplantation both prevents

TABLE 500–1. PHARMACEUTICAL AGENTS ASSOCIATED WITH GENERALIZED NEUROPATHY

Chloramphenicol	Nucleosides (ddC, ddI)
Dapsone*	Nitrofurantoin*
Disulfiram	Nitrous oxide
Ethionamide	Phenytoin
Gold	Platinum (cis-platin)†
Glutethimide	Pyridoxine†
Hydralazine	Sodium cyanate
Isoniazid†	Taxol
Metronidazole-misonidazole	Thalidomide†
	Vincristine

*Predominantly motor.
†Predominantly sensory.

TABLE 500–2. AGENTS CAUSING SYMPTOMS ASSOCIATED WITH TOXIC NEUROPATHY

Acrylamide (truncal ataxia)
Allyl chloride
Arsenic (sensory, brown skin, Mees' lines)
Buckthorn toxin
Carbon disulfide
Cyanide
Dimethylaminopropionitrile (urinary complaints)
Biologic toxin in diphtheritic neuropathy (pharyngeal neuropathy)
Ethylene oxide
n-Hexane
Lead (wrist drop, abdominal colic)
Lucel-7 (cataracts)
Mercury
Methyl bromide
Organophosphates (cholinergic symptoms, delayed onset of neuropathy)
Thallium (pain, alopecia, Mees' lines)
Trichloroethylene (facial numbness)
Vacor

and reverses uremic polyneuropathy. Patients with mild cases display prompt relief of paresthesias and a steady return of strength. Recovery is more prolonged in advanced cases and is not always complete. Chronic hemodialysis is less helpful and often ineffective in reversing the neuropathy.

PHARMACEUTICAL AGENTS

GENERAL. New pharmaceutical agents are constantly being implicated on clinical-epidemiologic grounds as causes of peripheral neuropathy. Except for isoniazid, pyridoxine, and vincristine, few careful experimental studies of these substances have been conducted. Since following prolonged use most of the offending agents produce an insidious-onset distal axonopathy, little in the clinical diagnostic profile helps to identify the specific offending agent. The most important diagnostic factor in these disorders is a meticulous history of drug use. Table 500–1 lists pharmaceutical agents that are associated with generalized neuropathy. Treatment consists of withdrawing the drug if symptoms are prominent or progressive.

OCCUPATIONAL, BIOLOGIC, AND ENVIRONMENTAL AGENTS

GENERAL. Many potentially toxic chemicals are deployed in the work place and general environment, and several have been implicated as causes of peripheral neuropathy, usually of the distal axonopathy type. Since the various agents result in similar clinical syndromes, a careful occupational and environmental history is often the most important clue for diagnosis. The various agents are listed in Table 500–2, with prominent clinical features included in parentheses. *Buckthorn* and *diphtheritic neuropathies*, which are demyelinating conditions, are the sole examples of diseases in which biologic toxins are consistently associated with neuropathy. Diphtheria is further discussed in Ch. 306.

Spencer PS, Schaumburg HH: Experimental and Clinical Neurotoxicology. Baltimore, Williams & Wilkins, 1980. *A multiauthored comprehensive text with special emphasis on the peripheral nervous system.*

501 Miscellaneous Disease-Specific Neuropathies

NEUROPATHY ASSOCIATED WITH MALIGNANCY AND DYSPROTEINEMIA

Direct compression of nerves by metastatic tumors occurs within the spinal canal or invertebral foramina and behind tight fascial sheaths. Bronchogenic, renal, prostatic, and breast carcinomas are especially prone to such metastases. The direct and nonmetastatic neurologic effects of cancer are described in Ch. 162.

TABLE 501–1. FAMILIAL AMYLOID POLYNEUROPATHIES

Type	Source of Amyloid
I (Portuguese)	met/val 30 TTR substitution
II (Indiana)	ser/ile 84 TTR substitution
III (Van Allen)	Variant apolipoprotein A1
IV (Finnish)	Not yet established
Other forms	
Jewish	ile/phe 33 TTR substitution
Appalachian	ala/thr 60 TTR substitution
German	tyr/ser 77 TTR substitution

Met = methionine; val = valine; ser = serine; ile = isoleucine; phe = phenylalanine; ala = alanine; thr = threonine; tyr = tyrosine.
From Schaumburg HH, Berger AB, Thomas PK: Disorders of Peripheral Nerves. Philadelphia, F. A. Davis Company, 1991; with permission.)

Polyneuropathy is more common in multiple myeloma than in most other malignancies; furthermore, subclinical neuropathy appears to be frequent. Recent evidence has demonstrated that the benign gammopathies are also associated with polyneuropathy; some resemble motor neuron disease.

AMYLOID NEUROPATHY

Extracellular deposition of the fibrous protein amyloid is associated with peripheral neuropathy in both hereditary (non–immunoglobulin-derived) amyloidosis and nonhereditary (immunoglobulin-derived) amyloidosis.

Seven different forms of familial amyloid polyneuropathy are currently recognized (Table 501–1), characterized by their clinical features and, except in two types, by a specific genetic mutation in the transthyretin (prealbumin) gene. The variant transthyretin (TTR) proteins have different amino acid substitutions; for example, in type I the variant TTR results from substitution of methionine for valine at position 30 in the molecule.

Hereditary amyloidosis is frequent only in endemic regions such as Portugal and Japan. In the Portuguese variety, which is inherited as an autosomal-dominant trait, the disorder usually begins in the third, fourth, or fifth decade and affects predominantly small sensory and autonomic fibers. Lumbosacral dermatomes show a syringomyelia-like loss of pain and thermal discrimination with preservation of touch-pressure sensation. Loss of potency in the male, postural hypotension, and bladder and bowel incontinence are common in advanced stages. The disorder tends to progress over a decade or so. Biopsied sural nerves show an endoneurial reduction in unmyelinated and small myelinated fibers with nodular deposits of amyloid among the nerve trunks.

Nonhereditary amyloidosis may be divided into primary and secondary varieties. The peripheral neuropathy of primary amyloidosis also affects the distal aspects of the lower extremities more than the upper and includes small fibers as much as or more than larger ones. When typical symptoms of neuropathy are associated with enlargement of the heart, nephropathy, and enlargement of the tongue, the diagnosis of primary amyloidosis should be strongly suspected and can be confirmed by histologic examination of rectal mucosa, kidney, carpal ligament, muscle, gingiva, nerve, or bone marrow. No effective treatment for the neuropathy is available.

Patients with multiple myeloma who develop a symmetric carpal tunnel syndrome should be investigated for systemic amyloidosis.

NEUROPATHY ASSOCIATED WITH NECROTIZING ANGIITIS AND RHEUMATOID ARTHRITIS

No fewer than nine disorders are associated with vasculitis and ischemic neuropathy. These include polyarteritis nodosa, rheumatoid arthritis, systemic lupus erythematosus (SLE), hypersensitivity angiitis, allergic granulomatosis (Churg-Strauss syndrome), Sjögren's syndrome, Wegener's granulomatosis, cranial arteritis (temporal arteritis), and nonsystemic vasculitic neuropathy.

Only polyarteritis nodosa, rheumatoid arthritis, and lupus erythematosus are encountered with any frequency in clinical practice. Although the fundamental expression of these conditions varies considerably, they all produce similar clinical and pathologic syndromes of ischemic mononeuritis multiplex. The pathogenesis of nerve fiber destruction in each condition presumably relates to focal ischemia from arteriolar occlusion. The clinical features are similar to those depicted for the mononeuropathies associated with diabetes (see Ch. 498).

Rheumatoid arthritis, in addition to producing a vascular mononeuropathy, may also cause entrapment neuropathy (reflecting prolonged immobilized postures and nerve compression by articular deformity) and a chronic symmetric sensory neuropathy. This latter disorder develops with long-term rheumatoid arthritis and is characterized by mild, distal, symmetric sensory loss. Although frequently painful, the condition is generally benign and improves spontaneously. Corticosteroid treatment is not indicated.

Neuropathy can accompany a variety of systemic illnesses other than those described in this chapter. Table 501–2 lists some of the more common conditions, and the text by Aminoff gives further details.

BELL'S PALSY (Idiopathic Facial Paralysis)

PATHOLOGY AND PATHOGENESIS. Neither the pathology nor the pathogenesis of this common illness is known. It is likely that mild cases with rapid recovery represent segmental demyelination and that axonal degeneration occurs in instances with prolonged dysfunction.

CLINICAL FEATURES. Idiopathic unilateral facial paralysis may develop rapidly within a few hours or evolve over 1 or 2 days and is often accompanied by pain behind the ipsilateral ear and excess tearing. Numbness of the face is a common complaint but inevitably refers to a proprioceptive sensation that accompanies weakness. Global facial muscle weakness is the hallmark of this condition. Hyperacusis, diminished lacrimation, and abnormal taste sensation are present to variable degrees. Untreated, 80 to 85 per cent of all patients with Bell's palsy recover completely or almost so. In a smaller number, persistent facial weakness ensues. Rarely, motor recovery fails completely. Aberrant regeneration is frequent. There may be embarrassing synkinetic movements (chewing producing eye winking) or excessive lacrimation.

Patients who are going to recover completely usually begin to show improvement during the first 2 weeks, while those destined to have permanent residual disability show no changes in status for 3 or more months. Except when paralysis is incomplete, there is little in the acute clinical profile to indicate prognosis. In patients who have complete paralysis from the onset, reliance must be placed on careful observation and electrodiagnostic tests of nerve excitability (performed at about 1 week after the onset).

Most authorities recommend treatment with prednisone, 1 mg per kilogram daily in two divided doses for 4 days, with dosage tapered to a total of 5 mg per day within 10 days. It is claimed that prednisone therapy should be instituted as soon as possible if it is to have an effect in decreasing residual paralysis and synkinetic movements. In any event, pain usually subsides promptly. Residual severe facial paralysis has a distressing cosmetic effect. Hypoglossal-facial nerve anastomosis will restore facial tone and is the operation of choice.

Hemifacial spasm, irregular clonic contractions of one side of the face, may be a temporary or permanent consequence of Bell's palsy. More commonly, hemifacial spasm develops without antecedent cause. In such cases, facial nerve compression by posterior fossa lesions (e.g., aberrant arterial loops, acoustic nerve tumors, aneurysms) may be present. Therapeutic choices include carbamazepine, botulinum toxin injection into the orbicularis oculi, and microsurgical nerve root decompression.

TABLE 501–2. OTHER MEDICAL CONDITIONS ASSOCIATED WITH NEUROPATHY

Herpes zoster (see Ch. 476.3)
Leprosy (see Ch. 334)
Sarcoidosis (see Ch. 67)
Human immunodeficiency virus (HIV) (see Ch. 414)
Lyme borreliosis (see Ch. 343)
Alcoholism, nutritional deficiency, malabsorption (see Ch. 456)

ACUTE BRACHIAL NEURITIS (Idiopathic Brachial Plexus Neuropathy)

Brachial neuritis is a syndrome wherein abrupt shoulder and neck pain is followed by a disabling upper limb weakness in a healthy individual.

PATHOLOGY AND PATHOGENESIS. There have been no thorough pathologic examinations of this condition, and the pathogenesis is unknown. Biopsy of cutaneous nerves has revealed nonspecific axonal degeneration. In most cases there is no common antecedent illness, immunization, or toxic exposure; some cases follow surgical procedures. The clinical profile is identical to that in certain serum vaccine paralyses, and a common immunologic basis has been suggested.

CLINICAL FEATURES. The condition arises as an acute, painful, and usually monophasic illness characterized by brachial plexus dysfunction. It is especially common in males aged 18 to 40. A cardinal feature is sudden severe shoulder girdle–scapular pain, occasionally extending into the arm or hand. The pain persists for a few days to a week and then subsides concomitantly with or shortly after the appearance of weakness, although it sometimes persists for several weeks. The serratus anterior is the single most commonly affected muscle. Distal weakness occurs less frequently. Rarely, the entire arm and ipsilateral diaphragm are affected. Uncommonly, weakness may appear in the other arm. Tendon reflexes are diminished in the involved extremity, but sensory loss is slight or negligible, being most commonly found at the apex of the shoulder. Involvement is usually restricted to muscles innervated by the brachial plexus. Weakness and atrophy of involved muscles lasts for months in many cases, but total recovery occurs in 90 per cent within 2 or 3 years. Treatment consists of physical therapy and orthotic devices to prevent joint damage. Corticosteroid therapy has no demonstrated value. There are occasional recurrences.

TRIGEMINAL NEUROPATHY

Rare cases are encountered of a slowly progressive bilateral sensory loss confined to the territory of the trigeminal nerve. This may lead to tissue destruction, particularly around the nostrils, as a result of repeated picking and scratching. High-level trichloroethylene exposure may cause this syndrome. Sjögren's syndrome, systemic sclerosis, and trigeminal neurilemomas should be excluded. Some cases have been found at autopsy to have infiltration of the trigeminal ganglion with amyloid. The explanation for other cases is obscure.

ACUTE PANDYSAUTONOMIA

Acute autonomic neuropathy is a poorly understood, rare condition. Pathologic studies are unavailable. The onset and time course are abrupt and progression is steady. Principal symptoms include postural hypotension, cramping abdominal pain, and varying amounts of diarrhea and constipation. Hypotension may be so severe that the patient cannot sit up without losing consciousness. Affected subjects reportedly improve with time, but few long-term follow-up studies are available.

Aminoff MJ (ed.): Neurology and General Medicine. New York, Churchill Livingstone, 1989.
Dyck PJ, Thomas PK (eds.): Peripheral Neuropathy, 3rd ed. Philadelphia, W. B. Saunders Company, 1991.
Halperin JJ, Luft BJ, Volkman DJ, et al: Lyme neuroborreliosis. Peripheral nervous system manifestations. Brain 113:1207, 1990. *A recent review of the many forms this disorder can take.*
Kelley JJ: Peripheral neuropathies associated with monoclonal proteins. A clinical review. Muscle Nerve 8:138, 1985. *A clear overview of this heterogeneous group of disorders.*
Moore PM, Cupps T: Neurological complications of vasculitis. Ann Neurol 14:155, 1983. *A comprehensive review of the protean neurologic complications of these disorders, especially the neuropathies.*

502 Acute Physical Injury and Chronic Compression-Entrapment Neuropathies

ACUTE PHYSICAL INJURY. The results of recent experimental studies suggest a simple classification for acute nerve injury in which the clinical features, including prognosis, closely

TABLE 502–1. TYPES OF NERVE INJURY

Type	Anatomic Lesion	Clinical Features	Course and Prognosis
Class 1	Either (A) transient conduction block due to ischemia or (B) demyelination	(A) Mild sensory loss and weakness (ischemic type) from transient abnormal posture (legs crossed) (B) Prolonged compression (Saturday night palsy) with paralysis and moderate sensory loss below site of lesion	(A) Rapid complete recovery (B) Gradual (lasting weeks) complete recovery
Class 2	Axonal interruption; connective tissue intact	Closed crush and percussion injury; loss of motor, sensory, and autonomic function below site of lesion; surgical exploration not indicated	Very slow recovery; prognosis best with distal lesions
Class 3	Transection of axons and connective tissue sheaths	Severe stretch injuries (heavy blows, motorcycle accidents) or penetrating wounds; total loss of all motor, sensory, and autonomic function; surgical intervention indicated for penetrating wounds	Little recovery even with surgical repair; poor prognosis

approximate the nature of the acute injury. Basically there are three different types (classes 1 through 3). In mild injury (class 1) axonal integrity is maintained but myelin may be damaged. In more severe injury (class 2) axonal continuity is lost but the connective tissue framework of the nerve is maintained. In the most severe injuries (class 3), nerve fibers and connective tissue are damaged to varying degrees. Table 502–1 depicts the types of nerve injury and their corresponding anatomic and clinical features.

COMPRESSION-ENTRAPMENT NEUROPATHY. The pathophysiologic features of chronic compressions and entrapment are still debated. It is widely believed that demyelination initially occurs and, if the condition persists, axonal destruction may follow. Several clinical forms are common, including carpal tunnel syndrome, ulnar palsy, and meralgia paresthetica (Table 502–2).

CARPAL TUNNEL SYNDROME. The median nerve becomes compressed at the wrist as it passes deep within the tissue to the flexor retinaculum. The usual symptoms include numbness, tingling, and burning sensations in hand and fingers. Pain sometimes radiates up the forearm as far as the elbow or even as high as the shoulder or root of the neck. These sensations are occasionally restricted to the radial fingers but may affect all digits. Pain and paresthesias are most prominent at night and often wake the patient from sleep. They may be relieved by shaking the hand. The hand tends to feel numb and useless on waking in the morning, but these sensations subside after brief use. The symptoms may recur following use or when the patient is sitting with the hands immobile. Such symptoms may persist for many years without objective signs of median nerve damage. In other patients, weakness of the thumb muscles develops in association with atrophy of the lateral aspect of the thenar eminence. Sensory loss may appear over the tips of the fingers. Occasionally, patients have motor symptoms of median nerve deficit in the hand without paresthesias, or motor and sensory signs may be discovered incidentally in the absence of symptoms, particularly in older individuals.

Most cases of carpal tunnel compression occur in middle-aged and often obese females. In younger women it is commonly

TABLE 502–2. COMPRESSION-ENTRAPMENT NEUROPATHIES

Common
Carpal tunnel
Ulnar palsy (cubital tunnel)
Lateral femoral cutaneous nerve of the thigh (meralgia paresthetica)
Rare
Cervical rib–thoracic outlet
Tarsal tunnel (tibial nerve at ankle)
Morton's neuroma (plantar nerve in anterior foot)

associated with excessive use of the hands, and it may develop in males after unaccustomed use of the hands, such as in housepainting. The disorder may be caused by tenosynovitis at the wrist, by involvement of the wrist joint in rheumatoid arthritis, or as a consequence of osteoarthritis of the carpus, perhaps in relation to an old fracture. Other predisposing causes are pregnancy, myxedema, acromegaly, infiltration of the transverse carpal ligament in primary amyloidosis, and chronic hemodialysis treatments. Diagnosis is based on clinical symptoms, Tinel's sign over the median nerve in the tunnel, and demonstration of slowed conduction at the wrist by motor nerve velocity studies. Individuals with muscle weakness and wasting or prominent sensory loss should undergo decompression of the nerve by section of the transverse carpal ligament. In patients with paresthesias alone or when the cause is probably tenosynovitis at the wrist, a reduction in hand activity may be sufficient to allow the symptoms to subside. Injection into the carpal tunnel of a long-acting corticosteroid preparation sometimes gives temporary relief, as does splinting of the wrist to reduce movement. When troublesome symptoms persist, decompression is advisable.

For most patients with paresthesias, symptoms are relieved by decompression. Sensory impairment and cutaneous hyperesthesia, however, may persist postoperatively, and there may not be recovery after prolonged denervation of the thenar muscles.

ULNAR PALSY. The ulnar nerve may be injured at the elbow, especially in persons with a shallow ulnar groove, those who rest their weight on their elbows excessively, and those who are cachectic and lie in bed. Injury may occur years following a previously malunited supracondylar fracture of the humerus with bony overgrowth (*tardive ulnar palsy*). Contrary to the findings in the carpal tunnel syndrome, muscle weakness and atrophy characteristically predominate over sensory symptoms and signs. Patients notice atrophy of the first dorsal interosseous muscle or difficulty in performing fine manipulation. There may be numbness of the small finger, the contiguous half of the proximal and middle phalanges of the ring finger, and the ulnar border of the hand. Treatment in mild cases consists of prevention of further injury. A doughnut cushion for the elbow may be helpful. Mobilizing and transplanting the nerve to a position in front of the medial epicondyle sometimes prevents further progression.

LATERAL CUTANEOUS NERVE OF THE THIGH. *Meralgia paresthetica* is an entrapment neuropathy resulting from compression of this nerve as it passes under the inguinal ligament. Although the case often remains unexplained, obese persons wearing tight girdles, individuals with gun belts, and those with pendulous abdomens are especially prone to develop numbness or burning sensations over the lateral thigh. Sometimes prolonged standing or walking provokes the symptoms. Weight reduction may help, and in many cases the condition subsides spontaneously. Surgical decompression is rarely necessary.

CERVICAL RIB AND THORACIC OUTLET SYNDROME.
Rarely, angulation of the brachial plexus over an abnormal rib or fibrous band can damage its lower fibers and lead to gradually progressive weakness and wasting of the small hand muscles. Numbness and pain may occur along the inner border of the forearm and hand. Surgical removal of the rib or fibrous band sometimes abolishes pain and paresthesias, but the small muscles of the hand often fail to recover strength. The overwhelming majority of individuals with paresthesias of the fingers prove to have either root compression from a cervical disc or carpal tunnel syndrome, not cervical rib or thoracic outlet.

Dawson D, Hallett M, Millender L: Entrapment Neuropathies, 2nd ed. Boston, Little, Brown and Co., 1990. *An extensive, excellently illustrated text covering all diagnostic and therapeutic aspects of these common disorders.*
Sunderland S: The anatomy and physiology of nerve injury. Muscle Nerve 13:771, 1990. *A concise review of the salient features of nerve injury.*

SECTION SEVENTEEN / DISEASES OF MUSCLE (MYOPATHIES) AND NEUROMUSCULAR JUNCTION

Andrew G. Engel

503 General Approach to Muscle Diseases

Muscle diseases are caused by derangements in the structure or function of the muscle fiber or in the innervation, blood supply, or connective tissue elements of muscle. A myopathy is a muscle disease not related to a demonstrable alteration in the innervation of muscle. Disorders that affect the innervation of muscle are considered in Ch. 495 through 502. Ch. 504 through 508 consider the myopathies. Ch. 509 deals with diseases of the neuromuscular junction. To facilitate the understanding of muscle diseases, this chapter begins with a brief overview of the structure and function of muscle.

BASIC STRUCTURE AND FUNCTION OF MUSCLE

Each voluntary muscle contains myriad muscle fibers. A small proportion of the fibers is confined to muscle spindles and innervated by γ or β motor neurons and by sensory neurons. These intrafusal fibers function as mechanoreceptors and participate in regulating the motor tone. Most muscle fibers are extrafusal and are innervated by α motor neurons. A *motor unit* consists of one α motor neuron and all muscle fibers innervated by that neuron. The peripheral axon of the motor neuron extends into muscle, where it divides into terminal branches that reach the neuromuscular junction on individual fibers. The number of motor units per muscle and the number of muscle fibers per motor unit vary from muscle to muscle. In general, motor units are smaller in small muscles subserving delicate movements (e.g., the external ocular, facial, and intrinsic hand muscles) than in large muscles maintaining posture or exerting strong force (e.g., biceps or quadriceps). The territory of a motor unit is a cylinder of the same length as the fibers and with a diameter that extends over a few millimeters. Muscle fibers belonging to different motor units intermingle with each other, so that the territories of individual motor units overlap. Many physiologic, biochemical, histochemical, and morphologic features of the muscle fibers are regulated by their innervation. Consequently, all muscle fibers in a motor unit share similar properties or are of the same type. Three major muscle-fiber (and motor-unit) types can be recognized: Type I, slow-twitch, fatigue-resistant fibers, high in oxidative enzymes but low in glycolytic enzymes; Type IIB, fast-twitch fatigable fibers, high in glycolytic enzymes and low in oxidative enzymes; and Type IIA, intermediate-twitch, fatigue-resistant fibers, high in glycolytic enzymes and with an intermediate content of oxidative enzymes. The myofibrillar ATPase, also different in the three fiber types, provides a convenient histochemical marker. In most human muscles the three fiber types occur in about equal proportions. Because the motor unit territories overlap, the fiber types intermingle randomly.

The muscle fibers of an adult are about 50 μm in diameter. Each fiber contains multiple subsarcolemmal nuclei. The myofibrils, which account for most of the fiber volume, are associated with mitochondria, glycogen granules, transverse (T) tubules, and sarcoplasmic reticulum (SR). The myofibrils, 0.5 to 1.0 μm wide, consist of repeating units, or sarcomeres, limited by Z disks. The latter anchor 1-μm-long thin filaments that extend from each Z disk toward the center of the sarcomere. The thin filaments interdigitate with 1.6-μm-long thick filaments in the central region (A-band) of the sarcomere. That part of the sarcomere which contains only thin filaments is referred to as the I band. It is the sarcomeres of adjacent myofibrils lying in register that give the striated appearance to the muscle fiber. The thin filaments are composed of actin, troponin, and tropomyosin. The thick filaments are made up nearly entirely of regularly arrayed myosin molecules. The head of each myosin molecule projects laterally from the thick filament and can serve as a cross-bridge between myosin and actin. The T-tubules are inward extensions of the muscle fiber surface membrane and propagate the action potential into the depth of the fiber. The SR abuts on the T-tubules and partially envelops individual myofibrils. In the resting state the SR sequesters calcium into its lumen by means of an ATPase and thereby maintains a very low calcium concentration (about 10^{-7} M) around the myofilaments.

When the T-tubules are depolarized by an action potential, voltage sensors embedded in their wall open calcium release channels positioned on the abutting SR surfaces and calcium escapes from the SR into the myofilament space. The released calcium binds to troponin on the thin filaments, which then acts on tropomyosin to allow repeated binding of the myosin cross-bridges to actin. Each binding is associated with a conformational change in the cross-bridge that exerts a force on the thin filament toward the center of the sarcomere. The cross-bridge cycle requires adenosine triphosphate (ATP), which is split by an ATPase on the cross-bridge. If ATP is depleted, the cross-bridges remain attached to the thin filaments and the muscle becomes stiff, as in rigor mortis. When ATP is available, the unloaded fiber shortens, the thin filaments are propelled into the A-band, and the Z disks are pulled closer together in every sarcomere. The active state subsides with calcium reuptake by the SR; interaction between actin and the cross-bridges ceases and relaxation sets in.

THE DIAGNOSIS OF MUSCLE DISEASES

The diagnosis of a muscle disease rests on a tripod: the clinical data, the electromyogram (EMG), and the muscle biopsy. None of the three approaches is entirely adequate by itself, but their combined use yields the correct diagnosis in a very high proportion of cases. Examples of disorders that are similar by clinical criteria but require muscle biopsy and EMG for accurate diagnosis are polymyositis, limb-girdle dystrophy, and adult acid maltase deficiency; distal muscular dystrophies, progressive muscular atrophy, and the slow-channel myasthenic syndrome; benign congenital myopathies, mitochondrial myopathies, and childhood or juvenile spinal muscular atrophies.

CLINICAL DATA. *The Genetic History.* This is relevant to diagnosis as well as counseling in the muscular dystrophies, congenital myopathies, and inherited metabolic myopathies. A negative family history, however, does not exclude autosomal recessive inheritance, an incompletely penetrant autosomal-dominant gene in one parent, or a new mutation. In autosomal dominant disorders (e.g., myotonic and facioscapulohumeral dystrophy or the familial periodic paralyses) a negative family history needs to be validated by examination of both parents. The clinical examination or biochemical tests may help in detecting heterozygotes in autosomal-recessive or X-linked recessive diseases. In Duchenne and Becker dystrophy, carrier detection and prenatal diagnosis are facilitated by dystrophin and DNA analysis.

The History of the Illness. Age at Onset, Duration, and Rate of Progression of Symptoms. Most benign congenital myopathies, congenital muscular dystrophy, congenital myasthenic syndromes, a number of inherited metabolic myopathies, and the acute form of spinal muscular atrophy present in infancy. Duchenne dystrophy usually presents in early childhood. Many inherited myopathies, inherited anterior horn cell diseases, and most hereditary peripheral neuropathies present in childhood or early adult life. Limb-girdle, Becker, and facioscapulohumeral dystrophy usually present in adolescence; myotonic, oculopharyngeal, limb-girdle, and distal dystrophies can present in adult life. Dermatomyositis and scleroderma can begin in childhood or adult life; pure polymyositis is unusual before adolescence; and inclusion body myositis seldom presents before the fifth decade.

Muscle weakness evolving over a few hours suggests an exogenous intoxication (e.g., organophosphorus or barium poisoning), periodic paralysis, or rhabdomyolysis. An abrupt onset of symptoms also can occur in myasthenia gravis or with other defects of neuromuscular transmission. Acute muscle weakness appearing during or after recovery from a Reye syndrome–like metabolic crisis suggests an enzyme defect in organic acid metabolism associated with secondary carnitine deficiency. Weakness evolving over a few days to a few weeks can occur in acute postinfectious polyneuropathy (Guillain-Barré syndrome), toxic neuropathies, and acute dermatomyositis. A subacute evolution, over a period of weeks to months, is seen in motor neuron disease; some metabolic myopathies, such as corticosteroid-induced or thyrotoxic myopathy; late-onset nemaline myopathy; and most cases of dermatomyositis and idiopathic polymyositis. A slow evolution over a number of years is typical of most dystrophies but can also occur in the inflammatory myopathies, such as inclusion body myositis, and in motor neuron disease.

Effects of Exercise, Rest After Exercise, Diet, and Temperature. Weakness appearing or increasing during exercise suggests a defect of neuromuscular transmission or in muscle energy metabolism. Weakness that decreases with exercise but increases during rest after exercise is typical of the periodic paralyses. Depending on the type of periodic paralysis, alterations in sodium, potassium, and carbohydrate intake can improve or exacerbate the symptoms. Fasting or a high-fat diet may provoke or worsen symptoms in patients with defects of fatty acid oxidation. Exposure to cold worsens myotonia and can provoke weakness in periodic paralysis and paramyotonia congenita. Exposure to heat can increase neuromuscular transmission defects.

Symptoms in Muscle Diseases. Relatively few symptoms are associated with diverse muscle diseases: weakness, decrease of muscle bulk, increased fatigability, muscle pain, cramps, stiffness, and discoloration of the urine caused by myoglobinuria. The cardinal symptom is muscle weakness, but patients often describe its consequences instead of speaking of weakness. Patients complaining of cramps sometimes suffer from contractures or tetany. The term *stiffness* is used to describe a variety of conditions, such as the stiff-man syndrome, neuromyotonia, and myotonia.

Muscle Weakness. Vague complaints, such as constant fatigue and exhaustion, or weakness of all muscles of uncertain duration in a patient who can carry out the tasks of everyday living suggest functional weakness. Patients with organic and evolving muscle weakness can always specify the tasks that they cannot do at present but could do a year, a month, or a few weeks before the examination.

Weakness of the cranial, cervical, torso, and limb muscles presents stereotypically. Weakness of muscles supplied by cranial nerves causes drooping of the eyelids (ptosis, third cranial nerve); double vision (diplopia, third, fourth, and sixth cranial nerves); failure of the eyelids to close at night, altered facial expression, difficulty in whistling or sucking from a straw (seventh cranial nerve); inability to close the jaw, difficulty in chewing hard food (fifth cranial nerve); difficulty in pronouncing words (dysarthria), hypernasal voice, nasal regurgitation of liquids, and difficulty in swallowing (dysphagia) (tenth and twelfth cranial nerves). Weakness of the cervical muscles is shown by difficulty in lifting the head from a pillow or holding the head erect, and weakness of the truncal muscles by difficulty in rolling over in bed or sitting up from the supine position. Weakness of the arm muscles is related as difficulty in holding the arms overhead, lifting heavy objects, or using the hands for motor tasks. Weakness of the pelvic girdle and of the proximal lower extremity muscles is reflected by difficulty in rising from sitting or squatting, climbing stairs, and stepping in or out of the bathtub. Weakness of the distal lower extremity may cause flopping of the feet or difficulty in rising on the toes.

Other Symptoms. In evaluating *abnormal fatigability*, it is important to define the duration and intensity of exercise that provokes it. Even mild exercise can induce fatigue in patients with defects of neuromuscular transmission or with mitochondrial myopathies that involve an electron transport complex. Brief periods of intense, anaerobic exercise precipitate fatigue in patients with glycolytic enzyme defects, but sustained exercise is required to induce fatigue in carnitine palmityltransferase deficiency.

Muscle pain (myalgia) at rest can occur in some of the inflammatory myopathies (especially dermatomyositis and the eosinophilia-myalgia syndrome), during acute viral infections, in polymyalgia rheumatica, myxedema, myotonic disorders, and necrotizing vasculitis, during attacks of myoglobinuria, and in neuropathies associated with vitamin-B$_1$ deficiency, arsenic intoxication, and alcoholism. *Muscle pain during and after exercise* is experienced when the energy supply to muscle is restricted, as with defects in glycolysis or fatty acid oxidation, AMP deaminase deficiency, ischemia (as in intermittent claudication, scleroderma, and amyloidosis involving muscle), or in normal subjects after unusually strenuous exercise.

Muscle cramps last from seconds to minutes, are associated with high-frequency (up to 150 Hz) discharges of the motor units, and can be initiated by strong contractions and stopped by stretching the muscle. They occur with dehydration, azotemia, hyponatremia, myxedema, in partially denervated muscles, and sometimes in normal individuals without known cause.

Muscle contractures are electrically silent, last from a few to more than 30 minutes, occur only in patients with glycolytic enzyme defects, are provoked only by exercise, and involve only those muscles that had been exercised.

The facial and carpopedal spasms of *tetany* occur with hypocalcemia or hypomagnesemia and are associated with high-frequency (up to 300 Hz) axonal discharges. High-frequency electrical discharges also occur in muscle in the *stiff-man syndrome*, *neuromyotonia*, and *myotonia*, arising in the spinal cord, the peripheral nerves, and in the muscle fiber surface membrane, respectively.

In *myotonic disorders* mechanical or electrical stimuli applied to any region of the muscle fiber surface membrane elicit repetitive spike discharges that wax and wane in amplitude and frequency. Mechanical deformation of the membrane during contraction acts as positive feedback, again depolarizing the membrane. This electrical activity, which is independent of the anatomic arrangement of the fibers in the motor unit, causes tetanic contraction of the individual fibers. The symptoms are stiffness, difficulty in relaxing muscles after a strong contraction, being muscle-bound at the beginning of exercise, and improvement with continued exercise.

Myoglobinuria follows the excessive release of myoglobin from muscle during a period of rapid muscle fiber destruction (rhabdomyolysis). Weakness, muscle pain, and malaise are associated features.

The Clinical Examination. Inspection. This can reveal muscle atrophy, hypertrophy, contractures, winging of the scapulas, fasciculations (twitching of portions of muscles at rest caused by single contractions of motor units), myokymia (fine undulating movements of muscles associated with sustained abnormal motor-unit activity). The examiner also notes the patient's stance and gait, ability to walk on toes and heels, hop on one foot, and rise from sitting, squatting, or lying supine.

Inspection provides information on the distribution of weakness, which is then confirmed by detailed manual muscle testing. For example, weakness of the pelvic girdle muscles causes a waddling gait; if there is also weakness of the back extensor muscles, the gait is also lordotic with hyperextension of the upper torso. Muscle atrophy consistently predicts muscle weakness, but not all weak muscles are atrophic, and muscle atrophy can be masked by obesity. Muscle hypertrophy not from voluntary exercise is common in myotonia congenita; it also occurs in the course of Duchenne and Becker and—less commonly—of limb-girdle dystrophy. Hypertrophy may appear with chronic partial denervation, acid maltase deficiency, the permanent myopathy of periodic paralysis, myxedema, sarcoidosis, amyloidosis, and cysticercosis. The nonspecific term *pseudohypertrophy* refers to enlargement of a weak muscle.

Manual Muscle Testing. This part of the examination requires knowledge of the origin, insertion, action, and innervation of the muscles tested, a consistent technique, and a generally accepted rating scale. A commonly used scale is that adopted by the British Medical Council: 5, normal power; 4, active movement against gravity and resistance; 3, active movement against gravity; 2, active movement with gravity eliminated; 1, trace contraction; 0, no contraction. Experienced examiners further differentiate among slight, mild, and moderate weakness within Grade 4. The results are recorded and used for following the patient's clinical course.

The distribution of the weakness can help in formulating the clinical diagnosis, as shown by the following examples. Weakness greater in proximal than distal muscles suggests a myopathy rather than a neuropathy. Predominantly distal muscle weakness suggests a neuropathy but can also occur in myotonic and other distal dystrophies and inclusion body myositis. Selective involvement of some muscles with sparing of others is more likely to occur in dystrophy than in inflammatory muscle disease, but it can also occur in such diverse entities as adult acid maltase deficiency, focal myositis, or the slow-channel myasthenic syndrome. The external-ocular and other cranial muscles can be affected by the Guillain-Barré syndrome, neuromuscular transmission defects, some mitochondrial myopathies, oculopharyngeal dystrophy, and myotubular myopathy. Diffuse, symmetric weakness of multiple cranial muscles with ptosis but with sparing of the ocular movements suggests myotonic dystrophy. Motor neuron disease can affect the bulbar muscles but spares the external ocular muscles except rarely in terminal stages. Selective weakness of the triceps, wrist extensor, finger extensor, iliopsoas, hamstring, anterior tibial, and peroneal muscles, with relative sparing of other muscles, suggests upper motor neuron involvement.

Other Findings. *Action myotonia* is observed as an inability to open the fist or the eyes promptly after closing them tightly for a few seconds. *Percussion myotonia* appears as a local postpercussion contraction followed by abnormally slow relaxation. It can best be observed in the tongue, deltoid, thenar, and extensor digitorum communis muscles. A local swelling appearing for a few seconds at the site of percussion is not myotonia but *myoedema*, seen in myxedema and emaciation.

The *deep tendon reflexes* are diminished in proportion to the weakness in most myopathies; an early loss of tendon reflexes is observed in neurogenic diseases of muscle, inclusion body myositis, the Lambert-Eaton myasthenic syndrome, and in a number of benign congenital myopathies. Slow relaxation of the reflexes is typical of myxedema.

A complete *examination of the nervous system* is also relevant

to the evaluation of muscle weakness. Table 503–1 lists clinical guidelines that differentiate nerve from muscle disease. Peripheral neuropathy, ataxia, neurosensory hearing loss, myoclonus, fluctuating neurologic deficits, and mental deterioration can be associated with mitochondrial myopathies.

Recognition of the *signs or symptoms of an associated illness* can point to the cause of the myopathy. Examples are collagen-vascular diseases, sarcoidosis, amyloidosis, the endocrine myopathies, and the mitochondrial myopathies with multisystem involvement. *Involvement of organs or tissues other than muscle* provides further diagnostic clues. For example, cardiomyopathy can be associated with myotonic dystrophy, Emery-Dreifuss dystrophy, certain types of periodic paralysis, thymomatous myasthenia gravis, familial limb-girdle myasthenia, and late-onset nemaline myopathy. Cardiomyopathy and/or hepatic enlargement can occur in sarcoidosis and in the myopathies associated with deficiencies of acid maltase, debranching enzyme, carnitine, acyl-CoA dehydrogenase, and of a mitochondrial electron transport complex.

Serum Enzymes of Muscle Origin. The serum creatine kinase (CK) level is elevated in many muscle diseases. The enzyme is released into serum from injured skeletal or cardiac muscle. CK is a dimer of muscle-specific (M) and brain-specific (B) monomers, and the different CK isoenzymes can be distinguished by electrophoretic analysis. Mature muscle contains predominantly the MM isoenzyme, whereas in mature cardiac muscle the MB form predominates. Accordingly, abnormal CK release from muscle increases mostly the MM isoenzyme, whereas CK release from heart increases the MB form in serum. Injured muscle releases other enzymes, such as aldolase, lactate dehydrogenase, and aspartate aminotransferase, but the increases are less marked and can derive from other tissues, such as the liver and erythrocytes. The serum CK level is a sensitive index of muscle fiber injury in a myopathy; it also can increase slightly or modestly in motor neuron disease, chronic peripheral neuropathies, after severe voluntary exertion, or following a convulsion.

ELECTROMYOGRAPHY (EMG). This test consists of the analysis of spontaneous, evoked, and voluntarily generated potentials from nerve and muscle. The procedure is useful in distinguishing between broad categories of disease, such as myopathy versus neuropathy, or demyelinating versus axonal neuropathy. In some instances the types of electrical potentials and the pattern of abnormality suggest a disease category, such as an inflammatory myopathy, a myotonic disorder, or a storage myopathy. A progressive decrease of the amplitude of the compound muscle action potential evoked by low-frequency repetitive nerve stimulation (decremental response) is observed with defects of neuromuscular transmission. Sequential assessment of an EMG abnormality can provide useful information of the distribution, degree of activity, and progression of a disease. For example, persistent fibrillation potentials in polymyositis reflect continuing disease activity; the decremental response can be used to monitor the course of myasthenia gravis; and alterations in nerve conduction velocities are a guide to the progression of peripheral neuropathies. Further details of the usefulness of EMG are given in Ch. 441.2, 496, and 509.

THE MUSCLE BIOPSY. Biopsy specimens are used for light microscopic, ultrastructural, and biochemical studies. In most

TABLE 503–1. CLINICAL CLUES DIFFERENTIATING MUSCLE FROM NERVE DISEASE

	Myopathy	Neuropathy-Neuronopathy
Distribution	Mainly proximal and symmetric	Distal if symmetric; nerve or root distribution if mono- or multifocal
Atrophy	Late and mild	Early and prominent
Onset	Usually gradual	Often rapid
Fasciculations	Absent	Sometimes present
Reflexes	Lost late	Lost early
Tenderness	Diffuse in myositis	Focal in nerve or root disease
Cramps	Rare	Common
Sensory loss	Absent	Often present
Muscle enzymes	Usually elevated	Usually not or slightly elevated

instances, light microscopic observations with enzyme histochemical studies are sufficient for diagnosis.

Muscles showing mild to moderate weakness are biopsied. Strong muscles may not show diagnostic pathologic change, and in more severely affected muscles excessive amounts of connective tissue may obscure the basic pathologic process. Muscles that have been injected (as is often the case for the deltoid) or recently examined by EMG are unsuitable for diagnosis.

Light Microscopy. The following pathologic alterations can be recognized in conventional paraffin sections of muscle: excessive variation in muscle fiber diameter; isolated or grouped atrophic fibers; target formations; increase in the number of internally located nuclei; focal loss of cross-striations; loss of myofibrillar markings; cytoplasmic inclusions; vacuolar change; fiber necrosis and phagocytosis; inflammatory exudates; invasion of non-necrotic fibers by mononuclear cells; regenerating fibers; ring fibers (caused by aberrant myofibrils); and proliferation of connective tissue elements. Histochemical studies of fresh-frozen sections reveal the dimensions of the muscle fibers in the native state; the distribution and abundance of mitochondria, lipid, and glycogen in the muscle fibers; myofibrillar integrity; increased lysosomal activity; the presence or absence of certain enzymes (phosphorylase, phosphofructokinase, cytochrome *c* oxidase, AMP deaminase); the histochemical profiles of the muscle fibers; and the distribution of the histochemical fiber types.

Neurogenic alterations in muscle consist of the appearance of atrophic fibers, singly or in groups of varying size; target formations; and grouping of histochemical fiber types caused by reinnervation of previously denervated fibers by collateral nerve sprouts. Central nuclei, loss of cross-striations, and hypertrophy and degeneration of nondenervated fibers also can occur in partially denervated muscle. Further details of muscle biopsy changes can be found in Dubowitz's monograph on the subject.

Electron Microscopy. This is primarily a research tool used in studying previously unrecognized syndromes and diseases of neuromuscular transmission or in analyzing mechanisms of muscle fiber injury. However, in some instances electron microscopy does have a role in diagnosis (e.g., in identifying the filamentous inclusions in inclusion body myositis or in revealing capillary microtubular inclusions and necrosis in dermatomyositis when inflammation and perifascicular atrophy are absent).

Biochemical Studies. These are essential for defining the biochemical basis of those metabolic myopathies in which the clinical or histologic data suggest a defect in carbohydrate, lipid, or mitochondrial metabolism. The direct measurement of the glycogen and carnitine content of muscle, assays of enzymes associated with glycolysis or fatty acid oxidation, determination of various aspects of mitochondrial respiration, analysis of cytochrome spectra, and a search for mitochondrial DNA deletions are examples of procedures currently used in the diagnosis of metabolic myopathies.

Dubowitz V: Muscle Biopsy: A Practical Approach. Philadelphia, Baillière Tindall, 1985. *A well-illustrated guide to the processing and interpretation of the muscle biopsy specimen.*
Engel AG, Banker BQ (eds.): Myology. New York, McGraw-Hill Book Company, 1986. *A multiauthored book on the anatomy, physiology, and biochemistry of skeletal muscle, the approach to muscle diseases, and the clinical aspects of muscle diseases.*
Walton J (ed.): Disorders of Voluntary Muscle. 5th ed. New York, Churchill-Livingstone, 1988. *A popular, multiauthored book with excellent chapters on the basic science and clinical aspects of muscle diseases.*

504 Muscular Dystrophies

DEFINITION AND BASIC CONCEPTS. Muscular dystrophies are inherited myopathies of unknown etiology associated with progressive muscle weakness, destruction and regeneration of the muscle fibers, and eventual replacement of the muscle fibers by fibrous and fatty connective tissue. There is no accumulation of metabolic storage material in the muscle fibers. Ultrastructural studies in Duchenne dystrophy indicate that breakdown of the muscle fiber plasma membrane is an early

abnormality in the course of muscle fiber destruction. The lesions are conditioned by a deficiency of dystrophin, a 400-kilodalton cytoskeletal protein that represents the primary product of the Duchenne/Becker gene. The membrane lesions result in the influx of calcium-rich extracellular fluid and complement components into the fiber, activation of intracellular proteases and complement, and, eventually, removal of the necrotic fiber by macrophages. It is not yet known whether membrane lesions initiate muscle fiber destruction in the other dystrophies. Recognition of the molecular basis of the other dystrophies awaits the identification of the primary product of the dystrophic genes.

The current classification of the muscular dystrophies is based on the mode of inheritance, age of onset and rate of progression, distribution of the involved muscles, and associated findings in muscle or other organs. This is not entirely satisfactory because some cases cannot be fitted into currently recognized groups, and some dystrophies, such as the limb-girdle, distal, and facioscapulohumeral types, are heterogeneous by clinical, pathologic, or genetic criteria. A classification of the muscular dystrophies based on the categories used by Gardner-Medwin (1980) is shown in Table 504–1. A more precise classification awaits the chromosomal assignment and mapping of the loci of dystrophic genes (thus far accomplished in Duchenne, Becker, facioscapulohumeral, and myotonic dystrophy) and the availability of probes that can identify the presence of a given dystrophic gene in a given patient.

DUCHENNE DYSTROPHY. This is a lethal, X-linked recessive disorder of childhood. The abnormal gene is positioned on band Xp21 of the X chromosome. In over 65 per cent of patients deletions have been detected in dystrophin gene which prevent the formation of translatable mRNA; and in nearly all patients immunoblotting or immunostaining shows complete absence of dystrophin from muscle. The incidence is close to 1 in 3300 male births, the mutation rate being about 1 in 10,000. The disease is present at birth, becomes symptomatic during early childhood, leads to failure of ambulation near the end of the first decade, and terminates fatally near the end of the second decade. Early symptoms are developmental delays, difficulty in running or climbing stairs, frequent falls, and enlargement of the calves. Initially the weakness is more proximal than distal. Except for the sternocleidomastoids, the cranial muscles and the external

TABLE 504–1. CLASSIFICATION OF THE MUSCULAR DYSTROPHIES

X-linked Recessive Dystrophies
Duchenne dystrophy
Becker dystrophy
Emery-Dreifuss dystrophy with joint contractures and atrial paralysis
   ? Scapuloperoneal syndrome variant
   ? Rigid-spine syndrome variant

Autosomal-recessive Dystrophies
Autosomal-recessive childhood (limb-girdle) muscular dystrophy
Scapulohumeral (limb-girdle) muscular dystrophy
Autosomal-recessive distal muscular dystrophy
   With necrotizing features
   With rimmed vacuoles
Congenital muscular dystrophy
   Without cerebral abnormalities*
? Autosomal-recessive rigid-spine syndrome

Autosomal-dominant Dystrophies
Facioscapulohumeral dystrophy
   With inflammatory changes in muscle
   With cochlear hearing loss and retinal telangiectasis
Autosomal-dominant scapuloperoneal dystrophy (? related to facioscapulohumeral dystrophy)
Dominantly inherited adult-onset limb-girdle dystrophy*†
Oculopharyngeal dystrophy
Myotonic dystrophy
Autosomal-dominant distal dystrophy
   With onset in upper limbs (Welander type)
   With onset in lower limbs

*Variable clinical phenotypes suggest genetic heterogeneity.
†X-linked dominant form may also exist.

anal sphincter are spared. The proximal deep tendon reflexes disappear in about half the cases by the age of 10. Joint contractures, caused by uneven weakness of agonist and antagonist muscles, appear in the majority of patients between 6 and 10 years of age. After ambulation is lost, all muscles decrease in size and paraspinal muscle weakness causes progressive kyphoscoliosis. Weakness of the respiratory muscles can be detected after the age of 10, but the diaphragm is relatively spared. Carbon dioxide retention and anoxemia occur terminally with respiratory infections. Pure respiratory failure without infection can also occur and is an irreversible terminal event. The heart is affected with scarring of the posterobasal portion of the left ventricle, producing tall right precordial R waves and deep left precordial Q waves in the electrocardiogram in 90 per cent of the patients. Clinically significant cardiomyopathy is uncommon and in only 10 per cent of cases is death related to cardiac dysfunction. Central nervous system involvement is indicated by lower than average intelligence and mild cerebral atrophy.

Infrequently, Duchenne dystrophy manifests in females who have Turner's (XO) or Turner's mosaic (X/XX or X/XX/XXX) syndrome, a structurally abnormal X chromosome, or an X-autosomal translocation. In a few female heterozygotes, the disease manifests because of incomplete inactivation of the maternal X chromosome.

BECKER DYSTROPHY. The disorder has an incidence of about 1 per 20,000 male births. The gene locus is the same as for Duchenne dystrophy, but the mutations do not prevent the formation of translatable mRNA, so that a dystrophin molecule smaller or larger than normal in size and/or reduced in amount is produced. The manifestations of the two diseases are also similar, but Becker dystrophy begins later and evolves more slowly. In Becker dystrophy the mean ages for onset of symptoms, becoming chair-bound, and death are 12, 30, and 42 years, respectively. All patients show marked enlargement of the calves until the terminal stage. The serum creatine kinase (CK) level is markedly elevated in preclinical and clinical stages of the disease but begins to decline after the age of 20. Contractures develop at the wheelchair stage. Only some patients show electrocardiographic abnormalities, and only a minority are mentally retarded. The disease usually can be distinguished from Duchenne dystrophy by its more benign course. Immunoblot analysis of dystrophin extracted from muscle reliably distinguishes between Becker and Duchenne dystrophy, as well as between sporadic cases of Becker and limb-girdle dystrophy.

X-LINKED MUSCULAR DYSTROPHY WITH EARLY JOINT CONTRACTURES AND CARDIOMYOPATHY (EMERY-DREIFUSS DYSTROPHY). The disease presents in childhood, progresses slowly, and involves distal or proximal muscles in the lower extremities and proximal muscles in the upper extremities. There is no muscle hypertrophy. The serum CK is moderately elevated. Contractures of the knees, elbows, and cervical and dorsolumbar spine appear early in the disease. Atrial conduction defects and paralysis, requiring treatment by pacemaker, appear later. The disorder has been referred to as Emery-Dreifuss dystrophy and as X-linked scapuloperoneal myopathy, the distinction depending only on whether the proximal or distal muscles are affected in the lower limbs. The lack of muscle hypertrophy, early contractures, slow progression, relatively low serum CK, and overt cardiac involvement distinguish this disease from Duchenne dystrophy; all these features but the slow progression differentiate it from Becker dystrophy. When cardiomyopathy cannot be detected or the pedigree of X-linked inheritance is not established, the disease can be difficult to distinguish from the rigid-spine syndrome or other heterogeneous scapuloperoneal syndromes.

LIMB-GIRDLE SYNDROMES. The term *limb-girdle dystrophy* was applied by Walton and Nattrass in 1954 to a group of 18 patients (11 males and 7 females). The shoulder girdle was first affected in 13 cases (Erb type) and the pelvic girdle in 5 (Leyden-Möbius type). The face was spared. The onset was in the second decade in 7 patients and later in the others. Severe disability appeared over the next 20 years. An autosomal-recessive inheritance was postulated, although in one family the inheritance appeared to be autosomal dominant. Subsequently, a number of incompletely defined disorders were called limb-girdle dystro-

phy. The following diseases now appear to be reasonably distinct entities.

Childhood Muscular Dystrophy of Autosomal-Recessive Inheritance. This disease presents in the first or second decade, progresses slowly, and involves pelvic and pectoral girdle muscles without muscle hypertrophy. The serum CK level is moderately elevated (up to tenfold). Ambulation is lost near the end of the second decade. Cardiac abnormalities are absent. More severe variants, with muscle hypertrophy and death before the age of 20, have been described in inbred Amish and Tunisian kinships.

Scapulohumeral Muscular Dystrophy of Autosomal-Recessive Inheritance. Phenotypically this entity resembles that described by Erb in 1884. The onset is usually in the second decade. The shoulder girdle is initially affected; weakness then slowly extends to the pelvic girdle and to distal limb muscles. Facial muscles are spared. There is no muscle hypertrophy. The serum CK is moderately elevated at the onset but decreases with progression of the disease.

Adult-Onset Limb-Girdle Dystrophy of Dominant Inheritance. This is a rare condition with onset from the second through the sixth decade of life. It begins proximally and remains restricted to limb-girdle muscles. The serum CK level is normal or elevated. In some families there are rimmed vacuoles in the muscle fibers. In some kindreds the expression of the disease is restricted to either males or to females. Thus, this disease is also heterogeneous.

The Differential Diagnosis of Limb-Girdle Syndromes. All patients with limb-girdle syndromes need to be further investigated by EMG and muscle biopsy. Only a minority have a pedigree consistent with autosomal-recessive or -dominant inheritance and can be fitted into one of the above clinically distinct syndromes. The differential diagnosis in these patients includes inherited metabolic myopathies (e.g., acid maltase deficiency or a lipid storage myopathy); morphologically distinct congenital myopathies or their late-onset variants (e.g., nemaline, central core, and myotubular myopathies); or progressive muscular atrophy. In sporadic cases of a limb-girdle syndrome the differential diagnosis includes the same diseases, and also inflammatory myopathies (polymyositis, inclusion body myositis, or sarcoidosis confined to muscle); endocrine myopathies, sporadic Duchenne dystrophy, Duchenne dystrophy manifesting in female carriers, sporadic Becker dystrophy, and sporadic Emery-Dreifuss dystrophy before the appearance of joint contractures or cardiomyopathy.

FACIOSCAPULOHUMERAL DYSTROPHY. The inheritance is autosomal dominant with high penetrance and variable expression. The gene resides at the tip of chromosome 4. The disease presents in childhood or adult life. It involves the facial muscles early and then descends to the scapular fixators, the muscles of the upper arm, and the anterior leg muscles. Early signs include failure to bury the eyelashes, an expressionless face, pouting lips, winging of the scapulas when the arms are raised, and an inward-sloping anterior axillary fold. The rate of progression and the extent to which pelvic girdle, forearm, and lower torso muscles are eventually affected vary considerably between and within families. There is no muscle hypertrophy; joint contractures are uncommon; and the serum CK level is normal or shows mild elevation. A number of variants have been described. In some families a conspicuous inflammatory reaction appears in affected muscles, but the course of the illness is unaltered by corticosteroid therapy. In other families an associated sensorineural hearing loss occurs, with or without retinal telangiectasis and progressive painless blindness (Coats syndrome). The differential diagnosis includes progressive muscular atrophy, congenital myopathies (e.g., nemaline, central core, and myotubular myopathy), mitochondrial myopathies, sporadic cases of Emery-Dreifuss dystrophy before the appearance of joint contractures or cardiomyopathy, the scapuloperoneal syndrome, the slow-channel myasthenic syndrome, and polymyositis.

MYOTONIC DYSTROPHY. Transmission is by dominant inheritance with high penetrance and variable expressivity. The gene resides on the proximal long arm of chromosome 19 and shows close linkage to the gene encoding the muscle isoform of creatine kinase. The incidence is about 1 in 7500 births. A typical distribution of the weakness, myotonia, and multisystem abnormalities characterizes the disease.

Myotonic dystrophy presents in childhood or adult life; the

mean age at onset is 19 years. Myotonic symptoms either precede or accompany the muscle weakness. As the disease evolves, the myotonia diminishes in those muscles severely affected by the dystrophic process. Distal limb, levator palpebrae, masticatory, facial, cervical, pharyngeal, laryngeal, and upper esophagus muscles are commonly affected. External ophthalmoplegia is rare. Weakness can also appear in the proximal limb and respiratory muscles. The latter, when severe, results in alveolar hypoventilation, hypercapnia, arterial oxygen unsaturation, and increasing somnolence. Action myotonia is commonly observed in facial, lid elevator, and hand muscles; percussion myotonia is usually found in tongue, thenar, finger extensor, and selected proximal limb muscles.

A congenital form of myotonic dystrophy can occur in infants born to affected mothers. The onset is at birth with hypotonia, respiratory distress, and cranial muscle weakness. Myotonic phenomena, absent at birth, appear later in childhood. Motor development is delayed and mental retardation common.

Myotonic dystrophy produces systemic abnormalities including frontal baldness, subcapsular cataracts, testicular atrophy and ovarian dysfunction in adult life, extrathyroidal hypometabolism, end-organ unresponsiveness to insulin, mental changes, and hypercatabolism of IgG. Cardiac conduction defects are common and can cause sudden death. Gastrointestinal smooth muscle involvement results in reduced lower esophageal and gastric motility and dilatation of segments of the colon. Some patients have bouts of diarrhea alternating with constipation and colicky abdominal pain. Less frequent manifestations are pigmentary retinal degeneration and cranial anomalies (hyperostosis cranii, small sella turcica, large paranasal sinuses, and prognathism).

The pathologic alterations in the affected muscles are relatively distinct. These consist of very large muscle fibers with numerous central nuclei, sarcoplasmic masses, ring fibers, and variable type 1 fiber atrophy. Necrotic fibers are uncommon, which may explain why the serum CK level is normal or only slightly elevated.

DISTAL DYSTROPHIES. A number of genetically distinct entities has been recognized. An *autosomal-dominant type*, initially described in a large Scandinavian kinship by Welander, presents between the fourth and sixth decades with selective weakness and atrophy of the forearm extensor and intrinsic hand muscles and then involves the anterior leg and small foot muscles. In patients homozygous for the dominant gene, the onset is earlier and proximal muscles are also affected. In other non-Scandinavian kinships with late onset and dominant inheritance, the disease first involves the lower extremities. The serum CK level is normal or slightly increased. Two varieties of *autosomal-recessive distal muscular dystrophies* have been described. In both there is a juvenile onset and the lower limbs are affected before the upper. In one type there is frequent fiber necrosis and regeneration and the serum CK level is markedly increased. In the other type the muscle fibers harbor rimmed vacuoles and the serum CK level is only slightly increased.

The differential diagnosis of the distal muscular dystrophies includes myotonic dystrophy, inclusion body myositis, debranching enzyme deficiency, distal mitochondrial myopathy, distal chronic spinal muscular atrophy, and the neuronal form of peroneal muscular atrophy.

OCULOPHARYNGEAL MUSCULAR DYSTROPHY. The disease, inherited as an autosomal dominant, presents in the fifth or sixth decade with progressive ptosis and dysphagia. Later, all external ocular and other voluntary muscles may become affected. Death usually results from starvation or aspiration pneumonia. The serum CK level is normal or slightly increased. Muscle biopsy discloses intranuclear tubular filaments and rimmed vacuoles in the muscle fibers. This syndrome needs to be distinguished from mitochondrial myopathies that involve the external ocular muscles with or without affecting facial and limb muscles, and with or without multisystem features. In the mitochondrial myopathies, as discussed below, the age of onset and mode of inheritance are variable, and the muscle biopsy displays ragged red fibers.

SCAPULOPERONEAL SYNDROMES. These are heterogeneous disorders identified by the distribution of the affected muscles. An X-linked recessive form of scapuloperoneal myopathy with early joint contractures which also involves the spine and produces late cardiac atrial paralysis is essentially identical with Emery-Dreifuss dystrophy. An autosomal-dominant scapulo-

peroneal myopathy resembles facioscapulohumeral dystrophy except that the face is spared. Other autosomal-dominant forms of the scapuloperoneal syndrome are associated with chronic anterior horn cell disease (Stark-Kaeser syndrome) or with a hypertrophic sensorimotor neuropathy (Davidenkow syndrome).

THE RIGID-SPINE SYNDROME. This is also a heterogeneous disorder in which muscle contractures involve the spine as well as other joints. The X-linked recessive form with cardiomyopathy and scapuloperoneal weakness appears to be identical with Emery-Dreifuss dystrophy. An autosomal-dominant form presenting with proximal muscle weakness in the first decade is also recognized. In most cases the disease is sporadic, begins in the first decade, and results in widespread muscle weakness and atrophy during the second decade.

CONGENITAL DYSTROPHIES. These present at birth with weakness and hypotonia, with or without multiple joint contractures. Most cases are sporadic; in some families several siblings are affected, suggesting autosomal-recessive inheritance. The weakness involves limb, torso, cervical, and sometimes the facial muscles. The serum CK level is normal or elevated. The subsequent course is one of slow or rapid progression, or the weakness increases only slightly during early childhood and then remains unchanged. The differential diagnosis includes Duchenne or autosomal-recessive limb-girdle dystrophy presenting at birth, morphologically distinct congenital myopathies, and acute infantile spinal muscular atrophy. The Fukuyama form of congenital dystrophy is associated with mental retardation, seizures, developmental abnormalities in the central nervous system, a progressive course, and death by the age of 10. The inheritance is autosomal recessive.

TREATMENT OF THE MUSCULAR DYSTROPHIES. There is no specific treatment of any of the muscular dystrophies. Physical therapy to prevent contractures, orthoses, and corrective orthopedic surgery can be used to improve the quality of life in some stages. The cardiac conduction defects in Emery-Dreifuss dystrophy and myotonic dystrophy may require treatment by pacemaker. The myotonia in myotonic dystrophy is rarely a clinical problem but can be treated with phenytoin (0.3 to 0.6 gram daily) or by quinine (0.3 to 1.5 grams daily).

Preventive treatment consists of prenatal diagnosis in families with known pedigrees, carrier detection, and genetic counseling. Some Duchenne carriers are recognized by immunostaining muscle for dystrophin, which may show scattered dystrophin-negative fibers. In some Becker carriers dystrophin of abnormal size or amount is detected by immunoblotting. Close to 65 per cent of Duchenne or Becker carriers and fetuses at risk can be identified by DNA analysis using cDNA probes or the polymerase chain reaction; carriers not identified this way may still be detected in families with known carriers by linkage analysis. In myotonic dystrophy, DNA markers closely linked to the locus of the disease allow prenatal diagnosis and detection of presymptomatic cases in 90 per cent of families.

Engel AG, Banker BQ (eds.): Myology. New York, McGraw-Hill Book Company, 1986. *An excellent, comprehensive description of the muscular dystrophies authored by multiple experts.*

Gardner-Medwin D: Clinical features and classification of the muscular dystrophies. Br Med Bull 36:109, 1980. *A revision of the classification proposed by Walton and Nattrass. Also contains concise and accurate summaries of the major clinical features of the different muscular dystrophies.*

Harper PS: Myotonic Dystrophy. Philadelphia, W.B. Saunders Company, 1979. *A modern classic—thorough in coverage, thoughtful in analysis, and written in a lively style.*

Kunkel LM, Hoffman EP: Duchenne/Becker muscular dystrophy. Br Med Bull 45:630, 1989. *A concise overview of current knowledge of the gene defective in Duchenne and Becker dystrophy, an account of normal and abnormal dystrophin, and a guide to newly available diagnostic tools.*

Miyoshi K, Kawai H, Iwasa M, et al.: Autosomal-recessive distal muscular dystrophy as a new type of progressive muscular dystrophy. Brain 109:31, 1986. *A well-documented study and a good review of the different types of distal muscular dystrophies.*

Shaw DJ, Harper PS: Myotonic dystrophy: Developments in molecular genetics. Br Med Bull 45:745, 1990. *Summary of recent progress in mapping the myotonic dystrophy gene and the application of this work to disease prediction.*

Wijmenga C, Frants RR, Brouwer OF, et al.: Location of facioscapulohumeral muscular dystrophy gene on chromosome 4. Lancet 336:651, 1990. *An important first step to cloning the gene and identifying its product.*

505 Morphologically Distinct Congenital Myopathies

DEFINITIONS AND BASIC CONCEPTS. The diseases in this group are characterized by the following features:

• The course is nonprogressive or relatively nonprogressive. The prognosis is generally benign except in reducing body myopathy and in the X-linked form of myotubular myopathy.

• A distinct pattern of inheritance is observed in some diseases (e.g., central core disease, nemaline myopathy); others are genetically heterogeneous (e.g., myotubular myopathy).

• Muscle weakness is present at birth or appears in early childhood. It is proximal or diffuse and may or may not involve the cranial muscles.

• The muscle bulk is normal or reduced. There is no muscle hypertrophy.

• The deep tendon reflexes are reduced or absent in most cases.

• Skeletal abnormalities related to the weakness, such as a high-arched palate, kyphoscoliosis, dislocated hips, and pes cavus, are common.

• The serum CK level is normal, except in some older patients with myotubular or sarcotubular myopathy.

• The EMG is normal or suggests a myopathy. Spontaneous electrical activity is absent in all cases, except for fibrillation potentials and myotonic discharges in some cases of myotubular myopathy.

• Each disease has one or more distinguishing, but not specific, morphologic features. Type I fiber preponderance and small type I fibers occur in most disorders.

Central Core Disease. The disease is transmitted by autosomal-dominant inheritance. The cranial muscles are usually not affected. The core formations can be central or peripheral, extend through the length of the fiber, are devoid of mitochondria, and may show focal myofibrillar degeneration. T-tubules, SR profiles, and glycogen are decreased in the cores.

Nemaline (Rod) Myopathy. An autosomal-dominant inheritance with variable expressivity has been demonstrated in some families. Facial, masticatory, oropharyngeal, neck flexor, respiratory, and proximal and distal limb muscles are typically affected. An oval face, micrognathia, and malocclusion are common. The disease is most severe in the first few years of life because of feeding difficulty and respiratory infections. Subsequently, some increase in strength takes place, and the clinical course remains stable. The nemaline bodies represent a replicative anomaly of the Z disk.

Myotubular (Centronuclear) Myopathy. X-linked recessive, autosomal-recessive, and autosomal-dominant forms of the disease have been described. The X-linked type is associated with severe respiratory muscle weakness and leads to death in early infancy. The autosomal-dominant form is relatively mild and may not present until adult life. External ocular, facial, oropharyngeal, and neck muscles are often affected. In each disorder the muscle fibers contain rows of central nuclei surrounded by cytoplasmic material, reminiscent of maturing myotubes. Type I fiber atrophy and type II fiber hypertrophy are common associated features.

Multicore Disease. The onset occurs in the first few months of life. Weakness is greater in proximal than distal muscles and in the upper than lower extremities. Ptosis as well as weakness of external ocular, facial, and neck muscles can occur. The inheritance is autosomal recessive with rare families manifesting heterozygotes or autosomal dominant with marked variation in penetrance. Individual muscle fibers contain myriad small core formations devoid of mitochondria.

Congenital Fiber Type Disproportion. The disease may occur in successive generations, suggesting an autosomal-dominant inheritance. Weakness is usually present at birth and tends to improve after the age of 2 years. Muscle contractures, skeletal deformities, and short stature are common. There is type I fiber atrophy and type II fiber hypertrophy with or without type I fiber predominance.

Other Morphologically Distinct Congenital Diseases. These less frequently encountered entities are identified by their morphologic abnormalities in muscle: fingerprint body myopathy, sarcotubular myopathy, reducing body myopathy, trilaminar myopathy, myopathy with focal lysis of the myofibrils in type I fibers, and spheroid body myopathy.

Late-Onset Variants. Adult-onset cases of central core disease, nemaline myopathy, myotubular myopathy, and multicore disease also exist. In some of these cases mild disease probably has been present since birth but is recognized only after additional progression in adult life or when discovery of an affected younger relative prompts investigation of other family members.

Two other forms of late-onset nemaline myopathy are noteworthy. One is sporadic, evolves subacutely or chronically, affects the proximal limb and torso but not the cranial muscles, and may cause death from respiratory failure. The CK level is normal. In some cases there is an associated monoclonal gammopathy. The EMG shows myopathic changes and fibrillation potentials. Histologically, there is progressive accumulation of nemaline rods and progressive atrophy of rod-containing fibers. Another late-onset form occurs in a familial setting, is associated with cardiomyopathy, and can result in sudden death.

Banker BQ: The congenital myopathies. In Engel AG, Banker BQ (eds.): Myology. New York, McGraw-Hill Book Company, 1986, pp 1527–1581. *A comprehensive, well-illustrated review. It raises numerous unanswered questions about etiology and nosology.*

506 Inflammatory Myopathies

DEFINITION AND CLASSIFICATION. Inflammatory myopathies represent a heterogeneous group of disorders. Most inflammatory myopathies are diffuse in distribution, but some are focal, affecting circumscribed regions in single or multiple muscles. Some are caused by or related to bacterial, parasitic, or viral infections. In most other inflammatory myopathies the etiology is undetermined, but an autoimmune etiology is suspected, and in inclusion body myositis both an autoimmune and a viral etiology have been postulated. A classification of the inflammatory myopathies is shown in Table 506–1. This section focuses on selected aspects of the idiopathic inflammatory myopathies not covered in other chapters.

Myopathies Related to Retrovirus infections. These can appear early or late in the course of immunodeficiency virus (HIV) infections. The most common form is HIV-associated polymyositis, which presents early in the infection and is mediated by T cells. Necrotizing myopathy without inflammation, or myopathies with nemaline rods or giant cells, necrotizing vasculitis, focal myositis in the form of pseudothrombophlebitis, and recurrent myoglobinuria without other predisposing factors can also occur. Attempts to immunolocalize HIV antigens in muscle fibers have consistently failed, and the manner in which the HIV virus induces myopathies is unclear. Zidovudine, an agent for treatment of the HIV infection, itself may induce a toxic mitochondrial myopathy that can coexist with the myopathy related to the HIV infection.

Human T-cell leukemia virus type I (HTLV-I), an agent associated with chronic spastic paraparesis, also can be associated with polymyositis, but the virus has not been shown to infect muscle fibers.

Autoimmunity in Idiopathic Inflammatory Myopathies. An autoimmune etiology in inflammatory myopathies has been inferred from one or more of the following observations: (1) The myopathy is associated with another identifiable autoimmune disease (e.g., systemic lupus erythematosus or rheumatoid arthritis). (2) Laboratory tests suggest an altered immune state (e.g., increased serum gamma globulins, decreased total hemolytic complement in serum, and positive tests for antibodies against native DNA, other nuclear or cytoplasmic antigens, or rheumatoid factor). (3) A predominantly mononuclear inflammatory exudate in muscle. (4) There is evidence of focal invasion and destruction of muscle fibers by antigen-specific cytotoxic T

TABLE 506–1. CLASSIFICATION OF INFLAMMATORY MYOPATHIES

Infections

Parasitic: toxoplasmosis, sarcosporidiosis, African trypanosomiasis, American trypanosomiasis, cysticercosis *(Taenia solium)*, trichinellosis

Bacterial: pyomyositis, septic myositis, gas gangrene *(Clostridium welchii)*, leprous myositis

Spirochetal: Lyme disease *(Borrelia burgdorferi)*

Viral: acute myositis following influenza or other viral infections, retrovirus-related myopathies (HIV, HTLV-I)

Idiopathic, autoimmune origin suspected

Pure polymyositis

Dermatomyositis

Inclusion body myositis

Scleroderma involving muscle

Inflammatory myopathy associated with another autoimmune disease (systemic lupus erythematosus, rheumatoid arthritis, Sjögren's syndrome, rheumatic fever, overlap syndromes, chronic graft-versus-host disease, polyarteritis nodosa)

Sarcoidosis involving muscle

Inflammatory myopathies with eosinophilia

  Eosinophilic polymyositis

  Localized eosinophilic myositis

  Eosinophilic perimyositis

  Diffuse fasciitis with eosinophilia

  Eosinophilia-myalgia induced by L-tryptophan preparations

Focal myositis

  Focal proliferative myositis

  Localized nodular myositis

    Pseudothrombophlebitis of a calf muscle

  Orbital myositis

Polymyalgia rheumatica*

Other inflammatory myopathies

Localized myositis ossificans

Generalized myositis ossificans

*There are no inflammatory changes in muscle.

---

cells. (5) The diseases respond to corticosteroids or other immunosuppressants. The first criterion, if fulfilled, represents strong, but indirect, evidence for an autoimmune origin of the myopathy. Laboratory tests suggesting an altered immune state are positive in a proportion of patients with dermatomyositis and in polymyositis. A mononuclear inflammatory exudate also can occur in some genetically determined muscle diseases (e.g., Duchenne or facioscapulohumeral dystrophy). Inclusion body myositis, in which an inflammatory exudate is often prominent, most cases of scleroderma, and some cases of pure polymyositis and dermatomyositis do not respond to immunosuppressants. Further, neither the factors that initiate self-sensitization nor the sensitizing antigen have been defined in any of the major inflammatory myopathies (idiopathic polymyositis, inclusion body myositis, dermatomyositis, and scleroderma). None has been transferred to an experimental animal.

Inclusion Body Myositis. This entity differs from the other idiopathic inflammatory myopathies in several respects. Clinically, it is not usually associated with another autoimmune disease and responds poorly to corticosteroids or other immunosuppressants. Most patients are older than 50, and there is male predominance. The disease evolves slowly, affecting the lower limbs first, involving both proximal and distal muscles, and resulting in selectively severe weakness and atrophy of the quadriceps. Facial, cervical, and pharyngeal muscles are spared. There is an early loss of deep tendon reflexes from the affected limbs. The serum CK level is mildly elevated or normal. The EMG indicates myopathic changes and abnormal electrical irritability, as in dermatomyositis or polymyositis, but there may be additional neurogenic features, such as an increase in the amplitude of motor unit potentials or mild slowing of nerve conduction velocities. Affected muscles show a typical pattern of histologic change: rimmed vacuoles in a significant proportion of the fibers; eosinophilic intranuclear and cytoplasmic inclusions in a few fibers; small groups of atrophic fibers without type grouping; and an endomysial and a lesser perivascular inflammatory exudate. The exudate is enriched in cytotoxic T cells that focally surround,

invade, and destroy non-necrotic fibers. Necrotic fibers also occur but are less common than in polymyositis. Ultrastructural studies show that the rimmed vacuoles contain myeloid structures and other cytoplasmic degradation products and that the inclusions consist of microtubular filaments resembling paramyxovirus nucleocapsids. The differential diagnosis of inclusion body myositis includes motor neuron disease, distal and other muscular dystrophies, peripheral neuropathies, and pure polymyositis. The diagnosis is usually clarified by a careful study of the muscle biopsy.

Differences Between Dermatomyositis and Pure Polymyositis. Dermatomyositis and pure polymyositis resemble each other in the predominantly proximal distribution of the muscle weakness, a mononuclear inflammatory exudate in muscle, myopathic changes and spontaneous electrical activity in the EMG, and responsiveness to corticosteroid therapy. Consequently, they are often treated as a single entity in evaluating their etiology, natural history, and therapy. However, several aspects of dermatomyositis differentiate it from pure polymyositis: (1) The characteristic rash of dermatomyositis is lacking in pure polymyositis. (2) Capillary injury and necrosis are early and constant findings in dermatomyositis. Many of the injured capillaries react to the membrane attack complex of complement, whereas other vessels are found to be occluded by platelet thrombi or to harbor microtubular inclusions. (3) Muscle fibers at the periphery of the fascicles undergo selective degeneration and atrophy. (4) The inflammatory exudate is concentrated at perimysial and perivascular sites and is enriched in B cells and helper T cells. (5) There is no evidence for T-cell–mediated cytotoxicity directed against the muscle fibers. These findings suggest that a humoral response against vascular elements plays an important role in the pathogenesis of dermatomyositis.

By contrast, in pure polymyositis there is no capillary necrosis or loss. The inflammatory exudate contains fewer B cells and helper T cells than in dermatomyositis, and B cells are virtually absent from the endomysium. There are focal invasion and destruction of non-necrotic muscle fibers by antigen-specific cytotoxic T cells accompanied by macrophages indicating cell-mediated cytotoxicity directed against the muscle fiber. Necrosis of isolated fibers also occurs. These findings suggest that a component of the muscle fiber surface membrane is a target of the immune effector response.

Differences Between Scleroderma and the Other Major Inflammatory Myopathies. In scleroderma, the serum CK level is either normal or only slightly elevated, spontaneous electrical activity is often absent from the EMG, and necrotic fibers are uncommon. The pathologic changes are those of fibrosis and inflammation involving the perimysium and the perimysial blood vessels. The inflammatory cells at these sites are predominantly T cells and macrophages. The findings suggest a cell-mediated immune response against a perimysial and/or vascular component in muscle.

Eosinophilia-Myalgia Related to L-Tryptophan Preparations. This syndrome appeared in 1989 in patients consuming L-tryptophan preparations. The features consisted of eosinophilia ($>10^9$ per liter), marked myalgias, fasciitis, and often a peripheral neuropathy. Interstitial pneumonitis, myocarditis, and encephalopathy occurred in some subjects. An autoimmune pathogenesis was implicated by onset or progression of the syndrome after withdrawal of the L-tryptophan preparation, inflammatory cells in the affected tissues, and responsiveness to immunotherapy in some cases. The pathologic substrate is an interstitial inflammation associated with an occlusive microangiopathy and fibroplasia. Thus far the triggering factor appears to be a contaminant of L-tryptophan produced by a single manufacturer, but the chance remains that this may not be the only source. Patients should be advised against L-tryptophan ingestion, at least until the matter is settled completely.

Myositis Ossificans. The *localized form* appears as a tender swelling after trauma to a muscle. After a few months this becomes hard and ossified. Therapy consists of excision. The *generalized form* represents an autosomal-dominant disease with variable expressivity that begins in childhood, involves many muscles, and causes progressive rigidity of body parts. The initial lesions appear in fascia and dermis and are associated with inflammation, local hemorrhage, and connective tissue proliferation. Cartilage and bone formation occur at a later stage. Other congenital malformations (microdactyly of the great toe, exostoses, absence of upper incisors or of ear lobules, and hypogenitalism) are found in most patients. There is no effective therapy.

Banker BQ: Other inflammatory myopathies. *In* Engel AG, Banker BQ (eds.): Myology. New York, McGraw-Hill Book Company, 1986, pp 1501–1524. *A well-illustrated review of the myopathies associated with eosinophilia, focal myositis, orbital myositis, and myositis ossificans.*

Dalakas MC, Illa I, Pezeshkpour GH, et al.: Mitochondrial myopathy caused by long-term zidovudine therapy. N Engl J Med 322:1098, 1990. *Excellent histologic analysis of the drug-induced mitochondrial myopathy, which is distinct from but can coexist with an HIV-related T-cell–mediated myopathy.*

Emslie-Smith A, Engel AG: Microvascular changes in early and advanced adult dermatomyositis. A quantitative study. Ann Neurol 27:343, 1990. *Presents evidence that the muscle microvasculature is an early and specific target of the disease process in dermatomyositis and highlights the differences between dermatomyositis and other inflammatory myopathies.*

Engel AG, Arahata K: Mononuclear cells in myopathies: Quantitation of functionally distinct subsets, recognition of antigen-specific cell mediated cytotoxicity in some diseases, and implications for the pathogenesis of the different inflammatory myopathies. Hum Pathol 17:704, 1986. *Describes antigen-specific T-cell–mediated cytotoxicity against the muscle fiber in polymyositis and inclusion body myositis, but not in dermatomyositis or scleroderma.*

Lotz B, Engel AG, Nishino H, et al.: Inclusion body myositis. Observations in 40 patients. Brain 112:727, 1989. *A summary of the clinical and morphologic features and a guide to the diagnosis of the disease.*

Martin RW, Duffy J, Engel AG, et al.: Eosinophilia myalgia syndrome associated with L-tryptophan ingestion: Clinical features and aspects of pathophysiology. Ann Intern Med 113:124, 1990. *A detailed account of the clinical and pathologic features of the syndrome in 20 patients.*

Simpson DM, Bender AN: Human immunodeficiency virus–associated myopathy. Ann Neurol 24:79, 1988. *A good description of several types of HIV-related myopathies.*

507 Metabolic Myopathies

GLYCOGEN STORAGE DISEASES. These are described in detail in Ch. 169. When muscle is involved, glycogen-filled vacuoles appear in the fibers; the glycogen excess can vary from slight to marked, and definitive diagnosis requires demonstration of a specific enzyme deficiency. Of the several glycogenoses, only glucose-6-phosphate dehydrogenase and liver phosphorylase deficiencies fail to affect muscle. All glycogenoses that affect muscle are transmitted as autosomal-recessive traits except phosphoglycerate kinase deficiency, which is X-linked recessive.

Acid Alpha-1,4-Glucosidase (Lysosomal Acid Maltase) Deficiency. The gene encoding the enzyme is mapped to chromosome 17. Various mutations affecting the synthesis, phosphorylation, and maturation of the enzyme have now been identified. Three major clinical variants exist. The *infantile type* presents in early infancy with generalized and rapidly progressive weakness and heart, tongue, and liver enlargement. There is widespread and marked glycogen excess in tissues, including lower motor neurons. Death occurs from cardiorespiratory failure before the age of 2 years. The *childhood type* presents in infancy or early childhood as a myopathy. Weakness is more proximal than distal, and there may be calf enlargement simulating muscular dystrophy. Glycogen excess is less marked and confined to muscle. Death occurs before age 20 of respiratory failure. The *adult type* presents between the second and seventh decade of life, either with slowly progressive limb muscle weakness that mimics limb-girdle dystrophy or polymyositis or with insidiously developing ventilatory insufficiency leading to respiratory failure. In all three types the serum CK level is increased, but to less than 10 times normal. The EMG in affected muscles shows myopathic changes and excessive abnormal electrical irritability, including myotonic discharges (but there is no clinical myotonia). The muscle biopsy demonstrates a vacuolar myopathy with high glycogen content and acid-phosphatase reactivity in the vacuoles, an appearance that otherwise occurs only in chloroquine myopathy and a rare cardioskeletal lysosomal storage disorder without acid maltase deficiency.

Debranching Enzyme Deficiency. A disabling myopathy affecting both proximal and distal muscles can appear in childhood or (more commonly) in adult life. Often there is a history of a protuberant abdomen and hypoglycemic episodes in childhood, along with muscle fatigue on exertion. Persistent hepatomegaly and biventricular cardiac hypertrophy are found in most cases. There is a diminished glycemic response to epinephrine and glucagon and an impaired rise of lactic acid after ischemic exercise. The EMG shows myopathic changes and abnormal electrical irritability in affected muscles.

Branching Enzyme Deficiency. The disease presents in infancy with progressive hepatosplenomegaly and failure to thrive. The abnormal starchlike glycogen, which resists diastase digestion, induces nodular cirrhosis and liver failure. Death occurs in early infancy from liver or heart failure. Muscle weakness is variable; if present, the tongue is severely affected.

Phosphorylase b Kinase (PBK) Deficiency. This syndrome shows marked clinical and genetic heterogeneity. Cardiac PBK deficiency is a fatal disease of infancy. An autosomal recessive form presents in childhood with weakness or hepatomegaly that improves with age; PBK is deficient in muscle, liver, and erythrocytes. An X-linked recessive disease presents in children with asymptomatic hepatomegaly or mild hypoglycemia; PBK is deficient in liver and erythrocytes. Another form of PBK deficiency which is restricted to muscle presents with exercise intolerance and myoglobinuria or a late-onset myopathy simulating muscular dystrophy.

Glycolytic Enzyme Defects: Myophosphorylase, Phosphofructokinase (PFK), Phosphoglycerate Kinase (PGK), Phosphoglycerate Mutase (PGM), and Lactate Dehydrogenase (LDH) Deficiencies. The common features are muscle cramps and periodic myoglobinuria on strenuous exertion since childhood; easy fatigability; a venous lactate level that fails to rise after ischemic exercise in myophosphorylase and PFK deficiencies, and fails to rise or rises by less than 100 per cent in PGK, PGM, and LDH deficiencies. Muscle cramps are prominent. They are caused by electrically silent contractures and are not associated with ATP depletion; their mechanism is not understood. The muscle glycogen excess is slight to modest. Permanent muscle weakness and atrophy are also slight, but they may increase with age. Fatal infantile variants have been identified in myophosphorylase and PFK deficiency. In PFK deficiency hyperuricemia and gout occur in some cases, and there is mild hemolytic disease caused by a partial erythrocyte enzyme defect. PGK mutations result in severe hemolytic anemia and neurologic deficits but no myopathy, or produce a myopathy with only the features described above.

DISORDERS OF FATTY ACID METABOLISM. Long-chain fatty acids taken up by muscle are utilized for energy metabolism or incorporated into triglycerides and stored as lipid droplets. Long-chain fatty acids entering the catabolic pathway are esterified with coenzyme A (CoA) to form acyl-CoAs. These react with carnitine to form acylcarnitines in a reaction catalyzed by carnitine palmityltransferase I, an enzyme positioned on the inner surface of the outer mitochondrial membrane. The acylcarnitines are transported through the inner mitochondrial membrane by a carnitine-acylcarnitine translocase and are then reconverted to acyl-CoAs by carnitine palmityltransferase II on the inner surface of the inner mitochondrial membrane. The acyl-CoAs undergo repeated cycles of β-oxidation, generating acetyl-CoAs that enter the citric acid cycle or form ketone bodies. The inner mitochondrial membrane is impermeable to long-chain fatty acids, CoA, and acyl-CoAs. Consequently, carnitine, carnitine-acyltransferases, and carnitine-acylcarnitine translocase jointly regulate the oxidation of fatty acids and modulate the intramitochondrial CoA/acyl-CoA ratio. Excessive intramitochondrial accumulation of an acyl-CoA compound leads to its conversion to a corresponding acylcarnitine. The acylcarnitine so formed leaves the mitochondrion via the translocase, diffuses out from the cell, and is preferentially excreted by the kidney. If this process continues, the muscle and body carnitine stores become depleted.

Derangements in fatty acid oxidation produce a variety of syndromes that affect muscle and other organs. The possible consequences include one or more of the following: intermittent energy shortage in muscle causing *rhabdomyolysis* and *myoglobinuria*; intramitochondrial acyl-CoA excess and CoA deficiency, secondary carnitine depletion, and inhibition of multiple mitochondrial enzyme systems (these events trigger a *Reye syndrome–like metabolic crisis* associated with hypoglycemia, acute fatty infiltration of the liver, hyperammonemia, marked release

TABLE 507–1. LIPID STORAGE MYOPATHIES ASSOCIATED WITH CARNITINE DEFICIENCY

Primary muscle or systemic carnitine deficiency
Organic acidurias with acyl-CoA dehydrogenase deficiencies*
  Long-chain acyl-CoA dehydrogenase deficiency
  Medium-chain acyl-CoA dehydrogenase deficiency
  Short-chain acyl-CoA dehydrogenase deficiency
  Multiple acyl-CoA dehydrogenase deficiency
  Long-chain 3-hydroxyacyl-CoA dehydrogenase deficiency
  Short-chain 3-hydroxyacyl-CoA dehydrogenase deficiency
Organic acidurias with defects in branched-chain amino acid metabolism*
  Isovaleryl-CoA dehydrogenase deficiency†
  Propionyl-CoA carboxylase deficiency
  Methylmalonyl-CoA mutase deficiency
  β-hydroxy-β-methylglutaric-CoA lyase deficiency
Defects in mitochondrial respiratory chain or energy utilization‡
  Block at NADH-coenzyme Q reductase (Complex I deficiency)
  Mitochondrial ATPase deficiency (Complex V deficiency)
Miscellaneous disorders‡
  Idiopathic Reye syndrome
  Valproate therapy
  Renal Fanconi syndrome
  Cirrhosis with cachexia

*Associated with secondary carnitine deficiency.
†This enzyme is also an acyl-CoA dehydrogenase.
‡Only some patients become carnitine deficient.

of enzymes from muscle and liver into serum, and encephalopathy); and triglyceride accumulation in muscle producing a *lipid-storage myopathy*. Many carnitine-deficiency syndromes are secondary to another metabolic defect in fatty acid oxidation, branched-chain amino acid metabolism, or the respiratory chain. A lipid storage myopathy can be caused by primary carnitine deficiency or by another defect of fatty acid oxidation with or without secondary carnitine deficiency (Table 507–1).

Carnitine Palmityltransferase Deficiency. The normal enzyme is a long-chain carnitine acyltransferase. The inheritance is autosomal recessive with reduced penetrance in women. The symptoms consist of muscle aching, fatigability, and periodic myoglobinuria on sustained exertion, especially if combined with fasting and exposure to cold. There are no symptoms between attacks, and the muscle lipid content is normal or only slightly increased. The mutant enzyme is not diminished in amount but is abnormally sensitive to inhibition by its own product and substrate, which explains why symptoms appear only when fatty acid metabolism is stressed and why little or no lipid accumulates in muscle.

Acyl-CoA Dehydrogenase Deficiencies. Deficiencies of the long-chain, medium-chain, and short-chain specific enzymes, and in the factors that transfer electrons from multiple acyl-CoA dehydrogenases to coenzyme Q (multiple acyl-CoA dehydrogenase deficiency), have been identified. Each syndrome causes secondary carnitine depletion, a lipid storage myopathy, and organic aciduria. The urinary organic acid and acylcarnitine profiles reflect the site of the metabolic block. *Short-chain acyl-CoA dehydrogenase deficiency* is associated with adult-onset lipid storage myopathy. Ketogenesis is not impaired and there are no metabolic crises. The other acyl-CoA dehydrogenase deficiencies produce intermittent metabolic crises resembling Reye syndrome. *Long-chain acyl-CoA dehydrogenase deficiency* usually has a neonatal onset and is associated with hepatomegaly and cardiomyopathy. *Medium-chain acyl-CoA dehydrogenase deficiency* presents in the first or second year of life with a metabolic crisis. Between attacks the patients are well or have mild weakness, easy fatigability, and mild hepatomegaly. *Multiple acyl-CoA dehydrogenase deficiencies* are genetically and biochemically heterogeneous. Severe neonatal forms with cardiomyopathy and milder late-onset cases have been described. Some cases respond to riboflavin therapy. The acyl-CoA dehydrogenase deficiencies are treated with a low-fat, high-carbohydrate diet and L-carnitine supplements (2 to 4 grams daily in adults and 100 mg per kilogram daily in infants and children). Crises can be prevented by avoiding fasting and maintaining alimentation at all times, especially during febrile illnesses. The crises are treated by intravenous therapy to correct the hypoglycemia and electrolyte abnormalities, and by L-carnitine, initially 100 mg per kilogram and then 25 mg per kilogram every 4 hours.

Primary Carnitine Deficiency Syndromes. Primary systemic carnitine deficiency is an autosomal recessive disease due to impaired carnitine transport in muscle, heart, kidney, and fibroblasts. A renal carnitine leak caused by the transport defect results in further tissue carnitine depletion. The disease is associated with cardiomyopathy, weakness, and episodes of hypoketotic hypoglycemic encephalopathy; it responds to carnitine replacement therapy. A myopathic form of primary carnitine deficiency also exists and may respond to prednisone therapy.

Other Lipid Storage Myopathies. Autosomal-recessive and -dominant lipid storage myopathies associated with lifelong weakness, myalgias, and electrical myotonia, but without carnitine deficiency, have been described. *Chanarin's disease* is a rare autosomal recessive condition with congenital ichthyosis, steatorrhea, and lipid storage in muscle fibers, hepatocytes, gastrointestinal epithelial cells, epidermal cells, monocytes, myelocytes, and fibroblasts.

MITOCHONDRIAL MYOPATHIES. These disorders are defined by a specific biochemical and/or a nonspecific morphologic abnormality in muscle mitochondria. The biochemical defects involve mitochondrial enzymes encoded by nuclear or mitochondrial DNA transmitted by, respectively, mendelian or vertical maternal inheritance. In many mitochondrial myopathies a substantial proportion of the muscle fibers appears ragged red in the trichrome stain. These fibers harbor accumulations of functionally defective mitochondria that are often large, contain abnormal cristae and various inclusions, and fail to react for cytochrome *c* oxidase. A current classification of mitochondrial myopathies is shown in Table 507–2.

From a clinical standpoint, in many mitochondrial myopathies there is slowly progressive weakness of limb and/or external ocular and other cranial muscles, abnormal fatigability on sustained exertion, and lactacidemia on exertion or even at rest. Some mitochondrial disorders affect multiple organs or systems, and the myopathy is but one facet of a multisystem disease.

Myopathies with Defective Energy Conservation. *Luft syndrome* is a hypermetabolic myopathy. Thyroid function studies exclude hyperthyroidism, but the basal metabolic rate is markedly elevated. The few patients observed to date had heat intolerance, hyperphagia, diaphoresis, polydipsia without polyuria, and progressive weakness since childhood. Oxidative phosphorylation was uncoupled, possibly because of abnormal recycling of calcium between the mitochondria and the cytosol.

TABLE 507–2. CLASSIFICATION OF MITOCHONDRIAL MYOPATHIES

Biochemically distinct disorders
  Defective energy conservation
    Hypermetabolic myopathy (Luft syndrome)
    Mitochondrial ATPase deficiency
  Impaired substrate utilization or transport
    Acyl-CoA dehydrogenase deficiencies
    Carnitine palmityltransferase deficiency
    Primary and secondary carnitine deficiency syndromes
    Defects in the pyruvate dehydrogenase complex
  Defects in the mitochondrial respiratory chain
    Coenzyme Q deficiency
    Complex I (NADH-coenzyme Q oxidoreductase) deficiency
    Complex II (succinate-coenzyme Q oxidoreductase) deficiency
    Complex III (coenzyme Q-cytochrome *c* oxidoreductase) deficiency
    Complex IV (cytochrome *c* oxidase) deficiency
      Fatal infantile type
      Benign infantile type
      Benign with external ophthalmoplegia
      Necrotizing encephalomyopathy (Leigh's syndrome)
      Trichopoliodystrophy (Menkes' disease)
Clinically distinct syndromes caused by mitochondrial DNA mutations
  Progressive external ophthalmoplegia with mitochondrial myopathy
  Kearns-Sayre syndrome (retinitis pigmentosa, heart block, external ophthalmoplegia plus other features)
  Myoclonus, generalized seizures, cerebellar syndrome, lactacidemia, plus other features (MERF)
  Encephalopathy with strokelike episodes and lactacidemia, plus other features (MELAS)
Recognizable only by morphologic criteria

2260 / XXIII NEUROLOGY

Mitochondrial ATPase deficiency is a multisystem disease that presents in childhood. It produces muscle weakness associated with a myopathy and peripheral neuropathy, high-tone hearing loss, frequent vomiting, increased spinal fluid protein, basal ganglia calcifications, retinopathy, ataxia, and dementia. Secondary carnitine deficiency and lipid storage in muscle can also occur. A point mutation of mitochondrial DNA affecting subunit 6 of complex V has been observed in one pedigree.

Impaired Substrate Utilization Caused by Transport or Enzyme Defects. These disorders include the primary carnitine deficiencies, acyl-CoA dehydrogenase deficiencies, carnitine palmityl-transferase deficiency (all dealt with above), and *defects in the pyruvate dehydrogenase complex.* The latter are associated with various neurologic syndromes that include movement disorders, ataxia, neuropathy, subacute necrotizing encephalomyelopathy (Leigh's syndrome), and fatal infantile lactic acidosis. The muscle biopsy shows ragged red fibers, lipid excess, or denervation atrophy.

Defects in the Mitochondrial Respiratory Chain. The mitochondrial respiratory chain includes four distinct enzyme complexes and also coenzyme Q and cytochrome *c.* The components are attached to the inner mitochondrial membrane and carry reducing equivalents from reduced nicotinamide adenine dinucleotide (NADH), flavin adenine dinucleotide ($FADH_2$), and electron-transferring flavoprotein (ETF) to molecular oxygen. A fifth complex, an ATPase, uses released energy to phosphorylate ADP to ATP in a tightly coupled process. Mitochondrial ATPase deficiency was discussed above. Defects in the electron transport complexes are associated with marked clinical, biochemical, and genetic heterogeneity. The reasons for this are that each complex is composed of multiple subunits, different subunits of a given complex are encoded by different genes, some subunits of a given complex are encoded by mitochondrial rather than nuclear DNA, some subunits are tissue specific, and some subunits are developmentally regulated. Mitochondrial DNA (mtDNA) can undergo point, deletion, or duplication mutations. With homoplasmic mutations, a single population of mutant mtDNA appears in all cells and produces a single clinical sydrome. With heteroplasmic mutations, normal and mutant forms of mtDNa coexist in the same cell, and subsequent cell replication leads to uneven segregation of normal and mutant DNA. The phenotypic expression depends on the proportion of mutant to normal mtDNA in cells of a given tissue, as well as tissue dependence on oxidative metabolism and the severity of the oxidation-phosphorylation defect.

Coenzyme Q Deficiency. A deficiency of mitochondrial coenzyme Q has been associated with a familial syndrome of marked lipid and mitochondrial excess in muscle, severe lactacidemia, intermittent myoglobinuria, progressive muscle weakness, cognitive deficits, cerebellar ataxia, and seizures. The activities of complex I, II, III, and IV and cellular cytochrome levels were normal.

Complex I (NADH-Coenzyme Q Oxidoreductase) Deficiency. Most of these begin in childhood and allow survival to adult life. Either muscular or central nervous system manifestations dominate the clinical picture. In the former group the findings include muscle weakness, exercise intolerance, exertional lactacidemia, and ragged red fibers in muscle. Headaches, progressive visual loss, hemiparesis, dysphasia, dementia, dystonia, and cerebral atrophy affect the latter group. A fatal infantile form also exists.

Complex III (Coenzyme Q–Cytochrome *c* Oxidoreductase) Deficiency. These also begin in childhood or adult life. Muscle weakness, exercise intolerance, exertional lactacidemia, and ragged red fibers are constant findings. Some patients also have external ophthalmoplegia and/or dementia, myoclonus, ataxia, pyramidal signs, and loss of proprioception. The muscle symptoms in one patient were improved by treatment with menadione and vitamin C, agents that can function as electron transfer mediators instead of complex III.

Complex IV (Cytochrome *c* Oxidase) Deficiency. Several syndromes are associated with this defect. A *fatal infantile mitochondrial myopathy* presents at birth or shortly thereafter with weakness, hypotonia, and lactacidemia. Renal Fanconi syndrome *or* cardiomyopathy *or* liver enlargement can be associated with the fatal infantile syndrome. Muscle contains large accu-

mulations of mitochondria, lipid, and glycogen. The phenotypic variability is attributed to the existence of tissue-specific subunits of complex IV. A *benign infantile myopathy* with reversible complex IV deficiency presents neonatally with profound weakness of all but the ocular muscles, hepatomegaly, macroglossia, and severe lactacidemia. Spontaneous improvement begins after 6 months, and only mild weakness persists into later life. Complex IV deficiency in muscle, liver, and brain also has been described in some cases of *necrotizing encephalomyelopathy* (Leigh's syndrome) and *trichopoliodystrophy* (Menkes' disease).

Progressive External Ophthalmoplegia with Mitchondrial Myopathy. In addition to the external ocular muscles, the disorder can affect other cranial, truncal, and limb muscles. More than half of the cases are sporadic and stem from a heteroplasmic mtDNA deletion arising in the maternal ovum or in early fetal life.

Kearns-Sayre Syndrome. The disease presents in childhood. Nearly all cases are sporadic, and are caused by large heteroplasmic mtDNA deletions arising in the maternal ovum or in early fetal life. Dominantly inherited nuclear DNA mutations affecting mtDNA have also been observed. The rate of progression, severity, and system involvement vary from case to case. The original description in 1958 was that of retinitis pigmentosa, heart block, and external ophthalmoplegia. Subsequently ataxia, hearing loss, short stature, and increased spinal fluid protein were noted in more than half of the cases. Muscle weakness, mental changes, pyramidal signs, hypogonadism, and diabetes occur in less than half of the cases. Serum and spinal fluid lactate and pyruvate levels are increased, and the muscle fibers contain morphologically abnormal mitochondria. The presence of heart block requires treatment by pacemaker.

Myoclonus, Generalized Seizures, Cerebellar Syndrome, Mitochondrial Myopathy, and Lactacidemia. The syndrome presents in childhood or adult life. A maternally inherited heteroplasmic point mutation of mtDNA involving transfer RNA has been observed in several pedigrees. Short stature, dementia, hearing loss, and optic atrophy are frequent; spasticity, central hypoventilation, endocrinopathies, and peripheral neuropathy occur less often.

Mitochondrial Myopathy, Encephalopathy, Lactacidemia, and Strokelike Episodes (MELAS). The main distinction between this syndrome and the preceding one is the occurrence in adolescence or young adulthood of strokelike episodes associated with intermittent vomiting. Brain imaging during the acute episodes discloses areas of encephalomalacia not in the territories of the main blood vessels. Other associated features include short stature, seizures, hearing loss, progressive dementia, macular degeneration, and calcification of the basal ganglia. Early development is normal, and the family history is often positive. MELAS is caused by a heteroplasmic mtDNA point mutation involving transfer RNA.

ENDOCRINE MYOPATHIES. Muscle weakness can be a symptom of any endocrine disorder. The serum CK level is normal, except in myxedema and in uremic hyperparathyroidism. The EMG is normal or myopathic without spontaneous electrical activity. The histologic alterations in muscle are often nonspecific, such as type II fiber atrophy, focal increases and decreases in mitochondria, and focal myofibrillar degeneration. Fiber necrosis and regeneration and connective tissue proliferation are uncommon.

Glucocorticoid-Induced Myopathy. Muscle weakness commonly occurs in Cushing's syndrome and in patients receiving relatively high doses of glucocorticoids. Fluorinated drugs (dexamethasone, triamcinolone) are more pathogenic than nonfluorinated ones (prednisone). Considerable variation exists in the minimal dosage that induces myopathy. However, daily treatment for 3 months with 60 mg prednisone in divided doses induces some weakness in nearly all patients. Women are more susceptible than men, and divided daily doses are more pathogenic than single or alternate daily doses. The onset is usually insidious but occasionally sudden with diffuse myalgias. The weakness is more proximal than distal and affects the lower more than the upper limbs. Hip and ankle flexors are selectively severely affected. The cranial muscles are spared. The serum CK level remains normal. The biochemical basis of the disease is poorly understood. Reduced protein synthesis, accelerated protein degradation, and enhanced lysosomal protease activity all may contribute. Therapy consists of reducing the steroid dosage to the lowest possible level. Muscle strength returns to normal within 1 to 4 months after therapy is stopped.

Adrenal Insufficiency. Weakness is a typical feature, closely related to derangements in fluid and electrolyte balance and possibly to the associated hypotension. Joint contractures, especially of the knees and not related to muscle weakness, may also occur. Hyperkalemia in chronic adrenal insufficiency can be a cause of secondary periodic paralysis (discussed below).

Thyrotoxic Myopathy. Both acute and chronic forms have been described. The acute form, seldom seen, appears during a thyroid storm and is associated with bulbar weakness. Some patients have responded to anticholinesterases and may have had acute myasthenia gravis beginning during thyrotoxicosis. The chronic form appears in 80 per cent of untreated cases of hyperthyroidism. The hyperthyroid state can be mild and of long duration or present for only a few weeks before the onset of the weakness. Weakness is predominantly proximal, less often both proximal and distal. The deep tendon reflexes are hyperactive or normal. The serum CK level remains normal. The EMG shows myopathic motor unit potentials but never fibrillation potentials.

Graves' ophthalmopathy is described in Ch. 216. Thyrotoxic periodic paralysis is considered below.

Hypothyroid Myopathy. Muscle aching, cramps, slow relaxation of the reflexes, ridging of the muscles on percussion (myoedema), and an increase of the serum CK level are common findings in myxedema. Muscle enlargement and limb-girdle weakness occur only occasionally. The Debré-Semelaigne syndrome consists of muscle hypertrophy, weakness, and slow movements in the cretinous child. The same features and painful spasms in hypothyroid adults constitute Hoffmann's syndrome.

Muscle Symptoms in Hyperparathyroidism and Osteomalacia. Parathormone and biologically active forms of vitamin D are important regulators of calcium metabolism and the serum calcium level. Vitamin D also affects calcium metabolism, protein synthesis, ATP stores, and force generation in muscle. Furthermore, conditions that lead to osteomalacia (vitamin D deficiency, renal tubular acidosis, or chronic renal failure) are associated with secondary hyperparathyroidism. Proximal muscle weakness, fatigability, and muscle pain and tenderness, usually with bone pain and tenderness, can occur in primary and secondary hyperparathyroidism and in osteomalacia.

A more malignant syndrome can appear in uremic hyperparathyroidism. Here, metastatic calcification of the media and proliferation of the intima of small blood vessels produce skin and visceral infarcts and a necrotizing myopathy with marked elevation of serum enzymes and myoglobinuria.

Muscle Symptoms in Hypoparathyroidism. The typical neuromuscular symptom is tetany. This is considered in Ch. 235.

Acromegaly and Hypopituitarism. Acromegaly initially causes muscle hypertrophy, particularly if the disorder begins before growth ceases. Later generalized weakness and atrophy develop. Muscle biopsies can show segmental muscle fiber degeneration, type I or type II fiber atrophy, or no pathologic change. The serum CK level remains normal. A hypertrophic distal neuropathy and nerve entrapment are common in acromegaly.

Hypopituitarism in children causes dwarfism and poor muscle development. Pituitary failure in adults results in weakness and fatigability with little muscle atrophy. The weakness itself may reflect the combined influence of thyroid, adrenal, and growth hormone deficiencies.

THE PERIODIC PARALYSES (PP). These disorders occur as either inherited (primary) or acquired (secondary) illnesses and can be further classified according to measurable alterations in the serum potassium level during attacks (Table 507–3). The primary types are transmitted by autosomal-dominant inheritance, but nearly a third of the cases arise sporadically. It is important to realize that in the primary forms the serum potassium decreases or increases but may still remain within the normal range during attacks and is normal or low-normal between attacks. By contrast, in secondary PP caused by potassium wastage or retention the serum potassium is always markedly reduced or elevated during and even between attacks.

In each type of PP the propagation of the muscle fiber action potential fails during an attack. Recent studies indicate the presence of distinct abnormalities in the sodium channel of the muscle fiber plasma membrane in the primary periodic paralyses

TABLE 507–3. CLASSIFICATION OF THE PERIODIC PARALYSES

Primary
Hypokalemic
Normokalemic
Hyperkalemic
   without myotonia
   with myotonia
   with paramyotonia
With cardiac arrhythmia (hyper-, hypo-, or normokalemic)

Secondary
Hypokalemic
   Thyrotoxic
   Urinary potassium wastage
   Gastrointestinal potassium wastage
   Barium intoxication
Hyperkalemic
   Renal insufficiency
   Adrenal insufficiency

that tend to reduce the resting membrane potential. The action potential mechanism fails during the attack because of diverse abnormalities residing in the voltage-sensitive sodium channel.

The different types of periodic paralysis share several common features: (1) The paralytic attacks last from less than an hour to as long as several days. (2) The weakness can be localized or generalized. (3) The deep tendon reflexes diminish and then disappear during attacks. (4) The muscle fibers become inexcitable to direct or indirect electrical stimulation during the attacks. (5) The generalized attacks begin proximally and spread distally. Respiratory and cranial muscles tend to be spared except in the most severe attacks. (6) Rest after exercise provokes weakness in the muscles that had been exercised. Continued mild exercise aborts attacks. (7) Exercise followed by rest of a single muscle can induce weakness of that muscle without any detectable change in the potassium level in the systemic circulation. (8) Exposure to cold can provoke weakness in the primary forms of the disease. (9) Complete recovery occurs after initial attacks. (10) In the primary disorders permanent weakness and a persistent vacuolar myopathy can develop after repeated attacks. Despite these similarities, the different forms of PP differ in their response to sodium, potassium, or carbohydrate loading, as well as their pattern of urinary electrolyte excretions during attacks, and in some of their clinical features.

Primary Hypokalemic Periodic Paralysis. The attacks begin in the first or second decade, increase in frequency during early adult life, and become less frequent or cease during the fourth or fifth decade. When attacks recur daily, the patient is weakest in the morning and becomes stronger as the day passes. High dietary sodium or carbohydrate intake as well as excitement provokes or exacerbates the episodes. Major attacks are associated with urinary retention of sodium, potassium, chloride, and water. The diagnosis is supported by a positive family history and a decrease in serum potassium during an attack. An abnormally low serum potassium level between attacks suggests secondary rather than primary PP. In diagnosing sporadic cases one must exclude potassium wastage and thyrotoxicosis. The oral or intravenous administration of glucose, 2 grams per kilogram of body weight, combined with 10 to 20 units of insulin given subcutaneously, may provoke an attack within 2 to 3 hours. Depression of the serum potassium during the attack and a favorable response to 2.5 to 7.5 grams of potassium chloride (KCl) given orally must be demonstrated. Provocative tests must never be done in patients already hypokalemic, and potassium chloride must not be given to patients unless they have adequate renal or adrenal reserve.

Thyrotoxic Periodic Paralysis. This disease resembles primary hypokalemic PP in the changes in serum and urinary electrolytes that accompany the attacks and in the response to glucose, insulin, potassium, and rest after exercise. However, 95 per cent of the cases are sporadic, the male to female ratio is six to one, most cases occur among Asians, the onset is usually in adult life, and correction of the hyperthyroidism prevents further attacks.

Barium-Induced Periodic Paralysis. The accidental ingestion of absorbable barium salts such as barium carbonate induces hemorrhagic gastroenteritis, hypertension, cardiac arrhythmias, convulsions, hypokalemia, and muscle paralysis. Barium blocks potassium channels and thereby reduces potassium efflux from muscle; potassium uptake by muscle, mediated by the sodium-potassium pump, continues, and hypokalemia results.

Periodic Paralysis Secondary to Urinary or Gastrointestinal Potassium Loss. The differential diagnosis of hypokalemia resulting from urinary or gastrointestinal potassium depletion is discussed in Ch. 74. Paralytic attacks do not occur unless the serum potassium falls below 3 mEq per liter, and during the attacks the serum potassium decreases even further. Other neuromuscular complications of severe potassium depletion include a necrotizing myopathy, myoglobinuria, and latent or manifest tetany.

Primary Hyperkalemic Periodic Paralysis. The attacks begin in the first or second decade. They are often brief but can last up to several days. Between attacks the serum potassium is normal or slightly lower than normal. During major attacks potassium moves out from muscle. The serum potassium increases but may not exceed the normal range, and the urinary potassium excretion increases. Myotonic, paramyotonic, and nonmyotonic forms of hyperkalemic PP can be distinguished. In *myotonic hyperkalemic PP* myotonia can be detected in facial, tongue, finger extensor, and thenar muscles between attacks. In *paramyotonic hyperkalemic PP* exposure to cold causes widespread and severe myotonia, and exercise in the cold is followed by prolonged weakness not reversed by rewarming. Paralytic attacks are provoked by orally administered KCl, 50 to 100 mg per kilogram, given in an unsweetened solution in the fasting state. The test is contraindicated in subjects already hyperkalemic or those without adequate renal or adrenal reserve. Paramyotonia congenita without hyperkalemic PP is discussed in the next chapter.

Secondary Hyperkalemic Periodic Paralysis. This can occur when the serum potassium level exceeds 7 mEq per liter. The usual cause is renal or adrenal insufficiency, but hyperkalemia from exposure to spironolactone and during attacks of malaria also have caused paralytic attacks. The diagnosis is suggested by the presence of a very high serum potassium level during attacks, persistent hyperkalemia between attacks, and the associated primary disorder.

Primary Normokalemic Periodic Paralysis. There are no consistent changes in the serum potassium during the attacks. The existence of the disease has been questioned because some patients are sensitive to potassium salts. The observations suggest that normokalemic PP is a heterogeneous entity.

Primary Periodic Paralysis with Cardiac Arrhythmia. Affected patients suffer from PP and tachyarrhythmias that can cause sudden death. The cardiac symptoms are provoked or worsened by hypokalemia and digitalis; are refractory to disopyramide phosphate, propranolol, or phenytoin; but may respond to imipramine. Dysmorphic features, such as short stature, clinodactyly, and microcephaly can also occur. The PP has been clearly related to hyperkalemia in some patients, but hypokalemic and normokalemic PP were diagnosed in others.

Therapy of the Periodic Paralyses. In all forms of primary PP, acetazolamide, from 250 mg to 2 grams daily, can prevent attacks or decrease their frequency. The metabolic acidosis induced by the drug may prevent sodium channel inactivation by small depolarizations. Prolonged exposure to the drug promotes the formation of renal calculi.

The treatment of attacks of *primary hypokalemic PP* consists of giving 2 to 10 grams of oral KCl. Preventive therapy includes acetazolamide, a low-carbohydrate and relatively low-sodium (2.3 grams per day) diet, and 2.5 grams of KCl taken orally three times daily. *Thyrotoxic PP* is treated by antithyroid therapy, KCl supplements, and a low-carbohydrate, low-sodium diet. Acetazolamide is ineffective.

In *primary hyperkalemic PP* one treats the acute attacks with 2 grams per kilogram of glucose by mouth and 15 to 20 units of crystalline insulin subcutaneously. The inhalation of 1.3 mg metaproterenol every 15 minutes for three doses, or of 0.18 mg albuterol repeated once after 10 minutes, has aborted acute attacks. Preventive treatment consists of acetazolamide or thiazide diuretics and frequent high-carbohydrate meals. Tocainide, 300 to 400 mg three to four times daily, prevents cold-induced

stiffness and weakness in paramyotonic hyperkalemic PP. The drug acts by blocking sodium channels in muscle.

The periodic paralyses caused by excessive wastage or retention of potassium are treated by correcting existing electrolyte abnormalities and, if possible, removing the existing cause. In acute barium poisoning, 10 ml of a 10 per cent solution of sodium sulfate is administered intravenously every 30 minutes until symptoms subside.

NUTRITIONAL AND TOXIC MYOPATHIES. Diffuse muscle atrophy and weakness associated with type II fiber atrophy are commonly observed in malnourished or cachectic patients. The muscle weakness in nutritional osteomalacia has been attributed partly to disuse and partly to malnutrition.

Vitamin E Deficiency. This has now been implicated in progressive gait and limb ataxia, sensorimotor neuropathy, extraocular muscle paresis, and a myopathy in which giant abnormal lysosomes accumulate in muscle. The cause is a malabsorption syndrome, as detailed in Ch. 102 and 456. High doses of vitamin E may be of benefit.

Myopathy in Alcoholism. An acute necrotizing myopathy associated with myoglobinuria occurs in chronic alcoholics after a bout of drinking. Hypokalemia caused by sweating, vomiting, diarrhea, and renal wastage may act as a precipitating factor. The hypokalemia may be followed by hyperkalemia as myoglobinuria and renal failure develop. A subacute alcoholic myopathy with proximal muscle weakness and elevation of the serum CK level may also exist. If so, it is usually associated with a chronic neuropathy.

Chloroquine Myopathy. The side effects of the drug include macular and corneal degeneration, peripheral neuropathy, and myopathy. Muscle weakness appears when the daily dosage is 500 mg for a year or longer. Pathologically, the condition produces a vacuolar myopathy and constitutes a prototype for myopathies due to an excited autophagic mechanism.

Emetine Myopathy. Emetine, an ipecac alkaloid, is used to treat amebiasis. Side effects include cardiotoxicity and muscle weakness. A reversible myopathy involving proximal limb muscles has been observed in patients with feeding disorders who abuse ipecac to induce vomiting and in alcoholics receiving emetine for aversion therapy. The pathologic findings include focal destruction of mitochondria and focal myofibrillar degeneration.

Other Toxic Myopathies. *Epsilon amino-caproic acid*, an inhibitor of fibrinolyis and of clot dissolution, infrequently causes myalgias, myonecrosis, and myoglobinuria. *Colchicine* in customary doses induces a vacuolar myopathy in patients with gout and renal insufficiency who attain elevated plasma drug levels. The antiarrhythmic agent *amiodarone* can induce an autophagic myopathy and a peripheral neuropathy. *Lovastatin*, an inhibitor of mevalonic acid and cholesterol biosynthesis, causes a necrotizing myopathy with or without myoglobinuria in less than 0.5 per cent of patients. Concomitant therapy with immunosuppressants increases the risk of myopathy. *Isoretinoic acid*, a vitamin A analogue for treating acne, infrequently causes myalgias, elevation of the serum creatine kinase, and reversible muscle damage. *Cocaine* abuse can result in a necrotizing myopathy and myoglobinuria. The myopathy induced by *zidovudine* is considered in Ch. 506.

MALIGNANT HYPERTHERMIA. This is an autosomal dominant disorder in which exposure to inhalation anesthetics (halothane, methoxyflurane, enflurane) or succinylcholine triggers an uncontrolled release of calcium from the sarcoplasmic reticulum (SR) into the myofilament space. The high intracellular calcium level activates phosphorylase kinase, saturates troponin, and overloads mitochondria with calcium. These events cause accelerated glycolysis, ATP consumption, uncontrolled muscle contraction, uncoupling of oxidative phosphorylation, and excessive production of heat, lactate, and carbon dioxide. The basic abnormality is a mutation involving the calcium release channel of the SR. The gene that encodes for the calcium release channel and causes the disease has been mapped to region q13.1 of chromosome 19. A similar syndrome also can occur in myotonic disorders, Duchenne dystrophy, branchial hypertrophic myopathy, central core disease, and a congenital myopathy with dysmorphic features. It is not yet known what proportion of patients with these disorders is at risk.

Warning signs of the attack include tachypnea, tachycardia,

increased carbon dioxide production, cyanosis, rising temperature, rigidity, sweating, and unstable blood pressure. Failure to obtain muscle relaxation with adequate doses of succinylcholine represents an early warning sign. Subsequently, body temperature rises rapidly (up to 1° C every 5 minutes), followed by a rapidly evolving lactic acidosis, respiratory acidosis from carbon dioxide overproduction, muscle rigidity, hyperkalemia, variable alterations in the serum calcium, and muscle fiber breakdown reflected by very high serum CK levels, myoglobinemia, and myoglobinuria.

Therapy of the acute syndrome consists of body cooling, hydration, sodium bicarbonate infusion, mechanical hyperventilation, and diuretics to maintain urine flow. More specific treatment consists of dantrolene, a medication that blocks excitation-contraction coupling between the T-tubules and the SR. The drug is given intravenously, 1 to 2 mg per kilogram, which may be repeated every 5 minutes to a total of 10 mg per kilogram. The mortality remains high. Screening of relatives of patients for the metabolic defect is important. Seventy per cent of those at risk have increased serum CK activity. If well standardized, an in vitro halothane contracture test on fresh muscle can also predict susceptibility. Preventive treatment of individuals at risk consists of dantrolene, 4 to 8 mg per kilogram per day in four divided doses for 1 to 2 days prior to surgery and, if possible, alternative methods of anesthesia.

Other Hyperthermic States. Two other syndromes are associated with hyperthermia, autonomic instability, abnormal muscle rigidity, and myoglobinuria. The *malignant neuroleptic syndrome* occurs in less than 1 per cent of all patients exposed to neuroleptics, and especially in young men. It evolves over 1 to 3 days and lasts 5 to 10 days after drug withdrawal. The mortality is about 25 per cent. A nearly identical *hyperthermic syndrome in Parkinson's disease* is precipitated by abrupt withdrawal of antiparkinson medications. The same treatment as in malignant hyperthermia, including the use of dantrolene up to 10 mg per kilogram per day, is beneficial in both disorders.

MYOGLOBINURIA. The clinical syndrome of myoglobinuria is associated with brown discoloration of urine by myoglobin and metmyoglobin. Myoglobin, a 17,000-molecular-weight protein with a prosthetic heme group, is present in muscle at a concentration of 1 gram per kilogram. It has a lower renal excretory threshold than hemoglobin. Small amounts of myoglobin not sufficient to discolor urine are excreted in various necrotizing myopathies. The visible discoloration of urine by myoglobin indicates both massive and acute muscle destruction (rhabdomyolysis) and warns of impending renal damage. The pigment has to be distinguished from hemoglobin and porphyrins. If there is no hemoglobinemia or hematuria, a positive benzidine test strongly suggests myoglobinuria. However, myoglobinuria itself can induce microhematuria, and certain identification of myoglobin must be made specifically. The immunoprecipitation assay has the virtue of being simple and quantitative but is so sensitive that it detects the pigment in the absence of overt myoglobinuria.

Muscle pain, swelling, and weakness precede overt myoglobinuria by a few hours. In addition to myoglobin, phosphate, potassium, creatine, and muscle enzymes are released into the circulation. The heme pigment in the glomerular filtrate and casts in the tubules cause proteinuria, hematuria, and tubular necrosis. Renal failure is more likely if there are also hypotension, acidosis, and hypovolemia. With increasing renal insufficiency, hyperphosphatemia, hypocalcemia, tetany, and life-threatening hyperkalemia appear. Death results from renal or respiratory failure. Otherwise, the myoglobinuria and proteinuria disappear in 3 to 5 days. The marked hyperenzymemia decreases gradually, and muscle strength returns relatively slowly after major attacks. EMG abnormalities, and especially fibrillation potentials, can persist for several months.

Myoglobinuria can have many causes: metabolic, infectious, toxic, ischemic and/or traumatic, secondary to another myopathy, and idiopathic. It is likely that many of the so-called idiopathic cases have a metabolic or infectious etiology.

Myoglobinuria Caused by a Metabolic Disturbance. The common denominator is impaired substrate utilization for energy metabolism, or a critical substrate deficiency in the face of excessive demands for energy. Most diseases in this group were considered earlier in this chapter. Deficiencies of phosphorylase kinase, myophosphorylase, phosphofructokinase, phosphoglycer-

ate mutase, phosphoglycerate kinase, and lactate dehydrogenase block anaerobic glycolysis; coenzyme Q and succinate dehydrogenase deficiencies interfere with oxidative phosphorylaton; and carnitine palmityltransferase deficiency impairs fatty acid oxidation when it is most needed. Substrate deficiency in the face of excessive demands and derangements of muscle metabolism account for the myoglobinuria associated with malignant hyperthermia, the malignant neuroleptic syndrome, and the abrupt withdrawal of antiparkinson drugs. Substrate deficiency may also account for the myoglobinuria that occurs after severe exercise in untrained individuals, as in military recruits.

Almost any severe metabolic insult can cause myoglobinuria. These include carbon dioxide poisoning, extreme hypoglycemia, severe hypokalemia, hypernatremia, or water intoxication.

Myoglobinuria with Infections. This can occur after influenza A, herpes simplex, Epstein-Barr, and coxsackievirus infections and early in the course of HIV infection. The precise mechanism of the rhabdomyolysis is not understood. Myoglobinuria also occurs with bacterial infections accompanied by high fever and sepsis, and with muscle gangrene caused by clostridial infection.

Toxic Myoglobinuria. The myoglobinuria associated with alcoholism was considered above. Intoxication with barbiturates, amphetamine, cocaine, and other narcotics, especially if associated with agitation or coma, can produce myoglobinuria. Myoglobinuria occurring with lovastatin, epsilon-amino-caproic acid, or amiodarone was discussed earlier in this chapter. The toxin of the Malayan sea snake, *Enhydrina schistosa*, induces myalgias, trismus, flaccid paralysis, and myoglobinuria.

Ischemic and Traumatic Myoglobinuria. Massive ischemia of muscle from any cause (e.g., major vessel occlusions, angiopathy in uremic hyperparathyroidism), crush injuries, or prolonged pressure on dependent muscles in the immobile comatose patient can induce myoglobinuria. Localized ischemic necrosis of muscle and sometimes myoglobinuria occur in severe forms of the anterior tibial syndrome.

Myoglobinuria Secondary to Other Myopathies. Myoglobinuria has been observed infrequently in acute dermatomyositis (where the cause is probably ischemia), systemic lupus erythematosus, and muscular dystrophies.

Treatment. The acute episode is treated by rest, maintenance of adequate urine flow by hydration and diuretics, and alkalinization of the urine with sodium bicarbonate. Other measures consist of treatment of the renal insufficiency as required and removal of the offending cause if possible.

Engel AG, Banker BQ: Myology. New York, McGraw-Hill Book Company, 1986. *Chapters by DiMauro and Bresolin, DiMauro and Papadimitron, Engel, Gronert, Morgan-Hughes, Penn, Ruff, and Victor provide detailed reviews of several of the metabolic myopathies.*

Fontaine B, Khurana TS, Hoffman EP, et al.: Hyperkalemic periodic paralysis and the adult muscle sodium channel α-subunit gene. Science 250:1000, 1990. *A linkage analysis study indicating that a mutation in the sodium channel α-subunit gene accounts for the myotonic form of primary hyperkalemic periodic paralysis.*

Goto Y, Nonaka I, Horai S: A mutation in the tRNA^Leu(UUR) gene associated with the MELAS subgroup of mitochondrial myopathies. Nature 348:651, 1990. *Clear evidence that MELAS, like MERRF and the Kearns-Sayre syndrome, is caused by a mitochondrial DNA mutation.*

Lehamn-Horn F, Küther G, Ricker K, et al.: Adynamia episodica hereditaria with myotonia: A non-inactivating sodium current and the effect of extracellular pH. Muscle Nerve 10:363, 1987. *This paper presents cogent reasons for recognizing three forms of hyperkalemic periodic paralysis and discusses aspects of the pathophysiology.*

McLennan DH, Duff C, Zorzato F, et al.: Ryanodine receptor gene is a candidate for predisposition to malignant hyperthermia. Nature 343:559, 1990. *Provides evidence that a mutation in the gene encoding the sarcoplasmic reticulum calcium release channel (which is a receptor for ryanodine) predisposes to malignant hyperthermia.*

Moxley RT, Ricker K, Kingston WJ, et al.: Potassium uptake in muscle during paramyotonic weakness. Neurology 39:952, 1989. *Presents clinical and physiologic criteria for distinguishing pure paramyotonia congenita from myotonic hyperkalemic periodic paralysis.*

Ogasahara S, Engel AG, Frens D, Mack D: Muscle coenzyme Q deficiency in familial mitochondrial myopathy. Proc Natl Acad Sci USA 86:2379, 1989. *The first report of selective and severe human coenzyme Q deficiency and its clinical and metabolic consequences.*

Roth D, Alarcon FJ, Fernandez JA, et al.: Acute rhabdomyolysis associated with cocaine intoxication. N Engl J Med 319:673, 1988. *Cocaine intoxication can cause acute myoglobinuria associated with renal failure, hepatic dysfunction, disseminated intravascular coagulation, and a high mortality.*

Shoffner JM, Wallace DC: Oxidative phosphorylation diseases. Disorders of two genomes. Adv Hum Genet 19:27, 1990. *An excellent overview of the genetic, biochemical, clinical, and therapeutic aspects of mitochondrial disorders affecting oxidative phosphorylation.*

Tein I, DeVivo DC, Bierman F, et al.: Impaired skin fibroblast carnitine uptake in primary carnitine deficiency manifested by childhood carnitine-responsive cardiomyopathy. Pediatr Res 28:247, 1990. *A description of the varied manifestations of primary systemic carnitine deficiency and the response to replacement therapy.*

508 Miscellaneous Myopathies

INFILTRATIVE MYOPATHIES. Systemic Amyloid Myopathy. The most common neurologic complication in various types of amyloidosis is a predominantly sensory-autonomic neuropathy. Amyloid deposition in muscle is frequent, but the muscle involvement is usually subclinical. Occasionally amyloidosis presents or is associated with an overt myopathy characterized by muscle enlargement, macroglossia, stiffness, exertional muscle pain, and proximal or diffuse weakness. Electromyography shows myopathic features in proximal muscles with or without changes of neuropathy distally. The amyloid deposits, identified by their metachromasia and affinity for Congo red stain, appear between and around the mural elements of the small vessels and extend into the interstitial spaces, where they tightly surround individual muscle fibers.

Hypertrophic Branchial Myopathy. This sporadic illness presents between the second and fourth decades of life and is restricted to muscles that derive from the embryonic branchial cleft. The disease evolves with slowly progressive, asymmetric, bilateral enlargement of temporalis, masseter, and pterygoid muscles. Weakness is minimal or absent. The swelling itself is painless but may lead to pain with jaw opening. The EMG and muscle biopsy show nonspecific myopathic alterations in the affected muscles. There is no satisfactory treatment. When chewing is impaired, partial excision of the enlarged muscles has proved beneficial.

SYNDROMES ASSOCIATED WITH ABNORMAL MUSCLE ACTIVITY. These can be caused by (1) abnormal neural activity in the central nervous system (e.g., dystonia, tetanus, stiff-man syndrome); (2) abnormal excitability of the peripheral nervous system (neuromyotonia, tetany, cramps); (3) abnormal excitability of the muscle fiber surface membrane (myotonic disorders); (4) a defect within the muscle fiber resulting in abnormal mechanical activity (e.g., malignant hyperthermia, contractures without electrical activity, and slow relaxation of electrically silent muscle fibers). Dystonia, tetanus, and tetany are considered in Ch. 235, 310, and 460. The remaining entities were discussed earlier in this section or will be discussed below.

Stiff-Man Syndrome. This is a disease of adult life affecting men more frequently than women. Initially intermittent spasms of axial and limb muscles are followed by continuous stiffness that immobilizes the patient. Agonist and antagonist muscles are simultaneously affected, preventing voluntary movement. The EMG shows constant firing of normal motor unit potentials in the stiff muscles. There are no signs of cerebral or spinal cord disease. Spinal anesthesia relieves the spasms. The disease is frequently associated with organ-specific autoimmune diseases, and especially insulin-dependent diabetes mellitus. Autoantibodies are detected in at least 60 per cent of patients against glutamic acid decarboxylase, the enzyme that converts glutamic acid to the inhibitory neurotransmitter gamma-aminobutyric acid (GABA). In tissue sections the autoantibodies bind to GABA-ergic neurons and pancreatic islet β cells. These findings suggest that the disease is caused by immune-mediated impairment of GABA-ergic inhibitory pathways. Relatively high doses of diazepam or baclofen, which increase GABA-mediated central inhibition, and clonidine, which prevents norepinephrine release from nerve terminals, may improve or relieve the symptoms.

Neuromyotonia. This can be generalized or focal. *Generalized* neuromyotonia is sporadic or familial. Some of the familial cases are associated with a peripheral neuropathy; some of the sporadic cases have an intrathoracic malignancy. Abnormal impulses arising in peripheral motor axons produce continuous muscle fiber activity that persists even during sleep. Depending on the site of origin in the axon, the abnormal activity is abolished by proximal nerve block or block of neuromuscular transmission. The EMG shows very high frequency (150 to 300 Hz) recurring bursts of motor unit potentials. The involuntary activation of multiple motor units causes stiffness and delayed relaxation of the affected muscles and continuous, small, undulating movements of the overlying skin (*myokymia*). Phenytoin or carbamazepine may inhibit the abnormal discharges and relieve the symptoms.

Similar high-frequency and rhythmically recurring bursts of motor unit potentials occur in *facial myokymia* seen with demyelinating or other lesions of the brain stem.

Focal neuromyotonia can occur following peripheral nerve lesions, but here the firing rate is slower (30 to 60 Hz). The delayed relaxation of an affected muscle after a willed contraction mimics action myotonia.

A benign syndrome of *muscle cramps, fasciculations, and myokymia* associated with low-frequency bursts of motor unit potentials also occurs and may incorrectly suggest the diagnosis of early motor neuron disease.

A syndrome associated with *myokymia, hyperhydrosis, mental symptoms, thymoma, and anti-acetylcholine receptor antibodies* but without symptoms of myasthenia gravis has been recently described.

Schwartz-Jampel Syndrome. This is an autosomal-recessive disease that begins in early childhood. It is characterized by chondrodystrophy, bone and joint deformities, short stature, a doleful facial expression with blepharospasm, hypertrichosis, muscle stiffness, and muscle hypertrophy or atrophy. There is delayed muscle relaxation suggesting myotonia. The EMG, however, shows high-frequency repetitive discharges, not myotonic discharges. Muscle biopsy reveals neurogenic and myogenic features.

Myotonia Congenita. Autosomal-dominant (Thomsen's disease) and autosomal-recessive forms are recognized. Both are benign and associated with diffuse muscle hypertrophy and diffuse action, percussion, and electrical myotonia. Cold increases the myotonia, and sustained exercise improves it. The membrane defect consists of a markedly reduced chloride conductance. Quinine, 0.3 to 1.5 grams daily, or phenytoin, 0.3 to 0.6 gram daily, relieves the myotonia.

Paramyotonia Congenita. This autosomal-dominant disease resembles myotonic hyperkalemic periodic paralysis. There are pure cases, however, in which potassium loading does not induce weakness. The myotonia is worsened rather than improved by exercise. Exercise in the cold causes prolonged electrically silent stiffness and weakness not relieved by rewarming. Although the membrane shows an abnormal increase in sodium conductance on cooling, this fails to explain the prolonged stiffness induced by cooling. Tocainide, 300 to 400 mg three to four times daily, prevents the cold-induced symptoms.

Slow Relaxation of Electrically Silent Muscle Fibers. This is a rare disease in which there is impaired muscle relaxation that is rapidly worsened by exercise. The slowly relaxing fibers are electrically silent. The defect lies within the calcium-pump ATPase of the sarcoplasmic reticulum.

Rippling Muscles. This is a benign and dominantly inherited disorder presenting in late childhood or adult life. Sporadic cases also occur. Local compression of a muscle evokes myoedema. This is replaced by a longitudinal depression parallel to the long axis of the muscle which then moves to the periphery of the muscle in 10 to 20 seconds in a wave that resembles the plucking of a chromatic scale on a harp. The response to percussion superficially resembles myotonia, but the rippling muscles are electrically silent. Mild muscle pain, stiffness at the beginning of exercise, and mild elevation of the serum CK level are associated features.

Auger RG, Daube JR, Gomez MR, et al.: Hereditary form of sustained muscle activity of peripheral nerve origin causing myokymia and muscle stiffness. Ann Neurol 15:13, 1984. *An excellent discussion of the differential diagnosis of neuromyotonias and related syndromes.*

Halbach M, Höberg V, Freund H-J: Neuromuscular, autonomic and central cholinergic hyperactivity associated with thymoma and acetylcholine receptor antibody. J Neurol 234:433, 1987. *The authors postulate that in this unique disorder anti-acetylcholine receptor antibodies facilitate rather than inhibit cholinergic action.*

Ii K, Hizawa K, Nunomura S, et al.: Systemic amyloid myopathy. Acta Neuropathol (Berl) 64:114, 1984. *A clear clinical and pathologic description and review of the relevant literature.*

Karpati G, Charuk J, Carpenter S, et al.: Myopathy caused by a deficiency of Ca²⁺-ATPase in sarcoplasmic reticulum (Brody's disease). Ann Neurol 20:38, 1986. *Provides an explanation for the slow relaxation of electrically silent muscle fibers.*

Mancall EL, Patel AN, Hirschhorn AM: Hypertrophic branchial myopathy. Neurology 24:1166, 1974. *A classic account of a neglected myopathy.*

Ricker K, Moxley RT, Rohkamm R: Rippling muscle disease. Arch Neurol 46:405, 1989. *A good description of an uncommon disease and a review of the literature.*

Rüdel R, Lehmann-Horn F: Membrane changes in cells from myotonia patients. Physiol Rev 65:310, 1985. *An up-to-date account of the clinical features and membrane abnormalities in the myotonic syndromes.*

Solimena M, Folli F, Aparisi R, et al.: Autoantibodies to GABA-ergic neurons and pancreatic beta cells in stiff-man syndrome. N Engl J Med 322:1555, 1990. *The report provides strong evidence that stiff-man syndrome is an organ-specific autoimmune disease and describes useful diagnostic tests.*

509 Disorders of Neuromuscular Transmission

DEFINITION AND BASIC CONCEPTS. Disorders of neuromuscular transmission can be acquired or inherited and are associated with abnormal weakness and fatigability on exertion. In each disorder the safety margin of neuromuscular transmission is compromised by one or more specific mechanisms. The following paragraphs provide a brief review of the anatomic and physiologic aspects of neuromuscular transmission.

The motor end-plate consists of a nerve terminal separated from the postsynaptic region by the synaptic space. Acetylcholine (ACh) is stored in quantal packets (6,000 to 10,000 molecules per packet) in synaptic vesicles in the nerve terminal. The vesicles release ACh into the synaptic space by exocytosis. The postsynaptic region has junctional folds containing on their terminal expansions acetylcholine receptor (AChR) molecules packed at a density of about 10^4 sites per square micrometer. The binding of two ACh molecules to an AChR molecule opens the AChR ion channel. After the ion channel closes, ACh dissociates from AChR. Acetylcholinesterase (AChE) is distributed throughout the basal lamina of the synaptic space at a density of about 2,500 sites per square micrometer.

In the resting state single ACh quanta are randomly released into the synaptic space. The high local ACh concentration saturates all nearby AChE sites so that most ACh molecules can reach postsynaptic AChR's. The AChR packing density is so high that ACh needs to diffuse only 0.3 μm along the top and 0.3 μm down along the junctional folds before it meets all the AChR it can saturate. The resultant resting depolarizations of the muscle fiber are known as miniature end-plate potentials (MEPP's). The MEPP amplitude depends on the number of ACh molecules in the quantum, the number of available AChR's, the geometry of the synaptic space, and the average depolarization generated by the opening of an AChR ion channel. When ACh dissociates from AChR it is hydrolyzed by AChE to choline and acetate. Choline is taken up by the nerve terminal and is reutilized for ACh synthesis.

Depolarization of the nerve terminal by nerve impulse opens voltage-sensitive calcium channels in the presynaptic membrane. The calcium influx increases the probability of synaptic vesicle exocytosis. The exocytosis occurs adjacent to active zones in the presynaptic membrane. The voltage-sensitive calcium channels are represented by regularly arrayed large membrane particles in the active zones.

The quanta released by a nerve impulse generate an end-plate potential (EPP), the amplitude of which depends on the MEPP amplitude and the number of quanta (m) released by the nerve impulse. The value of m depends on the probability of release

(p) and the number of quanta readily available for release (n) according to the relationship $m = np$. *The safety margin of neuromuscular transmission is defined as the difference between the actual EPP amplitude and the EPP amplitude required to trigger the muscle fiber action potential.*

Repetitive stimulation results in a frequency-dependent depression of the EPP amplitude and of the safety margin to a certain plateau. The decrease is mainly due to a decrease in n. Repetitive stimulation also can facilitate transmitter release by increasing p, or n, or both. The temporal profiles of the opposing processes are such that (1) a defect of neuromuscular transmission is most readily detected by a train of five to ten stimuli delivered at a low (2 to 3 Hz) frequency; (2) tetanic stimulation results in transient improvement and then a worsening of the defect.

Table 509–1 shows a classification of currently recognized defects of neuromuscular transmission. Botulism is described in Ch. 309, the others in this chapter.

MYASTHENIA GRAVIS (MG). This is an acquired autoimmune disorder in which pathogenic autoantibodies induce AChR deficiency at the motor end-plate. The safety margin of neuromuscular transmission is compromised by the small amplitude of the MEPP and consequently of the EPP. Circulating AChR antibodies are present in 80 to 90 per cent of the cases, and IgG and complement components are deposited on the postsynaptic membrane. AChR deficiency results from complement-mediated lysis of the junctional folds, accelerated internalization and destruction of AChR cross-linked by antibody (modulation), and, to a lesser extent, by antibodies blocking the binding of ACh to AChR.

Clinical Features. The incidence is two to five per year per million and the prevalence 13 to 64 per million. The female to male ratio is six to four. The disease may present at any age, but the incidence in females peaks in the third decade and in males in the sixth or seventh decade.

The disease can involve either the external ocular muscles selectively or the general voluntary muscle system. The symptoms may fluctuate from hour to hour, day to day, or over longer periods. They are provoked or worsened by exertion, exposure to extremes of temperature, viral or other infections, menses, and excitement. Ocular muscle involvement is usually bilateral, asymmetric, and typically associated with ptosis and diplopia. Weakness of other muscles innervated by cranial nerves results in loss of facial expression, everted lips, a smile that resembles a snarl, jaw drop, nasal regurgitation of liquids, choking on foods and secretions, and a slurred, hypernasal speech of a reduced volume. Abnormal fatigability of the limb muscles causes difficulty in combing the hair, lifting objects repeatedly, climbing stairs, walking, and running. Depending on the severity of the disease, dyspnea appears on moderate or mild exertion or is present even at rest. The abnormal fatigability can be demonstrated by asking the patient to look up without closing the eyes for a minute, to count loudly from one to one hundred, to hold the arms abducted to the horizontal position for a minute, or to perform repeated

TABLE 509–1. CLASSIFICATION OF DISORDERS OF NEUROMUSCULAR TRANSMISSION

Autoimmune
  Myasthenia gravis
  Lambert-Eaton myasthenic syndrome
Congenital
  Familial infantile myasthenia*
  End-plate acetylcholinesterase deficiency*
  Slow-channel syndrome†
  End-plate AChR deficiency*
  High-conductance fast-channel syndrome*
  Paucity of synaptic vesicles and reduced quantal release‡
  Putative abnormality of ACh-AChr interaction‡
Toxic
  Botulism
  Drug-induced
  Pesticide poisoning

*Autosomal-recessive inheritance
†Autosomal-dominant inheritance
‡Autosomal-recessive inheritance suspected

deep knee-bends. The deep tendon reflexes are normally active even in weak muscles. Atrophy of masseter, temporal, facial, or tongue muscles, and less often of other muscles, occurs in about 15 per cent of patients.

Initially, the symptoms are purely ocular in 40 per cent, are generalized in 40 per cent, and involve only the extremities in 10 per cent and only the bulbar or bulbar and eye muscles in another 10 per cent. Subsequently, the weakness can spread from ocular to facial to lower bulbar muscles and then to torso and limb muscles, but the sequence may vary. Proximal limb muscles are affected more than distal ones. In the most advanced cases the weakness is universal. By the end of the first year, the ocular muscles are affected in nearly all patients. The symptoms remain ocular in only 16 per cent. In nearly 90 per cent of those in whom the disease becomes generalized, this occurs within the first year after the onset. Progression is most rapid within the first 3 years, and more than half of the deaths caused by MG occur in that period. Spontaneous remissions lasting from weeks to years can occur. Long remissions are uncommon, and most remissions occur during the first 3 years.

Two thirds of patients with MG have thymic hyperplasia and 10 to 15 per cent have thymoma. A few with thymoma also develop myocarditis or giant cell myositis. In about 10 per cent the MG is associated with another autoimmune disease, such as hyperthyroidism, polymyositis, systemic lupus erythematosus, Sjögren's syndrome, rheumatoid arthritis, ulcerative colitis, pemphigus, sarcoidosis, pernicious anemia, and Lambert-Eaton myasthenic syndrome.

A clinical classification of MG, originally proposed by Osserman, is based on the distribution and severity of symptoms: group 1, ocular; group 2A, mild generalized; group 2B, moderately severe generalized; group 3, acute fulminating; group 4, late severe. Another classification, proposed by Vincent and Newsom-Davis, is according to the age of onset and the presence or absence of thymoma: Type 1, MG with thymoma: The disease is usually severe and the AChR antibody level is high; there is no association either with sex or HLA antigen. Type 2, no thymoma, onset before age 40: The AChR antibody level is intermediate; there is female preponderance and an increased association with HLA-A1, HLA-B8, and HLA-DRw3 antigens (HLA-B12 in Japan). Type 3, no thymoma, onset after age 40: The AChR antibody level tends to be low; there is male preponderance and increased association with HLA-A3, HLA-B7, or HLA-DRw2 antigens (HLA-A10 in Japan). Striated muscle antibodies are found in 90 per cent, 5 per cent, and 45 per cent, respectively, in the three types. The association with other autoimmune diseases is highest in Type 3 and lowest in Type 1. Both classifications are discussed further in the Engel chapters cited in the references.

Transient Neonatal MG. Circulating AChR antibodies can be detected in most infants born to myasthenic mothers, but only 12 per cent of such children develop MG, usually during the first few hours of life. The findings are feeble cry, feeding and respiratory difficulty, general or facial weakness, and ptosis. The mean duration is 18 days. There is no relation between the severity of MG in mother and infant. The disease is caused by the transfer of AChR antibodies or immunocytes from mother to infant, or perhaps fetal AChR damaged by maternal antibodies triggers a transient immune response in the infant.

Diagnosis. This is based on the characteristic history, physical examination, anticholinesterase tests, and laboratory studies. The latter include EMG studies, tests for AChR antibodies, and in selected cases, microelectrode studies in vitro of neuromuscular transmission and ultrastructural and cytochemical studies of the end-plate.

Anticholinesterase Tests. Edrophonium given intravenously acts within a few seconds, and its effects last for a few minutes. One to 2 mg of the drug is injected intravenously over 15 seconds. If there is no response in 30 seconds, an additional 8 to 9 mg is injected. The evaluation of the response requires objective assessment of one or more signs, such as degree of ptosis, range of ocular movements, and the force of the hand grip. Possible cholinergic side effects of the drug include fasciculations, flushing, lacrimation, abdominal cramps, nausea, vomiting, and diarrhea. The drug must be given cautiously to patients with cardiac disease, for it may cause sinus bradycardia, atrioventricular block, and, rarely, cardiac arrest. Atropine is used to reverse toxicity. Intramuscular neostigmine, 0.5 to 1.0 mg, acts maximally in about 30 minutes, and its effects last up to 2 hours, allowing a more leisurely evaluation of changes in clinical status.

Electromyography. Supramaximal stimulation of a motor nerve at 2 to 3 Hz results in a 10 per cent or greater decrement of the amplitude of the evoked compound muscle action potential from the first to the fifth response. The test is positive in nearly all patients, provided that two or more distal and two or more proximal muscles are examined. The decrement is caused by a normally occurring decrease in the number of quanta released from the nerve terminal, and hence in the amplitude of the EPP, at the beginning of low-frequency stimulation. In MG the EPP amplitude is already reduced by the AChR deficiency, and the additional decrease during stimulation results in blocking of transmission at an increasing number of end-plates. Single-fiber EMG compares the timing of action potentials between pairs of closely adjacent muscle fibers in the same motor unit during a willed contraction. In MG the low amplitude and relatively long rise time of the EPP cause abnormally long interpotential intervals and intermittent blocking of action potential generation at some fibers.

Serologic Tests. The usual AChR antibody test measures the binding of antibody to AChR labeled with radioactive α-bungarotoxin. The toxin itself is attached irreversibly to the ACh binding site of AChR. The antibody binding test is positive in nearly all patients with moderately severe or acute severe MG, in 80 per cent with mild generalized MG, in 50 per cent with ocular MG, but in only 25 per cent of those in remission. In a few patients only antibodies that block the binding of ACh to AChR can be detected. The antibody titer correlates only loosely with disease severity but in individual patients a greater than 50 per cent decrease in titer for more than 12 months is nearly always associated with sustained clinical improvement. Striated muscle antibodies also occur in MG patients. Their role remains unknown but they often are associated with thymoma.

Other Diagnostic Studies. Immune complexes can be localized at the MG end-plate in cryostat sections even when circulating AChR antibodies cannot be detected. C3 localization is technically the easiest and most convenient way to confirm the suspected diagnosis. Electrophysiologic studies of neuromuscular transmission in vitro can distinguish between atypical cases of MG, the Lambert-Eaton myasthenic syndrome, and some of the congenital myasthenic syndromes.

Differential Diagnosis. This includes neurasthenia, oculopharyngeal dystrophy, mitochondrial myopathies involving the external ocular and/or other cranial and limb muscles, intracranial mass lesions compressing cranial nerves, drug-induced myasthenic syndromes, and other disorders of neuromuscular transmission listed in the table. Neurasthenia is recognized by giving way on muscle testing and the lack of objective clinical and laboratory findings. In myopathies involving the ocular muscles, the weakness does not fluctuate, diplopia is seldom a symptom, the muscle biopsy may show distinct morphologic abnormalities, and pharmacologic and laboratory tests for MG are negative. Drug-induced and other myasthenic syndromes are considered below.

Therapy. Anticholinesterases, alternate-day prednisone treatment, azathioprine, thymectomy, and plasmapheresis are currently used to treat MG. Anticholinesterases are useful in all clinical forms of the disease. Pyridostigmine bromide (Mestinon) (60-mg tablets) acts for 3 to 4 hours, and neostigmine bromide (15-mg tablets) for 2 to 3 hours. The former drug has fewer muscarinic side effects and is therefore more widely used. One half to four tablets of pyridostigmine bromide are given every 4 hours in the daytime. This medication is also available in 180-mg "time-span" tablets for use at bedtime and as a syrup for children and patients requiring nasogastric feeding. If troublesome muscarinic side effects occur, these can be treated with 0.4 to 0.6 mg atropine given orally two or three times daily. Postoperatively or in critically ill patients intramuscularly injectable pyridostigmine bromide (the dose is one thirtieth of the oral dose) and neostigmine methylsulfate (the dose is one fifteenth of the oral dose) can be used.

Progressive weakness despite increasing amounts of anticholinesterases signals the onset of a myasthenic or cholinergic crisis.

Cholinergic crises are associated with muscarinic effects, such as abdominal cramps, nausea, vomiting, diarrhea, miosis, lacrimation, increased bronchial secretions, diaphoresis, and bradycardia. In a myasthenic crisis the muscarinic effects are not conspicuous, and 2 mg edrophonium given intravenously improves rather than worsens the weakness. In practice, however, the two types of crises often are difficult to distinguish, and overmedication of a myasthenic crisis can convert it into a cholinergic crisis. Therefore, patients who have increasing difficulty with respiration, feeding, or handling secretions and who are not responding to relatively high doses of anticholinesterases are best treated by drug withdrawal, tracheal intubation or tracheostomy, support with respirator, and intravenous feeding. Refractoriness to drug therapy usually disappears after a few days.

In patients with generalized disease not responding adequately to modest doses of anticholinesterases, other forms of therapy must be employed. Thymectomy increases the remission rate and improves the clinical course of MG. Although controlled clinical studies of thymectomy according to age, sex, and severity of disease have never been carried out, there is general agreement that the best response occurs in young women with hyperplastic thymus glands and high antibody titer. Thymoma represents an absolute indication for thymectomy because the tumor is often locally invasive. Computed tomography of the mediastinum is a sensitive screening test, but it can give false-positive results.

Alternate-day prednisone treatment induces remission or significantly improves the disease in more than half the patients. The treatment is relatively safe provided that one institutes the usual precautions for patients taking corticosteroid therapy. With an average dose of 70 mg on alternate days, the average time for significant improvement is 5 months. After the improvement reaches a plateau the dose must be lowered gradually over several months to establish the minimum maintenance dose.

Azathioprine in doses of 150 to 200 mg per day also induces remissions or measurable improvement in more than half the treated patients. The minimum time for improvement is 3 months. Surveillance to detect side effects (pancytopenia, leukopenia, serious infection, and hepatocellular injury) must be maintained during therapy.

Plasmapheresis is indicated in severe generalized or fulminating MG refractory to other forms of treatment. Daily exchanges of 2 liters of plasma result in objective improvement and lower the AChR antibody titer in a few days. Plasmapheresis, however, is expensive and does not confer greater long-term protection than immunosuppressants alone.

LAMBERT-EATON MYASTHENIC SYNDROME. This is an acquired autoimmune disease in which pathogenic autoantibodies cause a deficiency of voltage-sensitive calcium channels at the motor nerve terminal. This deficiency restricts calcium ingress into the terminal when it is depolarized by nerve impulse and thereby reduces the probability of quantal release. Among patients over 40 years, 70 per cent of males and 30 per cent of females have an associated carcinoma, usually a small-cell carcinoma of the lung. The syndrome may predate tumor detection by up to 3 years. In one third of patients the syndrome is non-neoplastic and occurs at any age. In these cases there is an association with other autoimmune disorders, HLA-B8 and DRw3 antigens, and organ-specific autoantibodies.

Patients have weakness and fatigability of proximal limb and torso muscles with relative sparing of extraocular and bulbar muscles. The lower limbs are more severely involved than the upper ones. On maximal voluntary contraction the force produced by a weak muscle increases for a few seconds and then again decreases. The tendon reflexes are hypoactive or absent in most patients. Autonomic manifestations (dry mouth, impotence, decreased sweating, orthostatic hypotension, or altered pupillary reflexes) occur in one half of the patients.

On EMG, the amplitude of the compound muscle action potential evoked by a single nerve stimulus from rested muscle is abnormally small. Repetitive stimulation at 2 Hz induces a further decrement, but stimulation at frequencies higher than 10 Hz or voluntary exercise for a brief period markedly facilitates the response so that the evoked potential attains normal amplitude.

Anticholinesterases are only slightly effective. Guanidine hydrochloride (10 mg per kilogram per day) or 3,4-diaminopyridine (1 mg per kilogram per day) increases quantal release from the nerve terminal and relieves the symptoms. However, the former drug has severe toxic side effects, and the latter is not yet available in clinical practice. Optimal treatment of non-neoplastic cases consists of modest doses of alternate-day prednisone and 2 mg per kilogram per day of azathioprine.

CONGENITAL MYASTHENIC SYNDROMES. *Familial Infantile Myasthenia.* This is an autosomal-recessive disorder characterized by fluctuating ophthalmoparesis since birth, feeding difficulty during early infancy, weakness after exercise, and attacks of apnea precipitated by crying, vomiting, or fever. The symptoms tend to improve with age. A decremental EMG response is present in muscles weak when examined. Weakness can be induced in some, but not all, muscles by exercise or repetitive stimulation at 10 Hz for a few minutes. Unlike in autoimmune MG, the postsynaptic region is intact and there is no AChR deficiency. The MEPP amplitude is normal in rested muscle but decreases to abnormally low values after 10-Hz stimulation for a few minutes. This suggests a presynaptic defect in ACh resynthesis or in ACh packaging into synaptic vesicles. Weakness, when present, responds to small or modest doses of anticholinesterases. Parenteral anticholinesterase therapy is indicated in crises. Parents of young patients must be taught to use a hand-assisted ventilatory device and to inject appropriate doses of neostigmine intramuscularly during crises.

Congenital End-Plate Acetylcholinesterase Deficiency. Sporadic and familial cases in males and females have been observed to date. Severe weakness refractory to anticholinesterases and a decremental EMG response are present in all voluntary muscles from birth. There is total absence of AChE from all end-plates. ACh-AChR interaction and the duration of the EPP are prolonged, so that a single stimulus applied to a motor nerve evokes two or more compound muscle action potentials. The motor nerve terminals are small and contain a reduced number of releasable ACh quanta. AChR is preserved or reduced at the end-plate. The AChR loss, if present, is caused by degenerative changes in the junctional folds, which can be accounted for by the ACh excess, but this in itself is mild because ACh release is also reduced. The safety margin of neuromuscular transmission is compromised by lack of releasable ACh quanta and by AChR deficiency.

Slow-Channel Syndrome. This is an autosomal-dominant disorder with high penetrance and variable expressivity. It presents in infancy or later life with selective weakness, fatigability, and atrophy of cervical, shoulder girdle, and forearm muscles. There is variable involvement of extraocular, other cranial, truncal, or limb muscles. The tendon reflexes are normal or hypoactive. Anticholinesterases are usually ineffective. A decremental EMG response appears in clinically affected muscles. The basic abnormality is slow closure of the AChR ion channel. This prolongs the duration of the EPP, causes a stimulus-linked repetitive compound action potential in all muscles, and allows abnormal accumulation of calcium in the postsynaptic region. The calcium excess results in destruction of the junctional folds, loss of AChR, and myopathic changes near the end-plates. The safety margin of neuromuscular transmission is compromised by the AChR deficiency and the altered end-plate geometry.

Congenital End-Plate AChR Deficiency. This is an autosomal-recessive disorder that presents during infancy. The symptoms and electrophysiologic abnormalities resemble those in autoimmune MG and respond to anticholinesterases. Circulating AChR antibodies are absent, and no immune complexes are found at the end-plate. The cause has not been established. It could stem from decreased synthesis, impaired membrane insertion or accelerated degradation of AChR, or abnormal ACh-AChR interaction.

Other Congenital Myasthenic Syndromes. These were recently recognized by in vitro electrophysiologic and ultrastructural analysis. In the *high-conductance fast-channel syndrome*, the conductance of the AChR ion channel is abnormally high but its open time is reduced. The disease is familial and is associated with mild fatigable weakness of ocular and limb muscles since birth. In another syndrome with *paucity of synaptic vesicles and reduced quantal release*, neuromuscular transmission is compromised by a decrease in m, which is due to a decrease in n. The disease presents in the neonatal period, involves all muscles, is moderately severe, and is partially responsive to anticholinesterase medications. In a syndrome caused by a *putative abnormality of ACh-AChR interaction*, the MEPP amplitude is markedly reduced without AChR deficiency, synaptic vesicles are of normal size, and analysis of ACh-induced current noise suggests abnormal interaction of ACh with AChR. The disorder presents in the neonatal period, is severely disabling, and responds poorly to anticholinesterase medications.

DRUG-INDUCED MYASTHENIC SYNDROMES. These are uncommon in clinical practice. Tetracycline, polymyxin and aminoglycoside antibiotics, antiarrhythmic agents (procainamide, quinidine), β-adrenergic blockers (propranolol, timolol), phenothiazines, lithium, trimethaphan, methoxyflurane, and magnesium given parenterally or in cathartics reduce the safety margin of neuromuscular transmission. However, overt myasthenic symptoms do not usually appear unless an overdose of the drug is administered or the renal or hepatic elimination of the drug is impaired. The same drugs and inhalation anesthetic agents also can potentiate neuromuscular blocking agents used during surgical procedures and both may worsen or unmask pre-existing disorders of neuromuscular transmission. Calcium channel blocking drugs can worsen the transmission defect in the Lambert-Eaton myasthenic syndrome.

Succinylcholine, a depolarizing blocking drug, is used to induce muscle relaxation during anesthesia. A single dose of the drug sufficient to cause transient apnea is eliminated by plasma pseudocholinesterase in 2 to 10 minutes. In approximately 1 of 2500 patients receiving the drug, prolonged apnea occurs and persists up to several hours. Most of these patients have an autosomal-recessive abnormality of the plasma pseudocholinesterase. In some genetic variants the plasma pseudocholinesterase activity is abnormally low; in others the enzyme shows increased sensitivity to inhibition by dibucaine.

PESTICIDE POISONING. Poisoning with pesticides containing long-acting anticholinesterases causes ACh accumulation at central, muscarinic, and nicotinic cholinergic synapses. The intoxication is associated with alterations in sensorium, severe muscarinic effects, and muscle weakness from desensitization of AChR at the neuromuscular junction. Therapy consists of respiratory support, large doses of atropine (2 to 4 mg intramuscularly and repeated as necessary) and pralidoxime (1 gram intravenously, repeated in 20 minutes if necessary).

Engel AG, Banker BQ (eds.): Myology. New York, McGraw-Hill Book Company, 1986. *Chapters by Engel and Magelby ably discuss the detailed anatomy, physiology, and clinical dimensions of neuromuscular transmission.*

Engel AG, Walls T, Nagel A, et al.: Newly recognized congenital myasthenic syndromes. Prog Brain Res 84:125–137, 1990. *An account of the clinical, morphologic, and electrophysiologic aspects of recently recognized congenital myasthenic syndromes.*

Grob D, Brunner NG, Namba T: The natural course of myasthenia gravis and effect of therapeutic measures. Ann NY Acad Sci 377:652, 1981. *A model clinical study.*

Nelson TC, Burritt MF: Pesticide poisoning, succinylcholine-induced apnea and pseudocholinesterase. Mayo Clin Proc 61:750, 1986. *A good description of pesticide poisoning and the different pseudocholinesterase deficiencies.*

Swift TR: Disorders of neuromuscular transmission other than myasthenia gravis. Muscle Nerve 4:334, 1981. *A thorough review of drug-induced myasthenic syndromes.*

Vincent A, Lang B, Newsom-Davis J: Autoimmunity to the voltage-gated calcium channel underlies the Lambert-Eaton myasthenic syndrome, a paraneoplastic disorder. Trends Neurosci 12:496, 1989. *A readable overview of the autoimmune etiology and immunopathology of the disease.*

PART XXIV
EYE DISEASES

John W. Gittinger, Jr.

Because many systemic diseases affect the eyes, ophthalmoscopy is a necessary skill for the physician. The pupil of the eye is a window opening onto the arterioles and venules of the retina, the optic disc, and the pigmented tissues of the fundus. Ch. 453 describes the autonomic and somatic motor disorders of ocular control and reviews the clinically important anatomy of the visual pathways.

The discussion that follows highlights the interrelationship between ocular and systemic disease, beginning with a discussion of visual loss, then a brief review of the two common ophthalmic disorders—cataract and glaucoma, before turning to ocular entities and ocular manifestations of medical disorders likely to present to nonophthalmic physicians.

510 Visual Loss

Visual loss may be either transient (see Ch. 453) or permanent, with most of the potential causes capable of producing either one. A major purpose of the ophthalmologic examination is to establish the etiology of visual loss. Except when it reflects a structural alteration in the eye, as in high myopia, the need for refractive correction is considered a variant of normal, not a disease process. Furthermore, when evaluating a patient for reduced vision, only the best-corrected acuity should be considered. Uncorrected acuity is of little interest in assessing the pathophysiology of eye disorders.

Many conditions can cause visual loss (Table 510–1). Normal visual development in an infant requires formed images on the retina and intact visual pathways in the rest of the brain. A neonatal eye with a dense opacity of the media such as a mature cataract (see below) does not develop useful vision unless the opacity is removed soon after birth and any resulting large refractive error is corrected quickly. Visual development proceeds through critical stages; any interruption of these stages during

early childhood can permanently prevent the normal capacity for processing visual information even if the causative condition is treated later on. If both eyes are involved, the development of nystagmus (rhythmic to-and-fro movements of the eye) at about 3 or 4 months of age signals that this critical period has been exceeded.

Normal adult levels of visual acuity can be measured electrophysiologically by 6 months of age, but the neural connections that permit fine visual processing become permanently established only later in childhood. During the first few years of life, strabismus—misalignment of the visual axes of the two eyes—may result in suppression of central vision in one eye. Such visual loss in an eye that appears anatomically normal is termed amblyopia. A large, uncorrected refractive error—ametropia—or a major difference in the refractive error in the two eyes—anisometropia—may also lead to amblyopia. (The term *amblyopia* is also sometimes applied to processes in which the ophthalmoscopic signs are subtle, e.g., toxic-nutritional amblyopia.) Strabismic amblyopia is potentially reversible until 6 to 10 years of age, when the neural processing networks for vision become fixed for life. With this final step in visual development, the visual system achieves adult inflexibility, and misalignment of the visual axes results in permanent diplopia rather than suppression.

Careful ophthalmic examination and appropriate testing should allow classification of reduced vision into one of the categories listed (Table 510–1): opacities of the media, chorioretinal disease, optic nerve disease, visual pathway disorders, amblyopia, or psychogenic visual loss. Two or more processes may affect the same eye.

PSYCHOGENIC VISUAL LOSS

Visual loss not attributable to an organic process is termed psychogenic. Alternative designations are functional, nonorganic, nonphysiologic, hysterical, and malingering. The last two are best avoided. Hysteria suggests to some a sexual bias and must be considered a psychiatric, not an ophthalmologic, diagnosis; malingering imputes motives that are difficult to prove. Functional visual loss, the usage currently preferred by some authorities, is potentially confusing because *functional amblyopia* refers to those forms of amblyopia in which the process is potentially reversible with treatment (strabismic, ametropic, and anisometropic). In these instances there is presumably an underlying physiologic alteration in the visual system itself.

Psychogenic visual loss is not necessarily a diagnosis of exclusion. Certain patterns of visual loss cannot represent organic disease. Concentric constriction of visual fields is a common finding in nonphysiologic visual loss but also occurs with advanced glaucoma and retinitis pigmentosa and after bilateral occipital infarctions. Failure of the visual field to expand to an appropriate stimulus with increased testing distance—tubular fields—is, however, diagnostic of psychogenic visual loss. Similarly, patients who claim to be completely blind in one eye but who have normal pupillary reactions, full stereopsis, and normal ipsilateral visual evoked responses must have a nonphysiologic component to their visual loss. Other testing techniques also may result in normal subjective responses from a supposedly blind eye.

Most cases of psychogenic visual loss occur in the setting of minor psychological reactions rather than major psychiatric disorders. Sometimes both organic and nonorganic components coexist. Unless the visual loss prevents the patient from working or attending school, simple reassurance and careful follow-up with treatment of intercurrent organic abnormalities constitute appropriate management, and spontaneous improvement occurs.

TABLE 510–1. DIFFERENTIAL DIAGNOSIS OF VISUAL LOSS

Opacities of the media	Corneal opacities (leukomas, edema, dystrophy) or irregularity; anterior chamber blood or inflammation; cataract; vitreous opacities
Chorioretinal disease	Macular and other retinal degenerations; retinal detachment; toxic, vascular, and traumatic retinopathies; infectious and inflammatory chorioretinitis; retinal tumors
Optic nerve disease	Glaucoma, other optic neuropathies (inflammatory, toxic, traumatic, vascular, hereditary); compressive and infiltrative neuropathy; optic nerve tumors
Visual pathway disorders	Vascular, inflammatory, infectious, degenerative, developmental, neoplastic
Amblyopia	Strabismic, nutritional deprivation, anisometropic, ametropic, idiopathic
Psychogenic	

Isenberg SJ: The Eye in Infancy. Chicago, Year Book Medical Publishers, 1989. *This monograph contains discussions of visual development and amblyopia.*
Thompson HS: Functional visual loss. Am J Ophthalmol 100:209, 1985. *An experienced clinician offers an approach to the problem.*

Jaffe NS, Jaffe MS, Jaffe GF: Cataract Surgery and Its Complications, 5th ed. St. Louis, The C. V. Mosby Company, 1990. *This profusely illustrated monograph addresses most of the issues of modern cataract surgery and includes extensive references.*

511 Cataract

A cataract is an opacity of the lens that produces painless, gradual loss of vision. Cataracts are described according to their location—nuclear (deep in the lens), cortical (more superficial), and subcapsular (immediately beneath the capsule). Cataracts are classified as immature, mature, or hypermature. An immature cataract has some clear cortex; a mature cataract is totally opaque—the pupil appears white (leukokoria). A hypermature cataract has liquefied cortex that leaks through the capsule and may excite destructive inflammation. Immature cataracts are usually removed for visual reasons. A mature or hypermature cataract in an eye with potentially useful vision should be removed to prevent irreversible damage.

ETIOLOGY. Congenital cataracts are a feature of rubella embryopathy and often are associated with other congenital malformations. Acquired cataracts may result from trauma, radiation, or metabolic disorder. Several examples of colorful cataracts have diagnostic, but little visual, significance. In Wilson's disease, orange copper deposits may appear on the anterior capsule—the sunflower cataract. Chlorpromazine administration may result in a brown or white dusting on the anterior lens surface. Red, green, and blue opacities in the lenticular cortex characterize myotonic dystrophy, but are occasionally encountered in its absence.

Hypocalcemia may be cataractogenic. Cataracts occur in disorders of carbohydrate metabolism: hypoglycemia, galactosemia, and diabetes mellitus. Diabetics do not necessarily have an increased incidence of cataracts, but theirs progress rapidly, perhaps because of variations in lens hydration.

Systemic corticosteroids promote formation of posterior subcapsular cataracts. Because of the path light takes through the lens, posterior subcapsular cataracts reduce vision more than similar, eccentric opacities. Central posterior opacities get in the way of light, especially when the pupil is small, as in bright light or with close work. Difficulties with driving and reading are often the first complaints.

Most cataracts have no known etiology. The common nuclear sclerotic cataract, or senile cataract, is often familial, but no specific factors have been proven to accelerate or retard its development.

TREATMENT. The treatment for cataract is surgical removal. With the exception of mature and hypermature cataracts and of immature cataracts that have swollen sufficiently to threaten to precipitate angle-closure glaucoma, most cataracts are removed for visual reasons. Considerations in planning cataract extraction are the patient's visual needs, the potential for improvement, and the risks of surgery. A person who drives requires surgery when the better eye is worse than 20/40, the legal minimum for a driver's license in most states. By contrast, an elderly patient with 20/200 vision and limited visual needs may be happy without intervention. Care must be taken to identify intercurrent ocular disease; removal of the lens of an eye with advanced glaucoma or macular degeneration does not improve vision.

The risk of cataract surgery itself is small. Despite the possibility of intraocular hemorrhage, postoperative infection, corneal decompensation, or problems with wound healing, the chances for a good visual outcome are excellent. Even successful cataract surgery, however, increases the likelihood of subsequent retinal detachment, and a small percentage of eyes postoperatively develop prolonged cystoid macular edema with reduced acuity.

General anesthesia constitutes a major portion of the risk. Cataract surgery, however, can usually be performed under local anesthesia, and this should be considered the method of choice in medically fragile patients.

512 Glaucoma

Glaucoma comprises a group of disorders in which elevated intraocular pressure damages the optic nerve. The major types of glaucoma are open-angle, angle-closure, congenital, and secondary.

The dynamics of aqueous humor control intraocular pressure. The aqueous humor is derived from blood by a process of secretion and ultrafiltration in the ciliary body. Aqueous humor then passes from the posterior chamber through the pupil to fill the anterior chamber, the space between the back of the cornea and the plane of the iris and pupil. The aqueous humor is reabsorbed through the trabecular meshwork, located in the angle between the cornea and the iris, to enter Schlemm's canal, which connects with the venous system (Fig. 512–1).

OPEN-ANGLE GLAUCOMA

In chronic open-angle glaucoma, the most common type, a block in aqueous humor reabsorption exists at the level of the trabecular meshwork. Intraocular pressure rises above its normal maximum of 21 mm Hg and gradually destroys axons and supporting tissue on the optic disc.

The prevalence of open-angle glaucoma varies with the population studied and the diagnostic criteria employed. A conservative estimate of unequivocal glaucoma in American and European adults is 0.5 per cent. Patients with increased intraocular pressure without signs of optic nerve damage are considered to have *ocular hypertension.* Treatment of ocular hypertension may be initiated if the pressure exceeds 30 mmHg.

Open-angle glaucoma is ordinarily asymptomatic until well advanced. Only rarely does the elevated intraocular pressure cause corneal edema, with the attendant perception of halos around lights. Pain is not characteristic of open-angle glaucoma. Initially only the peripheral visual field is lost; visual acuity remains normal until late in the course of the disease. Diagnosis is made by measurement of intraocular pressure, examination of the optic disc, and testing of the visual fields. Gonioscopy, the visualization of the angle structures under high magnifications with special contact lenses, can distinguish an angle-closure from an open-angle mechanism.

The treatment of open-angle glaucoma is primarily medical. Topical administration of parasympathomimetics (pilocarpine and carbachol), β-adrenergic blockers (timolol, betaxolol, and levobunolol), and sympathomimetics (epinephrine and dipivefrin) decreases intraocular pressure. When these medications—individually and in combination—are ineffective in arresting progressive disc damage and visual field loss, topical indirect parasympathomimetics (echothiophate) and systemic carbonic anhydrase inhibitors (acetazolamide and methazolamide) may be prescribed.

If maximum tolerated medical therapy fails to halt progression, surgery is indicated. *Laser trabeculoplasty* opens aqueous outflow channels by burning the surface of the trabecular meshwork. If all else fails, a surgical fistula can be created between the anterior chamber and the subconjunctival space, allowing direct absorption of aqueous humor by subconjunctival and episcleral vessels.

The management of open-angle glaucoma depends upon early recognition, careful follow-up, and patient compliance with therapeutic regimens. Routine measurement of intraocular pressures *(tonometry)* at general physical examinations is often advocated, but careful ophthalmoscopy with referral of patients whose central excavation ("cup") exceeds one third of the disc's area may be an equally effective screen.

ANGLE-CLOSURE GLAUCOMA

Angle-closure glaucoma develops when the normal path of aqueous flow is interrupted in an eye with a shallow anterior

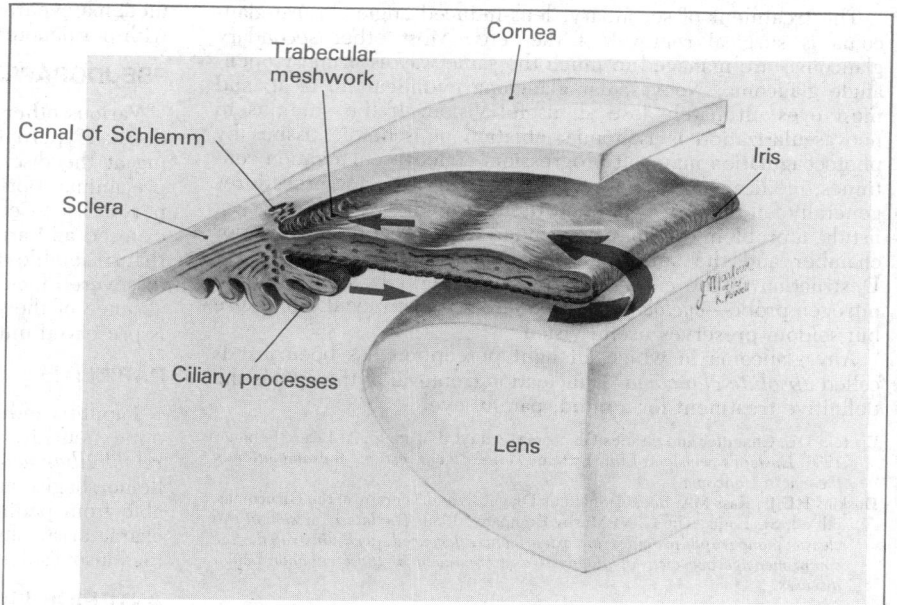

FIGURE 512–1. Circulation of aqueous humor in the normal eye. Aqueous is produced in the ciliary body and its processes, fills the posterior chamber (which also contains the lens), passes through the pupil *(large arrow)*, and is reabsorbed through the trabecular meshwork into the canal of Schlemm.

chamber, the consequence of a structurally anomalous anterior segment. Intraocular pressure is normal until resistance to aqueous flow through the pupil—pupillary block—bows the iris forward to obstruct the resorptive surfaces in the angle. The pressure then rises precipitously, often to above 50 mm Hg (Fig. 512–2).

Acute angle-closure glaucoma is generally monocular. The eye is red and painful and the pupil is about 6 mm and fixed. Vision is decreased. The patient is diaphoretic, nauseated, and often vomits.

Typical angle-closure glaucoma is easy to recognize. Occasionally, chronic or subacute angle-closure mimics open-angle glaucoma. Gonioscopy then distinguishes between the two mechanisms. The elderly do not necessarily develop the full set of clinical signs and symptoms. Always consider angle-closure glaucoma in patients with a fixed, mid-dilated pupil and decreased vision.

Angle-closure can be precipitated in predisposed eyes by dilating the pupils. The risk of pharmacologic dilation is assessed by noting the depth of the anterior chamber. Eyes with shallow anterior chambers are at risk for angle-closure. This distinction is not always easy to observe, and even an experienced ophthal-

mologist sometimes cannot determine whether an angle will close with dilation. The risk of dilation increases with age, and everyone over the age of 50 whose anterior chamber is less than full depth should be considered to have the potential for angle-closure. This does not mean that most patients should not be dilated, but rather that dilation should be performed with a short-acting mydriatic agent such as tropicamide or hydroxyamphetamine, and the patient observed until the mydriatic begins to wear off.

A nonophthalmologist should probably not routinely dilate adult outpatients. Children and in-patients may be dilated if there is no other contraindication such as recent head trauma, an iris-fixated intraocular lens, or impending general anesthesia. With these exceptions, the diagnostic benefits of dilation outweigh the risk of precipitating angle-closure. Should angle-closure glaucoma develop, it can be recognized and promptly treated.

An acute angle-closure attack creates an emergency. Initial management consists of administration of parenteral acetazolamide, oral glycerol, isosorbide (in diabetics) or intravenous mannitol, plus topical pilocarpine and a β-adrenergic antagonist. Once the attack has been broken, the anatomic predisposition can be circumvented by connecting the posterior and anterior chamber through the peripheral iris, either with a laser—*laser iridotomy*—or by surgical iridectomy. The anterior segment abnormality that underlies angle-closure glaucoma is bilateral, and prophylactic surgery on the other eye is usually indicated.

CONGENITAL GLAUCOMA

Congenital glaucoma is an open-angle glaucoma that results from dysgenesis of the angle structures. Increased intraocular pressure enlarges the immature eye *(buphthalmos)*; a corneal diameter greater than 12 mm suggests congenital glaucoma. Progressive corneal enlargement disrupts the deeper layers of the cornea, with resulting corneal edema and loss of transparency. The cornea of a child with advanced congenital glaucoma is enlarged, with a ground-glass translucency.

Treatment of congenital glaucoma is both surgical and medical. The condition is fortunately rare, as the prognosis for preservation of vision is only fair.

SECONDARY GLAUCOMA

Secondary glaucoma develops as the consequence of another ocular disease. Examples of secondary glaucomas are angle-closure glaucoma precipitated by intumescence of the lens, glaucoma developing as a result of formation of new vessels in the angle, and glaucoma in a chronically inflamed eye. Severe blunt trauma to the eye damages angle structures, predisposing to the subsequent development of open-angle glaucoma.

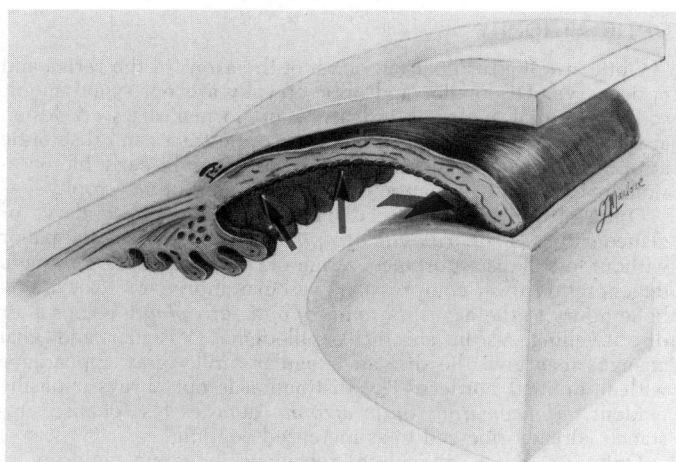

FIGURE 512–2. Angle-closure glaucoma. Owing to an anatomic anomaly in the anterior segment of the eye, the aqueous becomes trapped behind the pupil, bowing the iris forward (iris bombé) to cover the trabecular meshwork, which lies in the angle between the iris and the cornea.

The treatment of secondary, lens-induced angle-closure glaucoma is surgical removal of the lens. Most other secondary glaucomas are managed in much the same way as primary open-angle glaucoma. Neovascular glaucoma is difficult to treat, and most eyes ultimately lose all useful vision. If the stimulus to neovascularization is ischemia, ablation of ischemic tissues by photocoagulation may halt progression. If neovascularization continues, medical control becomes ineffective. Filtering procedures generally fail because exuberant tissue growth closes the surgical fistula, a problem that may be avoided by connecting the anterior chamber and the subconjunctival space with a plastic valve. Destruction of the ciliary body by an externally applied liquid nitrogen probe—*cyclocryotherapy*—controls intraocular pressure but seldom preserves useful vision.

Any glaucoma in which all light perception has been lost is called *absolute glaucoma*. Enucleation (removal of the eye) is the definitive treatment for a blind, painful eye.

Epstein DL: Chandler and Grant's Glaucoma, 3rd ed. Philadelphia, Lea & Febiger, 1986. *Epstein's revision of this text adds an excellent section on examination of the eye in glaucoma.*

Hoskins HD Jr, Kass MA: Becker-Shaffer's Diagnosis and Therapy of the Glaucomas, 6th ed. St. Louis, The C. V. Mosby Company, 1989. *The latest revision of this classic monograph provides an extensively referenced, well-illustrated, and comprehensive overview of diagnosis and treatment of these common ocular diseases.*

513 Disc Swelling and Optic Atrophy

The optic disc marks the transition from retina to optic nerve. The central retinal artery and vein pass through the disc and bifurcate on its surface. There is considerable normal variation in the disc's ophthalmoscopic appearance. A central excavation or cup occupies a variable portion of its substance; vessels are often seen curving over the edge of this cup.

Over one million axons originate in the ganglion cells of the retina and pass through each optic disc. Although these axons are nearly transparent, a bright ophthalmoscope will visualize fine reflective striations on the disc's surface and the immediately surrounding retina. Disc swelling can be a consequence of ischemia, infarction, infiltration, or local changes in tissue pressures (Table 513–1).

PAPILLEDEMA (See Color Plate 13*B*)

Disc swelling from increased intracranial pressure is termed papilledema. The swelling reflects primarily accumulation of axoplasm in and around the disc, appearing ophthalmoscopically as a protrusion of the disc, most obvious just adjacent to its normal borders. With rapid increases in intracranial pressure, the veins become engorged and hemorrhages may appear on the disc and adjacent retina.

TABLE 513–1. CAUSES OF DISC SWELLING

Increased intracranial pressure (papilledema)	Compressive optic neuropathy Graves' disease
Inflammatory optic neuropathy (papillitis)	Sphenoid wing meningioma
Infiltrative optic neuropathy Sarcoidosis	Vasculopathies Anterior ischemic optic neuropathy
Leukemia and other malignancies	Central retinal vein occlusion Malignant hypertension
Optic nerve tumors Angioma	Toxic-metabolic optic neuropathy Idiopathic
Optic nerve meningioma	Pseudopapilledema
Childhood optic nerve glioma	Optic disc drusen
Malignant optic nerve glioma	Hyperopia
Metastatic carcinoma	Other anomalies

Papilledema is usually bilateral but may be asymmetric. Visual acuity remains normal in acute papilledema. Long-standing papilledema eventually leads to secondary optic atrophy, sometimes with permanent loss of vision (see below).

PSEUDOPAPILLEDEMA

Various other disc appearances may be confused with papilledema. Hyperopic (farsighted) eyes are small, with axonal crowding at the disc. Drusen, depositions of hyaline material in the prelaminar optic nerve, can produce swollen discs in young persons (see Color Plate 13*D*). In time, the buried drusen become exposed and are visible ophthalmoscopically as refractile bodies that resemble rock crystals. Such anomalous discs are often discovered incidentally. One clue to their nature is the frequent absence of the physiologic cup, for in true papilledema the cup is preserved until the disc swelling is far advanced.

PAPILLITIS

Papillitis indicates an anterior inflammatory or demyelinating optic neuritis. In many instances the disc appears normal—*retrobulbar neuritis*. In papillitis, the disc is swollen and may be hemorrhagic, an appearance ophthalmoscopically indistinguishable from papilledema. Unlike papilledema, however, acuity is characteristically reduced, and the condition is usually unilateral. (See also Tables 452.2 and 452.3.)

ANTERIOR ISCHEMIC OPTIC NEUROPATHY

Papillitis is largely a disease of the young. In older persons, acute disc swelling and loss of vision suggest infarction—anterior ischemic optic neuropathy. Often only the superior or inferior half of the disc is involved, with consequent loss of function in the inferior or superior visual field. Most instances of ischemic optic neuropathy are idiopathic, but the disorder may be the initial manifestation of giant cell or temporal arteritis, a disease of the elderly described in Ch. 267.

OTHER CAUSES OF DISC SWELLING

Bilateral disc swelling may accompany severe hypertension. The relative roles of local vascular changes and of increased intracranial pressure in the pathogenesis are uncertain. Markedly decreased intraocular pressure, encountered after ocular surgery or injury, also produces disc swelling, and the disc may swell acutely during an attack of angle-closure glaucoma. Disc swelling is also a feature of some toxic and hereditary optic neuropathies.

Compression causes disc swelling only when the nerve is constricted. This occurs in some patients with the orbitopathy of Graves' disease (Ch. 516), pseudotumor of the orbit (Ch. 516), and sphenoid wing meningioma. Intrinsic tumors of the optic nerve, the most common being glioma and meningioma, may present as disc swelling and visual loss. Infiltration of the optic nerve heads is also encountered in leukemia, metastatic carcinoma, and sarcoid.

OPTIC ATROPHY

Optic atrophy results from death of the axons in the retina and optic nerve. Disc pallor and optic atrophy are not synonymous; some temporal pallor is a feature of normal discs. A lesion anywhere from the retina through the optic tract can cause optic atrophy. Lesions behind the lateral geniculate in early life occasionally cause trans-synaptic degeneration and optic atrophy.

Optic atrophy may be classified as primary, secondary, or glaucomatous. *Primary optic atrophy* refers to progressive pallor without loss of disc substance, a sign of retrograde or anterograde degeneration from compression, vascular injury, or toxic metabolic injury to the axons. *Secondary optic atrophy* develops after disc swelling, as in chronic papilledema. Vascular and glial changes may give the disc an irregular, milky gray appearance with ill-defined borders. The distinction is not always clinically evident. *Glaucomatous optic atrophy* denotes loss of disc substance, already referred to as increased cupping.

Optic atrophy is difficult to recognize in young children, in whom the discs may have a pale appearance normally. In adults with nuclear sclerotic cataracts, pallor may be masked by the lens acting as a yellow filter. The diagnosis of optic atrophy should not be made unless there is evidence of alteration in visual function: decreased acuity or field—or, in infants, nystagmus.

Ultimately, optic atrophy is not a clinical finding but a pathologic entity. In retinitis pigmentosa there is a primary dystrophy of the rods and cones. The ganglion cells remain intact, but secondary vascular and gliotic changes produce a waxy pallor of the disc, but not a true optic atrophy, since the axons are preserved.

LEBER'S HEREDITARY OPTIC NEURORETINOPATHY (LEBER'S DISEASE)

This disorder, sometimes called Leber's optic atrophy (see Color Plate 13C), produces acute or subacute visual loss in men around the age of 20 years. Women are much less often affected, with onset at age 30 or above. Initially the discs appear swollen because of opacification of the peripapillary nerve fiber layer, but the swelling does not represent edema, since fluorescein angiography demonstrates only telangiectatic vessels that do not leak dye. With time central vision is lost in both eyes, and optic atrophy evolves. Although no effective treatment exists, vision occasionally improves spontaneously. The disorder is transmitted via an abnormality in maternal mitochondrial DNA, explaining the sex-linked heredity. Most cases can be diagnosed by study of mitochondrial DNA from peripheral leukocytes.

Miller NR: Walsh and Hoyt's Clinical Neuro-Ophthalmology, 4th ed. Baltimore, Williams & Wilkins Company, 1982, Vol 1, pp 175–271, 311–317, 329–342. *The pages cited contain a comprehensive review of the entities discussed here.*
Singh G, Lott MT, Wallace DC: A mitochondrial DNA mutation as a cause of Leber's hereditary optic neuropathy. N Engl J Med 320:1300, 1989. *Describes the genetic analysis that identifies a point mutation in three families with Leber's disease.*

514   Uveitis

Uveitis denotes inflammation of the uveal tract—the iris, ciliary body, and choroid. There are two major clinical types, anterior and posterior (Table 514–1). Anterior uveitis, also known as *iritis* or *iridocyclitis,* has as its hallmark cells in the anterior chamber. Curiously, it is the rare case of iritis that displays any recognizable iris abnormality. Posterior uveitis may take the form of *chorioretinitis.* The choroid and retina are so intimately connected that it is difficult to have inflammation of one without the other.

Acute anterior uveitis presents with congestion of the eye, often in a perilimbal distribution described as ciliary flush. Frequently, the eye is painful, vision reduced, and the pupil small and poorly reactive. The diagnosis is confirmed on slit lamp examination by the presence of free cells in the aqueous humor, visible as bright points as the slit beam passes through the anterior chamber. In more severe inflammation, *keratitic precipitates,* cellular aggregates on the back of the cornea, appear.

Anterior uveitis may be a manifestation of a systemic inflammatory disease such as sarcoid, an infection such as syphilis or

TABLE 514–1. DISEASES ASSOCIATED WITH UVEITIS

	Infectious	Other
Anterior (iridocyclitis)	Herpes zoster *Herpesvirus hominis* Hansen's disease	Ankylosing spondylitis Rheumatoid arthritis Reiter's syndrome
Posterior (chorioretinitis)	Toxoplasmosis Toxocariasis Histoplasmosis Measles	
Both anterior and posterior	Syphilis Coccidioidomycosis Onchocerciasis Brucellosis	Sarcoid Behçet's syndrome Vogt-Koyanagi-Harada syndrome Inflammatory bowel disease

tuberculosis, or idiopathic. In some instances inflammation may be marked, with large, oily keratitic precipitates, a variant termed *granulomatous iritis.*

UVEITIS AND ARTHRITIS

Juvenile rheumatoid arthritis (see Ch. 258) and ankylosing spondylitis (see Ch. 259) are especially apt to be associated with uveitis. Young men with this disorder may have recurrent episodes that respond to standard treatments (see below). A majority are HLA-B27 positive. By contrast, the uveitis accompanying juvenile rheumatoid arthritis is chronic and may initially be subclinical. Young women with the pauciarticular form of juvenile rheumatoid arthritis who develop uveitis often have white and quiet eyes. With time, however, adhesions, called posterior synechiae, form between the iris and lens, potentially causing secondary pupillary block glaucoma or occlusion of the pupil. The inflammation may lead to cataract formation and ectopic calcification in the corneal epithelium—band keratopathy. Physicians treating seronegative pauciarticular arthritis should schedule slit lamp and dilated examinations several times a year. Posterior synechiae are visible with a hand light after instillation of mydriatics, as the pupil does not fully dilate and develops an irregular, scalloped border.

REITER'S SYNDROME

The triad of arthritis, urethritis, and conjunctivitis suggests Reiter's syndrome (see Ch. 259). This develops most often in men between the ages of 20 and 40 as a nonbacterial urethritis followed by polyarthritis and ocular inflammation. The initial ocular manifestation is usually a mucopurulent conjunctivitis, followed in many cases by an anterior uveitis. Keratitis and episcleritis also occur. As in ankylosing spondylitis, with which it shares similarities, HLA-B27 is often positive.

BEHÇET'S SYNDROME

Uveitis (or retinitis) is a cardinal feature of Behçet's syndrome (see Ch. 269). In some cases a characteristic layer of white cells forms in the lower portion of the anterior chamber (*hypopyon*). In other patients the primary ocular manifestation is a retinal vasculitis and vitritis. Rarer neuro-ophthalmic manifestations such as cranial nerve palsies or homonymous hemianopias are part of a wider central nervous system involvement.

UVEOMENINGITIS—THE VOGT-KOYANAGI-HARADA SYNDROME

Another systemic disease with characteristic ocular inflammation is uveomeningitis (the Vogt-Koyanagi-Harada syndrome). This disease affects the uvea, retina, meninges, and skin and is more common in Asians. Manifestations include meningeal signs, alopecia, poliosis, vitiligo, tinnitus, and dysacousis. There may be an anterior or a posterior uveitis with exudative retinal detachment.

MALIGNANCY MASQUERADING AS UVEITIS

A steroid-responsive exudative process simulating uveitis can occur in adults over the age of 40 as part of a lymphoreticular neoplasia (variously called reticulum cell sarcoma, histiocytic sarcoma, or—when the brain is involved—primary CNS lymphoma). Diagnosis may be made from the cytology of a vitreous aspirate. Radiation treatment has palliative value.

An apparent iritis developing during a course of treatment for leukemia may represent infiltration of the anterior segment. Diagnosis and therapy are similar to those for reticulum cell sarcoma.

TREATMENT

The treatment of uveitis consists largely of topical or, when the inflammation is prolonged or severe, systemic immunosuppression. Prednisolone or dexamethasone topically, or prednisone orally, is the preferred drug. Cytotoxic immunosuppressive agents are sometimes used in chronic, intractable uveitis. Topical administration of mydriatic-cycloplegics in anterior uveitis reduces discomfort and retards posterior synechiae formation.

Dinning WJ: Systemic Inflammatory Disease and the Eye. Bristol, Wright, 1987. *Describes the medical and ophthalmologic findings in a variety of systemic disorders.*

Kanski JJ: Uveitis: A Colour Manual of Diagnosis and Treatment. London, Butterworths, 1987. *Briefly considers and illustrates many entities.*

Nussenblatt RB, Palestine AG: Uveitis: Fundamentals and Clinical Practice. Chicago, Year Book Medical Publishers, 1989. *Contains chapters on Vogt-Koyanagi-Harada syndrome and other unusual uveitides.*

Rosenthal AR: Ocular manifestations of leukemia: A review. Ophthalmology 90:899, 1983. *This paper covers the retinal, orbital, optic nerve, and uveal manifestations of leukemia.*

Smith RE, Nozik RA: Uveitis: A Clinical Approach to Diagnosis and Management. Baltimore, Williams & Wilkins, 1989. *After a practically oriented discussion of uveitis in general, Smith and Nozik address both clinical syndromes and diagnostic entities, offering specific therapeutic recommendations.*

515 Ocular Infections

Ocular infections (or inflammations) are most sensibly grouped according to their locations. The most common superficial infection is a *blepharoconjunctivitis* or, more simply, *conjunctivitis*. Infection of the lacrimal gland is a *dacryoadenitis;* infection of the lacrimal drainage system, a *dacryocystitis*. Corneal involvement is called *keratitis*. *Uveitis, scleritis,* and *episcleritis*, which are seldom infectious, are discussed elsewhere (see Ch. 514, 518). Infection or inflammation inside the eye is an *endophthalmitis*. An infectious *vitritis* is a form of endophthalmitis. Some *chorioretinitis* is infectious. *Panophthalmitis* refers to infection that extends through the sclera or cornea and involves adjacent orbital tissues.

CONJUNCTIVITIS

The etiologies for the conjunctivitides include allergic, viral, bacterial, chlamydial, and chemical. Mild acute viral conjunctivitis, with a watery discharge and lids that are sealed closed upon awakening, usually requires only symptomatic treatment—warm or cool compresses and a topical vasoconstrictor to whiten the eye. Antibiotics have no clear efficacy. Any severe or chronic conjunctivitis should be managed by an ophthalmologist.

GONOCOCCAL CONJUNCTIVITIS. Purulent conjunctivitis is usually bacterial and amenable to antibiotics. An important variety is gonococcal conjunctivitis, a disease of the newborn (*gonococcal ophthalmia neonatorum*) and of sexually active adults. The eye is markedly inflamed with a copious discharge and swollen lids, a picture described as hyperpurulent conjunctivitis.

The discharge should be Gram stained and cultured on Thayer-Martin medium. Treatment consists of parenteral antibiotics and saline lavage of ocular secretions. Because of the emergence of penicillinase-producing strains, use of a β-lactamase–resistant cephalosporin such as ceftriaxone may be warranted. Untreated gonococcal infection can penetrate the intact eye and destroy it; treatment should be immediately initiated if there is a reasonable suspicion of the diagnosis.

CHLAMYDIAL CONJUNCTIVITIS. In some parts of the world, chronic chlamydial conjunctivitis leads to conjunctival scarring and corneal vascularization, a disease known as *trachoma*. The resulting blindness is an important international public health problem. In developed countries, chlamydial infection manifests as a subacute conjunctivitis, frequently with associated urethritis. Although a keratitis may be present, severe corneal damage does not ensue. Chlamydial conjunctivitis, also called *inclusion blennorrhea* because of the cytoplasmic inclusions found in Giemsa-stained conjunctival scrapings, is difficult to eradicate in adults unless treated with systemic tetracycline or erythromycin.

HERPETIC KERATITIS (See Color Plate 13A)

Viral keratitis is a common and potentially serious consequence of infection with herpes simplex. The corneal involvement may be recognized by the characteristic *dendrite*, a branching epithelial ulcer. Topical antiviral agents promote healing but recurrence is frequent with increasing risk of corneal stromal involvement

and scarring. Topical steroids activate epithelial herpes infections and should not be used without ophthalmologic consultation. Herpes zoster also can produce an acute dendritic keratitis.

CORNEAL ULCERS

Bacterial and fungal infections of the cornea are a serious threat to vision. Corneal ulcers tend to develop in the context of ocular trauma or contact lens wear, after surgery, or with pre-existing corneal disease. Corneal ulceration appears as an area of white, gray, or yellow infiltrate that stains with fluorescein. Such patients should be referred promptly to an ophthalmologist for evaluation and treatment with topical antibiotics and other measures.

ENDOPHTHALMITIS

Infection inside the eye most often follows accidental or surgical perforation of the eye. Epidemics have occurred following use of contaminated solutions in intraocular surgery. Only rarely do infections elsewhere metastasize to the eye.

Bacterial endophthalmitis must be treated aggressively if there is to be any chance of preserving vision. When the infection is recognized, cultures and smears are taken from the anterior chamber and vitreous cavity by aspiration, and a course of intravitreal and, sometimes, systemic, topical, and periocular antibiotics is begun. The choice of antibiotics depends on what organisms, if any, are found on the Gram stain. Surgical vitrectomy may be warranted.

CANDIDA ENDOPHTHALMITIS. *Candida albicans* is the most prevalent organism causing metastatic (endogenous) endophthalmitis. Fungemia after prolonged use of intravenous catheters or parenteral drug abuse results in colonization of the eye, with multiple white, fluffy chorioretinal infiltrates. These often involve the macula, reducing central vision. Careful direct ophthalmoscopy through a dilated pupil is indicated in patients at risk. Most *Candida* endophthalmitis requires systemic or intravitreal administration of antifungal agents, although spontaneous resolution has been observed.

INFECTIOUS CHORIORETINITIS

CONGENITAL TOXOPLASMOSIS (see Color Plate 13H). A common type of infectious chorioretinitis is *toxoplasmosis*, acquired in utero. This protozoan parasite can remain dormant in large, pigmented chorioretinal scars for many years and then become active, with white infiltration at the border of the scar and an overlying vitritis. If a previously uninvolved macula is threatened, treatment with pyrimethamine and sulfa or with clindamycin may be indicated.

CYTOMEGALOVIRUS CHORIORETINITIS (see Color Plate 14G). Cytomegalovirus chorioretinitis appears in immunosuppressed hosts as a discrete area of white or yellow retinal opacification with associated hemorrhage and vascular sheathing. The ophthalmoscopic picture resembles that of a branch retinal vein occlusion (see Ch. 519), but in this instance, one eye often has multiple foci, and there is a tendency for bilaterality.

Diagnosis can be made clinically and by culture of throat and urine. Dosages of immunosuppressive drugs should be reduced, if possible. The efficacy of treatment with antiviral agents is being actively evaluated.

OTHER INFECTIOUS CHORIORETINITIDES. Syphilis and tuberculosis are now rarely encountered as chorioretinitis. Herpes simplex retinitis resembles that of cytomegalovirus. Cryptococcal meningitis may have an associated chorioretinitis. Focal chorioretinitis can accompany subacute sclerosing panencephalitis (Ch. 478).

Darrell RD (ed.): Viral Diseases of the Eye. Philadelphia, Lea & Febiger, 1985. *Individual chapters on herpesvirus, cytomegalovirus, and measles, among others.*

Elliott AJ: Endophthalmitis in systemic disease: A review of *Candida albicans* endophthalmitis. Semin Ophthalmol 2:229, 1987. *While Elliott concludes that systemic therapy is necessary, some clinicians report successful management of intravitreal infection with vitrectomy and intravitreal amphotericin B alone (see Brod RD, Flynn HW Jr, Clarkson JG, et al.: Endogenous* Candida *endophthalmitis: Management without intravenous amphotericin B. Ophthalmology 97:666, 1990.)*

Stern GA, Engel HM, Driebe WT Jr: The treatment of postoperative endophthalmitis: Results of differing approaches to treatment. Ophthalmology 96:62, 1989. *Reviews 26 cases and makes therapeutic recommendations for bacterial endophthalmitis.*

Tabbara KF, Hyndiuk RA: Infections of the Eye. Boston, Little, Brown and Company, 1986. *Forty-three chapters cover most known infectious entities.*
Wilhelmus KR: Bacterial corneal ulcers. Int Ophthalmol Clin 24:1, 1984. *This practical clinical review can serve as a manual of diagnosis and management.*

516 Orbital Disease and Tumors

GRAVES' ORBITOPATHY

The orbitopathy of Graves' disease consists of inflammation and infiltration of orbital tissues, with characteristic enlargement and scarring of the extraocular muscles. The varied clinical manifestations include lid retraction, exophthalmos, and limitation of eye movement.

Graves' orbitopathy frequently develops in persons previously treated for hyperthyroidism. When the orbitopathy first appears, the patient may be hyperthyroid, euthyroid, or hypothyroid. A classic Graves' orbitopathy in the absence of a demonstrable thyroid abnormality, even to sophisticated testing, is referred to as *ophthalmic Graves' disease.* Coronal computed tomography demonstrating enlarged ocular muscles is probably the most sensitive diagnostic maneuver.

Graves' orbitopathy is the most frequent cause of both unilateral and bilateral exophthalmos. Retraction of the upper lid to expose sclera above the cornea exaggerates the appearance of exophthalmos and predisposes to a major complication, corneal exposure. Tethering of the eye by fibrotic muscles produces a mechanical ophthalmoplegia. Movement up and out is often restricted; pure loss of abduction mimicking sixth nerve palsy occurs. Ophthalmoplegia is not necessarily accompanied by exophthalmos.

Enlargement of the ocular muscles at the apex of the orbit may lead to another major complication of Graves' orbitopathy—compressive optic neuropathy. Severe exposure or major visual loss from compressive optic neuropathy is an indication for treatment. Systemic steroids reduce exophthalmos and relieve optic nerve compression temporarily. Surgical decompression of the orbit by one of several routes is one definitive therapy; orbital irradiation is also used. Direct surgery on the ocular muscles relieves diplopia and permanent lid retraction.

INFLAMMATORY PSEUDOTUMOR OF THE ORBIT

Orbital pseudotumor is an idiopathic inflammation that falls within the spectrum of lymphoproliferative disorders. Its clinical manifestations are pain, exophthalmos, and limitation of eye movement. There may also be erythema and swelling of the lids. Orbital pseudotumors can mimic orbital infection, true tumors, or the orbitopathy of Graves' disease. The major site of inflammation is muscle (myositis), nerve (perineuritis), sclera (scleritis), or lacrimal gland (dacryoadenitis).

If the inflammation is posterior to the orbital apex in the walls of the cavernous sinus, the painful ophthalmoplegia that results is called the *Tolosa-Hunt syndrome.* Orbital pseudotumor merges pathologically and clinically with orbital lymphoma, which in turn merges with systemic lymphoma.

Initial evaluation of a patient with clinical signs and symptoms of orbital pseudotumor includes orbital ultrasonography and computed tomography. A trial of high-dose systemic corticosteroids is usually indicated prior to biopsy. Orbital biopsy is not a trivial undertaking and should be reserved for steroid-unresponsive or recurrent processes. Some histologically benign infiltrations do not respond to corticosteroids. Biopsy in such cases reveals fibrous tissue—*sclerosing pseudotumor.* Occasionally, a patient with a histologically benign pseudotumor subsequently develops a systemic lymphoma.

A necrotizing vasculitis, Wegener's granulomatosis, must also be included in the differential diagnosis of orbital pseudotumor, especially when the inflammation is bilateral. Most cases of Wegener's granulomatosis involve contiguous sinus structures, but local ocular forms of the disease have been reported. The combination of progressive proptosis and sinus disease also sug-

gests orbital aspergillosis, especially in residents of warmer climates.

RHABDOMYOSARCOMA

Rhabdomyosarcoma is the most common malignant tumor of the orbit during the first decade of life and occurs during the second and third decades. The initial presentation is usually ptosis with lid infiltration and proptosis. Progression may be extremely rapid, the clinical picture mimicking trauma or cellulitis. Biopsy and prompt treatment with irradiation and chemotherapy result in a high percentage of survival, although vision in the eye on the side of the tumor is seldom preserved.

OTHER ORBITAL TUMORS

The variety of primary, secondary, and metastatic tumors in the orbit is large. Most present with exophthalmos, visual loss, and limitation of eye movement. High degrees of malignancy are rare with meningiomas, gliomas, hemangiomas/lymphangiomas, and dermoids. Carcinomas of the lacrimal or meibomian glands represent a serious threat to life, and some cases require the most distressing of all ophthalmologic surgery—*exenteration,* removal of the orbital contents. Carcinoma from contiguous sinuses invades the orbit, and breast carcinoma is especially likely to metastasize to the orbit.

Char DH: Thyroid Eye Disease. Baltimore, Williams & Wilkins, 1985. *Char reviews his subject comprehensively and recommends treatment emphasizing short-term steroids and high-voltage radiotherapy.*
Goldberg RA, Rootman J, Cline RA: Tumors metastatic to the orbit: A changing picture. Surv Ophthalmol 35:1, 1990. *An orbital tumor was the presenting sign of cancer in 42 per cent of cases. In women breast was the most common primary, followed by carcinoid; in men prostate, then melanoma and renal cell carcinoma.*
Kennerdell JS, Dresner SC: The nonspecific orbital inflammatory syndromes. Surv Ophthalmol 29:93, 1984.
Mauriello JA Jr, Flanagan JC: Management of orbital inflammatory disease. A protocol. Surv Ophthalmol 29:104, 1984. *Consecutive papers that provide an overview of pseudotumor of the orbit.*

517 Intraocular Tumors

RETINOBLASTOMA

Retinoblastoma, a malignancy of the retina, is the most common intraocular tumor of childhood (and one of the more common tumors at any site). One third are bilateral. About 6 per cent of retinoblastomas are inherited as an autosomal dominant disease; half of these are bilateral. Ninety per cent of retinoblastomas are discovered before the age of three.

MALIGNANT MELANOMA

Primary melanomas develop in the conjunctiva, iris, ciliary body, or choroid; skin melanomas have a predilection for metastasis to the eye and orbit. Malignant melanomas of the choroid are the most common primary intraocular tumor of adulthood. Most occur in middle-aged Caucasians.

The prognosis of malignant melanoma of the choroid depends upon size, cytology, and the presence or absence of extrascleral extension. Choroidal malignant melanomas often metastasize to the liver.

The differential diagnosis of a pigmented intraocular mass includes benign choroidal nevus, senile disciform macular degeneration (also known as central exudative hemorrhagic retinopathy), peripheral exudative hemorrhagic chorioretinopathy, choroidal hemangioma, and hypertrophy or hyperplasia of the retinal pigment epithelium. Many eyes have been removed because of the suspicion of malignant melanoma when the pathology revealed a benign condition.

Enucleation is the traditional treatment for malignant melanoma of the choroid. Other approaches include photocoagulation, radiotherapy, and local resection. Many pigmented choroidal tumors can be followed safely without intervention, especially when they are found incidentally in the seeing eyes of elderly patients.

METASTATIC CARCINOMA TO THE EYE

Once considered rare, metastatic cancer has become the most common ocular malignancy of adulthood, its incidence exceeding that of choroidal melanoma. Most are carcinomas invading the choroid (see Color Plate 13E), the most common coming from the breast. Next in frequency are carcinomas of the lung, followed by kidney, gastrointestinal tract, testis, and prostate. With lung or renal carcinoma, the primary site may be inapparent at the time the metastasis is detected.

If tumor is identified elsewhere, removal of the eye is seldom indicated. Enucleation should be performed only if the eye is completely blind and painful, as palliative radiotherapy or chemotherapy may preserve vision.

Char DH: Clinical Ocular Oncology. New York, Churchill Livingstone, 1989. *Extensively referenced and illustrated, this monograph provides an overview of ocular oncology.*
Yanoff M, Fine BS: Ocular Pathology: A Text and Atlas, 3rd ed. Philadelphia, Harper Medical, 1989. *A comprehensive textbook with clinicopathologic correlations.*

518 Episcleritis, Scleritis, and the Dry Eye

To a neurologist, the eye is an anterior extension of the brain; to a rheumatologist, the eye is a joint. Medicine and ophthalmology come together in the diagnosis and management of rheumatoid and connective tissue disorders. Uveal manifestations are discussed in Ch. 514; the toxicity of drugs used in treatment in Ch. 520; and the retinal changes in Ch. 519.

EPISCLERITIS AND SCLERITIS

Inflammation of the collagenous shell of the eye is either superficial (*episcleritis*) or deep (*scleritis*). The transparent, avascular cornea is continuous with the opaque, vascular sclera and may be secondarily involved.

Episcleritis resembles a localized conjunctivitis. The inflammation is deeper, however, and the dilated vessels do not always blanch with topically applied phenylephrine 2.5 per cent, as in a pure conjunctivitis. Episcleritis usually is self-limited (although it may be recurrent) and does not permanently damage the eye. Most episcleritis is idiopathic, but it may be encountered in rheumatoid arthritis, polyarteritis nodosa, Wegener's granulomatosis, systemic lupus erythematosus, dermatomyositis, progressive systemic sclerosis, and relapsing polychondritis.

Scleritis is more likely than episcleritis to accompany a systemic disease, although the list of associations is about the same for the two disorders. Any portion of the sclera may be affected. The diagnosis is especially difficult with posterior scleritis, which may present as ocular pain or as an exudative retinal detachment. Anterior scleritis often consists of a prolonged, indolent inflammation with eventual permanent structural alteration of tissues. Pain may be prominent and severe.

Initially in scleritis the inflammation is localized and may be nodular or diffuse. With prolonged inflammation, scleral thinning results in a localized bluish discoloration as the underlying choroid becomes visible. Scleral necrosis with perforation is possible; this is especially frequent in rheumatoid arthritis. The adjacent cornea may melt away.

Management of scleritis is difficult. Local steroid injections may predispose to perforation. Systemic corticosteroids and other antirheumatic drugs are useful in some patients. The ocular process often closely parallels the activity of the underlying disease, and the best approach is systemic therapy.

KERATOCONJUNCTIVITIS SICCA

Corneal inflammation as the result of drying is referred to as *keratoconjunctivitis sicca*. Keratoconjunctivitis sicca, a dry mouth (xerostomia), and a connective tissue disorder constitute *Sjögren's syndrome*. The underlying pathophysiology appears to be an autoimmune reaction affecting the lacrimal and salivary glands. Sjögren's syndrome is common in patients with rheumatoid arthritis, especially middle-aged women. Complaints of burning, irritation, or excessive secretions suggest a dry eye but are notoriously nonspecific.

Diagnosis depends upon demonstration of tear hyposecretion (usually by decreased wetting of a strip of litmus or filter paper placed between the lower lid and the eye in the inferior cul-de-sac) accompanied by corneal and conjunctival epithelial damage. Once epithelial cells start to slough, the corneal surface will take up fluorescein instilled into the conjunctival sac. Devitalized cells that have not yet been sloughed stain with rose bengal, making this dye an even more sensitive test for keratitis sicca.

Treatment consists of tear replacement and reduction of tear turnover. Various preparations of artificial tears are available. Other therapeutic maneuvers include occlusion of the lacrimal puncta to reduce tear outflow and placement of contact lenses, moisture chambers, or goggles over the eyes to decrease evaporation. Such measures are reserved for severe keratitis.

Baum J: Clinical manifestations of dry eye states. Trans Ophthalmol Soc UK 104:415, 1985. *Outlines the clinical and laboratory signs and associations. Other papers in the same issue are relevant.*
Benson WE: Posterior scleritis. Surv Ophthalmol 32:1, 1988. *Discusses the clinical manifestations of both posterior and other forms of scleritis.*

519 Ocular Vascular Disease

SYSTEMIC HYPERTENSION AND ARTERIOSCLEROSIS

Although the retinal vascular abnormalities in hypertension are nonspecific and variable, they can be important diagnostically and therapeutically. The effects of blood pressure on the retinal vessels depend upon both its absolute level and duration. Although essential hypertension is a disease of arterioles, the retinal vascular bed lacks sympathetic innervation, and the fundus changes must be considered secondary.

Arteriolar narrowing is the commonest hypertensive change and the most difficult to differentiate as abnormal. The normal ratio of the diameters of the arteriolar and venous blood columns is 2:3 or 3:4. A decrease in this ratio can best be appreciated in the smaller branches away from the disc.

Other findings include microaneurysms, hemorrhages, lipid deposits, and edema. Retinal and disc edema usually follows a rapid increase in systemic blood pressure. Disc edema defines the entity *malignant hypertension*. By contrast, opacification (or sclerosis) of the vessel walls—described ophthalmoscopically as copper or silver wiring—accompanies longstanding hypertension.

Thickening of the arteriolar wall explains arteriovenous nicking and venous dilation distal to the crossing. Cotton-wool spots are signs of local ischemia; hemorrhages and hard exudates reflect vascular leakage. Microaneurysms indicate irreversible structural alterations in the capillary beds. Retinal vascular occlusions (see below) and ischemic optic neuropathy are potential consequences of hypertensive vascular changes.

The only pure arteriosclerotic funduscopic change is atheroma of the retinal arterioles. These are seen as yellow-white plaques in the central retinal artery or its first branches, where the arteries still have an internal elastic lamina. The plaques must be differentiated from calcific or lipid emboli, which are usually smaller or more peripheral. Hypertension accelerates atherosclerosis, but atherosclerosis does not require hypertension.

DIABETIC RETINOPATHY (see Color Plate 14E and F)

Diabetic retinopathy, the most common of the vascular retinopathies, shares many features with hypertensive retinopathy. The pathophysiologic defect in diabetic retinopathy appears to lie at the level of the retinal capillaries. Progressive degeneration of the capillary walls results in leakage (hemorrhages and exudates), diffuse and focal expansion (microaneurysms), and closure of small vessels. The ischemic retina in the focal areas of nonperfusion elaborates factors stimulating new vessel and fibrous ingrowth. (A similar retinopathy can follow radiotherapy given as part of the treatment for head and neck cancers, which damages the capillary wall cells.)

Diabetic retinopathy is classified as *background* or *proliferative*. Background retinopathy is further subdivided into *simple background*—with microaneurysms, dot/blot hemorrhages, and hard exudates—and a *preproliferative* form. In preproliferative background retinopathy there is beading of veins, cotton-wool spots, and many hemorrhages. Also characteristic is intraretinal new vessel pathology, so-called *intraretinal microvascular anomalies.*

In proliferative retinopathy, neovascularization appears on the disc and elsewhere, especially along the major vascular arcades. There may be fibrovascular proliferation and vitreous hemorrhages. Proliferative diabetic retinopathy confers a poor visual prognosis.

Background retinopathy alone reduces visual acuity when there is edema or exudation in the macula. More new cases of blindness result from background retinopathy with macular edema than from proliferative retinopathy, because the former is much more prevalent. Background retinopathy with macular edema is common in type 2 diabetics over age 50.

TREATMENT. Good diabetic control appears to retard the progression of retinopathy. Ablation of ischemic retina by panretinal photocoagulation helps preserve central vision in patients with early proliferative retinopathy, making this the current treatment of choice. Advanced proliferative retinopathy may require major intraocular surgery—*vitrectomy.* In such cases the visual prognosis is guarded but an estimated 50 to 75 per cent of operated patients experience some visual improvement.

OTHER VASCULAR RETINOPATHIES (See Color Plate 14)

SYSTEMIC LUPUS ERYTHEMATOSUS. The retinopathy is common but nonspecific; the most frequent findings are retinal hemorrhages and cotton-wool spots. Cotton-wool spots are not exudations but, rather, localized areas of axoplasmic stasis caused by ischemia, which may indicate active vasculitis. Patients with lupus often also have hypertensive retinopathy. Central nervous system involvement may be associated with optic and chiasmal neuropathy, papilledema, ocular motor cranial nerve palsies, hemianopias, and a migraine-like syndrome.

HEMATOLOGIC DISEASE. Anemia and thrombocytopenia predispose to retinal and subconjunctival hemorrhages. When these are the result of leukemia, the hemorrhages often have a white center—the classic but nonspecific *Roth spot.* Roth spots also are encountered in subacute bacterial endocarditis (see Color Plate 14B) and other conditions.

Leukemia can cause hyperviscosity retinopathy, characterized by venous tortuosity and dilation, retinal hemorrhages, and vascular occlusions. A chronically elevated leukocyte count also predisposes to capillary drop out and microaneurysm formation, but proliferative retinopathy is rare. Other causes of hyperviscosity retinopathy are Waldenström's macroglobulinemia, multiple myeloma, polycythemia, and sickle cell anemia. In extreme cases sludging of blood in the veins is visible ophthalmoscopically.

PERIPHERAL RETINAL NEOVASCULARIZATION. Diabetic retinopathy affects largely the posterior pole of the eye. The retinopathy of prematurity (retrolental fibroplasia) and sickle cell disease have their major impact on the peripheral retina.

The ocular and systemic manifestations of sickling hemoglobinopathies correlate poorly. In patients with sickle cell anemia, proliferative retinopathy is rare. Peripheral neovascularization is more common in sickle cell hemoglobin C disease (SC) and sickle cell thalassemia (S-thal). Patients with sickle cell trait usually have no ocular symptoms, although hypoxia encountered at high altitudes may precipiatate hemorrhages and vascular occlusions.

The ocular findings in sickle hemoglobinopathies include small, dark red, comma-shaped conjunctival vascular segments, best seen on the inferior bulbar conjunctiva after instillation of a topical vasoconstrictor. Ischemic infarction of iris segments is also

observed. In addition to the "sea fan" peripheral neovascularization, other characteristic retinal findings include hemorrhages that have a salmon pink coloration from hemoglobin breakdown products and black chorioretinal scars with irregular borders in the equatorial periphery.

About one fifth of proliferative sickle retinopathy regresses spontaneously. The rest, if untreated, progress to retinal detachment and vitreous hemorrhage. Treatment consists of photocoagulation or trans-scleral cryotherapy or diathermy.

RETINAL VASCULAR OCCLUSIONS

CENTRAL RETINAL ARTERY OCCLUSION (CRAO) (see Color Plate 14C). The central retinal artery is a branch of the ophthalmic artery, in turn a branch of the internal carotid artery. Occlusion of the central retinal artery causes sudden, usually nearly complete, visual loss in one eye. Ophthalmoscopy reveals arteriolar narrowing and vascular stasis (most obvious as segmentation of the venous blood column—"boxcar" pattern).

Within hours the infarcted superficial layers of the retina lose their normal transparency to assume a milky white translucency. Because the thin retina over the fovea receives its oxygen from the underlying choroid, this region retains its normal reddish pink color. This contrasts with surrounding tissue, producing an appearance described as a cherry red macula. (A similar appearance is encountered in certain lipid storage diseases, in which abnormal metabolic products partially opacify the ganglion cell layer.)

Eventually arterial flow is restored, the edema resolves, and the fundus appearance returns to near normal. The disc, which is initially normal because it derives its blood supply from the surrounding choroid, gradually becomes pale and atrophic. After several weeks it is difficult to distinguish a central retinal artery occlusion from other causes of primary optic atrophy.

Acute central retinal artery occlusion is an emergency. Rarely, prompt action may dislodge an embolus and restore circulation in time to prevent retinal death and thus preserve vision. For a nonophthalmologist this action consists of firm, intermittent pressure on the globe with the heel of the hand to alternately raise and lower intraocular pressure. Ophthalmologists use other measures: retrobulbar injection of anesthetic and anterior chamber paracentesis to lower the pressure in the ocular vascular bed. Seldom does treatment save vision.

In some persons, portions of the retina are supplied by vessels arising from the choroidal circulation, and such areas may be spared if the central retinal artery alone is occluded. Most eyes with CRAO are deprived of useful vision.

CRAO's are the result of emboli (atheromatous, myxomatous, and material from diseased or artificial heart valves), of local small vessel disease, or of carotid occlusion. A CRAO is sometimes the initial sign of giant cell arteritis or polyarteritis nodosa. CRAO has been reported in patients with sickle cell trait after trauma or other stress.

BRANCH RETINAL ARTERY OCCLUSION (BRAO) (see Color Plate 14D). Branch arterial occlusions present as sudden loss of vision in a sector of the field affected. Ophthalmoscopically one observes a wedge-shaped area of infarcted retina spreading outward from an arteriolar bifurcation. Branch retinal artery occlusions are almost always embolic in origin. By far the most common source of emboli in older adults is the ipsilateral carotid artery. In children and young adults, migraine, coagulation abnormalities, increased intraocular pressure, and oral contraceptives may predispose to vascular occlusions.

CENTRAL RETINAL VEIN OCCLUSION (CRVO) (see Color Plate 14H). The dramatic ophthalmoscopic findings of dilated, tortuous veins, extensive retinal hemorrhages, and disc swelling in one eye have classically been called a central retinal vein occlusion. Actually there is evidence that such *hemorrhagic retinopathy* is the consequence of both arterial ischemia and venous disease.

A CRVO presents as sudden unilateral visual loss in older adults, but unlike a CRAO, a CRVO is not an emergency, as there is no accepted immediate therapy. There are also no specific accompanying diseases, although hypertension and diabetes are loosely associated, and hypercoagulable states must be considered.

Visual prognosis varies. In the fully developed form usually encountered in older persons, vision is poor and generally remains so. Panretinal photocoagulation may decrease the risk of subsequent neovascular glaucoma. A less severe ophthalmoscopic picture is encountered in younger patients. Acuity in such *partial central retinal vein occlusion* or *venous stasis retinopathy* is only slightly reduced, and the visual prognosis is good. Ischemic oculopathy after carotid occlusion produces a similar retinopathy; retinal arterial pressures measured by ophthalmodynamometry or oculopneumoplethysmography are low in such cases.

BRANCH RETINAL VEIN OCCLUSIONS. Patients with branch vein occlusions complain of blurred vision. In the fundus, hemorrhages and cotton-wool spots spread out in a wedge from an arteriovenous crossing. As in CRVO, there are few specific systemic associations. Neovascular glaucoma is rare, but vision may be persistently reduced by macular edema. Branch retinal vein occlusion must be distinguished from viral retinitis (see Ch. 515).

Catalano RA, Tanenbaum HL, Majerovics A, et al.: White centered retinal hemorrhages in diabetic retinopathy. Ophthalmology 94:388–392, 1987. *This paper considers the differential diagnosis of Roth spots and reports their common appearance in diabetic retinopathy.*

Hall S, Buettner H, Luthra HS: Occlusive retinal vascular disease in systemic lupus erythematosus. J Rheumatol 11:846, 1984. *Two cases with large retinal vessel occlusion.*

Kearns TP: Differential diagnosis of central retinal vein obstruction. Ophthalmology 90:475, 1983. *This paper is one of four in the same issue that describes the work-up, differential diagnosis, and management of CRVO.*

Little HL, Jack RL, Patz A, et al.: Diabetic Retinopathy. New York, Thieme-Stratton Inc., 1983. *A collection of 31 position papers on various aspects of diabetic retinopathy.*

McCrary JA III: Venous stasis retinopathy of stenotic or occlusive carotid origin. J Clin Neuro Ophthalmol 9:195, 1989. *Reviews the findings and differential diagnosis.*

520 The Eye and Medications

DRUGS WITH OCULAR SIDE EFFECTS

ANTICHOLINERGICS. A variety of systemic drugs have ocular side effects. Any medication with anticholinergic properties can dilate the pupil and diminish accommodation (the ability to focus at close range). The possibility of angle-closure is the basis for the caution that such medications are contraindicated in glaucoma. Patients on therapy for open-angle glaucoma are at little risk, as mydriasis will not usually affect intraocular pressure. If the patient has known angle-closure, previous iris surgery all but eliminates the danger of dilation. Only when there is a potential for angle-closure are such drugs contraindicated, and this is usually unrecognized. Of the systemic anticholinergic drugs, only transdermal scopolamine can dilate and fix pupils and paralyze accommodation, even in young persons.

CORTICOSTEROIDS. Prolonged administration of systemic dosages of corticosteroids often leads to the formation of posterior subcapsular cataracts. Topical corticosteroids increase intraocular pressure in genetically predisposed persons. Topical steroids also activate herpes simplex keratitis and should be administered only under the supervision of an ophthalmologist.

QUININE AND CHLOROQUINE. Quinine may cause acute blindness, with narrowing of the retinal arterioles. An overdose increases the probability of toxic effects, but rare persons are sensitive even to therapeutic doses. Other symptoms of quinine toxicity include dizziness, tinnitus, and hearing loss. Central vision may improve, with persistent constriction of peripheral field and evolution of optic atrophy.

The synthetic antimalarials chloroquine and hydroxychloroquine have a specific retinal toxicity. This usually appears only after prolonged administration in doses exceeding 250 mg per day for chloroquine and 400 mg per day for hydroxychloroquine. Reduced visual acuity is the usual initial symptom, the parafoveal

retina being most affected. Chloroquine binds to pigmented tissues, exerting a toxic effect on the retinal epithelium with loss of pigmentation in a target-like or bull's-eye pattern around the fovea. Discontinuation of the drug may result in improvement, but if the process is moderately advanced, visual loss may be progressive.

Chloroquine, hydroxychloroquine, and a variety of other drugs including the antiarrhythmic amiodarone cause whorl-like corneal epithelial deposits that are usually asymptomatic. Such deposits disappear after discontinuation of the drug.

THIORIDAZINE. Phenothiazines are potentially toxic to retina and retinal pigment epithelium, producing a coarse pigmentary degeneration. Of those now in common use, only thioridazine has clinically significant toxicity, and then only with dosages exceeding 1 gram per day for prolonged periods.

ETHAMBUTOL. Various drugs have been implicated in optic neuropathies. Only with ethambutol is the incidence of such side effects high enough that monitoring is considered mandatory. The physician administering ethambutol should perform monthly checks of acuity and color vision, especially when dosages exceed 15 mg per kilogram.

AMIODARONE. Amiodarone represents a class of drugs having the property of cationic amphiphilia. Amiodarone binds to polar lipids and accumulates within lysosomes, producing whorl-like depositions of pigment in the corneal epithelium which resemble the keratopathy of Fabry's disease (see Ch. 173). Amiodarone keratopathy seldom causes symptoms, but instances of disc swelling and visual loss resembling ischemic optic neuropathy have been reported. The visual effects of amiodarone papillopathy must be balanced against the risk of cardiac arrhythmia in deciding whether to decrease the dosage.

OCULOCUTANEOUS DISORDERS

A variety of related disorders (including erythema multiforme, Stevens-Johnson syndrome, and toxic epidermal necrolysis, or Lyell's syndrome) arise as idiosyncratic responses to drugs or infections. Their ocular manifestations are a bullous conjunctival eruption followed by a cicatricial conjunctivitis. Adhesions may obliterate the conjunctival sacs and prevent the normal production and distribution of tears. A severe dry eye may be the most disabling sequela.

Early treatment with topical steroids (and perhaps antibiotics to prevent secondary infection) sometimes limits damage. Sweeping the conjunctival fornices several times a day with a sterile glass rod inhibits adhesions.

SYSTEMIC SIDE EFFECTS OF TOPICAL OCULAR MEDICATIONS (Table 520–1)

Medications in solution are easily absorbed from the nasal mucosa, and systemic side effects are more likely with drops than ointments. Dilation of the pupil with 10 per cent phenylephrine solution can precipitate hypertension; topical epinephrine may increase ventricular extrasystoles, and timolol maleate can cause bronchospasm in asthmatics.

Topical anticholinergics such as atropine, scopolamine, and cyclopentolate may contribute to confusional states in the elderly.

TABLE 520–1. SYSTEMIC SIDE EFFECTS OF TOPICAL OCULAR HYPOTENSIVES

β-Blockers (timolol, betaxolol, levobunolol)
  Bronchospasm
  Bradycardia/hypotension
  Light-headedness/depression/fatigue
  Neuromuscular blockade in myasthenia gravis
Miotics
  Pilocarpine
    Brow ache (usually transient)
    Cholinergic overdose
  Echothiophate
    Prolonged action of succinylcholine or procaine
Sympathomimetics (epinephrine, dipivefrin)
  Tachycardia
  Atrial and ventricular arrhythmias
  Hypertension
  Headache

Cyclopentolate is occasionally a cause of acute hallucinations and even psychosis in the young. Pilocarpine, used in large doses in the treatment of acute angle-closure glaucoma, has resulted in cholinergic overdose—nausea, vomiting, salivation, and gastrointestinal cramps. As these are also symptoms of the angle-closure attack itself, such toxicity may not be immediately recognized, leading to continued administration and cardiovascular collapse.

Echothiophate iodide, an organophosphate used in the treatment of some forms of childhood strabismus and of open-angle glaucoma, predisposes to cholinergic crisis, mimicking an acute surgical abdomen. Also, patients receiving echothiophate have impaired metabolism of succinylcholine. Use of succinylcholine during the induction of general anesthesia in a patient receiving echothiophate has caused death.

Drug information inserts for tranquilizers, bronchodilators, vasoconstrictors, and other medications that alter autonomic nervous system function often include a caution against their use in glaucoma. Such warnings generally refer to the potential for precipitating angle-closure glaucoma by pupillary dilation and do not apply to most patients being treated for glaucoma (see Ch. 512). The actual risk affects persons with narrow angles, who would be unlikely to carry the diagnosis of glaucoma, as a determination of the potential for angle-closure should have been made by the examining ophthalmologist.

CARBONIC ANHYDRASE INHIBITORS

Acetazolamide and methazolamide inhibit aqueous production and are used systemically to reduce intraocular pressure when topical medications are inadequate. Most patients experience paresthesias; their absence is thought by some to indicate noncompliance. Carbonic anhydrase inhibitors also induce a systemic acidosis, with a syndrome of malaise and anorexia, depression, and weight loss that responds to concurrent administration of sodium bicarbonate and may rarely cause blood dyscrasias. Acetazolamide increases the incidence of urolithiasis. The combination of a carbonic anhydrase inhibitor and a thiazide diuretic depletes body potassium. Carbonic anhydrase inhibitors should not be given to people with known allergy to sulfonamides.

Everitt DE, Avorn J: Systemic effects of medications used to treat glaucoma. Ann Intern Med 112:120, 1990. *This brief review addresses internists.*

Fraunfelder FT, Meyer SM: Drug-Induced Ocular Side Effects and Drug Interactions, 3rd ed. Philadelphia, Lea & Febiger, 1989. *A compendium based on the experience of the National Registry of Drug-Induced Side Effects and the literature.*

Grant WM: Toxicology of the Eye, 3rd ed. Springfield, IL, Charles C Thomas, 1986. *An enormous review with component parts that are coherent and readable.*

Imperia PS, Lazarus HM, Lass JH: Ocular complications of systemic cancer chemotherapy. Surv Ophthalmol 34:209, 1989. *Tables and text elucidate the article's title.*

PART XXV
SKIN DISEASES
Frank Parker

521 Introduction

An understanding of how the skin functions in health and disease is relevant to every physician for several reasons: First, the skin is the interface with our environment and serves many functions crucial to survival, such as protection against the elements and thermoregulation. Second, the psychological roles the skin and its appendages, the hair, and nails, play in our appearance cannot be overestimated. Third, skin problems are exceedingly common, as some 30 per cent of Americans have dermatologic conditions requiring a physician's care, and indeed patients expect their physician to have a working knowledge of cutaneous disorders. Ten common skin problems constitute 76 per cent of the burden of skin disease as established by population survey (Table 521–1). Fourth, the skin can be readily examined and biopsied and frequently provides evidence of internal disease. The trained examiner recognizes certain apparently insignificant skin findings as subtle signs of life-threatening disease.

Chapter 522 reviews the functions subserved by the skin and the local variations in skin structures which help to explain the localization of certain disease processes to specific areas. Chapter 523 discusses the examination of the skin and presents an approach to diagnosing skin diseases based upon clinical morphology. Nine major disease groupings are described, and the common dermatologic conditions and their etiologies are discussed (Ch. 525). Chapter 524 contains a guide to general principles of therapy. Chapter 525 describes skin diseases of general medical importance as well as specific therapy for each disease.

Arnold HL, Odom RB, James WP: Andrews' Diseases of the Skin. Philadelphia, W.B. Saunders Company, 1990. *An up-to-date text covering cogent aspects of clinical dermatology.*

Callen JP: Cutaneous Aspects of Internal Disease. Chicago, Year Book Medical Publisher, 1981. *Discussions of skin disorders that confront the clinician which*

have underlying systemic disorders. Discussion of the pathogenesis of these disorders is provided by a number of contributing authorities.

Fitzpatrick TB, Eisen AZ, Wolff K, et al.: Dermatology in General Medicine. New York, McGraw-Hill Book Company, 1987. *A detailed and well-illustrated textbook covering all aspects of dermatology. Two volumes.*

Hurwitz SH: Clinical Pediatric Dermatology. Philadelphia, W. B. Saunders Company, 1981. *A well-written and well-illustrated book of dermatology of children and adolescents.*

Lookingbill DP, Marks JG: Principles of Dermatology. Philadelphia, W. B. Saunders Company, 1985. *A concise, well-illustrated textbook covering major topics in general dermatology.*

Rook A, Wilkinson DS, Ebling FJG, et al.: Textbook of Dermatology. Oxford, Blackwell Scientific Publication, 1986. *This three-volume multiauthored text covers every aspect of dermatology in great detail. It is well written and referenced.*

522 The Structure and Function of Skin

The skin serves a variety of functions crucial to survival and health. In general, the functions may be correlated with specific properties of epidermal or dermal regions. The epidermis differentiates to form anucleate cornified cells that act as a relatively impermeable protective barrier to the outward loss of body fluids and the inward penetration of various substances and microorganisms. These lamellae of cornified surface cells together with the brown pigment melanin also play an important role in protecting against the carcinogenic effects of ultraviolet radiation. Two components of the dermis, the unique circulatory system and the specialized cutaneous appendages, the sweat glands, play a vital role in the body's thermoregulation. Finally, the skin is important immunologically. Both the epidermis (Langerhans' cells) and dermis (epidermodermal junction structures) are sites at which a number of immunologic reactions occur that can give rise to unique inflammatory skin diseases.

ANATOMIC CONSIDERATIONS

The skin is composed of two mutually dependent layers: the outer *epidermis* and inner *dermis*, both cushioned on the fat-containing subcutaneous tissue, the *panniculus adiposus* (Figs. 522–1 and 522–2).

EPIDERMIS. The stratified cellular epidermis contains two main zones of cells (keratinocytes), an inner region of viable cells, the *stratum germinativum*, and an outer layer of anucleate cells known as the *stratum corneum*, or horny layer. Three strata of cells are recognized in the germinativum: the *basal, spinous,* and *granular* layers, each representing progressive stages of differentiation and keratinization of the epidermal cells as they evolve into the dead, tightly packed stratum corneum cells on the skin surface.

The epidermis is derived from the mitotic division of the basal cells resting on the basement membrane (*basal lamina*), with the daughter cells moving outward to the surface, where they become polyhedral as they synthesize increasing quantities of intracellular insoluble protein, keratin. These *stratum spinosum cells* attach to one another mechanically by desmosomes, complex modifications of the cellular membranes that impart a spinous or quill-like appearance to the cells. Desmosomes play a crucial role in maintaining the adherence of the epidermal cells to one another.

TABLE 521–1. PREVALENCE OF COMMON DERMATOLOGIC DISEASE IN THE UNITED STATES*

	Rate per 1000	Numbers (in 1000's)
Fungus infections	81.1	15,733
Tinea pedis	38.7	7509
Tinea unguium	21.8	4232
Tinea versicolor	8.4	1623
Tinea cruris	6.7	1301
Acne vulgaris	68.1	13,217
Cystic acne	1.9	375
Acne scars	1.7	321
Seborrheic dermatitis	28.2	5476
Verruca vulgaris	8.5	1684
Folliculitis	8.0	1553
Atopic dermatitis	6.9	1332
Lichen simplex chronicus	4.5	882
Hand eczema	1.6	311
Dyshidrotic eczema	2.1	405
Psoriasis	5.5	1070
Vitiligo	4.9	957
Herpes simplex	4.2	824

*Persons 1 to 74 years of age—noninstitutionalized.
Reprinted from the chapter by Dr. Marie-Louise Johnson in the 17th edition of the Cecil Textbook of Medicine, with her permission.

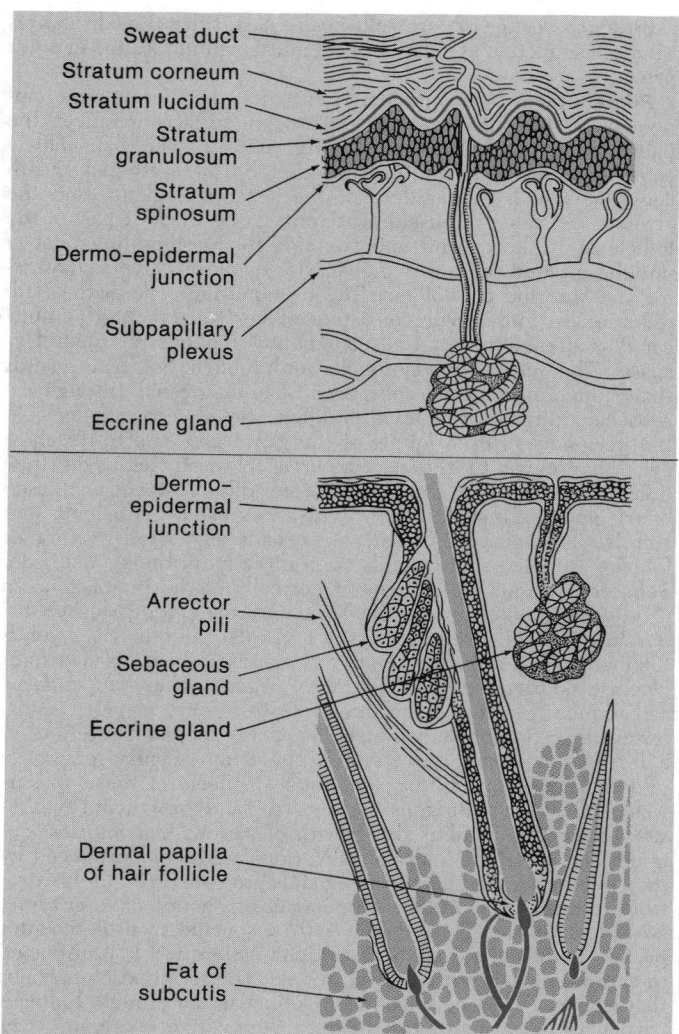

FIGURE 522–1. Structure of the skin. (Adapted from the 17th edition of the Cecil Textbook of Medicine with the permission of Dr. Marie-Louise Johnson.)

With further outward displacement the differentiating cells of the spinous layer become flattened, and refractile keratohyalin granules appear in the cytoplasm, accounting for the designation of *granular layer* that rests just below the stratum corneum.

The transformation from viable granular cells to anucleate, nonviable cornified cells is abrupt. The cornified layer consists of up to 25 layers of tightly packed, highly flattened horny cells.

The differentiation of the epidermal cells involves the formation of fibrous proteins known as *keratin*. The process of maturation of the epidermis (cornification) is complete in the stratum corneum, yielding cells with mature keratin, namely, a system of filaments embedded in a continuous matrix (which is probably derived from the keratohyalin granules) within a thickened cell membrane. The stratum corneum limits the rate of passage of ions and molecules into and out of the skin.

The basal layer of epidermis has a permanent population of germinal cells whose progeny undergo the specific pattern of differentiation just described. The new keratinocytes require about 14 days to evolve into stratum granulosum cells and another 14 days to reach the surface of the stratum corneum and be shed. Proper control of proliferation of basal cells and their subsequent orderly differentiation into keratinized stratum corneum cells produces the smooth, pliable surface of the skin. Alterations in the homeostatic state of cell division, defects in differentiation, or changes in exfoliation from the surface can lead to irregularities in the skin surface, characterized as roughening, scaling, and hyperkeratosis (accumulation of excessive layers of stratum corneum).

Two other cell types are found in the epidermis, the *melanocyte*

and the *Langerhans' cell.* Both are dendritic cells with cytoplasmic arms that stretch out to contact the keratinocytes in their vicinity. The melanocytes are pigment (melanin)-producing cells that are arrayed in the basal epidermal layer and hair follicles, whereas the Langerhans' cells are usually found in the suprabasal layers of the epidermis, and at times in the dermis. Each dendritic cell has a different origin and function.

Melanocytes evolve in the neural crest of the embryo and migrate to the skin in early embryonic life. These cells synthesize brown, red, and yellow melanin pigments that give us our distinctive skin coloration. Melanocytes contain distinctive submicroscopic organelles (melanosomes) within which melanin is synthesized. A specific enzyme, tyrosinase, found within the melanosome, oxidizes tyrosine to dihydroxyphenylalanine (DOPA) and then to DOPA quinone. Additional nonenzymatic oxidation and polymerization occur to form the final product, melanin. Two kinds of melanin are recognized: eumelanin (brown-black biochrome) and phaeomelanin (yellow-red biochrome that contains large quantities of cysteine). The genetic make-up of the individual determines which melanin is produced, thus providing the various colors and hues of our skin and hair. Once the melanosomes are fully melanized, the resulting melanin granules are transported out the dendritic processes of the melanocyte and transferred into the adjacent epidermal cells (or into hair in the case of hair follicles).

Langerhans' cells, derived from bone marrow, contain a unique submicroscopic racket-shaped organelle (Birbeck granule) and are now recognized as playing a major immunologic role in the skin (Fig. 522–2). They contain surface receptors for immunoglobulins,

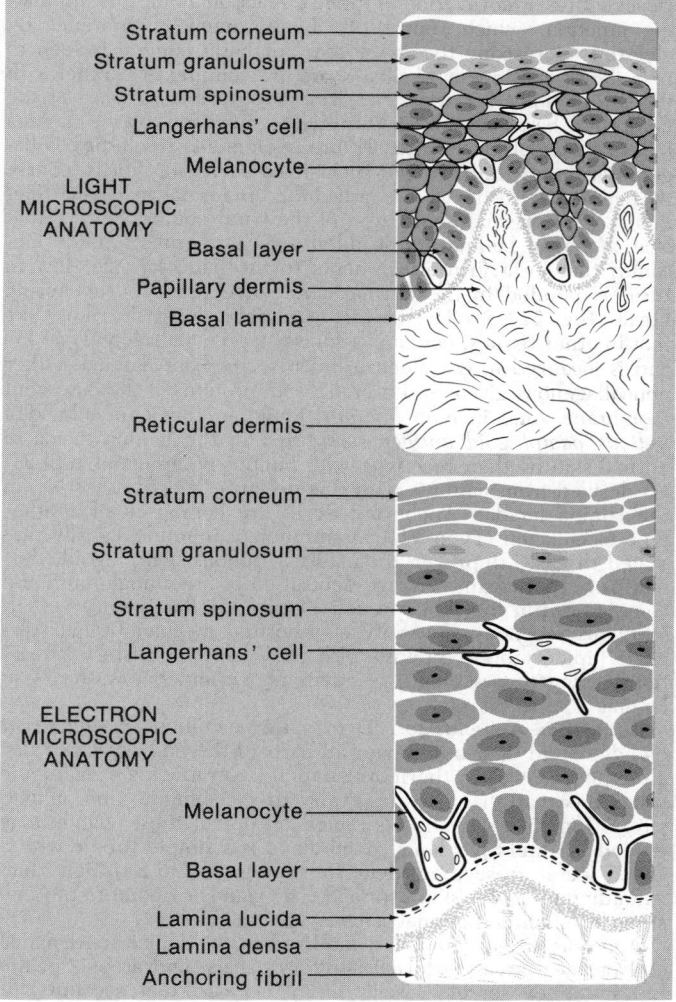

FIGURE 522–2. Diagrammatic representation of the light microscopic and electron microscopic anatomy of the skin.

complement, and Ia-antigens and are able to capture external antigenic materials that contact the skin and to circulate to draining lymph nodes and there induce specific sensitization of immunocompetent T cells. Langerhans' cells thus play a central role in delayed hypersensitivity reactions of the skin (allergic contact dermatitis).

DERMIS. Beneath the epidermis is the principal mass of the skin, the dermis, which is a tough, resilient tissue with viscoelastic properties. It consists of a three-dimensional matrix of loose connective tissue composed of fibrous proteins (collagen and elastin) embedded in an amorphous ground substance (glycosaminoglycans). At the microscopic level the collagen fibers resemble an irregular meshwork oriented somewhat parallel to the epidermis. Coarse elastic fibers are entwined in the collagenous fibers, being particularly abundant over the face and neck. This fibrous and elastic matrix serves as a scaffolding within which networks of blood vessels, nerves, and lymphatics intertwine and the epidermal appendages, sweat glands, and pilosebaceous units rest.

Dermoepidermal Junction. The structures situated at the interface between the epidermis and dermis constitute an anatomic functional unit of complex membranes and lamellae laced by divergent types of filaments that together serve to support the epidermis, weld the epidermis to the dermis, and act as a filter to the transfer of materials and inflammatory or neoplastic cells across the junction zone. At the level of light microscopy, this boundary zone is seen as an undulating pattern of rete ridges (downward finger-like or ridge-like extensions of the epidermis) and dermal papillae (upward projections of the dermis into the epidermis) (Fig. 522–2). Periodic acid–Schiff (PAS) staining discloses a thin uniform zone of intense reaction along this undulating junction, which represents the basement membrane. By electron microscopy the membrane (or basal lamina) is seen to be a dense continuous fibrillar structure running in parallel with the undulations but separated from the dermal surfaces of the epidermal basal cells by a thin clear amorphous space (lamina lucida). Several substructural fibrous elements, including collagen, elastic microfibrils, and specialized anchoring fibrils, course perpendicular to the lamina attaching epidermal to dermal elements. The plasma membranes of the basal epidermal cells that face the basal lamina are studded with numerous hemidesmosomes that form firm attachments to the basal lamina; this, in turn, is bonded to the dermal connective tissue by anchoring fibrils (Fig. 522–2). The basement membrane in the skin, like that in other tissues, contains a special type of collagen (Type IV) and is localized to the electron microscopic basal lamina. Other noncollagenous glyco- and proteoglycan proteins of the basement membrane zone include *laminin* (found in the lamina lucida), *bullous pemphigoid antigen* (identified in the lamina lucida of normal skin by their reactivity with bullous pemphigoid antibodies derived from patients with this disease), and *fibronectins* (in the lamina lucida). Anchoring fibrils are composed of another type of collagen (Type VII). A number of immunologically mediated diseases (lupus erythematosus, bullous pemphigoid, dermatitis herpetiformis) involve deposition of immunoglobulin and complement in the junction zone, causing inflammatory vesiculobullous reactions; a variety of inherited mechanobullous diseases (epidermolysis bullosa) also cause serious blistering reactions owing to pathologic reactions above and below the basal lamina.

Cutaneous Appendages. Two to three million *eccrine sweat glands*, found distributed over all parts of the body surface, play an important part in thermoregulation by producing a hypotonic solution (sweat) that provides evaporative cooling in times of heat stress (Fig. 522–1). The combined output of these glands may exceed 1.5 liters per hour. Each gland is a simple tubule with a coiled secretory segment deep in the dermis and a straight duct extending up to the skin's surface. The glands respond to thermal stimulation and emotional stress.

Apocrine sweat glands are localized to the axillae, circumanal and perineal areas, external auditory canals, and areolae of the breasts. They secrete viscid, milky material that accounts for axillary odor when bacteria degrade the secretion. Apocrine secretion occurs with both adrenergic and cholinergic stimulation. The exact function of these sweat glands is unclear, but they may

represent a vestige of our evolutionary past, since the odoriferous secretions function as cutaneous chemical communicators in other primates.

Pilosebaceous Appendages. Hair units, or pilosebaceous appendages, are found over the entire skin surface except on the palms, soles, and glans penis (Fig. 522–1). The hair follicle consists of the hair shaft surrounded by an epithelial sheath continuous with the epidermis, the sebaceous gland, and the arrector pili smooth muscle. The bulb is the thickest part of the follicle at its lower end and contains the proliferating pool of undifferentiated cells, which gives rise to various layers comprising the hair and the follicle. The proliferating cells in the bulb differentiate into a hair consisting of keratinized, hard, imbricated, flattened cortex cells surrounding a central medullary space. The sebaceous glands are multilobular holocrine glands that connect into the pilosebaceous canal (hair canal) through the sebaceous duct. Germinative undifferentiated sebaceous cells at the periphery of each lobule of the gland give rise to daughter cells that move to the central areas of each acinus as they differentiate and form sebum (a complex oily substance composed of tri- and diglycerides, fatty acids, wax esters, squalene, and sterols). The sebaceous glands are usually associated with a hair follicle, although some glands open directly on the skin surface. Sebaceous glands are also found normally in the buccal mucosa (Fordyce's spots), around the female areola (Montgomery's tubercles), on the prepuce (Tyson's glands), and in the eyelids (meibomian glands). The sebaceous glands and certain hair follicles are androgen-dependent target organs. These appendages can reduce testosterone to dihydrotestosterone, convert testosterone to estradiol, and metabolize dehydroepiandrosterone to androstenedione and testosterone. The action of androgen on the pilosebaceous units is the sum total of effects of these various weak and strong androgens. Sebaceous gland growth and synthesis of sebum, as well as the growth of various hair follicles, are under the control of androgens. Various androgens produced by the testes, ovaries, and adrenal glands are converted to dihydrotestosterone (DHT) in these appendages by action of an enzyme, 5α-reductase. DHT combines with a specific cytosol receptor protein found in androgen-dependent tissues and is transported to chromosomal DNA where it initiates transcription of enzymes that stimulate sebaceous gland and follicular hair growth. Follicles particularly responsive to androgen stimulation are found over the frontal and vertex areas of scalp, beard, chest, axillae, and upper and lower pubic triangles.

The rate at which hair grows and the size of the hair shaft are modulated in some hair follicles by androgens. Hair follicles are formed in early embryonic life, and no more develop after birth. Males and females have approximately the same number of hair follicles distributed over the body, but the degree of hairiness depends on two distinct features of hair growth—the *hair cycle* and the *hair pattern*. Hair growth consists of recurring cycles of growth (anagen phase), regression (catagen phase), and resting (telogen phase). Throughout telogen the resting hair lies high in the follicle, where it forms a stubby hair bulb that is easily shed. When anagen begins there is a burst of mitotic activity and the follicle grows downward to reconstitute a new hair bulb. The hair bulb cells divide rapidly and keratinize to form a new hair shaft that dislodges the old resting club telogen hair. With a hand lens a fallen or plucked hair can be identified by inspection as having been resting (telogen, root of the hair is a rounded fine bulb) or actively growing (anagen, elongated root with fine white sheath). Catagen is the brief respite when mitosis ceases and the hair follicle pulls upward in the dermis as the hair shaft evolves into a telogen club hair. In the adult scalp 85 per cent of the hairs are in anagen at any given time, 14 per cent in telogen, and 1 per cent in catagen. Considerable variation in timing of the cycle occurs from one region of the body to another, and the length of anagen determines the length of hairs. Thus, short hairs are found on the arms and eyebrows with relatively short anagen periods (few months), while long anagen periods are seen in the scalp (up to 6 years).

Hair cycles also vary with the second important feature of hair growth, namely, hair pattern or the type of hair growing in each follicle. Two types of hairs are seen: vellus hair (fine, soft, short, nonpigmented, and common on "nonhairy" areas of the body) and terminal hair (coarse, long, pigmented, and found on hairy areas of the body).

The dramatic changes in both hair cycle and hair pattern which occur at puberty are selectively mediated by either testosterone or dihydrotestosterone. The characteristic increase in hairiness at puberty is not the result of formation of new follicles. Rather, the increased hairiness results from the conversion of vellus hair follicles to large terminal follicles. In the axillae and lower pubic triangle this conversion is mediated by testosterone and androstenedione. In other regions such as the beard, chest, upper pubic triangle, nostrils, and external ears, this conversion is mediated by dihydrotestosterone. Paradoxically, DHT also mediates the reverse process, namely, the miniaturization of large terminal follicles into vellus hairs. Such physiologic miniaturization occurs with the reshaping of the frontal hairline from a straight line to an M-shaped configuration at puberty. This occurs in all men and in the majority of women.

Maternal androgens ensure full development and function of sebaceous glands at birth. The vernix caseosa covering the neonate is mostly sebum. Normally sebaceous glands atrophy after birth, until puberty, when androgens again stimulate their activity. Acne is often one of the earliest signs of puberty. Disorders of androgen excess in adult women (e.g., polycystic ovary syndrome) are also associated with increased sebaceous activity and acne. Estrogens in large amounts decrease gland size and secretion.

FUNCTIONS OF THE SKIN

PROTECTION. Several structures in the skin, including the stratum corneum, melanin, cutaneous nerves, and the dermal connective tissue, provide protective functions of importance to our survival. The skin protects against the loss of essential fluids, the entrance of toxic agents and microorganisms, and damage from ultraviolet radiation, mechanical shearing forces, and extreme environmental temperatures.

The *stratum corneum* serves as a low-permeability barrier that not only retards water loss from the inner epidermal hydrated layers, but also shields against damage from the environment. The barrier properties of the horny layer are of practical importance from several points of view: First, excessive drying or inflammatory reactions in the skin (e.g., eczema) lead to roughness and scaling as the normally compact layers of horny cells are disrupted. This leads to increased transepidermal water loss and, if extensive areas of the horny layer are disrupted (as in generalized exfoliative dermatitis, erythroderma, or burns), the total water loss can contribute to fluid and electrolyte imbalance. Second, with breaks in the horny layer, external substances more readily gain entrance to the underlying epidermis. Thus, various chemical substances, including medications placed on injured skin, have a greater opportunity for systemic absorption or a greater propensity to act as haptens or antigens, increasing the possibility of allergic contact dermatitis. This is a particularly common event when neosporin is used topically on chronically inflamed skin (such as in areas of stasis dermatitis or otitis externa), leading to superimposed allergic contact dermatitis. Third, the disruption of the barrier increases the chance of colonization of pathologic bacteria in the skin, especially in the presence of tissue fluid exudates, which serve as excellent culture media. Fourth, percutaneous absorption of various topical medications used in treating skin conditions, such as topical steroids, can be enhanced by hydrating the stratum corneum with the use of occlusive plastic wraps.

The stratum corneum not only serves as a barrier to the invasion of various bacteria, it also harbors a number of aerobic and anaerobic resident organisms (i.e., *Staphylococcus epidermidis*, diphtheroids, *Proprionibacterium acnes*, and *Pityrosporon*). Breaks in the stratum corneum, poor hygiene, and excessive humidity with maceration (especially in intertriginous areas) all contribute to cutaneous infections such as impetigo, erysipelas, folliculitis, furunculosis, and ecthyma.

A second structural component that provides protection is the *melanocyte*, which produces melanin pigment. Melanin is a large polymer that has the unique capability of absorbing light over the broad range of 200- to 2400-nm wave lengths. It serves as an excellent screen against the untoward effects of solar ultraviolet radiation, such as aging and wrinkling of the skin and the development of cutaneous neoplasms. The importance of melanin is dramatically illustrated by the high incidence of skin cancers

in sun-exposed areas of the body, particularly in light-skinned, blue-eyed, easily sunburned individuals and in albinos. Ultraviolet light exposure also causes aging and wrinkling of the skin. Neither sex nor race affects the number of melanocytes in the epidermis. Negroid skin contains the same number of melanocytes as Caucasian skin, but the pigmentation is more intense as a result of the synthesis of more melanin that is dispersed throughout the melanocytes and adjacent keratinocytes. Accordingly, black skin is much less likely to form skin cancers, and it ages more slowly than white skin.

A third structural component in the skin which plays a part in protection is the dermal *nerves*. Nerve endings are extensively distributed in the skin in two general morphologic types: free nerve endings and specialized endings (Pacini's and Meissner's corpuscles), which mediate many sensations including pain, pressure, and itch. Pain is important to our survival, since we pull away from the source of pain and avert further injury. Loss of sensation (e.g., diabetic neuropathy) may result in deep traumatic ulcers (trophic ulcers) without the patient's awareness of them. Damage to the dermatomal nerves (e.g., herpes zoster) may result in prolonged burning pain and hypesthesias (postherpetic neuralgia).

Itch is another important sensation mediated by cutaneous nerves. It is the most common symptom in dermatology and may occur in conjunction with a number of dermatologic diseases or without clinically evident skin disease (pruritus) (Tables 522–1 and 522–2). Itch and pain are carried on unmyelinated C fibers found in the upper portion of the dermis of the skin, mucous membranes, and cornea. The afferent C fibers enter the dorsal horn of the spinal cord, synapse, cross the midline, and ascend the spinothalamic tracts to the thalamus. Then the impulse proceeds to the sensory area of the postcentral gyrus of the cortex. Cutting the spinothalamic tract, as in an anterolateral hemichordotomy, abolishes pain and itch. A variety of peripheral mediators stimulate the C fibers and induce itching. These include histamine, trypsin, proteases, peptides (bradykinin, vasoactive intestinal peptide, substance P—all potent histamine releasers), and bile salts. Prostaglandins are modulators of pruritus rather than primary mediators, lowering the threshold to itching evoked by both histamine and pain. Central modulators of pruritus, such as systemic morphine, cause itch while relieving pain by acting on central opiate receptors.

Generalized itching in the absence of primary skin disease (pruritus) may be an important sign of internal disease (Table 522–2). Such diverse conditions as uremia, cholestatic biliary disease, lymphoma and myeloproliferative diseases, thyrotoxicosis, diabetes, carcinoma, iron deficiency anemia, and psychiatric disorders may cause severe pruritus. An important cause of pruritus is psychic stress. Some patients with psychogenic pruritus believe the itching is caused by invisible parasites in the skin. Such patients scratch until excoriations and prurigo papules (thickened papular areas of skin due to constant rubbing) evolve in areas that the patient can readily reach (extremities, scalp, upper back). Dry skin (xerosis) is a common cause of itching in older individuals. Certain drugs (aspirin, opiates) can cause itching without a visible rash. Patients with polycythemia vera display a unique type of pruritus, namely, itching triggered by sudden changes in temperature, especially as the patient emerges from a warm bath. The itch is prickly in nature and lasts minutes to hours.

The tough, viscoelastic properties imparted to the skin by the

TABLE 522–1. SKIN DISEASES ASSOCIATED WITH ITCHING

Xerosis (dry skin)
Insect infestations (scabies, pediculosis, insect bites)
Dermatitis (atopic, contact, nummular) including poison ivy contact
Drugs (opiates, aspirin, quinidine)
Lichen planus
Urticaria
Dermatitis herpetiformis (burning itch)
Sunburn
Fiber glass dermatitis

TABLE 522–2. PRURITUS ASSOCIATED WITH SYSTEMIC DISEASE

Systemic Disease	Postulated Etiology
Uremia	Secondary hyperparathyroidism, high skin calcium concentration, proliferation of mast cells, xerosis
Obstructive biliary disease	High concentrations of bile salts in skin
Primary biliary cirrhosis	
Cholestatic hepatitis secondary to drugs (chlorpropamide)	
Intrahepatic cholestasis of pregnancy	
Extrahepatic biliary obstruction	
Hematologic and myeloproliferative disorders	Unknown
Lymphoma including Hodgkin's disease	
Mycosis fungoides	
Polycythemia vera	
Iron deficiency anemia	
Endocrine disorders	Unknown
Thyrotoxicosis	
Hypothyroidism	
Diabetes	
Carcinoid	Serotonin
Visceral malignancies	Unknown
Breast, stomach, lung	
Psychiatric disorders	Unknown
Stress	
Delusions of parasitosis	
Neurologic disorders	Unknown
Multiple sclerosis (paroxysmal itching)	
Notalgia paresthetica—local itch of back, medial shaft scapula (local neuropathy)	
Brain abscess	
CNS infarct	

fibrous proteins (collagen and elastin) and amorphous ground substance that make up the dermis provide protection from shearing forces applied to the skin. The viscous and elastic properties of the ground substance allow it to resist compression and accept molding, thus serving to reduce point pressure on more sensitive skin structures.

THERMOREGULATION. Thermoregulation is subserved concomitantly by the cutaneous vasculature and the sweat glands. A massive network of interconnecting musculocutaneous arteries and venules, as well as capillaries, arteriovenous shunts, and small venules, plays a crucial role in the maintenance of body temperature (Fig. 522–1). The major fraction of the blood volume of the skin is contained in the large venous plexus, in which the blood moves with low velocity close to the surface, enabling maximal dissipation of heat. Equally important in thermoregulation is the formation of eccrine sweat, which provides cooling by evaporation from the skin's surface. For every gram of water that is evaporated from the skin, 580 calories of heat are lost.

Blood flow through the skin is 10 to 20 times that required to supply needed metabolites and oxygen. Under basal conditions 8.5 per cent, or 450 ml per minute of the total blood flow, passes through the skin, the control of flow being primarily by the sympathetic nervous system (via epinephrine and norepinephrine). Blood flow can increase up to 3.5 liters per minute with exercise in a warm environment. Because the heat conductivity and specific heat of blood are high, large amounts of heat can be dissipated through the skin. Both central (hypothalamic heating) and peripheral thermoreceptors stimulate sweating via the sympathetic nervous system, but in the case of sweat glands, acetylcholine is the postganglionic transmitter. Increase in body core temperature is the strongest stimulus for inducing sweating, whereas peripheral (cutaneous) thermoreceptors are only one tenth as effective in eliciting perspiration.

Response to cold begins when blood cooler than normal passes to the hypothalamus, which then elicits both heat conservation and heat production mechanisms. The sympathetics are excited, constricting cutaneous blood vessels and thereby reducing the transfer of heat to the body surface. Impulses from the hypothalamus also activate the motor center for shivering, which increases heat production by as much as 50 per cent. Conversely, when blood warmer than normal passes to the hypothalamus, the central heat production mechanism becomes inoperative, and cutaneous blood vessels dilate, allowing blood to accumulate near the skin surface and heat to be lost by conduction and convection. Vasodilatation also occurs reflexly through direct warming of the skin surface (in warm environments). In addition, stimulation of the hypothalamus produces sweating and increases evaporative heat loss. With periodic exposure to heat or to heat and work stresses (i.e., daily 1- or 2-hour exposures for 10 to 14 days), the secretory capacity of the eccrine sweat glands is enhanced (i.e., acclimatization).

One example of the crucial role of cutaneous vasculature in thermoregulation and in cardiovascular homeostasis is widespread inflammatory conditions of the skin causing *erythroderma*. In such diseases as generalized dermatitis, psoriasis, drug reactions, and underlying lymphomas, the inflammatory response in the skin can cause generalized cutaneous vasodilatation with diversion of 10 to 20 per cent of cardiac output through the skin. Central blood volume may be decreased. To maintain blood pressure, cardiac output must increase and in older individuals with impaired cardiac reserve high-output failure may occur in association with tremendous loss of body heat with wide swings in temperature and shivering.

THE SKIN AS AN ENDOCRINE ORGAN. Many metabolic activities of the skin are under hormonal regulation to the extent that the skin is recognized as an important hormone end organ. Indeed, not only do sebaceous glands and certain hair follicles respond readily to androgens, but they are capable of many diverse steroid transformations, as described above.

Dihydrotestosterone causes sebaceous glands to enlarge at puberty, the growth of certain hair (male sexual hair of the beard, chest, upper pubic triangle, nose, and ears), and the growth and development of the external genitalia. Antiandrogens, drugs that block the conversion of testosterone to DHT, do this by competitively inhibiting either 5α-reductase or the cytosol receptor protein for DHT. Drugs such as cimetidine and spironolactone have antiandrogenic activity and have been used to treat acne and hirsutism. In addition, thyroid hormones can regulate hair growth and alter the texture of the skin (fine, sparse hair and smooth, soft skin in hyperthyroidism; coarse hair and cool, rough, thick skin in hypothyroidism). Further, hormones affect melanin pigment formation, melanocyte-stimulating hormone, and estrogen-stimulating skin pigmentation.

THE SKIN AS AN IMMUNOLOGIC ORGAN. The epidermis and the dermoepidermal junctional area serve as active participants in immunologic reactions. The skin is composed of immunologically important cells including keratinocytes, Langerhans' cells, and melanocytes as well as immunologic structures such as the lamina lucida and basal lamina that are involved in a variety of bullous reactions of the skin.

Epidermal Immunologically Important Cells. Perhaps the most important immunologic cell in the epidermis is the Langerhans cell, comprising 2 to 5 per cent of the total epidermal cell population. Langerhans' cells play a role in a number of immunologic reactions, including macrophage–T cell interaction, T and B lymphocyte interactions, graft-versus-host (GVH) reactions, and skin graft rejection. The Langerhans cell synthesizes and expresses Ia antigens (Class II antigens, immune response gene–associated antigens) that are crucial in processing and presenting allergens to sensitized T lymphocytes critical in the elicitation of delayed hypersensitivity contact dermatitis. Lymphokines, made by the Langerhans cells during these immunologic reactions, augment and enhance these processes and also contribute to the accompanying inflammatory response.

Keratinocytes also play a role in immunologic responses by expressing Ia antigens on their surfaces in such conditions as GVH reaction, mycosis fungoides, allergic contact dermatitis, lichen planus, and tuberculoid leprosy. In these conditions the keratinocytes make lymphokines, particularly interleukin 1 (ETAF, epidermal cell thymocyte factor), which provides a second signal supplementing macrophages (Langerhans' cells) in mitogen- and antigen-induced T cell activation. In addition, epidermal cells make other cytokines such as prostaglandin E_2 and leukotrienes that participate in inflammatory reactions in the skin. Keratinocytes are the immunologic target in the pemphigus group of diseases where circulating autoantibodies against intercellular antigen of the epidermis and mucous membrane epithelium initiate intraepidermal acantholytic bullae.

The Dermoepidermal Junction as an Immunologic Structure. A variety of inflammatory diseases often characterized by bullous reactions seem to be mediated by immunoreactants, including IgG, IgA, and IgM, and complement deposition along the dermoepidermal junctional area. The anatomic site of blister formation correlates with the position of deposition of these immunoreactants. The antigens in several diseases have been isolated and partially characterized. The use of immunofluorescent techniques at the light microscopic and especially the ultrastructural level has been very helpful in more precisely diagnosing these bullous conditions. These are summarized in Table 522–3, along with immunofluorescent skin findings in connective tissue diseases.

INFLAMMATORY REACTIONS IN THE SKIN AND WOUND HEALING. Cutaneous inflammation reflects the sum of the effects of biologic products of cells (mast cells, infiltrating neutrophils, monocytes/macrophages, lymphocytes) as well as the effects of the products of the complement system, membrane-derived arachidonic acid metabolic pathways (prostaglandins and leukotrienes) and the Hageman factor–dependent pathways of coagulation, fibrinolysis, and kinin generation. Early phases of wound healing also encompass many of these reactions.

Cutaneous Inflammation. A variety of pathophysiologic reactions initiate inflammation, including infectious, immunologic, and toxic processes that affect the epidermis or dermis, or both. Mast cells in the skin not only function as the sentinel cells in immediate-type hypersensitivity reactions but also as major effector cells in inflammatory reactions releasing (1) histamine, prostaglandin D_2, and leukotrienes, which cause vascular dilation and increased permeability, redness, swelling, pain, and itch; (2) chemotactic factors for eosinophils and neutrophils; (3) proteases that interact with the complement, kinin, and fibrinolytic pathways; and (4) heparin, which may play a role in local angiogenesis. Degranulation of mast cells occurs in response to various antigens that cross-link IgE on the mast cell surface

(immediate hypersensitivity reactions), to by-products of complement activation C3a and C5a (as occurs in leukocytoclastic vasculitides), as well as to radiocontrast media, aspirin, insect venom, and various physical stimuli. Circulating peripheral blood cells infiltrate local tissue sites in response to chemotactic factors released by mast cells and other infiltrating cells. Basophils release histamine and chemotactic substances, such as those involved in allergic contact reactions, bullous pemphigoid, erythema multiforme, and inflammatory responses. Neutrophils release myeloperoxidase, acid hydrolases, and neutral proteases that are active against microbes and cause tissue destruction (dermatitis herpetiformis, psoriasis, leukocytoclastic vasculitis, and bacterial infections of the skin). Eosinophils release major basic protein and peroxidase (allergic drug reactions in the skin, bullous pemphigoid). Lymphocytes release lymphokines that modulate immunologic and inflammatory responses (lichen planus, lupus erythematosus, allergic contact dermatitis, tuberculoid leprosy). Monocytes and macrophages engulf foreign proteins and microorganisms (granulomatous reactions in the skin such as sarcoidosis, deep fungus and acid-fast bacilli infections, and cutaneous foreign body responses). In addition, both classic and alternate complement pathways release products that induce mast cell degranulation and induce inflammation. (The activation of the system seems to play a role in inflammatory reactions in hereditary complement deficiencies causing lupus erythematosus–like syndromes or pyodermas, as well as necrotizing vasculitis.)

Wound Healing in the Skin. Healing proceeds temporally in three phases: substrate, proliferative, and remodeling. The initial substrate phase, encompassing the first 3 to 4 days after wounding, is so named because the cellular and other interactions lead to preparation for subsequent events. During this phase vascular and inflammatory components prevail (vascular clotting in the severed vessels; leukocyte and macrophage chemotaxis into the area to ingest bacteria, debride the wound, and degrade collagen). The proliferative phase (10 to 14 days after wounding) results in regeneration of epidermis, neoangiogenesis, and proliferation of fibroblasts with increased collagen synthesis and closure of the skin defect. The final remodeling phase takes place over 6 to 12 months, during which time a more stable form of collagen is laid

TABLE 522–3. IMMUNOFLUORESCENT CUTANEOUS FINDINGS IN IMMUNOLOGICALLY MEDIATED SKIN DISEASE

Diseases	Biopsy Findings of Direct Immunofluorescence Immunoreactants (DIF)	Ultrastructural Localization of Immunoreactants	Site of Blister Formation on Routine Light Microscopic Pathology	Serum Findings: Indirect Immunofluorescence (IIF)
Bullous Diseases				
Pemphigus (all forms)	Deposits of IgG intercellular areas between keratinocytes	Between keratinocytes	Suprabasilar in pemphigus vulgaris; substratum corneum in pemphigus foliaceus	IgG antibodies to intracellular areas of keratinocytes in 95% of patients
Bullous pemphigoid	IgG and/or complement (C) in basement membrane zone (BMZ)	Lamina lucida and hemidesmosomes—upper part lucida and sub-basal cells	Subepidermal	IgG Ab to BMZ in 70%
Cicatricial pemphigoid	IgG and/or C in BMZ	Lamina lucida	Subepidermal	IgG antibodies to BMZ in 10%
Herpes gestationis	Complement in BMZ—occasionally IgG	Lamina lucida—close to lamina densa	Subepidermal—sub-basal cell—above lamina densa	IgG antibodies to BMZ in 20% (HG factor in 25%)
Dermatitis herpetiformis	IgA and C in dermal papillae (granular deposits)	Granular IgA associated with microfibril bundles in dermal papilla	Subepidermal in dermal papillae—papillar dermal microabscesses	No circulating antibodies
Epidermolysis bullosa acquisita	IgG in BMZ	Sublamina densa amorphous granular deposits	Subepidermal	No circulating antibodies
Linear IgA bullous dermatosis in childhood	IgA and complement in linear deposition in BMZ	—	Subepidermal	No circulating antibodies
Connective Tissue Diseases				
Bullous SLE	IgG, IgM, and complement in BMZ in involved and normal skin—linear homogeneous	Just beneath lamina densa (basal lamina)	Subepidermal	No circulating antibodies to BMZ; ANA found in 90%
Discoid LE	IgG, other Ig, and C in lesional skin at BMZ	—	—	No circulating antibodies to BMZ; ANA titers normal
Systemic LE	IgG band at BMZ in normal skin (over 90% in sun-exposed areas)	—	—	Elevated ANA titers
Systemic sclerosis	Nucleolar IgG	—	Epidermal thinning and increased dermal collagen	ANA, speckled, 85%, centromere + in CREST syndrome
MCTD	IgG/IgM in BMZ in some patients; nuclear IgG in epidermis	—	—	Speckled ANA and ENA (extractable nuclear antigens)
Dermatomyositis	Negative	—	—	ANA often normal range

down to form a scar of progressively increasing tensile strength. In some instances so much collagen is deposited in the healing wound that an elevated *hypertrophic scar* (red, raised scar within the boundaries of the original wound) or keloid (scar tissue extending beyond the boundaries of the original injury into surrounding normal tissue) is produced. Keloids, which occur most commonly over the anterior chest, upper back, and deltoid regions, rarely regress, and they recur after excision. Fibroblasts from keloid areas synthesize collagen at significantly greater rates than normal skin, even in tissue culture.

THE COSMETIC IMPORTANCE OF SKIN. With age virtually all the structures and functions of the skin change. Environmental insults, especially chronic sun exposure, cause far greater damage to the skin than time itself. Sun exposure over a lifetime, especially in fair-skinned, easily sunburned individuals, accelerates the aging process, resulting in thin, wrinkled skin in exposed areas. The major age changes in gross appearance of skin include roughness, wrinkling, laxity, uneven pigmentation, and a variety of benign and malignant proliferative lesions.

Changes with aging at the structural, physiologic, and biochemical levels are as follows: (1) A decrease in epidermal turnover rate of approximately 50 per cent occurs between the third and seventh decades. Concurrent loss of dermal elastic and collagen fibers accounts for the paper-thin, transparent quality of aged skin and the easy rupture of dermal vessels. Further, with age there is increasing cross-linkage of collagen and elastin, making the dermis more rigid and therefore less able to withstand shearing forces. Aged skin, when "tented up," only slowly returns to its original form, whereas young skin readily snaps back. (2) Sun-damaged aged skin shows microscopic collagen damage. Dermal collagen is replaced by amorphous basophilic staining material. This condition, termed *elastosis*, results in deep wrinkling and furrowing, especially over the face and back of the neck, and yellow papules and nodules in a reticular pattern on the face. (3) Decreases in the number of functioning sebaceous and sweat glands contribute to the dryness of aged skin and to impaired thermoregulation in aged persons. (4) Reduction in the vascular network in the skin surrounding hair bulbs and eccrine and sebaceous glands may be responsible for the atrophy of these appendages with age. (5) A 50 per cent reduction in the number of Langerhans' cells may account in part for the age-associated decrease in immune responsiveness and allergic contact dermatitis reactions in the elderly. (6) Loss of enzymatically active melanocytes (10 to 20 per cent per decade) causes irregular pigmentation of the skin and graying of the hair. (7) Gradual reduction occurs in the number of body hairs, especially in the scalp, axillary, and pubic regions (related in part to decreased androgen production). (8) Linear growth of nails also decreases by 30 to 50 per cent between early and late adulthood. Often nails become brittle and thickened. (9) A number of proliferative growths are associated with aging skin, including skin tags (acrochordon), cherry angiomata, seborrheic keratosis, lentigines, and sebaceous hyperplasia.

523 Examination of the Skin and an Approach to Diagnosing Skin Diseases

General considerations in history taking and physical examination:

THE DERMATOLOGIC HISTORY

A proper history includes the following: where the patient's skin condition first appeared; what it looked like and what symptoms, if any, were associated with it initially; how the skin disease progressed and changed and what has been done to treat the condition (by the patient or by other physicians).

A careful review of the systemic medications (both proprietary and prescribed) that the patient is taking is in order. The relationship of the onset of the skin rash to the use of systemic internal medications is particularly crucial in evaluating the possibility of a drug reaction.

A history of atopic diseases or skin cancer and a careful family history of skin problems help to alert the physician to genetic and familial aspects of dermatosis.

If contact dermatitis is suspected, a detailed work and hobby history can identify exposure to allergens or irritants, for instance by noting the waxing of the skin condition in relation to time on the job and waning during time away from work, such as weekends and vacations. Environmental exposure to the elements such as sun, cold, and heat may be important in provoking skin reactions. Also, when dealing with possible infectious and parasitic processes of the skin, it is useful to determine whether family members or sexual partners are similarly affected.

Psychological stress, although seldom a sole cause of cutaneous conditions, can exacerbate many dermatoses (e.g., acne, psoriasis, seborrhea, atopic eczema).

THE PHYSICAL EXAMINATION

Dermatology is a visual specialty, and because the identification of skin lesions is a crucial aspect of dermatologic diagnosis the examiner's eye and a magnifying lens are the most important tools. Good lighting is essential, either daylight or fluorescent light simulating daylight. At times side lighting in a darkened room is also useful for detecting minimally raised or depressed lesions.

The skin should be examined from head to toe in a systematic manner, so that all regions of the integument, including the nails and the mucous membranes, are evaluated. It is not unusual for the informed and observant physician to find some significant skin lesion, such as a basal cell carcinoma or even a melanoma, of which the patient is unaware. The general assessment of the entire skin, then, allows the examiner to determine the pattern of the skin problem before focusing on specific lesions. Distribution of the skin problem may follow neural (as in a dermatome) or vascular patterns (as in livedo reticularis). In addition, factors related to the patient's general medical condition can also be discerned in the skin by noting signs of aging, pigmentation, trauma, nutrition, and hygiene. Color changes related to underlying systemic conditions (e.g., jaundice with hepatobiliary conditions, cyanosis with various cardiopulmonary diseases, diffuse hyperpigmentation with Addison's disease, paleness with anemia) are important to the assessment.

In each region of the body the physical examination includes three maneuvers: (1) *Observation* for color or surface changes. It is extremely important when observing skin lesions to use an alcohol sponge to wipe off cosmetics or any oil or foreign material that might be present on the skin. (2) *Touch or light stroking* to perceive texture changes, warmth, and moisture. Smoothness or roughness of the skin depends on such things as normal keratinization, proper hydration of the stratum corneum, and normal cutaneous blood flow. (3) *Palpation* to determine the consistency and pliability of the skin by stretching the integument between the fingers. Plasticity depends on the normal structure and function of dermal connective tissue and ground substance.

Because there are many hundreds of dermatoses, a logical process of elimination is required to narrow the possibilities, first to specific groups of diseases and finally to one condition. Such a diagnostic approach is based on specific morphologic descriptions of the skin lesions that the physician sees and feels, together with an appropriate history and laboratory tests. Three steps are involved in this systematic approach. First, the entire skin is examined for primary and secondary skin lesions that allow the examiner to place the patient in one of nine diagnostic groups (the second step) (Table 523–1). Many skin conditions are found in each group, but all of the conditions in a given group manifest the same primary and secondary lesions. The third step involves differentiating the one disease the patient has from the others in the group. This is done by looking for several specific features, such as the distribution of skin lesions, any unusual shapes of the lesions or arrangement of several lesions (annular, serpiginous, dermatomal), color of the lesion including dominant hue and the color pattern, and the surface characteristics (particularly the appearance of scales or verrucous or vegetative changes).

STEP 1: DESCRIPTION OF PRIMARY AND SECONDARY SKIN LESIONS. Primary skin lesions are uncomplicated lesions that represent the initial pathologic change, uninfluenced by secondary alterations such as infection, trauma, or therapy. Secondary skin lesions are changes that occur as consequences of progression of the disease or scratching or infection of the primary lesions (Fig. 523–1). Most of the primary changes can also, at times, occur as secondary manifestations; for example, pustules may appear as primary lesions of folliculitis or as secondary lesions when scaling, itching lesions are scratched and infected. The trick is to recognize any single primary skin lesion as the initial change characteristic of the disease.

The terminology used to describe primary and secondary skin changes is the basic language of dermatology, the means by which one can accurately describe skin diseases to a colleague. If this terminology is not used correctly it will be difficult to arrive at the precise diagnosis of skin diseases. Each descriptive word is not only a short account of what is seen on the surface of the skin but also relays specific information about processes within the skin. A diagrammatic representation and description of primary and secondary skin lesions are presented in Figure 523–2.

STEP 2: ASSIGNMENT OF THE LESION TO A MAJOR GROUP OF DISEASES. Each disease within a given group shares the same primary and secondary skin lesions. Some diseases have overlapping traits so they may be assigned to more than one group. An arbitrary grouping that has proved to be of practical value is listed below and is used later in this chapter to discuss specific diseases within each group (Table 523–1).

STEP 3: NARROWING THE POSSIBILITIES TO THE EXACT DIAGNOSIS. Of great importance is the distribution of the skin disease, for many conditions have typical patterns or affect specific regions. For example, psoriasis commonly affects extensor surfaces and atopic eczema flexor areas of the extremities (Fig. 523–2). Photoreactions are confined to parts of the body exposed to sunlight. Involvement of the palms and soles is seen in erythema multiforme, secondary syphilis, psoriasis, and eczema. Contact dermatitis to exogenous allergens or irritants often presents with unusual patterns and distributions corresponding to the areas where the offending material came in contact with the skin. The best way to examine for distribution is to step away from the patient and view from a few feet away.

Another important clue in differentiating diseases in a given group is to consider the shape of the individual lesions and the arrangement of several lesions in relation to each other. A *linear* arrangement of lesions may indicate a contact reaction to an exogenous substance brushing across the skin, a pathologic process involving a vascular or lymphatic vessel, or a cutaneous nevus (Fig. 523–2). *Zosteriform* refers to lesions arranged along the cutaneous distribution of a spinal nerve. It is thus bandlike and unilateral and denotes herpes zoster and, occasionally, metastatic carcinoma of the breast or the dermatomal hemangiomatous growths of Sturge-Weber syndrome. *Annular* lesions are circular with normal skin in the center. Annular macules are observed in drug eruptions, secondary syphilis, and lupus erythematosus. Resolving hives may leave annular configurations. Annular lesions with scale suggest dermatophytosis or pityriasis rosea. *Iris* lesions are a special type of annular lesion in which an erythematous annular macule or papule develops a second red ring or a purplish papule or vesicle in the center (target or bull's-eye lesion). Iris lesions are seen in erythema multiforme. *Arciform* lesions form partial circles or arcs and may be seen in dermatophyte infections. *Polycyclic* patterns evolve when numerous annular lesions enlarge and run together. *Serpiginous* (snakelike, undulating, linear) patterns are seen in creeping eruptions and in psoriasis. *Herpetiform* refers to a grouping of lesions such as occurs in herpes simplex or dermatitis herpetiformis.

Other physical features are important in diagnosing skin diseases: Dry, lichenified lesions suggest a chronic state of a disease, whereas wet, weeping, macerated lesions suggest acute reactions. Abscesses are soft and fluctuant, whereas nodules are usually firm. Redness caused by dilatation of superficial blood vessels blanches with pressure, whereas erythema caused by extravasated blood as occurs in petechiae and purpuric lesions does not blanch. Hues of brown to black usually indicate melanin, although some drugs (e.g., tetracycline) cause brown-black pigmentation in the skin. The variation in color from melanin is related to the depth of the pigment in the skin—the deeper the pigment the more blue-black the color.

DIAGNOSTIC TESTS AND AIDS IN EXAMINATION OF THE SKIN

Certain technical, clinical, and laboratory aids and procedures, when combined with the history and physical examination, are indispensable in arriving at the correct diagnosis.

VISUAL AIDS. Magnification. Certain diagnostic findings are revealed by magnification of the skin lesions, for example, the follicular plugging seen in discoid lupus erythematosus, or fine telangiectasias in the pearly, opalescent borders of basal cell cancers.

Transillumination. Oblique lighting in a darkened room can be useful in detecting slight degrees of elevation or depression of lesions as well as fine wrinkling or atrophy of the epidermis. In addition, the application of a penlight directly to nodular lesions in a dark room may give clues as to the density and make-up of

TABLE 523–1. MAJOR GROUPS OF DERMATOLOGIC DISEASES BASED ON THE CLINICAL MORPHOLOGY OF THE SKIN CONDITION

Group	Clinical Morphology	Examples of Diseases in the Group
Eczema or dermatitis	Macules (erythema), papules, vesicles, lichenification, fine scaling, excoriations, crusting	Contact dermatitis, atopic dermatitis, stasis dermatitis, photodermatitis, scabies, dermatophytoses, exfoliative dermatitis, candidiasis
Maculopapular eruptions	Macules, erythema, papules	Viral exanthems, drug reactions, verruca vulgaris, Kawasaki's disease, vasculitic and purpuric eruptions
Papulosquamous dermatoses	Papules, plaques, erythema with unique scales	Psoriasis, Reiter's syndrome, pityriasis rosea, lichen planus, seborrheic dermatitis, ichthyosis, secondary syphilis, mycosis fungoides, parapsoriasis
Vesiculobullous diseases	Vesicles, bullae, erythema	Herpes simplex and zoster, hand-foot-and-mouth disease, insect bites, bullous impetigo, scalded skin syndrome, pemphigus, pemphigoid, dermatitis herpetiformis, porphyria cutanea tarda, erythema multiforme
Pustular diseases	Pustules, cysts, erythema	Acne vulgaris and rosacea, pustular psoriasis, folliculitis, gonococcemia
Urticaria, persistent figurate erythemas, cellulitis	Wheals and figurate, raised erythema, scaling	Urticaria, erythema annulare centrifugum, erysipelas, necrotizing fasciitis
Nodular lesions	Nodules and tumors, some associated with erosions and ulceration	Benign and malignant tumors—basal cell cancer, squamous cell cancer, rheumatoid nodules, xanthomas
Telangiectasias, atrophic, scarring, ulcerative diseases	Atrophic, sclerotic telangiectasias and ulcerative changes	Connective tissue diseases, radiation dermatitis, lichen sclerosus et atrophicus, vascular insufficiency (arterial and venous), pyoderma gangrenosum
Hyper- and hypomelanosis	Increased and decreased melanin deposition in skin	Acanthosis nigricans, café au lait spots, vitiligo, tuberous sclerosis, xeroderma pigmentosum, chloasma, freckles

such lesions. Cystic lesions allow transmission of some light, whereas nodules composed of cellular infiltrates do not.

Diascopy. Firm pressure with a microscope slide against skin lesions differentiates erythema of capillary dilatation from that of extravasated blood. Sarcoidosis, tuberculosis, and other granulomatous inflammatory reactions in the skin are suggested if diascopy of the lesions shows a characteristic "apple-jelly" or glassy, fawn-colored appearance.

Long-wave Ultraviolet or Wood's Light Examination. Long-wave ultraviolet light (UVA) (360 nm) is useful in evaluating several conditions of the skin. Wood's light is of great help in estimating subtle variations in pigmentation. It exaggerates the differences in the degree of pigmentation when the skin is examined with the lamp in a dark room. Melanin is a universal absorber of UV light, so decreased melanin shows more reflection (light color) and increased melanin less reflection (darker color).

Pigment in the epidermis is exaggerated with UVA light, but that in the dermis is not, so a reasonable guess as to the site of melanin in the skin can be made. Wood's light may be the only means of recognizing the hypomelanotic ash leaf–shaped macules in tuberous sclerosis. The extent of vitiligo and melanotic nevi (which appear darker than surrounding normal skin) can also be determined. Some superficial fungal infections of the scalp fluoresce blue-green; erythrasma, a superficial intertriginous bacterial infection that produces a porphyrin, fluoresces a brilliant coral red; *Pseudomonas* infections may give off yellow-green color under a Wood's light.

CLINICAL TESTS. *Patch Tests.* Patch testing is used to validate a diagnosis of allergic contact sensitization and to identify the causative allergen. Since the entire skin of sensitized humans is allergic, the test reproduces the dermatitis in one small area where the allergen is applied, usually on the back. The suspected allergen is applied to the skin, occluded, and left in place 48 hours. A positive test reproduces an eczematous response at the

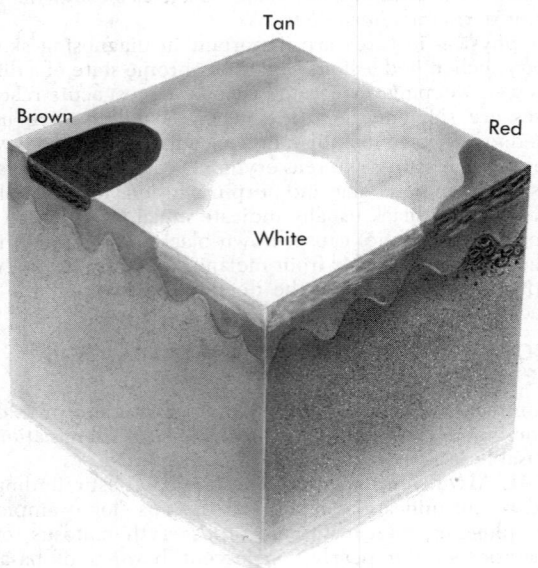

MACULE
A circumscribed color change

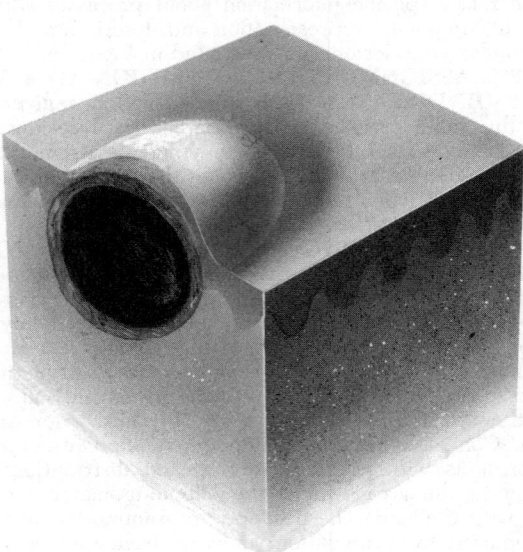

CYST
Semi-solid sac
Resilient

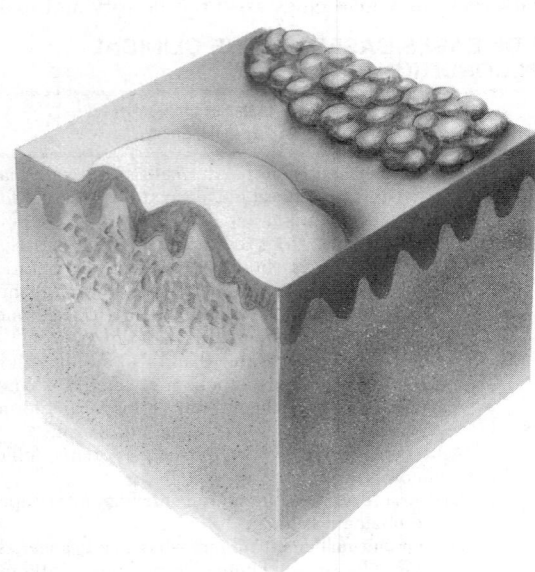

PAPULE
A solid elevation 1 cm or less
skin colored or not

PLAQUE
Raised, circumscribed,
extensive

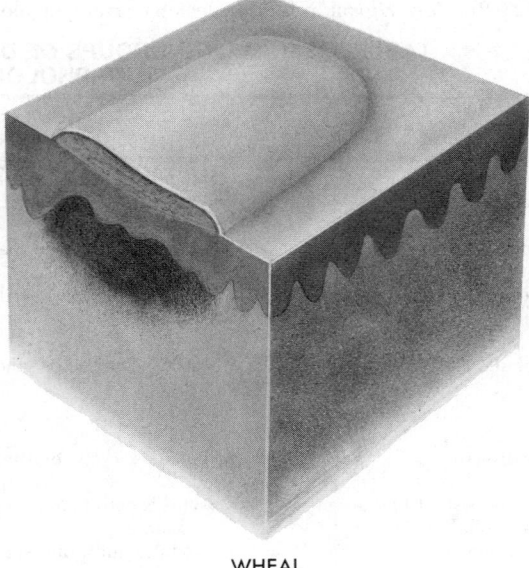

WHEAL
Evanescent
Edematous
Erythematous

FIGURE 523–1. Lesions of the skin. (From the 17th edition of the Cecil Textbook of Medicine, with the permission of Dr. Marie-Louise Johnson.)

test site from 48 hours up to a week after the test. The latter is a delayed hypersensitivity reaction. Considerable experience is required to accurately perform and interpret patch tests. *Photopatch testing* is performed to detect photocontact allergy. Suspected photoallergens are placed on the skin in two sets. One set of allergens is irradiated with appropriate wavelengths of light after the patches are in place on the skin 24 hours; the second set of the same photoallergens is kept covered to serve as controls. Photoallergens cause an erythematous reaction that will be evident 24 hours after exposure to light.

Physical Contact Testing. *Darier's sign* is the development of an urticarial and flare reaction after vigorously rubbing cutaneous mast cell (urticaria pigmentosa) lesions of the skin. The rubbing degranulates the mast cells, releasing histamine.

Nikolsky's sign demonstrates disadherence of the epidermal cells to one another. Pushing, rubbing, or rotating normal skin near bullous lesions causes the epidermis to be dislodged, leaving a moist, glistening defect. This sign is present in various forms of pemphigus and in toxic epidermal necrolysis.

The *Koebner phenomenon* occurs in certain skin diseases that tend to evolve new skin lesions after traumatic injury in areas of apparently normal skin. Thus, psoriasis may evolve within surgical scars and after sunburn or in the wake of a drug reaction involving the skin. Lichen planus may also exhibit this phenomenon.

Pathergy, the development of pustular and ulcerative lesions

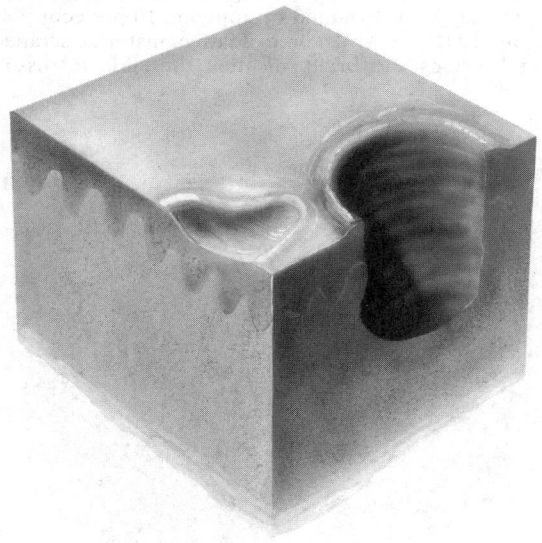

 EROSION
Superficial denudation

ULCER
Defect penetrates dermis

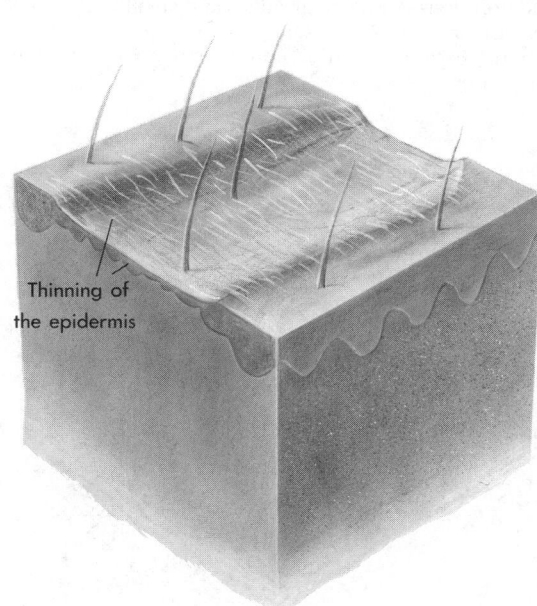

Thinning of the epidermis

ATROPHY

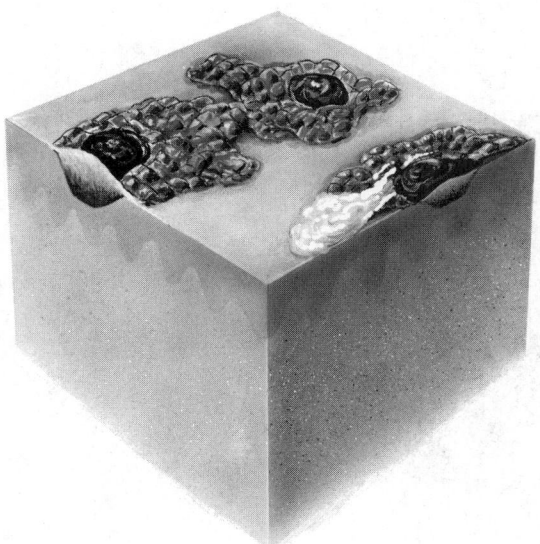

CRUST
Coagulated blood elements

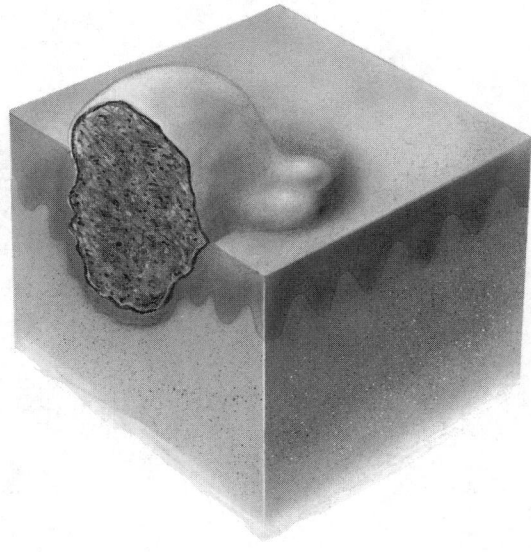

PUSTULE
Fluid-filled sac with neutrophils

FIGURE 523–1 *Continued*

Illustration continued on following page

at the site of needle puncture, is suggestive of Behçet's syndrome and pyoderma gangrenosum.

Hair-pull examination is done to assess hair loss in the scalp. It is often useful to pull vigorously on scalp hairs to (1) determine whether there is an increased number of falling hairs (normally only one or two can be removed with a tug of a group of hairs between the thumb and forefinger); (2) ascertain the ratio of anagen to telogen hairs; and (3) examine the hairs under a microscope for various congenital malformations of the shaft. Normally 10 to 15 per cent of scalp hairs are in telogen, whereas in telogen effluvium the percentage is greatly increased.

Paring Hyperkeratotic Lesions to Differentiate Warts from Calluses. After the hyperkeratosis is pared away, the wart displaces and obliterates epidermal ridges and small bleeding points, and black and red dots are seen in the wart. In calluses the epidermal ridges are not interrupted, and no vessels are seen within the callus.

LABORATORY PROCEDURES. ***Gram's Stain and Cultures.*** Gram's stain for bacteria and bacteriologic cultures are extremely important when the primary lesion is a pustule or furuncle or appears to be impetigo. When an unusual cutaneous infection is considered in an immunosuppressed patient, a skin biopsy specimen can be minced or ground in a sterile mortar and cultured for aerobic and anaerobic bacteria, including typical and atypical mycobacteria, deep fungi, and *Candida*. A more rapid method of screening for infectious agents in a skin infection in immunosuppressed patients (often the first sign of septicemia in such patients is pustules, nodules, or ulcerative lesions) is to perform frozen sections on a skin biopsy specimen taken from the lesion and to obtain Gram's stains, acid-fast bacterial stains, and PAS stains (to identify fungal and yeast elements). This may provide a diagnosis within a few hours.

Examination and Culture for Fungi and Candida. The presence of mycelia may be ascertained by applying 10 per cent potassium hydroxide (KOH) to scale or exudative material scraped from suspected lesions and briefly heating the slide to dissolve the

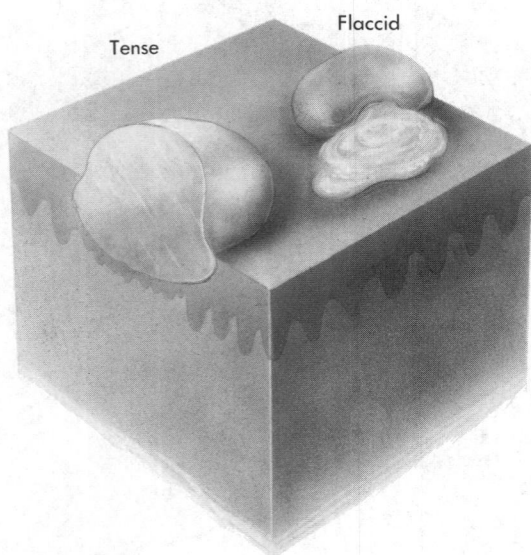

BULLAE
Fluid-filled
0.5 cm or larger

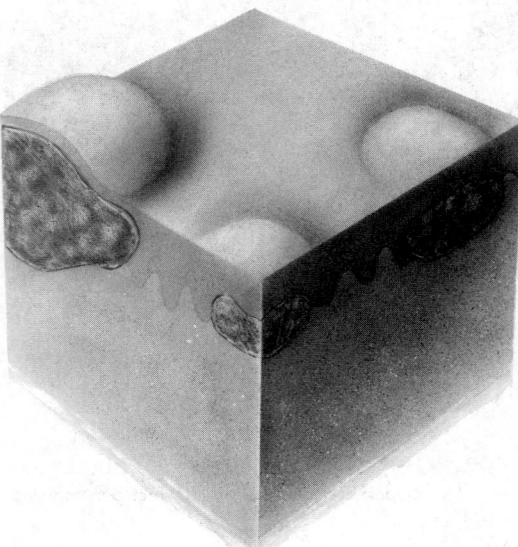

NODULE
Solid deeper lesion

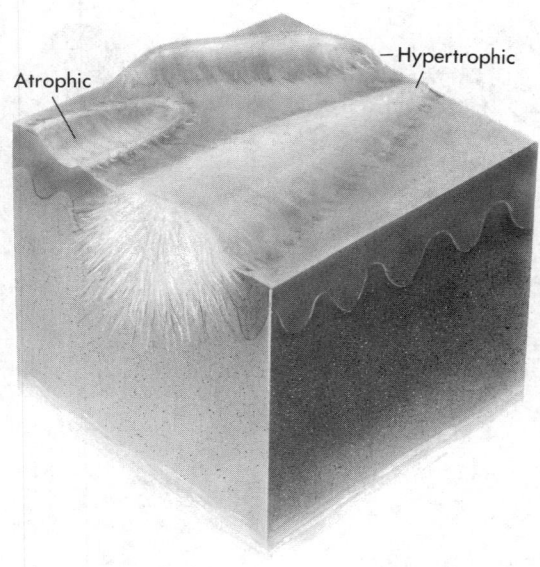

SCAR

FIGURE 523–1 *Continued*

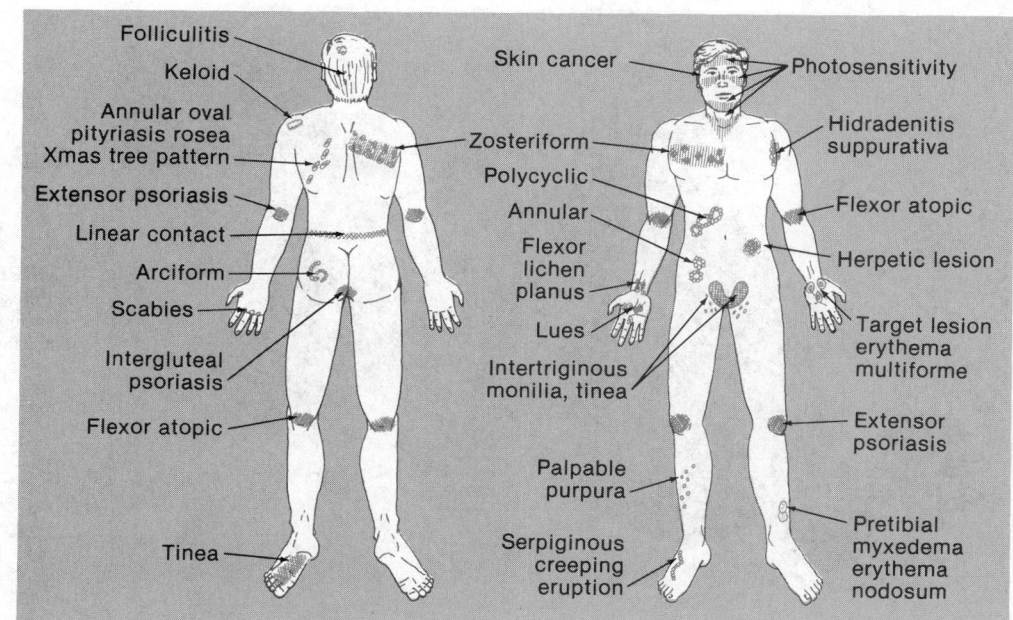

FIGURE 523–2. Configurational and regional diagnostic aids for the diagnosis of primary and secondary skin lesions.

keratin. Hyphal elements can be observed by direct microscopic examination (Fig. 523–3). Dermatophyte hyphae appear as long, branching, refractile, walled structures; *Candida* appears as shorter, linear hyphae in association with budding yeast forms (see Fig. 523–2); tinea versicolor is seen as round yeast forms with short, club-shaped hyphae (so-called spaghetti and meatballs pattern) (see Fig. 525–4). KOH examination of skin scrapings is mandatory to rule out tinea. A classic dictum is "if the skin lesion is scaly, scrape it."

Tzanck Smear. The microscopic examination of cells from the base of vesicles reveals the presence of giant epithelial cells and multinucleated giant cells in herpes simplex, herpes zoster, and

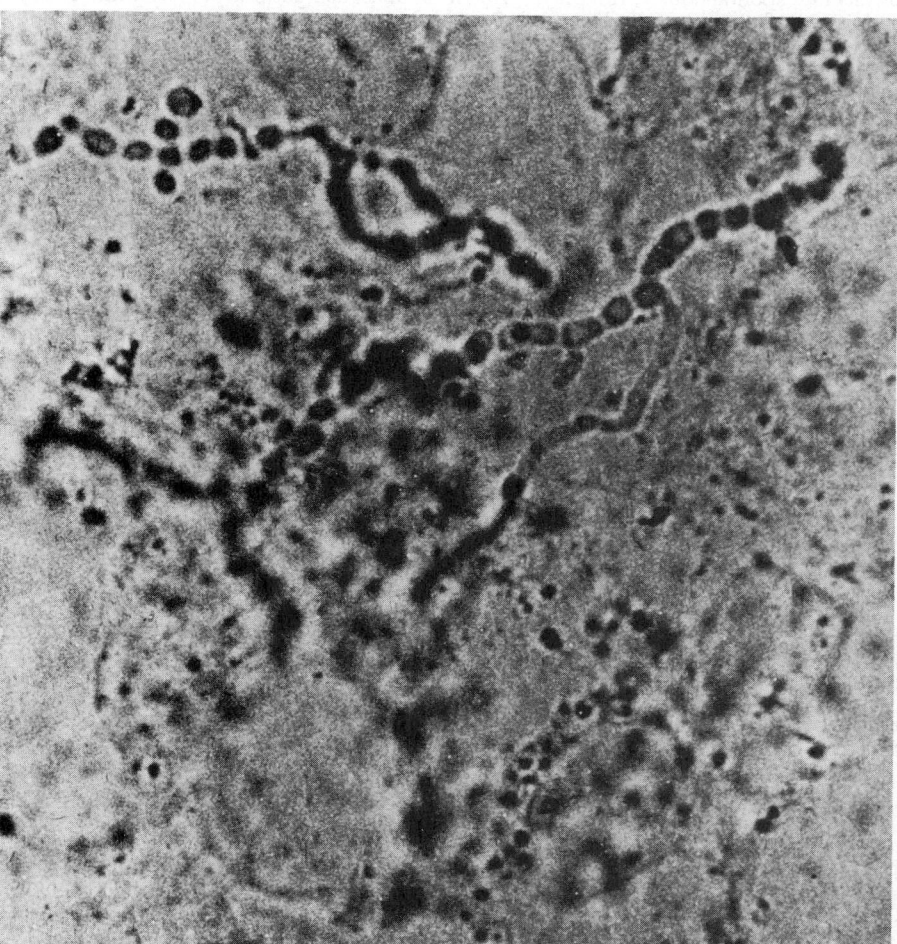

FIGURE 523–3. KOH preparation of mycelial hyphae, high power. (From the 17th edition of the Cecil Textbook of Medicine, with the permission of Dr. Marie-Louise Johnson.)

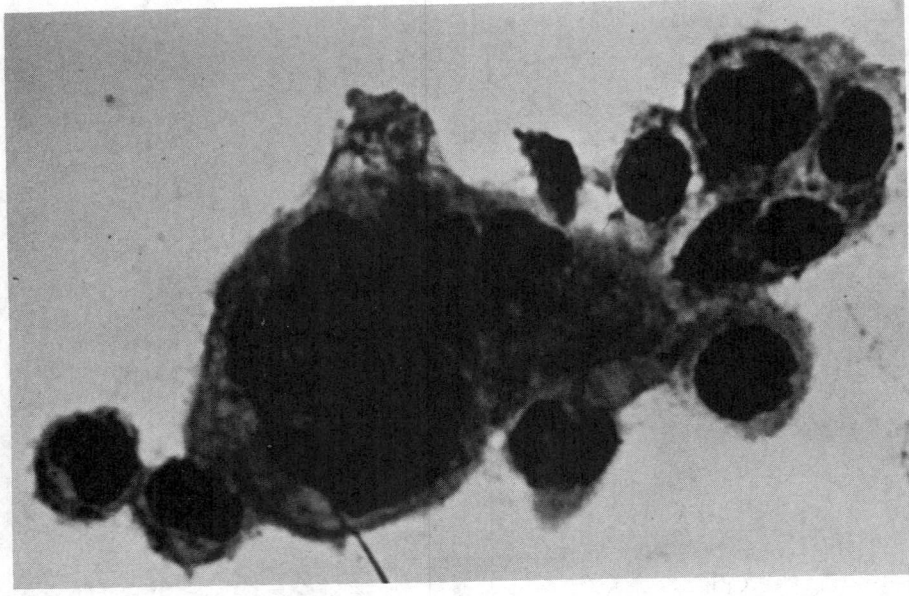

FIGURE 523–4. Positive Tzanck smear, herpes simplex. (From the 17th edition of the Cecil Textbook of Medicine, with the permission of Dr. Marie-Louise Johnson.)

varicella. Material is obtained from the base of a vesicle by gentle scraping with a scalpel and is spread on a glass slide and stained with Giemsa's or Wright's stain for the examination (Fig. 523–4).

Skin Biopsy. Lesions characteristic of the eruption (primary lesions) should be biopsied. Lesions altered by scratching, infection, crusting, or lichenification are not likely to provide useful information.

Clinical indications for biopsy include lesions thought to be malignant; lesions that fail to heal, increase in size, bleed easily, or ulcerate spontaneously; tumors or growths of uncertain nature; and many inflammatory conditions, especially those for which the diagnosis is uncertain.

Four types of biopsies can be performed. The choice of technique determines the size and shape of the specimen obtained (Fig. 523–5). The procedure selected should secure the tissue most likely to contain the pathologic alterations and leave the smallest cosmetic defect. For the most complete histopathologic assessment an *elliptical, full-thickness excision* is best because, in one procedure, the entire lesion is removed and secured for diagnosis and the remaining defect is easily sutured. The excisional biopsy technique is indicated when malignant melanoma is suspected or when a lesion is deep in skin or subcutaneous tissue and its orientation in surrounding tissue is relevant for diagnosis. A second procedure is the *paramedian incisional biopsy*, in which a thin but deep elliptical section is taken through the center of the lesion including normal skin at each end. This is especially useful in diagnosing large keratoacanthomas. A third biopsy method is the *shave*, or *parallel incision*, in which Xylocaine is injected locally under the lesion to lift it above the skin surface, and a scalpel (the knife horizontal to the skin surface) is used to "shave" off the protruding part of the skin and lesion. This technique is useful for diagnosing malignant and benign tumors when subsequent treatment by curettage and electrodesiccation is anticipated. It should never be used when melanoma is suspected, because the specimen obtained is too superficial for adequate histologic grading. Shave biopsy is convenient for removing superficial benign tumors such as seborrheic keratoses or skin tags. The fourth technique, *punch biopsy*, utilizes a tubular blade to cut out a circular plug of skin by slightly rotating and pushing the cutting edge deep into the dermis. The specimen is clipped off at its base with scissors, and the defect can be readily closed with sutures. Punch biopsies are used to diagnose inflammatory diseases and tumors.

If at first a skin biopsy does not provide an answer and there is a diagnostic dilemma, it is necessary and appropriate to rebiopsy. It is useful to give the pathologist adequate clinical history so that the specimen may be properly interpreted.

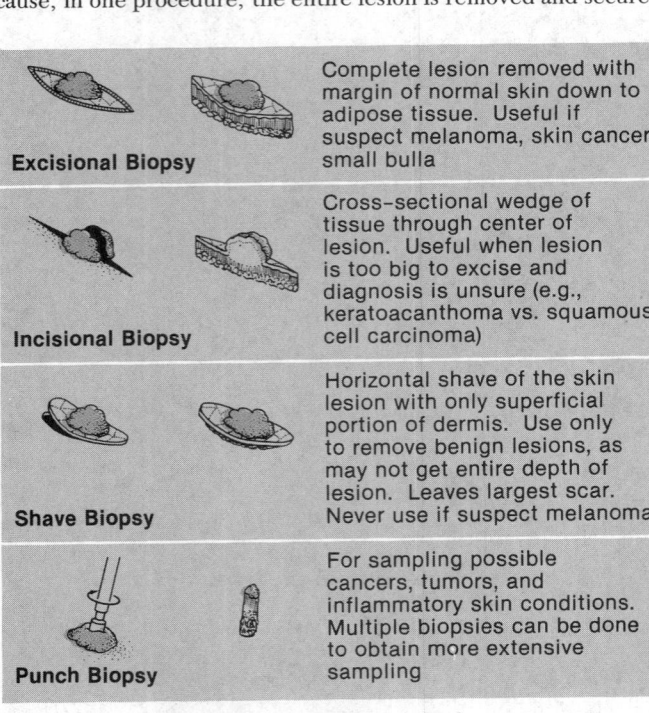

Excisional Biopsy	Complete lesion removed with margin of normal skin down to adipose tissue. Useful if suspect melanoma, skin cancer, small bulla
Incisional Biopsy	Cross-sectional wedge of tissue through center of lesion. Useful when lesion is too big to excise and diagnosis is unsure (e.g., keratoacanthoma vs. squamous cell carcinoma)
Shave Biopsy	Horizontal shave of the skin lesion with only superficial portion of dermis. Use only to remove benign lesions, as may not get entire depth of lesion. Leaves largest scar. Never use if suspect melanoma
Punch Biopsy	For sampling possible cancers, tumors, and inflammatory skin conditions. Multiple biopsies can be done to obtain more extensive sampling

FIGURE 523–5. Methods of skin biopsy.

524 Principles of Therapy

GENERAL CONSIDERATIONS

The skin is uniquely susceptible to topical as well as systemic forms of therapy. Significant progress has been made in controlling and curing some infectious and inflammatory skin diseases, although the pathogenesis of many skin conditions remains unknown, and only palliative and supportive therapies are available.

The goals of therapy are to define and remove the cause of the disorder, restore the structural and functional integrity of the skin, and relieve symptoms. Relief of such symptoms as itching, pain, or cosmetic disfigurement is an important goal. Damaged skin needs protection, as its barrier function is impaired. This can be assured with dressings and by minimizing scratching and avoiding abrasive clothing and soaps or chemicals. Removal of debris, such as excessive scale, hyperkeratoses, crusts, and infection, is also a crucial goal of therapy if the skin is to heal. Topical and systemic medications, dressings, and other treatments can alter skin temperature and blood flow and thus favorably affect the metabolism of the skin.

Some topical and systemic forms of therapy that have proven beneficial are discussed in this chapter.

TOPICAL MODES OF THERAPY

SOAKS AND WET DRESSINGS. The use of water, with or without various additives, can provide many benefits to the skin, including soothing comfort, antipruritic effects, and increased rate of epidermal healing with hydration and debridement of crusts, dead skin, and bacteria.

Baths. When the area of involvement is too large to apply compresses, a bath is useful. Baths with whirlpool action are particularly useful for debridement of large or deep ulcers. Medicated baths can evenly distribute soothing antipruritic and anti-inflammatory agents to widespread lesions. Starch and oatmeal complexes are commercially available in forms suitable for tub baths. Tar bath preparations are available for use in conjunction with ultraviolet light treatments. Bath oil prevents drying by leaving a thin film of emollient on the skin. The tub should be one-half full, and the soak should last no longer than 20 to 30 minutes, to avoid maceration. Warm baths cause vasodilation and may increase itching; cool baths constrict vessels and usually sooth pruritus. The best time to apply lubricants is immediately after the bath so that they may hold water in the hydrated stratum corneum.

Wet Dressings. Water and medication can be applied to the skin with dressings (finely woven cotton, linen, or gauze) soaked in solution. As water evaporates, the skin is cooled and pruritus is soothed. For maximal benefit from evaporation, the dressing should be no more than a few layers thick and should be dipped in the solution and reapplied to the area of treated skin every few minutes for 15 to 30 minutes several times a day. Wet compresses, especially with frequent changes, provide gentle debridement, the cleansing resulting from transfer of crusts, scales, and cutaneous debris to the compress. If the compresses are permitted to dry (wet to dry compresses) and to become adherent, the debriding effect is greater and can even damage the skin. The dressing may need to be remoistened in place to facilitate removal. Wet compresses also leach water-binding proteins from the stratum corneum and epidermis, causing drying, a desirable effect for moist, oozing and weeping lesions. Wet compresses are therefore useful in treating acute vesicular, bullous, oozing or weeping conditions as well as crusty, swollen, and infected skin. There are two types of wet dressings, open or unoccluded and closed or occluded.

The *open wet dressing* is applied directly to the skin, leaving the dressing exposed to the air. The fluid is allowed to evaporate, providing a cooling, antipruritic effect. Frequent reapplication of the compresses debrides exudate, crust, and bacterial contamination and dries out the skin, rapidly decreasing oozing and weeping.

Closed wet dressings, in which the moist fabric dressings are applied to the skin and covered with an impervious material such as plastic, oil cloth, or Saran wrap, may be useful when some degree of maceration and heat retention is required. For example, if there is excessive keratin of the palms or soles or when an early abscess needs heat to help localize the infection, this form of dressing may be appropriate. Closed dressings are less frequently used than open dressings.

Dry dressings protect the skin, hold medications against the skin, keep clothing and sheets from rubbing, and keep dirt and air away. Such dressings also prevent patients from scratching and rubbing. In the case of neurodermatitis or stasis dermatitis, they are often left in place for several days. Soft casts or castlike boots (e.g., Unna boot) serve the same purposes.

The medication most commonly added to baths and dressings is aluminum acetate, which serves to coagulate bacterial and serum protein. As a 5 per cent preparation it is known as Burow's solution, and it must be further diluted for use. Burow's solution can be readily made by dissolving tablets or powder packets in

appropriate amounts of water. (One tablet or packet in 500 ml = 1:20 concentration.) Potassium permanganate and silver nitrate are occasionally added to soak solutions for their antimicrobial properties, but they stain the skin, may be absorbed if used over large raw areas of skin, and may burn the skin if used in high concentrations. The question is often raised about the use of antimicrobial agents in wet dressings, but the quantities needed for adequate concentration in the dressing would make their use exceedingly inefficient and wasteful.

"Occlusive dressings" are being used with increasing frequency in the treatment of acute wounds and chronic venous, diabetic, and pressure ulcers. A variety of dressings is available including *films* (e.g., Op-Site, AcuDerm), *nontransparent adhesive hydrocolloids* (e.g., DUODERM), and *semitransparent nonadhesive hydrogels* (e.g., VIGILON), all of which enhance wound healing.

TOPICAL MEDICATIONS. Topical medications are the mainstay of dermatologic therapy. In general, topical medications consist of two major agents, the active ingredient or specific medication and the vehicle or base in which the active material is dissolved. Both are important in treating skin conditions.

Bases or Vehicles. Bases come in a variety of forms. *Powders* promote dryness by absorbing evaporative moisture. They are used to reduce moisture, maceration, and friction in intertriginous areas. Powders may be inert chemicals (corn starch, talcum), or they may contain medications. *Lotions* are suspensions of insoluble powders in water. As water on the skin surface evaporates, it cools, creating a feeling of dryness and leaving a uniform film of powder on the surface. The addition of alcohol increases the cooling effect. *Creams* are emulsions of oil in water (more water than oil). They seem to vanish into the skin because water evaporates and the residual oil is spread thinly and imperceptibly over the skin. *Ointments* consist of oils with variable smaller amounts of water added in suspension. They have a pleasant lubricating effect on dry or diseased skin, but they may also give a greasy feeling to the skin and clothing. Oils in bases give a softening effect to the skin by forming an occlusive layer that traps water and retards evaporation through the stratum corneum. Thus, ointments with large amouts of oil in them give a more sustained, softening effect to the skin than creams or lotions. In fact, ointments with large percentages of inert oil in them may be occlusive and thereby retain heat, increase pruritus, and increase percutaneous absorption of added active ingredients. The more occlusive ointments should not be used on oozing or infected areas, as the resulting occlusion and warmth may increase bacterial growth. *Pastes* are mixtures of powder and ointment (e.g., zinc oxide paste). *Sprays*, another form of base, are Freon-propelled aerosols.

Bases thus represent a spectrum of varying amounts of water and oil in emulsion. At one end of the spectrum are lotions with less than 5 or 10 per cent oil in water; creams are composed of relatively more oil dispersed in water, but water is still the continuous phase. As the oil-water ratio reverses and oil becomes the continuous phase, the preparation, considered an ointment, is more lubricating, leaving a noticeable greasy film on the skin. At the far end of the spectrum is inert mineral oil or petrolatum.

Selection of a base or emollient depends on the condition being treated and the needs of the patient. A powder in water, such as calamine lotion, permits evaporation and cooling with some drying. Lotions are useful for pruritic, oozing reactions. Petrolatum, by contrast, retains heat and promotes hydration and even maceration of the stratum corneum. Ointments are used most often on dry, scaling conditions in which endogenous hydration of the stratum corneum is defective. Between these two extremes there is a spectrum of possibilities that permit some cooling but add lubrication. Choice depends on the needs of and cosmetic acceptance by the patient.

Active Agents—Specific Agents. Having made a judgment about the base or vehicle required, the physician makes a separate selection of active ingredients to be added.

Topical steroids have revolutionized the practice of dermatology, providing effective local anti-inflammatory and antipruritic effects. Topical steroids have two basic anti-inflammatory actions. First, they cause immediate and profound constriction of cutaneous blood vessels. This is believed to prevent mobilization of polymorphonuclear leukocytes and monocytes into the reaction site. Second, they directly interfere with the inflammatory activities of cells that are already present (e.g., mast cells). Corticosteroids used in topical preparations are intrinsically active without need for further metabolism; this accounts for their rapid effect on cutaneous blood vessels as manifested by blanching of the skin. Therapeutic action is also rapid. Topical steroids slow the mitotic rate of fibroblasts, decreasing collagen synthesis, and possibly enhance collagen catabolism. They further interfere with phagocytosis and the skin's ability to fight off bacterial, viral, and fungal infections. Topical corticosteroids that are effective in treating skin diseases all have the basic hydrocortisone structure. A 1 per cent concentration of hydrocortisone ointment or cream continues to serve as a norm for comparing potency of subsequently modified topical steroids. By fluorinating hydrocortisone or adding acetonide, the potency of the steroid is greatly enhanced. Occlusion increases the efficacy of most topical steroids. Topical corticosteroid preparations may be classified in a general way as of low, intermediate, or high potency (Table 524–1). The potency corresponds closely to the degree of anti-inflammatory effectiveness as well as to the incidence and severity of associated side effects. Although some corticosteroids (particularly fluorinated compounds) are more topically active than others, the potency of a preparation is also related to the concentration of active drug in the vehicle and to the nature of the vehicle in which the steroid is mixed. Since corticosteroids are poorly soluble in most vehicles, many preparations deliver only a fraction of the drug to target cells. Of the various types of vehicles used in steroid preparations, ointments are the most efficient by virtue of the excellent solubility of steroids in ointments and because the occlusive nature of ointments increases stratum corneum permeability. Second in order of efficiency is acetone-alcohol gel, whereas creams and lotions are less useful. Some examples of topical steroids and their grouping according to potency are listed in Table 524–1.

The adverse effects of topical steroids relate almost exclusively to the intermediate and high-potency compounds. Epidermal and dermal atrophy can be a pronounced effect; decreased collagen synthesis and reduced stromal support for dermal blood vessels lead to telangiectasia, purpura, and striae. These are especially likely to occur in intertriginous "occluded" areas of the skin and on the face. Fluorinated steroids can cause a perioral scaling, papular and pustular dermatitis (perioral dermatitis), or facial redness, telangiectasia, and acne rosacea–like eruption. Potent topical steroids applied for prolonged periods around the eyes can occasionally cause glaucoma and even cataracts. Topical steroids can predispose to or worsen skin infections such as folliculitis, tinea, and candidiasis. Systemic absorption of potent topical steroids may lower plasma cortisol levels when they are used with occlusion over as little as 20 per cent of the body, but this is unusual.

The combined characteristics of drug potency and vehicle type should be used to advantage in treatment. Intermediate-potency steroids are useful in most dermatologic conditions. Ointments are useful for thickened skin or for dry, exposed areas where creams or gel preparations rapidly evaporate. Low-potency steroids are used to treat the face and the thin and occluded skin of the groin and genital area. Lotions and gels are best for hairy

TABLE 524–1. POTENCY RANKING OF SOME COMMONLY USED TOPICAL STEROIDS

Potency	Generic Name	Clinical Applications
High	Fluocinonide 0.05%; betamethasone dipropionate 0.05%; halcinonide 0.1%	Recalcitrant psoriasis; discoid lupus erythematosus; recalcitrant lichen planus
Intermediate	Triamcinolone acetonide 0.1%; betamethasone valerate (cream) 0.1%; fluocinolone acetonide 0.01%	Dermatitis—allergic contact, atopic; psoriasis; neurodermatitis
Low	Desonide 0.05%; hydrocortisone 1.0% or 2.5%	Intertrigo; pruritus ani; seborrheic dermatitis

TABLE 524–2. GUIDELINES FOR SELECTING TOPICAL STEROIDS

Location or Type of Lesion	Suggested Potency of Steroid	Suggested Vehicle
Areas of Body		
Trunk, arms, legs	Intermediate or low	Ointment or cream
Palms, soles	Intermediate or high	Ointment
Scalp	Intermediate or low	Lotion, gel, aerosol
Intertriginous areas	Low	Cream, lotion
Face	Low	Cream, lotion
Area around eyes	Low	Cream or ophthalmic preparation
Ears	Intermediate or low	Cream, gel or lotion
Types of Lesion		
Dry, scaling, fissuring, lichenified lesion	Intermediate	Ointment
Thickened, hyperkeratotic skin patches	High	Ointment
Oozing, weeping lesions	Intermediate	Lotion, cream
Ulcerative lesions. Do not use topical steroids		

areas. High-potency steroid preparations should not be used to treat most dermatologic conditions. Their use is primarily reserved for areas of skin that have been substantially thickened by disease, such as dense plaques of psoriasis or chronic dermatitis. There is a substantial risk of local side effects with these high-potency steroids, and the onset of these effects is more rapid than with less potent drugs. Table 524–2 gives some guidelines for selecting the steroid potency and vehicle most useful in various areas of the body.

Topical steroids are usually applied once or twice a day. The stratum corneum acts as a reservoir and continues to release topical steroid into the skin after the initial application. Chronic dermatoses become less responsive after prolonged use of topical steroids. This phenomenon is referred to as *tachyphylaxis*. Changing to another topical steroid often overcomes this phenomenon.

Intralesional corticosteroids are used to shrink inflammatory acne cysts and hypertrophic scars and keloids. They are occasionally injected into unresponsive, localized dermatoses such as alopecia areata, granuloma annulare, discoid lupus erythematosus, psoriasis, and lichen simplex chronicus. Several types of steroids are used for this purpose, varying in their duration of action. Triamcinolone acetonide is the most widely used, and its maximal duration of action is 4 to 6 weeks. Triamcinolone hexacetonide is longer acting (6 to 8 weeks); injectables of shorter duration (2 to 4 weeks) include Celestone and Decadron. The steroids should be diluted to less than 5 mg per milliliter to avoid the risk of causing significant skin atrophy. Since intralesional steroid preparations are crystalline and dissolve in the tissues very slowly over weeks to months, great care is necessary in using low concentrations and in shaking the diluted material just prior to injecting into the dermis to avoid the often disfiguring side effects of atrophy that can occur if precipitates settle in the solution.

Topical Antibiotics. These are used to help suppress bacteria in erosions or superficial infections and occasionally in chronic leg ulcers. Silver sulfadiazine preparations are particularly useful as an adjunct to currently accepted principles of burn wound care. The commonly used topical antibiotics are bacitracin, neomycin, clindamycin phosphate, erythromycin, and tetracycline hydrochloride. The latter three are used to treat acne vulgaris. All topical antibiotics have the potential to sensitize, but neomycin is particularly prone to do so, especially after long-term use on chronic stasis dermatitis and leg ulcers. Mupirocin, a new topical antibiotic ointment, is particularly useful in treating staphylococcal and streptococcal infections of the skin; when used three times a day for a week it eliminates 87 per cent of skin pathogens and may decrease nasal staphylococcus carriers.

Topical Antifungal Agents. Antifungals are used to treat localized infections by superficial dermatophytes, *Candida*, and tinea versicolor. Topical broad-spectrum antifungal preparations effective against all of these organisms include clotrimazole, econazole, and miconazole creams and lotions used two times a day. Topical agents useful against dermatophytes but not *Candida* include haloprogin and Tinactin. Over-the-counter preparations, perhaps less effective against dermatophytes, are undecylenic acid and Verdefam. No topical preparations are useful against nail infections with these fungal organisms. Nystatin creams, oral suspensions, and vaginal tablets are effective against *Candida* infections in various areas of the body. Ketoconazole is a broad-spectrum imidazole antifungal agent highly effective against dermatophytes, *Candida*, and tinea versicolor. It is available in cream and oral forms.

Tars and Anthralin. Crude coal tar is often applied directly to the skin to treat psoriasis. Tars increase the effectiveness of ultraviolet light and reduce the accelerated mitotic rate of keratinocytes in psoriasis. Tars are often incorporated into shampoos for control of seborrheic dermatitis and in bath oils for use in psoriasis.

Anthralin is a synthetic coal tar derivative that is used in the treatment of psoriasis. Both tar and anthralin cause staining of clothing and skin. They can also be irritating. Anthralin must be started at the lowest concentrations (0.1 per cent) and initially left on the skin for short periods of time (0.5 hour) to avoid irritation.

Antiparasitic Topical Medications. Antiparasitics are employed for the treatment of pediculosis capitis, pediculosis pubis, and scabies. The lice of pediculosis corporis live in the seams of clothes and bedding. These must be disinfected by washing or dry cleaning. One per cent gamma benzene hexachloride (lindane), cromatiton, and pyrethrin compounds (RID) all are useful in treating pediculosis and scabies. Lindane is not suggested for children less than 6 years of age or for pregnant or lactating women.

Sunscreens. Sunscreens help protect the skin from the acute and chronic effects of UV radiation. They are rated by their sun protective factor (SPF). The SPF, which ranges from 3 to 50, is the factor by which the product extends the period of exposure to reach the sunburn reaction that would have taken place without the sunscreen. The action of topical photoprotectives is to reduce penetration of photoactive nonionizing radiation. Such protection can be achieved by either absorbing or reflecting the radiation. No sunscreen enhances tanning. Rather, if partial block is achieved, it permits melanin production relative to the radiation transmitted and the inherent capacity of the partially protected skin to respond. Most sunscreens are less effective in blocking UVA (320 to 400 nm) than UVB (290 to 320 nm). Para-aminobenzoic acid and its esters protect the skin from UVB and allow UVA to pass. Other non-PABA chemical sunscreens such as benzophenones and cinnamates are also useful against UVB and, to some extent, UVA. If protection against UVA is required, a sunscreen containing benzophenones or anthranilate compounds should be sought. For complete protection or total blockade of UVB and UVA, physical sunscreens containing titanium dioxide, zinc oxide, or iron oxide are available as heavy creams or pastes that reflect ultraviolet light.

SYSTEMIC MODES OF THERAPY FOR DERMATOLOGIC CONDITIONS

ANTIHISTAMINES. By occupying histamine-receptor sites on various cell membranes, antihistamines interfere with one or more of the actions of histamine. Their most specific use is in the control of allergic disorders mediated by histamine, such as urticaria, angioedema, and allergic rhinitis. Non–histamine-induced itching is also suppressed by antihistamines by virtue of their sedative, soporific side effects. Antihistamines are of two major classes, the classic H_1 blockers and the newer H_2 blockers, which also decrease gastric acid secretion. H_1 blockers have three problems: (1) They don't block all the effects of histamine. (2) They provide only limited protection against anaphylaxis because mediators other than histamine are involved in this reaction. (3) They are not selective in their effects (i.e., they also have anticholinergic and sedative effects). Antihistamines (H_1 blockers) can be arranged into several groups depending on their molecular configurations (Table 524–3).

An effective agent for a given patient may be selected from one group or from a combination of groups, but its effects are

TABLE 524–3. ANTIHISTAMINES ARRANGED ACCORDING TO THEIR MOLECULAR CONFIGURATIONS

Antihistamine Group	Generic Name (Proprietary Name)
H_1 receptor antagonists	
Ethanolamines	Diphenhydramine (Benadryl)
	Bromodiphenhydramine (Ambenyl)
	Clemastine (Tavist)
Piperidines	Cyproheptadine (Periactin)
	Azatadine (Optimine)
Phenothiazines	Promethazine (Phenergan)
	Trimeprazine (Temaril)
Alkylamines	Chlorpheniramine (Chlortrimeton)
	Dexchlorpheniramine (Dimetane)
Ethylenediamines	Tripelennamine (Pyribenzamine, PBZ)
	Pyrilamine (Neoantergan)
Piperazines	Hydroxyzine (Atarax)
	Meclizine (Bonamine)
Miscellaneous H_1 receptor antagonists	
Tricyclic compounds	Doxepin (Sinequan)
H_2 receptor antagonists	Cimetidine (Tagamet)
	Ranitidine (Zantac)

unlikely to be enhanced by combining antihistamines within a given group. If response to one antihistamine is minimal, another from a different group should be added or substituted. Evidence that blood vessels in human skin have H_2 as well as H_1 receptors has led to the evaluation of H_2-receptor antagonists such as cimetidine in combination with an H_1 antagonist, and the combination has proved to be effective in the treatment of some cases of chronic urticaria otherwise unresponsive to H_1 antagonists.

Antihistamines should be started in moderate doses until sufficient improvement occurs or until troublesome side effects develop. Generally, they are administered three or four times a day. Low doses should be given to elderly patients, as they are unusually sensitive to central nervous system side effects such as confusion, dizziness, and syncope, as well as to urinary retention, dry mouth, and blurred vision. In children, paradoxically, antihistamines may induce hyperactivity.

SYSTEMIC STEROIDS. Systemic steroids are used for a number of dermatologic conditions, but they have several drawbacks: (1) Prolonged administration leads to adrenal suppression and susceptibility to infection. (2) Many diseases such as psoriasis and atopic dermatitis may worsen after steroid withdrawal. (3) Safer and simpler therapy is available for most common dermatoses. Systemic corticosteroids are used in three types of situations. First, patients severely ill with life-threatening diseases known to be responsive to corticosteroids (anaphylactic reactions, extensive erythema multiforme, acute exfoliative dermatitis, pemphigus vulgaris) are initially given high doses—80 to 100 mg daily. Second, patients with conditions that are acute and severe but self-limited are treated with steroids to control or suppress the condition during a predicted period of activity. Examples include widespread poison ivy dermatitis, extensive sunburn, and acute generalized urticaria of known cause. Intermediate doses of 60 to 80 mg of prednisone daily are used initially and then tapered over 1 to 2 weeks. Third, steroids are used for patients with chronic dermatologic conditions that, because of periodic exacerbations, intermittently require low doses (15 to 20 mg) of prednisone together with supportive topical therapy. Examples include flares of chronic atopic dermatitis, pemphigoid, and some connective tissue diseases.

SYSTEMIC ANTIFUNGAL AGENTS. Two systemic agents are available for superficial fungal infections: griseofulvin and ketoconazole. *Griseofulvin* is active against dermatophytes but not against tinea versicolor or *Candida*. It is fungistatic, entering the horny layer of the skin via the sweat and the nails by incorporation into the keratinizing cells at the nail matrix. The entire nail must grow out with the griseofulvin incorporated into it before tinea at the distal end of the nail is affected. It is for this reason that griseofulvin must be given for many months before dermatophytic infections of the toenails are cleared. Less time is required for infections of fingernails and glabrous skin.

TABLE 524–4. SUGGESTED DOSAGE AND LENGTH OF TREATMENT WITH GRISEOFULVIN FOR DERMATOPHYTE INFECTIONS

Region of Dermatophyte Infection	Dose of Griseofulvin Ultrafine	Length of Treatment
Extensive or resistant tinea corporis	500 mg b.i.d.	30 days
Tinea pedis	500 mg b.i.d.	2–4 months
Onychomycosis		
fingernails	500 mg b.i.d.	4–6 months
toenails	500 mg b.i.d.	12–18 months, but frequently cannot clear toenail involvement
Tinea capitis	500 mg b.i.d.	4–6 weeks

Griseofulvin is the treatment of choice for tinea capitis, onychomycosis, and tinea corporis too extensive for topical therapy and for superficial fungal infections in immunosuppressed patients (Table 524–4).

Ketoconazole, a broad-spectrum imidazole antifungal agent, is effective against dermatophytes and, unlike griseofulvin, also against tinea versicolor and *Candida.* Several instances of anaphylactic reactions to ketoconazole have been recorded, as well as fatal hepatocellular toxicity, so ketoconazole should be used only for extensive cutaneous or systemic *Candida* infections and extensive dermatophyte infections unresponsive to griseofulvin. Liver enzyme levels should be determined before starting treatment and monitored at monthly intervals during treatment.

RETINOIDS. Retinoids are derivatives of natural vitamin A compounds. Two retinoids, isotretinoin and etretinate, are available for use in the treatment of dermatologic conditions. Retinoids decrease epidermal cell proliferation and keratinization and inhibit sebaceous gland activity. Etretinate has been found to be useful in severe psoriasis, especially the erythrodermic and pustular forms, as well as in several forms of ichthyosis. Isotretinoin has proved to be especially useful in severe cystic acne, often inducing prolonged remissions for several years after the drug is given for the usual 3- to 4-month course. The retinoids have many side effects, including cheilitis, conjunctivitis, dryness and fragility of skin, congenital malformations (heart defects, hydrocephalus, microtia), osteophytic growths on the vertebrae, epiphyseal closure in growing youngsters, corneal opacities, night blindness, and elevations of very low density and low density lipoproteins.

SYSTEMIC GOLD SALTS. Chrysotherapy has been useful in the treatment of autoimmune bullous disease, particularly pemphigus vulgaris. Intramuscular compounds have been used in the same manner as in rheumatoid arthritis. Remissions with a mean duration of 21 months or longer have been obtained in some patients with these bullous diseases. Generally a total dose of 400 to 600 mg of gold must be given before bullae respond.

SYSTEMIC ANTIBIOTICS. These are frequently used to treat cutaneous bacterial infections and conditions aggravated by bacterial overgrowth such as acne vulgaris, acne rosacea, and acute dermatitis. Because most bacterial infections of the skin involve *Staphylococcus aureus* or *Streptococcus pyogenes* (erysipelas, cellulitis, folliculitis, furunculosis, carbunculosis), the penicillins, cephalosporins, and erythromycins are commonly used in treating these conditions. In addition, erythromycin and tetracyclines are effective in controlling acne vulgaris and acne rosacea. Trimethoprim-sulfamethoxazole is used for pyodermas in patients allergic to penicillin, for pyodermas caused by methicillin-resistant *S. aureus,* as an alternative therapy for gonorrhea, and occasionally for the treatment of acne vulgaris. The sulfone antibiotic dapsone is occasionally used successfully in treating noninfectious diseases such as dermatitis herpetiformis, pyoderma gangrenosum, and leukocytoclastic cutaneous vasculitis. How dapsone brings about improvement in these conditions is not known.

ANTIMALARIALS. Chloroquine, hydroxychloroquine, and quinacrine are beneficial for cutaneous lupus erythematosus, polymorphic light eruption, solar urticaria, and porphyria cutanea tarda. Antimalarials bind DNA, inhibit the LE cell phenomenon and antinuclear antibody reactions, block chemotaxis, and antag-

onize histaminic responses, all of which may be related to the therapeutic effects on the diseases mentioned above. Cutaneous and mucous membrane pigmentation, nausea, diarrhea, and cycloplegia are common toxic effects, but retinopathy is the adverse reaction of greatest concern. Quinacrine does not cause retinopathy.

SYSTEMIC ANTIVIRAL AGENTS. Acyclovir and vidarabine are used for treating herpes simplex and zoster skin and systemic infections. These drugs can be given intravenously, and acyclovir is also administered orally. Intravenous acyclovir is used in severe primary genital herpes simplex, in neonatal herpes simplex, and in cutaneous herpes simplex and zoster infections in immunosuppressed patients. Oral acyclovir is also effective in primary and recurrent genital herpes simplex and eczema herpeticum. The usual oral dose is 200 mg five times a day for 5 to 10 days; IV acyclovir is usually given at a dose of 15 mg per kilogram per day. Oral acyclovir is also effective in herpes zoster infections, but higher doses are required—800 mg 5 times a day orally for 10 days. Acyclovir is activated to acyclovir monophosphate by herpes simplex virus–coded thymidine kinase; the monophosphate is further phosphorylated to acyclovir triphosphate, which inhibits viral DNA synthesis. This antiviral agent is thus selectively activated only by virus-infected cells with little disruption of host cellular metabolism. This accounts for the low incidence of side effects. Acyclovir ointment is also available for mild primary genital and labial infections and for localized, chronic cutaneous lesions in immunosuppressed patients.

SYSTEMIC CYTOSTATIC DRUGS. Cytotoxic drugs such as methotrexate, cyclophosphamide, azathioprine, and hydroxyurea are used in a number of skin conditions when they cannot be controlled by more conventional means. Thus, psoriasis, when it is generalized, severe, and life-ruining, may be treated with modest doses of methotrexate, azathioprine, or hydroxyurea; life-threatening bullous diseases such as pemphigus vulgaris are occasionally treated with these agents as an alternative to high doses of corticosteroids.

ULTRAVIOLET LIGHT AS A THERAPEUTIC AGENT. UV phototherapy is used primarily in patients with psoriasis and vitiligo, but it may also help patients with nummular and atopic eczema, pityriasis rosea, the pruritus of uremia, and mycosis fungoides. UV light units are available in two wavelength ranges, UVB (the sunburn range of 280 to 320 nm) and UVA (long wavelength spectrum of 320 to 400 nm). The use of topical tar preparations, which "photosensitize" the skin to UVB wavelengths, adds to the effectiveness of treatment (the so-called Goeckerman regimen). This method used over many weeks to months is highly effective in controlling psoriasis.

UVA light units are employed by dermatologists (and also commercial suntan centers) to cause tanning rather than burning. The ability of UVA to evoke a sunburn is 1000 times less than that of UVB. The primary use of UVA is in the treatment of severe, extensive psoriasis and vitiligo, for which it is used in combination with topical or oral psoralen, a drug that binds to DNA in the skin and sensitizes it to the effects of UVA. The combination of psoralen with UVA light is called PUVA. The long-term side effects of PUVA therapy are unknown, although it seems to induce squamous and basal cell cutaneous carcinomas. The unprotected cornea and retina can be damaged by UV light, especially PUVA. Stringent guidelines for protecting the eyes, such as wearing special protective eye glasses for 24 to 48 hours after taking the psoralens as well as regular eye examinations, must be observed.

Shelley WB, Shelley GD: Advanced Dermatologic Therapy. Philadelphia, W.B. Saunders Company, 1987.

525 Skin Diseases of General Importance

In Chapter 523, an approach to diagnosing skin diseases was discussed in which the specific morphologic descriptions of primary and secondary skin lesions are used to place the condition into one of nine large diagnostic groups. These nine groups, encompassing the majority of skin diseases, are listed in Table 523–1. In this chapter, some of the diseases in each of these groups are discussed, providing the clinician with a differential diagnosis of conditions within each group. As stressed in Ch. 523, the differential diagnosis within each major group depends on such things as variations in distribution; specific location and symmetry of lesions; and shape, arrangement, color, and texture of lesions.

THE ECZEMAS (DERMATITIS)

The term *eczema* is derived from the Greek word that means "to boil out," a reference to the fact that eczematous reactions may be vesicular and oozing. Eczematous dermatitis is an inflammatory response of the skin to multiple exogenous and endogenous agents, although often the etiology is not clear. Eczemas are defined by their clinical appearance and are subdivided either by their pattern of distribution or by etiologic factors (when known). Many eczematous processes are related to immunologic reactions (Table 525–1).

The term *eczema* or *eczematous dermatitis* is applied to eruptions characterized histologically by epidermal intercellular edema, termed *spongiosis*. Eczemas can be acute, with marked spongiosis causing red papules and vesicles and oozing, weeping, and crusting, or they may be chronic, with redness, scaling, fissuring, and especially lichenification. Indeed, both acute and chronic forms of eczema may be seen in the same patient, with the acute reaction progressing to oozing and crusting; with

continued pruritus, the patient's rubbing and scratching converts the eczema to the chronic, dry, lichenified form. The hallmarks, then, of all types of eczematous dermatitis are (1) marked pruritus and (2) varying degrees of erythema along with papules, vesicles, fine scaling, or lichenification.

A number of the eczematous processes are listed in Table 525–1, along with some useful diagnostic findings that help to differentiate one from another. Histology of various types of eczemas is the same; skin biopsies identify a lesion as an eczematous reaction, but it does not differentiate among the various types of eczema.

CONTACT DERMATITIS. Contact dermatitis is the best understood cause of eczematous reactions and potentially the most correctable. For any eczematous rash, the clinician should first determine whether it could be a contact reaction. If the cause can be identified, avoidance of the offending substance will be curative. There are two types of contact dermatitis, *irritant* and *allergic*. Irritant contact dermatitis is produced by substances that simply irritate or have a direct toxic effect on the skin, such as acids, alkalis, solvents, and detergents; no immunologic process is involved. Allergic contact dermatitis, on the other hand, is a delayed-type hypersensitivity reaction that occurs in response to a wide variety of allergens commonly found in the environment. The allergens consist of small molecular weight substances that act as haptens and bind to proteinaceous components of the skin to form the sensitizing antigen. The antigen is processed by

TABLE 525–1. ECZEMATOUS DERMATITIS SKIN ERUPTIONS

Clinical Type	Etiology or Suspected Cause	Distinctive Diagnostic Findings
Eczemas with Known Causes		
Contact dermatitis		
Irritant contact	Chemical agents that have direct toxic effects on skin	Contact precedes rash by hours to days
Allergic contact	Chemical agents that elicit type IV delayed hypersensitivity reaction on skin	Contact precedes rash by 2 or more days; in both instances site and configuration of eczema reaction conforms to site of contact with exogenous substances (plants, medicaments, cosmetics, metals); patch tests
Photodermatitis	Ultraviolet light exposure plus topical or systemic substances induce type IV delayed hypersensitivity	Eczematous reaction in sun-exposed areas of skin with sharp "cut off" borders, i.e., face, ears, V of neck, dorsum of hands, extensor surfaces of arms
Eczematous drug-induced reaction	Drugs such as penicillin taken internally	Generalized eczema reaction evolves after taking medications (usually 10 or more days after first beginning drug; sooner if previously exposed) and clears with stopping drugs
Dermatophyte and *Candida* eczematous reactions	Dermatophytes and *Candida* induce eczematous inflammatory reaction	Dermatophyte or yeast found in scales or exudate
Infectious eczematoid dermatitis	Products from draining infected skin areas induce eczema reaction—linear infections, leg ulcers	Occurs near site of infection or other draining lesion; clears with treatment of infection
Dermatophytid	Hypersensitivity reaction occurring on distant areas of skin in response to products from fungal infection of other areas of skin	Often vesicular eruption of palms or fingers with dermatophyte infection of feet
Autosensitization	Hypersensitivity reaction to cutaneous or bacterial antigens released from area of acute dermatitis	Generalized dermatitis following localized acute dermatitis
Xerotic eczema or eczema craquelé	Dry skin or xerosis	Can lead to redness and fissuring of skin that appear as cracks in dried mud
Eczemas with Unknown or Unclear Etiologies		
Atopic eczema	Hereditary disposition in association with familial tendency for asthma and allergic rhinitis	Eczematous reaction often localized to face, neck, antecubital, and popliteal areas
Stasis dermatitis	Chronic venous insufficiency	Associated with varicosities, leg edema, hyperpigmentation, and ulcers
Lichen simplex chronicus (neurodermatitis)	Repeated scratching leads to eczema	Lichenified patches in areas within reach of fingers (nape of neck, lower legs)
Nummular eczema	Dry skin, underlying infections	Coin-shaped patches on extensor areas of extremities and trunk
Seborrheic dermatitis	Occurs in areas of high concentrations of sebaceous glands; may be related to intrinsic yeast in skin (*Pityrosporon ovale*)	Inflammatory, yellow, greasy, scaling patches on scalp, retroauricular areas, eyebrows, nasolabial fold, and presternal areas
Dyshidrotic eczema	Emotional stress—unrelated to disturbances in sweating	Pruritic vesicles on palms, soles
Nonspecific eczematous dermatitis	No obvious cause—diagnosis of exclusion after above eczemas ruled out	Acute and chronic eczema patches anywhere on body; severe itching

Langerhans' cells in the epidermis (see Ch. 521), which then present the antigen to T lymphocytes to elicit sensitization. Sensitization to the allergen requires 10 to 14 days to develop after the first encounter; subsequent exposure to the allergen elicits the eczematous response in 1 to 7 days (delayed hypersensitivity).

The onset of irritant reactions after exposure to the topical substance is variable. Skin damage is evident within hours after contact with a strong irritant. Weaker irritants may require multiple applications and days or weeks before the development of the eczema (e.g., housewife's eczema of the hands due to chronic exposure to water and detergents). Contact dermatitis accounts for more than 50 per cent of all occupational illnesses (excluding injury). In the industrial setting, approximately 70 per cent is irritant and 30 per cent allergic contact dermatitis.

Both irritant and allergic contact eczemas are initially confined to sites of contact, and therefore unique patterns of distribution and configuration suggest contact dermatitis as well as provide clues to the contactant. Thus, allergic reactions to plants, such as poison oak or ivy, appear as linear, red, papular and vesicular streaks where the plant brushes across the skin. Allergies to metals (especially nickel) cause eczematous reactions under rings or watchbands or on the lobes of ears (earrings). Dermatitis under a ring may also stem from trapped water and irritating soap residues.

The most common allergens causing allergic contact dermatitis are pentadecylcatechol (allergen in poison oak, ivy, and sumac as well as in cashews, mangos, and ginkgo trees), paraphenylenediamine (a substance in hair dyes which cross-reacts with benzocaine and hydrochlorothiazide), nickel, mercaptobenzothiazol and thiuram (components in rubber), and ethylenediamine (a preservative in many medications and also found in industrial dyes and insecticides). Other common sources of contactants include topical medications (neomycin, anesthetics such as benzocaine, topical antihistamines), preservatives (ethylenediamine, merthiolate, parabens), vehicles (propylene glycol), and cosmetics (fragrances, preservatives, paraphenylenediamines). It is obvious that a detailed history of the patient's occupation, hobbies, habits, clothing, cosmetics, and medications applied to the skin is necessary to find the contactant. Careful detective work on the part of the physician and the patient often brings to light the etiologic factor. One must not overlook the possibility that a topical medicine is perpetuating or exacerbating a pre-existing dermatitis.

There is no standard testing method available for diagnosing irritant contact dermatitis. For allergic contact eczema, the causative agent can be identified by patch tests, but these must be properly performed and interpreted by trained dermatologists.

Therapy of contact dermatitis is avoidance of the irritant or allergen if possible. This may require a change in lifestyle or occupation. Sometimes protective clothing is curative. Barrier creams are of little benefit. Acute, severe generalized contact dermatitis is treated with a short (10- to 14-day) course of systemic steroids and wet dressings or baths. Milder eczematous reactions respond to topical steroids and systemic antihistamines.

PHOTODERMATITIS. A variety of skin reactions, termed photosensitivity reactions, may occur in response to exposure to ultraviolet light. Some appear as eczematous reactions, so-called photoallergic dermatitis, which may occur in response to topical as well as systemic substances in the presence of UV light. The distribution of the eczematous eruption in light-exposed areas is an important feature in the differential diagnosis, with the cheeks, nose, forehead, and tips of ears as sites of predilection. The backs of hands and forearms are also frequently involved and, of course, the history of exposure to UV light prior to the onset of the reaction is important in identifying light sensitivity (see Fig. 523–2).

Photoallergic dermatitis is immunologic. Absorption of a specific wavelength of ultraviolet light by a topical substance or a systemic drug (which is deposited in the skin from the cutaneous circulation) causes chemical conversion of the substance or drug to a hapten that binds cutaneous proteins to become a complete antigen capable of eliciting a type IV delayed hypersensitivity reaction similar to an allergic contact dermatitis reaction. Photoallergic reactions appear only where the UV light hits the skin,

even though the systemic drug or topical photoallergen is present in the skin all over the body; i.e., the reaction depends on UV light hitting the skin with the allergen in it. Long wavelength UVA light is usually responsible for these reactions. UVA light penetrates window glass (UVB light is blocked by glass), so the reaction often occurs even though the patient remains indoors. Such drugs as thiazides and phenothiazines can cause photoeczematous reactions; a number of topically applied substances, such as methylcoumarin, musk ambrette, halogenated salicylanilids, and topical sunscreening agents, can cause a similar reaction. Photopatch testing can identify substances in materials causing these reactions. Avoidance of the offending material is often curative. Oral or topical steroids relieve the inflammatory reaction.

ATOPIC DERMATITIS. This chronic, eczematous condition of the skin is often associated with a personal or family history of atopic disease (asthma, allergic rhinitis, and atopic eczema). Pruritus is a prominent symptom, and the consequent scratching and rubbing lead to lichenification, most typically in the antecubital and popliteal flexural areas. The eczema usually manifests itself after the first few months of life, appearing on the face and extensor areas of the extremities as acute and subacute, red, vesicular and oozing dermatitis. Many cases resolve spontaneously by puberty only to recur in adolescence and adulthood as a chronic dermatitis with scaling, dryness, and lichenification over the face, neck, upper chest, and characteristically the antecubital and popliteal fossae (flexural dermatitis). Atopics have a readily identifiable facies with diffuse erythema, perioral pallor, and a redundant crease or fold below the lower eyelids (Dennie-Morgan fold). The palms often have an increased number of skin markings, noticeable as fine cross-hatched lines. Stroking the skin in atopic dermatitis causes a white line, or dermatographism, probably due to dermal edema and vasoconstriction.

The exact cause of atopic dermatitis is not known, but a number of immunologic and pharmacologic abnormalities are seen in association with the skin condition. For example, IgE reaginic antibodies are increased in 80 per cent of atopic patients, especially those with extensive skin disease (and such patients respond to many antigens applied by skin prick testing), but these antibodies seem to play no definitive role in *causing* atopic eczema. Avoiding antigens to which these patients react by scratch test does not improve the eczema. Patients with atopic eczema also have depressed cell-mediated immunity, with deficient T suppressor cells. This may account for the overproduction of IgE, resulting in unusual susceptibility to cutaneous herpes simplex, vaccina, molluscum contagiosum, and wart infections. Neutrophil and monocyte chemotaxis is reduced during exacerbations of eczema, explaining the frequent staphylococcal skin infections in these patients. Treatment with oral antibiotics to reduce staphylococcal flora (or overt staphylococcal infections such as folliculitis, furuncles, or cellulitis) often results in marked improvement in the eczema.

Atopic individuals are often tense, resentful, aggressive, and restless, but it is not clear whether this is a basic characteristic of the diathesis or the result of living with chronic, unremitting itching and skin inflammation. Whether these personality traits are primary or secondary, the physician must help the patient meet the stresses of life.

Keratoconjunctivitis and stellate anterior subcapsular cataracts are associated with atopic eczema, particularly in patients with extensive skin changes. The conjunctivitis and keratitis usually start in childhood. The cataracts may also begin at a young age and form rapidly, often by age 20. Keratoconus is seen in 25 per cent of atopics.

The treatment of atopic dermatitis is the same as for other eczematous eruptions and includes topical steroids, emollients, and systemic antihistamines. In some children (less than 2 years of age) food allergy can cause atopic dermatitis, but dietary factors remain controversial. Skin tests or RAST tests help identify which foods may be responsible. Positive results must be confirmed with controlled food challenges and elimination diets. Allergic immediate skin testing and desensitization have been of little value in atopic dermatitis.

Skin irritation must be avoided by wearing soft cotton clothing. Counseling, psychotherapy, and stress reduction may sometimes be helpful. Patients often worsen during the autumn and winter seasons when decreased humidity in homes associated with the

PLATE 13 EYE DISEASES

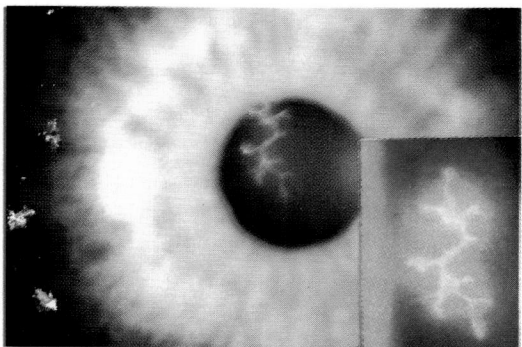

A, Herpes simplex corneal epithelial keratitis in diffuse light and *(inset)* in light passed through a cobalt blue filter after fluorescein staining.

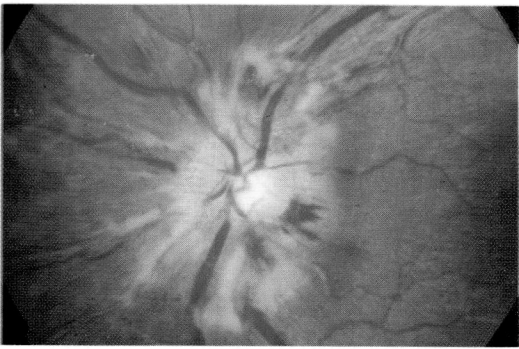

B, Papilledema in a young person. Note disc swelling, hemorrhages, and exudates, with preservation of the physiologic cup.

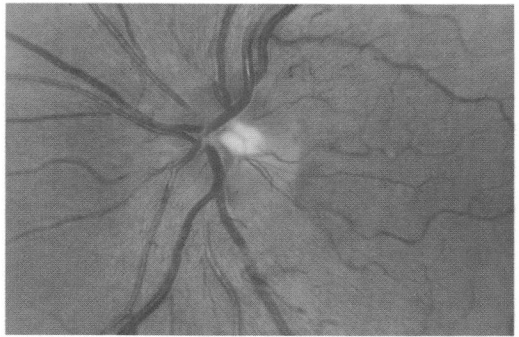

C, Disc in acute Leber's hereditary optic neuropathy. The disc tissue appears hyperemic, with peripapillary telangiectasia and opacification of the nerve fiber layer. Fluorescein angiography revealed no dye leakage.

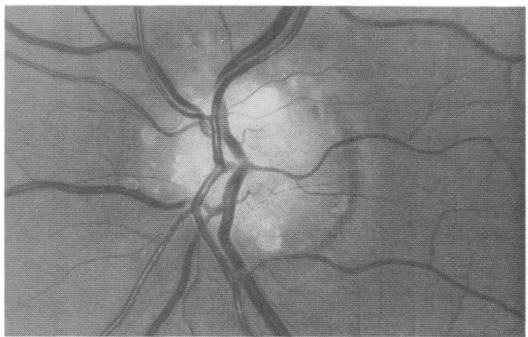

D, Optic disc drusen (also called hyaline bodies). Although obvious here, these calcified excrescences may be difficult to see in young persons, in whom the disc elevation they produce is mistaken for papilledema. (Also, they should be distinguished from retinal drusen—see *F* below.)

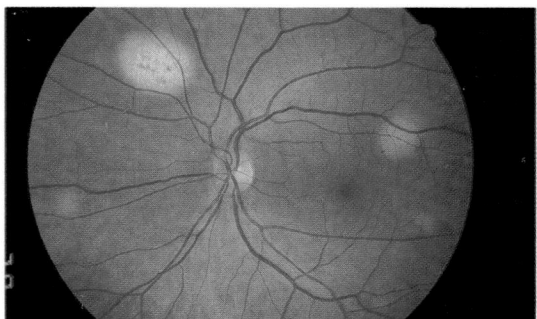

E, Multiple white choroidal metastases in a man with lung carcinoma.

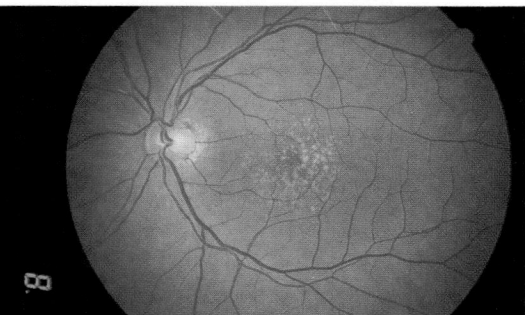

F, Retinal drusen. Multiple small white dots in the macula that represent abnormal accumulations in the retinal pigment epithelium basement (Bruch's) membrane. Such drusen are often precursors to visual loss from senile macular degeneration. (These should be distinguished from optic disc drusen—see *D* above.)

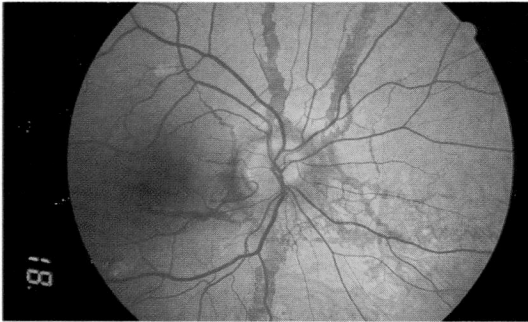

G, Angioid streaks in pseudoxanthoma elasticum. Breaks in the retinal pigment epithelium basement (Bruch's) membrane radial and circumferential to the disc indicate an underlying defect in elastic tissue formation.

Photographs taken by Mr. Harry Kachadoorian, C.R.A., University of Massachusetts Medical School, Worcester, Massachusetts.

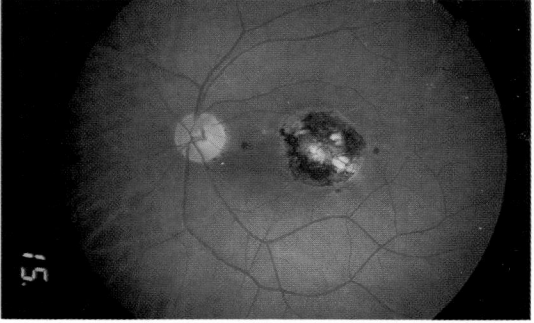

H, Macular chorioretinal scar. The appearance is typical of congenital toxoplasmosis, although other causes of chorioretinitis are included in the differential diagnosis.

PLATE 14 EYE DISEASES

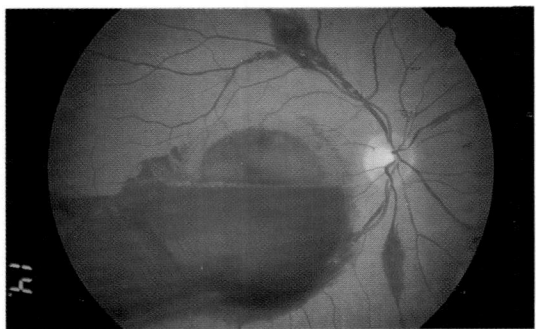

A, Preretinal (subhyaloid) hemorrhage. This occurred after a difficult intubation in an asthmatic woman with a previously normal eye examination. Similar findings are seen as a manifestation of diabetic retinopathy and in association with subarachnoid hemorrhage. The blood forms a meniscus with the patient in the upright position.

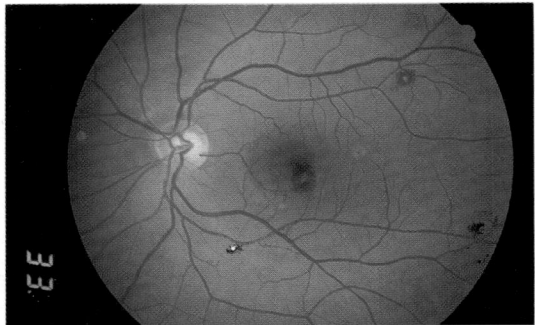

B, Roth spots. Multiple white centered hemorrhages in a man with recurrent subacute bacterial endocarditis. White centered hemorrhages are also seen with leukemia and diabetes. The small white scars are probably the residua of previous episodes.

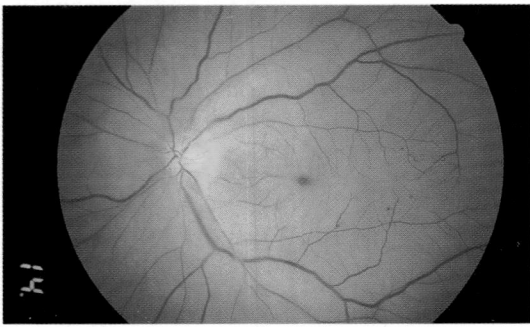

C, Central retinal artery occlusion. The retina is diffusely pale, lending a prominence to the normal coloration of the central fovea, often described as a cherry red spot.

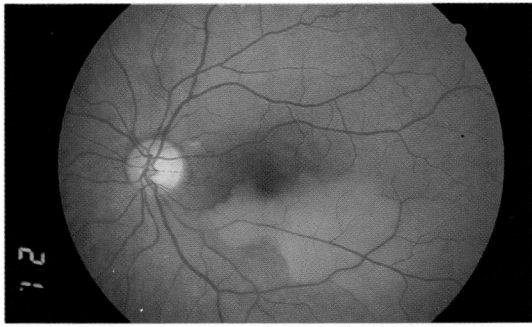

D, Inferior branch retinal artery occlusion. A pie-shaped sector of pale, infarcted retina extends from the embolic occlusion at the first branch of the arteriole of the inferior temporal arcade.

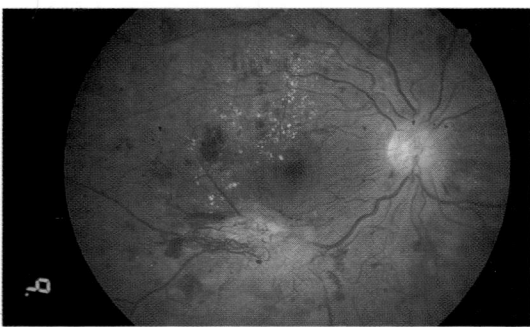

E, Proliferative diabetic retinopathy. Multiple hemorrhages, exudates, and new vessels are visible, with chorioretinal striae extending toward an area of fibrovascular proliferation along the inferior temporal arcade.

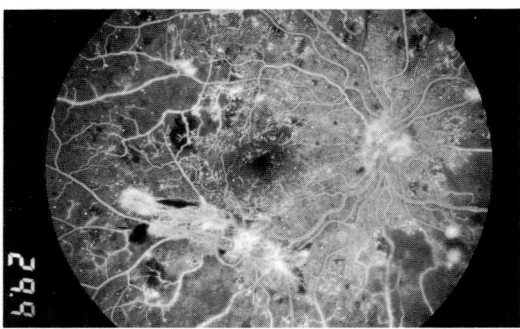

F, Fluorescein angiogram of the same fundus pictured in *E.* The new vessels, especially at the disc and the area of fibrovascular proliferation, are seen to leak fluorescein. Many of the "dot hemorrhages" are revealed as microaneurysms that fill with dye.

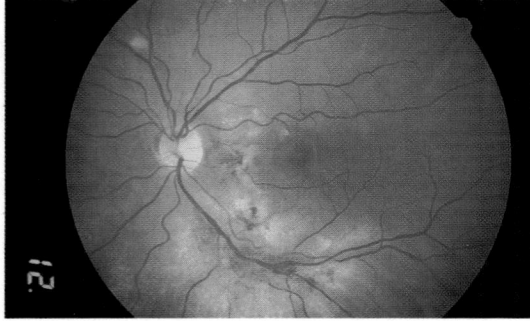

G, Cytomegalovirus retinitis in a patient with AIDS. There is a sector of retinal necrosis and hemorrhages along the inferior temporal arcade.

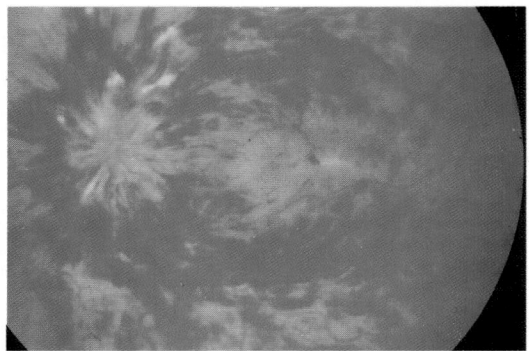

H, Central retinal vein occlusion. The disc is swollen with diffuse retinal hemorrhages and cotton-wool spots.

Photographs taken by Mr. Harry Kachadoorian, C.R.A., University of Massachusetts Medical School, Worcester, Massachusetts.

PLATE 15   SKIN DISEASES

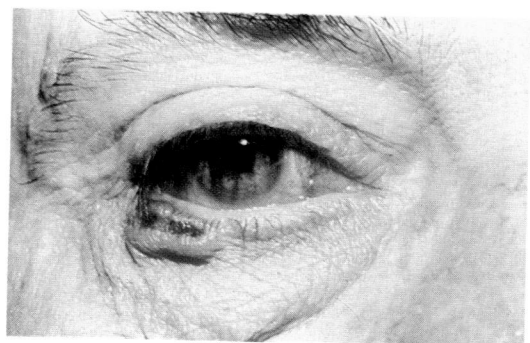

A, Basal cell cancer. Tumor with rolled, opalescent borders and central "rodent" ulcer.

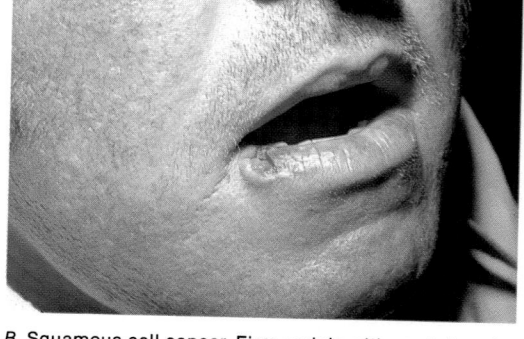

B, Squamous cell cancer. Firm nodule with eroded surface on the lower lip.

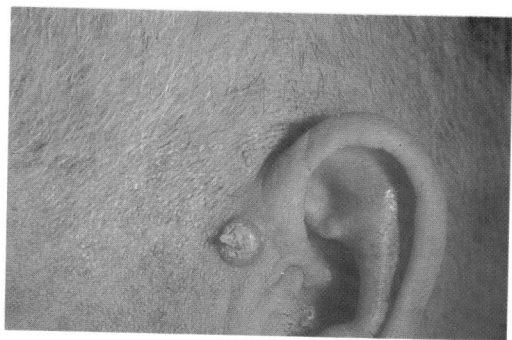

C, Cutaneous horn. Keratotic horn evolving from red nodule at base. These commonly are squamous cell cancers.

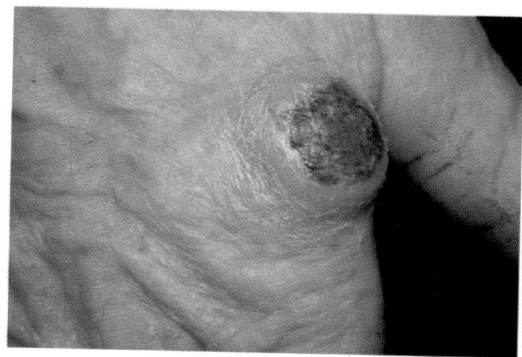

D, Keratoacanthoma. Large nodular lesion with central keratotic crater.

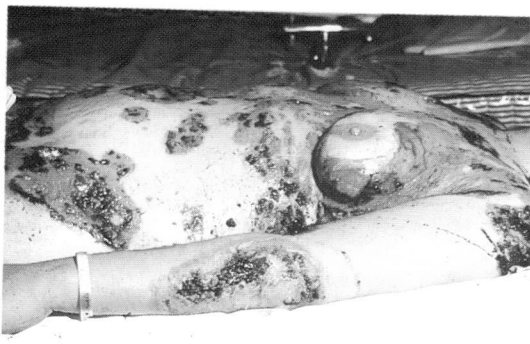

E, Pemphigus vulgaris. Intraepidermal bullae are easily ruptured, leaving superficial crusted erosions with thin shreds of blister roof along the edges. Careful examination reveals some intact blisters (primary lesions) below the breast.

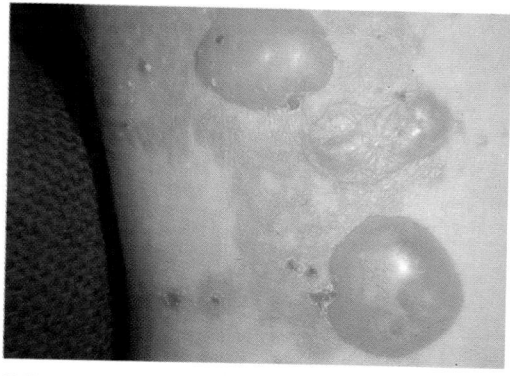

F, Bullous pemphigoid. Tense subepidermal bullae on an erythematous base.

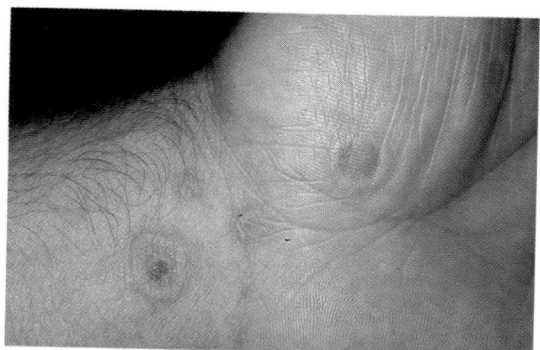

G, Erythema multiforme. Target or "bull's-eye" annular lesions with central vesicles and bullae.

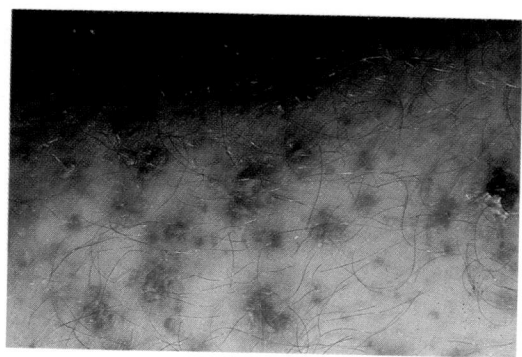

H, Palpable purpura. Leukocytoclastic vasculitis commonly causes raised purpuric and ulcerated lesions on legs.

PLATE 16 SKIN DISEASES

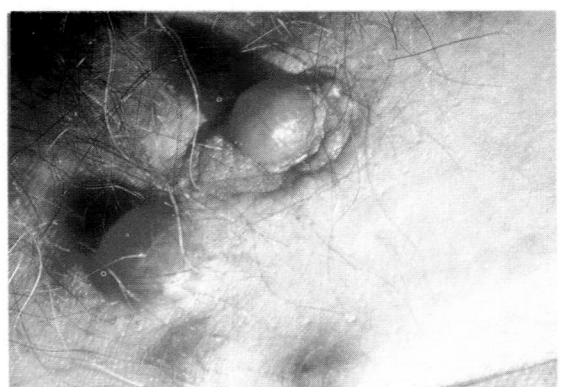

A, Skin metastases. Firm, hard, red nodules.

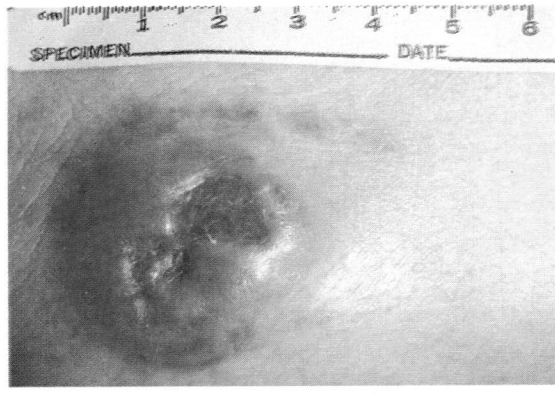

B, Mycosis fungoides, tumor stage.

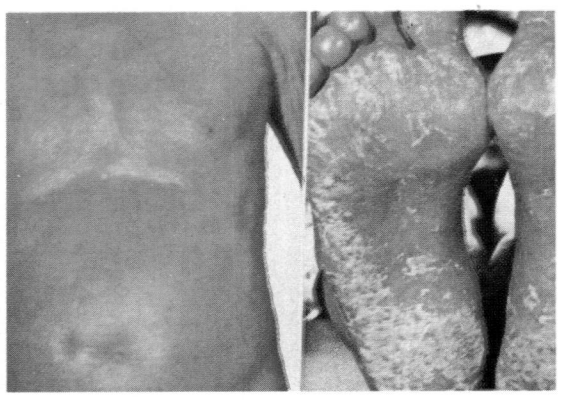

C, Sézary syndrome, exfoliative dermatitis stage.

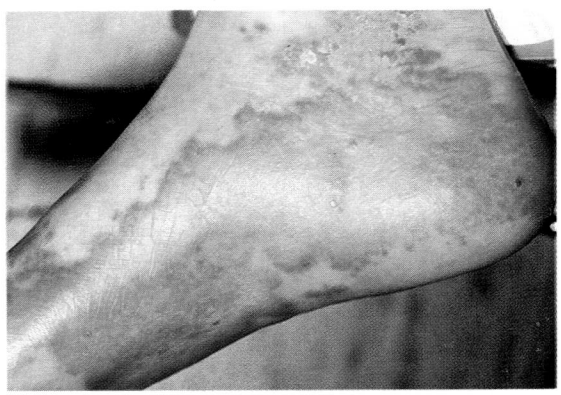

D, Classic Kaposi's sarcoma.

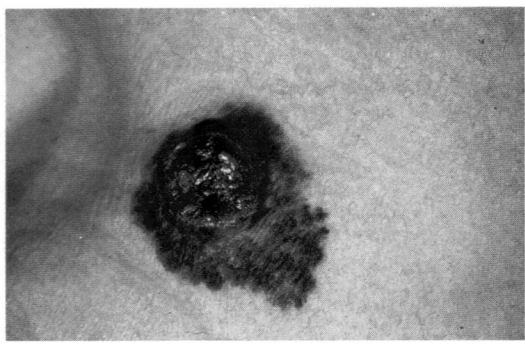

E, Malignant melanoma. Darkly pigmented, nodular lesion with irregular outline, irregular shades of dark pigmentation, and irregular surface configuration.

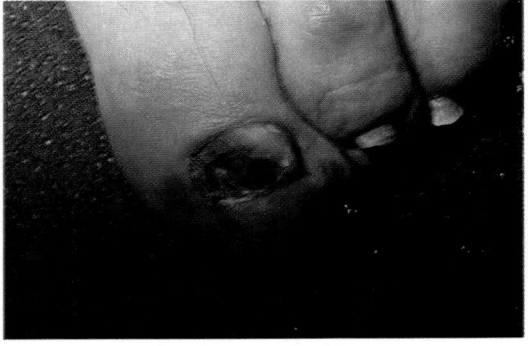

F, Subungual melanoma. Dark blue-black pigment within nail bed, with irregular dark pigment on the tip of the great toe.

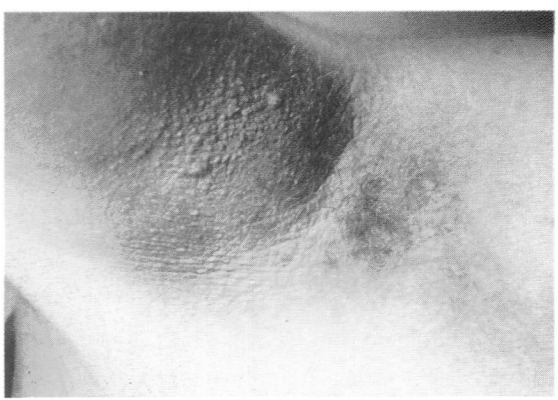

G, Acanthosis nigricans. Axillary lesion.

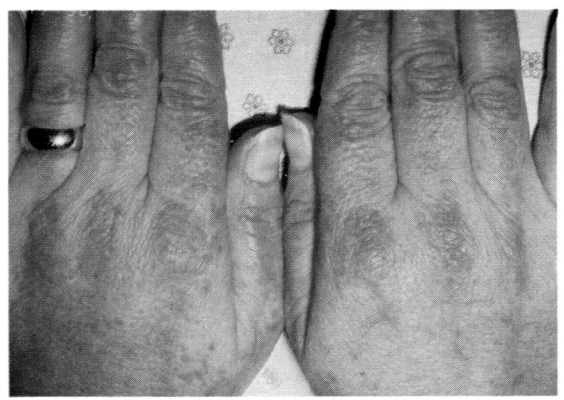

H, Dermatomyositis. Gottron's papules over the knuckles.

use of central heating causes increased skin dryness and itching. The frequent use of emollients is the best treatment for skin dryness, especially immediately after bathing when the skin is hydrated. Topical corticosteroids are the most important means of controlling the inflammatory response, and the least potent forms should be utilized, usually in an ointment base. Systemic steroids should be used only in short courses to overcome exacerbations not controlled by topical steroids.

STASIS DERMATITIS. This is an eczematous eruption of the lower legs secondary to peripheral venous insufficiency. Venous incompetence causes increased hydrostatic pressure and capillary damage with extravasation of red blood cells and serum. These conditions seem to trigger an inflammatory, brawny, edematous, red, and hyperpigmented petechial scaling or weeping reaction, usually around the medial malleolus or distal one third of the lower leg. Secondary allergic contact dermatitis frequently complicates this problem when neomycin is used chronically to treat accompanying stasis ulcers. The cornerstone of managing stasis dermatitis is prevention of venous stasis and edema with the use of supportive hose while the patient is ambulatory. Weight reduction is helpful in obese patients. The eczema is treated with topical steroids and wet compresses when oozing and crusting are present. Occasionally chronic stasis dermatitis, when secondarily infected, can undergo exacerbation with spread of the acute inflammation to distant areas of the body, a condition known as *autosensitization dermatitis*. These secondary eczematous patches evolve on the face, neck, and extensor areas of the extremities. Control is achieved with topical steroids (occasionally oral steroids if the reaction is severe) and antibiotics to control the cutaneous infection.

NUMMULAR ECZEMATOUS DERMATITIS. This condition is defined by coin-shaped patches predominantly on the extensor surfaces of the arms and legs, but the trunk is often involved as well. Lesions appear as patches of minute vesicles and papules that spread to become scaling and thickened, occasionally clearing in the center so that they may resemble superficial fungal infections. Mild to severe pruritus accompanies the eczematous patches. Although the cause is unknown, many factors acting alone or in combination may play a role. Dry skin is a frequent accompaniment, and the disease reaches a peak in the winter months. Irritating substances such as wool and soap and frequent bathing may also contribute to the condition. The combination of topical steroids (usually of intermediate potency), 3 per cent crude coal tar, and ultraviolet light treatments is helpful in controlling this form of eczema. The condition tends to persist with remissions and recurrences.

LICHEN SIMPLEX CHRONICUS. Also known as neurodermatitis, this is a chronic, pruritic, lichenified eczematous eruption that results from constant scratching. Pruritus often precedes the scratching, and rubbing induces lichenification, initiating a vicious circle of itch-scratch-itch. In most patients it is a nervous habit. Patches of neurodermatitis commonly are found on the nape of the neck, lower legs, groin, or other regions of the body within easy reach of the hands. Occasionally constant scratching results in scaling, thickened, excoriated papules and nodules (prurigo nodularis). Treatment consists of explaining to the patient the cause and the need to stop rubbing. Topical steroids and antihistamines may also be helpful, and steroids injected into the lesion will break the itching cycle more successfully than topically applied steroids.

SEBORRHEIC DERMATITIS. Seborrheic dermatitis is characterized by erythematous, eczematous patches with yellow, greasy scales localized to hairy areas and regions of the skin with high concentrations of sebaceous glands, especially the middle of the face, nasolabial folds, eyebrows, ear canals, retroauricular folds, and presternal areas. Dandruff is scaling of the scalp without inflammation. In severe cases the axillae and groin regions can also be involved. Seborrheic dermatitis may appear in infants until about 6 months of age ("cradle cap"); after that it does not appear until after puberty. Patients with neurologic disorders, such as Parkinson's disease or stroke, may have a dramatic flare of their seborrhea. Although the precise cause of seborrhea is unknown, the exacerbations associated with emotional stress and neurologic disease suggest a role of the central nervous system. Some studies suggest that the condition is related to excessive growth of yeast organisms (*Pityrosporum*) on the skin. It is sometimes difficult to differentiate seborrhea from psoriasis when the latter is localized to the scalp, ears, and face.

Antiseborrheic shampoos containing tar, sulfur, salicylic acid, selenium sulfide, or zinc pyrithione are the most useful form of treatment. The shampoo should be used daily, rubbed into the scalp and left on for 5 minutes before rinsing. Inflammatory seborrhea that does not respond to shampoos alone will benefit from a topical steroid lotion or gel in hairy areas and hydrocortisone cream for facial glabrous skin. Continual use of shampoo and topical steroids is required to control this chronic dermatitis. The use of topical or oral antiyeast medication, ketoconazole, may be of help in controlling seborrhea in some patients.

XEROTIC ECZEMA AND ECZEMA CRAQUELÉ. These conditions are characterized by chapping and symptomatic dryness that may lead to visible fissuring through the stratum corneum, giving criss-crossing cracks that resemble dried mud. Such changes occur most commonly in winter, and they respond to the frequent use of emollients and/or hydrocortisone ointments.

HAND ECZEMA. Hand eczema is most common in housewives, cooks, food handlers, and medical personnel. The most common etiologic factors are constant exposure to mild primary irritants (soap, water), frequent hand washing, atopy, and nummular dermatitis. Allergic contact dermatitis may be another cause. *Dyshidrotic eczema* (pompholyx), a relatively noninflammatory, recurrent, pruritic, vesicular eruption of the palms and soles of unknown etiology, differs from other hand eczemas in that the primary involvement is on the palm instead of the dorsum of the hands. The term *dyshidrotic eczema* suggests malfunction of the sweat ducts, but this is a misnomer. Pompholyx, from the Greek meaning bubble, is a more apt term. Emotional stress tends to be a trigger. Vesicles on the palms can also represent *dermatophytid*, an allergic reaction to a dermatophyte infection on the feet. If potassium hydroxide (KOH) examination of the feet is positive, treatment of the fungus will clear up the palmar reaction as well.

Treatment of hand dermatitis involves avoidance of primary irritants such as soap, solvents, detergents, and frequent exposure to water. The use of cotton gloves with rubber gloves over them is useful in protecting the hands in water. Topical steroids and emollients are also beneficial, and potent topical steroids are often required.

EXFOLIATIVE DERMATITIS (ERYTHRODERMA). Total body cutaneous erythema, edema, scaling, and fissuring may occur as an idiopathic entity without preceding dermatologic or systemic disease, or it may be the result of a variety of cutaneous diseases (atopic or contact dermatitis, psoriasis, seborrheic dermatitis, autosensitization, pityriasis rubra pilaris) or systemic disorders (mycosis fungoides, lymphomas, leukemias) as well as a reaction to a number of drugs (antibiotics, barbiturates, antiepileptic agents, gold) (Fig. 525–1). Other organ systems are affected by the general erythroderma and changes in the stratum corneum barrier function. For example, the diffuse redness and warmth of the skin reflect vasodilation and increased blood flow through the immense cutaneous vasculature. Blood flow may be increased 100-fold in erythroderma, and 5 to 8 per cent of the total cardiac output may be directed to the dilated, inflamed, cutaneous vasculature. This has two consequences. First, a compensatory increase in cardiac output occurs. In older individuals with underlying cardiac disease, heart failure may ensue. The second consequence is defective thermoregulation. Increased heat loss leads to decreased core temperature, shivering, and swings in temperature. When high-output failure occurs and/or thermoregulation is impaired, oral steroids decrease the cutaneous inflammation and correct the abnormalities. In less acute situations total body applications of topical steroids with plastic sauna suit occlusion reverse the erythroderma.

FUNGAL INFECTIONS OF THE SKIN. Fungal infections may be confused with eczematous conditions. These infections include dermatophytosis, candidiasis, and tinea versicolor. *Dermatophytes* are a homogeneous group of fungi that live on the keratin of the stratum corneum, nails, and hair and frequently provoke an inflammatory reaction in the skin with pruritus, redness, scaling, and vesiculation. Three genera of dermatophytes cause these infections: *Trichophyton*, *Microsporum*, and *Epidermophyton*. Dermatophytosis of the trunk (tinea corporis) can be caused by several species (*T. rubrum* and *T. mentagrophytes* are

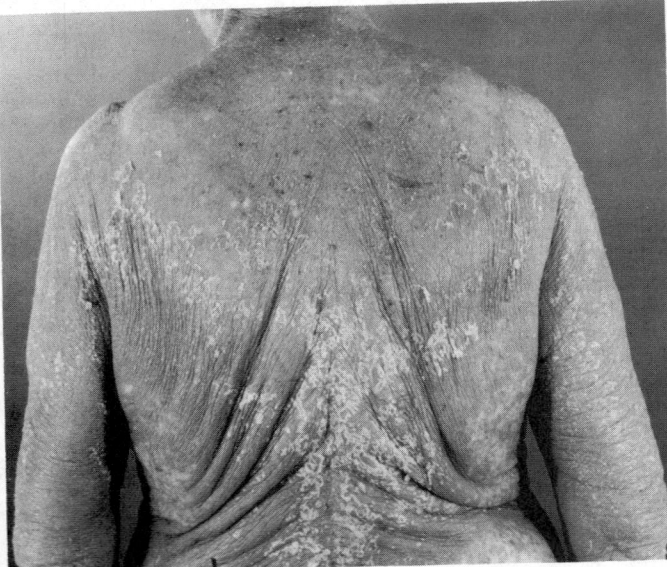

FIGURE 525–1. Exfoliative erythroderma. (From the 17th edition of the Cecil Textbook of Medicine, with permission of Dr. Marie-Louise Johnson.)

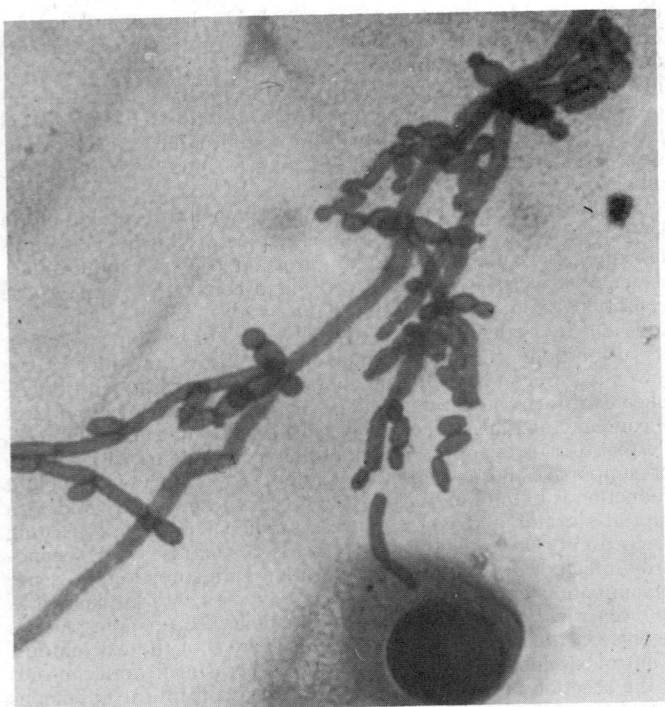

FIGURE 525–2. *Candida albicans.* (From the 17th edition of the Cecil Textbook of Medicine, with the permission of Dr. Marie-Louise Johnson.)

most common), resulting in annular inflamed patches with elevated scaling and, at times, vesicular borders with a tendency for central clearing. The eruption may be widespread and may mimic nummular eczema. Very extensive, red, scaling lesions with elevated serpiginous borders may occur in diabetic and immunosuppressed patients. The usual ringworm of the scalp appears as scaling areas of hair loss with black dots indicating breakage of hair shafts. Most infections are now due to *T. tonsurans* or *M. canis*. The latter agent may fluoresce under Wood's light, but this should not be used for diagnosis. Rather, examination with KOH preparations and cultures for fungi should be performed (using plucked hairs and scales from the affected areas in the scalp). Tinea cruris infection in the groin appears as red patches with elevated serpiginous and scaling borders. The scrotum is seldom involved. Erythrasma is still another type of intertriginous erythema caused by a *Corynebacterium* infection. It appears as velvety red patches with fine scale which, under Wood's light examination, fluoresce a diagnostic coral pink color. Erythromycin clears this infection. Tinea of the feet (pedis) and hands (manus) often present together. Infections of the feet appear in three forms: (1) interdigital maceration, scaling, and fissuring (*T. rubrum* and *T. mentagrophytes*); (2) diffuse, dry, scaling and mild erythema of the plantar surface, often extending onto the sides of the feet in a "moccasin" distribution, occasionally associated with dry scaling of one palm ("two foot–one hand syndrome"); (3) vesiculopustular lesions on the insteps of the feet. Involvement of the nails—onychomycosis—often accompanies hand and foot dermatophytosis.

Candidiasis, particularly involvement by *C. albicans* (Fig. 525–2), causes inflammatory skin reactions. Intertriginous moniliasis occurs in the groin, perineum, gluteal folds, inframammary areas, axillae, and digital webs. Typically, the folds become macerated and erythematous with small satellite papules and erosions around the periphery of the main lesion. Obesity, diabetes, and use of antibiotics may play a role in *Candida* infection. Chronic mucocutaneous candidiasis is a rare condition characterized by superficial *Candida* infection of the skin, nails, and oral and genital mucosal surfaces complicating a variety of systemic immunodeficiencies (see Ch. 405). *Tinea versicolor*, a common superficial fungus infection caused by *Pityrosporon orbiculare*, is identified by scaling, red to brown or white, oval patches over the neck, trunk, and upper arms. As the name versicolor implies, the lesions vary in color (Fig. 525–3). During the summer months when the skin is exposed to ultraviolet light, the lesions appear hypopigmented, as the infection prevents the involved skin from forming pigment. Examination of the lesion with KOH reveals budding yeast forms and club-shaped hyphae (Fig. 525–4).

Treatment of fungal infections of the skin can be accomplished with topical or systemic agents. If the dermatophytic or candidal glabrous skin infection is localized, econazole, miconazole, clotrimazole, and ciclopirox creams, ointments, and lotions are effective when applied two to three times a day for 3 to 4 weeks. Tinea versicolor also responds to these agents, but selenium sulfide antidandruff shampoo is less expensive and also effective. Application of the shampoo to the involved areas of skin for 10

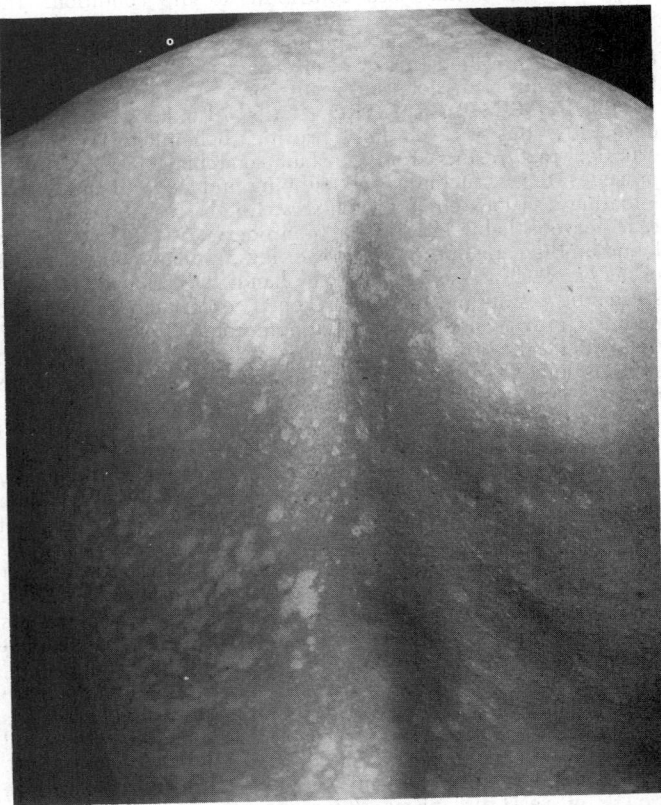

FIGURE 525–3. Tinea versicolor. (From the 17th edition of the Cecil Textbook of Medicine, with the permission of Dr. Marie-Louise Johnson.)

minutes each night for 3 to 4 weeks will clear the disease, although the hypopigmentation will not resolve until the patient is exposed to the sun. Regular shampooing with selenium sulfide reduces reinfection rates. Widespread fungal lesions, or those resistant to topical therapy, may require systemic agents. Griseofulvin is an effective, safe agent and the treatment of choice for dermatophyte infections, but it is not effective for *Candida* infections. The drug must be given for varying periods of time, depending on the site of infection. The micronized form (Ultra-fine, U/F) seems to be most consistently effective. Approximately 10 mg per kilogram per day is used in children and 1 gram per day in adults (see Table 524–4).

Ketoconazole is a second oral medication useful for dermatophytes, but it is also effective in *Candida* infections. Because ketoconazole occasionally causes severe liver damage, it should not be used initially for dermatophyte infections. It is useful in mucocutaneous candidiasis at a dose of 200 to 400 mg per day in adults. Because of its toxicity, liver function tests should be performed every 2 to 4 weeks.

MACULOPAPULAR SKIN DISEASES

The rashes included in this group represent diverse cutaneous and systemic conditions characterized by widespread erythematous macules and papules. Some of the conditions also have associated petechiae or purpura (Table 525–2).

VIRAL EXANTHEMS. Because many *viral exanthems* are maculopapular, this group of skin diseases is often termed morbilliform, or measles-like. The clinical appearance of virus-induced erythema is not specific for a given etiologic agent; other signs and symptoms help to suggest a particular viral agent. Most viral exanthems are preceded by a prodrome of fever and constitutional symptoms. A history of previous exposure to infected individuals may be obtained. Incubation times vary from days to weeks depending on the virus. Drug history may also be important, especially with infectious mononucleosis, in which only 3 per cent of patients have a maculopapular or petechial eruption, but with the administration of ampicillin the frequency approaches 100 per cent. In measles (rubeola) and rubella, the erythematous macules and papules begin on the face and spread to the trunk and extremities, fading with desquamation in 6 days in rubeola and on the third day in rubella. The rashes associated with enterovirus infection are most commonly rubella-like but occasionally are purpuric. Exanthem subitum (roseola infantum) displays fleeting, discrete, red papules surrounded by a whitish halo that begins on the trunk and then evolves on the neck. Erythema infectiosum (fifth disease) is an alarming-appearing red, "slapped cheek" rash over the face with reticulate maculopapular lesions on the extremities that clear in 3 to 6 days. Mucous membranes are sometimes involved. In rubella, red spots occur on the soft palate. In measles, Koplik's spots, tiny gray-white papules on an erythematous base, are found on the buccal mucosa opposite the molars. An erythematous, maculopapular rash that begins peripherally on the palms and soles and spreads to the trunk, often with a petechial component, is seen in *atypical measles*. This is a hypersensitivity reaction to wild measles virus in a partially immune host (one who has been vaccinated with killed measles virus).

SCARLETINIFORM ERUPTIONS. Scarlet fever, *Kawasaki's syndrome*, and *toxic shock syndrome* also present with erythematous macular and papular eruptions. Group A streptococcal pharyngitis or tonsillitis with a strain producing erythrogenic toxin initiates a confluent, papular eruption with sandpaper texture that begins on the neck and upper chest and evolves over the abdomen and extremities. The face is flushed, and circumoral pallor is prominent. Extensive desquamation occurs in 4 to 5 days. Punctate redness of the palate is seen in scarlet fever along with strawberry tongue.

Kawasaki's syndrome, a condition of unknown cause, displays a morbilliform or scarletiniform eruption more prominent on the trunk than on the face. Most distinctive are magenta red discolorations of the palms and soles associated with indurative edema of the hands and feet. The skin and extremity changes occur within 3 to 4 days of the onset of fever, along with mucous membrane inflammatory changes consisting of conjunctivitis and strawberry tongue. Palm, sole, and fingertip desquamation occurs 10 to 18 days after the onset of fever. Asymmetric lymphadenopathy, especially in the cervical area, is seen in 75 per cent of patients—hence the name *mucocutaneous lymph node syndrome*. This is a disease of young children and occasionally young adults, and 1 to 2 per cent of these individuals develop coronary aneurysms or myocardial infarction, sometimes fatal.

Toxic shock syndrome is a serious condition arising from toxins elaborated by *Staphylococcus aureus* infections, often in menstruating women using tampons but also in patients with post-surgical infections. The rash is an erythematous, macular, diffuse eruption that blanches readily with pressure followed by desquamation of the affected skin, in association with fever, strawberry tongue, hypotension, vomiting, and renal insufficiency. The rash often spares the skin where clothing fits tightly with pressure on the skin, e.g., waistline where underwear elastic and belt press tightly.

DRUG REACTIONS. The most common forms taken by drug eruptions are hives and morbilliform rashes (Fig. 525–5). The erythematous macules and papules that often become confluent usually begin within a week of initiating the drug. Unfortunately,

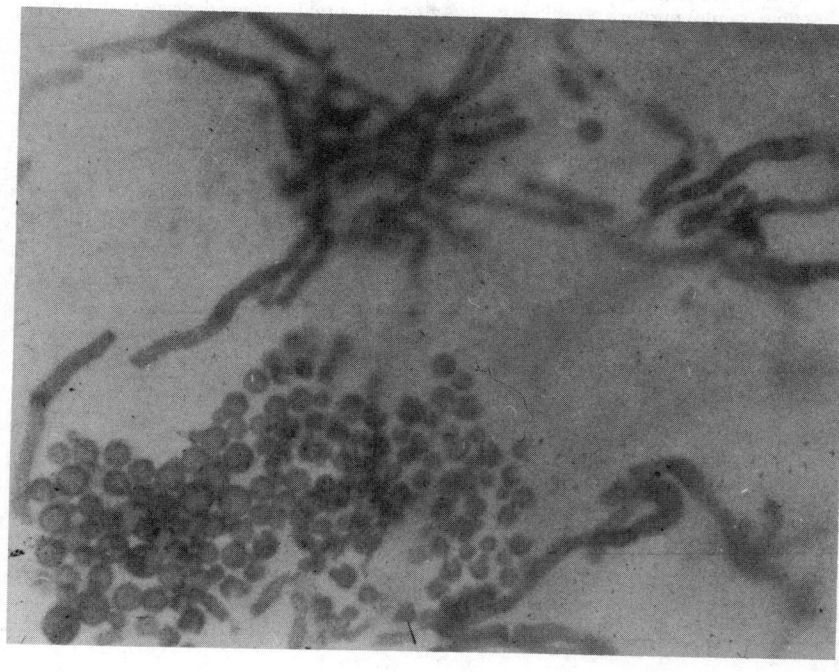

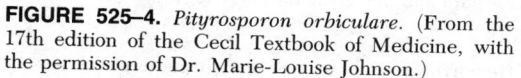

FIGURE 525–4. *Pityrosporon orbiculare.* (From the 17th edition of the Cecil Textbook of Medicine, with the permission of Dr. Marie-Louise Johnson.)

there are no laboratory tests to identify a responsible drug, so heavy reliance must be placed on the history. Often patients are taking several drugs. In trying to select the offending medication from the list, two variables to consider are (1) the temporal relationship between the initiation of the drug and the rash and (2) the odds that a given drug is likely to cause an eruption. Drugs most likely to cause maculopapular eruptions include trimethoprim-sulfamethoxazole, penicillin G, semisynthetic penicillins, ampicillin, quinidine, gentamicin sulfate, and blood products. Itching is common with drug reactions, and fever may occur. It is difficult to differentiate the maculopapular drug rash from viral exanthems except that viral prodromata and viral mucous membrane lesions are lacking in drug rashes (see section on drug reactions at the end of this chapter).

Verruca vulgaris and *molluscum contagiosum* are two examples of viral infections confined to the skin which elicit unique papular lesions. Wart papilloma virus induces various forms of warts: *common warts*, dome-shaped papules with corrugated, hyperkeratotic surfaces; *flat warts*, slightly raised, smooth, flat-topped papules often on the hands and face; *plantar warts*, painful papules on the soles of the feet covered by a thick callus with black puncta within the lesion; *condylomata acuminata*, or veneral warts, soft, moist, sessile, pedunculated and verrucous papules involving the perianal and genital areas. *Molluscum*

contagiosum is caused by a DNA poxvirus that infects epidermal cells to induce smooth, dome-shaped, translucent papules with a central umbilication from which a cheesy core can be expressed. These lesions occur most commonly on the trunk, face, and genitals. The treatment of warts relies on a variety of nonspecific destructive techniques, including liquid nitrogen cryotherapy, salicylic and lactic acid combinations, cantharidin, and podophyllin. Molluscum contagiosum lesions are removed by curettage of the central core, liquid nitrogen freezing, or cantharidin application for short periods of time (30 to 60 minutes).

Purpuric maculopapular skin lesions should cause the physician to consider a different group of conditions (Table 525–2). Purpura, because it represents extravasation of red blood cells outside the cutaneous vessels, cannot be blanched as erythema can. Purpura can be classified as nonpalpable (macular) and palpable (papular). Nonpalpable purpura results from bleeding into the skin without associated inflammation of the vessels and indicates either a bleeding diathesis or blood vessel fragility. Nonpalpable purpura can be *petechial* (macules less than 3 mm) or *ecchymotic* (macules larger than 3 mm). Thrombocytopenia causes petechiae, whereas abnormalities in the blood-clotting cascade commonly cause ecchymoses. Necrotic ecchymoses are found when thrombi form in dermal vessels, leading to infarction and hemorrhage as in disseminated intravascular coagulation (DIC). Palpable purpura results from inflammatory damage to cutaneous blood vessels, the inflammation causing elevated lesions as in vasculitis (see Color Plate 15H).

TABLE 525–2. SOME MACULAR AND PAPULAR SKIN CONDITIONS

Clinical Condition	Etiology	Distinctive Diagnostic Features
Nonpetechial or Nonpurpuric		
Viral exanthem	Hematologic dissemination of virus to skin where vascular response is elicited	Rubella, rubeola—begin on face; mucous membranes often involved—Koplik's spots; palate petechiae rash preceded by fever and prodromata
Scarlet fever	*Streptococcus* erythrogenic toxin	Sore throat preceding rash; bright erythema that feels like sand paper; desquamates; strawberry tongue
Kawasaki's disease	Unknown	Morbilliform or scarletiniform rash; red palms and soles; desquamation of hands and feet 10 to 18 days after fever
Toxic shock syndrome	*Staphylococcus aureus* toxin	Diffuse, maculopapular rash sparing areas where clothing presses on skin; associated with strawberry tongue, fever, vomiting, and renal insufficiency
Drug eruptions	Drugs	Often rash begins proximally and proceeds distally—legs involved last; no prodromata
Verruca vulgaris	Papillomavirus	Corrugated, hyperkeratotic papule
Molluscum contagiosum	Poxvirus	Smooth, dome-shaped, translucent papules with central umbilication
Petechial or Purpuric Component		
Nonpalpable Purpura Thrombocytopenic and blood clotting abnormalities	Thrombocytopenia	Petechiae and ecchymoses in dependent areas
Actinic (senile) purpura	Aging and chronic actinic damage to dermal collagen	Flat ecchymoses, usually on arms
Steroids	Thin dermis by decreasing dermal collagen	Flat ecchymoses on arms, legs
Amyloidosis of skin	Infiltration of dermal vessels by amyloid makes them more fragile	Petechiae and purpura with or without waxy papules around eyes; can be precipitated by trauma, including pinching ("pinch" purpura)
Ehlers-Danlos syndrome	Several variants, all with defects in collagen formation leading to decreased support and increased fragility of cutaneous blood vessels	Easy bruising of skin and joint hyperelasticity
Shamberg's disease	Capillaritis of dermal vessels—usually unknown cause, occasionally due to drugs	Hyperpigmentation with petechiae superimposed, usually on legs
Hypergammaglobulinemic purpura	Hypergammaglobulinemia of variety of causes associated with immune complex damage to blood vessels	Purpura and petechiae on lower legs
Disseminated intravascular coagulation	Intravascular clotting causes thrombosis in blood vessels with subsequent purpura and skin necrosis; induced by infections, malignancies	Hemorrhagic and purpuric star-shaped ecchymoses with skin necrosis and deep hemorrhagic crusts
Infections Causing Purpura Meningococcemia, disseminated gonococcemia, Rocky Mountain spotted fever, subacute bacterial endocarditis	Direct invasions of blood vessels by infective organisms or hypersensitivity vascular damage to vessels—Shwartzman reaction or immune complex reactions	Varying forms of petechiae and purpura in skin and mucous membranes
Palpable Purpura Vasculitis	Immune complex disease	Palpable purpuric lesions, ulcers on legs can be seen with drugs, infections, collagen vascular disease and underlying malignancies

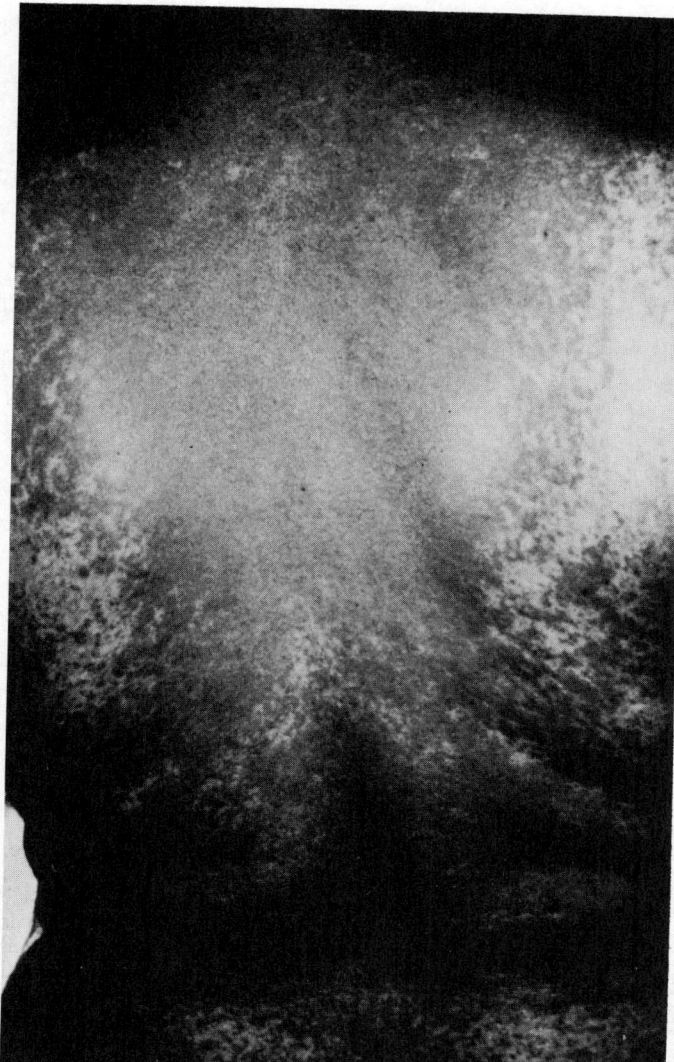

FIGURE 525–5. Drug eruption. (From the 17th edition of the Cecil Textbook of Medicine, with permission of Dr. Marie-Louise Johnson.)

shaped) purpuric ecchymoses with necrotic centers. The center of the lesion is dark gray, indicative of necrosis and impending slough. Petechiae are seen, and hemorrhagic bullae, acral cyanosis, mucosal bleeding, and prolonged bleeding from wound sites can occur. Patients may be systemically ill with fever, shock, and renal failure.

A variety of infectious diseases cause cutaneous petechiae, purpura, or ecchymoses. Already mentioned is *meningococcemia*, in which the organisms produce acute vasculitis or local Shwartzman-like reactions with erythematous macules, petechiae, purpura, and ecchymosis on the trunk and legs. These may become confluent, often with central necrosis. Patients with acute meningococcemia are ill with fever, malaise, headache, meningeal signs, and hypotension. The skin lesions of *disseminated gonococcemia* begin as tiny red papules and petechiae and then evolve into painful purpuric pustules and vesicles scattered on the distal extremities. Fever, polyarthritis, or monoarticular arthritis may be present. The rash of *Rocky Mountain spotted fever* appears between the second and sixth day of the illness, initially as small, erythematous macules that blanch on pressure but then evolving into petechiae, purpura, and ecchymoses. The rash first occurs on the acral areas and then spreads to the extremities and trunk. Small areas of necrosis may occur on the fingers, toes, and ear lobes. Fever, severe headache, toxicity, confusion, and myalgias commonly occur. *Infective endocarditis* is associated with petechial and purpuric skin lesions. Petechiae appear in crops in the conjunctivae, buccal mucosa, upper chest, and extremities. Splinter hemorrhages (linear, red to brown streaks under the fingernails or toenails); Osler nodes (2- to 15-mm, tender, red nodules on the pads of the fingers and toes); and Janeway lesions (small, painless plaques and palpable, purpuric nodules on the palms or soles) may be seen. The skin lesions are related to immune complex vasculitis or septic emboli.

PALPABLE PURPURAS. *Vasculitis* and *necrotizing angiitis* are terms used in disorders in which there is segmental inflammation in the blood vessel wall with accumulation of neutrophils and fibrinoid necrosis. The vascular reaction is mediated by immune complexes. Papules with purpura result from extravasation of blood from the damaged vessels. Although all sizes of blood vessels may be affected, the vasculitis in the skin involves venules. If the process is extensive or if large vessels are involved, skin necrosis and ulceration may occur. Depending upon the size of the blood vessels affected, at least five types of vasculitis may involve the skin. The size and type of vessels in the skin, in turn, determine the kind of morphologic lesion (Table 525–3).

In general, as the vasculitis involves progressively larger and more deeply situated vessels, the skin lesions become more nodular, with larger ulcerative or gangrenous processes. The term *granulomatous vasculitis* refers to angiitis associated with a histiocytic proliferation that also involves necrotizing granulomas in the connective tissue of multiple organs, causing rhinorrhea, sinusitis, cough, arthralgias, and ocular and neurologic symptoms (Churg-Strauss vasculitis).

Necrotizing leukocytoclastic vasculitis can occur in a variety of settings including (1) sepsis, (2) connective tissue disease—especially systemic lupus erythematosus and rheumatoid arthritis, (3) cryoglobulinemia, (4) drug reactions, and, occasionally, (5) underlying carcinomas, lymphomas, or leukemias. In many instances no apparent cause is found.

Circulating immune complexes have been demonstrated in patients with necrotizing angiitis. Immunoglobulins and complement are found in the affected vessel wall by direct immunofluorescence. The immune complexes lodge in the small vessel walls and activate the complement system, forming the anaphylatoxins C3a and C5a, which recruit neutrophils that induce inflammatory and necrotic damage to the vessel with accompanying fragmented nuclei of the neutrophils (so-called nuclear dust).

Several syndromes are associated with leukocytoclastic vasculitis, depending on the organ systems affected. *Henoch-Schönlein syndrome* occurs most often in children, frequently preceded by an upper respiratory infection and accompanied by arthralgias, abdominal pain, and renal vasculitis. IgA is usually found along with complement in the involved vessels on direct immunofluorescence. *Hypocomplementemic vasculitis* is characterized by urticaria-like lesions, arthritis, and low serum complement. IgG

NONPALPABLE PURPURAS. Nonpalpable purpuras include thrombocytopenic conditions, senile or actinic purpura, blood clotting abnormalities, Schamberg's disease, hypergammaglobulinemic conditions, and disseminated intravascular coagulation. *Actinic (senile) purpura* is a common problem in older individuals, the result of increased vessel fragility reflecting dermal connective tissue damage from chronic sun exposure and aging. Minor trauma induces ecchymoses, usually on the dorsum of the hands and forearms. The skin in these areas is thin and fragile. Topically or systemically administered steroids can induce similar purpura. Other causes of vascular fragility of the skin include *amyloidosis* and the *Ehlers-Danlos* syndrome. *Schamberg's disease*, or *pigmented purpuric dermatitis*, is an idiopathic capillaritis that causes petechial lesions of the lower legs (occasionally the arms and trunk) in association with hyperpigmentation. The lesions have the appearance of cayenne pepper. Occasionally Schamberg's disease is secondary to a drug reaction. Petechiae and purpura also occur in *hypergammaglobulinemic purpura*, a syndrome characterized by episodes of fever and arthralgias, which appear to be the result of immune complex–mediated damage to small blood vessels. *Disseminated intravascular coagulation* (DIC) refers to uncontrolled clotting within blood vessels with the formation of diffuse thrombosis. The skin is frequently involved with hemorrhage, ecchymosis, and infarction. DIC occurs in association with bacterial sepsis (particularly meningococcemia), as a postviral or poststreptococcal infection phenomenon (*purpura fulminans*), or in conjunction with malignancies such as prostatic carcinoma and acute myelocytic leukemia. The most distinctive hemorrhagic skin lesions are stellate (star-

and C3 are present in vessels taken from early skin lesions. Facial and laryngeal edema may also occur. A third form consists of purpura, arthralgia, weakness, and *mixed cryoglobulinemia* (mixed cryoglobulins contain IgG and IgM with anti-IgG or rheumatoid factor activity), which may be idiopathic or occasionally associated with systemic lupus erythematosus, infectious mononucleosis, lymphomas, or primary biliary cirrhosis.

If the vasculitis is idiopathic and cutaneous, the skin responds to prednisone (60 to 80 mg per day) or dapsone (100 to 150 mg per day). Systemic vasculitides may require prednisone and cyclophosphamide (2 mg per kilogram per day).

Necrotizing cutaneous vasculitis may occur in association with *hepatitis B* and in patients with *intestinal bypass surgery* for morbid obesity or in patients with jejunal diverticula or other gastrointestinal conditions characterized by bacterial overgrowth. An *arthritis-dermatitis syndrome* with intestinal bypass surgery may occur with polyarthritis and palpable purpura or purpuric nodules and pustules on the trunk, legs, feet, and arms. Antigenic components of the intestinal bacterial overgrowth lead to the formation of cryoprotein immune complexes that deposit in the skin and joints, causing a hypersensitivity vasculitis and nondeforming arthritis. Antibiotics such as chloramphenicol, sulfamethoxazole-trimethoprim, tetracycline, and metronidazole have been reported to improve the condition.

PAPULOSQUAMOUS SKIN DISEASES

Unique scales are the common characteristic of diseases in this group. *Squamous* refers to scaling that represents thickened stratum corneum and thus implies an abnormal keratinization process. The lesions, in addition to being scaly, are characterized by sharply demarcated, red to violaceous papules and plaques that result from thickening of the epidermis and/or underlying dermal inflammation.

The papulosquamous disorders have diverse etiologies and include psoriasis, Reiter's syndrome, pityriasis rosea, lichen planus, pityriasis rubra pilaris, secondary syphilis, mycosis fungoides, and ichthyosiform eruptions (Table 525–4).

PSORIASIS. Psoriasis is a genetically determined, chronic epidermal proliferative disease of unpredictable course. Onset is most frequent in early adult life, but it may begin at any age. Once the disease becomes manifest, it may remain localized to a few areas or may cause intermittent or continuous generalized disease.

The lesions appear as erythematous papules and plaques surmounted by silvery, thick scales that resemble mica (micaceous) and that are easily removed and may accumulate in the patient's clothing or bed (Fig. 525–6). In intertriginous areas maceration prevents scales from accumulating, but the lesions remain red and sharply defined. Classically, lesions are distributed symmetrically over areas of bony prominence such as elbows and knees. They also commonly occur on the trunk and scalp and in the intergluteal cleft. The latter two areas are frequently overlooked.

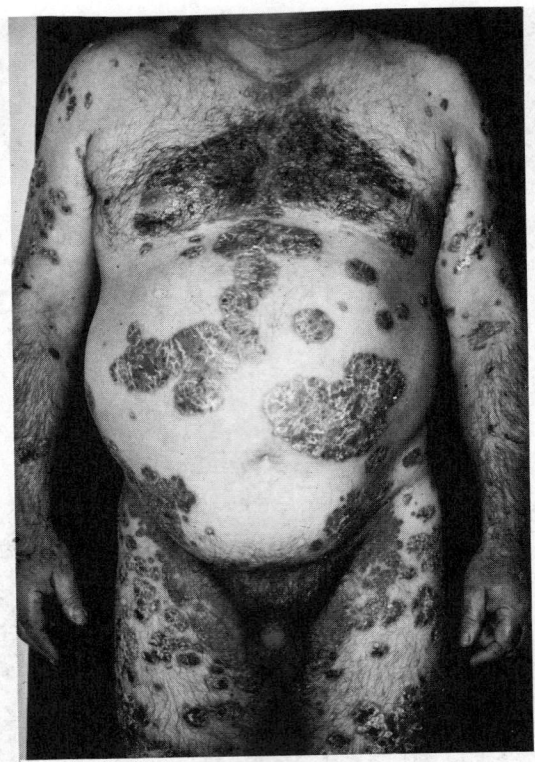

FIGURE 525–6. Psoriasis. (From the 17th edition of the Cecil Textbook of Medicine, with the permission of Dr. Marie-Louise Johnson.)

Palms and soles may be involved, with diffuse redness, scaling, and, at times, pustular lesions. Nail involvement occurs in up to 50 per cent of patients. The nails may be pitted with small ice pick–like depressions on the surface of the nail plate. Onycholysis can also occur, in which a plaque of psoriasis in the distal nail bed causes a red-brown discoloration that is reminiscent of an oil stain under the nail. Another helpful diagnostic feature is the Koebner phenomenon, in which intense trauma to the skin induces new skin lesions. Thus, scratches or surgical incisions elicit linear papulosquamous lesions that should alert the physician to the diagnosis. This may also explain the high incidence of psoriasis on the elbows and knees. Other aggravating factors include streptococcal infections, emotional stress, overuse of alcohol, and drugs, including lithium and beta blockers. Several common variants of psoriasis may also be seen: (1) *guttate psoriasis*, in which numerous, small papular lesions with silvery scales evolve suddenly over the body, often 1 to 3 weeks following streptococcal pharyngitis; (2) *inverse psoriasis*, in which plaques evolve in intertriginous areas and thus lack the typical silver scale because of maceration and moisture; (3) *pustular psoriasis*, a form

TABLE 525–3. TYPES OF VASCULITIS AND ASSOCIATED SKIN LESIONS

Type of Vasculitis	Blood Vessels Involved	Type of Skin Lesion
Leukocytoclastic or hypersensitivity angiitis: Henoch-Schönlein purpura, cryoglobulinemia, hypocomplementemic vasculitis	Dermal capillaries, venules, and occasional small muscular arteries in internal organs	Purpuric papules, hemorrhagic bullae, cutaneous infarcts
Rheumatic vasculitis: systemic lupus erythematosus; rheumatoid vasculitis	Dermal capillaries, venules, and small muscular arteries in internal organs	Purpuric papules; ulcerative nodules; splinter hemorrhages; periungual telangiectasia and infarcts
Granulomatous vasculitis		
Churg and Strauss allergic granulomatous angiitis	Dermal small and larger muscular arteries and medium muscular arteries in subcutaneous tissue and other organs	Erythematous, purpuric, and ulcerated nodules, plaques, and purpura
Wegener's granulomatosis	Small venules, arterioles of dermis, and small muscular arteries	Ulcerative nodules; peripheral gangrene
Periarteritis: classic type limited to skin and muscle	Small and medium muscular arteries in deep dermis, subcutaneous tissue, and muscle	Deep subcutaneous nodules with ulceration; livedo reticularis; ecchymoses
Giant cell arteritis: temporal arteritis, polymyalgia rheumatica, Takayasu's disease	Medium muscular arteries and larger arteries	Skin necrosis over scalp

of the disease in which superficial pustules occur in one of three presentations—pustules studding typical plaques; pustules confined to the palms and soles; and a rare generalized eruption in which pustules evolve abruptly on large areas of erythematous skin accompanied by fever and leukocytosis; (4) *erythroderma*—occasionally the psoriasis can become generalized to involve erythema and scaling of the entire integument. This may occur secondary to a general Koebner phenomenon with overvigorous therapy, a drug reaction, or withdrawal of oral steroids; (5) *psoriatic arthritis*—arthritis may accompany psoriasis in 10 to 15 per cent of cases.

At times Reiter's syndrome may be confused with psoriasis. The skin lesions of the two disorders are indistinguishable clinically and histologically. In Reiter's syndrome pustular and hyperkeratotic papules and plaques commonly occur on the palms and soles (keratoderma blenorrhagica) and scaling, red patches evolve encircling the glans penis and within the groin (balanitis circinata). The presence of asymptomatic erosions on the tongue and buccal mucosa, urethritis, iritis or conjunctivitis, arthritis, and occasionally diarrhea should suggest the diagnosis.

The pathogenesis of psoriasis is unknown, but it appears to be a multifactorial disease in patients who are genetically predisposed. There is an increased prevalence of psoriasis in individuals with HLA antigens BW17, B13, and BW37. Thirty per cent of patients have a family history of disease. The basic alteration represents an accelerated cell cycle in an increased number of dividing cells, culminating in rapid epidermal cell proliferation. Cellular turnover is increased sevenfold, and the transit time from the basal layer to the top of the stratum corneum is 3 or 4 days rather than the usual 28 days. This rapid turnover of keratinocytes alters keratinization, resulting in thickened epidermis (seen as papules and plaques) and parakeratotic stratum corneum (silvery scales). The basic mechanism underlying this benign proliferative reaction is unknown.

The goal of therapy is to decrease epidermal proliferation and underlying dermal inflammation. There is no curative agent for psoriasis, and treatment suppresses the condition only as long as it is administered. Three types of topical therapies are employed: (1) topical steroids, usually with intermediate and strong potency agents administered once or twice a day; (2) topical tars and anthralin preparations, often used once a day in combination with topical steroids; (3) ultraviolet light, either UVB with tar or UVA with oral psoralens (see Ch. 524).

Two systemic types of therapy are available, but because of their side effects these should be reserved for severe widespread disease that is unresponsive to topical measures: (1) antimetabolites or antimitotic agents, including methotrexate, azathioprine, and hydroxyurea. The most commonly used is methotrexate in low doses, usually given on a weekly basis. Because these agents affect bone marrow and liver (in the case of methotrexate), complete blood counts and liver function tests should be performed regularly, together with intermittent liver biopsies. (2) Etretinate, a retinoid, is particularly useful in pustular and erythrodermic forms of psoriasis. Careful monitoring of blood counts, plasma triglycerides, and liver function is required, and avoidance of pregnancy during the use of this drug is mandatory.

PITYRIASIS ROSEA. Oval or round, tannish pink or salmon colored, scaling papules and plaques appear rapidly over the

TABLE 525–4. PAPULOSQUAMOUS SKIN DISEASES

Disease	Appearance of Lesion	Distribution	Mucous Membrane Involvement	Other Features
Psoriasis	Erythematous plaques with silvery, mica-like scales, usually nonpruritic	Anywhere: scalp, knees, elbows, intergluteal cleft favored; symmetric	None	Koebner phenomenon, nail involvement, arthritis
Reiter's syndrome	Erythematous, silvery scaled plaques; hyperkeratotic papules of palms and soles (keratoderma blennorrhagicum)	Similar to psoriasis	Frequent: mouth, genitals; balanitis circinata	Nail involvement, arthritis, urethritis, conjunctivitis, iritis
Pityriasis rosea	Tannish pink, oval papules and plaques with delicate collarette scale; may or may not be pruritic	Rash preceded by herald patch, Christmas tree pattern on trunk; spares face, extremities	None	May be associated with upper respiratory infection; drugs may cause similar rash
Secondary syphilis	Ham red or copper colored scaling papules and plaques, sometimes annular	Generalized: palms and soles often involved	Mucous patches, often white or red; condyloma warts of anal area	Condylomata in genital area; serologic test for syphilis positive
Lichen planus	Violaceous polygonal, flat-topped papules with white scale or Wickham's striae. May be hyperkeratotic, annular, or bullous lesions; pruritic	Often on wrists and ankles, but can be generalized; Koebner reaction	Frequent reticulated white patches or erosive lesions in mouth or genital areas	Occasionally involves nails; drugs can cause similar reaction
Pityriasis rubra pilaris	Red, scaling plaques and patches with follicular horny excretions, especially on dorsum of hands and fingers; diffuse, yellow hyperkeratoses of palms and soles	Often diffuse, rough scaling erythema involving entire body with islands of normal skin	Occasionally lacy white plaques in mouth	Remits spontaneously in 2–4 years; nail changes as in psoriasis
Pityriasis lichenoides et varioliformis acuta (Mucha-Habermann disease)	Red, discrete, palpable papules that vesiculate and then become hemorrhagic, crust, scale, and leave a scar	Scattered lesions over trunk and extremities	May resemble leukocytoclastic vasculitis	May resolve in a few months or persist for years
Pityriasis lichenoides et varioliformis chronica (chronic parapsoriasis)	Guttate to larger, red, slightly scaling papules and plaques; nonpruritic	Usually on trunk	Some forms may represent early stages of mycosis fungoides	Responds to UVB light treatments
Mycosis fungoides	Persistent, pruritic, red, thickened plaques with fine scales as seen in eczema, or thick mica-like scales suggestive of psoriasis; may ulcerate	Scattered asymmetrically over trunk, extremities; girdle area often first area involved	Neoplastic T-cell lymphoma	May show islands of normal skin within red areas
Ichthyosis	A variety of syndromes with variation in scaling skin; fine, light scales to large, thick, coarse, verrucous scales that resemble fish skin; hyperkeratosis of palms and soles	Variable distribution but can involve flexural or extensor surfaces of extremities or trunk	Autosomal dominant, recessive, and X-linked recessive conditions	See Table 525–5

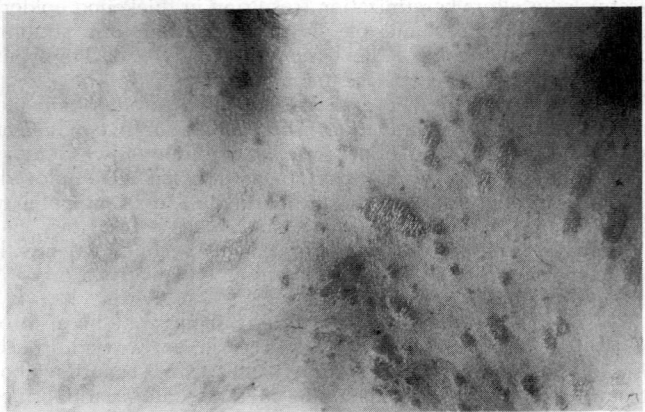

FIGURE 525–7. Pityriasis rosea. (From the 17th edition of the Cecil Textbook of Medicine, with the permission of Dr. Marie-Louise Johnson.)

trunk, neck, upper arms, and legs (Fig. 525–7). Several features of this self-limited papulosquamous condition are unique. First, the generalized eruption is preceded by a single lesion, termed the "herald patch," that is commonly misdiagnosed as "ringworm." The herald patch can occur anywhere but often appears on the neck or lower trunk area and precedes the general rash by several days to a week. Second, the oval patches have an unusual fine, white scale located near the border of the plaques, forming a collarette. Third, the lesions follow skin cleavage lines, in a pattern likened to a Christmas tree. Last, the condition spontaneously involutes in 1 to 2 months. Recurrences are rare. Itching occasionally is a prominent symptom.

Pityriasis rosea occasionally is preceded by a mild upper respiratory infection, and its greatest incidence is in the winter months, suggesting a viral etiology. However, the disease does not occur endemically and is not transmitted person to person.

Such conditions as tinea corporis and guttate psoriasis may be considered in the differential diagnosis, but two possibilities should always be entertained: drug eruption and secondary syphilis. If the rash persists longer than 2 or 3 months or generalizes to involve the trunk, extremities, and especially the face, a drug reaction should be considered. Such medications as gold compounds, barbiturates, captopril, clonidine, and tripelennamide can cause such a rash. Secondary syphilis should be suspected and a serologic test obtained if the rash involves palms and soles and if fever, coryza, or mucous membrane erosions (socalled mucous patches) are present.

Treatment of pityriasis rosea is usually not necessary, although topical corticosteroids and antihistamines may relieve itching and decrease erythema. Ultraviolet light (UVB), given as three to five treatments eliciting a mild erythema reaction, often clears the rash.

LICHEN PLANUS. This idiopathic, pruritic, inflammatory condition of the skin is included in the papulosquamous group of diseases because the primary lesion is a unique papule. The papules are flat topped (planus) and polygonal in configuration (i.e., the sides conform to normal fine skin folds) and have a lilac or purple hue. They may have visible scales on their surface, but more characteristic are subtle, fine white dots or white reticulated lines (Wickham's striae) surmounting the shiny, flat tops (resembling the appearance of a lichen). Wickham's striae are more visible under a hand lens after the application of a drop of mineral oil to the surface of the papule. The Koebner phenomenon occurs

in lichen planus, so linear streaks of papules at the sites of skin trauma may be noted.

Although lichen planus can occur anywhere on the body, typical locations are the ankles, wrists, mouth, and genitalia. There may be only a few papules or innumerable ones in a generalized distribution. Mucous membranes are commonly involved, the lesions appearing most frequently as asymptomatic white streaks in a reticulated pattern on the buccal mucosa, tongue, gums, or lips. At times blisters and erosions are superimposed (erosive lichen planus), causing severe discomfort. Lichen planus involving the male genitalia may appear as violaceous annular lesions. Rarely, lichen planus may appear as violaceous annular and polycyclic lesions on the legs and arms, or as hyperkeratotic, follicular, scarring alopecia. All lichen planus lesions leave residual hyperpigmented macules in their wake.

The etiology of lichen planus is not known, but two conditions may mimic lichen planus skin lesions and thus offer clues to an immune etiology. Certain drugs such as thiazides, phenothiazines, gold, quinidine, and antimalarials can cause lichen planus–like, generalized eruptions. Second, some patients with graftversus-host disease also develop a skin reaction that closely resembles lichen planus. The eruption can evolve into the usual chronic graft-versus-host sequelae of diffuse dermal sclerosis, cicatricial alopecia, reticulated pigmentation, and ulceration.

Lichen planus tends to be a chronic condition lasting for months to years. Perhaps two thirds of patients experience spontaneous resolution in 1 to 2 years. In general, the more acute, intense, and widespread the eruption, the more likely it is that an early remission may occur.

Treatment is nonspecific and often unsuccessful. Topical steroids help suppress the inflammatory reaction and itching. Severe oral lichen planus may respond to etretinate.

PITYRIASIS RUBRA PILARIS. This idiopathic papulosquamous and keratotic disease has an uncertain and often chronic course. The condition can appear in a familial form (autosomal dominant) with onset in infancy or childhood or as an acquired disease evolving during the fourth to sixth decades. In either form the following features help in diagnosis: (1) diffuse salmon color of involved skin with sharply bordered residual areas of normal skin (so-called island sparing), (2) waxy, yellow keratoderma of palms and soles similar to carnauba wax, and (3) erythematous hyperkeratotic papules on the dorsal surfaces of the proximal portions of the phalanges. The condition remits spontaneously in 2 to 4 years in 80 per cent of patients. Differentiation from psoriasis may be difficult. The cause of this disease is unknown, although low serum levels of retinol-binding protein have been found. High doses of vitamin A have been reported to help the condition, as has etretinate.

PITYRIASIS LICHENOIDES ET VARIOLIFORMIS ACUTA (MUCHA-HABERMANN DISEASE OR PLEVA). This unusual condition of unknown cause usually begins as widely scattered, red papules that may be purpuric and/or vesicular. Although not initially papulosquamous, the lesions evolve into scaling, eroded, and crusted papules that leave depressed scars in their wake. Lesions develop in crops, often in association with malaise and fever, and persist for months or years. Acute lesions show a lymphocytic vasculitis. No therapy is effective, although tetracycline, systemic corticosteroids, and cytotoxic agents may give short-lived remissions.

ICHTHYOSIS. A variety of inherited and acquired conditions cause rough, dry skin with retained scale simulating fish skin. On close inspection there may be fine scales with keratin-plugged follicles or large, polyhedral, loosely adherent scales.

A number of inherited ichthyosis conditions are recognized (Table 525–5), the most common being *ichthyosis vulgaris*, a dominant trait in which the cells of the stratum corneum are

TABLE 525–5. ICHTHYOSIFORM DERMATOSES

	Inheritance	Onset	Distribution	Clinical Associations	Kinetics
Lamellar ichthyosis	Autosomal recessive	Birth	Body, palms, soles	Ectropion	Increased
Epidermolytic hyperkeratosis	Autosomal dominant	Birth	Predominant flexural involvement	Blisters	Increased
X-linked ichthyosis (steroid sulfatase deficiency)	X-linked	Birth	Trunk	Corneal opacities	Normal
Ichthyosis vulgaris	Autosomal dominant	Childhood	Spares flexural areas	Atopy	Normal

Reprinted from the chapter by Dr. Marie-Louise Johnson in the 17th edition of the Cecil Textbook of Medicine, with her permission.

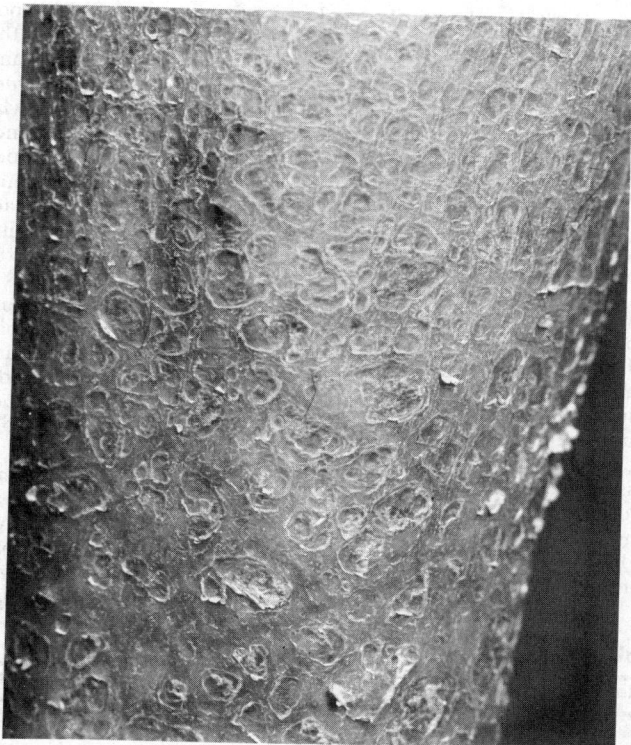

FIGURE 525–8. Ichthyosis. (From the 17th edition of the Cecil Textbook of Medicine, with the permission of Dr. Marie-Louise Johnson.)

retained, forming fishlike or reptilian scales on the extensor surfaces of the extremities (Fig. 525–8). Other forms of ichthyosis such as *lamellar* and *epidermolytic hyperkeratoses* may be associated with considerable erythema and blistering of the skin. Lamellar ichthyosis may be present at birth (collodion baby). A deficiency of steroid sulfatase has been found in association with *X-linked ichthyosis*. Mothers of such babies often have a prolonged labor, as steroid sulfatase appears to play an important role in the parturition process.

Emollients and keratolytic agents (propylene glycol, salicylic acid, lactic acid) are often useful in softening the skin. In severe ichthyosis oral retinoids, such as 13-*cis*-retinoic acid and etretinate, have been beneficial.

VESICULOBULLOUS DISEASES

Vesicles and bullae, when intact, are readily recognized primary skin lesions. Crusts or superficial erosions are secondary lesions that lead one to suspect a preceding fluid-filled primary lesion. The etiology of blistering disease includes bacterial and viral infections, contact dermatitis, and autoimmune and metabolic diseases. The pathogenesis of the blister formation is often helpful in understanding its anatomic location: Blisters occur either within the epidermis (intraepidermal) or at the dermoepidermal junction (subepidermal) (Table 525–6).

Intraepidermal vesicles or bullae usually contain clear fluid (but may become filled with purulent material secondarily) and have very thin roofs, so they are flaccid in appearance and are easily broken. At times the blisters are difficult to recognize, and only erosions, crusts, or the thin shreds of the epidermal blister roofs remain. Subepidermal blisters, on the other hand, have an epidermal roof and are tense and remain intact. Hemorrhagic fluid is common in subepidermal blisters because of their location close to dermal capillaries.

Biopsy of early vesicles or blisters is imperative in diagnosis. Immunofluorescence studies on biopsy material may differentiate certain immunologically mediated diseases. Pathologic studies are most informative when performed early, before therapy has been initiated.

INTRAEPIDERMAL VESICULOBULLOUS DISEASES. Pathologic processes involved in epidermal blister formation include spongiosis, primary cell damage, and acantholysis. Spongiosis, a common form of blister formation in eczematous proc-

esses, represents edema between cells of the prickle layer and liquefaction of cells, which gradually increases the size of the fluid spaces. Primary epidermal cell damage with fluid accumulation is seen in viral infections and friction damage. Blisters may also occur when cellular desmosomal attachments and intercellular cementing substances are immunologically or chemically altered, causing dyshesion referred to as acantholysis (pemphigus).

Bullous impetigo, a subcorneal infection of the skin with staphylococcal and/or streptococcal organisms, causes large, fragile, clear or cloudy bullae that form thin, honey-yellow crusts and a delicate collarette-like remnant of blister roof after the blisters rupture. Autoinoculation results in satellite lesions. The superficial epidermal blistering is caused by the toxic effects of an epidermal toxin elaborated by certain strains of these bacterial organisms.

A more serious variant of bullous impetigo is *staphylococcal scalded skin syndrome,* usually affecting infants and characterized by the formation of rapidly progressive, painful, erythematous patches in which large flaccid bullae evolve and shed as large sheets of skin, leaving a denuded, scalded-appearing surface. With only slight trauma the skin readily slides off, much like wet wallpaper slides off a wall (Nikolsky's sign—see Ch. 523). In contrast to localized bullous impetigo in which the *Staphylococcus aureus* may be recovered in the skin lesions, the bullae of scalded skin syndrome are sterile, although a staphylococcal infection may be found in the conjunctiva, nose, or pharynx. The widespread intraepidermal blistering results from an epidermal toxin elaborated by specific strains of *Staphylococcus* and hematogenously carried to the skin. These are penicillinase-resistant strains of *Staphylococcus* and therefore require methicillin-type antibiotics.

A somewhat similar condition, *toxic epidermal necrolysis* (TEN), occurs in adults, often secondary to drugs (e.g., ampicillin, allopurinol) and occasionally to *Staphylococcus* infections in an immunosuppressed patient. TEN is a reaction to a variety of antigenic materials that cause a suprabasilar split in the epidermis with necrosis of much of the overlying epidermis. Because of the more extensive destruction of epidermis and barrier stratum corneum layer (as opposed to staphylococcal scalded skin syndrome, in which the split is subcorneal), TEN is often fatal and, when extensive, should be treated as a widespread burn would be cared for. TEN also often involves the mucous membranes and therefore may be confused with Stevens-Johnson syndrome (see below).

Viral infections of the skin may cause vesicles and bullae by virtue of direct infection of the keratinocytes and the destructive effect on the cells. Vesicles caused by viruses often display two important characteristics: (1) they tend to occur in groups on an indurated erythematous base, and (2) they often take on an umbilicated appearance.

Herpes simplex is caused by two strains of DNA *Herpesvirus* (type 1, which commonly causes infections above the waist, and type 2, which most frequently is responsible for those in the genital region). Primary infections, gingivostomatitis, and vulvovaginitis, are extensive vesicular eruptions that quickly become necrotic, leaving painful, purulent erosions. The herpesvirus is highly contagious, spread by direct contact with infected individuals. The virus penetrates the epidermal cells, undergoes replicative cycles, and eventually lyses the host cell membrane. The virus is neuropathic, traveling up cutaneous nerves to dorsal nerve root sensory or autonomic ganglia, where it resides in a nonreplicative state. Reactivation of the replicative cycle triggers recurrence, and the virus spreads back down the nerve to induce grouped, umbilicated vesicles on an indurated, red base in areas of the skin innervated by the infected ganglia. Periods of latency vary, and recurrences have a shorter course than primary infections (1 to 2 weeks versus 3 weeks). A number of factors seem to induce recurrences, including fever, ultraviolet light, physical trauma, menstruation, and emotional stress. Recurrences are most common on the lips and face (herpes labialis), genital regions (herpes genitalis), and fingers (herpetic whitlow). *Eczema herpeticum* is a generalized herpes simplex skin infection in areas of atopic dermatitis. Recurrent herpes infections are contagious from the time the vesicular lesions develop to the time the vesicles re-epithelialize. Between attacks there is little chance of causing infection, although perhaps 1 or 2 per cent of individuals may be chronically shedding the virus in the saliva or genital excretions (women may also have active herpes simplex infections of the cervix and be unaware of them).

A complication of herpes simplex infection, *erythema multiforme*, is a hypersensitivity skin and mucous membrane reaction that evolves 1 to 2 weeks following herpetic recurrences as a result of an immune complex reaction to the herpes antigen. Herpes infection is only one etiologic stimulus leading to erythema multiforme (see below).

Diagnosis of herpes infections (including zoster and varicella) is made with a Tzanck preparation of material taken from the roof of vesicles. The contents are smeared onto a slide and stained with Wright's or Giemsa's stain to reveal multinucleated giant cells (see Ch. 523).

Acyclovir administered orally and intravenously is the most frequently used form of therapy for primary and recurrent forms of herpes (see Ch. 371 and Fig. 523–4).

Varicella infection, when initially encountered, causes chickenpox, a generalized pruritic eruption with widespread, delicate vesicles on an erythematous base which have been likened to a dew drop on a rose petal. They often become umbilicated, hemorrhagic, and pustular and may leave scars. Chickenpox lesions occur predominantly on the trunk but also involve the head, extremities, and mucous membranes of the mouth and conjunctiva. Successive crops of lesions evolve for a week. *Herpes zoster* is a recrudescence of latent varicella virus in persons who previously had varicella. It appears as grouped, umbilicated, and, at times, hemorrhagic vesicles and pustules on an erythematous base situated unilaterally along the distribution of cranial or spinal nerves. Frequently several immediately adjacent dermatomes are involved. Bilateral involvement is rare. Zoster is frequently associated with a prodrome of severe radicular pain in the involved areas. A common useful sign in making the diagnosis is hypesthesia of the dermatomal areas—the patient often bitterly complains that the rubbing of clothing on the area is intolerable. Most patients with herpes zoster are over 50 years of age, and cancer patients (especially those with lymphomas such as Hodgkin's disease) are particularly prone to this infection. In such patients or in immunocompromised individuals, cutaneous dissemination from the original dermatome may occur, as well as visceral involvement of liver, lung, and central nervous system. Postherpetic neuralgia is common in individuals over 50. Treatment of herpes zoster is usually symptomatic with Burow's compresses, analgesics, and acyclovir, especially in immunocompromised patients (800 mg five times per day orally for 10 days).

Insect bites including flea and fire ant bites may also induce

TABLE 525–6. VESICULOBULLOUS DISEASES

Location of Blister in Skin	Etiology if Known	Important Physical Findings	Other Facts of Note in History of Laboratory Results
Intraepidermal Blisters			
Bacterial infectious processes			
Bullous impetigo (subcorneal)	Staph toxin	Large, fragile, clear or cloudy bullae that break to leave honey-yellow crusts on face, neck, extremities; erythematous areas that slough as superficial blisters	An initial site may be followed by multiple pruritic autoinoculated sites
Staph scalded skin syndrome—upper epidermal blisters	Staph toxin		
Viral infections			
Herpes simplex, eczema vaccination, herpes zoster varicella (ballooning degeneration)	Direct cell damage	Grouped umbilicated vesicles on erythematous base anywhere on body; diffuse umbilicated vesicles in sites of atopic eczema; unilateral grouped umbilicated, clear or hemorrhagic vesicles in dermatomal distribution	Frequently recurrent; respond to acyclovir
Insect bites	Insect toxins or proteases, delayed hypersensitivity	Papules, bullae—pruritic	Associated with radicular pain and hypesthesia of involved dermatome; respond to acyclovir
Eczema–acute contact (spongiosis)	Type IV hypersensitivity or irritant	Vesiculobullous lesions on red base; often form unusual patterns of contact with substances	
Autoimmune diseases			
a) Pemphigus vulgaris and vegetans (suprabasilar split)	a) Autoimmune interepidermal cell IgG and C3	a) Superficial, flaccid bullae that readily rupture, leaving nonhealing erosions over the body that can cause death; Nikolsky's sign prominent	a) 100% of patients develop mucous membrane blisters, erosions
b) Pemphigus foliaceus and erythematosus (subcorneal split)	b) Autoimmune IgG and/or C3 between cells in upper epidermis	b) Superficial blisters crusting, oozing over scalp and face in seborrhea distribution or butterfly-like rash	b) Seldom see mucous membrane involvement
c) Hailey-Hailey disease (suprabasilar split)	c) Genetically inherited—dominant	c) Superficial erosive blisters, vesicles, pustules in flexural areas of body	c) No mouth lesions
Subepidermal Blisters			
Autoimmune or immunologic			
Bullous pemphigoid	C3 in lamina lucida	Tense bullae on normal or erythematous skin	
Herpes gestationis	C3 in basement membrane zone	Erythematous plaques, tense vesicles, and pruritic bullae that evolve first on abdomen and then on extremities; often polycyclic	Develops during 2nd or 3rd trimester of pregnancy—clears with delivery; increased fetal wastage
Erythema multiforme	Hypersensitivity reaction in blood vessels of dermis to number of antigens—immune complexes seen	Multiforme lesions of red urticaria, papules and target lesions on extremities, palms	Can involve mouth, eyes (Stevens-Johnson syndrome)
Cicatricial pemphigoid	Subepidermal IgG linear in basement membrane zone	Scarring blisters in the mucous membrane; 25% have blisters on skin	Causes blindness; stenosis of urethra, anal areas
Dermatitis herpetiformis (vesicles in dermal papillae)	Immunologic deposition of IgA in dermal papillae	Grouped, symmetrically distributed vesicles and urticarial papules on scalp, scapulae, buttocks, elbows, knees	Intense burning, itch; high incidence of asymptomatic celiac sprue
Metabolic			
Porphyria cutanea tarda	Metabolic defect in porphyrin metabolism	Tense bullae that leave scars in sun-exposed areas; bullae induced by sun, trauma	May also see facial hirsutism and hyperpigmentation
Bullous disease of renal disease	Unknown	Bullae usually in extremities	
Bullous disease in diabetics	Unknown	Large bulla on acral areas	
Mechanicobullous diseases			
Epidermolysis bullosa (split above, below, and within dermal-epidermal zone)	Variety of inherited conditions	Tense blisters that erode and scar, especially in recessively inherited forms; can lead to severe scars covering digits	Severe forms may involve mouth, esophagus
Epidermolysis bullosa acquista (blister below lamina densa)	Linear IgG and C3 deposits below lamina densa	Tense blisters that lead to scars and milia in pressure and trauma sites on hands, feet; scarring mucous membrane lesions also occur	Circulating antibody to sublamina densa antigen found

vesicles or bullae, a response to injected toxins or foreign chemicals or proteins in the bite or an allergic reaction to them.

Several unusual conditions, the *pemphigus diseases*, cause blistering in the epidermis by virtue of the process of acantholysis. Nikolsky's sign is commonly present in these conditions. *Pemphigus vulgaris* (see Color Plate 15*E*) and a variant, *pemphigus vegetans*, which heals with hypertrophic, "vegetative" surfaces, are acquired autoimmune diseases of the skin and mucous membrane. The superficial bullae, evolving just above the basal layer, readily rupture, leaving denuded, bleeding, weeping and crusted erosions over the body which do not heal. The oral mucosa is almost always involved and is frequently the presenting site. The painful erosions characteristically spill over the vermilion border of the lips and onto the skin. Lesions of the skin occur anywhere but often in pressure and friction areas. The blisters arise on normal-appearing skin. The usual course of untreated pemphigus vulgaris is slow progression with extensive denudation, leading to fluid and electrolyte imbalance, sepsis, and death. Pain from mouth lesions prevents adequate food intake. Skin biopsy of early vesicles should be obtained for routine histologic examination. The edge of a bulla, including adjacent normal skin, should be examined by direct immunofluorescence to make the diagnosis. Immunofluorescence shows deposits of immunoglobulins (usually IgG) and/or C3 in the intercellular spaces around keratinocytes (see Table 522–3). Antibodies to the intercellular areas of the epidermis are found in the serum of patients with pemphigus vulgaris. High doses of systemic steroids (100 to 200 mg of prednisone per day) over prolonged periods usually control the disease. Methotrexate and other cytotoxic agents are useful as steroid-sparing agents. Treatment with intramuscular gold is often successful, occasionally inducing long-term remissions (Ch. 524).

Pemphigus foliaceus is a less severe disease in which the acantholytic separation within the epidermis is in the upper portion of the prickle layer. *Pemphigus erythematosus* may be a localized variant of pemphigus foliaceus presenting with superficial blisters, erosions, and crusting and oozing over the scalp and face in a seborrheic dermatitis–like rash or often simulating the butterfly rash of systemic lupus erythematosus. Mucous membrane involvement in pemphigus foliaceus and pemphigus erythematosus is unusual, and lower doses of systemic steroids generally control these conditions. Immunofluorescent studies on skin from the edge of lesions reveal immunoglobulin and/or C3 in the intercellular areas of the upper portions of the epidermis.

Familial benign pemphigus, or Hailey-Hailey disease, is a dominantly inherited disorder with suprabasal cell acantholysis, the groups of bullae arising on erythematous skin in the flexural areas (neck, axillae, groin). Spreading erosions display vesicles and pustules at the borders with a moist, granular center. Warm weather and superficial bacterial infections seem to cause flares with spontaneous exacerbations and remissions continuing for years. Familial benign pemphigus differs from other forms of pemphigus in its genetic pattern, absence of mouth lesions, benign course, and absence of intercellular antibodies. Antibiotics, both topical and systemic, may improve acute flares of the disease.

DERMAL-EPIDERMAL VESICULOBULLOUS DISEASES. Separation of the epidermis from the dermis occurs in a variety of bullous diseases resulting from autoimmune and immunologic reactions, metabolic disturbances, and a number of inherited mechanicobullous conditions (Table 525–6).

Bullous pemphigoid (see Color Plate 15*F*), a disease of the elderly, is an autoimmune disorder in which tense, large blisters occur on normal or erythematous skin, often in the groin, axillae, and flexural areas. Nikolsky's sign is not present, and only one third of patients have oral blisters. Healing usually occurs in some blisters without scarring while new lesions evolve. Itching may be severe or absent. Skin biopsy specimens display a subepidermal blister through the lamina lucida (at the electron microscopic level), and direct immunofluorescence reveals deposition of the IgG immunoglobulin and complement. Circulating antibodies to the lamina lucida zone are found in 70 per cent of patients (see Table 522–3). The prognosis is good, and the disease usually subsides after months or years. Widespread bullae require therapy with 40 to 60 mg of oral prednisone per day and occasionally with immunosuppressive agents.

Another subepidermal blistering disease, *herpes gestationis*, is a rare autoimmune condition that occurs during pregnancy and the postpartum period. The name of the disease is misleading, for it is not associated with *Herpesvirus* infection. The blisters develop at any time throughout the course of pregnancy, although they most often begin during the second and third trimesters and subside a few weeks post partum. Some patients may experience transient flares or recurrences with each menstrual period or following the use of oral contraceptives. There are recurrences with subsequent pregnancies. Herpes gestationis is a pruritic condition with numerous tense vesicles arising on both normal-appearing and erythematous areas of skin. Arcuate and polycyclic red plaques with peripheral blistering are seen. The lesions first appear on the abdomen and then spread to involve the entire integument. Skin biopsy findings are indistinguishable from those of bullous pemphigoid by light microscopy, and examination of perilesional skin by direct immunofluorescence reveals C3 and less often an IgG linear band just below the epidermis. There is associated fetal mortality as high as 30 per cent, and there is also an increased rate of premature live births. Transient vesiculobullous lesions may infrequently occur in some otherwise healthy infants of affected mothers. Occasionally the patients' intractable pruritus and extensive bullae respond to high-potency topical steroid ointments and diphenhydramine, but most patients require oral prednisone (20 to 60 mg daily) throughout pregnancy with intermittent tapering.

Cicatricial pemphigoid (benign mucosal pemphigoid), another subepidermal blistering disease, has a predilection for mucous membranes, especially the conjunctiva where it causes scarring that leads to synblepharon and blindness. Subepidermal blisters also occur on the skin in one quarter of patients. Subepidermal IgG staining is seen on direct immunofluorescence, but circulating immunoglobulin antibodies are infrequently found. Therapy is unsatisfactory, although dapsone and gold may slow this chronic and progressive condition. Ophthalmologic care should be sought for the eye involvement.

Dermatitis herpetiformis is a chronic, intensely pruritic, vesicular disease that is identified by the bilaterally symmetric (herpetiform) grouping of papules, urticarial plaques, and vesicles over the elbows, knees, buttocks, low back, scapular areas, and scalp. The itching often has a burning quality. The blisters occur just below the epidermis, where collections of neutrophils are found in the dermal papillae. Direct immunofluorescence testing of perilesional normal-appearing skin reveals granular deposits of IgA at the tips of the dermal papillae. Approximately 75 per cent of patients have an associated gluten-sensitive enteropathy that is usually asymptomatic. A gluten-free diet strictly followed for at least 12 months causes remissions or significantly reduces the required dose of dapsone or sulfapyridine, either of which promptly clears the disease. The rash recurs when therapy is stopped.

Erythema multiforme (see Color Plate 15*G*) is an immunologic reaction in the skin and mucous membranes often mediated by circulating immune complexes that evolve in response to a number of antigenic stimuli (infections, drugs, connective tissue disease). As the name implies, the skin reaction is characterized by a variety of lesions, namely, erythematous plaques, blisters, and target or bull's-eye lesions. The mucous membranes of the mouth and eye may also be involved, and this is referred to as *Stevens-Johnson syndrome*. Typically the cutaneous lesions favor the extremities (often the palms) and are symmetric. Target lesions are diagnostic and are recognized by a central, dark purple area or a blister surrounded by a pale, edematous, round zone, surrounded in turn by a peripheral rim of erythema. In Stevens-Johnson syndrome the skin disease is more widespread, with blisters and painful erosions in the mouth and eyes. The patients look and feel ill with fever, prostration, and difficulty in eating. Histologically, subepidermal separation is found in the blistering center of the target lesion, and when early lesions are biopsied, immunofluorescence reveals immunoglobulin and complement in the walls of the small dermal blood vessels; the inflammation and bullae form in response to vascular damage and leaking. In one half of cases no etiology is found for the reaction, but a cause should be sought in all cases, especially drugs (penicillins, barbiturates, phenytoin [Dilantin], and sulfonamides) and infections (herpes simplex, *Streptococcus*, *Mycoplasma pneumoniae*). Recurrent herpes simplex infection is the most common cause of recurrent erythema multiforme. It is not clear whether medical therapy favorably alters the course of idiopathic erythema multiforme, although treatment of a precipitating infection seems appropriate and acyclovir may prevent recurrences of herpes-associated erythema multiforme. Stopping suspected drugs is also imperative. The value of systemic steroids in erythema multiforme and Stevens-Johnson syndrome is controversial. In addition, IV fluids may be required in patients with severe oral involvement, and topical anesthetics (viscous Xylocaine) may help to decrease mouth discomfort.

An example of a bullous disease caused by a metabolic disorder is *porphyria*. Porphyria is a group of disorders characterized by abnormalities in the heme biosynthetic pathway, resulting in the excessive accumulation of various porphyrins (see Ch. 191). In several types of porphyria light reacts with photosensitizing porphyrins in the circulation and skin to cause both acute and chronic alterations in the integument. The onset of photosensitivity in childhood and severe scarring, hair loss, and discolored red teeth are recognized findings in the very rare *congenital erythropoietic porphyria*. Adult porphyrias causing skin changes are, at times, more subtle. Photodistributed skin fragility, with bullae and erosions that leave scars over the dorsum of the hands, forearms, and face, is a frequently missed sign of *porphyria cutanea tarda* (a familial or acquired deficiency in the enzyme uroporphyrinogen decarboxylase). Urinary uroporphyrins and coproporphyrins are markedly elevated, causing the urine to appear dark brown and fluoresce an orange-red color under Wood's light. Both sun exposure and mild trauma to the skin induce subepidermal bullae that leave scars (Fig. 525–9). Facial hair, predominantly on the temples and lateral cheeks, mottled facial pigmentation, and, at times, diffuse scleroderma-like changes on the face and neck also occur. Porphyria cutanea tarda is worsened by alcohol and birth control pills. There seems to be an associated iron overload syndrome with elevated liver stores and serum iron. The treatment of choice is phlebotomy to reduce hepatic iron. When used carefully, antimalarials are also effective.

Other metabolic bullous diseases are those seen with chronic renal disease and diabetes mellitus. Subepidermal bullae occasionally occur in association with hemodialysis in chronic renal

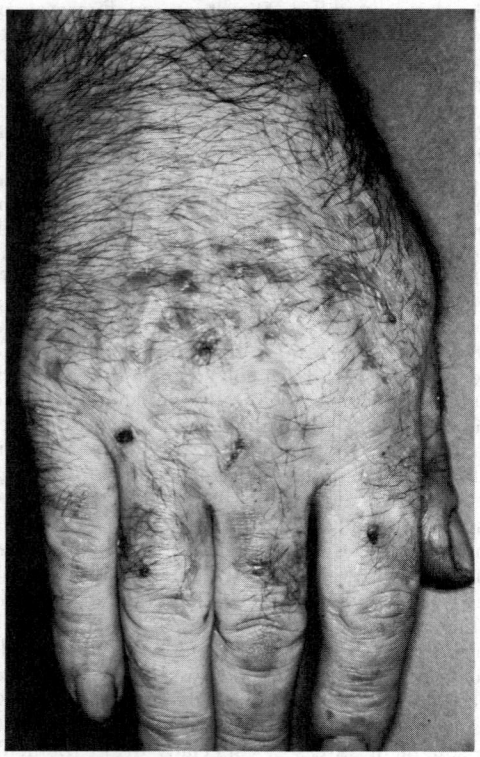

FIGURE 525–9. Porphyria cutanea tarda. (From the 17th edition of the Cecil Textbook of Medicine, with the permission of Dr. Marie-Louise Johnson.)

failure. The bullae are found on light-exposed areas, primarily the dorsa of hands, and may be worsened by sunlight. A few such patients have elevated uro- and coproporphyrins, suggesting that porphyria cutanea tarda is unmasked by dialysis, but most patients have had no alterations in porphyrin metabolism. These latter patients with *bullous dermatosis of hemodialysis* have scarring, tense, asymptomatic bullae without surrounding erythema. High doses of furosemide have also been reported to produce a bullous eruption on light-exposed skin of patients on hemodialysis. *Bullosis diabeticorum* appears as tense, bullous lesions on a noninflammatory base, usually localized to the lower extremities. These are related to trauma in diabetic patients with small vessel disease. A "pseudoporphyria" syndrome with skin changes identical to those seen in porphyria but without abnormalities in porphyrin metabolism is also being recognized with increasing frequency in patients receiving nonsteroidal antiinflammatory drugs.

The last group of subepidermal bullous diseases is the *mechanobullous conditions*, a variety of inherited defects in various structures found within and above the dermal-epidermal junction (*epidermolysis bullosa*). Blisters, erosions, ulcers, and varying degrees of scarring result from minor trauma to the skin. The forms vary by inheritance pattern, level of blister formation, and degree of scarring. Scars and milia at sites of repeated trauma are more common in the recessive dystrophic variants (anchoring fibrils are missing in these epidermolysis bullosa dystrophica patients). In severe forms the mouth and esophagus are involved, adhesions cover the digits, and growth is retarded. The more serious forms appear at birth, whereas milder types occur later in life. No therapy is available except in the severe dystrophic form in which two thirds of patients may be helped by phenytoin (Dilantin), which decreases the excess production of collagenase found in this condition.

An acquired type of epidermolysis bullosa (EB), *EB acquisita* (EBA), has recently been recognized. EBA occurs in adult life and is easily confused with EB dystrophica and/or bullous pemphigoid. It presents with bullous lesions and skin fragility to minor trauma over pressure points and on the hands and feet, which heal with wrinkled scars and milia (yellow-white inclusion cysts). Oral lesions as well as extensive esophageal, laryngeal, and ocular scarring, features of cicatricial pemphigoid, may also be seen. The blisters occur below the lamina densa zone, where linear deposits of IgG and complement react with an EBA autoantigen. Circulating antibodies to this sublamina densa antigen are found in many patients. No satisfactory therapy is available.

PUSTULAR DISEASES OF THE SKIN

Pustules usually bring to mind infection, but not all pustular dermatoses are caused by pathogenic microorganisms. Pustular conditions often occur in association with erythematous papules, cysts, and nodules and may open to form crusts (Table 525–7).

NONINFECTIOUS PUSTULAR SKIN DISEASES. *Acne* is the most common pustular condition of the skin. It is an inflammatory disorder affecting pilosebaceous units and hence is usually found over the face and upper trunk where the greatest concentration of these skin appendages is found. Several factors play a pathogenic role in acne as individuals enter puberty: (1) androgenic stimulation of the sebaceous glands and increased sebum production (see Ch. 522); (2) abnormal keratinization and impaction in the pilosebaceous canal (comedones) causing obstruction to sebum flow; (3) proliferation of anaerobic bacteria, *Propionibacterium acnes*, which predispose to rupture of the pilosebaceous unit with extravasation into the surrounding dermis, resulting in sterile, inflammatory papules, pustules, and cysts. The inflammatory lesions lead to disfiguring scarring. Therapy of acne is usually successful in controlling the disease until the patient "grows out" of this condition. Treatment is directed at correcting the three major factors that seem to cause acne. Thus, topical agents that remove comedones such as benzoyl peroxide and topical vitamin A preparations are particularly effective because their action allows sebum to flow freely onto the surface of the skin. Topical and oral antibiotics (tetracycline and erythromycin) are indicated in patients with inflammatory papules and pustules. Last, decreasing sebum production has beneficial effects, and oral 13-*cis*-retinoic acid decreases sebaceous gland size and sebum production. This drug should be used primarily for severe cystic

TABLE 525-7. PUSTULAR DISEASES OF THE SKIN

Name of Skin Condition	Etiology	Important Physical Findings	Other Facts of Note in History or Laboratory Results
Noninfectious Pustular Diseases of the Skin			
Acne	Androgens; follicular orifice keratinization problem; *Propionibacterium acnes*	Open and closed comedones; red papules, pustules, cysts; scarring of face and upper trunk	Rule out acneiform eruptions such as caused by drugs, greasy cosmetics, endocrinologic abnormalities
Rosacea	Unknown	Red papules, pustules on background of erythema, telangiectasia; central face flushing is a common problem; rhinophyma; eye involvement	Seen in patients usually older than those with acne
Perioral dermatitis	May be caused by potent topical steroids; variant acne	Perioral and periorbital red scaling patches, papules, and pustules	
Pustular psoriasis	Variant of psoriasis	Sterile pustules localized to palms and soles or generalized over body	Patient is toxic with fever, leukocytosis; can die of generalized form
Miliaria pustulosa	Occlusion of sweat glands in hot environment	Discrete red papules or pustules with red base over trunk, especially back	
Infectious Pustular Diseases of the Skin			
Localized to the skin			
Folliculitis, carbuncles, furuncles	*Staphylococcus aureus* invasion of hair follicles	Discrete pustules with red base with centrally placed hairs on buttocks, thighs, beard, scalp	Gram's stain, culture
Candidiasis	*Candida* organisms	Satellite pustules around beefy red patches in moist intertriginous areas	KOH preparation; culture
Hot tub folliculitis	*Pseudomonas aeruginosa*	Widely scattered, pruritic pustules with red base over trunk and extremities	Gram's stain, culture; folliculitis resolves spontaneously in 10-14 days; *Pseudomonas* contaminates hot tubs, whirlpools, and swimming pools
Dermatophytes-kerion	Dermatophyte	Boggy patch with pustules in scalp	KOH, culture
Tinea barbae	Dermatophyte	Pustular inflammatory reaction in beard area	
Systemic infectious (septicemias)			
Bacterial septicemia (gonococcal, streptococcal, fungal—*Candida*)	Gonococcus	Purpuric pustules—acral lesions in gonococcus; *Staphylococcus aureus; Candida*	Associated with arthritis in gonococcus; patients usually ill

acne. The clinician should recognize that other factors may play a role in exacerbating acne, including oil-based cosmetics and drugs (androgenic hormones, antiepileptics [phenytoin], high-progestin birth control pills, systemic corticosteroids, when taken in high doses, and iodide- and bromide-containing agents). Occasionally endocrinologic conditions characterized by excess androgen secretion may cause acne, i.e., polycystic ovarian disease, adrenal or ovarian tumors.

Rosacea is a chronic inflammatory disorder affecting the blood vessels and pilosebaceous units of the face in middle-aged individuals. Patients with rosacea have papules and pustules superimposed on diffuse erythema and telangiectasia over the central portion of the face. An important component of the patients'

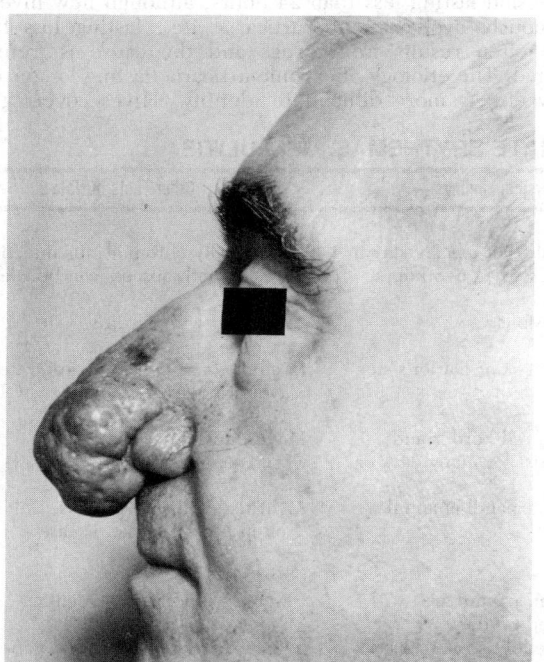

FIGURE 525-10. Rhinophyma. (From the 17th edition of the Cecil Textbook of Medicine, with the permission of Dr. Marie-Louise Johnson.)

history is easy flushing and blushing of the face, and this is often accentuated when alcohol, caffeine-containing, or hot spicy foods are ingested. Hyperplasia of the sebaceous glands, connective tissue, and vascular bed of the nose sometimes causes *rhinophyma* or a large, red, bulbous nose (Fig. 525-10). Ocular complications occur in a small but significant number of rosacea patients; these include blepharitis, chalazion, conjunctivitis, and keratitis. Progressive keratitis can lead to scarring and blindness. Rosacea and the eye complications are usually dramatically responsive to tetracycline, but the antibiotic must be continued for life (at the lowest dose that suppresses the condition) because rosacea recurs when therapy is interrupted. High-potency topical corticosteroid preparations may induce or aggravate pre-existing rosacea and should not be used for long periods of time on the face.

Perioral dermatitis, as the name suggests, is a conspicuous affliction consisting of red papules, pustules, and fine scaling erythema in a concentric oval about the mouth, sparing the skin immediately adjacent to the lips. Perioral dermatitis is probably a variant of rosacea or acne, and is most often seen in women between 18 and 40 years of age. Tetracycline is the mainstay of therapy, usually requiring 250 mg twice a day for 6 to 8 weeks.

Hidradenitis suppurativa is a chronic suppurative and scarring problem of the apocrine glands appearing as tense, draining lesions with retracted scars in the axillae and anogenital regions (Fig. 525-11).

Psoriasis can occasionally present in a pustular form, either localized to the palms and soles or as a generalized, total body reaction associated with fever and leukocytosis.

Miliaria, or heat rash, represents an inflammatory reaction caused by occlusion of sweat ducts with extravasation of their contents into the surrounding tissue. Occlusion of the duct at the level of the epidermal granular layer results in *miliaria rubra* (discrete, small, red papules), especially on the trunk and back. The presence of discrete lesions not associated with hair follicles suggests the diagnosis. In more deeply situated occlusion of the duct, *miliaria pustulosa*, or pustules with surrounding erythema, is seen. In the ambulatory patient miliaria results from exposure to a hot, humid environment, while in bedridden patients fever, sweating, and occlusion of the skin on bed sheets are predisposing factors. The problem usually remits with cooling and ventilation of the patient's skin.

INFECTIOUS CAUSES OF SKIN PUSTULES. *Folliculitis,* a *Staphylococcus aureus* infection of the hair follicle, appears as pustules with a red rim with hair emanating from the center of

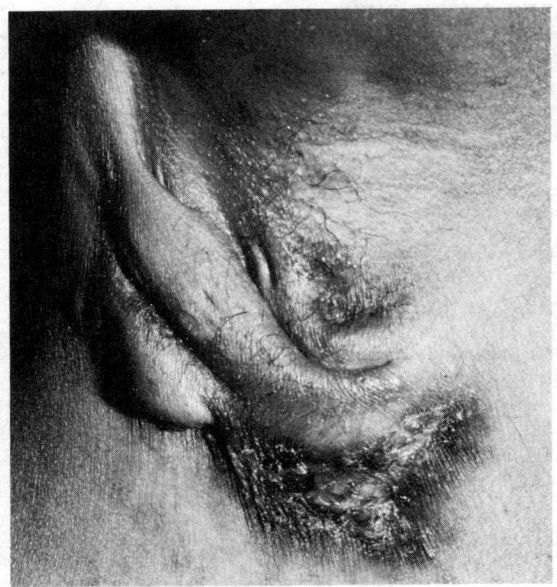

FIGURE 525–11. Hidradenitis suppurativa, axilla. (From the 17th edition of the Cecil Textbook of Medicine, with the permission of Dr. Marie-Louise Johnson.)

the pustule. Folliculitis typically occurs in hairy regions where clothing rubs (buttocks, thighs) or on the face. The key to diagnosis is finding a central hair in the pustule. Occasionally the follicular infection can extend more deeply to form a larger, red, fluctuant nodule that "points" to drain pus from one (furuncle) or more follicles (carbuncle). Systemic antibiotics such as erythromycin or dicloxacillin usually clear extensive infections; topical antiseptic cleansers such as povidone-iodine or chlorhexidine can resolve mild folliculitis and may be useful in preventing recurrences.

Candidiasis appears as beefy red patches in intertriginous, moist areas characteristically surrounded by satellite pustules. Paronychia, a painful red swelling in the periungual regions of the finger, may also drain pus in which *Candida* can be found with a KOH preparation. Topical agents such as clotrimazole and miconazole are used two or three times a day. These must be used for many weeks before the infection is cleared.

Hot tub folliculitis is a generalized, pruritic folliculitis caused by *Pseudomonas aeruginosa* that is acquired in hot tubs, whirlpools, or swimming pools contaminated by this organism. It usually begins 6 hours to 5 days after hot tub soaking and affects many people using the facility. It appears as a vesicular and then pustular eruption over the trunk, buttocks, legs, and arms but spares the head and neck. *Pseudomonas* can often be cultured from fresh pustules. In most instances the folliculitis resolves within 7 to 10 days without specific treatment. The tubs and pools implicated in causing this type of folliculitis should be cultured for *Pseudomonas* and disinfected.

Dermatophytes can, at times, infect hair follicles and result in pustules, particularly in the beard (tinea barbae) and scalp (kerions). These are readily confused with a bacterial folliculitis. Kerions appear as indurated, boggy, inflammatory plaques studded with pustules. These intense inflammatory reactions to superficial dermatophytes (especially *T. verrucosum*) respond to griseofulvin therapy, although a short course of oral corticosteroids is also useful.

Deep fungal infections such as *blastomycosis, sporotrichosis,* and *coccidioidomycosis* may cause pustules, as well as verrucous, ulcerative papules and nodules. Sporotrichosis characteristically spreads up cutaneous lymphatics and appears as nodular, pustular lesions in a linear distribution.

SYSTEMIC INFECTIONS CAUSING PUSTULES ON THE SKIN. A variety of septicemias including gonococcemia, staphylococcal septicemia, and *Candida* septicemia (in immunosuppressed patients) cause pustular lesions associated with purpura.

URTICARIA, PERSISTENT FIGURATE ERYTHEMAS, CELLULITIS

This group of skin lesions is of disparate appearance and etiology. The common feature is a raised edematous, red plaque with a sharply demarcated border (Table 525–8).

URTICARIAL REACTIONS. Urticaria, the most common condition in this group, appears as wheals, transient erythematous and edematous swellings of the dermis caused by local increase in permeability of capillaries and small venules. This increased permeability results from histamine and other chemical substances released from cutaneous mast cells by Type I IgE hypersensitivity reactions, as well as by nonimmunologic mechanisms (see Ch. 245). Certain agents such as aspirin, opiates, and some foods degranulate mast cells directly without an allergic mechanism. Other urticarial reactions are immunologically mediated by such allergens as infections (viral, i.e., hepatitis, sinus and tooth infections), infestations (systemic parasites), drugs, pollens, and injections (blood products, vaccinations). Other hives are caused by physical modalities: light (solar urticaria), cold (cold urticaria), heat or exercise (cholinergic urticaria), or pressure or rubbing of the skin (dermatographism). Hives are transient, any given lesion lasting less than 24 hours, although new hives may continuously evolve. Acute urticaria (i.e., lasting less than 6 weeks) often results from drugs and the cause is frequently identified. The etiology of chronic urticaria (lasting longer than 6 to 8 weeks) is more difficult to identify. Hives covering large

TABLE 525–8. URTICARIA, PERSISTENT FIGURATE ERYTHEMAS, CELLULITIS

Skin Condition	Etiology	Important Physical Findings	Other Facts of Note
Urticaria-like Reactions			
Urticaria	Drugs, foods, infections, physical modalities (heat, cold, light)	Transient, red wheals that usually stay in one area of skin less than 6–8 hours	Occasionally chronic sinus infection or apical tooth abscess can be silent cause
Erythema marginatum	Associated with rheumatic fever	Transient annular lesions	Associated with carditis
Urticaria pigmentosa	Abnormal accumulation of mast cells	Pigmented papules of skin; Darier's sign present	In adult, mast cells may infiltrate lymph nodes, liver, spleen, GI tract
Figurate Erythemas			
Erythema annulare centrifugum	Occasionally an "id" reaction to tinea infection elsewhere on the body	Annular lesions with red border and trailing scale; persist for many days or months	May mimic ringworm
Erythema chronicum migrans	Part of Lyme disease caused by bite of tick and spirochete infection	One or more slowly expanding annular lesions	Arthritis, cardiac problems, Bell's palsy often part of Lyme disease
Cellulitis			
Erysipelas	Streptococcal infection of dermis	Erythematous, warm, painful area with sharply demarcated border	Responds readily to penicillin
Necrotizing fasciitis	Mixed, aerobic, and anaerobic infection in fascial plane	Deep red, painful cellulitis that causes purpura and then tissue necrosis; moves rapidly	Seen in immunosuppressed patients and diabetics

areas and producing deep tissue swelling are termed *angioedema*. This condition can involve the tongue and throat and threaten to close off the airway. In such patients a careful history about medications (including over-the-counter drugs, especially cold tablets or medications containing aspirin) should be elicited. Infections such as "silent" sinusitis or apical abscess of teeth must be looked for. In addition, physical types of urticaria should be considered: *cholinergic* urticaria is characterized by evanescent multiple, small wheals surrounded by a wide pink flare induced by heat and exercise; *solar* urticaria by large plaques in sun-exposed areas; *cold* urticaria by wheals that evolve with exposure to cold. Urticaria accompanied by fever and arthralgias occurs in serum sickness reactions and in the prodromata of viral hepatitis. Occasionally urticaria occurs in conjunction with internal conditions such as malignancies or connective tissue diseases. Hereditary angioedema, an autosomal dominant disorder, causes recurrent urticaria, angioedema, intestinal colic, and life-threatening laryngeal edema.

If the cause for the urticaria cannot be found or avoided, symptomatic control is achieved with antihistamines or oral steroids. Acute angioedema or laryngeal edema requires rapid systemic treatment with epinephrine and diphenhydramine (see Ch. 245).

Other urticaria-like skin lesions include *erythema multiforme* (see above); *juvenile rheumatoid arthritis skin lesions*—small, 2- to 3-mm, salmon-colored hives that last only a few hours appearing with fever spikes; *erythema marginatum*—lesions found in 10 per cent of patients with acute rheumatic fever (Ch. 298). *Urticaria pigmentosa* (mastocytosis), a disease caused by increased accumulations of mast cells in the skin and at times in lymph nodes, liver, spleen, bones, and gastrointestinal tract (see Ch. 252), presents with multiple tan to brown, papular spots that urticate when rubbed (Darier's sign) owing to the release of histamine from the mast cells. A skin biopsy specimen stained with Giemsa's stain will readily identify increased numbers of mast cells in the dermis. When the lesions in the skin develop in early childhood, the condition is usually limited to skin and the lesions resolve by puberty, leaving only hyperpigmented macules. If the skin lesions evolve in adulthood there is a greater chance for mast cell infiltration of the organ systems noted above, and the skin lesions persist. Symptoms and findings in mastocytosis depend on the organ systems involved and the release of various vasoactive substances contained in the increased masses of mast cells. Hepatosplenomegaly, lymphadenopathy, and bone pain may occur secondary to infiltrates. Patients may experience flushing, palpitations, headache, syncope, hypotension, abdominal pain, and diarrhea, all related to histamine and prostaglandin release from the mast cells.

FIGURATE ERYTHEMAS. This is a group of uncommon conditions characterized by annular, polycyclic, and geographic erythematous skin lesions. These conditions, in contrast to the urticarial reactions, persist for many days or even years, moving slowly or rapidly over the skin surface (hence, the term sometimes used for these reactions—persistent figurate erythema).

The most common of these diseases, *erythema annulare centrifugum*, appears as one or more annular lesions with an elevated erythematous border and a fine scale on the inner aspect of the border (trailing scale).

Erythema chronicum migrans is the unique annular skin lesion found in Lyme disease caused by a spirochete inoculated by infected tick bites (see Ch. 343 and Color Plate 10A).

CELLULITIS. Although superficially resembling urticaria, these inflammatory infections of the dermis are readily distinguished from hives by their persistent, slowly enlarging nature as well as their pain and warmth. Group A streptococci and *Staphylococcus aureus* are the organisms most commonly responsible. *Erysipelas* is sometimes identified separately from cellulitis. It displays a sharply demarcated painful border and an "orange-peel" epidermal surface. Group A *Streptococcus* is the usual cause. Patients usually feel ill and are febrile. Cellulitis on the lower legs in adults may develop from fissures between the toes from tinea pedis. Systemic antibiotics, erythromycin, dicloxacillin, or the cephalosporins are the drugs most commonly used.

Necrotizing fasciitis is a special form of cellulitis involving the deep fascial structures underlying the skin. Rapidly evolving in enclosed fascial spaces, usually in diabetics or immunosuppressed patients, these infections are caused by a mixture of aerobic and anaerobic gram-negative organisms and must be diagnosed early by deep fascial biopsy and treated immediately with a broad spectrum of antibiotics and surgical debridement.

NODULES AND TUMORS OF THE SKIN

Nodular and tumorous lesions of the skin may evolve within the epidermis or the dermis and subcutaneous tissue, arising in various skin appendages and structures, including melanocytes. Such nodular lesions may represent benign or malignant growths, infiltrative or inflammatory reactions. In many instances the structures giving rise to the nodule reflect the colors of these structures; i.e., vascular lesions appear red to purple, whereas lesions involving melanocytes appear pigmented.

In general, epidermal nodules are recognized by localized thickening of the epidermis or corneum with hyperkeratosis or scale. Dermal or subcutaneous nodules appear as lumps, often with no alteration in the overlying epidermis.

Of primary concern in every patient with a nodule is whether it is benign or malignant. This is not always easy to discern, and therefore skin nodules and tumors often must be biopsied. Some clinical generalizations can be made in distinguishing benign from malignant tumors (Table 525–9).

Common nodular lesions of the skin are listed in Table 525–10.

NONPIGMENTED NODULES—BENIGN. *Warts* are benign epidermal growths caused by papilloma viruses (see above, under Maculopapular lesions).

Sebaceous hyperplasia occurs as papular and occasionally nodular lesions on the faces of individuals past 50 years of age. This proliferation of sebaceous glands surrounding a hair follicle appears as groups of yellow papules evolving in an annular configuration with a central pore. Sebaceous hyperplasia is sometimes clinically difficult to differentiate from basal cell cancers, although the yellow discoloration and central pore may help. At times skin biopsy may be necessary. No treatment is generally required.

Keratoacanthomas (see Color Plate 15D), or self-healing epitheliomas, are rapidly growing neoplasms of epidermal keratinocytes that are biologically benign. These lesions resolve spontaneously, leaving a scar. Keratoacanthomas are usually found on sun-exposed areas and begin as flesh-colored papules that rapidly grow over a period of 6 weeks, evolving a central keratin-filled crater. The lesions remain for 6 to 8 weeks and then subside. Such lesions are best excised because they leave unsightly scars and are difficult to differentiate from squamous cell cancer, even histologically.

Epidermal inclusion cysts appear as flesh-colored, firm nodules in the skin, particularly over the scalp and trunk. A helpful diagnostic sign is a central enlarged pore where the epidermis has invaginated to form the cyst. If the central pore is patent, slight squeezing will express white, cheesy, foul-smelling keratin and sebum. If the cyst is bothersome it can be excised.

Lipomas are more deeply situated than epidermal inclusion cysts; although they can feel firm and even rubbery, like a cyst, they usually are multilobulated and softer in consistency. If the diagnosis is in doubt and especially if the lesion is firm, a biopsy is indicated. Lipomas may be multiple, and familial multiple epidermal cysts and lipomas, fibromas, and osteomas associated with intestinal polyps are recognized as Gardner's syndrome.

Neurofibromas, focal proliferations of neural tissue within the dermis, may present in two forms: (1) soft, flesh-colored, pro-

TABLE 525–9. CLINICAL FEATURES HELPFUL IN DISTINGUISHING BENIGN FROM MALIGNANT TUMORS

Clinical Feature	Benign	Malignant
Configuration	Symmetric, sharp borders	Asymmetric, irregular borders
Rate of growth	Slow	Slow or rapid
Friability	No friability	Often friable
Bleeding or ulceration	Seldom bleed or ulcerate	Often bleed and ulcerate
Consistency	Firm or soft	Usually firm to hard
Color	Uniform color and pigmentation	Irregularity of color and pigmentation

TABLE 525–10. NODULAR LESIONS OF THE SKIN

Lesion	Appearance	Distribution	Etiology	Other Factors
Nonpigmented Nodules–Benign				
Warts	Skin-colored, corrugated hyperkeratotic surface	Anywhere on body	Papillomavirus	Appearance may vary, depending on location of wart; i.e., plantar warts are flat with callus on surface; condylomata acuminata are soft, moist, cauliflower-like nodules
Sebaceous hyperplasia	Yellow, papular nodules around hair follicles	Face	Benign hyperplasia of sebaceous glands	
Keratoacanthoma	Rapidly growing nodule with keratin-filled central crater	Sun-exposed areas	Benign hyperplasia of keratinocytes	Resolves spontaneously leaving scars
Epidermal inclusion cyst	Flesh-colored, firm nodules with rubbery consistency and enlarged pore on surface	Often scalp, face, trunk	Epidermally lined cysts	Occasionally becomes secondarily infected
Lipoma	Multilobulated, firm nodule with normal overlying epidermis	Extremities, trunk	Benign localized hypertrophy of adipose tissue	
Neurofibroma	Soft, flesh-colored, protruding nodules that can be invaginated deeper into skin—buttonhole sign	Extremities, trunk	Hyperplasia of neural tissue in dermis	Can be associated with von Recklinghausen's disease and café au lait spots and axillary freckling
Nonpigmented Nodules—Malignant				
Basal cell carcinoma	Opalescent, waxy nodule often with ulceration	Sun-exposed areas, 97% face, neck, arms	Ultraviolet light and genetics play a role	Locally invasive—seldom metastasizes
Squamous cell cancer	Hard, smooth or verrucous nodules that often show hyperkeratinization	Sun-exposed areas	Ultraviolet light and genetics play a role	May be metastatic, especially those on lower lip
Pigmented Nodules—Benign				
Seborrheic keratosis	Light brown to black verrucous lesions with stuck-on appearance	Face, trunk	Seen in older people	Individual lesions of uniform color
Dermatofibroma	Firm dermal papules and nodules with overlying brown hyperpigmentation; dimple sign—dimpling of epidermis with pinching of skin	Usually legs	Trauma, insect bites induce dermal fibrosis	Can be flesh-colored or red
Nevi	Uniformly pigmented, flat to nodular symmetrically shaped lesions	Anywhere on body	Accumulation of benign pigmented nevus cells	Itching nevi or changes in color, size, or configuration are danger signs of melanoma
Pigmented Nodules—Malignant				
Melanoma	Flat to nodular, pigmented lesions with asymmetry of growth, irregular borders, variegation of pigmentation, and diameter greater than 6 mm	Anywhere on body	Probably ultraviolet light exposure; genetic predisposition	Itching may be early sign of melanoma; melanoma can arise from pre-existing nevi
Vascular Tumors of Skin				
Hemangiomas	Flat to nodular, red, blue, purple, soft lesions	Anywhere on body	Proliferation of blood vessels of dermis	Strawberry hemangiomas usually regress; port-wine stains persist
Pyogenic granuloma	Bright red nodules that readily bleed	Extremities, hands, fingers	Proliferation of blood vessels following trauma	
Kaposi's sarcoma	Red, purple, brown papules and plaques	Legs, neck, trunk	Cytomegalovirus, AIDS	Seen most often with AIDS or immunosuppression
Inflammatory Nodules of Skin				
Erythema nodosum	Multiple, red, painful nodules; do not ulcerate; involute leaving bruises	Pretibial areas	Hypersensitivity reaction in subcutaneous fat	Number of antigenetic stimuli: drugs, infections, intestinal inflammatory disease
Subcutaneous fat necrosis	Red nodules, tender	Lower legs, thighs	Fat necrosis secondary to release of pancreatic lipase	Pancreatitis, pancreatitic cancer
Rheumatoid nodules	Nonpainful, firm nodules	Elbows, knees, fingers	Unknown	Rheumatoid arthritic changes with high rheumatoid factor titer
Nodules Associated with Metabolic Conditions				
Xanthomas	Nontender, firm, yellow to red papules and nodules	Elbows, knees, Achilles tendons	Hyperlipoproteinemias	Xanthomas related to genetic disorder of lipoprotein metabolism (primary) or secondary to underlying diseases

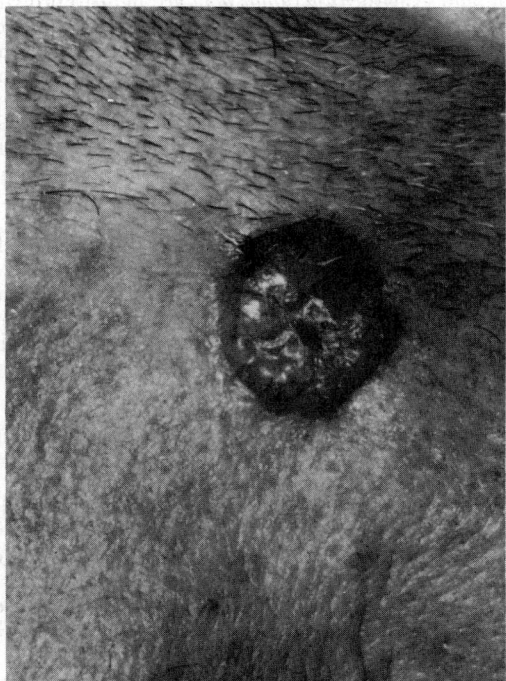

FIGURE 525–12. Basal cell epithelioma. (From the 17th edition of the Cecil Textbook of Medicine, with the permission of Dr. Marie-Louise Johnson.)

truding nodules that, on compression, can be invaginated into what feels like a defect in the skin (buttonhole sign), and (2) deep, firm, dermal or subcutaneous nodules. Neurofibromas may be solitary, but when they are multiple *von Recklinghausen's disease* should be considered, especially when café au lait spots (light brown macules) and axillary freckling are seen.

NONPIGMENTED NODULES—MALIGNANT. Malignant tumors of the epidermis—*basal cell* and *squamous cell carcinomas*—are related to the amount and intensity of electromagnetic radiation, including ultraviolet light and x-radiation, the skin has received over a lifetime. Such cancers are therefore found most commonly on sun-exposed areas, especially the face, neck, arms, and hands. The cancers are more common in patients living in southern latitudes of the northern hemisphere and in Australia in those with light complexions who sunburn easily, and especially in patients whose occupations keep them outdoors. In addition, these epidermal cancers are more common in immunosuppressed patients, attesting to the importance of the immune surveillance system in cancer etiology. A personal or family history of skin cancer should always make the physician more alert to the possibility of cancer.

Basal cell carcinoma (see Color Plate 15A) is a malignancy arising from the basal cells of the epidermis. These tumors rarely metastasize, but they have considerable potential for extensive, local destruction. Four clinical forms should be recognized: (1) The *nodular* type, the most common, appears as a pearly or opalescent, irregularly shaped papule or nodule with a central depression or crater; telangiectasias and a rolled, waxy border are often in evidence. When ulceration and crusting occur, it is referred to as a rodent ulcer (Fig. 525–12). Many times the raised, waxy border is subtle and is observed more readily by stretching the skin. (2) *Superficial* basal cell carcinoma is recognized as a red, slightly scaling, eczematous plaque that may be slightly eroded and crusted. Careful examination reveals a threadlike, pearly, rolled edge. This is an easily overlooked neoplasm, frequently confused with psoriasis or eczematous patches, so that a high index of suspicion, along with skin biopsy, is needed to make the diagnosis. (3) *Pigmented* basal cell carcinoma appears as a blue-black nodule or plaque with a pearly, opalescent sheen as seen in other basal cell cancers. Melanocytes are not histologically involved in these cancers, merely stimulated to make more pigment, and the prognosis of these pigmented forms is the same as for other basal cell cancers. (4) *Scarring* or *sclerosing* basal cell cancers present as atrophic, white, sometimes slightly eroded

or crusted plaques with telangiectasia. This is the most difficult form to cure because of its indistinct borders. The diagnosis of basal cell carcinoma should be confirmed by biopsy. Treatment depends on the location of the lesion, the morphologic type, the size of the tumor, and whether it is primary or recurrent. Treatment modalities include curettage and electrodesiccation, scalpel excision, radiotherapy, and cryotherapy. When these are selected properly each modality has a cure rate of greater than 90 per cent. A specialized form of excision using careful histologic orientation and detailed mapping of the extent of the tumor is the Mohs surgical technique. This tedious form of surgery is used for recurrent basal cell cancers, sclerosing basal cell cancers, and large primary basal cell cancers in regions in which recurrences are likely (particularly in the nasolabial folds and the periorbital and immediate preauricular areas).

Squamous cell carcinoma (see Color Plate 15B), a malignant neoplasm of the keratinocytes, is a less common but more aggressive type of cancer than basal cell cancer. Squamous cell carcinoma is locally invasive and has the potential to metastasize. It occurs primarily on the head and neck, upper extremities, and trunk, presenting as firm, red, smooth or verrucous nodules. Hyperkeratoses may be prominent, and indeed "cutaneous horns" are often squamous cell carcinomas (see Color Plate 15C). The cancers also display increased friability, ulceration, and crusting (Fig. 525–13). *Bowen's disease* is a squamous cell cancer in situ, appearing as red, scaling, crusted, sharply demarcated plaques. Squamous cell cancer in situ on the penis in uncircumcised males evolves as velvety red patches on the glans and foreskin (erythroplasia of Queyrat). Bowen's disease and erythroplasia are banal, easily overlooked conditions that can metastasize if not diagnosed early. *Actinic keratoses*, precancerous lesions of atypical keratinocytes, appear as red, ill-marginated macules and papules with yellow-brown, adherent scales in sun-damaged skin. They may evolve into squamous cell cancers. Any lesion suspected of being a squamous cell cancer should be biopsied. Excision is the treatment of choice in squamous cell cancers. Actinic keratoses are treated with liquid nitrogen freezing or, if numerous, with topical 5-fluorouracil applied as 1 or 5 per cent cream or solution over 2- to 4-week period.

PIGMENTED NODULES—BENIGN. *Seborrheic keratoses* are neoplasms of the epidermal cells that appear on the face and trunk in middle age. These 2-mm to 5-cm, elevated, tan to brown or occasionally black, round to oval lesions have a verrucous or crumbly, greasy surface and a stuck-on appearance. No therapy is necessary unless they are of cosmetic concern, and then liquid nitrogen cryotherapy or curettage is an effective means of removal.

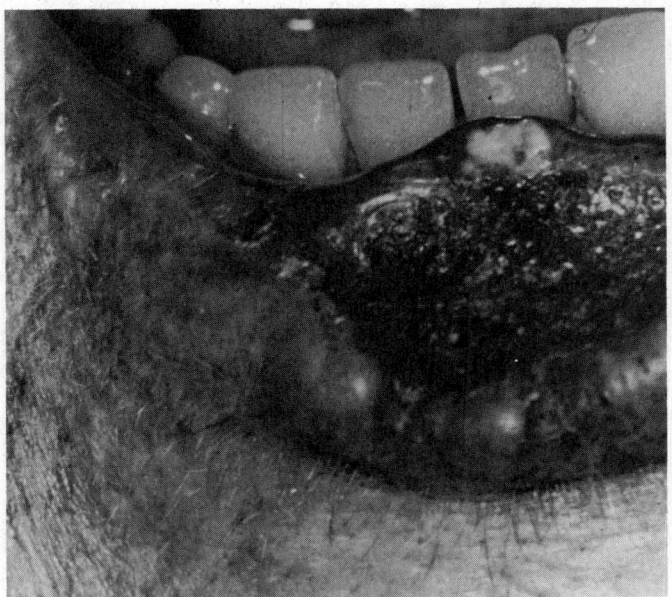

FIGURE 525–13. Squamous cell carcinoma. (From the 17th edition of the Cecil Textbook of Medicine, with the permission of Dr. Marie-Louise Johnson.)

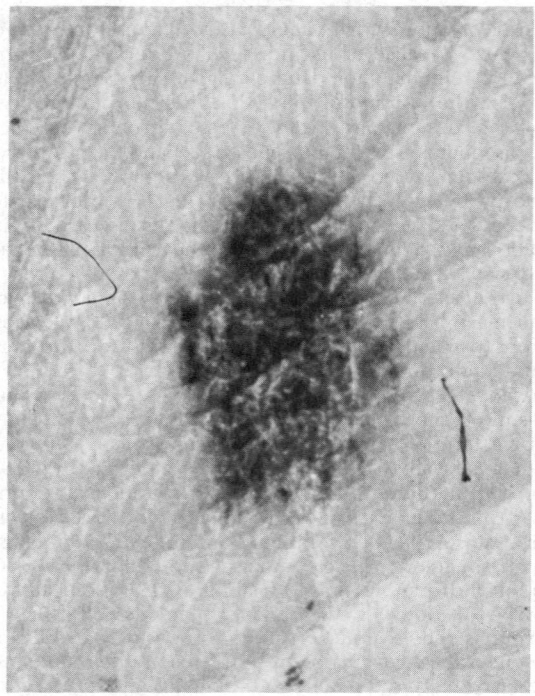

FIGURE 525–14. Junctional nevus. (From the 17th edition of the Cecil Textbook of Medicine, with the permission of Dr. Marie-Louise Johnson.)

Dermatofibromas are areas of focal dermal fibrosis accompanied by overlying epidermal thickening and hyperpigmentation, appearing clinically as brown papules or nodules. A useful diagnostic test is the "dimple sign," in which pinching the lesion results in central dimpling of the overlying epidermis. Some dermatofibromas are dark brown in color and occasionally raise the concern of melanoma, but the fibromas are symmetric and uniform in color. The lesions occur frequently on the lower extremities and less often on the arms, and they may be multiple. Although therapy is usually not required, simple excision can be done.

Nevi, or *moles,* are benign accumulations of pigment-forming nevus cells. They may be congenital or acquired, and most nevi evolve before age 35, appearing sometime after the first year of life. There are three forms, representing various stages of biologic

evolution and growth: *Junctional nevi* are light to brown macular lesions (Fig. 525–14). *Compound nevi* have flat, junctional portions along with brown papules with a smooth or rough surface; these evolve from junctional nevi in older children and young adults. Later, *intradermal nevi* evolve from the compound nevi as flesh-colored to brown papules or sessile growths (Fig. 525–15). Although nevi vary in appearance and color, individually they are uniform in color, symmetric in their growth and configuration, and usually less than 6 mm in diameter. Occasionally nevi darken in color or may itch, and new nevi may develop during pregnancy, but symptomatic nevi that change should be regarded suspiciously.

PIGMENTED NODULES—MALIGNANT. Malignant melanoma (see Color Plate 16E and F) is the cutaneous neoplasm of melanocytes and nevus cells. Four important clinical features are useful in recognizing malignant melanoma, the so-called A-B-C-D's of diagnosis:

A = Asymmetry of the lesion is due to irregular, random growth of the malignant cells associated with irregular surface topography and papules and nodules.

B = Borders of the tumors are irregular with notching and pigment "spilling" out beyond the edges.

C = Color variegation consists of browns, blacks, blues, and even shades of red and white. The variations in color represent different depths of invasion of pigment cells along with inflammatory reaction and immunologic response to the malignant cells.

D = Diameter or size of melanomas tends to be greater than 6 mm before they are recognized.

Several clinical forms or presentations of melanoma can be identified, each of these forms demonstrating the above characteristics. *Lentigo maligna melanoma* is a slowly evolving, multicolored lesion on the head and neck. It is preceded by lentigo maligna (in situ melanoma), which extends peripherally and is an unevenly pigmented, dark brown to black macule that can grow to a size of 5 to 7 cm over a period of many years before nodules develop, signifying dermal invasion (Fig. 525–16). *Superficial spreading melanoma* may occur on any area of the body, appearing as irregularly pigmented lesions with papules, nodules, and notched borders (Fig. 525–17). Invasion into the dermis occurs more rapidly than in lentigo maligna melanoma. *Nodular melanoma* appears as a rapidly growing, blue-black, smooth or eroded nodule (Fig. 525–18). It invades dermis early in its evolution, so it is less likely to be diagnosed in a premetastatic stage. *Acral lentiginous melanoma* occurs on the palms, soles, and digits. It evolves as an irregular, enlarging, variegate-colored, brown to black growth similar to lentigo maligna melanoma but more aggressive in its propensity for dermal invasion early in its course. Only minor degrees of papular elevation may be associated with deep invasion.

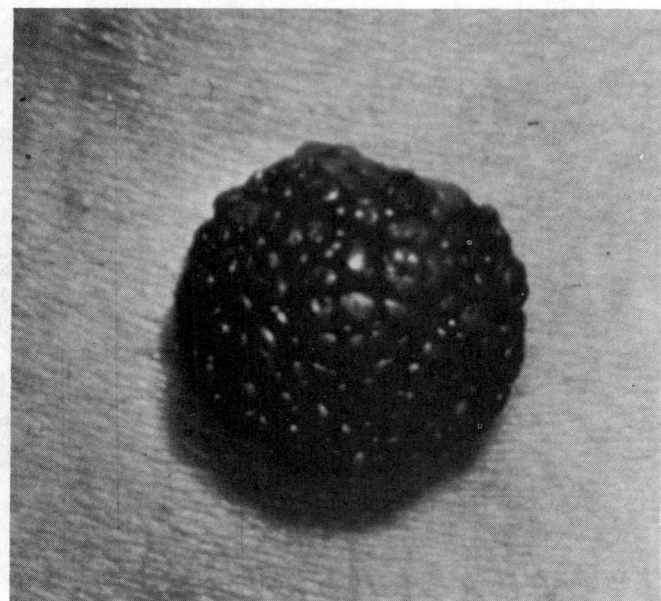

FIGURE 525–15. Intradermal nevus. (From the 17th edition of the Cecil Textbook of Medicine, with the permission of Dr. Marie-Louise Johnson.)

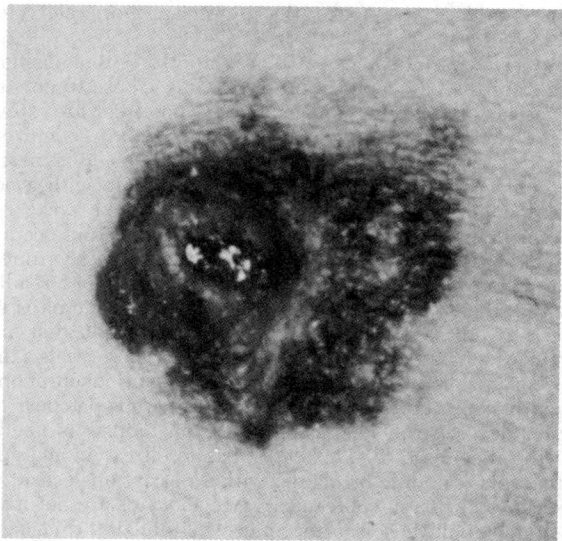

FIGURE 525–16. Lentigo maligna. (From the 17th edition of the Cecil Textbook of Medicine, with the permission of Dr. Marie-Louise Johnson.)

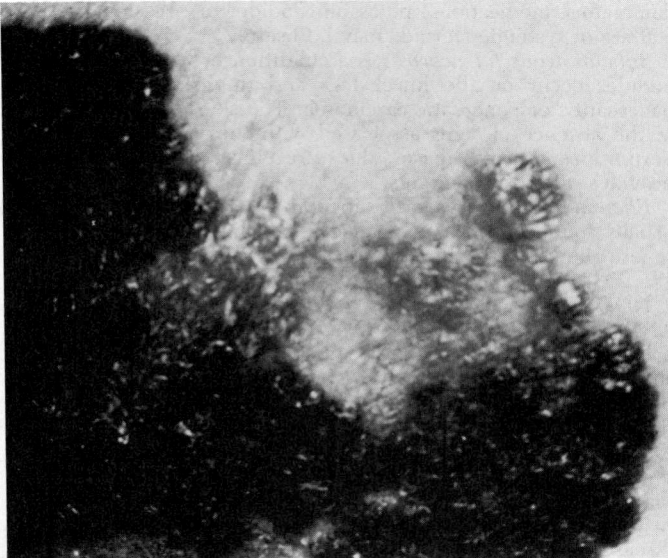

FIGURE 525–17. Superficial spreading melanoma. (From the 17th edition of the Cecil Textbook of Medicine, with the permission of Dr. Marie-Louise Johnson.)

One third of melanomas may arise from existing nevi, so that a change in size, shape, and color or itching of a pigmented lesion (a common symptom in melanomas) should be carefully investigated. Early diagnosis is the key to survival of patients with melanoma. The deeper the malignant cells invade the dermis, the more likely is metastasis. The depth of dermal invasion can be microscopically measured from the granular cell layer in the epidermis to the deepest penetration of melanoma cells into the dermis. If the melanoma is thin (< 0.76 mm), there is a virtually 100 per cent cure rate. If the depth is greater than 1.6 mm, only a 20 to 30 per cent 5-year survival is seen.

Any suspicious pigmented lesion must be biopsied, preferably by excision. Definitive, wide surgical excision should be undertaken only after confirmation of melanoma is established histologically. In large lesions such as lentigo maligna, it is acceptable to do incisional biopsy prior to definitive therapy. Suspicious pigmented lesions should never be shave-biopsied or shave-excised, nor should they be electrocauterized. Full-thickness tissue through the lesion is required for diagnostic and prognostic evaluation.

The precise cause of melanoma is unknown, but sunlight and heredity have been suggested as risk factors. The occurrence of melanoma has been increasing during the past few decades. Familial occurrence of malignant melanoma is seen in families with the *dysplastic nevus syndrome*. Numerous atypical, haphaz-

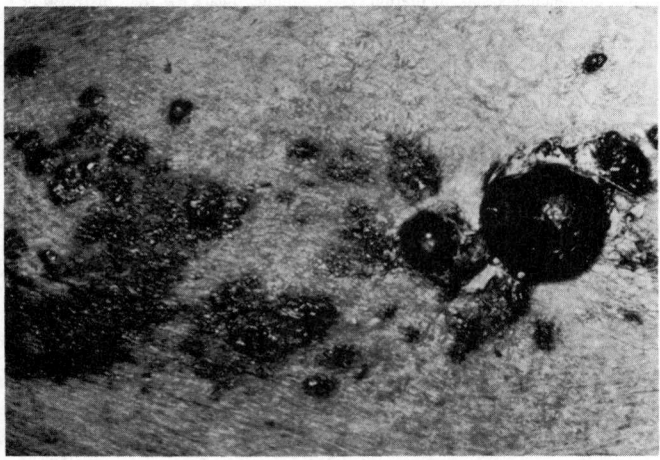

FIGURE 525–18. Nodular melanoma. (From the 17th edition of the Cecil Textbook of Medicine, with the permission of Dr. Marie-Louise Johnson.)

ardly colored, red-brown nevi with irregular borders are found over the trunk, extremities, and scalp. Biopsy of these atypical nevi reveals disordered melanocytic proliferation. The nevi may have an increased risk of developing melanoma, although the melanomas can also arise from normal skin in these individuals. Close clinical follow-up and excision of suspicious nevi are important.

VASCULAR TUMORS OF THE SKIN. *Hemangiomas,* benign proliferations of dermal vessels, appear as red, blue, or purple, flat to papular and nodular lesions present at or soon after birth. Their appearance depends upon the number, size, and depth of the proliferating vessels. Thus, capillary angiomas are composed of small, superficial vessels causing *nevus flammeus* and *strawberry hemangiomas. Cavernous hemangiomas* are made up of larger and deeper vessels. Cavernous and strawberry angiomas often enlarge at an alarming rate over the first year or two and then usually involute by age nine or ten. Cavernous hemangiomas are less likely to resolve and at times may be deeply situated, large lesions that, when located in strategic locations (around the eye and mouth), may require systemic steroids that, in some instances, shrink these tumors. Platelet consumption by large cavernous hemangiomas may occur in the *Kasabach-Merritt syndrome*. Ordinarily no therapy is required for hemangiomas; watchful waiting allows the lesions to resolve spontaneously, the cosmetic result usually being superior to that obtained by therapeutic intervention. When large hemangiomas ulcerate, bleed, or impinge on vital structures or functions (e.g., around the ears, eyes, nose, mouth), oral steroids given over short periods of time in the dose of 1 to 2 mg per kilogram body weight shrink the tumor temporarily while awaiting the natural involution.

Pyogenic granuloma, a bright red, raspberry-like growth that can reach a centimeter in size, is friable and bleeds easily when traumatized. These lesions occur most often on arms, legs, fingers, and hands. They enlarge rapidly within weeks but have no malignant potential; they represent capillary hemangiomatous proliferation and occur following injury or surgery. The term *pyogenic* is a misnomer, as no infectious process is involved. These lesions are treated with excision, curettage and electrocauterization, or cryotherapy. Occasionally amelanotic melanoma may present as a pyogenic granuloma, so pathologic examination of pyogenic granulomas should be performed.

Kaposi's sarcoma (see Color Plate 16D) is a rare neoplasm of multifocal origin which presents as red-purple to blue-brown macules, plaques, and nodules of the skin and other organs. The cutaneous lesions may be firm or compressible, solitary or numerous, and may even appear initially as a dusky stain, especially about the toes.

These round-cell and spindle-cell sarcomas are also found in viscera and until their association with AIDS was recognized, seemed to occur predominantly in older men, leading to their demise. In Europe and North America, where Kaposi's sarcoma is more frequently seen among Jews and those of Mediterranean descent, the lesions commonly affect the lower extremities, are indolent, and often are associated with chronic lymphedema, indicating tumor infiltration of the lymphatics. Men are affected 10 to 15 times more often than women, are usually in their seventh decade, and have an average survival time of approximately 10 years. The incidence of such Kaposi's sarcoma reported for the United States is less than 0.1 per 100,000 population and fewer than 0.02 per cent of all malignancies.

In tropical Africa, however, there is an endemic belt at an altitude of 1200 to 1500 meters where the disease accounts for 3 to 9 per cent of all malignancies, afflicting the black population while sparing white people and Indians. It has a peak incidence in the first decade, with most patients less than 20 years of age, and with survival of less than 3 years. Visceral rather than cutaneous involvement and marked lymphadenopathy are the predominant clinical signs in these African children, who exhibit a unique form of Kaposi's sarcoma found in no other population.

The selective geographic distribution of the lymphadenopathic type of Kaposi's sarcoma is remarkably similar to that of Burkitt's lymphoma. With electron microscopic studies that affirm an association between cytomegalovirus and Kaposi's sarcoma, another parallel is made with Burkitt's lymphoma, the malignancy so closely linked to the Epstein-Barr virus. In the acquiring of Kaposi's sarcoma, therefore, it would seem that infectious agents and immune status are of significance, as well as genetic and environmental factors. Kaposi's sarcoma has been observed to complicate systemic lupus erythematosus being treated with immunosuppression and to appear along with tumors of lymphoreticular origin in the immunosuppressed recipients of renal transplants. It is known to coexist with other primary malignancies. However, its appearance as an aggressive lethal tumor in the young male homosexual is the stunning observation of grave concern. Those affected have a mean age in the fourth decade. Their skin lesions are generalized in distribution and are smaller, softer, and lighter in color than the classic firm, indurated lesions of the legs. Mucous membrane tumors or symptomatic visceral or lung lesions may appear before the hemorrhagic sarcomas of the skin. Average survival time from onset of the disease is less than 2 years.

Such fulminant Kaposi's sarcoma appears alone or with *Pneumocystis carinii* pneumonia and other opportunistic infections in increasing numbers in male homosexuals and drug abusers. A small painless red nodule of the skin, easily overlooked, can signal a profoundly compromised immune state and grave prognosis (see Ch. 417 and Color Plate 12D).

INFLAMMATORY NODULES OF THE SKIN. *Erythema nodosum* is an inflammatory reaction in subcutaneous fat which represents a hypersensitivity response to a number of antigenic stimuli. These well-localized, multiple, tender, red, deep nodules, 1 to 5 cm in size, usually develop bilaterally over the pretibial areas. They eventually involute, leaving yellow-purple bruises. Ulceration does not occur. Immunoglobulin and complement deposition has been found in deep blood vessels in early lesions, and in some patients circulating immune complexes have been detected. The localization of the painful nodules to the lower legs may be related to hemodynamic factors. Although no cause can be found in many patients, the following etiologic factors have been identified: drugs (especially oral contraceptives), pregnancy, inflammatory bowel disease, sarcoidosis, streptococcal infection, *Yersinia* enterocolitis, deep fungus infections, and tuberculosis. If the etiology cannot be identified and eliminated, symptomatic therapy with aspirin, nonsteroidal anti-inflammatory medications, potassium iodide, or occasionally short courses of systemic steroids may be useful.

Subcutaneous fat necrosis is a condition in which tender, red nodules occur on the lower legs and thighs in patients with pancreatitis or pancreatic carcinoma. The skin lesions may occur in the absence of signs associated with the internal carcinoma. Serum amylase and lipase values are elevated, and skin biopsy provides diagnostic findings.

Rheumatoid nodules are subcutaneous inflammatory lesions usually found over elbows, knees, and fingers in patients with severe rheumatoid arthritis and high rheumatoid factor titer (see Ch. 258).

NODULES ASSOCIATED WITH METABOLIC DISEASES AND MISCELLANEOUS CONDITIONS. *Xanthomas* are focal collections of lipid-containing histiocytes in the dermis and tendon sheaths which appear as yellowish papules (eruptive xanthomas), plaques (xanthelasma), nodules (xanthoma tuberosum), and xanthomas in tendons and tendon sheaths (xanthoma tendinosum). Xanthomas often arise in association with inherited hyperlipoproteinemias (see Ch. 172) or in a variety of underlying metabolic diseases that alter lipoprotein metabolism, such as diabetes, hypothyroidism, cholestatic liver disease, pancreatitis, and renal disease, and in reaction to some drugs (e.g., 13-*cis*-retinoic acid). Xanthelasma usually develops in the absence of hyperlipidemia, although hypercholesterolemia (and increased low density lipoproteins) may be present.

Patients with gout occasionally deposit sodium urate in the skin, forming firm, hard papules and nodules (tophi) that may discharge whitish crystals in the pinnae of the ears and periauricular areas.

ATROPHIC SKIN CONDITIONS WITH SCARRING, INDURATION, ULCERATION, AND TELANGIECTASIAS

Connective tissue diseases are the most common conditions that lead to this spectrum of cutaneous changes.

SCARRING. *Lupus erythematosus* may be localized to the skin (discoid lupus) or present as a systemic condition (see Ch. 261) (Table 525–11). Discoid lupus skin lesions appear as red plaques with white, cohesive scales that often are accentuated in the follicular openings (follicular plugging). The plaques eventu-

TABLE 525–11. ATROPHIC SKIN CONDITIONS WITH SCARRING, INDURATION, ULCERATION, AND TELANGIECTASIAS

Condition	Etiology	Important Physical Findings	Other Facts of Note
Connective Tissue Diseases			
Discoid lupus	Autoimmune conditions	Plaques with atrophic centers, erythematous and telangiectatic borders; follicular plugging prominent	May rarely be associated with systemic LE
Systemic lupus	Unknown	Erythematous, scaling, telangiectatic rash in sun-exposed areas; butterfly configuration on face; periungual telangiectasias	Antinuclear antibodies plus arthritis and serositis
Dermatomyositis	Unknown	Heliotrope of eyelids; Gottron's papules on knuckles, poikilodermatous changes on face, V of neck, elbows	Proximal muscle weakness; occasionally associated with underlying cancer
Morphea	Unknown	Localized patches of induration with erythematous borders	Seldom related to systemic sclerosis
Progressive systemic sclerosis	Unknown	Hidebound, indurated, tight skin over acral areas and face; periungual and matlike telangiectasias; ulceration of fingertips	Raynaud's phenomenon common; lungs, heart, GI tract may also be involved
Lichen sclerosus et atrophicus	Unknown	Porcelain white, indurated plaques commonly on genitalia but may occur on trunk; follicular plugging may be seen	
Cutaneous Ulcers of Extremities			
Venous and arterial insufficiency	Impairment of vascular flow	Arterial insufficiency causes ulcers; gangrene acrally with associated claudication; venous ulcers usually around malleoli in association with stasis dermatitis	Lower leg and foot edema common in venous insufficiency
Hemoglobinopathies	Poor oxygenation of tissue	Sickle cell anemia and other hemoglobinopathies can cause ulcerations on lower third of leg	
Pyoderma gangrenosum	Hypersensitivity reaction	Deep, necrotic ulcer with undermined violaceous borders, usually on the legs	Associated with ulcerative colitis, rheumatoid arthritis, dysproteinemia
Ecthyma gangrenosum	*Pseudomonas* septicemia	Ulcers with erythematous borders, usually in body folds	Often early sign of *Pseudomonas* septicemia
Genital Ulcers			
Venereal diseases			
Herpes	*Herpesvirus hominis*	Grouped vesicles that leave superficial erosions	
Syphilis	*Treponema pallidum*	Superficial, indurated, painless ulcer	VDRL may or may not be positive
Chancroid	*Haemophilus ducreyi*	Multiple, soft, painful ulcers with undermined edges	
Lymphogranuloma venereum	*Chlamydia trachomatis*	Transient, painless skin ulcer—inguinal bubo	
Granuloma inguinale	*Donovania granulomatis*	Nodules that erode with granulation tissue ulcer	
Behçet's disease	Autoimmune disease	Multiple shallow genital ulcers in association with oral aphthae and iritis	Erythema nodosum, arthritis, and CNS symptoms also seen

ally atrophy, with depression and scarring along with hypopigmentation in the center of the lesions and a hyperpigmented rim. The lesions usually occur in sun-exposed areas and, when they involve the scalp, cause scarring alopecia. Systemic lupus erythematosus presents as an erythematous rash with a violaceous hue, accentuated in sun-exposed areas, especially the malar area, producing a butterfly configuration. Telangiectasias may also be prominent, and, at times, fine scaling is seen. Occasionally bullae, erosions, and ulcers also occur. Periungual telangiectasia is a prominent finding in systemic lupus as well as in other connective tissue diseases. Subacute lupus is a form in which psoriasiform skin patches are found on the face and trunk. Skin biopsy for both routine and direct immunofluorescence pathologic examination is useful in confirming the diagnosis (see Table 522–3).

Dermatomyositis (see Ch. 268 and Color Plate 16*H*) findings include violaceous edema of eyelids (heliotrope), flat-topped papules over the knuckles (Gottron's papules), and reticulated patches of hyper- and hypopigmentation, erythema, and telangiectasia (poikiloderma) found on the V of the neck, face, elbows, and knees.

X-radiation can cause chronic skin changes of atrophy, telangiectasias, irregular pigmentation, and eventually ulceration. Within these areas malignant changes may later appear.

DERMAL INDURATIONS (SCLEROSIS). *Scleroderma* is a condition in which excessive collagen is found in the dermis (see Ch. 262). *Morphea* is localized scleroderma confined to the skin, whereas *systemic scleroderma*, or *progressive systemic sclerosis*, is a more extensive form in which fibrosis diffusely involves the skin as well as internal organs (see Ch. 262). Morphea lesions are asymptomatic, oval to irregular, whitish, firm, thickened patches with an erythematous border. The plaques are most often found on the trunk. The thickened skin in progressive systemic sclerosis is not sharply demarcated, but rather causes indurated, "hidebound" tight skin over the fingers, toes, and extremities (acrosclerosis). Thickening of the facial skin causes smoothness and loss of wrinkles except for furrowing around the mouth. Ulcerations followed by pitted scars occur on the fingertips. Telangiectasia may be prominent, appearing as periungual telangiectasias and multiple, small punctate macules on the face and hands (matlike telangiectasia). A variant of systemic scleroderma, the *CREST syndrome*, displays extensive telangiectasias over face and hands. Patients with *hereditary hemorrhagic telangiectasia* also display telangiectasia, particularly around the mouth and nose and on the fingers, as well as vascular malformations in the gastrointestinal tract and, at times, the lung. No cutaneous induration is found in this condition.

Lichen sclerosus et atrophicus may be confused with morphea, presenting as porcelain white, atrophic, indurated plaques most commonly on the vulva or on the male genitalia (balanitis xerotica obliterans). At times it occurs as scattered patches on the trunk. Purpuric areas may also be seen within the lesions.

Myxedema may cause a doughy thickening of the skin from deposition of glycosaminoglycans in the dermis. This may be localized to the pretibial areas (pretibial myxedema) as firm, nonpitting plaques and nodules with accentuation of the follicular orifices giving a peau d'orange appearance.

CUTANEOUS ULCERS. Primary skin ulcers are caused by a wide variety of etiologies and conditions. The location of the ulcers, the symptoms associated with them, and the rapidity of their appearance are important clues in diagnosing their various etiologies.

Ulcers of the extremities are frequently associated with vascular disease. Sudden pain associated with numbness of an extremity and ulceration suggest arterial occlusion. Ulceration of digits associated with a purplish red color with dependency and pallor when the extremity is elevated suggests arteriosclerotic peripheral vascular disease. Brawny edema, brown discoloration, and dermatitis over the lower legs in association with ulcers around the malleoli are seen with venous insufficiency. Sickle cell anemia causes ulcerations in the lower third of the leg. Areas of pressure and trauma, particularly on the foot, in patients with peripheral neuropathy, are susceptible to neurotrophic ulcers (mal perforant), as in diabetes and leprosy. The skin around the ulcer is anesthetic and calloused. Pressure sores or decubitus ulcers occur in immobilized debilitated patients. Shearing forces, friction, moisture, and pressure contribute to the development of these sores. The sacral and coccygeal areas, ischial tuberosities, and greater trochanters are favored sites. The best treatment of

pressure sores is prevention by frequently moving immobilized patients, keeping the skin clean, and using air mattresses.

An unusual and dramatic ulcerative condition, *pyoderma gangrenosum*, often begins as an inflammatory nodule or pustule resembling a furuncle which breaks down, ulcerates, and gradually enlarges peripherally. Fully developed, the lesions are moderately deep, red, necrotic ulcers with undermined, violaceous, edematous borders. These lesions, which typically evolve on the lower legs, are postulated to represent a Shwartzman-like hypersensitivity reaction to a number of underlying internal conditions, including chronic ulcerative colitis, regional ileitis, rheumatoid arthritis, dysproteinemias, and occasionally leukemia or lymphoma. In over one half of the cases no etiology is identified.

Ecthyma gangrenosum is characterized by ulcerative lesions, often in the body folds (anogenital and axillary areas), in immunosuppressed patients with *Pseudomonas* septicemia. The painless lesions begin as hemorrhagic bullous patches that become necrotic and ulcerate and are surrounded by considerable erythema with a central gray to black eschar. *Pseudomonas* can be cultured from these skin lesions.

Ulcerations on the genitalia are suggestive of venereal disease, including herpes simplex (multiple grouped vesicles and erosions), syphilis (indurated, painless, round ulcer with a clean base), chancroid (single or multiple, soft, painful, purulent ulcers with undermined erythematous edges), lymphogranuloma venereum (transient, painless skin ulcer with associated inguinal bubo-adenopathy), and granuloma inguinale (small nodules on genitalia which erode and become filled with velvety red granulation).

Multiple genital ulcers also occur in *Behçet's syndrome* in association with oral ulcers and ocular disease (iridocyclitis). Erythema nodosum, arthritis, and neurologic and intestinal involvement may also occur. The oral and genital ulcers are small, painful aphthae. Occasionally sterile pustules and ulcers at the site of minor trauma such as blood sampling can occur (pathergy) (see Ch. 269).

Geometric, bizarre-shaped, angular ulcers are characteristic of a self-inflicted, factitial cause.

HYPER- AND HYPOPIGMENTATION OF THE SKIN

Disorders of melanin pigmentation can be classified as hypomelanoses (decreased or absent epidermal melanin) or hypermelanoses (increased epidermal or dermal melanin). Hyper- and hypomelanosis can be further subdivided into localized or generalized (total body) alterations of pigmentation (Table 525–12).

Hyperpigmentary Conditions

LOCALIZED PIGMENTARY CONDITIONS. *Freckles* (ephelides) are light brown-red macules found in sun-exposed areas which are caused by increased melanin production in normal numbers of melanocytes. These occur in fair-complexioned individuals with red or sandy hair. Ultraviolet radiation increases melanin production in these lesions.

Lentigines are also hyperpigmented macules, but they occur because of increased numbers of melanocytes in the basal layer of the epidermis. Two types are recognized: (1) *lentigo simplex*, which occurs in early life and is congenital, and (2) *actinic lentigines*, which are acquired in middle age and are related to sun damage over the face, arms, and dorsum of the hands. Actinic lentigines are sometimes difficult to distinguish from early lentigo maligna on the face, but actinic lentigines have no malignant potential. The *multiple lentigines syndrome* is a rare, dominantly inherited condition characterized by hundreds of Lentigines on the trunk, head, extremities, palms, and soles, and it is associated with Electrocardiographic abnormalities, Ocular hypertelorism, Pulmonary stenosis, Abnormal genitalia, Retarded growth, and Deafness (thus the acronym LEOPARD syndrome). Another dominantly inherited condition is *Peutz-Jeghers syndrome*, distinctive for its numerous lentigines occurring around the mouth, eyes, hands, and feet in association with gastrointestinal polyps, gastrointestinal hemorrhage, and occasionally malignant degeneration of the polyps.

Melasma (chloasma) of the face usually affects women, and in this instance the melanocytes produce more melanin than normal in response to hormonal factors (occurs during pregnancy or while on birth control pills) in association with ultraviolet radiation. This type of pigmentation occurs symmetrically over the malar eminences, forehead, and upper lip (Fig. 525–19). The lesions may fade with delivery but often persist and are accentuated when birth control pills are used. Hydroquinone, a bleaching agent (2 to 4 per cent creams), may help reduce the pigmentation but many authorities believe these are of no value and that they may worsen the problem. Sunscreens are also useful.

Postinflammatory hyperpigmentation is the term given to macular pigmentation following inflammatory skin diseases (lichen planus typically causes brown to blue pigmentation).

Café au lait spots are light brown (coffee-with-cream hue) macules that occur on the trunk and extremities in neurofibromatosis (Fig. 525–20). Six or more such lesions, each greater than 1.5 cm in diameter, are diagnostic for this dominantly inherited disease. Axillary freckling, discrete neurofibromas (Fig. 525–21), and large plexiform neurofibromas along with bony abnormalities combine to make this a disfiguring condition. Ten per cent of the normal population have isolated café au lait spots. In *Albright's disease* (polyostotic fibrous dysplasia) three or four large, irregularly shaped (so-called "coast-of-Maine" configuration), hyperpigmented macules are usually found unilaterally distributed on the buttocks or cervical area.

Xeroderma pigmentosum is a rare, heterogeneous group of diseases with hereditary deficiencies of enzyme systems in the skin that repair ultraviolet-induced damage to keratinocyte and melanocyte DNA. This inability to maintain the integrity of DNA leads to extreme sun sensitivity and multiple freckles over the face, lips, conjunctivae, and extremities which evolve into varia-bly sized pigmented patches interspersed with hypopigmented areas. Keratoses, keratoacanthomas, basal and squamous cell cancers, and malignant melanomas evolve and frequently lead to early death. This entity should be thought of whenever one finds otherwise unexplained extreme sensitivity to the sun or excessive freckling in youngsters. This disease can be subtle in its initial presentation, and total avoidance of the sun from early life may prevent subsequent fatal skin cancers.

GENERALIZED HYPERPIGMENTATION. Diffuse brown hyperpigmentation is a feature of *Addison's disease* with accentuation of the pigment in body folds (palmar creases), pressure points (knuckles, elbows), and gingival mucous membrane. A similar type of diffuse hyperpigmentation is seen following adrenalectomy in patients with Cushing's disease due to a pituitary tumor, as well as in patients with pancreatic and lung carcinomas. In all of these instances the generalized hypermelanosis results from overproduction of melanocyte-stimulating hormone (MSH) and adrenocorticotropic hormone (ACTH). These trophic hormones share common amino acid sequences. Both MSH and ACTH secretions are increased in Addison's disease as a result of diminished output of cortisol by the adrenals. Oat cell cancers of the lung and pancreatic carcinomas have been found to excrete increased amounts of MSH, thus causing similar hyperpigmentation. Melanocyte MSH receptors bind MSH, which stimulates intracellular cyclic AMP, and this, in turn, increases tyrosinase activity and pigment formation in melanocytes.

A number of drugs can cause Addisonian-like hypermelanosis including busulfan, cyclophosphamide, and nitrogen mustard. Blue-gray pigmentation may occur either diffusely or in localized patches following use of chlorpromazine, minocycline, and antimalarial drugs. In addition, inorganic trivalent arsenicals (found in insecticides and contaminated water) may also produce a

TABLE 525–12. HYPER- AND HYPOPIGMENTATION OF THE SKIN

	Etiology	Important Physical Findings	Other Facts of Note
Hyperpigmentation			
Localized			
Freckles	Increased melanin synthesis in skin	Light brown macules on sun-exposed areas	UV light accentuates
Lentigines	May be congenital or related to chronic sun exposure	Flat, light brown, uniformly pigmented lesions	No malignant potential
Melasma	Hormonal changes (pregnancy, birth control pills) plus sunlight	Irregular, flat, light brown areas on malar areas, cheeks, forehead	May fade after delivery or coming off birth control pills
Café au lait spots	Dominantly inherited pigmented lesion	Single to multiple coffee-with-cream-colored macules; may be associated with neurofibromatosis	Six or more such lesions suggest neurofibromatosis
Generalized			
Addison's disease	Increased MSH, ACTH	Diffuse hyperpigmentation with accentuation in body folds, palmar creases	Similar pigmentation with lung cancer; Cushing's disease with pituitary tumor
Hemochromatosis	Deposition of iron in skin and increased melanin in skin	Metallic gray-brown hyperpigmentation	
Chronic arsenic exposure	Stimulation of melanin synthesis in skin	Generalized hyperpigmentation studded with small depigmented macules	Keratosis on palms and soles
Hypopigmentation			
Localized			
Vitiligo	Immunologically mediated loss of melanocytes	Symmetrically distributed depigmented macules around body orifices and over bony prominences	In small percentage of cases associated with pernicious anemia, diabetes, thyroiditis, hyperthyroidism, Addison's disease
Piebaldism	Failure of melanocytes to migrate to skin in embryologic development	White forelock and depigmented patch—midline forehead, thorax	
Pityriasis alba	Dry skin	Pink, oval hypopigmented patches that often scale on face, trunk	Often accompanies atopic eczema, dry skin
Tuberous sclerosis	Dominantly inherited condition	Ash leaf–shaped, white macules on trunk, extremities; often present at birth	Associated with adenoma sebaceum, tuberous sclerosis
Generalized			
Oculocutaneous albinism	Autosomal recessive traits with variable degrees of tyrosinase insufficiency	White skin, hair; no pigment in fundi oculi; translucent irides	Nystagmus and eye problems common
Phenylketonuria	Deficiency of enzyme converting phenylalanine to tyrosine, so decreased precursor for melanin synthesis	Generalized depigmentation of hair, skin, eye color	Severe mental developmental defects if not diagnosed early and treated with special diet

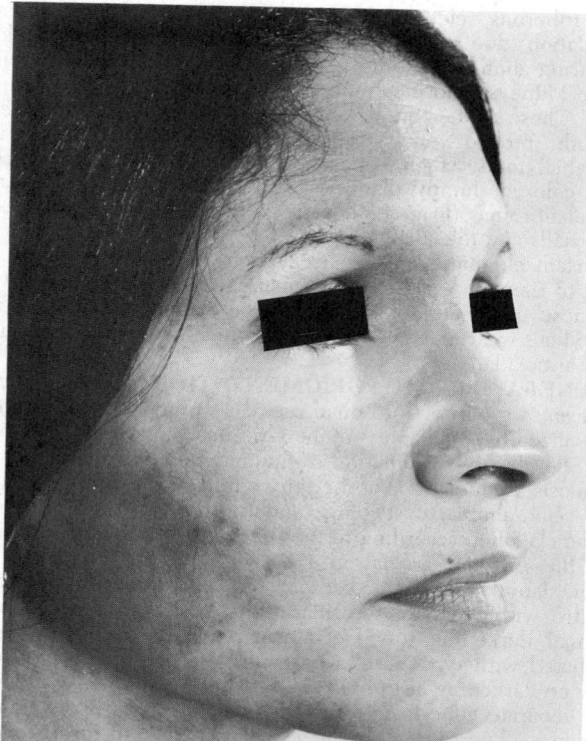

FIGURE 525–19. Melasma. (From the 17th edition of the Cecil Textbook of Medicine, with the permission of Dr. Marie-Louise Johnson.)

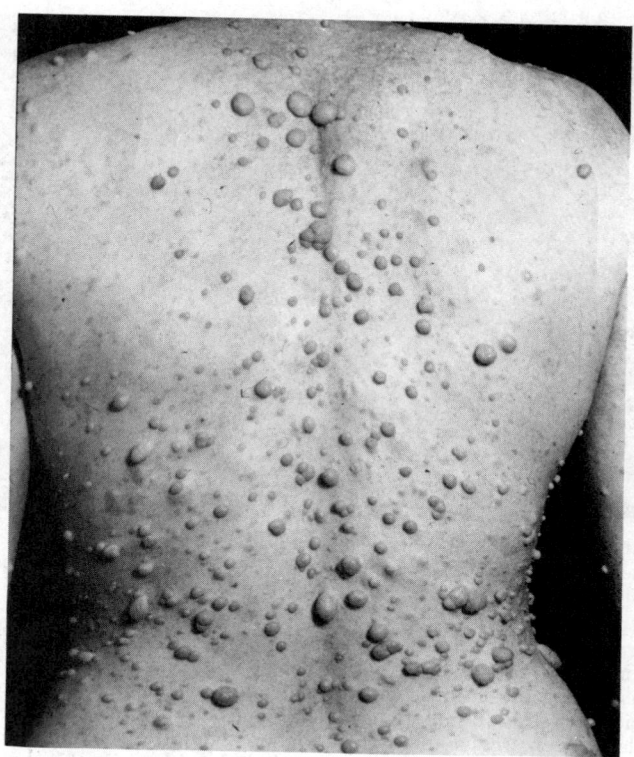

FIGURE 525–21. Neurofibromatosis—von Recklinghausen's disease. (From the 17th edition of the Cecil Textbook of Medicine, with the permission of Dr. Marie-Louise Johnson.)

generalized brown pigmentation, but in this instance the hyper-melanosis is studded with small, scattered, depigmented macules (likened to rain drops on a dusty road) and punctate keratoses on the palms and soles. *Hemochromatosis* causes a metallic gray-brown, generalized hyperpigmentation resulting from the combination of increased pigment formation in the skin and iron deposition.

Hypopigmentary Conditions

LOCALIZED PIGMENTARY CHANGES. *Vitiligo,* a circumscribed hypomelanosis of progressively enlarging amelanotic macules in a symmetric distribution around body orifices and over bony prominences (knees, elbows, hands), is familial in 36 per cent of cases. In one third of cases some spontaneous repigmentation occurs, particularly in sun-exposed areas. White hairs are common in the vitiliginous areas. Although most patients with vitiligo are healthy, there is an increased association with certain autoimmune conditions such as thyroiditis, hyperthyroidism, Addison's disease, pernicious anemia, and diabetes mellitus. Melanocytes are absent from the vitiliginous macules. Circulating complement-binding antimelanocyte antibodies have been found in some vitiligo patients. The use of PUVA may give some repigmentation, but it may require 200 or more such treatments.

Piebaldism is a local hypopigmentary condition representing an autosomal dominant hypomelanosis on the extremities, anterior surface of the thorax, and especially over the midline of the forehead and central scalp. A white forelock is typical. The hypomelanosis stems from the lack of normal migration of the melanocytes to these regions during embryologic development.

Waardenburg's syndrome, another autosomal dominant condition, may be confused with piebaldism, as a white forelock is seen, but other abnormalities are also found at birth, including perceptive deafness, heterochromia, and hypertelorism.

A common localized form of hypopigmentation, *pityriasis alba,* appears as slightly pink and hypopigmented, oval to round patches with mild, fine scaling. These occur on the cheeks of children, but they may also be found on the trunk, mimicking the hypopigmented, scaling patches seen in tinea versicolor (a KOH examination of the scales may be necessary to differentiate these two conditions). Pityriasis alba is most frequently seen in atopic dermatitis patients.

Tuberous sclerosis, an autosomal dominant condition, displays white macules in 98 per cent of cases. These depigmented macules characteristically are found on the trunk or buttocks in an oval or mountain ash–leaf configuration (Fig. 525–22). The presence of three or more of these macules is strongly suggestive of tuberous sclerosis, and because the hypomelanotic patches are

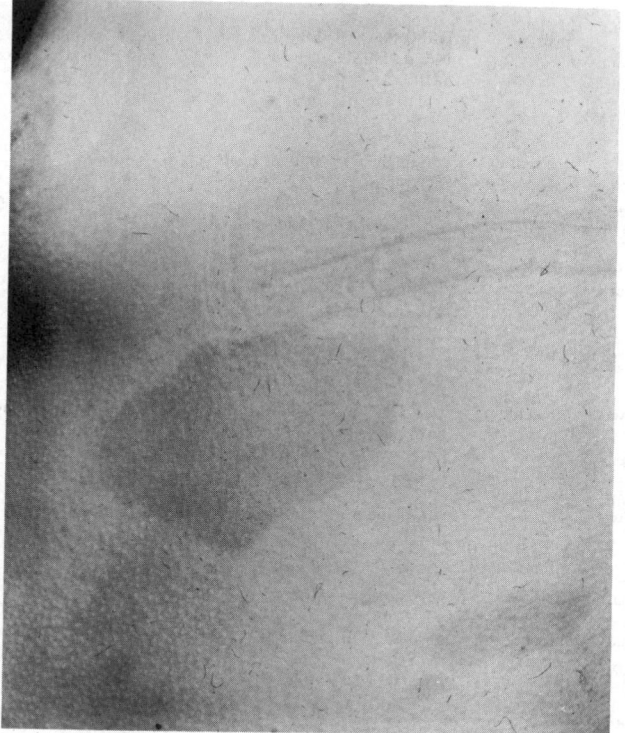

FIGURE 525–20. Café au lait spot. (From the 17th edition of the Cecil Textbook of Medicine, with the permission of Dr. Marie-Louise Johnson.)

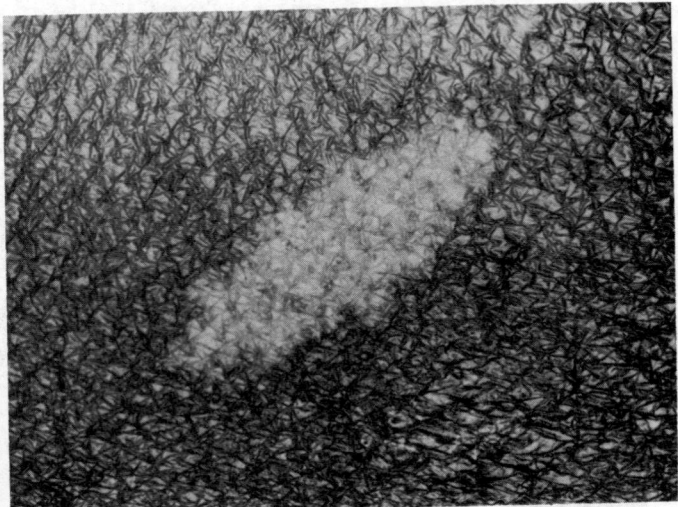

FIGURE 525–22. Tuberous sclerosis ash leaf. (From the 17th edition of the Cecil Textbook of Medicine, with the permission of Dr. Marie-Louise Johnson.)

present at birth, they represent one of the earliest signs of the condition. Examination with Wood's light is often useful in visualizing the lesions, which histologically contain melanocytes with decreased numbers of melanosomes. Newborns with unexplained seizures or mental retardation should be screened with a Wood's light for the presence of the white spots. CT brain scans are also useful in defining the tumorous dysplasia. Patients

with tuberous sclerosis (epiloia) suffer from seizures, mental retardation (due to hamartomatous gliomas), phakomas (yellow-appearing gliomatous tumors of the retina), bilateral hamartomas of the kidneys, and a number of hamartomatous tumors of the skin. These cutaneous lesions include *adenoma sebaceum* (smooth, red to yellow papules over the butterfly area and nasolabial folds which appear by age four), shagreen patches (flesh-colored, lumpy plaques over the lumbosacral area), and ungual fibromas (firm, pink papules in the periungual areas of fingernails and toenails).

Certain chemicals, particularly phenol derivatives, when applied to the skin, may cause permanent depigmentation. Hypomelanosis has been observed on the hands of black-skinned individuals wearing rubber gloves in which hydroquinone is used as an antioxidant.

GENERALIZED HYPOPIGMENTATION. *Oculocutaneous albinism*, a group of autosomal recessive traits, is recognized by generalized hypomelanosis of the skin, hair, and eyes (Table 525–13). The classic constellation of findings includes marked hypomelanosis or amelanosis of the skin, white or faintly yellow-blond hair, photophobia, nystagmus, and translucent irides. Albinism can be classified according to the presence or absence of tyrosinase, the enzyme crucial in the synthesis of eumelanin and pheomelanin. Normal plucked hair bulbs darken when incubated in vitro with tyrosine; tyrosinase-positive albinos display some minimal darkening (but not normal) of the hair bulb when incubated with tyrosinase, whereas tyrosinase-negative patients show no darkening of the hair bulb. These two types of albinism have separate gene loci. Although melanogenesis is deficient in both forms, persons with the tyrosinase-positive form develop some pigmented nevi and less eye damage than tyrosinase-negative albinos. Persons with *phenylketonuria* have diffuse hypopigmentation, with light hair and blue eyes. This is an autosomal recessive disorder in which the enzyme that converts

TABLE 525–13. ALBINISM

			Skin			Eyes	
	Inheritance	Frequency	Color	Pigmented Nevi Freckles	Hair	Color	Red Reflex
Oculocutaneous Albinism							
Tyrosinase-negative	AR*	1 in 34,000	pink/wte	none	white	gray-blue	present
Tyrosinase-positive	AR	blk: 1 in 15,000 wte: 1 in 40,000	wte-cream	present	wte-yellow red: darkens	blue-yellow brown	present but may be absent in dark races
Yellow-mutant	AR	rare—Amish, Polish, German-American; blacks (American, Ceylonese, African)	wte at birth, slgt tan pos	present	wte-birth red/yellow 6 mos	blue at birth: darkens	present
Hermansky-Pudlak syndrome	AR	rare—cases from Puerto Rico; Southern Holland; Madras	cream-lgt normal	present	wte-red dk brown	blue-gray to brown	wte—present blk—absent
Cross-McKusick-Breen syndrome (oculocerebral hypopigmentation syndrome)	AR	extremely rare—3 in Amish family	pink/wte	present	wte-lt yel	gray-blue	?, cataracts
Chédiak-Higashi syndrome	AR	rare in most countries; none in blacks	pink/wte	present	blond-dk brown-steel gray	blue to brown	present but diminishes with time
Oculocutaneous Albinoidism	AD†		pink/wte	?	wte blond	blue	present
Ocular Albinism							
Vogt	X-linked	uncommon	normal	present	normal	blue	
Forsius-Eriksson	X-linked	less common	normal	present	normal	blue	
Autosomal recessive	AR	10 families	normal	present	normal	blue	present

*AR = Autosomal recessive.
†AD = Autosomal dominant.
Reprinted from the chapter by Dr. Marie-Louise Johnson in the 17th edition of the Cecil Textbook of Medicine, with her permission.

phenylalanine to tyrosine is deficient. Consequently, melanin synthesis is decreased (see Ch. 177).

REGIONAL DIAGNOSIS OF SKIN DISEASES—COMMONLY ENCOUNTERED PROBLEMS BY ANATOMIC REGION

Many skin diseases have a predilection for certain areas or regions of the body, often related to variations in the structure and function of the integument (Table 525–14).

Disorders of the Nails

The nail is a plate of hard keratin synthesized from an invagination of the epidermis. The proximal nail fold houses the matrix of the nail where basal cells rapidly proliferate and differentiate into the nail plate, which grows over the nail bed. Nails grow continuously throughout life. The average fingernail grows 0.5 to 1.2 mm per week, whereas toenails grow at one half to one third this rate. It takes a fingernail about 5.5 months and the toenails 12 to 18 months to regrow from the matrix, although rate of growth slows as the individual gets older. Defects in nail formation go by various terms useful in describing nail disorders:

1. *Brittleness*—easy breaking of nail tips
2. *Leukonychia*—white discoloration of nails
3. *Striations*—longitudinal ridges running parallel or perpendicular to the length of the nail
4. *Onycholysis*—separation of the nail plate from the bed
5. *Onychogryphosis*—hypertrophy and thickening of the nail
6. *Onychomycosis*—dystrophy, destruction of the nail due to yeast and fungal infections
7. *Pitting*—discrete pitlike depressions in the nail surface
8. *Koilonychia*—spoon-shaped deformity of the nails (concave nail with everted edges)
9. *Pterygium formation*—growth of cuticle onto the nail plate.

SKIN DISEASES INVOLVING NAILS. Nail changes in *psoriasis* have been described above. Fingernails are more frequently involved than toenails. Fungal infection must be ruled out.

Therapy of psoriatic nail changes is not satisfactory, although topical tar and steroid preparations may be of some help.

In 10 per cent of *lichen planus* patients, accentuated longitudinal nail ridging occurs as well as pterygium formation resulting from destructive focal scarring of the matrix. Early treatment with oral steroids is indicated to arrest the cicatricial course.

Nail pitting frequently occurs in *alopecia areata* along with onycholysis. The nail is susceptible to deformities when *eczematous* processes involve the periungual regions and matrix. *Atopic eczema* and other eczematous entities may cause pitting, transverse striations, and onycholysis.

Onychomycosis, or fungal infections of the nail, may be caused by dermatophyte (tinea unguium) or candidal infections. Infection of toenails is more frequent than fingernails, but all nails may be involved. The nail plate is discolored (cloudy, yellowish or brown), thickened, crumbly, and onycholytic with accumulation of debris under the nail. White superficial onychomycosis appears as white patches in the toenail plate due to organisms growing on the surface barely penetrating the nail. Scrapings reveal hyphae upon KOH examination. An unusual condition, *chronic mucocutaneous candidiasis*, is caused by widespread *Candida albicans* infection leading to diffuse white thickening of all nails.

Topical antifungal therapy is ineffective, so oral griseofulvin is given for dermatophyte infection until the nails appear clear. Ketoconazole (200 mg daily) is an alternative should griseofulvin fail or when *Candida* is the causative agent. Oral therapy requires 4 to 6 months for fingernails and 12 to 16 months for toenails. In older individuals toenail problems may never be eradicated because the nails grow so slowly. Residual fungal spores in the patient's shoes and environment are no doubt responsible for the high frequency of recurrence, and for this reason topical antifungal powders may be helpful in long-term prophylaxis.

Paronychia, or painful, red swelling of the nail fold, is usually caused by *Candida albicans*. At times a small abscess or purulent discharge is seen. This infection usually occurs in hands constantly exposed to a wet environment (bartenders, janitors). Therapy

TABLE 525–13. ALBINISM Continued

Nystagmus	Photophobia	Eyes — Visual Acuity	Eyes — Pigment in Fundus	Eyes — Other	Hair Bulb Incubation (Tyrosine)	Defect	Melanosome Maturation by Stage	Complications or Associated Problems
marked	severe	legally blind	none	—	negative	no tyrosinase	I-unmelanized II	skin malignancy basal cell ca squamous cell ca
present but less	present but variable	severe defect in children; may improve with age	none; some with age	pigment cartwheel pupil, limbus	positive	no access of enzyme to tyrosine	I, II, some III, rare IV	skin malignancy basal cell ca squamous cell ca
present but variable	present but variable	marked defect; may improve with age	none; some with age	pigment cartwheel effect	neg to pos ?	unknown ? pheomelanogenesis	I, II, III	unknown
present but variable	present, may be severe	normal or slight decrease	none; some with age	may have pigment cartwheel	positive	pleiotropic effect— single gene mutation	I, II, III	storage-pool defect platelets; ceroid-like material in RE system, oral mucosa, urine
marked	—	blind	?, cataracts	?, cataracts	weakly positive	decreased melanocytes	I, II, III, IV	oligophrenia, athetosis, severe mental retardation
absent or slight	absent or slight	normal or slight decrease	some; increase with age	normal for cartwheel effect	positive	giant melanosomes, lethal defect in leukocytes	I, II, III, IV	infections; hematologic and neurologic abnormalities; lymphoreticular malignancy
no	no	normal or slight decrease	punctate		positive	unknown	unknown	none
present	severe	marked decrease	reduced		positive			
latent	absent or slight	color blind			positive			
present	severe	marked decrease			positive			

TABLE 525–14. REGIONAL DERMATOLOGY

Region of Skin	Type of Skin Group	Disease Process
Scalp	Papulosquamous and eczematous	Psoriasis, seborrheic dermatitis, tinea capitis, eczema (atopic, contact)
	Pustular	Folliculitis, kerion
	Nodular	Nevi, seborrheic keratosis, pilar cysts, verruca
	Atrophic and telangiectatic	Connective tissue disease, scleroderma, discoid LE
Face	Pustular	Acne, rosacea, folliculitis, tinea
	Papulosquamous and eczematous	Psoriasis, seborrheic dermatitis, contact dermatitis (cosmetics), atopic dermatitis, impetigo, lupus erythematosus, photodermatitis
	Vesicular	Herpes zoster and herpes simplex, insect bites
	Nodular	Basal cell cancers, squamous cell cancers, melanomas, keratoacanthomas, nevi, actinic keratosis, tuberous xanthomas
Trunk	Papulosquamous and eczematous	Psoriasis, atopic and contact eczema, tinea versicolor, pityriasis rosacea, scabies
	Vesiculobullous	Pemphigus, bullous pemphigoid
	Maculopapular	Secondary syphilis, drug reaction, viral exanthems
	Nodular	Nevi, seborrheic keratosis, lipoma, basal cell cancer, keloid, neurofibroma, angiomas, melanoma
	Pustular	Acne
	Urticarial	Hives
Arms and forearms	Eczematous and papulosquamous	Contact dermatitis—plants; atopic dermatitis, lichen planus
	Nodular	Nevi, warts, seborrheic keratosis, actinic keratosis
	Atrophic telangiectasia	Scleroderma, dermatomyositis
Legs	Eczematous and papulosquamous	Contact dermatitis, stasis dermatitis, atopic dermatitis, psoriasis, lichen planus
	Nodular	Erythema nodosum, dermatofibromas, nevi, melanoma, Kaposi's sarcoma, lipoma
	Maculopapular	Vasculitis, Schamberg's disease, actinic purpura, pretibial myxedema
	Atrophic, telangiectatic, and ulcerative	Scleroderma, dermatostasis ulcers, arterial insufficiency
Genitalia and groin	Eczematous and papulosquamous	Contact dermatitis, seborrheic dermatitis, scabies, pediculosis pubis, psoriasis, Reiter's syndrome, erythrasma, tinea, candidiasis, lichen planus, intertrigo, lichen simplex chronicus
	Vesiculobullous	Herpes simplex, Stevens-Johnson syndrome
	Ulcerative and atrophic	Syphilis, chancroid, lymphopathia venerum, Behçet's syndrome
	Nodular	Verrucae vulgaris, erythroplasia of Queyrat, squamous cell cancer, sebaceous cyst, molluscum contagiosum
	Pustular	Hidradenitis suppurativa
Hands	Eczematous and papulosquamous	Allergic contact and irritant contact dermatitis, dyshidrosis, pyoderma, tinea, dermatophytids, scabies, atopic dermatitis, secondary syphilis
	Vesiculobullous, pustular	Erythema multiforme, hand-foot-and-mouth disease, porphyria cutanea tarda, psoriasis
	Nodular	Warts, squamous cell cancer, actinic keratosis, keratoacanthoma, pyogenic granuloma, granuloma annulare, synovial cysts
	Hypopigmented	Vitiligo
	Atrophic-telangiectatic	Scleroderma, dermatomyositis
Feet	Eczematous and papulosquamous	Contact dermatitis, atopic dermatitis, tinea, psoriasis, lichen planus
	Vesiculobullous	Tinea, epidermolysis bullosa, erythema multiforme
	Nodules	Verruca, corn, nevus
	Atrophic-telangiectatic	Scleroderma

consists of avoidance of water and the use of antifungal solutions two or three times a day for a month or two.

EXOGENOUS FACTORS CAUSING NAIL CHANGES. Cosmetics, trauma, and occupational influences can all cause nail deformities. Nail hardeners, enamel removers, and stick-on nails all may cause reactions including onycholysis, subungual hyperkeratoses, paronychia, and contact dermatitis around the nails. Nail manipulation, biting, and tight-fitting shoes may induce nail injury. A variety of systemic drugs may induce color changes or other alterations in the nails (e.g., chronic arsenic ingestion causes transverse white lines—Mees' lines; antimalarials, blue-brown coloration; minocycline, variable brown discoloration).

NAIL DISTURBANCES IN SYSTEMIC DISEASES. *Splinter hemorrhages* result from the extravasation of blood from longitudinally oriented vessels of the nail bed. Although often thought to be associated with bacterial endocarditis, they are much more commonly associated with trauma to the nails. *Beau's lines* are commonly associated with systemic disease, but they are nonspecific, appearing as transverse depressions across the nail plates of all nails following any severe disability that temporarily interferes with nail growth, including systemic infections, myocardial infarction, and use of chemotherapeutic agents. *Longitudinal pigmented bands* occur most often in response to trauma or a nevus located in the matrix, but in white individuals a melanoma must be ruled out. *Yellow nail syndrome* exhibits yellow thickening of all the nails with absence of the lunula and variable degrees of onycholysis in association with a number of pulmonary conditions such as bronchiectasis, pleural effusion, and chronic obstructive pulmonary disease. Lymphedema of the extremities may be a third component of the syndrome. *Clubbing* of the nails (increased bilateral curvature of the nails with enlargement of the soft connective tissue of the distal phalanges resulting in the flattening of the obtuse angle formed by the proximal end of the nail and the digit) occurs most often with respiratory ailments, including bronchiectasis, lung abscess, and pulmonary neoplasms. Cardiovascular disease and chronic gastrointestinal diseases (ulcerative colitis, sprue) are also associated with clubbing. When clubbing is found with bone pain and proliferative periostitis, it is termed *hypertrophic osteoarthropathy*, and the condition is most often associated with bronchogenic squamous cell carcinoma. *Nail-patella syndrome* is a dominantly inherited condition affecting both mesodermal and ectodermal structures which causes defective growth of nails (often the nails are missing) in association with hypoplasia or absence of the patellae and enlarged, palpable iliac horns. *Hereditary ectodermal dysplasia* appears in two forms, hidrotic and anhidrotic. The teeth and hair are involved similarly in both (anodontia, hypodontia, and peg-shaped teeth in association with soft, downy, scant hair in the scalp and eyebrows), but in the hidrotic form sweat gland function is normal and the nails are small, thickened, and longitudinally striated.

TUMORS OF THE NAIL. A variety of benign tumors occur around the nail unit. These include *periungual fibromas*, *myxoid cysts*, and *subungual exostoses*. Surgical removal of the benign tumors is the only certain means of cure.

The main malignant tumor involving the nails is *melanoma*, which appears as a pigmented area at the base of the nail or as a longitudinal pigmented streak in the nail. Nevi can give the same appearance, and biopsy of the lesion in the matrix is the only absolute way of making a diagnosis.

Disorders of the Mucous Membranes

Any abnormality of color, texture, or appearance of the mucous membranes should be investigated. Malignant changes should be suspected in infiltrated or ulcerated lesions and a biopsy performed.

ULCERATIVE AND BULLOUS LESIONS. *Acute ulcerative lesions* may be caused by trauma (from jagged teeth or ill-fitting dentures); bacterial infections such as acute necrotizing ulcerative gingivostomatitis (Vincent's angina; infection with *Borrelia vincentii* and fusiform bacilli which cause punched-out ulcers in the interdental papillae and gingival inflammation); infections with *Staphylococcus* and gram-negative organisms in patients receiving chemotherapy; viral infections such as primary herpetic gingivostomatitis with small vesicles that rupture leaving shallow, discrete ulcers anywhere in the mouth; infectious mononucleosis, which frequently causes exudative tonsillitis and aphthous ulcers of the buccal and labial mucosae; a coxsackievirus infection termed herpangina which results in vesicles that rupture, leaving 1- to 2-mm ulcers with a grayish base over the pharynx; *Candida* infections causing white pseudomembranous lesions; drug reactions that can elicit oral ulcerations (salicylates, barbiturates, antiepileptic drugs, and particularly drugs used for chemotherapy such as methotrexate, actinomycin-D, and daunorubicin, which are extremely toxic to mucosal epithelium).

Chronic oral ulcerations are most frequently caused by bullous diseases (pemphigus, cicatricial pemphigoid, bullous pemphigoid—see above). Both discoid and systemic lupus erythematosus may have associated mouth lesions with central depressed erosions and elevated keratotic borders. Reiter's syndrome may include superficial erythematous erosions anywhere in the oral cavity. Any chronic, localized, erosive lesion in the mouth should be viewed with concern as a possible carcinoma.

Recurrent ulcerative conditions of the mouth are most commonly aphthous stomatitis or herpes simplex stomatitis. *Aphthous stomatitis* is manifested by multiple punched-out ulcers on the buccal and labial mucosae that may be grouped, simulating herpes. A severe form of aphthous stomatitis (periadenitis mucosa necrotica recurrens) with large, deep, recurrent painful ulcers may involve any area of the mouth. An immunologic reaction to intrinsic mouth bacteria may play a role in aphthous ulcers, as tetracycline suspension mouthwashes may reduce the duration, size, and pain of the oral ulcers.

Recurrent *herpes simplex* of the oral mucosa is unusual but should be differentiated from aphthous stomatitis by Tzanck preparation and herpes cultures. Another recurrent condition is Behçet's syndrome (see above). Erythema multiforme may present as an acute, recurrent, erosive stomatitis in association with target lesions of the skin.

WHITE PATCHES. Thrush (*Candida albicans* infection of the oral epithelium) appears as curdy white membranes that can be scraped away, leaving an inflamed base. It is most common in newborns and in immunosuppressed adults and is a common presenting symptom in AIDS, especially in Africa. KOH examination of material scraped from the white patch is diagnostic. Clotrimazole troches dissolved in the mouth twice a day are very successful in clearing such infections. The white oral lesions of lichen planus have been mentioned above. Leukoplakia is discussed in Ch. 95.

GLOSSITIS AND DISEASES AFFECTING THE TONGUE. Two common clinical varieties of glossitis (see Ch. 95) are geographic tongue and black hairy tongue. *Geographic tongue* is a recurrent condition characterized by loss of filiform papillae on the dorsum of the tongue. Typically, a white margin of desquamating epithelium surrounds a central, red, atrophic area. Lesions often migrate across the surface of the tongue, giving a maplike appearance. The lesions may be uncomfortable but are often asymptomatic. The cause is unknown, and no treatment is available. *Black hairy tongue* is a condition recognized by elongated black or brown filiform papillae that grow on the posterior tongue and extend toward the tip. The condition is seen in patients using systemic antibiotics and in those who smoke or chew tobacco and have poor oral hygiene, allowing an overgrowth of pigment-producing bacteria. Gentle brushing of the involved area with a soft tooth brush and hydrogen peroxide several times a day may be of some value. *Strawberry tongue* is the name applied to the white exudative glossitis with prominent red papillae poking through the exudate. After several days the tongue becomes beefy red. Typically a strawberry tongue is found in scarlet fever, Kawasaki's disease, and toxic shock syndrome.

Atrophy of the filiform papillae occurs as a response to iron-deficiency anemia and vitamin B_{12} and folate deficiency.

Glossodynia, or burning tongue syndrome, occurs in elderly women and is usually a psychological condition without mucosal abnormalities. Occasionally glossitis or stomatitis occurs as a result of irritant reactions to chewing gum, mouthwashes, and dentifrices.

CARCINOMA OF THE MUCOUS MEMBRANES. Squamous cell carcinoma is the most common oral malignancy, and its incidence increases with age (see Ch. 95). The sites of origin in order of decreasing frequency are the tongue, lower lip, oropharynx, floor of the mouth, gingiva, buccal mucosa, and hard

palate. Predisposing factors include use of all forms of tobacco (especially smokeless) and alcohol. AIDS patients may develop Kaposi's sarcoma on the palate, and such patients have an increased number of squamous cell cancers, especially on the tongue. Premalignant and malignant mucous membrane cancers are usually painless and appear most commonly as red, erythroplastic lesions in two distinct forms. The first is a granular, red, velvety lesion with either stippled or patchy areas of (white) keratin within or peripheral to the lesion. The second appears as a smooth, nongranular lesion, primarily red, with minimal or no keratosis. Leukoplakia or white lesions may also be precancerous, but only 4 per cent of leukoplakias develop into cancer. Less than 5 per cent of patients have attendant bleeding, ulceration, or induration with early cancers. It is incumbent upon the practitioner finding such red or white lesions to remove irritants that might cause keratoses; if the lesions do not resolve over a 2- to 4-week period, they should be biopsied.

DISEASES OF THE LIPS. Irritant or allergic contact cheilitis with redness, scaling, and fissuring can result from topical medications (lip salves), cosmetics (lipsticks), mouthwashes and dentifrices, and various dental materials. A careful history may establish the probable cause, which must be confirmed by patch testing.

Angular cheilitis, or *perlèche*, is an acute or chronic inflammation of the skin and contiguous labial mucous membrane at the angles of the mouth. Causative factors include poorly fitting dentures that permit saliva to accumulate at the angles of the mouth, riboflavin and iron deficiencies, and *Candida* infections.

Actinic cheilitis is a dry, scaling premalignant reaction, often with white, leukoplakic plaques most pronounced on the lower lip, in individuals chronically exposed to ultraviolet light.

Alterations of Hair Growth

The evaluation of patients with alopecia or hirsutism requires a detailed history, physical examination, and, at times, laboratory and biopsy examination. Important points in the history include age of onset, medications taken, recent emotional or physical stress, diet, grooming techniques, and family history of baldness or hair disorders.

HAIR LOSS (ALOPECIA)

In the growth phase, scalp hair grows about 10 to 15 mm every month. Physical, chemical, and emotional events cause fluctuations in hair growth and if severe enough may stop growth entirely. The physical examination is important in noting the pattern of hair loss and whether or not scarring is present. Nonscarring alopecia may be a temporary phenomenon, whereas scarring is indicative of permanent hair loss.

NONSCARRING ALOPECIA. *Localized Alopecia.* *Alopecia areata* is characterized by well-circumscribed, round or oval patches of nonscarring hair loss, usually over the scalp or in the beard, eyebrows, or eyelashes. Erythema may be present early in the course of the patches. Characteristically the periphery of patches of hair loss is studded with "exclamation point hairs," so named because these hairs are fractured, with tapered shafts resembling punctuation marks. Histologic features of this disease include small dystrophic hair follicles and a lymphocytic infiltrate around the hair bulbs. Occasionally all the scalp hair is lost (alopecia totalis), and all the body hair may fall out (alopecia universalis). Alopecia areata has a variable, unpredictable course. Most patients regrow hair within a few months, but one fourth of individuals experience recurrences. The more extensive the alopecia, the poorer the prognosis. Alopecia involving the occipital region or eyebrows, lashes, and nasal hairs portends a poor prognosis. Alopecia areata may be an autoimmune disease and is occasionally associated with Hashimoto's thyroiditis and pernicious anemia. Topical, intralesional, and systemic steroids give variable benefits. Recent modes of therapy include induction of allergic or irritant contact dermatitis (1 per cent anthralin, or topical dinitrochlorobenzene), photochemotherapy with PUVA, and topical minoxidil.

Tinea capitis is most likely to be confused with alopecia areata. However, tinea infection appears as one or more patches of hair loss with mild scaling and erythema and broken hair shafts leaving residual black stumps (black dot ringworm). Although Wood's light examination causes hairs to fluoresce bright green with *Microsporum audouini* and *M. canis* infections, these are now rare causes of tinea capitis; rather, nonfluorescing *Trichophyton tonsurans* is the usual etiology. Griseofulvin is the drug of choice in treating these infections.

Trichotillomania refers to traumatic, self-induced alopecia and results from compulsive twisting and rubbing, which causes breaking and epilation of the hair shafts. The scalp is usually affected, less often the eyebrows and lashes. If the patient can be given insight into the nature of the condition it is self-limited, but when more severe emotional problems underlie the trichotillomania, referral for psychiatric evaluation should be considered.

Women who develop hair thinning at the margins of the scalp may be using excessive traction or other traumatic hair styling techniques (*traction alopecia*). Traction from overtight hair curling such as corn rowing and the use of hot combs to straighten hair leads to progressive hair thinning and even scarring.

Hair loss is sometimes seen in the scalp of patients with *secondary syphilis*. The hair loss is spotty, often "moth-eaten" in appearance.

Androgenic alopecia, or male pattern baldness, involves the frontal, vertex, and upper occipital regions of the scalp while sparing the posterior and lateral margins. The process may begin at any age after puberty, with temporal recession of hair usually noted first. There is no actual loss of hair but rather the conversion of thick terminal hairs to fine, unpigmented, poorly seen vellus hairs. Common baldness is genetically predetermined and androgen dependent. Males who are castrated prepubertally or men born with low testosterone production, as in Klinefelter's syndrome, do not become bald, regardless of their genetic predisposition to balding. Women may also show balding, but it is milder with only diffuse thinning. However, women with elevated androgen levels, as occur in masculinizing disorders, have baldness in a pattern similar to that in men. Topical minoxidil may slow androgenic hair loss. Surgical techniques such as hair transplants (plugs of hair-bearing areas from the sides of the scalp placed in the thinned frontal and crown areas) or scalp reduction may be useful in some patients.

Diffuse or Generalized Alopecia. *Stress alopecia*, or *telogen effluvium*, is a transient, reversible, diffuse hair loss of scalp hair that results from alterations in the normal hair cycle. Normally 80 to 85 per cent of scalp hair follicles are in the growing anagen stage, while 15 to 20 per cent are in the resting (telogen) stage of growth (Ch. 522). Severe emotional and physiologic stress (high fever, systemic illness, major surgery with general anesthesia, crash diet) and certain drugs (heparin, coumarin, allopurinol, amphetamines, β-blocking agents, lithium, probenecid, thiouracil) may cause growing anagen hairs to convert prematurely to resting telogen hairs, which are subsequently shed. Pregnancy and oral contraceptives cause hairs to grow continually, rather than cycling at programmed times to telogen. After childbirth or discontinuation of oral contraceptives, anagen follicles "catch up" by simultaneously entering telogen, and shedding follows 2 to 4 months later. If the stress resolves, the hair regrows in 4 to 6 months. Diffuse hair loss may not be noticeable until there is greater than 50 per cent scalp hair loss. The patient may become aware of increased hair shedding (greater than 125 to 150 hairs per day) without thinning. Gentle pulling of the hair verifies the degree of shedding; if more than five hairs come out when a dozen are grasped, excessive shedding is present. All the hair bulbs that come out are telogen (i.e., a white bulb at the end of the shaft instead of an elongate white sheath as seen in anagen hairs).

Toxic alopecia, or *anagen effluvium*, occurs if hair growth is disrupted during anagen. The newly synthesized hair shaft is weakened and the hair breaks readily. Thinning may be extreme, occurring within a few weeks of an insult, involving all 80 per cent of follicles in anagen on the scalp. Chemotherapeutic agents, especially doxorubicin and related agents, exert their effect on rapidly growing cells in the hair bulb and commonly cause anagen hair damage in cancer patients receiving chemotherapy. Radiotherapy to the scalp area does the same thing. *Retinoids* and *hypervitaminosis A* cause hair loss owing to their interference with keratinization.

Diffuse hair loss over the scalp occurs in *hypothyroidism*, associated with hair that is dry and brittle. Nutritional deficiency (essential fatty acid, biotin, zinc, iron deficiency anemia) also causes diffuse alopecia.

Seborrheic dermatitis, with erythema and yellow, greasy scales throughout the scalp, may also be associated with mild, diffuse hair loss. Treatment of the seborrhea with tar shampoos and topical steroids to control the inflammatory response reverses the hair loss.

Diffuse scalp hair loss also occurs because of *hair shaft weakness*, either acquired (due to braiding, permanent wave solutions, or excessive heat when drying or straightening hair) or resulting from congenital hair shaft weakness. Patients with congenital hair shaft weakness have sparse fine or wiry hair from early childhood. A few of the more common conditions that can be identified with the naked eye, hand lens, or microscope include short beaded hair—monilethrix; twisted hair—pili torti; banded hair—low sulfur hair syndrome; and trichorrhexis nodosa—multiple hair shaft fractures.

SCARRING ALOPECIA. Scarring alopecias display atrophy of the scalp and absence of hair follicles. These cicatricial areas of hair loss can be the result of a variety of pathologic processes that permanently destroy the hair follicles.

Localized Scarring Alopecia. *Systemic lupus erythematosus* causes diffuse, nonscarring alopecia of the scalp in 20 per cent of patients, along with short, broken (lupus) hairs in the frontal margin, whereas *discoid lupus erythematosus* causes oval scarring areas of alopecia. Typical plaques have an active erythematous margin, white atrophic center, and telangiectasias and keratin-filled follicles.

Morphea, when it involves the scalp, causes firm, hairless, ivory colored, indurated lesions. At times morphea takes on linear patterns that simulate saber wound (en coup de sabre).

Aplasia cutis is a developmental, rectilinear defect in skin formation anywhere on the scalp but usually on the vertex in the newborn.

A number of *physical injuries* such as mechanical trauma, burns, and radiodermatitis may also cause local scarring alopecias.

Nonlocalized Scarring Alopecia. *Lichen planus* may cause diffuse, patchy scarring alopecia (*lichen planopilaris*). Typical lichen planus lesions are often found in other areas of the body. Biopsy of the affected areas may help in the diagnosis.

Poorly understood conditions of the scalp, *pseudopelade* and *folliculitis decalvans* cause oval, scarred, bald areas that are often multiple and may coalesce to form large, irregular, noninflammatory plaques, most often on the vertex. Pseudopelade may be the result of a variety of entities, including lupus erythematosus, lichen planus, or scleroderma. Folliculitis decalvans is characterized by follicular inflammation that leads to destruction of follicles and permanent alopecia. Small follicular pustules are usually seen.

HIRSUTISM (EXCESSIVE HAIR GROWTH)

Excessive hair growth, usually a complaint of females, may be due to either endocrinologic or nonendocrinologic conditions. When women are affected in those areas of the body which normally develop hair as a secondary sex characteristic in males, their hirsutism generally reflects treatable endocrinopathy, as it is these follicles that are responsive to high concentrations of testosterone and are capable of converting various androgens to dihydrotestosterone (Ch. 522).

NONENDOCRINE HIRSUTISM. *Ethnic* or *racial hirsutism* is characterized by excessive hair growth on the upper lip, beard area, chest, nipples, or lower abdomen in women without menstrual abnormalities or masculinization. Type of hair, rate of hair growth, and distribution of hair over the body differ among the races, relating to variations in the sensitivity of follicles to circulating androgens. A male pattern of hirsutism is more common in females whose ancestors came from the southern parts of Europe. Orientals and American Indians have less body hair. If endocrinologic abnormalities are not found (serum testosterone, dehydroepiandrosterone, and androstenedione are normal), bleaching or shaving may be sufficient to make the hair less noticeable. Electrolysis permanently destroys hair follicles but is time consuming and costly. Spironolactone,* which has antian-

---

*This use is not listed in the manufacturer's directive.

drogenic properties (200 mg per day), used for a period of 12 months is also useful in decreasing hair growth.

Certain *drugs* may also increase hair growth. Androgenic or steroidal medications, such as anabolic steroids, corticosteroids, and contraceptives, may cause increased hair growth in the beard, chest, and groin areas. Drugs such as phenytoin, phenothiazines, cyclosporine, and minoxidil cause excess hair in both men and women anywhere on the body.

Porphyria cutanea tarda causes increased hairiness of the face, especially on the temples and pinnae of the ears. Treatment of the condition results in decrease of hair growth.

ENDOCRINE HIRSUTISM. A distinction must be made between hirsutism caused by increased androgen production with and without virilization. In general, virilization is a sign of markedly elevated androgens derived from the adrenal glands or ovaries, especially adrenogenital syndrome, congenital adrenal hyperplasia, Cushing's disease or syndrome, Stein-Leventhal syndrome (polycystic ovarian syndrome), and occasionally malignant adrenal or ovarian tumors. Any woman with hirsutism and accompanying virilization should be tested for excess cortisol and androgen production.

Simple or *idiopathic hirsutism* is the designation given to those hirsute women in whom a specific etiologic diagnosis cannot be made and in whom normal or slightly elevated adrenal or ovarian androgens are found. The cause may be slightly increased production and metabolism of androgens or increased sensitivity of hair follicles to normal levels of androgens. Such patients have been successfully treated with cyclically administered birth control pills or with spironolactone.

PHOTOSENSITIVITY AND OTHER REACTIONS TO LIGHT

Certain wavelengths of light are capable of inducing a number of undesirable cutaneous reactions, including sunburn, skin aging, carcinogenesis, and a variety of photosensitivity reactions.

Clinically, photorelated conditions occur in a typical distribution of light-exposed areas, which should make the diagnosis of light-related reactions apparent (see Fig. 523–2). Thus, maximal changes occur over the forehead, malar eminences, bridge of the nose, and pinnae of the ears, with sparing of the upper lip (shaded by the nose), periorbital areas, and submental region. The V of the neck, dorsum of the hands, and forearms are often involved, with a sharp demarcation where clothing and watch bands cover the skin. In addition, light must be suspected from historical evidence. Seasonal recurrences are seen, especially in the spring or early summer. The evoked reaction may be to light alone, to light in association with exogenous substances (taken internally, such as drugs or externally applied materials), or to abnormal metabolites as in porphyria.

The incidence of photoreactions depends on a number of factors such as the amount of light reaching the earth's surface, season of the year, latitude and weather conditions, and thickness of the ozone layer, as well as topographic features of the environment. There are some useful climatologic and environmental factors to keep in mind which have bearing on the amount of sunlight hitting the skin. For example, 50 per cent of the daily ultraviolet light is emitted between 11 A.M. and 2 P.M., so avoiding exposure to sunlight during this time may be useful in minimizing photoreactions. Sitting in the shade does not protect against UV exposure, because 50 per cent of the ambient ultraviolet light is received; 90 per cent of ultraviolet light penetrates clouds, so one can get sunburns even in the shade and on cloudy days.

Electromagnetic radiation (EMG) from the sun has been arbitrarily classified into spectral regions measured in nanometers, ranging from short cosmic rays to long radiowaves. The solar spectrum that commonly affects human skin is in the ultraviolet light range (290 to 400 nm), which is subdivided into three bands designated as UVC (shorter than 290 nm), UVB (290 to 320 nm), and UVA, or long-wave ultraviolet light (320 to 400 nm). UVC does not reach the earth, being absorbed by ozone; UVB, or the sunburn spectrum, causes burning, tanning, aging, and carcinogenic changes in the skin. UVA is melanogenic and erythrogenic, but the amount of energy required to produce these effects is 1000 times greater than UVB. UVA causes skin reactions through window glass, and these wavelengths are often responsible for photoreactions in which chemical photosensitizers and UV radiation interact to cause inflammatory skin reactions.

The amount of UV light reaching various levels of the skin depends on wavelength. The longer wavelengths penetrate deeper into the dermis. Thus, depending on the wavelength of light and depth of penetration, the reactions may involve absorption by cellular DNA, RNA, and cutaneous proteins (keratin, collagen, etc.).

Direct Photo Effects on the Skin

ACUTE EFFECTS. Sunburning and tanning are common acute reactions to sun exposure and are attributed primarily to UVB light, although prolonged exposure to UVA can produce mild burn and marked hyperpigmentation. The sunburn reaction is a complex inflammatory process causing dyskeratotic cells, spongiosis, vacuolation of keratinocytes, and edema from capillary leakage, 12 to 24 hours after exposure to light. Occasionally, in addition to redness and pain, blisters may evolve. Prostaglandins may play a role in the burn reaction, as they are found in increased quantities in UV sunburned skin, and aspirin or indomethacin, prostaglandin synthesis inhibitors, can reduce the burn.

Three to four days after a sunburn, new melanin pigment is formed. Several cellular and molecular changes occur in the skin after each sunburn reaction which, if repeated, may lead to the chronic effects of UV light. A few days after UV light burning, epidermal mitosis and hyperplasia occur and DNA, RNA, and proteins in the skin are damaged.

CHRONIC EFFECTS. Degenerative changes of the skin consisting of wrinkling, telangiectasias, and keratoses are the long-term effects of chronic exposure to UV light. A furrowed and leathery condition of the skin may develop along with yellow papules and plaques due to solar degeneration of the dermal collagen, especially in fair-skinned individuals. These changes are caused by both UVB and UVA radiation. Such changes can be minimized by daily topical applications of effective sunscreens (see Ch. 524).

A number of malignant and premalignant skin lesions are associated with chronic sun exposure, including actinic keratoses, keratoacanthomas, basal cell and squamous cell carcinomas, and probably melanomas (see above).

Indirect Photo Effects on the Skin

Photoreactions that occur when systemic or topical chemicals induce photosensitivity or when there is an underlying immunologic, biochemical, or genetic abnormality that predisposes to sun sensitivity are considered indirect reactions; i.e., the sun alone does not cause photoreactions.

EXOGENOUS FACTORS CAUSING PHOTOSENSITIVITY. Chemical agents either taken systemically or placed topically on the skin can cause one of two general types of photoreactions: phototoxic and photoallergic. In these photosensitivity reactions, the absorption spectrum of a given drug, substance, or chemical is maximal at a certain wavelength of light that induces molecular changes in the exogenous material, which, in turn, initiates the cutaneous reaction. In most of the drug or chemical photosensitivity reactions, the wavelengths that evoke abnormal reactions are in the 320 to 400 nm (UVA) region. The reactions include acute, abnormal sunburn responses and eczematous and urticarial reactions.

Phototoxic reactions are those nonimmunologic cutaneous responses that occur in most individuals when enough light energy of a specific wavelength is absorbed by an appropriate concentration of drug or chemical in the skin. Free radicals are generated in the photosensitizer which damage cell membranes and lysosomes, inducing an exaggerated sunburn reaction, with intense redness, swelling, pain, and occasionally blistering. Most phototoxic agents absorb UVB light.

Photoallergic reactions to topical chemicals or internal drugs represent an acquired, altered response to light which involves immunologic mechanisms. Absorption of specific wavelengths of light by chemicals or drugs causes changes in their chemical configuration so that these substances become haptens that bind to proteins in the skin to become a complete antigen capable of eliciting a type IV delayed hypersensitivity immunologic response. The clinical manifestations of such photoallergic reactions

TABLE 525–15. CHARACTERISTICS OF PHOTOTOXIC AND PHOTOALLERGIC REACTIONS OF THE SKIN

Reaction	Phototoxic	Photoallergic
Clinical changes	Prolonged sunburn	Eczema or urticaria
Relative incidence	All people receiving chemical and exposed to appropriate wavelength of light	Few individuals exposed to chemical and appropriate wavelength of light
Concentration of drug necessary for reactions	High	Low
Reaction possible on first exposure	Yes	No
Incubation period necessary after first exposure	No	Yes
"Flares" at distant, previously involved sites possible	No	Yes
Cross-reaction to structural related agents	No	Frequent
Immunologic mechanism involved	No	Yes—type IV delayed hypersensitivity

are usually eczematous in nature (occasionally urticarial), evolving 24 hours after exposure to the sun in sun-exposed areas of the skin. The action spectrum is generally long-range UVA light, and less energy is required to elicit the reaction than for the production of phototoxic reactions.

Table 525–15 summarizes the differences between phototoxic and photoallergic reactions.

SYSTEMIC PHOTOSENSITIZERS. Drugs may cause either phototoxic or photoallergic reactions. Table 525–16 lists some of the drugs and chemicals that may induce photosensitivities and the type of reaction and action spectrum thought to induce them.

TOPICAL AGENTS CAUSING PHOTOSENSITIVITY. Most topical photosensitizing agents respond to the UVA action spectrum. Drugs and chemicals that induce *phototoxic contact reactions* include coal tar derivatives, topical drugs (phenothiazines, sulfonamides), dyes (eosins, methylene blue), and plant derivatives (furocoumarins). The photosensitive properties of coal tar

TABLE 525–16. SYSTEMIC PHOTOSENSITIZERS

Name	Type of Photoreaction	Action Spectrum (nm)
Sulfonamides	Phototoxic and photoallergic	290–320
Sulfonylureas (tolbutamide, chlorpropamide)	Phototoxic	290–360
Chlorothiazides	Phototoxic and photoallergic	290–320 320–400
Phenothiazines	Phototoxic, urticaria eruption, gray-blue hyperpigmentation	290–400
Antibiotics (tetracyclines, griseofulvin, nalidixic acid)	Phototoxic and photoallergic bullae	320–400
Furocoumarins (psoralens)	Phototoxic	
Nonsteroidal anti-inflammatory agents	Phototoxic and photoallergic	Unknown
Anticancer drugs (DTIC, fluorouracil, methotrexate, vinblastine)	Phototoxic	Unknown
Estrogens, progestins, and other drugs	Phototoxic, melasma	?290–320
Chlordiazepoxide (Librium)	Photoallergic	290–360
Cyclamates	Phototoxic and photoallergic	290–360
Quinidine, quinine	Photoallergic	320–400

derivatives and furocoumarins (psoralens) are utilized in treating certain skin diseases with ultraviolet light.

When plants, vegetables, or fruits containing a phototoxic chemical cause phototoxicity, the reaction is referred to as a *phytophotodermatitis.* Photocontact dermatitis develops with contact with plants in the Umbelliferae family, such as figs, cow parsnip, fennel, parsley, parsnip, and gas plant. Phytophotodermatitis also occurs in individuals exposed to Persian limes and celery. Such reactions are caused by furocoumarin compounds found in the plant which readily penetrate the epidermis. Two things are needed for initiation of phytophotodermatitis: (1) contact with a sensitizing furocoumarin and (2) subsequent exposure to UV radiation greater than 320 nm. Phytophotodermatitis may take on unique clinical forms: (1) berloque dermatitis presents as streaky erythema followed by hyperpigmentation in areas where perfumes containing oil of Bergamot (a psoralen) are applied to the skin (e.g., on the neck); (2) criss-cross linear streaks of erythema, vesicles, and bullae that heal with hyperpigmentation where meadow grass or other related plants rub on the skin; (3) oil of the rind of a Persian lime causes erythema and pigmentation on the hands of bartenders.

Photoallergic contact dermatitis, a form of delayed allergic hypersensitivity, evolves in some individuals after exposure to such chemicals as fragrances (methylcoumarin and musk ambrette), halogenated salicylanilides, sunscreens, and blankophores, or optical whitening agents, used in laundry soaps and bleaches. These photoallergic responses appear as eczematous reactions. A number of perfumes (after-shave lotions, colognes, etc.) contain musk ambrette, a synthetic fragrance fixative that causes a photoeczematous reaction over the face and hands. Paradoxically, sunscreening agents containing PABA esters and cinnamates that readily absorb UV light may cause eczematous photoallergic reactions. A small number of individuals have persistent chronic eczematous dermatitis after all exposure to the photosensitizing agent has ceased—so-called persistent light reactivity. Such patients may be so photosensitive that they react to artificial fluorescent light.

Identifying the cause of contact photoallergic reactions can be done with photopatch testing (Ch. 523). Treatment of photocontact sensitivity obviously begins by eliminating the photosensitizing agent and minimizing sunlight exposure (avoiding sun and use of sunscreens). Topical and, at times, oral steroids may be needed to decrease the cutaneous inflammatory response.

ENDOGENOUS CONDITIONS ASSOCIATED WITH PHOTOSENSITIVITY. Certain immunologic, biochemical, and genetic diseases display photoreactions as a prominent feature.

Immunologic diseases with photosensitivity include connective tissue conditions such as lupus erythematosus, both discoid and systemic, and solar urticaria. Solar urticaria, hives with itching and burning, evolves within minutes of sunlight exposure and lasts an hour or more. The inciting wavelength of light differs among patients.

Biochemical conditions associated with photosensitivity include two forms of porphyria: porphyria cutanea tarda and erythropoietic protoporphyria. These are discussed above (see Vesiculobullous Diseases).

Pellagra, once a common disease, especially in the southeastern United States, is caused by an inadequate diet and a deficiency of nicotinic acid. It is still seen occasionally with alcoholism, poor dietary intake in the elderly, and malabsorption. The carcinoid syndrome may also be associated with pellagra because tryptophan, the precursor of nicotinic acid, is diverted to serotonin production by the tumor. A scaly dermatitis on sun-exposed parts of the skin, especially on the face, the neck, and the back of the hands, is seen in association with diarrhea and dementia (the three D's). Low serum vitamin levels establish the diagnosis of this condition, and dietary replacement clears the skin and other signs of the disease.

Other Photosensitivity Conditions

A condition known as *polymorphous light eruption* (PML) presents with a variety of skin lesions, including eczematous patches, red to violaceous papules or plaques, and urticarial lesions over the face, the nape and V of the neck, and the back of the hands. The rash characteristically arises hours to days after sun exposure. The onset is frequently in early summer with some degree of resistance being acquired with continued sun exposure. Recurrences each spring and summer are common, and the eruption remits during the winter. The disease may begin at any age, but it is most frequent during the first half of life. The etiology is unknown, and its diagnosis is one of excluding other photosensitivity conditions.

PML may respond to the use of sunscreens with an SPF of 15 and, if elicited by UVA light, sunscreens with benzophenone or anthranilate to improve protection against the UVA spectrum. If sunscreens fail, the induction of tolerance by tanning with PUVA or UVB light or a short course of antimalarial agents or oral steroids may occasionally be needed.

Actinic reticuloid is another form of persistent photodermatitis of unknown etiology which occurs in middle-aged males and causes a most distressing photoreaction of red papules and pruritic eczematous patches. Both UVB and UVA appear to play a role. PUVA chemotherapy may help control the condition.

DERMATOLOGIC MANIFESTATIONS IN THE IMMUNOCOMPROMISED HOST

Immunosuppression causes an increase in benign and malignant skin growths as well as a variety of infections in the skin (see Ch. 287). Cutaneous neoplasms such as squamous cell and basal cell carcinomas occur with a much higher frequency than would be expected. Transplant patients have an estimated risk of skin cancer that is 7.1 times greater than normal. Most patients have multiple skin cancers.

Any skin lesion, no matter how innocuous, should be carefully evaluated in the immunosuppressed host. The gross morphology of infections is so frequently modified by the altered inflammatory response in the immunocompromised patient that early skin biopsies are essential for diagnosis. The array of potential pathogens is imposing in these patients, and even common infectious processes are greatly modified or obscured by immunocompromising illness. Skin infections are common, accounting for 22 to 33 per cent of infections in immunosuppressed patients.

Microbial involvement of the skin and subcutaneous tissue can be grouped into two major categories in immunocompromised patients: (1) *primary skin infections* that are typical of those occurring in nonimmunocompromised hosts, widespread involvement with infectious agents that commonly cause localized skin infection, and primary skin infections from opportunistic agents that rarely cause skin infection in normal patients; and (2) *disseminated systemic infections* metastatic to the skin from a noncutaneous portal of entry.

PRIMARY SKIN INFECTIONS. Typical primary skin infections, including group A streptococcal and *Staphylococcus aureus* cellulitis, are frequent, although more unusual causes of cellulitis in granulocytopenic patients must also be considered (*Pseudomonas*, anaerobic bacteria). Skin biopsy of the cellulitic areas for Gram's stain and culture is often helpful.

Unusually widespread, primary cutaneous infections by viruses and skin dermatophytes are also common. Warts caused by papillomavirus may be numerous, disfiguring, and difficult to remove. Malignant transformation has been documented in such warts in immunosuppressed individuals. Herpes simplex infections may present as chronic, large, ulcerated lesions persisting for weeks to months (herpes phagedena, especially in the genital areas), and there may be internal dissemination from cutaneous sites. Reactivation of herpes zoster infections is common in immunocompromised hosts, with systemic dissemination. Widespread dermatophyte infections of the skin appear as scaling, red patches that provide a portal of entry for bacterial infection.

Unusual opportunistic primary skin infections with atypical *Mycobacterium*, *Aspergillus*, *Rhizopus*, and *Candida* organisms cause cellulitis-like reactions that form a central pustule and eschar. Skin biopsy of such lesions with a portion of the biopsy processed by frozen section and specially stained for AFB and fungi may identify the pathologic organisms rapidly.

DISSEMINATED INFECTION METASTATIC TO THE SKIN. Hematogenous dissemination of infection to the skin from distant primary sites frequently occurs in patients with impaired host defenses. Three groups of organisms are responsible for this:

TABLE 525–17. CUTANEOUS DRUG REACTIONS

Type of Skin Reaction	Drugs Likely to Cause Skin Reaction
Eczematous (allergic contact reaction)	Antihistamines, neomycin, formaldehyde, sulfonamides
Photodermatitis	
Phototoxic	Chlorpromazine, psoralens, demeclocycline, doxycycline
Photoallergic	Promethazine, griseofulvin, Diuril, hypoglycemic drugs
Exfoliative dermatitis	Carbamazepine, hydantoins, nitrofurantoin, isoniazid, gold, allopurinol, phenothiazines
Maculopapular eruption (exanthematous)	Penicillin, sulfonamides, hypoglycemic drugs, phenothiazines, allopurinol, phenytoin, quinine, gold salts, captopril, meprobamate
Papulosquamous reactions Psoriasiform, lichen planus, pityriasis rosea–like	Beta blockers, lithium (psoriasiform), thiazides, gold, phenothiazines, quinidine, antimalarials (lichen planus–like); gold (PR-like); others—practolol, dapsone, ethambutol, furosemide
Vesiculobullous reactions	Azapropazone, captopril, clonidine, furosemide, gold, psoralens, barbiturates, phenytoin, Hydrodiuril, penicillamine
Toxic epidermal necrolysis	Acetazolamide, allopurinol, barbiturates, carbamazepines, gold, hydantoin, nitrofurantoin, pentazocine, tetracycline, quinidine
Pustular—acneiform reactions	Androgen hormones, corticosteroids, iodides, bromides, hydantoin, lithium
Urticaria and erythemas	
Urticaria	May occur with anaphylaxis; penicillin, xenogenic sera, cephalosporins, sulfonamides, barbiturates, hydralazine, phenylbutazone, hydantoin, quinidine, x-ray contrast media
Erythema multiforme	Sulfonamides, hydantoin, barbiturates, penicillin, carbamazepines, allopurinol, amikacin, phenothiazides
Nodular lesions	
Erythema nodosum	Birth control pills, sulfonamides, diuretics, gold, clonidine, propranolol, furosemide, opiates, penicillin
Vasculitis reaction	Allopurinol, barbiturates, carbamazepine, chlorothiazide, cimetidine, gold, indomethacin, hydantoin, piperazine, sulfonamides
Telangiectatic and LE reactions	Procainamide, hydralazine, phenytoin, penicillamine, trimethadione, methyldopa, carbamazepine, griseofulvin, nalidixic acid, oral contraceptives, propranolol
Pigmentary reaction	Anticonvulsants, antimalarials, antitumor agents (bleomycin, busulfan, cyclophosphamide, doxorubicin, melphalan), oral contraceptives, corticotropin, tetracyclines, phenothiazines, amiodarone
Other cutaneous reactions	
Fixed drug reactions	Phenolphthalein, barbiturates, gold, sulfonamides, meprobamate, penicillin, tetracyclines, analgesics
Alopecia	Alkylating agents, antimetabolites, heparin, coumarin, hydantoin, accutane, gold, nitrofurantoin, propranolol, colchicine, allopurinol
Hypertrichosis	Anabolic agents, diazoxide, minoxidil, phenytoin

(1) *Pseudomonas* and other gram-negative bacilli; (2) endemic systemic mycoses (*Histoplasma, Coccidioides*); and (3) opportunistic fungi (*Aspergillus, Candida,* Mucoraceae). The range of cutaneous clinical presentations of these infections is varied and mimicked by all of these infections, namely (a) *vesicles and bullae* that become hemorrhagic, (b) *gangrenous cellulitis* with necrotic ulcerations, and (c) widespread, red, warm, fluctuant *nodules* with pustules and purpura. Prompt biopsy of these lesions with frozen sections stained for bacterial and hyphal elements may provide rapid diagnosis.

CUTANEOUS DRUG REACTIONS

Rashes are among the most common adverse reactions to drugs and occur in 2 to 3 per cent of hospitalized patients. Any drug can potentially produce a rash, and over-the-counter preparations should be considered when defining drug reactions.

The causes of adverse drug reactions are multiple, including *toxic* (too much drug is given or degradation of the drug is slow owing to an underlying disease or action of another drug), *idiosyncratic* (unanticipated side effects), and *allergic* reactions. Because tests for drug allergy are not available, it is often difficult to be sure one is dealing with an allergic reaction. However, a hypersensitivity reaction can be suspected when (1) rechallenge or re-exposure to small amounts of the drug elicits the same response, (2) the reaction appears following several days to weeks of administration of the drug, (3) the reaction occurs when the patient is exposed to a structurally similar drug, and (4) the clinical response does not resemble the general pharmacologic effects of the drug.

Some of the most common drugs causing skin reactions in hospitalized patients are amoxicillin, trimethoprim-sulfamethoxazole, ampicillin, penicillin G, allopurinol, dipyrone, gentamicin sulfate, mefruside, nitrazepam, and barbiturates. Drugs least likely to cause allergic skin reactions include digoxin, antacids, promethazine, acetaminophen, nitroglycerin, aminophylline, propranolol, antihistamines, cromolyn, and emollient laxatives.

Table 525–17 lists the various morphologic types of drug reactions and some of the drugs capable of inducing each reaction.

Fixed drug eruptions are unique reactions that appear in the same area of the skin each time the responsible drug is administered. These appear as macular, eczematous, or even bullous, pink to dark red patches occurring as few or many lesions. When the drug is stopped the lesions fade, leaving postinflammatory hyperpigmentation. The lesions return in the same place within a few hours of taking the drug again.

Nonsteroidal anti-inflammatory drugs are being used with increasing frequency and may cause cutaneous reactions including vesiculobullous photosensitivity reactions, serum sickness, erythroderma, fixed drug reactions, and toxic epidermal necrolysis.

The treatment of drug reactions is discontinuation of the suspected agent. Often the patient is taking many drugs, and generally once a drug reaction is suspected all nonessential drugs should be stopped and appropriate substitutes used for the necessary medications. An asymptomatic eruption may require no therapy, or a mild reaction with pruritus may be controlled with topical steroid applications and antihistamines. In severe conditions such as exfoliative dermatitis, oral steroids are often indicated. Most drug eruptions resolve in 1 to 2 weeks after withdrawal of the drug, but some reactions take months to clear. While an occasional reaction may be fatal (e.g., toxic epidermal necrolysis), patients with drug eruptions usually have an excellent prognosis.

526 Principles of Occupational Medicine

Charles E. Becker

Occupational medicine is concerned with the physical and emotional safety and health of workers. It encompasses issues of public concern, particularly the quality of air and water, the degree of environmental pollution, and the complex mosaic of legal, economic, social, and ethical questions that are raised whenever human action produces human disorders.

Among the 100 million workers in the United States today, approximately 100,000 deaths per year are attributed to the workplace. Yet there are only 10,000 physicians whose self-determined primary specialty is occupational medicine, and only 500 of these have subspecialty board certification. Primary care internists, family physicians, and emergency physicians constitute the "front line" for identification of work-related disorders. Therefore, they must learn to target the medical history and to recognize classic signs and symptoms of occupational and environmental disorders.

Occupational medicine deals almost exclusively with diagnosis and prevention, not treatment. The diagnosis of an occupational disease may be difficult, since occupational diseases (1) may simulate many other disorders, (2) often lack unique pathology, and (3) may be marked by a long latency period between exposure and the manifestation of the disease.

Problems from chemical contamination do not always remain exclusively in the workplace; they may extend into the community: polychlorinated biphenyls (PCB's) in Japan; dioxin in Seveso, Italy; radiation exposure at Three Mile Island; mercury contamination in Minamata Bay; lead pollution in cities and around smelting plants; and nervous system, liver, and reproductive toxicity from chlordecone (Kepone) in Virginia. These events give rise to important political, social, and economic considerations that emphasize the need for specialized training in occupational medicine.

Competency in occupational medicine is best acquired from a base of general training in internal medicine, with extended knowledge and experience in epidemiology, industrial hygiene, biostatistics, and toxicology. The relationship between workplace-environmental exposure and disease centers on four basic concepts: recognition, prevention, exacerbation, and latent manifestation. Workplace-associated diseases are presumed to be preventable when recognized and fully understood. Since the signs and symptoms of occupational diseases may be identical to those of many other diseases, a high level of suspicion is required for the recognition that allows prevention. Rather than causing an illness, occupational environmental conditions may, in fact, exacerbate or compound a pre-existing condition. For example, a patient with toxicity from aminoglycoside antibiotics may have additional otologic injury from loud noises occurring at work. Although some environmental and occupational diseases become manifest acutely, many have a long latency period and may extend from the workplace into the family or society and thus present important considerations in diagnostic and preventive strategies (e.g., asbestos exposure).

In occupational medicine there are four basic categories of hazard: physical, biologic, psychological, and chemical. Physical hazards may include vibration, heat, noise, radiation, and trauma. Occupational injuries account for approximately 14,000 deaths, 245 million lost work days, and $25 billion in direct and indirect costs annually in the United States. Biologic hazards include the well-known occupational risks of hepatitis, human immunodeficiency virus (HIV) infection, or tuberculosis. Psychological hazards of stress and work-shift changes are complex and will be discussed subsequently. Chemical hazards involve exposure to solvents, dusts, vapors, and gases. It is important here to distinguish between toxicity and hazard. *Toxicity* is the inherent capability of a material to cause injury to a living cell. *Hazard* is the chance of a resultant injury from use of such a material in a given setting. Asbestos, for example, is a useful fire retardant construction material with known basic toxicity that may become hazardous only during repair or demolition work or fire, which may cause its release into the air.

In occupational medicine one is also concerned with the difference between exposure and dose. Exposure is determined by surveillance of the environment with the knowledge that a toxic agent has had the potential of being delivered into the body. For example, environmental measurements of lead can provide an index of exposure. These environmental measurements are often made by experts called industrial hygienists. Dose, however, can be assessed only by biologic monitoring of blood, urine, and hair and by indices of enzyme systems that may be affected. In the case of lead, the total dose delivered is dependent on the amount that is respirable and the amount absorbed from the gastrointestinal tract. Figure 526–1 depicts the complex interactions in the field of occupational medicine.

This chapter outlines some of the basic concepts and a few selected disorders encompassed in occupational medicine. Other chapters in this section describe at length occupational diseases of the lung (Ch. 527) and of the skin (Ch. 529) and a variety of chemical and physical sources of injury. Some chapters in other parts of the book contain useful information related to the discipline: toxic nephropathies (Ch. 80), epidemiology of cancer (Ch. 158), painful back and painful shoulders (Ch. 274 and 275), and neuropathies associated with the workplace (Ch. 533).

THE OCCUPATIONAL-ENVIRONMENTAL HISTORY

Key elements of an occupational and environmental history should be added to the data base collected on all patients. In every problem-oriented assessment of a current illness, individual problem lists should include such questions concerning the occupational health history: Are symptoms associated with work, or do they improve during vacations and weekends? Are other workers similarly affected? Is there or has there been direct exposure to dust, fumes, and chemicals? Have there been work-related injuries? Is periodic testing and medical surveillance or routine industrial hygiene sampling of the workplace performed?

A careful work history should include a chronologic list of all previous jobs with a reasonably detailed description of the work site, the scope of a typical work day, and such pertinent factors as protective equipment, ventilation, and pre-employment examinations.

A specific listing of the total number of days missed on each job and the reasons for the absences may be useful. Has a worker compensation claim been filed in the past? Does the worker perform additional jobs, i.e., is he or she moonlighting? A patient may not relate work to health, so the physician should obtain initially, on each examination, specific answers to common occupational problems, such as the following: Have you ever been exposed to loud noises, excessive vibration, or heat? Do you work with asbestos? Have you been exposed to radioactive chemicals? Have you had previous chemical exposure? During the military, what were your duties? Recent "right-to-know" legislation often allows workers to receive a written description of their chemical exposures, which the physician can help interpret.

The environmental health history should include information about industries located in the neighborhood, exposure to hazardous waste or toxic spills, jobs of the spouse, degree of air pollution, and types of hobbies and recreational activities that also may contribute to health-related problems, such as painting, sculpturing, welding, or woodworking.

In addition, it may be important to elicit a description of home insulation or heating as well as exposure to cleaning agents and insecticides. Special questions should be directed toward unique workplace problems, such as working hours and job schedule (Do these affect your sleep pattern? Are you bored on the job?). The reproductive history is essential: the number of miscarriages, children, stillbirths, previous pregnancies; difficulty in conceiving; and changes in libido and menses.

SIGNS AND SYMPTOMS OF OCCUPATIONAL AND ENVIRONMENTAL DISORDERS. Because occupational and environmental diseases have a long latency and may be synergistic with other causes of disease, the clinician should always consider that the signs and symptoms may be caused by occupational or environmental conditions. Sometimes it may be useful to identify all the signs and symptoms that could be associated with disease caused by the environment or the workplace. Knowledge of exposure to certain substances may implicate or suggest the cause: chlorinated hydrocarbons and acne; arsenic and thallium and alopecia; solvent exposure and anosmia; chlorinated hydrocarbons and arrhythmias; and aniline dyes and bladder or other cancers.

Reproductive hazards, noise-induced hearing abnormalities, work-shift changes, and ergonomics are discussed as important occupational entities not covered specifically by other chapters in this section.

REPRODUCTIVE HAZARDS

Seven per cent of all newborns in the United States have birth defects, approximately 70 per cent of which are of unknown cause. The relationship between exposure to environmental and occupational agents and consequent development of male and female reproductive abnormalities is an area of intense study and interest. Animal studies have demonstrated the transmission to

subsequent generations of chemically induced abnormalities of sperm and at a rate determined by mendelian principles. These observations have sparked interest in predicting and thereby preventing reproductive hazards from environmental agents. Short-term bioassays for mutagenesis, such as the Ames test, have been used to screen agents to predict reproductive outcome. These relatively inexpensive and rapid initial screening tests of chemicals can be performed in animals or bacteria. Agents encountered in the environment or the workplace can clearly cause reproductive hazards, e.g., testicular toxicity of dibromochloropropane (DBCP) recognized in California chemical workers. Male workers with sterility suffered no systemic illness and were working in an environment that was alleged to be safe. Previous laboratory tests in animals had suggested reproductive hazards from this chemical. The controversy surrounding this event sparked great interest in this subject. To date, the following environmental and occupational agents have been shown to cause adverse reproductive effects in men: anesthetic gases, carbon disulfide, diethylstilbestrol, toluene diamine, ethylene dibromide, chlordecone, and ionizing radiation. A much stronger data base is required to assess environmental effects on pregnancy outcome, spontaneous abortion, and stillbirth.

NOISE-INDUCED HEARING LOSS

More than 5 million people in the United States have noise-induced hearing loss. This most common form of hearing loss is associated with damage to, and loss of, hair cells in the organ of Corti. Early or moderately advanced noise-induced hearing loss is associated with normal hearing in the low frequencies but gradually increasing loss of hearing at higher frequencies (with a maximum of 3, 4, or 6 kHz). There may be some return toward normal function at 8 kHz. The audiometric shape of this curve is not pathognomonic because other otologic disorders (e.g., that caused by aminoglycoside antibiotic therapy) can result in an identical audiogram. Some of the hearing loss attributed to aging (presbycusis) may be due to the nearly ubiquitous noise pollution in modern society. Epidemiologic studies suggest that aging individuals in a nonindustrialized society have much better hearing preservation than older Americans. Major individual differences in susceptibility to noise-induced hearing loss occur. Men are much more susceptible to noise-induced hearing loss than women. Smoking and lack of skin pigmentation may also be risk factors for noise-induced hearing loss. Hearing impairment from occupational and environmental factors is a major and entirely preventable public health problem.

WORK-SHIFT CHANGES

Twenty per cent of American workers work evenings or nights. In some industries, such as automobile production, petrol chemicals, and textile manufacturing, shift workers number nearly 50 per cent. There is growing evidence to suggest clinically significant health effects from shift work on health care workers who work many hours without sleep. Twenty per cent of workers are unable to tolerate shift work, tolerance for which also diminishes with increasing age. Daily physiologic variations known as circadian rhythms are distorted by shift work, which in turn alters the quality of sleep and causes important disturbances of the gastrointestinal tract and other organs. Diabetes mellitus and epilepsy may be aggravated by shift work, and the risk of accidents

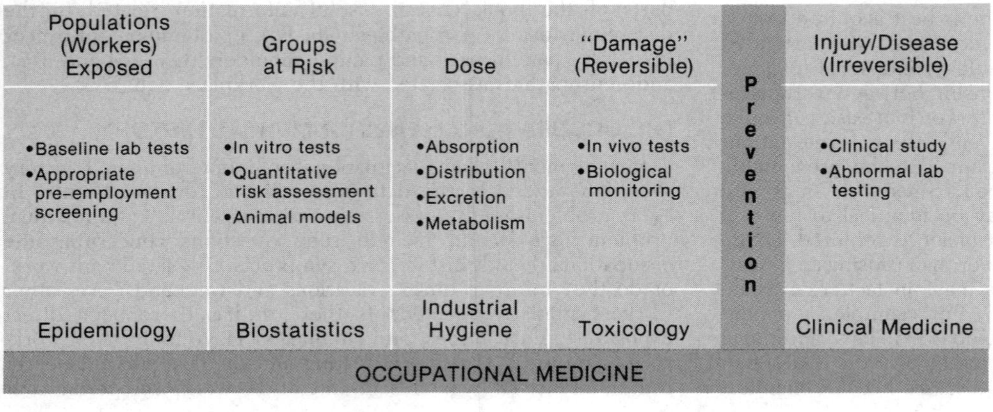

Populations (Workers) Exposed	Groups at Risk	Dose	"Damage" (Reversible)	Prevention	Injury/Disease (Irreversible)
•Baseline lab tests •Appropriate pre-employment screening	•In vitro tests •Quantitative risk assessment •Animal models	•Absorption •Distribution •Excretion •Metabolism	•In vivo tests •Biological monitoring		•Clinical study •Abnormal lab testing
Epidemiology	Biostatistics	Industrial Hygiene	Toxicology		Clinical Medicine
OCCUPATIONAL MEDICINE					

FIGURE 526–1. Multidisciplinary approach to occupational (environmental) medicine.

may be increased. Shift workers tend to have an increased number of subjective health complaints in general and may have enhanced risk factors complicating management of other medical disorders.

ERGONOMICS

Ergonomics is the interface of a worker with his or her work station, machine, or work environment. This interface may create physical and psychological stresses that present as common diseases to internists. Physical factors may include repetitive motion disorders, back injuries, and musculoskeletal problems. Psychological factors involve attention span, memory, vigilance, and behavior. They may play an important role in safety in the workplace and are often called *human error*. Ergonometric problems may progress from chronic discomfort of aches and pains to temporary disabling conditions, such as sprains, strains, tendinitis, and fibromyositis syndromes. These syndromes ultimately lead to long-term disabilities—nerve entrapment, chronic back pain, and musculoskeletal disorders. Careful history taking will suggest an ergonometric problem that frequently involves highly repetitive, monotonous work or fast-paced production jobs. Sometimes extremely sedentary work, such as word processing or microscopic inspection, may also cause a disability. It may be essential to make a visit to the plant to observe the work station in order to assist the patient in resolving an ergonometric problem. Reducing physical and psychological stresses may have beneficial effects that seem out of proportion to the magnitude of the changes in the work practice.

CONCLUSIONS

Strictly speaking, all diseases that are not genetic in origin are "environmental." Even genetic disorders are not totally endogenous, since they most frequently alter the ability of the host to accommodate to the environment. Broadly conceived, even the infectious diseases and nutritional disorders are environmental in origin. In practice, however, the term *environmental medicine* is used in a much more restrictive sense to reflect the chemical and physical hazards to which an individual is exposed and the injuries that may result from that exposure. Occupational medicine is that subset of environmental medicine directly concerned with the hazards of the workplace. The following chapters describe in greater detail some of the specific hazards and injuries incident to modern occupations. The topics selected cannot be inclusive, since the boundaries of occupational and environmental medicine are indistinct, merging into the traditional domains of internal medicine, epidemiology, toxicology, surgery, orthopedics, and many other clinical and basic science disciplines.

Ladou J: Current Occupational Medicine: Diagnosis and Treatment. Los Altos, Calif., Lange Medical Publications, 1990. *A full review of key occupational topics.*

Morgan WK, Seaton A: Occupational Lung Diseases. 2nd ed. Philadelphia, W.B. Saunders Company, 1984. *Useful, conservative approach with easy readings for occupational lung disease.*

Olsen K: Poisoning and Drug Overdose. Appleton-Lange, 1990. *A useful, up-to-date reference on acute and chronic chemical exposure.*

Proctor N, Hughes J, Hathaway GJ: Chemical Hazards of the Workplace. 3rd ed. Norwalk, Conn., Van Nostrand Reinhold, 1991. *Updated classic reference on workplace exposure.*

Rosenstock A, Cullen M: Clinical Occupational Medicine. Philadelphia, W.B. Saunders Company, 1986. *Useful, inexpensive guide to common occupational health problems.*

Selikoff I: The role of the internist in occupational medicine. Am J Indust Med 8:95, 1985. *An elder statesman of occupational medicine puts everything in perspective.*

527 Occupational Pulmonary Disorders

Dean Sheppard

The lung is the major interface between the human and the external environment. As such, the lungs and airways have evolved an elaborate system to filter out the myriad of potentially

toxic particles and gases present in inspired air in order to protect the delicate gas-exchanging apparatus of the alveolar surface. This system is remarkably durable. The irritant gases and approximately 2 mg of dust inhaled daily by urban dwellers generally have no effect on lung function. Even the high concentrations of dust, irritants, and carcinogens present in cigarette smoke, inhaled daily for periods of 50 years or more, fail to cause disease in most smokers. Given the continuing contact between the lungs and the environment, however, it is not surprising that the lungs are the most common site of serious environmentally induced disease. Environmental pollutants are generally present in highest concentration at sites of industrial use or production. Thus, environmentally induced lung disease usually results from occupational exposure.

The major determinants of disease in a given individual are the toxicity of the material inhaled, the dose and duration of exposure (including the duration of lung retention, which may be several years for some inhaled particles), and the individual's host defenses. One would like to be able to identify host factors that predispose to the development of occupational disease in order to advise individuals at risk to avoid particular occupations, but unfortunately this is rarely possible. A few notable exceptions are the increased susceptibility of cigarette smokers to asbestos-induced carcinoma of the lung and the increased susceptibility of atopic individuals to some types of occupational asthma. In general, a more fruitful approach to the prevention of occupational lung disease is protection of all workers from exposures that can be anticipated to cause disease in any. This approach is most likely to be effective if it includes a significant margin of safety, limiting exposures to levels considerably less than the exposure anticipated to cause disease. These principles underlie the workplace exposure standards promulgated by the American Council of Government Industrial Hygienists and more recently by the U.S. Occupational Safety and Health Administration. However, the standard-setting process is a slow one, and in the absence of adequate data, the assessments of disease probability on which they are based are necessarily subjective. Furthermore, as new data emerge, standards need to be continually revised, but this process too can take many years. Keeping these shortcomings in mind, physicians cannot assume that a given occupational exposure is not responsible for causing a disease, even if the exposure level was below the current standard.

Even if workplace standards could be set instantaneously with the emergence of new scientific data, individual practicing physicians would still play a critical role in the identification and ultimate prevention of occupational lung disease. Onset of occupational disease is often delayed long after exposure (e.g., up to 60 years for mesothelioma caused by asbestos exposure). Furthermore, the first cases of an occupational disease are rarely recognized as being caused by work exposure, especially when the disease is a common one, such as asthma or carcinoma of the lung. Thousands of new chemicals are introduced into the workplace each year without systematic screening for their ability to cause disease. Therefore, new causes of occupational lung disease will undoubtedly continue to emerge. Identification of these new causes of lung disease and prevention of additional cases will continue to be the responsibility of practicing physicians.

Even when adequate workplace standards exist, they are hard to enforce, especially for workers who are self-employed or who work in small shops. Under these circumstances the identification of an individual worker with an occupationally induced lung disease can be the first indication of unsafe working conditions. Thus, a diagnosis of occupational lung disease necessitates a report to the appropriate public health agency and a thorough investigation of the workplace to identify additional cases and prevent future ones.

The lung responds to injury in a limited number of ways. Virtually any type of lung disorder can be caused by an occupational exposure. The specific type of disorder is determined by the site of deposition of the responsible agent, the dose and duration of exposure, the susceptibility of specific lung cells to the agent's toxic effects, and the nature of the interaction between the agent and local host defense mechanisms.

Gases are deposited in the respiratory system based on their water solubility. Water-soluble gases, such as ammonia and sulfur dioxide, are nearly entirely removed from inspired air by the aqueous layer lining the nose, oropharynx, and upper airways. These gases thus are most likely to cause disease in the airways. Relatively water-insoluble gases, such as nitrogen dioxide and phosgene, bypass the upper airways and injure the distal airways and alveoli. In contrast, particles are deposited based on size or, more accurately, on "aerodynamic diameter," which means that a particle is deposited out of a moving airstream in the same fashion as would be a perfect sphere of that diameter. During quiet breathing through the nose, essentially all particles with aerodynamic diameters in excess of 10 μm are deposited on the nasal mucosa. During strenuous exercise, however, because of increased airflow and mouth breathing, up to 20 per cent of particles between 10 and 20 μm in diameter are deposited within the airways. Particles between 3 and 10 μm in diameter can be deposited throughout the tracheobronchial tree. More central deposition is favored by high inspiratory flow rates, by airway obstruction, and by the presence of increased quantities of mucus. Particles between 0.1 and 3 μm in diameter can also be deposited in the airways but are preferentially deposited within the alveoli. Smaller particles are mainly exhaled. A fiber is also deposited on the basis of aerodynamic diameter and not length. This explains why fibers up to 25 μm long are often deposited in alveoli.

GENERAL APPROACH TO A PATIENT WITH SUSPECTED OCCUPATIONAL LUNG DISEASE

HISTORY. A thorough occupational history is the most important step in diagnosing any occupationally induced disease. The history must go beyond the patient's present job to a complete list of each job done throughout the patient's lifetime. Job titles often are not helpful. Rather, a detailed description of what the patient actually did and what materials he or she worked with should be elicited. The relationship of the patient's work site to other associated jobs is important, as is the use and adequacy of exhaust ventilation and personal protective devices. For instance, one electrician could develop asbestosis from working near insulators in the holds of ships, while another electrician working outdoors on new-building construction might have no significant asbestos exposure. The presence or absence of special work clothes, lockers, and showers should be noted, since hazardous materials (e.g., asbestos) brought home by workers who have worked in their street clothes can cause disease in family members. Hobbies should also be described in detail; hazardous exposures in home workshops can cause disease (e.g., asthma from exposure to isocyanate varnishes). Each job and hobby should be recorded in chronologic order to ensure that all working years are accounted for. The temporal relationship between symptoms and exposure can also be important. This is especially true for disease with acute symptomatic exacerbations, such as occupational asthma and hypersensitivity pneumonitis. In all cases, it is important to determine that symptoms did not precede exposure. Because of the high prevalence of cigarette smoking, the important toxic effects of cigarette smoke itself on the lungs, and the possible interactions between smoking and occupational exposures, a careful quantitative smoking history is also important. Finally, it is important to seek out historical information that would suggest a nonoccupational cause for the patient's lung disease. For instance, a history of uveitis and parotid enlargement might suggest that sarcoidosis rather than asbestos exposure was responsible for a given patient's interstitial lung disease.

ROENTGENOGRAPHIC TECHNIQUES. Chest roentgenographs are important in the evaluation of patients suspected of having parenchymal lung disease and in detecting pleural abnormalities in workers exposed to asbestos. They can also be useful in surveillance of workers in hazardous occupations to detect subclinical abnormalities. For standardization of epidemiologic surveys, roentgenographic abnormalities should be characterized by trained and certified readers using the International Labor Office (ILO) classification system. In this system small parenchymal opacities are described by shape (irregular or rounded) and size. Profusion (the concentration of opacities) is scored on a 12-point scale (0/−, 0/0, 0/1, up to 3/3, 3/+). Large parenchymal opacities and the extent and width of pleural thickening are also quantified. This scoring system allows the clinician to make a

reasonable assessment of prognosis in individual patients. Computed tomography (CT) is more sensitive and specific than standard chest radiographs in detecting pleural abnormalities. Nonetheless, this technique is seldom necessary in symptomatic individuals, and its expense does not justify its use in screening. Similarly, although CT may be more sensitive than standard radiographs in detecting parenchymal infiltrates, the clinical significance of infiltrates detected by CT only is uncertain. Roentgenographs are not useful in evaluating patients with suspected occupational airway diseases.

PULMONARY FUNCTION TESTS. Tests of static lung function are important in evaluating patients suspected of having occupationally induced interstitial lung diseases or those with dyspnea of undetermined etiology. When these tests are abnormal, they provide information about the pattern and extent of lung dysfunction. Tests of static lung function do not provide information about the *cause* of lung dysfunction (occupational or not) or about dynamic abnormalities (e.g., bronchospasm or decreased pulmonary vascular reserve). Thus, for instance, many, if not most, patients with occupational asthma will have normal screening pulmonary function tests between symptomatic episodes. Special studies such as bronchial provocation tests (see below) may be required before a diagnosis of occupational lung disease can be excluded. An additional problem of tests of static lung function is the wide range of normal values seen among healthy individuals. For example, if an individual worker starts with a vital capacity near the upper limit of normal (120 per cent of predicted), his or her vital capacity would need to fall by one third (to 80 per cent of predicted) before it would be considered abnormal. If, as is often the case, a single measurement is made after many years of employment and a vital capacity of 90 per cent of predicted is recorded, a significant occupationally induced loss of lung function could easily be overlooked. To avoid this problem, serial measurements of lung function should be performed on the same equipment for surveillance of workers in occupations suspected of causing occupational lung disease. Accelerated rates of decline of lung function can thus be detected before the test results deviate from the predicted normal range.

In addition to tests of static lung function, pulmonary exercise testing can provide important information for the evaluation of any patient with unexplained dyspnea. This test can distinguish between cardiovascular and pulmonary limitations to exercise and can identify pulmonary vascular dysfunction (as occurs with interstitial fibrosis) in some patients with normal static lung function. In addition, exercise limitation can be measured and compared with the patient's actual job requirements.

EVALUATION OF THE JOB SITE. In the clinical evaluation of a worker suspected of having any occupationally induced disorder, it is important to inspect and monitor his or her workplace. It is essential to do so if a diagnosis of an occupationally induced disorder has been established. Inspections usually require the assistance of a trained industrial hygienist who may be employed by the worker's company, the worker's compensation insurance company, a state or federal agency (e.g, the Occupational Safety and Health Administration), or a specialized occupational health clinic. In addition to a visual walk-through inspection and direct observation of each of the worker's job tasks (and adjacent workers' tasks), an inspection should include air sampling for agents suspected of being released by the work processes involved. Even if for some reason air sampling cannot be obtained, direct site inspection can provide important clues to the occupational etiology of a worker's disease. For example, a maintenance worker with asthma may be found to be working in a warehouse in which toluene di-isocyanate is used in manufacturing.

Morgan WKC, Seaton A: Occupational Lung Disease. 2nd ed. Philadelphia, W. B. Saunders Company, 1984. *A reasonably priced, up-to-date textbook.*
Parkes WR: Occupational Lung Disorders. 2nd ed. London, Butterworths, 1982. *A detailed and very well-referenced textbook by a single author.*
Rom WN (ed.): Environmental and Occupational Medicine. Boston, Little, Brown & Company, 1983. *A comprehensive review of occupational medicine with excellent introductory chapters covering issues of assessment and control of workplace hazards and broad coverage of individual exposures and diseases.*

AIRWAY DISORDERS
Occupational Asthma

Occupational asthma is defined as asthma that occurs in a previously healthy individual as a result of occupational exposure.

TABLE 527–1. COMMON CAUSES OF OCCUPATIONAL ASTHMA

Agents	Occupational Exposure
Low Molecular Weight Chemicals	
Isocyanates	Plastics, varnishing, spray painting, foundries
Anhydrides: phthalic, trimellitic, tetrachlorophthalic	Plastics, epoxy resins
Soldering fluxes	Electronics, aluminum plants
Metal salts: platinum, chromium, nickel	Metal plating, refining, tanning
Wood dusts: red cedar, redwood, zebrawood	Sawmills, carpentry
Complex Organic Materials	
Plant dusts: grain, coffee bean, castor bean	Grain handlers, bakers, agricultural workers
Laboratory animals	Laboratory workers, animal handlers
Shellfish: crab, prawn, oyster	Shellfish processors
Biologic enzymes	Detergents, pharmaceuticals, chemical industry

This is usually distinguished from an exacerbation of pre-existing asthma on the basis of pre-employment history. Work-induced exacerbations of pre-existing asthma are also an important cause of morbidity and may qualify the affected worker for worker's compensation. Asthma is a common disease (affecting 3 to 6 per cent of the U.S. population), but most patients with mild disease can function normally under most circumstances (Ch. 57). Thus, virtually every occupation includes a significant number of workers with asthma. Patients with asthma are extremely sensitive to bronchoconstrictor stimuli and may develop symptomatic attacks from exposure to occupational irritants (e.g., low concentrations of sulfur dioxide gas) that have no effect on their nonasthmatic coworkers. In this circumstance, although the worker's asthma may have antedated occupational exposure, management would be the same as for patients with true occupational asthma, including application for compensation and job retraining if these are required to avoid further exposure.

CAUSATIVE AGENTS. Well over 100 causative agents are now recognized, and the list continues to grow (Table 527–1). This list can be roughly divided into highly reactive low molecular weight chemicals (such as toluene di-isocyanate and trimellitic anhydride) that share the ability to cause acute airway injury and complex organic materials such as animal dander and grain dust. Since asthma is common and usually of unknown cause, the occupational etiology of asthma is often missed. In addition, thousands of new chemicals are introduced into the workplace each year, but it takes many years for any association between exposure to a chemical and induction of asthma to be recognized. Finally, many workers are simultaneously exposed to dozens or even hundreds of different chemicals, so determining the single one responsible for causing asthma is often difficult. For all these reasons, a diagnosis of occupational asthma must often be considered on the basis of clinical characteristics even if a worker is not exposed to any agent already known to cause asthma. On the other hand, if it can be determined that a worker with asthma of recent onset *is* exposed to an agent known to commonly cause asthma (for instance, toluene di-isocyanate, grain dust, and western red cedar dust cause asthma in approximately 5 per cent of exposed workers), this information should increase the suspicion that the worker's asthma is occupationally induced.

PATHOPHYSIOLOGY. Organic materials such as animal excreta, green coffee beans, and shellfish extracts probably serve as antigens and cause asthma primarily as a result of repeated immediate hypersensitivity responses in the airways. Some of these agents (e.g., animal excreta) are most likely to affect individuals with a previously demonstrated predisposition to atopy. Most of the low molecular weight chemicals that cause asthma are too small to serve as antigens by themselves. These chemicals could trigger immediate hypersensitivity responses by combining with tissue proteins or by altering tissue proteins to create new antigenic determinants. Some of these agents (e.g., toluene di-isocyanate) can cause acute airway injury and inflammation in the absence of immune sensitization. Asthma appears to be more common in workers exposed to repeated accidental spills, suggesting that this acute airway injury may contribute to the development of asthma.

CLINICAL MANIFESTATIONS. *Cough* is the most common initial manifestation of occupational asthma. This is often preceded by symptoms of *rhinitis,* which is associated with asthma in up to 70 per cent of affected workers. Intermittent *chest tightness, dyspnea,* and *wheezing* may be present initially or develop weeks to months after the onset of cough and rhinitis. Initially, these symptoms occur with a distinctive temporal relationship to work exposure. The three most common temporal patterns are an immediate response characterized by short-lived symptoms occurring at the time of work exposure, a late response characterized by symptoms that begin 4 to 12 hours after exposure, and a dual response that combines elements of the first two (Fig. 527–1). Unfortunately, the immediate response—the pattern most commonly recognized as due to work exposure—is the least common. Furthermore, workers who experience dual responses are much more likely to notice the late response than the immediate one, because the late response is usually longer in duration and more difficult to treat. Thus, a typical history of occupational asthma would include symptoms that are most prominent in the evening or at night. Initially, improvement in these symptoms during weekends and vacations is the most important clue to their occupational origin. Eventually, however, as the worker's asthma becomes more severe, any temporal relationship with work may disappear, and an affected worker may complain of persistent asthma indistinguishable from asthma of any other etiology.

Symptoms of occupational asthma can develop at any time after the onset of employment but usually appear after months to years of exposure to the responsible agent. When the diagnosis is suspected soon after the onset of symptoms and further exposure to the responsible agent is prevented, most affected workers gradually improve. Workers who are diagnosed after several years of symptomatic asthma, however, or who continue to be exposed after the diagnosis has been established can develop

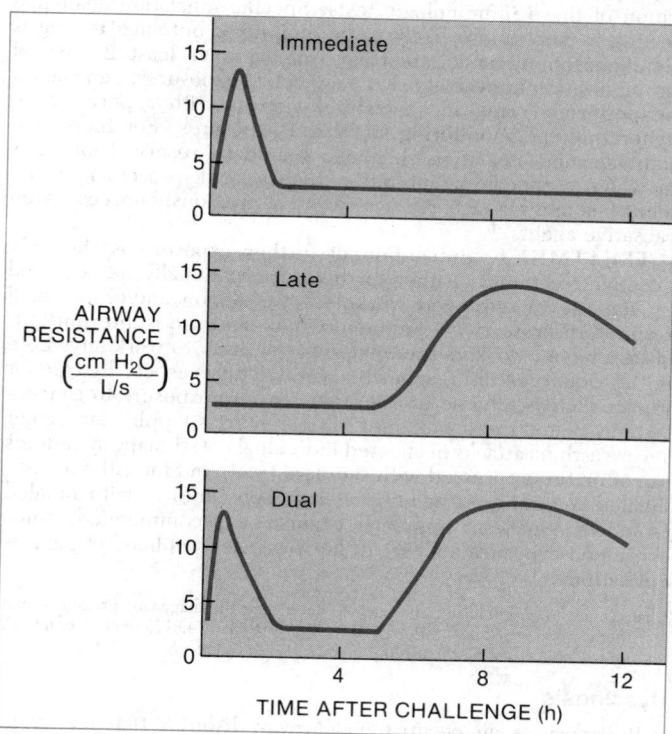

FIGURE 527–1. Temporal patterns of bronchoconstriction (as indicated by increases in airway resistance) after exposure to agents responsible for causing occupational asthma. Delayed responses that can begin from 4 to 12 hours after exposure tend to be more prolonged than immediate responses and thus often cause more prominent symptoms. (Reprinted by permission of the Western Journal of Medicine, from Sheppard D: Occupational asthma. West J Med 137:480, 1982.)

asthma that may persist for years (and perhaps indefinitely) even if further exposure ceases.

DIAGNOSIS. As noted above, a history of new-onset rhinitis, cough, chest tightness, dyspnea, and/or wheezing in a previously healthy worker is essential. Screening pulmonary function test results are usually normal between symptomatic episodes but may reveal reversible (or fixed) airway obstruction. Measurement of spirometry (forced expiratory volume in 1 second [FEV_1] and forced vital capacity [FVC]) before and after a work shift may reveal a more than 10 per cent decrease, but this test is insensitive because of inconsistent exposures over a single work shift and varied temporal patterns of response. If the worker is still actively employed, repeated measurements of peak expiratory flow can be performed and symptoms recorded at 2-hour intervals over a 2-week period that should ideally include at least two weekends. This method is sensitive to intermittent airway obstruction and provides information on the temporal relationship between obstruction and exposure. A 20 per cent difference between the best and worst values of peak flow during any 24-hour period is abnormal. If symptoms are recorded but peak flow does not vary, an explanation for the symptoms other than asthma should be sought.

A single measurement of nonspecific airway responsiveness (e.g., by methacholine or histamine challenge) can confirm a diagnosis of asthma but does not provide information about the occupational etiology. Furthermore, nonspecific airway responsiveness can be normal in workers with occupational asthma, especially during periods of minimal exposure to the responsible agent. Demonstration of a dramatic *increase* in airway responsiveness in association with work exposure does provide strong supportive evidence of an occupational etiology.

Skin testing and/or measurement of specific immunoglobulin E (IgE) antibody can be useful for selected causes of occupational asthma. These include animal exposures, green coffee beans, platinum salts, and trimellitic anhydride. For most causes of occupational asthma, however, the responsible antigens have not been sufficiently well characterized to allow definitive interpretation of these immunologic tests. Specific inhalation challenge testing is much more likely to be definitive, but such testing is time consuming and expensive, requiring at least 2 days of hospitalization to evaluate sham and actual exposures, and should be performed only in specialized centers with experience in generating and monitoring simulated exposures. For these reasons, specific inhalation challenge should be reserved for cases in which a specific agent rather than a work process must be identified and for research evaluation of previously unrecognized causative agents.

TREATMENT. Prevention of further exposure is the only effective treatment. Although this can occasionally be achieved by the use of improved workplace ventilation and/or personal respiratory protective equipment when exposure is intermittent, often affected workers are unable to continue to work anywhere in the vicinity of the responsible agent. This is especially true for vapors such as toluene di-isocyanate, where exposure to concentrations below the lower limit of detection (<1 ppb) can trigger severe asthma attacks in affected individuals. Asthmatic symptoms can often be suppressed with standard treatment for asthma (e.g., inhaled β-adrenergic agonists and theophylline) or with inhaled cromolyn. Such an approach cannot be recommended, since continued exposure appears to increase the likelihood of persistent asthma.

Chan Yeung M: A clinician's approach to determine the diagnosis, prognosis, and therapy of occupational asthma. Med Clin North Am 74:811, 1990. *A practical, up-to-date review by the leading investigator in this field.*

Byssinosis

Byssinosis is an occupational airway disorder that occurs in workers exposed to dust generated during the handling of crude cotton, hemp, or flax. This disorder differs from other forms of occupational asthma in that symptoms of chest tightness and dyspnea are most prominent during the initial work shift following a weekend or vacation and tend to diminish over the course of each work week. Although the dust component responsible for these symptoms has not been definitively identified, contaminants

such as bacterial endotoxins may play a prominent role. Steam cleaning crude cotton before it is carded and engineering controls to reduce airborne dust concentrations can both markedly reduce the incidence of acute symptoms. Long-term chronic exposure to cotton dust also appears to cause productive cough and accelerated loss of lung function in some workers.

Holt PG: Current trends in research on the etiology and pathogenesis of byssinosis. Am J Ind Med 12:711, 1987.
Mundie TG, Ainsworth SK: Etiopathogenic mechanisms of bronchoconstriction in byssinosis: A review. Am Rev Respir Dis 133:1181, 1986.

Industrial Bronchitis

Workers in a number of dusty industries have an increased prevalence of chronic daily productive cough. This effect of occupational dust exposure has been most clearly demonstrated in workers exposed to coal, grain, and cotton dusts. A similar increased prevalence of productive cough has been reported in workers chronically exposed to high concentrations of sulfur dioxide gas in smelters and paper pulp mills and in welders who are chronically exposed to a variety of irritant gases. The high prevalence of cigarette smoking among industrial workers and the potent effect of smoking in causing bronchitis often make establishing an occupational cause of bronchitis difficult. Each of the exposures noted above has been reported to cause bronchitis even in nonsmokers. In the absence of smoking, lung function is usually normal in workers with industrial bronchitis. Nonetheless, the prospective demonstration of accelerated loss of lung function in grain workers and data demonstrating a high prevalence of airway obstruction in cotton workers suggest that these exposures can cause chronic airflow limitation.

PARENCHYMAL LUNG DISORDERS

Disorders Caused by Inorganic Dusts

SILICOSIS

DEFINITION. Silicosis is the parenchymal lung disease caused by inhalation of particles of crystalline silicon dioxide (SiO_2). Free silicon dioxide is usually encountered in nature as quartz. Other crystalline forms, cristobalite and tridymite, are most often encountered in industry as by-products produced when amorphous silicates are heated to high temperature. More complex silicates such as asbestos, talc, and kaolin, cause clinically distinct pulmonary responses and will be discussed separately.

OCCUPATIONAL EXPOSURE. Silicon dioxide is widely deposited through the rock that makes up the earth's surface. Industrial activities that involve cutting, polishing, or shearing rock are thus all potential sources of respirable silica. These include mining, tunneling, quarrying, and stone cutting. Industrial uses of sand, which is largely composed of quartz, can lead to exposure to high concentrations of respirable silica, especially the use of sand for abrasive blasting. Sand is also widely used in foundry work, glass blowing, and pottery making.

PATHOLOGY AND PATHOGENESIS. Three different forms of silicosis are roughly related to the intensity of exposure to respirable silica. *Chronic silicosis* is defined as radiographic abnormalities that are first noted 15 years or more after the onset of exposure. *Accelerated silicosis* resembles the chronic disease but occurs 5 to 15 years after the onset of exposure to high concentrations of silica. *Acute silicosis* occurs within 5 years of the onset of exposure, is virtually always caused by massive exposure, and is clinically and pathologically quite different from the other two forms.

Chronic silicosis is characterized by small nodules that may be diffusely distributed or present primarily in the upper lobes (Fig. 527–2). Nodules are also present in hilar lymph nodes. The nodules have an acellular core composed of concentric swirls of hyalinized collagen and are surrounded by a cellular capsule containing macrophages, plasma cells, and fibroblasts (Fig. 527–3). Silica crystals are often present in these nodules. In a minority of patients, small nodules coalesce to form large masses that can compress and obliterate normal lung structures (so-called progressive massive fibrosis). These nodules occasionally cavitate in the absence of infection, but most often cavities result from infection with *Mycobacterium tuberculosis* and other mycobacteria. The appearance of accelerated silicosis is similar, but conglomerate nodules occur more commonly and giant cells may

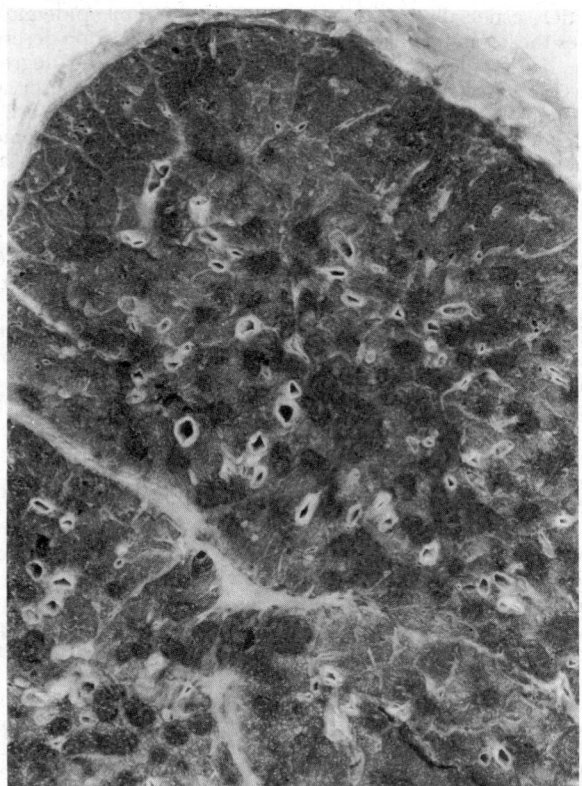

FIGURE 527–2. Close-up of the upper lobe of a slice of lung with marked simple silicosis. The rounded, sharply circumscribed black spots are silicotic nodules. The surrounding parenchyma is normal. (From Warnock ML, Kuwahara TJ, Wolery G: The relation of asbestos burden to asbestosis and lung cancer. Pathol Annu 18:109, 1983 [Part 2], reprinted with permission of Appleton-Century-Crofts, Norwalk, CT.)

be seen. Acute silicosis is characterized by an eosinophilic exudate that fills alveolar spaces and resembles alveolar proteinosis.

Tissue injury from silica is probably initiated by the interaction between silica crystals and alveolar macrophages and appears to involve disruption of phagolysosomes and release of lysosomal contents into the extracellular space. Macrophages stimulated by silica also secrete factors that are chemotactic for other macrophages and neutrophils and that stimulate fibroblasts to proliferate and lay down collagen.

CLINICAL MANIFESTATIONS. Chronic silicosis most commonly causes radiographic abnormalities without symptoms. When symptoms do develop, dyspnea is the most common, but it is usually severe only in patients with progressive massive fibrosis. Cough is commonly seen but is often attributable to chronic bronchitis in cigarette smokers or to superimposed infection. Patients with silicosis have an increased susceptibility to both tuberculous and nontuberculous mycobacterial infections; these should be suspected in affected workers who develop fever, weight loss, asymmetric upper lobe infiltrates, or cavitary lesions. Susceptibility to fungal infections is also increased. Chest pain and clubbing are not features of silicosis.

Chest radiographs usually show multiple small nodules that may be diffusely distributed but are often primarily in the upper lobes and are occasionally calcified. This pattern is called *simple silicosis*. Enlarged hilar lymph nodes may contain outer rims of calcium called *eggshell calcification*. In patients with progressive massive fibrosis, large masses are usually seen in the upper lobes, often symmetrically distributed around the hilar regions in a so-called angel's wing distribution. In these patients, compensatory emphysema is also common. Severe abnormalities in lung function are generally seen only in patients with conglomerate shadows who are said to have *complicated silicosis*. Because the airways and the pulmonary vascular bed are often distorted by these conglomerate masses, pulmonary function tests often reveal airway obstruction and a decrease in pulmonary diffusing capacity as well as the decrease in lung volumes commonly seen in patients with interstitial fibrosis.

Patients with rheumatoid arthritis who develop silicosis can present with multiple large pulmonary nodules that pathologically resemble extrapulmonary rheumatoid nodules. This presentation, called *Caplan's syndrome*, can also occur in workers with asbestosis or in coal workers' pneumoconiosis.

DIAGNOSIS. The diagnosis of silicosis is based on a history of significant occupational exposure to free silica and appropriate radiographic abnormalities. Pulmonary function tests are usually normal in patients with simple silicosis; they are not helpful in establishing the diagnosis. Pulmonary function tests are useful in evaluating and quantifying pulmonary impairment in symptomatic workers. In patients with simple silicosis, severe airflow obstruction is usually due to another coexisting disorder (e.g., bronchitis and/or emphysema) not caused by silica. However, recent evidence suggests that the adverse effects of cigarette smoking on lung function are probably exacerbated by exposure to silica. In accelerated or chronic silicosis, other causes of interstitial fibrosis should be considered in the differential diagnosis. In patients with progressive loss of lung function in whom the diagnosis is uncertain, lung biopsy should be performed to look for other treatable causes. Silica crystals can be seen as birefringent by plane polarizing microscopy, but this feature is not specific for free silica. In patients with mixed dust exposure, energy-dispersive x-ray analysis can identify silicon dioxide and other elements associated with silicates (e.g., calcium, magnesium, iron). Acute silicosis resembles other forms of alveolar proteinosis, but the history of massive silica exposure is usually obvious.

Antinuclear antibodies may be present in up to 40 per cent of patients with silicosis. This test is of no diagnostic value, however, since antibodies are also seen in a high percentage of exposed workers without silicosis. Rapid progression of conglomerate lesions, especially if this is unilateral, suggests coexisting mycobacterial infection or neoplasm and justifies aggressive efforts at diagnosis, as does the appearance of a new cavity. Some epide-

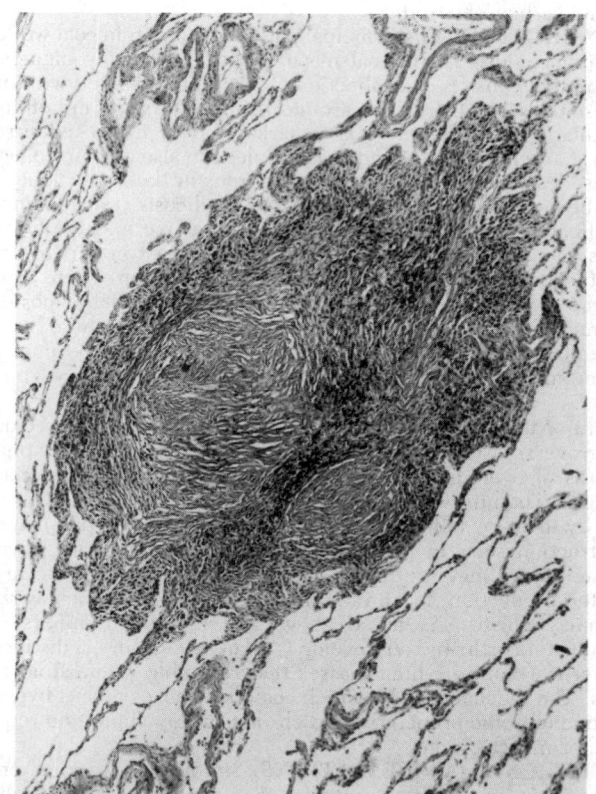

FIGURE 527–3. Light microscopic view of a typical silicotic nodule (original magnification, ×70). Note the whorled fibrous core. The surrounding alveoli are normal. (From Warnock ML, Kuwahara TJ, Wolery G: The relation of asbestos burden to asbestosis and lung cancer. Pathol Annu 18:109, 1983 [Part 2], reprinted with permission of Appleton-Century-Crofts, Norwalk, CT.)

miologic studies suggest that silica exposure increases the risk for pulmonary neoplasms, but most of these studies have involved workers exposed to other potential carcinogens, so the role of silica itself in pulmonary carcinogenesis remains controversial.

TREATMENT. There is no proven effective treatment for any form of silicosis. Patients with acute silicosis should probably be treated with sequential whole lung lavage, as are other patients with alveolar proteinosis. Mycobacterial infections should be treated with standard chemotherapy (Ch. 332). Patients with silicosis and a positive purified protein derivative (PPD) should receive a year of prophylactic therapy with isoniazid (300 mg daily).

The major hope for reducing the prevalence of silicosis lies with prevention. Industrial processes that generate respirable free silica should be enclosed or modified; dust containing silica should never be swept dry, and workers should always use personal respiratory protective devices for unavoidable short-term exposures. In many countries (not including the United States), sand is no longer allowed for use in abrasive blasting because of the large quantities of respirable silica produced. Such a ban should be instituted worldwide, since a number of acceptable replacements are available (e.g., steel grit and coal ash).

Davis GS: Pathogenesis of silicosis: Current concepts and hypothesis. Lung 164:139, 1986.

Silicosis and Silicate Disease Committee. Diseases associated with exposure to silica and nonfibrous silicate minerals. Arch Pathol Lab Med 112:673, 1988. *A recent consensus report focusing on the pathologic effects of silica.*

COAL WORKERS' PNEUMOCONIOSIS

DEFINITION. Coal workers' pneumoconiosis is the parenchymal lung disorder caused by inhalation of coal dust. A similar disorder occurs in workers exposed to graphite or carbon black. Coal dust inhalation also causes chronic bronchitis. These disorders occur primarily in coal miners but can occur in coal trimmers, graphite miners and millers, and workers involved in manufacturing carbon electrodes.

PATHOLOGY. The principal pathologic lesion in coal workers' pneumoconiosis is the coal macule, a small, heavily pigmented lesion that consists of a collection of macrophages filled with dust. These cells are distributed around terminal airways and often fill alveolar spaces, but there is remarkably little initial tissue reaction. Larger macules called coal nodules can also contain collagen. These lesions are usually more numerous in the upper lobes but can be found throughout the lungs. As in silicosis, a small minority of affected workers (~1%) develop progressive massive fibrosis. This complication appears to be related at least in part to heavy dust loads. Pathologically, large rubbery masses are seen, usually in the superior segments of the lower lobes and the posterior segments of the upper lobes. Microscopically, these masses resemble large coal nodules but contain considerably more collagen and are frequently associated with compensatory emphysema.

The pathogenesis of coal workers' pneumoconiosis remains controversial. The coal macules are probably produced by phagocytosis of overwhelming quantities of dust by air space macrophages. The interaction between coal dust and macrophages may not by itself be sufficient to explain the fibrosis and parenchymal destruction seen in patients with progressive massive fibrosis. Tissue injury may require concomitant exposure to silica, mycobacterial infection, or an immunologic abnormality such as rheumatoid arthritis. As noted above for silica, coal miners with rheumatoid arthritis can develop Caplan's syndrome, a distinctive pattern of multiple lung masses that resemble rheumatoid nodules. The mechanisms by which coal dust causes mucus hypersecretion (chronic bronchitis) and chronic airflow limitation require further investigation.

CLINICAL MANIFESTATIONS. Simple coal workers' pneumoconiosis most often consists of radiographic abnormalities without symptoms. Patients with complicated pneumoconiosis (progressive massive fibrosis) can develop progressive dyspnea, pulmonary hypertension, and respiratory failure. The risk of mycobacterial infection may be increased in patients with coal workers' pneumoconiosis, but not to the same extent as in patients with silicosis. Chest radiographs usually show small, irregular opacities, especially in the upper lung zones. For epidemiologic studies these can be quantified by the ILO classification described above. In simple coal workers' pneumoconiosis, the degree of profusion is well correlated with the dust burden, an observation that is not surprising, since radiographic abnormalities are primarily due to retained dust. In complicated pneumoconiosis, radiographs show large conglomerate shadows and compensatory emphysema.

Chronic sputum production and chronic airflow limitation are also complications of coal mining related to the quantity of dust exposure but not to radiographic abnormalities. Abnormalities in airflow tend to be mild in nonsmoking miners in the absence of complicated pneumoconiosis. In an individual coal miner who smokes, it is not possible to determine the relative contributions of coal dust and cigarette smoking to the development of chronic bronchitis and airway obstruction.

Pulmonary function tests in patients with simple coal workers' pneumoconiosis are usually normal. In patients with complicated pneumoconiosis, both airway obstruction (characterized by decreases in the FEV_1 and other tests of maximal flow) and lung restriction (characterized by a decrease in total lung capacity) can occur. In these patients, the diffusing capacity for carbon monoxide is often reduced as a result of obstruction or destruction of the pulmonary vascular bed. Some epidemiologic studies in coal miners have shown an increase in residual volume and a decrease in flow measured at low lung volumes in comparison to matched nonexposed control populations. These findings are consistent with mild airway obstruction caused by coal dust exposure.

DIAGNOSIS. The diagnosis of coal workers' pneumoconiosis is made on the basis of a history of exposure and appropriate radiographic abnormalities. In patients with large conglomerate shadows, mycobacterial infection needs to be excluded. Affected patients do not have an increased risk of lung cancer, but in smokers with unilateral enlarging masses, neoplasm must be excluded. The lesions of simple coal workers' pneumoconiosis do not generally progress or regress after the end of exposure, so a changing radiograph in a retired worker suggests another diagnosis.

TREATMENT AND PREVENTION. There is no effective treatment for coal workers' pneumoconiosis. Impending depletion of the world's oil reserves has stimulated an increased demand for coal, ensuring continued exposure to coal dust for years to come. Prevention of pneumoconiosis requires minimizing the airborne respirable dust concentration at each step in the extraction and processing of coal.

Heppleston AG: Prevalence and pathogenesis of pneumoconiosis in coal workers. Environ Health Perspect 78:159, 1988.

Disorders Caused by Asbestos

Inhaled asbestos is a more potent stimulus to tissue injury than is silica or coal. Furthermore, asbestos causes a broader range of clinical disorders besides pulmonary fibrosis: pleural fibrosis and effusion; mesothelioma of the pleura and peritoneum; and cancer of the lung, larynx, and gastrointestinal tract. The term *asbestosis* is usually reserved for the nonmalignant response of the lung parenchyma to inhaled asbestos fiber (pulmonary fibrosis).

OCCUPATIONAL EXPOSURE. Asbestos is not a single chemical entity, but rather a group of mineral silicates that have in common their fibrous nature and the potential to be woven. Worldwide use of asbestos increased dramatically throughout most of this century before beginning to decline in the late 1970's. Asbestos fibers have been widely used in ship building, construction, insulating, and automotive vehicle clutch and brake manufacturing because they are highly resistant to heat, acid, and chemical degradation. For the same reasons, asbestos has also been used in the manufacture of textiles and building supplies. In the past, the heaviest occupational exposures have occurred in miners, millers, shipyard workers, and insulation workers; but because of the diverse uses of asbestos, cases of asbestos-induced disease are seen among a wide variety of other occupations. As the use of asbestos in new construction has been nearly eliminated in the United States, continued exposure is likely to be due to demolition and renovation of buildings and ships containing asbestos. In developing countries, application of new asbestos continues to be widespread. Since most asbestos-induced diseases have a long latency, the prevalence of asbestos-induced diseases is not likely to fall for many years despite a marked decrease in exposure. Nonoccupational exposure can also cause disease. For instance, cases of mesothelioma and an increased prevalence of pleural thickening have been reported among household contacts of asbestos workers (presumably due to exposure to fibers brought home on work clothes).

PATHOLOGY AND PATHOGENESIS. *Pleural Disease.* Asbestos can cause localized or diffuse areas of acellular pleural fibrosis that are usually bilateral and primarily on the parietal pleura. Asbestos fibers are often found in the adjacent visceral pleura, suggesting that asbestos fibers that migrate out to the visceral pleural surface may injure the adjacent parietal pleura. Asbestos exposure can also cause benign exudative pleural effusions that usually contain a mixed population of inflammatory cells. The exudative lesion is nonspecific.

Pulmonary Fibrosis. Macroscopically, in advanced cases the lungs are small and stiff, and fibrous streaks are most prominent in the lower lobes and in subpleural locations. Honeycombing is occasionally seen (Fig. 527–4). Microscopically, asbestosis is indistinguishable from other causes of pulmonary fibrosis, except for the presence of asbestos fibers. A small percentage of asbestos fibers become coated with hemosiderin and form asbestos bodies that are visible under the light microscope. Identification of the more numerous uncoated fibers requires electron microscopy. The number of asbestos bodies recovered from dried lung correlates well with the total number of fibers (though there are several orders of magnitude more uncoated fibers). However, because asbestos bodies are not uniformly distributed throughout the lungs, examination of standard lung sections by light microscopy may not reveal asbestos bodies even from patients with a heavy asbestos burden and asbestosis. On the other hand, occasional asbestos bodies can be seen in urban dwellers without occupational exposure and are of little significance in the absence of associated pulmonary fibrosis.

In experimental animals exposed to asbestos, the earliest pathologic abnormality is an accumulation of inflammatory cells (especially macrophages) around asbestos fibers in the terminal

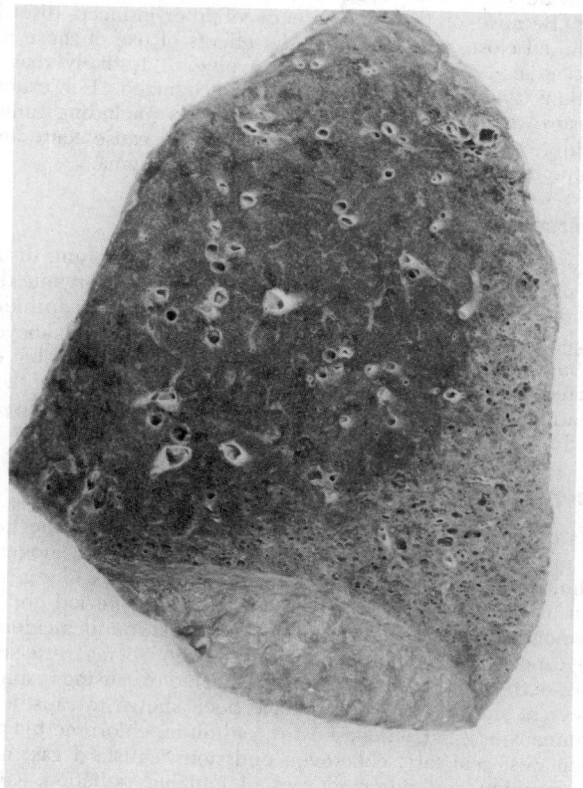

FIGURE 527–4. Slice of lower lobe from a patient with asbestosis. Note the thick pleural opacity at the base and the marked subpleural fibrosis with honeycombing. (From Warnock ML, Kuwahara TJ, Wolery G: The relation of asbestos burden to asbestosis and lung cancer. Pathol Annu 18:109, 1983 [Part 2], reprinted with permission of Appleton-Century-Crofts, Norwalk, CT.)

airways. Similar lesions are also common in asbestos-exposed workers and may explain why exposure to asbestos reduces airflow at low lung volumes.

Malignant pleural mesotheliomas are bulky, slow-growing tumors that spread by local extension to encase the lung and mediastinum. They vary histologically and can be difficult to distinguish from metastatic adenocarcinoma even in large specimens obtained by open pleural biopsy. Lung cancer can be of any cell type. Asbestos exposure and cigarette smoking act synergistically in causing lung cancer, so that heavily exposed smoking workers have a risk of lung cancer 30 to 90 times higher than that of unexposed nonsmokers (Ch. 68).

Asbestos fibers appear to cause tissue injury by stimulating alveolar macrophages to secrete cytotoxic materials, inflammatory cell chemoattractants, and at least one factor that stimulates fibroblast proliferation. Recent evidence suggests that reactive oxygen species are important in asbestos-induced lung injury. Because of their durability, individual fibers can repeatedly stimulate macrophages for many years without being degraded. This helps to explain the continued progression of asbestos-induced disease after exposure ceases and points out why the effective intensity of exposure depends on *time* from first exposure as well as total lung fiber burden. Nonetheless, the enormous variability in disease severity seen among individuals with equivalent exposure histories and lung fiber burdens suggests an important role for as yet uncharacterized host factors. One possibly important cofactor is cigarette smoking, which has been shown to increase the severity of radiographic abnormalities in workers exposed to asbestos.

CLINICAL MANIFESTATIONS. Pleural plaques are the most common manifestation of asbestos exposure. Patients with only pleural involvement are usually asymptomatic and have normal pulmonary function. Occasionally, patients with extensive pleural thickening develop extrapulmonary lung restriction that can cause dyspnea. The major significance of pleural plaques is that their appearance on a chest radiograph confirms a history of exposure. Diaphragmatic plaques are especially likely to calcify, and bilateral diaphragmatic calcification is almost always caused by asbestos exposure. Diffuse unilateral pleural thickening and/or pleuritic chest pain suggests the possibility of mesothelioma.

Asbestosis presents as do other forms of pulmonary fibrosis, with dyspnea that is initially most prominent with exertion and is often associated with cough. Bibasilar rales are a common finding, and clubbing can occur. The chest radiograph reveals linear and irregular opacities that are most prominent in the lower lung fields. Pleural thickening is often present but may not be radiographically apparent. As with other forms of pulmonary fibrosis, up to 10 per cent of patients with asbestos-induced fibrosis severe enough to cause lung restriction have normal chest radiographs. Progressive massive fibrosis is not seen. In patients with pulmonary fibrosis severe enough to cause dyspnea, pulmonary function tests usually show lung restriction (a symmetric reduction in all lung volumes) and a reduction in diffusing capacity. Flow-volume curves show reduced flow at low lung volumes, but marked airway obstruction, as manifested by a marked reduction in per cent of FEV_1, usually has other causes, such as cigarette smoking. In an asbestos-exposed smoker, a decrease in total lung capacity cannot be caused by smoking, but decreases in diffusing capacity and flow at low lung volume could be due to cigarettes, asbestos, or the combined effects of both.

DIAGNOSIS. The diagnosis of asbestos-induced pleural plaques is made on the basis of the typical bilateral appearance and a history of exposure. In approximately 80 per cent of patients with bilateral pleural plaques, asbestos exposure is responsible. Oblique radiographs increase the likelihood of detecting plaques, and CT is more sensitive than standard radiography and allows distinction between true plaques and subpleural fat. Since plaques themselves are rarely clinically significant, the considerable cost of these studies and the additional radiation exposure are difficult to justify, except for research purposes. The diagnosis of asbestos-induced pleural effusion depends on a history of exposure and exclusion of other causes of a pleural exudate.

Asbestosis is usually diagnosed on the basis of significant exposure, radiographic abnormalities, and pulmonary function studies showing lung restriction. Occasionally, in patients with early disease, radiographs or lung function studies may be normal, but exercise testing reveals abnormalities in pulmonary gas exchange. Lung biopsy should be performed only in patients with progressive disease to exclude causes of pulmonary fibrosis that might respond to treatment. If sufficient lung tissue is available (from open lung biopsy or autopsy), asbestos burden should be estimated by counting asbestos bodies from ashed tissue or asbestos fibers by electron probe analysis. In patients with stable lung function, lung biopsy should not be performed merely to establish asbestos exposure as the cause of lung fibrosis, since such a diagnosis does not lead to any specific therapy and all biopsy procedures are associated with some risk.

Asbestosis usually does not develop before 15 years after the first exposure to asbestos and usually requires several years of exposure. However, workers have been reported to develop the disease 15 to 30 years after periods of very heavy exposure as short as 6 months.

A diagnosis of asbestos-induced lung cancer is based on a history of heavy exposure that should ideally be confirmed by quantification of asbestos fiber burden from resected lung or autopsy specimens. Like pulmonary fibrosis, lung cancer does not develop within 15 years of first exposure and has its peak incidence within 25 to 40 years. The distribution of tumor cell types is the same as that seen in the general population. Epidemiologic evidence suggests that an increased incidence of lung cancer requires an intensity of asbestos exposure similar to that required to increase the incidence of pulmonary fibrosis. These data do not imply that both abnormalities would occur in the same individuals. Thus, lung cancer of any cell type in an individual with a well-documented history of heavy exposure can be reasonably considered to be due, at least in part, to asbestos exposure irrespective of coexistent pulmonary fibrosis.

TREATMENT AND PREVENTION. There is no proven effective treatment for asbestosis. The major strategy for prevention is worldwide elimination of new asbestos use and replacement with synthetic substitutes that appear to be considerably less toxic. Continuing exposure to asbestos currently in use needs to be minimized by use of engineering controls, personal protection, and public education. For prevention of lung cancer, individuals with past exposure should be strongly encouraged to stop smoking, since the risk of lung cancer falls dramatically (but is not eliminated) within a few years of smoking cessation.

American Thoracic Society, Medical Sectionof the American Lung Association: The diagnosis of nonmalignant diseases related to asbestos. Am Rev Respir Dis 143:363, 1990. *A concise review of the recommendations from a committee of experts in the evaluation of asbestos-related diseases.*
Becklake MR: Pneumoconiosis. *In* Murray JF, Nadel JA (ed.): Textbook of Respiratory Medicine. Philadelphia, W.B. Saunders Company, 1988, pp 1556–1592. *An excellent, comprehensive review of asbestos-induced diseases and other disorders induced by inorganic dusts.*

Beryllium Disease

Beryllium is a rare metal that can cause both acute and chronic disease. Acute beryllium disease results from intense exposure and resembles acute lung injury from other massive toxic exposures. Clinical manifestations include upper airway injury, bronchiolitis, and pulmonary edema. Mortality has been reported to be as high as 10 per cent. Chronic beryllium disease can follow acute disease but more often occurs without antecedent symptoms from months to years after first exposure. Because beryllium salts are absorbed through the respiratory tract and distributed throughout the body, exposure causes a systemic disease. Pathologically, chronic beryllium disease is characterized by noncaseating granulomas in lung, lymph nodes, liver, spleen, adrenal glands, and kidneys. Granulomas in the skin are thought to be due to direct exposure.

Before 1949, most cases of beryllium disease were due to the use of beryllium in fluorescent lights. Since such use was discontinued, most cases have occurred in the manufacturing of metal alloys and x-ray tubes and in the mining and milling of beryllium. The number of new cases has progressively fallen as industrial hygiene measures have been improved in these industries, but occasional cases continue to occur.

The diagnosis of chronic beryllium disease is made on the basis of a history of exposure and demonstration of granulomas on tissue biopsy. The lung pathology is nonspecific and indistinguishable from sarcoid and hypersensitivity pneumonitis (Ch. 67). Involvement of the uvea, salivary glands, or central nervous system and the presence of erythema nodosum favor sarcoid. Demonstration of beryllium in urine confirms exposure but does not correlate with disease. The disease is thought to be due to a cell-mediated immune response directed at beryllium-protein complexes. Lymphocyte transformation in response to beryllium has been demonstrated in vitro from peripheral blood lymphocytes and lung lymphocytes obtained by bronchoalveolar lavage from some patients with chronic beryllium disease. Transformation of blood lymphocytes is relatively insensitive, however, and can also be seen in exposed workers with no evidence of disease. The clinical course of chronic beryllium disease is quite variable. Most patients remain stable if exposure ceases, but the disease can remit or progress in some individuals. Treatment with corticosteroids has been recommended but has not been systematically studied.

Kriebel D, Brain JD, Sprince NL, et al.: The pulmonary toxicity of beryllium. Am Rev Respir Dis 137:464, 1988.
Newman LS, Kreiss K, King TE Jr, et al.: Pathologic and immunologic alterations in early stages of beryllium disease. Am Rev Respir Dis 139:1479, 1988.

Diseases Caused by Other Inorganic Dusts

Silicates other than asbestos can also cause pneumoconiosis. Kaolin, mica, and vermiculite, for example, cause radiographic abnormalities and pathologic lesions similar to those caused by coal dust. Talc inhalation causes pulmonary fibrosis with features of both asbestosis and silicosis, as well as foreign body granulomas. Pleural plaques have also been noted in workers exposed to talc, but they may be due to contamination of talc with asbestos. A severe granulomatous lung disease, sometimes associated with pulmonary hypertension, can occur in intravenous drug addicts from intravenous injection of talc. Synthetic vitreous fibers, such as fiberglass and glass wool, are physically similar to asbestos, but evidence to date suggests that they are considerably less toxic. Because of the long latency of fiber-induced disorders, continued close surveillance of the effects of use of these fibers is essential. As new technologies evolve, it is likely that new reactions to inorganic dusts will be recognized. For example, exposure to the dust of a variety of metals (including tungsten carbide, cobalt, titanium, and tantalum) may cause acute and/or chronic injury to the airways and lung parenchyma.

Hypersensitivity Pneumonitis

Hypersensitivity pneumonitis is a parenchymal lung disorder that usually results from occupational exposure to organic dusts. The disease is characterized clinically by recurrent episodes of cough, dyspnea, and signs of systemic illness (fever, leukocytosis, and myalgias). After long-term exposure to the responsible dust, affected workers can develop pulmonary fibrosis often with noncaseating granulomas in lung tissue. This disorder is discussed in detail in Ch. 59.

Occupational Lung Cancer

As the site of entry of most airborne carcinogens, the lung is the organ most often affected by occupational carcinogenesis. Definitive identification of an occupational agent as a lung carcinogen is made difficult by the long latency period for most carcinogens (20 to 40 years), the high background incidence of lung cancer, and the potent confounding effect of cigarette smoke. Thus, of the more than 100 agents suspected of causing respiratory cancer in animals, only a few have been shown to cause cancer in humans, e.g., arsenic, asbestos, cadmium, chloromethyl ether, chromates, coal tars, coke-oven emissions, mustard gas, nickel, and uranium and other sources of ionizing radiation. Chloromethyl ether appears to be especially likely to cause oat cell carcinoma, but most occupational carcinogens increase the risk for lung cancer of all common cell types. Prevention of occupational lung cancer requires minimizing exposure to suspected carcinogens *before* they are definitively shown to cause cancer in exposed workers.

528 Physical, Chemical, and Aspiration Injuries of the Lung

Claude A. Piantadosi

PHYSICAL AND CHEMICAL INJURIES OF THE LUNG

The lung has a large and delicate surface area that is protected from toxic substances in the environment by extensive defense mechanisms. Under normal conditions, inspired gas is fully humidified and warmed to body temperature, and all large particulate substances are cleared by the upper airways. These normal defenses are not adequate to handle exposure to many physical and chemical substances that cause lung injury. This chapter discusses lung disorders initiated by inhalation or aspiration of injurious chemicals or by exposure to potentially harmful physical environments.

Thermal Injuries and Smoke Inhalation

Approximately 130,000 patients per year require hospitalization in the United States for thermal injuries. After major burns, about one third of patients have pulmonary complications; these complications account for the majority of burn-related deaths. Thermal injury to the lung is associated with three groups of complications: (1) *immediate reaction*—direct thermal injury to upper airways, leading to upper airway obstruction, carbon monoxide poisoning, and smoke inhalation (potent bronchoconstrictors and edematogenic substances); (2) *adult respiratory distress syndrome* (ARDS) developing 24 to 48 hours after the thermal injury; and (3) *late-onset pulmonary complications*, which include pneumonia, atelectasis, thromboembolism, and chest wall restriction caused by circumferential thoracic burns.

The constituents of smoke are by-products of pyrolysis and incomplete combustion. Many of these products are potent mucosal irritants and bronchoconstrictors and contribute to both upper and lower lung lesions. Certain constituents of smoke have been identified consistently as contributors to respiratory injury. These are listed in Table 528–1. Smoke inhalation rarely causes thermal injury to the lung parenchyma; the large capacity of the upper airways to humidify and modify the temperatures of inhaled air protects the alveolar tissue from heat. Exceptions are steam burns and explosions in an enclosed space.

CLINICAL MANIFESTATIONS. The initial signs and symptoms of smoke inhalation are tachypnea, cough, dyspnea, wheezing, cyanosis, hoarseness, and stridor (an ominous sign). Facial burns may provide a clue to smoke inhalation and thermal injury to the upper airway. During the 12 to 48 hours immediately after the injury, the patient can manifest increasing hypoxemia, and lung compliance may decrease owing to noncardiogenic pulmonary edema. Roentgenograms of the chest may reveal a pattern of diffuse, patchy infiltrates. A major complication is infection, often caused by *Pseudomonas aeruginosa* or *Staphylococcus aureus*. The lung defenses against infection are compromised by thermal and chemical injury to the airway epithelium as well as by the presence of an endotracheal or tracheostomy tube. The pathway for infection is either by inhalation of airborne organisms or by hematogenous spread from cutaneous burns.

The ARDS may develop 24 to 48 hours after the initial injury. The causes of ARDS are controversial in burn patients, but possibilities include a chemical pneumonitis from constituents in smoke, a circulating burn toxin, disseminated intravascular coagulation, microembolism, and neurogenic pulmonary edema. The extent of surface thermal injury does not correlate with the degree of respiratory distress that occurs subsequently.

TREATMENT. The most immediate life-threatening complications in the patient presenting with major burns or with a history of smoke inhalation are upper airway obstruction and carbon monoxide intoxication. The patient should be closely observed for evidence of these complications. Laryngeal and tracheobronchial inflammation may be detected by fiberoptic bronchoscopy. Arterial blood gases should be measured and prompt intubation or tracheostomy performed if there is evidence of significant airway obstruction. Corticosteroids may be helpful to treat edema of the upper airways but must be used with caution, since infection is a major concern for managing both skin and pulmonary injury. Prophylactic antibiotics are of no value in preventing pneumonia and may predispose to infection with resistant organisms. Careful pulmonary toilet, humidification, and sterile suctioning should be used to reduce the risk of pneumonia. Serial bronchoscopy may be necessary to remove mucous plugs and thereby prevent segmental atelectasis and postobstructive infection.

Late-onset pulmonary burn complications—atelectasis, thromboembolism, and pneumonia—are discussed in Ch. 59, 65, and 292 to 295, respectively.

Haponik EF, Summer WR: Respiratory complications in burned patients: Pathogenesis and spectrum of inhalation injury. J Crit Care 2:49, 1987.
Haponik EF, Summer WR: Respiratory complications in burned patients: Diagnosis and management of inhalation injury. J Crit Care 2:121, 1987.

Carbon Monoxide Poisoning

Smoke inhalation is invariably accompanied by the uptake of carbon monoxide (CO) by the body. In some fires, CO exposure is complicated by cyanide poisoning from the combustion of plastic compounds. Carbon monoxide poisoning also is encountered frequently after exposure to automobile exhaust, and in the winter when victims are exposed to fumes from faulty furnaces. As a result, CO is the leading cause of accidental poisoning in the United States.

Carbon monoxide toxicity is a consequence of tissue hypoxia created by the displacement of oxygen from hemoglobin. Carbon monoxide competes with oxygen for binding at the iron-porphyrin centers of hemoglobin. These centers bind CO reversibly, but with an affinity more than 200 times greater than that for oxygen. The oxygen affinity of centers not occupied by CO is also increased in the presence of carboxyhemoglobin (HbCO). This HbCO-related increase in oxygen affinity shifts the oxyhemoglobin dissociation curve to the left and impairs the release of oxygen to the tissues. These two effects of CO on hemoglobin decrease the partial pressure of oxygen in the tissues. Tissue hypoxia has serious functional consequences for organ systems that require a continuous supply of oxygen, such as the brain and the heart. In addition, when tissue Po_2 is low, CO may bind more readily to intracellular hemoproteins such as myoglobin and cytochrome *c* oxidase, potentially inhibiting their functions.

CLINICAL MANIFESTATIONS. The clinical features of acute CO poisoning are diverse but most often related to the central nervous system. In normal, nonsmoking individuals, symptoms may appear when HbCO levels reach 10 per cent. Patients with chronic obstructive pulmonary disease (COPD) and coronary artery disease are more sensitive to the effects of HbCO. Smokers often maintain HbCO levels of 3 to 10 per cent, and they may tolerate slightly higher levels without symptoms. Common symptoms of CO poisoning include headache, nausea, vomiting, confusion, and visual disturbances. More severe CO poisoning can produce seizures, transient unconsciousness, coma, and death. Metabolic acidosis, pulmonary edema, and rhabdomyolysis may also accompany serious CO poisoning. The "classic" clinical findings of cherry red lips and nail beds are rare. The differential diagnosis includes drug overdoses, other poisonings (e.g. cyanide), and cerebrovascular accidents. The clinical diagnosis is confirmed by an elevated blood HbCO level measured by CO-oximetry. The severity of the clinical illness, however, may not correlate well with the HbCO level but may relate instead to the duration and extent of the exposure.

TABLE 528–1. TOXIC BY-PRODUCTS OF SMOKE IMPLICATED IN RESPIRATORY INJURY

Source	By-products
Cotton, paper, wood	Acrolein, CO, acetaldehyde
Petroleum products	Acrolein, CO, benzene
Polyvinyl chloride (PVC)	Hydrocyanic acid, CO, chlorine, phosgene
Nylon, silk, wool	Hydrocyanic acid, ammonia
Nitrocellulose	Oxides of nitrogen
Sulfur compounds	Sulfur dioxide

TREATMENT AND OUTCOME. Symptoms of mild CO poisoning generally subside within minutes to a few hours after removing the patient from the noxious environment. Patients with more severe forms of CO intoxication benefit from high inspired concentrations of oxygen to hasten the removal of CO from hemoglobin. In obtunded or comatose patients, 100 per cent oxygen should be administered via an endotracheal tube until the HbCO level is less than 5 per cent. Pure oxygen reduces the halftime for HbCO elimination from the body from approximately 240 minutes to 60 minutes. Patients with loss of consciousness or other neurologic impairment, cardiac symptoms or signs, or HbCO levels above 25 per cent should receive hyperbaric oxygen if it is readily available. Hyperbaric oxygen at 2.5 atmospheres absolute (ATA) reduces the HbCO halftime to approximately 30 minutes. Oxygen dissolved in plasma under hyperbaric pressure also bypasses the impairment of oxygen transport to tissues imposed by HbCO. As a result, potentially serious neurologic sequelae may be averted if the therapy can be instituted promptly. Adjunctive therapy, such as corticosteroids, hyperventilation, mannitol, and hypothermia, has been recommended for treatment of serious cases of CO intoxication, but benefit from these modalities is unproved.

Neurologic recovery in patients with mild to moderate CO poisoning is good. The prognosis after severe CO intoxication is variable and correlates with the extent and duration of the insult. Short-term memory impairment, depression, and syndromes related to lesions of the basal ganglia are well described. A syndrome of delayed neurologic deterioration occurs in approximately 3 per cent of victims of serious CO intoxication. Risk factors for the delayed syndrome include age over 40, prolonged exposure, and abnormalities of the brain on computed tomography (CT). Hyperbaric oxygen therapy has been reported to decrease the incidence of the delayed syndrome.

Piantadosi CA: Carbon monoxide intoxication. *In* Vincent JL (ed.): Update in Intensive Care and Emergency Medicine. Vol. 10. New York, Springer-Verlag, 1990, pp 460–471.

Other Toxic Inhaled Gases

A large number of gases and chemicals, to which exposures most frequently occur in an industrial setting, can cause acute and sometimes chronic injury to the respiratory system. A few agents cause an "asthma-like" reaction with cough, chest pain, and wheezing. Toluene di-isocyanate and other isocyanates (liberated as a gas during the manufacture of polyurethane foams), aluminum soldering flux, and platinum salts are typical examples. Reaginic and precipitating antibodies against platinum salts and soldering flux have been found in symptomatic individuals, suggesting an immunologic basis for the reaction. An allergic basis has not been demonstrated for the reaction to toluene di-isocyanate. The symptoms usually subside after removal from exposure; however, chronic lung injury may occur if the exposure is prolonged.

A number of highly irritating gases cause an *acute chemical pneumonitis.* Such gases include chlorine (used in the chemical and plastic industries and to disinfect water), ammonia (used in refrigeration), sulfur dioxide (used in paper manufacture and smelting of sulfide-containing ores), ozone (generated in welding and in photochemical smog), nitrogen dioxide (released from decomposed corn silage), and phosgene (used in production of aniline dyes).

An important injury of this type is *silo-filler's disease* (nitrogen dioxide). During the initial exposure, there may be no symptoms, there may be tracheobronchitis with cough and shortness of breath, or there may be the immediate onset of acute pulmonary edema. Signs of ocular and oropharyngeal mucous membrane irritation may be present. The symptoms can rapidly progress, but commonly the initial symptoms resolve and are followed by a period of minimal symptoms (cough) lasting up to 48 hours. Fever, myalgias, dyspnea, and progressive hypoxemia then occur, and the radiographic picture is that of pulmonary edema. These severe symptoms can resolve, only to recur 2 to 5 weeks later and lead to progressive pulmonary insufficiency with a picture of bronchiolitis obliterans. Treatment with corticosteroids (prednisone, 1 mg per kilogram per day) can dramatically improve the

acute illness. Bronchodilators, mechanical ventilation, and supplemental oxygen may be necessary. Since improvement after the initial exposure may be temporary, observation for a period of 48 hours is advisable.

The clinical response caused by each irritant gas varies but appears to be closely related to the degree of acute irritation it causes and to its water solubility. The less irritating gases, such as ozone and the oxides of nitrogen, phosgene, mercury, and nickel carbonyl, can be inhaled for prolonged periods and thereby cause injury throughout the respiratory system. Highly irritating and soluble gases, such as ammonia and hydrochloric acid, are less likely to be inhaled deeply and tend to result in immediate injury to the upper airways and have potential for obstruction secondary to mucosal edema. Less soluble substances, such as chlorine, cadmium, zinc chloride, osmium tetroxide, and vanadium, can cause injury to the entire tracheobronchial tree and generally do not produce upper airway obstruction as the initial presentation. Bronchiolitis and pulmonary edema are common, ultimately leading to bronchiolitis obliterans. Long-term consequences vary with the gas. Cadmium, for example, can cause diffuse emphysema and severe airway obstruction but only minimal fibrosis.

Different mechanisms are involved in the injury caused by irritant gases. Most of them cause injury by acting as a strong acid, a strong base, or an oxidant. Gases of chemicals that are strong acids or bases in water solution, such as hydrogen chloride, sulfuric acid, sulfur dioxide, and ammonia, tend to react more in the upper airways, where they change tissue pH and thereby cause cell damage.

Evans MJ: Oxidant gases. Environ Health Perspect 55:85, 1984. *A review of the effects of ozone, nitrogen dioxide, and oxygen on lung structures and the factors that can modulate the degree of damage.*

Pulmonary Oxygen Toxicity

Oxygen is toxic to the lungs when used in high concentrations for prolonged periods. This toxicity occurs clinically in patients in intensive care units who are on mechanical ventilators. The toxic effects of hyperoxia are believed to result from excessive generation of superoxide, an unstable free radical produced by the single electron reduction of oxygen. Superoxide is produced as a normal by-product of oxidative metabolism and scavenged by a protective enzyme, superoxide dismutase, that catalyzes its dismutation to hydrogen peroxide. If not scavenged by superoxide dismutase, this free radical can react with hydrogen peroxide to form hydroxyl radical (OH•), and free radical chain reactions can be initiated, resulting in the destruction of cell lipids and proteins (Fig. 528–1).

In the adult, the major site of oxygen injury is the pulmonary capillary endothelium. Pathologically, the lungs are atelectatic, congested, and edematous and have hyaline membranes. The most serious injury appears to be destruction of the capillary bed with resultant interstitial and alveolar edema, hypoxemia, and sometimes death. Alveolar epithelium is also injured, causing hyperplasia of type II cells. An acute tracheobronchitis also occurs, and histologic changes have been found in the ciliated epithelium and Clara cells in the small airways.

CLINICAL MANIFESTATIONS. Oxygen toxicity usually occurs in acutely ill patients who are receiving oxygen in high concentrations and mechanical ventilation for lung injuries that obscure the onset of pulmonary toxicity. Lung compliance progressively falls; the alveolar-arterial oxygen gradient gradually widens, and increasing concentrations of oxygen are needed to maintain adequate oxygenation of arterial blood. This cycle progresses to pulmonary edema, respiratory failure, and death.

The earliest symptoms of oxygen toxicity are those of acute tracheobronchitis. A dry, hacking cough and substernal pain may occur after 6 to 12 hours of breathing pure oxygen. Vital capacity decreases, and respiratory rate increases. The flow of tracheal mucus decreases after short exposures to excess oxygen, probably reflecting functional injury of airway epithelium. These patients are therefore more susceptible to mucus impaction and to infection caused by failure to clear inhaled pathogens adequately.

TREATMENT AND OUTCOME. The only proven therapy is prevention of the insult by judicious use of high oxygen concentrations. The physician often faces a dilemma in which increasing concentrations of oxygen are essential for immediate survival but eventually contribute to the demise of the patient. Alternative methods to enhance tissue oxygen delivery without using high inspired partial pressures of oxygen should be used whenever possible. These include positive end-expiratory pressure (PEEP), transfusion of packed red cells to raise the hematocrit to nearly normal levels, maintenance of cardiac output, and measures to decrease the tissue oxygen demand by reducing fever or agitation.

The safe maximal concentration of oxygen is not known. Many authors recommend 40 to 50 per cent oxygen as a safe limit because little injury has been demonstrated in normal animals or human volunteers breathing such concentrations for prolonged periods. The diseased lung, however, may be more susceptible to oxygen injury. A rational therapy is to use only enough oxygen to provide adequate arterial blood saturation, e.g., an Sa_{O_2} of 90 per cent. Corticosteroids have no benefit and may actually enhance the lung injury caused by hyperoxia. If the patient survives oxygen toxicity, some residual damage to the lung parenchyma may remain, with septal fibrosis replacing areas where the pulmonary capillary bed was destroyed by the hyperoxia.

Crapo JD: Morphologic changes in pulmonary oxygen toxicity. Annu Rev Physiol 48:721, 1986. *A detailed review of the time course and patterns of injury to the lung during exposure to hyperoxia.*

Jamieson D, Chance B, Cadenas E, et al.: The relationship of free radical production to hyperoxia. Annu Rev Physiol 48:703, 1986. *A review of the pathogenesis of hyperoxia-mediated cell injury.*

Radiation Lung Injury (See also Ch. 530)

The predominant factors determining the incidence of radiation pneumonitis are the total radiation dose, the number of fractions, and the duration of time over which the total dose is given. Some chemotherapeutic drugs may potentiate the damage from radiation. A total lung dose of less than 2000 rads generally is not associated with severe radiation pneumonitis, whereas a total dose in excess of 4000 rads, even if distributed over as many as 30 fractions, has virtually a 100 per cent risk of radiation pneumonitis.

The reaction of the lung to radiation injury can be divided into three phases. (1) An *acute phase*, occurring 1 to 2 months after radiation exposure, is characterized by vascular damage, congestion, edema, and mononuclear cell infiltration. Alveolar type II cells and alveolar macrophages are increased in number. (2) A *subacute phase* occurs 2 to 9 months later. The alveolar walls become infiltrated with mononuclear inflammatory cells and fibroblasts. (3) The *chronic* or *fibrotic phase* generally occurs more than 9 months after irradiation. Alveolar fibrosis and capillary sclerosis are its predominant histologic features.

CLINICAL MANIFESTATIONS. Signs of bronchial irritation, e.g., cough, may appear immediately after radiation therapy, followed shortly thereafter by esophagitis. Some patients may have no symptoms for 6 to 12 weeks. If large volumes of lung have been irradiated, or if high radiation doses have been given over short periods, the patient can develop dyspnea, tachypnea, and fever. These symptoms can be severe and will either progress to severe dyspnea and death or gradually subside, leaving varying degrees of respiratory impairment resulting from chronic lung fibrosis. Permanent fibrosis takes 6 to 24 months to evolve and then usually remains stable after 2 years if no further exposure occurs. Auscultation of the chest is usually normal, although rales, signs of consolidation, and pleural rubs may be found. Clubbing does not develop after radiation injury. Laboratory findings include a mild leukocytosis and an increased erythrocyte sedimentation rate. If the irradiated area is extensive, arterial hypoxemia may develop. Radiographic changes generally appear 1 to 3 months after treatment. The affected areas are generally demarcated by a "straight edge" defining the margins of the radiation portal and have a "ground-glass appearance"—a hazy increase in density with indistinct pulmonary markings. In the later phases of the radiation injury, fibrosis and contraction of the irradiated region are the predominant radiographic findings. Pulmonary function tests do not change until clinical symptoms appear, and then a restrictive ventilatory defect may be noted. Capillary sclerosis is associated with a decrease in blood flow to the affected region and a decrease in CO transfer capacity. Severe radiation injury is associated with a decrease in lung compliance and hypoxemia.

The diagnosis of acute radiation pneumonitis may be difficult to establish because of coincidental disease. The clinical picture is often complicated by the immunocompromised state of many of the patients, resulting in increased risk of bacterial or opportunistic pneumonias, e.g., that caused by *Pneumocystis carinii*, or by the signs and symptoms of the original neoplasm. Radiation pneumonitis has not been documented adequately in parts of the lung outside the radiation portal; however, a few patients have developed suspicious radiographic changes outside the field. Complications of radiation pneumonitis include small pleural effusions and, occasionally, spontaneous pneumothorax.

TREATMENT AND OUTCOME. The patient who develops radiation pneumonitis requires supportive care, including cough suppression, antipyretics, and supplemental oxygen for hypoxemia. Corticosteroids (prednisone, 1 mg per kilogram of body weight) have been advocated for treatment of severe cases of radiation pneumonitis, although there have been no controlled

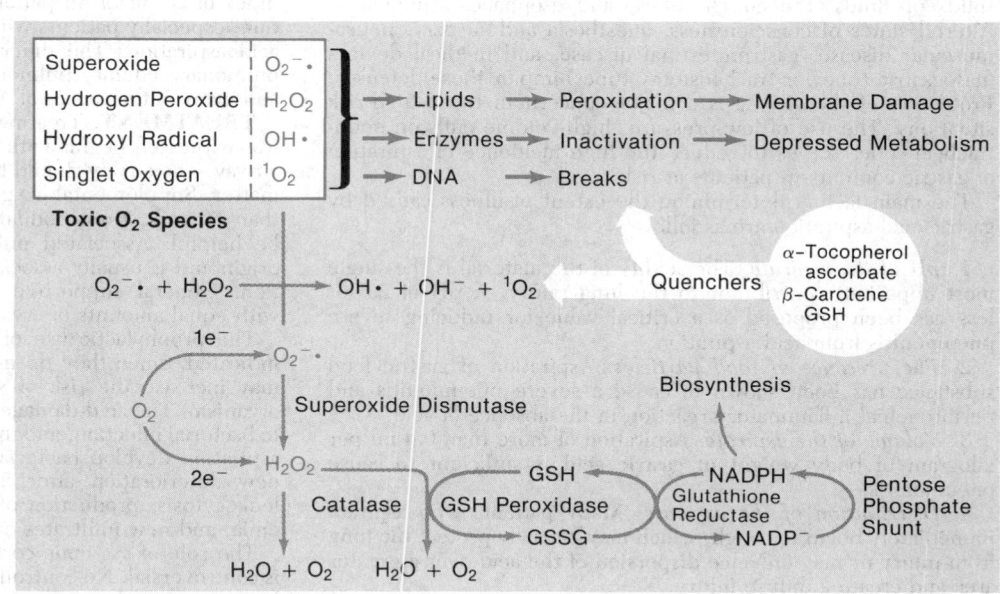

FIGURE 528–1. Toxic oxygen species and antioxidant defense systems. The incomplete reduction of oxygen produces superoxide and/or hydrogen peroxide. These species can react together in the presence of metal salts to form the hydroxyl radical and singlet oxygen. Free radical chain reactions can be initiated in lipid membranes, with enzymes and DNA also attacked by these reactive O_2 species. Quenchers interact with the oxygen species or with oxidized tissue components to block further tissue oxidation and to terminate free radical chain reactions. The antioxidant defense systems—superoxide dismutase, catalase, and glutathione peroxidase—function to detoxify superoxide and hydrogen peroxide, thus preventing the formation of other toxic O_2 species and the subsequent reactions with tissue. Glucose-6-phosphate dehydrogenase is the rate-limiting enzyme in the pentose phosphate shunt and thereby controls the availability of NADPH. This cofactor is essential both for the reduction of glutathione and for the biosynthetic pathways critical for repair processes. Net tissue injury represents the balance between the rate of production of partially reduced oxygen species, the rate at which these species are scavenged, and the rate of repair of any injury that occurs.

clinical trials. There is no evidence to support use of prophylactic corticosteroids, but their administration at the very onset of pneumonitis appears to be more effective than later therapy. On occasion, the response may be dramatic, with complete resolution of symptoms within 24 hours. Corticosteroids should be tapered carefully after achieving maximal clinical benefit. Pneumonitis has been reported occasionally after steroid withdrawal. No other effective therapeutic strategies are known. Antibiotic therapy should be reserved for patients in whom the clinical findings suggest infection. Since the lesion involves occlusion and thrombosis of many small blood vessels, anticoagulation has been tried, but there is no evidence of its effectiveness.

Gross NJ: The pathogenesis of radiation-induced lung damage. Lung 139:115, 1981. *A review of the biochemistry and cell biology of irradiated lung and how these factors relate to the clinical syndrome.*

Rosiello RA, Merrill WW: Radiation-induced lung injury. Clin Chest Med 11:65, 1990. *A summary of the clinical features of radiation-induced lung disease; with 51 references.*

ASPIRATION-RELATED INJURIES
Chemical Aspiration Pneumonitis

Injury to the respiratory system by aspiration can be categorized by the nature of the aspirate as (1) *infectious material,* (2) *chemical* or *inflammatory substances,* and (3) *inert material.* Contamination of the lungs by aspiration of oropharyngeal bacterial flora is discussed in Ch. 62. Aspiration of gastric acid is the most common example of chemical aspiration in adults; hydrocarbon aspiration occurs predominantly in children but is encountered occasionally in adults. Both of these injuries can cause fulminant illness. By contrast, lipids (mineral oil, vegetable and animal fats) most often provoke a chronic inflammatory reaction. Aspiration of inert material such as water causes injury (e.g., drowning), predominantly by asphyxia. Food particles can cause a fibrotic, granulomatous lesion or, if large enough to occlude the larynx or trachea, sudden death by asphyxiation ("café coronary").

GASTRIC ACID ASPIRATION

Aspiration pneumonitis refers to pulmonary injury caused by gastric acid. This condition is in contrast to "aspiration pneumonia," an infectious process caused by the contamination of the tracheobronchial tree by oropharyngeal flora. Aspiration of gastric acid can occur during vomiting or regurgitation, and in the latter instance the event may go unnoted—i.e., "silent aspiration." The normal protective mechanisms of the upper airway include epiglottic closure during deglutition, glottic closure on contact with solids or fluids, the cough reflex, and esophageal sphincters. Altered states of consciousness, anesthesia and surgery, neuromuscular disease, gastrointestinal disease, and medical devices (nasogastric tubes or tracheostomy tubes) impair these defenses. Protection of the airway is a major concern in these high-risk situations. The use of low-pressure, high-volume cuffs on endotracheal tubes serves to reduce the high incidence of aspiration of gastric contents in patients at risk.

The main factors determining the extent of illness caused by gastric acid aspiration are as follows:

1. *pH of the aspirate.* The acidity of the material is the single most important contributor to the lung injury. A pH of 2.5 or less has been proposed as a critical value for inducing severe pneumonitis from acid aspiration.

2. *The presence of food particles.* Aspiration of gastric food substance has been shown to cause a severe pneumonitis and peribronchial inflammatory reaction in the absence of acid.

3. *Volume of the aspirate.* Aspiration of more than 0.4 ml per kilogram of body weight of gastric acid is sufficient to cause pneumonitis.

4. *Distribution of the aspirate.* Many patients who aspirate immediately begin to cough, which may partially protect the lung from injury or may enhance dispersion of the acid over a greater area and create a diffuse injury.

After intratracheal instillation, acid is rapidly distributed in the lungs and can reach the pleura in 12 to 18 seconds. It is rapidly neutralized by bronchial secretions; in less than 30 minutes, the pH at the bronchial surface will have returned to normal. Acid causes chemical burns of the bronchi, bronchioles, and alveolar walls, with subsequent exudation of fluid into the lungs. Plasma volume may decrease by as much as 35 per cent in severe injury without fluid replacement, and cardiac output and systemic arterial blood pressure may fall. Pulmonary artery wedge pressure is normal or low, indicating a nonhydrostatic cause of the pulmonary edema. The characteristics of phospholipids in the alveolar surface lining layer (surfactant) are altered, causing increased surface forces and promoting early airway and alveolar closure. Lung compliance decreases secondary to the increase in interstitial fluids and the alteration of surface forces. These disturbances of airways, alveoli, and vascular elements cause profound imbalance of the normal ventilation-perfusion relationships. Increased intrapulmonary shunting is also common. As a result, hypoxemia is invariably present and usually severe.

CLINICAL MANIFESTATIONS. Some patients aspirate a large volume of gastric acid and almost immediately become apneic and hypotensive and die. More often, the patient survives the initial crisis but later develops a fulminant illness marked by dyspnea, cough, and frothy sputum. Alternatively, aspiration may be secondary to regurgitation and not accompanied by immediate coughing and agitation. After such silent aspiration, the patient may develop acute respiratory failure without an obvious reason for a precipitous deterioration in gas exchange. Within 1 to 5 hours after aspiration of gastric acid, tachypnea, rales, and rhonchi occur, and wheezing, cyanosis, cough, and hypotension may be present. Fever in the first 36 hours occurs in about 50 per cent of patients.

Laboratory tests are nonspecific. A moderate leukocytosis with left shift develops early. Arterial blood gases, the best variable to follow, show hypoxemia, and the arterial oxygen tension does not reach predicted levels after the patient has been breathing 100 per cent oxygen for several minutes, indicating increased intrapulmonary shunting of blood. The arterial PCO_2 may be slightly elevated, normal, or mildly reduced, and the pH will vary reciprocally. Abnormalities on chest roentgenograms are extremely variable, and no characteristic pattern is present. Radiographic abnormalities do not correlate with clinical outcome, although about 50 per cent of patients have changes consistent with pneumonitis. The acid is sometimes distributed preferentially to dependent areas, but usually the radiographic abnormalities are diffuse, presumably from enhanced dispersion of the acid during coughing. Pleural effusions and cavitation of infiltrates are not seen in uncomplicated cases. Bronchoscopic findings are diagnostic if food particles or other gastric contents are seen in the trachea or bronchi.

The diagnosis of aspiration pneumonitis begins with a high index of suspicion in patients with abrupt respiratory deterioration, especially patients with conditions that predispose to gastric acid aspiration. The differential diagnosis includes cardiogenic pulmonary edema, pulmonary embolism, bacterial pneumonia, and many of the causes of ARDS, such as sepsis and hypotension.

TREATMENT. Treatment of the individual whose aspiration was witnessed begins with prompt establishment of an adequate airway. The airway should be suctioned to remove any particulate matter. Supplemental oxygen is given to maintain a Pa_{O_2} of more than 60 torr. Bronchodilators (intravenous aminophylline) may be helpful. Associated pulmonary edema is noncardiogenic in origin and is usually associated with intravascular volume depletion. General supportive measures include fluid replacement with equal amounts of crystalloid and colloid solutions.

The prophylactic use of antibiotics for acid aspiration is not indicated, since they do not reduce morbidity or mortality and may increase the risk of subsequent infection with a resistant organism. The acid-damaged respiratory tract is more susceptible to bacterial infection, and up to one half of patients with significant aspiration develop bacterial pneumonia. Such patients undergo new deterioration after 2 or 3 days, with increasing fever, leukocytosis, production of purulent sputum, worsening hypoxemia, and new infiltrates on the chest radiograph.

The role of systemic corticosteroids in aspiration pneumonitis is controversial. No controlled human trials have been conducted. Early anecdotal reports supported their use, but more recent retrospective and prospective but uncontrolled series totaling approximately 250 patients have failed to show any decrease in morbidity or mortality.

Positive-pressure ventilation is helpful, particularly when it is initiated early after a major episode of aspiration. Arterial oxygen tensions improve, and mortality rates probably decrease with its use. Positive end-expiratory pressure to improve oxygenation has been beneficial in other forms of ARDS and is commonly used in the management of gastric acid aspiration. Caution should be used in applying PEEP, since it can increase extravascular water content in the acid-injured lung.

Aspiration pneumonitis carries a high mortality rate despite treatment, and because it largely occurs in a defined population at increased risk, efforts should be made at prevention. Elevation of the head of the bed will retard regurgitation. In intubated patients, placement of a nasogastric tube should be considered to keep the stomach decompressed. Aspiration may occur even in the presence of a cuffed endotracheal tube. Elective general anesthesia should be given with the stomach empty, after at least a 12-hour fast. Preoperatively, the pH of gastric contents can be raised by a single dose of an H_2 receptor blocker or by a single 10-ml oral dose of antacid given 2 to 4 hours before surgery.

OUTCOME. Mortality from aspiration pneumonitis is high, reaching 28 to 62 per cent of cases. Factors associated with highest mortality are age greater than 50 years, the early development of shock or apnea, severe and prolonged hypoxemia, very low pH of gastric contents at the time of aspiration, and the development of secondary bacterial pneumonia. Most patients survive the early moments but deteriorate over 12 to 24 hours. Some then show steady improvement, with radiographic resolution within a week. Others have a second episode of deterioration, an event that should suggest a new problem, such as bacterial infection, pulmonary embolism, heart failure, or another aspiration. Still others pursue a relentlessly worsening course to death. Few data exist regarding long-term clinical follow-up, but pulmonary fibrosis of varying degrees may occur in some of the survivors.

Bynum LJ, Pierce AK: Pulmonary aspiration of gastric contents. Am Rev Respir Dis 114:1129, 1976. *A retrospective analysis of the clinical features and outcome in 50 patients observed to aspirate gastric contents.*
Campbell JC, O'Donohue WJ Jr: Aspiration of gastric contents. Curr Pulmonol 8:163, 1987.

HYDROCARBON PNEUMONITIS

Hydrocarbon pneumonitis results from the direct toxic effects of volatile hydrocarbons on the respiratory epithelium and vasculature. It occurs in individuals who, having ingested the hydrocarbons, aspirate them into the respiratory tract. The problem occurs most often in children, particularly those below the age of 5 years. It is an uncommon problem in adults, occurring most often in industrial accidents, in patients attempting suicide, in siphoning of gasoline, and in uninformed alcoholics seeking an ethanol substitute.

Different hydrocarbons cause respiratory injury of varying extent, depending on the viscosity and volume of the aspirate. The lower the viscosity or the larger the volume, the worse the lesion. As lipid solvents, these compounds are directly toxic to respiratory tissues. The lungs of children dying of hydrocarbon pneumonitis demonstrate hemorrhage, pulmonary edema, atelectasis, hyaline membrane formation, and necrosis of airway epithelium and alveolar septa. These compounds also have systemic toxicity, and in fatal cases, degenerative changes have been seen in the liver and kidneys.

CLINICAL MANIFESTATIONS. Aspiration usually occurs at the time of hydrocarbon ingestion, although a history of vomiting after hydrocarbon ingestion is obtained in fewer than half the patients. Dyspnea, tachypnea, tachycardia, and high fever quickly ensue. Sputum may be bloody. Lethargy is common, but more severe disturbances of consciousness also occur, such as confusion, coma, and seizures. Auscultation is frequently normal, but rales and rhonchi may be present.

Laboratory tests give nonspecific results. A moderate leukocytosis with left shift is common. Arterial hypoxemia of various degrees develops owing to shunting and to ventilation-perfusion mismatching. The chest radiograph is particularly helpful, as infiltrates may occur within 20 to 30 minutes after aspiration of some types of hydrocarbons. The multiple, fluffy, ill-defined infiltrates favor dependent areas of the lungs. Some patients present a picture of bilateral perihilar infiltrates, a pulmonary

edema pattern. Pleural effusions, pneumothorax, and pneumomediastinum occur but are uncommon. Pneumatoceles can form later, especially in children.

The differential diagnosis is that of respiratory distress of abrupt onset, frequently in a patient with an impaired sensorium at the time of presentation. The adult patient is often an alcoholic. Gastric acid aspiration, cardiogenic pulmonary edema, pulmonary embolism, and acute bacterial pneumonia can all manifest similarly. The correct diagnosis requires the history of hydrocarbon ingestion or aspiration. The diagnosis is also suggested by the odor of the patient's breath and by extensive radiographic abnormalities in a patient with a clear chest on auscultation.

TREATMENT. Emesis to remove ingested hydrocarbons is contraindicated. Gastric lavage by nasogastric tube may cause vomiting and should be performed only after placement of a cuffed endotracheal tube in the patient who has recently ingested a large volume of hydrocarbons. Supplemental oxygen should be given to maintain a Pa_{O_2} greater than 60 torr. Mechanical ventilation and PEEP may be necessary. No data support the routine use of antibiotics. The use of systemic corticosteroids (prednisone, 1 mg per kilogram per day) during the acute illness is supported by anecdotal reports of improvement after their use in children and adults.

OUTCOME. Hydrocarbon pneumonitis in adults is rare, so that estimates of morbidity and mortality are not available. In children, death occurs in about 10 per cent of cases, but most children have a prompt clinical recovery. Bronchiectasis, recurrent bronchitis, and/or pulmonary fibrosis ensues in an unknown portion of cases. After recovery, children frequently have normal chest examinations and radiographs, although pulmonary function abnormalities suggestive of small airway (<2-mm diameter) disease have been found in asymptomatic patients as late as 8 to 14 years after hydrocarbon pneumonitis.

Klein BL, Simon JE: Hydrocarbon poisonings. Pediatr Clin North Am 33:411, 1986. *A review showing that most ingestions can be managed by careful observation and respiratory support.*

LIPOID PNEUMONIA

Lipoid pneumonia is a chronic inflammatory reaction of the lungs that results from the aspiration of vegetable, animal, or (most commonly) mineral oils. This exogenous material differs greatly from the excessive accumulation of endogenous lipids in the lungs occurring in fat embolism, cholesterol pneumonitis, pulmonary alveolar proteinosis, and the lipid storage diseases.

The most frequently implicated agent is mineral oil used as a laxative and to reduce dysphagia, either in clear liquid form or as petroleum jelly. Mineral oil is bland and, when introduced into the pharynx, can enter the bronchial tree without eliciting the cough reflex. It also mechanically impedes the ciliary action of the airway epithelium. The risk of mineral oil aspiration is increased in debilitated or senile patients, in those having neurologic disease that interferes with deglutition, and in patients with esophageal disease. Mineral oil taken as nose drops to relieve nasal dryness has caused lipoid pneumonia and in earlier years was a frequent cause of the illness. Inhalation of mineral oil mist by airplane and automobile mechanics has also been implicated as a cause of the problem.

Mineral oils, which are relatively inert, cannot be hydrolyzed in the body and provoke a chronic inflammatory reaction that may not become clinically overt until years later. The fat is emulsified in the alveolar spaces, where macrophages accumulate and phagocytize it. Some macrophages disintegrate, releasing their lysosomal enzymes and fat. The alveolar septa become thickened and edematous, containing lymphocytes and lipid-laden macrophages. Oil droplets are seen in the pulmonary lymphatics and hilar nodes. Later, fibrosis develops, and the normal lung architecture is effaced. It is usual in a single specimen to find both the early inflammatory and the later fibrotic picture, in keeping with repetitive aspirations over many months or years. If nodular, the lesion may grossly resemble tumor and is called a paraffinoma.

CLINICAL MANIFESTATIONS AND TREATMENT. Most patients are asymptomatic, coming to the physician's attention because of an abnormal chest radiograph. When patients are symptomatic, cough and exertional dyspnea are the most frequent complaints. Chest pain (sometimes pleuritic), hemoptysis, fever (usually low grade), chills, night sweats, and weight loss may occur. The physical examination may be completely normal, or fever, tachypnea, dullness on percussion of the chest, bronchial or bronchovesicular breath sounds, rales, and rhonchi may be found. Clubbing and cor pulmonale are rare.

In mild lipoid pneumonia, arterial blood gas values may be normal with the patient at rest but may show hypoxemia after exercise. In more severe disease, resting hypoxemia, hypocapnia, and mild respiratory alkalosis develop. Pulmonary function testing reveals a restrictive ventilatory defect; static compliance of the lungs is decreased. The only specific laboratory finding is the presence in sputum or bronchoalveolar lavage of macrophages with clusters of vacuoles 5 to 50 μm in diameter that stain deep orange with Sudan IV and extracellular droplets that stain similarly.

Radiographically, the earliest abnormalities are air space infiltrates, unilateral or bilateral, localized or diffuse, but most often in the dependent portions of the right lung. Air bronchograms may be seen. Hilar adenopathy and pleural reaction are rare. As fibrosis develops, volume loss occurs and linear and nodular infiltrates appear. A solid lesion that closely resembles bronchogenic carcinoma may develop, and lipoid pneumonia may carry an increased risk for bronchoalveolar cell carcinoma..

The differential diagnosis is extensive, particularly in the late phase, when multiple other causes of pulmonary fibrosis must be considered. The key to the correct diagnosis before biopsy is the history of chronic oral or intranasal use of an oil- or a lipid-based product, or an occupational exposure to oil mists. The presence of lipid-laden macrophages in the sputum confirms the diagnosis.

Once the diagnosis has been made and the aspiration stopped, the subsequent course is variable. Some patients have no change in symptoms. Others improve in some or all parameters, whereas a few patients deteriorate, with worsening pulmonary function and cor pulmonale. Since the only way the lung can dispose of mineral oil is by expectoration, the patient should be instructed in coughing exercises to be performed many times each day for months. Expectorants have not been shown to help. Systemic corticosteroids are recommended by some on the basis of improvement seen in a few uncontrolled reports. The rationale has been that the cellular reaction, rather than the oil itself, is the destructive factor. Because of the well-recognized side effects of systemic corticosteroids, their use for lipoid pneumonia should be limited to those patients who have significant symptoms, and then for as brief a period as possible to "buy time" while decreasing the lipid burden by expectoration.

Blondal T, Hartvig P, Bengtsson A, et al.: An unnecessary case of paraffin oil pneumonia. Acta Med Scand 213:227, 1983. *The problems in diagnosis of mineral oil pneumonia are illustrated.*

Near-Drowning

Drowning accounts for about 9000 deaths annually in the United States, mostly in children and young adults. It is one of the three leading causes of accidental death. In adults, alcohol consumption and shallow water blackout during breath-hold diving are common aggravating factors. Pathophysiologically, drowning can be of two types: (1) "wet" drowning—initial laryngospasm but early relaxation and subsequent aspiration of copious amounts of fluid; the majority of drownings are of this sort: (2) "dry" drowning—asphyxiation secondary to intense glottic spasm that persists beyond the point of apnea, so that when the muscles relax, little or no water is aspirated; this accounts for 10 to 20 per cent of drownings. The immediate cause of death in many victims of drowning is cardiac arrhythmia. Victims who survive the initial episode frequently develop ARDS a few hours to a few days after the event (secondary drowning).

The most important consequences of near-drowning are attributed to asphyxia. Asphyxia results in severe hypoxemia, hypercarbia, and metabolic acidosis. The metabolic consequences of drowning in fresh water or salt water appear to differ little except for drowning in water with very high mineral content (e.g., the Dead Sea). In both cases, hypoxemia is caused by the occlusion of airways with water and particulate debris, by changes in

surfactant activity, by direct injury to the alveolar septa, and by bronchospasm. Right-to-left shunting is markedly increased, and physiologic dead space is increased. Life-threatening electrolyte disturbances caused by water aspiration in humans are rare. Cardiac arrhythmias and central nervous system and renal insufficiency often occur after near-drowning. Brain anoxia is usually global anoxia, and if it is of sufficient duration and magnitude, it will lead to diffuse cerebral edema.

Autopsies of drowned persons demonstrate wet, heavy lungs with varying amounts of hemorrhage and edema and some disruption of alveolar walls. In about 70 per cent of victims, vomitus, sand, mud, and aquatic vegetation have been aspirated. Specimens from victims dying of secondary drowning show desquamation of alveolar epithelial cells, hemorrhage, hyaline membrane formation, acute inflammatory infiltrates, and foreign body reactions to particulate matter. Cerebral edema and diffuse neuronal injury are seen. Changes of acute tubular necrosis are found in the kidneys.

CLINICAL MANIFESTATIONS. The initial appearance of the patient can vary widely, from coma to agitated alertness. Cyanosis, coughing, and the production of frothy pink sputum are common. Tachypnea, tachycardia, and a low-grade fever in the first few hours are seen if the patient did not become hypothermic during submersion. Rales, rhonchi, and, less often, wheezes are heard. Neurologic signs vary and can fluctuate in any given patient but usually derive from diffuse cerebral dysfunction. Signs of associated trauma to the head and neck should be sought.

Laboratory studies reveal mild hypokalemia, hypernatremia, and hyperchloremia. A moderate leukocytosis may be present. Hematocrit and hemoglobin usually are normal at first measurement; in fresh water aspiration, the hematocrit may fall slightly in the first 24 hours owing to hemolysis. An isolated increase in serum free hemoglobin without a change in hematocrit is more common. Occasionally, the clinical picture of disseminated intravascular coagulation occurs in near-drowning. Arterial blood gas values, usually obtained after preliminary resuscitation, show severe hypoxemia and metabolic acidosis. The most common electrocardiographic changes are sinus tachycardia and nonspecific ST segment and T wave changes, which revert to normal within hours; however, other, more ominous abnormalities may occur—ventricular arrhythmias, complete heart block, or myocardial infarction. The chest radiograph may be normal initially despite severe respiratory disturbances. It often shows patchy infiltrates, and sometimes a classic pattern of pulmonary edema is seen.

TREATMENT. Treatment of the near-drowning victim begins with establishing an adequate airway and, if necessary, emergency cardiopulmonary resuscitation. Oxygen in high concentrations is necessary, since hypoxemia is present in essentially all victims. Even the patient who quickly becomes apparently normal should be hospitalized for 24 hours to watch for a subsequent clinical picture of ARDS. During transportation to a hospital, supplemental oxygen should be continued and precautions taken for potential head and neck injuries and other serious trauma.

In the hospital, therapy is dictated largely by the arterial blood gas values and the degree of respiratory failure. Continuous positive airway pressure or PEEP is particularly helpful for managing hypoxemia. Bronchospasm should be treated with nebulized β-agonists and intravenous theophylline. Patients with persistent localized atelectasis or localized wheezing should undergo bronchoscopy to exclude a foreign body as the etiology. Prophylactic antibiotics have not been shown to be beneficial, although many victims of near-drowning develop pneumonia, sometimes caused by unusual microorganisms. The use of corticosteroids for the pulmonary lesions of near-drowning remains controversial, and there have been no controlled prospective human studies to support their use. Animal models and retrospective studies in humans have failed to demonstrate any benefit.

The therapeutic approach to brain resuscitation after near-drowning is also controversial. If evidence of cerebral edema exists, intracranial pressure (ICP) monitoring may be useful to guide therapy. In the event of increased ICP, PEEP should be minimized, since it may increase ICP. Hyperventilation to maintain a Pa_{CO_2} of 25 to 30 torr decreases ICP at the expense of cerebral blood flow. Mannitol may decrease cerebral edema. It should be used to maintain the serum osmolarity near 300 mOsm per liter. Corticosteroids are used widely (e.g., dexamethasone, 10 mg given intravenously initially and then 4 to 6 mg given intravenously every 4 hours) but are not of proven benefit for the central nervous system injury. Seizures should be treated with anticonvulsants. Shivering or random, purposeless movements can increase ICP and should be aborted with muscle relaxants. If these maneuvers fail to lower ICP, then barbiturate coma can be undertaken for 24 to 48 hours.

OUTCOME. Outcome in near-drowning is best judged by the neurologic status, i.e., the presence or absence of coma. The shorter the interval between recovery from the water to first spontaneous gasp, the better the prognosis for recovery. The absence of spontaneous respiration after resuscitation from near-drowning is an ominous sign associated with severe neurologic sequelae. Permanent neurologic sequelae persist in about 20 per cent of comatose victims. Common sequelae include minimal brain dysfunction, spastic quadriplegia, extrapyramidal syndromes, optic and cerebral atrophy, and peripheral neuromuscular damage. Survival without neurologic damage is best in children who are hypothermic when recovered and may occur even after 40 minutes of submersion. Similar reports of survival after prolonged immersion in adults are very rare.

Hoff BH: Multisystem failure: A review with special references to drowning. Crit Care Med 7:310, 1979. *A complete review of the evaluation and care of the nearly drowned patient with attention to all critical organ systems.*
Redding JS: Drowning and near-drowning. Can the victim be saved? Postgrad Med 74:85, 1983. *A review of current therapy.*

DISORDERS CAUSED BY ALTERED BAROMETRIC PRESSURE

Significant alterations in environmental pressure are encountered by humans during ascent to altitude and during underwater diving. As altitude increases, barometric pressure falls from approximately 760 mm Hg at sea level to 380 mm Hg (0.5 ATA) at 18,000 feet. In seawater, the pressure of the water column increases by an amount equal to the barometric pressure for every 33 feet of depth. Hence at 33 feet of seawater, the absolute pressure is doubled (2 ATA). As a result, participants in activities such as mountaineering and scuba diving are often exposed to extremes of environmental pressure. Rapid pressure changes produce notable physiologic effects related to the behavior of atmospheric gases in the lungs and body tissues.

Diseases of High Altitudes

At high altitudes, the low barometric pressure causes physiologic effects due primarily to the decrease in the partial pressure of inspired oxygen. Physiologic changes begin to occur at 8000 to 10,000 feet. These changes become more apparent at altitudes above 10,000 feet owing to the shape of the oxygen-hemoglobin dissociation curve, which has a steep downslope below a P_{O_2} of approximately 60 mm Hg. A small drop in P_{O_2} below this level results in a relatively large decrease in arterial saturation. At 10,000 feet (3048 meters), the alveolar P_{O_2} is approximately 60 mm Hg, and some individuals manifest impairment of memory, judgment, and the ability to perform complex calculations. At 18,000 feet (5486 meters), the alveolar P_{O_2} is 40 mm Hg, and unacclimatized individuals may become unconscious after several hours.

Exposure to high altitude occurs most commonly in commercial aviation. In general, aircraft cabins are maintained at a pressure equal to or greater than that encountered at 8000 feet, so that supplemental oxygen is not required. Some patients with reduced cardiac reserve or with COPD may have difficulty tolerating even a small drop in arterial oxygen saturation and may require oxygen during flights. Aircraft regulations require that the flight crew receive supplemental oxygen when the cabin pressure drops below that at 10,000 feet and that passengers receive supplemental oxygen, should the cabin pressure drop below that at 15,000 feet.

ACUTE MOUNTAIN SICKNESS (AMS). Ascent to high altitude produces a wide spectrum of illness that depends on factors such as the absolute altitude, the rate of ascent, the length of stay, and individual susceptibility. Altitude illness may be classified into several syndromes, as shown in Table 528–2. The acute syndromes probably reflect a common pathophysiology initiated by a relatively abrupt lack of oxygen, although the

precise mechanisms remain uncertain. The ventilatory response to hypoxia and poor physical conditioning may play a role in susceptible individuals. The most common malady is AMS, and self-limited symptoms of headache, anorexia, malaise, and disturbed sleep may appear within a few hours of arriving at altitudes above 8000 feet. Mild AMS may affect half of unacclimatized visitors to 14,000 feet. At altitudes above 9500 feet, AMS may be severe and followed sometimes by the more serious conditions of high-altitude pulmonary edema (HAPE) and high-altitude cerebral edema (HACE) (Table 528–2), which frequently coexist. High-altitude retinal hemorrhages (HARH) are prevalent above 14,000 feet and probably share a similar pathophysiology with cerebral edema. Retinal hemorrhages are not significant unless they produce visual symptoms; the latter circumstance usually indicates involvement of the macula and mandates immediate descent. The more serious forms of AMS are discussed below.

HIGH-ALTITUDE PULMONARY EDEMA (HAPE). Acute noncardiogenic pulmonary edema is a potentially fatal complication of rapid ascent to altitudes above 9500 feet. Symptoms begin after 6 to 36 hours at high altitude and may follow an episode of AMS. Dyspnea at rest, tachypnea, and crackles are characteristic features of HAPE. Cyanosis, orthopnea, and hemoptysis commonly develop in more advanced cases.

At autopsy, the lungs are typically heavy, congested, and edematous and have hyaline membranes in small airways and alveoli. The cause of hyaline membrane formation is not known; this is not a characteristic finding in death caused by other forms of hypoxia. Hemodynamic studies have shown elevated pulmonary artery pressure with normal pulmonary venous pressure. The pulmonary edema may be due to an increase in pulmonary capillary pressure in small regions of the pulmonary capillary bed or to increased permeability in lung capillaries.

HIGH-ALTITUDE CEREBRAL EDEMA (HACE). HACE is relatively uncommon, occurring in perhaps 1.5 per cent of individuals affected by AMS. Hypoxemia produces cerebral vasodilation and increased cerebral blood flow, which may lead to mild brain edema and produce the symptoms of AMS. Cerebral edema may also be aggravated by hypoxic inhibition of the adenosine triphosphate (ATP)–dependent sodium pump. By factors yet to be defined, the brain edema may progress and become life threatening. Signs and symptoms of HACE include severe, progressive headache, ataxia, confusion, anxiety, hallucinations, and coma. Papilledema and meningeal signs occur. Examination of the cerebrospinal fluid reveals high opening pressures and perhaps hemorrhage or leukocytosis. Pathologically, the pattern of cerebral edema appears to be heterogeneous, and focal areas of capillary damage, red cell sludging, and platelet aggregation are seen.

TREATMENT OF ACUTE HIGH-ALTITUDE DISEASE. The simplest approach to the prevention and treatment of acute

TABLE 528–2. HIGH-ALTITUDE SYNDROMES

Syndrome	Clinical Description
Acute mountain sickness (AMS)	Common, self-limited; characterized by headache, anorexia, and malaise after ascent to altitudes >8000 ft; "normal puna"
High-altitude pulmonary edema (HAPE)	Noncardiac pulmonary edema recognized by dyspnea and tachypnea at rest, cough, and bibasilar crackles; usually at altitudes >9500 ft; "pulmonary puna"
High-altitude cerebral edema (HACE)	Uncommon, severe central nervous system dysfunction following AMS, characterized by severe headache, memory loss, ataxia, hallucinations, and confusion; may progress to coma and death; "nervous puna"
High-altitude retinal hemorrhages (HARH)	Dilated retinal vessels and peripheral flame-shaped or dot hemorrhages; occasionally cause visual symptoms
Chronic mountain sickness (Monge's disease)	Cor pulmonale with minimal lung disease in long-term residents of high altitude

altitude illness is to ascend to altitude gradually and to descend when troubling symptoms appear. Gradual ascent allows time for the body's adaptive responses to be recruited. If possible, the rate of ascent should be limited to approximately 1000 feet per day between altitudes of 7000 and 10,000 feet. Slower ascent (500 feet per day) is recommended for altitudes above 10,000 feet. If slow ascent is impractical, prophylactic treatment with acetazolamide is effective for prevention of AMS. Acetazolamide increases renal bicarbonate excretion and lessens the degree of respiratory alkalosis. The recommended regimen is 250 mg every 8 hours the day before, during, and for 1 day after the ascent. Some authors use one half to one third of this amount of acetazolamide to avoid dehydration and potassium depletion. Other diuretics have not been proved to be effective, and in practice, liberal water intake appears to hasten bicarbonate excretion and prevent hemoconcentration. Dexamethasone (4 mg every 6 hours) has also been shown to reduce the incidence and early symptoms of AMS; however, it is not recommended widely because of potential side effects.

The management of AMS consists of rest, mild analgesics, alcohol avoidance, and adequate hydration. The symptoms usually abate within a few days. The definitive treatment for HAPE, HACE, and severe HARH is oxygen administration and descent to lower altitude. High-altitude pulmonary edema has been reported to improve dramatically with a descent of only a few thousand feet. If the descent is delayed, the combination of oxygen and PEEP or continuous positive airway pressure, or placing the victim in a pressurized bag or chamber, is effective.

CHRONIC MOUNTAIN SICKNESS (MONGE'S DISEASE). Chronic mountain sickness occurs in people living at high altitudes, usually at over 14,000 feet, for many years. These "highlanders" have a blunted respiratory drive in response to hypoxia and have a lower minute ventilation at high altitudes than do those who normally reside at lower altitudes. Chronic mountain sickness is characterized by an exaggerated response to hypoxia resulting in cor pulmonale. Physiologic responses include erythrocytosis with hemoglobin levels as high as 25 grams per deciliter, a decreased minute ventilation with an elevated P_{CO_2}, hypoxemia, and impaired sensitivity of the respiratory center to hypoxia. Clinical manifestations are similar to those of polycythemia rubra vera and include cyanosis, dyspnea, cough, palpitations, headache, giddiness, muscular weakness, pain in the extremities, sensory and motor changes, and episodic stupor. The only therapy is to move the patient to a lower altitude. Subacute forms of this illness, in which cyanosis and alveolar hypoventilation are absent, also occur. A similar syndrome, brisket disease, has been described in cattle.

Houston C: Altitude illness and pulmonary edema. Curr Pulmonol 7:227, 1986. *An excellent review of high-altitude disorders; with 82 references.*

Decompression Sickness

Variations in the ambient pressure outside the body must be reflected across the lungs by proportional changes in the partial pressures of various gases dissolved in the tissues of the body. This condition is a consequence of the physical behavior of gases and their interactions with solutions. Since the quantity of gas dissolved in tissue varies directly with atmospheric pressure, changes in gas concentrations in the body are most pronounced during diving with compressed air, when, in order for the diver to expand his or her lungs, the density of the breathing gas must be increased in proportion to the column of water around him or her. Nitrogen uptake is most important in this respect because it comprises 80 per cent of the atmosphere and, unlike oxygen, it is inert (not metabolized). Inert gases like nitrogen must be eliminated from the body after a decrease in ambient pressure, e.g., return from a compressed air dive or rapid ascent to high altitude. The process of inert gas elimination is called decompression.

During decompression, inert gas dissolved in the tissues may come out of physical solution if the fall in environmental pressure is too rapid. Bubbles of inert gas form within the tissues and venous blood and produce various clinical manifestations known as decompression sickness (DCS), or caisson disease. Decompression sickness, however, is not entirely explained by gas bubbles

TABLE 528–3. CLASSIFICATION OF DECOMPRESSION SICKNESS (DCS)

Organ System	Signs and Symptoms
Mild DCS (Type 1)	
Skin	Pruritus, mottling, urticaria
Musculoskeletal	Pain (bends) usually in the joints, numbness, edema
Serious DCS (Type 2)	
Central nervous system	
Cerebral	Loss of consciousness, ataxia, vertigo, aphasia, hemiparesis
Audiovestibular	Vertigo, nystagmus, auditory symptoms
Spinal cord	Back pain, paraparesis, bladder and bowel dysfunction
Cardiopulmonary	Cough, substernal pain, tachypnea, asphyxia (chokes)
Systemic	Extreme fatigue, hypovolemic shock

in blood and tissue, and not all bubbles cause symptoms. Bubbles produce a number of secondary manifestations attributed to surface activity at the interface between the bubble and the blood or tissue. These secondary effects, such as activation of complement, platelet aggregation, and release of vasoactive mediators, may lead to ischemia and some of the manifestations of DCS.

CLINICAL MANIFESTATIONS. Decompression sickness can occur during decompression after diving to more than 25 feet of seawater (1.75 ATA) or during rapid ascent from sea level to 18,000 feet (0.5 ATA). Decompression sickness is most commonly encountered in compressed air (or gas) divers after prolonged or repetitive dives or after severe exercise and in divers with excessive body fat, poor physical conditioning, and increasing age. The signs and symptoms of DCS usually appear within a few minutes to a few hours after the end of the dive. Clinically, DCS is classified as either mild (type 1) or serious (type 2). This distinction is somewhat arbitrary because both mild and serious manifestations of DCS occur simultaneously in about one third of patients. The common clinical features of DCS are outlined in Table 528–3.

TREATMENT AND OUTCOME. The first step in the treatment of DCS is the administration of high concentrations of oxygen by face mask. Prompt recompression in a hyperbaric chamber with 100 per cent oxygen usually relieves symptoms in a matter of minutes. Even mild symptoms of DCS, with the exception of skin manifestations, should be treated with recompression. If recompression therapy is delayed for more than a few hours, the illness is more difficult to treat. The rationale for recompression is based on (1) enhancing the dissolution of gas bubbles by compression and (2) lowering the concentration of inert gas in venous blood with oxygen, thus increasing the rate of removal of nitrogen from body tissues and bubbles. With prompt treatment, complete recovery is to be expected. If therapy is delayed for more than 24 hours, the outcome is less certain, although many patients, even those with serious neurologic disease, respond to recompression after delays of several days.

Pulmonary Barotrauma and Arterial Gas Embolism

Pulmonary barotrauma and arterial gas embolism (AGE) may occur in compressed air divers during ascent to the surface, particularly with failure to exhale normally. They are also encountered during explosive decompression at high altitude and in blast injury of the thorax. Under these circumstances, ambient hydrostatic or barometric pressure decreases rapidly, and gas within the lungs expands reciprocally according to Boyle's law. Under water near the surface, small decreases in depth result in large increases in gas volume. If the expanding gas is not allowed to escape, it may create a pressure gradient exceeding the compliance of lung tissue. This positive-pressure gradient between alveolar gas and the pulmonary interstitium may lead to alveolar disruption and pulmonary interstitial emphysema and then to soft tissue or mediastinal emphysema, pneumothorax, or pneumopericardium. This condition is known as pulmonary barotrauma. Free gas may also enter pulmonary venous blood and travel through the left side of the heart to the systemic circulation. Air can be embolized throughout the arterial system, including the cerebral, coronary, and renal arteries.

CLINICAL MANIFESTATIONS. The clinical manifestations of AGE usually occur within minutes after the diver surfaces. Signs and symptoms that suggest distribution of gas to the carotid arteries frequently develop. This condition leads to acute cerebral dysfunction characterized by severe headache, blindness, loss of consciousness, seizures, or paralysis. Depending on the amount of pulmonary barotrauma, the quantity of embolized gas may be very large. This serious complication of ascent can occur in compressed air diving after very brief exposures or at very shallow depths, when DCS is not a diagnostic consideration.

TREATMENT AND OUTCOME. Severe central nervous system deficits from AGE are more likely to be permanently disabling or lethal in the absence of adequate treatment than is DCS. Recompression therapy should commence within minutes if good neurologic recovery is to be ensured. The management is similar to that of DCS, but the magnitude, length, and number of recompression treatments are generally greater. If treatment is delayed more than 24 hours, the likelihood of benefit from recompression therapy is low.

529 Occupational Diseases of the Skin

Edward A. Emmett

Occupational skin diseases are a group of heterogeneous conditions that share a common occupational etiology. They account for about one half of reported occupational disease in the United States. Occupational contact dermatitis, the prototypical disorder, makes up about 95 per cent of all occupational skin diseases; infections, about 2.5 per cent; and a large number of different, infrequent diseases, the remainder. The relative frequency of each of these diseases in any location depends largely on the pattern of industrialization.

Almost all occupational skin disease is due to external contact with chemical, physical, and biologic agents. The cause is often multifactorial. In relatively few instances are systemically (rather than locally) absorbed agents responsible.

OCCUPATIONAL CONTACT DERMATITIS

DEFINITION. Occupational contact dermatitis is an erythematous or eczematous response of the skin as a result of local contact with one or more irritating, allergenic, or photosensitizing chemical agents.

ETIOLOGY. Many chemicals from a wide variety of classes—alkalies, acids, volatile organic solvents, metallic salts, organic prepolymers, and many others—are capable of inducing contact dermatitis. The cause is often multifactorial; in addition to one or more chemicals, friction, abrasion, changes in temperature and humidity, and ultraviolet (UV) radiation may play a role. Superinfection may occur. Severe and persistent occupational contact dermatitis, particularly from irritants, is more frequent in those with an atopic diathesis.

INCIDENCE AND PREVALENCE. Bureau of Labor Statistics reports put the incidence in the United States at about 0.9 per 1000 full-time workers per year; because of substantial underreporting, the true incidence is estimated to be from 10 to 50 times higher.

EPIDEMIOLOGY. The incidence of occupational contact dermatitis is generally highest in agriculture/forestry/fishing, followed by the manufacturing industries. The highest risks occur in poultry-dressing plants, meat-packing plants, fabrication of rubber products, leather tanning and finishing, manufacture of ophthalmic goods, plating and polishing, production of frozen fruits and vegetables, internal combustion engine manufacture, machining operations, and canning and curing of seafoods. Virtually no industry is immune.

PATHOGENESIS. Contact dermatitis may result from direct local irritation, cell-mediated immune reactions, or photosensitivity.

Direct local irritation may be immediate, as in irritation from strong acids or alkalies, or may be delayed and occur only after repeated or prolonged local application as cumulative insult dermatitis. The latter can occur from one or more relatively mildly irritating substances that are termed marginal irritants.

Allergic contact dermatitis occurs as a result of sensitization to specific haptens through a process of cell-mediated immunity. The hapten combines with protein in the skin to form a complete antigen that is processed and presented to T lymphocytes by epidermal Langerhans cells, specialized macrophages that form an intraepidermal network. Among the most frequent allergens are poison ivy or oak; rubber additives, particularly accelerators and antioxidants; monomers of plastics and resins, such as epoxies, acrylates, and di-isocyanates; nickel; chromium salts; paraphenylenediamine and derivatives; and formaldehyde. There are many more possible allergens. The number of substances reported to cause allergic contact dermatitis is very large.

Chemical photosensitivity results from the photochemical excitation of a UV-absorbing molecule with resultant tissue damage. In a photoirritant reaction there is direct damage to cellular components, for example, when psoralens irradiated with long UV bind covalently to DNA. Coal tar pitch, certain aromatic dyes, and UV absorbers used in printing processes also cause photoirritation. In the rarer photoallergic reaction, photochemical alteration of the inciting chemical either forms a hapten or leads to a hapten-protein combination in the skin; the subsequent steps are identical with those for allergic contact dermatitis.

A major factor in the human's resistance to environmental chemicals is the barrier provided by the outer stratum corneum layer of the epidermis. Damage to this barrier by trauma, inflammation, or skin disease or by altering barrier conditions, e.g., by occlusion, may play an important role in the development of contact dermatitis.

CLINICAL MANIFESTATIONS. The clinical presentation is dominated by dermatitis that is confined, at least initially, to the region of contact. The morphology varies according to the concentration and duration of the exposure, the pathogenesis, and individual constitutional differences. Acute irritant dermatitis is characterized by erythema, perhaps edema, papules and vesicles, or, in the more extreme instance, one or more large bullae filled with purulent fluid. Postinflammation hyperpigmentation and hypopigmentation may occur; necrosis may leave scars. The cause of acute irritant dermatitis is usually obvious because of the rapidity with which the reaction develops.

Cumulative insult dermatitis may develop only after a long period of contact. On the hands it tends to start under rings or watchbands and to be somewhat patchy in distribution. Individual susceptibility varies widely. Initially, drying and fissuring may be seen, with subsequent development of an eczematous response with papules and vesicles. Excoriations and lichenification are frequent if the process persists. Relapse may occur on relatively brief exposure to mild irritants, even when the dermatitis is clinically healed, especially if the epidermal barrier has not yet been fully re-established.

Allergic contact dermatitis most often presents as an acute or chronic eczematous reaction with erythema, papules, vesicles, scaling, and pruritus. Characteristically there is a latent period of at least 7 to 10 days before the development of dermatitis following first exposure to the allergen. Recurrence usually occurs 24 to 72 hours after an eliciting exposure. Certain allergens, e.g., epoxy resin monomers, have a tendency to produce severe acute reactions with significant edema.

Localization is important for diagnosis. Over 90 per cent of occupational contact dermatitis involves the hands, sometimes in conjunction with other sites. When the eruption is due to contact with objects or contaminated surfaces, the pattern of contact determines localization. Reaction to immersion of the hands in liquids generally involves the dorsum of the hands and palmar aspects of the wrists. Photosensitivity reactions on exposed sites may be distinguished from airborne contact dermatitis by the relative sparing of shaded areas, such as the eyelids or behind the ears.

DIAGNOSIS. A good occupational history is the cornerstone of diagnosis. It is most useful to get a description of the worker's daily activities, including nonoccupational activities, with particular attention to contact of the skin with chemicals. The localization of the eruption at its onset, initial appearance of lesions, nature of progression, and circumstances of remissions and recurrences help determine an occupational etiology. A personal or family history or both confirm the presence of atopy, in which there is increased susceptibility to irritants, changes in heat and humidity, and other factors. A complete examination of the skin helps rule out dermatoses other than contact dermatitis, including id reactions of the hands secondary to dermatophytosis of the feet. Allergic contact dermatitis is confirmed by diagnostic patch testing; photoallergy, by photopatch testing. Patch testing is relatively easy to perform, but the interpretation requires skill. There is no clinically useful confirmatory test for irritant contact dermatitis.

Other information may be necessary to make a precise diagnosis and formulate appropriate management. Toxicity information on industrial compounds can be obtained from Material Safety Data Sheets, which reveal the composition and properties of industrial materials. In the United States these are available to most employees and their physicians. A visit by the physician to the workplace allows the physician to view the work firsthand. If such a visit is made, opportunity for skin contact with hazardous agents should be explored, as well as the use of protective measures.

Epidemiologic surveys to establish the prevalence of dermatitis in workers at similar jobs and industrial hygiene surveys to characterize the nature and amount of chemical exposure may occasionally be helpful. Public health authorities, university centers for occupational and environmental health, and sometimes concerned employers may be able to assist in such investigations.

TREATMENT. Symptomatic treatment is similar to that for dermatitis of other types. Acute contact dermatitis is treated with cold wet dressings of Burow's solution. Systemic steroids in rapidly tapering doses are indicated in severe acute widespread disabling eruptions; topical steroids and emollients, for dry and chronic eczema. Superinfection requires appropriate systemic antibiotics. Antihistamines may be given for sedation and are mildly antipruritic. The patient should be given careful instruction to avoid casual exposures and should be alerted to the fact that even when the skin has apparently healed, the barrier may not have returned to normal. A temporary or permanent change of job tasks may be necessary. If a permanent job change is necessary, vocational rehabilitation should be considered. Some states require reporting of occupational diseases.

PROGNOSIS. The prognosis of occupational contact dermatitis is surprisingly poor, especially if effective treatment is not given early and if the dermatitis is prolonged. The reasons for this are not entirely clear; however, surveys have shown that a high percentage of individuals still have dermatitis several years later, in many cases despite a change of employment. Those with atopy appear to have the worst prognosis. In allergic contact dermatitis, the prognosis is dependent on the ease with which the allergen can be avoided.

PREVENTION. Preventive measures serve both to prevent recurrences and to halt the development of new disease. These include elimination of or substitution for strong irritants and sensitizers; education of workers regarding skin care; avoidance of overly harsh skin cleansers; prompt reporting and treatment of dermatitis; engineering controls to minimize skin contact with potential hazards; appropriate impervious protective clothing; good personal hygiene with rapid, effective removal of contaminants; and counseling of individuals with predisposing conditions, such as atopy, regarding career selection.

OTHER OCCUPATIONAL DERMATOSES

A relatively large number of other dermatoses can result from occupational exposure. In large part, management is dependent upon diagnostic recognition and on discontinuing further exposures, using measures outlined above.

Chemical burns result from corrosive agents that produce necrosis, ulceration, and subsequent scarring. Prompt removal

of these agents (such as strong acids, alkalies, phenol, alkyl metal compounds, and metal chlorides) from skin, eyes, and mucous membranes is essential. Water is generally best for removal. Quicklime, tin tetrachloride, and titanium tetrachloride should be removed with mineral oil. Specific antidotes are few; these include topical or injected calcium gluconate for hydrofluoric acid burns.

Urticaria may occur from local contact with or systemic absorption of agents that elicit an immediate hypersensitivity reaction or directly release histamine and other vasoactive substances.

Fiber glass dermatitis causes intense pruritus; there may be no visible changes, or it may be accompanied by excoriations, pinpoint petechial papules, or both. Microscopy of a cellophane tape stripping from the skin, which had been treated with 10 per cent potassium hydroxide, reveals the fibers.

Relatively deep indolent *ulcers* of skin and mucous membranes result from contact with arsenic, chromates, and lime.

Chemical acne and folliculitis may result from contact with greases and oils, coal tar pitch, creosote, and a number of cosmetics (acne cosmetica) and from ingestion of bromides, iodides, and isoniazid. These forms of acne typically commence with comedones or inflammatory papules.

Chloracne is due to halogenated aromatic compounds with specific molecular shape, including dioxin and related chlorinated aromatic hydrocarbons. The illness is characterized by small straw-colored cysts and comedones that first involve the malar crescent and behind the ear and may not spread beyond these areas. Inflammatory pustules, abscesses, and large cysts may be seen in severe cases. Chloracne is the first and most constant finding in chronic dioxin poisoning. More variable findings may include porphyrinuria, hyperpigmentation, hypertrichosis, central and peripheral nervous system effects, alteration of lipid metabolism, and mild hepatotoxicity. Experimentally observed effects include teratogenicity, immunosuppression, and tumor induction.

Cutaneous granulomas occur as slightly erythematous grouped flesh-colored papules, with or without inflammatory changes, from foreign body reactions at the site of contact with talc and silica or as an immunologic response to beryllium and zirconium.

Chemical leukoderma, which may mimic vitiligo but which is confined to the areas of skin contact, may result from a number of phenols and catechols, including hydroquinone, monobenzyl, and monomethyl ethers of hydroquinone (used as rubber additives) and *p*-tertiary butyl and related phenols (in disinfectants).

Basal and squamous cell carcinomas and keratoacanthomas result from prolonged exposures to UV radiation, ionizing radiation, polycyclic aromatic hydrocarbons (including coal tar pitches and related products), and arsenic. Exposures to arsenic may be associated with various internal malignant neoplasms.

Cutaneous T cell lymphoma (mycosis fungoides) may be more frequent in those who have worked in heavy industry or who have industrial chemical exposure, but the particular causal agents are uncertain.

INFECTIONS AND INFESTATIONS

The development of infections and infestations frequently depends on occupational factors, individual susceptibility, and the geographic distribution of the causal organism. Occupational associations include the following:

Viral. Herpes simplex (dentists, medical personnel), milkers' nodules and papular stomatitis (veterinarians, milk handlers), orf (farmers, shepherds, abattoir workers), viral warts (butchers), Rift Valley fever (shepherds).

Bacterial. Staphylococcal infections of hands (abattoir workers and butchers), erysipeloid (fish, fowl, rabbit, and pig handlers), anthrax (wool, hair, and hide handlers), tularemia (farmers), nontuberculous mycobacterial infections (aquarium workers and pet shop attendants). Bacterial and yeast infections and tinea versicolor are prominent where there is heat, humidity, and lack of hygiene.

Fungal. Dermatophyte infections are more frequent in farm workers, surveyors, zoo attendants, animal care technicians, and certain others. Particular examples include tinea verrucosum (farmers); infection due to *Trichophyton rubrum* (miners), *Microsporum canis* (pet shop workers), *Trichophyton violaceum* (wrestlers), and *Candida albicans* (those in wet work, particularly those in contact with sugar and fruit); sporotrichosis (mine workers); chromomycosis (agricultural workers); and actinomycosis (agricultural workers).

Protozoal. South American leishmaniasis (foresters).

Helminths. Creeping eruption (plumbers, gardeners, farm workers in the tropics), ankylostomiasis (miners), schistosomiasis and cercarial dermatitis (rice planters and canal workers).

In addition, bites and stings of arthropods and other creatures are common in those who work out of doors and in certain other occupations.

Adams RM: Occupational Skin Disease. New York, Grune & Stratton, 1983. *A comprehensive review of contact dermatitis and related conditions, with descriptions of skin diseases caused by a variety of agents and with detailed lists of agents encountered in various occupations.*

Maibach HI (ed.): Occupational and Industrial Dermatology. Chicago, Year Book Medical Publishers, 1987. *A multiauthor text that broadly covers occupational dermatoses and dermatotoxicology and describes the skin diseases caused by a number of specific agents.*

530 Radiation Injury

Theodore L. Phillips

DEFINITION. Radiation injury may be defined as any somatic or genetic disruption of function or form caused by electromagnetic waves or accelerated particles. Common sources of such injury include ultraviolet radiation from the sun and man-made sources; microwave radiation from radar, ovens, and other appliances; high-intensity ultrasound; and ionizing radiation from natural and man-made sources.

Ultraviolet radiation, produced by the sun, is largely absorbed by the atmosphere of the earth. It penetrates tissue poorly and so is a threat only to exposed body surfaces. Injury occurs through direct chemical effects in molecules with high ultraviolet absorbance. Ultrasound and microwaves exert their effects by generating heat during absorption.

Radiation with wavelengths shorter than that of light has an additional property: the ability to displace electrons from their normal orbits. As these electrons traverse tissue, they generate ions and free radicals, which then react with biologically important molecules, leading to cell death. High-energy rays have the ability to penetrate and cause severe biologic damage after deposition of small amounts of energy.

Ionizing radiation, both natural and man-made, is of two types—photons (or waves) and accelerated particles. Photons, called *gamma rays,* are given off in many types of nuclear decay. Man-made ionizing rays, called *x-rays,* occur when an electron is stopped in a dense material. Accelerated particles include protons from solar radiation, heavy nuclei in cosmic rays, and beta and alpha particles given up in nuclear decay. These particles are charged, and they cause direct ionization. Neutrons are given off in nuclear decay and cause damage through secondary reactions in tissue in which protons are produced.

Radiation dose is defined in terms of energy deposition. The basic unit is the *gray* (Gy), equal to 1 joule per kilogram. Radioactivity is defined in terms of the rate of decay; one disintegration per second is a becquerel (Bq) (Table 530–1).

Because radiations differ in the density of the ionization they cause, their biologic effects vary; densely ionizing radiations have profound biologic effects. Thus, a unit called the sievert (Sv) is used to express risk estimates in which a *quality factor* is applied to the absorbed dose. Additional weight may be applied, depending on the specific organ or organs irradiated.

Absorption of charged particles and their range in tissue are determined by their charge and mass. Particles with high charge and mass give up their energy rapidly and penetrate only short distances, unless they are of high energy. Photons are absorbed exponentially by electron or nuclear interactions. Because photons diverge as they leave the source, the dose decreases as the square of the distance from the source.

Injury from radiation may be either thermal or ionizing. Ionizing radiation injury expressed within a few hours or days is called *acute;* when expressed after months or years, it is called *delayed.*

ETIOLOGY. *Biology of Ultraviolet Radiation.* Ultraviolet light photons are capable of generating chemical changes in DNA and other molecules, the most important of which is the production of pyrimidine dimers. Although these dimers may be excised and the DNA repaired, if unrepaired, these lesions lead to reproductive cell death and desquamation after skin irradiation. Ultraviolet exposure also causes immediate effects, such as vasodilatation and erythema. The limited penetration and the absorption by melanin limit human injury to the superficial layers of the skin and the eye. Solar carcinogenesis in the skin and eye is a major problem.

Biology of Ionizing Radiations. When electrons traverse a cell, they cause the formation of ion pairs both in cell water and in the DNA. During such events, reactive radicals containing unpaired outer electrons are formed. These radicals react with DNA or occur in the DNA itself. A radical may be repaired by reduction by SH groups or fixed by oxidation or electron transfer. If a free radical persists, it leads to a break in the DNA strand. Single-strand breaks are generally repaired, but if two occur side by side, a double-strand break occurs. Unrepaired double-strand breaks lead to chromosome aberrations that are lethal.

Chromosome injury is expressed at the time of cell division, which causes most mammalian cells to die a mitotic death. Deletions and dicentric chromosomes lead to loss of genetic information at each cell division. Some cells may survive a few divisions but will be incapable of sustained reproduction. Intermitotic death occurs in some lymphocytes and gonadal cells, even after low radiation doses, but most cells will survive 10 to 30 Gy until mitosis occurs.

Dose-Response Relationships. The percentage of cells that survive after exposure to ionizing radiation decreases logarithmically with dose. There are two components to the injury, reparable and irreparable, so that most dose survival plots show a shallow slope at small doses and become steeper with increasing dose. Low-level effects are thus generally less than one would expect based on observations at high doses. Cells can repair radiation damage very effectively. Repair is primarily of single- and double-strand DNA breaks and requires only a few hours.

The radiation dose required to reduce survival in mammalian cells to 10 per cent is relatively uniform. The most sensitive cells require 1 Gy to reduce survival to 10 per cent and the most resistant, about 5 Gy. Changes in sensitivity by a factor of 3 occur under hypoxia and as cells traverse the mitotic cycle.

INCIDENCE AND PREVALENCE. *Background Radiation.* Both ionizing and ultraviolet radiations are ubiquitous in the universe because of the fusion processes in stars. Gamma rays, x-rays, and highly energetic particles are emitted by stars and by nuclear decay of isotopes produced by stellar processes. On the earth, radiation comes from isotopes in the earth, water, human body, and construction materials and from the sun and other sources in space. The dose of radiation that one receives from this natural radiation depends on the altitude and the geologic nature of the region. The average annual exposure is 3.6 millisieverts (mSv), about four fifths of which is natural radiation and two thirds of which is due to radon (Table 530–2).

TABLE 530–1. RADIATION DOSE SPECIFICATION

Type	Dose Unit	Definition
Radioactivity	Becquerel (Bq)	One disintegration/second
Absorbed dose	Gray (Gy)	Energy deposited in tissue (1 joule/kg)
Dose equivalent	Sievert (Sv)	Absorbed dose weighted for the quality (damaging effect) of the radiation
Effective dose equivalent	Sievert	Dose equivalent weighted for the sensitivity of the organs
Collective effective dose equivalent	Man sievert	Effective dose equivalent applied to a population

TABLE 530–2. AVERAGE ANNUAL EFFECTIVE DOSE EQUIVALENT OF IONIZING RADIATIONS TO A MEMBER OF THE U.S. POPULATION

Natural		Artificial	
Source	Dose (mSv*)	Source	Dose (mSv*)
Radon	2	Medical	0.53
Cosmic	0.27	Consumer products	0.10
Terrestrial	0.28	Occupational	<0.01
Internal	0.39	Nuclear power	<0.01
		Fallout	<0.01
Total natural	3.0	Total artificial	0.63

*MilliSieverts, including quality factor.

Medical Exposure. Shortly after the discovery of x-rays by Roentgen in 1895 and the subsequent discovery of radioactivity, the first medical injuries occurred. The early workers were unaware of the injurious properties of the rays until damage to hands, eyes, and bone marrow became evident. After World War II, the full hazards of radiation exposure were recognized, and exposures were strictly limited. Currently, injury of the acute and chronic types is rare after medical diagnostic exposure but is a side effect of radiation therapy.

Radiation is used in the treatment of 50 to 60 per cent of patients with malignancy; 300,000 to 400,000 patients are exposed annually. Although every precaution is taken to avoid clinically important delayed effects, acute reactions to radiation therapy are common. Since most tumors require doses for cure close to organ tolerance, the risk of injury is always present.

Rarely, injuries occur to medical workers or patients during machine malfunction or repair operations. Workers and patients, as well as the general public, are also exposed to low-level radiation either while obtaining diagnostic studies or while working in medical radiation environments. Permissible exposures have been reduced to 50 mSv for workers and 5 mSv for the public; less than half that exposure is highly recommended. These rules keep the additional medical exposure of the population as a whole to less than one-fifth that of the background level.

Industrial and Military Exposure. High-level radiation exposure to the largest populations occurred at the Hiroshima and Nagasaki fission weapon explosions in World War II. Although most casualties were due to blast and burns, 40 to 50 per cent of the survivors had radiation injury. Late effects have included several hundred cases of leukemia and other malignancies. Atomic weapons testing has led to the inadvertent exposure of 300 or more persons, about 25 per cent of whom show clinically detectable effects. The fallout from nuclear tests initially added about 0.02 mSv to the annual background radiation exposure, but this has now dropped to less than 0.01 mSv.

Radiation accidents can be divided into two groups, depending on whether they involve large groups of the population exposed to relatively low doses or a small number of individuals receiving high doses. In general, accidents involving large numbers of individuals are related to the dispersion of radioactive elements through large areas of environment. Although these accidents may have different causes, the source is extremely important in determining the nature of the radionuclides released.

Most radiation accidents that have occurred have originated in civilian installations. Two reactor accidents can be considered to have had essentially no human consequences, the accidents in the United Kingdom in 1957 (Windscale) and in the United States in 1979 (Three Mile Island). The Chernobyl accident in the Soviet Union in 1986, however, resulted in very extensive releases of radioactivity and contamination with significant doses to a large population in the vicinity of the reactor as well as large collective doses, i.e., small doses multiplied through a large population, in much of the Northern Hemisphere.

Secondary to an explosion and then fire in a graphite reactor of poor design, a cloud of effluent continuing 40 million Ci of iodine-131, 3 million Ci of cesium-137, and 50 million Ci of xenon radioisotopes was released. Thirty per cent of the material was deposited within a 30-km radius of the plant. The majority

of the radiation dose to the exposed population came from cesium-137. To put things in perspective, 15 Ci of iodine-131 was released in the Three Mile Island incident.

Of 237 workers showing radiation sickness, 31 individuals died in the Chernobyl accident, 2 of whom were killed by the initial explosion and 29 of whom died of various combinations of thermal and radiation burns as well as gamma radiation injury. An estimated 50,000 Soviets received at least 0.5 Sv of exposure, and 4000 had an average of 2 Sv. The average dose in the United States was 0.002 mSv.

Accidents with sealed medical and industrial sources with high-energy gamma emissions have killed 28 persons. The most recent accident in Brazil involved improper disposal of a medical cesium source, leading to four deaths. In addition, nine persons have been killed in reactor criticality accidents.

Ingestion or inhalation of long-lived isotopes is also potentially injurious. About 5000 persons have been exposed to ingested radium, and at least 400 malignancies have occurred, with increased incidence in the sinuses and in bone. Inhalation of plutonium and other alpha emitters is a problem in the nuclear industry. Eleven deaths due to ingestion of radioactive isotopes other than radium have occurred.

EPIDEMIOLOGY. Radiation injury is not caused by a vector, and the source and nature of the exposure should be obvious. Persons may be exposed without awareness, and clinical symptoms must be identified before an exposure is suspected. In other cases, a psychologically deranged person may have access to radioactive materials and ingest them or expose himself or herself but deny the exposure.

It is important to determine the nature of the exposure and to reconstruct the dose distribution to predict the level of injury and the required treatment.

PATHOGENESIS. *Cell Kinetics and Radiation Effects.* Cells not subject to intermitotic death can live out their normal lifespan after irradiation, and their injury becomes apparent only because the dying cells cannot be replaced owing to mitotic death. Organs are made up of several populations of cells, some of which do not normally divide and persist for many years after a radiation exposure. Other cells, such as those in the renal tubules and the liver, are replaced slowly, and eventually depopulation occurs. The endothelial cells of the capillary system are slowly replaced. Radiation causes gradual loss of capillary patency, and the number of capillaries decreases.

Specific Tissue Radiobiology. The tissues of the body can be divided into those critical to life and those whose injury by radiation may cause morbidity but is not fatal. The critical tissues for survival are discussed below. *The doses quoted are single exposures to high-energy photons. Because of repair, doses two to four times higher are required for the same effect after fractionated exposures.*

Bone Marrow. Because of the short lifespan and rapid renewal of most peripheral blood and marrow cells, this organ shows the most dramatic clinical syndrome. Small lymphocytes die an intermitotic death, and depletion is seen in a few hours. The half-life of platelets and granulocytes is 1 week, and depletion is maximal at 3 weeks. The half-life of red cells is about 100 days. There is a dynamic balance between the declining numbers of mature cells and regeneration. The marrow regenerates after single whole-body exposures up to at least 6 Gy and may be repopulated by transplantation in some cases after doses up to 10 Gy.

Intestines. The mature surface and villus cells of the intestinal mucosa are replaced by the division of cells in the crypts that migrate up the villus. In contrast to this rapid renewal system, the muscular wall contains a slowly renewing capillary network. Doses as low as 1 Gy can reduce crypt cell survival to 50 per cent, but histopathologically detectable injury requires 10 Gy or more. After 15 Gy, the cell kill in the crypt is sufficient to cause complete loss of the villus and in some cases denudation, followed by repopulation. Higher local doses produce these acute changes but also lead to late fibrotic changes in the muscular layer and serosa caused by capillary injury.

Central Nervous System. The central nervous system has no rapid cell renewal systems, but the glial cells and the endothelial cells cycle slowly and can show injury. The neurons are not injured, except secondarily, at doses below 60 Gy. Large exposures of 50 to 500 Gy can produce acute functional changes and, at the highest doses, immediate death. After 15 Gy, changes begin in 4 to 5 months and persist in development over 1 to 2 years. Focal necrosis and calcification, demyelinization, and gliosis are seen, particularly in the white matter (see Ch. 162).

Skin. After exposure to between 3 and 9 Gy, the skin can show transient vasodilatation, cessation of mitosis in the basal layer, and thinning of the prickle cell layer. At doses above 20 Gy, denudation and ulceration occur before repopulation begins from either surviving basal cells or cells at the periphery of the exposed area. The cells of the hair follicles and sweat glands are often depleted and will not regenerate after 20 Gy. Late vascular damage can cause a second wave of ulceration.

Lung. In the lung, both the type II pneumocytes and the capillary cells, as well as the mucosal cells of the bronchial tree, regenerate slowly. About 90 days after a dose of 10 Gy, acute pneumonitis occurs, capillaries occlude, and endothelial cells are lost. This situation is preceded by depletion of surfactant and type II cells. Secondary influx of alveolar macrophages is seen. The acute phase is followed over the ensuing 9 months by replacement of the capillaries and alveoli by collagen. Acute pneumonitis is reversible only at the lowest doses, 6 to 10 Gy in a single exposure.

Heart. The cardiac muscle cells do not proliferate, so almost all radiation changes occur primarily in the endothelium of the capillaries. Four to 6 months after exposure of up to 15 Gy or more, the capillaries become occluded and show a dose-related reduction in number. This situation can lead to a secondary loss of muscle cells. The pericardium is also injured, with resulting effusion and fibrotic thickening.

Liver. The hepatocytes are normally replaced very slowly, but injury to the liver can induce a wave of cell division. The sinusoidal endothelium in the lobules is also continuously replaced. Six weeks after exposure to 10 Gy, central lobular occlusion occurs, and there is secondary hepatocyte loss and portal hypertension.

Kidney. After 10 Gy, the tubule cells are reduced in number and exhibit flattening in the tubule lining. Whole nephrons are lost over a period of 4 to 18 months after exposure. At the same time, many capillaries are occluded. At 1 year and beyond, damage in the glomerulus, with loss of foot processes and thickening of the basement membrane, can be seen. Secondary hypertension is common.

Gonads. In contrast to most other tissues during fractionated exposure, the gonads are quite sensitive to complete depopulation of the reproductive cells. Sterilization can occur after exposure to as little as 5 to 10 Gy, and prolonged hypospermia after even a smaller exposure. The hormone-secreting cells of the gonads are much more resistant, but, of course, ovarian hormone secretion is dependent on ovulation and is obliterated by sterilization.

CLINICAL MANIFESTATIONS. *Acute Whole-Body Exposures.* The classic acute whole-body radiation syndrome is usually seen after reactor accidents, after malfunction of large treatment or research accelerators or industrial radiation facilities, and after nuclear explosions. It is also seen after total-body irradiation for bone marrow transplantation and treatment of malignancy. In the subsequent discussion, doses quoted are for single exposures. *For fractionated exposures, doses two to four times higher are needed for the same effect because of repair.*

The initial symptoms are directly related to the radiation dose. After 2 Gy, about half the patients exhibit nausea and vomiting 2 to 6 hours after exposure. After 3 Gy, the incidence is 100 per cent. With doses above 3 Gy, three syndromes occur:

1. *The hematologic syndrome* occurs in patients who receive up to 10 or 12 Gy. At these doses, although the small intestine is affected, there is usually little or no diarrhea, and the bowel is not denuded. The chief effects are in the bone marrow, although patients who survive the acute phase can develop lung or kidney injury months to years later. In the hematologic syndrome, the patient experiences the prodromal symptoms of nausea and vomiting, and in the most serious cases these are often associated with malaise and weakness. These symptoms subside over the first 24 hours and may be followed by salivary gland swelling in some patients. If the dose has been less than 5 Gy, there will then be a quiescent period of 2 to 3 weeks. At that point, depopulation of the marrow and the resultant fall in granulocyte and platelet levels lead to infection and hemorrhage.

Purpura, petechiae, and fever are common. Skin erythema and desquamation can occur, particularly if there are local areas that have received higher doses. Temporary epilation occurs if the patient survives. If the dose is 3 Gy or below, recovery is the rule, and patients who have received doses up to 5 or 6 Gy can recover if they have medical support.

2. *The gastrointestinal syndrome* occurs at doses of 12 to 30 Gy. When the dose exceeds that needed to denude the small bowel, the gastrointestinal syndrome occurs before the hematologic syndrome and, since it is usually fatal, is the dominant manifestation. After initial symptoms similar to those of the hematologic syndrome, a brief asymptomatic period ensues, although malaise and diarrhea may be persistent. Five to 7 days after exposure, severe diarrhea and fluid loss occur, followed by infection with enteric bacteria. It is not possible to survive this syndrome after whole-body exposure, even with modern support techniques.

3. *The cardiovascular–central nervous system syndrome* occurs after very large doses and is uniformly fatal. After 20 to 50 Gy, the patient experiences immediate nausea, vomiting, and diarrhea. This condition is followed rapidly by ataxia, sweating, prostration, and shock. Huge doses, such as 300 to 500 Gy, can cause immediate death due to generalized central nervous system dysfunction.

Local or Regional Radiation Injury. The clinical syndromes following whole-body irradiation are all associated with acute effects that subside within 2 months of exposure. Local or regional exposures to very high doses may not be immediately fatal, and delayed effects can be seen. Local irradiation of the bone marrow does not usually produce a detectable clinical syndrome. The peripheral white and red cell counts are depressed, but more than half the marrow must be exposed to doses over 4 Gy before any clinical symptoms similar to those of the acute whole-body syndrome appear. Doses over 10 Gy in a single exposure or 25 Gy in a fractionated exposure produce prolonged aplasia of the marrow in the irradiated area. When the percentage of marrow irradiated is large, clinical symptoms of marrow hypoplasia will occur if additional radiation exposure, infection, or cytotoxic chemotherapy occurs. Abdominal irradiation can lead to signs and symptoms from the liver, kidney, and small bowel. The stomach and colon can be injured by doses of fractionated radiotherapy over 50 Gy. Radiation hepatopathy results in ascites, with other signs of portal hypertension 6 to 8 weeks after the exposure. Renal injury leads to proteinuria and edema 6 to 8 months later. Hypertension, occasionally severe, can be seen 1 to 10 years after exposure, as can renal failure. The acute small bowel or gastrointestinal syndrome can occur after abdominal exposure, but it is usually not fatal after local exposures. Delayed injury to the small bowel results in signs of intestinal obstruction, malabsorption, or diarrhea. Gastric irradiation produces signs of hypochlorhydria and at 15 Gy can lead to large greater curvature ulcers. Local irradiation of the central nervous system produces late signs. Whole-brain irradiation with 10 Gy in a single exposure causes edema with transient nausea and vomiting. Doses of 15 to 20 Gy can be fatal in 6 to 18 months, with generalized dementia. More focal irradiation can produce a mass lesion, with focal signs, headache, and vomiting. Injury to the skin results from local or regional exposures. This injury produces transient erythema the first day. After 3 weeks, erythema, dry desquamation, or moist desquamation can occur. Epidermolysis and chronic ulceration occur with single exposures over 25 Gy.

Thoracic irradiation can lead to symptoms due to either cardiac or pulmonary damage. Pulmonary damage is first seen 3 to 4 months after a single exposure or 6 weeks to 2 months after a fractionated exposure. The patient experiences fever, dyspnea, and cyanosis. If the acute phase is survived, chronic signs of pulmonary constriction and fibrosis will appear. Somewhat higher doses cause acute pericarditis, producing symptoms similar to those of a viral pericarditis, with fever, malaise, and some dyspnea 7 to 24 months after irradiation. Paradoxical pulse and cardiac tamponade can be seen with large pericardial effusions. Myocardial infarction and chronic myocarditis are sometimes seen.

Gonadal irradiation in the male rarely leads to symptoms. The patient becomes oligospermic after low doses and aspermic after higher doses about 6 weeks later. In the female, ovarian effects usually occur by the next menstrual cycle and result in amenorrhea, which is rarely reversible after doses of 5 Gy in single exposures or 20 Gy in fractionated exposures.

Systemic Exposure to Radionuclides. Systemic isotopes cause whole-body exposure and specific organ exposure, depending on the concentration of the isotope by the organ and the nature and energy of the radioactivity. Ingestion of iodine-131 leads to a whole-body exposure and high doses in the normal thyroid. There can be symptoms of nausea and vomiting, as well as the hematologic syndrome followed by hypothyroidism and pharyngitis. Plutonium concentrates in the pulmonary macrophages, causing local fibrosis and malignancy. For each isotope, it is necessary to know the distribution to predict the symptoms.

Delayed Effects of Low-Level Exposure. These effects are genetic and carcinogenic. If an exposure does not lead to sterilization, genetic damage can persist in the spermatogonia and oocytes. Experiments have shown point mutations in mice, but they have been difficult to prove in humans because of the background of about 10 per cent spontaneous abortions. The risk is estimated as being about one congenital abnormality per million live births per millisievert of exposure. The risk of carcinogenesis varies by organ and ranges from 70 to 1000 cases per sievert per million people exposed per year of follow-up.

DIAGNOSIS. It is essential that any facility likely to treat radiation injuries have a trained team on call. The physician should obtain as clear a history as possible about the exposure, including the nature of the radiation, the distance from the source, and any documentation such as monitors, badges, and witnesses. A preliminary estimate of the dose should be made from the history as well as from the symptoms. Malaise, nausea, and vomiting suggest an exposure over 1 Gy and occur in all patients who have been exposed to 3 Gy or more (Table 530–3). The physical examination should pay particular attention to the skin, conjunctivae, mucous membranes, and salivary glands. After high local doses, there may be acute erythema; 2 to 3 weeks after exposure, signs of infection or hemorrhage may be present.

Laboratory tests should include a complete blood count with differential. The total lymphocyte count directly reflects the whole-body dose within 24 hours. Elevation of the granulocyte count can occur transiently at 24 to 48 hours. If possible, a lymphocyte culture should be done by a cytogeneticist to determine the number of chromosome aberrations, which allows calculation of the dose received. Pulmonary function tests are useful after thoracic irradiation, as are lung scans and chest computed tomographs (CT's). Blood counts are essential 1 to 3 weeks after exposure to follow the pancytopenia and to direct therapy. In the gastrointestinal syndrome, there may be findings of dehydration and electrolyte imbalances.

Whole-Body Exposure. The total granulocyte count may rise transiently to 10,000 or more 24 to 48 hours after exposure, while the total lymphocyte count falls close to zero with doses of 3 Gy or more. The granulocyte count hits a nadir at 4 weeks and then returns toward normal at 8 weeks. The lymphocyte count may remain low for many years.

Local or Regional Exposure. Clinical findings after such exposure vary widely and reflect injury to the specific organ involved. Central nervous system damage will be reflected in an abnormal neurologic examination, with signs of edema and enhancing areas on the CT scan months to years after irradiation.

Radiation injury to the thorax is usually detected on the chest radiograph, although CT yields more accurate information on the volume of lung affected. Initially, areas of patchy or confluent pneumonitis conform to the shape of the exposed area. This condition progresses to stranded fibrosis and retraction. Cardiac injury may lead to transient electrocardiographic abnormalities, pericarditis with effusion detectable on ultrasound scans, and signs of myocardial ischemia.

Abdominal exposure leads to abnormal kidney and liver function test results. High doses to the pancreas can lead to diabetes and decreased pancreatic enzymes. Chronic diarrhea can occur owing to malabsorption and bile salt irritation.

Systemic Exposure to Radioisotopes. Large doses of gamma ray–emitting isotopes can cause symptoms and signs similar to those seen in the acute whole-body syndrome or local skin or mucosal injury. The most important diagnostic tests that must be obtained are radioactivity counts and spectroscopy to identify the isotope or isotopes, predict the dose, and localize the injury. Urine and blood samples should be obtained (and, if possible, a whole-body count in a suitable counter).

TREATMENT. ***Acute Whole-Body Exposure.*** The initial symptoms of whole-body exposure can be treated with antiemetics. The profound weakness seen at doses above 3 Gy can be reduced by a short course of intravenous corticosteroids. Further therapy is not needed for patients who have received 2 Gy or less. Above that, and up to 10 Gy, survival is possible with active medical management. Support similar to that used for the patient with pancytopenic leukemia is required, including reverse isolation or life island–type support. Trauma and burns complicate the situation and may dominate in terms of survival. Antibiotics should be used if the granulocyte count is below 1000 per microliter or if infection is present, in which case granulocyte transfusions should be used as well. Platelet transfusions should be given if the platelet count is below 10,000 per microliter. The diarrhea seen at doses below 10 Gy is usually mild but may require intravenous fluid and electrolyte replacement. Bone marrow transplantation may be a useful adjunct at doses of 5 Gy or more.

The experience after the Chernobyl accident, however, indicates that bone marrow transplantation in this kind of situation is only marginally effective. All the persons exposed to radiation doses at the level of 3 to 10 Gy or higher sustained significant trauma as well as thermal and superficial radiation burns. The effects of these injuries complicated the medical management. Bone marrow transplantation was used after Chernobyl in 13 patients, with 2 surviving. The donor marrow take was only transient in three patients who survived. Five died of burns, three of gastrointestinal damage, and three of pneumonitis, two of which were graft-versus-host related. Support with antibiotics, blood, platelets, and fluids seems the most effective treatment. Colony-stimulating factors and interleukins may be of great use in patients exposed to 6 to 10 Gy. Bone marrow transplantation can be considered for those exposed to 7 to 10 Gy if a good donor match is found.

Bone marrow samples and peripheral blood for tissue typing

TABLE 530–3. SYMPTOMS, THERAPY, AND PROGNOSIS AFTER RADIATION INJURY IN HUMANS

Dose range	0–1 Gy	1–2 Gy	2–6 Gy	6–10 Gy	10–20 Gy
Therapeutic needs	None	Observation	Specific treatment	Possible treatment	Palliative
Vomiting	None	5–50%	3 Gy = 100%	100%	100%
Time delay, nausea, and vomiting		3 hr	2 hr	1 hr	30 min
Main organ damaged	None	Lymphocytes	Bone marrow	Bone marrow	Small bowel
Symptoms and signs	—	Moderate leukopenia	Leukopenia, purpura, hemorrhage, epilation	Leukopenia, purpura, hemorrhage, epilation	Diarrhea, fever, electrolyte imbalance
Critical period	—	—	4–6 wk	4–6 wk	5–14 days
Therapy	Psycho-therapy	Observation	Transfusion of granulocytes, platelets; antibiotics	Transfusion; antibiotics; bone marrow transplant	Fluids and salts; possible bone marrow transplant
Prognosis	Excellent	Excellent	Guarded	Guarded	Poor
Lethality	None	None	0–80%	80–100%	100%
Time of death	—	—	2 mo	1–2 mo	2 wk
Cause of death	—	—	Infection, hemorrhage	Hemorrhage, infection	Enteritis, infection

should be obtained early, before depletion occurs. Techniques should be similar to those used for leukemia (Ch. 153). Exposures above 12 Gy (which will lead to the gastrointestinal or central nervous system syndrome) are uniformly fatal. Palliative support with fluids is indicated, as is the treatment of infection or hemorrhage.

Local or Regional Exposure. Skin reactions are the most common injury requiring treatment. Dry or moist desquamation occurs and can be ameliorated with cleansing, using an antibacterial soap. Crusts should be soaked off and the open areas dressed with petroleum jelly or bacitracin ointment. Large areas can benefit from temporary lanolin closed dressings, which should be changed daily, with the wound being washed before each redressing (Table 530–4).

The electrolyte imbalances seen with nausea and vomiting must be corrected. Radiation pneumonitis can be reversed at borderline doses with prednisone, 60 mg per day tapered the ensuing month. The acute symptoms of pericarditis can be relieved by aspirin or other anti-inflammatory agents. Cardiac tamponade should be treated by pericardiocentesis or a pericardial window. Delayed effects of doses of 20 Gy or more may require skin grafts, resection of necrotic bone, and other surgical procedures, including resection of necrotic brain tissue.

Systemic Exposure to Radionuclides. After the victim has been given urgent first aid and has been decontaminated, the dose and nature of the exposure should be determined, making use of a whole-body counter if possible. Large body burdens should be treated by specific methods designed to remove the isotope or to block uptake. After iodine exposure, stable iodine should be given as 5 drops of potassium iodide. One gram of soluble phosphate should be given to patients ingesting phosphorus-32. Radium ingestion can be treated with magnesium sulfate or epsom salts, 10 grams in 100 ml of water. Strontium exposure is treated with 100 ml of aluminum phosphate gel.

Pulmonary exposures to aerosols or dust can be treated by bronchial lavage, expectorants, or diethylenetriamine penta-acetic acid (DTPA) aerosol mist. DTPA products are available from the U.S. Department of Energy.

Gastrointestinal absorption can be reduced with mild laxatives. Sodium alginate and aluminum hydroxide gel may reduce strontium uptake. Certain heavier isotopes, including plutonium, americium, yttrium, lanthanum, cerium, scandium, and zinc, as well as other fission products can be partially removed from the body by DTPA. A dose of 0.5 to 1.0 gram should be given intravenously in 250 ml of normal saline.

PROGNOSIS. Acute Radiation Syndromes. Survival with little or no treatment other than good hygiene and treatment of infections can be expected after exposures to 3 Gy or less. Between 3 and 6 Gy, therapy with antibiotics, platelets, and granulocytes allows for a high survival rate. Leukemic patients show 80 per cent survival after 10 Gy of whole-body exposure at a dose rate of 4 Gy per hour when bone marrow transplantation is used. The use of all available methods may allow a high rate of survival after 5 Gy and some survival after acute exposures to 9 Gy.

The presence of traumatic and thermal injuries reduces the chances of survival across the whole range of radiation doses above 3 Gy. Of the 200 people receiving the highest doses at Chernobyl, 105 had received 1 to 2 Gy. All survived. Eight persons had higher doses but less than 6 Gy; seven survived. There were 25 patients thought to have received more than 6 Gy. Of these, 13 were given a bone marrow transplant, and 11 died. The other 12 did not undergo transplantation because of injuries (10), mismatch (1), or refusal (1) or because they were given fetal liver cells (6); all died. Thus, bone marrow transplantation in this group was less effective than that in patients undergoing transplantation for aplasia or leukemia.

Local Radiation Effects. Acute skin reactions usually heal completely. If the exposure has been over 20 Gy, late ulceration can be expected. Most delayed radiation injury is irreversible and slowly progressive as depopulation of stromal and capillary cells occurs.

Systemic Exposure. The prognosis depends on the whole-body radiation dose and the isotope. Large whole-body doses result in a prognosis similar to that for whole-body external exposure. Thyroid ablation occurs after 50 to 100 mCi of iodine-125, and bone marrow ablation occurs after smaller doses of phosphorus-32.

PREVENTION. Because radiation injury always has an irreversible component not subject to repair, prevention is essential. The largest exposure to the population is from the natural background and can be limited by careful selection of building materials and good ventilation of the home.

The next largest exposure is medical. This can be limited by careful selection of diagnostic tests. Optimal techniques and shielding of the gonads must be employed. Substitution of CT at some sites is helpful. The design of facilities must limit the exposure of public and monitored personnel to less than recommended levels. Proper training of workers using radiation is essential. Radiation treatment must be carried out by highly skilled specialists who limit the dose as much as possible to tumor areas.

Baramov A, Gale RP, Guskova A, et al.: Bone marrow transplantation after the Chernobyl nuclear accident. N Engl J Med 321:205, 1989. *A complete report on the attempts to treat persons exposed to high radiation doses at Chernobyl.*

Champlin RE, Kastenberg WE, Gale RP: Radiation accidents and nuclear energy: Medical consequences and therapy (clinical conference). Ann Intern Med 109:730, 1988. *A valuable general discussion of the handling of nuclear accidents.*

Hall EJ: Radiobiology for the Radiobiologist. 3rd ed. Philadelphia, J. B. Lippincott, 1988. *The best introductory text on the biologic effects of radiation for the medical worker.*

Health Effects of Exposures to Low Levels of Ionizing Radiation. Washington, D.C. BEIR V, National Academy Press, 1990. *The most up-to-date survey of health risks to populations from low-level radiation.*

Johns HE, Cunningham JR: The Physics of Radiology. 4th ed. Springfield, Ill., Charles C Thomas, 1983. *The most comprehensive text in the field of medical radiation physics.*

Nenot JC: Overview of the radiological accidents in the world, updated December 1989. Int J Radiat Biol 57:1073, 1990. *The most complete and most recent discussions of the world's major military, industrial, and medical accidents.*

TABLE 530–4. ORGAN DAMAGE, DYSFUNCTION, TREATMENT, AND PROGNOSIS AFTER IRRADIATION

Organ	Acute Lesion	Delayed Lesion	Clinical Signs	Treatment	Prognosis
Bone marrow	Pancytopenia	Vascular occlusion Myelofibrosis	Infection Hemorrhage	Antibiotics Transfusion	Good if percent of total marrow irradiation is small
Intestine	Flattened villi	Fibrosis, obstruction	Diarrhea	Fluid and electrolytes for acute symptoms Resection for obstruction	Good for acute Obstruction can be fatal
Central nervous system	Edema	Necrosis	Headache Focal neurologic	— Resection	Poor Fair
Skin	Desquamation	Ulcer, necrosis	Pain, oozing	Cleansing, ointments, graft	Good
Lung	Pneumonitis	Fibrosis	Cough, fever, cyanosis, dyspnea	Corticosteroids	Good at low dose Good if small volume
Heart	Pericarditis	Carditis	Fever dyspnea	— Anti-inflammatory agents, pericardiocentesis	Fair
Liver	Central venous thrombosis	Fibrosis	Ascites	Diuretics	Fair
Kidney	Tubular degeneration	Fibrosis	Proteinuria Hypertension, renal failure	Dialysis Transplantation	Fair

Principles and general procedures for handling emergency and accidental exposures of workers. Ann ICRP 2:1, 1978. *Detailed instructions and useful references for physicians who may be required to deal with victims of accidental exposure.*

Protection against ionizing radiation from external sources used in medicine. Ann ICRP 9:1, 1982. *The basic international manual that sets dose limits, protection standards, and monitoring standards. Essential for anyone employing radiation equipment.*

Shapiro J: Radiation Protection: A Guide for Scientists and Physicians. 3rd ed. Cambridge, Mass., Harvard University Press, 1990. *The standard introductory text for all radiation workers.*

Sources, Effects and Risks of Ionizing Radiation. New York, United Nations Publications, 1988. *A detailed compendium of radiation units, dose assessments, and risk assessments, with a review of the present situation.*

531 Electrical Injury

Cleon W. Goodwin

DEFINITION AND PREVALENCE. Electrical injury manifests in a variety of forms, ranging from cardiopulmonary arrest and minimal tissue damage to devastating electrocution and vaporization of major body parts. Tissue damage is a direct consequence of thermal injury generated by the flow of electrical current. The extent of injury is proportional to current, voltage, duration of exposure, and whether the electricity is alternating current or direct current. Alternating current is more dangerous than direct current because it can produce tonic muscle contractions and the victim may be unable to release the source of electricity. Further, cardiac arrest and coma frequently accompany electrocution with alternating current, and these events are most likely to occur at current frequencies of 50 to 60 cycles per second. As frequency increases above 60 cycles per second, tissue damage and risk of cardiac arrest decrease. Tissue damage caused by line voltages less than 1000 volts arbitrarily is designated as low-voltage injury. High-tension electrical injury is caused by line voltages above 1000 volts.

Electricity causes injury by four mechanisms: direct contact, conduction, arc, and secondary ignition. Low-voltage electrical sources produce direct injury at the point of contact. Skin and subcutaneous tissue are involved most commonly, although occasionally muscle and bone beneath the cutaneous burn may be damaged. High-voltage current not only causes direct injury at the point of contact but also damages tissues that conduct the electricity through the body. Arc burns occur without actual contact of the body surface with the source of electricity. Very high voltages are required to produce charge transfer, and when arcing occurs, extremely high temperatures are produced. The duration of the arc is brief, and the "flash" injury produced is usually limited to the body surface. A variant of arc injury occurs when electrical current being conducted along a body part flashes directly to an adjacent body part; such injuries are frequently observed in the axilla and other flexion creases. Finally, burns occur when the electrical source ignites clothing and other flammable materials. Very deep flame burns may occur, especially if the patient is unconscious. The victim may not be able to verify whether direct contact has occurred, and patient evaluation and management must assume that diverse multisystem effects of electrical injury may be present.

In an adult, electrical burns are occupational hazards. However, in recent years, the increasing number of electrical injuries reflects the technologic sophistication of society. Sport parachuting and hot air ballooning and installation of home radio and television antennas have become common causes of electrical injuries. In urban environments, electric-powered mass transit conduits are one of the most common sources of such injuries. Household appliances cause most electrical injuries in children. Lightning injury affects all age groups, especially in rural areas. Electrical injuries comprise 1 to 5 per cent of burn center admissions and up to 15 per cent of deaths.

PATHOGENESIS. Meticulous laboratory investigations have verified that tissue damage associated with electrical injury occurs when electrical energy is converted to thermal energy. The resulting injury is a thermal burn that produces physiologic responses similar to those caused by other mechanisms of thermal injury. Skin represents the initial barrier to current flow and is an effective insulator to deeper tissues. After electrical contact and the onset of current flow, the skin undergoes coagulation necrosis and desiccates. With low-voltage injuries, the charred skin at the point of contact terminates current flow and limits the extent of injury. The skin surrounding the contact point may sustain an arc burn as the increase in skin resistance terminates current flow (Fig. 531-1). At high voltages (over 1000 volts) skin resistance initially is overcome, and current flow through deep tissue in the body is unimpeded. Except for bone, these internal tissues act as a volume conductor, offering little resistance to flow. Current flow is terminated when the tissue at the point of electrical contact desiccates and resistance increases markedly. At this point, electrical arcing frequently occurs. The charred tissue now acts as an electrical insulator. No further tissue damage is possible.

Deep tissue damage is related to the density of current flow through these tissues. Heat production and, hence, thermal injury depend on the density of current flow. In body parts with small cross-sectional areas, such as an extremity, current density is high, and tissue destruction is severe. In areas of large cross-sectional areas, such as the trunk, current density is reduced, and deep injuries are unusual. Superficial tissues cool faster than deep tissues. Because bone has high resistance to current flow, it heats to higher temperatures than does surrounding soft tissue. As a result, the most severely damaged soft tissues are usually muscle and nerves directly adjacent to the bone, a position almost impervious to clinical detection. The most severe cutaneous and deep injuries are adjacent to contact sites, and damage decreases with increasing distance from contact points.

The extent of tissue injury appears to be determined at the time of electrical contact. Progressive soft tissue injury probably does not occur in spite of the clinical observation that muscle that appears to be viable immediately after electrical injury becomes necrotic several days later. In addition, electrical energy may cause lesser degrees of damage without producing coagulation necrosis. This phenomenon may explain the transient abnormalities of visceral organ function that follow electrical injury. In the heart, this minor damage may have disastrous consequences. In electrically injured patients who experience fatal cardiac arrest, focal necrosis of the myocardium and the specialized tissue of the sinus and atrioventricular nodes and contraction band necrosis of smooth muscle cells of the coronary arteries are widespread.

CLINICAL MANIFESTATIONS. High-voltage electrical injuries commonly involve multiple organ systems and dictate treatment in specialized burn treatment centers with broad multidisciplinary capabilities. Many of the abnormalities produced by electrocution may not be reflected by the surface appearance of the electrical burn and may not manifest clinically until long after admission. Consequently, meticulous serial ex-

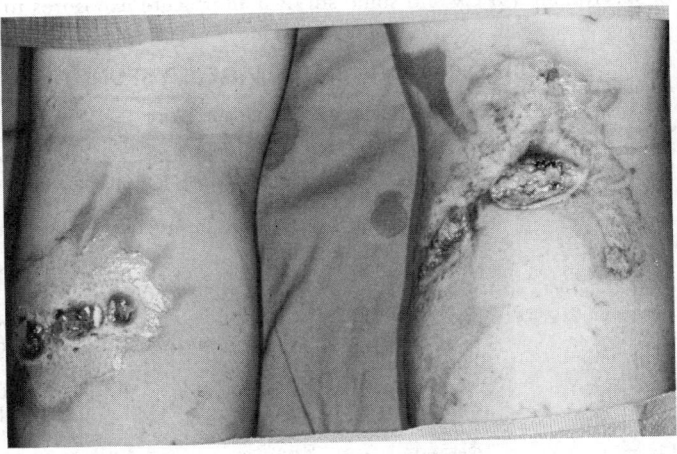

FIGURE 531-1. Charring of the skin of both calves indicates the points of contact with a high-voltage electrical current. These contact points are surrounded by full-thickness cutaneous burns caused by arcing of current. The extent of deep tissue destruction is often not related to the size of the cutaneous presentation of the injury.

aminations and documentation of electrically injured patients are necessary for both medical and legal assessment and for planning.

Cardiopulmonary Resuscitation. Cardiopulmonary arrest is common in patients with high-voltage electrical injuries, particularly lightning injury. Arrhythmias, conduction disturbances, and infarct patterns may be present on the admission electrocardiogram. Most arrhythmias are transitory, while conduction delays and infarct patterns are likely to be permanent. In those few patients who have undergone long-term cardiac function studies and angiography, these permanent electrocardiographic findings appear to represent no physiologic abnormalities.

Burn Wound. In patients who survive to be admitted to the hospital, the electrical burn itself becomes the major focus of treatment. Most high-voltage electrical injuries present with contact burns at the locations where the electrical current has entered or left the body. These contact burns typically are charred and excavated, and deeper anatomic structures may be visible in the depths of the wound. These contact areas are usually surrounded by less severe burns of variable depth. If ignition of clothing has occurred, the patient may have extensive cutaneous burns unrelated to the site of electrical contact.

Underlying injury to major muscle compartments is accompanied by edema formation, which may be accentuated by concomitant fluid resuscitation. When the tissue pressure beneath the muscle fascia increases, signs of vessel and nerve compression appear. Loss of sensation, pain, and decreased pulses indicate the presence of a compartment syndrome. Palpation often demonstrates tense muscle compartments, especially when the affected extremity is compared with an opposite unburned extremity. Even with good flow, the burned extremity may be cool to the touch and have no palpable pulse. Therefore, circulatory integrity is best judged by Doppler ultrasonography of distal pulses.

Acute Renal Failure. Acute renal failure presenting as early oliguria or anuria is not uncommon after electrical injury and is caused by two mechanisms. Gross underestimation of the extent of injury and of fluid resuscitation requirements rapidly leads to hypovolemia and oliguria. In many patients, the majority of severely damaged tissue is muscle that is hidden from view, and the need for fluid replacement may not be appreciated immediately. Second, necrotic muscle releases myoglobin, which is directly toxic to renal tubular cells. Hypovolemia potentiates the toxicity of myoglobin in the tubules unless high urine flow is maintained. Myoglobin causes the urine to appear reddish-brown. Deeply pigmented, concentrated urine typical of oliguric states may be mistaken for myoglobinuria. If uncertainty exists about the cause of urine pigments, a dipstick analysis will identify the heme nature of myoglobin. Visible myoglobinuria indicates massive acute muscle necrosis and impending renal failure. Life-threatening hyperkalemia may accompany massive muscle injury and myoglobinuria.

Nervous System. The electrical injury may involve both the central nervous system and the peripheral nervous system. A thorough neurologic examination on admission is essential, and because of the delayed presentation of neurologic complications, serial examinations should continue for several months. Both normal and abnormal function should be documented. Because extremities sustain the majority of direct electrical injuries, associated peripheral nerves are most often damaged at the time of contact. Such injuries are usually permanent and may determine the ultimate salvageability of the extremity. Some patients may also present with signs of peripheral neuropathy in locations anatomically distant from the sites of electrical injury. The mechanism responsible is not known, but fortunately these deficits usually are reversible. Motor involvement is more common than are sensory abnormalities. Several days to weeks following electrical injury, a syndrome of polyneuritis affecting nerves away from the sites of injury may occur. Associated deficits may only partially resolve. Immediate signs of spinal cord symptoms tend to be temporary and readily reversible. Spinal cord injuries of delayed onset are more often permanent or only partially reversible and manifest as transverse myelitis, ascending paralysis, hemiplegia, or related syndromes.

Fractures. Early evaluation should include assessment for skeletal trauma. Long-bone fractures frequently accompany falls, and fractures of the vertebral column may be produced by the tetanic contraction of the paraspinous muscle at the time of electrocution.

Both types of fractures can be identified on appropriate roentgenograms.

Internal Organs. Electrical injuries to the major viscera most commonly occur when the body wall overlying an organ is in direct contact with the electrical current. Otherwise, the volume of the torso is large by comparison with the extremities and allows the electrical current to be distributed over a large cross-sectional area at relatively low resistance. As a result, direct injury to internal organs rarely occurs. Dysfunction of the liver, pancreas, and gut may occur during hospitalization but probably reflects the patient's underlying condition rather than the unique effects of electrical injury.

TREATMENT. Cardiopulmonary Resuscitation. Cardiopulmonary arrest is common following electrical injury, and resuscitative effort should be instituted immediately. Patients in whom cardiac arrest has occurred frequently respond to cardiopulmonary resuscitation, particularly after lightning injury. All patients should be placed on cardiac monitors or telemetry for 48 hours, and continued monitoring is needed only if arrhythmias persist. The choice of antiarrhythmic agents is dictated by the nature of the rhythm disturbance. All persistent electrocardiographic alterations should receive thorough cardiologic investigation once the acute electrical injury has healed.

Fluid Therapy. As with any other tissue injury, fluid loss into damaged tissue is one of the major physiologic derangements after electrical burns. Intravascular volume is replenished with lactated Ringer's solution sufficient to maintain a urinary output of 50 to 75 ml per hour. If the patient has grossly visible myoglobinuria, urinary output should be increased to 100 to 150 ml per hour by raising the fluid infusion rate. The increased urine production facilitates dilution of myoglobin and its washout from renal tubules. If myoglobinuria is severe or urinary output remains low in spite of an increased rate of fluid administration, mannitol, 12.5 grams, is added to each liter of lactated Ringer's solution. In such cases, the addition of sodium bicarbonate to the resuscitation solution alkalinizes the urine and increases the solubility of myoglobin.

Wound Management. Wound care involves treatment of both cutaneous and deep soft tissue injuries. Immediately after electrical injury, second- and third-degree cutaneous wounds are debrided, cleansed, and placed in topical antimicrobial burn creams. Sulfamylon (mafenide acetate) is preferred for electrical injuries because of its superior ability to penetrate injured tissue deeply and its anticlostridial and antibacterial properties. Tetanus prophylaxis is brought up to date. Prophylactic antibiotics have not been shown to decrease episodes of infection and are not used. Extremity muscle compartment pressures are monitored by physical palpation and by Doppler ultrasonography of major arterial pulses. Tissue manometry using needle-tipped transducers appears to reflect compartmental pressures, and measurements of over 30 to 40 torr are indications for surgical decompression. If the extremity has been injured by a circumferential third-degree burn, escharotomy is carried out. If the compartment symptom persists, fasciotomy involving all major compartments is performed (Fig. 531–2). Since blood loss may be difficult to control, fasciotomy should be carried out in an operating room. While fasciotomy may allow preservation of nutrient blood flow to potentially viable tissue, it is likely that the ultimate extent of tissue damage is determined at the time of electrical injury and that progression tissue loss seldom, if ever, occurs.

Dead tissue promotes infection, which may be life threatening, and definitive therapy of the electrical burn is directed toward the timely removal of necrotic tissue. At the present time, the amputation of electrically injured extremities is not automatic. The availability of several diagnostic tools may allow definition of viable and nonviable tissue in wounds whose surface appearance may not reflect deeper injuries. Technetium-99m pyrophosphate scintigraphy is the most common diagnostic technique employed for evaluation of injured extremities and provides useful results within the first 24 hours. Normal isotopic uptake reflects normal perfusion, while totally nonviable tissue exhibits no uptake. Areas of potentially reversible injury demonstrate increased isotope uptake, and serial scanning may be useful in determining the need for debridement. In extremities with intact flow of the major arteries, arteriography may be helpful. Truncation of flow

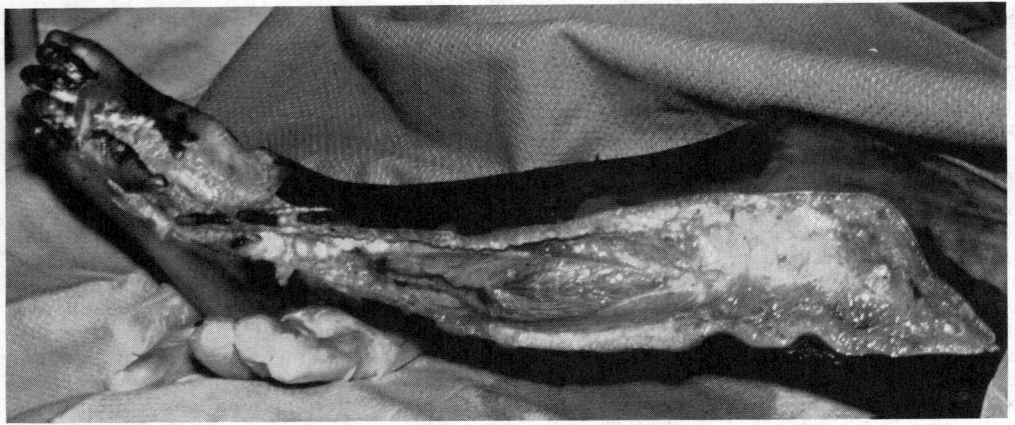

FIGURE 531-2. This severely burned lower extremity presented with no evidence of arterial circulation. Fasciotomy incisions were placed along the mid-medial and mid-lateral planes to decompress all muscle compartments. The incisional margins have separated because of massive edema in the proximal region of the incision. Necrotic muscle with overlying vessel thrombosis is seen distally. Following stabilization of the patient, exploration and debridement were carried out in the operating room.

to nutrient muscle branches indicates irreversible injury. Finally, the viability of deep tissue is determined most accurately by serial surgical exploration of the injured extremity.

The timing of surgical intervention and the extent of debridement are determined by the stability of the patient and the nature of the burn wound. Generally, initial exploration and debridement may commence at the end of the resuscitation phase, within 24 to 48 hours of injury. Distal portions of electrocuted extremities that are desiccated and mummified should be amputated. More proximally, it may be impossible to determine grossly the extent of deep tissue injury. These areas should be explored thoroughly, utilizing fasciotomy incisions if previously placed. All muscle groups should be inspected, especially those against bone. Only obviously necrotic tissue is removed, and every attempt should be made to salvage viable tissue. This approach requires daily wound examination and sequential operative debridements until all necrotic tissue is removed. Intervening complications, such as intractable hyperkalemia, severe myoglobinuria, or infection, may force abandonment of this sequential approach and require urgent amputation at a relatively high level. It is rarely advisable to proceed to early closure following amputation, and definitive closure of the debrided wound is carried out only when all necrotic tissue has been removed. Similarly, excision or grafting of full-thickness cutaneous burns may be delayed until this time. Long-term care requires multidisciplinary rehabilitation and prosthetics services.

LATE COMPLICATIONS. Patients sustaining electrical injuries may develop a number of apparently unrelated late complications that develop from a few months to several years after injury. As with cutaneous burns, more than half of electrically injured patients develop posttraumatic stress disorders, especially if a body part has been lost. Associated psychiatric symptoms respond well to psychotherapy and medication. Contractures require extensive rehabilitation care and reconstructive surgery. Cholelithiasis occurs with increased frequency in patients who have sustained electrical burns. Cataracts are particularly troublesome and occur in up to 6 per cent of electrically injured patients. The physical examination done on the admission of such patients should include a careful ophthalmologic evaluation to identify pre-existing cataracts. Although vision loss may be extensive, surgical correction is highly effective.

Amy BW, McManus WF, Goodwin CW Jr, et al.: Lightning injury with survival in five patients. JAMA 253:243, 1985. *The presentation and treatment of lightning injury are described, with emphasis on the primary role of first responder care.*

Baker MD, Chiaviello C: Household electric injuries in children. Am J Dis Child 143:59, 1989. *As with other forms of thermal injury, the household is the most common location of electrical injuries occurring in children. Similarly, most childhood electrical injuries can be prevented by utilization of inexpensive safety devices.*

Housinger TA, Green L, Shahangian S, et al.: A prospective study of myocardial damage in electrical injuries. J Trauma 25:122, 1985. *This report correlates serial electrocardiographic and cardiac enzyme determinations with radionuclide cardiac function studies in electrocuted patients. MB-creatine kinase values correlated poorly with other measurements of cardiac injury.*

Hunt JL, Mason AD Jr, Masterson TS, et al.: The pathophysiology of acute electric injury. J Trauma 16:335, 1976. *This classic experimental study demonstrates that electrical injury is caused by direct thermal damage to tissue. Further, the characteristic arteriographic findings of early occlusion of nutrient vessels to muscle and other tissues are related to subsequent necrosis.*

Hunt JL, Sato RM, Baxter CR: Acute electric burns: Current diagnostic and therapeutic approaches to management. Arch Surg 115:434, 1980. *An excellent description of electrical injury in a large series of patients. The use of technetium-99m pyrophosphate scans was introduced by these authors, and its efficacy in defining injured and nonviable tissue is confirmed.*

James TN, Riddick LR, Embry JH: Cardiac abnormalities demonstrated postmortem in four cases of accidental electrocution and their potential significance relative to non-fatal electrical injuries of the heart. Am Heart J 120:143, 1990. *This report provides an exhaustive review of the effects of electricity on the heart and describes a detailed pathologic study of postmortem damage in young men presenting with fatal cardiac arrest.*

Saffle JR, Crandall A, Warden GD: Cataracts: A long-term complication of electrical injury. J Trauma 25:17, 1985. *Cataracts occur in 5 to 10 per cent of patients with electrical injury. This report emphasizes the importance of early ophthalmologic examination, documentation, and long-term follow-up in determining disability in such patients.*

532 Disorders Due to Heat and Cold

James P. Knochel

To maintain a normal body temperature requires that heat gain equal heat loss. Heat is produced by metabolism or gained from the environment. Thermoregulation is heavily dependent upon blood flow to cutaneous vessels. Cutaneous flow is regulated by hypothalamic centers. Vasoconstriction reduces and vasodilatation increases delivery of heated blood to the skin. Heat is exchanged between the skin and the environment by radiation, conduction, or convection. If heat loss is inadequate by these means, active sweating begins, and cooling occurs by vaporization of sweat. If heat gain is necessary, metabolic heat production rises by a voluntary increase of physical activity or involuntarily by shivering. Body heat thus produced is retained by cutaneous vasoconstriction. *Acclimatization*, a term defining critical cardiovascular, endocrine, exocrine, and other physiologic adaptations to heat stress, requires 1 to 2 weeks to develop. Such adaptations permit one to work comfortably and safely under conditions of heat stress that were previously intolerable.

DISORDERS DUE TO HEAT

HEAT CRAMPS. Workers who sweat profusely and consume water with inadequate salt may experience excruciating muscle cramps. They are more common in acclimatized, physically fit men who are able to sweat voluminously. The cramps tend to occur in muscles used while working and often do not appear until the person relaxes after work. Cooling the muscles during a cold shower may precipitate the attack. Cramps in the abdominal wall may suggest a perforated viscus. Mild hyponatremia is the rule. Severe cramps may cause modest rhabdomyolysis and elevations of muscle enzymes in serum (creatine phosphokinase, CK). Salted liquids orally or saline intravenously leads to rapid improvement. Heat cramps are preventable by replacement of sweat with a hypotonic salt solution (40 mmol per liter or 0.5 teaspoon of salt per liter) or merely by increasing dietary salt intake.

HEAT EXHAUSTION. Heat exhaustion is a common disorder occurring after sustained heat stress that causes water and/or salt depletion.

Dehydration sharply increases the risk of heat stroke. It occurs most often in the elderly, infirm, obtunded, or very young who are unable to communicate their thirst. It is also seen in active persons who take salt supplements without adequate water. Deliberate efforts should be made to ensure water intake by patients in nursing homes where summertime room temperatures are often too high. Hypernatremia of several days' duration may itself reduce secretion of antidiuretic hormone and recognition of thirst. Symptoms of heat exhaustion due to water loss include intense thirst, fatigue, paresthesias, weakness, anxiety, and impaired judgment. Signs may include dehydration, hyperventilation, tetany, agitation, hysteria, muscular incoordination, and psychotic behavior. Body temperature may rise to 38.9°C. Delirium, rising temperature, coma, and frank heatstroke may follow. Laboratory findings include hemoconcentration, hypernatremia, mild azotemia, and oliguria.

Salt depletion heat exhaustion occurs mainly in unacclimatized persons in whom losses of thermal sweat are replaced with water but not adequate salt. Dehydration, weight loss, and thirst are absent in the pure form. Sweating and urinary output remain normal. Symptoms include profound weakness, fatigue, severe headache, giddiness, and muscle cramps. In some patients, anorexia, myalgia, nausea, vomiting, and diarrhea may masquerade as a viral illness. Such patients appear haggard, with pale, clammy skin. Hypotension and tachycardia are common. Fever is notably absent.

Treatment of heat exhaustion should be individualized. Most patients can be treated with lightly salted fluids, rest, and elimination of heat stress. Hypernatremic dehydration should be treated with isotonic dextrose at a rate sufficient to reduce serum sodium about 2 mEq per liter per hour. It is seldom necessary to administer hypertonic salt solutions to patients with hyponatremic heat exhaustion.

HEATSTROKE. Heatstroke is a catastrophic illness requiring immediate treatment for survival. It is subdivided into two forms, classic and exertional (Table 532–1).

Classic heatstroke occurs especially in the poor, the elderly, infants, the chronically ill, alcoholics, patients with advanced heart disease, and the obese. Hot, humid weather usually precedes this disorder. Deaths due to heart disease increase sharply during heat waves because of demands placed upon the heart by heat stress. Certain medications also increase the propensity to develop heatstroke. These include drugs that impair sweating (anticholinergics, phenothiazines, beta blockers, antihistamines), diuretics, drugs that may increase heat production (amphetamines, cocaine, neuroleptics), and butyrophenone, which may depress thirst. Rarely, victims may recall a prodrome resembling heat exhaustion or cessation of sweating. Once sweating stops, body temperature mounts and collapse soon follows. Typical findings include central nervous system dysfunction, especially coma or bizarre behavior; hot, dry, flushed skin; and hyperpyrexia. Rectal temperature exceeds 40.6°C and may reach 44°C or more. Hypotension is common. It is probably due to redistribu-

tion of blood from the central to the peripheral circulation, since it often responds to cooling alone. Convulsive seizures, fasciculations, and muscle rigidity are absent until active cooling is under way.

Exertional heatstroke is more likely in laborers, farmers, military recruits, football players, long-distance runners, and those who work in boiler rooms or foundries. They display physical findings in the acute phase similar to those of classic heatstroke, with one common exception: About half of these patients continue to sweat. If this occurs, the skin may be deceptively cool despite a high core temperature.

Other major differences between classic and exertional heatstroke become apparent from laboratory measurements. In the classic form, respiratory alkalosis is usual. (Blood pH, P_{CO_2}, and P_{O_2} should be corrected for temperature; cf. Table 532–2.) Circulatory collapse may cause modest increases of lactate, a particularly ominous sign. In contrast, *lactic acidosis* is the rule in exertional heatstroke, may exceed 20 mol per liter, and is not a foreboding finding in this condition. Serum CK activity may be slightly increased in classic heatstroke (usually not greater than 1000 to 2000 IU per liter). However, clinically important rhabdomyolysis is rare unless the patient has a pre-existing myopathy. Major *rhabdomyolysis* and its associated complications, such as hyperkalemia, hyperphosphatemia, hypocalcemia out of proportion to hypoalbuminemia, hyperuricemia, and myoglobinuria, are almost invariable findings in exertional heatstroke. Both forms of heatstroke may be complicated by *hemorrhage* (resulting from *disseminated intravascular coagulation*, fibrinolysis, clotting factor deficiency due to hepatic injury, or *thrombocytopenia* due to bone marrow injury); *jaundice*; *acute renal failure*; *pancreatitis*; *brain damage*; *spinal cord infarction*; *peripheral neuropathy*; *myocardial necrosis and arrhythmias*; and pulmonary capillary damage with *adult respiratory distress syndrome*. Mounting evidence suggests that gut ischemia during exercise in the heat permits endotoxin absorption and production of tumor necrosis factor and interleukins. These substances may underlie the multiple systems organ failure (MSOF) syndrome seen in severe cases of heatstroke. Hypokalemia in heatstroke usually results

TABLE 532–2. TEMPERATURE CORRECTION FACTORS FOR BLOOD pH AND GAS MEASUREMENTS

Patient's Temperature		pH	Pco₂	Po₂
°F	°C	(Add to observed values)		
110	43	− .09	+ 22%	+ 35%
109	42.5	− .08	+ 21%	+ 32%
108	42	− .07	+ 19%	+ 30%
107	41.5	− .07	+ 17%	+ 27%
106	41	− .06	+ 16%	+ 25%
105	40.5	− .05	+ 14%	+ 22%
104	40	− .04	+ 12%	+ 19%
103	39.5	− .04	+ 10%	+ 16%
102	39	− .03	+ 8%	+ 13%
101	38.5	− .02	+ 6%	+ 10%
100	38	− .01	+ 4%	+ 7%
98–99	37	None	None	None
97	36	+ .01	− 4%	− 7%
96	35.5	+ .02	− 6%	− 10%
95	35	+ .03	− 8%	− 13%
94	34.5	+ .04	− 10%	− 16%
93	34	+ .04	− 12%	− 19%
91	33	+ .06	− 16%	− 25%
90	32	+ .07	− 19%	− 30%
88	31	+ .09	− 22%	− 35%
86	30	+ .10	− 26%	− 39%
84	29	+ .12	− 29%	− 43%
82	28	+ .13	− 32%	− 47%
81	27	+ .15	− 34%	− 51%
79	26	+ .16	− 37%	− 54%
77	25	+ .18	− 40%	− 57%
75	24	+ .19	− 43%	− 60%
73	23	+ .21	− 45%	− 63%
72	22	+ .22	− 48%	− 65%
70	21	+ .24	− 50%	− 67%
68	20	+ .25	− 53%	− 70%

TABLE 532–1. MAJOR DIFFERENCES BETWEEN CLASSIC AND EXERTIONAL HEATSTROKE

	Classic	Exertional
Persons at risk	Infants, chronically ill, elderly	Laborers, soldiers, farmers, athletes
Skin	Usually hot, dry	Sweating may be present
Acid-base status	Respiratory alkalosis	Metabolic (lactic) acidosis
Rhabdomyolysis	Unusual	Major
Acute renal failure	Less than 5%	30% or more
Disseminated intravascular coagulation	Mild to moderate	Severe

from respiratory alkalosis, but it may represent potassium deficiency in those who have performed hard work in the heat for 1 or 2 weeks. Hypoglycemia may also occur.

Treatment of heatstroke is aimed at anticipation, prompt recognition, and rapid cooling. The importance of educating paramedical personnel, nurses, athletes, coaches, and trainers to prevent and accurately recognize heatstroke as well as to initiate immediate cooling cannot be overestimated. Common mistakes include administration of fluids to comatose patients or delay of cooling.

Proper emergency management includes removal from direct sunlight, removal of clothing, wetting the body surface, and fanning to move air and thereby promote vaporization. When such simple measures are undertaken on the spot, some victims awaken. Most require aggressive cooling in the hospital. A thermistor probe temperature device should be inserted high in the rectum to record core temperature. Tracheal intubation is advisable.

Conventional cooling techniques include immersion in ice water while the skin is rubbed briskly or placing the patient on a stretcher, rubbing the skin with ice bags while keeping the skin wet, and moving air over the skin to promote vaporization of the water. Rapid cooling by ice water immersion may cause cutaneous vasoconstriction, shivering, and convulsions. Immersion in cool water (11°C) may facilitate cooling with equal speed by avoiding cutaneous vasoconstriction. Ice water by gavage or enema is hazardous and may cause water intoxication.

Hypotension often responds to cooling alone, but if it persists, 0.5 liter of normal saline should be infused. Hypotension not responding to such quantities of saline suggests myocardial or capillary injury, and vasopressor support may be necessary. The stomach should be emptied, since vomiting and aspiration often occur during cooling. Cooling should be stopped when core temperature reaches 39°C to avoid progressive hypothermia.

Steroids are generally unnecessary. Hypokalemia and hypophosphatemia are very common in the acute phase but usually resolve quickly without treatment. Glucose may be necessary for hypoglycemia. Although lactic acidosis usually responds to volume expansion, if it persists in the absence of hypotension, 44 to 88 mEq of sodium bicarbonate may be helpful. Other complications described earlier should be anticipated, and appropriate measures taken as necessary.

MALIGNANT HYPERTHERMIA. This rare but serious disorder, representing an idiosyncratic reaction to general anesthesia, is discussed in Ch. 507.

MINOR DISORDERS RELATED TO HEAT STRESS. *Heat edema* is a transient, benign disorder that occurs during initial exposure to hot weather. It appears to result from aldosterone-mediated salt and water retention (a physiologic adaptation) and usually disappears spontaneously with continued heat exposure. It seldom, if ever, requires treatment. Diuretics should not be administered. *Miliaria* (heat rash) is caused by sweat gland occlusion. Its medical importance is enhanced, since it may impair sweat formation and evaporative heat loss.

Heat syncope is typified by simple fainting after prolonged standing in the heat. Salt and water losses induced by sweating and heat-induced vasodilatation of the superficial blood vessels contribute. When acclimatization occurs, the associated retention of salt and water corrects the problem. Besides syncope, findings usually include slight tachycardia and moist skin. Fever is absent. Recovery occurs rapidly if the patient is allowed to remain supine. Removal from the heat and administration of lightly salted liquids are helpful.

Hart GR, Anderson RJ, Crumpler CP, et al.: Epidemic classical heat stroke: Clinical characteristics and course of 28 patients. Medicine 61:189, 1982. *A detailed presentation of classic heatstroke, emphasizing the important roles of medications that impair heat loss and pre-existent disease in its pathogenesis. It also presents a detailed analysis of laboratory abnormalities commonly observed in this illness.*

Jones TS, Liang AP, Kilbourne EM, et al.: Morbidity and mortality associated with the July 1980 heat wave in St. Louis and Kansas City, Mo. JAMA 247:3327, 1982. *A report illustrating increased death rates during heat waves.*

Knochel JP: Catastrophic medical events with exhaustive exercise: "White collar rhabdomyolysis." Kidney Int 38:709, 1990.

Knochel JP, Reed G: Disorders of heat regulation. *In* Maxwell MH, Kleeman CR, Narins RG (eds.): Clinical Disorders of Fluid and Electrolyte Metabolism.

4th ed. New York, McGraw-Hill Book Company, 1986, pp 1197–1232. *A review of environmental heat illness, pharmacologic and endocrine hyperthermia, malignant hyperthermia, and hypothermic disorders.*

HYPOTHERMIA

Hypothermia, defined as a core temperature of less than 35°C, is a medical emergency that occurs in both temperate and cold environments. Its prompt recognition is critical to avoid serious morbidity or death. When body temperature declines, heat production increases by shivering, and heat loss is reduced by decreasing cutaneous blood flow. Reduction of core temperature decreases the rate of chemical reactions, so that cooling proceeds until a new equilibrium is established between the body and its environment.

As hypothermia develops, cerebral blood flow declines. The resulting fall in nutrient availability is offset by a reduction in brain metabolism. This fall in metabolic demand permits successful cerebral resuscitation of hypothermic patients even after prolonged periods of anoxia and circulatory arrest.

PATHOGENESIS. The causes of hypothermia seen in clinical practice are summarized in Table 532–3. Advanced age, disorders causing hypometabolism, central nervous system disease, malnutrition, a variety of drugs, and exposure commonly cause hypothermia. In elderly persons, hypothermia, hyperventilation, hypotension, and thrombocytopenia are common signs of bacteremia and sepsis.

CLINICAL MANIFESTATIONS. A decline in mental status, ataxia, tremulous speech, and hyperreflexia appear as temperature falls to about 32°C. At lower temperatures, hyporeflexia, stupor, dysarthria, and sluggish pupillary responses appear. Shivering usually stops below 32°C. Muscle rigidity becomes prominent. Established hypothermia reduces heart rate, blood pressure, peripheral vascular resistance, cardiac output, and central venous pressure. Creatine phosphokinase (MB isoenzyme) may increase with severe hypothermia without evidence of myocardial infarction, suggesting myocardial cellular damage. Atrial arrhythmias are usually benign. Ventricular ectopic beats may herald ventricular fibrillation, an imminent danger if core temperature becomes less than 28°C. Stimulation, such as urethral catheterization, movement, endotracheal intubation, and vascular catheterization, also predisposes to the development of this arrhythmia. Osborn waves, characterized by a widening of the base of the QRS complex and J point deflection, are the most characteristic ECG findings. They can be seen with hypothermia from any cause and do not herald the onset of ventricular fibrillation. Early tachypnea and respiratory alkalosis are replaced by progressive hypoventilation. Advancing hypothermia leads to carbon dioxide retention and respiratory acidosis. Shivering increases lactic acid production and hypoxia in muscles and may cause severe lactic acidosis.

In early hypothermia, hypokalemia may be caused by respiratory alkalosis. At lower temperatures, potassium becomes trapped inside cells despite acidosis and hypercarbia. During therapeutic rewarming, hyperkalemia may become important and contribute to arrhythmias.

TREATMENT. Significant hypothermia is a medical emergency. When it is suspected, an estimate of core temperature should be obtained by inserting a thermistor probe high into the rectum. Esophageal temperature probes are difficult to place

TABLE 532–3. CAUSES OF HYPOTHERMIA

Exposure plus:

I. Central nervous system disease	III. Interference with muscle movement
Brain tumor, injury, seizure	Paralysis, paresis
Cord transection	Extremes of age
Hypoglycemia	Drugs
Thiamine deficiency	Alcohol
Uremia	Phenothiazines
Hepatic failure	Hypothyroidism
II. Interference with vasoconstriction	IV. Mixed causes
Drugs	Starvation
Alcohol	Adrenal insufficiency
Phenothiazines	Hypothyroidism
Sepsis	Hypopituitarism
Erythroderma	

properly and may precipitate ventricular arrhythmias or fibrillation.

Airway patency must be ensured in comatose patients, and steps should be taken to prevent aspiration of gastric contents. A large intravenous catheter should be inserted, and thiamine and glucose given immediately in appropriate situations. Stimulation of the patient should be minimized to avoid precipitating ventricular fibrillation. Blood pressure, pulse, temperature, electrocardiogram, neurologic status, and urine output should be monitored frequently during rewarming.

A warming rate of about 0.5°C per hour is generally accepted as optimal. Most shivering patients spontaneously rewarm at a rate equal to or greater than this. *Passive* rewarming with blankets is ideal for hemodynamically stable, moderately hypothermic patients. This method allows a rise of 0.5 to 1°C per hour if the initial core temperature is greater than about 27°C. It is especially effective in patients with acute hypothermia who do not have underlying disease. *Active* rewarming becomes necessary in patients with severe hypothermia or cardiopulmonary arrest or both. This is especially important in patients with ventricular fibrillation or asystole because the hypothermic myocardium is resistant to mechanical or pharmacologic intervention until temperatures are above 28°C to 30°C. In such instances, warming by extracorporeal perfusion has been employed.

"Rewarming shock" and accentuated lactic acidosis have been most commonly encountered with active external rewarming techniques, i.e., heat applied to the surface of the body with hot water bottles or immersion in warm water. To avoid these problems, rapid rewarming of core blood has been attempted by several means in patients with severe hypothermia or cardiac arrest. Most patients with hypothermia tolerate warm intravenous fluids and heated oxygen. If rapid rewarming is required, peritoneal lavage with solutions warmed to about 40°C is effective.

Supportive measures may be very important. Because of the wide diversity of electrolyte derangements in hypothermic patients, no general recommendations can be made regarding fluid management other than warming the fluid to 37 to 40°C before administration. Plasma volume expanders may be given if the central venous pressure is low. Oxygen and bicarbonate should be given if serious metabolic acidosis exists. Subsequent metabolic alkalosis and its adverse effects on oxyhemoglobin dissociation, calcium, and ventricular irritability must be avoided. As patients are rewarmed, metabolic acidosis may worsen as lactate is washed out of previously hypoxic tissues. Recognition and treatment of this phenomenon are important to reduce the risk of ventricular fibrillation and cardiovascular collapse. Severe respiratory impairment with significant carbon dioxide retention should be treated with assisted ventilation. Ventilatory adjustments should be made with respect to reduced carbon dioxide production. Hypoglycemia should be suspected in any patient with hypothermia. Hyperglycemia should be treated only if severe and potentially life threatening. Vasopressors should be avoided if possible because of their ability to induce ventricular arrhythmias. Drugs with significant depressing effects on the myocardium, such as quinidine and propranolol, should be avoided. Thyroxine should be given only if significant hypothyroidism is suspected.

Burnet RW, Noonan DC: Calculations and correction factors used in determination of blood pH and blood gases. Clin Chem 20:1499, 1974.
Fitzgerald FR, Jessop C: Accidental hypothermia: A report of 22 cases and review of the literature. Adv Intern Med 27:127, 1982. Reuler JB: Hypothermia: Pathophysiology, clinical settings, and management. Ann Intern Med 89:519, 1978. *These two articles are excellent clinical reviews of hypothermia as seen in medical practice, with discussions of differential diagnosis, clinical manifestations, and treatment.*
Matz R: Hypothermia: Mechanisms and countermeasures. Hosp Pract 21:45, 1986. *This is a comprehensive presentation of the pathophysiology of hypothermia and its management.*

533 Trace Metal Poisoning

Donald B. Louria

Many trace elements, both metals and nonmetals, are capable of causing human disease. In some cases poisoning is a consequence of workplace exposure. In others the disease results from

use of prescription or nonprescription medicines or as an adverse effect of medical procedures such as hemodialysis or insertion of prosthetic devices. Occasionally trace element poisoning results from attempts at suicide or homicide.

Over the past few decades, increased awareness of the health consequences of industrial substances, more stringent federal and state regulations, and fear of lawsuits have resulted in a healthier workplace. However, the majority of the potentially exposed work force is employed by small industries that may not have plant physicians or insist on proper worker protection.

We know a great deal about overwhelming exposure that results in acute illness, but our knowledge of the subtle consequences of chronic, low-level trace element exposure is still grossly inadequate. This is well illustrated by lead exposure. Acute lead poisoning in children or adults is readily diagnosed, but we are only beginning to understand the consequences of increased body lead burdens in the absence of the anemia, colic, or clinically apparent encephalopathy.

The interrelationships between trace elements are also poorly understood. For example, copper smelter workers are exposed not only to copper but also to lead, zinc, arsenic, gold, silver, cadmium, and mercury; in these workers pneumonitis or other acute illnesses may result from two or more metals acting in concert. In other instances excesses or deficits of a trace element may act indirectly by inducing deficiency or toxicity of another trace element.

LEAD

ETIOLOGY. In the past lead poisoning was ascribed to pica (abnormal ingestion) among children living in dilapidated houses with peeling layers of lead-based paints. In the past two decades lead intoxication has occurred with increasing frequency in less socioeconomically deprived areas of the cities, as well as in more affluent suburbs. This may in part be related to environmental contamination from leaded gasoline; several studies relate environmental lead contamination to traffic density patterns. Contaminated soil is also a well-described source of lead.

In the United States, hundreds of occupations entail potentially significant exposure. It is estimated that more than 800,000 American workers have potentially significant lead exposure. Lead and other metal smelter workers or miners, welders, storage battery workers, and pottery makers are particularly heavily exposed. Workers in auto manufacturing, ship building, paint manufacture, and printing industries are also at substantial risk, as are house painters and those who repair old houses.

Lead-soldered kettles and cans and lead-glazed pottery can release lead when acidic fluids are stored or cooked in them; the latter appears to be a particularly worrisome problem in nursing homes and on psychiatric units. Demolition workers and those employed in firing ranges have become poisoned from intensive aerosol exposure. In the southern United States, moonshine whiskey is an important cause of poisoning. The stills are connected with lead solder, and old radiators containing lead are used as condensers; 20 to 90 per cent of moonshine samples contain lead in the potentially toxic range.

In past centuries lead was added to wine to sweeten it, a deception that was eventually made punishable by death. Recently, addition of lead to aphrodisiacs and various herbal and folk medicines has resulted in poisoning. Retained bullets can result in lead poisoning, especially if host metabolic changes favor lead mobilization or if a joint or bone is involved, since synovial fluid appears to be a good solvent for lead. The interval between lodging of the bullet and clinical evidence of lead poisoning has ranged from 2 days to 40 years. Lead poisoning has also occurred in adults who have eaten fowl and inadvertently ingested lead pellets that have lodged in the appendix. Children have been poisoned by swallowing lead household objects, such as lead curtain weights, that are then retained in the gastrointestinal tract for a prolonged time.

Gasoline sniffing for hedonistic purposes can produce lead poisoning; the organic tetraethyl lead appears to have a proclivity for the nervous system.

In a sense we are all lead poisoned; prior to the Industrial Revolution the total body burden of lead was about 2 mg, whereas currently in industrialized societies the whole body content is about 200 mg. One hundred fifty to 250 µg per day is ingested, 5 to 10 per cent of which is absorbed. In children the percentage is higher and absorption is facilitated by iron, calcium, magnesium, and perhaps zinc deficiency. Aerosol exposure is especially likely to result in poisoning, since approximately 40 per cent of inhaled lead is absorbed.

CLINICAL MANIFESTATIONS. The major toxic effects of lead are referable to the abdomen, the blood, and the nervous system.

Gastrointestinal Tract. The exact pathogenesis of lead colic remains uncertain; in part it appears to be due to a direct effect of lead on smooth muscle. The crampy, diffuse, often intractable abdominal pain may be accompanied by nausea, vomiting, anorexia, constipation, or occasionally diarrhea. The pain may be confined to the epigastric, periumbilical, or other areas of the abdomen and may simulate a variety of surgical and nonsurgical diseases. Lead-induced megacolon has been reported.

Blood. Lead interferes with a variety of red cell enzyme systems, including delta-aminolevulinic acid dehydratase and ferrochelatase. The former is needed for the conjugation of levulinic acid to form porphobilinogen; the latter facilitates the incorporation of iron into protoporphyrin IX (see Fig. 131–2). The red cell abnormalities include punctate basophilic stippling and clover leaf morphology. Anemia is frequent in severe acute lead poisoning and may be normocytic normochromic or microcytic hypochromic. An inherited deficiency in delta-aminolevulinic acid dehydratase can sensitize the individual to lead intoxication and result in the appearance of symptoms of acute lead poisoning at modest blood lead levels.

Nervous System. Either the brain or the peripheral nerves may be involved. The central nervous system (CNS) symptoms at first are vague and are often mistakenly disregarded. These manifestations include irritability, incoordination, memory lapses, labile affect, sleep disturbances, restlessness, listlessness, paranoia, headache, lethargy, and dizziness. In more serious cases manifestations include syncope-like attacks, disorientation, flaccidity, more intense headache, severe mental impairment, ataxia, vomiting, cranial nerve palsies, localized neurologic signs, psychosis, somnolence, seizures, blindness, and coma. Severe lead encephalopathy is not restricted to children. Occasionally the brain manifestations mimic a space-occupying lesion. The cerebrospinal fluid may be under increased pressure and may show an increased protein content, a modest pleocytosis (predominantly lymphocytic), and, rarely, diminished glucose levels. Papilledema has been reported, as have grayish deposits surrounding the optic disc and optic atrophy. Frank encephalopathy is an ominous prognostic sign in regard to both mortality and persistent brain damage. Most children who experience two or more bouts of clinically evident encephalopathy have neurologic residua.

The peripheral nerve involvement, seen more often in adults than in children, is almost always exclusively motor and involves muscle groups used extensively. Wrist drop and foot drop are seen most often; the former, depending on type of occupation, may be asymmetric, and there may be paresthesias.

The spinal cord may also be involved, manifestations having some similarity to those of amyotrophic lateral sclerosis.

Tetraethyl lead poisoning causes euphoria, nervousness, insomnia, hallucinations, convulsions, and sometimes frank psychosis.

There is increasing evidence of subtle brain damage in the absence of clinical evidence of encephalopathy. Inordinate body burdens of lead may result in mentation difficulties, emotional lability, deficits in intelligence and memory, impaired psychomotor and visual motor function, slowed nerve conduction, and behavioral aberrations in both children and adults, even in the absence of overt evidence of poisoning. These changes may occur at blood levels of 25 to 60 µg per deciliter (or even less in young children). Long-term effects of low-level exposure in childhood include poor performance in school.

Other Clinical Manifestations. In adults the kidneys are often involved (see Ch. 80), the characteristic lesion being interstitial nephritis; as the disease progresses, glomerular filtration rate falls. In children, Fanconi's syndrome, characterized by glycosuria, aminoaciduria, and phosphaturia, may occur transiently; and occasionally, asymptomatic renal failure supervenes. Lead

TABLE 533–1. POSITIVE SCREENING TESTS INDICATING UNDUE LEAD ABSORPTION

Whole-blood lead	Children	> 25 µg/dl
	Adults	> 40 µg/dl*
Whole-blood erythrocyte protoporphyrin or zinc protoporphyrin	Children	> 35 µg/dl*
	Adults	> 50 µg/dl

*This value is unsettled.

poisoning appears to be responsible for some cases of renal failure associated with either gout or hypertension, and there is increasing suspicion based on epidemiologic studies that the level of systolic or diastolic blood pressure may be in part related to blood lead concentrations.

Polyarthralgias, mild hepatic dysfunction, and dysuria may occur. Occasionally arrhythmias and cardiomegaly have been reported, as have abnormalities of liver function. A gingival blue, blue-black, or gray line is found in up to 20 per cent of adult patients but is infrequent in children.

Lead readily crosses the placenta and is thought to be responsible for an increased incidence of spontaneous abortion and miscarriage. Some studies suggest lead poisoning may result in hypospermia and other sperm abnormalities. Teratogenic effects occur in lead-treated animals, but congenital abnormalities have not been convincingly documented in humans. Lead exposure may also result in transient chromosomal breakage. Placental transfer of lead stored in the maternal skeleton can reduce neonatal growth.

DIAGNOSIS. A high index of suspicion and a careful examination of the peripheral blood for basophilic stippling are mandatory. The interference with delta-aminolevulinic acid dehydratase results in marked increase in delta-aminolevulinic acid in the urine. Urinary coproporphyrin levels are also increased. Lead interferes with incorporation of iron into heme and zinc and then replaces the iron to form zinc protoporphyrin (ZPP). The latter or its hydrolysis product, erythrocyte protoporphyrin (EP), can be measured rapidly fluorometrically; both EP and ZPP are reliable indicators of lead poisoning. EP and ZPP elevations also occur in patients suffering from iron deficiency anemia or erythropoietic protoporphyria. Table 533–1 lists some indications of undue lead absorption.

Blood aminolevulinic acid dehydratase activity can also be measured directly. Blood lead levels are readily determined by atomic absorption spectrophotometry or anodic stripping voltometry. Specimens can be obtained by either venipuncture or finger stick; the latter technique is often difficult to interpret because of skin contamination. Urine lead concentrations can also be measured; if concentrations are normal, increased body burdens can still be detected by measuring urinary lead excretion after administration of calcium disodium edetate (Table 533–2). This test is particularly useful in assessing lead storage in bones.

Additional industrial exposure should not be permitted if blood levels exceed 40 µg per deciliter or if there is any increase in EP or ZPP.

More than 90 per cent of the body stores of lead are retained in bone, with a biologic half-life of several decades. Blood lead,

TABLE 533–2. CaNa₂ EDTA LEAD MOBILIZATION TEST

	Children	Adults
Normal premobilization test	< 100 µg/day	< 150 µg/day
	Normal	
Post-CaNa₂ EDTA, 50 mg/kg IM or IV or 500–1000 mg/m² (children); or 1 gm IM* × 2, 12 hours apart, or 1–2 gm IV (adults)	< 0.60 µg Pb/mg CaNa₂ EDTA† administered over 8- to 24-hour collection period	< 650 µg/day
	Increased Body Burden	
	> 0.60 µg Pb/mg CaNa₂ EDTA administered	> 650 µg/dl

*Procaine must be used with intramuscular injections.
†EDTA = edetate.

TABLE 533-3. LEVELS OF CHRONIC LEAD EXPOSURE BODY BURDENS IN ADULTS

Exposure	Blood Pb (μg/dl)	EDTA Test (μg Pb/day)	Tibial* [Pb] (μg/g)
1. Low ambient	< 25	< 600	< 20
2. Moderate (intermittent)	25–50	600–1000	20–40
3. High (industrial)	> 50	> 1000	> 40

*Wet weight. Determined by in vivo tibial KXRF.

on the other hand, has a biologic half-life of only a few weeks. Bone lead is therefore a better indicator of cumulative lead absorption. The bone lead concentration can be measured in vitro in biopsy samples or in vivo noninvasively using x-ray fluorescence (XRF). The relationship between blood lead (assuming relatively constant exposure), chelatable lead, and bone lead in adults is illustrated in Table 533-3.

TREATMENT. Three agents are used that form tight complexes with lead and thus promote its elimination from tissues (Table 533-4). Dimercaprol (British antilewisite, BAL) is given in oil intramuscularly; calcium disodium edetate (calcium versenate) can be given either intramuscularly or intravenously; and D-penicillamine is administered by mouth. Chelation should be undertaken only after careful consideration in those with milder evidence of poisoning, because each of the agents may be associated with significant adverse effects. Because most of the body lead is stored in the bones, clinical improvement and reduction in blood lead levels (or reduction in EP or ZPP) may be followed by increases in blood lead concentrations and clinical evidence of repoisoning owing to mobilization of lead from bone. In such cases chelating agents should again be administered. The newer, less toxic oral dimercaprol analogues dimercaptosuccinic acid and dimercaptopropanesulfonate may be effective.

Treatment is ordinarily successful in extra-CNS disease but is not predictably effective in patients with encephalopathy. Various degrees of mentation deficits may remain in both children and adults. Among adults the frequency of residual brain deficits is not clearly established.

Current acceptable blood concentrations of lead for children are 25 μg per deciliter, and permissible levels for adults are up to 40 μg per deciliter, including those industrially exposed (30 μg per deciliter or less is recommended for pregnant women); but there is mounting evidence that significant toxicity can occur at lower levels and that acceptable concentrations should be further reduced to 15 μg per deciliter or less for children and pregnant women and less than 30 μg per deciliter for adults. Blood lead levels have fallen in the United States (and some other countries) in the past 15 years, but millions of children and

TABLE 533-4. CHELATION REGIMENS

	Children*	Adults*	Duration
CaNa₂ EDTA	50 mg/kg/day IM† or IV, or 1500 mg/m²/24 hr (severe disease); 1000 mg/m²/day (mild-moderate intoxication)	1.0 gram IV in 5% dextrose twice daily, or 2.0 grams/day IM in divided doses; longer term, 1 gram IM 3× per week† until lead burden reduced to satisfactory levels	3 to 5 days
BAL	3 mg/kg/dose IM, or 300–450 mg/m²/24 hr IM	2.5 mg/kg/dose IM	3 to 5 days
	(Given in divided doses every 4 hr)		
Penicillamine	30 mg/kg/day PO	1.0–1.5 grams/day PO	Until blood lead and FEP‡ levels approach normal§

*CaNa₂ EDTA and BAL are ordinarily used together for symptomatic illness.
†Procaine must be used for IM injections of CaNa₂ EDTA.
‡FEP = free erythrocyte protoporphyrin.
§Must be monitored carefully, since toxicity occurs in up to 20% of cases.

adults are still exposed to potentially toxic levels that could be responsible for subtle mental changes, hyperactivity, aggressiveness, and antisocial behavior.

More than 20 years ago, the extraordinary scientist and philosopher Rene Dubos observed: "The problem is so well-defined, so neatly packaged with both causes and cures known, that if we don't eliminate this social crime, our society deserves all the disasters that have been forecast for it." Amen.

Agency for Toxic Substances and Disease Registry, Public Health Service, U.S. Department of Health and Human Services: The nature and extent of lead poisoning in children in the United States. A Report to Congress, 1988. *This is a comprehensive and authoritative review of the sources and implications of lead poisoning in childhood.*

Baker EL, White RF, Pothier LJ, et al.: Occupational lead neurotoxicity: Improvement in behavioral effects after reduction of exposure. Br J Indust Med 42:507, 1985. *This is one of a growing number of articles that together offer a reasonably persuasive argument that significant defects in brain function occur in lead-exposed persons who do not exhibit evidence of obvious poisoning and whose blood lead levels in the past would have been considered in the acceptable range. Thirty-one references.*

Batuman V, Landy E, Maesaka JK, et al.: Contribution of lead to hypertension with renal impairment. N Engl J Med 309:17, 1983. Batuman V, Maesaka JK, Haddad B, et al.: The role of lead in gout nephropathy. N Engl J Med 304:520, 1981. *These two articles present reasonably compelling evidence that renal dysfunction associated with either hypertension or gout may be related to lead intoxication in a small but important percentage of such cases.*

Landrigan PJ: Toxicity of lead at low dose. Br J Indust Med 46:593, 1989. *A brief but solid analysis. Fifty-nine references.*

Needleman HL: The persistent threat of lead: Medical and sociological issues. Curr Probl Pediatr 18:703, 1988. *Another good article on toxicity at "low levels," with a major focus on societal effects. One hundred ten references.*

Needleman HL, Schell A, Bellinger D, et al.: The long-term effects of exposure to low doses of lead in childhood. An 11 year follow-up report. N Engl J Med 322:83, 1990. *This important, although still controversial, article gives substantial support for the notion that subtle lead poisoning in childhood can result in significant psychosocial defects later in life.*

Wedeen RP: In vivo tibial XRF measurement of bone lead (editorial). Arch Environ Health 45:69, 1990. *A summary of currently available methods for assessing cumulative lead absorption.*

Whitfield CL, Ch'ien LT, Whitehead JD: Lead encephalopathy in adults. Am J Med 52:289, 1972. *Twenty-three adults exposed to moonshine developed encephalopathy, manifestations ranging from confusion to coma, seizures, and death. This article emphasizes that encephalopathy can be a major problem in adults. Chelation therapy appeared to be effective.*

MERCURY

ETIOLOGY. Mercury has been used for at least 2000 years. At present more than 60 occupations involve mercury exposure. These include chloralkali work; manufacture of pesticides, insecticides, and fungicides; manufacture of mercury-containing instruments, lamps, neon lights, batteries, paper, paint, dye, electrical equipment, and jewelry; and dentistry. The exposure in dental offices has diminished substantially in recent years.

In addition to occupational or industrial exposure, poisoning has resulted from inadvertent contamination of grains by mercury-containing pesticides as well as from accidental or intentional ingestion or injection of elemental mercury or mercury-containing compounds. In the past, mercury was administered medicinally as a component of cathartics, teething powders, and anthelmintics. Mercury compounds are now rarely used as diuretics.

CLINICAL MANIFESTATIONS AND TREATMENT. The biologic effects, tissue distribution, and toxicity of mercury depend on the form in which it is introduced into the body. Mercury possesses a strong affinity for sulfhydryl, amine, phosphoryl, and carboxyl groups and inactivates a wide variety of enzymes. Mercury poisoning can be conveniently divided into four categories.

Metallic Mercury. Elemental mercury is a liquid at environmental temperatures but vaporizes with agitation as well as gentle heating. Bulk mercury is used in dental amalgams; up to 10 per cent of dental offices have been found to have excessive mercury vapor levels; and accidental spillage has occurred occasionally in homes or offices. There is increasing concern about the potential health consequences from slow intraoral leakage of mercury from dental amalgams. The greatest exposure to metallic mercury is in industry. Additionally, many workers are potentially exposed because of the widespread use of mercury in electrical equipment. Heavy aerosol exposure to mercury produces chills, fever, cough, chest pain, and hemoptysis; roentgenograms show diffuse pulmonary infiltrates. Inhaled elemental mercury is readily absorbed from the alveoli; thereafter the target tissue is the brain. With mild exposure the manifestations are likely to be subtle and diagnosis is difficult. Insomnia, nervousness, mild tremor, impaired judgment and coordination, decreased mental efficiency, emotional lability, headache, fatigue, loss of sexual drive, and depression are early manifestations and are often mistakenly ascribed to psychogenic causes. These symptoms have been referred to as micromercurialism. Abdominal cramps, dermatitis, and diarrhea may also occur, and the victim may complain of a metallic taste. As the poisoning becomes more severe, persistent involuntary tremors of the extremities are noted. Thereafter, other signs of mercury poisoning may appear, including amblyopia, polyneuropathy, erythroderma, acrodynia, joint pains, swollen gums with a blue line around the teeth, sialorrhea, and paresthesias. The major manifestation of mercury vapor exposure may be renal damage, including the nephrotic syndrome.

Blood and urine levels may be unreliable, and clear evidence of poisoning may be documented only after administration of drugs that augment mercury excretion in the urine.

In most cases improvement occurs after removal from exposure or treatment with either dimercaprol (BAL) or N-acetyl penicillamine.

The effects of ingestion of even large amounts of metallic mercury range from no clinical disturbance to local gastrointestinal irritation to CNS damage. Aspiration of liquid mercury is also usually benign, although roentgenologic visualization of mercury globules may be evident for many years. After intravenous injection of mercury, there may be no abnormalities other than roentgenologic densities or an illness ranging from mild to lethal, with hepatic, renal, lung, and CNS dysfunction.

The wide range of clinical findings after elemental mercury exposure appears to relate in part to the rate of oxidation to mercuric salts and the rapidity of their subsequent excretion through the kidneys, saliva, and urine.

Inorganic Mercury. Exposure to $HgCl_2$ and Hg_2Cl_2 occurs primarily in industry and results from ingestion. $HgCl_2$ is far more toxic than Hg_2Cl_2. The major manifestations are renal and include proteinuria, granular casts in the urinary sediment, the nephrotic syndrome, and pyuria from tubular damage. In some cases severe oliguria, and even anuria, may occur. Additionally, diarrhea, abdominal pain, hepatic dysfunction, and lesser evidence of CNS disease may be found (micromercurialism). Rhabdomyolysis with striking muscle enzyme elevation and acrodynia have also been reported. In this type of mercury poisoning, BAL or penicillamine is usually effective.

Organomercurials with Rapid Metabolism to Inorganic Mercury. Included are phenyl and methoxyethyl mercury salts found in diuretics and fungicides. Toxicity is limited and usually renal.

Short-Chain Alkyl Mercury Compounds. Methyl mercury is far more toxic than ethyl or diethyl mercury; the latter produces primarily renal abnormalities.

Methyl mercury is well absorbed from the intestinal tract, is widely distributed in the body, and readily passes through the placenta into the fetus and also into breast milk. About 10 per cent localizes in the brain, and the ensuing damage is largely irreversible. Major epidemics have resulted from industrial contamination of water, with subsequent biotransformation of elemental and inorganic mercury into methyl mercury, followed by ingestion by fish and then by humans. Other epidemics have resulted from use of grains contaminated by organic mercurial pesticides or animal ingestion of seeds treated with mercury. The epidemics in the Minamata and Niigata regions of Japan and in Iraq, Guatemala, Pakistan, and the United States have resulted in a high death rate and an appalling amount of permanent brain damage. In addition to the milder symptoms listed under elemental mercury poisoning, CNS manifestations include severe paresthesias, dysarthria, ataxia, visual field constriction, hearing loss, blindness, microcephaly, spasticity, paralysis, and coma. Some of the children of methyl mercury–poisoned mothers show various degrees of cerebral palsy–like abnormalities and mental retardation, and some die.

Chang LW: Neurotoxic effects of mercury—a review. Environ Res 14:329, 1977. *A very useful review with good clinical-pathologic correlations.*

Elhassani SB: The many faces of methylmercury poisoning. J Toxicol Clin Toxicol 19:875, 1982–1983. *A very nice, thorough review with 133 references.*

Joselow MM, Louria DB, Browder AA: Mercurialism: Environmental and occupational aspects. Ann Intern Med 76:119, 1972. *A useful summary with 149 references.*

Magos L: Mercury and mercurials. Br Med Bull 31:241, 1975. *A concise, valuable summary of the clinical manifestations and tissue localization after exposure to different chemical forms of mercury.*

Scarlett JM, Gutenmann WH, Lisk DJ: A study of mercury in the hair of dentists and dental-related professionals in 1985 and subcohort comparison of 1972 and 1985 mercury hair levels. J Toxicol Environ Health 25:373, 1988. *Exposure, currently reduced in intensity, can apparently result either from inhalation or by a direct nose-brain pathway.*

ARSENIC

ETIOLOGY. Arsenic is ubiquitous in nature; it is present in the earth's crust in concentrations of 2 to 5 parts per billion. It is found in inordinately high concentrations in some well water. It is used in the glass, pigment, textile, tanning, and bronze-plating industries; in wood preservation; in a variety of metal alloys; in veterinary medicines; in some herbicides, insecticides, and rodenticides; in fire salts to produce multicolored flames; and by farmers and vintners. American industry uses about one half of the world's production of arsenic trioxide. Arsenic poisoning has also resulted from using certain herbal preparations, from the ingestion of illegal (moonshine) whiskey, from the burning of arsenate-treated wood, and from the administration of arsenic-containing prescription medicines.

Elemental arsenic is not toxic even if ingested in substantial amounts. There are three toxic forms of arsenic: pentavalent salts, trivalent salts, and arsine gas. The arsenic in the earth's crust and in most foods is in the pentavalent form. Trivalent arsenic, which is far more toxic, accumulates in the body more readily than the pentavalent form. Arsenic gas (arsine) is extraordinarily toxic; it is formed by the hydrolysis of metallic arsenide or by the action of acids or nascent hydrogen on arsenical compounds, especially in the refining of certain metals. Arsine is also manufactured for and used in the electronics industry. Arsine can be liberated in sewage plants, and in one small cluster of cases, eight children were poisoned while cleaning out a cattle dip in Australia.

CLINICAL MANIFESTATIONS. *Arsine gas* poisoning is usually overwhelming and frequently fatal. The onset of symptoms after exposure is usually between 1 and 12 hours. Fever, headache, muscle pains, nausea, vomiting, epigastric pain, dysuria, and explosive diarrhea characterize the acute episode. Because arsenic preferentially binds to red blood cells, hemolytic anemia and hemoglobinuria occur early, and red cell ghosts may be seen in the peripheral blood. There may also be cyanosis and profound hypoxia. Renal failure due to acute tubular necrosis (occasionally due to cortical necrosis) occurs in the first few days after onset of symptoms. This may be accompanied by shock and encephalopathy, characterized by agitation and disorientation. Both bone marrow depression and myocardial damage may occur. Those who do not die of intractable vascular collapse often develop subacute manifestations of arsenic poisoning, described below. Those who recover may develop chronic renal failure.

Arsenic Ingestion. Although arsine gas poisoning can be mimicked by arsenic ingestion, the latter is usually more insidious and less overwhelming. Cramping abdominal pain and diarrhea are characteristic. Other acute manifestations include nausea, vomiting, dysphagia, cyanosis, headache, hematuria, and weakness. Hyperesthesia, muscle cramps, conjunctivitis, syncope, excessive thirst, periorbital swelling, epistaxis, and tinnitus may also occur. The patient may complain of a metallic taste, and there may be a garlic odor to the breath, but the latter is not pathognomonic, since it also may be observed in selenium, tellurium, and phosphorus poisoning.

Leukopenia occurs frequently, but in some cases moderate leukocytosis is found and both monocytosis and eosinophilia have been described. Anemia and thrombocytopenia may supervene.

Shortly after the initial red cell binding, arsenic can be found in liver, spleen, heart, kidneys, brain, and intestinal tract. Skin, nails, and hair do not usually contain arsenic until 2 to 4 weeks after exposure, but occasionally hair accumulation can occur more rapidly.

Other manifestations that may occur in the first week include jaundice; hepatomegaly with hepatic enzyme abnormalities; electrocardiographic abnormalities; a cardiomyopathy that can be lethal; pericarditis; rhabdomyolysis; pulmonary edema; evidence of encephalopathy, including headache, irritability, confusion, delusions, and hallucinations; seizures; renal dysfunction; kidney failure with acute tubular necrosis; and respiratory muscle paralysis. Megaloblastic changes may be seen in the bone marrow. Optic neuritis with visual field constriction has been reported after pentavalent arsenic exposure.

The most prominent manifestation after the first week of illness is symmetric polyneuropathy. At first, sensory manifestations predominate, the patient complaining of a burning sensation in a stocking-glove distribution. Motor involvement follows almost immediately with diminished or absent reflexes and severe weakness. Occasionally the neuropathy is unilateral. Prolonged encephalopathy and/or psychosis has been reported in a few instances.

In cases of subacute poisoning, Aldrich-Mees lines (transverse white bands) may be seen in the nails; like the garlic odor, these may be seen in other trace element intoxications. Erythroderma and exfoliative dermatitis may also supervene.

Chronic exposure is associated with several abnormalities. The most characteristic of these are the cutaneous lesions, particularly hyperpigmentation (arsenic melanosis) and hyperkeratoses located primarily on the palms and soles. Alopecia and so-called raindrop depigmentation may also occur. In about 5 to 10 per cent of those chronically exposed, skin cancers appear after latent periods of 5 to more than 25 years; these tend to be multiple, are situated mainly on the trunk and upper extremities, and show either intraepithelial squamous cell (Bowen's disease) or basal cell morphology on histologic examination. In the United States the most frequent cause of such skin lesions in past years was the medicinal use of Fowler's solution, an inorganic trivalent arsenical. Currently most cases arise after occupational exposure, but a small number have been ascribed to chronic exposure to well water with high arsenic content.

Epidemiologic studies on gold ore and tin miners, vineyard workers, laborers in sheep-dip factories, and smelter workers show a clear increase in the incidence of squamous cell carcinoma of the lung, the risk of bronchogenic cancer correlating with the intensity and duration of arsenic trioxide exposure.

Several types of liver disease may occur; these include postnecrotic cirrhosis, hepatocellular carcinoma, and hemangioendothelioma. Additionally, portal fibrosis and/or sinusoidal collagenosis may be found, which can lead to a form of noncirrhotic portal hypertension with splenomegaly and esophageal varices but normal hepatic artery wedge pressure. Like the skin cancers, the liver abnormalities may occur many years after exposure to arsenic has been discontinued, and the exposure period can have been relatively brief.

Arsenic exposure is also thought to induce chromosomal aberrations, but the significance of these abnormalities is not clear.

In Taiwan, high concentrations in well water have been associated with peripheral vascular (blackfoot) disease and various cancers.

DIAGNOSIS. If the diagnosis is suspected, there is a qualitative urine test (Gutzeit test) employing sulfuric acid, zinc, and silver nitrate. Arsenic concentrations can be measured in blood, urine, hair, or nails by atomic absorption spectrophotometry or neutron activation techniques.

TREATMENT. The treatment of choice is dimercaprol (BAL), but it should be given within the first 24 hours after exposure. If the BAL is given later, it is less likely that improvement will be observed, and in most cases the peripheral neuropathy is refractory to treatment. Exchange transfusion or dialysis shortly after the onset of acute illness has also been reported to be beneficial. Penicillamine may also be useful, as may orally administered 2,3-dimercaptosuccinic acid.

The neuropathy and renal failure may slowly resolve completely, or there may be residual abnormalities that range from mild to severe.

Massey EW, Wold D, Heyman A: Homicidal intoxication. South Med J 77:848, 1984. *Four cases and a comprehensive review in four packed pages. Thirty-two references.*

Schoolmeester WL, White DR: Arsenic poisoning. South Med J 73:198, 1980. *A fine comprehensive review with 102 references. Includes 10 illustrative case reports.*

Wu MM, Kuo TL, Hwang YH, Chen CJ: Dose response relation between arsenic

concentration in well water and mortality from cancers and vascular diseases. Am J Epidemiol 130:1123, 1989. *A solid epidemiologic study. Fifty-three references.*

Zaloga GB, Deal J, Spurling T, et al.: Case report: Unusual manifestations of arsenic intoxication. Am J Med Sci 289:210, 1985. *The case (with facial palsy and pericarditis) is interesting, and the review is terrific. Twenty-eight references.*

TRACE ELEMENTS WHOSE TOXICITY IS IN LARGE PART ASSOCIATED WITH HEMODIALYSIS

ZINC. The normal adult body zinc content is 1.5 to 3.0 grams. Daily intake ranges from 5 to 35 mg. Zinc is bound to metallothioneins synthesized in the liver and kidney and is excreted by both the urine and the gastrointestinal tract. Particularly high concentrations are found in the uveal tract, choroid plexus, and prostate; substantial amounts are also found in bone, brain, skeletal muscles, and other tissues of the eye.

Zinc has a strong affinity for red cells and plasma proteins. Consequently, there is no loss across dialysis membranes; instead, blood zinc concentrations may increase markedly during hemodialysis. There appear to be two well-documented zinc sources: adhesive plaster (containing zinc oxide) used to prevent dialysis coils from unwinding and the water of the dialysis fluid. Even if water has an initially low zinc content, galvanized iron pipes or tanks may release substantial amounts. This can be prevented by using deionized or distilled water.

The manifestations of zinc toxicity do not necessarily correlate well with plasma or whole-blood zinc levels. Nausea, vomiting, anorexia, lethargy, irritability, weakness, abdominal pain, and anemia are the most frequent manifestations. The mechanisms responsible for the anemia are not well understood, but in many cases the anemia is microcytic and may be associated with copper deficiency. Zinc can decrease copper absorption in the gut and also promote urinary copper excretion. Fever may accompany zinc toxicity. Other manifestations may include diarrhea, muscle pain, lymphadenopathy, hyperamylasemia with or without pancreatitis, intestinal bleeding, thrombocytopenia, oliguria, hypotension, and renal failure with tubular necrosis. Injection of large amounts of zinc has resulted in death. Intestinal manifestations may supervene after either orally or parenterally induced zinc intoxication.

Welders, smelter workers, and solderers are exposed to aerosolized zinc and may experience zinc fume fever, characterized by chills, fever, myalgias, a metallic taste, cough, nausea, lethargy, and occasionally hemoptysis. There may be diffuse roentgenologic infiltrates and pulmonary dysfunction. Ordinarily all manifestations disappear rapidly after cessation of exposure. If more prolonged pulmonary dysfunction occurs, it is thought to result from the effects of other metals to which the workers are simultaneously exposed.

ALUMINUM. Aluminum-induced dialysis dementia is an often fatal disease. The tap water used during dialysis is often to blame. Some waters naturally contain high concentrations of aluminum. In other cases aluminum sulfate had been added to the community water supply to remove organic materials. In still other cases the dialysis fluid appeared to be less responsible than aluminum-containing gels administered by mouth to reduce phosphate levels. Indeed, if oral aluminum hydroxide is administered to nondialyzed patients suffering from renal failure, the encephalopathy syndrome can occasionally occur; young children appear to be particularly at risk. Dialysis encephalopathy occurs only after repeated dialyses, usually spanning at least several months. Peritoneal dialysis can also be complicated by encephalopathy. Use of parenteral nutrition solutions containing aluminum can also be followed by aluminum poisoning.

Early manifestations include malaise, memory loss, and a characteristic speech disturbance. As the disease progresses, dysarthria, asterixis, myoclonic twitches, dementia, somnolence, and seizures occur. The electroencephalogram shows slowing, together with bursts of delta activity and high-voltage, symmetric spikes. Among those who die, aluminum levels are markedly increased in the gray matter. The use of reverse osmosis or deionization treatment has markedly reduced the incidence of severe dialysis dementia, but there is increasing evidence of a mild form of encephalopathy in chronic dialysis patients, characterized by psychomotor dysfunction, memory defects, weakness, and mild myoclonus.

Other manifestations of aluminum intoxication include myalgias, proximal myopathy, and severe skeletal pain caused by profound osteodystrophy that is unresponsive to vitamin D and is followed by fractures. Aluminum is deposited at the calcified bone-osteoid junction, and bone formation is impaired (Ch. 234, 237). Aluminum also interferes with parathyroid function, and it may be associated with cardiomyopathy.

Aluminum toxicity is also characterized by a poorly understood microcytic anemia that may be related in part to aluminum binding to transferrin and interference with iron incorporation into heme.

Although frequently lethal, in some cases the encephalopathy has regressed after intake of oral aluminum is stopped or the aluminum content of the dialysis water is reduced or following renal transplantation. Treatment with deferoxamine (DFO), which complexes with aluminum, may be beneficial. Those suffering from uremia should avoid food additives and nonprescription drugs that contain substantial amounts of aluminum. Citrates may increase aluminum absorption, as may the H_2 receptor antagonist cimetidine. Those with uremia should also be wary of community water supplies with inordinately high concentrations of aluminum.

Serum aluminum levels often do not reflect body loads; intoxication may be documented by a DFO mobilization test. Although DFO treatment can be beneficial in both aluminum-induced encephalopathy and osteodystrophy, it can temporarily exacerbate the encephalopathy and can cause hearing and vision impairment, hypotension, and iron deficiency; it also has been associated with superinfection with Zygomycetes. DFO treatment appears to be less successful in parathyroidectomized persons. It has been suggested that Alzheimer's disease and amyotrophic lateral sclerosis may be related to brain aluminum deposition, but available data are unconvincing.

Those involved in aluminum processing or manufacturing, pottery or explosive making, or welding may be exposed to aluminum aerosols. Pulmonary granulomas, fibrosis, and in some cases postfibrosis emphysema may supervene. In bauxite smelters this is known as Shaver's disease. Those involved in aluminum smelting may develop wheezing, chest tightness, and evidence of airway obstruction (potroom asthma).

COPPER. Since the late 1960's, copper tubing in dialysis equipment has been known to release copper when exposed to acid water. Copper levels may also be inordinately high in the dialysis water if the water is supplied through copper plumbing. Copper is a potent red cell poison, damaging cell membranes and inhibiting a variety of red cell enzymes. Major manifestations of toxicity include hemolysis and gastrointestinal disturbances. Nausea, vomiting, diarrhea, abdominal pain, fever, chills, hemolytic anemia, jaundice, hemoglobinuria, and severe myalgias all occur frequently. Myoglobinemia, necrotizing pancreatitis, hepatic necrosis, and profound leukocytosis may also occur.

Copper poisoning during dialysis is fortunately readily avoidable, since copper is no longer a component of the tubing.

Copper poisoning may also occur after intentional or accidental ingestion. There may be a metallic taste, vomiting, and abdominal pain. In more severe cases, hematemesis, melena, hepatic necrosis, and shock supervene.

In Wilson's disease rapid increases in circulating copper concentrations may be followed by acute hemolytic anemia.

Those exposed to metallic copper industrially may develop transient pulmonary manifestations (metal fume fever) and, rarely, green hair. These disappear rapidly when exposure is stopped.

COBALT. Patients with renal failure may have elevated tissue cobalt levels. In some cases cobaltous chloride has been given by mouth to patients on maintenance hemodialysis to combat anemia. This has been associated with increased blood and myocardial cobalt levels and suggestive evidence of cardiomyopathy. Toxicity included nausea, vomiting, anorexia, tinnitus, peripheral neuropathy, goiter resulting from blockage of iodine uptake, neurogenic deafness, hyperlipidemia, optic atrophy, and renal tubular damage.

Cobalt was added to beer in the 1960's as a foam stabilizer. This resulted in cardiomyopathy, often accompanied by pericardial effusion. Mortality from heart failure or arrhythmias ranged from 5 to 47 per cent (see Ch. 50).

Persons exposed to cobalt industrially may also occasionally develop cardiomyopathy. Workers exposed to finely powdered cobalt may develop pulmonary interstitial fibrosis and cor pulmonale. Cobalt is often a component of alloys that are used in joint prostheses. Cases have been reported of joint pains, spontaneous dislocation of the prosthesis, and bone necrosis starting 9 months to 4 years postoperatively, apparently caused by a reaction to the cobalt in the alloy.

OTHER METALS. In one group of dialysis patients, *nickel* toxicity occurred when nickel leached from a stainless steel water heater tank into the dialysis fluid. Manifestations included nausea, vomiting, weakness, and headache. Symptoms developed within a few hours after dialysis and disappeared within 24 hours.

Tissue *tin* concentrations, especially in the liver, are increased in patients undergoing hemodialysis. However, tin levels are even higher in uremic patients who have not been dialyzed. No definite clinical disease has been associated with these increased body tin burdens.

Patients undergoing maintenance hemodialysis are often treated with *iron* for anemia. In such patients parenteral and occasionally oral iron administration may be followed by hemosiderosis and occasionally hemochromatosis. Serum ferritin concentrations exceed 500 ng per milliliter. A proximal myopathy has been described. The severity of the tissue iron overload and the likelihood of hemochromatosis may be related to the histocompatibility antigens A-3, B-7, and B-14. Iron overload has been complicated by porphyria cutanea tarda and by a variety of infections, including those due to species of *Yersinia* and *Vibrio* and to the yeast *Trichosporon cutaneum*. Treatment with deferoxamine may reduce the body iron burden.

Aggett PJ, Harrison JT: Current status of zinc in health and disease states. Arch Dis Child 54:909, 1979. *This is a superb review with 110 references. Only a small section is devoted to toxicity.*

Fosmire GJ: Zinc toxicity. Am J Clin Nutr 51:225, 1990. *A nice review; emphasizes problems inherent in self-administration of 50 to 300 mg a day for "health" purposes. Thirty-one references.*

Gruskin AB: Aluminum: A pediatric overview. Adv Pediatr 35:281, 1988. *A superb, comprehensive review with 255 references.*

O'Hare JA, Callaghan NM, Murnaghan DJ: Dialysis encephalopathy. Clinical, electroencephalographic and interventional aspects. Medicine 62:129, 1983. *A marvelous summary article and a careful analysis of 14 patients who developed encephalopathy 16 to 92 months after starting dialysis.*

Ott SM, Maloney NA, Klein GL, et al.: Aluminum is associated with low bone formation in patients receiving chronic parenteral nutrition. Ann Intern Med 98:910, 1983. *The toxicity of aluminum to bone is clearly shown in 14 patients receiving casein hydrolysate.*

Sandstead HH: Trace elements in uremia and hemodialysis. Am J Clin Nutr 33:1501, 1980. *A very good review article in which the author urges caution in ascribing the dialysis encephalopathy syndrome solely to aluminum.*

Sherrard DJ, Andress DL: Aluminum-related osteodystrophy. Adv Intern Med 34:307, 1989. *A very nice review with 81 references.*

Simon P, Allain P, Ang KS, et al.: Prevention and treatment of aluminum intoxication in chronic renal failure. Adv Nephrol 14:439, 1985. *This is as good a review as there is; with 179 references.*

Taylor A, Marks V: Cobalt: A review. J Hum Nutr 32:165, 1978. *A nice review with 73 references.*

Webster JD, Parker TF, Alfrey A, et al.: Acute nickel intoxication by dialysis. Ann Intern Med 92:631, 1980. *Nausea, vomiting, weakness, and headache were the predominant manifestations among 37 patients. Symptoms remitted 3 to 13 hours after dialysis was concluded.*

CADMIUM

ETIOLOGY. Over 10 million pounds of cadmium are used industrially every year in the United States. The metal is a component of alloys; it is used in the manufacture of electrical conductors and in electroplating; and it is present in ceramics, pigments, dental prosthetics, plastic stabilizers, and storage batteries. It is also a by-product of zinc smelting and is used in the photographic, rubber, motor, and aircraft industries. Smelters, metal-processing furnaces, and the burning of coal and oil are responsible for much of the cadmium in air.

CLINICAL MANIFESTATIONS. *Acute intoxication* by cadmium fumes produces a characteristic clinical picture. Four to 10 hours after exposure, dyspnea, cough, and substernal discomfort supervene, often accompanied by prominent myalgias, fatigue, headache, and vomiting. In more severe cases, wheezing, hemoptysis, and progressive dyspnea caused by pulmonary edema may occur and may be accompanied by hypotension and renal failure.

In most cases, the pulmonary manifestations resolve rapidly, but pulmonary function abnormalities may not disappear for months; in these cases vital capacity is reduced, and there is a restrictive defect. Occasionally pulmonary edema is lethal.

Ingestion of large amounts of cadmium results in nausea, vomiting, and abdominal pain, often accompanied by weakness, prostration, and myalgias. The onset of the gastroenteritis occurs one half to 5 hours after ingestion, and the condition lasts for less than 24 hours.

Chronic cadmium exposure by aerosol for at least 10 years has resulted in emphysema in a small number of cases. The emphysema is not accompanied by bronchitis and may appear many years after industrial exposure has stopped. Workers exposed for at least 10 years also may suffer olfactory nerve damage; in some cases this progresses to total anosmia. The most frequent long-term consequence of aerosol or oral exposure is proteinuria. After prolonged and heavy contact, cadmium urinary excretion continues for years and is associated with damage to the proximal tubule. The major urinary protein is a low molecular weight β_2 microglobulin. Urinary retinal-binding protein and N-acetyl-D-glucosaminidase levels also increase.

On occasion the proteinuria may be accompanied by glycosuria and aminoaciduria. Only infrequently is the proteinuria and tubular damage followed by progressive renal failure. An exception to the relatively benign course of the renal damage is the disease in Japan known as itai-itai (ouch-ouch), which affected almost exclusively multiparous women of ages 40 to 70 who lived in an area contaminated by industrial cadmium waste. Manifestations included striking back and joint pains, a waddly gait, osteomalacia, bone deformities, and fractures, all presumably secondary to cadmium-induced renal tubular damage.

Some studies on workers exposed to cadmium have suggested an increased risk of lung or prostatic carcinoma, but the data are not convincing.

Brenner I: Cadmium toxicity. World Rev Nutr Diet 32:165, 1978. *Interactions with calcium, zinc, copper, and selenium are emphasized. Additionally, there is a detailed analysis of the role of metallothioneins. Contains 183 references.*
Lauwery RR, Roels AA, Buchet JP, et al.: Investigations on the lung and kidney function of workers exposed to cadmium. Environ Health Perspect 28:137, 1979. *Three epidemiologic studies were conducted on more than 200 workers. The kidneys were affected to a much greater extent than the lungs. Both tubular and glomerular aberrations were found, mainly in persons with substantially increased blood and urine cadmium concentrations.*

NICKEL

ETIOLOGY. Nickel is used widely industrially in various alloys, iron shell casings, ball bearings, and heart and joint prostheses. It is also used in nickel plating; as a catalyst; in magnetic tapes, dyes, and paints; and in acrylic plastics. It is found in petroleum and coal, in diesel fuels, and in soil and air. Municipal incinerators may contribute to the ambient air nickel concentrations.

Nickel is a potent contact allergen; the most frequent adverse effect for humans is nickel dermatitis, which may be both persistent and severe. Serious systemic reactions have occurred in allergic persons from nickel-containing dental prostheses, jewelry, pacemakers, or even fluids given intravenously through a nickel-containing needle. Prosthetic joints and heart valves have failed because of a reaction to the nickel in the prosthesis. In cases of recalcitrant nickel dermatitis, restriction in dietary nickel may be helpful.

CLINICAL MANIFESTATIONS AND TREATMENT. By far, the most toxic of the nickel compounds is nickel carbonyl, created by a reaction between nickel and carbon monoxide. Industrial aerosol exposure is followed immediately by headache, drowsiness, substernal pain, nausea, and vomiting. This is followed by a latent period of 1 to 5 days, after which the victim experiences fever, chills, dyspnea, a feeling of chest tightness, cough that is sometimes productive of blood-tinged sputum, muscle pains, weakness, and fatigue. Hepatic enzyme concentrations may be considerably elevated. In severe cases cyanosis, progressive respiratory difficulties, and convulsions ensue, and death may follow in 4 to 23 days. At autopsy the lungs show hemorrhage, atelectasis, fibroblastic proliferation, and hyaline membrane formation. The treatment of choice is diethyl dithiocarbamate (Dithiocarb); dimercaprol (BAL) is an alternative but less effective therapeutic agent. Although overwhelming pneumonitis caused by nickel carbonyl is now rare, milder pulmonary toxicity in occupations such as welding probably occurs quite commonly and goes unrecognized under the general rubric of metal fume fever. Nickel exposure may also be followed by Löffler's syndrome.

CARCINOGENESIS. Nickel is considered a potent respiratory tract carcinogen. Studies of nickel refinery workers have shown a fivefold increase in risk of lung cancer, a 150-fold increase in the risk of nasal cancer, and a substantially increased risk of larynx cancer. Those occupations most at risk among nickel workers are roasting, smelting, and electrolysis. Workers developing lung, laryngeal, and nasal cancers have usually been exposed for at least 10 years. Biopsies of nasal mucosa show potentially precancerous epithelial dysplasia in a substantial percentage of nickel workers. The cancer risk is so great that workers heavily exposed for over 10 years should probably have annual nasal mucosa biopsies as well as sputum cytologic studies and roentgenologic examinations every 4 to 6 months in an attempt at secondary prevention. The incidence of respiratory tract cancer in nickel workers is dependent on both the extent of nickel exposure and the effects of cocarcinogens, in particular, cigarette tobacco. Except for nickel miners and refinery workers, industrial nickel exposure has not been convincingly associated with increased risk of cancer.

Sunderman FW Jr: A review of the metabolism and toxicity of nickel. Ann Clin Lab Sci 7:377, 1977. *An excellent review by one of the world's leading authorities (with 177 references).*
Sunderman FW Sr: Efficacy of sodium diethyldithiocarbamate (Dithiocarb) in acute nickel carbonyl poisoning. Ann Clin Lab Sci 9:1, 1979. *The data presented strongly suggest that this is currently the agent of choice.*

OTHER TOXIC METALS

Thallium

ETIOLOGY AND PATHOGENESIS. Thallium is used in optical lenses, jewelry, low-temperature thermometers, semiconductors, luminescent tubes, dyes and pigments, scintillation counters, and fireworks. It forms a stainless alloy with silver and a corrosion-resistant alloy with lead and may be a by-product of lead and zinc production. In some areas it is still a component of rodenticides, pesticides, and insecticides. Thallium can enter the body through the respiratory tract, gastrointestinal tract, or skin. Like many other trace metals, thallium has a strong affinity for sulfhydryl groups and thus interferes with many enzyme systems. Additionally, it enters the cell, exchanging for intracellular potassium.

CLINICAL MANIFESTATIONS. Poisoning can be acute and overwhelming after suicidal ingestion, or it can be chronic and subtle. In acute poisoning, manifestations include nausea, vomiting, hematemesis, headache, lethargy, abdominal pain, diarrhea that may be bloody, insomnia, myalgias, muscle weakness, fever, hyperhidrosis, excessive thirst, confusion, delirium, seizures, coma, and respiratory failure. At least 10 per cent of acutely poisoned persons die.

Among those who survive at least a week or in those exposed to smaller amounts of thallium, the most predictable manifestations are a combined sensory and motor, often painful, peripheral neuropathy and alopecia. Although the head alopecia is total, the facial, axillary, and pubic hair is spared, as is the inner one third of the eyebrows. Motor manifestations may predominate, and the ascending, predominantly motor paralysis may mimic Guillain-Barré syndrome. The abdominal colic, nausea, and vomiting that occur frequently in both the acute and the subacute forms of thallium toxicity may so dominate the clinical picture that a diagnosis of acute appendicitis is made. Other manifestations of subacute intoxication include dementia, headache, fatigue, sleep disorders, intractable thirst, hallucinations, blindness caused by optic neuritis, impotence, amenorrhea, a blue discoloration of the gingivae, centrilobular hepatic necrosis, renal tubular necrosis, orthostatic hypotension, paralytic ileus, and myoclonic twitches. Multiple cranial nerves may be involved, but the eighth nerve is almost always spared. The electrocardiogram may show arrhythmias and changes similar to those associated with hypokalemia.

DIAGNOSIS. Thallium can be measured in blood and urine, but blood levels are often deceptively low even during clinically apparent poisoning. Since thallium is excreted in the urine, thallium determinations on 24-hour specimens are more reliable. A qualitative urine test is available. Urine is mixed with 0.4 per cent sodium bismuth in 20 per cent nitric acid and 10 per cent sodium iodide; if thallium is present, a red precipitate forms.

In some cases there is no history of occupational, environmental, or intentional exposure. Unexplained abdominal pain, neurologic abnormalities, and alopecia suggest the diagnosis.

TREATMENT. Treatment consists of hemodialysis, which can remove up to half the thallium body burden, potassium, forced diuresis, and administration of Prussian blue. Prussian blue, or activated charcoal given by mouth, absorbs thallium, so that fecal thallium concentrations increase. The half-life of thallium in the body is about 1 month, and repeated dialyses are usually needed. During potassium administration, thallium is displaced from its intracellular site, and this may cause transient exacerbations of clinical manifestations. Barbiturates may increase the severity of the disease, and their use should be avoided.

PROGNOSIS. As many as 30 per cent of those poisoned suffer some residual effects. The neuropathy may persist for many months before resolving, and some are left with variable amounts of dementia, neuropathy, ataxia, visual impairment, alopecia, and myoclonus.

Selenium

ETIOLOGY. Selenium is well absorbed from both the gastrointestinal tract and the lungs. The amount normally ingested varies markedly, depending on the local soil selenium content and on the geographic provenance of foods consumed. Grains, pork, kidney, seafoods, garlic, mushrooms, radishes, beef, egg yolk, and chicken frequently contain substantial amounts of selenium. The element is widely used in pigment, glass, electronics, ceramics, and steel industries.

CLINICAL MANIFESTATIONS. Both deficiency and toxicity syndromes are well described in animals. Deficiency, resulting from foraging on grains grown in soil deficient in selenium, produces white muscle disease, a diffuse, often severe myopathy. Excess caused by chronic ingestion of grains containing more than 10 parts per million of selenium results in two syndromes, alkali disease and the staggers. The former is milder and is characterized by anemia, emaciation, alopecia, and hoof deformity. The staggers is manifested by visual difficulties, anemia, liver cell degeneration, paralysis, and respiratory failure. In sheep, excessive selenium intake can produce severe cardiomyopathy.

In humans a *selenium deficiency syndrome* has not been clearly defined. However, in the Republic of China, diffuse cardiomyopathy (Keshan disease) has been associated with low soil and blood selenium levels, and the incidence of the disease apparently has been strikingly reduced by selenium supplementation.

Selenium toxicity syndromes in humans can be divided into acute and chronic poisoning. Subjects with inordinate exposure to selenium fumes experience one or more of the following: intestinal disturbances, giddiness, apathy, lassitude, pallor, nervousness, depression, hair and nail loss, a garlic odor to the breath, and a metallic taste. Sore throat, dyspnea, and cough may also be noted. Symptoms usually disappear after removal from the occupational exposure. Among those ingesting excessive selenium, the following symptoms and signs have been reported: nausea, vomiting, abdominal pain, diarrhea, anorexia, fatigue, sore throat, arthralgias, emotional lability, a metallic taste, a garlic odor to the breath, brittle nails, brittle hair, hair loss, a bronze color to the skin, hepatic dysfunction, and diffuse dermatitis. Increased selenium burdens may be associated with an increased prevalence of dental caries.

EPIDEMIOLOGY. A most impressive epidemic of chronic selenium intoxication was observed in China in the 1960's. Subacute and chronic selenium toxicity will likely be seen with an increasing frequency because selenium is being promoted as a nonprescription supplement. In experimental studies oral selenium in dosages of 0.1 to 2.0 parts per million diminishes the frequency of or delays the appearance of a variety of spontaneous or induced tumors. Some epidemiologic data suggest an inverse relationship between selenium blood levels and the incidence of

certain cancers, particularly of the intestinal tract, but at present the evidence that increased selenium intake modifies or prevents human cancer is unpersuasive.

Manganese

Manganese toxicity occurs primarily in miners who have been exposed to manganese dioxide aerosols for prolonged periods. The manifestations, known as manganic madness, are limited to the CNS. The manganese is concentrated primarily in the basal ganglia and cerebellum, accounting for the extrapyramidal Parkinson-like facies, the rigidity, and the difficulty in walking. Other manifestations include compulsive behavior (including singing, dancing, fighting, and running), explosive and involuntary laughter, headache, muscular weakness, tremors, somnolence, dystonia, hypotonia, retropulsion and propulsion, dementia, speech disturbances, irritability, sialorrhea, impotence, hypersomnia, and memory defects. In some cases psychosis may be the dominant feature. There is no effective therapy. After removal from manganese exposure or following attempts to reduce the body manganese load by treatment with calcium versenate or L-dopa, the mental aberrations usually improve but the neurologic abnormalities persist. Manganese contamination of dialysates or manganese ingestion has been associated with abdominal pain, liver dysfunction, and evidence of pancreatitis.

Barium

Barium compounds are used in printing; in the production of paints, glass, paper, leather, soap, and rubber; in ceramics, plastic, steel, oil, textile, and dye industries; as fuel additives; and in insecticides, rodenticides, and depilatories. There are two major adverse effects. After accidental or intentional ingestion of large amounts, abdominal pain, vomiting, and increased peristalsis occur. If enough is absorbed, potassium is displaced intracellularly, resulting in profound hypokalemia, which in turn may produce flaccid paralysis, potentially dangerous cardiac arrhythmias, renal failure, and respiratory paralysis. Poisoning has also been described after barium chloride skin burn. Treatment consists of administration of potassium and forced diuresis to promote barium excretion. Severe allergic reaction has followed barium enema; whether this is due to the barium or preservatives is not clear.

The other adverse effect from contact with barium is a benign pneumoconiosis that may supervene after 1 or more years of aerosol exposure. Chest roentgenograms show extensive, very dense bilateral nodules up to 4 to 5 mm in diameter. There is no prominent fibrosis and no clinically significant disease; the nodules often regress after occupational exposure is stopped.

Boron

Borates are used in soaps, detergents, fertilizers, wood preservatives, fungicides, and fire-retardant paints. There are few reports of boron toxicity. Ingestion of boric acid or absorption from local application can result in nausea, vomiting, diarrhea, anemia, and seizures; a variety of skin eruptions characterized by intense erythema, desquamation, and exfoliation; and striking alopecia. In acute boric acid poisoning, forced diuresis and/or dialysis may be helpful. In addition, occupational aerosol exposure to diborane (B_2H_6) in high-energy fuels can produce acute pulmonary edema that resolves after the exposure is discontinued. Exposure to pentaborane or decaborane can produce headache, nausea, drowsiness, vertigo, coma, dementia, cortical blindness, deafness, seizures, muscle spasms, acidosis, and cardiac arrest. A subacute mild organic brain syndrome has also been observed.

Antimony

Industrial antimony toxicity is very rare, as is intentional ingestion or inadvertent poisoning from release of antimony from inexpensive enamelware. Manifestations of acute poisoning include nausea, abdominal pain, weakness, headache, vomiting, diarrhea, hematemesis, myalgias, liver function abnormalities, acute renal tubular dysfunction, electrolyte abnormalities, and circulatory collapse. Gaseous SbH_3 (stibine) is as toxic as arsine, producing CNS abnormalities and hemolysis. After antimonial injection for medicinal purposes, adverse effects include nausea, vomiting, cough, and muscle and joint pain. Hepatic dysfunction can occur, as can cardiac arrhythmias, including Adams-Stokes syndrome. Antimony is also considered one of the metals capable of causing metal fume fever. Treatment of oral ingestion consists of lavage, administration of activated charcoal, and administration of dimercaprol or the less toxic analogues dimercaptosuccinic acid or dimercaptopropanesulfonic acid.

Chromium

Chromium is used extensively in metal and galvanizing industries and in the manufacture of dyes, enamel, and paints. Hexavalent chromium exposure is associated with an increased incidence of lung and certain upper respiratory tract cancers. Additionally, chromium-exposed workers may show evidence of proximal renal tubule dysfunction and may suffer nasal septum perforations.

Molybdenum

In animals, molybdenum produces diarrhea, anemia, alopecia, diminished growth, and bone and joint abnormalities. No clearly defined molybdenum toxicity syndrome has been reported in humans.

Platinum

The major adverse effects observed in platinum workers are allergic pulmonary reactions, including bronchial asthma.

Plutonium

In experimental models, plutonium, because of its radioactivity, is a potent carcinogen. Workers have been generally well protected, but recent data suggest that occupational exposure may be a significant problem. Some still controversial epidemiologic studies have suggested that accidental community exposure has resulted in an increase in frequency of certain cancers and fetal malformations.

Tellurium

Used particularly in rubber, metallurgic, and electronics industries, tellurium can cause giddiness, headache, nausea, a metallic taste, and a garlic smell to the breath. In animals tellurium causes neuropathy, but this has not been convincingly demonstrated in humans.

Tin

Tin can be released into beverages or foods from tin cans; ingestion can produce nausea, vomiting, abdominal pain, and diarrhea. Such toxicity occurs infrequently. Additionally, there have been occasional reports of neurologic abnormalities following exposure to organic tin, including the triethyl, trimethyl, and triphenyl tins. These are used primarily in agriculture for their

bactericidal, fungicidal, antiparasitic and molluscacidal properties. Manifestations include ataxic dysmetria, disorientation, seizures, nystagmus, impaired vision, hearing loss, headache, vertigo, paresthesias, intracranial hypertension, paresis, and polyneuropathy. Aerosol exposure to tin may result in stannosis, a mild pneumoconiosis in which there may be dense bilateral infiltrates but usually no pulmonary dysfunction.

Vanadium

Vanadium is used in alloys and in the steel and chemical industries. Its inhalation can result in neurasthenia, anorexia, vertigo, throat pain, nasal irritation (even nasal hemorrhage), and acute bronchitis characterized by a cough that is sometimes accompanied by a whoop. The nasal mucosa of vanadium-exposed workers shows vascular hyperemia and round cell infiltration. Recent studies also suggest that vanadium can interfere with heme synthesis.

Bencko V, Cikrt M: Manganese: A review of occupational and environmental toxicology. J Hyg Epidem Microbiol Immunol 28:139, 1984. *All you wanted to know about manganese and then some (77 references).*

Doig AT: Baritosis: A benign pneumoconiosis. Thorax 31:130, 1976. *Nine cases are described. Despite dense infiltrates, no significant clinical disease or physiologic abnormalities occurred.*

Lauwers LF, Roelants A, Rosseel PM, et al.: Oral antimony intoxications in man. Crit Care Med 18:324, 1990. *Four cases due to eating cake inadvertently spiked with antimony potassium tartrate; plus a nice review.*

Locatelli C, Minoia C, Tonini M, et al.: Human toxicology of boron with special reference to boric acid poisoning. Ital Med Lav 9:141, 1987. *It is difficult to find good reviews of boron toxicity. This is one of them; with 105 references.*

Nordberg GF: Factors influencing metabolism and toxicity of metals: A consensus report. Environ Health Persp 25:3, 1978. *This marvelous analysis covers the toxicity and interactions with other metals of arsenic, cadmium, lead, and mercury. Highly recommended. Contains 312 references.*

Silverman JJ, Hart RP, Garrettson LK, et al.: Post-traumatic stress disorders from pentaborane intoxication. JAMA 254:2603, 1985. *Fourteen persons exposed to B_5H_9 suffered neuropsychological deficits (33 references).*

Wainwright AP, Kox WJ, House IM, et al.: Clinical features and therapy of acute thallium poisoning. Q J Med 69:939, 1988. *A single case accompanied by an excellent discussion of clinical manifestations and treatment.*

Wilkinson GS, Tietjen GL, Wiggs LD, et al.: Mortality among plutonium and other radiation workers at a plutonium weapons facility. Am J Epidemiol 125:231, 1987. *Although confirmatory studies are needed, this very careful analysis of 5413 men suggests increased risks for several types of cancers.*

Wu RM, Chang YC, Chiu HC: Acute triphenyltin intoxication: A case report. J Neurol Neurosurg Psychiatry 53:356, 1990. *A brief report of a suicide attempt; with a useful literature review.*

Yang G, Wang S, Zhou R, et al.: Endemic selenium intoxication of humans in China. Am J Clin Nutr 37:872, 1983. *This is an excellent review of selenium intoxication based on a very significant epidemic in China. Selenium-laden vegetables and coal combined with a drought that reduced the rice crop were the major culprits. Seventeen references.*

PART XXVII
LABORATORY REFERENCE INTERVAL VALUES OF CLINICAL IMPORTANCE

534 Reference Intervals and Laboratory Values of Clinical Importance*

Ronald J. Elin

Reference intervals are valuable guidelines for the assessment of health and disease by the clinician, but they should not be used as absolute indicators of health and disease. For essentially every test, there is a significant overlap between the normal and diseased populations. Many factors may influence the determination of the reference interval. The method and mode of standardization are variables for the reference interval, particularly for immunologic and enzymatic tests. The selection of the "normal" population is also important, since factors such as age, sex, race, diet, personal habits (e.g., alcohol consumption, smoking), and exercise may influence the reference interval for a given analyte. Last, the statistics chosen to define the reference interval are also a factor. These multiple variables for the determination of the reference interval indicate why there are differences among institutions for the same analyte.

The values in this chapter are primarily for adults in the fasting state. Values for other groups, when included, are clearly identified. For convenience, this chapter is divided into the following three sections: clinical chemistry, toxicology, and serology; hematology and coagulation; and drugs—therapeutic and toxic. The list includes reference intervals for the most common tests used in the practice of internal medicine. For more information about the reference interval for a given test or a test not included in the list, I recommend *Clinical Guide to Laboratory Tests*, second edition, edited by Dr. Norbert W. Tietz. This book contains literature citations for most of the tests listed in this chapter.

All laboratory values are given in conventional and international units. If the value and units for a reference interval are the same for conventional and international units, the interval is listed only in the column for international units. The temperature for all enzyme assays listed in the chapter is 37°C. The pertinent prefixes denoting the decimal factors are listed.

---

*The material in this chapter was partially extracted from Tietz NW (ed.): Clinical Guide to Laboratory Tests. Philadelphia, W.B. Saunders Company, 1990. The material for the section on Therapeutic Drug Concentrations was partially extracted from Tietz NW: Textbook of Clinical Chemistry. Philadelphia, W.B. Saunders Company, 1986. The main contributors to this section of the book are NW Tietz and NM Logan. Other sources are listed under references for this chapter.

PREFIXES DENOTING DECIMAL FACTORS

Prefix	Symbol	Factor
mega	M	10^6
kilo	k	10^3
hecto	h	10^2
deka	da	10^1
deci	d	10^{-1}
centi	c	10^{-2}
milli	m	10^{-3}
micro	μ	10^{-6}
nano	n	10^{-9}
pico	p	10^{-12}
femto	f	10^{-15}

ABBREVIATIONS

AU	Arbitrary units
EU	Ehrlich unit
GD	General diagnostics
IFA	Immunofluorescent assay
IU	International unit (of hormone activity)
RIA	Radioimmunoassay
RID	Radial immunodiffusion
S	Substrate
U	International unit (of enzyme activity)

Beutler E: Hemolytic Anemia in Disorders of Red Cell Metabolism. New York, Plenum Publishing Company, 1978.

Brown SS, Mitchell FL, Young DS (eds.): Chemical Diagnosis of Disease. Amsterdam, Elsevier/North-Holland Biomedical Press, 1979.

Conn RB (ed.): Current Diagnosis. 7th ed. Philadelphia, W.B. Saunders Company, 1985.

Gilman AG, Rall TW, Nies AS, Taylor P (eds.): Goodman and Gilman's The Pharmacological Basis of Therapeutics. 8th ed. New York, Pergamon Press, 1990.

Henry JB (ed.): Clinical Diagnosis and Management by Laboratory Methods. 18th ed. Philadelphia, W.B. Saunders Company, 1991.

Hoeg JM, Gregg RE, Brewer HB: An approach to the management of hyperlipoproteinemia. JAMA 255:512, 1986.

Mabry C, Tietz NW: Tables of normal laboratory values. In Nelson WE, Vaughan VC, McKay JR, et al. (eds.): Nelson Textbook of Pediatrics. 23rd ed. Philadelphia, W.B. Saunders Company, 1983.

Miale JB: Laboratory Medicine: Hematology. 6th ed. St. Louis, The C.V. Mosby Company, 1982.

Tietz NW (ed.): Textbook of Clinical Chemistry. Philadelphia, W.B. Saunders Company, 1986.

Tietz NW, Blackburn RH (eds.): Reference Ranges and General Information. Clinical Laboratories, A.B. Chandler Medical Center, University of Kentucky, Lexington, Kentucky, 1984.

Tietz NW (ed.): Clinical Guide to Laboratory Tests. Philadelphia, W.B. Saunders Company, 1990.

Williams WJ, Beutler E, Erslev AJ, et al.: Hematology. 3rd ed. New York, McGraw-Hill Book Company, 1983.

CLINICAL CHEMISTRY, TOXICOLOGY, SEROLOGY

Test	Specimen	Reference Interval (Conventional Units)	Reference Interval (International Units)
Acetoacetate Semiquantitative	Serum or plasma (fluoride/oxalate)	Negative (<1 mg/dL)	Negative (<0.1 mmol/L)
Acetone Semiquantitative	Urine	Negative	Negative
Semiquantitative	Serum or plasma (fluoride or oxalate)	Negative (<1.0 mg/dL)	Negative (<0.17 mmol/L)
Acid phosphatase (S:p-nitrophenylphosphate)	Urine Serum	Negative	Negative M: 2.5–11.7 U/L F: 0.3–9.2 U/L
Adrenocorticotropic hormone (ACTH)	Plasma (heparin)	0800 h: 8–79 pg/mL 1600 h: 7–30 pg/mL	8–79 ng/L 7–30 ng/L
Alanine aminotransferase (ALT, SGPT)	Serum		8–20 U/L
Albumin Nephelometric, colorimetric	Serum	3.5–5.0 g/dL	35–50 g/L
Turbidimetric	CSF	15–45 mg/dL	150–450 mg/L
	Urine	<80 mg/d at rest <150 mg/d ambulatory	<80 mg/d <150 mg/d
Aldolase	Serum		1.0–7.5 U/L
Aldosterone	Plasma (heparin EDTA) or serum	Adult, average sodium diet supine: 3–10 ng/dL upright: 5–30 ng/dL	0.08–0.28 nmol/L 0.14–0.83 nmol/L
Alkaline phosphatase (S:4–NPP)	Serum		Adult (>18 y) F: 42–98 U/L M: 53–128 U/L
δ-Aminolevulinic acid (δ-ALA)	Serum	15–23 µg/dL	1.1–8 µmol/L
	Urine	1.5–7.5 mg/d	11.4–57.2 µmol/d
Ammonia nitrogen Resin or enzymatic	Serum or plasma (Na-heparin)	Adult 15–45 µg N/dL	11–32 µmol/L
	Urine, 24-h	140–1500 mg/d	10–107 mmol/d
Amylase (S:Beckman, defined substrate)	Serum		25–125 U/L
	Urine, timed specimen		1–17 U/h
Angiotensin I	Peripheral venous plasma (EDTA)	11–88 pg/mL	11–88 ng/L
Angiotensin II	Plasma (EDTA) Arterial blood	10–60 pg/mL	10–60 ng/L
α₁-Antitrypsin (nephelometry)	Serum	78–200 mg/dL	0.78–2.00 g/L
Anion gap [Na − (Cl⁻ + HCO₃⁻)]	Plasma (heparin) or serum	7–14 mEq/L	7–14 mmol/L
Arsenic	Whole blood (heparin)	0.2–2.3 µg/dL Chronic poisoning: 10–50 µg/dL Acute poisoning: 60–93 µg/dL	0.03–0.31 µmol/L 1.33–6.65 µmol/L 7.98–12.37 µmol/L
	Urine, 24-h	5–50 µg/d	0.067–0.665 µmol/d
Ascorbic acid (see Vitamin C)			
Aspartate aminotransferase (AST, SGOT)	Serum		10–30 U/L
Base excess	Whole blood (heparin)	−2 to 3 mEq/L	−2 to 3 mmol/L
Bicarbonate	Serum	18–23 mEq/L	18–23 mmol/L
Bile acids, total	Serum, fasting	0.3–2.3 µg/mL	0.74–5.64 µmol/L
	Serum, 1-h postprandial	1.8–3.2 µg/mL	4.41–7.84 µmol/L
	Feces	120–225 mg/d	294–551 µmol/d
Bilirubin Total	Serum	0.2–1.0 mg/dL	3.4–17.1 µmol/L
	Urine	Negative	Negative
Conjugated (direct)	Serum	0–0.2 mg/dL	0–3.4 µmol/L
Calcium, ionized (iCa)	Serum	4.65–5.28 mg/dL	1.16–1.32 mmol/L
Calcium, total	Serum	8.4–10.2 mg/dL	2.10–2.55 mmol/L
	Urine, 24-h	100–300 mg/d	2.5–7.5 mmol/d
	CSF	4.2–5.4 mg/dL	1.05–1.35 mmol/L
Carbon dioxide, total (TCO₂)	Serum or plasma (heparin)	23–29 mEq/L	23–29 mmol/L
Carcinoembryonic antigen (CEA)	Serum	Nonsmokers: <2.5 ng/mL	<2.5 µg/L
β-Carotene	Serum	10–85 µg/dL	0.19–1.58 µmol/L
Catecholamines, total	Urine, 24-h	<100 µg/d	<5.91 nmol/d
Ceruloplasmin (RID)	Serum	18–45 mg/dL	180–450 mg/L
Chloride	Serum or plasma (heparin)	98–106 mEq/L	98–106 mmol/L
	CSF	118–132 mEq/L	118–132 mmol/L
	Urine, 24-h	110–250 mEq/d	110–250 mmol/d

Table continued on following page

CLINICAL CHEMISTRY, TOXICOLOGY, SEROLOGY *Continued*

Test	Specimen	Reference Interval (Conventional Units)	Reference Interval (International Units)
Cholesterol, total	Serum or plasma (EDTA)	Recommended: <200 mg/dL Moderate risk: 200–239 mg/L High risk: ≥240 mg/dL	<5.18 mmol/L 5.18–6.19 mmol/L ≥6.22 mmol/L
Chorionic gonadotropin, β-subunit (β-HCG)	Serum or plasma (EDTA)	M and nonpregnant F: <5.0 mU/mL	<5.0 IU/L
Complement Total hemolytic Complement activity	Plasma (EDTA)	75–160 U/mL	75–160 kU/L
Copper	Serum	M: 70–140 μg/dL F: 80–155 μg/dL	10.99–21.98 μmol/L 12.56–24.34 μmol/L
	Erythrocyte (heparin) Urine, 24-h	90–150 μg/dL 3–35 μg/d	14.13–23.55 μmol/L 0.047–0.55 μmol/d
Coproporphyrin	Urine, 24-h Feces, 24-h	34–234 μg/d <30 μg/g dry wt 400–1200 μg/d	51–351 nmol/d <45 nmol/g dry wt 600–1800 nmol/d
Corticosteroid-binding globulin (CBG) (see Transcortin)			
Corticosterone	Serum	0800 h: 130–820 ng/dL 1600 h: 60–220 ng/dL	4–24 nmol/L 2–6 nmol/L
Cortisol	Serum or plasma (heparin)	0800 h: 5–23 μg/dL 1600 h: 3–15 μg/dL 2000 h: ≤50% of 0800 h	138–635 nmol/L 82–413 nmol/L Fraction of 0800 h: ≤0.50
Cortisol, free	Urine, 24-h	10–100 μg/d	27–276 nmol/d
C-Peptide	Serum	0.78–1.89 ng/mL	0.26–0.62 nmol/L
C-Reactive protein	Serum	68–8200 ng/mL	68–8200 μg/L
Creatine kinase (CK)	Serum		M: 38–174 U/L F: 26–140 U/L
Isoenzymes	Serum	Fraction 2 (MB) <4–6% of total (method-dependent)	Fraction of total: <0.04–0.06
Creatinine Jaffe, kinetic or enzymatic	Serum or plasma	M: 0.7–1.3 mg/dL F: 0.6–1.1 mg/dL	62–115 μmol/L 53–97 μmol/L
	Urine, 24-h	M: 14–26 mg/kg/d F: 11–20 mg/kg/d	124–230 μmol/kg/d 97–177 μmol/kg/d
Creatinine clearance (endogenous)	Serum or plasma, and urine	M: 90–139 mL/min/1.73 m² F: 80–125 mL/min/1.73 m²	0.87–1.34 mL/s/m² 0.77–1.20 mL/s/m²
Dehydroepiandrosterone serum (DHEA)	Serum	M: 1.8–12.5 ng/mL F: 1.3–9.8 ng/mL	6.2–43.3 nmol/L 4.5–34.0 nmol/L
Dehydroepiandrosterone sulfate (DHEA-S)	Serum	M: 1.7–6.7 μg/mL F: Premenopausal: 0.5–5.4 μg/mL Postmenopausal: 0.3–2.6 μg/mL	4.6–18.2 μmol/L 1.4–14.7 μmol/L 0.8–7.1 μmol/L
11-Deoxycortisol (compound S)	Serum	12–158 ng/dL	0.3–4.6 nmol/L
Estrogens, total	Serum	M: 20–80 pg/mL F, cycle: Follicular phase: 60–200 pg/mL Luteal phase: 160–400 pg/mL Postmenopausal: ≤130 pg/mL	20–80 ng/L 60–200 ng/L 160–400 ng/L ≤130 ng/L
	Urine, 24-h		M: 15–40 μg/d F: Preovulation: 4–25 μg/d Ovulation: 28–100 μg/d Luteal peak: 22–80 μg/d Pregnancy, term: <45,000 μg/d Postmenopausal: <20 μg/d
Fat, fecal	Feces, 72-h		<7 g/d fat-free diet: <4 g/d
Fatty acids, nonesterified (free)	Serum or plasma (heparin)	8–25 mg/dL	0.28–0.89 mmol/L
Ferritin	Serum	M: 20–250 ng/mL F: 10–120 ng/mL	20–250 μg/L 10–120 μg/L
α₁-Fetoprotein	Serum	<10 ng/mL	<10 μg/L
Fibrinogen (see Hematology and Coagulation section)			
Folate	Serum Erythrocytes (EDTA)	3–16 ng/mL 130–628 ng/mL packed cells	7–36 nmol/L 294–1422 nmol/L packed cells
Follitropin (FSH)	Serum or plasma (heparin)	M: 4–25 mIU/mL F: Follicular phase: 1–9 mU/mL Ovulatory peak: 6–26 mU/mL Luteal phase: 1–9 mU/mL Postmenopausal: 30–118 mU/mL	4–25 IU/L 1–9 U/L 6–26 U/L 1–9 U/L 30–118 U/L
	Urine, 24-h		4–18 U/d 3–12 U/d
Free thyroxine index (FT₄I)	Serum		4.2–13.0
Gastrin	Serum	<100 pg/mL	<100 ng/L

CLINICAL CHEMISTRY, TOXICOLOGY, SEROLOGY *Continued*

Test	Specimen	Reference Interval (Conventional Units)	Reference Interval (International Units)
Glucose	Serum	Adult: 70–105 mg/dL	3.9–5.8 mmol/L
		>60 y: 80–115 mg/dL	4.4–6.4 mmol/L
	Whole blood (heparin)	65–95 mg/dL	3.6–5.3 mmol/L
	CSF	40–70 mg/dL	2.2–3.9 mmol/L
Quantitative, enzymatic	Urine	<0.5 g/d	<2.8 mmol/d
Qualitative	Urine		Negative
Glucose, 2-h postprandial	Serum	<120 mg/dL	<6.7 mmol/L
Glucose tolerance test (GTT), oral	Serum	mg/dL	mmol/L

	Normal	Diabetic	Normal	Diabetic
Fasting:	70–105	>140	3.9–5.8	>7.8
60 min:	120–170	≥200	6.7–9.4	≥11
90 min:	100–140	≥200	5.6–7.8	≥11
120 min:	70–120	≥140	3.9–6.7	≥7.8

Test	Specimen	Reference Interval (Conventional Units)	Reference Interval (International Units)
γ-Glutamyltransferase (GGT)	Serum		M: 9–50 U/L F: 8–40 U/L
Glycerol, free	Plasma	0.29–1.72 mg/dL	0.032—0.187 mmol/L
Growth hormone (HGH, somatotropin)	Serum or plasma (EDTA, heparin)	Adult, M: <2 ng/mL	<2 µg/L
		F: <10 ng/mL	<10 µg/L
		>60 y, M: 0.4–10 ng/mL	0.4–10 µg/L
		F: 1–14 ng/mL	1–14 µg/L
Haptoglobin (see Hematology and Coagulation section)			
HDL-cholesterol (HDLC) (5th percentile from Lipid Research Clinics)	Serum or plasma (EDTA)	M: >29 mg/dL	>0.75 mmol/L
		F: >35 mg/dL	>0.91 mmol/L
Hemoglobin A₁c (electrophoresis)	Whole blood (heparin, EDTA, or oxalate)	5.6–7.5% of total Hb	Fraction of Hb: 0.056–0.075
Homovanillic acid (HVA)	Urine, 24-h	1.4–8.8 mg/d	8–48 µmol/d
17-Hydroxycorticosteroids (17-OHCS)	Urine, 24-h	M: 3.0–10.0 mg/d	8.3–27.6 µmol/d
		F: 2.0–8.0 mg/d	5.5–22.1 µmol/d
5-Hydroxyindole acetic acid (5-HIAA)			
Qualitative	Fresh random urine		Negative
Quantitative	Urine, 24-h	2–6 mg/d	10.4–31.2 µmol/d
17-Hydroxyprogesterone (17-OHP)	Serum	M: 0.5–2.5 ng/mL	1.5–7.5 nmol/L
		F: Follicular: 0.2–1.0 ng/mL	0.6–3.0 nmol/L
		Luteal: 1.0–5.0 ng/mL	3.0–15.5 nmol/L
		Postmenopausal: ≤0.7 ng/mL	≤2.1 nmol/L
Immunoglobulin A (IgA)	Serum	40–350 mg/dL	400–3500 mg/L
Immunoglobulin D (IgD)	Serum	0–8 mg/dL	0–80 mg/L
Immunoglobulin E (IgE)	Serum	0–380 IU/mL	0–380 kIU/L
Immunoglobulin G (IgG)	Serum	650–1600 mg/dL	6.5–16 g/L
	CSF	0.5–5 mg/dL	5–50 mg/L
Immunoglobulin M (IgM)	Serum	55–300 mg/dL	550–3000 mg/L
Insulin (12-h fasting)	Serum	6–24 µIU/mL	42–167 pmol/L
Intrinsic factor (see Vitamin B₁₂)			
Iron	Serum	M: 65–175 µg/dL	11.6–31.3 µmol/L
		F: 50–170 µg/dL	9.0–30.4 µmol/L
Iron-binding capacity, total (TIBC)	Serum	250–450 µg/dL	44.8–80.6 µmol/L
Iron saturation	Serum	M: 20–50	Fraction of iron saturation: 0.20–0.5 (M)
		F: 15–50	0.15–0.5 (F)
17-Ketogenic steroids (17-KGS)	Urine, 24-h	M: 5–23 mg/d	17–80 µmol/d
		F: 3–15 mg/d	10–52 µmol/d
Ketone bodies			
Qualitative	Serum	Negative (0.5–3.0 mg/dL)	Negative (5–30 mg/L)
	Urine, random		Negative
17-Ketosteroids, total (17-KS)	Urine, 24-h	M: 18–30 y 9–22 mg/d	31–76 µmol/d
		>30 y 8–20 mg/d	28–70 µmol/d
		F: 6–15 mg/d	21–52 µmol/d
L-Lactate	Whole blood (heparin)	Venous: 4.5–19.8 mg/dL	0.5–2.2 mmol/L
		Arterial: 4.5–14.4 mg/dL	0.5–1.6 mmol/L
Lactate dehydrogenase (LDH)	Serum		208–378 U/L
LDH isoenzymes (Electrophoresis, agarose)	Serum	%	Fraction of total:
		Fraction 1: 18–33	0.18–0.33
		Fraction 2: 28–40	0.28–0.40
		Fraction 3: 18–30	0.18–0.30
		Fraction 4: 6–16	0.06–0.16
		Fraction 5: 2–13	0.02–0.13
Lead	Whole blood (heparin)	<40 µg/dL	<1.93 µmol/L
		Toxic: ≥100 µg/dL	≥4.83 µmol/L
	Urine, 24-h	<80 µg/L	<0.39 µmol/L

Table continued on following page

CLINICAL CHEMISTRY, TOXICOLOGY, SEROLOGY Continued

Test	Specimen	Reference Interval (Conventional Units)	Reference Interval (International Units)
Lipase (turbidimetric)	Serum		Adult: 10–140 U/L
			>60 y: 18–180 U/L
LDL-Cholesterol (LDLC)	Serum or plasma (EDTA)	Recommended: <130 mg/dL	<3.37 mmol/L
		Moderate risk: 130–159 mg/dL	3.37–4.12 mmol/L
		High risk: ≥160 mg/dL	≥4.14 mmol/L
Lutropin (LH)	Serum or plasma (heparin)	M: 1–8 mU/mL	1–8 U/L
		F: Follicular phase: 1–12 mU/mL	1–12 U/L
		Midcycle: 16–104 mU/mL	16–104 U/L
		Luteal: 1–12 mU/mL	1–12 U/L
		Postmenopausal: 16–66 mU/mL	16–66 U/L
	Urine		M: 9–23 U/d
			F: non-midcycle, 4–30 U/d
Lysozyme	Serum, plasma	0.4–1.3 mg/dL	4–13 mg/L
Magnesium	Serum	1.3–2.1 mEq/L	0.65–1.05 mmol/L
	Urine, 24-h	6.0–10.0 mEq/d	3.00–5.00 mmol/d
Mercury	Whole blood (EDTA)	<5.0 μg/dL	<0.25 μmol/L
	Urine, 24-h	<20 μg/L	<0.1 μmol/L
		Toxic: >150 μg/L	<0.75 μmol/L
Metanephrine, total	Urine, 24-h	0.05–1.20 μg/mg creatinine	0.03–0.69 mmol/mol creatinine
Myelin basic protein	CSF		<2.5 ng/mL
Myoglobin	Serum		M: 19–92 μg/L
			F: 12–76 μg/L
	Urine, random		Negative
Osmolality	Serum		275–295 mOsmol/kg
	Urine, random		50–1400 mOsmol/kg, depending on fluid intake
			After 12-h fluid restriction: >850 mOsmol/kg
	Urine, 24-h		~390–900 mOsmol/kg
Oxalate	Serum	1–2.4 μg/mL	11–27 μmol/L
		Ethylene glycol poisoning: >20 μg/mL	Ethylene glycol poisoning: >228 μmol/L
Oxygen (Po₂)	Whole blood, arterial (heparin)	83–100 mm Hg	11–14.4 kPa
Oxygen saturation	Whole blood, arterial (heparin)	95–98%	Fraction saturated: 0.95–0.98
pH (37°C)	Whole blood, arterial (heparin)		7.35–7.45
Phosphorus, inorganic	Serum	2.7–4.5 mg/dL	0.87–1.45 nmol/L
		>60 y, M: 2.3–3.7 mg/dL	0.74–1.2 nmol/L
		F: 2.8–4.1 mg/dL	0.90–1.3 nmol/L
	Urine, 24-h	0.4–1.3 g/d	13–42 mmol/d
Porphobilinogen (PBG)			
Quantitative	Urine, 24-h	0–2.0 mg/d	0–8.8 μmol/d
Qualitative	Urine, fresh random		Negative
Potassium	Serum	3.5–5.1 mEq/L	3.5–5.1 mmol/L
	Plasma (heparin)	3.5–4.5 mEq/L	3.5–4.5 mmol/L
	Urine, 24-h	25–125 mEq/d	25–125 mmol/d
Pregnanediol	Urine, 24-h	M: 0–1.9 mg/d	0–5.9 μmol/d
		F: Follicular: <2.6 mg/d	<8 μmol/d
		Luteal: 2.6–10.6 mg/d	8–33 μmol/d
		Postmenopausal: 0.2–1.0 mg/d	0.6–3.1 μmol/d
Progesterone	Serum	M: 0.13–0.97 ng/mL	0.4–3.1 nmol/L
		F: Follicular: 0.15–0.70 ng/mL	0.5–2.2 nmol/L
		Luteal: 2.0–25 ng/mL	6.4–79.5 nmol/L
Prolactin (hPRL)	Serum	0–20 ng/mL	0–20 μg/L
Protein			
Total	Serum	6.4–8.3 g/dL	64.0–83.0 g/L
Electrophoresis	Serum	Albumin: 3.5–5.0 g/dL	35–50 g/L
		α₁-Globulin: 0.1–0.3 g/dL	1–3 g/L
		α₂-Globulin: 0.6–1.0 g/dL	6–10 g/L
		β-Globulin: 0.7–1.1 g/dL	7–11 g/L
		γ-Globulin: 0.8–1.6 g/dL	8–16 g/L
Total	Urine, 24-h		50–80 mg/d at rest
Total	CSF	Lumbar: 15–45 mg/dL	150–450 mg/L
Protoporphyrin	Whole blood (heparin or EDTA)	17–77 μg/dL RBC	0.30–1.37 μmol/L RBC
	Feces, 24-h	≤60 μg/g dry wt or <1500 μg/d	≤0.11 mmol/kg dry wt or <2.67 μmol/d
Pyruvic acid	Whole blood (heparin)	0.3–0.9 mg/dL	0.03–0.10 mmol/L
Renin (normal diet)	Plasma (EDTA)	ng/mL/h ± 1 SE	μg/L/h ± 1 SE
		Supine: 1.6 ± 1.5	1.6 ± 1.5
		Standing: (4-h): 4.5 ± 2.9	4.5 ± 2.9

CLINICAL CHEMISTRY, TOXICOLOGY, SEROLOGY *Continued*

Test	Specimen	Reference Interval (Conventional Units)	Reference Interval (International Units)
Riboflavin (see Vitamin B$_2$)			
Sediment	Urine, fresh, random		
Casts			Hyaline: occasional (0–1) casts/hpf
			RBC: not seen
			WBC: not seen
			Tubular epithelial: not seen
			Transitional and squamous epithelial: not seen
Cells			RBC: 0–2/hpf
			WBC: M: 0–3/hpf
			F: 0–5/hpf
			Epithelial: few
			Bacteria:
			Unspun: no organisms/oil immersion field
			Spun: <20 organisms/hpf
Sodium	Serum or plasma (heparin)	136–146 mEq/L	136–146 mmol/L
	Urine, 24-h	40–220 mEq/d	40–220 mmol/d
Specific gravity	Urine, random	1.002–1.030	
	Urine, 24-h	1.015–1.025	
		% of total	Fraction of total
Testosterone, free	Serum	M: 52–280 pg/mL 1.5–3.2	180.4–971.6 pmol/L 0.015–0.032
		F: 1.6–6.3 pg/mL 0.8–1.4	5.6–21.9 pmol/L 0.008–0.014
Testosterone, total	Serum	M: 300–1000 ng/dL	10.4–34.7 nmol/L
		F: 20–75 ng/dL	0.69–2.6 nmol/L
	Urine	20–50 y,	
		M: 50–135 µg/d	173–470 nmol/d
		F: 2–12 µg/d	7–42 nmol/d
		>50 y,	
		M: 40–60 µg/d	139–210 nmol/d
		F: 2–8 µg/d	7–28 nmol/d
Thiamine (see Vitamin B$_1$)	Serum		
Thyroglobulin (Tg)	Serum	3–42 ng/mL	3–42 µg/L
Thyroglobulin antibodies	Serum		<1:10
Thyroid microsomal antibodies	Serum		Nondetectable (hemagglutination) or <1:10 (IFA)
Thyrotropin (hTSH)	Serum or plasma	2–10 µU/mL	2–10 mU/L
Thyrotropin-releasing hormone	Plasma	5–60 pg/mL	5–60 ng/L
Thyroxine, free (FT$_4$)	Serum	0.8–2.4 ng/dL	10–31 pmol/L
Thyroxine (T$_4$), total	Serum	5–12 µg/dL	65–155 nmol/L
		>60 y, M: 5.0–10.0 µg/dL	65–129 nmol/L
		F: 5.5–10.5 µg/dL	71–135 nmol/L
Thyroxine-binding globulin (TBG)	Serum	15.0–34.0 µg/mL	15.0–34.0 mg/L
Thyroxine index, free (see Free thyroxine index)			
Transcortin	Serum	M: 18.8–25.2 mg/L	323–433 nmol/L
		F: 14.9–22.9 mg/L	256–393 nmol/L
Transferrin	Serum	200–400 mg/dL	2.0–4.0 g/L
		>60 y: 180–380 mg/dL	1.80–3.80 g/L
Triglycerides (TG)	Serum, after ≥12-hr fast	Recommended:	
		M: 40–160 mg/dL	0.45–1.81 mmol/L
		F: 35–135 mg/dL	0.40–1.52 mmol/L
Tri-iodothyronine, free	Serum	260–480 pg/dL	4.0–7.4 pmol/L
Tri-iodothyronine, total (T$_3$)	Serum	100–200 ng/dL	1.54–3.08 mmol/L
Tri-iodothyronine resin uptake test (T$_3$RU)	Serum	24–34%	24–34 AU (arbitrary units)
Urea nitrogen	Serum or plasma	7–18 mg/dL	2.5–6.4 mmol/L
	Urine	12–20 g/d	0.43–0.71 mol/d
Urea nitrogen/creatinine ratio	Serum	12/1–20/1	
Uric acid (uricase)	Serum	M: 3.5–7.2 mg/dL	0.21–0.42 mmol/L
		F: 2.6–6.0 mg/dL	0.15–0.35 mmol/L
	Urine, 24-h	250–750 mg/d	1.48–4.43 mmol/d
Urinary sediment (see Sediment)			
Urobilinogen	Urine, 2-h	0.1–0.8 EU	0.1–0.8 U
	Urine, 24-h	0.5–4.0 EU	0.5–4.0 U
	Feces	75–275 EU/100 g	750–2750 U/kg
		75–400 EU/d	75–400 U/d
		40–280 mg/d	67–473 µmol/d
Uroporphyrin	Urine, 24-h	<50 µg/d	<60 nmol/d
	Feces, 24-h specimen	10–40 µg/d	12–48 nmol/d
	Erythrocytes (heparin or EDTA)		Negative

Table continued on following page

CLINICAL CHEMISTRY, TOXICOLOGY, SEROLOGY *Continued*

Test	Specimen	Reference Interval (Conventional Units)	Reference Interval (International Units)
Vanillylmandelic acid (VMA)	Urine, 24-h	2–7 mg/d	10.1–35.4 μmol/d
Viscosity	Serum		1.10–1.22 centipoise
Vitamin A	Serum	30–80 μg/dL	1.05–2.8 μmol/L
Vitamin B_1 (Thiamine)	Serum	0–2 μg/dL	0–75 nmol/L
Vitamin B_2 (Riboflavin)	Serum	4–24 μg/dL	106–638 nmol/L
Vitamin B_6	Plasma (EDTA)	5–30 ng/mL	20–121 nmol/L
Vitamin B_{12}	Serum	100–700 pg/mL	74–516 pmol/L
Vitamin C	Plasma (oxalate, heparin, or EDTA)	0.5–1.5 mg/dL	28–85 μmol/L
Vitamin D_3, 1,25-dihydroxy	Serum	25–45 pg/mL	60–108 pmol/L
Vitamin D_3, 25-hydroxy	Plasma (heparin)	Summer: 15–80 ng/mL	37.4–200 nmol/L
		Winter: 14–42 ng/mL	34.9–105 nmol/L
Vitamin E	Serum	5.0–18.0 μg/mL	12–42 μmol/L
Zinc	Serum	70–150 μg/dL	10.7–22.9 μmol/L

HEMATOLOGY AND COAGULATION

Test	Specimen	Reference Interval (Conventional Units)	Reference Interval (International Units)
Activated partial thromboplastin time (APTT)	Whole blood (Na citrate)		25–35 sec
Bleeding time (BT)			
Ivy	Blood from skin		Normal: 2–7 min
			Borderline: 7–11 min
Simplate (G-D)			2.75–8 min
Blood volume	Whole blood (heparin)		M: 52–83 mL/kg
			F: 50–75 mL/kg
Bone marrow	Bone marrow aspirate	% (mean)	Number fraction (mean)
Differential count			
Myeloblasts		0.3–5.0 (2.0)	0.003–0.05 (0.02)
Promyelocytes		1.0–8.0 (5.0)	0.01–0.08 (0.05)
Myelocytes:			
Neutrophilic		5.0–19.0 (12.0)	0.05–0.19 (0.12)
Eosinophilic		0.5–3.0 (1.5)	0.005–0.03 (0.015)
Basophilic		0.0–0.5 (0.3)	0.00–0.005 (0.003)
Metamyelocytes		13.0–32.0 (22.0)	0.13–0.32 (0.22)
Polymorphonuclear neutrophils		7.0–3.0 (2.0)	0.07–0.30 (0.20)
Polymorphonuclear eosinophils		0.5–4.0 (2.0)	0.005–0.04 (0.02)
Polymorphonuclear basophils		0.0–0.7 (0.2)	0.0–0.007 (0.002)
Lymphocytes		3.0–17.0 (10.0)	0.03–0.17 (0.10)
Plasma cells		0.0–2.0 (0.4)	0.00–0.02 (0.004)
Monocytes		0.5–5.0 (2.0)	0.005–0.05 (0.02)
Reticulum cells		0.1–2.0 (0.2)	0.001–0.02 (0.002)
Megakaryocytes		0.03–3.0 (0.1)	0.0003–0.03 (0.001)
Pronormoblasts		1.0–8.0 (4.0)	0.01–0.08 (0.04)
Normoblasts		7.0–32.0 (18.0)	0.07–0.32 (0.18)
Clot lysis, 37°C	Whole clotted blood		48–72 h
Clot retraction screen	Whole blood (no anticoagulant)		Retraction begins at 1 h, maximum at 24 h
Clotting time, Lee-White, 37°C	Whole blood (no anticoagulant)		5–8 min
Differential count (see Bone marrow differential count or Leukocyte differential count)			
Eosinophil count	Whole blood (EDTA); capillary blood	50–400 cells/μL (mm³)	50–400 × 10⁶ cells/L
Erythrocyte count (RBC count)	Whole blood (EDTA)	millions of cells/μL (mm³)	× 10¹² cells/L
		M: 4.3–5.7	4.3–5.7
		F: 3.8–5.1	3.8–5.1
Erythrocyte sedimentation rate (ESR), Wintrobe			M: 0–15 mm/h
			F: 0–20 mm/h
Ferritin (see Chemistry section)			
Fibrin degradation products (Agglutination, Thrombo-Wellco test)	Whole blood: special tube containing thrombin and proteolytic inhibitor	<10 μg/mL	<10 mg/L
	Urine: 2 mL in special tube (see above)	<0.25 μg/mL	<0.25 mg/L
Fibrinogen	Plasma (Na citrate)	200–400 mg/dL	2.00–4.00 g/L
Glucose-6-phosphate dehydrogenase (G6PD) in erythrocytes	Whole blood (ACD, EDTA, or heparin)	12.1 ± 2.09 U/g Hb (1 SD)	0.78 ± 0.13 MU/mol Hb (1 SD)
Haptoglobin (Hp) RID	Serum; avoid hemolysis	26–185 mg/dL	260–1850 mg/L
Hematocrit (HCT, Hct)	Whole blood (EDTA)		
Calculated from MCV and RBC (electronic displacement or laser)		M: 39–49%	0.39–0.49 volume fraction
		F: 35–45%	0.35–0.45 volume fraction

HEMATOLOGY AND COAGULATION *Continued*

Test	Specimen	Reference Interval (Conventional Units)		Reference Interval (International Units)	
Hemoglobin (Hb)	Whole blood (EDTA)	M: 13.5–17.5 g/dL F: 12.0–16.0 g/dL		2.09–2.71 mmol/L 1.86–2.48 mmol/L	
	Plasma (heparin, ACD)	<3 mg/dL		<0.47 µmol/L	
	Urine, fresh, random			Negative	
Hemoglobin electrophoresis	Whole blood (EDTA, citrate, or heparin)			Mass fraction	
		HbA >95%		HbA >0.95	
		HbA₂ 1.5–3.5%		HbA₂ 0.015–0.035	
		HbF <2%		HbF <0.02	
Leukocyte count (WBC count)	Whole blood (EDTA)	4.5–11.0 × 10³ cells/µL (mm³)		4.5–11.0 × 10⁹ cells/L	
Leukocyte	CSF	0.5 mononuclear cells/µgL		0.5 × 10⁶ cells/L	
Differential count	Whole blood (EDTA)	%	Cells/µL (mm³)	Number fraction	Cells × 10⁶/L
Myelocytes		0	0	0	0
Neutrophils—bands		3–5	150–400	0.03–0.05	150–400
Neutrophils—segmented		54–62	3000–5800	0.54–0.62	3000–5800
Lymphocytes		23–33	1500–3000	0.25–0.33	1500–3000
Monocytes		3–7	285–500	0.03–0.07	285–500
Eosinophils		1–3	50–250	0.01–0.03	50–250
Basophils		0–0.75	15–50	0–0.0075	15–50
Leukocyte	CSF	%		Number fraction	
Differential count					
Lymphocytes		62 ± 34		0.62 ± 0.324	
Monocytes (includes pia-arachnoid mesothelial cells)		36 ± 20		0.36 ± 0.20	
Neutrophils		2 ± 5		0.02 ± 0.05	
Histocytes				Rare	
Ependymal cells				Rare	
Eosinophils				Rare	
Mean corpuscular hemoglobin (MCH)	Whole blood (EDTA)	26–34 pg/cell		0.40–0.53 fmol/cell	
Mean corpuscular hemoglobin concentration (MCHC)	Whole blood (EDTA)	31–37% Hb/cell or gHb/dL RBC		4.81–5.74 mmol Hb/L RBC	
Mean corpuscular volume (MCV)	Whole blood (EDTA)			80–100 fL	
Methemoglobin (MetHb)	Whole blood (EDTA, heparin, or ACD)	0.06–0.24 g/dL		9.3–37.2 µmol/L	
Partial thromboplastin time (PTT)	Whole blood (Na citrate)			60–85 sec	
Plasma volume	Plasma (heparin)	M: 25–43 mL/kg F: 28–45 mL/kg		0.025–0.043 L/kg 0.028–0.045 L/kg	
Platelet count (thrombocyte count)	Whole blood (EDTA)	150–450 × 10³/µL (mm³)		150–450 × 10⁹/L	
Prothrombin consumption	Whole blood (no anticoagulant)			>30 sec	
Prothrombin time, two-stage modified	Whole blood (Na citrate)			18–22 sec	
RBC count (see Erthyrocyte count)					
Red cell volume	Whole blood (heparin)	M: 20–36 mL/kg F: 19–31 mL/kg		M: 0.020–0.036 L/kg F: 0.019–0.031 L/kg	
Reticulocyte count	Whole blood (EDTA, heparin, or oxalate)	0.5–1.5% of erythrocytes		0.005–0.015 (number fraction)	
Sulfhemoglobin	Whole blood (EDTA, heparin, or ACD)	≤1.0% of total Hb		<0.010 of total Hb (mass fraction)	
Thrombin time	Whole blood (Na citrate)			Time of control ± 2S when control is 9–13 sec	
Thromboplastin time, activated (see Activated partial thromboplastin time [APTT])					

DRUGS—THERAPEUTIC AND TOXIC

Drug	Specimen	Reference Interval (Conventional Units)		Reference Interval (International Units)
Acetaminophen	Serum or plasma (hep or EDTA)	Therap:	10–30 µg/mL	66–199 µmol/L
		Toxic:	>200 µg/mL	>1324 µmol/L
Amikacin	Serum or plasma (EDTA)	Therap:		
		Peak	25–35 µg/mL	43–60 µmol/L
		Trough (severe infection):	4–8 µg/mL	6.8–13.7 µmol/L
		Toxic:		
		Peak	>35 µg/mL	>60 µmol/L
		Trough	>10 µg/mL	>17 µmol/L
ε-Aminocaproic acid	Serum or plasma (hep or EDTA); trough	Therap:	100–400 µg/mL	0.76–3.05 mmol/L
Amitriptyline	Serum or plasma (hep or EDTA); trough (>12 h after dose)	Therap:	120–250 ng/mL	433–903 nmol/L
		Toxic:	>500 ng/mL	>1805 nmol/L
Amobarbital	Serum	Therap:	1–5 µg/mL	4–22 µmol/L
		Toxic:	>10 µg/mL	>44 µmol/L
Amphetamine	Serum or plasma (hep or EDTA)	Therap:	20–30 ng/mL	148–222 nmol/L
		Toxic:	>200 ng/mL	>1480 nmol/L
Bromide	Serum	Therap:	750–1500 µg/mL	9.4–18.7 mmol/L
		Toxic:	>1250 µg/mL	>15.6 mmol/L

Table continued on following page

DRUGS—THERAPEUTIC AND TOXIC *Continued*

Drug	Specimen		Reference Interval (Conventional Units)	Reference Interval (International Units)
Caffeine	Serum or plasma (hep or EDTA)	Therap:	3–15 µg/mL	15–77 µmol/L
		Toxic:	>50 µg/mL	>258 µmol/L
Carbamazepine	Serum or plasma (hep or EDTA); trough	Therap:	4–12 µg/mL	17–51 µmol/L
		Toxic:	>15 µg/mL	>63 µmol/L
Carbenicillin	Serum or plasma	Therap:		Dependent on minimum inhibition concentration of specific organism
		Toxic:	>250 µg/mL	>660 µmol/L
Chloramphenicol	Serum or plasma (hep or EDTA); trough	Therap:	10–25 µg/L	31–77 µmol/L
		Toxic:	>25 µg/L	>77 µmol/L
Chlordiazepoxide	Serum or plasma (hep or EDTA); trough	Therap:	700–1000 ng/mL	2.34–3.34 µmol/L
		Toxic:	>5000 ng/mL	>16.7 µmol/L
Chlorpromazine	Serum or plasma (hep or EDTA); trough	Therap:	50–300 ng/mL	157–942 nmol/L
		Toxic:	>750 ng/mL	>2355 nmol/L
Cimetidine	Serum or plasma (hep or EDTA); trough	Therap:	0.5–1.2 µg/mL	2–5 µmol/L
Clonazepam	Serum or plasma (hep or EDTA; trough	Therap:	15–60 ng/mL	48–190 nmol/L
		Toxic:	>80 ng/mL	>254 nmol/L
Clonidine	Serum or plasma (hep or EDTA)	Therap:	1.0–2.0 ng/mL	4.4–8.7 nmol/L
Clorazepate	Serum or plasma (hep or EDTA)	As desmethyldiazepam:		
		Therap:	0.12–1.0 µg/mL	0.36–3.01 µmol/L
Cocaine	Serum or plasma (hep or EDTA); on ice	Therap:	100–500 ng/mL	330–1650 nmol/L
		Toxic:	>1000 ng/mL	>3300 nmol/L
Cyclosporine	Serum (12 h after dose)	Therap:	100–400 ng/mL	83–333 nmol/L
		Toxic:	>400 mg/mL	>333 nmol/L
Desipramine	Serum or plasma (hep or EDTA); trough (≥12 h after dose)	Therap:	75–300 ng/mL	281–1125 nmol/L
		Toxic:	>400 ng/mL	>1500 nmol/L
Diazepam	Serum or plasma (hep or EDTA); trough	Therap:	100–1000 ng/mL	0.35–3.51 µmol/L
		Toxic:	>5000 ng/mL	>17.55 µmol/L
Digitoxin	Serum or plasma (hep or EDTA) ≥6 h after dose	Therap:	20–35 ng/mL	24–46 nmol/L
		Toxic	>45 ng/mL	>59 nmol/L
Digoxin	Serum or plasma (hep or EDTA); trough (≥12 h after dose)	Therap:	0.8–1.5 mg/mL	1.1–1.9 nmol/L
		CHF: Arrhythmias:	1.5–2.0 ng/mL	1.9–2.6 nmol/L
		Toxic:	>2.5 ng/mL	>3.2 nmol/L
Diphenylhydantoin (see Phenytoin)				
Disopyramide	Serum or plasma (hep or EDTA); trough	Therap:		
		Arrhythmias:		
		Atrial	2.8–3.2 µg/mL	8.3–9.4 µmol/L
		Ventricular	3.3–7.5 µg/mL	9.7–22 µmol/L
		Toxic:	>7 µg/mL	>20.7 µmol/L
Doxepin	Serum or plasma (hep or EDTA); trough (≥ 12 h after dose)	Therap:	30–150 ng/mL	107–537 nmol/L
		Toxic:	>500 ng/mL	>1790 nmol/L
Ethchlorvynol	Serum or plasma (hep or EDTA)	Therap:	2–8 µg/mL	14–55 µmol/L
		Toxic:	>20 µg/mL	>138 µmol/L
Ethosuximide	Serum or plasma (hep or EDTA); trough	Therap:	40–100 µg/mL	283–708 µmol/L
		Toxic:	>150 µg/mL	>1062 µmol/L
Fenoprofen	Plasma (EDTA)	Therap:	20–65 µg/mL	82–268 µmol/L
Flecainide	Serum or plasma (hep or EDTA); trough	Therap:	0.2–1.0 µg/mL	0.5–2.4 µmol/L
		Toxic:	>1.0 µg/mL	>2.4 µmol/L
Furosemide	Serum (30 min after dose)	Therap:	1–2 µg/mL	3–6 µmol/L
Gentamicin	Serum or plasma (EDTA)	Therap:		
		Peak (severe infection)	8–10 µg/mL	16.7–20.9 µmol/L
		Trough (severe infection)	2–4 µg/mL	4.2–8.4 µmol/L
		Toxic:		
		Peak	>10 µg/mL	>21 µmol/L
		Trough	>4 µg/mL	>8.4 µmol/L
Glutethimide	Serum	Therap:	2–6 µg/mL	9–28 µmol/L
		Toxic:	>5 µg/mL	>23 µmol/L
Imipramine	Serum or plasma (hep or EDTA); trough (≥12 h after dose)	Therap:	125–250 ng/mL	446–893 nmol/L
		Toxic:	>500 ng/mL	>1784 nmol/L
Isoniazid	Serum or plasma (hep or EDTA)	Therap:	1–7 µg/mL	7–51 µmol/L
		Toxic:	20–710 µg/mL	146–5176 µmol/L
Kanamycin	Serum or plasma (EDTA)	Therap:		
		Peak	25–35 µg/mL	52–72 µmol/L
		Trough (severe infection)	4–8 µg/mL	8–16 µmol/L
		Toxic:		
		Peak	>35 µg/mL	>72 µmol/L
		Trough	>10 µg/mL	>21 µmol/L
Lidocaine	Serum or plasma (hep or EDTA); ≥45 min following bolus dose	Therap:	1.5–6.0 µg/mL	6.4–26 µmol/L
		CNS or cardiovascular depression	6–8 µg/mL	26–34.2 µmol/L
		Seizures, obtundation, decreased cardiac output	>8 µg/mL	>34.2 µmol/L
Lithium	Serum or plasma (hep or EDTA); (>12 h after last dose)	Therap:	0.6–1.2 mEq/L	0.6–1.2 nmol/L
		Toxic:	>2 mEq/L	>2 mmol/L
Lorazepam	Serum or plasma (hep or EDTA)	Therap:	50–240 ng/mL	156–746 nmol/L
Meperidine	Serum or plasma (hep or EDTA)	Therap:	400–700 ng/mL	1620–2830 nmol/L
		Toxic:	>1 µg/mL	>4043 nmol/L
Meprobamate	Serum	Therap:	6–12 µg/mL	28–55 µmol/L
		Toxic:	>60 µg/mL	>275 µmol/L

DRUGS—THERAPEUTIC AND TOXIC *Continued*

Drug	Specimen	Reference Interval (Conventional Units)	Reference Interval (International Units)
Methadone	Serum or plasma (hep or EDTA)	Therap: 100–400 ng/mL	0.32–1.29 µmol/L
		Toxic: >2000 ng/mL	>6.46 µmol/L
Methaqualone	Serum or plasma (hep or EDTA)	Therap: 2–3 µg/mL	8–12 µmol/L
		Toxic: >10 µg/mL	>40 µmol/L
Methotrexate	Serum or plasma (hep or EDTA)	Therap: variable	variable
		Toxic:	
		Low-dose therapy (1–2 wk) >9.1 ng/mL	>20 nmol/L
		High-dose therapy (48 h) >454 ng/mL	>1000 nmol/L
Methsuximide (N-desmethyl methsuximide)	Serum	Therap: 10–40 µg/mL	53–212 µmol/L
		Toxic: >40 µg/mL	>212 µmol/L
Methyldopa	Plasma (EDTA)	Therap: 1–5 µg/mL	4.7–23.7 µmol/L
		Toxic: >7 µg/mL	>33 µmol/L
Methyprylon	Serum	Therap: 8–10 µg/mL	43–55 µmol/L
		Toxic: >50 µg/mL	>273 µmol/L
Mexiletine	Serum or plasma (hep or EDTA)	Therap: 0.7–2.0 µg/mL	3.9–11.2 µmol/L
		Toxic: >2.0 µg/mL	>11.2 µmol/L
Morphine	Serum or plasma (hep or EDTA)	Therap: 10–80 ng/mL	35–280 nmol/L
		Toxic: >200 ng/mL	>700 nmol/L
N-Acetylprocainamide	Serum or plasma (hep or EDTA); trough	Therap: 5–30 µg/mL	18–108 µmol/L
		Toxic: >40 µg/mL	>144 µmol/L
Nitroprusside	Serum or plasma (EDTA)	As thiocyanate:	
Normethsuximide	Serum	Therap: 6–29 µg/mL	103–499 µmol/L
		Therap: 10–40 µg/mL	53–212 µmol/L
		Toxic: >40 µg/mL	>212 µmol/L
Nortriptyline	Serum or plasma (hep or EDTA); trough (≥12 h after dose)	Therap: 50–150 ng/mL	190–570 nmol/L
		Toxic: >500 ng/mL	>1900 nmol/L
Oxazepam	Serum or plasma (hep or EDTA)	Therap: 0.2–1.4 µg/mL	0.70–4.9 µmol/L
Paraquat	Whole blood (EDTA)	Toxic: 0.1–1.6 µg/mL	0.39–6.2 µmol/L
	Urine	Occup exp: 0.3 µg/mL	1.17 µmol/L
		Toxic: 0.9–64 µg/mL	3.50–249 µmol/L
Pentobarbital	Serum or plasma (hep or EDTA); trough	Therap:	
		Hypnotic 1–5 µg/mL	4–22 µmol/L
		Therap coma 20–50 µg/mL	88–221 µmol/L
		Toxic: >10 µg/mL	>44 µmol/L
Phenacetin	Plasma (EDTA)	Therap: 1–30 µg/mL	6–167 µmol/L
		Toxic: 50–250 µg/mL	279–1395 µmol/L
Phencyclidine	Serum or plasma (hep or EDTA)	Toxic: 90–800 ng/mL	370–3288 nmol/L
Phenobarbital	Serum or plasma (hep or EDTA); trough	Therap: 15–40 µg/mL	65–170 µmol/L
		Toxic:	
		Slowness, ataxia, nystagmus 35–80 µg/mL	151–345 µmol/L
		Coma with reflexes 65–117 µg/mL	280–504 µmol/L
		Coma without reflexes >100 µg/mL	>430 µmol/L
Phensuximide (both parent and N-desmethyl metabolites)	Serum or plasma (hep or EDTA)	Therap: 40–60 µg/mL	228–324 µmol/L
Phenylbutazone	Plasma (EDTA)	Therap: 50–100 µg/mL (not well defined)	162–324 µmol/L
		Toxic: >100 µg/mL	>324 µmol/L
Phenytoin	Serum or plasma (hep or EDTA); trough	Therap: 10–20 µg/mL	40–79 µmol/L
		Toxic: >20 µg/mL	>79 µmol/L
Primidone	Serum or plasma (hep or EDTA); trough	Therap: 5–12 µg/mL	23–55 µmol/L
		Toxic: >15 µg/mL	>69 µmol/L
Procainamide	Serum or plasma (hep or EDTA); trough	Therap: 4–10 µg/mL	17–42 µmol/L
		Toxic: >10 µg/mL	>42 µmol/L
		Also consider effect of metabolite, N-acetylprocainamide	
Propoxyphene	Plasma (EDTA)	Therap: 0.1–0.4 µg/mL	0.3–1.2 µmol/L
		Toxic: >0.5 µg/mL	>1.5 µmol/L
Propranolol	Serum or plasma (hep or EDTA); trough	Therap: 50–100 ng/mL	193–386 nmol/L
Protriptyline	Serum or plasma (hep or EDTA); trough (≥12 h after dose)	Therap: 70–250 ng/mL	266–950 nmol/L
		Toxic: >500 ng/mL	>1900 nmol/L
Quinidine	Serum or plasma (hep or EDTA); trough	Therap: 2–5 µg/mL	6–15 µmol/L
		Toxic: >6 µg/mL	>18 µmol/L
Salicylates	Serum or plasma (hep or EDTA); trough	Therap: 150–300 µg/mL	1086–2172 µmol/L
		Toxic: >300 µg/mL	>2172 µmol/L
Secobarbital	Serum	Therap: 1–2 µg/mL	4.2–8.4 µmol/L
		Toxic: >5 µg/mL	>21.0 µmol/L
Theophylline	Serum or plasma (hep or EDTA)	Therap: 8–20 µg/mL	44–111 µmol/L
		Toxic: >20 µg/mL	>110 µmol/L
Thiocyanate	Serum or plasma (EDTA)	Nonsmoker: 1–4 µg/mL	17–69 µmol/L
		Smoker: 3–12 µg/mL	52–206 µmol/L
		Therap, after nitroprusside infusion: 6–29 µg/mL	103–499 µmol/L
	Urine	Nonsmoker: 1–4 mg/d	17–69 µmol/d
		Smoker: 7–17 mg/d	120–292 µmol/d
Thiopental	Serum or plasma (hep or EDTA); trough	Hypnotic: 1.0–5.0 µg/mL	4.1–20.7 µmol/L
		Coma: 30–100 µg/mL	124–413 µmol/L
		Anesthesia: 7–130 µg/mL	29–536 µmol/L
		Toxic conc: >10 µg/mL	>41 µmol/L
Thioridazine	Serum or plasma (hep or EDTA)	Therap: 1.0–1.5 µg/mL	2.7–4.1 µmol/L
		Toxic: >10 µg/mL	>27 µmol/L

Table continued on following page

DRUGS—THERAPEUTIC AND TOXIC *Continued*

Drug	Specimen	Reference Interval (Conventional Units)		Reference Interval (International Units)
Tobramycin	Serum or plasma (hep or EDTA)	Therap:		
		Peak (severe infection)	8–10 µg/mL	17–21 µmol/L
		Trough (severe infection)	<4 µg/mL	<9 µmol/L
		Toxic:		
		Peak	>10 µg/mL	>21 µmol/L
		Trough	>4 µg/mL	>9 µmol/L
Tocainide	Serum or plasma (hep or EDTA)	Therap:	4–10 µg/mL	21–52 µmol/L
Valproic acid	Serum or plasma (hep or EDTA); trough	Therap:	50–100 µg/mL	347–693 µmol/L
		Toxic:	>100 µg/mL	>693 µmol/L
Vancomycin	Serum or plasma (hep or EDTA); trough	Therap:	5–10 µg/mL	3–7 µmol/L
		Toxic: (not well established)	>80–100 µg/mL	>55–69 µmol/L
Verapamil	Serum or plasma (hep or EDTA)	Therap:	100–500 ng/mL	220–1100 nmol/L
Warfarin	Serum or plasma (hep or EDTA)	Therap:	1–10 µg/mL	3–32 µmol/L

Note: Page numbers in **boldface** indicate major discussions; page numbers in *italics* indicate illustrations; page numbers followed by t refer to tables.

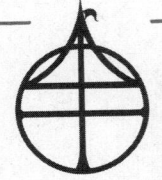

The colophon on the front cover and spine is an abstraction which symbolizes the universal aspects of medicine. The circle represents the world. The stylized triangle in the upper area is the classic image of positive and negative forces—the Law of Life. The vertical line with the upper right staff suggests the staff of Æsculapius and Hermes, and the horizontal bar connects all three symbols into the total summation of medicine as Art and Science.

The Integral Urban House